To students of Surgery, at all levels, in their quest for knowledge

PRINCIPLES OF
SURGERY
FIFTH EDITION

PRINCIPLES OF SURGERY

2 3 4 5 6 7 8 9 0   DOWDOW   9 4 3 2 1

ISBN 0-07-055822-1   1 VOL EDITION
ISBN 0-07-079979-2   2 VOL SET EDITION
ISBN 0-07-055826-4   VOLUME ONE
ISBN 0-07-055829-9   VOLUME TWO

This book was set in Times Roman by York Graphic Services, Inc.
The editors were Ray Moloney and Mariapaz Ramos-Englis.
The production supervisor was Elaine Gardenier.
The index was prepared by Philip James.
The cover was designed by Edward R. Schultheis.
Front cover art courtesy of: Yale Historical Library.

R. R. Donnelley & Sons Company was printer and binder.

Library of Congress Cataloging-in-Publication Data

Principles of surgery.

    Available as 1 v. and as a 2-v. set.
    Includes bibliographies and index.
    1. Surgery. I. Schwartz, Seymour, I., 1928–
II. Title. [DNLM: 1. Surgery. WO100 P957]
RD31.P88 1989   617   88-9158
ISBN 0-07-079979-2 (set)
ISBN 0-07-055826-4 (v. 1)
ISBN 0-07-055829-9 (v. 2)
ISBN 0-07-055822-1 (single v.)

PRINCIPLES OF SURGERY

FIFTH EDITION

EDITOR-IN-CHIEF

SEYMOUR I. SCHWARTZ, M.D.

Professor and Chair
Department of Surgery
University of Rochester School of Medicine and Dentistry

ASSOCIATE EDITORS

G. Tom Shires, M.D.

Professor and Chair
Department of Surgery
Cornell University Medical College

Frank C. Spencer, M.D.

Professor and Director
Department of Surgery
New York University School of Medicine

WITH

Wendy Cowles Husser, M.A.

University of Rochester
School of Medicine and Dentistry

McGraw-Hill, Inc.

Health Professions Division

New York St. Louis San Francisco Colorado Springs Oklahoma City
Auckland Bogotá Hamburg Lisbon London Madrid Mexico Milan Montreal
New Delhi Paris San Juan São Paulo Singapore Sydney Tokyo Toronto

Contents

PART I Basic Considerations

PART II Specific Considerations

Contributors

James T. Adams, M.D.
Professor of Surgery
Department of Surgery
University of Rochester school of
Medicine and Dentistry (35)

R. Peter Altman, M.D.
Rudolph N. Schullinger Professor of Surgery
College of Physicians and Surgeons
Columbia University (39)

Joseph F. Amaral, M.D.
Fellow in Surgery
Brown University (1)

Kathryn D. Anderson, M.D.
Professor of Surgery and Child Health
George Washington University
Attending Surgeon, Children's Hospital
Washington, D.C. (39)

Richard M. Bergland, M.D.
Clinical Professor of Surgery (Neurosurgery)
SUNY Downstate
Beth Israel Hospital (37)

George H. Bornside, Ph.D.
Professor Emeritus of Surgical Research
and Microbiology
Departments of Surgery and Microbiology
Louisiana State University
Medical Center (5)

Richard I. Burton, M.D.
Professor and Chair
Department of Orthopaedics
University of Rochester
School of Medicine and Dentistry (45)

Peter C. Canizaro, M.D.
Professor and Chairman
Department of Surgery
Texas Tech University Health Sciences
Center (2, 4)

C. James Carrico, M.D.
Professor and Chairman of Surgery
University of Washington School of
Medicine (4)

Douglas Chyatte, M.D.
Assistant Professor
Section of Neurological Surgery
Yale University School of Medicine (42)

Isidore Cohn, Jr, M.D.
Professor and Chairman
Department of Surgery
Louisiana State University
School of Medicine (5)

William F. Collins, M.D.
Harvey and Kate Cushing
Professor and Chairman
Department of Surgery
Yale University School of Medicine (42)

Robert E. Condon, M.D.
Ausman Foundation Professor
and Chairman, Department of Surgery
The Medical College of Wisconsin (34)

Alfred T. Culliford, M.D.
Associate Professor
Department of Surgery
New York University Medical Center (19)

Numbers in parentheses refer to contributors' chapters.

P. William Curreri
Professor and Chairman
Department of Surgery
University of South Alabama
College of Medicine *(7)*

Louis R. M. Del Guercio, M.D.
Professor and Chairman
Department of Surgery
New York Medical College, Valhalla *(13)*

Eric J. DeMaria, M.D.
Resident in Surgery
Brown University *(37)*

Charles C. Duncan, M.D.
Associate Professor of Surgery
Section of Neurosurgery
Chief, Pediatric Neurosurgery
Yale University School of Medicine *(42)*

Robert B. Duthie, M.D. M.B.
Nuffield Professor of Orthopaedic Surgery
Nuffield Orthopaedic Center
Oxford, England *(43)*

James S. Economou, M.D.
Assistant Professor of Surgery
Division of Surgical Oncology
UCLA School of Medicine and
Jonsson Comprehensive Cancer Clinic *(9)*

Martin R. Eichelberger, M.D.
Associate Professor of Surgery
and Child Health
George Washington University
Attending Surgeon, Children's Hospital
Washington D.C. *(39)*

Irwin N. Frank, M.D.
Professor of Surgery
Department of Urology
University of Rochester
School of Medicine and Dentistry *(40)*

Richard E. Fry, M.D.
Assistant Professor of Surgery
The University of Texas Southwestern Medical
School at Dallas *(23)*

William J. Fry, M.D.
Professor and Chairman
Department of Surgery
The University of Texas Southwestern Medical
School at Dallas *(23)*

Donald S. Gann, M.D.
J. Murray Beardsley Professor and
Chairman, Department of Surgery
Brown University *(1, 37)*

Stanley M. Goldberg, M.D.
Clinical Professor of Surgery
Director, Division of Colon and Rectal Surgery
Department of Surgery
University of Minnesota Medical School *(28)*

Lazar J. Greenfield, M.D.
Professor and Chairman
Department of Surgery
University of Michigan, Ann Arbor *(22)*

Philip C. Guzzetta, M.D.
Associate Professor of Surgery
and Child Health
George Washington University,
Attending Surgeon, Children's Hospital
Washington D.C. *(39)*

Charles M. Haskell, M.D.
Professor of Medicine and Surgery
UCLA School of Medicine
Director, Wadsworth Cancer Center
Chief, Hematology and Oncology Section
of the Medical and Research Services
W. Los Angeles V.A. Medical Center *(9)*

Richard H. Hatch, M.D.
Assistant Clinical Professor
Department of Obstetrics and Gynecology
University of Utah *(41)*

Arthur L. Herbst, M.D.
Chairman and Joseph Bolivar DeLee
Distinguished Service Professor
Department of Obstetrics and Gynecology
University of Chicago *(41)*

Franklin T. Hoaglund, M.D.
Professor of Orthopaedic Surgery, Department
of Orthopaedic Surgery
University of California at San Francisco
(43, 44)

Anthony M. Imparato, M.D.
Professor of Surgery
Director, Division of Vascular Surgery
New York University Medical Center *(21)*

Ronald C. Jones, M.D.
Clinical Professor of Surgery
University of Texas Health Science Center
and Chief of Surgery
Baylor University Medical Center, Dallas *(6)*

M. J. Jurkiewicz, M.D.
Professor of Surgery
Section of Plastic Surgery
Emory University School of Medicine *(46)*

Edwin L. Kaplan, M.D.
Professor of Surgery
Pritzker School of Medicine
University of Chicago   (38)

Thomas C. King, M.D.
Ferrer Professor of Surgery
Columbia Presbyterian Hospital   (17)

Stephen F. Lowry, M.D.
Associate Professor of Surgery
Director, Hyperalimentation Unit
Department of Surgery
Cornell University Medical College   (2)

Arnold Luterman, M.D.
Ripps-Meisler Professor of Surgery
Director
University of South Alabama Burn
Center   (7)

Robert N. McClelland, M.D.
Professor of Surgery
The University of Texas
Southwestern Medical School at Dallas   (6)

James M. McGreevy
Associate Professor of Surgery
University of Utah Medical School   (26)

Laura Ment, M.D.
Associate Professor
Department of Pediatrics and Neurology
Yale University School of Medicine   (42)

Richard J. Migliori, M.D.
Medical Fellow in Surgery
Department of Surgery
University of Minnesota Medical
Center   (10)

Ronald D. Miller, M.D.
Professor and Chairman of Anesthesia
and Professor of Pharmacology
Department of Anesthesia
University of California, San Francisco   (11)

Thomas A. Miller, M.D.
Professor of Surgery
Department of Surgery
University of Texas Health Science Center
at Houston   (26)

Frank G. Moody, M.D.
Denton A. Cooley Professor and Chairman
Department of Surgery
University of Texas Health Science Center
at Houston   (26)

Donald L. Morton, M.D.
Professor and Chief, Surgical Oncology
Director, John Wayne Cancer Clinic
UCLA School of Medicine
and Jonsson Comprehensive Cancer
Center   (9)

John H. Morton, M.D.
Professor of Surgery
Department of Surgery
University of Rochester School of Medicine
and Dentistry   (36)

John S. Najarian, M.D.
Jay Phillips Professor and Chairman
Department of Surgery
University of Minnesota Hospital   (10)

Kurt D. Newman, M.D.
Assistant Professor of Surgery and
Child Health
George Washington University
Attending Surgeon, Children's Hospital
Washington D.C.   (39)

Santhat Nivatvongs, M.D.
Associate Professor of Surgery
Senior Associate Consultant
General and Colon and Rectal Surgery
Mayo Medical School   (28)

Peter C. Pairolero, M.D.
Associate Professor of Surgery
Mayo Medical School   (25)

Robert G. Parker, M.D.
Professor and Chairman
Department of Radiation Oncology
UCLA School of Medicine
and Jonsson Comprehensive Cancer
Center   (9)

W. Spencer Payne, M.D.
James C. Masson Professor of Surgery
Mayo Medical School   (25)

Erle E. Peacock, Jr., M.D.
Chapel Hill
North Carolina   (8)

Malcolm O. Perry, M.D.
Professor of Surgery
Vanderbilt University School of Medicine   (6)

Joseph M. Piepmeier, M.D.
Associate Professor
Section of Neurological Surgery
Yale University School of Medicine   (42)

Judson G. Randolph, M.D.
Professor of Surgery and Child Health
George Washington University
Surgeon-in-Chief, Children's Hospital,
Washington D.C.   (39)

Keith Reemtsma, M.D.
Valentine Mott and Johnson and Johnson
Professor and Chairman
Department of Surgery
Columbia Presbyterian Hospital   (10)

Thomas S. Riles, M.D.
Associate Professor of Surgery
Department of Surgery
New York University Medical Center   (21)

Franklin Robinson, M.D.
Clinical Professor
Section of Neurological Surgery
Yale University School of Medicine   (42)

David A. Rothenberger, M.D.
Associate Professor
Division of Colon and Rectal Surgery
Department of Surgery
University of Minnesota Medical School   (28)

Benjamin F. Rush, Jr., M.D.
Professor and Chairman
Department of Surgery
University of Medicine and Dentistry
of New Jersey at Newark   (15, 16)

Kimberlee J. Sass, M.D.
Associate Research Scientist
Section of Neurological Surgery
Clinical Neuropsychologist
Yale University School of Medicine   (42)

John A. Savino, M.D.
Professor of Surgery
Department of Surgery
New York Medical College   (13)

Seymour I. Schwartz, M.D.
Professor and Chair
Department of Surgery
University of Rochester School of Medicine
and Dentistry   (3, 12, 24, 29, 30, 31, 33, 44)

G. Tom Shires, M.D.
Lewis Atterbury Stimson Professor and Chairman
Department of Surgery
Cornell University Medical College   (2, 4, 6)

G. Tom Shires III, M.D.
Assistant Professor
Department of Surgery
Cornell University Medical College   (2, 4, 6)

William Silen, M.D.
Johnson & Johnson Professor of Surgery
Harvard Medical School   (32)

Richard L. Simmons, M.D.
Professor of Surgery and Microbiology
Department of Surgery
University of Minnesota Medical Center   (10)

Craig R. Smith, M.D.
Assistant Professor of Surgery
Department of Surgery
Columbia Presbyterian Hospital   (10, 17)

William H. Snyder III, M.D.
Professor of Surgery
The University of Texas Southwestern Medical
School at Dallas   (6)

Dennis D. Spencer, M.D.
Nixdorff-German Professor of Neurosurgery
Professor and Chief
Section of Neurological Surgery
Yale University School of Medicine   (42)

Frank C. Spencer, M.D.
Professor and Chairman
Department of Surgery
New York University School of Medicine
(18, 19, 20)

Michael L. Steer, M.D.
Professor of Surgery
Harvard Medical School   (32)

Thomas R. Stevenson, M.D.
Assistant Professor of Surgery
Section of Plastic Surgery
University of Michigan Hospitals   (46)

Erwin R. Thal, M.D.
Professor of Surgery
The University of Texas Southwestern
Medical School at Dallas   (6)

James C. Thompson, M.D.
James Woods Harris Professor and Chairman
of Surgery
Department of Surgery
The University of Texas Medical Branch   (27)

Courtney M. Townsend, Jr., M.D.
Robertson-Poth Professor
Department of Surgery
The University of Texas Medical Branch,
Galveston   (27)

Victor F. Trastek, M.D.
Instructor
Mayo Medical School   (25)

Alonzo P. Walker, M.D.
Assistant Professor of Surgery
Medical College of Wisconsin   (34)

R. Christie Wray, Jr., M.D.
Professor and Chair
Division of Plastic Surgery
University of Rochester School of Medicine
and Dentistry   (14)

Preface

The publication of the 5th edition of this textbook constitutes a meaningful milestone. As with many anniversaries, the anniversary of the remaining editors' 25-year association with *Principles of Surgery* prompts reminiscence and reflections. Many events have occurred since six younger surgeons, David Hume, Richard C. Lillehei, G. Tom Shires, Frank C. Spencer, Edward H. Storer, and I, agreed to embark on a new venture—the creation of a new textbook of surgery that would be readily different from those already available. Drs. Hume, Lillehei, and Storer all died tragically during their intellectual prime. The three remaining editors have been privileged to witness extraordinary changes and refinements in the science of surgery. As a consequence, we have felt obliged to impart a presentation of these changes with the publication of subsequent editions. We are particularly gratified by the favorable reception of our extended efforts. The major reward that we have realized from these five editions is the sense that we have contributed to the education of a generation of students of surgery.

Seymour I. Schwartz, M.D.

Preface to the First Edition

The raison d'être for a new textbook in a discipline which has been served by standard works for many years was the Editorial Board's initial conviction that a distinct need for a modern approach in the dissemination of surgical knowledge existed. As incoming chapters were reviewed, both the need and satisfaction became increasingly apparent and, at the completion, we felt a sense of excitement at having the opportunity to contribute to the education of modern and future students concerned with the care of surgical patients.

The recent explosion of factual knowledge has emphasized the need for a presentation which would provide the student an opportunity to assimilate pertinent facts in a logical fashion. This would then permit correlation, synthesis of concepts, and eventual extrapolation to specific situations. The physiologic bases for diseases are therefore emphasized and the manifestations and diagnostic studies are considered as a reflection of pathophysiology. Therapy then becomes logical in this schema and the necessity to regurgitate facts is minimized. In appreciation of the impact which Harrison's PRINCIPLES OF INTERNAL MEDICINE has had, the clinical manifestations of the disease processes are considered in detail for each area. Since the operative procedure represents the one element in the therapeutic armentarium unique to the surgeon, the indications, important technical considerations, and complications receive appropriate emphasis. While we apprecite that a textbook cannot hope to incorporate an atlas of surgical procedures, we have provided the student a single book which will satisfy the sequential demands in the care and considerations of surgical patients.

The ultimate goal of the Editorial Board has been to collate a book which is deserving of the adjective "modern." We have therefore selected as authors dynamic and active contributors to their particular fields. The au courant concept is hopefully apparent throughout the entire work and is exemplified by appropriate emphasis on diseases of modern surgical interest, such as trauma, transplantation, and the recently appreciated importance of rehabilitation. Cardiovascular surgery is presented in keeping with the exponential strides recently achieved.

There are two major subdivisions to the text. In the first twelve chapters, subjects that transcend several organ systems are presented. The second portion of the book represents a consideration of specific organ systems and surgical specialties.

Throughout the text, the authors have addressed themselves to a sophisticated audience, regarding the medical student as a graduate student, incorporating material generally sought after by the surgeon in training and presenting information appropriate for the continuing education of the practicing surgeon. The need for a text such as we have envisioned is great and the goal admittedly high. It is our hope that this effort fulfills the expressed demands.

Seymour I. Schwartz, M.D.

Contents of Volume One

Endocrine and Metabolic Responses to Injury

Donald S. Gann and Joseph F. Amaral

Introduction

Systemic Neuroendocrine Reflexes
Stimuli
Integration of Stimuli and Modulation of Output
Efferent Output

Hormonal Response to Injury

Metabolic Changes Induced by Injury
Metabolic Response Consequent to Starvation
Metabolism in Injured Human Beings
    Energy Metabolism following Injury
    Lipid Metabolism during Injury
    Carbohydrate Metabolism during Injury
    Protein Metabolism during Injury

Fluid and Electrolyte Metabolism during Injury
Renal Conservation of Salt and Water following Injury
Blood Volume Restitution

INTRODUCTION

Injury occurs in so many forms and is of such varying intensities that it is not surprising that the response to injury may also be quite variable. There are metabolic changes that are common to virtually all injuries and that when taken together constitute one aspect of the body's response to trauma. These metabolic changes may be broadly divided into: (1) those concerned with whole body energy and substrate metabolism; (2) those concerned with fluid and electrolyte metabolism; and (3) those concerned with local wound metabolism. The changes in whole body energy and substrate metabolism and those in fluid and electrolyte metabolism are for the most part the result of the systemic neuroendocrine environment. By contrast, local wound metabolism is to a large extent independent of the systemic neuroendocrine environment.

Although it has been customary to view the neuroendo-crine environment consequent to injury as a response to injury per se, it is now clear that the pattern of hormonal response seen is the result of a set of physiological reflexes initiated by specific aspects of the injury. Each of these aspects of injury may be viewed as a stimulus initiating the reflex. The stimuli are alterations in "homeostasis" that are perceived by specialized receptors that are located peripherally and centrally. These receptors transduce the stimulus into a discrete set of neural inputs (afferent signals) that are transmitted to the central nervous system via specific neural pathways. In the central nervous system, these inputs are integrated with other signals, resulting in the production of a discrete set of neural outputs (efferent signals). In turn, the efferent signals result in the stimulation or inhibition of the release of numerous neuroendocrine effectors that produce physiologic changes aimed at correcting the alterations in homeostasis. The response to these stimuli may be modulated by a number of factors including concurrent medical illness, the quality and quantity of fluid replacement, concurrent medications, presence of ethanol or other commonly abused drugs, and the age of the individual.

In the absence of major injury, sepsis, or starvation, the alterations in homeostasis are small and the response is directed at fine tuning and integrating the physiologic functioning of the organism. In the presence of major injury, sepsis, or starvation, the stimuli are multiple and intensified and the reflexes are directed at an integrated attempt by the organism to restore cardiovascular stability, to preserve oxygen delivery, to mobilize energy substrates, to increase the supply of critical substrates, primarily glucose, directed at healing the wound, and to minimize pain.

In order to clarify the mechanisms underlying the response to injury, we will break the injury into its potential components (stimuli), the interactions and modulations of these components in the central nervous system, and the metabolic results of the neuroendocrine effectors. We will separate the metabolic responses of the whole body, of the kidney, and of the wound.

1

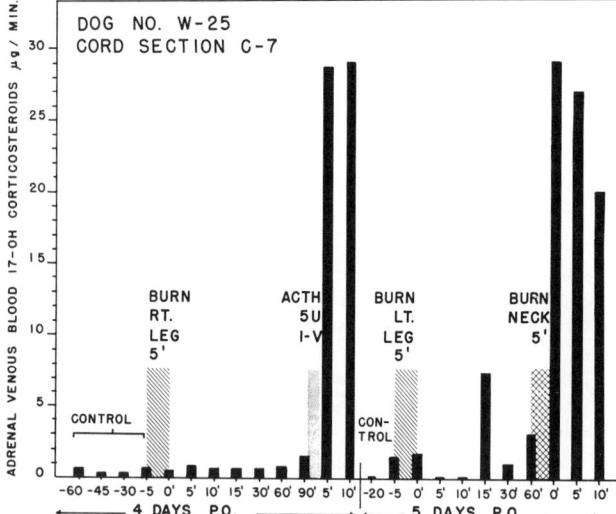

Fig. 1-1. Adrenocortical response to a burn following section of the cord at the level of C_7. A 5-min burn of the right leg, which was below the level of section, produced no increase in adrenocorticosteroid secretion over the control values. Five units of ACTH given intravenously produced an immediate and marked rise in adrenocortical output. With the dog under pentobarbital anesthesia, a burn of the left hindlimb produced no significant increase in adrenocorticosteroid output, but in marked contrast, a burn of the neck, which was above the level of cord section, produced an immediate and marked increase in adrenocortical secretion. (From: *Hume DM, Egdahl RH: Ann Surg 150:697, 1959, with permission.*)

SYSTEMIC NEUROENDOCRINE REFLEXES

Stimuli

In order for a reflex to be initiated, the stimulus must be perceived by specialized receptors that transduce the stimulus into electrical activity and transmit it to the brain. As shown in Fig. 1-1, dogs subjected to a 5-min burn of an area below the level of cord transection do not demonstrate any increase in corticosteroid secretion, whereas the same animals subjected to a 5-min burn above the level of cord transection demonstrate a response similar to that seen following the intravenous injection of five units of ACTH (maximum adrenal stimulation). Similarly, paraplegics do not respond to injuries below the level of the cord transection. As shown in Fig. 1-2, a paraplegic patient, from spinal cord transection at T_4, undergoing gastrectomy fails to release ACTH in response to the operation but is capable of producing corticosteroids in response to intravenously administered ACTH. In both examples, the denervation prevents afferent impulses from reaching the brain. This is exemplified by the experiments of Hume and Egdahl in which one hindlimb of a dog was left attached to the body only by the femoral nerve, artery, and vein (Fig. 1-3). Trauma to the innervated but otherwise detached hindlimb continued to evoke an increased secretion of ACTH and cortisol. When the nerve was severed, however, leaving only the artery and vein intact, the response to trauma was

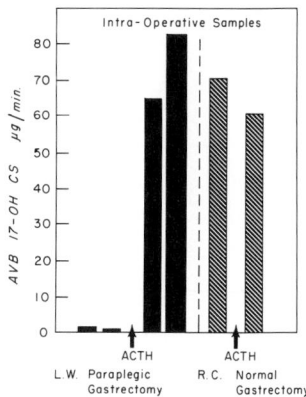

Fig. 1-2. Comparison of the adrenal venous blood content of 17-hydroxycorticosteroid (17-OHCS) in response to a gastric operation in a patient with spinal cord transection at T_4 and in a normal patient. The paraplegic patient fails to demonstrate an increase in 17-OHCS. This presumably results from the absence of ACTH production in response to surgery, since the ability of paraplegic patient's adrenal glands to respond to ACTH is demonstrated by the marked increase in 17-OHCS content of adrenal venous blood in response to intravenously administered ACTH. In contrast, the normal patient shows maximal secretion of 17-OHCS in response to the operation and no further increase is seen with intravenous ACTH. (From: *Hume DM et al: Surgery 52:174, 1962, with permission.*)

eliminated. Similarly, patients undergoing hip replacement under spinal anesthesia do not demonstrate an increase in vasopressin secretion during the procedure when compared with patients undergoing the same procedure under general anesthesia (Fig. 1-4). As the effect of spinal anesthesia wears off, the response for vasopressin is the same in both groups. Laparotomies or burns, in the absence of diminished circulatory volume, do not result in adrenocortical stimulation if the traumatized area is denervated. Similarly, local anesthetics, by blocking the

Fig. 1-3. The effect of limb denervation on ACTH secretion following trauma. The hind leg has been isolated so that it is attached to the body by only one artery, one vein, and one nerve. The burn of the isolated leg produces a marked and immediate response in adrenal venous corticosteroid secretion. During the height of this response the nerve was cut and the secretion dropped promptly to control values. A second burn of the leg now produced no adrenocortical response. ACTH injected subcutaneously into the isolated leg produced a prompt and marked increase in adrenocortical secretion. (From: *Hume DM et al: Surgery 52:697, 1962, with permission.*)

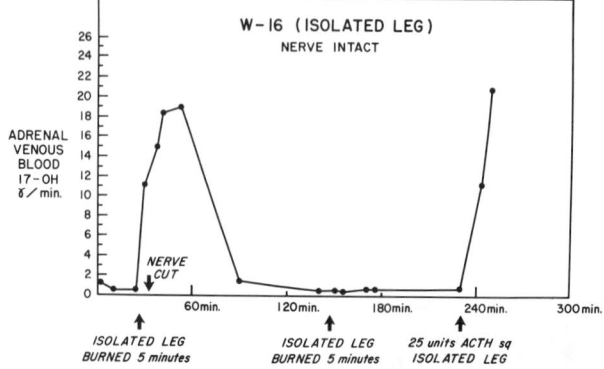

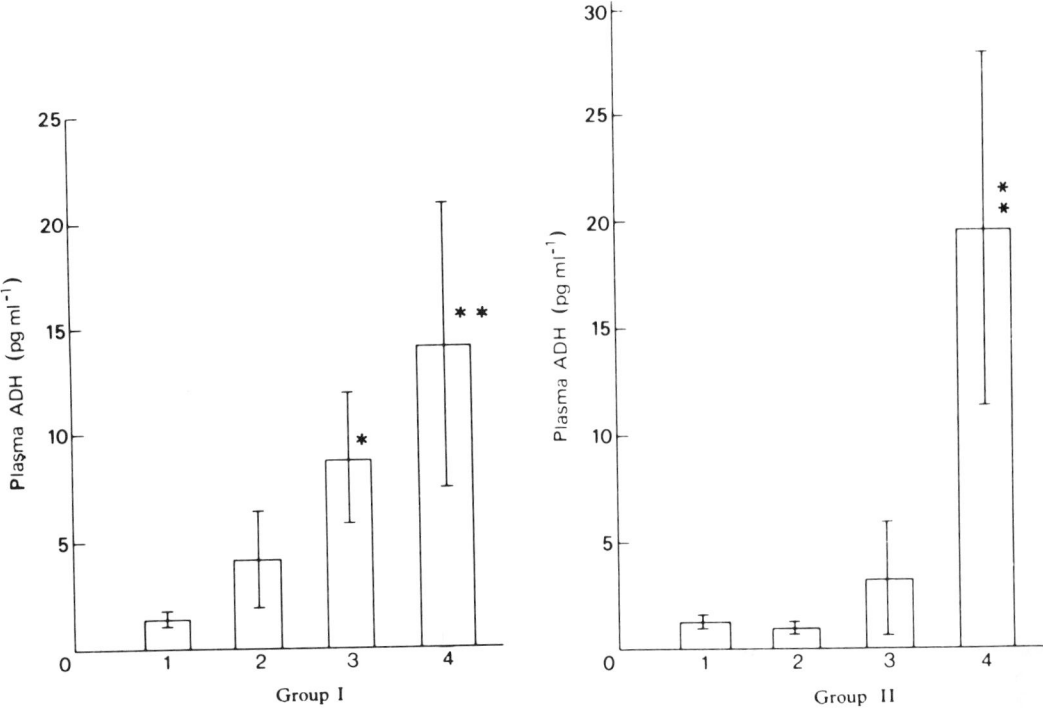

Fig. 1-4. Plasma vasopressin concentrations in 14 patients undergoing total hip replacement under general anesthesia (7 patients—Group I) or epidural anesthesia (7 patients—Group II). Patients who underwent surgery under general anesthesia developed a progressive increase in plasma vasopressin, whereas those under epidural anesthesia demonstrated an increase only 4-h after surgery and presumably as the anesthetic wore off. (From: *Bonnet F et al: Br J Anaesth 54:29, 1982, with permission.*)

transmission of afferent impulses from the area of injury, inhibit the neuroendocrine response to operative trauma elicited by stimuli present at the operative site.

The perception of the stimulus need not be conscious, as evidenced by the ability of individuals to respond to stimuli present in injury despite the presence of general anesthesia. The response may not be the same that would have occurred had anesthesia not been present. This difference arises, at least in part, through the ability of general anesthetics themselves to initiate, inhibit, or augment neuroendocrine reflexes. No operative trauma ought to be thought of without a consideration of the particular anesthetic agent employed and the depth and duration of anesthesia.

The primary stimuli to the neuroendocrine reflexes include (1) changes in effective circulating volume; (2) changes in the concentrations of oxygen, carbon dioxide, or hydrogen ions of tissues or blood; (3) pain; (4) emotional stimuli such as anxiety and pain; (5) alterations in the availability of substrates, particularly glucose; (6) changes in core or ambient temperature; and (7) sepsis (Fig. 1-5).

EFFECTIVE CIRCULATING VOLUME. Virtually all injuries are characterized by the loss of effective circulating volume that may result from the direct loss of blood, as in hemorrhage, from the loss or sequestration of plasma vol-

ume, as in dehydration and third space losses, and from the inability of the body fluids to circulate, as in cardiac failure or pulmonary embolism. The loss of the effective circulating volume is sensed by high-pressure baroreceptors in the aorta, carotid arteries, and renal arteries, which are sensitive to the arterial pressure and its rate of change, and by low-pressure stretch receptors in the atria, which are sensitive to the atrial volume and its rate of change. The total circulating volume and the effective circulating volume are not the same in that the total circulating volume is effective only to the extent that it is sensed by these receptors. Therefore, pump failure or sequestration of fluid behind an obstruction (e.g., tension pneumothorax, cardiac tamponade, and cirrhosis) leads to an effective circulating volume that is less than the total circulating volume. Even though the total circulating volume may be increased, as in congestive heart failure, the effective circulating volume as sensed by high- and low-pressure receptors is decreased. This results in the initiation and maintenance of the baroreceptor reflex such that salt and water continue to be conserved and total peripheral resistance is increased.

The afferent signals from high-pressure baroreceptors and from low-pressure stretch receptors exert a tonic inhibition over the release of many hormones and the activities of the central and autonomic nervous systems (Fig. 1-6). A decrease in effective circulating volume produces a decrease in baroreceptor and stretch receptor activities that leads to a release of the tonic inhibition of the neuroendocrine system. This leads to the increased secretion of ACTH, vasopressin, renin, growth hormone, beta-endorphin, and catecholamines. In turn, these neuroendocrine effectors bring about further neuroendocrine

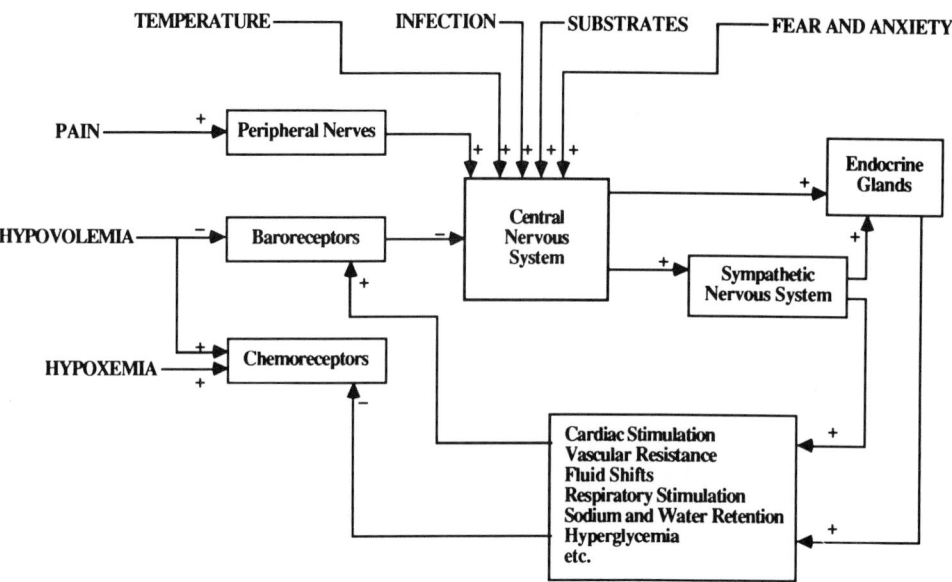

changes, including stimulation of cortisol secretion by the adrenal gland in response to ACTH, stimulation of the conversion of angiotensinogen to angiotensin in the vascular space by renin; stimulation of aldosterone secretion by the adrenal gland in response to ACTH and angiotensin II; stimulation of glucagon secretion by the pancreas in response to epinephrine, and inhibition of insulin secretion by the pancreas in response to epinephrine. Decreases in the effective circulating volume that are sensed by high-pressure stretch receptors in the juxtaglomerular complexes of the kidney also lead to the secretion of renin and, therefore, to the formation of angiotensin and to the secretion of aldosterone. The decrease in baroreceptor

Fig. 1-5. Overview of the neuroendocrine reflexes induced by shock and injury. There are at least seven stimuli consequent to injury that elicit neuroendocrine reflexes. These include hypovolemia; pain; changes in pO_2, pCO_2, pH; infection; emotional arousal; changes in substrate availability; and changes in temperature. The most common of these are hypovolemia and pain.

Fig. 1-6. Efferent limb of baroreceptor and chemoreceptor activation. Inactivation of baroreceptors or activation of chemoreceptors results in the stimulation of the hypothalamus and of the vascular component of the sympathetic nervous system. However, in contrast to the inactivation of baroreceptors, activation of chemoreceptors produces a decrease in cardiac sympathetic nervous system activity and an increase in parasympathetic activity.

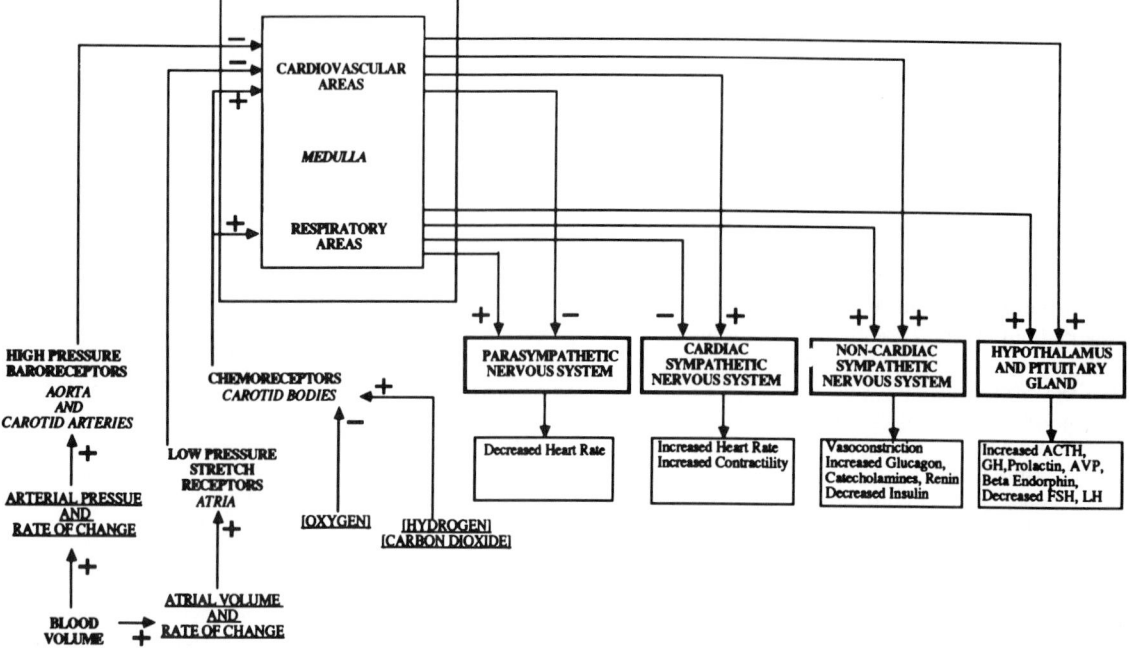

and in stretch receptor discharge also stimulates the vascular component of the sympathetic nervous system, leading to peripheral vasoconstriction and to an increase in cardiac sympathetic and a decrease in cardiac parasympathetic nervous activities, which in turn lead to an increase in heart rate and cardiac contractility.

The neuroendocrine and autonomic responses initiated by a decrease in effective circulating volume are proportional to the magnitude of the decrease. The neuroendocrine response to a 20 percent hemorrhage is greater than that observed following a 10 percent hemorrhage. Many of the neuroendocrine and cardiovascular responses have maximal responses that are achieved usually when the effective circulating volume has been decreased by 30 to 40 percent. Further decreases in the effective circulating volume cannot be compensated for, and hypotension ensues.

CHEMORECEPTOR REFLEX. Changes in the concentration of oxygen, hydrogen ions, and carbon dioxide in the blood initiate cardiovascular, pulmonary, and neuroendocrine responses through the activation of peripheral chemoreceptors. Under normal circumstances, these receptors, which are located in the carotid and the aortic bodies, are not activated. Decreases in the concentration of oxygen or, to a lesser extent, increases in the concentrations of hydrogen ions and carbon dioxide are sensed by these receptors, leading to the activation of neuroendocrine reflexes. As a result of the extremely high blood flow through the chemoreceptors, the pO_2 of arterial blood, chemoreceptor tissue, and venous blood is nearly the same. A decrease in arterial blood flow or in arterial oxygen tension increases the extraction of oxygen by the chemoreceptor tissue, decreases the venous pO_2, and through an unknown mechanism, activates the chemoreceptor.

Similar to the inactivation of baroreceptors and stretch receptors, the activation of chemoreceptors results in the stimulation of the hypothalamus and of the vascular component of the sympathetic nervous system (Fig. 1-6). In contrast to the inactivation of baroreceptors and stretch receptors, the activation of chemoreceptors produces a decrease in cardiac sympathetic nervous system activity and an increase in parasympathetic nervous system activity, thereby leading to a decrease in heart rate and cardiac contractility. Chemoreceptor activation stimulates the respiratory center, leading to an increase in respiratory rate. Hypovolemia is usually accompanied by hyperventilation because the decrease in the effective circulating volume activates the chemoreceptor through a reduction in blood flow.

PAIN AND EMOTION. Pain and emotional arousal are characteristic of any injury and lead to the activation of the neuroendocrine system. Pain, acting through projections of peripheral nociceptive fibers to the central nervous system, results in the stimulation of the thalamus and of the hypothalamus. Emotional arousal is produced by the perception or threat of injury and through the limbic areas of the brain invokes an emotional response resulting in anger, fear, or anxiety. In turn, these emotional changes stimulate the neuroendocrine reflexes through projections from the limbic system to hypothalamic and lower brain stem nuclei. As a result, both pain and emotion arousal produce an increase in the secretion of vasopressin, ACTH, endogenous opiates, catecholamines, cortisol, and aldosterone and changes in the activity of the autonomic nervous system.

Emotional factors have an effect on epinephrine release (sweating, tremor, tachycardia, dry mouth, pallor, etc.), the so-called fight or flight response described by Cannon. This factor may contribute to some of the differences between the effects of injury in the conscious state versus those of the same type of injury in the anesthetized patient. As noted by Wiggers when discussing the role of emotional factors in the investigation of hemorrhagic shock, ''The writer cannot be convinced that a subject with an indwelling catheter in his arm vein and auricle and forewarned that an experiment is to be conducted which will probably lead to uncomfortable experiences, is entirely free from psychic reactions which may influence the course of events.''

SUBSTRATE ALTERATIONS. Changes in the plasma glucose concentration are the primary substrate alterations that activate neuroendocrine reflexes. The plasma glucose concentration is sensed by receptors in the hypothalamus (ventromedial nucleus) and in the pancreas. A decrease in the plasma glucose concentration stimulates the release of catecholamines, growth hormone, cortisol, ACTH, beta-endorphin, and vasopressin through central pathways (hypothalamus and autonomic nervous system) and stimulates the release of glucagon both by central (autonomic nervous system) and by peripheral pathways (direct pancreatic activation). In addition, the secretion of insulin is inhibited by central pathways (autonomic nervous system) and by the pancreas itself.

Although changes in the concentrations of individual amino acids produce alterations in the secretion of various hormones, their potency varies from amino acid to amino acid and the mechanisms by which they produce these alterations are not entirely understood. For example, arginine is a potent stimulus to the secretion of insulin and of glucagon, but leucine, which also stimulates the secretion of insulin, does not stimulate the secretion of glucagon. The stimulation of hormonal secretion by amino acids is, at least in part, directed through cell surface receptors, since nonmetabolizable analogs of leucine and arginine are effective. The intracellular metabolism of amino acids may also be important. Amino acids also exert an important role in the neuroendocrine response because they are the parent compound for a number of hormonal agents and neurotransmitters (e.g., thyroxine, catecholamines, histamine, serotonin, and all peptide hormones).

TEMPERATURE. Changes in the core temperature of the body are sensed in the preoptic area of the hypothalamus and lead to alterations in the secretion of many hormones including ACTH, vasopressin, cortisol, epinephrine, growth hormone, catecholamines, aldosterone, and thyroxine. The core temperature may change as a result of alterations in ambient temperature, as a result of the loss of the normal thermal insulating barrier (burns), as a result of inadequate hepatic blood flow (hypovolemia) or substrate supply (starvation), or as a result of inadequate peripheral vasoconstriction or vasodilation (sepsis).

Changes in the ambient temperature stimulate neuroendocrine reflexes, either directly or through changes in the core temperature. Similarly, infection may stimulate the neuroendocrine system directly through the action of endotoxin, or indirectly through secondary changes in blood volume, oxygen concentration, substrate concentrations, and pain or through monokines released from inflammatory cells such as tumor necrosis factor and interleukin-1.

Integration of Stimuli and Modulation of Output

As indicated above, the principal signals to initiate the neuroendocrine response to injury are those of hypovolemia and of pain. The hormonal response is diffuse and includes the release of ACTH, cortisol, growth hormone, epinephrine, norepinephrine, glucagon, renin, angiotensin, and aldosterone (Table 1-1). In each case, the prompt initiation of hormonal release depends upon a reflex activated by afferent nerves. Although the reflex initiation of increased sympathetic activity may take place at the level of the medulla or spinal cord alone, it appears that even these reflexes require hypothalamic coordination similar to that observed in the control of the release of the anterior pituitary hormones. The precise pathways from afferent nerve endings to the hypothalamus have been studied in detail primarily for ACTH and to a lesser degree for vasopressin and catecholamines. Data for the control of other hormones, where they are available, seem analogous, and it is highly likely that the afferent pathways are shared to a considerable extent. This provides a basis for a coordinated response of the neuroendocrine system to injury.

The central pathways have been best delineated for the neural control of ACTH and vasopressin in response to hypovolemia and to a lesser extent in response to pain. The principal afferent receptors for blood volume lie in the right atrium and in the carotid arteries and for nociception in the substantia gelatinosa of the dorsal horn

Table 1-1. NEUROENDOCRINE RESPONSE

Increased release		Decreased release or unchanged
Epinephrine	Beta-endorphin	Insulin
Norepinephrine	Growth hormone	Estrogen
Dopamine	Prolactin	Testosterone
Glucagon	Somatostatin	Thyroxine
Renin	Eicosanoids	T_3
Angiotensin	Histamine	TSH
Vasopressin	Kinins	FSH
ACTH	Serotonin	LH
Cortisol	Interleukin-1	IGF
Aldosterone	TNF	

and nucleus caudalis of cranial nerve V. The afferent nerves from volume receptors converge on the nucleus tractus solitarius (NTS) and related structures in the dorsolateral medulla (Fig. 1-7). From this point, they project without synapsing to the nuclei of the locus ceruleus, parabrachial nucleus, and periaqueductal gray area in the dorsal pons, to the locus subceruleus and dorsal raphe nucleus of the dorsal pons and to the A1 region of the caudal, ventrolateral medulla. The pathway to A1 appears to constitute the principal projection from NTS. Nociceptive fibers also project to A1 neurons by nonsynaptic projections from the nucleus caudalis of cranial nerve V and the substantia gelatinosa of the dorsal horn. The A1 region of the medulla appears to be the first possible site for the interaction of pain and volume signals. Nucleus caudalis also projects to the region of the dorsal pons mentioned above, and interaction of nociception and volume stimuli has been observed in this region.

Fibers from A1 project, again without synapsing, to the nuclei of the locus ceruleus, parabrachial nucleus, and periaqueductal gray area in the dorsal pons and via the median forebrain bundle to the ventral hypothalamus and to the paraventricular nucleus. The dorsal pons area is critical to the generation of the classic neuroendocrine response to injury, since a lesion in the periaqueductal gray area of the dorsal pons will eliminate the response. This response appears to arise from fibers that project from the nuclei of the dorsal pons to the hypothalamus in three principal pathways, two stimulatory and one inhibitory. A dorsal stimulatory pathway courses through the dorsal longitudinal fasciculus to end in the dorsal hypothalamus, including the paraventricular nucleus. A ventral stimulatory pathway courses through the ventral tegmental area of the midbrain to enter the medial forebrain bundle and terminate in the anteroventral hypothalamic nuclei, including the suprachiasmatic and ventromedial nuclei and in the dorsal hypothalamus, including the paraventricular nucleus. An intermediate inhibitory pathway passes up the central tegmental tract and mammillary peduncles to terminate in the posterior hypothalamic area. Output from the paraventricular nucleus includes the release of corticotropin releasing factor (CRF), the agent that controls pituitary release of ACTH from the median eminence and arginine vasopressin (AVP). By contrast, output from the posterior hypothalamic area produces inhibition of CRF and AVP release either through the release of a specific factor or through inhibitory projections to the paraventricular nucleus and other hypothalamic areas.

Although the previous discussion has focused on the importance of the paraventricular nucleus in neuroendocrine reflexes, other nuclei in the hypothalamus play a central role in these reflexes by controlling the release of releasing factors, which in turn govern the secretion of various anterior pituitary hormones or autonomic nervous system activity. There is no clear overlap of function among the various hypothalamic nuclei. For example, the posterior hypothalamic area is involved in the control of ACTH and of the descending sympathetic activity. The paraventricular nucleus is involved in the con-

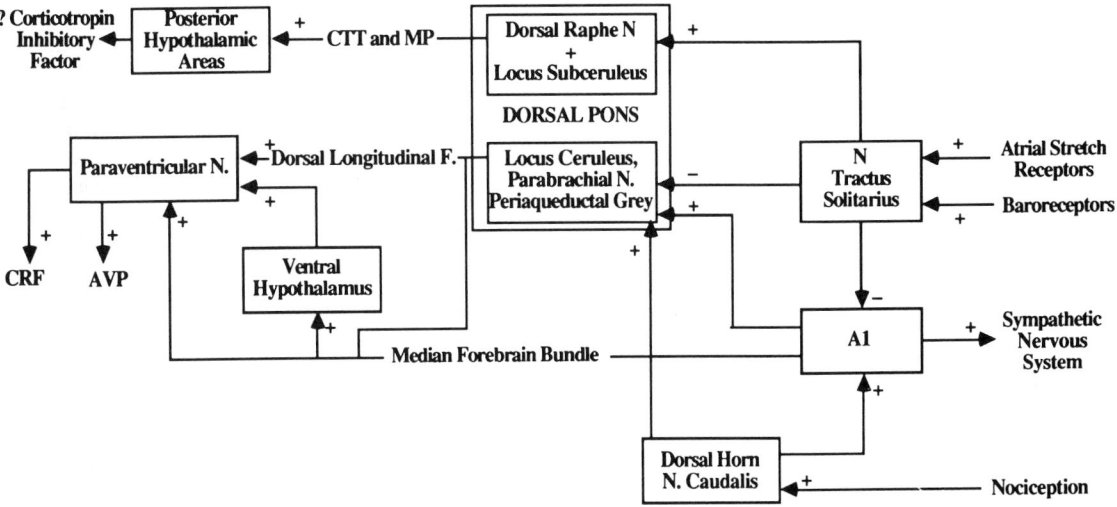

Fig. 1-7. The proposed neural organization for the control of ACTH and vasopressin in response to hemodynamic change and nociception. Three principal areas of the hypothalamus receive signals from the principal pontine areas, projecting through the areas defined in the midbrain to inhibit or facilitate release of vasopressin and of corticotropin releasing factor (CRF) by the median eminence and thus of ACTH. Thus, the principal pathways from atrial and carotid receptors to the median eminence for control of release of CRF and vasopressin are multiple. Symbols: N, nucleus; F, fasiculus; +, stimulates; −, inhibits.

trol of vasopressin, of oxytocin, and of ACTH. The ventromedial nucleus is involved in the control of growth hormone and ACTH. The supraoptic nucleus has been shown to be active in the control of vasopressin and of oxytocin. The suprachiasmatic nucleus appears to control the circadian rhythms of ACTH and of gonadotropins. In turn, hypothalamic control of the anterior pituitary is accomplished by the secretion of neurohormones into the capillary loops in the median eminence. Although this view focuses on the role of the hypothalamus in neuroendocrine control, it is clear that this region of the brain is important in the coordination of other autonomic functions as well as in the control of other hormones that appear to be less affected by injury.

As a result of the similar pathways through which sensory inputs enter into the central nervous system, integration of afferent signals can occur in the CNS with a resultant modulation of efferent signals from the CNS. Consequently, the neuroendocrine response to a given stimulus is not an all or none phenomenon nor is it always the same. The response depends to a large extent upon the intensity and the duration of the stimulus, the presence of simultaneous and sequential stimuli that are qualitatively the same or different, the status of the receptor at the time of stimulation, and the time of day during which the stimulus occurs.

The dependence of the response to a stimulus upon the intensity and duration of the stimulus, as well as the importance of central nervous system integration, is well described for cardiopulmonary reflexes and adrenomedullary secretion of catecholamines. Despite the potent activation of the sympathetic nervous system by small nonhypotensive hemorrhages, adrenomedullary secretion of catecholamines occurs only when hypotension develops. Since nonhypotensive hemorrhages have little if any effect upon arterial baroreceptors, this finding suggests that inactivation of cardiac stretch receptors alone is not sufficient for the activation of catecholamine release. Similarly, activation of chemoreceptors alone or inactivation of baroreceptors in isolation produces potent sympathetic nervous system activity but little adrenal catecholamine secretion. Adrenal catecholamine secretion does occur during hypotensive hemorrhages in which both receptors are activated, suggesting that high-pressure baroreceptors and low-pressure volume receptors both must be inactivated for adrenomedullary stimulation to occur. Afferent fibers from baroreceptors travel via the sinus branch of the glossopharyngeal nerve and via the vagus nerve to the nucleus tractus solitarius (NTS). Similarly, the afferent fibers from the cardiac stretch receptors travel via the vagus nerve to the NTS, from which secondary projections are sent to higher brain centers. Therefore, the interaction of arterial baroreceptor and cardiac stretch receptor inputs may occur as early as the NTS.

In addition to the intensity and the duration, the rate at which a stimulus is presented is also an important parameter in the modulation of efferent signals that are elicited by the stimulus. For example, Bereiter et al. have demonstrated that the serum epinephrine concentration in the cat following hemorrhage is a function of the rate and the magnitude of the hemorrhage (Fig. 1-8). Whereas small hemorrhages, equivalent to 10 to 20 percent of the blood volume, elicited the same increase in serum epinephrine concentrations independent of the rate of hemorrhage, large hemorrhages, equivalent to 30 percent of the blood volume, elicited a greater response when they were performed rapidly (10 percent/min) than when they were performed slowly (2 percent/min). Similar findings have also been reported for aldosterone, renin, and vasopressin (Fig. 1-9). Thus the neuroendocrine response of a trauma-

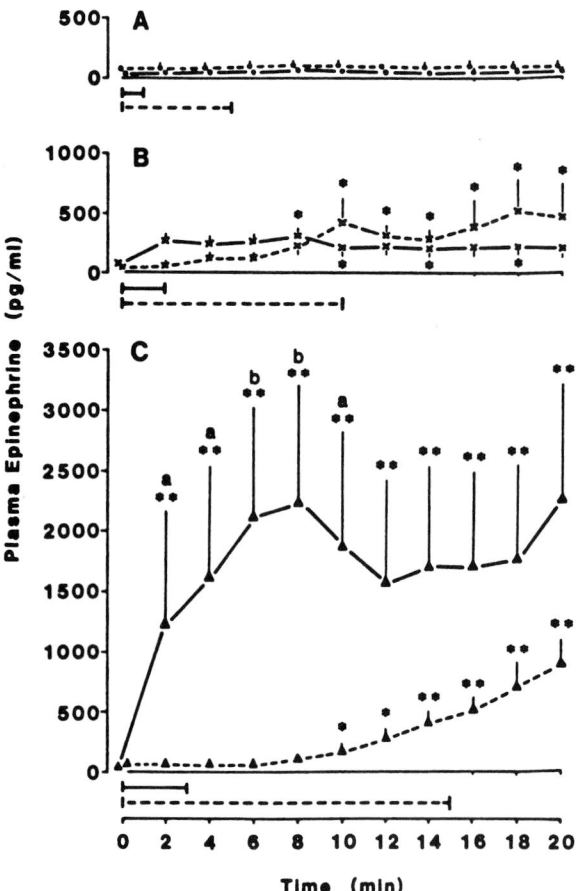

Fig. 1-8. Plasma epinephrine concentrations in response to graded blood loss in the cat at rapid and slow rates of hemorrhage. *A.* 10 percent hemorrhage, rapid rate = ●———● (*n* = 6), slow rate = ●————● (*n* = 7). *B.* 20 percent hemorrhage, rapid rate = ×———× (*n* = 11), slow rate = ×————× (*n* = 7). *C.* 30 percent hemorrhage, rapid rate = △———△ (*n* = 8), slow rate = △————△ (*n* = 8). The horizontal bars under each figure represent the period of blood removal for each hemorrhage magnitude. **p* < 0.05, ***p* < 0.01 vs. control group. a. *p* < 0.05; b. *p* < 0.01 vs. slow rate of hemorrhage. (From: *Bereiter DA et al: Am J Physiol 1986, with permission.*)

tized individual with a ruptured spleen who loses 30 percent blood volume in 1 h may be considerably different from the response seen in a patient with multiple long bone fractures who loses 30 percent blood volume over 1 day.

The responsiveness of receptors themselves to the transduction of the stimulus into neural activity is itself variable. For example, central osmoreceptors located in the hypothalamus, near the third ventricle, change their set point in response to other neural inputs. Alterations both of plasma osmolality and of effective circulating volume are potent stimuli to the secretion of vasopressin. Inputs from receptors monitoring these parameters interact in the central nervous system such that a change in the set point of the osmoreceptor occurs when the secretion of vasopressin is altered by neural inputs from baroreceptors. As a result, changes in the effective circulating volume do not eliminate the influence of the osmoregulatory system. Instead, the change in the set point of the osmoreceptor makes it more or less sensitive to a given osmotic stimulus. Clinically, this situation is observed in the hypervolemic, hyponatremic patient who despite an increased effective circulating volume produces vasopressin in response to the low plasma osmolality.

Similarly, the set point and the gain of baroreceptors may be altered by the convergence of other sensory inputs, such as viscerosomatic and somatosensory afferents, with baroreceptor inputs in the cardiovascular areas of the medulla. The responsiveness of baroreceptors themselves may be increased by the response they initiate, since baroreceptor responsiveness is increased by catecholamines, vasopressin, and angiotensin. Furthermore, the sensitivity of some receptors, such as those of the adrenal cortex, changes as a function of the time of day. For example, despite a similar response of ACTH to hemorrhage when it occurs in the morning or at night, the secretory response of cortisol to ACTH is significantly greater at night (Fig. 1-10). The latter finding may have particular significance for the traumatized patient, since severe trauma is much more likely to occur at night than during the day, but its importance in recovery from injury remains unknown. A particular stimulus of the same magnitude, rate, and duration may have less effect under certain circumstances than under others.

The stimuli accompanying injury, sepsis, and starvation rarely occur singly. Upon injury, the individual is likely to perceive multiple stimuli simultaneously. The neuroendocrine response to injury is the summation of all the stimuli the individual perceives and processes, and it is often different from the response to any single stimulus given alone (Fig. 1-11). For example, Egdahl and coworkers found hypothermic dogs responded with smaller increases in the secretions of ACTH, corticosteroids, and catecholamines than did normothermic dogs; Redding and Mueller found an increase in the survival of dogs that were hemorrhaged at lower ambient temperatures than dogs at normal or increased temperatures; Bereiter et al. demonstrated that the secretion of ACTH was greater to hemorrhage and noxious stimulation than to hemorrhage or noxious stimulation alone (Fig. 1-12); Wood et al. have demonstrated that dogs with an elevated rectal temperature (and presumably infection) respond with a greater decrease in blood pressure and a greater increase in the secretion of ACTH, corticosteroids, and vasopressin than do dogs who are normothermic; and Overman and Wang reported that although a 40 percent hemorrhage alone produced a 50 percent mortality, a 30 percent hemorrhage produced a similar mortality only when combined with sciatic nerve stimulation.

In addition to multiple stimuli occurring simultaneously, it is not uncommon for multiple stimuli to occur sequentially as well. A patient involved in a motor vehicle accident may first experience pain from fractured ribs, then hypovolemia from a ruptured spleen, and then hypoxia from a slowly developing tension pneumothorax. According to classic endocrine feedback mechanisms, one might expect that the elevation of serum cortisol, for

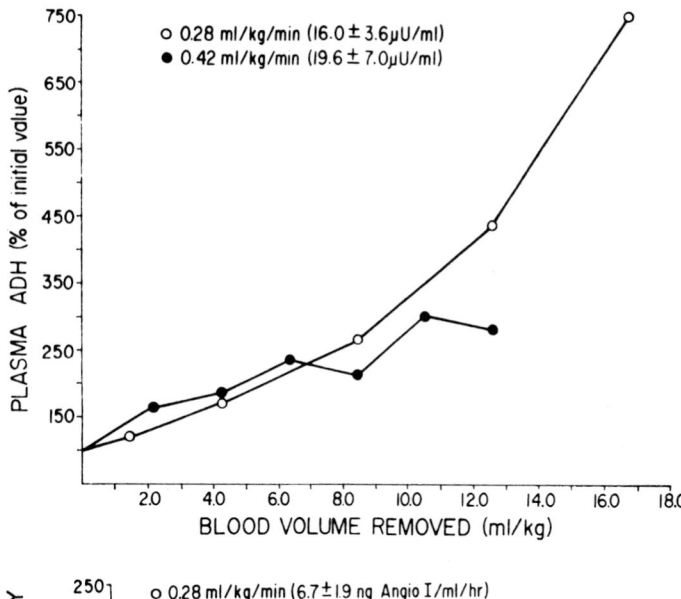

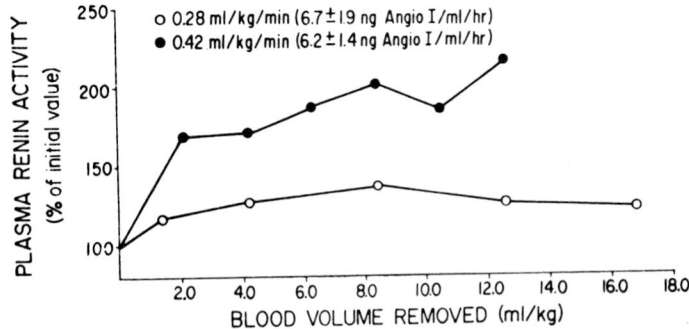

Fig. 1-9. The effect of rate of hemorrhage on vasopressin secretion and renin activity. There was no difference in plasma vasopressin when hemorrhages of 12 percent or less were performed either slowly (0.28 mL/kg/min) rapidly (0.42 mL/kg/min) in dogs. However, hemorrhages of greater than 12 percent were associated with a greater plasma vasopressin concentration if they were performed slowly. In contrast, renin activity was greater for fast hemorrhages. (From: *Claybaugh JR, Share L: Am J Physiol 224:519, 1973, with permission.*)

example, resulting from one set of stimuli would inhibit the release of ACTH by the second set. Under most circumstances this is not true and the response is unchanged or may actually be greater than the initial response (potentiation). The mechanism of this physiologic facilitation is not known, but it appears to take 60 to 90 min to offset the feedback inhibition of cortisol, and it lasts for at least 24 h. Gann, Lilly, and colleagues have demonstrated physiologic facilitation and potentiation for cortisol and catecholamines in response to sequential hemorrhages of the same magnitude and to sequential operations (Fig. 1-13). Similarly, Raff et al. have demonstrated potentiation of the adrenocortical response to hypoxia when an operation has been performed 2 h prior to the hypoxic stimulus but not 24 h prior (Fig. 1-14). The neuroendocrine response to trauma, shock, and sepsis may modify the response to subsequent operation, and the response to a second injury, such as posttraumatic operation, may

be considerably different from what it would have been had it occurred first.

The response to the stimuli consequent to injury may be modified by a variety of factors present in the individual prior to injury such as (1) ethanol and other recreational drugs, (2) concurrent medications, (3) drug withdrawal, (4) preexisting illness, and (5) the age of the individual.

Of these modifiers ethanol deserves special emphasis, since ethanol intoxication is a common finding in the multiply injured patient. According to *The Injury Fact Book* by Baker, O'Neill, and Karpf, over 75 percent of fatally injured motorcycle and auto accident victims between the ages of fifteen to sixty are intoxicated (blood ethanol > 100 mg percent) when the accident occurs at night and over 50 percent when it occurs during the day. Furthermore, over 50 percent of nighttime and 25 percent of daytime pedestrian deaths among people fifteen to sixty-five years old involves an intoxicated individual.

The significance of alcohol intoxication on the overall response to injury has not been well studied but the ability of alcohol to alter metabolic and endocrine events is well recognized. For example, ethanol impairs hepatic gluconeogenesis by decreasing the concentration of NAD+ in the liver and thereby producing a more reduced state. This action of ethanol probably explains the find-

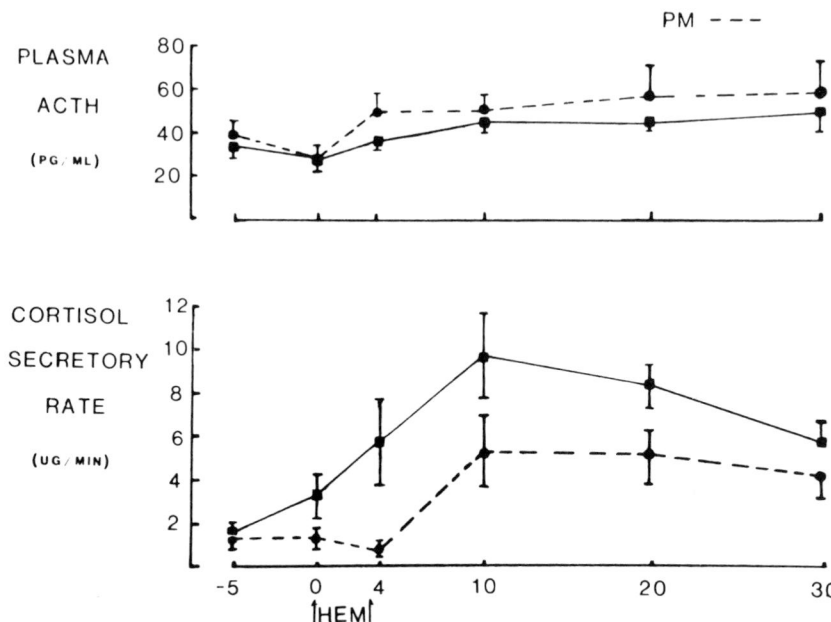

Fig. 1-10. Plasma ACTH concentration and cortisol secretory rates in dogs after a 10 mL/kg hemorrhage for 3 min in the morning ($n = 9$) or at night ($n = 7$). Although there was difference in plasma ACTH when the hemorrhage was performed in the morning or at night, cortisol secretion was greater in the morning. (From: *Engeland WC et al: Endocrinology 110:1856, 1982, with permission.*)

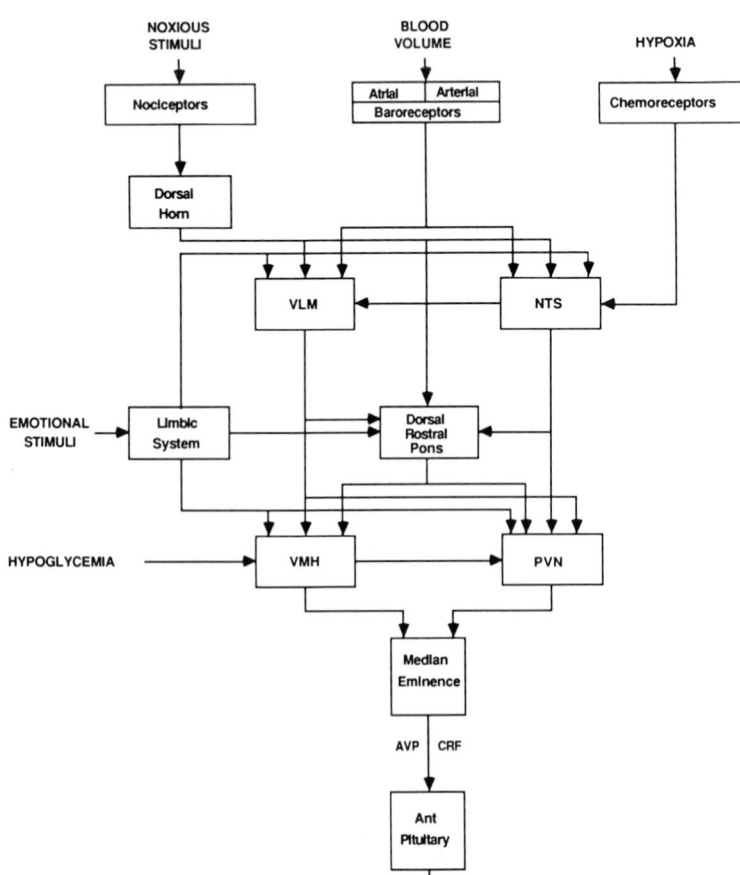

Fig. 1-11. Possible sites for the integration of the various stimuli elicited by injury are schematically represented. For example, noxious stimuli, hypovolemia, and hypoxia may first interact at NTS. Symbols: NTS, nucleus tractus solitarius; PVN, paraventricular nucleus; VLM, ventrolateral medulla; VMN, ventromedial hypothalamus (dorsomedial, arcuate, suprachiasmatic, periventricular, and premammillary nuclei). The dorsal rostral pons contains the loci ceruleus and subceruleus, the parabrachial nucleus, the periaqueductal gray and the dorsal raphe nucleus. Although this figure shows the release of ACTH, it is likely that other anterior pituitary hormones are controlled in a similar manner.

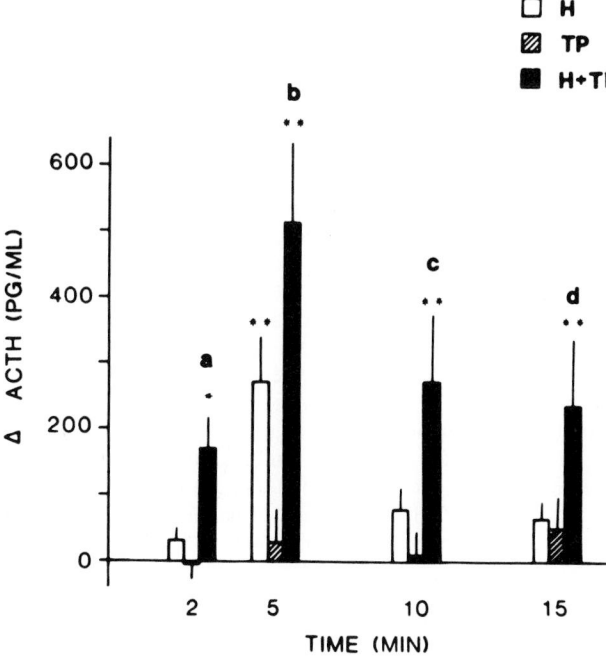

Fig. 1-12. Potentiation of the ACTH response to hemorrhage by nerve stimulation. H = hemorrhage, TP = tooth pulp, * = $p < 0.05$ vs. baseline, ** = $p < 0.01$ vs. baseline. (Letters above each sample time point denote intragroup individual comparisons: a = $p < 0.05$ H + TP vs. TP, b = $p < 0.01$ H + TP vs. TP or H, c = $p < 0.05$ H + TP vs. H, d = $p < 0.05$ H + TP vs. TP or H.) At all time points, the response of ACTH to hemorrhage and tooth pulp stimulation was greater than the response to either hemorrhage or tooth pulp stimulation alone. (From: *Bereiter DS et al: Endocrinology 113:1439, 1983, with permission.*)

ings of Stoner et al. in which the plasma glucose and pyruvate concentrations were lower and the plasma lactate concentrations were higher in intoxicated than in nonintoxicated patients at a given injury severity score. In addition, ethanol is capable of altering the neuroendocrine response as evidenced by an increase in central and urinary catecholamines, an increase in adrenal medullary catecholamine turnover, and by increasing plasma concentrations of cortisol and ACTH. Similarly, narcotics such as heroin and other recreational drugs such as cocaine produce potent metabolic and endocrine alterations and because of their anesthetic properties may serve to alter the response to injury. Withdrawal from these agents in the postinjury period may have profound metabolic and endocrine consequences that serve to prolong or alter the response to the injury. The latter is also true for commonly used drugs such as insulin which may be withheld from an unconscious patient who is not known to be diabetic.

Efferent Output

There are three major branches to the efferent limb of the reflex neuroendocrine response to injury, the autonomic response, the hormonal response, and the local tis-

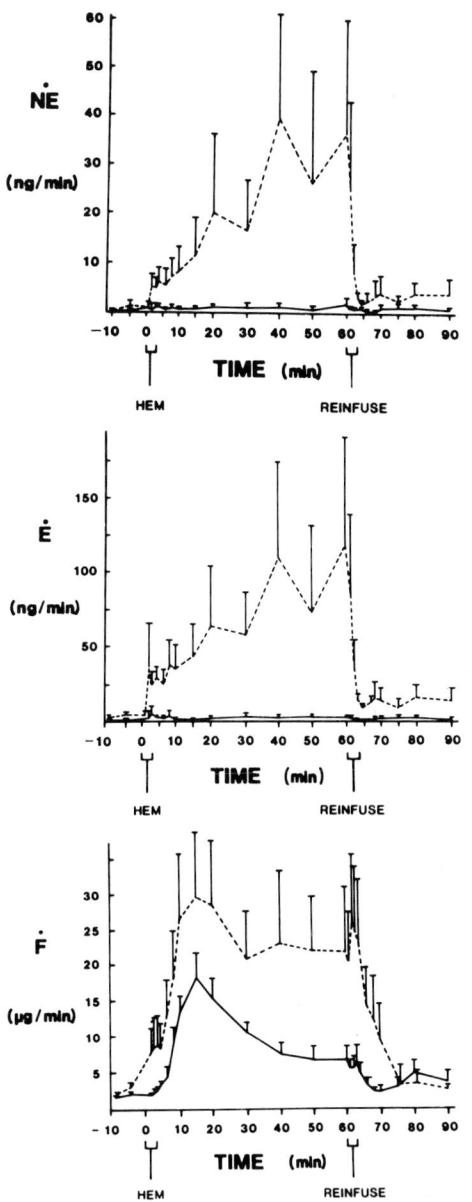

Fig. 1-13. Potentiation of the secretory rates of epinephrine (E), norepinephrine (NE), and cortisol (F) to a 7.5 mL/kg hemorrhage in dogs when a hemorrhage of the same magnitude was performed on the previous day. The pattern of response between E and NE is the same, but that for NE is at a lower absolute rate than that for E. Hemorrhages took place at 0 min; reinfusion occurred at 60 min. _____ = mean response on day 1; –––– = mean response on day 2. (From: *Lilly MP et al: Endocrinology 111:1917, 1982; 112:681, 1983, with permission.*)

sue response. The former two responses arise in two distinct areas of the brain: the autonomic regions of the brain stem and the hypothalamic-pituitary axis. Output from the former changes the activities of the sympathetic and parasympathetic nervous systems, whereas outputs from both areas change the rates of hormonal secretion. As such, the endocrine response may be divided into hor-

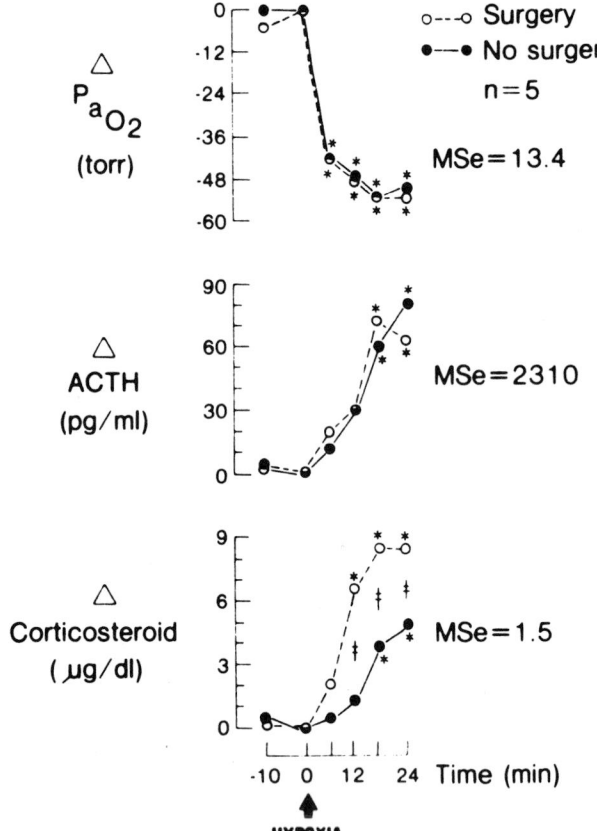

Fig. 1-14. Potentiation of plasma corticosteroids in dogs who are made hypoxic after surgery when compared with dogs made hypoxic without previous surgery. (* = different from 0 min sample; ‡ = difference between surgery and no surgery.) (From: *Raff H et al: Proc Soc Exp Biol Med 172:400, 1983, with permission.*)

mones whose secretion is primarily under hypothalamic-pituitary control (cortisol, thyroxine, growth hormone, and vasopressin) and hormones whose secretion is primarily under autonomic control (insulin, glucagon, and catecholamines). The local tissue response is composed of numerous small peptides (tissue factors, monokines, and autocoids) whose release may be mediated by the local inflammatory response in an injured area or by the injured tissue itself.

The hormones secreted by endocrine organs, the autocoids and monokines produced by tissues and inflammatory cells, and the neurotransmitters released at nerve terminals fall into one of five chemical classes. These are the fatty acid derivatives of cholesterol (cortisol, aldosterone) or arachidonic acid (prostaglandins, leukotrienes), proteins (insulin, glucagon), glycoproteins (thyroid stimulating hormone, follicle stimulating hormone), small polypeptides (vasopressin, enkephalin), and the amines (catecholamines, thyroxine, serotonin). All these agents act as cellular receptors that are either on the surface of cell membranes or in the cytoplasm of the cell. These cellular receptors are neither fixed nor unchangeable. Instead, they are in a dynamic state in which the number of recep-

tors on cells can be increased (up regulation) or decreased (down regulation) according to need. In addition, the affinity of these receptors for their specific hormone can also be changed.

By and large, the chemical nature of these agents determines the mechanism through which they exert their effects. Steroid hormones and possibly thyroxine, which are freely permeable to cell membranes, bind to cytosolic receptors in target cells. Although there are some rapid actions of steroid hormones that may be mediated by their binding to receptors on the plasma membrane, for the most part the interaction of steroid hormones and of thyroid hormones with receptors on the cell surface does not appear to be an important step in the initiation of the actions of these hormones since they appear to diffuse rapidly and freely across the cell membrane. Upon entering the cell, steroid hormones bind to cytosolic receptors that are specific for each hormone in a process that may be modulated by vitamin B_6. Once bound to the receptor, the receptor-hormone complex is activated and translocated to the nucleus. In the nucleus, the receptor-hormone complex binds to the nonhistone protein of nuclear chromatin, thereby modulating the transcription of genes into specific mRNA molecules that ultimately direct the synthesis of enzymatic, structural, and regulatory proteins (Fig. 1-15). This explains the 1- to 2-h delay in onset of most of the primary actions of steroid hormones. In addition, recent evidence suggests that the receptor hormone complex binds tRNA species. This may be a posttranscriptional mechanism through which steroid hormones are capable of modulating gene expression, i.e., by altering the efficiency of the translation of mRNA to proteins.

In contrast to steroid hormones, the action of most peptide and amine hormones, which generally bind to cell surface receptors, is faster and of shorter duration. In general, these hormones act either through alterations in the intracellular concentrations of cyclic adenosine monophosphate (cAMP) or calcium, the so-called second messengers, or through other intermediates (growth hormone via somatomedins). The second messenger system of hormonal action operates primarily through the activation and inactivation of regulatory proteins and enzymes rather than through the synthesis of new proteins (Fig. 1-16); this explains the faster onset of action and shorter duration of the effect of hormones that operate via this system versus those of steroid and other lipid soluble hormones.

The adrenergic receptor system may be considered the prototype for examining the mechanisms of action of second messengers since all the second messenger pathways known are represented in the four adrenergic receptors (alpha$_1$, alpha$_2$, beta$_1$, beta$_2$). Beta$_1$ and beta$_2$ receptors (differentiated on the basis of radioligand binding affinity) both function via the activation of membrane bound adenylate cyclase, which in turn leads to the production of cAMP. The increased intracellular concentration of cAMP activates an inactive protein kinase that then phosphorylates an inactive phosphorylase kinase to an active form. In turn, the active phosphorylase kinase phosphory-

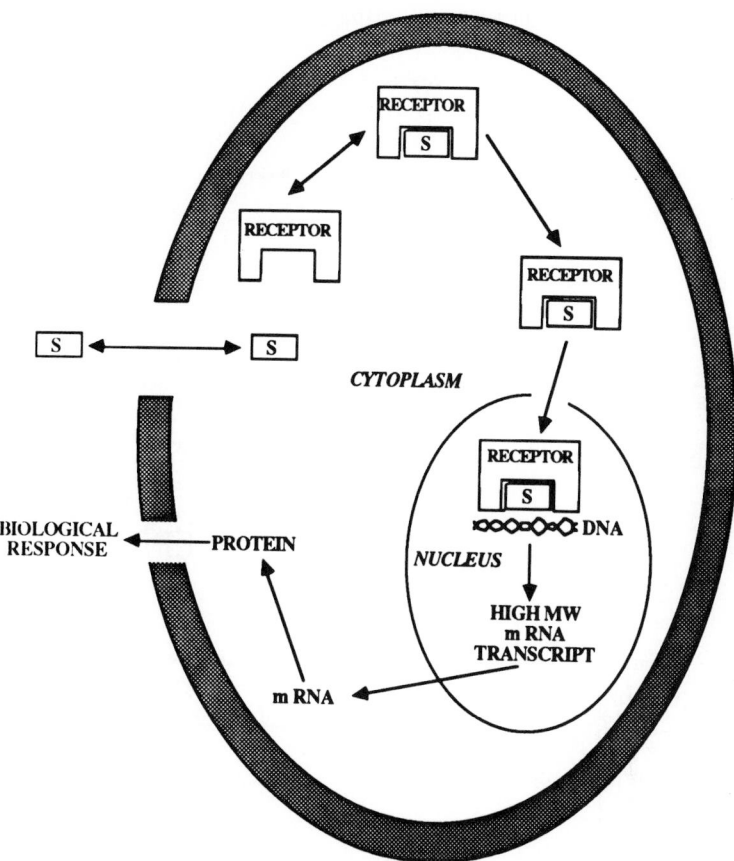

Fig. 1-15. The mechanism of action of steroid hormones. Steroids, which permeate the cell membrane freely, bind to cytosolic receptors and are then translocated to the nucleus, where the receptor hormone complex interacts with DNA to modulate transcription.

Fig. 1-16. Hormonal action mediated by cAMP or calcium. Alpha-1 receptors, through activation of phosphatidylinositol turnover, increase the intracellular concentration of calcium. Beta receptors, through activation of adenylate cyclase, increase the intracellular concentration of cAMP. An increase in either cAMP or calcium is then able to convert inactive protein kinase to active protein kinase.

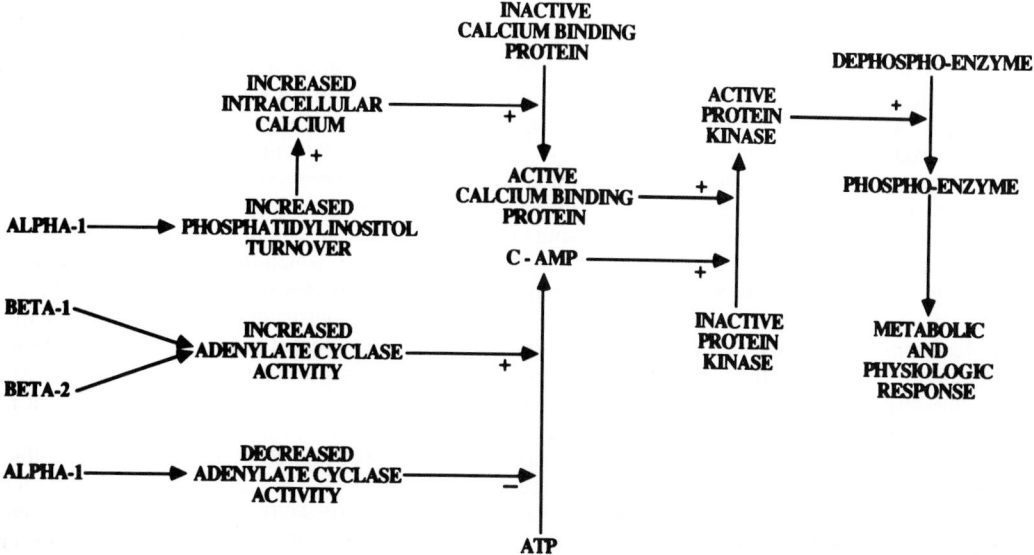

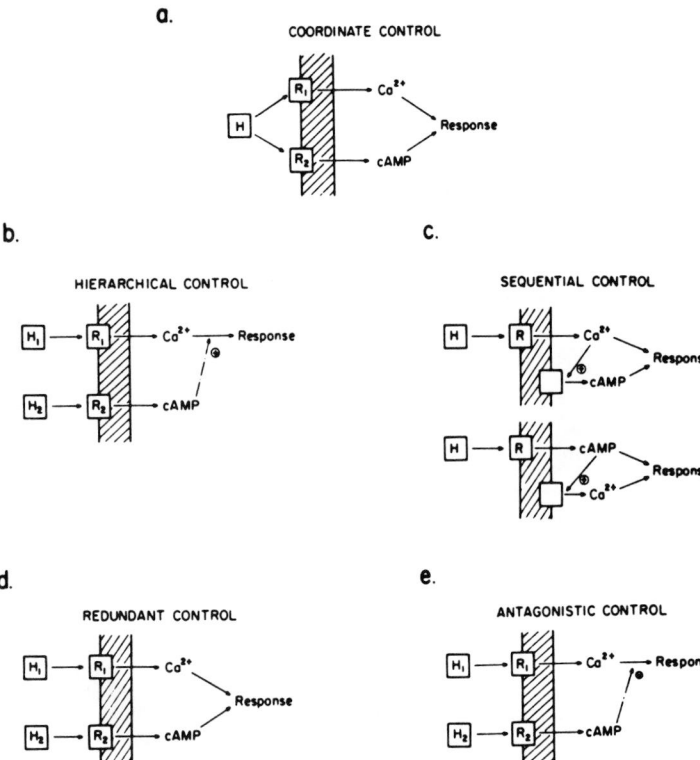

Fig. 1-17. The patterns of synarchic regulation by calcium and cAMP second messengers. See text for description of these patterns. (From: *Rassmusen H: Calcium and c-AMP as Synarchic Messengers. New York, Wiley Intersciences, 1981, Chap 4, with permission.*)

lates dephosphoregulatory enzymes, which may result in the activation of the regulatory enzyme (e.g., glycogen phosphorylase) or in its inactivation (e.g., glycogen synthetase). By contrast, alpha$_2$ receptor activation inhibits membrane bound adenylate cyclase, thereby decreasing the concentration of cAMP and active protein kinase.

Alpha$_2$ receptor activation results in an increase in phosphatidylinosital turnover that then mediates an increase in intracellular calcium concentration from intracellular and extracellular sources. The increase in intracellular calcium activates a calcium binding protein, calmodulin, which in turn activates an inactive protein kinase or phosphorylase kinase. It should also be noted that calcium is utilized as a second messenger for stimulus-response coupling of many other key biological processes including excitation-contraction coupling in muscle, excitation-secretion coupling at nerve endings and in exocrine and endocrine glands, maintenance of oxidative phosphorylation, activation of contractile and motile cell systems (microtubules and microfilaments), platelet activation, regulation of plasma membrane permeability, tight gap junction, and cell-to-cell communication.

The actions of intracellular cAMP and calcium in the coupling of receptor activation with hormonal action (stimulus-response coupling) are not independent. Instead, the actions of calcium and cAMP in stimulus-response coupling are highly interrelated and have been termed synarchic by Rassmusen. There are five basic patterns to the synarchic control of hormone-response coupling that cAMP and calcium (Fig. 1-17). In coordinate control, a hormone activates both a calcium activating receptor and a cAMP activating receptor, either one of which may produce the response alone. In hierarchical control, separate stimuli activate independently the calcium and cAMP pathways that are both necessary for a given response. In sequential control, the activation of one of the two limbs of the system leads to the activation of the other limb. Although the first limb can produce the response, activation of the second limb augments the response. In redundant control, two separate stimuli independently activate the two different limbs of the messenger system, either one of which can produce the response. Finally, in antagonist control one stimulus activates one limb of the messenger system that leads to the response and a second stimulus activates the second limb, which inhibits the ability of the first limb to produce the response. Although each of these control mechanisms can occasionally be found in cells in pure form, most of the presently known hormone-response coupling mechanisms involve mixed patterns.

HORMONAL REPONSE TO INJURY

CRF-ACTH-CORTISOL. Most types of trauma are characterized by an increased secretion of CRF, ACTH, and

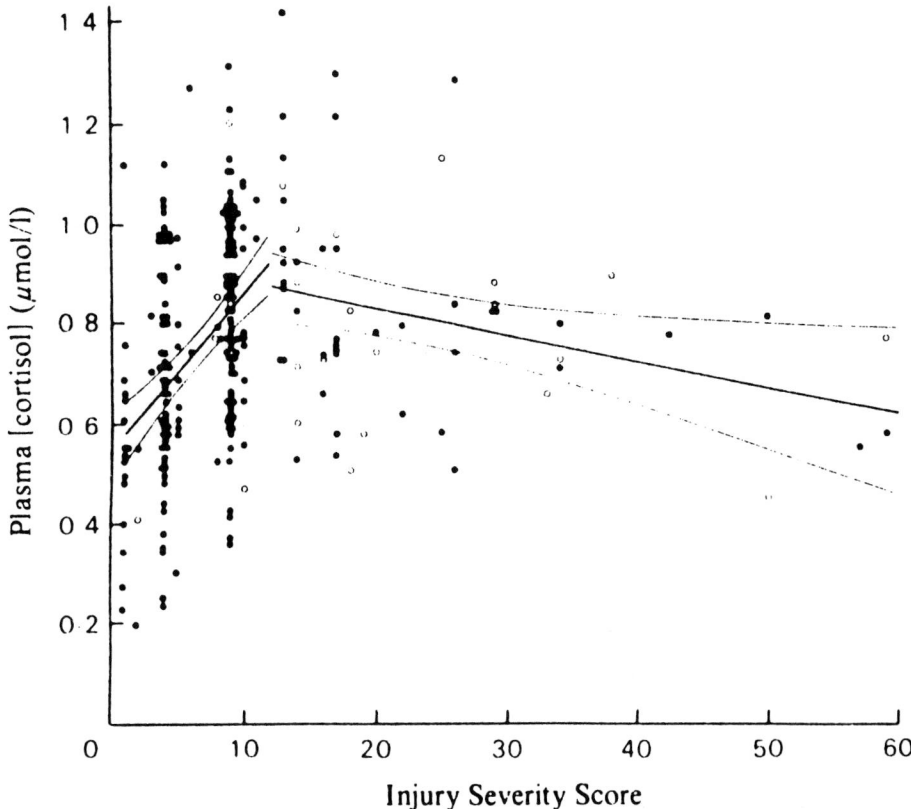

Fig. 1-18. The relationship between plasma cortisol and injury severity score (ISS) in initial samples from multiply injured patients studied within 8-h of injury. The regression lines and their 95 percent confidence limits between ISS 1 to 12 and ISS 13 to 59 are shown for ethanol negative (●) and ethanol positive (○) patients combined. (From: *Stoner HB et al: Clin Sci 56:563, 1979, with permission.*)

Fig. 1-19. There is a strong correlation between the extent of thermal injury, as determined by the percentage of body surface area burned and the plasma cortisol concentration in human beings. (From: *Vaughn GM et al: J Trauma 22:263–273, 1982, with permission.*)

cortisol that correlates with the severity of the injury (Fig. 1-18) and with the body surface area that is burned (Fig. 1-19). The plasma concentration of cortisol, which loses its normal circadian rhythm after injury, remains elevated for up to 4 weeks following thermal injury, for less than 1 week following soft tissue trauma, and for a few days following hemorrhage. In fact, in pure hypovolemia the plasma cortisol concentration returns rapidly to normal once the blood volume has been restored. Super-

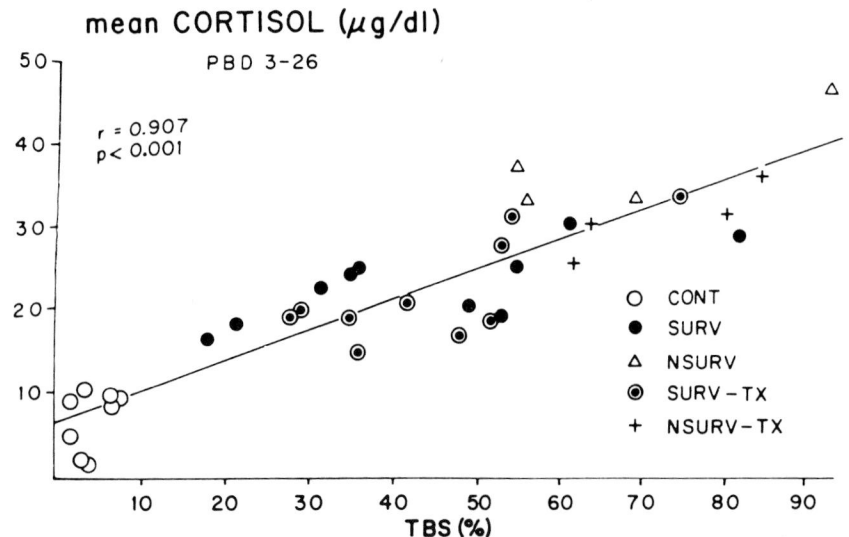

vening infection, however, will prolong the increase in plasma cortisol in all these injuries.

The synthesis and the release of cortisol from cells of the adrenal zona fasciculata is primarily under the control of adrenocorticotropin (ACTH) and is mediated by an increase in the intracellular concentration of cAMP that is produced by the binding of ACTH to surface receptors on the adrenal cells. ACTH is synthesized and stored in chromophobe cells of the anterior pituitary gland as a fragment of a larger molecule, pro-opiomelanocortin, that also contains gamma- and beta-lipotrophin, alpha-melanocyte stimulating hormone and beta-endorphin. The release of ACTH from these cells is stimulated by corticotropin releasing factor (CRF) from the paraventricular nucleus of the hypothalamus and may be potentiated by angiotensin II, vasopressin, and possibly oxytocin. Recent evidence also suggests that interleukin-1 may stimulate the production of ACTH by pituitary cells. By contrast, the release of ACTH is inhibited by cortisol (long feedback) and by ACTH itself (short feedback). In general, ACTH is increased following injury in a pattern that closely parallels that observed for cortisol. Cortisol may remain elevated for prolonged periods following injury despite an early return of ACTH to normal as demonstrated in the studies of burn victims by Vaughan and colleagues.

Corticotropin releasing factor is synthesized primarily in cells of the paraventricular nucleus that are near but distinct from those that secrete vasopressin. The release of CRF into the hypophyseal-portal venous system is induced primarily by neurogenic inputs into the hypothalamic cells. Vasopressin potentiates the release of CRF, as well as its action on the anterior pituitary gland; the release of both CRF and vasopressin may be potentiated by angiotensin II.

Cortisol has widespread effects upon the metabolism and utilization of glucose, amino acids, and fatty acids. In the liver, cortisol inhibits the pentose phosphate shunt, the action of insulin, and several regulatory glycolytic enzymes, including glucokinase, phosphofructokinase, and pyruvate kinase, and it stimulates the uptake of amino acids, the activities of amino acid transaminases, the activity of glycogen synthetase, and the activities and de novo synthesis of several regulatory gluconeogenic enzymes, including pyruvate carboxylase, phosphoenolpyruvate carboxykinase, fructose-1,6-bisphosphatase and glucose-6-phosphatase. Cortisol also potentiates the actions of glucagon and epinephrine on the liver. In skeletal muscle tissue, cortisol appears to have no direct effect on glucose uptake or glucose metabolism but it does inhibit insulin mediated glucose uptake. In addition, cortisol reduces the uptake and increases the release of amino acids by skeletal muscle. In the absence of cortisol, amino acid release and tissue concentrations of amino acids are decreased. Therefore, cortisol appears to exert an important role in maintaining, at least, euglycemia during stressful conditions by increasing the availability of gluconeogenic substrates to the liver. As a result of these actions, it is no surprise that there is a close correlation between the plasma concentrations of glucose and cortisol following injury.

In adipose tissue, cortisol increases lipolysis directly and indirectly through the potentiation of other lipolytic hormones such as epinephrine and growth hormone. As a result, the concentrations of free fatty acids in the plasma increase. Cortisol also decreases glucose uptake in adipose tissue.

Cortisol, at least in excess concentrations, inhibits immunologic and inflammatory responses, as reflected by impaired lymphocyte, monocyte, and polymorphonuclear cell functioning. In particular, the administration of corticosteroids increases the circulating concentrations of lymphocytes and neutrophils and decreases the circulating concentrations of monocytes and eosinophils. At inflammatory sites, corticosteroids reduce markedly the number of polymorphonuclear cells, monocytes, macrophages, and lymphocytes that accumulate. The reduction of the inflammatory response is, at least in part, the result of these alterations in white cell mobilization and migration. In addition, cortisol decreases glucose uptake and amino acid release by lymphocytes, inhibits phospholipase A (an enzyme necessary for prostaglandin and leukotriene synthesis), and stabilizes lysosomal membranes, actions that may alter the function of inflammatory cells by decreasing their metabolism and their release of prostaglandins and of proteolytic enzymes. Therefore, it is not surprising that patients receiving steroids have impaired wound healing and that they may frequently have a serious infection with little systemic manifestation.

Because of their potent anti-inflammatory properties, corticosteroids are administered for a variety of inflammatory disease states. The exogenous administration of corticosteroids partially inhibits ACTH, as described previously, and leads to decreased adrenal stimulation, atrophy, and finally very little production of corticosteroid. If the adrenal is sufficiently atrophic, even a large dose of ACTH, such as that which might occur following severe injury, will fail to stimulate the adrenal cortex acutely to produce an increased output of corticosteroids. Patients who have been on steroid administration for prolonged periods of time, whose adrenals have become atrophic, and who are not given corticosteroids to support them during an operation or following trauma may die because of the failure of cortisol to be released from an adrenal rendered temporarily inactive by atrophy. If acute adrenal insufficiency does occur, the most prominent features are fever and hypotension. In the past, when bilateral adrenalectomy was attempted prior to the availability of cortisone, it was universally fatal as a result of adrenal insufficiency. Similarly, if a patient with unsuspected adrenal insufficiency is operated upon without being supported with exogenous corticosteroids, death is likely to ensue. Thus, cortisol is necessary for the normal response to trauma.

Death resulting from adrenal insufficiency in an injured patient is generally associated with hypoglycemia, hyponatremia, and hyperkalemia. The latter two findings result from the loss of the sodium retaining and kaliuretic properties of aldosterone and to a lesser extent of cortisol. Hyponatremia in posttraumatic adrenal insufficiency is also exaggerated by increased concentrations of vasopressin (and therefore decreased free water clearance)

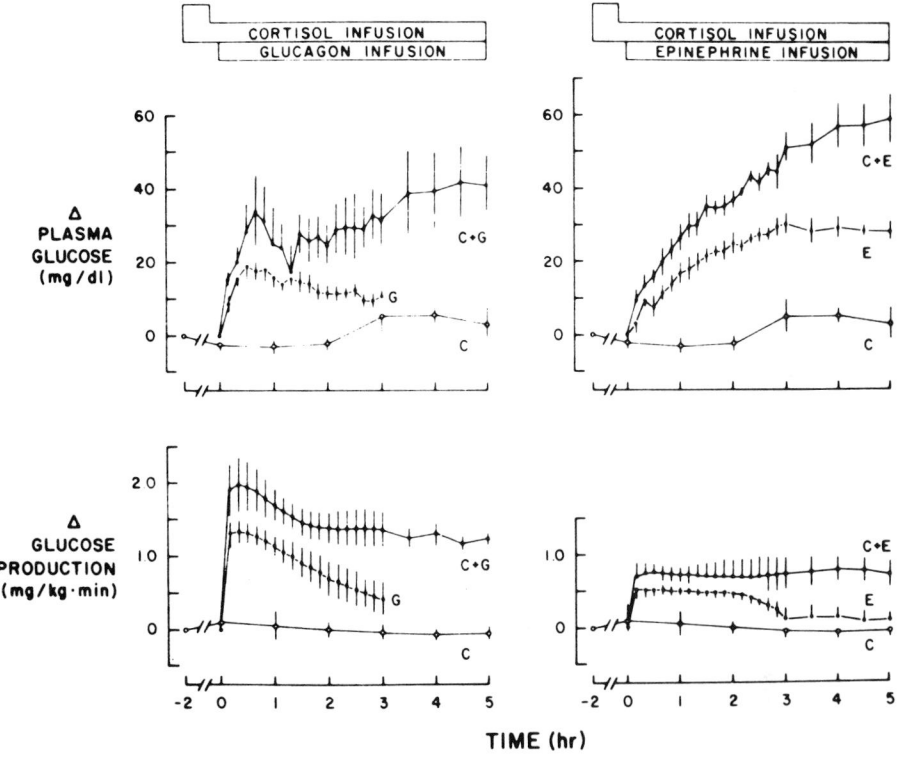

Fig. 1-20. The influence of cortisol (C) on the response of plasma glucose and glucose production to glucagon (G) or epinephrine (E). Cortisol, which by itself did not alter plasma glucose or glucose production, had the effect of increasing and more importantly prolonging the stimulatory effects of glucagon and epinephrine on glucose production. As a result, the effects of the combined hormone infusions on plasma glucose were more than additive. (From: *Eigler NJ et al: Clin Invest 63:114, 1979, with permission.*)

consequent to injury. Hypoglycemia arises because of the important effects cortisol exerts on hepatic glucose production. It is noteworthy that despite the major effects of cortisol on hepatic carbohydrate metabolism, adrenalectomized animals and man do not exhibit marked alterations in carbohydrate metabolism if food is constantly available. However, in the presence of injury or of starvation, adrenalectomized animals and man do exhibit marked alterations in hepatic carbohydrate metabolism that result in rapid and fatal hypoglycemia. The absence of cortisol mediated induction of de novo synthesis of hepatic enzymes is not sufficient to explain the reduction in serum glucose, since enzyme synthesis requires several hours. Perfusion of the livers of adrenalectomized animals in the absence of any gluconeogenic hormones, such as epinephrine or glucagon, reveals no difference in the gluconeogenic conversion of lactate or alanine to glucose when compared with normal animals. Total glucose release is impaired and glycogen stores are virtually absent. In the presence of glucagon or epinephrine, the perfused livers of adrenalectomized animals do exhibit a marked impairment in gluconeogenesis. Thus, stress-induced hypoglycemia in adrenalectomized animals and man appears to be, at least in part, the result of the inability to store glycogen and the absence of the permissive

action of corticosteroids on glucagon and epinephrine mediated gluconeogenesis.

The permissive action of cortisol was first proposed by Ingle to explain the finding that adrenalectomized animals given maintenance doses of corticosteroids showed some of the metabolic changes formerly ascribed to an increased secretion of corticosteroids. He proposed that the primary role of cortisol in trauma was to permit or augment the action of other hormones. Glucagon and epinephrine stimulated hepatic gluconeogenesis are markedly enhanced in the presence of cortisol, lending credence to this hypothesis (Fig. 1-20). Not all the beneficial effects of cortisol following trauma can be ascribed to their permissive action. For example, studies of blood volume restitution following hemorrhage have demonstrated that maintenance concentrations of cortisol are not sufficient for complete blood volume restitution and that increased concentrations of cortisol are necessary (Fig. 1-21).

Paraplegic patients who fail to respond to the operative trauma with an increase in cortisol secretion generally tolerate the operative procedure well. There are at least three possible explanations for this apparent paradox. First and foremost, the secretion of cortisol remains low in the paraplegic patient despite trauma because of the absence of afferent nerve impulses from the area of injury, but the response to uncompensated hemorrhage, supervening infection, or hypothalamic stimulation from hypoglycemia remains intact. Paraplegic patients are able to respond to a reduction in the effective circulating volume should it occur because the baroreceptor reflexes are mediated by cranial nerves. In severe trauma, the hepatic

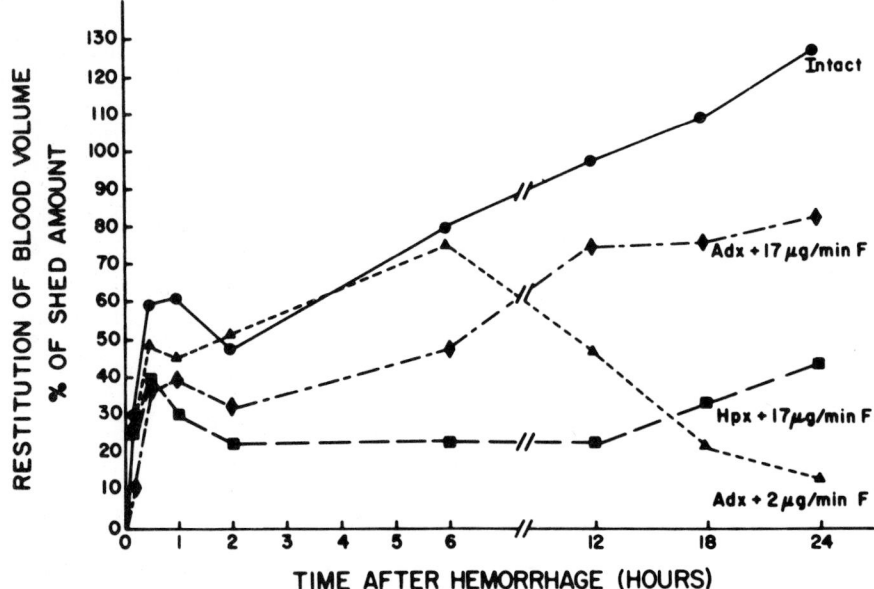

Fig. 1-21. Restitution of blood volume after 10 percent hemorrhage in four groups of splenectomized dogs: intact (●) adrenalectomized infused with cortisol at 2 μg/min (Δ); adrenalectomized infused with cortisol at 2 μg/min prior to hemorrhage, then at 17 μg/min (◆); hypophysectomized infused with cortisol at 17 μg/min (°). The response of each group differed significantly from that of each other group ($P < 0.01$, analysis of variance). (From: *Gann et al: Recent Prog Horm Res 34:357, 1978, with permission.*)

conjugation of corticosteroids to inactive forms may be reduced, so that larger amounts of the unconjugated (active) form are suddenly available even though the rate of secretion remains constant. An operative trauma is far better tolerated in patients whose body cells have not been deprived of the adrenal corticosteroids preoperatively than in those in whom preexisting deficiency is present.

Adrenal exhaustion, which was once thought to occur following prolonged trauma, probably never occurs, and isolated instances of adrenal insufficiency after severe injury are most likely the result of pituitary infarction secondary to hypotension. By contrast, most patients who die following injury, sepsis, burns, infection, and other forms of severe prolonged trauma die with very high blood levels of corticosteroids (Fig. 1-22). The very existence of continued high concentrations of plasma corticosteroids in the severely burned patient is usually a bad prognostic sign, suggesting that the trauma of burns is continuing and severe and that death may ensue.

TSH-THYROXINE. Since most injuries are associated with hypermetabolism in the immediate postoperative or posttraumatic period, it would be reasonable to postulate that the activity of thyroid hormones, agents known to dramatically increase the metabolic rate, would be increased following injury. This is not the case, however, and in most injuries the concentrations of thyroid hormones are normal or decreased (Fig. 1-23). Therefore, even though the presence of thyroid hormones is necessary for the normal functioning of organs in response to a traumatic stress, an increased secretion is not necessary.

The thyroid hormones, thyroxine (T_4) and triiodothyronine (T_3), are synthesized and released from the thyroid gland in response to thyroid stimulating hormone (TSH). Inhibition of thyroid hormone release occurs through the actions of T_4 and T_3 themselves on the hypothalamus and pituitary and thyroid glands. Upon stimulation by TSH,

the thyroid gland releases primarily T_4 which, in turn, is converted in the periphery to T_3. As a result, most of the circulating T_4 is derived from the thyroid gland and most of the circulating T_3 from peripheral conversion. Both T_4 and T_3 are bound to plasma proteins so that free and bound forms exist in the circulation. Following injury, burns, and a major operation the peripheral conversion of T_4 to T_3 is impaired, resulting in reduced circulating concentrations of both free and total T_3. In part this is the result of a cortisol mediated block of the conversion of T_4 to T_3 and of an increased conversion of T_4 to the biologically inactive molecule, reverse T_3. An increase in reverse T_3 is also characteristic of injury (Fig. 1-24). The plasma concentrations of total T_4 also are frequently decreased after injury, but free T_4 concentrations usually remain normal. In fact, depressed concentrations of free T_4 appear to be an ominous clinical finding associated with death in traumatized, burned, and critically ill medical patients (Fig. 1-23).

TSH is synthesized and released by basophilic cells of the anterior pituitary in response to the stimulatory action of the hypothalamic hormone, thyrotropin releasing hormone (TRH). Inhibition of TSH release is the result of the inhibitory influences of T_4 and T_3 on the pituitary gland and hypothalamus. The release of TSH is also stimulated by estrogens and inhibited by corticosteroids, somatostatin, growth hormone, and fasting. Physiologically, T_3 is much more potent than T_4. In addition, available evidence suggests that the inhibition of TSH secretion by the anterior pituitary gland occurs primarily through T_3.

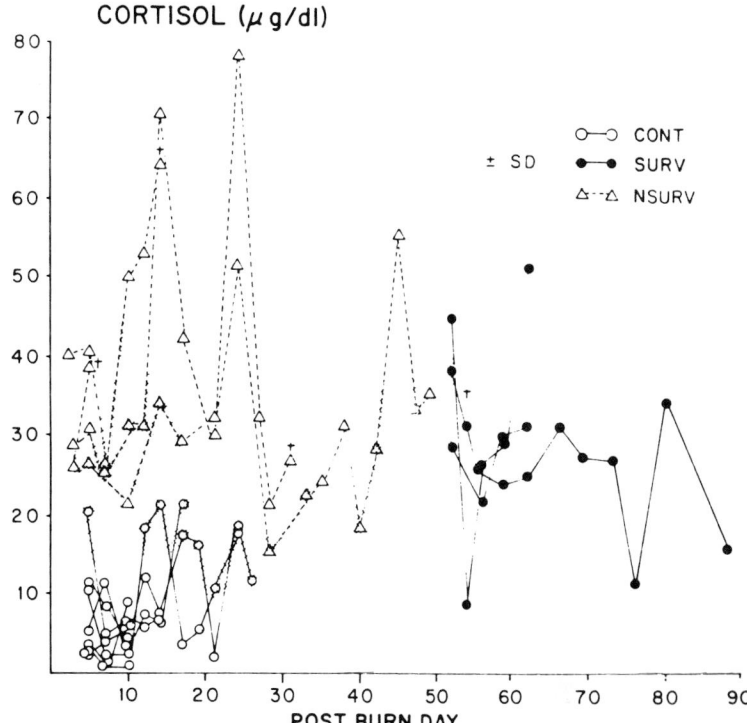

Fig. 1-22. There appears to be a negative correlation between survival after major thermal injury and plasma cortisol concentration with survivors (surv) having plasma cortisol concentrations below those of nonsurvivors (nsurv). Both groups had cortisol concentrations greater than controls. (From: *Vaughan GM et al: J Trauma 22:263–273, 1982, with permission.*)

However, despite this, TSH secretion is not increased after injury or surgery even though the plasma concentrations of free and total T_3 are frequently decreased. This appears to result from the rapid conversion of T_4 to T_3 by pituitary cells, such that T_4 and T_3 are equipotent inhibitors of TSH secretion. It appears that following injury the normal circulating concentrations of free T_4 are sufficient to inhibit the secretion of TSH. Burn patients, however, have recently been noted to have a reduction in the serum concentration of TSH that paradoxically is associated with low serum concentrations of both free T_4 and free T_3. This situation is similar to the euthyroid sick syndrome observed in critically ill nonsurgical patients and may be the result of an impairment in the pituitary's ability to secrete TSH, the hypothalamus's ability to secrete TRH, or an alteration in the peripheral binding of these hormones to their carrier molecules. The exact etiology is not known.

The synthesis of TRH is not limited to the hypothalamus and TRH is not specific for the release of TSH. TRH appears to be the primary agent responsible for the secretion of TSH by the pituitary gland. Recent evidence suggests TRH may be important in the response to shock, as evidenced by the improvement of blood pressure, respiratory rate, heart rate, and survival in animals who have been administered TRH during hemorrhagic shock. These improvements are thought to be mediated by TRH

stimulation of central pathways that modulate sympathoadrenal function, but the precise mechanisms for these phenomena are not known.

The thyroid hormones have numerous effects on cellular metabolism, growth, and differentiation. Among these are their ability to increase oxygen consumption, heat production, and the activities of the sympathetic nervous system. The thyroid hormones may also have profound metabolic effects when present in excess, including an increase in glucose oxidation, gluconeogenesis, glycogenolysis, proteolysis, lipolysis, and ketogenesis. Despite these actions, thyroid hormones do not appear to be important in the moment-to-moment regulation of plasma substrates, such as glucose.

GROWTH HORMONE. As is the case for most pituitary hormones, the secretion of growth hormone is under the control of a number of inputs including neural, hormonal, and nonneuroendocrine signals, such as substrate supply. The hypothalamic mechanisms controlling the synthesis and the release of growth hormone from acidophilic cells of the adenohypophysis involve both stimulation and inhibition. Pituitary release of growth hormone is stimulated by growth hormone releasing factor, a substance produced in the ventromedial, arcuate, and possibly dorsomedial nuclei of the hypothalamus. Inhibition of growth hormone release is primarily mediated by somatostatin, which is derived from the preoptic area and the amygdyla. Despite the presence of both stimulatory and inhibitory properties, the primary influence of the hypothalamus upon the release of growth hormone is stimulatory. This is evidenced by the inhibition of growth hormone secretion when the hypophyseal-portal circulation con-

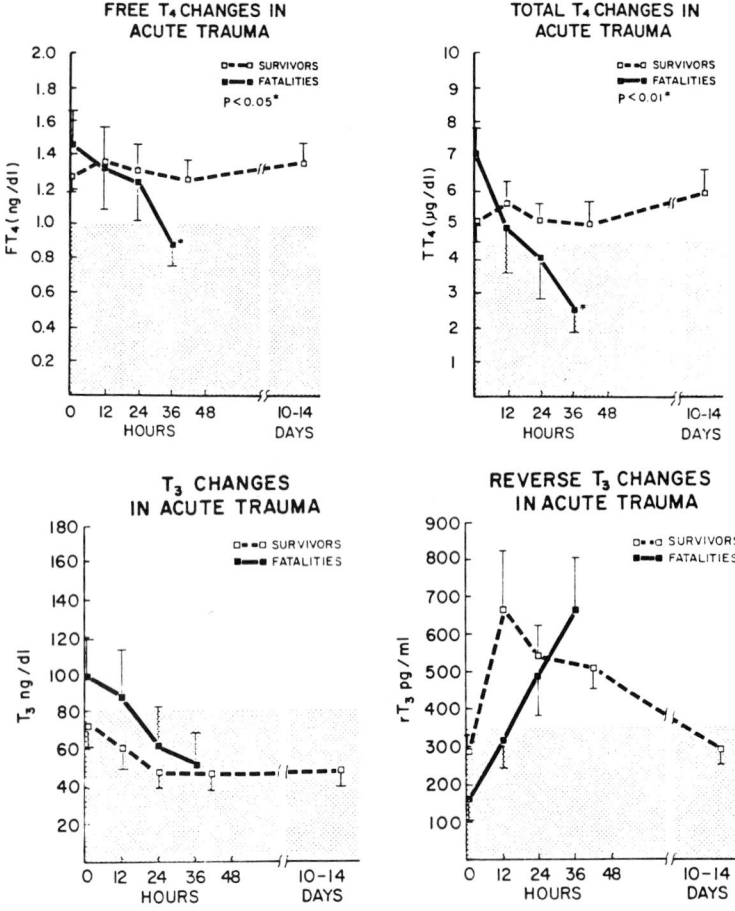

Fig. 1-23. Alterations in total T_4, free T_4, total T_3, and reverse T_3 in 19 acutely traumatized patients. Results are reported as mean ± SEM and statistically significant deviations are noted at matched time samples. Shaded regions denote subnormal levels of free T_4, total T_4, and total T_3 and normal range of reverse T_3. All patients had subnormal values of total T_3 and elevated values of reverse T_3 at some time point. Patients who died had subnormal values of total and free T_4, whereas survivors did not. (From: *Phillips RH et al: J Trauma 24:116, 1984, with permission.*)

necting the hypothalamus and pituitary gland is transected or injured. Other hormonal agents capable of stimulating growth hormone release include thyroxine, vasopressin, ACTH, alpha-MSH, testosterone, estrogen, and alpha-adrenergic stimulation. By contrast, only cortisol, growth hormone itself, and beta-adrenergic stimulation, in addition to somatostatin, suppress growth hormone release. Growth hormone secretion can also be stimulated by nonhormonal stimuli such as decreased effective circulating volume, fasting hypoglycemia, decreasing plasma fatty acid concentrations, increasing amino acid concentrations, exercise, and stress or inhibited by nonhormonal stimuli such as hyperglycemia and rising plasma fatty acid concentrations.

The ability of a decrease in effective circulating volume to stimulate growth hormone production results in the increased secretion of growth hormone following virtually all forms of injury. For example, Carey et al. found war wounds as well as hemorrhage to be potent stimuli for growth hormone release in human beings, and Chartiers et al. demonstrated an increased secretion of growth hormone following surgical stress such as an operation and anesthesia. Plasma concentrations of growth hormone remain elevated for approximately 24 h following these injuries and then return to normal (Fig. 1-25).

Growth hormone has numerous metabolic functions that lead to an increase in plasma glucose, by an inhibition of glucose transport in liver and skeletal muscle; an increase in plasma fatty acids and ketone bodies, by stimulation of lipolysis in adipose tissue and potentiation of the actions of catecholamines on adipose tissue; an increase in plasma ketone bodies, by stimulation of ketogenesis in the liver, and in the accumulation of nitrogen by the synthesis of proteins in skeletal muscle and in liver. In addition, growth hormone promotes linear growth. Thus the actions of growth hormone on protein metabolism are anabolic whereas on carbohydrate and lipid metabolism they are catabolic.

Although not completely understood, growth hormone appears to produce its effects either through direct action on target cells or through the release of a group of intermediary compounds, the somatomedins, which act as second messengers in a manner somewhat analogous to calcium and cAMP.

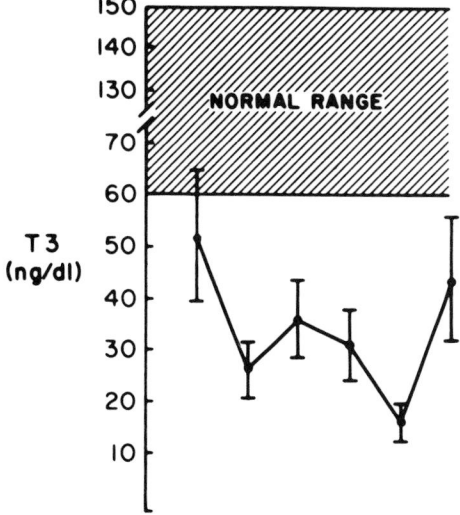

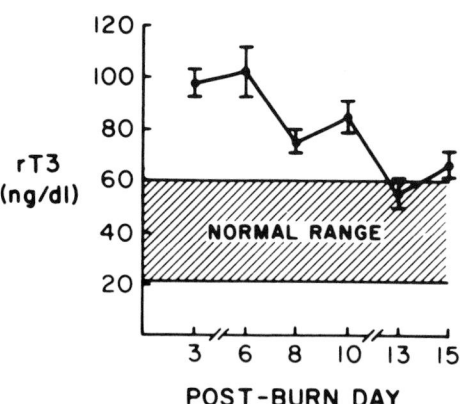

Fig. 1-24. Serum values (mean ± SEM) for T_3 and reverse T_3 in five male patients with a mean body surface area burn of 66.5 percent. Normal range represented by shaded area. T_3 values were decreased and reversed T_3 values increased following thermal injury. (From: *Becker RA et al: J Trauma 20:713, 1980, with permission.*)

GONADOTROPINS AND SEX HORMONES. Follicle stimulating hormone (FSH) and luteinizing hormone (LH) are synthesized and secreted by basophilic cells of the adenohypophysis. Both these hormones are released in response to luteinizing hormone releasing hormone. Estrogens, progestins, prolactin, and androgens and CRF inhibit their release. The secretion of LH and FSH is suppressed after but not during an operation and emotional stress. Following burns, there appears to be an initial increase during the first day following injury followed by a prolonged decrease of about 2 weeks. In part, the suppression of gonadotropin release following injury may result from the increased secretion of CRF that is consequent to injury. Although the changes in gonadotropin secretion presumably account for the menstrual dysfunction and diminished libido that are frequently seen after injury, the physiologic importance of alterations in gonadotropin secretion following injury remains unclear.

There are few data on the secretion of androgens and estrogens in the posttraumatic period, but at least in one study the concentration of testosterone following injury was decreased. Little is known regarding the significance of the physiologic changes that occur in the secretion of estrogens and androgens following injury; however, the pharmacologic administration of testosterone or conjugated estrogens shortly before shock has been demonstrated to improve survival.

PROLACTIN. Elevated concentrations of prolactin have been documented in adults following thermal injury, chest wall trauma, and surgery. By contrast, children and adolescents have been found to have decreased prolactin concentrations following thermal injury. This difference may reflect the changes that occur in reproductive function with aging. In the adult burn patients studied by Brizio-Molteni et al., hyperprolactinemia correlated with the severity of injury. Although they found no association of hyperprolactinemia with galactorrhea, other investigators have noted this association, particularly following chest wall trauma.

Prolactin is synthesized and released by acidophilic cells of the anterior pituitary gland in response to various emotional and physical stressors. Although the control of prolactin release, like that of growth hormone, is under the stimulatory and inhibitory influence of the hypothalamus, the inhibitory rather than stimulatory mechanisms predominate. This is evidenced by the hypersecretion of prolactin by a transplanted pituitary gland or one in which the hypophyseal portal circulation has been transected. The inhibitory response is mediated by a dopaminergic pathway that may be dopamine itself.

Prolactin appears to act primarily upon the breast to induce lactation and mammary development. In addition, prolactin receptors have also been identified in the kidney and in the liver. The presence of these receptors may explain the stimulation of salt and water retention by the kidney in several mammalian species, but not in man, and the increased retention of nitrogen, increased mobilization of lipids, and carbohydrate intolerance observed in man and in other mammals. Despite these functions, the physiologic importance of prolactin in man following injury is uncertain.

ENDOGENOUS OPIATES. Interest in opioid peptides has resulted from the finding that naloxone improves the hemodynamic response and survival in hemorrhagic, septic, and spinal shock. Subsequently, it has become apparent that elevated concentrations of endogenous opiates are common to a major operation, sepsis, trauma, shock, and stress (Fig. 1-26).

The endogenous opiates derive from three precursors: pre-proopiomelanocortin, pre-proenkephalin A, and pre-prodynorphin. Pre-proopiomelanocortin is found primarily in the anterior pituitary. Pre-proopiomelanocortin also possesses the sequences for ACTH and gamma-melanocyte stimulating hormone in addition to containing the amino acid sequences for the opiates, beta-lipotrophin and beta- and gamma-endorphin. Consequently, ACTH and beta-endorphin are cosecreted by the pituitary gland in response to a variety of stressors. Pre-proenkephalin-A,

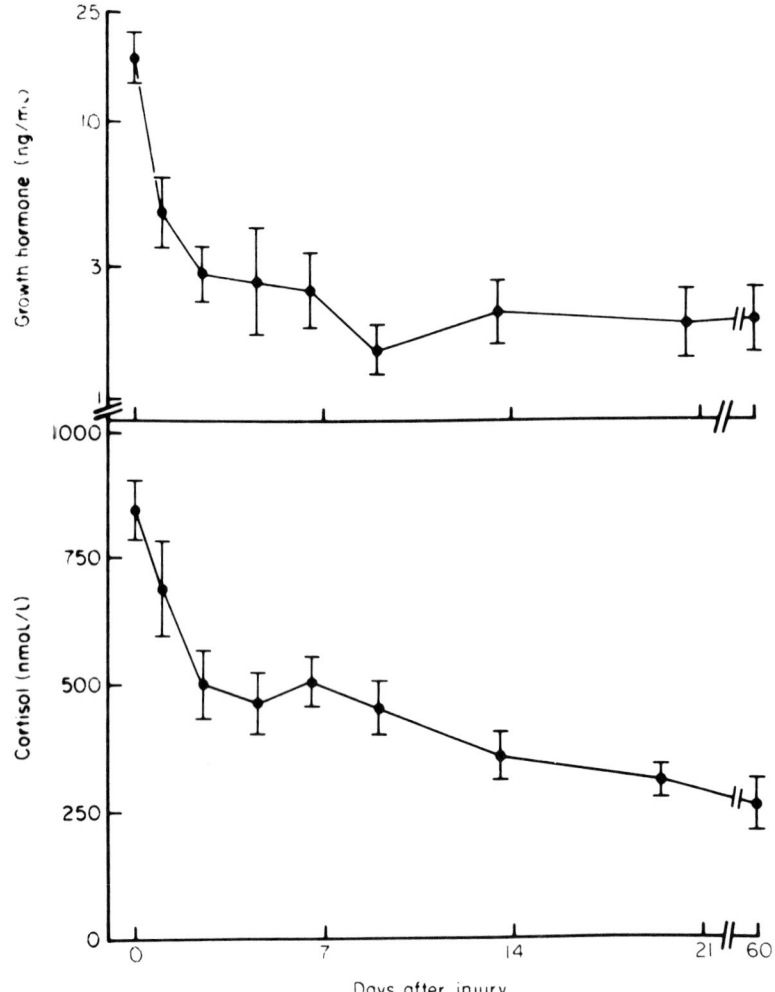

Fig. 1-25. Plasma growth hormone activity in 12 patients who sustained nonfatal musculoskeletal injuries. Plasma growth hormone concentrations were elevated acutely but then rapidly returned to normal in a pattern similar to that observed for cortisol. (From: *Frayn KN et al: Clin Endocrinol 20:179, 1984, with permission.*)

a poly-enkephalin from which the pentapeptides methionine and leucine enkephalin derive, is located in the adrenal medulla, brain, gut, and sympathetic ganglia. Preprodynorphin is found in the brain, spinal cord, and gut, and its cleavage results in the production of neo-betaendorphin and dynorphin. Thus, the endogenous opiates are composed of a variety of compounds that derive from numerous sites in the body.

Opiate compounds appear to act at three receptor subtypes: mu, delta, and kappa. Morphine and fentanyl act almost exclusively at mu receptors, met- and leu-enkephalin at delta receptors, and dynorphin at kappa receptors. The activity of opioid compounds at their receptors is similar to that of catecholamines in that a specific opiate compound may act at more than one receptor. For example, beta-endorphin acts at both mu and delta receptors. In fact, few endogenous opiates have 100 percent specificity for a single receptor subtype.

In addition to analgesic activity, endogenous opiates have cardiovascular effects, metabolic effects, and neuroendocrine modulating properties. The cardiovascular effects of opiates include a hypotensive effect of beta-

endorphin and morphine and a hypertensive effect of enkephalins. The action of beta-endorphin appears to be mediated through a serotonergic pathway, and it is much more potent that morphine. Neuroendocrine properties of opiates include the ability of beta-endorphin to increase catecholamine release from the adrenal medulla, to potentiate the action of ACTH on the adrenal cortex, and to inhibit the release of ACTH by the pituitary gland.

The metabolic effects of opiates have been primarily described for carbohydrate metabolism. Hyperglycemia following the administration of morphine is well recognized, and similar findings have been noted for centrally administered beta-endorphin. In addition, beta-endorphin, which does not appear to have any direct effect upon glucose uptake in skeletal muscle or upon glucose production by the liver, stimulates the release in vivo of glucagon and insulin by the pancreas. Finally, beta-endorphin appears to have an important role in the central

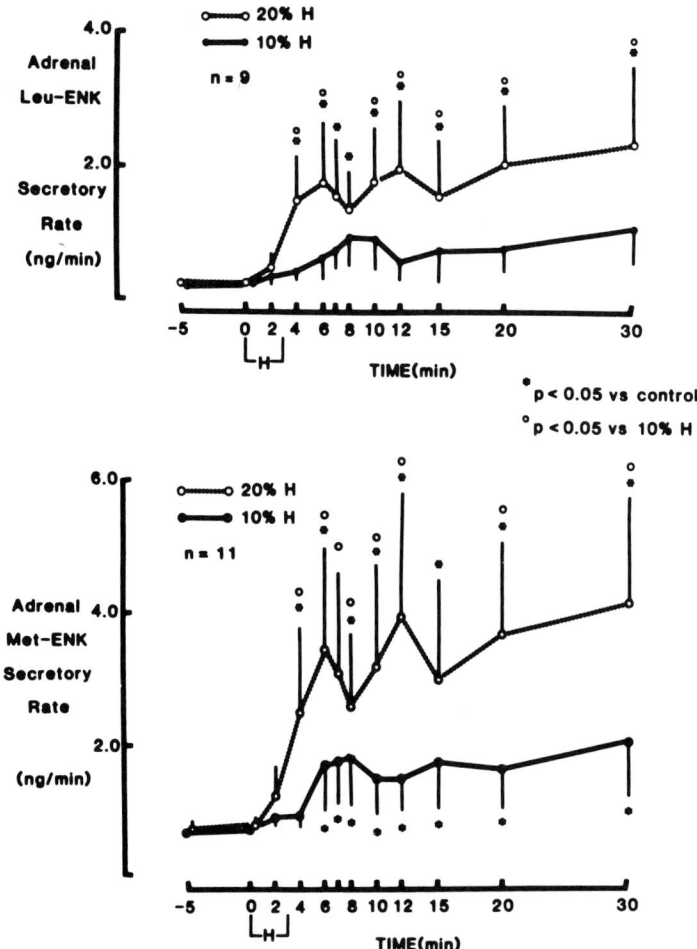

Fig. 1-26. Adrenomedullary secretion of methionine-enkephalin and leucine-enkephalin in dogs subjected to 10 or 20 percent hemorrhages. As shown, the secretion of met-enkephalin by the adrenal was always greater than that of leu-enkephalin, and although the ratio of secretory rates of met-enkephalin and leu-enkephalin varied from 2.8 to 4.9, it did not change in response to hemorrhage. (From: *Engeland WC, Dominique FB, Gann DS: Am J Physiol 251:R341, 1986, with permission.*)

regulation of glucose as evidenced by the substantial increase in the plasma concentrations of beta-endorphin during insulin induced hypoglycemia. Endogenous opiates may exert an important role in the response to injury through their analgesic, cardiovascular metabolic and neuroendocrine modulating activities. Their precise role in the response to injury remains ill defined at present.

VASOPRESSIN. Arginine vasopressin (antidiuretic hormone) and oxytocin are the primary hormones of the neurohypophysis in human beings. These hormones are synthesized in the hypothalamus and then transported to the neurohypophysis, where they are stored until neural signals to the neurohypophysis stimulate their release. For arginine vasopressin, synthesis takes place in cells of the supraoptic and paraventricular nuclei located in the anterior hypothalamus. An increase in plasma osmolality is the primary stimulus for vasopressin secretion. Alterations in plasma osmolality are sensed by cerebral osmoreceptors located in the hypothalamus near the third ventricles that are sentivie to sodium and its anions but not to glucose or other solutes. There is evidence to suggest the existence of extracerebral osmoreceptors located in the liver or the portal circulation. Although glucose and urea have little effect on the osmotic pathways for vasopressin release, hyperglycemia does increase vasopressin secretion through a nonosmotic pathway.

Changes in effective circulating volume also are important stimuli for vasopressin release. For example, a decrease of approximately 10 percent in effective circulating volume, which is equivalent to a change from the supine to the upright position, results in a two- to threefold increase in the plasma vasopressin concentration. A variety of other stimuli and hormones also can alter the secretion of vasopressin either directly by acting at the neurohypophysis (pain, emotional arousal, angiotensin II) or indirectly through peripheral alterations in blood volume, plasma osmolality, and blood glucose concentration (exercise, catecholamines, opiates, insulin, cortisol, and histamine).

Most of these stimuli occur to some extent during injury and stress. Therefore, it is no surprise that the secre-

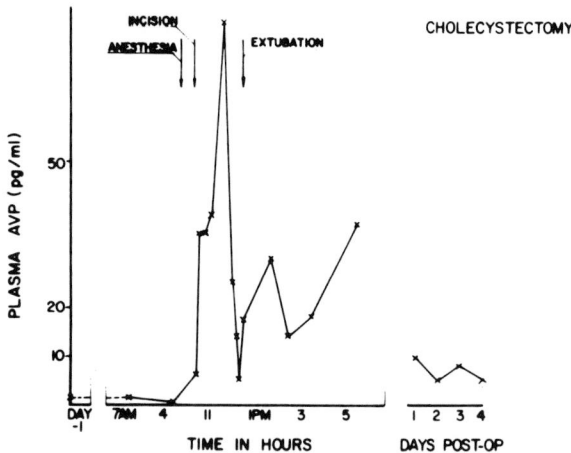

Vasopressin levels before, during, and after surgery.

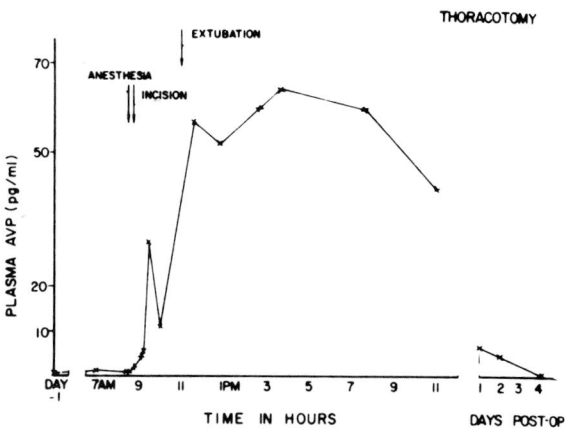

Vasopressin levels before, during, and after surgery.

Fig. 1-27. Plasma vasopressin concentrations during cholecystectomy and thoracotomy. (From: *Haas M, Glick SM: Arch Surg 113:597, 1978, with permission.*)

tion of vasopressin is increased after a major operation, trauma, hemorrhage, sepsis, and burns (Fig. 1-27). Moran et al. have identified four phases of vasopressin secretion following surgery. The first phase is the normal preoperative control period in which plasma vasopressin concentrations are within the normal range. The second phase consists of a mild elevation that results from the overnight fast. This phase can be abolished by the administration of fluids during the preoperative period. The third phase results from cutaneous and visceral stimulation (i.e., pain) and lasts from the skin incision to closure. This phase is characterized by transient elevations of the ADH concentration that return to normal values. The fourth phase corresponds to the postoperative phase in which there is an early increase in the plasma vasopressin concentration followed by a return to normal values by the fifth postoperative day. Similar patterns have been noted in patients placed on cardiopulmonary bypass and in thermally injured patients.

Moran et al. also hypothesized that there are four afferent reflexes controlling vasopressin release, each of which can override the preceding ones. Three of these reflexes, osmoreceptor, baroreceptor, and left atrial stretch receptor reflexes, are negative feedback loops. The fourth reflex is thought to be mediated through painful stimuli and is not a feedback loop. Therefore, in the presence of pain, vasopressin secretion can occur in the face of hypo-osmolality or hypervolemia, conditions that would normally inhibit vasopressin secretion and may explain the persistent elevation of vasopressin secretion seen for 5 to 7 days following surgery and thermal injury despite the presence of normovolemia and normal plasma osmolality (Fig. 1-4). It is apparent that the secretion of vasopressin following any injury or stressful condition cannot be considered inappropriate until all possible stimuli, particularly pain, have been eliminated. Recent evidence suggests inappropriate vasopressin secretion may occur late following thermal injury.

Inappropriate vasopressin secretion, also known as the syndrome of inappropriate antidiuretic hormone secretion (SIADH), is the term used to describe the excessive secretion of vasopressin beyond that needed to promote homeostasis. The persistent secretion of vasopressin produces a low urinary output with high osmolality and a profound dilutional hyponatremia. Although this situation occurs not infrequently after head injury, the converse situation of diabetes insipidus, in which there is an absence of vasopressin secretion, is more common. Diabetes insipidus following head injury may be either temporary or permanent and results from damage to the supraopticohypophyseal system. It is characterized by the production of large amounts of dilute urine and by a urine osmolality that is less than an abnormally high plasma osmolality. Since it frequently arises in comatose patients who cannot express thirst or regulate intake of water, the continued excessive polyuria associated with diabetes insipidus leads to hypernatremia and eventually to hypotension if not corrected by the administration of free water and exogenous vasopressin.

The actions of vasopressin may be broadly classified as osmoregulatory, vasoactive, and metabolic. Osmoregulation occurs through the reabsorption of solute-free water in the distal tubules and in the collecting ducts of the kidneys, an action mediated through cAMP. Vasoactive properties of vasopressin mediate an increase in peripheral vasoconstriction, especially in the splanchnic bed. This action is important in the regulation of blood pressure after hemorrhage, and it has been implicated in the pathophysiology of hypertension and of mesenteric infarction. Metabolic actions of vasopressin include the stimulation of hepatic glycogenolysis and gluconeogenesis. These actions may be important in increasing plasma glucose after injury, since on a molar basis, vasopressin is more potent than glucagon. In addition, vasopressin may alter the metabolism of fatty acids. Williamson and colleagues, using isolated hepatocytes from fed rats, have noted an inhibition of ketogenesis from oleate and an increase in the esterification of oleate in the presence of vasopressin. These investigators have also noted a de-

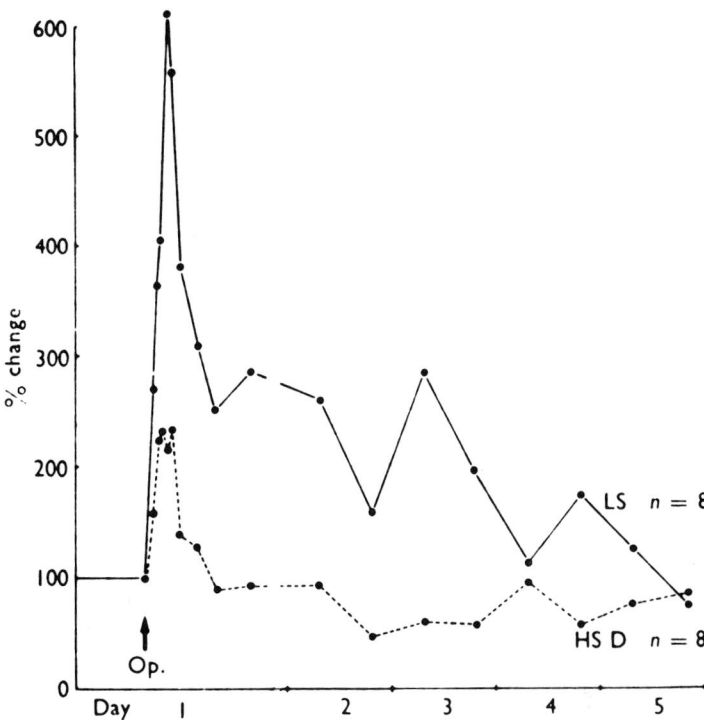

Fig. 1-28. Plasma aldosterone values in patients undergoing routine cholecystectomy. Patients who either had a conventional preoperative salt intake (LS) or a high salt intake (HS) both demonstrated an increase in plasma aldosterone secretion at the time of surgery. However, only patients with a normal salt intake preoperatively demonstrated a persistent elevation in plasma aldosterone, whereas patients on a high salt diet demonstrated an immediate return to normal values in the postoperative period. (From: *Cochrane JPS: Br J Surg 774, 1978, with permission.*)

crease in the release of nonesterified fatty acids from adipose tissue of starved rats in the presence of vasopressin. Vasopressin may act to lower the plasma concentrations of ketone bodies and nonesterified fatty acids following injury, but its role in lipid metabolism in man remains uncertain.

ALDOSTERONE. Plasma aldosterone concentrations, like those of cortisol, demonstrate a circadian rhythm in which the peak concentrations occur at midmorning and the lowest concentrations at late afternoon and night. Following injury, the circadian rhythm is lost and elevated concentrations of both these hormones are observed during the entire 24-h period. Plasma concentrations of aldosterone also increase following anesthesia alone but not to the extent seen following injury and a major operation (Fig. 1-28). The highest concentrations of aldosterone have been noted in the agonal period following injury.

Cells of the adrenal zona glomerulosa synthesize and secrete aldosterone in response to at least three stimuli. Angiotensin II stimulates aldosterone secretion through a calcium dependent, cAMP independent enhancement of the conversion of cholesterol to pregnenolone and of corticosterone to 18-hydroxycorticosterone and aldosterone. ACTH stimulates aldosterone secretion through a cal-

cium dependent, cAMP dependent pathway that enhances the early conversion of cholesterol to pregnenolone. Elevation of the serum potassium concentration stimulates the release of aldosterone through a calcium dependent, cAMP independent increase in the conversion of cholesterol to pregnenolone. There is also evidence suggesting the existence of a pituitary produced aldosterone stimulating factor (ASF) in human beings (not similar to ACTH) that is a glycoprotein present in the urine of normal but not of hypophysectomized human beings. This factor produces hypertension and hyperaldosteronism when given to rodents.

Following injury, the two most important mechanisms for aldosterone secretion appear to be through ACTH and angiotensin. ACTH is considerably more potent on a molar basis than angiotensin with regard to aldosterone secretion. For example, nephrectomized dogs produce aldosterone in response to hemorrhage despite the absence of angiotensin. Stress-induced elevations in aldosterone are probably mediated primarily through ACTH. The stimulatory effects of ACTH on aldosterone production are short-lived. As a result of this short-lived potency, ACTH probably has a minor role in the overall control of aldosterone secretion in chronic states during which angiotensin II is probably the most important stimulus. Angiotensin II appears to exert a role in early as well as late aldosterone production following injury, since hypophysectomy does not completely abolish aldosterone secretion following injury, aldosterone concentrations are elevated well after ACTH concentrations have returned to normal, plasma concentrations of aldosterone demonstrate a strong correlation with angiotensin II fol-

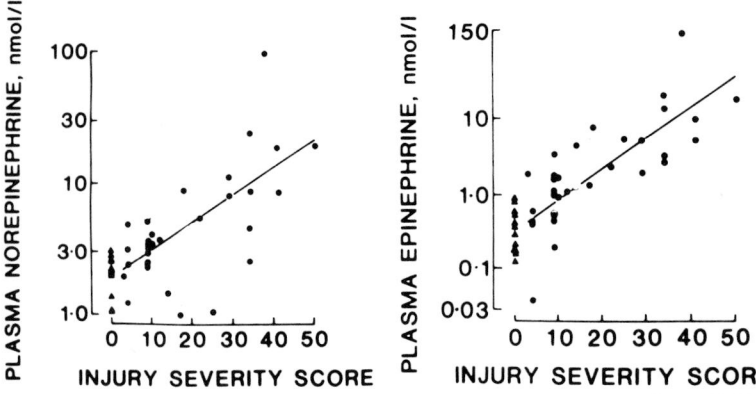

Fig. 1-29. The relationship between plasma concentrations of nor-epinephrine and of epinephrine with injury severity score in 40 multiply injured patients. There was a positive correlation between injury severity score, plasma norepinephrine, and plasma epinephine. (From: *Frayn KN, Little RA, Maycock PF: Circ Shock 16:229, 1985, with permission.*)

lowing injury, and nephrectomized dogs produce only 50 percent of the aldosterone they normally produce in response to hemorrhage when the kidneys are intact.

In addition to the three or four stimulatory pathways for the synthesis and the secretion of aldosterone, there is considerable evidence suggesting the presence of an inhibitory pathway that appears to involve a tonic inhibition terone secretion by dopamine. For example, metaclopropramide, a dopamine antagonist, produces an increased secretion of aldosterone, whereas bromocriptine, a dopamine agonist, decreases the secretion of aldosterone stimulated by ACTH or by angiotensin II but does not alter the basal secretory rate of aldosterone. This pathway may be important in mediating changes in the secretion of aldosterone in response to alterations in the plasma sodium concentration or the effective circulating volume.

The primary actions of aldosterone are related to fluid and electrolyte metabolism. In the early distal convoluted tubule, aldosterone increases the reabsorption of sodium and of chloride and in the late distal convoluted tubules and in the early collecting ducts it promotes the reabsorption of sodium and the secretion of potassium. The latter process is not an obligatory, one to one exchange of sodium ions for potassium ions and of sodium ions for hydrogen ions as has been previously thought. Instead, experimental evidence suggests that the secretion of potassium and of hydrogen ions results from an increase in the electronegativity of the luminal tubular fluid as sodium reabsorption is stimulated by aldosterone. In turn, the increase in tubular electronegativity drives potassium and hydrogen ions across the tubular membrane into the tubular fluid in order to restore electrical neutrality.

CATECHOLAMINES. Catecholamines increase immediately after injury and achieve peak concentrations at about 24 to 48 h after injury, from which time they decrease to base line. This increase appears to be related to the severity of injury (Fig. 1-29) and changes in norepinephrine and epinephrine are qualitatively and quantitatively the same. Changes in norepinephrine are generally thought to reflect changes in the activity of the sympathetic nervous system, i.e., spillover into the blood, whereas changes in epinephrine are generally thought to reflect changes in the activity of the adrenal medulla. In

this regard, epinephrine, produced almost exclusively by the adrenal medulla, functions primarily as a hormone whereas dopamine and norepinephrine, produced for the most part by nerve terminals, function primarily as neurotransmitters.

Plasma catecholamine concentrations have been extensively studied in numerous forms of injury in human beings. Among the most extensive studies are those of Benedict and Grahame-Smith, who examine plasma catecholamine concentrations in patients with shock due to septicemia, trauma, and hemorrhage (Figs. 1-30 and 1-31). In these studies, plasma norepinephrine (noradrenaline) and epinephrine (adrenal) concentrations were increased above normal irrespective of the type of shock (septic, hemorrhagic, and traumatic) whereas there was no difference in the plasma dopamine concentration between patients with shock and normal controls. In most of the nonsurvivors, irrespective of the type of shock, high plasma norepinephrine and, to a lesser extent, epinephrine concentrations were sustained until just before death, when they rapidly declined. The association between sustained norepinephrine concentrations and death is not well established, however, and was not seen in the studies of Davies et al. in which plasma catecholamine concentrations were measured in accident victims.

Numerous stimuli have been identified that lead to an increase in catecholamine secretion including hypovolemia, hypoglycemia, hypoxemia, pain, and fear, which are all present to some degree following injury. Among these stimuli, plasma catecholamine concentrations following injury are best correlated with the volume of blood lost. It is also important to note that part of the response following injury appears to be psychologically mediated since plasma catecholamine concentrations are greater in patients who sustained minor injuries in a motor vehicle accident than in those who sustained minor injuries by other means.

The exact mechanisms involved in the adrenomedullary control of catecholamine secretion remain poorly

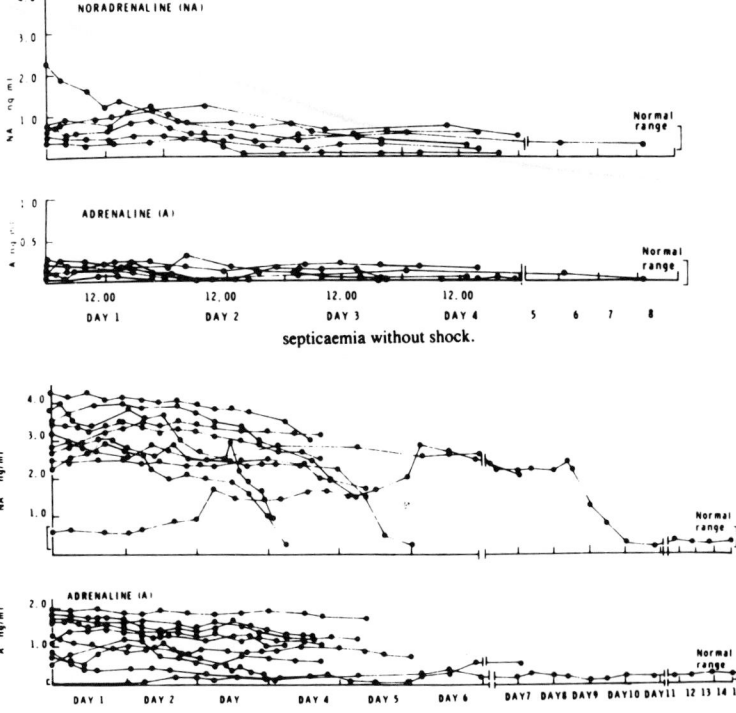

Fig. 1-30. Plasma noradrenaline and adrenalin concentrations in septic patients with or without shock. The concentrations of noradrenaline and adrenalin were greater in patients with shock than in those without. (From: *Benedict CR, Grahame-Smith DG: Q J Med 185:1, 1978, with permission.*)

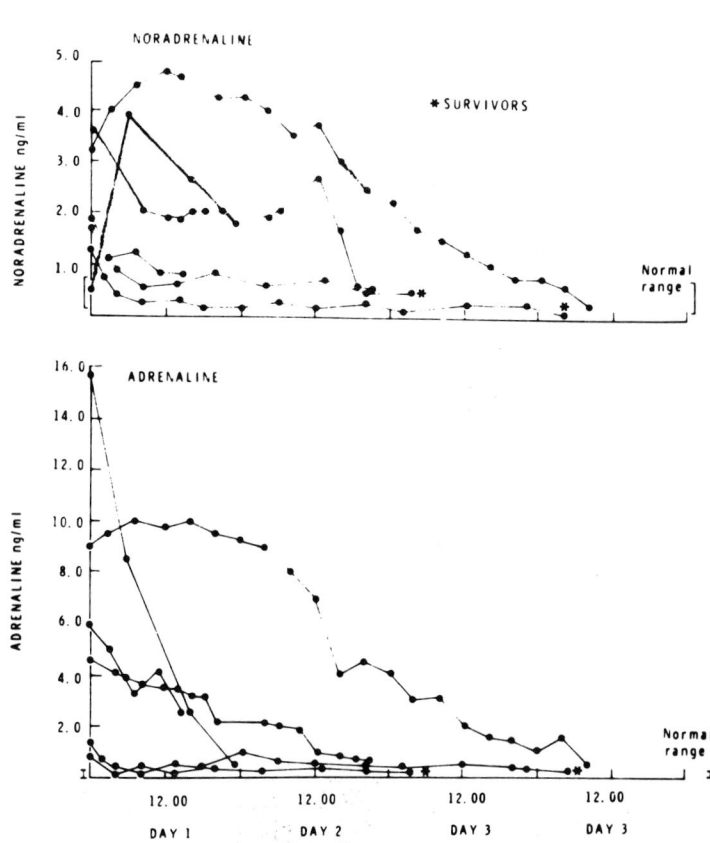

Fig. 1-31. Plasma noradrenaline and adrenalin concentrations in patients with hypovolemic shock. The concentrations of noradrenaline and adrenalin returned to normal values in survivors whereas they remained elevated in nonsurvivors. (From: *Benedict CR, Grahame-Smith DG: Q J Med 185:1, 1978, with permission.*)

understood. In this regard, it is of note that the activation of the sympathetic nervous system does not occur in an all or none fashion and that is not equivalent to adrenomedullary activation. Adrenomedullary activation is not equivalent to complete activation of the sympathetic nervous system. For example, sympathetically mediated adrenomedullary secretion of catecholamines can occur in the absence of increased cardiac or renal sympathetic nervous system activity. Conversely, small nonhypotensive hemorrhages lead to activation of the sympathetic nervous system but do not increase the adrenomedullary secretion of catecholamines. The latter occurs only when some degree of hypotension develops.

The actions of epinephrine and norepinephrine as hormones may be broadly classified as metabolic, hemodynamic, or modulatory. Metabolic actions of epinephrine include stimulation of glycogenolysis (alpha$_1$), gluconeogenesis (alpha$_1$), lipolysis (beta$_1$), and ketogenesis (beta$_1$) in the liver; stimulation of lipolysis (beta$_1$) in adipose tissue; and stimulation of glycogenolysis (alpha$_1$) and inhibition of insulin stimulated glucose uptake (beta$_2$ and alpha$_1$) in skeletal muscle. As a result of these actions, epinephrine appears to exert a major role in stress-induced hyperglycemia by increasing glucose production by the liver and by decreasing glucose uptake in peripheral tissues. There is a strong correlation between plasma glucose concentrations following injury and plasma catecholamine concentrations (Fig. 1-32).

Hormonal modulations produced by catecholamines include a beta receptor mediated increase in the release of renin and parathyroid hormone and an alpha receptor mediated inhibition and beta receptor mediated stimulation of insulin and glucagon secretion. The hormonal modulations produced by catecholamines are to a large extent dependent upon the adrenergic receptor density present on the secretory cells they act upon. For example, alpha and beta islets cells in the pancreas that secrete

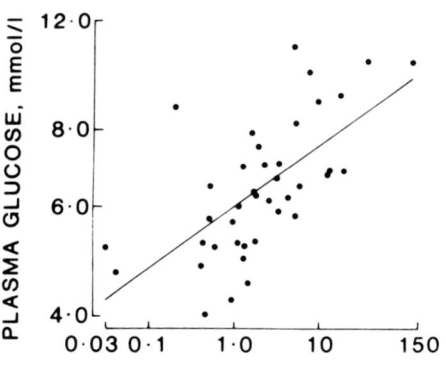

Fig. 1-32. The relationship between plasma concentrations of glucose and of epinephrine in 40 multiply injured patients. There was a positive correlation between plasma glucose and plasma epinephrine ($r = 0.64$, $p < 0.001$). (From: *Frayn KN, Little RA, Maycock PF: Circ Shock 16:229, 1985, with permission.*)

glucagon and insulin, respectively, contain both alpha- and beta-adrenergic receptors but beta islet cells have a greater number of alpha-adrenergic receptors than do alpha islet cells. As a result stimulation of the pancreas by catecholamines and by the sympathetic nervous system results in an increased secretion of glucagon and a decreased secretion of insulin (Fig. 1-33).

Hemodynamic effects of catecholamines include alpha$_1$ mediated venous and arterial vasoconstriction; beta$_2$ mediated arterial vasodilation; and beta$_1$ mediated increases in myocardial rate, contractility, and conductivity. Pharmacologically, the particular hemodynamic effect produced by catecholamines is dose dependent. For example, in low doses epinephrine acts primarily at beta$_1$ and beta$_2$ receptors whereas at high doses it acts primarily at alpha$_1$ receptors. Physiologically, it appears that

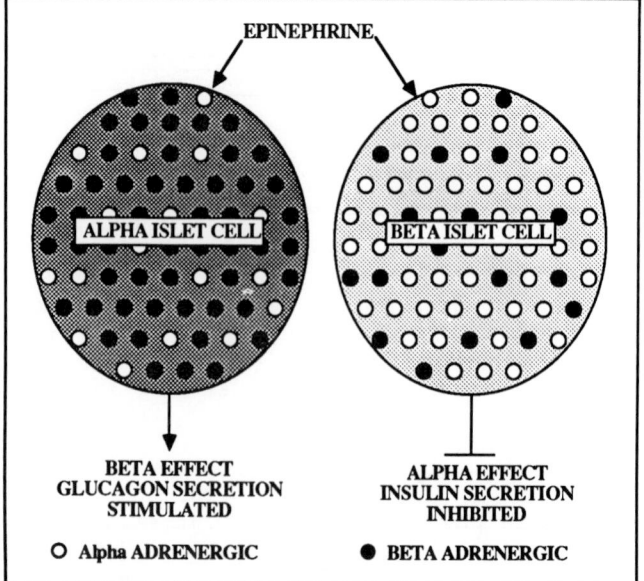

Fig. 1-33. Adrenergic receptor density of alpha and beta pancreatic islets. Beta islet cells have a greater density of alpha-adrenergic receptors and alpha islets have a greater density of beta-adrenergic receptors. As a result, stimulation of pancreatic islets by epinephrine or norepinephrine results in a decreased secretion of insulin and an increased secretion of glucagon.

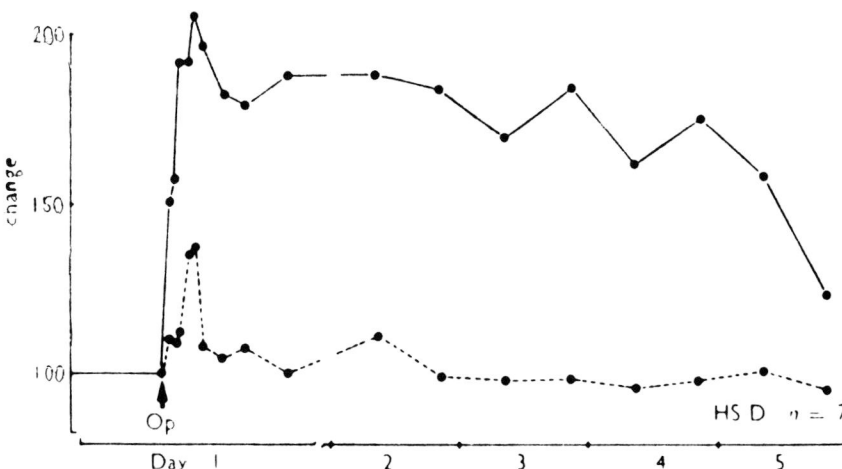

Fig. 1-34. Plasma renin activity in patients undergoing routine cholecystectomy. Patients who either had a conventional preoperative salt intake (LS) or a high salt intake (HS) both demonstrated an increase in plasma renin activity at the time of surgery. However, only patients with a normal salt intake preoperatively demonstrated a persistent elevation in plasma renin activity whereas patients on a high salt diet demonstrated an immediate return to normal values in the postoperative period. (From: *Cochrane JPS: Br J Surg 65:744, 1978, with permission.*)

norepinephrine is most important in the beta$_1$ and alpha$_2$ actions of catecholamines, whereas epinephrine is responsible for the beta$_2$ effects. The hemodynamic effects of dopamine are mediated through dopaminergic receptors as well as adrenergic receptors. In low circulating concentrations (<10 μg/mL), dopamine acts primarily through dopaminergic receptors, but at higher concentrations it acts at beta and eventually at alpha receptors. Because of dopamine's renal vasodilating effects at low concentrations, low-dose dopamine is frequently used following injury to improve urine output.

RENIN-ANGIOTENSIN. Plasma renin activity demonstrates a circadian rhythm in which the peak activity occurs at midmorning and the lowest activity at late afternoon and night. Following injury, the circadian rhythm is lost and an increased renin activity is observed during the entire 24-h period. The highest activity of renin has been noted in the agonal period following injury. It can be suppressed in the immediate postoperative period by salt and water loading (Fig. 1-34).

Renin exists in an inactive form, prorenin, in the myoepithelial cells of the renal afferent arterioles. The proteolytic cleavage of the zymogen and the release of renin are under the control of three intrarenal receptors (the macula densa, the juxtaglomerular neurogenic receptor, and the juxtaglomerular cell) and the influences of several hormones and ions (ACTH, vasopressin, prostaglandins, glucagon, potassium, magnesium, and calcium). The macula densa receptor senses the concentration of chloride in tubular fluid as it passes through the distal nephron such that a decrease in the concentration of chloride in the tubular fluid results in an increase in the release of renin. The neurogenic receptor of the juxtaglomerular apparatus responds to beta-adrenergic stimulation by in-

creasing the release of renin and the juxtaglomerular cell itself, which acts as a stretch receptor, responds to a decrease in stretch (and therefore blood pressure) with an increased secretion of renin.

In the circulation renin converts renin substrate, which is produced by the liver, into angiotensin I. Angiotensin I acts primarily as the precursor for the formation of angiotensin II, a process mediated in the pulmonary circulation by the carboxypeptidase, angiotensin converting enzyme. In addition, it potentiates the release of catecholamines by the adrenal medulla and it redistributes renal blood flow to the cortex by decreasing blood flow to the medullary areas of the kidney.

The actions of angiotensin II may be broadly classified according to its effects upon hemodynamics, fluid and electrolyte balance, hormonal regulation, and metabolism. Angiotensin II is a potent vasoconstrictor with additional hemodynamic activity including an increase in heart rate and contractility and an increase in vascular permeability. Angiotensin II affects fluid and electrolyte homeostasis through its potent stimulation of aldosterone synthesis and secretion, its ability to increase vasopressin secretion, and its participation in the regulation of thirst. Endocrine modulatory effects of angiotensin II, in addition to those noted on the secretion of aldosterone and vasopressin, include potentiation of the release of epinephrine by the adrenal medulla, increase in the release of CRF, and increase in sympathetic neurotransmission. Metabolic actions of angiotensin II include the stimulation of glycogenolysis and gluconeogenesis in the liver.

Plasma concentrations of angiotensin II are elevated immediately after injury. During slow hemorrhages, angiotensin levels are elevated prior to alterations in blood pressure or catecholamines. Angiotensin II production is increased during hemorrhage in baroreceptor deinnervated animals, presumably by the activation of renal receptors. The presence of angiotensin II during shock has been thought to be essential to survival, since nephrectomized animals do not withstand hypovolemia as well as nonnephrectomized animals. Recent studies with renin-angiotensin inhibitors suggest that inhibition of

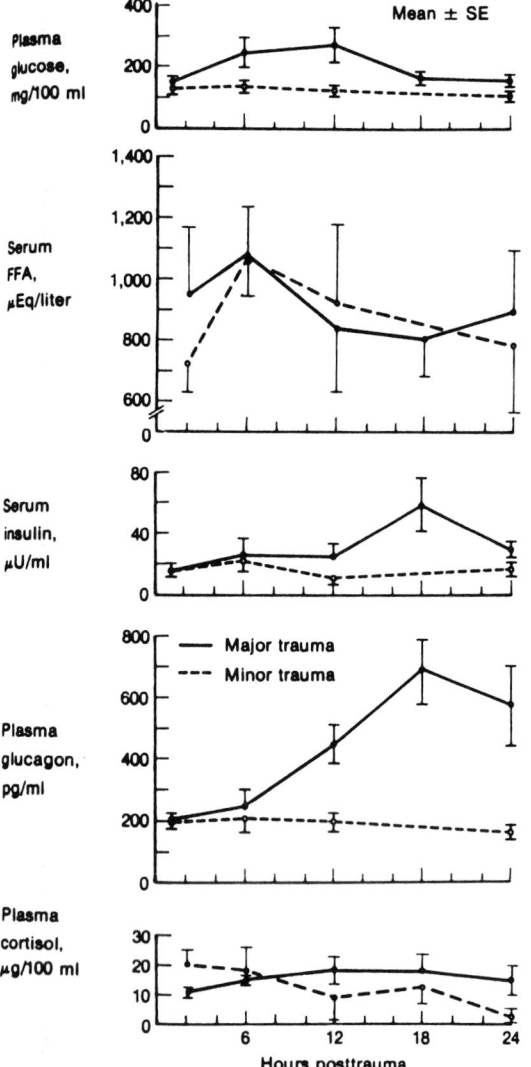

Fig. 1-35. Plasma concentrations of insulin, glucagon, cortisol, glucose, and free fatty acids in seven major and seven minor trauma patients observed over 24-h. The most significant findings were an early elevation of plasma glucose in association with a low-normal insulin concentration and a normal but gradually rising glucagon concentration that reached three times the normal value in 18-h. (From: *Meguid MM et al: Arch Surg 109:776, 1974, with permission.*)

the renin-angiotensin system may improve survival during severe hemorrhage. In part, the benefits obtained from inhibition of the renin-angiotensin system may be related to an improvement in renal blood flow and cardiac output consequent to a reduction in vascular resistance.

INSULIN. Studies examining the plasma concentration of insulin following injury in human beings have noted a biphasic pattern of insulin release (Fig. 1-35). The first period, lasting only a few hours, is characterized by the suppression of insulin secretion, which is mediated by the high concentrations of catecholamines released by stress. This is followed by a period of normal to increased insulin secretion, the so-called phase of insulin resistance. Early

increases in plasma insulin concentrations after injury in human beings have been noted by some investigators. For example, Vitek et al. in a study of road traffic accidents noted a 31.5 percent increase in the insulin concentration above controls by 3 h after injury and a 51.7 percent increase approximately 6 h after injury. As a result of the inconsistent response of the plasma insulin concentration to injury, plasma insulin concentrations correlate poorly with injury severity. In this regard, the insulin-glucose ratio appears to be a better predictor of survival than either the plasma glucose or plasma insulin concentration alone.

The synthesis and secretion of insulin by beta islet cells of the pancreas are controlled by the concentration of circulating substrate (glucose, amino acids, and free fatty acids), the activity of the autonomic nervous system, and the direct and indirect effects of several hormones. Increases in the plasma concentration of glucose, amino acids, free fatty acids, and ketone bodies stimulate the secretion of insulin. Under normal physiologic conditions, the plasma concentration of glucose is the most important stimulus for insulin secretion. During injury and stress, however, the effect of glucose is blunted by neural and humoral mechanisms, so-called insulin resistance. As noted previously, the effect of the autonomic nervous system on a target cell depends to a large extent on the adrenergic receptor density present. Beta islet cells have a greater density of alpha-adrenergic receptors, which inhibit insulin secretion, than of beta-adrenergic receptors, which stimulate insulin secretion. Stimulation of the sympathetic innervation of the pancreas or an increase in the circulating concentration of epinephrine or norepinephrine produce an inhibition of insulin secretion. Hormonal modulators of insulin secretion include somatostatin, glucagon, gastrointestinal hormones, and beta-endorphin, which act through a direct action on the B-islet cells, and cortisol, estrogen, and progesterone, which act indirectly by interfering with the peripheral actions of insulin.

Insulin is the primary anabolic hormone in human beings that promotes the storage of carbohydrate, protein, and lipid through its actions primarily on the liver, skeletal muscle, and adipose tissue, and secondarily on almost all other tissues in the body. Notable exceptions include hemopoietic, central nervous system, and wounded tissues. The major actions of insulin on carbohydrate metabolism are to promote the entry of glucose into cells by stimulating membrane transport of glucose, to promote glycogenesis and glycolysis, and to inhibit gluconeogenesis in the liver. The major action of insulin in protein metabolism is to promote protein synthesis, which is accomplished by increasing the transport of amino acids into the liver and other peripheral tissues and by inhibiting gluconeogenesis and amino acid oxidation. The actions of insulin on lipid metabolism are directed toward the stimulation of lipid synthesis and inhibition of lipid degradation.

GLUCAGON. Although an immediate increase in the plasma glucagon concentration that correlated with the plasma glucose concentration has been noted by Wilmore and colleagues following thermal injury, most studies of

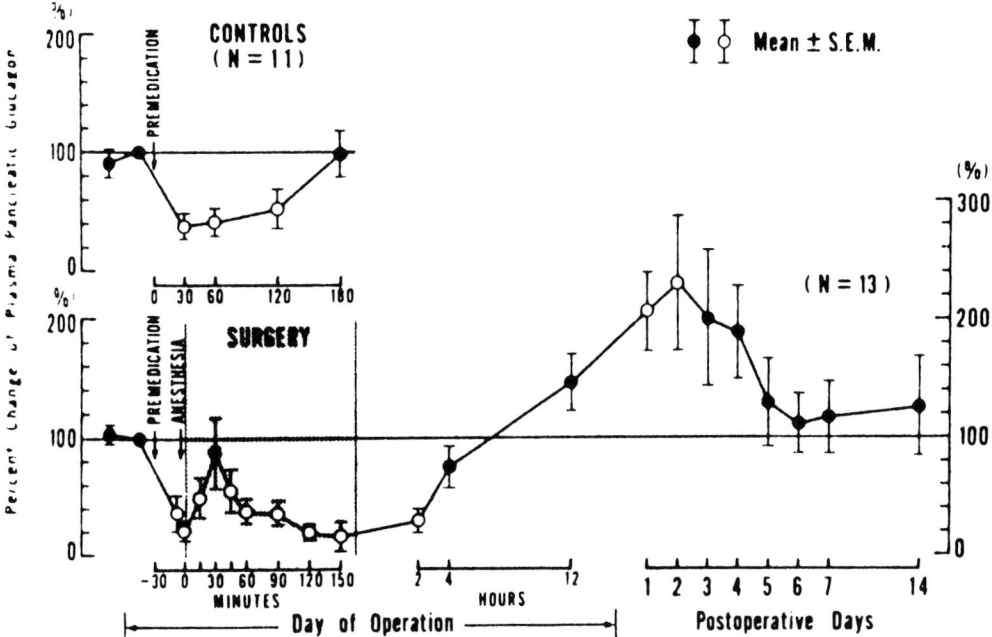

Fig. 1-36. Changes in plasma glucagon during and after elective surgery in 13 patients. Open circles represent significant differences when compared with the fasting value on the day of surgery. (From: *Miyata M, Yamamoto T, Nakao K: Horm Metab Res 8:239, 1976, with permission.*)

glucagon metabolism following nonthermal injury and hypovolemia have noted no increase in the plasma concentration of glucagon until 12 h after injury. During an operation, the plasma concentration of glucagon has been shown to decrease followed by a return to base line 12 h after injury, an increase above base line at 1 day, and a return to base-line values by 3 days (Fig. 1-36). Similarly, Meguid and colleagues, in a study of 14 injured patients, noted no increase in the plasma glucagon concentration immediately after injury, a peak increase at 18 h, and a return to base line by 36 h (Fig. 1-35). Following hemorrhage, portal venous delivery of glucagon also does not increase until well after hyperglycemia has ensued (Fig. 1-37). Despite the apparent difference between thermal and nonthermal injury, glucagon concentrations are generally increased at some point in the immediate postinjury period for all forms of injury.

The synthesis and secretion of glucagon by the alpha islet cells of the pancreas are under the control of the concentrations of circulating substrates (glucose, amino acids, and fatty acids), the activity of the autonomic and the central nervous systems, and the action of circulating and local hormones. Under normal conditions, the primary stimuli are the plasma concentrations of glucose and of amino acids and exercise. Glucose alters glucagon secretion in an inverse manner that appears to result primarily from a direct action of glucose on the alpha cell.

The potency of different amino acids to stimulate glucagon secretion is variable and unrelated to their ability to stimulate insulin secretion, but, in general, the gluconeo-

genic amino acids have a greater stimulatory effect than the nongluconeogenic amino acids. The ability of amino acids to stimulate glucagon secretion is critical for the maintenance of euglycemia when a protein meal is ingested. If this did not occur, the unopposed stimulation of insulin secretion by amino acids after a protein meal would result in hypoglycemia. In the presence of glucagon, however, the liver increases its production of glucose, thereby allowing the action of insulin to be opposed and glucose homeostasis to be maintained. Unger has proposed the insulin/glucagon (I/G) ratio in plasma as a quantitative measure of hepatic glucose balance. When the I/G ratio is greater than 5, glycogenesis, lipogenesis, and protein synthesis are favored. When the I/G ratio is less than 3, glycogenolysis, gluconeogenesis, and lipolysis are favored. The validity of this relationship in vivo is not certain.

The potency of glucose and of amino acids in altering glucagon and insulin secretion depends upon the route of administration, with a greater increase in glucagon and insulin secretion occurring following the ingestion of a protein meal than following the intravenous administration of similar concentrations of amino acids. Similarly, the ingestion of glucose results in a greater increase in insulin and decrease in glucagon than a similar glucose load administered intravenously. This phenomenon may be mediated through the presentation of a greater concentration of substrate to the pancreas when the substrates enter through the gastrointestinal tract, through the potentiation by gastrointestinal hormones of substrate induced pancreatic secretion, or through the effects of neural inputs to the pancreas that are activated by eating.

The autonomic nervous system mechanisms controlling glucagon release are similar to those for insulin; i.e., activation of alpha-adrenergic receptors stimulates gluca-

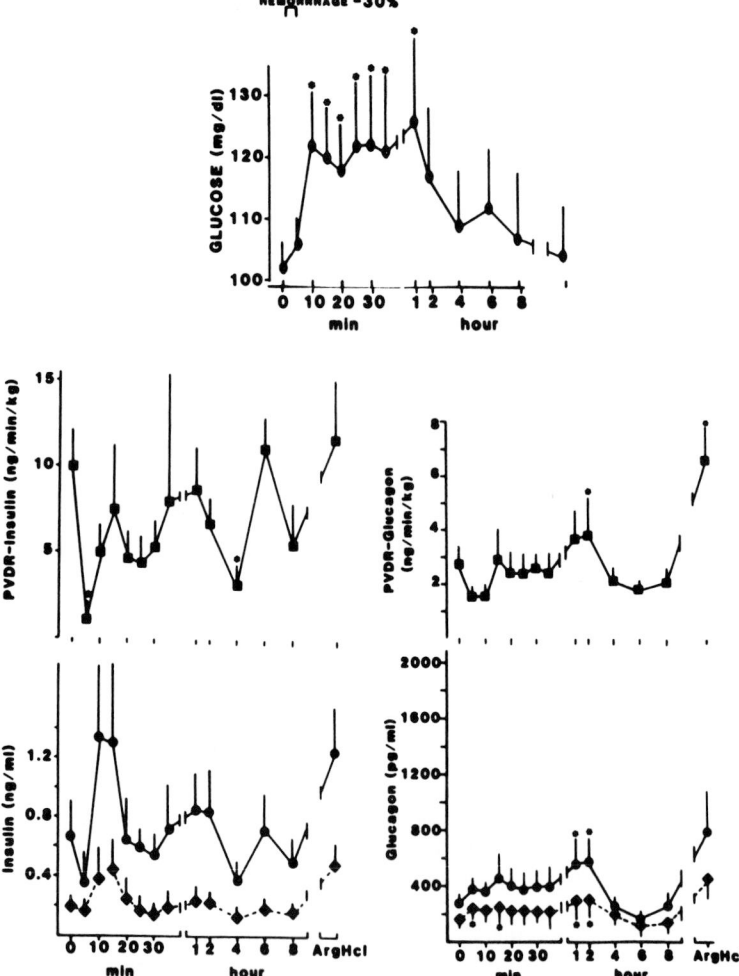

gon secretion whereas the activation of beta-adrenergic receptors or the parasympathetic efferents to the pancreas inhibit glucagon release. Unlike the beta islet cell, however, the alpha islet has a much greater density of alpha-adrenergic receptors than of beta-adrenergic receptors. As a result, increased circulating concentrations of epinephrine or norepinephrine, or sympathetic nervous system stimulation of the pancreas, increase rather than decrease the secretion of glucagon.

The physiologic actions of glucagon are limited primarily to the liver and include stimulation of glycogenolysis and gluconeogenesis. The net result is an increase in hepatic glucose production that under basal conditions accounts for approximately 75 percent of the glucose produced by the liver. Although in the absence of cortisol the peak action of glucagon is very brief, in the presence of cortisol the action of glucagon is longer and the initial increase in hepatic glucose production is greater. Nevertheless, the effects of glucagon are not long-lasting and after 30 to 60 min the activity assigned to glucagon decreases, even if the plasma glucagon concentration remains elevated. If the concentration of glucagon increases further, however, the activity of glucagon does

Fig. 1-37. Arterial (circles) and portal venous (diamonds) concentrations of glucagon and insulin, portal venous delivery (squares) of glucagon and insulin and arterial concentrations of glucose (ovals) in response to a 30 percent hemorrhage in dogs. These results suggest that alterations in glucagon occurred too late to participate in the immediate hyperglycemia that followed hemorrhage. (From: *McLeod MK, Carlson DE, Gann DS: Am J Physiol 251:E597, 1986, with permission.*)

increase because it appears that an increase in the concentration of glucagon rather than the absolute amount of glucagon present is what determines its physiologic activity.

Despite the increase in hepatic glucose production under normal circumstances, glucagon does not appear to exert an important role in the immediate hyperglycemia that follows injury. For example, McLeod et al. noted an immediate increase in plasma glucose following hemorrhage that was not associated with increases in peripheral glucagon concentrations or in the delivery of glucagon to the liver by the portal vein. In addition, Lautt and coworkers have demonstrated the abolition of the hyperglycemic response to hemorrhage in adrenalectomized and hepatic denervated cats and the restitution of this response when either the adrenals or the liver are left intact.

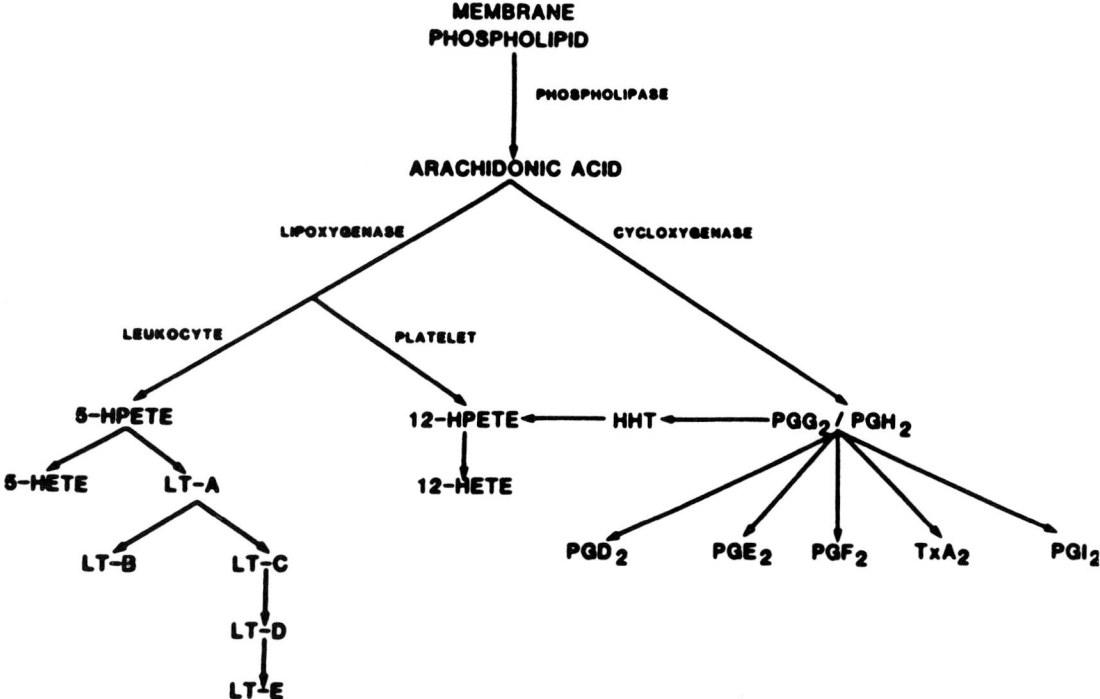

Fig. 1-38. Eicosanoid synthesis. Cortisol inhibits phospholipase A. As a result, the synthesis of all eicosanoids is decreased. In contrast, aspirin and indomethacin inhibit cyclooxygenase. As a result, the synthesis of leukotrienes may be increased. (From: *Gann DS, Amaral JF: The pathophysiology of trauma and shock, in Zuidema GD et al (eds): The Management of Trauma. Philadelphia, Saunders, 1985, with permission.*)

In addition to its effects on carbohydrate metabolism, glucagon stimulates lipolysis in liver and adipose tissue and stimulates ketogenesis in the liver. As a result, glucagon is very important during starvation and injury because of its ability to mobilize fatty acids and to increase ketogenesis.

SOMATOSTATIN. Somatostatin, which is present in pancreatic D cells, hypothalamus, limbic system, brain stem, spinal cord, other neural tissue, salivary glands, parafollicular thyroid cells, kidney, and gastrointestinal tissue, is a potent inhibitor of both insulin and glucagon secretion. Although somatostatin was originally named for its ability to inhibit growth hormone secretion, it is now recognized to also inhibit the secretion of TSH, renin, calcitonin, gastrin, secretin, and cholecystokinin as well as insulin and glucagon.

EICOSANOIDS. Plasma concentrations of eicosanoids, which compose a group of 20 carbon, cyclic fatty acids derived primarily from arachidonic acid, are increased during hemorrhagic, septic, and endotoxic shock and following thermal and nonthermal injury. The presence of these substances in increased concentrations has been implicated in pathologic conditions such as ARDS and renal failure.

The arachidonic acid used in eicosanoid synthesis is derived from cell membrane phospholipids (phosphatidylcholine and phosphatidylinositol) and is converted by a series of enzymatic reactions into four major eicosanoid groups composed of the classic prostaglandins (PGE, PGF), the prostacyclins (PGI), the thromboxanes (TxB), and the leukotrienes (Fig. 1-38). Cortisol inhibits phospholipase A and therefore inhibits the synthesis of all eicosanoids. By contrast, aspirin and indocin inhibit cyclooxygenase and therefore prostaglandin synthesis but they may increase leukotriene synthesis.

The eicosanoids are tissue-specific. For example, vascular endothelium converts arachidonic acid primarily to prostacyclin (PGI_2) whereas platelets convert it primarily to thromboxane (TxA_2). The eicosanoids have a very short half-life and duration of action of 30 s to 5 min once released. Their metabolism into inactive fragments occurs primarily at the site of release and secondarily in the lung. Since they are not stored in cells, the release of these agents requires de novo synthesis. Although there are numerous stimuli for prostaglandin synthesis and release, many of which are not recognized at present, the better-known stimuli include hypoxia, ischemia, tissue injury, pyrogen, endotoxin, collagen, thrombin, neural stimulation, and hormonal stimulation (serotonin, acetylcholine, histamine, norepinephrine, vasopressin, angiotensin II, and bradykinin). These stimuli are relatively nonspecific because they result in the release of several prostaglandins whose structures depend upon the tissue stimulated and not the stimulus itself.

Prostaglandin synthesis has been linked to phosphatidylinositol breakdown in calcium-dependent hormonal regulation (alpha₁). The increase in prostaglandins may, in turn, increase the breakdown of phosphatidylinositol, thereby augmenting the hormonal response. The biological actions of prostaglandins are closely linked to alterations in the intracellular concentration of cAMP. In general, a prostaglandin mediated increase in the concentration of cAMP in a target cell results in stimulation of a target cell action, whereas a prostaglandin mediated decrease in cAMP results in inhibition of a target cell action. In this regard, the most potent prostaglandins capable of producing changes in cAMP are prostacyclin and thromboxane. A specific prostaglandin does not always lead to a specific change in the intracellular cAMP concentration of all target tissues, so that the same prostaglandin that inhibits cAMP formation in one tissue may stimulate it in another.

The eicosanoids have widespread effects on systemic and pulmonary vasculature, on neurotransmission, and on the local effects of hormones. For every action produced by a given eicosanoid there is another that produces an antagonistic action. For example, thromboxane A_2 is a potent vasoconstrictor released by platelets that stimulates platelet aggregation, whereas prostacyclin is a potent vasodilator released by vascular endothelium that inhibits platelet aggregation. Because of their antagonistic actions, an increase in the release of TxA_2 or a decrease in the production of PgI_2 would favor platelet aggregation and vasoconstriction. These features are characteristic of the adult respiratory distress syndrome, and in fact, the ratio of TxB_2 (the major metabolite of TxA_2) to 6-keto-$F_{1\alpha}$ (the major metabolite of PgI_2) is greater in the plasma of patients with sepsis and ARDS than in patients with sepsis alone. Some investigators believe that the primary event in ARDS is platelet aggregation and thromboxane release that in turn produce pulmonary vasoconstriction, leukocyte trapping, free oxygen radical release, and endothelial damage.

The E family of prostaglandins, PGE_1 and PGE_2, produce bronchodilation, whereas $PGF_{2\alpha}$ produces bronchoconstriction. PgE_2 and $PgF_{2\alpha}$ increase pulmonary vascular resistance and capillary permeability, whereas they decrease systemic vascular resistance. These agents have also been implicated in the development of systemic sepsis, since the major hemodynamic feature of sepsis is an increase in pulmonary vascular resistance with a concomitant decrease in systemic vascular resistance.

The prostaglandins are major components of the inflammatory response, whose importance has been repeatedly documented by the resolution of inflammatory conditions such as bursitis, arthritis, and tenosynovitis with treatment with antiprostaglandin agents. The inflammatory response is characterized by increased vascular permeability, leukocyte migration, vasodilation, which lead to the classic manifestations of rubor, dolor, tumor, and calor (redness, pain, swelling, and heat). PgE compounds are capable of inducing all these local changes as well as systemic manifestations such as fever and headache. Prostaglandins of the PgD and PgG families also participate in the response, but members of the PgF family probably do not because they are venoconstrictors and much weaker than members of the PgE group. The PgF group is thought to be involved in the termination of the inflammatory response.

The leukotrienes are also important mediators of the inflammatory response, produced by a variety of cell types (pulmonary parenchymal cells, macrophages, mast cells, leukocytes, smooth muscle cells, and connective tissue cells) that may exert an important role in the development of cell and tissue injury during shock and ischemia. Included in this group of compounds is the slow-releasing substance of anaphylaxis. These compounds increase postcapillary leakage with 1000 times the potency of histamine and also produce leukocyte adherence, bronchoconstriction, and vasoconstriction. Although the concentrations of leukotrienes in the plasma increase only moderately during shock, their intense biologic activities suggest they may exert an important role in the pathophysiology of shock.

KALLIKREINS-KININS. There are two kinins in human beings, bradykinin and kallidin, that are produced through the action of the serine protease kallikrein on high (Fitzgerald factor) and low molecular weight kininogens in plasma and in tissues, respectively. As a result, bradykinin is present primarily in the circulation and kallidin in tissues. Kallikrein itself exists in plasma in an inactive form as prekallikrein (Fletcher factor), whose activation depends upon activation of the clotting system through Hageman factor. The plasma kinins are rapidly broken down by two enzymes: kinase I and kinase II. Kinase I is a carboxypeptidase that is identical to the anaphylatoxin inactivator that degrades C_{3a}, C_{4a}, and C_{5a} anaphylatoxins, and kinase II is a dipeptidase that is identical to angiotensin converting enzyme, which converts angiotensin I to angiotensin II. During ARDS, the resultant endothelial damage may inhibit the formation or action of kinase II, thereby producing an accumulation of bradykinin and a reduction of angiotensin II. These changes may be important in the systemic as well as the local manifestations of ARDS.

Increased plasma concentrations of kallikrein and bradykinin and decreased plasma concentrations of prekallikrein have been noted during hemorrhagic shock, endotoxic shock, septic shock, and tissue injury. For example, Aasen and colleagues have demonstrated in septic patients that the plasma concentration of prekallikrein decreases and the activity of kallikrein increases. Furthermore, these changes appeared to correlate with survival and severity of injury, since there was a gradual increase in the concentrations of prekallikrein in survivors but not in nonsurvivors and a greater activity of kallikrein in patients with septic shock than in patients with sepsis but no hypotension.

The kinins are potent vasodilators that increase capillary permeability, produce edema, evoke pain, increase bronchial resistance, and enhance glucose clearance. As such they appear to be important mediators of the inflammatory response. They have been implicated in the regulation of fluid and electrolytes by the kidney by causing renal vasodilation, a reduction in renal blood flow, an increase in the formation of renin, and an increase in sodium and water retention when administered in pharmacologic doses.

SEROTONIN. Serotonin (5-hydroxytryptamine), which is released by enterochromaffin cells of the gut and by platelets, is a neurotransmitter formed from tryptophan that acts primarily on smooth muscle and nerve endings. It is a potent vasoconstrictor and bronchoconstrictor that increases platelet aggregation, myocardial inotropy, and myocardial chronotropy. The action of serotonin on smooth muscle is considerably greater on venous smooth muscle than on precapillary sphincter muscle. As a result it is primarily a venoconstrictor rather than an arterial constrictor. It is released by tissue injury and is an important mediator of the inflammatory response.

HISTAMINE. Histamine has long been implicated in the pathophysiology of tissue injury and shock and elevated concentrations have been demonstrated after hemorrhagic shock, septic shock, endotoxemia, and thermal and nonthermal injury. The highest levels of histamine seem to occur with sepsis and endotoxemia. Following the administration of endotoxin to dogs, there is an immediate explosive release of histamine that correlates with the amount of endotoxin administered and with the decline in arterial blood pressure and circulating platelets consequent to the administration of endotoxin. Histamine levels have been inversely correlated with survival in patients with septic shock and after endotoxin administration in rats. By contrast, there is no association between the concentration of histamine and survival following thermal injury.

Histamine is synthesized from histidine and stored primarily in mast cells in tissue and in basophils in blood. It is also stored in the gastric mucosa, neurons, platelets, and epidermis. Release of histamine from these tissues is associated with a decrease in the intracellular concentration of cAMP and an increase in intracellular calcium. Histamine acts on cell surface receptors that are divisible into H_1 and H_2. Receptors of the H_1 type mediate an increase in the uptake of L-histidine (precursor of histamine) into cells as well as actions such as bronchoconstriction, increased myocardial contractility, and intestinal contraction, whereas receptors of the H_2 type inhibit histamine release and mediate changes in gastric secretion cardiac rate and immunologic function. Both receptor types appear to mediate small vessel vasodilation and increased vascular permeability. Exogenously administered histamine leads to a variety of effects common to septic shock including hypotension, peripheral pooling of blood, increased capillary permeability, decreased venous return, and myocardial failure.

SOMATOMEDINS AND THE INSULINLIKE GROWTH FACTORS. The somatomedins are a family of polypeptides that stimulate proteoglycan synthesis in cartilage and DNA synthesis and cell replication in a variety of cell types and that demonstrate insulinlike activity including increasing glucose uptake and protein synthesis in skeletal muscle, increasing glucose uptake, glucose oxidation, and lipid synthesis in adipose tissue, and increasing protein synthesis and glycogenesis in the liver. Human plasma also contains large amounts of insulinlike activity that does not reside in insulin itself, so-called nonsuppressible insulinlike activity, NSILA. It is divisible into two chemically and biologically related polypeptides, NSILA-I and NSILA-II, which in addition to their in-

sulinlike effects have marked effects on cell growth. They are now referred to as insulinlike growth factor I (IGF-I) and insulinlike growth factor II (IGF-II), and it appears that somatomedin-C, somatomedin-A, and IGF-I are the same molecule.

The plasma concentration of IGF-I is decreased after injury. This may be the result of the starvation that accompanies injury, since the plasma concentration of IGF-I is also depressed during fasting. Nonetheless, the concentration of insulinlike growth factors is increased during the late stages of endotoxicosis. This increase may explain the paradoxical increase in peripheral glucose utilization and depression in hepatic gluconeogenesis that has been noted during late endotoxicosis in association with a reduction in the plasma concentration of insulin.

INTERLEUKIN-1. Interleukin-1, or leukocyte endogenous mediator as it was called in the past, is a proteinlike molecule with a molecular weight of approximately 15,000 that is released primarily by activated monocyte-macrophage cell types. (It is also probably the same molecule as lymphocyte activating factor and endogenous pyrogen.) Activation of these cell types may result from the ingestion of cellular and tissue debrides, from contact with immune complexes, or by an interaction with chemicals such as endotoxin. Thus, nearly all infections, immunological reactions, and inflammatory processes stimulate the synthesis and release of leukocyte endogenous mediator by phagocytic cells. Once released, it circulates to various tissues in the body, having a profound influence upon the metabolism of the reticuloendothelial system, the liver, the brain, and skeletal muscle. For example, the fever that accompanies the acute phase response to injury or infection is thought to be the result of an interleukin-1 mediated alteration in the set point of the hypothalamic thermoregulatory center. As such, it can be considered a hormone. Many of the primary actions of interleukin-1 occur in the tissues from which it originates.

In the liver, interleukin-1 stimulates protein synthesis, resulting in the production of acute phase reactants, the accumulation of iron and zinc, and the release of copper. As a result, the plasma concentrations of iron and of zinc decrease, whereas the concentration of copper increases. The copper is released primarily with ceruloplasmin, a protein that is important in clearing oxygen radicals from injured and infected tissues and in donating copper groups to copper-dependent enzymes. An example of the latter is lysyl oxidase, an enzyme that is critical in wound healing because of its ability to form cross links between collagen molecules. The decrease in serum iron is thought to be important in the inhibition of bacterial growth and in the genesis of anemia in chronic infections. Other acute phase reactants that increase in response to interleukin-1 include fibrinogen, haptoglobin, C-reactive protein, and components of complement and alpha$_2$ macroglobin. The latter is a protease inhibitor that may exert an important role at the site of injury or infection by inhibiting the proteases that are released by leukocytes and by macrophages.

It is apparent that this burst in hepatic protein synthesis requires a great deal of energy and amino acid. This, in

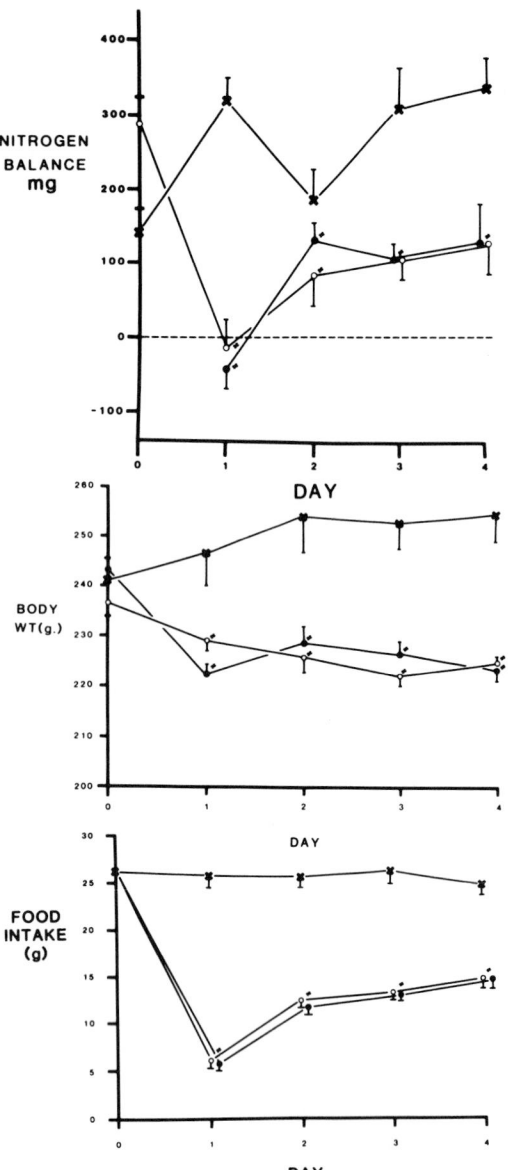

Fig. 1-39. Effect of wounding on food intake, nitrogen balance, and body weight. Food intake by wounded animals (●) was considerably less than that of animals allowed to eat ad libitum (×). When animals were pair-fed (○) to the reduced food intake of the wounded animals, negative nitrogen balance and weight loss were the same in these two groups. In contrast, there was a marked difference in nitrogen balance and body weight between wounded animals and animals allowed to eat ad libitum. (From: *Shearer JD et al: Am J Surg 147:456, 1984, with permission.*)

part, may be provided by an interleukin-1 mediated increase in protein degradation and amino acid release from skeletal muscle tissue that precedes the increase in hepatic protein synthesis. The amino acids released appear to be used by the liver for energy as well as for protein synthesis, since an appreciable amount of the amino acids released is oxidized. The skeletal muscle wasting and negative nitrogen balance that accompanies injury may be a direct result of interleukin-1. In addition, the increase in hepatic protein synthesis produced by interleukin-1 is not global. Albumin synthesis decreases during the acute phase response, and there is suggestive evidence that overall protein synthesis in the liver is decreased.

TUMOR NECROSIS FACTOR. Tumor necrosis factor (TNF), or cachectin, is a monokine released by macrophages that is capable of inducing hemorrhagic necrosis of tumors. In addition, it may be in large part responsible for the wasting associated with chronic illness and malignancy. Recent evidence suggests that TNF may exert an important role in the response to injury and infection. For example, the lethal effects of endotoxin including fever, hypotension, metabolic acidosis, hemoconcentration, hyperglycemia, and hypokalemia appear to be mediated by TNF. Tumor necrosis factor also mediates a decrease in the transmembrane potential of skeletal muscle that may be important in the sequestration of fluid and electrolytes during injury.

METABOLIC CHANGES INDUCED BY INJURY

The immediate postinjury period is characterized by starvation, immobilization, restoration of homeostasis, and repair. The metabolic events consequent to injury are the result of stimuli present in the injury and starvation and are presumably directed at restoration of homeostasis and at repair. For example, the nitrogen balance and weight loss that follow injury appear to be, in large part, the result of the starvation that accompanies the injury (Fig. 1-39). Recent evidence from our laboratories also suggests that the metabolic response to injury may be altered to some degree by the inflammatory response to the injury. For example, temporal alterations in plasma ketone body and lactate concentrations of wounded animals appear to correlate with the inflammatory infiltrate of wounded tissue. Tumor necrosis factor appears to be responsible for many of the manifestations of endotoxemia. An understanding of the metabolic response consequent to starvation and the metabolic alterations produced by the inflammatory infiltrate is central to an understanding of the metabolic response to injury.

Metabolic Response Consequent to Starvation

SUBSTRATE METABOLISM. The average resting, 70-kg human being using 1800 kcal/day of energy requires 180 g of glucose for the metabolism of the nervous tissue (144 g) and other glycolytic tissue (RBC, WBC, renal medulla) (36 g) (Fig. 1-40), energy for obligate daily activity, amino acids for protein synthesis, and fatty acids for lipid synthesis. In the absence of food, a fasting human being must supply these substrates from existing body stores.

Glucose and energy are obtained from the 75 g of glycogen stored in the liver (Table 1-2). However, this is not sufficient for the energy or the glucose requirements of a fasting human being. Free glucose cannot be provided to the circulation from the 150 g of glycogen present in skel-

FASTING MAN
(24 hours, basal :-1800 calories)

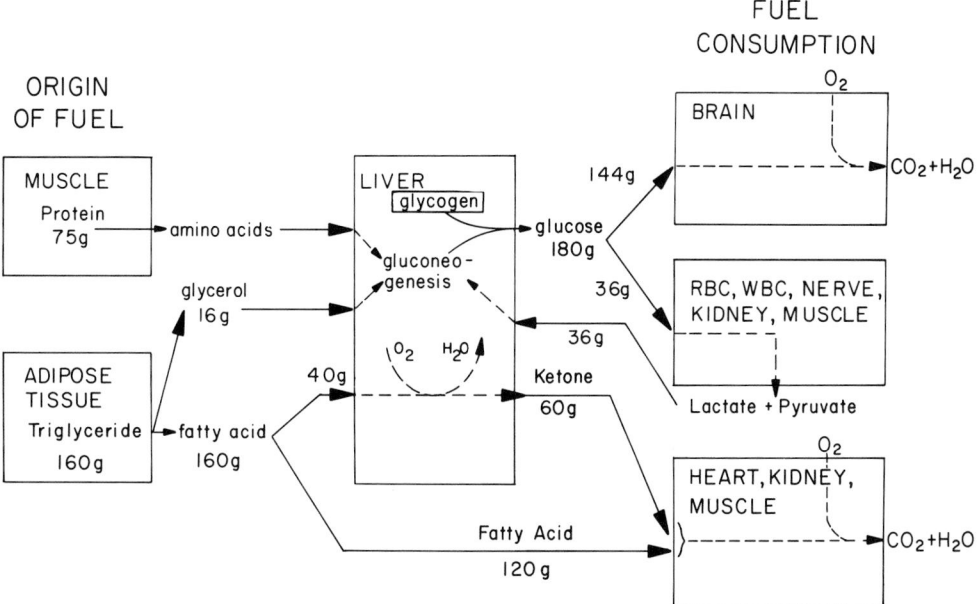

Fig. 1-40. Scheme of fuel utilization in a normal fasted man. The two primary sources are muscle protein and fat. The brain oxidizes glucose completely, the glycolyzers break down glucose by aerobic or anaerobic glycolysis into lactate and pyruvate, which are then remade in the liver in glucose, and the rest of the body burns fatty acids and ketones. (Adapted from: *Cahill GF: N Engl J Med 282:668, 1970, with permission.*)

etal muscle since it lacks glucose-6-phosphatase, the enzyme necessary for the release of free glucose from a cell. Thus, the primary stimulus to the metabolic events that occur during fasting and starvation is a reduction in the serum glucose concentration that occurs as the glucose needs of glucose-dependent tissues can no longer be met by the breakdown of glycogen (Fig. 1-41). The reduction in serum glucose, which occurs within 15 h of fasting, results in a decrease in the secretion of insulin and an increase in the secretion of glucagon, cortisol, growth

hormone, and catecholamines, changes that stimulate an increase in hepatic gluconeogenesis and glycogenolysis. The changes in insulin and glucagon secretion appear to be the primary response, since significant increases in the secretion of the counterregulatory hormones, particularly catecholamines, are not usually seen until the reduction in the serum glucose concentration is severe. Furthermore, an increase in the secretion of catecholamines, growth hormone, and cortisol is not necessary, since the basal concentrations of the counterregulatory hormones will be unopposed by the reduction in insulin. The glucose required for glucose-dependent tissues during starvation is provided by glycogenolysis and gluconeogenesis (Fig. 1-42). This requires the provision of gluconeogenic precursors to the liver.

There are three primary gluconeogenic precursors used by the liver and to a lesser extent by the kidney for the synthesis of glucose. These are lactate, glycerol, and amino acids such as alanine and glutamine (Table 1-3). There are two main sources for lactate. The first is from the metabolism of glucose by erythrocytes and white cells that do not oxidize the glucose they require. Although most cells that require glucose such as the brain and nervous tissue metabolize glucose completely to carbon dioxide, erythrocytes and white cells convert glucose to lactate by aerobic glycolysis and release the newly formed lactate into the circulation. In turn, this lactate can be reconverted to glucose in the liver and again made available for use by peripheral tissues, a process described by the Coris (Fig. 1-43). The lactate made available from these sources does not provide any new carbon skeleton for glucose synthesis, since the carbon is derived from preexistent molecules of glucose. If glucose use by

Table 1-2

Fuel	Weight, kg	Calories
Tissues:		
Fat (adipose triglyceride)	15	141,000
Protein (mainly muscle)	6	24,000
Glycogen (muscle)	0.150	600
Glycogen (liver)	0.075	300
Total		165,900
Circulating fuels:		
Glucose (extracellular fluid)	0.020	80
Free fatty acids (plasma)	0.0003	3
Triglycerides (plasma)	0.003	30
Total		113

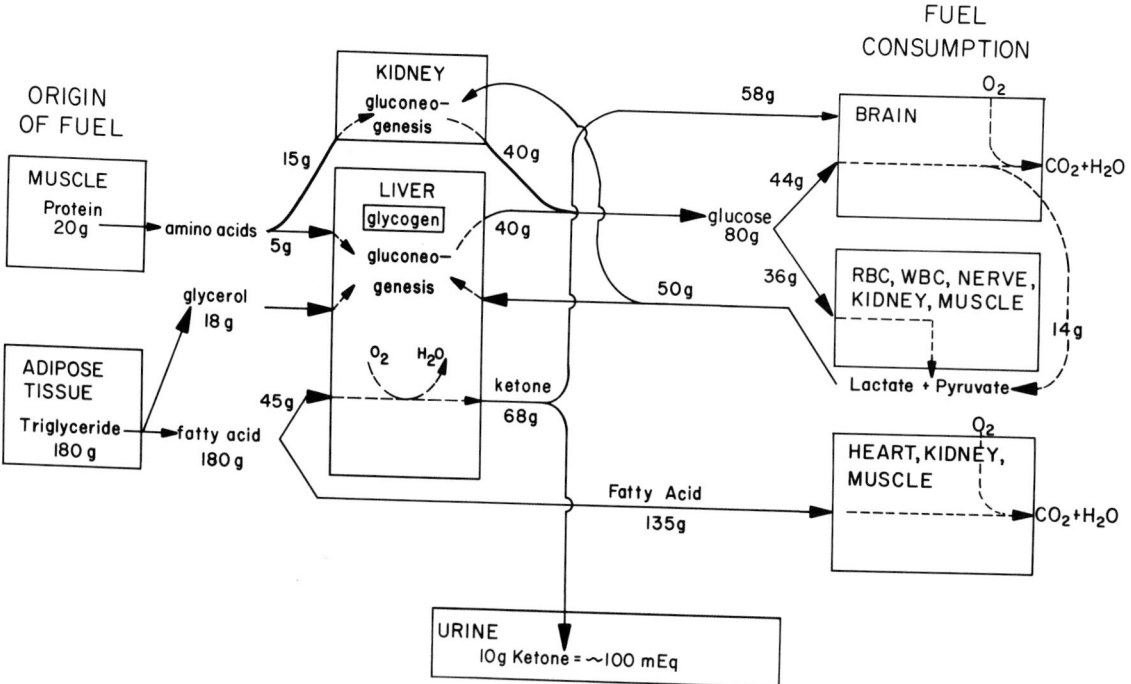

FASTING MAN ADAPTED (5-6 wks.)
(24 hours, basal : ~1500 calories)

Fig. 1-45. Schema of fuel metabolism after 5 to 6 weeks of starvation. Liver glycogen sources are depleted, there is a diminished utilization of muscle protein, the brain is burning ketones, and gluconeogenesis from amino acids is taking place to a large extent in the kidney. (Adapted from: Cahill GF: N Engl J Med 282:668, 1970, with permission.)

process before the carbon skeleton can be made available for gluconeogenesis. Although under normal circumstances, urea synthesis is the primary mechanism, the synthesis of urea in the liver requires a considerable amount of energy and the enzymes required for ureagenesis are decreased during prolonged starvation. Consequently, the renal excretion of ammonium ion becomes the primary route of elimination of alpha amino nitrogen during starvation. Additionally, the kidney also assumes an increasing role in gluconeogenesis since glutamine and glutamate serve as the primary amino acids for transport of the amino groups to the kidney for ammonia formation and for gluconeogenesis in the kidney. The kidney may account for up to 45 percent of glucose production during late starvation.

The rapid proteolysis of body protein cannot proceed at a rate of 75 g/day for very long. The total amount of protein in a 70-kg man is approximately 6000 g, and the continued degradation of protein results in continued loss of function such that death will ensue well before all the protein is broken down. Fortunately, proteolysis does slow down by about the fifth day of starvation and eventually reaches a nadir of 20 g of protein per day. This is reflected in a decline in urinary excretion of nitrogen to a minimum of approximately 2 to 4 g of nitrogen per day.

The reduction in protein breakdown is in large part made possible through ketoadaptation of the brain. Although the brain can metabolize ketone bodies, the limited transport of ketone bodies through the blood-brain

barrier under normal conditions limits their utilization. In the presence of adequate glucose concentrations, glucose is used preferentially. During starvation, transport systems in the blood-brain barrier increase the rate of ketone body transport, and the metabolism of the brain is adapted to utilize ketone bodies. Consequently, there is a significant reduction in the amount of glucose needed by the brain and therefore in the amount of protein that must be degraded for gluconeogenesis (Fig. 1-45 and Table 1-5).

Table 1-5. GLUCOSE AVAILABLE IN LATE
STARVATION STATE IN A 70-KG MAN

Origin	Amount of glucose, g/24 h
New glucose (gluconeogenesis):	
Fat (glycerol)	18
Protein	12
Stored or recycled glucose:	
Glycogen	0
Recycled glucose	50
Total	80

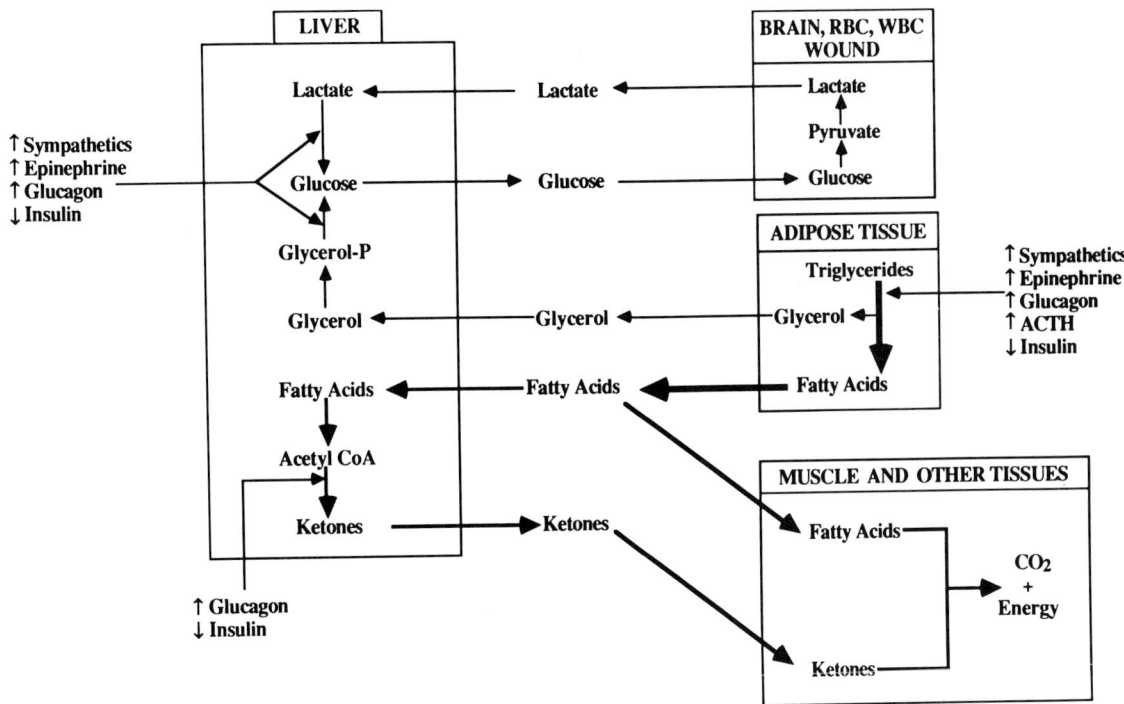

Fig. 1-46. Mobilization of fatty acids from adipose tissue during starvation provide fatty acids to various tissues that can be used for energy. In addition, fatty acids presented to the liver can be converted to ketone bodies for use throughout the body, and glycerol released during the degradation of triglycerides can be used by the liver to form new glucose. The primary hormones for lipolysis are catecholamines and for ketogenesis, glucagon.

The synthesis of glucose is an anabolic process that requires energy. Necessary enzymatic and muscular function such as neural transmission and cardiac contraction also requires energy. These daily energy requirements in a resting, fasting 70-kg human being can be met by the mobilization of approximately 160 g of triglycerides from adipose tissue in the form of free fatty acids (Fig. 1-46). The release of free fatty acids from adipose tissue is stimulated by a reduction in the serum insulin concentration and an absolute or relative increase in the concentrations of glucagon and other counterregulatory hormones. These endocrine alterations also stimulate ketogenesis. The free fatty acids and ketone bodies produced by the liver are used throughout the body by nonglycolytic tissues such as the heart, kidney, muscle, and liver as a source of energy. Consequently, the main source of energy in starvation is fat, accounting for up to 90 percent of the calories used during starvation.

The use of lipids during starvation not only can provide glucose from the 16 g of glycerol released in the breakdown of 160 g of triglycerides, it also decreases the overall amount of glucose required. For example, skeletal and cardiac muscle use fatty acids at a rate proportional to their concentration in the serum. The use of fatty acids by these tissues in turn decreases the amount of glucose required, the so-called Randle effect. Similarly, the use of ketone bodies inhibits glucose uptake in most tissues by inhibiting pyruvate dehydrogenase. The switch to fat as a main fuel source decreases the amount of glucose used and, therefore, the amount of gluconeogenesis and protein degradation required.

Concurrent with these alterations in metabolism there is a reduction in the resting energy expenditure by up to 31 percent. This is exemplified by the classic studies of total starvation of Benedict in which energy expenditure decreased from an average of 1650 cal/day in the first week to an average of 1290 cal in the third week. The reduction in resting energy expenditure is multifactorial and derives in part from a decrease in lean body cell mass, voluntary work, body temperature, cardiac work, sympathetic nervous system activity, and metabolic activity of muscle. Through a reduction in the resting energy expenditure, the utilization of protein for gluconeogenesis, the utilization of lipid for energy, and the ketoadaptation of the brain, human beings are able to survive during prolonged periods of starvation. Nonetheless, this does not occur without the impairment or loss of important body functions, and if starvation persists to a point at which 30 to 40 percent of the body weight has been lost, death ensues.

WATER AND ELECTROLYTE METABOLISM. Metabolic alterations induced by starvation are not limited to substrates. Major changes also occur in fluid and electrolyte metabolism. Initially, there is a loss of sodium, potassium, and water that accounts for the rapid and relatively large loss of weight observed in people who fast for a few days. This accounts for the greater amount of weight lost during early starvation than during late starvation. The loss of sodium during this period is obligate, since patients who were previously on a low-sodium diet lose salt

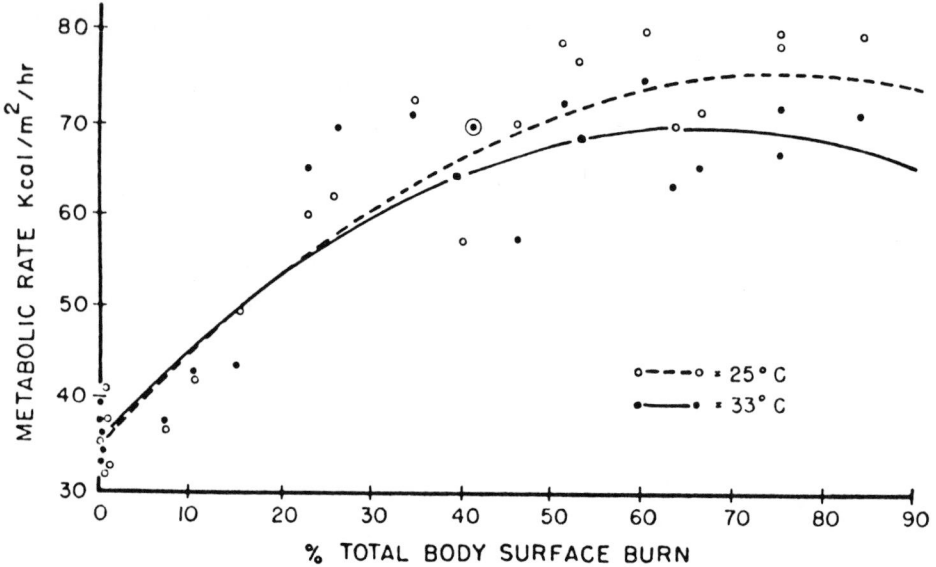

Fig. 1-47. Burned patients have a metabolic rate that correlates linearly with the size of the burn until massive thermal injuries are achieved, at which point the metabolic rate plateaus. This plateau suggests that patients with massive burns are at or near maximal rates of heat production. In addition, the increase in metabolic rate is secondary to endogenous heat production and not to a cold environment, since patients placed in a warm environment do not demonstrate a significant reduction in metabolic rate. (From: *Wilmore DW: Surg Clin North Am 56:999, 1976, with permission.*)

during fasting and starvation and the administration of salt and water to patients who are fasting does not stop the loss of sodium. The sodium loss appears to be related to the abrupt decrease in availability of carbohydrates, since the feeding of small amounts of glucose will decrease the amount of sodium lost. Although initially on the order of 150 to 250 meq/day, it gradually declines to 1 to 15 meq/day as the starvation persists. Alterations in sodium and water metabolism may also be the result of alterations in plasma membrane potential consequent to starvation. Parenthetically, the reduction in membrane potential following starvation is not corrected by total parenteral nutrition but is corrected by the administration of glutamine or catecholamines. Reductions in total body water and sodium are associated with a reduction in the plasma volume. A starved patient is less likely to tolerate hypovolemia than a well-fed patient.

Metabolism in Injured Human Beings

The alterations in substrate metabolism that occur following injury may be divided into three phases. The first phase, which occurs during the first several hours after injury, is characterized by hyperglycemia and by the restoration of circulating volume and tissue perfusion. The second phase, which occurs after tissue perfusion has been restored, may last from days to weeks, depending on the severity of injury, previous health of the individual, and medical intervention. It is characterized by generalized catabolism, negative nitrogen balance, hyperglycemia, and heat production. The third phase occurs once volume deficits have been corrected, infection has been controlled, pain has been eliminated, and complete oxygenation has been restored. This is associated with a slow but progressive reaccumulation of protein followed by the reaccumulation of body fat. It is usually considerably longer than the catabolic phase since the rate of protein synthesis cannot exceed 3 to 5 g/day. These three phases

correspond to the ebb, flow, and anabolic phases described by Cuthbertson and Moore.

ENERGY METABOLISM FOLLOWING INJURY

ENERGY EXPENDITURE. Injury of any type is associated with immobilization, starvation, and repair. Although starvation and immobilization are both associated with a reduction in energy requirements, reparative processes are associated with an increase in the energy needed. Overall, the energy requirements of traumatized, septic, and burned individuals are increased as reflected in the characteristic loss of body weight and increase in basal metabolic rate. The increase in the energy needed varies directly with the severity of injury. For example, the increase in resting energy expenditure following thermal injury is proportional to the size of the burn (Fig. 1-47). Kinney and coworkers have determined that healthy individuals undergoing an uncomplicated elective operation demonstrate no greater than a 10 percent increase in their resting energy expenditure (Fig. 1-48). This is increased to 10 to 25 percent in patients with multiple skeletal injuries. Febrile complication increases these requirements significantly, with an increase in resting energy expenditure of approximately 7 percent for each degree Fahrenheit of fever noted by Dubois. Severe infections, such as peritonitis or intraabdominal abscesses, are associated with an increase in resting energy expenditure of 20 to 75 percent. This increase is greater than one would predict on the basis of temperature elevation alone, and it appears to be related to the inflammatory

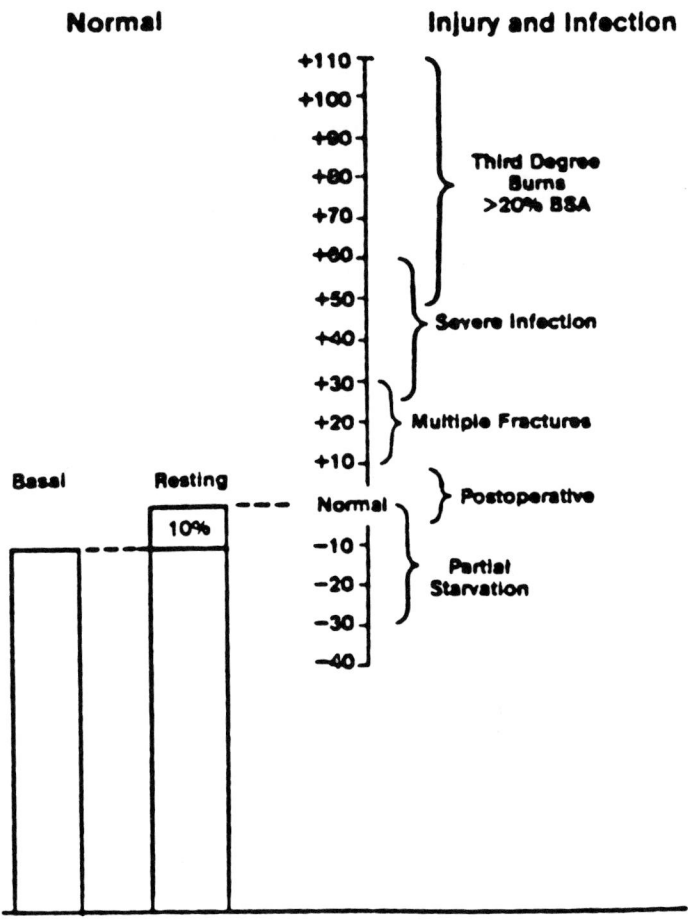

Fig. 1-48. Resting energy expenditure of adult patients during injury, stress, and starvation. The highest resting energy expenditures are seen following thermal injuries and severe infections. (From: *Kinney JM: The application of indirect calorimetry to clinical studies, in Assessment of Energy Metabolism in Health and Disease. Columbus, OH, Ross Laboratories, 1980, p 42, with permission.*)

process itself since it persists for as long as inflammation is present. The most severe injury is a thermal burn, in which sustained increases in resting energy expenditure of greater than 100 percent have been noted.

In large part, the increase in energy expenditure following injury appears to result from the increased activity of the sympathetic nervous system and the increased circulating concentrations of catecholamines. Wilmore and colleagues have demonstrated that the metabolic rate can be decreased in severely burned patients by the administration of alpha- and beta-adrenergic blockers or beta-adrenergic blockers alone. Conversely, the administration of epinephrine or norepinephrine to normal human beings increases the basal metabolic rate.

The increase in resting energy expenditure is also dependent upon the size of the individual and to some extent upon the environmental temperature. The largest increases in energy expenditure are seen in heavily muscled, well-nourished young men who have large body cell masses, and the smallest increases are in elderly, poorly nourished women who have small body cell masses. This is a reflection of the linear relationship between body cell mass and resting energy expenditure.

Although energy can be derived from carbohydrates, proteins, or fat, following injury the available stores of carbohydrate are small, nutritional intake of carbohydrates and proteins is reduced or absent, glucose required for glucose-dependent tissues persists, and degradation of protein for energy will require the loss or reduction of some body function. As a result, the primary source for energy during injury is fat, a finding that is reflected in the low respiratory quotients (0.7 to 0.8) that are noted after injury and sepsis. There is also evidence to suggest that the dependence on lipids after septic injury is greater than that observed following nonseptic injury. These findings argue in favor of the use of intralipids during parenteral nutrition.

ENERGY METABOLISM IN TISSUES. A significant reduction in energy charge and ATP content has been noted

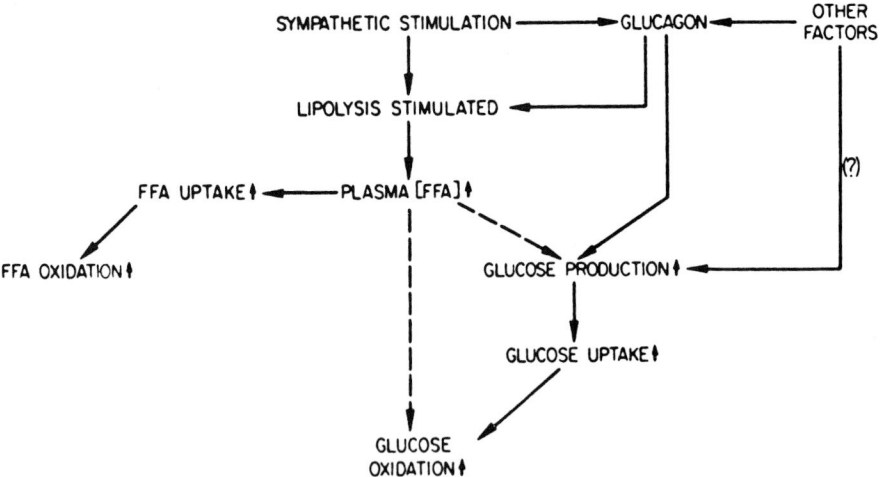

Fig. 1-49. The role of sympathetic stimulation in substrate kinetics during stress. (From: *Lefer AM, Schumer W: Molecular and Cellular Aspects of Shock and Trauma. New York, Alan R. Liss, 1983, with permission.*)

during severe hemorrhagic shock; hypoxia; total ischemia in the liver, kidney, skeletal muscle, and cardiac muscle; sepsis; and following wounding. The reduction in energy charge and high-energy phosphates is proportional to the severity of the injury.

The reduction in high-energy phosphates may be the result of anaerobic metabolism consequent to hypoperfusion or hypoxia or to a dilutional effect from inflammatory cells. For example, hypovolemia and sepsis demonstrate a reduction in tissue high-energy phosphate concentrations that appear to result from anaerobic metabolism in poorly perfused and hypoxemic tissues. The reduction in high-energy phosphates during shock usually occurs in the liver and kidneys prior to the reductions in cardiac and skeletal muscle and is related to the severity of the hemorrhagic, septic, or hypoxic insult. The different response between tissue types, in part, may be the result of the differences in blood flow and in the resting metabolic activity of the specific tissue examined. A reduction in the energy charge ATP and creatine phosphate content of all tissues eventually occurs if there is insufficient compensation to the hemorrhage or septic insult.

Wounded tissue also demonstrates a reduction in its energy charge, ATP, and creatine phosphate content during early healing that traditionally has been attributed to a decrease in the production of high-energy phosphate compounds from anaerobic metabolism in wounded tissue. Recent evidence suggests that the metabolism of wounded tissue is aerobic rather than anaerobic, a finding that implies wounded tissue has the same capacity for the production of high-energy phosphates as nonwounded tissue. A reduction in the energy charge of wounded tissue could be an artifact resulting from varying high-energy phosphate contents in the component cells of wounded tissue. Inflammatory cells that account for up to 50 percent of the DNA (and therefore 50 percent of the cells) present in wounded tissue contain very few high-energy compounds. As a result, the presence of these cells in wounded tissue can dilute the overall high-energy phosphate content measured in wounded tissue even though the high-energy phosphate content of the resident tissue is normal or actually increased. That is, the muscle present in wounded skeletal muscle may have the same high-energy phosphate content as that seen in normal skeletal muscle. This appears to be the case since the addition of macrophages to normal skeletal muscle results in a high-energy phosphate content similar to that observed in wounded muscle. Similarly, the high-energy phosphate content of septic tissue is usually reduced. Although this reduction also has been attributed to a decrease in high-energy phosphate production secondary to anaerobic metabolism, this reduction also may be dilutional, since septic tissue as well as wounded tissue has a marked inflammatory cell infiltrate.

LIPID METABOLISM DURING INJURY

LIPOLYSIS. The primary source of energy following injury is lipids. It is not surprising that rate of lipolysis is generally increased immediately following injury and during the reparative phase. Immediately after injury, elevated concentrations of cortisol, catecholamines, glucagon, growth hormone, and ACTH, increased sympathetic nervous system activity, and depressed concentrations of insulin favor lipolysis. Among these agents, the best-known stimulus for hormone-sensitive lipase is catecholamines. The sympathetic nervous system is of paramount importance in the lipolytic response to stress, since adrenergic blockade produces a marked reduction in lipolysis (Fig. 1-49). Evidence suggests that norepinephrine released by the sympathetic nervous system is more important in this response than the release of adrenal epinephrine, since the response appears to be primarily mediated through beta$_1$ receptors.

The net lipolysis observed during the ebb phase results in elevated concentrations of glycerol and free fatty acids in plasma. If the reduction in effective circulating volume is severe, such as might be seen in severe hemorrhage or sepsis, an elevation in plasma free fatty acids may not occur. This may result from intense vasoconstriction in peripheral tissues and therefore minimal blood flow in adipose tissue, such that neuroendocrine agents cannot act on adipose tissue. Because the net production of free fatty acids is dependent upon the balance between lipolysis and reesterification of fatty acids, an increase in the reesterification rate, such as that seen in the presence of high concentrations of lactate, may decrease net free fatty acid release. The latter is supported by the rise in plasma concentrations of glycerol noted after injury, which suggests that lipolysis is occurring, and by increased concentrations of lactate in studies in which there is no change in the concentration of free fatty acids. Other factors that may alter the mobilization of lipids after injury include a decrease in pH, hyperglycemia, and the anesthesia received. For example, lipolysis is directly inhibited by pentobarbital anesthesia, and hemorrhage in the presence of pentobarbital usually results in a fall in the plasma free fatty acid and ketone body concentrations. By contrast, hemorrhage experiments using other types of anesthesia or in awake animals produce a rise in the free fatty acid and ketone body concentrations.

During the reparative or flow phase, net lipolysis persists despite an increase in the concentration of insulin. This is reflected by an increased concentration of plasma free fatty acids and increased clearance of fatty acids. In the presence of oxygen, the fatty acids released can be oxidized by most tissues in the body, including cardiac and skeletal muscle, to produce energy, and normal or elevated rates of fatty acid oxidation have been noted during sepsis, endotoxemia, wounding, and thermal injury. If the rate of clearance of fatty acids is equal to or greater than their rate of appearance, no change or a decrease in the plasma fatty acid concentration may be noted. Even though there is an increase in the rate of appearance and oxidation of free fatty acids during sepsis and endotoxemia, a rise in the plasma free fatty acid concentration is not always noted. An analogous situation is also true for the hypertriglyceridemia that is characteristic of sepsis and endotoxemia. The latter may either be the result of an increase in the release of triglycerides that is in excess of the ability of tissues to clear them or the result of a normal rate of release in the face of a decrease in the ability of tissues to break down the molecules.

Controversy exists whether fatty acids can inhibit glycolysis following injury. Wolfe and colleagues have recently provided evidence in conscious burned dogs that the Randle effect does occur and that it may be a major mechanism for the reduction in glycolysis that occurs in nonseptic injury during the flow phase. An increase in the cytoplasmic concentration of citrate is seen during mild inflammation and injury but not after shock and major injury such as sepsis. Since fatty acid induced inhibition of glycolysis is mediated through citrate, the absence of an increase in citrate may in part explain the persistence of glycolysis and net proteolysis after injury.

KETOGENESIS. The high concentrations of intracellular fatty acids and the elevated concentration of glucagon during the ebb and flow phases inhibit fatty acid synthesis. In hepatocytes, this also stimulates the transport of acetyl CO-A into the mitochondria for oxidation and ketogenesis. The activity of ketogenesis after shock, injury, and sepsis is variable and correlates inversely with the severity of injury. After major injury, severe shock, and sepsis, ketogenesis is low or absent, whereas after minor injury or mild infection, it is increased but to a lesser extent than that seen during nonstressed starvation. Injuries in which ketogenesis is low also appear to be associated with a small or absent increase in plasma free fatty acid concentrations, suggesting that the absence of ketogenesis in these situations results from the absence of an increase in the intracellular concentrations of free fatty acids.

CARBOHYDRATE METABOLISM DURING INJURY

GLUCOSE METABOLISM. By contrast to fasting and starvation, characterized by hypoglycemia, injury, sepsis, and stress are characterized by hyperglycemia. Hyperglycemia following hemorrhage was first reported by Claude Bernard in 1877 and has subsequently been confirmed in different species such as the dog, cat, pig, rat, and human beings and for different injuries such as sepsis, trauma, and thermal injury. It occurs immediately after injury and persists into the reparative period. The increase in plasma glucose is proportional to the severity of injury as reflected in a positive correlation between injury severity score and glucose concentration trauma victims (Fig. 1-50).

The presence of hyperglycemia provides a ready source of energy to the brain and may be important to early survival. It also appears quite possible that, as suggested by Jarhult and by ourselves, the principal homeostatic significance of increased plasma glucose may be the resulting osmotic transfer of fluids from cells to the interstitium that it induces leading to the restitution of blood volume. Elevated concentrations of glucose may be necessary for adequate delivery of this substrate to wounded tissue.

The alterations in carbohydrate metabolism that occur during injury include an increased hepatic glucose production and an impaired peripheral uptake of glucose that result from an increase in the secretion of catecholamines, cortisol, glucagon, growth hormone, vasopressin, angiotensin II, and somatostatin and a reduction in the secretion of insulin. The primary source of glucose that is released immediately after injury is hepatic glycogen. By contrast, glucose production during the flow phase appears to result primarily from hepatic and renal gluconeogenesis.

Differences also exist in the mechanism through which these alterations occur. Although an immediate increase in the plasma glucagon concentration that correlated with

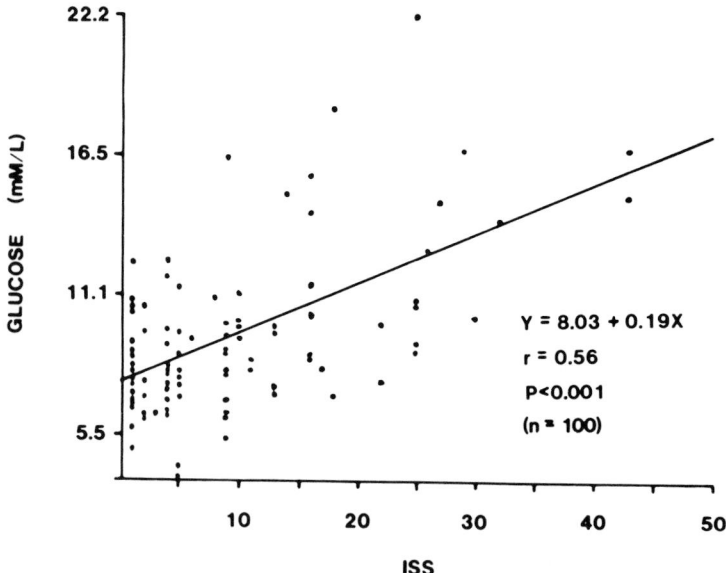

$$Y = 8.03 + 0.19X$$
$$r = 0.56$$
$$P < 0.001$$
$$(n = 100)$$

Fig. 1-50. There is a positive correlation between the serum glucose concentration and the severity of injury in multiply injured patients. (From: *Kenney PR, Allen-Rowlands CF, Gann DS: J Trauma 23:712, 1983, with permission.*)

the plasma glucose concentration following thermal injury was noted by Wilmore and colleagues, most studies of glucagon metabolism following nonthermal injury and hypovolemia have noted no increase in the plasma concentration of glucagon immediately after injury. This suggests that an increase in the peripheral concentration of glucagon or the delivery of glucagon to the liver is not required for the initial hyperglycemia after hemorrhage and injury. This is further supported by the studies of Lautt and coworkers who demonstrated the abolition of the hyperglycemic response to hemorrhage in adrenalectomized and hepatic denervated cats and the restitution of this response when either the adrenals or the liver were left intact. These data imply a redundant system for the control of the hyperglycemic response to hemorrhage and injury in which either of two effectors (hepatic nerves or adrenals) can effectively produce the hyperglycemic response. Thus, the immediate hyperglycemia that occurs following injury appears to be related primarily to the actions of catecholamines and cortisol with little contribution from glucagon, whereas during the flow phase, glucagon becomes more important.

The hyperglycemia that occurs following injury in diabetic patients may be different. Cryer and colleagues have documented the relevance of the counterregulatory hormones in patients with diabetes mellitus. Diabetic patients with insulin-dependent diabetes (IDDM) exhibit greater hyperglycemic responses to counterregulatory hormones, including glucagon, epinephrine, and cortisol, than nondiabetic patients; and acquired deficiencies in the secretion of some of the counterregulatory hormones occur commonly in patients with IDDM. For example, glucagon secretory responses to decrements in plasma glucose concentration occur early in the course of IDDM and deficiencies in epinephrine secretory responses frequently occur late in the disease. Patients with IDDM who have deficiencies in counterregulatory response may develop hypoglycemia following injury and patients with

normal responses may develop marked hyperglycemia as a result of the greater response to counterregulatory hormones when present.

INSULIN RESISTANCE. Another important difference in the mechanism of hyperglycemia following injury is related to the secretion of insulin. Immediately after injury, the plasma insulin concentration is depressed in relation to the degree of hyperglycemia. This results from a reduction in beta islet cell sensitivity to glucose that is mediated by catecholamines, somatostatin, reduced pancreatic blood flow, and the increased activity of the sympathetic nervous system. An intact adrenal gland is also necessary for this response since the blunting of the insulin secretion can be eliminated by adrenalectomy. During the flow phase, beta islet cell sensitivity returns to normal and insulin concentrations rise to more appropriate values but hyperglycemia still persists.

In part this is related to the delayed rate of assimilation of a glucose load, glucosuria, and a resistance to exogenously administered insulin noted in both the ebb and flow phases of injury. This diabetes of injury, first noted by Drucker, should not be interpreted as an actual reduction in glucose uptake and utilization, since glucose uptake and utilization by peripheral tissues in both the ebb and the flow phases is consistently greater than under normal circumstances. Instead the resistance to insulin is manifested in a decreased glucose clearance. The high-plasma glucose concentration and the attendant increase in the plasma to tissue glucose concentration gradient appear to overcome the resistance of peripheral tissues to glucose entry, thereby allowing for normal or increased rates of glucose uptake in peripheral tissues.

During the flow phase, gluconeogenesis persists despite near normal concentrations of insulin, another mani-

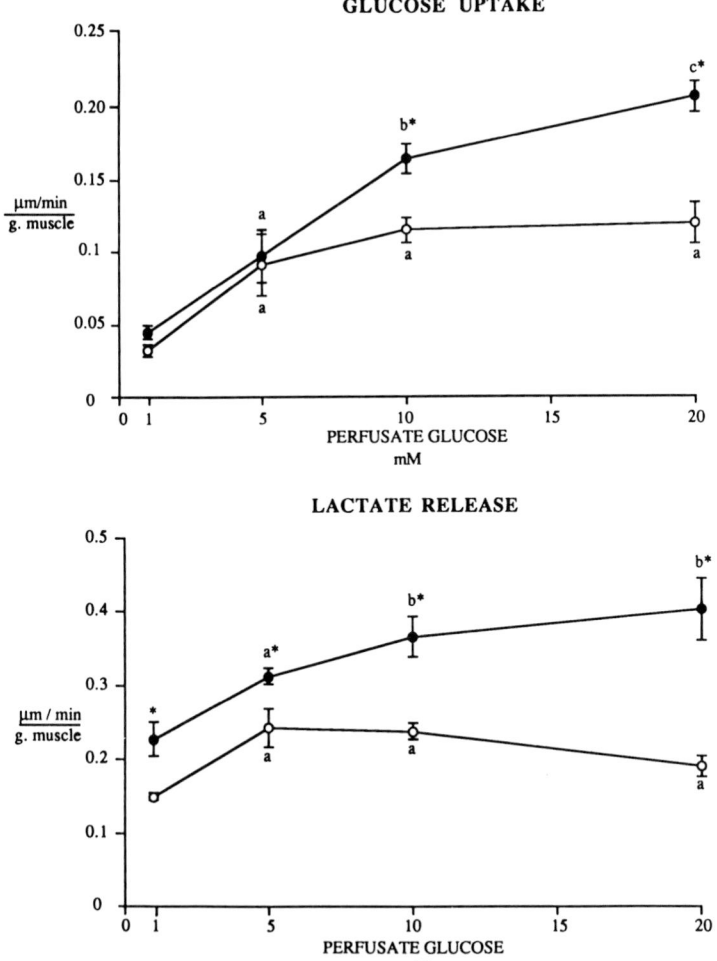

Fig. 1-51. Glucose uptake and lactate production by wounded (●) and nonwounded (○) hindlimbs of rats in response to increasing external glucose supply. Glucose uptake and lactate production by wounded hindlimbs increased as the concentration of external glucose increased. In contrast, glucose uptake and lactate production by nonwounded hindlimbs reached a plateau at an external glucose concentration of 5 mmol. *$p < 0.05$ wounded vs. nonwounded; a. = $p < 0.05$ intragroup difference vs. 1 mmol; b. = $p < 0.05$ intragroup difference vs. 5 mmol; c. = $p < 0.05$ intragroup difference vs. 10 mmol. (From: *Amaral JF et al: in preparation.*)

festation of the insulin resistance that occurs with injury. Therefore, the hyperglycemia that occurs after injury results from a combination of increased hepatic glucose production and release and from a peripheral resistance to the entrance of glucose. Since production supersedes utilization, hyperglycemia persists. If the rate of gluconeogenesis decreases through a reduction either in gluconeogenic precursors or in gluconeogenic enzymatic function, hepatic glucose production will decrease and hypoglycemia will ensue, a finding of terminal injuries and prolonged sepsis.

The insulin resistance that develops following injury is thought to arise from a reduction in the release of insulin from the pancreas and from an inhibition of insulin action on peripheral tissue that is mediated by the sympathetic nervous system, catecholamines, and cortisol. In vitro and in vivo studies have consistently demonstrated the ability of these agents to blunt the release and action of insulin; other unidentified factors are thought to be involved in this response. A reduction in insulin action on adipose tissue by a macrophage mediated monokine suggests a possible role of the inflammatory response in the diabetes of injury. This would not be surprising, since hyperglycemia is one of the earliest and best-recognized features of sepsis.

GLUCOSE METABOLISM IN WOUNDED TISSUE. Glucose must be provided not only to red cells, white cells, renal medulla, and neural tissues following injury, but also to wounded tissue. In fact, glucose uptake and lactate production in wounded tissue are increased by up to 100 percent and are proportional to the circulating concentration of glucose present (Fig. 1-51). The increase in glucose uptake in wounded tissue is associated with an increase in the activity of phosphofructokinase, a major rate limiting enzyme in glycolysis. Despite the increase in glucose uptake and phosphofructokinase activity, wounded and

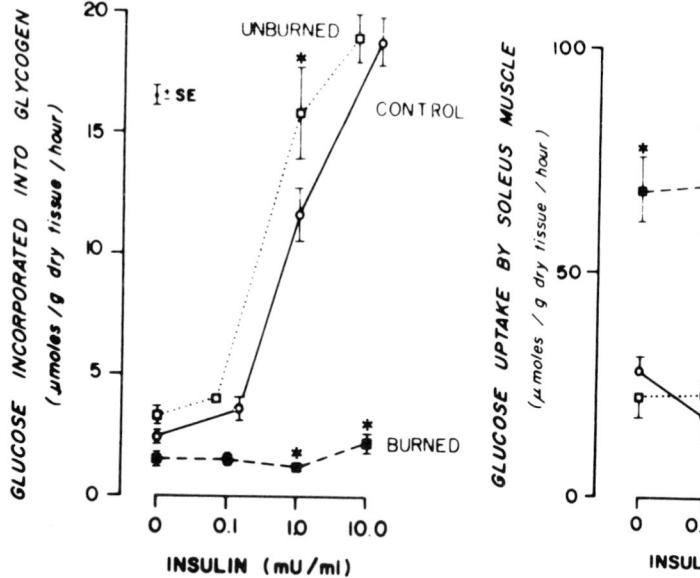
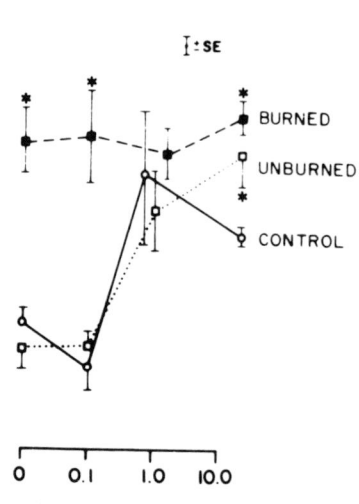

Fig. 1-52. Glucose uptake and glycogen synthesis by the soleus muscles from the burned and unburned limbs of rats 3 days after scald injury. Soleus muscles from the injured limb did not respond to insulin, whereas muscles from the uninjured limb responded to insulin in a dose-dependent fashion with an increase in glucose uptake and glycogen synthesis. (From: *Nelson KM, Turinsky J: J Surg Res 31:292, 1981, with permission.*)

burned tissues demonstrate a lack of insulin sensitivity and do not increase their glucose uptake or glycogenesis in response to insulin (Fig. 1-52).

The accelerated glucose uptake in wounded and burned tissue correlates with the degree of inflammatory cellular infiltrate present. It has been shown that much of the increase above the resting rate of glucose uptake in nonwounded muscle can be explained by glucose uptake in the inflammatory cells. The inflammatory infiltrate may actually mediate an increase in glucose uptake of the wounded noninflammatory tissue itself since the uptake of glucose by muscle in the presence of macrophages is greater than that of muscle not exposed to macrophages.

The increase in glucose uptake and lactate production by wounded, burned, and septic tissue has been attributed to anaerobic glycolysis that results from local tissue hypoxia and a reduction in local tissue perfusion. Although early after injury disruption of blood flow in the injured area may lead to aerobic glycolysis, glucose metabolism in wounded and burned tissue 3 to 5 days after injury appears to be primarily aerobic since oxygen consumption and CO_2 production are normal but lactate production is increased. Aerobic glycolysis is characteristic of the cellular inflammatory infiltrate that accompanies wounds and burns. Metabolic derangements suggestive of aerobic glycolysis have also been observed in septic and endotoxic tissue. An important source of glucose consumption following injury of all types may be the activation of white cells.

LACTATE METABOLISM. There is an increase in the plasma concentration of lactate following most injuries that correlates with the severity of injury (Fig. 1-53). The accumulation of lactate following shock accounts in part for the progressive acidosis of shock and derives from anaerobic metabolism in ischemic tissues. Under these circumstances, the likelihood of survival of patients in profound shock can be estimated from the excess levels

of lactate present in the blood. For example, Broder and Weil noted an 82 percent survival in patients in shock with an initial excess lactate concentration of 1 mmol/L, a 60 percent survival with 2 mmol/L, and a 26 percent survival when the excess lactate was 2 to 4 mmol/L. A better prognosticator of survival appears to be the serial change in total plasma lactate. Excess lactate should not be confused with total plasma lactate since the excess lactate is the amount of lactate present in the blood that increases the lactate-pyruvate ratio from normal.

Elevated plasma lactate concentrations may result from local tissue ischemia such as in mesenteric infarction, from diminished hepatic clearance of lactate, and from increased lactate production by inflammatory cells. The latter mechanism may account for the elevation in plasma lactate concentrations seen in burned and wounded tissue well after the effective circulating blood volume has been restored. The differential diagnosis of any injured patient with hyperlactacidemia should include systemic hypoperfusion, regional hypoperfusion, hepatic dysfunction, and severe inflammation.

PROTEIN METABOLISM DURING INJURY

NITROGEN BALANCE. The daily intake of protein for a healthy young adult is usually about 80 to 120 g, or 13 to 20 g of nitrogen. About 2 to 3 g of this nitrogen is excreted per day in the stool and 13 to 20 g in the urine. Following injury, nitrogen excretion in the urine increases greatly and rises to 30 to 50 g of nitrogen per day. This is nearly all in the form of urea nitrogen and results from net proteolysis since nitrogen intake immediately

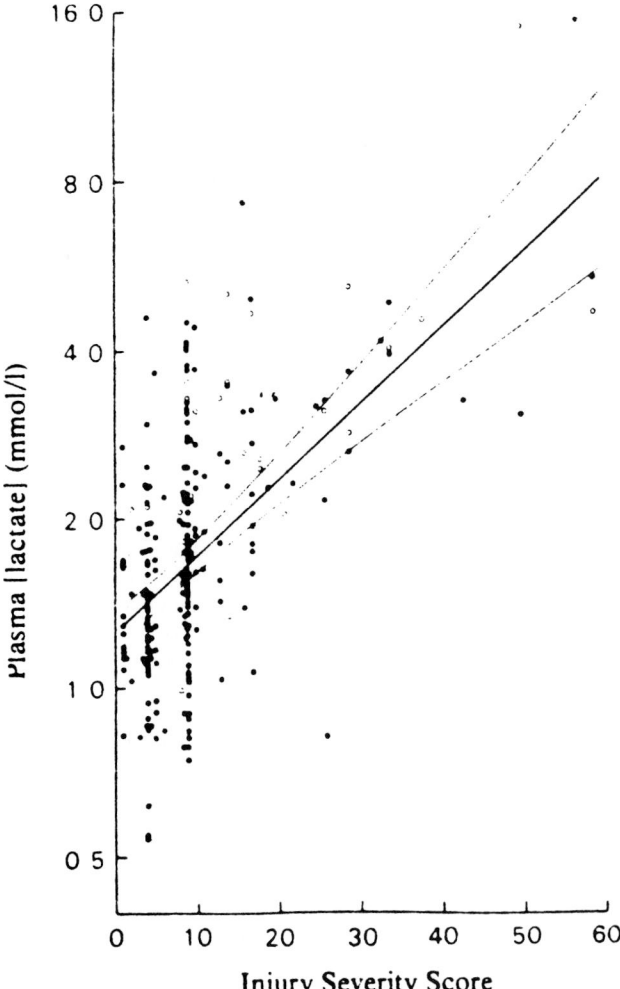

Fig. 1-53. Relationship between plasma lactate and the injury severity score in multiply injured patients. There was a positive correlation between ISS and plasma lactate in both patients who had ingested ethanol (○) and those who had not (●). (From: *Stoner HB, Frayn KN, et al: Clin Sci 56:563, 1979, with permission.*)

tein content and the incorporation of radiolabeled amino acids in visceral tissues and skeletal muscle confirm that it is skeletal muscle that is depleted while visceral tissues (liver, kidney) are spared, a finding contrary to starvation, in which visceral protein is used to a greater extent than muscle.

The net catabolism of protein can result from either increased catabolism, decreased synthesis, or a combination of these factors. Available data on total body protein turnover suggest that after injury, the net changes in catabolism and synthesis depend on the severity of the injury. Elective operations and minor injury appear to result in a decreased rate of synthesis with a normal rate of protein catabolism. Severe trauma, burns, and sepsis appear to be associated with increases in both synthesis and catabolism, but a greater increase in the catabolism occurs resulting in net catabolism. Accelerated proteolysis and a high rate of gluconeogenesis persist after major injury and during sepsis. This appears to result from an inhibition of ketoadaptation after major injury and sepsis since, unlike starvation, ketogenesis is not prominent and does not fuel the brain in significant amounts. As a result, a high requirement for glucose and therefore for gluconeogenesis persists. The mechanisms for inhibition of ketoadaptation are not known. Barocos et al., based on in vitro muscle incubations, have proposed that interleukin-1 may be responsible for the accelerated proteolysis that accompanies fever and sepsis, and Clowes et al. have presented evidence suggesting the involvement of a circulating peptide (proteolysis inducing factor-PIF) containing 33 amino acids in this response that may also represent interleukin-1 or that may be distinct.

The rise in urinary nitrogen and negative nitrogen balance begins shortly after injury, reaches a peak about the first week, and may continue for 3 to 7 weeks. The degree and duration of negative nitrogen balance is related to the severity of injury with elective operative procedures having a brief period of small degree and thermal injuries having long periods of major negative nitrogen balance. The degree of negative nitrogen balance and net protein catabolism also depends on the age, sex, and physical condition of the patient. Young healthy males lose more protein in response to an injury than do women or the elderly, presumably as a result of the smaller body cell mass present in the latter group. In addition, the urinary excretion of nitrogen is less after a second operation if it closely follows the first, presumably the result of a reduction in available protein stores consequent to the first operation. Negative nitrogen balance can be reduced or virtually eliminated by high caloric nitrogen supplementation as with enteral or parenteral nutrition. The loss of protein that occurs after injury is not entirely obligatory to the injury, and it is in large part a manifestation of acute starvation and the increased need for gluconeogenetic precursors during periods of stress.

The evidence that increased nitrogen metabolism following injury is related to the need for carbohydrates has been summarized by Kinney et al. as follows: (1) the caloric contribution of protein to the fuel mixture of normal and injured human beings is less than 20 percent; (2) two-

after injury is minimal or absent. Despite the large amount of protein that is broken down, only 20 percent is used for calories even with major increases in nitrogen excretion. The remainder is used by the liver and the kidneys to produce glucose and is reflected in the accelerated ureagenesis that is noted after injury. This results primarily from an increase in the circulating concentrations of cortisol, glucagon, and catecholamines and the decreased effectiveness of insulin.

The increased excretion of urea following injury is also associated with the urinary loss of sulfur, phosphorus, potassium, magnesium, and creatinine. This suggests the breakdown of intracellular materials. Isotope dilution studies point to a decrease in cell mass rather than in cell number as the source of the protein breakdown. The nitrogen-sulfur and nitrogen-potassium ratios suggest that this loss occurs mainly from muscle. Analysis of the pro-carbon fragments are readily available from adipose tissue as the major energy source; (3) the body has a continuous requirement for carbohydrate intermediates for synthetic purposes, for which the deamination of amino acids is the primary endogenous source; and (4) fatty acids cannot directly yield a net gain of carbohydrate intermediates, glucose, or glycogen.

AMINO ACID METABOLISM. The alterations in plasma amino acids in response to injury are not well defined. Immediately after injury there is little or no change in the total amino acid concentration. Increases have been noted, however, in the concentrations of alanine, cystine, taurine, and the aromatic acids. This may be the result of varying levels of nutrition prior to the insult, of hypoperfusion, of starvation, and of physical activity. Negative nitrogen balance, weight loss, and plasma amino acid concentrations of wounded animals are in the same direction and of the same magnitude as those that occur in nonwounded animals pair-fed to the reduced food intake of the wounded group. Although this suggests that the alterations in proteolysis and in amino acid metabolism are solely the result of starvation, in the same study, the intracellular skeletal muscle concentrations of specific amino acids differed markedly between groups. During the flow phase of injury, alterations in plasma amino acids also appear to be related to the time from injury when they are measured. This is best exemplified by the plasma concentration of alanine, which early in the flow phase is increased but as the injury persists is decreased, presumably as a result of lack of its availability in peripheral tissues and its continued hepatic uptake. This pattern for alanine is noted in most forms of injury.

The type and severity of injury may also have an effect on the alterations seen in amino acid metabolism, although no consensus is established. On the one hand, the direction of changes in the plasma concentrations of specific amino acids are similar in many studies of thermal injury, elective operations, trauma, and sepsis, but the degree of their magnitude is often greater in sepsis. This suggests that changes in amino acid metabolism are not dependent upon the type or the severity of injury. By contrast, other studies have noted marked differences in plasma and muscle amino acid patterns during sepsis and other injuries that suggest the changes seen are related to the severity of the injury or infection and to the offending microorganism.

Despite these opposing points of view, the intracellular muscle concentrations and the muscle to plasma ratios of glutamine are reduced markedly in most studies of sepsis, wounding, and thermal injury. In general, the release of glutamine is greater than can be predicted from its relative abundance in muscle tissue protein, and evidence for its synthesis in muscle has been presented. Glutamine release from wounded and nonwounded muscle is not different and if the release of glutamine is expressed as a ratio to the phenylalanine released, there is a lower release rate in wounded than in nonwounded tissue. Since phenylalanine is neither catabolized nor synthesized in muscle, a lower glutamine-phenylalanine ratio suggests that either the synthesis of glutamine in wounded tissue is reduced or the local catabolism in wounded muscle is increased. Glutamine is a major energy source for lymphocytes and fibroblasts. As a result, the accelerated utilization of glutamine by the cellular infiltrate in wounded or in septic tissue could explain the decreased concentrations noted at the site of injury and in the plasma. Souba and colleagues have recently shown that the gastrointestinal tract is a major consumer of glutamine following injury. The increased use of glutamine by the gastrointestinal tract may contribute further to the reduction in plasma glutamine concentrations during injury.

The importance of leukocyte and lymphocyte interactions with parenchymal cells in protein metabolism has been demonstrated by Keller, West, and colleagues. In their studies, isolated hepatocytes cultured in the presence of nonparenchymal hepatic (Kupffer) cells, peritoneal macrophages, or conditioned media in which nonparenchymal cells had been previously cultured demonstrated a marked reduction in protein synthesis as evidenced by a reduced rate of incorporation of radiolabeled leucine. This response was even greater when the hepatocyte–nonparenchymal cell mixture was coincubated with endotoxin. These data suggest that there may be a macrophage–Kupffer cell mediated factor that alters protein metabolism in hepatocytes.

WOUND HEALING. It is particularly astounding that most wounds heal despite the presence of negative nitrogen balance, negative energy balance, and reduced tissue and plasma concentrations of zinc, thiamine, riboflavin, vitamin C, and vitamin A. Moore has termed this ability of wound healing to proceed in the presence and absence of abundant substrate supply the biologic priority of wound healing. Levenson has noted that, "whereas the healing of a wound after injury appears satisfactory, it may be neither normal nor optimal." For example, there is a distinct delay in the wound healing of an incisional wound on burned animals when compared with incisional wounds on normal animals, and rodents with a fractured femur do not heal a skin incision as well as rodents with a skin incision alone. The biologic priority of wound healing does not mean that wound healing is normal in the severely injured patient.

The biologic priority of wound healing also does not mean that wound healing cannot be improved in severely injured patients. For example, large open wounds, such as burns, are associated with an inhibition of nitrogen anabolism of the host and may result in protein malnutrition and death if the substrate demands of the wounds are not met exogenously. Although it is not clear if the administration of protein improves wound healing per se, it has been shown to reduce negative nitrogen balance. Some investigators have also noted an improvement in wound healing with protein supplementation, but others have been unable to document any change.

SUMMARY. Generalized catabolism, hyperglycemia, persistent gluconeogenesis, protein wasting, negative nitrogen balance, heat production, and loss of body mass are characteristic of all significant injuries. The degree of these metabolic alterations is directly related to the severity of injury, with the largest and most sustained changes

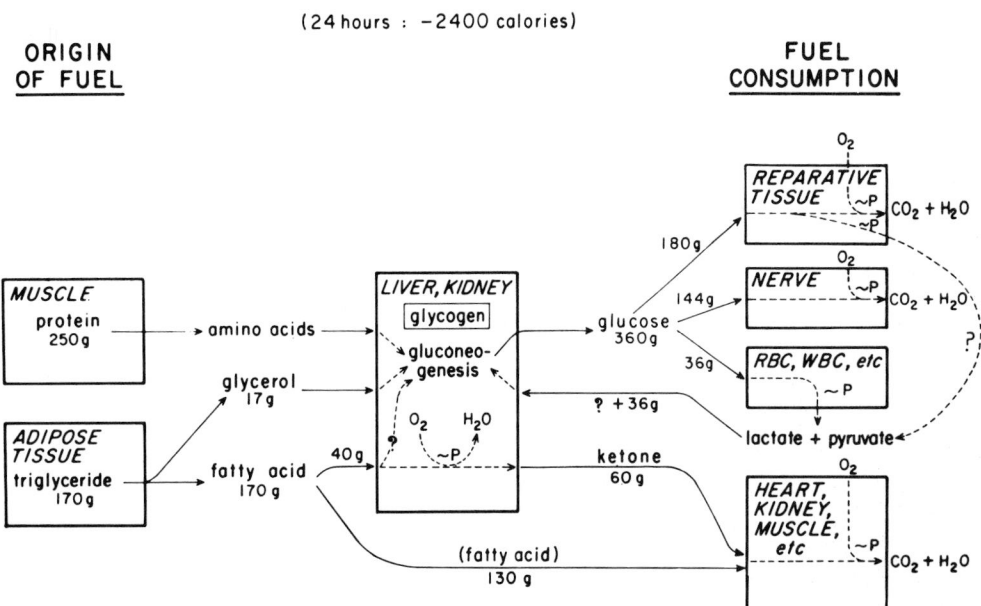

Fig. 1-54. Hypothetical scheme of rates of substrate flow in a traumatized individual excreting 40 g of nitrogen per day. Presumably reparative tissues are glucose utilizers, but the amount of glucose terminally combusted to carbon dioxide and that metabolized to lactate would depend both on the maturity of the tissue and on adequate perfusion and oxygenation. Fat still provides the bulk of the calories. (From: *Cahill GF et al, in Fox CL Jr, Nahas GG (eds): Body Fluid Replacement in the Surgical Patient, New York, Grune and Stratton, 1970, p 286, with permission.*)

being noted after sepsis and burns. Most of the energy required during the posttraumatic period is obtained from the oxidation of lipids; the net catabolism of 300 to 500 g of lean body cell mass per day is required as a source of amino acids for gluconeogenesis (Fig. 1-54). The persistence of the injury, particularly sepsis, through unknown mechanisms produces inhibition of the usual adaptive mechanisms that occur in starvation to reduce the amount of glucose needed per day. As a result, a highly catabolic state persists that in turn leads to protein wasting and malnutrition and ultimately to multiple organ failure and death if the stimuli are not eliminated.

FLUID AND ELECTROLYTE METABOLISM DURING INJURY

Almost all acute injuries are associated with changes in fluid and electrolyte metabolism, acid-base status, and renal function. In part, these alterations arise because patients do not usually have free access to water and electrolytes and frequently do not perceive thirst as a result of sedation, anesthesia, or head injury. A reduction in the effective circulating volume is characteristic of almost all injuries as a result of blood loss as in hemorrhage, loss of vascular tone as in sepsis, pump failure as in cardiac tam-

ponade, excessive unreplaced extrarenal losses as in diarrhea, vomiting, and the drainage of fistulae or from the sequestration of fluids.

The sequestration of fluids or third space is the result of an alteration in capillary permeability consequent to injury, ischemia, or inflammation. Since the fluid present in the third space has the same composition as the extracellular fluid (150 meq of sodium, 112 meq of chloride, 4.6 meq of potassium), one might think of this as an obligatory expansion of the total extracellular space. Although it is true that the total extracellular fluid space is expanded, the functional extracellular volume (that which can contribute to the maintenance of the effective circulating volume) is actually reduced because the fluid present in the third space is itself derived from the functional extracellular volume. Therefore, a liter of fluid trapped in the third space cannot be used, for example, during hemorrhage to replace the effective circulating volume lost. For this reason, the use of diuretics to mobilize fluid in an edematous postoperative patient who is not in congestive heart failure is pointless and potentially harmful, since it will result in a further reduction in the functional or exchangeable extracellular space and effective circulating volume but not in the volume of the third space. "Exchangeable" is not synonymous with "equilibrium" since the constituents of the third space are in dynamic equilibrium with those of the functional extracellular fluid volume. For example, fluid and electrolytes in a pleural effusion are in a constant state of recycling with the plasma and antibiotics administered to a patient will enter the pleural effusion. The volume of the third space cannot be used to replace the volume of the functional extracellular space.

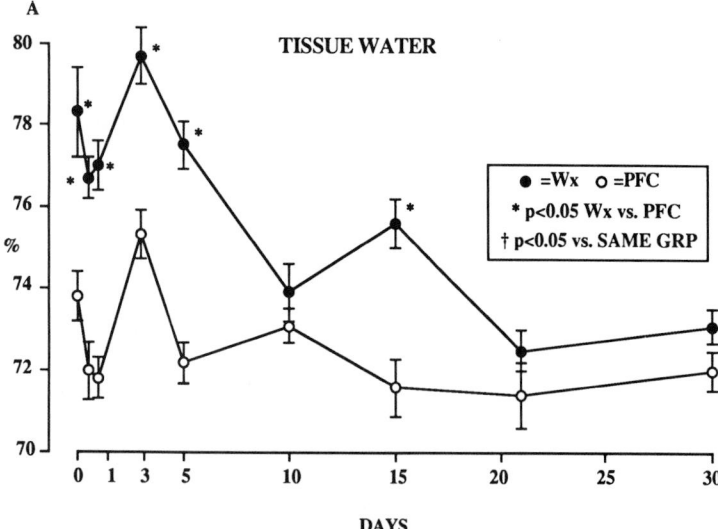

Fig. 1-55. The tissue water content of wounded hindlimbs was greater than that of the hindlimbs from pair-fed control animals at 0, ½, 1, 3, 5, and 15 days. The water content of wounded hindlimbs reached its maximum on day 3 (79.7 ± 0.7 percent). It then decreased to control values at day 10, from which time no further differences were noted between the two groups after day 15. (From: *Amaral JF et al: J Trauma, in press.*)

Blalock was the first to demonstrate that traumatic injury to an extremity resulted in the mobilization of fluid and electrolytes to an area of injury, thereby reducing the functional extracellular fluid volume. As shown in Fig. 1-55, even though the formation of the third space after nonthermal traumatic injury occurs immediately and is maximal by 5 to 6 h, the resolution of the third space is slower and may take longer than 10 days. Since the volume of third space is directly proportional to the severity of injury, minor operative procedures, such as an appendectomy, are associated with considerably less fluid sequestration than are major operative procedures such as an extensive retroperitoneal dissection. Similarly, minor traumatic injuries, such as an isolated simple limb fracture, are associated with less fluid sequestration than are those seen following major injuries, such as burns. If there is no intake of fluid into the functional extracellular space by either the oral or the intravenous route, the effective circulating volume will decline to a point at which hypotension ensues.

Hypovolemic shock is also associated with a reduction in the functional extracellular fluid volume in excess of the amount lost from the body by hemorrhage or by dehydration. Shires and colleagues have demonstrated that even though the return of shed blood alone after hemorrhage results in the return of the red cell mass and blood volume to normal, a deficit in the functional extracellular fluid volume persists. This deficit can be eliminated by the return of crystalloid solutions as well as shed blood. For this reason, patients who have sustained a major blood loss should receive blood or packed cells and crystalloid during their resuscitation. The site of this third space formation appears to be the intracellular space as evidenced by a contraction of the intercellular space and an increase in the intracellular volume following hemorrhages of greater than 30 percent of the total blood volume and is thought to be the reason for the irreversible shock encountered in some patients. The mechanism for its formation remains unknown.

Major burns produce an alteration in the capillary permeability of the burned tissue that results in an exudation of plasma and an evaporative loss of water. There is also an increase in fluid flux across capillaries in nonburned tissue that appears to result from hypoproteinemia rather than an alteration in capillary permeability. The formation of edema occurs primarily in the first 24 h with the greatest losses being incurred during the first 8. It is for this reason that thermally injured patients should receive 50 percent of their estimated fluid losses in the first 8 h. Colloid should be given on the second day to minimize edema formation in the nonburned tissue.

Sepsis produces a generalized capillary leak that again produces an increase in the total extracellular fluid volume but a decrease in the functional or exchangeable extracellular fluid volume. As sepsis persists, protein malnutrition produces hypoproteinemia, which in turn may increase the formation of edema. Therefore, the administration of colloid solutions during early sepsis when a capillary leak is present in the absence of hypoproteinemia may be unadvisable, since it may serve to further increase tissue edema. Once hypoproteinemia ensues, colloid administration may theoretically be helpful.

Any traumatic injury produces rapid changes in the functional extracellular fluid volume, effective circulating volume, extracellular osmolality, and electrolyte composition that result in the stimulation of the neuroendocrine system. In turn, the neuroendocrine response induces alterations in renal and circulatory function aimed at improving salt and water balance. Ultimately, the degree of impairment in fluid and electrolyte balance incurred following injury depends in part upon the amount of functional extracellular volume lost, the ability of the neuroendocrine, renal, and circulatory systems to respond, the severity of the injury, the quality and quantity of fluid given, the age of the patient, preexistent illness, concurrent medications, and the anesthetic agents used.

Despite the potentially large number of variables noted, the overall response to the loss of effective circulating volume and electrolytes may be simplified as a coordinated physiologic effort to prevent further unnecessary losses of circulating volume and to replace the volume lost. The former involves the renal conservation of salt and water to minimize excretion and the latter the restoration of blood volume.

Renal Conservation of Salt and Water Following Injury

SODIUM REABSORPTION. The regulation of fluid and electrolytes by the kidney involves the formation of a large glomerular ultrafiltrate from which variable amounts of these substances are reabsorbed or into which they are secreted. The formation of tubular fluid at the glomerulus is dependent upon the forces described in Starling's hypothesis of capillary equilibrium (Fig. 1-56). Thus, the quantity of filtrate formed is dependent upon the renal perfusion pressure at the glomerulus. Under normal circumstances approximately 25 percent of the cardiac output is directed to the kidneys, resulting in the filtration of approximately 180 L of plasma water per day from the 1584 L of blood that pass through the kidneys. Although a reduction in the effective circulating volume and therefore in renal perfusion pressure should result in a reduction in the amount of glomerular ultrafiltrate that is formed, glomerular filtration remains unchanged despite a reduction in the renal perfusion pressure to 80 mmHg (Fig. 1-57). This occurs through the maintenance of renal blood flow, a process referred to as intrinsic autoregulation. The latter is thought to involve tubuloglomerular feedback in which individual nephrons sense their tubular fluid flow and alter the rate of glomerular filtration by changing the glomerular capillary pressure, primarily at the efferent arteriole. Decreases in tubular fluid flow lead to an increase in the efferent arteriolar resistance that, in turn, results in an increase in the fraction of peritubular blood that is filtered at the glomerulus. Thus, the rate of glomerular filtration is maintained.

An increase in the amount of blood filtered at the glomerulus relative to the amount that passes through it produces an increase in the oncotic pressure of the peritubular capillary blood perfusing the proximal tubule (Fig. 1-58). This results from the impermeability of the glomerular basement membranes to protein such that the glomerular filtrate is an ultrafiltrate of plasma. The increase in peritubular oncotic pressure, in turn, produces an increase in the net transfer of water, sodium, chloride, and bicarbonate from the proximal tubular filtrate to the peritubular blood. Sympathetic nervous system activity may directly increase the proximal tubular transport of sodium and suppress the release of cerebral natriuretic hormone and atrial natriuretic factor.

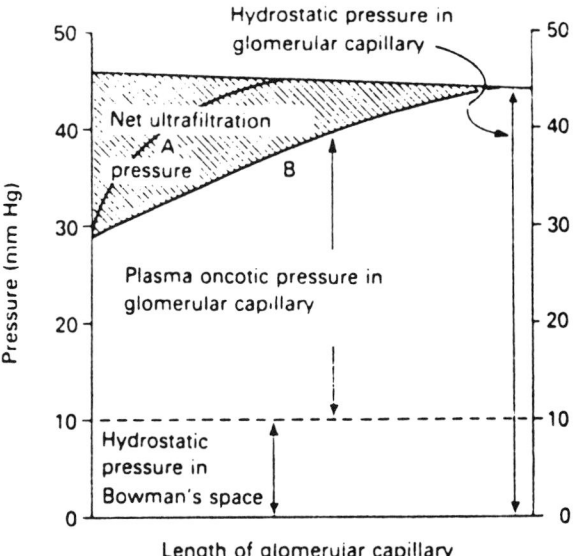

Balance of Mean Values

Hydrostatic pressure in glomerular capillary	45 mm Hg
Hydrostatic pressure in Bowman's space	10
Plasma oncotic pressure in glomerular capillary	27
Oncotic pressure of fluid in Bowman's space	0*
Net ultrafiltration pressure	8 mm Hg

Fig. 1-56. The Starling forces involved in the formation of the glomerular ultrafiltrate. Glomerular filtration pressure declines in the glomerular capillaries primarily as a result of a decrease in plasma oncotic pressure. In contrast, a decrease in the filtration pressure of extrarenal capillaries results primarily from a decrease in hydrostatic pressure. (From: *Valtin H: Renal Function: Mechanisms Preserving Fluid and Solute Balance in Health. Boston, Little, Brown, 1983, with permission.*)

Fig. 1-57. Despite a reduction in renal arterial pressure to 90 mmHg, renal blood flow and glomerular filtration rate are maintained through intrinsic autoregulation. (From: *Powers RS: In Sabiston DC (ed): Davis-Christopher Textbook of Surgery. Philadelphia, Saunders, with permission.*)

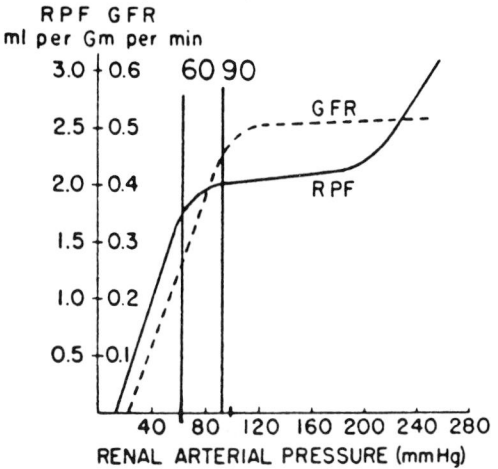

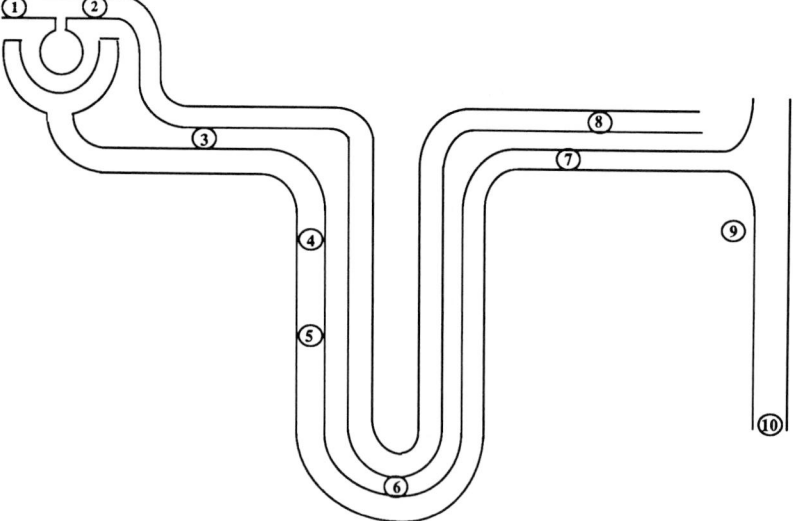

The net result of these alterations is that the delivery of sodium, chloride, and filtered fluid to the loop of Henle is decreased. Since the maintenance of the normal medullary osmotic gradient requires the adequate delivery of sodium and particularly of chloride to the long loops of Henle, a fall in medullary hyperosmolality frequently follows injury. A fall in medullary hyperosmolality may produce a defect in the ability of the kidneys to concentrate urine since the medullary gradient is essential to the renal countercurrent mechanism and the proper functioning of vasopressin. As a result, a larger amount of urine is necessary to eliminate the same amount of solute. This paradoxical increase in free water clearance secondary to a defect in the inner medullary interstitial solute has been termed polyuric prerenal failure and has been implicated in the genesis of nonoliguric renal failure.

Concomitant with the increase in filtration fraction, there is a redistribution of blood flow from glomeruli of the superficial cortical nephrons to those in the juxtamedullary region that further increases sodium reabsorption. The ability of the juxtamedullary nephrons to further increase sodium reabsorption is related to the much longer loops of Henle they possess when compared with those in the superficial cortical area (Fig. 1-59). The ability of the loops of Henle to reabsorb sodium is dependent on the presence of chloride, since the reabsorption of sodium in the loops of Henle passively follows the active reabsorption of chloride. The increase in the filtration fraction consequent to a reduction in the renal perfusion pressure produces an increased movement of sodium and of chloride to the peritubular fluid. As a result, the amount of chloride in the loop of Henle is low following injury and a large amount of sodium is delivered to the distal tubules. The increase in the distal delivery of sodium produces potassium wasting and metabolic alkalosis as sodium is reabsorbed and potassium and hydrogen ions secreted, a process that is augmented by the increased secretion of aldosterone that accompanies hypovolemia and injury. Conversely, if sodium delivery to the distal tubules is in-

Fig. 1-58. Alterations in nephron function during injury. 1. Decreased renal perfusion pressure. 2. Increased efferent arteriolar resistance leading to a maintenance of GFR (autoregulation). 3. Increased peritubular capillary oncotic pressure from an increase in filtration of blood leads to increased proximal tubular reabsorption. 4. Shift from cortical nephrons to juxtamedullary nephrons. 5. Increased proximal reabsorption leads to decreased delivery of chloride to loop of Henle. 6. Diminished medullary gradient secondary to impaired sodium reabsorption. 7. Increased presentation of sodium to the distal tubules. 8. Increased exchange of sodium for hydrogen and potassium that is enhanced by aldosterone. 9. Increased free water reabsorption mediated by vasopressin that may be impaired by a fall in medullary osmotic gradient. 10. Kaliuresis, acid urine, and possibly loss of free water if action of vasopressin is impaired.

adequate as a result of a marked decrease in glomerular filtration, potassium will not be excreted, even in the presence of aldosterone, and hyperkalemia and metabolic acidosis may ensue.

Sodium retention is a hallmark of injury that results in part from the increased secretion of corticosteroids and aldosterone. It is also clear that the larger the sodium load given to the postoperative patient the greater the amount retained. The amount of sodium retained depends more on the amount of sodium given than on the magnitude of injury. Sodium retention after injury cannot be solely explained on the basis of increased aldosterone and cortisol secretion since positive sodium balance persists well after the return of these hormones to normal concentrations (Fig. 1-60). Other factors that are known to contribute to positive sodium balance include an increase in the glomerular filtration fraction with an attendant increase in the proximal reabsorption of sodium and an increased blood flow to juxtamedullary nephrons.

ALKALOSIS. The increased delivery of sodium to the distal tubules is in part responsible for the metabolic alkalosis that commonly accompanies injury. Lyons and Moore have pointed out that the most common acid base disturbance in mild to moderately injured patients who have not deteriorated to severe renal circulatory or pulmonary decompensation is either metabolic or respira-

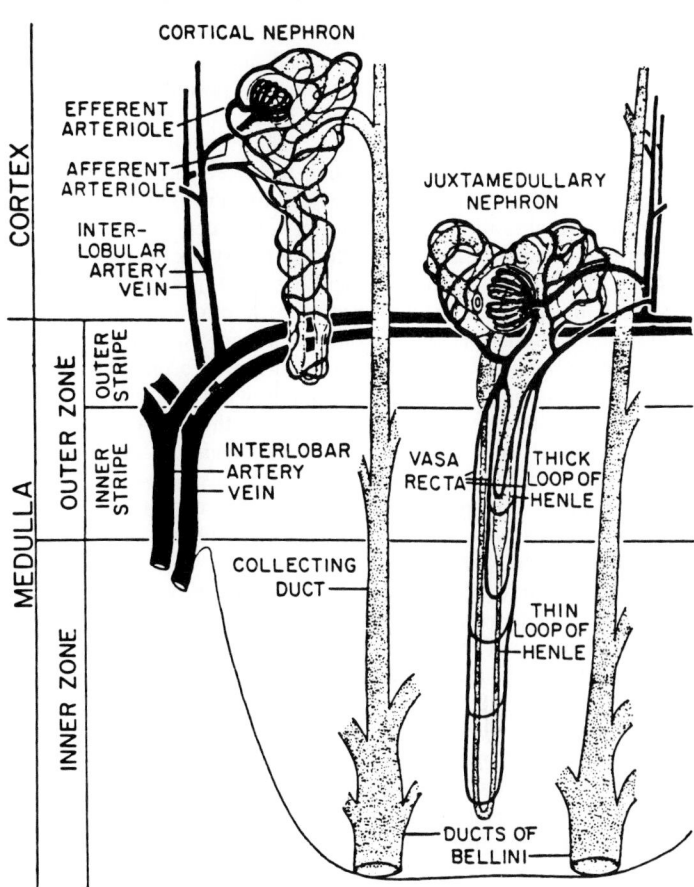

Fig. 1-59. The juxtamedullary nephrons have much longer loops of Henle than those of the cortical area. As a result they have a much longer surface area for reabsorption of sodium chloride and water. (From: *Pitts RF: Physiology of the Kidney and Body Fluids, Chicago, Yearbook Medical, 1974, with permission.*)

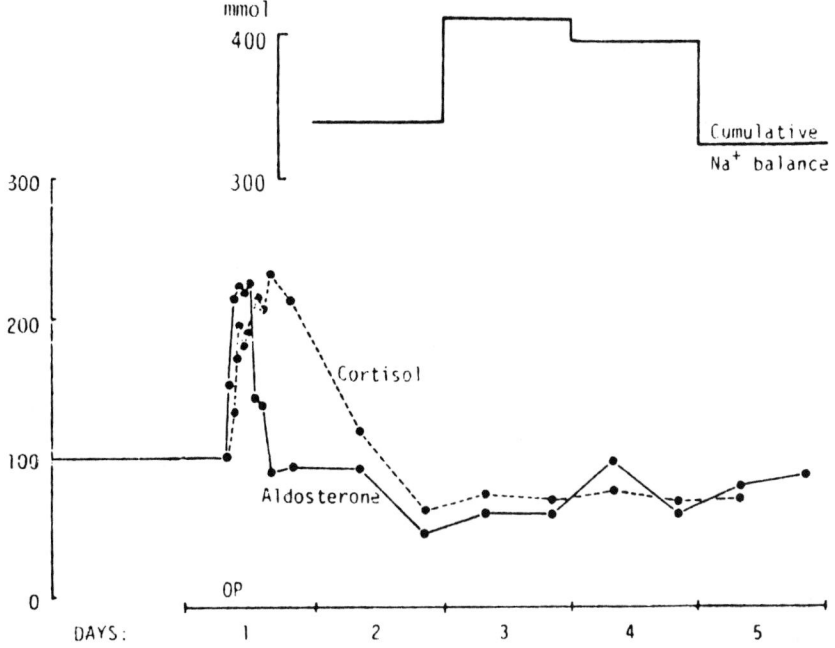

Fig. 1-60. Relationship of plasma aldosterone and plasma cortisol responses to postoperative sodium retention. The results are the median values for eight patients undergoing cholecystectomy at the start of day 1. All patients were in Na+ and K+ balance at the time of operation and the hormone changes are expressed as a percentage of the basal preoperative level. Intravenous intake was 259 mmol Na+ on day 2, and 152 mmol Na+ and 80 mmol K+ on days 3 to 5, with a total of 3 L of water on each day. The periods run from 0800 h. (From: *LeQuesne LP et al: Br Med Bull 1985, with permission.*)

tory alkalosis. In their study, 64 percent of the 105 patients who were operated on developed alkalosis on at least one determination in the postoperative period. It is important to prevent severe alkalosis in the surgical patient because of its potential hazards. These include the production of tissue hypoxia through the effect of alkalosis on the oxygen-hemoglobin dissociation curve, hypokalemia, and alterations in vasomotor tone such as the cerebral vasoconstriction seen with respiratory alkalosis.

ACIDOSIS. The most common acid base disturbance in severely injured patients or those who deteriorated to severe renal circulatory or pulmonary decompensation is either metabolic or respiratory alkalosis. Foremost among the etiologies for acidosis for following injury is shock. The metabolic acidosis that ensues is the result of tissue hypoperfusion and anaerobic metabolism and not the cause of it. Metabolic acidosis may also ensue in patients who have a respiratory alkalosis if hypoventilation suddenly occurs, since the rise in blood lactate that accompanies respiratory alkalosis will be unbuffered. Acidosis has profound effects on the cardiovascular system, producing a decrease in myocardial contractility, a decreased response of the myocardium and peripheral vasculature to catecholamines, and a predisposition to cardiac arrhythmias.

WATER REABSORPTION. Injury and hypotension are also characterized by an increase in water reabsorption. In part, this is related to the increase in sodium reabsorption since the reabsorption of sodium is associated with the passive reabsorption of water. The increase in water reabsorption is also the result of the stimulation of vasopressin secretion during hypotension and injury by osmotic and nonosmotic (baroreceptor) pathways. The increase in plasma vasopressin usually lasts for 3 to 5 days after injury. Under most circumstances it results in water retention and in oliguria unless specific steps are taken to prevent it. Postoperative oliguria was originally believed to be a normal accompaniment of injury that did no particular harm. Although it is certainly well tolerated in most forms of mild to moderate surgical trauma, it is a potentially harmful condition in two ways: the first is that it predisposes to acute tubular necrosis in patients with severe trauma in whom hypovolemia and hypotension are apt to occur, and the second is that it sets the stage for the development of water intoxication (severe hyponatremia) if large volumes of non-solute-containing fluids are given to the patient before, during, or immediately after the operative event. The most common electrolyte abnormality seen following surgery and injury is hyponatremia as a result of the administration of hypotonic fluids under conditions that favor salt and water retention.

The action of vasopressin in effecting water retention requires the presence of an intact countercurrent mechanism in the loop of Henle. If the countercurrent mechanism is disrupted by a fall in medullary osmolality, the action of vasopressin is impaired, resulting in a defect in urinary concentrating ability. Consequently, a normal or increased urine output in a hypotensive or injured patient does not necessarily reflect an adequate blood volume. In order to prevent a fall in the medullary gradient following

injury, adequate tubular fluid flow must be ensured and maximal sodium reabsorption in the proximal nephron must be avoided. This is accomplished by the administration of liberal amounts of salt solutions such as Ringer's lactate or normal saline in the postoperative period. The administration of the solutions may result in marked positive sodium and solute balance and in edema as noted previously. During this period of increased vasopressin secretion the urine volume cannot be increased by the administration of water alone. It is the solute load that determines urine volume, and free water clearance will occur only when the extracellular fluid space has been expanded (Fig. 1-61). By increasing the solute load and the extracellular fluid volume, the urine output can be maintained. Although this may result in a "puffy" patient postoperatively, it will maximize the protection of renal function. The effectiveness of treatment can be monitored by the maintenance of urine output at a rate of 30 mL/h or greater.

The return of vasopressin secretion to normal is signaled by the brisk diuresis of free water and resolution of tissue edema that is usually seen in most surgical patients on the third to fifth postoperative days. This is the so-called fluid mobilization phase of injury. This period may take considerably longer in the presence of pain, hypoxia, or other stimuli to vasopressin secretion. The presence of a diminished urine output and hyponatremia several days after injury is not necessarily related to the inappropriate secretion of vasopressin. The diagnosis of inappropriate secretion of vasopressin cannot be established until all possible stimuli to the secretion of vasopressin have been ruled out.

POSTOPERATIVE PATTERNS. The two patterns most commonly seen in the postoperative period are illustrated in Figs. 1-62 and 1-63. The first is that of a mild to moderate dilutional hyponatremia with hyperkalemia. This is primarily brought about by the secretion of vasopressin plus the overhydration of the patient with non-solute-containing fluids. The potassium level may be somewhat elevated, because potassium is lost from cells as a consequence of corticosteroid and starvation-induced catabolism, is infused in the form of high-potassium-containing old blood, is absorbed from blood left in the peritoneal cavity or wound, and is not well excreted because of impaired renal perfusion.

The hyponatremia and hyperkalemia are made much worse if the trauma is severe and prolonged or if the patient has had a chronic wasting illness prior to operation. Other factors that can make the response worse include starvation, which as previously noted can itself produce hyponatremia through natriuresis, preexisting renal impairment, which predisposes to a further elevation of potassium level and depression of sodium level, cardiac disease with edema, preexisting hyponatremia, a pronounced shift of sodium into the cell with severe trauma, and episodes of hypotension, which further impair renal function. Consequently, cardiac patients may still need sodium replacement postoperatively, even though they may have an elevated total body sodium and total body water.

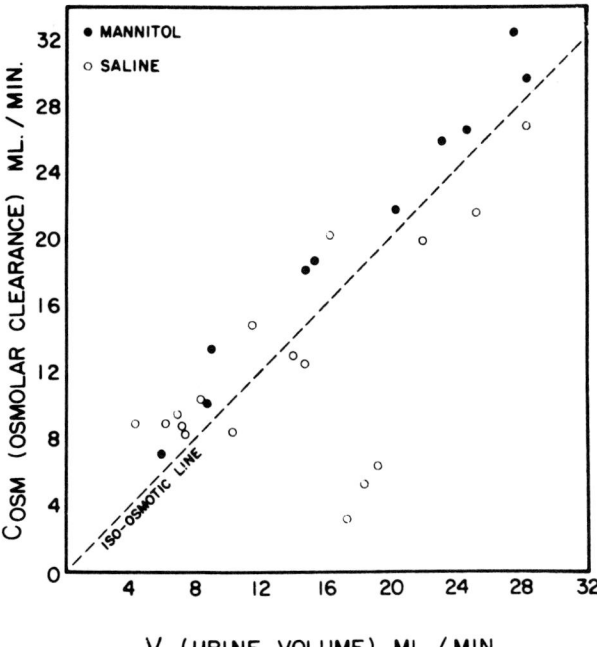

V (URINE VOLUME) ML./MIN.

Fig. 1-61. Postoperative patients failed to excrete a water load when given 5 percent dextrose in water. These patients were then given either saline or mannitol. As shown, patients with high urine flow rates given saline were able to excrete free water whereas those with mannitol did not. This suggests that acute expansion of ECF volume in postoperative patients leads to suppression of the high antidiuretic hormone activity normally seen during this period, and thus to excretion of hypotonic urine. (From: *Wright HK, Gann DS: Ann Surg 158:70, 1963, with permission.*)

Fig. 1-62. Pattern of hyponatremia in the postoperative patient. Solute is diluted principally by excessive administration of water without salt. In addition, in severe trauma sodium will move into cells in exchange for potassium. The hyperkalemia may be further aggravated by acidosis, by the action of cortisol, and by the breakdown of blood and may be opposed by the action of aldosterone.

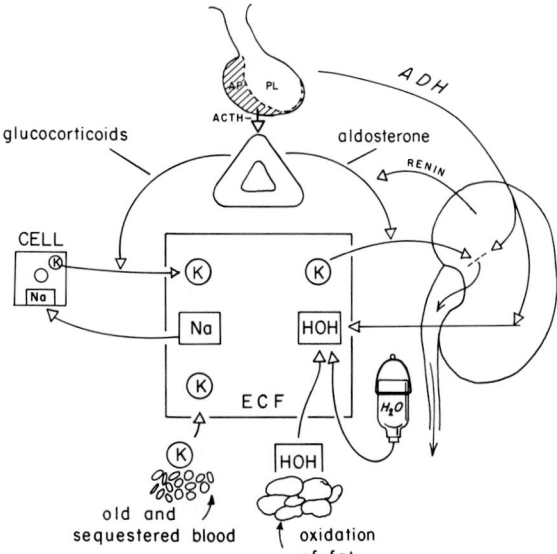

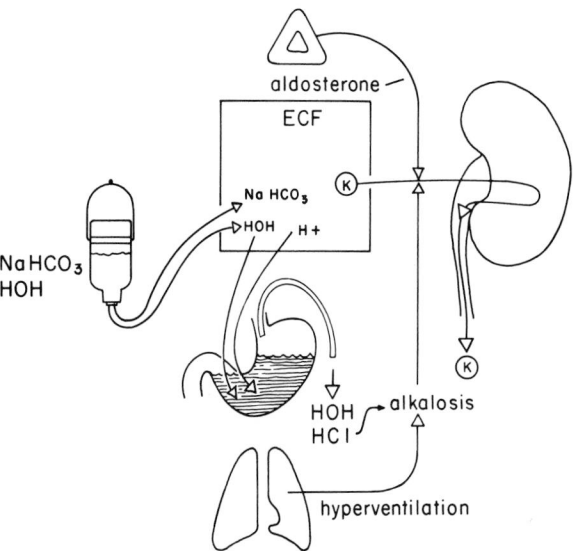

Fig. 1-63. Pattern of hypokalemic alkalosis in the postoperative patient. This is most commonly seen in patients who are alkalotic at the time of operation. The alkalosis produces an additional potassium loss in the urine. Hyperventilation increases the alkalosis and promotes further potassium loss. The administration of sodium bicarbonate, sometimes given in circumstances that are thought likely to be the result of acidosis, may further augment the alkalosis. These events then conspire to produce a severe hypokalemic alkalosis that, if renal function is good, may be made worse by the action of aldosterone in promoting potassium excretion.

These changes can be prevented or minimized by the use of sodium chloride–containing solutions in the preoperative, intraoperative, and postoperative periods and by the replacement of third space losses with normal saline. Potassium administration should be avoided unless the patient has unusual potassium losses or a declining serum potassium concentration.

The second pattern is one of hypokalemic alkalosis, classically seen in the patient with obstructing duodenal ulcer on continuous nasogastric suction or in the infant with hypertrophic pyloric stenosis with protracted vomiting. The alkalosis created by the loss of hydrogen ion from the stomach and the dehydration produced by the loss of water produces marked potassium losses in the urine since sodium reabsorption in the distal tubule must occur primarily in exchange for potassium rather than bicarbonate. The large quantities of chloride lost in the gastric juice limit the ability of the kidney to proximally reabsorb sodium. As a result, a large amount of sodium is delivered to the distal tubules for reabsorption there. Because of the large amount of sodium presented to the distal tubules and the increased secretion of aldosterone, patients with this condition usually have a paradoxically acidic urine from the exchange of hydrogen ion for sodium.

This condition is made worse by starvation, the intravenous administration of non-chloride- and non-potassium-containing solutions, the administration of proximal or loop diuretics, the administration of corticosteroids, the presence of diarrhea or a fistula, hyperventilation al-

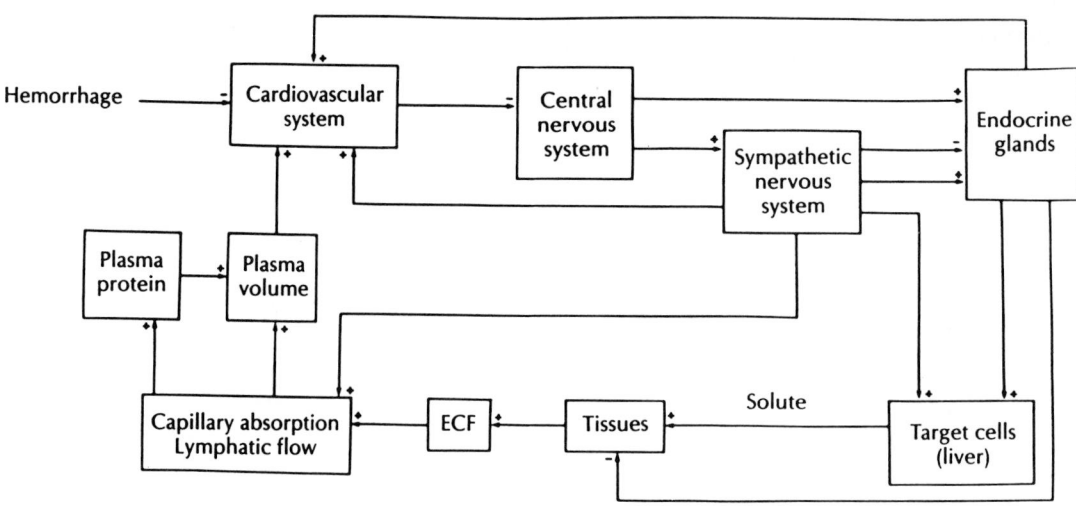

Fig. 1-64. Schematic representation of the restitution of blood volume. [From: *Gann DS, Amaral JF: The pathophysiology of trauma and shock, in Zuidema GD et al (eds). The Management of Trauma. Philadelphia, Saunders, 1985, with permission.*]

kalosis, the preexistence of hypokalemia, or the administration of sodium bicarbonate. These changes can be eliminated by the administration of potassium chloride. Chloride is the most important of these two electrolytes, since without chloride the delivery of sodium to the distal tubules will remain increased and potassium and bicarbonate will be continued to be wasted.

Blood Volume Restitution

Despite the renal conservation of salt and water following injury, an increase in the functional extracellular fluid volume cannot occur even in the complete absence of renal excretion. In order for the functional extracellular fluid volume and effective circulating volume to return to normal following injury, the blood volume must be restored.

The restitution of blood volume can be brought about by exogenous or endogenous fluids. The exogenous restitution of blood volume involves the administration of fluids. These fluids may be given intravenously, in which case the increase in blood volume is direct or they may be given orally, in which case the increase in blood volume is indirectly mediated through intestinal absorption. The endogenous restitution of blood volume involves the movement of fluids present in the interstitial fluid and in cells to the effective circulating volume. This process may be thought of as occurring in two overlapping phases: the first involves the movement of essentially protein-free fluid from the interstitium to the plasma and the second involves the restitution of plasma protein which in turn mediates the movement of additional fluid from the interstitium to the vascular space (Fig. 1-64).

A fall in capillary pressure mediates the net movement of protein-free fluid from the interstitium to the vascular

space. The decrease in capillary pressure is initiated by hypotension and augmented by reflex sympathetic vasoconstriction. As capillary hydrostatic pressure decreases, the steady-state flux of fluid described in Starling's hypothesis of capillary equilibrium is changed. This results in the net movement of fluid into the capillary bed and in the restoration of approximately 20 to 50 percent of the blood volume lost. Because this fluid is protein-free, interstitial colloid oncotic pressure and interstitial hydrostatic pressure also decrease, resulting in the establishment of a new steady state in which further net movement of fluid into the vascular space cannot occur.

The further movement of fluid and ultimately the complete restitution of blood volume depends upon the movement of protein from the interstitium to the vascular space. The resultant increase in capillary oncotic pressure and decrease in interstitial oncotic pressure, in turn, mediates a shift of fluid from cells via the interstitial space to the capillary bed. The protein involved in this process is primarily in the form of albumin. This albumin must derive from the interstitium itself, since the restitution of blood volume is complete by 24 h, whereas albumin synthesis takes at least 48 h. The movement of albumin and protein from the interstitium to the capillary space may occur through either the lymphatics or the fenestrae of the capillary membrane. In order for either to be effective, interstitial pressure must increase. The latter can be accomplished through an increase in interstitial volume, since the compliance of the interstitium is fixed. The increase in interstitial volume cannot be derived from the plasma volume since it is already decreased. Water will

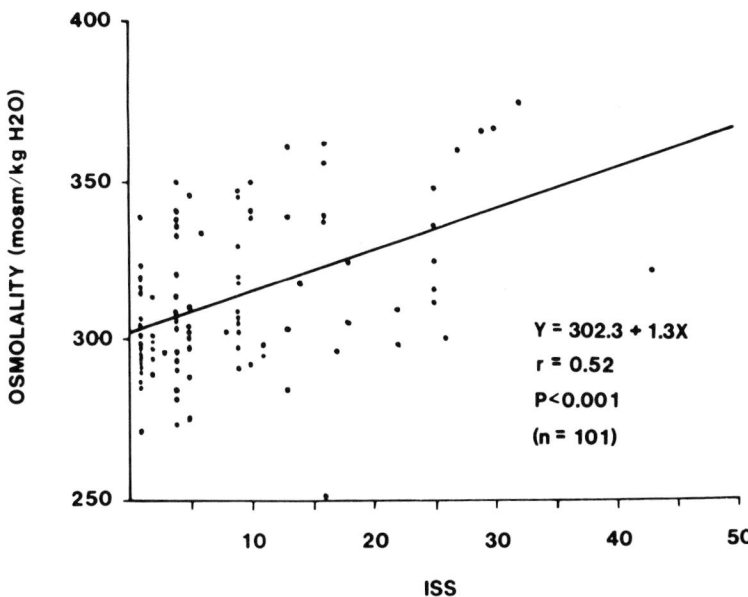

Fig. 1-65. There is a positive correlation between the plasma osmolality and the injury severity score in multiply injured patients. (From: *Kenney PR et al: J Trauma 23:712, 1983, with permission.*)

move out of cells only down an osmotic gradient. Thus, an osmotic gradient between the intracellular and the extracellular space must exist in order for the interstitial volume to increase.

The movement of water from cells to the interstitium appears to be mediated by a hormonally induced increase in extracellular osmolality that was first described by Bergentz and Brief in experimental animals and later confirmed in human beings by Boyd and Mansberger. The increase in serum osmolality occurs promptly after hemorrhage and correlates with the rate and degree of hemorrhage and the severity of the injury (Fig. 1-65). An increase in cortisol is necessary but not sufficient to produce the increase in osmolality. An adrenal factor (probably catecholamines), a pituitary factor (probably vasopressin), and glucagon are required. The solutes, which are derived primarily from the liver, include glucose, phosphate, lactate, and pyruvate. Since these molecules are permeable to the capillary membrane but relatively impermeable to cell membranes, an osmotic gradient is established between interstitium and cells that moves fluid from the cells to the interstitium. In turn, the increase in interstitial volume results in an increase in interstitial pressure, thereby allowing protein to move through the capillary membrane and the lymphatics. The rise in osmolality also appears to contribute to the phase of transcapillary refill, since the increase in interstitial pressure requires the movement of water to the vascular space in order for the equilibrium between the interstitium and capillaries to be maintained.

Nutritional status plays an important role in the hyperosmolality seen after hemorrhage. Fasted animals exhibit a lower degree of hyperglycemia and a slower rise in plasma osmolality than fed animals. As a result, the ca-

pacity for blood volume restitution is greater in animals who are fed than in those who are fasted. This difference presumably results from the depletion of hepatic glycogen stores during fasting since the difference can be eliminated by the administration of hyperosmolar glucose to the fasted animals.

One would predict that the higher the serum glucose the more favorable the response. This is in marked contrast to the studies of combat victims by Carey et al. in which a high glucose concentration was associated with a high mortality. It is important to recognize that the changes described result from an increase in the production of solute by the liver and its subsequent delivery to the interstitium bathing skeletal muscle. Given the same increase in solute production, changes in plasma solute concentrations will be smaller if muscle perfusion is adequate than if it is decreased by intense vasoconstriction. A very high increase in the serum glucose may be the result of inadequate tissue perfusion rather than an accelerated rate of glucose production. In this setting, restitution would be significantly impaired and an increase in mortality would be expected. Although the second phase of restitution is present during all hemorrhages, the restitution in very large hemorrhages (>25 percent of the total blood volume) is no greater than that seen in small hemorrhages of 10 percent. This finding correlates with the appearance of a decrease in transmembrane potential, cell swelling, and eventually cell death.

Bibliography

NEUROENDOCRINE REFLEXES
Stimuli, Integration, and Modulation

Achtel RA, Downing SE: Ventricular responses to hypoxemia following chemoreceptor denervation and adrenalectomy. *Am Heart J* 84:377, 1972.

Baertschi AJ, Ward DG, Gann DS: Role of atrial receptors in the control of ACTH. *Am J Physiol* 231:692, 1976.

Bereiter DA, Plotsky PM, Gann DS: Tooth pulp stimulation potentiates the ACTH response to hemorrhage in cats. *Endocrinology* 111:1127, 1982.

Bereiter DA, Zaid AM, Gann DS: Adrenocorticotropin response to graded blood loss in the cat. *Am J Physiol* 247:E398, 1984.

Bereiter DA, Zaid AM, Gann DS: The effect of rate of hemorrhage on sympathoadrenal catecholamine release in the cat. *Am J Physiol* 250:E69, 1985.

Bereiter DA, Gann DS: Caudolateral areas of medulla-mediating release of ACTH in cats. *Am J Physiol* 251:R934, 1986.

Blessing WW: Central neurotransmitter pathways for baroreceptor-initiated secretion of vasopressin. *NIPS* 1:90, 1986.

Brown AM: Receptors under pressure: an update on baroreceptors. *Circ Res* 46:1, 1980.

Claybaugh JR, Share L: Vasopressin, renin, and cardiovascular responses to continuous slow hemorrhage. *Am J Physiol* 224:519, 1973.

Egdahl RH: Pituitary-adrenal response following trauma to the isolated leg. *Surgery* 46:9, 1959.

Egdahl RH: The differential response of the adrenal cortex and medulla to bacterial endotoxin. *J Clin Invest* 38:1120, 1959.

Egdahl RH, Nelson DH, Hume DM: Adrenal cortical function in hypothermia. *Surg Gynecol Obstet* 101:15, 1955.

Engeland WC, Byrnes GJ, Gann DS: The pituitary adrenocortical response to hemorrhage depends on the time of day. *Endocrinology* 110:1856, 1982.

Gann DS, Cryer GL, Pirkle JC Jr: Physiological inhibition and facilitation of adrenocortical response to hemorrhage. *Am J Physiol* 232:R5, 1977.

Gann DS, Dallman MF, Engeland WC: Reflex control and modulation of ACTH and corticosteroids, in McCann SM (ed): *Endocrine Physiology,* III International Review of Physiology. University Park Press, Baltimore, 1981, vol 24, pp 157–199.

Gann DS, Berieter DA, et al: Neural interaction in control of adrenocorticotropin. *Fed Proc* 44:161, 1985.

Goldman WF, Saum WR: A direct excitatory action of catecholamines on rat aotic baroreceptors in vitro. *Circ Res* 55:18, 1984.

Grizzle WE, Dallman MF, et al: Inhibitory and facilitatory hypothalamic areas mediating ACTH release in the cat. *Endocrinology* 95:1450, 1974.

Hensel H: Neural processes in thermoregulation. *Physiol Rev* 53:948, 1973.

Heymans C, Neil E: *Reflexogenic Areas of the Cardiovascular System.* Boston, Little, Brown and Company, 1958.

Holmes AE, Ledsome JR: Effect of norepinephrine and vasopressin on carotid sinus baroreceptor activity in the anesthetized rabbit. *Experentia* 40:825, 1984.

Hume DM, Egdahl RH: The importance of the brain in the neuroendocrine response to injury. *Ann Surg* 150:697, 1959.

Hume DM, Egdahl RH: Effect of hypothermia and of cold exposure on adrenal cortical and medullary secretion. *Ann NY Acad Sci* 80:435, 1959.

Hume DM, Bell CL, Bartter FC: Direct measurement of adrenal secretion during operative trauma and convalescence. *Surgery* 52:174, 1962.

Kircheim HR: Systemic arterial baroreceptor reflexes. *Physiol Rev* 56:100, 1976.

Korner PI: Integrative neural cardiovascular control. *Physiol Rev* 51:312, 1971.

Lambertson CJ: Neural control of respiration, in Mountcastle,

VB (ed): *Medical Physiology.* St Louis, Mosby, 1980, 114th ed, p 1749.

Lefcort AM, Ward DG, Gann SD: Electrolytic lesions of the dorsal rostral pons prevents adrenocorticotropin increases after hemorrhage. *Endocrinology* 114:2148, 1984.

Lilly MP, Engeland WC, Gann DS: Adrenomedullary responses to repeated hemorrhage in the anesthetized dog. *Endocrinology* 111:1917, 1982.

Lilly MP, Engeland WC, Gann DS: Responses of cortisol secretion to repeated hemorrhage in the anesthetized dog. *Endocrinology* 112:681, 1983.

Longnecker DE, McCoy S, Drucker WR: Anesthetic influence on response to hemorrhage in rats. *Circ Shock* 6:55, 1979.

O'Berg B, White S: Circulatory effects of interruption and stimulation of cardiac vagal afferents. *Acta Physiol Scand* 80:383, 1970.

Overman RR, Wang SG: The contributory role of the afferent nervous factor in experimental shock: sublethal hemorrhage and sciatic nerve stimulation. *Am J Physiol* 148:289, 1947.

Quest JA, Gebber GL: Modulation of baroreceptor reflexes by somatic afferent nerve stimulation. *Am J Physiol* 222:1251, 1972.

Raff H, Shinsako J, Dallman MF: Surgery potentiates adrenocortical responses to hypoxia in dogs. *Proc Soc Exp Bio Med* 172:400, 1983.

Redding M, Mueller CB: Effect of ambient temperature upon responses to hypovolemic insult in the unanesthetized unrestrained albino rat. *Surgery* 64:110, 1968.

Sato A, Schmidt RF: Somatosympathetic reflexes: Afferent fibers, central pathways, discharge characteristics. *Physiol Rev* 53:916, 1973.

Wigger CJ: *Physiology of Shock.* New York, Commonwealth Fund, 1950.

Wood CE, Shinsako J, et al: Hormonal and hemodynamic responses to 15mL/kg hemorrhage in conscious dogs: Responses correlate to body temperature. *Proc Soc Exp Biol Med* 167:15, 1981.

Zimpfer M, Manders WT, et al: Pentobarbital alters compensatory neural and humoral mechanisms in response to hemorrhage. *Am J Physiol* 243:H713, 1982.

Mechanism of Hormone Action

Ali M, Vedeckis WV: The glucocorticoid receptor protein binds to transfer RNA. *Science* 235:467, 1987.

Cheung WY: Calmodulin. *Sci Am* 7:62, 1982.

Compton MM, Cidlowski JA: Vitamin B6 and glucocorticoid action. *Endocr Rev* 7:140, 1986.

Fain JN: Involvement of phosphatidylinositol breakdown in elevation of cytosol Ca^{++} by hormones and relationship to prostaglandin formation, in Kohn LD (ed): *Hormone Receptors.* New York, Wiley, 1982, vol 6, p 237.

Fain JN, Garcia-Sainz JA: Adrenergic regulation of adipocyte metabolism. *J Lipid Res* 24:945, 1983.

Farese RV: Phosphoinositide metabolism and hormone action. *Endocr Rev* 4:78, 1983.

Greengard P: Phosphorylated proteins as physiological effectors. *Science* 199:146, 1978.

Jensen EV: Interaction of steroid hormones with the nucleus. *Pharmacol Rev* 30:477, 1979.

Means AR, Lagace L, et al: Calmodulin as a mediator of hormone action and cell regulation. *J Cell Biochem* 20:317, 1982.

Motulsky JJ, Insel PA: Adrenergic receptors in man: Direct identification, physiologic regulations and clinical alterations. *N Engl J Med* 307:18, 1982.

Muldoon TG: Regulation of steroid hormone receptor activity. *Endocr Rev* 1:339, 1980.

O'Malley BW, Schrader WT: The receptors of steroid hormones. *Sci Am* 234:32, 1976.

Oppenheimer JH: Thyroid hormone action at the cellular level. *Science* 203:97, 1979.

Rassmusen H: *Calcium and C-amp as Synarchic Messengers.* New York, Wiley Intersciences, 1981.

Spiegel AM, Gierschik P, et al: Clinical implications of guanine nucleotide binding proteins as receptor effector couplers. *N Engl J Med* 312:26, 1985.

Sterling K: Thyroid hormone action at the cell level. *N Engl J Med* 300:117, 173, 1979.

Endocrine Effectors

Aasen AO, Smith-Erichsen N, Amundsen E: Plasma kallikrein-kinnin system in septicemia. *Arch Surg* 118:343, 1983.

Aguilera G, Mendelsohn AO, Catt KJ: Dopaminergic regulation of aldosterone secretion, in Martini L, Ganong WF: *Frontiers in Neuroendocrinology.* New York, Raven, 1984, p 265.

Amir S, Berstein M: Endogeneous opiates interact in stress-induced hyperglycemia in mice. *Physiol Behav* 28:575, 1982.

Aono T et al: Influence of surgical stress under general anesthesia on serum gonadotropin levels. *J Clin Endocrinol Metab* 42:144, 1976.

Aun F, Medeiros-Neto GA, et al: The effect of major trauma on the pathways of thyroid hormone metabolism. *J Trauma* 23:104, 1983.

Averill DB, Scher AM, Feigl ED: Angiotensin causes vasoconstriction during hemorrhage in baroreceptor-denervated dogs. *Am J Physiol* 245:H667, 1983.

Baer PG, McGiff JC: Hormonal systems and renal hemodynamics. *Annu Rev Physiol* 42:589, 1980.

Barakos V, Rodemann HP, et al: Stimulation of muscle protein degradation and prostaglandin E2 release by leukocyte pyrogen (interleukin-1). *N Engl J Med* 308:553, 1983.

Barton RN: Neuroendocrine mobilization of body fuels after injury. *Br Med Bull* 41:218, 1985.

Bauer WE, Vigar SNM, et al: Insulin response during hypovolemic shock. *Surgery* 66:80, 1969.

Baylis PH, Zepre RL, Robertson GL: Arginine vasopressin response to insulin-induced hypoglycemia in man. *J Clin Endocrinol Metab* 53:935, 1981.

Becker RA, Wilmore DW, et al: Free T4, free T3 and reverse T3 in critically ill, terminally injured patients. *J Trauma* 20:713, 1980.

Benedict CR, Grahame-Smith DG: Plasma noradrenaline and adrenaline concentrations and dopamine-B-hydroxylase activity in patients with shock due to septicaemia, trauma and hemorrhage. *Q J Med* 47:1, 1978.

Bernton EW, Long JB, Holaday JW: Opioids and neuropeptides; mechanisms in circulatory shock. *Fed Proc* 44:290, 1985.

Berry HE, Collier JG, Vane JR: The generation of kinins in the blood of dogs during hypotension due to hemorrhage. *Clin Sci* 39:349, 1970.

Besedovsky H, DelRey A, et al: Immunoregulatory feedback between interleukin-1 and glucocorticoid hormones. *Science* 233:652, 1986.

Beutler B, Cerami A: Cachectin and tumour necrosis factor as two sides of the same biological coin. *Nature* 320:584, 1986.

Bie P: Osmoreceptors, vasopressin and control of renal water excretion. *Physiol Rev* 60:961, 1980.

Bonnet F, Harari A, et al: Suppression of antidiuretic hormone hypersecretion during surgery by extradural anaesthesia. *Br J Anesth* 54:30, 1982.

Brizio-Molteni L, Molteni A, et al: Prolactin, corticotropin and gonadotropin concentrations following thermal injury in adults. *J Trauma* 24:1, 1984.

Buckingham J: Hypothalamic-pituitary responses to trauma. *Br Med Bull* 41:203, 1985.

Caldwell MD, Lacy WW, Exton JH: Effects of adrenalectomy on the amino acid and glucose metabolism of perfused rat hindlimbs. *J Biol Chem* 253:6837, 1978.

Carey LC, Cloutier CT, Lowery BD: Growth hormone and adrenal cortisol response to shock and trauma in the human. *Ann Surg* 174, 1971.

Carey LC, Lowery BD, Cloutier CT: Blood sugar and insulin response in human shock. *Ann Surg* 172:342, 1970.

Carey RM, Sen S: Aldosterone-stimulating factor: a new aldosterone secretagogue, in Ganong WF, Martini L: *Frontiers in Neuroendocrinology.* New York, Raven, 1986, p 191.

Caromona RH, Tsao RC, Trunkey DD: The role of prostacylin and thromboxane in sepsis and septic shock. *Arch Surg* 119:189, 1984.

Carretero OA, Scicli AG: The renal kallikrein-kinin system, in Dunn MJ (ed): *Renal Endocrinology.* Baltimore, Williams and Wilkins, 1983, p 96.

Carstensen H, et al: Testosterone, luteinizing hormone and growth hormone in blood following surgical trauma. *Acta Chir Scand* 138:1, 1972.

Cavalieri RR, Rappooport B: Impaired peripheral conversion of thyroxine to triiodothyronine. *Ann Rev Med* 28:57, 1977.

Chaisson JL, Shikama H, et al: Inhibitory effect of epinephrine on insulin-stimulated glucose uptake by rat skeletal muscle. *J Clin Invest* 68:706, 1981.

Chan TM: The permissive effects of glucocorticoids on hepatic gluconeogenesis. *J Biol Chem* 259:7426, 1984.

Charters AC, O'Dell MWD, Thompson JC: Anterior pituitary function during surgical stress and convalescence. *J Clin Endocrinol Metab* 29:63, 1969.

Clowes GHA, George BC, et al: Muscle proteolysis induced by a circulating peptide in patients with sepsis or trauma. *N Engl J Med* 308:545–552, 1983.

Cochrane JPS, Forsling ML, et al: Arginine vasopressin release following surgical operations. *Br J Surg* 68:209, 1981.

Cooper CE, Nelson DH: ACTH levels in plasma in preoperative and surgically stressed patients. *J Clin Invest* 41:1599, 1962.

Cowley AW, Quitlen EW, Skelton MM: Role of vasopressin in cardiovascular regulation. *Fed Proc* 42:3170, 1983.

Cox BM, Baizman ER: Physiological functions of endorphins, in Malick JB, Bell RMS (eds): *Endorphins: Chemistry, Physiology, Pharmacology and Clinical Relevance.* New York, Marcel Dekker, 1982, p 116.

Cryer, PE: Physiology and pathophysiology of the human sympathoadrenal neuroendocrine system. *N Engl J Med* 303:436, 1980.

Cryer PE: Diseases of the adrenal medulla and sympathetic nervous system, in Felig P, Baxter JD, Broadus AE, Frohman LA (eds): *Endocrinology and Metabolism,* 2d ed. New York, McGraw-Hill, 1987, p 651.

Curtis T, Lefer A: Protective actions of naloxone in hemorrhagic shock. *Am J Physiol* 239:H416, 1980.

Daughaday WH: The adenohypophysis, in Williams RH: *Textbook of Endocrinology*. Philadelphia, Saunders, 1981, p 73.

Davies CL, Newman RJ, et al: The relationship between plasma catecholamines and severity of injury in man. *J Trauma* 24:99, 1984.

Dinarello CA: Interleukin-1 and the pathogenesis of the acute phase response. *N Engl J Med* 311:1413, 1984.

Edelman IS, Ismail-Beigi F: Thyroid thermogenesis and active sodium transport. *Rec Prog Horm Res* 30:235, 1974.

Eigler N, Sacca L, Sherwin RS: Synergistic interactions of physiologic increments of glucagon, epinephrine and cortisol in the dog. *J Clin Invest* 63:114, 1979.

Emerson TW: Participation of endogenous vasoactive agents in the pathogenesis of endotoxic shock. *Adv Exp Med Biol* 23:25, 1974.

Engeland WC, Demsher DP, et al: The adrenal medullary response to graded hemorrhage in awake dogs. *Endocrinology* 109:1539, 1981.

Engeland WC, Bereiter DF, Gann DS: Sympathetic control of adrenal secretion after hemorrhage in awake dogs. *Am J Physiol* 251:R341, 1986.

Engels FL, Fredricks J: Contribution to understanding of mechanism of permissive action of corticoids. *Proc Soc Exp Biol Med* 95:593, 1957.

Fater DC, Sundet WD, et al: Arterial baroreceptors have minimal physiological effects on adrenal medullary secretion. *Am J Physiol* 244:H194, 1983.

Feldman M, Kiser RS, et al: Beta-endorphin and the endocrine pancreas. *N Engl J Med* 308:350, 1983.

Felig P: The endocrine pancreas: Diabetes mellitus, in Felig P, Baxter JD, Broadus AE, Frohman LA (eds): *Endocrinology and Metabolism*, 2d ed. New York, McGraw-Hill, 1987, p 1043.

Felig P, Sherwin RS, et al: Hormonal interactions in the regulation of blood glucose. *Recent Prog Horm Res* 35:501, 1979.

Fletcher JR, Ramwell PW, Herman CW: Prostaglandins and the hemodynamic course of endotoxin shock. *J Surg Res* 20:589, 1976.

Fletcher JR, Short BL, et al: Prostaglandins as mediators of the hemodynamic abnormalities in endotoxemia and sepsis, in McConn R (ed): *Role of Chemical Mediators in the Pathophysiology of Acute Illness and Injury*. New York, Raven, 1982.

Franchimont P: The regulation of follicle stimulating hormone and lutenizing hormone secretion in humans, in Martini L, Ganong WF (eds): *Frontiers in Neuroendocrinology*. New York, Oxford University Press, 1971, p 3331.

Fray JCS, Lush DJ, Valentine AND: Cellular mechanisms of renin secretion. *Fed Proc* 3250, 1983.

Frayn KN, Prete DA, et al: Plasma somatomedin activity after injury in man and its relationship to other hormonal and metabolic changes. *Clin Endocrinol* 20:179, 1984.

Frayn KN, Little RA, et al: The relationship of plasma catecholamines to acute metabolic and hormonal responses to injury in man. *Circ Shock* 16:229, 1985.

Frohman LA: CNS peptides and glucoregulation. *Annu Rev Physiol* 45:95, 1983.

Gann DS, Amaral JF: The pathophysiological response to injury, in Zuidema G, Rutherford R, Ballinger WF: *The Management of Trauma*. Philadelphia, Saunders, 1985, pp 35–100.

Gerich JE, Charles MA, et al: Regulation of pancreatic insulin and glucagon secretion. *Ann Rev Physiol* 38:353, 1976.

Goetel EJ: Leukocyte recognition and metabolism of leukotrienes. *Fed Proc* 42:3128, 1983.

Guillmen R, Vargo T, et al: B-Endorphin and adrenocorticotropin are secreted concomitantly by the pituitary gland. *Science* 197:1367, 1977.

Haberich FJ: Osmoreception in the portal circulation. *Fed Proc* 27:1137, 1968.

Haberland GL: The role of kininogenases, kinin formation and kininogenase inhibition in post traumatic shock and related conditions. *Klin Nochenschr* 56:325, 1978.

Halmagyi DFJ, Gillet DJ, et al: Blood glucose and serum insulin in reversible and irreversible post hemorrhagic shock. *J Trauma* 6:623, 1966.

Halmagyi DFJ, Neering IR, et al: Plasma glucagon in experimental posthemorrhagic shock. *J Trauma* 9:320–326, 1969.

Hammarstrom S: Leukotrienes. *Annu Rev Biochem* 52:355, 1983.

Handlers JS, Orloff J: Antidiuretic hormone. *Annu Rev Physiol* 43:611, 1981.

Hass M, Glick SM: Radioimmunoassayable plasma vasopressin associated with surgery. *Arch Surg* 113:597, 1978.

Hiebert JM, Kieler E, et al: Species differences in insulin secretion responses during hemorrhagic shock. *Surgery* 79:451, 1976.

Holaday JW, Black LE, Long JB: Neuropeptides in shock and trauma, in Gelhoed GW, Chernow B (eds): *Endocrine Aspects of Acute Illness*. Churchill Livingstone, 1985, p 257.

Hollt V: Multiple endogenous opioid peptides. *Trends Neurosci* 6:24, 1983.

Ingenbleck Y: Thyroid function in non-thyroid illness, in DeVisscher M (ed): *The Thyroid Gland*. New York, Raven, 1980.

Ippe E, Dobbs R, Unger RH: Morphine and beta endorphin influence the secretion of the endocrine pancreas. *Nature* 276:190, 1978.

Jackson I: Thyrotropin-releasing hormone. *N Engl J Med* 306:245, 1982.

Kampschmidt RF: Leukocytic endogenous mediator. *J Reticuloendothel Soc* 23:287, 1978.

Kaplan AP: Hageman factor-dependent pathways: mechanisms of initiation and bradykinin formation. *Fed Proc* 42:3123, 1983.

Kendler KS, Weitzman RE, Fisher DA: The effect of pain on plasma arginine vasopressin concentrations in man. *Clin Endocrinol* 8:89, 1978.

Kraus-Friedmann N: Hormonal regulation of hepatic gluconeogenesis. *Physiol Rev* 51:312, 1984.

Landgraf R, Landgraf-Leurs MMC: Prolactin: a diabetogenic hormone. *Diabetologia* 13:99, 1977.

Lang RE, Bruckner UB, et al: Effect of hemorrhagic shock on the concomitant release of endorphin and enkephalin like peptides from the pituitary and adrenal gland in the dog, in Costa E, Trabucchi R (eds): *Regulatory Peptides: From Molecular Biology to Function*. New York, Raven, 1982.

Larsen PR: Thyroid-pituitary interaction. *N Engl J Med* 23:32, 1982.

Lautt WW, Dwan PD, Singh RR: Control of the hyperglycemic response to hemorrhage in cats. *Can J Physiol Pharmacol* 60:1630, 1982.

Lautt WW, Martens ES, Legare: Insulin and glucagon response during hemorrhage induced hyperglycemia. *Can J Physiol Pharmacol* 60:1624, 1982.

Lee JB: The prostaglandins, in Williams RH (ed): *Textbook of Endocrinology*. Philadelphia, Saunders, 1981, p 1047.

Lefer AM: Eicosanoids as mediators of ischemia and shock. *Fed Proc* 44:275, 1985.

Levinsky NG: The renal kallikrein-kinin system. *Circ Res* 44:441, 1978.

McIntosh TK, Faden AI: Thyrotropin-releasing hormone and circulatory shock. *Circ Shock* 18:241, 1986.

McLeod MK, Carlson DE, Gann DS: Hormonal responses associated with early hyperglycemia after graded hemorrhage in dogs. *Am J Physiol* 251:E597, 1986.

Markley K, Horakova Z, et al: The role of histamine in burn, tourniquet and endotoxic shock in mice. *Eur J Pharmacol* 33:255, 1975.

Meguid MM, Brennan MF, et al: Hormone-substrate interrelationships following trauma. *Arch Surg* 109:776, 1974.

Merimer TJ, Zapf MJ, Froesch ER: Insulin-like growth factors in the fed and fasted states. *J Clin Endocrinol Metab* 55:999, 1982.

Miyata M, Yamomoto T, Nakao K: Suppression of glucagon secretion during surgery. *Horm Metab Res* 8:239, 1976.

Molteni A, Warphea RL, et al: Circadian rhythms of serum aldosterone, cortisol and plasma renin activity in burn injuries. *Ann Clin Lab Sci* 9:518, 1979.

Moran WH, Miltenberger FW, et al: Relationship of antidiuretic hormone to surgical stress. *Surgery* 56:99, 1964.

Morgan RJ, Martyn JAJ, et al: Water metabolism and antidiuretic hormone response following thermal injury. *J Trauma* 20:468, 1980.

Mortensen RF, Johnson AA, Eurenius K: Serum corticosteroid binding following thermal injury. *Proc Soc Exp Biol Med* 139:877, 1979.

Moss GS, Cerchio GM, et al: Serum insulin response in hemorrhagic shock in baboons. *Surgery* 68:34, 1970.

Munck A, Guyre PM, Holbrook NJ: Physiological functions of glucocorticoids in stress and their relation to pharmacological actions. *Endocr Rev* 5:25, 1984.

Nagy S, Nagy A, et al: Histamine level changes in the plasma and tissues in hemorrhagic shock. *Circ Shock* 18:227, 1986.

Nakao K, Nakai Y, et al: Substantial rise of plasma beta endorphin levels after insulin-induced hypoglycemia in human subjects. *J Clin Endocrinol Metab* 49:838, 1979.

Nelson DH: Corticosteroid-induced changes in phospholipid membranes as mediators of their action. *Endocr Rev* 1:180, 1980.

Newsome HH, Rose JC: The response of adrenocorticotrophic hormone and growth hormone to surgical stress. *J Clin Endocrinol Metab* 33:481, 1971.

Novelli GP, Marsili M, Pieraccioli E: Anti-shock action of steroids other than cortisone. *Eur Surg Res* 5:169, 1973.

Ono N, Lumpkin MD, et al: Intrahypothalamic action of corticotropin-releasing factor to inhibit growth hormone and LH release in the rat. *Life Sci* 35:118, 1984.

Otsuki M, Dakoda M, Baba S: Influence of glucocorticoids on TRF-induced TSH response in man. *J Clin Endocrinol Metab* 36:945, 1973.

Parrillo JE, Fauci AS: Mechanisms of glucocorticoid action on immune processes. *Annu Rev Pharmacol Toxicol* 19:179, 1979.

Paterson SJ, Robson LE, Kosterlitz HW: Classification of opioid receptors. *Br J Med* 39:31, 1983.

Peach MJ: Renin-angiotensin system: Biochemistry and mechanisms of action. *Physiol Rev* 57:313–370, 1977.

Perdue JF: Chemistry structure and function of insulin-like growth factors and their receptors: A review. *Can J Biochem Cell Biol* 62:1237, 1984.

Pfeffer MA, Pfeffer JM, et al: Systemic hemodynamic effects of leukotrienes C4 and D4 in the rat. *Am J Physiol* 244:H628, 1983.

Pfeiffer A, Herz A: Endocrine action of opioids. *Horm Metab Res* 16:386, 1984.

Phillips LS, Vassilopoulou-Sellin R: Somatomedins. *N Engl J Med* 302:371, 1980.

Phillips RH, Valente WA, et al: Circulating thyroid hormone changes in acute trauma: Prognostic implications for clinical outcome. *J Trauma* 24:116, 1984.

Porte D Jr, Smith PH, Ensinck JW: Neurohumoral regulation of the pancreatic islet A and B cells. *Metabolism* 25:1453, 1976.

Powanda MC, Bersil WR: Hypothesis: Leukocytic endogenous mediator/endogenous pyrogen/lymphocyte activating factor modulates the development of nonspecific and specific immunity and affects nutritional status. *Am J Clin Nutr* 35:762, 1982.

Raptis S, Dollinger HC, et al: Differences in insulin, growth hormone and pancreatic enzyme secretion after intravenous and intraduodenal administration of mixed amino acids in man. *N Engl J Med* 288:1199, 1973.

Rees M, Bowen JC, et al: Plasma beta endorphin immunoreactivity in dogs during anesthesia surgery, escherichia coli sepsis, and naloxone therapy. *Surgery* 93:386, 1983.

Regoli D, Barabe J: Pharmacology of bradykinin and related kinins. *Pharmacol Rev* 32:1, 1980.

Reichlin S: Somatostatin. *N Engl J Med* 309:1495, 1983.

Rizza RA, Mandarino LJ, Gerich JE: Cortisol-induced insulin resistance in man: Impaired suppression of glucose production and stimulation of glucose utilization due to a postreceptor defect of insulin action. *J Clin Endocrinol Metab* 54:131, 1982.

Samuelsson B: Prostaglandins and thromboxanes. *Recent Prog Horm Res* 34:239, 1978.

Sawchenko PE, Friedman MI: Sensory functions of the liver—a review. *Am J Physiol* 236:R5, 1979.

Schachter M: Kallikreins (kinninogenases)—a group of serine proteases with bioregulatory actions. *Pharmacol Rev* 31:1, 1980.

Schrier RW, Berl WT, Anderson RJ: Osmotic and non-osmotic control of vasopressin release. *Am J Physiol* 236:F321, 1979.

Share L: Control of plasma ADH titer in hemorrhage: Role of atrial and arterial receptors. *Am J Physiol* 215:1384, 1968.

Shirani KZ, Vaughan GM, et al: Inappropriate vasopressin secretion in burned patients. *J Trauma* 23:217, 1983.

Shirani KZ, Vaughan GM, et al: Reduced serum T4 and T3 and their altered transport binding after burn injury in rats. *J Trauma* 25:953, 1985.

Silverberg AB, Shah SD, et al: Norepinephrine: Hormone and neurotransmitter in man. *Am J Physiol* 234:E252, 1978.

Skillman JJ, Hedley-White J, Pallotta JA: Hormonal, fuel and respiratory relationships after acute blood loss in man. *Surg Forum* 21:23, 1970.

Skillman JJ, Lauler DP, et al: Hemorrhage in normal man: Effect on renin, cortisol, aldosterone, and urine composition. *Ann Surg* 166:865, 1967.

Sklar AH, Schrier RW: Central nervous system mediators of vasopressin release. *Physiol Rev* 63:1243, 1983.

Slotman GJ, Burchard KW, Gann DS: Thromboxane and prostacyclin in clinical acute respiratory failure. *J Surg Res* 1986.

Swerlick RA, Drucker NA, McCoy S: Insulin effectiveness in hypovolemic dogs. *J Trauma* 21:1013, 1981.

Tracey KJ, Lowry SF, et al: Cachectin/tumor necrosis factor

mediates changes of skeletal muscle plasma membrane potential. *J Exp Med* 164:1368, 1986.

Tracey KJ, Beutler B, et al: Shock and tissue injury induced by recombinant human cachectin. *Science* 234:470, 1986.

Unger RH, Dobbs RE: Insulin, glucagon and somatostatin secretion in the regulation of metabolism. *Annu Rev Physiol* 40:307, 1978.

Vaughan GM, Becker RA, et al: Cortisol and corticotrophin in burned patients. *J Trauma* 22:263, 1982.

Vitek V, Lang DJ, Cowley RA: Admission serum insulin and glucose levels in 247 accident victims. *Clin Chim Acta* 95:93, 1979.

Vitek V, Shatney CH, et al: Thyroid hormone responses in hemorrhagic shock: Study in dogs and preliminary findings in humans. *Surgery* 93:768, 1983.

Wahl R, Grusseudorf M, et al: Changes of thyroid hormone concentrations after severe trauma and in hemorrhagic shock. *Eur Surg Res* 9:suppl 1, 1977.

Williams GH: Aldosterone, in Dunn MJ (ed): *Renal Endocrinology*. Baltimore, Williams and Wilkins, 1983, p 205.

Williamson DH: Regulation of ketone body metabolism and the effects of injury. *Acta Chir Scand* 22-9, 1981.

Wilmore DW, Long JM, et al: Catecholamines: mediators of the hypermetabolic response to thermal injury. *Am Surg* 180:653, 1974.

Wilmore DW, Mason AD, Pruitt BA: Insulin response to glucose in hypermetabolic burn patients. *Ann Surg* 183:314, 1976.

Wilmore WD, Moylan DA, et al: Hyperglucagonemia after burns. *Lancet* 1:73, 1974.

Wise L, Margraf HW, Ballinger WF: Adrenal cortical function in severe burns. *Arch Surg* 105:213, 1972.

Woloski BM, Smith EM, et al: Corticotropin releasing activity of monokines. *Science* 230:1035, 1985.

Wright PD, Henderson K: Cellular glucose utilization during hemorrhagic shock in the pig. *Surgery* 77:322, 1975.

Wright PD, Johnston IDA: The effect of surgical operation on growth hormone levels in surgery. *Surgery* 77:479, 1975.

Yates FE, Marsh DJ, Maran JW: The adrenal cortex, in Mountcastle, VB (ed): *Medical Physiology*. St Louis, Mosby, 1980, 14th ed, pp 1588–1601.

SUBSTRATE METABOLISM FOLLOWING INJURY

Amaral JF, Shearer JD, et al: The temporal characteristics of the metabolic and endocrine response to trauma. *J Trauma,* 1988. (In press.)

Cuthbertson DP: The metabolic response to injury and its nutritional implications: Retrospect and prospect. *J Parenter Enter Nutr* 3:108, 1979.

Engels FL: The significance of the metabolic changes during shock. *Ann NY Acad Sci* 55:383, 1956.

Frayn KN: Substrate turnover after injury. *Br Med Bull* 41:232, 1985.

Moore FD, Brennan MF: Surgical injury: Body composition, protein metabolism and neuroendocrinology, in Ballanger WF, Collins JA, Drucker WR (eds): *Manual of Surgical Nutrition*. Philadelphia, Saunders, 1975, p 169.

Oppenheim W, Williamson D, Smith R: Early biochemical changes and severity of injury in man. *J Trauma* 20:135, 1980.

Siegel JH, Cerra FB, et al: Physiological and metabolic correlations in human sepsis. *Surgery* 86:163, 1979.

Stoner HB, Frayn KN, et al: The relationships between plasma substrates and hormones and the severity of injury in 277 recently injured patients. *Clin Sci* 56:563, 1979.

Stoner HB: Metabolism after trauma and sepsis. *Circ Shock* 19:75, 1986.

Volenec FJ, Clark GM, et al: Metabolic profiles of thermal trauma. *Ann Surg* 190:694, 1979.

Wilmore DW: Hormonal responses and their effect on metabolism. *Surg Clin North Am* 56:999–1018, 1976.

Starvation

Abbott NE, Anderson K: The effect of starvation, infection and injury on the metabolic processes and body composition. *Ann NY Acad Sci* 110:941, 1963.

Addis T, Poo LJ, Lew W: The quantities of protein lost by the various organs and tissues of the body during a fast. *J Biol Chem* 115:111, 1936.

Ahnefeld FW, Burri C, et al: *Parenteral Nutrition*. Springer-Verlag, New York, 1976.

Ashour B, Hansford RG: Effect of fatty acids and ketones on the activity of pyruvate dehydrogenase in skeletal muscle mitochondria. *Biochem J* 214:715, 1983.

Cahill GF: Starvation in man. *N Engl J Med* 235:668, 1970.

Cahill GF: Ketosis *J Parenter Enterol Nutr* 5:281, 1981.

Carter WJ, Shakir KM, et al: Effect of thyroid hormone on the metabolic adaptation to fasting. *Metabolism* 24:1177, 1975.

Chaisson JL, Liljenquist JE, et al: Gluconeogenesis from alanine in normal postabsorptive man: Intrahepatic stimulatory effect of glucagon. *Diabetes* 24:574, 1975.

Chopra IJ, Smith SR: Circulating thyroid hormones and thyrotropin in adult patients with protein caloric malnutrition. *J Clin Endocrinol Metab* 40:221, 1975.

Exton JH: Gluconeogenesis. *Metabolism* 21:945, 1972.

Felig P: The glucose-alanine cycle. *Metabolism* 22:17, 1973.

Hems DA, Whitton PD: Control of hepatic glycogenolysis. *Physiol Rev* 60:1, 1980.

Hers HG: The control of glycogen metabolism in the liver. *Annu Rev Biochem* 45:167, 1976.

Keys A, Brozek J, et al: *The Biology of Human Starvation*. University of Minnesota Press, 1950.

Korchak HM, Masoro EJ: Changes in the level of the fatty acids synthesizing enzymes during starvation. *Biochem Biophys Acta* 58:354, 1962.

Krebs HA: The metabolic fate of amino acids, in Munro HN, Allison JB (eds): *Mammalian Protein Metabolism*. New York, Academic, 1964, vol 1, p 125.

McGarry JD, Foser DW: Hormonal control of ketogenesis: Biochemical considerations. *Arch Intern Med* 137:495, 1977.

Mallette LE, Exton JH, Park CR: Control of gluconeogenesis from amino acids in the perfused rat liver. *J Biol Chem* 244:5713, 1969.

Masoro EJ: Lipids and lipid metabolism. *Annu Rev Physiol* 39:301, 1977.

Morgan HE, Earl DCN, et al: Regulation of protein synthesis in heart muscle. *J Biol Chem* 251:2151, 1971.

Munro HN, Crim MC: The proteins and amino acids, in Goodhart RS, Shils ME (eds): *Modern Nutrition in Health and Disease*. Philadelphia, Lea & Febiger, 1980, p 51.

Newsholme EA, Start C: *Regulation in Metabolism*. New York, Wiley, 1973.

Owen OE, Organ AP, et al: Brain metabolism during fasting. *J Clin Invest* 46:1589, 1967.

Palmblad J, et al: Effects of total energy withdrawal (fasting) on the level of growth hormone, thyrotropin, cortisol, adrenaline, noradrenaline, T4, T3 and rT3 in healthy males. *Acta Med Scand* 201:16, 1977.

Pozefsky T, Tancredi RG, et al: Effect of brief starvation on muscle amino acid metabolism in non-obese man. *J Clin Invest* 57:444, 1976.

Randle PJ, Newsholme EA, Garland PB: Regulation of glucose uptake by muscle: B. Effects of fatty acids, ketone bodies and pyruvate, and of alloxan-diabetes and starvation on the uptake and metabolic fate of glucose in rat heart and diaphragm muscles. *Biochem J* 93:652, 1964.

Sherwin RS, Hendler RG, Felig P: Effect of ketone infusion on amino acid and nitrogen metabolism in man. *J Clin Invest* 55:1382, 1975.

Energy Metabolism following Injury

Atkinson DE: The energy charge of the adenylate pool as a regulator parameter interaction with feedback modifiers. *Biochemistry* 7:4030, 1966.

Chaudry IH, Sayeed MM, Baue AE: Depletion and restoration of tissue ATP in hemorrhagic shock. *Arch Surg* 108:208, 1974.

Chaudry IH, Wichterman KA, Baue AE: Effect of sepsis on tissue adenine nucleotide levels. *Surgery* 85:205, 1979.

Dubois EF: The mechanism of heat loss and temperature regulation, in Dubois EF (ed): *Lane Medical Lectures,* Stanford University Press, 1937.

Duke JH, Jorgensen SB, et al: Contribution of protein to caloric expenditure following injury. *Surgery* 68:168, 1970.

Hems DA, Brosnan JT: Effects of ischemia on content of metabolites in rat liver and kidney in vivo. *Biochem J* 120:105, 1970.

Illner HP, Shires T: Membrane defect and energy status of rabbit skeletal muscle cells in sepsis and septic shock. *Arch Surg* 116:1302, 1981.

Im MJC, Hoopes JE: Energy metabolism in healing skin wounds. *J Surg Res* 10:459, 1970.

Kinney JM: Energy metabolism in Fischer JE (ed): *Surgical Nutrition.* Boston, Little, Brown and Co., 1983, p 97.

Kinney JM, Roe CF: Caloric equivalents of fever. Patterns of postoperative response. *Ann Surg* 156:610, 1962.

Kinney JM, Lister J, Moore FD: Relationship of energy expenditure to total exchangeable potassium. *Ann NY Acad Sci* 110:722, 1963.

Kinney JM, Long CL, et al: Tissue composition of weight loss in surgical patients. I. Elective operations. *Ann Surg* 168:459, 1968.

LePage GA: Biological energy transformations during shock as shown by tissue analysis. *Am J Physiol* 146:267, 1946.

Liaw KY, Askanazi J, et al: Effect of injury and sepsis on high energy phosphates in muscle and red cells. *J Trauma* 20:755, 1980.

Moore FD: Bodily changes during surgical convalescence. *Ann Surg* 137:289, 1953.

Moore FD: Energy and the maintenance of the body cell. *J Parenter Enterol Nutr* 4:22, 1980.

Morris A, Henry W, et al: Macrophage interaction with skeletal muscle: a potential role of macrophages in determining the energy state of healing wounds. *J Trauma* 25:751, 1985.

Nanni G, Siegel JH, et al: Increased lipid fuel dependence in the critically ill septic patient. *J Trauma* 24:14, 1983.

Pass LJ, Schloerb PR, et al: Liver adenosine triphosphate (ATP) in hypoxia and hemorrhagic shock. *J Trauma* 22:730, 1982.

Pruitt BA: Postburn hypermetabolism and nutrition in burn patients, in Ballinger WF, Collins JA, Drucker WR, Dudrick SJ, Zeppa R (eds): *Manual of Surgical Nutrition.* Philadelphia, Saunders, 1975, p 396.

Ryan NT: Metabolic adaptations for energy production during trauma and sepsis. *Surg Clin North Am* 56:1073, 1976.

Wilmore DW, Aulick LH, et al: Influence of the burn wound on local and systemic responses to injury. *Ann Surg* 186:444, 1977.

Wilmore DW, Long JM, et al: Catecholamines: Mediators of the hypermetabolic response to thermal injury. *Am Surg* 180:653, 1974.

Lipid Metabolism following Injury

Allison SP, Hinton P, Chamberlain MJ: Intravenous glucose tolerance, insulin and free fatty acid levels in burn patients. *Lancet* 2:1118, 1968.

Bagby GJ, Corll CB, Martinez RR: Triglyceride and free fatty acid turnover in E. coli endotoxin treated rats. *Circ Shock* 16:76, 1985.

Birkhain RN, Long CL, et al: A comparison of the effects of skeletal trauma and surgery on the ketosis of starvation in man. *J Trauma* 513, 1981.

Froholm BB: The effect of lactate in canine subcutaneous adipose tissue in situ. *Acta Physiol Scand* 81:110, 1971.

Kaufman RL, Matson CE, Beisel WR: Hypertriglyceridemia produced by endotoxin: Role of impaired triglyceride disposal mechanisms. *J Infect Dis* 133:548, 1976.

Kovach AGB, Russell S, et al: Blood flow, oxygen consumption and free fatty acid release in subcutaneous adipose tissue during hemorrhagic shock in control and phenoxybenzamine-treated dogs. *Circ Res* 26:733, 1970.

Smith R, Fuller DJ, et al: Initial effect of injury on ketone bodies and other blood metabolites. *Lancet* 1:1, 1975.

Wolfe RR, Shaw HF, Durkot MJ: Energy metabolism in trauma and sepsis: the role of fat, in *Molecular and Cellular Aspects of Shock and Trauma.* New York, AR Liss, 1983, p 89.

Carbohydrate Metabolism following Injury

Amaral JF, Shearer J, Caldwell M: Kinetics of glucose uptake in wounded tissue. *Fed Proc* (Abst), 1986.

Amaral JF, Shearer JD, et al: High dose endotoxin decreases glucose uptake in skeletal muscle. *Arch Surg* 1988. (In press.)

Amaral JF, Shearer J, et al: Macrophage insulin like activity increases glucose uptake and hepatic production in skeletal muscle. *Circ Shock* 1988. (In press.)

Amaral JF, Shearer JD, et al: Can lactate be used as a fuel by wounded tissue? *Surgery* 100:252, 1986.

Askanazi J, Elwyn DH, et al: Respiratory distress secondary to a high carbohydrate load. *Surgery* 86:596, 1980.

Black PR, Brooks DC, et al: Mechanisms of insulin resistance following injury. *Ann Surg* 196:420, 1982.

Caldwell MD, Shearer J, et al: Evidence for aerobic glycolysis in λ-carrageenan wounded skeletal muscle. *J Surg Res* 37:63, 1984.

Cannon WB: *The Wisdom of the Body.* New York, W.W. Norton, 1939.

Clark EJ, Rossiter R: Carbohydrate metabolism after burning. *Q J Exp Physiol* 32:279, 1944.

Cryer PE, White NH, Santiago JV: The relevance of glucose counterregulatory systems to patients with insulin-dependent diabetes mellitus. *Endocr Rev* 7:131, 1986.

Drucker WR, Dekieweit JC: Glucose uptake by diaphragms from rats subjected to hemorrhagic shock. *Am J Physiol* 206:317, 1964.

Drucker WR, Gallie BL, et al: In Kovach AGB, Stoner HB,

Spitzer JJ (eds): *Neurohumoral and Metabolic Response to Injury*. New York, Plenum, 1978, p 1870.

Filkins JP: Insulin-like activity (ILA) of a macrophage mediator on adipose tissue glucose oxidation. *J Reticuloendothel Soc* 25:595, 1979.

Forster J, Morris AS, et al: Increased PFK activity in wounded tissue. *Am J Physiol* 1988. (In press.)

Halmagyi DFJ, Irving MH, Varga D: Effect of adrenergic blockade on the metabolic response to hemorrhagic shock. *J Appl Physiol* 25:384, 1968.

Hiebert JM, Celik Z, et al: Insulin response to hemorrhagic shock in the intact and adrenalectomized primate. *Am J Surg* 125:501, 1973.

Hinton P, Allison SP, et al: Insulin and glucose to reduce catabolic response to injury in burned patients. *Lancet* 1:767, 1971.

Hunt TK, Conolly WB, et al: Anaerobic metabolism and wound healing: An hypothesis for the initiation and cessation of collagen synthesis in wounds. *Am J Surg* 135:328, 1978.

Jordan GL, Fischer EP, Lefiak EA: Glucose metabolism and traumatic shock in the human. *Ann Surg* 175:685, 1972.

Kahn CR: Insulin resistance, insulin insensitivity and insulin unresponsiveness: a necessary definition. *Metabolism* 27:1893, 1973.

Long CL, Spencer JL, et al: Carbohydrate metabolism in men: Effect of elective operations and major injury. *J Appl Physiol* 31:110, 1971.

Morris AS, Shearer J, Caldwell MD: The role of the cellular infiltrate on glucose metabolism in wounded tissue. *Surg Forum* 36:95, 1985.

Nelson KM, Turinsky J: Local effect of burn on skeletal muscle insulin responsiveness. *J Surg Res* 31:288, 1981.

Palmer BQ, Brooks DC, et al: Epinephrine acutely mediates skeletal muscle insulin resistance. *Surgery* 94:172, 1983.

Pekala P, Kawakami M, et al: Studies of insulin resistance in adipocytes induced by a macrophage mediator. *J Exp Med* 157:1360, 1983.

Romanosky AJ, Bagby GJ, et al: Increased muscle glucose uptake and lactate release after endotoxin administration. *Am J Physiol* E311, 1980.

Ryan NT, George BC, et al: Chronic tissue insulin resistance following hemorrhagic shock. *Ann Surg* 80:402, 1974.

Shangraw RE, Turinsky J: Local response of muscle to burns: Relationship of glycolysis and amino acid release. *J Parenter Enteral Nutr* 5:193, 1981.

Stoner HB: Studies on the mechanism of shock: The quantitative aspects of glycogen metabolism after limb ischemia in the rat. *Br J Exp Pathol* 39:635, 1958.

Swerlick RA, Drucker NA, McCoy S: Insulin effectiveness in hypovolemic dogs. *J Trauma* 21:1013, 1981.

Turinsky J: Glucose metabolism in the region recovering from burn injury. *Endocrinology* 113:1370, 1983.

Wilmore DW, Mason AD, Pruitt BA: Insulin response to glucose in hypermetabolic burn patients. *Ann Surg* 183:314, 1976.

Protein Metabolism following Injury

Albina JE, Shearer JD, et al: Amino acid metabolism following λ-carrageenan injury to rat skeletal muscle. *Am J Physiol* 250:E24, 1986.

Albina JE, Henry W, et al: Glutamine metabolism in rat skeletal muscle wounded with λ-carregeenan. *Am J Physiol* 250:E24, 1986.

Andrews RP, Morgan HC, Jhrkiewitz MJ: Relationship of dietary protein to the healing of experimental burns. *Surg Forum* 6:72, 1955.

Ardawi MSM, Newsholme EA: Glutamine metabolism in lymphoid tissue, in Haussinger D, Sies H (eds): *Glutamine Metabolism in Mammalian Tissues*. New York, Springer-Verlag, 1984, p 235.

Askanazi S, Elwyn DH, et al: Muscle and plasma amino acids after injury: The role of inactivity. *Ann Surg* 188:797, 1978.

Askanazi I, Carpentier YA, et al: Muscle and plasma amino acids following injury: Influence of intercurrent infection. *Ann Surg* 192:78, 1980.

Aulick LH, Wilmore DH: Increased peripheral amino acid release following burn injury. *Surgery* 85:560, 1979.

Bilmazer C, et al: Quantitative contribution by skeletal muscle to elevated ratio of whole-body protein breakdown in burned children as measured by 3-MEH output. *Metabolism* 27:671, 1978.

Birkhain RH, et al: Effects of major skeletal trauma on whole body protein turnover in man measured by [14C] leucine. *Surgery* 888:294, 1980.

Calloway DH, Grossman MI, et al: Effect of previous level of protein feeding on wound healing and on metabolic response to injury. *Surgery* 37:935, 1955.

Calwell FT Jr: Metabolic responses to thermal trauma. II: Nutritional studies with rats at two environmental temperatures. *Ann Surg* 155:119, 1962.

Chassin JL, McDougall HA, et al: The effect of adrenalectomy on wound healing in normal and in stressed rats. *Proc Soc Exp Biol Med* 86:446, 1954.

Clowes G, Randall H, Cha C: Amino acid and energy metabolism in septic and traumatized patients. *J Parenter Enteral Nutr* 4:195, 1980.

Crane CW, et al: Protein turnover in patients before and after elective orthopedic operations. *Br J Surg* 64:129, 1977.

Crowley CV, Seifter E, et al: Effects of environmental temperature and femoral fracture on wound healing in rats. *J Trauma* 17:436, 1977.

Cuthbertson DP: Observations on the disturbances of metabolism by injury to the limbs. *Q J Med* 1:233, 1932.

Cuthbertson DP, Tilstone WJ: Effects of environmental temperature on the closure of full thickness skin wounds in the rat. *Q J Exp Physiol* 52:249, 1967.

Dale G, et al: The effect of surgical operation on venous plasma free amino acids. *Surgery* 81:295, 1977.

Elwyn DH, Parikh HC, et al: Inter-organ transport of amino acids in hemorrhagic shock. *Am J Phys* 231:377, 1976.

Engels FL, Winton MG, Long CNH: Biochemical studies on shock. I. The metabolism of amino acids and carbohydrates during hemorrhagic shock in the rat. *J Exp Med* 77:397, 1942.

Frawley JP, Artz CP, Howard JM: Muscle metabolism and catabolism in combat casualties. *Arch Surg* 71:612, 1955.

Freund HR, Ryan JA, Fischer JE: Amino acid derangements in patients with sepsis: Treatment with branched chain amino acid rich infusions. *Ann Surg* 188:423, 1978.

Furst P, Bergstrom S, Chao L: Influence of amino acid sulphur on nitrogen and amino acid metabolism in severe trauma. *Acta Chir Scand Suppl* 494:136, 1979.

Howard JE, Bingham RS Jr, Mason RE: Studies on convalescence: In nitrogen and mineral balances during starvation and graduated feeding in healthy young males at bed rest. *Trans Assoc Am Physicians* 59:242, 1946.

Keller GA, West MA, et al: Multiple systems organ failure: Modulation of hepatocyte protein synthesis by endotoxin activated Kuppfer cells. *Ann Surg* 201:87, 1985.

Kien CL, et al: Increased rates of whole body protein synthesis and breakdown in children recovering from burns. *Ann Surg* 187:383, 1978.

Kinney JM, Elwyn DH: Protein metabolism and injury. *Ann Rev Nutr* 3:433, 1983.

Kline DL: The effect of hemorrhage on the plasma amino acid nitrogen of the dog. *Am J Physiol* 146:654, 1946.

LaBrosse EH, Beech JA, et al: Plasma amino acids in normal humans and patients with shock. *Surg Gynecol Obstet* 125:516, 1967.

Levenson SJ, Howard J, Rosen J: Studies of the plasma amino acids and amino conjugates in patients with several battle wounds. *Surg Gynecol Obstet* 101:35, 1955.

Levenson SM, Green RW, et al: Ascorbic acid, riboflavin, thiamine, and nicotinic acid in relation to severe injury, hemorrhage and infection in the human. *Ann Surg* 124:840, 1946.

Levenson SM, Pirani CL, et al: The effect of thermal burns on wound healing. *Surg Gynecol Obstet* 99:74, 1954.

Levenson SM, Seifter E, Van Winkle W: Nutrition, in Hunt TK, Dunphy JE (eds): *Fundamentals of Wound Management.* New York, Appleton Century Croft, 1979, p 286.

Long CL, Schiller WR, et al: Muscle protein catabolism in the septic patient as measured by 3-methylhistidine exertion. *Am J Clin Nutr* 30:1349, 1977.

Lund CL, Levenson SM, et al: Ascorbic acid, thiamine, riboflavin and nicotinic acid in relation to acute burns in man. *Arch Surg* 55:557, 1947.

McCoy S, Case SA, et al: Determinants of blood amino acid concentration after hemorrhage. *Ann Surg* 43:787, 1977.

Miller JDB, Bistran BR, Blackburn GL: Failure of postoperative infection to increase nitrogen excretion in patients maintained on peripheral amino acids. *Am J Clin Nutr* 30:1523, 1977.

Moore RN, Goodrum KJ, Berry LJ: Mediation of an endotoxic effect by macrophages. *J Reticuloendothel Soc* 17:187, 1976.

Odessey R, Khairallah EA, Goldberg AL: Origin and probable significance of alanine production by skeletal muscle. *J Biol Chem* 249:7623, 1974.

O'Donnell TF, Clowes GHA, et al: Proteolysis associated with a deficit of peripheral energy fuel substrates in septic man. *Surgery* 80:192, 1976.

O'Keefe SJD, Sender PM, James WPT: Catabolic loss of body nitrogen in response to surgery. *Lancet* 2:1035, 1974.

Ruderman NB, Berger M: The formation of glutamine and alanine in skeletal muscle. *J Biol Chem* 249:5500, 1974.

Russell JA, Long CH, Engel FL: Biochemical studies of shock: The role of peripheral tissues on the metabolism of protein and carbohydrate during hemorrhagic shock in the rat. *J Exp Med* 79:1, 1944.

Shearer J, Morris A, et al: Effect of starvation on the local and systemic metabolic effects of the λ-carrageenan wound. *Am J Surg* 147:456, 1984.

Shizgal HM, Milne CA, Spainer HA: The effect of nitrogen-sparing intravenously administered fluids on postoperative body composition. *Surgery* 86:60, 1979.

Souba WW, Wilmore DW: Postoperative alteration of arteriovenous exchange of amino acids across the gastrointestinal tract. *Surgery* 94:342, 1983.

Stein TP, Leskin MJ, et al: Changes in protein synthesis after trauma: Importance of nutrition. *Am J Physiol* 233:E348, 1976.

Vinnars E, Bergstrom J, Furst P: Influence of postoperative state in the intracellular free amino acids in human muscle tissue. *Ann Surg* 182:665, 1975.

West MA, Keller GA, et al: Mechanism of hepatic insufficiency in septic multiple system organ failure. *Surg Forum* 35:44, 1984.

Williamson MB, McCarthy TH, Fromm HJ: Relation of protein nutrition to the healing of experimental wounds. *Proc Soc Exp Biol Med* 77:302, 1957.

Williamson OH, et al: Muscle-protein catabolism after injury in man, as measured by urinary excretion of 3-methyl histidine. *Clin Sci Mol Med* 52:527, 1977.

Wilmore DM, Goodwin CW, et al: Effect of injury and infection on visceral metabolism and circulation. *Ann Surg* 192:491, 1980.

Woolfe LIU: Arterial plasma amino acids in patients with serious postoperative infections and in patients with major fractures. *Surgery* 79:283, 1976.

FLUID AND ELECTROLYTE METABOLISM

Andersson B: Regulation of body fluids. *Ann Rev Physiol* 39:185, 1977.

Arturson G: Microvascular permeability to macromolecules in thermal injury. *Acta Physiol Scand* 463:111.

Baxter CR, Shires T: Physiological response to crystalloid resuscitation of severe burns. *Ann NY Acad Sci* 150:874, 1968.

Blalock A: Experimental shock: The cause of low blood pressure caused by muscle injury. *Arch Surg* 20:959, 1930.

Demling RH, Kramer G, Harms B: Role of thermal injury-induced hypoproteinemia on fluid flux and protein permeability in burned and unburned tissue. *Surgery* 136–143, 95.

Elder JM, Miles AA: The action of the lethal toxins of gas gangrene clostridia on capillary permeability. *J Pathol* 74:133–145, 1957.

Harms B, Bodai B, et al: Microvascular fluid and protein flux in pulmonary and systemic circulations after thermal injury. *Microvas Res* 23:77, 1982.

Shires GT, Carrico J, Cannizaro P: Response of the extracellular fluid, in *Shock. Modern Problems in Clinical Surgery.* Philadelphia, Saunders, 1973.

Shires GT III, Peitzman AB, et al: Change in red blood cell transmembrane potential in hemorrhagic shock. *Surg Forum* 32:5, 1981.

Shires T, Williams J, Brown L: Acute changes in extracellular fluids associated with major surgical procedures. *Ann Surg* 154:803, 1961.

Tom WW, Villalba M, et al: Fluorophotometric evaluation of capillary permeability in gram negative-shock. *Arch Surg* 118:636, 1983.

Renal Salt and Water Conservation

Anderson RJ, Gordon JA, et al: Renal concentration defect following nonoliguric acute renal failure in the rat. *Kidney Int* 21:583, 1979.

Anderson RJ, Linas SL, et al: Nonoliguric renal failure. *N Engl J Med* 296:1134, 1977.

Cantin M, Genest J: The heart and atrial natiuretic factor. *Endocr Rev* 6:1, 1985.

Cochrane JPS: The aldosterone response to surgery and the relationship of this response to postoperative sodium retention. *Br J Surg* 65:744, 1978.

Gill JR Jr, Casper AGT: Role of sympathetic nervous system in the renal response to hemorrhage. *J Clin Invest* 48:915.

Gill JR Jr, Casper AGT: Effect of renal alpha-adrenergic stimulation on proximal sodium resorption. *Am J Physiol* 223:1201, 1972.

Hall JE, Guyton AC, Cowley AW Jr: Control of glomerular filtration rate by renin-angiotensin system. *Am J Physiol* 232:F215, 1979.

Itskovitz HD, McGriff JC: Hormonal regulation of renal circulation. *Circ Res* 34/35 (suppl I), 1974.

Johnson MD, Park CS, Malvin RL: Antidiuretic hormone and the distribution of renal cortical blood flow. *Am J Physiol* 232:F111, 1977.

LeQuesne LP, Cochrane JPS, Fieldman NR: Fluid and electrolyte disturbances after trauma: the role of adrenocortical and pituitary hormones. *Br Med Bull* 41:212, 1985.

Miller PD, Krebs RA, et al: Polyuric prerenal failure. *Arch Intern Med* 140:907, 1980.

Navar AG: Renal autoregulation; perspectives from whole kidney and single nephron studies. *Am J Physiol* 234:F357, 1978.

Navar LG, Ploth DW, Bell PD: Distal tubular feedback control of renal hemodynamics and autoregulation. *Ann Rev Physiol* 42:557, 1980.

Schrier RW: Effects of adrenergic nervous system and catecholamines on systemic and renal hemodynamics, sodium and water excretion and renin secretion. *Kidney Int* 6:291, 1974.

Stein JH, Boonjaren S, et al: Mechanism of the redistribution of renal cortical blood flow during hemorrhagic hypotension in the dog. *J Clin Invest* 52:3, 1973.

Valtin H: *Renal Function: Mechanisms Preserving Fluid and Solute Balance in Health.* Little, Brown and Company, 1983, 2d ed.

Blood Volume Restitution

Bergentz SE, Brief DD: The effect of pH and osmolality on the production of canine hemorrhagic shock. *Surgery* 58:412, 1965.

Boyd DR, Mansberger AR: Serum water and osmolal changes in hemorrhagic shock. *Am Surg* 34:744, 1968.

Brooks DK, Williams WG, et al: Osmolar and electrolyte changes in hemorrhagic shock. *Lancet* 1:521, 1963.

Byrnes GJ, Pirkle JC Jr, Gann DS: Cardiovascular stabilization after hemorrhage depends upon restitution of blood volume. *J Trauma* 18:623, 1978.

Casley-Smith JR: The functioning and interrelationships of blood capillaries and lymphatics. *Experientia* 32:1, 1976.

Chien S: Role of the sympathetic nervous system in hemorrhage. *Physiol Rev* 47:214, 1967.

Cope O, Litwin SB: Contribution of the lymphatic system to the replenishment of plasma volume following a hemorrhage. *Ann Surg* 156:655, 1962.

Drucker WR, Chadwick CDJ, Gann DS: Transcapillary refill in hemorrhage and shock. *Arch Surg* 116:1344, 1981.

Friedman SG, Pearce FJ, Drucker WR: The role of blood glucose in the defense of plasma volume during hemorrhage. *J Trauma* 22:86, 1982.

Gann DS: Endocrine control of plasma protein and volume. *Surg Clin North Am* 56:1135, 1976.

Gann DS, Carlson DE, et al: Impaired restitution of blood volume after large hemorrhage. *J Trauma* 21:598, 1981.

Gann DS, Carlson DE, et al: Role of solute in the early restitution of blood volume after hemorrhage. *Surgery* 94:439–446, 1983.

Haddy FJ, Scott JB, Molnar JJ: Mechanisms of volume replacement and vascular constriction following hemorrhage. *Am J Physiol* 208:169, 1965.

Jarhult J: Osmotic fluid transfer from tissue to blood during hemorrhagic hypotension. *Acta Physiol Scand* 1973.

Jarhult J, Lundvall J, et al: Osmolar control of plasma volume during hemorrhagic hypotension. *Acta Physiol Scand* 85:142, 1972.

Kenney PR, Allen-Rowlands CF, Gann DS: Glucose and osmolality as predictors of injury severity. *J Trauma* 23:712, 1983.

Leaf A, Cotran R: *Renal Pathophysiology.* New York, Oxford University Press, 1976.

Menguay R, Master YF: Influence of hyperglycemia on survival after hemorrhagic shock. *Adv Shock Res* 1:43, 1979.

Pirkle JC Jr, Gann DS: Expansion of interstitial fluid is required for full restoration of blood volume. *J Trauma* 16:937, 1977.

Pitts RF: *Physiology of the Body Fluids.* Chicago, Yearbook Medical Publishers, 3d ed, 1974.

Quiros G, Ware J: Modification of cardiovascular responses to hemorrhage by induced hyperosmolality in the rat. *Acta Physiol Scand* 117:391, 1983.

Ware J, Ljanquist O, et al: Osmolar changes in hemorrhage. The effect of an altered nutritional status. *Acta Chir Scand* 148:8, 1982.

Weil M, Afifi AA: Experimental and clinical studies on lactate and pyruvate as indicators of the severity of acute circulatory failure. *Circulation* XLI: 989–1001, 1970.

Wright FS, Briggs JP: Feedback control of glomerular blood flow, pressure and filtration rate. *Physiol Rev* 59:958, 1979.

Wright HK, Gann DS: A defect in urinary concentrating ability during postoperative anti-diuresis. *Surgery Gynecol Obstet* 121:47, 1965.

Wright HK, Gann DS: Correction of defect in free water excretion in postoperative patients by extracellular fluid volume expansion. *Ann Surg* 158:70, 1963.

Chapter 2

Fluid, Electrolyte, and Nutritional Management of the Surgical Patient

G. Tom Shires, Peter C. Canizaro, G. Tom Shires III, and Stephen F. Lowry

ANATOMY OF BODY FLUIDS

One of the most critical aspects of patient care is management of the body composition of fluid and electrolytes. Most diseases, many injuries, and even operative trauma impose a great impact on the physiology of fluid and electrolytes within the body. These changes often exceed those brought about by acute lack of alimentation. Therefore, a thorough understanding of the metabolism of salt, water, and electrolytes and of certain metabolic responses is essential to the care of surgical patients.

The anatomy of body fluids and the physiologic principles that maintain normal fluid and electrolytes will be defined. In addition, a classification of derangements will be outlined to allow an organized therapeutic approach.

A prerequisite to the understanding of fluid and electrolyte management is knowledge of the extent and composition of the various body fluid compartments. Early attempts to define these compartments were relatively accurate, but a more precise definition has been obtained by many investigators through the use of isotope tracer techniques. The wide range of normal values is a function of body size, weight, and sex, but these compartments are relatively constant in the individual patient in the normal steady state. The figures used in this section, therefore, are approximate and presented as a percentage of body weight.

Total Body Water

Water constitutes between 50 and 70 percent of total body weight. Using deuterium oxide or tritiated water for

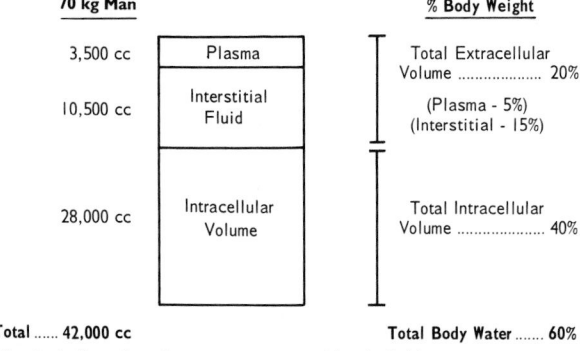

Fig. 2-1. Functional compartments of body fluids.

measurement of total body water, the average normal value for young adult males is 60 percent of body weight and 50 percent for young adult females. A normal variation of ±15 percent applies to both groups. The actual figure for each healthy individual is remarkably constant and is a function of several variables, including lean body mass and age. Since fat contains little water, the lean individual has a greater proportion of water to total body weight than the obese person. The lower percentage of total body water in females correlates well with a relatively large amount of subcutaneous adipose tissue and small muscle mass. Moore et al. have shown that total body water, as a percentage of total body weight, decreases steadily and significantly with age to a low of 52 and 47 percent in males and females, respectively. Con-

versely, the highest proportion of total body water to body weight is found in newborn infants, with a maximum of 75 to 80 percent. During the first several months following birth there is a gradual "physiologic" loss of body water as infants adjust to their environment. At one year of age, the total body water averages approximately 65 percent of the body weight and remains relatively constant throughout the remainder of infancy and childhood.

The water of the body is divided into three functional compartments (Fig. 2-1). The fluid within the body's diverse cell population represents between 30 and 40 percent of the body weight. The extracellular water represents 20 percent of the body weight and is divided between the intravascular fluid, or plasma (5 percent of body weight), and the interstitial, or extravascular, extracellular fluid (15 percent of body weight).

Intracellular Fluid

Measurement of intracellular fluid is determined indirectly by subtraction of the measured extracellular fluid from the measured total body water. The intracellular water is between 30 and 40 percent of the body weight, with the largest proportion in the skeletal muscle mass. Because of the smaller muscle mass in the female, the percentage of intracellular water is lower than in the male.

The chemical composition of the intracellular fluid is shown in Fig. 2-2, with potassium and magnesium the

Fig. 2-2. Chemical composition of body fluid compartments.

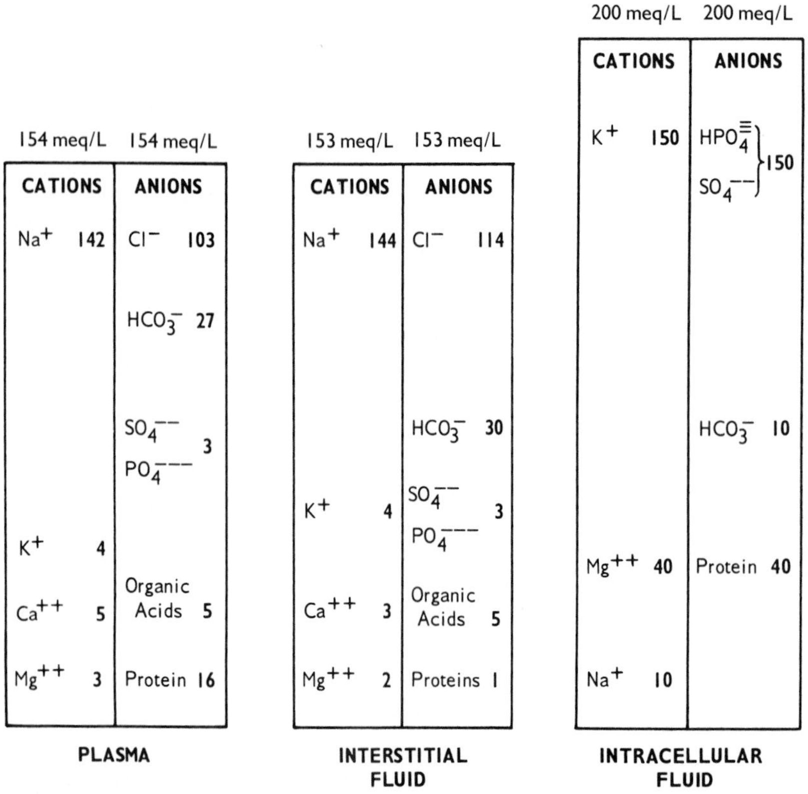

principal cations, and phosphates and proteins the principal anions. This is an approximation, since so few data concerning the intracellular fluid are available.

Extracellular Fluid

The total extracellular fluid volume represents approximately 20 percent of the body weight. The extracellular fluid compartment has two major subdivisions. The plasma volume comprises approximately 5 percent of the body weight in the normal adult. The interstitial, or extravascular, extracellular fluid volume comprises approximately 15 percent of the body weight.

The interstitial fluid is further complicated by having a rapidly equilibrating functional component, as well as several more slowly equilibrating nonfunctioning components. The nonfunctioning components include connective tissue water as well as water that has been termed *transcellular,* which includes cerebrospinal and joint fluids. This nonfunctional component normally represents only 10 percent of the interstitial fluid volume (1 to 2 percent of body weight) and is not to be confused with the *relatively* nonfunctional extracellular fluid, often called a "third space," found in burns and soft tissue injuries.

The normal constituents of the extracellular fluid are shown in Fig. 2-2, with sodium the principal cation, and chloride and bicarbonate the principal anions. There are minor differences in ionic composition between the plasma and interstitial fluid that are primarily due to the difference in protein concentration. Because of the higher protein content (organic anions) of the plasma, the total concentration of cations is higher and the concentration of inorganic anions somewhat lower than in the interstitial fluid, as explained by the Gibbs-Donnan equilibrium equation (i.e., the product of the concentrations of any pair of diffusible cations and anions on one side of a semipermeable membrane will equal the product of the same pair of ions on the other side). For practical consideration, however, they may be considered equal. The total concentration of intracellular ions exceeds that of the extracellular compartment and would seem to violate the concept of osmolar equilibrium between the two compartments. This apparent discrepancy is due to the fact that the concentration of ions is expressed in milliequivalents (meq) without regard to osmotic activity. In addition, some of the intracellular cations probably exist in undissociated form.

Osmotic Pressure

The physiologic and chemical activity of electrolytes depend on (1) the *number of particles* present per unit volume [moles or millimoles (mmol) per liter], (2) the *number of electric charges* per unit volume (equivalents or milliequivalents per liter), and (3) the *number of osmotically active particles* or ions per unit volume [osmoles or milliosmoles (mO) per liter]. The use of the terms *grams* or *milligrams per 100 milliliters* expresses the weight of the electrolytes per unit volume but does not allow a physiologic comparison of the solutes in a solution.

A mole of a substance is the molecular weight of that substance in grams, and a millimole is that figure expressed in milligrams. For example, a mole of sodium chloride is 58 grams (Na—23, Cl—35), and a millimole is 58 milligrams. The expression, however, gives no direct information as to the number of osmotically active ions in solution or the electric charges that they carry.

The electrolytes of the body fluids then may be expressed in terms of chemical combining activity, or "equivalents." An equivalent of an ion is its atomic weight expressed in grams divided by the valence, whereas a milliequivalent of an ion is that figure expressed in milligrams. In the case of univalent ions, a milliequivalent is the same as a millimole. In the case of divalent ions, such as calcium or magnesium, one millimole equals two milliequivalents. The importance of this expression is that a milliequivalent of any substance will combine chemically with a milliequivalent of any other substance; in any given solution, the number of milliequivalents of cations present is balanced by precisely the same number of milliequivalents of anions.

When the osmotic pressure of a solution is considered, it is more descriptive to employ the terms osmole and milliosmole. These terms refer to the actual number of osmotically active particles present in solution, but are not dependent on the chemical combining capacities of the substances. Thus, a millimole of sodium chloride, which dissociates nearly completely into sodium and chloride, contributes two milliosmoles, and one millimole of sodium sulfate (Na_2SO_4), which dissociates into three particles, contributes three milliosmoles. One millimole of an un-ionized substance such as glucose is equal to one milliosmole of the substance.

The differences in ionic composition between intracellular and extracellular fluid are maintained by the semipermeable cell membrane. The total number of osmotically active particles is 290 to 310 mO in each compartment. Although the total osmotic pressure of a fluid is the sum of the partial pressures contributed by each of the solutes in that fluid, the *effective* osmotic pressure is dependent on those substances which fail to pass through the pores of the semipermeable membrane. The dissolved proteins in the plasma, therefore, are primarily responsible for effective osmotic pressure between the plasma and the interstitial fluid compartments. This is frequently referred to as the *colloid oncotic pressure.* The effective osmotic pressure between the extracellular and intracellular fluid compartments would be contributed to by any substance that does not traverse the cell membranes freely. Thus, while sodium as the principal cation of the extracellular fluid contributes a major portion of the osmotic pressure, other substances that fail to penetrate the cell membrane freely, such as glucose, also increase the effective osmotic pressure.

Since the cell membranes are completely permeable to water, the effective osmotic pressures in the two compartments are considered to be equal. Any condition that alters the effective osmotic pressure in either compartment will result in redistribution of water between the compartments. Thus, an increase in effective osmotic pressure in the extracellular fluid, which would occur most frequently as a result of increased sodium concentration, would cause a net transfer of water from the intracellular to the extracellular fluid compartment. This transfer of water would continue until the effective osmotic pressures in the two compartments were equal. Conversely, a decrease in the sodium concentration in the extracellular fluid will cause a transfer of water from the extracellular to the intracellular fluid compartment. Depletion of the extracellular fluid volume without a change in the concentration of ions will not result in transfer of free water from the intracellular space.

Thus, the intracellular fluid shares in losses that involve a change in concentration or composition of the extracellular fluid but shares only slowly in changes involving loss of isotonic volume alone. For practical consideration, most losses and gains of body fluid are directly from the extracellular compartment.

NORMAL EXCHANGE OF FLUID AND ELECTROLYTES

Knowledge of the basic principles governing both the internal and external exchanges of water and salt is mandatory for care of the patient undergoing major operative surgery. The stable internal fluid environment, which is maintained by the kidneys, brain, lungs, skin, and gastrointestinal tract, may be compromised by severe surgical stress or direct damage to any of these organs.

Water Exchange

The normal individual consumes an average of 2000 to 2500 mL water/day; approximately 1500 mL water is taken by mouth, and the rest is extracted from solid food, either from the contents of the food or as the product of oxidation (Table 2-1). The daily water losses include 250

mL in stools, 800 to 1500 mL as urine, and approximately 600 mL as insensible loss. A patient deprived of all external access to water must still excrete a minimum of 500 to 800 mL urine/day in order to excrete the products of catabolism, in addition to the mandatory insensible loss through the skin and lungs.

Insensible loss of water occurs through the skin (75 percent) and the lungs (25 percent) and is increased by hypermetabolism, hyperventilation, and fever. The insensible water loss through the skin is not from evaporation of water from sweat glands but from water vapor formed within the body and lost through the skin. With excessive heat production (or excessive environmental heat), the capacity for insensible loss through the skin is exceeded, and sweating occurs. These losses may, but seldom do, exceed 250 mL/day per degree of fever. An unhumidified tracheostomy with hyperventilation increases the loss through the lungs and results in a total insensible loss up to 1.5 L/day.

A frequently overlooked source of gain is the water of solution, which is the water that holds carbohydrates and proteins in solution in the cell. Normally, gain of water from this source is zero, but after 4 to 5 days without food intake, the postoperative patient may begin to gain significant quantities of water (up to 500 mL daily) from excessive cellular catabolism.

Salt Gain and Losses

In the normal individual, the salt intake per day varies between 50 and 90 meq (3 and 5 g) as sodium chloride (Table 2-2). Balance is maintained primarily by the normal kidneys that excrete the excess salt. Under conditions of reduced intake or extrarenal losses, the normal kidney can reduce sodium excretion to less than 1 meq/day within 24 h after restriction. In the patient with salt-wasting kidneys, however, the loss may exceed 200 meq/L of urine. Sweat represents a hypotonic loss of fluids with an average sodium concentration of 15 meq/L in the acclimatized patient. In the unacclimatized individual, the sodium concentration in sweat may be 60 meq/L or more. Insensible fluid lost from the skin and lungs, by

Table 2-1. WATER EXCHANGE (60- to 80-KG MAN)

Routes	Average daily volume, mL	Minimal, mL	Maximal, mL
H$_2$O gain:			
Sensible:			
Oral fluids	800–1500	0	1500/h
Solid foods	500–700	0	1500
Insensible:			
Water of oxidation	250	125	800
Water of solution	0	0	500
H$_2$O loss:			
Sensible:			
Urine	800–1500	300	1400/h (diabetes insipidus)
Intestinal	0–250	0	2500/h
Sweat	0	0	4000/h
Insensible:			
Lungs and skin	600	600	1500

Table 2-2. SODIUM (SALT) EXCHANGE (60- to 80-KG MAN)

Sodium exchange	Average	Minimal	Maximal
Sodium gain:			
Diet	50–90 meq/day	0	75–100 meq/h (oral)
Sodium loss:			
Skin			
(sweat)	10–60 meq/day*	0	300 meq/h
Urine	10–80 meq/day	<1 meq/day†	110–200 meq/L‡
Intestines	0–20 meq/day	0	300 meq/h

* Depending on the degree of acclimatization of the individual.
† With normal renal function.
‡ With renal salt wasting.

Table 2-3. COMPOSITION OF GASTROINTESTINAL SECRETIONS

Type of secretion	Volume (mL/24h)	Na (meq/L)	K (meq/L)	Cl (meq/L)	HCO₃ (meq/L)
Salivary	1500 (500–2000)	10 (2–10)	26 (20–30)	10 (8–18)	30
Stomach	1500 (100–4000)	60 (9–116)	10 (0–32)	130 (8–154)	
Duodenum	(100–2000)	140	5	80	
Ileum	3000 (100–9000)	140 (80–150)	5 (2–8)	104 (43–137)	30
Colon		60	30	40	
Pancreas	(100–800)	140 (113–185)	5 (3–7)	75 (54–95)	115
Bile	(50–800)	145 (131–164)	5 (3–12)	100 (89–180)	35

definition, is pure water. For practical considerations, then, normal losses may be relatively free of salt in the healthy individual with normal renal function.

The volume and composition of various types of gastrointestinal secretions are shown in Table 2-3. Gastrointestinal losses are usually isotonic or slightly hypotonic, although there is considerable variation in the composition. These should be replaced by an essentially isotonic salt solution. It is also important to reiterate that distributional or sequestration losses of extracellular fluid at any point in the operative or postoperative course also represent isotonic losses of salt and water.

CLASSIFICATION OF BODY FLUID CHANGES

The disorders in fluid balance may be classified in three general categories: disturbances of (1) volume, (2) concentration, and (3) composition. Of primary importance is the concept that although these disturbances are interrelated, each is a separate entity.

If an isotonic salt solution is added to or lost from the body fluids, only the *volume* of the extracellular fluid is changed. The acute loss of an isotonic extracellular solution, such as intestinal juice, is followed by a significant decrease in the extracellular fluid volume and little, if any, change in the intracellular fluid volume. Fluid will not be transferred from the intracellular space to refill the depleted extracellular space as long as the osmolarity remains the same in the two compartments.

If water alone is added to or lost from the extracellular fluid, the *concentration* of osmotically active particles will change. Sodium ions account for 90 percent of the osmotically active particles in the extracellular fluid and generally reflect the tonicity of body fluid compartments. If the extracellular fluid is depleted of sodium, water will pass into the intracellular space until osmolarity is again equal in the two compartments.

The concentration of most other ions within the extracellular fluid compartment can be altered without significant change in the total number of osmotically active particles, thus producing only a *compositional* change. For instance, a rise of the serum potassium concentration from 4 to 8 meq/L would have a significant effect on the myocardium, but it would not significantly change the effective osmotic pressure of the extracellular fluid compartment. Normally functioning kidneys minimize these changes considerably, particularly if the addition or loss of solute or water is gradual.

An internal loss of extracellular fluid into a nonfunctional space, such as the sequestration of isotonic fluid in a burn, peritonitis, ascites, or muscle trauma, is termed a *distributional* change. This transfer or functional loss of extracellular fluid internally may be extracellular (e.g., peritonitis) or intracellular (e.g., hemorrhagic shock) or both (e.g., major burns). In any event, all distributional shifts or losses result in a contraction of the *functional* extracellular fluid space.

Volume Changes

Volume deficit or excess generally must be diagnosed by clinical examination of the patient. There are no readily available laboratory tests of benefit in the acute phase except measurement of the plasma volume. Changes secondary to long-standing derangements in volume, however, may be discernible by laboratory tests. For example, the blood urea nitrogen (BUN) level slowly rises with a long-standing extracellular fluid deficit of sufficient magnitude to reduce glomerular filtration. The concentration of serum sodium is *not* related to the volume status of extracellular fluid; a severe volume deficit may exist with a normal, low, or high serum level.

VOLUME DEFICIT. Extracellular fluid volume deficit is by far the most common fluid disorder in the surgical patient. The loss of fluid is not water alone, but water and electrolytes in approximately the same proportion as they exist in normal extracellular fluid. The most common disorders leading to an extracellular fluid volume deficit include losses of gastrointestinal fluids due to vomiting, nasogastric suction, diarrhea, and fistular drainage. Other common causes include sequestration of fluid in soft tissue injuries and infections, intraabdominal and retroperi-

Table 2-4. EXTRACELLULAR FLUID VOLUME

	Deficit		Excess	
Type of sign	Moderate	Severe	Moderate	Severe
Central nervous system	Sleepiness Apathy Slow responses Anorexia Cessation of usual activity	Decreased tension reflexes Anesthesia distal extremities Stupor Coma	None	None
Gastrointestinal	Progressive decrease in food consumption	Nausea, vomiting Refusal to eat Silent ileus and distention	At operation: Edema of stomach, colon, lesser and greater omenta, and small bowel mesentery	
Cardiovascular	Orthostatic hypotension Tachycardia Collapsed veins Collapsing pulse	Cutaneous lividity Hypotension Distant heart sounds Cold extremities Absent peripheral pulses	Elevated venous pressure Distention of peripheral veins Increased cardiac output Loud heart sounds Functional murmurs Bounding pulse High pulse pressure Increased pulmonary 2d sound Gallop	Pulmonary edema
Tissue	Soft, small tongue with longitudinal wrinkling Decreased skin turgor	Atonic muscles Sunken eyes	Subcutaneous pitting edema Basilar rales	Anasarca Moist rales Vomiting Diarrhea
Metabolic	Mild decrease temperature, 97–99°R	Marked decrease temperature, 95–98°R	None	None

toneal inflammatory processes, peritonitis, intestinal obstruction, and burns. The signs and symptoms of this state are easily recognized and are listed in Table 2-4. The central nervous system and cardiovascular signs occur early with acute rapid losses, whereas tissue signs may be absent until the deficit has existed for at least 24 h. The central nervous system signs are similar to barbiturate intoxication and may be missed by the casual observer if the volume deficit is mild. The cardiovascular signs are secondary to a decrease in plasma volume and may be associated with varying degrees of hypotension in the patient with a severe extracellular fluid volume deficit. Skin turgor may be difficult to assess in the elderly patient or in the patient with recent weight loss and is not diagnostic in the absence of other confirmatory signs. The body temperature tends to vary with the environmental temperature. In a cool room, the patient may be slightly hypothermic and the febrile response to illness may be suppressed. This occurs frequently and can be very misleading during clinical evaluation of the septic patient. After partial correction of the volume deficit, the temperature will generally rise to the appropriate level.

VOLUME EXCESS. Extracellular fluid volume excess may be generally iatrogenic or secondary to renal insufficiency, cirrhosis, or congestive heart failure. Both the plasma and interstitial fluid volumes are increased. In the healthy young adult, the signs are generally those of circulatory overload, manifested primarily in the pulmonary circulation, and of excessive fluid in other tissue (Table 2-4). In the elderly patient, congestive heart failure with pulmonary edema may develop rather quickly with a moderate volume excess.

Concentration Changes

Sodium is primarily responsible for the osmolarity of the extracellular fluid space: determination of the serum concentration of sodium generally indicates the tonicity of body fluids. Hyponatremia and hypernatremia can be diagnosed on clinical grounds (Table 2-5), but signs and symptoms are not generally present until the changes are severe. Clinical signs of hyponatremia or hypernatremia tend to occur early and with greater severity if the rate of change in extracellular sodium concentration is very rapid. Changes in concentration should be noted early by laboratory tests and corrected promptly.

HYPONATREMIA. Acute symptomatic hyponatremia (sodium less than 130 meq/L) clinically is characterized by central nervous system signs of increased intracranial pressure and tissue signs of excessive intracellular water. The hypertension is probably induced by the rise in intracranial pressure, since the blood pressure generally returns to normal with the administration of hypertonic solutions of sodium salts. Of importance with severe

Table 2-5. ACUTE CHANGES IN OSMOLAR CONCENTRATION

Type of signs	Hyponatremia (water intoxication)		Hypernatremia (water deficit)	
Central nervous system	Moderate: Muscle twitching Hyperactive tendon reflexes Increased intra-cranial pressure (compensated phase)	Severe: Convulsions Loss of reflexes Increased intra-cranial pressure (decompensated) phase)	Moderate: Restlessness Weakness	Severe: Delirium Maniacal be-havior
Cardiovascular	Changes in blood pressure and pulse secondary to increased intracranial pressure		Tachycardia Hypotension (if severe)	
Tissue	Salivation, lacrimation, watery diarrhea "Fingerprinting" of skin (sign of intracellular volume excess)		Decreased saliva and tears Dry and sticky mucous membranes Red, swollen tongue Skin flushed	
Renal	Oliguria progressing to anuria		Oliguria	
Metabolic	None		Fever	

hyponatremia is the relatively rapid development of oliguric renal failure, which may not be reversible if therapy is delayed.

Many chronic hyponatremic states are asymptomatic until the serum sodium level falls below 120 meq/L. One important exception is the patient with increased cerebrospinal fluid pressure, following closed head injury, in whom mild hyponatremia may be fatal, because of the progressive increase in intracellular water as the extracellular fluid osmolarity falls.

HYPERNATREMIA. Central nervous system and tissue signs characterize acute symptomatic hypernatremia. This is the only state in which dry, sticky mucous membranes are characteristic. This sign does not occur with pure extracellular fluid volume deficit alone, and may be misleading in the patient who breathes through his mouth. Body temperature is generally elevated and may approach a lethal level, as in the patient with heatstroke.

While volume changes occur frequently without a change in serum sodium, the reverse is not true. The disease states that cause a significant acute alteration in the serum sodium frequently produce a concomitant change in the extracellular fluid volume.

Mixed Volume and Concentration Abnormalities

Mixed volume and concentration abnormalities may develop as a consequence of the disease state or occasionally may result from inappropriate parenteral fluid therapy. Moyer noted that the clinical picture associated with a combination of fluid abnormalities will tend to be an algebraic composite of the signs and symptoms of each state. Like signs produced by both abnormalities will be additive, and opposing signs will tend to nullify one an-

other. For example, the tendency for the body temperature to fall with an extracellular volume deficit may be counteracted by the tendency for it to rise with severe hypernatremia.

One of the more common mixed abnormalities is an extracellular fluid deficit and hyponatremia. This state is readily produced in the patient who continues to drink water while losing large volumes of gastrointestinal fluids. It may also occur in the postoperative period when gastrointestinal losses are replaced with inadequate volumes of only 5% dextrose in water or a hypotonic sodium solution. An extracellular volume deficit accompanied by hypernatremia may be produced by the loss of a large amount of hypotonic salt solution, such as sweat, in the absence of fluid intake.

The prolonged administration of excessive quantities of sodium salts with restricted water intake may result in an extracellular volume excess and hypernatremia. This may also occur when pure water losses (such as insensible loss of water from the skin and lungs) are replaced with sodium-containing solutions only. Similarly, the excessive administration of water or hypotonic salt solutions to the patient with oliguric renal failure may rapidly produce an extracellular volume excess and hyponatremia.

Normally functioning kidneys may minimize these changes to some extent and compensate for many of the imprecise replacements associated with parenteral fluid administration. In contrast, the patient in anuric or oliguric renal failure is particularly prone to develop these mixed volume and osmolar concentration abnormalities. Fluid and electrolyte management in these patients, therefore, must be precise. Unfortunately, the fact that a patient with normal kidneys who develops a significant volume deficit may be in a state of "functional" renal failure is often not appreciated. As the volume deficit progresses, the glomerular filtration rate falls precipitously, and the kidneys' unique functions for maintaining fluid homeostasis are lost. These changes may occur with only a mild volume deficit in the elderly patient with borderline renal function. In these elderly patients, the blood urea nitrogen level may rise higher than 100 mg/dL in response to the fluid deficit with a concomitant rise in the serum creatinine level. Fortunately, these changes are usually reversible with early and adequate correction of the extracellular fluid volume deficit.

Composition Changes

Compositional abnormalities of importance include changes in acid-base balance and concentration changes of potassium, calcium, and magnesium.

ACID-BASE BALANCE

The pH (the negative logarithm of the hydrogen ion concentration) of the body fluids is normally maintained within narrow limits in spite of the large load of acid produced endogenously as a by-product of body metabolism. The acids are neutralized efficiently by several buffer systems and subsequently excreted by the lungs and kidneys.

The important buffers include proteins and phosphates, which play a primary role in maintaining intracellular pH, and the bicarbonate–carbonic acid system, which operates principally in the extracellular fluid space. The proteins and hemoglobin have only minor influence in the extracellular fluid space, but the latter is of prime significance as an intracellular buffer in the red cell.

A buffer system consists of a weak acid or base and the salt of that acid or base. The buffering effect is the result of the formation of an amount of weak acid or base equivalent to the amount of strong acid or base added to the system. The resultant change in pH is considerably less than if the substance were added to water alone. Thus, inorganic acids (e.g., hydrochloric, sulfuric, phosphoric) and organic acids (e.g., lactic, pyruvic, keto acids) combine with base bicarbonate producing the sodium salt of the acid and carbonic acid:

$$HCl + NaHCO_3 \longrightarrow NaCl + H_2CO_3$$

The carbonic acid formed is then excreted via the lungs as CO_2. The inorganic acid anions are excreted by the kidneys with hydrogen or as ammonium salts. The organic acid anions generally are metabolized as the underlying disorder is corrected, although some renal excretion may occur with high levels.

The functions of the buffer systems are expressed in the Henderson-Hasselbalch equation, which defines the pH in terms of the ratio of the salt and acid. The pH of the extracellular fluid is defined primarily by the ratio of the amount of base bicarbonate (majority as sodium bicarbonate) to the amount of carbonic acid (related to the CO_2 content of alveolar air) present in the blood:

$$pH = pK + \log\frac{BHCO_3}{H_2CO_3} = \frac{27 \text{ meq/L}}{1.33 \text{ meq/L}} = \frac{20}{1} = 7.4$$

pK represents the dissociation constant of carbonic acid in the presence of base bicarbonate and by measurement is 6.1. At a body pH of 7.4, the ratio must be 20:1, as depicted. From a chemical standpoint, this is an inefficient buffer system, but the unusual property of CO_2 to behave as an acid or change to a neutral gas subsequently excreted by the lungs makes it quite efficient biologically.

As long as the 20:1 ratio is maintained, regardless of the absolute values, the pH will remain at 7.4. When an acid is added to the system, the concentration of bicarbonate (the numerator in the Henderson-Hasselbalch equation) will decrease. Ventilation will immediately increase to eliminate larger quantities of CO_2 with a subsequent decrease in the carbonic acid (the denominator in the Henderson-Hasselbalch equation) until the 20:1 ratio is reestablished. Slower, more complete compensation is effected by the kidneys with increased excretion of acid salts and retention of bicarbonate. The reverse will occur if an alkali is added to the system. Respiratory acidosis and alkalosis are produced by disturbances of ventilation, with an increase or decrease in the denominator and a resultant change of the 20:1 ratio. Compensation is primarily renal, with a retention of bicarbonate and increased excretion of acid salts in respiratory acidosis and the reverse process in respiratory alkalosis.

The four types of acid-base disturbances are listed in Table 2-6. Use of the CO_2 combining power (approximates the plasma bicarbonate) or CO_2 content (includes bicarbonate, carbonic acid, and dissolved CO_2) and knowledge of the patient's disease may allow an accurate diagnosis in the uncomplicated case. Use of the serum CO_2 content or CO_2 combining power alone is generally inadequate as an index of acid-base balance. This test principally reflects the level of plasma bicarbonate, since dissolved CO_2 and carbonic acid contribute no more than a few millimoles under most circumstances. In the acute phase, therefore, respiratory acidosis or alkalosis may exist without any change in the serum CO_2 content; determinations of the pH and P_{CO_2} from a freshly drawn arterial blood sample are necessary for diagnosis.

Unfortunately, more complex acid-base disturbances are frequently encountered. Combinations of respiratory and metabolic changes occur and may represent compensation for the initial acid-base disturbance or may indicate two or more coexisting primary disorders (Table 2-7).

As previously noted, a knowledge of the pH, bicarbonate concentration, and P_{CO_2} will allow an accurate diagnosis of most acid-base disturbances. However, the clinical interpretation of these measurements is associated with some inherent problems. Although the arterial P_{CO_2} is considered an accurate index of primary respiratory disturbances, changes in the level may represent compensation for a primary metabolic alteration. Thus, a depressed P_{CO_2} (below 40 mmHg) is characteristic of respiratory alkalosis but also represents the normal compensatory response to a metabolic acidosis. Similarly, the level of plasma bicarbonate cannot be regarded exclusively as an index of metabolic disturbances. An elevated plasma bicarbonate level may indicate a primary metabolic alkalosis or a compensatory response to chronic respiratory

Table 2-6. ACIDOSIS-ALKALOSIS

Type of acid-base disorder	Defect	Common causes	$\dfrac{BHCO_3}{H_2CO_3} = \dfrac{20}{1}$	Compensation
Respiratory acidosis	Retention of CO_2 (Decreased alveolar ventilation)	Depression of respiratory center—morphine, CNS injury Pulmonary disease—emphysema, pneumonia	↑ Denominator Ratio less than 20:1	Renal Retention of bicarbonate, excretion of acid salts, increased ammonia formation Chloride shift into red cells
Respiratory alkalosis	Excessive loss of CO_2 (increased alveolar ventilation)	Hyperventilation: Emotional, severe pain, assisted ventilation, encephalitis	↓ Denominator Ratio greater than 20:1	Renal Excretion of bicarbonate, retention of acid salts, decreased ammonia formation
Metabolic acidosis	Retention of fixed acids or Loss of base bicarbonate	Diabetes, azotemia, lactic acid accumulation, starvation Diarrhea, small bowel fistulae	↓ Numerator Ratio less than 20:1	Pulmonary (rapid) Increase rate and depth of breathing Renal (slow) As in respiratory acidosis
Metabolic alkalosis	Loss of fixed acids Gain of base bicarbonate Potassium depletion	Vomiting or gastric suction with pyloric obstruction Excessive intake of bicarbonate Diuretics	↑ Numerator Ratio greater than 20:1	Pulmonary (rapid) Decrease rate and depth of breathing Renal (slow) As in respiratory alkalosis

acidosis. Astrup and colleagues proposed the use of the standard bicarbonate and base excess values. Base excess (or deficit) directly expresses, in meq/L, the amount of fixed base (or acid) added to each liter of blood. This defines the *metabolic* component of acid-base disorders.

One useful approach to defining pure, combined, or compensated disturbances relates measured changes in P_{CO_2} and pH to calculated changes that would be expected from pure etiologies. Within reasonable physiologic ranges, a 10-torr change in P_{CO_2} yields a 0.08 change in pH from the normal values of P_{CO_2} (40 torr) and pH (7.4).

RESPIRATORY ACIDOSIS. This condition is associated with retention of CO_2 secondary to decreased alveolar

Table 2-7. RESPIRATORY AND METABOLIC COMPONENTS OF ACID-BASE DISORDERS

Type of acid-base disorder	Acute (uncompensated)			Chronic (partially compensated)		
	pH	P_{CO_2} (respiratory component)	Plasma HCO_3^-* (metabolic component)	pH	P_{CO_2} (respiratory component)	Plasma HCO_3^-* (metabolic component)
Respiratory acidosis	⇊	⇈	N	↓	⇈	↑
Respiratory alkalosis	⇈	⇊	N	↑	⇊	↓
Metabolic acidosis	⇊	N	⇊	↓	↓	↓
Metabolic alkalosis	⇈	N	⇈	↑	↑?	↑

* Measured as standard bicarbonate, whole blood buffer base, CO_2 content, or CO_2 combining power. The *base excess value* is positive when the standard bicarbonate is above normal and negative when the standard bicarbonate is below normal.

tration of approximately 150 meq/L, and it is the major cation of intracellular water. Although the total extracellular potassium in a 70-kg male would approximate only 63 meq (4.5 meq/L × 14 L), this small amount is critical to cardiac and neuromuscular function. In addition, the turnover rate in the extracellular fluid compartment may be extremely rapid.

The intracellular and extracellular distribution of potassium is influenced by many factors. Significant quantities of intracellular potassium are released into the extracellular space in response to severe injury or surgical stress, acidosis, and the catabolic state. A significant rise in serum potassium may occur in these states in the presence of oliguric or anuric renal failure, but dangerous hyperkalemia (greater than 6 meq/L) is rarely encountered if renal function is normal. After severe trauma, however, normal or excessive urinary volumes may not reflect the ability of the kidney to clear solutes or to excrete potassium. (See the section High-Output Renal Failure.)

HYPERKALEMIA. The signs of a significant hyperkalemia are limited to the cardiovascular and gastrointestinal systems. The gastrointestinal symptoms include nausea, vomiting, intermittent intestinal colic, and diarrhea. The cardiovascular signs are apparent on the electrocardiogram initially, with high peaked T waves, widened QRS complex, and depressed ST segments. Disappearance of T waves, heart block, and diastolic cardiac arrest may develop with increasing levels of potassium.

Treatment of hyperkalemia consists of immediate measures to reduce the serum potassium level, withholding of exogenous potassium, and correction of the underlying cause if possible. Temporary suppression of the myocardial effects of a sudden rapid rise of potassium level can be accomplished by the intravenous administration of 1 g of 10 percent calcium gluconate under ECG monitoring. Serum potassium levels may be transiently decreased by administration of bicarbonate and glucose with insulin (45 meq $NaHCO_3$ in 1000 mL/D_{10}W with 20 units regular insulin), both of which promote cellular uptake of potassium. However, the definitive treatment of hyperkalemia requires either the enteral administration of cation exchange resins (kayexalate) or dialysis.

HYPOKALEMIA. The more common problem in the surgical patient is hypokalemia, which may occur as a result of (1) excessive renal excretion, (2) movement of potassium into cells, (3) prolonged administration of potassium-free parenteral fluids with continued obligatory renal loss of potassium (20 meq/day or more), (4) total parenteral hyperalimentation with inadequate potassium replacement, and (5) loss in gastrointestinal secretions.

Potassium plays an important role in the regulation of acid-base balance. Increased renal excretion occurs with both respiratory and metabolic alkalosis. Potassium is in competition with hydrogen ion for renal tubular excretion in exchange for sodium ion. Thus, in alkalosis, the increased potassium ion excretion in exchange for sodium ion permits hydrogen ion conservation. Hypokalemia itself may produce a metabolic alkalosis, since an increase in excretion of hydrogen ions occurs when the concentra-

tion of potassium in the tubular cell is low. In addition, movement of hydrogen ions into the cells as a consequence of potassium loss is partly responsible for the alkalosis. In metabolic acidosis the reverse process occurs, and the excess hydrogen ion exchanges for sodium with retention of greater amounts of potassium.

Renal tubular excretion of potassium ion is increased when large quantities of sodium are available for excretion. The more sodium ion available for resorption, the more potassium is exchanged for it in the lumen. Potassium requirements for prolonged or massive isotonic fluid volume replacement are increased, probably on this basis.

The renal excretion of potassium may be small when compared with the amount of potassium that may be lost in gastrointestinal secretions. The amount per liter in various types of gastrointestinal fluids is shown in Table 2-3. Although the average potassium concentration of some of these fluids is relatively low, significant hypokalemia will result if potassium-free fluids are used for replacement.

Hypokalemia also may be a serious problem in the patient maintained on intravenous nutrition. Large quantities of supplemental potassium generally are necessary to restore depleted intracellular stores and to meet the requirements for tissue synthesis during the anabolic phase.

In summary, most of the factors that tend to influence potassium metabolism result in excess excretion, and a tendency toward hypokalemia occurs frequently in the surgical patient except when shock or acidosis interferes with the normal renal handling of potassium.

The signs of potassium deficit are related to failure of normal contractility of skeletal, smooth, and cardiac muscle and include weakness that may progress to flaccid paralysis, diminished to absent tendon reflexes, and paralytic ileus. Sensitivity to digitalis with cardiac arrhythmias and electrocardiographic signs of low voltage, flattening of T waves, and depression of ST segments are characteristic. Signs of potassium deficit may be masked by those of a severe extracellular fluid volume deficit. Repletion of the volume deficit may further aggravate the situation by lowering the serum potassium level secondary to dilution.

The treatment of hypokalemia involves, first, prevention of this state. In the replacement of gastrointestinal fluids, it is safe to replace the upper limits of loss, since an excess is readily handled by the patient with normal renal function. No more than 40 meq should be added to a liter of intravenous fluid, and the rate of administration should not exceed 40 meq/h unless the electrocardiogram is being monitored. In the absence of specific indications, potassium should not be given to the oliguric patient or during the first 24 h following severe surgical stress or trauma.

CALCIUM ABNORMALITIES

The majority of the 1000 to 1200 g of body calcium in the average-sized adult is found in the bone in the form of phosphate and carbonate. Normal daily intake of calcium is between 1 and 3 g. Most of this is excreted via the gastrointestinal tract, and 200 mg or less is excreted in the urine daily. The normal serum level is between 8.5 and 10.5 mg/dL, and approximately half of this is not ionized and is bound to plasma protein. An additional nonionized fraction (5 percent) is bound to other substances in the plasma and interstitial fluid, whereas the remaining 45 percent is the ionized portion that is responsible for neuromuscular stability. Determination of the plasma protein level, therefore, is essential for proper analysis of the serum calcium level. The ratio of ionized to nonionized calcium is also related to the pH; acidosis causes an increase in the ionized fraction, whereas alkalosis causes a decrease.

Disturbances of calcium metabolism generally are not a problem in the uncomplicated postoperative patient, with the exception of skeletal loss during prolonged immobilization. Routine administration of calcium to the surgical patient, therefore, is not needed in the absence of specific indications.

HYPOCALCEMIA. The symptoms of hypocalcemia may be seen at serum levels less than 8 mg/dL, and include numbness and tingling of the circumoral region and the tips of the fingers and toes. The signs are of neuromuscular origin and include hyperactive tendon reflexes, positive Chvostek's sign, muscle and abdominal cramps, tetany with carpopedal spasm, convulsions (with severe deficit), and prolongation of the Q-T interval on the electrocardiogram.

The common causes include acute pancreatitis, massive soft tissue infections (necrotizing fasciitis), acute and chronic renal failure, pancreatic and small intestinal fistulas, and hypoparathyroidism. Transient hypocalcemia is a frequent occurrence in the hyperparathyroid patient following removal of a parathyroid adenoma, owing to atrophy of the remaining glands and avid bone uptake. Asymptomatic hypocalcemia may occur with hypoproteinemia (normal ionized fraction), whereas symptoms may appear with a normal serum calcium level in a patient with severe alkalosis. The latter is due to a decrease in the physiologically active or ionized fraction of total serum calcium. Calcium levels also may fall with a severe depletion of magnesium.

Treatment is directed toward correction of the underlying cause with concomitant repletion of the deficit. Acute symptoms may be relieved by the intravenous administration of calcium gluconate or calcium chloride. Calcium lactate may be given orally, with or without supplemental vitamin D, in the patient requiring prolonged replacement. The routine administration of calcium during massive transfusions of blood remains controversial and reflects a paucity of studies where calcium *ion* levels are measured. In the majority of studies, calcium ion concentrations have been estimated from measured *total* serum calcium levels. Presently, available data indicate that the majority of patients receiving blood transfusions do not require calcium supplementation. The binding of ionized calcium by citrate is generally compensated for by the mobilization of calcium from body stores. For patients receiving blood as rapidly as 500 mL every 5 to 10 min, however, calcium administration is recommended. An appropriate dose, from the data of Moore, is 0.2 g of calcium chloride (2 mL of 10% calcium chloride solution), administered intravenously in a separate line, for every 500 mL of blood transfused. To avoid dangerous levels of hypercalcemia, this dose of calcium is recommended only while blood is being transfused at the rate noted above. Additionally, the total dose of calcium generally should not exceed 3 g unless there is objective evidence of hypocalcemia. Larger doses are rarely indicated since there is some mobilization of calcium and citrate breakdown with release of calcium ion even with shock and inadequate peripheral perfusion. During massive transfusions, some attempt should be made to monitor the calcium level. A rough approximation of calcium ion concentration can be obtained by monitoring the Q-T interval on the ECG, although techniques for the rapid measurement of calcium ion concentration are now available.

HYPERCALCEMIA. The symptoms of hypercalcemia are rather vague and of gastrointestinal, renal, musculoskeletal, and central nervous system origin. The early manifestations of hypercalcemia include easy fatigue, lassitude, weakness of varying degree, anorexia, nausea, vomiting, and weight loss. With higher serum calcium levels, lassitude gives way to somnambulism, stupor, and finally coma. Other symptoms include severe headaches, pains in the back and extremities, thirst, polydipsia, and polyuria. The critical level for serum calcium is between 16 and 20 mg/100 mL, and unless treatment is instituted promptly, the symptoms may rapidly progress to death. The two major causes of hypercalcemia are hyperparathyroidism and cancer with bony metastasis. The latter is most frequently seen in the patient with metastatic breast cancer who is receiving estrogen therapy.

The treatment of acute hypercalcemia crisis is an emergency. Measures to lower the serum calcium level are instituted immediately while preparations are being made for more definitive treatment. Rapid correction of the associated extracellular fluid volume deficit will immediately lower the serum calcium level by dilution and by increased renal clearance that may be augmented by furosemide administration. Other measures that may be of temporary benefit include the use of calcitonin, mithramycin, steroids, or hemodialysis. The definitive treatment of acute hypercalcemic crisis in patients with hyperparathyroidism is immediate surgery.

Treatment of hypercalcemia in the patient with metastatic cancer is primarily that of prevention. The serum calcium level is checked frequently; if it is elevated, the patient is placed on a low-calcium diet, and measures to ensure adequate hydration are instituted.

MAGNESIUM ABNORMALITIES

The total body content of magnesium in the average adult is approximately 2000 meq, about half of which is incorporated in bone and only slowly exchangeable. The distribution of magnesium is similar to that of potassium, the major portion being intracellular. Serum magnesium concentration normally ranges between 1.5 and 2.5 meq/L. The normal dietary intake of magnesium is approximately 20 meq (240 mg) daily. The larger part is excreted in the feces, and the remainder in the urine. The kidneys show a remarkable ability to conserve magnesium; on a magnesium-free diet, renal excretion of this ion may be less than 1 meq/day.

MAGNESIUM DEFICIENCY. Magnesium deficiency is known to occur with starvation, malabsorption syndromes, protracted losses of gastrointestinal fluid, and prolonged intravenous fluid therapy with magnesium-free solutions, and during total parenteral nutrition when inadequate quantities of magnesium have been added to the solutions. Other causes include acute pancreatitis, treatment of diabetic ketoacidosis, primary aldosteronism, chronic alcoholism, amphotericin B therapy, and a protracted course following thermal injury.

The magnesium ion is essential for proper function of most enzyme systems, and depletion is characterized by neuromuscular and central nervous system hyperactivity. The signs and symptoms are quite similar to those of calcium deficiency, including hyperactive tendon reflexes, muscle tremors, and tetany with a positive Chvostek sign. Progression to delirium and convulsions may occur with a severe deficit. A concomitant calcium deficiency occasionally is noted, and will be refractory to treatment in the absence of magnesium repletion.

The diagnosis of magnesium deficiency depends on an awareness of the syndrome and clinical recognition of the symptoms. Laboratory confirmation is available but not reliable, as the syndrome may exist in the presence of a normal serum magnesium level. The possibility of magnesium deficiency should always be considered in the surgical patient who exhibits disturbed neuromuscular or cerebral activity in the postoperative period. This is particularly important in patients who have had protracted dysfunction of the gastrointestinal tract with long-term maintenance on parenteral fluids and in patients on parenteral hyperalimentation. Routine magnesium is always indicated in the management of these patients.

Treatment of magnesium deficiency is by the parenteral administration of magnesium sulfate or magnesium chloride solution. If renal function is normal, as much as 2 meq of magnesium/kg of body weight can be administered daily by the intravenous or intramuscular route in the face of severe depletion. The intravenous route is preferable for the initial treatment of a severe symptomatic deficit. The solution is prepared by the addition of 80 meq of magnesium sulfate (20 mL of 50% solution containing 4 meq/mL magnesium) to a liter of intravenous fluid and is administered over a 4-h period. If the patient is not symptomatic, the infusion should be given over a longer period of time. The possibility of acute magnesium toxicity should be kept in mind when giving this ion intravenously. When large doses are given, the heart rate, blood pressure, respiration, and ECG should be monitored closely for signs of magnesium toxicity, which could lead to cardiac arrest. It is advisable to have calcium chloride or calcium gluconate available to counteract any adverse effects of a rapidly rising serum magnesium level.

Partial or complete relief of symptoms may follow this infusion as a result of increased concentration of magnesium ion in the extracellular fluid compartment, although continued replacement over a 1- to 3-week period is necessary to replenish the intracellular compartment. For this purpose and for the asymptomatic patient who may have significant magnesium depletion, 10 to 20 meq of 50% magnesium sulfate solution may be given daily by the intramuscular route, in intravenous fluids, or orally as magnesium oxide (800 mg). When intramuscular magnesium sulfate is used, it should be given in divided doses or at multiple sites, since the intramuscular injection of this salt is painful. Following complete repletion of intracellular magnesium and in the absence of abnormal loss, balance may be maintained by the administration of as little as 4 meq of magnesium ion daily. The amount of magnesium supplementation required for patients on parenteral hyperalimentation varies but approximates 12 to 24 meq daily for the average patient.

Magnesium ion should not be given to the oliguric patient or in the presence of severe volume deficit unless actual magnesium depletion is demonstrated. If given to a patient with renal insufficiency, considerably smaller dosages are used, and the patient is carefully observed for signs or symptoms of toxicity.

MAGNESIUM EXCESS. Symptomatic hypermagnesemia, although rare, is most commonly seen with severe renal insufficiency. Retention and accumulation of magnesium may occur in any patient with impaired glomerular or renal tubular function, and the presence of acidosis may rapidly compound the situation. Serum magnesium levels tend to parallel changes in potassium concentration in these cases. In patients on ordinary dietary intakes of magnesium, increased serum concentrations of the ion do not occur until the glomerular filtration rate falls below 30 mL/min. Magnesium-containing antacids and laxatives (milk of magnesia, epsom salts, Gelusil, Maalox) are commonly administered in quantities sufficient to produce toxic serum levels of magnesium where impaired renal function is present. Other conditions that may be associated with symptomatic hypermagnesemia include early thermal injury, massive trauma or surgical stress, severe extracellular volume deficit, and severe acidosis.

The early signs and symptoms include lethargy and weakness with progressive loss of deep tendon reflexes. Interference with cardiac conduction occurs with increasing levels of magnesium and changes in the electrocardiogram (increased P-R interval, widened QRS complex, and elevated T waves) resemble those seen with hyperkalemia. Somnolence leading to coma and muscular paralysis occur in the later stages, and death is usually caused by respiratory or cardiac arrest.

Treatment consists of immediate measures to lower the serum magnesium level by correcting coexisting acidosis, replenishing preexisting extracellular volume deficit, and withholding exogenous magnesium. Acute symptoms may be temporarily controlled by the slow intravenous administration of 5 to 10 meq of calcium chloride or calcium gluconate. If elevated levels or symptoms persist, peritoneal dialysis or hemodialysis is indicated.

A readily available isotonic salt solution for replacing gastrointestinal losses and repairing preexisting volume deficits, in the absence of gross abnormalities of concentration and composition, is lactated Ringer's solution. This solution is "physiologic" and contains 130 meq/L sodium balanced by 109 meq/L chloride and 28 meq/L lactate. This fluid has minimal effects on normal body fluid composition and pH even when infused in large quantities. In a study of 52 patients in hemorrhagic shock, Canizaro et al. demonstrated a significant decrease in serum lactate levels and a return toward normal in serum pH during resuscitation with Ringer's lactate solution. The chief disadvantage of lactated Ringer's solution is the slight hyposmolarity with respect to sodium. Each liter of lactated Ringer's solution furnishes approximately 100 to 150 mL free water. This rarely presents a clinical problem if it is considered in calculating water replacement.

Normal saline is an isotonic solution of 0.9 percent sodium chloride and contains 154 meq/L sodium and 154 meq/L chloride. The high concentration of chloride above the normal serum concentration of 103 meq/L imposes on the kidneys an appreciable load of excess chloride that cannot be rapidly excreted. As such, infusion of a large volume of isotonic sodium chloride solution may induce or aggravate a preexisting acidosis by reducing the amount of bicarbonate anion in the body relative to the carbonic acid content. This solution is ideal, however, for the initial correction of an extracellular fluid volume deficit in the presence of hyponatremia, hypochloremia, and metabolic alkalosis.

A frequent choice for maintenance fluid in the postoperative period, 0.45% sodium chloride in 5% dextrose, provides free water for insensible losses and some sodium for renal adjustment of serum concentration. Potassium (10 to 30 meq/L) may be easily added and is increasingly provided as a prepackaged infusion with this solution for easy administration in the uncomplicated patient requiring a short period of parenteral fluids.

Solutions of 3% sodium chloride, 5% sodium chloride, or molar sodium lactate may be used to correct symptomatic hyponatremic states. The choice of anion (lactate or chloride) is determined by the accompanying acid-base derangement. The need for hydrochloric acid solutions in the treatment of an uncompensated metabolic alkalosis is extremely rare. Indications for its use include very shallow or slow breathing with cyanosis, severe tetany, or pH greater than 7.55. Following the correction of concentration or compositional abnormalities using specific electrolyte solutions, a balanced salt solution is used to replenish the remaining volume deficit.

FLUID AND ELECTROLYTE THERAPY

Parenteral Solutions

There are many electrolyte solutions of varied compositions that are available for parenteral administration (Table 2-8). Several of the more commonly used solutions are discussed below. Choice of a particular fluid depends on the volume status of the patient and the type of concentration or compositional abnormality present.

Preoperative Fluid Therapy

Preoperative evaluation and correction of existing fluid disorders is an integral part of surgical care. An orderly approach to these problems requires an understanding of the common fluid disturbances associated with surgical illness and adherence to a few simple guidelines.

The analysis of a particular fluid disorder may be facilitated by categorizing the abnormalities into volume, concentration, and compositional changes. Although some disease states produce characteristic changes in fluid balance, much confusion may be avoided by regarding each disturbance as a separate entity. There are no shortcuts; close observation of the patient and frequent reevaluation of the clinical situation is the most rewarding approach. For example, volume changes cannot be accurately predicted from a knowledge of the level of serum sodium, since an extracellular fluid volume deficit or excess may exist with a normal, low, or high sodium concentration. Similarly, any of the four primary acid-base disturbances may be associated with any combination of volume and concentration abnormalities.

CORRECTION OF VOLUME CHANGES

Changes in the volume of extracellular fluid are the most frequent and important abnormalities encountered in the surgical patient. Depletion of the extracellular fluid

Table 2-8. COMPOSITION OF PARENTERAL FLUIDS
(Electrolyte Content, meq/L)

Solutions	Cations				Anions		Osmolality, mO
	Na	K	Ca	Mg	Cl	HCO₃	
Extracellular fluid	142	4	5	3	103	27	280–310
Lactated Ringer's	130	4	3	—	109	28*	273
0.9% sodium chloride	154	—	—	—	154	—	308
D₅ 45% sodium chloride	77	—	—	—	77	—	407
D₅W	—	—	—	—	—	—	253
M/6 sodium lactate	167	—	—	—	—	167*	334
3% sodium chloride	513	—	—	—	513	—	1026

* Present in solution as lactate that is converted to bicarbonate.

compartment without changes in concentration or composition is a common problem. The diagnosis of volume changes is made almost entirely on clinical grounds. The signs that will be present in an individual patient depend not only on the relative or absolute quantity of extracellular fluid that has been lost but also on the rapidity with which it is lost and the presence or absence of signs of associated disease.

Volume deficits in the surgical patient may result from external loss of fluids or from an internal redistribution of extracellular fluid into a nonfunctional compartment. Generally, it involves a combination of the two, but the internal redistribution is frequently overlooked.

The phenomenon of internal redistribution or translocation of extracellular fluid is peculiar to many surgical diseases; in the individual patient, the loss may be quite large. Although the concept of a "third space" is not new, it is generally considered only in relation to patients with massive ascites, burns, or crush injuries. Of more importance, however, is the "third space" loss into the peritoneum, the bowel wall, and other tissues with inflammatory lesions of the intraabdominal organs. The magnitude of these losses may not be fully appreciated without realization of the fact that the peritoneum alone has approximately 1 m^2 of surface area. A slight increase in thickness from sequestration of fluid, which would not be appreciated on casual observation, may result in a functional loss of several liters of fluid. Swelling of the bowel wall and mesentery and secretion of fluid into the lumen of the bowel will cause even larger losses. Similar deficits may occur with massive infection of the subcutaneous tissues (necrotizing fasciitis) or with severe crush injury.

These "parasitic" losses remain a part of the extracellular fluid space and may be measured as a slowly equilibrating volume. The term *nonfunctional* is used because the fluid is no longer able to participate in the normal functions of the extracellular compartment and may just as well have been lost externally. Any transfer of intracellular fluid to the extracellular compartment for replenishment of the loss is insignificant in the acute phase. The patient with ascites may have an enormous total extracellular fluid volume although the functional component is severely depleted. The same is true of extensive inflammatory or obstructive lesions of the gastrointestinal tract, although the loss is not as obvious. These losses will evoke the signs and symptoms of an extracellular fluid volume deficit with or without the concomitant external loss of fluids.

Exact quantification of these deficits is impossible and, at the present time, probably unnecessary. The defect can be estimated on the basis of the severity of the clinical signs. A mild deficit represents a loss of approximately 4 percent of body weight, a moderate loss is 6 to 8 percent of body weight, and a severe deficit is approximately 10 percent of body weight. It is important to reemphasize the fact that cardiovascular signs predominate when there is acute rapid loss of fluid from the extracellular fluid compartment with few or no tissue signs. In addition to the estimated deficit, fluids lost during the period of treatment must be replaced.

Immediately following diagnosis of a volume deficit, prompt fluid replacement with a balanced salt solution should be started. Continuing thereapy is tailored to the response of the patient, based on frequent clinical examination. Reliance on a formula or single clinical sign to determine adequacy of resuscitation is fraught with danger. Rather, reversal of the signs of the volume deficit, combined with stabilization of the blood pressure and pulse, and an hourly urine volume of 30 to 50 mL are used as general guidelines. An adequate hourly urine output, although usually a reliable index of volume replacement, may be totally misleading. The excessive administration of glucose (over 50 g in a 2- to 3-h period) may result in osmotic diuresis, while an osmotic agent such as mannitol tends to produce urine at the expense of the vascular volume. Patients with chronic renal disease or incipient acute renal damage from shock and injury also may have inappropriately high urinary volumes. In addition, the rapid administration of salt solutions may transiently expand the intravascular volume, increase the glomerular filtration rate, and result in an immediate outpouring of urine, although the total extracellular fluid space remains quite depleted.

The choice of the proper fluid for replacement depends on the existence of concomitant concentration or compositional abnormalities. With pure extracellular fluid volume loss or when only minimal concentration or compositional abnormalities are present, the use of a balanced salt solution, such as lactated Ringer's, is desirable.

RATE OF FLUID ADMINISTRATION. This varies considerably, depending on the severity and type of fluid disturbance, the presence of continuing losses, and the cardiac status. In general, the most severe volume deficits may be safely replaced initially with isotonic solutions at rates up to 2000 mL/h, reducing the rate as the fluid status improves. Constant observation by a physician is mandatory when the administration exceeds 1000 mL/h. At these rates, a significant portion may be lost as urinary output owing to a transient overexpansion of the plasma volume.

In elderly patients, associated cardiovascular disorders do not preclude correction of existing volume deficits, but they do require slower, more careful correction with constant monitoring of the cardiopulmonary system. If urinary output is not promptly restored, this may require measurements of central filling pressures and cardiac output to prevent ongoing renal injury from overcautious volume restoration.

CORRECTION OF CONCENTRATION CHANGES

If severe *symptomatic* hyponatremia or hypernatremia complicates the volume loss, prompt correction of the concentration abnormality to the extent that symptoms are relieved is necessary. Volume replenishment should be accomplished with slower correction of the remaining concentration abnormality. For immediate correction of severe hyponatremia, 5% sodium chloride solution or molar sodium lactate solution is used, depending on the patient's acid-base status. In any case, the sodium deficit can be estimated by multiplying the decrease in serum sodium concentration below normal (in milliequivalents per liter) by the liters of total body water. Initially, up to one-half of the calculated amount of sodium may be administered slowly, followed by clinical and chemical reevaluation of the patient before any additional infusion of sodium salts.

Note that this estimate is based on total body water, since the effective osmotic pressure in the extracellular compartment cannot be increased without increasing this function proportionately in the intracellular compartment. Although absolute reliance on any formula is undesirable, proper use of this estimate will allow a safe quantitative approximation of the sodium deficit. Generally, only a portion of the total deficit is replaced initially to relieve acute symptoms. Further correction is facilitated when renal function is restored by correction of the volume deficit. If the total calculated deficit were given rapidly, severe hypervolemia might occur particularly in patients with limited cardiac reserve. In practice, the infusion of small, successive increments of hypertonic saline solution with frequent evaluation of the clinical response and serum sodium concentration is recommended.

In the treatment of moderate hyponatremia with an associated volume deficit, volume replacement can be started immediately with concomitant correction of the serum sodium deficit. Isotonic sodium chloride solution (normal saline) is used initially in the presence of metabolic alkalosis, whereas M/6 sodium lactate (167 meq/L each of sodium and lactate) is used to correct an associated acidosis. Only a few liters of these solutions may be necessary to correct the serum sodium concentration; the remainder of the volume deficit may be replaced with lactated Ringer's solution.

Treatment of hyponatremia associated with volume excess is by restriction of water. In the presence of severe symptomatic hyponatremia, a small amount of hypertonic salt solution may be infused cautiously to alleviate symptoms. As this will cause additional volume expansion, it is contraindicated in patients with limited cardiac reserve; peritoneal dialysis or hemodialysis is preferred in this situation.

For the correction of severe, symptomatic hypernatremia with an associated volume deficit, 5% dextrose in water may be infused slowly until symptoms are relieved. If the extracellular osmolarity is reduced too rapidly, however, convulsions and coma may result. For this reason, correction of hypernatremia concomitant with repletion of the volume deficit by half-strength sodium chloride or half-strength lactated Ringer's solution is safer in most cases. In the absence of a significant volume deficit, water should be administered cautiously since dangerous hypervolemia may result; constant observation and frequent determinations of the serum sodium concentration are indicated. The problem is somewhat simplified once a sufficient quantity of fluid has been given to permit renal excretion of the solute load.

COMPOSITION AND MISCELLANEOUS CONSIDERATIONS

Correction of existing potassium deficits should be started *after* an adequate urine output is obtained, particularly in the patient with metabolic alkalosis since this may be secondary to or aggravated by potassium depletion. Calcium and magnesium rarely are needed during preoperative resuscitation but should be given as indicated, particularly to patients with massive subcutaneous infections, acute pancreatitis, or chronic starvation.

Fluid abnormalities also must be suspected in the patient for whom an elective procedure is planned. Chronic illnesses frequently are associated with extracellular fluid volume deficits, and concentration and compositional changes are not uncommon. Correction of anemia and recognition of the fact that a concentrated blood volume may exist in the chronically debilitated patient is of obvious importance. The hematocrit increases approximately 3% following the infusion of one unit of packed cells into the adult of average size. The increase may be significantly greater in the patient with a contracted intravascular volume, indicating the need for concurrent volume replacement. Of additional importance is the prevention of volume depletion during the preoperative period. Prolonged periods of fluid restriction in preparation for various diagnostic procedures, the use of cathartics and enemas for preparation of the bowel, and osmotic diuresis from contrast agents may cause a significant acute loss of extracellular fluid. Prompt recognition and treatment of these losses before surgery is necessary to prevent complications during the operative period.

Of additional importance is the prevention of volume depletion during the preoperative period. Prolonged periods of fluid restriction in preparation for various diagnostic procedures, and the use of cathartics and enemas for preparation of the bowel may cause a significant acute loss of extracellular fluid. Prompt recognition and treatment of these losses is necessary to prevent complications during the operative period.

Intraoperative Fluid Management

If preoperative replacement of extracellular fluid volume has been incomplete, hypotension may develop promptly with the induction of anesthesia. This can be quite insidious, as the ability of the awake patient to compensate for mild volume deficit is revealed only when the compensatory mechanisms are abolished with anesthesia. This problem is prevented by maintaining base-line requirements and replacing abnormal losses of fluids and electrolytes by intravenous infusions in the preoperative period.

Blood lost during the operative procedure should be replaced steadily. It is usually unnecessary to replace blood loss of less than 500 mL, but after the loss has exceeded this, replacement should begin. The warnings against the use of a single transfusion during operation have been somewhat confusing. There may be a very definite need for a single-unit transfusion in the patient who loses between 500 and 1000 mL of blood during operation.

In addition to blood losses during operation, there appear to be extracellular fluid losses during major operative procedures. Some of these, including edema from extensive dissection, collections within the lumen and wall of the small bowel, and accumulations of fluid in the peritoneal cavity, are clinically discernible and well recognized. They generally are felt to represent distributional shifts, in that the functional volume of extracellular fluid is reduced but not externally lost from the body. These functional losses are often referred to as "parasitic losses, third space edema, or sequestration" of extracellular fluid. Another source of extracellular fluid loss during major operative trauma is the wound itself. This is a relatively smaller loss and very difficult to quantify except in extensive and major operative procedures.

At the beginning of this century, surgeons became aware that many changes occurred in urinary output, blood volume, and fluid and electrolyte composition during and after surgery. Assessment of these changes, however, awaited the development of analytic techniques and their application to patient studies. In the following 25 years, saline solutions in varying combinations were given to patients undergoing operation, often in excessive amounts. Work in the late 1930s and early 1940s by Moyer and by many others indicated that during and after operative procedures, saline and water solutions should be withheld entirely, because most of the fluid administered was retained.

The possibility existed that the operative and postoperative retention of salt and water administered in relatively small amounts might simply be physiologic retention to replace a deficit of salt and water incurred by the operative procedure. Subsequent studies have revealed that functional extracellular fluid decreases with major abdominal operations, largely as sequestered loss into the operative site. This extracellular fluid volume deficit can be replaced during the operative procedure. These data have led to the conclusion that the need for an extracellular "mimic" in the form of balanced salt solution now can be clinically estimated. Intraoperative correction of the volume deficit with salt solution markedly reduces postoperative oliguria, but is not intended to substitute for blood replacement. Rather, it is felt to be a physiologic supplement, or adjunct, to replace sequestered losses.

Thus, the pendulum has swung from indiscriminate use of salt solutions in the first quarter of this century to almost total withholding of fluid and electrolytes from surgical patients in the second quarter of the century; indications at present are that proper management lies somewhere between these two extremes. Some guidelines are necessary for the intraoperative administration of saline solutions as a "mimic" for the sequestered extracellular fluid. Since this varies from an almost imperceptible minimum to a high of approximately 3 L during an uncomplicated procedure, quantification is extremely difficult with the presently available means of measuring functional extracellular fluid. Consequently, no accurate formula for intraoperative fluid administration can yet be derived. Some arbitrary but clinically useful guidelines are the following: (1) Blood should be replaced as lost, irrespective of any additional fluid and electrolyte therapy. (2) The replacement of extracellular fluid should begin during the operative procedure. (3) Balanced salt solution needed during operation is approximately 0.5 to 1 L/h, but only to a maximum of 2 to 3 L during a 4-h major abdominal procedure, unless there are other measurable losses.

Using a similar fluid regimen, Thompson and associates reported experiences in a series of 670 patients undergoing major aortoiliac reconstructive procedures. In this group of patients, the average amount of Ringer's lactate solution administered was 3555 mL, giving an average intraoperative replacement of salt solution of 677 mL/h of operative procedure. In the last 6 years of this study there were only two deaths in 298 operations, an operative mortality of 0.67 percent. Among the entire 670 patients, only two patients died of renal failure, an incidence of 0.3 percent. No patient died of pulmonary insufficiency. This extremely low incidence of renal failure, even in the presence of extensive operative trauma, is similar to the authors' data for major abdominal operative procedures.

Data by Virgilio and others have indicated that in the previously healthy surgical patient, the addition of albumin to intraoperative blood and extracellular fluid replacement is not only unnecessary but potentially harmful. Operative measurements of cardiac function and extravascular lung water indicate optimal function with replacement of blood and an extracellular "mimic" without the addition of extra albumin.

In summary, the addition of crystalloid fluid resuscitation, in appropriate volume, to blood replacement in the last quarter century has markedly improved the ability to maintain intraoperative homeostasis and avoid organ injury associated with inadequate volume replacement.

Postoperative Fluid Management

IMMEDIATE POSTOPERATIVE PERIOD

Orders for postoperative fluids are not written until the patient is in the recovery room and the fluid status has been assessed. Evaluation at this point should include a review of preoperative fluid status, the amount of fluid loss and gain during operation, and clinical examination of the patient with assessment of the vital signs and urinary output. Initial fluid orders are written to correct any *existing* deficit, followed by maintenance fluids for the remainder of the day. For the patient with complications who has received or lost large amounts of fluid, it is frequently difficult to estimate the fluid requirements for the ensuing 24 h. In this situation, intravenous fluids are ordered 1 L at a time and the patient is checked frequently until the situation is clarified. Proper replacement of fluids during this relatively short period will facilitate subsequent fluid management.

Immediately after operation, extracellular fluid volume depletion may occur as a result of continued losses of fluid at the site of injury or operative trauma—for example, into the wall or lumen of the small intestine. Several liters of extracellular fluid may be slowly deposited in such areas within a few hours or more during the first day or so from the time of the injury. Unrecognized deficits of extracellular fluid volume during the early postoperative period are manifest primarily as circulatory instability. The signs of volume deficiency in other organ systems may be delayed for several hours with this type of fluid loss. Postoperative hypotension and tachycardia require prompt investigation, followed by appropriate therapy. The generally accepted adequate blood pressure of 90/60 and a pulse of less than 120 in postoperative patients may not be sufficient to prevent renal ischemia unless, in addition to lack of signs of shock, urine flow is adequate. Evaluation of the level of consciousness, pupillary size, airway patency, breathing patterns, pulse rate and volume, skin warmth, color, body temperature, and a 30- to 50-mL hourly urine output, combined with critical review of the operative procedure and the operative fluid management, usually is recommended. Since operative trauma frequently involves loss or transfer of significant quantities of whole blood, plasma, or extracellular fluid that can be only grossly estimated, circulatory instability is most commonly caused by underestimated initial losses or insidious, concealed continued losses. Operative blood loss is usually estimated by the operating surgeon to be 15 to 40 percent less than the isotopically measured blood loss from that patient. For a patient with circulatory instability, further volume replacement of an additional 1000 mL isotonic salt solution, while determining whether continuing losses or other causes are present, often resolves the problem.

It is unnecessary and probably unwise to administer potassium during the first 24 h postoperatively, unless a definite potassium deficit exists. This is particularly important for the patient subjected to prolonged operative trauma involving one or more episodes of hypotension and for the posttraumatic patient with hemorrhagic hypotension. Oliguric renal failure or the more insidious high-output renal failure may develop, and the administration of even a small quantity of potassium may be quite detrimental.

LATER POSTOPERATIVE PERIOD

The problem of volume management during the postoperative convalescent phase is one of accurate measurement and replacement of all losses. In the otherwise healthy individual, this involves the replacement of measured sensible losses, which are generally of gastrointestinal origin, and the estimation and replacement of insensible losses.

The insensible loss is usually relatively constant and will average 600 mL/day. This may be increased by hypermetabolism, hyperventilation, and fever to a maximum of approximately 1500 mL/day. The estimated insensible loss is replaced with 5% dextrose in water. This loss may be partially offset by an insensible gain of water from excessive tissue catabolism in the complicated postoperative patient, particularly if associated with oliguric renal failure.

Approximately 1 L of fluid should be given to replace that volume of urine required to excrete the catabolic end products of metabolism (800 to 1000 mL/day). In the individual with normal renal function, this may be given as 5% dextrose in water, since the kidneys are able to conserve sodium with excretion of less than 1 meq daily. It is probably unnecessary to stress the kidneys to this degree, however, and a small amount of salt solution may be given in addition to water to cover urinary loss. In the elderly patient with salt-losing kidneys or in patients with head injuries, an insidious hyponatremia may develop if urinary losses are replaced with water. Urinary sodium in these circumstances may exceed 100 meq/L and result in a daily loss of significant amounts of sodium. Measurement of urinary sodium will facilitate accurate replacement.

Urine volume is not replaced on a milliliter-for-milliliter basis. A urinary output of 2000 to 3000 mL on a given day may simply represent diuresis of fluids given during surgery or may represent excessive fluid administration. If these large losses are completely replaced, the urine output will progressively increase, and this may logically progress to a unique situation resembling diabetes insipidus with urinary outputs in excess of 10 L/day.

Sensible losses, by definition, can be measured or, as in the case of sweating, the amount can be estimated. Gastrointestinal losses are usually isotonic or slightly hypotonic, and they are replaced with an essentially isotonic salt solution. When the estimated loss is slightly above or below isotonicity, appropriate corrections can be made in the daily water administration, while isotonic salt solutions are used to replace these losses volume for volume. Sweating is not usually a problem except with the febrile patient in whom losses may, but seldom do, exceed 250 mL/day per degree of fever. Excessive sweating may, in addition, represent a considerable loss of sodium in the unacclimatized individual.

Determination of serum electrolyte levels is generally unnecessary in the patient with an uncomplicated postoperative course maintained on parenteral fluids for 2 to 3 days. A more prolonged period of parenteral replacement or one complicated by excessive fluid losses requires frequent determinations of the serum sodium, potassium, and chloride levels, and carbon dioxide combining power. Adjustments then can be made with intravenous fluids of appropriate composition.

Daily maintenance fluid should be administered at a steady rate as the losses are incurred. If given over a shorter period of time, renal excretion of the excess salt and water may occur while the normal losses continue over the full 24-h period. For the same reason, fluids of different composition are alternated, and additives to intravenous fluids (e.g., potassium chloride and antibiotics) are evenly distributed in the total volume of fluid given.

In summary, daily fluid orders should begin with an assessment of the patient's volume status and a check for possible concentration or compositional disorders as reflected by proper laboratory determinations. All measured and insensible losses are replaced with fluids of appropriate composition, allowing for any preexisting deficit or excess. The amount of potassium replacement is 40 meq daily for renal excretion of potassium in addition to approximately 20 meq/L for replacement of gastrointestinal losses. Inadequate replacement may prolong the usual postoperative ileus and contribute to the insidious development of a resistant metabolic alkalosis. Calcium and magnesium are replaced when needed, as previously discussed.

SPECIAL CONSIDERATIONS IN THE POSTOPERATIVE PATIENT

VOLUME EXCESSES. The administration of isotonic salt solutions in excess of volume losses (external or internal) may result in overexpansion of the extracellular fluid space. The otherwise normal person in a postoperative state tolerates an acute overexpansion extremely well. Excesses administered over a period of several days, however, will soon exceed the kidney's ability to excrete sodium. Therefore, it is important to determine as accurately as possible from intake and output records and serum sodium concentrations the actual needs of the patient managed over several postoperative days. Attention to the signs and symptoms of overload usually prevents this fluid abnormality. It arises most frequently with attempts to meet excessive volume losses that are not measurable, such as those occurring from incompletely controlled fistula drainage.

The earliest sign is a weight gain during the catabolic period, when the patient should be losing ¼ to ½ lb day. Heavy eyelids, hoarseness, or dyspnea on exertion may rapidly appear. Circulatory and pulmonary signs of overload appear late and represent a rather massive overload. Peripheral edema may be a sign, but it does not necessarily indicate volume excess. In the absence of additional evidence for volume overload, other causes for peripheral edema should be considered. Overexpansion of the *total* extracellular fluid may coexist with *depletion* of the functional extracellular fluid compartment, along with decreased effective circulating plasma volume.

HYPONATREMIA. Significant postoperative alterations in serum sodium concentration are infrequent if the fluid resuscitation during operation has included adequate volumes of isotonic salt solutions. The kidneys retain the ability to excrete moderate excesses of salt water administered in the early postoperative period if functional extracellular fluid has been adequately replaced during the operative or immediate postoperative period. Previous studies of sodium balance have revealed that patients do excrete sodium after the functional deficit incurred by the shift of extracellular fluid has been replaced. Wright and Gann have demonstrated normal capacity to excrete water postoperatively when isotonic salt solutions are administered prior to a challenge with a water load. Thus, the commonly described hyponatremia associated with surgical procedures and traumatic injury is prevented by the replacement of extracellular fluid deficits. The daily maintenance of normal osmolarity is simplified by the replacement of observable losses of known sodium content.

Hyponatremia may easily occur when water is given to replace losses of sodium-containing fluids or when water administration consistently exceeds water losses. The latter may occur with oliguria or in association with decreased water loss through the skin and lungs, intracellular shifts of sodium, or the cellular release of excessive amounts of endogenous water. Severe or refractory hyponatremia, however, is difficult to produce if renal function remains normal.

In the presence of hyperglycemia, determination of the glucose concentration is necessary to evaluate the significance of a depressed serum sodium level. Since glucose does not enter cells by passive diffusion, it exerts an osmotic force in the extracellular compartment. This contribution to osmotic pressure is normally small, but with an elevated glucose concentration, the increased osmotic pressure causes the transfer of cellular water into the extracellular compartment, resulting in a dilutional hyponatremia. Hyponatremia may therefore be observed when the total effective osmotic pressure in the extracellular compartment is normal or even above normal. Each 100 mg/dL rise in the blood glucose above normal results in a decrease in the serum sodium concentration of approximately 1.6 to 3 meq/L.

Endogenous Water Release. The patient maintained on intravenous fluids without adequate caloric intake will, between the fifth and tenth days, gain significant quantities of water (maximum, 500 mL/day) from excessive cellular catabolism, thus decreasing the quantity of exogenous water required per day.

Intracellular Shifts. Systemic bacterial sepsis is often accompanied by a precipitous drop in serum sodium concentration. This sudden change is poorly understood but usually accompanies loss of extracellular fluid as either interstitial or intracellular sequestrations. This can be treated by withholding free water, restoring extracellular fluid volume, and initiating treatment of the sepsis.

HYPERNATREMIA. Hypernatremia (serum sodium concentration above 150 meq/L), although uncommon, is a dangerous abnormality. In contradistinction to decreased serum sodium concentration, hypernatremia is easily produced when renal function is normal. The extracellular fluid hyperosmolarity results in a shift of intracellular water from within the cell to the extracellular fluid compartment; in this situation, a high serum sodium level may indicate a significant deficit of total body water. In surgical patients hypernatremia arises most often from excessive or unexpected water losses, although it may result from use of salt-containing solutions to replace water losses. Classification of water losses may be helpful in preventing and treating this abnormality.

Excessive Extrarenal Water Losses. With increased metabolism from any cause, but particularly associated with fever, the water loss through evaporation of sweat may reach several liters daily. Patients with tracheostomy in dry environments can (with high minute volumes) lose as much as 1 to 1.5 L of water/day by this route. Increased water evaporation from a granulating surface is of significant magnitude in the thermally injured patient, and losses may be as great as 3 to 5 L/day.

Increased Renal Water Losses. Extremely large volumes of solute-poor urine may result from hypoxic damage to the distal tubules and collecting ducts or loss of antidiuretic hormone stimulation from damage to the central nervous system. In both instances, facultative water resorption is impaired. The former occurs in high-output renal failure; in our experience, this is the most common type of renal failure following severe injury or operative trauma. The latter occurs with extensive head injuries accompanied by temporary diabetes insipidus.

Solute Loading. High protein intake may produce an increased osmotic load of urea, which necessitates the excretion of large volumes of water. Hypernatremia, azotemia, and extracellular fluid volume deficits follow. In general, these can be prevented by an intake of 7 mL of water/g of dietary protein.

Excessive glucose administration results in the need for a large volume of water for excretion. Osmotic diuretics such as mannitol and urea also result in the obligatory excretion of a large volume of water as well as increasing urinary sodium losses. In addition, isotonic salt solutions, if used to replace pure water losses, rapidly produce hypernatremia.

HIGH-OUTPUT RENAL FAILURE. Acute renal insufficiency following trauma or surgical stress is a highly lethal complication. The diagnosis is based on persistent oliguria and chemical evidence of uremia after stabilization of the circulation. The clinical course is characterized by oliguria lasting from several days to several weeks, followed by a progressive rise in daily urine volume until both the excretory and concentrating functions of the kidney are gradually restored.

Uremia, occurring without a period of oliguria and accompanied by a daily urine volume greater than 1000 to 1500 mL/day, is a more frequent but less well recognized entity. Clinical experience and laboratory experiments suggest that high-output renal failure represents the renal response to a less severe or modified episode of renal injury than that required to produce classic oliguric renal failure. It is a milder form of renal insufficiency and its presence, by serial measurement of blood urea nitrogen and serum electrolytes, permits intelligent chemical and fluid volume management with a much greater latitude because of the daily urine volume excretion. Normal extracellular fluid volume and normal serum sodium concentration, therefore, are quite easily maintained when accurate daily outputs of each are obtained and replaced accordingly. The sodium-containing fluids may be administered as lactate to control the mild metabolic acidosis that occurs. Severe acidosis may develop if isotonic losses from the gastrointestinal tract or renal excretion of sodium are replaced with sodium chloride.

The chief danger of high-output renal failure is the failure to recognize its existence because of normal output.

The inappropriate administration of intravenous potassium in this setting may result in hyperkalemia. Good urinary output and gastrointestinal involvement requiring suction usually indicate the need for daily potassium replacement. With this type of renal failure, however, potassium intoxication may be produced. As little as 20 meq of potassium chloride given intravenously may rapidly produce myocardial potassium intoxication requiring exchange resin or hemodialysis treatment.

The typical course of high-output renal failure begins without a period of oliguria. The daily urine volumes are normal or greater than normal, often reaching levels of 3 to 5 L/day while blood urea nitrogen is increasing. An attempt to decrease urine output by water restriction rapidly results in hypernatremia without a change in urine volume. On the average, urea nitrogen continues to increase for 8 to 12 days before a downward trend occurs. The blood urine urea ratio is about 1:10 until a decrease occurs in the blood urea concentration.

Functionally, the lesion is characterized by a glomerular filtration rate of less than 20 percent of normal and complete resistance to vasopressin for 1 to 3 weeks after the blood urea nitrogen has declined. During the next 6 to 8 weeks, the glomerular filtration rate gradually rises, and the response to vasopressin becomes normal.

NUTRITION IN THE SURGICAL PATIENT
Stephen F. Lowry

The majority of patients undergoing elective surgical operations withstand the brief period of catabolism and starvation without noticeable difficulty. Maintaining an adequate nutritional regimen may be of critical importance in managing seriously ill surgical patients with pre-existing weight loss and depleted energy reserves. Between these two extremes are patients for whom nutritional support is not essential for life but may serve to shorten the postoperative recovery phase and minimize the number of complications. Not infrequently a patient may become ill or even die from complications secondary to starvation rather than the underlying disorder. Therefore, it is essential that the surgeon have a sound grasp of the fundamental metabolic changes associated with surgery, trauma, and sepsis and an awareness of the methods available to reverse or ameliorate these events. A detailed discussion of the neuroendocrine and metabolic response to injury has been presented in Chap. 1.

Body Fuel Reserves

The body must mobilize appropriate nutrients from fuel reserves in order to withstand the necessary periods of partial or complete starvation and to meet the additional requirements imposed by surgery, trauma, or sepsis. The extent and availability of these reserves may be of critical importance for successful recovery from an illness. Available information concerning body fuel composition and

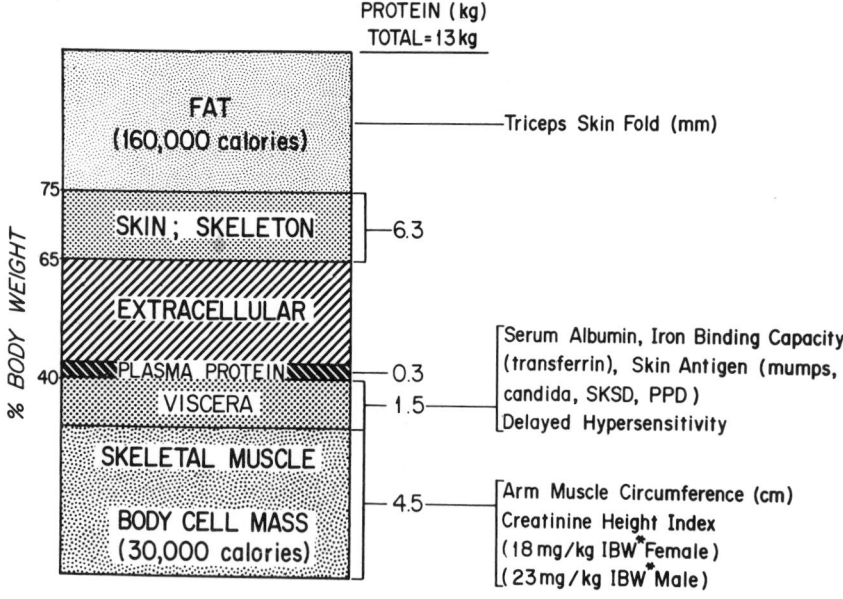

*Ideal Body Weight

Fig. 2-3. Body fuel composition, exclusive of glycogen (900 kcal), in a normal individual. Nutritional assessment techniques corresponding to components of body composition. (From: *Blackburn GL, Bothe A Jr: Cancer Bulletin 30:90, 1978, with permission.*)

the rate of fuel consumption in human beings has recently been reviewed by Cahill and is summarized below.

Carbohydrates, proteins, and fats are the three sources of fuel in human beings. Their relative contributions by both weight and caloric potential are illustrated in Fig. 2-3. Carbohydrate stores, primarily in the form of liver and muscle glycogen, are relatively small and could supply basal caloric requirements for less than 1 day. However, this relatively small quantity is absolutely essential in the emergency situation for the production of high-energy phosphates during anaerobic metabolism. Although glucose yields approximately 4 kcal/g, its storage as glycogen requires the addition of 1 or 2 g of intracellular water and electrolytes. Therefore, it yields only 1 or 2 kcal/g of wet weight.

Protein represents a considerably larger source of fuel, but, as emphasized by Cahill, every molecule of protein in the body has a specific purpose, such as an enzyme, a structural component, or a contractile protein in muscle. Thus, any protein loss represents loss of an essential function. Additionally, the amount of total body protein is relatively fixed in the normal healthy individual, and any additional protein is metabolized, the excess calories being stored as fat. Protein, like glycogen, represents an inefficient energy source relative to its wet weight, since it exists in an aqueous environment.

In contrast to glycogen and protein, fat is stored in a relatively anhydrous state. By weight, then, it is a relatively rich source of energy, supplying approximately 9 kcal/g. Most of the fat in the body serves as a readily available energy source; the few areas where fat serves a specific function (e.g., mechanical fat pads) are the last to be mobilized during starvation.

In summary, protein and fat are the only major sources of fuel. Total protein mass is relatively fixed in amount, and caloric excess or deficiency is met by an increase or decrease in the body's fat mass. Fat depots serve as sources of energy, protein stores represent *potential* sources of energy but only through the loss of some important function, and the small stores of carbohydrates are generally protected except for emergency use during anaerobic glycolysis.

Starvation

During the first several days of complete starvation, caloric needs are supplied by body fat and proteins: the small glycogen reserve is largely spared. Previous studies have shown an obligatory loss of approximately 10 to 15 g of nitrogen daily in the urine during this period, indicating the utilization of approximately 60 to 90 g of protein (each gram of nitrogen represents approximately 6.25 g of muscle protein). The majority of this protein, which is largely derived from skeletal muscle, is converted to glucose in the liver by the process of gluconeogenesis; most of this endogenously produced glucose is used by the brain. The remainder is used by certain tissues such as red blood cells and leukocytes which convert the glucose to lactate and pyruvate. These are returned to the liver and resynthesized into glucose (the Cori cycle). This obligatory nitrogen loss, then, reflects the use of amino acids derived from muscle protein for gluconeogenesis to supply glucose to the brain. No patient, however, should be allowed to starve completely. The administration of at least 100 g of glucose will obviate most of this gluconeogenesis and reduce the nitrogen loss by at least one-half—the well-known ''protein-sparing effect'' described by Gamble.

Available evidence from Cahill indicates that this protein-sparing effect is regulated by insulin, which is released when exogenous glucose is infused for use by the brain. The slightly elevated insulin level reduces amino acid release from the muscle, amino acid extraction by the liver, and gluconeogenesis. In the diabetic with an absolute or relative lack of insulin, the infusion of glucose does not inhibit gluconeogenesis, and muscle breakdown to amino acids continues unabated. The liver derives its energy by oxidizing fatty acids to ketones, and the remainder of the body utilizes both fatty acids and ketones to meet caloric requirements. Generally a small quantity of the ketones is excreted into the urine.

If complete starvation continues for more than a few days, the obligatory nitrogen loss progressively decreases, as the brain begins to use fat as its fuel source. Unlike other body tissues, however, the brain cannot utilize free fatty acids, since they do not cross the blood-brain barrier. Instead, use of keto acids that are produced by the liver and readily cross the blood-brain barrier gradually displaces the use of glucose by the brain. After prolonged starvation, the net effect of this adaptation to ketone utilization is a protein-sparing effect with reduction of urinary nitrogen excretion to approximately 4 g/day. This 4 g of nitrogen represents approximately 25 g of protein, or about 100 g of lean wet muscle. Thus, the normal individual with an average supply of fat and muscle may survive total starvation for several months. Insulin again may be the signal for the reduction in muscle catabolism and gluconeogenesis (coincident with the increased use of keto acids by the brain), according to Cahill. However, changes in the blood level of alanine, which is quantitatively one of the more important amino acids, may also play a role. A fall in the blood level of this amino acid appears to decrease gluconeogenesis and glucose production by the liver.

Surgery, Trauma, Sepsis

In contrast to the whole-body and tissue-specific energy and protein conservation response exhibited during unstressed starvation, the injured patient manifests variable, but obligatory, increases in energy expenditure and nitrogen excretion (Fig. 2-4, Table 2-9). While the extent and duration of this response to injury are modified by a variety of factors, including the adequacy of resuscitation, infection, and medication, the inability to downregulate body energy expenditure and nitrogen losses may rapidly deplete both labile and functional energy stores. The postinjury metabolic environnment precludes the efficient oxidation of fat and ketone production, thereby promoting the continued erosion of protein pools. This enhanced net protein catabolic process, if unchecked by effective disease-specific therapy and allowed to progress for an extended period without nutritional intervention, eventuates in critical organ failure.

The sequence of metabolic and endocrine events occasioned by surgery, trauma, or sepsis may be divided into several phases. As pointed out by Moore (1960), the magnitude of the changes and the duration of each phase vary

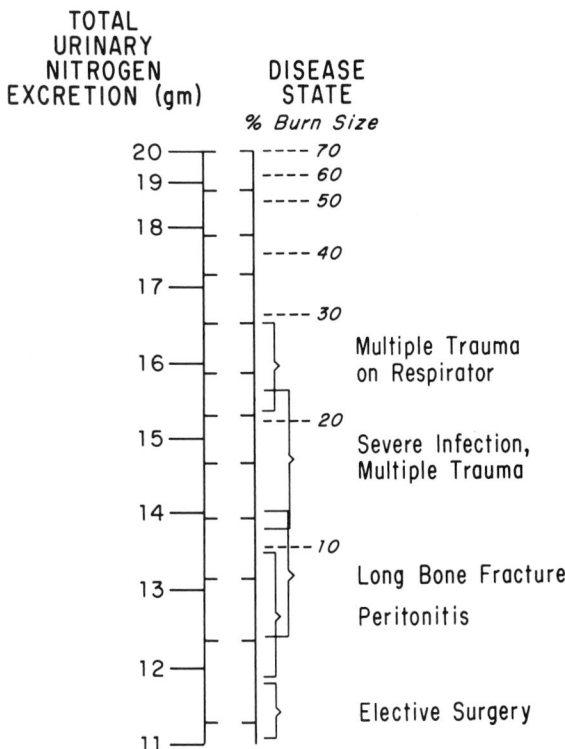

Fig. 2-4. The *minimum* anticipated daily urinary nitrogen excretion of adult patients in relation to the injury stimulus. These losses may be modulated by a number of variables including the age and nutritional status of the patient. (Adapted from: *Grant JP: Handbook of Total Parenteral Nutrition, Philadelphia, Saunders, 1980, with permission.*)

considerably and are directly related to the severity of the injury.

CATABOLIC PHASE. This phase has also been termed the *adrenergic-corticoid phase* since it corresponds to the period during which changes induced by adrenergic and adrenal corticoid hormones are most striking. Immediately following surgery or trauma, there is a sudden in-

Table 2-9. CORRELATION OF INCREASED ENERGY EXPENDITURE AND URINARY NITROGEN EXCRETION AFTER INJURY AND ILLNESS

	% Increase above basal energy expenditure	Daily urinary N excretion per kg
Normal	—	0.09
Elective, major surgery	24	0.21
Skeletal trauma	32	0.32
Blunt trauma	37	0.32
Head trauma/steroids	61	0.34
Sepsis	79	0.37
40% thermal injury	132	0.37

SOURCE: Adapted from Long CL et al: *J Parenter Enterol Nutr* 3:452, 1979.

crease in metabolic demands and urinary excretion of nitrogen beyond the levels associated with simple starvation. Patients generally cannot eat, cannot lower their metabolic rate, and cannot effectively alter the source of endogenous fuels to spare protein utilization. This is in distinct contrast to events in the normal individual subjected to prolonged starvation, where most body tissues use fat as their main source of fuel, thereby sparing protein. Trauma apparently results in an obligatory and excessive mobilization of protein in an attempt to provide skeletons for gluconeogenesis, acute phase, and wound repair proteins. The administration of moderate amounts of glucose to these individuals produces little or no change in the rate of protein catabolism, although recent evidence using isotopic determinations of protein kinetics suggests that provision of sufficient nonprotein calories in combination with amino acids does reduce the rate of body protein breakdown.

Glucose turnover is increased, while Cori cycle activity is stimulated and three-carbon intermediates are converted back to glucose in the liver by pyruvate carboxylase and phosphoenolpyruvate carboxylase. Increased synthesis of these two enzymes occurs in the presence of elevated levels of glucagon, glucocorticoids, and catecholamines and low concentrations of insulin—the hormonal environment present during the catabolic phase of injury. Lipolysis also is stimulated by this hormonal milieu, and an obligatory oxidation of fatty acids is evident.

Efforts directed at interruption of afferent neurogenic stimuli by extradural anesthesia have met with partial success in attenuating some of these abnormalities of energy substrate turnover. The impact of such therapy upon nitrogen loss has been far less dramatic, suggesting that circulating or tissue paracrine factors other than classical neuroendocrine hormones are of major importance in early postinjury metabolic responses. Recent evidence would suggest that a class of macrophage and lymphocyte-produced peptides (cytokines), some of which, such as cachectin/tumor necrosis factor and interleukin-1, are already known to enhance hepatic acute-phase protein mRNA and tissue glucose transporter protein production, are likely participants in the derangements of catabolic phase responses. The extent of the negative nitrogen balance in these patients varies considerably and is largely related to the magnitude of the injury.

EARLY ANABOLIC PHASE. Depending on the severity of injury, the body turns from a catabolic to an anabolic phase. This may occur within 3 to 8 days after uncomplicated elective surgery or after weeks in patients with extensive cross-sectional tissue injury, sepsis, or ungrafted thermal injury. This turning point, also known as the *corticoid-withdrawal phase,* is characterized by a sharp decline in nitrogen excretion and restoration of appropriate potassium-nitrogen balance. Generally, this transition period lasts no more than a day or two and coincides with diuresis of retained free water. Renewed interest in oral nutrition and the patient's immediate environment promotes greater muscular activity.

The early anabolic phase may last from a few weeks to a few months depending upon the capacity to ingest adequate nutrition and the extent to which erosion of protein stores has occurred. Nitrogen balance is positive, indicating synthesis of proteins, and there is a rapid and progressive gain in weight and muscular strength. Positive nitrogen balance reaches a maximum of approximately 4 g/day, which represents the synthesis of approximately 25 g of protein and the gain of over 100 g of lean body mass day. The total amount of nitrogen gain will ultimately equal the amount lost during the catabolic phase, although the rate of gain will be much slower than the rate of initial loss.

LATE ANABOLIC PHASE. The final period of convalescence or the late anabolic phase may last from several weeks to several months after a severe injury. This phase is associated with the gradual restoration of adipose stores as the previously positive nitrogen balance declines toward normal. Weight gain is much slower during this phase because of the higher caloric content of fat and can be realized only if intake is in excess of caloric expenditure. In most individuals, the phase ends with a gradual return to the previously normal body weight. The patient who is partially immobilized during this period of time, however, may exhibit a marked gain in weight due to decreased energy expenditure.

Assessment and Requirements

Nutritional homeostasis presupposes that proper timing and administration of nutrients will impact favorably upon the outcome of therapy. Muller has reported a randomized, prospective trial documenting a significant reduction of postoperative morbidity and mortality following intravenous nutritional support. Similar reductions in the complication rate following nutritional support have been observed by other groups in a variety of surgical and traumatic illnesses. Reports that up to 50 percent of selected surgical populations may manifest evidence of protein-calorie malnutrition underscores the importance of identifying patients at increased risk from nutritional morbidity.

Nutritional assessment is undertaken to determine the severity of nutrient deficiencies or excess and to aid in predicting nutritional requirements (Fig. 2-3). Important information is obtained by determining the presence of weight loss and of chronic illnesses or dietary habits that influence the quantity and quality of food intake. Social habits predisposing to malnutrition and the use of medications that may influence food intake or utilization should also be investigated. Physical examination seeks to assess loss of muscle and adipose tissues, organ dysfunction, and subtle change in skin, hair, or neuromuscular function reflecting a frank or impending nutritional deficiency. Anthropometric data (weight change, skin fold thickness, and arm circumference muscle area) and biochemical determinations (creatinine excretion, albumin, and transferrin) may be used to substantiate the historical and physical findings. It is imprecise to rely upon any single or fixed combination of the above findings to accurately assess nutritional status or morbidity. Appreciation for the stresses and natural history of the disease process, in

Table 2-10. ELEMENTAL REQUIREMENTS FOR
DEPLETED ADULT SUBJECTS

Element	Daily infusion, per kg*
N	0.4 g
PO_4^{2-}	0.018 g
K^+	0.65 meq
Na^+	0.74 meq
Cl^-	0.56 meq
Ca^{2+}	0.13 meq

* Requirements listed are based on kilogram of ideal body weight; appropriate adjustment to current body weight may be necessary.
SOURCE: Adapted from Rudman D et al: *J Clin Invest* 55:94, 1975.

combination with nutritional assessment, remains the basis for identifying patients in acute or anticipated need of nutritional support.

Balance studies have documented the basal requirements for nonstressed, depleted patients who are undergoing nutritional support (Table 2-10). These guidelines must be considered in relation to goals for gradual repletion of a malnourished patient or for maintenance of lean tissue stores in an otherwise well-nourished subject.

The above basal requirements are inadequate for patients who have undergone major surgery or who have suffered severe trauma or sepsis. The exact caloric and nitrogen requirements necessary to maintain an individual in balance after severe injury are dependent upon the extent of injury, the source and route of administered nutrients, and, to some extent, the degree of antecedent malnutrition.

A fundamental goal of nutritional support is to meet the energy requirements for metabolic processes, core temperature maintenance, and tissue repair. Failure to provide adequate nonprotein energy sources will lead to dissolution of lean tissue stores. The requirement for energy may be measured by indirect calorimetry or estimated from urinary nitrogen excretion which is proportional to resting energy expenditure (REE) (Table 2-9). Basal energy expenditure (BEE) may also be estimated by the equations of Harris and Benedict:

$$BEE \text{ (men)} = 66.47 + 13.75(W) + 5.0 \, (H) - 6.76 \, (A)$$
$$\text{kcal/day}$$
$$BEE \text{ (women)} = 655.1 + 9.56(W) + 1.85 \, (H) - 4.68 \, (A)$$
$$\text{kcal/day}$$

where W = weight, kg
H = height, cm
A = age, years

These equations are suitable for estimating energy requirements in 80 percent of hospitalized patients. A suitable correction for the degree of operative or traumatic stress may then be applied as in Table 2-9 to determine the resting energy expenditure. Nonprotein calories are supplied in excess of energy expenditure because the uti-

lization of exogenous nutrients is decreased and energy substrate demands are increased after traumatic or septic insult. Appropriate nonprotein caloric needs are 1.2 to 1.5 times REE during enteral nutrition and 1.5 to 2.0 times REE during intravenous nutrition.

The second objective of nutritional support is to meet the substrate requirements for protein synthesis. Maintenance of protein synthesis is dependent upon many factors, including the nature and degree of insult, the source and amount of exogenous protein, and prior nutritional status. As a consequence, no single nutritional formulation is appropriate for all patients. An appropriate calorie-nitrogen ratio (150 to 200:1) should be maintained, although recent evidence suggests that increased protein intake (and a lower ratio) may be efficient in selected hypermetabolic patients. In the absence of severe renal or hepatic dysfunction precluding the use of standard nutritional regimens, approximately 0.25 to 0.35 g of nitrogen/kg of body weight should be provided daily.

Amino acid formulations designed to improve protein kinetics in the posttraumatic or organ failure setting are under investigation. Solutions enriched in branched-chain amino acids are being used to preserve or enhance muscle protein synthesis. Branched-chain amino acids are also used in combination with reduced aromatic amino acid concentrations to alleviate encephalopathy secondary to hepatocellular dysfunction. Formulations designed to improve nitrogen utilization by providing intact or keto analogs of essential amino acids have gained wide acceptance in the management of acute renal failure.

The requirements for vitamins and essential trace minerals usually can be easily met in the average patient with an uncomplicated postoperative course, and vitamins usually are not given in the absence of preoperative deficiencies. Patients maintained on elemental diets or parenteral hyperalimentation require complete vitamin and mineral supplementation. The commercial defined-formula enteral diets contain varying amounts of essential minerals and vitamins (Tables 2-11 and 2-12). It is necessary to ensure that adequate replacement is available in the diet or by supplementation. Numerous commercial vitamin preparations are available for intravenous or intramuscular use, although most do not contain vitamin K and some do not contain vitamin B_{12} or folic acid. Supplemental trace minerals may now be given intravenously by commercial preparations. Essential fatty acid supplementation may also be necessary, especially in patients with depletion of adipose stores. Patients receiving intravenous feeding will require all of the above micronutrients to prevent evolution of deficiencies.

Indications and Methods for Nutritional Support

The selection of patients who require partial or complete nutritional support has become increasingly important. The ability to provide complete nutritional support in the starving patient and to counteract the nitrogen losses in catabolic states with elemental diets or parenteral hyperalimentation represents a substantial contribu-

Table 2-11. CASEINATES AND WHOLE PROTEIN FORMULAS*

Formula	Critcaire HN§	Ensure	Ensure HN	Ensure plus	Ensure plus HN	Entriton	Isotein HN	Isocal	Isocal HCN	Magnacal	Nutri-Aid	Osmolite	Osmolite HN	Precision isotonic	Precision HN	Precision LR	Renu	Sustacal	Sustacal HC	Traumacal	Travasorb MCT
NP, kcal/mL†	0.85	0.86	0.88	1.28	1.25	0.86	0.93	0.92	1.70	1.72	0.94	0.91	0.88	0.84	0.87	0.99	0.87	0.76	1.26	1.17	1.45
Nitrogen, g/L	6.00	5.92	7.10	8.80	10.0	5.60	10.8	5.44	12.0	11.2	6.29	5.92	7.10	4.64	7.04	4.16	5.60	9.60	9.76	13.20	5.92
Osmolality, mO/kg	650	450	470	600	650	300	300	300	740	590	350	300	310	300	557	525	330	625	650	550	312
Na, meq/L	27	32	40	46	50	61	27	23	34	43	33	23	40	34	42	30	21	40	36	52	32
K, meq/L	33	32	40	48	46	61	27	33	35	32	33	27	40	24	23	22	32	52	38	36	32
Cl, meq/L	30	30	40	46	45	56	27	30	34	26	30	23	40	28	33	31	18	44	36	45	30
Ca, meq/L	26	26	37	32	52	50	28	31	33	50	27	26	37	32	17	29	25	50	42	38	26
P, mmol/L	17	17	24	20	33	32	18	17	21	32	18	17	24	20	11	18	16	29	27	24	17
Mg, meq/L	17	17	25	26	34	33	19	17	22	33	17	17	25	21	11	19	16	31	28	17	17
Zn, mg/L	10	16	17	24	16	15	8.5	10	20	15	16	16	17	10	5	9	10	14	13	15	16
Cu, mg/L	1	1	1.5	1.6	1	2	1.1	1	2	2	1.1	1	1.5	1	0.7	1	2	2	2	1.5	1
Vitamins, 1/RDA/day‡	1.9	1.9	1.4	1.6	1.0	2.0	1.6	2.0	1.5	1.0	2.0	1.9	1.4	1.6	2.9	1.8	2.0	1.1	1.8	2.0	2.0

* Lactose-free.
† NP = nonprotein kilocalories per milliliters of solution.
‡ Volume in liters needed to meet the U.S. RDA per day.
§ This formula also contains synthetic amino acids.
SOURCE: Adapted from Legaspi A, Lowry SF: Agents affecting nutrition and homeostasis, in *Manual of Drug Therapy*. New York, Raven Press, 1985.

Table 2-12. ELEMENTAL AND PEPTIDE DIETS*

Formula	Vivonex	Vivonex HN	Vivonex TEN	Vital	Travasorb STD	Travasorb HN
NP, kcal/mL†	0.92	0.82	0.85	0.83	0.88	0.82
Nitrogen, g/L	3.36	6.72	6.08	6.72	4.80	7.20
Osmolality, mO/kg	550	810	630	460	560	560
Na, meq/L	20	23	20	16	40	40
K, meq/L	30	30	20	30	30	30
Cl, meq/L	20	23	23	19	42	38
Ca, meq/L	28	16	25	33	25	25
P, mmol/L	18	10	49	21	16	16
Mg, meq/L	18	10	17	22	16	16
Zn, mg/L	8	5	10	10	7.5	7.5
Cu, mg/L	1	0.7	1	1.3	1	1
Vitamins (1/RDA/day)‡	1.8	3.0	2.0	1.5	2.0	2.0

* Lactose-free.
† NP = Nonprotein kilocalories per milliliter of solution.
‡ Volume in liters needed to meet the U.S. RDA per day.
SOURCE: Adapted from Legaspi A, Lowry SF: Agents affecting nutrition and homeostasis, in *Manual of Drug Therapy.* New York, Raven Press, 1985.

tion. The need for nutritional support should be assessed during the preoperative and postoperative course of all but the most routine cases. However, it should be emphasized that the majority of surgical patients do not require special nutritional regimens. The reasonably well-nourished and otherwise healthy individual who undergoes an uncomplicated major surgical procedure has sufficient body fuel reserves to withstand the catabolic insult and partial starvation for at least 1 week. Adequate quantities of parenteral fluids with appropriate electrolyte composition and a minimum of 100 g of glucose daily to minimize protein catabolism will be all that is necessary in most patients. Assuming that the patient has a relatively uncomplicated postoperative course and resumes normal oral intake at the end of this period, defined-formula diets or parenteral hyperalimentation are probably unnecessary and inadvisable because of the associated risks. During the early anabolic phase, the patient must be provided with an adequate caloric intake of proper composition to meet the energy needs of the body and allow protein synthesis. A high calorie-nitrogen ratio (optimal ratio approximately 150 kcal/g nitrogen) and an adequate supply of vitamins and minerals are necessary for maximum anabolism during this period.

In contrast to this group, there are populations of surgical patients for whom an adequate nutritional regimen may be of critical importance for a successful outcome. These categories include preoperative patients who are chronically debilitated from their diseases or malnutrition and patients who have suffered trauma, sepsis, or surgical complications and cannot maintain an adequate caloric intake.

Specialized nutritional support can be given by enteral, enteral plus peripheral vein, and by central venous routes. The enteral route should be initially considered because it is simple, economical, and usually well toler-

ated in most patients. Nasopharyngeal, gastrostomy, and jejunostomy tube feedings may be considered for alimentation in patients who have a relatively normal gastrointestinal tract but cannot or will not eat. Elemental diets may be administered by similar routes when bulk and fat-free nutrients requiring minimal digestion are indicated. Finally, parenteral alimentation may be used for supplementation in the patient with limited oral intake or, more commonly, for complete nutritional management in the absence of oral intake.

Despite the failure to document clinical differences between the enteral and parenteral feeding routes with respect to the utilization of exogenous nutrients, the gastroentestinal tract serves a number of synthetic and immunologic functions that bear consideration in the design of nutritional support regimens. Toward this end, a number of approaches for preserving gastrointestinal mucosal integrity and gut mass, including luminal stimulation by digestible or nondigestible substrates, as well as infusion of critical intestinal fuel sources such as glutamine, are currently undergoing clinical trials.

The patient's ability to tolerate and absorb enteral feedings is determined by the rate of infusion, the osmolality, and the chemical nature of the product. Enteral feedings are often begun at a rate of 30 to 50 mL/h and are increased by 10 to 25 mL/h a day until the optimal volume is delivered. After full volume is attained, the concentration of the solution is increased slowly to the desired strength. If esophageal or gastric feedings are given, residual gastric volume should be monitored to reduce the risk of a major aspiration episode. If abdominal cramping or diarrhea occurs, the rate of administration or the concentration of the solution should be decreased. All feeding tubes should be thoroughly irrigated clear of solutions if feedings are interrupted or medications are given by this route.

NASOENTERIC TUBE FEEDING

The development of mercury-weighted silastic feeding tubes has improved the ability to provide safe and effective enteral nutrition. Use of such tubes represents a safer alternative to the practice of nasoesophageal or gastric feeding by large-bore red rubber or plastic tubes. Exceptions to this rule include patients with head and neck malignancies who will tolerate a blenderized diet that cannot easily be administered by smaller diameter tubes.

Nasoesophageal or gastric feedings should be used only in alert patients. The foremost contraindication for nasoesophageal or gastric tube feeding is unconsciousness or lack of protective laryngeal reflexes, which may result in life-threatening pulmonary complications due to aspiration. Even with a tracheostomy, it is inadvisable to feed mentally obtunded patients via such route, since feedings often can be recovered from tracheostomy suction, indicating continued aspiration of gastric contents. Pharyngeal tube feedings may be indicated for patients with oropharyngeal tumor; irritation may be prevented by inserting the tube into the pyriform sinus.

The nasojejunal tube may allow feeding beyond dysfunctional gastric stomas and high gastrointestinal fistulas. In such cases, it may be possible to maintain nutrition without a jejunostomy tube until stomal dysfunction relents or the fistula heals. Such tubes may be positioned in the upper small intestine by positioning the patient in a manner that promotes passage of the mercury-weighted tube into the desired intestinal segment. If this technique proves unsuccessful, placement may be effected by fluoroscopic guidance or by an experienced endoscopist. Proper position of the tube must be confirmed radiographically (with water-soluble opaque medium if necessary).

Whenever dietary preparations are administered into the gastrointestinal tract via tubes, it is advisable to employ bedside infusion pumps to ensure a constant rate of delivery over each 24-h period. The utilization of such pumps decreases the incidence of gastrointestinal side effects induced by too rapid delivery of hyperosmolar solutions, while at the same time allowing safer administration of larger daily volumes of nutrients, since gastric distention is minimized. Investigation is required for all abdominal complaints in such patients in view of reports of intussusception around feeding tubes placed more distally in the small intestine.

GASTROSTOMY TUBE FEEDING

The administration of blended food through a gastrostomy tube is a good method for feeding patients with a variety of chronic gastrointestinal lesions arising at or above the cardioesophageal junction. However, gastrostomy tube feedings are contraindicated for mentally obtunded patients with inadequate laryngeal reflexes. This feeding method should be used only in alert patients or in patients with total obstruction of the distal esophagus.

Generally, gastrostomies of the Stamm (serosa-lined, temporary) or modified Glassman (mucosa-lined, permanent) type are constructed. Percutaneous endoscopic gastrostomies (PEG) have proved to be a safe and effective method for pursuing enteral nutritional support. The feeding mixture may be ordinarily prepared food converted by a blender into a semiliquid. Hyperosmolarity of the feeding formula is not generally a problem as long as the pylorus is intact.

JEJUNOSTOMY TUBE FEEDING

Jejunostomy tube feedings are generally required for patients in whom nasoesophageal or gastrostomy tube feedings are contraindicated, e.g., comatose patients or patients with high gastrointestinal fistulas or obstructions, or in whom a nasojejunal feeding tube cannot be placed. The jejunostomy may be of the Roux en Y (permanent) or the Witzel (temporary) type. The latter is constructed by inserting a #18 French rubber catheter into the proximal jejunum approximately 12 in. distal to the ligament of Treitz. The wall of the jejunum is inverted over the tube for about 3 cm as it emerges from the bowel to create a serosa-lined tunnel that allows rapid sealing of the jejunal opening when the tube is removed. An alternative procedure is the placement of a smaller-bore polyethylene or silastic catheter. The tube is brought out through a stab wound in the left upper quadrant of the abdomen. The jejunum is sutured to the anterior abdominal wall at the point of tube entry to seal it from the peritoneal cavity.

Alternate methods that have gained wide acceptance include the needle catheter jejunostomy that is available in commercial kit form or may be constructed using subclavian catheter materials. In selected instances, jejunostomies may be placed endoscopically or converted from PEG catheters.

If the jejunostomy tube is inadvertently removed, blind attempts at reinsertion are contraindicated. If discovered within a few hours, the tube may be reinserted under fluoroscopic control to be sure it is in the bowel before feedings are resumed. The patient is observed for signs of peritonitis for 12 to 18 h after feedings are restarted. If there is any doubt about the position of the tube, it should be replaced surgically.

Feedings are safely begun 12 to 18 h after jejunostomy construction, even though peristalsis is not audible. Jejunostomy tube feedings are usually initiated with one of the many commercially available defined formula diets (Tables 2-11, 2-12). Such formulas, when provided by continuous infusion, are usually well tolerated.

With proper care, about 85 percent of jejunostomy patients tolerate their feedings. Diarrhea is usually controlled if the concentration and volume of formula are temporarily reduced. Failing this, feeding is halted for a day, then resumed from the beginning of the feeding regimen, progressing somewhat more slowly than before. If mild diarrhea or cramping persists, a pulverized Lomotil tablet or 8 to 10 drops of tincture of belladonna may be given through the tube 30 min prior to formula infusion. At times it may be necessary to give 5 mL paregoric 15 to 30 min before the formula to control cramping and diarrhea, but this should be employed sparingly and for as short a period as possible. In many cases, symptoms are relieved if the rate and volume of infusion are reduced and cold formula avoided. Failing control of diarrhea by the above means, or as an alternative method to opiates, the periodic administration of bulk-forming agents (Metamucil) may be helpful.

If the patient with a jejunostomy has a proximal bowel or biliary fistula draining more than 300 mL daily for prolonged periods, the fistular drainage may be collected by sump suction, cooled in an ice basin at bedside, and promptly refed in small increments throughout the day. To avoid jejunal overloading, the fistular fluid is refed between formula feedings. It is not advisable to refeed aspirated gastric juice, for this may cause jejunal irritation and profuse diarrhea. If the fistular drainage is profuse, it is usually not possible to refeed more than 2 L/day, and fluid and electrolyte losses must be replaced by appropriate intravenous supplements. Additional water may be given with the feedings or administered between the feedings as indicated. Occasionally, an elemental diet, as discussed below, may be indicated when other jejunostomy formulas are not tolerated.

ELEMENTAL DIETS

Commercial production of nutritionally complete liquid diets, derived in purified form either from natural foods or from foods prepared synthetically, has been given such designations as chemically defined or elemental diets.

Clinical experience with chemically formulated bulk-free elemental diets has been encouraging. These diets may be used for complete nutritional support or as dietary supplements for patients who are unable to eat or digest enough food to meet their energy requirements. They may be preferable to high-caloric parenteral feedings for patients who have at least part of the small bowel available for the absorption of simple sugars and amino acids. Elemental diets have been found useful for patients with depleted protein reserves secondary to gastrointestinal tract disease, such as ulcerative or granulomatous colitis and malabsorption syndrome, and for patients with only partial function of the gastrointestinal tract, such as the short bowel syndrome or gastric or small bowel fistulas with feeding distal to the fistula. The diets also have been used during preoperative bowel preparation.

As commercially prepared, these diets also contain base-line electrolytes, water- and fat-soluble vitamins (except vitamin K), and trace minerals. They contain no bulk and therefore produce a minimum of residue. Products such as Carnation Instant Breakfast and Meritene contain intact protein derived from milk products, eggs, or both and are designed for oral consumption in lactose tolerant patients. Other preparations contain intact protein from semipurified isolates of milk, soybean, or egg (Table 2-11). These do not contain lactose and are more readily tolerated in such lactase-deficiency states as gastroenteritis, intestinal resection, radiation, or genetic predisposition. Finally, there are several products whose protein content is either partially hydrolyzed or completely hydrolyzed to amino acids or dipeptides (Table

2-12). When digestion and absorption are normal, there appears to be little therapeutic advantage to the use of crystalline amino acid formulas. A listing of the basic constituents for several commercial preparations, as well as the volume necessary to achieve minimal daily requirements, is given in Table 2-11.

Special products designed for use in the presence of organ dysfunction are also available (Table 2-13). Amin-Aid provides essential amino acids and histidine with minimal electrolytes, vitamins, or bulk, but does yield 2 kcal/mL for use in the setting of renal failure. Hepatic Aid, which may be used in the presence of severe liver insufficiency, is enriched with branched-chain amino acids and is deficient in aromatic, ringed amino acids.

Fat may contribute less than 1 or as much as 47 percent of the calories in these commercial formulas. Most contain long-chain fats as corn oil, soy oil, or safflower oil. Some include medium-chain triglycerides, such as Precision-LR and Vital. Despite the high caloric density of fat, it does not increase the osmolality of the formula. When significant maldigestion or malabsorption is present, a diet low in fat or one supplemented with medium-chain triglycerides may be useful.

Specific products are limited in their overall clinical usefulness by virtue of the fixed content of nutrients. In recent years, there has been a trend in preparing enteral diets in modular form, where certain critical items, such as sodium, potassium, and fat, can be modified in concentration as dictated by clinical circumstances.

The amount of elemental diet required to maintain weight and nitrogen balance varies with the individual patient. In severe catabolic states the standard diet often fails to achieve positive nitrogen balance. Careful attention to water and electrolyte balance is mandatory, particularly when large quantities of fluid are being lost through fistulas or other routes. Additional sodium and potassium may be added to the mixture (not to exceed a total of 100 meq), although they should be given in intravenous fluids when larger quantities are needed. Water may be added to the mixture in the face of excessive pure water losses.

Complications include nausea, vomiting, and diarrhea which develop because of the high osmolarity of the diets. This generally can be controlled by decreasing the rate and or concentration of the mixture. Hypertonic nonketotic coma may occur in the presence of excessive water losses or if the diets are administered at concentrations above those recommended. Hyperglycemia and glycosuria may occur in any severely ill patient, particularly latent diabetics, and insulin may be indicated.

PARENTERAL ALIMENTATION

Dudrick et al. have demonstrated the clinical practicality of providing complete nutritional needs for an extended period of time using high-caloric parenteral feedings. Parenteral alimentation involves the continuous infusion of a hyperosmolar solution containing carbohydrates, proteins, fat, and other necessary nutrients through an indwelling catheter inserted into the superior

Table 2-13. SPECIALIZED FORMULATIONS FOR ENTERAL NUTRITION DURING ORGAN FAILURE*

Formula	Amin Aid	Hepatic Aid	Travasorb Hepatic	Travasorb Renal	TraumAid	Stresstein
NP, kcal/mL†	1.88	1.47	0.98	1.26	0.83	0.93
Nitrogen, g/L	2.35	6.47	4.4	4.4	7.58	11.2
Osmolality, mO/kg	1095	1150	690	590	675	910
EAA, g/L‡	18.6	22.15	20.0	13.8	26.2	89.6
BCAA, g/L§	7.5	15.3	14.5	6.67	15.0	61.6
Protein, g/L	19.4	42.6	29.0	23.0	43.0	70.0
Na, meq/L	<15	<15	19	0	23	28
K, meq/L	<6	<6	29	0	30	28
Cl, meq/L	0	0	19	0	23	29
Ca, meq/L	0	0	19	0	20	25
P, mmol/L	0	0	16	0	13	16
Mg, meq/L	0	0	15	0	11	17
Zn, mg/L	0	0	6.6	0	6.7	7.5
Cu, mg/L	0	0	0.8	0	0.7	1.0
Vitamins (1/RDA/day)‖	—	—	2.1	—	3.0	2.0

* Lactose-free.
† NP = nonprotein kilocalories per milliliter of solution.
‡ Essential amino acids, branched-chain amino acids included.
§ Branched-chain amino acids only; leucine, isoleucine, and valine.
‖ Volume in liters needed to meet the U.S. RDA per day.
SOURCE: Adapted from Legaspi A, Lowry SF: Agents affecting nutrition and homeostasis, in *Manual of Drug Therapy*. New York, Raven Press, 1985.

vena cava. In order to obtain the maximum benefit, the ratio of calories to nitrogen must be adequate (at least 100 to 150 kcal/g nitrogen) and the two materials must be infused simultaneously. When the sources of calories and nitrogen are given at different times, there is a significant decrease in nitrogen utilization. These nutrients can be given in quantities considerably greater than the basic caloric and nitrogen requirements, and this method has proved to be highly successful in achieving growth and development, positive nitrogen balance, and weight gain in a variety of clinical situations.

INDICATIONS FOR THE USE OF INTRAVENOUS HYPER-ALIMENTATION. The principal indications for parenteral alimentation are found in seriously ill patients suffering from malnutrition, sepsis, or surgical or accidental trauma when use of the gastrointestinal tract for feedings is not possible. It has been used in many instances either where it is not needed or where use of the gastrointestinal tract is more appropriate. In some instances, intravenous nutrition may be used to supplement inadequate oral intake. The safe and successful use of this regimen requires proper selection of patients with specific nutritional needs, experience with the technique, and an awareness of the associated complications. The fundamental goals are to provide sufficient calories and nitrogen substrate to promote tissue repair and to maintain the integrity or growth of the lean tissue mass. Listed below are situations in which parenteral nutrition has been used to successfully achieve these goals.

1. Newborn infants with catastrophic gastrointestinal anomalies, such as tracheoesophageal fistula, gastroschisis, omphalocele, or massive intestinal atresia

2. Infants who fail to thrive nonspecifically or secondarily to gastrointestinal insufficiency associated with the short bowel syndrome, malabsorption, enzyme deficiency, meconium ileus, or idiopathic diarrhea

3. Adult patients with short bowel syndrome secondary to massive small bowel resection or enteroenteric, enterocolic, enterovesical, or enterocutaneous fistulas

4. Patients with high alimentary tract obstructions without vascular compromise, secondary to achalasia, stricture, or neoplasia of the esophagus; gastric carcinoma; or pyloric obstruction

5. Surgical patients with prolonged paralytic ileus following major operations, multiple injuries, or blunt or open abdominal trauma, or patients with reflex ileus complicating various medical diseases

6. Patients with normal bowel length but with malabsorption secondary to sprue, hypoproteinemia, enzyme or pancreatic insufficiency, regional enteritis, or ulcerative colitis

7. Adult patients with functional gastrointestinal disorders such as esophageal dyskinesia following cerebral vascular accident, idiopathic diarrhea, psychogenic vomiting, or anorexia nervosa

8. Patients who cannot ingest food or who regurgitate and aspirate oral or tube feedings because of depressed or obtunded sensorium following severe metabolic derangements, neurologic disorders, intracranial surgery, or central nervous system trauma

9. Patients with excessive metabolic requirements secondary to severe trauma, such as extensive full-thickness burns, major fractures, or soft tissue injuries

10. Patients with granulomatous colitis, ulcerative colitis, and tuberculous enteritis, in which major portions of the absorptive mucosa are diseased

11. Paraplegics, quadriplegics, or debilitated patients with indolent decubitus ulcers in the pelvic areas, particularly when soilage and fecal contamination are a problem

12. Patients with malignancy, with or without cachexia, in

whom malnutrition might jeopardize successful delivery of a therapeutic option

13. Patients with potentially reversible acute renal failure, in whom marked catabolism results in the liberation of intracellular anions and cations, inducing hyperkalemia, hypermagnesemia, and hyperphosphatemia

Conditions *contraindicating* hyperalimentation include the following:

1. Lack of a specific goal for patient management, or where instead of extending a meaningful life, inevitable dying is prolonged
2. Periods of cardiovascular instability or severe metabolic derangement requiring control or correction before attempting hypertonic intravenous feeding
3. Feasible gastrointestinal tract feeding; in the vast majority of instances, this is the best route by which to provide nutrition
4. Patients in good nutritional status, in whom only short-term parenteral nutrition support is required or anticipated
5. Infants with less than 8 cm of small bowel, since virtually all have been unable to adapt sufficiently despite prolonged periods of parenteral nutrition
6. Patients who are irreversibly decerebrate or otherwise dehumanized

INSERTION OF CENTRAL VENOUS INFUSION CATHETER. The successful use of intravenous hyperalimentation generally depends upon the proper placement and management of the central venous feeding catheter. A 16-gauge, 8- or 12-in radiopaque catheter is introduced percutaneously through the subclavian or internal jugular vein and threaded into the superior vena cava. Although the technique for subclavian vein puncture (Fig. 2-5) has been quite popular, the internal jugular approach may be used (Fig. 2-6).

For insertion of the intravenous catheter through the subclavian vein, the patient is placed on his back in a 15° head-down position with a small pad placed between the shoulder blades to allow the shoulders to drop posteriorly. This allows expansion of the subclavian vein and easier penetration. The skin is scrubbed with ether or acetone to defat the surface and then with an iodophor compound. Drapes are carefully placed, and *scrupulous* aseptic precautions are observed. Local anesthetic is infiltrated into the skin, subcutaneous tissue, and periosteum at the inferior border of the midpoint of the clavicle. A 2-in-long, 14-gauge needle attached to a small syringe is

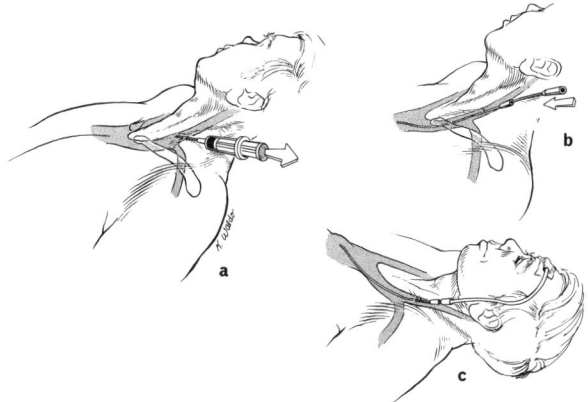

Fig. 2-6. Use of internal jugular vein for insertion of central venous catheter.

inserted, beveled down through the wheal, and advanced toward the tip of the operator's finger, which is pressed well into the patient's suprasternal notch. The needle should hug the inferior clavicular surface and go over the first rib into the subclavian vein. With slight negative pressure applied to the syringe, entrance into the vein will be noted by the appearance of blood. The needle is advanced a few millimeters further to be sure that it is entirely within the lumen of the vein. The patient is asked to perform a Valsalva maneuver, or the thumb is held over the needle hub as the syringe is removed to avoid air embolism. A 16-gauge, 8- or 12-in radiopaque catheter is then introduced through the needle and threaded into the superior vena cava. The needle is then withdrawn from the patient, and a small plastic splint is fitted over the junction of the catheter and needle to prevent catheter severance by the needle. The catheter is connected to a sterile intravenous administration tubing, and a slow infusion is begun while the catheter is sewn to the skin with a small synthetic suture. Antibiotic ointment is applied around the entrance of the catheter into the skin, and an occlusive dressing is applied over it including the junction of the intravenous tubing with the catheter. A chest film is immediately obtained to confirm the position of the radiopaque catheter in the vena cava and to check for a possible pneumothorax.

Every 2 or 3 days, the intravenous tubing is changed at the catheter entry site, the catheter site is scrubbed as for an operative procedure, and antibiotic ointment and a new occlusive dressing are applied. In general, withdrawal or administration of blood through the catheter or the use of the catheter for central venous pressure measurements should be avoided, since the risk of contamination and catheter occlusion are significantly increased.

The use of the internal jugular approach has also been quite satisfactory, especially for the pediatric age group. It is probably unwise, unless absolutely necessary, to place catheters into the inferior vena cava from the lower extremities because of the greater likelihood of sepsis and thromboembolic phenomena. Additionally, cutdown catheter insertions into the cephalic or basilic veins have not proved satisfactory.

Fig. 2-5. Use of the subclavian vein for insertion of central venous catheter.

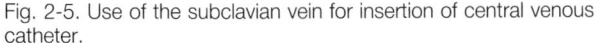

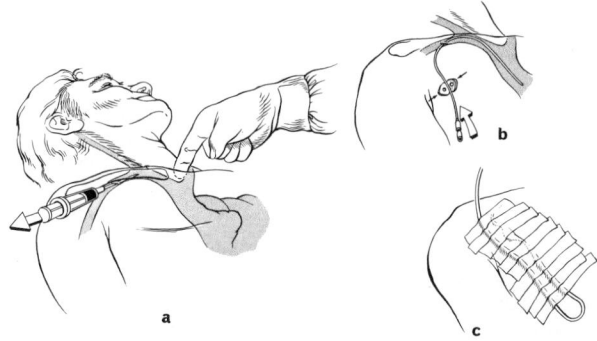

Table 2-14. DEXTROSE–AMINO ACID FORMULAS DELIVERED VIA A CENTRAL LINE

Formula	Aminosyn			Freamine III		Novamine		Travasol	
	10%	*8.5%*	*7%*	*10%*	*8.5%*	*11.4%*	*8.5%*	*10%*	*8.5%*
Osmolality, mO/L	1000	850	700	950	810	1049	785	1000	1322
Total AA, g/100 mL*	9.86	8.53	6.97	9.70	8.25	11.41	8.50	10.00	8.50
Total EAA, g/100 mL†	4.70	4.06	3.32	4.63	3.94	5.11	3.80	4.05	3.34
PE, g/L‡	100	85	70	96	82	113	84	103	89
N§	15.7	13.4	11.0	15.3	13.0	18.0	13.4	16.5	14.3

Vitamins are usually supplemented with a multiple vitamin preparation containing: vitamin A, 10,000 units; ergocalciferol, 1000 units; vitamin E, 5 units; thiamine HCL, 50 mg; riboflavin, 10 mg; pyridoxine HCL, 15 mg; niacinamide, 100 mg; dexpanthenal, 25 mg; ascorbic acid, 500 mg.

 * Total AA = total amino acids.
 † Total EAA = total essential amino acids.
 ‡ PE = protein equivalent.
 § N = nitrogen.
SOURCE: Adapted from Legaspi A, Lowry SF: Agents affecting nutrition and homeostasis, in *Manual of Drug Therapy*. New York, Raven Press, 1985.

PREPARATION AND ADMINISTRATION OF SOLUTIONS.
The basic solution contains a final concentration of 20 to 25% dextrose and 3 to 5% crystalline amino acids. The solutions are usually prepared in the pharmacy from commercially available kits containing the component solutions and transfer apparatus. Preparation in the pharmacy under laminar flow reduces the incidence of bacterial contamination of the solution. Proper preparation with suitable quality control is absolutely essential to avoid septic complications.

Since the formulation of commercially available alimentation solutions varies considerably with regard to amino acid and electrolyte concentration, it is imperative that the physician become thoroughly familiar with the levels of the components within the solution utilized (Table 2-14). Only in this manner may additives, in the form of additional electrolytes, be rationally planned to meet specific metabolic needs of the patient. One should recognize that the recommended concentrations of electrolytes are only estimates and that actual requirements may vary considerably (Table 2-10) between individual patients, dependent on routes of fluid and electrolyte loss, renal function, metabolic rate, cardiac function, and the underlying disease state.

Intravenous vitamin preparations should be added as recommended in Table 2-10. In addition, phytonadione (vitamin K_1) 10 mg and folic acid 5 mg should be administered intramuscularly once a week, since these are unstable in the hyperalimentation solution. Cyanocobalamin (vitamin B_{12}) 1 mg is given by intramuscular injection once a month. Intramuscular administration of iron may be required for patients with iron deficiency anemia although adequate mobilization of iron stores may occur once the patient is anabolic. During prolonged fat-free parenteral nutrition essential fatty acid deficiency may become clinically apparent, manifested by a dry, scaly dermatitis and loss of hair. The syndrome may be prevented by periodic infusion of a fat emulsion at a rate equal to 4 to 5% of total calories. Essential trace minerals may be required after prolonged total parenteral nutrition and may be supplied by direct addition of commercial preparations to dextrose amino acid solutions. The most frequent presentation of trace mineral deficiencies is the eczamatoid rash developing both diffusely and at intertriginous areas in zinc-deficient patients. Other rare trace mineral deficiencies include a microcytic anemia associated with copper deficiency and glucose intolerance presumably related to chromium deficiency. The latter complications are seldom seen except in patients receiving parenteral nutrition for extended periods of time. The daily administration of commercially available trace mineral supplements will obviate most such problems.

Depending upon fluid and nitrogen tolerance, parenteral nutrition solutions can generally be increased over 2 to 3 days to achieve the desired infusion rate. Insulin may be supplemented as necessary to ensure glucose tolerance. Wolfe and Elwyn have demonstrated that maximum efficiency of glucose utilization occurs at an infusion rate of 7 mg/(kg · min). Dextrose infusions above this level result in increased fat synthesis and provide no additional suppression of amino acid gluconeogenesis.

Rarely, additional intravenous fluids and electrolytes may be necessary with continued abnormal large losses of fluids. The patient should be carefully monitored for development of electrolyte, volume, acid-base, and septic complications. Vital signs and urinary output are regularly observed, and the patient should be weighed daily. Frequent adjustments of the volume and composition of the solutions are necessary during the course of therapy. Electrolytes are drawn daily until stable and every 2 or 3 days thereafter, and the hemogram, blood urea nitrogen, liver functions, phosphate, and magnesium are determined at least weekly.

The urine sugar level is checked every 6 h and blood sugar concentration at least once daily during the first few days of the infusion and at frequent intervals thereafter.

Relative glucose intolerance may occur following initiation of parenteral alimentation. Insulin may be supplemented as necessary to improve carbohydrate tolerance. The response of blood glucose to exogenous insulin is evaluated by frequent capillary blood determinations, rather than reliance upon glycosuria. If the blood sugar levels remain elevated or glycosuria persists, the dextrose concentration may be decreased, the infusion rate slowed, or regular insulin added to each bottle. The rise in blood glucose concentration observed after initiating an intravenous alimentation program may be temporary, as the normal pancreas increases its output of insulin in response to the continuous carbohydrate infusion. In patients with diabetes mellitus, additional crystalline or human insulin may be required.

The administration of adequate amounts of potassium is essential to achieve positive nitrogen balance and replace depleted intracellular stores. In addition, a significant shift of potassium ion from the extracellular to the intracellular space may take place because of the large glucose infusion, with resultant hypokalemia, metabolic alkalosis, and poor glucose utilization. In some cases as much as 240 meq of potassium ion daily may be required. Hypokalemia may cause glycosuria, which would be treated with potassium, not insulin. Thus, before giving insulin, the serum potassium level must be checked to avoid compounding the hypokalemia.

By virtue of the stress response following major trauma, sepsis, or burns, some patients may remain extremely insulin resistant.

Patients with insulin-dependent diabetes mellitus may exhibit wide fluctuations in blood glucose during parenteral nutrition. Partial replacement of lipid emulsions for dextrose calories may alleviate these problems in selected patients.

FAT EMULSIONS. Lipid emulsions derived from soybean or safflower oils are widely used as an adjunctive nutrient to prevent the development of essential fatty acid deficiency. Recent attention has also focused on their use as a major energy source in parenteral alimentation. Fat emulsion, dextrose, and amino acid combinations appear equally effective to carbohydrate and amino acid solutions in the repletion of nonstressed patients. The efficiency of fat as a caloric source in the traumatized, hypermetabolic patient is not well documented. There appears to be a theoretical advantage to the utilization of lipid emulsions in some septic and trauma patients where nonsuppressible fat oxidation and increased norepinephrine excretion accompany glucose infusion. Patients with abnormal fat transport or metabolism, lipoid nephrosis, coagulopathy, or serious pulmonary disease should not receive fat emulsions. Most investigators advise limitation of administered fat emulsions to between 2.0 and 2.5 g/kg of body weight per day.

SPECIAL FORMULATIONS. Numerous studies have documented the safety of parenteral alimentation in patients with renal failure. For this purpose, special formulations of essential amino acids may be indicated. Selection of the appropriate calorie and nitrogen concentrations must be judged by fluid tolerance, associated illnesses, and the frequency of dialysis. Appropriate use of dialysis is addi-

tive to nutritional support in improving survival of these patients. Solutions for patients with acute, oliguric renal failure contain a final dextrose concentration of 40 to 45% and only essential L-amino acids. In patients with nonoliguric renal failure, it may be possible to use both essential and nonessential amino acids to further promote protein synthesis.

Solutions designed for patients with hepatic failure contain increased levels of branched-chain amino acids and decreased concentrations of aromatic amino acids. Such solutions appear to improve encephalopathy but may not improve survival, which is dictated by the underlying hepatic pathology. Patients with moderate hepatic reserve and alcoholic hepatitis may also be treated with standard parenteral formulas to control encephalopathy and ascites.

Cachexia related to severe cardiac disease may be judiciously treated with highly concentrated dextrose and amino acid formulas that are low in sodium content.

COMPLICATIONS. Problems may arise either in the placement and maintenance of venous access or in the formulation and delivery of parenteral solutions. One of the more common and serious complications associated with long-term parenteral feeding is sepsis secondary to contamination of the central venous catheter. Contamination of solutions should be considered but is rare when proper pharmacy protocols have been followed. This problem occurs more frequently in patients with systemic sepsis and in many cases is due to hematogenous seeding of the catheter with bacteria. Usually, it is due to failure to observe strict aseptic precautions during preparation and administration of the solutions. One of the earliest signs of systemic sepsis may be the sudden development of glucose intolerance (with or without temperature increase) in a patient who previously has been maintained on parenteral alimentation without difficulty. When this occurs or if fever develops without obvious cause, a diligent search for a potential septic focus is indicated. Other causes of fever should also be investigated. If fever persists, the infusion catheter should be removed and cultured. Some centers are now replacing catheters considered at low risk for infection over a J-wire. Should evidence of infection persist over 24 to 48 h without a definable source, the catheter should be replaced in the opposite subclavian vein or into one of the internal jugular veins and the infusion restarted. It may be advisable to wait a short period of time before reinserting the catheter, especially if bacteremia or hemodynamic instability are present.

Other complications related to catheter placement include the development of pneumothorax, hemothorax, or hydrothorax; subclavian artery injury; cardiac arrhythmias if the catheter is placed into the atrium or the ventricle; air embolism or catheter embolism; and, rarely, cardiac perforation with tamponade. Clinically evident thrombophlebitis or thrombosis of the superior vena cava has been rare, but radiographically proved thrombophlebitis has been noted in up to 25 percent of selected patients. All these complications may be avoided by strict adherence to the techniques previously outlined.

Although there is a trend for increased utilization of

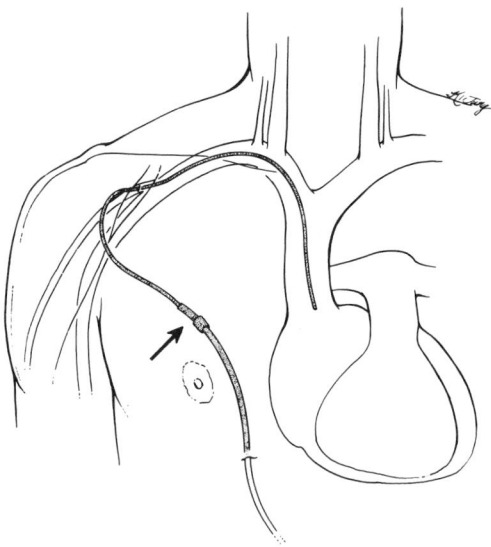

Fig. 2-7. A silastic catheter of the Hickman or Broviac type may be placed by percutaneous means into the superior vena cava or, as shown, by a venotomy in the cephalic, external, or internal jugular veins. The dacron cuff (arrow) may be positioned closer to the skin exit site than is demonstrated above. (Modified from: *Hickman RO et al: Surg Gynecol Obstet 148:871, 1979, with permission.*)

multiple lumen catheters for purposes of infusion therapy and monitoring critically ill patients, the risks, particularly of sepsis and of venous thrombosis, attending the prolonged use of such catheters may be increased. Efforts should be directed at replacing these catheters with standard single lumen intravenous feeding catheters at the earliest possible time. The acute nutritional management of surgical patients seldom requires the use of permanently implanted catheters (Fig. 2-7). Use of these catheters should be restricted to those nonseptic or high-risk patients requiring prolonged periods of nutritional and/or fluid therapy or for selected patients requiring frequent blood sampling.

Hyperosmolar nonketotic hyperglycemia may develop with normal rates of infusion in patients with impaired glucose tolerance or in any patient if the hypertonic solutions are administered too rapidly. This is a particularly common complication in latent diabetics and in patients following severe surgical stress or trauma. Treatment of the condition consists of volume replacement with correction of electrolyte abnormalities and the administration of insulin. This particularly serious complication can be avoided with careful attention to daily fluid balance and frequent determinations of urine and blood sugar levels and serum electrolyte content.

A number of volume, concentration, and compositional abnormalities may also develop, but these are largely avoided by careful attention to the details of patient management. This is particularly important for elderly patients and for patients with significant cardiovascular, renal, or hepatic disorders. Increasing experience has emphasized the importance of not "overfeeding" the parenterally nourished patient. This is particularly true of the depleted patient in whom excess calorie infusion may result in carbon dioxide retention and respiratory insufficiency. In addition, excess feeding has also been related to the development of hepatic steatosis or marked glycogen deposition in selected patients. Mild abnormalities of serum transaminases, alkaline phosphatase, and bilirubin may occur in many parenterally nourished patients. Failure of the tests to plateau or return toward normal over 7 to 14 days should suggest another etiology.

HOME PARENTERAL NUTRITION

Patients who do not require a hospital environment for management of their primary disease, yet cannot tolerate adequate enteral or oral feeding, *may* be candidates for home parenteral nutrition. Silastic catheters placed in the superior vena cava by the cephalic or internal jugular vein and tunneled over the chest wall to exit near the sternum have proved effective for this purpose (Fig. 2-7). Alternatives to this technique include the placement of subcutaneous infusion ports, which in preliminary trials have proved to be effective for long-term intravenous nutritional support. An absolute catheter-related infection rate of 0.3 per year per patient may be anticipated.

While home parenteral nutrition is generally more cost effective than similar inpatient methods, criteria for selection of patients must be more stringent than those listed above for hospitalized patients. Patients with terminal illnesses, lack of self-care ability, or a supportive home environment are *not* candidates for this method. The majority of patients will suffer from inflammatory bowel disease, motility disorders, or ischemic bowel infarction and resection.

An extended period of inpatient training is necessary to acquaint the patient and family with appropriate methods of solution preparation and delivery. This is best done in a multidisciplinary setting where professionals are thoroughly familiar with the acute and chronic complications of home parenteral nutrition. All patients on home parenteral nutrition should be placed on the registry maintained by Howard at the Oley Foundation (Albany Medical College). This will allow continued refinements in the clinical and technical management of these patients.

Bibliography

Fluid and Electrolyte Therapy

Agus ZS, Wasserstein A, Goldfarb S: Disorders of calcium and magnesium homeostasis. *Am J Med* 72:473, 1982.

Arieff AI, Leach W, Park R, et al: Systemic effects of NaHCO₃ in experimental lactic acidosis in dogs. *Am J Physiol* 242:F586, 1982.

Astrup P, Jorgensen K, Andersen OS, et al: The acid-base metabolism: a new approach. *Lancet* 1:1035, 1960.

Baxter CR, Zedlitz WH, Shires GT: High-output acute renal failure complicating acute traumatic injury. *J Trauma* 4:467, 1964.

Bishop RL, Weisfeldt ML: Sodium bicarbonate administration during cardiac arrest: effect on arterial pH, pCO₂ and osmolality. *JAMA* 235:506, 1976.

Canizaro PC: Oxygen transport in shock, in Shires GT (ed.): *Shock and Related Problems.* New York, Churchill Livingstone, 1984, pp 95–110.

Canizaro PC, Prager MD, Shires GT: The infusion of Ringer's lactate solution during shock. *Am J Surg* 122:494, 1971.

Carrico CJ, Canizaro PC, Shires GT: Fluid resuscitation following injury. *Crit Care Med* 4:46, 1976.

Collins JA: Problems associated with the massive transfusion of stored blood. *Surgery* 75:274, 1974.

Gamble JL: Chemical anatomy, physiology and pathology of extracellular fluid. In lecture syllabus. Cambridge, MA, Harvard University Press, 1949.

Kwun BK, Boucherit T, Wong J, et al: Treatment of metabolic alkalosis with intravenous infusion of concentrated hydrochloric acid. *Am J Surg* 146:328, 1983.

Mattar JA, Weil MH, Shubin H, et al: Cardiac arrest in the critically ill. II. Hyperosmolal states following cardiac arrest. *Am J Med* 56:162, 1974.

Mengoli LR: Excerpts from the history of postoperative fluid therapy. *Am J Surg* 121:311, 1971.

Moore FD, Olesen KH, McMurrey JD, et al: *Body Cell Mass and Its Supporting Environment: Body Composition in Health and Disease*. Philadelphia, Saunders, 1963.

Moyer CA: *Fluid Balance*. Chicago, Year Book Medical Publishers, Inc, 1954.

Narins RG, Emmett M: Simple and mixed acid-base disorders: a practical approach. *Medicine* 59:161, 1980.

Roberts JP, Roberts JD, Skinner C, et al: Extracellular fluid deficit following operation and its correction with Ringer's lactate; a reassessment. *Ann Surg* 202:1, 1985.

Shires GT, Cunningham JN, Baker CRF, et al: Alterations in cellular membrane function during hemorrhagic shock in primates. *Ann Surg* 176:288, 1972.

Shires GT, Jackson DE: Postoperative salt tolerance. *Arch Surg* 84:703, 1962.

Shires GT III, Peitzman AB, Albert SA, et al: Response of extravascular lung water to intraoperative fluids. *Ann Surg* 197:515, 1983.

Stewart AF: Therapy of malignancy-associated hypercalcemia: 1983. *Am J Med* 74:475, 1983.

Thompson JE, Vollman RW, Austin DJ, et al: Prevention of hypotensive and renal complications of aortic surgery using balanced salt solution: thirteen year experience with 670 cases. *Ann Surg* 167:767, 1968.

Virgilio RW, Rice CL, Smith DE, et al: Crystalloid vs. colloid resuscitation: is one better? *Surgery* 85:129, 1979.

Wang C, Guyton SW: Hyperparathyroid crisis: clinical and pathologic studies of 14 patients. *Ann Surg* 190:782, 1979.

Wong ET, Rude RK, Singer FR, et al: A high prevalence of hypomagnesemia and hypermagnesemia in hospitalized patients. *Am J Clin Pathol* 79:348, 1983.

Wright HK, Gann DS: Correction of defect in free water excretion in postoperative patients by extracellular fluid volume expansion. *Ann Surg* 158:70, 1963.

Nutrition

Abel RM, Beck CH Jr, Abbott WM, et al: Improved survival from acute renal failure after treatment with intravenous essential 1-amino acids and glucose. *N Engl J Med* 288:695, 1973.

Alexander JW, MacMillan BG, Stinnert JD, et al: Beneficial effects of aggressive protein feeding in severely burned children. *Ann Surg* 192:505, 1980.

Askanazi J, Rosenbaum SH, Hyman AI, et al: Respiratory changes induced by the large glucose loads of total parenteral nutrition. *JAMA* 243:1444, 1980.

Baker JP, Detsky AS, Stewart S, et al: Randomized trial of total parenteral nutrition in critically ill patients: metabolic effects of varying glucose-lipid ratios as the energy source. *Gastroenterology* 87:53, 1984.

Bartlett RH, Dechert RE, Mault JR, et al: Measurement of metabolism in multiple organ failure. *Surgery* 92:771, 1982.

Bessey PQ, Watters JM, Aoki TT, Wilmore DW: Combined hormonal infusion simulates the metabolic response to injury. *Ann Surg* 200:264, 1984.

Cahill GF Jr: Starvation in man. *N Engl J Med* 282:668, 1970.

Clague MB, Keir MJ, Wright PD, et al: The effects of nutrition and trauma on whole-body protein metabolism in man. *Clin Sci* 65:165, 1983.

Cuthbertson DP: The disturbance of metabolism produced by bony and non-bony injury, with notes on certain abnormal conditions of bone. *Biochem J* 24:1244, 1930.

Dahn MS, Lange P, Lobdell K, et al: Splanchnic and total body oxygen consumption differences in septic and injured patients. *Surgery* 101:69, 1987.

Dudrick SJ, Wilmore DW, Vars HM, et al: Long-term parenteral nutrition with growth, development, and positive nitrogen balance. *Surgery* 64:134, 1968.

Fischer JE (ed): *Surgical Nutrition*. Boston, Little, Brown, 1983.

Grant JP (ed): *Handbook of Total Parenteral Nutrition*. Philadelphia, Saunders, 1980.

Heymsfield SB, Bethel RA, Ansley JD, et al: Enteral hyperalimentation: an alternative to central venous hyperalimentation, *Ann Intern Med* 90:63, 1979.

Lindmark L, Bennegard K, Eden E, et al: Resting energy expenditure in malnourished patients with and without cancer. *Gastroenterology* 87:402, 1984.

Lowry SF: Host metabolic response to injury, in Shires GT, Davis JM (eds): *Host Defenses Advance in Trauma and Surgery*. New York, Raven Press, 1986.

Lowry SF, Brennan MF: Intravenous feeding of the cancer patient, in Caldwell MD, Rombeau JL (eds): *Clinical Nutrition*. Philadelphia, Saunders, 1985, vol II.

Mirtallo JM, Schneider PJ, Mavko K, et al: A comparison of essential and general amino acid infusions on the nutritional support of patients with compromised renal function, *J Parenter Enterol Nutr* 6:109, 1982.

Moore FD: *Metabolic Care of the Surgical Patient*. Philadelphia, Saunders, 1960.

Muggia-Sullam M, Bower RH, Murphy RF: Postoperative enteral versus parenteral nutritional support in gastrointestinal surgery: a matched prospective study. *Am J Surg* 149:106, 1985.

Mullen JL, Buzby GP, Matthews DC, et al: Reduction of operative morbidity and mortality by combined preoperative and postoperative nutritional support. *Ann Surg* 192:604, 1980.

Muller JM, Dienst C, Brenner V, et al: Pre-operative parenteral feeding in patients with gastrointestinal carcinoma. *Lancet* 1:68, 1982.

Rapp RP, Young B, Twyman D, et al: The favorable effect of early parenteral feeding on survival in head-injured patients. *J Neurosurg* 58:906, 1983.

Smith RC, Burkinshaw L, Hill GL: Optimal energy and nitrogen for gastroenterological patients requiring intravenous nutrition. *Gastroenterology* 82:445, 1982.

Twomey PL, Patching SC: Cost-effectiveness of nutritional support. *J Parenter Enterol Nutr* 9:3, 1985.

Wilmore WW (ed): *The Metabolic Management of the Critically Ill*. New York, Plenum Press, 1977.

Chapter 3

Hemostasis, Surgical Bleeding, and Transfusion

Seymour I. Schwartz

BIOLOGY OF HEMOSTASIS

Hemostasis is a complex process that prevents or terminates blood loss from the intravascular space, provides a fibrin network for tissue repair, and ultimately, removes the fibrin when it is no longer needed. Four major physiologic events participate, both in sequence and interdependently, in the hemostatic process. Vascular constriction, platelet plug formation, fibrin formation, and fibrinolysis occur in that general order, but the products of each of these four processes are interrelated in such a fashion that there is a continuum and multiple reinforcements (Fig. 3-1.).

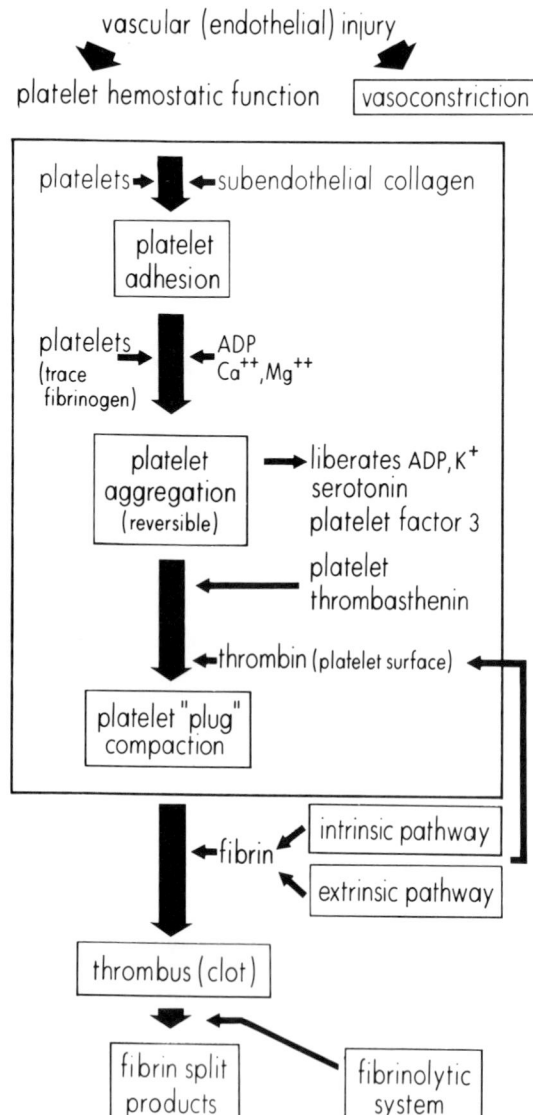

Fig. 3-1. Schematic representation of hemostasis.

tent vasodilator. Serotonin, 5-hydroxytryptamine (5-HT), released during platelet aggregation, is another vasoconstrictor, but it has been shown that when platelets have been depleted of serotonin in vivo, constriction is not inhibited. Bradykinin and fibrinopeptides in the coagulation schema are also capable of contracting smooth muscle. Some patients with mild bleeding disorders and a prolonged bleeding time have, as their only abnormality, capillary loops that fail to constrict in response to injury.

A lateral incision in a small artery may remain open because of physical forces, while complete transection of a similarly sized vessel contracts to the extent that bleeding may cease spontaneously. The vascular response factor should also include the contribution of pressure provided by surrounding tissues. Bleeding from a small venule ruptured by trauma, in the thigh of an athlete, may be negligible because of the compressive effect of surrounding muscle. In the same individual, bleeding from a similar vessel in the nasal mucosa may be significant. When there is low perivascular pressure, as seen in patients with muscle atrophy accompanying aging, prolonged steroid therapy, and in patients with the Ehlers-Danlos syndrome, bleeding tends to be more persistent.

Platelet Function

Platelets are 2-μm diameter fragments of megakaryocytes and number 200,000 to 400,000/mm^3 in circulating blood with a life span of 7 to 9 days. They play an integral role in hemostasis along two pathways. Platelets, which normally do not adhere to each other or to the normal vessel wall, form a plug that stops bleeding when vascular disruption occurs. Injury to the intima exposes subendothelial collagen to which platelets adhere within 15 s of the traumatic event. This requires von Willebrand factor (vWF), a protein that is lacking in patients with von Willebrand's disease. The platelets then expand and develop pseudopodal processes and also initiate a release reaction that recruits other platelets from the circulating blood. As a consequence, a loose platelet aggregate forms, sealing the disrupted blood vessel. The aggregation up to this point is reversible and is not associated with secretion. This process is known as *primary hemostasis*. The administration of heparin does not interfere with this reaction, and that fact explains why hemostasis can occur in the heparinized patient. Adenosine diphosphate (ADP) and serotonin are principal mediators in this process of adhesion and aggregation. Various prostaglandins have opposing activities. Arachidonic acid, released from platelet membranes, is converted by cyclooxygenase to PGG$_2$ and PGH$_2$, which, in turn, are converted to TXA$_2$, a potent platelet aggregator and vasoconstrictor. By contrast, PGE$_1$ (prostacycline) and PGE$_2$ inhibit aggregation and act as vasodilators.

ADP, released from damaged tissues and stimulated platelets, plus platelet factor 4 and trace thrombin on the platelet surface in the face of Ca^{2+} and Mg^{2+}, stimulate a platelet release reaction by which the content of the platelet and its granules is discharged. Fibrinogen is required for this process. The release reaction results in compac-

Vascular Constriction

Adherence of endothelial cells to adjacent endothelial cells may be sufficient to cause cessation of blood loss from the intravascular space. Vasoconstriction is the initial vascular response to injury even at the capillary level. It is dependent upon local contraction of smooth muscle that has a reflex response to various stimuli. The initial vascular constriction occurs prior to platelet adherence at the site of injury. Vasoconstriction is subsequently linked to platelet plug and fibrin formation. Thromboxane A$_2$ (TXA$_2$), that results from the release of arachidonic acid from platelet membranes during aggregation, is a powerful vasoconstrictor. By contrast, prostacycline, which is also secreted during the platelet release reaction, is a po-

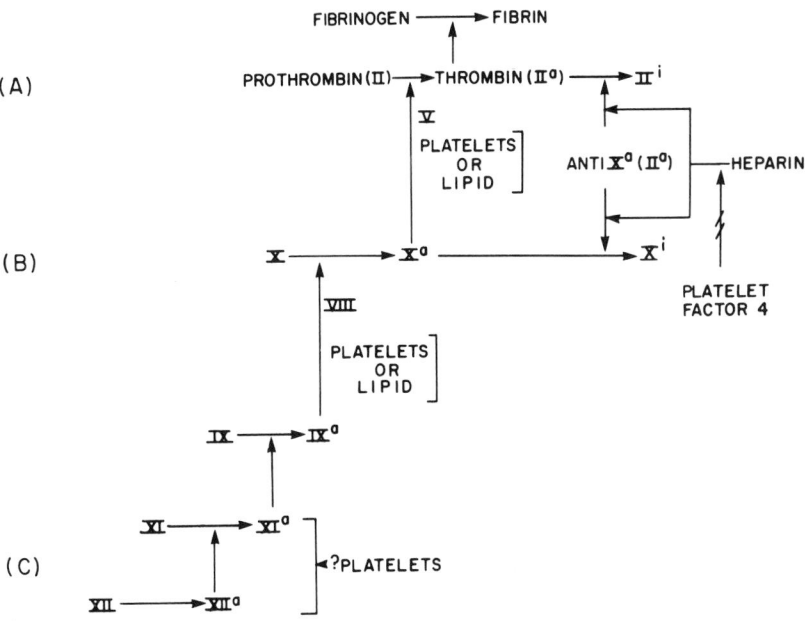

Fig. 3-2. Role of platelets in coagulation. Platelets or phospholipid accelerate reactions *A* and *B*. In addition, the role of platelets may be more complex in reaction *B* and may serve to protect factor X_a from inactivation by plasma inhibitors. Platelets may also play a part in activating the contact system *C*. Platelet factor 4 is the heparin-neutralizing substance (i = inactivated clotting factor). (From: *Weiss HJ: 1975, with permission.*)

tion of the platelets and the formation of an "amorphous" plug, wich is no longer reversible. This process is inhibited by cyclic AMP. As a consequence of the release reaction, platelet factor 3 is made available and contributes phospholipid to several stages of the coagulation cascade.

The lipoprotein surface provided by platelets catalyzes reactions that are involved in the conversion of prothrombin (factor II) into thrombin (Fig. 3-2). Platelet factor 3 is involved in the reaction by which activated factor IX (IXa), factor VIII, and calcium activate factor X. It is also involved in the reaction by which Xa, factor V, and Ca^{2+} activate factor II. Platelets may also play a role in the initial activation of factor XII and the activation of factor XI. Platelet factor 4 and β-thromboglobulin are also made available during the release reaction, and they may inhibit the activity of heparin and modify fibrin formation. The platelets also play a role in the fibrinolytic process by releasing an inhibitor of plasminogen activation.

Coagulation

Coagulation is the process by which prothrombin is converted into the proteolytic enzyme thrombin, which, in turn, cleaves the fibrinogen molecule to form insoluble fibrin in order to stabilize and add to the platelet plug. Coagulation consists of a series of zymogen activation stages in which circulating proenzymes are converted in sequence to activated proteases (Fig. 3-3). The traditional concept of the clotting system evolved from test tube

analysis and follows two pathways. The two pathways are the *intrinsic* pathway, which involves components normally present in blood, and the *extrinsic* pathway that is initiated by the tissue lipoprotein. In the intrinsic pathway factor XII is activated by binding to subendothelial collagen. Prekallikrein and high molecular weight kinogen amplify this contact phase. Activated factor XII (XIIa) proteolytically cleaves factor XI and also prekallikrein to form XIa and kallikrein. In the presence of Ca^{2+}, XIa activates factor IX (IXa). This, in turn, complexes with factor VIII, which can be activated to a more potent form by thrombin, and, in the presence of Ca^{2+} and the phospholipid platelet factor 3, activates factor X. In the extrinsic pathway, the tissue phospholipid, thromboplastin, reacts with factor VII and Ca^{2+} to activate factor X.

Activated factor X (Xa), produced by the two pathways, proteolyzes prothrombin (factor II) to form thrombin. This process is accelerated by factor V, tissue lipoproteins, platelet surface phospholipids, and Ca^{2+}. Thrombin activates the fibrin stabilizing factor (XIII) and cleaves fibrinopeptides A and B from fibrinogen (factor I) to form fibrin, a monomer that is cross-linked with XIIIa, to form a stable clot (Table 3-1).

All the coagulation factors except thromboplastin, Ca^{2+}, and most of factor VIII are synthesized in the liver. Factors II, VII, IX, and X require vitamin K for their production.

Fibrinolysis

Fibrinolysis is a natural process directed at maintaining the patency of blood vessels by lysis of fibrin deposits. Also involved in the maintenance of vascular patency is circulating ATIII which neutralizes the action of thrombin and other proteases in the coagulation cascade.

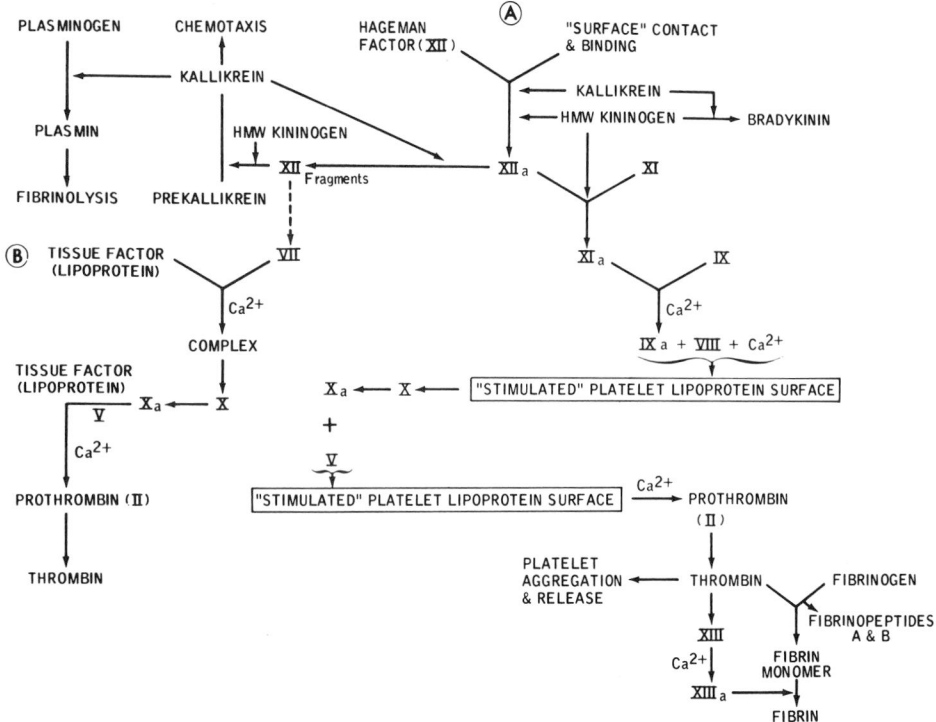

Fig. 3-3. Outline of the intrinsic (A) and extrinsic (B) pathways of fibrin formation. These interactions, which represent "secondary hemostasis," occur simultaneously with development of the hemostatic plug, i.e., primary hemostasis. The subendothelial blood vessel surface exposed by vascular damage or severance serves as a nidus for platelet adhesion and simulation. Factor XII (Hageman factor) also binds to the subendothelium and in so doing is converted from its precursor (zymogen) form to an activated molecule (XII$_a$). This interaction by itself (known as the contact phase) is relatively prolonged and inefficient. Amplification and enhancement occur by virtue of participation of prekalikrein and high-molecular-weight kininogen. The contact phase is also involved in initiation of fibrinolysis, kinin generation, and chemotaxis. Subsequent stages of intrinsic and extrinsic coagulation may be conceptualized as a biphasic catalytic system in which activated zymogens such as IX$_a$ form a complex with factor VIII. In the presence of calcium the complex catalyzes activation of factor X on the platelet lipoprotein surface. The X$_a$ receptor site on the platelet surface is known to be coagulation factor V (not phospholipid). Tissue factor lipoprotein (B) probably functions in a manner analogous to the stimulated platelet membrane. During activation of prothrombin by the X$_a$–V surface complex, prothrombin is bound via a calcium-mediated interaction. Three pairs of adjacent γ-carboxyglutamic acid residues are present on the prothrombin molecule, and each pair binds a calcium ion. In the absence of vitamin K an abnormal prothrombin molecule is synthesized containing glutamic but not γ-carboxyglutamic acid. Thus, calcium-mediated binding of prothrombin to the X$_a$–V-platelet lipoprotein complex is defective (these reactions have not yet been studied with platelets or platelet membranes, and the last statement is an assumption). Thrombin, a two-chain serine protease, cleaves arginine-glycine bonds of fibrinogen. One chain of thrombin (the B chain) closely resembles the serine proteases produced in the pancreas. Thrombin in concentrations that do not interact with fibrogen induces platelet aggregation and release. The stimulatory effect of the platelet surface may not be confined to coagulation proteins per se. It has been shown that tissue factor–type activity generated by leukocytes in the presence of endotoxin is enhanced by platelet membranes. (From: *Marcus AJ: 1978*, with permission.)

Fibrinolysis is initiated at the same time as the clotting mechanism under the influence of circulating kinases, tissue activators, and kallikrein present in many organs including venous endothelium. Fibrinolysis is dependent upon the enzyme, plasmin, which is derived from a precursor plasma protein (plasminogen) (Fig. 3-4). Plasminogen levels are known to rise as a consequence of exercise, venous occlusion, and anoxia. Plasminogen activation is also initiated by the activation of factor XII. The plasminogen is preferentially absorbed on fibrin deposits. The enzyme plasmin lyses fibrin and acts on other coagulant proteins, including fibrinogen, factor V, and factor VIII, as well. The smaller fragments of polypeptide products of fibrin that are produced interfere with normal platelet aggregation; the larger fragments are incorporated into the clot in lieu of normal fibrin monomers and result in an unstable clot. Human blood also contains an anti-plasmin that inhibits plasminogen activation, and platelets are believed to possess anti-fibrinolytic activity.

CONGENITAL HEMOSTATIC DEFECTS

Inheritance

The modes of inheritance of hemostatic disorders, with only rare exceptions, are three in type: (1) autosomal dominant, (2) autosomal recessive, and (3) sex-linked recessive. Since one chromosome of each of the 22 autosomal pairs normally is derived from each parent, any gene inherited as a part of an autosomal chromosome nor-

Table 3-1. NOMENCLATURE OF COAGULATION FACTORS

Factor I	Fibrinogen
Factor II	Prothrombin
Factor III	Thromboplastin (tissue or platelet factors)
Factor IV	Calcium
Factor V	Proaccelerin
Factor VI	(Same as factor V)
Factor VII	Proconvertin
Factor VIII	Antihemophilic factor A
Factor IX	Plasma thromboplastin component
Factor X	Stuart-Prower factor
Factor XI	Antihemophilic factor C
Factor XII	Hageman factor
Factor XIII	Fibrin stabilizing factor (Laki-Lorand)

mally will occur with equal frequency among males and females. Each child of a parent carrying an autosomal dominant gene has one chance in two of inheriting that trait. The most common hemostatic disorder transmitted by the autosomal dominant mode is von Willebrand's disease. Hereditary hemorrhagic telangiectasia and factor XI deficiency also appear to be transmitted in this fashion.

A normal individual should transmit no disease to his progeny. Occasionally, in a pedigree with an autosomal dominant gene, an *apparently* normal person may transmit disease to his or her child. The parent clearly carried the gene, which clinically expressed no defect. Explanation of this phenomenon is not at hand. The gene activity in the parent is referred to as "incompletely penetrant."

In inherited hemostatic disorders, the difference in clinical expression between dominant and recessive genes is a graded one rather than an "all-or-none" phenomenon. The heterozygous individual with an autosomal recessive trait may have a measurable deficiency of the factor governed by that gene, but no clinical disease. In order to demonstrate clinical expression of disease, the individual must be homozygous. This appears to be the case, for example, in factor X deficiency. The homozygote with clinical disease has less than 5 percent of factor X activity, while heterozygotes have levels ranging from 21 to 50 percent. Since the presumed heterozygotes within the same pedigree vary in factor X activity, it is convenient to suggest that the gene shows variable expression. Other hemostatic disorders probably inherited in this mode are factor V, factor VII, and factor I deficiencies.

Sex-linked recessive inheritance governs true hemophilia (factor VIII deficiency) and factor IX deficiency (Christmas disease). The genes for these diseases are recessive in expression and are carried on the female (X) chromosome. When paired with the normal X chromosome (the female carrier state), clinical disease is not present. When the affected X chromosome is paired with the normal male (Y) chromosome, clinical disease is expressed.

Theoretically, with the "graded" expression, the female carrier should be detectable in the laboratory. In fact, since the range of factor VIII activity normally is so broad, most female carriers *appear* to fall in the low-normal range. Estimates vary, but possibly as many as 50 percent of female carriers can be identified. Although the sex-linked recessive mode of inheritance has been confirmed repeatedly in true hemophilia, it seems likely that an *autosomal* gene also may influence factor VIII activity. This probability is emphasized by the autosomal dominant mode of inheritance of von Willebrand's disease, characterized by low factor VIII activity, and also by the patterns of variation in factor VIII activity among individuals within the same normal family and among different normal families.

Platelet Deficiencies

The most common congenital platelet deficiency is an abnormality seen in *von Willebrand's disease* (see material below). In this disorder, the von Willebrand factor (vWF), which is missing, has been shown to be required for platelet adhesion to subendothelial collagen. Also, unlike platelets of normal patients that aggregate in vitro when ristocetin is added, platelets from patients with von Willebrand's disease fail to aggregate with the addition of ristocetin. Another inherited disorder affecting platelets is the rare *Bernard-Soulier syndrome*. Patients with Bernard-Soulier syndrome have normal levels of vWF and the addition of that factor does not affect aggregation of platelets in the presence of ristocetin. In Bernard-Soulier syndrome, the platelet membrane receptor for vWF, a portion of the glycoprotein I complex, is missing.

Glanzmann's thrombasthenia is a rare congenital disorder in which platelets fail to aggregate in the presence of ADP, and mediation of factors involved in clot retention is impaired also. Patients with *congenital afibrinogenemia* also have impairment of platelet aggregation because fibrinogen is required for this process to occur. Patients with congenital afibrinogenemia have disturbed platelet function, manifested by a prolonged bleeding time correctable by fibrinogen administration.

Fig. 3-4. Fibrinolytic system.

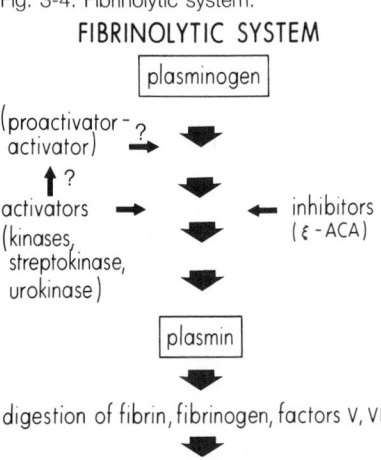

FIBRINOLYTIC SYSTEM

plasminogen

(proactivator - activator) ?

↑ ?

activators (kinases, streptokinase, urokinase) → ← inhibitors (ε - ACA)

plasmin

digestion of fibrin, fibrinogen, factors V, VIII

split products

Congenital disorders of platelet secretion include *storage pool disease,* in which the platelets lack the storage capability of ADP required for aggregation. The Hermansky-Pudlak syndrome (occulocutaneous albinism, ceroidlike deposits in macrophages, and bleeding diathesis) is classified in this category. Congenital *primary release defects* have also been described and are responsible for prolonged bleeding time.

Congenital Defects of Coagulation Factors

FACTOR VIII DEFICIENCY (CLASSICAL HEMOPHILIA)

Classical hemophilia (hemophilia A) is a disease of males. The failure to synthesize normal factor VIII activity is inherited as a sex-linked recessive trait. Spontaneous mutations account for almost 20 percent of cases. The incidence of the disease is approximately 1:10,000 to 1:15,000 population, and the clinical manifestations can be extremely variable. The accuracy for detecting the carrier state now approaches 90 percent.

CLINICAL MANIFESTATIONS. Characteristically, the severity of clinical manifestations is related to the degree of deficiency of factor VIII. Spontaneous bleeding and severe complications are the rule when virtually no factor VIII can be detected in the plasma. When plasma factor VIII concentrations are in the range of 5 percent of normal, the patient may have no spontaneous bleeding yet may bleed severely with trauma or surgical treatment. Patients with levels greater than 5 percent of normal (greater than $0.05\mu m/mL$) are considered mild hemophiliacs. Patients whose factor VIII levels fall between 1 and 5 percent of normal are considered moderately severe hemophiliacs. Typically, members of the same pedigree with true hemophilia will have approximately the same degree of clinical manifestations.

While the severely affected patient may bleed during early infancy, significant bleeding typically is noted first when the child is a toddler. At that time, in addition to the classic bleeding into joints, epistaxis and hematuria may be noted. Bleeding that is life-threatening may follow injury to the tongue or frenulum. Tracheal compression and retropharyngeal bleeding may follow tonsillar infection. Intracranial bleeding, associated with trauma in half the cases, accounts for 25 percent of deaths. Vascular and neural compromise may occur in relation to pressure secondary to bleeding into a soft tissue closed space. Equinus contracture deformity may be seen in severely hemophilic patients secondary to bleeding into the calf. Volkmann's contracture of the forearm and flexion contractures of the knees and elbows are also disabling sequelae of deep soft tissue bleeding.

Hemarthrosis is the most characteristic orthopaedic problem. Bleeding into the joint may cause few symptoms until distention of the joint capsule occurs. A large hemarthrosis generally is manifested by a tender, swollen, warm, and painful joint. Muscle spasm and pain around the joint arise from involvement of periarticular structures. These signs may mimic infection. The same ortho-

paedic problems are noted in association with severe factor IX deficiency (Christmas disease).

Retroperitoneal bleeding may follow lifting of a heavy object or strenuous exercise. Signs of posterior peritoneal irritation and spasm of the iliopsoas suggest the diagnosis. Hypovolemic shock may occur, since the amount of blood loss that can take place in this setting is enormous. The clinical manifestations of intramural intestinal hematoma are nausea and vomiting, crampy abdominal pain, and signs of peritoneal irritation mimic those of appendicitis. Fever and leukocytosis may be noted. Radiographs of the abdomen may fail to reveal an abnormality or may display a modest amount of ileus. Upper gastrointestinal examination may demonstrate a uniform thickening of mucosal folds which has been described as a "picket fence" or "stack of coins" appearance (Fig. 3-5). Intramural hematomas of the intestine occur with other hemostatic disorders and, therefore, should be considered

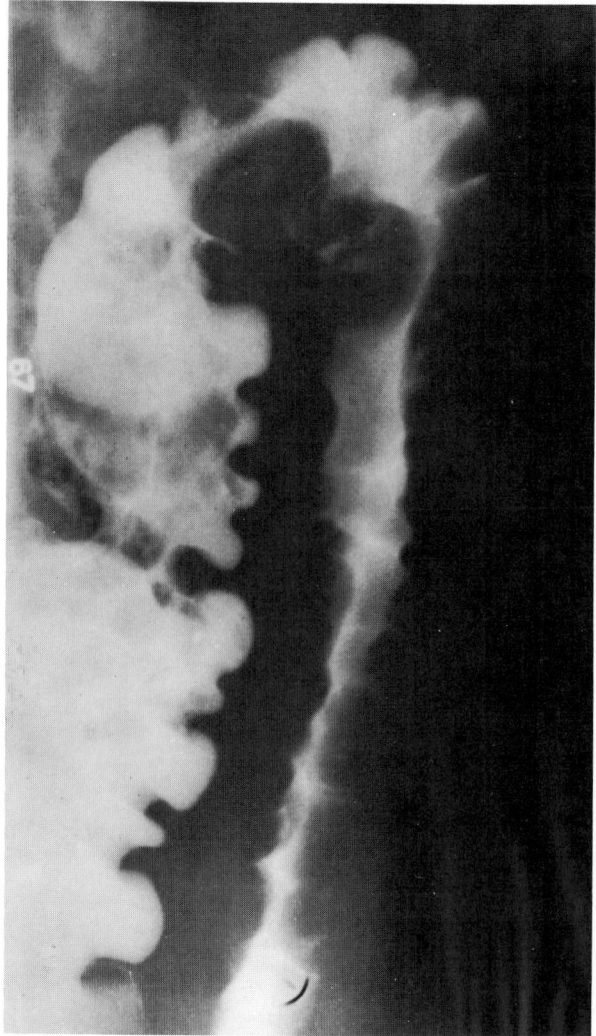

Fig. 3-5. Radiograph of patient with hemophilia. Note thickening of mucosal folds indicative of an intramural hematoma.

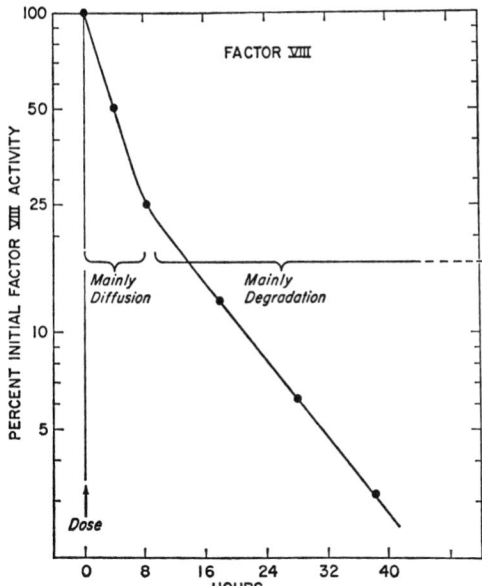

Fig. 3-6. Schematic representation of in vivo decay of a single dose of factor VIII. (From: *Shulman NR: 1968, with permission.*)

when any patient with a hemostatic problem presents with findings suggesting an acute intraabdominal process.

TREATMENT. Replacement Therapy. The plasma concentration of factor VIII necessary for maintenance of hemostatic integrity is normally quite small. Patients with as little as 2 to 3 percent of factor VIII activity usually do not bleed spontaneously. Once serious bleeding begins, however, a much higher level of factor VIII activity, probably approaching 30 percent, is necessary to achieve hemostasis.

The half-life of factor VIII is 8 to 12 h. Following administration of a given dose of factor VIII, approximately one-half of the initial posttransfusion activity disappears from the plasma in 4 h. This early disappearance is thought to be due, in large part, to diffusion from the intravascular space. The period of equilibration can extend for as long as 8 h, at which time only about one-quarter of the initial level remains in the circulating blood. From that time on, the slope of disappearance is less steep (Fig. 3-6). Twenty-four hours after a given dose, no more than 7 to 8 percent of administered factor VIII activity remains within the circulation.

One unit of factor VIII activity is considered that amount present in 1 mL of normal plasma. Actually, fresh frozen plasma contains 0.60 unit/mL. Theoretically, in a patient with 0 percent activity, to achieve an initial posttransfusion level of 60 percent of normal, using fresh plasma, a volume of plasma equal to 60 percent of the patient's estimated plasma volume would have to be administered. Table 3-2 shows approximate levels of factor VIII required for hemostasis in different lesions. The minimum hemostatic level of factor VIII for mild hemorrhages is 30 percent; for joint and muscle bleeding and major hemorrhages, it is 50 percent. For major surgery and life-threatening bleeding, levels of 80 to 100 percent

should be reached preoperatively and maintained above 30 percent for 2 weeks. Remembering the loss from the circulation, one-half the initial dose would need to be supplied every 12 h. The use of fresh plasma in such a circumstance would require a volume that is excessive. Factor VIII concentrates now available circumvent this problem. Cryoprecipitate concentrates of factor VIII can be regarded as containing 9.6 units/mL. The amount of material to be given can be computed from the formula

$$\frac{\text{Patient's weight (kg)} \times \text{desired rise of factor VIII (\% average normal)}}{\text{Total units of factor VIII in dose}} = R$$

where R is a factor that is fairly constant for any given type of material and represents the rise of factor VIII obtained in the patient's plasma for every unit of transfused factor VIII per kilogram of the patient's body weight. Half that amount is subsequently administered every 4 to 6 h to maintain a safe level. There is now a variety of factor VIII concentrates available. Regardless of the preparation employed, continued laboratory assessment of circulating factor VIII level is an important element in the control of these patients. Wet-frozen cryoprecipitate is preferred for replacement in patients with mild hemophilia since the risk of hepatitis is less than it is with factor VIII concentrates. The latter are preferred for major replacement problems. In mild hemophilia A and in mild von Willebrand's disease, DAVP (1-desamino-8-D-arginine vasopressin), a synthetic derivative of vasopressin, has been used to effect a dose-dependent increase of all factor VIII activities and to effect release of plasminogen activator. Patients undergoing orthopaedic or neurosurgical procedures should also receive a fibrinolytic inhibitor.

Following major surgical treatment of the hemophiliac, transfusion replacement of factor VIII should be continued for at least 10 days. Wounds should be well healed and all drains removed prior to the termination of therapy. If sutures remain, transfusion should be reinstituted prior to their removal. Many recent reports document the safety of major surgical procedures in hemophilic patients receiving replacement therapy. But in one large series, the incidence of postoperative hemorrhage did not improve over a 16-year period despite a threefold increase in dosage of factor VIII, suggesting that circulating factor VIII levels are not the sole determinant of bleeding in these patients.

The virus of homologous serum hepatitis is transmitted by the various concentrates of plasma. Other complications of replacement therapy include the appearance of inhibitors of factor VIII, which may arise in the hemophiliacs who have had transfusion. These inhibitors have been characterized as antibodies of the γ G variety. They tend to diminish in several weeks if further transfusion is not employed. Laboratory search for these factors should be carried out in every hemophilic patient who is considered a candidate for elective surgical treatment, as their presence complicates transfusion management. Paradoxical bleeding may occur in patients transfused to an appro-

Table 3-2. PRINCIPLES OF SUBSTITUTION THERAPY IN SURGERY IN PATIENTS WITH SEVERE BLEEDING DISORDERS

Type of operation and disease	Day of operation — Desirable level of (%)	Dosage — Initial units/kg	Dosage — Maintenance BW*	Dosage — Interval (h)	Day 2–7 postoperatively — Desirable level of (%)	Dosage — Maintenance units/kg BW	Dosage — Interval (h)	Day 8 postoperatively — Desirable level of (%)	Dosage — Maintenance units/kg BW	Dosage — Interval (h)
Hemophilia A	VII:C	VIII:C			VIII:C			VIII:C		
Major surgery	50–150	50–60	25–30	4–6	40–60	20–40	4–8	15–25	10–15	12–24
Minor surgery	40–50	25–40	20–30	4–8	30–50	15–20	6–12			
Hemophilia B	IX:C	IX:C			IX:C			IX:C		
Major surgery	50–150	60–70	30–40	8–12	40–60	30–40	12–24	15–25	10–20	24–48
Minor surgery	40–50	40–40	20–30	8–12	30–50	15–20	24			
von Willebrand's disease	VIII:C	VIII:C			VIII:C			VIII:C		
Major surgery	50–70 BT† < 5 min	30–40	30–40	4–5	> 40 BT < 10 min	10–20	12	20–40	5–10	24–48
Minor surgery	VIII:C 20–50 BT < 5 min	10–20	10–20	4–5	VIII:C > 40 BT < 10 min	5–10	12			

* Body weight.
† Bleeding time according to Duke.
SOURCE: Nilsson IM, Larsson SA, Bergentz SE, 1987, with permission.

priate factor VIII level due to the development of abnormal platelet function.

Adjunctive Management. Treatment of soft tissue bleeding is directed at the prevention of airway obstruction and vascular and neural damage. These are accomplished best by the administration of sufficient factor VIII. Bed rest and cold packs can be of some assistance. In general, results of fasciotomy to relieve pressure have varied from disappointing to disastrous. The occasional development of large cysts has resulted in sufficient deformity and disability to require amputation.

The primary treatment of hemophilic hemarthrosis is directed at maintaining full range of motion and minimal destruction of the cartilage. Aspiration of blood from the hemophilic joint is not uniformly endorsed, and when regarded as necessary, it should be considered a major surgical event. Elevation of factor VIII level by transfusion is necessary. The procedure should be carried out in the operating room under strict sterile precautions. In most instances, aspiration is not required, and the combination of factor VIII replacement and local cold packing proves sufficient. Physiotherapy plays a critical role and should consist of *active* exercises, since the patient is unlikely to move the extremity to a point where bleeding will recur. Passive exercises often result in recurrence of bleeding. The reader is referred to the review by Curtiss for details of orthopaedic management.

The management of intramural intestinal hematoma and retroperitoneal bleeding is predicated on appropriate transfusion therapy and avoidance of surgical treatment. Even when a relatively minor procedure, such as trache-ostomy, is performed, the plasma level of factor VIII should be raised above 25 to 30 percent. Since dental hygiene usually is poor in hemophilic patients, dental and oral surgical treatment frequently are necessary. The same principles of transfusion therapy pertain, and the procedures should be delegated to well-trained personnel working where optimal care can be provided.

FACTOR IX DEFICIENCY (CHRISTMAS DISEASE)

Factor IX deficiency clinically is indistinguishable from factor VIII deficiency and also has an X-linked recessive mode of inheritance. These two entities were considered a single disease until 1952, when their unique deficiencies were documented. Factor IX deficiency accounts for 20 percent of hemophiliacs. Christmas disease, like classical hemophilia, can occur in severe, moderate, or mild forms according to the level of factor IX activity in the plasma. The severe form has a factor IX level of less than 1 percent; one-half of the patients belong to this group.

TREATMENT. Most patients with severe factor IX deficiency require substitution therapy on a regular basis. All patients require substitution therapy whenever minor or major surgery is performed. Currently, therapy is generally based on the administration of factor IX concentrates. Initially the rate of disappearance of factor IX from the circulation is more rapid than that of factor VIII; subsequently factor IX, with a half-life of 18 to 40 h, has a slower disappearance rate. A variety of factor IX concentrates is available. Good therapeutic results have been achieved with each of the concentrates and minimal side effects have been noted. Konyne, which contains 10 to 60 units of factor IX/mL, has produced good results, but thromboembolic complications had been reported. More recently, the preparations have had other activated clotting factors removed, and the incidence of thromboembolic complications has decreased. During severe hemorrhage, treatment should be directed at achieving plasma factor IX levels of 20 to 50 percent of normal for the first 3 to 5 days, and then maintaining the plasma level at 10 to 20 percent of normal for approximately 10 days. The usual daily dose is 30 to 50 μm/kg of body weight, followed by 20 μm/kg of body weight/24 h. When an operation is required, the plasma level of approximately 50 to 70 percent of normal should be achieved. Sixty microns per kilogram of body weight every 24 h is recommended during the operation and the first postoperative day, followed by 30 to 40 μm/kg every 24 h for the next 2 to 3 days, and 20 μm/kg every 24 h for the remainder of the week. In all instances, the levels should be monitored by laboratory determinations. The development of antibodies against factor IX represents a serious complication that is difficult to deal with. This occurs in about 10 percent of patients with Christmas disease. These patients are managed by withholding all infusion therapy with blood or plasma. High doses of factor IX concentrates combined with cyclophosphamide have been effective.

VON WILLEBRAND'S DISEASE

von Willebrand's disease occurs as commonly as true hemophilia. The increasing recognition of this disease is related to more reliable factor VIII assays. This hereditary disorder of hemostasis is usually transmitted as an autosomally dominant trait but recessive inheritance may occur. The disease is characterized by a diminution of the level of factor VIII:C (procoagulant) activity that corrects the clotting abnormality in hemophilia A plasma. The reduction of factor VIII:C activity usually is not as great as that seen in classical hemophilia. Also unlike classical hemophilia, where factor VIII:C activity remains constant, in the patient with von Willebrand's disease variation in the level of circulating factor VIII:C activity may be noted. Characteristically, these patients also have a prolonged bleeding time, but this is less constant than the factor VIII:C reduction. A given patient may have an abnormal bleeding time on one occasion and a normal bleeding time on another. The level of factor VIII–related antigen (factor VIII:Ag) is disproportionately lower than that of factor VIII:C, and ristocetin fails to cause platelet aggregation in about 70 percent of patients with the disease.

CLINICAL MANIFESTATIONS. The manifestations of bleeding usually are mild and often overlooked until trauma or the stress of surgical treatment makes them apparent. A careful clinical history is, therefore, of great importance in these patients. Spontaneous manifestations often are limited to bleeding into the skin or mild mucous membrane bleeding. Epistaxis and menorrhagia have been relatively common in our personal experience. Serious bleeding following dental extractions and tonsillec-

tomy also are not uncommon. Fatal bleeding from the gastrointestinal tract has been described.

TREATMENT. Treatment is directed at correcting the bleeding time and factor VIII R:WF (the von Willebrand factor). Only cryoprecipitate is reliably effective. High-purity concentrates of factor VIII:C lack the required factor VIII R:WF. Ten to forty units per kilogram of cryoprecipitate are administered every 12 h to correct the bleeding time. Replacement therapy should be begun 1 day prior to a surgical procedure. Aspirin *must* be avoided for 10 days before an elective operation. Duration of treatment should be the same as that described for the patient with classical hemophilia.

FACTOR XI (PTA) DEFICIENCY (ROSENTHAL'S SYNDROME)

This uncommon and relatively mild disorder is inherited in an autosomally dominant fashion. Without careful laboratory testing, the affected males and females may be confused with von Willebrand's disease patients. A majority of patients are of Jewish ancestry.

Epistaxis is a common spontaneous clinical manifestation. The disease usually is recognized as a result of bleeding during and after operation. The bleeding usually is minor. Some patients have undergone major procedures without significant hemorrhage.

TREATMENT. Fresh frozen plasma is a suitable therapeutic medium. This factor disappears slowly from the circulation, and its biologic half-life may be as long as 80 h. An initial dose of 10 to 20 mL of plasma/kg of body weight can be given 6 or 8 h prior to anticipated surgical treatment, followed by a maintenance dose of 5 mL/kg administered every 24 h. Therapy usually can be discontinued several days earlier than with patients with more serious hemostatic disorders.

FACTOR V (PROACCELERIN) DEFICIENCY (PARAHEMOPHILIA)

This extremely rare deficiency usually is associated with mild bleeding, but serious bleeding may be encountered. The disease is transmitted as an autosomal recessive trait and is found in males and females alike. Only patients who presumably inherit the gene from both parents seem to be bleeders.

Factor V is synthesized in the liver but differs from prothrombin and factors VII, IX, and X in that factor V synthesis is not dependent upon vitamin K or inhibited by the administration of the coumarin drugs. Patients with severe parenchymal liver disease may be deficient in factor V. Both the prothrombin time (PT) and the partial-thromboplastin time (PTT) are prolonged, and the disorder is diagnosed by a specific assay. About one-third of patients have a prolonged bleeding time.

TREATMENT. Excessive bleeding may occur at the time of operation, usually in patients who have levels of less than 1 percent of normal factor V concentration. No more than 25 percent of normal activity is necessary for hemostasis during operative procedures. This level can be achieved by administering 15 mL of fresh frozen plasma per kilogram of body weight 12 h prior to operation. The administration of 7 to 10 mL/kg every 24 h will suffice to maintain hemostasis until healing has occurred. Once again, it is wise to administer the factor at the time of suture removal. Factor V, also known as labile factor, loses its activity during storage. Only plasma freshly frozen is applicable as therapy. Aspirin should be avoided in these patients.

FACTOR VII (PROCONVERTIN) DEFICIENCY

Factor VII (stable factor) deficiency is an uncommon but not rare disease. Mild clinical manifestations are the rule. The deficiency is inherited as an autosomal gene of "intermediate penetrance." The homozygous state results in significant deficiency and may be associated with serious bleeding. In these patients, spontaneous epistaxis, genitourinary and gastrointestinal bleeding, and even hemarthroses may be seen. The heterozygotes have minimal, if any, clinical manifestations. However, the correlation between factor VII level and bleeding is not good.

Factor VII, like factors II, IX, and X, requires vitamin K for synthesis. The synthesis is blocked by coumarin administration. Coumarin inhibition of synthesis is reversed by vitamin K administration. The administration of vitamin K to patients *congenitally* deficient in these activities will *not* result in synthesis and increased plasma levels.

As is also true for factor V–deficient patients and in patients with deficiencies of factors II and X, the one-stage prothrombin time is prolonged in patients with factor VII deficiency. Since factor VII is active only in the "extrinsic" blood-clotting system, deficient patients have a normal PTT and thrombin clotting time. A laboratory distinction between factor VII and factor X deficiency can be made by the use of the Stypven time test. Factor X is necessary for the effect of this viper venom in blood coagulation, while factor VII is not. Accordingly, the factor VII–deficient patient has a normal Stypven time.

TREATMENT. The biologic half-life of factor VII probably is the briefest of any of the blood-clotting factors— between 2 and 5 h. The initial half-life, thought to be due to equilibration between the intravascular and extravascular compartments, probably is no more than 30 min. The remainder of the disappearance time presumably represents catabolism and is estimated at between 5 and 6 h. Despite this relatively rapid disappearance, the transfusion management of patients with factor VII deficiency is not a great problem. Factor VII levels of less than 10 percent of normal are necessary before significant bleeding occurs. Even at these low levels of plasma activity, replacement transfusion is not always necessary for surgical procedures. Although the one-stage PT time recognizes deficiency of factor VII, this test is not an effective guide to the treatment of factor VII–deficient patients. The test is markedly abnormal at factor VII levels at which the deficient patient may not bleed. Transfusion of banked plasma, 10 mL/kg of body weight, on the day of

the operation, followed by half that amount daily for the next 5 or 6 days, provides adequate factor VII for hemostasis during major surgical treatment.

FACTOR X (STUART-PROWER) DEFICIENCY

This relatively rare deficiency is inherited as a highly penetrant incompletely recessive autosomal recessive trait and has been described in amyloidosis. An association between factor X deficiency and familial carotid body tumors has been reported. Clinically, affected patients are homozygotes, while the heterozygotes are clinically well and only minimally affected. The latter may demonstrate mild abnormalities with the one-stage PT and the PTT and the thromboplastin generation test. An assay is available.

TREATMENT. Little experience has been acquired in the surgical management of patients with factor X deficiency. Plasma levels of 10 to 40 percent of normal have proved sufficient to prevent significant bleeding following dental extractions. Plasma transfusion experiments in patients with factor X deficiency have demonstrated an 8- to 10-h first-phase disappearance time of half the administered activity, followed by a disappearance time estimated at 40 h. Applying these data, plasma levels of 15 percent or greater could be achieved by infusing 15 to 20 mL of frozen or normal plasma per kilogram of body weight initially, followed by half that amount per 24 h for 5 days. Prothrombin complex concentrates may be used. It is always prudent to give an additional infusion at the time of removal of the operative sutures.

INHERITED HYPOPROTHROMBINEMIA (FACTOR II DEFICIENCY)

This deficiency, inherited as an autosomal recessive trait, is perhaps the most rare of the inherited disorders of hemostasis. The prothrombin levels reported in affected patients have averaged about 10 percent of normal and are almost always less than 50 percent. Although the level of prothrombin activity required for hemostasis following surgical treatment is not precisely established, it seems likely that a level of 15 percent of normal is effective. The PTT is variably prolonged. An assay is available.

TREATMENT. The disappearance time of prothrombin from the intravascular compartment approximates that of factor X. An initial equilibration time of 9 h has been estimated, followed by a much slower disappearance of activity with another half-life of up to 3 days. Stored plasma contains factor II. Surgical treatment without faulty hemostasis should be possible in affected patients if an initial plasma infusion of 15 mL/kg of body weight is administered 12 to 24 h prior to the scheduled operation. This can be followed by an infusion of half this amount once daily until healing has occurred. Prothrombin complex concentrates may be used but are usually not warranted because they increase the risk of hepatitis and thromboembolic complications. Vitamin K is ineffective.

When the transfusion programs outlined above for deficiency of the prothrombin group of factors (factors II, V,

VII, and X) are employed, the one-stage prothrombin time does not return to normal. Rather, a one-stage prothrombin time slightly less than twice the control value is achieved. This is sufficient to result in normal hemostasis. Of the four "prothrombin" factors, only factor V must be provided as fresh or freshly frozen plasma. Stored plasma is equally effective as therapy for factors II, VII, and X.

INHERITED FIBRINOGEN ABNORMALITIES

Included in this category are patients with congenital afibrinogenemia, hypofibrinogenemia, and dysfibrinogenemia. Fewer than 200 cases of afibrinogenemia have been reported. This disorder is ascribed to an autosomal, recessive mode of inheritance. The affected individuals are presumably homozygous for the trait. Bleeding time may be markedly prolonged in some patients because fibrinogen is required for platelet aggregation. Conventional methods for measuring fibrinogen in the plasma give a zero value, but immunologic techniques may detect trace amounts of a fibrinogen-like protein. Patients have an indefinitely prolonged whole blood coagulation time, which can be corrected by the addition of fibrinogen. The deficiency, however, usually is less a clinical problem than is classical hemophilia. Bleeding usually begins early in life, and bleeding from the umbilical cord is a characteristic symptom. Bleeding may follow operations, dental extraction, and trauma but the most feared complication is intracranial bleeding following minor injury to the head.

Less profound inherited deficiencies of fibrinogen have been observed and categorized as congenital hypofibrinogenemia. Two groups of hypofibrinogenemic patients have been differentiated: those with fibrinogen values below 50 mg/dL and those with higher levels. The clinical manifestations depend on the fibrinogen concentration. Another congenital disorder is dysfibrinogenemia, in which there are structural defects in the fibrinogen molecule. Both the hypofibrinogenemia and the dysfibrinogenemia have a dominant mode of inheritance. Dysfibrinogenemic patients are frequently asymptomatic but may have moderate or severe bleeding associated with an operation. They have a propensity for thromboembolic disorders and have a higher incidence of wound dehiscence following operative intervention. The thrombin clotting time is diagnostic for this general category of abnormalities but definition of the precise abnormality requires a series of complex laboratory studies.

TREATMENT. Although the hemostatically optimal level of fibrinogen is not known, a level greater than 100 mg/dL is generally required during an operation. The patient's fibrinogen level should be raised above this prior to the procedure. Substitution therapy may be affected by the infusion of fresh frozen plasma or cryoprecipitate. In order to achieve a fibrinogen level near 100 mg/dL for 24 h, an initial dose of 20 to 25 mg fibrinogen/kg of body weight should be administered, followed by one-third the initial amount given on a daily basis throughout the postoperative period. But appropriate corrections must be based on actual fibrinogen measurements. Normal fibrinogen concentration should be maintained until wound healing is shown to be adequate.

CONGENITAL FACTOR XIII DEFICIENCY

This rare disorder is manifest by umbilical bleeding in the newborn and slow wound healing following an operation. In general, most of the bleeding manifestations are mild, but intracranial bleeding may result as a consequence of minor trauma. The mode of inheritance is an autosomal recessive trait. Immunologic assays have demonstrated deficiency of the protein. Therapy is accomplished with fresh frozen plasma, cryoprecipitate, or factor XIII concentrates. With major bleeding, or accompanying surgical intervention, the desired concentration of the recipient's plasma is 0.3 to 0.5 μm/mL. With minor bleeding or as prophylaxis, a level greater than 0.05 μm/mL is all that is required.

ACQUIRED HEMOSTATIC DEFECTS

Platelet Abnormalities

Thrombocytopenia is the most common abnormality of hemostasis that results in bleeding in the surgical patient. The patient may have a reduced platelet count due to a variety of disease processes such as idiopathic thrombocytopenic purpura, thrombotic thrombocytopenic purpura, and systemic lupus erythematosus, or secondary hypersplenism and splenomegaly of sarcoid, Gaucher's disease, lymphoma, and portal hypertension. In these circumstances the marrow usually demonstrates normal or increased number of megakaryocytes. By contrast, when thrombocytopenia occurs in patients with leukemia or uremia, and in those patients on cytotoxic therapy, there is generally a reduced number of megakaryocytes in the marrow.

Thrombocytopenia may occur acutely as the result of massive blood loss followed by replacement with stored blood. Exchange of one blood volume (11 units in a 75-kg man) decreases the platelet count from approximately 250,000/mm^3 to approximately 80,000/mm^3. Thrombocytopenia may be induced acutely by the administration of heparin and may be associated with thrombohemorrhagic complications. This situation, which is thought to have an immunologic basis, has been reported in 0.6 percent of patients receiving heparin. The lowest platelet counts occur after 4 to 15 days of treatment in patients given heparin for the first time and after 2 to 9 days in those given subsequent courses.

Thrombocytopenia is often accompanied by impaired platelet function. Impaired aggregation following the addition of ADP has been demonstrated in patients receiving a blood transfusion of more than 10 units. Uremia may be associated with increased bleeding time and an impaired aggregation, which can be corrected by hemodialysis or peritoneal dialysis. Defective aggregation and platelet secretion can occur in patients with thrombocythemia, polycythemia vera, or myelofibrosis. A variety of drugs interferes with platelet function. These include: aspirin, indomethacin, ibuprofen, dipyridamole, phenothiazides, penicillins, chelating agents, lidocaine, and cocaine.

The presence and extent of thrombocytopenia can be defined rapidly by a platelet count. In general, 60,000/mm^3 platelets are adequate for normal hemostasis, but if there is associated platelet dysfunction, there may be a poor circulation between the platelet count and the extent of bleeding. The template bleeding time is the most reliable in vivo test of platelet function.

When thrombocytopenia is present in a patient in whom an elective operation is entertained, it is managed based on the extent of the reduction of platelet count and the etiology. A count greater than 50,000/mm^3 requires no specific therapy. If thrombocytopenia is due to acute alcoholism, drug effect, or viral infection, the platelets will return to near normal levels within one to three weeks. Occasionally, severe thrombocytopenia may be secondary to vitamin B_{12} or to folic acid deficiency, in which case it is associated with a megaloblastic bone marrow. This condition generally occurs 2 to 3 years after total gastrectomy or in association with severe intestinal malabsorption. In either case, supplying the appropriate nutrient will correct the thrombocytopenia in 2 to 3 days.

If the patient has idiopathic thrombocytopenia or lupus erythematosus, and a platelet count less than 50,000 per mm^3, an attempt to raise the platelet count with steroid therapy or plasmapheresis may prove successful (see Chap. 33). The administration of platelet transfusions in these patients with the spleen in place is generally ineffective. In an unusual circumstance, a preemptive splenectomy may be in order in a thrombocytopenic patient in whom a potentially bloody procedure is anticipated. Splenectomy alone should not be performed to correct the thrombocytopenia associated with splenomegaly secondary to portal hypertension.

Prophylactic platelet administration as a routine accompaniment to massive blood transfusion is not required or indicated to prevent a hemostatic defect. Platelet packs are administered preoperatively to rapidly increase the platelet count in surgical patients with thrombocytopenia due to marrow depression or in association with massive bleeding and replacement with banked blood. Special platelet transfusion sets are used to reduce the loss of platelets due to adherence. One unit of platelet concentrate contains approximately 5.5×10^{10} platelets and would be expected to increase the circulating platelet count by about 10×10^9/L in the average 70-kg man. Thus, a transfusion of 4 to 8 pool platelet concentrates should raise the count by 40 to 80×10^9/L and should provide adequate hemostasis, as documented by bleeding time and control of the hemorrhagic manifestations. Fever, infection, hepatosplenomegaly, and the presence of antiplatelet alloantibodies decrease the effectiveness of platelet transfusions. In patients refractory to standard platelet transfusions, the use of HLA-compatible platelets coupled with special processors has proved effective.

Platelet aggregometry has been applied to screening for potential donors.

Acquired Hypofibrinogenemia

DEFIBRINATION SYNDROME

The largest proportion of patients with fibrinogen-related problems of surgical concern are in this group. The fibrinogen deficiency rarely is an isolated defect because thrombocytopenia and factors II, V, and VIII deficiencies of variable severity usually accompany this state.

The majority of patients with acquired hypofibrinogenemia suffer from intravascular coagulation, more properly known as *defibrination syndrome* or *consumptive coagulopathy,* and it is to this group of patients that the term *disseminated intravascular coagulation* (DIC) has been applied. The syndrome, now recognized with increasing frequency, is caused by the introduction of thromboplastic materials into the circulation. Because this material is found in most tissues, many disease processes may activate the coagulation system. The hemorrhagic disasters of the perinatal period, e.g., retained dead fetus, premature separation of the placenta, and amniotic fluid embolus, primarily are due to this pathophysiologic mechanism. The hemorrhagic state following hemolytic transfusion reaction is also related to this process. Defibrination has been observed as a complication of extracorporeal circulation, disseminated carcinoma, lymphomas, thrombotic thrombocytopenia, rickettsial infection, snakebite, and shock. Release of thromboplastic material has long been a recognized complication of gram-negative sepsis and has been attributed to the effects of circulating endotoxin on platelets. Septicemia due to gram-positive organisms may also be associated with DIC.

The differentiation of DIC with secondary protective fibrinolysis from primary fibrinolytic states can be extremely difficult because the TT is prolonged in both cases, as is the PT and PTT. There is no laboratory test to confirm or exclude the diagnosis. The combination of a low platelet count, a positive plasma protamine test indicating the presence of fibrin monomer–fibrinogen complexes in the plasma, and reduced fibrinogen accompanied by increased fibrin degradation products viewed in the context of the patient's underlying disease is highly suggestive of the diagnosis.

TREATMENT. The most important facets of treatment are relieving the patient's causative, primary medical or surgical problem and maintaining adequate capillary flow. The use of intravenous fluids to maintain volume and, at times, vasodilators to open the arterioles is indicated. If blood flow deficiency is related to the inability of a damaged heart to pump, the use of drugs such as digitalis or Isuprel may be indicated. Viscosity may be affected by an increased hematocrit, and, therefore, a plasma expander may be beneficial.

If there is active bleeding, hemostatic factors should be replaced with fresh frozen plasma, cryoprecipitate, and platelet concentrates. There is little evidence that this replacement therapy will "fuel the fire" and accelerate the pathophysiologic process. Most studies show that heparin is not helpful in acute forms of DIC, but the drug is indicated for purpura fulminans or venous thromboembolism. Fibrinolytic inhibitors such as ϵ-aminocaproic acid (EACA) may be used to block the accumulation of degradation products but are dangerous if the thrombotic process is still active. They should not be used without prior effective antithrombotic treatment with heparin.

FIBRINOLYSIS

The acquired hypofibrinogenemic state in the surgical patient also can be due to pathologic fibrinolysis. This may occur in patients with metastatic prostatic carcinoma, shock, sepsis, hypoxia, neoplasia, cirrhosis, and portal hypertension and in those patients on extracorporeal bypass.

The pathogenesis of this bleeding disorder is complex. Secondary to shock or hypoxia, a release of excessive plasminogen activator into the circulation occurs. This is thought to consist of endogenous kinases which can be released from vascular endothelium and other tissues. Pharmacologic activation of plasminogen also occurs with pyrogens, epinephrine, nicotinic acid, and acetylcholine. Electric shock and pneumoencephalography have also been reported to cause activation. Patients with cirrhosis and portal hypertension have a diminished ability to clear normal amounts of plasminogen activator from the blood.

In addition to the reduction in levels of plasma fibrinogen, diminution of factors V and VIII also occurs, since they also serve as substrates for the enzyme plasmin. Thrombocytopenia is not an accompaniment of the purely fibrinolytic state. Polymerization of fibrin monomers, a step in normal fibrin formation, is interfered with by the proteolytic residue of fibrinogen and fibrin. The fibrin and fibrinogen breakdown products usually disappear from the circulation in a matter of hours.

Streptokinase and urokinase have been used to induce therapeutic fibrinolysis, but enthusiasm for these drugs as treatment for venous thrombosis, pulmonary embolism, and clotted hemothorax is not widespread. As there is a limited endogenous supply of activator available, it is soon exhausted by the injections, and later injections fail to achieve the desired effect. Also, treatment with these drugs is frequently accompanied by chills and fever. Excessive bleeding has been noted in almost half the patients treated, and anemia has appeared beyond that anticipated by the amount of bleeding. At present, results of urokinase therapy for deep venous thrombosis should be regarded as encouraging but not conclusive.

TREATMENT. The successful treatment of the underlying disorder usually is followed by rapid spontaneous recovery, since the severity of fibrinolytic bleeding is dependent upon the concentration of breakdown products in the circulation. ϵ-Aminocaproic acid (EACA), a synthetic amino acid, interferes with fibrinolysis by inhibiting plasminogen activation. The drug may be administered intravenously or orally. An initial dose of 5 g for the average-sized adult is followed by another 1 g every 1 to 2 h until the hemorrhagic state subsides. Treatment rarely is required for more than 2 or 3 days. Just as the administration of EACA in a patient with consumptive coagulopathy is potentially dangerous, the administration of heparin in the patient who has a primary pathologic fibrinolysis is fraught with danger. Thus, fine clinical judgment and reliable laboratories are needed to avoid therapeutic complications. Restraint in definitive treatment of both fibrinolysis and consumptive coagulopathy is recommended, while measures designed to reverse the shock and stabilize the patient are emphasized.

Myeloproliferative Diseases

TREATMENT. Thrombocytosis can be reduced by the careful administration of alkylating agents such as busulfan or chlorambucil. These measures are time consuming. Surgical procedure should be delayed weeks to months following institution of treatment. Ideally, the hematocrit should be kept below 48 percent and the platelet count less than 400,000/mm^3. The blood volume also can be reduced more rapidly by phlebotomy. Prior to operation, a thorough laboratory investigation of hemostatic function should be conducted. Any gross defect, such as deficiency of vitamin K–dependent factors or low plasma fibrinogen values, should be corrected. When surgical treatment is imperative in these patients, the erythremic state should be reduced by phlebotomy. Operation, at all times, must be performed fastidiously. Postoperative fibrinolysis also has been known to occur, further complicating the postoperative course.

In one series reported from a clinic with considerable experience, 46 percent of polycythemic patients undergoing major procedures had complications at the time of operation or during the postoperative course, and a 16 percent mortality was associated with the surgical procedures. Significantly, 80 percent of the deaths were encountered in patients on whom operations were performed while the disease was not under control. In operations on patients in whom hematocrit and platelet count had been reduced prior to operation, the mortality and incidence of complications decreased. Hemorrhage is the most common complication occurring during or following operation and accounts for greater than two-thirds of the deaths. Thrombosis, either venous or arterial, is the next most frequent complication. Infection is also common, occurring in approximately 20 percent of patients.

POLYCYTHEMIA VERA

Surgical treatment of the patient with polycythemia vera is complicated by distinctly increased morbidity and mortality. This is particularly true for the untreated patient but also applies, to some extent, to the patient who has been treated successfully. Spontaneous thrombosis is a complication of polycythemia vera and can be explained, in part, by increased blood viscosity, increased platelet count, and increased tendency toward stasis. Paradoxically, a significant tendency to spontaneous hemorrhage also is noted in these patients. Approximately one-third of patients with polycythemia vera have some form of hemorrhagic complaint at the time of initial diagnosis. Patients with spontaneous bleeding characteristically have a platelet count of 1,500,000/mm^3 or greater. The bleeding time may be prolonged. Evidence has been offered that the platelets in these patients may be qualitatively defective.

The polycythemic patient with marked thrombocytosis is a major surgical risk. Operation should be considered only for the most grave surgical emergency. If possible, operation should be deferred until medical management has returned the blood volume, hematocrit, and hemostatic process to normal.

MYELOID METAPLASIA

Myeloid metaplasia frequently represents part of the natural history of polycythemia vera. Approximately 50 percent of patients with myeloid metaplasia are postpolycythemic, while in the remainder the condition apparently occurs as a separate, possibly related, disease entity. Myeloid metaplasia is characterized by many of the features of polycythemia vera. Splenomegaly usually is more prominent and may be massive. Laboratory features include leukocytosis, which may be severe, or, at times, severe leukopenia. Young myeloid forms may be present. Platelets may be strikingly increased in number, but thrombocytopenia also may be present. The latter is usually characteristic of the patient who has myelofibrosis rather than a hyperplastic bone marrow. Examination of the peripheral blood smear may reveal large, bizarre platelets, fragments of megakaryocyte nuclei, occasional nucleated red cells, and bizarre variations in red cell shape. Evidence suggesting qualitative platelet abnormalities has been described. This is considered a factor in bleeding in some myeloid metaplasia patients. Abnormalities of platelet factor 3 release have been demonstrated, as have abnormalities in platelet aggregation with ADP.

Relatively innocuous surgical procedures have been accompanied by nearly uncontrollable bleeding. Spontaneous bleeding from esophageal varices in patients with myeloid metaplasia and massive splenomegaly has also been reported. Preparation for an operation is similar to that described for polycythemia vera.

Other Diseases

Illnesses resulting in severe impairment of hepatic function may limit synthesis of plasma factors essential to normal coagulation. The patient with advanced cirrhosis may be lacking in factors of the prothrombin complex (II, V, VII, X), as well as factor XIII. In addition, there may be increased fibrinolysis due to failure of the liver to clear plasminogen activators.

Accelerated removal of plasma factors necessary for coagulation occurs in consumptive coagulopathies. Some illnesses are characterized by the production of sub-stances that interfere with the normal hemostatic mechanism. These diseases are associated with the production of abnormal proteins that may coat the platelets, as in macroglobulinemia, or bind with certain of the normal blood-clotting factors, as in multiple myeloma or in states associated with the production of cryoglobulin.

Anticoagulation and Bleeding

Spontaneous bleeding may be a complication of anticoagulant therapy with either heparin or the coumarin and indanedione derivatives. The incidence of bleeding complications related to heparin is reduced with a continuous infusion technique, regulating the PTT between 60 to 100 s (control: 30 to 35). An exaggerated response to oral anticoagulants may occur if dietary vitamin K is inadequate. The anticoagulant effect of coumarin is consistently reduced in patients receiving barbiturates, and increased coumarin requirements have also been documented in patients taking contraceptives, other estrogen-containing compounds, corticosteroids, and ACTH. Therefore, reduced anticoagulant dosage should be instituted following discontinuance of any of these drugs. Medications known to increase the effect of oral anticoagulants include phenylbutazone, the cholesterol-lowering agent clofibrate, anabolic steroids (norethandrolone), D-thyroxine, glucagon, quinidine, and a variety of antibiotics.

Unexplained bleeding in medical and paramedical personnel occasionally is due to surreptitious anticoagulation. The onset of hematuria or melena in the patient receiving anticoagulants should be investigated, since it has been shown that anticoagulants may unmask underlying tumors. Patients with bleeding secondary to anticoagulation may present only with epistaxis, gastrointestinal hemorrhage, or hematuria. Physical examination, however, almost always reveals other signs of bleeding such as ecchymoses, petechiae, or hematoma. Bleeding secondary to anticoagulation is not an uncommon cause of rectus sheath hematoma, simulating appendicitis, and intramural intestinal or retroperitoneal hematoma.

Surgical intervention may prove necessary in patients receiving anticoagulant therapy. The typical example is the patient with rheumatic heart disease receiving long-term anticoagulation because of repeated arterial emboli, who then is seen subsequent to a critical embolic episode. Increasing experience suggests that surgical treatment can be undertaken without discontinuing the anticoagulant program. The risk of thrombotic complications reportedly is increased when anticoagulant therapy is discontinued suddenly. If so, this may not be related to what has been called the "rebound phenomenon" but may represent an event in a patient who has an underlying thrombotic tendency. When the clotting time is less than 25 min in the heparinized patient or when the prothrombin time is greater than 20 percent of normal in a patient on coumarin, reversal of anticoagulant therapy may not be necessary. Meticulous surgical technique is mandatory, and the patient must be observed closely.

Certain surgical procedures should not be performed in the face of anticoagulation. In sites where even minor bleeding can cause great morbidity, e.g., the central nervous system and the eye, anticoagulants should be discontinued and, if necessary, reversed. Because of the added problem of local fibrinolysis, prostatic surgical treatment should not be carried out in a patient on anticoagulants. Procedures requiring blind needle introduction should be avoided. Deaths have been reported following sympathetic block for peripheral vascular disease in patients receiving anticoagulation.

Emergency operation occasionally is necessary in patients who have been heparinized as treatment for deep venous thrombosis. Reversal of heparinization may be desirable. The patient with repeated episodes of pulmonary embolization while fully heparinized is a potential candidate. Reversal of heparinization also can be a problem in cardiac and vascular surgical procedures. When the heparin has been given intravenously, its anticoagulant effect can be rapidly counteracted with protamine sulfate. Protamine sulfate also is administered intravenously. Theoretically, 1.28 mg should neutralize 1 mg of heparin. In fact, 1 mg of protamine may be given for each milligram of heparin given, provided the intravenous heparin was not given more than 2 h previously. Protamine sulfate in large doses also has an anticoagulant activity. The formation of both extrinsic and intrinsic prothrombinase can be retarded, prolonging the one-stage prothrombin time test and the partial thromboplastin time test. Some patients exhibit the phenomenon of "heparin rebound" following apparently adequate heparin neutralization with protamine. Prolongation of the clotting time again recurs after adequate postoperative antagonism of the heparin. This can contribute to postoperative bleeding. In our experience, this is the major cause of "unexplained" postoperative bleeding following cardiac and vascular surgical procedures. Activation of fibrinolysis and thrombocytopenia may also contribute to this problem.

Bleeding infrequently is related to hypoprothrombinemia if the prothrombin concentration is greater than 15 percent. In the elective surgical patient receiving coumarin therapy sufficient to effect anticoagulation, the drug can be discontinued several days prior to operation, and the prothrombin concentration then checked. A level greater than 50 percent is considered safe. If emergency surgical treatment is required, parenteral injection of vitamin K_1 can be used. Since the reversal effect may take 6 h, transfusion of whole blood or, preferably, freshly frozen plasma may be required. Parenteral administration of vitamin K also is indicated in elective surgical treatment of patients with biliary obstruction, malabsorption, and hypoprothrombinemia. The drug should result in a normal prothrombin time. In contrast, if the hypoprothrombinemia is related to hepatocellular dysfunction, vitamin K therapy is ineffective and should not be prolonged over a week if no response is noted. Vitamin K is an oxidant, and one must be aware that patients with red cell enzyme deficiencies may sustain hemolysis following its administration.

TESTS OF HEMOSTASIS AND BLOOD COAGULATION (Table 3-3)

The most important assessment of hemostasis is a careful history and physical examination. Only the history can indicate whether the patient has a hemorrhagic diathesis. Rather than asking a patient if he or she is a "bleeder," specific questions should be asked. These should include queries to determine if there was untoward bleeding during a major surgical procedure, or if there was *any* bleeding after a minor operation such as tonsillectomy, circumcision, or dental extraction, or if spontaneous bleeding was ever experienced. If there is a suggestion of bleeding diathesis, the age of onset and family history is helpful to determine whether a hereditary or acquired defect should be investigated. Questions should uncover a his-

Table 3-3. SCREENING TESTS IN ADULTS, HEALTHY TERM INFANTS, AND PREMATURE INFANTS

	Adults	*Term infants*	*Premature infants (32–35 weeks gestation)*
Platelet count (10^3/cm)*	300±50	259±35	239±50
Bleeding time (min)*	4±1.5	4±1.5	4±1.5
Prothrombin time (PT) (s)*	12–14	13–17	18
Partial thromboplastin time (PTT) (s)*	45	71	100
Thrombin time (TT) (s)*	10	14	14
Fibrinogen (mg/dL)†	200–350	117–225	—

* Values published by Hathaway and Bonnar.
† Values obtained in this laboratory.
Values for infants 35 to 39 weeks' gestation lie between those of term and 32 to 35 week infants.
Values for older children (>3 months) are the same as those for adults.
SOURCE: Karpatkin M, 1980, with permission.

tory of exposure to toxic agents, oral anticoagulants, and drugs that might interfere with hemostasis. Aspirin and ibuprofen are two of the more common medications in this category. A history of a recent regimen of broad spectrum antibiotics should alert the physician to the possibility of a deficiency of vitamin K–dependent clotting factors. Patients with malignancy may have a variety of abnormalities, such as compensated intravascular coagulation, and increased circulating fibrin complexes. Complex hemostatic disorders may accompany liver and renal failure.

PLATELET COUNT. Because thrombocytopenia is the most common abnormality of hemostasis in the surgical patient, determination of the level of circulating platelets is a critical screening test. Direct enumeration of blood platelets can be accomplished quite accurately. *Spontaneous* bleeding only rarely can be related to thrombocytopenia with platelet counts greater than 40,000/mm³. Platelet counts of 60,000 to 70,000/mm³ usually are sufficient to provide adequate hemostasis following trauma or surgical procedures if other hemostatic factors are normal. An abnormal count should be confirmed by inspection of the blood smear.

When an area where the red blood cells display their customary central pallor and where few of the red blood cells overlap one another is examined, 15 to 20 platelets per oil immersion field should be noted. If the blood is not anticoagulated before the smear is prepared, as many as half of these may be in clumps of three or four platelets. A well-stained blood smear that fails to display more than three or four platelets in at least every other oil immersion field can be considered significantly thrombocytopenic. In this situation, the patient's platelet count generally is less than 75,000/mm³. Blood smears which must be searched because platelets appear in only every four or five oil immersion fields usually represent platelet counts of fewer than 40,000/mm³. If cover slip smears have been prepared, the cover slips always should be mounted as matched pairs. Platelets occasionally stick to one of the cover slips, and examination of both will obviate a false impression of thrombocytopenia. Lightly stained blood smears may appear thrombocytopenic in that the platelets are not prominent enough to attract the examiner's attention.

Inspection of the blood smear has the other obvious advantage of permitting the examiner to identify additional pathologic features which may have meaning in the care of the patient. The presence of nucleated red blood cells or abnormal white cells can provide information important to the diagnosis. The presence of giant platelets or large fragments of megakaryocyte cytoplasm will also alert the examiner to possible pathologic platelet function.

BLEEDING TIME. This assesses both the interaction between platelets and a damaged blood vessel and the formation of the platelet plug. Bleeding time may be abnormal in thrombocytopenia, qualitative platelet disorders, von Willebrand's disease, and also in some patients with factor V deficiency, or hypofibrinogenemia. Aspirin ingested within one week will affect the results. The tests

can be performed by a variety of techniques that do not have the same normal times or the same degree of accuracy. The Duke bleeding time, performed by incising the most dependent portion of the earlobe and measuring the time lapse until the bleeding ceases, normally should not exceed 3½ min. The Ivy method is performed on the forearm after a blood pressure cuff has been inflated to 40 mmHg. It has an upper limit of normal of 5 min. The Mielke template technique, a modification of the Ivy method, provides more accurate results but may leave a scar.

OTHER TESTS OF PLATELET FUNCTION. Platelet aggregation can be assessed with a variety of induction agents to uncover specific abnormalities. The results may be affected by venipuncture, blood pH, temperature, duration of storage, and the equipment itself. The degree of abnormality detected by the test does not correlate with the extent of untoward bleeding. Aspirin is the most common cause of platelet aggregation abnormality. Failure of platelets to aggregate with the addition of arachidonate defines an aspirin effect. The failure of platelets to aggregate with ADP, epinephrine, and collagen is characteristic of Glanzmann's thrombasthenia. Abnormal platelet aggregation with ristocetin occurs in von Willebrand's disease and in Bernard-Soulier syndrome.

The ability of the platelets to liberate platelet factor 3 (phospholipid), essential in tiny amounts at several stages of the blood-clotting process (see Fig. 3-2), also can be measured. Impairment of platelet factor 3 release has been reported in conditions described as *thrombocytopathia*. This defect can represent a primary disease entity, but similar impairment has been described as a secondary phenomenon in uremia and liver disease. The inability of the platelet to make platelet factor 3 available for the clotting process may be a part of a more fundamental surface membrane abnormality. The ability of ADP, epinephrine, collagen, and arachidonic acid to liberate serotonin β-thromboglobulin, or platelet factor 4 can be measured.

PROTHROMBIN TIME (PT). This test measures the speed of the events described earlier as the extrinsic pathway of blood coagulation. A tissue source of procoagulant (thromboplastin), a lipoprotein, is added with calcium to an aliquot of citrated plasma and the clotting time determined. The laboratory should establish a normal dilution curve and normal values daily. The PT will be prolonged in the presence of even minute amounts of heparin. The presence of heparin, by its antithrombin action, will artificially prolong the clotting time of the mixture so that it appears that the prothrombin complex is low. Accordingly, an accurate prothrombin determination cannot be carried out in a patient receiving anticoagulation treatment with heparin until the heparin has disappeared from the plasma. This should be at least 5 h following the last intravenous dose. The amount of heparin used to maintain patency of an intravenous line is usually insufficient to alter the PT.

The use of tissue procoagulants in the test eliminates the roles of factors VIII, IX, XI, XII, and platelets. Properly done, the test will detect deficiencies of factors II, V, VII, X, and fibrinogen. The one-stage PT is the preferred method of controlling anticoagulation with the coumarin and indanedione drugs.

PARTIAL THROMBOPLASTIN TIME (PTT). The partial thromboplastin time is a screening test for the intrinsic clotting pathway. The in vitro clotting system now is sensitive to factors VIII, IX, XI, and XII, as well as the factors normally detected by the one-stage PT. The range of normal with this test varies with the product used. Each laboratory should establish a normal dilution curve daily, and the patient's plasma must be compared with a normal control.

The PTT, when used in conjunction with the one-stage prothrombin time, can help to place a clotting defect in the first or second stage of the clotting process. If the PTT is prolonged and the one-stage prothrombin time is normal, factors VIII, IX, XI, or XII may be deficient. If the PTT is normal and the one-stage PT is prolonged, a single or multiple deficiency of factors II, V, VII, or X or of fibrinogen may be present. The PTT is also abnormal in the presence of circulating anticoagulants or during heparin administration. It may be prolonged when heparin is used to maintain the patency of an intravenous line. The sensitivity of the test is such that only extremely mild cases of factor VIII or IX deficiency may be missed. In one study of over 600 patients with clotting abnormalities, only two mild abnormalities were not detected with this test.

THROMBIN TIME (TT). This test is of value in detecting qualitative abnormalities in fibrinogen and in detecting circulating anticoagulants and inhibitors of fibrin polymerization. The clotting time of the patient's plasma is measured following the addition of a standard amount of thrombin to a fixed volume of plasma. Controls of normal plasma must be run in parallel. Failure of the clot to form, in the absence of circulating inhibitors such as heparin or the fibrinolytic degradation products of fibrin and fibrinogen, is consistent with severe diminution of fibrinogen, usually well below 100 mg/dL. It is also prolonged when fibrinolysis is taking place.

OTHER TESTS OF COAGULATION. The fibrinogen level can be determined by clotting time measurements or gravimetrically. Specific assays of coagulation factors are performed by measuring clotting time of plasma congenitally lacking in one of these factors. Relatively simple tests permit identification of circulating anticoagulants. The simplest of these are based on the retardation of clotting of normal recalcified plasma by varying mixtures of the test plasma. The sensitivity of such tests usually can be increased by incubating the test plasma with the normal plasma for 30 min at body temperature prior to recalcification. Detection of factor XIII deficiency requires a special test.

TESTS OF FIBRINOLYSIS. Fibrin degradation products (FDP) can be measured by immunologic methods. The plasma protamine paracoagulation test (PPP) specifically detects fibrin monomers, but may be falsely positive in liver disease, thromboembolic disorders, renal disease, or pregnancy. Normally, dissolution of a recently formed blood clot will not occur for 48 h or more. When fibrinolysis is a significant factor in hemostatic failure, dissolution of the whole blood clot is observed in 2 h or less. The test has the disadvantage of being time consuming in a circumstance where time may be of the essence. In addition, a false impression of increased fibrinolytic activity may be gained from clots formed in patients with high hematocrits or in thrombocytopenia, where red cells may fall away from the clot. The euglobulin clot lysis time and dilute whole blood or plasma clot lysis time are more sensitive indices and permit more rapid evaluation of fibrinolysis.

The *thromboelastogram* is a graphic representation of clotting obtained by employing a special instrument, the thromboelastograph. The record obtained provides information about the clotting time, the speed of fibrin polymerization, and the strength and tendency toward dissolution of the clot. The instrument has provided information of research value but has not, in our experience, greatly aided the studies of clinical problems.

EVALUATION OF THE SURGICAL PATIENT AS A HEMOSTATIC RISK

Preoperative Evaluation of Hemostasis

The patient's history provides meaningful clues for the presence of a bleeding tendency. It is reasonable to use a questionnaire on which the patient indicates: (1) prolonged bleeding or swelling after biting the lip or tongue, (2) bruises without apparent injury, (3) prolonged bleeding after dental extraction, (4) excessive menstrual bleeding, (5) bleeding problems associated with major and minor operations, (6) medical problems receiving a physician's attention within the past 5 years, (7) medications including aspirin or remedies for headache taken within the past 10 days, and (8) a relative with a bleeding problem. Rapaport indicates that, based on the answers to these questions, one of the following conclusions can be reached: (1) hemostasis is apparently normal, (2) the history contains insufficient tests of hemostasis, or (3) there is a possibility or likelihood of a defect. He also proposes that this information, coupled with an appreciation of the planned operation, can be used to establish four levels of concern to determine the extent of preoperative testing.

In Level I, the history is negative and the procedure contemplated is relatively minor, e.g., breast biopsy or hernia repair: no screening tests are recommended. In Level II, the history is negative, screening tests may have been performed in the past, and a major operation is planned, but the procedure is usually not attended by significant bleeding: a platelet count and blood smear and PTT are recommended to detect thrombocytopenia, a circulating anticoagulant, or intravascular coagulation. Level III pertains to the patient whose history is suggestive of defective hemostasis and also to the patient who is to undergo an operative procedure in which hemostasis may be impaired, for example, operations using pump oxygenation or cell savers, or procedures in which a large, raw surface is anticipated. Level III also pertains to situations, such as intracranial operations, in which minimal postoperative bleeding could be injurious. In this level, a platelet count and bleeding time test should be performed to assess platelet function; a PT and PTT should be used to assess coagulation, and the fibrin clot should be incubated to screen for abnormal fibrinolysis. Level IV pertains to patients who present with a history highly suggestive of a hemostatic defect. A hematologist should be consulted, and, in addition to the tests prescribed for Level III patients, the bleeding time test should be repeated in 4 h following the ingestion of 600 mg of aspirin, provided that the operation is scheduled to take place 10 or more days after this study. In the case of an emergency procedure, platelet aggregation tests using ADP, collagen, epinephrine, and ristocetin should be performed, and a TT is indicated to detect dysfibrinogenemia or a circulating, weak, heparin-like anticoagulant. Patients with liver disease, renal failure, obstructive jaundice, and the possibility of a disseminated malignancy should have a platelet count, PT, and PTT performed preoperatively.

Evaluation of Excessive Intraoperative or Postoperative Bleeding

Excessive bleeding during or shortly after a surgical procedure may be due to one or more of the following factors: (1) ineffective local hemostasis, (2) complications of blood transfusion, (3) a previously undetected hemostatic defect, (4) consumptive coagulopathy and/or fibrinolysis. Excessive bleeding from the field of the procedure, unassociated with bleeding from other sites, e.g., central venous pressure or intravenous line or tracheostomy, usually suggests inadequate mechanical hemostasis rather than a defect in the biologic process. An exception to this rule applies to operations on the prostate, pancreas, and liver because operative trauma may stimulate local plasminogen activation and lead to increased fibrinolysis on the raw surface. In this circumstance 24 to 48 h interruption of plasminogen activation by the administration of EACA may prove effective.

Although one may be reasonably certain on clinical grounds that surgical bleeding is related to local problems, laboratory investigation must be confirmatory. Prompt examination should be made of the blood smear to determine the number of platelets, and an actual platelet count should be done if the smear is equivocal. A PTT, one-stage PT, and a TT all can be determined within minutes. Correct interpretation of the results should confirm the clinical impression or identify the problem.

As pointed out previously, massive blood transfusion is a well-documented cause of thrombocytopenia. Although most patients who receive 10 units or more of banked blood within a period of 24 h will be measurably thrombocytopenic, this is usually *not* associated with hemostatic failure. Therefore, prophylactic administration of platelets is not indicated, but if there is evidence of diffuse bleeding, 8 to 10 packs of fresh platelet concentrates should be given empirically, because no clear association has been documented between the platelet count, bleeding time, and the occurrence of profuse bleeding.

Another cause of hemostatic failure related to the administration of blood is a hemolytic transfusion reaction. The first hint of a transfusion reaction in an anesthetized patient may be diffuse bleeding in an operative field that had previously been dry. The pathogenesis of this bleeding is thought to be related to the release of ADP from hemolyzed red cells, resulting in diffuse platelet aggregation, following which the platelet clumps are swept out of the circulation. Release of procoagulants may result in progression of the clotting mechanism and intravascular defibrination. In addition, the fibrinolytic mechanism may be triggered.

Transfusion purpura is an uncommon cause of thrombocytopenia and associated bleeding following transfusion. In this circumstance, the donor platelets are of the uncommon Pl^{A1} group. These platelets sensitize the recipient, who makes antibody to the foreign platelet antigen. The foreign platelet antigen does not completely disappear from the recipient circulation but seems to attach to the recipient's own platelets. The antibody, which attains a sufficient titer within 6 or 7 days following the sensitizing transfusion, then destroys the recipient's own platelets. The resultant thrombocytopenia and bleeding may continue for several weeks. This uncommon cause of thrombocytopenia should be considered if bleeding follows transfusion by 5 or 6 days. Platelet transfusions are of little help in the management of this syndrome, since the new donor platelets usually are subject to the binding of antigen and damage from the antibody. Corticosteroids may be of some help in reducing the bleeding tendency. Posttransfusion purpura is self-limited, and the passage of several weeks inevitably leads to subsidence of the problem.

Disseminated intravascular coagulation (DIC) and disseminated fibrinolysis occur intraoperatively or postoperatively when control mechanisms fail to restrain the hemostatic process to the area of tissue damage. Either process can cause diffuse bleeding and can be caused by trauma, incompatible transfused blood, sepsis, necrotic tissue, fat emboli, retained products of conception. toxemia of pregnancy, large aneurysms, and liver diseases. It is important to distinguish between the two processes or the dominant element causing intraoperative or postoperative bleeding. No single test can confirm or exclude the diagnosis or distinguish between the two disorders. The combination of thrombocytopenia, defined by smear or platelet count, positive plasma protamine test for fibrin monomers, a low fibrinogen level and elevated fibrin degradation product (FDP) provides strong indications for DIC.

The simple single-tube clotting time test is helpful. Normally a clot forms within 10 min if there is periodic tilting of the test tube, and in 1 h the retraction begins. With DIC, formation occurs in a normal time and the clot promptly undergoes dissolution. The PT, PTT, and TT should be determined; this may be the most sensitive indicator of the three tests. Serial thrombin times, when used with the protamine sulfate test, have been used to differentiate the opposing mechanisms affecting hemostasis, i.e., DIC from fibrinolysis. The euglobulin lysis time provides a method of detecting diffuse fibrinolysis. The management of DIC and fibrinolysis has been presented previously.

A hemostatic defect may be imposed iatrogenically during surgical treatment employing extracorporeal bypass. Many etiologic factors may be involved, but the most commonly implicated is the introduction of heparin into the circulation. Bleeding after discontinuation of extracorporeal bypass may be due to inadequate neutralization of heparin with protamine sulfate. Since protamine sulfate is itself an anticoagulant when large doses are used, bleeding can be caused by these drugs. This is a rare occurrence. Rapid tests can be performed in vitro by adding small amounts of protamine sulfate to see if the clotting time is shortened. Other abnormalities attributed to extracorporeal circulation are defibrination and fibrinolysis. Fibrinolytic activity is often increased. These changes usually are related to the duration of pumping. Frequently there is a *lack* of clinical bleeding in the patients with laboratory evidence of fibrinolysis. Thrombocytopenia, hypofibrinogenemia, and reduction in factors V and VIII have been demonstrated. The thrombocytopenia usually is not severe, and the platelet count generally remains above $50,000/mm^3$. Evaluation of the patient with intraoperative or postoperative bleeding suspected of being due to hemostatic defect follows the same course previously outlined for preoperative evaluation of these patients.

Diffuse intraoperative and postoperative bleeding is a complication of biliary tract surgery in cirrhotic patients. This has been related to portal hypertension and coagulopathy associated with chronic liver disease. The tests used to distinguish DIC from fibrinolysis pertain. The therapeutic approach includes the intravenous administration of vasopressin to effect a temporary reduction in portal hypertension, and EACA to correct the increased fibrinolysis.

At times, an operation performed in a patient with sepsis is attended by continued bleeding. Severe hemorrhagic disorders due to thrombocytopenia have occurred consequent to gram-negative sepsis. The pathogenesis of endotoxin-induced thrombocytopenia has been studied in detail, and it has been suggested that a labile factor, possibly factor V, is necessary for this interaction. Defibrination and hemostatic failure also may occur with meningococcemia, *Clostridium welchii* sepsis, and staphylococcal sepsis. Hemolysis appears to be one mechanism in sepsis leading to defibrination. Evaluation of these patients includes platelet count, PT, PTT, and TT.

LOCAL HEMOSTASIS

Surgical bleeding, even when alarmingly excessive, is usually caused by ineffective local hemostasis. The goal of local hemostasis is to prevent the flow of blood from incised or transected blood vessels. This may be accomplished by interrupting the flow of blood to the involved area or by direct closure of the blood vessel wall defect. The techniques may be classified as mechanical, thermal, or chemical.

Mechanical Procedures

The oldest mechanical device to effect closure of a bleeding point or to prevent blood from entering the area of disruption is digital pressure. When pressure is applied to an artery proximal to an area of bleeding, profuse bleeding is reduced, permitting more definitive action. The Pringle maneuver of occluding the hepatic artery in the hepatoduodenal ligament as a method of controlling bleeding from a transected systic artery or from the surface of the liver is a classic example. Direct digital pressure over a bleeding site, such as a lateral rent in the inferior vena cava, is also effective. The finger has the advantage of being the least traumatic vascular hemostat. All clamps, including the so-called atraumatic vascular clamps, do result in damage to the intimal wall of the blood vessel. The obvious disadvantage of digital pressure is that it cannot be used permanently.

The hemostat also represents a temporary mechanical device to stem bleeding. In smaller and noncritical vessels, the trauma and adjacent tissue necrosis associated with the application of a hemostat are of little consequence. These minor disadvantages are outweighed by the mechanical advantage that the instrument offers to subsequent ligation. When bleeding occurs from a vessel that should be preserved, relatively atraumatic hemostats should be employed to limit the extent of intimal damage and subsequent thrombosis.

In general, a ligature replaces the hemostat as a permanent method of effecting hemostasis in a single vessel. When a vessel is transected, a simple ligature usually is sufficient. For large arteries with pulsation and longitudinal motion, transfixion suture to prevent slipping is indicated. When the bleeding site is from a lateral defect in the blood vessel wall, suture ligatures are required. The adventitia and media constitute the major holding forces within the walls of large vessels, and therefore multiple fine sutures are preferable to fewer larger sutures.

Historically, Aulus Cornelius Celsus devised the use of ligatures in the first century A.D. Because of the strong influence of Galen, who was inclined to cautery, this method did not gain popularity. Paré, in 1552, rediscovered the principle of ligature. In 1800, Physick used absorbable sutures of buckskin and parchment. In 1858, Simpson introduced the wire suture, and in 1881 Lister employed chromic catgut. Halsted, in the early 1900s, emphasized the importance of incorporating as little tissue as possible in the suture and indicated the advantages of silk. In 1911, Cushing reported on the use of silver clips to effect hemostasis in delicate vessels in critical areas. Recently, a wide variety of staples made of different metals, which are relatively inert in tissue, has been employed.

All sutures represent foreign material, and their selection is based on the characteristics of the material and the state of the wound. Nonabsorbable sutures, such as silk, polyethylene, and wire, evoke less tissue reaction than absorbable materials, such as catgut, polyglycolic acid (Dexon), and polygalactin (Vicryl). The latter are preferable, however, in the face of overt infection. The presence of nonabsorbable material in an infected wound can lead to extrusion or sinus tract formation. Wire is the least reactive of the nonabsorbable sutures but the most difficult to handle. Monofilament wire and coated sutures have an advantage over multifilament sutures in the presence of infection. The latter tend to fragment and permit sinus formation due to the interstices.

Diffuse bleeding from multiple transected vessels may be controlled by mechanical techniques which employ pressure directly over the bleeding area, pressure at a distance, or generalized pressure. These techniques are based on the premise that as pressure and flow are decreased in the area of vascular disruption, a clot will occur. As a standard procedure of military surgeons in the seventeenth century, pressure at a distance was effected by application of tourniquets and other pressure devices at pressure points proximal to bleeding sites. Now it is generally felt that direct pressure is preferable and is not attended by the danger of tissue necrosis associated with prolonged use of tourniquets. Gravitational suits have been employed to create generalized pressure and to decrease temporarily bleeding from ruptured major intraabdominal vessels.

Direct pressure applied by means of packs affords the best method of controlling diffuse bleeding from large areas. Rarely is it necessary to leave a pack at the bleeding site and remove it at a second sitting. If this is done, several days should elapse before removal, and the possibility of recurrent bleeding should be anticipated. The question as to whether hot wet packs or cold wet packs should be applied has been investigated. Unless the heat is so great as to denature protein, it may actually increase bleeding, whereas cold packs promote hemostasis by inducing vascular spasm and increasing endothelial adhesiveness. Bleeding from cut bone may be controlled by packing beeswax in the area. This material effects pressure and is relatively nonirritative to the body.

Thermal Agents

Galen's favoring of cautery influenced medicine for 1500 years, until the teachings of Paré were appreciated. The use of cautery was revitalized in 1928, when Cushing and Bovie applied this technique for effecting hemostasis of delicate vessels in recessed areas, such as the brain. Heat achieves hemostasis by denaturation of protein, which results in coagulation of large areas of tissue. With actual cautery, heat is transmitted from the instrument by conduction directly to the tissue; with electrocautery, heating occurs by induction from an alternating-current source.

When electrocautery is employed, the amplitude setting should be high enough to produce prompt coagulation but not so high as to set up an arc between the tissue and the cautery tip. This avoids burns outside the operative field and prevents exit of current through electrocardiographic leads or other monitoring devices. A negative plate should be placed beneath the patient whenever cautery is employed to avoid severe skin burns. The advantage of cautery is that it saves time; its disadvantage is that more tissue is necrosed than with precise ligature.

Certain anesthetic agents cannot be used with electrocautery because of the hazard of explosion.

A direct current can also result in electrical hemostasis. Since the protein moieties and cellular elements of blood have a negative surface charge, they are attracted to the positive pole, where a thrombus is formed. Direct currents in the 20- to 100-mA range have been applied to control diffuse bleeding from large serous surfaces. High-power argon-laser treatment has been applied successfully to the control of bleeding from superficial erosions.

At the other end of the thermal spectrum, cooling has been applied to control bleeding, particularly from the mucosa of the esophagus and stomach. Generalized hypothermia is of little avail, since, in order to reduce the blood flow to visceral organs, the systemic temperature must be brought down to the level of 35°C. At this point shivering and ventricular fibrillation may be encountered. Thrombocytopenia may also be a consequence of generalized cooling. Direct cooling with iced saline is effective and acts by increasing the local intravascular hematocrit and decreasing blood flow by vasoconstriction.

Extreme cooling, i.e., cryogenic surgery, has been applicable particularly in gynecology and neurosurgery. Temperatures ranging between -20 to -180°C are used, and freezing occurs around the tip of the cannula within 5 s. At temperatures of -20°C or below, the tissue, capillaries, small arterioles, and venules undergo cryogenic necrosis. This is caused by dehydration and denaturation of lipid molecules. The muscular walls of large arteries are an exception. Although the major arteries and blood may be frozen solid, the blood contained in these vessels does not clot. When thawing occurs, normal circulation is resumed.

Chemical Agents

Chemical agents vary in their hemostatic action. Some are vasoconstrictive, while others have coagulant properties. Still others are relatively inert but possess hygroscopic properties which increase their bulk and aid in plugging disrupted blood vessels.

Epinephrine, applied topically, induces vasoconstriction, but extensive application can result in considerable absorption and systemic effects. The drug generally is used on oozing sites in mucosal areas, during tonsillectomy, for example.

Historically, skeletal muscle was one of the first materials with locally hemostatic properties to be employed, its use having been introduced by Cushing in 1911. Shortly thereafter, hemostatic fibrin was manufactured. The properties required for local hemostatic materials include handling ease, rapid absorption, nonirritation, and hemostatic action independent of the general clotting mechanism. The most widely used of the commercially available materials are gelatin foam (Gelfoam), oxidized cellulose (Oxycel), oxidized regenerated cellulose (Surgicel), and micronized collagen (Avitene). All these materials act, in part, by transmitting pressure against the wound surface, and the interstices provide a scaffold on which the clot can organize (Table 3-4).

Gelfoam is made from animal skin gelatin which has

Table 3-4. ABSORBABLE HEMOSTATIC AGENTS

	Material	Time to hemostasis	Absorption time	Handling characteristics	Bactericidal property
*Surgical,** *absorbable hemostat*	Oxidized regenerated cellulose	2–8 min	1–2 weeks	Flexible conformable fabric does not adhere to wet gloves or instruments	Yes
*Surgical Nu Knit,** *absorbable hemostat*	Oxidized regenerated cellulose	1–5 min	1–2 weeks	Dense, strong material provides strong suture base. Does not adhere to wet instruments and gloves	Yes
Oxycel,[a] *oxidized gauze*	Oxidized gauze	2–8 min	3–4 weeks	Cotton fabric fibers may adhere to wet instruments and gloves	No
Gelfoam,[b] *absorbable gelatin sponge*	Purified gelatin	Not specified in labeling	4–6 weeks	Foam sponge softens when saturated with sodium chloride	No
Avitene,[c] *microfibrillar collagen hemostat*	Purified bovine corium collagen	1–5 min	12 weeks or less	Powder or nonwoven-web may adhere to wet instruments or gloves	No
Thrombin,[d] *thrombostat*	Bovine origin	Dependent upon concentration, usually less than 1 min	N/A	Can be used in powder form or as a solution (sprayed on or applied with a sponge)	No
*Instat,** *collagen absorbable hemostat*	Bovine dermal collagen	2–5 min	8–10 weeks	Sponge-like material maintains integrity when wet	No
*Collastat,** *absorbable collagen hemostatic sponge*	Collagen from bovine deep flexor tendon (achilles tendon)	2–4 min	8 or more	Sponge-like material does not adhere to wet instruments or gloves	No
Helistat,[f] *absorbable collagen hemostatic sponge*	Collagen from bovine deep flexor tendon (achilles tendon)	2–4 min	8 or more weeks	Sponge-like material does not adhere to wet instruments or gloves	No

* Johnson & Johnson Products, Inc.
[a] Deseret
[b] Upjohn
[c] Alcon Laboratories
[d] Parke-Davis
[e] Kendall
[f] American Biomaterials Corp.

been denatured. In itself, Gelfoam has no intrinsic hemostatic action, but it can be used in combination with topical thrombin, for which it serves as an absorbable carrier. Its main hemostatic activity is related to the contact between blood and the large surface area of the sponge and to the pressure exerted by the weight of the sponge and absorbed blood. Prior to application of Gelfoam, the sponge should be moistened in saline or thrombin solution, and all the air should be removed from the interstices.

Oxycel and Surgicel are altered cellulose materials capable of reacting chemically with blood and producing a sticky mass which functions as an artificial clot. These substances are relatively inert and are removed by liquefaction in 1 week to 1 month. They should be dry when they are applied. Like Gelfoam, these materials are nontoxic and relatively nonirritating but are somewhat detrimental to wound healing and require phagocytosis to be removed. Surgicel has been shown to have an antibacterial effect. Microcrystalline collagen has been shown to be as effective as other materials as a topical hemostatic agent where a large surface is oozing.

TRANSFUSION

Background

In 1967, the tercentennial anniversary of the transfusion of blood into human beings was celebrated. In June of 1667, Jean-Baptiste Denis and a surgeon, Emmerez, transfused blood from a sheep into a fifteen-year-old boy who had been bled many times as treatment for fever. The patient apparently improved, and a successful experience was reported simultaneously in another patient. Because of two subsequent deaths associated with transfusion from animals to humans, criminal charges were brought against Denis. In April of 1668, further transfusions in humans were forbidden unless approved by the Faculty of Medicine in Paris. It was not until the nineteenth century that human blood was recognized as the only appropriate replacement. In 1900, Landsteiner and his associates introduced the concept of blood grouping and identified the major A, B and O groups. In 1939, the Rh group was recognized. Numerous other groups have been uncovered since that time. Development of sensitive cross-matching procedures took place in the 1940s, and with the impetus of World War II, blood transfusion became a common procedure. The introduction of various preservative solutions, such as acid citrate dextrose (ACD), citrate-phosphate-dextrose (CPD), and, recently, citrate-phosphate-double-dextrose adenine (CP2D-A), has been the major advance in blood banking.

As the scope of surgery has expanded, the requirement for larger amounts of blood for transfusion has increased. Approximately 14 percent of all patients operated upon, exclusive of procedures performed in the outpatient department or emergency area, are transfused. Of 604 adults who received blood at a university medical center in association with surgical treatment, 125 required over

5000 mL. The record administration in this hospital in a patient who survived was 100 units within a 36-h period. Preservation of blood and its constituents has been achieved by freezing, and emphasis has been placed on the use of plasma expanders and component therapy.

Characteristics of Blood and Replacement Therapy

BLOOD

Blood has been described as a vehicular organ that perfuses all other organs. It provides transportation of oxygen to satisfy the body's metabolic demands and removes the by-product carbon dioxide. Blood also transports chemical nutriments for, and waste products from, metabolic activity. Homeostatic governors, including hormones, coagulation factors, and antibodies, are carried to and from appropriate sites within the fluid portion of the blood. Red blood cells, with their oxygen-carrying capacity, white blood cells, which function in body defense processes, and platelets, which contribute to the hemostatic process, comprise the formed elements.

REPLACEMENT THERAPY

BANKED WHOLE BLOOD. Whole blood generally is collected in CPD or CP2D-adenine solution and stored at 4°C. Such blood is considered suitable for administration any time up to 35 days of storage. At least 70 percent of the transfused erythrocytes remain in the circulation 24 h posttransfusion and are viable. Normal survival of red blood cells is 110 to 120 days. Sixty days after transfusion, approximately 52 percent of the cells will survive if the transfusion uses fresh blood. The major loss occurs in the first 24 h after transfusion, and subsequent to that time the survival slope for red cells from fresh blood and stored blood is identical. Red cell changes include reduction of intracellular ATP and 2,3-diphosphoglycerate (2,3-DPG), which alters the curve of oxygen dissociation from hemoglobin, decreasing the oxygen transport function.

Banked blood is a poor source of platelets, since platelets lose their ability to survive transfusion after 24 h of storage, and those that survive are functionally defective. Among the clotting factors, factor II (prothrombin), factor VII, factor IX, and factor XI are stable in banked blood. Factor V levels are adequate for 1 to 2 weeks in banked blood, while factor VIII rapidly deteriorates during storage.

During the storage of whole blood, red cell metabolism and plasma protein degradation result in certain chemical changes in the plasma (Table 3-5). Lactic acid increases from 20 to 150 mg/dL, an amount which is insignificant. The pH decreases from 7 to 6.68 within 21 days. Little change in the sodium occurs, but the potassium concentration rises steadily to 32 meq at the end of 21 days. This must be considered when transfusing patients with anuria, oliguria, or hyperkalemia. In these cases, fresher blood or frozen red cells obviously are preferable. The ammonia concentration also rises steadily during storage,

Table 3-5. CHARACTERISTICS OF PLASMA STORED IN ACD SOLUTION
AT 4 ± 1°C

Constituents	Unit value	Days stored				
		0	*7*	*14*	*21*	*28*
Dextrose	mg/dL	350	300	245	210	190
Lactic acid	mg/dL	20	70	120	140	150
Inorganic phosphate	mg/dL	1.8	4.5	6.6	9.0	9.5
pH*		7.0	6.85	6.77	6.68	6.65
Hemoglobin	mg/dL	0–10	25	50	100	150
Sodium	meq/L	150	148	145	142	140
Potassium	meq/L	3–4	12	24	32	40
Ammonia	μg/dL	50	260	470	680	

* Determined with glass electrode.
SOURCE: Strumia MM, Crosby WH, et al: *Transfusion.* Philadelphia, Lippincott, 1963, with permission.)

from 50 to 680 μg at the end of 21 days. This may be of significance for the patient with hepatic disease. The high citrate content may reduce plasma ionized calcium if large volumes of stored blood are administered rapidly. This is most pertinent in children, in patients with hepatic dysfunction, and in patients undergoing cardiopulmonary bypass. The hemolysis that occurs during storage for 21 days is insignificant, since lysis of only about 1 percent of the red cells occurs and the free hemoglobin is rapidly cleared from the circulation following transfusion. Patients receiving large amounts of banked blood frequently have an elevation of the serum bilirubin for several days.

Typing and Cross Matching. In selecting blood for transfusion, serologic compatibility is established routinely for the recipients' and donors' A, B, O, and Rh groups. Cross matching between the donors' red cells and recipients' sera (the "major" cross match) is performed. As a rule, Rh-negative recipients should be transfused only with Rh-negative blood. Since this group represents 15 percent of the donor population, the supply may be limited. If the recipient is an elderly male who has not been transfused previously, the transfusion of Rh-positive blood is reasonable if Rh-negative blood is unavailable. Anti-Rh antibodies form within several weeks of transfusion. If further transfusions are needed within a few days, more Rh-positive blood can be used. Rh-positive blood should not be transfused to Rh-negative females who are capable of childbearing. Administration of hyperimmune anti-Rh globulin to Rh-negative women shortly after Rh sensitization largely eliminates Rh disease in subsequent offspring.

A variety of cell-serum interactions may be detected by careful cross matching. Incompatibility may be due to the fact that either the donor or recipient has been wrongly grouped.

In the patient who is receiving repeated transfusions, serum drawn not more than 48 h prior to cross matching should be utilized for matching with cells of the donor. Emergency blood transfusion can be performed with group O blood. If it is known that the prospective recipient is group AB, group A blood is preferable. The O donor blood should have low titers of anti-A and anti-B.

Such emergency cases are extremely rare, with the exception of battlefield casualties, and it should be possible to wait 10 min, during which time the patient's group can be determined and type-specific blood used. The use of plasma expanders in the meantime makes this delay particularly feasible.

When the blood of multiple donors is to be transfused, such as in the case of extracorporeal circulatory procedures, the question arises as to whether all samples should be cross-matched with each other. In determining compatibility, screening is performed in the usual fashion. Major cross matches are performed. In patients with malignant lymphoma and leukemia, cryoglobulins may be present, and the blood should be administered at room temperature. If these antibodies are present in high titer, hypothermia may be contraindicated.

In patients with thalassemia and, more particularly, with acquired hemolytic anemia, typing and cross matching may be difficult, and sufficient time should be allotted during the preoperative period to accumulate blood that may be required during the operation. Cross matching should always be carried out prior to the administration of dextran, since dextran interferes with the typing procedure.

Because banked blood may be stored for up to 35 days, the use of autologous predeposit transfusion is growing. In otherwise healthy, nonanemic patients, up to 5 to 6 units of blood may be collected for use in elective surgical procedures.

FRESH WHOLE BLOOD. This term refers to blood that is administered within 24 h of its donation. Due to the requirements for HB_sAg, HTLV-III, and syphilis testing, fresh blood is available only untested for such agents. Fresh whole blood is now believed an inadequate source of platelets and factor VIII.

PACKED RED CELLS AND FROZEN RED CELLS. Concentrated suspensions of red cells can be prepared by removing most of the supernatant plasma from the blood following settling of the cells or centrifugation. A small amount of plasma is left, so that the packed cell volume is approximately 70 percent.

Frozen red cells have an advantage in that their use

markedly reduces the risk of infusing antigens to which the patient has been previously sensitized. The red cell viability is improved and the ATP and 2,3-DPG concentrations are maintained. Either packed or frozen red cells are applicable in the treatment of anemia without hypovolemia. Their use reduces the danger of circulatory overload. Reactions secondary to allergens in plasma to which the recipient is sensitive also can be minimized.

LEUKOCYTE AND PLATELET-POOR RED CELLS. These are prepared by aspirating the buffy coat and supernatant plasma, following slow centrifugation or settling. The red cells then are washed with sterile isotonic solution. This should be done only for patients with demonstrated hypersensitivity to either leukocytes or platelets (buffy coat reactions). Usually this syndrome is manifest by fever, chilly sensations, and urticaria in the absence of hemolysis.

PLATELET CONCENTRATES. The indications for platelet transfusion are as follows: thrombocytopenia due to massive blood loss and replacement with stored blood, thrombocytopenia due to inadequate production, and qualitative platelet disorders. The preparations should be used within 120 h of blood donation. One unit of platelet concentrates has a volume of approximately 50 mL. The recovery of platelets in the recipient usually is no more than 60 percent of those present in the donor blood. The platelet concentrate consists of platelets prepared from a unit of platelet-rich plasma. These are resuspended in 30 mL of fluid and should be administered without a filter. The platelet concentrate has the advantage of obviating circulatory overload. Both preparations may harbor the hepatitis virus and account for allergic reactions similar to those due to whole blood. When treating thrombocytopenic bleeding or preparing some thrombocytopenic patients for surgery, it is advisable to elevate the platelet levels to the range of 50,000 to 100,000/mm^3 to provide continued protection. The development of isoimmunity remains one of the most important factors limiting usefulness of platelet transfusion. Isoantibodies are demonstrable in about 5 percent of patients after 1 to 10 transfusions, in 20 percent after 10 to 20 transfusions, and in 80 percent after more than 100 transfusions. The use of HL-A–compatible platelets addresses this problem.

FROZEN PLASMA AND VOLUME EXPANDERS. Frozen plasma prepared from freshly donated blood or fresh plamsa is necessary to provide factors V and VIII. The other plasma clotting factors are present in banked preparations. The use of plasma for therapy in patients with hypovolemia rarely is indicated. The risk of hepatitis is the same whether fresh frozen plasma or whole blood/red cells is administered. Ringer's lactate or buffered saline solution, administered in amounts two to three times the estimated blood loss, is effective in an emergency and is associated with fewer complications. Dextran or a combination of Ringer's lactate solution and normal human serum albumin are preferred for rapid plasma expansion. Commercially available dextran preparations probably should not be administered in amounts exceeding 1 L per day, since prolongation of bleeding time and hemorrhage can occur. Low-molecular-weight dextran, i.e., molecu-

lar weight of 30,000 to 40,000, has achieved recent popularity because it possesses a higher colloidal pressure than plasma and effects some reversal of erythrocyte agglutination.

CONCENTRATES. *Antihemophilic concentrates* are prepared from plasma and are available for the treatment of factor VIII deficiency. Some of these concentrates are twenty to thirty times as potent as an equal volume of fresh-frozen plasma. The simplest factor VIII concentrate is the plasma cryoprecipitate. *Albumin* also has been concentrated, so that 25 g may be administered and provide the osmotic equivalent of 500 mL of plasma. The advantage of albumin is that it is a hepatitis-free product.

Indications for Replacement of Blood or Its Elements

VOLUME REPLACEMENT. The most common indication for blood transfusion in diseases of surgical interest is the replenishment of the circulating blood volume. It is difficult to evaluate the volume deficit accurately.

A variety of techniques employing dyes or isotopically tagged colloids has been introduced to determine the blood volume more precisely. Values for "normal blood volume" are variable, and the techniques are relatively inaccurate when there is a rapidly changing situation, such as hemorrhage. Chronically ill and elderly patients may have a diminution of blood volume. In patients with cardiac decompensation, the blood volume may be greater than normal. Many patients with chronically reduced blood volume are well accommodated to that volume. Blood volume, in itself, does not serve as an absolute indication for transfusion. Measurement of hemoglobin or hematocrit is also used to interpret blood loss. This measurement is misleading in the face of acute blood loss, since the hematocrit may be normal in spite of a severely contracted blood volume. It has been shown that, after a healthy adult male lost approximately 1000 mL of blood rapidly, the venous hematocrit fell only 3 percent during the first hour, 5 percent at 24 h, 6 percent at 48 h, and 8 percent at 72 h, thus indicating the time required for the body to restore blood volume.

A healthy person can lose 450 mL in 15 min with only minor effects on the circulation and little change in blood pressure or pulse, as evidenced by the normal blood donor. The normal person may lose 1 L of blood rapidly without a fall in blood pressure as long as he remains supine. About 40 percent of blood volume, or 2 L of blood, usually is lost before significant hypotension develops. Loss of blood may be evaluated in the operating room by estimating the amount of blood in the wound and on the drapes and by weighing sponges. The loss determined by weighing sponges is only about 70 percent of true loss. In patients who have normal preoperative blood values, blood loss up to 20 percent of total blood volume (TBV) is replaced with crystalloid solutions. Blood loss up to 50 percent TBV is replaced with crystalloids and red blood cell concentrates. Blood loss above 50 percent TBV is replaced with crystalloids, red blood cells, and albumin or plasma. Continued bleeding above 50 percent TBV should receive the same components and fresh frozen plasma. If electrolyte solutions are used to replace blood volume, an amount three to four times the lost volume is required because of immediate diffusion into the interstitial space.

IMPROVEMENT IN OXYGEN-CARRYING CAPACITY. This is primarily a function of the red cell. When anemia can be treated by specific therapy, transfusion should be withheld. Acute anemias, such as hemolytic anemia, are more disabling physiologically than chronic anemia, since most patients with chronic anemia have undergone an adjustment to the situation. In pregnancy, there is a moderate drop in hematocrit, and transfusions are not indicated to correct the physiologic anemia of pregnancy prior to surgical treatment. The correction of chronic anemia prior to surgical treatment, though often performed, is difficult to justify, and there is no indication that anemia predisposes to wound dehiscence. Blood volume may be replaced with dextran solution or Ringer's lactate solution with a reduction of the hemoglobin to levels below 10 g and little demonstrable change in the effects of a reduction in oxygen-carrying capacity or the capacity to remove metabolic gaseous by-products. A stroma-free hemoglobin solution has been shown to have

ability to carry and exchange oxygen. Also, a whole blood substitute, Fluosol-DA, has been proposed as a solution with oxygen-handling capabilities.

REPLACEMENT OF CLOTTING FACTORS. Transfusion of platelets and/or proteins contributing to coagulation may be indicated in specific patients either prior to or during operation (Table 3-6). In the treatment of certain hemorrhagic conditions, it is to be appreciated that the clotting defects may be multiple and the injection of substitutes and extracts may be less effective than transfusion of fresh blood or fresh frozen plasma. Efficacy of fresh frozen plasma (FFP) in the management of coagulopathy in patients with liver disease and in patients receiving large amounts of stored blood is not well defined. There are insufficient data to specify criteria for transfusion of FFP. The initial volume of FFP needed for an effect on coagulation ranges between 600 to 2000 mL administered in 1 to 2 h. The rigid use of the PT and PTT to anticipate the effect of FFP is not justified.

When transfusion with fibrinogen is deemed necessary, a plasma level greater than 100 mg/dL should be maintained. The hypofibrinogenemia encountered during surgical treatment is frequently related to excessive consumption. Adequate levels of fibrinogen frequently will

Table 3-6. REPLACEMENT OF CLOTTING FACTORS

Factors	Normal level	Life span in vivo ($\frac{1}{2}$ life)	Fate during coagulation	Level required for safe hemostasis	Stability in ACD bank blood (4°)	Ideal agent for replacing deficit
I (fibrinogen)	200–400 mg/ 100 mL	72 h	Consumed	60–100 mg/ 100 mL	Very stable	Bank blood; concentrated fibrinogen
II (prothrombin)	20 mg/100 mL (100%)	72 h	Consumed	15–20%	Stable	Bank blood; concentrated preparation
V (proaccelerin, accelerator globulin labile factor)	100%	36 h	Consumed	5–20%	Labile (40% at 1 week)	Frozen fresh plasma; blood under 7 days
VII [proconvertin, serum prothrombin conversion accelerator (SPCA) stable factor]	100%	5 h	Survives	5–30%	Stable	Bank blood; concentrated preparation
VIII [antihemophilic factor (AHF), antihemophilic globulin (AHG)]	100% (50–150)	6–12 h	Consumed	30%	Labile (20–40% at 1 week)	Fresh frozen plasma; concentrated AHF; cryoprecipitate
IX [Christmas factor, plasma thromboplastin component (PTC), hemophilia B factor]	100%	24 h	Survives	20–30%	Stable	Fresh frozen plasma; bank blood concentrated preparation
X (Stuart-Prower factor)	100%	40 h	Survives	15–20%	Stable	Bank blood; concentrated preparation
XI [plasma thromboplasma antecedent (PTA)]	100%	Probably 40–80 h	Survives	10%	Probably stable	Bank blood
XII (Hageman factor)	100%	Unknown	Survives	Deficit produces no bleeding tendency	Stable	Replacement not required
XIII [fibrinase, fibrin-stabilizing factor (FSF)]	100%	4–7 days	Survives	Probably less than 1%	Stable	Bank blood
Platelets	150,000–400,000/ mm^3	8–11 days	Consumed	60,000–100,000/ mm^3	Very labile (40% at 20 h; 0 at 48 h)	Fresh blood or plasma; fresh platelet concentrate (not frozen plasma)

SOURCE: Salzman EW: Hemorrhagic disorders, in Kinney JM, Egdahl RH, Zuidema GD (eds): *Manual of Preoperative and Postoperative Care*. Philadelphia, Saunders, 1971, p 157, with permission.

return within hours without replacement therapy if the precipitating cause is corrected. Cryoprecipitate is a source of concentrated fibrinogen (250 mg/10 mL). Deficiency of factor V, per se, is relatively rare; although transfusion will increase the level, there is suggestion that the biologic half-life is short and may not exceed 12 h.

Hypoprothrombinemia and deficiency of factor VII in patients on anticoagulant therapy can be reversed with injection of vitamin K_1. In patients who are deficient in prothrombin, such as those with cirrhosis, and who require surgical treatment, transfusion with frozen plasma may effect immediate benefit.

Transfusion therapy for patients with hemophilia subjected to trauma or surgical procedure requires sufficient quantities to raise and maintain the level of factor VIII in the plasma to above 30 percent of normal. Transfusion of small amounts of factor VIII is not justified. If a life-threatening situation exists, large amounts must be used. The factor IX–deficient patient subjected to surgery or trauma also requires levels of 20 to 30 percent for secure hemostasis. Such levels are difficult to attain with plasma infusions despite the stability of factor IX in stored plasma. Factor IX concentrates are preferable. The biologic half-life of factor IX is appreciably longer than that of factor VIII.

Usually, the hemostatic mechanism is not markedly altered with platelet counts greater than 50,000/mm³. If thrombocytopenia is more pronounced, however, the transfusion of platelet concentrates may be indicated to prevent or treat active bleeding. The life span of freshly infused platelets is only about 10 days, and in some instances the recipient represents a hostile environment, and the survival is reduced to several hours. The usual dose is 1 unit/10 kg.

SPECIFIC INDICATIONS

SINGLE-UNIT TRANSFUSION. There has been a general trend toward condemning all single-unit transfusion on surgical services. As has been previously mentioned, they are usually uncalled for. The Committee on Blood of the American Medical Association found it necessary to oppose this trend, however, pointing out that it is a poor practice to order 2 units of blood to escape criticism for using a single unit, and an appropriate volume of blood should be given whenever transfusion is required.

MASSIVE TRANSFUSION. The term *massive transfusion* implies a single transfusion greater than 2500 mL, or 5000 mL transfused over a period of 24 h. The approximate percentages of *original* blood volume remaining after varying degrees of hemorrhage and transfusion are shown in Table 3-7. A variety of problems may attend the use of massive transfusion. Dilutional thrombocytopenia, impaired platelet function, and deficiencies of factors V, VIII, and XI may occur. The acid load present in stored blood may have an additive effect in a patient with preexisting acidosis. Routine alkalinization is not advisable, since this could have an adverse effect on the oxyhemoglobin dissociation curve and presents an additional so-

Table 3-7. PERCENTAGE OF ORIGINAL BLOOD VOLUME REMAINING IN A PATIENT WITH A 5-L BLOOD VOLUME TRANSFUSED WITH 500-ML UNITS

Situation*	Magnitude of hemorrhage and transfusion		
	1 Blood volume (10 units)	2 Blood volumes (20 units)	3 Blood volumes (30 units)
Best	37	14	5
Usual	25–30	10	2–4
Worst	18	3	0.4

* The "best" situation requires simultaneous and equal replacement during hemorrhage; the "worst" situation means initial loss of one-half blood volume not replaced until the hemorrhage has stopped.
SOURCE: After Collins, 1976.

dium load to a compromised patient. The increased potassium content of multiple units of stored blood does not provide clinical effects unless the patient is severely oliguric.

Citrate toxicity may be associated with massive transfusion, particularly in young children and patients with severe hypotension or liver disease. This is related to an excessive binding of ionized calcium and is usually corrected by spontaneous mobilization of calcium from bone. The physiologic consequences of citrate toxicity rarely have a significant effect. The function of hemoglobin is altered by storage in that the concentration of 2,3-DPG (diphosphoglyceric acid) falls to a negligible level by the third week. This results in an increased affinity of the red blood cells for oxygen and a less efficient oxygen delivery system. In itself, reduction of 2,3-DPG may not have a significant effect but when combined with acute anemia it may be an important factor.

When large transfusions are administered, a heat exchanger may be used to warm the blood, since hypothermia may cause a decrease in cardiac rate and output and a reduction in the blood pH. Warming the blood decreases significantly the frequency of intraoperative cardiac arrest.

The use of blood from many donors increases the possibility of hemolytic transfusion reaction due to incompatibility. This can be reduced by screening each potential donor in the pool and eliminating those who show possible incompatibility. Paradoxically, patients who survive a massive transfusion do not have a high probability of developing isoantibodies subsequently, and the risk is no greater than that from a single transfusion. The risk of posttransfusion hepatitis increases progressively with each succeeding unit. When administering massive transfusions, the pH, blood gases, and potassium should be measured regularly. Acidosis and abnormalities should be corrected. If diffuse bleeding occurs, coagulation screening tests and platelet counts should be performed, and deficits corrected with frozen plasma and platelet concentrates.

EXTRACORPOREAL CIRCULATION. The heparin used to prevent the blood from clotting is usually neutralized with protamine. A variety of physiologic compatible fluids, such as Ringer's lactate solution, buffered saline solution, and dextran, may be applied to prime the pump during extracorporeal circulation and reduce the need for blood. The platelet count falls progressively during the initial intraoperative and bypass period, in part due to dilution by non-blood-priming solutions. In general, the platelet count remains about half baseline but exceeds 100,000 per mm^3 during the postoperative period, and, therefore, platelet therapy is usually not required.

Methods of Administering Blood

ROUTINE ADMINISTRATION. The rate of transfusion depends upon the patient's status. Usually, 5 mL/min is administered for 1 min, following which 10 to 20 mL/min may be administered to complete routine transfusion. When marked oligemia is being treated, the first 500 mL may be given within 10 min, and the second 500 mL may be given equally rapidly in most cases. Cold blood may be used for this amount, but when larger amounts are administered, warm blood is desirable.

The gauge of the needle is a critical factor in the rate of flow. Flow also is determined by the height at which the bottle is suspended. In patients with peripheral circulatory failure, the veins may be constricted with resultant increased resistance to flow, necessitating raising the bottle. Positive pressure may be applied with an inflated blood pressure cuff surrounding the plastic bag.

When large transfusions are administered, it is important not to overload the circulation, and the use of central venous pressure monitoring is particularly pertinent. There is no practical advantage in the use of intraarterial transfusion over the intravenous route in the treatment of oligemia. It has been shown that coronary flow and systemic arterial pressure respond as rapidly and to the same extent whether the blood is administered intravenously or intraarterially. The theoretical advantage of intraarterial infusion for patients in whom the blood cannot pass from the venous to the arterial side of the circulation because of cardiac arrest or ineffective ventricular contraction is offset by the delay in setting up an intraarterial transfusion.

OTHER METHODS. Blood may be instilled intraperitoneally or into the medullary cavity of the sternum and long bones. Intrasternal and intramedullary transfusion may be painful, and the rate of administration is limited. Approximately 90 percent of red cells injected intraperitoneally enter the circulation, but uptake is not complete for at least a week, and therefore the method is not suitable when immediate transfusion is required.

Intraoperative autotransfusion has become increasingly popular; it is a potentially life-saving adjunct to the management of trauma and is useful in elective operations in which multiple transfusions are likely to be required, e.g., liver resection. A variety of devices is commercially available, but none satisfies all the requirements. The cell savers wash the blood and separate the cells and reinfuse washed red cells, but they are limited by the constraints of time and do not provide a rapid reinfusion. Others are directed toward retrieving blood and returning it directly in order to avoid the time lapse. A major disadvantage of autotransfusion is the associated hemolysis and accumulation of cellular debris; the red cell survival is normal. Blood suctioned gently from the peritoneal cavity and reinfused through a filter has been shown effective, and in one series of 123 transfusions using intraperitoneal blood in patients with ruptured ectopic gestation, there was only one death.

COMPLICATIONS

HEMOLYTIC REACTIONS. Hemolytic reactions due to incompatibility of A, B, O, and Rh groups or many other independent systems may result from errors in the laboratory of a clerical or technical nature or the administration of the wrong blood at the time of transfusion. Hemolytic reactions are characterized by intravascular destruction of red blood cells and consequent hemoglobinemia and hemoglobinuria. Circulating haptoglobin is capable of binding 100 mg of hemoglobin/dL of plasma, and the complex is cleared by the reticuloendothelial system. When the binding capacity is exceeded, free hemoglobin circulates, and the heme is released and combines with albumin to form methemalbumin. This is detected by a positive Schumm's test. When free hemoglobin exceeds 25 mg/dL of plasma, some is excreted in the urine, but in most subjects hemoglobinuria occurs when the total plasma level exceeds 150 mg/dL. The renal lesions that may occur consist of tubular necrosis and precipitation of hemoglobin within the tubules. Red cell stromal lipid is liberated, and this may initiate a disseminated intravascular coagulation. The kallikrein-bradykinin system may be activated and affect the circulatory system. Minor incompatibilities may occur, causing hemolysis within the reticuloendothelial system manifested by fever, a mild decrease in hemoglobin, and an increase in bilirubin. If the recipient has a low antibody titer at the time of transfusion, reaction may be delayed for several days.

Clinical Manifestations. There is an increased hazard in patients with a previous transfusion reaction. If the patient is awake, the most common symptoms are the sensation of heat and pain along the vein into which the blood is being transfused, flushing of the face, pain in the lumbar region, and constricting pain in the chest. The patient may experience chills, fever, and respiratory distress, hypotension, and tachycardia from amounts as small as 50 mL. In patients who are anesthetized and undergoing operation, the two signs which may call attention are abnormal bleeding and continued hypotension despite adequate replacement. The mortality and morbidity resulting from hemolytic reactions is high if the patient receives a full unit of incompatible blood. Acute hemorrhagic diatheses occur in 8 to 30 percent of patients. There is a sudden fall in the platelet count, an increase in fibrinolytic activity, and consumption of coagulation factors, especially V and VIII, due to disseminated intravascular clotting.

Rudowski reported the following incidences of clinical manifestations in a large series with hemolytic posttransfusion reactions: oliguria, 58 percent; hemoglobinuria, 56 percent; arterial hypotension, 50 percent; jaundice, 40 percent; nausea and vomiting, 30 percent; flank pain, 25 percent; cyanosis and hypothermia, 22 percent; dyspnea, 20 percent; chills, 18 percent; diffuse bleeding, 16 percent; neurologic signs, 10 percent; and allergic reaction, 6 percent. The laboratory criteria are hemoglobinuria with a concentration of free hemoglobin over 5 mg/dL, a serum haptoglobin level below 50 mg/dL, and serologic criteria to show antigen incompatibility of the donor and recipient blood. The simplest clinical diagnostic test is insertion of a bladder catheter and evaluation of the color and volume of the excreted urine, since hemoglobinuria and oliguria are the most characteristic signs. A positive Coombs' test indicating transfused cells coated with patient antibody also provides evidence.

Treatment. If a transfusion reaction is suspected, the transfusion should be stopped immediately, and a sample of the recipient's blood should be drawn and sent along with the suspected unit to the blood bank for comparison with the pretransfusion samples. The serum bilirubin should be determined in the recipient. Each gram of hemoglobin is converted to about 40 mg of bilirubin. The hemolytic reaction is characterized by an increase in the indirect reacting fraction.

A Foley catheter should be inserted and the hourly urine output recorded. Since renal toxicity is affected by the rate of urinary excretion and the pH and since alkalinizing the urine prevents precipitation of hemoglobin within the tubules, attempts are made to initiate diuresis and alkalinize the urine. This can be accomplished with 40 mg of furosemide plus 45 meq of bicarbonate. If marked oliguria or anuria occurs, the fluid intake and potassium intake are restricted, and the patient is treated as a case of renal shutdown. In some instances, dialysis is required. Following recovery from oliguria or anuria, diuresis is often copious and may be associated with significant losses of potassium and sodium that require replacement.

FEBRILE AND ALLERGIC REACTIONS. These are relatively frequent, occurring in about 1 percent of transfusions. Reactions are usually mild and are manifested by urticaria and fever and occur within 60 to 90 min of the start of transfusion. In rare instances, the reaction may be severe enough to cause anaphylactic shock. Allergic reactions are caused by transfusion of antibodies from hypersensitive donors or the transfusion of antigens to which the recipient is hypersensitive. Reactions may occur following the administration of whole blood, packed red cells, plasma, and antihemophilic factor. Treatment consists of antihistamines, epinephrine, and steroids, depending on the severity of the reaction. Repeated reactions can be prevented by use of leukocyte-depleted or washed red cells.

BACTERIAL SEPSIS. Bacterial contamination of infused blood is rare and may be acquired either from the contents of the container or the skin of the donor. Gram-negative organisms, especially coliform and *Pseudomonas* species, which are capable of growth at 4°C, are the most common cause. Clinical manifestations include fever, chills, abdominal cramps, vomiting, and diarrhea. There may be hemorrhagic manifestations and increased bleeding if the patient is undergoing surgical treatment. In some instances, bacterial toxins can produce profound shock. If the diagnosis is suspected, the transfusion should be discontinued and the blood cultured. Emergency treatment includes adrenergic blocking agents, oxygen, antibiotics, and, in some cases, judicious transfusion.

EMBOLISM. Although air embolism has been reported as a complication of intravenous transfusion, healthy animals tolerate large amounts of air injected intravenously at a rapid rate. In experimental animals, the minimum lethal dose averages 7.5 mL/kg, and the mortality rate accompanying this amount of air injection can be halved by placing the animal on the left side at the time of injection. This displaces the air away from the outflow tract in the right ventricle. It has been suggested that the normal adult generally will tolerate an embolism of 200 mL of air. Smaller amounts, however, can cause alarming signs and may be fatal. Manifestations of venous air embolism include a rise in venous pressure and cyanosis, a "mill wheel" murmur heard over the precordium, hypotension, tachycardia, and syncope. Death usually is related to primary respiratory failure. Treatment consists of placing the patient on the left side in a head-down position with the feet up. Arterial air embolism is manifested by dizziness and fainting, loss of consciousness, and convulsions. Air may be visible in the retinal arteries, and bubbles of air may flow from transected vessels.

Plastic tubes used for transfusion have also embolized after they have broken off within the vein. Plastic tubes have passed into the right atrium and the pulmonary artery, resulting in death. Embolized catheters have been removed successfully.

THROMBOPHLEBITIS. Prolonged infusions into peripheral veins using either needles, cannulae, or plastic tubes are associated with superficial venous thrombosis. Intravenous infusions which last more than 8 h are more likely to be followed by thrombophlebitis. There is an increased incidence in the lower limb as compared to upper limb infusions. Treatment consists of discontinuation of the infusion and local compressing. Embolism from superficial thrombophlebitis of this nature is extremely rare.

OVERTRANSFUSION AND PULMONARY EDEMA. Overloading the circulation is an avoidable complication. It may occur with rapid infusion of blood, plasma expanders, and other fluids, particularly in patients with heart disease. In order to prevent this complication, the central venous pressure should be monitored in these patients and whenever large amounts of fluid are administered.

Circulatory overloading is manifested by a rise in the venous pressure, dyspnea, and cough. Rales generally can be heard at the bases of the lungs. Treatment consists of stopping the infusion, placing the patient in a sitting position, and, occasionally, venous section for removal of blood.

Although acute pulmonary edema occurs more frequently following large transfusions, it has been reported in patients receiving small transfusions. A syndrome which can be confused with pulmonary edema consists of postoperative hypoxia seen in patients who have undergone cardiac surgical treatment and extracorporeal bypass procedures. A damaging factor apparently is carried by the perfusing blood, and immature plasma cells are found in the interalveolar tissue. The lesion represents an immune response to blood. The incidence is reduced by employing the hemodilution technique of pump priming.

TRANSMISSION OF DISEASE. Malaria, Chagas' disease, brucellosis, and syphilis are among the diseases that can be transmitted by blood transfusion. Syphilis has been reported following the transfusion of platelets. The storage temperature used for all other blood components (4°C or lower) kills the spirochete. The incubation period ranges from 4 weeks to 4 months. The first manifestation is the skin rash of secondary syphilis. Cure is readily achieved with brief penicillin therapy. Malaria can be transmitted by all blood components, including platelets, fresh frozen plasma, and frozen or deglycerolized red cells. The species most commonly implicated is *Plasmodium malariae*. The incubation period ranges between 8 to 100 days; the initial clinical manifestation is shaking chill and spiking fever. Cytomegalovirus (CMV) infection, causing a syndrome resembling infectious mononucleosis, was commonly observed following open heart surgery when large amounts of heparinized blood were used to prime the pump. The most significant morbidity and mortality occurs following transfusion of CMV-infected blood in low-birthweight infants born of mothers who were CMV antibody negative.

Posttransfusion viral hepatitis remains the most common fatal complication of blood transfusion. It is estimated that for every case of icteric posttransfusion viral hepatitis there are four anicteric cases, many of which are asymptomatic. Hepatitis is caused either by hepatitis B virus, or the non-A, non-B virus. The incubation period of the former is up to 6 months, the latter's may be as short as 2 weeks. A serologic marker for hepatitis B surface antigen (HB_sAg) is detectable, and since 1975, blood collecting agencies have been required to test all units of blood for this antigen. As a result, hepatitis B virus transmission has been reduced. Because there is no specific test for the non-A, non-B virus, careful screening of volunteer donors remains the only preventive measure.

The clinical manifestations of hepatitis include lethargy and anorexia as part of anicteric disease, icterus, and chronic liver disease. HB_sAg persists in about 35 percent of patients who develop serum hepatitis of type B. There is no risk from human serum albumin and other plasma protein fractions.

Immune serum globulin is effective in preventing type A hepatitis but is inconsistent in regard to type B. Accidental self-inoculation with material that is definitely known to contain HB_sAg, or transfusion of blood which is HB_sAg-positive, constitutes an indication for immediate use of human specific immunoglobulin (HSI) anti-HB_sAg. The presently recommended dose is 0.5 IgG given as an intramuscular injection. Recently, a vaccine has been developed against HB_sAg, and it is recommended that all surgeons undergo vaccination. Originally it was felt that a determination of the presence of antibody should be performed prior to undergoing the vaccination regimen, but this policy is no longer adhered to.

Acquired immunodeficiency syndrome (AIDS) is thought to be caused by a transmissible agent. One percent of all cases fall into none of the groups regarded as at high risk. This one percent had received a blood transfusion within 5 years of their illness. The risk of AIDS following blood transfusion has been estimated to be one case per million patients transfused and blood collecting agencies have taken measures to preclude donors to high-risk groups and to apply screening techniques. Blood donors are *not* at risk.

Bibliography

General

Colman RW, Hirsh J, Marder VJ, et al (eds): *Hemostasis and Thrombosis*. Philadelphia, Lippincott, 1982.

Rudowski WJ (ed): *Disorders of Hemostasis in Surgery*. Hanover, New Hampshire, The University Press of New England, 1977.

Biology of Hemostasis

Davie EW, Ratnoff OD: Waterfall sequence for intrinsic blood clotting. *Science* 145:1310, 1964.

Jackson CM, Nemerson Y: Blood coagulation. *Annu Rev Biochem* 49:765, 1980.

Macfarlane RG: Enzyme cascade in the blood clotting mechanism and its function as a biochemical amplifier. *Nature (Lond)* 202:498, 1964.

Marcus AJ: The role of lipids in platelet function: With particular reference to the arachidonic acid pathway. *J Lipid Res* 19:793, 1978.

Rodman NF: The morphologic basis of platelet function, in Brinkhous KM, Shermer RW, Mostofi FK (eds): *The Platelet*. Baltimore, Williams & Wilkins, 1971.

Shattil AJ, Bennett JS: Platelets and their membranes in hemostasis: Physiology and pathophysiology. *Ann Intern Med* 94:108, 1980.

Sherry S: Present concept of the fibrinolytic system. *Ser Haemat* 7:70, 1965.

Weiss HJ: Platelet physiology and abnormalities of platelet function. *N Engl J Med* 293:531, 1975.

Weiss HJ, Platelet physiology and abnormalities of platelet function. *N Engl J Med* 293:580, 1975.

Congenital Hemostatic Defects

Brown B, Steed DL, et al: General surgery in adult hemophiliacs. *Surgery* 99:154, 1986.

Curtiss PH Jr: Orthopedic management of patients with hereditary disorders of blood coagulation. *Mod Treat* 5:84, 1968.

Kasper CK, Bowlen AL, et al: Hematologic Management of hemophilia A for surgery. *JAMA* 253:1279, 1985.

Nilsson IM, Larsson SA, Bergentz S-E: The use of blood components in the treatment of congenital coagulation disorders. *World J Surg* 11:14, 1987.

Ratnoff OD: Hereditary disorders of hemostasis, in Stanbury JB, Wyngaarden JB, Fredrickson DS (eds): *The Metabolic Basis of Inherited Diseases,* 2d ed. New York, McGraw-Hill, 1966.

Rudowski WJ: Major surgery in haemophilia. *Annu Rev Coll Surg Engl.* 63:111, 1981.

Shulman NR: Surgical care of patients with hereditary disorders of blood coagulation. *Mod Treat* 5:61, 1968.

Acquired Hemostatic Defects

Bell WR: Disseminated intravascular coagulation. *Johns Hopkins Med J* 146:289, 1980.

Bennett B, Towler HMA: Haemostatic response to trauma. *Br Med Bull* 41:274, 1985.

Feinstein DI: Diagnosis and management of disseminated intravascular coagulation: The role of heparin therapy. *Blood* 60:284, 1982.

Griner PF: Drug effects on oral anticoagulants, in Weed RL (ed): *Hematology for Internists.* Boston, Little, Brown, 1971.

Hoak JC, Koepke JA: Platelet transfusions. *Clin Haematol* 5:69, 1976.

Klingensmith W: Surgical implications of hemorrhage during anticoagulant therapy. *Surg Gynecol Obstet* 125:1333, 1967.

Schwartz SI: Myeloproliferative disorders. *Ann Surg* 182:464, 1975.

Schwartz SI, Hoepp LM, Sachs S: Splenectomy for thrombocytopenia. *Surgery* 88:497, 1980.

Silver D, Kapsch DN, Tsoi EKM: Heparin-induced thrombocytopenia, thrombosis, and hemorrhage. *Ann Surg* 198:301, 1983.

Slichter SJ: Identification and management of defects in platelet hemostasis in massively transfused patients. *Prog Clin Biol Res* 108:225, 1982.

Tests of Hemostasis and Blood Coagulation

Bowie EJ, Owen CA Jr: The significance of abnormal preoperative hemostatic tests. *Prog Hemost Thromb* 5:179, 1980.

Karpatkin M: Screening tests in hemostasis. *Pediatr Clin North Am* 27:831, 1980.

Mielke CH, Kaneshiro MM, et al: The standardized normal ivy bleeding time and its prolongation by aspirin. *Blood* 34:204, 1969.

Nye SW, Graham JB, Brinkhous KM: The partial thromboplastin time as a screening test for the detection of latent bleeders. *Am J Med Sci* 243:279, 1962.

Quick AJ: Clinical interpretation of the one-stage prothrombin time. *Circulation* 24:1422, 1961.

Rapaport SI: Preoperative hemostatic evaluation: Which tests, if any? *Blood* 61:229, 1983.

Reid WO, Henry RL, et al: Hemostasis: The balance concept of procoagulant and inhibitor systems and use of the serial thrombin time (STT). *Medical Hypotheses* 15:169, 1984.

Evaluation of the Surgical Patient as a Hemostatic Risk

Biggs R, Macfarlane RG: *Human Blood Coagulation and Its Disorders,* 3d ed. Philadelphia, Davis, 1962.

Colman RW, Hirsh J, et al, (eds): *Hemostasis and Thrombosis.* Philadelphia, Lippincott, 1987.

Hougie C: *Fundamentals of Blood Coagulation in Clinical Medicine.* New York, McGraw-Hill, 1963.

Shulman NR, Aster RH, et al: Immunoreactions involving platelets. V. Posttransfusion purpura due to complement-fixing antibody against genetically controlled platelet antigen: Proposed mechanism for thrombocytopenia and its relevance. *Clin Invest* 40:1597, 1961.

Local Hemostasis

Abbott W, Austen WG: The effectiveness and mechanism of collagen-induced topical hemostasis. *Surgery* 78:723, 1975.

Cushing H: The control of bleeding in operations for brain tumor. *Ann Surg* 54:1, 1911.

Evans BE: Local hemostatic agents (and techniques). *Scand J Haematol* (suppl 40) 33:417, 1984.

Halsted WS: The employment of fine silk in preference to catgut and the advantages of transfixing tissues and vessels in controlling hemorrhage. *JAMA* 60:1119, 1913.

Jenkins HP, Clarke JS: Gelatin sponge: A new hemostatic substance. *Arch Surg* 51:253, 1945.

Sawyer PN, Wesolowski SA: Electrical hemostasis, in *Conference on Bleeding in the Surgical Patient. Ann NY Acad Sci* 115:455, 1964.

Schechter DS: History of the evolution of methods of hemostasis and the study of blood coagulation, in Ulin AW, Gollub SS (eds): *Surgical Bleeding: Handbook for Medicine, Surgery, and Specialties.* New York, McGraw-Hill, 1966.

Silverstein FE, Auth DC, et al: High power argon laser treatment via standard endoscope. I. A preliminary study of efficacy in control of experimental erosive bleeding. *Gastroenterology* 71:558, 1976.

Waltz JM, Cooper IS: Cryogenic surgery, in Ulin AW, Gollub SS (eds): *Surgical Bleeding: Handbook for Medicine, Surgery, and Specialties.* New York, McGraw-Hill, 1966.

Willman VL, Hanlon CR: The influence of temperature on surface bleeding: Favorable effects of local hypothermia. *Ann Surg* 143:660, 1956.

Transfusion

American Medical Association Committee on Blood: Single unit transfusions. *JAMA* 189:955, 1964.

Brzica SM, Pineda AA, Taswell HF: Autologous blood transfusion. *Mayo Clin Proc* 51:723, 1976.

Bunker JP, Stetson JB, et al: Citric acid intoxication. *JAMA* 157:1361, 1955.

Caceres E, Whittembury G: Evaluation of blood losses during surgical operations: Comparison of the gravimetric method with the blood volume determination. *Surgery* 45:681, 1959.

Case RB, Sarnoff SJ, et al: Intra-arterial and intravenous blood infusions in hemorrhagic shock: Comparison of effects on coronary blood flow and arterial pressure. *JAMA* 152:208, 1953.

Chaplin H Jr, Brittingham TE, Cassell M: Methods for preparation of suspensions of buffy coat–poor red blood cells for transfusion, including a report of 50 transfusions of suspensions of buffy coat-poor red blood cells prepared by a dextran sedimentation method. *Am J Clin Pathol* 31:373, 1959.

Collins JA: Massive blood transfusions, in *Clinics in Hematology.* Philadelphia, Saunders, 1976.

Glover JL, Broadie TA: Intraoperative autotransfusion. *World J Surg* 11:60, 1987.

Ham JM: Transfusion reactions, in Condon RE, DeCosse JJ (eds): *Surgical Care*. Philadelphia, Lea & Febiger, 1980, chap 12, pp 178–186.

Harrigan C, Lucas CE, et al: Serial changes in primary hemostasis after massive transfusion. *Surgery* 98:836, 1985.

Hoff HE, Guillemin R: The tercentenary of transfusion in man. *Cardiovasc Res Cent Bull* 6:47, 1967.

Hogman CF, Bagge L, Thoren L: The use of blood components in surgical transfusion therapy. *World J Surg* 11:2, 1987.

Ingram GIC: The bleeding complications of blood transfusion. *Transfusion* 5:1, 1965.

Katz R, Rodriguez J, Ward R: Posttransfusion hepatitis: Effect of modified gamma-globulin added to blood in vitro. *N Engl J Med* 285:925, 1971.

Keeling MM, Gray LA, et al: Intraoperative autotransfusion: Experience in 725 consecutive cases. *Ann Surg* 197:536, 1983.

Krevans JR, Jackson DP: Hemorrhagic disorder following massive whole blood transfusions. *JAMA* 159:171, 1955.

Krugman S, Giles JP, Hammond J: Viral hepatitis, type B (MS-2 strain): Prevention with specific hepatitis B immune serum globulin. *JAMA* 218:1665, 1971.

Lalich JJ, Schwartz SI: The role of aciduria in the development of hemoglobinuric nephrosis in dehydrated rabbits. *J Exp Med* 92:11, 1950.

Maloney JV Jr, Smythe CMcC, et al: Intra-arterial and intravenous transfusion. *Surg Gynecol Obstet* 97:529, 1953.

Messmer KFW: Acceptable hematocrit levels in surgical patients. *World J Surg* 11:41, 1987.

Peskin GW, O'Brien K, Rabiner SF: Stroma-free hemoglobin solution: The "ideal" blood substitute? *Surgery* 66:185, 1969.

Phillipps E, Fleischner FG: Pulmonary edema in the course of a blood transfusion without overloading the circulation. *Dis Chest* 50:619, 1966.

Pruitt BA Jr, Moncrief JA, Mason AD Jr: Efficacy of buffered saline as the sole replacement fluid following acute measured hemorrhage in man. *J Trauma* 7:767, 1967.

Reed RL, Ciavarella D, et al: Prophylactic platelet administration during massive transfusion. *Ann Surg* 203:40, 1986.

Rizza CR: Coagulation factor therapy. *Clin Haematol* 5:113, 1976.

Rudowski WJ: Complications associated with blood transfusion, in Allgower M, Bergentz SE, Calne RY, Gruber UF (eds): *Progress in Surgery*. New York, Karger, 1971.

Schwartz SI, Adams JT, Bauman AW: Splenectomy for hematologic disorders. *Curr Probl Surg,* May 1971.

Shires T, Coln D, et al: Fluid therapy in hemorrhagic shock. *Arch Surg* 88:688, 1964.

Snyder EL (ed): *Blood Transfusion Therapy: A Physician's Handbook*. Arlington, VA, American Association of Blood Banks, 1983.

Tocantis LM, O'Neill JF: Infusion of blood and other fluids into the general circulation via the bone marrow: Technique and results. *Surg Gynecol Obstet* 73:281, 1941.

Wallace J: Blood transfusion and transmissible disease. *Clin Haematol* 5:183, 1976.

Wilson RF, Bassett JS, Walt AJ: Five years experience with massive blood transfusions. *JAMA* 194:851, 1965.

Yankee RA: HL-A antigens and platelet therapy, in Baldini MG, Ebbe S (eds): *Platelets: Production, Function, Transfusion, and Storage*. New York, Grune and Stratton, 1974.

Chapter 4

Shock

G. Tom Shires III, Peter C. Canizaro, C. James Carrico, and G. Tom Shires

CLINICAL MANIFESTATIONS OF SHOCK

Classification; Clinical and Physiologic Manifestations of Shock

DEFINITION AND WORKING CLASSIFICATION

The scope of modern medicine is increasing steadily. As understanding of physiologic and biochemical derangements is broadened, so is the horizon of possibilities for the relief of illness. As more seriously ill patients are presented, the symptom complex of shock is more frequently encountered by the physician.

Although shock has been recognized for over 100 years, a clear definition and dissection of this complex and devastating state has emerged only slowly. Many attempts have been made over the years to define adequately the entity known as shock. In 1872, the elder Gross defined shock as a "manifestation of the rude unhinging of the machinery of life." Although the accuracy of this definition is unquestioned, it is obviously far from precise. In 1942, Wiggers, on the basis of an exhaustive examination of available evidence at that time, offered the definition: "Shock is a syndrome resulting from a depression of many functions, but in which reduction of the effective circulating blood volume is of basic importance, and in which impairment of the circulation steadily progresses until it eventuates in a state of irreversible circulatory failure." Blalock offered the definition in 1940: "Shock is a peripheral circulatory failure, resulting from a discrepancy in the size of the vascular bed and the volume of the intravascular fluid." A more modern definition has been devised by Simeone, who stated that shock may be defined as "a clinical condition characterized by signs and symptoms which arise when the cardiac output is insufficient to fill the arterial tree with blood under sufficient pressure to provide organs and tissues with adequate blood flow."

Shock of all forms appears to be invariably related to *inadequate tissue perfusion*. The low-flow state in vital organs seems to be the final common denominator in all forms of shock.

For purposes of a working clinical classification, the etiologic classification offered by Blalock in 1934 is still a useful and functional one. Blalock suggested four categories:

1. Hematogenic (oligemic)
2. Neurogenic (caused primarily by nervous influences)
3. Vasogenic (initially decreased vascular resistance and increased vascular capacity)
4. Cardiogenic
   a. Failure of the heart as a pump
   b. Unclassified category (including diminished cardiac output from various causes)

It is now clear that shock results from one or more of four separate but interrelated dysfunctions, involving (1) the pump (heart), (2) the fluid that is pumped (blood volume), (3) the arteriolar resistance vessels, and (4) the capacity of the venous vessels. These dysfunctions may be correlated as follows with Blalock's etiologic classification:

1. Cardiogenic shock implies failure of the heart as a pump and may be brought about by primary myocardial dysfunction from myocardial infarction, serious cardiac arrhythmias, or a variety of causes resulting in myocardial depression; or by miscellaneous causes, including mechanical restriction of cardiac function or venous obstruction such as occurs in the mediastinum with tension pneumothorax, vena cava obstruction, or cardiac tamponade.

2. Reduction in blood volume may take the form of loss of whole blood, of plasma, or of extracellular fluid in the extravascular space or a combination of these three.

3. Changes in arterial resistance or venous capacity may be brought about by specific disorders. A decrease in resistance may result from spinal anesthesia or from neurogenic reflexes, as in acute pain, or may accompany the end stages of hypovolemic shock. Septic shock may produce changes in peripheral arterial resistance and in venous capacity, as well as peripheral arteriovenous shunting.

Therapy of shock will obviously revolve around the etiologic type or combination of types of shock present in a given patient who has undergone trauma.

CLINICAL MANIFESTATIONS

The signs and symptoms of hypovolemic shock, when they are well established, are classic and usually easy to recognize. Most of the signs of clinical shock are characteristic of low peripheral blood flow and are contributed to by the effects of excess adrenosympathetic activity.

On first inspection the patient in shock presents an anxious, tired expression, which early is that of restlessness and anxiety and later becomes a picture of apathy or exhaustion. Typically, the skin feels cool and is pale and mottled, and there is evidence of decreased capillary flow exhibited by easy blanching of the skin, particularly the nail beds.

There are varying discrepancies in the classic picture of shock. In neurogenic shock, particularly that in response to spinal anesthesia, the pulse rate is normal or, more often, decreased; the pulse pressure is wide, and the pulse feels strong rather than weak. The rapid pulse characteristic of early hemorrhagic or wound shock may be absent, even if the patient has lost blood rapidly. This is also true if the position is supine or prone, in which case a rapid pulse may not appear until the patient is moved or elevated to a sitting position. The varying clinical picture in septic shock is discussed subsequently.

In observing a large number of patients in hemorrhagic hypovolemic shock, one sees remarkably varied but typical responses of the sensorium to the shock episode. Most young, healthy patients who sustain wound or hemorrhagic shock, when seen early after the wounding, will appear to be restless and anxious and give the appearance of great fear. Shortly after being seen by a physician and started on treatment, this restlessness frequently gives way to great apathy and the patient appears sleepy. When aroused, the patient may complain of weakness or of a chilly sensation, although not actually having a chill. If blood loss is unchecked, the patient's apathy and sleepiness will rapidly progress into coma. In treating a large number of accident victims, it has been our experience that patients who have bled into frank coma from which they cannot be aroused, resulting simply from blood loss alone (unassociated with other injuries such as brain damage), have usually sustained lethal blood loss. This sign usually indicates rapid massive hemorrhage for which compensations are inadequate to maintain sufficient cerebral blood flow to sustain consciousness.

Thirst seems to be a characteristic of the injured person and is found in most emergency room patients brought in acutely ill from trauma with or without shock. The studies carried out to elucidate the nature of the thirst are many and varied. Most of these patients have intense adrenal medullary stimulation from trauma, not necessarily accompanied by shock. Consequently caution must be used in allowing water intake, since dangerous water intoxication may be induced by this intense stimulus to imbibe liquids in the face of altered renal function.

Another characteristic of the patient in hemorrhagic shock is the low peripheral venous pressure, manifested on inspection by empty peripheral veins. Indeed, the starting of a simple intravenous infusion in a patient in hemorrhagic shock can be quite difficult. Obviously there are exceptions, such as shock due to cardiac tamponade, in which there is restriction to inflow of blood to the right side of the heart. In this instance the peripheral veins, including the neck veins, are distended.

Nausea and vomiting from hypovolemic shock are common. It is true that other causes should be sought, but shock alone may be first manifested in this manner.

Another classic finding in hemorrhagic hypovolemia is a fall in body "core" temperature. Whether this is due to a lowered metabolic rate or to lower perfusion in areas where body temperature is measured is unclear; recent animal studies suggest a protective effect of this hypothermia.

PHYSIOLOGIC CHANGES

BLOOD PRESSURE. Arterial blood pressure is normally maintained by the cardiac output and the peripheral vascular resistance. Thus, when the cardiac output is reduced because of loss of intravascular volume, the blood pressure may remain normal so long as the total peripheral vascular resistance can be increased to compensate for the reduction in cardiac output. The vascular resistance varies in different organs and in different parts of the same organ, depending on the local conditions that determine the state of vasoconstriction or vasodilatation at the time of the loss of intravascular volume. An example of the differential increase in peripheral resistance with reduction in cardiac output is seen in the change in distributional total blood flow to organs such as the heart and the brain, as opposed to that of most other organs that are not essential for immediate survival. In hemorrhagic shock the heart may receive 25 percent of the total cardiac output, as opposed to the normal 5 to 8 percent. The great increase in peripheral resistance in such organs as the skin and the kidney causes significant reduction in flow in these organs while providing a lifesaving diversion of the cardiac output to the brain and the heart. Consequently the blood pressure may not fall until the reduction in cardiac output or loss of blood volume is so great that the adaptive homeostatic mechanisms can no longer compensate for the reduced volume. As the deficit continues, however, there is a progressive hypotension.

PULSE RATE. Characteristically, reduction of the volume in the vascular tree is associated with tachycardia. A fall in pressure within the great vessels results in excitation of the sympathicoadrenal division of the autonomic nervous system and, simultaneously, inhibition of the medullovagal center (Marey's reflex). Consequently, with hemorrhage or loss of circulating blood volume, the resulting fall in arterial blood pressure should cause an increase in heart rate.

This compensatory mechanism is variable in its effectiveness. Obviously, the degree of loss of intravascular volume, the amount of reduction in venous return, and other variables such as ventricular function may markedly influence the ability of Marey's reflex to compensate for the reduction in blood volume. Work with slow hemorrhage in normal healthy volunteers by Shenkin et al. has shown that, as long as the supine position is maintained, as much as 1000 mL of blood may be lost without significant increase in pulse rate. Similarly, the pacemaker system of the heart within the sinoatrial node is obviously influenced by other stimuli, such as fear and anxiety, that may also accompany the trauma producing the loss of intravascular volume.

Consequently, during the course of observation and treatment of shock, changes in pulse rate are of value only when followed over an extended period. Change in pulse rate may indicate response to volume therapy once other external sources that may have changed cardiac rate are diminished or removed.

VASOCONSTRICTION. Increase in peripheral vascular resistance by production of peripheral vasoconstriction rapidly becomes maximal in an effort to compensate for the reduced cardiac output. Vascular resistance can be measured only indirectly in human beings and in animals. There is good evidence that early disproportionate reduction in vascular resistance in the heart occurs while there is still little change in vascular resistance in many organs. Subsequently, maximal vasoconstriction occurs in the skin, kidneys, liver, and finally, the brain. Concomitantly, there is generalized constriction of the veins in response to reduction in intravascular volume. Venoconstriction is a necessary homeostatic mechanism, since over half the total blood volume may be contained within the venous tree.

These vascular responses to hemorrhage are immediate and striking. Within seconds following the onset of hemorrhage there are unequivocal signs of sympathetic and adrenal activation. Serum catecholamine levels show prompt elevation, indicative of action of the adrenal medulla. The adrenocortical and pituitary hormones also show prompt increase in serum levels following shock. Many of the clinical signs associated with shock are simply signs of response of the sympathetic and adrenal medullary system to the insult sustained by the organism.

HEMODILUTION. All the responses to reduction of intravascular volume eventually result in decreased flow to tissues and initiation of compensatory mechanisms directed at correction of the low-flow state. One such compensation is movement of fluid into the circulation, resulting in hemodilution. This fluid, commonly known as extracellular fluid, has the composition of plasma but a lower protein content.

It is now clear, however, that the hematocrit or hemoglobin concentration in shock is simply an index of the balance between the amount of whole blood or plasma lost and the amount of extravascular extracellular fluid gained. For example, in hemorrhagic hypovolemia there is generally progressive hemodilution, which increases with the severity of the shock state. Obviously, in this circumstance there has been a greater movement of fluid from the extravascular to the intravascular space with progression of the shock. This is in contradistinction to shock associated with loss of intravascular volume due primarily to plasma loss. High-hematocrit shock may occur with massive losses of plasma and extravascular extracellular fluid, such as is associated with peritonitis, burns, large areas of soft tissue infection, and the crush syndrome.

The mechanism of hemodilution following hemorrhage is initially on the basis of the Starling hypothesis: that is, the reduction in hydrostatic pressure in the capillaries because of hypotension and arterial and arteriolar vasoconstriction results in a shift of the pressure gradient to favor the passage of fluid from the tissue extracellular space into the intravascular capillary bed. In addition,

Gann and others have shown a second phase of blood volume restitution via a hormonally mediated increase in extracellular osmolality.

BIOCHEMICAL CHANGES

The measurable biochemical changes that occur as a response to the stress invoked by shock fall into three fairly well-defined categories. These are (1) the changes invoked by the pituitary-adrenal response to stress, (2) the changes produced by a net reduction in organ perfusion imposed by a low rate of blood flow, and (3) the changes brought about by failing function within specific organs.

PITUITARY-ADRENAL. The immediate effects seen from adrenosympathetic activity are those associated with high circulating epinephrine levels. Characteristically, these include eosinopenia and lymphocytopenia along with thrombocytopenia. This doubtless represents the laboratory reflection of increased circulating epinephrine that can be measured and has been found to be elevated as an early response to shock. These changes are nonspecific and are found early in a patient with shock or severe trauma. The phenomena usually disappear rapidly. Other evidences of the pituitary and hormonal response to shock are seen in the well-known stress reaction or metabolic responses so well described by Moore. These include a striking negative nitrogen balance, retention of sodium and water, and an increase in the excretion of potassium.

LOW-FLOW STATE. Those changes incident to the low rate of blood flow during shock are now becoming better understood. More evidence is accumulating to support the observation that, as a result of a decreased blood flow or low rate of perfusion, there is a reduction in oxygen delivered to the vital organs and, consequently, a mandatory change from aerobic to anaerobic metabolism. In the switch from aerobic to anaerobic metabolism, energy made available by the oxidation of glucose is greatly reduced during shock. The most striking example of a shift in metabolism is the production of lactic acid as the end product instead of the normal aerobic end product, carbon dioxide. This is reflected in a metabolic acidosis with a reduction in the carbon dioxide–combining power of the blood. The available buffer base is progressively decreased by combining with the increased lactic acid, and the respiratory compensation that occurs early in the course of hemorrhagic shock is frequently inadequate. Consequently the progressive decline in pH toward a striking acidosis is hastened. Indeed, in several studies the ability of animals as well as human beings to recover from shock has been found to correlate with the degree of lactic acid production and the decrease in the alkali reserve and pH of the blood.

In some cases determination of blood pH may not accurately reflect changes in pH at the cellular level. After the induction of hemorrhagic shock in experimental animals, skeletal muscle surface pH changes precede those in blood, and minimal changes may be masked by the efficient blood buffer systems. Lactate and excess lactate

levels correlate well with the clinical impression of the depth of shock, but the injuries producing the shock state have a much greater bearing on ultimate prognosis.

ORGAN FAILURE. The biochemical changes that appear incident to organ failure seem to be dependent in large part on the duration and severity of the shock. The changes in renal function induced by hypovolemia may vary from simple oliguria with a concentrated and acid urine to high-output renal failure with a urine of low specific gravity and high pH, or frank anuric renal failure. Similarly, the blood nonprotein nitrogen content depends on the degree of impairment in renal function. This may vary from slight or no retention of nitrogenous products to a steep and progressive rise that may require therapy.

Changes in ion concentration, including a rise of serum potassium, are dependent on many things, among them adrenal cortical response, the change in metabolism from aerobic to anaerobic with resultant release of potassium, and specific changes within tissues invoked by the shock. If renal function is maintained, the rise inevitably seen in serum potassium soon after the onset of shock is short-lived, in that the renal excretion of potassium is high during recovery from hemorrhagic shock. If renal function is impaired, the concentration of potassium and magnesium as well as creatinine can rise to high levels in the serum.

Although the kidney is quite sensitive to the physiologic alterations in shock, other organs vary in their response to various shock states. The lung is resistant to dysfunction induced by hemorrhage alone (see Pulmonary Responses). Concurrent direct lung injury or septic shock frequently lead to profound impairment in pulmonary function. Shock-induced changes in hepatocyte function may be reflected in early alterations in glucose metabolism and later alterations in bilirubin and protein metabolism. Loss of homeostasis in skeletal muscle, which represents a large proportion of body mass, produces major changes in fluid and electrolytes, as discussed below.

PATHOPHYSIOLOGIC RESPONSES TO SHOCK

Experimental Studies of the Response of Extracellular Fluid

EARLY RESULTS

Hypovolemic shock is the most common form seen clinically and is also the form that has been studied most intensively both clinically and in the laboratory. Most of our own studies have been carried out using hypovolemic shock produced by external blood loss as the model. A method has been developed that allows the simultaneous measurement of total-body red cell mass with the use of ^{51}Cr-tagged red blood cells and total-body plasma volume with the use of ^{131}I-tagged and, later, ^{125}I-tagged human serum albumin. In addition, total-body extracellular fluid can be measured simultaneously with the use of ^{35}S-tagged sodium sulfate. The three isotopes are simultaneously injected intravenously, and with the use of appropriate energy-differentiating counting instruments, all three isotopes can be traced after equilibration. Volumes are then determined by the dilution principle, using multiple sampling.

In an early study the three volumes were measured; splenectomized dogs were then bled a sublethal, sub-shock amount of 10 percent of the measured blood volume. After hemorrhage the three volumes were again measured. The loss of the amount of red blood cells and plasma removed during the hemorrhage could be detected by the method described. It was shown that the decrease in extracellular fluid volume was only the amount lost as plasma removed during the hemorrhage.

By use of the same model, volumes were measured before and after hemorrhage of 25 percent of the measured blood volume. This hemorrhage was again sublethal but produced hypotension. In this group of animals also the loss of the amount of red blood cells and plasma removed could be detected. In addition, however, the functional extracellular fluid volume as measured by the ^{35}S-tagged sodium sulfate was found to have decreased by 18 to 26 percent of the original volume. Since there was no measurable external loss of ^{35}S sulfate, this reduction was presumed to be an internal redistribution of extracellular fluid. Subsequent studies of external bleeding of 35, 45, and even over 50 percent hemorrhage always produced the same reduction in functional extracellular fluid as long as the animal was in shock.

In subsequent studies, splenectomized dogs were subjected to "irreversible" hemorrhagic shock according to a modified method of Wiggers, which utilizes a reservoir. Return of shed blood in this severe preparation resulted in the return of blood pressure to near control levels, followed by a fall in blood pressure within 1 to 16 h; death

resulted in 80 percent of the dogs, i.e., a standard mortality rate.

In one group of animals the three volumes were measured and the dogs were then subjected to shock by the Wiggers method. The three volumes were remeasured by reinjection during the period of shock; then shed blood was returned. The decrease in blood volume was the amount that had been removed. Concurrently, the functional extracellular fluid exhibited a decided reduction. Immediately after the return of the shed blood, the red cell mass returned to essentially normal levels, as did the plasma volume; however, there remained a deficit of functional extracellular fluid. In dogs treated with shed blood plus plasma (10 mL/kg), the losses during shock were again similar. After therapy with plasma, plus return of shed blood, there was a return of blood volume to normal. There remained, however, a decrease in functional extracellular fluid volume.

Dogs treated with an extracellular "mimic," such as a balanced salt solution plus shed blood, had comparable losses during shock. As in the previous groups, the blood volume returned essentially to normal after treatment. But dogs treated with salt solution plus shed blood exhibited return of functional extracellular fluid volume to control levels.

In this study only 20 percent of those dogs treated with shed blood alone survived longer than 24 h. When plasma was used in addition to whole blood as therapy, 30 percent of the dogs survived. Of the animals treated with lactated Ringer's solution plus shed blood, 70 percent survived (Fig. 4-1). The 80 percent mortality rate of a standard "irreversible" shock preparation was reduced to 30 percent by restoration of functional extracellular fluid volume in addition to return of shed blood.

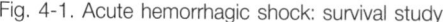

Fig. 4-1. Acute hemorrhagic shock: survival study.

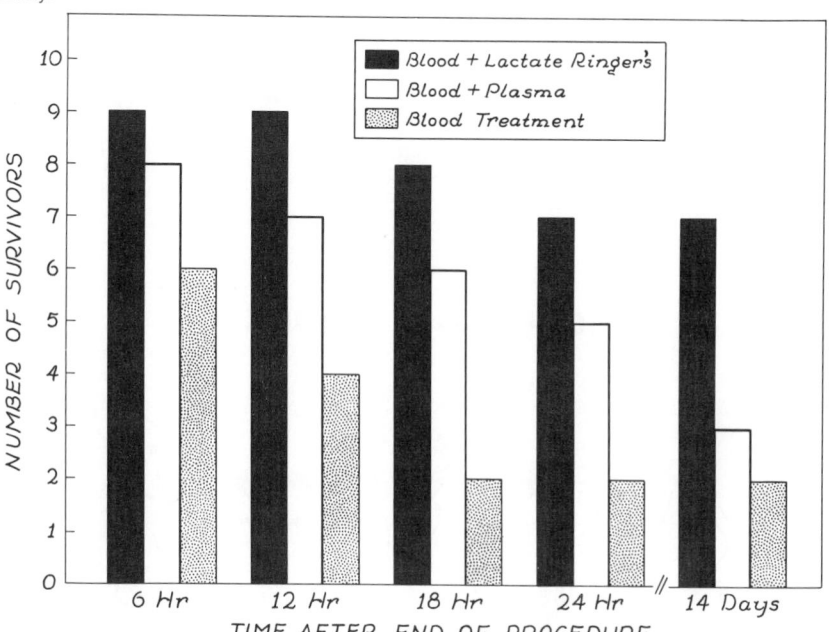

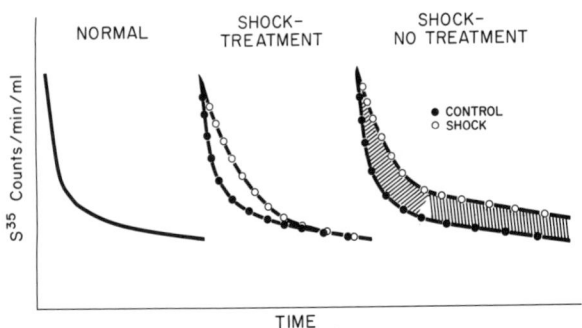

Fig. 4-2. Radiosulfate equilibration curve: semilogarithmic plot, summary model.

All these early studies of the measurement of the functional extracellular fluid were based on volume distribution curves of sulfate measured for approximately 1 h. At any point in the course of the curve there is a reduction in extracellular fluid in the untreated state of shock. Subsequent work has continued these volume distribution curves for many hours. In true untreated hemorrhagic shock there is a reduction in the total extracellular fluid, or final diluted volume of radiosulfate, when compared with preshock volumes (Fig. 4-2).

Even when a less severe shock preparation is used, there is still a reduction in early equilibrating extracellular fluid or early available extracellular fluid, whereas the total anatomic extracellular fluid may remain normal. Subsequent studies have shown that if shock is not of sufficient duration to produce reduction in both functional and total extracellular fluid, the reduction may be only in functional extracellular fluid. Furthermore, if therapy is instituted quickly and blood pressure is returned to normal, a long sulfate equilibration curve may fail to reveal the acute reduction that was corrected early.

Consequently, the current status of sulfate as a measure of the functional extracellular fluid must be interpreted as indicating that early sulfate volume measurement reveals functional or available extracellular fluid and that prolonged measurement of the volume distribution curves gives total extracellular fluid values. If therapy has been instituted or has been completed, the reduction in total or even in the available extracellular fluid may not be measurable.

Unquestionably, some plasma, or transcapillary, refilling occurs in response to hemorrhage and to hemorrhagic shock. This response, however, is initially rather limited and, in severe hemorrhagic shock, is grossly inadequate to explain the reduction seen in interstitial fluid. Since there is no source for external loss, the question arose as to whether interstitial fluid might move into the cell mass in an isotonic fashion (Fig. 4-3).

Fig. 4-3. Interstitial fluid response to hemorrhagic shock.

NORMAL

VASCULAR TREE   INTERSTITIAL FLUID   CELL FLUID

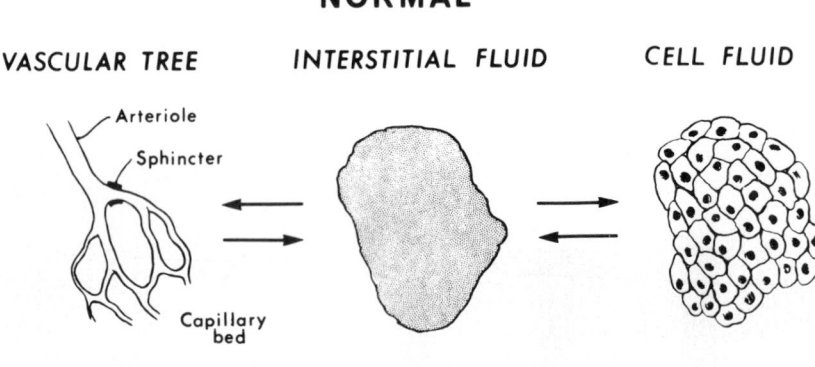

HEMORRHAGIC SHOCK

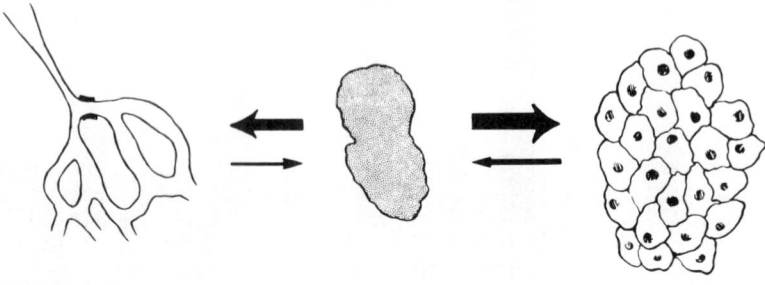

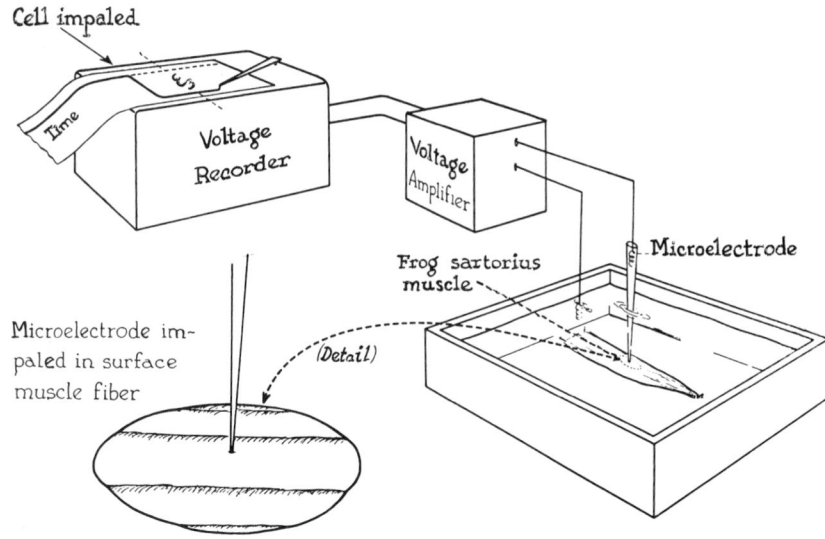

Fig. 4-4. Schematic of intracellular recording. [From: *Ruch and Fulton (eds): Medical Physiology and Biophysics, 18th ed, Philadelphia, Saunders, 1960, with permission.*]

CELLULAR STUDIES

Subsequently, studies of ion transport across the cell membrane were undertaken in order to determine the possibility of intracellular swelling in skeletal muscle in response to hemorrhagic shock. Using a Ling-Gerard ultramicroelectrode with glass tip diameter of less than 1 μm (Fig. 4-4), intracellular transmembrane potential

recordings were made. The electrode was modified to record intracellular transmembrane potentials in vivo before, during, and after shock (Fig. 4-5).

Skeletal muscle measurements in acute hemorrhagic shock demonstrate a constant and sustained fall in the normally negative intracellular transmembrane potential. This may represent a reduction in efficiency of the sodium pump induced by tissue hypoxia; it is present only during shock-producing hypotension. Additional studies in splenectomized dogs showed that changes in variables such as pH, P_{CO_2}, and bicarbonate do not influence the transmembrane potential in shock. Even with progressive

Fig. 4-5. In vivo transmembrane potential measurement in rat skeletal muscle.

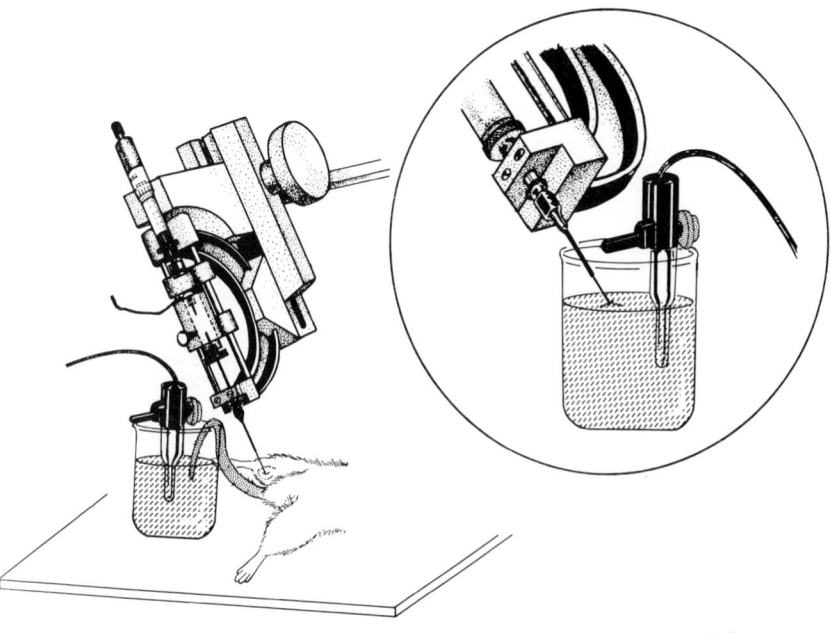

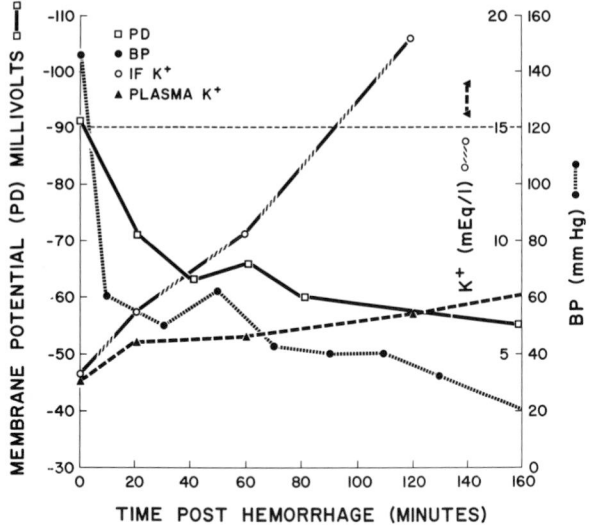

Fig. 4-6. Changes in membrane potential and interstitial K$^+$ in rats with hemorrhagic shock.

metabolic acidosis and its subsequent correction, the potential still follows the blood pressure and shock state.

Studies have been reported that utilized the ultramicroelectrode measurement of transmembrane potential combined with direct aspiration of skeletal muscle interstitial fluid by a modification of the technique of Hagberg. Using this technique, it was found that as blood pressure fell and transmembrane potential was reduced, plasma potassium rose slowly during the shock period (Fig. 4-6). The directly aspirated interstitial fluid potassium during the same period of time rose to a height of more than 15 meq/L of interstitial fluid. This explained where potassium, moving out of skeletal muscle cells, was being sequestered as sodium chloride and water moved into muscle cells.

Additional studies have been performed in primates that show essentially the same phenomenon (Fig. 4-7). These studies also reveal that this cellular membrane transport is a reversible phenomenon; i.e., once the shock state is treated, transmembrane potential recovers. Concomitant muscle biopsies show clearly that muscle cells gain sodium, water, and chloride while losing potassium. Thus the data reveal an isotonic swelling of skeletal muscle cells in response to shock injury (Fig. 4-8).

Studies in human beings reveal the same response to shock injury. Interesting corroborative changes in action potentials of single cells in skeletal muscles have been revealed in primates (Fig. 4-9). One study shows a decrease in resting membrane potential, a decrease in amplitude of action potential, and prolongation of both repolarization and depolarization times. Resuscitation quickly reversed these changes, except for repolarization time, which remained prolonged for several days. This confirms in vitro the alterations in intracellular sodium and potassium concentrations that were measured by skeletal muscle biopsy and resting membrane potential measurements.

Maintenance of the transmembrane potential difference (PD) is an important cellular function of both excitable and nonexcitable tissues. The resting PD is generally agreed to depend upon an energy-dependent Na$^+$-K$^+$ transport mechanism. The specific energy substrate of this membrane-bound complex is adenosine triphosphate (ATP).

Changes in muscle and liver PD have been shown to be reliable indicators of cellular dysfunction in prolonged hemorrhagic shock. This cell membrane depolarization

Fig. 4-7. Changes in membrane potential and blood pressure in primates during hemorrhagic shock and after resuscitation.

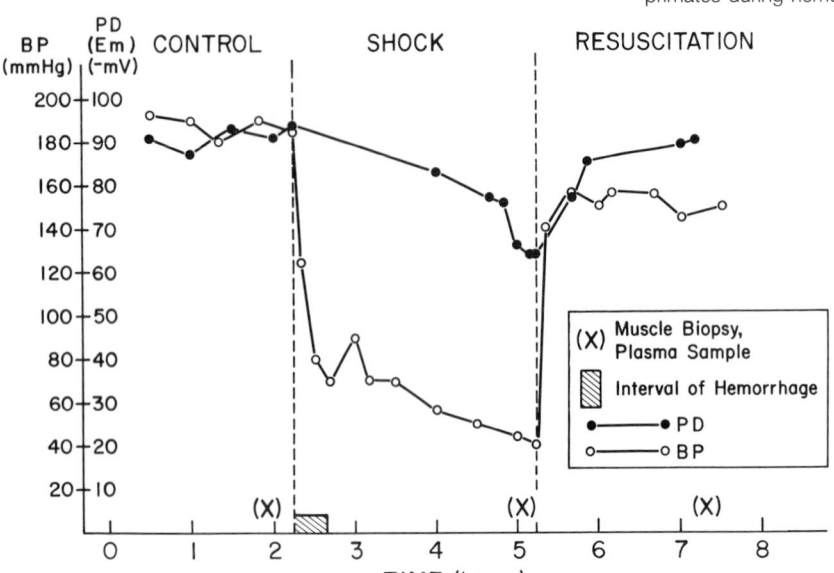

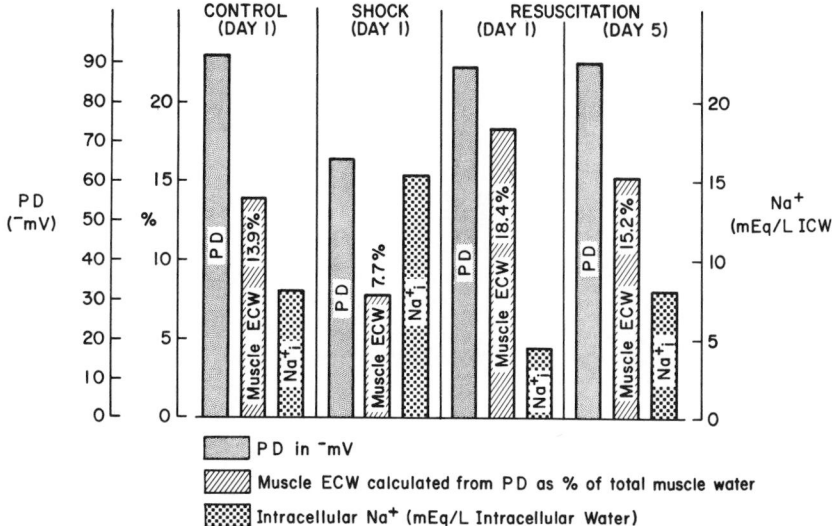

Fig. 4-8. Changes in membrane potential, extracellular water, and intracellular Na$^+$ in primates after resuscitation from hemorrhagic shock.

has been associated with cellular swelling, cellular uptake of sodium and chloride, and loss of potassium. Previous studies indicate that these abnormalities are due to failure of the active transport mechanism. The depletion of ATP in skeletal muscle, liver, and kidney in a hemorrhagic shock model in rats led to the proposal that the cellular dysfunction observed in hemorrhagic shock was secondary to inadequate energy stores. Subsequent studies reported markedly improved survival rates after hemorrhagic shock in animals that were administered ATP-MgCl$_2$ intramuscularly, intraperitoneally, or intravenously. In addition, restoration of tissue ATP levels was reported in the ATP-MgCl$_2$ resuscitated animals and was interpreted to be a result of entry into the cells of intact ATP molecules.

Our recent studies indicate that skeletal muscle ATP levels were maintained during prolonged hemorrhagic shock. Depletion of liver ATP or skeletal muscle creatine phosphate was not prevented by administration of intravenous ATP-MgCl$_2$. Cellular dysfunction in liver and muscle, indicated by depolarization of PD, was not ameliorated by infusion of ATP-MgCl$_2$.

Exogenously administered ATP is rapidly degraded in the plasma. In addition, several studies have demonstrated that ATP in the intact state does not cross the muscle cell membrane. Thus, late changes in cell energy contents appear to be the result of failing cellular function, rather than the primary cause of membrane failure in shock.

INTERPRETATION

Concisely stated, reduction in extracellular fluid in reversible hemorrhagic shock can consistently be shown (1) with extracellular fluid markers that enter cells slowly or not at all in the shock state when (2) reinjection of the extracellular fluid markers is utilized in the shock state, (3) extracellular fluid markers or tracers are allowed sufficient time for equilibration, (4) shock measurements are obtained while hemorrhagic shock is sustained, and (5) the shock preparation is sufficiently severe and is maintained until there is a change in cellular membrane transport.

Fig. 4-9. Action potentials in primates in hemorrhagic shock.

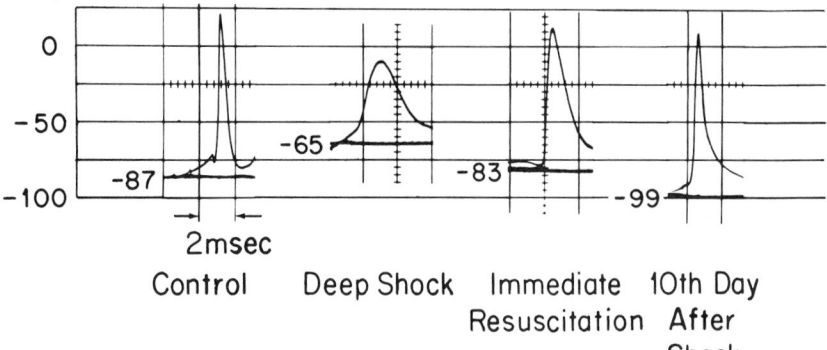

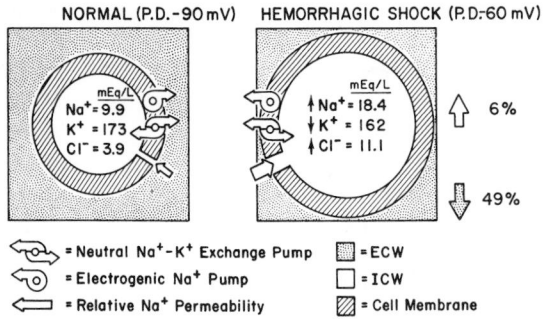

Fig. 4-10. Theoretic transport mechanisms responsible for alterations in potential difference *(PD)* and fluid-electrolyte distribution in hemorrhagic shock.

The data obtained from prior experiments support the use of transmembrane potential measurements as an accurate indicator of cellular alterations resulting from the low-flow state of hemorrhagic shock. Severe hypotension is associated with depression of transmembrane potential difference (PD) which is sustained in the presence of a continued shock state.

Transmembrane PD is generally agreed to be the result of either an electrogenic sodium pump (with active outward extrusion of sodium from muscle cells by a redox system) or a coupled sodium-potassium exchange pump with diffusion of sodium and potassium down their respective chemical gradients. In the latter theory the relative permeabilities of the membrane to the two ions must be considered and the potential interpreted on the basis of the Hodgkin-Katz-Goldman equation in which pNa^+ (relative permeability to sodium) is 0.01. Since permeability to potassium is assumed to be much greater than permeability to sodium in the cell membrane, the PD is essentially a potassium diffusion potential.

The present data thus suggest that skeletal muscle cells may be a principal site of fluid and electrolyte sequestration after severe, prolonged hemorrhagic shock. The exact mechanism for the production of electrolyte changes as well as for the notable diminution in extracellular water that occurs after hemorrhagic shock is not known. It appears that the changes may well represent a reduction in the efficiency of an active ionic pump mechanism or a selective increase in muscle cell membrane permeability to sodium, or both (Fig. 4-10).

With a reset membrane potential, extracellular fluid electrolyte concentrations are unchanged. Consequently, from the Nernst equation, intracellular Cl^- must rise from 3.5 to 10 meq and intracellular Na^+ from 10 to 22 meq. Transposition of these data to the previously cited measurements in hemorrhagic shock is shown (Fig. 4-10). This model shows that only a 6 percent isotonic swelling of muscle cells will explain the major reduction in extracellular fluid measured in hemorrhagic shock. Studies are under way to determine the involvement of cell masses other than muscle during the course of hemorrhagic shock. One such study indicates that severe hemorrhagic shock of significant duration is associated with elevation of the internal sodium concentration of the red blood cells. The magnitude of these changes appears to be a function of both the severity and the duration of the shock process and seems to be well correlated with changes in clinical course when sequential sampling procedures are utilized.

There is a measurable reduction in extravascular extracellular fluid in response to sustained hemorrhagic shock. The cellular response to hypovolemic hypotension is characterized by a consistent change in active transport of ions. Evidence obtained directly from living cells indicates that sodium and water enter muscle cells, with resultant loss of cellular potassium to the extracellular fluid. The interstitial fluid holds the extruded potassium. Replenishment of the depleted extracellular fluid counteracts these changes at the cellular level and is an important feature of therapy in patients with hypovolemic shock.

Some interesting new data on the cellular transport mechanism indicate that the endorphins play an integral role in the pathophysiology of hemorrhagic shock. Blockade of these endogenous opiates by naloxone can significantly alter the course of this syndrome. While naloxone administration to normal rats had no effect on the circulation or cellular function, it improved the hemodynamic status of animals subjected to hemorrhagic shock, resulting in improved tissue perfusion. In addition, the administration of this drug prevented the cellular dysfunction normally seen in hemorrhagic shock.

Much current research in shock physiology addresses the role of not only endorphins but also other endogenous compounds that may exert effects on cardiovascular performance and membrane function. Thyrotropin-releasing hormone, arachidonic acid metabolites of both the cyclooxygenase and lipoxygenase pathways, and monochines, particularly cachectin, have all been implicated in the host response to shock. Further delineation of the complex actions of and interactions among these mediators should allow even more specific adjunctive therapies, in addition to fluid resuscitation, to be developed in the future.

Renal Responses

The observation was made long ago that during severe shock, from any cause, renal function essentially stops in human beings. The kidneys, like the skin and the liver, share in the relative oligemia which is a rapid compensatory mechanism in shock to divert blood flow to those organs, such as the brain and the heart, most vital for maintaining life. Consequently the relative oligemia suffered by the kidneys in response to shock is severe and immediate.

The development of oliguria and even anuria is apparently a direct function of the severity and duration of the renal ischemia during shock. In human beings, under normothermic conditions, normal kidneys will tolerate renal ischemia for periods varying from 15 min to a maximum of approximately 90 min. After this degree of ischemia, some functional and anatomic changes inevitably occur. With the use of hypothermia, the period of renal ischemia tolerated during hemorrhagic shock can be considerably prolonged.

SUBCLINICAL RENAL DAMAGE FOLLOWING INJURY AND SHOCK

In civilian and military practice, improved resuscitation with balanced electrolyte solution and blood and immediate corrective surgery have resulted in a great reduction in the incidence of primary oliguric renal failure. Recognition of nonoliguric renal failure as a less severe form of renal insufficiency suggested that graded renal damage might occur in association with systemic injury. Identification of patients with subclinical renal damage should be important in their postinjury care.

PATIENT STUDIES. A study was recently undertaken to determine the presence and degree of such renal damage during the early course of severely injured civilian patients. During the period of this study, 96,000 patients were treated in the emergency department, 988 of whom were admitted to the hospital for care of their injuries. Forty of the most severely injured were selected for continued care in a Trauma Research Unit after resuscitation and operative treatment of injuries. The criteria for inclusion in the study were hypotension following trauma and multiple long bone fractures.

All 40 patients showed generalized depression of renal function initially. Within 24 h of admission, 30 demonstrated return of clearances to normal ranges. The patients were divided into groups according to blood urea nitrogen (BUN) values (Fig. 4-11). Group I, considered to show a characteristic renal response to trauma, was selected on the basis of BUN values continuously below 20 g/dL after the first hospital day. This group included 30 of the 40 patients. Eight patients with renal dysfunction (Group II) showed persistent moderate elevation of BUN values above 20 g/dL. Two patients showed frank renal failure with rapidly progressing azotemia. One of these patients had sustained a gunshot wound of the renal

vein and vena cava and had had the renal pedicle on the involved side clamped for 1 h. The other patient, with a gunshot wound of the aortic bifurcation, represented failure of resuscitation. These two patients with renal failure are not considered in the subsequent comparisons between patients with the characteristic renal response (Group I) and those with renal dysfunction (Group II). Three patients with direct renal injury requiring suture or partial nephrectomy were included in Group I.

As would be expected on the basis of the selection criteria for the groups, glomerular filtration rate (GFR) was quite different for the two groups. Urea clearance (C_{urea}), another clearance primarily related to filtration, was depressed in both groups initially, with a rapid return to and above normal in the dysfunction group. Urine/plasma (U/P) urea ratio and osmolar clearances (C_{osm}) were different in the two groups only subsequent to 12 h after admission (Fig. 4-12).

Tubular resorption of water (TcH_2O) was significantly different in the two groups only at 18 and 24 h after admission. The trend in Group I was toward excretion of free water, while the trend in the dysfunction group was toward continued retention of free water. Cardiac output was not significantly different in the two groups.

Sodium clearances (C_{Na}) were similar in the two groups until after 12 h following admission. Subsequently C_{Na} fell in Group II. Postoperative sodium balance, represented as the difference between daily sodium intake and urinary sodium excretion, was different in the two groups. Group I showed positive sodium balance during day 1, balance during day 2, and negative balance during day 3. In Group II, the dysfunction group, increasing sodium retention occurred during each of the 3 days of the study.

There were no discernible differences between the two groups in age, type of injury, length of hypotensive episode, fluid administration, positive-pressure ventilation,

Fig. 4-11. Renal function after trauma: blood urea nitrogen values.

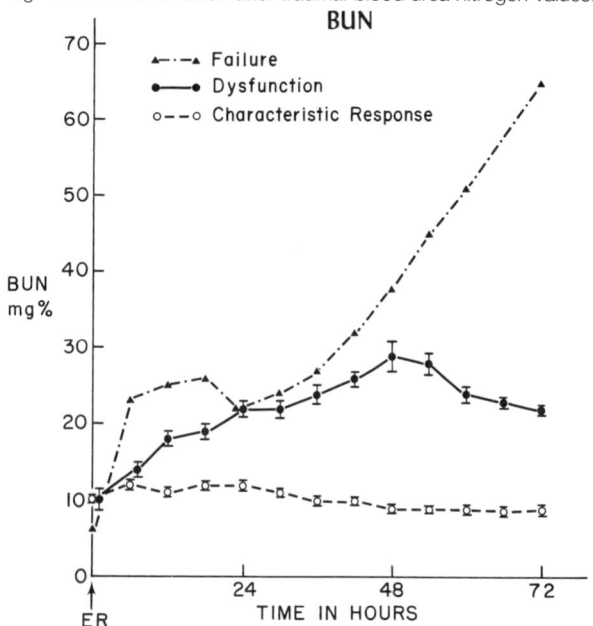

Fig. 4-12. Renal function after trauma: urine/plasma urea ratio.

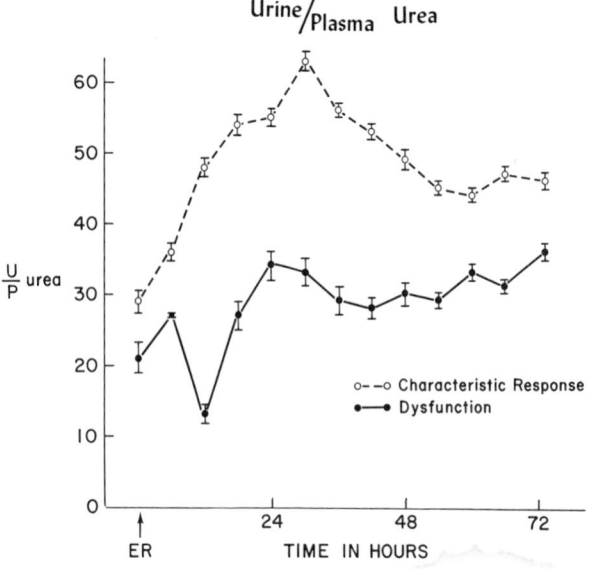

nephrotoxic antibiotics, minute urine volume, blood volume, or arterial P_{O_2} and pH.

Discussion

Classic renal clearance techniques have been used infrequently in surgical patients, partly because of errors inherent in the methods. All renal clearances are urine flow–sensitive. An increase in urine flow leads to a decrease in mean urine transit time. Consequently new filtrate washes out tubular and collecting system contents at a more rapid rate, yielding a factitiously high clearance. Conversely, a decrease in urine flow may lead to a factitiously low clearance. Errors in clearance measurements can be minimized by using constant mechanical infusion, long collection periods, and bladder washes. The long collection periods may obscure fluctuations during the period, but they provide accurate mean clearances.

In the normal human kidney, GFR may promptly increase 30 percent above basal level during diuresis. In the above-mentioned study, GFR was measured without fluid loading, and yet six of the patients in Group I showed a GFR above 150 mL/min, suggesting the presence of postinjury stimuli in the patients tending to increase GFR maximally. The patients with renal dysfunction (Group II) were presumably subject to similar stimuli but were unable to respond with any elevation in GFR because of renal damage or persistent neural or humoral influences affecting GFR.

Of interest is a study by Lucas et al. of the effects of albumin supplementation on renal function in 46 severely injured patients. Compared with a similar group of patients who received only crystalloid solutions and blood during resuscitation from hypovolemic shock, patients who received the additional albumin showed a decrease in GFR, C_{Na}, C_{osm}, and urine output. The authors postulated that these changes were due to increases in serum oncotic pressures in the glomerular tufts and peritubular vessels.

Endogenous creatinine clearance (C_{cr}) in both groups was always higher than GFR. Notable variation in C_{cr} in the injured patient was noted by Ladd, who concluded that endogenous C_{cr} was unsuitable for evaluation of GFR in battle casualties. Creatinine as determined by the Jaffe reaction overestimates the true creatinine in plasma, and since creatinine is secreted in human beings, the usual agreement of endogenous C_{cr} with inulin or iothalamate ^{125}I clearance is coincidental. Twofold and threefold increases in endogenous C_{cr} occur in association with the changes in muscle metabolism following severe trauma. Apparently normal values for C_{cr} may lead to a false sense of security when, in fact, the GFR may be reduced by a factor of 2 or 3 in the severely injured patient.

Muscle metabolism is profoundly altered in the injured patient, resulting in increased loads of creatinine and creatine presented to the kidney. In the early postinjury period, many patients had metabolic changes similar to those found in patients placed on a high protein diet. Even with increases in urea nitrogen load from tissue injury, multiple transfusions, and gluconeogenesis, these patients did not undergo azotemia and creatinemia. Azotemia and creatinemia are not inevitable consequences of severe tissue injury, and other factors are operative in the injured patient who exhibits such changes.

Small transient increases of GFR were apparent after administration of diuretics in some patients. In view of the demonstrated slow improvement in GFR that occurs after resuscitation and injury repair, it is difficult to ascribe increases in GFR during this early hospital period to furosemide. Further study of changes in GFR after administration of furosemide is indicated, however, in view of reports suggesting a beneficial effect of furosemide on renal function.

In a more recent study, Lucas et al. indicated that furosemide does not protect against renal failure by altering or increasing renal blood flow but may cause renal failure by producing hypovolemia. They were unable to demonstrate an increase in GFR, renal plasma flow, renal blood flow, or renal blood flow distribution in 54 critically ill surgical patients who received furosemide. Despite marked increases in urine output, C_{osm}, and C_{Na}, six of the patients developed renal failure, and five became hypotensive 2 to 10 h after administration of this diuretic.

C_{urea}, C_{cr}, C_{osm}, and U/P urea, U/P creatinine, and U/P osmolarity ratios have each been proposed as good clinical determinants of renal damage. Objections to the use of creatinine determinations alone have been noted above. Otherwise there is little to recommend any one of these tests over the others, since all relate filtration to some aspect of tubular function. Recognition of the need to measure at least one of the foregoing in urine and plasma simultaneously is important. U/P ratios approaching unity and clearances below 10 mL/min are diagnostic of some form of renal failure. Such determinations are of limited clinical use because many of the most difficult patients fall in an indeterminate group. Recently, Miller et al. have demonstrated the usefulness of comparing the fractional excretion of sodium with creatinine in oliguric patients. They demonstrated good separation of patients with prerenal oliguria from those with acute renal failure. There was very little overlap. The simplest such calculation comparing these two functions is the renal failure index ($U_{Na} \times PLCR$)/U_{cr}. An index of less than 1 usually indicates prerenal oliguria. An index of greater than 1 correlates well with acute renal failure.

A spectrum of secondary renal injury exists after severe trauma, varying from oliguric renal failure to transient depression of glomerular filtration and tubular function. Tissue trauma and multiple transfusions do not lead to azotemia in the injured patient with normal renal function. Conversely, even minimal persistent elevations of BUN are uniformly associated with significant renal dysfunction and sodium and water retention.

The more severely injured patient can be readily identified in the early postoperative phase by serial evaluation of the renal metabolism of urea or sodium. Identification of such patients should lead to meticulous supportive care, since the general metabolic reserve of the more severely injured patients is diminished and further insults are poorly tolerated.

HIGH-OUTPUT RENAL FAILURE

Posttraumatic acute renal insufficiency is well recognized as a highly lethal complication. The diagnosis is classically based on persistent oliguria and chemical evidence of uremia after stabilization of the circulation. The clinical course is characterized by oliguria of several days' to several weeks' duration, followed by a progressive rise in daily urine volume until both the excretory and concentrating functions of the kidney are gradually restored.

It is less well recognized that renal insufficiency may occur without an observed period of oliguria. This variant of renal insufficiency has been reported infrequently after burns, head injury, and soft tissue trauma. The reported cases are characterized by increasing azotemia, while the daily urine volume remains normal or increased. Many of these patients have an apparently inappropriate increase in urine volume, and the term *high-output renal failure* may best describe this entity, despite a theoretical objection. Until recently, this type of renal failure has not been noted frequently after trauma, nor has the clinical course been described in sufficient detail for recognition or management.

PATIENT STUDIES. This study describes the clinical course of acute renal failure without oliguria, emphasizing the problems encountered in management and suggesting renal ischemia as the basic causative mechanism (Fig. 4-13).

After severe abdominal trauma, the patients were in shock an average of 3.5 h, the individual times varying from 1 to 6 h. The average blood loss was 4.2 L and average blood replacement 3.6 L. The recorded blood loss was the amount measured at the time of operation. In most patients external bleeding was minimal. In addition to whole blood, they were given an average of 4 L of Ringer's lactate solution per patient prior to and during the operative procedure.

After operation the diagnosis of renal failure was not immediately suspected, since urine volumes were above 30 mL/h and few abnormalities were present in the initial values of blood urea nitrogen, potassium, sodium, carbon dioxide–combining power, and chlorides obtained on the first postoperative day.

In all cases not involving direct damage to the urinary tract, the urinalysis after operation showed specific gravities between 1.003 and 1.010, pH of 5.5 to 6.5, and urinary sediments containing at most a few red blood cells per high-power field and an occasional cast. The urine/plasma ratio of urea nitrogen was found to be slightly less than 20:1.

On the day of operation the minimum urinary output was 730 mL. This represented the output for less than 12 h in each case. There was a progressive increase in the mean urine volume for the first 6 to 8 days, reaching a peak of 2350 mL and returning gradually to normal between the sixteenth and seventeenth days. The continued high output of 3 L/day after the sixteenth day occurred in only one patient; the BUN in this patient did not return to normal for 37 days. Extremely high outputs were noted in some patients compared with the relatively normal values in others during the period of azotemia. The highest urine volumes were found in patients with the highest BUN values.

A progressive rise of the mean BUN during the 6 to 8 days after injury was followed by a gradual return to normal between the sixteenth and eighteenth days. The serum creatinine levels paralleled the azotemia, the highest value being 6.8 mg/dL. In all patients the increasing BUN level was paralleled by an increasing daily urinary volume. Similarly, the stepwise decline in blood urea was paralleled by a decreasing urinary volume.

In most instances the initial serum potassium values after operation were slightly below normal. In some the serum potassium levels were above 6 meq/L by the second or third postoperative day, while the remaining patients showed a slow but sustained rise. All the accelerated rises resulted from intravenous administration of potassium salts (not more than 60 meq/day). When the serum potassium reached 6 meq/L, treatment with cation exchange resins was instituted. This proved effective in preventing further rises in serum potassium. An increase in serum potassium from 5.5 to 9.2 meq/L was caused by the intravenous administration of 60 meq of KCl in a 12-h period. Extracorporeal hemodialysis was necessary to reduce the potassium intoxication that occurred.

Moderately low values for the carbon dioxide–combining power were present for the first 4 or 5 days after injury and represent a mild to moderate metabolic acidosis. All isotonic losses were replaced with lactated Ringer's solution when acidosis persisted. In most patients the acidosis was well controlled by the administration of isotonic lactate solutions, which occasionally resulted in a mild metabolic alkalosis, although two patients had carbon dioxide–combining power values between 15 and 18 meq/L despite lactate therapy and died on the tenth and twelfth postoperative days. After the eighth postoperative day carbon dioxide–combining powers were within a normal range without lactate administra-

Fig. 4-13. High-output renal failure.

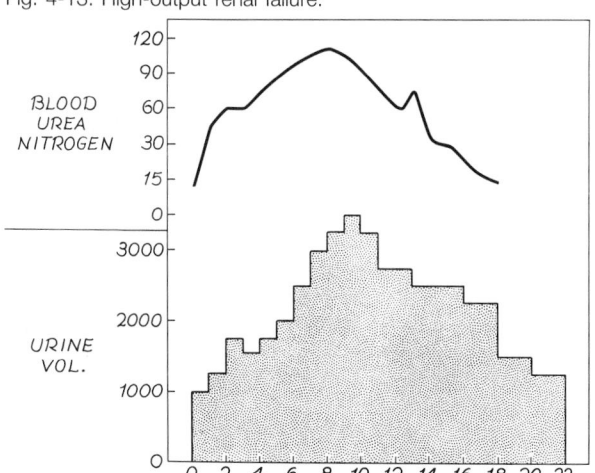

tion. The serum chlorides did not show a reciprocal relationship to the carbon dioxide–combining powers.

Serum sodium determinations were made throughout the period of renal failure. The highest values of 150 to 154 meq occurred during a trial of fluid restriction to determine whether the high urinary outputs were being induced by excessive administration of fluids. On these two occasions, hypernatremia was readily produced, indicating that the kidney was excreting a solute-poor urine.

Surviving patients were available for follow-up. Evaluation of renal function was carried out 1 to 1½ years after injury. Determinations of blood urea nitrogen, creatinine, sodium, potassium, carbon dioxide, and chloride were normal. Intravenous pyelography was normal. The lowest urinary concentration obtained was 1.020, and excretion of phenolsulfonphthalein (PSP) exceeded 30 percent in 30 min in all patients studied. Within 3 months both tubular and glomerular functions had returned to normal.

Autopsy was performed on patients who died. Microscopic examination of the kidneys from these patients showed regenerating patchy tubular necrosis. The damage in each instance was principally to the distal nephron; less severe changes were seen in the proximal segments.

A typical course of high-output renal failure shows an increasing urea nitrogen that parallels the increasing urine volume, a mild metabolic acidosis, and an acute hyperkalemia produced by the administration of potassium salts. Recognition of the disease entity permits control of these abnormalities.

ANIMAL STUDIES. Animal experiments using dogs were carried out to determine the modifying effect of hypothermia on renal ischemia. After contralateral nephrectomy, the remaining renal pedicle was clamped for 2 h and released.

As seen in Fig. 4-14, Group A consists of normothermic controls. Group B dogs had regional renal hypothermia

produced by irrigation of the peritoneal cavity with cold saline solution. Group C dogs had profound renal hypothermia to 25°C produced by circulating cold saline solution continuously around the kidney. This cooling technique has been previously described.

The results show progressive azotemia and death in untreated animals that are not cooled (Group A). There was only transient elevation of the BUN when the kidneys were cooled to 25°C (Group C). In Group B, regional hypothermia, the BUN rose to an average height of 60 mg/dL by the sixth to tenth day and gradually returned to normal between the twelfth and sixteenth days.

Utilizing this same model in six dogs with exteriorized ureters, minimum urine volumes of 400 mL/day were obtained without an observed period of oliguria. Usually the daily urine volume increased to between 600 and 900 mL/day before the BUN began to decline. Microscopic examination of these and six similarly treated animals, sacrificed between the fifth and tenth days, showed the tubular lesion to be confined principally to the distal tubules but with some proximal tubular involvement. These changes, both degenerative and regenerative, were scattered and irregular in distribution.

Consequently it can be seen that high-output renal failure in animals is an intermediate form of renal failure. With severe renal ischemia, unmodified oliguric renal failure inevitably resulted. When the kidney was protected with profound hypothermia, no significant renal failure resulted. On the other hand, with modest but practical protection to the kidney afforded by peritoneal sluicing with cold saline solution, moderate elevation of BUN associated with high urine volume was obtained. This protection resulted in recovery of the animal in each instance.

Discussion

Renal insufficiency without oliguria is important from the standpoint of recognition and clinical management of a variant of classic acute renal failure.

The clinical course of patients has been shown to be qualitatively the same as that occurring when oliguria is present. Quantitatively, however, these patients retain a limited ability to excrete acid products of metabolism, potassium, and urea. It is of primary importance that renal insufficiency of itself was not sufficient in terms of acidosis, uremia, potassium intoxication, or fluid volume control to cause death in this series.

The normal or high daily output of urine, although solute-poor, permits administration of fairly large quantities of water daily, in addition to replacement of isotonic salt losses such as those from gastrointestinal suction. The maintenance of normal extracellular fluid volume and normal serum sodium concentration is, therefore, easily accomplished when accurate daily outputs of each are obtained and losses are replaced accordingly. The quantity of fluids containing sodium may be administered as lactate to control the mild metabolic acidosis that occurs. The observations of Moore indicate that if the acidosis is not treated, it may become so severe as to become the outstanding abnormality in these cases.

Fig. 4-14. Blood urea levels in dogs with renal ischemia, showing effect of hypothermia.

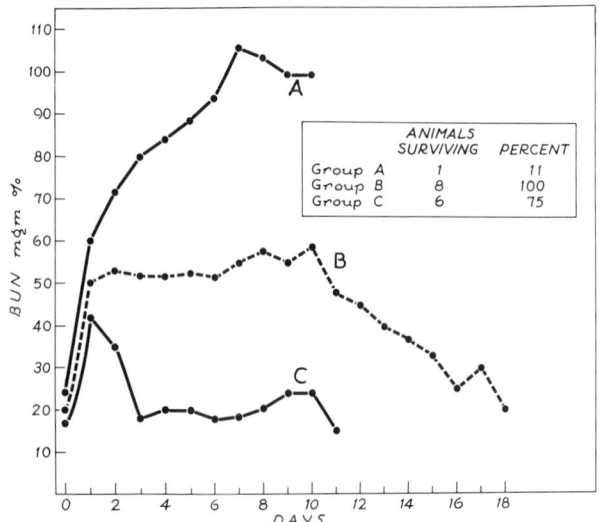

	ANIMALS SURVIVING	PERCENT
Group A	1	11
Group B	8	100
Group C	6	75

The chief dangers of high-output renal failure are (1) failure to recognize the existence of renal failure because of normal output and (2) the administration of potassium salts intravenously. Good urinary output and gastrointestinal involvement requiring suction would usually indicate the need for daily replacement of potassium. When this type of renal failure exists, however, potassium intoxication may be produced. In the early patients studied, five of nine required therapy for hyperkalemia. One required emergency hemodialysis for control of excessively high serum potassium levels. It is important that the serum level be determined daily and prior to the administration of any potassium-containing solutions.

The factors involved in the production of acute renal failure following trauma are incompletely understood, but renal ischemia is of unquestioned importance. This concept implies that the ischemia produces damage to the nephrons, which results in failure of the kidneys to excrete urine. Diuresis is felt to represent the recovery phase. Allowing for the physiologic variation between individuals and between given degrees of renal ischemia, a spectrum of the length of the oliguric phase should occur. This has been well documented by Teschan and Mason.

The frequency with which these cases occurred in relation to the small number of oliguric renal failures that were seen during the same period may represent differences in the therapy given during the ischemic episode. There are two outstanding differences in the therapy that we have routinely used. One is the administration of balanced salt solution along with whole blood in the resuscitation from hemorrhagic shock. It is well recognized that prolonged or severe extracellular fluid deficits are necessary for the production of renal failure in animals and may contribute to renal damage in human beings. The second difference in treatment is the use of renal hypothermia of a moderate degree to modify or prevent ischemic renal damage.

Clinical experience and laboratory experiments suggest that high-output renal failure represents the renal response to a less severe (or modified) episode of renal injury than that required to produce classic oliguric renal failure.

Pulmonary Responses

Acute respiratory failure following severe injury and critical illness has received increasing attention over the last two decades. With advances in the management of hemorrhagic shock and support of circulatory and renal function in injured patients, it has become apparent that 1 to 2 percent of significantly injured patients (with previously normal lungs) develop acute respiratory failure in the postinjury period. Initially this lung injury was thought to be specifically related to the shock state and its resuscitation. This is implied by such names as "shock lung" and "traumatic wet lung," which have been applied to acute respiratory insufficiency following injury. It is now recognized that there are many similarities in the pathophysiology and clinical presentation of acute lung injury following a variety of insults. This has resulted in the realization that the lung has a limited number of ways of reacting to injury and that several different causes of acute diffuse lung injury result in a similar pathophysiologic response. The common denominator of this response appears to be damage at the alveolar-capillary interface, with resulting leakage of proteinaceous fluid from the intravascular space into the interstitium and subsequently into alveolar spaces.

CLINICAL PRESENTATION. This injury with its resulting interstitial (and alveolar) edema produces a clinical picture ranging in severity from mild pulmonary dysfunction to progressive, eventually fatal, pulmonary failure. It differs from "classic" pulmonary failure in that the patients *are usually hypocarbic* rather than hypercarbic. The severe form has been labeled *adult respiratory distress* syndrome (ARDS) and is characterized by

1. Hypoxemia, which is relatively unresponsive to elevations of inspired oxygen concentration (indicating ventilation perfusion imbalance and shunting);
2. Decreased pulmonary compliance (progressively increased airway pressure required to achieve adequate tidal volume);
3. Chest x-ray changes, which are characteristically minimal in the early stages; with progression of the syndrome interstitial edema and diffuse bilateral infiltrates appear that may progress to widespread areas of consolidation;
4. Pulmonary edema due to cardiogenic causes or increased hydrostatic pressure, which should be ruled out, and this is generally done by the measurement of filling pressures.

The clinical criteria are summarized in Table 4-1.

Originally, four clinical stages were described. The first is quite subtle and is characterized by spontaneous hyperventilation with hypocarbia, diminished pulmonary compliance, and respiratory alkalosis. If the process continues, the patient progresses to the second stage, during which respiratory problems become more apparent. Persistent hyperventilation (with hypocarbia), progressive hypoxemia, decreased compliance, and an increase in pulmonary shunt fraction indicate that further pulmonary deterioration is occurring. Changes in chest roentgenograms are characteristically subtle during the early stages. As the syndrome advances to stage three (progressive pulmonary insufficiency) and stage four (terminal hypoxia with cardiac asystole), interstitial edema and diffuse infiltrates are observed on the roentgenograms.

Table 4-1. CLINICAL CRITERIA FOR POSTINJURY PULMONARY INSUFFICIENCY (ARDS)

Major
A. Hypoxemia (unresponsive)
B. Stiff lung (low compliance)
C. ↓ Resting volume (functional residual capacity)
D. X-ray (diffuse interstitial pattern)
E. ↑ Dead space ventilation

Minor
A. ↑ Cardiac output
B. Hyperventilation
C. R/O cardiogenic pulmonary edema

While these initial clinical descriptions are useful, several qualifying points are important. First, the early changes are nonspecific. Similar findings result from a variety of causes (e.g., early pneumonia, atelectasis, pulmonary edema). Second, the progression can be rapid and the stages are not clearly distinguishable. Studies of the incidence of ARDS have shown that >75 percent of patients developing "full-blown" ARDS do so within 24 h of the inciting cause and that 95 percent do so within 72 h. In these studies the diagnosis of ARDS required the following:

1. $Pa_{O_2} \leq 75$ mmHg while receiving $F_{I_{O_2}} \geq 0.5$
2. Diffuse pulmonary infiltrates
3. Pulmonary artery wedge pressure ≤ 18 mmHg
4. No alternate explanation for the above

Third, with currently available pulmonary support, progression to "stage four" is rare. While the mortality *associated with* ARDS remains high, death is rarely the result of respiratory failure alone.

PATHOPHYSIOLOGY. A review of basic terminology is shown in Table 4-2. The prominent derangements in pulmonary function associated with ARDS are (1) hypoxia that is unresponsive to increased inspired oxygen concentrations, (2) decreased pulmonary compliance (compliance defined as the amount of volume increase in the lungs obtained by a given increase in pressure), which clinically appears as "stiff lungs," and (3) a fall in resting lung volume, specifically a fall in the functional residual capacity. The functional residual capacity, as shown in Fig. 4-15, is the amount of air remaining in the lungs after a normal expiration.

The possible causes of hypoxia (decreased arterial P_{O_2}) are shown in Table 4-3. All clinicians are familiar with hypoventilation as a cause of hypoxia, as seen in the recovery room, but it is unlikely that hypoventilation is responsible for the hypoxia in this syndrome. Hypoventilation significant enough to produce hypoxia is associated with a rise in the P_{CO_2}. These patients, however, have an abnormally low P_{CO_2}.

Although diffusion defects can theoretically result from interstitial edema, they should respond to the administration of 100% oxygen. This is not the case in the patients in question, so diffusion defects alone appear to be unlikely causes of the clinical syndrome.

Ventilation/perfusion inequalities could explain the hypoxia seen in these patients, and shunting represents the ultimate ventilation/perfusion abnormality. This

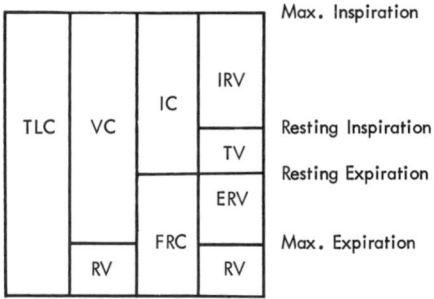

Fig. 4-15. Lung volumes and capacities: *TLC*, total lung capacity; *VC*, vital capacity; *IC*, inspiratory capacity; *FRC*, functional residual capacity; *RV*, residual volume; *ERV*, expiratory reserve volume; *TV*, tidal volume; *IRV*, inspiratory reserve volume.

statement deserves further explanation. Normally, there is autoregulation of ventilation and perfusion within the lung so that a balance exists between ventilation and perfusion of alveolar groups. When a group of alveoli become nonventilated or have decreased ventilation, compensatory mechanisms bring about a reflex decrease in blood supply to these alveoli. This, in its extreme, results in no ventilation and no perfusion to these alveolar units; thus no abnormality in terms of dead space ventilation or shunting occurs. The effects of loss of this normal balance or loss of compensatory mechanisms are shown in Fig. 4-16. On the left, alterations in blood flow are demonstrated. It can be seen that progressive decrease in blood flow with continued ventilation affects primarily carbon dioxide elimination. This can be defined as high ventilation/perfusion ratio and is usually reflected by increases in dead space ventilation. Such changes do not result in hypoxia. On the right side of Fig. 4-16 is shown the effect of reduction in ventilation while perfusion is maintained. It can be seen that progressive lowering of ventilation can result in hypoxia until the ultimate reduction, i.e., nonventilation, occurs. In theory, as long as any ventilation of the alveolus occurs, the hypoxia should be responsive to oxygen. This, then, is generally referred to as a ventilation/perfusion abnormality characterized by a low V/Q ratio. When alveolar collapse or nonventilation occurs for any reason, the hypoxia secondary to this is no longer responsive to oxygen; this is defined as a shunt.

Causes of pulmonary shunting are shown in Fig. 4-17. Shunting normally takes place, to the extent of about 3 percent of the cardiac output, through both intrapulmonary and extrapulmonary routes. Although pathologic shunts occur from extrapulmonary causes, intrapulmonary shunting appears to be the problem in ARDS. Basically, there is perfusion of alveoli that are collapsed or for

Table 4-2. BASIC TERMINOLOGY AND SYMBOLS

$\overline{V}_{O_2}$	Oxygen consumption
Q_T	Cardiac output
V_D/V_T	Physiologic dead space ventilation as fraction of tidal volume
Q_s/Q_t	Physiologic shunt as fraction of total cardiac output
AaD_{O_2}	Alveolar arterial gradient—oxygen
$F_{I_{O_2}}$	Fraction of inspired O_2
$V/\dot{Q}$	Ratio of ventilation to perfusion
Pa_{O_2}	Partial pressure, arterial, oxygen

Table 4-3. CAUSES OF HYPOXEMIA

1. Hypoventilation
2. Diffusion defects
3. V/Q abnormalities
4. Shunting

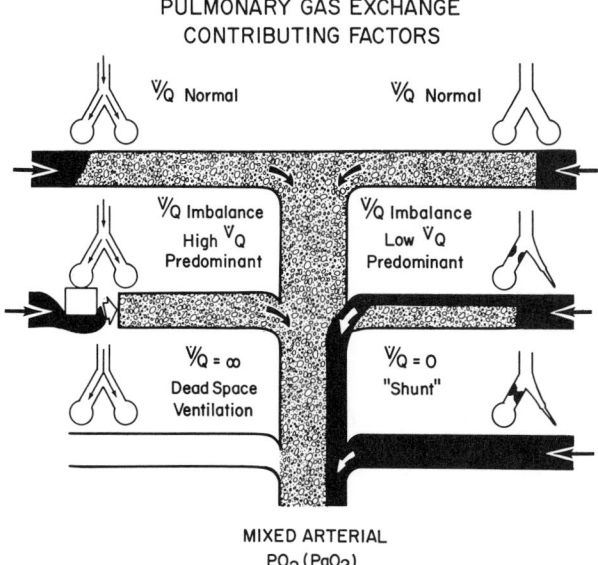

PULMONARY GAS EXCHANGE
CONTRIBUTING FACTORS

MIXED ARTERIAL
PO$_2$ (PaO$_2$)

Fig. 4-16. Diagrammatic representation of ventilation/perfusion ratio *(V/Q)* abnormalities.

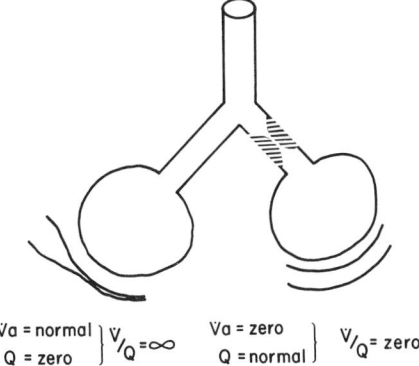

Fig. 4-18. Diagrammatic representation of mismatched ventilation and perfusion.

other reasons cannot be ventilated. The alveoli, for example, may be filled with secretions, exudate, blood, or edema.

Whatever the cause, the clinical picture appears to result from a distortion of the normal ventilation/perfusion balance. This concept is shown in Fig. 4-18. In some areas of the lung there is perfusion with poor ventilation; in other areas there is ventilation of nonperfused alveoli. This combination of abnormalities will produce decreased resting lung volume (functional residual capacity, or FRC), shunting, and increased dead space ventilation.

The common denominator producing the abnormalities in ventilation and perfusion and other abnormalities seen in ARDS is thought to be injury to the pulmonary capillary endothelium or alveolar epithelium. Injury to the capillary endothelium results in loss of integrity of the membrane, with increased permeability to albumin. The

Fig. 4-17. Mechanisms of arteriovenous admixture in pulmonary shunting.

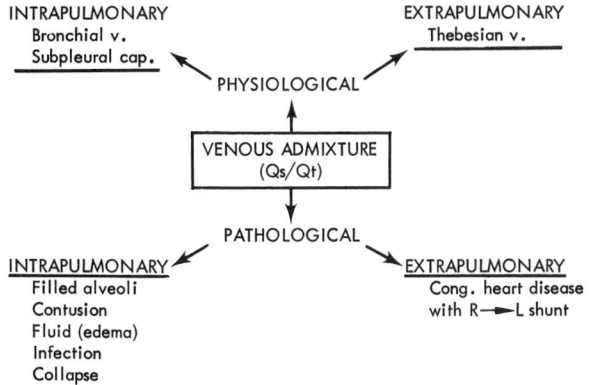

consequent leak of protein-rich fluid leads to *interstitial pulmonary edema* and decreased pulmonary compliance. With continued leakage, the alveolar units become fluid-filled and hypoxia (shunting) ensues. Thus the entire clinical picture of ventilation of poorly perfused segments (capillary injury), decreased compliance (interstitial edema), perfusion of poorly ventilated segments, and loss of lung volume (partially and completely fluid-filled alveoli) appears to result from capillary injury with a "capillary leak."

ETIOLOGY. A variety of factors have been suggested as capable of producing ARDS (Table 4-4). Several of these are specific to, or frequently present in the trauma patient. Some of these have been clearly shown to predispose patients to the development of ARDS as shown in Table 4-5. The definition of these factors and possible mechanism of production are discussed below.

Blood-Borne Injury. Among individual conditions, *sepsis syndrome* is the most frequent single precipitant of ARDS. Sepsis syndrome has been defined as evidence of serious infection (temperature $\leq 35°C$ or $\geq 39°C$, white blood cell count <2000 or >12,000 cells/mm^3, positive blood cultures, or source of infection) accompanied by a deleterious systemic response (unexplained arterial hypotension with systolic blood pressure <90 mmHg for greater than 2 h, systemic vascular resistance less than 800 dyne · s/cm^5, or unexplained metabolic acidosis).

The risk of ARDS after bacteremia alone, on the other hand, is relatively low, increasing markedly if bacteremia is accompanied by a deleterious systemic response such as hypotension or thrombocytopenia. While sepsis can serve as an example of a number of factors that appear to produce ARDS as a result of blood-borne injury, the precise mechanism by which this occurs has not yet been elucidated and is the subject of extensive investigation. Some propose that the injury is a direct result of bacterial products on the capillary endothelium. Others present evidence for extensive injury resulting from products of activated leukocytes or platelets. This raises the challenging issue of host defense mechanisms activated and out of normal physiologic control. Several possibilities proposed are worthy of investigation (and are not mutually exclusive) and well may lead to enhanced understanding

Table 4-4. DISORDERS ASSOCIATED WITH (CAUSING) ADULT RESPIRATORY
DISTRESS SYNDROME

Blood-borne or vascular source of injury

Trauma (soft tissue or skeletal)*	Drug overdoses:
Sepsis*	Heroin, methadone, ethchlorvynol,
Fat embolism	acetylsalicylic acid, propoxyphene
Pancreatitis	Drug idiosyncratic reaction
Shock	Thrombotic thrombocytopenic purpura
Multiple transfusions:	Leukemia
Microemboli	Venous air embolism
Leukoagglutinin reaction	Head injury
Disseminated intravascular coagulation	Paraquat
Surface burns	Cardiopulmonary bypass/hemodialysis
Miliary tuberculosis	

Inhalation or airway source	*Direct or physical source*
Aspiration of gastric contents*	Lung contusion
Diffuse infectious pneumonia:* viral,	Radiation
mycoplasma, Legionnaires', pneumocystis	High altitude
Near-drowning*	Hanging
Irritant gas inhalation: NO_2, Cl_2, SO_2, NH_3	Reexpansion
Smoke inhalation	
O_2 toxicity	

---

* Common cause of ARDS.

of ARDS and of the multiple organ failure syndrome following injury and associated with sepsis. Whatever the precise mechanisms, it is becoming clearer that the end result of this blood-borne injury is massive disruption of the capillary endothelium and alveolar epithelium. The end result is loss of selectivity of the endothelium for albumin, interstitial edema, and eventual alveolar flooding and the clinical picture of ARDS.

Other predisposing factors for ARDS that probably operate in a similar fashion include massive soft tissue and skeletal trauma (with microemboli as a possible circulating agent); multiple blood transfusions (with particulate or activated humoral agents causing capillary injury); fat embolism; disseminated intervascular coagulation; and activation (or lack of metabolism) of other circulating agents as might occur in pancreatic injury, pancreatitis, and massive hepatic injury.

The role of hypotension (shock) alone as a precipitating factor continues to be questioned. It appears probable that the presence of severe hypotension may augment injury from other causes but that hypotension alone is rarely the sole cause.

Inhalation or Airway Injury. Aspiration of gastric contents is among the most common causes of ARDS in several series. The clinical picture and roentgenographic findings that we now call ARDS were described by Mendelson in a classic paper in which he also presented animal studies on the pathophysiology of lung injury, stressing the role of acid pH. As in sepsis, the precise mechanism remains under investigation. Although a pH of 2.5 or less was originally suggested as being necessary to produce lung injury in human beings, data now exist that suggest that aspiration of substances with pHs greater than 2.5 can also produce this clinical picture.

Table 4-5. INCIDENCE OF ARDS AFTER PREDISPOSING CLINICAL
CONDITIONS

	Single condition present			Multiple conditions present		
		Number			*Number*	
Clinical condition	*Number*	*with ARDS*	*Incidence, %*	*Number**	*with ARDS*	*Incidence, %*
Sepsis syndrome	46	18	39	21	8	38
Aspiration	64	8	13	20	8	40
Multiple transfusions	31	8	26	37	12	32
Lung contusion	57	6	11	40	17	43
Multiple fractures	34	3	9	32	10	31
Near-drowning	5	2	40	6	4	67
Total	237	45	19	69	30	43

* Number with given condition as one of multiple risk conditions.

Despite the need to further define the mechanism, there is little question that aspiration of large amounts of gastric contents is a clear cause of ARDS. This has clinical significance, and in addition aspiration can serve as an example of other airway sources of injury. These include near-drowning, inhalation of toxic products (from burning wood, plastic, or chemical agents), oxygen toxicity, and diffuse infectious pneumonias.

Direct or Physical Lung Injury. Thoracic trauma with lung contusion is a well-established cause of ARDS. Here again, the mechanism requires continued investigation. ARDS can occur as a result of bilateral lung contusion due to chest trauma or blast injury. Lung contusion is usually localized and unilateral. Even a localized contusion can produce significant intrapulmonary shunting. The severe ARDS picture associated with bilateral contusions is more likely if the thoracic trauma is bilateral, although a severe unilateral blast injury can also result in ARDS involving both lungs. It has been suggested that significant increases in intrathoracic pressure occur with thoracic or abdominal injuries that produce much more extensive damage than initially appreciated on roentgenogram. There is little doubt that whatever the mechanism, "pulmonary contusions" are a predisposing factor in this devastating clinical picture. It is particularly important to recognize that this may not require evidence of extensive chest wall trauma. This is particularly true in children with their compliant chest walls.

Type and Amount of Resuscitative Fluid. The role of resuscitative fluids and the questions of the benefits of colloid versus crystalloid solutions have been a major area of controversy. Much of this concern has been based on knowledge of fluid exchange in the normal lung. This information is described mathematically in the following formula: $Q_f = K_w[(P_c - P_i) - \sigma_s(\pi_c - \pi_i)]$. A description of the symbols is as follows:

Q_f = net exchange of fluid across membrane
K_w = filtration coefficient of water
P_c = capillary hydrostatic pressure
P_i = interstitial hydrostatic pressure
σ_s = reflection coefficient of solute (factor by which ideal osmotic pressure is reduced owing to membrane permeability to solute; range of σ is 0 to 1.0)
π_c = capillary osmotic pressure
π_i = interstitial osmotic pressure

This concept is represented diagrammatically in Fig. 4-19.

If the pulmonary vasculature is normal, a fall in serum oncotic pressure renders the lungs more susceptible to pulmonary edema. Some authors reason that if crystalloid solutions are used in resuscitation, a fall in oncotic pressure might occur and cause or compound a pulmonary abnormality. If this were the case, the administration of colloid might be beneficial to the patient. The crucial flaw in the reasoning hinges upon the word "normal." Whether the injury leading to ARDS is to the endothelium or to the alveolar epithelium, the selectivity of the capillary for albumin and other large molecules is lost or impaired. Thus, the potential benefit of solutions containing high-molecular-weight compounds and the potential det-

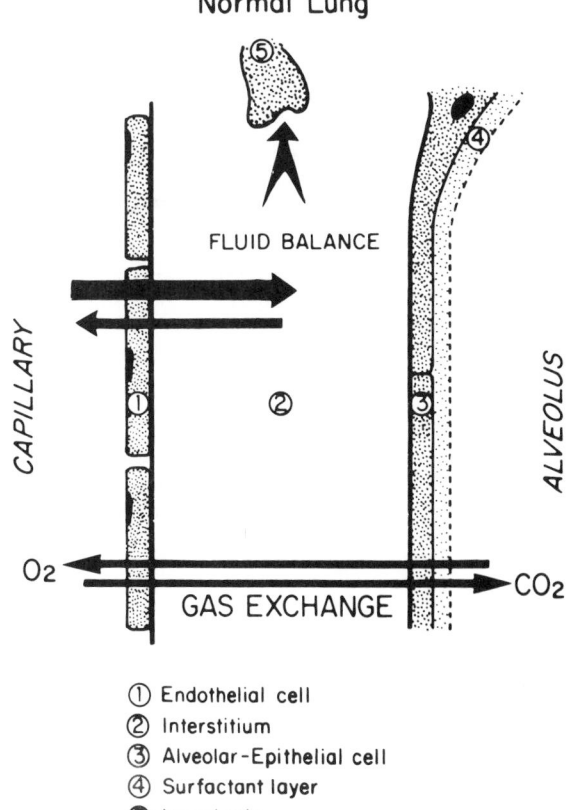

Normal Lung

FLUID BALANCE

CAPILLARY

ALVEOLUS

O₂ ← GAS EXCHANGE → CO₂

① Endothelial cell
② Interstitium
③ Alveolar-Epithelial cell
④ Surfactant layer
⑤ Lymphatic

Fig. 4-19. Dynamic processes occurring in the normal lung.

riment of reasonable amounts of electrolyte-containing solutions become a nonissue. This will be discussed in more detail in the section on fluid therapy.

DIAGNOSIS. Rigid criteria for the diagnosis of ARDS have been previously outlined. It is generally agreed that if one waits until patients meet these criteria, any opportunity for preventive or early therapeutic measures is lost. The general approach to these patients is to attempt to identify high-risk patients, place them in an intensive care area, and carefully observe them for signs of ARDS. Particular emphasis is placed on changes in oxygenation, changes in respiratory rate or arterial P_{CO_2}, and changes in lung mechanics.

Assessment of the adequacy of pulmonary function should begin immediately after injury in those patients at risk for developing ARDS. Endotracheal tubes inserted for airway control during surgery should not be removed prematurely. In many patients an additional 4 to 6 h of intubation postoperatively will be sufficient to allow the physician to determine that ARDS is not a threat. Extubation should not be considered until adequate lung function has been demonstrated (described below). If several days of intubation are contemplated, a nasotracheal tube may be substituted for the endotracheal tube in the operating room. This will allow for greater patient comfort and acceptance.

Table 4-6. ASSESSMENT OF PULMONARY FUNCTION

Function	Acceptable	Consider institution of therapy*
Oxygenation:		
Partial pressure oxygen arterial blood	$Pa_{O_2} > 90$ mm or 40% $F_{I_{O_2}}$	<90 mmHg on 40% $F_{I_{O_2}}$ or decreasing
Partial pressure oxygen arterial blood to fraction inspired oxygen ratio ($Pa_{O_2}/F_{I_{O_2}}$)	$Pa_{O_2}/F_{I_{O_2}} > 250$	<250 or decreasing
Alveolar-arterial oxygen gradient (breathing 100% O_2 for 10 to 15 min)	50–200 mmHg	>200 mmHg or increasing
Ventilation:		
Partial pressure carbon dioxide arterial blood	35–40 mmHg	30 or decreasing
Minute volume	<12 L/min	Increasing
Mechanics:		
Rate	12–25/min	25 or increasing
Effective compliance	50 cm³/cmH₂O	50 or decreasing

* Trends over a period of time are useful in marginal situations.

A prerequisite for optimal lung function is normal cardiovascular status. Hemodynamic monitoring, therefore, should be instituted routinely. This includes recording of heart rate, arterial pressure, electrocardiogram, central venous pressure, and pulmonary artery pressure if indicated. Serial body weight, intake and output balance, bacteriologic studies, coagulation profile, and chest x-rays are important data.

Monitoring of pulmonary function can be conveniently divided into three general areas: evaluation of oxygenation, ventilation, and lung-thorax mechanics. Table 4-6 details the most easily obtained tests and includes normal values. As a general principle, isolated determinations are not as valuable as serial measurements obtained at regular intervals. Hypoxemia is often detected in apparently normal patients who appear to be doing well clinically.

The partial pressure of oxygen in the arterial blood (Pa_{O_2}) is the hallmark of adequacy of oxygenation. This must be considered in the light of the inspired oxygen concentration ($F_{I_{O_2}}$). A simple means of establishing a measurable relationship between Pa_{O_2} and $F_{I_{O_2}}$ is their ratio ($Pa_{O_2}/F_{I_{O_2}}$). Ratios between 250 and 500 are considered adequate, while a value of less than 250 is definitely abnormal. This ratio provides the clinician with a gross estimate of the efficacy of oxygenation at the bedside during rapid changes in therapy. It appears to be most reliable when the $F_{I_{O_2}}$ is between 0.3 and 0.7.

The alveolar-arterial oxygen difference (AaD_{O_2}) may allow rapid differentiation of the cause of hypoxemia. Of the four causes of hypoxemia (hypoventilation, diffusion defects, ventilation/perfusion abnormalities, and pulmonary shunt), only the intrapulmonary shunt should affect their index if the patient is breathing pure oxygen. The AaD_{O_2} is affected by cardiac output, O_2 consumption, the position of the hemoglobin/O_2 dissociation curve, and the magnitude of the pulmonary shunt. In particular, as the $F_{I_{O_2}}$ varies, the AaD_{O_2} varies widely. This greatly limits its value as an initial screening test.

The adequacy of ventilation is measured by the arterial partial pressure of carbon dioxide (Pa_{CO_2}). By definition, hypoventilation occurs when the Pa_{CO_2} is elevated. Post-injury pulmonary failure is usually associated with hypocapnia (hyperventilation). Therefore, the patient with a decrease in both Pa_{CO_2} and Pa_{O_2} probably has ARDS. Tidal volume (VT)—the amount of air breathed during one respiratory cycle—is another indication of the adequacy of ventilation. This is readily measured with a modestly priced respirometer. VT multiplied by the respiratory rate is called the *minute ventilation*. This value is easily derived but by itself is only a rough guide to adequate ventilation. In many postinjury patients, high minute ventilations are recorded. It is not established whether this is a compensatory response or an indicator of a pathologic condition.

The effective compliance (C_{eff}) may be quite valuable as an assessment of the ease of distensibility of lung and thoracic cage. This derived value is obtained by dividing the VT by the peak airway pressure. C_{eff} indicates the "stiffness" of the lungs, i.e., how difficult they are to ventilate (low C_{eff} means increased stiffness). A decreased C_{eff} may indicate increased extravascular lung water, airway constriction, or increased chest wall resistance (impaired bellows activity). Low values are usually found in patients with ARDS.

An adequate assessment of pulmonary function can be achieved by serial measurement of arterial blood gases, tidal volume, minute ventilation, and effective compliance. Several other monitoring devices have been advocated. The work of breathing is almost always increased in ARDS. This value is a measure of the mechanical cost of achieving adequate ventilation. The major disadvantage of this test is that it requires an intraesophageal balloon to measure transthoracic pressure and the availability of an analog computer for usable results. Although highly desirable, the measurement of the work of breathing is difficult in the critically ill patient.

Table 4-6 is intended as a guide for identifying patients who require increased attention. Careful investigation for causes of pulmonary deterioration (pneumothorax, fluid excess, lobar atelectasis, etc.) is indicated, and more extensive monitoring may be required prior to instituting therapy for ARDS.

MANAGEMENT. Support of Pulmonary Function, (Support of Oxygenation, and CO_2 Elimination). The most common indication for beginning ventilatory therapy is hypoxemia. Initial management should be to increase the $F_{I_{O_2}}$ both as a diagnostic test and to temporarily relieve hypoxemia if the Pa_{O_2} is less than 65 mmHg. For effective therapy, control of the airway must be achieved. The most rapid and reliable way to do this is the insertion of an endotracheal or nasotracheal tube. Mechanical ventilation may then be applied. Since a defect in the matching of ventilation to perfusion is present, therapy is directed at maintaining ventilation to marginally ventilated alveoli and recruiting collapsed or partially occluded alveoli. This will directly increase the FRC of the lungs.

Technique. The volume ventilator is the device most often chosen for the treatment of ARDS. The initial tidal volume setting may be 10 to 15 mL/kg body weight at a rate of 12 to 14 breaths per minute, with an inspiration: expiration ratio of 1:2. The ventilator is adjusted so that the patient can "trigger" additional ventilator breaths. This can be described as assisted mechanical ventilation (AMV). An $F_{I_{O_2}}$ of 0.4 should be applied initially and blood-gas determinations used to indicate the efficacy of this treatment. Humidification of the inspired air via a heated nebulizer is essential to avoid drying airway secretions.

Blood gases are checked within 10 to 20 min of beginning respiratory treatment to determine the patient's response. If hypoxemia persists on 40 percent oxygen, increasing the VT still further may be warranted in an effort to increase the FRC. The effect of this maneuver is best assessed by following serial compliance changes. If the C_{eff} is improving, benefit from increased VT may be expected. If C_{eff} decreases with an increase in VT, too much volume is being given to the patient. Lower tidal volume ventilation will then be required to minimize the risk of complications of ventilatory therapy. The compliance curve is shaped somewhat like the Starling curve of cardiac function, i.e., a plateau is reached, after which any increase in volume is achieved only at the expense of a marked increase in airway pressure.

Alternative methods of mechanical ventilatory support are available. One that is being used more frequently is intermittent mandatory ventilation (IMV). This is a technique of mechanical ventilation that allows the patient to breathe spontaneously and at the same time to receive periodic support from the ventilator.

Acceptable levels of Pa_{O_2} are between 65 and 80 mmHg. If this cannot be achieved with the treatment outlined above, there are two alternatives: manipulation $F_{I_{O_2}}$ and support of lung volume.

The $F_{I_{O_2}}$ may be increased to higher levels. Since pulmonary shunting is caused by continued perfusion of nonventilated alveoli, simply increasing the concentration of oxygen will have no significant effect on the shunt. In addition, washout of nitrogen from poorly ventilated alveoli will make them more susceptible to collapse, thus converting low V/Q areas to areas of shunt resulting in more atelectasis. Although there is still controversy over the role of O_2 toxicity in the genesis of ARDS (see above), the literature clearly indicates that prolonged use of high O_2 concentrations can produce a clinical picture similar to ARDS. A concentration of more than 50% O_2 is required to produce deleterious effects in patients with normal lungs, depending on the amount of time alveolar hyperoxia is maintained. The higher the O_2 concentrations, the less the time required to produce damage. Therefore every effort should be made to limit the $F_{I_{O_2}}$ to less than 0.5.

Since acceptable manipulation of the $F_{I_{O_2}}$ is limited, the second alternative is to recruit collapsed or partially collapsed alveoli with some modification of ventilatory therapy. This can be done by applying continuous positive end-expiratory pressure (PEEP) to the airway. PEEP may be achieved by either inserting an airflow resistance during expiration or using a ventilator with an end-expiratory plateau of positive pressure. Providing positive pressure throughout the respiratory cycle prevents alveolar and small airway collapse and may recruit lung units that were previously collapsed. The beneficial effects of this modality are (1) increased FRC, compliance, and Pa_{O_2}; (2) increased V/Q ratio (when initially low); (3) decreased pulmonary shunting; and (4) decreased mortality from ARDS.

Technique of PEEP. The commonly used volume ventilators have the capability of instituting PEEP without modifying the equipment. Although there is some controversy about the absolute level required, incremental increases in pressure are advocated. The usual beginning level is 5 cmH_2O of PEEP. Cardiorespiratory function is monitored after 10 to 15 min to assess the effects. If no beneficial effect is noted, further increases in PEEP follow in increments of 3 to 5 cmH_2O pressure.

There may be variable response to PEEP. While some patients respond with an immediate increase in Pa_{O_2}, others may not show improvement for $\frac{1}{2}$ to 1 h or longer. Therefore, absence of immediate response should not be interpreted as an absolute failure of PEEP. Each patient has a different but demonstrable optimal PEEP level that correlates well with the highest compliance. Thus a practical bedside monitor of the effectiveness of PEEP may be compliance.

Complications of PEEP. It has been shown that cardiac output may be decreased secondary to an increase in intrathoracic pressure and decreased venous return. This is usually significant only when the intravascular volume is decreased. Therefore, fluids should be given to assure a normal volume status before beginning PEEP therapy. Monitoring of the pulmonary wedge pressure is valuable in the assessment of volume prior to and during the administration of PEEP. Cardiac output may also be measured to assure normal values.

Excessive pressure applied to the terminal airways may overdistend and rupture normal alveoli, leading to pneumothorax. This complication of PEEP is uncommon below 20 cmH_2O pressure.

Close attention to the effective compliance can prevent excessive airway and alveolar pressure being applied during PEEP therapy. PEEP is most beneficial when FRC is low initially. In patients with a high FRC from preexisting lung disease (Chronic Obstructive Pulmonary Disease), any level of PEEP may be detrimental. This can be determined only by closely monitoring the patient's response to treatment, noting compliance especially.

Control of Pa_{CO_2}. Hyperventilation is a common problem in patients who are being artificially ventilated. Hypocarbia has been shown to be deleterious to the cerebral circulation (vasoconstriction) and the pulmonary circulation. Therefore, ventilatory therapy should be set to maintain normal levels of Pa_{CO_2}. With high tidal volume ventilation, a compensatory decrease in respiratory rate is necessary to maintain a normal Pa_{CO_2}. Increasing the inspired concentration of CO_2 or adding dead space have both been advocated as methods of increasing the Pa_{CO_2} but are rarely effective in patients with ARDS. Effective control of the Pa_{CO_2} requires heavy sedation or muscle relaxation and control of the patient's respiration. Decrease of the Pa_{CO_2} below 30 is an indication for instituting respiratory control.

Oxygen-Carrying Capacity of Blood. Although the Pa_{O_2} can be increased by higher levels of $F_{I_{O_2}}$, it is the red blood cell that carries almost all the O_2 to the tissues. One unit of packed red cells carries more O_2 than plasma exposed to pure O_2 at hyperbaric pressure. Therefore, the hemoglobin (Hgb) concentration should be maintained between 12 and 14 g/dL. Attention should also be given to the acid-base status of the patient. Both acidosis and alkalosis produce shifts of the Hgb-O_2 dissociation curve that can affect the ability of Hgb to off-load O_2 at the tissue level.

Fluid Management. Fluid therapy can arbitrarily be divided into two phases when one is dealing with the acutely traumatized or critically ill patient. In the initial phase, or resuscitation phase, careful control of fluid volumes is important but may be difficult. Later, in the maintenance phase of fluid therapy, careful regulation of intake and output can be accomplished more easily. In both phases, the ideal would be the complete normalization of pulmonary vascular pressure. This can best be accomplished by invasive monitoring of pulmonary artery and central venous pressures. To avoid the complications of hydrostatic edema with resultant pulmonary dysfunction, continued monitoring of these parameters in acutely ill patients is essential. The values of these hemodynamic indices can guide the minute-by-minute volume replacement in the resuscitation phase and the hourly rates in the maintenance phase.

The type of fluid used for resuscitation and maintenance therapy is controversial. The two most common asanguinous fluids are isotonic balanced salt solutions and solutions containing albumin (colloid). Proponents of colloid therapy have stressed the sound physiologic principle of maintaining colloid osmotic pressure of the plasma (π_c) in the prevention of interstitial edema. Others

have argued that little or no change in plasma oncotic pressure occurs despite large volumes of balanced salt solutions. It is reasonable to assume that if the pulmonary membranes are injured the effect of oncotic pressure will be reduced, owing to the increased mobility of the protein species.

Randomized trials of crystalloid versus colloid therapy in acutely ill patients have been recently reported. Lowe and associates report no difference with regard to survival, incidence of pulmonary failure, or postresuscitation pulmonary function. Similarly, Virgilio and his colleagues have demonstrated the greater ease with which isotonic fluid therapy can be managed, despite its large volumes, as opposed to colloid therapy. On the other hand, others have suggested that the use of colloid solutions enhances the function of the myocardium and oxygen transport in patients with high cardiac indexes, whereas crystalloid tends to worsen pulmonary gas exchange.

Detrimental effects of albumin treatment have been proposed by several groups. It has been repeatedly demonstrated that albumin in the first several days of resuscitation has a negative inotropic effect and promotes fluid retention by limiting salt and water excretion. This same group has also suggested that albumin therapy may alter blood coagulation. Other investigators demonstrated an increased extravasation of albumin in the lungs after resuscitation with colloid solutions. This extravascular albumin may adversely affect fluid and protein movement in the lung.

Despite the conflict in the literature regarding the pros and cons of colloid therapy (albumin solutions), several points should be emphasized. Clinical and experimental studies generally find balanced salt solutions satisfactory for volume replacement. A second point is that massive volumes of isotonic salt solutions are necessary before severe changes in plasma osmotic pressure occur. A third point is that the changes that occur in colloid osmotic pressure may not be of importance in the injured lung because of the increased permeability of protein at the membrane level. Finally, the cost of albumin-containing solutions can be up to fifty times that of balanced salt solutions.

Based on the above, our approach is to treat the acutely ill or traumatized patient with blood and/or isotonic salt solutions, depending on the clinical status. Pulmonary vascular pressures are closely monitored to prevent the sequelae of overzealous therapy or hypovolemia.

Diuretics. Administration of diuretics has been proposed as a method for indirectly decreasing the amount of interstitial edema. Reports claiming a therapeutic role for diuretics in treating ARDS are not conclusive. There is no study that has randomly and prospectively shown that diuretics are as effective or more effective than ventilatory therapy alone. Our practice is to give small doses of furosemide *when hemodynamic studies indicate that fluid overload has occurred,* e.g., an elevated pulmonary artery wedge pressure. No attempt is made to "dry out" the patient by the long-term administration of diuretics. There is no solid evidence to suggest that lowering fluid volumes below normal will decrease the leak from injured capillaries. Such decreases in volume may have serious deleterious effects.

Corticosteroids and Anti-inflammatory Agents. Despite extensive interest in their use, there is no conclusive proof that pharmacologic doses of steroid should be part of the specific therapy of the ARDS syndrome. Data do exist to indicate that steroids may be effective in treating pulmonary fat embolism, and in selected patients with extensive acute fibrosis. Thus, we reserve steroid therapy for these clinical entities. Similarly, the use of other anti-inflammatory agents is unproved and should be confined to carefully constructed experimental trials.

Antibiotics. Phophylactic use of broad-spectrum antibiotics has no place in the primary therapy of ARDS. Indiscriminate use of these agents may allow the emergence of resistant strains of bacteria that are very difficult to treat. Many patients will already have been given antibiotics because of certain types of injury. Specific antibiotics are used to treat pulmonary sepsis. Their choice is determined by serial cultures of the sputum.

Ancillary Pulmonary Care. Patients treated in the intensive care unit tend to be bound to the bed by numerous tubes, wires, and catheters. Change in position then becomes a difficult problem. It has been shown, however, that significant improvement in oxygenation can result from frequent position changes. Maintenance of one position is likely to compound pulmonary abnormalities.

Routine pulmonary toilet, suctioning with sterile technique, and attempts to prevent pulmonary infection are very important. These must all be done on a routine basis.

PREVENTION. It has been suggested that early application of PEEP in high-risk patients could reduce the incidence of ARDS several-fold. This concept has been challenged by others. In a recent study we prospectively randomized 92 patients meeting entry criteria for ARDS risk factors to receive mechanical ventilation either without PEEP (control) or with 8 cm water PEEP (early PEEP). These therapies were continued for 72 h unless (1) ARDS developed or (2) the Pa_{O_2} was greater than 140 ($F_{I_{O_2}} = 0.5$) at 24 h and continued so following PEEP removal. This group included 65 trauma patients. The groups were comparable for age, severity of injury, number and types of ARDS risk factors, and additional oxygenation. Eleven of the 44 early PEEP patients (25 percent) and 13 of the 48 control patients (28 percent) developed ARDS. The incidence of atelectasis, pneumonia, and baro-trauma was the same in both groups as was mortality. Thus, we were unable to demonstrate any effect of early application of 8 cm of PEEP to high-risk patients on the incidence of ARDS. While this study does not rule out any potential benefit from early PEEP application, it effectively eliminates the possibility of a major reduction in the incidence of ARDS on a statistical basis. While there may be valid reasons for intubation and early mechanical support of injured patients, the probability that such treatment will significantly decrease the incidence of true ARDS is low. This is commensurate with the concept that a physical injury to the alveolar capillary interface has occurred. The impact of ventilatory support

Table 4-7. EARLY AND LATE MORTALITY IN ARDS PATIENTS BY IMMEDIATE CAUSE OF DEATH

	Early deaths (≤72 h)	Late deaths (>72 h)
Sepsis	3*	8
Respiratory	1	4†
Cardiac	1	5‡
Neurologic	3	4
Other	2	1

* Sepsis present prior to ARDS.
† All four with sepsis as a contributory cause.
‡ Three with sepsis as a contributory cause.

on the long-term progress of the disease remains debatable.

OUTCOME. Despite advances in ventilatory support and fluid management, the mortality associated with ARDS remains high. Most centers report mortalities of 50 percent or greater in patients who sustain rigidly defined ARDS. The causes of death, however, are rarely respiratory failure. In a recent review of ARDS patients at our institutions, we found that surprisingly few patients die as a direct consequence of respiratory failure (Table 4-7). Most of the early deaths (less than 72 h) are related to the underlying illness or injury. In contrast, sepsis was directly responsible for 38 percent of the late (greater than 72 h) ARDS deaths and was a contributing factor in 76 percent. This supports the intuitive impression that long-term survival in surgical patients with ARDS frequently depends on identification and elimination of the septic focus.

Summary. Acute pulmonary failure (ARDS) occurring in the injured patient has a variety of potential causes. Infection with systemic sepsis is the most common cause and the most amenable to definitive treatment. The chief functional defect, hypoxemia unresponsive to increased $F_{I_{O_2}}$, is treated with ventilatory therapy and support of lung volume (PEEP) on an empiric basis. Attempts at prevention with ventilatory means are of marginal value at best. Despite advances in ventilatory and fluid management, mortality has decreased little since the introduction of PEEP and long-term improvements in survival depend on identification and elimination of septic foci and on pharmacologic developments anticipated in the future.

Alterations in Oxygen Transport

Cell hypoxia and eventually cell death may result from the complex changes induced by shock, regardless of the type, and restoration of delivery of oxygen to the tissues at an adequate concentration and pressure forms the basis for treatment. In the past, attention was directed primarily toward the factors affecting oxygen transport capability, including the concentration and partial pressure of oxygen in the inspired air, alveolar ventilation, ventilation/perfusion relationships, cardiac output, blood volume, and hemoglobin concentration. The demonstration that the level of organic phosphates in the red blood cell has a significant effect on the position of the oxygen/hemoglobin dissociation curve has served to focus attention on the processes responsible for release of oxygen at the tissue level. Because of the clinical implication of these findings, a knowledge of factors regulating both uptake and release of oxygen has assumed increasing importance in the care of critically ill patients.

OXYGEN TRANSPORT

The oxygen transport system consists of several component processes that function collectively to extract oxygen from inspired air and deliver it at a partial pressure sufficient to allow rapid diffusion from blood into the body cells. Each of the component processes has its own internal controls, and failure of any one may be compensated for by adjustments in the remainder of the system. The functions of the oxygen transport system are summarized in the following formula:

$$\text{Oxygen consumption} = \text{arteriovenous oxygen difference} \times \frac{\text{cardiac output (L/min)}}{100}$$

The amount of oxygen in whole blood includes that bound to hemoglobin (1.38 mL O_2/g of hemoglobin) and a small amount dissolved in plasma (0.003 mL/mm of oxygen tension). The oxygen content of arterial (Ca_{O_2}) and venous blood (Cv_{O_2}) are calculated by the formula

$$\text{Oxygen content} = (1.38 \times Hb_{conc} \times Hb_{sat}) + (0.003 \times P_{O_2})$$

Consider a person with a hemoglobin of 15 g/dL, an arterial oxygen tension of 100 mmHg, a venous oxygen tension of 40 mmHg, arterial and venous hemoglobin saturations of 97 and 75 percent, respectively, and a cardiac output of 6 L/min. Substituting these values in the formulas above, arterial oxygen content is 20.4 vol%, venous oxygen content is 15.6 vol%, arteriovenous oxygen difference is 4.8 vol%, and oxygen consumption is 288 mL/min.

Changes in any one of these factors are of variable significance regarding oxygen delivery. For instance, pulmonary gas exchange with 20 percent inspired oxygen concentration ($F_{I_{O_2}}$) normally produces an arterial oxygen tension (Pa_{O_2}) of approximately 100 mmHg, slightly less than average alveolar oxygen tension. Increasing the $F_{I_{O_2}}$ to 100 percent would raise Pa_{O_2} to approximately 650 mmHg. This would increase the amount of dissolved oxygen in the plasma from 0.3 to 2.0 vol% but would only increase the hemoglobin saturation from 97 to 100 percent. In contrast, even moderate changes in hemoglobin concentration or cardiac output have a strong influence on oxygen transport capability. A hemoglobin concentration of 10 g/dL (instead of 15) in the example above would reduce the oxygen-carrying capacity of the blood by one-third ($Ca_{O_2} = 13.7$ vol%). Coupled with a fall in cardiac output from 6 to 3 L/min, assuming that other variables remain unchanged, oxygen consumption theoretically would fall from 288 to 96 mL/min. This is a not infrequent

clinical occurrence, although oxygen consumption would be maintained at a higher level by adjustments in other parts of the system (e.g., increase of arteriovenous oxygen difference).

Therapy designed to improve tissue oxygenation, therefore, includes an evaluation of all factors affecting the oxygen transport system. Adjustment of inspired oxygen concentration and efforts to improve alveolar ventilation are of obvious importance; however, therapeutic attempts to maintain a normal hemoglobin concentration and cardiac output deserve special attention.

OXYGEN/HEMOGLOBIN DISSOCIATION CURVE

Another aspect of oxygen transport that deserves emphasis is the relationship between hemoglobin oxygen saturation and oxygen tension. The oxyhemoglobin dissociation curve describes hemoglobin affinity for oxygen, and its unusual sigmoid shape reflects the phenomenon of heme-heme interaction. Each of four heme groups in the hemoglobin molecule reacts with oxygen in a prescribed order, and uptake of an oxygen molecule by one heme group facilitates the oxygenation of the next heme group. The sigmoid configuration of this curve is particularly suitable for the uptake, transport, and subsequent release of oxygen. Since the upper portion of the dissociation curve is relatively flat, oxygen loading by hemoglobin may remain relatively normal despite wide variations in the alveolar oxygen tension. As oxygenated blood traverses the peripheral capillary, however, P_{O_2} drops from approximately 100 to 40 mmHg, hemoglobin saturation falls from 97 to 75 percent, and the blood releases just over 22 percent of its oxygen load (Fig. 4-20). Since P_{O_2} values at the peripheral capillary level fall on the steep portion of the curve, significant changes in oxygen release are produced by only small alterations in oxygen tension.

The position of the oxyhemoglobin dissociation curve along the horizontal axis is characteristically termed the P_{50} value. This reflects the oxygen tension necessary to saturate 50 percent of the hemoglobin with oxygen; the normal value is approximately 27 mmHg.

The importance of positional changes of the curve is also related to its sigmoid shape. Within limits, rightward or leftward shifts have little effect on arterial oxygen saturation if Pa_{O_2} is above 80 mmHg. At the peripheral capillary level, however, even small shifts of the curve may be important. A rightward shift of the dissociation curve (P_{50} above 27 mmHg) indicates decreased hemoglobin affinity for oxygen, while a leftward shift (P_{50} below 27 mmHg) is associated with an increase of hemoglobin/oxygen affinity. Compared with the normally positioned curve, more oxygen is released at any given P_{O_2} with a rightward-shifted curve and less is released with a leftward-shifted curve. Therefore, if arterial and venous oxygen tensions remain constant, arteriovenous oxygen difference increases with a rightward shift of the curve and decreases with a leftward shift (Fig. 4-21).

Changes in position of the oxygen/hemoglobin dissociation curve are significant in at least two respects. The

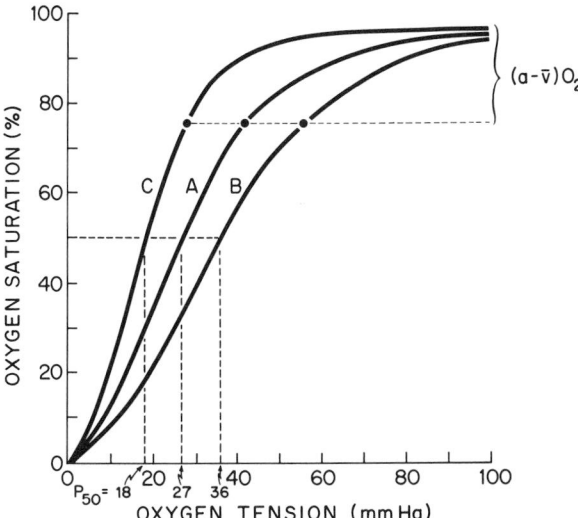

Fig. 4-20. Oxygen-hemoglobin dissociation curves in *(A)* normal, *(B)* rightward-shifted, and *(C)* leftward-shifted positions. The P_{50} value denotes the position of the curve along the horizontal axis and represents the oxygen tension (in mmHg) necessary to saturate 50 percent of available hemoglobin with oxygen. Note that as the curve moves toward the left, the arteriovenous oxygen difference, (a-v̄) O_2, can be maintained only by decreasing venous oxygen tension. (Adapted from: *Shappell SD, Lenfant CJM: Anesthesiology 37:127, 1972, with permission.*)

transfer of oxygen from the blood to the sites of intracellular utilization is directly related to the oxygen pressure differential. Thus a rightward shift of the curve is theoretically advantageous, since an equivalent amount of oxygen is released at a higher P_{O_2} than with a leftward-positioned curve. (Note that in curve *B* of Fig. 4-20, half of the oxygen would be released at a P_{O_2} of 36 mmHg; in curve

Fig. 4-21. Oxygen-hemoglobin dissociation curves similar to those in Fig. 4-20. Note that if arterial and venous oxygen tensions remain constant, arteriovenous oxygen difference decreases as the curve moves toward the left.

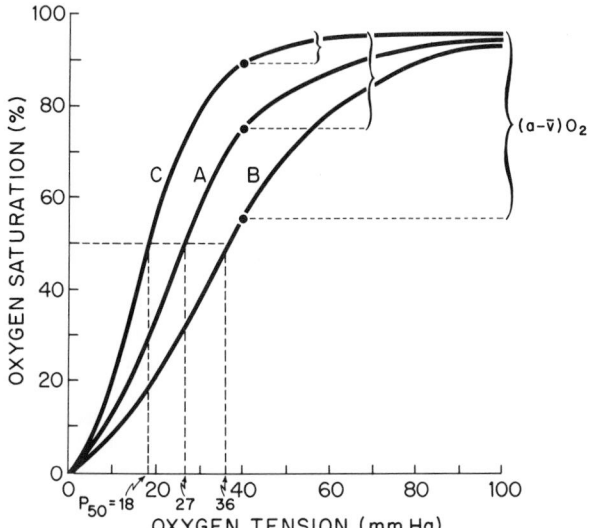

C, less than 10 percent of the oxygen would be released at the same P_{O_2}.) Second, the ability to maintain or enlarge the arteriovenous oxygen difference is dependent to some extent on the position of the curve. Normally, arterial hemoglobin saturation is near the upper limit and cannot be increased appreciably. Any enlargement of the arteriovenous oxygen difference necessitates reduction in venous hemoglobin saturation and venous oxygen tension Pv_{O_2}. As the curve moves to the left, maintenance of any given arteriovenous oxygen difference requires a progressive decrease in Pv_{O_2}. The fall in Pv_{O_2} is finally limited by the fact that a certain partial pressure is necessary for transfer of oxygen from the blood to the tissue cell. That level of oxygen pressure below which diffusion may be theoretically impaired and cellular function disturbed has been termed the "critical P_{O_2}."

Available data concerning the critical P_{O_2} are limited but suggest that it varies in individual organ systems and may depend on the level of activity of the tissues. Opitz and Schneider showed that oxygen uptake by the brain is impaired when venous oxygen tension falls below 20 to 25 mmHg, while Berne et al. indicated loss of myocardial function at oxygen tensions between 10 and 12 mmHg. With a leftward movement of the curve, therefore, maintaining or enlarging the arteriovenous oxygen difference is theoretically limited as the Pv_{O_2} approaches this critical level. Tissue oxygen delivery may be sustained in this instance by other mechanisms, principally by increasing cardiac output.

During hypovolemic shock, cardiac output is low and relatively fixed. Normally, enlargement of arteriovenous oxygen difference will partially compensate for the diminished blood flow; however, the response may be totally inadequate with a leftward shift of the dissociation curve. Continued survival and maintenance of essential organ function may be obtained only by shunting blood from tissues that tolerate a limited period of severe hypoxia (skin, skeletal muscle) to organs that require high oxygen flow rates (brain, heart).

FACTORS INFLUENCING THE POSITION OF THE OXYGEN/HEMOGLOBIN DISSOCIATION CURVE

Attempts to ensure a normal or rightward-positioned dissociation curve may be essential during treatment of patients with low-flow states. Factors affecting the position of the curve have been summarized by Shappell and Lenfant and are outlined in Table 4-8. The main in vivo influences include changes in pH, temperature, partial pressure of carbon dioxide, and level of red blood cell organic phosphates. Changes in hydrogen ion concentration and temperature have predictable and instantaneous effects on the position of the curve, while P_{CO_2} exerts its influence both by changing pH and by a pH-independent effect. The quantitative effects of these influences on the dissociation curve have been reviewed in several excellent publications.

The position of the dissociation curve is also influenced by interaction of hemoglobin with organic phosphates in the red blood cell. Both ATP and 2,3-diphosphoglycerate

Table 4-8. FACTORS THAT ALTER HEMOGLOBIN/
OXYGEN AFFINITY

Increase P_{50}	*Decrease P_{50}*
By direct effect:	By direct effect:
Increased [H$^+$]	Decreased [H$^+$]
temperature	temperature
P_{CO_2}	P_{CO_2}
DPG, ATP	DPG, ATP
Hb conc	Hb conc
Ionic strength	Ionic strength
Abnormal hemoglobin	Abnormal hemoglobin
Aldosterone	Carboxyhemoglobin
	Methemoglobin
By increasing DPG:	By decreasing DPG:
Decreased [H$^+$]	Increased [H$^+$]
Thyroid hormone	Decreased thyroid
Pyruvate kinase deficiency	hormone
Increased inorganic	Hexokinase deficiency
phosphate	Decreased inorganic
Cortisol	phosphate
Cell age (young)	Cell age (old)

SOURCE: Adapted from Shappell SD, Lenfant CJM: Adaptive, genetic and iatrogenic alterations of the oxyhemoglobin dissociation curve. *Anesthesiology* 37:127, 1971.

(DPG) bind to hemoglobin and lower the affinity of hemoglobin for oxygen, i.e., shift the dissociation curve to the right. In a quantitative sense, DPG is the more important of the two phosphates and exerts an additional influence in the intact red blood cell by lowering intracellular pH via Donnan equilibrium. Significant concentrations of DPG are found only in the red blood cell, and DPG is present in a concentration approximately equimolar with that of hemoglobin. DPG is a product of erythrocyte glycolysis, formed via a branch of the Embden-Myerhof pathway by conversion of 1,3-DPG to 2,3-DPG, catalyzed by diphosphoglycerate mutase.

Erythrocyte DPG undergoes considerable changes in response to several stimuli, with parallel changes in the position of the dissociation curve. Investigations have revealed that hypoxia increases erythrocyte DPG in conditions such as exercise, anemia, exposure to high altitude, cardiac failure, and various pulmonary diseases. The concomitant rightward shifts of the dissociation curve are thought to represent significant compensatory responses, allowing release of more oxygen at a higher P_{O_2}.

The regulation of DPG synthesis is complex and as yet not fully clarified. Although numerous factors influence the level of DPG (Table 4-8), the principal *mechanism* for increasing or decreasing its concentration appears to be related to the level of hydrogen ions in the red cell. DPG concentration increases as the red blood cell pH rises and decreases as the pH falls. These changes are due, in part, to the differential effects of pH on the activity of two red cell enzymes, DPG mutase and phosphatase. For instance, alkalosis stimulates DPG synthesis by increasing DPG-mutase activity and reducing the breakdown of DPG by DPG-phosphatase. The rise in red cell pH may be secondary to elevation of whole blood pH or, as in hypoxic states, a relative increase in the amount of deoxyhemoglobin. The pH also influences DPG binding to hemoglobin and may affect other enzymes in the glycolytic cycle. The net effect of pH changes on DPG concentration, therefore, probably represents a combination of these (and other unknown) influences. It should be noted that the pH-induced changes in DPG concentration tend to counteract the direct pH effects on the curve via the Bohr effect. Therefore, the immediate rightward shift of the curve secondary to acute acidosis is eventually offset by a pH-induced reduction in DPG concentration.

DPG synthesis is also responsive to hormonal influences and the level of inorganic phosphate. The phosphate level is directly related to DPG concentration, and maintenance of a normal inorganic phosphate level during intravenous hyperalimentation is necessary to prevent a reduction in the level of erythrocyte 2,3-DPG. Thyroid hormone acts directly to increase DPG synthesis, a fact that probably explains the elevated levels of this compound in hyperthyroid patients. Cortisol and aldosterone both shift the dissociation curve to the right, thereby decreasing hemoglobin/oxygen affinity. The effects of cortisol are probably secondary to direct stimulation of DPG synthesis. Hemoglobin/oxygen affinity also increases as the erythrocyte ages, presumably owing to a decreasing DPG concentration.

BLOOD TRANSFUSIONS, ERYTHROCYTE DPG, AND OXYGEN DELIVERY

The acceptability for transfusion of blood that has been stored in ACD (acid citrate dextrose) solution for up to 3 weeks is based on survival of at least 70 percent of the cells in the recipient's circulation. During this 3-week period, however, there is a rapid decline in erythrocyte DPG and a progressive increase in hemoglobin/oxygen affinity. Following transfusion, several hours are required for the DPG levels to return to normal. These findings suggest that oxygen delivery may be impaired after the administration of large quantities of stored blood and have led to a reevaluation of transfusion practices.

Several studies in both experimental animals and human beings have failed to show significant impairment of tissue oxygenation with markedly reduced levels of erythrocyte DPG and leftward shifts of the oxygen dissociation curve. Similar findings were noted in our study of 45 injured patients who received more than 5 units of whole blood stored in ACD solution during resuscitation and the subsequent operative procedure. Erythrocyte DPG levels were below normal in a majority of these patients and correlated well with the amount and storage time of the transfused blood. There were no consistent correlations, however, between DPG concentration and the measured parameters of oxygen delivery. This lack of correlation may be explained by two observations. First, the position of the dissociation curve cannot be reliably predicted from a knowledge of the DPG concentration alone. DPG represents only one of several factors that affect the curve, and the final P_{50} represents a composite of these influences. Normal or elevated P_{50} values noted in several patients with low DPG concentrations were probably due to other factors (e.g., pH and temperature) that tended to counteract the influence of DPG. A second observation is the lack of a consistent relationship between the P_{50} value and oxygen consumption. The majority of patients with leftward shifts of the dissociation curve had reasonably normal arteriovenous oxygen difference and oxygen consumption. Additionally, several of the patients with narrowed arteriovenous oxygen differences maintained oxygen delivery simply by increasing the cardiac output.

These findings do not imply that the position of the dissociation curve and the factors that influence it are unimportant. They do suggest that a person with reasonably intact cardiovascular and pulmonary systems is able to tolerate rather significant leftward shifts of the oxygen dissociation curve. The consequences may be quite different, however, in a patient with limited compensatory mechanisms and in some therapeutic regimens followed without understanding of their effects on the position of the curve. An example of this is shown in Fig. 4-22. Despite the sharp reduction in cardiac output following hemorrhage to a mean blood pressure of 50 mmHg, the control dog with a normal P_{50} value was able to maintain normal oxygen delivery by increasing the arteriovenous oxygen difference from 4.5 to 10.6 mL. In contrast the DPG-depleted dog was unable to expand the arteriovenous oxygen difference sufficiently (P_{50} value 15 mmHg). The problem was compounded by attempts to correct pH to normal by infusion of sodium bicarbonate solution. The dissociation curve moved farther to the left (P_{50} value 8 mmHg), the hemoglobin concentration fell secondary to hemodilution, and oxygen consumption fell to near zero. Although extreme, the experimental conditions are not unlike those which may be found in the clinical setting.

Fig. 4-22. Effects of hemorrhagic shock and sodium bicarbonate infusion on oxygen consumption after exchange transfusion with fresh blood (dog A) and DPG-depleted blood (dog B). I, Control period; II, after exchange transfusion (DPG concentration 6.20 μM/mL RBC in dog B); III, after induction of hypotension; IV, continued hypotension and sodium bicarbonate infusion.

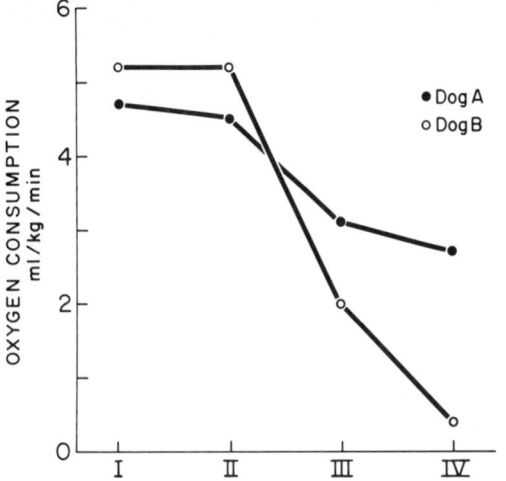

In summary, available evidence suggests that changes in hemoglobin/oxygen affinity, as reflected by the position of the oxygen dissociation curve, may be important in several circumstances. The elevated DPG concentrations and rightward shifts of the dissociation curve observed in hypoxic states (pulmonary disease, cardiac failure, anemia, exposure to high altitude, and so on) probably represent compensatory responses that facilitate oxygen unloading in the tissue capillaries. Oxygenation can be maintained in these instances by other mechanisms (e.g., increasing cardiac output) but at greater expense to body economy.

Leftward shifts of the dissociation curve observed following transfusions of stored blood, acute alkalosis, hypothermia, and so forth are, at best, undesirable phenomena and may significantly impair oxygen unloading. Although leftward shifts are tolerated in many circumstances, maintenance of a normally positioned dissociation curve may be of singular importance in patients with hypoxia, anemia, or hypotension when compensatory responses are limited.

THERAPEUTIC IMPLICATIONS

Obtaining a sufficient quantity of fresh blood for resuscitation of patients in hemorrhagic shock is difficult, and attempts are being made to find a suitable storage medium that will maintain the levels of organic phosphates (DPG, ATP) in red blood cells. In addition to DPG, maintenance of a sufficiently high ATP level is essential to maintain a flexible and highly deformable red cell membrane. The biconcave disc shape of a normal red blood cell is transformed toward a nondeformable spherocyte during storage. This loss of deformability hinders passage through the microcirculation and increases susceptibility of the cell to destruction. Although both DPG and ATP levels rapidly return to normal within 6 to 24 h, restoration may be delayed in the critically ill and massively transfused patient who is least able to tolerate increased microvascular resistance to flow and depression of tissue oxygenation. At the time of this writing, storage of blood in CPDA-1 (citrate phosphate dextrose adenine) solution seems to be the most practical alternative. Survival of red blood cells is similar after transfusion of blood stored in either ACD or CPDA-1 solution. Compared with blood stored in ACD solution, however, blood stored in CPDA-1 media has a higher pH, and DPG, ATP, and P_{50} are maintained at consistently higher levels. Additionally, use of CPDA-1 has increased the useful shelf storage life up to 35 days. Conversion from ACD to CPDA-1 solution for blood storage is a simple matter for blood banks and has been accomplished in most areas.

When large quantities of blood are administered, particularly in critically ill patients, some attention should be paid to the storage age of each unit of blood. If a significant portion of the blood administered has been stored for more than 7 to 10 days, every attempt should be made to obtain fresh blood for additional transfusion requirements. In our experience the institution of these simple changes, including conversion to CPDA-1 storage media, has been rewarding. The large reductions in DPG and P_{50} noted in the past are rarely seen today, even after massive transfusions.

Other factors that influence the position of the dissociation curve (Table 4-8) may also be important in the individual patient. For instance, the induction of respiratory alkalosis may produce an abrupt increase in hemoglobin/oxygen affinity. This is a common occurrence during operations and in patients requiring ventilatory assistance in the postoperative period; coupled with other factors that limit oxygen transport, the capacity to maintain tissue oxygenation may be sharply reduced. Similarly, the sudden correction of an acidosis, whether metabolic or respiratory, may have undesirable effects. In this regard the indiscriminate use of sodium bicarbonate during resuscitation of patients in hypovolemic shock is discouraged. The presence of a mild metabolic alkalosis is a common finding after resuscitation, owing in part to the alkalinizing effects of blood transfusions and the administration of lactated Ringer's solution. After infusion (and partial restoration of hepatic blood flow), the citrate and lactate contained in transfused blood and the lactate in lactated Ringer's solution are metabolized and bicarbonate is formed. If excessive quantities of sodium bicarbonate are administered simultaneously, a severe metabolic alkalosis may result. The alkaline pH may be highly undesirable, particularly in patients with hypoxia or low fixed cardiac output. Combined with other factors incident to blood replacement that increase hemoglobin/oxygen affinity (low DPG concentration and hypothermia), significant interference with oxygen unloading at the cellular level may occur.

The immediate and direct pH influences on the curve (via the Bohr effect) are eventually offset by reciprocal changes in DPG concentration. There is, however, a lag period of approximately 4 h before any change in DPG concentration is noted, and the final level is not reached until 48 h after induction of acidosis or alkalosis. The fact that the effects of sudden large changes in pH may persist for several hours should be considered during therapy. Correction of a metabolic acidosis, therefore, is properly directed toward correction of the underlying disorder. Bicarbonate therapy may be reserved for the treatment of severe metabolic acidosis, particularly following cardiac arrest, when *partial* correction of pH is essential to restore myocardial function. Similarly, pH correction in more protracted states of metabolic acidosis may be indicated but should be accomplished slowly.

Lowering body temperature also causes a leftward shift of the dissociation curve and an increase in hemoglobin/oxygen affinity, but any interference in oxygen delivery may be countered effectively by the hypothermia-induced reduction in metabolic requirements.

Rightward shifts of the curve are usually desirable and, unless extreme, rarely interfere with oxygen uptake in the lungs. Rightward shifts generally occur as a compensatory response to hypoxia, regardless of the cause. Nevertheless, in patients with severe arterial desaturation (exposure to high altitude, congestive failure, right-to-left cardiac shunts), any potential benefit from shifting the curve farther to the right may be offset by interference with oxygen loading.

In a complex clinical setting, multiple factors that influence hemoglobin/oxygen affinity may be operative at any given time, and abrupt changes secondary to therapy or the disease process itself may occur. Evaluation of these multiple influences may be difficult, since few data concerning their cumulative effects are available. Nevertheless their *net* effect can be estimated by determining the position of the oxygen dissociation curve.

Techniques for constructing an oxygen dissociation curve are time-consuming and not readily available in most hospitals. For this reason we have developed a rapid, though less precise, method for estimating the position of the curve (the P_{50} value). Since the shape and slope of the curve do not change appreciably with changes in position, determination of a single point of the steep part of the slope should allow a rough estimate of the entire curve. To obviate the use of a tonometer, a single sample of venous blood is drawn anaerobically and the P_{O_2} and oxygen saturation is measured. (An arterial sample is unsuitable, since the values fall on the upper flat portion of the curve.) An estimated P_{50} value may then be obtained using the Severinghaus slide rule or a nomogram as depicted in Fig. 4-23. The nomogram represents a computer plot of a family of O_2 dissociation curves, using the correction factor for pH as suggested by Severinghaus. The point on the nomogram corresponding to the measured P_{O_2} and saturation values is found and traced to the

Fig. 4-23. Nomogram for estimation of P_{50} value (position of the oxygen-hemoglobin dissociation curve). The point on the nomogram corresponding to the measured P_{O_2} and saturation of a sample of venous blood is traced to the line representing 50 percent oxygen saturation. This intersect represents the estimated P_{50} (normal value approximately 27 mmHg). In the example shown, the venous blood sample P_{O_2} is 39 mmHg, the oxygen saturation 65 percent, and the P_{50} value 31 mmHg (a rightward-positioned dissociation curve).

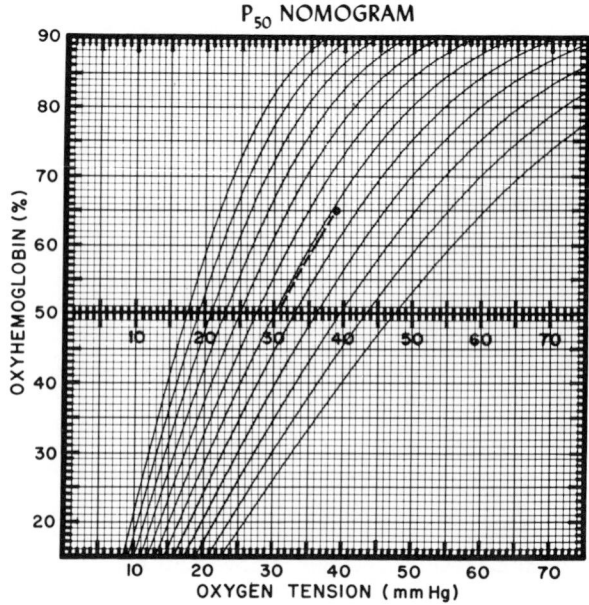

P_{50} NOMOGRAM

OXYHEMOGLOBIN (%) vs OXYGEN TENSION (mmHg)

line representing 50 percent oxygen saturation. This intersect represents the estimated P_{50}; the normal value is approximately 27 mmHg. A P_{50} above this level represents a rightward shift of the oxygen dissociation curve, while a lower value represents a leftward shift.

To test the validity of this technique, oxygen dissociation curves were constructed using a standard mixing technique on 50 occasions in 27 acutely ill patients. In each instance an estimated P_{50} was obtained from the nomogram using a single sample of venous blood drawn at the same time. Correlation between the two values was excellent (correlation coefficient .92).

Estimates of P_{50} have become routine in our care of critically ill patients. Combining this with measurements of both arterial and venous blood gases, a considerable amount of information may be obtained about the state of oxygenation and oxygen transport capability.

THERAPY OF SHOCK

Hypovolemic Shock

It is apparent from the previously described etiologic classification of shock that therapy will depend on detection of the causative mechanisms while providing support to the patient. Correction of the underlying causative factors can then be carried out. Consequently one sees again the usefulness of a practical clinical classification that includes (1) oligemic shock, (2) cardiogenic shock, and (3) shock caused by changes in peripheral resistance and capacity vessels (neurogenic shock and septic shock). In a patient who has undergone trauma, more than one causative factor may be operating. Once the diagnosis of shock has been made and supportive therapy begun, a diligent search can be made for the causative factor or factors. Treatment of shock, therefore, can best be thought of in relation to the type of shock that is present. As pointed out earlier, the pathogenesis of hypovolemic hypotension is varied. Recognition of deficits of total body water and electrolytes is usually subtle, and correction requires specific therapy with crystalloid solutions. Reductions in the extracellular fluid volume (plasma and interstitial fluids) primarily, as in burns, peritonitis, and some forms of crush injury, are more easily recognized. Specific therapy should be started with electrolyte solutions and rarely may require the use of plasma or some source of protein. External blood loss as seen in lacerations should be corrected immediately, as fluid therapy is begun, with first-aid measures, including pressure tamponade. Surgical procedures may then be carried out. Similarly, an external loss, such as bleeding from a duodenal ulcer, should be treated with the usual measures, including decompression of the stomach, while supportive therapy is begun.

The only other immediate concern in addition to control of the causative wounds is maintenance of an open airway. Pulmonary insufficiency rarely occurs from shock alone, but concomitant injuries may include crush injuries of the chest, pneumothorax, hemothorax, or spe-

cific obstruction of the airway from injuries to the head and neck. In these circumstances adequate respiratory exchange must be restored promptly.

VOLUME. The treatment of hemorrhagic shock continues to be the adequate replacement of whole blood, since this is the fluid that has been lost. Early use of properly cross-matched, type-specific whole blood is still the primary therapy when shock is due to whole blood loss. When available, type-specific or Rh-negative "universal donor" type O blood with low anti-A titer can be administered.

Extracellular Fluid Replacement

An effective therapeutic regimen for the treatment of hemorrhagic shock has now been used successfully in several thousand patients, taking into account the previously described changes in the peripheral circulation and interstitial fluid.

When patients are admitted to the emergency room in hemorrhagic shock, at least two large-gauge catheters are inserted into appropriate veins and an infusion of lactated Ringer's solution is begun immediately. At the same time, blood is drawn for typing and cross matching. The lactated Ringer's solution is run at a rapid rate so that in a period of 45 min between 1000 and 2000 mL of lactated Ringer's solution is given intravenously. This approach has several advantages.

The procedure is a highly effective therapeutic trial to determine the preexisting amount of blood loss or the presence of continuing blood loss. It is often observed that blood pressure will return to normal, become stable, and remain so in patients with initially severe hypotension after infusion of 1 or 2 L of a balanced salt solution. When such a response is correlated with measurements of red blood cell mass, plasma volume, and extracellular fluid volume, the preexisting blood loss is shown to be relatively minimal. If blood loss has been minimal and hemorrhage is not continuing, hemorrhagic hypotension can be alleviated simply by the infusion of a balanced salt solution.

If blood loss has been severe or hemorrhage is continuing, the elevation of blood pressure and decrease in pulse rate that occur with rapid intravenous infusion of lactated Ringer's solution is usually transient. When this occurs, whole blood that has been accurately typed and cross-matched is available and can be given immediately. Consequently, the initial use of the balanced salt solution allows time for accurate typing and cross matching.

In view of the disparate reduction in the extravascular, extracellular fluid as demonstrated in animals and human beings, it is felt that even though blood is needed, as it is in the majority of patients admitted in hemorrhagic hypovolemia, alleviation of the reduction in functional extracellular fluid is desirable.

Lactated Ringer's solution as initial therapy, both from the standpoint of a therapeutic trial and as a therapeutic adjunct, is a procedure that has been found to be effective. This is understandable, since lactated Ringer's solution is isotonic, essentially free from side reactions, and virtually harmless from the standpoint of aggravation of other fluid and electrolyte imbalances that may be present.

Further, it appears that the use of a balanced salt solution in this fashion significantly reduces the requirement of whole blood in the patient with hemorrhagic hypotension. This is true not only from the standpoint of proper hemoglobin and hemoconcentrations following therapy, but also from the standpoint of prevention of, or recovery from, renal failure.

A concern that Ringer's lactate solution may aggravate the existing lactate acidosis when used to treat patients in shock has been expressed by several investigators, but previous studies in both experimental animals and patients do not support this view. The use of blood plus Ringer's lactate solution to treat hemorrhagic shock in experimental animals results in a more rapid return to normal of lactate, excess lactate, and pH than does treatment with return of shed blood alone. Similar serial determinations of lactate, excess lactate, pH, and base excess have been obtained in 52 patients in hemorrhagic shock. All patients received Ringer's lactate solution in addition to whole blood during the period of resuscitation. There was a significant reduction in lactate and excess lactate levels and a return of pH and base excess values toward normal during the period of shock while Ringer's lactate solution was being infused. After resuscitation, all of these values rapidly returned to normal levels as increased tissue perfusion restored aerobic metabolism.

Blood Transfusions. Blood transfusions have been discussed above under Blood Transfusions, Erythrocyte DPG, and Oxygen Delivery.

Albumin Solutions. In the absence of whole blood, many substances have been proposed as transient substitutes for the combination of red blood cells and plasma available in whole blood. The most popular and commonly used substitute has been human plasma. Historically, in some circumstances, e.g., battlefield conditions, plasma has been a highly serviceable substitute. Currently, there appears to be little justification for the addition of albumin to balanced salt solutions for volume resuscitation in hypovolemic shock.

The primary hypothetical advantage of albumin resuscitation concerns the transient increase in intravascular colloid oncotic pressure. It had been felt that this might protect the lung from interstitial edema. However, an excellent review by Civetta points out that the lung does not function according to classic Starling forces. There is a rapid albumin flux across the normal pulmonary capillary membrane, and lung lymphatics rapidly clear the interstitium. Substantial evidence from Moss, Trunkey, and our laboratory has failed to show increases in lung water induced by hemorrhagic shock, crystalloid resuscitation, or the hypooncotic state. It is unlikely that a transcapillary oncotic gradient can be manipulated to produce change in extravascular lung water.

Well-controlled clinical trials have repeatedly documented the hemodynamic efficacy of crystalloid resuscitation without the induction of pulmonary complications. Albumin infusion does transiently produce a greater increase in intravascular volume, per unit volume adminis-

tered, than Ringer's lactate. The administered albumin rapidly disperses to the extravascular space. Thus, improvements in physiologic parameters rather than a calculated volume formula must remain the end points for the titration of fluid administration. Practical and potential disadvantages of colloid administration include postresuscitation hypertension, described by Lucas and Ledgerwood, increased intravascular volume at the expense of necessary interstitial fluid resuscitation, depression of circulating immunoglobulins, and suppression of albumin synthesis.

In summary, balanced salt solution is preferable to plasma for hemodynamic resuscitation for several reasons. It restores measured losses of extracellular fluid and reverses documented membrane dysfunction without inducing deleterious end-organ side effects. Crystalloid resuscitation avoids the potential problems outlined above and is both less expensive and easier to titrate safely, by repeated bolus infusion, than plasma.

Artificial Plasma Substitutes. Artificial colloid solutions have been devised to replace human albumin for plasma expansion. Hydroxyethyl starch (hetastarch), an amylopectin, and dextran, a polysaccharide, are the most commonly employed. Both are reasonably safe and inexpensive drugs, although both hetastarch and dextran have been associated with rare anaphylactoid reactions and ill-defined transient coagulopathies. A hypothetical concern of reticuloendothelial depression during blood clearance of these unphysiologic compounds has also been raised. In any case, these solutions have colloidal properties and physiologic impact that are similar to albumin. The above concerns regarding the administration of albumin solutions to unstable patients in shock also argue against the use of these artificial colloid solutions in this setting.

Blood Substitutes. Synthetic oxygen-carrying blood substitutes and stroma-free hemoglobin solutions have received considerable attention in the past few years. The Japanese have reported successful use of perfluorocarbons (Fluosol-DA) in chronic anemic states, but the solutions have found limited use in this country because of their short half-life and toxicity. Additionally, use in patients in hemorrhagic shock would be limited by the long preparation time that is necessary prior to use. Stroma-free hemoglobin solutions hold more promise for this purpose, but despite some rather remarkable advances recently, the solutions have not yet been approved for clinical use.

VASODILATORS. In 1948 Wiggers and his associates predicted that a significantly increased survival rate in animals treated with an adrenergic blocking agent and subjected to hemorrhagic shock would indicate the detrimental influence of protracted vasoconstriction in shock. Subsequently, in 1950, Remington and his associates reported an increased survival rate in dogs pretreated with Dibenamine before the induction of hemorrhagic shock. Zweifach similarly found that Dibenamine protected rats against lethal-graded hemorrhage if the animals were pretreated, and Boba and Converse reported that ganglionic blocking agents increased the survival of experimentally shocked animals. Webb noted hydralazine was deleterious during the hypotensive phase of hypovolemia. In practice, the use of vasodilators in the treatment of hemorrhagic shock has disappeared from clinical usefulness.

HEMODYNAMIC MEASUREMENTS. A patient in hemorrhagic or oligemic shock may rarely fail to respond to vigorous management as outlined above. Such a patient usually presents a complicated clinical picture. Frequently surgical procedures have been carried out for correction of the underlying causes of shock. Thus the problem is often compounded by massive fluid and blood administration, general anesthesia, and surgical trauma. At this point a comprehensive but rapid reevaluation of the patient must be carried out in order to institute effective therapy.

The basic defect underlying this "refractory shock" must be corrected. Possible causes are multiple: (1) continuing blood loss from the primary injury or disease or from another source, (2) inadequate replacement of fluids, (3) massive trauma and other derangements secondary to the trauma, especially cardiac tamponade and pneumothorax, (4) myocardial insufficiency either as a direct result of inadequate perfusion for a prolonged period or secondary to anesthetic agents, and (5) concomitant septic shock, as with intraperitoneal contamination from bowel perforation. The answers to this problem can best be obtained by careful clinical evaluation of the patient and evaluation of a few relatively simple hemodynamic parameters that may serve as a guide to satisfactory treatment.

POSITIONING. Positioning of the patient in shock has long been thought to be an adjunct in the treatment of hypovolemic shock. Most first-aid courses teach that the patient in shock should be placed in the head-down position. Although it is true that some forms of shock, particularly neurogenic shock, will respond to the head-down position, the effect of posture on the cerebral circulation in the face of true hypovolemia has not been defined. Frequently the patient with multiple trauma has sustained other injuries, within both the abdomen and the chest, so that the routine use of the Trendelenburg, or head-down, position may interfere with respiratory exchange far more than when the patient is left supine. The beneficial effect of the head-down position is probably the result of transient autotransfusion of pooled blood in the capacity or venous side of the peripheral circulation. This beneficial effect can be obtained easily by elevating both legs while maintaining the trunk and the remainder of the patient in the supine position. This is probably the preferable position, then, for the treatment of hypovolemic shock.

MAST GARMENT. There has been recent enthusiasm for the in-the-field application of military antishock trousers, the MAST garment. When applied to the extremities in modest pressures, the garment functions well as a splint and may control some venous bleeding. When applied at high pressures, the resultant increase in total peripheral resistance may elevate the systemic pressure while decreasing cardiac output and peripheral perfusion. In addition, inflation of the abdominal bolster may compress the inferior vena cava, impairing venous return to the heart by further increasing the venous resistance. Several re-

ports of reperfusion injury with compartment syndromes in uninjured limbs have appeared. Thus the MAST device may be of value when utilized strictly as a temporizing device or rarely as specific treatment of bleeding pelvic fractures. Its use must not delay the immediate repletion of intravascular and extravascular volume by fluid therapy or interfere with rapid transport of the injured patient.

PULMONARY SUPPORT. In the past, most writings on the treatment of hypovolemic shock stated that breathing high oxygen concentrations is probably of little value during a period of hypotension. These conclusions were based on the concept that the principal defect is in volume flow to tissues and decreased cardiac output. The oxygen saturation in the majority of patients with uncomplicated hypovolemic shock is generally normal, and the small increase in dissolved oxygen in the blood contributed by raising the P_{O_2} above this level is insignificant, particularly in the face of a markedly decreased cardiac output. This concept continues to be valid in terms of improvement of the shock state or tissue oxygenation itself. Nevertheless, in the small but significant group of patients in hypovolemic shock in whom the oxygen saturation is not normal, the *initial* use of increased oxygen concentrations may be extremely important, since the fall in cardiac output accompanying hemorrhagic shock has been shown to compound existing defects in oxygenation. This may occur in patients with preexisting defects, such as chronic obstructive lung disease. More frequently problems in oxygenation arise directly from the patient's injury and may include a coexisting pneumothorax, pulmonary contusion, aspiration of gastric contents or blood, or airway obstruction. Thus, although oxygen is not routinely administered to patients in shock, if any doubt exists as to the possibility of one of these circumstances or as to the adequacy of oxygenation of arterial blood, the initial administration of oxygen until the injuries to the patient have been diligently assessed is certainly justified. If oxygen is to be administered to patients under these circumstances, it should be delivered through loose-fitting face masks designed for this purpose. If controlled airway is indicated for other reasons, an endotracheal tube is ideal. The use of nasal catheters, particularly those passed into the nasopharynx, is avoided because of potential complications of pharyngeal lacerations and gastric distention. Gastric rupture has been recorded secondary to such a catheter being inadvertently placed in the esophagus.

ANTIBIOTICS. Antibiotics were used in the treatment of hypovolemic shock for many years and were thought to exert a protective mechanism against the ravages of hypovolemia. Subsequent data fail to support this hypothesis. The use of antibiotics in patients who have open or potentially contaminated wounds, however, continues to be sound practice, when combined with good surgical debridement and care. Consequently the use of wide-spectrum antibiotics is advisable as a preventive measure in the severely injured patient. Cefoxitin, 2 g I.V., has proved to be a safe and effective single agent in multiorgan abdominal injuries.

TREATMENT OF PAIN. Treatment of pain in the patient

with hypovolemic shock is rarely a problem from the standpoint of shock itself. If, however, the causative injury produces severe pain, as in fracture, peritonitis, injury to the chest wall, and the like, control of pain becomes mandatory. Generally, when the patient is moved to the emergency facility where physicians and care are available, simple supportive measures (administration of intravenous fluids, passing of catheters) will give reassurance. The need for analgesics is greatly reduced, since the need to allay fear and anxiety is decreased. If, however, the patient continues to have severe pain, the observations made by Henry K. Beecher in World War II become extremely pertinent. Beecher pointed out that many battle casualties received morphine or other narcotic agents by subcutaneous administration soon after wounding. Since these analgesics were not put into the circulation immediately, the pain continued and the patient ultimately received several doses that were poorly absorbed. Once effective therapy was begun for shock, the doses previously administered were absorbed and profound sedation resulted. As a result, the recommendation was made that small doses of narcotics be given *intravenously* for the management of pain in the patient with shock. This has been standard practice for 40 years and relieves pain without contributing significantly to the potentiation of the shock syndrome.

STEROIDS. Adrenocorticoid depletion was commonly regarded as a contributory factor in shock after it was learned that the presence of hypovolemic shock could in itself deplete the adrenal cortex of adrenocortical steroids. Subsequent studies, however, have shown that adrenocortical steroid production is stimulated maximally by the presence of hypovolemic shock. Steroid depletion with hypovolemic shock may possibly occur in the elderly patient or in patients who have specific adrenocortical diseases such as incipient Addison's disease, postadrenalectomy patients, or patients who have had adrenal suppression with exogenous adrenocortical steroids. In these specific instances the intravenous administration of hydrocortisone is desirable. In the general patient, with hypovolemic shock, however, administration of adrenocorticoids is probably not indicated. The use of steroids in more complicated unresponsive shock states, particularly when septic shock is suspected, remains controversial.

DIGITALIS. Digitalis has been advocated in the treatment of hypovolemic shock. There is no doubt that in some patients, particularly elderly ones, the stress of hypovolemic shock will in itself induce or aggravate cardiac failure. In these patients, digitalis is found to be helpful. Over the years many have investigated the role of the heart as a cause of the irreversible form of hemorrhagic shock, but experimental data obtained in patients indicate that heart failure in response to hypovolemic shock is merely a terminal event. Further evidence of this is supplied by the fact that the central venous pressure does not rise except terminally in hypovolemic shock.

VASOPRESSORS. In the past the use of drugs that cause vasoconstriction in hypovolemic shock has been popular because blood pressure in human beings can usually be elevated by these agents. However, the objective in treating hypovolemic shock is to increase tissue perfusion. Vasopressors raise blood pressure by increasing peripheral vascular resistance and decreasing tissue perfusion. Therefore, the injurious effects of shock may be aggravated.

As experience has accumulated with the use of vasopressors, it is obvious that the alpha and beta stimulating functions of the vasopressors must be separated during clinical evaluation.

The vasopressors generally have a threefold action consisting of central inotropic and chronotropic effects as well as a peripheral vasoconstricting effect.

In 1923, Cannon condemned the use of vasopressors on this physiologic basis: "Damming the blood in the arterial portion of the circulation, when the organism is suffering primarily from a diminished quantity of blood flow, obviously does not improve the volume flow in the capillaries." In 1940, Blalock also condemned the use of vasopressors in treating shock. More recent studies have more clearly defined the hazards of using vasopressors in hypovolemic shock. This is especially true since those studies show benefit only after volume has been restored.

There is other available evidence that the administration of vasopressors during hypovolemia reduces the already depleted plasma volume.

As more data becomes available, it is doubtful that the use of vasopressors in the treatment of hypovolemic shock is ever warranted.

In order to be of value, hemodynamic measurements should include an evaluation of several parameters. First, some estimate of fluid available for circulation is imperative. Second, the ability of the cardiovascular system to circulate this fluid adequately must be evaluated. This includes an evaluation of the efficacy of the heart and of the resistance of the vascular system.

Direct measurement of the blood volume initially seemed to be the appropriate approach; for several reasons, acute blood volume measurements have proved to be unreliable as a guide for therapy for hemorrhagic shock. If the plasma volume alone is measured, an estimate of the total blood volume requires the use of the hematocrit for calculation. These estimated volumes are no more reliable than the hematocrit itself, which has been established to be erratic in hemorrhagic shock. Furthermore, the anatomic blood volume has little relation to that available for circulation if a large portion of this is involved at the site of injury or inflammation or trapped in some vascular pool.

Determination of the extracellular fluid volume would seem extremely useful; this remains largely a research tool since a rapid bedside method is not practical. Use of central venous pressure monitoring has been popularized. This technique can be performed easily, and measurements can be repeated often. The central venous pressure is a relatively reliable approximation of the efficacy of venous return. The information gained by this method is enhanced if the venous pressure response to the rapid administration of fluids is assessed. The second of the two parameters requires evaluation of arterial blood pressure by either cuff or arterial cannulation, and estimation of cardiac output. Cardiac output can be estimated by using arteriovenous oxygen difference.

As with any patient who is at risk of developing serious cardiovascular complications, continuous monitoring of the crucial hemodynamic variables (heart rate, arterial pressure, central venous pressure, urinary output, electrolyte fluid balance) by using reliable equipment and accurate techniques will be required for the severely injured patient. In addition to the above "conventional" monitoring, the introduction into clinical practice of the thermodilution method for the determination of cardiac output at bedside by using the Swan-Ganz flow-directed catheter has made possible the continuous evaluation of cardiac function during various therapeutic interventions. Through the Swan-Ganz catheter, the pulmonary artery pressure and pulmonary capillary wedge pressure can be recorded concurrently with the injection of saline for the measurement of cardiac output. The diastolic pulmonary artery pressure or pulmonary capillary wedge pressure closely approximates the left atrial pressure, and either one can be taken as the left ventricular filling pressure. Stroke volume can be derived from cardiac output and heart rate. By plotting stroke volume versus left ventricular filling pressure, left ventricular curves can be constructed and myocardial performance can promptly be assessed under control conditions and during drug or fluid administration. With the above techniques, the main determinants of cardiac output (preload, blood pressure, and systemic arteriolar resistance) can instantaneously be monitored. Since generalized infection may adversely affect the outcome of the severely injured patient, care should be taken to introduce and maintain monitoring catheters under sterile conditions. For the same reason, pulmonary complications related to the Swan-Ganz catheter should be avoided, and the latter should not be introduced into the pulmonary circulation when contraindications exist (pulmonary rupture, pneumothorax, etc.).

With the use of these measurements the best method for treatment of a patient with hypotension and a complicated clinical picture can frequently be discerned. A depressed or normal central venous pressure that does not rise with rapid administration of a balanced salt solution usually indicates continuing hypovolemia. The diagnosis is supported by the presence of a measured decrease in cardiac output. If the hypovolemia is secondary to inadequate fluid replacement, a gradual and sustained rise in arterial pressure and cardiac output results from the administration of appropriate fluids. If continued fluid loss or acute bleeding is the cause, then fluid administration produces either a transient rise or no rise in the blood pressure and cardiac output.

The presence of an elevated central venous pressure or a central venous pressure that rises with the rapid administration of fluids (and produces either no change or a decrease in cardiac output) is indicative of impairment of the pumping mechanism. Usually this represents primary myocardial deficiency and must be treated accordingly; the defect in the pumping mechanism may occasionally be due to mechanical obstruction as with cardiac tamponade or mediastinal compression by intrapleural fluid or air. The possible presence of these surgically correctable lesions must be kept in mind, especially in the patient who has multiple injuries. Pulmonary embolism can produce a similar response but is rarely seen early in the course of the injured patient.

A normal or slightly increased central venous pressure with a normal or high cardiac output and disproportionate hypotension is usually due to a loss of peripheral vascular resistance. In this situation, the physician should suspect a "septic" component. Increased peripheral vascular resistance is the rule in oligemic shock. If accompanied by deficient myocardial function, the use of an inotropic agent (with minimal vasoconstrictor or preferably with vasodilator effects) may be beneficial. This should be done only after more direct therapy, such as volume replacement or digitalization, has been pursued. Hemodynamic measurements usually fail to show any indication for use of a vasoconstrictive agent in the treatment of hemorrhagic shock.

Several authors have questioned the value of central venous pressure measurements and pointed out that left ventricular overload and pulmonary edema can occur while right ventricular function (and the central venous pressure) remains adequate. This is particularly true after myocardial injury. In patients with normal cardiac reserve, however, *changes* in the central venous pressure with fluid infusion do indicate the ability of the myocardium to pump the volume presented to it. Properly applied, the central venous pressure remains a useful clinical tool in early resuscitation. Its interpretation can be augmented by measurement of pulmonary artery pressure and pulmonary wedge pressure, the latter approximating left atrial pressure. Such techniques are usually reserved for patients with more complicated problems, and the use of a balloon-tipped Swan-Ganz catheter is necessary.

A flow-directed pulmonary artery catheter is now available that provides continuous mixed venous oximetry. The potential benefits of this catheter in monitoring critically ill patients continue to be explored.

The ultimate hemodynamic criterion in the treatment of shock is the response of the patient. Adequate resuscitation is indicated when adequate cerebration and urine output are restored. Although diuresis by any means may be beneficial when a large pigment load is presented to the kidneys, the object of treatment in hypovolemic shock is to reestablish urine flow by adequate restoration of circulation and not to force urine flow in spite of inadequate resuscitation. The use of osmotic diuretics in uncorrected oligemic shock to produce "urine for urine's sake" would seem to have no physiologic basis and may, in fact, be detrimental by further depleting intravascular and extravascular extracellular fluid.

Cardiogenic Shock

In this form of shock the heart fails as a pump. Consequently primary therapy is directed toward the heart. Cardiac arrhythmias, whatever their origin, should be treated promptly. Cardiac tamponade, if this is the cause, should be relieved by pericardiocentesis. When the origin of the pump failure is myocardial infarction or myocarditis, the primary therapy again is directed toward the myocardial damage. If the myocardial damage is sufficiently severe to produce reduction in blood pressure, and indeed in organ perfusion, to the point that organ functions begin to fail, drugs with positive inotropic action may be efficacious.

HEMODYNAMIC MEASUREMENTS

Hemodynamic measurements play an important role in the management of postoperative patients with this type of hypotension. As previously described, the classic finding is a central venous or pulmonary artery pressure that is elevated or rises briskly with fluid administration. This is accompanied by a cardiac output that is depressed and fails to respond to fluid administration. In evaluating postoperative hypotension, as after an extensive procedure in the elderly or especially after cardiac surgery, the measurement of hemodynamic parameters may be of great benefit in differentiating hypovolemic hypotension from hypotension due to depressed myocardial function.

When hemodynamic measurements suggestive of deficient pumping action are found, myocardial insufficiency is usually at fault. It should be stressed again, however, that this can be due to mechanical obstruction (e.g., cardiac tamponade or mediastinal compression in the injured patient or pulmonary embolism in the postoperative patient), and treatment directed at primary myocardial insufficiency can lead to unnecessary delay and catastrophic results. Although identification of abnormalities causing mechanical obstruction to venous return or myocardial function must rest largely on clinical grounds, hemodynamic measurements may be of some benefit in that one may find a slow increase in cardiac output and arterial blood pressure accompanying the rising venous pressure produced by rapid fluid administration. This is in contrast to the picture usually seen in pure myocardial insufficiency, in which the cardiac output frequently falls in the face of a rising venous pressure. The rise in cardiac output probably occurs because the rising venous pressure is partially effective in overcoming the obstruction and maintaining a nearer to normal cardiac filling.

It has been demonstrated that with myocardial injury and after cardiac surgery, differences in functional reserve of the two ventricles occur and the central venous pressure alone loses a great deal of its reliability. Thus in these patients the use of pulmonary artery pressure, pulmonary wedge pressure, and, when feasible, left atrial pressure have their greatest value. Left atrial pressure (or left ventricular end-diastolic pressure) is not necessarily the same as right atrial pressure (or central venous pressure, or right ventricular end-diastolic pressure) under these circumstances.

In patients with low cardiac output from low blood volume who also have certain forms of heart disease, left atrial pressure may be considerably higher than right atrial pressure. Examples of such conditions are mitral stenosis and insufficiency, aortic stenosis and insufficiency, severe hypertension, and coronary artery disease. In such patients, unless one is actually measuring left atrial pressure, rapid infusion should probably be stopped when right atrial or central venous pressure reaches 12 mmHg (150 mm saline solution). The relation between changes in atrial pressure and changes in stroke volume or cardiac output at relatively high atrial pressures is not known. In most patients, however, when atrial pressures are about 15 mmHg (230 mm saline solution), further increases do not seem to increase cardiac output. Thus when central venous or right atrial pressure is less than 6 mmHg (80 mm saline solution), augmentation of blood volume is indicated. As the infusion proceeds, if central venous pressure rises rapidly and there is little evidence of increase in cardiac output, the infusion should probably be discontinued as being ineffective.

ABNORMALITIES IN CONTRACTILITY

In the condition in which there is low cardiac output and high atrial pressures and in which tamponade and ventricular outflow obstruction have been ruled out, there is probably an acute reduction of myocardial contractility. Treatment must therefore be directed toward improving contractility.

1. *Digitalis.* If time permits, digitalis is given, and digoxin is recommended. The estimated digitalizing dose given intravenously to a child or adult is 0.9 mg/m^2 of body surface area (1.5 mg for average adult). During digitalization, it is important to note that hypokalemia, hypercalcemia, and shock tend to increase the sensitivity of the heart to digitalis. Half or two-thirds of this may be given initially intravenously. An effect can be seen in 10 to 20 min, and the peak effect is reached in about 2 h. After 1 to 3 h, if no contraindication develops and further effect is desired, an additional one-sixth of the estimated digitalizing dose is given. This may be repeated after another 2 to 3 h. In less acute situations the same drug may be given orally; the digitalizing dose is then 1 mg/m^2. The estimated daily maintenance dose is one-quarter of the estimated digitalizing dose, usually given in divided doses.

2. *Inotropic Agents.* Dopamine in doses of 5 to 25 μg/(kg · min) intravenously may help restore the mean arterial blood pressure to a level of 70 to 80 mmHg to ensure adequate flow through cerebral and coronary vessels, particularly if they are partially occluded. The use of dopamine may result in an increase in cardiac output, without inducing an undesirable tachycardia. In doses less than 25 μg/(kg · min), there is either no change or a slight decrease in systemic vascular resistance and an increase in renal blood flow. At higher doses, alpha-adrenergic effects become predominant, resulting in systemic vasoconstriction and a decrease in renal blood flow.

Isoproterenol is rarely used today, particularly in patients with acute myocardial infarction, since it tends to increase myocardial oxygen consumption more than it increases coronary blood flow. In addition, it is not infrequently associated with tachyarrhythmias, particularly in a patient who has been digitalized.

The use of a vasopressor such as norepinephrine to

maintain a mean arterial blood pressure of approximately 70 to 75 mmHg may occasionally be indicated when other therapy has failed, including the use of dopamine.

Prior to treating patients with low cardiac output and high atrial pressures with these drugs on the basis that the cause is poor myocardial contractility, one must rule out pericardial tamponade. If high intrapericardial pressure exists in patients with high atrial and ventricular end-diastolic pressure, transmural pressure is low, and the poor output is due to end-diastolic ventricular volume and fiber length. The treatment is relief of the pericardial tamponade, which is about the only acute cause of high atrial pressures and small end-diastolic ventricular volume. A clinical analysis and chest x-ray are helpful in establishing the diagnosis. The presence of a paradoxic pulse should suggest strongly the presence of tamponade, and needle aspiration or open pericardiotomy is indicated.

3. *Ganglionic Blocking Agents.* Some patients with low cardiac output and high atrial pressures have relatively high arterial blood pressure. Systemic arteriolar resistance is high (*afterload-load* resisting shortening of myocardial sarcomeres). In these circumstances systolic left ventricular pressure is relatively high, as is systolic ventricular wall stress. Theoretically, reducing arterial blood pressure and systolic ventricular wall stress increases cardiac output. This can be done with an agent such as sodium nitroprusside. One should measure cardiac output before and during administration of this drug, and only if a significant increase in cardiac output has accompanied the decrease in arterial blood pressure should the drug be continued. Because of present uncertainties with the use of vasodilators (such as the effect on coronary, cerebral, liver, and renal blood flow) in this situation, it should be given only under special circumstances, and generally not in patients with hypovolemia.

In summary, attempts to diagnose and treat extramyocardial causes such as cardiac tamponade and pulmonary embolus should be made early in the course of cardiogenic shock. If the cause of shock is from primary failure of the myocardium as seen following acute myocardial infarction, the following modified guidelines suggested by Johnson and Gunnar seem reasonable.

After the diagnosis of cardiogenic shock has been made, an arterial line to measure direct arterial pressure and arterial blood gases, a Swan-Ganz catheter for measuring pulmonary artery and wedge pressures, and a Foley catheter should be inserted. Measurements of cardiac output by the thermal dilution technique can also be made using a specially constructed Swan-Ganz catheter. The response to treatment can then be effectively monitored by using these hemodynamic measurements.

1. If the patient is hypotensive and the wedge or pulmonary artery diastolic pressure is low, volume expansion with a suitable fluid is initiated.

2. If arterial pressure is low but pulmonary wedge pressure is 18 mmHg or above, an infusion of dopamine or dobutamine should be started. Dopamine is the preferable agent if arterial blood pressure can be maintained with low dosage levels without excessive tachycardia.

3. If the arterial systolic blood pressure is above 110 mmHg, the wedge pressure is above 18 mmHg, and there are signs of intense vasoconstriction with inadequate tissue perfusion, the cautious use of sodium nitroprusside may be indicated. It is emphasized that this form of therapy can be quite dangerous and careful monitoring of the effects of this agent is absolutely mandatory.

4. If the arterial pressure can be maintained with dopamine but wedge pressure remains elevated, the patient should be digitalized slowly and preload reduction considered.

5. If the patient's condition does not stabilize rapidly or if increasing amounts of pressor agents are necessary to maintain arterial pressure, and if the pulmonary wedge pressure remains elevated, the use of intraaortic balloon counterpulsation and cardiac catheterization should be considered.

Mechanical Assistance

The use of intraaortic balloon counterpulsation to maintain circulation in patients with severe cardiogenic shock due to failure of the myocardium is an established and effective form of therapy. The use of mechanical assistance should be considered early in the course of a patient with an acute myocardial infarction and pump failure who does not respond to the usual pharmacologic manipulations. Intraaortic balloon assistance can offer excellent temporary support of the circulation without increasing oxygen demands of the myocardium. While the patient is being supported in this manner, attempts should be made to find surgically correctable causes for the failure by evaluation of coronary artery anatomy and ventricular function. Patients not considered salvageable in the past may obtain excellent functional results with well-timed cardiac surgery following stabilization with the intraaortic balloon assistance device.

ABNORMALITIES IN RATE

Rapid ventricular rates (over 150 to 180 beats/min) are usually deleterious to cardiac output. Ventricular end-diastolic pressure is small because of the short period of ventricular filling with tachycardia, and ventricular extensibility is probably decreased because ventricular relaxation is not complete by the end of the extremely short diastolic period. Both tend to reduce stroke volume more than can be compensated for by the rapid heart rate, and cardiac output falls. If atrial fibrillation is the cardiac mechanism, digoxin is the drug of choice. Atrial flutter is more difficult to treat but should likewise be treated with digoxin. If no progress has been achieved with the drug after two-thirds of the digitalizing dose has been given, electroversion should be considered. Atrial tachycardia and premature atrial contractions as causes of excessively rapid heart rates are still more difficult to treat. Propranolol (Inderal) has been used with considerable success when the tachycardia was due to a resistant sinus tachycardia. Similarly, verapamil (Isoptin) has been used successfully for resistant tachyarrhythmias that are of atrial origin.

PVCs may on occasion cause fast ventricular rates.

Their tendency to cause ventricular fibrillation is of even greater concern. Lidocaine (Xylocaine) should be given intravenously in a single injection of 50 mg. If further lidocaine is needed, a solution containing 2 mg/mL of lidocaine can be given (1 to 4 mg/min) continuously. If it is used excessively, central nervous system irritability and depression of myocardial contractility may result. If protection against premature ventricular contractions is needed later, Pronestyl (procainamide hydrochloride) can be given orally in doses of 250 to 500 mg every 3 h. Bretylium tosylate has been useful in treating any resistant ventricular arrhythmias.

Low output associated with ventricular rates of less than 60 to 70 beats/min may occur in patients in whom cardiac performance is impaired. Because the myocardium is impaired, stroke volume cannot increase sufficiently to compensate for the slow rate. Regardless of whether the mechanism is sinus rhythm, atrial fibrillation with slow ventricular rate (too much digitalis or too little potassium), or complete atrioventricular dissociation, electrical pacing of the heart at a rate of 80 to 110 beats/min is advantageous. If there is a sinus mechanism, atrial pacing is preferred. Otherwise, direct ventricular pacing is indicated.

Neurogenic Shock

Neurogenic shock, or, by the older classification, "primary shock," is that form of shock which follows serious interference with the balance of vasodilator and vasoconstrictor influences to both arterioles and venules. This is the shock that is seen with clinical syncope, as with sudden exposure to unpleasant events such as the sight of blood, the hearing of bad tidings, or even the sudden onset of pain. Similarly, neurogenic shock is often observed with serious paralysis of vasomotor influences, as in high spinal anesthesia. The reflex interruption of nerve impulses also occurs with acute gastric dilatation.

The clinical picture of neurogenic shock is quite different from that classically seen in oligemic or hypovolemic shock. While the blood pressure may be extremely low, the pulse rate is usually slower than normal and is accompanied by dry, warm, and even flushed skin. Measurements made during neurogenic shock indicate a reduction in cardiac output, but this is accompanied by a decrease in resistance of arteriolar vessels as well as a decrease in the venous tone. Consequently there appears to be a normovolemic state with a greatly increased reservoir capacity in both arterioles and venules, thereby inducing a decreased venous return to the right side of the heart and subsequently a reduction in cardiac output.

If neurogenic shock is not corrected, a reduction of blood flow to the kidneys and damage to the brain result, and subsequently all the ravages of hypovolemic shock appear. Fortunately, treatment of neurogenic shock is usually obvious. Gastric dilatation can be rapidly treated with nasogastric suction. Shock in high spinal anesthesia can be treated effectively with a vasopressor such as ephedrine or phenylephrine (Neo-Synephrine), which will increase cardiac output as well as produce peripheral vasoconstriction. With the milder forms of neurogenic shock, such as fainting, simply removing the patient from the stimulus or relieving the pain will in itself be adequate therapy so that the vasoconstrictor nerves may regain the ability to maintain normal arteriolar and venous resistance.

There is rarely need for hemodynamic measurement in this usually benign and frequently self-limited form of hypotension. The exception to this occurs when this form of shock results from injury, as with spinal cord transection from trauma. In this instance there may be significant loss of blood and extracellular fluid into the area of injury surrounding the cord and vertebral column. Considerable confusion can arise as to the relative need for fluid replacement, as opposed to the need for vasopressor drugs, under these circumstances. Similarly, if surgical intervention for any reason becomes necessary, hemodynamic measurements may be of great value in the management of these patients. In uncomplicated neurogenic shock, central venous pressure should be normal or slightly low, with a normal or elevated cardiac output. If hypovolemia ensues, central venous pressure decreases, as does cardiac output. Thus, careful monitoring of central venous pressure may be necessary. Fluid administration without vasopressors in this form of hypotension may produce a gradually rising arterial pressure and cardiac output without elevation of central venous pressure, by gradually "filling" the expanded vascular pool; therefore, caution must be utilized during fluid administration.

In management of these patients balancing the two forms of therapy, slight volume overexpansion is much less deleterious than excessive vasopressor administration. The latter decreases organ perfusion in the presence of inadequate fluid replacement. Balance can best be obtained by maintaining a normal central venous pressure that rises slightly with rapid fluid administration (thus ensuring adequate volume) and using a vasopressor such as phenylephrine judiciously to support arterial pressure.

Septic Shock

During the past several years there has been a progressive increase in the incidence of shock secondary to sepsis, and the mortality rate remains in excess of 50 percent. This has occurred despite a better understanding of this entity, use of newer treatment regimens, and development of more potent antimicrobial agents. The most frequent causative organisms are gram-positive and gram-negative bacteria, although any agent capable of producing infection (including viruses, parasites, fungi, and rickettsiae) may initiate septic shock. Because of effective antibiotic control of most gram-positive infections, the majority of septic processes that result in shock are now caused by gram-negative bacteria. Among other causes, Altemeier and associates attribute this rising incidence of gram-negative sepsis to (1) the widespread use of antibiotics, with development of a reservoir of virulent and resistant organisms; (2) concentration in hospitals of large numbers of patients with established infections; (3) more extensive operations on elderly and poor-risk patients; (4) an increasing number of patients suffering from severe trauma; and (5) the use of steroids and immunosuppressive and anticancer agents.

GRAM-POSITIVE SEPSIS AND SHOCK

The shock state may be caused by gram-positive infections that produce massive fluid losses (necrotizing fasciitis) by dissemination of a potent exotoxin without evident bacteremia *(Clostridium perfringens, Clostridium tetani)* or, most often, by a fulminating infection from staphylococcus, streptococcus, or pneumococcus organisms. In the latter instance, shock is theoretically related to the release of exotoxins that many strains of staphylococcus and streptococcus (but not pneumococcus) are known to produce. The hemodynamic changes that occur are different from those seen in shock due to gram-negative organisms. Kwaan and Weil have noted hypotension of comparable severity in shock from both gram-positive and gram-negative infections, but their patients with gram-positive infections failed to show the other clinical manifestations of shock. Arterial resistance fell, but there was little or no reduction in cardiac output even with progressive hypotension. Urine flow was normal, sensorium clear, and perfusion of other organs was not grossly impaired, since neither acidosis nor a significant increase in serum lactic acid concentration appeared.

Treatment consists in the use of appropriate antibiotics, surgical drainage when indicated, and correction of any fluid volume deficit. A rapid and favorable response may be anticipated in many patients, and survival is substantially better than with gram-negative infections.

GRAM-NEGATIVE SEPSIS AND SHOCK

Gram-negative sepsis as a cause of shock is a more frequent and difficult problem. The highest incidence occurs during the seventh and eighth decades of life, and the response to treatment depends to a large extent on the age and previous health of the patient. There have been significant advances in the understanding of this entity, although much of the available information is still subject to controversy.

SOURCE. The most frequent source of gram-negative infections is the genitourinary system; almost half the patients have had an associated operation or instrumentation of the urinary tract. The second most frequent site of origin is the respiratory system, and many of the patients have an associated tracheostomy. Next in frequency is the alimentary system, with diseases such as peritonitis, intraabdominal abscess, and biliary tract infections; and then diseases of the integument, including burns and soft tissue infections. Indwelling venous catheters for monitoring and hyperalimentation are an increasing source of contamination, particularly with prolonged use. The reproductive system continues to be a significant source of infection (principally from septic abortions and postpartum infections), although the incidence is variable, depending on the hospital population.

The severity of septic shock varies considerably and appears to be a time-dose phenomenon, depending on the type and site of infection. For instance, mild hypotension following instrumentation of the genitourinary tract may represent nothing more than a transient bacteremia that is self-limited or responds to minimal therapy. In contrast, the patient with necrotizing pneumonia or multiple intraabdominal abscesses may have sepsis from an overwhelming number of organisms for a period of several days, and a much poorer prognosis. Similarly, the outlook is more favorable when the source of infection is accessible to surgical drainage, as in septic abortion, in which the infected products of conception can be removed readily. Variations in these factors must be considered when interpreting reported mortality rates and during the evaluation of new therapeutic regimens.

ASSOCIATED CONDITIONS. The presence of underlying disorders that limit cardiac, pulmonary, hepatic, or renal function increases the susceptibility to gram-negative infections and adversely affects the response to treatment. In Altemeier's reported series of 398 patients with gram-negative sepsis, almost half the patients had serious associated disease, including diabetes mellitus, malignant neoplasms, uremia, cirrhosis, burns, and malignant hematologic disorders. Of these conditions, cirrhosis of the liver appeared to have the most unfavorable prognosis. In addition, a small but significant number of patients were on corticosteroids or immunosuppressive agents, and corresponding mortality rates were 74 and 83 percent, respectively.

BACTERIOLOGY. The common causative organisms are similar to those found in the human gastrointestinal tract and include the coliform species and anaerobic bacilli. Recently the *Klebsiella*-Enterobacteriaceae-*Serratia* groups have been isolated with increasing frequency, and many are resistant to more conventional antibiotics. *Bacteroides* species are the predominant organisms in the fecal flora. These anaerobic organisms are difficult to culture and may account for a far greater number of infections than was previously reported. The majority of infections are caused by a single gram-negative organism, although in 10 to 20 percent of cases more than one organism may be isolated, particularly from intraabdominal sources. The isolates may be two or more gram-negative organisms or mixed cultures containing both gram-negative and gram-positive bacteria.

CLINICAL MANIFESTATIONS. Gram-negative infections are often recognized initially by the development of chills and elevated temperature above 101°F. The onset of shock may be abrupt and coincident with the signs and symptoms of sepsis or may occur several hours to days after recognition of an established infection. The complex hemodynamic abnormalities that follow are incompletely understood but are probably initiated by endotoxins from the cell walls of gram-negative bacteria. Intravenous injection of this lipopolysaccharide-protein complex into experimental animals will produce a shock state, but the hemodynamic responses vary in different animal species. The use of experimental animal models has contributed to our understanding of this entity, but direct extrapolation of the findings to human septic shock is difficult. A single injection of endotoxin into dogs causes pooling of blood in the splanchnic circulation, decreased venous return to the heart, reduction in cardiac output, and an abrupt fall in blood pressure. This initial response is transient and apparently due to hepatic venous outflow obstruction. Shortly thereafter the blood pressure rises toward normal but then slowly declines over the next several hours until death of the animal. This pattern is different from that seen in the subhuman primate and in human beings. Injection of *E. coli* endotoxin into human volunteers has been shown to produce (1) no response; (2) chills, fever, and vasoconstriction; or (3) peripheral vasodilation and a rise in cardiac output. These observations emphasize our lack of understanding of the effects of gram-negative infections and septicemia on the human circulation and the need for the development of more realistic experimental animal models.

Clinically, the shock state may be characterized by a primary adrenergic response, as seen in hypovolemic shock, with hypotension, peripheral vasoconstriction, and cold, clammy extremities. Earlier in the course, however, there may be an absence of adrenergic effects, with warm, dry extremities and decreased peripheral resistance. These diverse responses, presumably to the same stimulus, have led to a considerable amount of confusion over the clinical manifestations of septic shock, although a report by MacLean and associates tends to shed some light on this subject. They have noted two distinct hemodynamic patterns, depending on the volume status of the patient, and believe that the natural history of septic shock is one of progression from respiratory alkalosis to metabolic acidosis. A syndrome of early septic shock occurs in patients who are *normovolemic* prior to onset of sepsis and exhibit a hyperdynamic circulatory pattern characterized by (1) hypotension, (2) high cardiac output, (3) normal or increased blood volume, (4) normal or high central venous pressure, (5) low peripheral resistance, (6) warm, dry extremities, (7) hyperventilation, and (8) respiratory alkalosis. A typical patient with this pattern is the young, previously healthy person with a septic abortion. The high cardiac output is often associated with a decrease in oxygen utilization per unit flow, i.e., a narrowed arteriovenous oxygen difference. These findings can be explained by any of several mechanisms, but the two most likely possibilities are arteriovenous shunting and a primary cellular defect in the utilization of oxygen due to a direct effect of sepsis. In either case the presence of oliguria, altered sensorium, and blood lactate accumulation reflects the need for a further increase in flow despite the high cardiac output. MacLean suggests that treatment include measures to increase the cardiac output even more, combined with appropriate antibiotic therapy and early surgical drainage. In his series all but 4 of 28 patients with this hemodynamic pattern survived the episode of shock. If control of the infection is delayed or unsuccessful, the patient may pass into an acidotic phase with evidence of cellular damage (narrowing arteriovenous oxygen difference, decreasing oxygen consumption) and become refractory to further therapy.

In contrast, if septic shock develops in a patient who is *hypovolemic,* a hypodynamic pattern emerges characterized by (1) hypotension, (2) low cardiac output, (3) high peripheral resistance, (4) low central venous pressure, and (5) cold, cyanotic extremities. This response is typically seen in a patient with strangulation obstruction of the small bowel and a moderate to severe extracellular fluid and plasma volume deficit. If seen early, these patients are also alkalotic and will respond favorably to treatment. In the absence of overt cardiac failure, prompt volume replacement will often increase cardiac output, and a more favorable hyperdynamic circulation may develop. If therapy to combat sepsis is delayed or unsuccessful, the patient will inevitably have cardiac and circulatory failure, with a low fixed cardiac output and a resistant metabolic acidosis. At this point the patient may not be salvageable.

Our own experience in the treatment of septic shock tends to confirm MacLean's findings, although the presence of a metabolic acidosis has not necessarily been an ominous finding. We have seen several patients with hypodynamic and hyperdynamic circulatory patterns and metabolic acidosis in the early phase who have responded satisfactorily to therapy. The clinical picture may also be influenced by the patient's ability to meet the increased circulatory requirements imposed by sepsis. The elderly patient with limited cardiac reserve may be unable to increase cardiac output and enter the hyperdynamic phase, even with prompt volume replacement and measures designed to increase cardiac efficiency. In this instance the typical adrenergic response may persist, and the patient may rapidly succumb to the disease process.

The laboratory tests of value for diagnosis will depend to a large extent on the specific disease causing sepsis. Generally, the white blood cell count is appropriately elevated, but in debilitated and hypovolemic patients, those on immunosuppressive agents, and those with overwhelming sepsis, the white blood cell count may be normal or low. However, there is usually a noticeable left shift in the white blood cell differential, with many immature cell types. A falling platelet count may be an early and sensitive indicator of gram-negative septicemia, particularly in pediatric and burn patients. It has been suggested that endotoxin reacts with platelets, producing platelet aggregates that are subsequently trapped in the microcirculation. Patients at risk for sepsis should have serial platelet counts; a fall in the platelet count below 150,000 suggests the presence of gram-negative septicemia, and measures to find and eradicate the source should be undertaken. Rarely, a sudden fall in the platelet count may be a manifestation of disseminated intravascular coagulation (DIC), a syndrome known to be initiated by several stimuli, including endotoxin.

Progressive pulmonary insufficiency is characteristically seen in many patients with septic shock. Mild hypoxia with compensatory hyperventilation and respiratory alkalosis are commonly seen early in the course of shock in the absence of clinical or x-ray evidence of pulmonary disease. The arterial desaturation has been attributed to a variety of causes, including the presence of physiologic arteriovenous shunts in the pulmonary circulation secondary to perfusion of atelectatic or nonaerated alveoli. Regardless of the cause, the picture is frequently that of rapid deterioration of pulmonary function, development of patchy infiltrates that become confluent, superimposed bacterial infection, severe hypoxemia, and death.

Finally, it is worth emphasizing that development of mild hyperventilation, respiratory alkalosis, and an altered sensorium may be the earliest signs of gram-negative infection. This triad may precede the usual signs and symptoms of sepsis by several hours to several days. The exact cause is not known, although the condition is thought to represent a primary response to bacteremia. Early recognition of these findings, followed by a prompt search for the source of infection, may allow proper diagnosis prior to the onset of shock.

TREATMENT. The only effective way to reduce mortality in septic shock is by prompt recognition and treatment of the associated infection prior to the onset of shock. Once shock occurs, the control of infection by early surgical debridement or drainage and use of appropriate antibiotics represents *definitive* therapy. Other recommended measures, including fluid replacement, steroid administration, and the use of vasoactive drugs, represent *adjunctive* forms of therapy and are useful to prepare the patient prior to surgical intervention or to support the patient until the infectious process is controlled. This point deserves special emphasis, since death of the patient is inevitable if the infection cannot be adequately controlled.

As soon as gram-negative sepsis and shock are apparent, a prompt and thorough search for the source of infection is made while instituting other supportive measures. Because of the multiple complicating factors that may accompany endotoxemia, the patient is preferably treated in an intensive care unit. Careful monitoring of direct arterial pressure, central venous pressure (preferably pulmonary artery and pulmonary wedge pressures measured via a Swan-Ganz catheter), urine output, and arterial and central venous blood gases may be essential for proper management.

If the infectious process is amenable to drainage, operation is performed as soon as possible after initial stabilization of the patient's condition. In some cases surgical debridement or drainage of the infection must be accomplished before the patient will respond. These procedures may be performed under local or general anesthesia. For example, a patient with ascending cholangitis and shock secondary to sepsis may respond temporarily to supportive treatment. Improvement may be short-lived, however, unless prompt drainage of the biliary tract is instituted. The importance of surgical drainage is emphasized by the experience of MacLean et al. in their treatment of 53 patients. Forty-eight percent of their patients with infections amenable to surgical drainage survived, while only 23 percent of those not amenable to surgical treatment survived. More recently, Fry et al. emphasized the importance of surgical drainage and/or debridement in patients with infections caused by *Bacteroides* species. In a group of 98 consecutive adult patients with positive blood cultures for a *Bacteroides* organism, 77 had a mechanically treatable cause; most were due to intraabdominal abscess or an acutely perforated viscus.

Antibiotic Therapy. The use of specific antibiotics based on appropriate cultures and sensitivity tests is desirable when possible. The results may not be available for several days, but useful information may be gained from previous wound and blood cultures obtained during an earlier phase of the septic process and Gram's stain of appropriate material. Antibiotics must often be chosen, however, on the basis of the suspected organisms and their previous sensitivity patterns. These patterns are sufficiently diverse to preclude selection of a single antibiotic agent that will be effective against all the potential pathogens.

At present an effective combination of antibiotics in our hospital population when gastrointestinal tract organisms are suspected includes cefazolin or penicillin and gentamicin. This combination is effective against a majority of gram-negative organisms, with the notable exception of *Bacteroides* species. If presence of these organisms is suspected, an antibiotic of known effectiveness (e.g., cefoxitin or metronidazole) should be added to the regimen. Other antibiotics that are currently receiving extensive trials include a variety of third-generation cephalosporins, piperacillin, and imipenim.

When culture and sensitivity reports are available, more specific antibiotic coverage may be initiated if the infection is not under control. Altemeier and associates reported a mortality rate of 54 percent from sepsis in patients receiving inappropriate antibiotics and 28 percent when appropriate antibiotics were given.

Fluid Replacement. Prompt correction of preexisting fluid deficits is essential. A majority of patients will incur fluid losses from the disease processes that initiate sepsis and shock. "Third space losses," with massive sequestration of plasma and extracellular fluid, are characteristic of many surgical conditions, including peritonitis, burns, strangulation obstruction of the bowel, and extensive soft tissue infections.

The type of fluid used will vary, although most "third space losses" are properly replaced with a balanced salt solution such as Ringer's lactate. Any deficits in red blood cell mass should be corrected by the administration of packed cells or whole blood in order to maintain optimal oxygen-carrying capacity of the blood. Large quantities of replacement fluids are often needed in order to maintain an effective circulating volume. However, a fine balance exists between the need for volume replacement and the harmful effects that fluid overload may have on lungs already injured by the septic process. In this regard, attempts to increase pulmonary capillary osmotic pressure by the infusion of large volumes of plasma or albumin, in the absence of a specific need, may be detrimental. Because of the increase in pulmonary capillary permeability associated with severe sepsis, the use of large quantities of colloid solutions may result in an increase in extravascular pulmonary water. Careful replacement of "third space losses" with crystalloid solutions on the basis of patient response and continuous monitoring of the central venous or pulmonary artery and pulmonary wedge pressures are indicated.

Properly interpreted, the central venous pressure (CVP) will give a reliable estimate of the ability of the right side of the heart to pump the blood delivered to it. It is best used as an upper-limit guide; a rapid increase in central venous pressure, regardless of the initial level, may indicate that fluid is being administered too rapidly or that the heart is unable to handle additional volume. If central venous pressure is below 10 cm of water, fluids may be administered as rapidly as tolerated. If central venous pressure is above this level, fluids are still administered but at a slower rate of infusion. The central venous pressure may fall as blood pressure rises, owing to better perfusion of the coronary arteries and improved myocardial function. An abrupt rise in the central venous pressure or a fall in arterial pressure may indicate inability of the heart to respond, and the use of drugs that increase myocardial performance should be considered in conjunction with the use of a Swan-Ganz catheter.

In these instances, measurement of the CVP alone during fluid resuscitation is not sufficient, since it gives no direct information regarding function of the left side of the heart. Insertion of a Swan-Ganz catheter for measurements of *both* pulmonary artery (PA) and pulmonary capillary wedge (PW) pressure, the latter a reflection of left ventricular end-diastolic pressure, is necessary. This is particularly true in patients on mechanical ventilation and positive end-expiratory pressure.

Many patients will respond favorably to fluid administration combined with prompt control of the infection with a rise in blood pressure, an increase in urine output, warming of the extremities, and clearing of the sensorium. In these instances no additional therapy may be indicated.

Steroids. The use of pharmacologic doses of corticosteroids in the treatment of septic shock is controversial. There is no direct evidence that steroids are beneficial in these cases, although favorable responses, with improvement in cardiac, pulmonary, and renal functions and better survival rates, have been reported. Large doses of steroids are known to exert a modest inotropic effect on the heart and produce mild peripheral vasodilation. Although these salutary effects may be desirable, there are other, more potent drugs available with similar actions. Others have suggested that steroids protect the cell and its contents from the effects of endotoxin, for example, by stabilizing cellular and lysosomal membranes. In a prospective study of 172 consecutive patients in septic shock, Schumer noted a mortality rate of 10.4 percent in the steroid-treated patients, compared with a mortality rate of 38.4 percent in patients not receiving steroids. In a retrospective study of an additional 328 patients, the results were similar. Although impressive, evidence regarding the beneficial effects of steroids remains presumptive, because of many variables present in the clinical situation, including causes, associated conditions, and treatment.

Steroids may be administered concomitant with volume replacement or reserved for use if the response to fluid administration is only temporary or produces a rapid rise in central venous pressure. Many dosage schedules have been recommended, and most stress the need for a large initial dose and cessation of therapy within 48 to 72 h. One regimen is based on guidelines suggested by Lillehei. An initial dose of 15 to 30 mg/kg of body weight of methylprednisolone (or equivalent dose of dexametha-

sone) is given intravenously over a 5- to 10-min period. The same dose may be repeated within 2 to 4 h if the desired effects have not been achieved. If a beneficial response is obtained, additional injections are not given unless the effects are only short-lived. When the drug is used in this manner, there is rarely a need for more than two doses. It should be noted, however, that the current studies on immunosuppression by steroids may show that this effect outweighs other possible benefits from steroid therapy.

Vasoactive Drugs. Vasopressor drugs with prominent alpha-adrenergic effects are of limited value in treatment of this type of shock, since artificial attempts to maintain blood pressure without regard to flow are potentially harmful. Furthermore, they are probably contraindicated in hypovolemic patients with increased peripheral resistance, in view of the known deleterious effects of prolonged vasoconstriction. Beneficial effects attributed to these agents are probably due to their inotropic effects on the heart, although better drugs are available for this purpose. Rarely, use of vasoactive drugs with mixed alpha- and beta-adrenergic effects may be indicated in a patient with an elevated cardiac output and pronounced hypotension due to very low peripheral resistance. The increase in resistance (and slight increase in cardiac output) may produce a desired rise in blood pressure and improvement in flow.

Vasodilator drugs such as phenoxybenzamine have enjoyed some popularity, particularly when combined with additional fluid administration. Their use is based in part on improved survival of dogs when vasodilator drugs are given prior to the onset of endotoxic shock. These observations probably represent a specific canine response and cannot be directly extrapolated to human septic shock. Vasodilator agents have also been used in conjunction with adrenergic agents (for their inotropic effects), but data on their usefulness are limited.

Since the heart is frequently unable to meet the increased circulatory demands of sepsis, the use of an inotropic agent such as isoproterenol or dopamine would seem ideal when volume replacement and other measures have failed to restore adequate circulation. Dopamine, a naturally occurring catecholamine biochemical precursor of norepinephrine, is similar to isoproterenol in exerting positive inotropic and chronotropic effects on the heart by stimulation of beta-adrenergic receptors. Because of its lower potential for tachyarrhythmias and the ability to enhance renal blood flow when infused at a dose below 3 µg/(kg · min), dopamine has virtually replaced isoproterenol as the agent of choice.

In summary, a "polypharmacy" approach is discouraged, although proper selection and use of vasoactive drugs may offer needed support until infection can be controlled or eradicated. If eradication is not possible, response to any of these drugs is only temporary. Determination of cardiac output, combined with arterial, pulmonary artery, and pulmonary wedge pressure measurements can be of great benefit in establishing the nature of the hemodynamic alterations and evaluating responses to therapy.

Digitalis. Although both Hinshaw and Greenfield have

shown that digitalis can prevent or reverse heart failure in animals following endotoxin injection, the clinical importance of this finding has yet to be established. We have not routinely administered digitalis to patients in septic shock in the absence of specific indications. Gram-negative sepsis and shock frequently occur in older patients with congestive failure or may precipitate cardiac failure in patients with limited cardiac reserve. In these instances digitalis can be administered cautiously in full doses, although toxicity may occur if the patient is hypokalemic or receiving isoproterenol.

Pulmonary Therapy. Many patients with sepsis and shock will develop significant pulmonary insufficiency and require maintenance of a controlled airway (via nasotracheal or endotracheal intubation) and assisted ventilation. (For a discussion of the adult respiratory distress syndrome as related to sepsis and the management of patients requiring ventilatory support, the reader is referred to the section Pulmonary Responses.)

Since inadequate tissue oxygenation is a consistent feature of shock, attention to all components of the oxygen transport system is essential (see the section Oxygen Transport). Efforts to maintain a normal or rightward-positioned oxygen/hemoglobin dissociation curve may be particularly important in view of reported reductions in red blood cell organic phosphates in late septic shock.

Bibliography

Clinical and Physiologic Manifestations of Shock

Baue AE, Wurth MS, Sayeed MM: The dynamics of altered ATP-dependent and ATP-yielding cell processes in shock. *Surgery* 72:94, 1972.

Bessey PQ, Brooks DC, Black PR: Epinephrine acutely mediates skeletal muscle insuline resistance. *Surgery* 94:172, 1983.

Blalock A: Shock: Further studies with particular reference to effects of hemorrhage. *Arch Surg* 29:837, 1937.

Blalock A: *Principles of Surgical Care, Shock and Other Problems.* St Louis, CV Mosby, 1940.

Canizaro PC, Prager MD, Shires GT: The infusion of Ringer's lactate solution during shock. *Am J Surg* 122:494, 1971.

Carey LC, Lowery BD, Cloutier CT: Treatment of acidosis. *Curr Probl Surg,* p 37, January 1971.

Gann DS, Carlson DE, et al: Impaired restitution of blood volume after large hemorrhage. *J Trauma* 21:598, 1981.

Gann DS, Dallman MF, Engelund WC: Reflex control and modulation of ACTH and corticosteroid. *Int Rev Physiol* 24:157, 1981.

Gross SG: *A System of Surgery: Pathological, Diagnostic, Therapeutic and Operative.* Philadelphia, Lea & Febiger, 1872.

Hiebert JM, McCormick JM, Egdahl RH: Direct measurement of insulin secretory rate: Studies of shocked primates and postoperative patients. *Ann Surg* 176:296, 1972.

Marey EJ: Loi qui preside a la frequence des battements du coeur. *CR Acad Sci* 52:95, 1861.

Mela LM, Miller LD, Nicholas GG: Influence of cellular acidosis and altered cation concentrations on shock-induced mitochondrian damage. *Surgery* 72:102, 1972.

Moore FD: *Metabolic Care of the Surgical Patient.* Philadelphia, Saunders, 1959.

Shamoon HM, Hendler R, Sherwin RS: Synergistic interactions among anti-insulin hormones in the pathogenesis of stress hyperglycemia in humans. *J Clin Endocrinol Metab* 52:1235, 1981.

Shenkin HS, et al: On the diagnosis of hemorrhage in man: A study of volunteers bled large amounts. *Am J Med Sci* 208:421, 1944.

Sherwin RS, Sacca L: Effect of epinephrine on glucose metabolism in humans: Contribution of the liver. *Am J Physiol* 247:E157, 1984.

Shires GT: Principles and management of hemorrhagic shock, in Shires GT: *Principles of Trauma Care,* 3d ed. New York, McGraw-Hill, 1985, pp 3–43.

Simeone FA: Shock, in *Christopher's Textbook of Surgery.* Philadelphia, Saunders, 1964, p 58.

Wiggers CJ: Present status of shock problem. *Physiol Rev* 22:74, 1942.

Wiggers HC, Ingraham RC, et al: Vasoconstriction and the development of irreversible hemorrhagic shock. *Am J Physiol* 153:511, 1948.

Response of Extracellular Fluid

Albert S, Shires GT III, et al: Effects of naloxone in hemorrhagic shock. *Surg Gynecol Obstet* 155:326, 1982.

Campion DS, et al: The effect of hemorrhagic shock on transmembrane potential. *Surgery* 66:1051, 1969.

Conway EJ: Nature and significance of concentration relations of potassium and sodium ions in skeletal muscle. *Physiol Rev* 37:84, 1957.

Cunningham JN Jr, Shires GT, Wagner Y: Cellular transport defects in hemorrhagic shock. *Surgery* 70:215, 1971.

Cunningham JN Jr, Shires GT, Wagner Y: Changes in intracellular sodium and potassium content of red blood cells in trauma and shock. *Am J Surg* 122:650, 1971.

Goldman DE: Potential, impedance and rectification in membranes. *J Physiol* 27:37, 1943.

Hagberg S, Haljamas H, Rockert H: Shock reactions in skeletal muscle: III. The electrolyte content of tissue fluid and blood plasma before and after induced hemorrhagic shock. *Ann Surg* 168:243, 1968.

Hodgkin AL, Katz B: The effect of sodium ions on the electrical activity of the giant axon of the squid. *J Physiol* 108:37, 1949.

Illner HP, Shires GT: The effect of hemorrhagic shock on potassium transport in skeletal muscle. *Surg Gynecol Obstet* 150:17, 1980.

Ling G, Gerard RW: The normal membrane potential of frog sartorius fibers. *J Cell Sci* 34:383, 1949.

Mela LM, Miller LD, Nicholas GG: Influence of cellular acidosis and altered cation concentrations on shock-induced mitochondrian damage. *Surgery* 72:102, 1972.

Middleton ES, Mathews R, Shires GT: Radiosulphate as a measure of the extracellular fluid in acute hemorrhagic shock. *Ann Surg* 170:174, 1969.

Peitzman AB, Shires GT III, et al: Effect of intravenous ATP-MgCl₂ on cellular function in liver and muscle in hemorrhagic shock. *Curr Surg* 300, September–October 1981.

Schloerb PR, Sieracki L, et al: Intravenous adenosine triphosphate (ATP) in hemorrhagic shock in rats. *Am J Physiol* 240: (1): R52, January 1981.

Shires GT, et al: Alterations in cellular membrane function during hemorrhagic shock in primates. *Ann Surg* 176:288, 1972.

Shires GT, Brown FT, et al: Distributional changes in extracellular fluid during acute hemorrhagic shock. *Surg Forum* 11:115, 1960.

Shires GT, Brown FT, Canizaro PC: *Shock.* Philadelphia, Saunders, 1973, chap 4.

Wilde WS: The chloride equilibrium in muscle. *Am J Physiol* 143:666, 1945.

Renal Responses

Baxter CR, Zedlitz WH, Shires GT: High output acute renal failure complicating traumatic injury. *J Trauma* 4:567, 1964.

Bush HL: Renal considerations in the injured patient. *Surg Clin North Am* 62:133, 1983.

Flear CTG, Clarke R: The influence of blood loss and blood transfusion upon changes in the metabolism of water, electrolytes and nitrogen following civilian trauma. *Clin Sci* 14:575, 1955.

Gerrick S, Ledgerwood AM, Lucas CE: Post-resuscitation hypertension: A reappraisal. *Arch Surg* 115:1486, 1980.

Hermreck AS: The pathophysiology of acute renal failure. *Surgery* 144:605, 1982.

Ladd M: *Battle Casualties in Korea*, vol 4. U.S. Army Medical Service Graduate School, Walter Reed Army Medical Center, 1956, p 193.

Lucas CE: Renal considerations in the injured patient. *Surg Clin North Am* 62:133, 1982.

Lucas CE, Ledgerwood AM, Higgins RF: Impaired salt and water excretion after albumin resuscitation for hypovolemic shock. *Surgery* 86:544, 1979.

Lucas CE, Weaver D, et al: Effects of albumin versus non-albumin resuscitation on plasma volume and renal excretory function. *J Trauma* 18:564, 1978.

Lucas CE, Zito JG, Carter KM: Questionable value of furosemide in preventing renal failure. *Surgery* 82:314, 1977.

Miller TR, Anderson RJ, et al: Urinary diagnostic indices in acute renal failure; a prospective study. *Ann Med* 89:47, 1978.

Stein JH, Lifschitz MD, Barnes LD: Current concepts on the pathophysiology of acute renal failure. *Am J Physiol* 234:171, 1982.

Teschan PE, et al: Post-traumatic renal insufficiency in military casualties: I Clinical characteristics. *Am J Med* 18:172, 1955.

Teschan PE, Mason AD: Reproducible experimental acute renal failure in rats. *Clin Res* 6:155, 1958.

Weissman C, Rosenbaum LM, et al: Massive perioperative polyuria. *J Trauma* 22:1028, 1982.

Wright HK, Gann DS: Correction of defect in free water excretion in postoperative patients by extracellular fluid volume expansion. *Ann Surg* 158:70, 1963.

Pulmonary Responses

Ashbaugh DG, Petty TL: Sepsis complicating the acute respiratory distress syndrome. *Surg Gynecol Obstet* 135:865, 1972.

Bell RC, Coalson JJ, et al: Multiple organ system failure and infection in adult respiratory distress syndrome. *Ann Intern Med* 99:293, 1983.

Burford TH, Burbank B: Traumatic wet lung: Observations on certain physiologic fundamentals of thoracic trauma. *J Thorac Surg* 14:415, 1945.

Clauss RH, et al: Effects of changing body position upon improved ventilation-perfusion relationships. *Circulation* (suppl II-37)38:214, 1968.

Dahn MS, Lucas CE, et al: Negative inotropic effects of albumin resuscitation for shock. *Surgery* 86:235, 1979.

Demling RH, Manohar M, et al: The effect of plasma oncotic pressure on the pulmonary microcirculation after hemorrhagic shock. *Surgery* 86:323, 1979.

Fowler AA, Hamman RF, et al: Adult respiratory distress syndrome: Risk with common predispositions. *Ann Intern Med* 98:593, 1983.

Fulton RL, Jones CE: The cause of post-traumatic pulmonary insufficiency in man. *Surg Gynecol Obstet* 140:179, 1975.

Greenfield S, Teres D, et al: Prevention of gram negative bacillary pneumonia using aerosol polymyxin as prophylaxis: I. Effect on the colonization pattern of the upper respiratory tract of seriously ill patients. *J Clin Invest* 52:2935, 1973.

Harken AH, Brennan MF, et al: The hemodynamic response to positive end-expiratory ventilation in hypovolemic patients. *Surgery* 76:786, 1974.

Herman CM: Detection and management of intraabdominal sepsis in ICU patients: Indications and outcomes. *Infect Surg* 2:737, 757, 1983.

Holcroft JW, Trunkey DD: Pulmonary extravasation of albumin during and after hemorrhagic shock in baboons. *J Surg Res* 18:91, 1975.

Horvitz JH, Carrico CJ, Shires GT: Pulmonary response to major injury. *Arch Surg* 108:349, 1974.

Liebman PR, Patten MT, et al: The mechanism of depressed cardiac output on positive end-expiratory pressure (PEEP). *Surgery* 83:594, 1978.

Lowe RJ, Moss GS, et al: Crystalloid vs. colloid in the etiology of pulmonary failure after trauma. A randomized trial in man. *Surgery* 81:676, 1977.

Lucas CE, Ledgerwood AM, Higgins RF: Impaired salt and water excretion after albumin resuscitation for hypovolemic shock. *Surgery* 86:544, 1979.

Mendelson CL: The aspiration of stomach content into the lungs during obstetric anesthesia. *Am J Obstet Gynecol* 52:191, 1946.

Montgomery AB, Stager MA, et al: Causes of mortality associated with the adult respiratory distress syndrome. *Am Rev Respir Dis* 132:485, 1985.

Moore FD, et al: *Post-traumatic Pulmonary Insufficiency*. Philadelphia, Saunders, 1969.

Pepe PE, Potkin RT, et al: Clinical predictors of the adult respiratory distress syndrome. *Am J Surg* 144:124, 1982.

Pepe PE, Hudson LD, Carrico CJ: Early application of positive end-expiratory pressure in patients at risk for the adult respiratory distress syndrome. *N Engl J Med* 311:281, 1984.

Peters RM, et al: Objective indications for respiratory therapy in post-trauma and post-operative patients. *Am J Surg* 124:262, 1972.

Pontoppidan H, et al: Acute respiratory failure in adults. *N Engl J Med* 287:690, 1972.

Robertson HT, Lakshminarayan S, Hudson LD: Lung injury following a 50 metre fall into water. *Thorax* 33:175, 1978.

Roscher R, Bittner R, et al: Pulmonary contusion: Clinical experience. *Arch Surg* 109:508, 1974.

Schwartz DJ, Wynne JW, et al: Pulmonary consequences of aspiration of gastric contents at pH values greater than 2.5. *Am Rev Respir Dis* 121:119, 1980.

Sinanan M, Maier RV, Carrico CJ: Laparotomy for intraabdominal sepsis in ICU patients: Indications and outcome. *Arch Surg* 119:652, 1984.

Staub NC: The forces regulating fluid filtration in the lung. *Microvas Res* 15:45, 1978.

Stothert JC, Weaver J, et al: Pulmonary vascular permeability after acid aspiration. *Surg Forum* 31:237, 1980.

Sturm JA, Carpenter MA, et al: Water and protein movement in the sheep lung after septic shock. Effect of colloid versus crystalloid resuscitation. *J Surg Res* 26:233, 1979.

Virgilio RW, Matildi LA, et al: Colloid vs. crystalloid volume resuscitation of patients with severe pulmonary insufficiency. *Surg Forum* 30:166, 1979.

Virgilio RW, Rice CL, et al: Crystalloid vs. colloid resuscitation. Is one better? *Surgery* 85:129, 1979.

Wahrenbrock ET: The effect of posture on pulmonary function and survival of anesthetized dogs. *J Surg Res* 10:13, 1970.

Weighelt JA, Mitchell RA, Snyder WH: Early positive end-expiratory pressure in the adult respiratory distress syndrome. *Arch Surg* 114:497, 1979.

Alterations in Oxygen Transport

Bellingham AJ, Detter JC, Lenfant C: Regulatory mechanisms of hemoglobin oxygen affinity in acidosis and alkalosis. *J Clin Invest* 50:700, 1971.

Benesch R, Benesch RE: The effect of organic phosphates from the human erythrocyte on the allosteric properties of hemoglobin. *Biochem Biophys Res Commun* 26:162, 1967.

Berne RM, Blackman JR, Gardner TH: Hypoxemia and coronary blood flow. *J Clin Invest* 36:1101, 1957.

Bowen JC, Fleming WH: Increased oxyhemoglobin affinity after transfusion of stored blood. *Ann Surg* 180:760, 1974.

Bunn HF, May MH, et al: Hemoglobin function in stored blood. *J Clin Invest* 48:311, 1969.

Canizaro, PC: Oxygen transport in shock, in Shires GT (ed): *Shock and Related Problems, Clinical Surgery International*. New York, Churchill Livingstone, 1984, vol 9, pp 127–147.

Canizaro PC, Nelson JL, et al: A technique for estimating the position of the oxygen-hemoglobin dissociation curve. *Ann Surg* 180:364, 1974.

Chaunutin A, Curnish RR: Effect of organic and inorganic phosphates on the oxygen equilibrium of human erythrocytes. *Arch Biochem Biophys* 121:96, 1967.

Collins JA: Problems associated with the massive transfusion of stored blood. *Surgery* 75:274, 1974.

Collins JA: Problems and perspectives in surgical hemotherapy. *Bibl Haematologica* 46:241, 1980.

Dennis RC, Vito L, et al: Improved myocardial performance following high 2-3 diphosphoglycerate red cell transfusions. *Surgery* 77:741, 1975.

Duvelleroy MA, Mehmel HC, Laver MB: Hemoglobin-oxygen equilibrium and coronary blood flow. *J Appl Physiol* 35:480, 1973.

Feola M, Gonzalez HF, et al: Development of a bovine stroma-free hemoglobin solution as a blood substitute. *Surg Gynecol Obstet* 157:399, 1983.

Fry DE, Woods M: The influence of oxyhemoglobin affinity on tissue oxygen consumption. *Ann Surg* 183:130, 1976.

Gould SA, Rosen AL, et al: Fluosol-DA as a red cell substitute in acute anemia. *N Engl J Med* 314(26):1653, 1986.

Harken AH: The surgical significance of the oxyhemoglobin dissociation curve. *Surg Gynecol Obstet* 144:935, 1977.

Holcroft JW, Trunkey DD: Extravascular lung water following hemorrhagic shock in the baboon; Comparison between resuscitation with Ringer's lactate and plasmanate. *Ann Surg* 180:408, 1974.

Hoyt DB, Greenburg AG, et al: Resuscitation with fluosol-DA 20%-tolerance to sepsis. *J Trauma* 26:8, 713, 1986.

Kalter ES, Carlson RW, Thijs LG: Effects of methylprednisolone on hemodynamics, arteriovenous oxygen difference, P$_{50}$, and 2,3-DPG in bacterial shock: A preliminary study. *Crit Care Med* 10:662, 1982.

Kovalik SG, Ledgerwood AM, et al: The cardiac effect of altered calcium homeostasis after albumin resuscitation. *J Trauma* 21:275, 1981.

Lenfant C, et al: Effects of altitude on oxygen binding by hemoglobin and on organic phosphate levels. *J Clin Invest* 47:2652, 1968.

Lenfant C, Ways P, Aucutt C: Effect of chronic hypoxic hypoxia on the O$_2$-Hb dissociation curve and respiratory gas transport in man. *Respir Physiol* 7:7, 1969.

Lucas CE, Ledgerwood AM, Huggins RF: Impaired salt and water excretion after albumin resuscitation for hypovolemic shock. *Surgery* 86:544, 1979.

Metsuno T, Ohyanagi H, Naito R: Clinical studies of a perfluorochemical whole blood substitute (Fluosol-DA). *Ann Surg* 195:60, 1982.

Opitz E, Schneider M: Über die Sauerstoffversorgung des Gehirns und den Mechanismus von Mangelverhungerung. *Ergeb Physiol* 46:126, 1950.

Oski FA, et al: The *in vitro* restoration of red cell 2,3-diphosphoglycerate levels in banked blood. *Blood* 37:52, 1971.

Oski FA, Marshal BE, et al: Exercise with anemia, the role of the left shifted or right shifted oxygen-hemoglobin equilibrium curve. *Ann Intern Med* 74:44, 1971.

Proctor HJ, Parker JC, et al: Treatment of severe hypoxia with red cells high in 2,3-diphosphoglycerate. *J Trauma* 13:340, 1973.

Severinghaus JW: Blood gas calculator. *J Appl Physiol* 21:1108, 1966.

Tremper KK, Friedman AE, et al: The preoperative treatment of severely anemic patients with a perfluorochemical oxygen-transport fluid, Fluosol-DA. *N Engl J Med* 307:277, 1982.

Valeri CR, Hirsch NM: Restoration *in vivo* of erythrocyte adenosine triphosphate, 2,3-diphosphoglycerate, potassium ion, and sodium ion concentrations following the transfusion of acid-citrate-dextrose-stored human red blood cells. *J Lab Clin Med* 73:722, 1969.

Valeri CR, Zaroulis CG: Rejuvenation and freezing of outdated stored human red cells. *N Engl J Med* 287:1307, 1972.

Woodson RD, Wranne B, Detter JC: Effect of increased blood oxygen affinity on work performance in rats. *J Clin Invest* 52:2717, 1973.

Therapy of Shock

Aeder MI, Crowe JP, et al: Technical limitations in the rapid infusion of intravenous fluids. *Ann Emerg Med* 14:307, 1985.

Altemeier WA, Todd JC, Inge WW: Gramnegative septicemia: A growing threat. *Ann Surg* 166:530, 1967.

Beecher HK: Preparation of battle casualties for surgery. *Ann Surg* 121:769, 1945.

Blaisdel FW: Controversy in shock research. Con: The role of steroids in septic shock. 8:673, 1981.

Canizaro PC, Praeger MD, Shires GT: The infusion of Ringer's lactate solution during shock. *Am J Surg* 122:494, 1971.

Civetta JM: A new look at the Starling equation. *Crit Care Med* 7(3):84, 1979.

Forrester JS, Diamond G, Chatterjee K: Medical therapy of acute myocardial infarction by application of hemodynamic subsets. *N Engl J Med* 295:1356, 1976.

Guntheroth WG, Abel FL, Mullins GL: The effect of Trendelenburg's position on blood pressure and carotid blood flow. *Surg Gynecol Obstet* 119:345, 1964.

Hagman CF, Bagge L, Thoren L: The use of blood components in surgical transfusion therapy. *World J Surg* 11, 2, 1987.

Holcroft JW: Impairment of venous return in hemorrhagic shock. *Surg Clin North Am* 62:25, 1982.

Holcroft JW, Trunkey DD: Further analysis of lung water in baboons resuscitated from hemorrhagic shock. *J Surg Res* 20:291, 1976.

Johnson SA, Gunnar RM: Treatment of shock in myocardial infarction. *JAMA* 237:2106, 1977.

Kolff J, Deeb GM: Artificial heart and left ventricular assist devices. *Surg Clin North Am* 65:3, 1985.

Krausz MM, Perel A, et al: Cardiopulmonary effects of volume loading in patients in septic shock. *Ann Surg* 185:429, 1977.

Loeb HS, Winslow EBJ, et al: Acute hemodynamic effects of dopamine in patients with shock. *Circulation* 44:163, 1971.

Lucas CE, Ledgerwood AM: The cardiopulmonary response to massive dose of steroids in patients with septic shock. *Arch Surg* 119:537, 1984.

Lucas CE, Ledgerwood AM, et al: Impaired pulmonary function after albumin resuscitation from shock. *J Trauma* 20:446, 1980.

MacLean LD, Mulligan WG, et al: Patterns of septic shock in man: A detailed study of 56 patients. *Ann Surg* 166:543, 1967.

Maier RV, Carrizo CJ: Development in the resuscitation of critically ill surgical patients, in Mannick JA, et al (eds): *Advances in Surgery*. Chicago, Year Book Medical Publishers, 1986, vol 19, pp 271–328.

Mason DT: Afterload reduction and cardiac performance: Physiological basis of systemic vasodilators as a new approach in treatment of congestive heart failure. *Am J Med* 65:106, 1978.

Messmer K: Blood substitutes in shock therapy, in Shires GT (ed): *Shock and Related Problems, Clinical Surgery International*. New York, Churchill Livingstone, 1984, vol 9, pp 192–205.

Myers ML, Austin TW, Sibbald WJ: Pulmonary artery catheter infections: A prospective study. *Ann Surg* 201:237, 1985.

Nelson LD: Continuous venous oximetry in surgical patients. *Ann Surg* 203:329, 1986.

Niarchos AP: Management of cardiovascular problems in the trauma patient, in Shires GT (ed): *Principles of Trauma Care*. New York, McGraw-Hill, 1985.

Schumer W: Controversy in shock research. Pro: The role of steroids in septic shock. *Circ Shock* 8:667, 1981.

Shatney CH, Deepika K, Militello PR: Efficacy of hetastarch in the resuscitation of patients with multisystem trauma and shock. *Arch Surg* 118:804, 1983.

Shires GT, Shires GT III: Hypovolemic shock, in Shires GT (ed): *Shock and Related Problems, Clinical Surgery International*. New York, Churchill Livingstone, 1984, vol 9, pp. 127–147.

Sprung CL, Caralis PV, Marcial EH: The effects of high dose corticosteroids in patients with septic shock. *N Engl J Med* 311:1137, 1984.

Swan HJC, et al: Catheterization of the heart in man with use of a flow-directed balloon-tipped catheter. *N Engl J Med* 283:447, 1970.

Trinkle JK, Rush BE, Eiseman B: Metabolism of lactate following major blood loss. *Surgery* 63:782, 1968.

Valeri CR: Optimal use of blood products in the treatment of hemorrhagic shock. *Surg Rounds* 4:38, 1981.

Wright CJ, Duff JH, et al: Regional capillary blood flow and oxygen uptake in severe sepsis. *Surg Gynecol Obstet* 132:637, 1971.

Chapter 5

Infections

Isidore Cohn, Jr., and George H. Bornside

INTRODUCTION

Infection is a dynamic process involving invasion of the body by pathogenic microorganisms and reaction of the tissues to organisms and their toxins. Soon after birth, a variety of microorganisms colonize the external and internal surfaces of the human body. This indigenous microflora usually does no harm; it produces no detectable pathologic effects in tissues and may be beneficial. Indeed, the normal intestinal flora functions as a barrier providing natural resistance against enteric infections with pathogens such as *Salmonella* and *Shigella* species.

Infection evolves into overt disease only when the equilibrium between host and parasite is upset. Of the thousands of species of microorganisms in nature, only a few hundred are known to be pathogenic for human beings.

Current thinking concerning clinical disease resulting from host and parasite interrelationships recognizes the role of the general health of the host, the previous contact with infectious microorganisms, the past clinical history, and various insults (toxic, traumatic, or therapeutic) of nonmicrobial origin. When the host's resistance is lowered, the indigenous microflora can become involved in infectious disease. This presents a dilemma to both the clinician and the microbiologist, as it must be decided which of the several microorganisms usually isolated from a clinical specimen are involved in the patient's disease. There are very few pathogenic species that cause disease at all times. Most organisms found in and on human beings often are harmless but are capable of causing disease in patients who are elderly, very young, or debilitated (Table 5-1).

Despite more than 80 years of aseptic surgery and more than 40 years of experience with antimicrobial agents, the surgeon finds that infections are as great a problem now as in the past. But the etiologic agents have changed. Streptococci and pneumococci are no longer the captains of death, because they can be controlled by antibiotics. Staphylococci *continue* to cause nosocomial (hospital-acquired) infections, but those gram-negative bacteria usually considered nonpathogens, opportunists, or secondary invaders have become a major problem. Nosocomial infection results from the transmission of pathogens to a previously uninfected patient from a source in the hospital environment (*cross infection*). Alternatively, the pathogens may come from patients themselves (*autoinfection*). They may be carriers of the pathogen or become colonized with virulent hospital strains during hospitalization. Many nosocomial infections have an iatrogenic basis (i.e., result from treatment by physicians and their professional collaborators). Frequent or prolonged use of supportive procedures such as indwelling vascular or urinary catheters, tracheostomies, and equipment for postoperative respiratory care are responsible for most iatrogenic infections. Nosocomial infection causes morbidity, mortality, expense to the patient, and increasing malpractice liability for the surgeon and hospital.

A *surgical infection* is an infection that requires surgical treatment and has developed before, or as a complication of, surgical treatment. Thus, a postoperative wound infection is also a specific nosocomial infection. Surgical infections may be analyzed in relation to procedures in clean or contaminated fields, the anatomic site or system involved, and the pathophysiologic activities of the causative microorganisms (Table 5-2). The microorganisms commonly encountered in surgical infections are the staphylococci, streptococci, clostridia, bacteroides, and the enteric bacteria. Most surgical incisions are contaminated but not infected with normal skin flora (bacteria such as coagulase-negative staphylococci and anaerobic diphtheroids). However, traumatic wounds are usually contaminated if not yet infected, and operations on infected or "contaminated" tissue usually result in infec-

Table 5-1. SOME INDIGENOUS MICROORGANISMS AND SOME INFECTIONS WITH WHICH THEY MAY BE INVOLVED

Microorganism	Infection
Aerobic or facultative:	
Achromobacter spp.	Bloodstream, burns, meningitis, urethritis
Acinetobacter spp.	Bloodstream, burns, meningitis, urethritis, pneumonia
Alkaligenes fecalis	Bloodstream, conjunctivitis, meningitis, respiratory tract, urinary tract
Candida albicans and other yeasts	Endocarditis, pneumonitis, septicemia, thrush, vulvovaginitis, candidosis
Corynebacterium spp.	Endocarditis, lung abscesses
Enterobacteriaceae (*Escherichia, Klebsiella, Enterobacter, Proteus,* etc.)	Abscesses, bloodstream, meningitis, peritonitis, pneumonia, wounds, urinary tract, endocarditis, pyelonephritis, cystitis
Haemophilus spp.	Bronchitis, conjunctivitis, meningitis, urinary tract
Moraxella spp.	Conjunctivitis
Nocardia spp.	Nocardiosis
Pseudomonas spp.	Bloodstream, burns, meningitis, urinary tract, wounds
Staphylococcus aureus	Abscesses, pneumonia, wounds, pseudomembranous enterocolitis
Staphylococcus epidermidis	Endocarditis, septicemia, thrombophlebitis
Streptococcus faecalis	Endocarditis, bloodstream, urinary tract, wounds, peritonitis, meningitis
Streptococcus viridans	Endocarditis
Anaerobic:	
Actinomyces spp.	Actinomycosis
Bacteroides spp.	Abscesses, endocarditis, peritonitis
Clostridium spp.	Cellulitis, myonecrosis, pseudomembranous enterocolitis
Fusobacterium spp.	Abscesses, myonecrosis, bacteremia
Lactobacillus spp.	Endocarditis
Peptostreptococcus spp.	Abscesses, myonecrosis
Veillonella spp.	Endocarditis

tion. Postoperative infections present a double hazard: First, the infection itself may result in toxemia or produce extensive tissue damage and perhaps septicemia. Second, the local effects of infection delay healing of the wound and may cause hemorrhage or disruption of the wound. In either case, the patient's hospitalization is extended.

GENERAL PRINCIPLES

Pathogenic species of bacteria have the capacity to invade and produce disease. However, disease is a biologic

Table 5-2. CLASSIFICATION OF
SURGICAL INFECTIONS

I. Relative to final outcome
  A. Self-limiting infections: The patient recovers completely without medical or surgical treatment, or despite it (e.g., a boil).
  B. Serious infections requiring treatment: The outcome depends largely on the nature of treatment, the time after outset that it is administered, and clinical judgment (e.g., septicemia, pneumonia, empyema, primary peritonitis).
  C. Fulminating infections: These prove to be fatal or permanently disabling (e.g., retroperitoneal cellulitis).
II. Relative to time of onset
  A. Anteoperative surgical infections: These include all infections in which the microorganisms have gained entrance to the body before any operative procedure.
    1. Time and portal of entry are known—accidents.
    2. Time and portal of entry are not known—disease (infection) is established before the surgeon treats the patient.
  B. Operative surgical infections: These include all in which microorganisms gain entrance to the body during an operative procedure or as an immediate result of it (i.e., surgery may be considered either directly or indirectly responsible for the development of infection).
    1. Preventable operative surgical infections—failure of the surgeon or operating-room personnel to adhere to the principles of sterile procedure and all accepted and accredited practices
    2. Nonpreventable operative surgical infections
      a. Pathogenic microorganisms already resident within body tissues (e.g., incision seeded with *Staphylococcus aureus* resident in ducts and glands of normal skin)
      b. Microorganisms from a deep focus of infection (e.g., peritoneal abscess, lung abscess, etc.)
      c. Microorganisms resident on the surface of normal mucous membranes (e.g., intestinal tract, respiratory tract, genitourinary tract)
      d. Microorganisms on dust particles and borne by air currents
  C. Postoperative surgical infections: These are complications of the operation or the postoperative management of the patient.
    1. Surgical wound infection
    2. Respiratory tract infection
    3. Urinary tract infection

SOURCE: Modified from Meleney FL: *Treatise on Surgical Infections,* New York, Oxford University Press, 1948.

---

accident and represents a complex interaction between the microorganism and the host that occurs only under special circumstances. Healthy people may harbor pathogenic bacteria and yet be unaffected clinically. They are referred to as carriers of the particular pathogen. The healthy carrier of pathogenic microorganisms is the principal reservoir of most diseases. Although species such as *Staphylococcus aureus* and *Escherichia coli* are examples of pathogens, individual strains may be too feeble to cause infection. Feeble or noninvasive strains may cause infection if the resistance of the host is extremely low or if tremendous numbers of bacteria are introduced. Some bacteria that are nonpathogenic under ordinary conditions are opportunistic and may be pathogenic when the host-parasite equilibrium is upset, e.g., when normal flora

is eliminated by antibiotics or when incision makes available a new area of the body. Antibiotic-resistant strains of *Staphylococcus aureus* of specific phage types, which cause nosocomial postoperative wound infections, may be endemic among carrier personnel of a particular hospital. Patients may become infected by direct contact with a carrier or may become infected with a hospital staphylococcus with which they have become colonized during hospitalization.

The term *virulence* refers to the tissue-invading powers of a specific strain of a pathogen and is used in two different ways: First, virulence describes quantitatively the smallest dose of a bacterial strain that will produce disease in a specified host. This assessment is usually conducted in experimental animals and may have no relation to human disease. Second, virulence describes an epidemiologic concept such as a given phage type of *Staphylococcus aureus* producing human disease more frequently than another. In this situation, virulence is based on ecologic advantage in the external environment but may not necessarily involve greater capacity to be virulent as measured by the critical dose of bacteria causing clinical infection.

A large infecting dose is favorable to the production of bacterial disease because only a small number of bacteria may actually reach a favorable site in the host. A sudden change to a different environment or to a new site may injure most of the inoculum. Moreover, the defense mechanisms of the host often destroy a large proportion of the invading organisms before they can become established. The greater the number of bacteria introduced into the host, the greater the amount of preformed toxins that will be carried along. Preformed toxins may protect bacteria from destruction during the period when they are adapting to the new environment and are incapable of producing additional toxin. The resistance of the host is shown in the ability to keep bacteria out of the body initially and, failing in this, to localize and destroy them. A healthy, unbroken skin is the first line of resistance. Although mucous membranes are less resistant, even here minute breaks usually provide for bacterial entry. It is then that active defensive measures come into play. Primary defenses include the system of fixed phagocytic cells (i.e., the histiocytes of the reticuloendothelial system) and mobile phagocytes. These are aided by antibacterial substances in blood plasma, lymph, and interstitial fluid, by physical barriers to the spread of bacteria (i.e., ground substances, serous and fibrous membranes), and by local and systemic reactions such as hyperemia, fever, and leukocytosis. Secondary defenses are dependent upon the presence of specific antigenic stimuli (bacteria and bacterial products). The antibodies formed in response to these antigens inhibit or destroy bacteria, or neutralize their toxins. In the presence of sufficient antibodies, the primary defenses are greatly accelerated, bacteria are phagocytized and digested more quickly than before, and the ability of serum to neutralize bacterial toxins is increased many thousandfold. The presence of other disease may greatly reduce resistance to microbial infection. For example, diabetes predisposes to infection of the skin and the genitourinary tract. Influenza, measles, and other viral infections markedly predispose to secondary bacterial infections of the respiratory tract. Malignant disease, malnutrition, chronic alcoholism, or metabolic disease may interfere seriously with an individual's resistance to infectious disease.

Bacteria cause disease by invading tissues and producing toxins. Bacterial invasion leads to demonstrable damage of host cells and tissues in the vicinity of the invasion, whereas bacterial toxins are transported by the blood and lymph to cause cytotoxic effects at sites removed from the initial lesion. Species such as *Streptococcus pyogenes* are both invasive and toxigenic. *Staphylococcus aureus* produces local damage but has little tendency to spread, although the local inflammatory response may be severe as in the case of carbuncles. *Clostridium tetani* is almost solely toxigenic. Generally, invasiveness and toxigenicity are not completely separable, since invasion involves some degree of toxin production and toxigenicity requires some degree of bacterial multiplication. *Exotoxins* are specific, soluble, diffusible proteins produced by certain bacteria as they multiply in a circumscribed area. Exotoxins lose their toxicity upon denaturation but retain much of their original antigenicity. Such modified exotoxins are called *toxoids*. Those prepared from *Clostridium tetani* are used to induce active immunity in man. The alpha toxin of *Clostridium perfringens* is a lecithinase that acts upon the membrane lipids of body cells and erythrocytes. *Endotoxins* are complex lipopolysaccharides of the bacterial cell wall produced by many gram-negative species. They are released only on partial or complete dissolution of the bacterial cell. Endotoxins are relatively heat-stable; many withstand temperatures of 60 to 100°C for 1 h. They do not form toxoids. Their toxicity is associated with the phospholipid moiety of the molecule, whereas their antigenic determinants are associated with the polysaccharide moiety.

Diagnosis

The classic signs and symptoms of infection are redness, swelling, heat, and pain. Redness of the skin is due to intense hyperemia. Swelling accompanies infection unless the infection is confined to bone that cannot swell. Heat results from hyperemia and may be detected even in the absence of redness. Pain is the most universal sign of infection. Along with pain goes tenderness, or pain to the touch, which is greatest over the area of maximal involvement. Loss of function is another sign of infection. It is brought about by reflex and by voluntary immobilization. The patient immobilizes the painful part in the most comfortable position. For example, a finger with an infected tendon sheath is kept flexed. In peritonitis, the abdominal muscles are maintained in a state of tonic contraction to keep the inflamed peritoneum beneath from moving. Fever and tachycardia are additional, albeit nonspecific, signs of infection. Fever and chills indicate septicemia, while an elevated pulse rate is a sign of a toxic state.

Leukocytosis accompanies an acute bacterial infection more often than a viral infection. The more severe the infection, the greater is the leukocytosis. In most surgical infections, the total leukocyte count is only slightly or moderately elevated. However, a high leukocyte count (35,000/mm^3) occurs as a result of suppuration. The endotoxin released by gram-negative bacilli is thought to contribute to the production of high leukocyte counts. However, in the elderly, in the severely ill, and during therapy with antibiotic, some anticancer, and immunosuppressive drugs, white cell counts may be normal or low. The leukopenia of overwhelming sepsis is probably due to exhaustion of the supply of leukocytes and to bone marrow depression. Although the total number of leukocytes is normal in some infections, there is a preponderance of immature granulocytes, which may be increased above 85 percent compared with the normal below 75 percent ("shift to the left"). A chronic infection may be evident only by fatigue, low-grade fever, and perhaps anemia. Moreover, massive pyogenic abscesses may occur without leukocytosis, fever, or tenderness.

Exudate from the area of infection should be examined for color, odor, and consistency. The microorganisms causing a surgical infection often may be seen microscopically on gram-stained smears. For each bacterial cell observed under the oil-immersion lens, there are approximately 10^5 similar organisms in each milliliter of exudate from which the smear was prepared. The staining and examination of slides are simple, rapid, inexpensive procedures that provide valuable and immediate information for the surgeon. Pus from deep-seated abscesses may be obtained by needle aspiration or at the time of definitive drainage. Exudate from surface infections may be examined directly. Specimens submitted to the bacteriologic laboratory should be collected before chemotherapy is begun and should be labeled adequately to identify the patient, the clinical diagnosis, and the nature and site of the specimen. The laboratory should be requested to do aerobic and anaerobic cultures and antibiotic-sensitivity tests. The surgeon must initiate treatment immediately upon clinical judgment, although the subsequent laboratory report will often make appropriate changes possible.

Biopsy is useful in establishing a diagnosis in granulomatous infections such as tuberculosis, syphilis, and mycoses. Additional sources of biopsy material are enlarged lymph nodes draining an area of infection or a sinus tract. Blood cultures are the single most definitive method of determining etiology in infectious disease and are often helpful in identifying the microorganisms causing surgical infection. Transient bacteremias accompany the early phase of many infections and may result from manipulation of infected or contaminated tissues (e.g., surgical incision of furuncles or abscesses, instrumentation of the genitourinary tract, and dental procedures). Bacteria usually enter the circulation via the lymphatic system. Consequently, when bacteria multiply at a site of local infection in tissues, the lymph drained from that area carries bacteria to the thoracic duct and eventually to the venous blood. However, a blood culture taken at the time of chill and fever may be negative for bacteria, as phagocytes promptly remove bacteria suddenly entering the bloodstream and chill and fever occur 30 to 90 min later. Thus, blood cultures should be taken at frequent intervals in a patient with febrile disease of unknown origin in an attempt to obtain blood before an expected chill and rise in temperature. A careful history and physical examination provide the basis for diagnosis and laboratory tests.

Surgical Therapy

It is necessary to distinguish between contamination and infection. Almost all wounds are contaminated with bacteria from the skin or from sources external to the patient. However, very few wounds become infected (i.e., exhibit disease manifested by inflammation, dehiscence, suppuration, and necrosis). The major clinical responses to wound infection are suppuration and invasion. Bacteria grow in the wound on substrates consisting of blood clots, lymph, leukocytes, and necrotic debris. Extension of the local inflammatory response to adjacent tissues is associated with a systemic reaction. The hazard of generalized infection is associated with all traumatic wounds. These and preoperative surgical infections are treated to overcome existing infection and to prevent postoperative infection. Local treatment consists of debridement of all necrotic or injured tissue, drainage of abscesses, removal of foreign bodies, and adjunctive therapy with antibiotics. Supportive measures governing the treatment of established surgical infections are bed rest, immobilization of the infected region, elevation to promote venous and lymphatic drainage, and relief of swelling and pain. Moist heat is applied to increase local blood supply, facilitate exudation, and hasten sloughing. The detailed management of wounds is discussed in Chap. 8 (Wound Healing and Wound Care).

Antibiotic Therapy

The adjunctive use of antibiotics in the treatment of infections is dependent upon an adequate blood supply and is most effective against acute infections such as cellulitis, septicemia, or peritonitis. Antibiotics have slight access to abscesses and penetrate by slow diffusion, if at all. In these situations, they should be used in conjunction with incision and drainage. Antibiotics are the primary treatment for acute spreading infections and should result in clinical improvement in 24 to 48 h. Change to a more effective antibiotic may be based on the culture and sensitivity report.

Although clinical judgment frequently must be used to select an antibiotic and although the causative microorganism often is revealed on microscopic examination of a gram-stained smear of exudate or pus, the infecting microorganisms should be identified and antibiotic sensitivities determined by the laboratory. Accordingly, the specimen for culture (pus, exudate, blood, or urine) should be obtained before chemotherapy is begun. In severe infections, exudate often can be inoculated on a blood agar plate and antibiotic sensitivity discs positioned so that rapid, presumptive sensitivity information can be obtained after incubation overnight or for several hours. This crude procedure does not replace the official pure culture studies of all microorganisms isolated from the specimen.

Hyperbaric Therapy

Brummelkamp and associates in Amsterdam introduced the hyperbaric oxygen chamber for operative procedures. In 1963 they reported the first use of hyperbaric oxygen for gas-producing infections. Both the patient and medical personnel were placed in a room-sized chamber in which the air pressure was raised to three times that of the normal atmosphere (i.e., 2280 mmHg, or 3 atm absolute). For seven periods of $1\frac{1}{2}$ h during 3 days, the pressurized patient inhaled 100 percent oxygen from a face mask. This increased the normal oxygen tension in plasma, lymph, and tissue fluids about fifteen to twenty times. Dramatic clinical improvement was described in most patients within the first day. Roding and colleagues advise that "operations be limited to opening the original wound and incising abscesses. Any further excision and removal of necrotic tissue can be done much later after clinical resolution. The advantage of postponement is that the operation can be performed in a dramatically improved patient who is no longer toxic." Large pressure chambers are available at only a few medical centers in the world and at special military and marine industrial facilities. In addition, much less expensive single-patient chambers are now available and are also used to treat patients. Therapy with hyperbaric oxygen, antibiotics, and surgical debridement has been effective for clostridial myonecrosis. Hyperbaric oxygenation appears to reduce toxemia and diminish the amount of tissue requiring excision. However, gas-producing infection due to anaerobic streptococci, *Escherichia coli,* and *Klebsiella* species showed no improvement after exposure to high-pressure oxygen. The use of hyperbaric oxygen is advocated as an adjunct to the surgical treatment of clostridial infections. In cases of clostridial myonecrosis, all conventional means of treatment should be employed, including early surgical debridement and administration of antibiotics. The reliability of immediate surgical treatment and adjunctive antibiotic therapy remains unquestioned.

SOME COMMON SURGICAL INFECTIONS

Cellulitis is a nonsuppurative inflammation of the subcutaneous tissues extending along connective tissue planes and across intercellular spaces. There is widespread swelling, redness, and pain without definite localization. Central necrosis and suppuration may occur at a later stage. In severe infections, blebs and bullae form on the skin. Although a variety of aerobic and anaerobic bacteria produce cellulitis, the hemolytic streptococci are the classic etiologic agents. Treatment consists of antibiotic therapy and rest. Failure of the inflammatory swelling to subside after 48 to 72 h of antibiotic therapy suggests that an abscess has developed, and that incision and drainage are needed.

Lymphangitis is an inflammation of lymphatic pathways that is usually visible as erythematous streaking of the skin. This is especially true in infections by hemolytic streptococci. Lymphangitis and the associated inflammatory swelling of lymph nodes *(lymphadenitis)* are a normal defense reaction against bacterial invasion and are frequently seen in the forearm of a patient with an infection of the hand or fingers. Most cases will respond to antibiotic therapy and rest.

Erysipelas is an acute spreading cellulitis and lymphangitis, usually caused by hemolytic streptococci that gain entrance through a break in the skin. There is a severe systemic as well as local reaction with abrupt onset, chills, fever, and prostration. The skin is red, swollen, and tender, and there is a distinct line of demarcation at the advancing margin of the infection. Erysipelas may develop on any cutaneous surface but commonly involves the face in a "butterfly lesion" over the nose and cheeks. Recurrent erysipelas in an extremity may lead to chronic lymphedema. Antibiotic therapy will usually halt the progress of the invasive infection, but the erythema disappears more slowly since it is a toxigenic consequence of bacterial invasion.

Infection in soft tissues is of paramount concern to the surgeon, and a variety of superficial infections will be discussed. An *abscess* is a localized collection of pus surrounded by an area of inflamed tissue in which hyperemia and infiltration of leukocytes is marked. A *furuncle,* or boil, is an abscess in a sweat gland or hair follicle. The inflammatory reaction is intense, leading to tissue necrosis and the formation of a central core. This is surrounded by a peripheral zone of cellulitis. An abscess beneath the corium of the skin is a *subepithelial abscess. Impetigo* is an acute contagious skin disease characterized by the formation of a series of intraepithelial abscesses. Gangrenous impetigo may occur as a complication in severe chronic debilitating diseases (e.g., chronic ulcerative colitis), and hemolytic streptococci and staphylococci can be cultured from the exudate. The lesions appear as multiple small pustules that extend and coalesce to form large areas of cutaneous gangrene and ulceration. Although management is similar to that of postoperative gangrene, favorable response is proportional to success in overcoming the primary disease.

A *carbuncle* is a multilocular suppurative extension of a furuncle into the subcutaneous tissues. The nape of the neck, dorsum of trunk, hands and digits, and hirsute portions of the chest and abdomen are apt to be involved. Individual compartments in a carbuncle are maintained through persistence of fascial attachments to the skin. As these numerous component locules rupture separately, individual fistulas appear. Most abscesses are caused by pyogenic cocci, usually *Staphylococcus aureus.* However, gram-negative bacilli and streptococci may be found coincidentally. Carbuncles may be more extensive than they appear and should be excised widely to prevent spread and to effect a cure. The wound contracts to a small scar, and a skin graft is not usually required.

The course of a furuncle is often self-limited and may require no specific therapy. However, furuncles can be serious and may become carbuncles. Large furuncles and abscesses should be incised and drained and the patient treated with antibiotics. Abscesses in the "dangerous" nasolabial area of the face bounded by the bridge of the nose and the angles of the mouth may become complicated by septic phlebitis with intracranial extension along the nasal veins to the cavernous sinus. The incidence of septic cavernous sinus thrombosis has declined since the introduction of antibiotics, and this lethal complication is now rare.

Bacteremia is defined as bacteria in the circulating blood with no indication of toxemia or other clinical manifestations. Bacteremia is usually transient and may last only a few moments, as the reticuloendothelial system localizes and destroys these organisms under favorable conditions. The normal individual probably experiences bacteremia, unknowingly, many times each year. This state follows dental procedures, major traumatic wounds, etc., and may be the means by which apparently isolated infections arise in internal organs, e.g., osteomyelitis, pyelonephritis (descending type), or subacute bacterial endocarditis.

Septicemia is a diffuse infection in which infectious bacteria and their toxins are present in the bloodstream. Septicemia may arise directly from the introduction of infecting organisms into the circulation but, as a rule, is secondary to a focus of infection within the body. The major routes by which bacteria reach the blood are (1) by direct extension and entrance into an open vessel, (2) by release of infected emboli following thrombosis of a blood vessel in an area of inflammation, (3) by discharge of infected lymph into the bloodstream following lymphangitis. Many specific diseases, e.g., typhoid fever and brucellosis, include a septicemic phase. In the absence of systemic disease, beta-hemolytic streptococci *(Streptococcus pyogenes)* are most frequently responsible. Septicemia caused by alpha-hemolytic streptococci *(Streptococcus viridans)* is usually a consequence of subacute bacterial endocarditis. The majority of bacteria that produce suppurative lesions may give rise to secondary septicemia. *Pyemia* is septicemia in which pyogenic microorganisms, most notably *Staphylococcus aureus,* and their toxins are carried in the bloodstream and sequentially initiate multiple focal abscesses in many parts of the body. Before the advent of chemotherapy, staphylococcic pyemia was almost always fatal; the mortality is still high. In *toxemia,* toxins are circulating in the blood, though the microorganism producing the toxin need not be. Toxemia is usually associated with infection by toxin-producing bacteria (e.g., the clostridia of gas gangrene and the diphtheria bacillus), but this is not always so. For example, botulinum toxin or staphylococcal enterotoxin may have been ingested directly to cause a profound toxemia without true infection.

PRINCIPLES OF ANTIBIOTIC THERAPY

Basic Considerations

Chemotherapeutic agents act primarily upon the parasite and not upon the host. They include antibiotics and metabolic antagonists such as the sulfonamides. An antibiotic is a chemical compound derived from, or produced by, living organisms and capable, at low concentrations, of inhibiting the life processes of microorganisms. *Bacteriostatic* agents prevent the growth of bacteria but do not destroy them. The defense mechanisms of the body then eliminate the bacteria which are unable to multiply. If the defenses are insufficient or if the bacteriostatic drug is withdrawn prematurely, then the bacterial population will resurge, and the patient will suffer a relapse. *Bactericidal* agents actively kill bacteria and must be employed in patients whose defense mechanisms are impaired or altered by disease or immunosuppressive therapy. The distinction between bactericidal and bacteriostatic effects is sometimes relative to duration of therapy and dosage. Some drugs are bacteriostatic at low concentrations and bactericidal at high concentrations. With most bactericidal drugs, the rate of killing increases with concentration. Antibiotic agents exert their effects in a variety of ways (Table 5-3). They may inhibit the synthesis of the bacterial cell wall and consequently interfere with the cell's osmotic defenses, or they may affect the barrier function of the cell membrane and cause loss of vital metabolites. An entirely different mode of action impairs the translation of genetic information and affects protein synthesis. Bacteriostatic drugs affect early stages of protein synthesis in the ribosome and result in an insufficiency, preventing growth and proliferation of bacteria without actually destroying them. However, bactericidal drugs cause the ribosome to miscode and consequently induce the manufacture of defective proteins or enzymes that poison the cell. Replication of deoxyribonucleic acid (DNA) in the chromosome at the level of the assembly of purine nucleotides may be affected by some antibiotics. Although their precise locus of action is not known, these drugs impede the replication of genetic information.

The addition of antibiotics to the armamentarium of the physician has revolutionized the practice of medicine but has been a double-edged sword. Antibiotics not only achieve a therapeutic effect but also alter the ecology of the patient's microflora. Excessive use of antibiotics may select for strains of bacteria whose resistance to antibiotics is transmitted by plasmids. It is pertinent to point out that the surgeon employs antibiotic drugs as adjunctive agents in the treatment of surgical infections, whereas the internist usually employs antibiotics as the primary treatment for medical infections. For the surgeon the aims of antibiotic therapy are much the same as those of surgical therapy, i.e., to control or eradicate bacterial infections acquired before or during hospitalization and to prevent infection from developing postoperatively. To obtain these goals, antibiotic agents are administered (1) systemically by either parenteral or oral routes, (2) preoperatively for preparation of the large intestine (intestinal antisepsis), or (3) locally by (a) topical irrigation, (b) topical application, (c) intraperitoneal, intrapleural, or intrathecal instillation or irrigation, and (d) intraluminal instillation into the large intestine or abscess cavity. Antibacterial drugs may be administered preoperatively, perioperatively, and postoperatively to prevent infection (prophylaxis) or to treat already established infection.

The fundamental principles governing the use of antibiotics are (1) administration of an agent active against the infecting microorganism, (2) adequate contact between the drug and the infecting microbe, (3) absence of (or minimal) toxic side effects or complications for the patient, and (4) utilization of host defenses to augment antibacterial effects of the antibiotic. The specificity of the antibiotic for the infecting microorganism is based upon laboratory identification and antibiotic-sensitivity studies. Clinical judgment is called upon in serious, rapidly developing infections, such as gram-negative shock. The surgeon must administer an antibiotic known to be effective against microorganisms that may be involved in the infection even though the specific microorganism is unknown. Many surgical infections are polymicrobic, and often it is necessary to choose a single antibiotic or a combination of antibiotics that will cover the broad range of probable pathogens. If possible, cultures should be taken before antibiotic therapy is initiated. The antibiotic is changed, if necessary, when culture and sensitivity reports become available from the laboratory.

The antibiotic must come in contact with the infecting microorganism. In an acute, diffuse infection, blood flow into the area of infection will usually deliver adequate levels of systemic antibiotic. A spreading cellulitis with lymphangitis and lymphadenitis often responds within 24 h to an appropriate antibiotic. However, since antibiotics cannot penetrate a thick-walled pyogenic abscess or an infected serous cavity, they should be used in conjunction with drainage of the abscess, debridement of necrotic tissue, and removal of any foreign bodies. These principles apply to every organ of the body. A spreading infection of the meninges responds to chemotherapy, but a brain abscess must be drained; a staphylococcal septicemia is treated by chemotherapy, but a pulp abscess of the fingertip must be drained.

The surgeon must be aware of toxic complications of antibiotics and should be prepared to treat them. Toxic effects range from minor skin rashes, drug fever, and gas-

Table 5-3. ANTIBIOTICS: MODES OF ACTION

Cellular site of inhibition	Bactericidal	Bacteriostatic
Cell wall synthesis	Penicillins Cephalosporins Vancomycin Bacitracin	
Barrier function of cell membrane	Polymyxin B Colistin Amphotericin B	Nystatin
Protein synthesis in ribosome	Streptomycin Aminoglycosides	Tetracyclines Chloramphenicol Erythromycin Clindamycin
DNA replication in chromosome	Griseofulvin	

trointestinal disturbances to renal tubular necrosis, loss of vision and hearing, irreversible blood dyscrasias, and anaphylactic shock. In addition, alterations in the normal flora of the body may occur in patients receiving prolonged antibiotic therapy. In most cases these changes produce no ill result, but in some the alterations of flora result in the rapid overgrowth of virulent, antibiotic-resistant bacteria that may have been present originally in small numbers (colonization). If the patient's general resistance to infection is depressed, a new infection may follow the antibiotic-induced alteration of flora (superinfection). The term *colonization* indicates an antibiotic-induced quantitative change in the resident microflora of the patient, a common consequence of antimicrobial therapy. There is no clinical evidence of secondary infection, and discontinuance of the antibiotic usually allows the normal flora to become reestablished. However, there is the risk that colonization will lead to superinfection, a clinical event that may be of great danger to the patient. The term *superinfection* usually refers to a new microbial disease induced by antibiotic therapy. Superinfection is most frequent with broad-spectrum antibiotics. Inhibition of the normal flora allows proliferation of species and strains of bacteria not inhibited by the antibiotic. Superinfection is often due to gram-negative bacilli and fungi that are more difficult to eradicate than are gram-positive streptococci and pneumococci. Superinfection may be fatal, usually occurs in elderly patients, and often follows therapy with aminoglycoside antibiotics (e.g., gentamicin and kanamycin) and other broad-spectrum drugs (either alone or in combination with penicillin). Clinical evidence of secondary infection (i.e., a rise in temperature, increased peripheral white blood cell count, and physical signs of a disease not present at the beginning of antibiotic therapy) indicates that colonization has progressed to superinfection. Serial superinfections with different antibiotic-resistant microbial species may occur in the same patient.

Secondary or opportunistic infections may also occur in patients with noninfectious diseases. For example, mycotic infections may develop in patients with lymphoma or leukemia. Deficiencies in host resistance as a result of disease (e.g., diabetes mellitus, hematopoietic disorders, renal failure, liver disease) or as a consequence of therapy with radiation, antimetabolites, or corticosteroids confer the potential for pathogenicity on many ordinary nonpathogenic microorganisms. Indwelling venous or urinary catheters also contribute to lowered host resistance. The term *suprainfection* designates a secondary infection unrelated to antibiotic therapy.

Chemoprophylaxis

A prophylactic antibiotic is administered to an uninfected patient who is in jeopardy of acquiring a surgical infection. There is controversy regarding prophylactic antibiotic therapy because prophylaxis has not always been as valuable as therapeutic use. In surgical patients, prophylactic antibiotics are administered to treat contaminated or potentially contaminated wounds before infec-

tion occurs. Bacterial contamination is a component of every surgical wound, and may arise exogenously from the operating team or the environment through a flaw in aseptic surgical technique, or endogenously from the patient's skin, respiratory, gastrointestinal, or genitourinary tracts. The administration of antibiotic agents to prevent infection cannot be substituted for either sound surgical judgment or strict aseptic technique. Prophylactic antimicrobial use has no place in clean operative procedures or in those carrying a minimal risk of sepsis, but should be considered for operations involving trauma or severe burns and for operations in infected tissues or those associated with heavy contamination (e.g., operations involving the large intestine). An equally beneficial role for chemoprophylaxis is prior to operations in patients especially prone to infection because of malnutrition, impoverished blood supply, or preexisting infection remote from the operative site. Other patient-risk factors are obesity, old age, immunodeficient states, and shock. The patient undergoing immunosuppressive therapy and/or requiring insertion of a permanent prosthetic device is particularly prone to surgical infections. Other treatment-specific factors include use of steroids and antineoplastic agents, radiotherapy, and operative procedures of long duration, such as cardiac and vascular procedures.

Surgical wounds may be designated as "clean," "contaminated," or "dirty" depending upon the presence or absence of prior infection and contact with the interior of the respiratory, urinary, or gastrointestinal tracts. Traumatic wounds are usually grossly contaminated, whereas elective clean surgical procedures may be slightly contaminated during the operative procedure. Infection does not necessarily follow contamination, since host factors as well as microbial factors are involved. However, the greater the contamination, the greater the possibility of consequent infection. Accordingly, in surgery of traumatic wounds or in elective "contaminated" or "dirty" surgery, antibiotic therapy should be started before the operation so that adequate levels of antibiotic may be obtained in tissue and body fluids during the operative procedure to prevent colonization during bacterial seeding of the operative field. In procedures of long duration it is necessary to maintain tissue levels of the antibiotic by intraoperative administration of the antibiotic agent.

Antibiotics also may be administered postoperatively, but should be limited to reduce the probability of adverse effects, the emergence of resistant microorganisms, and superinfection.

A prophylactic antibiotic regimen may not be successful if the drug is not effective against all potential pathogens or if the agent does not come in contact with susceptible pathogens at the site of infection. The antibiotic should be administered parenterally and in sufficient dosage to achieve high circulating blood levels.

Prophylactic antimicrobials are currently used in the following areas:

Cardiovascular (valve and open heart, coronary artery bypass)
Orthopaedic (hip-fracture repair involving implantation of foreign material, total hip replacement)

Obstetric and gynecologic (vaginal hysterectomy, cesarean section)

Biliary tract (acute cholecystitis, obstructive jaundice, or stones in common duct without jaundice, when the patient is more than seventy years of age)

Gastrointestinal (gastric ulcer or carcinoma, colonic procedures in patients with unobstructed gastrointestinal tract, resection of oropharyngeal or laryngeal carcinoma)

Urologic (bacteriuric patients prior to urologic procedures)

Neurosurgical procedures of long duration

Intestinal Antisepsis

Intestinal antisepsis is a form of antimicrobial prophylaxis employed by the surgeon to lower the high rate of infectious complications after colorectal surgery. Intestinal antisepsis reduces the patient's normal intestinal flora so that there will be fewer microorganisms present in the large intestine to gain access to sterile tissues during minor, inadvertent intraoperative spills. In addition, the reduction of the patient's normal microflora provides a measure of protection to anastomoses during the immediate postoperative period.

The protocol for preoperative preparation of the unobstructed large intestine includes the specific prophylactic use of oral antibiotics. Bacterial infection following elective colonic surgery results from unavoidable seeding of the wound with contents of the colon. This is manifested by intraabdominal abscesses and anastomotic disruption with resultant peritonitis and fistula formation. The ideal antibiotic agent for preoperative preparation of the colon has rapid bactericidal activity against pathogens in the gastrointestinal tract, minimal absorption, and the absence of undesirable or toxic side effects.

The traditional protocol for intestinal antisepsis is now of historical interest only. It involved a 3-day period of hospitalization during which the patient was placed on a low-residue (or clear liquid) diet, given a cathartic and daily enemas, and administered suitable oral antibiotics for 72 h prior to operation. Although mechanical cleansing alone diminishes the volume of bulk feces and, consequently, the total number of fecal bacteria, the remaining feces contain the usual large number of bacteria (on the order of 10^{11} bacteria per gram of feces). Thus, the potential for postoperative sepsis remains a major hazard. We believe that oral prophylactic antibiotics and mechanical cleansing are both essential for effective preoperative preparation of the large intestine. The Nichols-Condon method is currently the most widely used. It consists of a 2-day fluid diet, mechanical preparation, and oral neomycin and erythromycin base administered on the second day to diminish aerobic and anaerobic colonic microflora. One gram of each antibiotic is given at 1, 2, and 11 P.M.; the operation is scheduled for 8 A.M. the next day.

Alternate methods of mechanical preparation include whole-gut irrigation with a polyethylene-glycol-electrolyte lavage solution (Golytely) beginning on the day before surgery. The patient ingests 1 L of chilled solution per hour for a maximum of 5 h or until the rectal effluent is completely clear. Moreover, intravenous antibiotics are used by some surgeons preoperatively and/or postoperatively as an adjunct to (or even as an alternative to) the oral preoperative antimicrobial agents. Reduction of colonic microflora by oral antibiotic and the provision of high tissue levels of antibiotic during the perioperative period are worthwhile objectives in aiding the patient to avoid wound sepsis.

Intestinal antisepsis has been shown to reduce the incidence of postoperative complications related to bacteria but does not protect against errors of surgical skill or judgment. Collected studies show that the average incidence of wound infection is 20 percent in patients placed on intestinal antisepsis as compared with 48 percent or less in patients not on any form of preoperative intestinal antisepsis. As new antibiotics become available it is likely that the optimal regimen for preoperative preparation of the bowel for colorectal operations will change, but the benefit of appropriate intestinal antisepsis in operations on the colon and rectum is well established.

Intraperitoneal Antibiotic Therapy

The most frequent indications for the intraperitoneal instillation of antibiotics are perforated and gangrenous appendicitis, perforated peptic ulcer, gangrenous intestinal obstruction, traumatic perforation of the gastrointestinal tract at any level, intraabdominal abscess, and excessive spillage associated with elective colonic, gastric, or small bowel surgery. Intraperitoneally administered antibiotics may be useful in pelvic inflammatory disease, acute pancreatitis, major intraabdominal vascular procedures, closure of evisceration, and repair of large abdominal incisional hernias. To be effective for routine intraperitoneal instillation, the antibiotic must provide adequate control of endogenous enteric bacteria that may be expected in the peritoneal cavity, with minimal accompanying pain and local or systemic reaction. Clinical success and safety have been achieved with kanamycin and also with cephalothin.

In recent years povidone-iodine and other iodophors have been used as antiseptic solutions to irrigate wounds as well as the peritoneal cavity in diffuse peritonitis. Subsequent laboratory studies, however, have demonstrated that intraperitoneal instillation of nonlethal doses of povidone-iodine antiseptic solution into the peritoneal cavity caused a uniformly fatal outcome within the succeeding 24 h. When saline solution was instilled in place of povidone-iodine antiseptic solution, the experimental animals survived an average of 96 h. The more rapid death after treatment with povidone-iodine was not associated with differences in peritoneal microflora but with peritoneal absorption of excessive amounts of iodine. Iodophors cannot be recommended for use intraperitoneally and have been shown to offer no therapeutic benefit when used to irrigate experimental wounds.

ANTIMICROBIAL AGENTS

Antibiotics and chemotherapeutic agents that are useful currently in surgical practice are described briefly in this section. It is important to use an antibiotic agent for a sensitive microorganism and not to treat a particular disease. Precise antimicrobial therapy is based upon the laboratory culture and sensitivity report. Table 5-4 is a guide to the activities of antibiotics against microorganisms commonly involved in surgical infections. Table 5-5 summarizes the routes of administration and the doses commonly employed. The selection of antibiotic and dosage for a specific infection depends upon clinical judgment, bacterial sensitivity tests, and awareness of the toxicity of the drug. The white blood cell count is important in evaluating the response to antibiotic treatment and the appearance of adverse reactions in patients with infections.

Penicillins

The penicillins all share the 6-aminopenicillanic acid nucleus in which the beta-lactam ring is essential for antibacterial activity. Penicillins are bactericidal for susceptible bacteria by binding to receptors and blocking the synthesis of bacterial cell wall mucopeptide, producing osmotic instability and causing lysis. At adequate concentrations, penicillins are bactericidal against sensitive microorganisms, and are most effective during the stage of active bacterial multiplication. Inadequate concentrations may produce only bacteriostatic effects. Microorganisms that are resistant to penicillins produce beta-lactamases that hydrolyze the beta-lactam ring of some penicillins and inactivate the drug. Penicillins can be arranged in several groups:

1. Those with highest activity against gram-positive microorganisms, but susceptible to hydrolysis by beta-lactamases (e.g., penicillin G)
2. Those relatively resistant to beta-lactamases, but of lower activity against gram-positive microorganisms, and inactive against gram-negative microorganisms (e.g., methicillin, nafcillin)
3. Those with relatively high activity against both gram-positive and gram-negative microorganisms, but destroyed by beta-lactamases (e.g., ampicillin, carbenicillin, ticarcillin)
4. Those stable to gastric acid and suitable for oral administration (e.g., penicillin V, cloxacillin, ampicillin)

Penicillin G (benzyl penicillin) is active against almost all gram-positive pathogens. It is well absorbed but is not suitable for oral administration because it is destroyed by gastric acidity. Penicillin G is injected intramuscularly or intravenously and becomes distributed throughout the body in a few minutes. Hypersensitivity to penicillin is an important problem and is usually manifested as urticaria, but almost any type of allergic response may develop. Anaphylactic reactions may occur in the highly sensitized patient within minutes after an injection, and will require subcutaneous epinephrine. Penicillin G is the drug of choice (provided hypersensitivity does not exist) for severe infections produced by pneumococci, streptococci, non-beta-lactamase-producing staphylococci, meningococci, gonococci, clostridia, actinomycetes, treponemata, and bacteroides (except *Bacteroides fragilis*).

Semisynthetic penicillins are prepared by adding side chains to the 6-aminopenicillanic acid nucleus. They combine one or more of the following advantages: (1) they are acid-resistant and suitable for oral use; (2) they exert prolonged action in the body; (3) they are resistant to the beta-lactamases produced by *Staphylococcus aureus* and some gram-negative bacteria. Cloxacillin or dicloxacillin are preferred for oral use against lactamase-producing staphylococci. For severe infections, however, a parenteral formulation of methicillin, oxacillin, or nafcillin should be used.

Ampicillin, amoxicillin, carbenicillin, and ticarcillin are hydrolyzed by beta-lactamases but have greater activity than penicillin G against gram-negative bacteria. Ampicillin is slightly less active than penicillin G against most gram-positive bacteria. It is bacteriostatic in vitro against *Streptococcus faecalis* but is bactericidal in combination with an aminoglycoside. This combination is widely used to combat surgical sepsis. The ampicillin covers gram-positive species, particularly *Streptococcus faecalis;* the aminoglycoside covers facultative gram-negative species. Amoxicillin is similar to ampicillin. Carbenicillin resembles ampicillin but is more active against *Pseudomonas* and *Proteus* species; *Klebsiella* species are usually resistant. Ticarcillin resembles carbenicillin but is more active in vitro, requiring one-fourth to one-half the concentration of carbenicillin to kill *Pseudomonas aeruginosa*. Timentin is a parenteral combination of ticarcillin with clavulanic acid (as the potassium salt), a beta-lactamase inhibitor. The addition of clavulanate protects the ticarcillin from inactivation and extends its antibacterial spectrum, giving coverage of some *Enterobacteriaceae* (especially *Klebsiella*) and *Staphylococcus aureus* while retaining coverage against gram-positive cocci, including enterococci. The combination of amoxillin and clavulanate (Augmentin) provides an oral drug with activity against *S. aureus, Haemophilus influenzae,* and penicillinase-producing neisseriae. Despite the extended coverage provided by these combinations with clavulanate, older drugs and drug combinations may be equally effective.

Other new extended-spectrum penicillins include azlocillin, mezlocillin, and piperacillin. These are more active in vitro than carbenicillin or ticarcillin against gram-negatives such as *Klebsiella, Serratia,* and *Pseudomonas aeruginosa*. These newer agents are indicated in the treatment of infections caused by ticarcillin-resistant microorganisms.

Cephalosporins

The cephalosporins and cephamycins are related to the penicillins. In place of a 6-aminopenicillanic acid nucleus they have a nucleus of 7-aminocephalosporanic acid. They are bactericidal, and their mode of action is similar to that of penicillins, namely, inhibition of bacterial cell wall synthesis. A bewildering number of new semisynthetic cephalosporins have been developed and have entered into clinical practice since cephalothin was introduced in 1964. They are arranged into generations based on their expanding activity against gram-negative bacteria

Table 5-4. ANTIBIOTICS USEFUL AGAINST MICROORGANISMS IN SURGICAL INFECTIONS

Microorganism	First choice	Alternative agents
Gram-positive cocci:		
Staphylococcus aureus		
Lactamase-producing	Methicillin, nafcillin, oxacillin	A cephalosporin, clindamycin, vancomycin
Non-lactamase-producing	Penicillin G or V	A cephalosporin, clindamycin, vancomycin
Streptococcus pyogenes	Penicillin G or ampicillin	An erythromycin, a cephalosporin, vancomycin
Streptococcus pneumoniae	Penicillin G or V	An erythromycin, a cephalosporin, chloramphenicol
Streptococcus viridans	Penicillin G	An erythromycin, a cephalosporin, vancomycin
Streptococcus faecalis	Ampicillin or penicillin G with gentamicin or streptomycin	Vancomycin with gentamicin or streptomycin
Peptostreptococcus spp.	Penicillin G	Clindamycin, a tetracycline, chloramphenicol
Gram-negative cocci:		
Neisseria gonorrhoeae	Amoxicillin or ceftriaxone	Ampicillin, cefoxitin, chloramphenicol
Neisseria meningitidis	Penicillin G	Chloramphenicol
Gram-positive rods:		
Clostridium spp.	Penicillin G	Clindamycin, metronidazole, a tetracycline
Clostridium tetani	Penicillin G	A tetracycline
Clostridium difficile	Vancomycin	Metronidazole
Gram-negative rods:		
Acinetobacter spp.	Gentamicin	Amikacin, doxycycline
Bacteroides spp.		
Oropharyngeal strains	Penicillin G	Clindamycin, metronidazole, cefoxitin
Gastrointestinal strains	Clindamycin or metronidazole	Chloramphenicol, cefoxitin, ticarcillin
Campylobacter fetus	An erythromycin	A tetracycline, chloramphenicol
Enterobacter-Klebsiella-Serratia group	Ampicillin alone or with an aminoglycoside	Carbenicillin, ticarcillin, mezlocillin, or piperacillin alone or with an aminoglycoside, chloramphenicol
Escherichia coli	Ampicillin alone or with an aminoglycoside	Carbenicillin, ticarcillin, mezlocillin, or piperacillin alone or with an aminoglycoside, chloramphenicol
Fusobacterium spp.	Penicillin G	Clindamycin, metronidazole, chloramphenicol
Proteus mirabilis	Ampicillin	An aminoglycoside, carbenicillin, ticarcillin, mezlocillin, or piperacillin; a cephalosporin, chloramphenicol
Proteus spp. (indol-positive)	An aminoglycoside	Carbenicillin, ticarcillin, mezlocillin, or piperacillin; a cephalosporin, chloramphenicol
Providencia spp.	An aminoglycoside	Carbenicillin, ticarcillin, mezlocillin, or piperacillin; a cephalosporin, chloramphenicol
Pseudomonas aeruginosa	Gentamicin, tobramycin, or netlimicin, with carbenicillin, ticarcillin, mezlocillin, or piperacillin	Amikacin with carbenicillin, ticarcillin, mezlocillin, or piperacillin
Salmonella spp.	Ampicillin or amoxicillin	Chloramphenicol, trimethoprim-sulfamethoxazole
Actinomyces:		
Actinomyces israelii	Penicillin G	A tetracycline
Nocardia spp.	Sulfonamides	Trimethoprim-sulfamethoxazole, ampicillin
Fungi:		
Blastomyces dermatitidis	Amphotericin B	Ketoconazole
Candida albicans and other yeasts	Amphotericin B (± flucytosine)	Ketoconazole, miconazole (topical), nystatin (oral or topical)
Coccidioides immitis	Amphotericin B	Miconazole, ketoconazole
Cryptococcus neoformans	Amphotericin B (± flucytosine)	Ketoconazole, miconazole
Histoplasma capsulatum	Amphotericin B	Ketoconazole
Mucor spp.; *Rhizopus* spp.; *Aspergillus* spp.	Amphotericin B	
Paracoccidioides brasiliensis	Amphotericin B	Miconazole, ketoconazole
Sporotrichus schenckii	Potassium iodide	Amphotericin B

Table 5-5. ROUTES OF ADMINISTRATION AND DAILY DOSAGE OF ANTIBIOTICS COMMONLY USED IN ADULT SURGICAL PATIENTS HAVING NORMAL RENAL FUNCTION

Drug (trade name)	Oral	Intramuscular	Intravenous
Amikacin (Amiken)		15 mg/kg/day	15 mg/kg/day
Amoxicillin (Amoxil; others)	750–1500 mg/day		
Amphotericin (Fungizone)			0.25–1.5 mg/kg/day
Ampicillin (Polycillin; others)	1.2 g/day	150–200 mg/kg/day	150–200 mg/kg/day
Azlocillin (Azlin)			225–300 mg/kg/day
Carbenicillin (Geopen)		200–500 mg/kg/day	200–500mg/kg/day
Cefamandole (Mandol)		4–12 g/day	4–12 g/day
Cefazolin (Ancef, Kefzol)		1–10 g/day	1–10 g/day
Cefonicid (Monocid)		2–4 g/day	2–4 g/day
Cefoperazone (Cefobid)		2–4 g/day	2–4 g/day
Ceforanide (Precef)		1–2 g/day	1–2 g/day
Cefotaxime (Claforan)		2–12 g/day	2–12 g/day
Cefotetan (Apacef)		1–2 g/day	1–2 g/day
Cefoxitin (Mefoxin)		4–12 g/day	4–12 g/day
Ceftazidime (Fortaz)		2–6 g/day	2–6 g/day
Ceftizoxime (Cefizox)		2–12 g/day	2–12 g/day
Ceftriaxone (Rocephin)		1–2 g/day	1–2 g/day
Cefuroxime (Zinacef)		3–6 g/day	3–6 g/day
Cephalexin (Keflex)	1–4 g/day		
Chloramphenicol (Chloromycetin)	50–100 mg/kg/day		50–100 mg/kg/day
Clindamycin (Cleocin)	600–1800 mg/kg/day	600–2700 mg/kg/day	600–2700 mg/kg/day
Cloxacillin (Tegopen)	1–2 g/day		
Doxycycline (Vibramycin)	100–200 mg/day		100–200 mg/day
Erythromycin (Erythrocin; others)	1–2 g/day		1–2 g/day
Flucytosine (Ancobon)	50–150 mg/kg/day		
Gentamicin (Garamycin)		3–5 mg/kg/day	3–5 mg/kg/day
Kanamycin (Kantrex)		15 mg/kg/day	15 mg/kg/day
Ketoconazole (Nizoral)	200–1000 mg/day		
Methicillin (Staphcillin; others)		4–6 g/day	4–6 g/day
Metronidazole (Flagyl)	30 mg/kg/day		30 mg/kg/day
Mezlocillin (Mezlin)		16–18 g/day	16–18 g/day
Miconazole (Monistat)			600–3600 mg/kg/day
Moxalactam (Moxam)		2–12 g/day	2–12 g/day
Nafcillin (Nafcil, Unipen)	Not recommended	2–6 g/day	2–6 g/day
Netlimicin (Netromycin)		3–6 mg/kg/day	3–6 mg/kg/day
Oxacillin (Prostaphlin)	2–6 g/day	2–6 g/day	2–6 g/day
Penicillin G		100,000–200,000 units/kg/day	100,000–300,000 units/kg/day
Piperacillin (Piperacil)		12–18 g/day	12–18 g/day
Streptomycin		2–4 g/day	Not recommended
Tetracycline (Achromycin; others)	1–2 g/day	Not recommended	1–2 g/day
Ticarcillin (Ticar)		200–300 mg/kg/day	200–300 mg/kg/day
Tobramycin (Nebcin)		3–5 mg/kg/day	3–5 mg/kg/day
Vancomycin (Vancocin)	1–2 g/day		2–3 g/day

(Table 5-6). All first-generation drugs have a similar spectrum, including activity against many gram-positive cocci (but not enterococci or methicillin-resistant *Staphylococcus aureus*), *Escherichia coli*, *Klebsiella pneumoniae*, and *Proteus mirabilis*. The presence of food in the stomach delays and reduces the peak serum level of the few oral cephalosporins by one-third. Most cephalosporins, however, are poorly absorbed from the gastrointestinal tract and must be given parenterally. Pain restricts intramuscular use for most of these drugs. The exception is cefazolin, which is best tolerated by this route. Cefazolin is as effective as cephalothin and is cheaper. Although all cephalosporins have activity against many gram-positive bacteria, the first-generation drugs are more active in this area than later drugs. On the other hand, the first-generation drugs have activity against only a few gram-negative

species, and of these many strains of *Escherichia coli*, *Klebsiella pneumoniae*, and *Proteus mirabilis* are now resistant to them. The first-generation cephalosporins are inactive against gram-negatives seen in nosocomial infections or against *Bacteroides fragilis*.

The second-generation cephalosporins have a wider spectrum against gram-negatives and are moderately active against many, including *E. coli*, *Klebsiella*, *Citrobacter*, *Enterobacter*, and *Proteus mirabilis*. Although cefamandole has been recommended for empiric therapy for patients having abdominal, pelvic, or cardiovascular surgery, other regimens provide better coverage and/or are less expensive. Cefamandole should not be used to treat intraabdominal infections caused by anaerobic bacteria. Cefoxitin can be used as a single agent in the treatment of most mixed aerobic-anaerobic infections of the skin and

Table 5-6. SOME CEPHALOSPORIN ANTIBIOTICS

Generic name	Trade name	Route of administration
First generation:		
Cephalothin	Keflin	I.M., I.V.
Cefazolin	Ancef, Kefzol	I.M., I.V.
Cephapirin	Cefadyl	I.M., I.V.
Cephadrine	Anspor, Velosef	P.O., I.M., I.V.
Cephalexin	Keflex	P.O.
Cefadroxil	Duricef, Ultracef	P.O.
Second generation:		
Cefamandole	Mandol	I.M., I.V.
Cefoxitin	Mefoxin	I.M., I.V.
Cefuroxime	Zinacef	I.M., I.V.
Ceforanide	Precef	I.M., I.V.
Cefonicid	Monocid	I.M., I.V.
Cefotetan	Apacef	I.M., I.V.
Cefaclor	Ceclor	P.O.
Third generation:		
Cefotaxime	Claforan	I.M., I.V.
Ceftizoxime	Cefizox	I.M., I.V.
Cefoperazone	Cefobid	I.M., I.V.
Moxalactam	Moxam	I.M., I.V.
Ceftazidime	Fortaz	I.M., I.V.
Ceftriaxone	Rocephin	I.M., I.V.

soft tissues, pelvic infections, and community-acquired abdominal sepsis. For nosocomial intraabdominal sepsis an aminoglycoside should be added to the regimen to expand the coverage for aerobic gram-negative bacilli. Neither cefamandole nor cefoxitin should be used to treat bacterial meningitis or infections caused by enterococci or methicillin-resistant *S. aureus*. Cefoxitin can be used in the prevention of infection after fecal soilage of the peritoneum due to trauma. It can be used to prevent infections in patients who cannot take oral neomycin-erythromycin bowel preparation owing to emergency operations or intestinal obstruction (Sanders et al.). The antibacterial spectrum of cefonicid is similar to that of cefamandole, but cefonicid has a half-life 6 to 10 times that of cefamandole. Accordingly, the typical dosing schedule with cefonicid is 1 to 2 g I.V. or I.M. q 24 h as contrasted to q 6 h for cefamandole.

The third-generation cephalosporins are newer and exhibit a wider spectrum against gram-negative bacilli than do the first- and second-generation drugs. For example, the third-generation drugs are a major therapeutic advance in the treatment of gram-negative meningitis, are very active against *Haemophilus influenzae* (including penicillinase-producing strains), and are more efficacious than the older cephalosporins in treating infection caused by gram-negative bacilli resistant to multiple antibiotics (i.e., nosocomial pathogens). This owes to their greater beta-lactamase stability and their high affinities for penicillin-binding proteins. These newer drugs, however, also display decreased activity against staphylococci, and their activity against gram-negative bacilli is often less predictable than that of the aminoglycosides. Their activity against anaerobes is inferior to that of cefoxitin, a

cheaper second-generation drug. Ceftizoxime, cefoperazone, and moxalactam have relatively long half-lives and may be administered on a q 8- to 12-h dosing schedule. Cefotaxime has a shorter half-life and should be administered on a q 4- to 6-h schedule. At our hospital ceftizoxime is restricted for use in treating infections due to gram-negative bacilli resistant to cefazolin and cefuroxime; cefoperazone may be used combined with an aminoglycoside in treating pseudomonal infections involving skin, soft tissues, and bones and joints in penicillin-allergic patients; cefotaxime is restricted for use in treating meningitis due to gram-negative bacilli; and ceftriaxone, which has a half-life of 6 to 9 h and may be administered once daily, is reserved for treating infections due to gram-negative bacilli resistant to cefazolin and cefuroxime. The third-generation cephalosporins have no place in the treatment of gram-positive or anaerobic infections, most community-acquired infections, or surgical prophylaxis. Based on their toxicities, moxalactam should be avoided and cefoperazone used with caution. The third-generation drugs are not cost-effective in most situations. Their economies in dosage because of long half-lives are offset by their high cost per gram and the frequent necessity of combining them with an aminoglycoside.

Erythromycins

Erythromycin is a macrocyclic lactone (i.e., a macrolide). It is active against pneumococci, beta-hemolytic streptococci, enterococci, many staphylococci, and clostridia. Erythromycin is bacteriostatic but may be bactericidal in higher concentrations, inhibiting bacterial protein synthesis. The antibiotic is uniformly distributed throughout the body and is excreted in the urine and bile. However, the major portion of the drug is metabolized in the body. Erythromycin base is generally well tolerated but may cause some gastrointestinal disturbance (nausea, vomiting, diarrhea, flatulence). Erythromycin is useful in pneumococcal and streptococcal infection, as a second choice in patients sensitive to penicillin, and for elimination of corynebacteria from the pharynx of carriers. Bacterial resistance to erythromycin is common during long-term treatment. Erythromycin is the agent of choice for treatment of mycoplasmal infections and Legionnaires' disease. It is useful in the treatment of actinomycosis.

Tetracyclines

The tetracyclines are a family of closely related antibiotics. Those now widely used are tetracycline, oxytetracycline, and doxycycline. There is no good evidence that tetracycline has any advantage over oxytetracycline in the treatment of disease or in the production of fewer side effects in the adult. Doxycycline possesses the advantage, because of its slower excretion, of requiring only one dose daily. Members of this group are broad-spectrum and active against those gram-positive species that are also sensitive to penicillin, against many gram-negative species that are not sensitive to penicillin, against *Treponema pallidum* and other treponemata, and against

Mycobacterium tuberculosis. They also inhibit the growth of actinomycetes, rickettsiae, mycoplasma, and agents of the psittacosis-lymphogranuloma venereum-trachoma group of *Chlamydia.* The tetracyclines are bacteriostatic. They interfere with protein synthesis by inhibiting amino acid transfer from RNA to microsomal protein. Resistance may be due to decreased permeability to the antibiotic. A microorganism resistant to one tetracycline is equally resistant to the others. Tetracyclines are usually administered orally; they become distributed throughout the body and appear to have affinity for fast-growing tissues, such as liver, tumors, and new bone. Tetracyclines (with the exception of doxycycline) are to be avoided in renal failure. Tetracyclines are deposited in teeth during early stages of calcification, causing a yellow to brownish discoloration that is undesirable cosmetically. Therefore, tetracycline treatment should be avoided in early childhood except for imperative reasons or when a short course will suffice. Liver damage has resulted from excessive doses. Replacement of suppressed normal flora by tetracycline-resistant microorganisms causes gastrointestinal disturbances such as nausea, vomiting, diarrhea, and flatulence. Superinfection with *Candida albicans* may produce soreness of the mouth and even thrush, which may spread to the pharynx and bronchi, or diarrhea and pruritus ani. Superinfection with *Proteus* and *Pseudomonas* species resistant to tetracycline commonly produces diarrhea. Superinfection with *Staphylococcus aureus* may produce a fatal staphylococcal enterocolitis. Activity against anaerobes is erratic. Tetracycline with penicillin is recommended for actinomycosis and, with sulfadiazine, for nocardiosis.

Chloramphenicol

Chloramphenicol is a broad-spectrum antibiotic; it is bacteriostatic and inhibits protein synthesis by interfering with messenger ribonucleic acid (mRNA). It is well absorbed orally and parenterally. About 90 percent can be detected in urine as an inactive conjugate with glucuronic acid; only about 10 percent appears as active antibiotic. Two different lethal toxic effects are known: First, a rare total aplasia of the bone marrow with aplastic anemia may occur during treatment or as long as 4 months afterward. Second, because of deficiency in detoxifying enzymes, premature infants may accumulate sufficient free chloramphenicol to cause an acute and usually fatal circulatory collapse (gray syndrome). Minor toxic effects include soreness of the mouth from overgrowth of *Candida albicans,* resulting from depression of normal flora due to antibiotic in the saliva, and optic neuritis in children with cystic fibrosis of the pancreas receiving treatment with chloramphenicol for pulmonary infection. Chloramphenicol should not be used for trivial infections or as a prophylactic agent to prevent bacterial infection. Chloramphenicol is the drug of choice for typhoid fever and other severe *Salmonella* infections, but since most *Salmonella* infections will respond to ampicillin, chloramphenicol should be used only if the patient does not respond to ampicillin or is allergic to it. Chloramphenicol is recom-

mended for patients who cannot tolerate tetracyclines and for those who have rickettsial disease, psittacosis, or lymphopathia venereum. It can be a life-saving drug in the treatment of patients with meningitis when penicillin cannot be administered. Chloramphenicol is the drug of choice in the treatment of severe infections caused by such microorganisms as *Haemophilus influenzae* in patients allergic to penicillin. Prolonged usage and repeated exposure should be avoided. White cell count and differential should be taken daily, and therapy should be discontinued if leukopenia occurs.

Aminoglycosides

The aminoglycosides are bactericidal antibiotics having similar structural, antimicrobial, pharmacologic, and toxic characteristics, and include streptomycin, neomycin, kanamycin, gentamicin, tobramycin, amikacin, and netlimicin. These agents inhibit protein synthesis in bacteria by disorganizing the proper attachment of mRNA to the bacterial ribosome. Resistance to aminoglycosides is based upon either (1) a deficiency of ribosomal receptor; or (2) enzymatic destruction of the drug (plasmid mediated) by adenylylation (nucleotidylation) of hydroxyl groups, acetylation of amino groups, and phosphorylation of hydroxyl groups; or (3) impermeability to the drug or failure of active transport across cell membranes. The aminoglycosides possess a wide range of bactericidal activity against gram-negative and gram-positive bacteria and mycobacteria. There is little absorption from the alimentary tract and fairly slow renal excretion in unchanged form after intramuscular injection. This affords therapeutic levels for 6 to 8 h. Aminoglycosides exhibit a high degree of mutual cross resistance, a strong dose-related tendency to damage the auditory branch of the eighth nerve, and some possibility of damage to the kidney. This nephrotoxicity is indicated with rising serum creatinine levels or reduced creatinine clearance.

The use of streptomycin is now limited by its toxicity to the initial treatment of tuberculosis as a second or third drug, and is the drug of first choice in the treatment of infections due to *Pasteurella* species (i.e., tularemia, plague). Neomycin is used now only topically in ointments and orally (in conjunction with erythromycin base) for intestinal antisepsis to prepare the colon for elective surgery.

Kanamycin is closely related to neomycin but is less toxic. It is bactericidal for most gram-negative bacilli and has a spectrum of usefulness similar to amikacin or gentamicin, with the exception of *Pseudomonas aeruginosa,* against which kanamycin is ineffective. Kanamycin is completely absorbed following parenteral injection and is rapidly excreted in the urine.

Gentamicin is produced by a *Micromonospora.* This is designated by the suffix "micin," whereas the suffix "mycin" indicates derivation from a *Streptomyces.* Gentamicin is used in severe infections caused by gram-negative bacteria that are likely to be resistant to other, less toxic drugs. It is administered by intramuscular or intravenous injection and becomes well distributed. Gentamicin is almost quantitatively excreted unchanged in the urine, principally by glomerular filtration. The drug may be synergistic with beta-lactam antibiotics, such as cephalosporins or carbenicillin, against *Klebsiella* and *Pseudomonas,* respectively. Tobramycin is virtually identical with gentamicin in antibacterial activity but is less nephrotoxic. Netlimicin is similar in activity to gentamicin and to tobramycin. Amikacin is a semisynthetic derivative of kanamycin. It is relatively resistant to several of the enzymes that inactivate gentamicin, tobramycin and netlimicin, and can therefore be used against many strains of gram-negative bacilli to which these aminoglycosides are resistant. Parenteral aminoglycosides are among the most valuable agents available for the treatment of life-threatening infections by enteric gram-negative bacteria. Because of the emergence of resistant strains of *Pseudomonas, Proteus, Providencia,* and *Serratia,* hospitals usually designate a single aminoglycoside antibiotic, such as gentamicin, for primary use and hold the others in reserve for use against infections caused by resistant bacteria. Amikacin is preferred for nosocomial infections by gram-negative pathogens in severely ill, hospitalized patients.

Polypeptide Antibiotics

The polymyxins are basic polypeptides especially useful against *Pseudomonas aeruginosa.* They are bactericidal for most gram-negative bacteria, except *Proteus* species and *Neisseria* species. Fungi and all gram-positive bacteria are resistant. Polymyxin B and colistimethate (polymyxin E) have similar antibacterial activities. They are not absorbed from the alimentary tract but are well absorbed following intramuscular injection. The polymyxins are toxic, usually producing paresthesias, dizziness, and flushing, and nephrotoxicity and respiratory arrest following high dosages. The introduction of broad-spectrum penicillins, cephalosporins, and aminoglycosides has lessened the importance of polymyxins in the treatment of pseudomonal infections, and practically eliminated their need in clinical medicine.

Bacitracin is a bactericidal, polypeptide antibiotic active against gram-positive bacteria, including beta-lactamase-producing staphylococci, but inactive against common gram-negative bacilli. It is absorbed to only a slight extent from the alimentary tract, skin, wounds, or mucous membranes. Systemic administration of bacitracin is no longer used because of severe nephrotoxicity, but it is useful for irrigating wounds, infected joints, or abscess cavities. Bacitracin in ointment base is used topically, combined with neomycin or polymyxin, in treating infected wounds, suppurative conjunctivitis, and superficial infections.

Specialized Drugs

Lincomycin and clindamycin are lincosamides. They closely resemble erythromycin (although different in structure) in antibacterial activity against gram-positive microorganisms, become widely distributed in tissues, and are excreted through the bile. Because lincomycin is less active in vitro and has no clinical advantage over clindamycin, its use is not recommended. Clindamycin is useful primarily in the treatment of anaerobic infections, including those caused by *Bacteroides fragilis.* Mixed intraabdominal infections caused by anaerobes and aerobic gram-negative bacilli may be treated with clindamycin and an aminoglycoside. Infections such as aspiration pneumonia and anaerobic pleuropulmonary infections are best treated with penicillin, but the alternate agent of choice is clindamycin. Although clindamycin is active in vitro against streptococci, including pneumococci, alternative agents, such as erythromycin, are potentially less toxic. Bloody diarrhea with pseudomembranous colitis has been associated with clindamycin (as well as other antibiotics). This is due to a necrotizing toxin produced by *Clostridium difficile,* which is resistant to clindamycin and which becomes the predominant clostridial flora of the intestine during oral as well as parenteral administration of clindamycin.

Vancomycin is bactericidal for gram-positive microorganisms, including staphylococci, streptococci, and clostridia. It inhibits the synthesis of bacterial cell walls, but by a mechanism different from that of the penicillins. Vancomycin is regarded as a reserve antibiotic that is valuable in the treatment of life-threatening infections with multiresistant staphylococci and with streptcocci (including *Streptococcus faecalis* endocarditis) in patients who are allergic to penicillin. The drug is administered intravenously. Since it is not absorbed from the gastrointestinal tract, oral administration is useful for the treatment of antibiotic-associated pseudomembranous colitis (caused by overgrowth of *Clostridium difficile*). Ototoxicity has been associated with prolonged serum concentrations greater than 60 to 80 μg/mL. Serum levels should be obtained. The serum half-life is prolonged in anuric patients.

Metronidazole (Flagyl) is a 5-nitroimidazole widely used in the treatment of trichomonal vaginitis, intestinal amebiasis, and giardiasis. It has become prominent because of its bactericidal action against all clinically important obligate anaerobic bacteria, such as *Bacteroides fragilis* and other species of bacteroides, fusobacteria, and clostridia. *Proprionibacterium, Actinomyces,* and microaerophilic streptococci are resistant. Metronidazole is the only drug exhibiting consistent bactericidal activity against *Bacteroides fragilis* at or close to the minimal inhibitory concentration. Its bactericidal activity depends on products resulting from the reduction of the 5-nitro group intracellularly at the low oxidation-reduction potential occurring within anaerobic microorganisms. This bactericidal metabolite is produced in both dividing and nondividing anaerobes.

Metronidazole has been used prophylactically in the perioperative period to prevent postoperative morbidity in patients undergoing elective colorectal and gynecologic operations. It has been given both intravenously and as a rectal suppository. Good results have been obtained in treating anaerobic and mixed aerobic-anaerobic infections, such as wound infections, abdominal abscesses, liver abscesses, perirectal abscesses, and decubitus ulcers. Metronidazole readily crosses the blood-brain barrier and has been effective in treating nontraumatic brain abscesses. Metronidazole may also be of value in dental surgery in decreasing the incidence of anaerobic infections. A combination of metronidazole and gentamicin is a relatively inexpensive, primary approach to treating intraabdominal and other polymicrobic infections. Metronidazole may cause peripheral neuropathy and convulsions in long-term therapy, and phlebitis if not buffered with sodium bicarbonate, but moderate reactions such as vomiting, diarrhea, and skin rash are more prevalent. Patients taking metronidazole should be warned against the use of alcohol because of the possibility of a disulfiram-like reaction. Although vancomycin is currently recommended for treating antibiotic-associated pseudomembranous colitis, metronidazole, which is much less expensive, may be used as an effective alternative treatment.

Imipenem is the first of a new class of beta-lactam antibiotics called carbapenems. It has the broadest antibacterial spectrum of any beta-lactam antibiotic now available (Barza). This includes gram-positive cocci (except methicillin-resistant staphylococci and some enterococci), gram-negative cocci, *Enterobacteriaceae, Pseudomonas aeruginosa,* and anaerobic bacilli including *Bacteroides fragilis.* Imipenem is administered intravenously in combination with an equal amount of cilastatin. The cilastatin inhibits renal tubular metabolism of imipenem, preventing the formation of potentially nephrotoxic compounds. Imipenem has been effective in treating mixed bacterial infections for which a combination of antibiotics, often including an aminoglycoside, are usually necessary—for example, pulmonary, gynecologic, and intraabdominal infections.

Antifungal Antibiotics

Antibiotics generally have no effect on pathogenic fungi, with the exception of the penicillins, which can be used to treat actinomycosis, and the sulfonamides, which can be used for nocardiosis. Pathogenic fungi are susceptible only to certain highly specialized drugs that usually have no antibacterial activity.

Amphotericin B is the only antifungal antibiotic effective in the treatment of systemic mycotic infections. It binds to sterols, specifically ergosterol, and interferes with the permeability of the fungal cell wall. Amphotericin B is the drug of choice for treatment of systemic candidosis, mucormycosis, disseminated active histoplasmosis, cryptococcosis, coccidioidomycosis, and pulmonary sporotrichosis. Amphotericin B is not appreciably absorbed from the gastrointestinal tract or the skin; it is administered intravenously or intrathecally, or instilled directly into the site of infection. Initial toxic effects commonly include fever, chills, nausea, vomiting, and headache. Toxic effects brought on by continued use may include anemia, thrombophlebitis at the site of injection, hypokalemia, rise of blood urea and serum creatinine levels, and permanent damage to the kidney.

Griseofulvin has its greatest activity against growing dermatophytes and is useful in treating superficial dermatomycoses of skin, hair, or nails due to species of *Mi-crosporum, Epidermophyton,* and *Trichophyton.* Griseofulvin is fungicidal, binds to RNA, impairs synthesis of nucleic acids and protein, and breaks down intracellular membranes of dermatophytes, but not of fungi causing systemic mycoses. This antifungal antibiotic is administered orally and is incorporated into liver, fat, keratin, and skeletal muscle. It is well tolerated even during long courses of treatment, and toxic effects (skin reactions, gastric discomfort, and neurologic reactions) are uncommon and rarely severe. Cultures are needed to determine that skin lesions are not due to *Candida* or bacteria, as these are not improved by griseofulvin and may be exacerbated by the antibiotic.

Nystatin is effective in the treatment of candidosis. It is fungistatic and damages the fungal cell membrane by binding to sterol sites in it. This antifungal antibiotic is not absorbed from the gastrointestinal tract, skin, or mucosal surfaces. It is used to treat gastrointestinal candidosis, which may result as a complication of therapy with broad-spectrum antibiotics. Such antibiotic-induced superinfection often disappears with discontinuance of the antibacterial therapy that provoked it. Nystatin is available in topical powders, creams, and ointments that may be useful in treating cutaneous and mucocutaneous candidosis. Nystatin tablets may be sucked for candida stomatitis; vaginal tablets are available for treatment of vaginal candidosis. Nystatin is harmless by local application. There have been rare cases of diarrhea, nausea, and vomiting after administration of large oral doses.

Flucytosine (5-fluorocytosine) is a halogenated pyrimidine inhibiting nucleic acid synthesis in yeastlike fungi. It is administered orally; there is good absorption and relatively low toxicity. Flucytosine may be effective for treatment of cryptococcosis and candidosis, but, when used alone, resistant organisms may emerge during therapy. However, the combination of amphotericin B plus flucytosine results in additive or even synergistic effects in systemic mycoses, reduces the dose requirement of amphotericin B alone, and may delay the emergence of resistance to flucytosine.

Miconazole and ketoconazole are imidazole derivatives having a broad spectrum of activity against dermatophytes, dimorphic fungi, yeast, and some bacteria. Miconazole is useful topically in the treatment of cutaneous and mucocutaneous candidal infections. Miconazole also can be given intravenously for the treatment of coccidioidomycosis, cryptococcosis, and candidosis when amphotericin B has failed or is contraindicated. Ketoconazole is clinically useful in the management of mucocutaneous candidosis, histoplasmosis, paracoccidioidomycosis, and dermatophytic infections. Therapeutic levels in blood are rapidly obtained after a single oral dose and are maintained for several hours.

Sulfonamides

Introduced in 1935, the sulfonamides initiated the modern antibacterial chemotherapeutic revolution in medicine. Their use antedates that of the antibiotics by several years, since penicillin did not become available until 1941. The sulfonamides are valuable agents in the management of some infections, particularly urinary tract infections due to *Escherichia coli,* and can be employed for the prophylaxis of recurrences of rheumatic fever. Although one of these compounds, mafenide acetate (Sulfamylon), has an important use in the topical therapy of severe burn wounds, the value of the sulfonamides in the treatment of surgical infections is severely limited by their inactivation by pus. The sulfonamides are bacteriostatic and active against both gram-positive and gram-negative bacteria. The drugs are strongly antagonized by *p*-aminobenzoic acid (PABA), an essential intermediate in the synthesis of folic acid by bacterial cells, and act as competitive inhibitors. Bacteria sensitive to the sulfonamides are unable to utilize preformed folic acid in the body and must synthesize it themselves. Folic acid acts as a coenzyme in the transfer of fragments containing one carbon atom, which are involved in the synthesis of amino acids (such as methionine and serine), purines, and thymine. These compounds also inhibit the activity of sulfonamides, but unlike PABA they are noncompetitive inhibitors, and their effect is not reversed by increasing the concentration of drugs. Accordingly, pus, which is rich in amino acids and purines made available by the breakdown of cellular protein and nucleic acids, inactivates the sulfonamides.

Some of the sulfonamides of use in surgical practice are sulfisoxazole (Gantrisin) and sulfamethoxazole (Gantanol), which are used for treating urinary tract infections, and mafenide (Sulfamylon), which is applied topically and used to treat burn wound infections. Mafenide is not inhibited by the products of tissue necrosis but causes pain. Of comparable value in the treatment of burns is the silver salt of sulfadiazine (Silvadene), which does not cause pain on application and is free of major toxicity.

Orally administered sulfonamides are rapidly absorbed in the stomach and duodenum and become distributed in all tissues and fluids. The sulfonamides are bound to either serum albumin or to tissue proteins, and they are detoxified in the liver. Both the drug and its less active metabolites are excreted by glomerular filtration. Sensitivity to one sulfonamide frequently confers sensitivity to others. Toxic reactions limiting sulfonamide therapy range from nausea, vomiting, and dermatitis to crystalluria, renal injury, hepatic damage, and hematologic disorders.

A fixed-dose combination of trimethoprim-sulfamethoxazole (Bactrim, Septra) is available in tablets for oral administration and also in a parenteral formulation. This combination is useful for the treatment of severe urinary tract infections, bronchitis in adults, pneumonia caused by *Pneumocystis carinii* (a presumed protozoan), and shigellosis. Trimethoprim-sulfamethoxazole is the drug of choice in typhoid fever with strains of *Salmonella typhi* resistant to both chloramphenicol and ampicillin.

STREPTOCOCCAL INFECTIONS

Streptococci form the dominant aerobic flora of the mouth and pharyngeal areas of human beings. They are gram-positive spherical or ovoid cells (rarely elongated

into rods) arranged in pairs (short chains). Long chains are observed when the organism is cultured in fluid media. Although most species are aerobic or facultatively anaerobic, there are also species that are obligately anaerobic (e.g., *Peptostreptococcus putridus* and *Peptostreptococcus micros*) or microaerophilic. They may be divided into those which produce a soluble hemolysin and those which do not. Aerobes producing a clear zone of hemolysis on blood agar (beta hemolysis) include most of the species associated with primary streptococcal infections in human beings and can be subdivided into 15 broad groups (Lancefield groups) that are identified by precipitin tests with group-specific antisera against specific carbohydrate haptens (C antigens) of the streptococci. Strains belonging to Lancefield group A (*Streptococcus pyogenes)* are responsible for over 90 percent of human streptococcal infections. These group A strains can be further subdivided for epidemiologic studies into Griffith types according to their surface protein antigens (M, T, and R) by capillary precipitin or slide agglutination tests.

Another group of streptococci produce an ill-defined zone of partial hemolysis having a green or brownish-green color (alpha hemolysis). These are strains of *Streptococcus viridans.* Streptococci that are without effect on blood agar (nonhemolytic) include the fecal enterococci (*Streptococcus faecalis).* Viridans and nonhemolytic streptococci are associated with chronic diseases or are nonpathogenic. *Streptococcus viridans* is part of the commensal flora of the mouth and throat and is dangerous in individuals with congenitally deformed or rheumatically damaged heart valves. It is the commonest cause of subacute bacterial endocarditis. *Streptococcus viridans* has been incriminated in apical tooth infections and is commonly found in carious teeth. Bacteremia frequently follows tooth extraction and even routine dental procedures. In otherwise healthy individuals the streptococci are rapidly removed from the circulation, but in those with heart lesions the organisms settle in or on the defective valves. Accordingly, patients with congenital or other valvular cardiac defects should be given penicillin prophylactically before and after any dental attention.

Nonhemolytic streptococci are always present in the colon and may be isolated from the terminal ileum and upper jejunum of 60 percent of surgical patients. These enterococci (*Streptococcus faecalis)* can cause suppurative lesions and urinary tract infections. Some strains of *Streptococcus faecalis* produce a true beta hemolysis; they belong to Lancefield group D.

Group A beta-hemolytic streptococci (*Streptococcus pyogenes)* are the principal causes of streptococcal pharyngitis, scarlet fever, and rheumatic fever. They also cause bacteremias following surgical procedures in patients with malignant disease. Groups B, C, D, F, and G are usually less virulent. Although group B streptococci are often isolated from patients with puerperal sepsis, with meningitis of the newborn, with diabetes mellitus, and/or with peripheral vascular insufficiency, they are also involved in pneumonias and infections of the male genitourinary tract. Since group C streptococci are part of the skin flora, they may be isolated from wounds and exudates more often than group B strains. The group G streptococci involved in infections usually originate in the genitourinary tract or skin, but they may also originate in the upper respiratory tract or gastrointestinal tract.

Streptococcus pyogenes is an invasive microorganism; it secretes two distinct hemolysins (streptolysins O and S) and several other products that aid in invasion. Streptolysin O is cardiotoxic and leukocidic and may be identical with leukocidin. Streptolysin S is a pure hemolysin responsible for beta hemolysis on blood agar plates. Hyaluronidase hydrolyzes hyaluronic acid and allows increased permeability of tissues. Streptokinase reduces fibrinolysis by activating the plasmin system. Streptodornase depolymerizes DNA. Erythrogenic toxin produces erythema when injected intradermally and is responsible for the punctate erythema of scarlet fever. The hyaluronidase and streptokinase produced by most strains of *Streptococcus pyogenes* are responsible for the spreading cellulitis (erysipelas) that is the typical streptococcal lesion. When abscess occurs, the pus is watery and often blood-stained due to the action of streptodornase and streptokinase, since the viscosity of pus is due to DNA and fibrin.

Erysipelas

Erysipelas is a spreading streptococcal cellulitis and lymphangitis with raised, sharply defined, irregular, reddish borders. Since erythrogenic toxin is produced in variable amounts by hemolytic streptococci, the development of cutaneous erythema is an inconstant manifestation of streptococcal infection. Minor skin abrasions and fissures predispose to these infections of the skin. The cutis is edematous and reddened, with a palpably raised border; the lesion is hot, tender, and painful. The classic lesion of erysipelas is a ''butterfly'' erythema centered around the nose and extending onto both cheeks. The systemic manifestations of erysipelas may be severe and suggest invasion via the lymphatics or bloodstream. Penicillin is usually effective against the invasive infection, but the erythema disappears more slowly.

Erysipeloid, a nonstreptococcal disease distinct from erysipelas, is a type of cutaneous cellulitis due to infection by *Erysipelothrix rhusopathiae,* a gram-positive, nonsporulating, facultative anaerobe in the family Corynebacteriaceae. The typical lesion is a violaceous nodule, often having a curved shape, which differs from that of erysipelas by its tendency to central clearing and the absence of suppuration. Human cases of erysipeloid may also occur as either a severe, generalized cutaneous disease or as septicemia with or without cutaneous involvement and often associated with endocarditis. Penicillin therapy is specific for most cases. Erysipelothrix infection is considered an occupational disease of abattoir workers, fish handlers, and others exposed to meat, poultry, and fish products.

Necrotizing Fasciitis

This is a life-threatening infection that may occur in only one or two patients a year in large city-county hospitals. The most significant manifestation of the infection is extensive necrosis of the superficial fascia with resultant widespread undermining of surrounding tissue and extreme systemic toxicity. The bacteria involved in about 90 percent of cases have usually been beta-hemolytic streptococci, or coagulase-positive staphylococci, or both. Gram-negative enteric pathogens alone have been associated with about 10 percent of cases of necrotizing fasciitis. The disease appears to be a clinical entity and not a specific bacterial infection. It has been described previously as hemolytic or acute streptococcal gangrene, gangrenous or necrotizing erysipelas, suppurative fasciitis, and hospital gangrene. Although necrotizing fasciitis may develop following surgical procedures such as appendectomy, the majority of cases have occurred outside the hospital following minor trauma such as abrasions, cuts, bruises, boils, injection of drugs, and insect bites on the extremities, particularly in individuals with diabetes and peripheral vascular disease. The chief diagnostic criterion for necrotizing fasciitis is superficial and widespread fascial necrosis. Cellulitis as well as edema (mild to massive) are present in most patients. The involved skin is pale red without distinct borders and with blisters or bullae. Pale red areas progress to a distinct purple. The diagnosis is confirmed by observation of (1) serosanguinous exudate; (2) swollen, stringy, dull gray, necrotic fascia with extensive undermining; and (3) a Gram-stained smear of the pus or fluid showing the types of bacteria involved and a substantial white blood cell response.

TREATMENT. This consists of multiple linear incisions over the affected area and debridement of all involved areas. In an open wound, the extent of undermining can be ascertained by passing a sterile hemostat along the plane just superficial to the deep fascia. In simple cellulitis or erysipelas, the hemostat cannot be passed. Before operation, the patient should be given a full dose of systemic antibiotic(s) effective against both hemolytic streptococci and penicillinase-producing staphylococci. The combination of an aminoglycoside and clindamycin and penicillin G or ampicillin covers the majority of pathogens involved. Therapy is continued postoperatively until the infection is controlled. Repeated debridement may be necessary if the patient continues to be febrile. With the appearance of clean granulation tissue after 5 to 10 days, the wound may be closed by skin graft or suture. Rea and Wyrick (1970) report a 30 percent mortality.

Peptostreptococci (anaerobic streptococci) are also pathogenic. They are normal inhabitants of the mouth, intestine, and vagina. They are abundant when oral hygiene is poor, and aspiration into the lungs and sinuses may lead to putrid lung abscess, empyema, and sinusitis. Brain abscesses often develop as complications of chronic or acute infections of the lungs, sinuses, or ears. *Peptostreptococcus putridus* has been isolated from cases of puerperal sepsis, brain abscess, and infected wounds. *Nonclostridial crepitant anaerobic cellulitis* is due to peptostreptococci, whereas *synergistic necrotizing cellulitis* with widespread involvement of deeper tissues is caused by the symbiotic activity of peptostreptococci, aerobic gram-negative rods, and frequently bacteroides.

Streptococcal Myonecrosis

Anaerobic streptococci can cause gas gangrene. Facultative streptococci and *Staphylococcus aureus* also may be isolated. *Streptococcal myonecrosis* resembles subacute clostridial gas gangrene and was not described until World War II. After an incubation period of 3 to 4 days, there is swelling, edema, and purulent wound exudate. These signs are followed by pain which rapidly becomes severe. Gas is present, and the infected muscle changes from pale and soft to bright red, striped with purple, and finally purple and gangrenous. The seropurulent discharge has a sour odor. In this disease, muscle is involved, in contrast to necrotizing fasciitis, in which the fascia is affected. Treatment consists of incision and drainage, antibiotic therapy, and supportive measures.

Progressive Synergistic Gangrene

As early as 1924, Meleney established the importance of microaerophilic and anaerobic streptococci in special wound infections known as progressive synergistic gangrene and chronic burrowing ulcer. *Meleney's progressive synergistic gangrene* characteristically develops in sutured, infected thoracic or abdominal incisions or around a colostomy, ileostomy, or simple abrasion. The initial lesion is a small, painful, superficial ulcer that gradually spreads. The central ulcerated area is surrounded by a rim of gangrenous skin, which in turn is encircled by a zone of purple erythema blending into a surrounding area of bright, painful erythema. There is seropurulent discharge. Cultures taken from the outer edematous part of the lesion yield microaerophilic or anaerobic nonhemolytic streptococci. Cultures taken from the central ulcerated area yield *Staphylococcus aureus* and sometimes gram-negative bacilli, such as *Proteus* species. However, clinical cases of progressive synergistic gangrene from which anaerobic or microaerophilic streptococci could not be isolated have been reported. Treatment involves wide excision and therapy with penicillin or chloramphenicol. Corticosteroids have been employed to aid healing. Ledingham and Tehrani find that the problem in acute dermal gangrene following surgery, such as necrotizing fasciitis and progressive synergistic gangrene, is no longer any apparent specificity of invading bacteria but rather a vicious cycle of infection, local ischemia, and diminished host defense mechanisms.

Meleney's Ulcer

Chronic burrowing or undermining ulcer, often designated as *Meleney's ulcer,* is caused by a nonhemolytic anaerobic or microaerophilic streptococcus. The lesion begins as a small, superficial ulcer following trauma or surgery and may also originate from an infected lymph node or subcutaneous abscess. The ulcer is only mildly painful, and systemic reaction is minimal. Slow, progressive enlargement of the lesion occurs over months or years. Infection of subcutaneous tissue is associated with ulceration of the overlying skin. Cutaneous gangrene is absent, and the edges of the undermined skin roll inward. The periphery of the lesion is erythematous, and the advancing edge of the lesion is characterized by pain and tenderness. Meleney's ulcer occurs most frequently after incision of a lymph node in the neck, axilla, or groin and after operations on the genital and intestinal tracts. As the lesion spreads, multiple ulcers and sinuses develop, producing epithelial strands and undermined bridges of skin. Treatment consists of debridement, drainage of sinuses, penicillin therapy, and split-thickness skin grafts over denuded areas as soon as the wound appears clean.

Peptostreptococci, either in pure culture or mixed with bacteroides, are frequently involved in appendiceal abscesses, peritonitis, abdominal wall sepsis, perirectal abscesses, and superficial abscesses related to infections of pilonidal and sebaceous cysts. Most abscesses are treated successfully by incision and drainage, and penicillin therapy. Peptostreptococcal infections, including septicemias, commonly occur in the female pelvic area following septic abortion and postpartum sepsis.

STAPHYLOCOCCAL INFECTIONS

Staphylococci form part of the permanent bacterial flora of the normal skin and nasopharynx and may cause a variety of infections, often characterized by suppuration, ranging from mild, localized pustules to lethal septicemias. Surgical and traumatic wounds are particularly susceptible to purulent infection. In stained preparations of pus, staphylococci appear as spherical cells occurring singly, in pairs, or in small clusters. They are gram-positive and nonmotile, and produce no spores. Staphylococci are aerobic or facultatively anaerobic and grow on ordinary unenriched bacteriologic media. They may produce pigmentation varying from white, orange, or yellow to golden. Blood agar is often hemolyzed (beta hemolysis). Two species are of medical importance: *Staphylococcus aureus* and *Staphylococcus epidermidis*. *Staphylococcus aureus* is usually associated with disease, and will be discussed subsequently. On the other hand, *Staphylococcus epidermidis* usually has not been considered a pathogen, but it has become recognized as an important cause of opportunistic infection following surgical procedures in which foreign materials and prostheses are placed in the patient. *Staphylococcus epidermidis* can cause endocarditis following open heart surgery and occasionally produces septicemia.

The criteria identifying staphylococci are colonial appearance on blood agar, gram stain reaction, microscopic morphologic features, production of coagulase, and fermentation of mannitol. *Staphylococcus aureus* is coagulase-positive and produces acid from mannitol. *Staphylococcus epidermidis* produces neither coagulase nor acid from mannitol. Filtrates of cultures of *Staphylococcus aureus* contain hemolysins, dermonecrotic and lethal factors, leukocidins, and enzymes. Strains of *Staphylococcus aureus* may be classified into groups on the basis of their susceptibility to various bacteriophages. Although phage typing of isolates is of value in epidemiologic investigations, it is not employed by the diagnostic laboratory for routine identification of clinical isolates.

Staphylococci are readily phagocytized by polymorphonuclear leukocytes, which may then be killed by the bacteria, presumably by their leukocidins. Although leukocidins, hemolysins, and coagulase are antigenic, antibodies to these antigens provide little or no protection. Since the antigenic components of staphylococci responsible for virulence are unknown, it has not been possible to make effective vaccines.

Staphylococcal infections in human beings depend upon many factors, including the type and number of staphylococci, the route of introduction, and the toxic substances produced by the staphylococci. Of equal importance are the susceptibility of the host, the previous exposure to specific strains, the general health and nutritional state, and the amount of trauma sustained. Factors such as toxemia, allergic reactions, starvation, and diabetes influence the onset and course of staphylococcal infections. Foreign body reaction as a consequence of sutures is an important factor in staphylococcal infection.

The skin is the most common site of staphylococcal infections. Lesions range from furuncles (boils) and carbuncles to surgical wound infections. Hospital-acquired staphylococcal infection by antibiotic-resistant strains reached epidemic proportion during the 1950s. The development and use of semisynthetic penicillinase-resistant penicillins has controlled these infections. However, the antibiotic-resistant staphylococci are now endemic in hospitals and pose a continual threat to the patient. A rapidly spreading cellulitis is sometimes seen with staphylococcal infections and should be treated vigorously with an appropriate antibiotic. Often there is pain, swelling, induration, patchy discoloration of the skin, and fever. Cellulitis may occur at the site of a venipuncture for intravenous cannulation. Staphylococcal abscesses characteristically begin in hair follicles or small sebaceous glands. An indurated area of cellulitis undergoes central necrosis and formation of an abscess having thick, odorless, and yellow or greenish pus. Staphylococci are a primary cause of acute wound sepsis and are involved in postoperative infections of "clean" incised wounds. The source of the infecting microorganisms is frequently exogenous. Virulent, antibiotic-resistant, hospital strains of *Staphylococcus aureus* may be carried in the nares and on the hands of physicians and hospital personnel, and these may be newly colonized on the skin of the patient. The air in the operating room may bear microorganisms from the nasopharynx, skin, hair, and clothing of the surgical staff and of the patient. Accordingly, it is essential to maintain strict, rigid rules for asepsis in the operating room.

Infected incisions should be opened widely and allowed to drain. Therapy with antistaphylococcal antibiotics should be initiated. Fulminating septicemias may arise from severe wound infections. The patient is ill with high fever, leukocytosis, toxemia, and evidence of irritation of the central nervous system. The mortality rate in fulminating untreated infections may be as high as 90 percent. If the infection persists, metastatic abscesses form in lungs, heart, kidneys, gallbladder, appendix, liver, peritoneum, and bone. Meningitis and brain abscesses hasten death. Endocarditis is a frequent complication of staphylococcal septicemia. Staphylococcal pneumonia is another nosocomial postoperative infection. It may be severe and is often associated with a tracheostomy. In fatal cases, the major finding at autopsy is marked pulmonary edema with little destruction of tissue.

Staphylococcal Enteritis

Enteritis with a drug-resistant staphylococcus following oral administration of a broad-spectrum antibiotic was first described by Kramer in 1948. Generally, this disease is benign with mild to moderate symptoms including nausea, vomiting, diarrhea, abdominal distention, fever, and weakness, but it may be fulminating and lead to septicemia and death. Discontinuance of the oral antibiotic usually leads to disappearance of symptoms. The prognosis is good so long as the intestinal mucosa remains intact.

Staphylococcal enterocolitis (pseudomembranous enterocolitis) is an acute inflammatory disease of the small and large intestine characterized by foci of epithelial necrosis and erosion of the mucosa. There is profuse, continuous diarrhea that soon becomes watery, contains desquamated, membranous patches, and often is greenish. The disease is a complication in debilitated surgical patients following therapy with broad-spectrum antibiotics. The use of neomycin in debilitated patients for preoperative intestinal antisepsis and for treatment of hepatic coma has resulted in staphylococcal enterocolitis. The major etiologic factors are suppression of normal gastrointestinal flora by a broad-spectrum antibiotic and acquisition of an enterotoxic strain of *Staphylococcus aureus* possessing multiple antibiotic resistance. Secondary factors are debilitation and an empty small bowel (as a result of preoperative starvation). Although stool cultures from some patients yield a pure culture of *Staphylococcus aureus,* pseudomembranous enterocolitis may exist without culturable *Staphylococcus aureus.* Conversely, *Staphylococcus aureus may exist in pure culture in the intestine of a patient with the symptoms of enteritis but in the absence of a pseudomembrane.* Discovery during the past decade of the role of toxin(s) of *Clostridium difficile* in antibiotic-associated pseudomembranous colitis explains some of these discrepancies. (Discussion is found under Clostridial Infections of the Gastrointestinal Tract.)

TREATMENT. Treatment consists of discontinuing previous antibiotics and employing a specific antistaphylococcal drug such as oral methicillin or oral vancomycin, hydration with intravenously administered fluids, replacement of electrolytes, intramuscular administration of corticosteroids, and attempts to reestablish a normal flora. The fulminating form of enterocolitis may be refractory to all forms of therapy and may result in death.

Peptococci and Disease?

Both obligately anaerobic staphylococci (peptococci) and facultatively anaerobic staphylococci grow in anaerobic cultures. However, the facultatives (e.g., *Staphylococcus aureus*) can be subcultured aerobically and separated from the peptococci that grow anaerobically only. In contrast to the role of pure cultures of staphylococci in disease, the peptococci may be found in wound infections, abscesses, and septicemias in association with bacteroides, clostridia, aerobic gram-negative bacilli, and aerobic cocci. These bacterial groups are major components of the normal flora of the skin and mucous membranes and can exert a role in mixed infections when these sites are disturbed. Peptococci (e.g., *Peptococcus magnus* and *Peptococcus asaccharolyticus*) account for approximately 20 percent of anaerobes found in clinical specimens from surgical patients (Holland et al.). Nevertheless, the peptococci have slight, if any, propensity to produce disease and seem unable to cause progressive infection in laboratory animals. This apparent nonpathogenicity is shared by many anaerobic species from normal flora found in anaerobic infections and has led to speculation that the unitarian theory of infection that has evolved from the monumental work of Koch and Ehrlich (one microbe, one disease, one drug) does not explain all infectious disease (Gorbach and Bartlett).

CLOSTRIDIAL INFECTIONS

The clostridia are large, gram-positive, rod-shaped microorganisms. They are ubiquitous. *Clostridium perfringens* is more widespread than any other pathogen. Its principal habitats are the soil and the intestinal tract of human beings and animals. The most characteristic feature of clostridia is the presence of an oval, central, or subterminal spore. In the case of *Clostridium tetani,* the spore is spherical and terminally located and produces a characteristic drumstick appearance. The clostridia are obligate anaerobes and can be cultured only on media having a low oxidation-reduction potential. This may be achieved by employing fresh media incubated in an anaerobic atmosphere in specially designed jars or with liquid media exposed to the atmosphere, but containing added reducing agents (such as sodium thioglycolate, powdered iron, or chopped meat).

The lesions produced by the pathogenic clostridia are due to their exotoxins. Gas gangrene is a necrosis of tissue along with putrefaction and is usually caused by clostridia derived from the intestine or soil. The infection is localized but its systemic effects are far-reaching. Gas gangrene is rarely a pure culture infection. It usually involves *Clostridium perfringens* along with other clostridial species, such as *Clostridium novyi, Clostridium septicum, Clostridium bifermentans (sordellii),* sometimes *Clostridium tetani* and *Clostridium botulinum,* and often nonpathogenic but proteolytic *Clostridium sporogenes* and *Clostridium histolyticum.* In addition, grampositive cocci and gram-negative enterobacteria are often present.

Clostridium perfringens is, nevertheless, the most important organism. Five types, A through F, have been described. They are differentiated on the basis of production of lethal toxins. All types produce alpha toxin, a le-

thal, necrotizing, hemolytic exotoxin, which is also a lecithinase. *Clostridium perfringens* type A produces the greatest amount of alpha toxin. In addition, some strains of type A produce variable amounts of hemolysin (theta toxin), collagenase (kappa toxin), hyaluronidase (mu toxin), and deoxyribonuclease (nu toxin).

Clostridial Wound Infection

MacLennan in 1962 described three types of anaerobic wound infection: simple contamination, clostridial cellulitis, and clostridial myonecrosis.

SIMPLE CONTAMINATION

Simple contamination of a wound by clostridia is common. It causes no discomfort to the patient and is of little concern to the surgeon. When anaerobes are digesting dead tissue, there may be a thin seropurulent exudate. If the necrotic material is removed, there will be no subsequent invasion of underlying tissues. The relatively common occurrence of clostridia in accidental wounds in the absence of anaerobic infection is probably due to the ubiquitous presence of these anaerobes and their spores. The absence of subsequent anaerobic infections is most likely due to unsuitable conditions for further multiplication of the contaminant and for toxin production. MacLennan estimated that between 10 and 30 percent of all severe civilian wounds were infected with spore-forming anaerobic bacilli. A high oxidation-reduction potential (Eh) due to the surrounding healthy tissues prevents colonization of the tissues. In the absence of treatment, however, cellulitis or myonecrosis may develop from the simple contamination, and the three types of anaerobic wound infection may be considered as ascending grades of severity.

CLOSTRIDIAL CELLULITIS

This is a gassy, crepitant infection involving necrotic tissue (killed by ischemia or trauma, but not by bacterial activity). Intact, healthy muscle is not invaded. The cellulitis is characterized as a foul-smelling, seropurulent infection of the depths and crevices of a wound. There is often local extension along fascial planes, but involvement of healthy muscle and marked toxemia are absent. Although *Clostridium perfringens* may be present, the predominant organisms are proteolytic and nontoxigenic clostridia, such as *Clostridium sporogenes* and *Clostridium tertium.* Clostridial cellulitis generally has a gradual onset; the incubation period is from 3 to 5 days; systemic effects are usually mild; there is no toxemia; the skin is rarely discolored; and there is little or no edema. This distinguishes the infection from gas gangrene. The spread of the cellulitis in the tissue spaces often has been rapid and extensive, necessitating immediate radical surgical drainage.

CLOSTRIDIAL MYONECROSIS (GAS GANGRENE)

This infection is rapid-spreading. It may be crepitant, or noncrepitant and edematous, mixed, or toxemic. The lesion also has been described as a "myositis," which is not as precise a term as is *myonecrosis*. The infection occurs in association with severe wounds of large muscle masses that have become contaminated with pathogenic clostridia, especially *Clostridium perfringens*. Such wounds are most commonly caused by the high-velocity missiles of modern warfare and by accidental trauma. Sometimes clostridial myonecrosis follows clean elective surgical procedures. Many patients with clostridial myonecrosis harbor a variety of anaerobic as well as aerobic bacteria. In fatal cases it is rare for only a single species to be present. Clostridial myonecrosis is most likely to develop in wounds in which there has been extensive laceration or devitalization of thick muscle masses, such as the buttock, thigh, and shoulder. Associated with such trauma is impaired arterial supply to the limb or muscle group and gross contamination of the wound by soil, clothing, and other foreign bodies. These conditions provide an ideal substrate for the development of clostridia. In anoxic muscle, glycolysis continues and the oxidation-reduction potential (Eh) of the muscle falls. With the accumulation of lactate, alkaline reservoirs become depleted, and the pH also falls. As a consequence of lowered Eh and pH, the proteinases present and the amino acids produced not only lower the pH further but provide substrate for the growth of clostridia. Once bacterial growth is established and toxins and other products of bacterial metabolism accumulate, the invasion of uninjured tissue is promoted, and the anaerobic infection is established. The infection is aided further by the fact that neither phagocytes nor antibodies can enter the necrotic lesion. Gas gangrene is considered to have begun when the infecting pathogenic anaerobes have produced sufficient toxins to overcome local defenses. Gas gangrene is relatively infrequent in clinical practice. The overall incidence is less than 2 percent, although from 4 to 40 percent of wounds may be contaminated with clostridia.

Clostridium septicum myonecrosis is related to malignancy. Debilitation and immunosuppression appear to underlie the resultant *Clostridium septicum* sepsis in patients with either hematologic or intestinal malignancy. Conversely, in a patient from whom *Clostridium septicum* is isolated, malignancy (e.g., hematologic or intestinal) should be suspected. In a patient with evidence of clostridial myonecrosis or sepsis and no external source, the cecum or distal ileum should be considered a likely site of malignancy.

TREATMENT. Early and adequate surgery is the most effective means of treating gas gangrene. Because of the rapid spread of the infection, a 24-h delay in treatment may be fatal. The diagnosis of gas gangrene is based on clinical evidence. Multiple longitudinal incisions for decompression and drainage and aggressive surgical debridement of all involved or devitalized tissues usually arrest the disease. If not or if early diagnosis was not made, then amputation is necessary. Antibiotic therapy with penicillin G and tetracycline has been most effective as an adjunct to operative treatment. Antitoxin is of no value therapeutically or prophylactically and should not be used. Adjunctive hyperbaric oxygenation has been used with success.

Infections of the Gastrointestinal Tract

Clostridia are usually present among the mixed flora in peritonitis, appendicitis, and strangulation intestinal obstruction. Quantitatively, the most numerous flora in peritoneal and loop fluids of dogs with experimental strangulation intestinal obstruction are clostridia, coliforms, bacterioides, and streptococci, in that order. Although it appears reasonable to assume that *Clostridium perfringens* actively participates in the pathophysiology of severe cases of appendicitis and acute cases of strangulated intestinal obstruction, direct clinical evidence is lacking. Experimental studies demonstrate that clostridial exotoxins contribute to the lethal activity of filter-sterilized strangulation fluids. However, this finding does not preclude a role for combinations of varying proportions of viable bacteria, bacterial endotoxins, and clostridial exotoxins. In biliary tract infections due to clostridia, acute emphysematous cholecystitis (gas gangrene of the gallbladder) and postcholecystectomy septicemia, it is generally believed that clostridia are transported to the liver from the gastrointestinal tract via the portal circulation and then excreted with the bile into the biliary tract. In postoperative gas gangrene of the abdominal wall, a rare complication of abdominal surgery, intestinal clostridia contaminate the abdominal wound at the time of operation. It occurs less often after operations on the stomach and duodenum than after those involving the lower intestinal tract. These infections are usually due to *Clostridium perfringens* and are fatal; they require awareness and early treatment. Gas gangrene of the abdominal wall must be distinguished from Meleney's progressive synergistic gangrene of the abdominal wall following drainage of appendiceal abscesses. Synergistic gangrene is a chronic, superficial progressive gangrene characterized by a slow, relentless progression, severe local symptoms, and absence of severe systemic symptoms. It is due to anaerobic cocci mixed with *Staphylococcus aureus, Streptococcus pyogenes, Pseudomonas aeruginosa,* or *Proteus* species.

ANTIBIOTIC-ASSOCIATED PSEUDOMEMBRANOUS COLITIS. In 1977 a toxin was first reported in the feces of patients with pseudomembranous colitis following antimicrobial therapy. Subsequent studies identified *Clostridium difficile* as the source of the toxin and suggested that antibiotic therapy altered the normal microflora of the colon and permitted overgrowth of *Clostridium difficile* in a previously colonized patient. The symptoms of antibiotic-associated colitis can appear during antimicrobial therapy or even as long as 2 or 3 weeks following its cessation. Watery diarrhea without gross blood is typical and may be accompanied by fever, abdominal pain, and leukocytosis. Sigmoidoscopy or colonoscopy reveals yellow-white, raised exudative plaques or pseudomembranes. The role of *Clostridium difficile* is demonstrated by isolating the microorganism from feces. Sterile filtrates of such feces produce cytotoxic effects when added to cell cultures. The cytotoxin(s) is neutralized by antitoxin produced from *Clostridium sordellii,* a closely related species.

Although almost all commonly used antibacterial agents have been implicated in antibiotic-associated colitis, those most frequently associated have been ampicillin, clindamycin, and cephalosporins. When diarrhea is not relieved by stopping the offending antibiotic, or when the diarrhea is severe, oral vancomycin is an effective treatment of *Clostridium difficile*-related colitis and diarrhea, and can be life-saving. Cholestyramine, an anion exchange resin that binds the toxins of *Clostridium difficile,* is an alternative for treatment of a patient who is not too seriously ill. However, if the drug fails or if the patient is seriously ill, oral vancomycin should be used. Oral metronidazole is also effective in treating *Clostridium difficile*-induced colitis.

Clostridium difficile is the most important cause of antibiotic-associated pseudomembranous colitis, which is most frequent in seriously ill, hospitalized patients. Only about 3 percent of healthy adults are reported to carry the microorganism in their stools, yet rates of antibiotic-associated colitis of 10 percent or higher have been found in some hospitals. This discrepancy suggests the possibility of nosocomial cross infection. Fekety et al. found that contamination with *Clostridium difficile* was common in the immediate environment of patients with the disease, and were able to isolate the microorganism from the hands and stools of asymptomatic hospital personnel. Therefore, such patients should be isolated.

Urogenital Infections

Postoperative infections due to *Clostridium perfringens* have occurred following procedures such as nephrectomy, lithotomy, and prostatectomy. Almost all uterine clostridial infections are due to *Clostridium perfringens.* They generally occur following criminal abortion and are rare following normal childbirth. Introduction of the organisms into the uterus is favored by instrumentation and manipulation. In modern obstetrics, the use of prophylactic antibiotic therapy and the wide use of cesarean section probably account for the decreasing frequency of this already rare form of uterine infection. In contrast, in cases of criminal abortion both endogenous and exogenous sources of contamination occur as the result of unskilled manipulations and the use of unsterile and unclean instruments and abortifacients. Once the interior of the puerperal or postabortal uterus has been contaminated, fragments of blood clot and necrotic tissue provide conditions favorable for multiplication of clostridia. Early diagnosis depends upon clinical recognition of such signs as jaundice, hypotension, tachycardia, shock, hemoglobinuria, uterine or perianal tenderness, and offensive vaginal discharge. The simplest method for the rapid detection of *Clostridium perfringens* is the demonstration of gram-positive rods with rounded ends in direct smears from the cervical os or canal. The treatment of uterine gas gangrene involves immediate chemotherapy, hyperbaric oxygenation, treatment of shock, hysterectomy, and management of renal failure. Penicillin is the antibiotic of choice.

Tetanus

This disease is a toxemia resulting from the growth of contaminating *Clostridium tetani* at a traumatized site and consequent production of exotoxin. In contrast to the clostridia of gas gangrene, *Clostridium tetani* is noninvasive, and neurotoxin is responsible for the symptoms of tetanus. The conditions necessary for the development of tetanus are the presence of the organisms or spores in the wound and favorable anaerobic conditions for bacterial growth and the elaboration of exotoxin. The presence of *Clostridium tetani* in soil and in the intestine of human beings and animals ensures that accidental wounds are exposed to the risk of contamination at the time of injury. However, as with other clostridial infections, the mere presence of *Clostridium tetani* or its spores in a wound is not followed always by tetanus, and the organism may be isolated from wounds in individuals who never develop tetanus. A low oxygen tension is necessary if *Clostridium tetani* is to grow. Currently, tetanus commonly follows mild injuries because the routine protective measures employed in severe cases may be omitted. The types of lesions leading to the development of tetanus are penetrating wounds due to splinters, thorns, rusty nails, and even dirty abrasions. In about 50 percent of cases, it is presumed that the wound was slight and healed before evidence of intoxication developed. Such mild injuries may not induce significant local anoxia, but they may be accompanied by other infections that lower the oxidation-reduction potential of the tissues to a point at which the spores of *Clostridium tetani* can germinate. For example, chronic ulcers of the leg, measles rash, boils, paronychia, and dental extractions have been implicated as modes of entry. In the United States, tetanus has become a disease primarily of unvaccinated adults. The median age of patients with nonneonatal tetanus varies from fifty-five to fifty-seven years; the median age for those dying from tetanus is from fifty-five to sixty years.

Currently, tetanus is seen in urban centers of the United States as a complication of narcotic addiction; *urban tetanus* has a mortality of 90 percent. *Tetanus neonatorum* results from contamination of the cut surface of the umbilical cord and is an important cause of infant mortality in developing countries where primitive unhygienic obstetric practices prevail. There is often continuous crying for hours followed by cessation of sucking and crying, convulsions, and fever. Severe spasm of the respiratory muscles is a common cause of death. *Postabortal tetanus* and *puerperal tetanus* result from unsterile manipulation or instrumentation of the genital tract. *Postoperative tetanus* sometimes follows elective surgical procedures, and is usually due to some breakdown in sterile technique, but it may also be caused by contamination from the patient's intestinal tract.

CLINICAL MANIFESTATIONS. The average incubation period for tetanus is from 7 to 10 days after injury, but it may range between 3 and 30 days. The incubation period is followed by the *period of onset,* that is, the time interval between the first symptom (usually trismus) and the onset of spasms. In severe cases reflex spasms may begin 12 h after onset, in moderately severe cases after 2 to 3 days, and in milder cases after 5 or more days. In general, the shorter the periods of incubation and onset, the worse the prognosis. Even with modern treatment, the mortality rate is rarely less than 30 percent.

Trismus is the most common early symptom. It often is combined with pain and stiffness in the neck, back, and abdomen. Occasionally dysphagia appears first. These symptoms increase according to the severity of the attack. Twenty-four hours after the onset, a patient with a moderately severe attack has a characteristically anxious expression (*risus sardonicus*) in which the eyebrows and the corners of the mouth are drawn up. The muscles of the neck and trunk are rigid to varying degrees, and the back is usually slightly arched. The patient is usually comfortable except for occasional pain in the neck or back, which tends to be made worse by movement. Manipulation of a limb or palpation of any part of the body tends to increase muscular rigidity and may bring on cramplike pain. Initially, reflex spasms are brought on by external stimuli, such as moving the patient or knocking the bed, but later they occur spontaneously at regular and increasingly shorter intervals until the height of the disease is reached. Spasms often begin with a sudden jerk. Every muscle in the body is thrown into intense tonic contraction, the jaws are tightly clenched, the head is retracted, the back is arched, the chest and abdomen are fixed, and the limbs are usually extended. A severe spasm may stop respiration. Spasms may last a few seconds or several minutes. When spasms occur frequently, they lead to rapid exhaustion and sometimes to death from asphyxiation. Without spasms, mortality is low; with severe spasms, few survive. Aspiration pneumonia is a common contributory cause of death.

Less common manifestations of the disease include local contracture of muscles in the neighborhood of the wound: *local tetanus*. This may precede the more generalized forms of involvement. *Cephalic tetanus* is a manifestation in which irritation or paralysis of cranial nerves appears early and dominates the picture. The facial nerve is affected most often, but ophthalmoplegia from involvement of the ocular nerves and spasm or paralysis of the tongue from involvement of the hypoglossal nerve may develop. Trismus and dysphagia may also be present. This condition, which is a type of local tetanus, follows wounds of the head and face, and the symptoms often appear first on the injured side.

Severe tetanus is terrible and often fatal, but those who recover do so completely. The patient who has survived tetanus is not immune and, unless immunized, is susceptible to a second attack. *Recurrent tetanus* in the same patient has been reported. Apparently a sublethal amount of tetanus toxin is not sufficient to provide an adequate antigenic stimulus for the production of active immunity.

The diagnosis of tetanus is a clinical one with bacteriologic confirmation sometimes possible. Frequently the presumed lesion has been so slight that it is not detectable at the time when clinical tetanus develops.

IMMUNIZATION. Prophylaxis with tetanus toxoid is the best means of preventing tetanus. For active immunization of individuals seven years old or over, the initial dose is 0.5 mL aluminum phosphate–adsorbed tetanus toxoid given intramuscularly, preferably in the left deltoid region, but it also may be given subcutaneously. This is repeated in 4 to 6 weeks, and a third injection is given in 6 to 12 months (or more). Only after this third injection is the basic series considered complete. For children six years old or under, diphtheria and tetanus toxoid combined with pertussis vaccine (DTP) is used. Delay in administering the second and third injections is not disadvantageous, and the series does not need to be restarted or repeated. Even after 25 years, a booster will rapidly recall complete active protection.

Following the initial dose of tetanus toxoid, nonimmunized individuals require approximately 30 days to acquire a safe antibody level (at least 0.01 I.U. of serum antitoxin per milliliter of blood). Patients are passively immunized in the interim by intramuscular administration of human hyperimmune globulin containing 250 units of tetanus antitoxin simultaneously with the toxoid. This protects for about 4 weeks. Passive immunization is not recommended for individuals who have received previous active immunization.

TREATMENT. Surgical care of wounds should be immediate. The most important features of surgical wound care are thorough cleansing and debridement. Foreign bodies and necrotic tissue can be contaminated massively with *Clostridium tetani* and establish wound conditions promoting growth and exotoxin production by *Clostridium tetani*. The wound should be left open until the patient has recovered from the convulsive stage of the disease. Antibiotic therapy with penicillin is effective against vegetative cells of *Clostridium tetani*. Tetracycline hydrochloride may be used if an allergy to penicillin exists. Antibiotics also are important as prophylaxis against respiratory infections, which are common in tetanus. Treatment of the patient with severe tetanus involves the use of muscle relaxants, sedation with Pentothal sodium, balance of fluid and electrolytes, control of respiratory secretions, and elimination of visceral stimuli such as distention of the urinary bladder and fecal impaction. A tracheostomy is performed if needed or when the period of onset is 1 day or less. Constant nursing care is required.

COMPLICATIONS. Tetanus is a particularly lethal disease, and death is generally due to respiratory arrest. Some complications of tetanus and its treatment are drug intoxication, especially from barbiturates; bronchopneumonia or other pulmonary infection; compression fracture of vertebrae, especially the thoracic vertebrae; anemia; and exhaustion, which may be so severe as a result of repeated convulsions that the patient lapses into coma and expires. Before human tetanus immune globulin was available, the risk of anaphylaxis complicated the use of bovine or equine tetanus antitoxin.

PROPHYLAXIS. The Committee on Trauma of the American College of Surgeons recommends the following guidelines (1979) for prophylaxis against tetanus in the management of wounds:

I. General principles
  A. The attending physician must determine for each patient with a wound, individually, what is required for adequate prophylaxis against tetanus.
  B. Regardless of the active immunization status of the patient, meticulous surgical care, including removal of all

devitalized tissue and foreign bodies, should be provided immediately for all wounds. Such care is essential as part of the prophylaxis against tetanus.

C. Passive immunization with Tetanus Immune Globulin-Human (called human T.I.G.) must be considered individually for each patient. The characteristics of the wound, conditions under which it was incurred, its treatment, its age, and the previous active immunization status of the patient must be considered. Passive immunization with human T.I.G. is not indicated, however, if the patient has ever received two or more injections of toxoid.

D. Every wounded patient should be given a written record of the immunization provided, with instructions to carry the record at all times, and if indicated, to complete active immunization. For precise tetanus prophylaxis, an accurate and immediately available history regarding previous active immunization against tetanus is required.

E. Immunization in adults requires at least three injections of toxoid. A routine booster of adsorbed toxoid is indicated every 10 years thereafter. In children under seven, immunization requires four injections of diphtheria and tetanus toxoids combined with pertussis vaccine. A fifth dose may be administered at four to six years of age. Thereafter, combined tetanus and diphtheria toxoid (adult type) is recommended for routine or wound boosters.

II. Specific measures for patients with wounds
   A. Previously immunized individuals
      1. When the attending physician has determined that the patient has been previously fully immunized and the last dose of toxoid was given within 10 years:
         a. For non-tetanus-prone wounds, no booster of toxoid is indicated.
         b. For tetanus-prone wounds and if more than 5 years has elapsed since the last dose, 0.5 mL adsorbed toxoid should be given. If excessive prior toxoid injections have been given, this booster may be omitted.
      2. When the patient has had two or more prior injections of toxoid and received the last dose more than 10 years previously, 0.5 mL adsorbed toxoid for both tetanus-prone and non-tetanus-prone wounds should be given. Passive immunization is not considered necessary.
   B. Individuals not adequately immunized, i.e., the patient has received only one or no prior injection of toxoid or the immunization history is unknown
      1. For non-tetanus-prone wounds, 0.5 mL adsorbed toxoid should be given.
      2. For tetanus-prone wounds:
         a. 0.5 mL adsorbed toxoid and 250 units (or more) of human T.I.G. (using different syringes, needles, and sites of injection) should be given.
         b. Administration of antibiotics should be considered, although the effectiveness of antibiotics for prophylaxis of tetanus remains unproved.

Medical students sometimes question on theoretical grounds the validity of administering toxoid and antitoxin (immune globulin) simultaneously to a previously unimmunized patient. The problem of interference during simultaneous active and passive immunization against tetanus has been studied quantitatively. There is some lowering of the antigenicity of toxoid, but the interference is not clinically significant if 250 units of tetanus immune globulin is injected. The antibody level in patients receiving immune globulin is protective for at least 4 weeks, and the second and third doses of toxoid produce an active antitoxin response. In addition, alum-adsorbed tetanus toxoid stimulates a quicker, higher, and more durable immunity than does plain toxoid because the aluminum in the preparation is an immunologic adjuvant. Use of the recommended adsorbed toxoid is, therefore, more reliable.

Wound Botulism

Botulism is an example of an intoxication resulting from the ingestion of exotoxin formed by *Clostridium botulinum* growing in improperly sterilized or inadequately preserved foods. Following gastrointestinal symptoms, botulism progresses to diplopia, blurred vision, and dysphagia and to a descending motor paralysis spreading to involve other cranial nerves and peripheral motor nerves. Although *C. botulinum* may be isolated from a wound as a simple contaminant, *wound botulism* is indicated by the presence of clinical signs of botulism. Wound botulism is a rare disease but should be suspected in any patient with a wound who presents with clinical signs of descending paralysis and a negative food history. Therapy of the wound is routine; therapy of the botulism is supportive, with respiratory care and assisted ventilation if required. Equine trivalent antitoxin should be given after testing for sensitivity to equine serum.

INFECTIONS CAUSED BY GRAM-NEGATIVE BACILLI

The gram-negative bacilli of importance to surgery are for the most part indigenous to human beings and often found in the intestinal tract. They are non-spore-forming rods, and they may be aerobes, facultative anaerobes, or obligate anaerobes. The role of some gram-negative bacilli as primary pathogens has long been known, e.g., *Pseudomonas aeruginosa* and *Salmonella typhi*. Others have been recognized only rarely as primary pathogens in human beings, e.g., *Serratia marcescens* and *Enterobacter aerogenes*. However, since the development of modern chemotherapy after World War II, the gram-negative bacilli have become increasingly important as causes of serious infection, particularly in hospitalized patients. Prior to the introduction of broad-spectrum antibiotics, the role of gram-negative bacilli as pathogens was usually overshadowed by the pneumococci, streptococci, and staphylococci. We now know that infection is most likely to occur when body defense mechanisms are either undeveloped or overtaxed, as in the case of infants and debilitated patients, and that therapeutic measures to combat one situation may provide an environment promoting the establishment of infection by almost any mixture of gram-negative bacilli. This situation prevails because of the great number of patients with impaired host defenses secondary to the use of multiple antibiotics, corticosteroids, immunosuppressive agents, antineoplastic drugs, and radiotherapy. Surgical procedures in which foreign bodies such as prosthetic valves or grafts are inserted appear to allow these less virulent species to become established

Table 5-7. TAXONOMY OF GRAM-NEGATIVE
BACILLI

Family	Tribe	Genus
Pseudomonaceae		*Pseudomonas*
Enterobacteriaceae	Eschericheae	*Escherichia* (*E. coli*, including *Alkalescens-Dispar* group)
		Shigella
	Edwardsielliae	*Edwardsiella*
	Salmonelleae	*Salmonella*
		Arizona
		Citrobacter (including Bethesda-Ballerup group)
	Klebsielleae	*Klebsiella*
		Enterobacter (including *Hafnia*)
		Pectobacterium
		Serratia
	Proteae	*Proteus*
		Providencia
Bacteroidaceae		*Bacteroides*
		Fusobacterium

and to produce infection. Indwelling venous and urethral catheters, endotracheal tubes and mechanical ventilators, peritoneal dialysis apparatus, and pump-oxygenators for extracorporeal circulation in cardiac surgery often serve as portals of entry for the gram-negative bacilli. The current taxonomic organization of gram-negative bacilli (aerobic, facultative, and anaerobic) is outlined in Table 5-7.

Aerobic and Facultative Bacteria

Pseudomonas aeruginosa is a strict aerobe; it is widely distributed and is frequently present in small numbers on healthy skin surfaces and in the normal intestinal flora of some individuals. *P. aeruginosa* is an opportunistic pathogen that can cause serious and lethal infections in debilitated or immunosuppressed patients, such as those with cancer, large burns, or cystic fibrosis, and is common in postoperative infections following the use of mechanical ventilators and indwelling urinary catheters. It is incriminated in primary infections such as meningitis resulting from lumbar puncture, traumatic injuries to the eye, and enteritis with associated bacteremia. Heroin addicts are subject to hematogenous pseudomonal osteomyelitis. Although *P. aeruginosa* is gram-negative and produces an endotoxin, its cell-wall lipopolysaccharides are not as toxic as those isolated from the enteric bacteria. It does, however, produce a variety of extracellular products that contribute to its pathogenicity, including hemolysins, proteases, an enterotoxin, and a heat-labile exotoxin. This exotoxin is more toxic than the other extracellular products or the endotoxin. *Pseudomonas* infections are treated with either tobramycin or gentamicin alone, or in

combination with carbenicillin or ticarcillin. Since resistant strains of *Pseudomonas* may be involved, antibiotic sensitivity tests should be performed.

Escherichia coli is found in the intestinal tract of human beings and animals and is the predominant facultative commensal in the normal intestinal flora. Although more than 145 different envelope capsular (K) antigens have been identified, the ability of a strain to be typed does not necessarily denote pathogenicity or virulence. Nevertheless, certain strains belonging to distinct antigenic types are *enteropathogenic,* others are *enterotoxigenic* by their capacity to produce toxins, and others are *enteroinvasive* by their ability to penetrate mucosal cells. These strains produce diarrheal disease, especially in infants. Stool isolates may have none, one, two, or all three of these pathogenic characteristics. *Escherichia coli* may produce meningitis, septicemia, endocarditis, appendiceal abscess, peritonitis, septic wounds, and pyogenic infections, chiefly urinary tract infections (pyelitis, cystitis, etc.) in pure culture or in association with fecal streptococci. *Escherichia coli* also has the capacity to produce a potent endotoxin that enters the circulation and induces shock. The antibiotic of choice in the treatment of the patient seriously ill with *Escherichia coli* sepsis is ampicillin alone or combined with gentamicin or tobramycin.

The *Salmonella* species are a large group of enteric pathogens transmitted via food and water. They cause enteric fevers (particularly typhoid fever), gastroenteritis, and septicemia. *Salmonella typhi* and *Salmonella enteritidis* pass from the small intestine by way of the lymphatics to the mesenteric glands. After multiplication there, they invade the bloodstream via the thoracic duct. Complications that may result from this hematogenous dissemination include thrombophlebitis, lymphadenitis, pneumonia, osteomyelitis, arthritis, endocarditis, and meningitis. Hemorrhage may occur from perforation of ulcers in lymphoid tissue of the intestine. The specific surgical treatment for perforation, i.e., simple closure or segmental resection, is determined by the pathologic findings encountered at operation. Chloramphenicol has long been advocated in the treatment of typhoid fever, but ampicillin is equally effective. Although postoperative wound infection due to *Salmonella typhi* is rare, recorded cases occur after gallbladder surgery in patients who are unsuspected typhoid carriers. Contaminated wound drainage and positive stools from such patients are distinct hazards to other hospitalized patients.

Before the introduction of modern chemotherapy, gram-negative bacilli of the tribe Klebsielleae were rarely noted as primary pathogens. However, along with other gram-negative bacilli, they have assumed increasing importance as causes of serious hospital-acquired infections. *Klebsiella pneumoniae* causes a severe pneumonia having a propensity for debilitated (frequently alcoholic) patients. *Klebsiella* has also been implicated in endocarditis, septic thrombophlebitis, septicemia, urinary tract infection, wound infection, crepitant cellulitis, and myonecrosis. *Enterobacter aerogenes* is a commensal in the intestinal tract of approximately 5 percent of healthy individuals. It has less pathogenic potential than strains of *Klebsiella* but is commonly involved in hospital-acquired sepsis. *Serratia marcescens* is another species formerly considered to be nonpathogenic for human beings. Although it too has low virulence for healthy individuals, it is now found primarily in hospitalized patients with some underlying disease. It may spread like other "hospital bacteria," and infection may not always produce clinical symptoms. Classically, *Serratia marcescens* has been recognized by its ability to produce a characteristic red pigment, and it has been thought to be an obligate pigment producer. However, the majority of strains of *Serratia marcescens* involved in hospital-acquired infections are nonpigmented and often have been mistaken for other enterobacteria. These nonchromogenic strains of *Serratia marcescens* now can be identified by appropriate biochemical tests. The *Klebsiella-Enterobacter-Serratia* species are often isolated in mixed culture from sputum, urine, blood, and wounds in which there are other potential pathogens such as streptococci, staphylococci, *Escherichia coli, Proteus* species, *Citrobacter* species, and *Pseudomonas aeruginosa*. Epidemiologic studies indicate that the particular strains and types of the gramnegative species producing infection are nosocomial and acquired in the intestinal tract of patients during hospitalization. They are often highly drug-resistant, and the overall mortality associated with bacteremia is approximately 50 percent. The risk of bacteremia appears to be related to the underlying disease of the patient and the nature of the infection (urinary tract, respiratory, wound infection, abscess, etc.). The antibiotic of choice in treatment of infections caused by the *Klebsiella-Enterobacter-Serratia* species is an aminoglycoside (gentamicin, tobramycin, netlimicin, or amikacin).

Gram-negative bacilli in the genera *Proteus* and *Providencia* also compete for prominence with the other aerobic gram-negatives in infections. Rapid and abundant urease production distinguishes *Proteus* from *Providencia*. These organisms often occur in abscesses, in infected wounds, and also in burns as one component of a mixed infection. They are resistant to most antibiotics, and what was originally a mixed infection may be converted into a pure proteus infection as a result of antibiotic therapy. Sepsis due to indol-negative *Proteus (Proteus mirabilis)* is treated with ampicillin, while that due to indol-positive species (*Proteus vulgaris, P. morganii,* and *P. rettgeri*) is treated with gentamicin, tobramycin, netlimicin, or amikacin. *Providencia* species are also sensitive to these aminoglycosides. The genus *Acinetobacter* includes gramnegative pleomorphic aerobes previously known by a wide variety of names. *Acinetobacter calcoaceticus* var. *anitratus* (formerly *Herellea vaginicola* and *Bacterium anitratum*) and *Acinetobacter calcoaceticus* var. *lwoffi* (formerly *Mima polymorpha*) are opportunists capable of causing therapy-potentiated infections in compromised patients. An aminoglycoside also constitutes appropriate therapy for these infections.

Anaerobic Bacteria

Obligately anaerobic bacteria, especially gram-negative bacilli, are found as normal flora on skin and all mucous membrane surfaces. They are by far the major component of the normal flora. In the normal oral cavity, anaerobes outnumber aerobes 10 to 1, and in the normal colon, 1000 to 1. When the mucous membrane barrier is disturbed by disease, trauma, or surgical procedures, these bacteria can invade adjacent tissue and may cause infection. In the upper respiratory tract and lungs, the major anaerobic pathogens are peptostreptococci, fusobacteria, and *Bacteroides melaninogenicus*. In intraabdominal infections, *Bacteroides fragilis* is the most frequent isolate; clostridia, peptostreptococci, and peptococci are also found. In infection of the female genital tract, the same anaerobes are also the principal pathogens. Although anaerobic infections often originate close to a mucosal surface, they may occur anywhere in the body as a result of direct or hematogenous spread. Clues to diagnosis include foulsmelling discharge, gas, necrotic tissue, abscess formation, and failure to obtain growth on aerobic culture despite the presence of organisms on Gram-stained direct smear. Anaerobes are associated with 90 percent of cases of intraabdominal abscess, 95 percent of appendiceal abscess, 90 percent of aspiration pneumonia, 95 percent of lung abscess, 85 percent of brain abscess, and 75 percent of upper tract female pelvic infections.

The bacteroides are obligately anaerobic, gram-negative, non-spore-forming bacilli. They are sometimes the only microorganisms found in clinical specimens but more often are found in association with other anaerobes and aerobes. Currently, human pathogens are assigned to the genus *Bacteroides* and the genus *Fusobacterium*. *Bacteroides* are rod-shaped cells with rounded ends and are sometimes coccobacillary; *Fusobacterium* may be bacilli with pointed ends or pleomorphic, filamentous forms with swellings and free, round bodies. Species causing infections in human beings are *Bacteroides fragilis, Bacteroides melaninogenicus, Fusobacterium fusiforme,* and *Fusobacterium necrophorus*.

In circumstances such as chronic illness, malignant disease, surgical treatment, and cystoscopy, the bacteroides may invade the bloodstream to cause septicemia and penetrate tissue and organs to produce abscesses. The clinical spectrum of infections varies from superficial infections to deep abscesses with overwhelming bacteremia and shock. The gastrointestinal tract, especially the colon and appendix, appears to be the most frequent source of bacteroides infection. Gynecologic infections involve the vagina, uterus, and contiguous structures, and are related to malignancy of pelvic organs, septic abortions, and postpartum complications. Upper respiratory tract infections and those of the nasopharynx, mouth, and jaw (tonsillar and peritonsillar abscesses, chronic otitis media, and dentoalveolar abscesses) have become relatively uncommon since the widespread use of antibiotics (penicillin or tetracycline) for the treatment of undiagnosed pharyngitis. Brain abscesses are a well-known complication of these upper respiratory tract infections in which bacteroides are involved along with other microorganisms, such as anaerobic streptococci.

Bacteroides bacteremia is characterized by a spiking fever, jaundice, and leukocytosis. In the patient more than forty years old, it is associated with chronic debilitating disease, hypotension, and a high mortality. Bacteremias have followed primary infection in the gastrointestinal, pelvic, and pharyngeal areas, and may originate from thrombophlebitis in these sites of infection. An indication of *Bacteroides* infection is the presence of a foul-smelling exudate from wounds or abscesses that contain gram-negative forms but produce no growth on aerobic culture. There appears to be a disposition toward *Bacteroides* infection in patients with underlying malignant disease. Often these patients have undergone elective intestinal surgery after preoperative intestinal antisepsis. This suggests that changes in the normal intestinal flora may predispose to *Bacteroides* infection. Therefore, the surgeon should be alert to the possibility of *Bacteroides* infection. A changing pattern of pyogenic abscesses of the liver has been characterized by an increased incidence of *Bacteroides* as the pathogen.

Treatment of anaerobic infections consists of surgical drainage of abscesses, excision of necrotic tissue, and appropriate antibiotic therapy. This should be based upon the results of sensitivity tests. Penicillin G is the drug of choice for most anaerobic infections, including those caused by oropharyngeal strains of *Bacteroides fragilis*. Infections caused by gastrointestinal strains of *Bacteroides fragilis*, however, require treatment with clindamycin. An alternative agent for either type of *Bacteroides* infection is metronidazole. (See Table 5-4 for other alternative agents.)

PSEUDOMYCOTIC INFECTIONS

Among the actinomycetes, *Actinomyces israelii* and *Nocardia asteroides* are isolated most frequently as human pathogens, although other species of each genus may also be implicated in human infections. Actinomycetes are true bacteria but traditionally have been studied and grouped with the fungi because of their resemblance to mycotic agents and their involvement in diseases resembling mycoses. Infections caused by these false fungi (pseudomyces) may be called pseudomycoses to separate them from true fungal infections. They will therefore be considered separately from the true mycoses.

Actinomycosis

Actinomyces israelii is a strict anaerobe present in normal oral flora. Actinomycosis is therefore an endogenous infection. There are three clinical types of actinomycosis: cervicofacial (the most common type), thoracic, and abdominal. A dense fibroblastic reaction is produced, and connective and granulation tissue tend to form a wall around the abscess. Wherever lesions occur, abscesses expand into contiguous tissue and form burrowing, tortuous sinuses to the outside, where they discharge pus and necrotic material. This pus contains dense clusters of organisms and hyphae appearing as macroscopic, yellow-brown "sulfur granules," which facilitate diagnosis when examined microscopically and cultured. Actinomycosis can be cured with massive doses of penicillin G or tetracycline. Surgical drainage of abscesses and aggressive

resection of damaged tissue are important adjuncts to long-term chemotherapy.

Nocardiosis

Nocardia, in contrast to actinomycetes, are aerobic inhabitants of soil and are not part of the normal flora of human beings. *Nocardia asteroides* and *Nocardia brasiliensis,* opportunistic pathogens for human beings, are less acid-fast than mycobacteria, and their filaments tend to branch. Nocardiosis tends to be progressive and fatal but is a rare disease. Pulmonary infection arises from inhalation of the organisms, while subcutaneous abscesses (mycetomas) result from contamination of skin wounds, usually of the hands and feet of laborers. Massive doses of sulfonamides, e.g., sulfadiazine 6 to 8 g/day orally for at least 4 to 6 months, is the preferred therapy; ampicillin is an alternate agent. Drainage of empyema and abscesses is an important surgical adjunct to chemotherapy.

MYCOTIC INFECTIONS

The relation of the surgeon to mycotic infection has changed in recent years. The need for surgical treatment has diminished because of more effective modern chemotherapy. However, the long-term use of cytotoxic agents, corticosteroids, and antibacterial drugs for patients with leukemia and neoplasms has increased the incidence of opportunistic mycotic infections. Among the pathogenic fungi to be discussed, *Blastomyces dermatitidis, Paracoccidioides brasiliensis, Histoplasma capsulatum, Cryptococcus neoformans,* and even *Coccidioides immitis* are frank pathogens but may be opportunistic to the extent that they cause progressive infections in debilitated patients more frequently than in healthy ones. Definite opportunistic infections are caused by species of *Mucor, Rhizopus, Aspergillus,* and *Candida.* Fungal infection threatens any compromised hosts, such as severely burned patients and those with implanted prosthetic devices and transplanted organs. Some of the symptoms of mycotic disease are chronic skin or mucous membrane lesions, low-grade fever, weight loss, chronic pulmonary or meningeal involvement, hepatosplenomegaly, and lymphadenopathy. Mycotic disease should be suspected unless another cause is clearly established. A mycosis may coexist with a lymphomatous disease, e.g., the association of histoplasmosis and cryptococcosis with Hodgkin's disease. A presumptive clinical diagnosis of a mycosis must be confirmed in the laboratory. Serologic tests are useful in reaching a presumptive diagnosis. The morphologic features of the fungus in tissue and culture are significant in identification.

The majority of patients with fungal infections seen by the physician have serious illness and present with typical symptoms of infection. Symptoms of pulmonary involvement frequently are present. Hematogenous dissemination of the disease produces manifestations such as tender swollen joints, draining subcutaneous abscesses, ulcerative lesions of the oropharynx, and meningitis. Many pa-

Table 5-8. MYCOSES IMPORTANT IN SURGICAL INFECTIONS

Type of disease	Mycosis	Representative fungus	Fungal morphology		
			Dimor-phism	Infected tissue	Laboratory culture
Systemic	Blastomycosis	*Blastomyces dermatidis*	Yes	Yeast	Mycelia
	Paracoccidioidomycosis	*Paracoccidioides brasiliensis*	Yes	Yeast	Mycelia
	Histoplasmosis	*Histoplasma capsulatum*	Yes	Yeast	Mycelia
	Coccidioidomycosis	*Coccidioides immitis*	Yes	Spherules	Mycelia
	Cryptococcosis	*Cryptococcus neoformans*	No	Yeast	Yeast
Subcutaneous	Sporotrichosis	*Sporotrichum schenckii*	Yes	Yeast	Mycelia
Systemic, particularly opportunistic	Phycomycosis	*Mucor corymbifera*	No	Mycelia	Mycelia
		Rhizopus oryzae	No	Mycelia	Mycelia
	Aspergillosis	*Aspergillus fumigatus*	No	Mycelia	Mycelia
	Candidosis	*Candida albicans*	Yes	Yeast and hyphae	Yeast and hyphae

tients with systemic mycoses, as well as those with dermatophytoses, have skin lesions that are painful, itching, weeping, crusting, malodorous, and disfiguring. Fungi of ever-increasing importance as agents of infection in surgical patients are grouped in Table 5-8 according to the type of disease they cause and will be discussed in the order shown.

Blastomycosis (North American Blastomycosis)

Blastomyces dermatitidis is a dimorphic fungus; it grows in tissues and in culture at 37°C as a spherical thick-walled, single-budding yeast and in culture at room temperature as a mold. Lateral, rounded conidia borne along hyphae are presumably the infectious spores. Demonstration of nonencapsulated, thick-walled, multinucleate yeast cells in pus, sputum, or tissue sections and their subsequent laboratory culture establish the diagnosis. Blastomycosis usually begins in the lungs as a subacute respiratory infection (pulmonary form) that gradually increases in severity over a period of weeks or months and sometimes resembles tuberculosis or carcinoma. Frequently, during the course of infection, patients develop skin lesions. These may be the only apparent signs of blastomycosis. Pulmonary blastomycosis spreads hematogenously to establish focal destructive lesions in other parts of the body. Spreading, ulcerated, crusted skin lesions in particular arise as metastases from the primary pulmonary lesions. Amphotericin B is indicated in treating all forms of blastomycosis. If surgery is indicated for diagnosis to rule out bronchogenic carcinoma, amphotericin is used both pre- and postoperatively to minimize operative spread.

Paracoccidioidomycosis (South American Blastomycosis)

Paracoccidioides brasiliensis is dimorphic and grows in tissue as a multiple-budding yeast, in contrast to the single-budding yeast in blastomycosis. Paracoccid-ioidomycosis is characterized by primary pulmonary lesions with dissemination to visceral organs, by conspicuous ulcerative granulomas of the buccal and nasal mucosa, and by generalized lymphangitis. In blastomycosis, visceral organs are *not* involved. Treatment with amphotericin B is usually effective.

Histoplasmosis

Histoplasma capsulatum is dimorphic; it appears characteristically in infected tissues as many small, oval yeast cells packed within macrophages and reticuloendothelial cells; at room temperature it forms slowly growing mycelial colonies. This pathogen is present in soil, especially that enriched by feces of birds and bats, and is endemic in the Mississippi and Ohio valleys and along the Appalachian mountains of the United States. Inhalation of conidia leads to pulmonary infection. The initial infection is mild and may be inapparent or may occur as a primary acute disease. Symptoms may include fever, cough, chest pain, dyspnea, and pleurisy with effusion. Localized pulmonary histoplasmosis resembles tuberculosis in its histopathology. In a few individuals the infection becomes progressive and widely disseminated and may simulate miliary tuberculosis. Disseminated histoplasmosis primarily involves the reticuloendothelial system in various tissues and organs and often coexists in individuals who have tuberculosis, leukemia, or Hodgkin's disease. Histoplasmosis is treated with high doses of intravenous amphotericin B. In chronic cavitary disease surgical resection should be performed, with amphotericin therapy given before and after surgery to reduce postoperative complications and avoid relapse.

Coccidioidomycosis

Coccidioides immitis is a somewhat different dimorphic fungus; it varies in structure between a hyphal form found in soil and a spherule or sporangium form found in infected tissues. The sporangia are thick-walled structures filled with globular endospores or sporangiospores. At maturity the sporangium bursts and releases hundreds of endospores, each of which can form a new sporangium in tissue. When sporangia are plated on Sabouraud agar, growth of the mycelial form occurs. Barrel-shaped arthrospores are formed in the mycelium. These arthrospores are highly infectious and become airborne easily. The mycelial (saprophytic) form is readily converted into the sporangium (parasitic) form in human beings. *Coccidioides immitis* is endemic in the southwestern United States and adjacent Mexico, where it grows as a saprophyte in desert soils. Infection is established by inhalation of airborne arthrospores.

About 60 percent of infected individuals remain asymptomatic but become skin-sensitive to coccidioidin. The acute and most common form of coccidioidomycosis resembles influenza. When confined to the lungs, the disease is usually self-limited and heals with scarring. However, a chronic, progressive, granulomatous disease occurs in fewer than 1 percent of infected individuals. Years may elapse between primary infection and the more serious disseminated disease. Patients with disseminated coccidioidomycosis appear to have some defect in their immune response to the fungus. The symptoms are similar to those seen in advancing tuberculosis. Any organ or tissue of the body may be involved. However, the infection shows predilection for bone, skin, and subcutaneous tissue. This disease is not contagious, since it is spread only by saprophytic arthrospores. The majority of patients with primary infection recover without therapy or with only symptomatic care. Amphotericin B is used to treat disseminated coccidioidomycosis but is less effective than with blastomycosis, histoplasmosis, and cryptococcosis.

Cryptococcosis

Cryptococcus neoformans is *not dimorphic;* in both infected tissue and in culture it appears as encapsulated yeast cells. The yeast cells are thin-walled, but the large, clear polysaccharide capsules surrounding them are distinctive. *Cryptococcus neoformans* is found in dust and bird droppings. Inhalation of yeast cells is thought to initiate pulmonary infection, which may be inapparent or mild. There is little inflammatory response of invaded tissues. Cryptococcosis is a subacute or chronic mycotic infection most frequently involving tissues of the central nervous system but occasionally producing lesions in the lungs or skin. Cryptococcal meningitis is the most frequent form of disseminated disease and mimics tuberculous meningitis, brain abscess, or brain tumor. Pulmonary lesions are usually found at autopsy. Many patients with pulmonary or dermal cryptococcosis respond to therapy with flucytosine. Surgical resection is indicated for both cavitary and nodular pulmonary disease. When diagnosis is established by surgery, therapy with amphotericin B is begun postoperatively to avoid meningitis and recurrence. Amphotericin B is the drug of choice for cryptococcosis of the central nervous system. Cryptococcosis is an opportunistic mycosis in debilitated patients, particularly those with Hodgkin's disease or leukemia.

Sporotrichosis

Sporotrichum schenckii is dimorphic. When found in tissues or exudate stained by the periodic acid–Schiff technique, this fungus appears as fusiform bodies or round budding cells, but these are rarely seen. When these materials are cultured on Sabouraud agar at room temperature, the mycelial form grows. Microscopically, hyphae are slender and septate, and conidia are individually attached by sterigmata to a common conidiophore. Hyphae are converted to the yeast form by injection into mice and by cultivation at 37°C on an enriched medium. Human beings become infected by accidental subcutaneous inoculation from thorns and splinters. Sporotrichosis is a chronic progressive infection of the skin and subcutaneous tissue that frequently begins as a primary lesion of the skin of the hand or forearm and secondarily involves lymphatic channels and lymph nodes draining the area, which become cordlike, resulting in a chain of ulcers. Generalized infection occurs in the compromised host by way of the blood, and any organ or tissue can be the site of lesions. Symptoms are then related to the region involved. Orally administered potassium iodide is specific in sporotrichosis and must be continued for several weeks after recovery seems complete. Intravenous amphotericin B is indicated for disseminated sporotrichosis. *Sporotrichum schenckii* has caused suprainfection in patients with underlying hematologic malignant disease who have been treated with antitumor agents and steroids.

Phycomycosis

Species of *Mucor* and *Rhizopus* are saprophytes common in nature and are *not dimorphic.* They can produce rapidly fatal disease when they invade the brain, lungs, or other organs of a compromised host. These fungi may also produce a superficial infection of the skin with occasional ulceration and granuloma or abscess formation. *Mucor* and *Rhizopus* are opportunistic pathogens, and are held in check by normal serum factors that become diminished in individuals suffering from uncontrolled diabetes mellitus, blood dyscrasias, endocrine disturbances, malnutrition, and burns. Corticosteroid therapy and prolonged use of broad-spectrum antibiotics may also enhance susceptibility to phycomycosis. The local cutaneous lesions heal with proper hygiene and fungicides; extensive lesions may require debridement. Amphotericin B and correction of the underlying disease is the therapy for the acute form of phycomycosis. Amphotericin should be used to treat any patient not responding to other measures. Surgery should be considered for patients with pulmonary lesions not responsive to amphotericin.

Aspergillosis

Aspergillus has become an important pathogen in patients with impaired host defenses. These mycelial fungi are saprophytic and are not dimorphic but can cause local as well as disseminated disease. *Aspergillus fumigatus* is the most commonly reported species. Two forms of pulmonary aspergillosis are frequently seen: (1) pulmonary or bronchial aspergilloma (fungus ball), due to secondary invasion of a tuberculous or coccidioidal cavity, and (2) allergic bronchopulmonary aspergillosis. In the compromised host these may proceed to disseminated infection. Otomycosis is secondary to bacterial infection of the ear. The fungus grows on ear wax and macerated tissue. Systemic aspergillosis may complicate severe underlying diseases that are being treated with steroids, immunosuppressive drugs, or broad-spectrum antibiotics. Local superficial lesions often heal spontaneously with hygienic care. Localized abscesses and granulomas should be excised. Systemic infection requires treatment with amphotericin B. The prognosis in disseminated aspergillosis is poor; the patient often succumbs to the underlying disease.

Candidosis

Candida albicans is indigenous in human beings and is dimorphic; both yeast and mycelial forms are seen in infected tissue. *Candida albicans* affects mucous membranes and causes diseases ranging from thrush (oral candidosis) and vulvovaginal candidosis to systemic candidosis. The former are common medical problems, the latter an opportunistic infection of the compromised host. Patients with hemopoietic and lymphoreticular neoplasms, as well as those being treated with immunosuppressives, glucocorticoids, and broad-spectrum antibiotics, are particularly prone to systemic fungal infections. Patients with burns and those undergoing intravenous hyperalimentation are also prone to systemic candidosis. Candidal endocarditis, especially that due to *Candida parapsilosis,* is seen in drug addicts using intravenous heroin.

Thrush and other clinically distinctive candidal infections frequently result from antibacterial therapy, and discontinuance of the therapy will usually cause the antibiotic-induced superinfection to disappear. Topical nystatin is effective in treating candidal infections of the skin, mouth, and vagina. Amphotericin B is the mainstay in treating systemic candidosis. Oral flucytosine is considerably less toxic than amphotericin, but 50 percent of *Candida* strains are initially resistant. The use of combination therapy with amphotericin B and flucytosine produces an antifungal synergism using a lower and less toxic dose of amphotericin. Combination therapy has resulted in successful treatment of candidosis and also cryptococcosis.

SURGICAL ASEPSIS

Surgical asepsis, the prevention of the access of microorganisms to an operative wound, is achieved by methods designed to destroy bacteria or remove them from all objects coming in contact with the wound. Modern surgery is aseptic in the use of sterile instruments, sutures, and dressings and in the wearing of sterile gowns and rubber gloves by the operating personnel. Although this is pres-

ently the extent of routine sterility in surgical asepsis, the technology of germ-free research is able to provide sterile flexible plastic isolation chambers in which neonates or antibiotic-decontaminated patients may be maintained in a sterile environment. Operations may be performed in ''surgical'' isolators cemented to the operative site of the patient. The surgeon makes his incision through the site of attachment of the isolator, and the operation may be conducted in the absence of all microorganisms. There is considerable interest in unidirectional (laminar) airflow systems as a less absolute means of limiting the number of bacteria to which a patient is exposed. These systems recirculate air through high-efficiency particulate air filters that assure unidirectional flow in either a downward or horizontal direction. However, the advantages or necessity of such systems in operating rooms are controversial, since there has not been substantial evidence to demonstrate their effectiveness in reducing postoperative infections. The Committee on Control of Operating Room Environment of the American College of Surgeons does not recommend laminar airflow for general use in operating rooms.

It is necessary to resort to the use of antiseptics to degerm the site of the operation on the patient's skin. The surgeon and operating-room personnel usually use soaps or detergents containing antiseptics for scrubbing their hands before donning gloves or else rinse in an antiseptic after the scrub. An *antiseptic* is a chemical agent that either kills pathogenic microorganisms or inhibits their growth so long as there is contact between agent and microbe. By custom as well as by federal law, the term ''antiseptic'' is reserved for agents applied to the body. The antiseptic may actually be a disinfectant used in dilute solutions to avoid damage to tissues. A *disinfectant* is a germicidal, chemical substance used on inanimate objects to kill pathogenic microorganisms but not necessarily all others. These germicidal agents are used to disinfect instruments and other equipment that cannot be exposed to heat. They are essential for good housekeeping practices in hospitals, where they are used to disinfect floors, fabrics, and excreta. The first step in any process of biologic decontamination is thorough mechanical cleansing with soap or detergent and water to remove all traces of blood, pus, proteins, and mucus before the antiseptic or disinfectant is employed.

Sterilization

Sterilization is the process of killing all microorganisms (bacteria, spores, viruses, mycotic agents, and parasites). It is the ultimate in disinfection. The practical criterion of sterility is the failure of microbial growth to appear on tests in suitable bacteriologic media. Sterilization can be achieved by either physical or chemical agents. *Steam under pressure* is the most reliable means of sterilizing surgical supplies because of its power of penetration, microbiologic efficiency, ease of control, and economy of operation. Application of steam under a pressure of 15 psi (pounds per square inch) for 15 to 45 min will destroy all forms of life. Free-flowing steam, like boiling water, has a temperature of 100°C, but the same steam under pressure of 15 psi exerts a temperature of 121°C. Steam gives up heat by condensing into water. Thus when a bundle containing surgical pads or sponges is sterilized, the steam contacts the outer layer. There a portion of it condenses into water and releases heat. The steam then penetrates to a second layer, where another portion condenses and gives up heat. The steam thus approaches the center of the package, layer after layer, until the whole package is sterilized. The time of exposure depends upon the size of the parcel and its wrappings. Sterilization by steam under pressure is carried out in an autoclave. A major caution to be recognized when operating an autoclave is that a mixture of air and steam has a lower temperature than does pure steam. Therefore, when air is present in the chamber, the killing power of the process is diminished in proportion to the amount of air present. Most autoclaves depend upon gravity displacement of air from the chamber and from within articles being sterilized. Thus, improperly packed and positioned articles in the autoclave may fail to become sterile even though all physical conditions of the run may be correct. A new development in autoclaves is the high-vacuum sterilizer. A vacuum pump is incorporated into the system, and a vacuum is pulled in the chamber at the beginning and end of the sterilizing cycle. There is a considerable shortening of the time needed for sterilization, as only 3 min are needed to achieve sterility rather than the 20 min on the regular systems. In addition, there appears to be less damage to rubber, fabrics, and sharp instruments because of reduced exposure to moisture. There is less danger of creating air pockets and less chance of the steam's failing to penetrate to the center of bundles. Materials emerge dry, and much greater tolerances in packing the chamber are afforded.

Dry-heat sterilization is commonly used for glassware, for items that are injured by moisture, and for materials that resist penetration by steam, such as talc, vaseline, fats, and oils. The process consists of baking the material to be sterilized in a hot-air oven. At a temperature of 121°C (250°F) it takes about 6 h to sterilize glassware, but at 170°C (340°F) the time required is about 1 h. *Gas sterilization* is practical with ethylene oxide, a gas employed as a sterilizing agent in specially designed chambers in which temperatures and humidity can be controlled and from which air can be evacuated. The killing action is slow, and an exposure period from 3 to 6 h is needed. Sterilization employing ethylene oxide is used for delicate surgical instruments with optical lenses, for tubing and plastic parts of heart-lung machines and respirators, for prepacked commercial plastic products such as disposable syringes, and for blankets, pillows, and mattresses. Ethylene oxide is most reliable when applied to clean, dry surfaces that do not absorb the chemical. The gas dissolves in plastic, rubber, fabric, and leather, and chemical burns may occur when materials laden with ethylene oxide are applied to tissue. The dissolved chemical escapes from materials when they are exposed to air, and a minimum of 24 h of aeration is necessary to ensure removal of the gas from sterilized articles. However, solid

metal or glass items may be used immediately after sterilization. *Radiation sterilization* refers to ionizing radiation by cobalt 60 sources (γ-radiation) and by electron accelerators (high-energy electrons). It is currently used commercially to sterilize disposable hospital supplies, such as plastic hypodermic syringes and sutures. Radiation sterilization of heat-sensitive pharmaceuticals has been recommended.

Chemical sterilization is currently achieved with a 2% aqueous solution of glutaraldehyde. This compound is an effective disinfectant for surgical, anesthetic, and dental equipment, rubber and plastic mouthpieces, catheters, and other heat-sensitive hospital equipment. Either a buffered alkaline solution (Cidex) or a potentiated acid solution (Sonacide) of glutaraldehyde may be used. They are equally bactericidal, sporicidal, and virucidal. Isopropyl alcohol may also be used for the chemical sterilization of instruments if they are first cleansed of all blood, pus, and body fluids. Only in the absence of spores is alcohol an effective sterilizing agent.

Degerming of Skin

Antiseptics incorporated into soaps are used for preoperative preparation of the skin at the operative site and for surgical hand scrubs by operating personnel. The bacteriologic content of normal skin consists of a resident flora, composed of coagulase-negative *Staphylococcus epidermidis* and anaerobic diphtheroides (e.g., *Propionibacterium acnes*), which reside on the surface of the skin, in hair follicles, and in the ducts of sebaceous glands. These bacteria can be diminished temporarily, but they cannot be permanently eradicated. They are not usually responsible for surgical infections. Superimposed upon the resident flora is a transient flora consisting of bacteria picked up as a result of temporary colonizing of the skin. In the hospital, this transient flora often consists of pathogens resistant to antibiotics and is likely to be composed of pathogenic strains of *Staphylococcus aureus* and gram-negative enterobacteria. Therefore, pathogenic bacteria on the hands of operating personnel at the time of operation must be removed by scrubbing and destroyed by an antiseptic agent. The patient's skin must be degermed in the area of operation prior to the incision. The most efficient method is a vigorous scrub with liquid soaps containing either hexachlorophene, an iodophor, or chlorhexidine.

Hexachlorophene is a bisphenol that disinfects the skin slowly. Commercial preparations containing 3% hexachlorophene, a detergent, and liquid soap are used for surgical scrubbing. Over a period of days, regular use of these surgical soaps brings about a progressive decrease in the number of bacteria on and in the skin. The hexachlorophene leaves an active film, which is renewed with each scrubbing. Consequently, its antibacterial activity persists so long as one continues to wash with soap containing hexachlorophene. A single washing with ordinary soap removes the antibacterial film. Hexachlorophene is effective against gram-positive pathogens such as *Staphy-*

lococcus aureus, but it is without activity against gram-negative bacteria, such as the pseudomonas and the enterobacteria. Significant blood levels have been found in frequent users, and vacuolar encephalopathy has been noted postmortem in premature infants bathed with hexachlorophene. It is also suspected of teratogenicity. Hexachlorophene preparations should be restricted for use only with specific indications, and removed from general use within a hospital.

Iodophors are organic complexes of iodine and a synthetic detergent. About 1% iodine is available in the formula, whose germicidal action results from the liberation of free iodine when the compound is diluted with water. The detergent in the complex enhances the bactericidal activity of the iodine. Advantages of iodophors are that they destroy both gram-positive and gram-negative bacterial cells, but not spores; they do not stain skin and clothing; and allergic reactions are reduced. However, they do not maintain adequate residual activity. Iodophors have been incorporated into surgical scrub soaps for hands and for the operative site, and are effective for this use, but they should not be used to lavage serous cavities. (Discussion is found under Intraperitoneal Antibiotic Therapy.)

Chlorhexidine gluconate is effective against gram-positive and gram-negative bacteria and fungi; it is sporicidal only at elevated temperatures. Chlorhexidine gluconate (4%) combined with 4% isopropanol in a sudsing base is used as a surgical hand scrub, a superficial skin wound cleanser, and a handwashing agent. Preoperative preparation of the skin is accomplished with a 0.5% solution of chlorhexidine in 70% isopropanol.

Other Surgical Antiseptics

No economical antiseptic or disinfectant is available to kill all microbial flora in a reasonable time at concentrations that will not irritate tissue or damage medical devices. However, there are several agents that have high reliability and low toxicity as surgical antiseptics. Among them are alcohol and iodine. The combination of inorganic iodine and alcohol, either as a tincture or as a mixture of 1 to 3% iodine with 70% ethyl or isopropyl alcohol, kills both gram-positive and gram-negative bacteria. Only a short contact time is needed, and the solution itself is not likely to be contaminated. Some patients, however, have adverse reactions to iodine, and most physicians hesitate to use this combination on mucous membranes or denuded skin. Aqueous iodophor solutions are available as an alternative. These also have a broad antimicrobic spectrum and are not likely to be contaminated, and they provoke adverse reaction less frequently than do inorganic tinctures of iodine. For patients sensitive to iodine, a thorough scrub with soap and water followed by a 2-min scrub with 70 to 90% ethyl or isopropyl alcohol is effective surgical antisepsis. Isopropyl alcohol is slightly more effective than ethyl alcohol when used as a 70% solution and is less expensive and more readily obtained because it is not potable. As a group, alcohols exhibit many desirable features. They are bactericidal, have a cleansing action, and evaporate readily. They do not, however, kill spores, and the best one can hope to accomplish with alcohol is to reduce the number of viable bacteria and destroy pathogens that may be on the skin as transients.

Aqueous quaternary ammonium compounds such as benzalkonium chloride (Zephiran chloride) are used diluted 1:750 for skin antisepsis for venipuncture and for disinfection of cystoscopes and bronchoscopes. They are less expensive than many other products and are nontoxic and nonallergenic but *must* be used with caution. Although they are potent bactericides in vitro and are particularly active against gram-positive cocci, benzalkonium antiseptics have been implicated in nosocomial infections by resistant *Pseudomonas capacia* and *Enterobacter* species that contaminate working solutions of these compounds. Accordingly, there are few applications for quaternary ammonium compounds in hospitals other than for environmental sanitation. Alternative surgical antiseptics such as iodine, iodophors, chlorhexidine, and alcohol have a broad antibacterial spectrum.

Bibliography

Introduction; General Principles; Surgical Infections

American College of Surgeons, Committee on Control of Surgical Infections: *Manual on Control of Surgical Infections,* 2d ed. Philadelphia, Lippincott, 1984.
Brummelkamp WH, Boerema I, et al: Treatment of clostridial infections with hyperbaric oxygen drenching: A report of 26 cases. *Lancet* 1:235–238, 1963.
Cruse PJE, Foord R: The epidemiology of wound infection: A 10-year prospective study of 62,939 wounds. *Surg Clin North Am* 60:27–40, 1980.
Hart GB, Lamb RC, et al: Gas gangrene: I. A collective review; II. A 15-year experience with hyperbaric oxygen. *J Trauma* 23:991–1000, 1983.
Holland JA, Hill GB, et al: Experimental and clinical experience with hyperbaric oxygen in the treatment of clostridial myonecrosis. *Surgery* 77:75–85, 1975.
Hunt TK: Surgical wound infections: An overview. *Am J Med* 70:712–718, 1981.
Meleney FL: *Treatise on Surgical Infections.* New York, Oxford University Press, 1948.
Meleney FL: *Clinical Aspects and Treatment of Surgical Infections.* Philadelphia, Saunders, 1949.
Polk HC Jr, Stone HH (eds): *Hospital-Acquired Infections in Surgery.* Baltimore, University Park Press, 1977.
Roding B, Groeneveld PHA, et al: Ten years of experience in the treatment of gas gangrene with hyperbaric oxygen. *Surg Gynecol Obstet* 134:579–585, 1972.

Basic Considerations of Antibiotic Therapy

Polk HC Jr, Ausobsky JR: The role of antibiotics in surgical infections. *Adv Surg* 16:225–275, 1983.
Pratt WB, Fekety R: *The Antimicrobial Drugs.* New York, Oxford University Press, 1986.
Yale CE, Peet WJ: Antibiotics in colon surgery. *Am J Surg* 122:787–791, 1971.

Chemoprophylaxis; Intestinal Antisepsis; Intraperitoneal Antibiotics

Bolton JS, Bornside GH, et al: Intraperitoneal povidone-iodine in experimental canine and murine peritonitis. *Am J Surg* 137:780–785, 1979.

Burke JF: Use of preventive antibiotics in clinical surgery. *Am Surg* 39:6–11, 1973.

Clarke JS, Condon RE, et al: Preoperative oral antibiotics reduce septic complications of colon operations: Results of prospective, randomized, double-blind clinical study. *Ann Surg* 186:251–259, 1977.

Cohn I Jr: *Intestinal Antisepsis.* Springfield, IL, Charles C Thomas, 1968.

Cohn I Jr: Intestinal antisepsis. *Surg Gynecol Obstet* 130:1006–1014, 1970.

Evans M, Pollock AV: Trials on trial: A review of trials of antibiotic prophylaxis. *Arch Surg* 119:109–113, 1984.

Fleites RA, Marshall JB, et al: The efficacy of polyethylene glycol-electrolyte lavage solution versus traditional mechanical bowel preparation for elective colonic surgery: a randomized, prospective, blinded clinical trial. *Surgery* 98:708–715, 1985.

Jagelman DG, Fazio VW, et al: A prospective randomized, double-blind study of 10% mannitol mechanical bowel preparation combined with oral neomycin and short-term, perioperative, intravenous flagyl as prophylaxis in elective colorectal resections. *Surgery* 98:861–865, 1985.

Nichols RL, Broido P, et al: Effect of preoperative neomycin-erythromycin intestinal preparation on the incidence of infectious complications following colon surgery. *Ann Surg* 178:453–462, 1973.

Nichols RL, Condon RE: Preoperative preparation of the colon. *Surg Gynecol Obstet* 132:323–337, 1971.

Rodeheaver G, Bellamy W, et al: Bactericidal activity and toxicity of iodine-containing solutions in wounds. *Arch Surg* 117:181–186, 1982.

Silverman SH, Ambrose NS, et al: The effect of peritoneal lavage with tetracycline solution in postoperative infection. *Dis Colon Rectum* 29:165–169, 1986.

Smith EB: A rationale for intraperitoneally administered antibiotic therapy. *Surg Gynecol Obstet* 143:561–564, 1976.

Antimicrobial Agents

Bartlett JG: Metronidazole. *Johns Hopkins Med J* 149:89–92, 1981.

Calderwood SB, Moellering RC Jr: Common adverse effects of antibacterial agents on major organ systems. *Surg Clin North Am* 60:65–81, 1980.

Conte JE Jr, Barriere SL: *Manual of Antibiotics and Infectious Diseases,* 5th ed. Philadelphia, Lea & Febiger, 1984.

Fry DE: Third generation cephalosporin antibiotics in surgical practice. *Am J Surg* 151:306–313, 1986.

Garrod LP, Lambert HP, et al: *Antibiotic and Chemotherapy,* 5th ed. Edinburgh, Churchill Livingstone, 1981.

Kagan BM (ed): *Antimicrobial Therapy,* 3d ed. Philadelphia, WB Saunders, 1980.

Sanders CV, Greenberg RN, et al: Cefamandole and cefoxitin. *Ann Intern Med* 103:70–78, 1985.

Streptococcal Infections

Aitken DR, Mackett MCT, et al: The changing pattern of hemolytic streptococcal gangrene. *Arch Surg* 117:561–567, 1982.

Altemeier WA, Culbertson WR: Acute non-clostridial crepitant cellulitis. *Surg Gynecol Obstet* 87:206–212, 1948.

Dellinger EP: Severe necrotizing soft-tissue infections: Multiple disease entities requiring a common approach. *JAMA* 246:1717–1721, 1981.

Dougherty SH: Role of enterococcus in intraabdominal sepsis. *Am J Surg* 148:308–312, 1984.

Giuliano A, Lewis R Jr, et al: Bacteriology of necrotizing fasciitis. *Am J Surg* 134:52–57, 1977.

Ledingham I McA, Tehrani MA: Diagnosis, clinical course and treatment of acute dermal gangrene. *Br J Surg* 62:364–372, 1975.

MacLennan JD: Streptococcal infection of muscle. *Lancet* 1:582–584, 1943.

Meleney FL, Friedman ST, et al: The treatment of progressive bacterial synergistic gangrene with penicillin. *Surgery* 18:423–435, 1945.

Rea WJ, Wyrick WJ Jr: Necrotizing fasciitis. *Ann Surg* 172:957–964, 1970.

Stone HH, Martin JD Jr: Synergistic necrotizing cellulitis. *Ann Surg* 175:702–711, 1972.

Staphylococcal Infections

Altemeier WA, Hummel RP, et al: Staphylococcal enterocolitis following antibiotic therapy, *Ann Surg* 157:847–858, 1963.

Elek SD: *Staphylococcus Pyogenes and Its Relation to Disease.* London, Livingstone Ltd., 1959.

Gorbach SL, Bartlett JG: Anaerobic infections: Old myths and new realities. *J Infect Dis* 130:307–310, 1974 (editorial).

Holland JW, Hill EO, et al: Numbers and types of anaerobic bacteria isolated from clinical specimens since 1960. *J Clin Microbiol* 5:20–25, 1977.

Kramer IRH: Fatal staphylococcal enteritis developing during streptomycin therapy by mouth. *Lancet* 2:646–647, 1948.

Clostridial Infections

Altemeier WA, Fullen WD: Prevention and treatment of gas gangrene. *JAMA* 217:806–813, 1971.

Altemeier WA, Hummel RP: Treatment of tetanus. *Surgery* 60:495–505, 1966.

Brooks GF, Buchanan TM, et al: Tetanus toxoid immunization of adults: A continuing need. *Ann Intern Med* 73:603–606, 1970.

Faust RA, Vickers OR, et al: Tetanus: 2,449 cases in 68 years at Charity Hospital. *J Trauma* 16:704–712, 1976.

Gerding DN, Olson MM, et al: *Clostridium difficile*-associated diarrhea and colitis in adults. A prospective case-controlled epidemiologic study. *Arch Intern Med* 146:95–100, 1986.

Kaiser CW, Milgram ML, et al: Distant nontraumatic clostridial myonecrosis and malignancy. *Cancer* 57:885–889, 1986.

Katlic MR, Derkac WM, et al: *Clostridium septicum* infection and malignancy. *Ann Surg* 193:361–364, 1982.

MacLennan JD: The histotoxic clostridial infections of man. *Bacteriol Rev* 26:177–276, 1962.

Matzkin H, Regen S: Naturally acquired immunity to tetanus toxin in an isolated community. *Infect Immun* 48:267–268, 1985.

Oakley CL: Gas gangrene. *Br Med Bull* 10:52–58, 1954.

Rubbo SD, Suri JC: Combined active-passive immunization against tetanus with human immune globlin. *Med J Aust* 2:109–113, 1965.

Willis AT: *Clostridia of Wound Infection.* London, Butterworth Scientific Publications, 1969.

Aerobic Infections

DiGioa RA, Kane JG, et al: Crepitant cellulitis and myonecrosis caused by Klebsiella. *JAMA* 237:2097–2098, 1977.

Doggett RG: *Pseudomonas Aeruginosa: Clinical Manifestations of Infection and Current Therapy.* New York, Academic Press, 1979.

Forkner CE Jr: *Pseudomonas Aeruginosa Infections.* New York, Grune & Stratton, 1960.

Reisig G, Schaffner W: Postoperative detection of *Salmonella typhi. Arch Surg* 104:349–350, 1972.

Steinhauer BW, Eickhoff TC, et al: The *Klebsiella-Enterobacter-Serratia* division: Chemical and epidemiologic characteristics. *Ann Intern Med* 65:1180–1194, 1966.

Sugerman HJ, Peyton JWR, et al: Gram-negative sepsis. *Curr Probl Surg* 18:405–475, 1981.

Wilkowske CJ, Washington JA II, et al: *Serratia marcescens:* Biochemical characteristics, antibiotic susceptibility patterns, and clinical significance. *JAMA* 214:2157–2162, 1970.

Anaerobic Infections

Anderson CB, Marr JJ, et al: Anaerobic infections in surgery: Clinical review. *Surgery* 79:313–324, 1976.

Finegold SM: *Anaerobic Bacteria in Human Disease.* New York, Academic Press, 1977.

Gorbach SL, Bartlett JG: Anaerobic infections. *N Engl J Med* 290:1177–1184; 1237–1245; 1289–1294, 1974.

Gorbach SL, Bartlett JG (eds): The role of clindamycin in anaerobic bacterial infections. *J Infect Dis* (suppl) 135: March 1977 (symposium).

Leigh DA: Wound infections due to *Bacteroides fragilis* following intestinal surgery. *Br J Surg* 62:375–378, 1975.

Sinkovics JG, Smith JP: Septicemia with bacteroides in patients with malignant disease. *Cancer* 25:663–671, 1970.

Stone HH, Kolb LD, et al: Incidence and significance of intraperitoneal anaerobic bacteria. *Ann Surg* 181:705–715, 1975.

Wilson SE, Finegold SM, et al: *Intra-abdominal Infection.* New York, McGraw-Hill, 1983.

Mycotic Infections

Bennett JE: Chemotherapy of systemic mycoses. *N Engl J Med* 290:30–32; 320–323, 1974.

Codish SD, Tobias JS, et al: Recent advances in the treatment of systemic mycotic infections. *Surg Gynecol Obstet* 148:435–447, 1979.

Emmons CW, Binford CH, et al: *Medical Mycology,* 3d ed. Philadelphia, Lea & Febiger, 1977.

Moss E, McQuown AL: *Atlas of Medical Mycology,* 3d ed. Baltimore, Williams & Wilkins, 1969.

Odds FC: *Candida and Candidosis,* Baltimore, University Park Press, 1979.

Schroter GPJ, Temple DR, et al: Crytococcosis after renal transplantation. *Surgery* 79:268–277, 1976.

Solomkin JS, Flohr A, et al: *Candida* infections in surgical patients: dose requirements and toxicity of amphotericin B. *Ann Surg* 195:177–185, 1982.

Stevens DA (ed): *Coccidioidomycosis: A Text.* New York, Plenum, 1980.

Surgical Asepsis

Block SS (ed): *Disinfection, Sterilization, and Preservation,* 3d ed. Philadelphia, Lea & Febiger, 1983.

Crowder VH Jr, Bornside GH, et al: Bacteriological comparison of hexachlorophene and polyvinylpyrrolidine-iodine surgical scrub soaps. *Am Surg* 33:906–911, 1967.

Kaul AF, Jewett JF: Agents and techniques for disinfection of the skin. *Surg Gynecol Obstet* 152:677–685, 1981.

Zamora JH: Chemical and microbiologic characteristics and toxicity of povidone-iodine solutions (review). *Am J Surg* 151:400–406, 1986.

way or bleeding from a gunshot wound. The primary treatment is to establish an airway and control the bleeding. This type of patient may require surgical treatment for massive internal bleeding within 5 to 10 min following arrival in the emergency room. The operating room should be alerted when the patient is admitted to the emergency room, and no time is wasted in getting the patient into "operative" condition. Often the control of hemorrhage is dependent on a rapid thoracotomy or laparotomy to occlude injured major vessels.

A second group of patients are those with injuries that offer no immediate threat to life. These include patients who have received gunshot wounds, stab wounds, or blunt trauma to the chest and abdomen but whose vital signs are stable. The majority of injured patients are in this category. Although they will require surgical procedures within 1 to 2 h, there is time for additional information to be obtained. Blood for typing and cross matching is drawn, and blood is made available if there is any possibility that the patient will require surgical intervention. If vital signs are stable, x-rays may be obtained to determine the course of the missile and the extent of possible associated injuries, such as fractures. Cystography and pyelography may be performed to assess hematuria. Since patients with penetrating and blunt abdominal injuries may develop shock at any moment, a physician must be in constant attendance during all evaluations. Patients who suddenly develop shock are immediately taken to the operating room without additional diagnostic procedures.

The third group of patients are those whose injuries produce occult damage. This group is composed primarily of patients who have sustained blunt trauma to the abdomen that may or may not require surgical intervention and in whom the exact nature of the injury is not apparent. These patients usually have time for extensive laboratory studies, x-rays, and more complete physical examination. Surgical intervention in this group may be delayed hours or days, as with delayed rupture of the spleen.

Patients who are severely injured are admitted to the emergency room in a trauma area equipped for emergency resuscitation. This room should contain such items as intravenous fluids, overhead operating-room light, oxygen, cardiac monitor and defibrillator, and a portable carriage that is suitable for an operating-room table in an emergency situation. A cabinet should be in the room containing equipment for endotracheal intubation, tracheostomy tray, closed drainage tray, venous section tray, central venous catheters, closed-chest drainage tubes, intravenous fluids with tubing, needles, and syringes for four-quadrant abdominal paracentesis, and pericardiocentesis and peritoneal lavage catheters. The cabinet shelf should have clearly visible labels under each tray or set of instruments. These trays and instruments should be kept in this trauma room and not in central supply, as a waiting period of even 5 min may prove fatal.

ADEQUATE AIRWAY. The first and most important emergency measure in the management of the severely injured patient is to establish an effective airway. A cabinet should be available at the head of the emergency room

carriage in which a laryngoscope and cuffed endotracheal tubes of various sizes are available. Endotracheal intubation is the most rapid method of obtaining an adequate airway. Once an airway is established, a means of positive-pressure breathing such as an Ambu bag or anesthesia machine should be available, and a cuffed endotracheal tube is desirable, so that positive-pressure breathing may be accomplished if needed in the resuscitation or in the administration of anesthesia. Either wall suction or a portable suction machine must be available in the trauma room to remove pulmonary secretions, foreign bodies, and frequently, blood from the upper respiratory tract. In the presence of suspected cervical spine injuries, when an endotracheal tube cannot be readily inserted, a tracheostomy may be required.

SHOCK AND HEMORRHAGE. Shock is usually controlled while the patient's airway is being cleared by another person. Internal hemorrhage will require immediate surgical intervention. Hypovolemic shock is best prevented or controlled by starting intravenous infusions in at least two extremities, using 18-gauge or larger catheters. A balanced salt solution such as Ringer's lactate solution is usually started until blood is available. Blood for typing and cross matching is drawn at the time the intravenous fluid is started, and the balanced salt solution is given in addition to the blood. Shock resulting from a blood loss of 750 mL can usually be corrected by rapid administration of 2 L of Ringer's lactate solution over a 15- to 20-min period. Blood loss in excess of 750 mL usually requires the administration of whole blood in addition to balanced salt solution. Often, 2 L of balanced salt solution will replace the volume and correct hypotension so that no blood is necessary, reducing the possibility of blood transfusion reaction. When a patient initially responds to 1 to 2 L of balanced salt solution, as evidenced by a normal blood pressure and decrease in pulse rate, but subsequently becomes hypotensive, blood administration usually is indicated. However, by this time, type-specific blood usually is available and often cross-matched, which reduces the chances for a transfusion reaction. Should a patient not respond to the rapid administration of 2 L of balanced salt solution, uncross-matched, type O, Rh-negative blood is administered without hesitation.

External bleeding is best controlled by direct finger pressure on the bleeding wound or vessel. Tourniquets are of little benefit in the control of major arterial bleeding and often injurious if they occlude collateral circulation. A frequent mistake is the placement of a tourniquet on an extremity tight enough to obstruct venous return but loose enough not to inhibit arterial flow; this only increases the blood loss and edema. The danger of tissue loss from tourniquet use is always present.

Superficial vessels may be ligated if they are readily seen; however, wounds are not probed in a blind attempt to place a hemostat on a vessel. As soon as bleeding is controlled, the wound is covered with a sterile dressing, and the patient is taken to the operating room, where the wound is more adequately visualized and proper instruments are available. The needless probing of wounds in the emergency room may lead to severe infection, which can be avoided by proper exploration including adequate irrigation and sterile surgical technique in the operating room.

NEUROLOGIC EVALUATION. After an adequate airway has been obtained and hemorrhage has been controlled, a gross neurologic evaluation of the patient is undertaken. Motor function in the four extremities should be verified. A progressing neurologic deficit following injury to the spinal cord may indicate the necessity for an emergency laminectomy. Decompression of a hematoma may result in return of function. Thoracoabdominal injuries usually take precedence over orthopaedic or neurologic injury.

CHEST INJURIES. Airway obstruction may be due to mucus, fragments of bone from facial fractures, dirt and debris, and, commonly, broken teeth or dentures. If the patient does not ventilate normally after an endotracheal tube is inserted, or a tracheostomy has been performed, several injuries should be considered. These include pneumothorax, hemothorax, cardiac tamponade, flail chest, and ruptured bronchus.

Pneumothorax. If a pneumothorax is questionable, an 18-gauge needle may be inserted into the chest in the anterior axillary line and aspiration done to reveal the presence of air. A chest x-ray is preferable, but often severe respiratory distress precludes time for x-ray confirmation. Tension pneumothorax with mediastinal shift is suggested by displacement of the trachea to the opposite side. Auscultation of the chest may reveal decreased breath sounds. The patient with a pneumothorax is treated with closed-chest drainage. As there is little danger from the insertion of a chest tube in the absence of a pneumothorax, an anterior chest tube should be inserted if there is doubt.

Hemothorax. Diagnosis of hemothorax is similar to that of pneumothorax. If the patient on the emergency-room cart is in distress, a needle may be inserted in the eighth interspace in the posterior axillary line and aspiration done to reveal a hemothorax. This is best drained with both anterior and posterior chest tubes. The anterior chest tube is placed in the second interspace in the midclavicular line and the posterior chest tube is placed in the eighth interspace in the posterior axillary line in the region between the midaxillary and posterior axillary line. Chest tubes are of large caliber so that adequate drainage may be maintained. Thoracotomy may be indicated, depending on the rate of bleeding or the presence of intrathoracic clots.

Cardiac Tamponade. During initial observation, an unsuspected cardiac tamponade may develop secondary to blunt or penetrating trauma. This is often not present on arrival in the emergency room but may develop after 1 to 2 h of observation. The clinical signs pathognomonic for cardiac tamponade are increased venous pressure, decreased pulse pressure, particularly with a paradoxical pulse and with or without cyanosis, and decreased heart sounds. The diagnosis may be subtle until the subsequent development of hypotension. Emergency treatment includes aspiration of the pericardial sac with an 18-gauge

needle through the xiphocostal angle. Decompression of as little as 20 mL of aspirated blood may make a remarkable difference in the patient's vital signs. The high incidence of false-positive and false-negative findings with pericardiocentesis has led to the use of subxiphoid pericardial window in some centers. Depending on the cause of cardiac tamponade, immediate thoracotomy is usually required to repair the cardiac wound. When a patient arrives at the emergency room in shock without evidence of blood loss, this diagnosis should be suspected.

Flail Chest. Paradoxical chest wall motion from major blunt trauma has historically been managed by endotracheal intubation and mechanical ventilation or operative stabilization of the rib fractures. However, this approach has been replaced by ventilatory management based upon the physiologic derangement of the associated lung injury. Although this requires the careful assessment of arterial blood gases and clinical parameters of pulmonary function combined with vigorous pulmonary toilet, it allows many patients to overcome the morbidity associated with prolonged intubation and ventilation.

Ruptured Bronchus. After rupture of a bronchus, respiratory distress, hemoptysis, cyanosis, and a massive air leak with both mediastinal and subcutaneous emphysema and/or tension pneumothorax may be observed. Often the diagnosis is not obvious. There is a close relationship between fractures of the first and second ribs and rupture of a bronchus. If extrapleural hematoma is noted, special views of the first ribs are indicated. A ruptured bronchus is treated initially with closed-chest drainage. If this does not effectively keep the lung expanded, bronchoscopy and open thoracotomy with repair of the bronchus is indicated.

Open Chest Wounds. The patient with a chest injury resulting in a sucking chest wound is best managed by immediately covering the open wound with whatever material is available, such as a large vaseline gauze bandage or a thin sheet of plastic wrap. This prevents further shifting of the mediastinum and allows ventilation of the opposite lung. Chest tubes are usually inserted prior to operation, and immediate surgical intervention is indicated.

Ruptured Thoracic Aorta. The diagnosis may be suspected from chest x-ray showing a widened mediastinum and confirmed by arteriography. Immediate operation usually is indicated.

PENETRATING WOUNDS OF THE ABDOMINAL WALL. All penetrating injuries to the abdominal wall are explored locally in the emergency room to determine if the peritoneal cavity is penetrated. Exploration is usually accomplished by extending the stab wound and determining its depth. In the event that the extent of penetration cannot be determined or if the stab wound violates the peritoneal cavity, the abdominal cavity is lavaged. The mortality and morbidity from a negative abdominal exploration is negligible, but failure to discover such injuries as colon or liver injury for several hours may allow peritonitis and other complications to develop. All gunshot wounds of the abdomen should be explored whether penetration is evident or not. Shock waves from nonpenetrating gunshot wounds of the abdominal wall can easily transect bowel or lacerate the liver or spleen without entering the abdominal cavity. Most gunshot wounds that enter the peritoneal cavity damage a vessel, organ, or hollow viscus.

THE UNCONSCIOUS PATIENT. Patients with closed head injuries who are unconscious must have an airway established immediately. Hypotension rarely results from a closed head injury but is almost always caused by blood loss, usually in the thorax or abdomen. The cause of the blood loss is most rapidly determined by using an 18-gauge needle for immediate abdominal and chest taps, which may reveal nonclotting blood. The absence of blood does not rule out an intraabdominal or thoracic injury. Extreme care should be used in moving unconscious patients until injuries of the spine have been ruled out.

Immediate Nonoperative Surgical Care

Hematuria. A Foley catheter is routinely inserted, particularly following blunt trauma to the abdomen, to determine the presence of hematuria as well as to follow the urinary output during and immediately following the surgical procedure. Gross hematuria is evidence of urinary tract injury resulting from contusion, laceration, or rupture. If the patient's vital signs are stable and hematuria is present, a combined cystogram and intravenous pyelogram should be done. A single 15-min film is usually adequate to determine kidney function as well as indicate extravasation from the bladder, ureter, or kidneys. Failure to demonstrate extravasation does not rule out the possibility of a ruptured bladder or kidney. Should a nephrectomy be required during a laparotomy, functioning of the kidney on the opposite side should be proved. It is useless to attempt to visualize the kidneys by intravenous pyelogram when the patient is hypotensive. X-rays are delayed until the patient has been resuscitated and bleeding has been controlled in the operating room. If time is not available preoperatively for an intravenous pyelogram, a cassette may be placed under the patient prior to the start of surgical procedures and a pyelogram obtained intraoperatively.

FRACTURES. Fractures of the extremities are best managed immediately with splints for the extremities. Immobilization may prevent additional nerve and blood vessel injury and conversion of a closed fracture to an open one. The presence or absence of pulses in the fractured extremities should be noted on initial examination. Intravenous infusions should not be started in an injured extremity. Massive thoracoabdominal bleeding takes precedence over fractures, unless there is an accompanying arterial injury of such magnitude that there is danger of loss of limb. In such instances, it is often necessary to have two surgical teams working simultaneously.

Unstable pelvic ring fractures are best treated by early stabilization. The immediate application of external pelvic fixation not only allows early mobilization and pain relief but also may be lifesaving by controlling bleeding into the fracture hematoma.

ARTERIAL INJURIES. Any penetrating injury in the region of a major blood vessel or nerve deserves evaluation by arteriography. On initial examination, 18 percent of subsequently proved arterial injuries are noted to have a normal pulse distal to the arterial injury, and one-third of the patients have a palpable but diminished distal pulse. Vessel exploration in the region of the neck should be done under endotracheal anesthesia and may require resection of a portion of the clavicle for adequate visualization. Early recognition of an arterial injury is the most important factor in preserving a viable extremity or functioning distal organ.

Diagnosis and Management of Unapparent Injury

Blunt trauma to the abdomen may produce severe intraperitoneal or retroperitoneal injury with minimal physical findings. Bowel sounds may not be lost for several hours, and evidence of retroperitoneal or intraabdominal injury may not become apparent for as long as 18 h.

An abdominal paracentesis may be performed early in the observation period in patients with injuries from blunt trauma to the abdomen who have equivocal physical findings or altered consciousness. A 95 percent diagnostic accuracy is associated with the positive abdominal tap. A negative abdominal tap does not rule out intraabdominal injury and should be followed by peritoneal lavage or CT scan. Patients with signs of peritoneal irritation require exploratory laparotomy even in the absence of a positive abdominal tap or peritoneal lavage.

RADIOGRAPHS. These are taken when a patient's vital signs remain stable but are omitted for patients in severe shock. X-rays of the chest and abdomen are routinely performed to rule out foreign bodies such as knife blades within the depths of the wound. Patients sustaining gunshot wounds should have x-rays when possible in an attempt to trace the course of the missile. Patients sustaining blunt trauma often require multiple x-rays to rule out obscure fractures of the vertebral spine and retroperitoneal injuries. X-rays of extremities will be of value in determining whether or not the missile struck bone, fractured bone, or passed near vital structures.

NASOGASTRIC INTUBATION. A Levin tube is routinely inserted in most severely injured patients; exceptions include those patients with penetrating neck wounds, complex facial injuries, or suspected cervical spine fractures. Passage of the tube may provoke vomiting and empty the stomach of large particles, preventing subsequent aspiration during anesthesia. Esophageal or gastric injury from penetrating or blunt trauma may be diagnosed by finding bright red blood in the Levin tube drainage. Gastric intubation prevents gastric dilation during tracheal intubation and aids in the prevention of postoperative distention of the small bowel.

PROPHYLACTIC ANTIBIOTICS. Antibiotics are administered preoperatively to all patients sustaining penetrating wounds of the abdomen, beginning as soon as possible after the injured patient arrives in the emergency room. They may be discontinued if exploratory laparotomy is negative. Considerable experimental evidence indicates that prophylactic antibiotics in trauma are of benefit if administered within the first 3 h following injury. A retrospective review of a group of patients who sustained penetrating abdominal injuries showed that there was a decrease in the incidence of infections in those patients who received antibiotics preoperatively or intraoperatively as opposed to those who received antibiotics in the immediate postoperative period or therapeutically. This was significant for gunshot but not for stab wounds. A prospective study now being conducted indicates coverage should be against both aerobes and anaerobes.

Tetanus Prophylaxis. Following injury, immunized patients are administered a tetanus toxoid booster. In unimmunized patients the wound is debrided, and 250 units of tetanus human immune globulin is administered. Patients who were previously immunized but are now taking steroids, immunosuppressive therapy, or chemotherapy or who have had extensive irradiation should receive human immune globulin, since they may not have normal antibody response. Severely contaminated wounds should be left open or converted to open wounds when feasible.

PRINCIPLES IN THE MANAGEMENT OF WOUNDS
Ronald C. Jones and G. Tom Shires

Primary Wound Management

The most important single factor in the management of contaminated wounds is adequate debridement. This old surgical principle frequently has been forgotten since the advent of antibiotics. All tissue that is dead, has a poor blood supply, or is heavily contaminated should be removed if at all possible. This is particularly true of subcutaneous fat and muscle. Skin with impaired blood supply should be removed initially because of its tendency to become infected. Granulation tissue formation and later grafting procedures are preferable. Following sharp debridement and hemostasis, the wound is irrigated with copious quantities of saline solution, depending on the area and degree of soft tissue injury and contamination. That the incidence of wound infection is inversely proportional to the amount of irrigation and debridement at the time of injury has been demonstrated by Singleton and by Peterson and confirmed clinically many times.

LOCAL CARE OF WOUNDS

Glass or sharp instruments usually carry a minimal amount of foreign material into a wound and cause a minimal amount of tissue trauma. X-rays should be taken of any area in which the depth of the wound cannot clearly be seen. It is not uncommon for the deep portion of a stab wound to contain the tip of a knife blade or other foreign body. Stab wounds of soft tissues are explored in the emergency room with the gloved finger or under local anesthesia by extending the length of the laceration to determine the direction and extent of the wound and to rule out any major vessel, nerve, or organ injury. The wound is then irrigated with copious amounts of saline solution. If the wound is found not to penetrate the peri-

toneal cavity, a small soft-rubber Penrose drain is inserted and the wound is left open for drainage. The drain is removed in 24 h. Gunshot wounds are debrided externally and left open for drainage. Suturing these wounds leaves a closed contaminated space, and the infection can easily spread to surrounding soft tissue structures. Deep lacerations involving the extremity with damage to major vessels and tendons and massive muscle injury are managed by controlling major vessel bleeding and immediately wrapping the wound in sterile dressings. An x-ray is taken, if indicated, but a severe laceration is not explored until the patient is in the operating room. This procedure prevents undue contamination of the wound in the emergency room before the patient is adequately prepared. Minor lacerations can be managed in the emergency room.

Fascia usually can be approximated, and, depending on the type of wound, the skin and subcutaneous tissue may or may not be closed initially. These wounds are often left open and have delayed primary closure in 3 to 5 days. Damaged muscle due to gunshot wounds is debrided, hemostasis is obtained, and the wound is irrigated as outlined above. The wounds are packed open and closed with delayed closure. All patients with such wounds receive antibiotics and tetanus toxoid.

Antibacterial soaps or detergent materials are not used to irrigate wounds when muscle, tendon, or blood vessels are visible. Severe chemical irritation to these structures may occur, with resultant structure impairment and delayed wound healing.

Many factors, such as the number and virulence of organisms, blood supply of tissue, host resistance, shock, adequacy of surgical debridement, tissue tension, dead space, hemostasis, age, and associated diseases, are responsible for infection. Condie demonstrated in dogs that obliterating dead space reduced the occurrence of wound infection in the presence of contamination. Viable bacteria can be demonstrated in many surgical wounds at the time of closure; however, few incisions become infected.

Cosmetic appearance is a secondary consideration; the primary aim is to avoid infection and cover vital structures. No attempt at plastic repair is made at the initial closure of a potentially contaminated wound. Jagged edges of skin with poor blood supply are trimmed, and any resulting unpleasant scar can be cared for at a later date when no infection is present. Most lacerations, regardless of location, will never need revision if they meet the criteria previously outlined for the primary closure.

PUNCTURE WOUNDS. The most frequent puncture injury is that caused by a rusty nail in the foot. The patient is administered antibiotics both to prevent secondary infection and to aid in the prevention of tetanus, since this wound is not completely open to the air. Puncture wounds are debrided conservatively if they involve only the skin and subcutaneous tissue. Human tetanus immune globulin is given (250 mg) to the unimmunized patient. Debridement with conversion to an open wound and the administration of antibiotics and tetanus toxoid, whether or not the patient has been previously immunized, is also performed.

POWER MOWER INJURIES. Injuries resulting from the use of power mowers have increased in recent years. These include injuries from flying objects thrown from the power mower and from the mower itself to the hands and feet, particularly the fingers and toes. Treatment has consisted of covering exposed bones with muscle and leaving the entire wound open. These injuries almost uniformly become infected if an attempt is made to close the wound primarily. Patients are treated with systemic antibiotics and tetanus prophylaxis, and the wounds are packed with fine-mesh gauze. Skin grafting and reconstructive procedures should be delayed.

Emergency Laparotomy

INCISIONS. A midline incision is regularly used for exploratory laparotomy in patients with abdominal trauma and does not endanger the abdominal muscle, blood supply, or nerve supply, or damage aponeuroses. Minimal ligatures are used on bleeders that are contained in small bits of tissue, as each extra ligature is a foreign body and enhances the chance of a wound infection. Tissues should be kept moistened and gently handled. Surgical technique governs the development of wound infection as significantly as any single factor.

SUTURE. Number 0-Prolene is the suture material of choice for closing the uncomplicated midline abdominal incision, particularly in operations for traumatic lesions. It has not been the cause of draining sinuses following postoperative wound infections. Suture placement is probably the most important factor in the prevention of wound dehiscence. Sutures should not be placed at equal distances from the edge of the fascia, as they will fall in the same group of fibers; should one suture tear the fascia longitudinally, the tear may extend from suture to suture until dehiscence occurs. Sutures should be staggered or placed at varying intervals from the edge of the fascia. With such a closure, there should be no fear in having a patient cough vigorously for adequate postoperative pulmonary care. An occasional patient with minimal subcutaneous tissue will complain of pain in the incision when the suture is under a pressure point such as a belt. These sutures are easily removed under local anesthesia.

Simple interrupted suture is used to close the fascia and peritoneum in a single layer. This is felt to be superior to the figure-of-eight suture, because less tissue is gathered and the suture can be placed faster, thus reducing anesthesia time. Interrupted sutures are used instead of running sutures because a break in the suture material will not loosen the entire incision. Regardless of the type of suture or method of placement, the fascia should be loosely approximated and not strangulated. Tightening fascial sutures may lead to necrosis with the suture subsequently cutting through the tissue. Retention sutures have not been regularly used. Routine antibiotic irrigation of the wound for the prevention of infection has not been necessary.

Through-and-Through Closure Several local and systemic factors noted at the time of the original operation may make through-and-through closure the procedure of

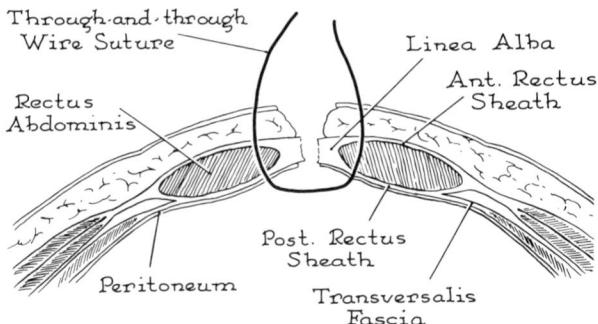

Fig. 6-1. Through-and-through wire closure. (From: *Shires GT: Care of the Trauma Patient. New York, McGraw-Hill, 1966, p 37, with permission.*)

choice (Fig. 6-1). This uses adjustable bridges and large braided nonabsorbable suture or German silver wire swaged on a large cutting needle. The bridges prevent cutting of skin by the wire and allow for swelling that occurs in the first 24 to 48 h postoperatively. The bridges can be adjusted to compensate for swelling of tissues. Wounds massively contaminated from shotgun wadding and fecal material, in patients with steroids, or associated with massive infection and peritonitis are best handled with through-and-through closure. Often a single patient may have several indications for this type of closure such as chronic pulmonary disease, obesity, and/or chronic debilitating disease. Occasionally through-and-through closure is used at the end of a lengthy operation with a long incision to shorten anesthesia time if the patient is not tolerating the procedure well. This type of closure is routinely used in the patient requiring reoperation in the early postoperative period because of gastrointestinal bleeding or intestinal obstruction. The wires are left in place for 3 weeks. This measure has proved to be sure, safe, timesaving, and often lifesaving.

INFECTION. Infection and severe abdominal distention are frequently mentioned as causative factors in dehiscence. Wound infection may be prevented in the markedly contaminated abdomen by leaving the skin and subcutaneous tissue open down to the fascia for delayed primary closure. This method is frequently used in long operations or with excessive contamination such as from feces. Abdominal wounds frequently harbor coliform organisms if bowel injury has been sustained. These wounds are packed open with fine-mesh gauze, changed daily for debridement, and either closed at 5 days or allowed to granulate until closure. This procedure will usually result in an excellent scar.

DRAINS. Subcutaneous drains will not substitute for good hemostasis. Failure to obtain hemostasis will give rise to a hematoma which is an excellent culture medium for an already contaminated wound. Drains from the abdominal cavity are usually brought out through a separate stab wound and by the most direct route. This is especially true for some liver and pancreatic injuries. Drainage of the free peritoneal cavity is not attempted.

Antibiotics

Following hemorrhage sepsis is the second most common cause of death in patients sustaining penetrating abdominal trauma and is a leading cause of postoperative mortality. Burke has demonstrated in animal models the relationship of time between contamination and implementation of antibiotic therapy. Experimentally, if antibiotics were delayed for greater than 3 h following contamination, the inflammatory response was unaltered, indicating antibiotics must be administered as soon after injury as possible. The incidence of infection following gunshot wounds is two or three times greater than following stab wounds.

Jones evaluated 257 patients sustaining penetrating abdominal trauma at Parkland Memorial Hospital in Dallas (PMH), 147 of whom had colon and small bowel injuries following penetrating abdominal trauma. Combination therapy using clindamycin/tobramycin was compared with single agents cefoxitin active against both aerobes and anaerobes and cefamandole active against aerobes but no anaerobes (Table 6-1). Cefoxitin was statistically more effective than cefamandole and comparable with clindamycin/tobramycin. Cefoxitin was also an effective agent in more serious infections including bacteremia, intraabdominal abscess, and severe operative soft tissue infections. Infection rate is higher in hypotensive patients than in normotensive patients (30 vs. 14 percent). Although Nichols could not correlate shock with infection, he did relate infection to number of units of blood transfused. In another report Gentry compared ticarcillin/tobramycin vs. cefamandole vs. cefoxitin and demonstrated cefoxitin to be comparable with combination therapy and superior to cefamandole. At PMH the usual dose of cefoxitin is 2 g q 6 h for 48 h following penetrating abdominal trauma. Nichols advocates 5 days of therapy in patients sustaining a colon injury. Oreskovich, administering penicillin and vibramycin or cefoxitin, was unable to demonstrate any difference in infection rate whether antibiotics were administered for 12 h or 5 days. However, these studies agree that it is important to cover *Bacteroides fragilis*.

Finegold and Gorbach have studied the microflora of the gastrointestinal tract, providing information regarding the bacteriology of intraabdominal injuries. They noted that the large intestine harbors predominantly anaerobic flora. These anaerobes have a total concentration of 10^{11} per gram and outnumber coliform organisms by 1000 to 10,000:1. Onderdonk using an animal model reported the concept of synergy between anaerobes and facultative bacteria as the mechanism for the abscess formation. Mortality related to coliform organisms injected into the peritoneal cavity, whereas abscess formation was associated with the combination of aerobes and anaerobes. Enterococcus strains alone did not produce mortality or abscess. Louie and Bartlett evaluated several single and combination antibiotics, and found that regimens most effective in reducing abscesses were those using clindamycin or cefoxitin, both of which are effective against anaerobes. They concluded in the animal model that the cefoxitin was superior to cefamandole.

Tally reported the sensitivities of 550 *Bacteroides fragilis* organisms and found none resistant to metronidazole. Approximately 7 or 8 percent were resistant to either clindamycin or piperacillin. Cefoxitin had 16 percent resistance. Over 40 percent of the *Bacteroides fragilis* were resistant to cefotaxime (Claforan) and cefoperazone (Cefobid).

Infection increases as the number of organ injuries increases and as the patient's age increases. Studies suggest that patients sustaining contamination of the peritoneal cavity with colonic contents probably benefit from antibiotic coverage effective against both aerobes and anaerobes. With colonic contamination the antibiotic is administered for a minimum of 48 h and, depending upon the condition of the patient and the number of associated injuries, may be administered for a longer period. Routine administration of an aminoglycoside is unnecessary following penetrating abdominal trauma and may contribute to renal damage.

Failure to debride nonviable tissue may result in infection and antibiotic failure. Surgical technique and appropriate surgical judgment such as whether or not to perform an intestinal anastomosis is just as important if not more so than the antibiotic chosen.

Following severe penetrating abdominal trauma, intraabdominal abscess formation remains common even with prophylactic antibiotic therapy. Jones retrospectively reviewed 50 patients who had sustained penetrating abdominal trauma and who subsequently developed intraabdominal abscess. Missile injuries were responsible for 92 percent of these injuries and 60 percent of these patients had associated colon injuries. The highest risk of infection follows missile injuries to the colon. The mortality in this review was 22 percent. The organisms recovered from these abscesses included *Escherichia coli*, *Klebsiella*, and *B. fragilis*. Gram-positive organisms included enterococcus, anaerobic streptococci, and *Clostridium*. Early diagnosis of intraabdominal abscess is usually easiest using a CT scan. Mortality from intraabdominal abscess has been reduced to 12 percent using the CT scan. With proper patient selection percutaneous drain-

Table 6-1. PENETRATING ABDOMINAL TRAUMA: COLON AND/OR SMALL BOWEL INJURIES AT PARKLAND MEMORIAL HOSPITAL ($N = 147$)

	Pt	Pt infections	Bacteremia abdominal abscess operative soft tissue
Cleocin/Tobra	51	15 (29%)	7 (14%)
Mandol	44	20 (45%)	11 (26%)
Cefoxitin	52	8 (15%)	5 (10%)
I vs. III		$p = 0.086$	$p = 0.515$
II vs. I and III		$p = 0.006$	$p = 0.048$

SOURCE: Jones RC, Thal ER, et al: *Ann Surg* 201:576, 1985, with permission.

age of intraabdominal abscess has had 80 percent satisfactory results. Following percutaneous drainage the patient may not respond as rapidly as with open surgical drainage and the drainage catheter may have to remain in place for several days, resulting in longer hospitalization. Gastrointestinal fistula and hemorrhage can occur with either approach.

INTRAPERITONEAL ANTIBIOTICS. Intraperitoneal antibiotic irrigation is not recommended. Toxic blood levels develop following intraperitoneal irrigation with kanamycin even with only 2 to 5 min of contact with the peritoneal cavity, and a significant amount of the irrigant cannot be recovered with suction. Patients with significant intraperitoneal contamination are given systemic antibiotics, the abdomen is irrigated with saline solution, which is of questionable value, and the fascia is closed. The skin and subcutaneous tissue may be left open for delayed primary closure, usually within 3 to 4 days following severe contamination. If the patient develops an infection following topical or intraperitoneal irrigation with antibiotics, the organisms isolated are often resistant to the antibiotic used.

BITES AND STINGS OF ANIMALS AND INSECTS
Ronald C. Jones and G. Tom Shires

Rabies

INCIDENCE. In the United States an estimated 2 million human beings are bitten by animals yearly, and one-half million are bitten by dogs. Any mammalian animal may carry rabies. In 1985 there were 5606 laboratory-confirmed cases of rabies. The animals most frequently reported infected and the percentage of the cases they accounted for were skunks (45 percent), raccoons (26 percent), bats (15 percent), foxes (3 percent), cattle (4 percent), dogs (2 percent), and cats (2 percent). Skunks, raccoons, and bats are the major hosts. Rabid skunks increased by 20 percent in 1985 to 2507. Raccoons represented 75 percent of all rabid animals in the mid-Atlantic states of Maryland, Pennsylvania, Virginia, West Virginia, and Washington, D.C. In 1981, for the first time, rabid cats outnumbered rabid dogs. Wildlife species accounted for 91 percent of the rabies in this country. Wildlife rabies has been reported in coyotes, opossum, otter, bobcats, bear, squirrel, deer, mink, woodchucks, coatis, ferrets, and a badger. Domestic rabies has been reported in cattle, dogs, cats, horses, mules, sheep, goats, swine, and guinea pigs. The Communicable Disease Center estimates that this represents less than 10 percent of the cases that actually exist. Mexico reported 10,756 cases of animal rabies of which 93 percent were in dogs. In the past 5 years, there has been an average of two cases of human rabies per year. Table 6-2 shows the incidence and frequency of reported rabies in the United States in various animals and in human beings by states or territory in 1985. Many of the cases of human rabies reported in the

past 10 years have resulted from exposure outside the United States.

RABIES CONTROL. Saliva from a rabid animal contains large numbers of the rabies virus and is inoculated through a bite, any laceration, or a break in the skin. Animal experiments and at least two human infections indicate that animals and human beings can become infected by bats, without being bitten, by inhalation of rabies virus. Girard examined bats and demonstrated rabies virus in the brain, kidney, urine, salivary gland, adrenal gland, and liver, using the fluorescent antibody test.

The maintenance of wild and exotic animals such as skunks, raccoons, ocelots, and bobcats as household pets is discouraged since many of these animals are infected with rabies. If people insist on maintaining wild and exotic animals as household pets, the animals should be quarantined for a minimum of 90 days after capture and vaccinated at least 30 days prior to being released to an owner. Annual vaccination is recommended.

Dogs and cats bitten by a known rabid animal should be destroyed immediately. If the owner refuses to have this done, the unvaccinated animal should be placed in strict isolation for 6 months and vaccinated 1 month before being released. If the animal has been vaccinated within the previous 3 years, it should be revaccinated immediately and confined for 90 days. Since cat rabies cases now exceed the annually reported cases in dogs, immunization of cats should be required.

DIAGNOSIS. Circumstances of the Bite. Circumstances surrounding the attack frequently furnish vital information as to whether or not vaccine is indicated. Most domestic animal bites are provoked attacks; if this history is obtained, rabies vaccine can usually be withheld if the animal appears healthy. Children are frequently bitten while attempting to separate fighting animals or while teasing or accidentally hurting the animal. Bites during attempts to feed or handle an apparently healthy animal should generally be regarded as provoked. Frequently the patient has attempted to handle a sick animal. Although vaccination of the animal does not totally rule out the possibility of transmitting rabies, it is over 90 percent effective.

Bites from rodents, including squirrels, gerbils, chipmunks, guinea pigs, rats, and mice, seldom require specific rabies prophylaxis. Each case of possible exposure must be studied individually before a conclusion can be reached as to whether antirabies therapy is indicated. An unprovoked attack is more likely to indicate that the animal is rabid.

Extent and Location of Bite Wound. The likelihood that rabies will result from a bite varies with its extent and location. For convenience in approaching management, two categories of exposure are widely accepted:

Severe. Multiple or deep puncture wounds, or any bites on the head, face, neck, hands, or fingers.

Mild. Scratches, lacerations, or single bites on areas of the body other than the head, face, neck, hands, or fingers. Open wounds, such as abrasions, suspected of being contaminated with saliva also belong to this category.

Table 6-2. RABIES IN THE UNITED STATES BY STATE AND ANIMAL TYPE, 1985

	Dogs	Cats	Cattle	Domestic animal total*	Skunks	Bobcats	Raccoons	Bats	Wild animal total*	Total
Totals	116	127	213	503	2507	7	1487	830	5103	5606
Ala.	2	1		5	4		85	27	119	124
Alaska	2			2					41	43
Ariz.	1		1	3	86	1		29	120	123
Ark.	1	1	4	7	131			13	144	151
Calif.	5	2	5	13	421	2	2	136	573	586
Colo.		1		1				25	25	26
Conn.								7	7	7
Del.								1	1	1
D.C.	3			3			4	1	5	8
Fla.	1	1		2	4	2	111	21	144	146
Ga.	7	5		12	9		158	10	188	200
Hawaii										0
Idaho								10	10	10
Ill.	2	1	2	6	20			23	43	49
Ind.	1		1	2	11			11	22	24
Iowa	5	9	19	35	96			17	114	149
Kan.		2	3	6	50			4	55	61
Ky.	10		1	13	19			9	29	42
La.					14			10	24	24
Maine								1	1	1
Md.	1	11	3	17	6		672	34	743	760
Mass.								14	14	14
Mich.		2		2	6			17	24	26
Minn.	10	11	34	57	155		1	5	162	219
Miss.								10	10	10
Mo.	1		2	3	35			20	56	59
Mont.	2	5	15	26	207	1	2	12	224	250
Neb.	1	1	3	5	30			1	31	36
Nev.								15	15	15
N.H.								1	1	1
N.J.								38	38	38
N. Mex.		1		1	2			9	11	12
N.Y.		5	12	17	24		2	43	136	153
N.C.								12	12	12
N. Dak.	2	8	28	45	97		2	2	104	149
Ohio	1		2	4	9			15	26	30
Okla.	3	4	8	16	88			6	95	111
Oreg.								6	6	6
Pa.	3	10	4	20	81		285	44	429	449
R.I.										0
S.C.	3	7		11			40	11	51	62
S. Dak.	8	9	44	63	274		2	6	284	347
Tenn.	3			3	58			10	71	74
Tex.	28	22	13	74	404	1	3	99	514	588
Utah								4	4	4
Vt.								1	1	1
Va.	1	3	1	6	43		102	16	173	179
Wash.								5	5	5
W. Va.		1		2	8		15		27	29
Wis.	5	3	4	12	39		1	13	54	66
Wyo.	1	1	1	3	76			6	82	85
Guam										0
P.R.	3		3	6					35	41
V.I.										0

* Not shown in the table, but included in the totals are other domestic animals: horses and mules 38, sheep and goats 7, swine 2; other wild animals: coyotes 2, foxes 181, rodents and lagomorphs 23, other 66.

The only documented cases of rabies from human to human transmission occurred in four patients who received corneas transplanted from persons who died of rabies undiagnosed at the time of death.

Laboratory Diagnosis. The direct focus inhibition test of brain material is the recommended technique to diagnose rabies. The intracerebral inoculation of mice combined with the microscopic examination of brain tissue for Negri bodies is still one of the most useful tests in the laboratory diagnosis of rabies and should be used whenever human beings have been bitten by suspect animals and the direct focus inhibition test is negative.

MANAGEMENT OF BITING ANIMALS. Most animal bites of human beings are caused by dogs and cats, and in most instances it is possible to observe the biting animal for the development of rabies. Domestic animals that bite a person should be captured and observed for symptoms of rabies for 10 days. If none develop, the animals may be assumed to be nonrabid. If the animal dies or is killed, the head should not be damaged but should be sent promptly to a public health laboratory for examination. The tissue requires refrigeration, but not freezing, and transportation to the laboratory following death of the animal must be rapid. Clinical signs of rabies in wild animals cannot be interpreted reliably; therefore, any wild animal that bites or scratches a person should be killed at once (without unnecessary damage to the head) and the brain examined for evidence of rabies.

Information from the county health department regarding which animals, both domestic and wild, have been reported to be rabid within the past 10 years in the particular area may indicate a possible specific animal transmitting rabies.

PATIENT MANAGEMENT. Exposed Persons Previously Immunized. For mild exposure of a person who has demonstrated an antibody response to antirabies vaccination received in the past, two I.M. doses (1.0 mL each) of human diploid cell vaccine (HDCV), one immediately and one 3 days later, is recommended. RIG should not be given in these cases.

If it is not known whether an exposed person has had antibody previously demonstrated, the complete postexposure antirabies treatment (RIG plus five doses) may be necessary. Because of variation in vaccine potency and individual response, immunization should not be considered complete until antibody is demonstrated in the serum. If antibody can be demonstrated in a serum sample collected before vaccine is given, treatment can be discontinued after at least two doses of HDCV.

Preexposure Prophylaxis. Those whose vocations or avocations result in frequent contact with dogs, cats, foxes, skunks, or bats should also be considered for preexposure prophylaxis.

A significant number of citizens of the United States have been and, with increasing frequency, will continue to be exposed to rabies in other countries where rabies in dogs is a major problem. Because rabies in animals is widespread in large areas of Asia, Africa, and Latin America, the Foreign Quarantine Program of the U.S. Public Health Service has advised that preexposure immunization against rabies be suggested for Americans traveling in these areas. The dog remains the major source of human exposure.

Three 1-mL injections of HDCV given intradermally in the deltoid area on days 0, 7, and 21 or 28 are required. This series of three injections can be expected to have produced neutralizing antibody in all patients. Rabies has been reported to develop in a patient following four doses of HDCV when human rabies globulin was not also given. Serologic testing is not necessary after preexposure prophylaxis with HDCV administered by either the intradermal or intramuscular route. The intradermal route should not be used for postexposure prophylaxis. Chloroquine phosphate (administered for malaria) chemoprophylaxis may interfere with the antibody response to HDCV in persons traveling to the developing countries. In persons receiving preexposure prophylaxis in preparation for travel to a rabies endemic area, the intradermal dose route should be initiated early enough to allow the three-dose series to be completed 30 days or more before departure. If this is not possible, the intramuscular dose route should be used.

The intradermal human diploid cell rabies vaccine (HDCV) was licensed for preexposure use in the United States on May 30, 1986. Fishbein recently demonstrated that 95 percent of previously immunized persons who had inadequate titers at the time of booster responded with a fivefold increase in titer by day 7 after a single booster dose of HDCV. In contrast, persons receiving the primary rabies immunization do not begin to respond for 7 days and do not obtain significant titers from 10 to 14 days. For other persons, such as veterinarians and animal control officers in areas of low rabies endemicity, primary immunization may be all that is necessary until an exposure occurs. Routine 2-year boosters in the latter groups appear to be unnecessary and probably risky. Bernard demonstrated that intradermal boosters at 1 year following preexposure immunization resulted in generalized reaction, consisting primarily of headache, malaise, fever, muscle aches, joint pain, or generalized itching in 26 percent of patients.

Intradermal HDCV has not been approved for postexposure use. Should an exposure occur in any one who has had a recommended primary preexposure regimen of HDCV, the individual should receive two intramuscular (I.M.) booster doses of HDCV, one each on days 0 and 3.

Accidental Human Exposure to Vaccine. Accidental inoculation may occur in individuals during administration of animal rabies vaccine. Such exposures to inactivated vaccines constitute no known rabies hazard. There have been no cases of rabies resulting from needle or other exposure to a licensed modified live virus vaccine in the United States; however, the local or state health department can be contacted.

Postexposure Prophylaxis. *Incubation Period.* It is generally accepted that the incubation period for rabies in human beings ranges from 10 days to 1 year, most cases occurring 20 to 90 days from exposure. In cases of exposure of the head, neck, or upper extremities, the incubation period is potentially less than 30 days.

Immediate Local Care. Not all persons bitten by rabid animals contract the disease. Vigorous local treatment to remove possible rabies virus may be as important as specific antirabies therapy. Free bleeding from the wound is encouraged. Local care of an animal bite should consist of:

1. Thorough irrigation with copious amounts of saline solution;
2. Cleansing with a soap solution;
3. Debridement;
4. Administration of antibiotic when indicated to prevent bacterial infection;
5. Administration of tetanus toxoid;
6. Immediate suturing of the wound generally is not advised, since it may contribute to the development of rabies, but a severe laceration secondary to a dog bite may be sutured if exposure to rabies is unlikely.

Passive Immunization. Rabies immune globulin, human (RIG) (Cutter Laboratories, Hyperaperab and Merieux Institutes, IMOGAM) is antirabies gamma globulin prepared from hyperimmunized human donors. Human rabies immune globulin (HRIG) in combination with HDCV is considered the best postexposure prophylaxis. HRIG, 20 I.U./kg of body weight, is recommended for most exposures classified as severe, for all bites by rabid animals or those suspected of having rabies, for unprovoked bites by wild carnivores and bats, and for nonbite exposure to animals suspected of being rabid. A portion of the HRIG is used to infiltrate the wound, and the remainder is administered intramuscularly. HRIG is given only once, as early as possible following exposure and up to the eighth day. After the eighth day RIG is not indicated, since an antibody response to the vaccine is presumed to have occurred. The use of human immune antirabies globulin is accompanied by five intramuscular 1.0-mL doses of HDCV. If HRIG is not available, the recommended dose of equine antibodies serum is 40 I.U./kg of body weight (Table 6-3).

Table 6-3. POSTEXPOSURE ANTIRABIES TREATMENT GUIDE

Species of animal	Condition of animal at time of attack	Treatment of exposed person
Skunk Fox Coyote Raccoon Bat	Regard as rabid	HRIG + HDCV
Dog Cat	Healthy	None
	Unknown (escaped)	HRIG + HDCV
	Rabid or suspected rabid	HRIG + HDCV*
Other	Consider individually—see Circumstances of the Bite	

These recommendations are only a guide. They should be applied in conjunction with knowledge of the animal species involved, circumstances of the bite or other exposure, vaccination status of the animal, and presence of rabies in the region.

* Discontinue vaccine if tests of animal killed at time of attack are negative.

Active Immunization, Primary Immunization. Over 25,000 people per year undergo postexposure prophylaxis after bites by suspected or proved rabid animals. HDCV is an inactivated virus vaccine prepared from fixed rabies virus grown in human diploid cell culture. Five intramuscular 1.0-mL doses of HDCV on days 0, 3, 7, 14, and 28 are administered. The WHO currently recommends a sixth dose 90 days after the first dose. All injections are given in the deltoid area. The routine serologic testing of persons who receive recommended preexposure or postexposure treatment regimens of HDCV is not necessary, nor is it necessary to perform routine serologic testing following booster doses of HDCV for persons given the recommended primary HDCV vaccination or those shown to have had an adequate antibody response to primary vaccination with duck embryo vaccine or other rabies vaccination. The vaccine may be stopped if the animal is proved nonrabid.

Evidence from laboratory and field experience in many areas of the world indicates that postexposure prophylaxis combined with local wound treatment, vaccine, and rabies immune globulin is uniformly effective when appropriately used. However, rabies has occasionally developed in human beings who have received postexposure rabies prophylaxis with the vaccine alone.

Booster Doses. In persons continuously exposed to the risk of rabies, booster doses of HDCV should be given at 2-year intervals. A previously immunized person who is exposed to rabies should receive two doses I.M. of 1 mL of HDCV, one immediately and one 3 days later. Laboratory workers in rabies biologic exposure areas should be tested for rabies antibody every 6 months and vaccinated when antibody as measured with the rapid fluorescent-focus inhibition test is low. HRIG is not indicated.

Side Reaction to Vaccine. Following vaccination with HDCV, reactions have included warmth, redness, pain, swelling, and itching at the infection site in approximately 15 to 25 percent of patients. Other side effects have included fever, nausea, vomiting and diarrhea, lymphadenopathy, headache, and dizziness. Rarely have systemic reactions including hives and anaphylaxis occurred. Two cases of illness resembling Guillain-Barré syndrome have been reported.

Precautions and Contraindications. Immunosuppression. Corticosteroids and other immunosuppressive agents and immunosuppressive illnesses can interfere with the active immunity in predisposed patients developing rabies. Immunosuppressive agents should not be administered during postexposure therapy, unless essential for the treatment of other conditions. When rabies and postexposure prophylaxis are administered to persons receiving steroids or other immunosuppressive therapy, it is especially important that serum be tested for serum antibody to ensure that an adequate response has developed.

Pregnancy. Because of the potential consequences of inadequately treated rabies exposure and limited data to indicate that fetal abnormalities have not been associated with rabies vaccination, pregnancy is not considered a contraindication to postexposure prophylaxis.

Allergies. Persons with histories of hypersensitivities should be given rabies vaccines with caution. When a patient with a history suggesting hypersensitivity to HDCV must be given that vaccine, antihistamines can be given; epinephrine should be readily available to counteract antiphylactic reactions, and the person should be carefully observed.

Manifestations and Treatment of Disease. Rabid dogs are noted to have purposeless movements with snapping, drooling, and vocal cord paralysis. Death usually occurs in 2 to 5 days. Human beings die essentially the same way. There are 2 to 4 days of prodromal symptoms before the patient reaches the excited stage. Paresthesia in the region of the bite is an important early symptom. Symptoms noted with the onset of clinical rabies include headaches, vertigo, stiff neck, malaise, lethargy, and severe pulmonary symptoms including wheezing, hyperventilation, and dyspnea. The patient may have spasm of the throat muscles with dysphagia. The outstanding clinical symptom of rabies is related to swallowing. Drooling, maniacal behavior, and convulsions ensue and are followed by coma, paralysis, and death.

Instead of sedation and symptomatic treatment only, it is now recognized that intensive respiratory supportive care may be beneficial, in view of a case of human rabies in which the patient survived. Strict attention was given to the management of airway, pulmonary care, cardiac arrhythmias, and seizures. This included tracheostomy, vigorous suctioning, Dilantin for seizures, close monitoring of blood gases, electrocardiograms, electroencephalograms, and a ventricular shunt. Nursing care is extremely important.

At least one case of human rabies has been treated with interferon in the United States. In animal studies interferon has been shown to offer protection against challenge by rabies virus only when it is administered before or shortly after virus challenge. Once clinical disease develops, the use of interferon is justified because clinical rabies is almost uniformly fatal despite active or passive immunization.

Snakebites

INCIDENCE. In North America all the poisonous snakes of medical importance are members of the family Crotalidae, or pit vipers, with the exception of the coral snake, of the Elapidae family. Coral snakes are scattered from Florida to southern Arizona, are biologically related to the Indian cobra, and produce a different envenomation syndrome from the crotalids. The pit vipers include the rattlesnake, cottonmouth moccasin, and copperhead.

Approximately 8000 persons are bitten each year by poisonous snakes. Over 98 percent of snakebites occur on the extremities. Thirty-five percent of snakebites occur in children less than ten years of age, usually in an area around their homes. Since 1960, an average of 14 victims have died annually as a result of snakebites. Five states account for 70 percent of these deaths: Texas, Georgia, Florida, Alabama, and southern California. Rattlesnakes are responsible for approximately 70 percent of all deaths due to snakebites. Death from the bite of a copperhead is extremely rare.

POISONOUS VERSUS NONPOISONOUS SNAKES. Pit vipers are named for the characteristic pit, a heat-sensitive organ, that is located between the eye and the nostril on each side of the head. As a rule, these snakes may be identified by their elliptical pupils, as opposed to the round pupil of harmless snakes. Nonpoisonous snakes do not have pits. However, the coral snake does have a round pupil and lacks the facial pit. Pit vipers have two well-developed fangs that protrude from the maxillae, whereas nonpoisonous snakes have rows of teeth without fangs. Pit vipers also may be identified by turning the snake's belly upward and noting the single row of subcaudal plates. Nonpoisonous snakes have a double row of subcaudal plates (Fig. 6-2). The coral snake is a brightly colored small snake with red, yellow, and black rings. This color combination occurs also in nonpoisonous snakes, but the alternating colors are different. Only the coral snake has a red ring next to a yellow ring; when red touches yellow, it is a coral snake. The nose of the coral snake is black.

The venoms of poisonous snakes consist of enzymatic, complex proteins that affect all soft tissues. Venoms have been shown to have neurotoxic, hemorrhagic, thrombogenic, hemolytic, cytotoxic, antifribin, and anticoagulant effects. Phospholipase A is probably responsible for hemolysis. Most venoms contain hyaluronidase, which enhances the rapid spread of venom by way of the superficial lymphatics. There may be considerable variation in the venom effect. Either neurotoxic features such as muscle cramping, fasciculation, weakness, and respiratory paralysis or hemolytic characteristics may predominate depending on the snake and the patient.

CLINICAL MANIFESTATIONS. Pain from the bite of a poisonous snake is excruciating and probably the symptom that most easily differentiates poisonous from nonpoisonous snakebites. Poisonous snakes characteristically produce one or two fang marks, whereas nonpoisonous snakes may produce rows of punctures. Local signs and symptoms may include swelling, tenderness, pain, and ecchymosis and may appear within minutes at the site of the venom injection. If no edema or pain is present within 30 min following the injury, the pit viper probably did not inject any venom. Swelling may continue to increase for 24 h. Hemorrhagic vesiculations, bullae, and petechiae may appear between 8 and 36 h, with thrombosis of superficial vessels and eventual sloughing of tissues. Systemic symptoms include paresthesias and muscle fasciculations. Muscle fasciculations are most common following a rattlesnake bite and often are in the perioral region. Fasciculations almost never follow a copperhead bite and rarely follow a cottonmouth bite. They are often seen in the face muscles and over the neck, back, and the involved extremity, and may occur within 10 min. Hypotension, weakness, sweating and chills, dizziness, nausea, and vomiting are other systemic symptoms.

Rattlesnake. Most rattlesnakes probably eject less than 50 percent of their venom during a single biting act. Following a rattlesnake bite, ecchymosis, hemorrhagic

CHARACTERISTICS OF SNAKES

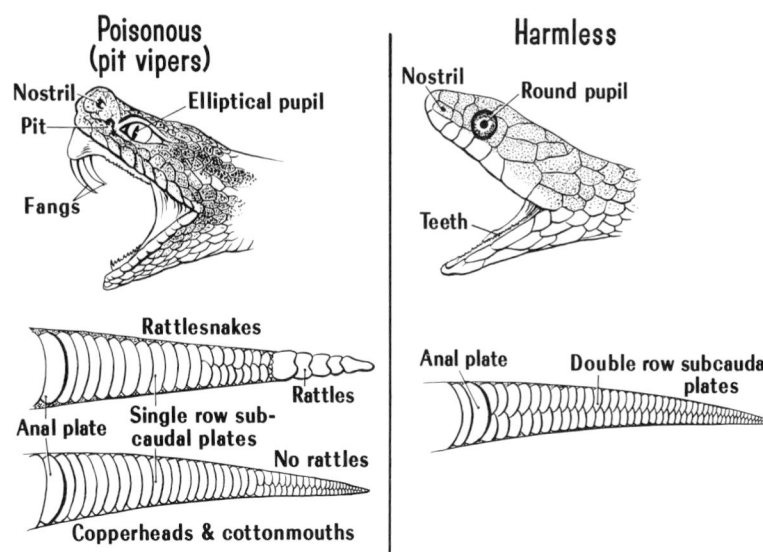

Fig. 6-2. Characteristics of poisonous and nonpoisonous snakes. (From: *Parrish HM: Texas State J Med 60:592, 1964, with permission.*)

vesiculations, swelling of the regional lymph nodes, weakness, fainting, and sweating commonly are reported. The venom produces deleterious changes in the blood cells, defects in blood coagulation, injuries to the intimal linings of vessels, damage to the heart muscles, alterations in respiration, and, to a lesser extent, changes in neuromuscular conduction. Pulmonary edema is common in severe poisoning, and hemorrhage into the lungs, kidneys, heart, and peritoneum may occur. Hematemesis, melena, changes in salivation, and muscle fasciculations may be seen. Urinalysis may reveal hematuria, glycosuria, and proteinuria. Red blood cells and platelets may decrease, and bleeding and clotting times are usually prolonged.

Coral Snakes. The coral snake contributes to only 3 percent of all bites and 1.5 percent of all deaths from poisonous snakes. Bites by the coral snake occasionally provoke blurred vision, ptosis, drowsiness, increased salivation, and sweating. The patient may notice paresthesia about the mouth and throat, sometimes slurring of speech, and nausea and vomiting. Pain is not a constant complaint, nor is edema a constant finding. Thus coral snake venom causes more extensive changes in the nervous system, but death may occur from cardiovascular collapse.

LABORATORY EVALUATION. Blood should be immediately drawn for typing and cross matching, because hemolysis may later make this difficult. Since hemolysis and injury to kidneys and liver may occur, it is important to follow alterations in clotting mechanism and renal and liver function as well as electrolyte status. Routine tests include a complete blood count, platelet count, prothrombin time, partial thromboplastin time, urinalysis, blood sugar, BUN, and electrolytes. Additional tests depending on the severity of the bite include fibrinogen, red cell fragility, clotting time, and clot retraction time.

LOCAL TREATMENT. The treatment of the bite of a poisonous snake varies considerably but is related to the length of time from the bite until treatment is instituted. Application of a tourniquet, incision, and suction are appropriate if employed within 1 h from the time of the bite. The Committee on Trauma of the American College of Surgeons in consultation with many experts in this field developed a poster for emergency department use entitled "Management of Poisonous Snakebites."

Immobilization. Patients are kept quiet, and the extremity is immobilized. Splinting the limb may inhibit the local diffusion of venom by stopping the movement of muscle bellies within their sheaths. Snyder and Knowles have shown in animals that exercise greatly enhances the absorption of venom and as much as 30 percent may be absorbed within 30 min following vigorous exercise.

Tourniquet. The snake injects venom into the subcutaneous tissue, and this is absorbed by the lymphatics. As almost none of the venom is absorbed through the bloodstream, the tourniquet is applied loosely to obstruct only venous and lymphatic flow. The index finger should be easily inserted beneath the tourniquet after its application. The distal pulse is checked and should be palpable after tourniquet application. The tourniquet is not released once applied and may be left in place during the 30 min that suction is being applied. Snyder and Knowles have injected ^{131}I-tagged venom into dogs and have demonstrated that if the tourniquet is applied promptly, less than 10 percent of the venom leaves the leg of the dog in 2 h. The tourniquet may be removed (1) as soon as an intravenous infusion is started, (2) when antivenin is ready for administration, and (3) if the patient is not in shock.

EMERGENCY DEPARTMENT MANAGEMENT OF POISONOUS SNAKEBITES

Clinical evaluation of the victim

1. Assess respiratory status.
2. Assess circulatory status.
3. Determine the extent of systemic reaction from the presence of hypotension; nausea; vomiting; sweating; weakness; or neurotoxic symptoms such as dizziness, perioral paresthesia, ptosis, paralysis, or muscle fasciculations.
4. Inspect the area of the bite, noting one or more fang marks (although a coral snake may leave none), swelling, pain, or ecchymoses.
5. Identify the snake if possible. Most bites are from nonpoisonous snakes.

Laboratory evaluation

1. Routine tests:
   a. Complete blood count
   b. Type and cross match
   c. Prothrombin time
   d. Partial thromboplastin time
   e. Platelet count
   f. Urinalysis
   g. Blood sugar; blood urea nitrogen (BUN); electrolytes
2. Additional tests, depending on the severity of the bite:
   a. Fibrinogen
   b. Red cell fragility
   c. Clotting time
   d. Clot retraction time

Grade of envenomation

The grade of envenomation will vary with time after the bite. (If the victim is seen early, severe envenomation may be underassessed.) Observe at least 6 h after the bite.

1. Indications of minimal envenomation:
   a. Local symptoms and signs
   b. Few systemic symptoms and signs
   c. Minimal laboratory abnormalities
2. Indications of moderate envenomation:
   a. Swelling that progresses beyond the area of the bite
   b. Some systemic symptoms and signs
   c. Abnormal laboratory findings—i.e., abnormal clotting factors; a fall in hematocrit or platelets
3. Indication of severe envenomation:
   a. Marked local symptoms and signs
   b. Severe systemic symptoms and signs
   c. Significant abnormalities in laboratory findings

Treatment

1. Start intravenous infusion of balanced salt solution if any evidence of envenomation exists.
2. Oxygen and appropriate vasopressors should be available.
3. Keep the bitten part level with the heart.
4. Release compression band (if one has been applied) only if:
   a. The patient is not in shock
   b. An intravenous line has been established
   c. Antivenin is available
5. Local care of the area of the bite:
   a. If the victim is treated within 30 min of the bite, incise at least full-thickness skin to the depth of the bite. Apply suction for 20 min.
   b. Some consultants with extensive experience and good results recommend early exploration of the snakebite area under local or general anesthesia as primary therapy, to diagnose the status of envenomation and to determine the depth and amount of tissue destruction.
   c. Cryotherapy is not indicated in the emergency department.
6. Update tetanus immunization.
7. Antivenin (see Grade of Envenomation):
   a. Withhold antivenin from patients without symptoms or signs of envenomation.
   b. Withhold antivenin from patients exhibiting local but not systemic symptoms or signs. Many patients will not require antivenin. (Copperhead venom is not usually very toxic, and rarely necessitates antivenin.)
   c. Admit all patients who receive antivenin.
   d. Administer antivenin intravenously in a continuous saline drip on the basis of grade of envenomation:
      • Minimal: 0 to 4 vials
      • Moderate: 5 to 9 vials, especially in children and the elderly
      • Severe: 10 to 15 or more vials
   Administer antivenin only after a skin test. Read product information carefully.

EMERGENCY DEPARTMENT MANAGEMENT OF POISONOUS SNAKEBITES (continued)

e. Epinephrine 1/1000 in a syringe should be available before antivenin is given.

f. Judge the amount of antivenin by improvement in symptoms and signs, not by the patient's weight. Children may need more antivenin than adults.

g. If systemic manifestations are severe, antivenin should be given rapidly, by intravenous drip, in large doses.

8. Watch for vascular insufficiency or compartment syndrome. Fasciotomy may be required if distal vascularity is impaired by swelling.

Additional antivenin considerations:

- Polyvalent antivenin (Wyeth Laboratories) is the current antivenin of choice for all North American rattlesnake, water moccasin (cottonmouth), and copperhead bites.
- North American coral snake antivenin (Wyeth Laboratories) should be used for eastern coral snakebites only—not for western or Arizona coral snakebites.

Incision and Suction. Incision and suction may be of benefit if accomplished within 30 min after snakebite. Approximately 50 percent of subcutaneously injected venom can be removed when the suction is started within 3 min. Treatment in the first 5 min is important, since half the value of suction is lost after 15 min and almost all after 30 min. A 30-min period of suction extracts about 90 percent of the venom that can be removed by this procedure. The incision should be $\frac{1}{4}$ in. long and $\frac{1}{8}$ to $\frac{1}{4}$ in. deep, longitudinal and not cruciate. When two fang marks are seen, the depth of the venom injection is generally considered to be one-third of the distance between the fang marks. A good rule of thumb has been to incise the skin and subcutaneous tissue in length the same distance as between the fang marks to ensure adequate drainage. A superficial incision may be easily accomplished by raising the skin with a pinch between two fingers. Severe bites may result in envenomations between the fascia, and surgical exploration may be indicated. Incisions made proximal to the bite do not usually recover enough venom to make the procedure worthwhile and thus are contraindicated.

When a suction cup is not available after incisions have been made, mouth suction may be used if the mucosa of the mouth is intact. Snake venom is not absorbed through an intact oral mucosa but may be absorbed when there is any denuded area or minor laceration of the mucosa. The digestive juices neutralize poisonous snake venom if it is swallowed.

Russell has demonstrated that the serosanguinous fluid removed during suction contains substances that when injected into animals produce a fall in systemic blood pressure and changes in respiratory rates and alterations in the electrocardiogram and electroencephalogram similar to those observed following injection of crude Crotalus venom. If exudate removed during suction contains venom, its removal should increase the chances of survival.

Excision. Snyder and Knowles showed that wide excision of the entire area around the snakebite within 1 h from the time of injection can remove most of the venom. Excision of the fang marks including skin and subcutaneous tissue should be considered in severe bites and in patients known to be allergic to horse serum who are seen within 1 h following the bite. However, the average snakebite does not require surgical excision. This procedure is reserved for the most severe envenomations. Most fatalities from snakebites do not occur for 6 to 48 h following the bite, giving time to institute other first aid measures. Excision often causes severe scarring and possible skin graft.

Cryotherapy. This form of therapy has been used but is not recommended, as it only increases the local area of necrosis. McCollough and Gennard analyzed cryotherapy in relation to amputation and noted that 75 percent of children requiring amputation following snakebite had received cryotherapy. Cooling or refrigeration experimentally produces intense vasoconstriction and thus decreases the amount of antivenin getting into the area of the bite. Gill found that dogs developed edema and ecchymosis just as rapidly and extensively with cryotherapy as without it. There was no evidence to suggest inactivation of venom by tissue temperature of 15°C and below.

SYSTEMIC TREATMENT. The most important treatment for a snakebite is antivenin, although many patients will not require it. Copperhead venom is not usually very toxic and rarely necessitates antivenin. In 1954 polyvalent Crotalidae antivenin became commercially available. Most snakebite fatalities in the United States during the past 20 years have involved either delay in obtaining treatment, no antivenin treatment, or inadequate dosage. Because antivenin contains horse serum, its administration requires prior skin testing. Epinephrine 1/1000 in a syringe should be available before antivenin is given.

Information concerning identification of a snake or proper antivenin frequently can be obtained from the nearest zoo herpetarium. A major problem with bites by exotic poisonous snakes is the choice and availability of suitable antiserum. Physicians confronted with this situation may obtain advice from the local poison control center or from the Antivenin Index Center of the Oklahoma Poison Information Center, Oklahoma City, Oklahoma (405-271-5454).

Because the rattlesnake, cottonmouth moccasin, and copperhead belong to the same biologic family, their bites can be treated by the same antivenin (antivenin Crotalidae polyvalent).

The coral snakebite is rare, and the antivenin is different from that for the pit vipers. A North American coral snake *(Micrurus fulvius)* antivenin has been developed. It effectively treats Micrurus coral snakebites but is not effective in treating bites of Micruroides, the genus native to Arizona and New Mexico. Coral snake antivenin can be obtained from many state health departments. Also, a large supply has been stocked at the U.S. Public Health Service National Communicable Disease Center in Atlanta, Georgia.

The time of antivenin administration depends upon the snake involved. If the bite is from a snake with a quick-acting venom, such as a king cobra or mamba, an initial dose of antivenin may be required as part of the first-aid treatment. However, for bites by most snakes, such as rattlesnakes and others with less virulent venom, antivenin should be withheld until a physician can determine if it is indicated. Approximately 30 percent of all poisonous snakebites in the United States result in no envenomation.

The indication for antivenin is governed by the degree of envenomation, as outlined by Wood et al. and modified by Parrish and by McCollough and Gennard:

Grade 0—no envenomation: One or more fang marks; minimal pain; less than 1 in. of surrounding edema and erythema at 12 h; no systemic involvement.

Grade 1—minimal envenomation: Fang marks; moderate to severe pain; 1 to 5 in. of surrounding edema and erythema in the first 12 h after bite; systemic involvement usually not present.

Grade II—moderate envenomation: Fang marks; severe pain; 6 to 12 in. of surrounding edema and erythema in the first 12 h after bite; possible systemic involvement including nausea, vomiting, giddiness, shock, or neurotoxic symptoms.

Grade III—severe envenomation: Fang marks; severe pain; more than 12 in. of surrounding edema and erythema in first 12 h after bite; grade II symptoms of systemic involvement usually present and may include generalized petechiae and ecchymosis.

Grade IV—very severe envenomation: Systemic involvement is always present, and symptoms may include renal failure, blood-tinged secretions, coma, and death; local edema may extend beyond the involved extremity to the ipsilateral trunk.

With frequent observations using this classification, the severity of the bite will be found to increase with time, and thus a change in grade is observed. Most bites will have reached a final staging within 12 h.

Antivenin usually is not required for grades 0 or 1 envenomation. Grade II may require 3 or 4 ampules, and grade III usually requires 5 to 15 ampules. If symptoms increase, several ampules may be required during the first 2 h. Because children are smaller, they receive relatively larger doses of venom, which places them in a higher-risk group. Thus, the smaller the patient, the relatively larger the required dose of antivenin. Proper dosage can be estimated by observing the clinical signs and symptoms. If systemic manifestations are severe, antivenin should be given rapidly, by intravenous drip, in large doses.

The injection of antivenin locally around the bite is not advised, as massive edema usually occurs in that area. Absorption from this area is poor, and additional anti-venin fluid will further decrease perfusion and perhaps increase tissue anoxia.

If any antivenin is indicated, 3 to 5 vials are given by intravenous drip in 500 mL of normal saline solution or 5 percent glucose solution. If severe systemic symptoms are already present, 6 to 8 vials are added. McCollough and Gennard have demonstrated in studies with radioisotopes that antivenin accumulates at the site of the bite more rapidly after intravenous than after intramuscular administration. The dose of intravenously administered antivenin can be more easily titrated with response to treatment, and the amount administered is based on improvement in signs and symptoms, not on weight of the patient. Antivenin is administered until severe local or systemic symptoms improve. When it is obvious that antivenin therapy will be instituted, the tourniquet should be left in place until antivenin is started intravenously. All patients who receive antivenin are admitted to the hospital.

If too much time has elapsed for excision to be effective and the patient is allergic to horse serum, a slow infusion of 1 ampule of antivenin in 250 mL of 5% glucose solution may be given in a 90-min period with constant monitoring of the blood pressure and electrocardiogram depending on the seriousness of the bite. This is accomplished in an active emergency department or an intensive care unit where resuscitation equipment and personnel trained in resuscitation are available. If an immediate reaction occurs, the antivenin is stopped, and a vasopressor, epinephrine, and perhaps an antihistamine may be required, depending on the severity of the reaction.

The incidence of serum sickness is directly related to the volume of horse serum injected. Of patients receiving 100 to 200 mL of horse serum, 85 percent will have some degree of sensitivity in 8 to 12 days following injection. This complication will have to be dealt with at a later time, since some patients may require from 1 to 5 ampules of antiserum every 4 to 6 h.

Steroids have been used but are of questionable benefit. Russell experimentally used doses of methylprednisolone up to 100 mg/kg in mice and noted that steroids neither affected survival nor prevented tissue damage and inflammation. When used in association with the antivenin, there is a decreased incidence of serum sickness. According to Parrish, cortisone and ACTH do not affect the survival rate of animals poisoned with pit viper venom. Tracheal intubation and prolonged ventilation may be required for respiratory failure. Acute renal failure may require renal dialysis.

Intravenous fluids are frequently required to replace the decreased extracellular fluid volume resulting from edema formation. Fascial planes may become very tense, with obstruction of venous and later arterial flow, requiring fasciotomy. Adequate antivenin treatment usually makes surgical intervention unnecessary. Roberts has advocated intracompartment pressure monitoring and found it to be elevated in two cases. However, careful monitoring of skin color, distal pulses, and capillary refill of the nail bed may prove helpful in determining if fasciotomy is indicated.

These patients may need blood, since anemia can develop from the hematologic effects. As afibrinogenemia has been reported, fibrinogen may be required. Vitamin K may also be required. Bleeding and clotting abnormalities are treated with antivenin in addition to blood components. Antibiotics are started immediately to prevent secondary infection, and tetanus toxoid is administered. The most common species of organisms isolated from rattlesnake venom are *P. aeruginosa, Proteus* species, *Clostridium* species, and *B. fragilis*.

Stinging Insects and Animals

HYMENOPTERA

The most important insects that produce serious and possibly fatal anaphylactic reactions are the arthropods of the order Hymenoptera. This group includes the honeybee, bumblebee, wasp, yellow and black hornet, and the fire ant. The venom of these stinging insects is just as potent as that of snakes and causes more deaths in the United States yearly than are caused by snakebites. Drop for drop, the venom of the bee is just as potent as that of the rattlesnake. Parrish noted that, of 460 deaths between 1950 and 1959, 50 percent were due to Hymenoptera, 30 percent due to poisonous snakes, and 14 percent due to spiders. Scorpions accounted for eight deaths. No other poisonous creature killed more than 5 persons.

Insects of the Hymenoptera group, except the bee, retain their stinger and are in a position to sting repeatedly, each time injecting some portion of the venom sac contents. The worker honeybee sinks its barbed sting into the skin, and it cannot be withdrawn. As the bee attempts to escape, it is disemboweled. The stinger with the bowel, muscles, and venom sac attached are left behind. The muscles controlling the venom sac, although separated from the bee, rhythmically contract for as long as 20 min, driving the stinger deeper and deeper into the skin, and continuing to inject venom.

Bee venoms contain histamine, serotonin, acetylcholine, formic acid, phospholipase A, hyaluronidase, and other proteins. Once the proteins of these insects are injected, the patient may become sensitized and be a candidate for anaphylactic response with the next sting.

CLINICAL MANIFESTATIONS. Symptoms consist of one or more of the following: localized pain, swelling, generalized erythema, a feeling of intense heat throughout the body, headache, blurred vision, injected conjunctivae, swollen and tender joints, itching, apprehension, urticaria, petechial hemorrhages of skin and mucous membranes, dizziness, weakness, sweating, severe nausea, abdominal cramps, dyspnea, constriction of the chest, asthma, angioneurotic edema, vascular collapse, and possible death from anaphylaxis. Fatal cases may manifest glottal and laryngeal edema, pulmonary and cerebral edema, visceral congestion, meningeal hyperemia, and intraventricular hemorrhage. Death apparently results from a combination of shock, respiratory failure, and central nervous system changes. Most deaths from insect stings occur within 15 to 30 min following the bite or sting.

TREATMENT. Early application of a tourniquet may prevent rapid spread of the venom. Affected persons should be taught to remove the venom sac if present, being careful not to squeeze the sac. It may be necessary for some patients to carry an emergency kit, which is commercially available, supplied with a tourniquet, sublingual isoproterenol in 10-mg tablets, epinephrine hydrochloride aerosol for inhalation to reduce bronchospasm and laryngeal edema, and tweezers to remove the sting and venom sac until a physician is available. Patients should be taught to give themselves an epinephrine injection. Patients having severe reactions should first receive 0.3 to 0.5 mL of a 1:1000 solution of epinephrine intravenously. Antihistamines also may be intravenously administered, and oxygen may be given. If wheezing continues, aminophylline may be given slowly intravenously. Occasionally, the patient may require a tracheostomy.

DESENSITIZATION. The Insect Allergy Committee of the American Academy of Allergy noted that 50 percent of people who had a severe generalized reaction to stings had no previous history of a severe reaction. A sharp rise was noted in the proportion of serious reaction after the age of thirty, suggesting increasing sensitivity as the total number of stings increase. Patients with a history of severe local or systemic involvement following insect stings should be desensitized. Venom immunotherapy is safe and is highly effective within a few weeks. Venom immunotherapy is the recommended form of prophylaxis for insect sting allergy.

It has been suspected that a refractory period of 10 to 14 days persists following an insect sting during which skin tests may be negative. Therefore, skin tests should be delayed several weeks after stinging and be performed with extreme caution. Cross reactions to the wasp, bee, and yellow jacket may occur.

STINGRAYS

Approximately 750 persons each year are stung by stingrays. However, during the past 60 years, only two deaths in this country have been attributed to the venom of the stingray.

As the spine, which is curved and has serrated edges, enters the flesh, the sheath surrounding the spine ruptures, and venom is released. As the spine is withdrawn, fragments of the sheath may remain in the wound. The wound edges are often jagged and bleed freely. Pain is usually immediate and severe, increasing to maximum intensity in 1 to 2 h and lasting for 12 to 48 h.

TREATMENT. This consists of copious irrigation with water to wash out any toxin and fragments of the spine's integumentary sheath. Russell noted that the venom is inactivated when exposed to heat. Therefore, the area of the bite should be placed in water as hot as the patient can stand without injury for 30 min to 1 h. After soaking, the wound may be further debrided and treated appropriately. Patients treated in this manner were shown to have rapid and uncomplicated healing of the wound. Patients not treated with heat had tissue necrosis with prolonged drainage and chronically infected wounds.

PORTUGUESE MAN-OF-WAR

This coelenterate is commonly found along our southern Atlantic coast. Its tentacles are covered with thousands of stinging cells, the nematocytes, capable of emitting microscopic organelles, the nematocysts, each of which consists of a small sphere containing a coiled hollow thread. When activated by touch, the thread is uncoiled with such force that it can penetrate skin and even rubber gloves. On contact, venom in the cyst is injected into the victim through the thread. This sting produces extreme pain and often signs of clinical shock; however, no deaths have been reported due to this sting alone.

Following a severe sting there may be almost immediate severe nausea, gastric cramping, and constriction and tightness of throat and chest with severe muscle spasm. There is intense burning pain with weakness and perhaps cyanosis with respiratory distress.

TREATMENT. The most important emergency treatment is to inactivate the nematocysts immediately, to prevent their continuous firing of toxins. This is accomplished by application to the involved area of a substance of high alcohol content, such as rubbing alcohol. This is followed by application of a drying agent, such as flour, baking soda, talc, or shaving cream. The tentacles may then be removed by shaving. Alkaline agents, such as baking soda, are then applied to the involved area in order to neutralize the toxins, which are acidic. Antihistamines may be helpful in controlling the inflammatory response after these emergency treatments. Demerol and Benadryl may dramatically relieve the pain and symptoms. Aerosol corticosteroid-analgesic balm is helpful.

Spider Bites

BLACK WIDOW SPIDER

The most common biting spider in the United States is the black widow *(Latrodectus mactans)* (Fig. 6-3). The spider is black and globular, with a red hourglass mark on the abdomen. Latrodectism is a syndrome characterized by severe muscular pain and stiffness, nausea, vomiting, and headache. The female spider has a reddish orange hourglass on its ventral surface. *Latrodectus* venom is primarily neurotoxic in action and appears to center on the spinal cord. Following a bite by the black widow spider, the majority of patients experience pain within 30 min and a small wheal with an area of erythema appears. Nausea and vomiting occurs in approximately one-third of patients, headache in one-fourth, and dyspnea may occur.

The time of onset of symptoms following the bite is from 30 min to 6 h. The severe symptoms last from 24 to 48 h. Generalized muscle spasm is the most prominent physical finding. Cramping muscle spasms occur in the thighs, lumbar region, abdomen, or thorax. Priapism and ejaculation have been reported.

Even if the bite is on an extremity, the spasm may involve the abdomen and chest. Although the abdomen is rigid, it is nontender and patients do not demonstrate signs and symptoms of generalized peritonitis. Less commonly the patient may have hypertension, hyperreflexia, and urinary retention. Most patients recover within 24 h.

TREATMENT. Treatment has consisted of narcotics for the relief of pain and a muscle relaxant for relief of spasm. Either methocarbamol (Robaxin) or 10 mL of a 10% solution of calcium gluconate relieves symptoms. It is believed that calcium acts by depressing the threshold for depolarization at the neuromuscular junctions. Calcium gluconate may give instant relief of muscular pain as well as relieving muscular spasm. Methocarbamol can be administered intravenously, 10 mL over a 5-min period with a second ampule started in a saline solution drip. Although antivenin *(Lactrodectus mactans)* is available, it is rarely required. The manufacturer recommends its use for patients younger than sixteen years or older than sixty years and for patients with underlying cardiovascular diseases. The antivenin is prepared from horse serum and is administered intramuscularly after appropriate skin tests. Hospitalization may be required for the young, elderly, and patients with significant chronic diseases or with severe signs and symptoms of envenomation.

NORTH AMERICAN LOXOSCELISM

The distinguishing mark of the *Loxosceles reclusa* is the darker violin-shaped band over the dorsal cephalothorax (Fig. 6-4). The spider is native to the south central United States and is found both indoors and outdoors. They are frequently found in attics, closets, old clothes, wood piles, boat docks, and in infrequently worn shoes. The first recognized and documented case in the United States by a *Loxosceles reclusa* was published in 1957.

CLINICAL MANIFESTATIONS. The body ranges from 7 mm to 1.2 cm and including the legs ranges from 2 to 3 cm. The initial bite may go unnoticed or be accompanied by a mild stinging sensation. Pain may recur 6 to 8 h afterward. A mild envenomation is associated with local urticaria and erythema. This usually resolves spontaneously. More severe bites result in progression to necrosis and sloughing of skin with residual ulcer formation. A generalized macular and erythematous rash may appear in 12 to

Fig. 6-3. Abdominal view of a female black widow spider showing the hourglass marking. (From: *Paton BC: Surg Clin North Am 43:537, 1963, with permission.*)

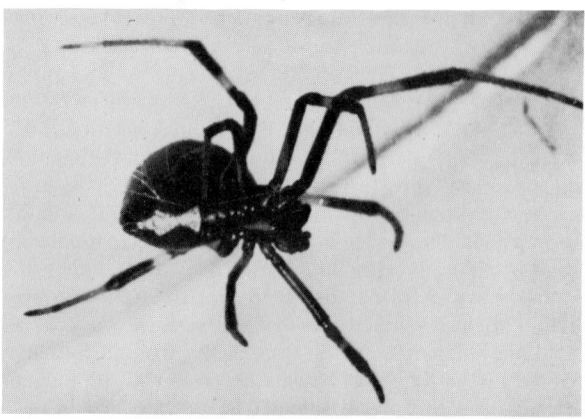

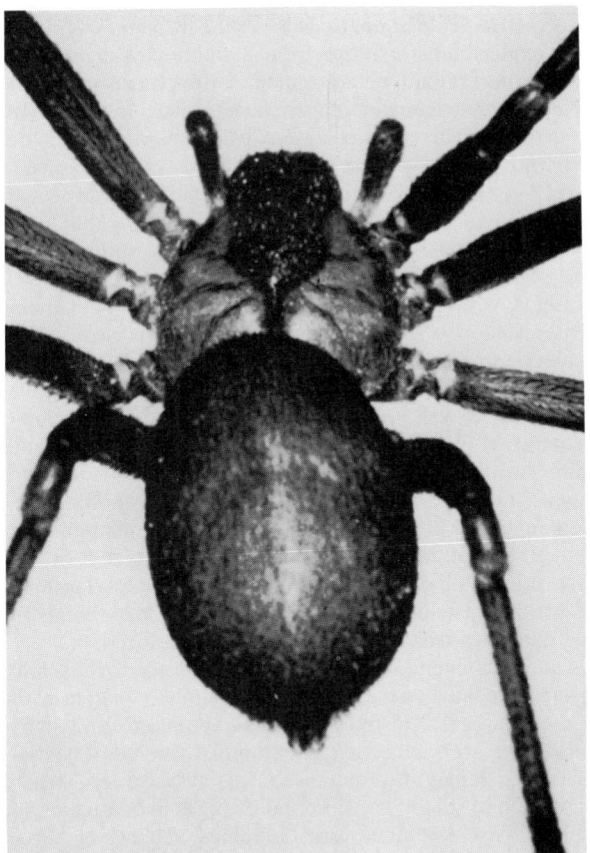

Fig. 6-4. The distinguishing mark of the *Loxosceles reclusa* is the darker violin-shaped band over the dorsal cephalothorax. (From: *Dillaha CJ, Jansen GT, et al: JAMA 188:33, 1964, with permission.*)

24 h. Erythema develops, with bleb or blister formation surrounded by an irregular area of ischemia. A zone of hemorrhage and induration and a surrounding halo of erythema may develop peripherally. The central ischemia turns dark, an eschar forms by the seventh day, and by the fourteenth day the area sloughs, leaving an open ulcer. Approximately 3 weeks is required for the lesion to heal. The pain may be out of proportion for the size of the area involved. The progression from blue to black gives the bite a necrotic appearance, and the more severe ones develop within a few hours to 2 days. Lesions found in areas of fatty tissue such as thigh, buttocks, and abdomen tend to be more extensive and result in severe scar formation. The necrotic lesions usually do not involve tendons or muscles.

Systemically, the patient may have fever, nausea, vomiting, arthralgia, and malaise. Severe systemic manifestations may occur in 24 to 48 h in small children, with fever, chills, malaise, weakness, nausea, vomiting, joint pain, and even petechial eruption. The two principal systemic effects, hemolysis and thrombocytopenia, have been responsible for deaths. Hemoglobinemia, hemoglobinuria, leukocytosis, and proteinuria may also occur. Renal failure can develop secondary to hemoglobinuria. *Loxosceles* venom is chiefly cytotoxic in action.

Laboratory studies are obtained in patients with severe envenomation including prothrombin time, PTT, platelet count, and urinalysis.

The current understanding of the pathophysiology of the bite is that intravascular coagulation and the formation of microthrombi within the capillary occur, leading to capillary occlusion, hemorrhage, and necrosis.

TREATMENT. Immediate excision with primary closure has been advocated as the treatment of choice. This usually is not possible since patients rarely can be certain that they were bitten by a brown recluse spider. Likewise, the excision may be inadequate, allowing venom to migrate in the residual tissue, resulting in ulcer formation requiring reexcision and often grafting. Treatment of loxoscelism seems to be conservative, because of the difficulty in predicting the severity of the bite. Various treatments have been advocated in addition to early excision such as corticosteroids, heparin, regitine, dextran, and infusion, but clinical studies have failed to identify the benefit of these agents. The dose for steroids has varied from 30 to 80 mg of methylprednisolone daily tapered over a period of several days. Excision of the necrotic area with skin grafting may be required at a later date.

Rees has recently reported using a leukocyte inhibitor, dapsone, used in leprosy, to be effective in reducing inflammation at the site of the brown recluse venom injection. Many of the patients were treated 48 h or more following the bite. Some received surgical excision and others were treated conservatively with dapsone 100 mg daily for 14 days before surgical excision, if required. They concluded that the incidence of scarring and deformity was much less in the dapsone treated group than with observation and subsequent surgical excision. Only one patient required hospitalization while on dapsone therapy compared with 50 percent in the observed group. These data imply that the high incidence of delayed wound healing, abscess formation, and objectionable scarring may be avoided if surgical therapy is delayed until the eschar has matured. The mechanism of action of dapsone is unclear. There are significant side effects associated with dapsone treatment including dose-dependent hemolytic anemia, methemoglobinemia, and rash. Rees suggests obtaining blood for G6PD levels and hematocrit before dapsone therapy. Complete blood counts are recommended weekly since reduction in leukocytes, platelets, or severe anemia due to hemolysis may develop. Hemolysis may be exaggerated in individuals with glucose-6-phosphate-dehydrogenate (G6PD) deficiency. Whether or not dapsone improves morbidity following brown spider bites awaits further clinical evaluation. Conservative therapy seems to be the preferred treatment. Excision of the necrotic area with skin grafting may be required at a later date.

PENETRATING WOUNDS OF THE NECK AND THORACIC INLET

Although penetrating injuries of the neck are uncommon in civilian surgical practice, the concentration of deep vital structures makes any cutaneous wound a potentially serious injury. Life-threatening consequences of unrepaired injuries of the larynx, trachea, pharynx, esophagus, and blood vessels of the neck and thoracic inlet mandate early diagnosis and operative correction. There is general agreement that penetrating wounds with overt evidence of deep injuries require urgent operations. A difference of opinion exists regarding the necessity for operative exploration of patients without evidence of such injuries. Numerous reports document similar results in patients treated by routine operative explorations and those observed, with or without adjunctive diagnostic studies, and operated upon for positive tests or evolving clinical findings.

GENERAL CONSIDERATIONS. Before World War II, the treatment of penetrating wounds of the neck was largely nonsurgical unless major bleeding or deep injuries were obvious. Reported mortality rates were 18 percent of 188 cases in the Spanish-American War and 11 percent of 594 cases in World War I. During World War II the mortality rate fell to 7 percent, probably because of a variety of factors, including earlier tracheostomy, more frequent and expedient surgical exploration, antibiotics, and improvements in surgical and anesthetic techniques.

Since 1960, numerous civilian series have been reported and mortality rates approximate 5 percent. Most deaths are due to spinal cord and blood vessel injuries, although tracheal and esophageal wounds account for some. Fogelman and Stewart pointed out that the mortality rate for their cases that were promptly explored was 6 percent, whereas for those in which surgical intervention was omitted or postponed the mortality rate was 35 percent.

Mandatory (Routine) Exploration. Based on the improved results of operative care of penetrating neck injuries, the policy evolved in many major trauma centers of "treating the platysma like the peritoneum" and exploring virtually all neck wounds that penetrated the platysma. In 1967, Jones et al. reviewed 274 penetrating neck wounds treated in this manner at Parkland Memorial Hospital. There were 11 deaths, for a mortality rate of 3.6 percent. Of the fatalities, four were due to complications from spinal cord injuries, three from massive hemorrhage, and the remainder from cerebral complications of vascular or laryngotracheal injuries. Of the 274 cases, 103 (38 percent) explorations were negative, i.e., with no hematoma, no significant bleeding, and no damage to any named structure in the neck, although the tract of the injury frequently was within millimeters of vital structures. In the negative explorations there were no deaths and the only complication was a superficial wound infection that cleared promptly with drainage. These patients usually were discharged within 72 h to clinic follow-up if there were no associated injuries. Similar results have been documented more recently in the series reported by Saletta et al. and Roon and Christensen. These three series represent 700 patients, 327 (47 percent) of whom had major structural injuries. Thirty-one (4.4 percent) of these patients with important injuries were considered preoperatively to be "clinically negative." Most of these silent injuries were not life-threatening, but many patients with serious injuries had soft signs indicating their presence.

Selective Exploration. Because of the frequency of negative explorations resulting from the policy of mandatory exploration, a number of trauma centers have begun the selective management of penetrating neck injuries. Patients with overt signs of vascular or visceral injuries are promptly operated upon and those with "clinically negative" penetrating wounds are monitored by repeated physical examinations, with or without radiographic and endoscopic diagnostic procedures. Reports summarizing the results of selective management of more than 1200 patients with penetrating neck trauma have been published since 1983. About half the patients in most series underwent explorations because of clinical or radiographic evidence of deep injuries, and the rate of negative explorations was in the range of 20 to 30 percent. Subsequent explorations were infrequently required and minimal morbidity occurred in observed patients. No significant differences in mortality or morbidity were demonstrated between series managed by mandatory or selective exploration, including the randomized single-institution study by Golueke. Variable cost saving may result from a selective management policy, depending on the extent to which diagnostic studies are used.

Clinical evidence of an underlying vascular or visceral injury mandates operative exploration in any patient with penetrating cervical trauma. Acute symptoms and signs suggesting cervical vascular injuries include arterial bleeding, hematoma, diminished distal pulsation, bruit, unexplained shock, and cerebral changes indicative of an ischemic or embolic event. Findings suggesting aerodigestive tract injuries include stridor, dysphonia, aphonia, hemoptysis, hematemesis, dysphagia, odynophagia, and subcutaneous emphysema. Most laryngotracheal injuries acutely cause symptoms and physical findings, while vascular and pharyngoesophageal injuries are more often initially occult.

In hemodynamically stable and "clinically negative" patients with penetrating neck trauma, careful examination of the wound is an important aspect of estimating the potential for morbid injuries. If the extent of the injury is not apparent, the wound is very gently probed with a small hemostat, only to the depth of the platysma muscle. If the platysma has been penetrated, the probing is discontinued. Neck wounds should not be probed beneath the platysma muscle because hemostasis may be disrupted. A valid appraisal of the likelihood of deep injury requires knowledge of the anatomic relationships of the visceral and vascular structures of the neck. Wounds in the posterior triangle are less often associated with serious visceral and vascular injuries than those in the anterior and lateral aspects of the neck. Directly anterior wounds infrequently injure the esophagus without an intervening tracheal injury that is usually manifest by subcutaneous emphysema or air escaping from the wound. Plain films of the neck may be useful diagnostically by demonstrating subfascial air or, in the case of missile wounds, may assist in defining the trajectory by revealing a retained bullet or metallic fragments in bone.

Because a penetrating wound may be the only sign indicating the presence of a major vascular injury, arteriography has become an important modality in the manage-

REGIONS OF THE NECK

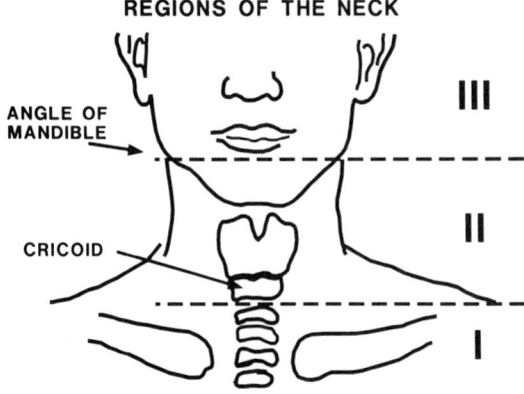

ANGLE OF
MANDIBLE

III

II

CRICOID

I

Fig. 6-5. Arbitrary division of the cervical region into three zones. Management of penetrating wounds of the neck is based on the area involved. (From: *Monson DO et al: 1969, with permission.*)

ment of neck injuries. The validity of biplane multifilm arteriography in the evaluation of peripheral arterial injuries was documented by Snyder et al. These studies may be useful in precisely defining the site of an arterial injury, as well as for the purpose of confirming arterial integrity. Monson's division of the neck into three zones is useful in considering the arteriographic evaluation of penetrating neck trauma (Fig. 6-5): Zone I—below a horizontal line 1 cm above the claviculomanubrial junction or inferior to the cricoid cartilage; Zone II—between Zone I and the angle of the mandible; and Zone III—between the angle of the mandible and the base of the skull. Zones II and III are considered the neck proper and Zone I is the base of the neck or thoracic inlet. Arteriography has been used extensively and successfully to exclude arterial injuries in the selective management of cervical trauma. Many authors recommend its routine use in stable patients with overt signs of arterial injury, especially in Zones I and III because of the potential technical problems with exposure and vascular control in these regions. This will be considered more thoroughly in the section on specific injuries.

The possibility of underlying pharyngoesophageal injury has remained a problem in the management of "clinically negative" penetrating neck trauma. Important laryngotracheal injuries are essentially always overt, arterial injuries can be accurately diagnosed arteriographically, and occult venous injuries are unlikely to have much morbid potential. The validity of nonoperative exclusion of pharyngoesophageal injuries has not been thoroughly addressed. In an attempt to resolve this issue, 118 patients with penetrating neck trauma in Zones II or III treated at Parkland Memorial Hospital were prospectively studied. Essentially all patients had cervical arteriography, barium esophagrams, and flexible and rigid endoscopies, followed by operative neck explorations. Esophageal injuries were found at exploration in 10 patients; barium swallows and rigid esophagoscopies detected the injuries in eight of the nine patients so studied. Flexible endoscopy was inaccurate, yielding falsely negative results in five of the eight patients with esophageal perforations having this examination. Of 108 patients in

whom esophageal injuries were operatively excluded, false-positive studies occurred in none of the 103 patients having barium swallows, one of the 98 patients having flexible esophagoscopies, and five of the 107 patients undergoing rigid endoscopies. The patient with a falsely negative barium swallow had a positive rigid endoscopy, and the esophogram demonstrated the injury in the single patient with a negative rigid endoscopic examination. Therefore, all patients with esophageal injuries had at least one positive study preoperatively. The sensitivity (ability of a test to detect an injury if present) for barium swallow and rigid esophagoscopy was 89 percent. The specificity (ability of a test to exclude an injury if absent) was 100 and 95 percent for barium swallow and rigid esophagoscopy, respectively.

Summary. Patients with clinical findings of vascular or visceral injuries are operatively explored in the operating room under general anesthesia. Patients with altered sensoriums in whom appropriate information, examinations, and diagnostic studies are impossible are also explored. Based on the above data, our current recommendations for stable patients with penetrating injuries in Zones II and III, without clinical evidence of vascular or aerodigestive tract injuries, include biplane four-vessel cervical angiography, barium esophagography in two projections with cineradiography, and rigid esophagoscopy. If arteriography reveals an injury requiring operation, no further studies are performed and the patient is operatively explored. If arteriography is negative, barium esophagography is performed. If esophagography is normal, important injury is considered unlikely and the patient is admitted for observation. If esophagography is positive, operative exploration is recommended, preceded by rigid esophagoscopy under general anesthesia. If esophagoscopy is negative, the judgment regarding proceeding with operative exploration is based on the certainty of the abnormality seen on esophagram. If any of the aforementioned studies cannot be adequately completed or are equivocal, operative exploration is recommended. Patients with injuries in Zone I are more liberally explored, despite the absence of objective clinical findings, because the site of injury is less amenable to observation, unexpected bleeding is difficult to control nonoperatively, and the validity of arteriographic exclusion is questionable.

Success with selective management of penetrating neck trauma requires surgeons and radiologists experienced in evaluating such injuries and the 24-h availability of precise radiologic studies. In addition, the necessary commitment of time and personnel for careful and repeated patient observation is substantially greater than is required for a cervical exploration. Routine exploration probably remains the safest approach to the management of penetrating neck injuries for surgeons working in hospitals caring for a limited number of traumatized patients.

The cost of observation without radiologic studies is clearly less than for an operative procedure and a brief postoperative stay. The expense of several radiologic studies makes the cost of the two modes of treatment more similar. Additional expenses mount related to the number of patients requiring operative procedures after the diagnostic studies. It seems that the total expense of a policy of mandatory exploration is likely to be at least equal to if not less than for selective management.

TREATMENT. Initial Evaluation and Management. On admission to the emergency room, all patients with neck injuries are immediately evaluated regarding their systemic condition, i.e., airway patency and adequacy of ventilation, blood pressure, pulse, and mental state. Peripheral signs of shock such as sweating, cold skin, and collapsed veins should be recorded. If there is external bleeding, pressure is applied for temporary hemostasis. Adequate ventilation may require endotracheal intubation in obtunded patients or tracheostomy if a laryngotracheal injury or a cervical hematoma has caused upper airway obstruction. One or two large-bore intravenous cannulas are inserted in peripheral veins and an infusion of Ringer's lactate solution is started while blood is drawn for typing and cross matching. If shock is present, the fluid is given rapidly; if there is no evidence of blood loss, the intravenous solutions are kept going by slow drip. When indicated, whole blood is administered as soon as it is available. Usually the salt solution will temporarily reverse the shock state until cross-matched blood is available. If shock is severe and is not improved promptly by the Ringer's lactate solution, type O, Rh-negative low-titer unmatched blood is infused rapidly until matched blood is available. Plasma has also been used but has no advantage over salt solutions; i.e., both are quite helpful temporarily, although neither is a substitute for whole blood. Tube thoracostomy is often necessary for intrathoracic bleeding or pneumothorax from the commonly associated pulmonary injuries. If there is no clinical evidence of pneumothorax or hemothorax and the patient's condition is stable, an upright chest film is obtained with a physician in constant attendance. No attempt is made to pass a nasogastric tube in the emergency room because of the danger of recurrent hemorrhage as a result of coughing or gagging.

The major initial risk is airway compromise for patients with injuries of the neck proper and exsanguinating hemorrhage for those with penetrating trauma entering the mediastinum. The clinical presentation of patients with superior mediastinal vascular injuries varies from innocuous-appearing cutaneous wounds to terminal hemorrhagic shock. Hemostasis may be transient and spontaneously break down, or it may be disrupted by changes in intravascular or intrathoracic pressure. Acute hemorrhage from these injuries can sometimes be controlled by external pressure, but occasionally control requires an anterolateral thoracotomy in the emergency room. The innominate and right subclavian vessels can be controlled through a right thoracotomy and the left subclavian artery controlled through a left chest incision.

Special x-ray studies such as contrast esophagography and arteriography may be useful but are considered only in hemodynamically stable patients. The use of these studies was previously summarized from the standpoint of diagnostic maneuvers, but arteriography as a preoperative study will be considered in more detail in this section. The potential benefits from preoperative arteriography

can be related, in part, to the location of the wound. The neck proper extends from the base of the skull to about the level of the cricoid cartilage. This area corresponds to Zones II and III described by Monson (Fig. 6-5) or to the middle and upper neck. Penetrating wounds coursing inferior to the cricoid are considered wounds of the thoracic inlet or base of the neck (Zone I). An upper neck wound whose course extends above the angle of the mandible (Zone III) often presents dangerous intraoperative problems. Arteriographic definition of the site and extent of arterial injury may importantly alter operative plans. Internal carotid injuries near the base of the skull are difficult to expose and cephalad control may be essentially impossible. Initial extracranial-intracranial arterial bypass (EC-IC) is a reasonable consideration in patients with such injuries. Cerebral protection, with an initial EC-IC, may occasionally be important in cephalad injuries with continued flow because intraluminal shunt insertion is often not possible. In addition, reconstruction of the internal carotid artery may not be technically feasible and ligation may be required. Operative control of mid-neck carotid wounds (between the mandible and the level of the cricoid cartilage—Zone II) is usually simple and arteriographic definition is less important. Vertebral artery injuries that may otherwise go undetected may be demonstrated if arteriography is performed on patients with injuries in this region.

Penetrating wounds in the low neck (Zone I) may involve vessels of the superior mediastinum and require thoracic incisions for adequate exposure. Arteriography is potentially helpful in such wounds, but the necessary delay poses substantial risk. In most anatomic sites, exacting arteriography accurately defines specific arterial lesions and confirms arterial integrity. In the superior mediastinum there are many important structures, and risk of occult hemorrhage argues against substituting arteriography for operative exploration. The concentration of major arteries increases the likelihood of missing minor arteriographic defects that indicate the presence of major injuries. Such inaccuracies result because of the superimposition of dye columns caused by the spatial orientation of these vessels. The validity of "exclusion" arteriography, established for extremity injuries, cannot be transposed to the diagnostic evaluation of mediastinal wounds. For these reasons, operative exploration is indicated for most penetrating injuries suspected of entering the mediastinum.

Although arteriography may not reliably exclude mediastinal vascular injuries, it can be helpful in defining the site of arterial wounds. The decision to use arteriography for planning the operation must take into account delay and the risk of cardiovascular deterioration. The bleeding may be tamponaded by soft tissues, but this is tenuous, as emphasized in a report by Flint of 146 patients with base-of-the-neck vascular injuries. Of the 90 patients initially normotensive, six (7 percent) became profoundly hypotensive en route to or shortly after arrival in the operating room. Rapid hemostasis was obtained operatively in all six patients and all survived, but the personnel and facilities available in the operating room played a major role. If these unanticipated events had occurred in the radiology suite, the outcome would most likely have been different. In summary, preoperative arteriography is frequently helpful in evaluating patients with potential arterial injuries of the neck and thoracic inlet, but it should not be used to obviate the need for operative exploration in patients with intrathoracic bleeding, and arteriograms should be considered only in stable patients.

The frequent absence of overt signs of vascular trauma and the minimal morbidity imposed by operative exploration was documented in the review by Flint et al. of 146 patients with base-of-the-neck vascular injuries. Thirty-two percent of these patients had no diagnostic signs of vascular injuries. Even innominate and subclavian vessel wounds had no overt manifestations in 29 percent of these patients with such injuries. Most of the injuries in these patients were adequately managed with cervical or transverse clavicular incisions, and very few of those without overt injury manifestations required thoracic incisions.

Anesthesia. Exploration is performed under general anesthesia, using an orotracheal airway with an inflatable cuff. The anesthetic agent varies considerably according to the specific problem, necessity for rapid induction, circulatory status, and preexisting disease. There are no specific contraindications in patients with neck injuries to any of the commonly used anesthetic agents or relaxants.

Anesthetic induction requires attention to different problems in patients with superior mediastinal injuries as compared with those with wounds of the neck proper. Intubation while awake is preferred in patients with wounds of the neck proper because difficulties imposed by cervical hematomas or upper airway edema may delay adequate oxygenation in paralyzed patients. In these wounds, disruption of existing hemostasis by retching or struggling with intubation is usually amenable to control by external pressure. On the other hand, intubation in patients with superior mediastinal wounds may produce major hemorrhage that cannot be controlled by local pressure. These patients less often have structural alterations of the upper airway, and intubation can more safely follow the infusion of muscle relaxants. Because gastric decompression is omitted to avoid sudden alterations in intrathoracic pressure, precautions are necessary in the technique of induction to minimize the aspiration risk. In either instance, preinduction preparation for emergency tracheostomy is essential.

The chest is again examined just before induction, because pneumothorax may develop slowly following a neck wound, appearing an hour or longer after an initially negative chest x-ray. Wounds in the base of the neck following a downward path may cause minimal apical pulmonary injuries so that a pneumothorax is not apparent initially and may not be manifest until after the patient is intubated. This should be kept in mind as a cause for hypotension or hypoxia during anesthesia.

Technique of Operation. With adequate control of the ventilatory and cardiovascular systems, the surgeon can now safely and adequately explore the structures that may be injured. Patient positioning and preparation of the sterile field require foresight concerning operative exposure and the need for venous autografts. The supine position with some cervical extension is used. The prepared operative field includes the neck, chest, anterior shoulders, and a separate site for harvesting saphenous vein.

The incision is planned to allow full exposure of the tract of injury. Proximal and distal control of the major blood vessels must also be considered in the length and position of the incision. Incisions commonly used are the oblique incision along the anterior border of the sternocleidomastoid muscle, the horizontal clavicular incision with resection of the medial portion of the clavicle, median sternotomy, and anterolateral thoracotomy. A collar incision is occasionally useful for bilateral injuries or those primarily involving the larynx or proximal trachea.

The tract of injury is followed to its depth, with systematic examination of each adjacent structure. Blast injury, especially from high-velocity missiles, may not be immediately apparent and requires careful evaluation. If injuries to the major blood vessels are suspected, tapes are passed around the vessels proximal and distal to the point of suspected injury before local clots are removed. Injured structures are repaired as outlined in the following paragraphs and muscles are anatomically approximated.

Most soft tissue neck wounds are drained for 24 to 48 h using Penrose drains or Silastic suction catheters to prevent the accumulation of blood and serum. If the pharynx or esophagus is injured, drainage is continued for 4 to 8 days. In the case of a massive gunshot wound, such as close-range shotgun injury, the wound is left open initially and, if possible, a delayed primary closure is performed 3 to 4 days later.

Specific Injuries

VASCULAR INJURIES. Clinical problems posed by acute vascular injuries are best considered by dividing the discussion into injuries of the neck proper (Zones II and III) and those of the base of the neck or thoracic inlet (Zone I). Cerebral ischemia and tracheal compression from contained bleeding are the major concerns with injuries of the middle and upper neck. External hemorrhage can usually be controlled by pressure, and the diagnosis is signaled by an adjacent penetrating wound, a bruit, or a neurologic deficit. The major problems of vascular injuries of the thoracic inlet are exsanguinating hemorrhage, early diagnosis, and operative exposure. Operative techniques of vessel repair are straightforward and infrequently pose important management problems. Although the specific vessel injured is sometimes defined by preoperative arteriography, the surgical management of potential vascular injuries must often proceed without this information.

Cervical Blood Vessels. Major vascular injuries in this region include the common carotid artery and its extracranial branches, the vertebral artery, and the internal jugular vein. Special attention is directed to preoperative neurologic evaluation because cerebral infarction may affect the intraoperative decision regarding flow restoration. Transient hypotension may exaggerate cerebral ischemia, but it does not appear to have a predictably deleterious effect on eventual neurologic status. Rapid fluid volume restitution and restoration of normal blood pressure is important for physiologic reasons and also allows a more accurate evaluation of the neurologic consequences of the injury. Thal and associates described the relationship between preoperative neurologic status, vascular procedure, and results in 60 patients with carotid injuries. Forty-one (68 percent) patients were neurologically intact preoperatively and 19 (32 percent) had deficits of varying severity. It was concluded from this review that vascular reconstruction was advisable in patients with mild deficits and in those with severe deficits in whom prograde flow was present preoperatively. Ligation was recommended in patients with severe neurologic deficits and no preoperative prograde flow. Ligation may occasionally be appropriate for patients with neurologic deficits and persistent prograde flow in whom thrombus exists in the cephalad vessel. If thrombectomy cannot be performed without risk of cerebral embolization, ligation may be the best choice. Arterial reconstruction, if feasible, was recommended in essentially all neurologically intact patients. The only exception is the patient with obstructed prograde flow and intraluminal thrombus in the cephalad vessel. If reconstruction risked cerebral embolization, ligation was suggested. Controversy continues regarding the therapeutic implications of preoperative neurologic deficits. Recent reviews by Unger et al. and by Liekweg and Greenfield support the recommendation that injured carotid arteries should be reconstructed, if technically feasible, in all except comatose patients with prograde flow. In these authors' opinion, flow should also be restored in patients without prograde flow, except those with severe or rapidly progressing deficits and seriously depressed sensoriums.

Operative Technique. Before the induction of anesthesia, preparations are made for the performance of emergency tracheostomy in the event of intubation difficulties. Stability of the cervical spine should be confirmed before intubation, particularly in high-velocity missile trauma. If an internal carotid injury near the base of the skull has been demonstrated arteriographically, exposure may be difficult and an additional 1 to 2 cm can be obtained by jaw dislocation or subluxation. The mandible is pulled inferiorly and anteriorly and held in place with dental wires.

Patients with potential or proved carotid injuries should be handled with consideration given to the tenuous hemostasis provided by soft tissue tamponade and the likelihood of intraluminal thrombus. A vigorous antiseptic scrub may dislodge a clot and cause either bleeding or embolization. Preparation of the operative field preferably includes the shoulder and anterior chest in case further exposure is required, as well as a site for harvesting a venous autograft.

Incision extensions that may be necessary are described with vascular injuries of the thoracic inlet. Shunts are rarely needed for repairs of common carotid injuries if the cephalad clamp does not occlude communication between the external and internal carotid arteries. Adequate collateral flow from the external carotid is easily verified by momentarily releasing the cephalad clamp. Following proximal and distal occlusion, with or without an intraluminal shunt, repair is carried out by standard vascular techniques. Injuries of the internal jugular vein are primarily repaired if this can be readily accomplished by lateral venorrhaphy, patch venoplasty, or end-to-end anastomosis. Unilateral ligation is well tolerated and the use of interposition grafts to restore venous continuity is not justified.

The common use of preoperative arteriography in recent years has uncovered an increasing number of vertebral artery injuries. In the past these injuries have been recognized infrequently, apparently because vertebral flow is not essential, and the size and course of the vessel make overt manifestations uncommon. Acute complications of vertebral artery injury are rare, but massive hemorrhage may be lethal. An AV fistula is the most common late complication, usually diagnosed months or years after injury. The incidence of these sequelae is unknown. Meier et al. described a series of 13 patients with acute vertebral artery trauma treated at Parkland Hospital during a 3-year period. During this time period 54 carotid injuries were treated, yielding a comparative incidence of about 20 percent for vertebral artery injuries.

Forty-one patients with penetrating vertebral artery injuries treated at the same institution during an 11-year period have recently been reviewed by Reid and Weigelt. Five of these patients were in shock on arrival but no patient presented with or developed neurologic signs attributable to the vertebral-basilar system. Three-quarters of these patients had no clinical findings of arterial injuries other than the penetrating wound or a stable hematoma. The remaining patients had expanding hematomas and four had overt arterial hemorrhage. The diagnosis was made arteriographically in 35 patients and during urgent operative explorations in the remainder. Proximal and distal vertebral artery ligations were performed in 28 patients; 13 had only proximal ligations and two were treated nonoperatively. Several complications developed in the patients having only proximal ligations and the authors recommend both proximal and distal ligations when feasible. Because the frequency of untoward sequelae of vertebral artery injuries is unknown, the indications for operations in asymptomatic patients are not clear. Reid and Weigelt recommended ligation of injured vertebral arteries in all patients with normal contralateral arteries if no spinal cord branches arise from the injured vessels but state that nonoperative management may be reasonable in asymptomatic patients with arteriographically minimal injuries. The site of proximal ligation is immediately distal to the subclavian origin of the vertebral artery. The site of distal ligation depends on the location of injury and can be performed as high as the C1-C2 interspace, when the artery is free of the bony canal.

Base of the Neck (Thoracic Inlet). Thoracic inlet injuries involve the vessels of the superior mediastinum that are proximate to the pleural spaces and separated from the surgeon by the claviculosternal "shield." The specific vessels include the innominate, the subclavian, and the proximal common carotid arteries and adjacent veins. Anatomic characteristics make the diagnosis of injured vessels difficult and impede rapid hemostasis and operative exposure for vascular control and repair. Exsanguinating hemorrhage is the predominant risk; bleeding may not be easily recognized because of free decompression into the pleural spaces. Abundant collateral blood supply generally protects against cerebral or upper extremity ischemia but also disguises the injury by maintaining distal perfusion and exaggerates blood loss during operative exposure. The major clinical differences between these injuries and those in the neck proper are obscure hemorrhage, difficulty obtaining immediate hemostasis, the extensive incisions that may be required for exposure, and the infrequency of cerebral ischemia.

Rapid resuscitation, liberal surgical exploration, and a thorough knowledge of the operative approach are the necessary ingredients of success. Indications to consider early surgical exploration are listed in Table 6-4. Diagnostic errors and subsequent inappropriately conservative management rarely occur with overt signs of major vascular injury. Unfortunately, many of these injuries appear innocuous at the time of presentation, and a high index of suspicion is necessary. In this circumstance platysmal penetration and proximity of the wound to a major vascular structure are used as indications for surgical exploration. As previously discussed, arteriography to modify the principle of proximity and penetration exploration remains controversial. It may prove useful if immediately available, but valuable time should not be wasted with studies if objective evidence of major vascular injury exists.

Important factors in the management of these injuries are emphasized by the series of Flint et al. During an 11-year period, 146 patients with 206 injuries of major vascular structures at the base of the neck were treated. Arterial injuries accounted for 49 percent, including 36 injuries to the subclavian artery, 29 to the common carotid, and 7 to the innominate artery. Of the 74 venous injuries, there were 31 to the subclavian vein, 32 to the internal jugular, and 11 to the innominate vein. Signs and symptoms of major vascular injury were equivocal in many patients and totally absent in 32 percent of the patients. These patients were explored on the basis of platysmal penetra-

Table 6-4. FINDINGS SUGGESTING MAJOR VASCULAR INJURY

Obvious or direct evidence of injury:
1. Circulatory instability
2. Excessive external bleeding
3. A large or progressing hematoma
4. Distal pulse deficit
5. Neurologic deficit involving nerves anatomically adjacent to major vascular structures
6. Massive or continued intrathoracic bleeding

Indirect evidence indicating injury:
1. A wound above the clavicle or manubrium that penetrates the platysma muscle
2. Thoracic wounds whose trajectory traverses the superior mediastinum or thoracic inlet.
3. Mediastinal widening demonstrated radiographically

tion and the proximity of the wound to a major vascular structure. The overall mortality was 7.8 percent and was generally related to the magnitude of associated injuries or the extent of blood loss before operation. Thirteen percent of the patients with arterial trauma died, compared with 3 percent of those with venous injuries. Early and liberal surgical exploration with emphasis on adequate exposure resulted in low mortality and morbidity rates in this large series.

Operative Technique. Vessel exposure and control of hemorrhage are the major problems in the operative management of thoracic inlet injuries. The varied vessels and adjacent structures that may be involved and the overlying bony shield are the basis of these problems. The inaccuracy of preoperative wound localization and the wide exposure often required for vascular control make a flexible operative approach essential. A variety of incisions may be needed, often involving the mobilization of overlying bony structures, as illustrated in Fig. 6-6. The initial incision may not provide adequate exposure and may require extension or another separate incision. Such extensions or additional incisions were required in 25 percent of 146 patients with these injuries reported by Flint et al. The supine position and a wide operative field including the entire neck, chest, and upper arms offers the most operative flexibility.

The approaches used to expose these injuries are the oblique cervical and horizontal clavicular incisions, median sternotomy, left anterolateral thoracotomy, and a musculoskeletal chest wall flap (Fig. 6-6). The right oblique cervical incision generally is adequate to expose the entire right common carotid artery. The horizontal clavicular incision with subperiosteal resection of the medial half of the clavicle adequately exposes the right subclavian vessels. Extension to a median sternotomy is necessary to expose the innominate artery. The distal left common carotid artery is easily exposed through a left oblique neck incision, but the proximal vessel requires a sternal extension. The distal left subclavian artery can be reached through a horizontal clavicular incision, but its proximal portion requires a sternotomy or, more appropriately, a left anterolateral thoracotomy. A musculoskeletal flap, or "trapdoor," may be used to expose the proximal left carotid and the entire left subclavian arteries and the left innominate vein. This is formed by combining horizontal clavicular, superior median sternotomy, and anterolateral thoracotomy incisions. Most base-of-the-neck injuries can be exposed through the oblique cervical and/or horizontal clavicular incisions. Major extensions should be made without hesitation when these incisions provide inadequate exposure. The vascular repair seldom is difficult and most often can be accomplished by lateral arteriorrhaphy or end-to-end anastomosis. When graft interposition is required, autogenous material is preferred.

The operative approach to penetrating injuries of the base of the neck is appropriately based on the presenting clinical picture, supplemented when possible by arteriography. The factors considered in choosing the primary incision are hemodynamic status, predicted wound course, site of the injury, and evidence of intrathoracic

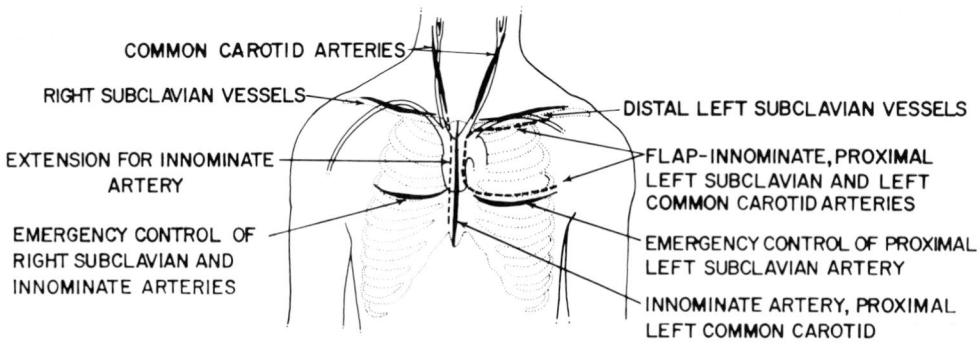

Fig. 6-6. Incisions and extensions for base-of-the-neck vascular injuries.

bleeding. Sound judgment and the flexibility to widely extend incisions result in maximal required exposure and minimal incisional complications and morbidity.

In unstable patients with suspected major mediastinal injuries, especially in the presence of large or continuing intrathoracic bleeding, initial thoracic incisions are advisable. This usually implies a median sternotomy, but if the wound is on the left and a proximal left subclavian injury is suspected, an anterolateral thoracotomy is performed. Anterolateral thoracotomy is performed on the side of injury in patients with massive intrathoracic bleeding if sternal splitting instruments are not immediately available.

Oblique cervical and horizontal clavicular incisions often provide adequate exposure without the added risk and morbidity of thoracotomy. One of these incisions is appropriate in stable patients with cervical, periclavicular, or supramanubrial wounds without evidence of deep mediastinal penetration or intrathoracic hemorrhage. A wide operative field is essential, however, and extension to a thoracic incision is made without hesitation.

The oblique cervical incision provides adequate exposure for most cervical wounds without evidence of mediastinal penetration. In the series of Flint et al., this incision provided adequate exposure for the control and repair of 84 percent of internal jugular vein and 76 percent of common carotid injuries. Lateral extension with resection of the medial half of the clavicle is sometimes necessary for additional exposure. Using this extension, satisfactory access was obtained in more than 90 percent of patients with common carotid and internal jugular injuries. If difficulty with proximal exposure is encountered during the dissection of either common carotid artery, a midsternal extension is made.

The horizontal clavicular incision is initially used in stable patients with periclavicular or supramanubrial wounds and suspected mediastinal penetration but without notable intrathoracic bleeding. Eighty-seven percent of subclavian vein injuries, 75 percent of innominate vein injuries, and 60 percent of subclavian artery injuries were

successfully repaired by Flint and associates using this incision.

If possible, complete proximal and distal vascular control should precede dissection into the immediate area of suspected injury and the tamponading hematoma. If exposure is inadequate during the dissection of either proximal common carotid artery or the right subclavian artery, a midsternal extension should be made without hesitation. If proximal exposure is inadequate during the transclavicular dissection of the left subclavian artery, a left anterolateral thoracotomy is performed and, if additional exposure is required, midsternal extension forms a musculoskeletal flap.

The repair of the vascular injury, once isolated, seldom presents a major problem and can usually be accomplished by lateral arteriorrhaphy or end-to-end anastomosis. When graft interposition is required, autogenous material is preferred. The use of shunts or extracorporeal circulation to maintain cerebral flow should be considered if flow is reduced in more than one of the vessels supplying the brain. Vascular reconstruction is desirable, but because of the rich collateral circulation, single arterial ligations can usually be safely performed, especially when survival depends on early completion of the operation. Measurement of "stump" pressures may be helpful in predicting the consequences of major arterial ligations. Venous ligation usually results in minimal morbidity and may be indicated when optimal repair is not possible, although both innominate veins should not be ligated.

LARYNX AND TRACHEA. The signs and symptoms of laryngeal and tracheal injuries include respiratory distress, hoarseness, hemoptysis, and subcutaneous emphysema. As emphasized earlier, essentially all penetrating laryngotracheal injuries are clinically obvious and this fact may be useful in predicting the course of a missile. Subcutaneous air is not diagnostic of such an injury since air may enter through the skin wound or be due to an injury of the esophagus, bronchus, or lung.

Whenever laryngeal or tracheal injury produces difficulty breathing in the emergency room, a tracheostomy is performed before transfer of the patient to the operating suite. If the patient is hoarse or the wound is near the thyroid or larynx, laryngoscopy is performed preoperatively, when feasible, to evaluate the larynx and function of the recurrent laryngeal nerves. Direct laryngoscopy, using a small-diameter flexible endoscope, is more often successful and less cumbersome than indirect laryngoscopy in the acutely traumatized patient.

Tracheal wounds are usually obvious during operative exploration, but if the injury cannot be identified the endotracheal tube cuff should be deflated to increase intratracheal pressure and enhance the air leak. Clean lacerations of the trachea or larynx are closed using synthetic absorbable suture such as Dexon or Vicryl. These materials result in less frequent problems with chronic granulation tissue postoperatively. Tracheal wounds can more often be primarily repaired than was previously thought. If a tracheostomy is not also performed, an endotracheal tube may be indicated for several days postoperatively to ensure an adequate airway. A tracheostomy may be required instead of or in addition to primary repair, depending on the site and size of the defect and the magnitude of associated injuries. Patients with laryngeal injuries should have normal anatomy reconstructed as accurately as possible to lessen subsequent airway and speech difficulties. If a tracheostomy is required, it is maintained until healing is complete and laryngeal or tracheal edema has subsided, usually in 4 to 8 days.

PHARYNX AND ESOPHAGUS. The clinical findings suggesting pharyngeal or esophageal injury are hematemesis, dysphagia, and subcutaneous emphysema. Carefully performed barium esophagography with cineradiography in two projections may be used to exclude esophageal injury in the asymptomatic patient with platysmal penetration. False-negative examinations occasionally occur, and all patients are closely observed in the hospital and without oral intake for at least 24 h. Pharyngoesophageal injuries are notoriously silent, and a high index of suspicion and a liberal attitude regarding operative exploration result in the lowest incidence of missed esophageal perforations.

After adequate debridement, injuries of the pharynx and esophagus usually may be primarily repaired using an inner layer of absorbable suture such as Vicryl or Dexon and an outer layer of silk, cotton, or Prolene. If a small esophageal injury is suspected but cannot be demonstrated during exploration, an anesthetic mask may be applied to the nose and mouth and positive pressure exerted while the wound is filled with saline solution. Bubbles may disclose the point of injury. It is vital to drain all such wounds, because infections and salivary leaks are potential complications. If there is massive loss of esophageal tissue, as with a close-range shotgun blast, it may be necessary to perform a cutaneous esophagostomy for feeding purposes and a cutaneous pharyngostomy for salivary drainage. A secondary reconstruction will be required after initial healing is complete. A small plastic nasogastric tube is used for feeding for 8 to 10 days following major esophageal injuries, unless a gastrostomy is deemed preferable.

NERVE INJURIES. A preoperative neurologic examination is performed, whenever possible, to identify injured nerves. The brachial plexus, deep cervical plexus, phrenic nerves, and the cranial nerves are systematically tested. The vagus and recurrent laryngeal nerves can be evaluated by examining the vocal cords. A hypoglossal or spinal accessory nerve injury is particularly easy to miss unless a preoperative neurologic examination is performed. An associated head injury or alcoholic intoxication often impedes an adequate neurologic examination. Whenever possible, severed or lacerated nerves are debrided and repaired primarily using interrupted fine silk sutures on the perineurium.

SALIVARY GLANDS. The diagnosis of salivary gland injury is usually made during operative exploration but, if suspected preoperatively, may be made with sialography. Debridement, hemostasis, and simple drainage provide effective treatment. In the absence of ductal obstruction, a salivary fistula rarely occurs after injury to the gland substance. When the major duct is injured, it may be repaired with fine silk over a ureteral catheter stent. The catheter should be removed after repair is completed. When repair is not feasible because of the patient's condition or for some other compelling reason, the duct may be ligated and the gland allowed to atrophy, or the duct may be reimplanted in the mucosa at a later time. If a salivary fistula does occur postoperatively and fails to close spontaneously, irradiation usually arrests salivary flow, but it is not advisable in children or young adults.

MISCELLANEOUS INJURIES. Thyroid injuries require only debridement of devitalized tissue, hemostasis, and adequate drainage. The thoracic duct may be injured with wounds near the left innominate-jugular venous bifurcation. Repair of the duct is not feasible because of its friability, but simple ligation is adequate. The duct may divide immediately before entering the vein or there may be tributaries from the head and arm and multiple ligations may be required for lymphostasis. The area should be thoroughly dried and inspected before closing, because a large collection of lymph may occur postoperatively from even a small leak. If lymph does accumulate, incision and drainage with the application of a bulky pressure dressing for a few days will usually effect closure of the lymphatic fistula. Injured right thoracic ducts, though less frequent, are treated similarly.

ABDOMINAL TRAUMA

Erwin R. Thal, Robert N. McClelland, Ronald C. Jones, Malcolm O. Perry, and G. Tom Shires

The incidence of abdominal trauma continues to increase. Each year about 3.5 million persons in the United States are injured in automobile accidents, and many of these injuries involve the abdominal contents. Mortality rates are generally higher in patients sustaining blunt trauma than in those with penetrating wounds. Although newer and better diagnostic techniques such as computed tomography are now available, blunt trauma still presents a difficult challenge to the clinician. The spleen, liver, kidneys, and bowel are the most frequently injured abdominal organs. In a review of several series of blunt ab-

Table 6-5. FREQUENCY OF INJURY IN
ABDOMINAL TRAUMA

Viscera injured	Frequency, %
Spleen	26.2
Kidneys	24.2
Intestines	16.2
Liver	15.6
Abdominal wall	3.6
Retroperitoneal hematoma	2.7
Mesentery	2.5
Pancreas	1.4
Diaphragm	1.1

dominal trauma the frequency of injury has been determined (see Table 6-5).

Early diagnosis facilitates optimal management. Initial evaluation serves as a baseline but is frequently difficult because of the masking of abdominal injury by other associated injuries. Often the patient is unconscious because of alcoholism, drug abuse, shock, or associated head injury. Chest trauma, orthopedic problems, and retroperitoneal injuries may further complicate the diagnostic process. Another misleading factor in diagnosis, often not recognized, is that relatively trivial injuries may rupture abdominal viscera. The index of suspicion must be high, even in cases of supposedly minor abdominal trauma, if diagnostic errors are to be avoided.

CLINICAL MANIFESTATIONS. The evaluation of the patient with blunt abdominal trauma begins with a careful history and physical examination. Knowing the mechanism of injury is essential in discerning the likelihood of abdominal injury. Information about the patient and the accident scene can be obtained from the paramedics, witnesses, family, police, and the patient as well. Factors such as rapid deceleration, impaling forces, and seat belt restraints make abdominal viscera prone to injury. Physical examination in the alert patient remains the most reliable predictor of injury, yet this will be misleading as either a false-positive or false-negative examination in 10 to 20 percent of patients. The entire patient must be examined as well as the abdomen because of the high incidence of associated trauma. Fitzgerald et al. reported extraabdominal injuries were present in 97 percent of patients with abdominal injuries who were dead upon arrival at the hospital and in 70 percent of those admitted alive. In spite of the explosion of diagnostic technology, if the diagnosis is unclear, one must depend on repeated physical examinations done at frequent intervals by the same examiner. One cannot overemphasize the importance of the bedside clinical evaluation in determining which patients will benefit from operative management of their injuries.

Abdominal pain and tenderness when present are very reliable findings. Abdominal rigidity, and/or involuntary guarding, are indicative of intraperitoneal injury, and even when present alone, warrant exploratory celiotomy without further diagnostic procedures. It is important to note that blood in the peritoneal cavity may or may not cause irritation; hence hemoperitoneum may or may not

produce significant physical findings. Patients with an altered state of consciousness resulting from closed head injuries, alcoholism, or drug abuse also may demonstrate evidence of abdominal discomfort. Injuries to organs in the retroperitoneal space such as pancreas, duodenum, kidney, and blood vessels, by virtue of their anatomic location, frequently do not produce signs of peritoneal irritation such as rebound tenderness, referred pain, and abdominal wall rigidity.

Newer diagnostic studies and better imaging techniques such as computed tomography have increased the clinician's ability to rapidly identify abdominal injuries. These studies have significantly helped to reduce the number of negative celiotomies. In a small number of cases it will be difficult to determine the extent of injury and occasional negative procedures will be performed. It is still preferable to perform a negative celiotomy on occasion with virtually no mortality and very little morbidity than to suffer the consequences of a missed injury.

In patients with blunt abdominal trauma, determinations of alterations in blood pressure are often useful. A valuable sign of continuing intraabdominal hemorrhage is transient elevation of the blood pressure to normal levels for a few minutes followed by return to hypotensive levels with the rapid infusion of 500 to 1000 mL of Ringer's lactate solution. Patients who are hypotensive from minimal blood loss or from neurogenic shock usually do not behave in this manner. The Ringer's lactate solution generally is infused over a period of 15 to 20 min while other measures, such as blood typing and cross matching, are being carried out. Postural hypotension, when the patient assumes the erect position, is another useful sign of continuing intraabdominal bleeding. Often subtle signs of hemorrhage such as mild to moderate tachycardia, tachypnea, narrowing of the pulse pressure, and cool skin temperature will be early manifestations of intraabdominal hemorrhage. Blood loss in the range of 30 to 40 percent of the blood volume will be necessary to produce sustained marked hypotension with a systolic blood pressure consistently below 60 to 70 mmHg.

DIAGNOSTIC PROCEDURES. Whereas history and physical examination remain the most reliable diagnostic modalities, other diagnostic aids will frequently confirm clinical suspicions. In general, laboratory determinations do not offer much help in the young, previously healthy traumatized patient.

Sudden acute blood loss may not be adequately reflected by early hemograms; hence, a normal hemoglobin and hematocrit shortly after injury may be misleading. Serum glucose and creatinine determinations may be helpful in elderly patients suspected of having diabetes or renal insufficiency. Whereas serum electrolytes are rarely abnormal, the serum potassium level is extremely important if operation is contemplated. Unrecognized hypokalemia may lead to disastrous consequences. A serum amylase level, when elevated, is a relatively reliable predictor of intraabdominal injury although not always an indication for operative intervention. In addition to being elevated with pancreatic injury, abnormal amylase levels are also seen in injuries to the duodenum and upper small bowel. Leakage of the amylase-containing fluid is rapidly absorbed into the blood from the peritoneal cavity.

Serum isoenzyme amylase analysis has been advocated by some authors to be more specific than total amylase for pancreatic injury; however, other reports refute this hypothesis.

Studies of urinary sediment are useful, since hematuria may indicate injury to the genitourinary tract. Recent studies indicate that dipstick urinalysis is very accurate in determining hematuria in addition to being very cost-effective. If the patient with abdominal injury cannot void, catheterization should be done to obtain urine for examination. Catheterization is contraindicated prior to obtaining an urethrogram, if there is a scrotal hematoma, perineal hematoma, blood at the tip of the male meatus, or a high-riding or floating prostate on rectal examination. In these instances injury to the urethra is suspected and additional damage may be done if a catheter is blindly inserted.

Levin tubes are inserted in all patients sustaining blunt abdominal trauma. The stomach contents are aspirated and the aspirate is examined for the presence of blood. In addition, a Levin tube provides decompression of the stomach, prevents gastric dilatation, and prevents aspiration with the induction of anesthesia. The instillation of 30 to 60 mL of an antacid in the Levin tube will neutralize the stomach contents and further minimize the ravages of aspiration, should it occur.

Blood-gas determinations should be obtained in all multiply injured patients and, in particular, those patients with a history of chronic pulmonary disease, chest injuries, or possible aspiration.

Radiologic Findings. For patients who have sustained severe abdominal injury and in whom other clinical signs obviously point to such injury, radiography, for diagnosis, may dangerously delay surgical intervention. For some patients with stable vital signs and questionable diagnoses of intraabdominal injury, x-ray studies may occasionally be helpful. When a patient is suspected of having intraabdominal injuries, upright films of the chest should be made, in addition to supine films of the abdomen. Occasionally additional information may be obtained from lateral and left lateral decubitus films. The skeletal system is surveyed for fractures or dislocations. Examination of the soft tissues may give information about changes in size, shape, or position of many viscera. Pneumoperitoneum may be diagnosed with the patient in the erect or lateral decubitus positions. Indirect evidence of solid viscera rupture with secondary hemorrhage may be presumed by an increase in density in the region, by displacement of neighboring viscera, or by accumulation of fluid between the gas shadows of bowel loops. If a gastric, duodenal, or upper jejunal rupture is suspected, the appearance of pneumoperitoneum may be facilitated by injecting 750 to 1000 mL of air into the nasogastric tube, after which the patient sits in a semierect position for 10 min before an upright chest film or left lateral decubitus film of the abdomen is made. Films should also be made prior to the air injection for purposes of comparison if the patient's condition permits.

Examination of the upper gastrointestinal tract by contrast radiography using a water-soluble opaque medium may identify an injury of the stomach, duodenum, or upper small bowel. Although rarely needed or used, it may be helpful in identifying an intramural duodenal hematoma. Contrast material is frequently used in conjunction with computed tomography. The use of barium mixtures for this is dangerous, since a severe peritoneal reaction may be caused by barium if it leaks through a gastrointestinal perforation. This is especially true if there is fecal contamination in the peritoneal cavity from a concomitant colon injury.

Intravenous pyelograms should be done if feasible for patients with hematuria or other evidence of genitourinary injury, not only to establish the nature of the injury but also to determine if both kidneys are functioning prior to surgical intervention in case an injured kidney must be removed. It is important to note that occasional renal injuries are not detected by intravenous pyelography and, if clinically suspected, may be better confirmed by arteriography or computed tomography. If arteriography is contemplated, the intravenous pyelogram and cystogram can be obtained at the conclusion of the angiogram, thereby eliminating one study and conserving time. If necessary, intravenous pyelograms may be done during the surgical procedure to determine the presence of a functional kidney on one side before removing the other kidney.

Cystograms using a minimum of 300 mL of contrast material to adequately distend the bladder may also be useful for diagnosing bladder injury or perforation from blunt abdominal trauma, but normal cystograms do not necessarily rule out bladder injury.

Computed tomography. As experience is gained, the CT scan and perhaps later the MRI will provide excellent images of intraabdominal viscera. Resolution is excellent for solid organs such as the liver and spleen as seen in Fig. 6-7. Whereas lavage is unreliable for retroperitoneal

Fig. 6-7. Markedly disrupted spleen with blood seen surrounding the splenic remnant.

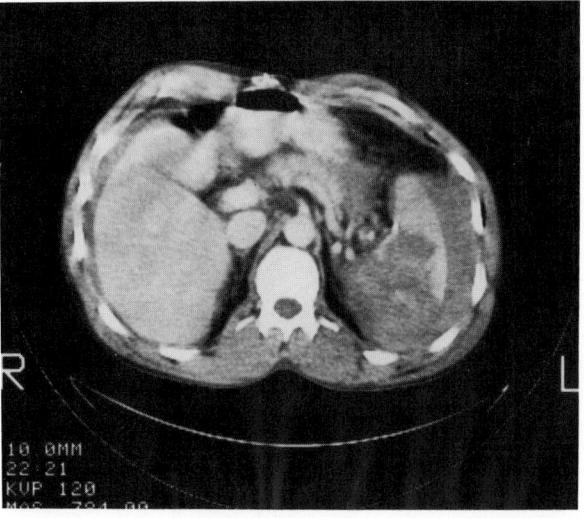

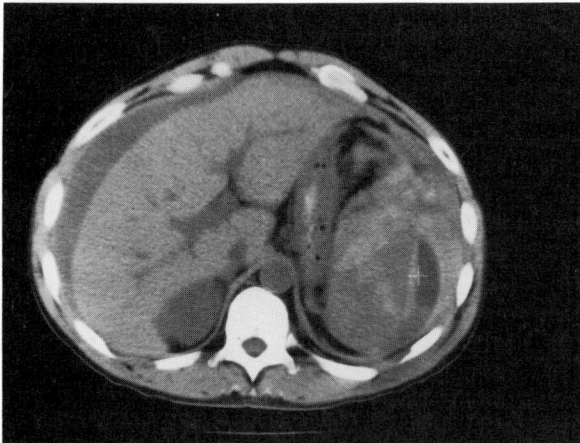

Fig. 6-8. Large spleen with inhomogeneous density representing blood in and around the spleen. Small fluid level seen within the spleen. Free fluid (blood) in the abdomen and surrounding liver. There are areas of high density (clotted blood) within lower-density fluid.

injuries the CT scan has a distinct advantage in this area. Pancreatic injuries are frequently identified with clarity.

Hollow organs are harder to evaluate unless contrast material is used. This is recommended and given both orally and intravenously. Intravenous contrast will permit assessment of the genitourinary system and possibly obviate the need for an intravenous pyelogram.

Fluid collections, usually blood, may be seen surrounding organs or in dependent places such as the pelvis (Fig. 6-8). Contained hematomas can be seen within solid organs that would be missed with lavage if there is no free blood in the peritoneal cavity (Fig. 6-9).

It must be emphasized that unstable patients are not candidates for computed tomography. The length of the procedure will vary according to whether contrast is used, experience with the technology, and the availability

Fig. 6-9. Patient fell two stories. Large intraparenchymal hematoma seen in right lobe of liver.

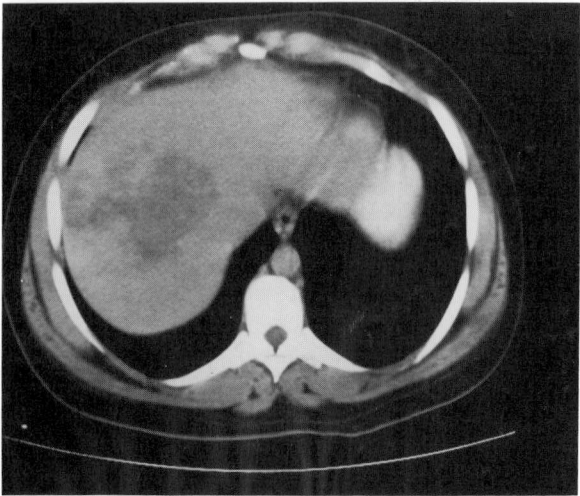

of the scanner. Again, valuable time should not be wasted if hemodynamic stability is in question.

Early reports are very enthusiastic, but caution must be given to the fact that significant injuries have been missed with CT scans and hence continued clinical evaluation is essential for optimal care in spite of a negative procedure.

The emergence of the CT scan has led to consideration of nonoperative management of some selected injuries. Until the natural history of these injuries is better defined, specific recommendations regarding nonoperative therapy should be withheld.

Arteriography. Selective arteriography is another available study occasionally used in diagnosis of blunt abdominal trauma. Selective catheterization of the celiac, mesenteric, or renal vessels may be performed. A film taken several minutes after injection can be used as an excretory urogram.

Arteriography is useful in assessing renal artery injury and is routinely employed if a kidney is not promptly visualized with intravenous pyelography. Intimal tears, aortic occlusion, and traumatic aneurysms are often seen in conjunction with seat belt injuries and are occasionally associated with serious lumbosacral trauma.

When continued pelvic bleeding occurs with extension into the retroperitoneal space secondary to pelvic fractures, arteriography may be beneficial in localizing the site of bleeding. Additionally, vasospastic agents or hemostatic agents such as autologous clot may be embolized to control bleeding. Again, it must be emphasized that time should not be wasted on adjunctive procedures when surgical intervention is indicated.

Scintiscanning. Both liver and splenic scanning have been described in conjunction with blunt abdominal trauma. This technique primarily is limited to those patients whose diagnoses are uncertain and whose conditions remain stable. The radionuclide most frequently used is ^{99mm}Tc sulfur colloid. Most series reporting results of this technique are small and emphasize the relative inaccuracy of the examination.

Paracentesis. Needle abdominal paracentesis is a useful diagnostic aid only for those cases of abdominal trauma in which, after physical examination, the examiner continues to suspect intraabdominal hemorrhage. The abdominal tap has been particularly useful as a diagnostic adjunct for comatose patients with head injury in whom adequate physical examination of the abdomen is not possible. A review of this procedure shows a diagnostic accuracy of 95 percent if blood is aspirated. A negative tap is extremely unreliable and should be followed by another diagnostic study such as peritoneal lavage. In female patients with suspected intraabdominal hemorrhage, culdocentesis may be positive for blood when abdominal taps are negative.

The technique was well described by Drapanas and McDonald and is illustrated in Fig. 6-10. The abdomen is prepped with an iodinated compound or other standard solutions. An 18-gauge short-bevel spinal needle is attached to a syringe and inserted through the abdominal wall after prior infiltration with a local anesthetic agent. Suction is applied to the syringe as the needle is slowly

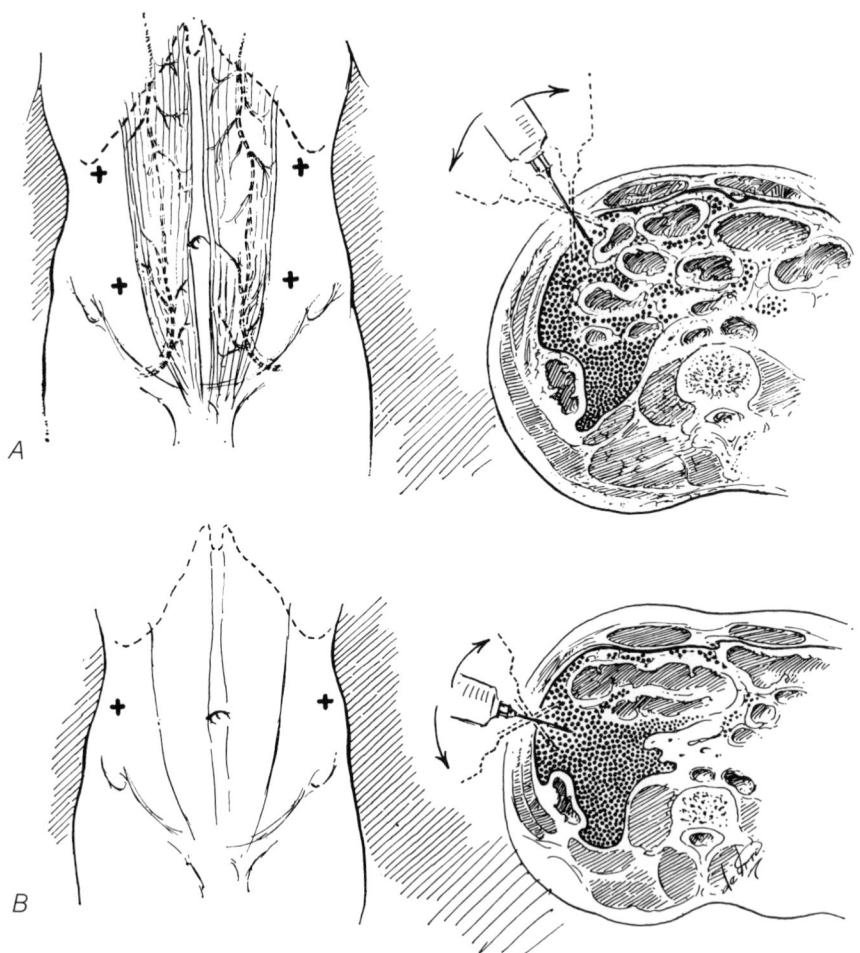

Fig. 6-10. *A.* Technique for four-quadrant peritoneal taps. Preferred location for aspiration of each quadrant is shown. Note that puncture through the rectus abdominis sheath is avoided. *B.* Technique for bilateral flank taps. Aspiration is performed in each flank midway between the costal margin and iliac spine. In our experience, bilateral flank taps are equally reliable as, and more easily performed than, four-quadrant taps in cases of abdominal trauma. (From: *Drapanas T, McDonald J: Surgery 50:742, 1961, with permission.*)

advanced into the abdomen at the sites illustrated. Return of a minimum of 0.1 mL of nonclotting blood constitutes a positive tap. Occasionally, an intraabdominal blood vessel may be entered, but this blood will clot and differentiate it from blood obtained from the free peritoneal cavity. Bilateral flank taps are as reliable as four-quadrant taps and may be more reliable if only small amounts of blood are present. Puncture of the rectus abdominis sheath anteriorly should be avoided. This will prevent a rectus abdominis sheath hematoma resulting from injury to the epigastric vessel and diminish the chance of penetrating the intestine, since gas-filled loops of bowel tend to float anteriorly in an abdomen containing fluid or blood. Actually, the danger of penetrating the intestine is slight; several studies have shown that penetration with an 18-gauge needle is harmless, as a hole in the bowel seals off quite rapidly with no leakage. Other technical

considerations include the following: (1) Areas of abdominal scars or other points of possible bowel fixation to the abdominal wall should be avoided. (2) The direction of the needle inside the abdominal cavity should be changed only by withdrawing the point of the needle superficial to the peritoneum, redirecting the needle, and reintroducing it into the peritoneal cavity. (3) Peritoneal taps should be avoided in the presence of markedly distended bowel, since abnormally elevated intraluminal pressure may cause continued leakage.

Paracentesis is simple, quick, and safe with relatively few complications. A positive needle tap is quite accurate, but the major drawback is the high percentage of false-negative results.

Peritoneal Lavage. Because of the poor reliability of paracentesis, if nonclotting blood is not aspirated, other procedures have been developed to detect intraabdominal injury. Canizaro et al. described the use of intraperitoneal saline infusions in animals. Root et al. first described the technique of peritoneal lavage in human beings in 1965 and subsequently reported a series of 304 patients with a 96 percent accuracy. Numerous reviews of this procedure have proved peritoneal lavage to be a safe and reliable adjunctive procedure for evaluating patients with blunt abdominal trauma. The indications for this technique are patients with closed head injuries, altered consciousness, spinal cord injuries, equivocal abdominal findings, and negative needle paracentesis. It is not recommended for patients with gunshot wounds to the lower chest or abdomen, stab wounds to the back, previous abdominal procedures, presence of dilated bowel, late pregnancy, or positive needle paracentesis.

Several techniques have been described. The Lazarus-Nelson approach utilizes a small Teflon catheter inserted over a previously placed flexible guide wire. The technique popularized by Perry selects a point in the lower midline below the umbilicus approximately one-third of the distance between that and the pubic symphysis. After decompression of the urinary bladder and the stomach by the use of a Levin tube, the skin is cleansed and prepared with an iodinated antiseptic solution. A wheal is raised with 1% lidocaine with epinephrine and the skin incised with a #11 scalpel. At this point a standard peritoneal dialysis catheter can be inserted, and the trocar advanced carefully until it just penetrates the peritoneum (Fig. 6-11). An alternative and perhaps safer method is to incise the abdominal wall to the peritoneum and insert the trocar under direct vision. Once the peritoneum is penetrated, the trocar is removed and the dialysis catheter advanced toward the pelvis. A syringe is then attached to the catheter and the peritoneal cavity is aspirated.

Nonclotting blood will often be aspirated through the larger catheter in spite of a negative needle paracentesis. If no blood is aspirated, a liter of balanced salt solution (Ringer's lactate) is rapidly infused into the peritoneal cavity over 5 to 10 min. For children and small adults 10 to 15 mL/kg is used. The patient is then turned from side to side in order to further mix the blood and fluid. If other injuries such as pelvic or long bone fractures are present, this step is eliminated.

The empty intravenous-fluid bottle is lowered and the fluid siphoned out of the peritoneal cavity. A sample is sent to the laboratory for quantitative analysis. In addition to obtaining red cell and white cell counts, it is important to determine the presence or absence of amylase,

Fig. 6-11. Insertion of catheter for peritoneal lavage in the lower midline below the umbilicus.

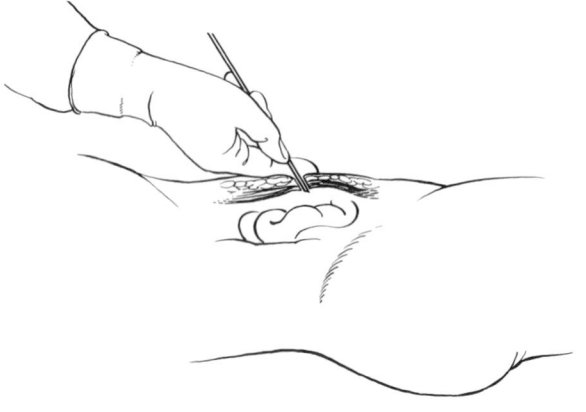

bile, or bacteria. Greater than 100,000 RBC/mm^3, 500 WBC/mm^3, or detection of bile, bacteria, food fibers, or amylase in excess of normal serum values is considered a positive study. Some have recommended colorimetric methods, but these do not appear to be as accurate as quantitative analysis of the fluid. Controversy exists regarding the number of red cells that constitute a positive study. Most authors agree with 100,000 for blunt trauma but figures as low as 1000 have been reported for penetrating trauma.

It must be emphasized that peritoneal lavage is very inaccurate in predicting retroperitoneal injuries. Unless the posterior peritoneum has been torn or considerable time has elapsed between the injury and lavage, most pancreatic injuries are not detected. The same is true for duodenal, urologic, and major vessel injuries that are retroperitoneal. Diaphragmatic injuries likewise are rarely detected by peritoneal lavage. Complications, although very rare (1 to 2 percent), occur frequently enough that lavage is not recommended for every patient suspected of abdominal injury. A negative lavage, however, may spare the patient an exploratory celiotomy. The role of peritoneal lavage is now being reassessed and its use redefined since the emergence of computed tomography. There clearly is a place for both diagnostic tests.

Other Procedures. Sonography has been used in the evaluation of blunt abdominal injury but is not nearly as accurate as computed tomography. Although some advocate laparoscopy, this technique as well as needleoscopy provides a less than complete examination and cannot be recommended at this time for the multiply injured patient.

Penetrating Trauma

STAB WOUNDS

Diagnosis of penetrating injuries of the abdomen does not usually present the difficult problem often posed by blunt abdominal trauma. Three methods of management have evolved: (1) routine exploration of all patients with abdominal stab wounds, (2) selective management, or (3) exploration following demonstration of peritoneal cavity and/or visceral injury.

Before 1960 there was little controversy, since essentially all surgeons agreed that penetrating trauma to the abdomen required exploratory celiotomy to rule out visceral injury. This agreement was first challenged by Shaftan in 1960, who recommended exploratory celiotomy only for patients with physical evidence of injury due to penetrating abdominal trauma and observation in the hospital for those without evidence of visceral injury. The major controversy now revolves around the following issues, which assume paramount importance: (1) How reliable are the various diagnostic criteria for visceral injury? (2) What is the effect of delayed celiotomy on the complication and mortality rate in patients who have no clinical manifestations of visceral injury after penetrating trauma, but who subsequently develop such manifestations? (3) Does negative celiotomy cause significant morbidity and mortality?

Some clinicians favor mandatory celiotomy for all patients who have sustained penetrating abdominal trauma. This point of view was supported by Bull and Mathewson, who found that 23 percent of 78 patients with significant intraabdominal injury confirmed at celiotomy and due to penetrating abdominal wounds had had no physical signs preoperatively. In contrast, 18 percent of 100 patients with possible penetrating injuries in whom the peritoneal cavity was not entered did have physical findings suggestive of visceral injury.

In spite of the fact that there is virtually no mortality associated with a negative celiotomy, most series report postoperative complications in the range of 10 to 20 percent. A recent review of 247 patients with negative celiotomies at Parkland Hospital revealed a 2 percent incidence of small bowel obstruction. Seventy-five percent of the patients had an average follow-up of 57 months. Because of the high incidence of negative celiotomy following routine exploration, most trauma centers have abandoned this approach.

Selective management of abdominal stab wounds is now recommended by many authors. Following clinical assessment, the decision to perform exploratory celiotomy is based on the following factors: (1) physical signs of peritoneal injury; (2) unexplained shock; (3) loss of bowel sounds; (4) evisceration of omentum or a viscus; (5) evidence of blood in the stomach, bladder, or rectum; and (6) evidence of visceral injury such as pneumoperitoneum or visceral displacement on x-ray films. Occasionally, other diagnostic studies are employed, including intravenous pyelography, cystography, arteriography, needle paracentesis, peritoneal lavage, or computed tomography (CT). In the absence of any indication of visceral injury, these patients are admitted to the hospital for a 24- to 48-h period of observation and are reevaluated frequently, preferably by the same observer. If the patient's condition deteriorates or changes significantly, exploratory celiotomy is performed. Nance and Cohn reported a reduction in the percentage of negative celiotomies following selective management from 53 to 11 percent; 4.8 percent of 210 patients initially observed subsequently required an operation when manifestations of visceral injury developed. This delay in surgical treatment caused no mortality or significant morbidity.

An alternative approach to either routine exploration or selective management involves the use of adjunctive methods to help determine whether penetration of the peritoneal cavity has occurred. The decision to operate is based upon confirmation of peritoneal penetration and/or visceral injury. Cornell et al. have described the diagnostic injection of radiopaque contrast material. Following aseptic preparation of the wound site, a small catheter is inserted into the wound and held tightly by a purse-string suture; 50 to 100 mL of contrast media is injected; and anteroposterior, lateral, and oblique films of the abdomen are obtained. Contrast media seen within the peritoneal cavity is an indication of peritoneal penetration. Objections to this technique are the following: (1) some patients are hypersensitive to the contrast material; (2) injection of this material may be quite painful, thereby masking further evaluation; (3) the incidence of false-positive and false-negative results is as high as 15 to 25 percent in some series; (4) the technique is impractical for multiple stab wounds.

Local exploration is another modality that may provide useful information. The abdominal wall is prepared with an antiseptic agent. Using local anesthesia, the wound is opened sufficiently to visualize the complete course and depth of the tract. Often with adequate light, instruments, assistance, and exposure, it is obvious that a wound thought to have penetrated the peritoneal cavity is actually superficial and not damaging to the viscera. These patients are managed by simple drainage and outpatient follow-up if other injuries do not require hospitalization. Local wound exploration must involve more than simple instrument probing to determine penetration. This blind probing may be misleading, since a tortuous wound tract may allow passage of the probe for only a short distance, creating a false impression of nonpenetration. If the end of the tract cannot be visualized or the peritoneum is penetrated, local exploration is considered positive. This technique is equally useful for stab wounds of the back, although the thickness of the paraspinous muscles may prevent visualization of the end of the wound tract. Frequently, innocuous small stab wounds of the back significantly damage such retroperitoneal structures as the inferior vena cava, ureter, pancreas, or duodenum. A recent review of over 300 abdominal stab wounds by the authors indicated that nearly 20 percent of the patients could be discharged from the emergency room without hospital admission based on a negative local exploration that clearly demonstrated the end of the tract.

The abdominal viscera are at risk to injury with stab wounds of the lower chest as well as the abdomen. Figure 6-12 indicates the diaphragmatic excursion with maximal inspiration and expiration and clearly demonstrates elevation of the diaphragm as high as the fourth to fifth intercostal space anteriorly. Wounds at or below this level are therefore evaluated for abdominal injury as well.

If the stab wound to the chest is located below the fifth intercostal space and medial to the anterior axillary line and there is no obvious indication for operation, peritoneal lavage is performed. If lavage is negative, the patient is admitted to the hospital and observed for 24 to 48 h. If lavage is positive, operation is performed.

Patients with stab wounds of the abdomen located medial to the anterior axillary line are evaluated clinically. If there is no indication for operation, local exploration is performed. If the end of the tract is not visualized or the peritoneum has been penetrated but the abdominal physical findings are considered negative, lavage is similarly performed. Since lavage is unpredictable in determining retroperitoneal injuries, this method of management is limited to lower chest and abdominal wounds that are located between the two anterior axillary lines. Whereas these wounds have previously been treated by routine celiotomy, a review of 123 patients treated in this manner successfully reduced the incidence of negative celiotomies from 25.6 to 4.1 percent; 70 percent of the patients in this series were spared operative procedures,

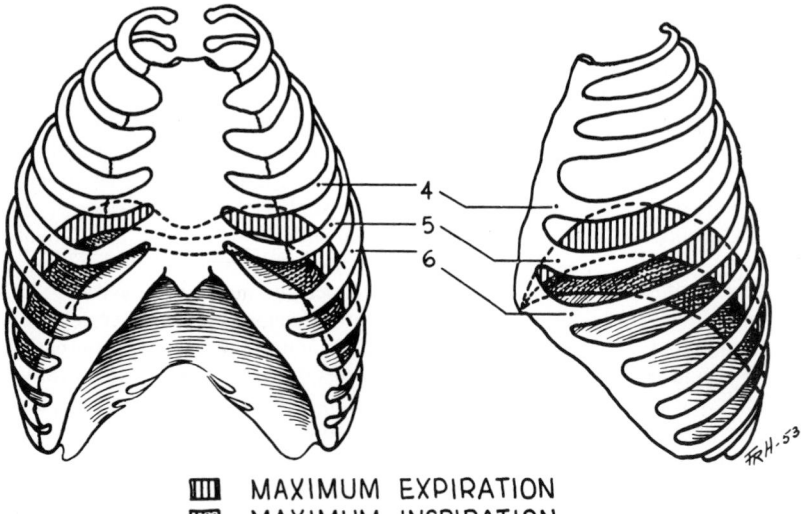

▥ MAXIMUM EXPIRATION
▨ MAXIMUM INSPIRATION

Fig. 6-12. Maximum diaphragmatic respiratory excursion. (From: *Shefts LM: Surg Clin North Am 38:1577, 1958, with permission.*)

while 2.3 percent of the 88 patients initially observed were subsequently operated upon but did not suffer any ill effects from delayed surgical treatment.

Patients with posterior wounds lateral to the anterior axillary line are not lavaged because of this method's unreliability with retroperitoneal injuries. In many centers these wounds are treated according to the criteria for selective management; other institutions recommend operative intervention to rule out visceral injury.

Since lower chest wounds may penetrate the diaphragm, it is important to evacuate air and blood from the pleural space with chest tubes prior to celiotomy. Although a pneumothorax may not be indicated by x-ray or physical examination, prophylactic insertion of an anterior chest tube will decrease the danger of a tension pneumothorax developing during induction of anesthesia and subsequent abdominal exploration.

GUNSHOT WOUNDS

The incidence of visceral injury in patients with abdominal gunshot wounds is at least 90 percent, as compared with 30 to 40 percent in patients with abdominal stab wounds. There is an eightfold to tenfold difference in mortality rates associated with gunshot wounds when compared with stab wounds.

It is not possible to predict the path of a missile by merely observing the entrance and exit wounds or connecting a line between an entrance wound and the appearance of a bullet on the x-ray film. These missiles may bounce, tumble, ricochet, and embolize.

Extraperitoneal gunshot wounds may produce intraabdominal injury by blast effect. In a report by Edwards and Gaspard, 14 percent of 35 patients sustaining gunshot wounds to the abdomen without penetration of the peritoneal cavity sustained at least one visceral injury.

Any bullet passing in proximity to the peritoneal cavity requires exploratory celiotomy. This includes all wounds of the lower chest and abdomen, flank, and back. Ap-

proximately 25 percent of lower chest wounds will produce intraabdominal injury. Celiotomy is recommended for patients with entrance wounds below the fifth intercostal space. If the patient's condition permits, anterior-posterior and lateral films of the abdomen should be made to locate the missile. Selective management, the use of radiopaque material, local exploration, or peritoneal lavage are not recommended for patients sustaining gunshot wounds in proximity to the abdomen. A review of 59 gunshot wound patients all of whom were taken to the operating room in spite of a negative physical examination and negative periotoneal lavage had a 25 percent incidence of visceral injury. Injuries not detected by either modality included the colon, diaphragm, kidney, pancreas, and aorta.

Once the diagnosis of intraabdominal injury is established and resuscitation is instituted, the abdomen is explored. A long midline incision is preferred for the following reasons: (1) It may be made much more rapidly than other incisions, a matter of vital importance when attempting rapid control of exsanguinating hemorrhage. (2) It gives wide access to all parts of the abdomen, which transverse incisions do not. (3) It may be readily extended into either side of the thorax or continued superiorly as a median sternotomy in case of combined thoracoabdominal injury or when better abdominal exposure is required. (4) It may be rapidly closed, which is or great importance in decreasing the anesthesia and operative time in gravely injured patients.

MANAGEMENT OF PATIENTS WITH EXSANGUINATING ABDOMINAL HEMORRHAGE. With improvement of prehospital care, more patients are arriving at the hospital in extremis. Frequently this condition is due to massive intraabdominal hemorrhage that is refractory to standard resuscitative measures. Ledgerwood and associates have advocated performing preliminary left thoracotomy and temporary thoracic aortic occlusion prior to opening the abdomen in patients with massive hemoperitoneum, tense abdominal distention, and persistent hypotension. The descending thoracic aorta is quickly and bluntly dissected circumferentially and occluded by a straight vascular clamp just above the diaphragm. Although this procedure may have occasional applicability, caution is expressed because it requires opening another major cavity, it increases afterload on the heart, the blood supply to the spinal cord may be interrupted, renal circulation is diminished, and it is ineffective in controlling major venous bleeding.

Once the abdomen is opened, the aortic clamp can be slowly released following stabilization of the patient, and proximal control gained at a lower level. A medium or large Richardson retractor may be used to obtain rapid temporary occlusion of the abdominal aorta just below the diaphragm. The lesser curvature of the stomach is pulled inferiorly, and the flat surface of the retractor blade is compressed firmly against the abdominal aorta, thus occluding it against the vertebra just beneath the diaphragm.

With effective control of massive hemorrhage, resuscitation can be successfully completed, ensuring continuous perfusion to the heart and brain and minimizing the possibility of sudden cardiac arrest.

Stomach

Injuries to the stomach from blunt trauma are infrequent, perhaps because of a relative lack of fixation of the stomach and its protected position; but penetrating injuries of the stomach from gunshot wounds occur frequently.

DIAGNOSIS. The diagnosis of gastric injury is generally suspected from the course of the penetrating object, and, at times, additional suspicion of gastric injury arises from the presence of bloody fluid aspirated from the Levin tube. Generally, wounds of the anterior stomach wall are easily seen at celiotomy. Because of the possibility of missing posterior stomach wall wounds, it is important in all cases of proved or possible gastric injury to open the lesser sac through the gastrocolic omentum. This permits the entire posterior aspect of the stomach to be searched for injury. The points of attachment of the greater and lesser omenta on the greater and lesser curvatures of the stomach, respectively, should also be carefully inspected. If a hematoma is noted at the mesenteric attachment, it should be evacuated and the stomach wall at that site carefully inspected for injury.

TREATMENT. Gastric wounds are repaired by first placing a continuous locked 2-0 suture through all layers of the gastric wall (Vicryl or Dexon suture material may be preferable to chromic catgut); a purse-string suture in the stomach does not provide adequate hemostasis. This hemostatic stitch is very important to control extensive bleeding that may occur from the rich submucosal network of blood vessels in the stomach. After this inner layer closure, an outer inverting row of interrupted nonabsorbable mattress sutures of the Lembert or Halsted type is placed. The outer row of sutures provides adequate serosal approximation of the stomach wall, seals off

readily, and prevents leaks. These sutures in the outer layer should not be through-and-through, as is the first row of sutures, but should extend through the seromuscular coat and the submucosal layer of the stomach. Wounds of the stomach are not drained externally, since they are unlikely to leak, as duodenal wounds may. However, it is very important to suction the peritoneal cavity, with special attention to the subhepatic and subphrenic spaces and the lesser sac, so that all food particles and gastric juice spilled into these areas are removed.

After operation for a gastric wound, nasogastric tube suction should be maintained for several days until active peristalsis resumes and the danger of postoperative gastric dilatation passes. The gastric aspirate should be observed for excessive bleeding, which may occur if the hemostatic suture line is inadequate. If bleeding is brisk or persists, the patient should be immediately reexplored to control the gastric bleeding point. After peristalsis resumes, gastric aspiration is discontinued and the patient is initially started on clear liquids and rapidly advanced to a normal diet.

COMPLICATIONS Complications that may develop after stomach injury are hemorrhage from, or leakage of, the suture line and development of subhepatic, subphrenic, or lesser sac abscesses secondary to spilling of contaminated gastric contents. Development of such abscesses is suspected after gastric wounds in patients who fail to do well postoperatively and who have unexplainable fever for more than a few days. If contamination seems heavy, the skin and subcutaneous tissue should be left open until the wound appears clean.

Duodenum

Injuries to the duodenum and small bowel comprise about one-quarter of blunt and penetrating abdominal trauma. In 1947, Lauritzen reported the mortality rate of retroperitoneal duodenal perforation as approximately 60 percent and related it to the difficulty in establishing an early diagnosis. Burrus et al., in 1961, reported a series of 86 duodenal injuries with an overall mortality of 26 percent.

Mortality rates for duodenal injuries have steadily decreased and are directly proportional to the number and severity of associated injuries as well as the time between injury and treatment. Lucas and Ledgerwood reported a mortality rate of 40 percent in patients who were not operated upon in the first 24 h after injury, in contrast to a mortality of only 11 percent among those operated upon within less than 24 h. The improving mortality rate among patients with duodenal injuries is indicated by four series of duodenal wounds reported since 1978. The total number of patients in these series was 677 and the mortality rates ranged from 10.5 to 14 percent. The mortality rate for simple stab wounds involving only the duodenum should be significantly less than 5 percent, while the mortality for severe blunt trauma or shotgun wounds to the duodenum ranges from about 35 to more than 50 percent, especially when such trauma is combined with serious pancreatic injuries.

DIAGNOSIS. The diagnosis of blunt trauma to the duodenum and small bowel is considerably more difficult than that of penetrating trauma to these organs. With duodenal or small bowel trauma, all the characteristic signs of injury to abdominal viscera may be minimal or absent for several reasons: (1) The injury of the duodenum following blunt trauma is frequently retroperitoneal, so that duodenal contents leak into the retroperitoneal area rather than into the free periotoneal cavity. (2) Duodenal and small bowel fluid may cause minimal contamination and may not lead to early signs of bacterial peritonitis. This is not true of injuries of the intraperitoneal duodenum, in which duodenal fluid freely flows into the peritoneal cavity. The highly alkaline pH of this fluid causes immediate chemical irritation of the peritoneum and physical signs of such irritation.

Injuries of the duodenum or upper small bowel should be suspected in any patient who receives a blow to the upper abdomen or lower chest, such as from a steering wheel. Testicular pain should raise suspicion of retroperitoneal duodenal rupture. Also, pain referred to the shoulders, chest, and back may be associated with perforation of the duodenum and small intestine.

Several diagnostic aids may be helpful in determining rupture of the duodenum or small bowel. First, needle paracentesis of the abdomen, especially in the right gutter region or in the upper quadrants, may be helpful if blood, bile, or abnormal amounts of small bowel contents are aspirated. Plain radiographs of the abdomen are helpful and may be diagnostic, but absence of free intraperitoneal air does not rule out bowel perforation. Retroperitoneal rupture of the duodenum is not often diagnosed by x-ray. However, the diagnosis may be based on detection of a large accumulation of air about the right kidney or along the psoas muscle margins. After x-ray films of the abdomen and upright chest films are made to search for intraabdominal air collections, it is helpful to inject air through the nasogastric tube to produce or enlarge these air collections so they are more readily detectable. The accuracy of radiographic studies may also be increased by giving the patient a water-soluble radiopaque contrast medium orally and making abdominal x-ray films to detect leakage of the medium from the duodenum or small bowel. Such diagnostic procedures are unnecessary if other clinical signs indicate the need for exploratory celiotomy. Federle et al. have shown that computerized tomography may be useful in the diagnosis of intraabdominal trauma, especially in the retroperitoneal area, where ruptures of the third and fourth portions of the duodenum are likely to occur.

When a celiotomy is done for suspected intraabdominal injury, duodenal lesions are often missed, especially retroperitoneal lesions of the third or fourth portions. This is due to superficial observation, inadequate exposure, and lack of persistence on the part of the surgeon. It has been reported that duodenal perforations have been missed initially in 33 to 50 percent of the various reported series of retroperitoneal duodenal injuries. To avoid overlooking duodenal trauma and contributing to the high mortality from duodenal wounds, it is important to inspect the entire duodenum during abdominal exploration for trauma. This is especially true if a retroperitoneal hematoma is noted near the duodenum or if there is crepitation or bile-stained fluid along the lateral margins of the duodenum retroperitoneally. If these signs are noted or if the duodenum is contused, it should be widely mobilized by the Kocher maneuver, incising the peritoneum along its lateral margin, so that the duodenum can be completely mobilized along with the head of the pancreas. Thus, small areas of perforation in the retroperitoneal aspect of the duodenum may be identified. Often retroperitoneal wounds of the duodenum that were missed at initial exploration are not recognized until several days later when bile-stained fluid drains from the abdominal wound of a patient who has continued to do poorly postoperatively. The following signs, in addition to those mentioned previously, require careful exploration of the duodenum and the retroduodenal area: elevation of the posterior peritoneum with glassy-appearing edema; petechiae or fat necrosis over the ascending and transverse colon or mesocolon; retroperitoneal phlegmon; hematoma over the head of the pancreas extending into the base of the mesocolon; fat necrosis of the retroperitoneal tissues; and/or discoloration of retroperitoneal tissues—dark from hemorrhage, grayish from suppuration, or yellowish from bile.

The third and fourth portions of the duodenum may be exposed by mobilizing the cecum, right colon, hepatic flexure of the colon, and mesenteries of these organs up to and including the ligament of Treitz, carrying the dissection of the mesocolon along the attachment at the root of the small bowel mesentery, as shown in Fig. 6-13.

TREATMENT. The local treatment of the duodenal perforation itself depends more on the size of the perforation than on any other single factor. In general, an attempt is made to close the duodenal perforation if this can be done without decreasing the lumen of the duodenum. This closure is carried out with a continuous locking 3-0 suture through all layers of the duodenal wall (preferably using Vicryl or Dexon suture material) followed by an outer layer of nonabsorbable interrupted mattress sutures in the seromuscular layer of the duodenum. After this, the duodenum is carefully palpated to exclude stenosis. If the perforation is so large that simple closure will cause a stricture of the duodenum, consideration should be given to (1) complete division of the duodenum and an end-to-end anastomosis or (2) division of the duodenum, closure of both ends, and a gastroenterostomy.

Kobold and Thal first reported a method of managing large duodenal defects that previously might have required one of the above techniques of duodenal division. Their method consisted of using a retrocolic loop of proximal jejunum that is sutured over a large defect in the duodenum, with an inner row of absorbable sutures taken between the torn edge of the duodenum and the seromuscular layer of the jejunum and an outer layer of nonabsorbable mattress sutures taken between the seromuscular coats of the duodenum and the jejunum. Animal studies, as well as clinical usage, have shown the feasibility of this "patching" technique in managing large duodenal defects (Fig. 6-14). Large duodenal wounds and duodenal wounds that have dehisced also have been managed

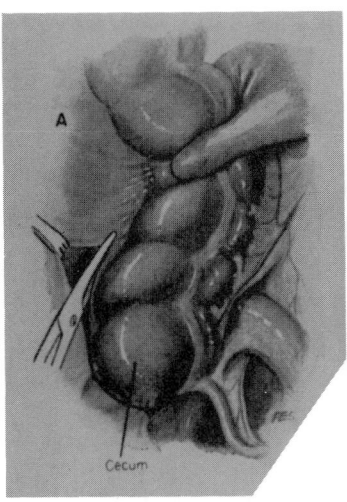
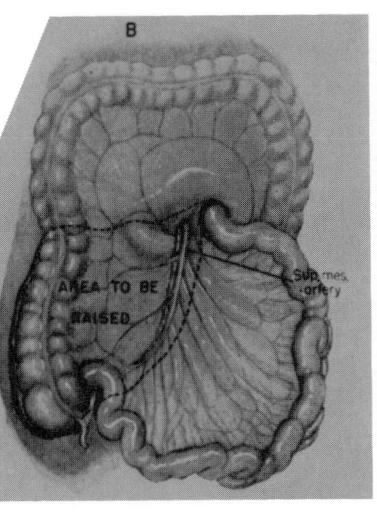
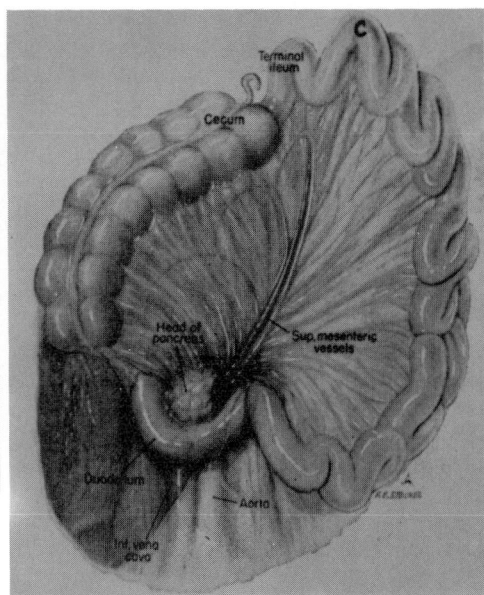

Fig. 6-13. A technique for the exposure of the third and fourth portions of the duodenum. *A* and *B*. Initial dissection for mobilization of the right side of the colon, small intestine, and mesentery. *C*. Exposure obtained of the third and fourth portions of the duodenum. (From: *Cattell RB, Braasch JW: Surg Gynecol Obstet 111:379, 1960, with permission.*)

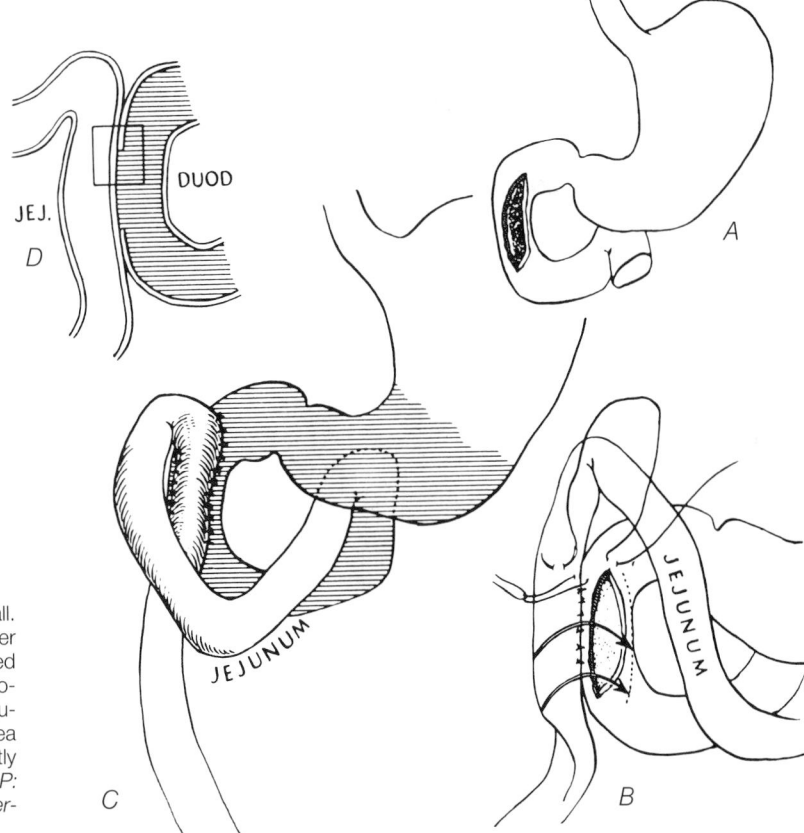

Fig. 6-14. *A*. Area of excision of duodenal wall. *B*. Technique of placement of intact jejunum over the wound to form a patch. *C*. The completed closure. *D*. Cross section of the completed closure showing the relationship of the intact jejunum to the duodenal perforation. The boxed area is the site from which tissue was subsequently removed for study. (From: *Kobold EE, Thal AP: Surg Gynecol Obstet 116:340, 1963, with permission.*)

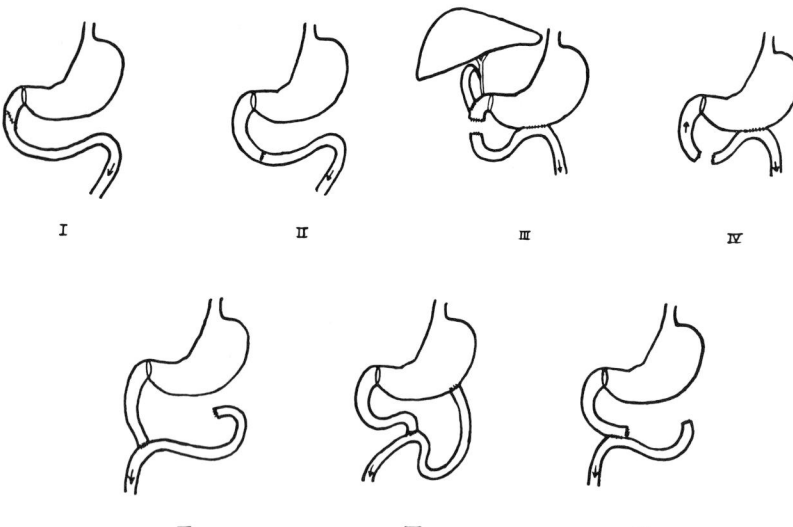

Fig. 6-15. Diagrammatic representation of various operative procedures in a series of cases. I, Simple closure; II, end-to-end duodenoduodenostomy; III and IV, closure of both ends of duodenum and gastroenterostomy; V, closure of distal duodenum and duodenojejunostomy; VI, duodenojejunostomy and gastroduodenostomy; VII, resection of fourth part of duodenum and duodenojejunostomy. (From: *Cleveland HC, Waddell WR: Surg Clin North Am 43:413, 1963, with permission.*)

by anastomosis of the open end or the side of a defunctionalized Roux en Y loop of proximal jejunum over the duodenal defect.

If the region of the ampulla is involved in a duodenal injury, the common bile duct should be identified by insertion of a T tube, since reimplantation of the common duct sometimes may be necessary. Approximately 75 to 80 percent of all duodenal injuries can be closed by debridement of the wound edges and simple suture. However, for the other 20 to 25 percent, one of the reparative procedures described above recommended by Cleveland and Waddell is used (Fig. 6-15). Rarely, even a pancreaticoduodenectomy may be necessary to manage extensive devitalizing trauma to the duodenum and periampullar region, especially when such injuries are combined with severe pancreatic trauma and it is difficult to control bleeding (see the section Combined Duodenum and Pancreatic Injuries).

Very severe injuries of the duodenum or combined severe injuries of the pancreas and duodenum may be treated by a Berne duodenal "diverticulization" procedure instead of by pancreatoduodenal resection unless the destruction and devitalization of the pancreas and duodenum is too extensive. The duodenal diverticulization procedure was first described by Berne and associates in 1960. This operation is illustrated in Fig. 6-16. This operation consists of diversion of the alimentary stream away from the injured duodenum and pancreatic head. This is achieved by removing the gastric antrum, closing the duodenal stump, and performing a Billroth II gastrojejunostomy and vagotomy. The duodenal laceration is closed with interrupted monofilament nonabsorbable sutures, and the duodenum is decompressed with a tube duodenostomy to reduce the possibility of disruption of the duodenal suture line from increased pressure within the duodenal stump. The tube duodenostomy is performed by inserting a #12 or #14 French straight rubber

catheter into the lateral duodenal wall through a stab wound, securing the tube with a purse-string suture. The area of the combined pancreatic and duodenal injuries is then extensively drained with several large Penrose drains and a soft suction drain. Closed suction drains may be preferable to Penrose drains if the area of tissue de-

Fig. 6-16. The essential components of duodenal diverticulization including gastric antrectomy, tube duodenostomy, gastrojejunostomy, and drainage of the biliary tract may be advisable. (From: *Berne CJ, Donovan AJ, et al: Am J Surg 127:503, 1974, with permission.*)

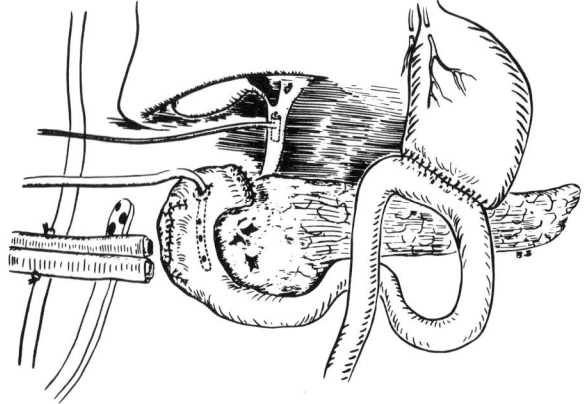

struction is not too extensive. The biliary tract is drained by inserting a T tube into the common duct or by performing a tube cholecystostomy. In 1974, Berne and associates reported the use of this operation in the treatment of 50 patients with severe pancreatic and duodenal injuries with a mortality rate of only 16 percent, which is gratifyingly low for patients with such grave injuries. Even though duodenal and pancreatic fistulae may develop in patients undergoing the Berne duodenal diverticulization procedure, these lesions are generally well tolerated since they are, in effect, end rather than lateral fistulae because the gastric contents are diverted from the duodenum and pancreas. In the experience reported by Berne and associates, there were seven duodenal fistulae and five pancreatic fistulae among their 50 patients, but all closed spontaneously.

An alternative method for diverting the gastric contents from severe duodenal injuries was reported by Vaughn and associates. This procedure consists of repair of the duodenal wound, followed by a gastrotomy on the greater curvature of the antrum of the stomach in a site selected for gastrojejunostomy. Through this opening, the pylorus is closed with sutures of chromic catgut (or Vicryl suture). Gastrojejunostomy, side-to-side, is then accomplished (Fig. 6-17). These surgeons used this procedure in 75 patients selected from 175 consecutive patients who had duodenal trauma. The mortality was 19 percent and the rate of fistula formation was 5 percent among the patients treated by pyloric exclusion and gastrojejunostomy, in contrast to a 14 percent mortality rate and a 2 percent fistulization rate in the entire series of 175 patients. The mortality and fistulization rates were somewhat higher in the pyloric exclusion group, probably because these patients had more severe duodenal injuries. Two of the three patients who developed duodenal fistulae after pyloric exclusion had spontaneous closure of the fistula, and the remaining patient required surgical closure. Vaughan and associates note that in other series of duodenal injuries the rate of lateral duodenal fistula formation has ranged between 6 and 14 percent regardless of the type of closure. This compares very favorably with

the 2 percent overall fistulization rate in their series of 175 patients with duodenal injuries. Kelly and associates have performed the same type of pyloric exclusion with gastrojejunostomy but have used staples instead of sutures as employed by Vaughan and associates to close the pylorus.

Prevention of Duodenal Fistulization after Duodenal Trauma. Various surgeons suggest that duodenal fistulas can be prevented by prolonged decompression of the duodenum after closure of the wound. This may be especially indicated in more severe injuries of the duodenum and can be accomplished in several ways. Snyder and associates performed duodenal tube decompression in 53 percent of the 190 of their patients with duodenal injuries who had duodenorrhaphies. The reasons for duodenal decompression in their series were difficult to determine retrospectively but were probably related to the surgeon's subjective impression of the severity of the duodenal wound. In this series, duodenal fistulae developed in 9 percent and caused death in 4 percent of those who had duodenal decompression. A review of their patients did not allow comment on the efficacy of tube duodenostomy in the prevention of fistulae. However, they did state that the morbidity and mortality might have been greater if tube decompression had not been used. These results suggest that decompression is not a complete safeguard against fistula formation. Stone and Fabian reported a series of 321 patients with duodenal wounds and the most recent 237 were all managed with duodenal decompression via a gastrostomy tube and twin jejunostomy tubes (one passing retrograde into the duodenum). Only one duodenal fistula (0.5 percent) occurred in 210 surviving patients. In contrast, failure to decompress the duodenum was associated with an 8 percent leak rate. Thus, tube decompression of the duodenum is a reasonable and probably effective adjunct in the management of selected duodenal wounds. However, decompression is not an effective substitute for careful reconstructions of severe duodenal injuries.

Reliance on an abdominal drain in the management of duodenal trauma has varied considerably, although several reports suggest that routine drainage of the duodenal suture line may favor fistula formation. However, other clinical analyses have reached the opposite conclusion and use of a drain has been urged to provide a tract for discharge of intestinal contents if a duodenal leak occurs. Objective data about drainage of duodenal wounds are lacking, and the argument remains unsettled about whether a soft rubber drain should or should not be used. Probably, in the opinion of most surgeons, drainage is considered advisable.

Postoperative Care. After repair of duodenal injuries, decompression with a nasogastric or gastrostomy tube is usually continued for about 5 to 7 days to protect the suture lines. If fistulae form, gastroduodenal decompression should be continued for prolonged periods and a sump drain should be inserted into the drain site for continuous active suction of the fistulous tract. This is done to prevent the possible spread of duodenal fluid throughout the peritoneal cavity, to prevent collapse and healing of the

Fig. 6-17. Duodenal injury and method of excluding the pylorus. (From: *Vaughan GD, Frazier OH, et al: Am J Surg 134:785, 1977, with permission.*)

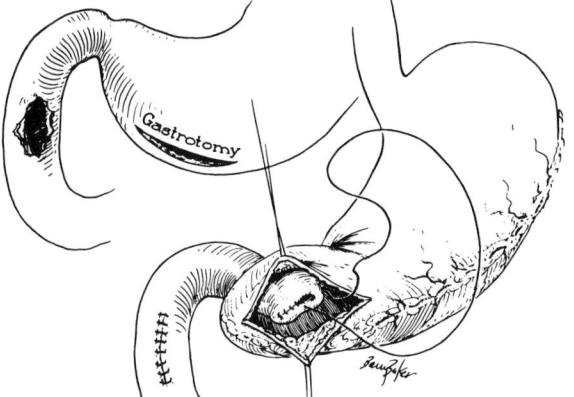

fistulous tract, to prevent digestion of the skin by duodenal fluid draining onto the skin, and to aid calculation and replacement of fluid and electrolyte losses from the fistula. Also, when a duodenal fistula develops, the patient is placed on central intravenous hyperalimentation according to the principles of Dudrick and associates, which are discussed in Chap. 2. This regimen maintains excellent nutrition and may reduce the volume of gastrointestinal secretions. Occasionally, the duodenal fistula does not spontaneously close despite adequate nonoperative treatment with intravenous hyperalimentation and sump drainage. In such cases, when a reasonable trial of conservative treatment has been made and the patient is in optimal condition for reoperation, the abdomen is opened and completely explored to rule out distal bowel obstruction that may be causing the fistula to persist. The fistula is exposed at its origin from the duodenum, and a Roux en Y defunctionalized limb of proximal jejunum is brought up to the fistula and anastomosed to it. This anastomosis may use either the end or the side (after closing the end of the jejunal limb) of the defunctionalized jejunum. This procedure permanently diverts the fistula drainage internally and is very effective.

INTRAMURAL HEMATOMA

Intramural hematoma of the duodenum is usually due to blunt abdominal trauma, including child abuse, which causes rupture of intramural duodenal blood vessels with formation of a dark, sausage-shaped mass in the submucosal layer of the duodenal wall. The hematoma may cause partial or complete duodenal obstruction, but the obstruction is usually partial. The patient has signs of a high small bowel obstruction, with nausea and vomiting associated with upper abdominal pain and tenderness, and sometimes a suggestion of a right upper quadrant mass on palpation of the abdomen. Plain films of the abdomen may show an ill-defined right upper quadrant mass and obliteration of the right psoas shadow. Felson and Levin have shown that an upper gastrointestinal tract series is generally diagnostic, showing dilation of the duodenal lumen with the appearance of a "coiled spring" in the second and third portions of the duodenum due to the crowding of the valvulae conniventes by the hematoma. The serum amylase level may be elevated. An intramural duodenal hematoma may also occur spontaneously in patients on anticoagulants.

Wooley and associates state that traditionally the recommended treatment for intramural duodenal hematoma has been surgical. The most common operation has been simple evacuation of the hematoma; however, gastroenterostomy as well as duodenal resection has been performed. Izant and Drucker in 1964 suggested that most infants and children with intramural duodenal hematomas could be successfully treated without surgical intervention. Nonsurgical treatment of these patients consists of cessation of oral intake, nasogastric suction, and intravenous replacement of fluids and electrolytes. Holgerson and Bishop in 1977 reported on nine patients with intramural duodenal hematomas, only one of whom was operated on. It is now increasingly evident that when there is no indication of bowel perforation, most patients with this condition will respond to the conservative treatment noted above.

Small Bowel

Injuries to the small bowel are more common than injuries to the duodenum or colon. Eighty percent of bowel injuries occur between the duodenojejunal junction and the terminal ileum, with approximately 10 percent each in the duodenum and the large intestine. The usual mechanism of small bowel injury from blunt trauma is crushing of the small bowel against the vertebral column. Rupture of the small bowel is also caused by shearing and tearing forces applied to the abdomen, and rarely by sudden elevation of the intraluminal pressure of the bowel with bursting from such sudden high pressure. Williams and Sargent have experimentally shown that rupture due to sudden elevation of pressure within the bowel is quite unusual.

In exploring the abdomen for injuries to the small bowel, it is important to inspect minutely the entire circumference of the small bowel and its attached mesentery from the ligament of Treitz to the ileocecal valve. The bowel may be completely transected in one or more places in blunt trauma with or without severe injury to the mesentery and its blood supply; at times, the mesentery may be torn from a segment of bowel, thus depriving the bowel of its blood supply. Penetrating trauma to the small bowel from a gunshot wound or stab wound is common, although, surprisingly, it has been noted at the time that in patients with a stab wound of the abdomen, the small bowel has been spared. This is probably because the great mobility of the small bowel allows it to slide away from the knife, a much less likely occurrence with gunshot wounds than with stab wounds.

TREATMENT. Small, single perforations of the small bowel may be closed safely with a single layer of interrupted nonabsorbable mattress sutures that include and invert the seromuscular and submucosal coats of the bowel. A hemostatic stitch, as required for stomach wounds, is not necessary for small bowel injuries, because the small bowel does not tend to continue bleeding from the submucosal plexus, as does the stomach. However, individual bleeders should be ligated with fine suture material. An advantage of a single-layer closure is its rapidity of performance, which is important in patients in precarious condition after multiple trauma.

Two small perforations of the bowel that are very close together may often be repaired by converting the wounds into one and closing the resulting defect as a single linear wound. This type of repair does not constrict the lumen of the bowel as much as two separate lines of suture placed close together and is more secure. Multiple perforations of the small bowel may occur after injury from shotgun pellets. Each one of these injuries should be carefully sought out and closed with interrupted rows of nonabsorbable mattress sutures.

Long linear lacerations of the small bowel lumen also should be closed with a single row of nonabsorbable sutures after ligating any persistent bleeders with small nonabsorbable sutures. Longitudinal lacerations may be closed in a longitudinal direction or transversely according to the Heineke-Mikulicz principle.

Small bowel injuries produced by high-velocity missiles cause severe contusions of tissue surrounding the actual perforation. Because the contusion is a site of potential tissue necrosis and bowel leakage caused by thrombosis of vessels in the area of blast injury, it should be debrided. The debridement should extend into viable bowel where active bleeding is obtained. If the wound is too large or is long and longitudinal, the bowel may not be adequately closed without compromising the lumen, and the damaged segment should be resected. Also, if there are multiple wounds in a short segment of bowel, it is much safer and easier to resect the injured segment than to attempt to suture each of the closely spaced wounds, with resulting impairment of the bowel lumen and blood supply and subsequent obstruction and/or necrosis and leakage. Perforations or lacerations to the mesenteric border, unless they are quite small, are difficult to repair and frequently are associated with vascular impairment. They also should be managed by resection of the involved bowel if an adequate closure cannot be obtained without impairment of the blood supply. Following transection the bowel should be reanastomosed after debriding contused and damaged areas on either side of the wound back to normal intestine that has a good blood supply. Careful attention should be given to leaving uninjured mesentery adjacent to the suture line of the reanastomosis.

Extensive segments of bowel may be avulsed from the mesentery, so that the bowel loses its blood supply. All the necrotic or potentially necrotic bowel and injured mesentery must be resected and an end-to-end anastomosis made between uninjured bowel attached to uninjured mesentery.

Contusions of the small bowel should be assumed to be larger than is apparent. Such injuries are dangerous, since they may lead to subsequent necrosis and perforation. Contusions up to 1 cm in diameter may be turned in with a row of fine nonabsorbable mattress sutures. Larger contusions should be resected.

Temporary control of bowel spillage can be quickly obtained by stapling either the perforation or both ends of a transection while attention is directed toward managing more serious problems. After stabilization has been accomplished the bowel can be repaired more leisurely as described above. Postoperative care of patients with wounds of the small bowel includes maintenance of nasogastric suction and low oral intake until adequate bowel activity returns. Leakage from suture lines and intestinal obstruction rarely occur if small bowel wounds are properly managed.

Colon Injuries

The morbidity and mortality from acute injuries to the colon and rectum have been significantly reduced by an aggressive surgical approach. This has been largely influenced by the experiences of military surgeons during World War II, the Korean conflict, and the Vietnam War.

In World War II, an impressive improvement in the mortality from wounds of the colon was noted. This was due to several factors including improved methods of triage and transportation, effective replacement of blood and fluid, and early surgical intervention combined with ancillary use of antibiotics.

The mortality rate for wounds of the colon of 37 percent in World War II was reduced to approximately 15 percent during the action in Korea. The majority of military surgeons treating acute injuries of the colon tended to exteriorize the wound as an artificial anus to prevent further soilage of the peritoneal cavity. This approach to these particular wounds was duly carried over into civilian practice and reflected in the subsequent reduction in mortality and morbidity. In the later phase of the Korean conflict, however, some modification of the aggressive technique was noted in that small, primary wounds treated early were handled by primary closure without exteriorization.

Acute wounds of the colon that occur in a civilian environment exhibit features that may modify the indications for exteriorization of the wound. The types of injury usually noted in a military situation resulted from either high-velocity missiles or fragmentation missiles in which there was massive destruction of tissue and usually gross soilage of the peritoneal cavity. In the civilian environment, the wounds more often are caused by low-velocity missiles and usually are unassociated with massive destruction of surrounding organs and tissue. The time from wounding to initial treatment in the civilian situation is generally somewhat less than that noted during military conflict. Similarly, associated injuries occurring in civilian accidents do not tend to be so numerous or so massive as those in a military environment, and this has a definite influence on morbidity and mortality.

ETIOLOGY. Acute injuries of the colon and rectum may be divided into penetrating wounds and wounds resulting from blunt trauma. In the former group, accidental colon injuries may be the result of industrial accidents involving explosions resulting in impalement, penetrating injuries from flying objects, or blast injuries.

These injuries may be either the direct result of explosives or the result of accidents involving sources of greatly compressed air. External acts of violence constitute an important source of injuries to the colon, and these are generally penetrating injuries caused by guns or knives or, on rarer occasions, blunt abdominal trauma. Wounds of the rectum, particularly, may be the result of instrumentation during the process of sigmoidoscopy, the administration of enemas, or unnatural sexual behavior. There may also be perforations of the colorectum by foreign bodies that pass through the alimentary canal into the colon. Inadvertent penetration of the colon or rectum may occur during difficult operations; this is especially true of pelvic operations for neoplastic or severe inflammatory disease. Falls resulting in impalement upon sharp objects may produce wounds of the rectum. Automobile accidents and other forms of blunt trauma may also produce acute injuries to the colon and rectum.

DIAGNOSIS. A systematic diagnostic approach to problems of abdominal trauma is necessary, but specific examinations of the colon and rectum may be necessary to delineate an injury. This is particularly pertinent in those instances in which instrumentation is the cause of suspected perforation. Rectal examination and sigmoidoscopy should occupy a prominent place in the examination of these patients. Diagnostic abdominal x-ray studies should be employed to determine if there is a perforation with leakage of air into the free peritoneal cavity. Anteroposterior and lateral decubitus views are particularly helpful in these instances. Contrast studies of the colon should be employed rarely and cautiously in view of the high morbidity and mortality associated with leakage of barium and feces into the free peritoneal cavity. Aqueous opaque media, such as Gastrografin, are preferable when penetration of the colon is suspected.

TREATMENT. The general principles of management of patients with abdominal trauma apply to those patients who have acute injuries of the colon. It is important that the time from wounding to definitive operation be as short as possible, and aggressive replacement of fluid and blood losses should be undertaken at once. Patients with penetrating abdominal trauma or suspected colon or rectal injury should have a broad-spectrum antibiotic with aerobic and anaerobic coverage begun prior to surgery.

A thorough and complete exploration of all abdominal viscera is made, for the morbidity and mortality vary directly with the number of associated injuries. Bleeding should be controlled as rapidly as possible and immediate efforts made to reduce peritoneal soilage from any penetrating wound of an abdominal viscus. The specific care of the wound of the colon should be approached by noting the anatomic differences between the intraperitoneal and extraperitoneal large intestine. Particular attention must be paid to the type of wound, its location, the amount of tissue destruction, the presence of associated injuries, and the time from wounding to definitive care.

Small primary wounds located on the antimesenteric border that are seen quite early, in which there is minimal tissue destruction, and minimal or no peritoneal soiling including those of the left colon, in the absence of associated injuries of other abdominal viscera, may often be adequately managed by a primary two-layer closure.

The mucosa is approximated with a running lock suture of 3-0 absorbable suture and the seromuscular layers are closed with interrupted permanent sutures using the Lembert technique. High-velocity missile wounds associated with shock, large fecal contamination, and significant associated injuries should rarely if ever be closed primarily. Tissue destruction in these cases is often excessive and may not be readily apparent.

A less well-accepted modification of primary closure in which the repaired colon wound is exteriorized and then returned to the abdominal cavity, usually about 10 to 14 days later, has been reported by several groups of surgeons. If the repaired colon wound fails to heal after exteriorization, it is converted to a colostomy and managed in the usual manner; otherwise the patient is returned to the operating room and, under general anesthesia, the repaired and well-healed segment of bowel is freed up and dropped back into the peritoneal cavity. In general, the colon wounds managed by exteriorization-repair are somewhat more severe than those managed by simple primary closure. Flint and associates have classified colon injuries into three grades. His classification has been used to determine the type of repair that is most appropriate. It includes: Grade 1—isolated colonic injuries with minimal fecal contamination, no shock and minimal delay (these injuries are most suitable for primary repair). Grade 2—through and through perforation, lacerations, moderate contamination, and associated injuries. Grade 3—severe tissue loss, devascularization of the colon, heavy contamination, prolonged hypotension, or significant delay in treatment (these wounds should routinely be managed by exteriorization as a colostomy, by primary repair and a proximal colostomy, resection and colostomy with mucous fistula, or a Hartmann closure of the distal colonic segment).

Favorable experiences with selective use of exteriorization-repair have been reported by Lou and associates and by Dang and associates. In 65 to 75 percent of the patients in these series the colon wound healed and could be returned to the peritoneal cavity after several days. The mortality rates were zero and the colon-related morbidity rates were 18 percent in both of these experiences. These two series consisted of a total of 88 patients who had exteriorization-repairs. Probably less than 15 percent of patients with colon injuries can be treated in this manner. It is important to emphasize that if exteriorization-repair is used, a generous opening must be made in the abdominal wall to permit exteriorization of the repaired wound without obstruction of the colon.

Burch and associates recently reported a series of 727 patients with colon injuries. Primary repair was accomplished in 52 percent, the majority of which were simple closure. Seventy-eight percent of right colon injuries, 62 percent of transverse colon injuries, and 32 percent of left colon injuries were closed primarily. The late mortality rate (>48 h) was 1.2 percent for primary repair compared with 9.2 percent for patients treated with a colostomy. It should be noted that more seriously injured patients had a colostomy, hence the higher mortality rate, but with careful selection primary repair can be safely accomplished.

Acute injuries of the intraperitoneal colon resulting from high-velocity missiles that are associated with extensive destruction of tissues or that are large and ragged in nature and are located near or involve the mesenteric border should not be closed primarily. If located in the ascending, transverse, or descending colon, the wound may be exteriorized as a colostomy. Similarly, if the time from wounding to definitive care is relatively long, allowing seeding of the peritoneal cavity with a large number of bacteria, some type of colostomy should be performed either as a wound exteriorization or as a proximal diverting colostomy. Primary closure of the distal wounds is then permissible. Although a loop colostomy may be done for expediency, a completely diverting double-barrel colostomy is favored. It is preferable to open the loop colostomy immediately, usually with the cautery in order to secure early, complete fecal diversion. This is performed in the operating room after all the wounds are closed and dressed. When there are associated massive injuries to other viscera, although the colon wound itself might fulfill the indications for primary closure, a colostomy is indicated. In some instances, there may be massive injury of the cecum or of the ileocecal area, in which case it will be necessary to resect the injured bowel and do an ileotransverse colostomy.

Recent enthusiasm for primary repair in part has been predicated on a feeling that there is an excessive morbidity associated with colostomy closure. Thal and Yeary reported their experience with 137 patients who had colostomy closures following trauma. The morbidity in their series was 10.2 percent, including wound infection 5.1 percent, bowel obstruction 2.9 percent, and fistula formation 1.5 percent. There was no mortality in their series. They concluded that the morbidity following colostomy closure was low enough so as not to be a factor in the consideration of primary repair versus colostomy as an initial operative procedure.

Localized minor wounds of the right colon and cecum that do not produce extensive destruction of the large bowel and are not associated with massive soilage or serious injuries to other viscera may often be managed by primary closure and appendicostomy. In these instances, after debridement and careful closure of the laceration of the cecum, tube appendicostomy is performed to decompress this segment. Seromuscular sutures are placed about the base of the appendix and secured to the lateral parietal peritoneum in order to prevent intraperitoneal leakage about the area of the tube insertion. By this technique, suitable decompression of the cecum and right colon may be obtained, and removal of the tube appendicostomy permits the vent to close spontaneously.

The extraperitoneal perforations of the rectum must be evaluated under the same principles employed for colon injuries within the peritoneal cavity. If clean lacerations with minimal spillage are seen early, primary bowel repair may be indicated if the wound is accessible. Presacral drains should then be inserted. Associated perineal wounds should be debrided and, if grossly contaminated, left open. If debridement is adequate and these wounds are clean, they may be closed with drainage. Any damage to the anal sphincter may be repaired at this time. When a perineal wound is present but not penetrating the colon, it should be debrided widely and if not grossly contaminated then may be closed with drainage. Where there is no perineal wound but there is significant tissue destruction about the extraperitoneal rectum, presacral drainage should be instituted.

For all injuries of the rectum, complete diversion of the fecal stream is mandatory and can be accomplished by constructing a proximal double-barrel colostomy. Even in those instances where the rectal wound has been closed and diverting colostomy performed, presacral drainage is necessary.

Drainage of the retrorectal area is extremely important. This can be established by making a curvilinear incision in the posterior perianal area, incising the anococcygeal ligament, and bluntly dissecting into the presacral space. Two Penrose drains will usually suffice, but with extensive injuries, it may be necessary to utilize sump drainage for a few days.

Lavenson and Cohen, on the basis of their experience in the Vietnam conflict, strongly recommended removal of all feces from the distal rectum. This is accomplished by irrigating copious amounts of saline solution through the defunctionalized segment until the return is clear. They report a significant decrease in mortality and complication rates when utilizing this technique. Military injuries are generally associated with higher-velocity missiles and cause more fecal contamination and blast injury to surrounding pelvic tissue. In civilian injuries, distal irrigation may not be as important, as evidenced by Trunkey and Shires, who report a lower morbidity and mortality rate in their series, in which distal irrigation was not employed but adequate drainage and diversion were used.

Serious perineal injuries are treated in a similar manner. Even in the absence of rectal injury, sepsis can be avoided by early fecal diversion. Failure to recognize this potential problem may lead to extensive soft tissue infections extending from the knee to the axilla, with potential involvement of the anterior and posterior abdominal wall.

Early closure of the colostomy is indicated in patients who have completely recovered and have no distal colon injury. It is desirable to close the simple colostomy in 2 or 3 weeks. Prior to closure, both limbs of the colon should be visualized radiographically to assure that no lesion persists. Mechanical and bacterial cleansing of the colon is effected preoperatively.

Liver

Injury to the liver is suspected in all patients with penetrating or blunt trauma that involves the lower chest and upper abdomen. Among patients with penetrating abdominal trauma, the liver is second only to the small bowel as the organ most commonly injured; among those with blunt trauma, the liver is second only to the spleen as the most commonly injured organ. About 80 percent of liver injuries occur as a result of penetrating trauma from stab wounds or gunshot wounds; only 15 to 20 percent occur from blunt trauma. In recent years, the incidence of stab wounds has diminished while the incidence of gunshot wounds, especially those caused by higher-velocity and larger-caliber missiles, and blunt trauma has increased. These changes in the types of liver injuries, the more rapid transport of patients with hepatic trauma to treatment facilities, and better resuscitation methods have caused an increase in the severity of liver injuries that are likely to confront the surgeon.

Early exploration, prompt replacement of blood and use of balanced electrolyte solution, antibiotics, proper choice of surgical treatment, and adequate drainage are all factors that have led to increased survival rates. The average overall mortality rate of patients with hepatic trauma is about 10 to 15 percent. However, this rate is directly related to the severity of the liver injury and the presence of associated visceral trauma. The mortality rate of stab wounds to the liver without associated organ injury is only about 1 percent. When significant liver trauma is associated with injuries of more than five other intraabdominal organs, or when major hepatic resection is required to control the bleeding, the mortality rate rises to about 45 to 50 percent.

TREATMENT. After initial resuscitation and diagnostic maneuvers, patients with suspected hepatic injuries are rapidly moved to the operating room. The entire abdomen and chest are "prepped" and draped, and a long upper midline abdominal incision is made. Sources of bleeding from the liver and abdomen are quickly appraised, and temporary control of the bleeding is obtained by manual compression or packs placed over the bleeding sites and by temporary occlusion of appropriate major vessels. Digital compression of the hepatic artery and portal vein to occlude temporarily the blood flow to the liver (the Pringle maneuver) may control or slow hepatic hemorrhage in some patients, but more often it is necessary to combine the Pringle maneuver with compression packs placed over the liver injury to control hemorrhage effectively. There is general agreement that, in the normothermic liver, blood flow to the liver can be completely occluded with safety for at least 15 min and probably longer without causing any hepatocellular damage. If it is necessary to occlude the hepatic blood supply for more than 15 min, the vascular occlusion can be briefly interrupted every 10 or 15 min to allow short periods of uninterrupted hepatic blood flow. In a small, uncontrolled clinical experience with 22 patients who had complex hepatic injuries, Pachter and Spencer gave an intravenous bolus of methylprednisolone (30 to 40 mg/kg) before hepatic inflow occlusion.

This use of steroids may have been responsible for increasing tolerance to inflow occlusion beyond 20 min in 82 percent; however, it is emphasized that this was an uncontrolled observation. In addition, Pachter and Spencer used 2 L of iced Ringer's lactate solution intraperitoneally to induce some degree of hepatic hypothermia. Again, this method of protection against warm ischemia was not adequately evaluated, since an intrahepatic temperature probe was not used to confirm the achievement of local hepatic hypothermia. Induced hypothermia may have adverse cardiac effects and should be used cautiously if used at all.

Definitive treatment of liver injuries may be accomplished by drainage alone, suture or hemostatic maneuvers and drainage, or variations of hepatic resection or resectional debridement.

Drainage Alone. Hepatic hemorrhage ceases spontaneously by the time the abdomen is opened or stops soon after compression of the bleeding site in about half of patients with liver injuries. In such patients, the only treatment necessary is adequate drainage of the injury. Suturing of nonbleeding liver injuries is unnecessary. This is emphasized by Trunkey, Shires, McClelland and by Lucas and Ledgerwood who reported no rebleeding among several hundred patients with liver injuries that stopped bleeding spontaneously or soon after temporary pack compression. Suturing of nonbleeding liver wounds may cause bleeding and needlessly traumatizes hepatic tissue.

In the opinion of most surgeons who manage large numbers of hepatic injuries, these injuries should be drained externally. A combination of Penrose drains and sump suction drains is often used when treating massive injuries. Large, 1-in.-wide Penrose drains should be brought out posterolaterally, as dependently as possible, through an abdominal stab wound to achieve the best drainage by gravity. It is important to make an adequate opening in the abdominal wall, sufficient to admit at least two fingers, to assure optimal function of the Penrose drains; otherwise, the drains act as plugs rather than drains. Adequate drainage of the perihepatic space in patients with liver injuries greatly reduces the formation of infected collections of bile, blood, and tissue fluid in the subphrenic and subhepatic spaces. The Silastic suction drains now available are generally very effective in providing aspiration drainage for most patients with liver injuries. It is preferable to bring suction drains out through small stab wounds in the abdominal wall that are separate from the Penrose drains if both types are used. In large patients with more extensive liver wounds, it may be preferable to resect the lateral half or two-thirds of the right twelfth rib to achieve more effective gravity drainage. The Penrose drains are left in place 5 to 10 days, thereafter being slowly removed over a 3-day period. Only at this time is a firm, fibrinous tract formed about the drains that ensures adequate external drainage of the material that accumulates in the abdomen after the drain is removed. Suction drains generally should remain in place until drainage is less than 25 to 30 mL of fluid daily. Some authors have suggested that minor injuries may be managed without drainage; however, the evidence is inconclusive at this time.

Suture, Hemostatic Techniques, and Drainage. Bleeding persists despite temporary compression packing of the injury site in approximately half of patients with liver injuries. Definitive hemostasis of persistently bleeding liver injuries usually can be achieved by liver sutures. Simple interrupted sutures are placed 2 cm from the wound margins, using 2-0 or 0 chromic sutures swaged onto a 2-in. blunt-tipped "liver needle." This allows gentle but firm approximation of the wound edges, thereby stopping most bleeding that originates from the outer 2 cm of the liver parenchyma immediately beneath the hepatic capsule. Passage of the suture through buttressing material such as Surgicel, Gelfoam, or omentum is seldom needed if the sutures are placed 2 cm from the margin of the injury and tied gently. However, if a bolster is needed, it is preferable to use a vascularized pedicle of omentum instead of foreign material. Trunkey, Shires, and McClelland have abandoned the technique previously described using interlocking mattress sutures for hemostasis. These authors now recommend direct suture ligation of the bleeding vessel as an attempt to reduce the chance of strangulation and subsequent necrosis by mattress sutures.

Microcrystalline collagen powder (Avitene) may be used in selected patients to control bleeding from minor liver wounds. Unlike other material such as Gelfoam, Avitene can be left in liver wounds without inciting significant foreign body reaction.

The use of liver sutures to obtain hemostasis from both the entrance and exit sites of long gunshot tracts in the liver is controversial. However, Lucas and Ledgerwood state that this technique was successfully used in several of their patients who otherwise would have required extensive surgery. Placement of the liver sutures at both ends of the bullet tract stops bleeding arising from the subcapsular area, which is the usual source. During their 5-year prospective review, Lucas and Ledgerwood found that only one patient developed an intrahepatic abscess following use of this technique, and no patients developed hemobilia after closure of both ends of a long gunshot tract. They noted that continued bleeding that persists after closure of both ends of a tract is usually identified at the initial operation by blood oozing between the liver sutures or by an increase in the size of the liver within 10 min after placement of the sutures. If there is persistent bleeding from the tract, hemostasis is best achieved by opening the tract and individually ligating the bleeding vessels.

Ligation of an appropriate major branch of the hepatic artery (i.e., the right or left branch) while reported in the past is now rarely advocated. Lucas and Ledgerwood did not find ligation of major branches of the hepatic artery as effective in arresting hemorrhage, possibly because some of these patients were bleeding from major venous injuries. It is suggested that the right or left hepatic artery should not be ligated if a simple temporary compression pack or suturing of a bleeding injury controls the hemorrhage.

Flint and Polk reviewed their large experience with hepatic artery ligation in the management of liver trauma. Critical reanalysis of their results showed that hepatic artery ligation was actually required in only 12.4 percent of their 540 patients with liver trauma rather than in the 17 percent who actually had this procedure. They also pointed out that the unrealistic expectation that hepatic artery ligation would control venous bleeding undoubtedly led to late recognition of hepatic and portal vein injuries in patients who continued to bleed after hepatic artery ligation. In their present approach to bleeding liver lacerations, Flint and Polk initially pack the liver wound and manually compress the liver while restoring blood volume and controlling other bleeding sites. Preparations are made and the packs are removed. If bleeding recurs, the porta is occluded temporarily with a vascular clamp. If hemorrhage continues after the Pringle maneuver, the wound is repacked and a search is made for hepatic venous injury. When porta compression controls hemorrhage, the laceration is gently explored for specific bleeding sites amenable to suture ligation. After this, devitalized liver tissue is debrided and the area is drained.

The use of a pedicle of omentum as an autogenous pack to control hemorrhage in major hepatic injuries has been recommended by Stone and Lamb and by Pachter and Spencer. The omental pedicle provides the necessary bulk to fill a traumatic crevice in the liver so as to obstruct further hemorrhage without causing pressure necrosis of the surrounding hepatic parenchyma. In large liver wounds, this viable pack of omentum may eliminate dead space as well as tamponading venous oozing from the liver.

Resection. Resectional debridement or limited wedge resection is recommended to control bleeding from ragged liver injuries that may be caused by shotgun wounds, high-velocity rifle wounds, and severe blunt injuries. Limited resectional debridement of shattered liver tissue usually achieves hemostasis from such injuries effectively and safely. The margins of resectional debridement should be 2 or 3 cm beyond the point of injury, and bleeding during debridement is controlled by digital parenchymal compression and/or temporary occlusion of the inflow of blood to the liver at the porta hepatis. The liver parenchyma is separated bluntly by finger fracture, a suction tip, or a scalpel handle. Vessels and bile ducts are secured by individual suture ligation or by metal hemoclips as these structures are encountered. It is not necessary to oppose the margins of the resection with interrupted liver sutures if bleeding from the resected surface is controlled. If such hemostasis is not achieved, the omental pack referred to above may be employed.

Anatomic hepatic lobectomy to control bleeding, especially from the right lobe, is preferably reserved for patients in whom (1) hepatic suturing is unsuccessful; (2) resectional debridement or hepatotomy with intraparenchymal hemostasis is precluded by the anatomic location of the injury; (3) occlusion of the hepatic artery fails to control hemorrhage. Although resectional debridement or sublobar hepatic resection may be required in about 4 or 5 percent of all patients with liver injuries, no more than 2 or 3 percent require anatomic, lobar resection to control hemorrhage. Most of the few patients with liver injuries who require major hepatic lobectomies to control bleeding have massive, shattering injuries to the major hepatic veins at or near the junction with the vena cava (Fig. 6-18). If it becomes apparent that major lobar resection is necessary, the hepatic bleeding is temporarily controlled by manual compression of packs placed over the liver wound and by a Pringle maneuver while the midline abdominal incision is extended by performing a median sternotomy.

A median sternotomy is much more quickly and easily made and closed than a right thoracoabdominal incision, causes considerably less diaphragmatic injury, provides much easier access to the vena cava and hepatic veins, permits easier insertion of a retrohepatic vena caval shunt if this is required, and causes less postoperative pain and pulmonary morbidity than a right thoracoabdominal incision.

After wide exposure is obtained by the median sternotomy extension of the midline abdominal incision, Rumel tourniquets are placed about the vena cava superior and inferior to the liver. The superior tape is placed about the vena cava superior to the central tendon of the diaphragm after this portion of the vena cava is exposed by opening the pericardium. These tapes permit temporary occlusion of the vena cava for insertion of an intracaval shunt if vascular isolation of the liver is required during hepatic lobectomy because of major retrohepatic vena cava or major hepatic vein injury near where these veins enter the vena cava. The hepatic artery, portal vein, and bile ducts supplying the lobe to be resected are then suture-ligated and divided. After this, hepatic resection can be done by

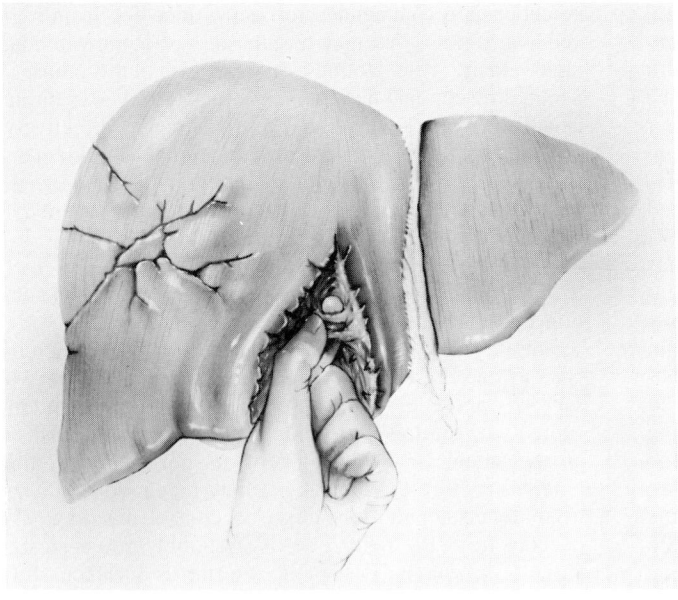

Fig. 6-18. Typical liver injury requiring hepatic resection.

dividing Glisson's capsule with a cautery along the line appropriate for the lobe being removed. The lobe is removed by fracturing through the liver substance along the line of resection with the thumb and forefinger or with the top of an abdominal suction tube from which the guard has been removed. As the blood vessels and bile ducts are encountered within the liver, they are isolated by passing a right-angle clamp around them and are then ligated and divided. After the larger vessels and ducts are suture-ligated, the smaller ones are secured with metal hemoclips. No attempt is made to secure the hepatic veins at their junction with the retrohepatic vena cava before beginning the resection; instead, it is much easier and safer to isolate and suture-ligate or oversew the appropriate major hepatic veins as they are encountered posteriorly during the liver resection. The resection begins anteriorly and progresses posteriorly toward the right or left side of the vena cava, keeping to the right or left of the middle hepatic vein (depending upon whether a right or left lobectomy is being done). The middle hepatic vein demarcates the right from the left lobe of the liver and passes in a line from the middle of the gallbladder bed posteriorly to the midportion of the retrohepatic vena cava. The hepatic veins and other large vascular structures must be oversewn, since simple ligatures on these large structures often slip off and cause catastrophic bleeding.

The Lin hepatic compression clamp may be helpful in performing resections. With the use of this clamp, there is considerable reduction in blood loss and operating time, but its availability should not cause a broadening of the strict indications for liver resection for trauma. The clamp can be used for resecting the liver only when the liver has been severely shattered and devitalized without injury to the retrohepatic vena cava or the major hepatic veins near the junction of the vena cava.

Vascular Isolation. Vascular isolation may be required in a highly selective group of patients with liver injuries.

This technique allows the surgeon to control bleeding from and to repair retrohepatic vena caval or major hepatic venous injuries. Vascular isolation of the liver is attained by using one of two techniques. The first of these techniques employs occlusive vascular clamps placed across the aorta just below the diaphragm, on the porta hepatis, and across the inferior vena cava above and below the liver. This technique may be associated with cardiac dysrhythmias and renal insufficiency. The second technique for obtaining vascular isolation of the liver was first described and reported by Schrock and associates and further successful experience with this reported by Yellin and associates. When this technique is used, retrohepatic vena caval and hepatic venous isolation is attained by inserting a #36 endotracheal tube with an inflatable balloon near the caudal end via the right atrial appendage of the heart. The tube is then passed down the retrohepatic cava and shunts blood around the liver from the lower portion of the body to the right heart. Control of vascular inflow to the liver is obtained by placing a Rumel tourniquet or vascular clamp on the porta hepatis. The introduction of the intracaval shunt via the right atrial appendage is most expeditiously done through a median sternotomy. Also, it is suggested that three equidistant "guy" sutures should be placed in the right atrial wall somewhat outside the atrial purse-string suture before making the atrial opening in the center of the purse-string suture to insert the shunt tube. These "guy" sutures are then spread apart and held up by assistants as the atrium is opened; this greatly facilitates insertion of the shunt by stabilization of the atrial wall. Defore and associates reported survival of 7 of 15 patients with major vena caval or hepatic vein injuries following vascular isolation and introduction of an intracaval shunt as described. Nevertheless, this technique is difficult and somewhat dangerous to perform and should be used only when it is certain that the vena caval and/or hepatic vein injuries are severe enough that bleeding can be controlled in no other way. In the latter instance, the shunt may be lifesaving. It is also emphasized that the results with the shunt probably can be improved if it is used promptly as soon as it becomes apparent that no other method will achieve hemostasis. In some experiences reporting poor results with the shunt, its use may have been delayed too long and the massive transfusions required in the interim may have led to an intractable coagulopathy. In reviewing 60 patients from several institutions in whom the shunt was used, Walt found a survival rate of 20 percent and very probably most of these patients would not have survived without the shunt.

Another method for controlling hemorrhage from the retrohepatic vena cava or major hepatic veins has been described by the authors. If the major venous laceration is in such a position in the suprahepatic vena cava or the extrahepatic portion of the hepatic veins, a Foley catheter may be quickly inserted into the exposed laceration. The balloon of the Foley catheter is then inflated and gently pulled up against the wall of the vena cava or hepatic vein to occlude the laceration, arrest the hemorrhage, and thus permit repair of the venous laceration with relatively good exposure and little blood loss.

It is again emphasized that these methods should not be used except by a skillful and experienced surgeon in whose judgment exsanguination will occur unless vascular isolation is carried out. If such is not the case, the temporary use of gauze packing to control intractable hemorrhage may still be indicated. A recent experience with the use of packs to control hemorrhage in patients with hepatic trauma was reported by Feliciano and associates. These surgeons recommend intraabdominal gauze packing for hepatic tamponade in patients with continued or uncontrollable hepatic parenchymal oozing despite all attempts at surgical control of extensive injuries. The packing can be removed at relaparotomy or on rare occasions through the abdominal drain site. Nine of the ten patients initially reported survived and there were no cases of rebleeding after removal of the packing. The packs were removed when their hemodynamic status was satisfactory, bleeding seemed to be under control, and other systemic problems did not preclude another general anesthetic to remove the packs. The packs are generally removed 3 to 4 days after the original operation. Feliciano and associates note that reoperation to remove the packs is not necessary, but a "second-look" operation is valuable since it permits further debridement of nonviable tissue, irrigation of the subphrenic and subhepatic spaces, and insertion of clean perihepatic drains. A warning must be given against indiscriminate packing as a primary treatment for liver injuries, as was often done with catastrophic results many years ago. In this regard, Feliciano and associates state that packing is a valuable adjunct for controlling hepatic hemorrhage in highly selected patients and should be performed early if indicated. Appropriate use of this packing technique will often preclude massive transfusions and subsequent fatal coagulopathy problems. Placing a steridrape between the liver surface and the pack has been recommended. This technical point will facilitate the removal of the pack without disturbing the hemostasis or clot formation that has been achieved at the injury site.

SUBCAPSULAR HEMATOMA. The treatment of subcapsular hematomas of the liver is somewhat controversial. Left alone, these may (1) resolve spontaneously, (2) expand and burst with delayed intraperitoneal bleeding, (3) cause a hepatic abscess, or (4) decompress into the biliary tree and cause hematobilia. The risk of inducing massive hemorrhage, at times uncontrollable, accompanies attempts at incision and evacuation.

Richie and Fonkalsrud reported a series of subcapsular hematoma patients who were treated nonoperatively. They emphasize that severe bleeding may result in some patients in whom hematomas of the liver are unroofed, and they further noted that since some hematomas are centrally located within the liver, they often do not lend themselves to resection or control by hepatic artery ligation. These authors recommended performing an emergency liver scan, although CT scans would be preferable now, on patients with probable blunt hepatic trauma who do not have persistent hemorrhage or shock and who do not have other indications for immediate laparotomy, such as positive needle paracentesis of the abdomen or positive peritoneal lavage. If the patient's condition remains stable, and a subcapsular hematoma is seen on liver scan, they recommend close observation in the hospital by means of frequent physical examinations, serial hematocrit determinations, and performance of liver function tests. The status of the hematoma is apprised by serial CT scans to be certain it is resolving and not increasing in size. Geis and associates have also reported a successful experience with the treatment of subcapsular and intrahepatic hematomas. These authors emphasize that serious sequelae of these lesions may occur approximately 1 to 28 days after injury. They also pointed out that one-quarter of their 16 patients with intrahepatic hematomas had palpable livers and all of these had large hematomas visualized by hepatic scan. Furthermore, three of the four with large hematomas had complications. Thus, they caution that a palpable liver is an ominous sign that indicates a large hematoma and a very high incidence of serious complications. Other recent favorable experiences with the nonoperative management of subcapsular hematomas of the liver have been reported by Cheatham and associates and by Lambeth and Rubin.

Emergency hepatic arteriography for patients in stable condition with probable subcapsular or intrahepatic hematomas due to blunt trauma may be used on rare occasions.

An advantage of hepatic arteriography in some stable patients with intrahepatic hematomas is that this technique can be used therapeutically as well as diagnostically. If a site of arterial hemorrhage is visualized arteriographically, the hemorrhage may be controlled nonoperatively and atraumatically by embolizing several 2-mm^2 pieces of Gelfoam through the hepatic arterial catheter. These emboli obstruct the bleeding site and prevent further bleeding.

Hematobilia. Hematobilia is caused by arterial hemorrhage into the biliary tract after liver trauma; classically it presents with a triad of findings consisting of upper or lower gastrointestinal hemorrhage, obstructing jaundice, and colicky abdominal pain. In the past, the standard treatment for this condition consisted of hepatic resection or hepatotomy with direct exposure and suture ligation of the bleeding artery. Such treatment is often associated with considerable blood loss and high operative mortality and morbidity. There are now several reports of successful management of traumatic hematobilia by ligation of the hepatic arteries supplying the involved lobe of the liver. Also, in 1976, Walter and associates first reported successful control of hematobilia by hepatic artery catheter embolization. Since that time, Heimbach and his colleagues and Perlberger have also successfully treated traumatic hematobilia with angiographic embolization.

COMPLICATIONS. Major nonfatal complications occur in approximately 20 percent of patients with liver injuries. Since the thorax is involved in many hepatic injuries, there is a high incidence of pulmonary complications. Also, the incidence of intraabdominal and perihepatic abscesses ranges from 4.5 to 20 percent. The probability of such abscess formation increases with more complex injuries of the liver and with the presence of associated colon injuries.

Patients with major lobar resections may be expected to have some postoperative bilirubin elevation, probably secondary to transient biliary obstruction by blood clots and temporary hepatic insufficiency (due to shock, loss of hepatic mass, operative trauma, and occasionally, postoperative sepsis). Hyperbilirubinemia usually disappears within about 3 weeks, with no further surgical treatment required for the relief of jaundice. Liver function studies generally show hepatic impairment but usually return to normal after several weeks. Glucose metabolism is altered after resection, and in the early postoperative period it may be necessary to give the patient supplemental glucose solutions. Studies indicate that survival is possible with only 20 percent of the normal hepatic mass, and that within 1 to 2 years, most of the resected hepatic tissue is replaced by hepatic regeneration.

Although Merendino and associates and Perry and LaFave suggested that T-tube drainage of the common bile duct should be carried out after hepatic resections, reports by Lucas and Walt and by Pinkerton and associates suggest that septic complications and bleeding from gastroduodenal stress ulcers are significantly increased by T-tube drainage. Lucas and Walt, in a well-controlled prospective study, supported the position that effective biliary decompression is not achieved by the T tube and that drainage of the common duct may increase the incidence of complications in patients with hepatic trauma, especially those due to infection and bile duct obstruction (i.e., jaundice, cholangitis, and bile duct stricture). T-tube drainage of the uninjured bile duct associated with hepatic injuries is no longer advocated.

Gallbladder

Although perforations of the gallbladder due to blunt trauma are very unusual, penetrating abdominal trauma frequently causes gallbladder injuries. Penetrating or avulsion injuries of the gallbladder are best managed by cholecystectomy, but in unstable patients with other severe injuries, when, in the surgeon's judgment, cholecystectomy is inadvisable, a tube cholecystostomy should be done, with placement of drains around the gallbladder and the subhepatic space. In general, simple suture of a gallbladder perforation is not recommended because of the probability of bile leakage. After about 4 weeks, if a patient who has had a tube cholecystostomy is doing well, a cholangiogram is performed through the cholecystostomy tube, and if this shows that the gallbladder and biliary ducts are normal, with free flow of contrast material into the duodenum, the cholecystostomy tube can be removed. Routine cholecystectomy after removal of the cholecystostomy tube in patients who have sustained gallbladder trauma is unnecessary, but it is probably advisable to perform an oral cholecystogram or sonogram several months after injury to determine the status of the gallbladder.

Extrahepatic Biliary Tree

PENETRATING INJURIES

The diagnosis of penetrating injuries of the extrahepatic biliary tree usually presents no problem as compared with the diagnosis of blunt trauma of the biliary tree, which may be difficult unless intraabdominal hemorrhage occurs. When the hepatic artery and portal vein are involved, the mortality rate is inordinately high because of massive hemorrhage that may be virtually impossible to control before irreversible hypoxic damage occurs to the brain and myocardium. Probably most patients with injuries to the extrahepatic biliary tree and one of the major vessels in the hepatoduodenal ligament do not survive to come to surgical exploration. This is especially true when the wounding agent is a large-caliber, high-velocity missile. In contrast, wounds of the gallbladder, which are seen frequently after penetrating abdominal trauma, have a low mortality rate and are not so commonly associated with injuries to the major vessels in the hepatoduodenal ligament.

While opening the abdomen, blood and bile seen issuing from the subhepatic region indicate possible injury to the biliary tree. At times, the amount of bile, blood, or contusion may be minimal, and the gallbladder, cystic duct, and hepatoduodenal structures must be carefully inspected to evaluate the significance of any subserosal hematoma or bile staining. If the patient has survived to be surgically explored, generally no massive bleeding from the subhepatic region will be noted initially. However, many times in obtaining exposure of the hepatoduodenal ligament structures, clots that have formed and tamponaded major bleeding sites may be dislodged, with recurrence of vigorous bleeding from the portal vein, hepatic artery, or their branches, which are so frequently injured when the bile ducts are injured.

Generally, the hemorrhage may be immediately arrested by lacing the fingers in the foramen of Winslow and compressing the hepatoduodenal ligament (the Pringle maneuver). Following this, after removing the free blood and obtaining good exposure while maintaining finger tamponade as above, more definitive control of the hemorrhage may be obtained by placing vascular or rubbershod clamps across all the structures in the hepatoduodenal ligament. One clamp should be placed as far distal as possible on the hepatoduodenal ligament, and this maneuver is aided by dividing the lateral serosal reflection of the duodenum and reflecting the duodenum and head of the pancreas medially. Another clamp is then placed on the hepatoduodenal ligament through the foramen of Winslow as near the liver hilus as possible.

After hemorrhage is controlled, the serosa of the hepatoduodenal ligament at the site of the hematoma formation is incised, and the disruption of the portal vein or hepatic artery is visualized by rapidly dissecting out these structures. When the defects in the major vessels are located, repair is carried out with 5-0 arterial sutures using the general principles and techniques of vascular surgery. The vascular repair should be done only after careful exposure of the defect, but also with dispatch, since the known safe occlusion period of hepatic vascular inflow is limited. As noted in the section on liver trauma, it may be possible to extend this period by giving an intravenous bolus of methylprednisolone according to Pachter and Spencer.

The management of blunt and penetrating injuries of the extrahepatic biliary tree was reviewed by Busuttil and associates who treated 21 patients with severe injuries to the porta hepatis over a 10-year period. Fourteen of these patients had bile duct injuries, eight had complete transection of the common duct, and five had a tangential or incomplete disruption with a portion of the duct wall remaining intact. Five of the eight patients who had complete transection had primary end-to-end repair with T-tube stenting, while three underwent primary Roux en Y choledochojejunostomy. All patients with incomplete disruptions had primary repairs with or without T-tube stenting. Of the five patients with complete disruptions who had primary end-to-end anastomosis of the bile duct with T-tube stenting, all required secondary biliary tract reconstruction by some type because of subsequent bile duct stricture. In contrast, no patient with complete transection treated by means of a primary Roux en Y choledochojejunostomy or choledochoduodenostomy required reoperation.

Busuttil and associates state that the most important factor in determining how to manage the bile duct injury is whether or not the duct is completely or incompletely transected. From their experience, complete transection almost always ends with stricture if the duct is primarily repaired end-to-end but has a favorable outcome if some type of duct-enteric anastomosis is done. These findings were reported by Belzer some years ago when he showed that an incomplete ductal injury could be successfully repaired by duct anastomosis or patch (vein or gallbladder graft); however, a complete division, when mobilized for primary anastomosis or patch, almost always ends in stricture Also, Longmire recommended duct-enteric anastomosis as the best method for the early treatment of injuries to the extrahepatic bile ducts.

Busuttil and his colleagues further state that if the duct has been perforated or incompletely divided, primary repair can be successfully performed. There seems to be no definitive evidence that the presence or absence of a T-tube stent makes any difference in the rate of success in these cases. However, Busuttil and associates believe that a T-tube stent should not be used if the duct is of small caliber.

If the patient is in poor condition and cannot tolerate a prolonged procedure for definitive repair of the bile duct, then the defects of the biliary duct may be repaired by simple bridging with a T tube fixed in place with a suture at either end of the ductal defect; secondary repair can then be done as soon as the patient can tolerate it. If possible, however, definitive repair should be done, since recurrent strictures are more likely after the more difficult secondary repairs of the bile ducts.

If the gallbladder and cystic duct are intact, the biliary-enteric bypass to repair a ductal injury also may be done between the gallbladder and jejunum with ligation of the distal and proximal limbs of the damaged common duct. Also, it may be more expedient at times to use a simple loop of jejunum instead of a Roux en Y limb to perform the bypass procedure.

BLUNT TRAUMA

Blunt trauma to the biliary tree deserves separate discussion, not because the surgical management differs, but because of its relative rarity and difficulty of diagnosis. Soderstrom and associates reported that through December 1979, there were 101 patients with gallbladder injuries due to blunt abdominal trauma reported in the English literature. This included 31 patients from their own experience; these 31 patients represented 2.1 percent of 1349 patients who had blunt intraabdominal injuries from 1973 through 1979 at the Maryland Institute for Emergency Medical Services System. The usual mechanism of closed injury to the extrahepatic biliary tree is a shearing force applied to the common duct.

When blunt trauma to the biliary tree is severe enough to result in a free flow of bile into the peritoneal cavity, the characteristic picture of bile peritonitis occurs. According to Sturmer and Wilt, the usual history involves a crushing injury to the right upper quadrant, the epigastrium, or the lower part of the chest, which results in severe pain and may be followed by shock. Bile or nonclotting blood may be found on peritoneal tap or lavage.

Shock is usually secondary to the marked outpouring of extracellular fluid into the peritoneal cavity due to the chemical irritation of the peritoneum by bile. The initial chemical peritonitis caused by bile may be followed shortly after by bacterial peritonitis. If biliary leakage is minimal, shock may be of relatively short duration or may be absent, and abdominal signs initially may be slight. This may be followed by the recovery and well-being of the patient, which may last for periods up to 5 or 10 days. However, the onset of jaundice on about the third day is a fairly constant sign. The appearance of clay-colored stools and the presence of bile in the urine may be noticed from the second to the fifth day after injury of the duct.

Carmichael reported that of 12 deaths due to common duct avulsion, delay in surgical treatment of the 22 survivors following common bile duct avulsion averaged 9 days.

A gradual increase in abdominal size may occur during the first 10 days that may be unattended by the usual signs of peritonitis in patients with bile duct rupture. This increasing abdominal girth is accompanied by progressive signs of extracellular fluid volume deficit and by evidence of infection manifest by fever and leukocytosis. In the reported cases of transection of the common duct, the site of transection was uniformly in the retroduodenal area of the superior margin of the pancreas. This serves to emphasize the importance of extensive medial reflection of the duodenum to explore the retroperitoneal duodenum as well as the distal common duct and pancreas in patients undergoing celiotomy for blunt abdominal trauma.

In reviewing the surgical treatment of the 34 patients reported to have blunt injuries of the common bile duct, Carmichael notes that 9 of the earlier patients were treated by simple external drainage and 7 of these 9 patients died. Of the two survivors of simple drainage, choledochoduodenostomy was required for stricture $2\frac{1}{2}$ months after injury in one and a primary repair of a stricture was done later in the other. Thus, simple drainage is unwise because of the high mortality and high stricture rate associated with this method of treatment. Although many surgeons recommend primary end-to-end repair, three developed strictures and one of these died with cholangitis and cirrhosis. Moreover, T-tube stents were used in the initial repair of the duct in all three of the patients who developed strictures after end-to-end reconstruction. Longmire has stated that primary repair of the common duct should be attempted only if there is an adequate lumen, no inflammation, and a short injured segment of the duct. Carmichael advocates choledochoduodenostomy when the distal duct is unsuitable for primary repair or is missing. Of eight choledochoduodenostomies in his review, all did well except one, who required a cholecystojejunostomy to reestablish bile flow. No duodenal fistulae occurred. Choledochojejunostomy with or without a Roux en Y jejunal limb was done in six patients, and all of these did well. Finally, Carmichael reported that cholecystoenterostomy was done in seven cases, with ligation of the distal bile duct. This operation was associated with one death and two revisions.

Thus, Carmichael concluded that the most successful procedures in reconstruction of the avulsed common bile duct are Roux en Y choledochojejunostomy or choledochoduodenostomy. Choledochojejunostomy offers a better exposure if a future operation is required, a tension-free anastomosis, and a technically easier mucosa-to-mucosa anastomosis. Also, this procedure avoids the lateral duodenal fistula that may occur after choledochoduodenostomy.

The postoperative therapy of biliary tract injuries, in which bile peritonitis is an important complicating feature, should include adequate replacement of extracellular fluid volume deficits, which may require intravenous infusion of several liters of balanced salt solutions in 24 h.

These solutions should be given as soon as possible preoperatively and continued throughout the surgical procedure and postoperatively to avoid extracellular fluid volume deficit. Broad-spectrum antibiotics should be given before the surgical procedure and continued during the operation and postoperatively until the chances of sepsis diminish.

The overall mortality in the collected series of common duct injuries reported by Carmichael was 35 percent; however, the mortality from biliary tract injuries probably should be below 5 to 10 percent if they are discovered early and treated appropriately.

Portal Vein

Approximately 90 percent of portal vein injuries occur because of penetrating trauma. They are frequently associated with other visceral injuries, most commonly to the inferior vena cava, liver, pancreas, and stomach. Mattox and associates reported a survival rate of 50 percent in their series of 22 patients with portal vein injuries. Lateral venorrhaphy, if possible, is the preferred method of treatment. Mattox suggests performing a portacaval or mesocaval shunt as an alternative treatment of portal vein injury if suture repair is impossible and patient's general condition is stable. In contrast, Fish reported that four of five patients who had portacaval shunts for portal vein reconstruction after trauma developed hepatic decompensation or encephalopathy, whereas those complications were not observed in patients undergoing portal vein ligation.

The insertion of an autogenous vein graft to bridge the defect in the portal vein (using the left common iliac vein, left renal vein, or a paneled saphenous vein graft) may be preferable to a portacaval shunt if the patient's condition is stable and the proximal and distal ends of the injured vein are suitable for the insertion of a graft. This procedure should prevent portal hypertension or hepatic deterioration that may occur if the vein is ligated. However, if associated injuries are severe, ligation of the portal vein may make it possible to save the patient. Even though portal vein ligation may cause portal hypertension, interruption of the vein is compatible with patient's survival in about 80 percent of the cases. It should, of course, be emphasized that in those with associated hepatic arterial injuries, a good repair of the hepatic artery must be achieved before accepting treatment of portal vein injuries by ligation. It has been reported recently that 80 percent of 20 patients survived portal vein ligation when lateral venorrhaphy was not possible. However, because of obstruction to portal outflow, acute splanchnic hypervolemia develops simultaneously with peripheral hypovolemia. Patients have died of such splanchnic pooling after portal vein ligation. Since this problem has been appreciated, these patients have been followed closely with either central venous or pulmonary artery pressure measurements to maintain a functionally normal peripheral blood volume. This may require overtransfusions of a volume of blood almost equal to the patient's own normal blood volume.

Pancreas

Ronald C. Jones and G. Tom Shires

Travers described the first pancreatic injury found in an intoxicated woman who was struck by a stage coach wheel in England in 1827. Approximately 70 percent of pancreatic injuries are caused by penetrating and 30 percent result from blunt trauma. Between 1950 and 1985, 500 patients were initially treated for penetrating and blunt pancreatic trauma at Parkland Memorial Hospital (PMH) in Dallas.

DIAGNOSIS. Diagnosis of pancreatic injuries is based upon a complete history, including the mechanism of injury, thorough physical examination, serum amylase level, and adequate visualization of the pancreas at surgical exploration.

Following isolated blunt pancreatic trauma, symptoms are often mild and delayed and physical signs may be absent or minimal. Usually, however, there is at least mild upper abdominal tenderness, but in the absence of a history of significant trauma or severe symptoms, this sign may be overlooked. Injuries to retroperitoneal organs such as the pancreas may not produce clinical findings of loss of bowel sounds, tenderness, guarding, or spasm for several hours.

Computed tomography of the abdomen may become the most specific method of diagnosing organ injury preoperatively, particularly following blunt trauma. It should not take the place of a good physical examination or close follow-up observation.

Serum Amylase Determination. Over 25 years ago, Matthewson and Halter advocated routine serum amylase determinations in patients sustaining blunt trauma and emphasized that pancreatic injury was more common than had been previously appreciated. Serum amylase elevation alone is not an indication for exploratory celiotomy. If signs of peritonitis are present (such as spasm, tenderness, and absent bowel sounds), then a celiotomy is performed. Unrecognized severe pancreatic injury can be a fatal lesion, particularly when it is accompanied by disruption of pancreatic tissue and leakage of pancreatic juice.

Many patients have been found to have an elevated serum amylase level but negative abdominal findings. These patients are closely observed for evidence of peritonitis or until the amylase level returns to normal. An amylase determination is performed on peritoneal lavage fluid, but the elevation is more often due to small bowel injury than to pancreatic injury.

Sometimes the serum amylase is elevated in less than 2 h following injury, but the longer the delay from injury to surgery, the more likely an elevation. A preoperative serum amylase determination was performed in 270 patients in the PMH study. Only 16 percent of the patients had preoperative elevations of serum amylase following penetrating trauma and 61 percent of patients had an elevation following blunt trauma. Even with complete transection of pancreas only 65 percent of the patients had elevated serum amylase levels. Berni noted that the serum amylase level was elevated in two-thirds of their

patients with blunt trauma compared with 10 percent of those with penetrating pancreatic injury. Amylase determinations may be misleading. Olsen stated that 33 percent of patients with hyperamylasemia had no significant intraabdominal trauma, and no patient in his series with hyperamylasemia had significant intraabdominal injury without other evidence of trauma. He reemphasized that hyperamylasemia alone without any other evidence of visceral injury is not an indication for exploratory celiotomy. Serum amylase is not a reliable indicator of pancreatic injury. The serum amylase is indicated as a diagnostic test following blunt trauma but is of no benefit following penetrating trauma and thus is not cost-effective. Though these various reports show that it is unwise to perform exploratory celiotomy on the basis of elevated amylase levels alone, the detection of hyperamylasemia in asymptomatic patients who have sustained abdominal trauma cannot simply be dismissed. These patients are admitted to the hospital and closely observed. Plain abdominal x-ray films may show evidence of retroperitoneal trauma. This is suspected when there is obliteration of the psoas margin, retroperitoneal air along a psoas margin or around the upper pole of the right kidney, or displacement of the stomach.

Since pancreatic injury is relatively uncommon it has been difficult to assess the true value of CT scan in preoperative diagnosis of transection of the pancreatic duct. Cook reported CT findings in 20 patients who subsequently underwent laparotomy or autopsy. In three patients a CT diagnosis of pancreatic contusion or traumatic pseudocyst was surgically proved; in four other patients the CT diagnosis was pancreatic contusion; however, at surgery the pancreas was normal. The CT can document gross pancreatic injury demonstrating parenchymal disruption, focal or diffuse enlargement, and peripancreatic fluid collection. The majority of missed diagnoses is due to unopacified bowel loops adjacent to the pancreas that may be mistaken for focal pancreatic swelling. Peripancreatic hematoma from trauma to the spleen, left kidney, and streak artifacts are other causes for diagnostic errors. Nasogastric tubes should be retracted to the gastroesophageal junction to more readily visualize the pancreas. Jeffrey correctly diagnosed 11 of 13 pancreatic injuries. However, three represented delayed diagnosis with pseudocysts formation. There were two false-negative results in the remaining 10 patients who had pancreatic fractures. Thus, 20 percent of acute pancreatic injuries were missed.

As more experience is gained with endoscopic retrograde pancreatography, it is possible that this technique may have a role in the diagnosis of pancreatic injury. Gougeon advocated transduodenal pancreatography using the fiberoptic duodenoscope intraoperatively to determine ductal injury. Taxier utilized endoscopic retrograde pancreatography to evaluate the pancreas after trauma, but primarily in patients with delayed diagnosis of pancreas injury. Emergency endoscopic retrograde cholangiopancreatography would require expertise and rapid availability to be of value in the critically ill patient.

Surgical Exploration. When preoperative diagnostic

studies indicate a probability of pancreatic injury, it is necessary to visualize the entire pancreas. The head of the pancreas and the duodenum are completely mobilized to the midline by performing a Kocher maneuver. The gastrocolic omentum is also divided in order to enter the lesser sac and view the entire body of the pancreas.

Any retroperitoneal hematoma in the upper part of the abdomen or a peripancreatic hematoma should be considered presumptive evidence of pancreatic injury and should be explored. Over 60 percent of patients sustaining penetrating trauma have an associated retroperitoneal injury, but pancreatic injury occurs in only 20 percent of patients following blunt trauma.

ASSOCIATED INJURIES. Isolated pancreatic injury is rare following penetrating trauma but occurs in 20 percent of blunt injuries. Associated injuries are usually more obvious indications for surgical exploration than suspected pancreatic injury. Death and serious complications are frequent in pancreatic trauma but are rarely caused by the pancreatic injury. Although the pancreas is a vascular organ, it is not often responsible for uncontrollable hemorrhage. When profuse bleeding occurs from the pancreatic area, the pancreas is mobilized and the superior mesenteric and the splenic vessels, the aorta, and the vena cava are inspected, since they are often the source of severe hemorrhage. Because of the location of the pancreas, injuries to the liver and the stomach are frequent following penetrating trauma whereas liver and spleen are more commonly injured following blunt trauma.

MANAGEMENT. Drainage. After bleeding from the pancreas or from adjacent major blood vessels is controlled, the extent of the pancreatic injury is determined. Simple pancreatic contusions without capsular or ductal disruption and without persistent hemorrhage require no suturing or debridement. These injuries are drained with a sump drain placed directly at the site of the pancreatic contusion and brought out along a short, direct tract at the tip of the twelfth rib. The drains are left in place for 10 days, since several patients have been observed to have minimal pancreatic drainage for up to 7 days and then have significant increase in drainage. Lack of drainage to such areas of unrecognized capsular injury may lead to complications associated with intraabdominal collections of pancreatic secretions such as pseudocysts, pancreatic abscesses, and lesser-sac abscesses. Simple drainage is a satisfactory method of management in 75 percent of patients sustaining either stab or gunshot wounds. In the last 100 patients evaluated for septic complications, 9 percent had an associated infection of the drain tract. As a result of this septic complication and intraabdominal abscess formation, closed sump drainage is now utilized in favor of combined Penrose and sump drainage. However, there are few data to support this conclusion.

Fistulae may develop following pancreatic contusion and 4 of the 10 fistulae that drained for greater than 1 month in the PMH series followed contusion injuries.

Distal Pancreatectomy. The most effective method of treatment for pancreatic injuries with obvious disruption of the pancreatic duct in the body or tail of the gland is distal pancreatectomy. This is performed at the point where the main duct is injured, and allows removal of the traumatized and devitalized tissue.

When performing a distal pancreatectomy, sutures are placed in the superior and inferior borders of the pancreas approximately 1.5 to 2 cm from the edge. This, along with isolation of the splenic vessels during distal pancreatectomy, prevents unnecessary blood loss and probably provides better visualization. In resecting the distal pancreas, the cut edge is beveled in a fish-mouth fashion. This enables a better closure of the proximal end of the pancreas. The transected duct of Wirsung in the remaining proximal gland is ligated with a transfixion suture of fine monofilament, nonabsorbable material such as Prolene, to discourage fistula formation. The cut surface of the transected proximal pancreas is oversewn with interrupted, interlocking mattress sutures, which facilitates hemostasis. The auto stapler has been used with excellent results. This method of management provides hemostasis and prevents fistula formation. The stump of the pancreas is extensively drained with a sump drain.

Most patients sustaining a stab or gunshot wound do not require surgical resection. A conservative approach in the absence of proved ductal injury results in a low mortality. Liberal use of resective debridement for only possible ductal injury contributes to a higher mortality. Simple drainage of the pancreas is the treatment of choice for most penetrating injuries, particularly in the unstable patient.

During the past 5 years less than 10 percent of patients at PMH have undergone distal pancreatectomy for penetrating and blunt trauma. Approximately 25 percent of patients undergoing a distal pancreatectomy develop an intraabdominal abscess.

Pseudocysts almost never develop following distal pancreatectomy and sump drainage. Approximately 10 percent of patients managed by distal pancreatectomy die usually secondary to sepsis and associated injuries. One disadvantage to distal pancreatectomy is the frequent iatrogenic associated splenic injury necessitating splenectomy. Patients who are extremely unstable and who have pancreatic injury can always be managed conservatively with drainage alone and if they survive the pancreatic injury can be managed at a later date. Four patients in the PMH series died intraoperatively while undergoing distal pancreatectomy, two of whom could have been managed with drainage. Some patients who initially appear to have pancreatic duct damage may do well with drainage alone, and obviously the suspected ductal injury has not occurred.

The integrity of the pancreatic duct can be determined by opening the duodenum and performing a pancreatogram or performing a distal pancreatectomy with pancreatogram. These diagnostic procedures are rarely indicated, particularly if the duodenum is intact and if the spleen is uninjured. Iatrogenic splenic injury associated with distal pancreatectomy is common. If pancreatic ductal injury is doubtful, simple drainage is performed. In an unstable patient with questionable ductal injury, drainage is the treatment of choice.

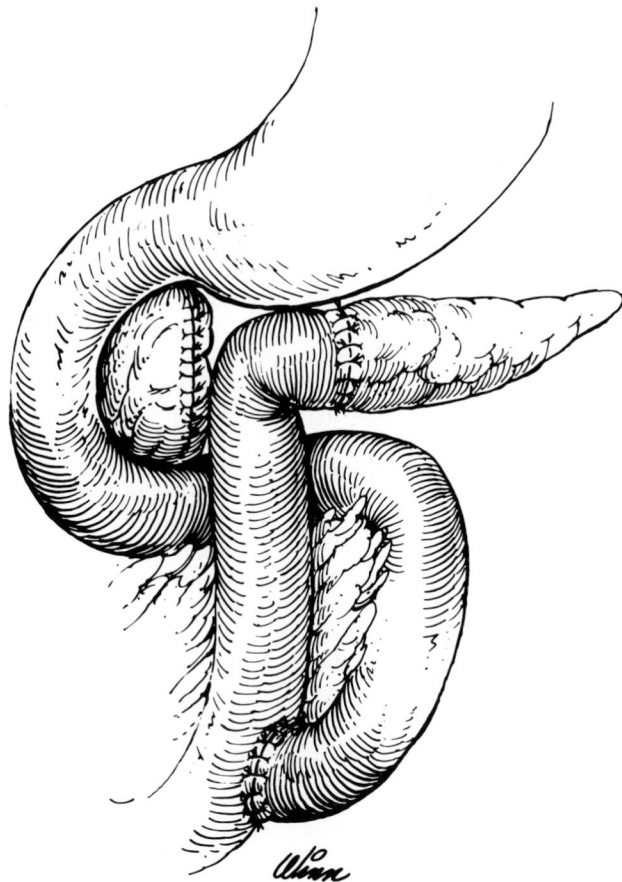

Fig. 6-19. Technique of Roux en Y anastomosis to the transected body of the pancreas.

Roux en Y Pancreaticojejunostomy. Several methods of treating pancreatic transection have been described. For the pancreas completely transected over the superior mesenteric vessels and to the right of these vessels, a Roux en Y anastomosis to the distal pancreas with over-sew of the end of the proximal segment may be used, particularly if the spleen is not injured (Fig. 6-19). This treatment has been recommended by Jones and Shires for treatment of injuries that require removal of 80 percent or more of the pancreas. Transections of less magnitude are treated by simple distal pancreatectomy. This method leaves all functioning pancreatic tissue, thereby avoiding the possibility of pancreatic insufficiency or diabetes. The risk of injury to the underlying splenic vessels is less with this mode of treatment than with resection. The possibility of fistula and pseudocyst formation is also minimized.

The Roux en Y anastomosis is accomplished using permanent sutures placed approximately 1 cm apart in a single-layer anastomosis. Once this anastomosis is accomplished, drainage is established with sump drains. Unless the completely severed pancreatic duct is managed with definitive surgery, a pseudocyst or fistula will almost always result. A Roux en Y anastomosis to one fragment of the severed pancreas is little more time-consuming than resection of the distal fragment, which often requires a splenectomy.

PANCREATIC INSUFFICIENCY. The normal pancreas is approximately 12 to 15 cm in length. Eleven patients in the Parkland Memorial Hospital series required 80 percent or more resection; three of these patients required from 35 to 100 units of insulin per day and an additional three patients had elevated blood sugar levels and abnormal glucose tolerance tests. A twelfth patient underwent a pancreaticoduodenectomy and developed pancreatic insufficiency and blood glucose elevations in excess of 500 mg/dL. Roux en Y drainage is considered only for patients who would otherwise require 80 percent or more resection of the distal pancreas which fortunately is an uncommon injury. Although implantation of both ends of the pancreas is no longer used at PMH, a modification described by Letton and Wilson remains an alternative; pancreaticojejunostomy may not be indicated when there is associated colonic contamination. Several authors have reported pancreatic insufficiency and diabetes as complications of extensive pancreatic resection.

Complete Transection. Approximately two-thirds of the patients with complete transection of the pancreas will have a preoperative elevation of serum amylase. The majority of patients are managed with distal pancreatectomy; however, the occasional patient without splenic trauma can be managed with a Roux en Y anastomosis to the distal portion of the pancreas. This anastomosis is not performed in the presence of colonic contamination or if the pancreas has poor consistency and will not securely hold sutures. If the surgeon is not accustomed to pancreatic anastomosis, a distal pancreatectomy may be a wiser choice.

Isolated Pancreatic Injuries. Isolated pancreatic injuries occurred in over 20 percent of patients sustaining blunt trauma in the PMH series and none died, although six had complete transections. There were eight penetrating injuries and none of these patients died. This supports the conclusion that pancreatic injury is rarely the cause of death.

Combined Duodenum and Pancreatic Injuries. Over 20 percent of penetrating pancreatic injuries are associated with duodenal trauma, but less than 10 percent of blunt injuries have duodenal trauma. The mortality for combined pancreaticoduodenal trauma is 20 percent, mostly from associated injuries, but excluding intraoperative deaths the mortality is only 15 percent.

These injuries are usually managed by drainage of the pancreas and suture of the duodenum. A duodenostomy tube may be inserted, but it is difficult to demonstrate that this decreases morbidity or mortality. Duodenal fistula following duodenostomy tube insertion was higher than without duodenostomy, but more severe injuries were treated with a duodenostomy tube.

Pyloric exclusion has been used by Vaughan resulting in only a 5 percent duodenal fistula rate. Berne diverticulization has been advocated for moderately severe injuries and pancreaticoduodenectomy for the most extensive injuries. Most patients in the PMH series with combined pancreaticoduodenal injuries treated with

Berne diverticularization have had major complications, such as duodenal, biliary, and pancreatic fistula with sepsis and death. Indications for Berne diverticulization have not been clearly delineated. Pyloric exclusion is a simpler and less time-consuming operation and prevents duodenal fistula formation.

Pancreaticoduodenectomy. Pancreaticoduodenectomy has been reported as a method of management in approximately 120 patients in over 30 series in the literature with a mortality rate of 30 percent following penetrating injuries and over 20 percent following blunt trauma for a combined mortality rate of 25 percent. Strict indications for pancreaticoduodenectomy include combined pancreaticoduodenal injuries in which the duodenum cannot be repaired or is not viable or there is uncontrollable hemorrhage from the pancreas. In the presence of colonic injuries, intraabdominal abscess is frequent. Prior to performing a pancreaticoduodenectomy the presence of a pancreatic ductal injury should be verified. With duodenal rupture cannulation of the pancreatic duct with pancreatogram is easily performed. An alternative method of determining ductal injury is by mobilizing the tail of the pancreas and performing a pancreatogram through the distal pancreatic duct. Hemostatic sutures are placed 2 cm into the superior and inferior portions of the pancreas prior to incising the tail. The common duct is identified and proved to be intact by operative cholangiogram or by passing a catheter through the common duct and into the duodenum. If the common bile duct and major duct system are intact and the duodenal injury can be closed, a pancreaticoduodenectomy is not indicated. Avulsion of the common duct from the duodenum with avascular duodenal wall, and stellate fracture with bleeding from a crushing injury of the head of the pancreas may be indications for pancreaticoduodenectomy. The overall condition of the patient and associated injuries must be considered prior to submitting the patient to several more hours of surgery. There are times when this procedure is necessary, but they are rare, particularly if the duodenum is intact. Complications following pancreaticoduodenectomy are common. Thus mortality rate of this procedure must be low to justify its use if any other form of management can be employed.

In addition to fistula formation and abscesses, marginal ulceration with upper gastrointestinal bleeding has occurred following pancreaticoduodenectomy in which a vagotomy or subtotal gastric resection was not performed. Symptoms of dumping, diabetes, and weight loss with diarrhea have occurred following pancreaticoduodenectomy for trauma. Postoperative bleeding into the intestinal tract from the pancreaticojejunostomy requiring reoperation has been reported.

COMPLICATIONS. Complications following pancreatic trauma include fistula, pancreatic abscesses, vascular necrosis with hemorrhage from the drain site, pseudocyst formation, and intestinal fistula secondary to suture line breakdown from pancreatic juice activation.

Fistula. Most pancreatic fistulae are minor and close within a period of 1 month. Major pancreatic fistulae have been arbitrarily defined as those which drain longer than 1 month. The frequency of pancreatic fistulae depends on definition, and the rate is higher if defined as drainage for 1 week rather than 1 month. The serum amylase level is frequently elevated while the fistula is present, probably because of transperitoneal absorption. Almost all pancreatic fistulae will eventually spontaneously close; therefore, treatment is conservative. Attention must be given to preventing autodigestion of the surrounding skin.

Many patients with pancreatic fistulae can continue oral intake of food, especially if the fistula drains less than 500 mL each day and the volume does not increase significantly when the patient eats. In the presence of large-volume pancreatic fistulae, it is preferable to institute intravenous hyperalimentation. Intravenous hyperalimentation has two beneficial effects on such patients: (1) It maintains excellent nutrition and nitrogen balance without stimulating the pancreas, as do oral feedings; and (2) intravenous hyperalimentation can significantly reduce the volume of pancreatic exocrine secretion by one-half or more.

Pseudocyst. A pancreatic pseudocyst is a false cyst the wall of which is inflammatory fibrous tissue that does not contain epithelium but is made of those structures surrounding the region of the pancreas in the retroperitoneum. The most frequent symptoms associated with a pancreatic pseudocyst are an abdominal mass, pain, nausea, and vomiting. The serum amylase level may be elevated for a long time prior to this diagnosis. Diagnosis is by sonography or computed tomography. The pseudocyst rarely spontaneously resolves. Pancreatic pseudocyst is now a rare complication following pancreatic trauma if the pancreas has been explored and managed appropriately, such management including adequate drainage. The preferred method of draining pancreatic pseudocysts is internally by either cyst gastrostomy or Roux en Y cyst jejunostomy.

Sepsis. Intraabdominal abscess is a common complication following multiple abdominal trauma and is the second most common cause of death. Although pancreatic fistulae rarely cause death, they occasionally give rise to lesser-sac abscesses and subphrenic abscess. Subphrenic abscess is frequently associated with injuries to the liver, spleen, and colon. The location of a right or left subdiaphragmatic abscess is predictable in most patients depending on whether the associated injury was to the spleen or to the liver. A lesser-sac abscess may contribute to either sepsis or retroperitoneal bleeding and death. In almost all patients in whom the pancreatic injury contributes to death, there is association with severe sepsis. Sepsis usually is associated with duodenal and colonic fistula, renal failure, and occasionally pulmonary embolus. Cultures of the abscess grow a predominance of mixed gram-negative organisms: however, staphylococci and enterococci may be present. The serum amylase level is not consistently elevated in patients with a pancreatic or lesser-sac abscess. The method of management of pancreatic abscess consists of adequate debridement and drainage, frequently with gastrostomy and feeding jejunostomy.

Hemorrhagic pancreatitis may present with massive

Table 6-6. PANCREATIC TRAUMA, 1950–1984

	Pt	*Died*	*Mortality, %*
Penetrating			
Stab	76	4	5
Gunshot	252	55	22
Shotgun	34	19	56
Blunt	138	26	19
Total	500	104	21

SOURCE: Jones RC: Management of pancreatic trauma. *Am J Surg* 150:698, 1985, with permission.

bleeding from the drain tract, probably from erosion of ligated retroperitoneal vessels.

Mortality. The mortality rate caused by pancreatic injury is variable and is chiefly related to hemorrhage from major blood vessels. The mortality following stab wounds is 5 percent, gunshot wounds 22 percent, and blunt trauma 19 percent (Table 6-6).

Recognition of pancreatic injury at the time of initial surgical exploration is the key to decreasing the morbidity rate of pancreatic injury. It is best accomplished by opening the lesser sac through the gastrocolic ligament and directly visualizing the pancreas. There are several reasons why the pancreatic injury appears not to be the cause of death. The mortality for isolated pancreatic injury is less than 1 percent. Patients developing shock following injury have a 40 percent mortality in association with pancreatic trauma whereas the normotensive patient with pancreatic injury had a 4 percent mortality, and no patient with an isolated pancreatic injury in the PMH series died. The mortality rate due to the pancreatic injury in the multiply injured patient is less than 3 percent.

SUMMARY. The majority of patients who sustain pancreatic injury can be managed with sump drainage including most with gunshot wounds to the head of the pancreas. Pancreaticoduodenectomy may be indicated in 2 to 3 percent. Patients who require resection of 80 percent or more of the pancreas and do not have splenic injuries should be considered for a Roux en Y anastomosis to the distal pancreas after ductal injury has been proved. The severity of injury often dictates the appropriate treatment. A conservative approach is indicated for most pancreatic injuries, resulting in shorter operating time and less blood loss in the unstable patient with multiple injuries. Most important is identification of ductal injury at the initial operation and institution of surgical drainage.

Spleen

The spleen is the abdominal organ most frequently injured by blunt trauma: such injuries to the spleen represent approximately one-quarter of all blunt injuries of the abdominal viscera. The spleen also is often injured by penetrating abdominal trauma and is frequently associated with blunt and penetrating thoracoabdominal injuries.

DIAGNOSIS. The diagnosis of splenic injury is usually easily made with penetrating trauma but is often more difficult in patients sustaining blunt trauma. The clinical manifestations are the systemic symptoms and signs of hemorrhage and local evidence of peritoneal irritation in the region of the spleen. Only about 30 to 40 percent of patients with splenic injury present with a systolic blood pressure below 100 mmHg. However, many patients with splenic trauma may develop hypotension and tachycardia when assuming the sitting position. A tender abdomen with guarding and distention is apparent in only about 50 to 60 percent of those patients with splenic rupture.

A history of injury, which may be seemingly slight, followed by abdominal pain, predominantly in the left upper quadrant, left shoulder pain, and syncope is very significant. Often the left shoulder pain, or Kehr's sign, occurs only when the patient is in a supine or head-down position. This is caused by irritation of the inferior surface of the left side of the diaphragm by free blood or blood clots. Elevation of the foot of the bed or pressure in the left subcostal region may occasionally reproduce pain at the top of the left shoulder. Ballance's sign, which refers to fixed dullness to percussion in the left flank and dullness in the right flank that disappears on change of position of the patient, thus indicating large quantities of clot in the perisplenic region and free blood in the remainder of the peritoneal cavity, may be helpful in establishing the diagnosis. Whereas a decreased or falling hematocrit, leukocytosis of more than 15,000, x-ray findings such as fractures of the left lower ribs, gastric displacement, loss of splenic outline, and splinting or elevation of the left diaphragm are useful diagnostic findings, they are frequently absent.

Abdominal paracentesis and diagnostic peritoneal lavage are extremely helpful in establishing the diagnosis in doubtful cases, particularly in patients whose sensibility is obtunded by other injuries. In patients with splenic trauma the incidence of false-negative diagnostic peritoneal lavage is reported, in repeated series, to be less than 1 percent.

Radionuclide scans are occasionally used to detect splenic injury and to follow patients who are treated by either nonoperative therapy or one of the many splenic preservation procedures. Computerized tomography is now a preferable procedure and has essentially replaced the nuclear scans for this purpose as a diagnostic aid. It is an accurate, simple way to diagnose subcapsular hematomas and more extensive transcapsular lacerations. Jeffrey et al. reported correct interpretation in 49 of the first 50 patients studied with 28 true-negatives and 21 of 22 true-positives being identified.

Delayed rupture of the spleen was first described by Baudet in 1902, and the asymptomatic interval between abdominal injury and rupture of the spleen is known as the latent period of Baudet. It was postulated that bleeding appeared several days after injury because (1) a subcapsular splenic hematoma gradually increased in size until it caused a delayed rupture of the splenic capsule and intraperitoneal hemorrhage or (2) there was initial bleeding from a splenic laceration that ceased spontaneously but began again in several days or weeks when the perisplenic hematoma became dislodged. This concept has been challenged by Olsen and Polley and by Benjamin and associates. These authors report a rate of delayed rupture of the spleen of less than 1 percent in over 600 patients. They suggest that delayed splenic rupture is an unusual occurrence and that the 15 percent incidence reported in older papers actually represents a delay in diagnosis rather than a delayed rupture in those patients.

TREATMENT. King and Shumacker in 1952 reported that all five patients under six months who had splenectomies developed meningitis or overwhelming septicemia. Two of these five patients died. This observation stimulated further investigation followed by considerable confusion and contradictory remarks into the relationship between splenectomy and what was later termed overwhelming postsplenectomy infection (OPSI). This syndrome is characterized by an abrupt onset of overwhelming sepsis, massive bacteremia, usually pneumococcal, followed by early death.

Eraklis and Filler reported a mortality rate of 0.8 percent in 342 patients under age sixteen who had splenectomy for trauma. Singer reviewed 23 series from the literature including 2795 patients. The risk of sepsis was 1.45 percent in the 688 patients (300 adults) who had splenectomy for trauma. Only four of these patients died for a mortality rate of 0.58 percent. This has been compared with the general population where a death rate due to sepsis is estimated at 0.01 percent. This comparison is not accurate as the two groups are dissimilar by virtue of the fact the former group have all sustained some type of trauma and undergone an operative procedure that is not accounted for in the control group.

O'Neal and McDonald reported a mortality rate of 2.7 percent in a series of 356 adult patients. There were no fatalities in the 115 patients with splenectomy for trauma. All of the deaths in the series occurred in patients whose spleen was removed in conjunction with other nontraumatic elective procedures or patients with proved malignancies.

The literature supporting this syndrome in the adult trauma patient is increasing but still is not as convincing as for pediatric and nontrauma patients. Nevertheless, stimulated by these and many other reports describing the immunologic abnormalities and pathophysiology of the overwhelming sepsis syndrome, a more conservative approach has evolved concerning the management of splenic trauma. Nonoperative therapy in the pediatric age group has been advocated by Aronson et al., Ein et al., and others. This approach has several distressing aspects. In assessing the patient with multiple trauma one cannot assume the spleen is the only injured organ; hence other injuries may be missed in as many as 30 percent of patients. Nonoperative therapy requires a prolonged hospitalization that is generally accomplished in an intensive care unit. Other drawbacks include a prolonged convalescence, increased hospital cost, and risk and complications associated with repeated blood transfusions, such as delayed autoimmune disease.

Based upon an extensive review of the literature, Luna

and Dellinger concluded that the 1 to 2 percent incidence figures for postsplenectomy infection represented a 10- to 20-fold overestimation of the true incidence. These authors quoted a 60 percent success rate in three series of nonoperative observation in adults who were initially stable without evidence of blood loss. Ninety-three percent of the patients who failed nonoperative management required a splenectomy, suggesting that splenic salvage rates were not improved by nonoperative observation when the initial injury was felt to be relatively minor.

Luna further states it has been estimated that 35 to 40 percent of patients who are successfully observed will require a blood transfusion that averages 40 to 50 percent of their blood volume. Although symptoms may occur in only 50 percent of patients with non-A non-B hepatitis and only 20 percent become icteric, it is estimated that the per unit risk for a single unit transfusion may approach 3 percent. The posttransfusion hepatitis death rate per unit of blood transfused is 0.14 percent.

Proper management of patients with splenic injuries is still controversial, and continued reevaluation of data is necessary. It is possible that failure of nonoperative therapy frequently results in splenectomy rather than splenorraphy (the preferable procedure) and the increased incidence of blood transfusion with its attendant disease transmission problems may outweigh any theoretic advantages of avoiding surgery. Luna and Dellinger also concluded that in adults 0.26 percent of the observed patients die (0.17 percent for pediatric patients) compared with 0.06 percent for those operated upon initially.

A more rational approach to the problem is splenic preservation in carefully selected patients at the time of operation. The procedures include (1) no therapy for nonbleeding capsular lacerations, (2) application of microfibrillar collagen or other hemostatic agents to minor lacerations with minimal bleeding, (3) suture repair of more extensive injuries, (4) partial splenectomy for splenic injuries that do not involve the hilus. Contraindications to splenic salvage procedures as recommended by Traub include (1) patient instability secondary to major associated injuries, (2) splenic avulsion or extensive fragmentation, (3) extensive hilar vascular injury, (4) failure to attain splenic hemostasis. Relative contraindications include significant peritoneal contamination from concomitant bowel injury and rupture of a diseased spleen.

Increasing experimental data and clinical evidence indicate that an intact spleen is required to produce important opsonic antibodies that are necessary for optimal function of the macrophage system and production of immunoglobulins. Sepsis is a rather frequent occurrence following splenectomy for certain hematologic disorders, many of which have diffuse reticuloendothelial abnormalities. Many of these patients, however, receive various forms of therapy that alter immunity and response to infection. Splenectomy is still a safe procedure and the indicated procedure of choice in many patients.

OPERATIVE TECHNIQUE (See Chap. 33). Although drainage of the splenic bed following elective splenectomy is controversial, there is little question that drainage should be employed when splenectomy is performed under most emergency conditions. The incidence of drain tract infections and subphrenic abscess has been reported to be as high as 25 to 50 percent when drains were used, in contrast to 5 to 12 percent when drains were not employed. Many of these infections, however, were related to the presence of associated injuries, usually in the gastrointestinal tract, or to the immunologic defects often present in patients requiring splenectomies for conditions other than trauma, and not to the drains per se. The routine use of drains following splenectomy for trauma is supported by the series reported by Naylor and Shires. These authors reported an incidence of subphrenic abscess of only 3.4 percent in 408 patients undergoing splenectomy for trauma. Among the 72 patients who had splenectomy for trauma involving the spleen alone, there were no subphrenic abscesses and an incidence of drain tract infection of only 1.3 percent. Thus, while it cannot be proved that drainage of the splenic bed after splenectomy for trauma reduces the incidence of subphrenic collections, it is most probable that drainage in such cases does not increase the incidence of subphrenic abscess. Also in those instances of splenic injury in which there is any question of associated pancreatic or gastric trauma, drainage of the splenic bed may prevent complications that could arise if such unrecognized injuries were not drained. Even those authors who incriminate the usage of splenic bed drains report no higher incidence of subphrenic abscess or other infections if the drains are removed before the sixth postsplenectomy day.

Another area of controversy is the issue of prophylactic antibiotics in the postsplenectomized patient, particularly in the pediatric age group. Most authors advocate prophylactic penicillin therapy until at least age five years, but it has been recommended that protection be extended into the teenage years, and isolated reports suggest indefinite protection. The use of long-term antibiotics is not without untoward effects, such as drug sensitivity, bacterial resistance, and suppression of natural immunologic defenses. Patient compliance over a long period of time is very poor. Patients who have undergone splenectomy are advised to contact their physician at the first sign of any febrile illness.

Pneumococcal vaccination is recommended following splenectomy. This should protect against 80 to 85 percent of the pneumococcal strains leading to sepsis. It must be stressed, however, that although pneumococcus is the most prevalent offending organism, the syndrome can be caused by other organisms such as meningococcus and *Haemophilus influenzae*. Currently there are no recommendations for a second or booster dose of pneumococcal vaccine. Asplenic patients should be considered immunocompromised, receive close follow-up, and be instructed about the potential risks of the asplenic state.

MORTALITY. Factors contributing to mortality following splenic injury include (1) associated injury, (2) mechanism of injury, (3) presence of shock on admission to hospital, and (4) advanced age. Naylor and associates reported an overall mortality rate of 11.2 percent in their series of 408 patients, which compares favorably with that in other reports.

Retroperitoneal Hematoma

The management of traumatic retroperitoneal hematoma is a controversial problem. The most common cause of retroperitoneal hemorrhage, according to Baylis et al. and according to the experience at Parkland Memorial Hospital, is pelvic fracture, which accounts for about 60 percent of all traumatic retroperitoneal hematomas. The diagnosis of retroperitoneal hematoma is most difficult following blunt, nonpenetrating trauma to the abdomen, and should be suspected in any patient following trauma who has signs and symptoms of hemorrhagic shock but no obvious source of hemorrhage. Hemorrhage within the retroperitoneal area may be massive and may exceed 2000 mL of blood. Experimental data have shown that as much as 4000 mL of fluid can extravasate into the retroperitoneal space under pressure equal to that in the pelvic vessels.

DIAGNOSIS. Abdominal pain occurs in approximately 60 percent of patients, and back pain in about 25 percent. The abdominal pain is usually vague and generalized but is occasionally localized over the hematoma. Local or generalized tenderness is present in about two-thirds of the patients, and shock occurs in approximately 40 percent. Occasionally, a tender mass is palpable through the abdomen or in the flanks, and in some cases, rectal examination will reveal a boggy mass anterior or posterior to the rectum. Dullness to percussion over the flanks or the abdomen that does not vary with changing positions of the patient has been recorded in some instances. At times, discoloration of the flanks from retroperitoneal hemorrhage has been noted after the lapse of a few hours (Grey Turner's sign). Progressive decreases in the hemoglobin and hematocrit is a consistent finding, and hematuria is found in 80 percent of patients. Hematuria may represent the first clue to the development of a retroperitoneal hematoma.

Somewhat more than half the patients produce free, nonclotting blood on diagnostic paracentesis or lavage of the abdomen; this blood is generally related to the presence of both retroperitoneal and intraabdominal hemorrhage. However, if the retroperitoneal hematoma that occurs without intraperitoneal hemorrhage is large enough to yield a so-called false-positive peritoneal tap or lavage from retroperitoneal hemorrhage alone, then the hematoma itself may require abdominal exploration to search for the persistent source of the retroperitoneal bleeding. If a large pelvic hematoma is suspected, special care should be taken when performing lavage so as not to inadvertently enter the hematoma, which may cause significant and difficult to control hemorrhage.

Radiography, according to Baylis et al., has been valuable in several respects; approximately two-thirds of the patients with peritoneal hematoma have had fractures of the pelvis, and other x-ray findings have included obliteration of the psoas shadow in 30 percent, abdominal mass in 5 percent, and paralytic ileus in 8 percent. Also, displaced bowel-gas shadows and fractured vertebrae have been noted. Intravenous pyelograms and/or retrograde cystograms are generally obtained in patients with sus-

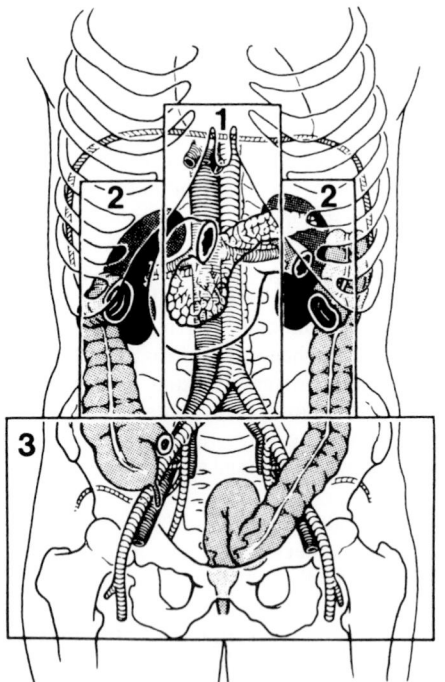

Fig. 6-20. Retroperitoneal classification. Zone 1 = central-medial retroperitoneal hematomas. Zone 2 = flank retroperitoneal hematomas. Zone 3 = pelvic retroperitoneal hematomas. [From: *Sheldon GF: Retroperitoneal hematoma, in Blaisdell WF, Trunkey DD (eds): Abdominal Trauma. New York, Thieme-Stratton, 1982, p·281, with permission.*]

pected retroperitoneal hematomas, if the patient's condition is stable. Arteriography and CT scan may be helpful in establishing the diagnosis of retroperitoneal injury. In the patient whose condition is deteriorating, however, immediate exploration is performed without obtaining such studies, in order to attempt rapid control of progressive bleeding. Many retroperitoneal hematomas from pelvic fractures will tamponade themselves within a short time, and the patient's condition will remain stable.

TREATMENT. One of the most frequently debated areas of abdominal surgery is that of the proper management of retroperitoneal injuries. The major controversy centers around the question of whether to open and explore retroperitoneal hematomas depending upon the anatomic location. The retroperitoneum has been divided into three areas in an attempt to clarify the various problems encountered (Fig. 6-20). Area 1 is the upper central area and extends from the diaphragmatic hiatus to the sacral promontory. Area 2 consists of the right and left flank, and area 3 consists of the pelvis.

The decision to open the hematoma is dependent upon several considerations. These include the wounding mechanism, the location, and the intraoperative evaluation of the size of the hematoma. There is general agreement that all penetrating injuries should be explored as well as all hematomas in the central medial area from the hiatus to the sacrum (area 1).

Injuries located in the flanks (area 2) are frequently individualized. The most common injury in this area is the

kidney, renovascular pedicle, and posterior colon. Once again, penetrating injuries in this area should be explored. Patients with blunt trauma are often managed selectively. If the evaluation of the kidney has been unremarkable, including an arteriogram, and the hematoma is lateral or contained in Gerota's fascia and not expanding, many authors recommend nonexploration. If, however, the hematoma is expanding or large and the preoperative evaluation is incomplete or inconclusive, it is best to investigate this area of potential injury. Prior to opening Gerota's fascia, it is extremely important to gain control of the renal artery and vein so that if massive hemorrhage is encountered the surgeon will be in a position to control it. If there is any question of a hematoma around the large bowel, it must be completely explored.

Large retroperitoneal hematomas that are located deep in the pelvis (area 3) and associated with pelvis fractures are best not explored. It is important to be certain there is no injury to the distal aorta, iliac vessels, or takeoff of the internal iliac vessels. If major vessels are not explored at the time that hematomas occur near them, major and sometimes fatal postoperative bleeding may occur. Present-day vascular surgical techniques obviate the fear of incurring massive hemorrhage as a contraindication to exploring retroperitoneal hematomas.

Ligation of one or both hypogastric arteries may, at times, control persistent bleeding in the pelvic retroperitoneal space from pelvic fractures that cannot be controlled by any other means. Certainly it is preferable to locate a single vessel that is bleeding and either ligate or repair it. Selective arteriography, either intraoperatively or in the x-ray department, and infusion of vasospastic drugs or the embolization of autologous clots or hemostatic agents may be beneficial in controlling this type of hemorrhage. On rare occasions it may be necessary to pack the pelvis with large lap packs for 24 to 48 h in order to achieve hemostasis.

Inferior Vena Cava

Inferior vena caval injuries associated with penetrating abdominal wounds are being seen with increasing frequency. It has been reported that 1 in every 50 gunshot wounds and 1 in every 300 knife wounds of the abdomen will injure the vena cava. These are serious injuries: one-third of the patients die before reaching the hospital, and up to half the remaining persons will die during hospitalization. Most deaths occur from bleeding because of the inherent difficulties in controlling injuries of large veins, but significant wounds of other structures, especially in the retroperitoneum, are common and often adversely affect therapeutic efforts.

ETIOLOGY AND DISTRIBUTION. Most injuries of the inferior vena cava are caused by gunshot wounds, but stab wounds or blunt trauma may also be involved (Table 6-7). Simple penetrating wounds produced by knives and low-velocity missiles are less lethal than those wounds caused by shotguns, high-velocity bullets, and especially blunt trauma. Widespread serious damage to other structures, particularly liver and major arteries and veins, are likely

Table 6-7. CAUSES OF INFERIOR VENA CAVAL
INJURIES

	Total	Died	Mortality, %
Bullet	69	23	33
Shotgun	8	6	75
Stab	12	2	17
Blunt	12	11	92
Total	101	42	42

to result from shotgun wounds and blunt trauma to the abdomen and lower part of the chest.

The infrarenal vena cava is most susceptible and most often injured (Table 6-8). The level of injury is a major determinant of survival, and injuries of the suprarenal, intrahepatic vena cava are extremely dangerous, especially when accompanied by wounds of hepatic and renal veins. Difficulties in exposure and control are invariably encountered, and adjunctive measures are often necessary.

DIAGNOSIS. Injuries of the inferior vena cava should be considered in all cases of penetrating wounds of the abdomen and lower part of the chest. Because of the vagaries of the trajectory of bullets, innocent-appearing small-caliber wounds may produce serious damage to retroperitoneal structures, without intraabdominal organ injury. Patients who have suffered stab wounds of the back or lower part of the chest may also harbor unsuspected caval injuries.

One of the major determinants of survival of these patients is the presence of hemorrhagic shock on admission. This is often a clue that despite the absence of identifying physical findings, major vascular injuries are present. Hemoperitoneum, hemothorax, subcutaneous blood staining from retroperitoneal bleeding, and evidence of distal vena caval obstruction may be helpful in diagnosis.

Except for direct venous studies with contrast media, radiographic examination is rarely specific. Routine x-ray studies, including anteroposterior and lateral films of the chest and abdomen, are useful and are recommended, but in a patient in unstable condition these should be obtained in the operating room as preparations for surgery are in progress. It is usually best not to delay surgery for elaborate studies if firm indications for exploration exist.

TREATMENT. As alluded to in the discussion of other vascular injuries, associated injuries are common and are a major factor in survival of these patients (Table 6-9).

Table 6-8. LOCATION OF INFERIOR VENA
CAVAL INJURY

	Total	Died	Mortality, %
Above renal veins	19	11	58
At renal vein level	21	13	62
Below renal veins	47	14	30
Bifurcation	14	4	29

Table 6-9. INJURIES ASSOCIATED WITH
INFERIOR VENA CAVAL INJURY

Aorta, iliac artery	13	Kidney	21
Major splanchnic vessel	26	Pancreas	18
Renal artery or vein	20	Spleen	10
Liver	46	Colon	27
Duodenum	27	Other	21

Prior to exploration, resuscitation and attention to other problems often are important. An adequate airway must be obtained, volume and blood deficits repaired, and fractures stabilized. Vena caval injuries that require clamping may reduce the effectiveness of using lower-extremity veins for fluid administration, and at least one large-bore catheter should be placed into the upper-extremity venous system. This line is best reserved for blood and fluid administration and should not be used for primary anesthetic manipulations.

Thoracotomy may be required, especially in patients with suprarenal caval injuries. If transatrial intracaval shunts are needed, a median sternotomy offers good exposure for this maneuver as well as for control of associated hepatic injuries.

Abdominal exploration is performed through a midline incision that can be extended as required, and median sternotomy can be added if necessary. Rapid abdominal exploration will usually expose major injuries and establish priorities of repair. It is usually wise to control the bleeding, pause, and complete volume and blood restoration before definitive repairs are begun. Attempts to complete bowel repairs while bleeding persists from other injuries often extend the hypotensive episode and increase blood loss.

Centrally located retroperitoneal hematomas above the pelvis often harbor significant injuries, and usually are explored. Damage to other retroperitoneal structures is common (79 percent) and not always evident without formal exploration. The size or stability of the hematoma does not offer reliable evidence as to the presence or absence of significant injuries. Continued bleeding from the vena caval injury, however, is ominous. Patients actively bleeding at the time of operation have a very high mortality rate, especially if the vena caval injury is at or above the renal arteries and veins (Table 6-10).

Initial control of bleeding can usually be obtained with pressure and packs. Occasionally temporary occlusion of the abdominal aorta at the diaphragmatic hiatus is useful in reducing blood loss from high caval injuries. Exposure

Table 6-10. RELATIONSHIP OF BLEEDING AND
MORTALITY FROM INFERIOR VENA CAVAL
INJURIES

	Total	Died	Mortality, %
Active bleeding	41	32	78
Tamponade	57	9	16
Not specified	3	0	0

Simple Anterior
Repair

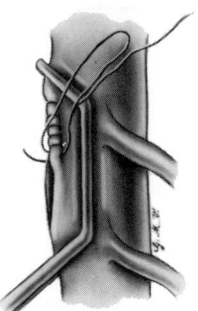

Fig. 6-21. Repair of anterior laceration of the inferior vena cava. Note the use of a partially occlusive clamp.

Anterior and Posterior Rotation Repair
Repair

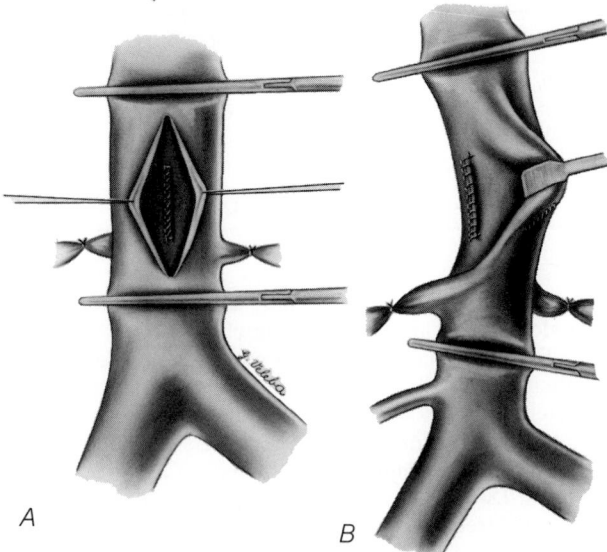

A   *B*

Fig. 6-22. Repair of through-and-through injury to the inferior vena cava. *A.* Anterior laceration is enlarged to permit closure of the posterior wall from within the lumen. *B.* Rotation of the posteroinferior vena cava.

of the inferior vena cava is obtained by reflecting medially the right colon, duodenum, and pancreas. Direct tamponade, manually or with sponge sticks, is usually effective in controlling bleeding. Simple lacerations or punctures are most common, but transections, avulsion, or multiple lacerations may be encountered, and control may be very difficult in the last group.

Simple lacerations can be controlled with gentle digital pressure and sutured by simply passing the needle under the occluding finger. In some cases the edge of the wound can be held gently in apposition with vascular forceps or blunt Allis clamps while repair is effected. Balloon catheter tamponade has also been employed for control of these wounds. Partial occlusion with vascular clamps is a useful technique and can be instituted after the initial use of other maneuvers (Fig. 6-21). These simple tangential wounds usually can be repaired without injury to lumbar veins, but occasionally ligation of gonadal and lumbar tributaries is required (Fig. 6-22).

Transections may be repaired by end-to-end vascular surgical techniques after mobilizing the vena cava. If there are multiple caval wounds requiring complicated repairs, or if repair poses an undue risk in a patient with multiple injuries, infrarenal ligation is preferable. In most cases construction of venous grafts is not required, and the time and effort necessary to perform these repairs may increase the operative morbidity and mortality.

Wounds at or above the renal veins are difficult to expose and repair. If bleeding from behind the liver is encountered and is not easily identified as coming from a laceration of the anterior cava wall below the caudate lobe, an intracaval shunt may be needed. The liver can be rotated medially after division of supporting ligaments, and if intrahepatic vena cava or combined hepatic vein lacerations are present, the shunt can be inserted as described by Schrock et al. The transatrial approach is easier than inserting the shunt from the intrarenal vena cava, and is very useful in managing these extremely dangerous wounds. A large chest tube (34 to 38 F tube) with a proximal side hole is inserted through the atrial appendage, and the tip is placed near the orifices of the renal veins. Umbilical tapes encircling the inferior vena cava within the

pericardium and above the renal veins secure the catheter. The side hole in the catheter is placed at a level to permit the return of blood via the tube into the right atrium. This shunt, occasionally combined with temporary occlusion of the portal triad, will usually allow sufficient control of bleeding to effect repairs. This technique is rarely required.

Unlike injuries of the infrarenal cava, most wounds above the renal veins should be repaired. Ligation of the inferior vena cava at this level produces serious complications. Some survivors have been reported, and those were usually in operations uncomplicated by hypotension, shock, or multiple injuries.

Those vascular procedures used in other areas are effective in repairing the suprarenal vena cava. Simple venorrhaphy often may suffice, but patch graft angioplasty or anastomosis may be needed (Fig. 6-23). If graft interposition is required, autogenous venous grafts obtained from the infrarenal cava or iliac vein are preferred (Fig. 6-24). Concomitant repair of hepatic vein injuries can be effected, but in some cases ligation may be preferable.

These repairs can usually be completed within 30 min, a period of ischemia well tolerated by the normothermic liver. Regional hypothermia may be induced with iced saline solution by irrigation techniques, thus conferring further protection of the liver during more prolonged ischemia.

COMPLICATIONS. In patients with isolated wounds of the inferior vena cava, repair is usually effective and complications are few. In these patients, two episodes of ileofemoral venous thrombosis have been encountered,

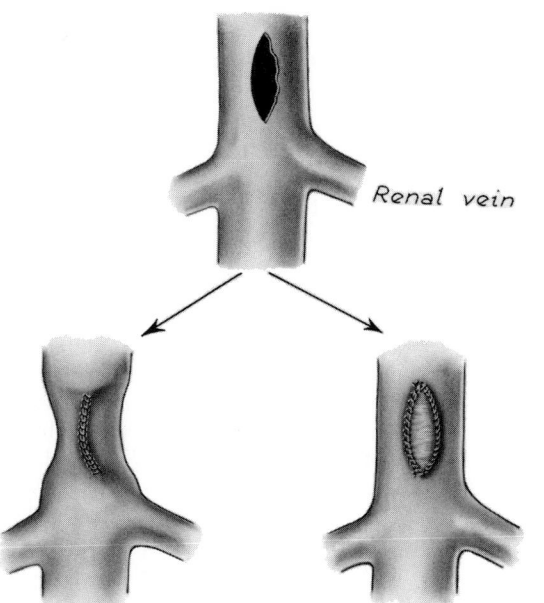

Fig. 6-23. Repair of the inferior vena cava using a patch graft to prevent stenosis.

and an additional patient had a pulmonary embolus. Pancreatitis has also been encountered, and recurrent retroperitoneal bleeding occurred in one patient.

The mortality in patients with isolated inferior vena caval injuries was 11 percent in the present series, but 67 percent of the patients with one or more major vessel injuries died. All the patients with inferior vena caval wounds at or above the renal veins had significant associated injuries, usually liver and bowel, occasionally pancreas, stomach, and lung. The mortality is high in this group of patients, especially if the inferior vena cava is actively bleeding at surgery.

Female Reproductive Organs

Injuries to the female reproductive organs are infrequently seen following either blunt or penetrating trauma

Fig. 6-24. Interposition of an excised segment of the infrarenal inferior vena cava to establish continuity of the suprarenal inferior vena cava.

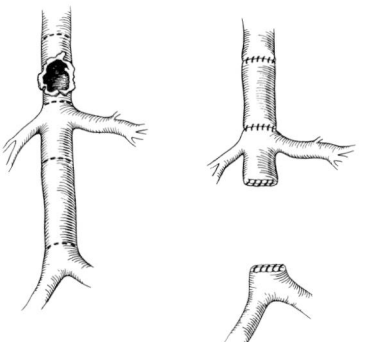

to the abdomen. A series reported by Quast and Jordan revealed only 27 patients with gynecologic injuries in a 16-year period at their hospital. Two of those injuries resulted from blunt trauma with rupture of the uterus in patients who were in the immediate postpartum period. These are apparently the only cases recorded of rupture of the nonpregnant uterus. The remaining injuries were penetrating wounds. An enlarged uterus was present in 10 of their patients. Six patients were pregnant, two had large uterine myomas, and two were in the postpartum period. No cases of rupture of an unenlarged uterus by blunt trauma have been recorded, however. Rupture of the pregnant uterus due to blunt trauma is rare but has occurred in a number of instances. The major threat to the fetus in blunt trauma is placental abruption, which if complete, will result in fetal demise. Of blunt and penetrating wounds to the female reproductive tract, 90 percent involve the uterine corpus and 10 percent involve the remaining adnexa.

In the past serious questions have been raised about the efficacy of pregnant patients wearing seat belts in automobiles. Crosby et al, have shown rather conclusively that more maternal and fetal lives have been saved by the use of lap belts, with or without shoulder harnesses, than by not using them.

The diagnostic evaluation of the pregnant patient sustaining traumatic injury should be undertaken with careful consideration for radiation exposure. Many procedures can be condensed to give maximum information with minimal exposure. On the contrary, no necessary procedure should be withheld because of a known or suspected pregnancy.

The most common cause of fetal death in automobile accidents is maternal death; therefore, important diagnostic and therapeutic measures designed to save the mother should be performed. In general, intrauterine exposure to diagnostic radiation is not an indication to terminate a pregnancy.

Pregnant patients sustaining penetrating trauma are managed the same as nonpregnant patients. It may be difficult to perform lavage in the late second and third trimester for stab wounds, but patients sustaining gunshot wounds should be formally explored in the operating room. In spite of the fact the gravid uterus may afford considerable protection to abdominal viscera, these organs are still at risk.

TREATMENT. The signs and symptoms from a ruptured pregnant uterus are those of abrupt and massive intraperitoneal hemorrhage. Associated with these findings are generalized abdominal pain and tenderness, abdominal distention, ileus, and the absence of fetal heart sounds and movements. If the patient arrives at the hospital alive (which is not often the case), immediate blood volume and extracellular fluid replacement must be instituted through several large-bore intravenous catheters, preferably placed in the upper extremities, since there may be an interference with venous return from lower extremities of those patients. Urgent celiotomy is necessary to control hemorrhage, even though the patient may still be in shock at the time. Probably the only anesthesia that will be required is assisted respiration with 100% oxygen administered through an endotracheal tube. Other agents may be added if and when shock abates. The treatment of choice is evacuation of the uterus, closure of the disruption with large chromic catgut sutures, and thorough peritoneal toilet with removal of all blood and foreign tissue.

Wounds of the uterus and adnexa are repaired by figure-of-eight chromic catgut sutures without drainage in most instances, although in occasional patients hysterectomy is indicated, as in injury of the lower uterine segment and major uterine vessels caused by high-velocity missiles. In these instances, hysterectomy is preferable to an attempted suture repair, since repair may cause stenosis of the cervical canal with resultant hematometra and dystocia. Also, hysterectomy for lower-uterine-segment injuries is indicated to obtain proper control of bleeding vessels and to help rule out uretheral injury at the point where the ureter and uterine artery are in juxtaposition.

It is best to leave the vaginal cuff partially open following hysterectomy for trauma, because of the likelihood of vaginal cuff or cul-de-sac abscess formation, especially if there is appreciable blast injury or concomitant colon injury. If abscesses occur and the vaginal cuff has been left open, it is usually a relatively simple matter to drain the abscess with a finger inserted through the vagina into the open cuff. If gross fecal contamination is present from colon injury, the cuff should be left open and a Penrose drain led out of the vagina from the cul-de-sac. This drain may be secured to the vaginal cuff by a single small chromic catgut suture.

If massive uncontrollable or recurrent bleeding occurs following trauma to the female pelvic organs, it may be rapidly and adequately controlled by bilateral in-continuity ligations of the hypogastric arteries with nonabsorbable suture material. This will not often be required but should be borne in mind as a very helpful and possibly lifesaving procedure.

Following injury to the pregnant uterus, the loss of the fetus is quite high. Quast and Jordan reported a salvage of only 1 of 10 pregnancies. One patient who was pregnant at the time of a tangential knife injury of the uterus had a uterine repair for penetrating trauma and subsequently delivered the child uneventfully per vagina.

Other instances have been reported in which penetrating uterine injury during pregnancy has been repaired with ensuing normal delivery. Quast and Jordan found that 81 percent of their patients with uterine injuries during pregnancy delivered subsequently per vagina with no difficulty. The cesarean section rate was 19 percent. Of the patients they followed after uterine injury, all who were in the childbearing age subsequently were able to conceive children. In this group, the abortion rate for these later pregnancies was 16 percent, with no apparent cause found.

By far the majority of pregnant patients with uterine injuries will abort shortly after the injury, frequently requiring curettage to control bleeding after spontaneous abortion. Others will require elective emptying of the uterine contents at the time of celiotomy in order to secure adequate hemostasis and uterine repair. Intravenous oxytocin should be given in such instances to aid in uterine contraction and hemostasis after hysterotomy.

Abdominal Wall

Injury to the abdominal wall without peritoneal injury is often difficult to diagnose. Muscular guarding and rigidity are frequently present, and it may be impossible to rule out intraabdominal injury from a hematoma of the abdominal wall. Such hematomas are usually due to rupture of the rectus abdominis or the epigastric artery by direct trauma or severe muscular exertion. The epigastric artery may also be injured by penetrating trauma, resulting in a hemoperitoneum. The patient may become hypotensive from such an injury because of the severe intraperitoneal bleeding that sometimes occurs.

The mass from the rectus abdominis hematoma is below the umbilicus in over 80 percent of the cases. To distinguish this mass from intraperitoneal masses, patients should be requested to raise their heads against resistance; the mass should disappear if it is intraperitoneal and remain the same if it is in the abdominal wall. This sign is not completely reliable, and if adjunctive diagnostic aids such as paracentesis and lavage are equivocal, then abdominal celiotomy should be performed.

On occasion missile injuries will appear to be limited to the abdominal wall. Depending upon the bullet caliber, distance at which it was shot, and body habitus blast effect may injure hollow and solid abdominal viscera without actual penetration of the peritoneum. Local wound exploration, peritoneal lavage, and computed tomography are unreliable in these cases. As stated above, these patients are best treated by celiotomy.

Bibliography

General Considerations

Shires GT: *Principles of Trauma Care*. New York, McGraw-Hill, 1985.

Principles in Wound Management and Antibiotics

Alexander JW, Kaplan JZ, Altemeier WA: Role of suture materials in the development of wound infection. *Ann Surg* 165:192, 1967.

Burke JF: The effective period of antibiotic action in experimental incisions and dermal lesions. *Surgery* 50:161, 1961.

Condie JP, Ferguson DJ: Experimental wound infections: Contamination versus surgical technique. *Surgery* 50:367, 1961.

Dunphy JE, Jackson DS: Practical applications of experimental studies in the care of the primarily closed wound. *Am J Surg* 104:273, 1962.

Finegold SM: Intestinal bacteria. *Calif Med* 110:455, 1969.

Gentry LO, Feliciano DD, Lea AS: Perioperative antibiotic therapy for penetrating injuries to the abdomen. *Ann Surg* 200:561, 1984.

Gorbach SL: Intestinal microflora. *Gastroenterology* 60:1110, 1971.

Jones RC: in Shires G Thomas (ed): *Care of the Trauma Patient,* 2d ed. New York, McGraw-Hill, 1978.

Jones RC, Thal ER, et al: Evaluation of antibiotic therapy following penetrating abdominal trauma 201:576, 1985.

Jones RC: Newer antibiotics for the surgeon. *Am J Surg* 152:577, 1986.

Louie TJ, Onderdonk AB, et al: Therapy for experimental intra-abdominal sepsis: Comparison of four cephalosporins with clindomycin plus gentamicin. *J Infect Dis* 135:5, 1977.

Mann LS, Spinazzola AJ, et al: Disruption of abdominal wounds. *JAMA* 180:99, 1962.

Nichols RL, Smith JW, Klein DB: Risk of infection after penetrating abdominal trauma. *N Engl J Med* 311:1065, 1984.

Onderdonk AD, Bartlett JG, Louie T: Microbial synergy in experimental abdominal abscess. *Infect Immun* 13:22, 1976.

Oreskovitch MD, Dellinger EP, Lennard S: Duration of preventive antibiotic administration for penetrating abdominal trauma. *Arch Surg* 117:200, 1982.

Thadepalli H, Gorbach SL, et al: Abdominal trauma, anaerobes and antibiotics. *Surg Gynecol Obstet* 137:270, 1973.

Thorngate S, Ferguson DJ: Effect of tension on healing of aponeurotic wounds. *Surgery* 44:619, 1958.

Wagner DH: Errors in the choice of abdominal wall incisions and in their closure. *Surg Clin North Am* 38:175, 1958.

Bites and Stings of Animals and Insects

Anderson LJ, Baer GM, Smith JS: Rapid antibody response to human diploid rabies vaccine. *Am J Epidemiol* 113:270, 1981.

Auer AI, Hershey FB: Surgery for necrotic bites of the brown spider. *Arch Surg* 108:612, 1974.

Berger RS, Addelstein GH, Anderson PC: Intravascular coagulation: The cause of necrotic arachnoidism. *Invest Dermatol* 61:142, 1973.

Bernard KW, Mallonie J, Wright JC: Preexposure immunization with intradermal human diploid cell rabies vaccine—Risks and benefits of primary and booster vaccinations. *JAMA* 257:1059, 1987.

Bernstein B, Erhlich F: Brown recluse spider bites. *J Emerg Med* 4:457, 1986.

Bitseff EL, Garoni WJ, et al: The management of stingray injuries of the extremities. *South Med J* 63:417, 1970.

CDC Rabies Surveillance Annual Summary 1985, U.S. Department of Health and Human Services, issued 1986.

Christopher DG, Rodning CB: Crotalidae Envenomation. *South Med J* 79:159, 1986.

Compendium of Animal Rabies Control. *Mortality and Morbidity Weekly Report* 35:53, 1987.

Davidson T: Inside world of the honeybee. *Natl Geograph* 154:188, 1959.

Dillaha CJ, Jansen GT, et al: North American loxoscelism. *JAMA* 188:33, 1964.

Emergency Department Management of Poisonous Snake Bites, American College of Surgeons Committee on Trauma, February 1981.

Fardon DW, Wingo CW, et al: The treatment of brown spider bites. *Plast Reconstr Surg* 40:482, 1967.

Fishbein DB, Bernard KW, Miller KD: Early kinetics of the antibody response after booster immunizations after human diploid cell vaccine. *Am J Trop Med Hyg* 35:663, 1986.

Golden DBK, Langlois J, et al: Treatment failures with whole-body extract therapy of insect sting allergy. *JAMA* 246(21):2460, 1981.

Golden DBK, Valentine MD, et al: Regimens of hymenoptera venom immunotherapy. *Ann Intern Med* 92:620, 1980.

Goldstein EJC, Citron DM, et al: Bacteriology of rattlesnake venom and implications for therapy. *J Infect Dis* 140(5):818, 1979.

Huang TT, Blackwell SJ, Lewis SR: Tissue necrosis in snakebite. *Tex Med* 77:53, 1981.

Huang TT, Lynch JB, et al: The use of excisional therapy in the management of snakebite. *Ann Surg* 179:598, 1974.

Human diploid cell rabies vaccine. *Med Let* 22(22):93, 1980.

Hunt KJ, Valentine MD, et al: A controlled trial of immunotherapy in insect hypersensitivity. *N Engl J Med* 299:157, 1978.

Ledbetter EO: What's new in the management of snakebite. *Tex Med* 77:41, 1981.

Levine MI: Insect stings. *JAMA* 217:964, 1971.

Marr JJ: Portuguese man-of-war envenomization. *JAMA* 199:115, 1967.

Marteic Z: Lactrodectism: Variations in clinical manifestations produced by Lactrodectus species of spiders. *Toxicon* 21:457, 1983.

Parrish HM: Incidence of treated snakebites in the United States. *Public Health Rept (US)* 31:269,1966.

Parrish HM, Carr CA: Bites by copperheads in the United States. *JAMA* 201:927, 1967.

Portuguese man-of-war. *JAMA* 192:994, 1965 (editorial).

Rabies prevention in the United States. Recommendations of the Public Health Service, Immunization Advisory Committee. *Mortality and Morbidity Weekly Report* 33(28):393, July 1984.

Rabies prevention: Supplementary statement on the preexposure use of human diploid cells rabies vaccine by the intradermal route. *JAMA* 257:1037, 1987.

Rees R, Shack RB, Withers E: Management of brown recluse spider bites. *Plast Reconstr Surg* 68:768, 1981.

Rees RS, Altenbern DP, et al: Brown recluse spider bites: A comparison of early surgical excision vs. dapsone and delayed surgical excision. *Ann Surg* 202:659, 1985.

Reisman RE, Arbesman CE, Lazell M: Clinical and immunological studies of venom immunotherapy. *Clin Allergy* 9:167, 1979.

Roberts RS: Csenscsitz TA, Heard CW: Upper extremity compartment syndromes following pit viper envenomation. *Clin Orthop* 193:184, 1985.

Russell FE: *Snake Venom Poisoning.* Philadelphia, Lippincott, 1980.

Russell FE, Carlson RW, et al: Snake venom poisoning in the United States—Experiences with 550 cases. *JAMA* 233:341, 1975.

Schwartz HJ, Lockey RF, et al: A multicenter study on skin test reactivity of human volunteers to venom as compared to whole-body hymenoptera antigens. *J Allergy Clin Immunol* 67:81, 1981.

Snyder CC, Knowles RP: Snake bite! *Consultant (SKF)* 3:44, 1963.

Sprenger TR, Bailey WJ: Snakebite treatment in the United States—Review. *Int J Dermatol* 25:479, 1986.

Strauss MB, Orris WL: Injuries to divers by marine animals: A simplified approach to recognition and management. *Milit Med* February 1974.

Timms PK, Gibbons RB: Lactrodectism—Effects of the black widow spider bites. *West J Med* 144:315, 1986.

Van Mierop LHS: Poisonous snakebite: A review. II. Symptomatology and treatment. *J Fla Med Assoc* 63(3):201, 1976.

Van Mierop LHS, Kitchesn CS: Defibrination syndrome following bites by the eastern diamondback rattlesnake. *J Fla Med Assoc* 67:31, 1980.

Wasserman GS, Anderson PC: Loxoscelism and necrotic arachnoidism. *J Toxicol Clin Toxicol* 21:451, 1984.

Penetrating Wounds of the Neck and Thoracic Inlet

Ayuyao AM, Kaledzi YL, et al: Penetrating neck wounds: Mandatory versus selective exploration. *Ann Surg* 202:563, 1985.

Dunbar LL, Adkins RB, Waterhouse G: Penetrating injuries to the neck: Selective management. *Am Surg* 50:198, 1984.

Flint LM, Snyder WH, et al: Management of major vascular injuries in the base of the neck: An 11-year experience with 146 cases. *Arch Surg* 106:407, 1973.

Fogelman MJ, Stewart RD: Penetrating wounds of the neck. *Am J Surg* 91:581, 1956.

Gewertz BL, Samson DS, et al: Management of penetrating injuries of the internal carotid artery at the base of the skull utilizing extracranial-intracranial bypass. *J Trauma* 20:365, 1980.

Golueke PJ, Goldstein AS, et al: Routine versus selective exploration of penetrating neck injuries: A randomized prospective study. *J Trauma* 24:1010, 1984.

Graham JM, Feliciano DV, et al: Management of subclavian vascular injuries. *J Trauma* 20:537, 1980.

Hiatt JR, Busuttil RW, Wilson SE: Impact of routine arteriography on management of penetrating neck injuries. *J Vasc Surg* 1:860, 1984.

Jones RF, Terrell JC, Salyer KE: Penetrating wounds of the neck: An analysis of 274 cases. *J Trauma* 7:228, 1967.

Jurkovich GJ, Zingarelli W, et al: Penetrating neck trauma: Diagnostic studies in the asymptomatic patient. *J Trauma* 25:819, 1985.

Larson DL, Cohn AM: Management of acute laryngeal injury: A critical review. *J Trauma* 16:858, 1976.

Liekweg WG, Greenfield LJ: Management of penetrating carotid artery injury. *Ann Surg* 188:587, 1978.

Meier DE, Brink BE, Fry WJ: Vertebral artery trauma: Acute recognition and treatment. *Arch Surg* 116:236, 1981.

Metzdorff MT, Lowe DK: Operation or observation for penetrating neck wounds? A retrospective analysis. *Am J Surg* 147:646, 1984.

Monson DO, Saletta JD, Freeark RJ: Carotid-vertebral trauma. *J Trauma* 9:987, 1969.

Narrod JA, Moore EE: Selective management of penetrating neck injuries. *Arch Surg* 119:574, 1984.

Noyes LD, McSwain NE Jr, Markowitz IP: Panendoscopy with arteriography versus mandatory exploration of penetrating wounds of the neck. *Ann Surg* 204:21, 1986.

Obeid FN, Haddad GS, et al: A critical reappraisal of a mandatory exploration policy for penetrating wounds of the neck. *Surg Gynecol Obstet* 160:517, 1985.

Ordog GJ, Albin D, et al: 110 bullet wounds to the neck. *J Trauma* 25:238, 1985.

Prakashchandra MR, Bhatti MFK, et al: Penetrating injuries of the neck: Criteria for exploration. *J Trauma* 23:47, 1983.

Reid JDS, Weigelt JA: Forty-three cases of vertebral artery trauma. Presented at the 47th Annual Meeting of The American Association for the Surgery of Trauma, Montreal, Quebec, Canada, September 1987.

Roon AJ, Christensen N: Evaluation and treatment of penetrating cervical injuries. *J Trauma* 19:391, 1979.

Rosoff L Sr, White EJ: Perforation of the esophagus. *Am J Surg* 128:207, 1974.

Saletta JD, Lowe RJ, et al: Penetrating trauma of the neck. *J Trauma* 16:579, 1976.

Snyder WH III, Thal ER, et al: The validity of normal arteriography in penetrating trauma. *Arch Surg* 113:424, 1978.

Symbas PN, Hatcher CR Jr, Boehm GAW: Acute penetrating tracheal trauma. *Ann Thorac Surg* 22:473, 1976.

Thal ER, Snyder WH III, et al: Management of carotid artery injuries. *Surgery* 76:955, 1974.

Thomas AN, Goodman PC, Roon AJ: Role of angiography in cervicothoracic trauma. *J Thorac Cardiovasc Surg* 76:633, 1978.

Unger WS, Tucker WS Jr, et al: Carotid arterial trauma. *Surgery* 87:477, 1980.

Weigelt JA, Thal ER, et al: Diagnosis of penetrating cervical esophageal injuries. Presented at the 39th Annual Meeting of the Southwestern Surgical Congress, San Diego, California, April 1987.

Abdominal Trauma

Ahmad W, Polk HC Jr: Blunt abdominal trauma. A prospective study with selective peritoneal lavage. *Arch Surg* 111:489, 1976.

Arango A, Baxter CR, Shires GT: Surgical management of traumatic injuries of the right colon; 20 years civilian experience. *Arch Surg* 114:703, 1979.

Aronson DZ, Scherz AW, Einhorn AH: Nonoperative management of splenic trauma in children: A report of six consecutive cases. *Pediatrics* 60:482, 1977.

Bach RD, Frey CF: Diagnosis and treatment of pancreatic trauma. *Am J Surg* 121:20, 1971.

Backwinkel K: Rupture of the rectus abdominis muscle. *Arch Surg* 90:35, 1965.

Balfanz JR, Nesbit ME, Jarvis C: Overwhelming sepsis following splenectomy for trauma. *J Pediatr* 88:458, 1976.

Barnes JP, Diamonon JS: Traumatic rupture of the gallbladder due to nonpenetrating injury. *Tex State J Med* 59:785, 1963.

Bartizal JF, Boyd DR, et al: A critical review of management of 392 colonic and rectal injuries. *Dis Colon Rectum* 17(3):313, 1974.

Bass EM, Crosier JH: Percutaneous control of posttraumatic hepatic hemorrhage by gelfoam embolization. *J Trauma* 17(1):61, 1977.

Baudet quoted by Terry JH, Self MM, Howard JM: A discussion of injuries of the spleen. *Surgery* 40:615, 1956.

Baylis SM, Lansing EH, Glas WW: Traumatic retroperitoneal hematoma. *Am J Surg* 103:477, 1962.

Beall AC, Bricker DL, et al: Surgical considerations in the management of civilian colon injuries. *Ann Surg* 173:971, 1971.

Benjamin CI, Engrav LH, Perry JF Jr: Delayed rupture or delayed diagnosis of rupture of the spleen. *Surg Gynecol Obstet* 142:171, 1976.

Berne CJ, Donovan AJ, et al: Duodenal "diverticulization" for duodenal and pancreatic injury. *Am J Surg* 127:503, 1974.

Bull JC Jr, Mathewson C Jr: Exploratory laparotomy in patients with penetrating wounds of the abdomen. *Am J Surg* 116:223, 1968.

Buntain WL, Lynn HB: Splenorrhaphy: Changing concepts for the traumatized spleen. *Surgery* 86:784, 1977.

Burch JM, Brock JC, et al: The injured colon. *Surg* 203(6):701, 1986.

Burrington JD: Surgical repair of a ruptured spleen in children: Report of eight cases. *Arch Surg* 112:417, 1977.

Burrington JD: Preservation of the traumatized spleen in children. *Contemp Surg* 15:11, 1979.

Busuttil RW, Kitahama A, et al: Management of injuries to the porta hepatis. *Ann Surg* 191(5):641, 1980.

Canizaro PC, Fitts CT, Sawyer RB: Diagnostic abdominal paracentesis: A proposed adjunctive measure. *US Army Surg Res Unit Annl Rept* June 1964.

Carmichael DH: Avulsion of the common bile duct by blunt trauma. *South Med J* 72(2):166, 1980.

Cassebaum WH, Bukanz SL, et al: Ligation of the inferior vena cava above the renal vein of a sole kidney with recovery. *Am J Surg* 113:667, 1967.

Cattell RB, Braasch JW: A technique for the exposure of the third and fourth portions of the duodenum. *Surg Gynecol Obstet* 111:379, 1960.

Cerise EJ, Scully JH Jr: Blunt trauma to the small intestine. *J Trauma* 10(1):46, 1970.

Cheatham JE Jr, Smith EI, et al: Nonoperative management of subcapsular hematomas of the liver. *Am J Surg* 140:851, 1980.

Cobb LM, Vinocur CD, et al: Intestinal perforation due to blunt trauma in children in an era of increased nonoperative treatment. *J Trauma* 26(5):461, 1986.

Cook A, Levine BA, et al: Traditional treatment of colon injuries. *Arch Surg* 119:591, 1984.

Cook DE, Walsh JW, et al: Upper abdominal trauma: Pitfalls in CT diagnosis. *Radiology* 159:65, 1986.

Cornell WP, Ebert PA, et al: A new nonoperative technique for the diagnosis of penetrating injuries to the abdomen. *J Trauma* 7:307, 1967.

Crosby W: Safety of lap belt restraints for pregnant victims of automobile collisions. *N Engl J Med* 248:632, 1971.

Crosby W: Committee on medical aspects of automobile safety belts during pregnancy. *JAMA* 221:20, 1972.

Curtis LE, Simonian S, et al: Evaluation of the effectiveness of controlled pH in management of massive upper gastrointestinal bleeding. *Am J Surg* 125:474, 1973.

Dang CV, Peter ET, et al: Trauma of the colon. Early drop-back of exteriorized repair. *Arch Surg* 117:652, 1982.

Dauterive AH, Flancbaum L, Cox EF: Blunt intestinal trauma. A modern-day review. *Ann Surg* 201(2):198, 1985.

Dawes LG, Aprahamian C, et al: The risk of infection after colon injury. *Surgery* 100(4):796, 1986.

Defore WW Jr, Mattox KL, et al: Management of 1,590 consecutive cases of liver trauma. *Arch Surg* 111:493, 1976.

Dickerman JD: Bacterial infection and the asplenic host: A review. *J Trauma* 16(8):662, 1976.

Dickerman JD: Splenectomy and sepsis: A warning. *Pediatrics* 63:938, 1979.

Dixon JA, Miller F, McCloskey D: Anatomy and techniques in segmental splenectomy. *Surg Gynecol Obstet* 150:516, 1980.

Donohue JH, Crass RA, Trunkey DD: The management of duodenal and other small intestinal trauma. *World J Surg* 9(6):904, 1985.

Douglas GJ, Simpson JS: The conservative management of splenic trauma. *J Pediatr Surg* 6:565, 1971.

Drapanas T, McDonald J: Peritoneal tap in abdominal trauma. *Surgery* 100:22, 1960.

Dudrick SJ, Wilmore DW, et al: Spontaneous closure of traumatic pancreatoduodenal fistulas with total intravenous nutrition. *J Trauma* 10(7):542, 1970.

Duke JH, Jones RC, Shires GT: Management of injuries to the inferior vena cava. *Am J Surg* 110:759, 1965.

Edwards J, Gaspard DJ: Visceral injury due to extraperitoneal gunshot wounds. *Arch Surg* 108:865, 1974.

Ein SH, Shandling B, Simpson JS: Nonoperative management of traumatized spleen in children: How and why. *J Pediatr Surg* 13:117, 1978.

Eraklis AJ, Filler RM: Splenectomy in childhood: A review of 1413 cases. *J Pediatr Surg* 4:382, 1972.

Fabian TC, Mangiante EC, et al: A prospective study of 91 patients undergoing both computed tomography and peritoneal lavage following blunt abdominal trauma. *J Trauma* 26(7):602, 1986.

Federle MP, Richard AC, et al: Computed tomography in blunt abdominal trauma. *Arch Surg* 117:645, 1982.

Feliciano DV, Jordan GL, et al: Management of 1000 consecutive cases of hepatic trauma (1979–1984). *Ann Surg* 204(4):438, 1986.

Feliciano DV, Mattox KL, Jordan GL Jr: Intra-abdominal packing for control of hepatic hemorrhage: A reappraisal. *J Trauma* 21(4):285, 1981.

Feliciano DV, Mattox KL, et al: Packing for control of hepatic hemorrhage. *J Trauma* 26(8):738, 1986.

Felson B, Levin EJ: Intramural hematoma of the duodenum: Diagnostic roentgen sign. *Radiology* 63:828, 1954.

Fischer RP, Beverlin BC, et al: Diagnostic peritoneal lavage: Fourteen years and 2586 patients later. *Am J Surg* 136:701, 1978.

Fish JC: Reconstruction of the portal vein: Case reports and literature review. *Am Surg* 32:472, 1966.

Fitzgerald JB, Crawford E, DeBakey ME: Surgical considerations of abdominal injuries: Analysis of 200 cases. *Am J Surg* 100:22, 1960.

Flint LM, Vitale GC, et al: The injured colon. Relationships of management to complications. *Ann Surg* 193:619, 1981.

Flint LM Jr, McCoy M, et al: Duodenal injury. Analysis of common misconceptions in diagnosis and treatment. *Ann Surg* 191:697, 1980.

Flint LM, Polk HC Jr: Selective hepatic artery ligation: Limitations and failures. *J Trauma* 19(5):319, 1979.

Foley WJ, Gaines RD, Fry WJ: Pancreaticoduodenectomy for severe trauma to the head of the pancreas and the associated structures: Report of three cases. *Ann Surg* 170:759, 1969.

Forde KA, Ganepola AP: Is mandatory exploration for penetrating abdominal trauma extinct? The morbidity and mortality of negative exploration in a large municipal hospital. *J Trauma* 14(9):764, 1974.

Freeark RJ, Corley RD, et al: Unusual aspects of pancreatoduodenal trauma. *J Trauma* 6:482, 1966.

Fullen WD, McDonough JJ, et al: Sternal splitting approach for major hepatic or retrohepatic vena cava injury. *J Trauma* 14(11):903, 1974.

Fullen WD, Selle JG, et al: Intramural duodenal hematoma. *Ann Surg* 179:549, 1974.

Geis WP, Schulz KA, et al: The fate of unruptured intrahepatic hematomas. *Surgery* 90(4):689, 1981.

Giddings WP, Wolff LH: Penetrating wounds of the stomach, duodenum, and small intestine. *Surg Clin North Am* 38:1605, 1958.

Giuliano A: Is splenic salvage safe in the traumatized patient? *Arch Surg* 116:651, 1981.

Gougon FW, Legros G, Archambaul TA: Pancreatic trauma, new diagnostic approach. *Surgery* 132:400, 1976.

Graham JM, Mattox KL, et al: Traumatic injuries of the inferior vena cava. *Arch Surg* 113:413, 1978.

Graham JM, Mattox KL, Jordan GL: Traumatic injuries of the pancreas. *Am J Surg* 136:744, 1978.

Green JB, Shackford SR, et al: Late septic complications in adults following splenectomy for trauma: A prospective analysis in 144 patients. *J Trauma* 26(11):999, 1986.

Haddad GH, Pizzi WF, et al: Abdominal signs and sinograms as dependable criteria for the selective management of stab-wounds of the abdomen. *Ann Surg* 172:61, 1970.

Heimbach DM, Ferguson GS, Harley JD: Treatment of traumatic hemobilia with angiographic embolization. *J Trauma* 18(3):221, 1978.

Holgerson LO, Bishop HC: Nonoperative treatment of duodenal hematoma. *J Pediatr Surg* 12:11, 1976.

Howman-Giles R, Gilday DL, et al: Splenic trauma—nonoperative management and long term follow-up by scinti-scan, *J Pediat Surg* 13:121, 1978.

Ivatury RR, Nallathambi M, et al: Liver packing for uncontrolled hemorrhage. *J Trauma* 26(8):744, 1986.

Izant RJ, Drucker WR: Duodenal obstruction due to intramural hematoma in children. *J Trauma* 4:797, 1964.

Jackson GL, Thal ER: Management of stabwounds of the back and flank. *J Trauma* 19(9):660, 1979.

Jeffrey RB, Federle MP, Goodman PC: CT of splenic trauma. *Radiology* 141:729, 1981.

Jeffrey RB Jr, Federle MP, Crass RA: Computed tomography of pancreatic trauma. *Radiology* 147:491, 1983.

Jones RC: Management of pancreatic trauma. *Ann Surg* 187(5):555, May 1978.

Jones RC: Management of pancreatic trauma. *Am J Surg* 150:698, 1985.

Jones RC, Shires GT: The management of pancreatic injuries. *Arch Surg* 90:502, 1965.

Jones RC, McClelland RN, et al: Difficult closures of the duodenal stump. *Arch Surg* 94:696, 1967.

Jones RC, Thal ER, et al: Evaluation of antibiotic therapy following penetrating abdominal trauma. *Ann Surg* 120(5):576, 1985.

Kelly G, Norton L, et al: The continuing challenge of duodenal injuries. *J Trauma* 18(3):160, 1978.

King H, Shumacker HB Jr: Splenic studies: I. Susceptibility to infection after splenectomy performed in infancy. *Ann Surg* 136:239, 1952.

Kobold EE, Thal AP: A simple method for the management of experimental wounds of the duodenum. *Surg Gynecol Obstet* 116:340, 1963.

Kudsk KA, Sheldon GF, Lim RC Jr: Atrial-caval shunting (ACS) after trauma. *J Trauma* 22(2):81, 1982.

Lambeth W, Rubin BR: Nonoperative management of intrahepatic hemorrhage and hematoma following blunt trauma. *Surg Gynecol Obstet* 148:507, 1979.

Lavenson GS, Cohen A: Management of rectal injuries. *Am J Surg* 122:226, 1971.

Ledgerwood AM, Kazmers M, Lucas CE: The role of thoracic aortic occlusion for massive hemoperitoneum. *J Trauma* 16(8):610, 1976.

Letton AH, Wilson JP: Traumatic severance of pancreas treated by Roux-y anastomosis. *Surg Gynecol Obstet* 109:473, 1959.

Lim RC, Glickman MG, Hunt TK: Angiography in patients with blunt trauma to the chest and abdomen. *Surg Clin North Am* 52(3):551, 1972.

LoCicero J III, Tajima T, Drapanas T: A half-century of experience in the management of colon injuries: Changing concepts. *J Trauma* 15(7):575, 1975.

Longmore WP: Early management of injury to the extrahepatic biliary tract. *JAMA* 165:822, 1966.

Lou Sister MA, Johnson AP, et al: Exteriorized repair in the management of colon injuries. *Arch Surg* 116:926, 1981.

Lucas CE: What is the role of biliary drainage in liver trauma? *Am J Surg* 120:509, 1970.

Lucas CE, Ledgerwood AM: Factors influencing outcome after blunt duodenal injury. *J Trauma* 15(10):839, 1975.

Lucas CE, Ledgerwood AM: Prospective evaluation of hemostatic techniques for liver injuries. *J Trauma* 16(6):442, 1976.

Lucas CE, Walt AJ: Analysis of randomized biliary drainage for liver trauma in 189 patients. *J Trauma* 12(11):925, 1972.

Lucas CE, Canizaro PC, Shires GT: Repair of hepatic venous intrahepatic vena caval, and portal venous injuries, in Madding GF, Kennedy PA: *Trauma to the Liver,* 2d ed. Philadelphia, Saunders, 1971, chap 10, p 146.

Luna G, Dellinger EP: Nonoperative observation therapy for splenic injuries. *Am J Surg* 153:462, 1987.

McLelland BA, Hanna SS, et al: Analysis of peritoneal lavage parameters in blunt abdominal trauma. *J Trauma* 25(5):393, 1985.

McClelland RN, Shires T: Management of liver trauma in 259 consecutive patients. *Ann Surg* 161:248, 1965.

McClelland RN, Shires T, Poulos E: Hepatic resection for massive trauma. *J Trauma* 4:282, 1964.

McInnis WD, Aust JB, et al: Traumatic injuries of the duodenum: A comparison of 1° closure and the jejunal patch. *J Trauma* 15(10):847, 1975.

Mahon PA, Sutton JE Jr: Nonoperative management of adult splenic injury due to blunt trauma: A warning. *Am J Surg* 149:716, 1985.

Malangoni MA, Levine AW, et al: Management of injury to the spleen in adults. Results of early operation and observation. *Ann Surg* 200(6):702, 1984.

Martin TD, Feliciano DV, et al: Severe duodenal injuries. Treatment with pyloric exclusion and gastrojejunostomy. *Arch Surg* 118(17):631, 1983.

Mattox KL, Espada R, Beall AC Jr: Traumatic injury to the portal vein. *Ann Surg* 181:519, 1975.

Maynard AL, Oropeza G: Mandatory operation for penetrating wounds of the abdomen. *Am J Surg* 115:307, 1968.

Mays ET: Lobar dearterialization for exsanguinating wounds of the liver. *J Trauma* 12(5):397, 1972.

Miller DR: Median sternotomy extension of abdominal incision for hepatic lobectomy. *Ann Surg* 175:193, 1972.

Moore FA, Moore EE, et al: Risk of splenic salvage after trauma. *Am J Surg* 148:800, 1984.

Moretz JA III, Campbell DP, et al: Significance of serum amylase level in evaluating pancreatic trauma. *Am J Surg* 130:739, 1975.

Morgenstern L: Microcrystalline collagen used in experimental splenic injury: A new surface hemostatic agent. *Arch Surg* 109:44, 1974.

Morgenstern L, Shapiro SJ: Techniques of splenic conservation. *Arch Surg* 114:449, 1979.

Morton JR, Jordan GL: Traumatic duodenal injuries: Review of 131 cases. *J Trauma* 8(2):127, 1968.

Mucha P Jr, Daly RC, Farnell MB: Selective management of blunt splenic trauma. *J Trauma* 26(11):970, 1986.

Nance FC, Cohn I Jr: Surgical judgment in the management of stab wounds of the abdomen: A retrospective and prospective analysis based on a study of 600 stabbed patients. *Ann Surg* 170:569, 1969.

Nance FC, Wennar MH, et al: Surgical judgment in the management of penetrating wounds of the abdomen: Experience with 2212 patients. *Ann Surg* 179:639, 1974.

Naylor R, Coln D, Shires GT: Morbidity and mortality from injuries to the spleen. *J Trauma* 14(9):773, 1974.

Nichols RL, Smith JW, et al: Risk of infection after penetrating abdominal trauma. *N Engl J Med* 311(17):1065, 1984.

Oakes DD: Splenic trauma. *Curr Probl Surg* 17:342, 1981.

Olsen WR: The serum amylase in blunt abdominal trauma. *J Trauma* 13(3):200, 1973.

Olsen WR, Polley TZ Jr: A second look at delayed splenic rupture. *Arch Surg* 112:422, 1977.

Olsen WR, Redman HC, Hildreth DH: Quantitative peritoneal lavage in blunt abdominal trauma. *Arch Surg* 104:536, 1972.

O'Neal BJ, McDonald JC: The risk of sepsis in the asplenic adult. *Ann Surg* 194:775, 1981.

Oreskovich MR, Carrico CJ: Stab wounds of the anterior abdomen. Analysis of management plan using local wound exploration and quantitative peritoneal lavage. *Ann Surg* 198(4):411, 1983.

Pachter HL, Pennington R, et al: Simplified distal pancreatectomy with the auto suture stapler: Preliminary clinical observations. *Surgery* 85:166, 1979.

Pachter HL, Spencer FC: Recent concepts in the treatment of hepatic trauma. Facts and fallacies. *Ann Surg* 190(4):423, 1979.

Pachter HL, Spencer FC, et al: The management of juxtahepatic venous injuries without an atriocaval shunt: Preliminary clinical observations. *Surgery* 99(5):569, 1986.

Parvin S, Smith DE, et al: Effectiveness of peritoneal lavage in blunt abdominal trauma. *Ann Surg* 181:255, 1975.

Peitzman AB, Makaroun MS, et al: Prospective study of computed tomography in initial management of blunt abdominal trauma, *J Trauma* 26(7):585, 1986.

Perlberger RR: Control of hemobilia by angiographic embolization. *AJR* 128:672, 1977.

Perry JF Jr, DeMeules JE, Root HD: Diagnostic peritoneal lavage in blunt abdominal trauma. *Surg Gynecol Obstet* 131:742, 1970.

Perry JF Jr, LaFave JW: Biliary decompression without other external drainage in treatment of liver injuries. *Surgery* 55:351, 1964.

Perry MO: *The Management of Acute Vascular Injuries*. Baltimore, Williams & Wilkins, 1981, p 105.

Perry MO, Thal ER, Shires GT: Management of arterial injuries. *Ann Surg* 173:403, 1971.

Printen KJ, Freeark RJ, Shoemaker WC: Conservative management of penetrating abdominal wounds. *Arch Surg* 96:899, 1968.

Quast DC, Jordan GL: Traumatic wounds of the female reproductive organs. *J Trauma* 4:839, 1964.

Reinhardt GF, Hubay CA: Surgical management of traumatic hemobilia. *Am J Surg* 121:328, 1971.

Reinhoff WF, Donahoo JS: Isolated complete rupture of the pancreas from non-penetrating abdominal trauma treated by distal resection. *Am Surg* 33:148, 1967.

Richie JP, Fonkalsrud EW: Subcapsular hematoma of the liver. *Arch Surg* 104:781, 1972.

Root HD, Hauser CW, et al: Diagnostic peritoneal lavage. *Surgery* 57:633, 1965.

Rosoff L, Cohen JL, et al: Injuries of the spleen. *Surg Clin North Am* 52(3):667, 1972.

Rydell WB Jr: Complete transection of the common bile duct due to blunt abdominal trauma. *Arch Surg* 100:724, 1970.

Ryzoff RI, Shaftan GW, Herbsman H: Selective conservatism in abdominal trauma. *Surgery* 59:650, 1966.

Salyer K, McClelland RN: Pancreaticoduodenectomy for trauma. *Arch Surg* 95:636, 1967.

Schrock T, Blaisdell FW, Mathewson C: Management of blunt trauma to the liver and hepatic veins. *Arch Surg* 96:698, 1968.

Schrock T, Christensen N: Management of perforating injuries of the colon. *Surg Gynecol Obstet* 135:65, 1972.

Seaver R, Lynch J, et al: Hypogastric artery ligation for uncontrollable hemorrhage in acute pelvic trauma. *Surgery* 55:516, 1964.

Shackford SR, Sise MJ, et al: Evaluation of splenorrhaphy: A grading system for splenic trauma. *J Trauma* 21(7):538, 1981.

Shaftan GW: Indications for operation in abdominal trauma. *Am J Surg* 99:657, 1960.

Shannon FL, Moore EE: Primary repair of the colon: When is it a safe alternative? *Surg* 98(4):851, 1985.

Sheldon GF, Cohn L, Blaisdell W: Surgical treatment of pancreatic trauma. *J Trauma* 10:795, 1970.

Sheldon GF, Lim RC Jr, et al: *Ann Surg* 202(5):539, 1985.

Shires GT, Jackson D, Williams J: Temporary duodenal decompression as an adjunct to gastric resection for duodenal ulcer. *Am Surg* 28:709, 1962.

Singer DB: Postsplenectomy sepsis, in Rosenberg HS, Bolande RP (eds): *Perspectives in Pediatric Pathology*. Chicago, Year Book Medical, 1973, vol 1, p 285.

Smiley K, Perry MO: Balloon catheter tamponade of major vascular wounds. *Am J Surg* 121:326, 1971.

Smithwick W III, Gertner HR Jr, Zuidema GD: Injection of hypaque (sodium diatrizoate) in the management of abdominal stab wounds. *Surg Gynecol Obstet* 127:1215, 1968.

Snyder WH III, Weigelt JA, et al: The surgical management of duodenal trauma. *Arch Surg* 115:422, 1980.

Soderstrom CA, Maekawa K, et al: Gallbladder injuries resulting from blunt abdominal trauma. An experience and review. *Ann Surg* 193(1):60, 1981.

Sparkman RS: Massive hemobilia following traumatic rupture of the liver. *Ann Surg* 138:899, 1953.

Starzl TE, Kaupp HA, et al: Penetrating injuries of the inferior vena cava. *Surg Clin North Am* 43:387, 1963.

Steele M, Lim RC: Advances in management of splenic injuries. *Am J Surg* 130:159, 1975.

Stone HH, Fabian TC: Management of duodenal wounds. *J Trauma* 19(5):334, 1979.

Stone HH, Lamb JM: Use of pedicled omentum as an autogenous pack for control of hemorrhage in major injuries of the liver. *Surg Gynecol Obstet* 141:92, 1975.

Strate RG, Grieco JC: Blunt injury to the colon and rectum. *J Trauma* 23(5):384, 1983.

Strauch GO: Preservation of splenic function in adults and children with injured spleens. *Am J Surg* 137:478, 1979.

Sturmer FC, Wilt KE: Complete division of the common duct from external blunt trauma. *Am J Surg* 105:781, 1963.

Taxier M, Sivak MV, et al: Endoscopic retrograde pancreatography in the evaluation of trauma to the pancreas. *Surg Gynecol Obstet* 150:65, 1980.

Thal ER: Evaluation of peritoneal lavage and local exploration in lower chest and abdominal stabwounds. *J Trauma* 17:642, 1977.

Thal ER: Peritoneal lavage. Reliability of RBC count in patients with stab wounds to the chest. *Arch Surg* 119:579, 1984.

Thal ER, May RA, Beesinger D: Peritoneal lavage: Its unreliability in gunshot wounds of the lower chest and abdomen. *Arch Surg* 115:430, 1980.

Thal ER, Shires GT: Peritoneal lavage in blunt abdominal trauma. *Am J Surg* 125:64, 1973.

Thal ER, Yeary EC: Morbidity of colostomy closure following colon trauma. *J Trauma* 20(4):287, 1980.

Thompson JS, Moore EE, Moore JB: Comparison of penetrating injuries of the right and left colon. *Ann Surg* 193:414, 1981.

Traub AC, Perry JF: Splenic preservation following splenic trauma. *J Trauma* 22(6):496, 1982.

Trunkey D, Hays RJ, Shires GT: Management of rectal trauma. *J Trauma* 13(5):411, 1973.

Trunkey D, Shires GT, McClelland RN: Management of liver trauma in 811 consecutive patients. *Ann Surg* 179(5):522, 1974.

Tuggle D, Huber PJ Jr: Management of rectal trauma. *Am J Surg* 148:806, 1984.

Turpin I, State D, Schwartz A: Injuries to the inferior vena cava and their management. *Am J Surg* 134:25, 1977.

Vannix RS, Carter R, et al: Surgical management of colon trauma in civilian practice. *Am J Surg* 106:364, 1963.

Van Stiegmann G, Moore EE, Moore GE: Failure of spleen repair. *J Trauma* 19:698, 1979.

Vaughan GD III, Frazier OH, et al: The use of pyloric exclusion in the management of severe duodenal injuries. *Am J Surg* 134:785, 1977.

Walt AJ: The mythology of hepatic trauma—or Babel revisited. *Am J Surg* 135:12, 1978.

Walter JF, Baaso BT, Cannon WB: Successful transcatheter embolic control of massive hematobilia secondary to liver biopsy. *AJR* 127:847, 1976.

Weichert RF III, Hewitt RL, Drapanas T: Blunt injuries to intrahepatic vena cava and hepatic veins with survival. *Am J Surg* 121:322, 1971.

Weinstein ME, Govin GG, Rice CL: Splenorrhaphy for splenic trauma. *J Trauma* 19:692, 1979.

Wilder JR, Habermann ET, Schachner SJ: Selective surgical intervention for stab wounds of the abdomen. *Surgery* 61:231, 1967.

Wilder JR, Lotfi MW, Jurani P: Comparative study of mandatory and selective surgical intervention in stab wounds of the abdomen. *Surgery* 69:546, 1971.

Witek JT, Spencer RP, et al: Diagnostic spleen scans in occult splenic injury. *J Trauma* 14:197, 1974.

Woolley MM, Mahour GH, Sloan T: Duodenal hematoma in infancy and childhood. Changing etiology and changing treatment. *Am J Surg* 136:8, 1978.

Yajko RD, Seydel F, Trimble C: Rupture of the stomach from blunt abdominal trauma. *J Trauma* 15(3):177, 1975.

Yellin AE, Chaffee CB, Donovan AJ: Vascular isolation in treatment of juxtahepatic venous injuries. *Arch Surg* 102:566, 1971.

Yasugi H, Mizumoto R, et al: Changes in carbohydrate metabolism and endocrine function of remnant pancreas after major pancreatic resection. *Am J Surg* 132:577, 1976.

Yasugi H, Rosoff L Sr: Pancreatoduodenectomy for combined pancreatoduodenal injuries. *Arch Surg* 110:1177, 1975.

Burns

P. William Curreri and Arnold Luterman

The complex pathophysiologic alterations that accompany major thermal injury present the surgeon with an extraordinary therapeutic challenge. During the past two decades, few areas of medical science have experienced more rapid development of new treatment modalities. As a result, marked improvement in the care of patients with major burn injury has been noted. Comprehensive treatment centers now utilize sophisticated, multidisciplinary teams to aid in the diagnosis of rapidly changing physiologic responses to the injury and to assist in providing the vast array of specialized therapeutic services that are necessary to minimize morbidity and mortality.

Burn injury constitutes a major national health problem. More than 2 million persons suffer thermal injury annually, of whom 100,000 must be hospitalized. Burn injuries are now exceeded only by motor vehicle accidents as a cause of accidental death. As in other types of trauma, thermal injury frequently afflicts children and young adults. Prolonged morbidity, as well as temporary or permanent disability, associated with thermal injury results in a staggering economic drain on social resources. Hospital and medical costs for the treatment of burn injuries are now estimated at greater than one billion dollars a year. Financial support is often required to defray expenses associated with prolonged hospitalization, loss of family income sources, and replacement of lost labor within the working force.

ETIOLOGY OF BURNS

Burns are caused by the application of heat to the body. The depth of the resulting burn injury will be dependent on the intensity and duration of heat application and the conductivity of the tissues involved. The most common heat sources are an open flame and hot liquid. In addition, thermal injury is frequently observed in patients who have been exposed to direct contact with hot metal, toxic chemicals, or high-voltage electric current. Damage as a result of heat rarely occurs below 45°C. Between 45 and 50°C, gradations of cell injury may occur; and above 50°C, denaturation of protein elements of the cell becomes apparent.

Laboratory accidents, civilian assaults, industrial mishaps, and inexpert application of agents used for medical purposes account for most of the chemical burns in the civilian population. At least 25,000 products capable of producing chemical burns are available for use in industry, agriculture, military science, and the home. The number of patients with chemical burns requiring professional medical care is estimated to exceed 60,000 per year. At least 3000 deaths annually in the United States can be attributed to cutaneous and gastrointestinal chemical injuries. A principal difference between thermal and chemical injury is the length of time during which tissue destruction continues, since the chemical agent causes progressive damage until inactivated by reaction with tissue, while thermal injury ceases shortly after removal of the heat source. Tissue destruction associated with exposure to chemicals may be limited by application of large volumes of water to dilute the offending agent and reduce its contact time. Compared with thermal injury, the severe, full-thickness chemical burn may appear deceptively superficial, with only mild bronze discoloration of intact skin during the first few postburn days.

Electrical injuries cause 2400 admissions to emergency rooms annually, accounting for 3 percent of all admissions to major burn centers and resulting in 1500 deaths per year. The number of accidents is steadily increasing. One-third of all major electrical accidents occur in electrical workers, one-third in construction workers, and the remainder in non-work-related settings such as home accidents. The extremities are the most common sites of contact with electric current, with the upper limbs involved more frequently than the lower limbs.

In contrast to both thermal and chemical burns, electrical injury usually results in minimal destruction of skin. The magnitude of the injury is directly related to the amount of current passing through tissue between the point of contact with the electrical source and the exit site at which the patient is grounded. The magnitude of current passing through various organs is indirectly related to the resistance of the tissue. Nerve, blood, and muscle offer the least resistance to electric current and thus sustain the maximum amount of tissue damage. As a result, cutaneous injury may be apparent only at the entrance and exit sites, although considerable deep tissue destruction of upper and lower extremity musculature may be present.

The cross-sectional area of different portions of the body will also determine the extent of damage produced. In those portions of the body with small cross-sectional areas (e.g., a distal limb), current density and the temperatures generated will be higher than in those areas of greater cross-sectional area.

The electrical resistance of skin can vary dramatically depending on its moisture, cleanliness, and thickness. The average resistance measurement for skin is 40,000 ohms. Calloused skin may have a resistance as high as 1 million ohms, while the resistance of moist skin may be as low as 300 ohms.

Small, deep burns in the antecubital space or in the axilla are often observed in the patient with severe electrical injury of the upper extremity. These burns result from the arcing of current across the joint via the path of least resistance, the skin moistened with perspiration. When arc burns are present, they are nearly always accompanied by extensive, deep muscular destruction. This type of injury is frequently associated with release of hemochromagens into the bloodstream that are excreted via the urinary tract. Thus, "port-wine" colored urine containing myoglobin is not unusual following major electrical injury.

IMMEDIATE THERAPY

Initial therapy of the patient with a major burn should be directed toward restoration of normal physiologic parameters and prevention of life-threatening complications. With the exception of chemical burns, in which the toxic agent must be diluted with water and physically removed as rapidly as possible to prevent further tissue destruction, the burn wound is of secondary importance during the first few hours after the injury.

Maintenance of Airway

Immediate pulmonary complications may become manifest in the thermally injured patient. Excessive exposure to smoke may result in carbon monoxide poisoning. Carbon monoxide is a colorless, odorless gas with an affinity for hemoglobin approximately 210 times greater than that of oxygen. Patients with carbon monoxide poisoning exhibit the signs and symptoms of hypoxia, which may range from pronounced tachypnea and agitation to respiratory arrest and coma.

The diagnosis may be quickly confirmed by analyzing the concentration of carboxyhemoglobin in the blood. Treatment includes the administration of 100% oxygen, with ventilatory support if necessary, in order to displace the tightly bound carbon monoxide from the hemoglobin molecule. Since carbon monoxide is not toxic to lungs per se, the syndrome is entirely reversible, provided anoxic damage to distant tissues (e.g., the central nervous system) has not occurred. Although several decades ago few patients with severe carbon monoxide poisoning survived long enough to reach the emergency room, the development of sophisticated paramedical teams trained to insert endotracheal tubes and administer ventilatory support in the field has allowed greater salvage of such patients in the last several years.

Upper airway obstruction in patients with burns of the head and neck may occur during the first 48 hours after injury. The obstruction is related to soft tissue edema of the oral pharynx and vocal cords following exposure to hot gases. Direct thermal injury to the lower respiratory tract is exceedingly unusual, since the nose and oral pharynx are extremely efficient heat exchangers, allowing cooling of inhaled hot gas prior to its entrance into the trachea. Since it is more difficult to extract heat from liquid, direct thermal injury of the lower respiratory tract is occasionally noted in patients injured by superheated steam.

Upper airway obstruction is usually heralded by an increase in the respiratory rate and progressive hoarseness. In addition, a patient may exhibit increased difficulty in clearing bronchial secretions as the vocal cords become more edematous. Confirmation of impending obstruction is made by direct visualization of the posterior oral phar-

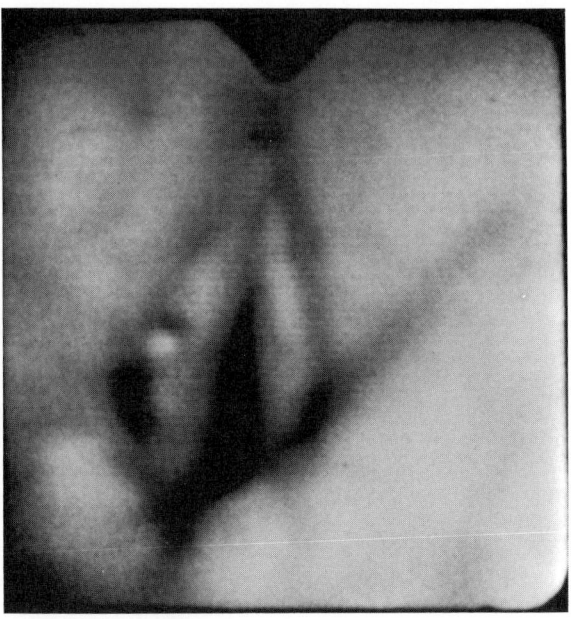

Fig. 7-1. Vocal cords seen through a fiberoptic bronchoscope shows swelling, vesicles, and carbonaceous deposits.

ynx and cords, utilizing either direct laryngoscopy or fiberoptic endoscopy (Fig. 7-1). The latter is usually preferred, since at the same time, assessment of smoke inhalation may be accomplished by visualizing the lower respiratory tract.

Impending upper airway obstruction is treated by the immediate insertion of an endotracheal tube. Tracheos-tomy is performed only when nasotracheal or endotracheal intubation is impossible. Soft tissue edema is maximal at between 24 and 48 h. Therefore, the endotracheal tube is usually not removed until the third postburn day. Direct visualization of the posterior pharynx and larynx is performed prior to extubation to determine if swelling has decreased. Reintubation, if required, often is technically difficult to perform.

Intravenous Resuscitation

Cardiovascular alterations occur almost immediately following burn injury. There is a massive shift of fluid and electrolytes from the intravascular and extracellular fluid space into the cells. Reversion of water and sodium from the intracellular fluid back into the extracellular fluid begins between 24 and 48 h but is not complete until the tenth postburn day. In general, these changes are directly proportional to the extent and depth of burn. Therefore, any consideration of fluid resuscitation to prevent hypovolemic shock requires an accurate estimation of the magnitude of burn injury. The burned wound is three-dimensional; therefore, not only the depth but the surface area involved must be estimated.

Burns are classified as first, second, or third degree (Table 7-1). First-degree burns are characterized by simple erythema of the skin, with only microscopic destruction of superficial layers of the epidermis. A mild sunburn is characteristic of a first-degree injury. The first-degree injury is of little clinical significance, since the water barrier of the skin is not disturbed. Systemic cardiovascular disturbances are rarely observed following first-degree

Table 7-1. CLASSIFICATION OF BURNS

Classification	Morphology	Clinical appearance	Cause
First degree	Only superficial layers of epidermis devitalized; dilatation and congestion of intradermal vessels	Erythema only—blanches on pressure	Ultraviolet exposure (ultraviolet light, sunburn), very short flash
Second degree	Destruction of varying depths of epidermis with coagulation necrosis; clefting of epidermis with fluid collection (blister formation); congestion and coagulation in subdermal plexus. Some skin elements remain viable (often only skin appendages), from which epithelial regeneration can occur*	Erythematous, weeping, painful. Blisters and bullae often present. Superficial layers of skin can be readily wiped away. Remaining skin elements waxy white, soft, dry, insensitive	Short flash, spill scald
Third degree	Destruction of all skin elements; coagulation of subdermal plexus	Dry, hard, inelastic, translucent, with thrombosed vein visible	Flame, immersion scald, chemical contact, electric current

* Initial injury may be partial-thickness, with only dermal appendages (hair follicles and glands) remaining, but these skin elements are readily destroyed by infection, with resulting conversion to full-thickness (third-degree) burn.

burn injury. The burns rapidly heal if the patient avoids further exposure to a heat source. First-degree burns are *not* considered when estimating the magnitude of burn injury for purposes of planning intravenous fluid replacement.

Second- and third-degree burns are of equal physiologic significance and may be summated in the estimate of total body surface burn injury. Second-degree burns extend through the epidermis into the dermis. By definition, viable epithelial elements from which epithelial regeneration can occur are retained in second-degree burn injury; thus the burn is often described as *partial-thickness*. Even when most of the epithelium is destroyed, regeneration may occur from epithelial cells surrounding hair follicles or sweat glands. On the other hand, third-degree burns are characterized by total irreversible destruction of all the skin, dermal appendages, and epithelial elements. Spontaneous regeneration of epithelium is not possible, and the burns are described as *full-thickness*. Such burns require the application of skin grafts if the development of scar tissue is to be avoided.

Since skin varies in thickness in different parts of the body, application of the same intensity of heat for a given period of time will result in a burn that will vary in depth, depending on the thickness of the skin itself in the local area, as well as the existence and degree of development of the dermal appendages (sweat glands and hair follicles) and dermal papillae. In the very old person, in whom dermal papillae and appendages are atrophic, and in the very young, in whom they have not yet fully developed, deep burns result from the same heat intensity that produces a moderate second-degree burn in the middle-aged adult. Since the skin of the back is thicker than that on any other part of the body, full-thickness burns are less common in this area. On the other hand, skin covering the inner arm is extraordinarily thin, thus full-thickness injury is frequently observed in this area.

The length and width of the burn wound is expressed as a percentage of the total body surface area displaying either second- or third-degree burns. The extent of the body surface involved is most commonly estimated by the "rule of nines" (Table 7-2). The major anatomic portions of the adult may be divided into multiples of 9 percent of the body surface area. The proportion of each of these areas with second- or third-degree burns is esti-

mated, and the summation of these estimates represents the percentage of the total body surface area burn. Because the surface area of the head and neck in childhood is significantly larger than 9 percent of the total body surface area and the surface area associated with the lower extremities is smaller, the rule of nines may not be used to estimate total body surface area burns in children. For example, a one-year-old child has 19 percent of the total body surface area associated with the head, as compared with only 7 percent in the adult patient. In contrast, each lower extremity represents only 13 percent of the total body surface area in the year-old infant. Thus the total body surface area burn in children is best estimated by the utilization of charts that relate regional body surface to age (Figure 7-2). A useful rule of thumb for estimating the amount of body surface area involved by a scattered burn injury is the *palm of hand rule*. The surface area of the patient's palm is roughly 1 percent of the total body surface area.

Over the past 20 years, many resuscitation formulas have been developed as guides to initial resuscitation in hypovolemic shock following thermal injury. Most utilize various combinations of crystalloid and colloid solutions but differ widely in the ratio of colloid to crystalloid, as well as the rate of fluid administration. The ideal resuscitation formula would rapidly restore normal hemodynamic stability. Such a response is dependent on the rate at which fluid is lost from the extracellular fluid compartment, the composition of the fluid lost, and the ability of various solutions to restore an effective circulating extracellular volume. Unfortunately, most formulas have been derived empirically from clinical experience, in which the amount of fluid required to restore renal function was accepted as optimal replacement therapy.

Although controversy still remains over "the solution" for resuscitation in burn shock, scientific investigation supports the need for both crystalloid and colloid solutions. *It is of relatively little consequence which formula is utilized to begin such therapy, as long as this is modified according to the patient's changing requirements.* The formula shown in Table 7-3 has been popularized by Baxter and is known as the *Parkland formula*. This formula has been adopted in most burn centers and is currently the standard against which new formulas must be compared. Data from numerous studies now suggest that both volume and the sodium ion are critical to providing adequate resuscitation in hypovolemic burn shock. Administration of crystalloid solution results in early expansion of depleted plasma and extracellular fluid volumes and return of the cardiac output toward normal. After 24 h, colloid remains the most effective solution to maintain plasma volume without further increasing edema formation. The Parkland formula was derived to provide specific replacement of known deficits measured by simultaneous determinations of red cell volume, plasma volume, extracellular fluid volume, and cardiac output during burn shock. The formula calls for the administration of 4 mL of lactated Ringer's solution/kg of body weight/percent of body surface area burn during the first 24 h postinjury. Fluid therapy during the second 24 h,

Table 7-2. "RULE OF NINES" FOR ESTIMATING PERCENTAGE OF BODY SURFACE INVOLVED IN BURNS

Anatomic area	Percent of body surface
Head	9
Right upper extremity	9
Left upper extremity	9
Right lower extremity	18
Left lower extremity	18
Anterior trunk	18
Posterior trunk	18
Neck	1

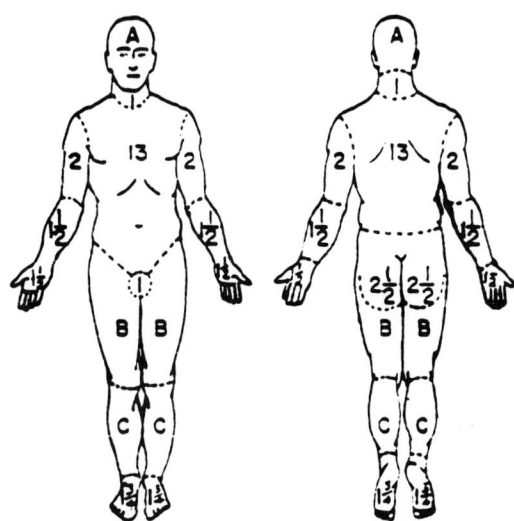

UNIVERSITY OF SOUTH ALABAMA MEDICAL CENTER
HOSPITAL AND CLINICS

BURN CHART

Relative Percentage of Areas Affected by Growth

Age	Age in Years					
	O	I	5	IO	I5	ADULT
A − ½ of head	$9\frac{1}{2}$	$8\frac{1}{2}$	$6\frac{1}{2}$	$5\frac{1}{2}$	$4\frac{1}{2}$	$3\frac{1}{2}$
B − ½ of one thigh	$2\frac{3}{4}$	$3\frac{1}{4}$	4	$4\frac{1}{4}$	$4\frac{1}{2}$	$4\frac{3}{4}$
C − ½ of one leg	$2\frac{1}{2}$	$2\frac{1}{2}$	$2\frac{3}{4}$	3	$3\frac{1}{4}$	$3\frac{1}{2}$

Total Percent Burned_____ 2°+ _____3°= ___

Fig. 7-2. Burn charts are used to determine exactly what percent of the total body surface area is involved.

Table 7-3. FLUID RESUSCITATION OF BURNED PATIENTS: PARKLAND FORMULA

First 24 h:
  Electrolyte solution (lactated Ringer's): 4 mL/kg body wt./% second- and third-degree burn
  Administration rate: ½ first 8 h, ¼ second 8 h, ¼ third 8 h
  Urine output: 30–70 mL/h

Second 24 h:
  Glucose in water (D_5W): To replace evaporative water loss, maintaining serum sodium concentration of 140 meq/L
  Colloid solution (plasma): To maintain plasma volume in patients with more than 40% second- and third-degree burns
  Urine output: 30–100 mL/h

according to this formula, consists in the administration of free water (5% dextrose in water) in quantities sufficient to maintain the serum sodium concentration at 140 meq/L (approximately 4 to 5 L in a 70-kg patient with a 50 percent burn) and plasma sufficient to return the plasma volume to normal and sustain adequate perfusion of peripheral organs and tissues (approximately 250 mL for each 10 percent total body surface area burn over 20 percent). Supplemental potassium replacement is usually not required during the first few days of management. The catabolic state caused by the burn injury results in increased urine levels of potassium with a decrease in total body potassium. The serum level of potassium remains normal or slightly elevated. When nutritional support is instituted and an anabolic state created, large amounts of potassium may be required to replenish this deficit and avoid acute decrease in serum potassium concentration.

During the first 24 h, the rate of fluid administration is adjusted to correspond as closely as possible with the rate of extracellular fluid loss. Baxter's studies have confirmed that extracellular deficits occur rapidly within the first 6 to 12 h postinjury. Therefore, one-half of the total calculated fluid volume is delivered during the first 8 h *from the time of injury* and the remaining fluids more slowly over the next 16 h.

The adequacy of resuscitation can best be judged by frequent measurements of vital signs, central venous pressure, hourly urine output, and observation of general mental and physical response. Urine output (normal, 30 to 100 mL/h in the adult) still remains one of the most reliable guides to adequacy of fluid therapy. Acute tubular necrosis, with resultant renal failure, is extremely rare in an adequately resuscitated patient, with the possible exception of a patient in whom there is extensive muscle damage (electrical burns) resulting in hemachromogen release and intratubular protein precipitation. Therefore, oliguria during the early postburn period is most often an indication of inadequate resuscitation, and increased fluid administration is the treatment of choice. Restriction of fluid is almost never indicated, and the administration of diuretics should be reserved for those cases in which tubular damage from circulating pigments appears likely, and then only after a sufficient amount of resuscitation fluids has been administered.

Urinary outputs of 30 to 100 mL/h should be maintained during the first 24 h in the adult patient. In the absence of hypoxia related to respiratory dysfunction, the patient's sensorium accurately reflects cerebral circulation. Well-resuscitated patients with major thermal injury rarely display hysteria, acute anxiety, or hostility.

The indications to use central venous catheters, Swan-Ganz catheters, and arterial lines in burn patients are identical to those for any trauma victim. The burn injury does not contraindicate their use (when needed) even if entrance through a burned site is necessary. Nonburned areas are preferred because of the difficulty in securing a catheter to eschar. All intravenous lines should be changed every 72 h whether or not they traverse burned tissue to lower the risk of septic thrombophlebitis and its sequelae.

Sedation

One of the most frequent therapeutic errors in the treatment of patients with major burns is the overuse of sedation. An insignificant burn of a minute area incurred during a common household mishap may be quite painful. Projection of such an experience by medical and paramedical personnel has resulted in marked overestimation of the pain associated with a major burn. If there is full-thickness skin destruction, the intrinsic sensory nerve endings have also been destroyed and the wound itself is painless. In contrast, the second-degree burn can be quite painful initially. Pain from a burn injury is markedly increased when the wound is roughly handled, or by exposing the wound to a cold environment. It is essential to completely examine the burn patient to determine if other injuries have occurred. When the physical examination is over, however, the wounds should be covered and the patient kept warm. This usually minimizes the pain from the burn sites, thereby decreasing the need for analgesics.

Sedative and analgesic medications must never be administered before hypoxia, hypovolemia, or both have been excluded, both states commonly producing an anxious, thrashing, disoriented patient. When given they should be kept at an *absolute minimum* to prevent depression of cardiopulmonary function and to allow evaluation of the sensorium, an important indicator of the adequacy of fluid resuscitation. Decreased peripheral circulation to muscle and skin is often associated with the hypovolemic state, so any narcotics administered intramuscularly or subcutaneously are subject to erratic uptake. Therefore, narcotics should always be administered in small doses by the intravenous route during the first 4 to 5 days. Administration by this route ensures rapid and predictable concentrations of the drug in the central nervous system and prevents the narcosis that may result following fluid resuscitation if repeated doses of narcotics have been administered by the intramuscular route.

Antibiotics

Subsequent to thermal injury, microorganisms contaminating the surfaces of the wound and persisting in the depth of the hair follicles and sweat glands begin to proliferate rapidly if topical chemotherapeutic agents are not applied. In the absence of topical chemotherapy, the superficial areas of the burn wound contain up to 100 million organisms per gram of tissue within 48 h following injury.

Characteristically, gram-positive organisms are responsible for this initial proliferation and colonization of the burn wound. At one time, most experienced clinicians prophylactically administered penicillin to patients with major burn injuries for a period of 3 to 4 days. Routine prophylactic administration of penicillin in the immediate postburn period is no longer recommended. Recent studies have demonstrated that the routine administration of prophylactic penicillin fails to lower the incidence of early gram-positive cellulitis, increases the incidence of yeast colonization of the gastrointestinal tract, and is associated with more rapid emergence of resistant gram-negative organisms in the burn wound. Penicillin prophylaxis, as a routine, has now been discontinued in most burn centers, and the incidence of early streptococcal cellulitis has not increased.

The full-thickness burn wound is relatively avascular. When it becomes infected, the avascular tissue may prevent the ingress of host defense factors and systemically administered antibiotics. The burn wound, once infected, may behave like an undrained abscess. Despite the current availability of newer antibiotic agents, some of which may penetrate to the eschar, one cannot rely totally on systemic agents as the sole mechanism of controlling microorganism proliferation in the burn wound. Other modalities such as topical antibiotics must be employed.

Systemic antibiotic agents are most useful in treating specific distant bacterial infections (e.g., pneumonia) that may complicate the burn victim's hospital course.

Tetanus Prophylaxis

All burn injuries must be considered contaminated, and tetanus prophylaxis is mandatory except in those patients actively immunized within the preceding 12 months. If a booster was received within the preceding 10 years, the intramuscular administration of 0.5 mL of absorbed tetanus toxoid will usually provide adequate prophylaxis. In the absence of active immunization within 10 years prior to the burn injury, 250 to 500 units of tetanus immunoglobulin (human) should be simultaneously administered at another site, utilizing a different syringe and needle so as to prevent inactivation of the immune globulin by toxoid.

Escharotomy

A principal characteristic of human skin is a remarkable degree of elasticity, which allows the skin to stretch with only minimum applied force. The elasticity of skin allows considerable edema of underlying soft tissues without increasing central limb pressure, which might impede either venous outflow or arterial inflow. If the skin were unyielding, a patient with a severely sprained ankle might lose blood flow to the distal foot as soft tissue edema occurred. Skin with second-degree injury retains its elastic properties. Full-thickness injury (third degree) is characterized by almost complete loss of elasticity. Thus circumferential third-degree burns are frequently associated with decreased peripheral blood flow as fluid resuscitation, accompanied by soft tissue edema, progresses. Failure to recognize this situation may result in unnecessary loss of distal extremities.

The usual clinical signs associated with poor peripheral blood flow in the nonburned patient, that is, diminished peripheral pulses and decreased skin temperature, are unreliable in patients with severe thermal injury. Hypovolemia with peripheral vasoconstriction usually results in decreased temperature of distal extremities in all patients with major second- and third-degree burns, and distal pulses often may not be felt as a result of overlying soft tissue edema preventing palpation of the underlying artery. More reliable signs of decreased peripheral flow in patients with circumferential third-degree burns are slow capillary refill (observed in the nail beds) and the onset of neurologic deficits. The most accurate monitoring device for assessing distal blood flow to extremities is the ultrasonic Doppler, which allows repetitive evaluation of both venous and arterial flow in the digital arteries and veins.

Patients with burns involving the extremities should have the affected limb elevated to minimize soft tissue edema. Should vascular impairment become apparent, however, escharotomies should immediately be performed. An escharotomy is simply an incision through the full depth of the eschar, thus relieving underlying pressure on the central arteries and veins. These incisions may be performed without anesthesia, since third-degree burns are anesthetic. Blood loss is minimal because of the extensive intracapillary coagulation that has occurred as a result of the thermal injury. The escharotomies are usually performed on the lateral and medial aspects of the extremity and must be carried across the joints, since the skin is most tightly adherent to the underlying fascia at these points and vascular obstruction is most likely to occur in these areas. In the upper extremity, the escharotomy should extend through all areas of third-degree burn down to and including the thenar and hypothenar spaces, in order to preserve the intrinsic muscles of the hand. Similarly, in the lower extremities, escharotomies should extend to the base of the large and small toes if the foot exhibits extensive third-degree burns. Escharotomies should only be performed once resuscitation is in progress and an adequate intravascular volume has been achieved. Once escharotomies have been performed, signs of adequate peripheral perfusion are to be expected. Persistent impairment of peripheral blood flow requires reassessment of intravascular volume status, and the extent and depth of the escharotomies. Fasciotomies may be considered at this stage.

Fasciotomy, a linear excision of the deep fascia surrounding the muscles, is rarely indicated in patients with severe burns. In rare instances of extensive incineration when burns involve not only the skin but the underlying fat and muscle, fasciotomy becomes necessary as a result of swelling within the muscle compartments. More frequently, fasciotomy is required in the treatment of electrical burns where there has been extensive muscle injury that appears potentially reversible.

Gastric Decompression

Most patients with more than 20 percent total body surface area burns will develop a reflex paralytic ileus some time during the first 24 h. Although bowel sounds are usually active for 6 to 10 h following the injury, intestinal motility is gradually lost for a short period of time during the latter half of the first 24 h. Unfortunately, the development of ileus frequently occurs at the time when medical and nursing surveillance has relaxed and the patient is asleep following sedation and restoration of fluid volume. Vomiting in such a patient carries a high risk of pulmonary aspiration, a complication associated with severe morbidity and high mortality. For this reason, patients with major burns require a nasogastric tube, so that the stomach may be effectively decompressed until normal gastrointestinal motility has been demonstrated.

The insertion of a nasogastric tube will also allow inspection of the gastric contents at periodic intervals. Patients with major burns are at risk of hemorrhagic gastritis as a result of increased stress. For this reason, gastric aspirates should be monitored frequently for the presence of frank blood or guaiac-positive material, and antacid should be instilled through the nasogastric tube at hourly intervals to prevent superficial erosions of the gastric mucosa.

Histamine H_2 receptor antagonists that suppress gastric acid secretion may also be used to prevent or treat stress gastritis. In elderly patients and at high doses, certain of these compounds may produce central nervous system changes such as confusion, slurred speech, delirium, and hallucinations. Fever, serum creatinine changes, leukopenia, bradycardia, and diarrhea have been reported to occur infrequently. Therefore, these compounds are usually used if stress gastritis develops despite adequate antacid administration.

Medical Evacuation

Although most hospitals are equipped to provide emergency therapy of the patient with a major burn, the majority of community hospitals have neither the nursing nor the paramedical expertise to comfortably care for a patient with massive burn injury. Furthermore, because of the special physical requirements necessary for optimal treatment of such patients, personnel in community hospitals often transfer such patients to special facilities as soon as appropriate arrangements can be made. Guidelines for hospitalization or transfer to a burn treatment facility are outlined in Table 7-4.

Extensive experience with medical evacuation of severely burned soldiers during the Korean and Vietnam wars has yielded valuable information that may assist in ensuring safe transfer of burned patients. In general, such patients tolerate evacuation best if they are moved within the first 24 to 48 h. Prior to transfer, a fluid resuscitation program should be started. Patients with a larger than 20 percent burn should have a Foley catheter inserted into the bladder, so that urinary output can be monitored during the evacuation and fluid administration appropriately adjusted. Pulmonary function should be assessed, and if impending upper airway obstruction or severe smoke inhalation is suspected, an endotracheal tube should be inserted prior to transfer. Extensive debridement or treatment of the burn wounds is unnecessary and is generally to be avoided, since it interferes with evaluation of the burn wound by the receiving hospital. Rather, the

Table 7-4. TRIAGE CRITERIA

Burn size	Admit to hospital	Transfer to burn treatment facility
Total	>15%	>20%
Third degree	>2%	>10%
Age	<5 or >60	<5 or >60
Airway or inhalation injury	Present	Severe
Electric injury	Present	Severe
Significant associated injury or preexisting disease	Present	Present
Deep burns of face, hands, feet, or perineum	Present	Present
Suspected child abuse	Present	Present

SOURCE: American College of Surgeons, *Bulletin,* October 1979.

wounds should be temporarily wrapped in sterile dressings to provide maximal comfort during the transfer. If air evacuation is to be utilized, it is especially important to insert a nasogastric tube, since air within the stomach will expand at increased altitude, often inducing acute gastric distention and vomiting. This, in turn, could result in aspiration pneumonitis, which would be particularly compromising in a patient with the smoke inhalation syndrome.

THERAPY OF THE BURN WOUND

Debridement and Excision

Second-degree wounds (partial-thickness burn injury) usually present as vesicular lesions. Unless very small, the overlying blister should be punctured and the nonviable skin removed. This permits the direct application of topical chemotherapeutic agents to the underlying viable dermal remnants. Failure to prevent secondary bacterial infection of deep second-degree burn wounds may result in conversion of the partial-thickness injury to a full-thickness injury. Debridement can usually be accomplished without anesthesia, utilizing careful surgical technique and modest amounts of sedation prior to removing the nonviable superficial epithelium.

The nonviable skin of the third-degree burn is referred to as the *eschar.* Usually the eschar remains tightly adherent to the underlying subcutaneous tissues and cannot be sharply debrided without severe hemorrhage and significant pain. Therefore, except in special circumstances, only loose eschar, which may be debrided without anesthesia or excessive blood loss, is removed initially. The remaining eschar is left intact, and efforts are made to prevent bacterial colonization and invasion by the use of topical chemotherapeutic agents. Topical chemotherapeutic agents do not sterilize the third-degree burn eschar, and eventually bacterial growth will occur. The topical agents are employed to control the rate of proliferation of bacteria within the burn wound, so as to prevent invasion of underlying viable tissue, with entrance of bacteria into the bloodstream. At about 18 to 24 days following burn injury, the third-degree burn eschar will separate from the underlying viable tissue as a result of the liberation of bacterial proteases. At this time, it is extraordinarily important that the eschar be promptly debrided, in order to prevent systemic sepsis as a result of localized abscess formation beneath the eschar. Normally, the patients are taken to a hydrotherapy area once or twice a day during the first 3 weeks in order to cleanse the surface of the eschar and to inspect the wound. Each day, the physician debrides any loose areas of eschar and carefully inspects the wound and unroofs any localized abscess pockets.

Modern surgical principles dictate the surgical debridement of nonviable tissue in the treatment of major injury. In the case of burn injury, however, immediate total debridement of nonviable eschar is not always possible. Some investigators have advocated the use of topical enzyme preparations to more rapidly remove the eschar. The advantages of such an approach include debridement without anesthesia and limitation of associated hemorrhage. The efficacy of currently available enzymes has not been conclusively demonstrated. Furthermore, most enzyme preparations require the use of overlying wet dressings to maintain the activity of the enzyme. Such dressings promote wound infection, since they provide a warm, moist environment. In addition, some of the enzyme preparations inhibit the effectiveness of topical chemotherapeutic agents in controlling the rate of proliferation of bacterial growth. Therefore, other authors have condemned the use of enzymatic debridement, maintaining that the risks of sepsis far outweigh the benefits of early debridement. In addition, some enzyme preparations do not effectively differentiate nonviable eschar from underlying normal tissues, and erosion of vessels in viable tissue occasionally induces unexpected bleeding from the wound.

Tangential excision of deep second- and third-degree wounds has become increasingly more popular in major burn centers in the past decade. The eschar is tangentially excised utilizing a specially designed knife or an air-driven dermatome to sequentially remove layers of the eschar in sheets approximately 0.010 in. in thickness until viable tissue, as evidenced by capillary bleeding, is encountered. Primary closure is achieved by immediate grafting with autograft (if adequate donor sites are available) or temporary closure with heterograft, homograft, or synthetic barrier dressings. The procedure, although technically easy to perform, requires experience in determining an adequate level of excision. This is especially true when full-thickness injury has occurred and the level of excision is into the subcutaneous fat. Viability of this relatively avascular layer is often difficult to appreciate. The decision to perform early tangential excision (within 72 h of admission) must depend on analysis of both potential risks and benefits of this technique. The major advantage is a shortened hospital stay and potentially improved function when wounds extend across joints. The major disadvantage is the risk of performing a major surgical procedure (with significant blood loss) requiring general anesthesia in an already critically injured patient. Most centers now employ tangential excision for deep second- or third-degree burns of functionally critical areas, such as hands and face, and to shorten the hospital course in relatively good risk patients.

Several investigators have utilized the carbon dioxide laser to excise third-degree burn eschar. The CO_2 laser allows removal of tissue with relatively little blood loss, and the level of excision can be readily selected by the surgeon. The procedure is very slow, because of the limited power that can be generated by the CO_2 laser with safety for both the patient and the operating room personnel. Thus the procedure results in prolonged operating time. Furthermore, the required equipment is expensive and somewhat cumbersome to use. Since the laser beam may cause serious damage to the retina following exposure, operating room personnel must wear protective glasses. Finally, the laser energy is partially dissipated in the underlying viable tissue (the graft recipient site), and the resulting injury to superficial cells may prevent acceptance of heterograft, homograft, and autograft.

When third-degree burns are relatively limited in size (less than 5 percent), as may occur following contact with a hot piece of metal, the full-thickness eschar may be excised primarily under anesthesia without excessive hemorrhage. The wound should be covered immediately with autograft. This approach markedly decreases postburn morbidity and often results in a better cosmetic appearance.

Children with massive injuries (greater than 70 percent of total body surface area being third degree) have been successfully treated with staged, extensive excision to fascia of all burned areas. The open wounds are immediately covered with viable homograft that is allowed to "take." Immunosuppression with antithymocytic globulin (ATG) has been utilized by at least two investigators. Immunosuppression has not been proved efficacious, however, and can only be recommended for use in specialized burn facilities actively involved in clinical investigation of skin transplant immunology. This approach has not proved to be of value in treating the massively burned adult.

Adult patients with massive burn injuries of more than 70 percent total body surface burns, of which at least 60 percent is third-degree, should undergo early, deep burn wound excision. Such procedures should be attempted only in major centers, since this approach requires enormous medical, paramedical, and nursing support. Prior to excision, the burn wound must be sterile or contain only a relatively low concentration of bacteria (less than 10^4 organisms per gram of tissue). Some authors advocate the preoperative infusion of antibiotics by subeschar clysis into the eschar that is to be excised. In this manner, maximum antibiotic concentration is achieved in the relatively avascular eschar, and the chances of seeding the bloodstream during the procedure are presumably reduced. Both the eschar and the underlying subcutaneous fat are excised. The exposed deep fascia must be immediately covered with homograft. Failure to provide immediate physiologic coverage results in desiccation of the fascia and subsequent secondary infection. Thus an unlimited bank of homograft, obtained from cadavers, must be maintained. Furthermore, excision of 20 percent of the total body surface is frequently associated with loss of the patient's complete blood volume. Centers using this approach must have blood banks capable of providing significant quantities of both stored and fresh blood. In some cases, the blood loss has been reduced by utilizing deliberate hypotensive anesthesia during the procedure. Obviously, the operative procedure inflicts great stress on the patient, who already will have evidenced marked pathophysiologic alterations. Extraordinary intensive care support by both physicians and specialized nursing personnel is therefore required postoperatively in the intensive care area.

Patients with electrical injuries often have injury to the muscle compartments of the extremity. Early surgical exploration, fasciotomy, and removal of nonviable muscle should be performed when motor dysfunction or massive edema of the extremity occurs. Repeat exploration within a few days may be required to further debride necrotic tissue. In the interim, the wounds can temporarily be closed with heterografts.

Cutaneous burns resulting from contact with hot tar or asphalt are not infrequently encountered. By the time the physician sees the patient, the tar has solidified on the burn wound as it has cooled. It may be removed by applying generous quantities of Neopolycin ointment to the burn wound, over which a large occlusive dressing is applied. The dressing may be removed 18 to 24 h later. At this time most or all of the tar will be dissolved, and a water-soluble topical chemotherapeutic agent may be applied.

Topical Chemotherapy

Modern antibacterial topical therapy was advocated by Monafo and Moyer in the early 1960s. These investigators used aqueous silver nitrate (0.5%) solution as a continuous wet soak, in combination with large, bulky dressings. The mode of action of silver nitrate is not specifically known but probably depends on the free silver ion, which is active at relatively low concentrations. Silver nitrate is effective against most gram-positive organisms and most strains of *Pseudomonas,* although it has limited effectiveness against other gram-negative bacteria such as *Enterobacter* and *Klebsiella.* The agent sterilizes the surface of the wound but has limited penetration of deeper tissues. Therefore, the eschar must be removed rapidly when deep bacterial colonization occurs, in order to prevent invasion of underlying viable tissue. The major complication associated with the use of silver nitrate solution is severe electrolyte depletion (primarily sodium and chloride), necessitating frequent monitoring of serum electrolytes, since specific replacement therapy is required. Silver nitrate therapy has been acclaimed as the most economical topical agent. The drug itself is inexpensive and available in most hospital pharmacies. The large quantities of dressings required, the increased nursing personnel requirements to effect the dressing changes, and the major housekeeping problems associated with discoloration caused on contact by precipitation of silver salts significantly increase the cost of this form of treatment. In addition, the necessity for bulky dressings inhibits the early active movement of extremities and therefore encourages less than optimum joint function.

In the mid-1960s, Lindberg, Moncrief, and Mason introduced mafenide acetate (Sulfamylon), a topically applied cream that allowed open treatment of burn wounds. Mafenide acetate has proved effective against a wide range of gram-positive and gram-negative organisms, as well as most anaerobes. This drug actively diffuses through the eschar, thus providing protection in the depth of the eschar at the interface between the viable and nonviable tissue. Since the burns remain exposed, wounds can be more readily examined. In addition, the treatment does not interfere with intensive physical therapy and allows uninhibited treatment of associated soft tissue inju-

ries. Unfortunately, the drug is a potent inhibitor of carbonic anhydrase and therefore may induce acid-base derangements. Acidosis may develop rapidly in the presence of pulmonary dysfunction. The use of the drug is associated with a pronounced reduction of the buffering capacity of the blood, as a result of increased bicarbonate excretion by the kidney, and simultaneous hypocapnea secondary to hyperventilation. Other disadvantages associated with the use of this drug include pain on application, an occasional hypersensitivity reaction (5 to 7 percent), delayed eschar separation due to improved bacterial control, and the emergence of opportunistic infections, including *Providencia, Serratia,* fungal, yeast, and viral infections.

Silver sulfadiazine (Silvadene), developed by Fox in the late 1960s, has essentially the same bacterial spectrum as mafenide acetate but is associated with fewer disadvantages. The major side effects are hypersensitivity reaction to sulfa (5 to 7 percent), delayed eschar separation, and emergence of opportunistic infections. The agent appears to desiccate the wound less than other topical drugs and consequently keeps the eschar soft, allowing for greater joint mobility. It does not inhibit carbonic anhydrase activity, and its application is soothing rather than painful.

Betadine, a water-soluble topical antiseptic complex of polyvinylpyrrolidone (povidone) iodine, is effective against a wide range of gram-positive and gram-negative organisms, as well as some fungi. The drug is manufactured as an ointment and as an aerosol cream. The drug readily diffuses through the eschar and is absorbed and excreted rapidly. Systemic toxicity is apparently rare. One major disadvantage of this agent is its propensity to cause rapid desiccation of the eschar, resulting in interference with progressive active physical therapy programs. In addition, its application to partial-thickness burns may be associated with mild to moderate pain. This agent has only recently been extensively used for the topical therapy of burns and, as in the case of other topical agents, emergence of opportunistic infections may be expected after more extensive experience.

The properties of each of the currently utilized topical chemotherapeutic agents are summarized in Table 7-5. Newer and even more effective topical agents are currently in clinical trial and may be expected to be marketed in the near future. It is important to emphasize that burn wounds treated with these topical agents are not sterilized; rather, the bacterial population is effectively suppressed and remains at levels below that associated with the development of invasive burn wound sepsis. Furthermore, the agents are effective in preventing bacterial conversion of second-degree burns to full-thickness injury, thus reducing the amount of skin that might be required had the agents not been employed.

Bacteriologic Monitoring

Despite the use of topical chemotherapeutic agents, some patients, particularly those with burns of more than 60 percent of the total body surface, will evidence pro-

Table 7-5. PROPERTIES OF TOPICAL CHEMOTHERAPEUTIC AGENTS

Agent	*Antibacterial spectrum*	*Dressings required?*	*Disadvantages*
Sodium mafenide (Sulfamylon)	Gram-positive and gram-negative organisms and most anaerobes	No	Pain on application; skin allergy; carbonic anhydrase inhibition; resistant organisms
Silver nitrate 0.5%	Most gram-positive organisms and some strains of *Pseudomonas*	Yes	Hyponatremia; hypochloremia; failure to penetrate eschar; methemoglobinemia
Silver sulfadiazine (Silvadene)	Gram-positive and gram-negative organisms and *Candida albicans*	No	Skin allergy; resistant organisms
Povidone-iodine (Betadine)	Gram-positive organisms and fungi; possibly less effective vs. some gram-negative organisms	Yes (cream) No (aerosol)	Pain on application; excessive drying of eschar

gressive colonization of the burn wound, with subsequent invasion of viable tissue and bloodstream dissemination of the bacteria. Therefore, clinical bacteriologic monitoring of the burn wound is imperative in order to diagnose incipient burn wound sepsis and effect immediate treatment.

In general, cultures of the burn wound surface have failed to accurately predict progressive bacterial colonization or incipient burn wound sepsis. Qualitative and quantitative correlation is poor between flora on the surface of the burn wound and bacterial colonization of the deep layers of the eschar. Blood cultures, although helpful if bacteral growth is demonstrated, have not proved particularly useful, since life-threatening sepsis may occur in the absence of bacteremia, and the presence of bacteria in the bloodstream is a relatively late phenomenon, often just preceding death. Bacterial growth in burn wounds is best monitored by semiquantitative burn wound biopsy cultures. Multiple full-thickness wound biopsies are obtained serially from representative areas of the burn wound. The tissue is weighed, homogenized, serially diluted, and inoculated on blood agar and eosin–methylene blue plates. In this manner, the precise number of viable organisms per gram of tissue can be calculated. When wound biopsy cultures reveal more than 10^5 organisms per gram of tissue or a hundredfold increase in the concentration of organisms per gram of tissue is observed within a 48-h period, it may be assumed that the organisms have escaped effective control by the topical chemotherapeutic agent and that burn wound sepsis is incipient.

Heterograft and Homograft

All terrestrial mammals require an intact epithelial covering in order to maintain water, electrolyte, and thermal homeostasis. Following spontaneous separation of eschar or after surgical removal by tangential or fascial excision, the wound can be temporarily covered with a biologic dressing. Either porcine heterograft or homograft obtained from cadavers is most commonly utilized. The application of these materials, providing early temporary wound closure, can contribute to the prevention and control of infection, the preservation of healthy granulation tissue, and maintenance of joint function. Specifically, the physiologic dressings decrease evaporative water loss and diminish heat loss secondary to evaporation; they cover exposed sensory nerves and therefore decrease pain associated with the open wound; and they protect neurovascular tissue and tendons that would otherwise be exposed. When the physiologic dressing adheres to the underlying granulation tissue, bacterial proliferation is readily inhibited, since the heterograft or homograft provides an acceptable surface against which neutrophils may entrap bacteria. Until the wound is ready for definitive autograft, deeper tissues are protected from desiccation. The physiologic dressings prevent the development of hypermature granulation tissue and promote a well-nourished recipient bed, and they act as an excellent test material to determine the optimal time for subsequent autograft. When adherence is observed, the bed may be assumed to be in optimal condition for autograft, and postoperative loss of split-thickness skin grafts (autografts) will rarely occur.

Heterograft and homograft are most commonly used for temporary coverage of open wounds, as described above. The grafts are removed within 5 days and replaced with new physiologic dressing until autografting has been accomplished. These physiologic dressings may also be utilized to debride untidy wounds immediately after eschar separation. The heterograft or homograft hastens separation of very tiny pieces of eschar left behind at the time of debridement. It should be emphasized, however, that physiologic dressings may be used for this purpose with safety only if more than 95 percent of the eschar has been mechanically removed in the course of daily debridement or by surgical excision.

Either heterograft or homograft may be used electively over reepithelializing deep second-degree burns, once superficial necrotic debris has been entirely removed (usually 5 to 7 days). Adherent physiologic dressings at this time will promote the rate of reepithelialization and decrease pain in the wound, allowing decreased hospitalization time. Some clinicians utilize heterograft or homograft to immediately cover very superficial second-degree burns. The advantages of such treatment include marked decrease in pain, decreased hospitalization, earlier return of joint function, and more rapid reepithelialization of the burn. Utilization of physiologic dressings in this manner must be undertaken with caution. One must be certain that the wound is indeed extremely superficial in depth with minimal necrotic tissue, since coverage of a deeper wound essentially closes an open abscess and may precipitate burn wound sepsis. In addition, the homograft or heterograft must be applied within hours after the burn injury, before colonization with microbial organisms occurs.

It is important that the physiologic dressing and burn wound be inspected within 24 h to ensure continued adherence to the dermal remnants. Should the physiologic dressing become dislodged or should fluid accumulate beneath it, the material should be removed immediately and the wound treated with topical chemotherapeutic agents in the conventional manner. If the heterograft or homograft remains adherent, it is important that it not be removed but rather be allowed to separate spontaneously as reepithelialization occurs. Frequent changing of physiologic dressings applied to second-degree burns results in sequential removal of epithelial cells at the time of removal and may convert them to full-thickness burn wounds.

Autograft

Definitive closure of burn wounds as soon as possible after injury is the ultimate objective of all burn wound care. There are, however, priorities of coverage dictated by functional and cosmetic considerations. In general, the hands, feet, joints, and face should be covered prior to nonfunctional surfaces. Autografts may be applied as sheets of skin without the need of suture fixation or "pie crusting" incisions to allow release of plasma. Fixation with bandaging is not required unless accidental dislodgment is likely, e.g., on circumferentially burned limbs or on burns of patients with uncontrollable motion. Exposure of the freshly applied autograft allows continuous graft inspection and early evacuation of any collections of blood or serum that may occur beneath the graft. When dressings are used, they should be removed 72 h following grafting. If the grafts are adherent, active motion of the burned area may be begun.

Patients with extensive burns often present a serious disproportion between the area requiring autografting and available donor sites. Mesh or expanded grafts may be utilized to cover large areas from limited donor sites. After harvest of the skin grafts, the grafts are placed on plastic carriers and passed through a Tanner-Vanderput mesh dermatome. A series of parallel incisions is made in the sheet graft, allowing expansion of up to six times the area of the original donor site. The small interstices are rapidly filled by epithelialization (4 to 8 days), resulting in a somewhat thinner but physiologically functional skin cover. When mesh grafts are used, moist protective dressings or dressings with material that will maintain a moisture barrier (semipermeable or impermeable) prevent the deeper tissues (exposed through the interstices

of the mesh graft) from desiccating. Once the epithelium has extended from the edges of the mesh across the interstices, the grafts may be exposed to room air and humidity. In general, mesh grafts are not used on the face, hands, feet, and flexion creases, since the healed grafts are not as cosmetically acceptable as intact autografts. In addition, mesh grafts are less able to withstand recurrent localized trauma.

Synthetics

Synthetic skin substitutes possess many theoretical advantages over their biologic counterparts (heterograft, homograft). Synthetic materials can be mass-produced, have an indefinite shelf life, are relatively inert, and are comparatively inexpensive. Numerous products are now available for very specific types of wounds; results are equal to those produced by biologic materials.

"Spray-on" polymeric dressings have, in general, been abandoned. In extensive testing they were found safe in treating superficial second-degree burns and donor sites. When used, however, they required daily inspection of the wound for purulence or nonadherence of the dressing, and their use on deeper second- or third-degree burns was contraindicated.

A variety of synthetic sheet dressings with varying water permeability and adherence properties are now available. These have proved useful in the treatment of donor sites and superficial second-degree burns and as temporary dressings after surgical excision of the eschar. Poor adherence remains a major problem with these materials, so their use for extended periods of time following major burn wound excision is not recommended.

Recently a bilayer artificial skin composed of a temporary silastic epidermis and a porous collagen chondroitin 6-sulfate fibrillar dermis has been developed. Following grafting, the dermal component is populated with fibroblasts and vessels from the wound bed. The silastic epidermis remains firmly adherent but can be removed weeks or even months later when autograft tissue is available for transplantation. When the silastic is removed, extremely thin (0.003 to 0.004 in. thick) epidermal grafts are placed on the newly formed dermal bed. The extremely thin donor sites heal rapidly, allowing earlier recropping if required.

The neodermis produced with the use of artificial skin microscopically resembles normal dermis. The gross feel and texture of the neodermis is more analogous to normal dermis than to scar tissue. Artificial skin currently is being tested in a number of centers in this country, and preliminary results are excellent.

GENERAL THERAPEUTIC CONSIDERATIONS

Metabolism and Nutrition

Hypermetabolism characterizes the human response to major injury. Several investigators have now shown a direct relationship between the magnitude and duration of the hypermetabolic response and the severity of the sustained trauma. Wilmore has demonstrated a curvilinear relationship between the resting metabolic expenditure and the magnitude of total body surface burn in human patients. Resting metabolic rate approached a maximum response of approximately twice normal in patients with burns of more than 60 percent of the total body surface. Both Reiss and Wilmore have documented caloric expenditure in excess of 60 kcal/($m^2 \cdot h$) in patients with major thermal injury. Total daily energy consumption during the nonresting state in severely burned patients approached 40 kcal for each percent of body surface burned, plus 25 kcal/kg of body weight.

Previously, the hypermetabolic response was attributed in part to obligatory energy losses in the form of heat associated with a marked increase in evaporative water loss. The increase in evaporative water loss results from destruction of the water barrier within the skin. If water evaporation is mechanically prevented, however, there is no significant decrease in the metabolic rate observed in the burn patient. Furthermore, one cannot reduce oxygen consumption in thermally injured patients to normal levels by manipulation of environmental temperature and humidity. This suggests that the hypermetabolic response is non-temperature-dependent. A close correlation has been demonstrated between oxygen consumption and urinary catecholamine excretion. In addition, hypermetabolic response has been partially blocked by the administration of alpha- and beta-adrenergic blocking agents. The hypermetabolic response in human beings is associated with increased rectal and skin temperatures, and animal experiments have demonstrated that burn injury is associated with a true increase in critical temperature. These studies suggest that the hypermetabolic response to burn injury is mediated through the hypothalamic temperature center, which emits an efferent signal expressed via catecholamine excretion.

In addition to elevated energy requirements, a marked catabolic response accompanies severe burn injury. The postburn catabolism is associated with weight loss, retarded wound healing, and negative nitrogen, potassium, sulfur, and phosphorus balance. Again, the magnitude and duration of the catabolic response roughly parallels the severity of the burn injury. Up to 30 g of nitrogen/day may be recovered from the urine of severely burned patients. If extraordinary means to provide excessive dietary nitrogen are not pursued, negative nitrogen balance may be observed for up to 2 months following the thermal accident. However, protein catabolism does not proceed uniformly in all tissues. Structural and functional integrity of vital organs such as the heart and liver is maintained at the expense of muscle protein.

Posttraumatic negative nitrogen balance can be ameliorated if sufficient caloric and nitrogen intake is provided. More than 20 g of nitrogen/m^2 of body surface per day is required in patients with major burns during the first postburn month in order to maintain positive nitrogen balance. During the second postburn month, nitrogen intake of 13 to 16 g/($m^2 \cdot$ day) will maintain nitrogen equilibrium. The catabolic response in burn patients is associated with increased levels of glucagon and catecholamine (catabolic hormones) in the plasma and depressed levels of insulin (anabolic hormone).

Total oxidation of a normal 70-kg male would yield approximately 166,000 endogenous kcal. It is estimated that healthy persons can tolerate acute losses of up to one-third of lean body weight before death ensues. Thus an extensively burned adult, with energy requirements of 5000 kcal/day, becomes a severe nutritional risk within 2 weeks, assuming no oral or parenteral caloric intake. Since most of the kinetic energy requirements of the supine, bedridden patient are associated with maintenance of normal respiratory function, the most common cause of death in these patients is pulmonary sepsis. An ineffective respiratory effort results in progressive atelectasis and subsequent lung infection by opportunistic pathogens.

The clinical consequences of inadequate nutritional replacement include profound weight loss, development of superior mesenteric artery syndrome, decreased immunologic response, diminished leukocyte function (host resistance), impaired wound healing, and severe inhibition of cellular active transport, resulting in cellular dysfunction.

Current knowledge of the hypermetabolic response following injury allows more rational therapy aimed at preventing morbid consequences of acute malnutrition. Control of the environment by maintaining an externally warm temperature (31°C) will alleviate patient discomfort and shivering associated with a cold environment and prevent further increases in the metabolic rate subsequent to cold stress (Fig. 7-3). Furthermore, apprehension and pain may be treated appropriately with narcotics and tranquilizers, since both these stresses are known to potentiate the release of catecholamines.

Effective prohylaxis against infection and timely closure of the burn wound will ameliorate both the catabolic and the hypermetabolic response to burn injury. A progressive physical therapy program will also enhance the deposition of protein into lean muscle mass, which allows performance of kinetic work required for maintenance of normal function.

The cornerstone of nutritional management of the burn patient is the provision of adequate exogenous calories and nitrogen to prevent prolonged catabolism. Whenever possible, the gastrointestinal tract should be used for the various dietary regimens designed to supply the nutritional needs of the patient. Maintenance of adequate nutrition is best monitored by accurate daily measurements of body weight. Postburn weight loss of less than 10 percent is usually well tolerated, provided the patient was not nutritionally depleted prior to the burn injury. Weight loss that exceeds 10 percent of the preburn weight is often associated with an increased incidence of morbidity.

When the voluntary food intake of the burned patient is insufficient to provide for positive energy balance, the physician must intervene with forced feedings, by either the parenteral or the enteral route. Enteral feedings may be accomplished by insertion of a small silastic nasogastric feeding tube through which nutrients are delivered

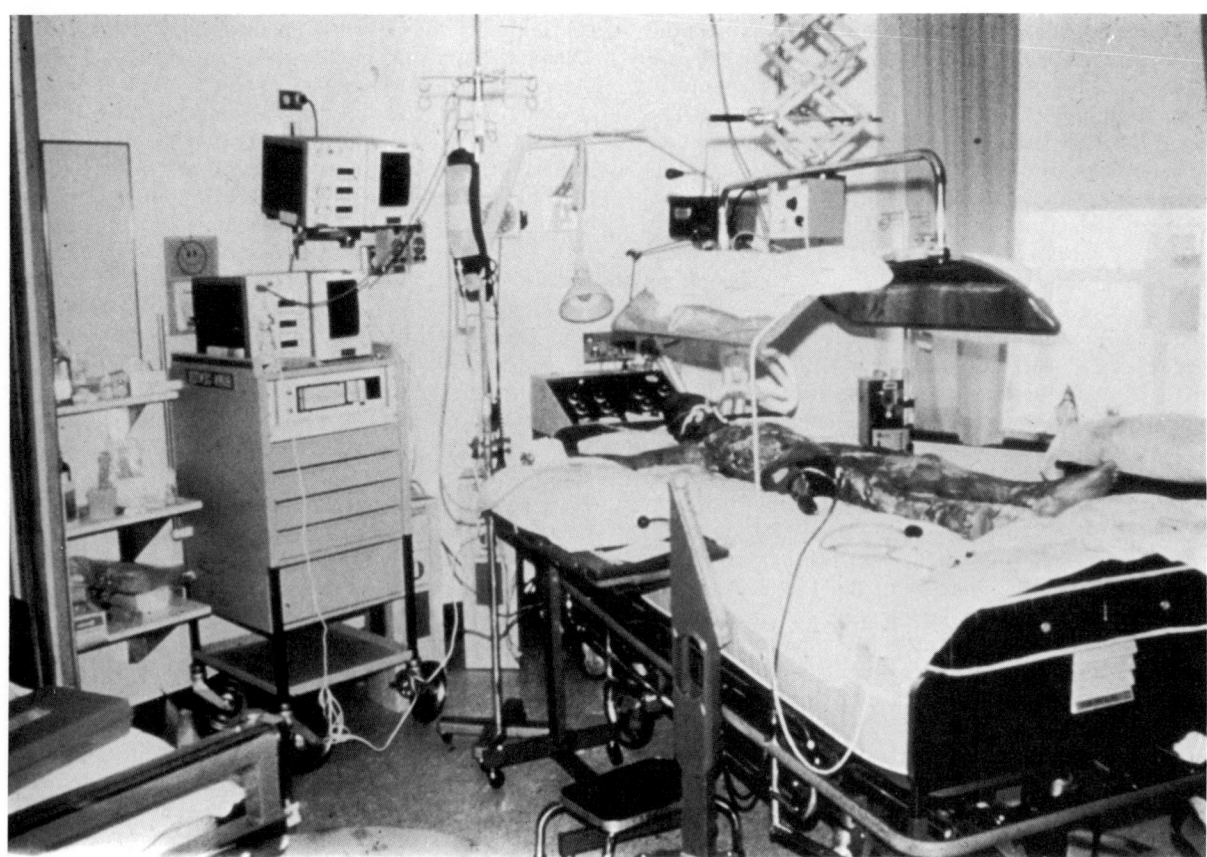

Fig. 7-3. Burn patients require well-equipped facilities for optimum care. The patient is maintained in a warm environment under a heat shield to minimize cold stress.

24 h a day via a constant delivery pump. Usually patients with major burns tolerate a complete homogenized diet. Partially digested or elemental diets are usually contraindicated, since the higher osmolality associated with these diets often results in gastric distention, profuse diarrhea, or dehydration when large caloric intakes are administered. When positive energy balance is unobtainable by utilization of the gastrointestinal route alone, intravenous hyperalimentation should be employed simultaneously in order to avoid prolonged periods of malnutrition. The intravenous administration of fat emulsions and amino acid solutions by peripheral vein may also be used to supplement enteral caloric intake, if necessary.

Physical Therapy, Splinting, and Rehabilitation

Contractures associated with serious loss of joint function may complicate severe thermal injury. It has now been documented that a progressive physical therapy program implemented immediately after hospital admission is associated with preservation of range of motion in joints with overlying burn injury. It should be emphasized that the program must begin on the day of admission and be continued until the burn wounds are healed and normal range of joint motion can be maintained by the patient. Major burn centers have found it necessary to employ full-time physical therapists to supervise active physical therapy at the bedside during waking hours. Repetitive exercises are conducted in the direction opposite that of any anticipated deformity.

Prolonged immobilization must be avoided, and early motion following skin grafting should be encouraged. In addition, proper positioning during bed rest must be monitored, and splints must be manufactured to maintain anticontracture positions during sleep. When a carefully supervised program of physical therapy is an integral part of burn wound care, 85 percent of the joints underlying surface burns should have a normal range of motion at the completion of therapy. The upper extremities are more susceptible to the deleterious effects of prolonged immobilization than the lower extremities. The ideal position for the lower extremities (knees extended, feet in neutral position) is comfortable to the patient and relatively easy to maintain in either the prone or supine position. The shoulders, however, are difficult to position or splint in patients with extensive burns. Elevation and abduction of the arm at the shoulder joint are often uncomfortable, and a patient with burns at the shoulder invariably assumes and maintains a position of adduction and extension if not carefully monitored by nursing personnel and therapists.

Many factors influence the success of a physical therapy program, including patient motivation, but no factor

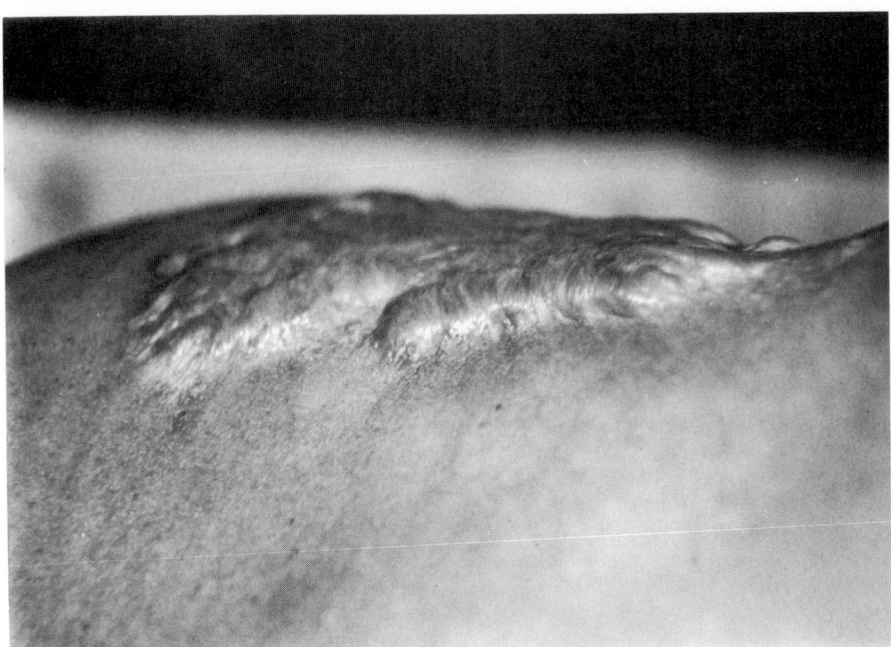

Fig. 7-4. Hypertrophic scarring usually develops in areas of second-degree burns that have spontaneously healed.

is more deleterious to the preservation of motion than delay of treatment. Daily range-of-motion evaluation and appropriate daily exercises to achieve maximum potential range of motion in joints underlying both second- and third-degree surface burns are of paramount importance. Goals should be established during the early postburn period, which must be rapidly achieved and thereafter maintained. The patient should be encouraged to pursue daily self-care activities as soon as possible. By the time of discharge, the patient should be as independent as possible and should have mastered a home physical therapy program to maintain function.

The development of hypertrophic scars may occur after hospital discharge (Fig. 7-4). The resultant scar overgrowth may inhibit function and often causes severe disfigurement. Larson and his associates have reported reduction of hypertrophic scar formation following the application of conforming isoprene splints and/or elastic garments during the convalescent period (Fig. 7-5). A variety of new materials are now available that can be placed deep to the pressure garments or splints to concentrate pressure on critical contoured areas (bridge of nose, chin, neck, web spaces of the hand). A new technique using clear high-temperature plastic is also available to control scarring about the face. An exact casting of the face is first made using plaster, over which the high-temperature plastic is molded. The resultant face mask is applied to the face as soon as the burns have healed.

All these devices exert pressure on the scar, causing better alignment of collagen fibrils and reduction of local interstitial edema. Splints and pressure devices are started when the patient is in the burn center, and the

Fig. 7-5. Form-fitted elastic compression garments may help to minimize hypertrophic scarring.

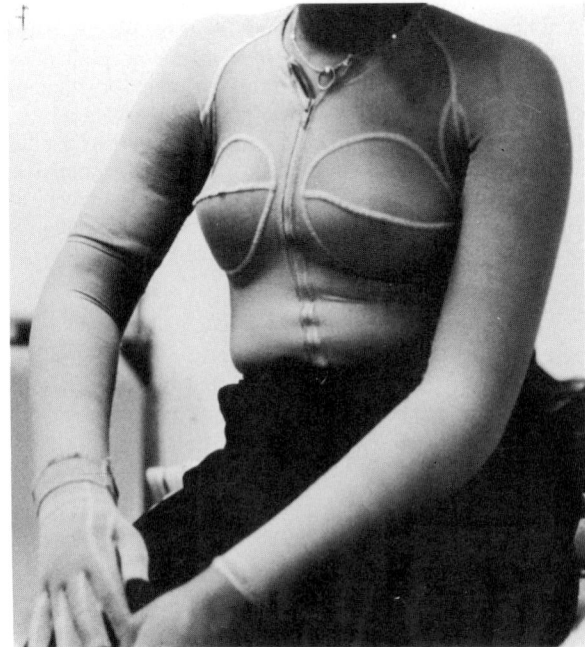

devices are continued for at least 6 months after discharge to discourage the delayed development of a hypertrophic scar.

COMPLICATIONS

Smoke Inhalation Syndrome

Smoke inhalation syndrome is an acute pulmonary dysfunction related to lower respiratory tract pathophysiology occurring within 72 h after exposure to gaseous products of incomplete combustion (primarily aldehydes). The severity of this syndrome is a function of the type of smoke inhaled, its amount, and the magnitude of the accompanying thermal injury. Patients with smoke inhalation syndrome frequently exhibit *no* physical signs or symptoms of injury during the first 24 h after sustaining a major burn. Smoke inhalation should be highly suspected in patients burned within an enclosed space, patients injured while under the influence of alcohol or drugs, and patients who lost consciousness at the time of the accident. Such patients are most likely to have inhaled large amounts of smoke prior to being evacuated from the scene of the fire.

Diagnosis is dependent on a high index of suspicion and careful physical and laboratory examination (Table 7-6). At the time of initial examination, sputum should be obtained from the lower respiratory tract and examined for the presence of carbon. When carbonaceous sputum is noted, the patient should be hospitalized and observed for the development of severe respiratory dysfunction within 18 to 36 h. Carboxyhemoglobin concentration should be measured as soon as the patient reaches the hospital. Normal carboxyhemoglobin levels are of relatively little value, since the patient may have been exposed to smoke containing low concentrations of carbon monoxide or may have been treated effectively with oxygen by paramedical personnel prior to arrival at the hospital. The presence of increased concentrations of carboxyhemoglobin suggests the inhalation of a significant amount of smoke, and the patient should be retained in the hospital for observation, since most such patients will later develop a pathophysiologic condition of the lower respiratory tract following recovery from carbon monoxide poisoning. Within 6 to 12 h after injury, the hospitalized patient should be subjected to fiberoptic bronchoscopy to assess the lower respiratory tract. Direct visualization of the trachea and bronchus provides approximately 86 percent accuracy in indicating significant smoke inhalation. Objective findings include the extramucosal appearance of carbonaceous material, bronchorrhea, mucosal edema, vesicles, erythema, hemorrhage, and ulceration.

The Pa_{O_2} while the patient is breathing 100 percent oxygen may also be utilized to monitor for the development of smoke inhalation syndrome. Patients with an initial Pa_{O_2} of less than 300 should be suspected of significant smoke inhalation. This test also has an accuracy of approximately 86 percent.

Other authors have utilized a ^{133}Xe scan to diagnose lower respiratory tract injury. An abnormal scan following the injection of ^{133}Xe into a peripheral vein is indicated by incomplete washout from the lungs within 90 s or the presence of local radioisotopic trapping. The test is 87 percent accurate but has been infrequently utilized, since it requires the movement of severely ill patients to special radioactivity-counting facilities.

Between 24 and 48 h after injury, the patient exhibits progressive bronchospasm with expiratory wheezes, rales, tachypnea, and progressive respiratory failure. The subsequent development of bronchopneumonia secondary to bacterial growth distal to occluding plugs (consisting of inspissated mucus and sloughed bronchial epithelium) is a fairly constant feature. Radiographic changes are usually not noted until 72 h after the injury (Fig. 7-6).

The treatment of smoke inhalation syndrome can be divided into nonspecific and specific therapy. Nonspecific modalities include rapid fluid resuscitation of burn shock, performance of escharotomies of the chest and the abdomen, the provision of external dry heat, and frequent monitoring of respiratory function. Prompt intravenous fluid resuscitation and restoration of normal intravascular volume prevents exacerbation of central nervous system hypoxia. When circumferential third-degree burns of the chest and abdomen are present, chest wall and diaphragmatic excursion are inhibited unless escharotomies are performed. The provision of an externally warm environment minimizes oxygen demand associated with an increased metabolic rate. Most important, however, is the frequent assessment of respiratory function by repetitive

Table 7-6. SMOKE INHALATION SYNDROME

History: Enclosed space, alcohol/drugs, unconsciousness
Physical Exam.: Altered mental status, carbon in sputum, delayed symptoms

Diagnostic tests	Advantages	Disadvantages
Carboxyhemoglobin	Simple, rapid	Nonspecific, rapid disappearance
Fiberoptic bronchoscopy	Simple, rapid, objective	
^{133}Xe scan	Objective	Complicated, expensive
AaD$_{O_2}$ gradient	Simple, rapid, ? objective	Unproved

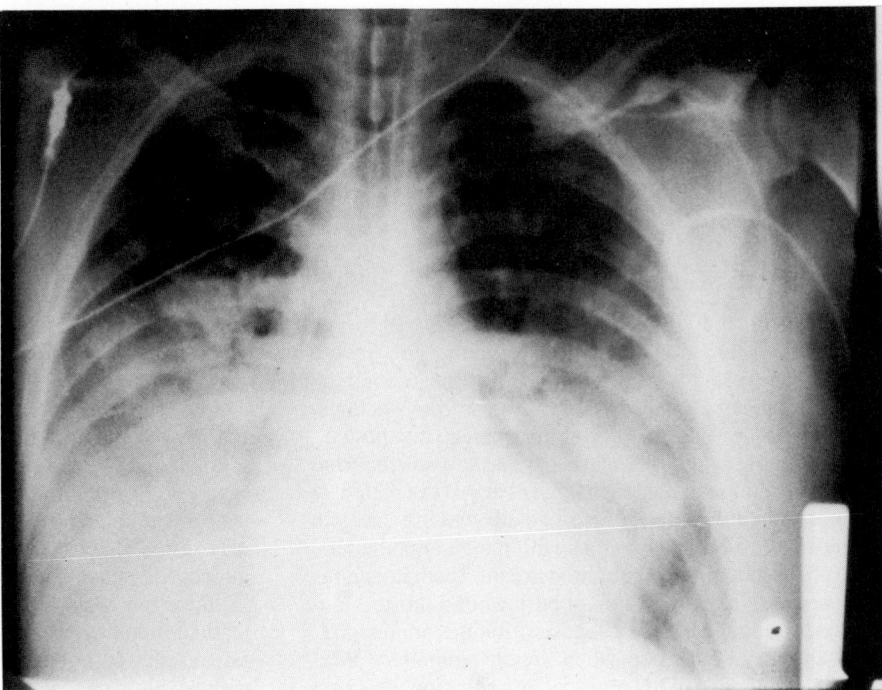

Fig. 7-6. Chest x-ray changes secondary to smoke inhalation may not be evident for 72 h. The clinical syndrome that develops is similar to the adult respiratory distress syndrome.

physical examination, serial determinations of arterial P_{O_2}, and pulmonary compliance, which often decreases prior to a significant fall in the arterial P_{O_2}.

Specific treatment includes the provision of humidified air and oxygen as required. If respiratory failure is incipient, endotracheal intubation should be performed and the patient supported with mechanical ventilation. Often it is necessary to institute positive end-expiratory pressure (PEEP) to prevent progressive respiratory failure. Intravenous administration of bronchodilators often alleviates the severe bronchospasm. Routine use of steroids should be avoided. Administration to patients with smoke inhalation may lead to up to three times higher incidence of infectious complications and increased mortality. When smoke inhalation syndrome is complicated by pneumonia, appropriate antibiotics should be administered by a parenteral route. Prophylactic antibiotics either parenterally or by aerosolization are contraindicated. They do not lower the incidence of subsequent infection and may result in the emergence of highly resistant strains of bacteria.

Burn Wound Sepsis

One of the principal causes of death following massive thermal injury is burn wound sepsis. Burn wound sepsis is characterized by the active invasion of microorganisms into viable subeschar tissue, with subsequent bacteremia. Third-degree burn wounds are essentially avascular, so systemic delivery of antibiotics via the bloodstream does not reliably suppress microbiological growth within the burn wound. Moreover, host resistance to infection is now known to be markedly diminished in patients with major thermal injury. Complement abnormalities, hypogammaglobulinemia, cell-mediated immunity, decreased neutrophil intracellular bacterial killing, and abnormalities in the inflammatory response within the burn wound have all been described. In addition, there is a marked decrease in neutrophil and monocyte chemotactic responsiveness. These two factors, markedly decreased perfusion of the eschar and severely compromised host resistance to infection, may result in rapid bacterial colonization if topical chemotherapeutic agents are not utilized. Although the topical agents have reduced the incidence of bacterial invasion of the viable subeschar tissue, bacterial proliferation may still escape the control of all currently used chemotherapeutic preparations particularly if they are used for prolonged periods. Early excision of eschar with closure obviates this problem. This technique may not always be feasible, however, necessitating a nonsurgical approach, i.e., spontaneous separation of eschar with delayed autografting. When bacterial escape is proved by quantitative wound biopsy, administration of antibiotics by needle clysis beneath the eschar has been employed with success. This therapy is most effective when initiated at the time wound colonization reaches 10^4 organisms per gram of tissue. Antibiotics administered by subeschar clysis should be selected after review of in vitro sensitivity of the offending organism. The entire daily "systemic" dose of the selected antibiotic should be dissolved in a solution of isotonic saline solution or half-strength saline solution of sufficient quantity to infuse each 44-cm^2 area of burn eschar with 25 mL of solution once daily.

Utilization of antibiotics administered by subeschar clysis has allowed recovery of children with documented *Pseudomonas* burn wound sepsis accompanied by ecthyma gangrenosum. Prior to the utilization of subeschar antibiotics, the complication of *Pseudomonas* septicemia was uniformly fatal in burn patients. Up to 50 percent survival was reported in such patients in 1974 by Loebl and his colleagues.

Distant Septic Complications

Because of decreased host resistance, distant septic complications are not unusual in patients with severe burn injury. Bronchopneumonia is the most common complicating infection. Sputum cultures from such patients usually reveal the same microorganism that has colonized the burn wound. Bacteria may be aerosolized from the burn wound and inhaled in large doses as the patient is manipulated during the course of daily wound care. In about one-third of burn patients with pneumonia the bacteria are seeded via the bloodstream (hematogenous pneumonia) as a complication of burn wound sepsis. Conventional treatment with systemic antibiotics and respiratory support is indicated when septic pulmonary infiltrates are diagnosed by physical examination or chest radiography.

Suppurative thrombophlebitis occurs more frequently in patients with massive thermal injury than in other hospitalized patients with severe illness. This complication follows prolonged venous cannulation with polyethylene catheters utilized for the delivery of intravenous fluid. In contrast to bland thrombophlebitis, this type often exhibits no abnormal physical signs. Calf tenderness and edema are only infrequently present. More commonly, the patient presents with bacteremia of unknown origin. Blood cultures often yield staphylococci. The diagnosis may be confirmed by surgical exploration of all peripheral veins that have been cannulated during hospitalization. The vein is opened and milked in a retrograde manner, and any effluent is observed. If pus can be identified, the diagnosis is confirmed. In the absence of liquefied suppurative material, the vein should be biopsied and subjected to frozen section. Bacterial colonization of the intima of the vein also strongly suggests the presence of suppurative thrombophlebitis. The incidence of suppurative thrombophlebitis may be markedly reduced in the burn population by limiting the duration of any single intravenous catheter to periods of 72 h or less. Should the complication occur, the offending vein must be excised in its entirety. Failure to employ prompt surgical treatment usually results in fatal bacteremia.

Thermally injured cartilage is another common site of bacterial infection. Cartilage is relatively avascular, and local host resistance to established infection is diminished as a result. The cartilage of the external ear is covered only by cutaneous tissue and thus frequently is injured when full-thickness burns of the ear are sustained. The development of suppurative chondritis often may be prevented in patients with severe ear burns by minimizing external pressure upon the ear. Such patients should sleep without bed pillows and be prevented from assuming a lateral position with the burned ear down. When suppurative chondritis occurs, either in the cartilage of the external ear or in other cartilaginous structures, surgical excision of the involved cartilage is necessary to arrest progressive septic destruction.

Gastrointestinal Complications

Gastric and duodenal ulcers have been reported previously as a common complication of major thermal injury. These ulcers were first described by Curling in 1842 and have been reported to occur in as many as 25 percent of hospitalized burn cases. The incidence of Curling's ulcers has been markedly reduced during recent years, and operative intervention for upper gastrointestinal bleeding following burn injury is only rarely necessary today. In the past, 85 percent of upper gastrointestinal hemorrhage was associated with bacteremia. The decreased incidence of Curling's ulcer is associated with the reduced frequency of major septic complications, the prophylactic introduction of antacids into the stomach via a gastrointestinal tube (maintenance of a neutral pH in gastric aspirates), and the improved provision of nutritional supplements, allowing more rapid healing of small acute mucosal erosions.

If major upper gastrointestinal hemorrhage should occur, the patient should be promptly treated with iced saline solution lavage and blood volume replacement begun. When hemorrhage cannot be controlled by conservative means, prompt surgical intervention is indicated, since these critically ill patients do not tolerate prolonged periods of hypovolemic shock. The abdominal cavity can be, and often must be, opened through the burn wound. At closure, the subcutaneous tissue and skin are left open to prevent soft tissue infection. Once the bleeding source is identified by gastrotomy or duodenotomy, hemostasis is obtained by oversewing the base of the ulcer. Blood volume replacement is continued until the patient's condition is stable, and then a vagotomy and hemigastrectomy should be performed. Lesser procedures are associated with an unacceptable incidence of rebleeding, and reoperation carries a prohibitive surgical risk.

SPECIAL PROBLEMS

Long Bone Fractures

Often physicians are confronted with a patient who has sustained a long bone fracture with overlying cutaneous burns. Such a patient cannot be treated with closed cylinder casts, since second-degree burns will rapidly convert to full-thickness injuries as a result of bacterial growth. Furthermore, bacterial growth will be unchecked in third-degree burns, resulting in subsequent burn wound sepsis. Open repair of the fracture is generally contraindicated unless simultaneous excision of all burn tissue and autograft closure is possible. The fracture should be immobilized by insertion of Steinman pins or Kirschner wires in order to effect suspension of the extremity in balanced skeletal traction. The burn wounds can then be left exposed and treatment with topical chemotherapeutic agents initiated. The wounds must be cleansed and inspected daily and the chemotherapeutic agent reapplied.

Following electrical burn, bone may be thermally injured at the entrance and exit sites. This is most likely to occur when the entrance or exit site is on the scalp, the sternum, or the anterior leg. In these locations the underlying bone is in close approximation to the overlying skin. The burn wound is debrided of nonviable soft tissue, and topical chemotherapeutic agents are applied to remaining soft tissue defects and the exposed nonviable bone. When granulation tissue has developed over the soft tissue, temporary coverage with physiologic dressings is instituted until the soft tissue is definitively grafted. After soft tissue wounds are closed, the devitalized bone is decorticated until bleeding bone is encountered. Granulation tissue will develop from the endothelium of the vessels and eventually cover the remaining viable bone. Split-thickness skin graft can then be successfully applied.

Burn Injury of Joints

Occasionally burn injury may extend down to and include the joint capsules. Such injuries are most likely to occur where the overlying skin and soft tissue are relatively thin. The interphalangeal joints of the dorsal surfaces of the fingers and toes are most commonly involved. When it is apparent that the joint capsule has been devitalized and the joint is open, the cartilage should be surgically removed and a formal arthrodesis performed to allow ankylosis of the joint in an optimal position. Interphalangeal joints should be fixed in the extended position or with just a few degrees of flexion. Crossed Kirschner wires are utilized to hold joint position until healing of adjacent bony surfaces has occurred at about 6 weeks. When arthrodesis of joints is necessary, it is particularly important to maintain maximal function of adjoining joints. Ankylosis of the interphalangeal joints results in little long-term disability as long as metacarpophalangeal and metatarsophalangeal joint function is maintained.

Occasionally patients with burns of the hand cannot be maintained in appropriate position by splints during the acute postburn period. This problem most frequently occurs in infants and young children, in whom the fingers are not long enough to allow application of appropriate pressure dressings to maintain optimal extremity position within the splint. In such patients the temporal insertion of a single axial wire through both interphalangeal joints of each finger prevents interphalangeal flexion contractures. The wires are removed at 3 weeks and aggressive active physical therapy is employed to regain finger flexion.

Burns of the Face

Because of its exposed position, the head, with its appendages and orifices, is an anatomic area frequently burned. The protective action of the lids and the constant moisture that surrounds the ocular structures prevents the eyes from being directly involved by thermal injury, except in cases of contact, chemical, or electrical burns. Injury due to these agents often results in perforation of the cornea or opacification of the cornea, which may require later correction with a corneal graft. Moreover, third-degree burn injury of the lids may cause retraction of the lids, allowing the cornea to be constantly exposed to the drying action of air. Thus extreme care must be directed toward protecting the cornea of the eye. The instillation of artificial tears (methyl cellulose) and the use of antibiotic ointments are often required to prevent corneal desiccation. When such third-degree burn injuries are present, it is often beneficial to perform tarsorrhaphies shortly after the burn injury, limiting subsequent lid contraction deformity. The upper and lower tarsal plates are sewn together in such a fashion as to allow union of the two cartilaginous structures. The patient is able to see through a small peephole in the center of the eye, where the upper and lower lids are not joined. The tarsorrhaphies are not released until long after autografting has been accomplished and further lid contraction is not expected. Skin should be grafted over the lids as soon as eschar separation is complete. If subsequent lid retraction still occurs, reconstruction of the eyelids is accomplished by blepharorrhaphy.

Patients with second- or third-degree burn injury of the face may develop microstomia as a result of gradual fibrosis of the circumoral tissues. Prophylactic treatment to prevent this complication is particularly cumbersome and of only limited success. Surgical reconstruction of the mouth may be carried out 1 year after the burn injury.

Frequently patients become very self-conscious about major or minor postburn scarring on the face. Most scars should be treated initially by conservative management, utilizing elastic pressure masks for a period of 1 to 2 years. Attempts at early surgical reconstruction are often unsuccessful, since the tissue remains extraordinarily hyperactive for a year or more. Scar revision for cosmetic purposes should generally not be attempted for an interval of 1.5 to 2 years following the burn injury.

MORBIDITY AND MORTALITY

Whereas survival after burns of 30 percent of the total body surface area was infrequent 25 years ago, today very few patients with injuries of this magnitude die. The size of a burn injury capable of producing a 50 percent mortality has steadily risen over the past 30 years. Currently the LD_{50} by age group is in the range of 62, 63, and 38 percent total body surface area for patients with ages from 0 to 14, 15 to 40, and 40 to 65 years, respectively. Patients over the age of 65 years have a 50 percent mortality with burns of only 25 percent total body surface area. Chronic disease states in this group frequently interfere with appropriate physiologic response to major thermal injury.

More importantly, the development of multidisciplinary teams to ensure total care of the burn patient has markedly reduced the morbidity associated with this severe injury. At several centers, more than 90 percent of surviving patients have been able to return to an occupation as remunerative as their preinjury employment. Self-respect and independence are preserved, and the quality of life experienced by the patient usually approaches, or in some cases exceeds, the preinjury level.

Bibliography

General

Artz CP, Moncrief JA, Pruitt BA Jr: *Burns: A Team Approach.* Philadelphia, Saunders, 1978.

Curreri PW, Luterman A, et al: Burn injury, analysis of survival and hospitalization time for 937 patients. *Ann Surg* 192:472, 1980.

Curreri PW, Marvin JA: Advances in clinical care of burn patients. *West J Med* 123:275, 1975.

Monofo WW: *The Treatment of Burns: Principles and Practice.* St. Louis, WA Green, 1971.

Pruitt BA Jr: The burn patient: I. Initial care. II. Later care and complications of thermal injury. *Curr Probl Surg* April–May 1979.

Shuck JM, Moncrief JA: The management of burns. *Curr Probl Surg* (monograph), February 1969.

Etiology of Burns

Baxter CR: Present concepts in the management of major electrical injury. *Surg Clin North Am* 50:1401, 1970.

Curreri PW, Asch MJ, Pruitt BA Jr: The treatment of chemical burns: Specialized diagnostic, therapeutic, and prognostic considerations. *J Trauma* 10:634, 1970.

Gruber RP, Laub DR, Vistnes LM: The effect of hydrotherapy on the clinical course and pH of experimental cutaneous chemical burns. *Plast Reconstr Surg* 55:200, 1975.

Jelenko C: Chemicals that burn. *J Trauma* 14:65, 1974.

Immediate Therapy

Baxter CR: Crystalloid resuscitation of burn shock, in Polk HC, Stone HH (eds): *Contemporary Burn Management.* Boston, Little, Brown and Company, 1971, p 7.

Baxter CR, Marvin JA, Curreri PW: Fluid and electrolyte therapy of burn shock. *Heart and Lung* 2:707, 1973.

Baxter CR, Marvin JA, Curreri PW: Early management of thermal burns. *Postgrad Med* 55:131, 1974.

Curreri PW, Marvin JA: Advances in the clinical care of burn patients. *West J Med* 123:275, 1975.

Hummel RP, MacMillan GB, Altemeier WA: Topical and systemic antibacterial agents in the treatment of burns. *Ann Surg* 172:370, 1970.

Loebl EC, Baxter CR, Curreri PW: The mechanism of erythrocyte destruction in the early post-burn period. *Ann Surg* 178:681, 1973.

Loebl EC, Marvin JA, et al: Erythrocyte survival following thermal injury. *J Surg Res* 16:96, 1974.

Salisbury RE, McKeel DW, Mason AD Jr: Ischemic necrosis of the intrinsic muscles of the hand after thermal injury. *J Bone Joint Surg* [Am] 56-A:1701, 1974.

Simon TL, Curreri PW, Harker LA: Kinetic characterization of hemostasis in thermal injury. *J Lab Clin Med* 89:702, 1977.

Therapy of the Burn Wound

Bromberg BE, Song IC, Mohn MP: The use of pig skin as a temporary biological dressing. *Plast Reconstr Surg* 36:80, 1965.

Burke JF, Quinby WC, et al: Immunosuppression and temporary skin transplantation in the treatment of massive third degree burns. *Ann Surg* 182:183, 1975.

Burke JF, Yannas IV, et al: Successful use of physiologically acceptable artificial skin in the treatment of extensive burn injury. *Ann Surg* 194:413, 1981.

Curreri PW, Desai MH, et al: Safety and efficacy of a new synthetic burn dressing. *Arch Surg* 115:925, 1980.

DiVincenti FC, Curreri PW, Pruitt BA Jr: Use of mesh skin autografts in the burn patient. *Plast Reconstr Surg* 44:464, 1969.

Durthschi MB, Orgain C, Counts CW, et al: A prospective study of prophylactic penicillin in acutely burned hospitalized patients. *J Trauma* 22:11, 1982.

Fox CL, Roppole BW, Stanford W: Control of *Pseudomonas* infection in burns by silver sulfadiazine. *Surg Gynecol Obstet* 128:1021, 1969.

Hummel RP, Kautz PD, et al: The continuing problem of sepsis following enzymatic debridement of burns. *J Trauma* 14:572, 1974.

James JH, Watson ACH: The use of OPSITE, a vapour permeable dressing on skin graft donor sites. *Br J Plast Surg* 28:107, 1975.

Lindberg RB, Moncrief JA, Mason AD Jr: Control of experimental and clinical burn wound sepsis by topical application of sulfamylon compounds. *Ann NY Acad Sci* 150:950, 1968.

Luterman A, Kraft E, Kookless S: Biologic dressings, an appraisal of current practices. *J Burn Care Rehab* 1:18, 1980.

MacMillan BB: Deep excision and early grafting, in Polk HC, Stone HH (eds): *Contemporary Burn Management.* Boston, Little, Brown and Company, 1971, p 357.

Monafo WW, Aulenbacher CE, Pappalardo E: Early tangential excision of the eschars of major burns. *Arch Surg* 104:503, 1972.

Monafo WW, Moyer CA: Effectiveness of dilute aqueous silver nitrate in the treatment of major burns. *Arch Surg* 91:200, 1965.

Pruitt BA Jr, Curreri PW: The burn wound and its care. *Arch Surg* 103:461, 1971.

Pruitt BA Jr, Curreri PW: The use of homograft and heterograft skin, in Polk HC, Stone HH (eds): *Contemporary Burn Management.* Boston, Little, Brown and Company, 1971, p 397.

Salisbury RE, Hunt JL, et al: Management of electrical burns of the upper extremities. *Plast Reconstr Surg* 51:648, 1973.

Snyder WH, Bowles BM, MacMillan GB: The use of expansion meshed grafts in the acute and reconstructive management of thermal injury: A clinical evaluation. *J Trauma* 10:740, 1970.

Travis MJ, Thornton J, et al: Current status of skin substitutes. *Surg Clin North Am* 50:1233, 1978.

General Therapeutic Considerations

Curreri PW: Long-term supranormal dietary programs in extensively burned patients, in Sheets WL, Cowan GSM Jr (eds): *Intravenous Hyperalimentation.* Philadelphia, Lea & Febiger, 1972, p 136.

Curreri PW: Metabolic and nutritional aspects of thermal injury. *Burns* 2:16, 1975.

Curreri PW, Hicks JE, et al: Inhibition of active sodium transport in erythrocytes from burn patients. *Surg Gynecol Obstet* 139:538, 1974.

Curreri PW, Richmond D, et al: Dietary requirements of patients with major burns. *J Am Diet Assoc* 65:415, 1974.

Curreri PW, Wilmore DW, et al: Intracellular cation alterations following major trauma: Effect of supranormal caloric intake. *J Trauma* 11:390, 1971.

Dobbs ER, Curreri PW: Burns: Analysis of results of physical therapy in 681 patients. *J Trauma* 12:242, 1972.

Larson DL, Abston S, Evans EB: Splints and traction, in Polk HC, Stone HH (eds): *Contemporary Burn Management.* Boston, Little, Brown and Company, 1971, p 419.

Larson DL, Abston S, et al: Techniques for decreasing scar formation and contractures in the burn patient. *J Trauma* 11:807, 1971.

Reiss E, Pearson E, Artz CP: The metabolic response to burns. *J Clin Invest* 35:62, 1956.

Rickler JM, Bruck HM, et al: Superior mesenteric artery syndrome as a consequence of burn injury. *J Trauma* 12:979, 1972.

Salisbury RE, Palm L: Dynamic splinting for dorsal burns of the hand. *Plast Reconstr Surg* 51:226, 1973.

Sawchuk RJ, Zaske DE: Drug kinetics in burn patients. *Clin Pharmakokinet* 5:548, 1980.

Wilmore DW: Hormonal responses and their effect on metabolism. *Surg Clin North Am* 56:999, 1976.

Wilmore DW, Curreri PW, et al: Supranormal dietary intake in thermally injured metabolic patients. *Surg Gynecol Obstet* 132:881, 1971.

Wilmore DW, Mason AD Jr, et al: Effect of ambient temperature on heat production and heat loss in burn patients. *J Appl Physiol* 38:593, 1975.

Wilmore DW, Mason AD Jr, Pruitt BA Jr: Insulin response to glucose in hypermetabolic burn patients. *Ann Surg* 183:314, 1976.

Wilmore DW, Orcutt TW, et al: Alterations in hypothalamic function following thermal injury. *J Trauma* 15:697, 1975.

Zawacki BC, Spitzer KW, et al: Does increased evaporative water loss cause hypermetabolism in burn patients? *Ann Surg* 171:236, 1970.

Special Problems

Achauer BM, Allyn PA, et al: Pulmonary complications of burns: The major threat to the burn patient. *Ann Surg* 177:311, 1972.

Achauer BM, Bartlett RH, et al: Internal fixation in the management of the burned hand. *Arch Surg* 108:814, 1974.

Alston DW, Kozerefski P, et al: Materials for pressure inserts in the control of hypertrophic scar tissue. *J Burn Care Rehab* January–February 1981.

Altman LC, Klebanoff SJ, Curreri PW: Abnormalities of monocyte hemotaxis following thermal injury. *J Surg Res* 22:616, 1977.

Asch MJ, Curreri PW, Pruitt BA Jr: Thermal injury involving bone: A report of 32 cases. *J Trauma* 12:135, 1972.

Asch MJ, Moylan JA Jr, et al: Ocular complications associated with burns: Review of a five-year experience including 104 patients. *J Trauma* 11:857, 1971.

Bartlett RH, Allyn PA: Pulmonary management of the burned patient. *Heart and Lung* 2:714, 1973.

Bruck HM, Pruitt BA Jr: Curling's ulcer in children: A 12-year review of 63 cases. *J Trauma* 12:490, 1972.

Curreri PW, Bruck HM, et al: *Providencia stuartii* sepsis: A new challenge in treatment of thermal injury. *Ann Surg* 177:133, 1973.

Curreri PW, Heck EL, et al: Stimulated nitroblue tetrazolium test to assess neutrophil antibacterial function: Prediction of wound sepsis in burned patients. *Surgery* 74:6, 1973.

Heck EL, Browne L, et al: Evaluation of leukocyte function in burned individuals by *in vitro* oxygen consumption. *J Trauma* 15:486, 1975.

Heimbach DM: Smoke inhalation. *Top Emer Med* 3:75, 1981.

Loebl EC, Marvin JA, et al: The method of quantitative burn-wound biopsy cultures and its routine use in the care of the burned patient. *Am J Clin Pathol* 61:20, 1974.

Loebl EC, Marvin JA, et al: Survival with ecthyma gangrenosum, a previously fatal complication of burns. *J Trauma.* 14:370, 1974.

Loebl EC, Marvin JA, et al: The use of quantitative biopsy cultures in bacteriologic monitoring of burn patients. *J Surg Res* 16:1, 1974.

Marvin JA, Heck EL, et al: Usefulness of blood cultures in confirming septic complications in burn patients: Evaluation of a new culture method. *J Trauma* 15:657, 1975.

Moncrief JA: Burns of specific areas. *J Trauma* 5:278, 1965.

Moylan JA: Inhalation injury—a primary determinant of survival following major burns. *J Burn Care Rehab* March–April 1981.

Moylan JA: Smoke inhalation and burn injuries. *Surg Clin North Am* 60:1533, 1980.

Pruitt BA Jr, Erickson DR, Morris A: Progressive pulmonary insufficiency and other pulmonary complications of thermal injury. *J Trauma* 15:369, 1975.

Pruitt BA Jr, Foley FD: The use of biopsies in burn patient care. *Surgery* 73:887, 1973.

Pruitt BA Jr, Goodwin CW: Stress ulcer disease in the burned patient. *World J Surg* 5:209, 1981.

Quan PE, Rau SB, et al: Control of scar tissue in the finger web spaces by use of graded pressure inserts. *J Burn Care Rehab* January–February 1981.

Reckler JM, Flemma RJ, Pruitt BA Jr: Costal chondritis: An unusual complication in the burned patient. *J Trauma* 13:76, 1973.

Rosenthal A, Czaja AJ, Pruitt BA Jr: Gastrin levels and gastric acidity in the pathogenesis of acute gastroduodenal disease after burns. *Surg Gynecol Obstet* 144:232, 1977.

Silverstein P, Peterson HD: Treatment of eyelid deformities due to burns. *Plast Reconstr Surg* 51:38, 1973.

Voorhis CC, Law EJ, MacMillan BG: Operative treatment of Curling's ulcer in children: Report of 4 cases with 3 survivors. *J Trauma* 14:175, 1974.

Wanner A, Cutchavaree A: Early recognition of upper airway obstruction following smoke inhalation. *Am Rev Respir Dis* 180:1421, 1973.

Warden JD, Mason AD, Pruitt BA Jr: Suppression of leukocyte chemotaxis *in vitro* by chemotherapeutic agents used in management of thermal injuries. *Ann Surg* 181:363, 1975.

Chapter 8

Wound Healing and Wound Care

Erle E. Peacock, Jr.

INTRODUCTION

During the course of human evolution a valuable defense mechanism—the ability to regenerate compound tissues—was replaced by a much less complicated and far less valuable process—the phenomenon of healing. Although ability to heal has been of enormous importance in natural selection, restoration of physical integrity by synthesis of scar tissue can be regarded, at best, as only a method of preserving homeostasis and cannot be compared with the more pristine function of multi-germ-layer regeneration. Moreover, the fibrous tissue synthesis stage of healing can be detrimental even to the extent of destroying the organism that it sought to preserve. Examples are the potentially fatal deformity of valve leaflets incurred during healing of rheumatic fever valvulitis, development of posthepatitic cirrhosis, and development of esophageal stenosis after swallowing a corrosive agent. The patient may survive the initial disease or injury only to succumb months or years later from complications of fibrous tissue synthesis during healing.

Posthepatitic cirrhosis is of special interest to students of biology of wound healing, because the liver is probably the only example of a compound organ in human beings in which almost embryonic propensity for secondary regeneration appears to be retained. Under most circum- stances, the liver can be counted upon to regenerate most, if not all, of preinjury mass; in fact, the failure of regeneration to occur with normal rapidity and effective- ness in severe nodular cirrhosis gives the impression that only overgrowth of fibrous tissue may have prevented hepatic regeneration. The significance of this hypothesis reflects the possibility that fibrous protein synthesis any- where in the body chokes or overpowers cellular regener- ation; from an evolutionary standpoint, such a hypothesis has some factual basis. The hydrozoan *Tubularia* will sometimes regenerate an amputated hydranth without forming a connective tissue scar; at other times the organ- ism will merely heal the wound by formation of scar tis- sue. When scar tissue is found, only an abortive attempt at regeneration can be identified. Another example can be found during development of newts when the ability to regenerate is disappearing. If during this time connective tissue synthesis is blocked by pharmacologic agents, the ability to regenerate a new limb will be prolonged.

With the possible exception of the liver, regeneration in human beings is essentially limited to simple tissue such as epithelium; compound structures such as skin, deep organs, and nervous system can heal only by sealing the wound in a manner to be described. The sealing process varies, depending upon whether structural integrity is in- terrupted or tissue substance is removed. In both types of wounds, epithelization is the fundamental process that seals the wound, and fibrous tissue synthesis and remod- eling is the process that provides structural strength. When tissue is missing, an additional process—con- traction—moves tissue edges into closer approximation so that epithelization and fibrous protein synthesis can accomplish their objectives. Simple as this description may sound, most of the mistakes made by physicians in treating wounds are attributable to failure to realize and understand the limitations and end results of these funda- mental processes and how they differ from pristine regen- eration. Thus optimal wound management requires de- tailed knowledge of epithelization, fibrous protein synthesis, and the biology of wound contraction. Study of these processes requires, in addition, some knowledge of the milieu in which they occur—the ground substance.

WOUND CONTRACTION

In 1793, John Hunter wrote, ''In the amputation of the thick thigh (which is naturally 7, 8, or more inches in diameter) . . . the cicatrix shall be no broader than a crown piece.'' The essence of this quotation is that full-thickness wounds of organs (including skin) do not heal by synthesis of fibrous scar with the exact dimensions of the original defect. A crown piece in Hunter's time was $1\frac{1}{2}$ in. in diameter, thus over 90 percent of the amputation wound was closed by centripetal movement of skin edges. This process is called *contraction*—a dynamic term denoting action, which should not be used interchangeably with ''contracture,'' the correct term for the end result (Fig. 8-1*A* and *B*). Just as loss of brain or stomach produces a permanent defect in human beings, loss of skin also is permanent, and when a defect in the integument occurs, restoration of integrity is dependent largely upon stretching surrounding skin to cover exposed subcutaneous tissue. Obviously, stretching skin will distort movable features such as lips, eyelids, breasts, or digits. The fundamental process in contraction can be illustrated perfectly and the end result predicted positively by simply grasping the edges of a gaping wound and manually coapting them. Such replication of the contraction process produces the exact deformity that will result from natural wound contraction over a longer period of time. If it is not physically possible to coapt the edges of a wound

by reasonable external force, one can be certain that natural processes also will not be effective, as the amount of skin present is all that will be available to be stretched over the wound. Unnatural stretching by an implanted expansion device, of course, is an exception to this statement. The area that remains uncovered will either remain as an open granulating wound or, if it is small, be covered by epithelium, which is a poor substitute for normal skin and establishes a potentially dangerous area for the development of epidermoid carcinoma.

Thus the effectiveness of the contraction process in producing complete wound closure and the cosmetic and functional deformity that closure by contraction produces are related to the amount of skin available in a given area of the body. Because the hands and face of a young person do not contain excess skin, closure of a defect by contraction causes distortion of facial features or restriction of joint motion. In areas where there is redundancy of skin, such as the cervical region or face of old people, wound contraction can be extremely effective in closing defects without producing cosmetic or functional abnormalities. Where an excess of skin is not present but flex-

Fig. 8-1. *A.* Severe contracture produced by full-thickness skin loss in burn wound of neck and face. Note ectropion of lower lip. *B.* Release of contracture in same patient shown in Fig. 8-1*A.* Contracture was released by excising scar tissue and resurfacing the defect with several split-thickness skin grafts. Note absence of wrinkling of graft and restoration of cervical profile. Facial scars ultimately excised and resurfaced.

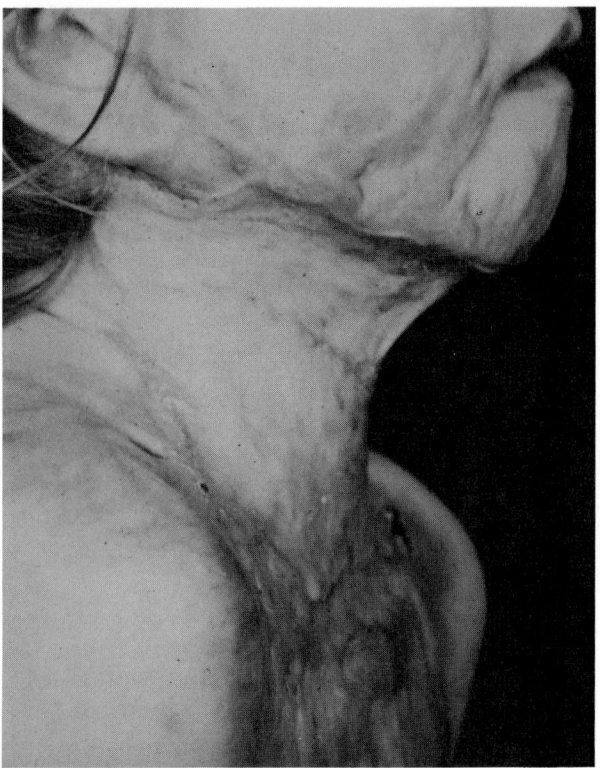

A   B

ion or extension of a joint will move wound edges together, wound contraction inexorably results in movement of the joint into an extreme position. After healing has occurred, the joint will be fixed because of lack of a satisfactory envelope. When loss of skin occurs over an area such as the malleolar surface of the lower leg and ankle, wound contraction simply cannot occur because there is not enough skin to stretch over the defect. In this instance the wound either becomes covered by a thin, almost gelatinous film of epithelium or remains open for an indefinite length of time.

Three questions immediately arise about the contraction process: What starts it? What stops it? What is the mechanism by which it occurs? On first consideration, the answer to the first question appears obvious, in that interruption of the integrity of skin always seems to be the initiating stimulus. Close examination of the series of events that occur following removal of a piece of full-thickness skin, however, reveals that wound contraction does not begin immediately; about 4 days elapse before movement of the edges is measurable. This so-called lag phase of healing seems to include the contraction phenomenon, and it can only be surmised that a set of conditions must be established or an assembly of cells or energy source completed before the actual work of mobilizing skin edges begins. One might surmise also that reestablishment of physical integrity is the stimulus that stops contraction; but again, measurement of the timing of other events reveals that contraction of a wound does not stop immediately with closure; indeed, wounds that were not caused by a loss of tissue and that have their edges approximated immediately will sometimes undergo considerable contraction. Even closure of a wound by the application of a free skin graft or pedicle flap does not stop the contracting process once movement of wound edges has begun (Fig. 8-2). An interesting observation is that the rate of wound contraction is not the same for all points on the circumference of a wound unless the wound is a perfect circle. The ultimate configuration of the scar produced by a contracting wound is the result of variations in the rate of movement of different segments as well as the firmness of attachment of different areas of the skin to both movable and immovable structures. From a practical standpoint, the surgeon may use such information to reduce the final extent of wound contraction. For example, a wound created by bringing ileum through the abdominal wall to form a permanent ileostomy can produce ileal obstruction if the skin opening undergoes contraction. One way to minimize skin wound contraction is to make the skin incision a perfect circle.

The first step in studying the mechanism of wound contraction is to try to define precisely where the fundamental process is located. In the crudest analysis it must be determined whether centripetal movement occurs because an energy or power source located outside the defect is pushing the skin edges in or whether a centrally located power source is pulling the skin edges to the center of the defect. Curiously, even after 35 years of intensive study, the answer is not entirely clear. There is good evidence that energy is being expended in both areas, and

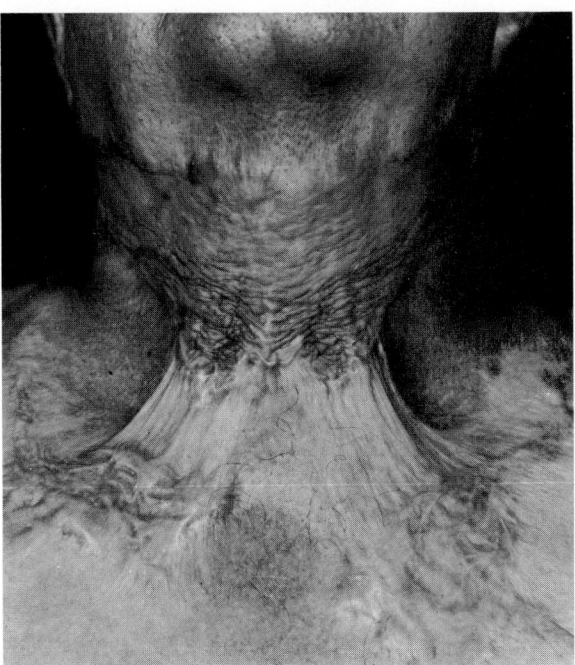

Fig. 8-2. Appearance of split-thickness skin graft applied to granulating wound while undergoing contraction. Note wrinkled appearance of graft and effect of continued contraction on surrounding skin.

the question becomes whether both processes are effective or whether only one is effective and the other either is reacting to wound contraction or is insufficient to produce effective tissue movement.

Over the years most investigators have assumed either that central granulation tissue in a contracting wound was retracting and pulling the normal skin over the granulating base or that contents of the wound were being absorbed as the skin edges moved toward the center. In 1958, Grillo et al. awakened interest in this question by reporting some experiments designed to determine whether changes in the central mass of wound tissue were pulling the skin edges together or whether central wound tissue was merely adjusting to movement of wound edges propelled by peripheral force. The commonly held opinion that dehydration of wound tissue was responsible for contraction was destroyed by Grillo's measurements, which showed that water content of central wound tissue at the beginning of wound contraction had not changed significantly at the end of contraction. The assumption that collagen synthesis and contraction might be responsible for drawing wound edges together also was disproved by direct measurement of collagen content of wound tissue during contraction. Although collagen content increases significantly between the fifth and eighth day of healing, total collagen in the wound falls significantly after 4 weeks and cannot be correlated with rate of wound contraction. Moreover, rate of wound contraction is not affected by suppressing collagen synthesis or interfering with cross linking.

The result of such studies was that attention became

focused upon living cells as the motor units in the contraction process. Wound contraction occurs only in living organisms, and the force that produces migration of wound edges is generated by living cells. As might be expected, a cytochrome poison, such as potassium cyanide, can be shown to impair wound contraction although it does not abolish the process completely. Migration of mesodermal cells in tissue culture also has been shown to be restricted by a cytochrome poison. These observations are readily reversible, which suggests an inverse relationship between inhibition of aerobic respiration and cell migration.

In an attempt to determine if cells responsible for wound contraction were located in granulation tissue, Grillo excised all central wound tissue from wounds in guinea pigs every day during the contracting process. Curiously, excision of central tissue did not affect rate of wound contraction. Such data are not conclusive in localizing the mechanism of wound contracture, however, because they cannot be correlated with results produced by other manipulations of the central mass of wound tissue. For instance, if a square of granulation tissue in the center of a healing wound is outlined by tattoo marks and then separated from the rest of the wound tissue by circumferential incision during wound contraction, two interesting observations can be made: The centrally migrating wound edge will retract peripherally, and the centrally circumcised area of granulation tissue will contract centrally. This finding leads one to the inescapable conclusion that granulation tissue between two wound edges was not being compressed by peripheral skin moving inward but was under considerable tension produced by the advancing wound edges. Moreover, in other experiments, wounds that were splinted for several days and then released did not show marked acceleration of wound contraction following removal of the splint if central granulation tissue was incised. Additional evidence that tension in granulation tissue is causally related to wound contraction is found in the ingenious experiments of James and Newcombe, who measured the contraction force of granulation tissue and plotted it against the length of tissue elements and the cross-sectional area of granulation tissue. No significant correlation between wound tension and overall wound area could be shown, but a highly significant correlation was found between cross-sectional area of granulation tissue and the tension that was developed during wound contraction. Such studies suggest that granulation tissue under tension resembles stretched elastic tissue, in that the amount of tension produced is related to cross-sectional area and not to overall length or surface area. These data, plus the demonstration that granulation tissue contains cells of a type that can exert migratory force of a magnitude necessary to mobilize skin edges, strongly suggest that the machinery for wound contraction is located in the central granulating mass. A recent discovery by Majno et al. of highly specialized cells (termed *myofibroblasts*) with smooth-muscle-like contracting powers lends additional support to this concept.

Grillo found that although wound contraction was not inhibited by excising the entire central mass of granulation tissue, it could be stopped decisively by excising a very limited zone of tissue just beneath the advancing dermal edge. The term "picture frame area" was developed to describe the strategic location of cells that appear to constitute the machinery for wound contraction. Histologic examination of the "picture frame area" reveals a collection of large, stellate, pale-staining cells that have been thought to be the cells responsible for moving the overlying dermis.

Presently it can be said only that recent investigations have eliminated changes in nonliving materials as the cause of wound contraction and have established that the movement of wound edges requires a high order of energy transfer performed by living cells. No unifying hypothesis exists by which all the available data can be explained or the exact site or mechanism of action of wound contraction identified. The apparently incompatible findings of Grillo and of Abercrombie and James concerning the importance of the central granulation tissue can probably best be resolved by hypothesizing that the wound margin makes its way over the surface of movable granulation tissue, and as it does so, it forces it by counteraction in a centrifugal direction, thus putting central granulation tissue under enough tension to cause retraction when it is excised or divided. Regardless of the exact location, however, the phenomenon of wound contraction is one of the most predictable and powerful of all biologic reactions and must be positively reckoned with in the management of wounds where tissue has been lost. The process is carried out by myofibroblasts. Under the microscope, myofibroblasts show characteristics of fibroblasts and smooth muscle cells including a rough endoplasmic reticulum, microfilament bundles similar to smooth muscle, and abundant microtubules that apparently perform a bracing function. In contrast to normal fibroblasts, myofibroblasts often are joined by hemidesmosomes, allowing the cells to "pull on each other." Histochemical studies indicate that the common contractile protein in smooth muscle cells and myofibroblasts is actin. Wound contraction can be controlled by topical application of smooth muscle inhibitors such as Trocinate. Inhibitors of microtubule formation such as colchicine and vinblastine also inhibit wound contracture under experimental conditions. Colchicine has been found to be too toxic to utilize clinically in the control of wound contraction in human beings.

EPITHELIZATION

An attempt to cover by regenerating epidermis any area of the body denuded of skin is the first irrefutable sign of wound repair and occurs long before any evidence of connective tissue synthesis. Factors that control movement of epidermal cells and the mechanism by which cells cover a denuded area are important to students of wound healing for two reasons. The first is that epithelization is necessary in the repair of all types of wounds if a watertight seal is to occur. Protection from fluid and particulate-matter contamination and maintenance of an internal milieu are dependent upon the physical characteristics of keratin. It should be pointed out, however, that just as the plastic liner of a home swimming pool contributes only a watertight seal while structural stability is maintained by concrete blocks, the epidermis, although essential to maintain a watertight seal, provides very little structural strength. It is the surrounding fibrous protein framework that gives strength to a scar (Fig. 8-3). Actually, no cellular structure or globular protein can impart much strength in the repair of a wound. When structural strength is needed, fibrous protein must be utilized. Thus highly cellular organs, such as liver, spleen, kidney, or brain, have almost no structural strength and cannot be sutured as effectively as fibrous tissue organs, such as dura, dermis, fascia, or peritoneum. A wound healed only by epithelium will stop "weeping" and be safe from bacterial invasion as long as the epithelium is intact, but the slightest trauma literally will wipe off what is hardly more than a gelatinous film; thus no degree of permanent protection has been achieved.

Second, epithelization is of great importance in the study of wound healing, because when certain variations in the control of cell division and cell movement occur, normal epithelization becomes uncontrolled growth, with awesome invasive potential. The recognized potential for development of cancer in certain types of wound scars (radiant-energy-induced wounds particularly) and in all wounds that are prevented from healing over a long period of time emphasizes the close similarity between cancer and the healing process (Fig. 8-4A and B). Actually, a histologic section from a 5-day-old healing wound can be interpreted as fibrosarcoma if none of the historical details are available. Healing is dependent upon what may be thought of as a return to embryonic status; at certain times in the healing process the overall picture—characterized by mitosis, pleomorphism, disorganization, and loss of polarity—resembles uncontrolled growth of a malignant neoplasm. A major difference exists, however: the factor of control. In a healing wound, the embryonic state is temporary and some controlling influence brings order out of disorder, a resting state to rapidly multiplying cells, and a remodeling of recently synthesized fibrous tissue to produce purposeful structural patterns. In a neoplasm, however, the situation is similar to a healing wound in which the factor of control never reappears, so that healing continues without purpose or control until the entire organism is consumed by direct extension or metastasis of the products of regeneration. Considered in this way, there may be only a fine distinction between healing and malignant growth; it may be that when we understand all the factors that influence cells to return to embryonic activity during healing, and even more important, the factors that control their growth and movement after healing has been accomplished, an important step will have been taken in solving the riddle of cancer. For now, however, it is important to remember that the stimulus following injury to overcome entropy and develop embryonic kinetics is one of the most powerful and predictable phenomena in biology.

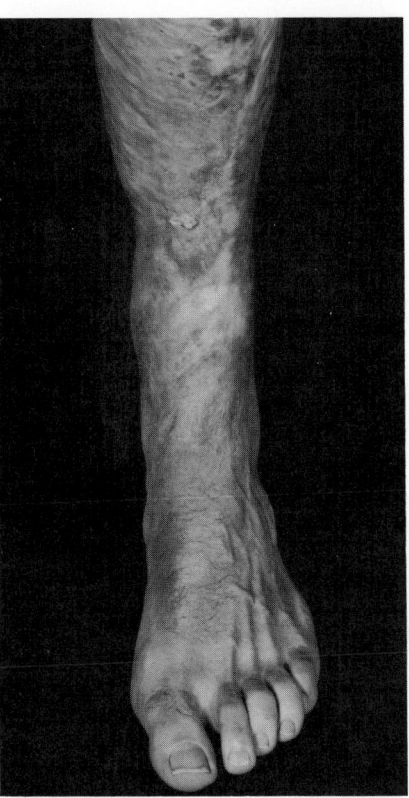

Fig. 8-3. Third-degree burn of lower leg following healing by epithelization. Absence of dermis accounts for shiny appearance and relative fragility of the surface.

Apparently cell division and ameboid movement cease only when cells are surrounded by other cells of their own type; this characteristic of cells has something to do with determining the direction in which a mass of cells will move. Weiss observed that when epithelial and mesenchymal cells are mixed and suspended in a proper medium, random movement of cells occurs, causing numerous collisions. Collisions of dissimilar cells (i.e., epidermal and mesenchymal) result in repulsion, whereas collision of similar cells results in two cells sticking together and developing protoplasmic bridges and protofibrils. Thus random movements and collisions over a sufficient period of time invariably result in cells of similar type becoming agglutinated on one side of the medium and the remainder becoming agglutinated on the other side. As increasing portions of the circumference of a cell membrane become satisfied by attaching to cells of similar lineage, the remaining unsatisfied sides become the exploring or searching surface; thus some degree of polarity for the whole mass is established. Failure to achieve complete surface contact with other cells results in a continued state of embryonic activity. One does not have to use much imagination to predict that as cells continue to be driven by an insatiable desire to contact cells of similar type, the risk of loss of control over replication and locomotion increases. Until more is known about the factors involved in control of cell growth and movement,

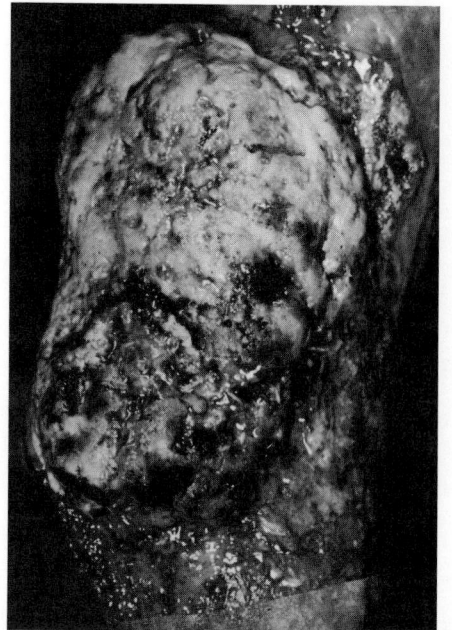

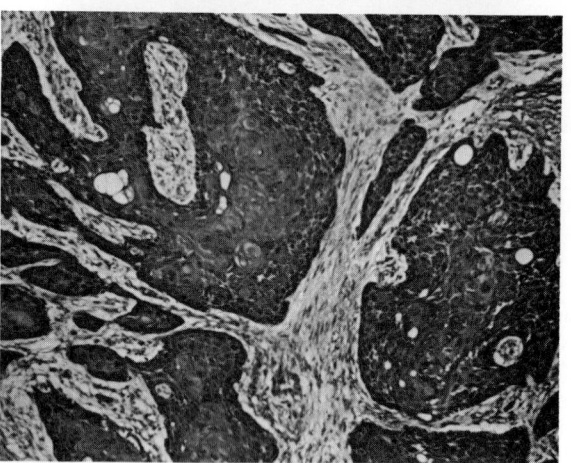

Fig. 8-4. *A.* Epidermoid carcinoma in open third-degree burn wound of thigh. Burn is 15 years old. *B.* Microscopic appearance. Carcinoma developing in burn wounds metastasizes by vascular routes more frequently than other carcinomas.

however, one can only take cognizance of the fact that any wound that is prevented from healing is potentially a malignant neoplasm.

Wounds caused by certain agents such as radiant energy or specific chemicals have unusual propensity for developing cancer in scars or chronic ulcers. In wounds induced by radiant energy, the length of time before cancer develops appears to be directly proportional to the wavelength of the damaging ray. Thus thermal burn wounds and scars may require 20 years for invasive cancer to develop, while in gamma- or x-ray-induced wounds cancer may develop in a few months. Solar and cosmic radiation, a causative agent in most human skin cancer, is short-wavelength radiation, but because it is filtered by

atmosphere and melanin, human development of epidermoid cancer from this source usually does not occur until late in life.

The development of cancer is more rare in surgical or traumatic wounds than in radiant-energy or chemical-induced wounds. No type of wound is exempt, however, when healing has been prevented by constant reinjury or inadequate skin replacement. Even in postphlebitic leg ulcer (a common chronic ulcer) cancer may develop over a long period of time.

The mechanism by which epithelium attempts to close a wound has caused considerable speculation. Previous descriptions of the process, based on the assumption that mitosis was not a prominent occurrence, are not correct. Although it is difficult to find mitotic figures in the advancing margin of epithelium, the works of Bullough and of Gillman and Penn have shown conclusively that mitosis does occur in several layers of epithelium and that it is a recognizable part of epithelization. Theoretically, it should be possible for a wound of any size to be epithelized, although there is a practical limit in clinical practice to the size of the area that will become epithelialized naturally.

Two important gross and histologic differences between normal epithelization in a healing wound and abnormal epithelial growth in epidermoid cancer are size and shape of the peripheral cell mass. A striking feature in a normally healing wound is diminishing thickness to monolayer proportions of the advancing cell front (Fig. 8-5*A* and *B*). In carcinoma, cells pile up and tumble over one another to produce a grossly umbilicated appearance (Fig. 8-6*A* and *B*). Loss of surface protein appears to be a key factor in changes in cell adhesiveness. Thus in normal epithelial regeneration, even though mitosis does occur, the most fundamental process is dedifferentiation and cell movement by development of ruffled membranes and pseudopods. The process begins early (within hours) and results in flat, thin, resting cells at the margin of the wound. These cells develop ruffled membranes and move across the center of the wound. When this occurs, the cell seems to adopt the characteristics of a typical basal cell; if it comes to rest in a more superficial position, it becomes a typical prickle cell.

In incised and sutured wounds, epithelization produces a watertight seal in 24 hours even though there is a dip where the cells have migrated into the crevice. Although the area of regeneration thickens with addition of more cells, the center of the wound remains somewhat inverted until underlying connective tissue synthesis pushes the epithelium into an everted position. Gillman and Penn have pointed out that the cutaneous tract of a skin suture on either side of the scar is also a wound of the epithelium, and that the inverted contour of epithelium over the wound also occurs along the path of a suture to the extent that a completely epithelized tract may be produced or a small cyst formed after a suture is removed.

Epithelization of a surface wound (whether partial thickness of skin such as an abrasion, or split-thickness skin-graft donor site, or full-thickness wound such as postphlebitic ulcer of the ankle) involves similar movement of epithelial cells but over a much more hazardous terrain and greater distance than incised and sutured wounds. The early escape of blood and serum in open wounds produces a scab, and the regenerating epithelium moves beneath the scab, literally detaching it from the underlying surface as it seals the wound. Actually, epithelium does not move along the interface between dermis or fat and the scab but seems to prefer to infiltrate or actually cut through the fibrous tissue substrate by elaborating an enzyme that renders collagen soluble. This phenomenon is the result of tissue collagenase elaborated at the interface between epithelium and mesenchymal tissue. Confirmation of the observation that epithelium literally cuts its own path through fibrous and fibrinous tissue may be extremely important in understanding the remodeling of deep fibrous tissue to produce a new dermalepithelial interface. A significant problem in recent attempts to grow epithelium on artificial collagen substrate for replacement of burned skin has been difficulty in reproducing rete pegs to provide stable adherence of cells to fibrous protein.

The protective influence of a scab or other cover (eschar, surgical dressing, etc.) to prevent physical trauma, drying, hemorrhage, contact with caustic materials, and the like is the basis for medical care of secondarily healing wounds. In the final analysis, successful epithelization occurs only if the cumulative effect of physical manipulation, drying, bacterial enzymes, wound area, etc., does not exceed the finite capacity of available cells to divide, dedifferentiate, and move across the surface. Considered in the simplest analysis, it may be that interruption of epidermis merely allows the epidermis to do what it normally would do if it had room, since cell movement and cell division are to a large extent prevented in the intact epidermis by the compression effect of surrounding cells.

Epidermal growth factor (EGF), a single polypeptide chain of 53 amino acid residues that contains three intramolecular disulfide bonds, has been identified and extracted from a number of tissues. EGF enhances a number of cellular events that are part of the mitogenic response during wound healing. Local application of EGF enhances the accumulation of cells and ground substances in experimental wounds. EGF has not been shown to be of any clinical value in the treatment of healing wounds in human beings.

GROUND SUBSTANCE

Even as late as 1952, some treatises on wound healing made no mention of the role of ground substance. The mystery surrounding ground substance is nowhere better exemplified than in the name itself, a mistranslation of the German *grundsubstance,* which referred to a mysterious matrix from which all the formed elements of connective tissue were believed to originate. A similar connotation was expressed by the French *substance fondamentale.* Modern definitions have done little to clarify the true nature of this amorphous material, and the best that can be said, even now, is that the term "ground substance" usu-

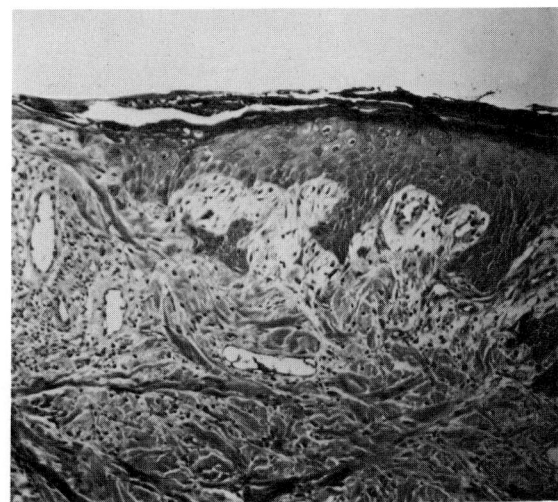

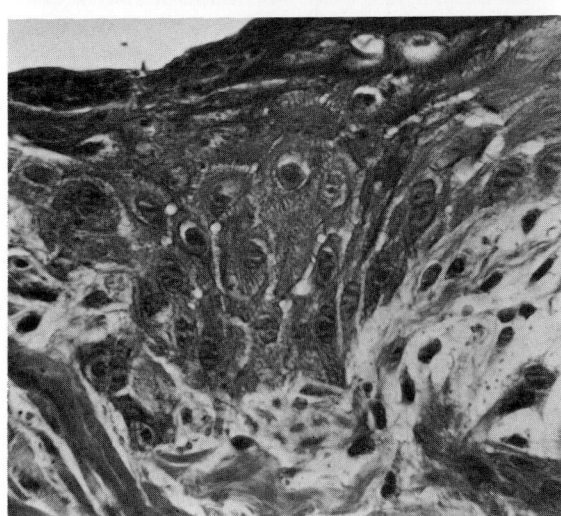

Fig. 8-5. *A.* Low-power view of epithelium advancing over granulating surface in a human wound. Note decreased thickness of advancing margin. *B.* High-power view of advancing epithelium in granulating human wound. Note dedifferentiation of cells, deep migratory activity suggesting subsurface enzyme activity at epithelial-mesenchymal tissue interface, and absence of visible mitotic activity.

ally refers to a continuous nonfibrillar matrix including water and electrolytes through which metabolites diffuse between blood vessels and cells. Recent investigations on the function of one component, fibronectin, have failed to reveal anything more specific than a general structural frame. Histologically, ground substance is identified by a remarkable propensity to absorb certain dyes such as toluidine blue and to undergo characteristic reactions with periodic acid. By such staining reactions it can be seen that ground substance is relatively organized in some areas, such as basement membrane, and undergoes, during inflammation and healing, characteristic changes in staining reaction called *metachromasia.* Such histochemical reactions seem to be due to reactions with mucopolysaccharides, many of which contain hexosamine. Be-

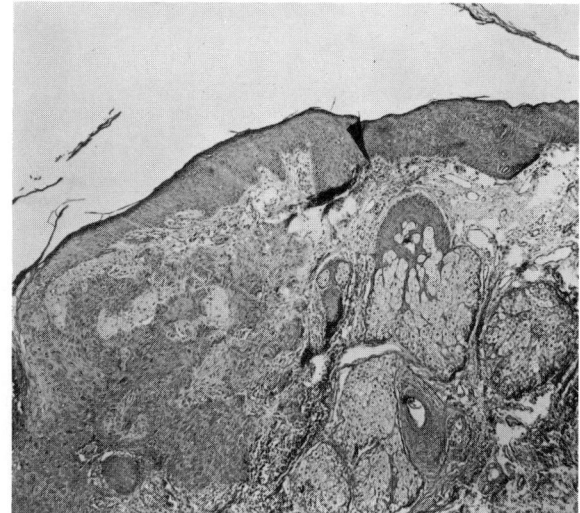

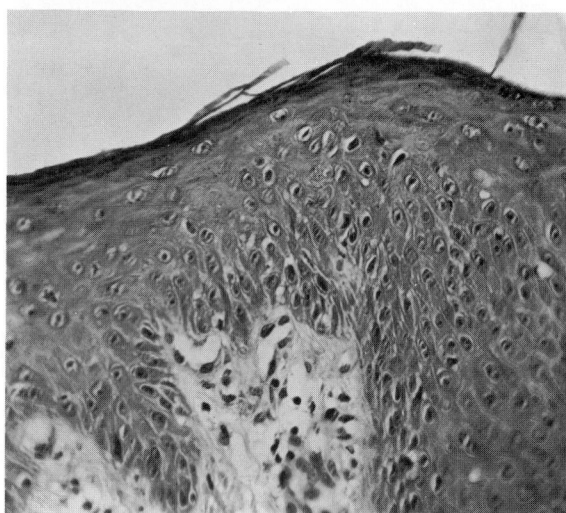

Fig. 8-6. *A.* Low-power view of epidermoid carcinoma of skin. Note accumulation of cells producing increased thickness of epithelium without purposeful migratory activity. *B.* High-power view of epidermoid carcinoma. Note numerous mitotic figures.

cause of characteristic staining reactions, attention has been focused on the acid mucopolysaccharides, even though it must be remembered that they account for only a small portion of ground substance. As a result, errors have been made by measuring hexosamine in connective tissues and drawing conclusions about the relative amount and importance of ground substance.

Meyer's division of the acid mucopolysaccharides into two major groups has been useful in the study of wound healing. These groups are nonsulfated mucopolysaccharides, of which hyaluronic acid and chondroitin can be easily identified, and sulfated mucopolysaccharides, of which chondroitin sulfate A, chondroitin sulfate B, chondroitin sulfate C, heparitin sulfate, and keratosulfate have been identified. Presently it seems that the nonsulfated group is the main component of the structureless gel fraction of ground substance and that the sulfated group is

most closely associated with the fibrillar elements of connective tissue. Thus changes in sulfated acid mucopolysaccharides are most likely to be of significance during the healing process, and, indeed, such substances are found to be increased during early stages of wound healing. Determination of actual amounts of any of the components of ground substance may be misleading, however, as synthesis and deposition involve polymerizing reactions and formation of giant molecules with molecular weight varying between 10,000 and 10,000,000.

Because the healing process is characterized by polymerizing aggregating reactions, it is interesting to speculate upon the role of mucopolysaccharides. Discovery that acid-sulfated mucopolysaccharides accumulate during healing raises the question of whether linkages between fibrillar proteins and ground substance occur. The same question has been raised about normal tissues such as tendons, where chondroitin C is a prominent portion of the ground substance; stabilization of tendon by cross linkages between collagen fibrils and chondroitin C has not been demonstrated conclusively. Chondroitin A protein complex seems important in stabilization of cartilage, and destruction of this complex by local injection of papain in a rabbit's ear will produce a lop-ear deformity that will return to normal as soon as the complex is reconstituted. It seems likely that ground substance is most important in the phenomenon of healing because of its relation to collagen synthesis and remodeling. Although chemical linkages between mucopolysaccharides and collagen have been extremely difficult to identify, chemical bonds are present that may be important in the development of strength or orientation of collagen fibers and fibrils. Certainly the assembly of collagen subunits into fibrils and fibers is dependent upon many environmental conditions, including a purely physical template or lattice. Variations in the relative amounts of sulfated fractions are believed by some to be instrumental in determining the configurations of collagen fibrils, but how much this complicated substance actually participates in the healing process is not clear.

COLLAGEN

As far as the questions that patients ask their physicians following repair of wounds are concerned, fibrous protein synthesis is the essence of healing. Accurate answers to such questions as "When do the stitches come out?" "When can I go back to work?" "How bad will the scar be?" and others are dependent upon a thorough knowledge of collagen synthesis, collagen degradation, and the factors that influence equilibrium between the two. Unfortunately, there are gaps in our knowledge about collagen metabolism; but enough is known so that the care of wounds does not have to be a mixture of craft and religion, as Paré expressed it, but can be, in most instances, a scientific exercise with a predictable outcome. Even such seeming trivia as the selection of a suture or dressing material can be the result of logical reasoning based upon factual knowledge.

Collagen is an extracellular secretion from specialized fibroblasts, and the monomeric particles or basic molecules that fibroblasts synthesize are frequently called *tropocollagen*. The tropocollagen molecule is one of the largest biologic macromolecules, with a molecular weight of about 300,000 and dimensions of 15 Å in width and 2800 Å in length. It is a stiff, elongated rod that can be visualized by an electron microscope and is soluble in cold salt solution. Thus tropocollagen is sometimes referred to as saline-extractable, or salt-soluble, collagen.

Recently it has become evident that genetic pleomorphism is expressed in subtypes of collagen molecules. Three types of collagens can be recognized by analyzing the composition of $\alpha 1$ and $\alpha 2$ chains. Type I collagen is the most prevalent type in the mature vertebrate organism. Type II collagen appears limited to cartilage and is found primarily in human articular and costal cartilages and in chick embryo bones. Type III collagen is found in association with Type I collagen and is most prevalent in tissue undergoing remodeling or fetal organogenesis. Type III collagen also appears to be an important component of tissues with an unusual degree of elasticity, such as those of the aorta, esophagus, and uterus. Other types and subtypes of collagen appear only in highly specialized tissue and do not appear important in wound healing biology.

The amino acids found only in collagen, and used to identify it in analytical procedures, are hydroxyproline and hydroxylysine. The amount of collagen in a specimen of tissue is determined by measuring the amount of hydroxyproline and multiplying the result by a factor of 7.8. Other fibrous tissues such as elastin do not contain significant amounts of hydroxyproline. Formerly it was believed that hydroxyproline in collagen had much to do with the formation of various intra- and intermolecular cross links that give collagen molecules, fibers, and fibrils their characteristic rigidity. The three-plane fixation of the triple-helix structure results, teleologically speaking, in being able to rely on collagen to transmit energy accurately in tendons or to support nonfibrous structures such as muscle. The supporting nonelastic properties of collagen can be destroyed by rupturing cross links within and between molecules, but fortunately, the destruction of cross links to this extent requires rather harsh treatment for mature collagen, such as temperatures over 70°C or exposure to strong acids or alkalies. Under these circumstances, what is produced is gelatin, which, of course, has no structural strength even though the essential amino acids are present. Hydroxylation of proline and lysine also are important in transport of collagen molecules across cell membranes.

Synthesis of collagen is an intracellular phenomenon that occurs on polysomes; a critical stage in construction of the molecule is the hydroxylation of proline to produce hydroxyproline. Externally administered hydroxyproline is excreted rapidly in the urine and apparently cannot be utilized by fibroblasts to synthesize collagen. Among other things, one of the metabolic defects that can be identified in collagen-deficiency diseases such as scurvy is accumulation of proline-rich precursors and deficiency of hydroxy-proline-containing polypeptides. During active collagen synthesis, rough endoplasmic reticulum in fibroblasts forms characteristic parallel lines, or canaliculi, and it appears that monomeric molecules are excreted into the extracellular milieu through these canaliculi. In ascorbic acid deficiency, the microsomes do not form parallel lines of canaliculi but are arranged, instead, in large cystic spaces. It is from these areas that proline-rich and hydroxy-proline-poor amorphous material is found.

Before aggregation and normal assembly can occur, a specific extracellular enzyme, procollagen peptidase, is needed to remove nonhelical terminal extensions from both the N-terminal and C-terminal ends of collagen molecules. The terminal peptide extensions of the collagen molecule are registration peptides facilitating triple-helix formation. These terminal peptides interfere with subsequent fibril aggregation and failure to remove them because of congenital absence of procollagen peptidase results in poorly assembled collagen with marked structural abnormalities. A type of Ehlers-Danlos syndrome has been found to be the result of persistent pro-α chains. A similar condition appears to be responsible for the structural malformations called dermatosparaxis in a disease first observed in Belgian cattle.

Monomeric collagen particles exposed to proper pH, temperature, osmotic conditions, etc., in the intercellular milieu aggregate or polymerize rapidly by the formation of cross links of various types. The most important such cross links are covalent ester bonds such as a Schiff's base between an amino group of one molecule and an aldehyde group of another. Oxidative deamination of lysine by an important enzyme, lysyl oxidase, is a necessary first step in formation of covalent ester cross links. In addition, other types of cross links, such as oppositely charged electrostatic groups and Van der Waals interactions, are involved in assembling monomeric particles into polymerized aggregates.

The rodlike collagen molecules appear to lie in staggered, overlapping, parallel formation, with one-quarter-length overlap. It is this staggered one-quarter-overlap arrangement of tightly packed units that gives collagen a typical repeating axial periodicity of 640 Å. Whenever collagen molecules are assembled under physiologic conditions such as those provided by the extracellular ground substance, typical fibrils with 640-Å repeating periods are produced. In certain laboratory preparations, however, it is possible to alter the characteristic 640-Å periodicity by forcing the monomeric particles to line up exactly parallel or end-on. This can be accomplished by adding glycoprotein to the milieu or by charging the preparation with a high-energy system such as adenosine triphosphate. Under these conditions, fibrils with band widths of 2000 Å can be produced; such atypical fibers are called *segment long-spacing fibers,* or *fibrous long-spacing fibrils.* These preparations have been extremely valuable in the laboratory, as they have revealed much about the size and method of polymerization of collagen molecules; they are not of any physiologic importance, however, as far as is known.

Although the collagen molecule basically is a triple

helix with a spiral configuration, heat-sensitive intramolecular cross links prevent it from having elastic or recoil properties. However, if a collagen fiber or fibril is placed in a water bath with a small weight suspended from one end and the temperature of the bath is elevated, a point will be reached when the heat-sensitive intramolecular cross links will be destroyed and recoil of the spiral polypeptide chain will occur. The temperature at which this phenomenon occurs is called the *thermal shrinkage temperature,* and the magnitude of this reaction is such that a fiber or fibril will shrink to one-third physiologic length. The thermal shrinkage temperature of collagen, therefore, is an excellent indicator of the strength and degree of inter- and intramolecular bonding. By measuring the thermal shrinkage temperature of various types of collagen, it has been possible to learn about variations in bonding under physiologic conditions and, in some instances, to correlate the development of physical properties of collagen with the extent of cross linking. From such studies it has become clear that cross linking, among other factors, is a function of aging; the older a specimen of collagen becomes, the firmer and more numerous the cross links are. Thus, collagen gel that is only a few minutes old has relatively few cross links, has low thermal shrinkage temperature, and is so flimsy that cold salt solution solubilizes it. If the gel is allowed to mature for 24 h, the number and strength of the cross links increase to the extent that a weak acid may be needed to depolymerize even a portion of it and a higher temperature will be required to cause it to undergo thermal shrinkage. If the aggregate is allowed to polymerize for several weeks, the maximum number and firmness of cross links will be realized, with the result that a strong acid may be needed to get even a portion of the collagen into monomeric units and the thermal shrinkage temperature will be the highest yet. In summary, therefore, both solubility and thermal shrinkage temperatures can be used to measure the age of collagen as represented by the effectiveness of the cross-linking process.

In addition to naturally occurring cross links such as ester bonds, artificial cross links can be added to change the physical properties of collagen. Just as adding an agent that shares electrons easily, such as a sulfur molecule, will increase the strength of rubber (vulcanization) sevenfold, addition of a similar agent such as the methyl group in formaldehyde will increase the number and kinds of cross links in collagen. Just how much the addition and destruction of cross links has to do with physical properties of wound-repair collagen in scar tissue is not known. It has been shown, however, that addition of methyl or amide cross links will increase the tensile strength of scar tissue in incised and sutured wounds in rats as much as threefold on the eighth postwound day. That variations in cross linking are partially responsible, however, for the final appearance, texture, or elasticity of human scars is becoming more certain.

At this point, other factors involved in tensile strength must be considered, for cross linking may have very little to do with tensile strength after fibrils and fibers have been formed. It is highly unlikely, in the opinion of the

author, that fibrils and fibers are cross-linked very efficiently, because the average distance between fibrils is of the order of 1 μm. Chemical cross links are approximately 2.8 Å, which means that the distance is roughly 500 times too great for the usual types of cross links to span the distance between fibrils. However, because addition of cross links such as methyl or amide bonds definitely increases tensile strength in wet scar tissue, the inescapable conclusion seems to be that rupture of scar tissue must occur, to some extent, along inter- and intramolecular planes. There is no uniform agreement on this point, and the question of the importance of cross linking in the development of strength in scar tissue must be investigated further.

After a certain amount of collagen has been synthesized, the most important factor in gain of strength may be the physical weave of fibrils and fibers. Certainly it is possible to vary the physical properties of other fibrous materials by varying the weave of the small components exclusive of any chemical bonds. A good example of this principle is to be found in the physical weave of a nylon stocking. Nylon thread is nonelastic, yet a nylon stocking can be made elastic by properly weaving the fibers. Transposed to a biologic system, nonelastic tendon or fascia shows physical characteristics similar to nylon thread, while elasticity of the wall of the aorta is similar to that of a nylon stocking.

The old concept of collagen as a static, adynamic substance—the excelsior of the body—is erroneous. Actually, as will be shown later, collagen in wound scar is a relatively dynamic structure that, like other tissues, is undergoing constant remodeling and replacement. After the forty-second day of wound healing there is no measurable increase in the amount of collagen in a healing wound, and yet the scar continues to gain strength for at least 2 years. Thus changes in collagen, such as increased cross linking and rearrangement of fibers and fibrils, must be occurring. Turnover of collagen in a healing wound is extensive. Most newly synthesized collagen is replaced as the scar matures and literally all of the collagen in a fibrous transplant, such as a skin graft, will be removed and replaced ultimately.

Before we leave the subject of remodeling, it is important to mention a disease, lathyrism, which has been useful in the study of collagen metabolism and which is beginning to have far-reaching implications for control of human scar tissue. The disease, recognized by Hippocrates, is caused by excessive ingestion of certain peas of the genus *Lathyrus.* Considerable differences exist between the human form of the disease, which is manifested by spastic paralysis, and the disease in laboratory animals, which is characterized by skeletal and cardiovascular abnormalities secondary to altered collagen metabolism. The active and highly potent fraction that produces altered collagen metabolism is beta-aminopropionitrile. Considerable data are available on the effect of this substance on both developing and mature tissues. Most such data support the hypothesis that the primary effect of beta-aminopropionitrile is to block the formation of inter- and intramolecular cross links during all stages of collagen aggregation. Thus beta-aminopropionitrile affects growing tissue more than adult tissue. Characteristically, beta-aminopropionitrile produces a significant increase in saline-extractable collagen, as it prevents the assembly of monomeric collagen units into stable fibrils and fibers. There is evidence that fibril formation is not stopped during lathyrism but that cross linking in fibrils is so unstable that cold saline will solubilize much of the collagen that was assembled during beta-aminopropionitrile poisoning. Growing embryos literally become saline-soluble under the effect of beta-aminopropionitrile, and mature animals will develop hernias or die suddenly of dissecting aneurysms. Wound healing, as might be predicted, is affected by beta-aminopropionitrile; there is cessation of gain in tensile strength within hours after the agent is administered; saline-extractable collagen increases approximately ten times. Clinical implications of the beta-aminopropionitrile effect are exciting, for it is a clear-cut demonstration that it is possible to alter the physical properties of collagen in dramatic fashion. Because some of the effects of fibrous tissue healing in specialized organs, such as the liver or heart, can be more ruinous to health than the disease or injury that preceded healing, the demonstration that some control over deep scar formation is possible is an exciting one. If, in addition, mature recently synthesized collagen also could be solubilized selectively, a major breakthrough in many disease processes could evolve. Highly purified beta-aminopropionitrile has been administered to human beings with scleroderma, urethral stricture, and keloid. It can be given safely to human beings, but is not available for treatment of human diseases. At this time, penicillamine, a lathyrogenic agent as well as a copper chelater previously utilized to treat Wilson's disease, is being used to treat arthritis in human beings and also is being studied as a treatment for undesirable scar tissue.

Several times in this chapter the term "remodeling" of scar tissue has been used. The thoughtful student is likely to be concerned over such a term, as it connotes not just synthesis of collagen but collagen breakdown as well. Because no enzyme able to lyse collagen had been identified in human beings until approximately 25 years ago, collagen turnover in either normal tissue or wound scar was suspect. Even though no such mechanism could be demonstrated, however, indirect evidence has been abundant that some enzyme or mechanism for solubilizing collagen must exist. There is always some extractable collagen in the skin of even the oldest and most depleted individuals. Obviously, if all tropocollagen were going into the skin, the dermis would soon be as thick as elephant hide. Some collagen must be coming out of dermis, and the relatively constant thickness of skin only attests to an equilibrium that exists between collagen synthesis and degradation. Cutaneous scars are raised above the surface 2 to 4 weeks after injury; yet they usually soften, become pliable, and decrease considerably in size with passage of time. The loss of 50 percent of collagen from the gravid uterus 36 hours after parturition and the rapid disappearance of dermis when tetraplegic patients are allowed to lie unattended attest that human beings possess

an effective enzyme capable of degrading mature collagen. Search for such an enzyme was unsuccessful for a long time because it was assumed that the enzyme could be extracted from tissue. In 1963, Gross, Lapiere, and Tanzer hypothesized that collagenolytic enzyme was the product of living cells and that contact with a living cell was necessary in order for collagenolysis to occur. In one of the most important experiments performed in the wound-healing field during that era, the hypothesis was tested by preparing culture plates of reconstituted collagen and amphibian Tyrode culture medium. Specimens of tissue from the rapidly absorbing tail of a metamorphosing tadpole (a structure containing mostly collagen that is absorbed and not broken off during metamorphosis) were placed on the collagen-Tyrode substrate, and the culture plates were incubated under tissue culture conditions. After several days a clear zone appeared around each implant, and if the tissues were kept alive long enough, the entire substrate became lysed by collagenolytic activity. Failure of the cells to survive stops collagenolytic activity immediately; even after lysis has begun, it can be stopped by killing the cells. Thus Gross and Lapiere demonstrated that collagenolytic enzyme is a product of living cells and that cells that produce enzyme need to be in close contact with collagen fibers for lysis to occur. Riley and Peacock cultured a variety of normal and pathologic human tissues and found collagenolytic enzyme to be widely distributed, particularly in epithelium-containing structures.

The most uniformly positive tissue for collagenolytic enzyme in human beings is cutaneous scar. Scar tissue reveals positive lytic activity approximately 10 days after closure of a cutaneous laceration, and a high level of activity has been found in dermal scars as long as 30 years after injury. Granulation tissue is only slightly active; burn eschar does not show any activity for about 2 weeks. Between 2 and 3 weeks after a third-degree burn, however, cultures of separating dermal eschar are strongly positive for collagenolytic activity. These findings suggest that invasion of dead eschar by underlying connective tissue cells or undermining epidermal cells is necessary for contact between cells and heat-tanned collagen. Retarded wound healing may be the result of excessive collagenolysis. Serum, cysteine, and progesterone have been shown to inhibit tissue collagenase acting at neutral pH. Progesterone in ophthalmic concentrations is the agent of choice in treating corneal injury, particularly alkali burns in which delayed tissue collagenase activity is the cause of rupture of the globe.

By measuring collagen synthesis and collagen breakdown, it is possible to study healing from the standpoint of variations in metabolic equilibrium. Considered as such, scar tissue is a product of opposing forces of collagen synthesis and collagen destruction, and the result of such forces will vary according to the relative rate and effectiveness of each. The maximum amount of total collagen in a healing wound is found by the forty-second day. Although increased amounts of saline-extractable collagen (compared with nonwounded resting dermis) can be extracted from scar tissue for as long as 18 months, there is no further gain in insoluble (or mature) collagen. The conclusion would seem to be that, even though remodeling of the collagen continues, equilibrium has been established between collagen synthesis and collagen destruction. Demonstration by Cohen of accelerated collagen synthesis and deposition and collagenolytic activity in human keloids probably represents an abnormality of such an equilibrium.

The concept that all collagen to some extent, and healing wound collagen particularly, is undergoing simultaneous construction and destruction can serve as a basis for speculation concerning some of the previously unexplainable findings in the healing process. One such enigma is the behavior of wounds during ascorbic acid depletion. In the classic descriptions of scurvy it is important to remember that sailors' wounds did not just fail to heal; they actually disrupted months after thay had healed perfectly. This observation has been verified in animals and raises the question of whether collagen is dependent upon ascorbic acid for structural integrity. It is known that collagen can be repeatedly depolymerized and reconstituted in the laboratory without contact with ascorbic acid, and artificially reconstituted collagen does not lose tensile strength. Therefore, the notion that vitamin C has anything to do with strength of mature scar tissue is untenable. Because synthesis of new collagen is blocked during ascorbic acid deficiency, and because collagenolytic activity probably proceeds normally, a possible explanation for old scar dehiscence would seem to be that tissue previously in equilibrium becomes unbalanced by having synthesis knocked out and lysis continue. Inexorably, the scar will become weaker until a point is reached where normal tissue tension produces disruption.

Although to some extent hypothetical (actual quantitative measurements of lysis and synthesis are not sensitive enough now to prove or disprove the equilibrium hypothesis), the theory is important as it relates to the whole field of conditions erroneously referred to in the past as "collagen diseases." The collagen in such diseases is precipitated under physiologic conditions and, as might be predicted, is normal as far as can be determined by electron or light microscopy, x-ray defraction, or amino acid analysis. Thus all the evidence supports the idea that so-called collagen diseases represent abnormal amounts of collagen in abnormal places but are not specific diseases of the collagen molecule or fibril. Such an explanation is entirely logical, as one cannot have a disease of a nonliving structure. Collagen is a crystalline protein in which the nearest thing that could be classified as a disease process is the abnormal construction of collagen during lathyrism. The collagen in such diseases as rheumatic fever, dermatomyositis, and scleroderma is more accurately considered as the ash or scar from a burnt-out primary wound or inflammatory process. In the other direction, destruction of collagen in diseases such as rheumatoid arthritis is, at least partially, the result of excessive tissue collagenase activity. The concept of the collagen system as a dynamic, constantly remodeling one opens the door for investigation of a large number of diseases of unknown cause that are characterized by deficient or excessive collagen formation.

SEQUENCE OF EVENTS: SUMMARY

Once the basic processes in the healing phenomenon have been mastered, the student has only to relate them to one another in proper sequence to be ready to start the study of what physicians can do to aid healing. The most important concept in this regard is the understanding that healing is not a series of events but is a concert of simultaneously occurring processes, some of which continue for many years after physical integrity of wounded tissue has been reestablished. The most dramatic events, such as sealing the wound, regaining tensile strength sufficient to permit normal stress, and acquiring a scar that is cosmetically and functionally acceptable, occur in a relatively short period of time. Long-term processes, such as remodeling of collagen and development of cancer in scar tissue, fortunately are not processes that cause patients much concern. Although the basic processes are much the same in an incised and sutured wound properly coapted (healing by primary intention) and a wound in which tissue has been lost so that healing must occur by contraction and epithelization (secondary healing, or healing by secondary intention), the time required for secondary healing is so much longer and the area involved usually so much greater that it is convenient to study the secondary healing process to see how the basic steps in wound healing relate to one another.

The first thing that happens after full-thickness skin loss is that normal elasticity of the skin and external tension produced in some areas by muscle pull enlarge the defect according to the amount of force exerted and the direction over which it acts. Thus the shape of a skin defect may have little relation to the size or shape of the fragment of tissue that was removed. If hemorrhage is not too severe, a clot forms quickly, then contracts and dehydrates to form a scab. Because a scab is essentially a dehydrated, fully contracted blood clot, it is less durable and effective in closing the wound than collagenous eschar. Nevertheless, a scab serves a useful purpose in providing limited protection from external contamination, satisfactory maintenance of internal hemostasis, and a surface beneath which cell migration and movement of wound edges can occur. Classically, the beginning of wound healing is described as the "lag" phase—an inaccurate term that carries the connotation that there is a period when nothing of importance is happening. Actually, a great number of important things are happening even though they usually are not considered part of the healing process. One soon recognizes, however, that almost instantly following infliction of an injury the stage for healing is set, and the props and background for the events that are to follow are essentially those of controlled inflammation. Study of the biology of repair has emphasized that the most successful reparative processes occur against a background of inflammation and that, up to the point of necrosis, how well the wound heals is related to the amount of inflammation present. Specifically, the release of various amines from connective tissue mast cells, perfusion of capillaries surrounding the defect, change in permeability of capillary walls, release of enzymes, fluid, and protein into extracellular spaces, accumulation of white blood cells and connective tissue cells, and formation of thrombi in peripheral lymphatic channels are well-known changes in general inflammation that are important in providing the best milieu for repair to proceed. It is only when bacteria, foreign bodies, medications, or accumulation of destructive enzymes cause necrosis of tissue that inflammation becomes a deterrent to healing. Therefore, the author prefers to see the term "lag" phase replaced by strong emphasis on inflammation as an active part of the reparative process.

Approximately 12 h after injury has occurred, and at a time when inflammation has been established, epithelial migration—the first clear-cut sign of rebuilding—occurs. In a primary wound, epithelization is complete in a few hours; in a secondary healing wound, migration of cells is rapid at first, but as the line of cells from the wound margin becomes extended and the epithelial probe dwindles to a monolayer, progress becomes slower, so that days or even weeks elapse before epithelization is complete. After 4 or 5 days, however, epithelization is assisted as the machinery of wound contraction begins, and the wound margins start central movement.

A great amount of activity takes place in the center of the wound after a scar or eschar has been removed and before epithelium has covered the surface. Grossly, the surface that was once gray or yellow-brown and smooth becomes bright red and granular. The reason for this is an extravagant proliferation of richly perfused capillary loops. The knuckles or loops of blood vessels impart a granular appearance to the surface, and it is because of them that the wound is often described as granulating or showing granulation tissue. Granulation tissue provides a good defense against invasion by surface contaminants, but it is fragile and produces a difficult terrain for advancing epithelial cells. This is particularly true if surface infection, edema, or deep fibrous tissue interfere with return circulation. When this happens, the fiery red granular dots will change to a purple, soggy, gray-black cluster that may fill the entire wound cavity and spill over the wound edge, thus eliminating the possibility of epithelization.

Although no visible signs of collagen synthesis can be found until the fourth to sixth day, biochemical evidence of collagen synthesis can be found between the second and fourth days. The level of hydroxyproline in wound tissue rises rapidly, and the saline-extractable-collagen level becomes elevated shortly thereafter. Before signs of collagen synthesis occur, the ground substance changes, as evidenced by accumulation of sulfated mucopolysaccharides and development of metachromasia. On or about the seventh day wounds will show a delicate fine reticulum of young collagen fibrils. Actually, the gelation that is occurring at this time is so random that polymerization of new collagen fibrils is much like that of a new gel in a laboratory beaker—without purposeful orientation or polarity. There is a short period when young fibrils and fibers take silver stains selectively, and it is thought that this property reflects the presence of large numbers of unsatisfied bonding sites; mature collagen fibers do not stain selectively with silver. As fibrogenesis proceeds, purposefully oriented fibers seem to become thicker, presumably because they are accruing more collagen particles; nonpurposefully oriented fibers disappear. The overall effect appears to be one of lacing the wound edges together by a three-dimensional weave. In secondary wounds the mass of scar tissue becomes dense, compact, and smaller in circumference but shows little in the way of purposeful organization. The overall direction is one of replacing granulation tissue, allowing the surface to become covered with epithelium, and filling in the remaining skin defect with scar tissue after contraction is complete. As far as filling the defect is concerned, contraction is the major influence; it exerts full potential before scar-tissue synthesis is complete. The central scar seems to remodel itself to fill the defect after contraction is over. Thus wounds surrounded by mobile and redundant skin will have a small central scar, while wounds surrounded with tight nonmovable skin will have relatively large central scars regardless of the size of the defect.

Development of tensile strength (strength per unit of scar tissue) and burst strength (strength of the entire wound) is the result initially of blood vessels growing across the wound, epithelization, and aggregation of globular protein. Later, collagen synthesis is important. The effect of vascularization and epithelization, although relatively small, is adequate on the fifth day to hold wound edges, if not under excessive tension, coapted without sutures. The really significant gain in tensile strength begins about the fifth day, however, when collagen synthesis becomes apparent; tensile strength measurements in laboratory animals usually are recorded from that day. Increase in strength is rapid for 17 days and slow for an additional 10 days; there is an almost imperceptible gain in tensile strength for at least 2 years. In spite of the measurable increase in tensile strength for such a long period, strength of scar in rat skin never quite reaches that of unwounded skin.

Collagen content of the wound tissue rises rapidly between the sixth and the seventeenth days but increases very little after the seventeenth day and none at all after the forty-second day. Gain in strength after the seventeenth day, therefore, is due primarily to remodeling of collagen and, hence, is not correlated with total collagen content except for a very short portion of the healing curve.

When a normally healing wound is disrupted mechanically after the fifth day and immediately resutured, the return of tensile strength is so rapid that within 2 days the burst strength is nearly what it would have been had the secondary wound not occurred. This phenomenon, commonly called the *secondary healing effect,* has been studied intensely to determine the exact mechanism of rapid gain of tensile strength following repair of a secondary wound. Curiously, it is neither more rapid collagen synthesis nor more rapid assembly of collagen subunits; secondary wounds contain slightly less collagen than primary wounds of the same age. Because the thermal shrinkage temperature of secondary wound collagen is significantly higher than that of primary wounds of the same age, it has been suggested that more effective cross linking or better physical weave of collagen subunits is responsible for the rapid gain in strength of secondary wounds. The demonstration by Madden and Smith that secondary healing is really nothing more than continued primary healing (without a lag phase) invalidates previous cross-linking theories of secondary wound healing. Whatever the explanation, however, the machinery for producing rapid gain in tensile strength in secondary wounds is limited to an area of 7 mm around the first wound. Excision of skin edges more than 7 mm circumferential to the primary wound results in secondary wound healing at the same rate as in a primary wound.

WOUND CARE

From a treatment standpoint, there are essentially two types of wounds: those which are characterized by loss of tissue and those in which no tissue has been lost. Lacerations are an example of wounds without tissue loss, and avulsions or burns are examples of wounds that, in addition to interruption of surface continuity, result in loss of tissue. A question that must be answered for both is whether immediate closure can be performed safely. Whether the wound can be closed by suturing the edges together or a graft of some sort is required, a decision must be reached about whether closure can be immediate or should be delayed until the danger of infection is past.

The key to deciding when a wound should be closed is an understanding of the difference between contamination and infection; the trick to determining when one has become the other is the ability to recognize and interpret signs of inflammation. A contaminated wound can be converted by skillfully performed surgery into a clean wound that can then be closed safely; an infected wound cannot be surgically debrided without high risk of failure, including the potentially lethal complications of interfering with natural localizing processes. The history and physical examination contribute valuable information, because the length of time needed for contamination to become infection reflects, among other things, the strength of the bacterial inoculum and the ability of the substrate to combat invasion. A clean razor slice of highly vascular skin of the face might be closed safely 48 h after injury, whereas a stable-floor-nail penetration of the foot of an elderly person might not be closed safely 1 min after injury. Laboratory data also are helpful, particularly when considering the time to close a secondary healing wound. Quantitative measurements of the number of bacteria in tissue samples have shown that concentrations greater than 10^5 organisms per gram of tissue are likely to cause abscess and wound breakdown following second-

ary closure. If the concentration of bacteria in tissue is significantly less than 10^5 organisms per gram of tissue, the chances of successful wound closure are much improved. Because contaminated wounds have bacteria only on the surface and ideally the surface will be mechanically or hydrodynamically cleansed, quantitative bacteriology is reserved primarily for diagnosis of granulating previously infected wounds.

Once the decision has been made to close a laceration, the surrounding skin should be prepared with suitable antiseptic and local anesthetic injected. A guide to application of antiseptic is never to put anything in a wound that could not be tolerated comfortably in the conjunctival sac. Any caustic solution that is capable of sterilizing the surface of the skin will also destroy delicate cells on the surface of the wound. Therefore, harsh antiseptics should be applied only to the edge of a wound, never within it. Recent popular use of povidone iodine solution to irrigate or soak wound tissues may offer some advantages over saline irrigation, but data presently are not convincing. Moreover, absorption following prolonged use in large wounds such as burns or in wounds containing serous membranes such as peritoneum or pleura has caused significant complications. Debridement of a wound can be done either hydrodynamically or mechanically. When the wound contains only surface contaminants not attached to wound tissues, a copious stream of saline will flush foreign bodies and undesirable organisms out of the wound cavity. When devitalized or contused tissue fragments are still attached to the wound tissues and external contaminants are partially driven into the tissues, however, surgical excision of affected tissues must be performed. When there is a redundancy of tissue and there are no important structures in the depth of the wound, such as nerve or tendon, the best type of debridement is excision of the entire wound to produce a new wound that is surgically clean. When there is a shortage of tissue or when a wound involves important structures that cannot be sacrificed without producing disability, damaged tissue must be carefully dissected until all dead tissue and extraneous material have been removed. In a wound of the hand involving numerous tendons and nerves, this type of debridement may be tedious and require several hours to perform.

After the wound has been debrided, proper suture materials must be selected for closure. There are two major types of sutures, absorbable and nonabsorbable, and selection of the proper suture should be based on what has been learned about the biology of the healing process. For the most part, absorbable sutures, which are made of sheep intestines or synthetic polymers, are used when infection is known to be present or when debridement has been difficult and thoroughness is in doubt.

Plain gut sutures will be solubilized by tissue collagenase in less than 10 days, while gut that has been tanned lightly with chromium salts will remain structurally intact for approximately 3 weeks. Gut sutures are usually not used when they can be avoided because the reaction to a foreign animal protein is considerably greater than the reaction to such substances as cotton, silk, and nylon.

Synthetic absorbable sutures are not as locally irritating as animal proteins but because the collagen-synthesis stage of wound healing is barely under way at 10 days and scar tissue is far from mature even at 3 weeks, a more permanent material may be needed.

Nonabsorbable sutures are usually preferable because they produce less tissue reaction and can remain permanently below the surface of the integument. The major disadvantage of permanent sutures is that if they are placed in areas where infection develops, the suture material can harbor organisms; hence infection will not subside until the sutures are removed. A nonabsorbable suture of steel or some alloy may be mechanically irritating, and sometimes an inflammatory reaction develops around nonabsorbable sutures that resembles a local allergic phenomenon. Sutures are placed in different types of tissue for different reasons; before a suture is selected and placed in a wound, the questions should be asked: What is the suture required to do? and How long does it need to do it? Sutures that are placed in tissues to hold wound edges together under tension should be placed in fibrous tissue. Sutures placed in cellular tissues such as fat, epidermis, liver, or kidney provide little structural strength, as they tend to cut through tissues, having no appreciable strength. Sutures in weak tissues usually are used to obliterate a potential cavity (dead space), provide hemostasis, or act as a fine-adjustment leveling device on the surface of the skin. Objectives for such sutures are met in a few hours; thus absorbable sutures can be used satisfactorily if they are desirable.

A typical facial wound involving skin, subcutaneous fat, fascia, and superficial muscle might be repaired in the following way: After local anesthesia has been administered, the skin prepared, contaminants flushed out with saline solution, and any dead fragments of tissue excised, closure is performed. The muscle, being primarily cellular, does not hold sutures well. Muscle is closed primarily to stop hemorrhage and to obliterate dead space. A synthetic absorbable suture is satisfactory for these purposes. Fibrous tissue surrounding muscle has significant strength, however, and should be closed with a permanent suture of silk or some synthetic substance. If the skin is closed in a single layer, the retracted subcutaneous fat might not come together completely, thus producing a cavity that would become filled with blood and possibly infected. A loosely tied suture in subcutaneous fat, although it contributes almost nothing to tensile strength because it does not pass through fibrous tissue, may be utilized to obliterate a subcutaneous cavity and discourage hemorrhage. After the subcutaneous tissue has been closed, a decision should be made about the desired final appearance of the surface scar. The width of the wound following closure of the subcutaneous tissue will be an accurate indicator of how wide the final cutaneous scar will be if the next sutures merely approximate skin edges and are tied on the outside. The reason is that, if suture marks are to be avoided, skin sutures should be removed in 6 to 8 days because of development of inflammatory reaction, epithelial lined tracts, or small stitch abscesses. Although the wound edges may be accurately coapted

with only a hairline scar at the time that cutaneous sutures are removed, the wound is held together only by epithelium, blood vessels, and globular protein. Even though it usually will not dehisce before collagen production takes over, the scar will stretch and widen during the ensuing 21 days while collagen formation and remodeling occur. The result usually is that a 7-day-old 1-mm-wide scar may become a 1-cm-wide scar 3 weeks after the sutures have been removed. One way to reduce widening of a scar after skin sutures are removed is to place permanent sutures in the fibrous protein layers of the skin to bring the edges together. This is accomplished by a subcuticular or intradermal suture of fine silk or synthetic material. The overlying epidermis is gently retracted, and sutures are placed in the lower part of the dermis. The knot is sometimes placed deep in subcutaneous tissue but can be tied superficially provided that the ends of the suture are cut close and the knot and suture ends are covered by overlying epithelium. It is important to use a very fine suture that will not be palpable beneath the epithelium and a clear or light-colored suture material that will not show through translucent epithelium. It has been shown recently that permanent subcuticular sutures will not eliminate completely secondary widening of a scar; such sutures will reduce the extent of transverse remodeling in many wounds, however.

After subcuticular sutures have been placed, the skin edges will be as close together as it is possible to bring them; yet the overlying epithelial edges may be vertically uneven. A final row of sutures of fine silk or synthetic material that serve as a fine adjustment or leveler of the epithelial edges is frequently utilized to produce an even surface. Because these sutures are in cellular tissue, they contribute little to the strength of the wound and should not be placed more than 1 mm from the wound edge. They should be tied loosely and removed before any epithelial reaction develops. Actually, external sutures in a wound closed in this manner probably can be removed in a few hours or as soon as the plasma clot seals the epithelial edges. For practical purposes, however, they are not removed until the first dressing, whenever that may be. In recent years the use of external cutaneous sutures has been partially eliminated by the development of various types of adhesive strips that can be used to hold skin edges together without producing epithelial sinuses or reaction.

When should sutures be removed? is a question frequently asked of surgeons. The answer is simple: when they have done the job they were put in to do, namely, hold the wound edges together until adequate tensile strength has developed. To set a finite period of time for removal of sutures is to imply that wounds heal at a standard rate; but the rate of healing is variable even in different parts of the body and under different conditions in a single individual. Instead of counting days until sutures can be removed, the wound must be examined; sometimes one or two sutures must be removed to see if the skin edges are sufficiently adherent to permit removal of all sutures. In wounds where a narrow scar is important and where some tension is unavoidable, it is advisable to splint the immature scar with adhesive strips for 2 or 3 weeks or until new collagen has attained sufficient strength and reliability.

The appearance of a linear scar frequently is worse between the third and fifth weeks after wound closure than it is at the time sutures are removed. The irregular, raised, purplish appearance of immature scar tissue can be a cause of great concern to young patients. Resorption of excess collagen, development of pliability, and the fading of undesirable color are called *maturation* of the scar, and maturation occurs more rapidly in older people than in the young. Children and teen-age patients, particularly, may have a distressing amount of red color in scars for several years. This condition is temporary, however, and redness should not be an indication for secondary surgical revision.

Scars should be revised secondarily only after they have undergone maximum maturation. Beefy, red, hypertrophic, immature scars usually recur after excision, and it is often amazing how much natural improvement will occur if sufficient time is allowed. It is seldom wise to attempt surgical improvement of a scar in less than 6 months; often natural improvement will continue for as long as 12 months.

Secondary revision should not be performed with the idea of changing the color of a scar or with the idea that a scar can be eliminated completely. All that secondary revision can accomplish is to take out a scar that resulted from unskilled closure or closure under unsatisfactory conditions and to close the defect as skillfully as possible under optimal conditions. Leveling uneven edges, changing the direction so that the scar does not cross lines of changing dimensions, and supporting a wide scar by the use of meticulously placed subcuticular sutures are the main improvements that can be accomplished. If scar tissue is elevated slightly above the level of surrounding skin, abrasion of that area with sandpaper or rotating brush will produce a smooth denuded surface over which new epithelium will spread in a more even plane.

Wounds characterized by a loss of skin can be allowed to heal by contraction and epithelization if there is sufficient skin to be stretched across the defect. This is usually permitted only when infection prevents primary closure and when contraction does not produce a contracture that would interfere with function or produce a cosmetically unacceptable scar. In all other wounds, a skin graft should be performed to replace the skin that has been lost.

At the moment, there is no known catalyst to accelerate normal wound healing; about all that a physician can do to aid normal healing is to protect the wound from physical, chemical, or bacteriologic complications that retard or prevent healing. Abnormal healing sometimes can be corrected as in the utilization of topical vitamin A to correct inhibition of epithelization caused by cortisone therapy. Vitamin A does not accelerate epithelization over normal expectation; it only corrects inhibition of epithelization caused by a specific drug effect. Platelet-derived growth factor, activated wound macrophages, *Staphylococcus aureus* bacterial strains, epidermal growth factor, and cartilage-derived growth factor are some of the biological substances that presently are being evaluated as wound-healing stimulants because of theoretical considerations or the early results of animal experiments. Protection usually means the use of an artificial dressing unless a natural dressing material, such as an eschar or scab, can serve the same purpose. Once the scab or eschar deteriorates, however, it, like any other dressing material, must be changed (debrided), and either definitive coverage provided or an artificial dressing applied. As in the selection of suture materials, choosing dressing materials involves a clear understanding of the objectives of each component of the dressing and the fundamental biologic processes that the dressing is supposed to protect. The first layer of a dressing is usually made of fine-mesh gauze, so that granulation tissue will not penetrate the interstices and cause hemorrhage when the dressing is removed. A long search for a pharmacologic substance to incorporate in the gauze to stimulate epithelial growth has been unsuccessful so far. Because certain by-products of the azo dye industry are carcinogenic, it was hoped that related dyes such as scarlet red might offer epithelial stimulation without being carcinogenic. All such substances have been disappointing, however, although most surgeons do use a gauze impregnated with some bland substance such as petroleum jelly or topical antibiotic in a water-soluble base. The main value of such medicated dressings is that there is less adherence of epithelium and vascular tissue to the dressing, hence less interference with wound healing when the dressing is changed. Dry gauze is a perfectly satisfactory dressing for most wound surfaces, however, and when carefully applied and removed, it can be as atraumatic as any other material. The usual coarse 4×4 hospital gauze sponge with cotton-filled center is not a good material to place against open wounds; the interstices permit permeation by vascular tissue, and the cotton lint that is included becomes embedded in the wound. Sponges, mechanics' waste, cotton, and the like are used to give bulk to a dressing after the fine-mesh gauze has been applied to make the dressing conform to a desired shape and immobilize the wounded part. Nonstretchable, firm, roller gauze bandage and adhesive tape are used to complete the dressing in a typical occlusive (erroneously called "pressure") dressing. The nonstretchable gauze and adhesive tape provide a compact and stable immobilizing influence. A clean wound has very little drainage and no odor, and does not have to be dressed very often.

Infected wounds have considerable drainage and odor and, therefore, must be dressed often to provide suitable drainage and tolerable appearance. It is common practice to use a wet dressing on infected wounds, which means that the inside layers of the dressing are intentionally moistened with saline solution or some other substance. The realization that there is no catalytic effect upon healing or any control of infection from water and that maceration of skin or eschar produces favorable conditions for bacterial or fungus growth throws doubt upon the beneficial effects to be obtained by applying a wet dressing. The usual answer is that drainage is increased by capillary action or that debridement is accomplished as detritus sticks to the dressing. Such reasoning has never seemed logical to the author; a dry dressing will absorb more wound drainage than a wet one, and debridement can usually be accomplished more efficiently by surgical means. It often appears that wounds become clean more quickly with the use of wet dressings, but in the author's experience this is partly because wet dressings are changed more often. Of course, less pain may be associated with wet-dressing changes than with dry-dressing changes. However, when dry dressings are changed frequently and skillfully, surface detritus may be removed more effectively by dry dressings than by wet ones. One sound reason for using a wet dressing, however, is that wet heat is more penetrating than dry heat, and when additional warmth is desirable to increase the local inflammatory response, a warm moist dressing is effective. Failure to keep a moist dressing warm by the addition of external heat, however, results in a cold soggy dressing that has no particular virtue and is definitely inferior to a frequently changed dry one. The objective is to keep wound secretions from accumulating and retarding repair by enzyme activity. Fibrinolysins, particularly, inhibit healing.

SKIN GRAFTS

Skin grafts are classified as free grafts (meaning that they are separated completely from their donor sites before being transferred to recipient areas) and pedicle grafts (which maintain a vascular connection with the general circulation). Free grafts are full-thickness (which means that the entire thickness of the skin, including epidermis and dermis, is transferred) and split-thickness (which means that the entire epidermis and only a portion of the dermis are transferred). The remainder of the dermis after split-thickness skin grafting remains at the donor site.

The "take" of a free graft refers to a pink appearance that occurs between the third and fifth days after transfer, signifying that vascular connections have developed between the recipient bed and the transplant. Before this time, free grafts are white (unless microvascular surgery has provided instantaneous restoration of circulation) and do not show any change in color when pressed upon and released. It is a matter of considerable conjecture whether there is diffusion of gases and nutrients between cells of the graft and underlying capillaries prior to development of actual vascular connections, and it has been assumed in the past that diffusion was necessary to keep cells nourished during the first few days. When grafts that include more than full thickness of the skin do not survive as free transplants, or when split-thickness grafts with pus or blood interposed between graft and capillary bed do not survive, it has been considered that diffusion could not occur through fat, pus, blood, etc. It seems more likely now, however, that diffusion is not important in the take of a graft and that mechanical barriers such as pus, blood, or fat prevent the take of a free graft by preventing

vascular connections from developing. Whatever the reason, the thicker the graft, the more likely will be the failure of take if mechanical or inflammatory conditions at the graft-wound interface are less than optimal. For this reason, thin grafts are used to cover less than ideally prepared wounds; full-thickness grafts are reserved for surgically produced wounds under optimal conditions.

In taking a full-thickness skin graft the surgeon produces a wound that will have to be closed by suturing the edges together or by applying a split-thickness skin graft from another donor site. If this is not done, closing a wound in one area with a graft will leave a wound of the same size and shape at the donor site. Full-thickness grafts are usually small grafts that can be taken from a place where there is an excess of thin skin, such as the inframammary fold or the groin, where the donor site can be closed by suturing the skin edges together.

It was once thought that split-thickness skin grafts must be taken through the level of the dermal-epidermal undulating interface so that small islands of stratum germinativum cells would remain to reepithelialize the denuded surface. Because of this notion, surgeons were careful to take grafts as thin as possible, and the taking of a split-thickness skin graft was relegated to only a few highly skilled individuals (Fig. 8-7). It seems obvious now that if it were possible to take a graft through only the epithelium, a satisfactory take would be unlikely. Most of the cells would be dead, and the covered wound would be resurfaced by cells that would provide no better coverage than that which would have occurred from normal epithelization. The qualities of skin other than waterproofing (strength, flexibility, appearance, etc.) that are desired in a graft are qualities provided by dermis. The final appearance of both recipient and donor sites, therefore, reflects the amount of dermis that has been transferred and the amount of dermis that is left behind. Epithelial cells migrate out of deep glands and hair follicles, and donor sites

Fig. 8-7. Removal of thick split-thickness skin graft with a freehand knife. The largest possible grafts can be taken by this method. Most grafts are taken with a dermatome.

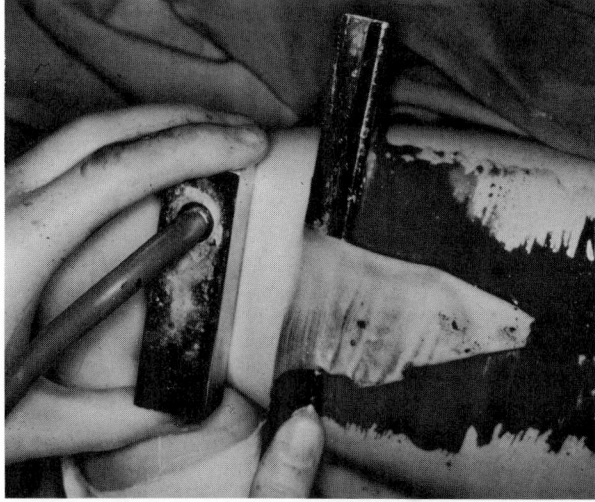

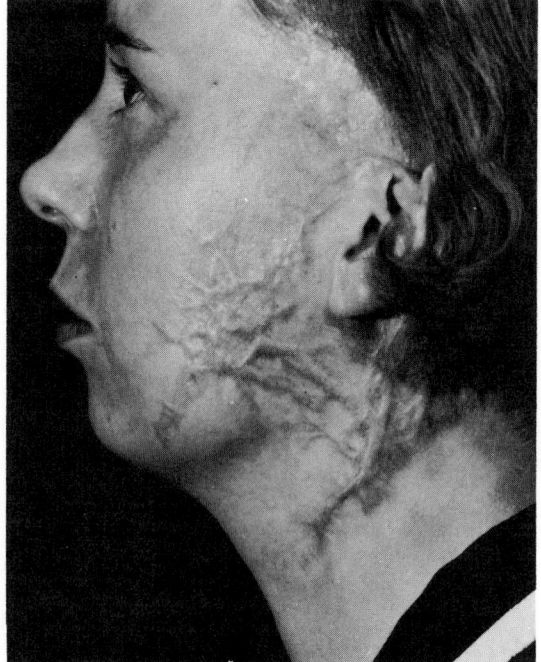

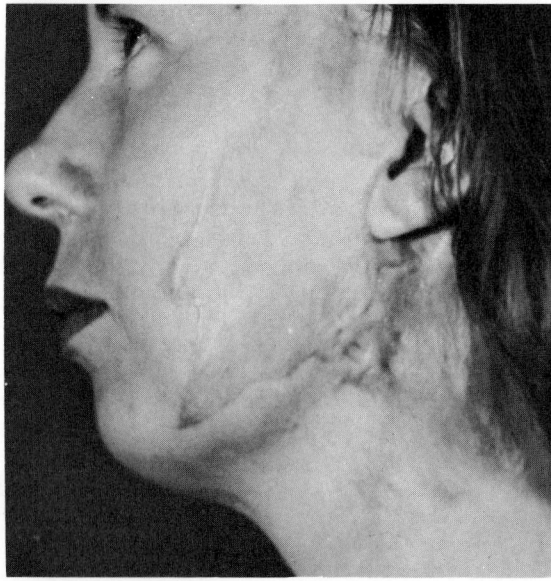

Fig. 8-8. *A.* Hypertrophic scar produced by deep second-degree burn. Although a significant amount of full-thickness skin has not been lost, overproduction of collagen has produced an unsightly scar. *B.* Patient shown in Fig. 8-8*A* following excision of facial portion of scar and application of a thick split-thickness skin graft. Cervical portion of scar resurfaced later. A single graft covering facial and cervical areas would obliterate submandibular groove. Note that scar at junction of graft and skin is most prominent near angle of mouth where motion and tension are unavoidable. Although different in texture, hue, and thickness from normal skin, the graft provides a smooth surface over which cosmetics can be applied more effectively than over previous scar.

that do not extend through the entire depth of the dermis will be reepithelialized from these sources. Dermis, being a complex organ and not a simple tissue, does not regenerate, however, and if all the properties of normal dermis are desired in the recipient area, full-thickness dermis must be transferred; if less than the full thickness is transferred, the resulting graft will be abnormal in appearance and function.

In choosing the thickness of a free skin graft, qualities that are desired in the recipient area must be balanced against cost incurred in the donor site. How such factors influence selection of graft thickness can be illustrated by comparing two extremes in wound and donor-site conditions. In a large thermal burn, the recipient area is not optimal in that usually it is infected, edematous, and involves a large area. The take of a graft therefore is uncertain, and revascularization is problematic. From the standpoint of the donor site, it may be necessary to procure several grafts from the same area to obtain enough skin for the entire wound; thus rapid healing, with remaining dermis thick enough for subsequent grafts to be taken, is mandatory. In this case, both donor-site and recipient conditions require thin grafts. In contrast, a 2-cm-diameter wound caused by loss of skin from the cheek of a young person presents an entirely different set of requirements for an optimal graft. The recipient bed should be optimal if excised immediately; the need for full-thickness dermis is mandatory so that normal texture, color, and thickness will produce the most cosmetically acceptable result. The graft usually is small, and so a variety of areas with a 2-cm redundancy of skin can be found for a donor site. Thus all factors point to the selection of a full-thickness graft. In other wounds the choice may not be quite so clear, but the principles involved in these two cases are the factors that must be considered in selection of any free graft (Fig. 8-8*A* and *B*).

Split-thickness skin grafts have a tendency to develop deep pigmentation after transfer. It is important to warn patients who recently have had split-thickness skin grafts placed on exposed areas of the body that protection from solar radiation is advisable for at least 6 months. Thick grafts have less tendency to develop undesirable pigment, and usually will blend into new surroundings more quickly than thin ones.

Finally, a word should be said about the concept of a "dressing graft." Split-thickness skin is the best possible dressing material for an open wound, and failure of surgeons to take advantage of this fact usually is based on the mistaken notion that placing a split-thickness skin graft on a wound is tantamount to closing the wound. Although the possibility that some portion or all of the graft may take and thus close the wound is the main advantage in using split-thickness skin grafts as a dressing material, placing the graft on a wound of questionable suitability for closure does not in itself produce a closed wound in the same manner as suturing two full-thickness skin edges together. Actually, a skin dressing does not close the wound any more than a petroleum jelly gauze dressing. If the wound has been inadequately debrided or infection is not yet controlled, the graft will slough in a few days and may disappear by the time of the first dressing. In such instances nothing will have been lost except a few square centimeters of split-thickness skin from the donor area. Dressing a questionable wound of relatively small size with split-thickness skin, therefore, is a sort of biologic test to determine suitability for closure, as well as providing some benefit if even a part of the graft survives. Xenografts of porcine skin, human allografts of split-thickness skin, and human amnion also are used as biologic dressings to test the suitability of the wound for definitive closure and to prevent metabolic and infectious complications of large wounds remaining open for protracted periods. Such grafts should be removed before take occurs and often are changed several times before optimum conditions for autograft application are obtained. In the judgment of the author, a porcine xenograft is a poor choice for a biologic dressing. Availability through a commercial source makes it easy for a surgeon to obtain porcine grafts, but expense and theoretical considerations of crossing major histocompatibility loci augur strongly for using human skin obtained from autopsy specimens or amnion obtained from the delivery room instead.

When more than the skin has been lost, and the skin plus some other tissue such as fat, tendon, muscle, or nerve must be replaced to restore function and appearance, transfer of skin by pedicle flap or direct vascular anastomosis is required (Fig. 8-9). As the name implies, pedicle transfers maintain vascular connection with the host, so that interruption of the capillary circulation never occurs. The vessels that are most important during transfer of tissue are the vessels in the subdermal plexus. These vessels are relatively large, frequently longitudinally oriented, and are located on the undersurface of the dermis superficial to subcutaneous fat. One frequently hears that a pedicle flap has been made thicker than actually needed for cosmetic or functional purposes in order to provide a safe blood supply. Fat on the undersurface of a flap does not add any appreciable blood supply, and it may be removed safely to produce as thin a pedicle as needed, provided the important vessels lying on the undersurface of the dermis are not injured. The problem in transplanting tissue by the pedicle method is to design a pedicle so that the base is as narrow as possible in relation to the length needed to cover the deficient area. It becomes a matter of considerable judgment, therefore, to gauge the shape and dimensions of a flap so that blood supply through the intact pedicle will be adequate to nourish the distal end of the flap. A great deal depends upon the natural profuseness of vascular beds; thus it is possible to move a pedicle flap on the face or cervical region that is three times as long as it is wide, while it may not be possible (without performing preliminary procedures to increase the blood supply) to transfer a flap on the leg that is no longer than it is wide. The blood supply in the base of a contemplated flap can be improved by performing a procedure commonly referred to as delay of the flap. The principle of delay is to reduce blood supply gradually to small segments of the circumference of the flap and thus improve the remaining blood supply to the point where a pedicle that was of insufficient width before

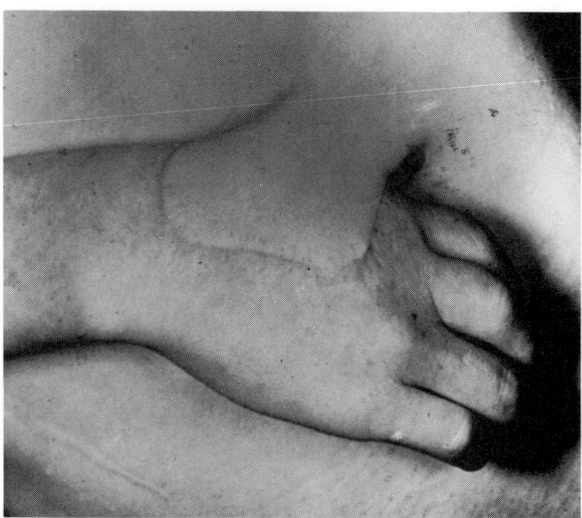

Fig. 8-9. Abdominal pedicle flap applied to dorsum of hand. Scar on hand has been turned back to resurface the raw side of pedicle and a portion of the donor site. Flap will be separated from the abdominal wall in 18 days.

the flap was delayed becomes adequate to nourish the flap. The mechanism by which delay (gradual interruption of a portion of the blood supply to a flap) improves circulation in the base is not completely clear. It seems doubtful that new blood vessels actually grow into the area, although casual observation of changes in the vessels at the base suggests that this is what may happen. The rapidity with which delay improves the circulation strongly suggests, however, that the release of various amines, probably in response to changes in pH secondary to increased anaerobic metabolism, causes a closure of normally open shunts that prevent perfusion of the entire capillary network. The effect is a substantial hyperemia at the base of the flap; over a period of several weeks and after several delaying procedures, the vessels in the pedicle base become racemose in appearance, and the amount of blood flow is increased to the extent that a relatively long flap can be transferred on a narrow pedicle. Following transfer of a flap, circulation must be observed carefully for the first 48 h, as signs of impending circulatory embarrassment occur before irreversible thrombosis and cell death. It is not unusual for the distal end of a flap to be dusky following transfer; venous spasm secondary to the trauma of rotation may be all that is involved. Improvement usually occurs in a few hours, but during this time the danger of venous thrombosis is increased; if there is progression of cyanosis and edema, the possibility that tension on veins is interfering with return circulation must be investigated by removing a few sutures. Perhaps the most serious, but still reversible, sign of impending venous thrombosis is development of a sharp line of color differentiation. A gradual change from normal pink to slight cyanosis is not so significant as a clearcut line demarcating the area of circulatory deficiency. Even if all sutures have to be removed and the flap returned to its original bed, the sign must be attended to, or

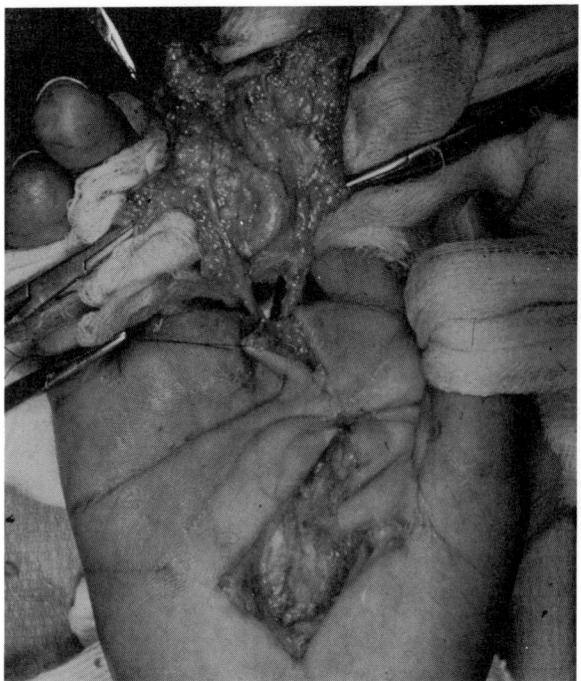

Fig. 8-10. Island pedicle flap developed during amputation of long finger. The flap is nourished by a single digital artery and nerve. Sensation is preserved by including a digital nerve in the vascular pedicle.

an irreversible demarcation will soon develop, signifying complete thrombosis and certain distal necrosis. In sensibly planned and adequately prepared flaps, one does not have to be particularly concerned about arterial insufficiency; venous drainage is the function that develops complications. Complications usually are the result of too much tension, poor dressing, hematoma, or infection.

The use of heparin and low-molecular-weight dextran has seemed to be beneficial in dangerously compromised circulation. Recently smoking has been shown to affect adversely circulation in face flaps. Hyperbaric oxygenation has been reported instrumental in saving flaps of laboratory animals, but is not practical for managing human flaps.

Advancement flaps and rotation flaps are the simplest pedicle transfers. They are dependent upon redundancy of soft tissue adjacent to a defect so that the donor defect can be closed by approximating the skin edges or applying split-thickness skin grafts. More complicated flaps require the use of an arm as a carrier to provide circulation during the period that skin is detached from the original donor site, such as abdominal wall, and transferred to a distant site, such as the lower leg. Because of similarity of tissue characteristics, safety in transfer, and expense and time involved, it is desirable to design flaps as close to the point where they are needed as possible.

One of the most sophisticated rotation flaps is an island pedicle flap (Fig. 8-10), which combines the pedicle principle of intact blood and nerve supply with some of the advantages of a free graft. The principle of the island pedicle is that careful dissection of the artery and vein (and sometimes the nerve) to a piece of skin can be performed so that the skin is detached from surrounding skin and remains attached to the body only by essentials for survival—an artery, a vein, and sometimes a nerve. Depending on the length of these structures, it is possible to move a full-thickness skin and fat graft, or an intact finger, or a portion of a finger or toe, a long distance. Transfer of hair-bearing portions of the scalp on a temporal artery-and-vein supported flap to the supraorbital region for eyebrow reconstruction and transfer of a finger to replace a missing thumb are examples of island pedicle transfers.

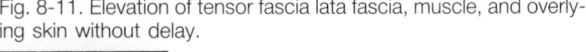

Fig. 8-11. Elevation of tensor fascia lata fascia, muscle, and overlying skin without delay.

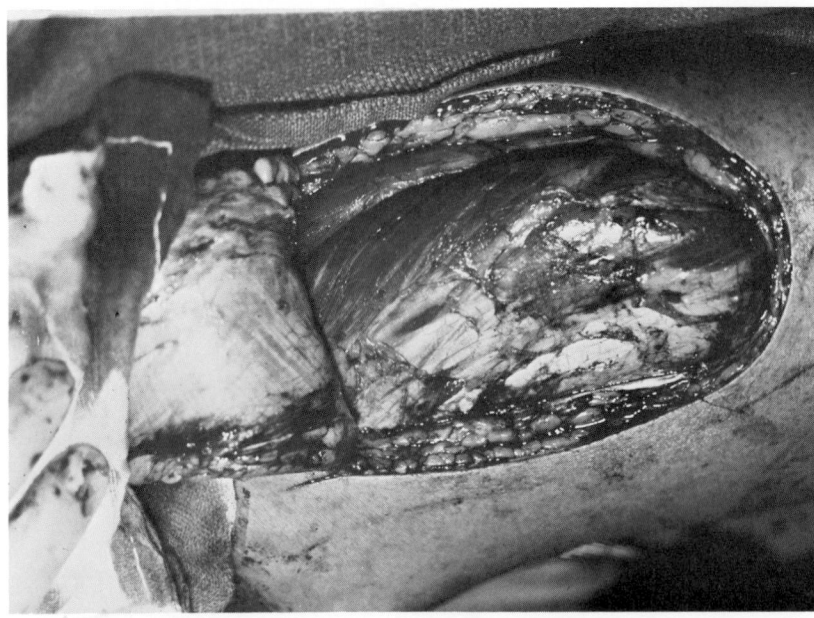

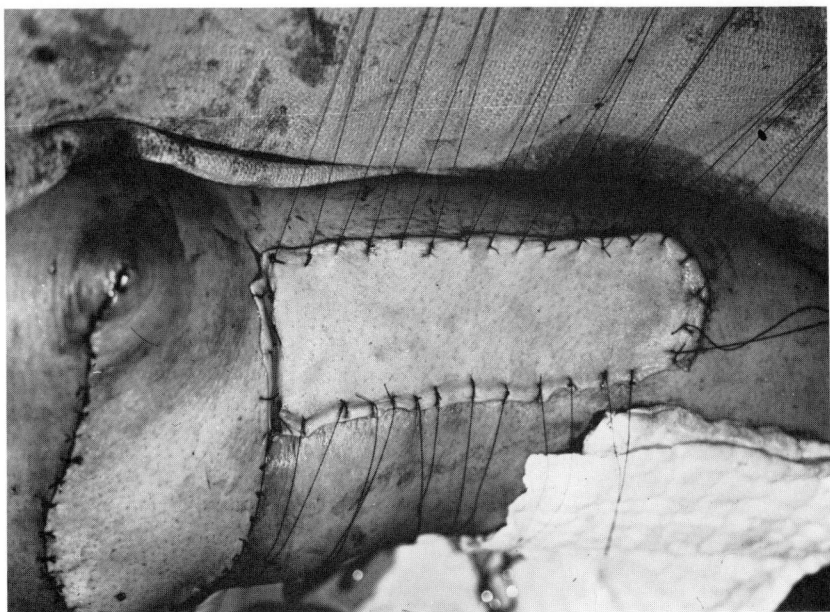

Fig. 8-12. Rotation of tensor fascia lata myocutaneous flap to cover debrided trochanteric decubitus ulcer.

The need to perform time-consuming and costly delay procedures has been reduced significantly by the development of myocutaneous and free microvascular transfer flaps. Discovery that muscle under skin supplies blood vessels sufficient to nourish skin is the basis for composite flaps, called myocutaneous, that transfer intact muscle, subcutaneous tissue, and overlying skin as a single unit rotated on the relatively narrow vascular supply of the muscle. Pectoralis major, latissimus dorsi, gracilis, and tensor fascia lata myocutaneous flaps are used fre-

quently to transfer skin and subcutaneous tissue without delay procedures. An example of a tensor fascia lata myocutaneous flap rotated 180° to a trochanteric defect on the single artery and vein nourishing the muscle is shown in Figs. 8-11 and 8-12. Perhaps the most elegant such transfer is a free flap in which muscle, muscle and skin, or skin alone is transferred to a distant site. After transfer, the blood vessels are sutured by microvascular technique to vessels in the recipient area, thus reestablishing active circulation. Latissimus dorsi, gracilis,

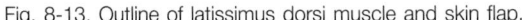

Fig. 8-13. Outline of latissimus dorsi muscle and skin flap.

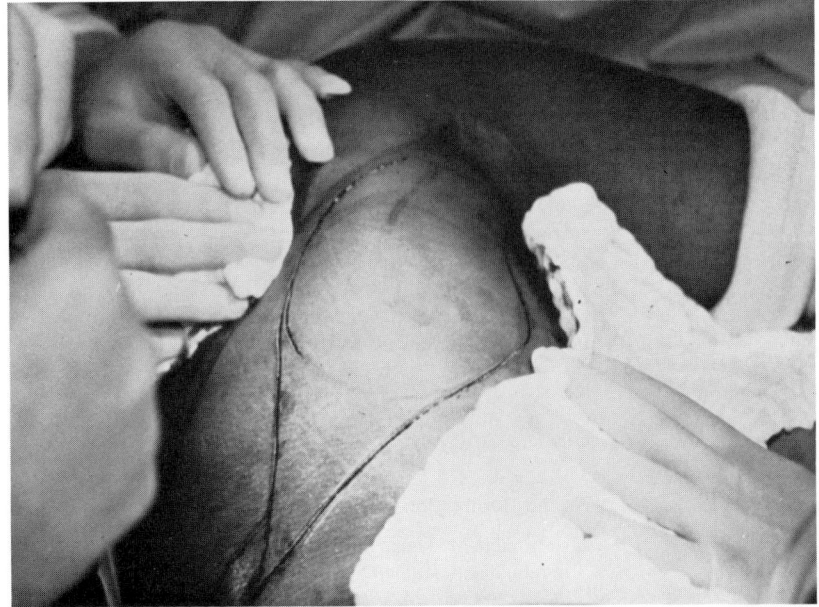

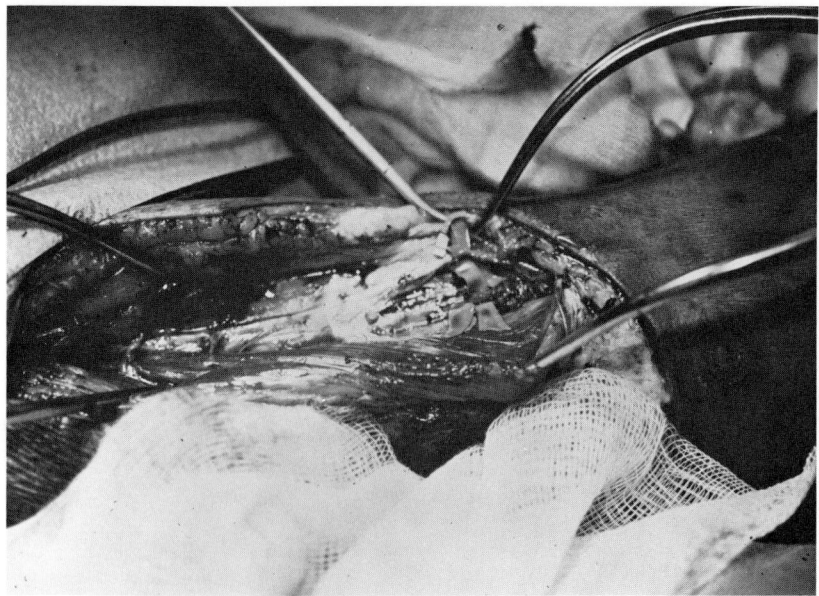

Fig. 8-14. Preparation of anterior tibial artery and veins to receive thoracodorsal vessels of latissimus free flap.

groin, and scapular skin flaps have been very successful in restoring surface defects in the lower leg and foot. Free jejunal and omental grafts have been utilized in the head and neck. Transfer of rib, subcutaneous tissue, and overlying skin by microvascular anastomosis of intercostal vessels to facial vessels has been useful in reconstructing composite defects of the face and lower jaw. An example of free-flap transfer of a latissimus dorsi and overlying back skin flap to the lower leg with anastomosis of the thoracodorsal vessels to the anterior tibial (end-to-side) artery and vein is shown in Figs. 8-13 to 8-15.

Finally, in the opinion of many, maturity in restorative surgery can be measured, in part, by how often one thinks

Fig. 8-15. Latissimus free flap on leg following microvascular anastomosis of thoracodorsal vessels to anterior tibial artery and vein.

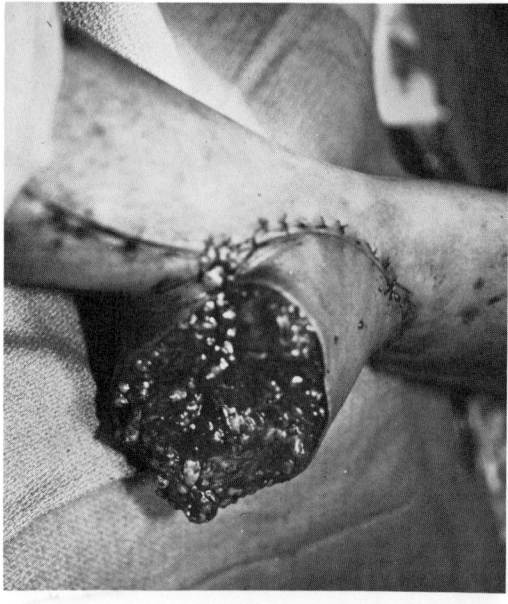

of a pedicle flap as the only means of rebuilding a damaged area and then devises a way to make a free graft suffice. Pedicles are dramatic, particularly as used by military surgeons to rebuild enormous tissue defects caused by high-explosive wounds; fortunately, however, civilian injuries are not often so devastating, and the practical points of expense, length of time away from work, utilization of hospital facilities, and the like have to be considered in each case where a pedicle could be used. In addition, although areas such as the face may appear in photographs to have been superbly restored by massive flaps, yet it must be remembered that flaps have no dynamic function; they are expressionless, and often look better in photographs than they do as part of the constantly moving facial features. A recent development that has reduced the need for distant pedicle flaps is local tissue expansion with an implanted inflatable device. Gradual stretching of skin for 4 to 6 weeks can be accomplished with such a device so that local rotation advancement flaps become possible in areas where local skin was not sufficient to resurface the defect before expansion. When a pedicle flap is needed, nothing else will suffice, and pedicles are an extremely valuable part of restorative surgery. The high cost of donor-site mutilation, length of time required for transfer, and adynamic features, however, make the pedicle flap definitely second choice to a free graft if a free graft can be used.

Bibliography

Wound Contraction

Abercrombie M, James DW, Newcombe JF: Wound contraction in rabbit skin, studied by splinting the wound margins. *J Anat* 94:170, 1960.

Ariyan S, Enriquez R, Krizek T: Wound contraction and fibrocontractive disorders. *Arch Surg* 113:1034, 1978.

Danes B, Leinfelder PJ: Cytological and respiratory effects of cyanide on tissue cultures. *J Cell Comp Physiol* 37:427, 1951.

Ehrlich HP, Grislis G, Hunt TK: Evidence for the involvement of microtubules in wound contraction. *Ann Surg* 133:706, 1977.

Grillo HC, Gross J: Studies in wound healing. III. Contraction in vitamin C deficiency. *Proc Soc Exp Biol Med* 101:268, 1959.

Grillo HC, Watts GT, Gross J: Studies in wound healing. I. Contraction and wound contents. *Ann Surg* 148:145, 1958.

Madden JW, Carlson EE, Hines J: Presence of modified fibroblasts in ischemic contracture of the intrinsic musculature of the hand. *Surg Gynecol Obstet* 140:509, 1975.

Madden JW, Morton D Jr, Peacock EE Jr: Contraction of experimental wounds. I. Inhibiting wound contraction by using a topical smooth muscle antagonist. *Surgery* 76:18, 1974.

Majno G, Babbiani G, et al: Contraction of granulation tissue *in vitro:* Similarity with smooth muscle. *Science* 173:548, 1971.

Phillips JL, Peacock EE: Importance of horizontal plane cell mass integrity in wound contraction. *Proc Soc Exp Biol Med* 117:539, 1964.

Rudolph R: Contraction and the control of contraction. *World J Surg* 4:288, 1980.

Rudolph R, Guber S, Woodward M: Inhibition of myofibroblasts by skin grafts. *Plast Reconstr Surg* 63:173, 1979.

Ryan GB, Cliff WJ, et al: Myofibroblasts in human granulation tissue. *Hum Pathol* 5:55, 1974.

Watts GT, Grillo HC, Gross J: Studies in wound healing. II. The role of granulation tissue in contraction. *Ann Surg* 148:153, 1958.

Epithelization

Alexander SA: Patterns of epidermal cell polarity in healing open wounds. *J Surg Res* 31:456, 1981.

Alexander SA, Gonoff RB: The glycosaminoglycans of open wounds. *J Surg Res* 29:499, 1980.

Alvarez OM, Mertz PM, Eaglstein WH: The effect of occlusive dressings on collagen synthesis and re-epithelialization in superficial wounds. *J Surg Res* 35:142, 1983.

Argyris TS: The regulation of epidermal hyperplastic growth, CRC critical review. *Toxicology* 9:151, 1981.

Franklin JD, Lynch JB: Effects of topical applications of epidermal growth factor on wound healing. *Plast Reconstr Surg* 64:766, 1979.

Gillman T, Penn J: Studies on the repair of cutaneous wounds. *Med Proc* 2(suppl 3): 121, 1956.

Laato M, Niinikoski J, et al: Stimulation of wound healing by epidermal growth factor. *Ann Surg* 203:379, 1986.

Sullivan DJ, Epstein WS: Mitotic activity of wounded human epidermis. *J Invest Dermatol* 41:39, 1963.

Collagen

Baur PS, Parks DH: The myofibroblast anchoring strand—the fibronectin connection in wound healing and the possible loci of collagen fibril assembly. *J Trauma* 23:853, 1983.

Bornstein P: Disorders of connective tissue function and the aging process: a synthesis and review of current concepts and findings. *Mech Ageing Dev* 5:305, 1976.

Cohen IK, Keiser HR, Sjoersdma A: Collagen synthesis in human keloid and hypertrophic scar. *Surg Forum* 22:488, 1971.

Dayer J, Russell RG, Krane SM: Collagenase production by rheumatoid synovial cells: stimulation by a human lymphocyte factor. *Science* 195:181, 1977.

Diegelmann RF, Cohen IK, Kaplan AM: The role of macrophages in wound repair: a review. *Plast Reconstr Surg* 68:107, 1981.

Duskin D, Bornstein P: Impaired conversion of procollagen to collagen by fibroblasts and bone treated with tunicamycin, an inhibitor of protein glycosylation. *J Biol Chem* 252:955, 1977.

Ellis H: Internal overhealing: The problem of intraperitoneal adhesions. *World J Surg* 4:303, 1980.

Ellis H, Lapiere CM: Collagenolytic activity in amphibian tissues: A tissue culture assay. *Proc Natl Acad Sci USA* 48:1014, 1962.

Fleischmajer R, Olsen BR, Kühn K (eds): Biology, chemistry, and pathology of collagen. *Ann NY Acad Sci* 460, 1985.

Hoffmann H, Olsen B, et al: Segment-long-spacing aggregates and isolation of COOH-terminal peptides from type I procollagen. *Proc Natl Acad Sci USA* 73:4304, 1976.

Madden JW: Some aspects of fibrogenesis during the healing of primary and secondary wounds. *Surg Gynecol Obstet* 115:408, 1962.

Miller ES: Biochemical characteristics and biological significance of the genetically-distinct collagens. *Mol Cell Biochem* 13:165, 1976.

Olsen B, Hoffmann H, Prockop DJ: Interchain disulfide bonds at the COOH-terminal end of procollagen synthesized by matrix-free cells from chick embryonic tendon and cartilage. *Arch Biochem Biophys* 175:341, 1976.

Peacock EE Jr: Collagenolysis: The other side of the equation. *World J Surg* 4:297, 1980.

Prockop DJ, Kivirikko KI, et al: The biosynthesis of collagen and its disorders. *N Engl J Med* (3001):13, 1979.

Raju DR, Jindrak K, et al: A study of the critical bacterial inoculum to cause a stimulus to wound healing. *Surg Gynecol Obstet* 144:347, 1977.

Riley WB Jr, Peacock EE Jr.: Identification, distribution, and significance of a collagenolytic enzyme in human tissue. *Proc Soc Biol Med* 214:207, 1967.

Wound Care

Ariyan S, Cuono CB: Use of the pectoralis major myocutaneous flap for reconstruction of large cervical, facial or cranial defects. *Am J Surg* 140:503, 1980.

Bucknall TE, Ellis H: *Wound Healing for Surgeons.* Philadelphia, WB Saunders, 1984.

Cutting CB, Bardach J, Finseth F: Hemodynamics of the delayed skin flap: A total blood flow study. *Br J Plast Surg.* 34:133, 1981.

Faulk WP, Stevens PJ, et al: Human amnion as an adjunct in wound healing. *Lancet* 1(8179): 1156, May 31, 1980.

Harii K: Myocutaneous flaps—clinical applications and refinements. *Ann Plast Surg* 40:440, 1980.

Hunt TK, Dunphy JE: *Fundamentals of Wound Management.* New York, Appleton-Century-Crofts, 1979.

Leighton WD, Johnson ML, Friedland JA: Use of the temporary soft tissue expander in post traumatic alopecia. *Plast Reconstr Surg* 77:737, 1986.

McGregor JC, Buchan AC: Clinical experience with the tensor fasciae latae myocutaneous flap. *Br J Surg* 33:270, 1980.

Mulliken JB, Healey NA: Pathogenesis of skin flap necrosis from an underlying hematoma. *Plast Reconstr Surg* 64:540, 1979.

Olivari N: Use of thirty latissimus dorsi flaps. *Plast Reconstr Surg* 64:654, 1979.

Peacock EE Jr: *Wound Repair,* 3d ed. Philadelphia, Saunders, 1984.

Peacock EE Jr: Wound healing, in *The Scientific Management of Surgical Patients.* Boston, Little, Brown, 1983, chap 2.

Serafin D, Riefohl R, et al: Vascularized rib-periosteal and osteocutaneous reconstruction of the maxilla and mandible: An assessment. *Plast Reconstr Surg* 66:718, 1980.

Sindelar WF, Mason GR: Intraperitoneal irrigation with povidone-iodine solution for the prevention of intraabdominal abscesses in the bacterially contaminated abdomen. *Surg Gynecol Obstet* 148:409, 1979.

Teh BT: Why do skin grafts fail? *Plast Reconstr Surg* 63:323, 1979.

Chapter 9

Oncology

Donald L. Morton, James S. Economou, Charles M. Haskell, and Robert G. Parker

INTRODUCTION

Oncology (from the Greek *onkos,* mass, or tumor, and *logos,* study) is the study of neoplastic diseases. Neoplasms are an altered cell population characterized by an excessive, nonuseful proliferation of cells that have be-

come unresponsive to normal control mechanisms and to the organizing influences of adjacent tissues. Malignant neoplasms are composed of cancer cells that exhibit uncontrolled proliferation and impair the function of normal organs by local tissue invasion and metastatic spread to distant anatomic sites. Benign neoplasms are composed of normal-appearing cells that do not invade locally or metastasize to other sites.

Cancer has plagued human beings since antiquity, and many of its clinical manifestations were described by Hippocrates (460–375 B.C.). Neoplasms have been identified in all species of animals including the lower vertebrates, such as amphibia and fish. The wide distribution of neoplasia in natural and human history suggests that cancer may be common to all multicellular organisms.

Neoplastic disease is the second most frequent cause of death in the United States. The magnitude of the cancer problem is exemplified by the fact that three of every ten persons living today has or will develop cancer. An estimated 73 million Americans, 30 percent of those presently alive, will develop cancer sometime during their lifetime. Approximately 40 percent of those who get cancer will survive for at least 5 years after treatment. Until recently such facts caused many physicians and surgeons to approach the cancer patient with feelings of pessimism and despair that frequently interfered with adequate therapy.

Fortunately, exciting developments in tumor immunology, viral oncology, and molecular biology and advances in the therapy of some neoplasms led to a rebirth of interest in the basic biologic and clinical problems posed by cancer. Specialty boards have been established in medical oncology and gynecologic oncology. A wide variety of scientists from many disciplines have been attracted to cancer research. As a result, more advances have been made in cancer therapy in the past 10 years than in all previous times. This chapter is designed to introduce the student to general principles that can be used as the basis for acquiring further knowledge in this rapidly growing field.

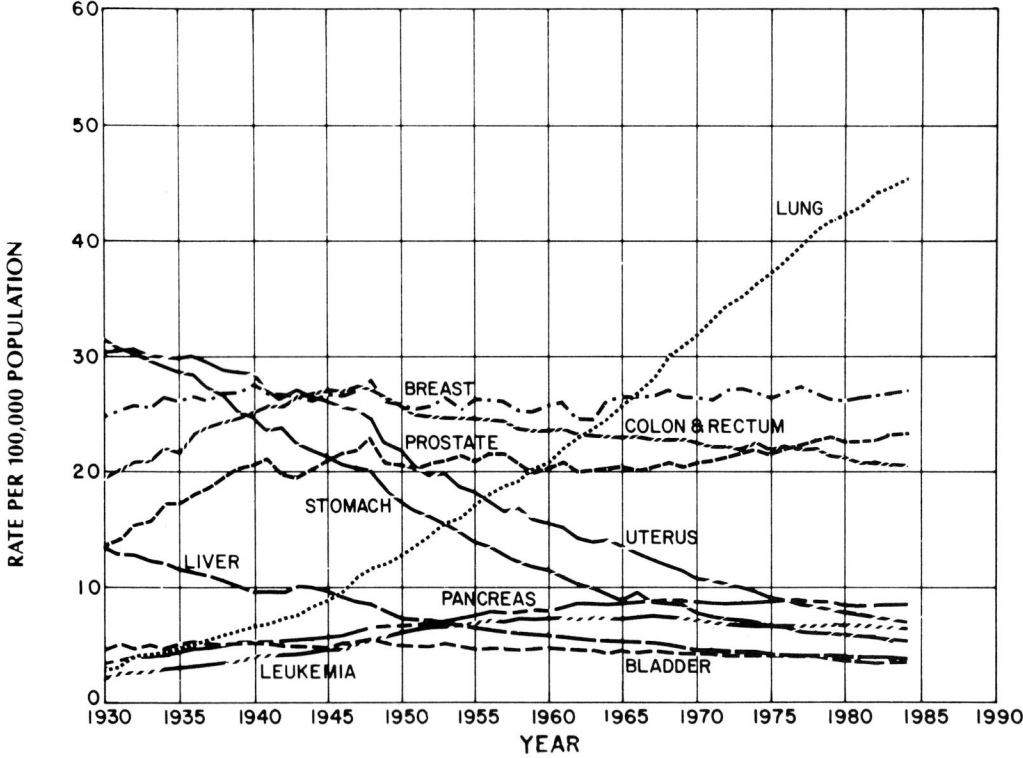

Fig. 9-1. Cancer death rates by site, United States, 1930–1984. (From: *National Vital Statistics Division and Bureau of the Census, United States.*)

EPIDEMIOLOGY

The changes in death rates from cancer by body site for males and females in the United States during the past 45 years are summarized in Fig. 9-1. Although there has been a decrease in mortality from certain neoplasms, the overall cancer death rates continue to show a slow, steady increase.

The mortality rates from lung cancer have increased steadily and probably represent the most dramatic change for any cancer site. There will be about 150,000 new cases of lung cancer in the United States in 1987, and the incidence in black males and females continues to rise. Thirteen percent of all lung cancer patients are alive 5 years after diagnosis. Compared with 40 years ago, the mortality has risen from 18.3 to 67.5 per 100,000 for men and from 4.6 to 16.6 for women. Lung cancer represents the leading cause of cancer death when both sexes are considered.

Pancreatic cancer death rates also have steadily increased through the years. Today, the rates are twice what they were in women and three times that in men when compared with 1930.

There has been a striking reduction during the past 50 years in death rates caused by cancers of the stomach and uterus. The stomach cancer death rate is now less than one-fourth the 1930 rate in men and less than one-fifth the 1930 rate in women, although there has been little im-

provement in the survival rates of stomach cancer. The reason for this declining incidence is unknown.

Death rates due to uterine cancer are only one-half what they were 40 years ago. In this case, the causes of the reduction are known to be earlier detection and improved treatment for cancer of the uterine cervix and corpus.

The incidence of cancer in different sites and the mortality rate in each sex are compared in Fig. 9-2. The sites most frequently causing death in males, in order of decreasing frequency, are (1) lung, (2) colon and rectum, and (3) prostate. The sites, in order of decreasing frequency in females, are (1) lung, (2) breast, and (3) colon and rectum.

The incidence of various types of neoplasms differs from the death rates for the same neoplasms (Fig. 9-2) because different forms of cancer are not equally lethal. The most significant 5-year survival rates are achieved in patients with cancer of the skin, cervix, uterus, and bladder; the lowest survival occurs in patients with pancreatic cancer. Lung cancer is the leading cause of cancer death even though skin cancer occurs more commonly.

Females tend to have a greater number of 5-year survivals with cancers of any given primary site than males, although the reasons are unknown at this time. The overall 5-year survival for women with cancer is 50 percent,

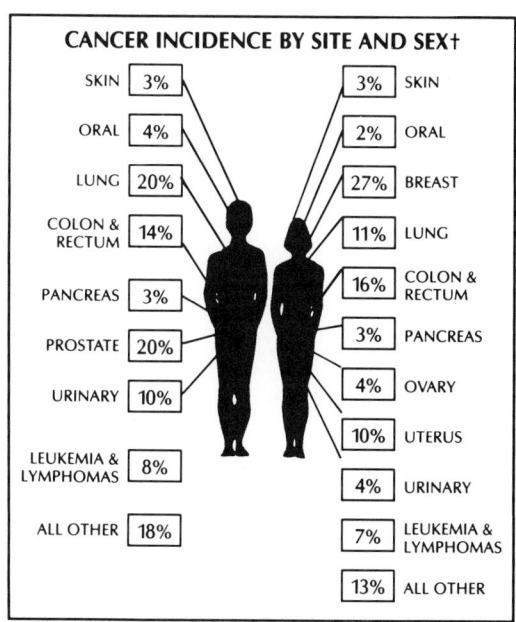

CANCER INCIDENCE BY SITE AND SEX†

	Male			Female	
SKIN	3%		3%	SKIN
ORAL	4%		2%	ORAL
LUNG	20%		27%	BREAST
COLON & RECTUM	14%		11%	LUNG
PANCREAS	3%		16%	COLON & RECTUM
PROSTATE	20%		3%	PANCREAS
URINARY	10%		4%	OVARY
			10%	UTERUS
LEUKEMIA & LYMPHOMAS	8%		4%	URINARY
ALL OTHER	18%		7%	LEUKEMIA & LYMPHOMAS
			13%	ALL OTHER

Fig. 9-2. Estimated cancer incidence by site and sex, 1987 estimates. *(American Cancer Society, Cancer Facts and Figures, 1987.)*

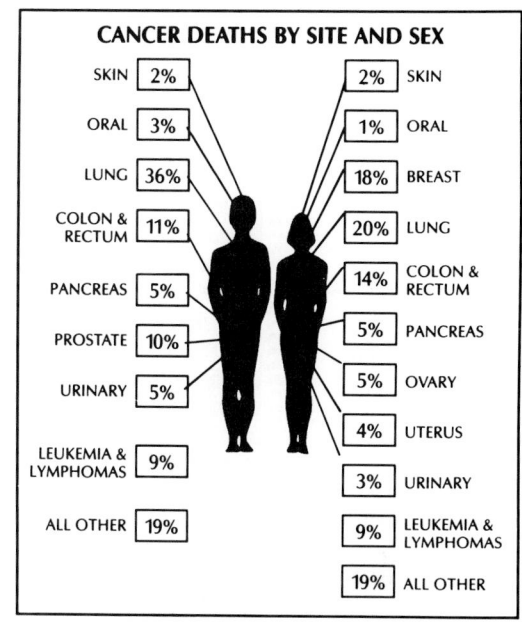

CANCER DEATHS BY SITE AND SEX

	Male			Female	
SKIN	2%		2%	SKIN
ORAL	3%		1%	ORAL
LUNG	36%		18%	BREAST
COLON & RECTUM	11%		20%	LUNG
PANCREAS	5%		14%	COLON & RECTUM
PROSTATE	10%		5%	PANCREAS
URINARY	5%		5%	OVARY
			4%	UTERUS
LEUKEMIA & LYMPHOMAS	9%		3%	URINARY
ALL OTHER	19%		9%	LEUKEMIA & LYMPHOMAS
			19%	ALL OTHER

compared with only 31 percent for men. The overall 5-year cancer survival rates for common malignant tumors of selected sites are shown in Fig. 9-3.

ETIOLOGY

While many etiologic agents for cancer have been recognized, some for centuries, the underlying molecular mechanisms have only recently been better understood. A discussion of current thinking about oncogenes and growth factors will be preceded by a review of classical etiologic agents and epidemiological factors.

CHEMICAL CARCINOGENS. The first cause-and-effect relation between a carcinogenic stimulus and the development of cancer in human beings was described by Percival Pott, an English surgeon, in 1775, when he described a cancer of the scrotum frequently occurring in chimney sweeps. Yamagiwa and Ichikawa, working from 1915 to 1918, identified the carcinogen when they experimentally produced cancers by painting the ears of rabbits with coal tar. Kennaway and Cook, in studies from 1924 to 1932, demonstrated that pure hydrocarbons, such as 1,2-dibenzanthracene and similar compounds isolated from coal tar, were carcinogenic agents. Subsequently, a variety of chemical agents have been found that are capable of inducing neoplasms in experimental animals and in human beings. These chemicals are called *carcinogens*. There may be many years separating the time of exposure to a carcinogen and subsequent development of a neoplasm. Consequently, the present-day evaluation of the safety of food additives or other products for human consumption that are chronically ingested over long periods of time is a most difficult task.

A variety of chemicals associated with different types of human neoplasms are shown in Table 9-1. Aromatic amines are known to cause tumors of the urinary tract; workers in the dye industry have a higher incidence of this type of cancer. Benzene has been associated with acute leukemia in shoe repairmen in Italy, solvent manufacturers, painters, and printers who use it as a solvent. Coal tar, pitch, creosote, and anthracene have been associated with cancer of the skin, larynx, and bronchus. A variety of paraffin oils, waxes, and tars are associated with cancer of the skin. Isopropyl oil has been associated with cancer of the sinuses, larynx, and bronchus in workers exposed to it. Mesotheliomas occur very frequently in miners and ship workers who have been exposed to asbestos. Certain metals have been associated with tumors, including chromium, nickel, and arsenic.

PHYSICAL CARCINOGENS. Ionizing radiation was found to be carcinogenic in the 1920s when subcutaneous sarcomas were induced by radium implants in experimental animals. The carcinogenic effects of radiation in human beings were recognized when radium dial painters who commonly licked brushes containing radioactive materials developed bone cancers. Since then, many examples of the carcinogenic effects of radiation have been recognized. Physicians and dentists exposed to multiple x-ray exposures develop recurrent skin cancer. Cancer of the thyroid in adults is frequently associated with neck irradiation in early childhood. The survivors of the atomic bomb detonations show an increased incidence of leukemia. Ultraviolet light on exposed areas may foster the

FIVE YEAR CANCER SURVIVAL RATES* FOR SELECTED SITES

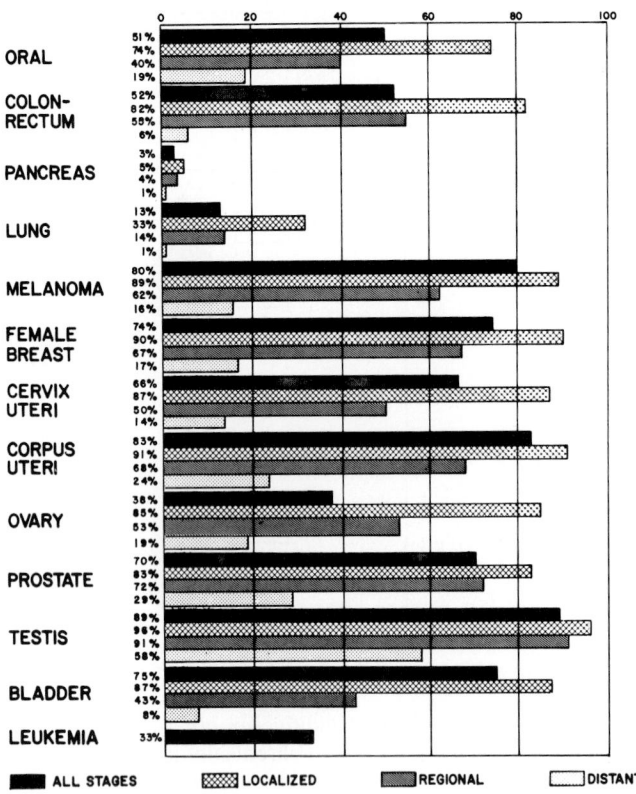

ORAL 51% 74% 40% 19%

COLON-RECTUM 52% 82% 55% 6%

PANCREAS 3% 5% 4% 1%

LUNG 13% 33% 14% 1%

MELANOMA 80% 89% 62% 16%

FEMALE BREAST 74% 90% 67% 17%

CERVIX UTERI 66% 87% 50% 14%

CORPUS UTERI 83% 91% 68% 24%

OVARY 38% 85% 53% 19%

PROSTATE 70% 83% 72% 29%

TESTIS 89% 96% 91% 58%

BLADDER 75% 87% 43% 8%

LEUKEMIA 33%

■ ALL STAGES   ▨ LOCALIZED   ▨ REGIONAL   ☐ DISTANT

*Adjusted for normal life expectancy
 This chart is based on cases diagnosed in 1974-1982

Source: Surveillance and Operations Research Branch,
        National Cancer Institute

Fig. 9-3. Five-year cancer survival rates for selected sites. *(American Cancer Society, Cancer Facts and Figures, 1987.)*

development of skin cancer. Farmers and sailors have an increased incidence of skin cancers from excessive exposure to sunlight, as do fair-skinned people living in tropical regions.

Mechanical Irritation. Chronic mechanical irritation may be associated with the development of cancer, although the exact mechanisms are unknown. Examples include the malignant degeneration in old burn scars (the chronic ulcer of Marjolin), and cancer of the liver and bladder subsequent to parasitic infestation by schistosomes.

Tumor viruses have become increasingly implicated as primary etiologic agents for a small number of human tumors. That viruses could cause cancers in animals and induce cell transformation in vitro was demonstrated many years ago. The study of retroviruses in particular has led to the discovery of oncogenes (see below) and provided the first clear insight into the molecular mechanisms of neoplasia.

Epidemiologic and molecular biologic evidence has circumstantially implicated a number of viruses with human malignancies: Hepatitis B and hepatocellular carcinoma, human T-cell leukemia virus and adult T-cell leukemia/lymphoma, Epstein-Barr virus with both Burkitt's lymphoma and nasopharyngeal carcinoma, and herpes simplex virus-2 and cervical cancer.

HEREDITARY FACTORS. Genetic factors are of major importance in determining the effectiveness of chemical, physical, and viral carcinogens in animals.

Clear-cut examples in human cancer development are demonstrated when the same type of cancer occurs in identical twins, when colon cancer develops in family members with familial polyposis, and with the familial patterns associated with breast cancer. Cancer of the breast is about three times more common in the daughters of women with premenopausal breast cancer and in women whose blood relatives have had at least two incidences of breast cancer. Furthermore, the daughters develop breast cancers at a younger age than did their mothers.

A more indirect genetic role is found in certain families who seem to have an increased incidence of neoplastic diseases. A clearly defined pattern of inheritance has been established for some of these tumors. It is often difficult to assess the importance of environmental factors in these cases. Substantiated examples include a pattern of dominant inheritance in some families for diseases such as retinoblastoma, lipomatosis, and colonic polyposis. In other families, there may be an association of multiple diseases that may include one or more neoplasms. An

Table 9-1. CHEMICAL AND PHYSICAL CARCINOGENS IN HUMAN BEINGS

Carcinogen	Site of neoplasm	Site exposed	Persons at risk
Chemical agents:			
Aromatic amines, especially β-naphthylamine	Urinary tract	Cutaneous and respiratory	Chemical workers producing dye stuffs, rodenticides, laboratory reagents
Benzol or benzene	Blood, lymphatic organs	Cutaneous and respiratory	Coal-tar refiners, solvent manufacturers, painters, printers, mechanics
Coal tar, pitch, creosote, anthracene, tobacco	Skin, larynx, bronchus	Cutaneous and respiratory	Coke-oven workers, coal-tar distillers, lumber industry workers, chemical workers, smokers
Petroleum, shale and paraffin oils, waxes, tars	Skin	Cutaneous	Workers in oil refineries, wax and asphalt producers, mechanics
Isopropyl oils	Sinus, larynx, bronchus	Respiratory	Producers of isopropyl alcohol
Asbestos	Bronchus, mesothelioma of pleura	Respiratory, generally >2 years	Asbestos miners, shippers, millers
Chromium	Bronchus	Respiratory and cutaneous	Workers engaged in chromate ore reduction
Nickel	Nasal cavity, sinus, bronchus	Respiratory	Nickel miners, shippers, and refiners
Arsenic	Skin, bronchus, bladder	Respiratory	Smelters, pesticide manufacturers
Physical agents:			
Ionizing radiation	Skin, thyroid, tongue, tonsil, sinus, bone, blood	Local or systemic, therapeutic (e.g., treatment of spondylitic polycythemia)	Radium dial workers
	Bronchus	Respiratory	Pitchblende miners
Ultraviolet radiation	Skin	Cutaneous	Farmers, other outdoor workers, sailors, fishermen, and fair-skinned people in tropical climates

example of this is the association of pheochromocytoma with medullary (amyloid-producing) carcinoma of the thyroid, cerebellocortical hemangioblastoma, or neurofibromatosis. Other examples include some cases of polyendocrine adenomas (pituitary, parathyroid, pancreas), including the Zollinger-Ellison syndrome and hereditary adenocarcinomatosis (adenocarcinoma of the colon, stomach, uterus, and ovary occurring in different members of the same family). There are also several relatively rare heritable nonneoplastic diseases that have been associated with malignant tumors with great frequency. An example is the high incidence of skin cancer in patients with xeroderma pigmentosa. There also is an association between dermal inclusion cysts and multiple carcinomas of the colon, polyposis, multiple bony exostoses, and benign connective tissue tumors (Gardner's syndrome).

There are marked differences in the frequency of certain neoplastic diseases with respect to age, sex, and other constitutional factors suggesting that additional host determinants may be important. Acute lymphocytic leukemia is essentially a disease of childhood, whereas malignant melanoma is essentially a postpubertal disease. Testicular tumors and Hodgkin's disease are more frequent in young adults, and breast cancer is far more common in women than in men. In many other tumors, the frequency in both sexes increases markedly with increasing age.

GEOGRAPHIC FACTORS. Neoplasms may be found in all human populations, but there are some striking racial and regional differences in the occurrence of specific types of cancer. Although it is difficult to separate the genetic from the environmental factors, such as diet or habits, it is important to be aware of certain particularly strong differences. In a comparison study with the Caucasian population of the United States, Shimkin noted the following differences in cancer incidence:

1. High incidence of cancer of the stomach in Scandinavia, Iceland, and Japan
2. High incidence of primary cancer of the liver in South and West Africa
3. High incidence of cancer of the nasopharynx in China
4. High incidence of cancer of the urinary bladder in Egypt
5. Low rate of colorectal cancer in black Africa
6. Low incidence of cancer of the prostate and breast in Japan
7. Low incidence of cancer of the uterine cervix in Israel and in Jewish women in general
8. Low incidence of cancer of the skin in blacks

Custom and environment obviously play an important role in the development of cancer. Migration of populations usually causes a shift toward the patterns of cancer incidence of the host country. For example, in Japan there is a very high incidence of stomach cancer and a relatively low incidence of lung cancer. However, a second generation Japanese-American has a low risk of stomach cancer, and if a heavy smoker, he has as high a risk of lung cancer as his American counterpart.

For unknown reasons, socioeconomic factors may also influence cancer incidence. Cancer of the stomach and of the cervix are three to four times more frequent in lower economic groups than in middle and higher economic groups. On the other hand, cancer of the breast, leukemia, and multiple myeloma are more frequent in higher socioeconomic groups.

PRECANCEROUS CONDITIONS. Some clinical disorders, such as leukoplakia, actinic keratosis, polyps of the colon or rectum, neurofibromas, dysplasia of the cervix or bronchial mucosa, and chronic ulcerative colitis, are described as precancerous because they are so frequently followed by the development of cancer. It is particularly important that the physician be aware of these conditions in order to conduct careful follow-up of these patients.

ONCOGENES AND GROWTH FACTORS. Many lines of research in the molecular mechanisms of cancer have led to the discovery of oncogenes, which, when improperly regulated, cause the cell to enhance or decrease essential products associated with growth and differentiation and to exhibit the unrestricted growth and dissemination characteristic of cancer.

Much of our insight into oncogenes comes from the study of retroviruses. These are RNA tumor viruses found in avian and mammalian systems that can cause carcinomas, sarcomas, leukemias, and lymphomas. Retroviruses have an enzyme, reverse transcriptase, which permits the single-stranded viral genomic RNA to be transcribed into complementary DNA (cDNA). This cDNA may then integrate very efficiently into the cellular genome (Fig. 9-4). There are two major subgroups of oncogenic retroviruses—acute and chronic. Acute transforming retroviruses induce tumors in experimental animals within a few weeks while chronic transforming viruses do so after many months.

The Rous sarcoma virus (RSV) is a classic acute transforming virus whose genome is depicted in Fig. 9-4. The GAG gene codes for a structural protein found in the viral core, the POL gene codes for reverse transcriptase, and ENV is the viral envelope glycoprotein. The RSV genome also contains a V-*Src* gene that is known as the viral oncogene. The V-*Src* gene is responsible for the in vitro and in vivo oncogenic potential of RSV.

Current evidence has shown that all viral oncogenes are derived from normal cellular genomes called proto-oncogenes or cellular oncogenes (C-onc). About 20 different cellular oncogenes have been characterized, and these genes are highly conserved in evolution. Homologous oncogene sequences can be found in the genomic DNA of mammals, fish, birds, yeast, invertebrates, and *Drosophila*. However, viral oncogenes are not exact copies of cellular oncogenes, and the difference may range from a single amino acid substitution, to deletions, insertions, or major truncations. These observations have led to the general theory that cellular oncogenes are normal and perhaps important genes that regulate growth and differentiation. Molecular alterations of the oncogene itself or of its regulation may result in abnormal growth and differentiation of the cell.

Our understanding of cellular oncogenes makes the behavior of chronic transforming retroviruses easier to understand. These viruses do not contain oncogenes. These viruses, however, may integrate near cellular oncogenes, placing these under the potent viral transcriptional control.

For several oncogene families (V-*abl*, V-*erb* B, V-*ets*, V-*mos*, V-*myb*, V-H-*ras*, V-k-*ras*, and V-*sis*) there is circumstantial evidence of their association with human malignancies, most of which belong to the *ras* family.

During evolution, families of cellular oncogenes with

Fig. 9-4. The genome organization of Rous sarcoma virus, the reverse transcription of viral genome into cDNA, and subsequent integration into the chromosome.

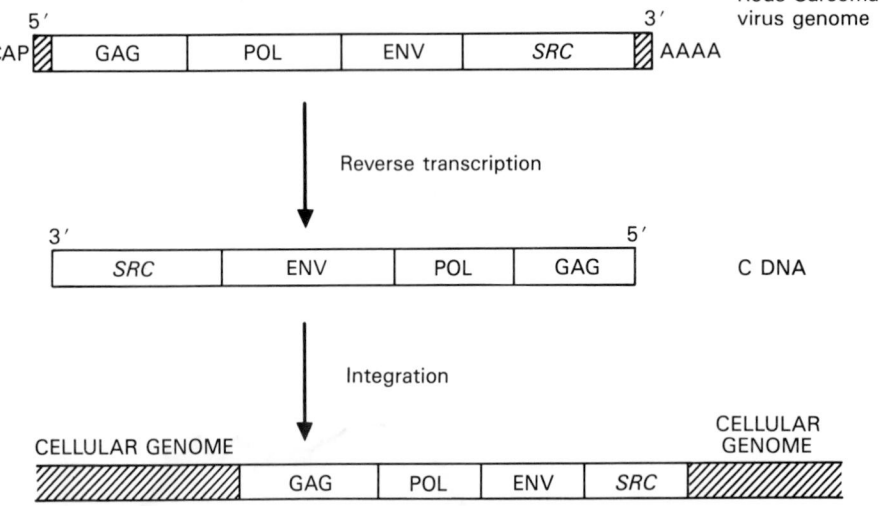

Rous Sarcoma virus genome

C DNA

similar structures seem to have arisen. The *ras* genes (Ha, K-, and N-*ras*) is one such family. The Ha-*ras* cellular oncogene is homologous to the Harvey murine sarcoma virus and has been circumstantially associated with human bladder, lung, and kidney cancers. Other *ras* oncogenes have been associated with other human cancers. *Ras* oncogenes code for a highly homologous series of proteins of 21,000 daltons called p21 proteins. Normal p21 proteins are located on the cytoplasmic surface of the cell membrane, have GTPase activity, and are thought to be intimately involved in some way with the regulation of cell proliferation. Malignant transformation by *ras* oncogenes is caused by a single point mutation in the amino terminal region of the *ras* gene. These mutations are confined to two "hot spots," codons 12 and 61, which result in a mutant p21 protein that lacks GTPase activity. Our understanding of the mechanism of transformation in a setting of a mutated *ras* gene product is still incomplete, but the mutational loss of GTPase activity gives the cell a growth-promoting signal in some way. It is interesting that such mutations can be caused by known carcinogens such as nitroso-methyl-urea and dimethyl nitrosamine.

Another major oncogene family specifies gene products that have tyrosine kinase activity. This oncogene family includes the *src* oncogene of the previously described RSV. Tyrosine kinases are capable of phosphorylating tyrosine residues on various proteins, and those oncogenes possessing this activity all share extensive homology around the kinase domains of their various gene products. Perhaps less than 0.1 percent of all protein phosphorylation occurs at tyrosine residues, but this enzymatic activity must be relevant to cell proliferation and oncogenesis. A number of receptors for normal growth factors—platelet-derived growth factor (PDGF), epidermal growth factor (EGF), and insulin-like growth factor (IGF 1)—have intrinsic tyrosine kinase activity when activated by an appropriate ligand. PDGF is a small glycoprotein stored in platelet alpha granules that can signal fibroblasts in the G0 phase to enter the cell-division cycle (G1-S-G2-M-G1). Progression through G1 to S (DNA replication) requires EGF and IGF. PDGF is highly homologous to the *sis* viral oncogene product, the oncogene of the simian sarcoma virus (Fig. 9-5). While normal fibroblasts do not have detectable c-*sis* messenger RNA, many human sarcomas do, and some release PDGF-like growth factors that may stimulate these tumors in an autocrine fashion. Normal fibroblast division appears to be regulated by the interaction of several cellular oncogenes (which code for normal growth factors and their receptors). These results provide a basis for understanding how mutations in any of these oncogenes could result in unrestricted proliferation. The V-*erb* B oncogene codes for a truncated form of the EGF receptor, a gene product that has the tyrosine kinase and transmembrane domains but lacks the normal ligand receptor. This mutant growth factor receptor may act as if it is persistently activated.

Myc-like oncogenes are associated with Burkitt's lymphoma, neuroblastoma, retinoblastomas, and other human tumors. The study of N-*myc* oncogene in neuroblastomas provides an example of another form of aberrant oncogene expression–oncogene amplification. In oncogene amplification, the cell increases the number of copies of the oncogene, and its expression may be greatly enhanced. N-*myc* amplification correlates closely with tumor progression. The absence of N-*myc* gene amplification (namely, one copy per tumor cell) was associated with a favorable response to conventional therapy, regardless of stage at diagnosis. The generally favorable

Fig. 9-5. *A.* Homology between V-*erb* B gene product and epidermal growth factor receptor. *B.* Homology between V-*sis* gene product and platelet-derived growth factor (PDGF).

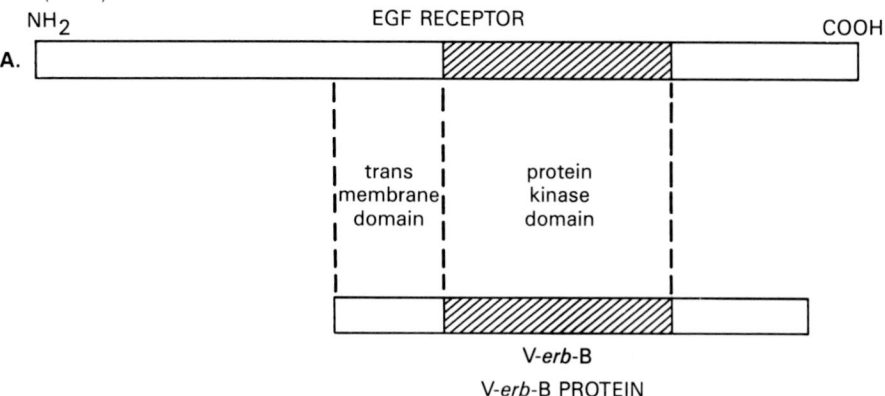

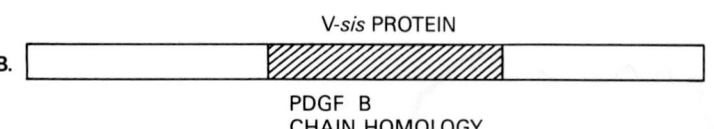

stage IV S, characterized by skin and liver metastases, also had single oncogene copies. Neuroblastomas with N-*myc* amplification (3 to 10 or > 10 copies) had a higher incidence of progression after conventional therapy. The N-*myc* oncogene appears to play a key role in determining the aggressiveness of neuroblastomas and is being used as an important intrastage prognostic factor. Early studies suggest that HER-2/*neu* oncogene amplification in breast cancer may also be correlated with prognosis.

Chromosomal abnormalities frequently occur in human cancers. Such gene rearrangements may activate or suppress important regulatory genes. A well-studied example is the gene translocation in Burkitt's lymphoma in which the long arm of chromosome 8 is translocated to number 14 (or occasionally 2 or 22). The long arm of 8 has the C-*myc* oncogene while 14, 2, and 22 have loci for various immunoglobulin genes. The result is an abnormal regulation and timing of C-*myc* expression. Also, the classic translocation involving chromosomes 9 and 22 producing the Philadelphia chromosome of chronic myelogenous leukemia involves repositioning the C-*abl* oncogene.

The clinical applications of oncogene research are only just being realized. The greatest benefit will be a molecular understanding of the mechanism of oncogenesis. Examining the oncogene activity of individual tumors even now permits intrastage prognostic assessment. Recently, a monoclonal antibody to the gene product of the N-*myc* oncogene is being used to histochemically stain neuroblastoma cells. A *ras*-specific monoclonal antibody has been found to intensely stain cells from areas of carcinoma in situ and invasive carcinoma in colon and breast cancer. Therapeutic strategies in the future may involve the creation of drugs that suppress oncogene expression or their products.

MULTIFACTORIAL ETIOLOGY. It is likely that all individual cancers are the result of multiple factors, such as an interaction of an oncogenic virus with a chemical or physical carcinogen. It is also possible that two chemical carcinogens may act synergistically to increase the incidence of cancer. A chemical may be a carcinogen only in a host with a hereditary susceptibility. When condensations of smog or cigarette smoke are applied separately to the cheek pouch of the golden hamster, there is a low but definite incidence of tumor. However, when they are applied together, there is a markedly increased incidence of tumors. Similarly, viruses have enhanced the oncogenic effects of smog and cigarette smoke in tissue culture. It is very possible that such synergistic interactions occur in human beings.

The possibility that multiple factors may be involved in the etiology of human neoplasia, rather than any one, may increase the chances of ultimate cancer prevention. For example, in carcinoma of the lung, it may be that in addition to heavy cigarette smoking (perhaps only chronic irritation), one requires a specific genetic background (since not all heavy smokers develop cancer of the lung), suitable male hormonal factors (since males are more frequently affected), and a virus. In addition, the latent period between start of smoking and high incidence of lung cancer is roughly 35 years. Although cigarette smoking may not be the only cause of lung cancer, it is the only factor that can be controlled. On the basis of present knowledge, lung cancer could be prevented by eliminating cigarette smoking altogether or by limiting cigarette smoking to a shorter period of time.

Custom and environment obviously are involved in the etiology of this cancer. Although cigarette smoking has been strongly implicated as a cause of squamous cell carcinoma of the lung, the habit is sufficiently ingrained in people in the United States to make its total elimination extremely difficult. Habits and customs in other parts of the world may be equally difficult to eliminate. The inhalation of snuff and the mastication of betel nuts have been associated with nasal and oral pharynx tumors, but the use of such materials continues despite their known carcinogenic effects. Nevertheless, efforts to identify the causative factors and to educate people regarding these factors must be continued.

BIOLOGY

Regardless of the etiologic agent, the cancer cell is a progeny of a normal cell that has lost its cellular mechanisms for controlling proliferation. The cancer cell differs from a normal cell in a variety of ways, but none of its new characteristics are absolutely indicative of malignancy. Cytogenetic studies of some cancer cells have revealed various abnormalities in chromosome number and appearance. However, these changes have not been shared by all cancer cells, and many cancer cells have normal chromosomal profiles.

Almost all malignant neoplasms seem to arise from a single cell that has undergone malignant transformation to form a malignant clone (group of cells); however, other human neoplasms such as the neurofibromas occurring in von Recklinghausen's disease may develop from multiple clones of cells. Simultaneously multifocal origins of carcinoma of the breast, oral pharynx, colon, and other organs also have been observed. Studies of patients with breast carcinoma have demonstrated that at least 30 percent have other areas involved with in situ carcinoma. Nevertheless, the primary tumor mass that was the cause for clinical presentation arises from a single cell alone.

Cancer cells generally proliferate faster than normal cells, except for leukocytes or cells of the intestinal mucosa. However, the proliferative rate decreases as the tumor mass grows; the proportion of cells undergoing mitosis is much greater when there are only a few cancer cells present than when there are many cells present in a large tumor mass. There are many rapid changes in the mitotic fraction of neoplasms during the initial growth phase, but after the tumor mass is 1 cm in diameter, the rate of division usually follows a predictable pattern.

After neoplastic transformation has occurred, the cancer cell differs from the normal cell not only in proliferative index but also in morphology, biochemistry, antigenic expression, and many other aspects.

MORPHOLOGIC CHANGES. Malignant cells tend to revert to more primitive cell types, that is, to dedifferentiate. The normal orderly tissue patterns are lost or replaced by the random piling up of malignant cells without definite pattern. Other histologic changes may include cellular pleomorphism, a high index of mitoses, and hyperchromatism in the nucleus and nucleoli. Invasion of adjacent normal structures also may be seen microscopically. These morphologic changes are the basis for histopathologic or cytologic diagnoses of cancer and usually allow very accurate diagnosis of neoplastic diseases.

BIOCHEMICAL CHANGES. The biochemical activity of cancer cells is similar, though not identical, to that of normal cells. A great diversity exists in the biochemical characteristics of different tumor cells, usually correlating with rate of proliferation. Changes in DNA, RNA, and the chemical architecture of the cellular membrane of malignant cells are associated with the loss of contact inhibition to proliferation and intercellular adhesiveness. However, no single biochemical alteration has yet been defined that is absolutely characteristic of malignant transformation.

Reversion of the normal cellular biochemistry to that of the embryonal cells produces distinctive embryonal substances whose presence in the adult may be used to diagnose cancer. The carcinoembryonic antigen associated with gastrointestinal cancers, and α-fetoglobulin associated with hepatoma and embryonal cancers are thought to be examples of this type. The synthesis of these substances may be due to depression of fetal gene function that occurs during oncogenesis.

Malignant cells may also produce biologically active substances that are normally produced by the cells from which the neoplasm originated. The release of these substances may cause symptoms similar to hyperfunction of that particular organ, for example, hyperparathyroidism produced by parathyroid carcinomas. Neoplasms may also produce biologically active substances that are not normally produced by the cells of origin. Some bronchogenic carcinomas may produce parathyroidlike hormones, ACTH, antidiuretic hormones, and other hormones.

The mechanism of this ectopic hormone secretion is based upon the hypothesis of variable genetic activity or *selective derepression* of a specific gene. All cells contain the same genes; however, only about 10 percent of these genes are expressed in any one cell type; the remainder are repressed. Cancer cells are primitive cells; with dedifferentiation, they acquire the ability to express some of these previously repressed genes. This new genetic expression is responsible for the production of a new specific-messenger RNA and the production of new polypeptides and hormones.

GROWTH RATES OF NEOPLASMS. Approximately two-thirds of the growth of human neoplasms occurs before they are clinically detectable. If one assumes that a cancer begins from a single cell, then it takes about 30 exponential divisions to produce a 1-cm nodule (1 billion cells). At 45 exponential divisions the patient is apt to be dead from the sheer bulk of the malignant tumor.

The growth rate of tumors can be expressed by the *tumor doubling time,* i.e., the time it takes for a tumor to double in volume. Tumor doubling times appear to be an accurate and precise method for comparing the biologic aggressiveness of neoplasms in different patients. This measurement is particularly applicable to metastatic pulmonary lesions, since these are usually peripheral in location and are discretely delineated on chest radiographs, so that accurate serial measurements are easily obtainable.

The method used in the measurement of the tumor doubling time is illustrated in Fig. 9-6. Briefly, the average of the greater and the lesser diameters of each metastatic nodule is determined from successive chest radiographs. The averages are plotted on semilogarithmic paper against the time in days between these points; the slope of this line represents the rate of tumor growth. Where this line crosses any two doubling lines, the horizontal distance between them represents the tumor doubling time in days. This measurement has been shown to be an accurate and reproducible method for the quantitation of the rate and pattern of tumor growth in individual patients.

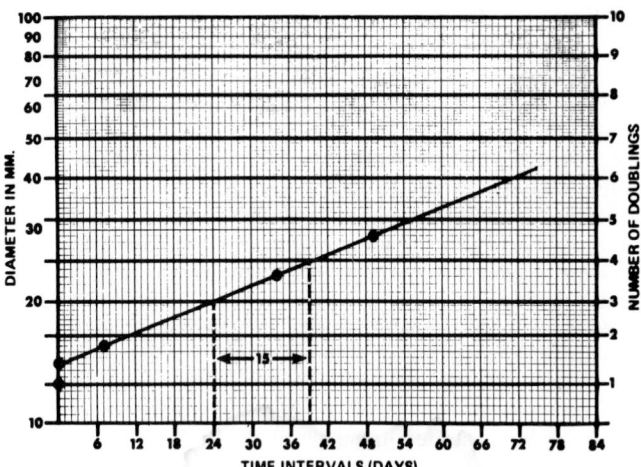

Fig. 9-6. Method of plotting tumor doubling time, based upon the direct measurement of the changing diameters of metastatic pulmonary nodules. (From: *Joseph WL et al: J Thorac Cardiovasc Surg 61:23, 1971, with permission.*)

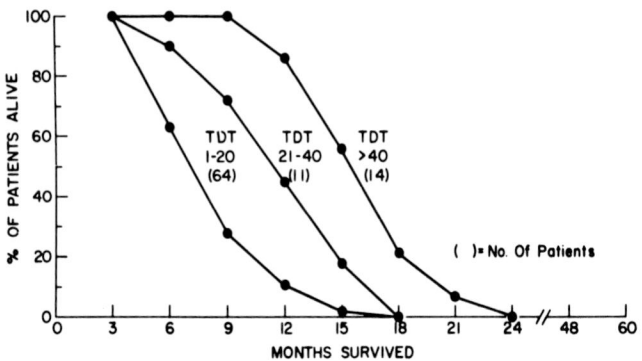

Fig. 9-7. Survival curves in 89 untreated patients following the onset of pulmonary metastases, showing three groups based upon tumor doubling time. (From: *Joseph WL et al: J Thorac Cardiovasc Surg 61:23, 1971, with permission.*)

The tumor doubling time varies from 8 to 600 days; most tumors double in 20 to 100 days. The measurement of tumor doubling times can be extremely helpful in determining prognosis, in evaluating response to chemotherapeutic agents, and in comparing responses to different therapeutic regimens.

In one study the tumor doubling times of a large series of patients with pulmonary metastases from tumors of different histologic types were measured. Wide variations within particular types of neoplasms were found. The tumor doubling time correlated closely with the length of survival in three distinct groups of patients. This is illustrated in Fig. 9-7. This correlation might be expected, because the tumor doubling time represents the balance between the intrinsic proliferative rate of the tumor cell and the patient's inhibiting defense mechanisms.

On the basis of growth dynamics, most human tumors have been present in the body for at least 1 year and many for as long as 10 years prior to their clinical detection. Thus, it appears that there is a long period of time between the inception of neoplastic transformation and the development of clinical cancer. During this time, detection may be possible and surgical treatment might result in cure. Tests must be perfected to detect cancer earlier, to shorten this preclinical interval and make surgical treatment more successful.

Immunobiology

The concept that cancer patients may develop an immune response against their neoplasms is not new. This view became very popular at the turn of the century when it was found that strong immunity could be induced against transplantable neoplasms in randomly bred laboratory rodents. A period of intense laboratory and clinical investigation followed, in anticipation that tumor immunity might lead to control of malignant disease. However, it soon became evident that the immunity was not directed against tumor-specific antigens (TSA), but instead was against normal tissue antigens in the neoplasm due to genetic differences between tumor donor and recipient. Thereafter, interest in tumor immunology declined because no antigens other than the transplantation antigens could be demonstrated in neoplasms.

Interest in the immunology of neoplastic diseases was reawakened in the 1950s when tumor-specific antigens were conclusively demonstrated in methylcholanthrene-induced sarcomas in mice. In order to eliminate any histocompatibility factors the investigators used inbred strains of rodents that, after many years of inbreeding, had the genetic homogeneity of monozygotic twins. Specific tumor transplantation resistance was induced by presensitization with a transplant of tumor tissue that was allowed to grow for a time and then was excised. The immunized rodents were then resistant to challenge with further transplants of the same neoplasm (Fig. 9-8). However, the immunity induced in these animals was relative, not absolute. Whereas a challenge with 100,000 tumor cells produced a growing tumor in control mice, it did not in the immune mice. Challenge with larger numbers of

Fig. 9-8. Mouse A, immunized with benzpyrene-induced tumor t, resists subsequent challenge with t tumor cells. Challenge with cells from another benzpyrene-induced tumor, t_2, leads to progressive tumor growth and death of the mouse.

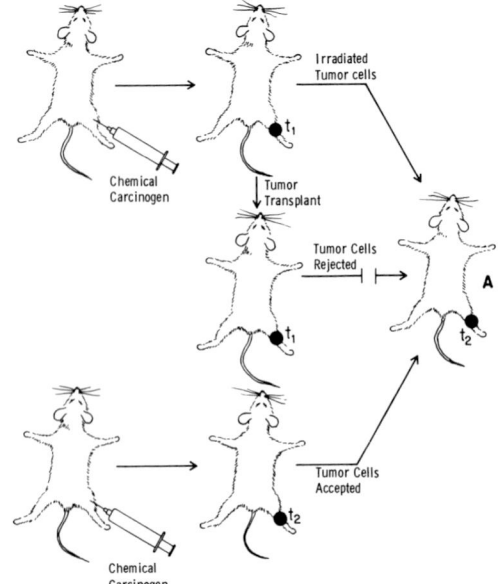

cells (1 to 10 million), however, usually overwhelmed the immunologic defense, and progressive tumor growth was observed.

Tumor-specific antigens have been demonstrated in most viral, chemical, and physical-carcinogen-induced neoplasms and possibly in some spontaneous tumors. During the past 25 years there has been tremendous progress in tumor immunology. Because tumor antigens were first identified by their ability to elicit rejection when transplanted from one animal to another, they became known as "tumor-specific transplantation antigens." Other assays have been developed, and these antigens are rarely referred to by this term. However, fundamental questions concerning the expression of tumor-specific antigens by human tumors, the host response to these antigens, and the ability to manipulate the response to achieve tumor regression continue to be the goals of human tumor immunology.

ANTIGENIC SPECIFICITY OF ANIMAL NEOPLASMS. The wide variety of viral-, chemical-, and physical-carcinogen-induced neoplasms for which tumor-specific transplantation antigens were originally demonstrated are summarized in Table 9-2. The antigenic specificities of these major types of carcinogenic agents have been found to be quite different.

Table 9-2. TUMOR-SPECIFIC ANTIGENS CAPABLE OF INDUCING REJECTION RESPONSES IN SYNGENEIC HOSTS

Inducing agent	*Antigenic specificity*
Chemical carcinogens:	
3-Methylcholanthrene	
1,2,5,6-Dibenzanthracene	
9,10-Dimethylbenzanthracene	
3,4,9,10-Dibenzpyrene	
3,4-Benzpyrene-dimethylam-	Antigens distinct for
inoazobenzene	each individual
Physical agents:	neoplasm
Films	
Millipore filter	
Cellophane film	
Radiation	
Ultraviolet	
^{90}Sr	
Virus:	
DNA	
Polyoma	
SV-40	
Adenovirus 12,18	
Shope papilloma	Common antigens in
RNA:	each neoplasm in-
Mammary tumor agent	duced by the same
Leukemia	virus
Gross	
Moloney	
Rauscher } Shared common	
Friend } antigens	
Graffi	
Rich	
Rous (Schmidt-Ruppin)	

Tumor-Specific Antigens of Neoplasms Induced by Chemical and Physical Carcinogens. These are individually distinct for each tumor, even if induced by the same carcinogen, in the same strain, and of the identical histologic type (Fig. 9-9). For example, injection of a chemical carcinogen such as benzpyrene in two inbred mice of the same strain will result in two antigenically different tumors, t_1 and t_2. If mouse *A* is immunized with irradiated tumor cells from t_1, it will subsequently reject tumor cells from the same tumor transplanted into an intermediate host. However, the same animal, immune to t_1, will develop a tumor when injected with the same number of tumor cells from t_2.

Tumor-Specific Antigens of Neoplasms Induced by Viral Carcinogens. In contrast to the unique tumor-specific antigens of chemical-carcinogen-induced tumors, the tumor-specific antigens of viral-induced neoplasms are common to all neoplasms induced by the same virus, but differ from those induced by other viruses (Fig. 9-9). For example, with inbred mice of the same strain, mouse *A* is immunized with SV-40 virus alone, mouse *B* is immunized with *irradiated* tumor cells from an SV-40 virus-induced mouse tumor, and mouse *C* is immunized with tumor cells from an SV-40 virus-induced rat tumor. All will reject challenge of tumor cells from SV-40 virus-induced tumor t. However, challenge with the same tumor cells in mice *D* and *E*, immunized with either polyoma virus alone or polyoma virus-induced tumor cells, leads to progressive tumor growth and death.

Although the generalization that virus-induced neoplasms contain common antigens and chemical-carcinogen-induced neoplasms contain individually distinct antigens is usually correct, more recent studies have demonstrated that this distinction is not as absolute as originally believed. Common antigens related to leukemia viral antigens have been found in chemical-carcinogen-induced sarcomas, and some carcinogen-induced neoplasms arising in the bladder have contained common antigens. Furthermore, spontaneous mouse mammary carcinomas induced by the mammary tumor virus contain individually distinct antigens in addition to the common antigens of the mammary tumor virus.

EFFECTOR MECHANISMS IN TUMOR IMMUNITY. The host provides a number of effector mechanisms with theoretical and proved effectiveness in the immune destruction of tumors. The important effectors include tumor-antigen-specific antibodies, mononuclear phagocytes, natural killer cells, and cytotoxic T lymphocytes, neutrophils, and K cells.

Antitumor Antibodies. There are five classes of immunoglobulin molecules (IgG, A, M, D, E) in human beings. The major antibody classes associated with tumor immunity are IgM and IgG. The antigen-binding region of the antibody molecule is located in the aminoterminal or Fab portion. Binding of antibody to the tumor target cell does not by itself result in growth suppression or destruction. It serves only as a recognition signal for cytolytic effectors such as complement, macrophages, or K cells to perform the cytotoxic event. Antitumor antibodies of the

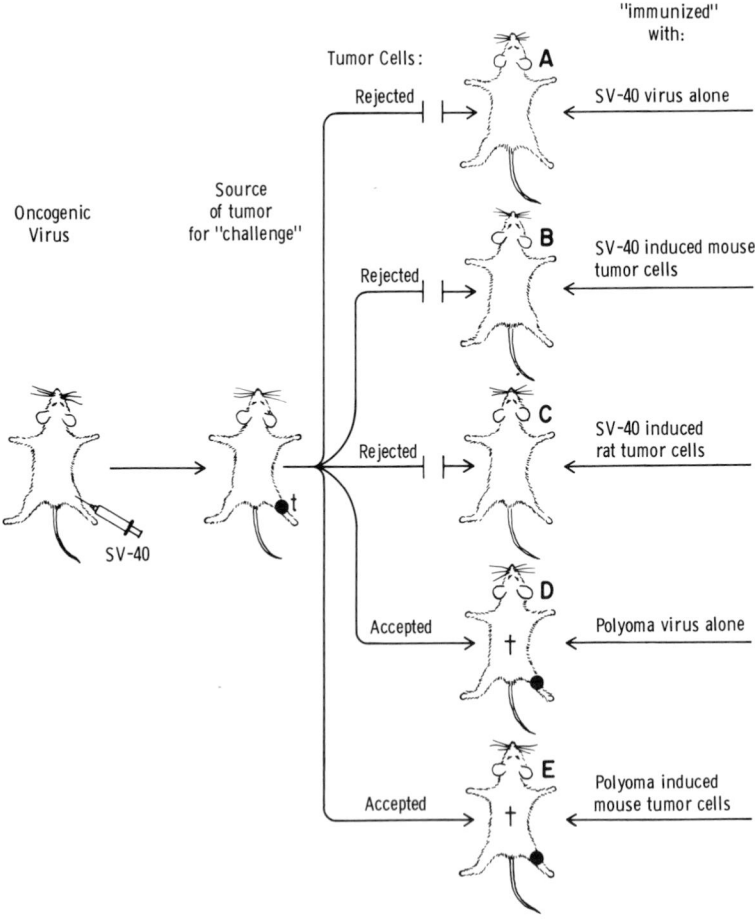

Fig. 9-9. Mice A, B, and C, immunized with SV-40 virus or SV-40 virus-induced tumor cells, reject challenge of tumor cells from SV-40 virus-induced tumor t. Challenge with the same tumor cells in mice D and E, immunized with polyoma virus or polyoma virus-induced tumor cells, leads to progressive tumor growth and death of the mouse.

appropriate subclass are effective in suppressing small numbers of tumor cells in certain experimental settings. Recently, the administration of human monoclonal antibodies specific for tumor-associated antigens to tumor-bearing patients has shown promising results.

Complement. The classical complement system is composed of a group of serum proteins (Cl-9), most of which are β-globulins. The binding of the C1 to the appropriate immunoglobulin subclass (IgG1, IgG3, IgM in human beings) initiates a cascade of component activation and macromolecular aggregation that results in (1) release of the anaphylatoxins C3a and C5a, which causes neutrophil chemotaxis, neutrophil activation, increased vascular permeability, release of histamine from mast cells, and smooth muscle contraction; and (2) assembly of the C5-9 membrane attack complex, which inserts in the lipid bilayer of the target cell membrane, forming a "doughnut" and thus providing for the free exchange of water and electrolytes and the consequent osmotic lysis of the cell. The alternative complement pathway provides for the assembly and activation of complement on target membranes without antibody or C1 fixation and appears to be more important in microbial immunity.

Antibody-Dependent Cell-Mediated Cytotoxicity (ADCC). Antibody-coated tumor cells may be killed by a variety of cellular effectors that are able to engage via Fc receptors on the effector cell surface. Thus, the antibody molecule provides the specific recognition signal while the otherwise quiescent and nonspecific effector cell is directed to the target cells to provide the cytotoxic event. Monocytes and macrophages are very efficient cytotoxic effectors in the ADCC system. The so-called K cell, a poorly defined lymphocyte of uncertain lineage that closely resembles the NK cell, is quite active. In addition, neutrophils and perhaps eosinophils and platelets are active in certain settings. The mechanisms of killing by these ADCC effectors are not fully defined.

Mononuclear Phagocytes. Cells of the mononuclear phagocytic system play a central role in immunity. They are composed of circulating monocytes, macrophages in the alveolus, spleen, and lymph node, Kupffer cells in the liver, and brain microglial cells. Circulating monocytes are the best studied of these cells and are of greater interest to the tumor immunologist because of their ability to migrate to sites of inflammation and tumor.

Macrophages have a number of important immunoregulatory and cytotoxic functions. They help to initiate immune response by serving as antigen-presenting cells. Such cells are especially abundant in germinal centers of lymph nodes and as Langerhans cells in the skin. In addition, macrophages have a wide range of regulatory, tumoricidal, and bactericidal properties. Elaboration of such lymphokines as interleukin-1 (IL-1) is important in T and B lymphocyte activation and the generation of fever. Macrophages also produce monocytotoxins that include tumor necrosis factor (TNF) which has a broad range of cytocidal and regulatory properties (see lymphokine section). Many other macrophage products—prostaglandins, complement components, proteolytic enzymes and hydrolases, hydrogen peroxide, superoxides—mediate other regulatory and cytotoxic functions. Macrophage function is initiated and enhanced by the process of "activation." Activation is a complex multistep process characterized by morphologic changes (maturation, spreading, pinocytosis, synthesis of lysosomal granules), elaboration of monokines and cytotoxins, and enhanced bactericidal activity. Macrophages may be activated by lymphokines (IFNY), bacterial products (endotoxin), and antibody-coated targets.

Natural Killer Cells. NK cells comprise about 5 percent of peripheral blood leukocytes and morphologically are large granular lymphocytes. NK cells, freshly isolated from the peripheral blood leukocytes and morphologically large granular lymphocytes, are capable of killing certain tumor target cells in short-term in vitro assays. This killing does not require immunologic memory or specificity and is not restricted by the major histocompatibility complex (as with cytolytic T lymphocytes). NK cells may be found in the peripheral blood, spleen, and bone marrow but are found infrequently in the thymus, lymph nodes, or lymph. NK cells can kill a selected repertoire of cultured and freshly isolated human tumor cells, but many appear to be resistant. The mechanism of NK lysis is not fully understood but requires cell contact and may be mediated by cytotoxins contained in their cytoplasmic azurophilic granules. The target structure recognized by NK cells as well as the lineage of NK cells is still being debated. A number of biologic response modifiers such as interleukin-2 (IL-2) and interferon (IFN) will augment NK activity in vitro and in vivo. Prostaglandin E2, which can be produced by macrophages and tumor cells, suppresses NK activity. There is much convincing circumstantial evidence to suggest that NK cells are important in immunologic surveillance and eradication of small numbers of tumor cells. It is unlikely that they play an effective role in the immune response against established tumors, and NK cells found within tumors have defective function. A current area of interest is the use of biologic response modifiers such as IL-2 to augment NK function in cancer patients.

Lymphokine-Activated Killer Cells. See below, section on Immunotherapy.

Cytolytic T Lymphocytes. The classic cytotoxic cell of cellular immunity is the cytotoxic T lymphocyte (Tc), the only one with intrinsic immunological specificity by virtue of its antigen-specific receptor. The T cell receptor is composed of two disulfide linked peptides (α and β) which recognize foreign antigens only in association with Class I major histocompatibility complex (MHC) antigens (HLA-A,B,C). Class I MHC antigens are glycoproteins with molecular weight of 44,000, are associated with $\beta2$-microglobulin, and are present on all cells except erythrocytes. This is an important concept since T cells sensitized to viral or tumor antigens of one MHC haplotype are unable to recognize and kill cells bearing the same foreign antigen in association with a different haplotype. Other MHC antigens such as Class II or D region antigens are important in cooperation and interaction between cells in the immune system.

Cytolytic T cells (Tc) induce ultrastructural lesions in the membrane lipid bilayer of nucleated target cells. As with the complement (C9) membrane lesion, these Tc-mediated lesions appear to be caused by polymerization of 18 to 20 precursor molecules (termed "perforins") into tubular complexes that perforate the cell membrane. These molecules and lymphotoxin, a cytotoxin similar in action to and sharing some homology with TNF, are under intense scrutiny as the effector molecules for Tc and other cytotoxic cells. Cytotoxic T lymphocytes may be clonally expanded in the presence of IL-2, and such cytotoxic T cell clones are valuable research tools and potential therapeutic agents.

Suppressor T cells can be induced by tumor antigen, products other than antigens (e.g., prostaglandins), and direct interactions with immune cells. There are also suggestions that there are natural suppressor cells that control immune reactions. Suppressor T cells are themselves regulated by countersuppressor T cells. It is logical that immunotherapy should consist of modulators of suppressor cells along with appropriate stimulation. In recent years emphasis in immunotherapy has been on biologic response modifiers. These agents include cyclophosphamide, cimetidine, and indomethacin which are used primarily to inhibit immune suppression and to augment tumor immunity.

BIOLOGIC RESPONSE MODIFIERS. Genetic engineering technology has permitted large-scale production of purified, homogeneous lymphokines. Some of these factors can be used in supraphysiologic doses to modify host tumor immunity in vivo or immune effectors in vitro.

Interleukin-1. Interleukin-1 (IL-1) is a lymphokine originally defined as a thymocyte mitogen produced by activated macrophages. It is now known that many different types of cells produce IL-1 (including monocytes, macrophages, dendritic cells, Langerhans cells, endothelial cells, neutrophils, NK cells, microglial cells), and that two IL-1 molecules exist that have broad ranges of immunologic, biologic, and inflammatory properties.

There are two IL-1 genes whose gene products—IL-1α

and IL-1β—both have molecular weights of 17,000. These two molecules have only a 20 percent amino acid sequence homology, although there are a number of regions of close homology between the α and the β forms that may represent common functional domains. Both IL-1α and IL-1β bind to the same surface membrane receptor on target cells to effect their hormonal action.

IL-1 has many biologic effects, and it has not yet been fully determined which, if any, of these properties segregate to the α or β species. IL-1 induces some T cells to produce IL-2 and others to express IL-2 receptors, which is important in the clonal expansion of T cell subsets. IL-1 may also have a maturation effect on pre-B cells and participate in the proliferation of mature B cells by inducing the production of interferon β_2. Thus, IL-1 has a vital and integral role in cellular and humoral immunity. In addition, IL-1 initiates the febrile response, directly acts on the bone marrow to cause release of neutrophils into the circulation, induces hepatic synthesis of acute-phase proteins, induces skeletal muscle catabolism, and promotes the degradation of cartilage matrix. IL-1 can cause the production and release of IL-2 and tumor necrosis factor (TNF) by appropriate target cells and is thereby able to initiate a cascade of important inflammatory and immunoregulatory functions, many of which remain to be fully defined.

Interleukin-2. Interleukin-2 (IL-2) is a glycoprotein with a molecular weight of 15,000 that is produced by helper T lymphocytes. Originally called "T-cell growth factor," IL-2 can support the long-term proliferation of T cells in culture. IL-2 has been cloned in *Escherichia coli* and the recombinant nonglycosylated form and is fully active and available in large quantities for experimental and clinical studies.

IL-2 augments the generation of cytolytic T lymphocytes, natural killer (NK) cells, lymphokine activated killer (LAK) cells, and alloantigen responsiveness. This lymphokine may help in restoring immunocompetence from certain immunodeficiency states. Human recombinant IL-2 is currently being used in clinical immunotherapy trials.

TUMOR NECROSIS FACTOR. Tumor necrosis factor (TNF) was originally described as a protein found in the sera of mice sensitized with *Corynebacterium parvum* or *Bacillus* Calmette-Guérin and then challenged with bacterial endotoxin. TNF causes hemorrhagic necrosis of certain experimental tumors in mice. It is likely that TNF was responsible for the occasional necrosis of human tumors induced by "Coley's toxins" when these bacterial toxins were used in the 1930s. It is now known that TNF has a broad range of biologic activities.

TNF is a peptide hormone whose subunit molecular weight is 17,000. TNF is produced by monocytes, macrophages, endothelial cells, large granular lymphocytes, and neutrophils. The TNF gene is closely linked to the lymphotoxin gene with which it shares 30 percent amino acid sequence homology. Properties of TNF include (1) direct cytotoxicity for certain cells, (2) stimulation of procoagulant activity by vascular endothelial cells (which may contribute to the phenomenon of in vivo hemorrhage

necrosis of tumors), (3) activation of neutrophil adherence and phagocytosis, and (4) induction of fever by direct effect on the hypothalamic thermoregulatory center. Shires has demonstrated that this protein can cause many of the effects of endotoxin shock. TNF is one of the major effector molecules of macrophage-mediated cytotoxicity of tumor cells, plays a central role in the pathogenesis of endotoxin-induced shock, and may account for the wasting and catabolic state associated with chronic illness and cancer. Some investigators who feel that the term "tumor necrosis factor" is misleadingly narrow have coined the term "cachectin" instead.

Interferons. Interferons (IFN) were discovered about 30 years ago as antiviral agents. There are three major classes of IFNs, α, β, γ, all of which have now been fully characterized and cloned using recombinant DNA technology. There are over a dozen physicochemically related IFN subtypes, all with a molecular weight of about 20,000. IFNα used to be called leukocyte IFN and is produced by monocytes. IFNβ (fibroblast IFN) has the same molecular weight as IFNβ. Only one species of IFNγ has been identified, and it is produced by immune T cells. IFNγ has also been called immune IFN and macrophage activating factor (MAF). IFNγ has a molecular weight of 25,000 and shares only 12 percent amino acid sequence homology with other IFNs.

IFNs have diverse effect on many different cell types. IFNs have a wide range of direct antitumor effects whose sensitivity may be related to IFN receptor expression. IFNs may augment expression of MHC antigens and alter membrane lipids and cytoskeleton. IFNs also may augment the activity of cytotoxic T lymphocytes, NK cells, K cells, and tumoricidal macrophages.

IFNs have been used in clinical trials since the early 1970s, but only recently have purified, recombinant IFNs become available for clinical use. IFNα A as a single agent can cause partial and occasionally complete responses in leukemia, Kaposi's sarcoma, breast carcinoma, renal cell carcinoma, lymphomas, malignant melanoma, and others. IFNβ may have some activity with multiple myeloma and lymphoma. Less is known about the therapeutic efficacy of IFNγ.

IFNs may act synergistically with other biologic response modifiers (other IFN classes, IL-2, etc.), and it may be in this setting that they will find more effective clinical applications.

IMMUNE SURVEILLANCE. The concept of immunologic surveillance is based upon the premise that carcinogenesis occurs frequently as a spontaneous mutation, from chemical carcinogens or from oncogenic viruses. Burnet postulated that the teleology of the immune system was to recognize the foreignness of tumor-specific antigens on the neoplastic cells and to mount an immune response capable of eliminating them. In this context, clinical cancer would represent a failure of the mechanisms for immunologic destruction, although it may be the exception rather than the rule. The NK cells may be the basis of the surveillance system because they can recognize new antigens, whereas the T cells do not seem to have this capability.

Mechanisms for Evasion of Immune Surveillance. If neoplastic cells are capable of eliciting a host immune response that leads to their specific destruction, it is pertinent to ask why or how cancer develops. A variety of possible ways by which cancer cells evade the immune surveillance mechanisms have been described:

Insufficient antigenicity to evoke an immune response may account for the growth of some neoplasms. Tumor antigens and tumor-associated antigens are usually weaker immunogens than transplantation antigens. Some neoplastic cells may have either an extremely weak tumor antigen or an extremely low density of tumor antigens on the cell surface. Thus, the tumor cell with the stronger tumor antigen may be recognized and eliminated, whereas those cells with weak tumor antigens may escape detection and destruction.

Antigenic modulation of a thymus leukemia (TL) antigen has been observed on a murine lymphoma cell. The TL antigen disappears when the cell is transplanted in immunized hosts or carried in tissue culture containing specific antibody, but it will reappear when the tumor cells are passed in tissue culture without antibody or transplanted in unimmunized hosts. Furthermore, antigenic shift may be another form of antigenic modulation whereby tumor cells escape control immunologic surveillance. This phenomenon has been described with certain animal neoplasms in which the lung metastases are antigenically different from the primary tumor.

Immunologic indifference may explain the observation by Old and associates that small numbers of tumor cells having tumor-specific antigens develop into progressively growing tumors although larger numbers of cells are rejected. In this instance the small number of cells may not be immunogenic enough and can "sneak through" the host immune response.

Immunosuppression by irradiation, neonatal thymectomy, chemotherapy, or steroid or antilymphocyte globulin administration usually increases the frequency and growth rate, and shortens the latency period, for both virus- and carcinogen-induced neoplasms in experimental animals. The incidence of cancer in human beings increases significantly with advancing years as the immune response to a variety of antigens decreases. Furthermore, in human beings with congenital immunodeficiency diseases, the incidence of spontaneous cancer is 10,000 times that of the general age-matched population. In human organ transplant recipients on immunosuppressive drugs, the incidence of spontaneous cancer is more than seventy times that of the general age-matched population. NK function may be depressed in patients who develop cancer. Renal transplant patients and patients with Chédiak-Higashi disease who have a high incidence of lymphoproliferative disorders appear to have abnormal NK cell function.

Immunologic tolerance that develops during the fetal or neonatal periods owing to exposure to tumor-specific antigens or an oncogenic virus may account for tumor growth in some animals when the immunologic surveillance system would otherwise afford protection. Bittner discovered in 1936 that C3H female mice transmitted mammary tumor virus (MTV) through the milk to their nursing young that later induced mammary tumors in a high percentage of their adult female progeny. Morton demonstrated that mice infected as neonates subsequently became tolerant to the tumor-specific antigens of the MTV-induced neoplasms and consequently could not be immunized against them as adults. Newborn mice foster-nursed on non-MTV-carrying mothers from another strain were not tolerant to the virus and, when adult, could be effectively immunized against the MTV-induced mammary tumors. The incidence of mammary tumors in these foster-nursed mice was much lower than in those nursed on MTV-infected mothers.

Low-dose immunologic tolerance similar to that seen with transplantation systems, but secondary to prolonged exposure to small amounts of weak tumor-specific antigens may account for the growth of some tumors. Low-dose tolerance may explain the development of metastases from breast cancer in immunocompetent patients many years after radical mastectomy.

CLINICAL EVIDENCE FOR TUMOR IMMUNITY IN HUMAN BEINGS

For obvious reasons the tumor transplantation techniques used to demonstrate these tumor-specific antigens of animal neoplasms were not applicable to the study of human tumors. Nevertheless, there are a number of well-documented clinical observations that suggest human host immune defenses against cancer. Although other physiologic, endocrinologic, and biologic explanations can be given for these observations, they are most easily explained on an immunologic basis:

1. Spontaneous regression of established tumors is a rare but well-documented phenomenon. Sometimes these regressions have followed a minor viral or bacterial infection. Although spontaneous regression has been observed in many different tumor types, it is most frequently seen in neuroblastomas of children, malignant melanoma, choriocarcinoma, adenocarcinoma of the kidney, and soft tissue sarcomas. However, spontaneous regression occurs less frequently than 0.5 percent in all types, except for neuroblastomas.

   Spontaneous regression of small pulmonary metastases following the surgical removal of the primary tumor has been observed and occurs most frequently in hypernephromas. Spontaneous regression also may account for the prolonged survival or cure of patients after incomplete surgical excision of the cancer.

2. Recurrence of tumor 10 years after successful treatment of the primary is often manifested by rapid tumor growth and death. Although endocrinologic changes may account for some of these observations in breast cancer, in other tumors this course suggests a host defense that inhibits the tumor growth during the disease-free interval.

3. Microscopic evidence of the histiocytic, plasmocytic, lymphocytic, and eosinophilic infiltration, which resembles that seen in an organ transplant or tumor transplant that is undergoing rejection in a human being, is associated with an improved prognosis. For example, in stomach cancer, these findings correlate better with survival than does adequate surgical removal of the tumor.

4. The presence of many tumor cells in the peripheral blood, lymphatics, pleural cavity, and operative wounds of patients

who subsequently never develop metastases suggests host immune defense.

5. There is a low incidence of successful growth of tumor tissue, or autotransplants in patients with advanced disease. The resistance against tumor growth was relative rather than absolute, since challenge with greater numbers of cancer cells usually resulted in tumor growth. The immune nature of this resistance was suggested when autologous leukocytes or plasma was mixed with these tumor cells, and cancer growth decreased in approximately half the patients studied.

IMMUNOLOGIC EVIDENCE FOR TUMOR-ASSOCIATED ANTIGENS IN HUMAN NEOPLASMS. During the past 20 years, a variety of sensitive immunologic techniques has demonstrated that many human neoplasms contained antigens that appear to be at least tumor-related if not uniquely specific. These antigens are capable of eliciting an immune response in human beings.

Humoral antibodies have been shown by the immunofluorescence, complement fixation, immunocytolysis, and immunodiffusion techniques. Cellular immunity has been demonstrated by lymphocyte-mediated cytotoxicity (the ability of lymphocytes to kill tumor cells in tissue culture), lymphocyte blastogenesis tests (the ability of lymphocytes to be stimulated to proliferate by tumor antigens), and migration inhibition tests (macrophages or other blood leukocytes inhibited in their migration by tumor-specific antigens). Finally, it has been found that cancer patients develop delayed cutaneous hypersensitivity reactions to tumor antigens. Thus, it has become increasingly apparent that some tumor antigens are capable of eliciting an immune response that can be monitored by the immunologic techniques used to study other types of immune reactions. The wide variety of human neoplasms in which tumor antigens have been detected are listed in Table 9-3. The precise specificity of these antigens remains controversial.

Various classes of antigens may be expressed by a malignant cell. For example, the fetal or differentiation antigens that are normal on the cells of the developing fetus, but not on adult normal cells, are expressed on many types of tumor cells. Group-specific antigens have been found on tumor cells of the same histologic type, on tumor cells of various histologic types, and on some normal cells. Individual-specific antigens appear to be like the highly restricted specific antigens on chemically in-

Table 9-3. HUMAN NEOPLASMS WITH DEMONSTRATED TUMOR-ASSOCIATED ANTIGENS

Burkitt's lymphoma
Malignant melanoma
Neuroblastoma
Osteosarcoma
Soft tissue sarcomas
Colon carcinoma
Breast carcinoma
Leukemia
Lung carcinoma
Bladder carcinoma
Renal carcinoma

duced sarcomas in animals. At issue is whether there are antigens on human tumors that are never expressed by the normal fetal or adult cells. These antigens would be truly tumor-specific. Most authorities agree that at the present time there is insufficient evidence for the existence of such tumor-specific antigens. Nevertheless, many types of *tumor-associated* antigens have been demonstrated whose specificity is restricted to human tumor and fetal tissues.

Differentiation, or Fetal, Antigens. Most tumor-associated antigens are located on the cell surface, where they are susceptible to immune attack by antibodies or lymphocytes. Thus, they are probably of considerable importance in the tumor-host relationship. However, there are other types of antigens that may not be located at the cell surface, although they are more or less specific for the neoplastic state. One such group is composed of the fetal, or carcinoembryonic, antigens.

Fetal antigens are produced by normal fetal organs during embryonic development. Their production is repressed shortly after birth, and they are not produced in significant quantities in normal adult organs. However, during neoplastic transformation, reversion of the cell to the embryonic state is accompanied by a renewed production of these fetal antigens. The fetal antigens are thought to represent the phenotypic expression of genes active during fetal life but not expressed during normal adult life. Their occurrence in tumors is thought to be secondary to alterations in the pattern of gene regulation as the result of the dedifferentiation and reversion of the cell to a primitive embryonic state.

The carcinoembryonic, or fetal, antigens initially were thought to be a useful means of detecting malignant disease before other clinical evidence of disease is apparent or as a detector of recurrence following therapy to provide a basis for further treatment. Fetal antigens that are common to many different histologic types of human neoplasms have been described, as have those that are restricted to the organ of origin.

α-Fetoglobulin. The α-fetoglobulin circulating in approximately 70 percent of patients with primary hepatomas is found in normal human fetal serum up to 1 year after birth. The fetal antigen also has been found occasionally in patients with gastric cancer, prostatic cancer, and primitive testicular tumors such as teratomas, although it appears to be relatively specific for hepatomas. The specificity of the test was demonstrated when adult monkeys were given hepatic carcinogens; α-fetoglobulin appeared in the serum of a high percentage of these monkeys prior to any histologic evidence of neoplastic change.

The α-fetoglobulin test has been clinically evaluated and found to be useful in the diagnosis of hepatomas. It is not positive in patients with rapidly dividing cells due to hepatic regeneration following liver resection or in those with cirrhosis.

Carcinoembryonic Antigen. The carcinoembryonic antigen (CEA) reported in 1965 by Gold and Freedman is another tumor-associated antigen occurring in fetal gut, liver, and pancreas during the first two trimesters of gestation. This antigen was originally thought to be specific for adenocarcinomas arising in the gastrointestinal tract and pancreas, but more recently it has been found in a variety of carcinomas, sarcomas, and lymphomas of many different histologic types.

Since the CEA appears in the bloodstream, it was initially thought to be of great importance as a diagnostic tool for malignant disease prior to other clinical evidence of cancer. A radioimmunoassay capable of detecting nanogram quantities of CEA in the blood was developed. However, elevated CEA levels were found in patients with a variety of nonmalignant conditions including alcoholic cirrhosis, pancreatitis, cholecystitis, colonic diverticulitis, and ulcerative colitis. This test has not been useful as a serologic method for the diagnosis of malignant tumor.

The serum levels of CEA do appear to correlate with the extent of known carcinomas of the colon. Metastasis to the liver is frequently associated with the highest levels. It has been shown that the CEA level drops during the postoperative period in those patients who have successful resection of the tumor. Patients who develop tumor recurrence often show a rise in CEA titer to the preoperative levels. Thus, CEA may be of some value for following the clinical course of patients with known malignant disease in order to detect evidence of recurrence prior to its becoming clinically detectable.

GENERAL IMMUNE COMPETENCE OF CANCER PATIENTS. A number of studies have tested the general functional capacity of the cancer patient's immunologic system. Such studies can be grouped into two categories— those concerned with humoral antibody production and those dealing with cell-mediated immune reactions.

Formation of humoral antibody to known antigenic substances has been studied by many investigators, who have found most cancer patients have the ability to form humoral antibodies against a variety of antigenic substances, even in the presence of advanced disease. There is no evidence to implicate a defect in humoral antibody production in most cancer patients.

The cell-mediated immune reactions have been measured by the cancer patient's ability to manifest delayed cutaneous hypersensitivity to a variety of common skin test antigens to which most normal persons are reactive by virtue of previous exposure such as to mumps, tuberculin, streptokinase, or streptodornase. In addition, a primary immune response was tested against a new antigen by studying the survival of skin allografts and by sensitizing patients to an antigen, such as the contact sensitizer dinitrochlorobenzene (DNCB). DNCB reacts with proteins in the skin and forms a hapten that sensitizes the immunocompetent patient (Fig. 9-10). Cell-mediated immunity can be studied with an in vitro test that requires lymphocyte recognition and proliferation in response to foreign tissue antigens or mitogens such as phytohemagglutinin.

These immunologic studies revealed that cell-mediated immune reactions are significantly impaired in patients with lymphoreticular neoplasia. Since these diseases usually diffusely involve the immune effector system, this

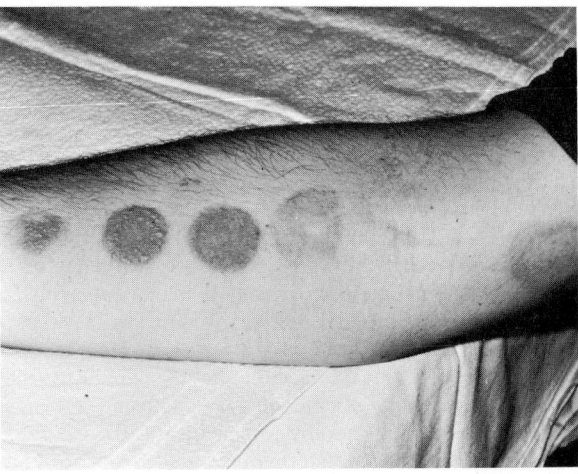

Fig. 9-10. Positive reaction to dinitrochlorobenzene (DNCB), showing initial exposure and subsequent challenges.

might be expected. In patients with solid tumors, the degree of immunologic impairment seems to vary with the extent of disease. Patients with localized tumors rarely have detectable defects in immunocompetence, whereas patients with advanced disease are often anergic.

The etiology of immunosuppression in cancer patients remains obscure. It is possible that immunosuppression could be the result of a humoral factor elaborated by the cancer cell or a complex physiologic response against the cancer cell that can depress normal cell-mediated immunity.

HYBRIDOMAS AND MONOCLONAL ANTIBODIES. Kohler and Milstein developed a method for producing large amounts of antibody with specificity against only one set of antigenic determinants. With this technique, plasma cells are fused to myeloma cells in such a way that a single clone of antibody-producing cells can be selected and grown in tissue culture indefinitely. This ability to produce a single clone of cells making huge quantities of a single antibody molecule has revolutionized immunology and, perhaps, tumor biology.

Much of the uncertainty and disagreement concerning tumor-specific antigens may be related to the assay systems used in their demonstration. The creation of hybridomas that produce antibodies against a single antigen makes the study of tumor immunology and tumor-specific antigens more precise.

Hybridomas have produced monoclonal antibody that appears to react with the tumor-specific antigens of target cells. Such antibody could be used to develop immunodiagnostic techniques. Radioimmunoassays for serum-borne tumor antigens and scans using labeled antibody have been reported. Specific monoclonal antibody has been used for immunotherapy of cancer patients with observed regressions in a significant proportion of treated patients. Attempts are being made to link specific monoclonal antibody to cytoxic agents such as Adriamycin or ricins in order to deliver lethal drugs to a tumor without affecting the normal tissues.

It is too early to assess the impact of hybridomas and monoclonal antibodies on human cancers. However, it is easy to envision a new age for immunodiagnosis and immunotherapy based on this technological advance.

POSSIBLE APPLICATIONS OF IMMUNOBIOLOGY TO CANCER THERAPY. There are many possible applications of cancer immunobiology to cancer therapy besides those of the immunotherapy. Immunoprevention by vaccine prepared from the common tumor antigens or tumor viral antigens is theoretically possible. However, because of the long latency period of most human neoplasms, it would require several decades to evaluate such a vaccine even if it were already in hand.

Immunobiology has great potential as a guide to standard cancer therapy. Immunologic monitoring of cancer patients undergoing therapy for malignant disease could be extremely useful in determining choice of therapy, as well as determining the patient's response to the therapy. Immunologic testing also may be useful in following the patient's response to certain therapeutic modalities that are known to be immunosuppressive, such as chemotherapy or radiation therapy, so that therapeutic regimens that are nonimmunosuppressive may be devised. Furthermore, with multiphase immune monitoring, it may become possible to carry out immunologic engineering in patients with defective immune responses. The deficiencies then might be corrected by appropriate adjunctive therapy once the site of the defect has been diagnosed.

PATHOLOGY

When confronted with a mass, the clinician must first determine whether it is neoplastic or inflammatory. If the mass is suspect for neoplasia, a biopsy is necessary before a specific diagnosis can be made.

In general, biopsy of a tumor must be obtained before therapy is instituted since the histology of the tumor will determine the mode of treatment. The pathologist's interpretation of materials submitted for microscopic examination depends not only upon experience and the quality of the material submitted but also upon the clinical history and findings on the patient and a review of any previous biopsy material. The features to which pathologists must direct their attention are partly histologic, that is, the arrangement of the tumor cells and their relation to the surrounding tissue, and partly cytologic, namely, the nature of the tumor cells and, in particular, the appearance of the nucleus and nucleoli.

The characteristics of benign and malignant neoplasms are listed in Table 9-4. *Anaplasia* means lack of differentiation. *Polarity* is the normal orderly alignment of epithelial cells, which are arranged in sheets. One of the early signs of malignant change is the loss of this normal polarity, so that the cells may present as a disorderly arrangement in relation to the surface and to each other. *Nuclear changes* of the malignant cells are often seen as enlarged and hyperchromic nuclei. These three features may all be seen before invasion of the deeper tissues has occurred. *Preinvasive carcinoma,* or *carcinoma in situ,* will demonstrate this change with no evidence of invasion of deeper histologic layers.

One of the most characteristic features of malignant disease is the ability to infiltrate and destroy deeper cellular layers and adjacent tissues, e.g., malignant colonic epithelial cells invading the muscular or serosal layers of the colon. In contrast, a benign tumor grows by expansion, compressing the surrounding tissues to form a capsule, but does not infiltrate these tissues.

On the basis of these microscopic criteria, the pathologist usually has no difficulty in determining whether the neoplasm is malignant or benign. Sometimes the microscopic diagnosis is difficult and opinions are divided among the different pathologists examining the tissue. When this happens, several options are open to the clinician: If the biopsy is not adequate, more material should be obtained. Special stains are sometimes helpful, such as oil red O, to show fat globules as in liposarcoma. Biopsy material may be examined by electron microscopy or even with immunologic stains to detect surface antigens such as those seen on subtypes of malignant lymphomas. Outside expert opinion may be useful, such as from the Armed Forces Institute of Pathology or the National Can-

Table 9-4. GENERAL CHARACTERISTICS OF BENIGN AND MALIGNANT NEOPLASMS

Characteristic	Benign neoplasms	Malignant neoplasms
Nuclear structure	Normal size, staining, and shape	Large, hyperchromatic with variation in size and shape
Mitotic figures	Usually rare	Frequent and perhaps atypical
Anaplasia	Absent	Varying degree
Polarity	Orderly arrangement	Disorderly arrangement
Local invasion or infiltration	Absent (except angioma)	Usually present
Capsule	Present	Absent or a pseudocapsule
Recurrence	Absent or rare	Frequent
Metastases	Absent	Frequent
Growth	Slow, self-limited	Often rapid
Systemic effects	Rare, except for neoplasms	Frequent

cer Institute, which act as referral centers for patients with unusual malignant neoplasms.

The electron microscope has been helpful in diagnosing some undifferentiated tumors, such as malignant melanoma and soft tissue sarcomas. Hormonal assay may be helpful, as in diagnosing a glucagon-producing alpha cell cancer of the pancreas. However, it is well to remember that sometimes tumors produce biologic substances that are not normally produced by the tissue from which they originated. For example, estrogen receptors have been found in neoplasms other than breast cancer.

It may not be possible, in certain situations, to differentiate histologically between a benign and a malignant neoplasm, as with the parathyroid carcinomas, giant cell sarcomas of bone, and thymomas. In these cases, clinical characteristics of the lesions in terms of the development of recurrence, metastases, and progressive growth may be the only differentiating criteria available to the clinician.

CLASSIFICATION OF NEOPLASMS. Many different classifications of tumors exist, but the most useful one is based upon the cell type of tissue of origin. When the neoplasm is undifferentiated, the special methods discussed above may help to classify it.

Neoplasms arising from epithelial cells regardless of whether in the ectoderm or the entoderm are known as carcinomas. Sarcomas arise from connective tissue and cells of mesenchymal origin and include tumors of fibrous, muscular, fatty, vascular, and skeletal origin. Teratoma signifies a neoplasm in which anaplastic, immature somatic cells, comparable with blastoderm, are usually dominant; it exhibits varying degrees of differentiation into mature somatic cells of ectodermal, mesodermal, and entodermal types. Teratomas occur in the testis, ovary, and mediastinum. A simplified classification of benign and malignant neoplasms arising from different sites is given in Table 9-5.

GRADING OF MALIGNANCY. Broders classified carcinomas into four grades according to their degree of differentiation, the appearance of cells, their nuclei, and the number of mitotic figures. On this basis, the least malignant are classified as grade 1, and the most malignant are grade 4. In general, the lower-grade, more differentiated neoplasms are less malignant and tend to metastasize less frequently than the higher-grade, more anaplastic ones.

CARCINOMA IN SITU AND PREMALIGNANT LESIONS. Carcinoma in situ is a lesion with the cytologic characteristics of malignant tumors but with no detectable invasion into the surrounding tissue or infiltration into deeper cell layers. Most likely these in situ lesions develop into invasive cancer after variable delay periods. The interval between the detection of carcinoma in situ of the cervix and invasive carcinoma may be 10 to 15 years. Carcinoma in situ also occurs in the skin, bronchus, stomach, and pharynx. When these lesions are adequately treated, a cure is assured.

ROUTES FOR SPREAD OF NEOPLASMS. There are few subjects of greater importance to the oncologist than the spread of cancer. Much is known about the routes of spread but little about the conditions that determine that spread. Some cancers are metastatic at the time of their clinical discovery, while others of the same type and in the same organ tissue may remain localized for years.

Metastases may entirely dominate the clinical picture, while the primary tumor remains latent and asymptomatic. Some patients present with metastatic cancer and no evidence of a primary site. For example, metastases to the brain secondary to silent cancers in the bronchus or the gastrointestinal tract are often mistaken for primary brain tumors.

Knowledge of the particular manner in which different types of cancer spread is important in planning therapy. In general, a malignant tumor may spread by four routes: directly by infiltrating surrounding tissue; via lymphatics;

Table 9-5. SIMPLE CLASSIFICATION OF NEOPLASMS

Tissue of origin	Site of origin	Benign	Malignant
Epithelial origin (ectoderm or entoderm)	Skin, mouth, larynx, lung, esophagus, urinary tract, cervix	Papilloma	Squamous cell carcinoma
	Breast, stomach, colon, pancreas, liver	Adenoma	Adenocarcinoma
Mesodermal origin	Fibrous tissue	Fibroma	Fibrosarcoma
	Muscular tissue	Leiomyoma, rhabdomyoma	Leiomyosarcoma, rhabdomyosarcoma
	Fatty tissue	Lipoma	Liposarcoma
	Vascular tissue	Angioma	Angiosarcoma
	Hemopoietic tissue		Leukemia, multiple myeloma, lymphoma
	Bone	Osteoma, chondroma	Osteogenic sarcoma, chondrosarcoma
Special types:			
Melanocytes	Skin, eye	Nevus	Malignant melanoma
Neural tissue	Brain, spinal cord nerve	Astrocytoma	Glioblastoma multiforme
		Ganglioneuroma	Neuroblastoma
Trophoblast	Placenta, testis	Chorioepithelioma	Choriocarcinoma
Notochord	Spine	Chordoma	Chordoma
Blastoderm	Mediastinum, ovary, testis	Teratoma	Teratoma

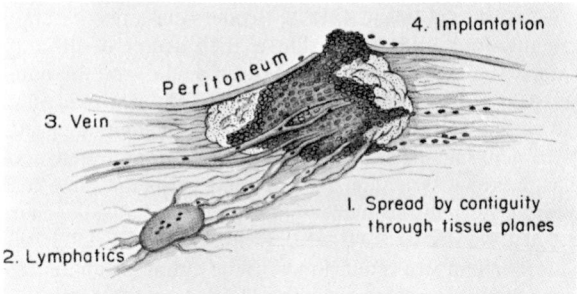

Fig. 9-11. Four mechanisms of the dissemination of cancer cells. This is a diagrammatic illustration; the original tumor could be one of many organs with cells disseminating by the four mechanisms. (From: *Cole WH et al: Dissemination of Cancer. New York, Appleton-Century-Crofts, 1961, with permission.*)

by vascular invasion; or by implantation in serous cavities (Fig. 9-11). Knowledge of the patterns of neoplastic spread in different types of cancer is important in planning definitive therapy. However, many cancers will spread by more than one route, and an orderly course of metastases cannot be relied upon. For example, many patients with breast cancer or melanoma may manifest distant metastatic disease in lungs or liver but will never develop evidence of lymph node metastases. Metastatic patterns of various types of human tumors are summarized in Table 9-6.

Direct Extension. Cancer cells may spread by direct extension through tissue spaces. Some neoplasms, such as soft tissue sarcomas and adenocarcinomas of the stomach or esophagus, may extend for considerable distances (10 to 15 cm) along tissue planes beyond the palpable tumor mass. Other neoplasms, such as basal cell carcinoma of

skin, rarely extend for more than a few millimeters beyond the visible margin. Even though some of the central nervous system tumors rarely spread, their location can cause death by interfering with vital CNS functions.

Lymphatic Spread. Tumor cells can readily enter lymphatics and extend along these channels by permeation or embolism through the regional lymphatics to lymph nodes. Permeation is the growth of a colony of tumor cells along the course of the lymph vessel. This occurs commonly in the skin lymphatics in carcinoma of the breast and in the perineural lymphatics in carcinoma of the prostate.

Spread along the lymphatics of embolism to the regional nodes or distant lymph nodes is of much greater importance. Lymph node metastases are first confined to the subcapsular space; at this stage the node is not enlarged and may appear normal to the naked eye. Gradually the tumor cells permeate the sinusoids and replace the parenchyma. There is little direct spread from node to node, because the capsule is not penetrated until a late stage. The tumor cells travel by anastomosing lymphatics, and the spread occurs in other nodes by way of collateral lymph channels. When a lymph node containing tumor is more than 3 cm in diameter, tumor has usually extended beyond the capsule into the perinodal fat.

The lymph from the abdominal organs and lower extremities drains into the cisterna chyli and then into the thoracic duct, which finally opens into the left jugular vein. Tumor cells probably freely pass from the lymph to the bloodstream. Originally, oncologists believed that solid neoplasms involved regional lymph nodes and then spread into the bloodstream by drainage through the lymphatics into the thoracic duct and to other parts of the body. An alternative explanation favored by many oncol-

Table 9-6. ESTIMATED FREQUENCY* OF PATTERNS OF NEOPLASTIC SPREAD FOR COMMON HUMAN NEOPLASMS

Neoplasm	Hematogenous	Lymphatic	Local infiltration (expressed as local recurrence)
Adenocarcinoma			
Breast	4	3	2
Colon	3	3	1
Stomach	4	4	3
Pancreas	4	4	3
Epidermoid carcinoma			
Lung	4	3	2
Oral pharynx	1	3	3
Larynx	1	3	2
Cutanteous neoplasm			
Squamous cell carcinoma	1	2	1
Melanomas	3	3	2
Basal cell carcinomas	0	0	1
Sarcomas			
Bones	4	1	1
Soft tissue	4	1	3
Brain neoplasms	0	0	4

* 0—Does not occur, 1—1 to 15 percent, 2—15 to 30 percent, 3—> 30 percent, and 4—> 50 percent.

ogists assumes that the presence of cancer cells in regional lymph nodes indicates an unfavorable host-tumor relationship and the likelihood of distant metastases.

Lymphatic involvement is extremely common in epithelial neoplasms of all types, except basal cell carcinoma of the skin, which does not metastasize to regional lymphatics. Sarcomas metastasize to lymph nodes only 2 to 5 percent of the time.

VASCULAR SPREAD. Cancer cells may reach the bloodstream either through the thoracic duct or by invasion of blood vessels. Capillaries are almost always invaded. The veins are invaded frequently, the arteries rarely. The chief reason for the striking differences in invasion characteristics between arteries and veins appears to be that lymphatics frequently penetrate the walls of the large veins from without and form a plexus reaching to the subendothelial region, thus providing a portal of entry for tumor cells through the vein wall. When the vascular endothelium is destroyed, a thrombus forms that is quickly invaded by tumor. This combination of thrombus and tumor may detach to form large tumor emboli. Vascular invasion is commonly seen in both carcinomas and sarcomas and is associated with a poor prognosis. Some types of neoplasms have a remarkable tendency to grow as a solid column along the course of veins, for example, renal carcinomas and sarcomas. Renal carcinomas have been known to grow out of the renal vein into the inferior vena cava and up the inferior vena cava to the right atrium.

Spread through Serous Cavities. Tumor cells occasionally gain entrance to serous cavities via direct growth of tumor through the wall of an organ. Many tumor cells are capable of growth in suspension without a supporting matrix and may grow and spread within the peritoneal cavity or attach to serous surfaces. In either case, it is common for tumor cells to spread widely when they encounter a space lined with a serous surface. Thus, widespread peritoneal seeding is commonly seen with gastrointestinal neoplasms and tumors of ovarian origin. A similar mechanism appears to operate in the case of malignant gliomas, which may spread widely within the central nervous system via cerebral spinal fluid.

CLINICAL MANIFESTATIONS OF CANCER

The clinical presentation of cancer is varied and inconstant. Cancer may appear as an asymptomatic lesion too small to be seen without magnification or special studies such as a mammogram. It may appear as an asymptomatic lump, or the patient may complain of symptoms that are subsequently found to be caused by an underlying malignancy. Often, symptoms are nonspecific and resemble those of nonmalignant diseases.

The clinical abnormalities produced by advancing neoplastic diseases may be grouped into two categories—those abnormalities which stem directly from the presence of a tumor mass and those physiologic derangements which are produced indirectly. By teaching patients those key symptoms of cancer which require medical evaluation, earlier diagnosis and treatment may be achieved.

Table 9-7. CANCER'S SEVEN WARNING SIGNALS

Change in bowel or bladder habits
A sore that does not heal
Unusual bleeding or discharge
Thickening or lump in breast or elsewhere
Indigestion or difficulty in swallowing
Obvious change in wart or mole
Nagging cough or hoarseness

The onset of the neoplastic state is difficult to date in human beings. As previously discussed, a prolonged latent or induction period is likely before clinically detectable disease evolves. Therefore, the use of the word "early" in describing a cancer may lead to confusion. To avoid this, we will use the terms "early" and "late" in relation to the clinical stage of a neoplasm rather than to indicate its duration in the body. When viewed in this manner, the curable cancer may have been present a long time prior to its diagnosis and therapy. The term *early* usually means a neoplasm that can be effectively treated. These neoplasms are small rather than large, do not extend into essential organs, and have not metastasized. Some lesions that have been present for years still may be early, whereas other lesions with more rapid growth rates may be *late* even if present for only a few months.

The "Seven Danger Signals of Cancer," as formulated by the American Cancer Society, are listed in Table 9-7. These may be helpful in the ongoing effort to educate people and increase the frequency of early diagnosis for certain major tumors. The more common patterns of clinical presentation, and some of the more common syndromes related to cancer will be discussed in detail in the paragraphs that follow.

Carcinoma in situ and other premalignant lesions were discussed earlier under pathology and will not be discussed further here.

SIGNS OF EXPANSILE GROWTH. The signs attributable to the expansile growth of a tumor depend upon its location. When the neoplasm is either on or near the surface of the body, it may present simply as a visible or palpable mass. In the gastrointestinal, biliary, respiratory, and urinary tracts, signs are frequently related to obstruction. Examples are vomiting, jaundice, cough, or urinary retention. Within the central nervous system, expansile growth may cause pain, paralysis, or sensory loss.

Expansile growth of a tumor may also result in destruction of host tissues. Examples are pathologic fractures, hepatic insufficiency, and Addison's disease.

SIGNS OF INFILTRATIVE GROWTH. Pain, numbness, and paralysis may result when tumor infiltrates nerves. Frequently, signs of nerve invasion are also signs of incurability. Examples are lumbosacral plexus pain in cancer of the cervix and rectum, dorsal and lumbar spine pain in cancer of the pancreas, and the shoulder and arm pain and palsy when carcinoma of the lung infiltrates the brachial plexus. Other signs of infiltration generally denoting incurability are thickening of the uterine ligaments

Table 9-8. UNKNOWN PRIMARY TUMORS
PRESENTING AS METASTASES

Site of metastasis	Primary neoplasm
Lymph nodes:	
Cervical nodes	Nasopharynx, pharynx, oral cavity, thyroid, larynx, lymphomas
Supraclavicular nodes	Bronchus, breast, stomach, esophagus, pancreas, colon, testis, ovary, cervix
Axillary nodes	Breast, melanoma, lymphoma
Inguinal nodes	Genitalia, anus, melanoma
Skin and subcutaneous tissues	Melanoma, breast, bronchus, stomach, kidney
Lung	Breast, colon, kidney, stomach, testis, melanoma, thyroid, sarcomas
Liver	Stomach, colon, breast, pancreas, bronchus
Ovary	Stomach, colon
Bones	Breast, bronchus, prostate, thyroid
Central nervous system	Breast, bronchus, kidney, colon
Serous cavities	Bronchus, breast, ovary, lymphoma

in cancer of the cervix and fixation to the chest wall in breast cancer.

SIGNS OF TUMOR NECROSIS: BLEEDING AND INFECTION. Tumors may become necrotic, ulcerate, and bleed. Fatigue and weakness may be the only symptoms or signs in cancer of the stomach or right colon, because the tumor ulceration and bleeding have resulted in anemia. If a cancer becomes ulcerated and infected, the signs of inflammation include edema, pain, tenderness, and fever. The inflammation caused by cecal cancer can mimic the clinical symptoms of acute appendicitis or cholecystitis. Therefore, response of such inflammation to antibiotics or the healing of an ulcer does *not* necessarily indicate a nonneoplastic lesion.

Tumor necrosis at any site may produce fever, leukocytosis, elevation of sedimentation rate, anorexia, and malaise. Such necrosis constitutes one of the causes of the "fever of unknown origin." Keller and Williams, in studies of 46 patients with unexplained fever, found that in 19 who underwent exploratory laparotomy the cause of the fever was intraabdominal malignant disease.

UNKNOWN PRIMARY TUMORS PRESENTING AS METASTASES. Usually the site of origin of a metastasis is known. However, the initial presentation of a tumor may be at a distance from its origin. In fact, the primary neoplasm giving rise to the metastases may have regressed completely and may never be detected in some neoplasms, such as malignant melanoma and carcinomas of the oral pharynx. Surgical resection of the metastatic lesions may result in long-term cure without the site of the primary ever being detected.

The most frequent sites of presentation of metastatic neoplasms are the cervical and supraclavicular lymph nodes, lungs, liver, bones, and brain. The most common metastatic sites for unknown primary neoplasms are listed in Table 9-8.

SYSTEMIC MANIFESTATION OF MALIGNANT DISEASE. Tumors may have a variety of remote and systemic effects that contribute to morbidity. Cancer patients frequently develop unusual symptoms and physiologic derangements that cannot be attributed to the mechanical presence of primary or metastatic disease, or to physiologic changes resulting from hormones normally secreted by the tissue of origin.

Some symptoms, such as the cachexia of carcinomatosis, may result from competition between the tumor and the host for basic components of the same metabolic pool. However, the pathogenesis of many of these disorders is unknown. Some of these nonmetastatic, systemic manifestations of malignant tumors are thought to result from (1) the ectopic production of known hormones; (2) the secretion of unidentified, physiologically active substances that do not resemble known hormones but that have hormonelike effects; (3) autoimmune phenomena in which the host is sensitized to an antigen from the tumor; and/or (4) toxic substances secreted from the tumor.

The nonmetastatic clinical manifestations of malignant disease and the neoplasms with which they are associated are presented in Table 9-9. Sometimes palliative surgery is indicated to treat these systemic manifestations, for example, resection of metastases that are producing hormones that induce hypercalcemia, or hypoglycemia.

CANCER DIAGNOSIS AND STAGING EXTENT OF CANCER

Diagnosis

Diagnosis of cancer should proceed in an orderly fashion: careful history, thorough physical examination with examination of the blood and urine, and investigation of suspicious findings by appropriate radiologic examinations and radioisotope scans.

A *history* of any of the following is suspicious and should prompt a search for cancer: weight loss; loss of appetite; bleeding or a discharge from any body orifice or nipple; a sore that is slow to heal; changing color or size of a mole; persistent cough or wheeze; change in voice; difficulty in swallowing; growing lump either in or under the skin, in the breast, in the abdomen, or in the muscles; and/or change of bowel habits.

Physical examination includes a thorough search of the entire skin surface for squamous cell and basal cell carcinomas, indurated lesions, ulcers, suspicious or irritated nevi, nodules, and other signs of malignant disease. Lymph nodes should be palpated for enlargement. Breasts should be carefully examined. All body orifices should be examined. A Papanicolaou smear from the cervix should be obtained prior to a bimanual pelvic exami-

Table 9-9. SYSTEMIC MANIFESTATIONS OF MALIGNANT DISEASE

Clinical manifestations	Associated neoplasms	Clinical manifestations	Associated neoplasms
Cutaneous		Hormonal and metabolic effects of nonendocrine tumors	
Acanthosis nigricans	Cancer of stomach, lung, and breast	Hypoglycemia (mechanism unknown)	Retroperitoneal or mediastinal mesenchymal tumors, hepatic tumors
Dermatomyositis	Cancer of stomach, breast, lung, and ovary	Cushing's syndrome (increased ACTH)	Cancer of the lung, malignant thymoma, pancreatic cancer
Erythema multiforme, exfoliative dermatitis, bullous pemphigoid	Allergic response to a variety of neoplasms, lymphoma, myeloma	Hypercalcemia (increased PTH, vitamin D-like substances or bone destruction)	Cancer of lung, kidney, breast, uterus, sarcomas, hemopoietic neoplasms
Peutz-Jeghers syndrome	Intestinal polyposis		
Hematologic		Hyponatremia (increased ADH)	Cancer of lung, intracranial tumors
Abdominal red cell mass		Hyperthyroidism (increased TSH)	Choriocarcinoma, testicular embryonal carcinoma
Erythrocytosis (increased erythropoietin)	Renal cell carcinoma, hepatoma, uterine myoma, cerebellar tumors, pheochromocytoma	Precocious puberty and/or gynecomastia (increased gonadotropin)	Hepatoma, lung, adrenal cancer, testicular tumors
Anemia:		Zollinger-Ellison syndrome (increased gastrin secretion)	Pancreatic nonbeta islet cell adenomas
Myelophthisic	All tumors	Elevated liver enzymes	Renal cell carcinoma
Hypoproliferative	Thymoma, renal cell carcinoma	Anorexia and weight loss	Most neoplasms
Hemolytic	Hemopoietic neoplasm	Hyperuricemia	Hemopoietic neoplasms
Miscellaneous causes (infection, bleeding, radiation effects, uremia, etc.)		Atypical carcinoid syndrome	Pancreatic duct, islet cell, gastric, thyroid, and oat cell cancer of lung
Abnormal leukocyte or platelet mass		**Nonmetastatic neuromuscular**	
Leukemoid reactions	Miscellaneous neoplasms	Multifocal leukoencephalopathy	Hemopoietic neoplasms
Leukopenia	Hemopoietic neoplasms, lung, pancreas	Subacute cerebellar degeneration	Multiple neoplasms, especially of lung, ovary, and breast
Thrombocytosis			
Coagulation and bleeding disorder		Polyneuropathy and/or myopathy	Multiple neoplasms, especially of lung, ovary, and breast
Disseminated intravascular coagulation (DIC)	Mucin-secreting adenocarcinoma	Myasthenia gravis	Thymoma
Vascular			
Thrombophlebitis	Cancer of lung, reproductive tract, pancreas, and breast		
Fibrinogen deficiency (increased fibrinolysis)	Cancer of prostate and lung		
Flushing, vasodilatation, violaceous skin, asthma	Carcinoid tumor		

SOURCE: Modified from Owens AH Jr: Neoplastic diseases, in Harvey AM et al: *The Principles and Practice of Medicine.* New York, Appleton-Century-Crofts, 1972, with permission.

nation. Rectal examination should include proctoscopic examination of patients who have hemorrhoids or rectal symptoms. The oral pharynx should be examined with special attention to the floor of the mouth. Indirect laryngoscopy should be performed if the patient is hoarse, has a neck mass, or is suspected of having an intrathoracic neoplasm or cancer of the thyroid gland.

Laboratory examination should include complete blood cell count, urinalysis, examination of stool for occult blood, and chest radiograph. Other tests should be ordered where indicated by symptoms. Before operating on a patient for cure or palliation, a metastatic work-up should be done, directed by symptoms and the most likely site of metastases. Prior to extensive disfiguring or disabling procedures, tomograms of the lungs, bone marrow biopsy, scalene node biopsy, isotope scans, or arteri-

ography may be useful in determining whether the neoplasm is still localized. Cytologic examination should be performed if a pleural effusion or ascites is present.

Diagnosis of solid tumors rests upon locating and performing a biopsy of the lesion. This goal is most easily fulfilled when the tumor is near the body surface or involves one of the orifices of the body that can be examined with appropriate visual instruments, such as a bronchoscope, proctoscope, or cystoscope. Carcinomas of the breast, tongue, or rectum can be seen or palpated, and a portion can be excised for definitive diagnosis.

The most difficult cancers to diagnose, and unfortunately the most lethal ones, occur in the internal organs. Space-occupying lesions in the internal organs may grow quite large before causing symptoms. Techniques that may be useful in localizing such lesions include barium examinations of the gastrointestinal tract; examination of the bronchial tree by endoscopy media; selective arteriography of major vessels supplying internal organs; radioisotopes and radiopaque dyes that concentrate in various organs such as the liver, gallbladder, kidney, and lymph nodes; and ultrasonography and abdominal computer-assisted tomography (CT scans are rapidly becoming the most useful investigative studies for intraabdominal tumors). Exploratory surgery is often required to confirm the diagnosis and to obtain biopsy.

CANCER DETECTION EXAMINATION. Any given individual stands approximately 1 chance in 4 of developing cancer during his or her lifetime. Therefore, in screening 1000 persons for an entire life span, we will find cancer in 250 of them. Since a person can harbor more than one primary cancer and a second lesion will develop with increasing frequency as the number of people who have survived the first one increases, we might count on a very crude estimate of 350 cancers in our population of 1000. Since we expect people to live an average of 72 years, we must carry out 72,000 annual examinations to discover 350 cancers, or less than 5 cancers per 1000 examinations. By directing our search to the middle and late adult years when the incidence is highest, we might conceivably double the yield to 10 per 1000. Thus, the chances of detecting cancer in a given annual examination are no more than 1 in 100 even under the most optimal circumstances.

The problem of cancer detection is further complicated by the relative insensitivity of our methods for clinical cancer detection. The earliest neoplasms must be at least 1 cm in size before they are detectable by physical examination, and often tumor masses up to 10 cm in diameter will go undetected if in the liver, retroperitoneum, or other "silent" areas.

Both physicians and patients have been rather slow to adopt the habit of periodic examinations to detect asymptomatic tumors. Although approximately 1 in 4 Americans will develop cancer in a lifetime, it is difficult to determine whether mass screening will have an impact on the cure rate for cancer. The problem most likely will be solved by selecting certain high-risk groups and screening those periodically. For example, Papanicolaou smears yearly in women over thirty have markedly decreased the death rate from carcinoma of the cervix. The use of mammography to screen postmenopausal women may also have an impact on reducing the death rate from breast cancer. However, periodic chest x-rays or proctoscopy may not affect the cure rate for carcinoma of the lung or colon. Much research remains to be done in the field of cancer detection and screening before routine screening examinations can be expected to improve survival.

Perhaps as more sensitive methods are developed for detection of cancers at an earlier stage, screening can be done more effectively. One hope for such a screening test has been the development of immunologic assays for detection of tumor antigens or antibodies in the patient's serum. Examples of these assays include those for α-fetoprotein and carcinoembryonic antigen.

BIOPSY. It is imperative that microscopic proof of malignant disease be obtained prior to institution of treatment, since significant morbidity and mortality may result from all forms of cancer therapy. The specific type of antitumor therapy will depend upon the histologic type of tumor which must be established by biopsy. Significant errors have been made when biopsies were not obtained; examples are radical mastectomies for fat necrosis and radiation therapy for renal cysts.

Even when biopsy reports from another hospital are available, the slides of the previous biopsy must be obtained and reviewed prior to the institution of therapy. This is essential because, not infrequently and particularly in rare neoplasms, an erroneous interpretation may have been made. *Definitive therapy cannot be planned rationally without knowing the nature of the neoplastic lesion.*

Three methods for biopsy of suspicious tissue are commonly used. They are the *needle,* the *incisional,* and the *excisional,* or open, biopsy; each has its advantages and disadvantages. Regardless of method used, the pathologic interpretation of the tumor mass can be valid only if a representative section of tumor is obtained. A problem of "sampling error" can occur with the needle and the incisional biopsies when only a small portion of the total tumor mass is submitted for pathologic examination.

Needle biopsy is the simplest method and may be used for biopsy of subcutaneous masses, muscular masses, and some internal organs, such as liver, kidney, and pancreas. Further, this method is inexpensive and causes minimal disturbance of the surrounding tissue. The danger of implanting tumor cells in a needle track during aspiration biopsy is extremely small and can be avoided if the location of the needle track is such that it can be excised easily at the time of the definitive surgical procedure. Needle biopsy may be disadvantageous when the specimen is quite small and not representative of the total tumor, or the needle may miss the space-occupying lesion. Hence, a needle or aspiration biopsy does require experience to interpret. A negative report for malignant disease is always viewed with skepticism and should be followed by incisional or excisional biopsy if there is any doubt. Some centers have used fine-needle aspiration cytology. In this procedure, a fine needle is inserted into the tumor, and strands of single cells are obtained for cytologic diagnosis. This procedure is extremely useful for a number of tumors but requires considerable skill to interpret and should only be done by an experienced pathologist.

Incisional biopsy involves removal of only a portion of a tumor mass for pathologic examination. It is best performed under circumstances where, if tumor cells are spilled at the time of biopsy, the incisional wound can be encompassed and totally excised at the time of the definitive surgical procedure. Incisional biopsy includes removal of portions of tumor with forceps during endoscopic examination of the bronchus, esophagus, rectum, and bladder. Incisional biopsy is indicated for deeper subcutaneous or muscular tumor masses when needle biopsy fails to establish a diagnosis.

The incisional biopsy is also used when a tumor is so large that total local excision would prejudice any subsequent adequate, wide, locally curative resection because of the wide tissue planes that are necessarily exposed by biopsy. Such biopsy should take a deep section of tumor, as well as a margin of normal tissue, if possible. Incisional biopsy does suffer from the same hazard as the needle biopsy in that the removed portion may not be representative of all the involved tissue; hence, a negative biopsy does not preclude the presence of cancer in the remaining mass. Another theoretic objection to the incisional method is the possibility that the surgeon may seed cancer cells into the operative wound or that exposed open lymphatics may transport the cells to distant sites. Despite these dangers, one must keep in mind that definitive surgical procedures cannot be planned rationally without knowing the nature of the neoplastic lesion.

Excisional biopsy is total local removal of the tumor mass. This is used for small, discrete masses, 2 to 3 cm in diameter, when local removal will not interfere with the wider excision required for permanent local control. A major advantage of an excisional biopsy is that it gives the entire lesion to the pathologist. However, this method is contraindicated in large tumor masses because, again, the biopsy procedure often scatters tumor cells throughout a large biopsy incision that must be widely and totally encompassed by subsequent definitive surgical procedures. Therefore, excisional biopsy is usually contraindicated for skeletal and soft tissue sarcomas, although it is ideally suitable for superficial squamous or basal cell carcinomas and malignant melanomas. Surgeons should always mark the excisional biopsy margins with sutures so that if removal is incomplete, they will know where tumor margin was positive should further excision be indicated.

Biopsy incisions should be closed with meticulous hemostasis, since it may be possible for a collecting hematoma to extend tumor cell contamination by widespread infiltration of tissue planes. Contaminated instruments, gloves, gowns, and drapes should be discarded and replaced with noncontaminated substitutes when the definitive procedure is to follow immediately after the biopsy procedure.

The excisional method is principally used for polypoid lesions of the colon, for thyroid and breast nodules, for small skin lesions, and when the pathologist cannot make a definitive diagnosis from tissue removed by incisional biopsy. An unbiopsied lump is surgically removed when the suspicious character of the lesion, the need for its removal whatever the diagnosis, and the nonmutilating nature of the operation make such an approach reasonably definitive. Examples of such procedures include hemithyroidectomy for thyroid nodules, partial colectomy for lesions at any point beyond the reach of the sigmoidoscope, or a right colectomy for a cecal mass that might be inflammatory or neoplastic.

Lymph nodes should be carefully selected for biopsy. Cervical lymph nodes should not be biopsied until a careful search for a primary tumor has been made. Indirect laryngoscopy, pharyngoscopy, esophagoscopy, bronchoscopy, and thyroid scan may be included in the workup. Enlargement of the upper cervical nodes is usually due to metastases from laryngeal, oropharyngeal, and nasopharyngeal neoplasms. Supraclavicular nodes are more frequently enlarged from metastases originating in the thoracic or abdominal cavity.

The specimen may be prepared for pathologic examination by either frozen or permanent sections. Frozen sections are made immediately, and pathologic diagnosis can be obtained within 10 to 20 min. Although frozen sections may be as adequate as permanent sections for diagnosis of some neoplasms, most pathologists would prefer to make a definitive diagnosis in questionable cases on permanent sections. Although such sections require 1 to 2 days for processing, it is usually best to have a definite diagnosis before discussing the therapeutic options. Therefore, frozen sections are used when the diagnosis is required at the time of major surgery and when it is in the patient's best interests to have the definitive resectional surgery carried out at that time.

Occasionally, an exploratory thoracotomy or laparotomy will be necessary to obtain tissue for microscopic examination and confirmation of diagnosis. As a general rule, regardless of the clinical picture, the neoplastic nature of the disease process must be confirmed by frozen section examination prior to closure of the wound. This is critical because the permanent sections may fail to confirm the neoplastic nature of the pathologic process, and the patient will have experienced the morbidity of operation without obtaining a diagnosis.

Exfoliative cytology constitutes one possible method for the early diagnosis of certain types of neoplasms. This technique is based upon the fact that cancer cells are shed from the surfaces of neoplasms arising in epithelial-lined body cavities and orifices, such as the vagina, bronchus, and stomach. These cells can be collected, stained, and recognized as malignant because of their individual morphologic changes.

Staging Extent of Cancer

The extent of the patient's tumor by clinical evaluation at the time of initial presentation is called the *clinical stage*. In addition to making an exact histologic diagnosis of cancer, it is essential that the clinical stage of the disease be determined prior to making a decision regarding therapy. This is especially important when the patient initially presents for treatment, but also it is often desirable to repeat some of the diagnostic procedures periodically during the patient's course in order to assess his or her true status. The recognized importance of this staging has led to a variety of international and national attempts to standardize the staging of the patient with cancer. To date, no single system has been universally accepted (Table 9-10). Stage I usually indicates a neoplasm confined to its primary site of origin, Stage II indicates metastases to the regional lymph nodes, and Stages III and IV indicate distant metastatic spread.

The Union Internationale Contre Cancrum (UICC) has attempted to standardize one system for all nations. This has been called the TNM system because it relies on a statement of tumor extent in terms of the primary tumor (T), presence or absence of node metastases (N), and the

Table 9-10. CHRONOLOGY AND TYPES OF STAGING RECOGNIZED BY THE AMERICAN JOINT COMMITTEE ON CANCER*

Stage	Comment
cTNM	*Clinical-diagnostic staging:* The extent of disease using all information available prior to first definitive treatment, including pathologic confirmation of extent of disease by biopsy or invasive techniques
pTNM	*Postsurgical resection-pathologic staging:* The extent of disease using all data available at the time of surgery and on examination of a completely resected specimen
sTNM	*Surgical-evaluative staging:* The extent of disease using all clinical information available plus that obtained on surgical exploration; usually done for a few inaccessible tumors that are not amenable to definitive resection
rTNM	*Retreatment staging:* The classification when restaging is necessary for additional or secondary definitive treatment after a (disease-free) interval following first treatment
aTNM	*Autopsy staging:* Used only when the cancer is first diagnosed at autopsy

* From Beahrs OH, Myers MH (eds): *Manual for Staging of Cancer,* 2d ed., published for the American Joint Committee on Cancer by Philadelphia, Lippincott, 1983, p 6, with permission.

presence or absence of distant metastases (M). The system was developed following careful analysis of the results of treatment in patients with various constellations of clinical findings. It was found that patients with larger tumors did less well than those with smaller tumors; hence, the separation of various stages on the basis of tumor size. For different tumors size criteria vary, but in this system decreasing prognosis is indicated by increasing numbers after the T, such as T_1, T_2, T_3, or T_4 for lesions of increasing sizes. The presence or absence of regional spread is usually indicated by variations in the secondary category, under N for nodes. The absence of nodal metastasis is designated as N_0; the presence of nodal metastasis is N_1; for more extensive nodal involvement, additional numbers may be used. Finally, distant metastases are indicated by adding a subscript 1 following M for metastases, or a subscript 0 for their absence. Thus, a small lesion that has neither spread to regional nodes nor metastasized would be designated as a $T_1N_0M_0$ lesion. A lesion that was larger and involved regional nodes but without distant metastases might be identified as a $T_2N_1M_0$ lesion. A larger neoplasm with both regional and distant metastases would be designated a $T_3N_1M_1$ lesion. For some tumor types such as soft tissue sarcoma a G for grade of malignancy is added. High-grade tumors are more anaplastic and tend to metastasize sooner.

The American Joint Committee on Cancer recognizes several types of cancer staging schemas (Table 9-10). The clinical-diagnostic staging (cTNM) represents the extent of disease prior to first definitive treatment. Postsurgical resection-pathologic staging (pTNM) provides additional information after operation, and is especially useful in planning adjuvant therapy for many types of tumors. Other staging types include surgical-evaluative staging (sTNM) usually for tumors that cannot be resected, retreatment staging (rTNM) usually after a disease-free interval, and autopsy staging (aTNM).

The importance of accurate staging when designating a therapeutic program for a patient with cancer cannot be overemphasized. It is an important consideration when comparing the results of therapy in different centers, and as therapeutic methods for cancer improve, it is only by careful staging that new forms of therapy can be appropriately evaluated. For example, only accurate staging can identify patients, such as those with Stage II breast cancer, whose more advanced disease is still potentially curable by adjuvant therapy. These patients probably have subclinical metastases at the time of operation.

Unfortunately, one of the great deficiencies of the present staging methods is their inability to detect subclinical microscopic metastatic lesions. Many patients who are treated for apparently localized cancers already have disseminated metastases. For example, about one-half of those patients who have cancer of the breast and who undergo mastectomy have subclinical distant metastasis at the time of the operation.

THERAPY

General Considerations

At present, approximately 55 percent of all cancer patients are treated by surgical resection (40 percent by surgery alone); 34 percent by radiation therapy (16 percent by radiation therapy alone); and 22 percent by chemotherapy alone or in combination with the other modalities. As the use of chemotherapy as an adjuvant to surgery increases, it is likely that a much larger percentage of patients will have chemotherapy as part of their cancer treatment. At the present time, most patients with potentially curable solid tumors are treated with surgery. In an effort to improve overall cure rates, radiation and chemotherapy can be added to the surgical procedure.

Surgery and radiation therapy today represent the most successful means of dealing with cancer as long as it remains localized to the primary site and regional lymph nodes. Since these forms of therapy exert their effect locally, neither can be considered curative once the disease has metastasized beyond the local region, although both methods of therapy may be useful as palliative treatment. Chemotherapy and immunotherapy, unlike surgery and radiation therapy, represent systemic forms of treatment effective against tumor cells already metastatic to distant organ sites. These systemic therapeutic modalities have a greater chance of curing patients with a minimum number of tumor cells than those with clinically evident disease. Thus, though surgery and radiation therapy cannot be curative unless the tumor is confined locally or regionally, they can decrease the patient's tumor burden so that chemotherapy or immunotherapy may become more effective. During the past several years, enough evidence has accumulated to suggest that treatment combining surgery, radiation therapy, chemotherapy, and, possibly, immunotherapy will significantly improve cure rates above those achieved with any single therapeutic modality.

Cancer treatment, therefore, should be approached in an interdisciplinary manner. Just as oncology should be approached as a unique field of study, so cancer should be regarded as a single but complex disease requiring a multidisciplinary approach. The practice of assigning certain types of neoplasms to surgery, radiation therapy, or medicine with a further division into various anatomically oriented specialties should be discontinued.

GOALS OF THERAPY—CURE OR PALLIATION. Once the diagnosis of malignant disease has been made and the extent of disease determined, a decision must be made about the specific therapy. *Is the patient curable?* This is the foremost question that must be answered before the physician recommends aggressive therapy with its attendant complications. The goals of therapy vary with the extent of the cancer. If the cancer is localized without evidence of spread, the goal is to eradicate the cancer and cure the patient. When the cancer is spread beyond local cure, the goal is to control the patient's symptoms and to maintain maximum activity for the longest possible period of time. Palliation should be measured in terms of useful life. Diabetes is not cured, but the manifestations of the disease are controlled so that a patient has many years of activity and useful life. Goals for the palliation of patients living with cancer are similar.

Patients are generally judged as incurable if they have distant metastases or evidence of extensive local infiltration of adjacent organs or structures. The most common criterion for incurability is distant metastases. However, some patients are potentially curable even if they have distant metastases. For example, patients with solitary pulmonary metastases may be curable by resection, and even those with widespread metastases who have choriocarcinoma may be curable with chemotherapy. Histologic proof of distant metastases should be obtained before the patient is assessed as incurable. Occasionally, an exploratory celiotomy or thoracotomy may be necessary to determine the nature of equivocal lesions in the lungs or liver. In some situations, e.g., multiple pulmonary metastases, the clinical situation may point so overwhelmingly to distant metastases that the patient may safely be considered incurable without biopsy.

Local extension may be a criterion of incurability. For each anatomic site, there are certain local criteria that place the patient unequivocally in an incurable status, while others imply a poor prognosis but are not absolutely indicative of incurability. In equivocal situations after extensive studies have failed to demonstrate metastatic or incurable local extension, the patient deserves the benefit of doubt and should be treated for cure.

CHOICE OF THERAPY. Surgery, radiation therapy, and chemotherapy are the most frequently used therapeutic

modalities in the fight against cancer. Each may play a role in both curative and palliative therapy. Immunotherapy is a new modality that has a limited role in cancer therapy at the present time, but one that may become increasingly useful in the future. In choosing therapy, a variety of factors must be considered regardless of whether the aim is cure or palliation. The natural history of the disease and the results obtained from each type of therapy must be known prior to choosing a modality or combination of modalities.

The patient's general condition and the presence of any coexisting disease must be considered in planning therapy. Surgery may be contraindicated in a patient who has recently experienced a myocardial infarction. A patient with preexisting diabetes will be much more susceptible to the toxic effects of hormonal therapy with corticosteroids. Renal disease may increase the toxicity of some of the chemotherapeutic drugs, such as methotrexate. In addition, any evidence of infection or bleeding in a patient may make any form of cancer therapy dangerous, requiring vigorous treatment prior to the initiation of definitive therapy.

The psychologic makeup of the patient and the patient's life situation must be considered. A patient who is unable to accept the realities of a given treatment should be offered an alternative approach when possible. This is particularly true of any surgical procedures that significantly alter appearance or that involve change of organ function requiring the patient's daily care, such as colostomy. Experimental forms of therapy, such as intraarterial infusion of drugs, should also be avoided in some patients. Obviously, a patient who is going to be unwilling to tolerate the inconvenience of an intraarterial catheter and who might remove it without medical approval should not undergo such treatment.

Adjuvant Therapy

Even though extensive staging procedures indicate that a tumor localized to the primary site and regional lymph nodes is potentially curable by local therapy (either surgery or radiation), about 60 percent of malignant tumors will ultimately recur. Obviously, patients whose tumors fall into this category have subclinical metastases at the time of diagnosis. The probability for cure may be improved if systemic therapy is coupled to the local treatment. This adjuvant treatment can consist of chemotherapeutic agents or, in some instances, immunotherapy using vaccines or nonspecific stimulants.

The rationale for chemotherapy under these circumstances relates to the principles of the log cell kill hypothesis—a given dose of drug kills a constant fraction of cells, the so-called first-order cell kill. However, the drugs must be given when the number of tumor cells is low enough to permit destruction but at doses that can be tolerated by the patient. The opportunity for cure probably occurs during the early stage of the disease or immediately after surgery when tumor burden is minimal. At the present time, most trials of adjuvant chemotherapy are experimental; however, the results of extensive breast cancer trials have convinced most clinicians that adjuvant chemotherapy for premenopausal patients with Stage II carcinoma of the breast can improve disease-free survival. Other subsets of breast cancer patients also may respond to adjuvant chemotherapy, although these results are less clear-cut. Other tumors that seem to respond to adjuvant chemotherapy are Wilms' tumor, osteosarcoma, Ewing's sarcoma, and ovarian carcinomas.

Surgical Therapy

Surgical treatment represents the most frequently used and the most successful single method of cancer therapy currently available. More patients are cured of cancer by surgery than by any other therapeutic modality. However, only about one-third of cancer patients are cured by surgery alone, since surgical therapy, with few exceptions, is curative only in those patients in whom the disease is localized to the primary site and regional nodes.

Cancer surgery has been based upon the concept that cancer begins as a local disease and spreads in an orderly fashion from the primary site to adjacent tissues by direct extension to the regional lymph nodes by lymphatics and through the blood vessels. The surgical procedure was designed to remove the primary neoplasms and the usual contiguous routes of spread with the aim of removing *every* cancer cell from the body. New evidence suggests that many malignancies have a relatively long latency period and probably shed cells throughout the body as they grow. Surgery, in these instances, would be considered as a means for local control of the disease. This decrease in tumor burden could alter the host-tumor balance to favor the patient with minimal metastases.

Advances in surgical techniques, anesthesia, and supportive care (blood transfusion, antibiotics, and fluid and electrolyte management) have permitted the development of more radical and extensive operative procedures. These advances have resulted in significant improvements in the cure rates for certain human neoplasms. Ultraradical operations have been extended to their anatomic limits, permitting the surgical removal of nearly all organs. Unfortunately, these more radical procedures have often failed to significantly increase cure rates.

There have been few significant improvements in the management of most human neoplasms by surgery alone during the past two decades. Furthermore, advances in cancer surgery techniques beyond those presently practiced are unlikely to significantly change the cure rates of most human neoplasms. It would appear, then, that any therapeutic advances must come from the combination of other modalities with cancer surgery.

PREOPERATIVE PREPARATION. Often, the patient's physical condition is relatively poor. Many malignant tumors seem to have a toxic effect on the host disproportionate to the size of the lesion. Patients may have a poor nutritional status because of interference with normal alimentary function as with cancers of the oral pharynx, esophagus, and intestinal tract. Pain may contribute to anorexia and severe electrolyte disorder. Anemia, vitamin defi-

ciencies, and defects in the coagulation mechanisms must be corrected before an operation can be safely performed.

Every effort should be made to correct nutritional deficiencies, restore depleted blood volumes, and correct hypoproteinemia prior to extensive surgical procedures. Total parenteral nutrition can be used to prepare the malnourished patient for a major operation. Otherwise the operative morbidity and mortality following extensive cancer operations will be excessive.

CANCER SURGERY

Once the decision has been made to proceed with surgical therapy, the operative procedure should be planned carefully. It is essential to realize that the best, and often the only, opportunity for cure is at the time of the first operation. If the neoplasm is incompletely excised at that time, tissue planes, lymphatics, and blood vessels are violated and tumor cells are seeded throughout the wound. Any recurrence that follows may be difficult to separate from the inflammatory reaction and scarring that can distort tissue planes to a point where tumor margins are indistinct. Therefore, enucleation or incomplete excision of tumor masses is *never* indicated as a therapeutic measure.

PREVENTION OF CANCER CELL IMPLANTATION DURING SURGERY. Local recurrence of cancer following surgery may be due to incomplete removal or spillage of cancer cells into the operative area (Fig. 9-12). The cancer surgeon constantly must be aware of the possible danger of transferring cancer cells by inoculation into the surrounding tissues during the course of an operation. As soon as the incision is made, all edges of the wound should be protected with a plastic drape to prevent tumor cell contamination. This precaution is exemplified best when laparotomy or thoracotomy is performed for malignant disease within the abdomen or thorax.

Fig. 9-12. During the operative procedure, cancer cells may be seeded in the wound by direct contact with the primary tumor, with lymph nodes containing metastatic tumor, or with contaminated gloves and instruments. Cancer cells may also enter the wound via cut lymphatics and divided blood vessels. (From: *Cole WH et al: Dissemination of Cancer.* New York, Appleton-Century-Crofts, 1961, with permission.)

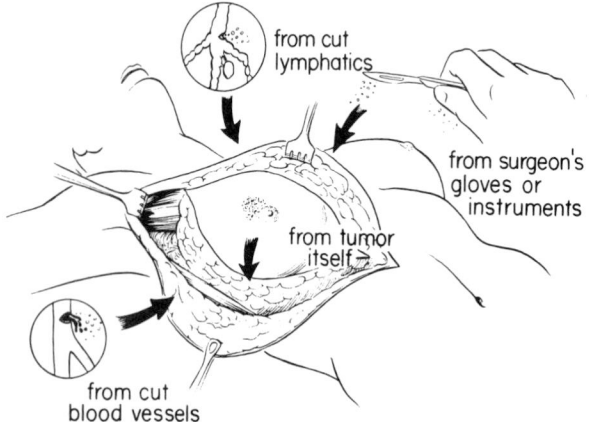

Tumor cells may be inadvertently transplanted from the primary site to other sites during the surgical procedure. When preliminary biopsy has been done, the entire operative field should be reprepared after the biopsy incision is closed. The instruments and gloves used during the biopsy are not used again, because they may have been contaminated. Even the basin of saline solution in which the surgeon's gloved hand is dipped may be contaminated with cancer cells. The importance of this is illustrated by a patient with breast cancer who had a skin graft taken from the thigh to close a skin defect after a mastectomy. Later tumor nodules having the same histologic characteristics as the primary neoplasm developed on the thigh at the skin graft donor site.

If the tumor is entered during the operative procedure, the risk of implanting cancer cells into the wound is greatly increased. Should this happen, the operative field must be isolated; the cut surface of the tumor must be cauterized with the electrocautery and isolated from the remainder of the wound; and the contaminated knife, instruments, and gloves must be discarded. Then, and then only, can the operation continue through a new plane of dissection allowing a much wider margin around the tumor.

Many different cytotoxic solutions have been used to irrigate the wound following cancer surgery in an effort to sterilize the operative site. None have been very effective in decreasing the local recurrence rate, with the exception of 0.5% formaldehyde used to prevent local recurrence from carcinoma of the cervix. Sodium hypochlorite solution, nitrogen mustard, and thiotepa have all been tried, with little success.

The rate of local recurrence in the suture line following resection for carcinoma of the colon is about 10 percent. There has been some success with various techniques to prevent this local recurrence. Ligation of the bowel with umbilical tape proximal and distal to the tumor, or anastomosis, or irrigation of the cut ends of the colon with bichloride of mercury solution and then excision of the edge of each end of the bowel have been used and have decreased the recurrence rate to less than 2 percent. The use of closed anastomosis and iodized sutures has decreased the anastomotic recurrence rate in the laboratory. Local recurrence can occur despite every effort to isolate the tumor or avoid spilling cancer cells into the operative field. For example, tumor in local lymphatics may be unrecognized at the time of the initial operation, or blood-borne cells may implant the fresh wound. Usually a local recurrence is associated with systemic disease and is an unfavorable prognostic factor.

PREVENTION OF VASCULAR DISSEMINATION AT SURGERY. Blood-borne metastases are a major factor in the death of patients with most tumors. Although cancer cells have been identified in the blood of many cancer patients, only a small number of these circulating cancer cells survive because of host resistance and other factors. Thus, tumor embolism and metastases are not synonymous. In fact, there appears to be little difference in the prognosis of patients with or without tumor cells in their blood preoperatively. However, there is a correlation between the presence of tumor cells seen in the blood during the operative procedure and prognosis. Furthermore, manipulation of the tumor at any time in the surgical procedure can greatly increase the number of cancer cells recovered from the blood.

Definite measures should be taken to prevent the dissemination of tumor cells during the operation. These can include (1) avoiding manipulation of the tumor ("no-touch" technique), (2) early ligation of the vascular pedicle, (3) the use of tourniquets on all extremity tumors.

Since any manipulation of the tumor mass may result in exfoliation of tumor cells into the lymphatics and blood, such manipulation must be kept to a minimum prior to the operative procedure, during preparation of the skin with antiseptic agents as well as during the operative procedure. Furthermore, it is imperative to use an incision of proper size to minimize unnecessary manipulation of the tumor. One that is too small will not permit the necessary wide excision without excessive handling. Turnbull and associates have reported a significant higher survival in left colon cancer using the no-touch technique, which combines minimal manipulation, early ligation of the vascular pedicle, and wide excision. However, the importance of early ligation of the vascular pedicle has been questioned by Stearns, who reported similar results without the early ligation.

TYPES OF CANCER OPERATIONS. Local Resection. Wide local resection in which an adequate margin of normal tissue is removed with the tumor mass may be adequate treatment for certain low-grade neoplasms that do not metastasize to regional nodes or widely infiltrate adjacent tissues. Basal cell carcinomas and the mixed tumors of the parotid gland are examples of such neoplasms. However, it is essential that at least some normal tissue surrounding the tumor is excised in order to prevent local recurrence.

Radical Local Resection. Some neoplasms may spread widely by infiltration into adjacent tissues. This is especially true for soft tissue sarcomas and esophageal and gastric carcinomas. For this reason, it is necessary to remove a wide margin of normal tissue with the neoplasm in these cases. The wide normal-tissue margin between the line of excision and the tumor mass also acts as a protective barrier against tumor cell spill into the severed lymphatics and vessels. The greater the thickness of normal tissue between the plane of dissection and the tumor, the greater likelihood of a complete local excision.

If the tumor was previously explored but not removed or if an incisional biopsy was performed, it is extremely important that a wide segment of skin and the underlying muscles, fat, and fascia be removed far beyond the limits of the original incision, because tumor cells may have been implanted in the incision at the time of this initial operation.

It must be constantly emphasized that malignant neoplasms are not well encapsulated. A pseudocapsule composed of a compression zone of neoplastic cells usually covers the tumor. This apparent encapsulation offers a great temptation for simple enucleation, because the tumor may be dislodged from its bed so easily. This temptation must be resisted. The surgeon must cut through normal tissue at all times and should never encounter the neoplasm during its removal. Dissection should proceed with meticulous care to avoid tumor cell spill. Retraction always should be away from, rather than toward, the tumor. It is important for the surgeon to remember to be as far as possible from the gross extent of the tumor on all sides including the deep aspect. Skin, subcutaneous fat, and muscle usually can be sacrificed with impunity and little functional loss. Involvement of major vessels, nerves, joints, or bones may require sacrifice of these structures and even amputation in order to obtain a curative result. During the surgical procedure, the extent of operation should be determined not only by the concern for cure, but also by functional considerations.

All deeply situated sarcomas lying between or within muscle groups require the removal of all muscle bundles from their origin to insertion within that particular fascial compartment; all surrounding or adjacent fascia, periosteum, vessels, nerves, and connective tissues; and all skin adjacent to the lesions. These procedures are imperative when surgery alone is used to treat sarcomas, because these lesions tend to infiltrate along fascial and muscle planes far beyond the palpable limits of the tumor. As surgeons proceed with the operation, they may be forced to alter their initial operative plan as they visualize the extent of tumor and as the pathology reports of frozen section examinations of surgical margins are made available. These decisions as to extent of resection are difficult and require experienced judgment. In borderline situations, it is usually better to proceed with a potentially curative resection of the tumor mass unless there is histologic confirmation that the lesion has extended beyond the boundaries of possible surgical resection. Advances in the use of combined modality therapy for skeletal and soft tissue sarcomas have permitted the salvage rather than amputation of extremities for selected patients (see the section on Combined Modality Therapy).

Radical Resection with en Bloc Excision of Lymphatics. Since many neoplasms commonly metastasize by way of the lymphatics, operations have been designed to remove the primary neoplasm and the regional lymph nodes draining that area in continuity with all the intervening tissues. Conditions are best for this type of operation when the collecting nodes of the lymphatic channels draining the neoplasm lie adjacent to the primary site or if there is a single avenue of lymphatic drainage that can be removed without sacrificing vital structures. It is important to avoid cutting across involved lymphatic channels because such action greatly increases the possibility of local disease recurrence.

This principle was applied to breast cancer by Meyer and by Halsted at the turn of the century and has formed the foundation of cancer surgery for many years. At the present time, it is generally agreed that such en bloc regional lymph node dissections should be performed in patients having clinical involvement of nodes by metastatic tumor. In many cases, the tumor has already spread beyond the regional nodes, and the cure rates following such procedures may be quite low. En bloc removal of the involved nodes offers the only chance for cure and provides significant palliation and local control. Therefore, the defeatist attitude toward metastatically involved regional nodes must be discouraged.

The high rate of local cancer recurrence following surgical resection when lymph nodes are grossly involved and the high error rate when palpation is used to assess the extent of the involvement have led to routine dissection of regional nodes close to the primary tumor even though they are not clinically involved. Microscopic examination of the excised lymph nodes in these patients who have no clinical evidence of palpable enlargement reveals evidence of tumor spread in 20 to 40 percent of carcinomas and melanomas. This concept is supported by comparison of the higher 5-year survival rate of patients showing microscopic involvement of lymph nodes with that of patients in whom lymph node involvement was clinically recognizable.

Recently some surgeons have challenged the concept of elective, or prophylactic, lymph node dissection in cases where the regional nodes are not obviously involved, because it is not clear whether cure rates are improved if the nodes are removed before they are palpable. However, in many types of cancer the foreknowledge of tumor in regional nodes does affect the staging of the patient and can alter the treatment modality. For example, patients with breast cancer who have metastases to regional nodes may benefit considerably from adjuvant chemotherapy as would some patients with deep melanomas. Furthermore, a comparison of experimental results from one institution with another depends upon accurate staging of each patient at the time of the initiation of therapy. For these reasons, the decision to recommend a prophylactic lymph node dissection must be based on the likelihood of benefit to the patient.

Randomized prospective studies will be necessary to answer the question of which patients do best after prophylactic dissection. Until then, the surgeon must weigh benefit against risk for each patient. Certainly, the argument against lymphadenectomy because it diminishes the host's immune system has not been proved by experimental studies, and should not be a consideration when planning therapy.

Extensive Surgical Procedures. Some slow-growing primary tumors may reach enormous size and may locally infiltrate widely without developing distant metastasis. Supraradical operative procedures can be undertaken for these extensive, nearly inoperable tumors, with cure of occasional patients. Although surgical care, anesthesia, blood replacement, and physiologic monitoring are much improved over the past, these operations should not be undertaken except by experienced surgeons who can select those patients most likely to benefit. Furthermore, these extensive surgical procedures sometimes offer a chance for a cure that is not possible by other means, and are justified in selected situations when extensive laboratory work-up shows no evidence of distant metastases. However, the surgeon must be willing to accept the responsibility for the postoperative emotional rehabilitation of the patient before undertaking such extensive procedures as the pelvic exenteration, hemipelvectomy, fore-quarter amputation, or mutilating operations for head and neck carcinomas.

Pelvic exenteration is a well-conceived operation capable of curing patients with radiation-treated recurrent cancer of the cervix and certain well-differentiated and locally extensive adenocarcinomas of the rectum. This operation removes the pelvic organs (bladder, uterus, and rectum) and all soft tissues within the pelvis. Bowel function is restored with colostomy. Urinary tract drainage is established by anastomosis of ureters into a segment of bowel (ileum or sigmoid colon). The 5-year relapse-free survival from pelvic exenteration is 25 percent in this situation.

Hemipelvectomy (resection of the lower extremity and iliac bone) can sometimes be curative for skeletal sarcomas limited to the head of the femur or acetabulum or to one-half of the pelvic structures, and in some slowly growing soft tissue sarcomas of the upper thigh and buttock that recur locally but metastasize slowly. Forequarter amputation (resection of the upper extremity and scapula) can offer similar results when the neoplasm is limited to the bones of the scapula and upper humerus or to the soft tissues of the shoulder girdle.

SURGERY OF RECURRENT CANCER. There is a definite role for surgical resection of localized recurrent neoplasms of low-grade malignancy and slow growth where further resection may produce a long period of remission. Additional surgical procedures are frequently successful in controlling recurrent soft tissue sarcomas, anastomotic recurrences of colon cancer, certain basal and squamous carcinomas of skin, and recurrent breast cancer.

Routine "second-look" operations to detect early recurrence of colon cancer were advocated by Gilbertsen and Wangensteen. The results of this second-look procedure have not been impressive and do not appear to justify its routine use. However, various tumor markers, such as CEA, have been extremely useful for selecting patients likely to benefit from reoperation. In general, a local recurrence can be treated surgically or with radiation. The surgeon must decide which form of treatment will achieve local control with the lowest morbidity.

RESECTION OF METASTASES. Although logic would suggest that once a neoplasm has metastasized to a distant site it should no longer be curable by surgical resection, removal of metastatic lesions in the lung, liver, or brain has occasionally produced a clinical cure. Therefore, in selected patients with slowly growing neoplasms, resections of the metastatic lesions may be indicated, especially if the metastasis is solitary. Prior to undertaking resection, an extensive laboratory work-up should rule out metastatic spread to other body areas.

Some patients with isolated liver metastases may benefit from surgical resection. Those patients with a solitary metastasis, or metastases located in one lobe, are often successfully treated with resection. Approximately 25 percent of these patients will survive for 5 years. However, less than 5 percent with colon cancer metastatic to the liver are candidates for this type of treatment. Most of these patients have diffuse disease and are best treated with systemic or intraarterial chemotherapy. Occasionally, resection is recommended for the patient whose primary tumor is controlled and who has no evidence of other metastases. As can be seen in Fig. 9-13, the result can be very gratifying.

The results of resection of pulmonary metastatic lesions have been much more satisfactory. In fact, resection of a solitary pulmonary metastasis provides a higher rate of 5-year survival than resection of primary bronchogenic carcinoma of the lung. Resection of pulmonary metastases may be indicated even when more than one metastatic lesion is present. Many patients die from their pulmonary metastases; resection could provide cure. Our experience has shown that patients with tumor doubling times greater than 40 days received significant palliation from their pulmonary resections and remained free of disease for as long as 5 years. In contrast, patients with tumor doubling times of less than 20 days did not significantly benefit from resection of their metastatic lesions (Fig. 9-14).

ADMINISTRATION OF CHEMOTHERAPY BY ARTERIAL INFUSION OR ISOLATED PERFUSION. The concentration of chemotherapeutic drugs can be greatly increased when the drug is administered directly into the artery supplying the neoplastic lesion. Continuous infusion of chemotherapeutic drugs over a period of weeks can be carried out

Fig. 9-13. Resected liver and smiling patient at 10-year anniversary of operation for hepatic metastases.

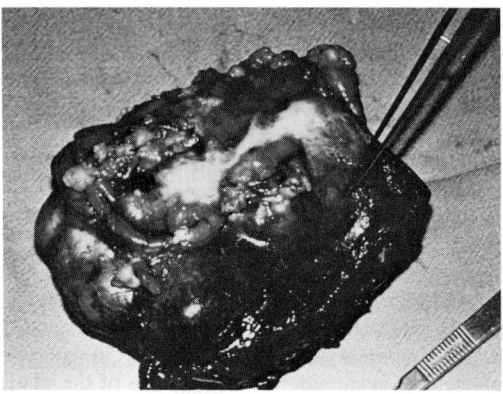
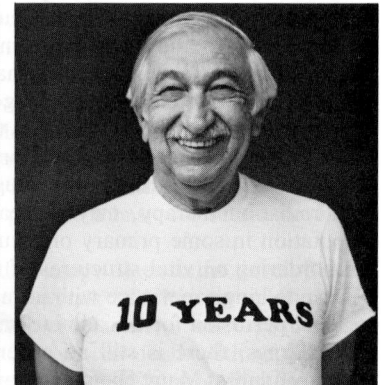

lian normal or tumor cells is remarkably similar, with doses of 110 to 240 cGy consistently reducing reproductive cell survival to 37 percent (D_0 dose). Therefore, differences in the rapidity and completeness of response of human tumors and normal tissues must be based on other factors such as the capacity to repair sublethal damage, cell cycle time, distribution of cells in the replication cycle, and repopulation.

The difference between radiosensitivity and radiocurability is important. Radiosensitivity is the measure of susceptibility of cells to injury by ionizing radiations. This injury may be lethal to the cell through interruption of the capacity to replicate indefinitely (reproductive death) or through metabolic incapacitation or structural degeneration independent of progression of the cell through the reproductive cycle (interphase death).

Radioresistance is the reciprocal of radiosensitivity and so both terms are relative. All mammalian cells are radiosensitive through a narrow range (D_{37} or D_0 = 110 to 240 cGy) when measured by reproductive death.

Radiocurability, which is permanent tumor control allowing survival of the host, is related primarily to tumor size, site, and type, and less to radiosensitivity. Most radiocurable tumors are only moderately responsive when measured by rate of gross decrease in size (epidermoid carcinomas of the oral cavity, pharynx, larynx, skin, cervic, and adenocarcinomas of the breast, prostate, and uterus). Indeed, except for seminoma, many of the rapidly responding tumors (non-Hodgkin's lymphomas, undifferentiated carcinomas) are not radiocurable, usually because of widespread extent.

Radiation-instigated cell killing can be modified in several ways. Inasmuch as molecular oxygen must be present for maximal cell killing by ionizing radiations, tumor cellular hypoxia can decrease the effectiveness of radiation therapy by as much as a factor of 3. This may explain the postirradiation persistence of tumor cells when there is necrosis or fibrosis.

Heat directly kills cells and alters radiosensitivity. Hyperthermia is an attractive adjuvant to radiation therapy because it is effective during the S-phase of the cell cycle and is not adversely influenced by hypoxia, and it blocks repair of sublethal damage (see section on Hyperthermia).

The intrinsic radiosensitivity of cells can be increased by altering the target DNA, such as by replacing thymidine with halogenated pyrimidine analogs (BUdR, IUdR) during cell replication. Cell killing can be increased by inhibiting the postirradiation repair processes. For example, the repair of DNA strand breaks can be inhibited by actinomycin D and Adriamycin, and by heat (42 to 45°C). Unfortunately, current methods of altering the target DNA and inhibiting postirradiation repair are not selective for tumor cells and so do not favorably alter the therapeutic ratio.

Cell killing can be modified by changes of the dose rate. As the dose rate decreases, cell killing, per unit of dose, decreases. Low dose rates, i.e., less than 10 cGy/min, may favor repair in normal cells. This is exploited clinically in improving lung tolerance in total body irradiation

and allowing very large total doses in interstitial and intracavitary treatments.

Inherent cellular radiosensitivity to photons varies by a factor of approximately 2, depending on position in the cell cycle. Thus, frequent doses of photons may decrease the radiosensitivity of a homogeneous population of cells by selectively killing cells in the most vulnerable phase of the cycle.

Such variations in radiosensitivity to photons related to cell age, repair of sublethal damage, and hypoxia are minimized by the use of high-energy particles (fast neutrons, heavy ions, pi mesons), thus providing a basis for investigation of these radiations.

CLINICAL BASIS. Like surgery and chemotherapy, radiation therapy has definite indications and contraindications. Irradiation may be the only anticipated treatment or it may be combined with surgery and/or chemotherapy.

Whether radiation therapy may be useful is based on factors related to both the tumor (type, primary site, extent) and the host (general condition, local and regional tissue status). Inasmuch as all forms of cancer treatment may cause serious morbidity and once used may enforce an initial diagnosis, it is essential that a diagnosis be positively established, if possible. This usually means identification of tumor by biopsy. An unfortunate historic activity, a trial of radiation therapy to determine "sensitivity," not only was biologically meaningless but was detrimental because of destruction of evidence necessary to identify the tumor properly. On a rare occasion, when biopsy may pose an unreasonable risk to the patient (brain stem, optic tract), treatment may be licensed by strong diagnostic evidence. The introduction of computerized tomography (CT) and magnetic resonance imaging (MRI) should reduce unfortunate diagnostic errors. Once the tumor identity has been established, reappearance after treatment, particularly in palliative situations, may require less potentially morbid diagnostic efforts.

Histologic tumor type and grade may be useful pretherapeutic predictors of biologic behavior and radiosensitivity (Table 9-11). However, this evidence is much less useful in predicting radiocurability.

The potential for tumor control by radiation therapy is more closely related to tumor size and primary site. Generally, as tumors increase in size, the likelihood of radiocurability decreases, presumably related to a direct correlation of tumor cell number and radiation dose required to kill all the tumor cells. The primary tumor site predicts biologic behavior and dictates which adjacent normal tissues must tolerate the incidental irradiation. For example, small epidermoid carcinomas of the uterine cervix and vocal cords are localized and can be eradicated by radiation doses tolerated by the surrounding normal tissues. Larger tumors at the same sites are less frequently controlled by similar doses and, in addition, are more likely to spread regionally, thus requiring treatment of a larger volume with consequent reduction of normal tissue tolerance.

After initial evaluation of the patient, the objective of radiation therapy must be defined. If the cancer is radio-

Table 9-11. RELATIVE RADIOSENSITIVITY OF MALIGNANT TUMORS

(Listed in order of decreasing radiosensitivity)

Malignant tumors arising from hemopoietic organs (lymphosarcoma, myeloma)
Hodgkin's disease
Seminomas and dysgerminomas
Ewing's sarcoma of the bone
Basal cell carcinomas of the skin
Epidermoid carcinomas arising by metaplasia from columnar epithelium
Epidermoid carcinomas of the mucous membranes, mucocutaneous junctions, and skin
Adenocarcinomas of the endometrium, breast, gastrointestinal system, and endocrine glands
Soft tissue sarcomas
Chondrosarcomas
Neurogenic sarcomas
Osteosarcomas
Malignant melanomas

SOURCE: From Ackerman LV, del Regato JA: *Cancer: Diagnosis, Treatment, and Prognosis,* 4th ed. St Louis, Mosby, 1970, with permission.

curable, patient inconvenience, relatively high cost, and a moderate risk of serious treatment-related morbidity should be considered in that fortunate perspective. If the objective is palliation of bothersome cancer-related symptoms or signs, these consequences of treatment usually are not acceptable.

Radiation treatment planning and delivery have become highly complicated. In most patients, the primary tumor and its regional spread are graphically displayed in three dimensions and incorporated in a planned treatment volume. The best method of delivery of the radiations is selected from a range of options including multiple beams of photons and/or electrons, sometimes augmented by interstitial and/or intracavitary applications. The dosimetry data are incorporated in computer-assisted programs, which allow rapid, accurate calculations of the desired options.

Repetitive treatment delivery can be accurate to within a few millimeters, if required (proton or heavy ion beam treatment of choroidal melanoma or linear accelerator treatment of retinoblastoma).

Doses to different sites in the same patient may vary according to need. The treatment plan may include the integration of different types of radiations. For example, a primary squamous cell cancer of the oral tongue or cervix may receive a high local dose from an isotope source, while regional lymph nodes, which may harbor metastases, may receive lower doses from a photon teletherapy source. The integration of all the components of such a comprehensive plan for radiation therapy is possible only when directed by a single, trained, responsible physician.

Even when seemingly indicated, radiation therapy may be inappropriate because of host factors. These may include general debility, making the tolerance to vigorous irradiation unlikely; or there may be local tissue changes

precluding high-dose local treatment; or the patient may fear the treatment, making its proper use impossible.

Radiation therapy is increasingly being used in planned combination with surgery and/or chemotherapy. Multidisciplinary treatment implies continuous cooperation of all physicians involved in planning, delivering, and monitoring a treatment program. The objective of combined surgery and radiation therapy is improved local and regional control of tumor. Both methods may be directed to the same site, as when resection of a cancer of the hypopharynx is followed by irradiation, or when irradiation of a soft tissue sarcoma in an extremity is followed by surgery; or each method may be directed to a different site, as when orchiectomy is followed by irradiation of the retroperitoneal lymph nodes, or when a neck dissection follows interstitial irradiation of a cancer of the oral tongue.

When surgery and radiation therapy are directed to the same site, the interval between their use depends on a range of facors, which should be decided by mutual agreement. Thus, low-dose irradiation of a soft tissue sarcoma may be followed by resection in 10 to 14 days, while rectosigmoid resection should be delayed 4 to 6 weeks after high-dose pelvic irradiation to allow for regression of edema and hyperemia. Most postoperative radiation therapy is with high doses directed to sites at high risk for persistent tumor and so should be delayed until wound healing is as complete as possible.

Such planned combined treatment is in stark contrast to the use of one method to rescue the failure of the other. In these circumstances, the effectiveness of the second method is reduced. Surgery in tissues heavily irradiated in a curative attempt many months before is difficult because of fibrosis, loss of tissue planes, and decreased vascularity, and the frequency and severity of complications are consequently increased. Irradiation of tumor regrowing in tissues altered by surgery is likely to be less effective, often because of decreased vascularity, and more morbid, as when bowel is fixed by adhesions, resulting in high doses to small segments.

Every effective anticancer therapy may produce undesirable and, occasionally, dangerous side effects. It is important to recognize that the potential to cause and avoid serious sequelae is much different today from in the past. Also, the incidence of treatment-related side effects varies with the philosophy of the radiation oncologist, who must answer whether the risks of frequent serious sequelae are worth slightly more frequent tumor control.

Early radiation-induced reactions, although undesirable, are self-limited. These include anorexia and even nausea, fatigue, diarrhea, esophagitis, skin and mucosal reactions, epilation, and hematopoietic suppression.

The clinically important severe sequelae of radiation therapy, such as bowel stenosis and bone necrosis, become evident months or years after treatment (Table 9-12). Often these are predictable and can be minimized by good modern treatment. Such developments, if the result of well-considered risks, can be correlated with unavoidable sequelae of other treatments. For example, is a colostomy, made necessary because of radiation-induced stenosis of bowel occurring during curative irra-

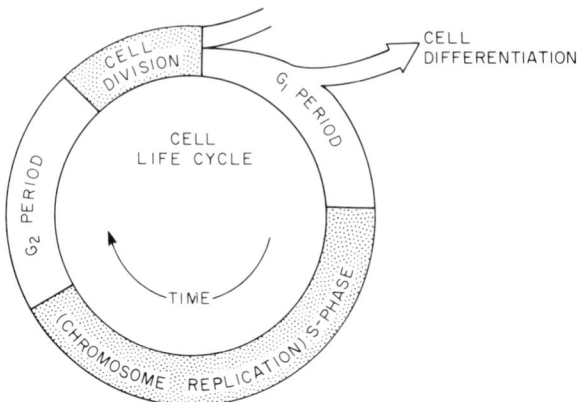

Fig. 9-15. Schematic diagram of the cell life cycle. G_1 is the first "gap" period, and G_2 is the second "gap" period. [From: *Baserga R (ed): The Cell Cycle and Cancer. New York, Marcel Dekker, 1971, with permission.*]

tion of DNA synthesis due to the lack of an essential building block.

Other major drugs appear to work primarily by affecting substrates. The usual substrate affected is the DNA macromolecule, although some of these agents will interfere with other substrates, such as proteins, and may have other diverse effects. Three major chemical classes of drugs appear to act by affecting specific substrates. The alkylating agents are extremely reactive compounds that can substitute an alkyl group (for example, $R—CH_2—CH_2^+$) for the hydrogen atoms of many organic compounds. The primary compounds affected appear to be the nucleic acids, especially DNA. Such alkylation produces breaks in the DNA molecule and cross linking of the twin strands of DNA, thus interfering with DNA replication and the transcription of RNA. Since these effects are somewhat similar to that seen with ionizing radiation, alkylating agents are sometimes called "radiomimetic." Another group of compounds that appear to work primarily on substrates are the *antibiotics.* These are natural products derived from certain soil fungi. They produce their antineoplastic effect by forming relatively stable complexes with DNA, thereby inhibiting the synthesis of DNA and RNA. The final class of drugs acting primarily on substrates is the *vinca alkaloids.* Although their total mechanism of action may not be completely defined, it is apparent that they can bind to microtubular proteins necessary for cell division. These proteins form the spindle apparatus that allows the chromosomes to separate to either end of the dividing cell; the vinca alkaloids appear to be able to dissolve this protein, leading to death of the cell during mitosis.

Table 9-14 lists representative examples of each group along with selected characteristics considered to be of clinical importance.

BIOLOGIC AND PHARMACOLOGIC FACTORS IN CANCER THERAPY. A major theme in pharmacology has been the study of variations in drug absorption, distribution, metabolism, and excretion as related to a stable, invariant biologic receptor. In cancer chemotherapy, however, the

biologic receptor, the cancer cell, is a variable and fluctuating target. Thus, the kinetics of tumor growth must be given as much attention as the kinetics of drug absorption or metabolism when considering cancer chemotherapy. Specifically, five general principles of tumor biology relevant to treatment appear to be extremely important. These include an understanding of (1) antineoplastic drug action as a function of the cell cycle, (2) tumor cell population growth, (3) tumor cell heterogeneity and drug resistance, (4) the log–cell kill hypothesis, and (5) the critical role of drug scheduling in optimizing therapy. These biologic factors will be reviewed first, followed by a brief discussion of clinical pharmacologic factors that are especially important in cancer chemotherapy.

Drug Action and the Cell Cycle. The life cycle of all cells, both normal and neoplastic, starts with mitosis, or cell division. This is followed either by differentiation or a series of biochemically distinct phases known, in sequence, as G_1 (the first "gap" phase), S phase (DNA synthesis), G_2 (second "gap" phase), and mitosis (Fig. 9-15). Although these events are similar in neoplastic and normal cells, there appear to be some quantitative differences in the duration of the cycle and the sensitivity of cells to drugs during various phases of the cell cycle. Because of these differences, one must differentiate between drugs that kill cells only during specific phases of the cycle *(phase-specific)*, and drugs that kill cells during all or most phases of the cell cycle *(phase-nonspecific)*. The distinction between a phase-specific and phase-nonspecific drug may not be absolute. Some authorities distinguish additional categories or use different names for these categories. In particular, some workers separate the phase-nonspecific drugs into an additional two categories: *cycle-specific* and *non-cycle-specific.* For this discussion, drugs that can affect multiple phases of the cell cycle or that appear to be effective against nondividing cells are grouped together under the term *phase-nonspecific,* since the clinical usefulness of this group appears to be correlated with their lack of phase specificity.

Gompertz and Cell Population Growth. The human organism consists of communities of cells, many of which are capable of self-renewal through cell division. Generally these renewable populations grow rapidly when they are small in number and slowly when they are large. Thus, the fetus grows rapidly, but the adult organism remains constant in size, thanks to a balance between cell production and cell loss. This relation between size and growth rate may be expressed quantitatively in either of two ways: (1) as a function of volume doubling times (time for any given number of cells to double in number) or (2) as a function of the growth fraction (that fraction of cells undergoing division at any one time). Figure 9-16 presents a logarithmic plot of human fetal and childhood growth against time and includes specific data on the volume doubling times during growth. Growth in the early years is clearly exponential with a high growth fraction and very short volume doubling times. As time passes, the doubling time lengthens and the growth fraction decreases. The general slope of this curve can be expressed mathematically as an exponentially decreasing function.

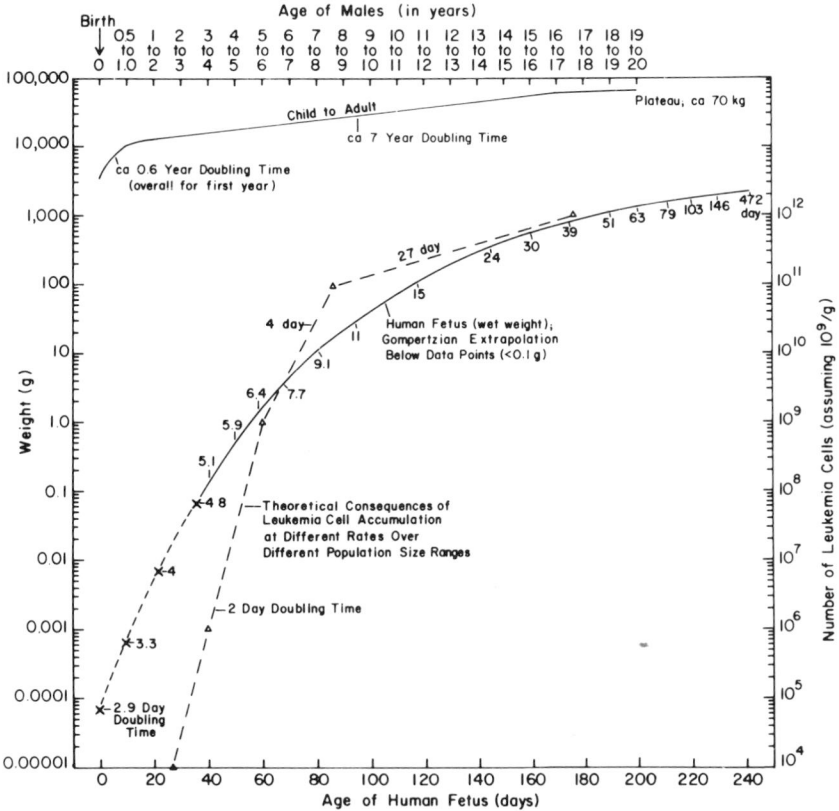

Fig. 9-16. Human fetal and childhood growth as a Gompertzian process, and the theoretic consequences of accumulation of leukemic cells at different rates over varying population ranges. (From: *Skipper HE, Perry S: Cancer Res 30:1883, 1970, with permission.*)

The specific equation describing this relationship was originally derived by the eighteenth century mathematician Gompertz; therefore, biologic growth that conforms to this pattern is referred to as *Gompertzian growth*. Interestingly, evidence that not only normal cell growth but neoplastic cell growth follows a Gompertzian pattern is increasing. At least 18 different animal tumors conform to a Gompertzian growth curve, and Sullivan and Salmon have shown that human myeloma follows a Gompertzian growth pattern.

Tumor Cell Heterogeneity and Drug Resistance. Tumor cells appear to be intrinsically unstable and highly susceptible to mutation. For some tumors, multiple clones of cells may arise through the process of mutation, leading to a highly heterogeneous population of cells with differing sensitivity patterns to various chemotherapeutic agents. This phenomenon, known as tumor cell heterogeneity, has important implications for cancer treatment. It implies that the larger the size of the tumor, the more likely there will be resistance to multiple chemotherapeutic agents. Since drug resistance is the most important reason for the failure of cancer chemotherapy, it implies that chemotherapy should be used as early as possible in the natural history of the cancer in order to assure the highest probability that the tumor will be sensitive to treatment.

The Clonogenic Assay. The search for an in vitro sensitivity test for malignant tumors, analogous to the culture and sensitivity tests in use for bacteria, continues to command the attention of oncologists. Most currently used chemosensitivity tests are based on the human tumor stem cell—or clonogenic—assay developed by Hamburger and Salmon. In this system, single-cell suspensions derived from a biopsied tumor are plated in vitro on a soft agar medium and exposed to various chemotherapeutic agents. Malignant cells alone possess the capability of sustained growth in the semisolid agar medium. The growth of the cultured malignant cells is measured either by the number of colonies formed (usually defined as 30 or more cells per colony as counted by an automated optical scanner) or by the incorporation of radioactive substrates such as tritiated thymidine. The two techniques have been shown to give equivalent results, with the latter technique having the advantages of shorter turnaround time (5 days versus 2 to 3 weeks) and elimination of clumping artifacts (clumps of nonviable tumor cells incorrectly scored as viable colonies). In either method, the in vitro growth of drug-treated tumor cells is compared with untreated "control" cells to determine in vitro sensitivity.

Numerous studies have demonstrated that clonogenic assays, regardless of the exact method employed, have similar predictive accuracies for sensitivity and resistance. Predictive accuracy for sensitivity, defined as the percent probability that a tumor that is sensitive in vitro will be responsive clinically, has consistently ranged from 50 to 65 percent in these studies. Predictive accuracy for resistance, the probability that a tumor that is resistant in vitro will not respond clinically, has been much higher—85 to 95 percent—suggesting that these assays may be particularly useful for determining which tumors will fail to respond to chemotherapy. Prospective trials have been carried out that confirm the ability of the clonogenic assay to direct chemotherapy. A prospective, randomized trial of the assay has recently been completed in which patients treated with single-agent chemotherapy selected by the assay had a significantly higher clinical response rate than those treated with the physicians's choice of drug.

Despite these favorable results, problems remain. Low in vitro growth rates are common for some tumor types, such as sarcomas and primary breast cancers. Heterogeneity of the chemosensitivity of a tumor, either in the same tumor deposit over time or between two different deposits of the same tumor (e.g., a primary and a metastasis) is a significant theoretical concern and probably a real factor in limiting the predictive accuracy of these assays. Chemotherapeutic combinations—clinically used far more than single-drug therapy—have not been tested as rigorously as single agents. More than any other factor, however, the lack of available active antineoplastic drugs limits the clinical usefulness of predictive testing for most common tumor types. For this reason, attempts have been made to use the clonogenic assay for screening potential new anticancer drugs, with some success.

At present, routine use of in vitro sensitivity testing cannot be advocated for all tumors. Such tests represent a potent research tool and a potential aid in the ongoing search for new antitumor agents. In selected cases, assay-directed chemotherapy can yield a higher likelihood of success than the clinician's best choice. As technical and methodological advances continue to improve in vitro growth rates, it is anticipated that the number of patients who can benefit from in vitro sensitivity testing will increase.

The Log–Cell Kill Hypothesis. Antineoplastic drugs are incapable of killing all cancer cells at any given exposure; rather, they will kill a variable fraction of cells from a very few up to a maximum of 99.99 percent. The fractional cell kill observed can usually be graphed on semilog paper as a line with a negative exponential slope, and so experimental chemotherapeutic data are usually expressed in logarithmic terms. Since the body burden of tumor cells in a human being with an advanced malignant tumor may be greater than 10^{12} cells, and since the best one can hope for with a single maximal exposure of tumor cells to a drug is 2 log–cell kill, it is apparent that treatment must be repeated many times in order to achieve even partial control. Theoretically, this hypothesis also suggests that chemotherapeutic drugs may not be capable of totally eradicating any given population of tumor cells. There is good evidence that immunotherapy does not face this restriction, since it can completely eradicate small numbers of tumor cells; however, it may be totally inef-

fective against larger tumor cell masses (greater than 0.1 mg of tumor in most model systems).

Drug Scheduling and Combination Therapy. Studies with experimental animal tumors have conclusively demonstrated the critical importance of drug scheduling in therapy. Cytosine arabinoside, an antimetabolite that kills only cells in S phase, must be given frequently in order to assure contact with cancer cells during this critical period. When this drug is so employed, it is possible to "cure" some forms of murine leukemia, whereas maximally tolerated doses of the drug given at less frequent intervals fail to prolong survival. On the other hand, cyclophosphamide (Cytoxan), which is phase-nonspecific, achieves optimal suppression of most experimental neoplasms when given on an intermittent schedule.

A second factor related to drug scheduling is the growth status of any given tumor. In general, solid tumors with a large tumor mass will be growing slowly, and will have a small growth fraction (less than 10 percent) and a prolonged tumor volume doubling time. Since relatively few of these cells are dividing, these tumors are generally resistant to phase-specific drugs. Thus, the usual treatment for advanced nonhematologic tumors has been with phase-nonspecific drugs, such as the alkylating agents or 5-FU. However, successful treatment with such phase-nonspecific drugs may render the tumor more susceptible to phase-specific drugs, by converting the tumor from one with a low growth fraction with few of the cells in S phase to one with a higher growth fraction with many cells in S phase.

It is clear that the optimal way to use chemotherapy against most forms of human cancer is by using combinations of drugs. Since cancer chemotherapy usually involves the use of toxic drugs, one must design programs of combination chemotherapy with care in order to minimize dangerous toxicity. In general, the successful programs of combination chemotherapy have been designed with the following criteria in mind: (1) only drugs active against the tumor in question are included; (2) drugs included have different mechanisms of action, in order to minimize the possibility of drug resistance; and (3) drugs chosen generally have different spectra of clinical toxicity, thus allowing the administration of full or nearly full doses of each of the active agents.

Clinical Pharmacology. In addition to the principles relating to tumor biology described above, numerous pharmacologic principles must be considered in cancer chemotherapy. The first such consideration relates to the route of administration of a drug or a combination of drugs. A variety of routes can be chosen, such as oral, intravenous, intramuscular, intraarterial, or local application. By using a carefully selected parenteral route of administration, difficulties related to absorption of drugs are avoided. It also may be possible to improve the antitumor effect of a given drug. Particularly promising in this regard has been the use of drugs by the intraarterial route, such as when the primary tumor is in the liver or on an extremity. Using a portable infusion pump, drugs can be continuously infused over weeks or months. An extension of this approach has been with isolation-perfusion of an extremity with high doses of chemotherapy. As newer drugs are developed, particularly drugs with very short half-life periods, it is likely that the choice of the route of administration will become increasingly important.

A second consideration relates to transport mechanisms for the drug in question. If the drug is transported on serum proteins, it is possible that other drugs may alter significantly the proportion of the bound and free anticancer drug. An example of this is the ability of salicylates to displace methotrexate from its binding site on albumin. In this setting, high doses of salicylates may result in augmented host toxicity from methotrexate.

Another consideration is the possible effect of drug interactions when drugs are given in combinations. One well-established drug interaction involves allopurinol, a xanthine oxidase inhibitor, when it is used with 6-mercaptopurine (6-MP). Since degradation of 6-MP is catalyzed by xanthine oxidase, the use of allopurinol along with full doses of 6-MP has been shown in the past to be dangerous. Normal function of organs important in drug metabolism or degradation may be critical to the biologic fate of a drug. For example, serious liver disease may increase the toxicity of drugs that are cleared by that route, such as vincristine or Adriamycin. Severe neurotoxicity has been observed in patients with concomitant liver disease when given otherwise clinically well-tolerated doses of vincristine.

The route of excretion of a drug may be critical. Methotrexate is primarily excreted by the kidney, and even modest elevation of the BUN (blood urea nitrogen) may be associated with major hematologic toxicity from the use of relatively low doses of methotrexate. For this reason the status of the kidneys must be observed very closely in all patients receiving methotrexate therapy. In fact, it is wise to observe renal function in all patients receiving cancer chemotherapeutic drugs, since nearly all of them have some extent of excretion by the renal route. In addition, it is not unusual for a brisk response to chemotherapy to result in elaboration of large amounts of uric acid, from the breakdown of the nucleic acids of the destroyed cancer cells. Uric acid nephropathy may result. Pretreatment with allopurinol may prevent this complication.

A final factor relates to the ability of a given drug to enter the cancer cell: many drugs require direct access to a specific biochemical pathway within the cell, and failure to gain entry will be associated with drug resistance. To some extent this effect may be overcome by giving very large doses of the drug; however, this is usually associated with unacceptable drug toxicity. An exception to this limitation may be the experimental use of large doses of methotrexate and its antidote, citrovorum factor. Cancer cells appear to lack this transport system. When normal and cancer cells are exposed to massive doses of methotrexate, a high intracellular drug concentration results. When the antidote is subsequently given in lower doses, the normal cells are "rescued" by virtue of the cell membrane transport system. Future work with this treatment

and with others that rely on the transport of drugs across cell membranes may result in further improvements in drug therapy.

The most common cause of treatment failure is the development of drug resistance by tumor cells. Recent studies with human tumors grown in short-term tissue culture suggest that clinical tests for such drug resistance may be possible. Salmon and coworkers have successfully used such "clonogenic assays" to predict drug resistance, and there is widespread interest in the use of such tests clinically. Further work with these assays is needed, but they are very promising as a useful clinical tool.

Ultimately, all factors that might alter either the concentration of the critical drug at its primary site of action or the duration of time available for such activity should be considered in the use of drugs. This may be expressed as a function of concentration times time, and because of its importance it is commonly referred to as the $C \times T$ function.

CHEMOTHERAPY AS AN ADJUVANT TO CANCER SURGERY. The proved ineffectiveness of surgical resection alone for many types of neoplasms has led many investigators to the use of cancer chemotherapeutic agents as adjunctive treatment. It was postulated that these agents might control microscopic foci of cancer already disseminated in the body. Controlled clinical trials have been carried out to determine the effectiveness of single chemotherapeutic agents when combined with surgical resection for carcinomas of the breast, lung, stomach, and colon. Very few significant benefits have been demonstrated thus far using single agents. However, the chemotherapeutic agents chosen for these studies, their dosage, and the duration of administration may not have been optimal for the desired result. It is likely that future applications of this concept using newer chemotherapeutic agents in combination for prolonged periods of time may well result in improved survival for these patients. This approach may be further enhanced by advances in immunotherapy and radiation therapy. An example of one approach to adjuvant chemotherapy as applied to breast cancer appears later in this chapter.

GUIDELINES FOR CHEMOTHERAPY IN PATIENTS WITH NONHEMATOLOGIC MALIGNANT TUMORS. The initial major question a physician must ask when considering chemotherapy for any patient with a neoplasm is whether benefit will result with tolerable toxicity. The physician must have all the facts regarding the patient, including the type, extent, and grade of the malignant tumor, its expected natural history, the results of current therapy, and the psychologic makeup of the patient. In addition, one must consider the following three principles:

1. The patient should have a histologic diagnosis of a malignant disease that is known to respond in a reasonable percentage of cases in a manner beneficial to the patient. Table 9-15 outlines the current status of cancer chemotherapy for a variety of nonhematologic neoplasms. Brief comment on specific drug-sensitive neoplasms will be presented subsequently. In general, patients in whom disease usually or often responds to chemotherapy should receive drug treatment, unless there is a specific contraindication. In addition, patients suspected of

Table 9-15. CURRENT STATUS OF CANCER
CHEMOTHERAPY FOR
NONHEMATOLOGIC NEOPLASMS

Disease	*Major drugs used*
Chemotherapy used alone with curative intent	
Gestational trophoblastic neoplasia	Methotrexate, actinomycin C, vinca alkaloids, alkylating agents, cisplatin
Testicular tumors	Cisplatin, vinblastine or etoposide, bleomycin
Chemotherapy used with curative intent as part of combined modality therapy	
Wilms' tumor	Actinomycin D, vincristine
Ewing's sarcoma	Cyclophosphamide, vincristine, actinomycin D, doxorubicin
Osteosarcoma	Doxorubicin, methotrexate, cisplatin
Breast cancer	Cyclophosphamide, methotrexate, 5-fluorouracil, doxorubicin
Ovarian cancer	Cisplatin, doxorubicin, cyclophosphamide
Medulloblastoma	Methotrexate
Chemotherapy used with major palliative intent	
Small-cell lung cancer	Cyclophosphamide, vincristine, doxorubicin, etoposide
Prostatic carcinoma	Estrogens
Endometrial carcinoma	Progestins
Adrenal carcinoma	o, p'-DDD
Islet cell carcinoma	Streptozocin
Soft tissue sarcomas	Doxorubicin, cyclophosphamide, cisplatin
Advanced poorly differentiated carcinoma of unknown primary origin	Cisplatin, bleomycin, vinblastine

Chemotherapy is experimental or is given with minimal hope of palliation

Epidermoid carcinomas of the head and neck, cervix, lung, and from an unknown primary site
Adenocarcinomas of the gastrointestinal tract, pancreas, liver, bile ducts, lung, and from an unknown primary site
Carcinomas of the bladder or kidney
Melanoma
Neuroblastoma
Brain tumors
Carcinoid tumors

having minimal residual disease (micrometastases) after local therapy also may be candidates for adjuvant chemotherapy. Such therapy would be questionable for those patients with a tumor known to be minimally inhibited by commercially available drugs. Experimental therapy may be warranted for these patients.
2. It is absolutely essential that there be adequate facilities to monitor the potential toxicity outlined in Table 9-14, and physicians should not initiate therapy unless they are adequately trained in the use of drugs and committed to monitoring the patient for drug therapy. Chemotherapy is generally contraindicated for patients with nonhematologic malignant conditions if they have major bleeding or infection, although patients with leukemia and, in some cases, lymphomas may require treatment even during such episodes in order to control life-threatening bleeding or infection. Patients with major dysfunction of an organ system particularly susceptible to the toxicity of a cancer chemotherapeutic drug must be followed carefully and may be more suitably treated with an alternative drug. An example of this latter situation would be a patient with a severe neuromyopathy, who might be better treated with drugs other than vinca alkaloids, as these may exacerbate the condition. Patients in whom a rapid response to therapy is possible or who have preexisting renal disease should be treated with allopurinol to prevent the complication of uric acid nephropathy. Finally, patients who are under active chemotherapy and develop severe toxicity may require aggressive support with platelets, red blood cells, antibiotics, or in some cases, white blood cells for control of infection.
3. Cancer chemotherapeutic drugs are toxic. In order to minimize unwarranted toxicity, the physician should conduct a diligent search for disease markers to assist in monitoring treatment. Ideally, several parameters of tumor response should be followed in order to objectively assess the response to therapy. Some factors that can be considered in assessing response to treatment are described in more detail in Table 9-16. As a general rule, tumor size is of particular importance. Most oncologists require a 50 percent reduction in the product of the greater and lesser diameters of any given tumor to accept the change as a "partial response."

The specific choice of a drug or drugs for a given patient with cancer and the precise choice of a dose and schedule for such single agent or combination therapy are best decided in the light of current therapeutic research. To some extent such choices can be determined by referring to Table 9-16 and the following section. Other useful sources of information include the *Medical Letter on Drugs and Therapeutics,* which period-

Table 9-16. CRITERIA FOR RESPONSES IN
PATIENTS WITH SOLID TUMORS

Tumor size	Palpation and measurement with calipers
	Radiologic measurement
	Radioisotope scans
	Ultrasound
	CAT scan
	Magnetic resonance imaging (MRI)
Tumor products	Quantitative level of chorionic gonadotropin (choriocarcinoma and certain testicular tumors)
	Quantitative level of carcinoembryonic antigen (CEA) in bowel cancer
	Quantitative level of α-fetoprotein in hepatoma or testicular tumors
	Serum or urine paraproteins in myeloma
	Urinary adrenal hormone (adrenal carcinoma treated with o,p'-DDD)
Improvement in symptoms or sign of tumor	Improvement in hypercalcemia (particularly with carcinoma involving bone)
	Improvement in obstruction due to tumor (such as bowel obstruction or obstructed ureter)
	Disappearance of effusions from tumors involving pleura, peritoneum, or obstructing lymphatics
	Subjective symptoms are important to patient but are generally poor indicators of antitumor response

ically publishes information on the choice of therapy in the treatment of cancer; books on the treatment of cancer (such as that edited by Haskell); and the specialty journals of cancer (*Cancer; Cancer Treatment Reports; The Journal of Clinical Oncology; Seminars in Oncology*).

ILLUSTRATIVE NEOPLASMS HIGHLY RESPONSIVE TO CHEMOTHERAPY. Trophoblastic Tumors of the Uterus. Metastatic gestational choriocarcinoma is curable in 80 to 90 percent of women using chemotherapeutic drugs alone. The discovery by Li et al. in 1956 that methotrexate could control metastatic disease in women with choriocarcinoma represents a landmark in the history of cancer chemotherapy. Subsequent systematic study of this disease has markedly increased our understanding about cancer and its treatment. Certain points are worthy of special mention.

1. Methotrexate must be started as soon as possible after the diagnosis has been made. This relates to the finding that the best prognosis, with cure rates of 95 to 100 percent, is seen in patients whose disease is treated within 4 months of onset, in whom metastases do not include the brain or liver, and in whom 24-h urine quantities of human chorionic gonadotropins (HCG) are less than 100,000 I.U.
2. Combination chemotherapy should be used if the initial response to chemotherapy is suboptimal or if the patient presents with high titers of HCG, with liver or brain involvement, or with symptoms present longer than 4 months. Second-line drugs for this disease include actinomycin D, vincristine, alkylating agents, and doxorubicin.
3. Therapy should be continued for 6 months after the chorionic gonadotropin titer has returned to normal. This is even more important than eliminating radiographic evidence of disease, since residual pulmonary lesions may be present despite cure of clinical growths. This is analogous to the residual changes of many nonneoplastic diseases, such as tuberculosis.

Germ-Cell Tumors of the Testis. All forms of testicular cancer are now considered to be highly responsive to chemotherapy. This was initially proved in patients with advanced embryonal cell carcinomas, yolk sac tumors, and choriocarcinoma using various combinations of cisplatin, bleomycin, and vinblastine. Subsequently, the same has been shown for patients with bulky or advanced seminoma. Currently, the major difference between the treatment of advanced seminoma and the various forms of "nonseminomatous germ-cell tumors" of the testis is how one utilizes combined modality therapy. Both groups of patients with advanced, bulky disease now receive immediate combination agent chemotherapy for at least 4 months. Patients with nonseminomatous tumors with persistently elevated levels of the tumor markers alpha-fetoprotein or beta-chorionic gonadotropin may be treated even longer. After the completion of chemotherapy, patients with seminoma may receive additional radiation therapy to areas of previously known disease or to residual masses. Masses that persist after this therapy are almost always scar tissue or necrotic tumor, so surgery plays no role in these patients. They are considered potentially cured with chemotherapy alone, or with the combination of chemotherapy and radiation therapy. The situation is very different, however, for the various forms of nonseminomatous tumor. These tumors tend to consist of a heterogeneous population of tumor cells, and it is not unusual for chemotherapy to eradicate the drug-sensitive population, leaving histologically benign teratomas. These "benign" tumors are resistant to radiation therapy, and they can be locally aggressive, so they must be surgically removed. Thus, patients with nonseminomatous tumors usually undergo surgical exploration rather than radiation therapy following the completion of combination chemotherapy.

Carcinoma of the Prostate. The mainstays of therapy for disseminated cancer of the prostate are orchiectomy and estrogen therapy. These modalities have increased survival of these patients modestly, and they are of major palliative value in controlling pain. Many different doses of the most commonly used estrogenic hormone have been employed. However, data from the Veterans Administration Cooperative Research Group have shown up to a 25 percent increased mortality from cardiovascular diseases in a group of patients treated with moderately high doses (5 mg daily) of diethylstilbestrol. A prospective study has since proved that a low dose of 1 mg daily results in good antitumor effects without significant cardiovascular toxicity.

Wilms' Tumor. Improvements in survival for patients with Wilms' tumor have developed steadily in recent years. Whereas this was once considered a hopeless tumor to treat, it is now possible to control the disease for substantial periods of time in 80 percent of children with the disease. This improvement involves the sequential use of optimal surgery, radiation therapy, and chemotherapy with actinomycin D and/or vincristine. A national study group is currently trying to resolve the optimal combination of these modalities; however, it is clear that the addition of effective chemotherapy has substantially improved the care of these patients.

Carcinoma of the Breast. Recent developments involving a combination chemotherapy, estradiol receptor protein, competitive inhibitors of estrogen, medical adrenalectomy, and adjuvant chemotherapy have substantially changed the contemporary treatment of this disease.

Most physicians are currently treating advanced breast cancer with multiple combinations of drugs. One such combination includes 5-FU, cyclophosphamide, vincristine, methotrexate, and sometimes prednisone (CMFVP). Another combination includes Adriamycin and cyclophosphamide (AC) or 5-FU, Adriamycin, and cyclophosphamide (FAC). Response rates for these combinations have been generally 50 percent or greater, compared with 20 to 35 percent for the same drugs used as single agents. The median duration of response with combination chemotherapy has been in the range of 9 months.

Changing concepts of the biology of breast cancer have stimulated a number of clinical trials of adjuvant chemotherapy using single or multiple agents given intermittently over prolonged periods after operation. Many such studies are currently in progress, and most have demonstrated a reduced early recurrence rate for patients treated with adjuvant chemotherapy. One study has also shown an improved 10-year survival rate for patients

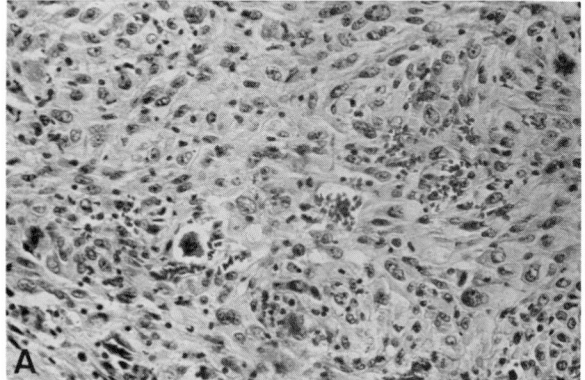

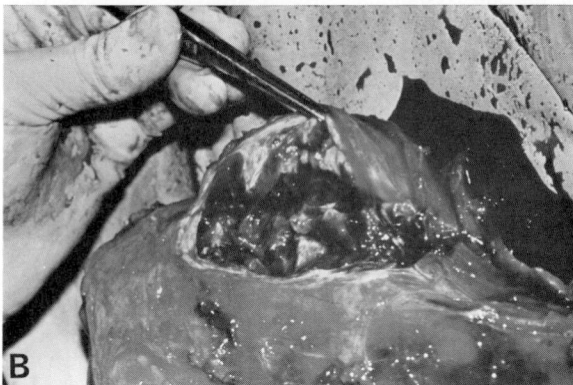

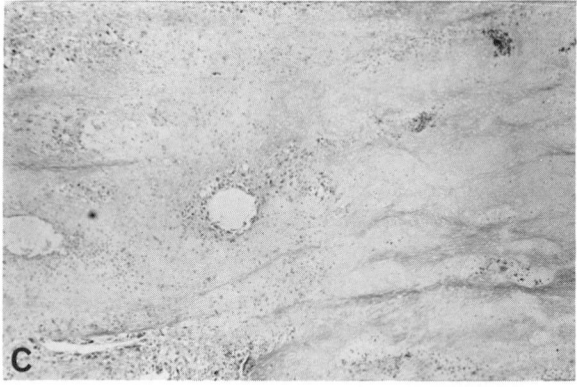

Fig. 9-17. *A.* Photomicrograph of pretreatment biopsy showing osteosarcoma with minimal necrosis (×250). *B.* Resected surgical specimen following preoperative treatment with intraarterial Adriamycin and radiation therapy. Note gross tumor liquefaction and necrosis. *C.* Photomicrograph of posttreatment specimen showing 99 percent tumor necrosis with loss of nuclei (×40). (From: *Morton DL et al: Ann Surg 184:268, 1976, with permission.*)

treated after operation with cyclophosphamide, methotrexate, and 5-fluorouracil (CMF). If these exciting preliminary results are confirmed, they will mark the first real impact on the natural history of breast cancer since the Halsted radical mastectomy.

A number of interesting therapeutic options in breast cancer are being evaluated by studies currently in progress. These include investigations to determine (1) the

optimal combination and sequence of drugs and/or hormonal agents; (2) the efficacy of adjuvant chemoimmunotherapy, chemohormonal therapy, or hormonal manipulation used alone in women with estradiol receptor–positive tumors; (3) whether surgical adrenalectomy and medical adrenalectomy using aminoglutethimide are comparable; and (4) the usefulness of the estrogen antagonist tamoxifen in different patient groups.

COMBINED MODALITY THERAPY. Pediatric oncologists pioneered the use of combined modality therapy—radiation in combination with chemotherapy and surgical therapy—to overcome childhood neoplasms. The cure rate for localized retinoblastoma and other sarcomas in children has been increased dramatically with combined therapy. Wilms' tumor can be cured 75 percent of the time if surgical therapy is followed by radiation and chemotherapy, an increase of 40 percent over operation alone. Embryonal rhabdomyosarcoma responds best to combinations of radiation, chemotherapy, and operation.

Until recently, the effectiveness of multimodality therapy had been demonstrated only occasionally for adult neoplasms. An example illustrates the complexity of such combined therapy for skeletal and soft tissue sarcomas.

Surgical therapy, the accepted method for management of most skeletal and soft tissue sarcomas of the extremity, has been associated with frequent treatment failure. Even with amputation, approximately 50 percent of patients with soft tissue sarcoma and 80 percent of those with sarcomas of bone eventually developed and died from their distant metastases. In an attempt to improve results of treatment for the sarcomas, a regimen of combined pre- and postoperative therapy was developed. Preoperative continuous intraarterial infusion of doxorubicin and radiation therapy followed by surgical resection achieved preservation of a functional extremity in most patients with no decrease in survival.

The preoperative therapy with intraarterial Adriamycin followed by radiation was found to produce extensive tumor cell necrosis as high as 88 percent (Fig. 9-17*A*, *B*, *C*). The effectiveness of this preoperative therapy permitted local resection of the sarcoma and salvage of a viable, functional extremity. Local recurrence rates are as low as with amputation, and long-term results are functionally and psychologically superior.

Early data suggest that multimodality therapy may be effective for small localized breast cancers. In several studies, radiation and minimal surgery were as effective as mastectomy for control of small breast cancers. Survival and local recurrence rates were the same for both groups, and patients treated with multimodality therapy were spared the physical deformity and the psychological problems of mastectomy.

Immunotherapy

One of the basic problems associated with all forms of cancer therapy is caused by the similarities in the biochemical and subcellular constituents of the cancer and normal cells. Although some cancer cells may have a rapid rate of cell division when compared with normal cells of the same organ, there are other normal cells in the body (e.g., those in the bone marrow and intestinal epithelium) that may grow even more rapidly. Hence, any therapy designed to inhibit the proliferation rate of cancer cells may also inhibit the function of these normal cells. Radiation and chemotherapy can injure the normal tissue as well as tumor cells. Similarly, cancer surgery often requires the sacrifice of normal tissues and organs to ensure an adequate margin around the cancer cells. In contrast, immunotherapy depends upon basic antigenic differences between neoplastic and normal cells for its therapeutic effect.

In contrast, immunotherapy is a logical adjunct for the treatment of subclinical microscopic disease following definitive cancer surgery, radiation therapy, or chemotherapy, for the following reasons: (1) Patients who have only small foci of cancer cells remaining after destruction of the major tumor bulk are the most likely to benefit from immunotherapy, because the tumor mass that must be destroyed is smallest at that time. (2) The specificity of the immune response provides a possible therapeutic tool that has selectivity for small numbers of cancer cells not possible with any other therapeutic modality. (3) Patients with disease in earlier stages are more likely to respond to immunotherapeutic maneuvers, since the cancer patient's general immune competence is greatest when the disease is localized and is often impaired after metastasis. (4) Immunotherapy should complement rather than interfere with currently available methods of cancer therapy. However, since both irradiation and chemotherapy are immunosuppressive, the use of immunotherapy in combination with these therapeutic modalities must be carefully controlled.

Numerous attempts at immunotherapy of cancer have been undertaken since the turn of the century. Although an occasional striking regression was obtained, in most cases the results were neither impressive nor consistent, and interest in this treatment modality declined until recently. With the availability of large quantities of purified biological response modifiers (such as interleukin-1 and -2, interferon, tumor necrosis factor) made available by recombinant DNA technology, a patient's immune defenses may be dramatically manipulated in a number of ways. These scientific advances, coupled with a clearer understanding of the regulation of tumor immunity, have ushered in a new era for the clinical immunotherapy of human cancer.

ACTIVE SPECIFIC IMMUNOTHERAPY. This form of immunotherapy is an effort to stimulate the host to generate a specific immune response to its tumor, generally with the use of tumor cell or tumor antigen vaccines. In this method of treatment, efforts are made to increase the patient's tumor immunity by altering the tumor antigen in such a way that it becomes more antigenic before immunizing the patient.

Most attempts at immunotherapy in human beings have involved vaccines composed of whole tumor cells inactivated by a variety of different methods to render the cells incapable of proliferation. These methods have included radiation, mitomycin C treatment, freezing and thawing,

or heat treatment. Although such techniques have prevented progressive tumor growth, they may have inactivated the tumor-specific antigens as well. For example, the same freezing and thawing technique frequently used to prepare human tumor vaccines has often inactivated tumor-specific antigens of carcinogen-induced animal neoplasms.

Studies with animal neoplasms demonstrate that living tumor cells administered intradermally in numbers insufficient for progressive tumor growth generally are the most effective immunogens. The possibility that living tumor cells might result in tumor growth at the inoculation site has inhibited the use of such vaccines in human beings. However, it would seem that with certain tumors that share common tumor-specific antigens, such as skeletal and soft tissue sarcomas, one patient could be immunized with an allogenic vaccine of living tumor cells from another patient. An immune response could be induced against the foreign HLA transplantation antigens on the tumor cells, causing their rejection. Theoretically this immunization should induce a strong immune response against a common cross-reacting tumor-specific antigen as well.

Repeated attempts have been made to increase the antigenicity of tumor vaccines by modifying the tumor cells in a variety of ways. These have included coupling highly antigenic carrier proteins such as rabbit γ-globulin to the tumor cells, and chemical treatment by agents such as iodoacetate and, more recently, with neuraminidase and concanavalin A. Regression of established tumors has been observed in animals following active immunotherapy with such vaccines (Fig. 9-18).

Many of these experiments have used immunological adjuvants as well, such as bacillus Calmette-Guérin

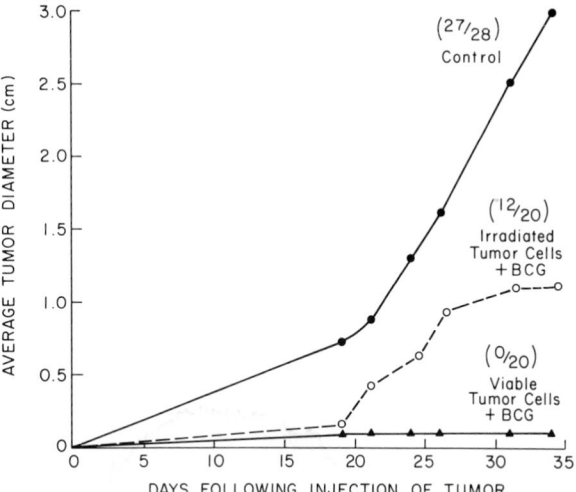

Fig. 9-18. Immunotherapy experiments with a transplantable liposarcoma in syngeneic strain 2 guinea pigs: 1×10^5 liposarcoma tumor cells were inoculated intramuscularly into the leg, and immunotherapy was initiated intradermally in four sites on the back with 1×10^6 living or 1×10^7 irradiated tumor cells mixed with bacillus Calmette-Guérin (BCG). (From: *Morton DL et al: Ann Surg 172:740, 1970, with permission.*)

(BCG) vaccine, *Corynebacterium parvum,* and Freund's adjuvant, in an attempt to enhance the host's immune response to the native or modified tumor antigens.

The ideal tumor vaccine in many respects, however, would be one composed of the isolated and purified tumor-specific transplantation antigens from the cell surface. Such vaccines would have the advantages of safety, stability, and ease of administration. Previous experience gained with guinea pig sarcomas from which isolated and partially purified tumor-specific antigen preparations induced good immunity to tumor challenge suggests that success can be anticipated for this approach. However, to date, there has been little progress along these lines with the human tumor-associated transplantation antigen.

In summary, active immunotherapy using vaccines prepared in a variety of ways combined with many different types of immunoadjuvants has been used in clinical trials. It can be demonstrated clearly that such autoimmunization procedures do enhance patients' immune responses to their own tumors. Results to date, however, have not been impressive, although newer knowledge about lymphokines that modulate the immune response suggests that active immunotherapy may become more effective in the future.

PASSIVE IMMUNOTHERAPY. In passive immunotherapy, tumor-specific antiserum is used systemically in an effort to suppress tumor. This approach is fraught with a number of theoretic and practical problems. Passive immunotherapy, for a number of reasons, is only effective in suppressing small numbers of tumor cells and must work in concert with host effectors (complement, macrophages, K cells, etc.) to effect a cytotoxic action on target cells. Moreover, only antibodies of certain classes and subclasses can interact effectively with certain cellular effectors. Finally, most of the better characterized human tumor-specific antisera are murine monoclonal antibodies that, because of their antigenicity, have limited applications in human beings. Recently, Irie and Morton have successfully used a human monoclonal IgM antibody specific for ganglioside GD2 to successfully treat human melanoma satellite lesions. The emerging field of human monoclonal antibodies will likely make these immunotherapy modalities more practical and effective.

IMMUNOTOXINS. Immunotoxins are tumor-specific antibodies to which are attached toxic molecules. This intuitively appealing concept, first proposed by Paul Ehrlich one century ago, employs the antibody molecule to preferentially localize anticancer agents in the vicinity of tumors. It obviates the need for the host to supply effector cells or complement to mediate tumor destruction. Monoclonal antibodies are preferred to heterologous antiserum since they permit the use of homogeneous, purified antibodies of defined specificity. A wide range of toxic molecules has been tested in vitro and includes radioactive isotopes, traditional cancer drugs, and plant and bacterial toxins. Recombinant DNA technology now permits the creation of hybrid or chimeric immunotoxin molecules in which the Fc portion of the immunoglobulin molecule has been replaced by a polypeptide toxin sequence. Immunotoxins are currently undergoing clinical trials, although their overall therapeutic efficiency in clinical oncology is unproved.

ADOPTIVE IMMUNOTHERAPY. In adoptive immunotherapy, immune lymphoid cells are transferred to a recipient to mediate tumor destruction. In many experimental murine tumors, in vivo transfer of lymphocytes from an immune mouse to a tumor-bearing mouse can cause dramatic tumor regression (Fig. 9-19). These immune lymphocytes are tumor-antigen-specific, display major histocompatibility complex restriction, and have classical T cell markers; thus, they are classical cytolytic T lymphocytes. In these animal models, it is necessary to use large numbers of cells from immunized, syngeneic (genetically identical) donor mice. This effective immunotherapeutic modality is unfortunately technically impractical in human beings.

Rosenberg and colleagues have pioneered the study of adoptive immunotherapy using so-called lymphokine-activated killer (LAK) cells. LAK cells are cytolytic lymphocytes that are generated in the presence of interleukin-2 (IL-2). Treatment of human lymphocytes from almost any source (peripheral blood, lymph nodes, spleen, thymus, bone marrow) results in the creation of cytolytic cells capable of killing a wide range of fresh and cultured human cancer cells but not normal cells. The biochemical nature of this tumor-specific recognition and killing is not fully defined. Human LAK cells do not have T cell markers and are not MHC or antigen-specific in their killing. It is not yet certain whether they represent a novel cell type or are expanded and modified from an NK precursor pool.

Extensive animal experiments demonstrate the ability of systemically administered LAK cells and IL-2 to cause dramatic regression of many different types of primary and metastatic tumors. Clinical trials using autologous LAK cells (obtained by repeated leukopheresis and in vitro IL-2 expansion) and systemically administered IL-2 have resulted in clear, objective responses in some patients with bulky metastatic cancer. Administration of high doses of IL-2 alone have some clinical efficacy but considerable toxicity. Even greater toxicity is seen with combined administration of LAK cells and IL-2 and includes fluid retention and renal dysfunction. Nevertheless, these impressive studies, in patients with large tumor burdens, are an exciting glimpse of the potential of properly manipulated immune systems.

NONSPECIFIC IMMUNOTHERAPY

The theoretic basis for nonspecific immunotherapy depends upon the observation that certain substances, such as mixed bacterial toxins and fractions of the tubercle bacillus, have the ability to nonspecifically enhance host resistance to most viral, fungal, and bacterial agents. Although the exact mechanism is unknown, these agents do appear to stimulate immune response to a wide variety of antigens, including tumor antigens.

Historically, a type of nonspecific immunotherapy was described by Bradford Coley at the turn of the century in one of the first reports of a tumor regression possibly in-

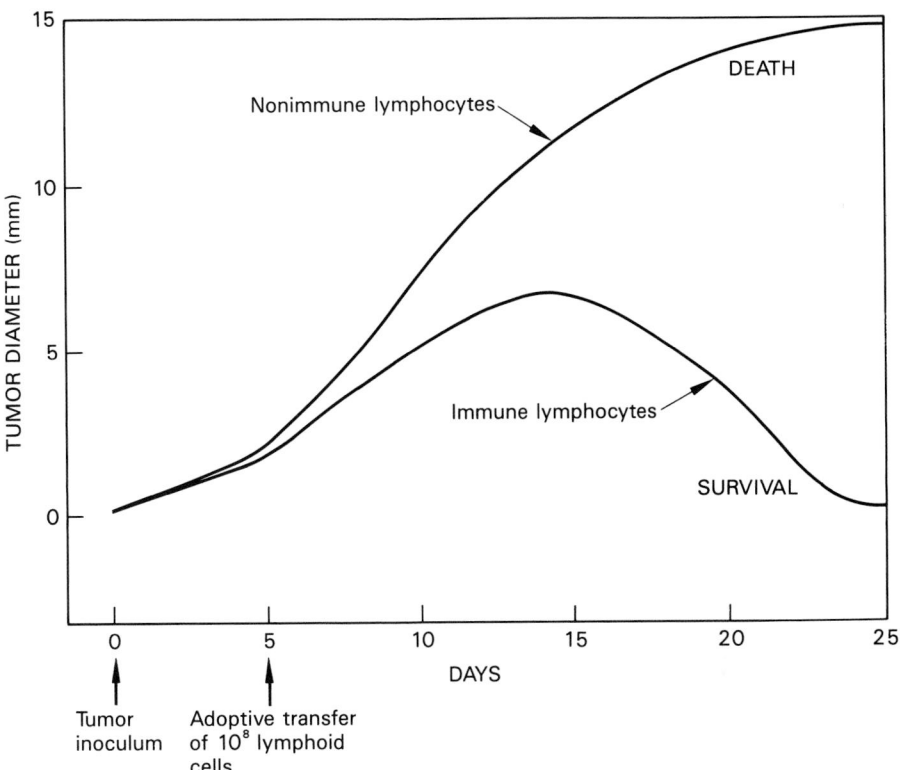

Fig. 9-19. Regression of experimental tumor upon adoptive transfers of immune lymphocytes.

duced by immunologic means. Coley's interest in the possible value of such therapy was stimulated when he observed a recurrent inoperable sarcoma of the neck regress completely for 7 years after the patient had had attacks of erysipelas. This observation led to the development of Coley's toxins, a mixture of killed bacterial vaccines. Coley injected this admixture directly into tumor lesions or gave it intravenously. Some impressive regressions of tumors and long-term cures resulted from these agents. Because the responses were inconsistent, Coley's toxins never received widespread use, and interest in them died out. Recent interest in a nonspecific immunotherapy of a similar type has been revived using attenuated bovine tuberculosis bacillus (BCG).

Our work with BCG began more than 20 years ago, when we injected BCG into metastatic nodules in the skin and subcutaneous tissues in patients with malignant melanoma. We observed that the intratumor injection of BCG caused 90 percent of the intradermal metastases to regress in patients who were immunologically competent. In addition, in about 20 percent of these patients, uninjected nodules were observed to regress. Satellite, intransit metastases, and local recurrence often can be controlled in the extremity by this technique; however, many of these patients still develop systemic metastases. Although the intratumor injection of BCG may not control systemic disease, it is nonetheless a very useful method to control local disease that avoids the side effects of chemotherapy and can result in long-term survival.

There are several possible mechanisms to explain tumor regression following BCG injection; both specific and nonspecific immune reactions were probably involved. The tumor cells may be killed as "innocent bystanders" during the delayed cutaneous hypersensitivity reaction that occurs when lymphocytes and macrophages attack BCG dispersed throughout the tumor nodule. This is supported by the observation that the intratumor injection of BCG works only in patients who can be sensitized to BCG, as shown by their delayed cutaneous hypersensitivity reaction to PPD.

In addition to the nonspecific effect, a specific immune response to melanoma-associated tumor antigens also occurs in some patients because an associated rising titer of antimelanoma antibody is observed following BCG immunotherapy. Sequential biopsies of tumor nodules following BCG inoculation reveals that the regression of these nodules is associated with a granulomatous infiltration of lymphocytes, monocytes, and fibroblasts surrounding and infiltrating the melanoma cells. Furthermore, the regression of melanoma nodules not given injection with BCG is accompanied by the appearance of lymphocyte infiltrates within the regressing melanoma tumor nodules (Fig. 9-20). The specific antitumor effect may result from more lymphocytes and macrophages coming into contact with the tumor cells so that the afferent limb of the immune response is increased. Conversely, it may work via the effector limb of the immune response by bringing greater numbers of both stimulated and unstimulated lymphocytes to the tumor.

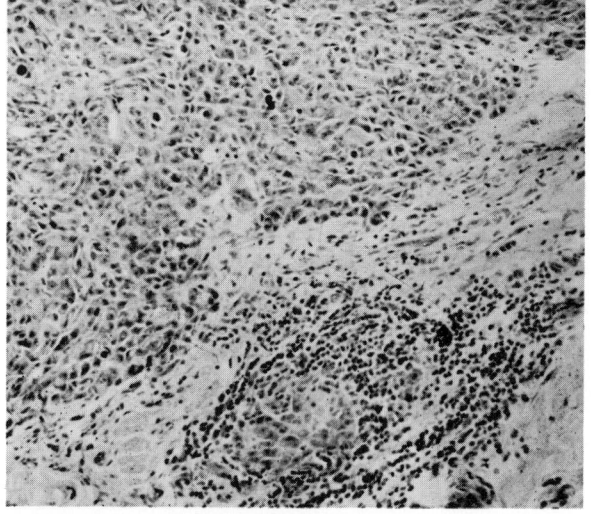

A

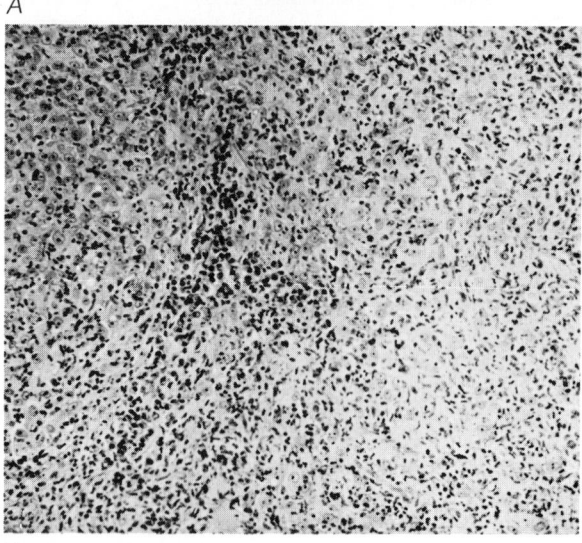

B

Fig. 9-20. *A.* Subcutaneous metastasis of malignant melanoma prior to immunotherapy with BCG. Note the absence of lymphocytic and monocytic infiltration among the tumor cells. *B.* Subcutaneous metastasis that has decreased in size from 10 to 5 mm during the 6-week period following immunotherapy with BCG injections into other melanoma nodules. BCG was *not* injected into this nodule. Note the marked lymphocytic and monocytic infiltration among the melanoma cells. (From: *Morton DL et al: Ann Surg 172:740, 1970, with permission.*)

Our results have now been confirmed by a number of investigators. The observation that the intratumor injection of BCG occasionally led to the regression of uninjected nodules suggested that BCG might be useful as an adjuvant to operation to control micrometastatic disease in human beings. BCG has been shown to prevent growth of spontaneous metastases in some animal tumor models where variables of tumor load and time of BCG vaccination can be carefully controlled. In human beings, a number of preliminary reports have suggested that intradermal BCG delays recurrence in patients with melanoma

who are at high risk because of metastases to regional nodes. However, in our prospective randomized trial of adjuvant immunotherapy, BCG did not diminish the recurrence rate, but did significantly extend survival once the disease recurred.

BCG is only one of a wide variety of agents that can nonspecifically stimulate the immune system's response to a variety of different types of antigens. Examples of other agents include *Corynebacterium parvum,* MER (methanol-extractable residue of BCG), bacterial antitoxins, and polynucleotides.

Other impressive results with nonspecific immunotherapy come from the studies of Klein in patients with basal and squamous cell carcinomas of the skin. Here the induction of delayed hypersensitivity reactions to DNCB resulted in the resolution of more than 90 percent of superficial basal or squamous cell carcinomas. Klein observed that the mixture of multiple antigens such as PPD, mumps, and *Candida* increased the delayed hypersensitivity and effectiveness of this form of immunotherapy.

Another form of nonspecific immunotherapy involves the use of agents capable of restoring depressed immune responses. Several agents have been proposed in such a context, including thymic hormones such as thymosin and the antihelminthic drug levamisole.

The rational application of immunotherapy to human cancer will depend, to a large extent, on a better knowledge of tumor-associated antigens in human neoplasms and methods for increasing the immune response against these antigens. Specificity for cancer cells cannot be achieved by any other known therapeutic means, but the potency of immunotherapy is limited.

Expectations of dramatic benefits from immunotherapy for malignant disease have been high; however, the results of many clinical trials have fallen short of these expectations. The theoretical advantages of a specific systemic antitumor adjuvant with minimal toxicity continues to make immunotherapy a promising avenue of future investigation. At the present time, its use should be limited to cancer facilities where the effects of this form of treatment can be scientifically evaluated.

SURGERY AS IMMUNOTHERAPY

A tumor may promote its own growth by a number of immune mechanisms. The cancer cell may act as a "factory" that is constantly producing both immunosuppressive factors and tumor-associated antigens (Fig. 9-21). The specific and nonspecific immunosuppression decreases the patient's immune defenses and facilitates growth of the tumor. In numerous studies, this immunosuppression appears to be related to the presence of the tumor.

The key to recovery of the balance in the host-tumor relationship depends on destruction or removal of the tumor cell "factory." Surgery appears to be the most efficient means of removing the factory. Once the mass of tumor is gone, the patient with cancer is more likely to be able to mount an immune response that may destroy any subclinical foci of tumor cells scattered through the body.

CANCER SURGERY AS IMMUNOTHERAPY

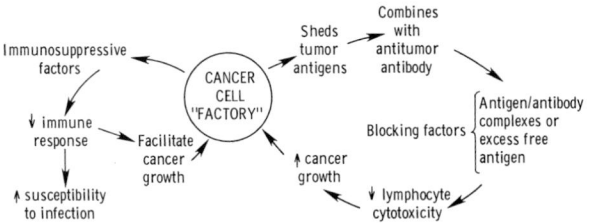

Fig. 9-21. Schematic of cancer cell factory as it might function to enhance its growth by producing immunosuppression in the host. Theoretically, cancer surgery removes the cancer factory and its associated immunosuppressants, which allows the host immune responses to return to normal. (From: *Morton DL et al: Chest 71:640, 1977, with permission.*)

However, if the recovery of the immune response is inadequate or if the number of tumor cells in any distant metastatic focus is too large, the patient may fail to regain control of the disease. Nonetheless, surgery for cancer becomes the first step in immunotherapy.

If this thesis is correct, it would follow that the approach to the surgical treatment for solid neoplasms must change dramatically. The future lies not in treating every patient with a solid neoplasm as one with localized disease but in assuming that the local disease is merely a manifestation of a systemic illness, whether or not the patient has overt metastatic disease. Not until we accept surgery as merely the first step in the treatment of cancer can we significantly improve our rates of cure. Therapeutic advances eventually must come from a multimethod combination of immunotherapy and chemotherapy with surgical therapy or radiotherapy. Unlike surgery and radiotherapy, both local treatments, the triple combinations represent a systemic treatment effective against tumor cells already metastatic to distant sites. However, at present, systemic therapeutic techniques have greater potential for curing those patients with a minimal number of tumor cells, rather than those with clinically evident disease. Surgery for apparently localized tumors can favorably affect the host-tumor relationship and may even cure the patient with subclinical distant metastases. However, debulking the unresectable or recurrent tumors in the patient with metastatic disease is usually unsuccessful and rarely indicated.

Hyperthermia*

National efforts are under way to establish additional safe and reliable forms of therapy. Results in laboratory models, animals, and initial human clinical trials have been very encouraging and suggest that thermal therapy—hyperthermia—may have a substantive role in future cancer treatment. In 1967, Cavaliere and his colleagues in Rome announced that tumor cells were apparently selectively thermosensitive compared with normal cells at

* Storm FK (ed): *Hyperthermia in Cancer Therapy*. Chicago, Year Book Medical Publishers, 1985.

temperatures from 42 to 45°C (108 to 113°F). During the late 1960s and early 1970s, evidence continued to suggest that at 42 to 45°C tumor cells were slightly more sensitive to heat than normal cells. When a cell subline derived from a non-tumor-producing line acquired high tumor-producing ability, it also acquired reduced thermotolerance. These and other investigations both in vitro and in vivo suggested that the acquisition of malignant potential was associated with increased thermosensitivity.

Investigators have found that a major factor in cell killing at 42°C is the irreversible damage to cancer cell respiration. Coincident alterations appear to take place in nucleic acid and protein synthesis that include a reduction of activity in many vital enzyme systems. These factors, associated with an increase in cell-wall membrane permeability and the liberation of lysozymes, probably account for the autolytic cell destruction after hyperthermia. The efficacy of thermocytotoxicity increased rapidly as temperatures were increased from 42 to 45°C, the threshold of thermal pain in human beings. At such temperatures, the differential thermosensitivity between malignant and normal cells is reduced and replaced by a linear cell kill from progressive protein denaturation. Thus, at 45°C, host tissue tolerance becomes a prime concern in the design of clinical trials.

It is well known from experiments on exposed tumors that energy concentrated within a tumor, from interstitial implants, focused ultrasound, or microwaves potentially provides enough local heat for tumor destruction. Less well known is the fact that nonfocused microwaves and capacitive, inductive, and magnetic-loop radio-frequency applicators can heat a region of the host that contains the tumor, providing "selective tumor heating," this having remarkable implications for the treatment of deep-seated tumors. Extensive temperature measurements during hyperthermia therapy in spontaneous animal and human tumors demonstrate that many tumors selectively retain more heat than normal tissues because their neovascularity is physiologically unresponsive to thermal stress and is incapable of regulating and augmenting blood flow. Thus effective independent tumor heating is possible deep within the body, even without the ability to focus such energy.

Interstitial hyperthermia has been achieved by passing a low-frequency current between electrodes implanted directly into tumors. While invasive, this technique has been useful for small accessible tumors where the full extent of the lesion was known (for example, oropharynx, vagina, and rectum). Liquid silicone impregnated with finely powdered iron particles has been used to occlude the vascular beds of tumors. The potential for selectively heating the metallic material that remains in the tumor in the vulcanized silicone offers promise. Ultrasound, a well-defined and spatially manipulative source of acoustic energy when focused, has potential for noninvasive selective heating of a target volume at depth. However, unlike electromagnetic energy, ultrasound does not propagate effectively through air and is ineffective near air-containing spaces (for example, oral-nasal cavity and respiratory and gastrointestinal tracts). Most clinical trials have been limited to superficial tumors heated to 43 to 45°C. Microwaves have produced effective noninvasive localized hyperthermia to large areas of surface tissues and have been quite useful for treatment of superficial tumors. Radio frequency (RF) has provided a means for both local and regional in-depth noninvasive hyperthermia, particularly when magnetic-loop applicators are employed. These create a strong electromagnetic field into which the body or limb is immersed. This approach permits safe and effective heating of visceral human tumors and has provided most of the available knowledge about the effects of localized heat therapy on deep internal human cancers.

Effective hyperthermia can be achieved in most superficial and visceral solid human tumors regardless of histopathologic type, although it is most effective for large tumors. Some tumors cannot be safely heated to 42°C and seem to retain their ability to regulate blood flow and dissipate heat. Distinct histologic changes occur in effectively heated tumor cells but not in stromal or vascular cells within the tumor, or in adjacent normal tissues. Rapid autolytic disintegration of heat-damaged tumor cells is observed, followed by a marked increase in connective stroma associated with progressive scar formation. Progressive coagulation necrosis occurs at 45°C, although its results appear to differ depending on the location of the tumor. Superficial tumors generally slough off, whereas visceral tumors may not significantly change in size after a transient increase in size during treatment. Therefore, biopsy or careful assessment of tumor doubling time (for example, stabilization of a previously progressive tumor) is necessary to determine the effects of high-temperature internal tumor therapy.

At temperatures greater than 45°C, tumors display extensive vascular thrombosis. Subsequent resection has been facilitated in some instances by the avascular nature of the tumor. Heat also sensitizes tissues to ionizing radiation. Hyperthermia has been combined with radiation therapy, both external beam and interstitial, in an effort to produce a synergistic or additive response. Several investigators have concluded that hypoxic cells may be at least as sensitive to hyperthermia as oxygenated cells, forming one rationale for combination therapy. Others have suggested that the primary effect of hyperthermia is to inhibit cellular recovery from sublethal radiation injury. As previously noted, heat seems to alter tumor cell membrane permeability. This finding suggested that enhanced intracellular drug uptake might occur at elevated temperatures, which has since been documented in in vitro studies. A recent review of laboratory investigations has shown an additional 2- to 3-log kill at 43 to 45°C over that at 37°C for thiotepa, bleomycin, phenylalanine mustard (L-PAM), amphotericin B, methyl-CCNU, CCNU, cisplatin, methotrexate, and Adriamycin. The best-known clinical example of this synergism can be found in regional hyperthermic chemotherapeutic limb perfusion for in-transit metastatic melanoma. Once hyperthermia therapy is optimized, it may be possible to achieve responses at lower drug doses, which, in turn, may reduce drug toxicity and prolong the duration of therapy. It also may be possible to reinstitute use of previously less effective drugs with the expectation of enhanced activity due to hyperthermia.

PROGNOSIS

Predicting the future course of a patient's malignant disease is one of the most difficult problems an oncologist faces. At the present time, it is impossible to predict the future course of a given patient except in general terms. However, a number of known factors are important in determining prognosis.

The *site of origin* of the primary tumor is one of the most important factors influencing prognosis. The propensity of a neoplasm to metastasize to distant sites varies according to its tissue of origin. Over 90 percent of carcinomas of the lung, pancreas, and esophagus spread beyond their primary site and cause death, whereas carcinomas of the skin, breast, and thyroid glands are frequently localized and curable, even when metastatic in some patients.

The *stage of disease* at the time of initial treatment is of considerable importance in determining survival for all types of neoplasms. The chance for cure is best when the neoplasm is confined to the organ of origin. The smaller the primary neoplasm, the better the prognosis, as well. Thus, in situ carcinoma of the cervix, carcinomas of the breast less than 1 cm in diameter, and small polypoid carcinomas of the colon are generally curable; larger neoplasms may not be curable. Direct extension into adjacent organs or metastases to regional nodes suggest a more guarded prognosis, although many patients are still curable at this stage of the disease. The spread of cancer by the bloodstream with metastases to distant sites portends a grave prognosis, and few patients are curable at this stage. As a general rule, lymph node involvement sharply reduces survival probability by about one-half that of patients without involved nodes. The total number of involved nodes is an important prognostic guide.

The *histopathologic features* of the neoplasm correlate in a general way to prognosis. The more undifferentiated, highly malignant-appearing neoplasms with frequent mitosis are more likely to develop early distant spread and local recurrence. However, some very malignant neoplasms still can be cured with adequate treatment. Venous invasion is a grave prognostic factor in all types of neoplasia.

Host immune factors, as previously discussed, may be an important factor in determining prognosis. Immunologic methods for monitoring immune responses are currently under development. It is already apparent that those patients who have spontaneous depression of their immune responses have a uniformly poor prognosis following therapy.

The *age of the patient* may be an important factor affecting prognosis. Some oncologists believe that neoplasms in younger patients carry a poorer prognosis than the same tumors in middle-aged or elderly patients, although elderly patients may have associated medical problems that do not permit adequate treatment of the cancer. While there may be some validity in this concept, it should not be overemphasized, because many young patients have a good prognosis. In fact, some have a much better prognosis than adults with the same neoplasms. Those neoplasms which occur prior to one year of age generally have a better prognosis than those which occur later in childhood. This can be determined in the following manner: The child is usually cured of the neoplasm if free of disease for 9 months after treatment, plus double the age at the time treatment was begun. This concept is based upon the supposition that if the earliest cancer cell started with conception and if the cancer grew at a constant rate, then it would reach a certain size at the time treatment was initiated. If treatment was successful in eliminating all cancer cells except one, then in a period equal to 9 months plus double the age of the child, the cancer size would again be equivalent to the original tumor mass. Therefore, if there is no recurrence after this time span, it can be assumed that the patient is cured.

The *adequacy of treatment* is most relevant to prognosis for certain types of neoplasms. The cure rate for some neoplasms, such as soft tissue sarcomas and certain childhood neoplasms, may be twice as high in sophisticated cancer centers when compared with cure rates in small community hospitals where experience and supportive systems are less extensive.

PSYCHOLOGIC MANAGEMENT OF THE CANCER PATIENT

The physician can ease the cancer patient's fear of the disease by free and open communication. Psychologic support and education are necessary in order for the patient to deal with any disability that may result from therapy. Examples include training in the care of a stoma following curative surgery for colonic and rectal cancer or referral to lay groups associated with the American Cancer Society for counseling the anxious patient with an altered body image resulting from mastectomy.

Despite the prognostic factors discussed previously, it is still impossible to predict the exact course of any malignant tumor. Patients with the most grim prognoses are occasionally cured by aggressive therapy, and spontaneous regressions are sometimes observed even in patients with metastases. In contrast, some patients with apparently localized disease may be dead of disseminated cancer in a few months. This uncertainty about the future is one of the most difficult adjustments faced by cancer patients and their families. Most reassuring in this regard is to emphasize that for each month that passes following successful treatment of the primary neoplasm, the chances for cure improve. This is particularly correct for tumors such as squamous cell carcinoma of the lung or oral pharynx. Although other, more slowly growing neoplasms, such as carcinoma of the breast and malignant melanoma, may recur after disease-free intervals of 10 or 20 years, the chances of recurrence also decrease with

time. Recognition that cancer is a chronic disease is an important aspect of management. Long-term, consistent follow-up provides opportunities for reassurance and usually can ensure detection of recurrence at an early stage.

Some patients do not want to know about their illness for fear of having their suspicions verified. Never lie to a patient, even if requested by the family. In general, gentle and optimistic truth is best. Untruths often create barriers between patients and their families that can lead to psychologic isolation of patients who are unable to discuss their fears and anxieties with those they need most.

With the patient for whom primary cancer therapy has failed, one of the most difficult problems faced by the physician is "What should the patient be told?" Most oncologists who deal exclusively with cancer patients agree that the incurable patient also must be told the truth as gently and optimistically as possible. Hope and reassurance as to the physician's continuing concern are best sustained by continuing active treatment until it is certain that the patient can no longer benefit. Realistic and consistent support is actually more important to the patient and the family at this stage of the disease than earlier. There is increasing evidence that patients tolerate the process of dying much better when cared for in this manner.

Some incurable patients are unable to accept the realities of the situation. In this case, it is essential that a responsible family member be informed. The life duration of the incurable patient is so uncertain that predictions should be avoided. If, as frequently happens, the relatives insist upon some estimate, a combined minimum-maximum prognosis, such as from 6 months to 2 years, will help the family accept this uncertainty.

The basic aim in caring for the patient with advanced cancer is to prolong useful life, but not useless suffering. The patient should be permitted to die with dignity when active therapy can no longer be of benefit.

Bibliography

Etiology

American Cancer Society: *Cancer Facts and Figures*. New York, 1987.

Barbocid M: Human oncogenes, in DeVita VY, Hellmen S, Rosenberg SA (eds): *Important Advances in Oncology*. Philadelphia, Lippincott, 1986, p 3.

Barratt RW, Tatum EL: Carcinogenic mutagens. *Ann NY Acad Sci* 71:1072, 1958.

Bishop JM: The molecular genetics of cancer. *Science* 235:305, 1987.

Bishop JM: Retroviruses and cancer genes. *Cancer* 55:2329, 1985.

Bister K, Jansen HW: Oncogenes in retroviruses and cells; biochemistry and molecular genetics. *Adv Cancer Res* 47:99, 1986.

Boice JD Jr, Fraumeni JF Jr (eds): *Radiation Carcinogenesis: Epidemiology and Biological Significance*. New York, Raven, 1984.

Boyland E: The history and future of chemical carcinogenesis. *Br Med Bull* 36:5, 1980.

Butlin HT: Cancer of the scrotum in chimney-sweeps and others: I. Secondary cancer without primary cancer. II. Why foreign sweeps do not suffer from scrotal cancer. III. Tar and paraffin cancer. *Br Med J* 1:1341; 2:1; 3:66, 1892.

Campisi J, Fingert HJ, Pardee AB: Basic biology and biochemistry of cancer, in Knapp RC, Berkowitz RS (eds): *Gynecologic Oncology*. New York, Macmillan, 1984, chap 2.

Doll R: The epidemiology of cancer. *Cancer* 45:2475, 1980.

Elson LE, Betts TE: Death rates from cancer of the respiratory and oral tracts in different countries in relation to the types of tobacco smoked. *Eur J Cancer* 17:109, 1981.

Garfinkel MA: Cancer mortality in nonsmokers; prospective study by the American Cancer Society. *J Natl Cancer Inst* 65:1169, 1981.

Heuper WC: Environmental cancer, in Homburger F (ed): *The Physiopathology of Cancer*. New York, Harper & Row, 1959, p 919.

Kennaway EC: The formation of a cancer producing substance from isoprene (2-methyl-butadiene). *J Pathol Bacteriol* 27:233, 1924.

Kindt TJ, Robinson MA: Major histocompatibility complex antigens, in Paul WE (ed): *Fundamental Immunology*. New York, Raven, 1984, pp 347–378.

Land H, Parada LF, Weinberg RA: Cellular oncogenes and multistep carcinogenesis. *Science* 222:771, 1983.

Lee Y-T (Margaret): Cancer statistics of Chinese versus Americans. *J Surg Oncol* 27:355, 1981.

Locke FB, King H: Cancer mortality risk among Japanese in the United States. *J Natl Cancer Inst* 65:1149, 1980.

Lorenz E: Radioactivity and lung cancer: a critical review of lung cancer in the miners of Schneeburg and Joachimstall. *Cancer Res* 5:1, 1944.

Martland HS: Occupational poisoning in manufacture of luminous watch dials: General review of hazard caused by ingestion of luminous paint with special reference to the New Jersey cases. *JAMA* 92:466, 1929.

Minz B, Fleischman RA: Teratocarcinomas and other neoplasms as developmental defects in gene expression. *Adv Cancer Res* 34:211, 1981.

Porter CD, White CJ: Multiple carcinomata following chronic x-ray dermatitis. *Ann Surg* 46:649, 1970.

Pott P: *Chirurgical Observations Relative to the Cataract, the Polypus of the Nose, the Cancer of the Scrotum, the Different Kinds of Ruptures, and the Mortification of the Toes and Feet*. London, Hawkes, Clarke and Collins, 1775.

Prehn RT: Specific isoantigenicities among chemically induced tumors. *Ann NY Acad Sci* 101:107, 1962.

Rous P: Transmission of a malignant new growth by means of a cell-free filtrate. *JAMA* 56:198, 1911.

Schottenfeld D: The epidemiology of cancer: an overview. *Cancer* 47:1095, 1981.

Schreiber MM, Bozzo PD, et al: Malignant melanoma in Southern Arizona: Increasing incidence and sunlight as an etiologic factor. *Arch Dermatol* 117:6, 1981.

Seeger RG, Brodeur GM, et al: Association of multiple copies of the V-mvc oncogene with rapid progression of neuroblastomas. *N Engl J Med* 313:1111, 1985.

Shimkin MB: Research on the causes and nature of cancer, in del Regato JA, Spjut HJ (eds): *Cancer*. St. Louis, Mosby, 1977, p 3.

Storer JB: Radiation carcinogenesis, in Becker FF (ed): *Cancer:* *A Comprehensive Treatise,* 2d ed. New York, Plenum, 1982, vol 1, pp 629–659.

Varmus HE: The discovery of cellular oncogenes and their role in neoplasia. *Cancer* 55:2324, 1985.

VanBeveren C, Vermal M: Homology among oncogenes. *Curr Top Microbiol Immunol* 123:73, 1986.

Waterfield MD, Scrace GT, Whittle N, et al: Platelet-derived growth factor is structurally related to the putative transforming protein p28 in sarcoma virus. *Nature* 304:35, 1983.

Wigle DT, Mae Y, et al: Relative importance of smoking as a risk factor for selected cancers. *Can J Publ Health* 71:269, 1980.

Biology and Immunobiology

Black PH: Shedding from the cell surface of normal and cancer cells. *Adv Cancer Res* 32:75, 1980.

Burnet FM: *Immunological Surveillance*. New York, Pergamon, 1970.

Drysdale BE, Zacharcheck CM, Shin HS: Mechanisms of macrophage mediated cytotoxicity: Production of a soluble cytotoxic factor. *J Immunol* 131:2362, 1983.

Eilber FR, Morton DL: Impaired immunologic reactivity and recurrence following cancer surgery. *Cancer* 25:362, 1970.

Eilber FR, Nizze A, Morton DL: Sequential evaluation of general immune competence in cancer patients: correlation with clinical course. *Cancer* 35:660, 1975.

Everson TC, Cole WH: *Spontaneous Regression of Cancer*. Philadelphia, Saunders, 1966.

Fidler IJ, Hart IR: Biological diversity in metastatic neoplasms: Origins and implications. *Science* 217:998–1003, 1982.

Foley EJ: Antigenic properties of methylcholanthrene-induced tumors in mice of the strain or origin. *Cancer Res* 13:835, 1953.

Gatti RA, Good RA: Occurrence of malignancy in immunodeficiency diseases: A literature review. *Cancer* 28:89, 1971.

Giuliano AE, Rangel DM, et al: Serum-mediated immunosuppression in lung cancer. *Cancer* 43:917, 1979.

Gold P, Freedman SO: Specific carcinoembryonic antigens of the human digestive system. *J Exp Med* 122:467, 1965.

Golightly MG, D'Amore P, et al: Studies on cytotoxicity generated in human mixed lymphocyte cultures. III. Natural killerlike cytotoxicity mediated by human lymphocytes with receptors for IgM. *Cell Immunol* 70:219, 1982.

Golub SH, D'Amore P, et al: Systemic administration of human leukocyte interferon to melanoma patients. II. Cellular events associated with changes in NK cytotoxicity. *J Natl Cancer Inst* 68:711, 1982.

Golub SH, Dorey F, et al: Systemic administration of human leukocyte interferon to melanoma patients. I. Effects of NK function and cell populations. *J Natl Cancer Inst* 68:703, 1982.

Goodwin WE: Regression of hypernephromas. *JAMA* 20:609, 1968.

Gupta RK, Morton DL: Clinical significance of tumor-associated antigens and anti-tumor antibodies in human malignant melanoma, in Reisfeld RA, Ferrone S (eds): *Melanoma Antibodies and Antigens*. New York, Plenum, 1982, p. 139.

Henney CS, Gillis S: Cell-mediated cytotoxicity, in Paul WE (ed): *Fundamental Immunology*. New York, Raven, 1984, pp 669–684.

Klein G: Tumor antigens. *Ann Rev Microbiol* 20:223, 1966.

Kohler PF: Human complement system, in Samter M (ed): *Immunologic Diseases,* 3d ed. Boston, Little, Brown, 1979, pp 244–280.

Morton DL: Acquired immunological tolerance and carcinogenesis by the mammary tumor virus. I. Influence of neonatal infection with the mammary tumor virus on the growth of spontaneous mammary adenocarcinomas. *J Natl Cancer Inst* 42:311, 1969.

Morton DL, Eilber FR, et al: Immunological factors in human sarcomas and melanomas: A rational basis for immunotherapy. *Ann Surg* 172:740, 1970.

Morton DL, Holmes EC, et al: Immunological aspects of neoplasia: a rational basis for immunotherapy. *Ann Intern Med* 74:587, 1971.

Old LJ, Boyse EA: Antigens of tumors and leukemias induced by virus. *Fed Proc* 24:1009, 1965.

Old LJ, Boyse EA, Stockert E: Antigenic properties of experimental leukemias: I. Serological studies in vitro with spontaneous and radiation-induced leukemias. *J Natl Cancer Inst* 31:977, 1963.

Old LJ, Stockert E, et al: Antigenic modulation: loss of TL antigen from cells exposed to TL antibody: Study of the phenomenon in vitro. *J Exp Med* 127:523, 1968.

Paul WE: *Fundmental Immunology*. New York, Raven, 1984.

Piessens WF: Evidence of human cancer immunity. *Cancer* 26:1212, 1970.

Pilch YH, Meyers GH, et al: Prospects for the immunotherapy of cancer: Part I, Basic concepts of tumor immunology. *Curr Probl Surg* January 1975, p 1.

Pitot HC: The natural history of neoplastic development: the relation of experimental models to human cancer. *Cancer* 49:1206, 1982.

Prehn RT, Main JM: Immunity to methylcholanthrene-induced sarcomas. *J Natl Cancer Inst* 18:769, 1957.

Reinherz EL, Meuner SC, Schlossman SF: The human T cell receptor: Analysis with cytotoxic T cell clones. *Immunol Rev* 74:83, 1983.

Skipper HE: In *The Proliferation and Spread of Neoplastic Cells*. Baltimore, Williams & Wilkins, 1968.

Southam CM, Brunschwig W, et al: The effect of leukocytes on transplantability of human cancer. *Cancer* 19:1743, 1966.

Stutman O: The immunological surveillance hypothesis, in Herberman RB (ed): *Basic and Clinical Tumor Immunology*. Boston, Martinus Nijhoff, 1983, pp 1–81.

Sugarbaker EV: *Cancer Metastasis: A Product of Tumor-Host Interactions*. Chicago, Year Book Medical Publishers, 1979, no 7, vol 3, pp 1–59.

Watson JD, Mochizuki DY, Gillis S: Molecular characterization of interleukin-2. *Fed Proc* 42:2747, 1983.

Watson JD, Tooze J, Kurtz DT: *Recombinant DNA*. Scientific American, New York, 1983.

Pathology

Anderson W: The general pathology of tumors, in *Boyd's Pathology for the Surgeon*. Philadelphia, Saunders, 1967, p 92.

Bloom HJG, Richardson WW, Harries EJ: Natural history of untreated breast cancer (1805–1933): Comparison of untreated and treated cases according to histological grade of malignancy. *Br Med J* 2:213, 1962.

Boyd W: *An Introduction to the Study of Disease*. Philadelphia, Lea & Febiger, 1971, p 210.

Cole WH, McDonald GO, et al: *Dissemination of Cancer*. New York, Appleton-Century-Crofts, 1961.

Collins VP, Leoffler RK, Tivey H: Observations on growth rates of human tumors. *Am J Roentgenol Radium Ther Nucl Med* 76:988, 1956.

Everson TC: Spontaneous regression of cancer. *Ann NY Acad Sci* 114:721, 1964.

Garland LH, Coulson W, Wollin E: The rate of growth and apparent duration of untreated primary bronchial carcinoma. *Cancer* 16:694, 1963.

Hawkins RS, Roberts MM, et al: Oestrogen receptors and breast cancer: Current status. *Br J Surg* 67:153, 1980.

MacMahon B, Feng MA: Prenatal origin of childhood leukemia: Evidence from twins. *N Engl J Med* 270:1082, 1964.

Moertel CG: Incidence and significance of multiple primary malignant neoplasms. *Ann NY Acad Sci* 114:886, 1964.

Pearson HA, Grello FW, Cane EC Jr: Leukemia in identical twins. *N Engl J Med* 268:1151, 1963.

Pund ER, Nettles TB, et al: Preinvasive and invasive carcinoma of the cervix uteri: Pathogenesis, detection, differential diagnosis, and pathologic basis for management. *Am J Obstet Gynecol* 55:831, 1948.

Rigler LB: Natural history of untreated lung cancer. *Ann NY Acad Sci* 114:755, 1964.

Russell WO, Ibanex ML, et al: Thyroid carcinoma: Classification, intraglandular dissemination, and clinicopathologic study based upon whole organ sections of 80 glands. *Cancer* 16:1425, 1963.

Slaughter DP: Multicentric origin of intraoral carcinoma. *Surgery* 20:133, 1946.

Viadana E, Kwai-Lung A: Patterns of metastases in adenocarcinomas of man. *J Med* 6:1. 1975.

Clinical Manifestations

Barrie JG, Knapper WH, Strong EW: Cervical nodal metastases of unknown origin. *Am J Surg* 120:466, 1970.

Bhattacharya SK, Sealy WC: Paraneoplastic syndromes resulting from elaboration of ectopic hormones, antigens, and bizarre toxins. *Curr Probl Surg* May 1972.

Giuliano AE, Moseley AS, et al: Clinical aspects of unknown primary melanoma. *Ann Surg* 191:98, 1981.

Greenberg BE: Cervical lymph node metastases from unknown primary sites. *Cancer* 19:1091, 1966.

Jesse RH, Neff LF: Metastatic carcinoma in cervical nodes with an unknown primary lesion. *Am J Surg* 112:547, 1966.

Keller JW, Williams RD: Laparotomy for unexplained fever. *Arch Surg* 90:494, 1965.

Myers WPL, Tashima CK, Rothschild EO: Endocrine syndromes associated with non-endocrine neoplasms. *Med Clin North Am* 50:763, 1966.

Diagnosis and Staging

Commission on Clinical Oncology of the Union Internationale Contre Cancrum: *TNM Classification of Malignant Tumors*. International Clinics against Cancer, Geneva, 1968.

Copeland MM: American Joint Committee on Cancer Staging and End Results Reporting: Objectives and progress. *Cancer* 18:1637, 1965.

Eilber FR, Holmes EC, Morton DL: Immunotherapy as an adjunct to surgery in treatment of cancer. *World J Surg* 1:547, 1977.

Finck ST, Giuliano AE, et al: Results of ilioinguinal dissection for stage II melanoma, *Ann Surg* 196:180, 1982.

Jones SE: Importance of staging in Hodgkin's disease. *Semin Oncol* 7:126, 1980.

Russell WO, Cohen J, et al: A clinical and pathological staging system for soft tissue sarcomas. *Cancer* 40:1562, 1977.

Williams PA: A productive history and physical examination in the prevention and early detection of cancer. *Cancer* 47:1146, 1981.

Surgery

Barnes JP: Physiologic resection of the right colon. *Surg Gynecol Obstet* 94:722, 1952.

Cole WH, Packard D, Southwich HW: Carcinoma of the colon with special reference to prevention of recurrence. *JAMA* 155:1549, 1954.

Deckers PJ, Ketcham AS, et al: Pelvic exenteration for primary carcinoma of the uterine cervix. *Obstet Gynecol* 37:647, 1971.

Eilber FR, Grant TT, et al: Internal hemipelvectomy—excision of the hemipelvis with limb preservation: an alternative to hemipelvectomy. *Cancer* 43:806, 1979.

Eilber FR, Mirra JJ, et al: Is amputation necessary for sarcomas? A 7-year experience with limb salvage. *Am J Surg* 192:431, 1980.

Flanagan L, Foster JH: Hepatic resection for metastatic cancer. *Am J Surg* 113:551, 1967.

Gilbertsen VA, Wangensteen OH: A summary of thirteen years' experience with the second look program. *Surg Gynecol Obstet* 114:438, 1962.

Giuliano AE, Eilber FR, et al: The management of locally recurrent soft tissue sarcoma. *Ann Surg* 196:87, 1982.

Halsted WS: The results of operations for the cure of cancer of the breast performed at the Johns Hopkins Hospital from June 1889 to January 1894. *Ann Surg* 20:297, 1894.

Huggins C, Bergenstal DM: Inhibition of human mammary and prostatic cancer by adrenalectomy. *Cancer Res* 12:134, 1952.

Kiselow M, Butcher HR, Bricker EM: Results of the radical surgical treatment of advanced pelvic cancer: A fifteen-year study. *Ann Surg* 166:436, 1967.

Miles WE: A method of performing abdomino-perineal excision for carcinoma of the rectum and the terminal portion of the pelvic colon. *Lancet* 2:1812, 1908.

Miller DR, Albritten FF Jr: Principles of surgery for cancer, in Nealon TF Jr (ed): *Management of the Patient with Cancer.* Philadelphia, Saunders, 1966, p 154.

Mockman S, Curreri AR, Ansfield FJ: Second-look operation for colon carcinoma after fluorouracil therapy. *Arch Surg* 100:527, 1970.

Mueller CB, Jeffries W: Cancer of the breast: Its outcome as measured by the rate of dying and causes of death. *Ann Surg* 182:334, 1975.

Patt YZ, Chuang VP, et al: The palliative role of hepatic arterial infusion and arterial occlusion in colorectal carcinoma metastatic to the liver. *Lancet* 1:349, 1981.

Pierce EH, Clagett OT, et al: Biopsy of the breast followed by delayed radical mastectomy. *Surg Gynecol Obstet* 103:559, 1956.

Ramming KP: Is partial hepatectomy, intrahepatic artery infusion of 5-FU, or systemic chemotherapy the best form of treatment for colon carcinoma metastatic to the liver? in O'Connell TX (ed): *Controversies in Surgical Oncology.* Philadelphia, Saunders, 1981, p. 246.

Ramming KP, Sparks FC, et al: Hepatic artery ligation and 5-fluorouracil infusion for metastatic colon carcinoma and primary hepatoma. *Am J Surg* 132:236, 1976.

Ramming KP, Sparks FC, et al: Management of hepatic metastases. *Semin Oncol* 4:71, 1977.

Roberts SS, Hengesh JW, et al: Prognostic significance of cancer cells in the circulating blood: A ten year evaluation. *Am J Surg* 113:757, 1967.

Stearns MW, Schottenfeld D: Techniques for the surgical management of colon cancer. *Cancer* 28:165, 1971.

Stehlin JS: Hyperthermic perfusion with chemotherapy for cancer of the extremities. *Surg Gynecol Obstet* 129:305, 1969.

Stehlin JS Jr, Giovanella BC, et al: Results of hyperthermic perfusion for melanoma of the extremities. *Surg Gynecol Obstet* 140:339, 1975.

Storm FK, Kaiser L, et al: Thermo-chemotherapy for melanoma metastases in liver. *Cancer* 49:1243, 1982.

Turnbull RB, Kyle K, et al: Cancer of the colon: the influence of the no-touch isolation technic on survival rates. *Ann Surg* 166:420, 1967.

Veronesi U, Saccozzi R, et al: Comparing radical mastectomy and quadrectomy, axillary dissection, and radiotherapy in patients with small cancers of the breast. *N Engl J Med* 305:6, 1981.

Watkins E, Khazei AM, Nabra KS: Surgical basis for arterial infusion chemotherapy of disseminated carcinoma of the liver. *Surg Gynecol Obstet* 130:581, 1970.

Wilkens EW Jr: The surgical management of metastatic neoplasms of the lung. *J Thorac Cardiovasc Surg* 42:298, 1961.

Radiation Therapy

Baker AR: Local procedure in the management of rectal cancer. *Semin Oncol* 7:385, 1980.

Harris JR, Recht A, et al: Time course and prognosis of local recurrence following primary radiation therapy for early breast cancer. *J Clin Oncol* 2:37, 1984.

Harris JR, Beadle GF, Hellam S: Clinical studies on the use of radiation therapy as primary treatment of early breast cancer. *Cancer* 53:705, 1984.

Higgens GS Jr, Conn JH, et al: Preoperative radiotherapy for colo-rectal cancer. *Ann Surg* 181:624, 1974.

Johns HE, Cunningham JR: In *The Physics of Radiology.* Springfield, Ill., Charles C Thomas, 1977.

Kaplan HS: Historic milestones in radiobiology and radiation therapy. *Semin Oncol* 6:479, 1979.

Kotalik JF: Multiple daily fractions in radiotherapy. *Cancer Treat Rev* 8:127, 1981.

Moss WT, Brand WN: *Therapeutic Radiology; Rationale, Technique, Results,* 3d ed. St. Louis, C. V. Mosby, 1969.

Paulson DL, Shaw RR, et al: Combined preoperative irradiation and resection for bronchogenic carcinoma. *J Thorac Cardiovasc Surg* 44:281, 1962.

Powers WE, Tolmach LJ: Preoperative radiation therapy: Biologic basis and experimental investigation. *Nature* 201:272, 1964.

Stevens KR: A review of the value of radiation therapy for adenocarcinoma of the rectum and sigmoid. *Fron Gastrointest Res* 5:93, 1979.

Till JE, McCulloch EA: A direct measurement of the radiation sensitivity of normal mouse bone marrow cells. *Radiat Res* 14:213, 1961.

Chemotherapy

Bailor JC, Byar DP: Estrogen treatment for cancer of the prostate. *Cancer* 26:257, 1970.

Baserga R: Molecular biology of the cell cycle. *Int J Radiat Biol* 49:219, 1986.

Bonadonna G, Brusamolino E, et al: Combination chemotherapy as an adjuvant treatment in operable breast cancer. *N Engl J Med* 294:405, 1976.

Bruce WR: The action of chemotherapeutic agents at the cellular level and effects of these agents on hematopoietic and lymphomatous tissue. *Can Cancer Conf* 7:53, 1966.

Calabresi P, Schein PS, Rosenberg SA: *Medical Oncology: Basic Principles and Clinical Management of Cancer.* New York, Macmillan, 1985.

Chabner B (ed): *Pharmacologic Principles of Cancer Treatment.* Philadelphia, Saunders, 1982.

Chabner BA: The oncologic end game (Karnofsky Memorial Lecture). *J Clin Oncol* 4:625, 1986.

De Vita VT, Hellman S, Rosenberg SA (eds): *Cancer Principles and Practice of Oncology,* 2d ed. Philadelphia, Lippincott, 1985.

Einhorn LH: Testicular cancer as a model for a curable neoplasm: The Richard and Hinda Rosenthal Foundation Award Lecture. *Cancer Res* 41:3275, 1981.

Erlichman C: Potential applications of therapeutic drug monitoring in treatment of neoplastic disease by antineoplastic agents. *Clin Biochem* 19:101, 1986.

Gilman A: The initial clinical trial of nitrogen mustard. *Am J Surg* 105:574, 1963.

Greco FA, Vaughn WK, Hainsworth JD: Advanced poorly differentiated carcinoma of unknown primary site: Recognition of a treatable syndrome. *Ann Intern Med* 104:547, 1986.

Haskell CM (ed): *Cancer Treatment.* 2d ed. Philadelphia, Saunders, 1985.

Huggins C, Hodges CV: Studies on prostatic cancer. I. The effect of castration, of estrogen and androgen injection on serum phosphatases in metastatic carcinoma of the prostate. *Cancer Res* 1:293, 1941.

Lewis JL: Chemotherapy of gestational choriocarcinoma. *Cancer* 30:1517, 1972.

Li MC, Hertz R, Spencer DB: Effect of methotrexate therapy upon choriocarcinoma and chorioadenoma. *Proc Soc Exp Biol Med* 93:361, 1956.

Salmon SE: Cloning of human tumor stem cells, in *Progress in Clinical and Biologic Research.* New York, A.R. Liss, 1980.

Schabel FM Jr: The use of tumor growth kinetics in planning "curative" chemotherapy of advanced solid tumors. *Cancer Res* 29:2384, 1969.

Schnipper LE: Clinical implications of tumor-cell heterogeneity. *N Engl J Med* 314:1423, 1986.

Skipper HE: Cancer chemotherapy is many things: GHA Clowes Memorial Lecture. *Cancer Res* 31: 1173, 1971.

Skipper HE, Perry S: Kinetics of normal and leukemic leukocyte populations and relevance to chemotherapy. *Cancer Res* 30:1883, 1970.

Strawitz JG: Cancer chemotherapy using isolation perfusion, in Brodsky I, Kahn SB, Moyer JH (eds): *Cancer Chemotherapy II.* New York, Grune & Stratton, 1972, p 443.

Sullivan PW, Salmon SE: Kinetics of tumor growth and regression in IgG multiple myeloma. *J Clin Invest* 51:1697, 1972.

Tannock IF: Experimental chemotherapy and concepts related to the cell cycle. *Int J Radiat Biol* 49:335, 1986.

Combined Therapy

Burk MW, Morton DL: Adjuvant cancer therapy: Rationale for its use. *Surg Clin North Am* 61:1245, 1981.

Eilber FR, Morton DL, et al: Limb salvage for skeletal and soft tissue sarcomas: Multidisciplinary preoperative therapy. *Proc Int Colloquium Cancer* 1981/2001, 1981.

Gilbert HA, Kagan RA, Winkley J: Soft tissue sarcomas of the extremities: Their natural history, treatment and radiation sensitivity. *J Surg Oncol* 7:303, 1975.

Haskell CM, Eilber FR, Morton DL: Adriamycin (NSC-12317) by arterial infusion. *Cancer Chemother Rep* 6:187, 1974.

Haskell CM, Silverstein MJ, et al: Multimodality cancer therapy in man: A pilot study of adriamycin by arterial infusion. *Cancer* 33:1485, 1974.

Jaffe N, Frei E, III, et al: Adjuvant methotrexate and citrovorum factor treatment of osteogenic sarcoma. *N Engl J Med* 291:994, 1974.

Lindberg RD: The role of radiation therapy in the treatment of soft tissue sarcoma in adults, in *Proceedings of 7th National Cancer Congress.* Philadelphia, Lippincott, 1972.

McNeer GD, Cantin J, et al: Effectiveness of radiation therapy in the management of sarcoma of the soft somatic tissues. *Cancer* 22:391, 1968.

Martin RG, Butler JJ, Albores SS: Soft tissue tumors: Surgical treatment and results, in *Tumors of Bone and Soft Tissue.* Chicago, Year Book Medical Publishers, 1965, p 333.

Morton DL, Eilber FR: Soft tissue sarcomas, in Holland JF, Frei E III (eds): *Cancer Medicine.* Philadelphia, Lea & Febiger, 1982, p 2141.

Morton DL, Eilber FR, Sondak VK, Economou JS (eds): *The Soft Tissue Sarcomas.* Orlando, Grune & Stratton, 1987.

Morton DL, Eilber FR, et al: Limb salvage from a multidisciplinary treatment approach for skeletal and soft tissue sarcomas of the extremity. *Ann Surg,* 184:268, 1976.

Murphy WT: The role of radiation therapy in the management of soft somatic tissue sarcoma. *Proc. 6th Natl. Cancer Congress* 1968, p 775.

Rosen G, Murphy ML, et al: Chemotherapy, en bloc resection and prosthetic bone replacement in the treatment of osteogenic sarcoma. *Cancer* 37:1, 1976.

Rosen G, Suwansirikal S, et al: High dose methotrexate with citrovorum factor rescue and Adriamycin in childhood osteosarcoma. *Cancer* 33:1151, 1974.

Rossi A, Bonodonna G: Current impact of adjuvant chemotherapy on resectable cancer. *Cancer Chemother Pharmacol* 3:17, 1979.

Storm FK (ed): *Hyperthermia in Cancer Therapy.* Chicago, Year Book Medical Publishers, 1985.

Suit HD, Russell WO: Radiation therapy of soft tissue sarcomas. *Cancer* 36:759, 1975.

Suit HD, Russell WO, Martin RG: Sarcoma of soft tissue: Clinical and histopathological parameters and response to treatment. *Cancer* 35:1478, 1974.

Townsend CM Jr, Eilber FR, Morton DL: Skeletal and soft tissue sarcomas: Results of treatment with adjuvant immunotherapy. *JAMA* 236:2187, 1976.

Immunotherapy

Bordon EC: Interferons and cancer: How the promise is being kept, in Gresser I (ed): *Interferon.* London, Academic, 1984, pp 43–83.

Buick RN, Salmon SE: Variables in the demonstration of human tumor clonogenicity: Cell interactions and semi-solid support, in Salmon SE (ed): *Cloning of Human Tumor Stem Cells.* New York, Alan R Liss, 1980, p 199.

Cobbald SP, Waldmann H: Therapeutic potential of monovalent monoclonal antibodies. *Nature* 308:460, 1984.

Deckers PJ, Pilch YH: RNA-mediated transfer of tumor immunity: A new model for immunotherapy of cancer. *Cancer* 28:1219, 1971.

Economou JS: The role of antibody in tumor immunity. *Surg Gynecol Obstet* 153:417, 1981.

(*isografts, isogeneic grafts,* or *syngeneic grafts*) or from individuals to themselves (*autografts,* or *autogenous grafts*) survive indefinitely after the vascular supply has been reestablished.

Allografts normally survive the transplant operation as well as isografts. If the recipient has not previously encountered the antigens present on the donor graft, the allograft is not morphologically or physiologically distinguishable from the isograft in the early posttransplant period—the rejection process normally takes several days. Medawar first noted that skin grafts between unrelated rabbits appeared normal until the fourth or fifth day. At that time inflammation appeared within the graft bed in the form of a dense leukocyte infiltrate that led to necrosis of the entire graft by about the tenth day. He further demonstrated that the rejection process is the result of immunologic mechanisms. Whereas the "first-set rejection" takes place in 10 or 11 days, a second graft from the same rabbit resulted in an accelerated "second-set rejection." The process of first-set and second-set rejection of an allogeneic graft takes place whether or not the graft is *orthotopic* (a graft placed in the anatomic position normally occupied by such tissue) or *heterotopic* (placed in other than the original location). The reaction is immunologically specific for the antigens involved, and the second-set rejections occur only when the recipient has been sensitized to antigens shared with the first graft.

Transplantation (Histocompatibility) Antigens

The rejection of an allograft is elicited by foreign histocompatibility antigens on the grafted tissue. Many antigens can serve as histocompatibility antigens. For example, the ABO blood group antigens will elicit rapid graft rejections in hosts with natural isoantibody. Similarly, xenografts between distant species are rejected rapidly because tissue incompatibilities are so profound between most species that preformed antibodies may exist in the recipient of the graft. Alloantigeneic incompatibilities between members of a species vary, however, and strong antigens can lead to graft rejection within 8 days, while weaker differences will permit graft survival of well over 100 days.

THE IMMUNOGENETICS OF HISTOCOMPATIBILITY

The strongest of the transplantation antigens is the expression of a single chromosomal region called the *major histocompatibility complex* (MHC) (Fig. 10-1). In human beings the MHC is located on chromosome 6. All mammals have a similar MHC, but the nomenclature varies among species. In human beings, the gene products of the MHC were first investigated on leukocytes and were named *human leukocyte antigens* (HLA). Naturally, the first-discovered antigens would be likely to be the major determinants.

The presence of HLA antigens on a cell surface can be detected in one of two ways. The serologic method uses antigen-specific antisera, which binds to cells carrying the antigen. A second method measures the reactivity of host lymphocytes to lymphocytes from potential graft donors. The responding lymphocytes are reacting to other cellular

Fig. 10-1. Gene map of chromosome 6 in human beings. This segment of the chromosome between the locus coding for the enzyme glyoxylase (GLO) and HLA-A is usually referred to as the HLA complex. The loci of HLA can be divided into two classes: Class I loci include HLA-A, HLA-B, and HLA-C, whereas the Class II loci include HLA-DR, HLA-DP, and HLA-DQ. Gene products of the Class I molecules are glycoproteins consisting of a heavy chain that penetrates the cell membrane. The heavy chain is folded into three immunoglobulin-like domains (α_1, α_2, and α_3). A B_2 microglobulin unit completes the structure. The Class II molecules consist of two polypeptide chains, both of which penetrate the cell membrane. The extracellular part of each chain is folded into two domains. The domains adjacent to the cell membrane are homologous with the α_3 and B_2M domains of the Class I antigens and the constant domain of the immunoglobulin molecule. [From: *deVries RRP, Van Rood JJ (eds): Immunobiology of HLA Class I and Class II Molecules. Basel (Switzerland), Karger, 1985, with permission.*]

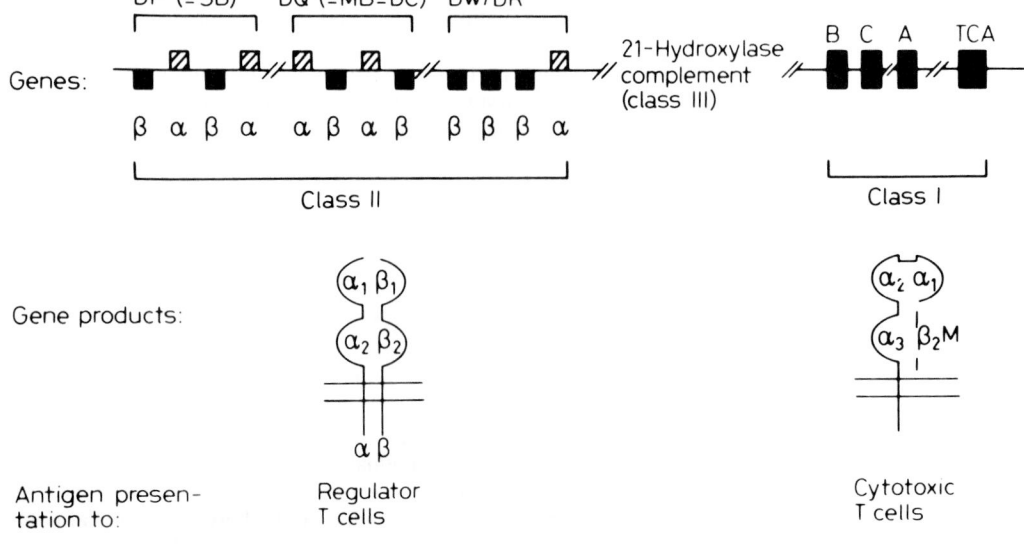

transplantation antigens. The antigens that can best trigger the proliferation of allogeneic lymphocytes were designated *Class II antigens*. The antigens that trigger allogeneic lymphocyte proliferation poorly were designated *Class I antigens*. Both Class I and Class II antigens can now be detected by specific antisera. The Class I antigens are expressions of those portions of the MHC supergene called HLA-A, HLA-B, and HLA-C. The Class II antigens are expressions of HLA-D, D, DQ, and DW/DR subloci.

HLA Class I molecules can be detected on the cell surfaces of almost all nucleated cells. In contrast HLA Class II molecules are found only on cells of the immune system—macrophages, dendritic cells, B cells, and activated T cells. Resting T lymphocytes do not express Class II antigens. Both Class I and Class II antigens each are composed of two polypeptide chains with variable and constant regions. The polymorphism is expressed in the variable regions of each molecule distant from the cell membrane. The portion of molecule closest to the cell membrane shows considerable homology between Class I and Class II molecules and also with the constant part of immunoglobulin molecules. This fact suggests that a common evolutionary origin exists between these three molecules (Fig. 10-1).

The HLA antigens have formed the basis for transplantation tissue typing for many years. Because of extreme polymorphism, only rarely do two unrelated individuals share all the antigens expressed. Relatives, on the other hand, often share some antigens because each person inherits one chromosome and, hence, one set of HLA antigens from each parent (Fig. 10-2), and because all the HLA antigens are expressed (codominant) on the cell surface.

The MHC subloci have been found to be closely linked but separable, and therefore genetic crossover between them, though unusual, can occur. As shown in Fig. 10-2, the parental HLA-A, -B, and -D pairs are usually inherited together, and the antigens originating from one chromosome are called *HLA haplotype*. Almost always the haplotype the child receives from each parent corresponds to the haplotype of one of the parental chromosomes. When crossover occurs during meiosis, however, the child receives a recombinant haplotype from a parent. (In the example shown, recombination occurred between A and B antigens. Recombination can occur between B and D also.)

Detection of the A, B, and D alleles for tissue typing requires banks of monospecific antisera. Typing was thought to be clinically useful because it seemed clear that survival of transplanted organs between family members correlated with the closeness of the HLA antigen match. The clinical results of organ transplantation have not, however, clearly demonstrated the importance of HLA-A and -B identity in organ transplantation between unrelated (cadaver) donor–recipient pairs. This apparent paradox seems caused by the fact that inheritance of the MHC in its entirety is important for graft survival rather than simple sharing of several HLA antigens.

It is important to recognize that there are genes on

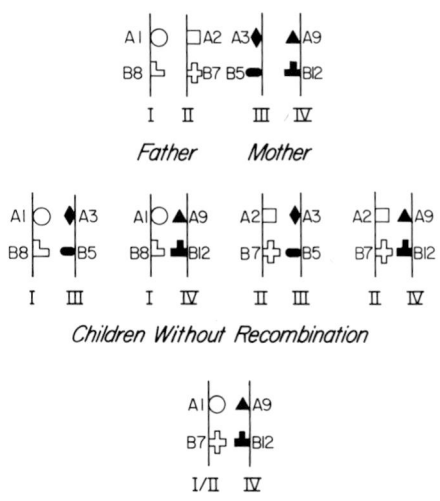

Fig. 10-2. Hypothetic examples of inheritance of serologically detectable HLA antigens of the A and B series. Four offspring of mating between parents with chromosomes labeled I-II and III-IV are shown, as well as one possible result of recombination within the HLA region and subsequent inheritance. The parental chromosomes are usually transmitted intact, and the offspring receive one chromosome containing an A and B pair from each parent. Occasionally, however, crossover occurs and the child receives a recombinant antigen pair from a parent. For simplicity, genes coding for the C and D series of antigens within the HLA complex are not shown. See Fig. 10-1 for the presumed location of the genes within the HLA complex.

other chromosomes outside the MHC that code for weaker histocompatibility loci. In human beings, such antigens are not well understood, but a graft from a sibling identical at the HLA locus will be rejected if immunosuppressive drugs are not utilized. Such rejections are the natural consequence of these minor histocompatibility loci.

NORMAL ROLE FOR THE MHC. The functions of histocompatibility antigens are not totally understood, but clearly they do not exist merely to thwart the efforts of transplant surgeons. Most likely they are important to the recognition phenomena during cell-cell interactions within the same organism. For example, the T lymphocyte can recognize certain microbial antigens and initiate immune responses against them most efficiently when those antigens are associated with certain of its own HLA determinants. Thus HLA polymorphism is useful to the host in antimicrobial immunity.

DISTRIBUTION OF HLA ANTIGENS. Not all cells and tissues express equivalent amounts of HLA antigens. Some cells even express greater or lesser quantities at different phases of the cell cycle. Most adult parenchymal cells express Class I antigens, but only passenger leukocytes have a full complement of Class II antigens. For this reason, it is possible to deplete experimental grafts of their passenger leukocytes and diminish the strength of the rejection response. In clinical practice, however, these techniques are not yet possible. Almost all transplanted organs contain enough HLA antigens to elicit prompt rejection by a normal host, and there is evidence that the expression of HLA Class II antigens can be induced on parenchymal cells in the presence of an immune response. This reaction seems to be the result of the action of interferon-gamma on parenchymal cells.

Histocompatibility Matching

It is obvious that, other things being equal, the less antigenic the graft, the less the host will react against it. In human transplantation, when the donor and recipient are identical twins, there is no antigenic difference, and the tissues are accepted. When the donor and recipient are siblings or when a parent donor is used for offspring, there is a greater statistical likelihood of antigen sharing between donor and recipient than when a cadaver or other unrelated donor is used.

Several methods have been developed for the purpose of demonstrating antigenic similarities between donor and recipient prior to transplantation, so that donor and recipient pairs that are relatively histocompatible may be selected.

The best current method is called leukocyte typing.

HLA antigens on circulating lymphocytes can be detected with antisera derived originally from multiply transfused patients or from women with multiple pregnancies. Some of the antisera seem to recognize groups of antigens, and others recognize single antigens (*monospecific antisera*). Using the patient's leukocytes and a group of standard antisera, it is thus possible to characterize most of the strong HLA antigens in both donor and host. Only HLA antigens can be routinely determined in this way. Weaker histocompatibility antigens at other loci have not been detected by serologic techniques in human beings.

Antigens are currently detected by isolating lymphocytes from the peripheral blood of potential donors or recipients. The cells are incubated with antisera of various specificities and rabbit serum as a source of complement. Cells that react with antibodies in the serum die in the presence of complement and can be stained with vital dyes. Typing sera is becoming increasingly standardized. A typical set of results from the University of Minnesota typing laboratories is illustrated in Table 10-1.

Histocompatibility typing is useful in determining the best match between donor and recipient when family donors are utilized. Siblings who share all HLA antigens

Table 10-1. LYMPHOCYTE ANTIGEN TYPING REPORT OF THEORETICAL FAMILY*

Family member	ABO	*HLA-A locus*											*HLA-DR locus*									
		A1	A2	A3	A9	A10	A11	A28	Aw19	Aw34	Aw36	Aw43	DR1	DR2	DR3	DR4	DR5	DRw6	DR7	DRw8	DRw9	DRw10
Father AB	A	+	−	+	−	−	−	−	−	−	−	−	−	−	+	+	−	−	−	−	−	−
Mother CD	A	−	+	−	−	−	−	+	−	−	−	−	−	+	−	−	−	−	+	−	−	−
Son AC (patient)	O	+	−	−	−	−	−	+	−	−	−	−	−	+	+	−	−	−	−	−	−	−
Son AD	A	+	+	−	−	−	−	−	−	−	−	−	−	−	+	−	−	−	+	−	−	−
Daughter BC	O	−	−	+	−	−	−	+	−	−	−	−	−	+	−	+	−	−	−	−	−	−
Daughter BD	A	−	+	+	−	−	−	−	−	−	−	−	−	−	−	+	−	−	+	−	−	−
Daughter AC	O	+	−	−	−	−	−	+	−	−	−	−	−	+	+	−	−	−	−	−	−	−

Family member	ABO	*HLB-B locus*																		
		B5	B7	B8	B12	B13	B14	B15	Bw16	B17	B18	Bw21	Bw22	B27	Bw35	B37	B40	Bw41	Bw42	Bw47
Father AB	A	−	−	+	−	−	−	−	−	−	−	−	−	−	+	−	−	−	−	−
Mother CD	A	−	−	−	−	−	−	−	−	−	+	−	−	+	−	−	−	−	−	−
Son AC (patient)	O	−	−	+	−	−	−	−	−	−	−	−	−	+	−	−	−	−	−	−
Son AD	A	−	−	+	−	−	−	−	−	−	+	−	−	−	−	−	−	−	−	−
Daughter BC	O	−	−	−	−	−	−	−	−	−	−	−	−	+	+	−	−	−	−	−
Daughter BD	A	−	−	−	−	−	−	−	−	−	+	−	−	−	+	−	−	−	−	−
Daughter AC	O	−	−	+	−	−	−	−	−	−	−	−	−	+	−	−	−	−	−	−

* The specifications for the A, B, C, and DR loci are those currently used at the University of Minnesota.

Son AC is the prospective transplant recipient. Daughter AC is a perfect match for all four antigens; she shares the inheritance of both HLA haplotypes and is the ideal donor. Both parents, son AD, and daughter BC share only one haplotype with the potential recipient and are theoretically not as good donors. Daughter BD shares no HLA haplotypes with the recipient and is the poorest donor in the family.

More important than the HLA type are the ABO blood types. The father, mother, son AD, and daughter BD *cannot* donate, because they are all blood group A and the recipient is blood group O and possesses anti-A antibodies in his serum.

are the best possible donor-recipient pair. But several points about histocompatibility matching deserve emphasis:

1. Recipients receiving grafts, even from donors who are HLA identical matches with them, will still reject the graft (although more slowly) unless immunosuppressive drugs are utilized. Only an identical twin is truly a perfect match.
2. Even with poor histocompatibility matches between relatives, the results are frequently good, which probably indicates it is sometimes possible to suppress even great degrees of antigenic incompatibility.
3. Even with a good histocompatibility match, the graft may fail if the host happens to have preformed antibodies against a donor's tissue. These antibodies can be recognized if recipient serum is allowed to react with donor lymphocytes in a cytotoxicity test. This test, called *cross matching,* should be performed with fresh serum as a final test of compatibility prior to transplant. Preformed cytotoxic antibodies to donor tissue cannot be detected by the usual typing procedure itself.
4. The presence of ABH isohemagglutinins will most often lead to the prompt rejection of tissue bearing incompatible blood group substances.
5. Despite the results of tissue typing, a related donor has generally produced better transplant results than an unrelated (cadaver) donor.
6. Tissue typing for unrelated cadaver donors has not been successful, with one exception: HLA-identity of all detectable antigens correlates with a higher incidence of graft success. But such identity is rare.

MIXED LYMPHOCYTE CULTURE (MLC). The other method capable of detecting degrees of histocompatibility between donor and recipient is the MLC test, which detects differences principally at the Class II locus. Lymphocytes of the recipient are mixed with lymphocytes of the donor in tissue culture. If significant antigenic differences exist between the two, they will respond by transformation into blast cells, DNA synthesis, and mitosis. The incorporation of tritiated thymidine into DNA can be quantified to assess the degree of stimulation. As the test was originally devised, it was a two-way test—cells of the donor were capable of reacting against cells of the recipient and vice versa. In order to isolate the response of the recipient cells to the donor antigens, the donor lymphocytes can be inactivated by irradiation. The test is not useful as a screening test for cadaver organ transplantation but retains usefulness in related bone-marrow transplantation.

The Immune Apparatus

The immune response to the histocompatibility antigens on the cells of transplanted organs triggers the rejection reaction. At birth, human beings are already immunologically competent and have undergone a complex developmental process. It is now agreed that there is a single hemopoietic stem cell, found in the extraembryonic yolk sac. The daughter stem cells migrate to various centers for further differentiation. Within these centers, progenitor cells for erythrocytes, eosinophils, basophils, neutrophils, and lymphoid cells arise, depending on the local microchemical environment. It is likely that further proliferation of these progenitor stem cells depends on the action of "poietins," which tend to expand the populations of specialized cells in the way that erythropoietin acts on the erythrocyte line (Fig. 10-3).

The lymphoid cell line first appears within two primary (or central) lymphoid tissues. The thymus governs the development of cellular immunity. In birds, the bursa of Fabricius governs the development of humoral immunity. The bursa exists as a clearly defined central lymphoid structure only in birds. The equivalent of the bursa of Fabricius has not been defined in mammals, but there is evidence that it exists—perhaps within the fetal liver or bone marrow. In human beings the characteristics of sex-linked agammaglobulinemia of the Bruton type—very low levels of immunoglobulins, with normal cellular immunity and thymus-derived lymphocytes—suggest that the bursa equivalent has failed to develop.

Both the thymus and the bursa (or its equivalent) are responsible for the further development of the peripheral lymphoid tissues, i.e., spleen, lymph nodes, Peyer's patches. Certain areas of the lymph node are dependent on the functional presence of the thymus and the bursa (Fig. 10-4). The paracortical regions between the cortical germinal centers and the medulla are dependent on the thymus, while the germinal centers themselves and the medullary cord lymphoid tissue are under the developmental control of the bursal equivalent. Therefore, thymectomy early in the neonatal period or congenital thymic deficiency results in failure of development of the paracortical regions of the lymph nodes. In chickens, bursectomy leads to failure of development of germinal centers and medullary cord lymphoid tissues.

All cells that were once dependent on the thymus for their development are called *T cells.* T cells represent the immunocompetent cell population responsible for the development of cellular rather than humoral immunity. These reactions include delayed hypersensitivity reactions, as well as many of the early reactions responsible for allograft rejection.

The *B cells* descend from stem cells in the bone marrow and become responsible for the manufacture of circulating immunoglobulins and thus for humoral immunity (Fig. 10-3). The B cells appear to be relatively sessile, but their end products, immunoglobulin antibodies, can interact with foreign antigens at distant sites. The T cells responsible for cell-mediated immunity are of necessity more peripatetic and must migrate to the periphery in order to neutralize foreign antigens.

The lymphoid system is the seat of the body's immunologic response and the small mature lymphocytes and the plasma cells are the immunocompetent cells. Once the lymphocytes (T or B cells) have migrated to the peripheral lymphoid tissue, they are fully immunocompetent. It is likely that Burnet's clonal selection theory holds true—i.e., a state of preparedness for a certain antigen or group of related antigens exists within a lymphoid cell so that it is only capable of responding to a narrow range of genetically determined antigenic specificities. For this reason only a small percentage of the lymphocytes in the body will respond to a specific antigen.

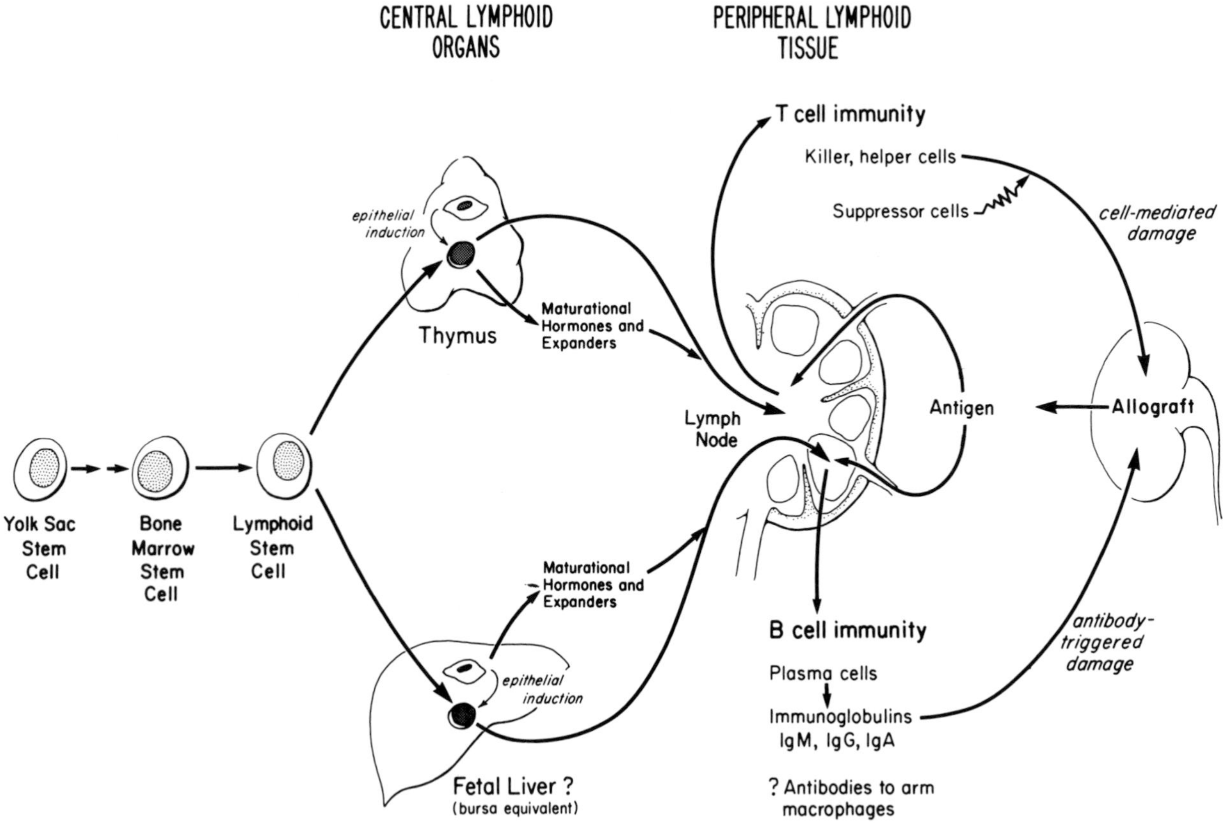

CENTRAL LYMPHOID
ORGANS

PERIPHERAL LYMPHOID
TISSUE

T cell immunity

Killer, helper cells

Suppressor cells

cell-mediated
damage

*epithelial
induction*

Thymus

Maturational
Hormones and
Expanders

Lymph
Node

Antigen

Allograft

Yolk Sac
Stem
Cell

Bone
Marrow
Stem
Cell

Lymphoid
Stem
Cell

Maturational
Hormones and
Expanders

*epithelial
induction*

Fetal Liver ?
(bursa equivalent)

B cell immunity

Plasma cells

Immunoglobulins
IgM, IgG, IgA

? Antibodies to arm
macrophages

*antibody-
triggered
damage*

Fig. 10-3. Encapsulation of the extraordinarily complex developmental sequences of the immune system. Certain of the known inducers, expanders, growth factors, and sites of maturation needed to establish the T and B cell lines are presented. Much of this takes place before birth, so transplant recipients are fully competent with established peripheral lymphoid populations in the lymph nodes, Peyer's patches, and spleen. Therefore, clinical immunosuppression consists principally of lymphocyte depletion and inhibition of the activation of antigen-stimulated lymphocytes. [From: *Foker JE, Simmons RL, Najarian JS: Principles of immunosuppression, in Sabiston DC Jr (ed): Davis-Christopher Textbook of Surgery. Philadelphia, Saunders, 1977, p 506, with permission.*]

In order for a lymphocyte to respond to its predetermined antigen, it must have a specific chemical receptor for that antigen on its cell surface (Fig. 10-5). B cells possess a receptor very similar to an immunoglobulin. T cells have receptor molecules whose structures share many structural similarities with immunoglobulin and also with both Class I and Class II histocompatibility antigens (see Figs. 10-1 and 10-5). Attached to these shared constant (c) regions close to the cell membrane are variable (v) por-

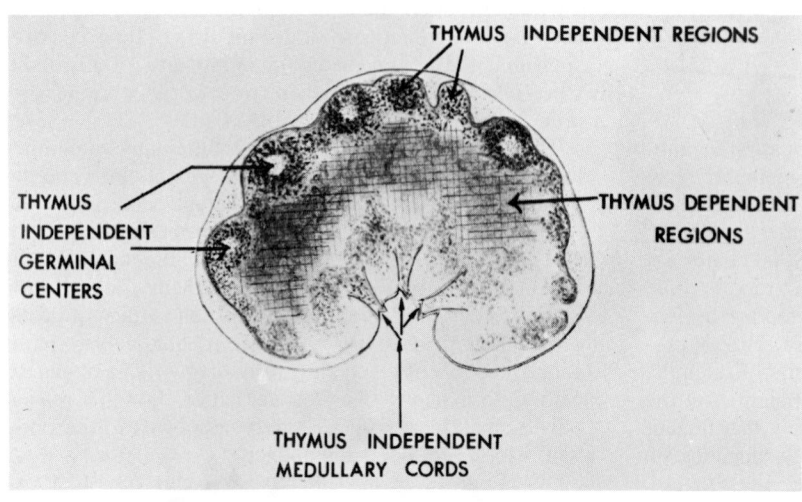

Fig. 10-4. The thymus-dependent and thymus-independent areas are illustrated in this schematic representation of a lymph node. [From: *Good RA, Finstad J: Structure and development of the immune system, in Najarian JS, Simmons RL (eds): Transplantation. Philadelphia, Lea & Febiger, 1972, p 26, with permission.*]

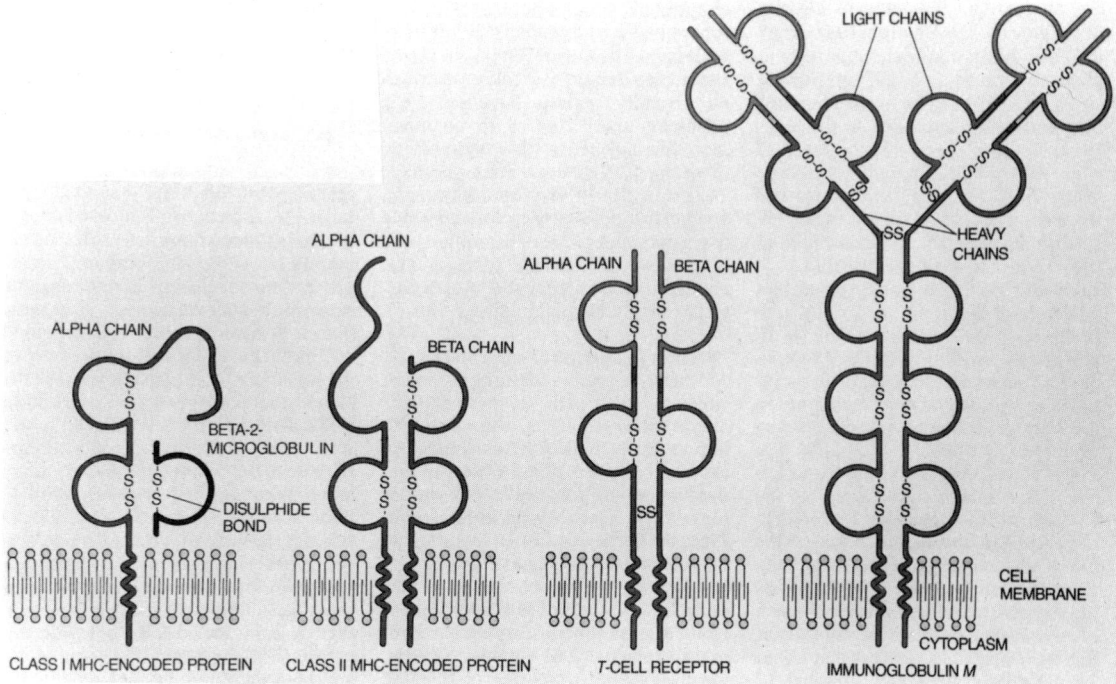

Fig. 10-5. Homology between HLA antigens and antigen binding molecules on the surfaces of lymphocytes. The molecular structures are similar and the molecules share similar amino acid sequences. (From: *Mannack P, Kappler J: The T cell and its receptor. Sci Am 254:36, 1986, with permission.*)

tions of the receptor molecule that permit it to bind and be activated by specific antigens. The variable portion of the T receptor molecule does not resemble an immunoglobulin, however.

Immunologic Events in Allograft Rejection

INDUCTION OF IMMUNITY

ROLE OF THE SMALL LYMPHOCYTE. Mature lymphocytes appear to sit in a state of immunologic readiness. The small lymphocyte can react to its bound antigen by proliferation, differentiation, maturation, and the production of molecules (antibodies, protein markers on the cell surface, lymphokines) that can react with the antigen and recruit other mediators of the immune response. After proliferation some of these cells have a life span of many years so that a much larger pool of antigen-reactive cells (memory cells) remains. Such cells also may be capable of a more rapid response.

THE AFFERENT ARC. The small lymphocyte thus recognizes the immunogenic determinants and translates that recognition into an immunologic response. The first phase of the immunologic response has been called afferent arc. It involves the grafting process itself, the release of the immunogenic histocompatibility antigens from the graft, the processing and recognition of the immunogens,

and the stimulation of the responsive lymphoid cell population. After organ allografting, this process takes place principally within the graft, and to a lesser degree in the lymphoid depots.

The immunogens of a grafted organ, being surface components of the cell membrane, are readily available to the recipient's T lymphocytes that percolate through the transplanted organ. In order for the lymphocyte to become sensitized, however, an accessory cell of the monocyte-macrophage lineage is necessary. In the case of protein antigens, the macrophage efficiently traps an antigen, processes it, and presents it in a form more easily recognized by the T cell receptor. For this to occur, the responding lymphocyte and the macrophage must share identical Class II antigens on their cell surfaces. This is strong evidence for the importance of self-recognition of cooperating cells in the immune response.

The accessory cell has a second function as well, namely, to provide a second signal by means of a secreted (monokine) molecule that enhances T cell responses in its immediate vicinity. The most important monokine in the activation of T cell responses is called interleukin-1 (IL-1) (Fig. 10-6). But interleukin-1 has many other functions including mediating the production of fever and metabolic change during inflammatory responses.

Within the microenvironment of the immune cellular response, however, IL-1 has well-defined functions. In cooperation with antigen binding by the T cell, IL-1 fosters the appearance of receptors for a second lymphokine on the cell surface of the antigen-reactive cell, namely, IL-2 receptors. Interleukin-2 (IL-2) is simultaneously secreted by antigen-responsive helper cells. Interaction of

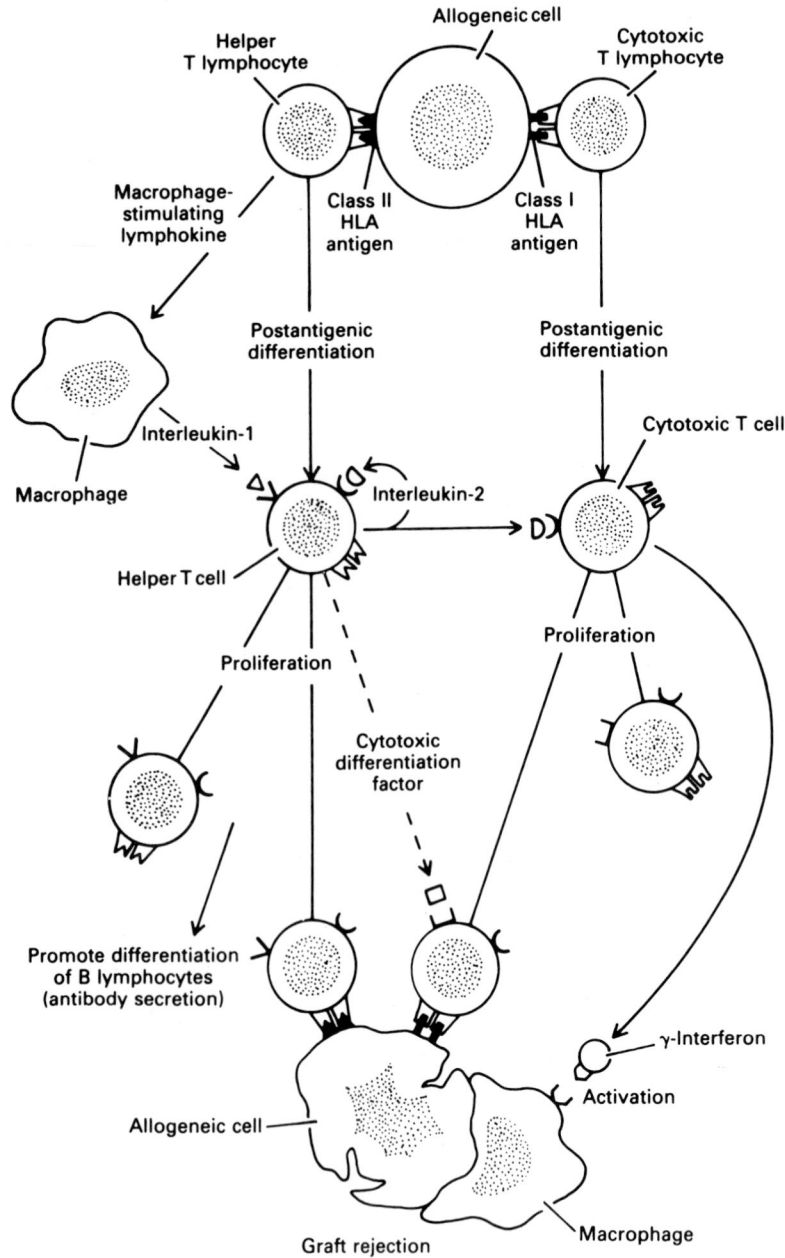

Fig. 10-6. Cellular immune response of T cells to transplantation antigens. The sequence leading to the proliferation of alloreactive T cells includes antigen, interleukin-1, and interleukin-2. (Adapted from: *Strom TB: Kidney Int 26:353, 1984, with permission.*)

IL-2 with its receptor allows the cell to proliferate and mature (Fig. 10-6).

CELL-CELL INTERACTIONS. During graft rejection, antigen-responsive clones of lymphocytes do not act alone. They not only require accessory cells plus interleukin, they also interact with other lymphocytes. Extensive lymphocyte-lymphocyte interaction is needed for the development of maximum lymphocyte proliferative and cytotoxic activity. The cooperation occurs both between T and B cells and between defined subpopulations of T cells.

The requirement for cooperation between T and B cells was established by showing that neither cell population alone could mount an immune response to certain antigens, whereas mixtures of the two cell types resulted in the production of high levels of antibody. Because B cells are the precursors of antibody-forming cells and T cells do not synthesize readily detectable amounts of immunoglobulin, certain T cells must serve as "helper cells" that assist B cells to differentiate into producers of antibody. An antibody response to the major histocompatibility antigens requires this cooperation, and suspensions of B cells alone in tissue culture will not effectively produce antibodies to these antigens unless T cells are added. Therefore, T-cell recognition of the antigen is necessary for the production of specific antibody by the B cell. Not all T cells can function in this role, only the subgroup of helper T cells (T_H). A full antibody response to most antigens seems to require aid from T_H cells.

Just as T_H cells are necessary for B-cell antibody response, T_H cells are needed for the development of lymphocyte-mediated cytotoxicity. The lymphocytes that produce direct cytotoxicity are also T cells: effector (T_E), or killer cells. The T_H cell is required for the T_E cell to develop fully the capacity to inflict cell damage. Cell-associated histocompatibility antigens are prominent among the antigens that require T_H-T_E cell cooperation for induction of maximum cytotoxicity.

There is evidence that yet another T-cell subgroup can inhibit either the development of antibody-producing B cells or the generation of T_E cells. These regulatory lymphocytes have been called suppressor T (T_S) cells.

The elucidation of these interactions has occupied many cellular immunologists during the past decade. Convincing experimental demonstration of lymphocyte-lymphocyte interaction required the various cells to be identified and separated from the bulk populations of lymphocytes in vitro. This was facilitated by the discovery of distinct antigenic proteins on the surfaces of the various subsets of lymphocytes. Antibodies to these surface marker proteins could then be used to deplete or enrich the bulk populations of a specific cell type and thereby clarify the function of each cell type. Table 10-2 lists the functional lymphocyte subtypes and the markers they possess.

Once the lymphocyte subpopulations were identified, the mechanisms of their interaction could be elucidated.

Table 10-2. FUNCTIONAL SUBPOPULATIONS OF LYMPHOCYTES

A. T lymphocytes
   1. Regulatory T lymphocytes
      a. Helper cells
      b. Suppressor cells
   2. Effector T lymphocytes
      a. Delayed hypersensitivity (DHT)
      b. Mixed lymphocyte reactivity
      c. Cytotoxic T lymphocyte (CTL or "killer" cells)
B. B lymphocytes
   1. Precursors of antibody-forming cells Bμ, Bγ, Bα, Bϵ
   2. Memory cells
   3. ? Regulatory B lymphocytes

SOURCE: From Katz DH: The immune system: An overview, in Fudenberg HH, Stites DP, Caldwell JL, Wells JV (eds): *Basic and Clinical Immunology,* 3d ed. Los Altos, CA, Lange Medical Publications, 1980, p 1.

Most interactions seem to involve the manufacture and release of soluble substances (*lymphokines*) by stimulated cells that trigger responder cells that bear receptors for these lymphokines. Table 10-3 lists some of the lymphokines that have been studied and their putative function.

The most powerful of the lymphokines secreted by activated T_H cells is called interleukin-2. T_E cells cannot secrete interleukin-2, but T_E cells require it in order to proliferate and mature. The interaction of the antigen-responsive T_H cell with the antigen plus interleukin-1 permits it to secrete interleukin-2, which acts on both T_H and T_E cells to permit expansion of the antigen-sensitive clones. A second set of lymphokines that act on antigen-stimulated B cells is necessary for B cells expansion (Fig. 10-6, Table 10-3).

Table 10-3. LYMPHOKINES RELEASED BY ANTIGEN-ACTIVATED T CELLS

Lymphokine		Target cell and function
		Other lymphocytes
Interleukin-2	IL-2	Maintains growth of activated T cells
B cell growth factor	BCGF	Maintains B cell growth
B cell differentiation factor	BCDF	Induces B cell differentiation
Suppressor factor		Suppresses T and B cell functions, not well characterized
		Macrophages
Macrophage activating factor	MAF	Activates macrophages, may be same as gamma-IFN
Migration inhibition factor	MIF	Inhibits macrophage mobility
Macrophage chemotactic factor	MCF	Attracts macrophages
Procoagulant induction		An activation activity, affects coagulation
Fc receptor induction		Induces elevated number of Fc receptors
		Polymorphonuclear leukocytes
Eosinophil chemotactic factor	ECF	Attracts eosinophils
Eosinophil stimulator		Induces eosinophilia
Chemotactic factor		Attracts PMN
		Donor tissue
Gamma-interferon	IFN	Induces elevated MHC expression and has antiviral activity, may be the same as MAF
Lymphotoxin	LT	May be involved in cell damage mediated by LC
		Bone marrow
Interleukin-3	IL-3	Promotes the growth and differentiation of stem cells
Colony stimulating factor	CSF	As above, may include IL-3

Most evidence supports the idea that B lymphoid differentiation to antibody-producing cells is accompanied by cellular proliferation. When the B cell proliferates, morphologic differentiation accompanies the proliferation, and the result is a plasma cell busily engaged in making specific antibody. Conversion from a transformed cell to a plasma cell is seen within a few days of grafting, in both organ allografts and the lymphoid tissue stimulated by these transplants.

The situation for T cells responding to Class I and Class II alloantigens during allograft rejection has proved to be a fascinating variation on the standard immunologic response. Class II alloantigens stimulate T_H cells preferentially and Class I alloantigens stimulate T_E cells preferentially (Fig. 10-6). The T_E cells, after proliferation under the influence of interleukin-2 from helper cells responding to Class II antigens, mature into cells that interact with cells bearing Class I antigens. Such an interaction leads to donor cell death. The T_E and T_H precursors respond to different alloantigens within the closely linked HLA complex, and different T-cell types appear to accomplish differentiation and proliferation. Differentiation requires proliferation, but quite unexpectedly they occur in different cells.

EXPRESSION OF IMMUNITY: GRAFT DESTRUCTION

Specifically sensitized T_E cells are present within most rejecting allografts and are capable of inflicting damage. Alloantigenically stimulated T_H cells are there as well, and can secrete lymphokines (Table 10-3) capable of mediating delayed hypersensitivity reactions. But specifically sensitized cells are in the minority and it is likely that a small number of specifically sensitized lymphoid cells initiate a rejection reaction but that the completion of reaction requires many nonsensitized cells as well. Polymorphonuclear eosinophils, leukocytes (PMNs), plasma cells, and unsensitized mononuclear cells are all part of the rejection process. Furthermore, there is convincing evidence that antibody can initiate graft destruction in the relative absence of a cellular reaction under appropriate circumstances.

In Vitro Lysis of Target Cells by Cytotoxic Lymphocytes. The specifically sensitized lymphoid cells that collect at the site of an allograft have long been known to damage the donor tissues directly in the absence of humoral antibody or complement. Direct contact between the sensitized lymphocyte and the target cell appears to be important. The mechanism of cell membrane damage has not been identified. Several cytotoxic agents have been found that may be released by the lymphocytes, but the specificity of the reaction in vitro favors the idea that interaction of cell surfaces is important to direct the damage of the target cell.

EFFECTOR MOLECULES (LYMPHOKINES) RELEASED BY ACTIVATED LYMPHOCYTES. The release of cytotoxic factors by lymphocytes infiltrating an allograft would be the most direct way to damage foreign cells, but probably not the most efficient, since nonspecific cell killing would result. Several other kinds of molecules are released by specifically sensitized T cells, and these products or lymphokines serve to activate and enlist macrophages, polymorphonuclear leukocytes (PMNs), lymphocytes, etc., so that the initial cellular response is amplified. Several lymphokines have been identified, but it is not yet clear whether there is a small number of molecules with multiple functions or whether a different molecule is specific for each function (Table 10-3).

Macrophages seem to be very active participants in graft rejection; their role does not end with antigen processing. Two of the most investigated lymphokines, migration inhibitory factor (MIF) and chemotactic factor (CF), may serve to attract macrophages and then inhibit their escape. Other lymphokines function to activate the macrophage. Macrophages resemble lymphocytes in that they have resting and activated states. In the later phase, the cytoplasm has the appearance of great activity, both morphologically and enzymatically. Phagocytosis, pinocytosis, and bacteriostatic and tumoricidal activities are increased. The levels of many intracellular enzymes, including the digestive enzymes found in lysosomes, are markedly elevated. Macrophages found at the site of graft rejection appear to be in the activated state and thus better able to participate in tissue destruction.

A host of other activities has been ascribed to the lymphokines. Neutrophils, basophils, and eosinophils are attracted by them (Table 10-3). Growth inhibitory and cytotoxic activities against target cells have been described in vitro. Several apparent lymphokines affect lymphocytes themselves and can be shown under suitable experimental conditions to stimulate mitoses and increase antibody production. Transformed lymphocytes also release a vascular permeability factor in addition to the cytotoxic lymphokines. Little is known about the permeability factor(s) and its possible effect on an allograft rejection. Tissue edema is, however, a prominent feature of graft rejection, and it may join the vascular permeability factors released by the complement activation and neutrophil and platelet participation in the efferent arc of rejection.

ROLE OF ANTIBODY IN ALLOGRAFT REJECTION. Circulating antibody is not an obligatory participant in the rejection of solid tissue allografts. In fact, the inability to make immunoglobulin does not preclude graft rejection. There is now no doubt, however, that rejection can be mediated by alloantibodies—especially the rejection of vascularized organ allografts.

Humoral antibody provides only the recognition portion of graft rejection. Unlike cell-mediated immunity, where the recognition system is intimately associated with the destruction of the target, humoral antibody must activate other systems in order to effect cell death.

Although antibodies bind to allografts, such binding is of no consequence by itself, and the antibody would probably be cleared during the course of normal cell membrane repair. The combination of antibody with the antigen produces an active complex, which triggers a number of nonspecific effector pathways (Fig. 10-7). Each effector pathway typically consists of a sequential activation of enzymes that attract and hold active cells, produce vascular permeability, release enzymes capable

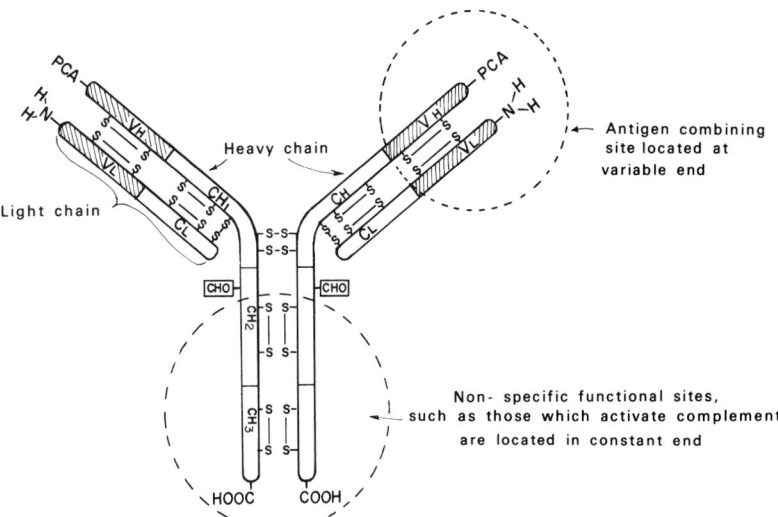

Fig. 10-7. Structure of the IgG antibody molecule. V_H and V_L are the variable portions of the heavy and light chains, respectively, and together they form the antigen-combining site. C_L is the constant portion of the light chain. CH_1, CH_2, and CH_3 are the subunits forming the invariable area of the heavy chain. The approximate positions of the inter- and intrachain disulfide bridges are shown. [From: *Foker JE, Simmons RL, Najarian JS: Allograft rejection: I. The induction of immunity: The afferent arc, in Najarian JS, Simmons RL (eds): Transplantation. Philadelphia, Lea & Febiger, 1972, p 63, with permission.*]

of degrading cell surfaces and other proteins, release factors causing smooth muscle contraction, and precipitate the formation of fibrin clots.

The immunologic response, therefore, can be both efficient and discriminatory. Relatively few specifically differentiated cells can produce molecules that will perform the recognition function. Since few cells are committed to each antigen, many more antigens can be discriminated. The antibodies in turn initiate a relatively general effector mechanism that can destroy the graft.

THE COMPLEMENT SYSTEM. The most important of the several effector molecular cascade systems triggered by antigen binding by antibody is the complement system. The combination of antibody (of IgG_1, IgG_2, IgG_3, or IgM classes) with antigen changes the conformation of the antibody molecule. Included in this change is the activation of a site on the constant (Fc) end of the antibody molecule, which then triggers the complement pathway. The alternate (properdin) pathway can be set off by the immunologically nonspecific serum proteins of the properdin system reacting with sugar structures found on bacterial surfaces and conceivably mammalian cells; its role in graft rejection, however, is unknown. The components of both pathways are circulating protein molecules that, when activated, react in a sequential fashion. At present, the system is known to be made up of a number of distinct molecules that are capable of interacting with one another, with antibody, and with cell membranes. Once activated they can act enzymatically on the next molecule in the sequence, which serves as the inactive substrate. Components C6 and C9 are nonenzymatic and bind to the

previous components, resulting in conformational and activity changes.

Most of the biologically significant activities of the complement system arise during activation of the last six reacting complement components, C3 and C5 through C9 (Fig. 10-8). The two parallel but entirely independent initial pathways—the classic and the alternate pathways—both lead to activation of the terminal, biologically important portion of the sequence, involving the reactions of C5 through C9. The terminal portion of the complement sequence may also be directly activated by certain noncomplement serum and cellular enzymes without participation of the early reaction factors. For example, fibrinolytic enzymes in plasma and certain lysosomal enzymes will activate the C3 and C5 stages.

The classic complement pathway (Fig. 10-8) appears to be the most important for immune reactions. Three biologic consequences of complement activation are most important in transplantation rejection.

1. Complement has been shown to be capable of mediating lytic destruction of many kinds of cells to which antibodies have bound. The active components are in the C8 and C9 complexes, but the mechanism of lysis is not clear; perhaps enzymatic activity of the complex damages the membrane directly.

2. Many kinds of cells possess receptors for the C3b or C4b (activated) components, including B lymphocytes, neutrophils, monocytes, and macrophages. If C3b or C4b attach to a damaged cell they may act as opsonins, bringing the target cells in contact with the phagocytic macrophages and monocytes or exposing the surface antigens of these cells to B lymphocytes.

3. Many of the complement cleavage products have biologic actions of their own. For example, C4a and C2b act as kinins. C3a has chemotactic activity for polymorphonuclear leukocytes, causes the release of histamine from mast cells (anaphylatoxin activity), has a kinin activity, and causes immune adherence. C5a is a very potent chemotactic factor, stimulates histamine release from mast cells, and attracts neutrophils and liberates lysosomes from them.

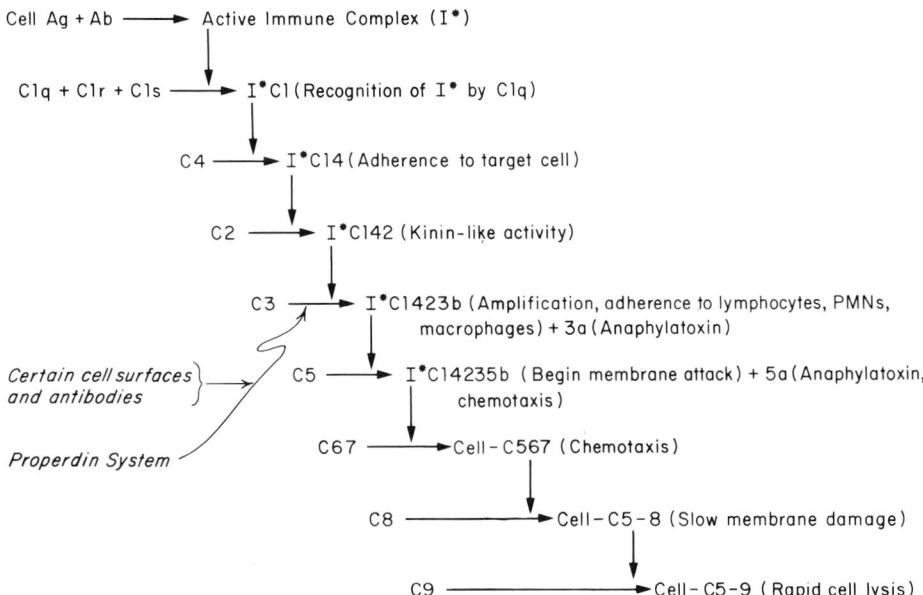

Fig. 10-8. The complement pathways and the biologic activity released at each step. The classic pathway begins with a specific antigen-antibody reaction. The properdin pathway is triggered by a more nonspecific interaction between cell surfaces and the molecules that make up the properdin systems. Both pathways, however, converge at the C3 step, where most of the biologic activity associated with complement activation begins. Amplification also occurs at several steps, but it is greatest at C3. The subsequent steps lead to the molecular condensation on the target cell surface, which ultimately results in membrane damage and lysis. There are several other important consequences of complement activation. The presence of these molecules on the target cell surface makes them adherent to other cells. Macrophages, platelets, polymorphonuclear leukocytes, and lymphocytes adhere and increase the damage to the graft cells. The steps through C5 are largely enzymatic in nature; the C3 and C5 components, for example, are split during activation, releasing chemotactic and vasoactive (anaphylatoxins) molecules. Attachment of the C5b molecule to the cell begins the condensation ending in membrane damage; this seems to occur away from the immune complex. Interaction of the C6,C7 components results, additionally, in the release of another chemotactic factor. The activation of the complement pathway, therefore, contributes to many of the features seen in allograft rejection; cellular infiltrates, adherent PMNs and platelets, thrombosed vessels, interstitial edema, and cellular damage.

Therefore, complement activation releases kinins that increase vascular permeability, leading to edema; attracts polymorphonuclear leukocytes that release other vasoactive compounds and lysosomal enzymes; encourages phagocytosis of damaged tissue; releases lysosomal enzymes from macrophages; opsonizes cells; binds cells to damaged cell surfaces (immune adherence); and leads to cell death.

An important biologic characteristic of the complement system as well as the other cascade systems discussed in this section is that they are capable of self-amplification. Thus, in one study 450 C4 molecules were found fixed to each sensitized sheep red blood cell, but each erythrocyte had approximately 100,000 C3 components on its surface. In addition, the C3 components were distributed over the cell membrane surface, rather than confined to the site of the antigen-antibody combination, thus enlarging the area of effect. Although this step produces the greatest numerical amplification, other steps in the complement pathway also expand the number of active molecules.

THE CLOTTING SYSTEM. Theoretically the deposition of fibrin in the allografted organ may arise in two ways: The first, the so-called *extrinsic pathway* of thrombin formation, requires tissue thromboplastin to initiate the sequence of events. The release of this cellular substance may follow damage to the endothelial cell membranes either by antibody and complement or through the direct cytotoxic effect of lymphocytes. The activation of complement through C3 would also promote the adherence of platelets, which, in turn, would stimulate platelet retraction and release of platelet phospholipids. These phospholipids have been shown to promote clotting.

The second method of inducing clot formation, the *intrinsic pathway*, has the potential to be activated directly by immunologic reaction. In the intrinsic pathway, Hageman factor (factor XII) begins a sequence that proceeds through factors XI, IX, VII, and V to the activation

of prothrombin factor to form thrombin with the eventual polymerization of fibrin. Antigen-antibody complexes will activate Hageman factor to trigger this cascade and produce clotting in vitro in the absence of platelets. Thus, an entry into the intrinsic pathway is present within the interactions of antigens and antibodies (Fig. 10-9).

As the reaction proceeds and tissue damage is produced, tissue thromboplastin is released, collagen fibers are exposed, and clotting is facilitated. It is now generally hypothesized that the progressive obliterative vascular reaction of a chronically rejecting allograft is a by-product of fibrin laid down along endothelium that has been damaged by immune mechanisms.

THE KININ SYSTEM. The kinin, or kallikrein, system is initiated by activation of coagulation factor XII, leading

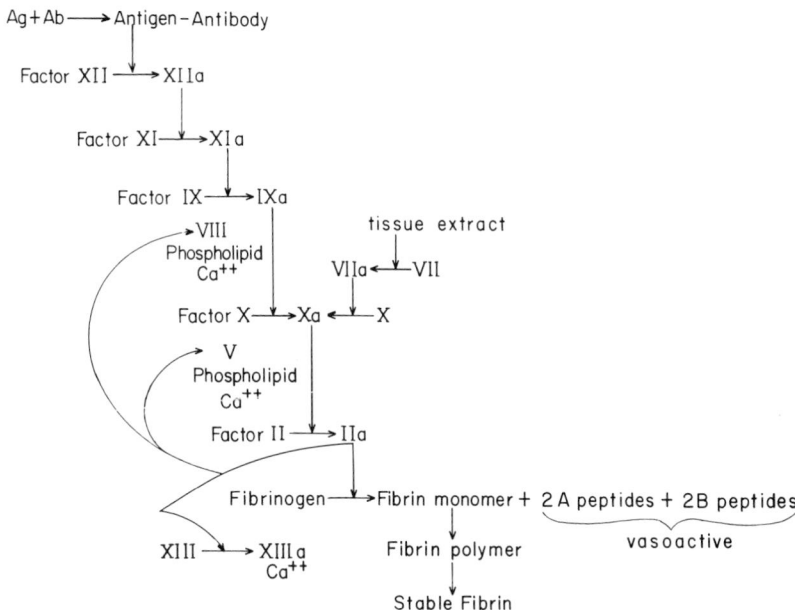

Fig. 10-9. The coagulation cascade system. Fibrin and two vasoactive peptides are the final products of the cascade. The two modes of activation of the system are diagrammed. Factor XII (Hageman factor) can be activated by immune complexes initiating the intrinsic pathway. Tissue damage (presumably produced by immunologic damage) could precipitate the extrinsic system. In both systems, the factors shown, with the probable exceptions of V and VIII, are enzymes. Activation of the pathways involves the sequential conversions of these enzymes to active forms (represented by XIIa, XIa, etc.). [From: *Najarian JS, Foker JE: Allograft rejection: II. The expression of immunity: The efferent arc, in Najarian JS, Simmons RL (eds): Transplantation. Philadelphia, Lea & Febiger, 1972, p 94, with permission.*]

eventually to the formation of kallikrein, which acts on kininogen, an α-globulin substrate in the plasma, and results in bradykinin. Bradykinin is one of the kinins, a group of active peptides that are rather rapidly inactivated, after formation, by kininases present in plasma. The kinins possess a variety of biologic activities, including chemotaxis of PMNs, smooth muscle contraction, dilatation of peripheral arterioles, and increase of capillary permeability. The involvement of the kinin system in graft rejection is likely but is as yet unproved.

INTERRELATIONSHIPS OF THE MOLECULAR CASCADE SYSTEMS (Fig. 10-10). Antigen-antibody complexes activate complement and Hageman factor. Hageman factor in turn produces clotting, activates plasmin, and perhaps directly activates complement. Plasmin in turn can activate C3 to produce, among other effects, chemotactic factors, immune adherence, and opsonization. Activation of Hageman factor also leads to kinin production. Activation of the complement system produces aggregation of platelets and, consequently, initiation of the clotting mechanism. Thrombin formation, in turn, stimulates the production of plasmin from plasminogen. Prostaglandin activity is released following complement activation, and may contribute to vascular permeability, although the significance of this in allograft rejection remains unclear.

Not only are the activators of these systems interrelated, but also the inhibitors are intertwined. The C1 esterase inhibitor also decreases the activity of the kinin and plasmin systems. Neither activation nor inhibition of one system can occur without affecting the other pathways.

The complexity of the allograft reaction is just beginning to be understood. Not only does it involve a variety of recognition molecules (antibodies) and presumably a similar variety of specifically sensitized cells; there is much recent evidence that unsensitized lymphocytes can be specifically directed and actively lyse target allogenic cells by a coating with antibody. In addition, the main force of the reaction may be produced by a bewildering array of amplifying chain reactions that include both molecular amplification schemes and cellular amplifiers. The activation of complement, the clotting system, kinin formation, and the stimulation of PMN, macrophages, and platelet assault produce a variety of damage to the transplanted organ. Included are occlusive phenomena within the graft vessels, induced permeability of these same vessels with interstitial edema accumulation, disruption of cellular basement membranes, and the infiltration of the graft with a profusion of cell types (Fig. 10-10).

AN INTEGRATED VIEW OF THE REJECTION OF ORGAN ALLOGRAFTS. Rejection morphology has two main components: The first component is the host response, and it is composed of effector cells and molecules, both immunologically specific and nonspecific. In rapid rejections these comprise most, if not all, of the pathologic picture so that the speed of the reaction virtually precludes response by the organ cells. The second component becomes prominent only with longer survival of the transplanted organ and encompasses morphologic alterations peculiar to the injured organ.

RECOGNITION

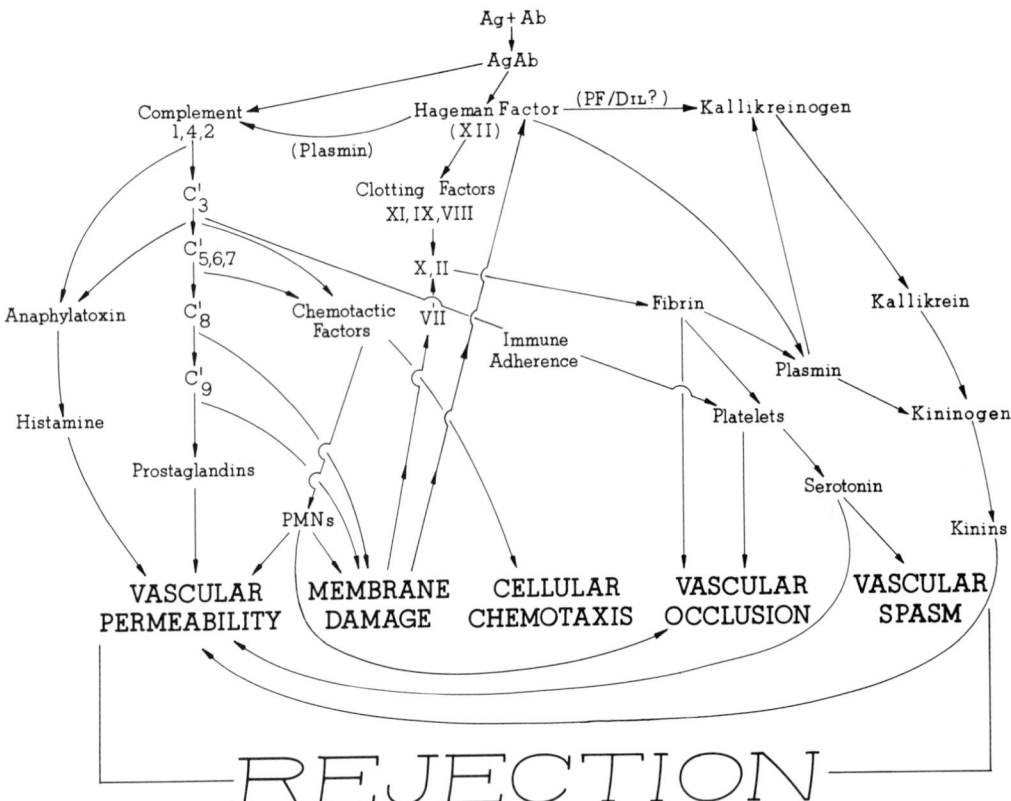

Fig. 10-10. Integration of the humoral amplification system in graft rejection. This diagram suggests the complexity of allograft rejection. The three main cascade pathways—complement, clotting, and kinin—generate many active molecules, including the kinins, chemotactic factors, anaphylatoxins, histamine, and serotonin. These molecules, together with platelets and polymorphonuclear leukocytes (PMNs), produce the destructive effects on the graft. The most prominent consequences include increased vascular permeability (edema), spasm, and occlusion, as well as cell and basement membrane damage and cellular chemotaxis (infiltration). It is clear that these systems do not operate singly but tend to activate each other. Not shown are the many interlocking inhibitory factors that keep these systems in check once they are activated. [From: *Najarian JS, Foker JE: Allograft rejection: II. The expression of immunity: The efferent arc, in Najarian JS, Simmons RL (eds): Transplantation. Philadelphia, Lea & Febiger, 1972, p 94, with permission.*]

A predictable series of events ensues when an unsensitized patient is allografted. The first visible change is a perivascular infiltration of round cells (Fig. 10-11). The accumulation of cells is not significant for several hours after transplantation but can reach considerable numbers within 48 h. The original enclaves around small vessels spread, and the interstitial space is further infiltrated. A potpourri of cells accumulates: cells resembling small lymphocytes are seen, as well as large transformed lymphocytes with basophilic cytoplasm. Large histiocytes or macrophages are just beginning to arrive in numbers. Plasma cells are still relatively scarce; as a terminal product of cellular differentiation, they may require several cell divisions before they appear in the organ (Fig. 10-12).

Antibody and complement are deposited in the area of the capillaries, and some of the infiltrating lymphoid cells are producing immunoglobulins by the third day. Recognition molecules (antibody) as well as sensitized cells are therefore present early in the allograft reaction.

Sensitized lymphoid cells, upon recognizing the foreign tissue, release several mediators of inflammation and cell damage. The release of cytotoxic factors directly injures membranes of adjacent cells. Mitogenic products stimulate division of lymphoid cells, perhaps expanding the immunocompetent population. Activated, phagocytic macrophages are effectively concentrated in the area by migration inhibitory factor and other chemotactic factors. In addition, vascular permeability agents are released.

Meanwhile, complement is fixed, thereby producing chemotactic factors, anaphylatoxins, and finally cellular damage when the terminal components are activated. Capillary permeability is increased by anaphylatoxins from the complement chain and probably by kinins. Interstitial edema becomes prominent. At the same time there are several additional inducements to cellular infiltration. The complement cascade generates molecules that produce immune adherence and others that have chemotactic activity. Damaged cells release additional compounds that contribute to infiltration by PMNs as well as other cells. PMNs in turn release vasoactive amines (including histamine or serotonin, depending on the species) and

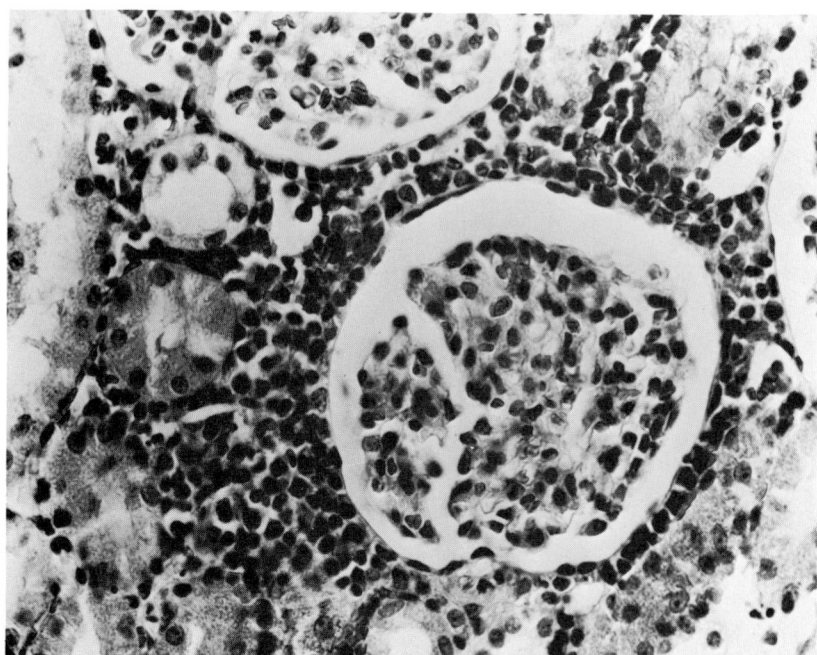

Fig. 10-11. Canine renal allograft 48 h after transplantation into unmodified recipient. Round cell infiltration, usually the first overt sign of host activity against the allograft, is apparent within 6 to 12 h after transplantation. By 48 h the number of invading cells is substantial. The original perivascular infiltrate has surrounded a glomerulus and adjacent tubules. [From: *Foker JE, Najarian JS: Allograft rejection: III. The pathobiology of organ rejection, in Najarian JS, Simmons RL (eds): Transplantation. Philadelphia, Lea & Febiger, 1972, p 122, with permission.*]

additional vascular permeability-promoting factors. The PMNs squeeze through the enlarged endothelial cell junctions and release proteolytic cathepsins D and E, causing basement membrane damage.

Fibrin and α-macroglobulins, whose contribution is not understood, are deposited by 7 days. During this time, lymphoid cells have continued to accumulate and, joined by significant numbers of plasma cells and PMNs, obscure the normal architecture. The round cell population presumably contains many macrophages and other immunologic nonspecific cells at this point. Increasingly frequent mitoses may indicate the production of immunocompetent cells within the graft.

The small vessels become plugged with fibrin and platelets, diminishing the perfusion and preventing function. In this relatively rapid sequence of events the organ has little chance to respond, and the pathologic process is dominated by the host effector pathways.

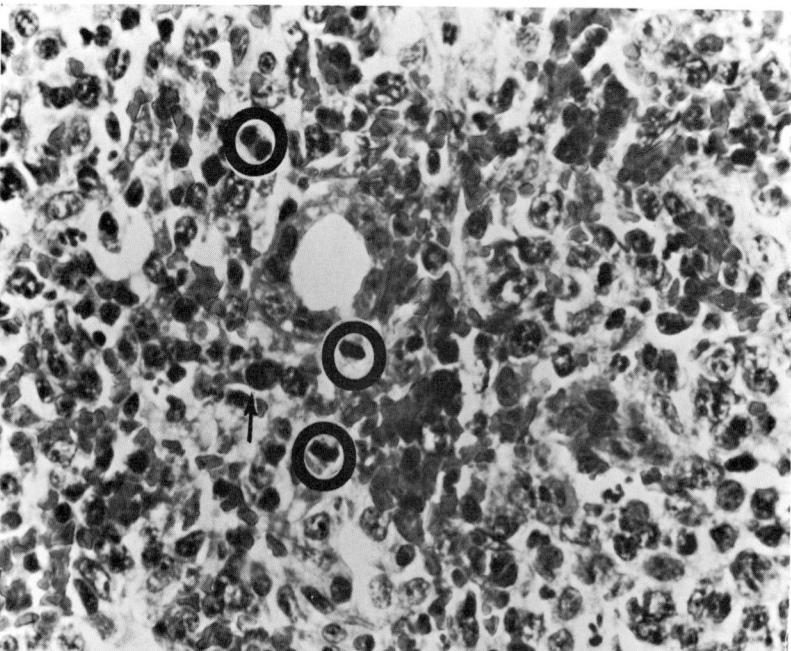

Fig. 10-12. Canine renal allograft 4 days after transplantation into an unmodified recipient. Invading cells all but obscure the architecture of the kidney. Numerous mitoses (circles) can be found, and this cellular proliferation may be producing immunologically competent cells within the graft. A plasma cell (arrow) is present, but most of the cells resemble lymphocytes and macrophages. [From: *Foker JE, Najarian JS: Allograft rejection: III. The pathobiology of organ rejection, in Najarian JS, Simmons RL (eds): Transplantation. Philadelphia, Lea & Febiger, 1972, p 122, with permission.*]

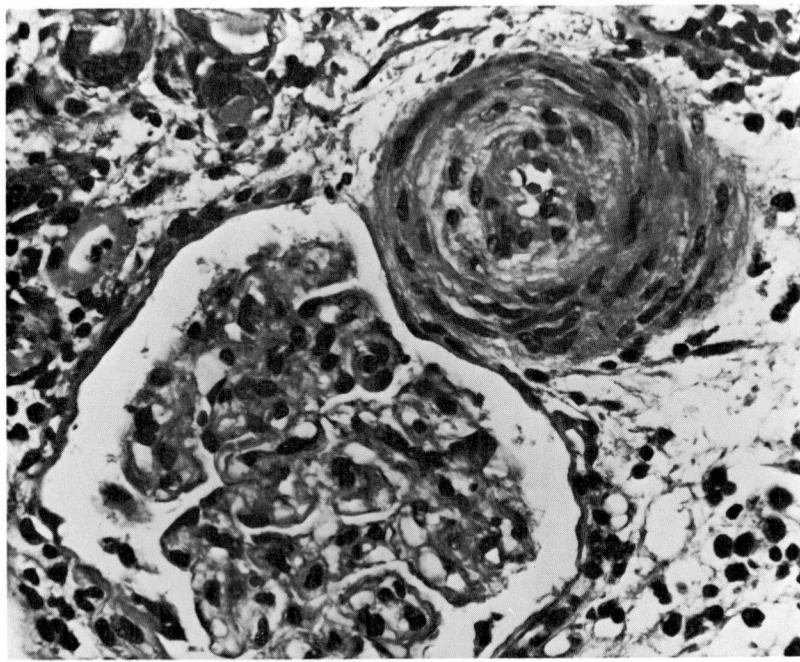

Fig. 10-13. A rejected human allograft removed 18 months post-transplant. The lumen of the arteriole has all but disappeared as a consequence of hyperplasia of the cells of the vessel. Most of the thickening of the wall is probably due to proliferation of smooth muscle cells, with spindle-shaped nuclei. Endothelial cells, with rounder nuclei, almost fill the lumen. [From: *Foker JE, Najarian JS: Allograft rejection: III. The pathobiology of organ rejection, in Najarian JS, Simmons RL (eds): Transplantation. Philadelphia, Lea & Febiger, 1972, p 122, with permission.*]

Obviously, rejection modified by immunosuppressive agents is not a distinct morphologic classification. The morphologic features associated with this more chronic rejection become dominated by the response of the organ tissue itself. Here the normal response of tissue to injury predominates in the pathologic picture. A good deal of endothelial cell damage occurs in the allograft, and the responses of cellular repair, hypertrophy and hyperplasia, follow.

Endothelial cell damage also elicits repair processes. Aggregations of platelets within the intimal layer are resolved, and the dissolution of the thrombi is accompanied by the infiltration of macrophages and foam cells. The result is a thickened intimal layer with the loss of smooth endothelial lining and the presence of vacuolated cells. The lumen narrows as a result. Narrowing of the vessel lumen is also a consequence of the medial thickening. Studies using nonimmunologic disease models have shown that most of the cells proliferating in response to the stimulus of injury are smooth muscle cells. A reasonable extrapolation is that hyperplasia of these cells produces much of the lumenal narrowing in the allograft (Fig. 10-13).

Although the exposed position of the endothelial cells and the striking proliferation of the smooth muscle cells argue for their being an important target of the immune reaction, there is evidence that the basement and elastic membranes of the vessel absorb a major portion of immune-mediated damage. Either immune complexes or antibodies to the vascular basement membrane activate complement and attract polymorphonuclear cells. These nonspecific effector cells release at least four protein factors that increase the permeability of the vessel and in addition produce cathepsins D and E, which digest base-

ment membranes. The PMNs are active in reaching the basement membrane and will lift the endothelial cells to gain this access.

Platelets may be of greater significance than PMNs in mediating damage. Immune complexes (which activate complement) will result in platelet adherence and the release of vasoactive substances. Platelet aggregation leads to the release of histamine, serotonin, and other capillary permeability factors that expose more basement membrane; the exposed collagen fibers of the basement membrane further enhance platelet aggregation. Platelets and PMNs drawn to these sites release cathepsins, elastases, and phosphatases that increase destruction and attract other nonspecific cellular effectors including macrophages.

The myocardial cell is the characteristic cell of the heart, the tubular cell of the kidney, the acinar and islet cell of the pancreas, etc. The differentiation and function of these cells demand an ample oxygen supply, and if destroyed, they cannot be replaced by further cellular division. Therefore, compromise of respiration by vascular endothelial and medial hypertrophy, intravascular aggregations of platelets, and interstitial accumulations of edema and mononuclear cells will have predictable consequences for these cells. They will atrophy, and death may be followed by replacement fibrosis (Fig. 10-14).

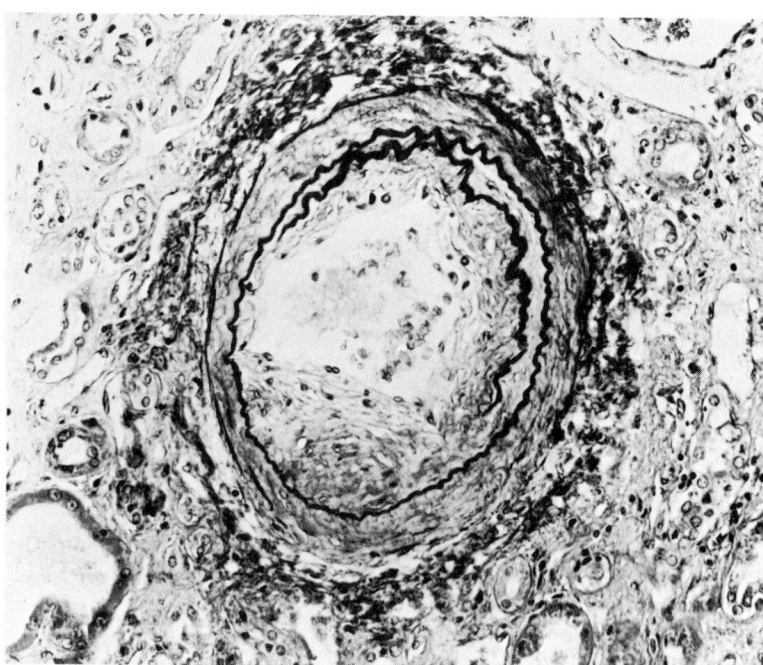

Fig. 10-14. Extensive damage to the small artery in a human renal allograft removed 14 months posttransplant is apparent. The elastic membranes are badly frayed, and the elastica interna has been destroyed entirely along half the circumference of the vessel. The intimal layer shows extensive disruption and loss of cells. The cells remaining are often vacuolated. The lumen is narrowed by tissue from several origins: proliferation of smooth muscle cells in the media, endothelial cell swelling and hyperplasia, and the presence of an organized thrombus. The adventitial area shows damage and edema formation. Note also that severe tubular atrophy and interstitial fibrosis are present. [From: *Foker JE, Najarian JS: Allograft rejection: III. The pathobiology of organ rejection, in Najarian JS, Simmons RL (eds): Transplantation. Philadelphia, Lea & Febiger, 1972, p 122, with permission.*]

The interstitial area concomitantly increases in size. The interstitial area, however, has much activity in its own right. Repair of immunologic damage stimulates many fibroblastic cells to proliferate, and it attracts macrophages. The persisting immunogenic capacity of the allograft is indicated by the inevitable presence of infiltrating plasma cells and lymphoid cells.

It is impossible to determine what proportions of these effects result from ischemia produced by vascular occlusion, interstitial edema, or cellular infiltrates. Similarly, the contribution made by the direct cytotoxic action of specific and nonspecific effector cells and molecules is unknown.

CIRCUMVENTING REJECTION

Clinical Immunosuppression

Theoretically, there are a number of methods by which the allograft rejection response can be suppressed including (1) destroying the immunocompetent cells prior to transplantation, (2) making the antigen unrecognizable or even toxic to the reactive lymphocyte clones, (3) interfering with antigen processing by the recipient cells, (4) inhibiting lymphocyte transformation and proliferation, (5) limiting lymphocyte differentiation into killer or antibody-synthesizing cells, (6) activating sufficient numbers of suppressor lymphocytes, (7) inhibiting destruction of graft cells by killer lymphocytes, (8) interfering with the combination of immunoglobulins with target antigens, or (9) preventing tissue damage by the nonspecific cells or antigen-antibody complexes.

In practice, a clinically useful immunosuppression largely depends on the destruction of the immunocompetent cells and on inhibiting the differentiation and proliferation of these cells. Methods of inducing specific immune tolerance by various antigen preparations prior to grafting, or by inhibiting sensitized cells and antibodies after they have produced, have not been clinically successful. It is more difficult to inhibit the immune response after it is underway, so less can be gained clinically after sensitization has occurred. To be most effective, immunosuppression must be present at the time of transplantation, or even before. Nevertheless, some success can be achieved in reversing the exacerbations of the rejection reaction seen in clinical transplantation.

ANTIPROLIFERATIVE AGENTS

Most traditional immunosuppressive agents act to impair the proliferation of lymphocytes. Such agents include the antimetabolites, alkylating agents, toxic antibiotics, and x-ray. They inhibit the full expression of the immune response by preventing the differentiation and division of the immunocompetent lymphocyte after it encounters the antigen. All of them, however, fall into one of two broad mechanistic categories. Either they structurally resemble needed metabolites or they combine with certain cellular components, such as DNA, and thereby interfere with cell function.

The former group, the antimetabolites, have a structural similarity to cell metabolites and either inhibit enzymes of that metabolic pathway or are incorporated during synthesis to produce faulty molecules. The antimetabolites include purine, pyrimidine, and folic acid analogs, which are most effective against proliferating and differentiating cells. They are given at the time of transplantation when the immunocompetent cells are first stimulated, and then for the life of the graft to interfere with the continuing stimulus to the immune system.

Alkylating agents and certain antibiotics include those compounds that combine with DNA and other cellular components. Although these agents would be useful in the pretransplant period to reduce the number of effective immunocompetent cells in the recipients, and thereafter to prevent proliferation, they are so toxic that their use has been limited to bone marrow transplantation and as occasional substitutes for azathioprine.

PURINE ANALOGS. The purine analog azathioprine (AZ) (Imuran) has been the most widely used immunosuppressive drug in clinical organ transplantation. Azathioprine is 6-mercaptopurine (6-MP) plus a side chain to protect the labile sulfhydryl group. In the liver, the side chain is split off to form the active compound, 6-MP. The mechanism of action would seem to be similar for these two compounds; however, azathioprine seems to enjoy the advantage of slightly lower toxicity.

Full metabolic activity comes in the cell with the addition of ribose 5-phosphate from phosphoribosyl pyrophosphate to form 6-MP ribonucleotide. The structural resemblance of this molecule to inosine monophosphate is obvious, and 6-MP ribonucleotide inhibits the enzymes that begin to convert inosine nucleotide to adenosine and guanosine monophosphate (Fig. 10-15). In addition, the presence of 6-MP ribonucleotides slows the entire purine biosynthetic pathway by fraudulent feedback inhibition of an early step. The steric similarity to either adenosine or guanine nucleotides is not great enough to allow significant incorporation into DNA or RNA and synthesis of

faulty molecules. The result of inhibiting these several enzymes, however, is to block the synthesis of cellular RNA, DNA, certain cofactors, and other active nucleotides.

The toxicity of azathioprine results from the same mechanisms. Its primary toxic effect is bone marrow suppression, leading to leukopenia. Liver toxicity can also result, possibly because of the high rate of RNA synthesis by these cells. The mechanism is unclear, however, because hepatic dysfunction does not seem to be dose-related.

Although pyrimidine analogs have been studied extensively as immunosuppressants in the laboratory, they have only limited clinical use.

FOLIC ACID ANTAGONISTS. The folic acid antagonists, aminopterin and methotrexate, inhibit the enzyme dihydrofolate reductase, and prevent the conversion of folic acid to tetrahydrofolic acid. This step is necessary for the synthesis of DNA, RNA, and certain coenzymes; again, proliferating cell systems are most affected.

Some of the toxicity of aminopterin and methotrexate can be abrogated by the administration of folinic acid some hours or even days after the use of the antagonist. Nevertheless, the ratio of immunosuppression to toxicity has not justified their use in clinical kidney transplantation. The immune reactions that accompany bone marrow transplantation are more difficult to control, and methotrexate is used to both prevent and reverse the severe graft-versus-host reactions that occur. Since methotrexate is usually used with one or more other drugs, its toxic effects can be difficult to identify. Megaloblastic hemopoiesis, mucosal breakdown with severe gastrointestinal bleeding, and liver damage seem to be related to methotrexate therapy. These effects, even with high dosages of

Fig. 10-15. Mechanism of antimetabolite action. 6-Mercaptopurine (6-MP) ribonucleotide resembles inosine monophosphate in its steric configuration. It thereby competes with inosine in its transformation into adenosine monophosphate and guanosine monophosphate and their subsequent incorporation into RNA and DNA. In addition, 6-MP inhibits the purine biosynthetic pathway, since it resembles a product of that biosynthetic pathway (feedback inhibition). [From: *Simmons RL, Foker JE, Najarian JS: Principles of immunosuppression, in Sabiston DC Jr (ed): Davis-Christopher Textbook of Surgery. Philadelphia, Saunders, 1972, p 471, with permission.*]

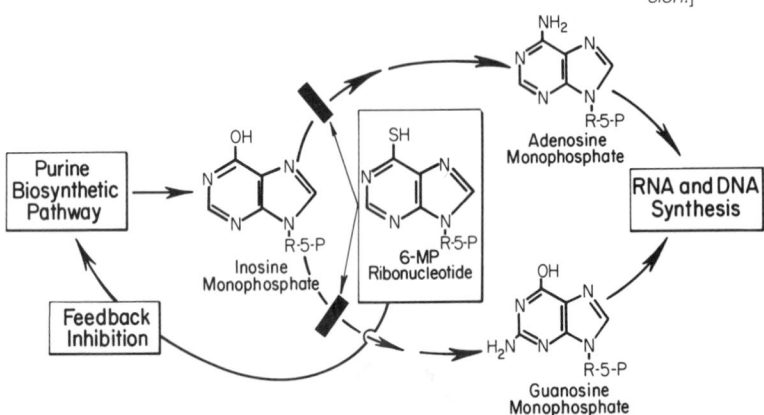

methotrexate, can usually be prevented by folinic acid (citrovorum rescue). Obviously, depression of the transplanted marrow may also result from the activity of methotrexate, although assigning the cause may be difficult in the complex clinical situation.

ALKYLATING AGENTS. The alkylating agents have highly reactive rings as part of the molecular structure. These unstable rings have electron-seeking points that combine with electron-rich nucleophilic groups such as the tertiary nitrogens in purines and pyrimidines, or with $-NH_2$, $-COOH$, $-SH$, and $-PO_3H_2$ groups on a variety of molecules. The high-energy rings of alkylating agents break and combine with these constituents to form stable covalent bonds. Obviously, many cell components have such groups, including DNA, RNA, and the enzymatic and structural proteins. Alkylation of DNA is probably the most detrimental. If the DNA strands are not repaired, chromosomal replication will be faulty in proliferating cells. Both DNA and RNA can be alkylated at several points, but a common site appears to be N-7 of the guanine ring (Fig. 10-16). Mispairing of DNA during replication may result from the presence of the alkylating agent itself, the clipping out of the alkylated guanine residue, or the cleavage of an alkylated guanine ring. Also chain breaks and cross-linkages frequently interfere with chain replication.

Since the damage to DNA can be repaired, these effects are apparently time-dependent. Consequently, the administration of alkylating agents just before and during stimulation by the antigen would most interfere with the ability of the immunocompetent cells to respond to that antigen. Continued use of the alkylating agents would also muffle the proliferative response of these cells in the face of a persistent stimulus. There are differences, however, in the response of T and B cells. The B cell seems to be more susceptible to cyclophosphamide than the T cell. This drug is a potent inhibitor of antibody formation, but its effect on skin or kidney rejection is much less spectacular. The reason for this apparent difference is unknown.

The usefulness of alkylating agents, which include nitrogen mustard, phenylalanine mustard, busulfan, and cyclophosphamide, is limited by their toxicity. Even so, cyclophosphamide has been used with good results in renal transplantation when liver toxicity prohibited the use of azathioprine. Cyclophosphamide is frequently used in clinical bone marrow transplantation, where it potentiates the effects of radiation and enhances the disruption of DNA. When cyclophosphamide is used, lower doses of radiation are required to deplete the recipient bone marrow population and provide space for donor cells. When leukemia is the indication for bone marrow transplantation, cyclophosphamide will aid in the destruction of these cells.

Toxicity is high, however, and predictable reactions occur, principally to rapidly replicating cell populations. Stomatitis, nausea, vomiting, diarrhea, skin rash, anemia, and alopecia are all common reactions. The more specific effects of cyclophosphamide administration are prompt fluid retention, occasionally severe hemorrhagic cystitis, and cardiac toxicity. The cardiac and edema problems suggest that even nonreplicating cell populations are adversely affected by this drug.

ANTIBIOTICS. The immunosuppressive antibiotics include the inhibitors of nucleic acid synthesis, and chloramphenicol and puromycin, which interfere with cellular protein synthesis. Actinomycin D binds to the guanine residue of DNA, thereby sterically interfering with RNA polymerase and, consequently, with DNA-directed RNA

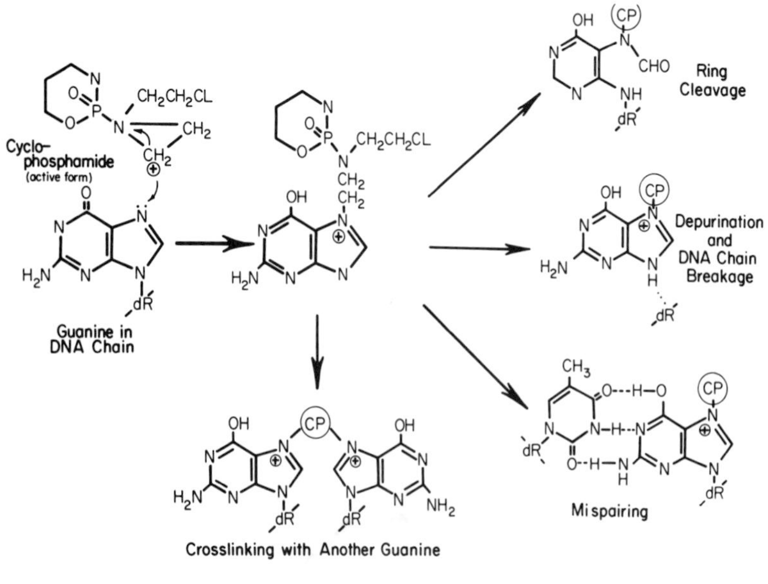

Fig. 10-16. Mechanism of the action of the alkylating agent cyclophosphamide (CP). CP binds to the guanine molecule within the DNA chain. The guanine-CP complex leads to further damage to the DNA molecule. Four examples of the damage to DNA are shown. [From: *Simmons RL, Foker JE, Najarian JS: Principles of immunosuppression, in Sabiston DC Jr (ed): Davis-Christopher Textbook of Surgery. Philadelphia, Saunders, 1972, p 471, with permission.*]

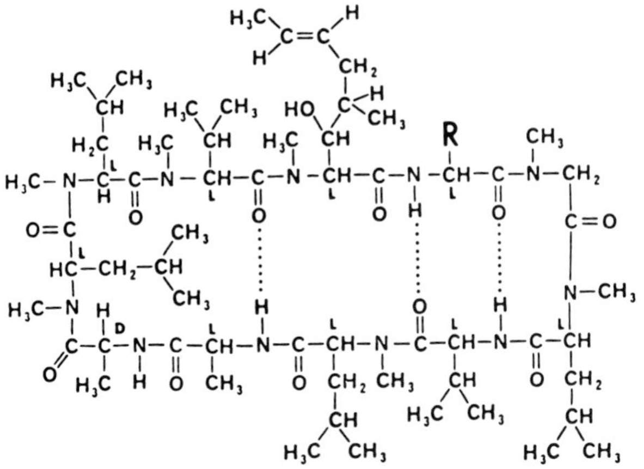

Fig. 10-17. Structure of cyclosporine. CyA,R = —CH$_2$CH$_3$; CyD,R = —CH(CH$_3$)$_2$.

synthesis. Mitomycin C combines with cellular DNA and hinders replication. None of these agents is clinically useful as an immunosuppressive agent for transplantation.

CYCLOSPORINE. Cyclosporine is a fungal cyclic peptide (Fig. 10-17) which represents an entire new class of clinically important immunosuppressive agents. It is not an alkylating, antimitotic, or lympholytic agent. Its action at the molecular level seems highly specific, not just for lymphoid cells, but rather for certain subpopulations of T cells.

Cyclosporine strongly inhibits the formation of cytotoxic T cells in mixed lymphocyte culture, and prophylactic administration is strongly suppressive of allograft rejection. Indeed, rejection or graft-versus-host disease can sometimes be overcome or reversed. Stopping the drug permits rejection to resume so that cyclosporine plus antigen does not lead to permanent tolerance.

Cyclosporine does not appear to affect precursor hematopoietic cells, resting or dividing lymphocytes, or macrophage functions. It acts by interfering with the production of the lymphokine interleukin II, which is normally essential for lymphocyte proliferation. Thus the expansion of antigen-responsive clones of T lymphocytes is suppressed. T suppressor cells, however, are not inhibited. Additive immunosuppressive effects can be achieved in combination with ALG, azathioprine, prednisone, irradiation, and other anti-inflammatory drugs.

Cyclosporine has virtually revolutionized clinical transplantation. In combination with modest doses of prednisone, it appears to be of equal clinical utility, or superior, to ALG-azathioprine and prednisone. Its renal toxicity is a serious disadvantage but can usually be controlled by reducing the dose or combining it with conventional immunosuppressive drugs. A minor disadvantage is that it can only be administered by mouth in a lipid-soluble medium (milk, oil), and its absorption is unpredictable. An intravenous formulation is also available but nephrotoxicity is a problem. In clinically useful doses, cyclosporine is no more likely to induce lymphoma formation than the older immunosuppressive agents.

IMMUNOSUPPRESSION BY LYMPHOCYTE DEPLETION

ADRENAL CORTICOSTEROIDS. Despite uncertainty about their mechanism of action, steroids are necessary for successful human organ transplantation and are commonly used to produce immunosuppression in other types of patients.

Many effects of steroids are known (Fig. 10-18). The problem is deciding which are primary and which are secondary actions. Steroids cross the cell membrane and bind to specific receptors in the cytoplasm of most cells, lymphocytes included. The steroid-receptor complex then enters the nucleus and interacts with DNA in an unknown way. In lymphocytes, DNA, RNA, and protein synthesis is inhibited, as is glucose and amino acid transport. At a sufficient dosage, lymphocyte degeneration and lysis occur. Cytolysis can readily be produced in vivo, and T cells appear to be most susceptible. The primary antilymphocyte action of steroids may be to deplete small lymphocytes before they are activated by antigen. Steroids also suppress most of the accessory functions of macrophages including the ability to secrete interleukin-1.

The functional effects of steroids are predictable, and all T-cell responses are depressed. Paradoxically, the steroid-resistant thymocytes that remain after an injection of steroids have increased activity, but the net immunologic capability of the treated animal is reduced.

Although B-cell activity and antibody production are relatively unaffected by steroids, many other cell types that participate in graft rejection are damaged. Both macrophage and neutrophil chemotaxis and phagocytosis are inhibited. The accumulation of neutrophils, macrophages, and monocytes at sites of immune and inflammatory activity is reduced. Steroids also increase the membrane stability of digestive lysosomal particles in these cells, which reduces their inflammatory activity. Inflammation is so intertwined with any substantial immune reaction that the various effects are inseparable. The variety of immunologic activities that steroids will suppress means that their effectiveness against the rejection reaction is probably the sum of many influences. Steroids alone cannot prevent clinical allograft rejection, but, together with other compounds, they are potent in both preventing and reversing rejection reactions.

Steroid toxicity of some degree is frequent and commonly includes a cushingoid appearance. Other characteristic problems from steroid therapy are hypertension; weight gain; peptic ulcers and gastrointestinal bleeding; euphoric personality changes; cataract formation; hyperglycemia, which may progress to steroid diabetes; and osteoporosis with avascular necrosis of bone. The appearance and severity of these complications vary considerably, but all too frequently they are life-threatening or disabling. Clinical transplantation will be improved tremendously when more specific means of immunosuppression are developed and present steroid dosages can be reduced.

ANTILYMPHOCYTE GLOBULIN. A variety of antibody preparations designed to react with immunoresponsive

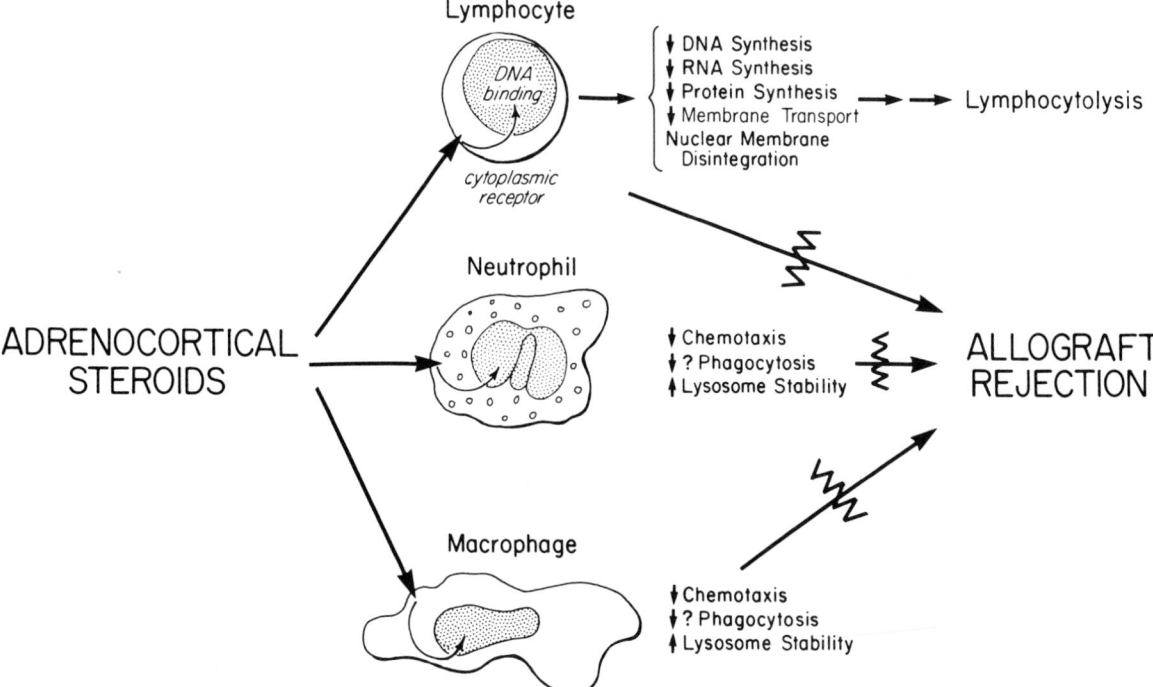

Fig. 10-18. Adrenocortical steroids play an important role in clinical allograft immunosuppression. Many apparent sites of action have been located experimentally. These compounds bind to cytoplasmic receptors, and this complex combines with DNA. How this relates to the many functional consequences of steroids presented in this diagram is unclear. In the complex clinical transplantation setting it is not possible to determine if the primary suppression of lymphocytes is more important than the anti-inflammatory effects on neutrophils and macrophages in the suppression of allograft rejection reactions. The suppression of interleukin-1 production by macrophages is probably a most important mechanism.

lymphocytes are available, and their number and variety will increase in the next few years. They are designed to prevent and to treat graft rejection.

Heterologous polyclonal antilymphocyte globulins (ALG) are produced when thoracic duct, peripheral blood, lymph nodes, thymus, or spleen lymphocytes are injected into animals of a different species. Cell membranes or cultured lymphocytes serve equally well to provide the antigenic stimulation. The addition of adjuvants, usually Freund's complete adjuvant, is used to enhance the immunogenicity of the foreign lymphocytes and produce sera that are consistently more immunosuppressive. The rabbit and the horse are commonly used to produce antisera for clinical transplantation.

The antibodies produced in this crude way are reactive with a number of different epitopes on the many subsets of lymphocytes injected. As a consequence, the immunosuppressive effect is the net result of the destruction of many lymphocyte subsets.

The action of heterologous polyclonal ALG seems to be directed mainly against the T cell. ALG therefore interferes most with the cell-mediated reactions-allograft

rejection, tuberculin sensitivity, and the graft-versus-host reaction. ALG can abolish preexisting delayed hypersensitivity reactions, and larger doses will prolong the survival of some xenografts. ALG has a definite, but lesser, effect on antibody production to T-cell-dependent antigens.

Although these preparations, purified and administered intravenously, have been widely used in clinical transplantation with beneficial results in both the prevention and treatment of organ allograft rejection, monoclonal reagents with more predictable reactivity are becoming available. Such antibodies are the products of cell fusions between antilymphocyte antibody-producing clones of mouse B cells and laboratory myeloma cells. The resulting hybridomas have become rendered immortal and each cell line produces a single antibody directed to a single antigen on a human lymphocyte. If the target cell is a cell type essential for the immune response, such as a T cell, severe degrees of immunosuppression can be induced in the recipient of the monoclonal antibody. Mouse monoclonal antibody directed against T cells is now available for clinical use in the treatment of rejection.

The toxicity of any heterologous antibody prepared against human tissue depends in part on its cross reactivity with other tissue antigens, and the ability of the patient to make antibodies against the protein itself. Polyclonal ALG can produce anemia and thrombocytopenia despite prior absorption with human platelets and red cell stroma. Monoclonal antibodies have few cross reactions, but fever, chills, nausea, diarrhea, and aseptic meningitis are frequently seen during the intravenous administration of the first few doses. All heterologous globulins can elicit allergic reactions against themselves. These are generally mild and infrequent, but monoclonal antibodies are strongly antigenic so that they are less effective after 1 or 2 weeks of use. Polyclonal antibody preparations seem to be repeatedly effective.

RADIATION. Radiation was probably the first agent used to produce immunosuppression. Ionizing radiation (x-rays, alpha rays, beta rays) affects both cellular proteins and nucleic acids. Despite the fact that relatively small dosages of irradiation may disrupt the secondary protein structure formed by hydrogen bonding and the tertiary conformation that results, biologically significant alterations of protein function seem to require very high dosages. Consequently, most of the immunosuppressive effects of x-radiation are caused by changes produced in nucleic acids. DNA is particularly vulnerable, and therefore so is cellular replication. The most important of the several modes of damage is the production of scattered breaks in the deoxyribose-phosphate backbone of DNA (Fig. 10-19). Disruption of either the carbon-carbon bonds of the deoxyribotides or the bonds involving the phosphate groups produces breaks in one of the DNA strands. Occasionally both strands are broken at the same point. Other sites of damage, such as the bases themselves, are even less frequent.

Repair mechanisms exist to mend the breaks, but insuf-

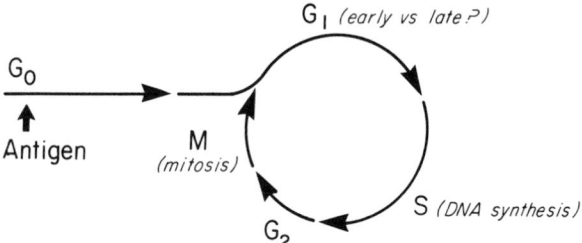

Fig. 10-20. The phases of the cell cycle. Following stimulation by an antigen, or other type of mitogen, small lymphocytes are activated. They are converted from the resting G_0 phase to the active G_1 phase. The G_1 phase lasts 10 h or longer before DNA synthesis (S phase) begins. The S phase lasts about 10 h and is followed by a short (2 to 4 h) G_2 phase before mitosis (M phase). M phase is relatively brief, usually less than 2 to 3 h, after which the cells are returned to the G_1 phase. The susceptibility of the cell to the immunosuppressive agents used in transplantation varies with the phase of the cycle. Periods of most intense nucleic acid synthesis, particularly S phase, are most vulnerable to the antimetabolites. As discussed in the text, the resting G_0 lymphocyte is also susceptible to several of the clinically used immunosuppressive agents. [From: *Foker JE, Simmons RL, Najarian JS: Principles of immunosuppression, in Sabiston DC Jr (ed): Davis-Christopher Textbook of Surgery. Philadelphia, Saunders, 1977, p 509, with permission.*]

Fig. 10-19. X-ray-induced damage of DNA molecule. Irradiation frequently induces single breaks in the deoxyribotide backbone of the DNA double helix. More rarely, irradiation induces double breaks within the backbone. [From: *Simmons RL, Foker JE, Najarian JS: Principles of immunosuppression, in Sabiston DC Jr (ed): Davis-Christopher Textbook of Surgery. Philadelphia, Saunders, 1972, p 471, with permission.*]

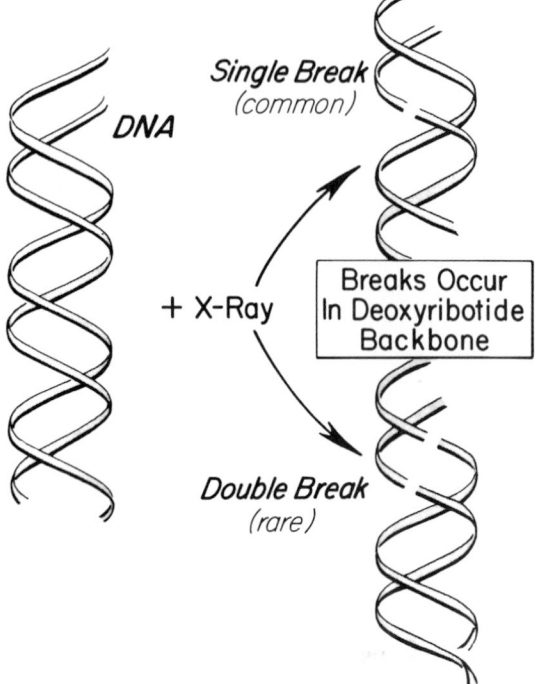

ficient time may be available in the dividing cell. Therefore, the effectiveness of radiation is dependent upon the phase of the cell cycle in which the cell is found (Fig. 10-20). Cells in the M or G_2 phase are most sensitive to irradiation. Presumably, DNA breaks that occur during these phases cannot be repaired quickly enough, and the synthetic events and precise apportionment of cellular components that occur during mitosis may become scrambled. Conversely, the early G_1 phase and the latter part of the S phase are the most resistant portions of the cell cycle. Although irradiation is, in general, most effective just prior to or during mitosis, lymphocytes are a special case. For reasons that are not known, these cells are also sensitive in their resting, or G_0, phase.

The effect of irradiation on the immune response depends greatly on its timing with relation to antigen exposure. When an antigen is given soon after irradiation, the immune response will be inhibited because there is insufficient time for the immunocompetent cell population to recover before the antigen is encountered. If radiation is given during the time of maximal proliferation of the immunocompetent population to an antigen (soon after antigen administration), the immune response will be strongly inhibited. On the other hand, if antigenic stimulation is delayed long enough for the precursor cells to recover from the radiation, there will even be a slight augmentation of the response. Radiation is ineffective if given long after the antigen, when a mature population of effector cells has been formed.

Total body irradiation has limited use in clinical transplantation because the toxicity is too great. Fractionated doses of radiation to the lymphoid tissues (total lymphoid irradiation), similar to that used in the treatment of Hodgkin's disease, is under investigation. Profound immunosuppression is produced, and low dosages of azathioprine and prednisone can maintain the effect. Local irradiation of the graft may also provide some immunosuppressive effects by damaging invading lymphocytes as well as producing nonspecific anti-inflammatory effects.

Both total body radiation and total lymphoid irradiation have been used to eliminate the immune reactivity of patients in preparation for bone marrow transplantation. Cytotoxic chemotherapy is used in combination. The toxicity is predictable. The rapidly replicating skin and gastrointestinal tract are universally affected, and nausea, vomiting, diarrhea, and skin changes occur.

THYMECTOMY. The atrophic adult mammalian thymus continues to play a small role in maintaining immunologic responsiveness. Its extirpation can enhance the effects of immunosuppressive agents or irradiation. Unfortunately, thymectomy has not been useful in clinical transplantation.

LYMPHOID EXTIRPATION AND SPLENECTOMY. Immunity becomes rapidly systemic. It is not confined for long to the regional lymph nodes or to a single major lymphoid organ like the spleen. Splenectomy, however, appears to be beneficial in combination with ALG, azathioprine, and prednisone in prolonging human organ allograft survival. Its effect may simply be to reduce the toxicity of the myelosuppressive drugs so that greater doses of azathioprine can be tolerated in splenectomized transplant recipients. Because splenectomy also increases the risk of subsequent infection, it is used less often in organ transplantation.

THORACIC DUCT DRAINAGE. Cannulation and drainage of the thoracic duct will deplete the body of a large proportion of its circulating T lymphocytes, and such depletion will lead to prolongation of allograft survival and to lesser decreases in the capacity for antibody synthesis. Thoracic duct cannulation and drainage have been used for clinical immunosuppression with great success, but the procedure is cumbersome. The indwelling cannula can become plugged or infected and protein depletion may result if the cell-free lymph is not reinfused. It is doubtful whether this complicated technique, which requires prolonged hospitalization, is superior to drug therapy.

ADVERSE CONSEQUENCES OF IMMUNOSUPPRESSIVE THERAPY

The complications of immunosuppressive therapy in recipients of organ allografts are difficult to distinguish from the complications of recurrent rejection. Patients who do not have rejection episodes generally do not suffer major complications of immunosuppressive therapy. Conversely, the patient who requires repeated large doses of prednisone to avoid further rejection episodes or who suffers diminished renal function in the presence of high doses of azathioprine will have potentially lethal complications. The major complications all relate to a relative inability to respond effectively to a large variety of pathogenic, and even to normally saprophytic, organisms. There may be, moreover, a decrease in the normal capacity to destroy mutant, potentially neoplastic cells.

PARAMETERS OF IMMUNOSUPPRESSION. Can immunosuppression be measured in any other way than by graft function? All methods of clinical immunologic monitoring are restricted to measuring the specific or nonspecific responses of peripheral blood lymphocytes—the spleen, thymus, and lymph nodes not being readily available. With this restriction in mind, an immunosuppressive effect can be detected during the first 2 weeks after kidney transplantation. The response of the patient's circulating lymphocyte to either the mitogen phytohemagglutinin (PHA) or to foreign leukocytes is depressed. In recipients of ALG, azathioprine, and prednisone, the loss of reactivity is proportional to the decrease in number of circulating T cells. The T-cell number in cyclosporine recipients is not diminished, but there may be some alteration in the relative proportions of helper and suppressor T cells. In some recipients of long-surviving grafts, peripheral blood lymphocytes may not respond to graft antigens in vitro. There is no other reliable way to monitor the level of immunosuppression achieved. Nor is it possible to predict incipient rejection accurately. Because the degree of immunosuppression cannot yet be measured, the dosages of immunosuppressive agents are regulated instead by toxicity produced.

BACTERIAL AND FUNGAL INFECTION. Immunosuppression understandably increases the risk of infection. The routine posttransplant immunosuppression regimen does not necessarily result in a higher bacterial infection rate. With suitable aseptic precautions and antibiotic perioperative prophylaxis, the postoperative wound infection incidence is very low. When there are no severe rejection reactions and the graft maintains good function, the day-to-day bacterial challenge to the recipient is handled. Although urinary tract infections are frequent, they are usually mild and easily controlled by antibiotics.

We do not mean to imply that bacterial infection is an insignificant problem for transplantation patients. On the contrary, infection is still the most common complication of immunosuppression, and overall it is the most common cause of death in transplant recipients (Fig. 10-21). Infections are the natural consequence of impaired healing of visceral anastomoses after renal, liver, or pancreatic transplantation. Increasing experience has reduced the incidence of perigraft infections, however, and the most common infections are now caused by organisms that are normally weakly pathogenic. Antibiotics will eradicate the more aggressive bacteria, but they leave opportunistic organisms free to colonize the susceptible transplant patient. The opportunistic organisms, which are normally eliminated by cellular mechanisms, can now blossom in the face of the relative T-cell depression. Fungi are prominent opportunists, and they can cause cutaneous, mucosal, pulmonary, and central nervous system infections, as well as generalized sepsis. *Candida* infections are probably the most common. The inevitable mucosal candidiasis can be satisfactorily prevented by oral mycostatin.

Aspergillus species are probably the second most common cause of fungal infection and typically produce upper lobe pulmonary cavities and brain abscesses. There have been many reports of hospital epidemics traceable to con-

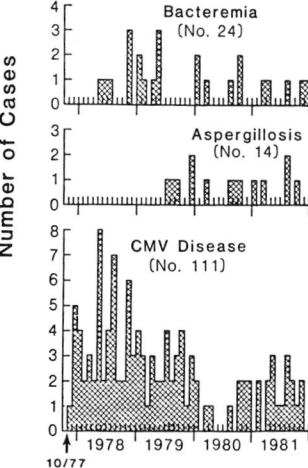

Fig. 10-21. Incidence of infections in 535 consecutive transplants performed between October 1977 and September 1981, at the University of Minnesota hospital, and followed until January 1982. The incidence varied widely, even though the rate of transplantation was the same, i.e., 10 to 15 transplants per month. The reasons for this variation are not clear. (From: *Peterson PK, Ferguson R, et al: Infectious diseases in hospitalized renal transplant recipients: A prospective study of a complex and evolving problem. Medicine, 61:360, 1982, with permission.*)

struction or ventilation problems. *Rhizopus oryzae, Histoplasma capsulatum,* and *Cryptococcus neoformans* also invade the lung, and the latter is the most common cause of meningitis. The indolent bacterium *Nocardia asteroides* occasionally infects, producing nodular pulmonary lesions. The protozoan *Pneumocystis carinii,* more commonly seen in patients undergoing cancer chemotherapy, usually causes a diffuse alveolar infiltrate.

Standard patient isolation precautions are of little use against these organisms, and prophylactic antibiotics are not available for most of them. Prevention is dependent upon avoiding excessive dosages of immunosuppressive agents in a futile attempt to prolong the function of a rejected graft. Some protection against *P. carinii, Nocardia,* the pneumococcus, *Listeria, Legionella,* and other susceptible organisms may be provided by the prophylactic trimethoprim and sulfamethoxazole. The pneumococcal vaccine may ultimately be useful.

VIRAL INFECTIONS. Viral infections seem to be almost ubiquitous among kidney transplant recipients. The herpes group of DNA viruses are most common etiologic agents. Infection or antibody response to cytomegalovirus (CMV) is found in 50 to 90 percent of patients after renal transplantation (Fig. 10-21). Herpes simplex infection occurs in about 25 percent and zoster in 10 percent of graft recipients; both can be prevented or treated with the antiviral agent acyclovir. Epstein–Barr virus (EBV) commonly infects transplant patients, but most infections are mild. EBV is associated with posttransplant malignancy in rare patients, however.

Antigenic evidence for hepatitis B virus infection can be detected in many transplant patients and non-A, non-B hepatitis is probably a cause of liver failure in some long-term survivors. Immunosuppressed patients have both typical and atypical patterns of infection. Hepatitis is particularly illustrative. Transplantation and hemodialysis patients may have no symptoms of acute hepatitis, but antibody responses and viral elimination are unusual. For this reason, persistent active hepatitis is a common finding in long-term survivors and a common underlying cause of death years after the transplant.

Cytomegalovirus (CMV) is the most important infectious illness that afflicts immunosuppressed transplant patients. CMV infection can produce a spectrum of illness typically characterized by fever, neutropenia, arthralgias, malaise, myocarditis, pancreatitis, or gastrointestinal ulceration. The most severe illnesses are acquired as primary infections from latent virus residing in the grafted tissue. Less often blood transfusions are the vector. Some cases of apparently new infection represent reactivation of latent intracellular viruses. Transplant recipients who do not have antibodies to CMV and who receive grafts from donors who do are at highest risk. The use of antilymphocyte antibody preparations for immunosuppression increases the risk. Recipients of cyclosporine appear to be at lower risk.

The typical CMV infection is a mild febrile illness, followed by an antibody response and regression of viral symptoms. A rejection episode sometimes accompanies the viral infection and raises the controversy of whether the virus triggers the rejection episode. These patients usually recover but may continue to excrete CMV in urine or saliva despite the presence of antibodies to CMV. In certain patients, however, there is no effective immune response, and the infection can be lethal. The virus itself induces a profound state of immunosuppression rendering these patients exquisitely susceptible to bacterial or fungal opportunists. Many serious infections are superinfections in patients already suffering CMV infections.

PREVENTION OF INFECTION. The incidence of severe, near-fatal infections has been reduced through a number of precautions. (1) The most important precaution is to eliminate all sources of infection prior to transplantation, especially those in the urinary tract and dialysis access site. Other sources of infection should be sought by routine preoperative cultures and careful examination. If any source is found, it should be eliminated by the appropriate use of surgical drainage or antibiotic therapy. (2) When technical problems are avoided, wound sepsis is uncommon. Urinary, biliary, or pancreatic anastomotic breakdown especially predisposes to wound infection. (3) Organs from related and well-matched cadavers elicit less frequent and less vigorous rejection reactions. If repeated rejection can be avoided, the doses of immunosuppressive drugs can be minimized and the rate and severity of infection will diminish. (4) Many patients who die of infection develop leukopenia (especially neutropenia) at some time. Some bouts of leukopenia can be attributed to cytomegalovirus infections. Leukopenia can be prevented by careful reduction in azathioprine doses when the leukocyte count or platelet count falls. The use of other bone marrow depressants (chloramphenicol) should be avoided in patients already on azathioprine therapy. Cyclosporine A is not myelosuppressive and should reduce the incidence of neutropenia. (5) Protective isolation protocols were formerly used to minimize infections in the initial postoperative care. Most transplant units have discontinued their use because they restrict access to the patients, impose psychologic stress, and are probably ineffective against viral, fungal, or endogenous bacteria.

MALIGNANCY. Cancer has been an unexpectedly frequent companion of clinical transplantation. The incidence of cancer is not high enough, however, to contraindicate the transplant procedure. Tumors in transplant recipients have come from two general sources. A rare cause is the inadvertent transplantation of a cancer from a cadaver donor in whom the cancer was unsuspected. These tumors can sometimes be treated simply by halting immunosuppression therapy and allowing rejection of the tumor tissue, as well as the transplant, to occur.

The more common cancers are the primary tumors that appear in the immunosuppressed recipient. Only certain tumors grow more readily in immunodepressed patients. Seventy-five percent of the spontaneous cancers are either epithelial or lymphoid in origin. Carcinoma in situ of the cervix, carcinoma of the lip, and squamous or basal cell carcinomas of the skin account for about half of this group, while B-cell lymphomas make up the remainder. It has been estimated that the risks to the transplant recipient of developing cervical cancer, skin cancer, or lymphoma are increased by 4, 40, and 350 times, respectively. The lymphomas are unusual both in their frequency and in their behavior. Almost 50 percent of the immunosuppressed patients with lymphomas have brain involvement, which occurs in only 1 percent of nontransplanted related cases of lymphoma. These lymphomas, although initially responsive to radiation therapy, are usually fatal.

Recent evidence suggests that all lymphomas are not true neoplasms. Immunologic analysis has indicated that these tumors secrete several different types of immunoglobulins, i.e., they do not have the monoclonal characteristics of cancer. Most evidence suggests that some may represent uncontrolled B-cell proliferative responses to EBV. At this stage, antiviral chemotherapy with acyclovir appears promising. Subsequently true lymphoid neoplasms seem to evolve from chromosomal abnormalities; such true monoclonal malignancies have not responded well to conventional cancer chemotherapy.

We do not know why transplant patients have an increased risk for these cancers. It has been postulated that the surveillance and elimination of tumor cells as they arise by lymphocytes is an important natural defense of human beings against cancer. Certainly this function might be abnormal in immunodepressed patients. Another possibility is the use of mutagens like azathioprine as immunosuppressive drugs. There is also growing evidence that herpes viruses, to which the immunosuppressed patient is manifestly susceptible, can induce these neoplasms. EBV is almost certainly the cause of the polyclonal B-cell lymphoproliferative disorder that evolves into a monoclonal lymphoma. All these lesions contain the EBV genome as part of the cellular DNA.

Less certain is the possibility that cancers of the epithelium may be a consequence of herpes virus transformation. This group of viruses is carcinogenic in animals and infects epithelial cells of lip, skin, and genital tissue. Circumstantial evidence exists for a role in human cervical cancer. Herpes viruses are usually dormant, but the stress of transplantation or the action of antimetabolite may activate them. The viruses might then either proliferate and cause a clinical viral illness or produce cellular transformation into cancer cells. Similarly, the Papova viruses are probably the cause of skin cancer in immunosuppressed patients.

CUSHING'S DISEASE. Most transplant patients who receive steroid therapy develop Cushing's syndrome. The appearance of the face is altered by rounding, puffiness, and plethora; fat tends to be redistributed from the extremities to the trunk and face. There is also an increased growth of fine hair over the thighs and trunk and sometimes over the face. Acne may appear or increase, and insomnia and increased appetite are noted. The underlying metabolic changes can be even more serious: The continuing breakdown of protein and diversion of amino acids to glucose increase the need for insulin and result in weight gain, fat deposition, muscle wasting, thinning of the skin with striae, and sometimes the development of steroid diabetes, cataracts, and osteoporosis. In some patients a myopathy develops, the nature of which is unknown. The cushingoid changes may represent such a problem that transplant nephrectomy will be necessary on that basis alone.

GASTROINTESTINAL BLEEDING. Gastrointestinal bleeding due to reactivation of a preexisting ulcer or diffuse ulceration of the gastrointestinal tract can be a fatal complication. The relative pathogenetic contribution of progressive uremia and steroid administration is unknown, but when bleeding appears, it can be difficult to control by nonoperative means. Occasionally the use of cimetidine or the intramesenteric arterial infusion of vasopressin is effective.

During moderate doses of steroid therapy, episodes of gastrointestinal bleeding can be almost totally prevented by the use of antacids between meals. In patients with rejection who require high steroid dosage, antacid therapy must be intensified with each increase in steroid administration. Pretransplant antiulcer operations have been used in patients with peptic disease.

OTHER INTESTINAL COMPLICATIONS. A number of colonic complications, including diverticulitis, bleeding, and ulceration, are associated with immunosuppressive treatment. A syndrome of acute cecal ulceration with gastrointestinal bleeding is due to cytomegalovirus. Cytomegalovirus underlies sporadic ulcer disease in other enteric locations as well.

CATARACTS. Cataracts are common in patients who require steroids. The cataracts, which develop slowly, appear to be independent of the absolute prednisone dosage.

THROMBOSIS AND THROMBOEMBOLIC PHENOMENA. Thrombophlebitis may occur in the renal transplant recipient, particularly on the side of the graft where the venous anastomosis may become partially or completely thrombosed. The diagnosis is difficult because swelling of the leg on the side of the transplant site is an occasional sign of rejection, associated with increases in weight, pulmonary infiltrates, and slight increases in serum creatinine level. When the differential diagnosis is difficult, a femoral venogram is indicated. The diagnosis of pulmonary embolism may also be difficult because clinical thrombophlebitis seldom precedes the embolus.

HYPERTENSION. Many of the patients who come to renal transplantation are already hypertensive. Hypertension can usually be controlled with dialysis or, in rare refractory cases, with nephrectomy. Hypertension in most patients will develop soon after transplantation, but posttransplant hypertension can be easily controlled with dietary salt restriction and drugs. The hypertension seems to be due not only to prednisone but also to failure to regulate the normal salt and water balance in the early posttransplant period and secretion of renin by the kidney. Hypertension may be aggravated by rejection. It should be remembered, however, that significant hypertension may be due to renal arterial stenosis, and arteriography may be necessary for the differentiation.

DISORDERS OF CALCIUM METABOLISM. Patients frequently come to renal transplantation with renal osteodystrophy. Alterations in vitamin D metabolism and secondary hyperparathyroidism are prominent factors in the pathogenesis of skeletal disease. Long-standing acidosis may likewise be contributory. The resulting osteoporosis, osteomalacia, and osteitis fibrosa cystica in the child can lead to growth restriction, epiphysiolysis, skeletal deformities, and pathologic fractures. The bone disease in some cases can be arrested with pharmacologic dosages of vitamin D or aluminum hydroxide.

Hemodialysis can correct the uremic state, but the bone disease may actually progress if the stimulus to parathyroid hormone secretion is not effectively eliminated. Great attention should be directed toward keeping the dialysate calcium concentration at a level (6 to 7 mg/dL) that does not promote calcium loss from the blood. Parathyroidectomy is sometimes required to help arrest progressive bone disease but is not indicated for hypercalcemia alone after transplant. Parathyroidectomy seems primarily indicated for patients on chronic hemodialysis in whom transplantation is not planned.

MUSCULOSKELETAL COMPLICATIONS. A disturbing complication of successful renal transplantation is avascular necrosis of the femoral heads and other bones. Its occurrence is most closely correlated with the dosage of steroid used. Transient rheumatoid symptoms precede changes visible by radiography by several months. The bone changes apparently occur secondarily to steroid osteopenia or osteonecrosis with resulting microfractures. Alterations in lipid metabolism caused by fluctuating high levels of steroids likewise appear to be important in the pathogenesis. The treatment is for the most part symptomatic. It is doubtful that bone lesions can revascularize sufficiently to restore normal architecture in the presence of maintenance steroids. Should symptoms increase, replacement arthroplasty is usually successful.

Migratory arthralgia, myalgia, and tendonitis are com-mon, but persistent joint pain and swelling are most often signs of intraarticular infection. Occasionally, an unexplained septic arthritis crops up in these patients; mycobacterial infections are most commonly reported.

PANCREATITIS. Pancreatitis may appear suddenly and unexpectedly in renal allograft recipients, and recurrent bouts may prove to be fatal. It has been attributed variously to corticosteroid therapy, azathioprine, cytomegalovirus, or hepatitis virus. Steroids are known to thicken pancreatic secretions.

ERYTHREMIA AND ANEMIA. The transplanted kidney is apparently fully capable of manufacturing erythropoietin. During rejection, the serum level may be increased. Erythremia also may appear, but apparently it is not related to elevated erythropoietin levels. Phlebotomy has been advised for hemoglobin levels greater than 16 g/dL.

Anemia usually is not present except in association with uremia or immunodepression secondary to azathioprine toxicity. A microangiopathic hemolytic anemia has also been thought to be induced by the vascular changes within the chronically rejecting kidney.

GROWTH. Since chronic renal failure itself is inhibitory to development, uremic children are usually far behind their peers in size. After successful transplantation their growth response is highly variable and may depend on age, previous growth rate, renal function, and immunosuppressive drug regimen. Many children return to a normal growth rate; unfortunately the growth that was lost during their original illness is not made up, so these children will always be smaller than their peers.

PREGNANCY. Many normal children have been born to renal transplanted women despite their use of mutagenic immunosuppressive drugs. The pregnancies of renal transplanted recipients are frequently complicated, however, by toxemia and bacterial and viral infections, particularly of the urinary tract. Both toxemia and infection may contribute to a higher incidence of premature labor and small neonates. Another important problem that must be faced is the decreased life expectancy of the transplant recipient. Parenthood is a long-term obligation, and counseling of these patients should include a discussion of these considerations.

CLINICAL TISSUE AND TRANSPLANTATION

Clinical allotransplants may be of several types: (1) temporary free grafts, such as skin allografts and blood transfusions; (2) partially inert struts that provide a framework for the ingrowth of host tissue, such as bone, cartilage, nerve, tendon, and fascial grafts; (3) permanent, partially privileged, structurally free grafts, such as cornea, blood vessels, and heart valves; (4) partially privileged functional free grafts such as parathyroid, ovary, and testes; (5) whole organ grafts, such as pancreas, kidney, liver, lung, and heart; and (6) bone marrow that acts as a functional replacement of the entire hemopoietic and lymphopoietic systems. Immunosuppression is warranted only for grafts essential for life. Tooth bud and thyroid grafts, which would require immunosuppression for any success, are trivial grafts and are easily replaced by prostheses or medication.

Clinical autotransplants have been carried out with hair, skin, teeth, kidney, legs, arms, veins, arteries, pericardium, valves, bone, cartilage, fascia, fat, tendons, nerves, stomach, bowel, parathyroid, thyroid, ovary, testis, adrenal, and hemopoietic tissue. Allotransplants have been carried out employing cornea, teeth, thyroid, parathyroid, adrenal, ovary, testis, pituitary, spleen, lymph node, bone marrow, skin, bone, cartilage, fascia, tendons, nerves, arteries, valves, veins, hemopoietic tissue, pancreas, duodenum, intestine, kidney, liver, lung, and heart. Xenografts of skin, heart valves, heart, kidney, testis, bone, and cartilage have been tried in the past.

Skin

Autotransplants of skin containing hair are used to reconstruct eyebrows or to replace the scalp after traumatic avulsion. Autotransplants of individual hair roots are sometimes used as a treatment for baldness. Skin autotransplants have been used to reconstruct the esophagus, urinary tract, vagina, and hernial weaknesses as well as the usual surface defects. The main use of skin autografts is to cover and replace areas destroyed by trauma, burn, or operation.

Skin allotransplants are also used quite extensively in burned patients when autochthonous skin is not available. The theory behind this is that the skin allograft provides a better coverage than any other material, and during the period of time when it is taking, it prevents the continued spread of sepsis. Skin allografts are commonly used in three different ways: In the first they are applied as a dressing to the freshly excised burned area and are removed after 10 to 14 days. At this time additional allografts are reapplied if the area does not appear to be clean enough to accept autografts. The second method is to place pinch grafts of autografted skin within defects created in a sheet allograft covering large defects. As the allografted skin is gradually rejected, it is replaced by epithelial cells that grow in from the autografts. In a modification of these techniques widely meshed autografts are covered with a sheet allograft to protect both the ungrafted areas and the fragile autograft. The allografts are eventually lifted off by the regenerating autograft.

Xenografts of skin are commonly used as temporary biologic dressings and are replaced at 1- to 5-day intervals. Fresh porcine skin is more physiologic and bacteriostatic but should be removed before it becomes vascularized. Commercial preparations of porcine skin are nonviable and do not become vascularized. A vast array of synthetic substitutes as well as animal collagenous materials are being developed, but their value must be compared with the present optimum temporary dressing, allograft.

Vascular Grafts

AUTOGRAFTS

Vein autografts have been used for over 50 years to replace segments of damaged arteries. This is still the best bypass graft for occluded vessels in the lower extremity.

After a period of time in the arterial circuit the vein wall thickens, and the vein becomes somewhat arterialized. Although there are occasional instances in which vein grafts weaken and rupture, by and large they make very satisfactory arterial substitutes. The two most common usages at the present time are in femoropopliteal artery–saphenous vein bypass grafts and coronary artery bypass grafts. Pieces of autologous vein are also used as patch grafts. It is possible too to carry out successful autologous vein grafts to bridge defects in veins, although veins are less likely to stay open than arteries.

Autografted arteries are also sometimes used as vascular replacements; most often the hypogastric artery is utilized. Pieces of pericardium are sometimes used to patch defects or divert flow in the repair of intracardiac defects.

ALLOGRAFTS

Allografted arteries are seldom used now. There are three reasons for this: (1) aneurysms sometimes occur, with rupture and a fatal outcome; (2) plastic prostheses have proved so suitable for the larger blood vessels; (3) for smaller blood vessels the use of the autologous saphenous vein has proved to be better than either prostheses or allografts. Arterial allografts, even if viable, do not survive but in part are replaced by host tissue and in part persist as semi-inert material.

When organs are transplanted, the artery supplying the organ becomes an arterial allograft. It has been shown that the epithelium of smaller blood vessels is antigenic and some degree of allograft rejection occurs.

Fresh, sterile aortic valve allografts have been used quite extensively. They appear to elicit a minimal antigenic response when compared with arterial allografts. Even so, gradual thickening, immobility, and calcification of these valves occur; their functional life expectancy is short. Preserved porcine valve xenografts are more useful, but loss of mobility sometimes indicates their replacement.

Vein allografts have been used for a number of years in sporadic fashion, and umbilical vein allografts have become commercially available for arterial bypass. Allografts have always been inferior to fresh autografts because of the rejection reaction that these grafts elicit. For some reason there has been a great reluctance among surgeons and others to accept the fact that arterial and venous allografts are antigenic. It is true that the antigenicity is relatively mild and that the graft can provide structural function even in the face of the immunologic response, but it eventually limits the life of the graft.

Fascia

Fascial autografts, either free or attached at one end, are used as living sutures for the repair of inguinal hernias; for the repair of chest wall defects, torn ligaments and tendons, abdominal wall hernias, and defects in the pleura, dura, diaphragm, trachea, and esophagus; for wrapping aneurysms; in arthroplasty; for fascial slings to correct paralysis of the facial muscles; in the stabilization of fractures and joints; in the construction of flexor sheaths; and to correct urinary incontinence. Fascial autografts have been used most commonly because of their convenience and ready availability. Some freeze-dried, preserved (nonviable) allografts have been used, however, and these dead grafts have united with muscle nearly as quickly as living fascia. Such allografts lose much of their histoincompatibility and serve as strong lattice for the ingrowth of autologous tissue.

Tendon

Free tendon autografts are used every day in standard surgical procedures. By far the most common use is that of repairing severed flexor tendons to the fingers. Usually the palmaris longus, plantaris, or extensor tendons of the toes are used, and the graft is inserted from the level of the midpalm of the hand to the distal phalanx. Tendon allografts are rarely of clinical use.

Nerve

Nerve autotransplants are used to bridge defects in important motor nerves or sometimes to transfer the function of one nerve into the distal end of another, to repair a severed facial or recurrent laryngeal nerve, for instance. The autografts undergo Wallerian degeneration with proliferation of Schwann cells and are penetrated by regenerating fibers of the host's nerve after a few weeks. When the nerve graft is thick, the center of the graft may develop a zone of avascular necrosis through which regeneration fails to occur. This does not happen with thin grafts. As a consequence of this, some investigators have advocated the use of cable grafts consisting of several strands of smaller nerves to bridge defects in nerves of larger caliber. Experimental work is being done to evaluate the function of vascularized nerve grafts transferred with microsurgical techniques. Motor recovery can occur as well as sensory recovery.

When allografts are used, the rate and intensity of nerve fiber penetration are less, and the outcome is far inferior to that obtained with autografts. In general they should probably be used only when autografts cannot be obtained. Xenografts have been tried but appear to be of no value to human beings. It is likely that the inflammatory rejection response interferes with the passage of autologous nerve endings down the transplanted nerve sheath.

Cornea

Perhaps the most common clinical allotransplant is that of the cornea. The eye should be harvested from cadavers within 6 h after death. Eyes removed more than 36 h after death are unsuitable for corneal transplantation. The whole eye is generally preserved in a sterile container at a temperature of 3 to 5°C, and the graft is cut from it at the time of use. The eye is suspended from a suture passed through the severed optic nerve to keep it from coming in contact with the sides of the vessel. Eye banks store the cornea in nutrient media at 4 or 34°C as long as 1 month.

Two types of corneal transplants are utilized: the full-thickness graft and the lamellar, or partial-thickness, graft. The full-thickness graft gives the best results, but infrequently complications such as secondary glaucoma, anterior synechiae, and a partial lifting off of the graft, causing astigmatism or opacification, occur. These complications are avoided in lamellar keratoplasty, which is the operation of choice when the corneal opacity does not involve the full thickness of the cornea. In order to achieve a successful graft there must be good apposition between the graft and the host, the graft must be in contact with healthy cornea at some point in the circumference if it is to remain transparent, and blood vessels must not invade the graft to any appreciable extent.

The best patients for grafting are those with central corneal scars and healthy surrounding cornea with no vascularization, keratoconus, especially if the apex of the cone is beginning to break down, and corneal dystrophy. Indolent corneal abscesses, perforating ulcers of the cornea, and descemetocele have less positive outcomes. The results are also somewhat less good in acne rosacea and herpetic keratitis because of the danger of recurrence of the disease.

Corneal grafts are apparently so successful because they remain effectively isolated from the host's cells so long as the graft itself and the cornea directly around it remain avascular. Systemic immunosuppression is used only on rare occasions. Many corneal grafts remain clear indefinitely, although occasionally a graft that has remained clear for several weeks becomes opaque. Apparently the fibrous barrier that is formed at the junction between the host and the graft is almost impervious to blood vessels and helps to maintain the isolation of the graft even when vessels have entered the host's cornea. The clouding over of a previously clear graft is due to the allograft reaction, usually because of vascularization.

Bone

Bone implants are used for the following indications: (1) to hasten the healing of defects and cavities, e.g., the use of cancellous bone chips in the residual defect after curettage of a unicameral bone cyst; (2) to supplement bony union in cases of delayed healing or pseudarthrosis arising after fracture, e.g., sliding or barrel stave grafts for nonunion of tibial shaft fractures, or to supplement the healing of certain fresh acquired or surgical fractures where skeletal continuity is problematic, e.g., cancellous autogenous implants for fractures of both bones of the forearm in an adult, (3) to reconstruct contour or major skeletal defects arising as a result of surgery trauma, disease, or congenital malformation, e.g., replacement of calvarial defects after surgery for trauma by compact bone implants.

Bone grafts are used to provide one or more of the following: (1) a source of viable osteoblasts (bone production); (2) a source of replacement for lost skeletal architecture (bone conduction); or (3) new bone formation (bone induction). Autografts of cancellous bone may provide all three: a source of living bone cells when harvested in thin strips where diffusion will provide cell nourishment, conduction of new bone formation along the cancellous surfaces, and bone induction from the matrix component diffusion that induces the differentiation of mesenchymal cells to form new bone. Autografts of cortical bone, such as fibular struts, may provide some small amount of living cells but primarily serve to reconstruct skeletal defects without the problems of antigenicity encountered in allografts. Allografts are generally reserved for large defects that cannot be filled or bridged by autografts without major disability at the donor site. Allografts will only provide for conduction and induction of a new bone. Combinations of autogenous cancellous grafts with cortical autografts or allografts are frequently used to hasten incorporation of these grafts to the recipient sites.

A variety of grafting techniques have been devised to meet the differing clinical requirements. The most frequent types of bone grafts are autogenous grafts with or without internal fixation. These may be applied as barrel stave grafts, sliding grafts, or cancellous chips. In addition, there are vascularized pedicle grafts of two types, those with a bony base, and muscle pedicle grafts. Microvascular anastomosis to provide free viable bone grafts or composite bone and soft tissue grafts has been useful in major defects of the limbs from trauma or neoplasia. Similarly, in some locations, vascularized grafts may be mobilized and rotated on their vascular pedicle to provide a viable graft without the requirement of anastomosis.

Autografts are preferred for clinical use, since the cellular elements of bone allografts usually elicit a rejection response. Bone allografts do elicit new bone formation (osteoinduction) and serve as struts for the ingrowth of autologous bone (osteoconduction). When properly prepared, the immune response to the allograft can be substantially reduced. As such, allografts are of great clinical use.

For the most part stored or processed bone allografts are used in clinical situations. Preservation methods include (1) refrigeration, (2) freezing, (3) freeze-drying, (4) decalcification, or (5) any one of the above plus irradiation for sterilization. Such nonviable grafts mainly serve to stimulate and conduct new autologous bone formation.

Cartilage

It has been long known that cartilage can be successfully transferred between individuals of different genetic backgrounds without the need for immunosuppression therapy. This immunologic privilege is attributable in adult articular cartilage to the absence of a blood supply. Under normal circumstances the fluid-nutritional needs are met via the synovial fluid. Thus, the absence of direct vascular contact and the presence of a dense proteoglycan-collagen matrix will insulate the chondrocytes from the host immune response.

Free autografts of cartilage have been used most extensively in plastic reconstructive surgery (1) to rebuild the contours of the nose after congenital or posttraumatic deformity, (2) to reconstruct the pinna, and (3) to fill out defects in the facial bones and the skull.

The fresh cartilage autograft comes closest to fulfilling the description of an ideal cartilage graft: it should maintain its structure, have the potential for growth and repair, provoke no untoward reaction, and form a firm union with host tissues, persisting without loss of viability or absorption. Recent experimental and clinical application of rib perichondral grafts as a source of new cartilage growth remains promising as an autograft technique for small joints.

The fresh cartilage allograft, however, has been reported to be a reasonable substitute for the autograft in particular circumstances because of its greater ease of procurement. The major drawback of such grafts is that despite the immunologic privilege of cartilage, the bulk of experimental and clinical evidence suggests that the tendency for late deterioration and absorption is somewhat greater than that of autografts. Furthermore, the potential for infection or transmission of viral-induced disease is similar to other living tissue transplants that are not proved sterile by culture or donor serology.

The preserved cartilaginous allograft has been used as a substitute for the fresh implant primarily because of the convenience that storage of such implants in cartilage banks provides. Refrigerated and chemically preserved frozen sections of cartilage have all been used with variable success.

COMPOSITE GRAFTS OF BONE AND CARTILAGE

Composite grafts involve the surgical transfer of entire functional units rather than the implantation of bits and pieces of cartilage or bone.

EPIPHYSEAL GROWTH PLATES. The object of the transplantation of epiphyseal growth plates is to restore longitudinal growth in hypoplastic limbs, whether congenital or acquired. This type of procedure has been used in efforts to improve the function of children with congenital deficiency of the radius. In these cases, autotransplantation of the proximal fibula has been used as a substitute for the radial deficiency. Although, in some cases, enlargement of the transplant could be demonstrated, this was always inferior to the natural growth potential and has not been sufficient to justify incorporation of this procedure into the surgical armamentarium. Microvascular transfer of epiphyseal growth plates shows continued growth and hypertrophy. This technique is now under clinical trial for restoring growth in damaged limbs.

OSTEOCHONDRAL GRAFTS. The diseases that destroy the articular cartilage are common. The osteochondral or osteoarticular graft might be a useful substitute. Transplants of articular cartilage, in conjunction with a very thin shell of subchondral supporting bone, are still in the experimental stage. Both allogenic and autogenous composites are now being applied in clinical trials in selected centers.

TRANSPLANT OF HEMIJOINTS OR WHOLE JOINTS. The experimental transplantation of joints was initiated by Judet in 1908. Autografts tend to heal their osteosynthesis sites, revascularize the bony component, and in general maintain the articular surfaces in a fair state of preservation. On the other hand, both fresh and preserved allogenic transplants give unpredictable results, sometimes healing well with good function, and other times showing progressive deterioration. The latter changes in the allogeneic groups are associated with delayed revascularization of the bony component, subchondral fracture and collapse, and synovial invasion of the joint surfaces. (Animal work suggests that immunosuppressive techniques can abort this phenomenon.) Artificial hemijoints or whole joints have superseded transplantation, at least for the present, but are more commonly used as composite replacements in major segmental defects. These composites generally use an allogeneic bone segment with an artificial joint implant to allow soft tissue reattachment around the joint for better function; host tendons and ligaments will generally reattach to the allograft and do not grow into a metal implant.

Extremity Replantation

Autotransplants or replantation of extremities have been carried out with increasing frequency in recent years. These procedures have usually involved the upper extremity, because the chances for good functional recovery are far greater in the arm than in the leg. Excellent prostheses exist for the lower extremity, but they are much less satisfactory for the upper. The major advantage of replantation is the development of useful sensation in the replanted extremity.

Shortening of the reimplanted extremity usually is necessary, and this produces much more incapacity in the leg than in the arm. Replantation of the leg might be considered when the opposite leg has been extensively damaged or lost or when the amputation has been so high that good prostheses are not available. Advances in microsurgery have made replantation of digits routine for the experienced microsurgeon.

The technique of limb replantation initially requires a general evaluation of the patient to assess other associated injuries. This should include radiography of the proximal stump as well as the amputated extremity itself, and particularly of the spine to be certain that the spinal roots to the extremity have not been avulsed. After securing hemostasis with pressure and being certain that no serious injury has been overlooked, the replantation can begin. During this initial phase the severed limb should be placed in a plastic container and packed in ice. The extremity should not be frozen, however, and for that reason, dry ice should be avoided. The limb may be replanted even though several hours have elapsed between its severance and the start of replantation. The exact critical period of ischemia has not definitely been established, but it appears that at least 12 h for a limb and up to 36 h for a finger can elapse with successful results after replantation. The more distal the amputation, the less ischemia-sensitive muscle tissue is in the extremity and prolonged cold ischemia is tolerated.

Prior to replantation a thorough debridement of grossly devitalized tissue is carried out. The bone is fixed first so that the limb will be stabilized before beginning the repairs of the vessels and nerve supply. Bones may require slight shortening to freshen up the ends and to gain additional length for relaxation of the arteries and nerves, and closure of soft tissue. Intramedullary fixation is used whenever possible.

After proper fixation of the bones, and repair of the tendons, the blood vessels are joined. In a distal amputation, a microsurgical team is required. The precise sequence of repair varies from surgeon to surgeon, but often the largest vein is joined first, so that there will be outflow available at the moment when the blood is ready to flow through the artery. It is important to join normal vessels beyond the zone of injury using vein grafts as necessary. If a nerve gap exists, nerve repair is delayed until healing is complete and a nerve graft can be done. If the nerve has been cleanly severed, immediate primary repair is carried out. A better result is obtained in distal nerve transections than in proximal ones, and in young people as compared with older ones. Distal sensory nerves give the most favorable results. Motor recovery in the median nerve is much more successful than in the ulnar nerve.

After completing the arterial and venous anastomoses and after either joining the ends of the nerves or deciding to perform a nerve graft as a secondary procedure, attention is turned to the soft tissues. With the blood supply restored, viability of tissues is easier to ascertain, and debridement can be completed. The shortening of the bone makes it possible to join several muscles together with a view to covering the blood vessels with living tissues. If soft tissue loss is minimal, the coverage can be achieved with the skin of the extremity, and other defects can be covered with split-thickness skin grafts. If the soft tissue defect is great and no covering is available, the defect must be covered by a pedicle flap. The newer microsurgical techniques permit the use of free revascularized myocutaneous flaps, usually as a secondary procedure.

In the postoperative period the patient's limb must be kept in an elevated position to minimize edema. It is important to do a fasciotomy, including carpel tunnel release, at the end of the replantation to avoid compartment swelling from ischemic damage to the arm musculature. Heparin and dextran are not generally used postoperatively. Some degree of hypotension may occur as a consequence of leakage of plasma into the replanted extremity and acute blood loss. This is particularly true of proximal extremity injuries. The hypotension is counteracted by the administration of plasma.

In a major limb amputation there is a period of acute acidosis as a consequence of absorption of metabolic products from the ischemic extremity and venous return begins. This acidosis is aggressively treated with the administration of bicarbonate. Both bicarbonate and mannitol are administered to protect against myoglobin renal damage and prophylactic antibiotics are also administered. If early severe sepsis supervenes, the extremity may have to be amputated. Low-grade late infection, usually consisting of osteomyelitis, is treated by drainage and irrigation. The fixation materials are left in place until the bone heals, even in the face of sepsis—because fixation must be achieved if possible.

Passive movement of all joints is begun immediately and continued throughout the course of treatment. Galvanic stimulation of the intrinsic muscles of the hand or foot can be utilized to maintain the tone of muscles. Extensive physical therapy is instituted as soon as wound healing is complete. If primary nerve suture has not been carried out, the nerves are reexplored 6 weeks or more after the injury, and grafting is carried out then. The long-term functional results have been good.

Muscle and Musculocutaneous Grafts

Occasionally, following a severe trauma or extirpative surgery, vital structures such as brain, bone periosteum, tendon, nerve, and major vascular structures become exposed in a wound. Such wounds require full-thickness flap coverage to preserve the viability of these important structures and promote functional recovery. In situations where no local or regional flaps are available for transfer, autogenous muscle or musculocutaneous flaps must be grafted using microsurgical techniques. The most commonly used muscles and musculocutaneous flaps are the rectus abdominis perfused on the inferior epigastric arterial pedicle, and the latissimus dorsi, perfused by the thoracodorsal artery and vein. Microsurgical transfer of these muscles results in minimal donor site functional morbidity, and provides a large volume of tissue for reconstruction of the wound.

Following harvest, the muscles are revascularized using appropriate recipient vessels in the region of wound. Care must be taken to perform the microsurgical anastomosis outside the zone of injury so that normal vessels are used to revascularize the flap. Utilization of an end-to-side anastomosis has a theoretically increased patency rate and does not jeopardize distal perfusion of an already injured extremity. These free flap transfers are commonly done by organized microsurgical teams where technical skills are maintained by a high volume of replantation and reconstructive surgery.

Other free flaps are occasionally employed for specialized situations. The skin and soft tissue of dorsum of the foot, perfused by the dorsalis pedis artery and thin skin of the volar forearm perfused by the radial artery are occasionally used for reconstructions in the head, neck, and face where their thinness and malleability are an asset. The great toe or the second toe perfused on the dorsalis pedis axis can be transferred to reconstruct the thumb or hand where no digits are available for opposition. These transfers are extremely complex, and require reconnection of tendons, nerves, and bone, as well as successful microvascular anastomosis.

Microsurgical techniques have significantly increased the reconstructive surgeon's armamentarium. Using microsurgery, a wide variety of autogenous transplants are possible and can provide functioning tissue where it is needed. Successful methods of immunosuppression are being developed and will ultimately allow microsurgeons to transfer functioning heterografts for reconstructive purposes.

Hemopoietic and Lymphoid Tissues

BONE MARROW

Bone marrow is easily destroyed by whole-body ionizing irradiation, drugs, or chemicals. In contrast, the mature peripheral blood cells are in most instances not sensitive to injury by irradiation or by chemical substances, but these cells have a relatively short life span, and a regular supply of new cells is needed. In leukemia, the bone marrow is replaced by tumor cells, a situation effectively the same as that existing when marrow is destroyed by other means.

Injury to bone marrow by drugs, chemicals, and diseases poses several clinical problems. Bone marrow transplants between identical twins have been successfully carried out in many cases of irradiation exposure, aplastic anemia, and leukemia. Autologous marrow transplantation has also been found useful after planned treatment with toxic levels of alkylating agents.

Marrow allotransplants are far less successful. Marrow is highly immunogenic and will be readily rejected by the immunologically normal host. If, however, the marrow is allotransplanted into an immunologically crippled (irradiated, immunosuppressed) host, a chimera is produced. The problem then becomes, not destruction of the marrow by the host, but the maturation of donor marrow stem cells that results in total immunological competence and rejection of the host by the graft. This graft-versus-host (GVH) phenomenon is not seen with skin, kidney, heart, and liver grafts, but it is a major unsolved problem in the transplantation of foreign bone marrow, white blood cells, and lymphoid tissues. GVH disease does not occur in bone marrow transplants between identical human twins, and the GVH reaction is less severe if the donor and recipient are identical at the entire HLA locus.

The major sites of injury in GVH reactions are the lymphatic tissues, the skin, the intestine, and the liver of the host. Dermatitis, diarrhea, loss of weight, poor liver function, and infection associated with immunoincompetence are intrinsic parts of the reaction. The GVH reactions in bone marrow transplantation in human beings have been of overwhelming importance and are the major problem in this growing clinical area. Some of the experimental and clinical approaches to the problem of the control of GVH disease are listed in Table 10-4. A combination of tissue typing and immunologic suppression is now used to control the GVH reaction in human beings, but selective deletion from the transplanted marrow of T-cell precursors responsible for GVH may soon be practical. Monoclonal antibodies directed against potentially immunoreactive cells in the mixed population of bone marrow cells are promising.

A long-range goal in marrow transplantation is the use of these grafts as a means of promoting acceptance of other organs, such as liver, heart, and kidney. Once the

Table 10-4. SOME APPROACHES TO THE CONTROL OF GRAFT-VERSUS-HOST DISEASE

A. Immunologic compatibility:* histocompatibility typing and matching of donor and recipient
B. Immunologic suppression
  1. Treatment of marrow recipient
     a. Methotrexate*
     b. Cyclophosphamide*
     c. Antilymphocyte serum*
     d. Cyclosporine*
  2. Treatment of marrow donor: antilymphocyte serum
C. Removal of immunologically active cells
  1. Treatment of the marrow in vitro with ALG or monoclonal antibodies against selected T-cell subpopulations
  2. Cell separation.
D. Innate absence of immunocompetent cells; use of fetal and newborn blood-forming tissue as the donor source

* Currently in clinical use.

foreign marrow is established, a state of relative or complete specific nonreactivity against donor antigens is conferred, and other tissues taken from the same donor as the marrow can be successfully transplanted without further immunosuppression.

In practice, human bone marrow allotransplantation has enjoyed increasing success. More than 2000 transplants are carried out yearly in the United States. HLA-identical marrow transplants (from matched siblings) are commonly used to treat aplastic anemias, combined immunodeficiency disease, and thalassemia major. The majority of patients enjoy long-term disease-free survival. Marrow transplantation is now used to treat other acquired and congenital disorders of hemapoietic stem cells and congenital enzymatic defects. Transplantation for leukemia is less successful. The best results are achieved in the treatment of chronic myelogenous leukemia in the chronic phase, and for acute nonlymphoblastic leukemia in first remission.

Aside from transplants between identical twins, transplantation with HLA-matched but nonidentical twin marrow is very successful with the best record of successful engraftment and the least severe GVH disease. The use of non-HLA-matched donors is far less successful. In these patients, marrow allotransplantation requires much larger doses of immunosuppressive cytotoxic drugs than those used to gain acceptance of kidney grafts. Furthermore, the GVH disease in these HLA-mismatched recipients has been difficult to control. Matching unrelated donors at the HLA locus is better than using mismatched relatives as donors.

THYMUS

The congenital absence of thymic tissue prevents the maturation of the entire T-cell system. Such patients are deficient in cell-mediated immune responses and those B-cell responses requiring T-cell interaction. Transplantation of an embryonic fresh or cultured thymus into such patients has resulted in considerable improvement in these normal defense mechanisms. The exact indications

Table 10-5. INDICATIONS FOR PARATHYROID TRANSPLANTATION

1. Autotransplantation
   a. Severe secondary hyperparathyroidism
   b. Primary generalized parathyroid hyperplasia
   c. Inadvertent removal of parathyroid tissue
2. Allotransplantation
   a. Congenital absence of parathyroid glands—DiGeorge's syndrome
   b. Iatrogenic aparathyroidism that is not controllable with a medical regimen

and success rates have not been fully defined, but this is a promising field of investigation.

Endocrine Grafts (Other than the Pancreas)

The placement of endocrine fragments as autografts into intramuscular pockets has been successful in several clinical situations. The indications for parathyroid autotransplantation are listed in Table 10-5. When it appears possible that a patient may have insufficient parathyroid tissue following removal of the thyroid gland, or of all four parathyroid glands for chief cell hyperplasia, the glands should be diced and implanted into intramuscular pockets. The volar forearm muscle is a useful site for autotransplantation because the parathyroids are readily available for subsequent excision if hyperparathyroidism recurs. Their function can be easily assessed by hormone assay of antecubital vein blood.

Similar indications for other endocrine organs have been suggested. None of these indications has been well defined, however, because hormonal replacement (parathyroids excepted) is simpler. The prognosis for endocrine allotransplants is in doubt for the same reason. Replacement therapy for endocrine deficiency (aside from insulin deficiencies) is generally adequate, and there is seldom an indication for the use of systemic immunosuppressive drugs to eliminate the need for endocrine replacement therapy. In the case of parathyroid allotransplants, there has been an insistent and recurrently hopeful effort. Parathyroid deficiency is not treated with specific hormone replacement, but rather with calcium and vitamin D, which give inadequate results. An occasionally successful parathyroid allotransplant in a patient with a functioning renal allograft already receiving immunosuppressive drugs has been reported.

ORGAN TRANSPLANTATION

Pancreas

The discovery of insulin in 1921 was hailed as the cure of diabetes; it prevented death from diabetic coma, controlled the overt symptoms of diabetes, and provided an increased life expectancy. As diabetic patients lived longer, however, previously unseen complications developed. Diabetes was responsible for at least 30,000 deaths in 1974, and it is the leading cause of new cases of blindness in adults. Diabetics are seventeen times more liable to kidney disease, five times more liable to gangrene of the extremities, and twice as likely to develop heart diseases. Obviously, new approaches to treatment are required. Pancreas and islet transplantation offer the possibility that the development and progression of diabetic lesions will be prevented by precise regulation of carbohydrate metabolism—control not yet achieved by injected insulin.

An unresolved question is whether juvenile-onset diabetics suffer only from a lack of insulin or whether the absence of insulin reflects other subcellular derangements. Whether normalization of carbohydrate metabolism in these patients will prevent the development of systemic lesions is still unanswered. Several observations, however, support the hypothesis that angiopathic lesions associated with diabetes are secondary to abnormal metabolism:

1. Nephropathy and retinopathy occur in patients who develop diabetes as a result of other disease states (e.g., hemochromatosis) or after total pancreatectomy.
2. Numerous longitudinal clinical studies have shown a relationship between duration of the disease, control of plasma glucose, and development of lesions.
3. Nephropathy and retinopathy occur in animals with induced diabetes.
4. Studies in animals have demonstrated that reduction of hyperglycemia by insulin therapy or by transplantation of whole pancreas or islets prevents or minimizes formation of diabetic lesions in the eye, kidney, and nerve.
5. Kidneys transplanted from normal to diabetic rats develop histologic lesions characteristic of diabetes in the rat, whereas kidneys transplanted from diabetic to normal rats showed disappearance or lack of progression of these lesions.

These observations suggest that it may be possible to prevent the systemic complications of diabetes by insulin released from transplanted pancreatic islets. Alternative methods to provide precise glucose homeostasis, such as an implantable glucose sensor coupled to an insulin pump, are also possible, however.

WHOLE ORGAN

Either whole organ or distal segmental pancreatic transplants will ameliorate experimental diabetes. In addition to the expected problems associated with the control of immunologic rejection and the need for immunosuppressive drugs, there are special technical concerns. Of these, the major problem is difficulty in establishing drainage of the pancreatic duct. Theoretically, ligation of the pancreatic duct should result in atrophy of exocrine tissue without affecting endocrine tissue. But in practice a severe inflammatory reaction occurs and leads to a constricting fibrosis that damages even the islets. Filling the ductal system with plastic is an alternative approach to the prevention of exocrine secretion. Unfortunately pancreatic fibrosis remains a problem with this technique as well.

All alternative approaches are less successful. Initial attempts used a combined pancreaticoduodenal approach, with the duodenum serving as a conduit for drainage of exocrine enzymes. When a generous segment of transplanted duodenum was used, however, it was particularly susceptible to rejection and to anastomotic leakage. These complications can be eliminated by direct anastomosis of the pancreatic duct to an enteric drainage site, but fistulas are common. Permitting the duct to drain freely into the peritoneal cavity for absorption has been successful in animals, but some patients develop ascites. The use of a short segment of duodenum anastomosed to the bladder seems to be the most successful solution. Graft thrombosis and other complications associated with graft pancreatitis continue to plague progress in this field. Despite these problems, more than 1000 clinical transplants have been performed. Usually cadaver organs are used, and most recipients already have diabetic end-stage renal disease; both kidney and pancreas are transplanted at a single operation. Increasingly, however, as success grows, pancreas transplantation will be carried out in patients before advanced renal disease occurs.

Successful whole-organ or segmental pancreatic transplants produce circulating insulin and normal plasma glucose levels. When the venous drainage of the pancreatic graft is hooked up to the systemic circulation, the circulating insulin levels are higher than when the venous anastomosis is made to the portal system, although the plasma glucose levels are similar. Rejection episodes are as difficult to reverse as they are to detect. By the time glucose levels become abnormal, rejection is usually too far advanced, and serum enzyme levels do not become elevated. When the pancreatic duct is anastomosed to the bladder, however, the urine amylase level falls early in the rejection response. Thus, the most successful technical solution seems to permit better immunologic monitoring of the rejection response.

Experience in human beings has shown that functioning vascularized pancreatic allograft will correct the metabolic deficiency in diabetes. The techniques (Figs. 10-22 and 10-23) are now safer and more successful. The results of transplant carried out between 1983 and 1986 are illustrated in Fig. 10-24. Most current clinical research continues to focus on methods of controlling pancreatic exocrine secretion without inducing pancreatitis in the transplant. Rejection, thrombosis, and fibrosis remain serious barriers to widespread clinical application, even though fistula formation is now an unusual problem.

ISLET TISSUE

It is not necessary to transplant the pancreas in order to cure diabetes; transplantation of the pancreatic islets will suffice. The current technique for isolation of islets from the pancreas involves mechanical disruption, enzymatic digestion, and density-gradient separation. Isolated adult islets infused into the portal vein will produce long-lasting control of diabetes in rats. This technique has also been successfully applied to the autotransplantation of islets in people who require total pancreatectomy for chronic painful pancreatitis.

Clinical islet allotransplantation has been frustrated by

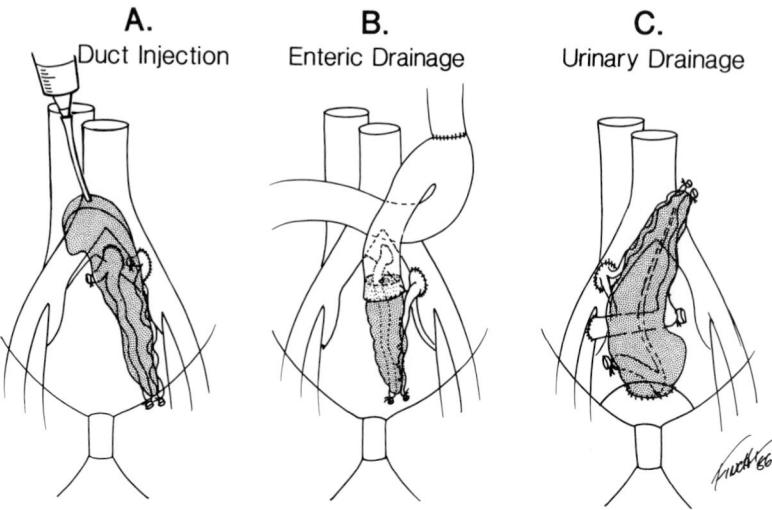

A.
Duct Injection

B.
Enteric Drainage

C.
Urinary Drainage

Fig. 10-22. Technique of pancreas transplantation. The body and tail can be transplanted with anastomoses of splenic vessels of donor pancreas to iliac vessels of recipient. The duct can be injected with a polymer to occlude it, or the duct can be anastomosed to a loop of bowel or the bladder. These techniques are still in use in some centers. (Adapted from: *Sutherland DER, Kendall D, et al: Surg Clin North Am 66:557, 1986, with permission.*)

the apparent increased susceptibility of islets to allograft rejection. Survival is difficult to achieve even when immunosuppression that will prolong skin, kidney, or heart allografts is used. The clinical application of islet transplantation will also require techniques such as cold storage or culture to preserve the cells.

The experimental evidence that islet tissue graft can prevent, halt, and even improve the vascular and neurological lesions of diabetes provides a tremendous impetus to continue research, despite these formidable difficulties.

Gastrointestinal Tract

Various segments of intestine can be autotransplanted by removal from the body and reimplantation. Stomach, small bowel, and colon can be used to replace esophagus, with reimplantation of the vascular supply. Allotransplantation of the small bowel and stomach has been carried out experimentally. These grafts are rejected in the usual fashion, and within the same general period as kidneys and other organs. There is some evidence that the lymphoid tissue within the intestinal wall can initiate a graft-versus-host reaction.

Although there is little apparent clinical use for a gastric transplant, there is a definite need for transplantation of the small bowel. Infarction of the bowel sometimes requires excision of the entire small bowel, and this leads to a nutritional deficiency that requires expensive and cumbersome parenteral alimentation. Patients with various nutritional and motility problems, as well as certain patients with Crohn's disease, might benefit from safe

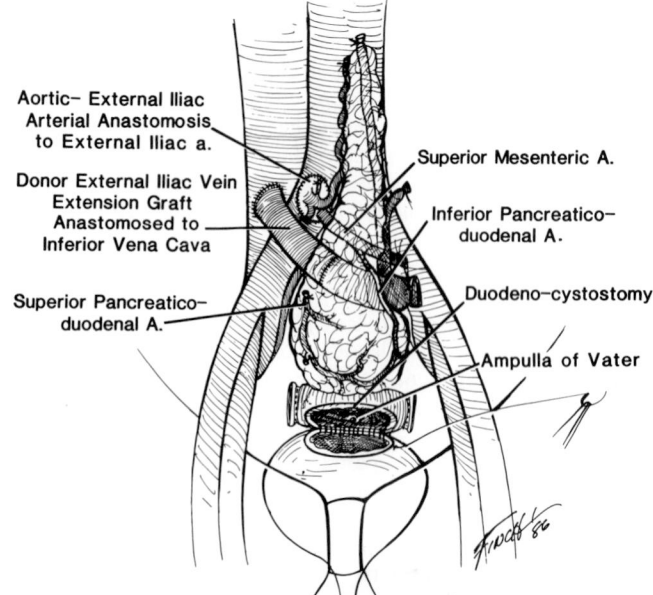

Aortic- External Iliac Arterial Anastomosis to External Iliac a.

Donor External Iliac Vein Extension Graft Anastomosed to Inferior Vena Cava

Superior Pancreatico-duodenal A.

Superior Mesenteric A.

Inferior Pancreatico-duodenal A.

Duodeno-cystostomy

Ampulla of Vater

Fig. 10-23. Preferred method of pancreatic-duodenal transplantation. The whole pancreas is used. The celiac axis and superior mesenteric arteries are anastomosed to the iliac artery. The portal vein provides venous drainage. The duodenum is anastomosed to the bladder. [From: *Sutherland DER, Najarian JS, in Simmons RL, Finch M, et al (eds): Manual of Vascular Access, Organ Donation, and Transplantation. New York, Springer-Verlag, 1984, with permission.*]

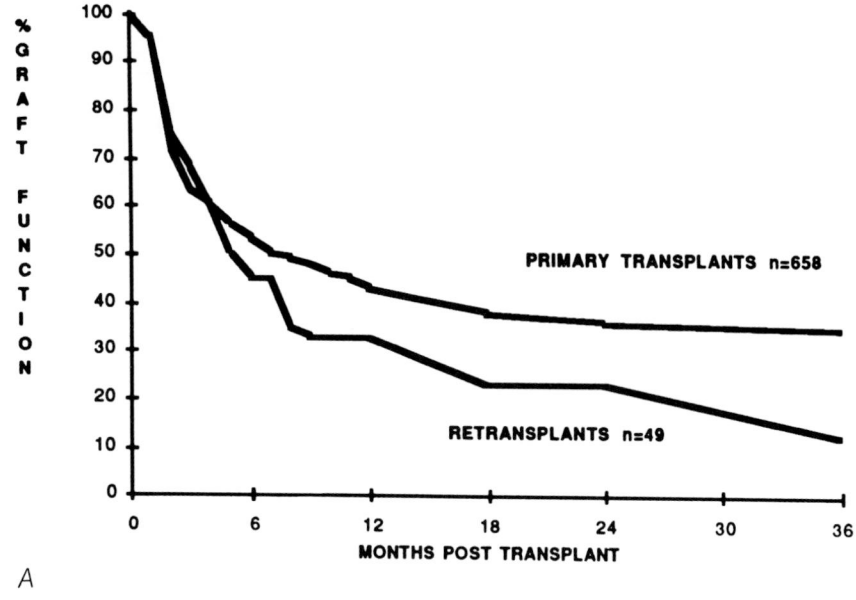

A

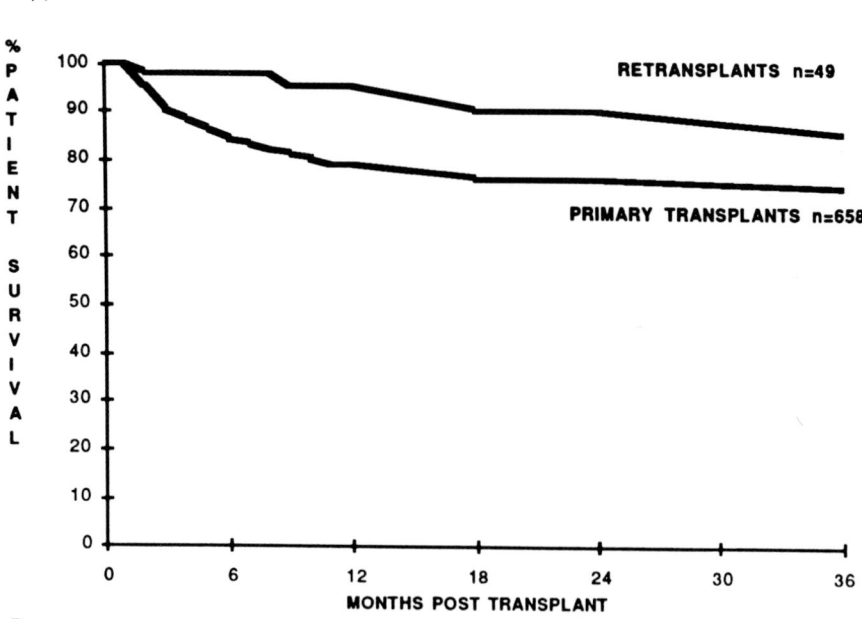

B

Fig. 10-24. Results from the World Pancreas Registry. *A*. Insulin-independent graft function. *B*. Recipient survival rate for primary transplants and retransplants reported between January 1, 1983, and August 31, 1986.

and successful bowel transplantation. A few attempts in human beings have been successful for several months, but no long-term survival has been achieved.

Liver

Liver transplantation has become a highly successful solution to a variety of congenital and acquired hepatic disorders in thousands of patients. A liver transplant may be positioned in the normal anatomic location (orthotopic transplantation) following a total hepatectomy of the recipient. Alternatively, the donor organ can be placed in an ectopic site (heterotopic transplantation), generally with retention of the host's liver (auxiliary transplantation). Orthotopic grafts are universally preferred by clinicians because experimental heterotopic grafts have been so unsuccessful.

INDICATIONS FOR LIVER TRANSPLANTATION. In theory, liver transplantation is appropriate for any disease that will cause total liver failure (Table 10-6). Chronic active hepatitis is the most common indication for liver transplantation in adults, followed by alcoholic cirrhosis, primary biliary cirrhosis, and secondary biliary cirrhosis.

Table 10-6. COMMON INDICATIONS FOR HEPATIC TRANSPLANTATION

Adult	*Children*
Chronic active hepatitis	Biliary atresia
Alcoholic cirrhosis	Chronic active hepatitis
Primary biliary cirrhosis	Hepatoma
Secondary biliary cirrhosis	Neonatal hepatitis
Secondary cholangitis	General hepatic fibrosis
α-1-Anti-trypsin deficiency	Secondary biliary cirrhosis
Hemachromatosis	Inborn errors of metabolism
Budd–Chiari syndrome	
Acute hepatitis B	

Modified from Ascher NL, Simmons RL, Najarian JS: Host hepatectomy and liver transplantation, in Simmons RL, Finch ME, Ascher NL, Najarian JS (eds): *Manual of Vascular Access, Organ Donation, and Transplantation.* New York, Springer-Verlag, 1984, pp 255–284.

Also, certain patients with rare types of malignancy confined to the liver may benefit from a liver graft.

In children the most common indication for transplantation is extrahepatic biliary atresia. Virtually all these patients previously have had one or more Kasai procedures. Transplantation is technically feasible in infants weighing as little as 5 kg; in patients smaller than this, the portal vein is usually too small to remain patent.

Naturally transplantation is contraindicated in any patient with (1) irreversible infection, (2) widespread malignancy, (3) concurrent disease (e.g., myocardial failure, old age) that would seriously impair survival, or (4) a high risk for recurrent disease in the transplant organ. Because active hepatitis also usually recurs, the presence of HBsAg or HBeAg antigenemia is a relative contraindication. The risk of recurrent alcoholism also makes alcoholic cirrhosis a relative contraindication unless the patient has abstained from alcohol for at least 2 years. In patients with sclerosing cholangitis, active ulcerative colitis also rules out liver transplantation. Patients with portal vein thrombosis cannot be successfully revascularized with orthotopic grafts.

PREOPERATIVE EVALUATION OF THE RECIPIENT. Intensive preoperative evaluation is designed to (1) characterize those physiologic defects in hepatic, pulmonary, renal, or cardiac function that will influence the patient's chance of survival, (2) determine whether the transplant is technically feasible for that particular patient, and (3) search out sites of occult infection and malignancy (Table 10-7).

During the complete history and physical examination, special attention is given to specific extrahepatic organ systems. For example, fluid overload and congestive heart failure are frequently present and must be treated with fluid restriction, diuretics, and lanoxin. In adults, roentgenograms of the chest and electrocardiograms are obtained, and a stress exercise test is done if recommended after a formal cardiology consultation.

Attention to respiratory reserve is important. Because all patients are respirator-dependent in the early post-transplant period, knowledge of their prior pulmonary

Table 10-7. WORK-UP OF POTENTIAL RECIPIENTS FOR LIVER TRANSPLANTATION

1. General
   a. History and physical examination
   b. Chest roentgenogram
   c. Electrocardiogram (ECG)
   d. Serum electrolytes
   e. Fasting blood sugar
2. Hematology
   a. Hemoglobin, leukocyte count, and differential count
   b. Platelet count, bleeding-clotting time, prothrombin time, partial thromboplastin time, thrombin time (factor analysis)
3. Hepatic
   a. Bilirubin, alkaline phosphatase, serum glutamic–pyruvic transaminase (SGPT), aspartate aminotransferase (AST)
   b. Protein electrophoresis
   c. Serum amino acid analysis
   d. α-Fetoprotein
   e. Ultrasound
   f. Ascitic cytology and culture
4. Nutritional evaluation
   a. Transferrin, prealbumin, serum amino acid analysis
5. Renal
   a. Urinalysis
   b. Blood urea nitrogen (BUN), serum creatinine
   c. 24-h creatinine clearance
6. Calcium metabolism (primary biliary cirrhosis)
   a. (Bone roentgenograms: hands, skull, clavical, lamina dura)
   b. (Ca, PO₄, Mg, alkaline phosphatase)
   c. (Parathormone)
7. Gastrointestinal
   a. Upper GI series
   b. Upper GI endoscopy
   c. (Variceal sclerotherapy)
8. Immunologic studies
   a. Blood type (ABO)
   b. Tissue typing including serial cytotoxic antibody determinations
9. Pulmonary function studies
   a. Chest roentgenogram
   b. Blood gases
   c. Pulmonary function tests
10. Infectious work-up
    a. Chest roentgenogram
    b. Blood, urine, throat, feces, ascites cultures
    c. Hepatitis screen
    d. Dental consult
11. Financial-social rehabilitation

The tests enclosed within parentheses are not administered routinely during the potential recipient work-up, but only when the circumstances indicate.

Modified from Ascher NL, Simmons RL, Najarian JS: Host hepatectomy and liver transplantation, in Simmons RL, Finch ME, Ascher NL, Najarian JS (eds): *Manual of Vascular Access, Organ Donation, and Transplantation.* New York, Springer-Verlag, 1984, pp 255–284.

function will help during the process of weaning from the respirator. Therefore, pulmonary function tests are obtained on all adult patients but only arterial blood gases and chest roentgenograms are necessary for pediatric patients. Postoperative ascites or a marginally oversized donor liver can further compromise respiratory function.

A variety of preoperative tests are obtained to assess hepatocellular function (Table 10-7). Hepatitis screening results will determine the need for hyperimmune globulin to prevent recurrent hepatitis, and unsuspected tumors are sought using a-fetoprotein, hepatic ultrasound, and computerized axial tomography (CAT). A coagulation profile is obtained to document functional capacity of the liver and predict the need for correction. An uncorrectible prothrombin time abnormality is a poor prognostic sign. A radionuclide hepatic excretion scan will reveal unsuspected biliary calculi that must be removed from the common bile duct at the time of recipient hepatectomy. An upper gastrointestinal series and upper gastrointestinal endoscopy will reveal the presence of gastric or esophageal varices. Sclerotherapy is used to treat bleeding esophageal varices while the patient is awaiting transplantation. Oral nystatin antifungal prophylaxis must be used to prevent invasive candidosis at the sclerotherapy site.

Patency of the portal vein system must be determined before transplantation because occlusion of the portal vein contraindicates liver transplant. CAT scans used to detect silent malignancy may also show portal vein patency. If either CAT scan or ultrasonography fails to visualize the portal vein, celiac angiography, with special attention to the venous phase, may be required.

The value of immunologic testing has not been determined, but most centers prefer that liver donors and recipients are ABO compatible. Liver donor organs are far too scarce, and the time before transplantation is too short for the time-consuming HLA matching tests to be performed.

While awaiting transplant a program of pretransplant management is set up to optimize the patient's general condition and to improve the suboptimal function of the multiple organ systems. Nutritional and respiratory functions receive special attention. All patients, especially those with pulmonary insufficiency, are begun on an intensive program of pulmonary toilet and exercise. For example, smokers must stop smoking, and postural drainage and short courses of broad-spectrum antibiotics may be necessary to treat bacterial infection.

The judicious use of furosemide and aldactone diuretic treatment of ascites is weighed against the possibility of exacerbating renal insufficiency. Blood volume is maximized using colloid to treat the prerenal component of the hepatorenal syndrome.

The patient's preoperative nutritional status may be enhanced by cautiously increasing dietary protein while monitoring the serum ammonia and serial amino acid profiles. Sclerotherapy is implemented as needed for bleeding varices.

IMMEDIATE PRETRANSPLANT MANAGEMENT. A rigidly defined protocol must be set up for the recipient as soon as a potential cadaver donor is located. Most of the procedures simply reassess the patient's condition while others are designed to prevent infection, replace blood loss, correct coagulation defects, and institute immunosuppression. Prophylactic antibiotics are begun to reduce colonization of the gastrointestinal tract, to minimize wound infection, or to provide protection against herpes virus infection.

Immediate preoperative exchange transfusion is indicated in all patients with impaired coagulation parameters, even though an effective exchange often results from the replacement of lost blood during the early stages of the operation. To effect rapid replacement of blood loss or perform exchange transfusion, central venous cannulation must be carried out. Systemic arterial and pulmonary artery pressure measurements should be monitored during the administration of fresh frozen plasma and load-reducing agents. This requires both arterial and pulmonary artery cannulation (Swan–Ganz catheter).

TECHNIQUE. Liver transplantation is a relatively straightforward procedure, although excessive bleeding, brought on by the extensive collateral venous system caused by the patient's portal hypertension, makes the native hepatectomy the most difficult part of the transplant process. Complications can occur if there is a septic focus, or if residual scars exist from prior operations (portosystemic shunts; attempts at biliary decompression). If technical difficulties prohibit the completion of the liver transplant, the patient will die.

The following eight precautions should be followed: (1) Do not remove the spleen (bleeding is excessive, removal obviates an important portosystemic collateral pathway, and splenic vein flow may be essential to maintain a patent portal vein); (2) minimize retroperitoneal dissection; (3) do not interfere with collateral vessels; (4) avoid thoracic incisions; (5) preserve the blood supply to the distal common duct by minimizing dissection in this region; (6) preserve as much length of suprahepatic vena cava, portal vein, hepatic artery, and infrahepatic vena cava as possible; (7) avoid clamp injury to the renal vessels; and (8) match the weights of donor and recipient ±20 percent. In children the donor can be smaller by as much as 20 percent but only minimally larger.

The most common incision for an orthotopic liver graft is a transverse abdominal incision. The diseased liver is dissected free and clamps are applied to the suprahepatic and intrahepatic vena cavas, the portal vein, and the hepatic artery. The liver can then be removed and replaced by the cadaver liver. Many surgeons perform a portal vein–to–superior vena cava temporary shunt so that the splanchnic venous bed does not become excessively congested during clamping of the vein. A concurrent temporary inferior vena cava–to–superior vena cava shunt minimizes renal venous congestion and permits the return of blood to the heart during the anhepatic phase.

The allograft anastomoses are shown in Fig. 10-25. The suprahepatic caval anastomosis is the most difficult to perform. The second anastomosis is usually the portal vein to minimize venous congestion of the intestine. After the portal vein anastomosis is completed, the inferior hepatic caval clamps should be briefly removed, leaving the suprahepatic vena cava clamped. The portal vein inflow should be opened to allow the liver to be perfused with warm blood. This sequence is useful to remove the cold perfusate from the liver and prevent systemic hypothermia and heparinization. As soon as the perfusate is

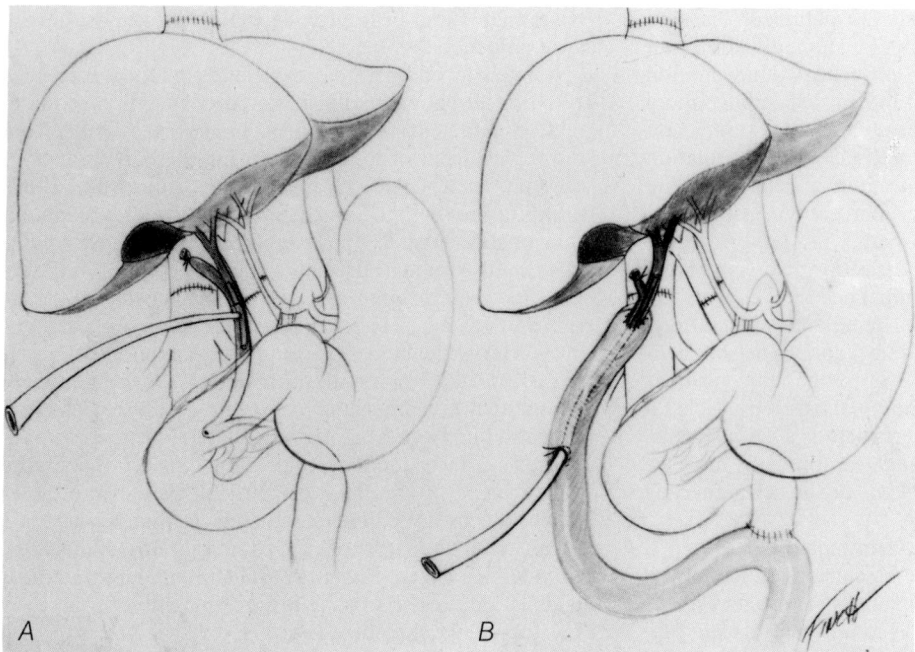

Fig. 10-25. Completed orthotopic liver transplant in *(A)* adults and *(B)* children. The two preferred methods of biliary reconstruction are illustrated. [From: *Ascher NL, Najarian JS, et al, in Simmons RL, Finch M, et al (eds): Manual of Vascular Access, Organ Donation, and Transplantation. New York, Springer-Verlag, 1984, with permission.*]

washed from the liver and it becomes firm and pink, the intrahepatic vena cava is clamped, and the suprahepatic vena cava clamp is removed. The remaining vascular anastomoses (hepatic artery, inferior vena cava) can then be accomplished.

Following the vascular anastomoses, biliary drainage must be obtained. A direct bile duct–to–bile duct anastomosis is preferred in adults. A choledochojejunostomy is preferred in children.

As many as 30 to 40 percent of patients have double hepatic arteries, and one of them may arise from the superior mesenteric artery. Care must be taken during the donor operation to preserve this arterial supply to the transplanted liver.

A common complication is paralysis of the right side of the diaphragm, which apparently results from crushing of the right phrenic nerve by the vascular clamp applied to the suprahepatic inferior vena cava. Enough length must be preserved during total hepatectomy for the clamp to be applied without impinging on the diaphragm.

POSTOPERATIVE MANAGEMENT. The early posttransplant management of liver recipients is so complex that protocols have been designed to guarantee that crucial details are not omitted. If renal function is satisfactory, cyclosporine and prednisone are preferred for immunosuppression. If renal function is poor, cyclosporine is omitted and antilymphoblast serum and azathioprine are used.

Some degree of acute tubular necrosis is common in the immediate postoperative period, probably because of poor perfusion due to blood loss and the clamping of the inferior vena cava with renal venous hypertension. If renal function is already compromised, the nephrotoxic effect of cyclosporine can be minimized by delaying its

use until 12 h after transplantation. Constant monitoring of renal function and cyclosporine levels will ensure the precise adjustment of the dosage.

Respiratory support is usually required for at least 24 to 48 h after extubation. Most patients can then be transferred to a regular nursing ward. Nasogastric suction is maintained until bowel function returns, and intravenous hyperalimentation is used until they can eat. Levels of BUN, creatinine, electrolytes, calcium, phosphate, white blood cell count, and hemoglobin are determined daily. Chest roentgenograms are taken daily for 5 days, and whenever the patient becomes febrile, to seek evidence for atelectasis, pneumonia, diaphragmatic paralysis, and pleural effusion. Culture samples are taken as indicated.

Monitoring liver transplant function with frequent chemical determination of coagulation parameters (especially prothrombin time, factor V levels, the serum bilirubin, transaminase, and alkaline phosphatase levels) is mandatory. Changes in these levels can signal rejection, ischemia, viral infection, cholangitis, or mechanical obstruction.

A radionuclide excretory cholangiogram is performed on postoperative day 3 and at weekly intervals; excretion of the radioisotope by the liver into the small bowel by 45 min is considered to be normal. A delay can reflect hepatocellular damage during death of the donor, complications of the donor operation, prolonged cold storage, vascular compromise, or rejection. Also, delayed excretion into the biliary tree can reflect rejection, hepatocellular damage from ischemia, or viral infection. Delayed passage into the small bowel can indicate mechanical obstruction or breakdown. A T-tube cholangiogram (performed with gravity) will diagnose breakdown at the site of biliary drainage, or if a T tube has not been used (e.g., with a cholecystojejunostomy), transhepatic cholangiography may be necessary to evaluate the biliary system.

During rejection lymphocytes infiltrate portal tracts and central veins, with varying degrees of bile duct epithelial damage; therefore, a percutaneous liver transplant biopsy and culture is the only way to differentiate among rejection, ischemia, viral infection, and cholangitis. Rejection is treated initially with intravenous steroids or with antilymphoblast globulin. The presence of polymorphonuclear leukocytes within the portal tracts indicates cholangitis. The patient is treated with antibiotics and a search is made for a mechanical obstruction as an underlying cause. Cytomegalovirus hepatitis is treated with ganciclovir.

Postoperative Complications. The most serious complication is primary nonfunction, in which the liver fails to function sufficiently well to support life. This may be a result of ischemia, technical factors, or accelerated rejection. Primary nonfunction is first suspected when factor V levels in the plasma fail to return to normal.

Intraoperative bleeding results from many causes: Extensive portasystemic shunts are almost always present and global coagulation defects always exist. Even when hemostasis appears adequate during operation, bleeding is a special hazard in the immediate postoperative period. Coagulation parameters, including platelet levels and serum calcium levels, must be measured during closure of the abdomen so that they can be corrected. Blood loss may continue into the postoperative period, although immediate normal transplant function will minimize these complications. A normal prothrombin time and factor V level are early signs that normal function has returned.

Thrombotic occlusion of either the hepatic artery or portal vein will cause sudden deterioration of hepatic function. The bilirubin and transaminase values rise rapidly, coagulopathy, hyperkalemia, and hypoglycemia appear, and the liver fails to extract radionuclides during liver scan. In many centers, these catastrophes are indications for retransplantation.

Vena caval stenosis (most often the suprahepatic anastomosis) leads to edema in the lower trunk and renal insufficiency. An angiogram of the vena cava will confirm the diagnosis. Operative repair must be undertaken. Milder degrees of stenosis of the suprahepatic vena cava anastomosis in children declare themselves by nonspecific alterations in hepatic function: persistent ascites, elevated bilirubin, and hepatic enzymes. Balloon angioplasty can be used for vena cava stenosis in the late postoperative period.

Respiratory complications are common. Liver transplant recipients have ascites, pleural effusion, paralyzed diaphragms, and a new edematous liver. The operative pain and spasms of the abdominal wall add to the high risk of pulmonary complications. The atelectasis can easily become complicated by pneumonia. Prophylaxis includes both training the prospective recipients to use their accessory respiratory muscles, and vigorous pulmonary toilet in the postoperative period. The liberal use of bronchoscopy to reexpand atelectatic lung segments and to remove (and culture) purulent material is also helpful. Function usually returns to a paralyzed diaphragm within 3 to 4 weeks. The ascites can be drained via peritoneal dialysis catheters if care is taken to maintain asepsis. Provided that liver function is good and infection does not supervene, almost all patients can be weaned from their often lengthy respirator dependence.

Renal malfunction is common both before and after transplantation, but the posttransplant problems can be minimized by attention to a number of details: (1) maintain renal perfusion in the preoperative period by maintenance of blood volume; (2) do not compromise the renal veins or the right renal artery as it courses behind the vena cava; (3) use a portasystemic shunt during the operation to reduce renal vein pressure during the anhepatic phase; (4) intravenous cyclosporine should be infused slowly in low doses during the initial periods of recovery so that peak blood cyclosporine levels remain below nephrotoxic levels; (5) stop the use of cyclosporine therapy with the first sign of renal compromise, and temporarily use conventional immunotherapy (ALG, azathioprine); (6) avoid nephrotoxic agents (aminoglycosides, amphotericin B); and (7) remove ascites to reduce intraabdominal pressure.

Although infectious complications are no longer the most common causes of death after liver transplantation, they continue to be a major problem. For example, the incidence of bacterial sepsis has diminished with the use of cyclosporine and newer methods of biliary drainage. Cholangitis and biliary anastomotic breakdown are now rare. Even so, perioperative antibiotics should be used in repeated doses during operation because the blood loss is great and the operation is long. Topical antibiotics (0.1% cephapirin) used repeatedly during the operation will obviate the need for repeated systemic doses. Postoperative antibiotics should be based on intraoperative culture results of contaminated material.

Oral trimethoprim sulfamethoxazole will reduce the postoperative incidence of *Pneumocystis carinii* and *Nocardia* infections, as it does in renal transplant patients.

Fungal infections remain a major problem in liver recipients but can be controlled by the preoperative and postoperative use of high-dose oral, esophageal, and gastric nystatin. Also, prompt institution of systemic amphotericin B for candidosis without fungemia will minimize the adverse consequences.

Central venous pressure lines should be removed as soon as possible to decrease the chance of their colonization.

Viral infections are a major problem the most serious of which is cytomegalovirus (CMV). CMV can be treated with ganciclovir, a new antiviral drug. Acyclovir will not prevent or cure CMV, but it will prevent herpes simplex.

Cholangitis in the absence of discernible biliary obstruction is more common than previously described. Only by biopsy of the transplant can it be diagnosed. Cul-

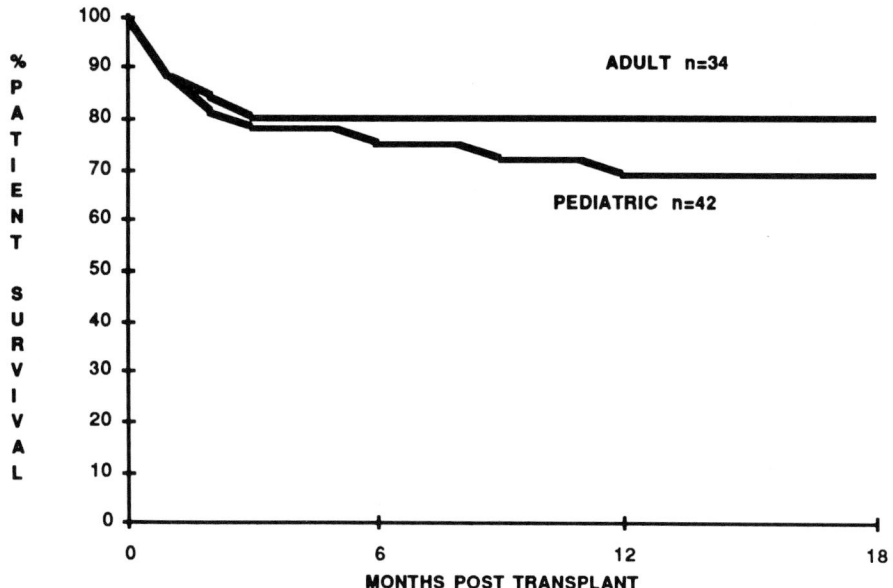

Fig. 10-26. Results of adult and pediatric liver transplants performed at the University of Minnesota between April 1984 and March 1987.

ture of the specimen permits rational antimicrobial therapy.

Subclinical and reversible rejection episodes are commonly detected if liver biopsies are carried out at weekly intervals. Rejection may occur at any time in the postoperative period including the first 24 h, but most cases occur at least several weeks after transplantation.

RESULTS. Although the first liver transplant in a human being was performed in 1963, the procedure was not successful until 1967. From then until 1978 the results were generally poor, with 1-year survival figures ranging from 25 to 30 percent. The longest-living survivor is well 12 years after transplantation. Since 1979, Starzl's group has enjoyed markedly improved survival, in the range of 70 to 80 percent for 1 year. The results of hepatic transplantation have improved with the use of cyclosporine. Currently, a combination of steroids, azathioprine, and cyclosporine are used for the prophylaxis of rejection following liver transplantation at the University of Minnesota. The results using this regimen are shown in Fig. 10-26.

Heart, Heart-Lung, and Single Lung

Craig R. Smith and Keith Reemtsma

HEART

HISTORICAL DEVELOPMENT. Cardiac transplantation is a young field that has progressed dramatically in the 1980s. Christiaan Barnard performed the first human heart transplant in 1967; this stimulated a flurry of imitation throughout the world. Disappointing results led to a backlash of public disparagement, and early eclipse into disfavor by 1970. More cardiac transplants were performed in 1968 (54) than were performed in any subsequent year until 1981.

Public discouragement with early clinical results tended to overshadow the substantial experimental foundations of the procedure. Heterotopic transplants, in which the heart is placed in parallel in the circulation, were done as early as 1905 by Carrel and Guthrie. Orthotopic transplants, in which the donor heart replaces the recipient heart, were first done successfully in dogs by Lower and Shumway in 1959. By 1967 the operative technique was well refined, and the procedure was reproducible in animals. Operative technique has changed remarkably little in 20 years. Because he was so actively involved in the experimental development of the field, Shumway persevered clinically, and nurtured the field through the 1970s. By 1982 the series at Stanford enjoyed 50 percent survival at 5 years.

With the clinical introduction of cyclosporine in 1982, cardiac transplantation entered a phase of exponential growth. More transplants were done in 1985 (984) than were done from 1967 to 1984. At the beginning of the 1980s, fewer than 10 centers were performing cardiac transplants, a number that has grown to more than 80.

SPECTRUM OF DISEASE. Patients requiring cardiac transplantation can be combined under a diagnosis of congestive cardiomyopathy, a broad category of diverse pathogenesis, defined by histopathology and functional characteristics. The "idiopathic" cardiomyopathies are a heterogeneous group of conditions sharing common end-stage pathology characterized by dilated cardiac chambers, myocardial degeneration, and fibrosis. Viral cardiomyopathy is thought to account for the majority of "idiopathic" cases. Specific diagnoses such as familial cardiomyopathy, alcoholic cardiomyopathy, or postpartum cardiomyopathy account for a small fraction of the group, since most are ultimately idiopathic. Idiopathic cardiomyopathy primarily attacks young and otherwise healthy patients.

Ischemic cardiomyopathy is loosely defined as an end-stage manifestation of coronary atherosclerosis. Compared with patients with idiopathic cardiomyopathy, patients with ischemic cardiomyopathy are generally older and have a higher frequency of associated problems such as diabetes and peripheral vascular disease. Patients with end-stage ventricular failure associated with valvular disease are infrequently transplanted and are difficult to classify. Congenital heart disease presents similar problems, and transplantation in childhood is elected for a combination of idiopathic cardiomyopathies and primary congenital lesions, such as hypoplastic left heart syndrome. However defined, such cases account for a small percentage of cardiac transplants.

The age range for all patients transplanted from 1967 through early 1986 is 4 days to 66 years, with a mean age of 40 plus or minus 12 years. The broad distribution of age over the middle decades reflects overlap between the differing age distributions of idiopathic and ischemic cardiomyopathy. If eligibility for transplant were not influenced by age, the distribution of diagnoses would shift toward those of coronary atherosclerosis, with all its associated problems, and the mean age would increase accordingly. At present, 57 percent of all patients transplanted have had idiopathic cardiomyopathy, 40 percent have had ischemic cardiomyopathy, and 3 percent have had congenital heart disease or other diagnoses. Eighty percent of patients transplanted have been men. It is not clear whether this is due to differences in the expression of cardiomyopathies by gender or to differences in selection criteria favoring men.

RECIPIENT SELECTION. Recipients are selected from among patients with end-stage ventricular failure, clinically NYHA Class III–IV, who are unlikely to survive more than 1 year, and for whom there is no alternative therapy. Selection criteria (Table 10-8) continue to be quite strict because of the belief that heart donors are a scarce resource that must be distributed preferentially to those with the greatest chance of benefit. The proper psychosocial profile includes evidence of ability to comply with an elaborate regimen of postoperative care. Until recently patients older than 55 years were excluded, but at present carefully selected older patients are being transplanted when the other essential criteria are met.

Contraindications include systemic diseases likely to compromise long-term survival, such as malignancy, severe peripheral vascular disease or autoimmune vasculitis, and renal or hepatic dysfunction not likely to respond to an improvement in cardiac output. Diabetes and peptic ulcer disease have been considered relative contraindications.

The level of pulmonary vascular resistance in a potential recipient is given particular attention. In all patients with left ventricular failure, regardless of etiology, pulmonary artery pressure (PAP) increases as left atrial pressure rises. Pulmonary vascular resistance (PVR) increases variably but can become extremely elevated and fixed. A normal donor heart, accustomed to low pulmonary artery pressure and resistance, will fail immediately if placed in a recipient with sufficiently elevated PVR. Therefore, right heart catheterization provides essential information regarding operative risk. PVR index equals mean PAP minus wedge pressure divided by cardiac index and is assigned dimensionless units called Wood's units (WU). The normal range is 0 to 3 WU. Cardiac output is frequently used for the denominator, but some accuracy in prediction is lost when the patient's body surface area is significantly greater or less than 1.0 m². At the time of catheterization, patients with elevated PAP and PVR receive a trial infusion of nitroprusside or prostaglandin E-1, observing the effect on PVR as the infusion rate is increased up to the point at which systemic pressure falls below an acceptable level. If the PVR can be reduced to less than 5 WU, the patient is considered an acceptable risk. At the same time, pulmonary artery systolic pressure that remains greater than 50 mmHg is reason for concern but not necessarily for exclusion.

DONOR EVALUATION. Estimates based on current recipient acceptance criteria suggest that about 14,000 people per year in the United States could benefit from cardiac transplant. Estimates of the number of potential heart donors suggest that a maximum of 2000 are available each year. Under such conditions the cornerstone of any cardiac transplant program is an effective system for identifying and managing potential donors.

Table 10-9 summarizes the process of donor evaluation. It must be emphasized that such listings are guidelines and not requirements, and a balance must be reached between the desire to use only ideal donors and the need to minimize the mortality on the recipient waiting list. Many of the exclusions made are not meant to imply that the heart is not functioning perfectly well in the donor but are based on concern about the ability of the donor heart to tolerate ischemia during the cold preservation period. The limits of an acceptable donor heart are still being defined, and extending the limits would be one way to increase the number of potential donors.

The donor heart is ischemic from the time the aortic cross clamp is applied in the donor until the cross clamp is

Table 10-8. SELECTION OF RECIPIENTS FOR CARDIAC TRANSPLANTATION

Indications:	End-stage ventricular failure
	NYHA Class III–IV existence
	Poor 6- to 12-month prognosis for survival
	Medically compliant psychosocial profile
	No alternative treatment
Contraindications:	Systemic disease (vascular, autoimmune)
	Irreversible renal/hepatic insufficiency
	Neoplasia
	High, fixed pulmonary vascular resistance
	Active infection
Relative contraindications:	Age > 55 years
	Diabetes mellitus
	Active peptic ulcer disease

Table 10-9. ELEMENTS OF DONOR EVALUATION

Travel time (major variable in ischemic time)
Age (male < 40, female < 50)
Size (approximately recipient weight ±20%)
ABO blood group
Lymphocyte cross match (controversial)
Etiology of brain death
  Blunt trauma: rule out myocardial contusion
  Penetrating trauma and primary neurologic:
    look carefully at medical history
Medical history
  Cardiac history
  Hypertension
  I.V. drug abuse
  Smoking
  Alcoholism
Hemodynamic history since admission
  Cardiac arrest or prolonged hypotension
  Cardioactive and vasoactive drug requirements
  Central venous pressure
Cardiac
  ECG: ST-T waves can be misleading in brain death
  Echocardiogram: contractility, regional wall motion
  Evaluation by cardiologist
Pulmonary
  Oxygenation
  Chest x-ray: contusion, pneumothorax, infiltrates, edema
Serology
  Hepatitis B
  HTLV-III
  Cytomegalovirus

removed from the recipient, and ideally this ischemic period is kept under 4 h. Travel time between the donor and recipient hospitals is usually the main determinant of ischemic time; so expedient transportation is arranged accordingly. Age criteria are set to minimize the risk of using a heart with silent coronary atherosclerosis. Size matching is designed to avoid extreme discrepancies in the atrial and great vessel anastomoses, and to avoid any predictable mismatch in hemodynamics, as might occur if a small female heart is placed in a man with borderline acceptable PVR.

Major blood group compatibility is essential. The importance of a prospective lymphocyte cross match remains controversial in the transplantation of solid organs other than the kidney. As a practical matter, time constraints usually prohibit prospective cross matching.

Victims of blunt trauma must be assessed carefully for myocardial contusion, which can be present with few objective findings. On the other hand many normal hearts will be thrown away if indirect evidence such as thoracic fractions and pulmonary contusions is overemphasized. Victims of penetrating trauma frequently have a social profile that makes attention to certain features of medical history such as I.V. drug abuse important. Patients with primary neurologic brain death (i.e., subarachnoid hemorrhage) require close scrutiny for evidence of major hypertension and its cardiac sequelae.

Features of the hemodynamic course that might be alarming in isolation, such as cardiac arrest or a high-dose dopamine infusion, need to be considered in context or good donors will be wasted. A common scenario is a patient on high-dose dopamine with diabetes insipidus and a low CVP, who can be taken off dopamine after volume replacement.

The ECG should be normal, but striking ST-T changes can be associated with cerebrovascular accidents, hypothermia and electrolyte abnormalities. Echocardiography is extremely helpful under such circumstances, as it is in the evaluation of blunt trauma, to assess contractility and search for focal wall motion abnormalities.

A fairly broad spectrum of pulmonary pathlogy can be tolerated as long as oxygenation is adequate and sepsis is avoided. Extensive traumatic injury should raise the index of suspicion for myocardial contusion but is not an independent exclusion.

Positive serology for HTLV-III or hepatitis B excludes a potential donor. The information can be difficult to obtain quickly but should be insisted upon if the donor's medical and social history suggests increased risk. Knowledge of the potential recipient's cytomegalovirus (CMV) titer is required to interpret a positive CMV titer in the donor. Acute CMV infection in an immunosuppressed seronegative recipient is very serious and appears to be transmissible with the heart. Although many CMV positive recipients will experience CMV reactivation infection after transplant, it is far less serious. Of course, use of a seronegative donor for a seronegative recipient does not guarantee safety, since the disease can be transmitted equally well through blood transfusion.

DONOR OPERATION. The procedure is timed in coordination with teams removing liver and kidneys, and with the team preparing for implantation in the recipient. The heart is exposed through a median sternotomy, and a final assessment is made by visual inspection. Heparin is given. Removal begins with ligation of the superior vena cava and division of the inferior vena cava and pulmonary veins (Fig. 10-27). This is done as the first step in order to decompress the heart and avoid any ventricular distention with the aorta occluded. An aortic cross clamp is applied just proximal to the innominate artery. Preservation is begun by infusing hyperkalemic cardioplegia solution at 4°C into the aortic root to produce a prompt arrest in diastole. The cooling provided by coronary perfusion is augmented by immersion in saline solution at 4°C. The heart is observed closely for distention, which can be relieved if necessary by passing a finger across the mitral valve from the opening in the pulmonary veins. Finally the aorta and pulmonary artery are divided distally (Fig. 10-28); the heart is removed from the pericardium and wrapped in ice for transport.

RECIPIENT OPERATION. The recipient operation begins with median sternotomy and cannulation for cardiopulmonary bypass, using two separate venous cannulae that can be snared in the cavae. The cannulae are inserted well away from the atrioventricular groove, where the right atrial anastomosis will eventually be made. To minimize ischemic time, close communication is maintained with the donor team so that implantation can proceed as soon as the donor heart arrives in the recipient operating room. The patient is placed on total cardiopulmonary bypass

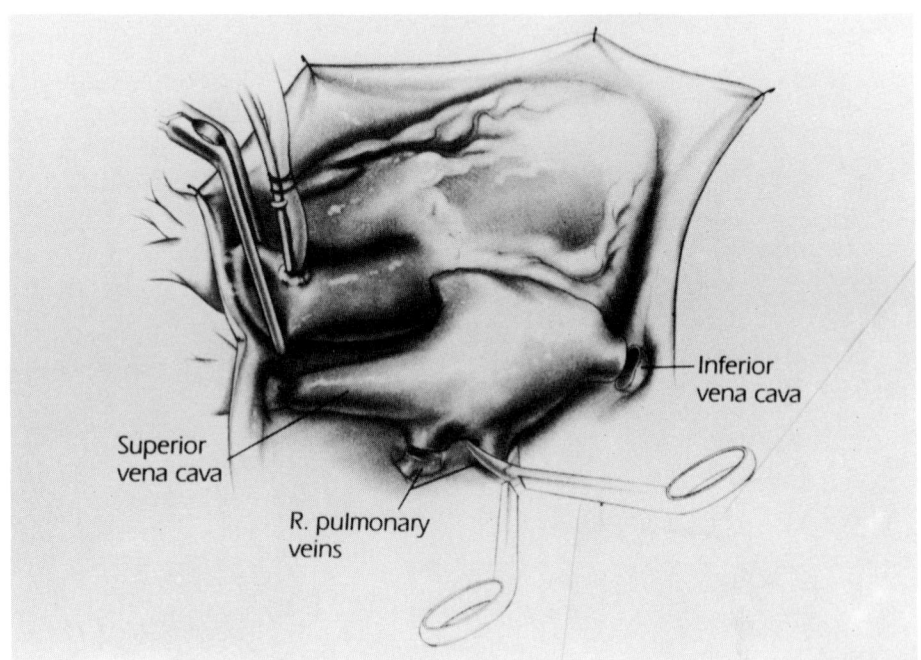

Fig. 10-27. Donor cardiectomy. The aortic cross clamp has been applied, and cardioplegia is being infused through a cannula in the aortic root. The superior vena cava has been ligated. The inferior vena cava and right superior pulmonary vein have been divided, and the scissors are about to divide the right inferior pulmonary vein. For the next few minutes attention is directed toward achieving a rapid arrest without ventricular distention, and beginning topical hypothermia with iced saline irrigation.

with moderate systemic hypothermia. The recipient aorta is cross-clamped just proximal to the innominate artery, and the heart is removed by dividing the great vessels at their commissures and separating the atria from the ventricles at the atrioventricular groove. Both atrial appendages are excised. The posterior aspects of both atria are left intact and connected by the interatrial septum. The donor heart is brought onto the field, trimmed appropriately, and carefully inspected, looking particularly for a patent foramen ovale. If a patent foramen is left open, a significant right-to-left shunt can occur in patients with residual pulmonary hypertension. Implantation proceeds with anastomosis of the left atria, followed by the right atria, pulmonary arteries, and aortae (Fig. 10-29). Size discrepancies are easily accommodated in the atrial suture lines. Significant aortic size discrepancy is quite common, especially when there is a large age difference between donor and recipient. Remarkably large mis-

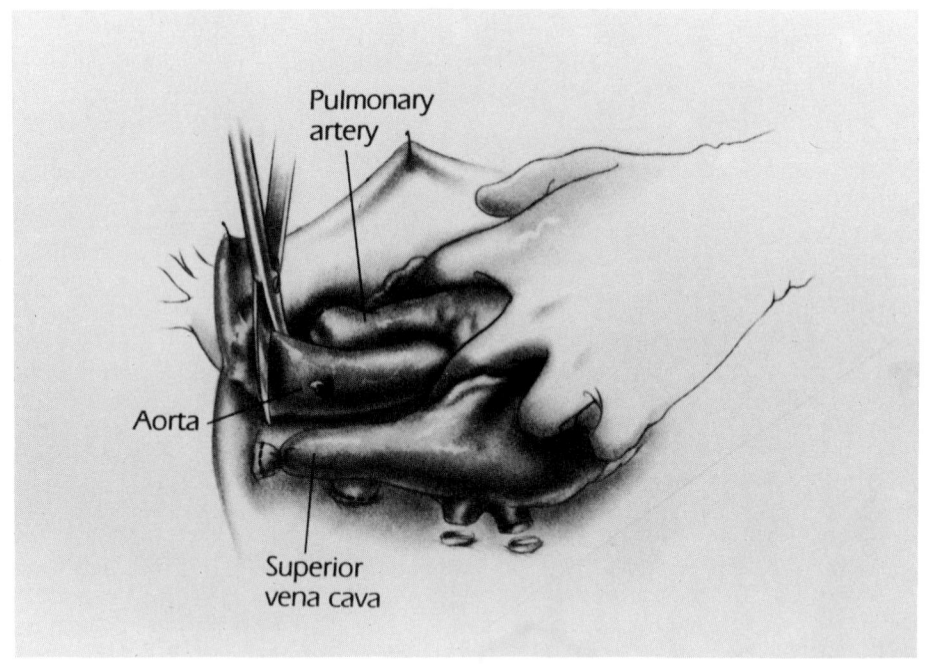

Fig. 10-28. Donor cardiectomy. The scissors are about to divide the aorta. The pulmonary artery and superior vena cava will be divided next and the donor heart removed for transport. The pulmonary artery is usually divided at or beyond the bifurcation to preserve all possible length. It is convenient to divide the right pulmonary artery just to the right of the superior vena cava (dotted line) and divide the left pulmonary artery at the pericardial reflection. (From: *Doty DB: Cardiac surgery: A looseleaf workbook and update service. "TRANSPL" section in Update 3. Chicago, Year Book Medical Publishers, 1986, with permission.*)

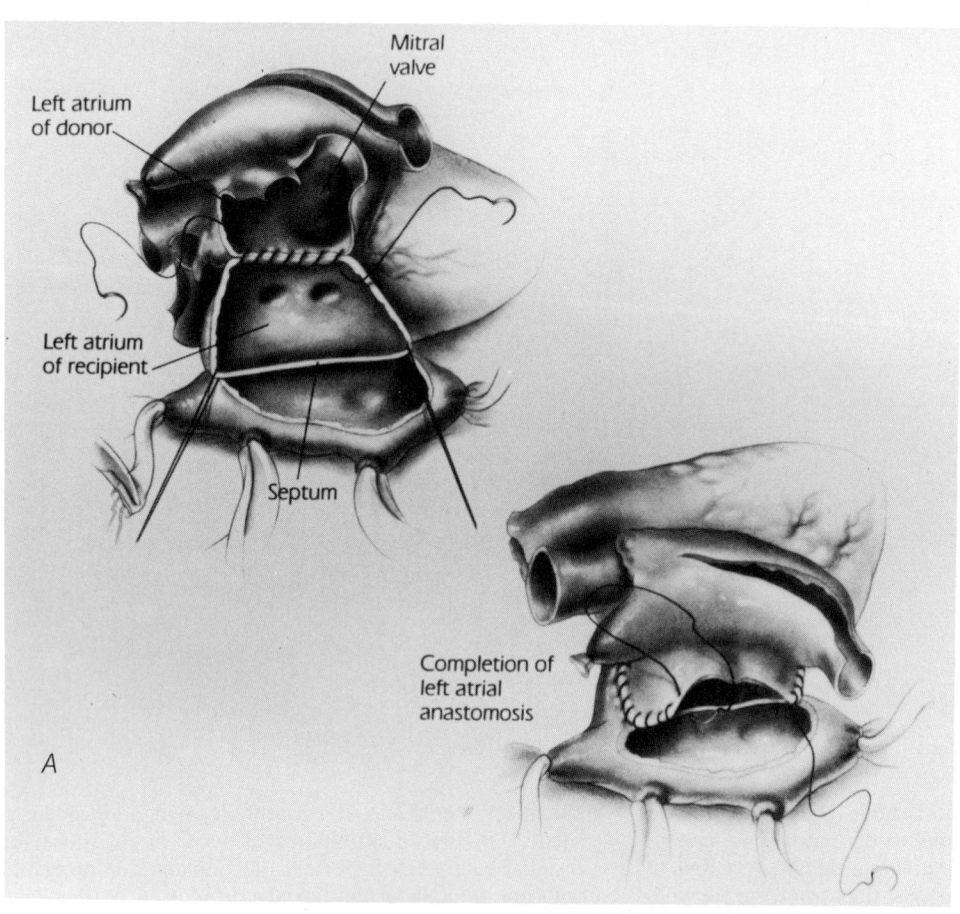

Left atrium
of donor

Mitral
valve

Left atrium
of recipient

Septum

Completion of
left atrial
anastomosis

A

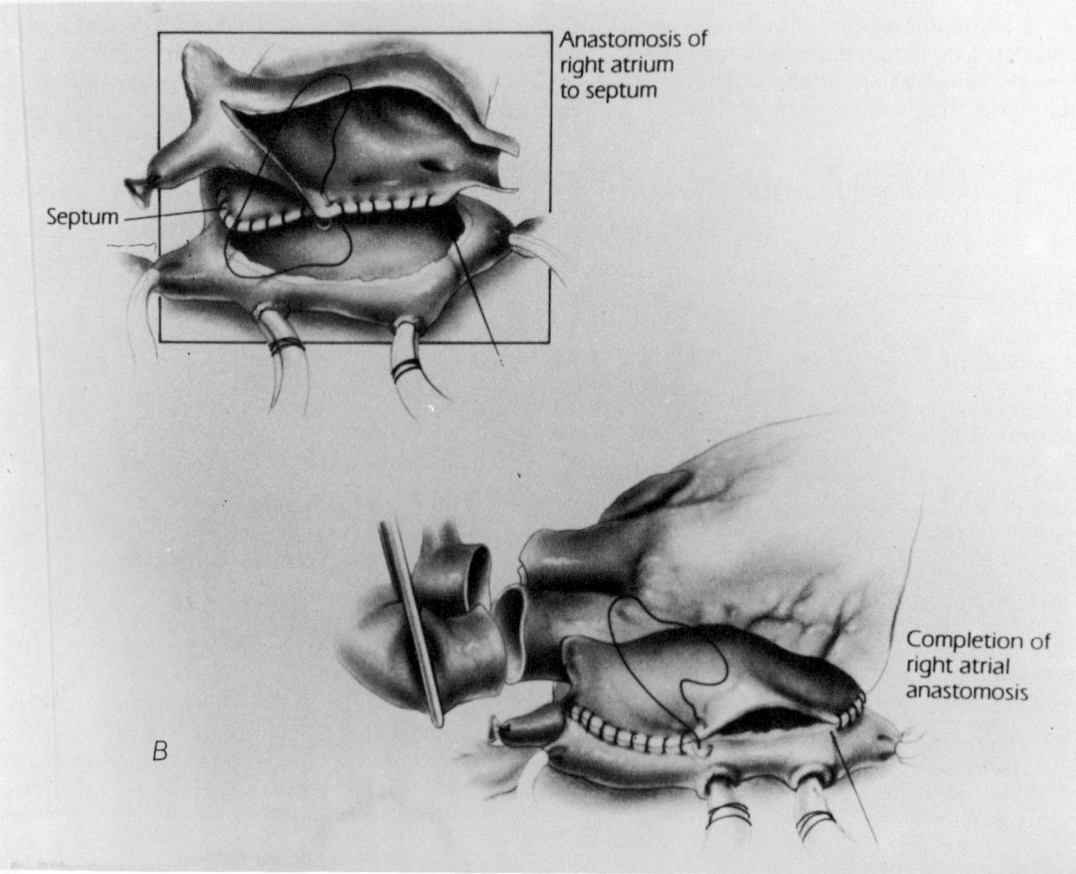

Anastomosis of
right atrium
to septum

Septum

Completion of
right atrial
anastomosis

B

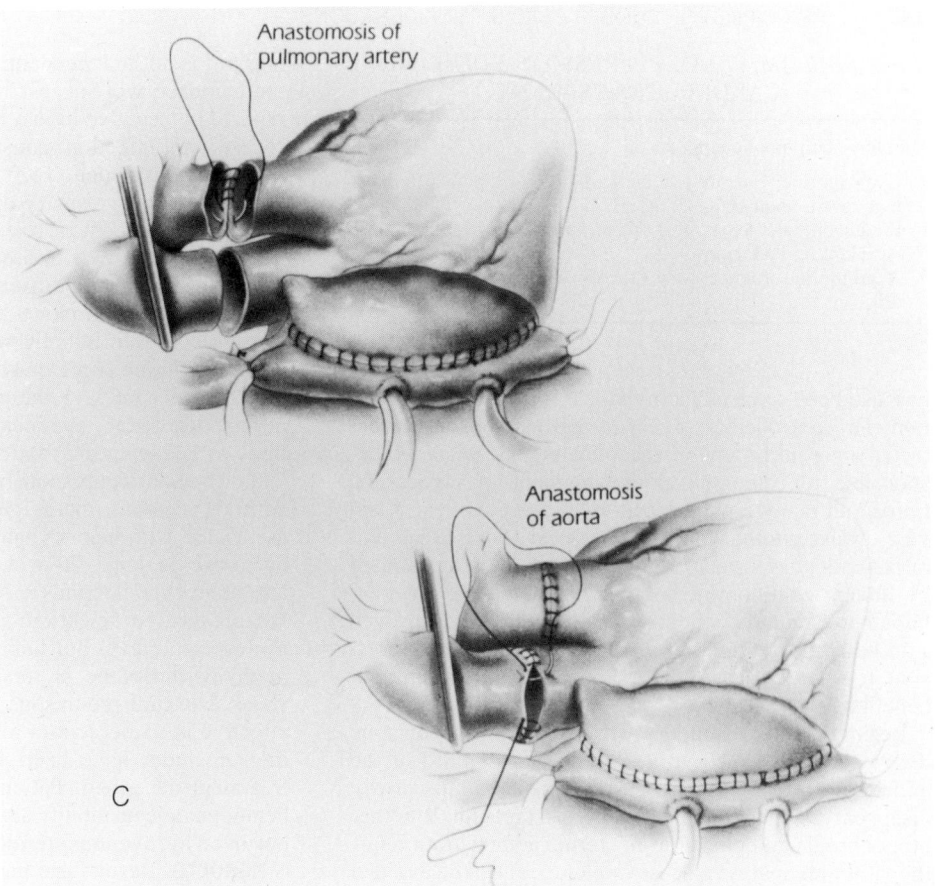

Anastomosis of
pulmonary artery

Anastomosis
of aorta

C

Fig. 10-29. *A.* Implantation of the donor heart. The left atrial anastomosis is begun adjacent to the left atrial appendage of the donor
and the confluence of the left pulmonary veins in the recipient
(upper figure). It is completed by joining the right edge of the donor
left atrium to the interatrial septum (lower figure). Note the opening
in the right atrium, which is directed from the inferior vena caval
orifice toward the middle of the right atrial appendage. *B.* Implantation of the donor heart. The right atrial anastomosis is begun by
rolling the posterior edge of the right atriotomy over to the interatrial
septum, where the suture line overlaps the septal segment of the
left atrial suture line just completed (upper figure). The closure diverges from the left atrium at the inferior and superior ends of the
septum and continues anteriorly (lower figure). *C.* Implantation of
the donor heart. The pulmonary artery (upper figure) and aorta
(lower figure) are trimmed and joined with a continuous suture, beginning posteriorly. Discrepancies in circumference are taken up
with careful suture spacing. (From: *Doty DB: Cardiac surgery: A
looseleaf workbook and update service. "TRANSPL" section in
Update 3. Chicago, Year Book Medical Publishers, 1986, with permission.*)

matches can be accommodated with a careful anastomosis, in part because of the elasticity of youthful aortic tissue. The cross clamp is removed, and a spontaneous
rhythm is restored. The sinus node of the donor heart
becomes the dominant pacemaker. The recipient's intrinsic rhythm frequently persists, producing regular noncon-
ducted contractions of the native atrial tissue and a second independent P-wave on the posttransplant ECG.

Early postoperative care is identical in most respects to
that given any patient following open heart surgery, ex-

cept that strict reverse isolation is observed. The denervated heart often requires a period of chronotropic support, which is usually provided by isoproterenol infusion
or epicardial pacing to maintain a heart rate of 90 to 110.
Virtually all patients demonstrate a degree of right ventricular decompensation as the donor right ventricle tries
to adapt to the residual elevated PVR in the recipient.
Clinical manifestations include a rising central venous
pressure, a right ventricular gallop, and edema. Echocardiography done during this period typically shows decreased right ventricular contractility with chamber dilation, and may show tricuspid insufficiency. In correctly
selected patients these findings will return to normal as
the PVR gradually falls, but inotropic and vasodilator
support may be required for many days.

IMMUNOSUPPRESSION. Maintenance immunosuppression (Table 10-10) consists primarily of oral cyclosporine
and prednisone, usually given twice daily. Cyclosporine
dosage is adjusted to maintain an appropriate blood or
serum level. Complex interactions with other medications
are frequently seen, especially with drugs metabolized in
the liver. Dilantin is a common example.

Unfortunately, in spite of its miraculous immunosuppressive effects, cyclosporine has significant renal and
other toxicity. A decrease in renal function and a rise in
systemic blood pressure are seen over time in a high percentage of patients, and appear to be dose-related. There

Table 10-10. IMMUNOSUPPRESSION FOLLOWING
CARDIAC TRANSPLANT

Maintenance immunosuppression:

1. Cyclosporine: Usually 4–8 mg/kg P.O. b.i.d., adjust to maintain serum level 100–300 ng/mL
2. Prednisone: 0.2 mg/kg P.O. b.i.d., taper after 3–6 months to ≤0.1 mg/kg P.O. b.i.d.
3. Azathioprine (optional—protocols vary): 1–2 mg/kg P.O. q.d.

---

has also been some concern that chronic low-grade rejection not controlled by cyclosporine and not easily detected by routine endomyocardial biopsy might be responsible for the gradual development of myocardial fibrosis in many patients, and for the appearance of severe diffuse coronary artery disease in about 10 percent of patients after 1 year. Many programs have responded by adding azathioprine to their maintenance regimen, hoping to gain a reduction in cyclosporine dosage as well as a boost in the level of maintenance immunosuppression. It is not yet clear that this approach will produce any benefits.

Beginning 3 to 6 months posttransplant the prednisone dose is tapered slowly to a level about one-third of the initial dose. Most features of a cushingoid habitus slowly disappear as the prednisone dose is tapered. Whether other chronic complications of steroid administration (arthopathy, myopathy, glucose intolerance) will be avoided remains to be seen.

REJECTION. Rejection is monitored by right ventricular endomyocardial biopsy, done at least weekly in the first month, then less frequently on a tapering schedule. At the time of each biopsy a right heart catheterization is performed. Most rejection episodes have normal hemodynamics, but a low cardiac output, low mixed venous oxygen saturation, and elevated right atrial or wedge pressures raise suspicion of rejection. The biopsy is performed through the same venipuncture with a flexible biopsy forceps passed into the right ventricle. Adequate sampling is important, since the false negative rate only drops below 5 percent when three or more pieces of muscle can be examined on the slide. The biopsy material can be fixed, stained, and examined microscopically within 24 h.

Histologic evidence of myocyte necrosis is considered diagnostic of significant rejection. Inflammatory cell infiltrates are considered abnormal but are usually not treated as rejection in the absence of myocyte necrosis in patients on cyclosporine. All suspected rejection episodes are considered in clinical context, especially if the histological diagnosis is ambiguous. Subjective signs are frequently subtle but may include malaise, fatigue, and frank dyspnea or orthopnea. Physical findings are usually absent but can include tachycardia, a ventricular gallop, rales, and edema. Diminution in ECG voltage is correlated with rejection in patients maintained on azathioprine and steroids but is without value in patients on cyclosporine. Echocardiography can add suggestive findings but is not independently diagnostic. Occasionally all the evidence will suggest rejection in the presence of a repeatedly negative biopsy. In such cases, once bacterial sepsis, viral infection, constrictive pericarditis, and tamponade are excluded, a left heart catheterization is likely to show diffuse coronary disease.

About 95 percent of rejection episodes can be treated initially with steroids. Many institutions prefer to give intravenous methylprednisolone (usually 1 g/day for 3 days) as initial treatment. At Columbia Presbyterian rejection is treated initially with an increase in oral prednisone to 50 mg twice daily for 3 days, followed by a 10 mg/day taper back to the maintenance dose, a protocol designed to reduce the incidence of infectious complications by reducing the total steroid dose (Fig. 10-30). Rejection episodes unresponsive to the oral pulse are treated with intravenous methylprednisolone, unless they are associated with hemodynamic instability or a low serum cyclosporine level, in which case intramuscular rabbit antithymocyte globulin (R-ATG) is added simultaneously. Uncomplicated rejection associated with an adequate cyclosporine level but failing to respond to intravenous methylprednisolone is treated with R-ATG as a third stage. The oral prednisone protocol described has been effective in 91 percent of all rejection episodes, and half the remainder have been salvaged with the adjunctive treatment described. Patients who present initially with hemodynamic instability are at high risk and are promptly begun on intravenous steroid and antithymocyte globulin.

RESULTS. Results are being carefully tabulated in the Registry of the International Society for Heart Transplantation, which presently includes just over 3500 cases (January 1987). With early (30-day) mortality included, 1-year survival expectancy is 79 percent (Fig. 10-31). Survival remains high thereafter, with 77 percent actuarial survival at 5 years. Improvement in results since the introduction of cyclosporine is evident when the curve for patients treated with cyclosporine is compared with that for noncyclosporine patients. One-year survival with cyclosporine is 79 versus 66 percent without cyclosporine, and at 5 years the difference is 77 versus 55 percent. The curves are significantly different ($p < 0.01$).

Although long-term survival appears to be excellent, perioperative mortality remains high. During 1985 there was 12 percent mortality during the first 30 days. In cyclosporine-treated patients, 30-day mortality was attributed to rejection in 22 percent, infection in 20 percent, and "cardiac" and other causes in the majority (58 percent). The most common cardiac causes of early mortality are poor donor selection, poor donor preservation, and prohibitive pulmonary hypertension in the recipient. In comparison with patients treated with azathioprine and steroids, cyclosporine has significantly reduced the frequency of early death due to rejection, from 32 to 22 percent, but has had no significant impact of deaths due to other causes.

For all patients risk falls dramatically during the first year. Three-quarters of the first-year mortality occurs during the first quarter of the year. Although the period of high risk coincides with the period having the greatest

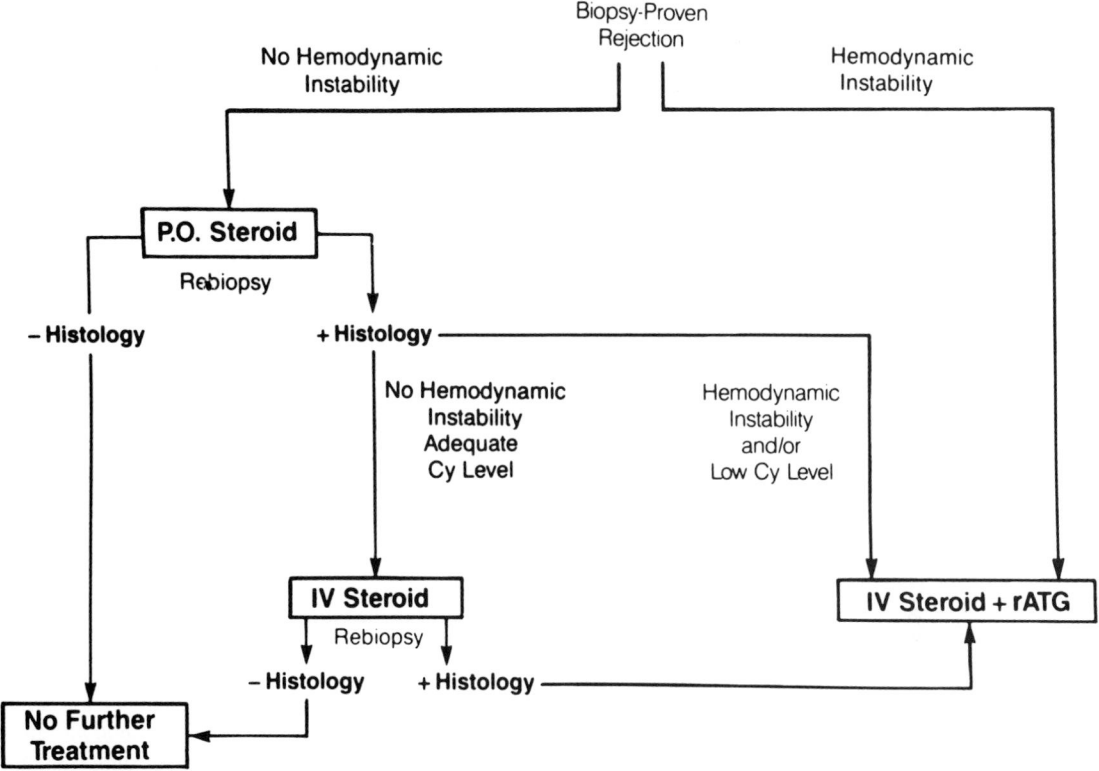

Fig. 10-30. Treatment algorithm for biopsy-proved rejection used at Columbia Presbyterian Medical Center. Ninety-five percent of all rejection episodes are treated initially with oral steroid. "Cy level" is the cyclosporine level. (From: *Michler, Smith, et al, with permission.*)

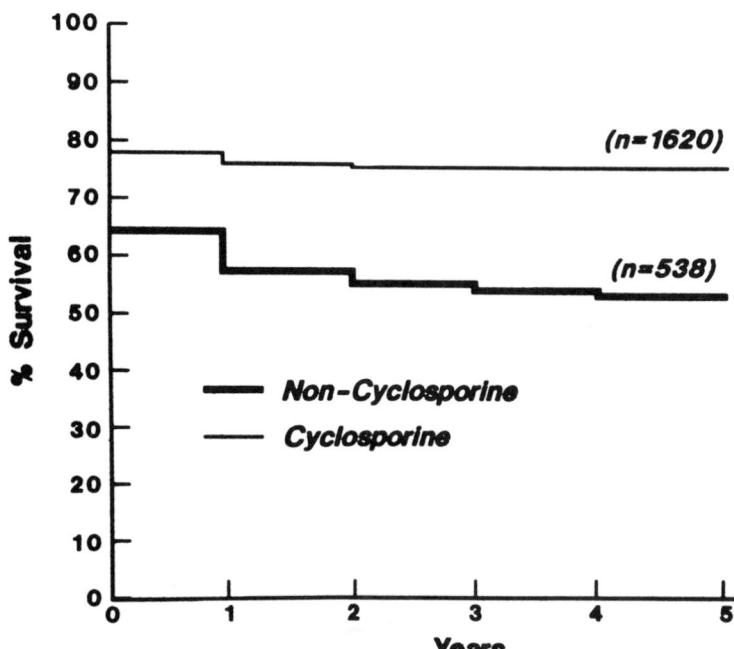

Fig. 10-31. Overall actuarial survival of patients transplanted from 1978 through 1985, compiled for the most recent Official Report of the Registry of the International Society for Heart Transplantation in June 1986. Early (30-day) mortality (about 10 percent) is included. The curves for cyclosporine-treated and non-cyclosporine-treated patients are significantly different (p < 0.01). (From: *Solis and Kaye, with permission.*)

frequency of rejection episodes, it is complications of immunosuppression, infection in particular, that accounts for the highest mortality. In patients treated with cyclosporine, the percentage of mortality due to infection increases from 20 percent at 30 days to 29 percent at 60 days, and eventually accounts for about 40 percent of the mortality in the registry. Death due to rejection remains relatively stable throughout at 20 to 25 percent.

Infectious complications in cardiac transplant recipients are most often pulmonary. Opportunistic pathogens predominate, and include *Pneumocystis carinii, Cytomegalovirus, Legionella,* and fungi. Antibacterial and antifungal agents will control most infections if the level of immunosuppression can be tightly controlled.

Most chronic complications can also be viewed as consequences of immunosuppression. Slowly progressive renal insufficiency and hypertension are still common in patients on long-term cyclosporine, although it appears that tighter control of dosage will arrest the problem. Malignancies occur in 2 to 5 percent of patients, and have a spectrum of pathology characteristic of immunosuppressed patients.

Lymphoma, especially non-Hodgkin's lymphoma, Kaposi's sarcoma, and other relatively unusual neoplasms predominate. Problems related to regulatory physiology in a denervated heart, which were the subject of much speculation and experimental modeling in the early years, do not appear to be major. The adaptive mechanisms are incompletely understood, and probably involve a combination of humoral control and receptor regulation. By whatever mechanism, the autoregulation of cardiac output is remarkably well preserved after cardiac transplantation.

One unfortunate consequence of denervation is that angina cannot occur as a premonitory symptom in patients developing graft atherosclerosis, so that these patients tend to present with sudden death or congestive heart failure. The coronary atherosclerosis seen in cardiac transplants is characteristically diffuse and progressive, frequently occurring in the first 1 to 2 years, with an incidence of about 10 percent. The leading suspicion regarding etiology is that the phenomenon reflects chronic low-grade rejection that is poorly detected by conventional means, and raises concern that the incidence may continue to increase. Every large series by now contains several patients who have required retransplantation for this problem.

The most impressive results are those measured by functional status. In Stanford's first 106 patients, 97 percent were restored to NYHA Class I existence. Assessments of employment status are complicated by the fact that many patients were originally students or housewives, but if return to a previous life-style is used as the criterion, 82 percent of the Stanford series did so. At Columbia Presbyterian, 62 percent of patients have returned to their previous life-style after 6 months, a figure that rises to 100 percent after 2 years.

Cardiac transplantation is now a well-established therapy for end-stage heart failure, but progress is needed in several areas. Age limits are being stretched in both directions. As yet there is no evidence to substantiate the intuitive notion that results in older patients will be less satisfactory, but only small numbers are available for analysis at present. At the other end of the spectrum, results in infants and children have been disappointing, with 1-year survival of only 49 percent in the 0- to 10-year age group recorded in the registry. Although the management of immunosuppression in infants and small children has proved to be very difficult, progress is anticipated with experience.

Endomyocardial biopsy is a reliable method for monitoring rejection, but it remains an invasive procedure with measurable risks. Noninvasive methods for the diagnosis of rejection are the focus of intensive research activity in echocardiography, nuclear scanning, magnetic resonance imaging, and labeled antimyosin monoclonal antibody, to name a few.

The most imposing problem of all is the rapid increase in demand for the procedure in the face of a limited inventory of replacement parts. The efficiency of human donor procurement efforts is increasing steadily but will inevitably lag behind, especially if age criteria are relaxed substantially. Use of the artificial heart as permanent replacement may regain popularity if the trend continues, and if use of the artificial heart as a temporary bridge to transplant continues to have encouraging results. Another alternative is the use of nonhuman donors (xenografts), which has received scant attention in the past but gained sudden notoriety recently when Bailey transplanted a baboon heart into a human infant with hypoplastic left heart syndrome. The child survived 20 days. In a heterotopic primate model recently developed at Columbia Presbyterian, 12-fold improvement in survival over controls was obtained with conventional (cyclosporine and steroid) immunosuppression. If success is achieved in the orthotopic position, it is hoped that chimpanzees and other species could be used to expand the donor pool.

Heterotopic Transplantation

In heterotopic transplantation, the donor heart is placed in parallel in the circulation. Experimentally this has been done in both sides of the thorax, in the abdomen, the neck, and the inguinal region. Clinically, it is placed in the right chest, with separate left atrial, right atrial, aortic, and pulmonary arterial anastomoses (Fig. 10-32). Advocates of the procedure have cited the advantage of having the native heart in place during severe rejection episodes, and the advantage of using donors smaller than could be used in the orthotopic position. Results obtained to date in the heterotopic position do not support wide application of this approach. The largest series in the world is at the Groote Schuur Hospital in South Africa, and a recent report (May 1986) documented a disappointing 55 percent 1-year survival and 22 percent 5-year survival in 49 patients. The authors currently recommend heterotopic transplantation only for certain conditions: patients with pulmonary vascular resistance too

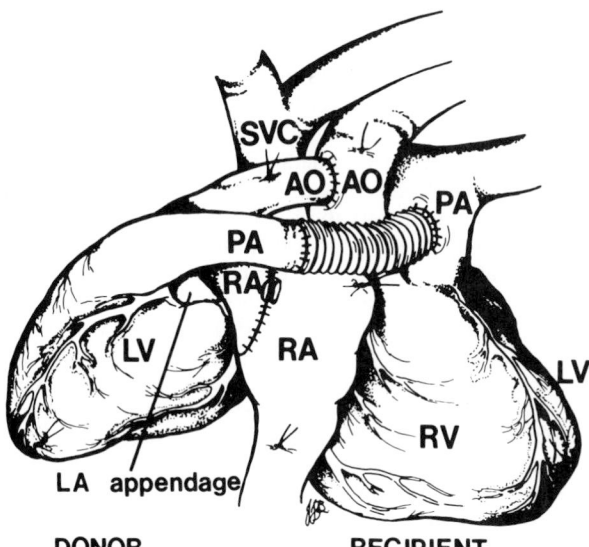

Fig. 10-32. A completed heterotopic cardiac transplant. The donor aorta (AO) crosses over the superior vena cava (SVC) and is anastomosed end-to-side to the recipient aorta. The donor pulmonary artery (PA) reaches the recipient PA by adding a segment of Dacron tube graft. The right atrial (RA) anastomosis lies partially obscured by the PA. The left atrial anastomosis, performed first because it is most posterior, is not visible, although the left atrial appendage can be seen (LA appendage). The procedure is performed on total cardiopulmonary bypass with aortic and bicaval cannulation. (From: *Novitzky D, Cooper DKC, et al: The surgical technique of heterotopic heart transplantation. Ann Thor Surg 36:476–482, 1983, with permission.*)

high for orthotopic transplantation, and patients whose critical condition demands use of a donor heart too small to be used orthotopically.

HEART-LUNG

The first successful human heart-lung transplant was performed by Reitz in 1981, following several years of work in the laboratory at Stanford spent developing the method in a primate model. Three previous attempts in human beings, in 1968 (Cooley), 1969 (Lillihei), and 1971 (Barnard) were all early failures. Reitz's first patient was a woman with primary pulmonary hypertension who was leading a virtually normal life until her death due to unrelated causes.

SPECTRUM OF DISEASE. Patients who might benefit from heart-lung transplant have suffered irreversible damage to both the heart and lungs. Such patients can be divided into two groups—those with pulmonary vascular disease and those with respiratory disease. In pulmonary vascular diseases the high-resistance circulatory disorder is primary, while in respiratory diseases chronic disturbance in gas exchange and alveolar mechanics leads to a secondary increase in pulmonary vascular resistance. Even though both pathways end in right ventricular failure, there is therapeutic relevance in this distinction. Pulmonary vascular diseases reach end stage with no significant tracheobronchial or alveolar abnormalities, and with no effect on chest wall mechanics, so that the entire disease process is removed at transplant. By contrast, respiratory diseases reach a cardiac end stage after years of worsening ventilatory mechanics, so that heart-lung transplant still leaves behind an older, nutritionally depleted patient with chronically infected secretions and distorted thoracic anatomy, with attenuated diaphragmatic and intercostal musculature. The results of heart-lung transplant have been very poor when performed for respiratory disease, although the total numbers are still small.

RECIPIENT SELECTION. The cardinal fact guiding selection of candidates for heart-lung transplant is the rarity of suitable donors, which makes it mandatory to select only patients with the greatest probability of a good outcome. Results have been best in young patients with end-stage primary pulmonary hypertension (PPH) or Eisenmenger's syndrome. In patients thought to have PPH it is important to exclude chronic pulmonary thromboembolism, both because of concern about recurrence after transplant, and because certain patients with thromboembolic occlusion of both pulmonary arteries can benefit from pulmonary thromboendarterectomy. In such cases there is no reliable substitute for pulmonary angiography, although magnetic resonance imaging is promising.

In patients with Eisenmenger's syndrome correctable lesions that may have been overlooked should be excluded, and any previous history of cardiothoracic operation carefully reviewed. Based on the limited experience accumulated to date, patients who have had previous operations have had nearly insurmountable bleeding problems, with operative mortality greater than 50 percent. The problem tends to be particularly severe in Eisenmenger's patients with primary cyanotic lesions, who usually have large systemic-pulmonary collaterals throughout the mediastinum, and form highly vascular adhesions. History of a previous cardiothoracic operation is very nearly an absolute contraindication to heart-lung transplant in 1987.

DONOR SELECTION. In addition to the familiar criteria for a satisfactory cardiac donor, heart-lung donors must have a clear chest x-ray, normal gas exchange, and clean tracheobronchial secretions (Table 10-11). The lungs tend to deteriorate quickly in most patients with brain death. Even if neurogenic pulmonary edema or contusion from blunt trauma are absent, the lungs remain susceptible to the insults of mechanical ventilation and airway colonization with nosocomial pathogens. It is also important to

Table 10-11. CRITERIA FOR A SATISFACTORY HEART-LUNG DONOR

1. Satisfactory heart donor
2. Clear chest x-ray
3. Normal gas exchange ($P_{O_2} > 90$ torr with $F_{I_{O_2}} \geq 40\%$, PEEP ≥ 5 cm)
4. Clean secretions (no more than a few colonizing organisms)
5. Close size match

have a close size match between the donor lungs and the recipient thorax, to avoid chronic basal atelectasis and infection when the lungs are too large, and to avoid large pleural effusions when the lungs are too small. After using height and weight as a rough guide, thoracic dimensions are carefully compared by overlapping comparable donor and recipient chest x-rays. Ideally, the overlap should be a centimeter or less in all dimensions.

DONOR OPERATION. Techniques for preservation of the heart and lungs have been very slow to develop, and dependence on the cumbersome transfer of an intact donor from another hospital to an adjacent operating room has greatly retarded the growth rate of the procedure. Methods for preservation that would allow distant procurement remain somewhat controversial. Cooling on cardiopulmonary bypass, cooling with pulmonary artery perfusion, topical hypothermia alone, and preservation in an autoperfusion apparatus all have advocates. A method developed at Stanford, attractive in its relative simplicity, has been used very recently and successfully for distant procurement in two patients at Stanford, two patients at the University of Pittsburgh, and one patient at Columbia Presbyterian, with ischemic times ranging up to 4 h and 45 min. The technique consists of high-volume pulmonary artery flush with modified Collin's solution at 4°C, preceded by pulmonary vasodilation with a prostaglandin E-1 infusion, and standard cardioplegic arrest of the heart. The technique seems to offer great hope for the future.

The heart and lungs can be removed from the donor through a median sternotomy or a bilateral anterior thoracotomy, which is preferred by Hardesty and Griffith. The anterior contents of the mediastinum are removed, and the major structures isolated. Heparin is given. Whatever method of lung preservation is to be used is begun, the aorta is clamped just proximal to the innominate artery, and the heart is arrested with cardioplegia. The trachea is divided several rings above the carina after clamping distally with the lungs partially inflated, and the organs are dissected free of their posterior mediastinal attachments, taking care to achieve hemostasis on the organ block. The organs are immersed in cold saline for transport.

RECIPIENT OPERATION. The recipient operation is performed through a median sternotomy. Both pleural cavities are entered. Both phrenic nerves are dissected free on pedicles of pericardium from the diaphragms to a point just above the pulmonary arteries. The trachea is exposed deep to the aorta and just superior to the pulmonary artery bifurcation, where it will later be divided just above the carina. The patient is placed on cardiopulmonary bypass with moderate systemic hypothermia, using aortic and bicaval cannulation, the heart is excised, leaving the posterior aspects of both atria, and the great vessels are divided at their commissures (Figs. 10-33 and 10-34).

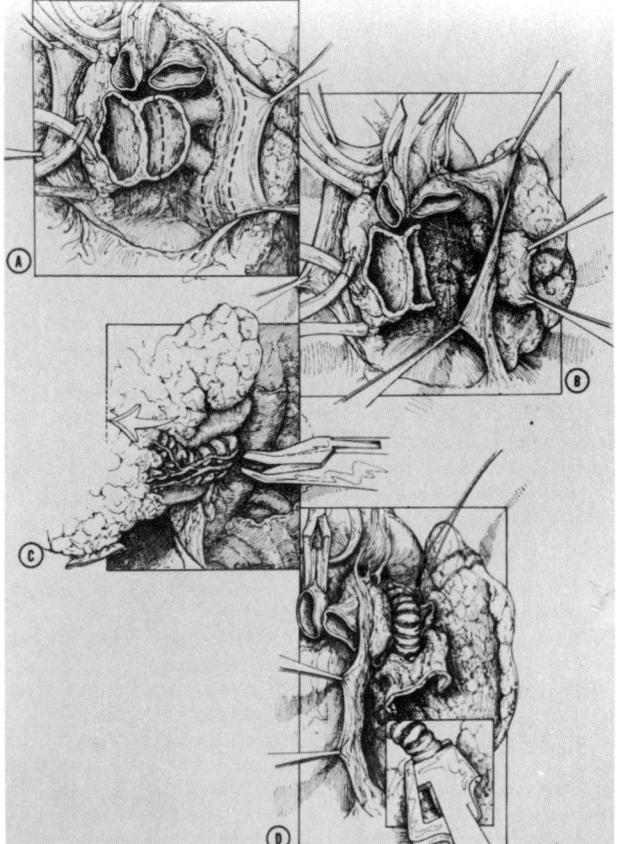

Fig. 10-33. *A.* The recipient atria after removal of the heart. Incisions are made so as to preserve the phrenic nerve in a "ribbon" of pericardium. The left and right pulmonary veins are separated by a longitudinal incision in the posterior left atrial wall and thus into the oblique sinus. *B.* The left pulmonary veins are withdrawn beneath the phrenic nerve. The vagus nerve is immediately posterior. *C.* The left lung is progressively mobilized, and the bronchial arteries are secured. *D.* The left pulmonary artery is divided and the bronchus is stapled and cut. (Copyright B. Hyams.) (From: *Jamieson, Stinson, et al, with permission.*)

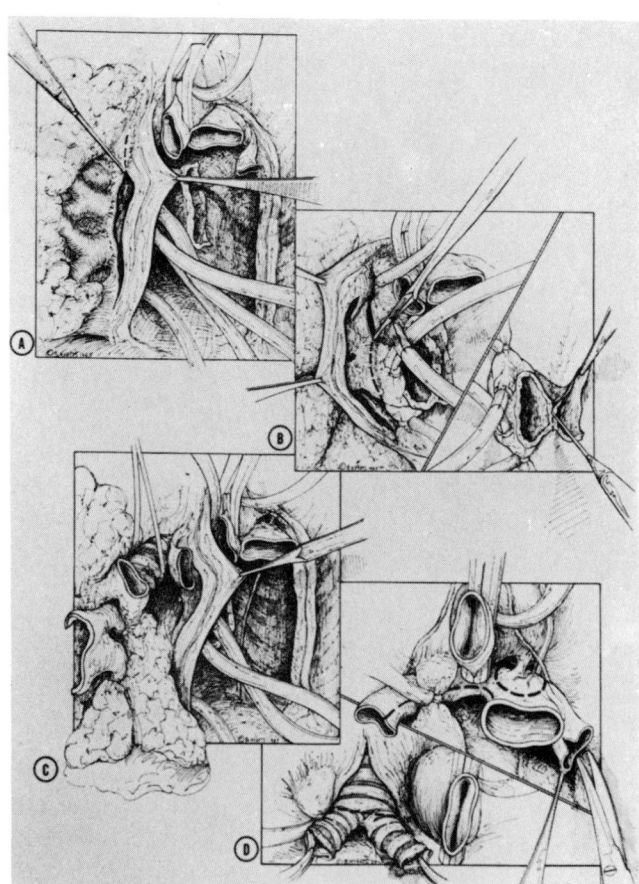

Fig. 10-34. *A.* The right phrenic nerve is separated from the hilum. *B.* The right pulmonary veins are separated from the right atrium. *C.* The right pulmonary ligament is divided, the lung is mobilized, and the pulmonary artery and bronchus are cut. *D.* The remnants of the pulmonary artery are removed, leaving the area around the ductus ligament and recurrent nerve. The trachea and bronchial remnants are exposed to the right of the aorta. The trachea is cut just above the carina. (Copyright B. Hyams.) (From: *Jamieson, Stinson, et al, with permission.*)

Removing the heart improves exposure for the difficult posterior hilar and mediastinal dissection that follows. The two lungs are excised separately along with the left atrium. Both cavae are mobilized to provide room for the new right lung to pass under the right atrium. The atrial septum becomes the posterior free wall of the new atrium; so a patent foramen or ASD must be closed securely. Any remaining pulmonary artery is removed, leaving a small patch containing the ligamentum arteriosum so that injury to the recurrent nerve can be avoided. The recipient trachea is divided just above the carina, the new organ block is brought onto the field, and the donor trachea is divided just above the carina. Implantation begins with anastomosis of the trachea, usually with a simple continuous suture, followed by right atrial and aortic anastomoses. The lungs are passed under each phrenic pedicle, with the right lung passing under the right atrium as well (Fig. 10-35).

The technical keys to operation are hemostasis in the middle mediastinum and protection of both phrenic nerves, both vagus nerves, and the recurrent nerve. Hemostasis can be very difficult to achieve, especially in patients with large bronchial collateral vessels. Postoperative bleeding has been a major problem, one that can begin a vicious cycle of massive transfusion and deteriorating pulmonary function. Paralyzed diaphragms and gastric dilatation can contribute to difficulties maintaining lung expansion. Pyloroplasty has been required in at least two patients.

POSTOPERATIVE CARE. The early postoperative challenge is to maintain full lung expansion and good gas exchange. Before and after extubation tracheobronchial secretions are managed with bronchoscopy and vigorous pulmonary toilet. Pleural effusions are common and can interfere with lung expansion; they are managed with thoracentesis or tube thoracostomy. During the first 2 weeks, before lymphatic drainage is reestablished and ischemic injury has healed, the lungs are kept as dry as possible with vigorous diuresis.

Immunosuppression is modified by problems unique to the lungs. Because steroid administration is known to impair bronchial healing, tracheal healing is carefully protected by withholding maintenance steroids for 2 to 3 weeks. Maintenance cyclosporine treatment is augmented during that period with azathioprine, and frequently with antithymocyte globulin as well. Steroid treatment for rejection is not withheld if indicated.

A greater problem is that diagnosis of rejection in the lungs is very difficult, and surveillance for cardiac rejection with endomyocardial biopsies cannot be relied upon to faithfully mirror activity in the lungs. Diagnosis of lung rejection is still a complex clinical judgment in most

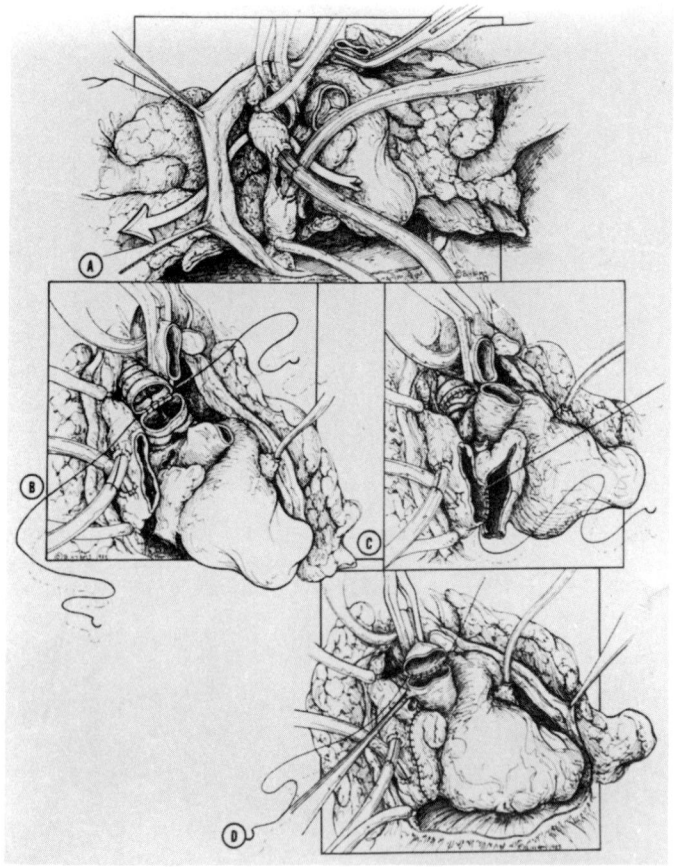

Fig. 10-35. Reimplantation: *A*. The right lung passes beneath the right atrial remnant and the phrenic nerve. *B*. The tracheal anastomosis is performed first, commencing with the posterior wall. *C*. The right atrial anastomosis. *D*. The aortic anastomosis. (Copyright B. Hyams.) (From: *Jamieson, Stinson, et al, with permission.*)

cases, based on an intuitive synthesis of evidence provided by arterial blood gases, chest x-rays, bronchoscopy, and airway cultures. At present, the more sophisticated methods brought to bear, such as bronchoalveolar lavage and labeled leukocyte scanning, can differentiate normal from abnormal but fail to make the crucial distinction between infection and rejection.

If fever, tachycardia, diffuse pulmonary infiltrates, and worsening oxygenation occur, the tracheobronchial tree is aggressively cultured, and an endomyocardial biopsy is obtained. If the cardiac biopsy and the cultures are negative, a trial course of intravenous methylprednisolone (1 g/day for 3 days) may be given, anticipating prompt improvement if the presumptive diagnosis of isolated pulmonary rejection is correct. If the response is inadequate and infection is still securely excluded, a course of antithymocyte globulin can be given. The most difficult distinction to make is between viral pneumonia and rejection, which can be clinically indistinguishable. Because viral pneumonia will become rapidly progressive when treated as rejection, it is necessary on occasion to resort to open lung biopsy in ambiguous situations. In the first few postoperative weeks it can be equally difficult to distinguish rejection from early ischemic/edematous changes, although the consequence of error is not quite as great.

Routine surveillance for cardiac rejection is carried out with endomyocardial biopsy on a regular basis, and cardiac rejection is treated with steroids and/or antithymocyte globulin. A curious feature of heart-lung transplantation is that cardiac rejection is seen with much lower frequency than in cardiac transplantation ($p < 0.01$).

RESULTS. In early 1986, with just 91 cases recorded in the Registry of the International Society for Heart Transplantation, 1-year survival was a rather disappointing 54 percent. On the other hand, the 3-year actuarial survival of 51 percent provides some reason for optimism, implying that the survival curve will remain quite flat. As with cardiac transplantation, the mortality is skewed heavily toward the early postoperative period, and survival in the first year should improve with experience. Patients who have done well have shown remarkable functional improvement comparable with that seen in cardiac transplant patients. The first 10 survivors in the Stanford series were restudied at an average of almost 2 years postoperatively, and were found to have essentially normal pulmonary function.

Some caution is still warranted because of the frequency with which bronchiolitis obliterans is being observed in late survivors. Obliterative bronchiolitis was detectable in half of Stanford's first 20 long-term survivors at a mean of 11 months, with similar experience beginning to emerge from other series. Mortality has been 30 to 50 percent with at least half the remainder demonstrating significant functional impairment. Retransplant has been successfully performed once at Stanford and once in England. The cause of bronchiolitis obliterans is not known. Opinion divides between those who believe the cause to be chronic inadequately treated rejection, and those who suspect a relationship to chronic infection, especially with *Pneumocystis*. The latter theory is supported by the high frequency of *Pneumocystis* colonization in survivors.

It is fair to conclude that heart-lung transplant offers an excellent therapeutic alternative in certain diseases for which no other treatment exists, but long-term durability remains uncertain, and the procedure is likely to remain a therapeutic frontier for the rest of the decade.

SINGLE LUNG

The first human lung transplant was performed in 1963, and was followed by more than 45 attempts around the world during the next 20 years, without a single long-term success. Average survival was less than 10 days. Bronchial healing seemed to pose an insolvable problem, since dehiscence of the bronchial anastomosis was a lethal complication seen in almost every patient surviving more than 7 days. The focus of effort shifted to the laboratory, where Cooper and other members of the Toronto Lung Transplant Group confirmed that steroids markedly inhibited bronchial healing, while cyclosporine and azathioprine did not. Directing their attention to the tenuous vascularity of bronchial anastomoses, the group found that placement of a pedicled omental wrap around the anastomosis restored systemic blood supply to the site within 4 days. Patient selection criteria also underwent refinement as it was recognized that single lung transplantation in patients with emphysema set the stage for major ventilation/perfusion mismatch, because of preferential ventilation and air trapping in the highly compliant native lung at the same time that perfusion was directed almost exclusively to the low compliance vascular bed of the transplanted lung.

Applying the lessons learned in their laboratory, the group in Toronto performed a successful single lung transplant in 1983 in a fifty-eight-year-old man with idiopathic pulmonary fibrosis. That patient returned to work in 3 months, and in 1986 had no difficulty tolerating emergency resection of a leaking abdominal aortic aneurysm. By the end of 1986 seven single lung transplants had been performed in Toronto with five long-term survivors, all demonstrating similar outstanding improvement in their quality of life. The criteria used to select recipients were highly restrictive, and their initial experience focused entirely on patients with pulmonary fibrosis, avoiding patients with emphysema and cystic fibrosis. All patients had to be weaned from steroids before transplant, and all had reasonably well preserved right ventricular function.

The procedures were done through a posterolateral thoracotomy, with a pulmonary artery anastomosis, a broad left atrial cuff anastomosis for pulmonary venous drainage, and a bronchial anastomosis reinforced with a pedicled omental wrap (Fig. 10-36). Heparinization and

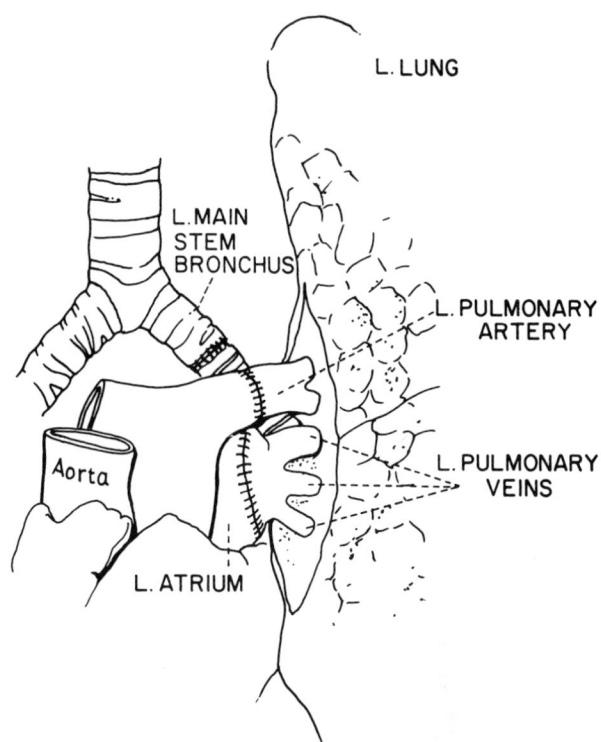

Fig. 10-36. Technique for single lung transplantation, left lung. A cuff of left atrium remains at the confluence of the donor pulmonary veins, so that the anastomosis can be made through the wall of the left atrial cuff rather than through each individual pulmonary vein. After completion of the anastomoses, omentum is brought into the pleural space and circumferentially wrapped around the bronchial anastomosis (not shown).

cardiopulmonary bypass were required in only one case. The left lung was transplanted in most cases, because the mobility of the left diaphragm allowed implantation of an oversized lung. Maintenance steroids were withheld for 3 weeks, although numerous intravenous doses of methylprednisolone were given in each case when a clinical diagnosis of rejection was made. Cyclosporine, azathioprine, and antilymphocyte globulin (ALG) were used initially for immunosuppression, discontinuing the ALG after 5 to 7 days. Perfusion lung scans appeared to be useful in the diagnosis of rejection, demonstrating a shift in perfusion away from the transplanted lung, presumably a reflection of increased pulmonary vascular resistance during rejection.

The results in Toronto are being followed internationally with great interest, and it is likely that the latter half of the 1980s will see a burst of activity in clinical single lung transplantation. It is not clear that the procedure can be extended to patients falling outside the highly selective criteria applied successfully in Toronto. It still appears that patients with end-stage pulmonary disease who have significant right ventricular failure will be operable only with combined heart-lung transplant, which requires extension of that procedure into a patient group in which results to date have been uniformly disappointing. Patients with preserved right ventricular function but with obstructive or septic bilateral pulmonary disease present additional problems. This category is potentially quite large, containing many patients with emphysema and cystic fibrosis, but single lung transplant would appear to be unsuitable because of the potential for ventilation-perfusion mismatching, and the risk of septic contamination of the transplanted lung. Double lung transplantation may prove suitable for such patients. During 1986 one such procedure was performed at Toronto, and three were performed in England, with encouraging early results.

Transplantation for pulmonary disease is still in an exciting embryonic stage that can be expected to demonstrate considerable differentiation during the next several years. The procedure will need to be tailored specifically to the underlying disease process. At present it appears that patients with preserved right ventricular function should receive a single lung transplant for pulmonary fibrosis, and double lung transplant for obstructive and septic diseases. Heart-lung transplant should be reserved for patients with pulmonary vascular disease, and possibly for selected patients with nonvascular pulmonary disease and significant right ventricular failure.

Kidney

The technical knowledge necessary to perform kidney transplants has been available since the turn of the century, when Carrel and Guthrie developed the techniques of vascular suture. Renal transplantation is now the treatment of choice for many patients with renal failure, although hemodialysis and peritoneal dialysis serve as an adequate substitute for most patients.

INDICATIONS AND CONTRAINDICATIONS. The precise indications for the selection of recipients of renal allotransplants have never been defined. In general, irreversible renal failure is the only indication necessary for the patient with a normal urinary outflow tract and without active infection, severe malnutrition, disseminated malignancy, or life-limiting systemic disease. Lower tract abnormalities can usually be corrected. The only absolute contraindications are active infection or malignant disease that cannot be brought under control. A partial list of diseases for which transplantation has been carried out is included in Table 10-12.

Transplantation, when successful, offers a greater degree of rehabilitation to the uremic patient than does either hemodialysis or peritoneal dialysis. The risks are also slightly greater because immunosuppression is required for the duration of graft function. Rigid guidelines that dictate certain therapies for individual patients have not been established. In general, however, children should be transplanted because growth is better after transplantation. Diabetics seem to have fewer problems after transplantation than during dialysis. Older patients without related donors, however, may survive longer on hemodialysis. All patients with HLA-identical sibling donors should certainly be transplanted. In other groups of patients, the indications are less clear, and the preference of the individual is the dominant factor. Most patients who have had a transplant—even one that has

Table 10-12. INDICATIONS FOR RENAL TRANSPLANTATION

Irreversible chronic renal failure	Irreversible acute failure
Chronic pyelonephritis	Cortical necrosis
Chronic glomerulonephritis	Hemolytic uremic syndrome
Diabetic nephropathy	Acute and subacute glomerulonephritis
Goodpasture's disease	Anaphylactoid purpura (Henoch–Schönlein)
Hypocomplementemic nephritis	Acute tubular necrosis
Steroid-resistant nephrotic syndrome	Trauma requiring nephrectomy
Hypertensive nephrosclerosis	Renal vascular diseases
Obstructive uropathy	Renal artery occlusion
Acquired	Renal vein thrombosis
Congenital	Tumors requiring nephrectomy
Congenital disorders	Renal carcinoma
Aplasia	Wilms' tumor
Hypoplasia	Tuberous sclerosis
Horseshoe kidney	Other
Hereditary nephropathies	Multiple myeloma
Alport's syndrome	Macroglobulinemia
Polycystic kidney disease	Wegner's disease
Medullary cystic disease	Scleroderma
Metabolic disorders	Lupus erythematosus
Hyperoxaluria	Polyarteritis (periarteritis nodosa)
Nephrocalcinosis	
Gout	
Oxalosis	
Amyloidosis	
Cystinosis	

Modified from Simmons RL, Ascher NL, Najarian JS: Host hepatectomy and liver transplantation, in Simmons RL, Finch ME, Ascher NL, Najarian JS (eds): *Manual of Vascular Access, Organ Donation, and Transplantation.* New York, Springer-Verlag, 1984, pp 255–284.

failed—prefer life with a kidney transplantation to life on dialysis.

A few renal diseases will recur in transplants but such diseases are only relative contraindications; foral glomerulosclerosis, hemolytic uremia syndrome, membranoproliferative glomerulonephritis of the dense-deposit type, and diabetes are among them.

A number of metabolic diseases (gout, oxalosis, cystinosis, hyperoxaluria, nephrocalcinosis, and amyloidosis) have very little in common except for the accumulation within the kidney of abnormal deposits associated with renal failure. Transplants in most of these diseases can be successful, although recurrence after oxalosis is common.

The psychologic disturbances exhibited by some patients with chronic renal failure are not contraindications to selection. It is extremely difficult to judge the psychologic and social stability of a patient with chronic illness. Similarly, one cannot exclude, out of hand, patients with coronary disease or cerebrovascular accidents. Patients with severe liver disease, however, are more susceptible to cyclosporine or azathioprine toxicity and sepsis. Liver disease, therefore, remains a relative contraindication.

More important than the actual selection technique of the potential recipient is the choice of time for the institution of treatment by dialysis or transplantation. Treatment by either technique should always be instituted prior to the development of uremic complications. Once hypertension, pericarditis, cardiac failure, severe anemia, and neuropathy appear, management is markedly complicated and rehabilitation compromised. Ideally, the conservative management of patients treated for progressive renal functional deterioration should be carried out in conjunction with nephrologists associated with both dialysis and transplant centers. In this way, the complication of severe uremia can be rapidly prevented by treatment without the delays inherent in the referral process.

The traditional indication for the institution of dialysis has been a serum creatinine level greater than 15 mg/dL or a creatinine clearance less than 3 mL/min despite meticulous conservative care. It is obvious that there are exceptions to this rule. Some patients, particularly patients with polycystic kidney disease, with serum creatinine levels greater than 15 mg/dL can be maintained well for months on dietary management. In other patients, especially diabetic patients, severe complications of uremia will develop long before the serum creatinine reaches that level. The most pernicious of these complications is peripheral neuropathy. If there are signs of motor involvement, the patient should have dialysis and transplantation without delay, since very rapid progression of the disease can make it impossible ever to rehabilitate such a patient. Another indication for early dialysis-transplantation is uncontrollable hypertension, or hypertension that can be controlled only at the expense of severe orthostatic hypotension and other side effects. Severe anemia with anemic symptoms (dyspnea at the mildest exertion), severe bone disease (especially in children), and the failure of the patient to maintain a diet or carry on social and family obligations all should lead to early dialysis and transplantation. There is little to be gained by a delay of 3 to 6 months, and lives may be lost in futile attempts at conservative management.

Since some of the complications of uremia may appear suddenly during conservative management, it is extremely important that the patient be fully evaluated as early in the course of progressive uremia as possible. In addition to the medical evaluation, this preparation should include interviews with the hospital, the rehabilitation clinic, and social service in order to ameliorate the financial and social difficulties that may accompany dialysis and transplantation. Rehabilitation of the patient can be actively pursued even prior to the institution of definitive treatment.

Although most patients with end-stage renal disease will undergo a period of dialysis prior to transplant, many patients who are carefully followed for progressive uremia can be transplanted without dialysis. In this way, the number of vascular or peritoneal access procedures necessary for dialysis can be reduced and care can be rendered more economically.

PREPARATION FOR TRANSPLANTATION. The pretransplantation studies are listed in Table 10-13. Most of these studies are used by many transplant groups and for patients on dialysis. A few deserve elaboration.

The urinary tract should be evaluated for patency of its outflow and absence of ureterovesical reflux. In general, a voiding cystogram suffices. That test makes it possible to determine that the urethra is unobstructed, that the bladder empties, that there are no abnormalities of the bladder wall, and that there is no ureteral reflux. It is almost impossible to evaluate bladder emptying in the presence of ureterovesical reflux. Contraction of the bladder wall leads to reflux of the urine into the ureters, which then empty back into the bladder when the bladder wall is relaxed. It may be necessary to remove both ureters at the ureterovesical junction prior to evaluation of the bladder for competence.

The upper gastrointestinal tract should be evaluated for the possibility of a preexisting peptic ulceration. Pretransplant treatment regimens have almost completely eliminated upper gastrointestinal tract bleeding as a complication of steroid administration after transplant.

Because so many patients with uremia also have hearing deficits, periodic audiograms should be carried out.

Tissue Typing and Cross Matching. The principles of transplantation immunogenetics have been presented in detail above. Prior to transplantation, tissue typing to match donor and recipient should be carried out—both for the selection for the most appropriate donor and for the determination of the prognostic implications of tissue matching. It is possible at present to type most patients completely at the HLA-A, -B, and -D/DR loci (Table 10-1). This is extremely valuable in family donor selection because HLA identity between siblings occurs 25 percent of the time. Transplants between such perfectly matched siblings have long-term success rates of 95 percent. There is controversy whether matching unrelated cadaver donors with recipients will have beneficial consequences for the outcome of renal transplantation. Whatever the con-

and long-term therapy. The principal disadvantages are the energy-consuming nature of the treatment that requires a continuous commitment of the patient and physician to details of daily care. For this reason, transplantation, if successful, is preferable for younger patients.

SELECTION AND EVALUATION OF LIVING DONOR. The principles of histocompatibility typing and matching have been described above. From the recipient's point of view it is generally preferable that the donor be a biologic relative. Even mismatched sibling and parent kidneys may survive with better function and for more prolonged periods than do closely matched cadaver kidneys. Before the advent of histocompatibility typing, it was shown that kidneys from sibling donors functioned better than kidneys from parental donors. Because the genes governing the expression of histocompatibility antigens are situated at one (complex) locus, there will always be one major allelic difference between the parent and the offspring, whereas one-fourth of siblings will be identical, one-half will have a one haplotype difference, and one-fourth will have both haplotypes different. Tissue typing can usually identify that sibling (if any) who shares all the serologically detectable antigens at the major histocompatibility complex (MHC). Such sibling grafts have a better than 95 percent chance for long-term success.

A living related donor offers other advantages to the recipient: the delay between renal failure and rehabilitation is shorter, posttransplant renal function is usually immediate, and there are fewer rejection episodes, so that smaller doses of immunosuppressive drugs are required.

The major blood group antigens (ABO) are strong transplantation antigens. Although a number of successful allotransplants have been carried out across isoantibody barriers, it is generally unwise to perform transplants into patients with known preformed isohemagglutinins against the donor blood type. The same rules apply to clinical transplantation that apply to transfusion, i.e., AB is the universal recipient and O the universal donor. When such blood type barriers are crossed, the most violent type of hyperacute rejection reaction may occur. There is some evidence to suggest that Lewis blood group factors (but not Rh, Duffy, Kell) act as histocompatibility antigens.

The living related donor should be in perfect health to minimize any risks inherent in an operation of this magnitude. Rare deaths following renal donation from a healthy person have been reported, and the utmost caution must be exerted not to harm or diminish the renal reserve of a healthy volunteer. Table 10-14 lists the examinations routinely carried out on volunteer related donors.

Ethical Problems. Selection of a related donor is made on the basis of histocompatibility testing when possible; often, however, there is only one volunteer. The ethical and social problems of donor selection have been extensively discussed elsewhere, but brief consideration is pertinent here.

In practice, the recipient should be informed of the risks and benefits of receiving a kidney from a related donor. The recipient knows best which relatives can be approached and which cannot. When a volunteer appears

Table 10-14. PROTOCOL FOR LIVING RELATED DONOR WORK-UP

1. History and physical examination.
2. Hematology: hematocrit, leukocyte count, differential count, platelet count
3. Coagulation: prothrombin time, partial thromboplastin time, thrombin time
4. Chemistry: serum Na^+, K^+, Cl^-, CO_2^{2-}, SGOT, bilirubin, uric acid, Ca^{2+}, P, BUN, creatinine, fasting blood sugar, glucose tolerance test
5. Urine: urinalysis, 24-h urine for creatinine clearance
6. Microbiology: clean-catch urine culture $\times 2$
7. Immunology: blood type (major and minor), tissue typing, leukocyte cross match for recipient antidonor and leukocyte antibodies; VDRL; screen for hepatitis
8. X-ray: chest x-ray, intravenous pyelogram (IVP), renal arteriograms
9. Isotope: bilateral renogram
10. Electrocardiogram

he or she is blood-typed and tissue-typed. If the volunteer is acceptable on these grounds, the risk of donor nephrectomy is explained to him or her. The risk to life in an otherwise perfectly healthy patient has been estimated to be 0.05 percent. The long-term risk has been estimated by actuarial statistics to that incurred by driving a car 16 miles every working day. Much evidence suggests that no long-term harm results from life with a single kidney. Although risks are small, the pain, anxiety, and loss of work time are real.

It is difficult to conceive of a living related donor who is not subject to some family pressure to donate. That such pressures exist, however, is evidence that people have feelings of family and role obligations within the society. When a person freely volunteers to donate, both the benefits to the recipient and the risks to the donor are explained. No pressure is exerted to persuade or dissuade potential donors. They are not subjected to extensive psychologic interviews or testing. Careful studies of actual donors indicate a remarkably favorable psychologic response in most donors, but some ambivalence and conflict within the family occur in a minority. On occasion, when the potential donor expresses anxiety concerning the donation, it is necessary to fabricate a medical excuse not to donate that can be used by the otherwise medically and immunologically compatible donor.

Sometimes it is necessary or advisable to use donors under the age of eighteen. This has frequently been necessary for identical-twin transplants. The use of such donors, however, should be restricted to those circumstances in which other donors are not available. A court of law will find it difficult to decide whether an adolescent should donate to parents or siblings when family pressure may exist. Teen-aged donors have been used when they have insisted on donation and the court has agreed to it.

Unrelated persons are not generally encouraged to donate, since the results are no better than those achieved with cadaver donors.

SELECTION OF CADAVER DONOR. The ideal cadaver kidney donor (1) is young, (2) has remained normotensive until a short time before death, (3) is free of transmissible infection and malignant disease, and (4) has died in the hospital after observation for a number of hours, during which time blood group and tissue type have been determined and urinary function has been assessed. Under these ideal conditions the donor kidneys can be removed within minutes to minimize the warm ischemia time. It is often necessary, however, to compromise with these ideal principles. The age of the donor is not of crucial importance but kidneys from young children have decreased survival. A donated kidney can recover from long periods of shock and anuria that occur while it is still in the donor. But not more than 1 h of warm ischemia time should elapse during donation.

Criteria of Brain Death. The procurement of cadaver organs for transplantation has raised some serious moral, ethical, legal, and psychologic problems. The first problem is to establish when death occurs. Since the decision is a clinical one, made by the physician in the interest of the patient (potential donor), it should be based primarily on clinical criteria of irreversible brainstem damage— fixed, dilated pupils; absent reflexes; unresponsiveness to external stimuli; and the inability to maintain vital functions such as respiration, heartbeat, and blood pressure without artificial means. The decision should be made by physicians who are not associated with the potential recipient in any way, either as the referring physician or as a member of the transplant team. The exact criteria vary among institutions. Table 10-15 lists the guidelines for the determination of death reported to the President's Commission for the Study of Ethical Problems in Medicine and Biomedical and Behavioral Research by a panel of medical consultants.

In the past, a falling blood pressure has been used as a criterion of brain death, but this sign is frequently the result of dehydration due to diabetes insipidus. This is aggravated by loss of vasomotor tone, which produces hypotension. Almost all patients with brain death can be maintained for prolonged periods with normal vital signs using plasma and vasopressors; cardiac stimulants are rarely required. Urinary output can likewise be maintained with hydration and diuretics. Even the head-injury patient who has been anuric and in shock for many hours can be restored to hemodynamic stability by restoration of a normal blood volume.

The principles of organ preservation are described in a subsequent section. The advances in organ preservation have alleviated the urgency of cadaver transplantation. It is possible to harvest kidneys at the moment of death and preserve them in iced solutions for more than 24 h until the transplant recipients are ready. Kidneys can now be routinely preserved by hypothermic perfusion for more than 48 h (see subsequent section). The use of machines for this purpose has increased the availability of cadaver kidneys because the kidneys can be transported for long distances. The development of preservation also allows for more careful typing, matching, shipping, and sharing of organs between various centers.

ORGAN HARVEST. Related Living Donor. The actual technique of the donor operation is not as crucial as those

Table 10-15. CRITERIA FOR DETERMINATION OF DEATH

An individual with the findings in either section A (cardiopulmonary) or B (neurologic) is dead.

A. Cardiopulmonary
   An individual with irreversible cessation of circulatory and respiratory functions is dead.
   1. Cessation is recognized by an appropriate clinical examination . . . absence of responsiveness, heartbeat, respiratory effort . . .
   2. Irreversibility is recognized by persistent cessation of functions during an appropriate period of observation and/or trial of therapy.
B. Neurologic
   An individual with irreversible cessation of all functions of the entire brain, including the brainstem, is dead.
   1. Cessation is recognized when evaluation discloses findings of *a* and *b*:
      a. Cerebral functions are absent.
      b. Brainstem functions are absent.
   2. Irreversibility is recognized when evaluation discloses findings of *a* and *b* and *c*:
      a. The cause of coma is established and is sufficient to account for the loss of brain functions.
      b. The possibility of recovery of any brain functions is excluded.
      c. The cessation of all brain function persists for an appropriate period of observation and/or trial of therapy.

SOURCE: From Report of the medical consultants on the diagnosis of death to the President's Commission for the Study of Ethical Problems in Medicine and Biomedical and Behavioral Research, Guidelines for the determination of death. *JAMA* 246:2184, 1981.

factors that maintain urinary output in the donated kidney and in the remaining donor kidney. An active diuresis in the donor at the moment of renal artery occlusion favors prompt function in the recipient. For these reasons, the urine output is monitored throughout the donor operation and should not fall below 1 mL/min per kidney. The patient is hydrated several hours prior to operation, and both colloid [5 mL/(kg · h)] and crystalloid [5 mL/(kg · h)] solutions are administered during the operation, with constant attention to the central venous pressure and the urine output. Mannitol and furosemide are given shortly before the kidney is removed. In addition, systemic heparinization is carried out a few minutes before the renal artery is occluded. The heparin is then counteracted with protamine.

The donor operation is carried out through a flank incision and a retroperitoneal approach. The peritoneum is retracted, the ureter identified, and a length of ureter is dissected free. The ureter is then transected (preserving its blood supply from the renal pelvis) so that the urinary output of the donor kidney can be observed throughout the operation. The remainder of the ureter is dissected free up to the renal vein. A large lumbar vein, the ovarian or testicular vein, and the adrenal branch of the renal vein are doubly ligated on the left side. There are no major branches of the renal vein on the right side. Dissection on the renal vein is carried down to the vena cava. The artery is not dissected free until the dissection of the renal vein is complete. The kidney is not removed until urinary output from the donor kidney itself is excellent. At that time the renal artery and vein are sequentially clamped and divided.

Minor complications of nephrectomy in healthy related donors are common, but serious complications are quite rare. The function of the remaining kidney increases to about 70 percent of the preoperative value. Prolonged follow-ups indicate that the health and life expectancy of the donor are not adversely affected by donation.

Cadaver Donor. The technique of kidney harvest from a cadaver donor depends to a large degree on the status of the donor's circulation. If the cadaver is brain-dead but with intact circulation and urine output, nephrectomy can be performed at leisure via the transperitoneal route.

If the donor has a sudden irreversible circulatory collapse, the kidneys must be removed more rapidly to minimize ischemia time. Heparin is administered, and both kidneys are removed together by clamping the aorta and vena cava above the origin of the renal arteries and veins and pulling the kidneys up together, prior to transection of the aorta and vena cava below the origin of the renal vessels and the ureters in the pelvis. Prompt cooling of the organs is required, and both kidneys can be perfused with iced crystalloid solution prior to storing them in the cold or perfusing them on preservation machines.

TECHNIQUE. Preparation. It is probably not necessary to remove the kidneys from most patients. Removal of the patient's diseased kidneys may be considered to control hypertension to eliminate a source of infection or eliminate the nephrotic syndrome. Recurrence of the glomerulonephritis in the transplanted kidney is not known to be aggravated by the presence of the diseased kidneys. Asymptomatic polycystic kidneys rarely present a problem.

When indicated, most transplantation centers perform the nephrectomy sometime prior to transplantation in order to minimize the surgical stress at transplantation when immunosuppressant drugs are utilized and optimal transplant function desired, or to completely eliminate urinary tract infection before immunosuppression is begun.

When two-stage transplantation is carried out (i.e., nephrectomy preceding the transplantation by a week or 10 days), the postnephrectomy management is simple. Hyperkalemia is a recurrent postnephrectomy problem, but it can usually be prevented if a 20 percent glucose solution is administered prophylactically (with insulin if the patient has diabetes). Rectal ion-exchange resins may be required to control hyperkalemia. Dialysis can usually be postponed 2 or 3 days with these techniques. Delay in reinstituting dialysis is preferred if heparinization is required. Peritoneal dialysis can be resumed immediately to avoid clotting of the catheter.

Splenectomy or thymectomy, or both, have also been performed in kidney recipients prior to transplantation but both have fallen into disuse.

During preparation for transplantation, sepsis from any source must be scrupulously removed. Frequent sources of sepsis are (1) the hemodialysis cannulae, if present, (2) the bladder in patients with preexisting urinary tract infections, (3) the skin of patients with uremic dermatitis, and (4) dental caries. The bladder of the totally anuric patient frequently becomes infected and should be irrigated with appropriate antimicrobial agents several times weekly prior to grafting.

Dialysis should be frequent and intense in the immediate pretransplantation period. Recipients of cadaver kidneys will have little preparation time prior to transplantation. Many patients will be maintained on systemic anticoagulants because of clotting problems in hemodialysis shunts; the anticoagulants must be discontinued, and vitamin K must be administered.

Transplantation. The operative technique of renal transplantation has become standardized. A retroperitoneal approach is used to the iliac vessels, and the renal artery and vein are anastomosed to the iliac vessels as shown in Figs. 10-38 and 10-39.

There must be no deficit in blood volume following the vascular anastomoses. Hypovolemia interferes with the rapid resumption of renal function. Urine usually appears within a few minutes of completion of the vascular anastomoses in related living donor kidneys; mannitol and furosemide may be helpful in hastening the appearance of urine, a useful sign that there are no serious technical deficiencies.

Fig. 10-38. Sites of anastomoses of renal vein to the side of the iliac vein. [From: *Simmons RL, Kjellstrand CM, Najarian JS: Kidney: II. Technique, complications, and results, in Najarian JS, Simmons RL (eds): Transplantation. Philadelphia, Lea & Febiger, 1972, p 445, with permission.*]

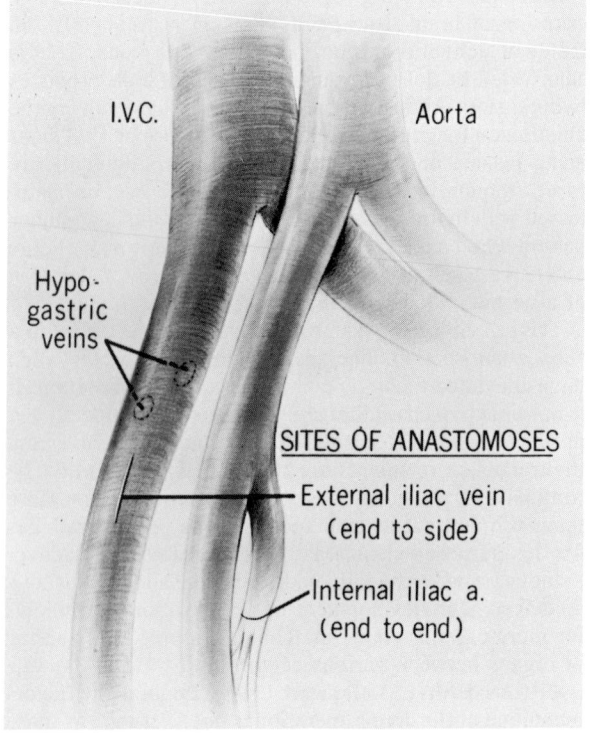

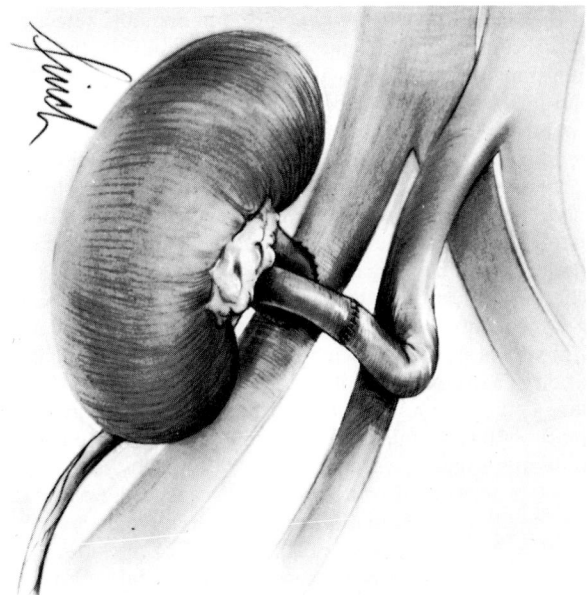

Fig. 10-39. Completed anastomosis of hypogastric artery to renal artery, and of renal vein to common iliac vein. [From: *Simmons RL, Kjellstrand CM, Najarian JS: Kidney: II. Technique, complications, and results, in Najarian JS, Simmons RL (eds): Transplantation. Philadelphia, Lea & Febiger, 1972, p 445, with permission.*]

Three methods are generally available for establishing urinary tract continuity. The preferred method involves ureteroneocystostomy. Pyeloureterostomy and uretero-ureterostomy have also been used. Systemic or topical perioperative antibodies will help prevent wound infections.

Anesthesia in the Anephric Patient. Certain precautions are necessary during any operation on an anephric patient. In particular, certain anesthetics are excreted almost exclusively by the kidney and should not be used. These include the muscle relaxant gallamine triethiodide. Both curare and succinylcholine are metabolized by the liver, but both may also be accompanied by prolonged paralysis in the postoperative period. In the case of succinylcholine, a number of investigators have found that serum cholinesterase is broken down during hemodialysis. In such patients, succinylcholine would be expected to have prolonged action. Conduction anesthesia has been used, but most anesthesiologists prefer general anesthesia.

In the administration of anesthetics and fluids, it should always be assumed that the kidney will not function immediately after transplantation, even if dialysis is rarely required after transplantation. Similar thinking should be employed with regard to hyperkalemia in the uremic patient. Other concerns of the anesthesiologist are the loss of the hypertensive state after induction of anesthesia to normal levels, and the low hematocrit in patients with chronic uremia. The hematocrit should be raised to 30 prior to transplantation, and hypovolemia due to excessive ultrafiltration during hemodialysis should be avoided.

POSTTRANSPLANTATION CARE. The management of kidney allograft patients in the early posttransplant period does not differ radically from the management of other postoperative patients. Vital signs are monitored frequently for the first day, and the central venous pressure is utilized as a guide to blood volume. A Foley catheter is left in the bladder, which is not irrigated unless clots are thought to be occluding the catheter. The urine output is measured at least every hour. The volume of urine should be replaced with intravenous fluids. A convenient replacement solution consists of one-half normal saline solution with 5% dextrose and water and 10 meq of sodium bicarbonate per liter. Potassium need not be added to the intravenous fluids except in small children, whose urinary electrolytes should be replaced milliequivalent for milliequivalent. Diabetic patients should receive continuous insulin infusion intravenously to maintain blood sugars in the slightly hyperglycemic range (150 to 200 mg/dL).

The urinary output in the early postoperative period may be enormous, partly because of tubular dysfunction but primarily because of the overhydrated state of even the best-dialyzed patient. A creatinine clearance obtained on the evening of transplantation will be helpful in assessing renal function.

The Foley catheter can be removed almost any time after the first day. The tip of the catheter should be cultured at that time. Moderate hypertension is frequently seen in the early posttransplant period, and a low-sodium diet and low doses of antihypertensive medication (α-methyldopa, hydrochlorothiazide, or hydralazine) are useful to counteract this tendency. Antacids are useful in preventing the appearance of gastrointestinal ulceration of patients on immunosuppressive drugs. The patient is allowed out of bed and oral fluids are begun on the first postoperative day.

The 2-h creatinine clearance determination can be useful in interpreting early oliguria, but the test is not routine. The hematocrit should be followed at 4-h intervals, since rebleeding is a rare but severe complication that can produce oliguria and the onset of acute tubular necrosis (ATN).

A base-line sonogram and [131]I Hippuran renogram are usually performed soon after transplantation. Intravenous pyelography (IVP) is rarely necessary. Determinations of blood urea nitrogen (BUN), serum creatinine, and creatinine clearance suffice to estimate daily renal functions. Serum electrolyte determinations can usually be discontinued after good renal function is established. Periodic leukocyte and platelet counts are necessary to assay the state of the bone marrow during immunosuppression. Rarely, hyperglycemia and hypercalcemia are complications, and therefore blood sugar and calcium levels should be determined from time to time. The diabetic patient will require frequent blood sugar determinations and adjustments of insulin dosage.

Prophylactic Immunosuppression. Standard immunosuppressive management at most clinical transplant centers now consists of cyclosporine and prednisone. Because of cyclosporine's nephrotoxic properties, ALG or azathioprine, or both are sometimes employed until renal

Table 10-16. PROPHYLACTIC IMMUNOSUPPRESSION FOR RENAL TRANSPLANTATION AT THE UNIVERSITY OF MINNESOTA

A. Antilymphoblast globulin (ALG)
   1. 20 mg/kg intravenously daily
B. Azathioprine (evening dose after checking leukocyte count)
   1. Preoperative dose is 5 mg/kg per day
   2. First and second postoperative days: 5 mg/kg
   3. Third through sixth postoperative days: 4 mg/kg
   4. Seventh postoperative day: 3 mg/kg; maintain at 2 to 3 mg/kg
   5. Adjust at all times with respect to WBC, platelet count, and renal function
   6. Caution: Reduce dosage to 1.5 mg/kg for severe renal functional impairment
C. Prednisone
   1. 0.25 mg/kg every 6 h for 1st week
   2. 0.25 mg/kg per day for 2d week
   3. 0.5 mg/kg per day for 3d week
   4. Reduce dose slowly to achieve a maintenance dose of 0.5 mg/kg per day
D. Cyclosporine
   1. Start at 8 mg/kg per day on day 5. Adjust dose to achieve whole blood levels approximating 200 mg/mL

function approaches more normal levels Table 10-16). Then ALG is stopped and cyclosporine started. Most centers are currently individualizing the concurrent use of all four of these drugs, but cyclosporine has replaced azathioprine as the backbone of the regimen. A higher dose of prednisone or methylprednisone is used for rejection episodes. Some centers reserve the use of ALG or monoclonal antilymphocyte antibodies to treat steroid-resistant rejection epidoses.

COMPLICATIONS. Renal Failure. The most serious complication of renal transplantation is the failure of the graft to initiate or maintain function. Although the causes of failure can easily be defined, the differential diagnosis may, at the time, be impossible. The functional failure of the kidney is best examined in relation to the time after transplantation. The kidney may (1) never function, (2) have delayed onset of functions, (3) fail to function after a brief or prolonged time, or (4) gradually lose its function over a period of months or years. In each phase, four general diagnoses should be considered: (1) ischemic damage to the kidney; (2) rejection of the kidney by reactions directed against histocompatibility antigens on the kidney; (3) technical complications; and (4) the development of renal disease, either a new disease or recurrence of the original.

The simplest and best assay for decreased renal function is the frequent determination of BUN and serum creatinine, and the determination of creatinine clearance. Sonograms and renograms are also useful. The differential diagnosis of renal malfunction, however, may require percutaneous pyelography, arteriography, and renal biopsy.

Early Anuria and Oliguria

Early anuria or oliguria is a major diagnostic problem. The possibilities include (1) hypovolemia, (2) thrombosis of the renal artery or renal vein, (3) hyperacute rejection of the kidney, (4) ischemic renal damage (ATN), (5) compression of the kidney (by hematoma, seroma, or lymph), and (6) obstruction of the urinary flow.

The investigation of early posttransplant anuria should be rapidly performed in a strict sequence. The Foley catheter should first be irrigated and/or changed to remove any question of catheter obstruction. Unfortunately, whatever the cause of anuria, a clot can be obtained by bladder irrigation in the first posttransplant day. The clot may not be the primary cause of anuria, however, because blood will clot within the bladder if the urine is not copious enough to wash it out prior to coagulation. Therefore, even if a clot is present within the urinary catheter, the urine output should be monitored for the first 10 to 15 min after emptying the bladder to determine urine output adequacy.

If the obstructed catheter has not caused the oliguria, one must rule out hemorrhage and hypovolemia combined with compression or displacement of the kidney by the hematoma. If hypotension and tachycardia are present and the central venous pressure is low, hypovolemia is very likely. A radiograph of the abdomen will reveal displacement of the intraperitoneal contents by a massive hematoma. Echography and repeated hematocrit determinations will confirm the diagnosis. The normal degree of ischemic damage to the transplanted kidney plus hypovolemia and compression of the kidney and vessels by a hematoma all conspire to impair renal function. If anuria or severe oliguria is present, restoration of the blood volume will seldom suffice to restore renal function, even if furosemide or other diuretics are used. Many patients will require reexploration to control the bleeding point. After exploration, if the period of hypovolemia and renal compression has been relatively brief and diuretics have been used during ischemia, prompt restoration of renal function usually occurs.

The diagnosis of bleeding is frequently apparent and obviates the need for the next step in the investigation sequence—an [131]I Hippuran renogram (Fig. 10-40). The renogram permits assessment of the blood flow to the kidney and the ability of the kidney to concentrate and excrete the Hippuran. The results are never diagnostic. If the vascular phase and concentration are near normal, however, the renal arterial and venous anastomoses are patent. If the Hippuran uptake by the kidney is severely depressed, a renal arteriogram should be done. Arteriography will assess the renal arterial anastomosis, and if it reveals the presence of intravascular thrombosis of the kidney the diagnosis of hyperacute rejection will be suggested.

Technical Complications. Thrombosis of the renal arterial anastomosis is rare. Partial obstruction due to torsion or kinking of the vessels is more common and should be promptly repaired. When the renogram demonstrated poor concentration of the [131]I Hippuran, an arteriogram should be performed to detect correctable technical complications (Fig. 10-41). Thrombosis of the renal vein occurs even more rarely than thrombosis of the renal artery. When it does occur, thrombosis of the artery ensues because the collateral venous circulation of the kidney has

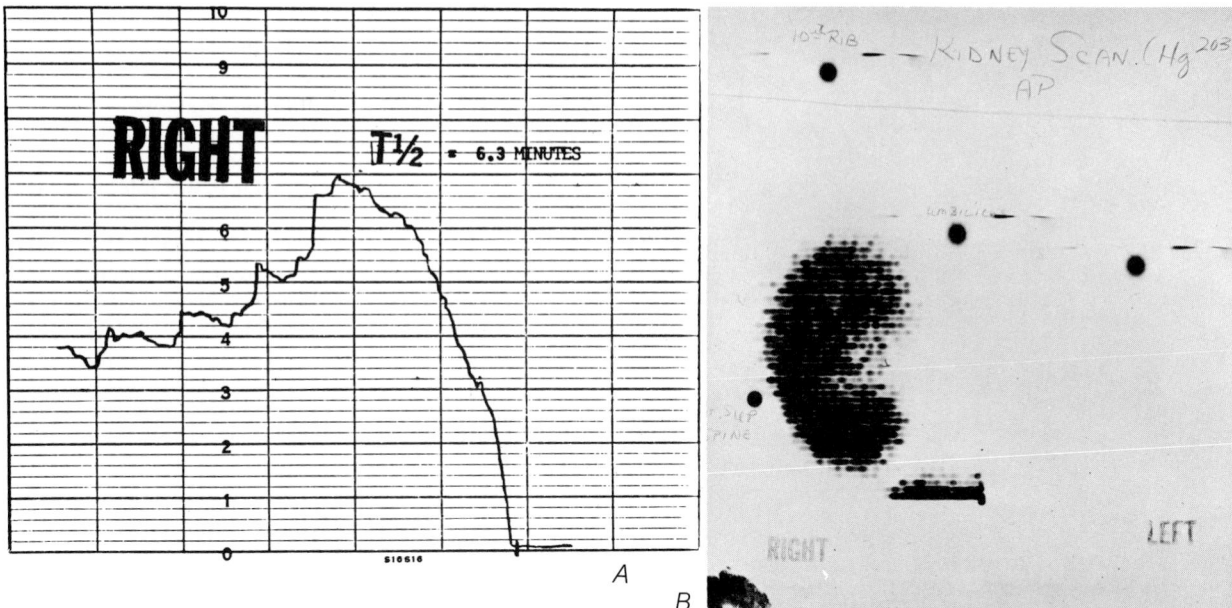

Fig. 10-40. Function of a homotransplanted kidney. *A.* A radiograph showing a half-life of 6.3 min and a completely normal-appearing curve. *B.* A scan of the same transplant showing excellent uptake in the kidney and the appearance of the radioactive material in the bladder. This transplant continued to have excellent function 5½ years later. (From: *Hume DM: Advances in Surgery, vol II. Chicago, Year Book Medical Publishers, 1966, with permission.*)

Fig. 10-41. Correctable arterial complications in the early posttransplant period. Oliguria was present in both patients. [131]I Hippuran revealed poor vascular phase. The arteriograms revealed torsion distal to the renal arterial anastomosis, which was corrected by a reanastomosis. [From: *Simmons RL, Kjellstrand CM, Najarian JS: Kidney: II. Technique, complications, and results, in Najarian JS, Simmons RL (eds): Transplantation. Philadelphia, Lea & Febiger, 1972, with permission.*]

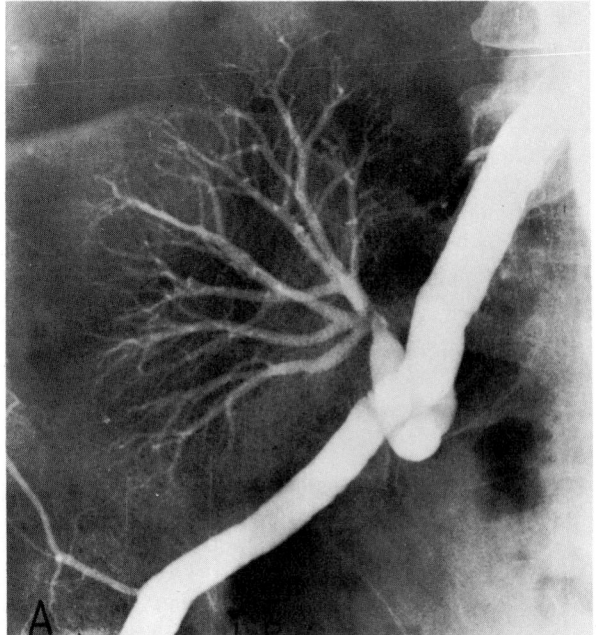

been interrupted by the transplant procedure. Partial thrombosis of the renal and iliac veins has occurred. Usually, this is accompanied by swelling of the ipsilateral lower extremity, fever, and evidence of pulmonary embolism.

Formerly, one of the most common, and most frequently fatal, complications following renal transplantation was urinary extravasation due to distal ureteral necrosis. Rejection was seldom at fault. The problem can generally be avoided by (1) using the ureter as short as possible; (2) avoiding tension at the ureteroneocystostomy site; (3) avoiding hematomas within the wound, which put tension on the ureter and also interfere with the developing collateral blood supply to the distal ureter; (4) avoiding transperitoneal "clotheslining" of the ureter by always placing the ureter in the retroperitoneal position where tension will be minimal and the collateral blood supply can develop.

Urinary extravasation is a serious complication that can lead to infection. It demands urgent reexploration with reimplantation of the ureter into the bladder, nephrostomy, or performance of a pyeloureterostomy to the host ureter. On occasion, the pelvis of the transplanted kidney may be involved, and nephrectomy may be required. Delay in definitive repair will frequently lead to infection, loss of the kidney, and death.

Technical errors can become manifest long after the immediate posttransplant period. Arterial stenosis, venous thrombosis, and late ureteral leaks and strictures are frequently confused with rejection (see below). Prior to any antirejection treatment, technical problems should be ruled out by echography, arteriography, renography, or percutaneous nephrostograms.

Hyperacute Rejection. Hyperacute rejection of the kidney is almost always mediated by humoral antibody, with the subsequent participation of the complement, coagulation, and kinin cascade systems. Platelets, PMNs, and

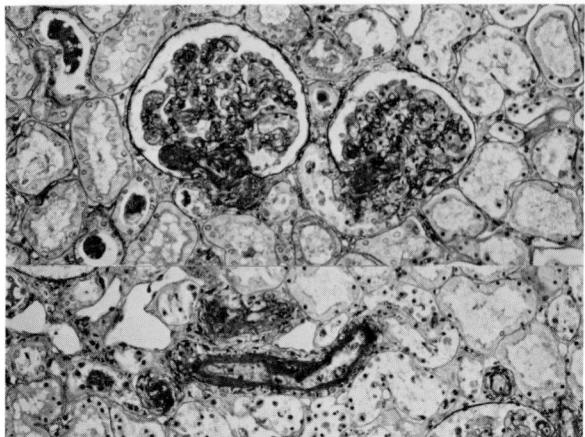

Fig. 10-42. Hyperacute renal rejection 20 h posttransplantation in a twenty-five-year-old male. Hyperacute rejection is characterized initially by fibrin and platelet thrombosis and fibrinoid necrosis of glomerular tufts, renal arterioles, and small arteries. A massive polymorphonuclear leukocyte reaction, interstitial hemorrhage, and tubular necrosis occur with subsequent cortical infarction 24 to 36 h posttransplantation. (×160.) (From: *Richard K. Sibley, personal communication*.)

vasospasm may also play a role. Classical hyperacute rejection is now rare because laboratory techniques can demonstrate cytotoxic antibody directed against donor histocompatibility antigens positive cross match. A rare patient will have a hyperacute rejection in the absence of demonstrable cytotoxic antibody. Indeed, detectable cytotoxic antibody will appear and disappear at intervals in patients awaiting transplantation. In the classic hyperacute rejection, the kidney will fail to regain its normal turgor and healthy pink color after anastomoses are established. Biopsy and histologic study at this time may reveal leukocytes in the glomerular capillaries, and intravascular renal thrombosis follows (Fig. 10-42). Definite evidence of a hyperacute rejection should be treated by immediate nephrectomy. A less acute rejection may occur, however, and renal function may not fail until a day or two following transplantation. Such rapid rejection has been differentiated by the term *accelerated rejection*.

Acute Tubular Necrosis. The diagnosis of ischemic renal injury is one of exclusion. If all other causes of renal functional failure in the early posttransplant period have been ruled out, one must assume that the diagnosis is ATN. "Acute tubular necrosis" in clinical parlance refers to kidneys whose function is impaired from ischemia or a variety of other causes. If kidneys from this clinical spectrum are biopsied, they most frequently show only hydropic changes. The more severe the insult, the more likely will be the presence of tubular necrosis. The correlation between tubule pathology and function, however, is not always good and suggests the interplay with other mechanisms, including prolonged vasoconstriction and vascular endothelial cell swelling. Most kidneys will recover, but sometimes disruption is so severe that cellular repair is not possible.

ATN occurs most commonly in cadaver recipients when the donor had undergone long periods of stress and hypotensive insult to the kidney to be transplanted. Another cause of recipient ATN is a long period of warm ischemia preceding transplantation. Kidneys with warm ischemic intervals greater than 1 h should not be utilized for transplantation, because function will seldom return to normal. Cold ischemia is much better tolerated, and preservation up to 48 h is now very satisfactory.

Almost all transplanted kidneys have undergone some degree of damage secondary to trauma and ischemia. A second trauma (hypovolemia, hypoxemia, renal compression, bacteremia, allergic reactions to ALG) that normally might not result in ATN in normal kidneys may cause oliguria in transplanted kidneys. One must not diagnose rejection and institute massive steroid therapy in the early posttransplant period without ruling out the possibility that an additional insult to an already damaged kidney has occurred and that the diagnosis is not acute rejection but ATN. Renal biopsy may be necessary to make this differentiation.

The management of the patient with ATN is simple. Urinary flow will resume in almost all cases within 2 or 3 weeks, but anuria for as long as 6 weeks with total recovery has been observed. [131]I Hippuran renograms are useful in following improvement prior to resumption of urinary flow. Dialysis is maintained intermittently during the period of oliguria. A number of studies have shown that the long-term function of renal transplants is independent of the presence or absence of oliguria in the early posttransplant period.

Rejection

Technical errors may not become evident for several weeks post grafting, and any trauma can aggravate the degree of ATN in a previously damaged kidney. Nevertheless most renal failure appearing after the first posttransplant week can be attributed to rejection.

With better immunosuppression, the acute rejection episodes that formerly appeared in the first month following transplantation are seen less and less frequently. The majority of patients, however, will sustain at least one acute rejection episode during the first 3 to 4 months following transplantation. Clinical rejection is rarely an all-or-nothing reaction, and the first episode seldom progresses to complete renal destruction. The functional changes induced by rejection appear to be in large part reversible; therefore, the recognition and treatment of the rejection episode prior to the development of severe renal damage is of extreme importance. Usually the rejection reaction responds to increased prednisone doses and local irradiation. Even with prompt treatment the creatinine clearance may be permanently impaired, however slightly, following each clinical rejection episode.

Differential Diagnosis. The clinical picture of a rejection reaction may be distressingly similar to several other problems: ureter leak or obstruction, hemorrhage with consequent ATN, infection, or stenosis or twist in the renal artery or vein. Classic renal rejection is characterized by oliguria, enlargement and tenderness of the graft, malaise, fever, leukocytosis, hypertension, weight gain,

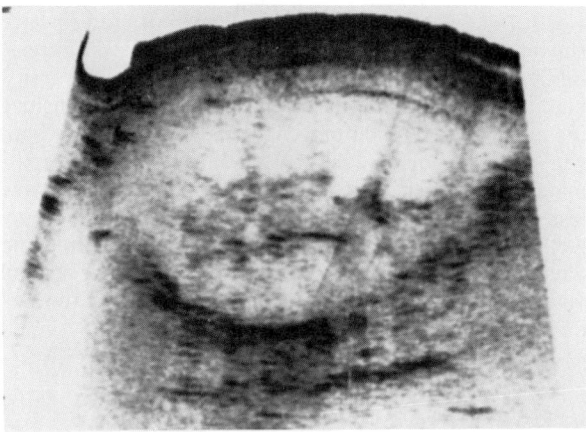

Fig. 10-43. Longitudinal sonogram of a renal transplant during episode of acute rejection (characterized clinically by anuria, fever, weight increase, and elevated creatinine levels to 0.079 mg/mL). Note enlarged pyramids of decreased echogenicity anteriorly. Interpyramidal cortex (septa of Bertin) shown as echogenic bands between pyramids. The kidney appears enlarged and more globular in shape compared with a base-line study 4 weeks earlier. Biopsy confirmed severe acute rejection requiring transplant nephrectomy 3 days after the sonogram. (From: *Frick MP, Feinberg SB, et al: Ultrasound in acute renal transplant rejection. Radiology 138:659, 1981, with permission.*)

Table 10-17. STANDARD ANTIREJECTION THERAPY AT THE UNIVERSITY OF MINNESOTA

1. Therapy
   a. Prednisone: 2 mg/kg × 3 days; then 1.5 mg/kg × 3 days; then 1.0 mg/kg × 3 days; thereafter reduce prednisone slowly to a maintenance dose.
   b. Azathioprine: Regulate dose to prevent leukopenia; do not increase.
   c. Irradiate kidney transplant: 150 rad every other day for three doses.
2. Adjuncts
   a. Reinstitute antacid therapy.
   b. Reinstitute oral nystatin (100,000 units twice daily) to prevent mucosal candidiasis.
   c. Reduce protein and fluid intake if renal function is significantly impaired.

and peripheral edema. Laboratory studies have shown lymphocyturia, red cell casts, proteinuria, immunoglobulin fragments, fibrin fragments in the urine, complementuria, lysozymuria, decreased urine sodium excretion, renal tubular acidosis, and increased lactic dehydrogenase in the urine. The level of the blood urea nitrogen increases, as does serum creatinine. Creatinine clearance is obviously decreased; renograms will show slow uptake of the Hippuran and slow urinary excretion. Echography can show edema of the renal papillae (Fig. 10-43).

The most important parameter to follow is the serum creatinine level. Unlike the BUN, which is sensitive to a number of changes (steroid administration, fever, and high-protein diet), serum creatinine levels are relatively stable for each patient. The creatinine clearance is more sensitive, but it depends on a carefully timed collection of urine.

The most reliable clinical signs of renal functional deterioration are a slight decrease in urinary output, slow weight gain, small increases in diastolic blood pressure, and edema of the lower extremity on the side of the graft. A peripheral leukocyte count and a serum creatinine level should be determined to confirm renal functional deterioration. A renogram and echogram should be promptly performed and compared with those obtained at the peak of renal function (usually prior to discharge from the hospital) to rule out urinary extravasation, urinary obstruction, or ureteral stenosis. Arteriography is seldom necessary but may reveal (1) characteristic changes of decreased concentration of dye flowing into the kidney, (2) decreased nephrogram effect, (3) an irregularity of the cortical vasculature and intralobar vasculature character-

istic of rejection, and (4) normal renal artery and anastomosis, eliminating the possibility of a technical problem.

Renal biopsy should be a definitive diagnostic tool. Both open biopsy and needle biopsy techniques have been described, and the histologic changes of rejection are characteristic (Figs. 10-11 through 10-14). A normal kidney biopsy is diagnostic, but a biopsy that reveals renal damage may merely reflect acute rejection, a chronic ongoing process, exacerbation of the pre-existing renal disease, or damage due to infection or radiation. With experience, however, needle biopsy of transplanted kidneys is a safe procedure and usually provides the diagnosis. Aspiration of the kidney to obtain cells for cytologic analysis can also be used to diagnose rejection.

Treatment. Most institutions have developed a standard rejection regimen for allografted kidneys (Table 10-17). This standard regimen can be repeated as many as three times within a 2-month period in patients for whom rejection appears to be unremitting. If it is repeated more often than that, infection may appear and be lethal. The decision to stop immunosuppression and sacrifice the transplant frequently depends on subtle factors and is difficult to make, particularly in patients who have deterioration of renal function over a period of months and years.

Renal Failure due to Recurrent Disease

Certain diseases are known to recur in the transplanted kidney. These are listed in Table 10-18. Transplantation is not necessarily contraindicated in these diseases since the recurrence is unpredictable and the transplant may provide long-term palliation that is superior in the individual case to dialysis. The best example is diabetes, in which the histologic features of diabetes often recur with only gradual deterioration of function.

RESULTS. Figure 10-44 shows the results of renal transplantation in adults at the University of Minnesota for the years since 1984 when a combination ALG, azathioprine, cyclosporine, and prednisone therapy was initiated.

TRANSPLANTATION IN CHILDREN. Renal failure in children is a common cause of death. Traditionally, young children have not been considered ideal candidates for renal transplantation, although excellent results have

Table 10-18. RISK OF RECURRENCE OF
PRIMARY RENAL DISEASE
FOLLOWING TRANSPLANTATION

High risk
  Focal sclerosis (proliferative type)
  IgA disease
  Membrano-proliferative glomerulonephritis
    (dense-deposit disease type)
  Hemolytic uremic syndrome
  Diabetes mellitus
  Oxalosis
Moderate risk
  Antiglomerular basement membrane disease
  Scleroderma
Low risk
  Membranous glomerulonephritis
  Amyloidosis
  Rapidly progressive crescentic
    AP nephritis
  Lupus
  Wegner's
No risk
  Congenital nephrosis
  Fabry's disease
  Cystinosis
  Myeloma kidney
  Polycystic kidney
  Pyelonephritis
  Glomerulonephritis
  Congenital renal disease (aplasia/dysplasia; valves)

been reported by a number of investigators. The small caliber of vessels and active social behavior of children make their management on hemodialysis extremely difficult. Long-term immunosuppressive therapy is also thought to interfere with normal growth with resultant social problems. Long-term hemodialysis is seldom satisfactory, and a parent is almost always willing to donate a kidney. Several infants have had transplants, and at least one has survived for more than 1 year. The growth of children following transplantation has been the subject of several studies. Most children with allografts grow slightly more slowly than normal. The adolescent growth spurt is absent in children with transplants and adolescent growth is particularly depressed in girls.

This early cessation of growth causes the typical appearance of girls with transplants, who are short and more cushingoid than the boys. Attempts to correlate the amount of first-year posttransplant growth with the kidney donor, renal function, or prednisone dosage have been unsuccessful. No such correlations can be made, even though it is generally felt that prednisone interferes with growth.

Sexual maturation in boys appears to be normal, although the period of observation has been short. Similarly, some girls have failed to menstruate at the usual age despite relatively normal renal function and only moderate doses of prednisone. Most girls have resumed menstruating if previously mature, or they undergo a normal menarche upon reaching age thirteen or fourteen.

MULTIPLE TRANSPLANTS. A number of studies have shown that second and third transplants are less successful than the first, if the first was rejected soon after transplantation. The rejection of one transplant may sensitize the patient to a number of weaker histocompatibility antigens that cannot be easily detected by sensitive cross-match techniques. In addition, such patients may have less compromised immune systems that permitted the rejection of the first transplant. By contrast, patients who have maintained a successful first transplant for several years will, after losing the first transplant, accept the second transplant more readily.

XENOGRAFTS

Xenografts between related species are rejected by the same immune mechanisms as are allografts. Xenografts between distant species are rejected by an additional mechanism—the reaction of the xenograft with preformed antibodies that then trigger the efficient complement and clotting cascades. In short, xenografts across distant species barriers are rejected like hyperacute rejections.

There is not much information about clinical xenografts, because, in general, they have not proved to be useful. Xenografts of calf skin have sometimes been used for burn dressings and appear to offer some advantage over other dressing material, although they are not as useful as allografts. Some xenograft calf heart valves have been placed in patients, although it seems likely that these will not be as successful as are allografts, and they might be expected to calcify and become incompetent over a period of years. One xenograft chimpanzee heart has been placed in a patient, but this functioned for only about an hour. Since allografted hearts are invariably rejected experimentally, it would be expected that cardiac xenotransplants would suffer the same fate even more quickly. Renal and heart xenografts using both chimpanzee and baboon donors have been done in a number of human beings, but this procedure has been abandoned. Surprisingly enough a few relatively long-term survivors were achieved with chimpanzee renal transplants that were considerably better tolerated than baboon transplants. Some testicular xenografts have been carried out in human beings in the past but have long since been abandoned. Bone and cartilage xenografts are still used from time to time but seem to offer no advantage over allografts. The use of organs from nonhuman species for extracorporeal perfusion, both kidneys and livers, has been tried but currently is of little value.

ORGAN PRESERVATION

The viable preservation of whole organs is one of the essential components of any transplantation program. Only cadaver donors can be used for some organs (heart

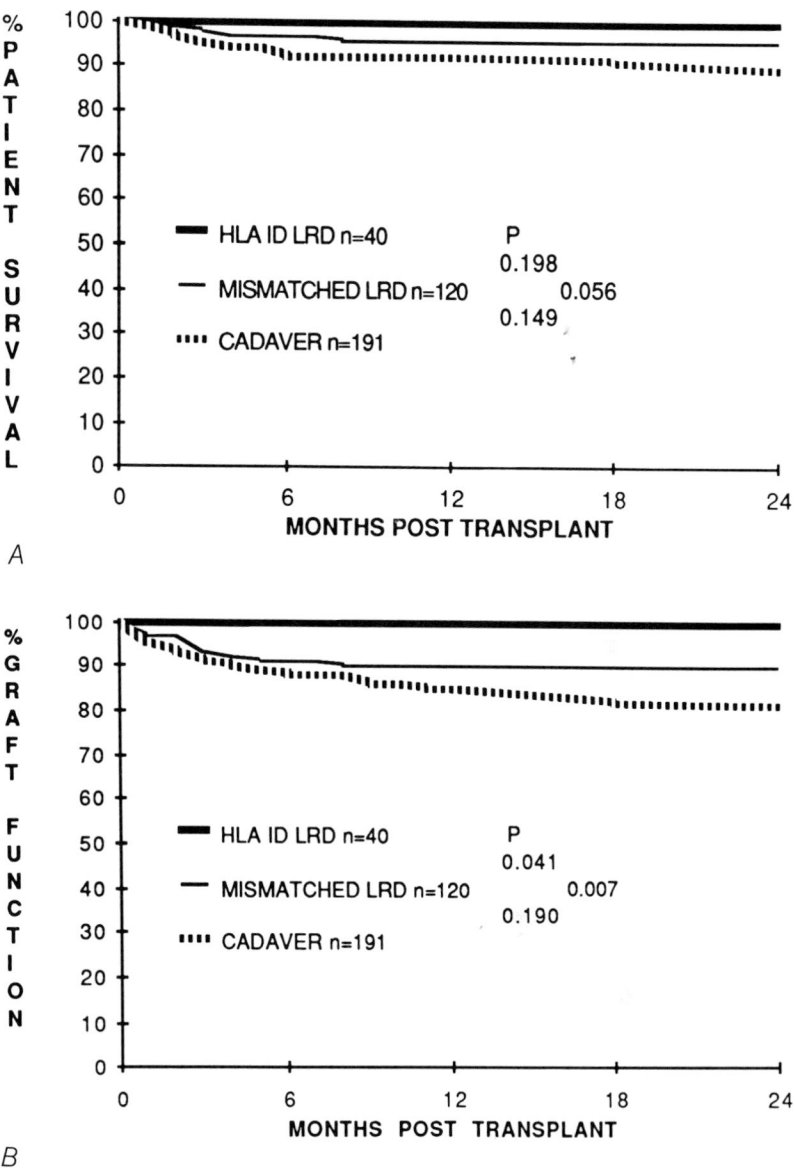

Fig. 10-44. *A* and *B*. Patient and graft survival rates in recipients according to donor source for all adult renal allografts transplanted from 1984 to 1986 at the University of Minnesota.

and liver), and even when the organ is expendable (as in one of a pair of kidneys), the use of cadaver donors avoids the risks inherent in surgical removal of the organ from living persons. If tissue typing and matching ever achieve their true potential, it may be necessary to store the organ until these matching procedures can be carried out. Even more time-consuming procedures, such as tolerance induction, may ultimately become available to pretreat the recipient and make him or her unresponsive to specific histocompatibility antigens. Table 10-19 lists some of those procedures that might be useful to carry out during organ preservation.

Methods of Viable Organ Preservation

The main problem associated with preservation of organs in a viable state seems to be hypoxia. When the organ is removed from its physiologic state, it is deprived of its normal oxygenation. The two major approaches to organ preservation have been what might be called metabolic inhibition and metabolic maintenance.

Metabolic inhibition seeks to prevent the normal catabolic processes from causing severe or irreversible damage to the tissues, during the period of preservation. It is currently best achieved by hypothermia, which protects the organ by slowing metabolic activity and decreasing oxygen need. Two techniques of cooling are currently available: (1) simple cooling of a kidney by immersing it

Table 10-19. PROCEDURES DURING
ORGAN STORAGE

A. Evaluation of the organ
   1. Typing and matching
     a. ABO typing
     b. Lymphocyte typing
     c. Organ cell typing
     d. Mixed lymphocyte culture with the recipient
   2. Diagnosis of disease in the donor or donor tissue
     a. Malignant tumors
     b. Infections
     c. Degenerative conditions
   3. Determination of functional state
   4. Restoration of normal function
B. Preparation of the recipient
   1. Induction of tolerance
   2. Immunosuppression
   3. Surgical procedures
C. Logistical procedures
   1. Stockpile various sizes and types
   2. Transport to a distant recipient
D. Modification of the immunogenicity of the organ

---

in, or flushing it with, a cold solution, which allows many hours of preservation and is almost always used for short periods of time, prior to transplantation of any organ; and (2) perfusion cooling, which allows longer periods of preservation.

Metabolic maintenance, the second approach to organ preservation, attempts to sustain a level of metabolic activity as close to physiologic normalcy as is feasible. Usually it implies perfusion of the organ in vitro with a carefully controlled fluid medium, although tissue oxygenation may be attempted. In practice metabolic maintenance is always best combined with perfusion cooling. The best system, at present, utilizes a pulsatile pump and pooled homologous plasma passed through a membrane oxygenator. Excellent transplantation results are obtained after perfusion as long as 72 h. These moderately long preservation periods provide adequate time for accurate matching of donors and recipients.

Not all organs can be perfused equally well by the same approach. Certain precautions are necessary. It is necessary *to maintain optimal organ function* up to and beyond the moment of clinical death. For kidneys, adequate hydration and maintenance of systemic blood pressure are recommended. Manipulation of the organ also contributes to vasospasm, and so surgical dissection should be as rapid and efficient as possible. The *period of time* between the cessation of blood flow through the organ and the establishment of the organ in its new environment (warm ischemia time) is critical in preservation studies. *Temperature* is also important. Successful perfusion systems have incorporated hypothermia to reduce the need for oxygen and metabolic nutrients. *Oxygenation* is also critical. Oxygen dissolves in aqueous solution more readily at lower temperatures; a membrane oxygenator is incorporated into the system.

The *flow rate* necessary at 37°C can be substantially reduced when metabolic activity is lessened by hypothermia; flow rates of one-fifth to one-third of normal have been satisfactory. The *viscosity of the perfusion fluid* may have some influence on perfusion pressure and flow rate. The perfusion pressure is significant. If the flow rate is adequate to provide the nutrients and waste removal, then the absolute level of pressure is not critical, but excessive perfusion pressure invariably causes transudation of the perfusate, tissue edema, and, ultimately, obstruction to the flow. Another factor is *pulsation.* Perfusion results in less damage when the flow is pulsatile, particularly at normothermic temperatures. The necessity for pulsatile flow during hypothermic perfusion is less well documented. It is probably not necessary to maintain any *venous pressure gradient.* The *perfusate composition* has apparent significance. Whole plasma probably is the most physiologic perfusate and contains most of the nutrient ingredients, including fatty acids, that might be required for the metabolic activity of organs. Many other formulations have been successful, including dextran, albumin, other plasma expanders, tissue culture media, and balanced salt solutions. *Osmolarity* is important. Crystalloids are poor perfusates and lead to edema. The perfusate must be maintained at "normal" pH range of 7.35 to 7.45. CO_2 buffering may be necessary with the addition of 2.5 to 5 percent of this gas to the oxygenator. Extremes of alkalosis and acidosis can be prevented with the addition of HCl or $NaHCO_3$ as necessary. A number of *additives* to the perfusate have been tried. These include membrane stabilizers, vasodilators, and anticoagulants. *Hyperbaric oxygenation* has also been used to prolong the viability and storage time of organs in conjunction with hypothermia or a combination of hypothermia and perfusion. Hyperbaric oxygenations will probably play no significant role in organ preservation, or at least its effects may not prove to be additive to those of hypothermia and perfusion.

There is evidence that an adequate flow rate during perfusion is a good prognostic sign of the viability and transplantability of the organ. The most significant indication of inadequate flow rate is the swelling caused by fluid retention. This edema is usually the result of anoxia with subsequent lysosomal and cellular damage. Poor perfusion itself can produce anoxia, so that a vicious cycle of edema-anoxia-edema can be started. Other possible causes of interstitial edema are perfusate osmolarity and excessive perfusion pressure. Even hypothermia alone may cause cellular swelling. Another important factor in the obstruction of flow is simple blockage of the microvasculature. The many causes of this blockage have been described in detail and include bubbles in the perfusion system, fibrin, red cell agglutination, the adherence of platelets and leukocytes to endothelial cells, cell breakdown due to mechanically imperfect pumps, crystal formation, and even agglutination of bacteria. Some of this blockage can be prevented with adequate filtration, but even blood-derived perfusion media like whole plasma have been shown to contain aggregates that appear during hypothermic perfusion. This aggregated material has been identified as lipoprotein. Fortunately, these substances can be removed from plasma quite easily by freezing, which causes flocculation of the lipoprotein, and by subsequent filtration and/or ultracentrifugation to remove the aggregates.

When plasma or plasma products are used as perfusates, immunologic damage is possible. This may be due to antibodies directed against organ antigens or to the precipitation of circulating antigen-antibody complexes within the organ. Although complement cannot be activated at hypothermic temperatures, bound antibody will activate complement within the recipient's body soon after transplantation. Although this has led to few recognized complications after renal transplantation, elimination of immunoglobulins from perfusates would be preferable.

One of the major problems in organ preservation research is the lack of methods to assay the functional state of organs in vitro and the consequent inability to measure the effectiveness of innovations in organ preservation techniques. Ultimately, of course, each preservation method must be tested by reimplantation of the organ. This is an all-or-none test that requires a large number of transplants in order to get statistically valid data. What is needed is an in vitro assay technique that can predict the transplantability of an organ and provide quantitative assessment of viability as the organ is subjected to the various preservation protocols. For practical purposes, such an assay should be utilized both before preservation (to determine whether postmortem changes have rendered the organ unfit for preservation) and immediately before transplantation (to determine whether the preservation efforts have been effective). As mentioned, the currently most popular technique involves the measurement of perfusate flow to the preserved kidney. Studies of enzymes or metabolites (like lactate) released from the graft appear promising.

Various pharmacologic agents have also been used as metabolic inhibitors. These include such drugs as magnesium sulfate, chlorpromazine, chloroquine, hydrocortisone, and diuretics such as mersalyl. Unfortunately, experiments utilizing such agents in addition to hypothermia show little additive effect. Most recently, however, allopurinol has been shown to protect against some of the anoxic damage to organs.

Storage of Nonviable Tissues by Freeze-Drying

Tissue grafts have been used in human reconstructive surgery for several decades. A majority of these grafts are from connective tissue and do not require that the graft be viable to function adequately. A major constituent of most of these tissues is collagen, which seems to maintain its integrity (or at least its strength) even after long-term storage by freezing or freeze-drying. Many thousands of patients each year receive bone, fascia, dura, tendon, heart valve, or skin grafts in treatment of traumatic or surgical defects. The architecture of these grafts is used as a framework for reconstruction as the host slowly replaces the tissue.

These tissues are probably best preserved by freeze-drying, which consists of rapid freezing of the tissue and the application of vacuum for removal of the water from the frozen state to the vapor state without permitting it to become liquid. Such a process usually results in maintenance of morphologic structure and therefore maintains the strength and structural integrity of the tissue. The rapidity of the initial freeze is important, as slow freezing can result in the formation of large ice crystals that can disrupt the tissue. This is apparently not a severe problem in tissues that consist largely of collagen. Other tissues, such as vascular grafts that contain elastic fibers, can show a disruption of these fibers due to crystal formation. In this instance, the most rapid freeze possible would be indicated to minimize crystal size. The graft is then dehydrated to a residual moisture of 5 percent. At this level it has been noted that tissues can subsequently be stored under vacuum at room temperature for years without further degradation or activation of metabolic processes. On reconstitution, it has been found preferable to inject water or saline solutions into a vacuum bottle containing tissue, so that the fluid can enter the tissue before it is exposed to air. Prior exposure to air apparently allows air molecules to enter the tissue and delays or prevents subsequent penetration of the water molecules necessary to rehydrate the tissue.

The usefulness of freeze-dried allografts is at least partly due to reduced antigenicity remaining in such grafts. The results of using freeze-dried allogeneic bone and autografting bone are not remarkably different. The dura has also been preserved by freeze-drying and functions extremely well when used to cover large cranial defects. Flexor tendon grafts of the hand have also been freeze-dried and used successfully, particularly when removed with their tendon sheaths intact. Many other freeze-dried tissues have been used with greater or lesser success. Cornea for nonpenetrating lamellar transplants, fascia, cartilage, heart valve, and nerve have all been tried.

Similarly, freeze-dried grafts have served as temporary biologic dressings to cover large burn wounds. In these instances the nonviable, freeze-dried graft "takes" and is even revascularized. It remains in place for several weeks or months, before it is finally sloughed. These grafts can be applied repeatedly without sensitization or acceleration of sloughing. Skin grafts have proved to be the best biologic dressing to prevent infection and to promote maximum granulation tissue formation in open skin wounds.

The usefulness of these techniques for the preservation of transplantable tissue has recently led to the organization of the American Association of Tissue Banks. The purpose of this organization is to encourage research into and to standardize successful methods for the harvest, storage, and distribution of tissues and organs to needy patients.

Bibliography

General

Abouna GM (ed): *Current Status of Clinical Organ Transplantation: With Some Recent Developments in Renal Surgery*. The Hague, Martinus Nijhoff, 1984.

Davis FD, Lucier JS, et al: Organization of an organ donation network. *Surg Clin North Am* 66:641, 1986.

Evans RS: Cost-effective analysis of transplantation. *Surg Clin North Am* 66:603, 1986.

Morris PJ (ed): *Kidney Transplantation: Principles and Practice*. New York, Grune and Stratton, 1984.

Morris PJ, Tilney NC (eds): *Progress in Transplantation*. Edinburgh, UK, Churchill Livingstone, 1985.

Najarian JS, Simmons RL (eds): *Transplantation*. Philadelphia, Lea & Febiger, 1972.

Park WE, Barber R, et al: Ethical issues in transplantation. *Surg Clin North Am* 66:663, 1986.

Penn I: Cancers following cyclosporine therapy. *Transplantation* 43:32, 1986.

Rapaport FT, Dausset J (eds): *Human Transplantation*. New York, Grune and Stratton, 1968.

Report of the Task Force on Organ Transplantation Issues and Recommendations: US Department of Health and Human Services, 1986.

Roberts AJ, Parnven GA (eds): Organ transplantation. *Surg Clin North Am* 55:1, 1986.

Simmons RL, Finch NL, et al (eds): *Manual of Vascular Access, Organ Donation and Transplantation*. New York, Springer-Verlag, 1984.

Simmons RG, Klein SK, et al: *Gift of Life: The Social and Psychological Impact of Organ Transplantation*. New York, Wiley, 1977.

Terasak PI (ed): *Clinical Kidney Transplants 1985*. Los Angeles, UCLA Tissue Typing Laboratory, 1985.

Tilney NL, Lazarus JM: *Surgical Care of the Patient with Renal Failure*. Philadelphia, Saunders, 1982.

Yunis EJ, Gatti RA (eds): *Tissue Typing and Organ Transplantation*. New York, Academic, 1973.

Transplantation Immunology

Calne RY (ed): *Transplantation Immunology: Clinical and Experimental*. Oxford, Oxford Medical, 1984.

deVries RRP, Van Rood JJ: Immunology of HLA class I and class II molecules. *Prog Allergy* 36:1, 1985.

Goldstein G: An overview of Orthoclone OKT3. *Transplant Proc* XVII:927, 1986.

Hayry P: Intragraft events in allograft destruction. *Transplantation* 38:1, 1984.

Hayry P, von Willebrand E: Transplant aspiration cytology. *Transplantation* 38:7, 1984.

Kahan BD: *Cyclosporine, Diagnosis and Management of Associated Renal Injury*. Orlando, FL, Grune and Stratton, 1985.

Kirkmon RL, Berrett LV, et al: Administration of anti-interleukin 2 receptor monoclonal antibody prolongs cardiac allograft survival in mice. *J Exp Med* 162:358, 1985.

Mason DW, Morris PJ: Effector mechanisms in allograft rejection. *Annu Rev Immunol* 4:119, 1986.

Murrach P, Kappler J: The T cell and its receptor. *Sci Am* 254:36, 1986.

Shevach EM: The effects of cyclosporine on the immune system. *Annu Rev Immunol* 3:397, 1985.

Strom TB: Clinical transplantation, in Stites DP, Stoles JD, et al (eds): *Basic and Clinical Immunology*. Los Altos, CA, Lange Medical, 1982.

Strom TB: Immunosuppressive agents in renal transplantation. *Kidney Int* 26:353, 1984.

Van Buren CT: Cyclosporine: Progress, problems and perspectives. *Surg Clin North Am* 66:435, 1986.

Liver Transplantation

Ascher NL, Simmons RL, et al: Host hepatectomy and liver transplantation, in Simmons RL, Finch ME, et al (eds): *Manual of Vascular Access, Organ Donation, and Transplantation*. New York, Springer-Verlag, 1984, p 255.

Cosmini AB, Cho SI, et al: A randomized clinical trial comparing OKT3 and steroids for treatment of hepatic allograft rejection. *Transplantation* 43:91, 1987.

Demetriou AA, Chowdrury NR, et al: New method of hepatocyte transplantation and extracorporeal liver support. *Ann Surg* 204:259, 1986.

Fath JJ, Ascher NL, et al: Metabolism during hepatic transplantations. Indicators of allograft function. *Surgery* 96:64, 1984.

Gordon RD, Shaw BW, et al: Indications for liver transplantation in the cyclosporine ERA. *Surg Clin North Am* 66:541, 1986.

Hood JM, Koep LJ, et al: Liver transplantation for advanced liver disease with alpha-1-antitrypsin deficiency. *N Engl J Med* 302:272, 1980.

Kam I, Lynch S, et al: Low flow venous bypasses in small dogs and pediatric patients undergoing replacement of the liver. *Surg Gynecol Obstet* 163:33, 1986.

Kretchtle SJ, Kolbeck PC, et al: Hepatic transplantation into sensitized recipients: Demonstration of hyperacute rejection. *Transplantation* 43:8, 1987.

Krom RAF, Kingma LM, et al: Choledococholedochostomy, a relatively safe procedure in orthotopic liver transplantation. *Surgery* 97:552, 1985.

Lerut J, Gordon RD, et al: Biliary tract complication following human orthotopic liver transplantation. *Transplantation* 43:47, 1987.

Perkins JD, Wiesner RH, et al: Immunohistologic labelling as an indication of liver allograft rejection. *Transplantation* 43:100, 1987.

So SKS, Platt JL, et al: Increased expression of class I MHC antigens on hepatocytes in rejecting human liver allografts. *Transplantation* 43:79, 1987.

Wall WJ, Grant DR, et al: Liver transplantation without veno veno bypass. *Transplantation* 43:56, 1987.

Pancreas Transplantation

Corry RJ, Nghiem DD, et al: Surgical treatment of diabetic nephropathy with simultaneous pancreatic duodenal and renal transplantation. *Surg Gynecol Obstet* 162:547, 1986.

Hullett DA, Faleny JL, et al: Human fetal pancreas—A potential source for transplantation. *Transplantation* 43:18, 1987.

Nghiem DD, Gonwa TA, et al: Metabolic effects of urinary diversion of exocrine secretion in pancreatic transplantation. *Transplantation* 43:70, 1987.

Prieto M, Sutherland DER, et al: Experimental and clinical experiences with urine amylase monitoring for early diagnosis of rejection in pancreas transplantation. *Transplantation* 43:73, 1987.

Sutherland DER: Pancreas and islet transplantation II. Clinical trials. *Diabetologia* 20:435, 1981.

Sutherland DER, Ascher NL, et al: Pancreas transplantation, in

Simmons RL, Finch ME, et al (eds): *Manual of Vascular Access, Organ Donation, and Transplantation*. New York, Springer-Verlag, 1984, p 237.

Sutherland DER, Kendall D, et al: Pancreas transplantation. *Surg Clin North Am* 66:557, 1986.

Bone Marrow Transplantation

Advisory Committee of the Bone Marrow Transplant Registry: Bone marrow transplantation from donors with aplastic anemia: A report from the ACS/NTH bone marrow transplant registry. *JAMA* 236:1131, 1976.

Beatty PG, et al: Marrow transplantation from related donors other than HLA identical siblings. *N Engl J Med* 313:765, 1985.

Bolman RM, Molina JE, et al: Heart transplantation, in Simmons RL, Finch ME, et al (eds): *Manual of Vascular Access, Organ Donation and Transplantation*. New York, Springer-Verlag, 1984, p 209.

Frazier OH, Cooley DA: Cardiac transplantation. *Surg Clin North Am* 66:477, 1986.

Gentry LO, Zelerff BJ: Diagnosis and treatment of infection in cardiac transplant patients. *Surg Clin North Am* 66:454, 1986.

Griffith BP, Trento AF, et al: Cardiac transplantation: Emerges from an experiment to a science. *Ann Surg* 204:308, 1986.

Modry DL, Oyer PE, et al: Cyclosporine in heart and heart/lung transplantation. *Can J Surg* 28:274, 1985.

Thomas ED: Bone marrow transplantation in hematologic malignancies. *Hospital Practice* 22:77, 1987.

Thompson CB, Thomas ED: Bone marrow transplantation. *Surg Clin North Am* 66:589, 1986.

Heart Transplantation

Andreone PA, Olivari MT, et al: Reduction of infectious complications following heart transplantation with triple-drug therapy. *J Heart Transplant* 5:13, 1986.

Bailey LL, Nehlsen-Cannarella SL, et al: Baboon-to-human cardiac xenotransplantation in a neonate. *JAMA* 254:3321, 1985.

Barnard CN: A human cardiac transplant. *S Afr Med J* 41:1271, 1967.

Baumgartner WA: Infections in cardiac transplantation. *J Heart Transplant* 3:75, 1983.

Bieber CP, Reitz BA, et al: Malignant lymphoma in Cyclosporin A treated allograft recipients. *Lancet* 1:43, 1980.

Billingham ME: Diagnosis of cardiac rejection by endomyocardial biopsy. *J Heart Transplant* 1:125, 1982.

Carrel A, Guthrie CC: The transplantation of veins and organs. *Am Med* 10:1101, 1905.

Cooper DKC, Novitzky D, et al: Are there indications for heterotopic heart transplantation in 1986? *Thorac Cardiovasc Surg* 34:300, 1986.

Dummer ST, White LT, et al: Morbidity of cytomegalovirus infection in recipients of heart or heart-lung transplants who received cyclosporine. *J Infect Dis* 152:1182, 1985.

Evans RW, Manninen DL, et al: Donor availability as the primary determinant of the future of heart transplantation. *JAMA* 255:1892, 1986.

Fuster V, Gersh BJ, et al: The natural history of idiopathic dilated cardiomyopathy. *Am J Cardiol* 47:525, 1981.

Hunt SA: Complications of heart transplantation. *J Heart Transplant* 3:70, 1983.

Lower RR, Shumway NE: Studies on orthotopic transplantation of the canine heart. *Surg Forum* 11:18, 1960.

Mammana RB, Peterson EA, et al: Pulmonary infections in car-

diac transplant patients: Modes of diagnosis, complications, and effectiveness of therapy. *Ann Thorac Surg* 36:700, 1983.

Meister ND, McAleer MJ, et al: Returning to work after heart transplantation. *J Heart Transplant* 5:154, 1986.

Michler RE, Smith CR, et al: Reversal of cardiac transplant rejection without massive immunosuppression. *Circulation* 74(suppl III):68, 1986.

Pennock JL, Oyer PE, et al: Cardiac transplantation in perspective for the future. *J Thorac Cardiovasc Surg* 83:168, 1982.

Sadeghi AM, Robbins RC, et al: Cardiac xenotransplantation in primates. *J Thorac Cardiovasc Surg* 93:809, 1987.

Solis E, Kaye MP: The Registry of the International Society for Heart Transplantation: Third Official Report, June 1986. *J Heart Transplant* 5:2, 1986.

Heart-Lung

Burke CM, Baldwin JC, et al: Twenty-eight cases of human heart-lung transplantation. *Lancet* 1:517, 1986.

Burke CM, Theodore J, et al: Post-transplant obliterative bronchiolitis and other late lung sequelae in human heart-lung transplantation. *Chest* 86:824, 1984.

Griffith BP, Hardesty RL, et al: Asynchronous rejection of heart and lungs following cardiopulmonary transplantation. *Ann Thorac Surg* 40:488, 1985.

Hardesty RL, Griffith BP: Autoperfusion of the heart and lungs for preservation during distant procurement. *J Thorac Cardiovasc Surg* 93:11, 1987.

Hardesty RL, Griffith BP: Procurement for combined heart-lung transplantation: Bilateral thoracotomy with sternal transection, cardiopulmonary bypass, and profound hypothermia. *J Thorac Cardiovasc Surg* 89:795, 1985.

Haverich A, Scott WC, et al: Twenty years of lung preservation—A review. *J Heart Transplant* 4:234, 1985.

Jamieson SW, Stinson EB, et al: Operative technique for heart-lung transplantation. *J Thorac Cardiovasc Surg*. 87:930, 1984.

Painvin GA, Reece IJ, et al: Cardiopulmonary allotransplantation, a collective review: Experimental progress and current clinical status, *Tex Heart Inst J* 10:371, 1983.

Reitz BA, Burton NA, et al: Heart and lung transplantation: Autotransplantation and allotransplantation in primates with extended survival. *J Thorac Cardiovasc Surg* 80:360, 1980.

Reitz BA, Wallwork JL, et al: Heart-lung transplantation: Successful therapy for patients with pulmonary vascular disease. *N Engl J Med* 306:557, 1982.

Solis E, Kaye MP: The Registry of the International Society for Heart Transplantation: Third official report, June 1986. *J Heart Transplant,* 5:2, 1986.

Starkey TD, Sakakibara N, et al: Successful six-hour cardiopulmonary preservation with simple hypothermic crystalloid flush. *J Heart Transplant* 5:291, 1986.

Theodore J, Jamieson SW, et al: Physiologic aspects of human heart-lung transplantation: Pulmonary function status of the post-transplanted lung. *Chest* 86:349, 1984.

Single-Lung Transplantation

Dark JH, Patterson GA, et al: Experimental en bloc double lung transplantation. *Ann Thorac Surg* 42:394, 1986.

Dubois P, Choiniere L, et al: Bronchial omentopexy in canine lung allotransplantation. *Ann Thorac Surg* 38:211, 1984.

Goldberg M, Lima O, et al: A comparison between cyclosporine A and methylprednisolone plus azathioprine on bronchial healing following canine lung autotransplantation. *J Thorac Cardiovasc Surg* 85:821, 1983.

Jamieson SW, Ogunnaike HO: Cardiopulmonary transplantation. *Surg Clin North Am* 66:491, 1986.

Montefusco CM, Veith FM: Lung transplantation. *Surg Clin North Am* 66:503, 1986.

Nelems JM, Rebuck AS, et al: Human lung transplantation. *Chest* 78:569, 1980.

Toronto Lung Transplant Group: Unilateral lung transplantation for pulmonary fibrosis. *N Engl J Med* 314:1140, 1986.

Veith FJ: Lung transplantation in perspective. *N Engl J Med* 314:1186, 1986.

Veith FJ, Kamkolz SL, et al: Lung transplantation. *Transplantation* 35:271, 1983.

Veith FJ, Norin AJ, et al: Cyclosporine A in experimental lung transplantation. *Transplantation* 32:474, 1981.

Kidney Transplantation

Burlingham WJ, Grailer A, et al: Improved renal allograft survival following donor specific transfusions. II. *In vitro* correlates of early DST type rejection episodes. *Transplantation* 43:41, 1987.

Calne RY, Wood AJ: Cyclosporine in cadaveric renal transplantation: 3 year followup of a European multicenter trial. *Lancet* 2:549, 1985.

Canadian Multicentre Transplant Study Group: A randomized trial of cyclosporine in cadaveric renal transplantation. *N Engl J Med* 314:1219, 1986.

Cast.eneda-Zuniga WR (ed): *Radiographic Diagnosis of Renal Transplant Complications.* Minneapolis, University of Minnesota, 1986.

Chandler ST, Buckels J, et al: Indium labelled platelet uptake in rejecting renal transplants. *Surg Gynecol Obstet* 157:242, 1983.

Cho SI, Zalneraetes BP, et al: The influence of acute tubular necrosis on kidney transplant survival. *Transplant Proc* XVII:16, 1985.

Fryd DS, Sutherland DER, et al: Results of a prospective randomized study on the effect of splenectomy versus no splenectomy in renal transplant patients. *Transplant Proc* XIII:48, 1981.

Keown PA, Stiller CB: Kidney transplantation. *Surg Clin North Am* 66:517, 1986.

Malkowicz SB, Perloff LJ: Urologic consideration in renal transplantation. *Surg Gynecol Obstet* 160:579, 1985.

Mauer SM, Barbosa J, et al: Development of diabetic vascular lesions in normal kidneys transplanted into patients with diabetes mellitus. *N Engl J Med* 295:916, 1976.

Mendez–Picon G, Posner MS, et al: The effect of delayed function on long term survival of renal allografts. *Surg Gynecol Obstet* 161:351, 1986.

Monoco AP: Clinical kidney transplantation. *Transplant Proc* XVII:5, 1985.

Najarian JS, Fryd DS, et al: A single institution, randomized, prospective trial of cyclosporine, versus azathioprine-antilymphocyte globulin for immunosuppression in renal allograft recipients. *Ann Surg* 201:142, 1985.

Najarian JS, So SKS, et al: The outcome of 304 primary renal transplants in children (1968–1985). *Ann Surg* 204:246, 1986.

Najarian JS, Sutherland DER: The impact of transplantation on the understanding and treatment of diabetes and the pancreas. *Transplant Proc.* XII:634, 1980.

Novick AC (ed): Renal transplantation. *Urol Clin North Am* 10:203, 1983.

Opelz G: Correlation of HLA matching with kidney graft survival in patients or without cyclosporine treatment. *Transplantation* 40:240, 1985.

Opelz G: Current relevance of the transfusion effect in renal transplantation. *Transplant Proc* XVII:1015, 1985.

Ortho Multicenter Study Group: A randomized clinical trial of OKT3 monoclonal antibody for acute rejection of cadaveric renal transplants. *N Engl J Med* 313:37, 1985.

Report of the medical consultants on the diagnosis of death: Guidelines for determination of death. *JAMA* 246:2184, 1981.

Simmons RG, Anderson CR: Related donors and recipients: Five to nine years post-transplant. *Transplant Proc* XIV:9, 1982.

Simmons RL, Najarian JS: Kidney transplantation, in Simmons RL, Finch ME, et al (eds): *Manual of Vascular Access, Organ Donation, and Transplantation.* New York, Springer-Verlag, 1984, p 292.

Simmons RL, Sutherland DER: Transplant nephrectomy, in Simmons RL, Finch ME, et al (eds): *Manual of Vascular Access, Organ Donation, and Transplantation.* New York, Springer-Verlag, 1984, p 329.

So SKS, Simmons RL, et al: Improved results of multiple transplantation in children. *Surgery* 98:729, 1985.

Sommer BG, Henry M, et al: Sequential antilymphoblast globulin and cyclosporine for renal transplantation. *Transplantation* 43:85, 1987.

Starzl TE, Hakala TR: Variable convalescence and therapy after cadaveric renal transplantation under cyclosporin A and steroids. *Surg Gynecol Obstet* 154:819, 1982.

Stiller CR, Keown PA: Immunologic monitoring: Current perspectives and clinical implications. *Transplant Proc* XIII:1699, 1981.

Sutherland DER: International human pancreas and islet transplant registry. *Transplant Proc* XII:229, 1980.

Sutherland DER, Fryd DS, et al: The high-risk recipient in renal transplantation. *Transplant Proc* XIV:19, 1982.

Wing AJ, Broyer M, et al: Renal transplantation in Europe—Some comparisons between national programs. *Transplant Proc* XIV:5, 1982.

Transplantation of Other Organs

Baird RN, Abbott WM: Vein grafts: An historical perspective. *Am J Surg* 134:293, 1977.

Cohen Z, Wassef R, et al: Transplantation of the small intestine. *Surg Clin North Am* 66:583, 1986.

Friedlander GE, Mankin HJ, et al (eds): *Osteochondral Allografts.* Boston, Little, Brown, 1983.

Pritchford TJ, Kirkman RL: Small bowel transplantation. *World J Surg* 9:860, 1985.

Quilici PJ, Vieta JO, et al: The use of dura mater allografts in the surgical repair of the abdominal wall. *Surg Gynecol Obstet* 161:47, 1985.

Vrist MR: Practical application of basic research on bone graft physiology. Instructional course lectures. *Am Acad Orthoped Surg* 25:1, 1976.

Chapter 11

Anesthesia

Ronald D. Miller

INTRODUCTION

Anesthesia care involves care for the entire perioperative period, including preoperative evaluation, selection of appropriate monitoring for the perioperative period, administration of anesthesia, and postoperative care as it relates to anesthesia and surgery. Anesthesiologists also serve as consultants in the areas of chronic pain, critical care medicine, and respiratory therapy. In this chapter, the discussion will be limited to those aspects of anesthesia related to the perioperative period.

ANESTHETIC RISK

Anesthetic risk, per se, is difficult to determine because perioperative complications are usually a result of multiple causes related to concurrent disease, the complexity of surgery, and perhaps anesthesia itself. Examples of complications solely related to anesthesia are vomiting and aspiration of gastric contents and hypoxemia due to the inability to maintain a patent airway and/or adequate ventilation. Increasing emphasis has been placed on rare anesthetic mishaps, such as anesthetic overdose, undetected intubation of the esophagus instead of the trachea, and accidental disconnection of the ventilator from the endotracheal tube. It is extremely difficult to determine the true incidence and, therefore, risks of pure anesthetic complications that occur at such a low frequency. Taking all studies into account and despite the above stated limitations, death rates of 1 in 10,000 due entirely to anesthesia and about 2 in 10,000 in major part due to anesthesia appear to be reasonable estimates of overall anesthetic risks. These figures obviously do not take into account the multiple causes of morbidity, such as postoperative neurological complication, broken teeth, and many others. Despite the problems listed above, with proper care, anesthetic risk is extremely low.

The patient's physical status is usually classified according to the criteria in Table 11-1. This system does not specifically identify anesthetic risk but is often utilized for epidemiologic and descriptive purposes.

Table 11-1. PHYSICAL STATUS CLASSIFICATION
OF THE AMERICAN SOCIETY OF
ANESTHESIOLOGISTS

Class	Physical status
1	Patient has no organic, physiologic, biochemical, or psychiatric disturbances
2	Patient has mild to moderate systemic disturbance that may or may not be related to the disorder requiring surgery (e.g., essential hypertension, diabetes mellitus)
3	Patient has severe systemic disturbance that may or may not be related to the disorder requiring surgery (e.g., heart disease that limits activity, poorly controlled essential hypertension)
4	Patient has severe systemic disturbance that is life-threatening with or without surgery (e.g., congestive heart failure, persistent angina pectoris)
5	Patient is moribund and has little chance for survival, but surgery is to be performed as a last resort (resuscitation effort) (e.g., uncontrolled hemorrhage, as from a ruptured abdominal aneurysm)
E	Patient requires emergency operation

PREOPERATIVE EVALUATION

History and Physical

The history and physical examination is not meant to duplicate the surgeon's evaluation, but rather it is to specifically examine those areas relevant to anesthesia. Preoperative evaluation by an anesthesiologist is considered to be the standard of care in anesthesia. The history should include a review of the patient's previous hospitalizations, surgeries, and anesthesia, in an effort to identify clues that may influence anesthesia care, such as allergic reactions, delayed awakening, and jaundice. Concurrent diseases can have a tremendous influence on perioperative care, especially certain endocrine diseases (i.e., diabetes), cardiovascular disease (i.e., hypertension and myocardial infarction), respiratory disease (i.e., obstructive airway disease), coagulopathies (i.e., hemophilia), and abnormalities of vital excretory organs (i.e., kidney and/or liver disease).

Concurrent drug therapy must be reviewed because many drugs influence the response to anesthetic drugs. For example, echothiophate may prolong the response to succinylcholine. Various antihypertensive and other vasoactive drugs can alter the circulatory response to anesthetics (e.g., beta-adrenergic blocking drugs). Many drugs can either increase or decrease anesthetic requirement, including acute cocaine intoxication, tricyclic antidepressants, and antihypertensive drugs. Other drugs may prolong the neuromuscular blocking properties of nondepolarizing muscle relaxants, such as antibiotics and local anesthetics. Still other drugs may influence the metabolism of anesthetic drugs, increasing the possibility of a toxic reaction.

The physical examination should focus on those aspects that are important to the particular anesthetic being planned. If regional anesthesia is being planned, examination of the landmarks (and their accessibility) should be ascertained. For example, an epidural anesthetic may not be appropriate in an extremely obese patient in whom the vertebra cannot be palpated. In a more general sense, a physical examination should most assuredly include the cardiovascular system, lungs, and upper airway. Arterial blood pressure should often be determined in both the supine and sitting positions to ascertain whether postural hypotension is present, which serves to assess the presence of autonomic dysfunction and/or an inadequate intravascular volume. If abnormalities are found, additional tests (e.g., pulmonary function tests) may be indicated. Laboratory tests should not be ordered unless a specific diagnostic and therapeutic end point is defined. For example, in a patient with obstructive airway disease, pulmonary function tests may be indicated to ascertain whether any additional preoperative respiratory care is indicated (e.g., the response to bronchodilators) and to provide a baseline with which postoperative pulmonary care can be compared. Lastly, a limited neurological examination should be performed depending on the position and the type of anesthesia to be chosen. Certain intraoperative positions are well known to be associated with postoperative neuropathies.

Laboratory Tests

Traditionally, hospital rules and regulations dictated that certain minimal laboratory tests be obtained. Recognizing the expense of routine testing and with sophisticated cost-benefit analyses, many of these regulations are now realized to be inappropriate. In general, the history and physical examination are the most important guides as to whether certain laboratory tests are needed. In a patient who has a completely normal history and physical examination, our practice (at the University of California, San Francisco Medical Center) is not to automatically order any laboratory tests in adult men who are under the age of 40 years and have no history of problems with anesthesia or no abnormal findings upon physical examination. Women of this age and health status usually only require a hemoglobin determination.

Informed Consent

In general, an "informed consent" is difficult to define for both anesthesia and surgery. Theoretically, the patient should know of all possible risks associated with anesthesia. Yet, in many patients this presents an undue concern, especially if the risk is particularly tragic and extremely rare. It is not practical and it may even be harmful to cause undue worry. Also, the extent to which the complications are described depend on the necessity for surgery and anesthesia (e.g., minor cosmetic surgery versus an exploratory laparotomy for a ruptured appendix). Despite the above-stated limitations, patients should know what to expect from the administration of anesthesia and possible adverse effects and risks. Those areas that should receive particular attention include the timing and administration of preoperative medication, anticipated time of transport to the operating room, sequence of events prior to induction of anesthesia, anticipated duration of surgery, a description of where awakening from anesthesia will occur and whether catheters will be present, expected time of return to the hospital room, the likelihood of postoperative nausea and vomiting, and the measures that will be taken to deal with postoperative pain. A signed consent form should be obtained from the patient, and all the risks discussed with the patient should be noted in the patient's medical records.

Recently, there has been increasing concern whether a separate informed consent should be obtained for blood transfusions. While it is this author's belief that such a separate consent is unwarranted, clearly complications of blood transfusions should be discussed with the patient, especially recognizing the relatively high risk of hepatitis (e.g., 3 to 15 percent) and the rare problem associated with the acquired immunodeficiency syndrome (AIDS).

IMMEDIATE PREOPERATIVE CARE AND PREPARATION

Preoperative Medication

Preoperative medication is usually given to provide sedation and possibly induced amnesia. This combination generally will result in also alleviating anxiety. Because of the concern of vomiting and aspiration of gastric contents, another goal of preoperative medication is to decrease secretion of saliva and gastric juices and to elevate gastric pH. For inpatients, medication is usually given 1 to 2 h prior to the induction of anesthesia. The value and the selection of preoperative medication is largely subjective. Most commonly, sedation is provided with the oral administration of diazepam, although other drugs such as barbiturates and narcotics are frequently given intramuscularly. Gastric secretion can be reduced by H_2 receptor antagonist, such as cimetidine. Drying agents such as atropine or scopalomine are rarely indicated and in fact make the patient uncomfortable by providing excessive drying of the mouth. These drugs historically were necessary when anesthetics markedly increased salivary secretions (e.g., diethyl ether). Modern anesthetics, however, do not increase salivary secretions to an unusual degree.

A thoughtful and concerned conversation with the patient preoperatively can attenuate the need for preoperative medications regarding anesthesia and surgery. For patients who arrive the morning of surgery, premedications, if needed, can be given immediately prior to being taken into the operating room. For example, it is common to give midazolam, 1.0 to 4.0 mg/70 kg intravenously to provide a calming effect and a high incidence of amnesia. Often, concomitant narcotics are given if regional anesthesia is about to be performed.

Preparation for Administration of Anesthesia

GENERAL CONSIDERATIONS

When the patient arrives in the operative theater, he or she should be properly identified and the nurses' notes from the preceding evening should be reviewed to ensure that any unexpected changes in the patient's condition have not occurred. Also, the administration of preoperative medication should be verified. Lastly, all personnel in the operating room should be specifically instructed as to what requirements will be needed during induction of anesthesia (e.g., cricoid pressure during a rapid sequence induction of anesthesia).

ANESTHETIC MACHINE

The anesthetic machine and all associated equipment (e.g., suctioning device) must be checked immediately prior to inducing anesthesia. Rare anesthetic mishaps have been related to an unexpected malfunctioning of the anesthesia machine. This should not happen if the machine has been properly checked prior to induction of anesthesia.

MONITORING

Increasingly, standards are being set for monitoring that should apply to nearly all administrations of anesthesia. Several hospitals in the Harvard Medical School have established the minimum requirements listed in Table 11-2. An anesthesiologist or nurse anesthetist should be present in the operating-room theater at all times during the administration of general anesthesia, regional anesthesia, and monitored intravenous anesthetics. Occasionally a brief exit is tolerated when a known hazard, such as radiation, is being applied. Under most circumstances, heart rate and blood pressure should be monitored at a minimum rate of every 5 min. It is highly desirable to have the electrocardiogram continuously displayed from the induction of anesthesia until the patient is prepared for leaving the operating-room theater. Even though heart rate and arterial blood pressure are recommended to be measured every 5 min, measures should be taken to ensure that cardiorespiratory function is continuously moni-

Table 11-2. BASIC MONITORING REQUIREMENTS*

Anesthesiologist's or nurse anesthetist's presence in the
  operating room
Blood pressure and heart rate
Electrocardiogram
Continuous monitoring for cardiorespiratory function
Breathing system disconnection monitoring
Oxygen monitor
Temperature

* Adapted from Eichhorn JH, Cooper JB, et al: *JAMA* 256:1017, 1986.

tored. This may include palpation or observation of the reservoir breathing bag, auscultation of breath and heart sounds, or more sophisticated monitoring such as a tracing of an intraarterial blood-pressure line. When ventilation is controlled by an automatic mechanical ventilator, a device should be present to warn the anesthesiologist when the ventilator becomes accidentally disconnected from the endotracheal tube. An oxygen analyzer should be functioning during the administration of general anesthesia to ensure that hypoxic mixtures are not being administered. Lastly, although not a requirement in every patient, a means to measure body temperature should be available, especially to detect intraoperative hypothermia or the rare case of malignant hyperthermia.

POSITION

The patient must be positioned properly on the operating table in order to avoid physical and physiologic complications. Nerve damage can be caused by placing the patient in a position that stretches or applies pressure to the nerve. The most common peripheral nerve injuries are related to the brachial plexus and especially the ulnar nerve. Also, the patient's position can cause cardiovascular changes, such as hypotension when the patient is rapidly shifted from the supine to the sitting or prone position. Lastly, complications can occur from improper application of the anesthetic mask strap, or endotracheal tube connector. Necrosis of the bridge of the nose has occurred when the mask is applied with excessive pressure. Removal of the mask every 5 min and massaging the nose should minimize this complication. Also, patients have had loss of hair when their head has been in one position for several hours. This complication can be minimized by changing the patient's head position every 1 or 2 h.

INTRAOPERATIVE ANESTHESIA

General Anesthesia

GENERAL CONSIDERATIONS

Although the various inhaled and intravenous anesthetics have marked differences in pharmacologic activity, especially circulatory changes, the selection of anesthesia has never been demonstrated to be an important factor regarding overall outcome. The lack of influence of choice of anesthesia on outcome may be related to the greater importance of the anesthesiologist's skill rather than the specific agent chosen. Conversely, perhaps small differences in outcome are related to the choice of anesthesia but have not been demonstrated because of the lack of availability of large epidemiologic outcome-related studies.

Until the early 1960s, the potency of anesthetic drugs had not been precisely determined because of a lack of a suitable technique. Since then, the minimum alveolar anesthetic concentration (MAC) has been developed and utilized as a measure of anesthetic potency for the inhaled anesthetics. MAC is defined as that alveolar concentra-

tion at which 50 percent of the subjects move in response to a noxious stimulus. MAC has been determined in anesthetized patients by finding that concentration at which half of the patients do not move in response to a skin incision. This concept and measurement has allowed comparison of the pharmacologic and physiologic effects of various anesthetic drugs at equipotent concentrations. Also, MAC has allowed a more precise determination of those physiologic factors that may influence anesthetic requirements, including increasing age, debility, and the concomitant administration of other drugs. The determination of MAC was greatly facilitated by being able to measure the end-tidal anesthetic concentration, which is a direct reflection of the alveolar concentration and, therefore, the brain concentration at steady state. Studies are being conducted to provide comparable measurements of anesthetic potency for the intravenously administered anesthetics.

INDUCTION OF ANESTHESIA

Anesthesia can be induced by giving drugs intravenously, by inhalation, or by a combination of both. Two major factors govern the method by which anesthesia is induced. One is the necessity to protect the airway if a patient has recently eaten or has a condition known to facilitate vomiting and aspiration of gastric contents (e.g., pregnancy or ascites). The other factor is the physiologic status of the patient. If a patient is very fragile (e.g., a reduced intravascular volume, or elderly), anesthesia probably should be given very slowly so that the known cardiovascular depressant effects of most anesthetics do not become excessive.

Other than an awake endotracheal intubation, the airway is most rapidly protected by using a "rapid sequence" method of inducing anesthesia. This method of inducing anesthesia has the disadvantage of needing to administer large doses of anesthetic drugs with known adverse cardiovascular effects. Anesthesia is most commonly induced by the administration of an ultra-short-acting barbiturate (e.g., thiopental) followed by a depolarizing muscle relaxant (e.g., succinylcholine). This allows anesthesia to be induced rapidly and the trachea intubated within 30 to 90 s. If cricoid pressure is concomitantly administered, theoretically the airway should be completely protected from aspiration of gastric contents. Cricoid pressure needs to be precisely applied in order to occlude the esophagus and prevent gastric contents from entering the pharynx, and therefore the trachea. Oxygen is usually given via mask before inducing anesthesia to allow maximum time for intubation while the patient is apneic.

Anesthesia can be induced by inhalation of a potent volatile anesthetic (e.g., halothane, enflurane, or isoflurane) with or without nitrous oxide. Anesthesia can be induced within 3 to 5 min. This technique has the advantage of allowing careful titration of the anesthetic and the immediate withdrawal of the anesthetic if adverse effects, such as hypotension, occur. This technique has the disadvantage that induction of anesthesia is longer than by the intravenous route and requires a skilled anesthetist to administer the anesthetic while avoiding coughing and the excitement stage (i.e., stage II of anesthesia). After anesthesia has been induced, the trachea can be intubated with or without administration of a neuromuscular blocking drug. Attempting endotracheal intubation in a spontaneously breathing, unparalyzed, anesthetized patient is difficult. Although conditions for intubation may not be as good with this method, the patient will still be breathing if some difficulties with intubation prolong the time before complete airway control is achieved. If severe difficulties with airway control are anticipated, an awake endotracheal intubation should be considered, possibly with the aid of a fiberoptic bronchoscope.

Anesthesia is usually induced by intravenously administered anesthetics with or without the concurrent administration of an inhaled anesthetic. Thiopental undoubtedly is the most commonly administered intravenous anesthetic, although various narcotics (e.g., fentanyl, morphine, sufentanil) and benzodiazepines (e.g., diazepam and midazolam) have become increasingly popular. The intravenously administered anesthetic has the advantage of minimizing the discomfort of the anesthetic mask and inducing anesthesia very rapidly.

AIRWAY MANAGEMENT (ENDOTRACHEAL INTUBATION)

Although general anesthesia can be given without intubating the trachea, this is very uncommon. While the complications of endotracheal intubation are avoided, this approach has many disadvantages. The airway is unprotected in case the patient vomits. Also, the anesthesiologist must hold the mask with one hand during the entire procedure, which hinders the performance of many other tasks, including monitoring and blood or drug administration.

Endotracheal intubation is usually performed during general anesthesia to ensure a patent airway, to prevent aspiration of gastric contents, and to facilitate tracheal or bronchial suctioning and positive-pressure ventilation. Also, if the patient is in a position other than the supine or Trendelenburg position, it is very difficult to provide adequate ventilation via a mask, and endotracheal intubation is usually indicated.

There are several complications of endotracheal intubation. On an immediate basis, complications from direct laryngoscopy and insertion of the endotracheal tube often involves injuries to the teeth. If a tooth is dislodged, it must be removed. If the tooth cannot be located, radiographs of the chest and abdomen should be obtained to ascertain that the tooth has not passed into the airway via the glottic opening. Because endotracheal intubation is very stimulating, hypertension and tachycardia can occur. However, this is so transient that it is of rare clinical significance. It can be minimized by assuring that the depth of anesthesia is adequate and/or by administration of 100 mg/70 kg of lidocaine intravenously.

Intraoperatively, the endotracheal tube can be obstructed or accidentally removed. If it has been incorrectly inserted (e.g., into the esophagus) hypoxemia will result. If this is not detected soon enough, permanent adverse complications can occur (i.e., hypoxic brain

damage). Auscultation of the lungs and stomach, and palpation of the endotracheal tube cuff in the trachea will assure proper placement of the endotracheal tube. Also, if too much pressure is applied to the balloon cuff of the endotracheal tube, the tracheal mucosa may be ischemic. This complication has been decreasing because of the use of "low-pressure cuffs," which adapt to the irregularities of the tracheal wall and produce a seal at pressures of 15 to 30 mmHg (previous endotracheal tube cuffs required 80 to 250 mmHg of pressure to occlude the trachea). Still, ciliary denudation can occur over the tracheal rings with only 2 h of intubation and tracheal pressure less than 25 mmHg.

Upon completion of anesthesia, extubation of the trachea can be complicated by laryngospasm, aspiration of gastric contents, pharyngitis, laryngitis, and laryngo- or subglottic edema. The incidence of these complications can be reduced by using the low-pressure endotracheal tube cuff and performing prompt extubation when clinically possible.

MAINTENANCE OF ANESTHESIA

Intraoperatively, anesthesia must provide analgesia, unconsciousness, skeletal muscle relaxation, and control of the sympathetic nervous system responses to noxious stimulation. The inhaled and intravenous anesthetics can be given alone or together to achieve these ends. Monitoring depth of anesthesia is relatively straightforward in an unparalyzed patient. Movement, depth and rate of respiration, and many other physiologic responses to anesthesia can be monitored. However, when a patient is paralyzed by neuromuscular blocking drugs, such as pancuronium, many of the signs of anesthesia are absent. It is essential that the anesthesiologist continue to attempt to assess the depth of anesthesia to avoid having a patient be awake, but paralyzed, during the surgical procedure.

A major challenge for anesthesia, especially during intraabdominal cases, is to provide adequate relaxation by the administration of proper anesthetic and neuromuscular blocking drug doses. Monitoring with a peripheral nerve stimulator will guide the anesthesiologist as to whether an adequate neuromuscular blockade is present and to avoid excessive doses of neuromuscular blocking drugs. If excessive doses of neuromuscular blocking drugs are given, the patient may have prolonged postoperative paralysis. If anesthesia is sufficient, elimination of 90 percent of the response to peripheral nerve stimulation will usually ensure adequate relaxation. The effectiveness of the neuromuscular blocking drug and anesthesia is facilitated when the surgical team takes other measures to maximize exposure, such as correct positioning.

Regional Anesthesia

GENERAL CONSIDERATIONS

Regional anesthesia has several advantages. The concept of anesthetizing only that part of the body upon which surgery is being performed (e.g., brachial plexus for arm or hand surgery), rather than subjecting the entire body to the problems of general anesthesia is an attractive concept, although it is not clear that regional anesthesia will improve mortality and morbidity. Furthermore, regional anesthesia has the advantage that skeletal muscle relaxation is usually excellent if an appropriate dose of local anesthetic is administered. A major disadvantage of regional anesthesia is the occasional failure to produce adequate anesthesia, necessitating that additional anesthesia be given, usually by the inhalation or intravenous route. As far as operating-room efficiency is concerned, proper plans and logistics must be made, or regional anesthesia has the possibility of increasing time between cases.

Despite the limitations described above, there are some suggestions that regional anesthesia indeed does have advantages in certain situations. Blood loss from total hip arthroplasty and prostatectomy is clearly reduced by spinal or epidural anesthesia. Thromboembolic complications following total hip arthroplasty may be reduced by the use of a local anesthetic. Also, regional anesthesia may reduce postoperative impairment of pulmonary function. More recently, regional anesthesia has been shown to prevent postoperative impairment of some immune functions, although the relationship to postoperative infection has not been established. Lastly, the time of convalescence may be less with regional anesthesia. These proposed advantages require an epidemiologic study involving hundreds or perhaps thousands of patients to ascertain whether these and other advantages of regional anesthesia are in fact true. As indicated with general anesthesia, regional anesthesia is facilitated by an anesthesiologist skilled with these procedures.

SPINAL AND EPIDURAL ANESTHESIA

Spinal anesthesia is usually produced by inserting the local anesthetic into the lumbar intrathecal space. The local anesthetic then blocks nerve conduction in the spinal nerve routes, dorsal route ganglia, and probably the periphery of the spinal cord. Epidural anesthesia is accomplished by injecting the local anesthetic into the extradural space, usually in the lumbar area. Another form of epidural anesthesia is "caudal" anesthesia, in which the local anesthetic is deposited into the epidural space when the needle is introduced into the sacral hiatus. The epidural space is that compartment between the dura mater and the bony ligamentous walls of the spinal canal. It is a potential space filled with fat and the internal vertebral plexus of veins. Either spinal or epidural anesthesia has the advantage of providing anesthesia selectively in regard to the surgical site. In addition, the patient may be awake or sedated. As indicated above, profound muscle relaxation can be achieved without the use of neuromuscular blocking drugs, such as pancuronium or d-tubocurarine. The gastrointestinal tract is usually contracted, which facilitates exposure within the abdominal cavity for the surgeon. Despite these advantages, bias often exists against the use of spinal or epidural anesthesia. Often these biases are based on the patient's fear of being awake and the surgeon's concern that the block may be inadequate, resulting in a delay in starting the operation while the anesthesiologist induces general anesthesia.

The circulatory responses to epidural and spinal anesthesia are a result of peripheral sympathetic nervous system blockade. Because the level of sympathetic blockade is about two dermatomes higher than that of a sensory blockade, a sensory level of T3 will result in a total sympathetic blockade. This will result in decreases in arterial blood pressure and central venous pressure. The decrease in blood pressure is primarily due to a decrease in cardiac output, secondary to pooling of blood in denervated veins. Treatment of hypotension during spinal anesthesia is to increase venous return, which facilitates cardiac output. This objective is best achieved by a modest Trendelenburg position, administration of crystalloids intravenously, or a small dose of a vasopressor, such as ephedrine, 10 to 25 mg/70 kg intravenously.

The most common complication of a spinal anesthetic is a postoperative headache. The mildest forms of postspinal headache can be treated conservatively by enforcing bed rest for 24 to 48 h. In severe cases, a "blood patch" epidural should be administered, in which 5 to 10 mL of the patient's own blood is introduced into the epidural space. This results in over 95 percent success of obliterating the postspinal headache. Urinary retention is also a complication; neurologic sequelae are extremely rare.

In most respects, epidural anesthesia is similar to spinal anesthesia, except that the circulatory responses are more gradual in onset. The major site of action of the local anesthetic placed in the epidural space is probably at the nerve roots and dorsal root ganglion beyond the point of the meningeal covering.

PERIPHERAL NERVE BLOCKS

The most common peripheral nerve blocks performed are those related to the upper extremity. The brachial plexus can be blocked by three approaches, namely, the axillary, supraclavicular, or interscalene. Also, the radial, ulnar, and median nerves can be blocked at the elbow or wrist. The upper and lower extremity can be blocked by the "Bier block." This block is performed by placing a tourniquet proximal to the site of an intravenous injection of an appropriate volume of local anesthetic. The local anesthetic effect can be terminated by releasing the tourniquet. Obviously a major hazard of this technique is the premature release of the tourniquet, allowing an excessive dose of local anesthetic to enter the circulation and, therefore, the brain, causing convulsions. However, if the tourniquet is properly applied, this complication is indeed rare.

Other nerve blocks performed less frequently include intercostal nerve blocks for postoperative pain relief and sciatic-femoral nerve block for surgery of the lower extremities. Unfortunately, peripheral nerve blocks are not a major component of anesthesia given intraoperatively because of the discomfort they cause when inexperienced individuals are administering them and the time they require.

Special Techniques

Several techniques that can be used in anesthesia may result in decreased blood loss and/or decreased metabolism. Recognizing the concern regarding the infectivity of blood transfusions (e.g., posttransfusion hepatitis and AIDS), the overall indications for blood transfusions intraoperatively have been reexamined, which is the subject of other chapters in this text. There are techniques that anesthesiologists can utilize to decrease the amount of blood lost, and therefore the amount of blood required during surgery.

METHODS TO DECREASE BLOOD TRANSFUSIONS

DELIBERATE HYPOTENSION. Deliberate (or controlled) hypotension is an anesthetic technique in which arterial blood pressure is decreased electively to decrease blood loss during surgery and to provide a dry surgical field for the surgeon. In certain operative procedures (e.g., plastic surgery) deliberate hypotension is said to facilitate the surgical procedure from a technical point of view. Numerous techniques and drugs have been used to lower arterial blood pressure, including ganglionic blockers and deep levels of general anesthesia. The most common operative procedures in which deliberate hypotension is used are neurosurgery, total hip arthroplasty, plastic surgery, and operations for head and neck cancer.

It is not known precisely what the absolute contraindications to this technique should be. For example, the brain can tolerate a mean arterial blood pressure of 55 mmHg, but the lower limits and the influence of specific diseases have not been defined. In general, patients who have had strokes, transient ischemic attacks, myocardial infarctions within the previous 3 years, renal disease, previous renal transplant, and untreated hypertension should not be considered for deliberate hypotension.

AUTOTRANSFUSION. Autotransfusion therapy is performed by using one of three approaches: preoperative removal and storage; immediate preoperative phlebotomy and hemodilution; and intraoperative blood salvage and retransfusion. The latter technique is of prime importance in terms of anesthesia involvement. The concept of transfusing a patient's own blood and retrieving it during surgery to maintain circulatory stability is attractive. However, this approach has been fraught with complications, including hemolysis, coagulation disorders, microembolism (fat, denatured protein, microaggregates such as platelets and leukocytes), air embolism, and sepsis and metastasis if used in patients with infection or malignancy.

The technology has improved so that the incidence of the first four complications listed above has been reduced or nearly eliminated with use of the appropriate blood-salvage apparatus. Obviously, the transmission of bacteria or cancer cells is still a problem.

HEMODILUTION. Hemodilution and autologous transfusions are now being used for open heart surgery. Basically, this is an extension of the preoperative form of autologous transfusion by infusion of a hemodiluent in one vein and simultaneous phlebotomy from another vein to produce a state of normovolemic anemia. Specifically, one or two units of blood from an arterial cannula can be withdrawn into plastic bags containing citrate phosphate dextrose solution. After phlebotomy, blood pressure and heart rate are maintained with crystalloid administration and, when needed, homologous blood. The autologous blood is then transfused at the end of perfusion after the administration of protamine. Many clinicians have reported successful use of this technique. Obviously, the value of hemodilution and autologous transfusion lies in the fact that significantly less homologous blood will be needed.

HYPOTHERMIA

When the body is cooled, the metabolism decreases at about 8 percent/°C to one-half normal at 28°C. Hypothermia is used clinically to reduce metabolic rate, rendering the brain and other metabolically active organs less susceptible to periods of ischemia or hypoxia. Hypothermia is used mainly for cardiac and neurosurgery.

Special Anesthetic Problems

ASPIRATION PNEUMONITIS

A major hazard of anesthesia is vomiting and aspiration of gastric contents during anesthesia. When the airway is unprotected, especially during induction and emergence from anesthesia, this complication is most likely to occur. Although undigested food may be aspirated, producing airway obstruction and respiratory distress, the more common problem is aspiration of gastric secretions, which have a pH below 2.5. Aspiration of such acid material can produce sudden bronchospasm, tachypnea, diffuse rales, cyanosis, and hypotension. Cardiac arrest may occur in severe cases.

The most important measure in preventing aspiration of gastric contents is to minimize the time that the airway is unprotected. Generally, any patient who has eaten within 8 h of surgery should be considered to have a full stomach and, therefore, to be at risk of vomiting during induction. In a patient who has pain or is pregnant, gastric emptying may be delayed, and the interval between eating and elective surgery probably should be lengthened to at least 12 h. Various antacids have been utilized to neutralize the gastric pH. Specifically, drinking sodium citrate will raise the gastric pH in most patients, but it must be given 45 to 75 min before induction of anesthesia. If time does not permit such a wait, either endotracheal intubation with the patient being awake or a rapid sequence induction of anesthesia should be performed.

MALIGNANT HYPERTHERMIA

Malignant hyperthermia can occur soon after the induction of anesthesia in patients with this inherited disease. The onset of malignant hyperthermia can be acute and rapid, particularly during induction of anesthesia with an inhaled anesthetic, or the use of succinylcholine. The course of malignant hyperthermia can be extraordinarily rapid, including a striking increase in metabolism, resulting in an intense production of heat, carbon dioxide, and lactate, and associated respiratory and metabolic acidosis. If untreated, the fatality rate is extremely high. Treatment should include all conceivable cooling measures and the administration of dantrolene up to 10 mg/kg intravenously.

Patients who require anesthesia and are known to be susceptible to malignant hyperthermia should be pretreated with dantrolene for 1 to 3 days, and given anesthetics known not to trigger the syndrome, which include narcotics, barbiturates, nitrous oxide, and ester local anesthetics.

HEPATOTOXICITY

Over 20 years ago, halothane administration was proposed to be unrelated to massive postoperative hepatic necrosis and to be safe for use in hepatobiliary surgery. Massive hepatic necrosis has been associated with other anesthetics and may be related to other conditions (i.e., blood transfusions, hypovolemic shock). Still, in the rare patient, halothane appears to cause a form of hepatitis. The most recent theory is that the cellular susceptibility to damage from halothane occurs after exposure to electrophilic drug metabolites. The predisposing factor is familial and constitutional, but presently there is no method of preoperatively identifying those rare patients who may be susceptible to developing massive hepatic necrosis from halothane.

RECURRENT MYOCARDIAL INFARCTION

If a patient has had a myocardial infarction preoperatively, he or she may have an increased risk of postoperative myocardial infarction. This increased risk is related to the time since the previous infarction. The risk of postoperative myocardial infarction decreases to about 5 percent (50 times the normal risk) 6 months after the first infarction. Therefore, elective surgery, especially thoracic and upper abdominal procedures, should be delayed for 6 months. The incidence of myocardial infarction is increased in patients having intrathoracic or intraabdominal operations lasting more than 3 h. There is no correlation between risk and the site of previous infarction, the site of surgery if less than 3 h in duration, or choice of anesthetic drugs or techniques. Close hemodynamic monitoring using intraarterial and/or pulmonary artery catheters and prompt treatment of hypotension or hypertension decrease the risk of periperative infarction in high-risk patients.

POSTANESTHETIC ROOM (RECOVERY ROOM)

General Considerations

The postanesthetic or recovery room is that area designated for the monitoring and care of patients who are recovering from the immediate physiologic derangements produced by anesthesia and surgery. This room should be staffed with specially trained nurses skilled in the prompt recognition of postoperative complications. Such complications include upper-airway obstruction, arterial hypoxemia, alveolar hypoventilation, hypotension, hypertension, cardiac dysrhythmias and agitation (emergence delirium). Location of the recovery room in close proximity to the operating rooms assures rapid access to physician consultation and assistance. Specifically, a qualified physician, usually an anesthesiologist, should be readily available and responsible to ensure the patient's safe recovery from anesthesia. Equipment and drugs must be available to provide routine care (supplemental oxygen, suction, monitoring of vital signs, electrocardiogram and advanced organ support, ventilators, transducers to monitor intravascular pressures, devices for continuous infusion of drugs). An electrical defibrillator and appropriate drugs to assist in the optimal provision of cardiopulmonary resuscitation must also be available. The recovery room should have good access to radiographic and arterial blood gas services. The size of the recovery room is determined by the number and type of operative procedures, with approximately 1.5 recovery room beds necessary for every operating room.

Pain Relief

Pain is a predictable response as the effects of anesthetic drugs wane in the early postoperative period. Postoperative pain is influenced by patient age and personal interaction of physicians and nurses with the patient. In general, greater personal contact between health care professionals and the patient will reduce the amount of pharmacologic pain relief required. Treatment of postoperative pain is usually with incremental doses of intravenous narcotics, usually morphine in a dose of 15 to 30 μg/kg. In the future, continuous intravenous infusion of a low dose of narcotic may be used to provide more consistent and optimal analgesia with minimal respiratory depression. Continuous thoracic or lumbar epidural blockade with a long-acting local anesthetic such as bupivacaine is also an effective method of providing postoperative analgesia.

The epidural administration of a narcotic, usually morphine, has proved to be an innovative method of producing postoperative analgesia. In this situation, patients can have complete relief of pain with no autonomic sensory or motor blockade. This technique has been limited because of the rare occurrence of postoperative respiratory depression several hours after the administration of the narcotic epidurally. Once this rare complication is eliminated, it is this author's opinion that this technique will become a dominant form of postoperative pain relief. Patient-controlled analgesia is frequently used, in which a dilute form of narcotic is infused by control of the patient using various devices that will not allow an excessive dose of narcotic to be administered.

MONITORED ANESTHESIA CARE (STANDBY ANESTHESIA)

Monitored anesthesia care, often termed standby anesthesia, refers to the intravenous administration of sedative hypnotics (e.g., diazepam or midazolam) and/or narcotics (e.g., fentanyl) while the surgeon uses local infiltration of local anesthetic. Often, these types of cases do not require an anesthesiologist. However, in the elderly or fragile patient (especially those with an unprotected airway), these cases can be as challenging or complex as those cases in which the patient undergoes general anesthesia. In such cases, anesthesiologists will monitor the patients and titrate the appropriate drugs to provide sedation. This is particularly challenging to administer the appropriate amount of sedative drugs in a patient whose airway is unprotected.

ANESTHESIA AND AMBULATORY SURGERY

Increasingly, surgery is being performed on a "come-and-go" basis. Approximately 20 to 40 percent of a hospital's inpatient surgery could be performed in an outpatient setting. Compared with inpatient surgery, the advantages of performing the same operation on an outpatient basis include a decrease in medical costs, increased availability of beds for patients who require hospitalization, protection from hospital-acquired infections, and avoidance of the disruption of the family unit attendant upon hospitalization. Patients who report to the hospital on the day of surgery must be given detailed instructions well in advance of surgery. Local or general anesthesia usually is used in ambulatory surgical procedures, although epidural anesthesia can be used. Spinal anesthesia is inadvisable because of the possibility of postanesthetic headache. Recovery from anesthesia is accompanied by a return of vital signs to a normal level of consciousness and the ability to walk without assistance. Nausea, vomiting, and vertigo should be absent, and the patient should not have excessive pain. The patient should be able to drink fluids.

The ambulatory surgical patient should be reminded that mental clarity and dexterity may remain impaired for a period of 24 to 48 h, despite an overall feeling of well-being. Driving motor vehicles or operating complex equipment should not be attempted during this period. Finally, the patient should be given the physician's telephone number and instructed to report any new symptoms or other concerns.

Bibliography

Anesthetic Risks

Davies JM, Strunin L: Anesthesia in 1984: How safe is it? *Can Med Assoc J* 131:437,1984.

Hamilton WK: Unexpected deaths during anesthesia: Wherein lies the cause? *Anesthesiology* 7:25, 1979.

Keats AS: What do we know about anesthetic mortality? *Anesthesiology* 50:387, 1979.

Keenan RL, Boyan CP: Cardiac arrest due to anesthesia: A study of incidences and causes. *JAMA* 253:2373, 1985.

Tinker JH, Roberts SL: Anesthetic risk, in Miller RD (ed): *Anesthesia,* 2d ed. New York, Churchill Livingstone, 1986, chap 10.

Preoperative Evaluation

Egbert LD, Battit GE, et al: The value of the preoperative visit by an anesthetist. *JAMA* 185:553, 1963.

Kaplan EB, et al: The usefulness of preoperative laboratory screening. *JAMA* 253:3576, 1985.

Immediate Preoperative Care and Preparation

Britt BA, Joy N, et al: Positioning trauma, in Orkin FK, Cooperman LH (eds): *Complications in Anesthesiology.* Philadelphia, Lippincott, 1983, chap 51.

Eichhorn JH, Cooper JB, et al: Standards for patient monitoring during anesthesia at Harvard Medical School. *JAMA,* 256:1017, 1986.

Roizen MF: Routine preoperative evaluation, in Miller RD (ed): *Anesthesia,* 2d ed. New York, Churchill Livingstone, 1986, chap 8.

Stone DR, Downs JB, et al: Adult body temperature and heated humidification of anesthetic gases during general anesthesia. *Anesth Analg* 60:736, 1981.

Intraoperative Anesthesia

Cutler BS: Avoidance of hemologous transfusion in aortic operations: The roles of autotransfusion, hemodilution, and surgical technique. *Surgery* 95:717, 1984.

El-Hassan KM: Venous pressure and arm volume changes during simulated Bier's block. *Anaesthesia* 39:229, 1984.

Fahmy NR: Nitroprusside versus nitroprusside-triemethophan mixture for induced hypotension: A comparison of hemodynamic effects and cyanide release. *Anesthesiology* 61:A40, 1984.

Farrell G, Prendergast D, et al: Halothane hepatitis: Detection of a constitutional susceptibility factor. *N Engl J Med* 313:1310, 1985.

Flacke JW, Bloor BC, et al: Comparison of morphine, meperidine, fentanyl, and sufentanil in balanced anesthesia: A double blind study. *Anesth Analg* 64:897, 1985.

Ghoneim MM, et al: Comparison of four opioid analgesics as supplements to nitrous oxide anesthesia. *Anesth Analg* 63:405, 1984.

Goldman L: Cardiac risk and complications of noncardiac surgery. *Ann Surg* 198:780, 1983.

Gronert GA: Malignant hyperthermia, in Miller RD (ed): *Anesthesia,* 2d ed. New York, Churchill Livingstone, 1986, chap 56.

Kehlet H: Does regional anesthesia reduce postoperative morbidity? *Intensive Care Med* 10:165, 1984.

Little PE, et al: Site of action of intravenous regional anesthesia. *Anesthesiology* 61:507, 1984.

Manchikanti L, Marrero TC, et al: Preanesthetic cimetidine and metoclopramide for acid aspiration phrophylaxis in elective surgery. *Anesthesiology* 61:48, 1984.

McAuley CE, Watson CG: Effective inguinal herniorrhaphy after myocardial infarction. *Surg Gynecol Obstet* 159:36, 1984.

Nilsson A, et al: Midazolam as induction agent prior to inhalational anesthesia: A comparison with thiopentone. *Acta Anaesthesiol Scand* 28:249, 1984.

Rao TKL, Jacobs KH, et al: Reinfarction following anesthesia in patients with myocardial infarction. *Anesthesiology* 59:499, 1983.

Rogers SN, Benumof JL: New and easy technique for fiberoptic endoscopy-aided tracheal intubation. *Anesthesiology* 59:569, 1983.

Schmidt JF, Schierup L, et al: The effect of sodium citrate on the pH and the amount of gastric contents before general anesthesia. *Acta Anaesthesiol Scand* 28:263, 1984.

Weymuller EA Jr, Bishop MJ, et al: Quantification of intralaryngeal pressure exerted by endotracheal tubes. *Ann Otol Rhinol Laryngol* 92:444, 1983.

Postanesthetic Room (Recovery Room)

Catley DM, Thornton C, et al: Pronounced, episodic oxygen desaturation in the postoperative period: Its association with ventilatory pattern and analgesic regimen. *Anesthesiology* 63:20, 1985.

Cucchieri RJ, Morran CG, et al: Postoperative pain and pulmonary complication: Comparison of three analgesic regimens. *Br J Surg* 72:495, 1984.

Glenski JA, Warner MA, et al: Postoperative use of epidurally administered morphine in children and adolescents. *Mayo Clin Proc* 59:530, 1984.

Rodriguez JL, Weissman C, et al: Morphine and postoperative rewarming in critically ill patients. *Circulation* 68:1238, 1983.

Slotman GJ, Jed EH, et al: Adverse effects of hypothermia in postoperative patients. *Am J Surg* 149:495, 1985.

Wallace LM: Surgical patients' expectations of pain and discomfort: Does accuracy of expectations minimize post-surgical pain and distress? *Pain* 22:363, 1985.

Anesthesia and Ambulatory Surgery

Carter JA, Dye AM, et al: Recovery from day-case anaesthesia: The effects of different inhalational anaesthetic agents. *Anaesthesia* 40:545, 1985.

Natof HE: Complications associated with ambulatory surgery. *JAMA* 244:1116, 1980.

Ryan JA Jr, Adye BA, et al: Outpatient inguinal herniorrhaphy with both regional and local anesthesia. *Ann J Surg* 148:313, 1984.

Chapter 12

Complications

Seymour I. Schwartz

GENERAL CONSIDERATIONS

Surgical care must encompass an appreciation and anticipation of postoperative complications that may result from the disease process per se, errors of omission, or errors of commission in technique. In regarding the patient postoperatively, any deviation from the anticipated norm for clinical evaluation and/or diagnostic findings should alert one to focus on complications of the disease and also to retrace the operative procedure. It is unusual, although certainly possible, that clinical and laboratory abnormalities may be caused by the chance occurrence of an unrelated disease during the postoperative period. Acute cholecystitis and appendicitis are two examples of diseases that may become manifest during the postoperative course of the patient.

CHRONOLOGIC CONSIDERATIONS. Fever that presents shortly after surgical treatment in a patient who was previously afebrile is generally related to atelectasis or aspiration. Fever may also appear early in the postoperative course secondary to urinary tract infection, particularly if the patient has been catheterized. Fever of wound infection and leakage of an intestinal anastomosis or closure more frequently become evident on the fourth to seventh postoperative day. Hypotension in the early postoperative phase may be due to continued hemorrhage or the effects of depressive drugs that have been administered during the recovery period. Hypotension later in the postoperative course in a patient with sepsis should alert one to the possibility of septic shock.

WOUND COMPLICATIONS

Wound Dehiscence

Wound disruption, or dehiscence, generally refers to a separation of an abdominal wound involving the anterior fascial sheath and deeper layers. The inaccuracy of computing the frequency of wound disruption is notorious; the incidence in the literature ranges from 0.5 to 3 percent, averaging 2.6 percent when all abdominal operations are considered collectively. The incidence is definitely related to age and is reported to be 1.3 percent for patients under forty-five years in contrast to 5.4 percent for those over forty-five years. There is a higher incidence in elderly, debilitated patients with poor nutrition and in the presence of significant ascites or jaundice. Carcinoma is also associated with an increased incidence. Over 5 percent of laparotomies in patients in whom cancer was found are reported to have wound disruption in contrast to a 2 percent incidence when laparotomy demonstrates a benign condition. Other general factors that have been implicated include hypoproteinemia and atelectasis with its associated coughing, which, along with retching and hiccuping, increases the intraabdominal pressure and puts a strain on the incision. Obesity is definitely associated with an increased incidence. A lack of correlation between anemia and wound disruption has been reported.

Local factors involved in wound disruption include hemorrhage, infection, excessive suture material, and poor technique. Several series have suggested that the incidence of wound dehiscence is increased with vertical incisions. Recently this has been refuted in a prospective randomized series. When an intestinal stoma or a drain is brought out through any incision, the incidence of wound dehiscence increases.

A multicentric randomized prospective trial compared continuous and interrupted sutures of polyglycolic acid with close midline abdominal incisions. The overall dehiscence rate was 1.6 percent in patients with continuous versus 2 percent in the patients with interrupted sutures. The dehiscence rate in the interrupted group was significantly higher than in the continuous group when the wounds were contaminated. No significant difference has been noted between polyglycolic acid and polygalactin sutures.

CLINICAL MANIFESTATIONS. Most disruptions are concealed in the deeper layers of the wound and do not manifest until the fifth postoperative day, although the separation may, in fact, occur in the operating room or recovery room. The presenting sign that precedes the diagnosis of dehiscence in about 85 percent of cases is serosanguineous drainage from the wound, and if this occurs more than 24 h postoperatively, it is virtually pathognomonic. Frequently, wound dehiscence becomes manifest when the skin sutures are removed and evisceration of intraperitoneal contents, either intestine or omentum, occurs. In some instances, wound disruptions remain concealed beneath an intact cutaneous closure and go unrecognized initially, only to become manifest later in the form of a postoperative ventral hernia.

TREATMENT. The management depends on the patient's condition. If the patient can tolerate the procedure, a secondary operative closure is indicated. The author prefers through-and-through horizontal mattress sutures placed

superficial to the peritoneum or buried figure-of-eight monofilament stainless steel sutures to approximate the muscle and fascial layers. In some instances, it is preferable to treat the patient conservatively with an occlusive wound dressing and binder and to accept the complication of a postoperative hernia. If evisceration occurs, sterile moist towels should be applied to cover the extruded intestine or omentum, and the patient should be taken directly to the operating room. After general irrigation, the abdomen is closed with one of the two previously mentioned techniques.

The mortality associated with wound disruption depends on the patient's age and original pathologic condition. Although one recent series reported that 34 percent of patients died after operative closure of an abdominal wound evisceration, most authorities report that the mortality has been reduced to 0.5 to 0.3 percent in recent years. The main morbidity is prolonged hospitalization. The incidence of postoperative hernia is hard to define but has been reported to be at least 32 percent.

Wound Infection

Postoperative wound infection results when bacteria within the wound multiply, exciting a local reaction and, frequently, a systemic response. Most wounds become infected in the operating room while they are open, but the presence of bacteria in the wound at the end of the surgical procedure does not usually result in a wound infection. The bacterium most frequently implicated is *Staphylococcus aureus*. Enteric organisms are the causative agents when bowel operation has been performed, and hemolytic streptococci account for about 3 percent of infections. Other common pathogens include enterococci, *Pseudomonas, Proteus,* and *Klebsiella.*

The reported incidence of wound infection has a wide range. The Public Health Laboratory Service of England and Wales reported an overall wound infection rate of 9.7 percent. In a combined study conducted by the Division of Medical Sciences, National Academy of Science-National Research Council, and reported in 1964, the overall incidence of infection in five participating hospitals varied from 3 to 11.1 percent. Clean atraumatic and uninfected operative wounds in which neither the bronchi, nor the gastrointestinal tract, nor the genitourinary tract was entered and which were elective, primarily closed, and undrained had an overall incidence of definite infection of 3.3 percent, while similar wounds that were either not elective, or not primarily closed, or drained mechanically through the incision or via a stab wound had a 7.4 percent incidence of wound infection. Operative wounds in which the bronchus, gastrointestinal tract, or oropharyngeal cavity were entered but without unusual contamination had an overall incidence of infection of 10.8 percent. Open, fresh traumatic wounds, operations with a major break in sterile technique, and incisions encountering acute nonpurulent inflammation were associated with an incidence of wound infections of 16.3 percent. Old traumatic wounds and those involving abscesses of perforated viscera had the highest rate of infection (28.6 percent).

A variety of factors other than the nature of the wound also influence the incidence of infection. Age is a definite factor; the rate of wound infection rises steadily from 4.7 percent in the fifteen- to twenty-four-year-old group to 10.7 percent in the sixty-five to seventy-four-year-old group. There is virtually no difference in sex and race. The presence of diabetes is associated with an increase in infection rate, but when this is adjusted for age, there is no statistical significance to this figure. Steroid therapy affects the wound infection rate adversely; an incidence of 16 percent for patients receiving steroids has been contrasted with 7 percent for those not on such drugs. Patients who are extremely obese also have a more than doubled rate of wound infection when compared with control groups. In the combined study, patients with severe malnutrition also displayed a markedly increased rate of wound infection, but this was distorted by other factors, which, if corrected, cast doubt on the widely held belief that malnourished patients are intrinsically more susceptible. Patients who harbor infections remote from the operative incision have an increased infection rate. The duration of operation exerts a profound influence on wound infection, the incidence rising steadily from 3.6 percent for procedures lasting less than 30 min to 18 percent for those lasting over 6 h. The urgency of operation only indirectly influences the wound infection rate.

The use of a drain was associated with an 11 percent infection rate, whereas undrained wounds had a rate of 5 percent, but it could not be concluded that the drains themselves were responsible for the infection. Patients hospitalized for fewer than 2 days preoperatively had an infection rate of 6 percent, whereas those hospitalized for periods greater than 3 weeks preoperatively had a rate of 14 percent, and this relationship could not be explained on the basis of other associated factors. The prophylactic use of antibiotics was paradoxically associated with a much higher wound infection rate in the combined series, and similar findings were reported for orthopaedic cases. In contrast, Ketcham et al., in a double-blind study, reported a reduction of wound infection in patients with extensive cancer who were placed on prophylactic antibiotics. In addition preoperative and early postoperative use of cephalosporin or metronidazole reduced the incidence of wound infection in patients in whom segments of stomach or intestine were opened.

The two factors of importance in the genesis of infection are breaks in surgical technique and the host-parasite relationship. Two potential sources of contamination are patients themselves, particularly the gastrointestinal tract, and the environment of the operating room including the operating team. Carriers of *Staph. aureus* in the hospital population have become an increasing source. It has been demonstrated that patients who are nasal carriers of *Staph. aureus* have a higher incidence of wound infection than noncarriers.

CLINICAL MANIFESTATIONS. In a typical situation about 3 to 4 days following operation, there is some increase in pulse rate, and about the fourth postoperative day, a low-grade, intermittent fever is noted. Usually there is edema and redness of the wound, but the most important early sign is undue pain. In some types, marked thrombosis of surrounding blood vessels is an important feature. Wound dehiscence is usually not caused by infection per se unless the infection is neglected. The diagnosis is usually made on the fifth to seventh day, but this interval may be extended if the patient has been on antibiotics. At that time, the wound is commonly seen as a suppurative process, essentially an abscess. Systemic features of septicemia may be present.

TREATMENT. The most important prophylactic measure is excellent technique. In human volunteers, Elek and Conen have shown that the presence of suture material enhances the infective power of *Staph. aureus* 1000 to 10,000 times. Therefore, fine sutures and accurate hemostasis should reduce the incidence. It is generally felt that prophylactic antibiotics do not contribute to a reduction in the incidence of wound infection. In patients undergoing intestinal resections, wound irrigation with a cephalosporin has reduced the incidence of infection. Irrigation of subcutaneous tissue with povidone-iodine significantly reduced the incidence of wound infection following a variety of surgical procedures in one series. Other studies, however, have shown no greater protection than that achieved with saline irrigation and less than that with local cephaloridine.

Once diagnosed, the treatment consists of surgical drainage. The skin sutures should be removed and the wound irrigated with saline solution and lightly packed. As a general principle, antimicrobial drugs are not required unless the offending organism is *Streptococcus pyogenes* or hemolytic streptococci, which should be treated with penicillin for a period of at least 1 week. Also, patients with wound infections around the central area of the face should receive antimicrobial therapy to prevent intracranial extension. Finally, if the wound sepsis is associated with bacteremia or spreading cellulitis, antimicrobial therapy is also indicated. The antibiotic used is determined by culture and sensitivity studies of the infected wound.

See Chap. 5 for a discussion of specific infections, i.e., staphylococcal infections, streptococcal infections, anaerobic clostridial cellulitis, clostridial myonecrosis, streptococcal myositis, and tetanus.

Wound Hemorrhage, Hematoma, and Seroma (Accumulation of Serum)

Wound hemorrhage is generally related to an error in technique in which hemostasis is not accomplished. There is a higher incidence in patients with polycythemia vera, myeloproliferative disorders, or coagulation defects and in patients receiving anticoagulant therapy (see Chap. 3). Postoperative hemorrhage usually becomes manifest with a sensation of pressure or pain within the wound shortly after the patient awakes from anesthesia. There may be leakage of sanguineous or serosanguineous material at that time. To control bleeding from the wound edges, pressure may be applied initially, but if the bleeding continues, additional sutures or reexploration of the wound may be required.

The placement of drains in areas of anticipated wound bleeding is usually not indicated. If the bleeding is trivial, the drain is unnecessary; if the bleeding is severe, it will not evacuate the material. Drains or catheters connected to closed suction are appropriately used to evacuate serous fluid from underneath skin flaps, such as that associated with mastectomy or neck or groin dissection, in order to prevent the vicious cycle in which an expanding serous collection produces significant bleeding as it separates the wound. If a large skin flap has been raised, fluid will develop, and in order to facilitate apposition between the subcutaneous tissue and deep fascia, drainage should be effected. This obviates formation of a seroma.

Once a seroma develops, it should be aspirated initially; if multiple aspirations are required, a polyethylene catheter may be inserted and attached to negative suction. Prompt treatment is indicated, since the presence of contained serous fluid increases the incidence of subcutaneous infection. The same situation pertains to a subcutaneous hematoma, and drainage is required, since the blood affords an excellent culture medium and also prevents apposition between the two surfaces.

POSTOPERATIVE PAROTITIS

Postoperative parotitis is a serious complication and is associated with a high mortality related to it and to the primary disease with which it is associated. Recent reviews indicate a real recrudescence related to the increasing age of the surgical population. The right and left glands are involved equally, and in 10 to 15 percent of cases, the disease presents bilaterally. Seventy-five percent of patients are seventy years or older, and the overwhelming majority have associated diseases. Patients having major abdominal surgical treatment, fractured hip, debilitating diseases, and severe injury are among the most commonly afflicted.

The factors implicated in the etiology include poor oral hygiene, dehydration, and the use of anticholinergic drugs. In one large series, one-third of the patients with acute suppurative parotitis had carcinoma, and one-half had preexisting major infection elsewhere in the body. In only one-third of the cases in this series the acute suppurative process developed in the postoperative period.

The pathogenesis is thought to be a transductal inoculation of the parotid, and the majority of infections are due to staphylococci. The combination of poor oral hygiene and lack of oral intake to stimulate parotid secretions predisposes to bacterial invasion of Stensen's duct. The inflammatory lesions of early parotitis are confined to an accumulation of cells within the larger ducts. The parenchyma of the smaller ducts are initially spared, but once penetration of the parenchyma occurs, multiple abscesses form and later coalesce. If the process continues, the purulent material penetrates the capsule and invades the surrounding tissue along one of three routes: downward into the deep fascial planes of the neck, backward into the external auditory canal, or outward into the skin of the face.

CLINICAL MANIFESTATIONS. The interval between operation and the onset of parotitis varies from a few hours to many weeks. The patient initially presents with pain in the parotid region. The pain is usually unilateral but may become bilateral in a short period of time. Initially, inspection shows the gland to be slightly swollen, and palpation demonstrates exquisite tenderness. Because of the septate anatomy of the gland, fluctuance is rarely demonstrable. The course of postoperative parotitis is rapid and fulminating with severe cellulitis developing on the affected side of the face and neck. The temperature and leukocyte count may be extremely high. Obstruction of the airway may necessitate tracheostomy, and the abscess may rupture into adjacent structures of the ear, mastoid, pharynx, or anterior and posterior triangles of the neck. Parotitis is to be differentiated from benign postoperative swelling of the parotids, which occurs more frequently in Blacks and may be related to straining, atropine, and neuromuscular depolarizing drugs.

TREATMENT. Prophylactic therapy consists of adequate hydration and good oral hygiene that can be aided by allowing the patient to take ice chips and stimulating salivary flow. Prophylactic antibiotics are of no apparent value.

Once the diagnosis is entertained, pus should be expressed from Stensen's duct and culture and sensitivity tests performed. A broad-spectrum antibiotic that acts against the staphylococci should be started while awaiting results. In one series of 66 glands cultured, 64 contained staphylococci. In some cases, these were combined with streptococci, gram-negative bacilli, and pneumococci. If there is considerable pain and the disease is less than 48 h old, irradiation of the gland in small doses is indicated. Irradiation may provide symptomatic relief by reducing the secretions of the obstructed gland, but this type of therapy does not affect the course of the disease as much as antibiotics or surgical drainage.

Frequent observation of the patient is essential. If the disease persists or progresses, drainage should be considered as early as the third day. If there is moderate improvement, drainage may be delayed for a day or two, but in no circumstance should it be delayed beyond the fifth day. An incision is made anterior to the ear, extending down to the angle of the mandible, and flaps are reflected, exposing the gland. A hemostat is inserted through the capsule and opened in the direction of the course of the branches of the facial nerve. Multiple drainage sites are thus established, and the wound is packed lightly open. Deferring drainage until fluctuation is apparent is unwise. Stimulation of the salivary flow by massage of the gland or other means is contraindicated, once the inflammatory process is established.

PROGNOSIS. In a recent series, the mortality rate approximated 20 percent, but this was frequently related to the patient's basic disease. Thirty-six percent of the patients who died demonstrated active parotitis. In 80 percent of patients treated with incision and drainage, the parotitis was palliated or cured.

POSTOPERATIVE RESPIRATORY COMPLICATIONS

Respiratory Failure

Respiratory failure is the major cause of death after surgical or accidental trauma, accounting for 25 percent of postoperative deaths. It is a significant contributory factor in another 25 percent of postoperative patients. It can be defined as a situation in which the partial pressure of oxygen in arterial blood (Pa_{O_2}) is below 50 torr while the patient is breathing room air, or when the Pa_{CO_2} is above 50 torr in the absence of metabolic alkalosis.

PATHOPHYSIOLOGY. Physiologic causes of acute respiratory insufficiency following surgery include (1) hypoventilation, (2) diffusion defects, (3) abnormalities in the ventilation-perfusion ratio, (4) shunting that is either anatomic or related to atelectasis, (5) reduction in cardiac output with concomitant persistent shunt, and (6) alteration in the hemoglobin level and/or dissociation curve. Respiratory failure occurs when the functional residual capacity (FRC), i.e., the amount of air present in the lung at the end of a normal expiration, is reduced to a level that is associated with alveolar collapse and consequent intrapulmonary shunting that leads to hypoxemia.

A variety of measurements of ventilation and oxygenation have been applied to assess the pathophysiologic events. Ventilatory mechanics are evaluated by measuring the ventilatory rate, the vital capacity (VC), total volume (VT), and dead space (VD). VD/VT, which is also influenced by cardiac output, is used to assess CO_2 elimination. Compliance is a measurement of the distensibility of the lung.

The partial pressure of CO_2 in arterial blood (Pa_{CO_2}) can be considered as a reciprocal function of ventilation and is normally 40 torr. The adequacy of intrapulmonary blood-gas exchange is determined by measuring the Pa_{CO_2} and the Pa_{O_2} in relation to the inspired $F_{I_{O_2}}$. One method of estimating the efficacy of oxygen exchange in the lung is to measure the alveolar-arterial oxygen tension difference [$(A-a)D_{O_2}$]. Factors that influence the $(A-a)D_{O_2}$ include the degree of mismatching of ventilation to perfusion, shunts around the lung, the difference between the arterial and mixed venous oxygen content, the mixed venous oxygen content itself, which may reflect oxygen consumption, the cardiac output, the inspired oxygen concentration ($F_{I_{O_2}}$), the position of the oxygen hemoglobin dissociation curve, and the position of the Pa_{O_2} on the curve. A nomogram can be used to define the calculated amount of blood shunted around the lung as a fraction of the total cardiac output ($\dot{Q}_S/\dot{Q}_T$) based on the measurement of Pa_{O_2} and pulmonary alveolar oxygen tension (PA_{O_2}), as shown in Fig. 12-1. As can be seen, small changes in the $\dot{Q}_S/\dot{Q}_T$ are more readily detected when the patient is breathing 100% oxygen for 20 to 30 min. This may result in absorption atelectasis that will increase

$\dot{Q}_S/\dot{Q}_T$. Therefore, "shunt fraction" is usually measured at the inspired O_2 concentration ($F_{I_{O_2}}$) required to maintain an adequate arterial P_{O_2} (60 to 70 torr or greater). The ratio of arterial P_{O_2} to alveolar P_{O_2} tends to be independent of inspired $F_{I_{O_2}}$. Determinations are affected by alterations in the cardiac output and pH.

PATHOGENESIS. Hypoventilation may be related to thoracic trauma, muscle weakness, and deleterious changes in the respiratory mechanics, which have been shown to exist for several days following thoracotomy and laparotomy. The defects also may be related to the aspiration of gastric content, which is now appreciated to occur more commonly; an incidence of 10 percent has been reported for intubated patients undergoing elective operations, and a higher percentage for patients undergoing emergency operations. There is no evidence that tracheostomy completely protects against such aspiration. Oxygen itself has intrinsic toxicity, and when $F_{I_{O_2}}$ is over 50% for more than 2 to 3 days, destruction of respiratory epithelium may occur. Therefore, it is preferable to maintain patients with respiratory insufficiency at the lowest $F_{I_{O_2}}$ that still maintains a Pa_{O_2} of 70 torr rather than expose the airway to 100% oxygen for a long period of time. Fluid overload with pulmonary edema decreases compliance and impairs gas exchange. Other intrapulmonary lesions that may contribute to interference with oxygenation include microemboli, fat emboli, and pulmonary in-

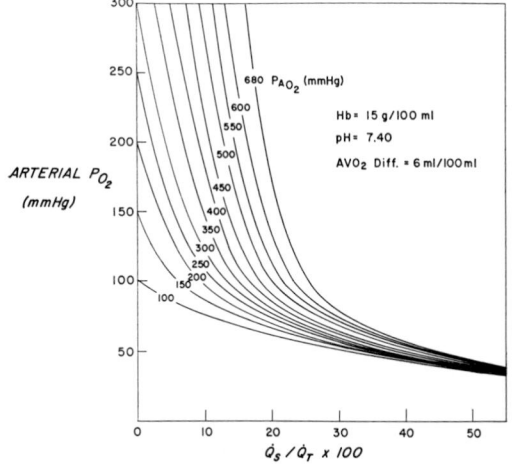

Fig. 12-1. Analog-computed relationship between percent right-to-left shunt ($\dot{Q}_S/\dot{Q}_T \times 100$), arterial P_{O_2}, and inspired oxygen or alveolar oxygen tension (PA_{O_2}). The alveolar-arterial oxygen tension gradient can be obtained by drawing a horizontal line from the ordinate (arterial P_{O_2}) to the appropriate PA_{O_2} line. For example, when $\dot{Q}_S/\dot{Q}_T \times 100 = 20$, and $PA_{O_2} = 680$ mmHg, then the arterial P_{O_2} is approximately 175 mmHg and the $(A-a)D_{O_2} = 680 - 175 = 505$ mmHg. Note that below a right-to-left shunt value of 30, small changes in $\dot{Q}_S/\dot{Q}_T \times 100$ can produce drastic alterations in arterial P_{O_2} particularly when the subject is breathing high concentrations of oxygen. The curves were drawn assuming a hemoglobin concentration of 15 g/100 mL, an arterial pH of 7.40, an $A - V_{O_2}$ difference of 6 mL/100 mL, and a standard oxyhemoglobin dissociation curve. (From: *Pontoppidan H et al: Adv Surg* 4:163, 1970. Copyright 1970 by Year Book Medical Publishers, Chicago. Used by permission. Graphs kindly prepared by Dr. M. A. Duvelleroy.)

fection. Abnormalities of the ventilation-perfusion ratio ($\dot{V}/\dot{Q}$) result when areas well perfused with blood are underventilated. Maintaining the patient in a supine position accentuates this maldistribution, and the resultant consequence of atelectasis is a significant contributor to increased $\dot{V}/\dot{Q}$. Other factors that alter the ventilation-perfusion ratio are obesity and upper abdominal operation with consequent collapse of the basal alveoli. Both atelectasis and reduced cardiac output result in intrapulmonary shunting. A shift in the oxygen-hemoglobin dissociation curve to the left decreases oxygen delivery to the tissues. This may be caused by respiratory alkalosis, by deficiency in 2,3-diphosphoglycerate, which results from transfusion of banked blood more than 3 days old, and by carbon monoxide poisoning, which is commonly present in patients with smoke inhalation associated with burns.

The term "shock lung" is inappropriate. Hemorrhagic shock unassociated with sepsis rarely causes acute pulmonary insufficiency. There is no distinct pathologic lung lesion in patients dying of hemorrhagic shock. $Na^+ - K^+$ transport and adenosine nucleotides in the lung are unchanged in hemorrhagic shock, indicating that cellular energy utilization or production in the lung is unchanged. Sepsis is the most common factor implicated in the development of adult respiratory distress syndrome (ARDS). Almost 20 percent of hospitalized patients with septicemia develop ARDS. The pulmonary insufficiency usually cannot be reversed unless sepsis is controlled. Severe pancreatitis and the fat embolism syndrome also are etiologic factors. ARDS in these patients is an ominous manifestation.

CLINICAL MANIFESTATIONS. Among the situations that should alert the observer to the development of the syndrome of postoperative pulmonary insufficiency are (1) congestive failure, (2) dyspnea, (3) cyanosis, (4) evidence of obstructive lung disease, (5) pulmonary edema, and (6) unexplained deterioration of arterial O_2 tension.

Tachypnea and hypoxemia are the earliest manifestations of respiratory insufficiency. Early in the evolution of the syndrome, the patient manifests hyperventilation associated with a reduction in Pa_{CO_2} below 35 torr that may minimize a significant reduction in Pa_{O_2}. Ultimately there is a reduction in Pa_{O_2} that becomes more significant when the patient does not respond to increases in $F_{I_{O_2}}$. Radiographic changes tend to occur late in the course of the condition and may represent the effects of therapy. These lesions are characteristically scattered, ill-defined, bilateral densities. A correlation exists between the extension of the densities and deterioration of pulmonary function. The diagnosis of ARDS is usually assigned when conservative measures such as oxygen by mask, pulmonary toilet, and/or bronchodilators fail to maintain the Pa_{O_2} above 60 torr.

TREATMENT. Control of postoperative pain can effect a significant reduction in the incidence of pulmonary complications following thoracic or upper abdominal operations. Epidural bupivacaine has been particularly effective. Continuous positive airway pressure (CPAP), administered with a mask, offers an advantage because it requires no effort from the patient, and it is not painful. But attention to respiratory therapy, regardless of the modality employed, may be the most important factor.

The treatment of acute respiratory insufficiency is based primarily on ventilatory support. Specific indications for ventilatory support are listed in Table 12-1. This is accomplished through either an endotracheal tube or a tracheostomy, since ventilation via a face mask or mouthpiece is rarely effective for more than short periods and puts the patient at risk for acute aspiration. Endotracheal intubation, preferably through the nose, is considered the technique of choice when control of airway is urgently required. Although endotracheal tubes are not tolerated as well as tracheostomy tubes and prolonged intubation is associated with laryngeal swelling, 6 days in adults and up to 3 weeks in children are regarded as reasonable periods

Table 12-1. INDICATIONS FOR RESPIRATORY SUPPORT

		Acceptable range	Chest physical therapy, oxygen, close monitoring	Intubation tracheostomy, ventilation
Mechanics	Respiratory rate	12–20	20–30	> 30
	Vital capacity, mL/kg	70–30	30–15	< 15
	Inspiratory force, cmH_2O	100–50	50–25	< 25
Oxygenation	$(A-a)D_{O_2}$, torr*	100–200	200–350	> 350
Ventilation	VD/VT	0.3–0.4	0.4–0.6	> 0.6
	Pa_{CO_2}, torr	35–45	45–50	> 50†
Functional residual capacity (% normal predicted value)		80–100	50–80	< 50
Pulmonary venous admixture (shunt) (Q_{SP}/Q_T) %		<5	15–20	> 20

* After 15 min of 100% O_2.
† Except in chronic hypercapnia.

of prolonged endotracheal intubation. In general, intubation via a nasotracheal route is tolerated better than via the orotracheal route, but insertion may be more difficult. Attempts at swallowing may make an oral tracheal tube advance into the right main stem bronchus, resulting in atelectasis of the left lung. The major advantage of endotracheal intubation is that the mortality is low, the complications are minimal, and the hazards associated with tracheostomy are avoided.

Tracheostomy is now generally reserved for the patient who requires prolonged ventilatory support and may be associated with the complications of stenosis generally related to cuff pressure. The introduction of low-pressure cuffs has reduced the incidence of this complication.

If patients have criteria that indicate the need for ventilatory support (Table 12-1), intubation is carried out and an $F_{I_{O_2}}$ greater than 0.5 may be temporarily required, but this should be rapidly reduced. PEEP is increased in 2 cmH$_2$O increments until a $Pa_{O_2}/F_{I_{O_2}}$ ratio of 250:1 is achieved or, preferably, until the intrapulmonary shunt fraction should be determined to be less than 25 percent. Civetta and associates advise the use of a pulmonary arterial catheter if there is compromise of cardiac function or if a PEEP of 15 cmH$_2$O does not achieve the desired $Pa_{O_2}/F_{I_{O_2}}$ ratio. Intermittent mandatory ventilation (IMV) is increased by two breaths per minute to maintain a pH of 7.35 to 7.45, and a Pa_{CO_2} of 45 torr or less. The ventilatory is set to deliver a volume of 12 to 15 mL/kg body weight. PEEP results in increased functional residual capacity, reduced normal negative intrathoracic pressure with, at times, conversion to positive values, increased venous pressure, and decreased venous return to the heart. PEEP ventilation is particularly effective in causing a rise in Pa_{O_2}, a fall in physiologic shunt, and a decrease in shunting across the lung. PEEP ventilation is preferred for patients with profound hypoxemia, significant physiologic shunting, atelectasis, and high cardiac output. It is particularly appropriate for patients with massive chest wall injuries. PEEP is usually contraindicated for conditions characterized by normal oxygenation, hyperexpansion of the lung, such as pulmonary emphysema, and low cardiac output. PEEP should be increased in increments of 2 to 3 cm of water until the intrapulmonary shunt is reduced to 15 percent. The Pa_{O_2} on 30 percent O$_2$ should reach about 100 torr.

Prolonged artificial ventilation has been characterized by the formation of edema and deterioration of blood-gas interchange, which is generally manageable by water restriction and the administration of diuretic agents. When there is objective evidence that lung function is adequate to permit transfer from artificial to spontaneous ventilation, a gradual weaning process is required. Difficulty in weaning can be attributed to abnormalities in blood-gas exchange, pulmonary mechanics, reduction in cardiac output, and general muscle weakness. A more gradual weaning, employing intermittent mandatory ventilation, may expedite the process. Weaning should be accomplished only with careful monitoring of blood-gas exchange; the pulmonary mechanics are indicated in Table 12-1.

In the weaning process the first priority is to reduce the $F_{I_{O_2}}$ to less than 0.5 to avoid maintaining the collapse of the alveoli. Next, the number of IMV breaths should be decreased to a level that permits a normal pH and a Pa_{CO_2} of 35 to 45 torr at a respiratory rate of less than 30 per min. This is continued until only two mechanical breaths per minute are required. PEEP is lowered in increments of 2 to 3 cmH$_2$O/min monitoring the Pa_{O_2}. When adequate oxygenation is maintained with a PEEP of 5 cmH$_2$O and the IMV is 0 and the CPAP is 5 cmH$_2$O, and the criteria in the early ARDS columns of Table 12-1 are met, the patient generally no longer requires ventilatory support.

Ancillary treatment consists of cardiovascular interventions directed at the preload, contractility, and afterload. Intravascular and extracellular fluid deficits should be corrected. Care is taken to avoid fluid overload of the patient and to maintain the colloidal osmotic pressure of serum. The administration of concentrated albumin solutions to reduce pulmonary edema is ill-advised because the albumin will merely pass into the extravascular spaces. If fluid therapy is necessary to restore ventricular filling pressure, balanced electrolyte solutions are preferable. The administration of diuretics may have a negative net effect on cardiovascular function.

Enhancement of cardiac contractility may be required. Dopamine and/or dobutamine are employed to increase contractility without causing a marked increase in oxygen requirements. Decreasing the afterload by reducing the impedance to cardiac outflow has an additive effect. Drugs such as sodium nitroprusside that decrease arteriolar resistance or venous capacitance may be required.

Atelectasis

Atelectasis comprises 90 percent of all postoperative pulmonary complications, but a lack of definition and difficulty in diagnosis has resulted in a wide range of reported incidences varying between 1 and 80 percent depending on the type of operation. It occurs more commonly after upper abdominal operations. The term "atelectasis" is derived from the Greek meaning "incomplete expansion" but is generally applied to the situation in which there are airless alveoli. Although collapse of alveoli may occur within definite anatomic units such as segments, lobes, or an entire lung, the most commonly encountered variety is platelike and subsegmental.

ETIOLOGY. The two major factors that have been implicated as causes of atelectasis are bronchial obstruction with distal gas absorption and hypoventilation or ineffectual respiration. The loss of chemical elements that stabilize the lung at low volumes by reducing alveolar surface tension, i.e., *surfactants*, has been implicated.

Obstruction of the tracheobronchial airway occurs secondary to changes in bronchial secretion, defect in the expulsion mechanism, and reduction in bronchial caliber. Subsequent to tracheobronchial obstruction by secretion, vomitus, blood, or tumor material, there is a period during which a change occurs in the composition of gases within the alveolus, following which the gas composition in the obstructed alveoli remains constant until absorption is complete. The rate of absorption is a function of the pressure difference between the gas in the alveoli and the gas in the blood, the absorption coefficient of the gas, and the rate and quantity of blood flow. Obstruction of a large conductive airway certainly leads to atelectasis of the distal lung segment. However, there are many observations that cast doubt on bronchial obstruction as the sole or major causative factor in postoperative atelectasis.

Currently, many feel that atelectasis usually consists of small and diffuse lesions that are nonobstructive in origin and are due to inspiratory insufficiency. Atelectasis has been thought to occur without airway obstruction as a result of a constant volume ventilation with volumes approximating normal tidal volume, and the process is reversible by hyperinflation.

A major cause of alveolar collapse is related to the surface forces acting at the gas-liquid interface within the alveolar units. Normally, there is a film, surfactant, which has the property of reducing surface tension when the alveolar volume is decreased. Increased surface tension of this film encourages collapse or decrease in the size of the alveolus and makes it more difficult to inflate. Regional changes in the pulmonary circulation may alter the characteristics of surfactant. Deep breathing mobilizes surfactant from within the alveolar cell to augment or replace the aging surfactant on the alveolar surface, maintaining stability and preventing atelectasis.

Many factors predispose to the development of postoperative atelectasis. There is an increasing incidence in patients who smoke and those who suffer from bronchitis, asthma, emphysema, or other chronic lung diseases. Anesthesia and postoperative narcotics depress the cough reflex, while chest pain, immobilization, and splinting with bandages reduce the effective nature of the cough. The incidence of atelectasis is related to the duration and depth of anesthesia, and although higher incidences have been reported with general anesthesia than with regional anesthesia, when the same postoperative care was applied to the two groups, the difference disappeared. Nasogastric tubes have been implicated because of the increased secretions and predisposition toward aspiration. Bronchospasm is a predisposing factor, but severe bronchospasm is rarely encountered during clinical anesthesia. Congestion of the bronchial walls due to edema represents another source of decrease in the bronchial lumen.

CLINICAL MANIFESTATIONS. Atelectasis usually becomes manifest in the first 24 h after an operation and rarely appears after 48 h. There is usually a sudden onset of fever and tachycardia. Frequently, the pulmonary manifestations are so minor that they are not recognized. Early findings include rales located posteriorly in the bases, diminished breath sounds, and bronchial breathing. With massive involvement, there may be a shift of the trachea, mediastinum, and heart to the involved side, but this is not present with the more common subsegmental lesions. Pronounced dyspnea and/or cyanosis are relatively uncommon. Radiographs may demonstrate areas of consolidation, but in early cases bronchial breathing is detected more frequently than radiographic changes. Determination of blood gases indicating intrapulmonary shunting of blood provides the diagnosis. Characteristically with atelectasis and significant shunting, the arterial Pa_{O_2} is decreased while the arterial Pa_{CO_2} may be normal or decreased. The ventilation is normal or increased.

If atelectasis persists, the clinical manifestations are those generally associated with pneumonia. The temperature increases to a greater extent, and there is increasing tachycardia, dyspnea, and cyanosis. It is felt that the great majority of postoperative pneumonias begin as atelectasis, since atelectatic areas are poorly drained and represent good sites for infection. In some instances, however, pneumonia may result from the aspiration of infected material. Another consequence of atelectasis is the development of lung abscess, which also may be initiated by the aspiration of foreign material, such as teeth or blood during tonsillectomy and purulent material from putrid abscesses in the mouth. Aspiration of gastric contents also represents a possible cause of lung abscess.

TREATMENT. Prophylaxis begins preoperatively by having the patient cease smoking, if possible, for at least 2 weeks prior to operation and instructing the patient in deep abdominal breathing and productive coughing. Postoperative prophylaxis includes the minimal use of depressant drugs, the prevention of pain that may limit respiration, frequent changes of body position, deep breathing and coughing exercises, and early ambulation. Sustained maximal inspiration, which can be accomplished with the aid of a variety of devices, is an important factor in the prevention and treatment of atelectasis.

Three groups of medications have been applied to the prophylaxis and therapy of atelectasis. These are (1) expectorants to provide more liquid and less viscous secretions, (2) detergents and mucolytic solutions to alter the surface tension of secretions and render their elimination more likely, and (3) bronchodilators used primarily by inhalation to provide increased size of the tracheobronchial tree and elimination of bronchospasm. The mucolytic agents, such as Mucomist or Alevaire, are indicated because inhaled air with a relative humidity lower than 70 percent inhibits ciliary activity and tends to desiccate secretions.

Once atelectasis becomes clinically manifest, coughing, clearing of secretions, and increase in depth of respiration may be stimulated by endotracheal suction with a soft rubber catheter or the instillation of 1 to 2 mL of saline solution directly into the trachea via an intracatheter polyethylene tube. If these measures are not successful, bronchoscopy may be required, and if multiple bronchoscopic aspirations are necessary, tracheostomy should be performed to facilitate subsequent aspiration.

Pulmonary Edema

Pulmonary edema may occur during or immediately after an operation. The increased use of massive blood transfusions, plasma expanders, and other fluids during operative procedures has resulted in an increased incidence of this complication. Circulatory overload represents the most common cause of pulmonary edema. Other factors that have been implicated include left ventricular failure, shift of blood from the peripheral to pulmonary vascular bed, negative pressure on the airway that increases the gradient between the transmural capillary pressure and the alveolar pressure favoring transudation, and injury to the alveolar membrane by noxious substances.

Although circulatory overload is most frequently due to infusion of fluid during operative procedure, it may also result from the absorption of solutions during irrigation of hollow viscera, such as the bladder, and is frequently associated with subclinical heart failure in those patients in whom pulmonary edema becomes manifest.

Incomplete cardiac emptying may be attributed to any anesthetic, narcotic, or hypnotic agent, since all are capable of decreasing myocardial contractility. Incomplete cardiac emptying may also be due to gross irregularities in rhythm. Left ventricular failure results in elevated left atrial and pulmonary artery blood pressures. Peripheral vascular beds may vasoconstrict, causing blood to shift centrally and result in pulmonary edema. A reflex mechanism of neurogenic origin that causes redistribution of blood from the periphery to the pulmonary bed has been reported to occur during manipulation of the brain and following head trauma.

Pulmonary edema caused by injury to the alveolar membrane is associated with the inhalation of noxious gases or vapors and the aspiration of gastric contents or chemicals, particularly kerosene, that are pulmonary irritants. Endotoxins released during gram-negative sepsis cause pulmonary edema by increasing pulmonary permeability. White blood cells sequestered in the lung with pulmonary emboli and hypoperfusion release vasoactive substances that effect these changes.

CLINICAL MANIFESTATIONS. The early disturbances of pulmonary edema are accumulation of fluid in the sheath around small pulmonary arteries and thickening of the capillary and alveolar membranes. In the early stage, the principal effect is widening of the $(A-a)O_2$ gradient. A reduction in lung compliance precedes evidence of carbon dioxide retention in the blood. Bronchospasm usually occurs and contributes further to reducing the compliance. As frank edema develops, a frothy pink-stained fluid appears in the alveoli, bronchi, and trachea, and at this time the problem is one of airway obstruction. Clinically, bronchospasm and marked reduction in lung compliance in a patient being ventilated should provide premonitory evidence and anticipate the development of dyspnea and cough. A few scattered rales may appear early, but as the process intensifies, bubbling rales and rhonchi are heard all over the chest. The systemic blood pressure is usually raised initially but may be normal or reduced, and characteristically there is a marked tachycardia. Shock may appear with signs of peripheral circulatory failure, and death may occur from asphyxia.

TREATMENT. Therapy is directed at (1) providing oxygen, (2) allowing oxygen access to the alveoli by removing obstructive fluid, and (3) correcting the circulatory overload if present. Arterial oxygen saturation can be restored by increasing the concentration of oxygen in inspired air.

Measures to reduce the pulmonary capillary pressure include venous occlusion tourniquets, placing the patient in a head-up or sitting position to reduce the flow of venous blood to the heart, and phlebotomy. Since systemic vasoconstriction has been shown to be a precipitating cause, therapy may be indicated to reverse this mechanism. Spinal anesthesia has been applied successfully in the treatment of pulmonary edema, as have the ganglionic blocking agent Arfonad and afterload reduction with sodium nitroprusside.

Drug therapy includes furosemide or ethacrynic acid for rapid diuresis and digitalis glycosides for situations where myocardial failure and lower output coexist (particularly in mitral stenosis) or where there is arrhythmia such as flutter or fibrillation. Morphine has been shown to be of value, though its mode of action remains unclear. If applied early, CPAP can reverse the process; in the intubated patient PEEP is most effective.

CARDIAC COMPLICATIONS

This section considers cardiac arrhythmias and myocardial ischemia and infarction related to surgery. A discussion of cardiac arrest and the postcardiotomy syndrome is presented in Chap. 19.

Arrhythmias

Although cardiac arrhythmias are frequently associated with operative repair of congenital and acquired lesions of the heart (see Chaps. 18 and 19), they represent a potential complication of any surgical procedure. As the age of the surgical population increases, one should encounter an increasing incidence of these disturbances.

INCIDENCE. The incidence varies and is somewhat determined by whether sinus tachycardia is included in the series. In a recent review, Reinikainen and Pontinen report that the incidence of cardiac arrhythmias occurring during extrathoracic operative procedures ranged between 30 and 100 percent. During thoracotomies carried out under general anesthesia, incidences as high as 77 percent have been recorded. Heart diseases increased the incidence; in one series, in 51 percent of cardiac patients as contrasted with 20 percent of other patients, arrhythmia developed during anesthesia. Kuner and associates, monitoring continuous electrocardiographic signals on magnetic tape for prolonged periods of time, found the incidence of cardiac arrhythmia during anesthesia to be 61 percent. The arrhythmias that they noted most frequently were wandering pacemaker, atrioventricular (AV) dissociation, and nodal rhythm and premature ventricular systoles. Relating intraoperative arrhythmias to type of anesthesia, Reinikainen and Pontinen recorded arrhythmias in 24 percent of patients in whom operations were carried out under local anesthesia. The majority of these were of vagal origin and caused by the occulocar-

treatment is required, though atropine will correct the abnormality, since it is related to vagal tone.

Sinoatrial Block. Either single beats drop out with regular sequence, or there are runs of two or three dropped beats. If the block is prolonged, nodal or ventricular escape occurs. The block is caused by increased vagal tone and depression of the sinus node impulse. It occurs during tracheobronchial suctioning, with carotid sinus pressure, and in hyperkalemia, and is associated with neostigmine administration. It may reverse itself spontaneously or with atropine administration.

Atrial Fibrillation. Atrial fibrillation with its characteristic irregular pulse most frequently appears postoperatively in arteriosclerotic patients subjected to thoracic surgical treatment. In early cases, the ventricular rate is usually rapid, but when digitalis has been given, a slow ventricular rate may be noted. In the absence of failure, no treatment is indicated, since spontaneous correction may occur. In the case of a paroxysmal atrial fibrillation, which may precipitate congestive heart failure, digitalis therapy is indicated. Quinidine or electric cardioversion may be used when there is no associated failure.

Premature Contractions. These represent the most common irregularities of the pulse, and they may originate from any portion of the conduction system. The premature beat characteristically occurs earlier than expected and is followed by a pause due to failure of the ventricle to respond to the next normal impulse. The abnormality occurs in 2 to 8 percent of postoperative patients. The occurrence has been associated with changes in posture, drug therapy with ephedrine and epinephrine, digitalis toxicity, and myocardial infarction. Usually premature contractions have no clinical significance and require no therapy, though if they occur with disturbing frequency, quinidine or lidocaine is recommended unless there is congestive failure, in which case digitalis is the drug of choice, provided it does not represent a possible cause.

Myocardial Infarction

The majority of patients who died suddenly during the operative and immediate postoperative period demonstrated coronary artery thrombosis or myocardial infarction at autopsy. The reported incidence for postoperative myocardial infarction is about 0.15 percent of all surgical patients; the incidence is ten times greater for patients over seventy years old. Eleven unsuspected acute myocardial infarctions were detected by routine postoperative electrocardiograms taken on 1000 patients in the recovery room.

Tarhan et al. recently assessed the significance of operative procedures under general anesthesia performed in patients who had previous myocardial infarction; 6.6 percent had another infarct in the first week after operation, and 54 percent of these died. Myocardial infarction after a major operation is more lethal than myocardial infarction alone. Reinfarction occurred most frequently after operations on the thorax or upper abdomen. In over one-third of patients operated on within 3 months of infarction, reinfarction occurred. This rate decreased to 16 percent in

patients at 3 to 6 months postinfarction and to 4 to 5 percent when infarction occurred more than 6 months prior to surgery. The cardiac risk of a noncardiac operation is definitely increased within 6 months following a myocardial infarction but may be lower than previously reported. Patients with congestive failure, significant valvular disease, and arrhythmias such as frequent premature ventricular contractions are also at increased risk, as are patients over seventy years. Stable angina and moderate hypertension are not significant risk factors. Goldman has developed a multifactorial assessment of risks in patients undergoing an operation (Table 12-2). High-risk patients have scores greater than 5. The risk of death from cardiac causes is increased in patients with scores exceeding 25.

CLINICAL MANIFESTATIONS. The majority of cases occur on the operative day or during the first 3 postoperative days, and although infarction has been associated with all anesthetics, the incidence is higher after general anesthesia for abdominal or pelvic surgical treatment. The most important precipitating factor is shock, either during the operation or in the early postoperative phase. The more prolonged the shock, the greater the risk of coronary thrombosis and myocardial ischemia. The electrocardiogram may show ST depression and T-wave flattening with the loss of as little as 500 mL of blood in patients with previous coronary occlusion.

The diagnosis may be difficult, because chest pain is often absent or obscured by narcotics. Chest pain occurred as a primary clinical manifestation in only 27 percent of patients, which is less than the 97 percent generally reported in patients in whom a coronary occlusion is

Table 12-2. COMPUTATION OF MULTIFACTORIAL INDEX SCORE TO ESTIMATE CARDIAC RISK IN NONCARDIAC SURGERY

	Points
S3 gallop or jugular venous distention on preoperative physical examination	11
Transmural or subendocardial myocardial infarction in the previous 6 months	10
Premature ventricular beats, more than 5/min documented at any time	7
Rhythm other than sinus or presence of premature atrial contractions on last preoperative electrocardiogram	7
Age over 70 years	5
Emergency operation	4
Intrathoracic, intraperitoneal, or aortic site of surgery	3
Evidence for important valvular aortic stenosis*	3
Poor general medical condition†	3

* Findings of a cardiologist's examination, noninvasive testing, or cardiac catheterization.

† As evidenced by electrolyte abnormalities (potassium, <3.0 meq/L: HCO_3, <20 meq/L), renal insufficiency (blood urea nitrogen, >50 mg/dL; creatinine, >3.0 mg/dL), abnormal blood gases (P_{O_2}, <60 mmHg; P_{CO_2}, >50 mmHg), abnormal liver status (elevated aspartate transaminase or signs at physical examination of chronic liver disease), or any condition that has caused the patient to be chronically bedridden.

SOURCE: Goldman L: *Ann Surg* 198:780, 1983, with permission.

not related to surgery. It is appropriate to consider routinely monitoring patients with previous infarction in an intensive care unit. The sudden appearance of shock, dyspnea, cyanosis, tachycardia, arrhythmia, or congestive failure should alert one to the diagnosis. The triad of dyspnea, cyanosis, and arterial hypotension requires a differential diagnosis between cardiac and respiratory problems. The electrocardiogram may provide the diagnosis with a characteristic infarction pattern. However, this is not an unequivocal finding, since, in older patients, ST segment and T-wave changes may be associated with myocardial ischemia, and the same changes may be observed with postoperative shock. A study of arterial gases may provide a differential diagnosis in reference to respiratory problems. Left ventricular failure with pulmonary edema is not generally accompanied by carbon dioxide retention, and, in contrast to airway obstruction and alveolar hypoventilation, there is usually a reduction in arterial carbon dioxide tension (Pa_{CO_2}) and respiratory alkalosis when cardiac failure accompanies myocardial infarction. The CPK-MB isoenzyme is the most precise method for detection of myocardial necrosis following operation. If myocardial infarction is suspected, serial studies, including ECG, SGOT, and CPK-MB, should be done daily. Isotope scanning of the myocardium using technetium pyrophosphate may detect a recent acute infarction.

TREATMENT (See Chap. 4). Preoperative preparation of patients with signs of cardiac insufficiency should include digitalization for patients with enlarged hearts or histories of previous cardiac failure. Routine digitalization is not indicated. Anemia, if present, requires treatment, and attention should be directed toward the regulation of fluid and electrolyte balance and hypovolemia. Patients on propranolol should continue to receive the drug until the morning of the operation. Operation is contraindicated for a period of at least 6 weeks and preferably 6 months following myocardial ischemia or infarction, except in an emergency. During the operation, a broad spectrum of factors that precipitate myocardial infarction should be avoided. These include anoxia, hypotension, hemorrhage, dehydration, electrolyte disturbance, and arrhythmias. The regulation of blood pressure during anesthesia is probably the most important measure in the prevention of myocardial ischemia and infarction. When the blood pressure falls significantly, in the absence of blood loss, the prompt correction of anoxia by adequate ventilation with oxygen and the administration of vasopressors is indicated. Digitalization may be required when shock is combined with heart failure. The administration of blood or fluid is indicated to maintain blood volume.

Treatment of myocardial infarction itself consists of relief of pain and anxiety using morphine and sedation. Relief of anoxia is accomplished with 33 to 50% oxygen delivered via a BLB mask or nasal catheter. Suctioning of the tracheobronchial tree may be required to clear obstructing secretions. Critically ill patients are best managed in an intensive care unit setting with invasive monitoring using arterial lines and a Swan-Ganz catheter. Shock is treated by vasopressor agents. Promptness in

instituting vasopressor therapy will increase the chances of its being effective. Rapid digitalization is applicable in treatment of shock when the myocardial insufficiency may be responsible for the severe hypotension. Digitalization is also indicated for the treatment of heart failure, which is a frequent manifestation of postoperative myocardial infarction. In addition to digitalization, parenteral diuretic therapy may be used in the treatment of cardiac failure. Some writers have advocated the use of anticoagulant therapy after the danger of excessive bleeding from an operative site ceases.

DIABETES MELLITUS

Diabetes mellitus occurs in 2 to 3 percent of the general population with a higher rate among older people. In two series, the disease was discovered in the perioperative period in 16 and 23 percent of patients. The most commonly associated operative procedures were related to vascular disease, but in a high percentage of patients diabetes was discovered prior to an emergency procedure. Diabetic patients represent a special challenge during total surgical care, because the impairment of the homeostatic mechanism for glucose may result in ketoacidosis if untreated or hypoglycemia if overtreated and also because of the associated incidence of generalized vascular disease.

PATHOPHYSIOLOGY. The basic defect is a lack of metabolically effective circulating insulin. The elevated blood sugar level is a result of deficient utilization on the part of peripheral tissues and an increased output of glucose by the liver. In diabetes, the breakdown of fatty acids is increased, and since the metabolism of the ketone bodies is limited, they accumulate in the bloodstream and are eliminated via the kidneys. Glycosuria itself produces an osmotic diuresis that is enhanced by the presence of ketone bodies and the associated loss of sodium and potassium. Evaluation of decompensated diabetes, therefore, includes not only measuring the blood glucose but also measuring acetone, electrolytes, and carbon dioxide–combining power of the serum.

The anesthetic agent may affect carbohydrate metabolism, in which case the hyperglycemia is related to an increased breakdown of liver glycogen and a concomitant catabolism of muscle glycogen with the formation of lactic acid. Also, the anesthetic agents affecting glucose catabolism cause an exaggerated hyperglycemic epinephrine response and an increased resistance to exogenously administered insulin.

The stress of surgical treatment aggravates hyperglycemia because of the increased secretion of epinephrine, growth hormone, and glucocorticoids. Increased epinephrine secretion results in an increased breakdown of liver glycogen to glucose, which is released into the general circulation. The glucocorticoids also increase hepatic glucose output via mobilized protein and exert an anti-insulin effect by stimulating a circulating insulin antagonist. The effects of both epinephrine and glucocorticoids are offset to some extent by an increased secretion of endogenous insulin in the normal person but may require the administration of larger doses of insulin in diabetic patients. Treatment is directed at preventing ketoacidosis, hyperosmolar nonketotic coma, decreased cardiac output with associated poor peripheral perfusion, electrolyte imbalance, impaired polymorphonuclear leukocyte phagocytosis, and decreased wound healing, all of which have been related to uncontrolled diabetes.

MANAGEMENT. In the diabetic patient, essential laboratory studies include hemoglobin determination, white cell count, urinalysis for sugar and acetone, fasting and timed postprandial blood glucose determination, blood urea nitrogen, and, in older patients, serum cholesterol determination and electrocardiography. Diabetic patients should have a preference for an early place on the operative schedule to minimize the effects of fasting and ketosis. Preoperative medication should be kept to a minimum, since diabetic patients, particularly elderly ones, are sensitive to narcotics and sedatives and there is a danger of hypercapnia and hypoxia. The choice of anesthesia should be determined by the operative procedure and the preference of the anesthesiologist. It should not be influenced by the presence of diabetes. Spinal anesthesia has little tendency to evoke hyperglycemia apart from the stress of the operation; among the inhalation anesthetics, nitrous oxide, trichloroethylene, and halothane have the least effect on carbohydrate metabolism. The degree of control during the perioperative period should be assessed by serial determination of the blood sugar and urinalysis for glycosuria and acetonuria. In general, it is safer to permit mild glycosuria and minimal elevation of the blood sugar level in the perioperative periods, particularly in the elderly and cardiac patients. In the patient with postoperative hypotension, blood glucose determination should be obtained to rule out hypoglycemia as an etiologic factor.

Mild diabetics frequently do not require insulin, and dietary control is sufficient. The cornerstone of all diabetic management is the dietary or parenteral intake. The preoperative diabetic intake should contain 140 to 200 g of carbohydrates, 60 to 100 g of protein, and adequate vitamins and minerals and should furnish 1200 to 2100 kcal daily. If parenteral fluids are required, there is a theoretical advantage to the use of fructose or sorbitol, which can be utilized in amounts up to 50 g daily in the diabetic patient. The goal of the dietary or parenteral fluid regimen is to keep the patient free of acetonuria and without excessive hyperglycemia. The patients in whom diabetes is well controlled with oral agents should continue the use of these drugs until the day prior to operation, particularly if the medication is tolbutamide or phenformin. With longer-acting agents, such as chlorpropamide, the drug should be discontinued 72 h preoperatively if the administration of insulin is contemplated. Galloway and Shuman stated that patients who take tolbutamide preoperatively usually require insulin during and immediately after major surgical treatment whereas patients receiving chlorpropamide usually do not require insulin during the immediate paraoperative period.

Insulin Therapy. A variety of programs for the administration of insulin have been proposed. One of the popular methods of treatment employs a regimen in which the daily carbohydrate requirement is divided into four equal doses and given parenterally as 5 to 10% dextrose in water every 6 h. This initiation of the parenteral glucose infusion is accompanied by the subcutaneous injection of unmodified regular insulin in doses equal to approximately one-fourth the dose of insulin that the patient required prior to operation. Urine is checked regularly, and supplementary doses of crystalline insulin are given as indicated. Based on the extent of glycosuria, 4 to 10 units of additional insulin is provided for each unit of positivity. Larger doses may be indicated when acetonuria, severe stress, infection, or marked hyperglycemia is present. The advantage of this method is that glucose and insulin are given at regular intervals, permitting adjustment in the dose during the day. It is preferable to monitor blood glucose levels. The major disadvantage is that inadvertent interruption of glucose infusion may result in hypoglycemia. With this regimen as with others, slight glycosuria is preferable provided there is no acetonuria.

The second basic regimen is directed at patients who are under control with single-injection therapy employing long-acting insulin and in whom a complicated postoperative course is not anticipated. On the day of operation, the patient receives 50 g of glucose in 1000 mL of solution, and at the time the intravenous solution is started, one-half the daily dose of insulin that previously was required is administered. Following operation and return to the recovery room or ward, the remainder of the usual daily dose of insulin is given subcutaneously. Thus, the amount of insulin given on the day of operation approximates that given the day before. On the day following operation, the usual dose of insulin is given in the morning prior to breakfast or at the time of starting an intravenous infusion. Modifications of this approach employ small doses of regular insulin subcutaneously during the postoperative period based on the extent of glycosuria or preferably the serum glucose level. In patients who have been treated with single daily injections and who are not under control prior to operation, conversion to a regimen of soluble insulin is indicated.

There is general agreement that severe hyperglycemia in patients undergoing major operations is more effectively managed with intravenous regular insulin. The problem of insulin absorption by the container has been overcome by the use of plastic containers, high concentrations of insulin, and flushing the system. A specific infusion protocol is outlined in Table 12-3.

A simplified protocol has been proposed by Woodruff et al. The patients receive their evening dose of insulin the preoperative day but no subcutaneous insulin on the morning of surgery. The patient is scheduled as the first case. Insulin and glucose are controlled with two separate infusion pumps; one infuses 5% dextrose in Ringer's lactate at 2 mL/(kg · h), while the other dispenses insulin from a plastic bag containing 250 mL sodium chloride to which 50 units of U-100 regular insulin was added. The rate of insulin infusion is based on the serum glucose level. Twenty units per hour is infused for glucose levels

Table 12-3. INSULIN INFUSION PROTOCOL IN MAJOR SURGERY IN DIABETIC PATIENTS

1. Day before surgery
    a. Obtain 5:00 P.M. plasma glucose STAT.
    b. Start intravenous infusion of 5% dextrose in water at the rate of 50 mL/h and maintain this rate until the patient is taking solid foods without difficulty postoperatively.
    c. "Piggy-back" to dextrose infusion an infusion of regular insulin using IVAC or other infusion pump. Preparation of insulin solution: 50 units in 250 mL 0.9% N saline; flush 60 mL of infusion mixture through system and discard before attaching.
    d. Set infusion rate with this equation:

$$\text{Insulin (units/hour)} = \frac{\text{plasma glucose (mg/dL)}}{100}$$

    (Divide by 150 rather than 100 if the patient is thin or is not taking corticosteroids.)
    e. Repeat glucose determination every 3 h as needed with appropriate insulin adjustments to obtain a plasma glucose level between 100 and 200 mg/dL.
2. Day of surgery
    a. Continue dextrose solution as above.
    b. Manage fluid and electrolyte requirements in peri- and postoperative periods with non-glucose-containing solutions *only*.
    c. Obtain plasma glucose STAT every 2 h during surgery and every 6 h for the rest of that 24-h period; adjust insulin accordingly.
3. Days after surgery
    a. Continue dextrose and other fluid replacement as on the day of surgery
    b. Obtain daily fasting and afternoon plasma glucose values to assess insulin treatment and adjust as necessary.
    c. Hypoglycemia contingencies (plasma glucose less than 50 mg/dL):
        (1) Obtain STAT plasma glucose; decrease insulin rate accordingly; treat orally.
        (2) Give 15 mL intravenous bolus of 50% dextrose in water if oral therapy is insufficient.
        (3) Repeat steps 1 or 2 at 15-min intervals if symptoms persist or recur.
        (4) Determine cause of hypoglycemia and treat promptly.
    d. Discontinue infusion when patient is tolerating solid food.
        (1) Reinstitute appropriate twice-a-day insulin dosage.
        (2) Do not stop infusion completely without switching to insulin injections.

SOURCE: From Meyer EJ, Lorenzi M, et al: *Am J Surg* 137:323, 1979, with permission.

greater than 200 mg/dL, no insulin for levels below 80 mg/dL. The surgical procedure is not begun until the level is below 200 mg/dL. Insulin therapy during emergent surgery or surgery complicated by infection will require greater amounts of insulin to maintain serum glucose levels below 200 mg/dL. In extreme cases, bolus injection of 0.1 to 0.4 unit/kg may be required as an additive.

Management of Ketoacidosis. The preparation for surgical treatment of a patient with ketoacidosis is critical, and one should keep in mind that ketoacidosis itself may masquerade as a surgical emergency. The patient with frank diabetic coma is no candidate for surgical treatment regardless of the indication. Crystalline insulin should be used in all cases to establish control. Page et al. reported effective management of diabetic coma with continuous low-dose insulin infusion using an average of 7.2 units/h. Plasma glucose, ketone bodies, and free fatty acids decreased 58 percent in 4 h. There is an associated deficiency of dehydration and electrolyte abnormality that must be corrected, and the ordinary patient with advanced coma will require an average of 2 to 4 or more liters of fluid to overcome the dehydration. The serum potassium should be determined at 6- to 8-h intervals and potassium added to the fluid in quantities of 40 meq/L administered at a rate of no greater than 25 meq/h. Usually the need for potassium does not exceed 80 meq. There is generally no need to add glucose to intravenous fluid unless the blood glucose level falls below normal. Gastric atony is a frequent accompaniment of diabetic ketoacidosis, and suction is frequently required to minimize pulmonary aspiration. It is usually possible to correct ketoacidosis in sufficient time so that the patient's surgical status is not compromised.

Nonketotic Hyperglycemic Hyperosmolar Coma. Hyperosmolar dehydration and coma is a relatively uncommon syndrome that usually occurs in elderly diabetic or nondiabetic obese patients and patients receiving total parenteral nutrition. The blood sugar level is frequently above 1000 mg/dL, and ketone bodies are absent from the plasma and urine. Treatment consists of large amounts of hypotonic solutions plus intravenous insulin. Marked lowering of the blood sugar level may result with small doses of insulin, and it is recommended that a test dose of 10 units be given to determine responsiveness.

FAT EMBOLISM SYNDROME

Fat embolism is one of the important causes of increased morbidity and mortality in patients with fractures and extensive trauma. A distinction must be made between fat as a pathologically demonstrable phenomenon and fat embolism as a clinical entity. The presence of pulmonary fat embolism is a relatively common accompaniment of trauma, while the clinical entity is an infrequent occurrence. The pathologic entity of fat emboli in the pulmonary capillaries following trauma was described initially by Zenker in 1862. In World War I, 112 cases in which fat embolism was implicated as the cause of death had been reported. Mallory et al. reported that 65 percent of 60 patients who died of battle wounds in World War II had pulmonary fat embolism, and a similar finding was noted in 39 percent of 79 patients dying from war wounds in the Korean conflict. In 1962, Sevitt described 100 cases of fat embolism, 82 percent of which were related to long bone fractures.

The occurrence of the pathologic entity of fat embolization is correlated with the degree of injury and survival time. In a study of 300 accident victims, 80 percent of those dying immediately had embolization of varying degrees. In those living up to 6 h after accident, fat embolism was found in 96 percent of autopsies, and 12 h after a fatal accident from mechanical trauma, there was not a single case without fat embolism. Massive fat embolism occurred in 26 percent of the cases with one fracture and 44 percent of those with multiple fractures. Chan and associates reported that 8.75 percent of patients with fractures of the femur, tibia, and pelvis, or multiple fractures presented with overt clinical manifestations of the fat embolism syndrome.

In addition to fat embolization associated with extensive trauma, the clinical syndrome has been reported in blast concussion, with liver trauma, in burns, in severe infection (particularly that due to clostridia, which mediate alpha-toxins that disintegrate fat), in closed-chest cardiac massage, with the use of extracorporeal circulation, and following renal transplantation and high-altitude flights.

PATHOGENESIS AND PATHOPHYSIOLOGY. In the fat embolism syndrome there is an interaction between platelet aggregation, a coagulopathy, and circulating fats that result in diffuse organ changes, particularly in the lungs and central nervous system. There is disagreement as to whether the embolized fat originates from bone marrow and soft tissue or from circulating blood lipids. The most popular theory, which implicates mechanical causes, proposes that with trauma there is a liberation of liquid fat and intravasation of fat into the vascular channels. Bone, with its high fat content, vascularity, and rigidity, provides an ideal setting. Most of the cases of fat embolism occur after fracture of major long bones with high fat content, and occasionally hemopoietic marrow fragments have been found within the lung as an accompaniment of fat embolization.

It is also proposed that the normal emulsion of fat within the plasma is altered to allow coalescence of the chylomicrons into larger fat droplets with subsequent embolization. This is supported by the fact that emboli may be found in nontraumatic conditions and that the chemical makeup of the embolic fat more closely resembles circulating lipids than marrow or depot fat. Several contributing factors are important in the pathogenesis. These include shock, disseminated intravascular coagulation, sepsis, local pressure, and release of kinins.

Circulating fat macroglobules larger than 20 μm in diameter are the offending elements. The lung usually acts as a very effective filter, as evidenced by the observation that 95 percent of patients dying of injury had pulmonary involvement while only 23 percent demonstrated systemic fat embolism. Thus, in approximately three-fourths of the patients with fat embolism the lesion is confined to the lung. The first stage is hypoperfusion due to the mechanical effects of the macroglobules and adherent platelets, red cells, and fibrin plus the chemical effects of released serotonin and kinins. Local lipolysis leads to the second stage, chemical pneumonitis. Damage to the alveolar wall interferes with lung surfactant activity. Pathophysiologically, early hyperpnea leads to a transitory respiratory alkalosis, but combined respiratory and metabolic acidosis evolves rapidly. The cardiac effects are related primarily to the increased pulmonary vascular resistance and, to a lesser degree, to diffuse fat embolism

within the myocardium itself. If the fat emboli pass through the pulmonary filter to reach the circulation, they may lodge in the cerebral vessels, accounting for central nervous system manifestations, and in the skin, producing the characteristic petechial changes. Although the kidneys are involved quite regularly when there is systemic fat embolism, they are usually not severely damaged.

CLINICAL MANIFESTATIONS. Although pathologic pulmonary fat embolization is a common occurrence, the clinical manifestations are rare. Symptoms characteristically occur within 12 to 48 h but have been noted as late as 10 days following injury. The main manifestations relate to pulmonary pathology. Before symptoms become apparent, blood-gas determinations may define significant hypoxemia. Tachypnea and tachycardia are characterisic. Pulmonary infection may ensue and lead to augmented respiratory symptoms plus manifestations of sepsis. Rarely, massive pulmonary embolization of fat will result in the sudden onset of right heart failure.

Cerebral fat embolism usually does not occur without evidence of pulmonary involvement. Symptoms that suggest cerebral involvement include changes in personality, drowsiness leading to coma, muscle weakness, spasticity, or rigidity, diplopia or blindness, and, rarely, extreme pyrexia. The cerebral manifestations must be differentiated from delirium tremens, cerebral contusion, and epidural hematoma. The lucid interval with cerebral contusion is usually absent, whereas it characteristically lasts 6 to 10 h with epidural hematoma and 24 h with fat embolism. Coma may be present immediately with cerebral contusion and evolves rapidly with fat embolism and slowly with an epidural hematoma. Decerebrate rigidity occurs early in fat embolism and is a terminal event with epidural hematoma. Tachypnea and tachycardia are characteristic of fat embolism, whereas the pulse and respiratory rate are slow with epidural hematoma.

The classic physical finding of fat embolism is the appearance of petechial hemorrhages in the capillary plexus of the dermis. They occur in a distinctive pattern over the shoulders, chest, axilla, and, rarely, the abdominal wall and extremities. They may also be noted in the subconjunctival region and on the palate. Petechiae occur as early as the second or third day and as late as the ninth day after injury and are present in 20 percent of patients found at autopsy to have fat embolism. A counterpart to the petechial hemorrhages is evident on funduscopic examination as emboli within the retinal vessels, and there may be streaks of hemorrhage throughout the retina and macular edema. Renal involvement usually does not produce severe damage, and both gross hematuria and impaired function are rare occurrences. Recently, an association with acute peptic ulceration has been noted.

DIAGNOSTIC STUDIES. A sudden and precipitous drop in the hematocrit is frequently noted and has been related to trapping of red cells and occasionally an associated DIC within the pulmonary parenchyma. It may occur as early as the second or third day following injury, just prior to the onset of dyspnea, disorientation, and the appearance of petechial hemorrhages. Thrombocytopenia

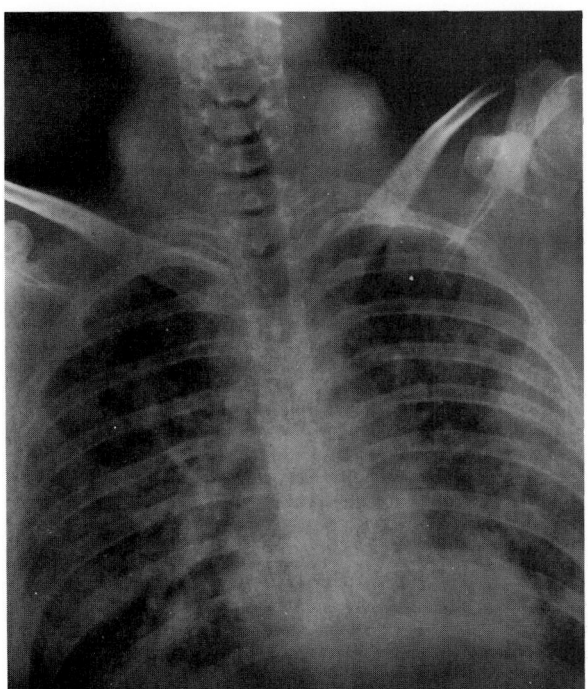

Fig. 12-2. Pulmonary fat emboli. Note bilateral extensive ill-defined nodular densities situated primarily in peripheral lung fields. Patient was in an automobile accident and fractured his femur and two metatarsals. Twenty-four hours after admission fever developed, and 3 days later hemoptysis and mental confusion. Changes were seen radiographically on the fourth day after trauma. There were lipid bodies in the urine, and the serum lipase level was elevated. The patient was treated with antibiotics, heparin, and dextran, and the symptoms subsided 7 days after therapy.

occurs less frequently. Radiographic pulmonary changes are noted in about 36 percent of the cases. The characteristic pattern is that of unevenly distributed areas of radiodensity, congestive hilar shadows, and increased bronchovascular markings with dilation of the right side of the heart (Fig. 12-2). Serial measurements of Pa_{O_2} offer a better index of the degree of pulmonary involvement. In one series, 64 percent of patients with clinical manifestations had a significant reduction in Pa_{O_2}. The electrocardiogram may reveal changes that reflect myocardial ischemia and right ventricular strain. These are usually noted 24 to 48 h after injury. The important findings are the sudden appearance of a prominent S wave in lead I and prominent Q waves in lead III. Inversion of the T wave indicates severe overloading of the right ventricle. Depression of the RS-T segments suggests subendothelial ischemia. There may be a right bundle branch block. Arrhythmias are frequent. The electroencephalogram may indicate a diffuse slow wave pattern.

Detection of Fat. A cryostat test has been applied to determine the presence of fat globules in blood. In one series the test was positive in 52 percent of symptomatic patients. Lipuria occurs in the first few days following injury and is usually associated with a serious degree of fat embolism. Free fat in the urine has been demonstrated in over 57 percent of cases in one series. Examination of

the urine is simple but must be precise. The collecting apparatus must be free of fat, and the bladder must be emptied completely, since the fat floats and the majority of globules remain in the bladder residue. The patient should be catheterized using a nonoily lubricant and the fluid collected in a volumetric flask. The meniscus may be skimmed, or, after centrifugation, the supranatant is smeared and stained with Sudan III. Deep-orange-colored droplets represent fat globules. Another method of demonstrating fat in the urine is the Scuderi "sizzle" test, which involves placing a wire loop containing the supranatant fluid over a flame and listening for a pop or sizzle produced by burning fat. The fat can be detected in concentrations as small as 1:1000. The demonstration of fat in the sputum has little diagnostic value, since it is a common phenomenon following trauma. Biopsy of petechiae may establish the diagnosis, and frozen section is mandatory to determine the presence of fat. Needle biopsy of the kidney also has been applied to demonstrate fat globules.

Serum Lipase. A serum lipase level elevation occurs in about 14 to 50 percent of the cases, the rise usually beginning on the third day and reaching a maximum on the seventh or eighth day after injury. An elevation greater than 1 mL is significant, and this determination is considered by Peltier to be the best laboratory test between the third and seventh day. The serum lipase level can be suppressed by the administration of ethyl alcohol and augmented by heparinization. Once elevated, the level is thought to reflect the prognosis, and elevations greater than 2 mL are associated with a higher incidence of favorable outcome. In a patient with extensive trauma, an elevated serum lipase level in the first 48 h is more suggestive of pancreatitis.

TREATMENT. Prophylaxis against potentiating fat embolization includes careful handling of the patient and early splinting of fractures. Vigorous applications of resuscitative measures are indicated to correct oligemic shock, since it has been demonstrated that fewer emboli may be lethal in the hypotensive than in the normotensive patient. High doses of corticosteroids (1.0 to 1.5 g hydrocortisone) administered during the first 2 days following injury may inhibit the pneumonitis or expedite its resolution. Pulmonary manifestations are treated with oxygen therapy, rapid digitalization, and intensive endotracheal suction to minimize the accumulation of secretions. IPPB or PEEP are frequently indicated. Pa_{O_2} should be monitored and maintained between 80 and 100 mmHg. Endotracheal intubation is preferred over tracheostomy, since the latter has been associated with a high mortality rate in these patients. Cerebral manifestations are treated with sedation and anticonvulsive therapy.

Trasylol, which inhibits the effects of kinins, has been beneficial in several instances. Heparin in doses that do not have an anticoagulant effect will clear lipemic plasma and stimulate lipase activity. A dose of 5000 units may be administered intravenously every 6 h. In the presence of acute systemic toxicity or a rapidly rising lipase level, the drug should be discontinued, since the release of fatty acids is undesirable. Low-molecular-weight dextran

(40,000) has been administered intravenously to counteract intravascular thrombosis. One thousand milliliters is administered per 24 h for 2 days. Ethyl alcohol, which may decrease the rate of hydrolysis of neutral fat and slow the release of toxic free fatty acids, has been used. Presently, this applicability of alcohol is debatable.

PROGNOSIS. Old age, preexisting lung disease, and reduced cardiac reserve have adverse effects. The early appearance of marked hypoxemia and the requirement of persistently high $F_{I_{O_2}}$ are bad prognostic signs, as is hypocalcemia resulting from ion binding by FFA, while a persistently high serum lipase level is a favorable sign. At the Birmingham Accident Hospital, a fatality rate of 12 percent has been reported for 25 cases diagnosed according to strict criteria (all had petechial rash). While the "pure" cerebral form of the fat embolism syndrome generally has a better prognosis, the presence of coma is a poor sign. Acute respiratory disease usually is self-limiting.

PSYCHIATRIC COMPLICATIONS

Severe psychiatric disturbances may occur any time during an illness, but their appearance in the postoperative period is particularly significant. The first account of postoperative psychiatric disturbance presented by a surgeon was that of Dupuytren who, in 1834, wrote that "the brain itself may be overcome by pain, terror, or even joy and reason leaves the patient at the instant when it is most necessary to his welfare that he should remain calm and undisturbed." In 1910, Da Costa indicated that the anticipated frequency for such complications is as high as 1 in 250 laparotomies, while Lewis, more recently, suggested an incidence of 1 in 1500. Scott described 11 cases in 2000 surgical procedures. The validity of any of these figures, however, is open to question, since "postoperative psychosis" per se does not appear in the standard nomenclature and is frequently not coded on the patient's record. Diagnostic criteria for psychosis have become more specific over the years. Also, surgeons may not be sensitive to the behavioral patterns that are psychodiagnostic.

The study of Titchener et al., who evaluated 200 patients admitted to the surgical service of the Cincinnati General Hospital utilizing interview and the Minnesota Multiphasic Personality Inventory to substantiate a psychiatric diagnosis, indicated that 86 percent of the sample had either distressing psychologic symptoms, disabling patterns of behavior, or both. The patients considered were in a municipal hospital and represented a lower socioeconomic group, but the figures of 21 percent having neuroses, 11 percent psychophysiologic reactions, 14 percent psychoses, 34 percent character behavior disorders, and 3 percent chronic brain syndrome are most impressive.

GENERAL CONSIDERATIONS. "Postoperative psychosis" cannot be considered as a distinct clinical entity. No single factor has been shown to be responsible, and the physical illness and operative procedure may merely bring to light a latent psychotic tendency. Both illness, particularly when prolonged, and surgical procedures represent threats to the integrity of the organism on somatic and psychologic grounds. In nearly every person informed of the need for a surgical procedure, some degree of anxiety arises. There may be fear of loss of life, of loss of body part or function, such as castration as with pelvic and hernia operations. The anxiety signal is assimilated and integrated by the patient in preparation for the surgical stress. Surgical intervention to cure, modify, or prevent illness is the beginning of a complicated and multifaceted process. The psychodynamic processes at work during the preoperative, postoperative, and convalescent periods may be classified as involving (1) psychophysiologic factors, (2) somatopsychic factors, or (3) psychosocial factors. Psychophysiologic factors represent processes originating from psychologic stress that act along neurogenic or humoral pathways to modify the healing process. A poorly functioning gastroenterostomy or marginal ulcer in a patient with emotional stress represents an example of this type. The somatopsychic factors have to do with the psychologic adaptation involved when the surgical procedure imposes a somatic defect, such as an ileostomy or colostomy. The psychosocial factors refer to patients' concern with the effects of their physical illness or surgical procedure on their ultimate position in society. All these may interplay and contribute to anxiety, neurotic symptoms, severe depression, and frank psychosis.

CLINICAL MANIFESTATIONS. The time of occurrence of psychiatric derangement during illness is variable, and the duration of latent interval between surgical treatment and the psychologic disturbance may be days to weeks. Winkelstein and associates reported that, in the recovery room, patients who had been subjected to surgical procedures under general anesthesia exhibited a lack of concern about the operation and an absence of affective response, despite the fact that they were sufficiently oriented to be interviewed. After 24 h the patients responded with these concerns and emotions that were so conspicuously absent in the immediate postoperative period. Both psychologic and pharmacologic factors are implicated in this response, since patients under spinal anesthesia exhibit immediate and overt emotional reaction.

The manifestations are extremely variable. Fear may be accompanied by depression or elation and overactivity. The clinical picture may be that of acute delirium with confusion and disorientation or merely a vague alteration in perception and mood. The manic type of reaction may incorporate psychomotor excitement, delirium, delusions, visual or auditory hallucinations, agitated depression, and feelings of persecution. The psychotic reactions that were observed in 44 of 200 patients in the Cincinnati series are indistinguishable from the range of psychoses observed under other circumstances. The acute brain syndrome, or delirium, was manifest in 20 patients.

Delirium may begin with an inappropriate remark or a dramatic agitated outburst and is frequently the first sign of continued mental deterioration leading to a chronic brain syndrome, particularly in an elderly patient. Therefore, delirium must be regarded as a potentially dangerous situation. It occurs most commonly in elderly patients who have lost closeness and support of family or friends and in patients who are immobilized for long periods of time.

Depressive reactions represented the second most important psychosis in surgical patients and occurred in 4.5 percent of patients in the Cincinnati series. The patient is characteristically uncooperative in an active way, or recovery may be impeded by listlessness, anorexia, and disinterest. The depressive reaction may be accompanied by physiologic changes; Moore et al. demonstrated the effects of emotion on the pituitary-adrenal axis during the immediate and subsequent postoperative period. Suicide is a major risk in patients with depressive reaction.

Another category includes the paranoid psychotic disorder. Although it is not rare for schizophrenic reaction to have its onset in the surgical patient, no acute breaks of the schizophrenic type were noted among the 200 patients studied by Titchener et al. Generally, there is no contraindication to surgical treatment of patients with schizophrenia. Manic excitement is a particularly difficult problem in the management of surgical patients and requires the close cooperation of psychiatrist, surgeon, and anesthesiologist.

MANAGEMENT. The first step in the management of psychiatric disturbances occurring in the course of the surgical illness or following surgical procedures is that of anticipation. Although Knox has indicated that the incidence of postoperative psychosis was not related to the duration of preoperative hospital stay, the duration of illness, particularly when prolonged, does determine the patient's psychologic reaction to surgical experience. At the other end of the spectrum, sudden emergency operation often results in reactions marked by acute anxiety, nightmares, insomnia, irritability, and protective withdrawal from all stimuli. Age is an important factor, the highest incidence occurring in children under the age of two and in the elderly patients. In the latter group, this is particularly true of patients who have lost their proximity to and support of family and friends, and who have not developed a close relation with the hospital personnel. Knox has presented evidence of constitutional predisposition, and although 17 percent of his patients had had previous surgical treatment uncomplicated by psychiatric disturbances, 11 percent did have a previous psychiatric illness. Twenty-two percent of patients had a family history of mental illness of serious proportion. There is an increasing incidence of delirium in response to anesthesia and surgical treatment in patients who are alcoholic, while patients suffering from extensive trauma may have organic psychosis. Acidosis, acetonuria, hyperglycemia, hypercalcemia, hypomagnesemia, and hepatic insufficiency may all cause postoperative mental aberrations, and cerebral hypoxia frequently results in behavioral changes. Medications, such as barbiturates, anticholinergics, and cortisone, also have been implicated.

There is an obvious need for integrating psychologic treatment with the management of surgical patients. As Titchener and Levine emphasize, it is not necessary, possible, or advisable for these needs to be turned over to psychiatrists, and it is frequently preferable that the measures be carried out by the surgeon in charge. Verbal communication between the surgeon and patient is the best means of overcoming emotional or mental difficulty. The anesthesiologist is regarded as an impersonal distant figure who carries out a task without emotional impact on the patient. The surgeon should become aware of the patient's feelings, attitudes, and needs for specific information, i.e., diagnostic procedures, operating approach, and postoperative possibilities. Information on expected feelings and sensations may have a direct effect on the adequacy of adjustment. Also, changes to increase the patients' positive adaptation to their illness should be constantly considered. The striking incidence of significant postoperative disturbance suggests the need for "mental check" to be incorporated into the usual postoperative surgical rounds. Efforts should be directed at removing toxic causes of the acute brain syndrome, removing undue stimuli without isolating the patient, and providing psychologic or pharmacologic tranquilization.

The physician's psychologic approach should include repeated explanation and inquiries about the patient's concerns. In some instances, specific counseling and directive treatment, which may require direct intervention in the patient's personal or family affairs and the assistance of the social service department, is indicated. The best prophylactic therapy, however, can be classified as supportive, in that surgeons allow themselves to be the object of dependency on the part of the patient. This relationship is fostered by interest on the part of the surgeon and trust on the part of the patient.

The provocative patient who emits anger or attempts to irritate others as a mechanism for covering fear or relieving guilt needs understanding of the emotional reason for the provocation and an attitude of firmness rather than anger from the physician. The attempt on the part of patients to sign out against advice is a mechanism of expressing anger or fear and should be handled by the surgeon in such a way that patients are allowed to change their minds without becoming embarrassed. In these and other situations, patients may hide their real feeling behind an intellectual screen. For understanding, patients should be encouraged to bring forth both the emotional and intellectual aspects of their personalities.

Consultation with a psychiatrist is indicated in the case of any acute and severe emotional disturbance, and the referral should be candidly discussed between the surgeon and the patient. Patients must come to the conclusion that they require expert help for their problems. Referral is also indicated for long-standing disturbances discovered during hospitalization and is frequently appropriate in patients with psychosomatic illness. Browning and Houseworth, in a study of patients with peptic ulcer, demonstrated that the removal of symptoms without altering the psychosomatic disorders led to the formation of a new spectrum of symptoms. The surgeon should be prepared to differentiate organic from functional disorders, psychosis, and depressive states since psychiatric consultation may not be available or may be refused by the patient. Specific drugs may be prescribed. Most postoperative traumatic neuroses, manifest by anxiety and reliving the operative experience, can be managed with minor tranquilizers, e.g., diazepam, lorazepam, or hypnotics such as flurazepam. Psychoses such as schizophrenia, mania, and depression may respond to a phenothiazine derivative. Benzodiazepine derivatives are preferable for nonpsychotic anxiety. Tricyclic antidepressants have an effect that can be delayed 1 to 3 weeks and are associated with acute cholinergic side effects and changes in cardiac conduction. These drugs are rarely used in the postoperative period.

Special Surgical Situations

The very young and old patients are particularly vulnerable to the development of psychiatric complications following surgical treatment. Psychotic disturbances have been found in 2 to 3 percent of patients following cataract extraction. The combination of surgical procedure and the awareness of the implications of the illness is critical in the patient with cancer. Because of the high incidence of emotional disorders following surgical procedures, special consideration is indicated for mastectomy and gynecologic procedures, cardiac surgical treatment, dialysis and transplantation, and prolonged periods in an intensive care unit. The management of drug addicts is assuming greater importance.

PEDIATRIC SURGERY

In children, severe anxiety states may be precipitated by the shock of operation. Levy reported that of a group of 124 children who had operations, 20 percent showed residual emotional disturbances. This occurred most frequently in the one- to two-year-old group; after the age of three there was a sharp decrease with age. The age distribution was attributed to a greater dependence on home and mother, and Levy went so far as to suggest postponement of elective surgical treatment until the child could comprehend something about the situation. Postoperative reactions consisted of negativism, disobedience, tantrums, defiance, destructive behavior, and dependency, as manifested by clinging to the mother or attendant. The responses have been related to a feeling of betrayal and the consequent desire for revenge and rebellion. When a child is suffering from fears engendered by an operation, a second operation usually intensifies the earlier fears.

Prophylactic therapy is important. The maturity of the child's emotional adaptation is more a factor in the response than the operation per se. Parental absence is frequently associated with emotional difficulty. Prugh and associates compared two groups, one treated without organized consideration for emotional needs and another in which these needs were considered and ample opportunity for play was provided. Moderate or severe anxiety reactions, immediately after leaving the hospital, were observed in 92 percent of the control group and in 68 percent of the experimental group, with a peak incidence in children under three. Three months after discharge, the incidence of persisting anxiety had fallen to 58 percent for the control group and 44 percent for the experimental group. The youngest children reacted more severely with apprehension, feeding disturbances, and depression. The pattern for the four- to six-year-old group was a tendency toward obsessive worries, phobias, and accentuated aches and pains. The six- to ten-year-olds manifested conversion symptoms, compulsive behavior, and restlessness.

SURGERY IN THE AGED

Elderly patients are more prone to become emotionally disturbed when confronted with new situations, especially if they have inadequate comprehension and a generalized feeling of insecurity. The operative procedure also presents an obvious physical threat to the integrity of the nervous system. Titchener and associates reported a 25 percent incidence of significant and, at times, irreversible change in cerebral function in the patients in their group over the age of sixty-five. Some degree of depression was observed in 90 percent of the older patients, and this was of a disabling nature in about 50 percent. Indifference of the family, friends, and society contributed to the evolution of a paranoid cycle.

Attempts should be directed at limiting the physical insult to the brain, and postoperative mental evaluation is indicated on a routine basis in order to detect the early changes of the organic brain syndrome and delirium. Efforts should be made to familiarize the patients with the hospital and personnel, and visitors should be encouraged to maintain a human contact and prevent withdrawal. Collaboration with a social worker is frequently indicated for long-term rehabilitation.

GYNECOLOGIC AND BREAST SURGERY

Removal of the breast and a variety of gynecologic procedures are highly represented in most series of postoperative psychosis. Maguire and associates found that 1 year after mastectomy the women reported a 20 percent incidence of depressed feelings, a 10 percent incidence of anxiety, and 38 percent incidence of sexual difficulties. Contact with other mastectomy patients expedites psychologic rehabilitation. Routine counseling lowered the postoperative psychiatric morbidity from 38 to 12 percent. Hysterectomy is associated with emotional disturbance more frequently than other gynecologic operations, and the more the procedure antedates the menopause, the more the likelihood of associated psychologic disturbance. The loss of menstrual function is perceived by the woman as a blow to normal feminine esteem. Hollender reported that of 203 women admitted to psychiatric hospital, 9 had pelvic surgical treatment as a precipitating event, and this was in contrast to a total of 5 women admitted following operations of all other kinds. Lindemann noted that the relative frequency of restlessness, insomnia, agitation, and preoccupation with depressive thoughts was greater after pelvic operations than after cholecystectomy.

CANCER SURGERY

Cancer patients are exposed to two major threats, disease and extensive surgical treatment. They are concerned with death or injury during operation and disruption of their pattern of living as a result of the effects of cancer or the surgical procedure. Patients with emotional problems involving self-destruction are particularly vulnerable to preoperative anxiety concerning death and mutilation. This may be manifest by anorexia, insomnia, tachycardia, fear, and panic. Acute depression with suicidal tendencies has been reported in anticipation of surgical procedures. Postoperatively, depression is related to an anticipated interference with valued activities. Sutherland and associates have demonstrated that colostomy imposed on almost all patients a new order of living, and the subjects were powerfully motivated to avoid social rejection. A rigid life arose from the fearful expectation of rejection because of the colostomy combined with the fear of death from cancer. There is a tendency toward seclusion, withdrawal, and nonparticipation. Spells of depression are frequent, and Sutherland and his associates are of the opinion that loss of an important bodily part or function is more depressing than the fear or expectation of death. The management of patients with carcinoma must be based on an appreciation that they frequently suffer a sense of isolation, guilt, and abandonment.

CARDIAC SURGERY

Serious psychiatric disturbances have been observed to occur with considerable frequency following mitral valvulotomy and open heart surgery. Fox and associates and Bliss et al. reported, respectively, a 19 and 16 percent incidence of serious emotional disturbance following mitral valve surgery. Bolton and Bailey, however, in an evaluation of 1500 consecutive patients, noted an incidence of psychosis of 3 percent with no relation to age, sex, severity of heart disease, duration of failure, or complications of surgical treatment. Egerton and Kay noted delirium in 25 of 60 adults following open heart surgery.

Manifestations generally occur after an initial lucid interval 3 to 5 days after operation and clear shortly after the patient is transferred from an intensive care unit to a standard hospital ward. Postoperative incapacitation and increased time on the heart-lung machine apparently are factors increasing the likelihood of delirium, while age and sex do not alter the incidence. Zaks has suggested that cardiac operation may produce organic brain damage, thus sensitizing patients and increasing the incidence of postoperative psychologic symptomatology. A prediction equation was successful in differentiating reactors from nonreactors. Using the ego strength variable of the Minnesota Multiphasic Personality Inventory, there is a significant inverse correlation between the reaction and the incidence of acute psychotic episodes following cardiac operation. The incidence of psychoses is greater in males, older patients, and those expressing minimal preoperative anxiety. A preoperative psychiatric interview reduces the incidence of postoperative psychosis by 50 percent.

Following operations on the heart, the patients with emotional disturbances manifest perceptual distortion, visual and auditory hallucinations, disorientation, and paranoia. Twenty-eight percent of adult patients subjected to open heart surgery, as reported by Egerton and Kay, had delirious states ranging in duration from several nights to several weeks, averaging 5 days. The delirious patients had no psychologic sequelae, and no relation could be established between the incidence of delirium and the duration of cardiac bypass, but open heart procedures were more likely to produce delirium than other intrathoracic operations. The writers felt that the precipitating factors for delirium included dehydration, hyponatremia, and the performance of a tracheostomy, while the predisposing factors included a familial history of psychosis, previous brain damage, overwhelming personal problems, and the presence of a rheumatic valvular lesion. Other psychiatric disturbances noted in patients following open heart surgery were disabling anxiety state, conversion hysteria, tension headaches, and, in a surprising 5 percent of the operative cases, exacerbation of peptic ulcer. The almost total absence of delirium and other emotional disorders in children is of particular interest and may be related to the fact that the concept of death as a permanent biologic process usually does not develop until the age of nine.

DIALYSIS AND TRANSPLANTATION

A variety of emotional disturbances have been observed in patients undergoing hemodialysis. The suicide rate is 300 times greater than for a comparable healthy population. Uremia, debilitating disease, and the repeated technical procedures that are performed all constitute etiologic factors. Wright et al. followed 11 patients on chronic dialysis and noted a number of stresses affecting them, such as unpredictability of well-being, tensions arising in the marital situation from guilt and anger, effects of separation on the families, and financial anxiety. Following each episode of dialysis, the main patient response was one of relief. Cramond and associates noted that their patients at first denied their illness and later realized that they had lost their health and independence and their futures were uncertain. This has been referred to as a "mourning reaction." From time to time the patients wished to be dead. They felt that life dependent on chronic dialysis was not worth living. Some patients passed from the mourning reaction to a state of active depression.

All patients undergoing dialysis become extremely dependent on the staff and emotionally attached to them. The patients often react emotionally to a sense of loss when any replacement of staff occurs. During the course of the dialysis program, regression occurs relatively frequently and the patient becomes withdrawn and pretends to sleep. Insomnia and frightening dreams also occur, and the frequency with which emotional disturbances have been noted suggests that psychiatric assistance plays an important role in a dialysis program.

Two distinct groups of patients, the donors and recipients, must be considered in a renal homotransplantation program. Psychologic screening of the potential donors is indicated, and selection should be from individuals who are stable and who have mature judgment. Individuals with psychopathologic motives such as sacrifice or exhibitionism should be excluded, particularly when they are unrelated donors. It is to be emphasized that those who refuse to cooperate risk being rejected by the family and are frequently made to feel guilty. Therefore, when potential donors are rejected on psychiatric grounds, the rejection should be ascribed to a minor physical variation. In four of five cases, Cramond noted an ambivalent relationship between donors and recipients. Donors experienced emotional and physical investment in the patient and, at times, sought to overprotect the patient. They felt that their sacrificial gift was in jeopardy if the patient behaved in a manner of which they did not approve.

The recipient has been shown to be aware of an obligation to the donor and resents the dependency relationship. At times feelings of shame and guilt must be considered. Kemph, in a follow-up of recipients of renal homotransplants, has noted periods of severe depression and concern with bodily damage and sexual damage. After the operation the donors also experience depression. Many expressed the feeling that they were not attentively supported by the hospital personnel.

Some recipients regard the operation as symbolic of rebirth and may undergo a religious conviction. In some recipients, a graft from a donor of an opposite sex is considered a threat to sexual identity. All recipients demonstrate anxiety in reference to injury of the grafted kidney. Although severe depressions and emotional reactions are uncommon, psychologic adjustment takes longer than a year to accomplish. When given a choice, patients who have rejected their kidney transplants have almost uniformly chosen a second transplant over return to dialysis.

INTENSIVE CARE DELIRIUM

Delirium manifested by a wide variety of behavior patterns, ranging from apathy to restlessness and combativeness, is a common occurrence in intensive care units. Drugs are a common cause, but both environmental and metabolic factors also have been implicated. The former can be corrected by transferring the patient to a regular hospital ward or room as soon as possible. Katz et al. indicated a physiologic abnormality, such as hypoxemia or electrolyte or acid-base abnormality, as the cause in the great majority of patients. Preoperative discussion and support lowered the incidence of postcardiotomy delirium from 37 to 14 percent in one series.

DRUG ABUSE

Beebe and Keats have shown that not all narcotic addicts require detoxification associated with an operation. Methadone is the drug of choice for treating withdrawal. Haloxone may be preferable in an emergency situation. For patients on methadone maintenance, this drug can be stopped temporarily and frequent doses of conventional narcotics substituted during the early postoperative period. Withdrawal from barbiturates prior to elective operation may take 2 to 3 weeks. There is no physiologic addiction requiring maintenance of amphetamines or hallucinogens.

COMPLICATIONS OF GASTROINTESTINAL SURGERY

The complications considered in this section are divided into (1) vascular complications, including hemorrhage and gangrene; (2) mechanical problems of gastroenterostomy and enteroenterostomy, including stomal obstruction, the afferent, or blind, loop syndrome, extrinsic obstruction and internal hernia, and inadvertent gastroileostomy; (3) leakage of an anastomosis, including the duodenal stump blowout; (4) external fistulas and stomal problems; and (5) damage to adjacent organs, including postoperative pancreatitis and jaundice.

Vascular Complications

HEMORRHAGE

Gastrointestinal hemorrhage that occurs subsequent to a gastrointestinal anastomosis may become manifest postoperatively by hematemesis, melena, hematochezia, or, most frequently, the passage of bright blood via a nasogastric tube positioned in the stomach. Bleeding from the suture line is most commonly associated with gastric surgery, occurring in approximately 1 to 5 percent of patients following gastric resection, with a higher incidence in those patients in whom operation is performed for a duodenal ulcer. Bleeding from the suture line is apt to occur either immediately after the operation or on the first postoperative day, but a second minor peak in incidence has been noted between the seventh and tenth postoperative days. Bleeding arising from the suture line on the first postoperative day is usually minimal or moderate and requires no specific therapy, but if it is continuous, the stomach should be aspirated and irrigated with ice-cold saline solution. Hemorrhage that does not stop following conservative measures constitutes an indication for endoscopy. Endoscopically directed coagulation or laser therapy may effect control of a bleeding site. If bleeding continues, reoperation is indicated, at which time the suture line should be inspected. It may be preferable to enter the stomach above the line of anastomosis and ligate vessels from within. Bleeding later in the course of convalescence is usually due to sloughing from the suture line and generally responds to iced saline lavage. Significant hemorrhage from the suture line of small intestinal and large intestinal anastomoses is extremely rare. Upper gastrointestinal bleeding following a surgical procedure in a patient who is debilitated or in whom sepsis develops frequently indicates a stress ulcer (see Chap. 26).

GANGRENE

Gangrene is a rare complication of resection of a segment of gastrointestinal tract, since the intestine is supplied with a rich network of arteries. Necrosis of the gastric remnant has been reported following a high subtotal gastrectomy, particularly if the procedure incorporates ligation of the left gastric artery and concomitant splenectomy. Devascularization of the areas to be anastomosed should not occur following small intestinal surgical procedures if attention is directed toward the vascular supply. A precautionary measure is to slant the lines of incision so that more intestine is resected on the antimesenteric aspect. Small intestinal gangrene is more frequently due to mechanical strangulation, obstruction secondary to postoperative adhesions, volvulus, internal hernias, or vascular thrombosis. Gangrene of the segment of intestine may be apparent in the case of a colostomy in which an inadequate vascular supply has been provided. In each instance, the recognition of gangrene requires resection of the gangrenous segment of intestine or stomach and reestablishment of intestinal continuity or a colostomy in bowel that is viable.

Mechanical Problems

STOMAL OBSTRUCTION

Although obstruction of the stoma may follow any intestinal anastomosis as a result of technical factors, postgastrectomy stomal obstruction represents the most common type and is frequently related to local edema. Factors that have been implicated in the etiology of edema include electrolyte depletion, hypochloremia, incomplete hemostasis, hypoproteinemia, leakage from the anastomosis, inadequate proximal decompression, and incorporation of too much tissue within the sutures. Other causes include rotation of the jejunum on its long axis, obstruction by the transverse mesocolon, particularly in an obese patient, obstruction by a fatty omentum, effect of vagotomy, and, rarely, jejunogastric intussusception, which has been reported as a complication in slightly over 100 cases of Billroth II procedures.

Postgastrectomy stomal obstruction is a most troublesome complication, and the reported incidence has ranged between 1 and 3 percent. In a review of 648 partial gastrectomies, an incidence of 4.6 percent for patients requiring further operative therapy, 4.1 percent for Billroth II operations, and 3.5 percent for Billroth I types was recorded. In most instances in their series, the efferent loop was obstructed by the transverse mesocolon.

Symptoms usually occur on the third to fourth postoperative day, at which time there is abdominal fullness and increased return from the nasogastric suction. If the patient has been on oral intake, nausea followed by vomiting of large quantities of bile-colored gastric fluid occurs. Instillation of barium or Gastrografin via the nasogastric tube may reveal stomal obstruction or a patent stoma with distal loop obstruction. The symptoms usually persist for only short intervals and cause little disability, but occasionally they are prolonged and then have severe metabolic effects.

Prophylaxis is directed at avoiding the factors that have been implicated. Therapy of established stomal obstruction consists of adequate decompression and replacement of fluids and nutrients, while waiting for the obstruction to become relieved spontaneously. The course may be prolonged, extending over a period of several weeks.

Metaclopramide or bethanechol may be administered for several days in an attempt to improve gastric atony. If there is not relief after extended conservative management or if the patient's condition is deteriorating, operative intervention is indicated. Rarely, a simple release of adhesions may be therapeutic, but more often the anastomotic site requires revision, a procedure that is frequently difficult in view of the extensive reaction around the stoma. It is generally preferable to transect the proximal and distal loops of intestine at their entrance to and exit from the indurated mass. These are then anastomosed to one another, and the short segment of intestine and a cuff of stomach are removed with the gastroenterostomy. Continuity is reestablished with a long antecolic gastrojejunostomy.

AFFERENT (BLIND) LOOP SYNDROME

The afferent loop syndrome represents a complication of subtotal gastrectomy with Billroth II gastroenterostomy. The afferent loop consists of duodenum and a segment of jejunum of variable length. Acute or chronic obstruction can occur at any point proximal to the gastrojejunostomy. Blomstedt and Dahlgren reported an incidence of 18 percent with mild to moderate symptoms (type I and type II). The symptom complex of partial obstruction of the afferent loop was reported by Magnuson et al. to occur following gastrectomy in 4.2 percent of patients with gastric ulcer in contrast to 0.9 percent of patients with duodenal ulcer.

PATHOGENESIS. Normally after partial gastrectomy, biliary and pancreatic secretions enter the afferent loop, pass through the gastrojejunostomy to mix with gastric juice, and then pass through into the efferent loop. During a 24-h period, approximately 1 to 1.5 L of secretion enters the afferent loop. The afferent loop syndrome is caused by partial and, rarely, total obstruction of flow from the afferent loop. The pressure within the duodenum and segment of jejunum rises, and the loop becomes dilated by bile and pancreatic juice. After the ingestion of food, particularly a fatty meal, the duodenal contents increase rapidly, thus explaining the postcibal nature of the syndrome. With incomplete obstruction, pressure within the intestine eventually becomes sufficient to overcome resistance, and the contents are emptied into the stomach, causing variable amounts to be vomited. With total obstruction, the loop no longer has any communication with the stomach, and vomitus is free of bile.

CLINICAL MANIFESTATIONS. The symptoms of partial obstruction of the afferent loop occur most commonly in the early postoperative period. Two-thirds of the cases occur during the first week, but in some instances the syndrome becomes apparent months to years following gastrectomy. The symptoms vary in intensity and are characterized by postcibal vomiting. Mild symptoms consist of eructation of a mouthful of green biliary fluid within an hour and a half after a meal. Vomiting is generally preceded by the sensation of fullness and, at times, pain in the epigastrium. In some instances, the symptoms of chronic obstruction persist for several months, and the amount of biliary vomiting and antecedent epigastric pain are appreciable. With persistence of partial obstruction, the stools become bulky and gray and contain much fat. Radiographic examination may show passage of contrast material into the efferent loop, while the afferent loop, as a rule, fails to fill. Chronic partial obstruction is associated with anemia. Urinary excretion of B_{12} is reduced or absent and is unaffected by the administration of intrinsic factor, in contrast to pernicious anemia. However, following a course of 3 to 5 days of tetracycline, B_{12} urinary excretion returns to normal.

In the rare situation of the acute complete obstruction of the afferent loop, the patient becomes acutely ill with severe epigastric pain, and bile is characteristically absent from the vomitus. A mass may be felt in the upper abdomen. The patient's condition may deteriorate rapidly, and shock may occur as a result of compromise of the circulation of the duodenal wall and/or perforation with generalized peritonitis. Radiographs are of little diagnostic assistance. There may be delayed emptying of contrast material from the gastric remnant, and no barium enters the afferent loop. The amylase level may be markedly elevated.

TREATMENT. Incomplete obstruction generally subsides on a conservative regimen. Capper and Welbourn collected 44 cases requiring surgical intervention and reported that 36 of them had a good outcome. Surgical decompression of the afferent loop may be accomplished by anastomosis between the afferent and efferent loops, by employing a Roux en Y anastomosis or converting a gastrojejunostomy to a gastroduodenostomy. In the case of acute total obstruction, early operation with decompression of the afferent loop is mandatory.

INTESTINAL OBSTRUCTION

Intestinal obstruction in the immediate postoperative period is most frequently due to ileus or fibrinous adhesions. Following laparotomy the stomach usually recovers motor activity in hours, the small intestine within a day, and the colon in 30 days. In the face of peritonitis or mesenteric or retroperitoneal hematoma, ileus is usually prolonged. It may be impossible to distinguish postoperative ileus and mechanical obstruction. Following the progression of radiopaque material instilled via a nasogastric tube may distinguish the two disorders. Internal herniation represents a complication of subtotal gastrectomy, generally following a Billroth II antecolic anastomosis. Internal herniation of the small intestine may also take place through improperly closed mesenteric rents or when the mesentery of the ileum or colon is not tacked to the peritoneum in the course of an ileostomy or colostomy. Closed-loop obstruction generally results and may rapidly progress to compromise the vascular supply with ultimate perforation. Operative reduction and repair of an internal hernia are required. Adhesions and/or volvulus may occur in the postoperative hospitalization and require surgical intervention for relief of obstruction. The incidence is particularly high following resection for congenital atresia in infancy, especially when the proximal dilated bowel is not resected. Postoperative intussusception, generally involving the small intestine, is also to be considered in the pediatric age group.

INADVERTENT GASTROILEOSTOMY

The error of anastomosing the stomach to the ileum rather than the jejunum is fortunately uncommon. The situation results in a malabsorption syndrome that begins as soon as the patient is allowed to eat solid food. Diarrhea, weight loss, and inanition in the absence of abdominal pain are characteristic. The stool contains a high percentage of undigested food and a large quantity of unabsorbed fat. Fecal vomiting and hemorrhage occasionally occur, and an ulcer may develop at the site of the ileum, in which case abdominal pain may be present. The diagnosis can be established radiographically by demonstrating a rapid transit and short distal intestine. The error should be avoided by using the ligament of Treitz as a landmark in establishing a gastroenterostomy; in the absence of a ligament of Treitz an anomaly of rotation should be suspected, and the loop of intestine for anastomosis should be selected by tracing the duodenum distad or the small bowel proximally from the cecum. The preoperative management of patients with gastroileostomy requires a vigorous preparation with TPN, or a preliminary feeding jejunostomy is of value. A block resection of the gastroileostomy is advocated for patients who have had subtotal gastric resection, while, in the absence of gastric resection, the ileostomy may be taken down directly. A gastrojejunostomy and reconstitution of intestinal continuity are then performed.

Anastomotic Leak

Suture line leakage represents a potential complication of any intestinal anastomosis. The three prime etiologic factors are (1) poor surgical technique, (2) distal obstruction, and (3) inadequate proximal decompression. Leak from an enteroenterostomy becomes manifest as localized or generalized peritonitis. Small leaks with localized response may be treated by proximal decompression and administration of appropriate antibiotics, while large leaks and diffuse peritonitis frequently require surgical intervention. Fistulization may develop as a tract becomes established between the point of leakage and the skin. A leak from the line of anastomosis is a relatively rare complication following gastroenterostomy. Such leakage occurs more frequently when there has been impairment of the blood supply of the residual gastric pouch and a concomitant splenectomy has been performed. A common point at which leaks develop has been referred to as the "angle du mort," where the residual gastric pouch of a Hofmeister closure meets the line of anastomosis of the small intestine.

Duodenal stump leakage (blowout) is a more frequent and critical complication of gastric resection. A review of gastrectomies performed at the Mayo Clinic in 1956 revealed that 4.5 percent of patients subjected to the procedure for gastric ulcer had some evidence of leak, while 5.6 percent of patients in whom the same procedure was carried out for duodenal ulcer revealed similar evidence. In that study, drains had been inserted into the stump region, and in many patients increased drainage represented the evidence of a leak. Edmunds et al. reported a 1.1 percent incidence of dehiscence of the stump, the mortality due to this cause was 0.6 percent.

Duodenal stump leakage occurs most commonly after operation for a duodenal ulcer and frequently when gastrectomy is performed as an emergency procedure to stop hemorrhage. In a great majority of cases, the leak arises as a result of technical error and failure of the suture line. A scarred and edematous duodenum predisposes to the complication as does obstruction of the afferent loop and local pancreatitis. Complications of duodenal leakage include peritonitis, subhepatic abscess, pancreatitis, sepsis, and establishment of an external fistula with fluid and electrolyte abnormalities.

Specific measures can be taken to avoid this complication. In the face of marked inflammatory disease in the duodenal region, vagotomy and gastroenterostomy definitely represent safer procedures. When resection has been undertaken and duodenal closure is difficult, catheter duodenostomy may be used as an adjunct. Rodkey and Welch reported that in 51 cases with difficult duodenal stump closures in whom planned duodenostomy was carried out, there was only one death, and only five patients had drainage from the fistula that lasted more than 48 h after the catheter was removed. As a compromise between primary closure and planned duodenostomy, some surgeons have advised drainage of the right upper quadrant placed in the region of the duodenal stump in the hope that if perforation occurs, the contents will discharge along the tract. However, this does not provide the safety factor of planned duodenostomy, since the drain tract may wall off from the stump before the perforation becomes established.

Duodenal blowout is a major catastrophe that is most likely to occur between the second and seventh postoperative day, and becomes manifest by sudden pain, elevation in temperature and pulse rate, and general deterioration of the patient's condition. Adequate drainage must be instituted at once and is best accomplished by an incision below the right costal margin and insertion of a large sump catheter that is passed down to the duodenal stump area, with constant suction applied. Attention must be directed toward fluid and electrolyte therapy, and TPN should be instituted. Fistula closure can be anticipated within 2 to 3 weeks. Another area in which leaks are a major concern is low colon anastomoses; incidences of 5 to 51 percent have been reported. Pedicled omentum may be applied to seal the anastomosis. The mortality rate in patients with major colon leaks is extremely high, and this has led to a resurgence of enthusiasm for protective transverse colostomy if the anastomosis appears compromised.

External Fistulas and Stomal Complications

FISTULAS

External fistulas may arise from the stomach and duodenum, the small intestine, or the colon. In one series of 157 patients, there was equal distribution of fistulas from the three major segments of the intraabdominal alimentary tract. Surgical procedures have been implicated as etiologic factors in 67 to 80 percent of cases.

Gastric and Duodenal Fistulas

The incidence of gastrojejunal or duodenal stump fistulas following subtotal gastrectomy has been reported to be 1 to 2 percent, approximately one-quarter of which originated from the gastrojejunostomy. Suture line failure accounted for 82 percent of all gastroduodenal fistulas. The causes of fistulas arising from the gastrojejunostomy may be related to the suture line containing tumor, ischemia of the gastric stump due to high ligation of the gastric artery and vasa brevia, stomal obstruction, and pancreatitis or tension on the suture line. The causes of duodenal stump fistula have been referred to in the previous section on stump leakage. The complications of an established gastric or duodenal fistula include electrolyte abnormalities and malnutrition, sepsis, intraperitoneal abscesses and wound infection, jaundice, and pancreatitis.

Treatment. Intensive fluid, electrolyte, and nutritional therapy is frequently required. This may be facilitated by TPN or enteral feeding with elemental diet delivered distally via a jejunostomy or a nasogastric tube advanced beyond the area of the fistula. Large amounts of drainage can usually be collected with a well-fixed appliance; continuous suction is rarely employed. Skin care is an essential factor; autodigestion can be prevented with a variety of barrier powders or sheets. The majority of fistulas that close spontaneously do so within 6 weeks.

An established gastric fistula may require resection and correction of distal obstruction if the latter is present. Fistulas arising at the site of a gastrojejunostomy generally require resection and establishment of a new gastroenterostomy. Duodenal fistulas are generally not amenable to direct closure. Tarazi and associates recently reported an experience with 47 patients, 18 with gastric and 29 with duodenal fistulas, and they reviewed other series. The mortality of gastric fistulas was 22 percent compared with reported percentages of 15 to 50 percent. The mortality of lateral duodenal fistulas was 25 percent compared with other reports of 0 to 67 percent. The mortality of duodenal stump fistulas ranged from 12 to 50 percent. The incidence of spontaneous closure ranged from 25 to 54 percent of gastric fistulas and from 37 to 100 percent for duodenal fistulas. When operation was performed for duodenal fistula, the authors noted a success rate of less than 50 percent; others have reported excellent results with a jejunal or ileal serosal patch or a Roux en Y anastomosis to the defect.

Small Bowel Fistulas

Seventy-two percent of the 46 fistulas in this group reported by Edmunds et al. represented surgical complications secondary to dehiscence of anastomoses or inadvertent injury during dissection or closure of an abdominal incision. Although jejunal and proximal ileal fistulas are frequently characterized by profuse drainage, the fluid loss is generally less than that associated with duodenal fistulas, and therefore fluid and electrolyte abnormalities occur less frequently. Malnutrition must be aggressively combated in these patients, and sepsis is a major complication. A large number of intraperitoneal abscesses develop. Skin digestion is a frequent occurrence, and many of these patients eventually develop a ventral hernia due to wound complications.

Many factors influence the outcome of treatment of enterocutaneous fistulas. Jejunal fistulas have a poorer prognosis than ileal fistulas; high-output fistulas are also associated with a greater mortality rate. Intraabdominal sepsis, anemia, and malnutrition all have adverse effects. Series reported since 1970 indicate medical regimens effect cures in an average of 62 percent of cases and are associated with an average mortality rate of 13 percent.

Treatment. Supportive management of small bowel fistulas is similar to that outlined for gastroduodenal fistulas. This includes maintenance of fluid and electrolyte balance and nutrition. An elemental diet may be applicable particularly for low output fistulas. TPN may be applicable. In the case of a proximal jejunal fistula, a distal feeding jejunostomy is frequently indicated to permit adequate fluid and nutritional intake. Oral feeding of low-residue diets is feasible with ileal fistulas. Control of fluid loss and diarrhea may be accomplished with the use of Lomotil, Kaopectate, and opiates plus nonabsorbable antibiotics when indicated. Protection of the skin in the region of the fistula is indicated.

Operative procedures include direct attack on a fistula with resection both of the fistula and the segment of intestine from which it arises or an indirect attack through a clean abdominal incision with a bypass operation or complete exclusion of the fistula by means of end-to-end anastomosis of the proximal and distal intestine. The excluded loop is then decompressed completely through a large fistula by exteriorizing the ends of the intestine to prevent later blowout. Definitive operations should be performed only in sepsis-free patients in wound nutritional status.

Colonic Fistulas (See Chaps. 27 and 28)

These are generally caused by anastomotic leaks or inadvertent trauma to the segment of intestine. Anastomosis in the region of tumor or inflammation and distal partial obstruction are predisposing factors. Fluid and electrolyte abnormalities are uncommon, while the incidence of infection is extremely high. This includes peritonitis, intraperitoneal abscesses, and wound infections. Significant skin digestion and irritation are rare.

Treatment. The patients can generally be managed on a low-residue or elemental diet, using enteric or parenteral antibiotics when indicated. Spontaneous healing of fistulas in these regions is the rule rather than the exception, but defunctionalizing colostomies for descending colon fistulas or ileal transverse colostomies for ascending colon and distal ileal fistulas may be indicated. Medical management is generally indicated for about 6 weeks to permit any active inflammation to subside. Definitive surgical treatment is indicated for fistulas that fail to progress satisfactorily after 6 weeks. If the fistula is accompanied by generalized peritonitis, early emergency resection is indicated and frequently should be accompanied by a proximal defunctionalizing procedure. Definitive operations include a turn-in procedure or resection that may be coupled with a temporary protective colostomy or bypass. Seventy-five percent of patients with no operation experienced spontaneous cure; 74 percent of chronic fecal fistulas treated by turn-in or resection were cured.

EXTERNAL STOMAL COMPLICATIONS (See Chap. 28)

Ileostomy

Ileostomy performed for ulcerative colitis may be associated with complications related to technical factors, presence of disease, and the nature of the intestinal contents that are discharged. The location of ileostomy is critical to permit application of an effective collecting device, while the method of fixation of the ileal mesentery is important to prevent internal herniation. Formation of the ileostomy itself is important in reducing the incidence of complications. The technique of operative maturation by everting the mucosa reduces the incidence of serositis and peritonitis. The liquid nature of the ileostomy discharge requires that measures be taken to avoid excoriation of the skin, which is usually due to delayed application of the bag and a poor fit. When excoriation appears, it is generally wise to discontinue the use of cement and apply a soothing powder. The patient may be placed in a prone position on a frame so that the ileal contents are allowed to drain into a container and contact with the skin is avoided. The complication of prolapse, which requires revision, should be seen infrequently if the mesentery has been fixed. Fistulas that develop at or below the skin level are an indication for early revision of the ileostomy.

Cecostomy and Colostomy

Cecostomies generally demand more attention than colostomies, and frequent irrigation is indicated. Subsequent to removal of the cecostomy catheter, spontaneous closure is to be anticipated, but in unusual circumstances, surgical closure is required. Complications following colostomy include ischemia, gangrene, bleeding, wound abscesses, stenosis, or retraction of the stoma. In the case of a terminal colostomy, fixation and maturation during the operative procedure should prevent retraction. If either retraction or gangrene becomes evident, immediate operation is indicated to revise the colostomy using viable bowel of sufficient length. A paracolostomy hernia may require direct fascial repair.

Bibliography

General Considerations

Artz CP, Hardy JD: *Complications in Surgery and Their Management.* Philadelphia, Saunders, 1967.

Wound Complications

Alexander HC, Prudden J: The causes of abdominal wound disruption. *Surg Gynecol Obstet* 122:1223, 1966.

Banerjee SR, Daoud I, et al: Abdominal wound evisceration. *Curr Surg* 40:432, 1983.

Elek SD, Conen PE: The virulence of *Staphylococcus pyogenes* for man: A study of the problems of wound infections. *Br J Exp Pathol* 38:573, 1957.

Fagniez J–L, Hay JM, et al: Abdominal midline incision closure. *Arch Surg* 120:1351, 1985.

Gammelgaard N, Jensen J: Wound complications after closure of abdominal incisions with Dexon or Vicryl. *Acta Chir Scand* 149:505, 1983.

Goligher JC, Irvin TT, et al: A controlled clinical trial of three methods of closure of laparotomy wounds. *Br J Surg* 62:823, 1975.

Greenburg AG, Saik RP, Peskin GW: Wound dehiscence. *Arch Surg* 114:143, 1979.

Halasz NA: Dehiscence of laparotomy wounds. *Am J Surg* 116:210, 1968.

Pemberton LB, Manax WG: Complications after vertical and transverse incisions for cholecystectomy. *Surg Gynecol Obstet* 132:892, 1971.

Pollock AV, Froome K, Evans M: The bacteriology of primary wound sepsis in potentially contaminated abdominal operations: The effect of irrigation, povidone-iodine and cephaloridine on the sepsis rate assessed in a clinical trial. *Br J Surg* 65:76, 1978.

Sindelar WF, Mason GR: Irrigation of subcutaneous tissue with povidone-iodine solution for prevention of surgical wound infections. *Surg Gynecol Obstet* 148:227, 1979.

Wolff WI: Disruption of abdominal wounds. *Ann Surg* 131:534, 1950.

Postoperative Parotitis

Hemenway WG, English GM: Surgical treatment of acute bacterial parotitis. *Postgrad Med* 50:114, 1971.

Krippaehne WW, Hunt TK, Dunphy JE: Acute suppurative parotitis: A study of 161 cases. *Ann Surg* 156:251, 1962.

Lary BG: Postoperative suppurative parotitis. *Arch Surg* 89:653, 1964.

Petersdorf RG, Forsyth BB, Bernake D: Staphylococcal parotitis. *N Engl J Med* 259:1250, 1958.

Postoperative Respiratory Complications

Adriani J, Zepernick R, et al: Iatrogenic pulmonary edema in surgical patients. *Surgery* 61:183, 1967.

Ashbaugh DG, Petty TL: Positive end-expiratory pressure: Physiology, indications, and contraindications. *J Thorac Cardiovasc Surg* 65:165, 1973.

Civetta JM, Augenstein JS: Acute respiratory failure following surgery and trauma, in Greenfield LJ (ed): *Complications in Surgery and Trauma*. Philadelphia, Lippincott, 1984, chap 21, pp 243–259.

Clements JA: Surface phenomena in relation to pulmonary function (sixth Bowditch lecture). *Physiologist* 5:11, 1962.

Cuschieri J, Morran G, et al: Postoperative pain and pulmonary complications: Comparison of three analgesic regimens. *Br J Surg* 72:495, 1985.

Davis HA, Pollak EW: Adult respiratory distress syndrome in postoperative patients: Study of pulmonary pathology in ''shock lung'' with prophylactic and therapeutic implications. *Am Surg* 41:391, 1975.

Joffe N: Roentgenologic findings in post-shock and postoperative pulmonary insufficiency. *Radiology* 94:369, 1970.

Laver MB, Bendixen HH: Atelectasis in the surgical patient: Recent conceptual advances. *Prog Surg* 5:1, 1966.

Neely WA, Robinson TW, et al: Post-operative respiratory insufficiency. *Ann Surg* 171:679, 1970.

Norwood SH, Civetta JM: Ventilatory support in patients with ARDS. *Surg Clin North Am* 65:895, 1985.

Peters RM, Hilberman M, et al: Objective indications for respiratory therapy in post-trauma and postoperative patients. *Am J Surg* 124:262, 1972.

Pontoppidan H, Geffin B, Lowenstein E: Acute respiratory failure in the adult: Trends in treatment of acute respiratory failure. *N Engl J Med* 287:690, 1972.

Pontoppidan H, Geffin B, Lowenstein E: Acute respiratory failure in the adult: Assessment of respiratory function. *N Engl J Med* 287:743, 1972.

Pontoppidan H, Geffin B, Lowenstein E: Acute respiratory failure in the adult: Effect of mechanical ventilation and airway pressures on circulation and blood gas exchange. *N Engl J Med* 287:799, 1972.

Pontoppidan H, Laver MB, Geffin B: Acute respiratory failure in the surgical patient. *Adv Surg* 4:163, 1970.

Rinaldo JE, Rogers RM: Adult respiratory distress syndrome. Changing concepts of lung injury and repair. *N Engl J Med* 306:900, 1982.

Sayeed MM, Chaudry IH, Baue AE: Na^+–K^+ transport and adenosine nucleotides in the lung in hemorrhagic shock. *Surgery* 77:395, 1975.

Shoemaker WC: Controversies in the pathophysiology and fluid management of postoperative adult respiratory distress syndrome. *Surg Clin North Am* 64:931, 1985.

Staub NC: Pulmonary edema due to increased microvascular permeability. *Annu Rev Med* 32:291, 1981.

Stock MC, Downs JB, et al: Prevention of postoperative complications with CPAP, incentive spirometry, and conservative therapy. *Chest* 87:151, 1985.

Cardiac Complications

Buckley JJ, Jackson JA: Postoperative cardiac arrhythmias. *Anesthesiology* 22:723, 1961.

Dreifus LS, Rabbino MD, et al: Arrhythmias in the postoperative period. *Am J Cardiol* 12:431, 1963.

Goldman L: Cardiac risks and complications of noncardiac surgery. *Ann Surg* 198:780, 1983.

Mauney FM Jr, Ebert PA, Sabiston DC Jr.: Postoperative myocardial infarction: A study of predisposing factors, diagnosis, and mortality in a high risk group of surgical patients. *Ann Surg* 172:497, 1970.

Merideth J: Cardiac arrhythmias in the postoperative patient. *Surg Clin North Am* 49:1083, 1969.

Reinikainen M, Pontinen P: On cardiac arrhythmias during anaesthesia and surgery. *Acta Med Scand Suppl* 457, 1966.

Singh BN, Ellrodt G, Peter CT: Verapamil: A review of its pharmacological properties and therapeutic use. *Drugs* 15:169, 1978.

Tarhan S, Moffitt EA, et al: Myocardial infarction after general anesthesia. *JAMA* 220:1451, 1972.

Wroblewski F, LaDue JS: Myocardial infarction as a postoperative complication of major surgery. *JAMA* 150:1212, 1952.

Diabetes Mellitus

Galloway JA, Shuman CR: Diabetes and surgery: A study of 667 cases. *Am J Med* 34:177, 1963.

Gastineau CF, Molnar GD: The care of the diabetic patient during emergency surgery. *Surg Clin North Am* 49:1171, 1969.

Kidson W, Casey J, et al: Treatment of severe diabetes mellitus by infusion. *Br Med J* 2:691, 1974.

Marble A, Steinke J: Physiology and pharmacology in diabetes mellitus: Guiding the diabetic patient through the surgical period. *Anesthesiology* 24:442, 1963.

Meyer EJ, Lorenzi M, et al: Diabetic management by insulin infusion during major surgery. *Am J Surg* 137:323, 1979.

Page M McB, Alberti KGMM, et al: Treatment of diabetic coma with continuous low dose infusion. *Br Med J* 2:687, 1974.

Woodruff RE, Lewis SB, et al: Avoidance of surgical hyperglycemia in diabetic patients. *JAMA* 244:166, 1980.

Fat Embolism Syndrome

Ashbaugh DG, Petty TL: The use of corticosteroids in the treatment of respiratory failure associated with massive fat embolism. *Surg Gynecol Obstet* 123:495, 1966.

Benoit PR, Hampson LG, Burgess JH: Value of arterial hypoxemia in the diagnosis of pulmonary fat embolism. *Ann Surg* 175:128, 1972.

Chan KM, Tham KT, et al: Post-traumatic fat embolism—its clinical and subclinical present status. *J Trauma* 24:45, 1984.

Evarts CM: The fat embolism syndrome: A review. *Surg Clin North Am* 50:493, 1970.

Palmovic V, McCarroll JR: Fat embolism in trauma. *Arch Pathol* 80:630, 1965.

Pazell JA, Peltier LF: Experience with sixty-three patients with fat embolism. *Surg Gynecol Obstet* 135:77, 1972.

Sevitt S: *Fat Embolism.* London, Butterworth Scientific Publications, 1962.

Shier MR, Wilson RF: Fat embolism syndrome: Traumatic coagulopathy with respiratory distress. *Surg Annu* 12:139, 1980.

Weisz GM: Fat embolism. *Curr Probl Surg* November 1974.

Psychiatric Complications

Altschule MD: Postoperative psychosis. *Surg Clin North Am* 49:677, 1969.

Beebe HG, Keats NM: Surgical patients and drug abuse syndrome. *Am Surg* 39:88, 1973.

Bolton HE, Bailey CP: Surgical aspects in psychosomatic aspects of cardiovascular surgery. in Cantor AJ, Foxe AN (eds): *Psychosomatic Aspects of Surgery.* New York, Grune & Stratton, 1955, chap 3.

Donovan JC: Some psychosomatic aspects of obstetrics and gynecology. *Am J Obstet Gynecol* 75:72, 1958.

Egerton N, Kay JH: Psychological disturbances associated with open heart surgery. *Br J Psychiat* 110:433, 1964.

Fox HM, Rizzo ND, Gifford S: Psychological observations of patients undergoing mitral surgery: Study of stress. *Psychosom Med* 16:186, 1954.

Hackett TP, Weisman AD: Psychiatric management of operative syndromes. I. The therapeutic consultation and the effect of noninterpretive intervention. *Psychosom Med* 22:267, 1960.

Hackett TP, Weisman AD: Psychiatric management of operative syndromes. II. Psychodynamic factors in formulation and management. *Psychosom Med* 22:356, 1960.

Howell JG: *Modern Perspectives and Psychiatric Aspects of Surgery.* New York, Brunner-Mazel, 1976.

Johnson JE, Leventhal H: Contribution of emotional and instrumental response processes in adaptation to surgery. *J Pers Soc Psychol* 20:55, 1971.

Katz NM, Agle DP, et al: Delirium in surgical patients under intensive care: Utility of mental status examination. *Arch Surg* 104:310, 1972.

Kemph JP: Renal failure, artificial kidney and kidney transplant. *Am J Psychiat* 122:1270, 1966.

Knox SJ: Severe psychiatric disturbances in the postoperative period: A five-year survey of Belfast hospitals. *J Ment Sci* 107:1078, 1961.

Kornfeld DS, Zimberg S, Malm JR: Psychiatric complications of open-heart surgery. *N Engl J Med* 273:287, 1965.

Layne OL Jr, Yudofsky SC: Postoperative psychosis in cardiotomy patients: The role of organic and psychiatric factors. *N Engl J Med* 284:518, 1971.

Maguire P, Tait A, et al: The effect of counselling on the psychiatric morbidity associated with mastectomy. *Br Med J* 281:1454, 1980.

Meyer BC: Some psychiatric aspects of surgical practice. *Psychosom Med* 20:203, 1958.

Prugh D, Staub E, et al: A study of the emotional reactions of children and families to hospitalization and illness. *Am J Orthopsychiatry* 22:70, 1953.

Spiro HR: Psychiatric reactions associated with surgery. in Condon RE, DeCosse JJ (eds): *Surgical Care.* Philadelphia, Lea & Febiger, 1980.

Titchener JL, Levine M: *Surgery as a Human Experience: The Psychodynamics of Surgical Practice.* Fair Lawn, NJ, Oxford University Press, 1960.

Titchener JL, Zwerling I, et al: Psychosis in surgical patients. *Surg Gynecol Obstet* 102:59, 1956.

Weiss SM: Psychological adjustment following open-heart surgery. *J Nerv Ment Dis* 143:363, 1966.

Winkelstein C, Blacher RS, Meyer BC: Psychiatric observations on surgical patients in recovery room: Pilot study. *NY J Med* 65:865, 1965.

Wright RG, Sand P, Livingston G: Psychological stress during haemodialysis for chronic renal failure. *Ann Intern Med* 64:611, 1966.

Zaks MS: Disturbances in physiologic functions and neuropsychiatric complications in heart surgery, in Luisada AA (ed): *Cardiology: An Encyclopedia of the Cardiovascular System.* New York, McGraw-Hill, vol 3, 1959.

Complications of Gastrointestinal Surgery

Blomstedt B, Dahlgren S: The afferent loop syndrome. *Acta Chir Scand* 120:347, 1961.

Brooke BN: Management of an ileostomy including its complications. *Lancet* 2:202, 1952.

Capper WM, Welbourn RB: Early postcibal symptoms following gastrectomy. *Br J Surg* 43:24, 1955.

Devlin HB, Elcoat C: Alimentary tract fistula: Stomatherapy techniques of management. *World J Surg* 7:489, 1983.

Dietel M: Elemental diet and enterocutaneous fistula. *World J Surg* 7:451, 1983.

Edmunds LH Jr, Williams GM, Welch CE: External fistulas arising from the gastro-intestinal tract. *Ann Surg* 152:445, 1960.

Fazio VM: Alimentary tract fistulas—an introduction. *World J Surg* 7:445, 1983.

Fischer JE: The pathophysiology of enterocutaneous fistulas. *World J Surg* 7:446, 1983.

Gleysteen JJ, Sillin LF, Condon RE: Delayed gastric emptying, in Condon RE, DeCosse JJ (eds): *Surgical Care.* Philadelphia, Lea & Febiger, 1980, chap 2.

Herrington JL Jr, Sawyers JL: Complications following gastric operations, in Schwartz SI and Ellis H (eds): *Maingot's Ab-*

dominal Operations. Norwalk, Appleton Century Crofts, 1985, pp 897–942.

Hill GL: Operative strategy in the treatment of enterocutaneous fistulas. *World J Surg* 7:495, 1983.

Johnson CL, McIlrath DC: Management of patients with enterocutaneous fistulas. *Surg Clin North Am* 49:967, 1969.

Malangoni MA, Madura JA, Jesseph JE: Management of lateral duodenal fistulas: A study of fourteen cases. *Surgery* 90:645, 1981.

Magnuson FK, Judd ES, Dearing WH: Comparison of postgastrectomy complications in gastric and duodenal ulcer patients. *Am Surg* 32:375, 1966.

Morgenstern L, Yamakawa T, et al: Anastomotic leakage after low colonic anastomosis. Clinical and experimental aspects. *Am J Surg* 123:104, 1972.

Pettersson S, Wallensten S: Leakage at suture lines after partial gastrectomy for peptic ulcer. *Acta Chir Scand* 135:229, 1969.

Rodkey GV, Welch CE: Duodenal decompression in gastrectomy. *N Engl J Med* 262:498, 1960.

State D: Immediate complications of gastric surgery. *Surg Clin North Am 44:371, 1964.*

Tarazi R, Coutsoftides T, et al: Gastric and duodenal cutaneous fistulas. *World J Surg* 7:463, 1983.

Woods JH, Kowalske M, DeCosse JJ: The new stoma: Ileostomy and colostomy, in Condon RE, DeCosse JJ (eds): *Surgical Care.* Philadelphia, Lea & Febiger, 1980, chap 6.

saved by monitoring. In this case, the electrocardiograph is an almost ideal monitor because it is safe, noninvasive, and specific for the physiologic aberration of cardiac arrhythmias that kills most myocardial infarction victims.

This chapter summarizes the usefulness and indications of various monitoring modes, from routine screening techniques to advanced cardiorespiratory monitoring of high-risk surgical patients preoperatively, intraoperatively, and postoperatively.

A review of the fundamental and basic monitoring techniques utilized in most intensive care units as well as an elaboration of physiologic principles regarding oxygen delivery to the tissues will be provided. Subsequently, invasive and noninvasive techniques will be discussed. Special emphasis will be placed on the use of invasive hemodynamic monitoring techniques to preoperatively evaluate high-risk surgical patients.

BASIC MONITORING

The ultimate improvement in patient outcome or decision-making ability results from increased information. The broad spectrum from noninvasive to highly invasive monitoring is shown in Table 13-1. Measurements that are appropriate for the surgical patient with multiple organ abnormalities and that directly or indirectly provide information about organ function in most ICU settings are listed in Table 13-2. Not all of these measurements are necessary in every surgical patient being monitored. Selection of tests should be made based on the likelihood that the information generated will be valuable for clinical decision making. Selected variables, their units, formulas, and normal values are presented in Table 13-3.

Table 13-1. MONITORING PROCEDURES

Noninvasive procedures
  Physical examination
  Electrical sensing with surface electrodes, e.g., ECG
    and EEG
  Impedance phlebography
  Arterial tonometry
  Gas sampling using skin surface probes
  Radiologic examination
  Bedside mass spectrometry
  Expired gas analysis
Invasive procedures
  Intravenous injection and blood sampling from
    capillaries and peripheral veins
  Cutaneous needle electrodes for ECG and EEG
  Rectal probe for temperature
  Bladder catheter for renal function
  Tissue oxygen probe
  Intraarterial and venous gas tension and pH analysis
Highly invasive procedures
  Arterial and central venous catheter
  Intracardiac probes
  Transcardiac probes for pulmonary artery catheter
    for pressures and flows
  Subarachnoid probes for pressure
  Intracranial probes for CSF pressures and flows

Table 13-2. PHYSIOLOGIC VARIABLES (IN ORDER OF INCREASED SPECIFICITY)

1. Arterial blood pressure
2. Heart rate, respiratory rate
3. Temperature
4. Hematocrit and hemoglobin concentration
5. Urine output rate
6. Central venous pressure (CVP)
7. Electrocardiogram (ECG), chest x-ray
8. Serum electrolytes: Na^+, K^+, Cl^-, HCO_3^-, BUN, creatinine
9. Arterial blood gases—pH
10. Tidal volume (V_T), respiratory rate (f), minute volume (MV)
11. FeNa, RFI, creatinine clearance
12. Plasma and urine osmolalities, osmolar and free water clearances
13. Electroencephalogram (EEG)
14. Intracranial pressure (ICP)
15. Pulmonary arterial and capillary wedge pressures (PAP and PCWP)
16. Cardiac output and hemodynamic variables
17. O_2 transport variables: O_2 delivery, O_2 consumption (V_{O_2}), and O_2 extraction rate
18. End-tidal CO_2 (PET_{CO_2}), V_{CO_2}, V_D/V_T, $P(A-a)D_{O_2}$
19. Mass spectrometry
20. Transcutaneous O_2 and CO_2

VITAL SIGNS. Arterial pressures, heart rate, temperature, and respiratory rate, the so-called vital signs, are the simplest, most easily measured, and most commonly monitored variables. They are a useful screening technique and, as such, are a part of the admission note, physical exam, and daily nursing routine. Vital signs are recorded more frequently during critical periods to provide a running graphic record for frequent evaluations of the patient's condition. Arterial pressures and the other vital signs are monitored in routine hospital and ICU admissions; in preoperative, intraoperative, and postoperative patients, in patients with suspected acute circulatory problems, and patients with myocardial infarction, sepsis, or blood loss; in cases of major trauma, head injury, or blunt injury to chest or abdomen; in shock syndromes; and in other life-threatening conditions or emergencies.

Frequent observation of a patient's mental status can provide important clues to the presence of hypoxemia, hypercapnia, and acidosis. Restlessness and confusion can be early warning signs of sepsis and low output status. Careful attention to the skin can yield valuable clues to the presence of anemia (pallor), severe hypoxemia (cyanosis), and decreased perfusion (decreased temperature or diaphoresis or both). These plus the fundamentals of physical examination can yield a tremendous amount of information rather inexpensively and without risk in an era of sophisticated ICU care.

ARTERIAL PRESSURE. Arterial pressure, the most frequently monitored circulatory variable, reflects the overall circulatory status but lacks diagnostic specificity. Pressures fall after hypovolemia from blood or fluid loss, during cardiac failure, and in the terminal stage of most

Table 13-3. SELECTED VARIABLES: THEIR UNITS, FORMULAS, AND NORMAL VALUES

Abbreviation	Variable name	Formula	Normal values	Units
MAP	Mean arterial pressure	MAP = diastolic + 1/3 pulse pressure	89–95	mmHg
CVP	Central venous pressure	Direct measurement	0–10	cmH_2O
Hb	Hemoglobin concentration	Direct measurement	12–15	g/dL
MPAP	Mean pulmonary arterial pressure	Direct measurement	10–18	mmHg
PCWP	Pulmonary capillary wedge pressure	Direct measurement	2–12	mmHg
CI	Cardiac index	Cardiac output/ body surface area	2.5–3.5	$L/min/m^2$
LVSW	Left ventrical stroke work	$LVSW = \dfrac{SI \times MAP \times 13.6}{HR}$	44–68	$g \cdot m/m^2$
TPR	Total peripheral resistance	TPR = 80 (MAP − CVP)/CI	1200–1800	$dynes \cdot s/cm^5 \cdot m^2$
PVR	Pulmonary vascular resistance	PVR = 80 (MPAP − WP)/CI	150–250	$dynes \cdot s/cm^5 \cdot m^2$
HR	Heart rate	Direct measurement	65–80	beats/min
Temp	Temperature	Direct measurement	98–98.6; 37	°F; °C
O_2	O_2 availability	O_2 avail = $CI \times Ca_{O_2} \times 10$	500–700	$mL/min/m^2$
V_{O_2}	O_2 consumption	$V_{O_2} = CI \times (Ca_{O_2} - Cv_{O_2}) \times 10$	180–200	$mL/min/m^2$
O_2 ext	O_2 extraction	$O_2 \text{ ext} = \dfrac{Ca_{O_2} - Cv_{O_2}}{Ca_{O_2}}$	20–30	
V_D/V_T	Dead space/tidal	$V_D/V_T = \dfrac{PA_{CO_2} - PE_{CO_2}}{PA_{CO_2}}$ or $\dfrac{Pa_{CO_2} - PE_{CO_2}}{Pa_{CO_2}}$	1.30	
P_{osm}	Plasma osmolality	Direct measurement	279–295	mO/kg
PA_{O_2}	Alveolar oxygen tension	$PA_{O_2} = (P_B - 47)\, F_{iO_2} - \dfrac{PA_{CO_2}}{R}$	5–20	mmHg
Q_s/Q_t	Physiologic shunt	$Q_s/Q_t = \dfrac{C_{CO_2} - Ca_{O_2}}{C_{CO_2} - Cv_{O_2}}$	3–5	Percent

diseases. Decreased blood pressure indicates circulatory decompensation or failure of a specific therapy; increased pressure may indicate improved circulatory function or sympathetic neurohormonal response, unless the elevation of pressure is produced by vasopressor therapy.

Arterial pressures do not directly measure reductions of blood flow and volume, but rather the failure of circulatory compensations. Since blood pressure, flow, and volume interactions are extremely complex, only the grossest aspects of the circulatory status are reflected by serial blood-pressure measurements. In short, arterial-pressure measurements are very useful for screening and for rapid assessment of trends in emergency conditions, especially trauma and gastrointestinal bleeding, but in and of themselves are of dubious physiologic import.

Normal arterial blood pressure taken by sphygmomanometer cuff is approximately 120/80 mmHg for healthy young adults; this increases gradually with age. As a rough estimate, the upper limit of normal for systolic pressures over 160 and diastolic pressures over 90 mmHg are considered hypertensive. Young adults, especially teenage females, may normally have pressures as low as 90/60 mmHg. It is important to know the patient's base-line preillness pressure to properly treat those individuals whose normal pressures are not within the standard range.

The pulse pressure, which is the difference between systolic and diastolic pressures, often is more informative than the latter two pressures. Decreased pulse pressure often precedes a decrease in diastolic pressure in patients developing hypovolemic shock and is one of the first clinical signs of blood volume loss; increased pulse pressure is an early sign of volume restoration.

Mean arterial pressure (MAP) is the diastolic pressure plus one-third of the pulse pressure; alternatively, it may be expressed as one-third the sum of the systolic pressure plus twice the diastolic pressure. MAP is also measured directly in various recording systems as a dampened electrical mean of the systolic and diastolic pressures.

Intraarterial pressure, obtained by a system of intraarterial catheters, pressure transducers, and a continuous recording system that has been zeroed and calibrated, is more accurate than cuff pressure. In normal conditions, pressures obtained from intraarterial catheters are about 2 to 8 mmHg higher than cuff pressures. In critically ill patients, intraarterial pressures may be 10 to 30 mmHg higher than cuff pressure. Furthermore, cuff pressures are often inaccurate when there is severe vasoconstriction with low stroke volume. Arterial pressures of 50 to 60 mmHg have been noted by intraarterial catheter and transducers when the cuff pressures were unobtainable.

Therefore, the indications for this type of continuous pressure recording are shock, critical illness, intraoperative and postoperative monitoring in extensive operations, marked peripheral vasoconstriction, and high-risk conditions. In these cases, accurate, continuous arterial-pressure display is needed for trend analysis and for assessment of therapy. Moreover, the presence of an arterial catheter allows frequent arterial blood-gas measurements.

Because specific unilateral arteriosclerotic or traumatic vascular lesions may produce 10 to 20 mmHg differences between the left and right sides, early in the patient's hospital course pressures should be taken in both arms. Similarly, in trauma to the aorta or femoral artery, there may be differences in the cuff pressures of each leg or each arm; usually the femoral arterial pressures are 5 to 10 mmHg higher than brachial pressures.

Arterial pressures decrease during shock and trauma states; however, these decreases are nonspecific and only poorly and belatedly reflect deficits in blood volume or cardiac function; this is because compensatory neurovascular reactions sustain pressures in the face of falling blood flow. Usually, arterial pressure decreases after the compensations are exhausted, which may be long after the precipitating event. Severely reduced cardiac output has been documented for periods of 40 min to 2 h before a significant reduction in arterial pressures was observed.

Intraarterial catheters may be placed in the femoral, radial, brachial, or axillary arteries. The femoral artery was frequently used in the past, but it makes nursing care difficult and limits and patient's ability to move about, sit up, or ambulate. Further, its placement near the groin risks infection. The radial artery is probably the most commonly used site for continuous arterial pressure monitoring. The brachial artery is most frequently used for cardiac catheterization; however, clotting at the catheter site is likely to jeopardize the limb's circulation during long-term monitoring.

Complications of arterial puncture or arterial catheterization are infrequent but may include hematoma and bleeding at the catheter site; puncture and penetration of the posterior arterial wall; dissection of the intima of the posterior wall by the needle or Seldinger wire; arteriovenous fistula and pseudoaneurysm; arterial spasm; arterial thrombosis; arterial occlusion, ischemia, or gangrene; arteritis; foreign body from sheared-off end of catheter; and cardiac arrest.

The rate of catheter-associated sepsis (demonstrated by positive cultures of blood and the catheter tip that yield the same organism, with no other of infection) is about 4 percent. Sepsis is more likely with surgical cut-downs if the catheter is left in place for more than 4 days or if evidence of local inflamation is present. The pressure transducer or flushing solution can also become infected if left in place more than 48 h.

To minimize the risks with arterial lines, one must perform Allen's test to ensure the patency of the ulnar circulation. Other procedures that will minimize the risk of thrombosis and infection include percutaneous insertion rather than surgical cut-down, changing the entire infusion apparatus every 48 h, using a No. 20 rather than a No. 18 catheter, and removing the catheter within 4 days if at all possible. Continual observation for skin mottling or decrease in temperature of the patient's hand mandates immediate catheter removal.

HEART RATE. The indications for measuring heart rate (pulse) are the same as those for arterial pressure. Arterial pressures and heart rate are routinely taken together and graphically recorded daily or twice daily on the vital signs sheet of the patient's chart.

Heart rate is usually counted by manual palpation of the radial artery just above the wrist, for at least 30 s. When there are premature ventricular contractions (PVCs), skipped beats, or other irregularities, the heart rate is counted by auscultation of the apex; the difference between apical and radial rates is the number of dropped beats. Heart rates may also be measured automatically from either the ECG wave or the arterial-pulse wave.

Heart rate is a very nonspecific cardiorespiratory variable. Its increase suggests blood flow and blood volume deficits; the faster the heart rate, the greater the hypovolemia or cardiac impairment. However, heart rate also increases with infection, anxiety, stress, nonspecific fever, exercise, pain, and discomfort. Tachycardia is a heart rate over 100 beats/min. With irregularities of heart rate, apical as well as radial rates should be compared.

A slow heart rate, or bradycardia, may occur with inferior myocardial infarction when occlusion of the right coronary artery produces ischemia and block of the sinatrial node, and with certain types of arteriosclerotic heart disease. Bradycardia during low cardiac output is an ominous sign suggesting inadequate coronary blood flow. Dysrhythmias associated with cardiac problems require ECG and other methods of specific diagnosis.

TEMPERATURE. Body temperature is taken routinely with the blood pressure, pulse, and respirations. Usually, it is taken rectally in ill patients or orally when significant elevations are not expected. On occasion, thermocouples may be used to take temperatures orally and at the skin of the big toe to obtain the toe-oral temperature gradient, and at the tympanic membrane or midesophagus to assess more accurately the central body core temperature. Pulmonary arterial temperatures, which also reflect core temperature, are routinely available with the pulmonary-artery thermodilution catheter. With a respiratory rate of 40/min, the oral temperature may underestimate the rectal temperature by 3°C.

Temperature elevations are most often associated with infection, tissue necrosis, late-stage carcinomatosis, Hodgkin's disease, leukemias, hyperthyroidism, and other hypermetabolic states. Low-grade fever is also present after accidental or surgical trauma, particularly with hematomas, foreign bodies, fistulae, urinary extravasation, or stasis of urinary or bronchial secretions. Hypothermia may occur in a small percentage of patients with septic shock, reduced metabolism associated with hypothyroidism, malnutrition, and cold exposure. Like arterial pressure and heart rate, temperature is a very useful but nonspecific screening test of little direct physiologic meaning.

RESPIRATORY RATE. One of the earliest responses to a decrease in Pa_{O_2} or a rise in Pa_{CO_2} is an increase in respiratory rate. The normal range is 10 to 16/min, and a rate over 20/min should be viewed as abnormal, particularly if an upward trend continues. Rates over 30/min indicate severe respiratory distress and may produce severe hypocarbia. A sudden increase in respiratory rate may be the first detectable sign of sepsis or a pulmonary embolization.

Observation of the patient's respiratory pattern can yield valuable information. Rapid, shallow respirations are common with interstitial edema, whereas large tidal volumes are typical of pulmonary vascular disease, metabolic acidosis, and sepsis. Rates of less than 12 suggest central-nervous-system depression. Irregular respiratory patterns (Cheyne-Stokes and Biot's respirations) may indicate central-nervous-system or cardiovascular disease.

BODY WEIGHT. An accurate record of daily weight is often the most important indicator of fluid balance. Patients receiving only intravenous fluids usually lose 0.3 to 0.5 kg (0.6 to 1 lb) per day. Weight loss greater than this amount is excessive. Unless a patient is receiving substantial intravenous or enteral alimentation, stable weight or a weight gain indicates retention of water.

HEMATOCRIT. The hematocrit, which is a measure of the percentage of red cells in a sample of venous blood, has been widely used to assess blood loss after trauma and surgery. In general, hematocrit values are decreased by hemorrhage and increased by dehydration.

The hematocrit is measured in routine admissions; emergency conditions, including trauma and hemorrhage or suspected hemorrhage; dehydration, fever, or other suggested water loss; suspected overtransfusion; suspected overhydration; hemolysis or destruction of red cells from fresh-water drowning, envenomation, or consumption coagulopathies, including disseminated intravascular coagulopathies, postoperative states, especially when intraperitoneal bleeding is suspected; and acute illnesses, circulatory shock, and sepsis.

A decreased percentage of red blood cells is an indirect effect of blood loss produced by compensatory transcapillary refilling of the plasma volume from the extracellular water. It takes time for this compensation to occur. If a patient rapidly exsanguinates in a few minutes, the first and last drops of blood will have nearly the same hematocrit. However, a 500-mL blood loss in human volunteers will be replaced by interstitial water over an 18-h period. Replacement occurs at about 1 mL/min for the first few hours and then at successively decreasing rates. For these reasons, serial hematocrits at 4-h intervals are useful in the early period of traumatic shock when covert blood loss is suspected.

Decreases in serial hematocrits of postoperative and posttraumatic patients can signal intraabdominal hemorrhage, but this test is nonspecific and has severe limita-

tions. Since the hematocrit represents a static measurement of red cell concentration in a sample of venous blood, it is affected by a gain or loss of plasma water as well as a gain or loss of red cells. However, it cannot distinguish among the effects of fluids administered intravenously, fluids leaking from the plasma to the interstitial space, red cells being transfused, and other red cells forming aggregates and microthrombi and dropping out of the circulation. Therefore, after the patient has been given large volumes of crystalloids and colloids, as well as multiple transfusions, changes in hematocrit may be misleading and are extremely difficult to interpret. Although the hematocrit may be a reasonably good screening test for gross changes in early stages of hemorrhage, it is not generally a reliable estimation of the blood volume status.

URINE OUTPUT RATE. The rate of urine output is easily measured at minimal expense. The patient is catheterized, preferably with a Foley catheter, and the urine is collected in a closed sterile system; output is usually recorded hourly. The catheter must be irrigated with aseptic precautions at regular intervals, since the most common cause of low urine output, or anuria, in the hospitalized patient is an occluded catheter. (Normal output = $\frac{1}{2}$ mL/kg/min.)

The hourly rate of urine output obtained using an indwelling urethral catheter is a reasonable measure of the perfusion of one vital organ, provided the patient has an adequate blood volume and no preexisting renal disease. In resuscitation from acute injury, decreased urine flow may reflect low blood volume, poor perfusion of the kidney, or the onset of acute renal failure. Other measures of renal function, such as osmolar and free water clearance, are presented below.

Urine output provides a good estimate of the adequacy of renal perfusion, and urine specific gravity reflects renal concentrating ability. Serum creatinine and blood urea nitrogen (BUN) levels are traditionally used to monitor renal function; however, other less frequently used tests may also be useful, since the BUN and creatinine values are not abnormal until 70 percent of renal function is lost. An early sign of relative hypovolemia may be a falling urine sodium concentration and/or a rising urine osmolality. Urine sodium less than 10 to 20 meq/L or urine osmolality greater than 450 mO/L suggests hypovolemia. A urine sodium greater than 40 meq/L suggests acute tubular necrosis and a urine osmolality less than 300 mO/L suggests antetubular necrosis (ATN).

Renal function also can be monitored by measurement of plasma (P_{osm}) and urine (U_{osm}) osmolality as well as calculation of osmolar and free water clearance. The U_{osm}/P_{osm} ratio is calculated, and if it is greater than 1.7, good concentrating ability is present. The osmolar clearance (C_{osm}) is calculated according to the following equation:

$$C_{osm} = \frac{U_{osm}}{P_{osm}} \times \text{Urine output (1 h)} \qquad N: 100–125 \text{ mL/h}$$

The osmolar clearance reflects the rate of removal of solutes from plasma. Normal osmolar clearance is 120 mL/h and is decreased in renal failure. Free water clearance is calculated by subtracting the C_{osm} from the 1-h urine output. The free water clearance (C_{H_2O}) usually is negative (-125 to -100 mL/h), and the values close to zero or above precede acute renal failure.

The creatinine clearance (C_{cr}) reflects the glomerular function, since this substance is neither excreted nor absorbed by the tubules. Clearance results are normalized and expressed as milliliter per minute per 1.73 m^2.

$$C_{cr}: \frac{U_{cr} \times U \text{ vol (1 h)} \times 1.73}{P_{cr} \times 60 \times \text{body surface area}}$$

$$N: 100\text{--}125 \text{ mL/min/1.73 m}^2$$

$$C_{Na}: \frac{U_{Na} \times U \text{ vol (1 h)} \times 1.73}{P_{Na} \times 60 \times \text{body surface area}}$$

$$N: 3\text{--}4 \text{ mL/min/1.73 m}^2$$

Excretion data include the fractional excretion of sodium (F_eNa) and renal failure index (RF_i), which allow differentiation between reversible prerenal azotemia and antetubular necrosis.

$$F_eNa(\%): \frac{U_{Na} \times P_{cr} \times 100}{P_{Na} \times U_{cr}} \quad \begin{array}{l} <1 = \text{prerenal} \\ >1 \text{ or } >3 = \text{ATN} \end{array}$$

$$RF_i(\%): \frac{U_{Na} \times P_{cr}}{U_{cr}} \quad \begin{array}{l} <1 = \text{prerenal} \\ >3 = \text{ATN} \end{array}$$

Urinary indices have long been utilized for diagnosis of prerenal failure, or ATN. In prerenal azotemia, tubular function remains intact, and reabsorption of sodium and water is characteristic of this period. Hence urinary sodium <20 meq/L, $U_{osm} > 450$ mO, U/P creatinine >40. In acute tubular necrosis the concentration ability is impaired owing to tubular damage, resulting in $U_{Na} >40$ meq/L, $U_{osm} < 300$ mO, U/P creatinine < 20. F_eNa and RF_i are found to be below 1 percent in prerenal azotemia and above 3 percent in ATN.

Normal osmolality of body fluids is 275 to 295 mO/L H_2O. Plasma osmolality is calculated by the following formula:

$$P_{osm} \text{ (mO/L)} = 2 \times \text{sodium (meq/L)}$$
$$+ \frac{\text{glucose (mg/dL)}}{18} + \frac{\text{BUN (mg/dL)}}{2.8}$$

An osmolality above 320 mO/L generally is tolerated poorly, and levels greater than 350 mO/L may be fatal. The calculated serum osmolality is normally 5 to 8 mO less than the measured osmolality. This difference is called the osmolar discriminant and is due to the presence of anions, e.g., lactate or phosphate. An increased osmolar discriminant is usually associated with increased lactate production and a poorer prognosis.

The advantages of utilizing a renal profile, especially if computerized, is that the clinician is provided with all the parameters that need to be evaluated to differentiate acute tubular necrosis from an oliguric prerenal state. By utilizing a multiple-parameter approach, an earlier diagnosis of acute tubular necrosis can be made. The comput-

erized method provides the clinician with all the parameters that usually require tedious calculations rapidly and expeditiously. Vo et al. have previously described the automated renal profile.

ARTERIAL BLOOD-GAS ANALYSIS AND PULMONARY MONITORING

Arterial blood-gas tensions are determined by the composition of alveolar gas and the efficiency of gas transfer between the alveoli and pulmonary capillary blood. Alveolar gas tension depends on the mixture of inspired gas, ventilation and blood flow (V/Q), and the composition of mixed venous blood gases. Because mixed venous P_{O_2} usually varies with cardiac output, significant arterial hypoxemia can result from shunting of venous blood with a low P_{O_2} through the pulmonary circulation. Failure to recognize this nonpulmonary cause of arterial hypoxemia may cause a clinician to falsely ascribe a falling Pa_{O_2} to deteriorating pulmonary function.

Pulmonary abnormalities that may result in hypoxemia, alone or in combination, include diffusion block, ventilation-perfusion inequality, intrapulmonary shunting, and hypoventilation. Diffusion abnormalities lead to hypoxemia if pulmonary end-capillary blood fails to equilibrate fully with alveolar gas. Such conditions are probably a very uncommon cause of hypoxemia except in patients with chronic lung disease during exercise or exposure to a decreased F_{iO_2} at high altitude.

Although bulk oxygen is carried in combination with hemoglobin, delivery to tissue depends on its partial pressure in the blood, which also reflects the amount of oxygen available to be delivered from hemoglobin. A fall in Pa_{O_2} without a change in Pa_{CO_2} suggests that blood oxygenation is deteriorating despite constant alveolar ventilation. In the acutely ill patient, this finding usually is due to ventilation-perfusion imbalance or intrapulmonary shunting. An important feature of shunting is that hypoxemia cannot be abolished by the administration of 100 percent oxygen because the chemoreceptors sense any elevation in Pa_{CO_2} and reflexly induce an increase of ventilation.

When patients hypoventilate while breathing ambient air, hypoxemia results from an increase in alveolar P_{CO_2}. Calculation of the alveolar oxygen tension and determination of the alveolar-arterial ($A-a$) oxygen tension difference $P(A-a)D_{O_2}$ allows separation of hypoventilation from other causes of hypoxemia. With hypoventilation, the $A-a$ oxygen gradient is normal; with other causes of hypoxemia, it is increased. The alveolar oxygen tension can be estimated from the following abbreviated formula, which is adequate for clinical purposes:

$$PA_{O_2} = P_{iO_2} - \frac{Pa_{CO_2}}{R}$$

P_{iO_2} is equal to the barometric pressure (P_B) minus the water vapor pressure (47 mmHg at 37°C) multiplied by the F_{iO_2}. The respiratory quotient (R) is approximately 0.8 in the steady-state resting condition. It is assumed to be

0.8 in respiratory failure, although this assumption is not always valid.

The correction for R varies depending on the inspired oxygen concentration (F_{iO_2}), as can be seen from the nonsimplified alveolar air equation:

$$PA_{O_2} = F_{iO_2} (P_B - 47) - PA_{CO_2} \left(F_{iO_2} + \frac{1 - F_{iO_2}}{R} \right)$$

Although this equation appears formidable, if Pa_{CO_2} is used rather than PA_{CO_2}, and 100 percent oxygen is inhaled, solution of the equation is simply the difference between inspired P_{O_2}. For clinical purposes, it is important to appreciate the small but definite error if PA_{O_2} is calculated using the abbreviated formula at different inspired oxygen concentrations.

The $P(A-a)D_{O_2}$ in normal human beings breathing room air varies between 10 and 15 mmHg. Half of this venoarterial admixture is caused by true shunting of desaturated blood into the left atrium, and the other half by ventilation-perfusion imbalance. When the patient with normal cardiorespiratory function breathes pure oxygen for 15 or 20 min, the alveolar-arterial gradient is between 25 and 65 mmHg. Barometric pressure, less carbon dioxide tension, less water vapor pressure, less the normal gradient yields a value of around 630 mmHg for arterial oxygen tension while breathing pure oxygen. In this condition the gradient represents both anatomic shunting and perfusion of total nonventilated alveoli. Patients are ready to begin to be reversed from the ventilator when their gradient of alveolar to arterial oxygen is less than 350 mmHg while they are receiving 100 percent oxygen (indicating that they could be maintained on 50 percent oxygen).

The arterial oxygen tension divided by the alveolar oxygen tension is called the a/A ratio. This ratio is relatively stable with a varying F_{iO_2}, unlike the classic alveolar-arterial gradient. Thus it is a useful index of changes in lung function when a patient's inspired oxygen concentration is changed. The normal a/A ratio is 0.75. The ratio can also be used to predict the new Pa_{O_2} that results from a change in inspired oxygen concentration.

Another nonpulmonary factor that can significantly affect gas exchange is the level of CO_2 production (V_{CO_2}). The amount of CO_2 produced by the body is a function of the metabolic rate and the substrate(s) used as fuel. CO_2 production varies from 70 to 100 percent of the O_2 consumption as the fuel is switched from fat to carbohydrate. When caloric input exceeds metabolic needs, excess calories are converted to fat, which further increases CO_2 production.

Measurements of CO_2 production by indirect calorimetry may be helpful in patients receiving hyperalimentation. Although nutritional support is vital in the critically ill patient, it may sometimes raise CO_2 production above base-line levels. Thus, patients may require higher levels of ventilation to eliminate CO_2. If the ventilation cannot be increased, arterial partial pressure of CO_2 will rise. Decreasing CO_2 production in the patient who is difficult to wean may make weaning easier by reducing the requirements for ventilation. Although one obviously does not want to eliminate essential nutrients, the administration of fat instead of some of the glucose will help to lower the CO_2 production.

Agarwal et al. have developed a computerized automated metabolic profile that provides the physician with a comprehensive review and graphic display of a patient's nutritional status, energy expenditure, substrate utilization, and nutritional requirements. Utilizing indirect calorimetry, the nutritional management of patients requiring ventilatory support can be optimized according to their needs with facility. Savino et al. have demonstrated with indirect calorimetric techniques that the work of breathing can be quantitated more accurately.

Monitoring P_{50} (P_{O_2} at 50 percent oxyhemoglobin saturation) may also be helpful in assessing oxygen delivery. A right-shifted curve (e.g., higher P_{50}) assists in delivery of oxygen to tissues. The significance of shifts of the oxyhemoglobin curve on overall tissue oxygenation remains a topic of active investigation. Rightward shifts are commonly seen in conditions associated with decreased oxygen delivery, e.g., anemia and chronic hypoxemia. Beneficial effects of decreased oxygen affinity are difficult to demonstrate experimentally. Increased mortality and decreased oxygen consumption and cardiac output have been associated with a low P_{50} in experimental studies. These findings are of clinical significance to patients receiving large transfusions of stored blood or others who develop respiratory alkalemia or metabolic alkalosis, resultant leftward shift of the oxyhemoglobin dissociation curve and decreased P_{50}. As these patients are more likely to have limited cardiac reserve because of acute illness, they are least able to compensate by an increase in cardiac output or a shift in blood flow to tissues utilizing high extraction ratios to meet required oxygen demands. Organs such as the heart and brain are particularly vulnerable.

Marked changes in Pa_{O_2} in critically ill patients that may be missed by intermittent sampling occur during the administration of drugs, suctioning, and changes in body position. The frequency with which arterial blood gases should be measured depends on the clinical situation. In patients with severe chronic obstructive pulmonary disease and impending respiratory failure, arterial blood gases may need to be measured every 30 to 60 min. Continuous monitoring of Pa_{O_2} by electrodes in the femoral, radial, and brachial arteries as well as the P_{O_2} in mixed venous blood in the pulmonary artery has been reported. Obviously these techniques have the same problems as other invasive techniques, and further experience is needed before it can be concluded that such monitoring is indicated in the management of critically ill patients.

Because of the intermittent nature of blood-gas measurement and the lag in reporting results, considerable effort has been directed to developing noninvasive continuous monitoring of blood- and tissue-gas values. On occasion, ear oximetry allows continuous monitoring of oxygen saturation, the values obtained reflecting changes in arterial oxygen saturation. Artificially low readings are recorded in patients with jaundice and when oxygen saturation is lower than 65 percent. Artificially high values are obtained when levels of carboxyhemoglobin are higher than 3 percent. When they are accurately calibrated, ear oximeters can markedly decrease the number of needed blood-gas measurements and reflect changes in the patient's hemodynamic status. Unfortunately, ear oximetry is less valuable in unstable patients with rapidly changing hemodynamic parameters. Transcutaneous oxygen measurements are less accurate because the values vary with skin thickness, blood volume, and flow. With a normal cardiac output, transcutaneous oxygen tracks partial pressure of arterial oxygen, whereas with diminished cardiac output, it tracks oxygen delivery.

The measurement of the peak expired CO_2 is directly related to the Pa_{CO_2}, which in turn is primarily related to the CO_2 production, alveolar ventilation, and pulmonary capillary blood flow. End-tidal CO_2 analysis allows the clinician to change Pa_{CO_2} during mechanical ventilation. Currently two methods of CO_2 analysis are commonly used, infrared spectroscopy and mass spectrometry. With infrared spectroscopy absorption of infrared energy by a given gas such as CO_2 produces an infrared spectrum consisting of a number of energy bands, whereby the identity and concentration of CO_2 are discerned by the end-tidal gas monitor. Mass spectrometers, unlike infrared monitors, typically monitor multiple different expired gas tensions simultaneously, including CO_2.

End-tidal CO_2 monitoring is extremely useful as a diagnostic tool in several situations unique to anesthesia. The most important role of end-tidal CO_2 monitoring is in the verification of intratracheal placement of breathing tubes, particularly in infants, obese patients, and patients with craniofacial or anatomical airway abnormalities. Once the tube has been inserted, if CO_2 is present in expired gases in the appropriate concentration of 4 to 6 volumes percent (28 to 42 mmHg), then intratracheal-tube placement and pulmonary ventilation are assured.

Blockage of the pulmonary circulation by air emboli results in an increase in dead space, thus reducing alveolar and end-tidal CO_2 concentration. This form of monitoring is recommended in neurosurgical cases requiring the sitting position.

End-tidal CO_2 monitoring can be an extremely valuable diagnostic tool for detecting malignant hyperthermia. In a number of documented cases the initial presenting sign of this pharmacogenic disease was an unexplained increase in the end-tidal CO_2 concentration in the face of unchanged ventilation.

Decreases in cardiac output are associated with corresponding decreases in the end-tidal CO_2. Thus capnography can serve as an additional monitor of cardiovascular function and signal the need for an appropriate therapeutic intervention. Certainly this form of monitoring is invaluable in detecting anesthesia-machine malfunction during surgery but it can also be utilized in the ICU environment as a ventilator disconnect alarm as well as a system to determine ventilator malfunction.

Unfortunately, with obstructive airway disease and resultant abnormalities in the distribution of ventilation, and with rapid shallow respirations, it is difficult to determine the end-tidal partial pressure of carbon dioxide accurately. As technology improves, this method may become a valuable noninvasive method of monitoring ventilation.

Two of the most practical instruments for measuring ventilatory parameters are the Wright and Drager respirometers. Low tidal volumes associated with tachypnea increase dead-space ventilation. The product of rate and tidal volume is minute volume, a useful measure of total ventilation. High minute ventilation suggests severe hypocarbia or decreased dead space and respiratory work that may lead to exhaustion. A tidal volume greater than 5 mL/kg and a vital capacity greater than 10 mL/kg may be useful guidelines for predicting successful weaning from mechanical ventilation. Vital-capacity levels below 15 mL/kg are often associated with an inadequate cough, and below 10 mL/kg hypercarbia develops. Measurement of minute volume and maximum inspiratory pressure is also employed. Sahn and Lakshminarayan showed that a resting minute volume of less than 10 L and the ability to double the resting minute volume on command predicts success in weaning patients on ventilators. Inspiratory force is normally less than −80 cm of water. Values below −20 cm of water are usually adequate to maintain normal minute ventilation.

In the spontaneously breathing patient it is important to monitor trends in blood gases and mechanics in order to predict and treat acute respiratory decompensation. In general there are four reasons to intubate a patient:

1. For oxygenation when a patient is unable to maintain a Pa_{O_2} of 70 mmHg with 100 percent O_2 administered through a face mask, nasal prongs, with a reservoir bag;
2. For ventilation when respiratory acidosis develops;
3. For protection of the airway from aspiration;
4. For management of excessive secretions. Patient selection is extremely important, but frequently in order to diminish stress one may opt for sedation and early controlled ventilation.

The ventilator in a patient who is intubated is a readily available source of monitoring of the patient's ventilatory mechanics and oxygenation. Physiologic dead space is the portion of the tidal volume that does not participate in gas exchange. In the healthy adult the physiologic dead space is approximately 150 mL at rest (about 20 to 30 percent of each tidal volume). This value represents the anatomic dead space from the mouth, pharynx, larynx, trachea, bronchi, broncholes, as well as a contribution from the alveoli that are overventilated with respect to perfusion. Positive pressure alone can increase dead space.

With respiratory failure the physiologic dead space is increased because of continued ventilation of the alveoli whose perfusion is either absent or decreased. The ratio of dead space to tidal volume (V_D/V_T) can be calculated by measuring the arterial and mixed expired CO_2 tension ($P_{\overline{E}CO_2}$) by the Bohr equation:

$$\frac{V_D}{V_T} = \frac{PA_{CO_2} - P_{\overline{E}CO_2}}{PA_{CO_2}}$$

The Enghoff modification of the Bohr equation is often used clinically:

$$\frac{V_D}{V_T} = \frac{Pa_{CO_2} - P\overline{E}_{CO_2}}{Pa_{CO_2}}$$

If the end-tidal P_{CO_2} is substituted for the Pa_{CO_2}, anatomic dead space can be calculated, requiring only expired air (eliminating arterial blood sampling). A correction for dead space due to the expansion of the tubing in mechanically ventilated patients should be made. Ratios of dead space to tidal volume reflect the amount of wasted ventilation; rising values are usually associated with respiratory failure and progressive involvement of the pulmonary vascular bed. Values above 0.6 are usually not compatible with adequate spontaneous ventilation.

Volume change per unit of pressure change is compliance, a useful measure of the elastic properties of the body. The compliance of the normal lung is approximately 200 mL/cmH$_2$O. Particularly important in monitoring pulmonary mechanics is peak inspiratory pressure, which should be monitored at least hourly. Increases in the peak inspiratory pressure and correspondingly in the dynamic compliance [tidal volume/(plateau pressure − PEEP)] may indicate the presence of an obstructed or misplaced endotracheal tube, mucous plugging, bronchospasm, and pneumothorax. Measurements of static compliance [tidal volume/(plateau pressure − PEEP)] can be obtained by adding a respiratory pause. Changes in static compliance can reflect atelectasis or an increase in the amount of lung water. Monitoring static compliance is useful in evaluating the course in patients with the adult respiratory distress syndrome and during PEEP trials in order to determine the appropriate levels of PEEP. Compliance measurements are a good indication of the patient's work of breathing.

Normal compliance of the lung and chest wall in the mechanically ventilated patient is about 70 mL/cmH$_2$O. When the static compliance of the lung and chest wall is less than 25 mL/cmH$_2$O, as in severe respiratory failure, difficulties in weaning are common because of the high work of breathing.

If one ventilates the lungs at various tidal volumes and records the peak and plateau pressure for each volume, dynamic and static curves can be quickly graphed; the former correlates with airway resistance and the latter is a measure of lung stiffness.

Two errors in these measurements are possible with unrelaxed respiratory muscles. If the patient is resisting mechanical ventilation, the total pressure developed by the ventilator will be greater than that required to inflate the lungs of the relaxed patient. Also, if the patient is actively inspiring, the pressure developed by the ventilator will be less than the total pressure required.

Elucidation of the mechanical function of the lung requires the continuous recording of pressure and flow during the respiratory cycle. Flow usually is measured by a pneumotachograph, which senses the differential pressure across a resistance in most cases. Inspiratory and expiratory pneumotachographs are a part of some single-patient monitoring systems, as in the Siemens-Elema ventilator. With in-line pneumotachographs, expired volume measurements that include volume expended by compression in the expansion of the ventilator circuit are less of a problem. Incorporation of pneumotachographs into the ventilator system introduces an entirely new set of problems, however, ranging from incorrect information because of mucous plugging of the pneumotachograph to problems of calibration changes caused by varying gas concentration. Because of problems with constant measurements using the Fleish pneumotachograph, other flow-measuring devices have been developed, including the variable-orifice flowmeter, ultrasonic flowmeter, and turbulent flowmeter. These flowmeters are presently undergoing clinical trials, and their accuracy and durability are still to be determined.

The pneumotachograph must be frequently calibrated to avoid error, usually with a 1- to 3-L syringe in line with a standard spirometer. Because pneumotachographs are sensitive to temperature, humidity, and flow, they should be calibrated under clinical conditions for reliable results. Flow rates should be linear over a range of 0 to 3 L/s, and appropriate pneumotachographs should be used in those patients. In automated systems, airway pressure is measured by reliable strain gauges that provide a linear electrical output spanning a range of 0 to 200 cmH$_2$O.

A Fleish pneumotachograph with pressure- and gas-sampling lines leading to a mass spectrometer and computer allows simultaneous measurement of inspired and expired gases and mechanics.

To measure lung compliance rather than lung and chest wall compliance, transpulmonary pressure must be determined. Respiratory pressure fluctuations reflected by an esophageal balloon or from the proximal port of a thermodilution Swan-Ganz catheter or a central venous catheter can be used for this purpose. Esophageal balloons are now available that attach to standard nasogastric tubes. If an esophageal balloon is used, a differential pressure transducer is needed to measure intrapleural pressure relative to mouth pressure. Lung plus chest wall compliance measured from airway pressure of the ventilated patient is affected by muscle contractions. The direct measurement of lung compliance thus adds both specificity and resolution.

Cardiovascular Physiology in Acute Illness

The overall assessment of oxygen transport, or the delivery of oxygen from the atmosphere to the mitochondria of the body cell mass, can be used as a model to evaluate the abilities of particular monitoring systems to detect critical events and trends. This process involves many organ systems and complicated feedback loops for regulation and compensation. It is imperative for the survival of the individual that the oxygen transport system continue in operation without interruption.

Many factors are capable of influencing an individual

patient's metabolic response to acute illness. The period immediately after acute injury is characterized by a systemic O_2 consumption (V_{O_2}) that may be less than normal. This period of initial resuscitation is quickly followed by a time when the metabolic rate, hence V_{O_2}, is increased and when the host's response is now primarily devoted to ensuring appropriate tissue repair. An increase in systemic V_{O_2} is, therefore, a characteristic response to injury and the early stages of sepsis. Wilmore has determined that the elevation in systemic V_{O_2} in such cases is related to a rise in body temperature, increased mechanical work (for example, heart and lungs), and increased synthetic work (for instance, protein). The range of changes noted in systemic V_{O_2} from base line depends upon the primary illness itself, as well as on associated complications. For example, patients with severe burns usually have the greatest increase in V_{O_2}, but, when these patients have the complication of acute respiratory failure, the systemic V_{O_2} will rise to even greater levels because of the additive metabolic load imposed on the patient secondary to an increase in mechanical work of the respiratory musculature.

Actively metabolizing cells require nutrients (for example, glucose) as well as O_2. Ranges in the internal milieu of the gluconeogenetic hormones usually favor maintenance of adequate glucose calories in the early hypermetabolic stages of trauma and sepsis. Hence, the concentration of essential nutrients may not be as potentially rate-limiting in the critically ill patient as is the supply of cellular oxygen. In summary, critically ill patients demonstrate a range of systemic V_{O_2} that depends upon the metabolic stress of the underlying illness. Traumatized patients and those with sepsis demonstrate a need for a greater oxygen delivery (D_{O_2}) than do cardiac patients because of the increased metabolic rate characteristic of the former groups compared with the latter.

To ensure survival, microcirculatory D_{O_2} must, therefore, balance systemic V_{O_2}. Anything less is reflected in the definition of heart failure, which is an inability of the ventricles to deliver adequate quantities of blood (e.g., oxygen) to the metabolizing tissues at rest or during normal activity. Failure to balance the metabolic demands of peripheral tissues will result in a shift from aerobic to the inefficient anaerobic use of O_2. If uncorrected, lactic acidosis will ensue as a result of cellular hypoxia, and a sequence of events will then develop that eventuates in cellular metabolic failure, characterized by an inability of the cell to use available O_2 and finally by death of the organism. Heart failure is functionally not defined in terms of the level of a cardiac output (CO) or of a pulmonary capillary wedge pressure (PCWP), but rather in terms of the heart's ability to support the metabolic needs of the body adequately, regardless of the demands imposed by the systemic V_{O_2}.

In the presence of an increased O_2 demand (V_{O_2}) by the periphery, there are local and systemic adaptive responses that will assist in increasing cellular O_2 availability. Locally, improved cellular O_2 transport may occur as a consequence of:

1. Peripheral vasodilation, with a consequent increase in the surface area of the microcirculatory bed across which oxygen may diffuse to the cell;
2. A rightward shift of the oxyhemoglobin dissociation curve, which will facilitate the peripheral unloading of oxygen from hemoglobin, both of which will result in increased oxygen extraction down the concentration gradient provided between oxygen tension within the cell and the microcirculation.

The natural affinity of hemoglobin for oxygen is decreased by heat, hydrogen ions, carbon dioxide (Bohr effect), and red cell diphosphoglycerate (DPG). These agents act at a stereochemical level to help form a hemoglobin molecule that is more stable in its unsaturated state. The heat of working tissues, hypoxic acidosis, and carbon dioxide from cellular metabolism all tend to shift the oxyhemoglobin dissociation curve to the right where more oxygen is released at a higher tissue oxygen tension. The relative position of the oxyhemoglobin dissociation curve is identified by the P_{50} value, the partial pressure of oxygen at which the hemoglobin is half saturated at 37° and pH 7.4.

When adaptation by the local factors to maintain cellular O_2 supply is exhausted, and compensatory acute changes in the systemic control of O_2 transport are likewise stressed, selective vasoconstriction in some organs will follow in order to divert O_2 to critical areas, such as the heart and brain, but at the expense of reduced O_2 supply to teleologically noncritical organs, such as skin and skeletal muscle. Other factors may also operate at a local level to enhance cellular O_2 availability (for example, changes in the rheologic properties of blood), although their role is not as well defined in the critically ill as the aforementioned.

Systemically, delivery of O_2 to the periphery is a direct function of the cardiac output and the arterial oxygen content (Ca_{O_2}) which represents the oxygen bound to hemoglobin (1.34 mL/g). O_2 delivery (D_{O_2}) = [flow (cardiac output)] $\times$ [(Hb)(Sa_{O_2}) + 0.0031(Pa_{O_2})]. The importance of three major organ systems in ensuring O_2 availability within the peripheral microvasculature is emphasized in this equation: the cardiovascular system to subserve tissue perfusion, the respiratory system to oxygenate venous blood, and the hematopoietic system to provide adequate hemoglobin to carry O_2. In patients with a normal hemoglobin and with a Pa_{O_2} greater than 70 mmHg, there is little remaining compensation acutely available to augment D_{O_2} by changes in Ca_{O_2}. Chronically, however, polycythemia and an increase in 2.3-diphosphoglycerate (2.3-DPG) would assist in improving CO (for instance, in chronic airflow limitation). Therefore, in acute disease states characterized by a heightened systemic V_{O_2}, in which an increase in CO is a requirement to ensure metabolic survival of the organism, an increase in the systemic flow, i.e., increased cardiac output, is likely to be the most important and immediate mechanism available to the organism to ensure an appropriate increase in systemic O_2 delivery. As a result, "the appropriate" hemodynamic response to any critical illness typified by a heightened systemic V_{O_2} may be defined as a high cardiac output, nonhypotensive state. Initial studies of patients with systemic sepsis complicated by adult respiratory distress syndrome (ARDS) identified a positive correlation between the ability of the myocardium to sustain a high cardiac output state and ultimate survival; regarding systemic sepsis, Weil and colleagues noted that the mortality rate was greater in patients with underlying cardiac disease than in those without preexisting ischemic heart disease.

The correlation between survival and a high cardiac output, or "hyperdynamic," response may be analyzed further in those disease states characterized by an increased systemic V_{O_2}. The appropriate cardiovascular response is the one that assists in improving D_{O_2} to the cell and hence prevents the development of an anaerobic state. In this regard, the need to match D_{O_2} with systemic V_{O_2} in patients with sepsis or trauma is no different from the systemic response to strenuous exercise. Strenuous exercise is not reflective of the sustained demand on D_{O_2} that diseases may be. In some acute disease states there seems to be a defect in the maximal use of the peripheral mechanisms potentially available to improve cellular D_{O_2}. Specifically, O_2 extraction may not be as sufficient within the periphery in patients with ARDS as in patients with acute cardiac illnesses. Therefore, to maintain the balance between cellular D_{O_2} and systemic V_{O_2}, and hence to prevent the development of anaerobiosis, more dependence is apparently placed on the systemic adaptive mechanisms for increasing cellular O_2 delivery. The correlation between survival and the level of the CO in the critically ill thereby reflects a positive correlation between survival and the ability of the host to increase systemic D_{O_2}, accomplished primarily by an elevation in the CO. In a description of the hemodynamic sequelae of critical illness, emphasis must, therefore, be placed on understanding those factors that may influence the biventricular response to the particular disease, since an appropriate response is the one that ensures that CO, hence D_{O_2}, will vary according to the total metabolic demands imposed on the patient by the underlying illness.

SERUM LACTATE LEVELS. Arterial blood lactate levels have been found to be of great assistance to the clinician in circumstances of impaired tissue perfusion by providing an index of the severity of shock. Serum lactate has also been found to be a prognostic indicator in the early stages of a clinical course, as well as a monitor of the success of various therapeutic maneuvers.

Blood lactate levels are normally 0.7 to 1.8 mmol/L. During impaired perfusion, tissue hypoxia stimulates anaerobic metabolism with subsequent overproduction of lactate from pyruvate, although reduced splanchnic renal flow may impair lactate clearance by the liver and kidneys. Studies of lactate levels have been performed in both hypovolemic and septic shock. In hemorrhagic shock lactate is an indicator of the degree of anaerobic metabolism consequent upon oxygen deficiency. The situation in septic shock is much more complex, with impaired tissue perfusion existing as only one factor together with biochemical alterations at the cellular level

that may influence lactate production, and hepatic effects that may determine lactate clearance.

In septic shock, a hyperdynamic circulation with elevated cardiac output frequently exists. Oxygen consumption in this situation may be normal, elevated, or reduced in the presence of raised serum lactate levels. This suggests that the tissues are unable to extract the optimum amount of oxygen from the blood in the face of increased demands related to fever, tissue inflammation, and increased circulating catecholamines. Anaerobic metabolism thus ensues despite increased oxygen delivery. This failure to utilize oxygen in sepsis has been attributed to an inhibiting effect of endotoxin, lysosomal enzymes, and acidosis on mitochondrial function together with the presence of arteriovenous shunts.

Although anatomical shunts have not been demonstrated, it is known that maldistribution of tissue perfusion may occur, with blood traversing preferred route capillaries rather than nutrient vessels.

Rashkin recently attempted to define the critical level of oxygen delivery in critically ill patients and found that survival was good, together with lactate concentration in or near the normal range of oxygen delivery greater than 8 mL/kg/min. Below this level survival was poor and blood lactate markedly increased. He suggested that an oxygen delivery of greater than 8 mL/kg/min is probably sufficient to sustain organ function. However, measurement of oxygen delivery necessitates invasive procedures and blood lactate is a more convenient indicator of tissue oxygenation and metabolism.

Recent studies have suggested that serial lactate measurements could be used as a useful adjunct to the clinical evaluation of the critically ill patient and that consideration should be given to a change in therapy should a fall in lactate not be demonstrated during the early stage of treatment.

Waxman and colleagues demonstrated that despite attempts to maintain cardiac output during the intraoperative period at or above preoperative levels, the magnitude of this increase appeared to correlate with the degree of intraoperative reduction in oxygen consumption. These data suggested that a metabolic debt usually accumulates intraoperatively from inadequate tissue oxygenation. The hyperdynamic and hypermetabolic postoperative period may then represent a compensatory state necessary to repair intraoperative cellular and organ damage resulting from inadequate cellular oxygenation.

In a subsequent study sequential arterial blood lactate concentrations were determined pre-, intra-, and postoperatively in 12 high-risk surgical patients. These levels were correlated with simultaneous measurements of arterial blood pressure, cardiac index, and oxygen consumption. There was a marked increase in lactate values intraoperatively. This increase did not correspond to decreases in either mean arterial pressure or cardiac index but did appear to correlate with decreased intraoperative oxygen consumption. Postoperatively lactate levels remained elevated, and this elevation appeared to correlate with an estimation of intraoperative oxygen deficit.

Postoperatively cardiac index and oxygen consumption were increased.

While decreased oxygen consumption during operation has been previously recognized, it has usually been attributed to decreased demands caused by anesthetic agents and intraoperative hypothermia. Elevated lactate values, however, suggest that the oxygen consumption may be reduced beyond the reduction in metabolic demands, such that inadequate tissue oxygenation may be occurring. This inadequate tissue oxygenation is occurring despite therapy to maintain systemic blood flow. This implies impaired cellular utilization of oxygen, caused by either microcirculatory flow maldistribution, impairment of oxyhemoglobin dissociation, or a direct impairment of mitochondrial functions. An alternative explanation is that lactate clearance decreased intraoperatively and that this represents the pathophysiology of the increased levels rather than increased lactate production.

The persistently elevated levels of lactate into the postoperative period suggests that the metabolic deficit may persist into that period. Presumably, this supports the concept of the hyperdynamic postoperative state based on increased circulatory and metabolic demands because of a persistent metabolic deficit from the operation. Athletes, similarly, have increased cardiac output and oxygen consumption after exercise. A quantitative relationship between intraoperative oxygen deficit and postoperative lactate concentration was demonstrated. Potentially, lactate levels postoperatively may indicate the degree of the metabolic insult that the patient has suffered intraoperatively. Patients with more intraoperative oxygen deficit and higher postoperative lactate levels may require higher and more prolonged increases in cardiac index and oxygen consumption to recover.

The Waxman data also imply that the commonly monitored intraoperative clinical signs such as arterial pressure, heart rate, ECG, and CVP appear to be inadequate in detecting deficiencies of tissue oxygenation. Monitoring methods and systems that more directly address tissue oxygenation are needed. Lactate determinations may be very useful both in assessing the degree of accumulated oxygen deficit and in titrating therapy to support the necessary physiologic compensations.

Cowan and colleagues supported the idea that serial lactate measurements were better at predicting outcome than single measurements, when they demonstrated a fall in blood lactate during the first 3 h of resuscitation from shock in association with an improvement in the clinical condition. Statistical analysis of results, however, suggested that serial measurements of simple hemodynamic variables such as urine output, core-peripheral temperature gradient, or mean arterial pressure may be more valuable in predicting outcome than serial blood lactate.

CARDIOVASCULAR MONITORING

In considering the physiology of body blood flow, two important points must be made: the cardiac output alone is not an indicator of myocardial contractility, and arterial blood pressure alone is not an indicator of blood flow. Myocardial contractility refers to the state of health of the heart muscle and the rate at which the muscle fibers can shorten circumferentially around the bolus of blood within the ventricles. As will be seen later, myocardial contractility is intimately involved with myocardial oxygen transport (Fig. 13-1).

Cardiac output, the actual amount of blood ejected by the heart, is related to three other factors besides contractility: preload, afterload, and pulse rate. The preload is the degree of muscle fiber stretch imposed by filling of the ventricles during diastole. According to Starling's law of the heart, this varies directly with cardiac output (Fig. 13-2). The afterload is the impedance to cardiac ejection during systole imposed by vascular resistance, blood pressure, and blood viscosity (Fig. 13-3). The stroke output of the heart varies inversely with the afterload. The cardiac output varies directly with the pulse rate up to a level of 160, at which point there is insufficient time for complete ventricular filling. Any monitoring system designed to assess the state of the myocardium must include these factors. The Sarnoff ventricular function curve is a plot of stroke work (the product of stroke volume and mean aortic blood pressure) against ventricular end-diastolic pressure or end-diastolic volume. It provides a good evaluation of myocardial contractility because it includes consideration of afterload and preload. The bedside determination of fundamental hemodynamic variables such as cardiac output and PCWP is essential for the proper management of severely ill surgical patients.

Catheterization of the central venous system or right side of the heart for manometry, injection of indicator, or mixed venous sampling is used as an integral part of many

Fig. 13-1. Determinants of stroke volume, cardiac output, and arterial pressure.

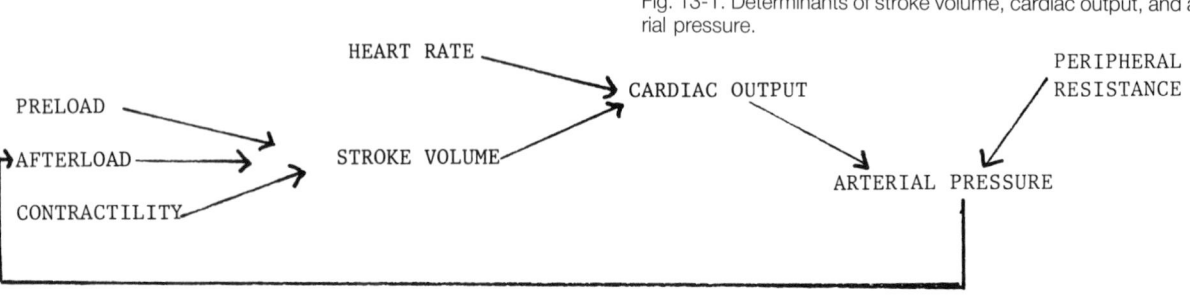

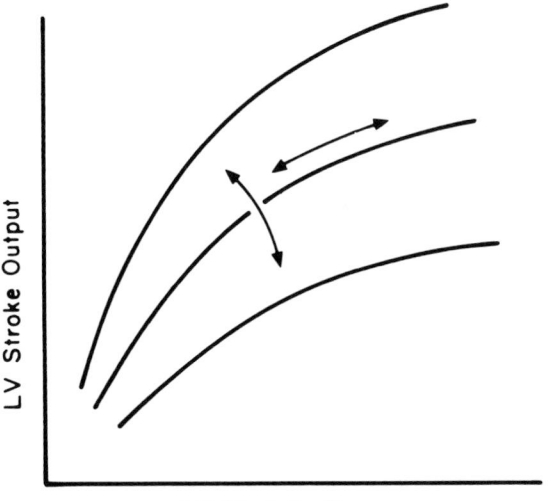

Fig. 13-2. Relationship between stroke output and diastolic pressure (Starling's law).

surgical monitoring systems. There are several routes of access to the central venous system. In order of increasing risk these are the median basilic vein in the the antecubital fossa, the external jugular vein, the internal jugular vein, and the subclavian vein. The femoral vein is seldom used because of contamination and thrombophlebitis. The median basilic vein directs the catheter directly into the subclavian vein and superior vena cava if the arm is extended laterally during the procedures, whereas the cephalic vein is difficult to negotiate at the shoulder. The external jugular vein is best approached with the neck extended, turned to the opposite side and lower than

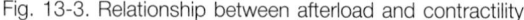

Fig. 13-3. Relationship between afterload and contractility.

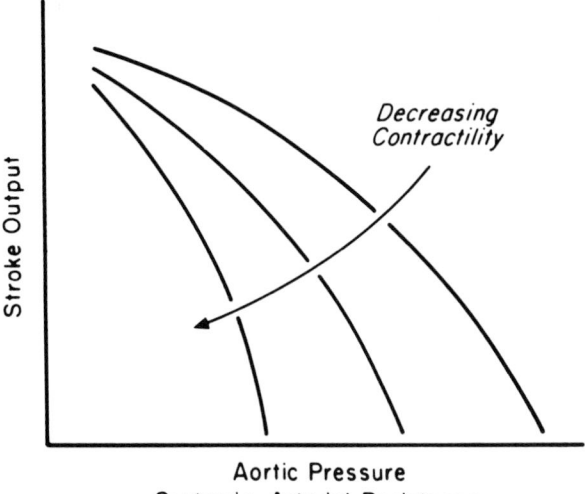

heart level (to fill the vein and prevent air embolism). The vein can also be steadied and distended by proximal pressure at the neck. As with the antecubital approach, venisection is best done before the vein is damaged with multiple puncture attempts. If there is difficulty passing the jugular-subclavian junction, the catheter may pass if the shoulder is depressed. The internal jugular vein can be cannulated percutaneously above the clavicle. The puncture is made immediately lateral to the pulsation of the common carotid artery through the lateral head of the sternocleidomastoid muscle. The distance to the proper position in the superior vena cava requires a catheter 20 cm long.

Puncture and catheter introduction into the subclavian vein involves a slightly greater risk of pneumothorax, but its ease of access makes it popular in emergency situations. As with the other sites, local anesthesia should be used as well as complete sterile precautions. Skin puncture is done just inferior to the clavicle at the junction of the middle and inner thirds, with the needle aimed at a point behind the manubrium. The catheter should not be threaded through or over the needle until venous blood is easily aspirated. When threaded through the needle, the catheter should never be withdrawn separately because of the danger of shearing it off with the sharp edge of the needle. Some commercial sets have protective sleeves that can be extended beyond the needle point to prevent cutting the catheter. A chest radiograph should always be obtained following central venous catheterization to check for pneumothorax and ascertain the position of the catheter tip. If a nonradiopaque catheter is used, it can be filled with contrast medium during the exposure. A number of commercial intravenous catheter sets are available that are ingeniously designed to facilitate advancement of the catheter without contamination or kinking (Fig. 13-4).

The proper interpretation of central venous pressure or pulmonary artery wedge pressure for monitoring surgical patients requires an understanding of all factors that may cause elevated readings. Artifacts such as inaccurate zero level, blockage, or kinking should be excluded by observation of 1- to 2-cm pressure fluctuations with the respiratory cycle and careful sighting of the zero level at the midaxillary line. The zero level should correspond to the point of projection of the posterior leaflet of the tricuspid valve on the right chest wall. Noncardiac factors that increase central venous pressure are hypervolemia, vasoconstrictor drugs (metaraminol and mephentermine constrict the veins as well as arterioles), positive-pressure ventilation, pneumothorax, hydrothorax, flail chest, and mediastinal compression. If none of these factors exists, normal readings vary between 0 and 9 cm of water for central venous pressure and 5 to 12 mmHg PCWP. Elevated values suggest the inability of either ventricle to handle its venous return. Filling pressure alone is not a measure of ventricular function or myocardial contractility, because afterload and ventricular work are unknown quantities. A high central venous pressure does serve as a warning that volume infusion should be continued with extreme caution. However, in situations such as pericardial tamponade or pulmonary embolism, a high central

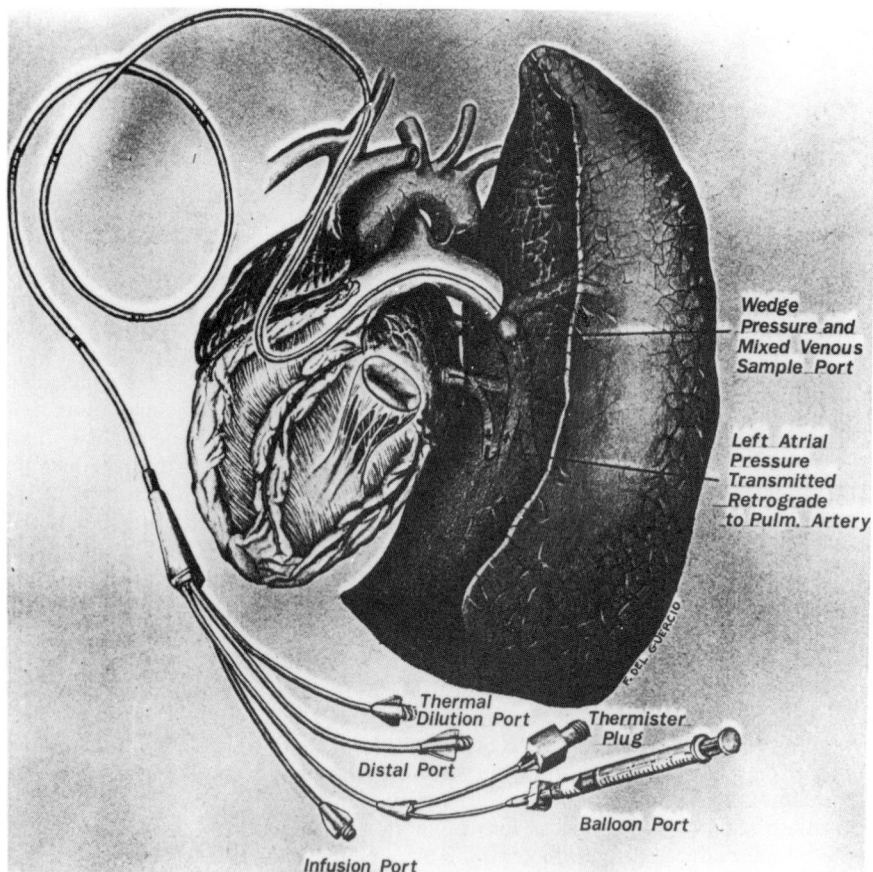

Wedge
Pressure and
Mixed Venous
Sample Port

Left Atrial
Pressure
Transmitted
Retrograde
to Pulm. Artery

Thermal
Dilution Port

Thermister
Plug

Distal Port

Balloon Port

Infusion Port

Fig. 13-4. Balloon catheter for invasive studies.

venous pressure is essential to maintain an adequate cardiac output until definitive therapy is used to relieve the obstruction. The most logical use of central venous pressure or PCWP as a guide to fluid replacement in seriously ill patients is the observation of the response to challenge with 100 mL increments of volume infusion. Infusion is stopped when a sharp rise in pressure occurs.

Equating wedge pressure with left atrial pressure assumes an open circuit from the catheter tip to the left atrium. This is not the case if the vessel is filled with blood clots or if the catheter is located in zones I and II in the pulmonary vascular bed, where alveolar pressure is greater than arterial pressure (zone I) or venous pressure (zones I and II) (Fig. 13-5).

In zone III, where both arterial and venous pressures exceed alveolar pressure, there is continuous flow, and conditions are met for accurate measurement of pulmonary-capillary wedge pressure. Fortunately, most of the lung enters zone III when the patient is supine, and most pulmonary-artery catheters will float into zone III since most of the blood is flowing into this zone. When vascular pressures are very low (hypovolemic shock) or when PEEP increases alveolar pressure, zone III may be converted to zone II. It has been shown that if the tip of the catheter is at or below the left atrium, the conditions in zone III exist even if PEEP values are as high as 30 cm

H_2O. If one finds that the wedge pressure has increased almost as much as the PEEP has, this increase suggests that the catheter has slipped into zone II or I. A cross-table, lateral chest film should confirm the location of the catheter tip relative to the left atrium. If the tip is above the atrium, the catheter should be repositioned.

Left atrial pressure does not equal left ventricular end-diastolic pressure in the presence of mitral-valve disease or markedly reduced ventricular compliance, in which atrial contraction can cause an appreciable increase in left ventricular end-diastolic pressure. In such a setting the pulmonary-capillary wedge pressure will still be an accurate monitor for cardiogenic pulmonary edema but will be less helpful in assessing left ventricular function. One must also realize that the left ventricular end-diastolic pressure may not be an accurate reflection of left ventricular end-diastolic volume. Very stiff noncompliant ventricles may allow a high end-diastolic pressure to accompany a normal end-diastolic volume. PEEP may increase end-diastolic pressure without increasing end-diastolic volume. Thus, although pulmonary-capillary wedge pressure usually reflects left ventricular end-diastolic pressure, it may not reflect actual preload.

There are additional problems due to PEEP-induced changes in vascular and pleural pressures. During spontaneous breathing the measured pulmonary-capillary wedge

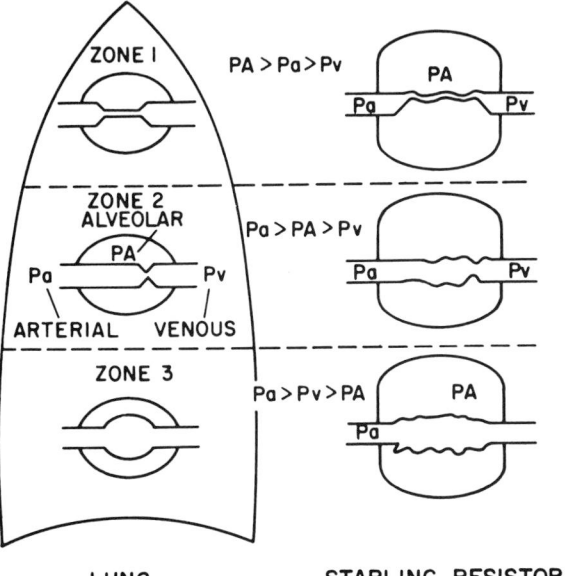

LUNG   STARLING RESISTOR

Fig. 13-5. The pulmonary capillary bed has flow characteristics of a Starling resistor, which consists of a length of flaccid collapsible tubing passing through a rigid chamber. In the Starling resistor, when chamber pressure (PA) exceeds the downstream pressure (pv), flow is independent of downstream pressure. However, when downstream pressure exceeds the chamber pressure, flow is determined by the upstream-downstream difference. The alveolar pressure is the same throughout the lung. The pulmonary artery pressure (Pa) increases down the lung. Zone 1 exists when alveolar pressure exceeds pulmonary arterial pressure and no blood flow occurs. This might occur when the pulmonary arterial pressure is decreased, as in hypovolemia, or when alveolar pressure is increased, as with the application of positive end-expiratory pressure. Zone 1 functions as alveolar dead space. In zone 2, pulmonary arterial pressure increases and exceeds alveolar pressure. In zone 2, blood flow is determined by the difference between arterial and alveolar pressures. In zone 3, blood flow is determined by the arteriovenous pressure difference. (From: *Bone RC: The treatment of severe hypoxemia due to the adult respiratory distress syndrome. Arch Intern Med 140:85, 1980, with permission.*)

pressure approximates the transmural pulmonary-capillary wedge pressure (measured value minus value for pleural pressure) because pleural pressure is small. This may not be true during breathing under PEEP, which may increase pleural pressures. Furthermore, some of the PEEP may be directly transmitted to the vessel itself. The application of PEEP can lead to artificially high intravascular-pressure readings if transmural pressures are falling. The amount of pressure transmitted to the pleural space and intrathoracic vessels depends on the compliance of the lungs and chest wall. When the lungs are very compliant and the chest wall is very stiff (e.g., as in emphysema), more pressure will be transmitted, making interpretation of pressure measurements quite difficult.

How does one cope with the above uncertainties? In general, if the level of PEEP is below 10 cmH$_2$O, there is no difference between pulmonary-capillary wedge pressures measured during ventilation and without ventilation. One study found that PEEP up to 30 cmH$_2$O did not markedly affect pressures in patients with very poor lung

compliance. Other studies, however, suggest that even in patients with stiff lungs, measured vascular pressures may increase with increasing PEEP and transmural pressures may actually decline.

There are two potential solutions to this problem, short of inserting pleural catheters in all patients. One is to disconnect the patient from the ventilator and measure all the pressures. This is not a practical approach. Although ventilation with 100 percent oxygen through one hand is probably safe, it may not always be. Moreover, the patient needs the ventilator. The second solution is to place the pulmonary-artery line in zone III of the lung and to keep the level of PEEP below 10 cmH$_2$O. If the PEEP level is higher, the measured vascular pressures may rise 1 to 2 mmHg for every 5 cm of PEEP applied to 10 cmH$_2$O. Although a pulmonary-capillary wedge pressure of 18 mmHg in a patient breathing spontaneously would be associated with interstitial pulmonary edema, it may be an acceptable value in a patient receiving PEEP at 20 cmH$_2$O. One must take readings consistently at end expiration, be sure that all the equipment is properly calibrated, and be careful not to overinterpret pressure readings in patients receiving PEEP.

Bedside monitoring of left ventricular dynamics by right-sided catheterization was facilitated by the development of the balloon-tipped Swan-Ganz catheter. With the balloon inflated, the catheter sails through the right side of the heart into a wedge position in the pulmonary artery in less than 1 min. In the absence of pulmonary vascular disease, pulmonary capillary wedge pressure is a reliable guide to left atrial and, in turn, left ventricular end-diastolic pressure. Without the wedge position, the pulmonary artery end-diastolic pressure is an acceptable indicator of mean left atrial pressure. Central venous pressure alone has been found to be an unreliable index of left ventricular function, since filling pressure in the left side of the heart may rise sharply and pulmonary edema may occur without significant increase in right atrial pressures.

The right ventricle is bound by a convex septal wall and a concave free wall, which enclose a crescent-shaped slit between them. In the right ventricular cavity a relatively narrow space is therefore confined between two broad surfaces, so that the surface area of the chamber is great in relation to the volume. Therefore, the configuration of the right ventricle is ideally suited to the ejection of large volumes of blood with minimal amounts of myocardial shortening. This architectural design is not conducive to the development of high intraventricular pressures. Anatomically, the pericardium surrounding the right and left ventricles may have a substantial effect on ventricular function, as this rather still membrane is not capable of acute rapid expansion.

Considerable "interdependence" exists between right and left ventricular function. In a noncompliant nondistensible pericardium, an acute increase in right ventricular end-diastolic volume may result in a shift of the interventricular septum toward the left ventricular cavity with a consequent reduction in the left ventricular end-diastolic volume. In this instance, assessment of left ventricular preload may not be accurately measured as the pulmonary artery wedge pressure due to the decrease in left ventricular compliance.

The development of pulmonary artery hypertension is a common denomination in severe cases of acute respiratory failure during critical illness. The pulmonary vascular bed provides the impedance to ejection (afterload) faced by the right ventricle. The physiologic consequences of increased impedance on right ventricular function have been well described. Initially an increase in systolic force of right ventricular contraction is noted with increased right ventricular systolic pressures. Subsequently, an increase in the right ventricular diastolic pressure may be followed by right ventricular failure.

Recently, some of the pathophysiologic consequences of pulmonary hypertension and right ventricular function have been defined. Initially, increased force of right ventricular ejection is allowed by an increase in right ventricular end-diastolic volume. The use of the Starling relationship in this circumstance results in a maintenance of right ventricular ejection. As the compliance characteristics of the right ventricle are altered, the increased end-diastolic volume results in increased intracavitary pressures. During diastole, such increased pressures exceed left ventricular end-diastolic pressures, and the septum will therefore be shifted toward the left ventricular cavity. Septal shift may then affect left ventricular function by reducing the volume (preload) of the left ventricle. Therefore, an adaptive response on the right side of the heart to pulmonary hypertension may result in left ventricular dysfunction.

The critically ill patient, most especially during sepsis, may show evidence of pulmonary hypertension associated with higher right ventricular end-diastolic volume, intracavitary pressure, septal shift, and reduced left ventricular function. The right and left ventricular dysfunction may be accentuated by the application of positive-pressure ventilation, particularly with use of positive end-expiratory pressure.

CENTRAL VENOUS OXIMETRY. The mixed venous oxygen level reflects the extent to which the body must call upon the blood oxygen stores in states of cardiovascular stress. The value of right heart oxygen saturation monitoring during surgery has been demonstrated (Fig. 13-3). Changes in cardiac output secondary to hemorrhage and other problems are reflected by early changes in right atrial oxygen saturation, usually before changes in arterial blood pressure, venous pressure, or heart rate. Changes in arterial oxygen content secondary to pulmonary shunting or decreased oxygen-carrying capacity also promptly affect mixed venous oxygen saturation. It was originally thought that pulmonary arterial samples would be necessary for this type of monitoring, but experience has shown that, in the stressed patient, right atrial or right ventricular samples correlate well with those from the pulmonary artery. Saturations below 50 percent from these sites are a bad prognostic sign and indicate either severe arterial hypoxemia or very significantly decreased cardiac output.

In a recent study by Nelson, continuously measured mixed venous oxygen saturation (Sv_{O_2}) was a reliable predictor of Sv_{O_2} measured intermittently by in vitro methods. In critically ill surgical patients, Sv_{O_2} does not correlate highly with the individual determinants of oxygen transport but rather correlates with the oxygen utilization coefficient (V_{O_2}/D_{O_2}) and therefore reflects the overall balance between oxygen consumption and delivery.

To understand this concept clearly, the components of the Fick equation must be analyzed and rearranged. The Fick equation relates cardiac output, tissue oxygen consumption, and the arterial-venous oxygen content difference.

$$V_{O_2} = C(a - v)_{O_2} \times CO \times 10$$

Other cardiopulmonary parameters that are calculated include:

$$Ca_{O_2} = (Sa_{O_2} \times Hb \times 1.34) + (Pa_{O_2} \times 0.0031)$$

$$Cv_{O_2} = (Sv_{O_2} \times Hb \times 1.34) + (Pv_{O_2} \times 0.0031)$$

$$C(a - v)_{O_2} = Ca_{O_2} - Cv_{O_2}$$

$$D_{O_2} = CO \times 10 \times Ca_{O_2}$$

$$OUC = V_{O_2}/D_{O_2}$$

where Ca_{O_2} = arterial oxygen content (mL/dL), Sa_{O_2} = arterial oxygen saturation (fraction), Hb = hemoglobin concentration (g/dL), Pa_{O_2} = arterial oxygen tension (mmHg), Cv_{O_2} = venous oxygen content (mL/dL), Sv_{O_2} = mixed venous oxygen saturation (fraction), Pv_{O_2} = mixed venous oxygen tension (mmHg), $C(a - v)O_2$ = arterial-venous oxygen content difference (mL/dL), D_{O_2} = oxygen delivery (mL/min), CO = cardiac output (L/min), V_{O_2} = oxygen consumption (mL/min), OUC = oxygen utilization coefficient (fraction).

When the terms of the Fick equation are rearranged, it may be seen that the determinants of Sv_{O_2} are the components of oxygen delivery and oxygen consumption:

$$\frac{V_{O_2}}{CO \times 10} = C(a - v)_{O_2}$$

$$\frac{V_{O_2}}{CO \times 10} = Ca_{O_2} - Cv_{O_2}$$

$$\frac{V_{O_2}}{CO \times 10} - Ca_{O_2} = -Cv_{O_2}$$

$$Cv_{O_2} = Ca_{O_2} - \left[\frac{V_{O_2}}{CO \times 10}\right]$$

$$\frac{Cv_{O_2}}{Ca_{O_2}} = 1 - \left[\frac{V_{O_2}}{CO \times 10 \times Ca_{O_2}}\right]$$

If $Sa_{O_2} = 1.0$, then

$$Sv_{O_2} = \frac{Cv_{O_2}}{Ca_{O_2}}$$

$$Sv_{O_2} = 1 - [V_{O_2}/(CO \times 10 \times Ca_{O_2})]$$

$$Sv_{O_2} = 1 - \frac{V_{O_2}}{D_{O_2}}$$

From the foregoing formulas only three mechanisms can account for a decrease in the venous oxygen content (Cv_{O_2}): a decrease in the arterial oxygen content (Ca_{O_2}), oxygen consumption (V_{O_2}), and total cardiac output (CO). Similarly, provided there is no change in the other components in the equation, an increase in the oxygen consumption (V_{O_2}) or a decrease in the cardiac output (CO), hemoglobin concentration (Hb), or arterial oxygen saturation (Sv_{O_2}) will produce a decrease in the Sv_{O_2}.

A major development in pulmonary-artery catheters has been the addition of a channel including two fiberoptic bundles for light transmission, allowing continuous measurements of oxygen saturation of the mixed venous blood by an oximeter. The insertion of fiberoptic catheters is not afflicted with additional difficulties, despite the fact that the optic fibers are relatively fragile and can easily be fractured. A major problem lies in the high cost of the catheter and the oximeter. Continuous Sv_{O_2} display, however, can limit the number of venous blood gas and cardiac output determinations. As an online parameter, it is undoubtedly an invaluable indicator of acute cardiorespiratory disturbance in severely ill patients.

While continuously measured Sv_{O_2} may correlate with hemodynamic changes (cardiac output) in some groups of patients, the nonsteady nature of critical illness has taught us not to expect that arterial oxygen saturation, hemoglobin concentration, or oxygen consumption will remain stable, and therefore changes in Sv_{O_2} will not necessarily reflect changes in cardiac output in these patients. Nelson indicated that, although there is some statistical correlation between Sv_{O_2} and both cardiac output and oxygen delivery, the correlation coefficients are so small that the use of Sv_{O_2} as a predictor of cardiac output is unreliable. Similarly, correlations could not be established between Sv_{O_2} and arterial oxygenation, oxygen consumption, or arterial-venous content difference as independent variables. The high degree of inverse correlation between Sv_{O_2} and oxygen utilization ratio makes this relationship clinically useful.

The goal of many interventions in critically ill patients is to ensure that oxygen delivery to the tissue meets or exceeds the oxygen demand of that tissue. Our clinical ability to monitor this relationship is severely lacking. While we can measure total body oxygen uptake by the patient with reasonable reliability, oxygen uptake is equal to oxygen consumption only in the steady state. To make matters worse, oxygen consumed by the patient is not necessarily equal to the oxygen demand by the tissues of the patient. Normally, oxygen consumption increases when oxygen demand increases. Oxygen consumption may increase through an increase in the extraction of oxygen from arterial blood as it traverses the capillary bed [(i.e., an increase in $C(a - v)_{O_2}$] or through an increase in blood flow (i.e., cardiac output). Both of these factors may increase by approximately threefold in normal subjects, allowing a ninefold increase in oxygen consumption to meet the oxygen demand of the tissue. Critically ill patients may not be capable of increasing cardiac output spontaneously and therefore may have a markedly diminished "safety factor" in regard to increasing oxygen

consumption. When oxygen demand exceeds oxygen consumption, anaerobic metabolism ensues and lactic acidosis results, as previously described.

In the normal resting state, the entire body consumes only 25 percent of the oxygen transported to it by the cardiac output. Normal mixed venous blood is found to be 75 percent saturated with a partial pressure of 40 mmHg. An additional complicating factor is the fact that oxygen consumed by the various tissues differs, and it is not possible at this time to measure clinically oxygen demand or consumption of individual organs. For example, at rest myocardial oxygen extraction is near maximal while renal oxygen extraction is very low. At times of stress when myocardial oxygen demand increases, oxygen consumption can increase only by increases in myocardial blood flow. During this same period of stress, renal blood flow may actually decrease dramatically and renal oxygen consumption may be maintained by increased oxygen extraction in the renal capillary bed. Mixed venous blood represents a "flow-weighted average" of the blood returning from all perfused tissues. That is to say, the magnitude of the effect of oxygen extraction by any organ on Sv_{O_2} is proportional to the blood flow to that organ so that low-consumption, high-flow organs (kidneys) have a greater effect on Sv_{O_2} than do high-consumption, low-flow organs (myocardium).

Since our goals are not necessarily to provide the highest oxygen delivery but rather to bring into balance the relationship between oxygen consumption and oxygen delivery, it seems apparent that continuously measured Sv_{O_2} is at this time the best indicator clinically available to assure that this goal has been attained.

A low or rapidly decreasing Sv_{O_2} indicates an imbalance between oxygen consumption and oxygen delivery that requires further investigation of the determinants of these parameters. A low or falling Sv_{O_2} does not tell us which therapy is appropriate in a given situation but rather tells us that more information is needed to assess the problem. The falling Sv_{O_2} may indicate a decrease in hemoglobin concentration, arterial oxygen content, or cardiac output, or an increase in tissue oxygen consumption. When a low or decreasing Sv_{O_2} is encountered, the clinician may obtain an arterial blood-gas analysis, hemoglobin value, and hemodynamic assessment of the patient to select the most appropriate intervention that may restore the balance between oxygen consumption and delivery. This function has been described by Watson as the "early warning system" of cardiorespiratory imbalance.

CARDIAC-OUTPUT DETERMINATIONS

Invasive Techniques

In spite of various questions regarding accuracy in high- or low-flow states, the description of indicator-dilution curves from central circulation remains the basic method for monitoring cardiac output. The technique involves the injection of an indicator into the right side of the heart and continuous determination of its concentration as it mixes with the cardiac output somewhere downstream. Any indicator can be used, as long as it does not affect hemodynamics or disappear from the blood before the concentration is measured. It can best be understood as a variation of the Fick principle, where the known amount of indicator is equivalent to a fixed amount of oxygen consumption, and the mean concentration of indicator after mixing is equivalent to the arteriovenous oxygen difference. It follows, then, that the faster the volume of blood flow, the lower the arteriovenous oxygen difference and mean concentration of indicator. All methods for the calculation of cardiac output from both continuous and single-bolus injection of indicator use this principle in analyzing the time-concentration curves to obtain the mean concentration of indicator. The number of milligrams of indicator injected divided by the mean concentration of indicator gives the volume of flow during the time of the indicator-dilution curve. Thermal dilution curves are similar in principle, with use of cold saline solution as the indicator. They are popular because of their simplicity and the availability of bedside computers, but the required flow-directed balloon-tipped thermistor catheters are expensive. Since cardiac output is usually expressed as flow per minute, the volume of flow during description of the curve is multiplied by 60 and divided by the number of seconds of duration of the curve.

Intracardiac and arterial blood-pressure data, cardiac output data, and electrocardiograph tracings combined with arterial and mixed venous blood-gas data permit calculation of a number of derived cardiorespiratory variables of physiologic significance. A microprocessor-controlled printer located right in the intensive care unit gives all professional personnel immediate access to a comprehensive display of cardiovascular performance, pulmonary function, and oxygen transport. A programmed instruction feature makes it easy to use.

Several hand-held calculators with program cards specifically made up for shock-cart calculating are available. The primary data obtained from the recorder and blood-gas machines are entered on the keyboard, and the derived values are immediately computed. Civetta's and Shoemaker's groups have made available magnetic card programs for the rapid automatic calculation of up to 27 derived cardiorespiratory variables, using Hewlett-Packard and Texas Instrument calculators, respectively.

Data become information only in the brain of the beholder. The average physician is "turned off" by a column of numbers representing cardiac index, stroke index, right and left ventricular stroke work, pulmonary and systemic vascular resistance, ventricular function indices, intracardiac and systemic pressures, arteriovenous oxygen difference, venoarterial admixture, oxygen consumption, P_{50}, serum lactate, and arterial base excess or deficit. In an attempt to make dull data attractive, Cohn and Del Guercio devised a system for displaying these derived variables on an easily scanned, logically organized, bar-chart format. Arterial and mixed venous blood-gas and saturation values along with cardiac output, temperature, height, weight, and inspired oxygen concentration are entered on the keyboard of a minicomputer, and within

seconds the derived variables are drawn on a preprinted sheet by an *X-Y* alphanumeric recorder. This system, called the automated physiologic profile, is a compromise between the hand-held calculator approach and the very expensive built-in digital computer monitors. The profile serves as a useful permanent record of cardiorespiratory status before and after therapeutic interventions.

The example shown in Fig. 13-6 demonstrates a number of points regarding monitoring of the critically ill patient. This was a study, with Swan-Ganz thermistor catheter and radial artery cannula, of a young man who suffered a 30 percent burn and smoke inhalation. The physiologic assessment was done 24 h after injury and showed a "normal" cardiac index and blood pressure with an increase in oxygen consumption resulting from a widened arteriovenous oxygen content difference. Why, then, was there evidence of anaerobic metabolism and hypoxic acidosis with twice normal serum lactate levels and a base deficit of 6 meq/L? Because the patient's oxygen needs were even greater, and had the state of increasing oxygen debt continued, the patient surely would have died. The ventricular function curve in the lower right quadrant shows why the patient could not increase his cardiac output enough to supply his increased oxygen needs. The plot, representing the Starling-Frank relationship, is significantly below the zone of normal ventricular function. The cause for this cardiac failure could have been circulating myocardial depressant factors, known to be associated with burns, early sepsis, or poisoning of myocardial mitochondrial cytochromes by the high level of carbon monoxide (S_{CO}), which probably had been much higher on admission. The high right atrial and pulmonary artery wedge pressures indicate that both ventricles had more than adequate preload. Since total peripheral vascular resistance was normal, that determinant of cardiac output (afterload) also was not the limiting factor. It was obvious from this physiologic profile (but not from the ECG, PCWP, or systemic BP) that the patient would not survive unless inotropic therapy could stimulate the myocardium to at least normal contractility. This was accomplished with digitalis, dopamine, and GIK (glucose, insulin, potassium).

At the same time, the profile also illustrated the need for a volume-cycled respiratory with PEEP to reduce the severe pulmonary shunting (venoarterial admixture) caused by the smoke inhalation. The most appropriate setting of end-expiratory pressure (optimum PEEP) was determined by performing automated physiologic profiles sequentially at increased levels of PEEP. Beyond a certain level, reduced cardiac output, resulting from restricted preload, produced a net decrease in oxygen transport, even though arterial oxygen content continued to improve. Had it not been for the information provided by the monitoring of these derived cardiorespiratory variables, it is unlikely that lifesaving therapeutic decisions could have been made in time.

The effect of the 15% carboxyhemoglobin concentration on the position of the oxyhemoglobin dissociation curve is also shown. The P_{50} STD value of 30.2 excludes the effect of carbon monoxide, and the P_{50} STDX value of

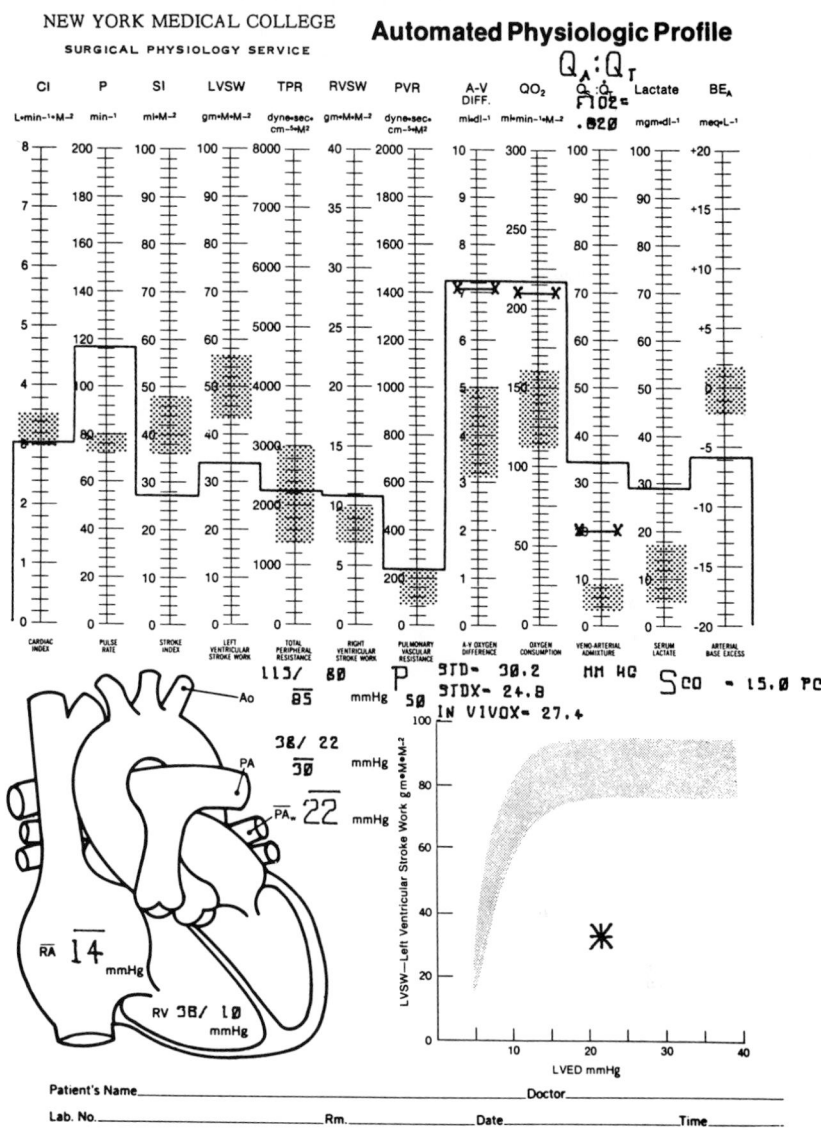

Fig. 13-6. Automated physiologic profile.

24.9 indicates the shift to the left caused by carboxyhemoglobin. The lines with the X's on the bar charts for "A-V Diff," Q_{O_2}, and Q_a/Q_t indicate those values at the patient's actual P_{50} compared with what they would have been had the P_{50} been normal (26 to 27 mmHg). This type of calculation is of value clinically, since it is possible to manipulate the P_{50} by pharmacologic means in order to improve oxygen transport. Harken's recent review of this aspect of monitoring emphasizes the importance of dissociation-curve shifts in clinical syndromes.

The automated physiologic profile is in use in many institutions, including a number of community hospitals, where it has been proved cost-effective, particularly when used for preoperative assessment and physiologic fine tuning in the high-risk patient, which will be discussed later (Fig. 13-7).

There are other monitoring systems that involve the use of catheter-tip sensors. One measures pressure and electromagnetic flow velocity. When threaded retrograde into the left ventricle, this sensor permits the on-line recording of the left ventricular pressures, left ventricular pressure acceleration (dp/dt), intracardiac heart sounds, ascending aortic blood velocity, and ascending aortic blood acceleration. If the cross-sectional area of the aorta is known, total flow can be calculated. All these serve as very useful indices of left ventricular function, particularly following myocardial infarction. The problem of calibration of the electromagnetic flowmeter probe without a zero-flow calibration point is a serious one, as it is for all clinical studies involving electromagnetic flowmeters.

A disposable, very thin polarographic oxygen-sensing electrode can be used for mixed venous oxygen tension

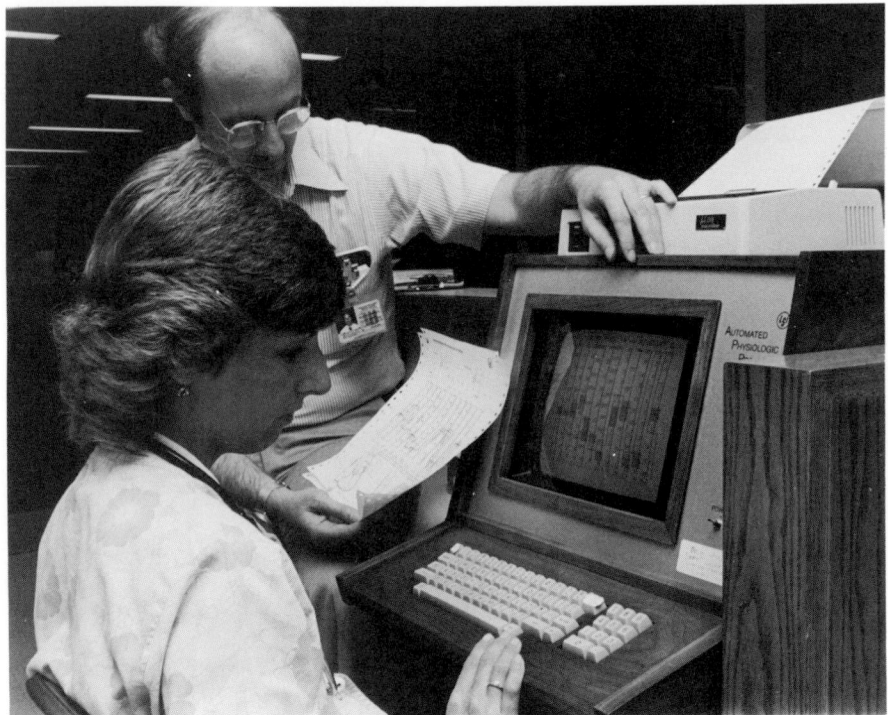

Fig. 13-7. Hardware for automated physiologic profile.

monitoring. The miniature sensor is fabricated by dip-coating or painting the various insulators, diffusion membranes, and buffers directly onto the central wire electrode. Other similar devices are available complete with compact solid-state battery-powered recorders for use at the bedside.

The insertion of a long catheter from the radial artery up to the region of the aortic arch permits a detailed analysis of the aortic pulse contour. Warner has perfected this technique for clinical monitoring. Stroke volume is computed from the pulse contour on a beat-by-beat basis. This, combined with pressure variables, provides an almost instantaneous cardiovascular assessment. Unfortunately, McDonald et al. have pointed out, the method depends upon a stable vascular impedance, which is seldom the case in critically ill patients. For this reason, the technique is not in general use.

Preoperative Hemodynamic Assessment

There is evidence that preoperative hemodynamic assessment of patients is applicable to specific situations. Using pulmonary-artery catheters, Corlon and associates have revealed seriously impaired hemodynamic function in many patients. Patients with abnormal cardiac function had a postoperative mortality rate approximately 100 times higher than the average for all patients in that institution. Patients readmitted to the ICU postoperatively who received extensive hemodynamic monitoring and management had substantially better results than those not readmitted.

Del Guercio and associates have used right-sided heart balloon flotation catheters for arterial sampling to determine the physiologic variables representing left and right ventricular function, oxygen transport, and metabolic parameters of ventricular function curves in a group of elderly patients. Invasive preoperative assessments of these elderly patients disclosed a high percentage of serious physiologic abnormalities requiring a delay of operation in some and cancellation in others. The frequent observation of subtle underlying defects in cardiac reserve in patients who otherwise appeared healthy to the clinician precipitated the opening of a preoperative assessment unit at the Westchester County Medical Center. Preoperative assessment of patients who underwent gastric partition procedures for morbid obesity demonstrated that although there was no clinical evidence of congestive heart failure and there was no evidence of abnormality in the arteriovenous oxygen content differences, the left ventricular function was reduced to 57 percent of normal.

Circulatory response to trauma of a major operation, performed with general anesthesia, consists of two phases—the operative phase and the postoperative phase. The first phase is characterized by depressed cardiac output and cardiac index, and the second by an elevation of the cardiac output and index, particularly in the immediate postoperative period. The first phase response is more marked in obese patients and the increase characteristic of the second phase is less than that noted for nonobese patients. The abnormal response of the second phase is an important contributing factor to the increased operative mortality in the morbidly obese patients. Vascular disorders in which there is frequent coexistence of heart disease, hypertension, diabetes, stroke, as well as the usual high-risk factors of advanced age also benefit from preoperative evaluation. The study by Barber et al. indicates that only one-third of patients undergoing preoperative evaluation for a vascular operation had normal left ventricular function and required no therapeutic intervention before the operative procedure. About one-quarter of patients with impaired left ventricular function responded to preload augmentation, 40 percent required inotropic support, 13 percent needed afterload reduction, and about 10 percent required a combination of a change in preload inotropic support and afterload reduction. It is also appropriate to perform a preoperative physiologic profile on patients with acute limb ischemia because low cardiac output with or without excessive SVR is present in about 10 percent. The ischemia resulting from the low flow portends a dire prognosis, and a discernible improvement in the circulatory status in the limbs coincided with the correction of low-flow states by appropriate hemodynamic maneuvers. Preoperative physiologic assessment of patients with hip fractures and optimizing the hemodynamic status reduce mortality and morbidity. This circumstance also pertains to elderly patients undergoing urologic procedures.

Studies have concluded that right heart catheterization is indicated for severely ill hemodynamically unstable patients who do not respond to therapy deemed appropriate after clinical evaluation. The clinical states that benefit most and have more clearly defined indications for the use of invasive pulmonary catheter monitoring are listed in Table 13-4.

Table 13-4. INDICATIONS FOR
PULMONARY-ARTERY CATHETERS

1. Myocardial infarctions complicated by
   a. Hypotension unresponsive to volume challenge
   b. Marked hemodynamic instability requiring intravenous inotropic or vasoactive drugs or mechanical assist devices
   c. Hypotension and congestive heart failure
   d. ?Cardiac tamponade (equalization of end-diastolic pressures)
   e. ?Acute mitral regurgitation (giant V waves)
   f. ?Ruptured interventricular septum (step-up in oxygen saturation)
2. Unstable angina requiring intravenous nitroglycerin (most patients)
3. Congestive heart failure unresponsive to conventional therapy, to guide preload and afterload therapy
4. Pulmonary hypertension, for diagnosis and monitoring during acute drug therapy
5. Distinguishing cardiogenic from noncardiogenic pulmonary edema
6. Optimizing PEEP and volume therapy in the adult respiratory-distress syndrome
7. Resolving doubts about volume or cardiovascular status if a diuretic or fluid challenge would be unsafe or would yield equivocal results
8. Preoperative assessment of high-risk patients

Noninvasive Techniques

As more sophisticated noninvasive techniques develop in the next decade, the use of invasive techniques will diminish. At the present time preoperative Swan-Ganz catheter insertion can be performed safely and efficiently, and also provides the surgeon and anesthesiologist an on-line continuous monitoring mode of hemodynamic parameters intraoperatively and postoperatively.

Assessment of right ventricular function is made difficult by the complex geometry and shape of the right ventricle. The thermodilution techniques used to measure cardiac output with the pulmonary-artery catheter can now also determine right ventricular ejection fraction quite easily if a fast-response thermistor is used. An essential advantage of this measurement is the ability to repeatedly evaluate right ventricular function during the course of disease, and also to assess the effects of therapeutic interventions. These catheters are about 20 percent more expensive than standard ones, and the cardiac-output computers needed for calculation of the right ventricular ejection fraction cost twice as much as standard cardiac-output computers.

All the methods of estimating cardiac output described thus far are invasive to varying degrees and therefore present some risk and considerable expense because they require skilled personnel for their application. A number of promising noninvasive adaptations of the indicator-dilution principle are in clinical use. Included in this category are gamma densitometry (quantitative angiography), videodensitometry, isotope-dilution analysis, fluorescence excitation analysis, and magnetic fluid tracer dilution.

Information regarding flow rates, vascular volumes, distribution of pulmonary transit times, intracardiac and pulmonary shunting, and right or left ventricular ejection efficiency is theoretically contained in the shapes of indicator-dilution curves. With the conventional indocyanine green dye technique, sampling rates are too slow, and the injection and sampling sites are too far apart for complete interpretation of the physiologic events that create the shape of the curve. Catheter lag between the sampling point and the densitometer cuvette also produces distortion of the curves and loss of potential information. Gamma densitometry, in which the indicator is a small bolus of radiopaque contrast medium and the blood vessels or cardiac chambers serve as the densitometer cuvettes, avoids these problems. Gamma rays or x-rays, projected through the cardiac silhouette, produce high-dynamic-response indicator time-concentration curves through the detection of changes in gamma photon density related, according to Beer's law, to the concentration of radiopaque indicator in the blood. In clinical practice, solid-state radiation detectors are placed behind the patient as in a portable x-ray unit. Five milliliters of Hypaque is then injected into the central venous catheter, and six simultaneous contrast dilution curves are recorded from the heart and great vessels. Analysis of these curves permits calculation of pulmonary circulation time, pulmonary blood volume, right and left ventricular ejection fraction, and other useful variables. More sophisticated interpretation requires electronic data processing for transfer-function analysis.

Videodensitometry and digital subtraction angiography are similar in principle to gamma densitometry, except that an actual angiocardiogram is performed and recorded. The advantages are that, at leisure, an infinite number of curves can be obtained from any point in the cardiac silhouette as the tape is played over and over. Disadvantages include great expense, lack of portability, and low signal-to-noise ratio requiring signal processing to obtain recognizable curves.

Isotope dilution analysis has made a great leap forward with the development of the Anger scintillation camera and other rapid-response isotope scanning devices. The ability to image and quantify the distribution of a radioactive tracer second by second through the heart and lungs adds a new dimension of considerable value to surgical cardiovascular monitoring. High-photon-yield isotopes are injected intravenously and the gamma camera images are recorded on magnetic tape. Later, specific areas can be analyzed to produce indicator-dilution curves that can be related to changes in size and position of the cardiac chambers. Jones et al. have produced good indicator-dilution curves for the right and left sides of the heart using an autofluoroscope. Spatial resolution and dynamic response, however, can never be as good as that obtained with the linear interrogating beams of radiation used in gamma densitometry.

With the advent of the radionuclide gated blood-pool scans, one could determine the left ventricular ejection fraction very accurately in critically ill patients in the intensive care unit. The scan relies upon technetium 99 pyrophosphate to label circulating erythrocytes, and the tracer quantity of radionuclide produces an image that is gated to an electrocardiogram to provide a very accurate measure of left ventricular ejection fraction and continuous motion of the heart chambers. The latter method allows one to evaluate ventricular wall motion by performing simultaneously a radionuclide scan and thermodilution cardiac index. One can calculate the end-diastolic volume index using the following formula:

$$\text{LV end-diastolic volume} = \frac{\text{stroke volume index}}{\text{LV ejection fraction}}$$

where LV is left ventricular, stroke volume index is determined from the thermodilution cardiac output, and the left ventricular ejection fraction is determined from the radionuclide scan. Because the tracer remains in the bloodstream for 6 or more hours with a single radionuclide injection, one can determine the left ventricular ejection fraction for this 6 h. Thus, if a base-line scan and output are performed, one can calculate the ventricular volumes serially for 6 h in response to a volume infusion, pressors, or vasodilator administration.

It is also possible to tag flowing blood in vivo by reversing the magnetic alignments of hydrogen nuclei in the water of the plasma by applying a powerful external magnetic field. These effects are detected farther downstream by means of magnetic resonance imaging. Magnetic resonance imaging devices are currently available. The technique, as described by Singer, is totally noninvasive.

It is obvious that noninvasive techniques for describing indicator-dilution curves will play a prominent role in surgical monitoring for years to come. Surgeons will be provided information regarding cardiac and circulatory function in their patients that will permit management of critical states on a firm physiologic basis.

The determination of systolic time intervals provides an external assessment of left ventricular function based entirely on intrinsic electrical and mechanical events. The methodology is gaining in popularity because it is physiologically sound and has been largely validated by extensive comparative clinical studies including catheterization of the left side of the heart.

Simultaneous recordings of the electrocardiogram, phonocardiogram, and external carotid pulse tracing are analyzed for the following time variables: total left ventricular systolic time (QRS complex to second heart sound), left ventricular ejection time (duration of carotid pulse upstroke), and preejection period (the difference between total left ventricular systolic and left ventricular ejection times). Although the calculations are straightforward, placement of the carotid pulse sensor and phonocardiogram microphone on the neck and chest is critical. With technical care in the performance of the recordings, remarkably good correlation with direct measures of the dynamics of the left side of the heart can be shown. Weissler et al. have found that the ratio of the preejection period to left ventricular ejection time (PEP/LVET) is relatively constant around 0.35 in patients with normal hearts. With failure of the left side of the heart, the PEP becomes longer and the LVET shorter, increasing the ratio. Serial studies reveal good correlation between the PEP/LVET ratio and left ventricular ejection fraction, end-diastolic volume, and end-diastolic pressure. This noninvasive approach, which requires inexpensive equipment, is useful for the continuous bedside monitoring of left ventricular function.

Alterations of left ventricular conduction, however, as in left bundle branch block, prolong the PEP selectively with no apparent change in LVET. Changes in peripheral impedance or vascular runoff, as occur in septic shock, may alter the relation between the PEP/LVET ratio and cardiac performance.

The application of ultrasound to clinical monitoring is undergoing a period of rapid growth according to Feigenbaum. Both industrial and academic sectors have developed methods for cardiovascular assessment based on interrogating beams of high-frequency sound waves (less than 1 mm wavelength). Ultrasonic energy can penetrate all tissues except bone and air-filled structures and provide good spatial resolution for diagnostic studies. Thus far, at the levels of energy needed for clinical work, there has been no suggestion of injury to living tissue, not even the fetus. The lack of hazard and the reasonable cost of the equipment required have led to more clinical studies than with any other technique aside from electrocardiography.

There are two basic methods of operation of ultrasound for diagnostic purposes—the pulse-echo mode (sonar) and the backscatter frequency-shift mode (Doppler effect). In the former, the distance between the emitter and any sound-reflecting interface deep within the body is measured in terms of the transit time of bursts of ultrasound to and from the tissue. An A scan device is held stationary against the body and a recording of the depth of structures in the path of the beam is made on the basis of the known speed of sound in tissue. The B scan is produced if the ultrasonic emitter is traversed across the body while echo-ranging, in order to produce a picture of the tissue cross section.

Not only is ultrasound less harmful than ionizing radiation, but it is capable of revealing internal surfaces that are invisible to x-rays. These include the internal structures of the heart and blood vessels. In addition, devices using the Doppler principle can detect rapid motions within the body. This makes them useful for studies of peripheral blood flow and cardiac valve function.

In echocardiography for ultrasonic determination of cardiac chamber size and stroke volume, a transducer is applied to the chest over the cardiac area. Sound in the 1- to 5-MHz frequency is delivered through the chest in on-off bursts about 1500 times per second. Echoes are detected during the off periods and recorded in terms of time lag (distance). The distances between the intraventricular septum and the posterior endocardial wall of the left ventricle are recorded at end diastole and end systole. The calculations of end-diastole and end-systolic volumes are made on the assumption that the shape of the chamber is a prolate ellipse. The results from a number of investigators are remarkable. The left ventricular volumes measured by echocardiography and by biplane angiocardiography were very similar over a wide range of values (correlation coefficient .97). The problem with this technique for surgical monitoring is that operators must be highly skilled and experienced in aiming the transducer and recognizing on the scan the exact structures they wish to measure. The device cannot be simply strapped on and left alone for 24 h to record left ventricular function. Some method will have to be devised for the ultrasonic beam to "lock on" to the left ventricular wall reflections.

The Doppler flowmeter has achieved considerable sophistication as a clinical tool in the past few years. Readout varies from a simple audible signal related to pulse velocity to signals combining vessel cross section and velocity to provide actual flow measurements. These techniques cannot yet be applied to aortic flow determination, but the entire field of ultrasonics offers many possibilities for the evolution of the perfect cardiovascular monitor.

The concept of measuring pulse volume on the basis of the electrical properties of blood goes back 40 years, but practical instruments for measuring electric impedance related to movement of electrolyte of the electromagnetic field have only recently been developed. In the instrument developed by Kubicek et al., two electrodes are placed around the neck and two around the abdomen just below the chest. The volume of blood between the electrodes decreases as the stroke volume flows up the carotids and down the aorta. This produces a decrease in electric impedance in the thorax. Since this cyclic change in impedance, compared with total chest impedance, is equivalent to less than one part in a thousand, considerable electronic sophistication is required for its detection. Alternating current is sent through the outer electrodes, and the change in voltage between the inner electrodes measured during cardiac systole indicates the impedance change due to left ventricular ejection. The problem is that venous inflow occurs more or less continuously, so that a net stroke volume during maximum ejection is measured. Great hopes were held for thoracic impedance plethysmography as a relatively inexpensive noninvasive means of monitoring cardiac output and ventricular function. Unfortunately, electrode motion artifacts and lack of correlation with other methods for the estimation of cardiac output in nonsteady states have dampened enthusiasm for this class of instruments.

There is no more consistently accurate method of measuring cardiac output than a properly calibrated electromagnetic flowmeter placed firmly around the ascending aorta. This approach is accepted as the standard against which other cardiac output monitoring equipment is evaluated for accuracy. Electromagnetic flowmeters can be used only for assessing vascular operations.

The nuclear probe (nuclear stethoscope, bios) has been developed as a modification of the equilibrium blood-pool scan (MUGA). This device consists of a collimated single-crystal nuclear probe or camera and a dedicated computer (Fig. 13-7).

The nuclear probe study has several advantages over other nuclear techniques—true portability, decreased cost, superior detector sensitivity and temporal resolution, and a reduced radionuclide dose requirement. There is, however, no imaging to guide the user to areas of interest. Instead, characteristics of the ventricular volume (or time activity) curve along with the length of an indicator bar are used to identify the left ventricle and background positions.

The nuclear probe or stethoscope provides a nonimaging assessment of left ventricular performance with a simple means of quantifying various systolic and diastolic parameters. Its portability and ease of handling add to the attractiveness of serial determinations over long- or short-term intervals. Accepted clinical applications have included arrhythmia analysis, assessment of myocardial infarction, shock, heart failure, and postoperative states, as well as drug-response patterns (e.g., doxorubicin toxicity).

MONITORING OF TISSUE METABOLISM

Under certain conditions, such as hypoxemia or septic shock, a high cardiac output is no guarantee of adequate delivery of oxygen to the cells. Couch and colleagues have succeeded in developing a practical and simple solution to the problem of an early warning system for tissue hypoxia. With an electrometer and right-angle pH electrode, skeletal muscle surface pH is continuously monitored. A 2-cm incision through skin, subcutaneous tissue, and fascia is required for placement of the electrode in gentle contact with the surface of the biceps muscle in adults and the quadriceps in children. Clinical monitoring by this technique has been continued for as long as 8 days.

The rationale for this approach is that with tissue deprivation of oxygen, oxidative phosphorylation ceases, and pyruvate is converted to lactic acid rather than carbon dioxide and water. Diffusion of the hydrogen ions and lactate across the cell membranes into the extracellular fluid is passive and rapid. Extracellular fluid acidosis related to anaerobic glycolysis precedes arterial pH depression because of a number of factors: in low-flow states there is a delay of acid metabolite washout into the peripheral circulation; arterial pH will change only after the hemoglobin-, bicarbonate-, and phosphate-buffering capacity of the blood is exceeded; and metabolism of lactate by the heart and liver tends to reduce the peripheral lactate levels until late in shock.

Skeletal muscle itself offers several advantages for surveillance of overall oxygen transport. Since it can tolerate hypoxia, its blood supply tends to get shut off early in critical states, and it tends to shift readily into anaerobic glycolysis and lactate production because of its high glycogen content. The surface of the muscle rather than the interior is monitored to avoid artifacts due to hematoma formation. Studies in human beings have shown that muscle surface pH is a sensitive indicator of muscle metabolism and as such is valuable as a practical monitoring instrument to alert against hypoxia of more vital tissues. The normal resting biceps pH is 7.38, slightly below arterial pH. When the normal oxygen gradient to the muscle cells is restored after the circulatory crisis is over, pH promptly returns to the normal resting level.

Couch's group has also done redox potential measurements of muscle as an indicator of balance between oxygen delivery and tissue needs. Redox potential of tissue reflects the overall balance of electron transfer, which shifts toward the negative or reduced state with prolonged hypoxia. Although the trends were found to be similar to the surface pH changes, absolute redox potential values were not as reliable indicators as pH changes. Muscle surface pH monitoring provides a good early warning of disaster during and after surgery. The small incision certainly can be justified in high-risk patients or those undergoing formidable operations.

Woldring et al. developed a mass spectrometer as previously described, which accurately records partial pressures of oxygen, carbon dioxide, or other gases, sampled through plastic or rubber membranes mounted on a catheter tip. Using a mass spectrometer, Owens et al. measured intracerebral gas tensions continuously across a heparinized silastic membrane on a perforated cannula. The measurements represent the gas tensions in the extracellular fluid surrounding local tissue injury rather than intact cells. Other problems are related to changes in membrane permeability due to fibrin deposits and protein denaturation.

Bioengineers are looking for noninvasive methods of scanning cellular bioenergetics. Huckabee had defined hypoxia as the "condition which exists when the supply of oxygen to the exterior of living cells is reduced to a rate insufficient for their current metabolic needs, with the result that various cellular oxidation-reduction systems must shift toward more reduced state." Detection of this state by a safe external sensor is the ultimate goal.

A number of attempts in this direction are in progress. One involves the stimulation of intracellular oxygen molecules with modulated soft x-rays. The stimulated emission of oxygen is in the microwave area of the 0.5-cm band and can be detected externally with a suitable waveguide and amplifier system. This approach would offer some degree of spatial discrimination of tissue hypoxia in specific organs. Another experimental method is a cross between Chance's fluorescence-emission technique and thermography. Energy transfers within living cells emit specific wavelengths of electromagnetic radiation according to quantum bioenergetic laws. Energy dissipation associated with inefficient anaerobic metabolism or uncoupling of oxidative phosphorylation should be detectable by suitable instrumentation. Such a system has been developed to detect and identify narrow-band and line spectra associated with abnormal tissue states. These signals in a physiologic situation are superimposed on the broad-band (black-body) radiation of the skin or organ surface along with the far-infrared spectral pattern of cellular water and carbon dioxide. The desired signals are somewhat analogous to the Fraunhofer lines of the solar spectrum due to absorption in the sun's mantle. The approach differs from conventional infrared thermography in that the strategy is to analyze the spectral pattern rather than to determine the energy level within a specified wavelength. A Fourier interferometer, which is about the size of a bread box, is used to scan the patient at the bedside. The recorded interferogram is then transmitted by a time-shared system over telephone lines to a computer for Fourier transform and a signature analysis. Emission power spectral density tracings have been obtained from human limbs as well as other tissues and superficial carcinomas. Cross-correlation techniques have been used to establish significant differences. Alterations in infrared emission spectra reflect changes in tissue metabolism from analysis of the frequencies of radiation corresponding to molecular vibrations and rotations. Although highly experimental, this is a good example of monitoring at the business end of the oxygen transport chain.

Biosensors are an emerging technology that combines advances in biology and electronics to produce devices capable of measuring minute quantities of substances within the body. The term refers to a broad base of devices that will enable the detection, in vivo and in vitro, of a variety of physiologic parameters that were previously either impossible to acquire or could be obtained only with difficulty. Additionally, these devices are likely to provide data in real time, so that biological activity can be continuously monitored—and on a remote basis if so desired. They will also be used for closed-loop drug-administration systems that deliver medication automatically in direct response to body requirements.

Biosensors generally rely on a selective mechanism such as an enzyme or antibody to selectively detect a substance or react with it to determine and quantify its presence. When the chemical or biologic detector is attached to a transducer, the chemical reaction is converted into electronic signals and passed along to a monitor. The electronic signal is proportional to the concentration of a substance within the body.

Biosensors offer the potential not only for detecting and quantifying the presence of various substances within the body but also for regulating the action of implantable devices that could deliver drugs or electrical charges selectively to various sites. Theoretically, in addition to the pacemaker-control function, coronary vasodilators could be delivered through a closed-loop system measuring myocardial oxygen consumption in angina. A barosensor implanted within the vascular system could measure blood pressure, causing release of antihypertensive medication from a reservoir implanted within the body in cases of severe hypertension, thus affording optimal control compared with present methods. Arrhythmias theoretically could be better controlled by pharmacologic means if medication could be immediately released from an internal reservoir at the instant one developed. Individuals known or thought to be at risk of acute sudden death are also likely to benefit from this type of technology.

Bibliography

Basic Monitoring

Baek SM, Brown RS, Shoemaker WC: Early prediction of acute renal failure and recovery. *Ann Surg* 177:253, 1973.

Band JD, Maki DG: Infections caused by arterial catheters used for hemodynamic monitoring. *Am J Med* 67:735, 1979.

Bedford RF: Wrist circumference predicts the risk of radial-arterial occlusion after cannulation. *Anesthesiology* 48:377, 1978.

Bedford RF, Wollman H: Complications of percutaneous radial-artery cannulation: An objective prospective study in man. *Anesthesiology* 38:228, 1973.

Brown RS, Babcock R, et al: Renal function in critically ill post-operative patients: Sequential assessment of creatinine, osmolar and free water clearances. *Crit Care Med* 8: 68, 1980.

Davis FM, Stewart JM: Radial artery cannulation: A prospective study in patients undergoing cardiothoracic surgery. *Br J Anaesth* 5241, 1980.

Dunea G, Freedman P: Renal clearance studies. *JAMA* 205:170, 1968.

Espinel CH: The FeNa test. *JAMA* 236:579, 1976.

Gardner RM, Schwartz R, et al: Percutaneous indwelling radial-artery catheters for monitoring cardiovascular function: Prospective study of the risk of thrombosis and infection. *N Engl J Med* 290:1277, 1974.

Hermreck AS: The pathophysiology of acute renal failure. *Am J Surg* 144:605, 1982.

Hilberman M, Meyers BD, et al: Acute renal failure following cardiac surgery. *J Thorac Cardiovasc Surg* 77:880, 1979.

Lucas CE: The renal response to acute injury and sepsis. *Surg Clin North Am* 56:953, 1976.

Maki DG, Hassemer C: Endemic rate of fluid contamination and related septicemia in arterial pressure monitoring. *Am J Med* 70:733, 1981.

Miller TR, Anderson RJ, et al: Urinary diagnostic indices in acute renal failure. *Ann Intern Med* 89:47, 1978.

Shoemaker WC: Monitoring of critically ill patient, in Shoemaker WC (ed): *Textbook of Critical Care*. Philadelphia, Saunders, 1984, pp 905–120.

Stott RB, Cameron JS, et al: Why the persistently high mortality in acute renal failure? *Lancet* 2:75, 1972.

Vo NM, Savino JA, et al: The automated renal profile. *J Clin Engr* 8:4, Oct–Dec 1983.

ABG and Pulmonary Monitoring

Agarwal NR, Savino JA, et al: The automated metabolic profile. *Crit Care Med* 11:546, 1983.

Askanazi J, Norderstrom J, et al: Nutrition for patients with respiratory failure: Glucose vs. fat. *Anethesiology* 54:373, 1981.

Askanazi J, Rosenbaum SJ, et al: Respiratory changes induced by the large glucose loads of parenteral nutrition. *JAMA* 243:1444, 1980.

Bland R, Shoemaker WC, Czor LSC: Evaluation of the biological importance of various hemodynamic and oxygen transport variables. *Crit Care Med* 7:424, 1979.

Bone RC: Diagnosis of causes for acute respiratory distress by pressure-volume curves. *Chest* 70:740, 1976.

Bone RC: Monitoring respiratory function in the patient with adult respiratory distress syndrome, in Decker BC (ed): *Adult Respiratory Distress Syndrome. Seminars in Respiratory Medicine*. Vol 2, 1981, p 140.

Bone RC: Treatment of respiratory failure due to advanced obstructive lung disease. *Arch Intern Med* 140:1018, 1980.

Danek SI, Lynch JP, et al: The dependence of oxygen uptake on oxygen delivery in the adult respiratory distress syndrome. *Am Rev Respir Dis* 22:387, 1980.

Downs JB, Douglas ME: Assessment of cardiac filling pressure occurring in continuous positive pressure ventilation. *Crit Care Med* 8:285, 1980.

Fox MG, Brady JS, Weintraub LR: Leukocyte larceny: A case of spurious hypoxemia. *Am J Med* 676:742, 1979.

Gilbert F, Keightley JF: The arterial/alveolar oxygen tension ratio: an index of gas exchange applicable to varying inspired concentrations. *Am Rev Respir Dis* 109:142, 1974.

Luterman A, Horowitz JH, et al: Withdrawal from positive end-expiratory pressure. *Surgery* 83:328, 1978.

Newell JC, Shah DM, et al: Pulmonary pressure-volume relationships in traumatized man. *J Surg Res* 26:114, 1979.

Peabody JL, Willis MM, et al: Clinical limitations and advantages of transcutaneous oxygen electrodes. *Acta Anesth Scand* (suppl) 68:76, 1978.

Popovich J, Bone RC, et al: Mass spectrometry. *Respir Ther* 10:50, 1980.

Sahn Sa, Lakshminarayan S: Bedside criteria for discontinuation of mechanical ventilation. *Chest* 63:1002, 1973.

Savino JA, Dawson J, et al: The metabolic cost of breathing in critical surgical patients. *J Trauma* 25:1126, 1985.

Savino JA, Vo N, et al: Monitoring respiratory complications in critically ill patients. *Infect Surg* 2(8):585, August 1983.

Savino JA, Vo NM, et al: Automated respiratory profile. *J Clin Engr* 9(1): Jan–Mch 1984.

Savino JA, Vo NM, et al: Systemic organ assessment using computerized profiles. *Med Instrum* 17(6):433, 1984.

Shimada Y, Yoshiga I, et al: Evaluation of the progress and prognosis of adult respiratory distress syndrome: Simple physiologic measurement. *Chest* 76:180, 1979.

Suwa K, Hedley-White J, Bendixen HH: Circulation and physiological dead space changes on controlled ventilation of dogs. *J Appl Physiol* 231:1855, 1966.

Sweet SJ, Glenney JP, et al: Effect of acute renal failure and respiratory failure in the surgical intensive care unit. *Am J Surg* 141:492, 1981.

Tremper KK, Waxman K, et al: Transcutaneous oxygen monitoring during arrest and CPR. *Crit Care Med* 8:377, 1980.

Tremper KK, Waxman K, Shoemaker WC: Effects of hypoxia and shock on transcutaneous PO$_2$ values in dogs. *Crit Care Med* 7:526, 1979.

Turney SZ, McAslan TC, Cowley RA: The continuous measurement of pulmonary gas exchange and mechanics. *Ann Thorac Surg* 13:229, 1973.

Versmold HT, Linderkamp O, et al: Limits of the tCPO$_2$ monitoring in sick neonates: Relation to blood pressure, blood volume, peripheral blood flow and acid base status. *Acta Anaesth Scand* (suppl) 68:88, 1978.

Wagner PD: Diffusion and chemical reaction in pulmonary gas exchange. *Physiol Rev* 57:257, 1977.

Wagner PD, West JB: Effects of diffusion impairment on O$_2$ and CO$_2$ time courses in pulmonary capillaries. *J Appl Physiol* 33:62, 1972.

Wagner PD, Saltzmann HA, West JB: Measurement of continuous distributions of ventilation-perfusion ratios: Theory. *J Appl Physiol* 36:588, 1974.

West JB, Wagner PD: Pulmonary gas exchange, in West JB (ed): *Bioengineering Aspects of the Lung*. New York, Marcel Dekker, 1977.

Wilson RS: Monitoring the lung: Mechanics and volume. *Anesthesiology* 45:135, 1976.

Zwillich CW, Pierson DJ, et al: Complications of assisted ventilation. *Am J Med* 57:161, 1974.

Cardiovascular Response to Acute Illness

Abraham E, Bland RD, et al: Sequential cardiorespiratory patterns associated with outcome in septic shock. *Chest* 85:65, 1983.

Aubier M, Viires N, et al: Respiratory muscle contribution to lactic acidosis in low cardiac output. *Am Rev Respir Dis* 126:648, 1982.

Braunwald E: Heart failure, in Wintrobe MM, Thorn G, Adams R et al (eds): *Harrison's Principles of Internal Medicine*, 7th ed. New York, McGraw-Hill, 1974, pp 1117–25.

Bursztein S, Taiterman U, et al: Reduced oxygen consumption in catabolic states with mechanical ventilation. *Crit Care Med* 6:162, 1978.

Cain SP: Peripheral oxygen uptake and delivery in health disease. *Clin Chest Med* 4:139, 1983.

Clowes GH, Del Guercio LRM, Braiunsky J: The cardiac output in response to surgical trauma. *Arch Surg* 81:212, 1960.

Connors AF Jr, McCafree DR, Gray BA: Evaluation of right-heart catheterization in the critically ill patient without acute myocardial infarction. *N Engl J Med* 308:263, 1983.

Cryan L, Ledingham IM: Significance of blood lactate in intensive care. *Intensive Crit Care Dig* 5:15, 1986.

Danek SJ, Lyncy JP, et al: The dependence of oxygen uptake on oxygen delivery in the adult respiratory distress syndrome. *Am Rev Respir Dis* 122:387, 1980.

Dawkins KD, Jamieson SW, et al: Long-term results, hemodynamics and complications after combined heart and lung transplantation. *Circulation* 71:919, 1985.

Enger EA: Cellular metabolic response to regional hypotension and complete ischemia in surgery. *Acta Chir Scand* (suppl) 178:481, 1977.

Finch CA, Lenfant C: Oxygen transport in man. *N Engl J Med* 268:407, 1972.

Forrester JS, Diamond G, et al: Filling pressures in the right and left sides of the heart in acute myocardial infarction: A reappraisal of central-venous pressure monitoring. *N Engl J Med* 285:190, 1971.

Greene NM: Lactate, pyruvate and excess lactate in anesthetized man. *Anesthesiology* 22:404, 1961.

Laver MB, Strauss HW, Pohost GM: Right and left ventricular geometry: Adjustments during acute respiratory failure. *Crit Care Med* 7:509, 1979.

Lowenstein E, Teplick R: To (PA) catheterize or not to (PA) catheterize—that is the question (editorial). *Anesthesiology* 53:361, 1980.

MacLean LD, Mulligan WG, et al: Patterns of septic shock in man—a detailed study of 56 patients. *Ann Surg* 166:543, 1967.

Rhodes GR, Newell JC, et al: Increased oxygen consumption accompanying increased oxygen delivery with hypertonic mannitol in adult respiratory distress syndrome. *Surgery* 84:490, 1978.

Robin ED: Of men and mitochondria: Coping with hypoxic dysoxia. *Am Rev Respir Dis* 122:517, 1980.

Schwager O, Howland WS, et al: The effect of ether and halothane on blood levels of glucose, pyruvate, lactate and metabolites of the tricarboxylic acid cycle in normotensive patients during operation. *Anesthesiology* 28:814, 1967.

Shoemaker WC: Cardiorespiratory patterns in complicated and uncomplicated septic shock: Physiologic alterations and their therapeutic implications. *Ann Surg* 174:119, 1971.

Shoemaker WC, Appel P, et al: Pathogenesis of respiratory failure (ARDS) after hemorrhage and trauma: 1. Cardiorespiratory patterns preceding the development of ARDS. *Crit Care Med* 8:504, 1980.

Shoemaker WC, Priten KJ, et al: Hemodynamic patterns after acute anesthetized and unanesthetized trauma. *Arch Surg* 95:492, 1967.

Shoemaker WC, Montgomery Ed, et al: Physiologic patterns in surviving and nonsurviving shock patients. *Surg Gynecol Obstet* 152:633, 1981.

Sibbald WJ: Myocardial function in the critically ill: Factors influencing left and right ventricular performance in patients with sepsis and trauma. *Surg Clin North Am* 65:867, 1985.

Silverman WA: *Retrolental fibroplasia: A Modern Parable*. New York, Grune & Stratton, 1980.

Waxman K, Nolan LS, Shoemaker WC: Sequential perioperative lactate determination. Physiological and clinical implications. *Crit Care Med* 10:96, 1982.

Waxman K, Lazrove S, Shoemaker WC: Physiologic responses to operation in high risk surgical patients. *Surg Gynecol Obstet* 152:633, 1981.

Weil MH, Nishijima H: Cardiac output in bacterial shock. *Am J Med* 64:920, 1978.

Wilmore DW, Aulick LH: Systemic response to injury and the healing wound. *J Parenter Enterol Nutr* 4:147, 1980.

Wilson RF, Thal A, et al: Hemodynamic measurements in septic shock. *Arch Surg* 91:121, 1963.

Cardiovascular Monitoring

Alderman EL, Glantz SA: Acute hemodynamic interventions shift the diastolic pressure-volume curve in man. *Circulation* 54:662, 1976.

Archer G, Cobb LA: Long term pulmonary artery pressure monitoring of mixed venous oxygen saturation in critically ill patients. *Anest Analg* 61:513, 1982.

Baele PL, McMichan JC, et al: Continuous monitoring of mixed venous oxygen saturation in critically ill patients. *Anest Analg* 61:513, 1982.

Birdman H, Haq A, et al: Continuous monitoring of mixed venous oxygen saturation in hemodynamically unstable patients. *Chest* 86:753, 1984.

Civetta JM: Continuous mixed venous saturation: Neither too little nor too much. *Soc Crit Care Med* (panel). May 1985, Chicago.

Civetta JM: Critical illness: The nonsteady state. *Surg Forum* 23:153, 1972.

DeCampo T, Civetta JM: The effect of short-term discontinuation of high-level PEEP in patients with acute respiratory failure. *Crit Care Med* 7:47, 1979.

Elliott CG, Zimmerman GA, Clemmer TP: Complications of pulmonary artery catheterization in the care of critically ill patients: a prospective study. *Chest* 76:647, 1979.

Feliciano DV, Mattox KL, et al: Major complications of percutaneous subclavian vein catheters. *Am J Surg* 138:869, 1979.

Forrester JS, Diamond G, et al: Filling pressures in the right and left sides of the heart in acute myocardial infarction: A reappraisal of central-venous pressure monitoring. *N Engl J Med* 285:190, 1971.

Gore JM, Sloan K: Use of continuous monitoring of mixed venous saturation in the coronary care unit. *Chest* 86:757, 1984.

Hynes JB, Carson SD, et al: Positive end-expiratory pressure shifts left ventricular diastolic pressure-area curves. *J Appl Physiol* 48:670, 1980.

Jamieson WRE, Turnbull KW, et al: Continuous monitoring of mixed venous oxygen saturation in cardiac surgery. *Can J Surg* 25:538, 1982.

Jernigan WR, Gardner WC, et al: Use of the internal jugular vein for placement of central venous catheter. *Surg Gynecol Obstet* 130:520, 1970.

Kazarian KK, Del Guercio LRM: The use of mixed venous blood gas determinations in traumatic shock. *Ann Emerg Med* 9:179, 1980.

Nelson LD: Continuous venous oximetry in surgical patients. *Ann Surg* 203:329, 1986.

Pinilla JC, Ross DF, et al: Study of the incidence of intravascular catheter infection and associated septicemia in critically ill patients. *Crit Care Med* 11:21, 1983.

Puri VK, Carlson RW, et al: Complications of vascular catheterization in the critically ill: A prospective study. *Crit Care Med* 8:495, 1980.

Qvist J, Pontoppidan H, et al: Hemodynamic responses to mechanical ventilation with PEEP: The effect of hypervolemia. *Anesthesiology* 42:54, 1975.

Roy R, Powers SR Jr, et al: Pulmonary wedge catheterization during positive end-expiratory pressure ventilation in the dog. *Anesthesiology* 46:385, 1977.

Shasby DM, Daube IM, et al: Swan Ganz catheter location and left atrial pressure determine the accuracy of the wedge pressure when positive-end-expiratory pressure is used. *Chest* 80:666, 1981.

Swan HJC, Ganz W, et al: Catheterization of the heart in man with use of a flow-directed balloon-tipped catheter. *N Engl J Med* 283:447, 1970.

Todd TRJ, Baile EM, Hogg JC: Pulmonary arterial wedge pressure in hemorrhagic shock. *Am Rev Respir Dis* 118:613, 1978.

Tooker J, Huseby J, Butler J: The effect of Swan-Ganz catheter height on the wedge pressure-left atrial pressure relationship in edema during positive-pressure ventilation. *Am Rev Respir Dis* 117:721, 1978.

Waller JL, Bauman DI, Craver JM: Clinical evaluation of a new fiberoptic catheter oximeter during cardiac surgery. *Anesth Analg* 61:676, 1982.

Watson CB: The PA catheter as an early warning system. *Anesth Rev* 10:34, 1983.

West JB, Dollery CT, Naimark A: Distribution of blood flow in isolated lung: Relation to vascular and alveolar pressures. *J Appl Physiol* 19:713, 1964.

Zapol WM, Snider MT: Pulmonary hypertension in severe acute respiratory failure. *N Engl J Med* 296:476, 1977.

Cardiac-Output Determinations—Invasive Monitoring

Askanazi J, Koenigsberg DI, et al: Echocardiographic estimates of pulmonary artery wedge pressure. *N Engl J Med* 305:1566, 1981.

Civetta JM: Cardiopulmonary calculations: A rapid, simple and inexpensive technique. *Intensive Care Med* 3:209, 1977.

Cohn JD, Engler PE, Del Guercio LRM: The automated physiologic profile. *Crit Care Med* 3:51, 1975.

Del Guercio LRM: Contrast dilution analysis. *Trans NY Acad Sci* 33:387, 1971.

Del Guercio LRM, Cohn JD: Monitoring methods and significance. *Surg Clin North Am* 56:977, 1976.

Ganz W, Swan HJC: Measurement of blood flow by thermal dilution. *Am J Cardiol* 29:241, 1972.

Shabot MM, Shoemaker WC, State D: Rapid bedside computation of cardiorespiratory variables with a programmable calculator. *Crit Care Med* 5:105, 1977.

Shoemaker WC, Chang P, et al: Cardiorespiratory monitoring in postoperative patients: II Quantitative therapeutic indices as guides to therapy. *Crit Care Med* 7:243, 1979.

Siegel JH, Fabian M, et al: Clinical and experimental use of thoracic impendance plethysmography in quantifying myocardial contractility. *Surgery* 67:907, 1970.

Siegel JH, Greenspan M, et al: A bedside computer and physiologic nomograms: Guides to the management of the patient in shock. *Arch Surg* 97:480, 1968.

Weissler AM, Harris WS, Schoenfield CD: Bedside techniques for the evaluation of ventricular function in man. *Am J Cardiol* 23:577, 1969.

Cardiac-Output Determinations—Noninvasive Monitoring

Berger HJ, Davis RA, et al: Beat-to-beat left ventricular performance assessed from the equilibrium cardiac blood pool using a computerized nuclear probe. *Circulation* 63:133, 1981.

Bourguignon MH, Wagner HN Jr: Noninvasive measurement of ventricular pressure throughout systole. *Am J Cardiol* 44:466, 1979.

Hansen RM, Viquerat CE, et al: Poor correlations between pulmonary arterial wedge pressure and left ventricular end-

visible sweating is about 500 to 700 mL daily. The insensible loss from both the skin and the lungs shows a linear relationship to the basal metabolic rate. Water intake has no effect on cutaneous loss in the adult but does increase it in children. In hypothyroidism, the water loss is conspicuously low, whereas in thyrotoxicosis, total insensible perspiration is greatly increased. The stratum corneum acts as the rate-determining layer.

THERMOREGULATION. The skin plays an important role in the regulation of body temperature. Heat is lost through the skin under the processes of radiation, convection, conduction, and evaporation. Sweating is a useful process only when the sweat can evaporate. It is therefore very efficient as a regulatory mechanism in a dry, hot environment, but with increased humidity the efficiency decreases markedly. Humidity begins to be of importance between 30 and 31°C (86 to 88°F) air temperature, at which point the difference between 50 and 100 percent relative humidity decides whether the person will be comfortable or hyperthermic. If heat production is raised or atmospheric temperature is raised, there is a shift of blood flow from the interior to the skin. The converse is also true, and this process is carried out reflexly.

Cold stimuli of a moderate degree result in the production of pallor. After the stimulus has ceased, there is reactive arterial vasodilatation. Cold stimuli of long duration are associated with livid discoloration as a result of paresis in the venous limbs of the capillaries. With extreme stimuli, there may be a reddish discoloration due to dilatation of the arterioles. The condition, however, is not associated with increased blood flow, and skin temperature does not rise. Further cooling causes the skin to become frostbitten. The reduction in temperature is also accompanied by interference with the utilization of oxyhemoglobin. Immersion foot, or "trench foot," occurs when the skin is exposed for long periods of time to cold water. There is vasoconstriction and capillary damage, and if the skin's temperature is returned to normal rapidly, reactive hyperemia and blistering result. Thrombosis may complicate the situation. Exposure to the cold (frostbite or immersion foot) should be treated by immersion of the involved portion of the limb in water at a temperature of 40°C. The role of sympathectomy early in the course of frostbite has been debated.

Heat exhaustion refers to a syndrome characterized by excessive loss of salt and water when people are exposed to high temperatures. A sweat retention syndrome has been recognized among troops in hot, humid climates. The common name "heat stroke" may be applied either to heat exhaustion or to the sweat retention syndrome. In the latter situation, the high humidity prevents the effective cooling of the body by evaporation of sweat. The patients develop exhaustion, headache, palpitation, dizziness, and confusion. Moderate hyperthermia may progress to extreme hyperthermia and death if environmental conditions are unchanged and insufficient salt and water intake persists. Treatment is immediate cooling by evaporation (pouring water on the victim and fanning) or by the application of ice. Simultaneously, intravascular volume replacement with fluids is indicated.

PRESSURE SORES

Pressure on an area of skin for 2 or more hours, particularly in patients with impaired nutritional status, may result in sufficient ischemia to cause a decubitus ulcer. The ulceration usually occurs over bony prominences. Preventive measures include a nutritive diet, correction of anemia, and relief of pressure over the area. Routinely turning the patient and using special mattresses is effective. Surgical therapy is indicated in most patients who are generally suitable for rehabilitation. This requires sharp debridement to excise the ulcer and underlying fascia and necrotic material. The bony prominence frequently requires modification; the aim is to remove the most prominent portion of the bone, thereby increasing the surface area and decreasing the pressure. Enough bone is removed to maximize the surface area of the remaining bone. Following hemostasis, the bony prominence is usually covered with a flap. Recently myocutaneous flaps have gained popularity. The muscular portion may be more effective in treating infected bone. The popularity of myocutaneous flaps compared with skin flaps is due to the lower necrosis rate of the former.

HIDRADENITIS SUPPURATIVA

This is a chronic acneform infection of the cutaneous apocrine glands, subcutaneous tissue, and fascia. It is generally confined to areas in which these glands are found, namely, the axilla, areola of the nipple, groin, perineum, and circumanal and periumbilical regions. The disease was first described by Velpeau in 1839, and clinical manifestations vary with the duration of the lesion. At first, there is a slight subcutaneous induration, and as the lesion enlarges, the process advances to the skin, which becomes inflamed and adherent. Suppuration eventually develops, and cellulitis surrounds the abscess. At this stage, pain is often severe. Incision and drainage at this point result in a few drops of thick, viscous, purulent material. The process may subside after 2 or 3 days, only to recur. In the chronic stage, the patient presents with multiple painful cutaneous nodules that coalesce and are surrounded by fibrous reaction. The pathologic picture is a combination of that seen in acute pyogenic infection and chronic inflammation of the skin, but involvement of the apocrine glands establishes the diagnosis. Culture of the pus yields a variety of saprophytic and pathogenic bacteria with a preponderance of staphylococci and streptococci.

Cures can be achieved early in the course of the disease by improved hygiene and incision and drainage. Mild cases respond to high dosages of tetracyclines. Once the chronic inflammation and pattern of recurrent, acute inflammation is established, curative treatment can be obtained only by operation. Complete excision of the involved area is necessary. In the axilla, advancement flaps combined with adduction of the arm obtain better results than skin grafting. Localized areas in the perineum can also be treated by excision and advancement flap or primary closure. More extensive areas require split-thickness skin grafting.

CYSTS

Epidermal Inclusion Cyst

When the epithelium of the skin is trapped subdermally as a result of trauma or for other reasons, it may continue to grow and desquamate. This creates a cyst lined by epidermal cells and filled with keratin and desquamated cells (Fig. 14-1). The cysts may occur anywhere in the body, but the vast majority of patients who desire removal have cysts on the head and neck. Occasionally cysts on the hand limit the ability to make a fist. If the cyst becomes infected, incision and drainage is indicated. Incision and drainage is temporarily beneficial, but cyst elements usually persist and repeat infection is likely. Both for the noninfected cyst and for those previously infected, cure is effected by complete removal of the cyst.

Sebaceous Cyst

Sebaceous glands are most numerous on the face and in the midline of the trunk, and they are generally associated with hair follicles and a keratinizing epithelium. They produce sebum, an oily material, which serves as a natural dressing for the hair and skin. If the exit of sebum is blocked, the material accumulates and a cyst is formed. True sebaceous cysts are very rare. In 15 years of practice I have removed over 1000 epidermal (or keratinous) cysts, but not a single sebaceous cyst. Sebaceous cysts are often incorrectly diagnosed; the presence of glandular epithelium lining is necessary for the diagnosis.

Dermoid Cyst

This is usually a congenital lesion that does not manifest until early childhood. The primary clinical differentiation between dermoid and epidermal cysts is age of presentation. Dermoid cyst present in the first few years of life and epidermal inclusion cysts appear in early to late adulthood. Cutaneous openings connecting to the cyst are somewhat more common in epidermal than in dermoid cysts. Dermoid cysts generally occur in the midline of the body, the lateral eyebrow (Fig. 14-2A and B), on the scalp over the occiput, on the nose, and in the abdominal and sacral regions. They are considered to be occlusion cysts, taking their origin from an embryonic process. Although it has been suggested that malignant degeneration may occur, no authentic case has been reported. Surgical excision is the treatment of choice. Communication of the dermoid with the central nervous system is extremely rare in any location but more common with those located in the nasal region. For this reason a CT scan should be obtained preoperatively before excision of a nasal dermoid.

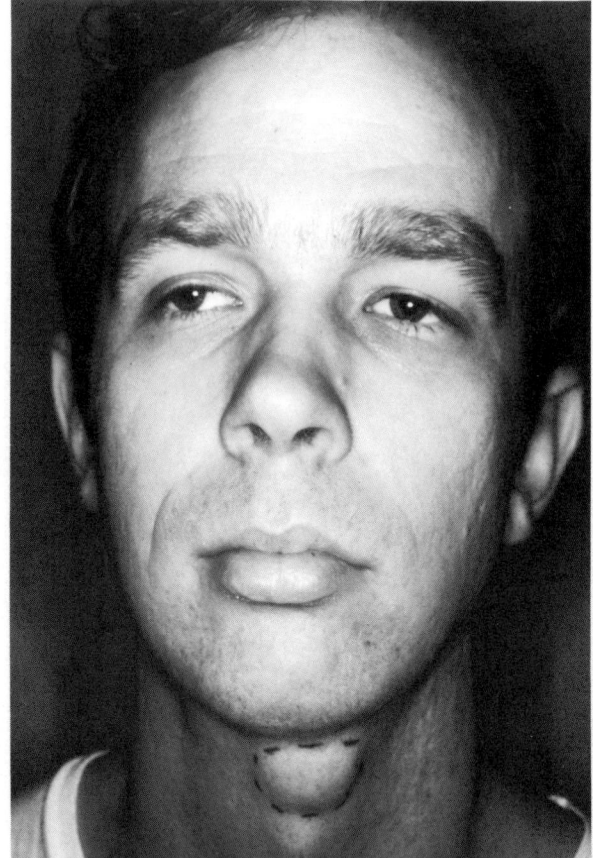

A

B

Fig. 14-1. *A.* Epidermal inclusion cyst. Subepidermal swelling in anterior neck is marked. *B.* Cut cross section of lesion on left and external surface of lesion on right.

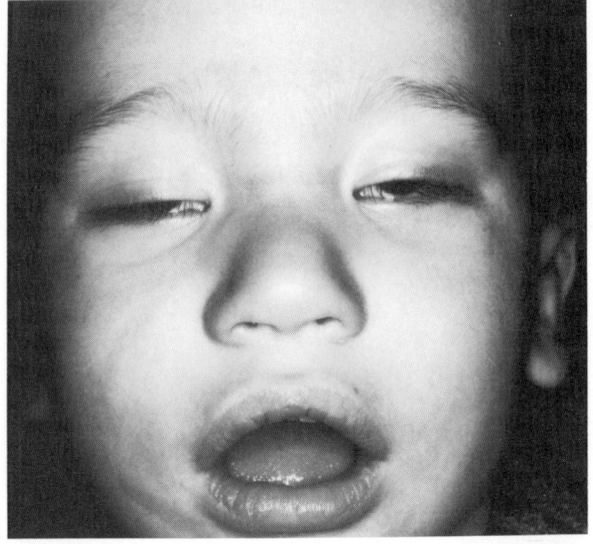

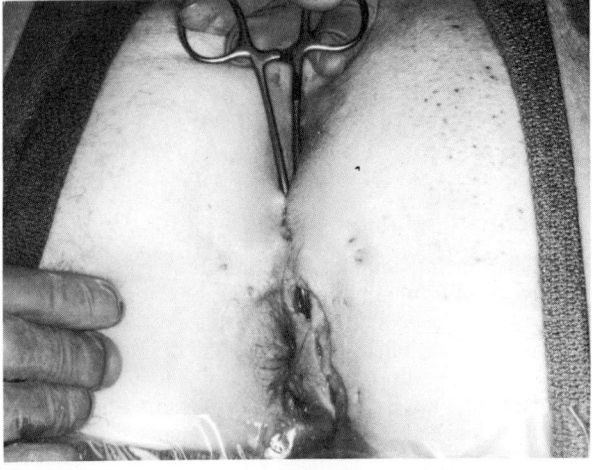

A

A

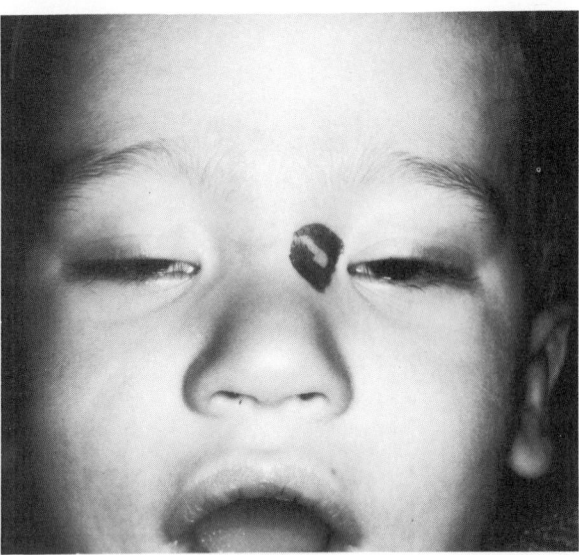

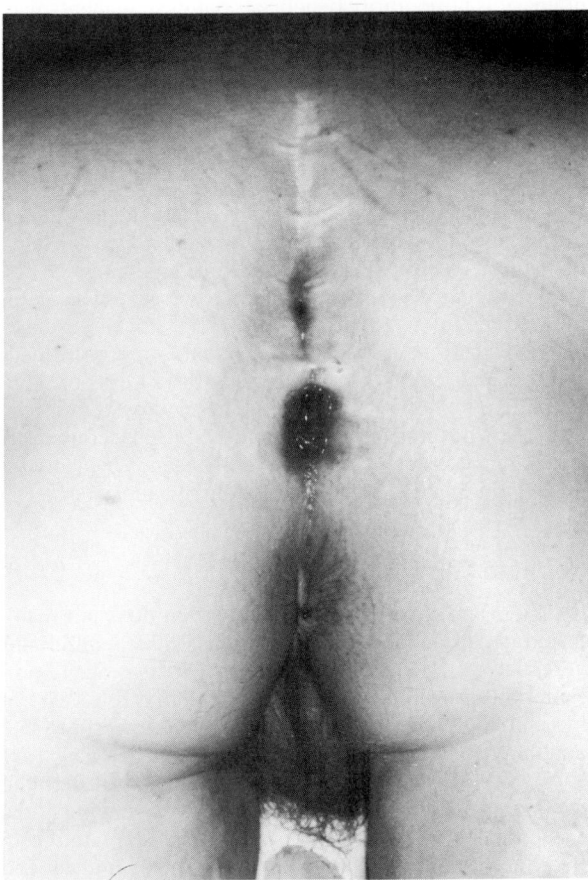

B

Fig. 14-2. *A.* Dermoid cyst. Note slight asymmetry of medial canthal region. *B.* Site of subepidermal mass marked.

Pilonidal Cyst and Sinus

These are common malformations that occur over the sacrococcygeal region. Their origin is associated with the neurenteric canal, and it is thought that their development is related to blockage of a congenital coccygeal sinus that is a vestige of this canal. This is substantiated by evidence that some of the pilonidal cysts and sinuses result from penetration of local skin by growing hairs (Fig. 14-3*A* and *B*). The ingrowth of such hairs sets the stage for cyst formation and repeated infection. The lesions may often be present from birth but are usually not manifest until the late adolescent or early adult years. The disease has been referred to as "jeep-driver's disease," and it is

B

Fig. 14-3. *A.* Typical interconnecting pilonidal disease with a clamp showing site of interconnection. *B.* Pilonidal disease recurrent despite six operations.

thought that the bumpy driving merely aggravates a congenital condition. Histologically, both the cysts and sinuses are lined with the stratified squamous epithelium.

The clinical manifestations vary from a barely perceptible dimple at the superior end of the buttock crease to an obvious sinus tract or cyst at this site. The sinus may chronically drain or become infected. The cyst also gradually increases in size and is susceptible to secondary infection. There have been rare reports of escape of cerebrospinal fluid from the pilonidal sinuses and equally rare instances of meningitis resulting.

TREATMENT. If the cyst is acutely infected, tender, and erythematous, incision and drainage are indicated. Secondary removal of the cyst or sinus is then planned after the infection has subsided. Elective surgical removal must be complete, and methylene blue may be injected as a guide to determine the extent of arborization of the sinus tract. Following excision of the sinus, closure may be accomplished either primarily or by granulation and epithelialization from the wound margins. If there is obvious infection, it is preferable to leave the wound open, unroofing all the tracts and allowing it to heal by secondary intention. In some instances, a very thin split-thickness graft (0.008 to 0.01 in.) may be used to achieve early closure. The thin skin graft permits the desirable contracture of the wound that accompanies the open technique. Primary closure of skin and subcutaneous tissue is usually successful for previously untreated patients. For treatment of recurrent lesions three additional approaches are useful. Simple gluteus muscle advancement and closure in the midline, gluteous myocutaneous flaps, or a z-plasty procedure to move the scar out of the midline are procedures of choice.

Ganglia

Ganglia are areas of mucoid degeneration of retinacular structures. They are tense, subcutaneous cystic masses occurring most commonly over the dorsum of the wrist and over tendon sheaths of the hands and feet (Fig. 14-4). They grow very slowly and are usually associated with only minimal discomfort. The lesions consist of a wall of collagenous tissue that may or may not have synovial cells. The cysts contain thin clear collagenous fluid similar to joint fluid. They have been related to trauma, either accidental or occupational.

Aspiration of the ganglion or deliberate rupture by the physician are temporarily effective but usually associated with about a 75 percent recurrence rate. The recurrence rate after iatrogenic rupture is very low for palmar ganglia or ganglia arising from the digital flexor sheath. For the latter lesions, destruction of the ganglion with a needle is usually curative. Surgical excision after exsanguination and application of a tourniquet to permit precise dissection is curative for the other ganglia. The ganglia that are closely adherent to a tendon sheath are relatively easy to remove, but those that communicate with the synovium of a joint require excision of a portion of the joint capsule to protect against recurrence.

BENIGN TUMORS

Warts

The common wart, or verruca vulgaris, is caused by a variety of viruses and is both contagious and autoinoculable (Fig. 14-5*A* and *B*). Lesions may occur on any part of the body but are most common on the hand and the soles of the feet. They appear as circumscribed intraepidermal tumors that may be elevated or flat. Verruca plantaris (plantar wart) is the most troublesome variety and is located on the soles of the feet in the region of the metatarsal heads or over the os calcis. These warts may become quite tender and painful.

Verruca vulgaris may be treated by a variety of simple methods including freezing with liquid nitrogen, and caustic agents, e.g., 40% salicylic acid plaster. In general, however, electrodesiccation under local anesthesia is the most efficacious treatment. All treatments have been fol-

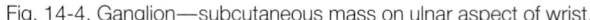

Fig. 14-4. Ganglion—subcutaneous mass on ulnar aspect of wrist.

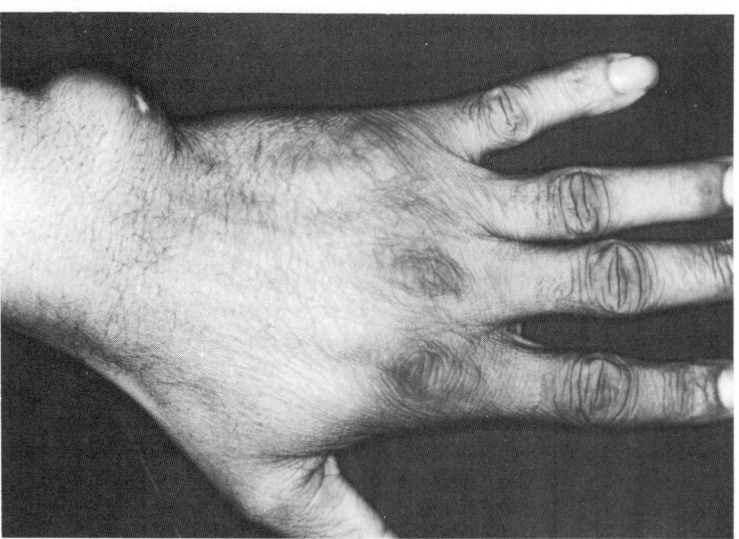

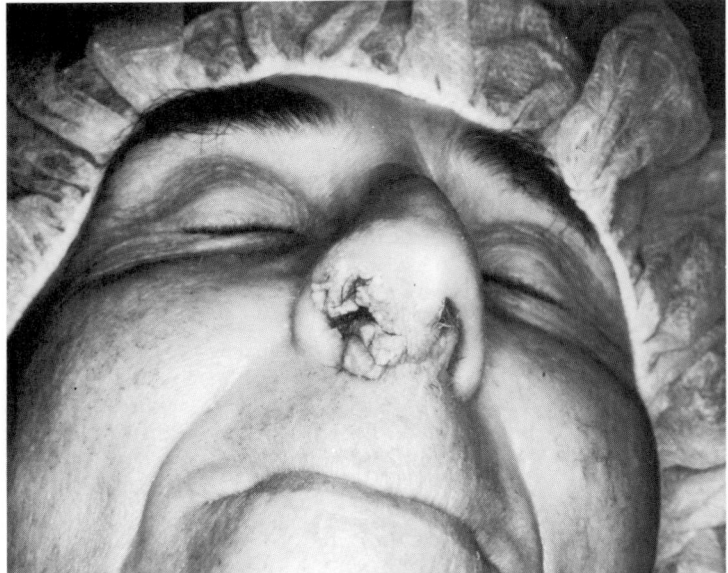

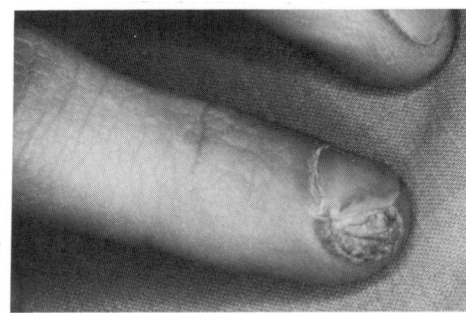

B

A

Fig. 14-5. *A.* Verruca vulgaris. Rough-surfaced lesion on inferior aspect of alar rim and columella. *B.* Recurrent verruca vulgaris on radial aspect of index finger after 10 previous attempts at removal.

lowed by a finite rate of recurrence due to the infectious nature of the lesion. The symptoms of plantar warts may be relieved by using pads or metatarsal bars to remove direct weight bearing from the wart area. Chemotherapy and surgical paring have also been used, and injection of local anesthesia into the base of the wart has achieved some success. Hyfercation has been very effective. It is difficult to evaluate therapy of these lesions, since the clinical course is extremely variable and spontaneous disappearance, formation of daughter warts, and recurrence challenge conclusions.

Keratosis

This represents hypertrophy of the epidermis and is considered a precancerous lesion. Clinical classification includes senile keratosis, arsenical keratosis, and seborrheic keratosis.

Senile keratoses develop most commonly in individuals with fair complexion and characteristically present as multiple lesions in the sixth, seventh, and eighth decades. Lesions proved benign by biopsy may be treated with liquid nitrogen, trichloracetic acid, topical 5-fluorouracil, or electricodesiccation. Lesions suspected of being malignant should be treated by surgical excision.

Seborrheic keratoses (Fig. 14-6) develop in middle-aged or older people as multiple lesions occurring chiefly on the trunk. They appear as thickened areas and are usually brown but may be gray or black. They are often great in number and may be confluent. The darker lesions have been mistaken for melanotic tumors. Histologically, they may be differentiated from senile keratoses and remain benign. Treatment is usually conservative, employing shaving and electrocoagulation.

Fig. 14-6. Seborrheic keratoses: pigmented, greasy lesions that, when solitary, may be mistaken for melanotic tumors.

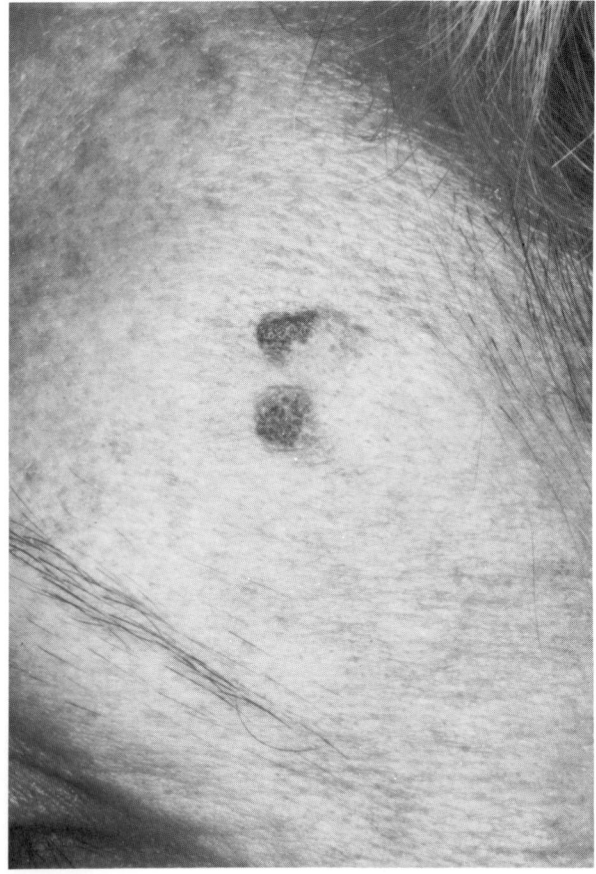

Keloid

The term is derived from the Greek word meaning "crab's claw" and refers to a dense accumulation of fibrous tissue that extends above the surface of the skin and also circumferentially beyond areas that were originally traumatized or incised and sutured. Keloids are usually erythematous in their early stages and hyperpigmented in the later stages (Fig. 14-7). Current research indicates the defect is a failure of collagen breakdown and not an increase in collagen production. Keloids are most common in blacks and progressively less common in Orientals, dark-skinned Caucasians, and light-skinned Caucasians. Keloids may occur anywhere in the body but are frequent in the skin over the shoulder and sternum particularly in young females. Because of their visibility, keloids on the head and neck are frequently presented for treatment. Keloids distal to the knee are rare and those of the palm and soles extremely rare. Recurrence following simple excision is common.

The first line of treatment of keloids or hypertrophic scars is steroid injection. Steroid injection is effective in relieving the burning and itching sensation and may produce actual shrinkage of the lesion. The most definitive treatment is excision combined with steroid injection at the time of operation and postoperatively. Formerly, intralesional excision (leaving a margin of keloid unexcised) was recommended. No data support intralesional excision, however. Admonitions against subcuticular sutures are voiced, but no study has clearly demonstrated them

Fig. 14-7. Keloid of ear originally following small laceration on helical rim. Three previous attempts at removal.

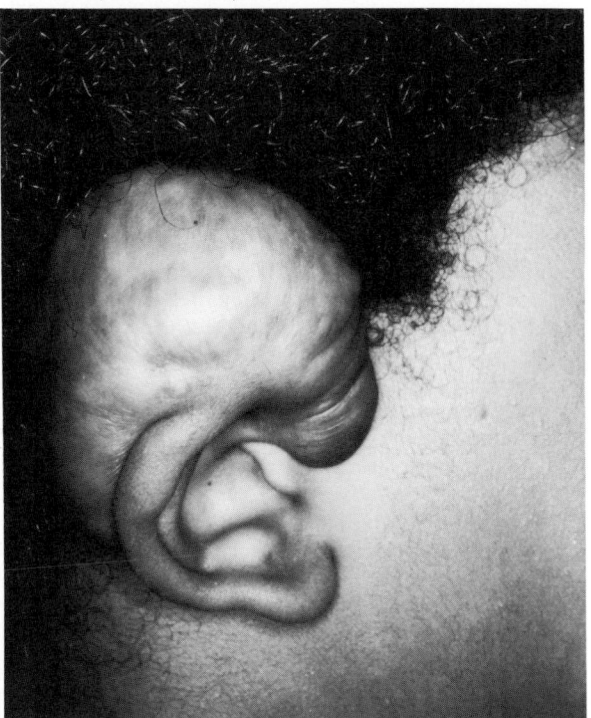

detrimental. If primary closure is not possible, split-thickness skin grafting may be needed. The use of postoperative radiation therapy is controversial. No controlled study has demonstrated benefits from postoperative radiation therapy. Knowledge of the long-term ill effects of radiation has mandated against its use in recent years.

Vascular Tumors

Classically the terminology of vascular tumors has been quite confusing. Different authors have used the same name for different lesions. Recently Mulligan has developed a more rational classification based on the endothelial features of cutaneous vascular tumors. This has allowed division into two major categories based on the rate of endothelial turnover. Hemangiomas are vascular tumors with increased endothelial turnover during their proliferative phase; they may have a normal endothelial turnover during their stable or involutional phase. Vascular malformations are tumors with a normal endothelial cell turnover rate throughout their lifetime.

CAPILLARY (PORT WINE) MALFORMATION

The lesion is made up of closely packed, dilated abnormal capillaries in the subpapillary, dermal, or subdermal region of the skin. Clinically, there is no elevation or contour change but rather a reddish or purplish patch of staining (Fig. 14-8). Growth parallels that of the involved area. If the lesion is small, it may be treated by excision and closure with excellent results. Larger lesions, however, are most difficult to treat, since the entire dermis is involved and excision results in a contour defect and scar. Argone laser treatment is currently accepted as the most useful for larger lesions. Results have ranged from marked to minimal improvement. The degree of improvement seems to increase when there are more vessels located just beneath the skin and the lesion is more nearly purple than pink. Owing to the development of hypertrophic scarring, laser treatment is generally recommended only in patients older than 14 years.

HEMANGIOMA (STRAWBERRY MARK) (Fig. 14-9)

This appears in infancy and undergoes a remarkable change with the growth of the child. The lesion generally enlarges, sometimes quite dramatically, during the first several months to 1 year, subsequent to which spontaneous regression usually occurs. Clinically, immature hemangiomas are raised and irregular, with some bright-red areas. They are compressible and may show superficial areas of opacity suggesting the beginning of regression. Regression takes the form of increasing opacity and whitening of the surface with progressive thickening and flattening. The hemangioma may become ulcerated if it is in an area subjected to trauma, but hemorrhage from these lesions is not common and is generally readily controlled by pressure. Such episodes of ulceration, minor hemorrhage, or superficial infection may actually hasten spontaneous resolution. Treatment in large part consists of

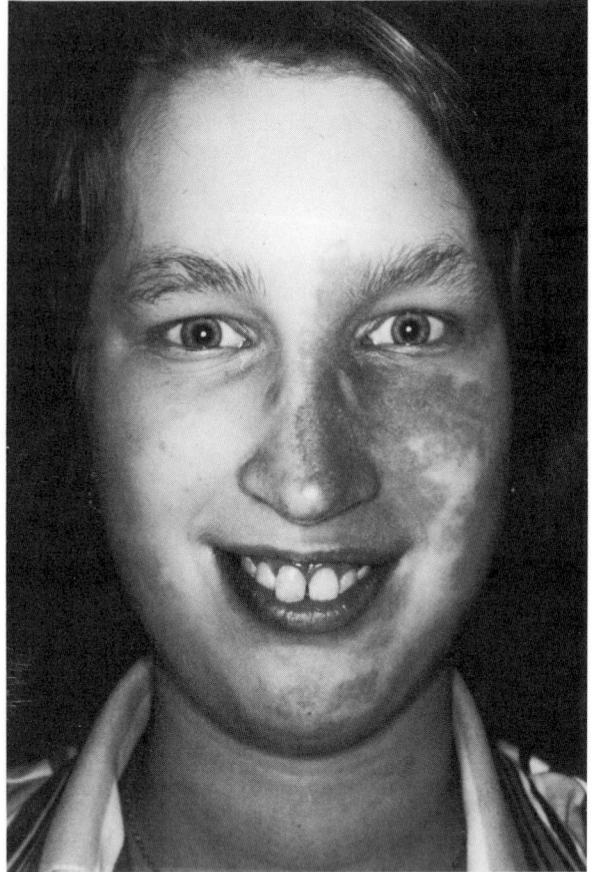

Fig. 14-8. Capillary (port wine) malformation. Note discoloration in forehead, nose, cheek, and upper lid area. Limited almost precisely to the midline.

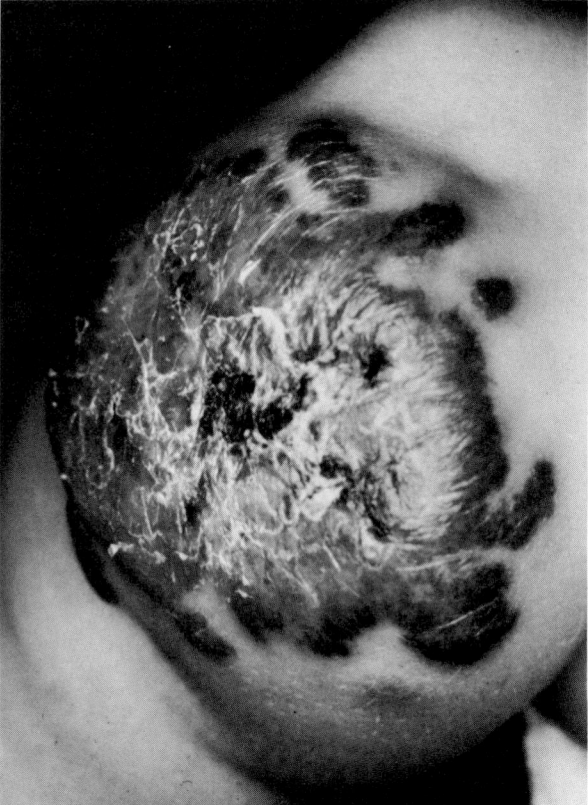

Fig. 14-9. Immature hemangioma (strawberry mark). Note opacification in the center. Lesion is undergoing spontaneous resolution.

reassuring the parents that spontaneous resolution will occur by about age seven in over 90 percent of the lesions. Rapidly growing tumors in childhood that involve the eyes, mouth, or ears may require treatment. These hemangiomas may stop expanding or regress on a high-dose oral prednisone regimen (2 to 3 mg/kg).

ARTERIOVENOUS MALFORMATION

These lesions have been called cavernous hemangiomas by many authors. The lesions are full-sized in proportion to the child at birth and do not undergo changes with rapid growth or spontaneous regression. They consist of mature vessels and may include multiple arteriovenous communications.

Arteriovenous malformations frequently involve deep tissues, such as muscles and even the central nervous system. They may also be combined with lymphatic malformation elements. Treatment of cavernous hemangiomas that invade deep to the subcutaneous tissue is extremely difficult. Wide local excision is the treatment of choice, but involvement of vital structures, particularly in the head and neck, frequently prevents complete excision. An encouraging new therapy involves preoperative embolization of feeding vessels using selective radiography followed by wide local excision. Despite this combination of techniques, incomplete excision is frequent. Incomplete excision almost inevitably leads to a recurrence equaling or exceeding the size of the original.

GLOMUS TUMOR

The glomus tumor is a benign, rare, and exquisitely painful small neoplasm of the skin and subcutaneous tissue occurring usually on the extremities and particularly in the nail beds of the hands and feet (Fig. 14-10). The tumor is derived from the glomic end organ apparatus consisting of arteriovenous anastomoses that function normally to regulate the blood flow in the extremity. The organ contributes to the regulation of local and general body temperature through the dissipation or conservation of heat.

The tumors vary in structure but resemble the normal glomus unit and have often been referred to as *angiomyoneuroma*. The layers of circular muscle of the vessels may be separated from the endothelium by collagenous membrane, or the endothelium may be bordered directly by the so-called glomus epithelioid cells. In some tumors, the blood vessels are so enlarged that they resemble true angiomas. The glomus cells are supplied by nonmyelinated nerve fibers, which accounts for the pain-

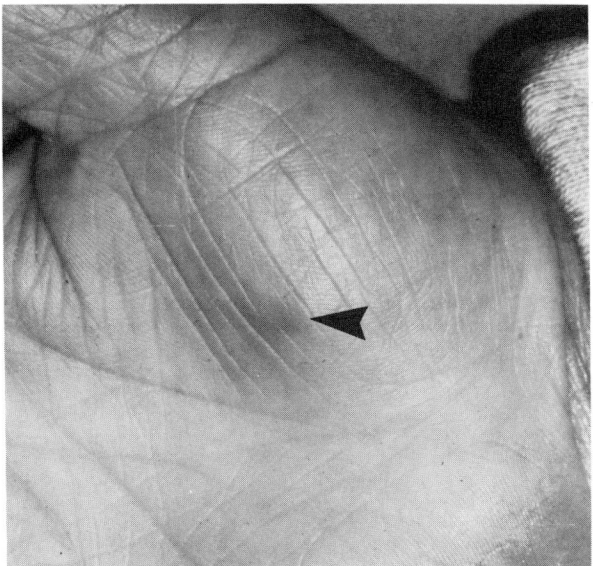

A

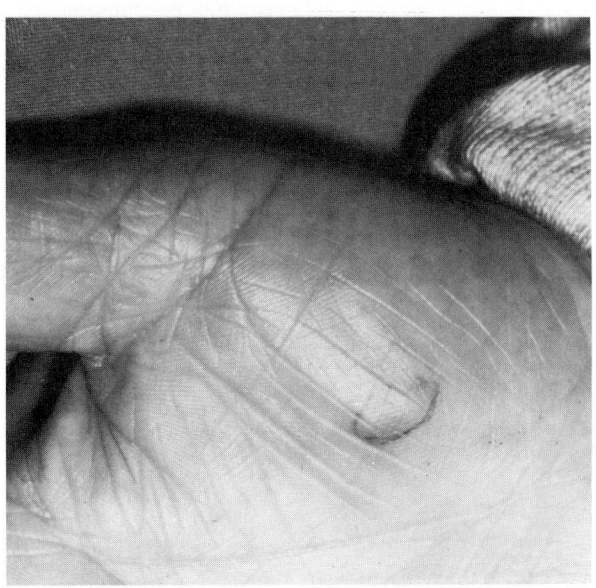

B

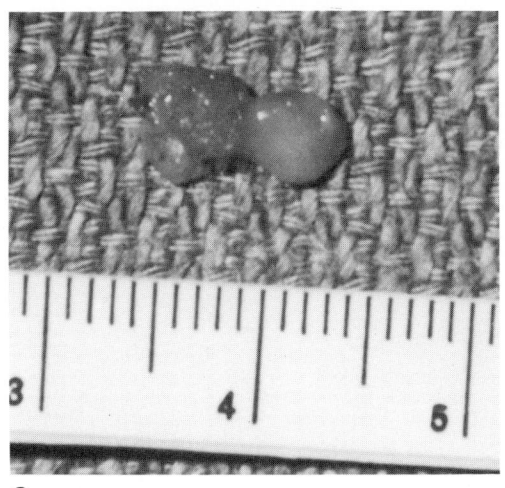

C

Fig. 14-10. *A.* Area glomous tumor—area of discoloration in proximal aspect of thenar eminence. *B.* Area of discoloration outlined. *C.* Cross section and external surface of tumor—scale in centimeters.

ful nature of the lesion. Although the tumor per se is benign, a malignant counterpart exists and is referred to as a *hemangiopericytoma.*

Glomus tumors are usually single, but a familial multicentric form, which is usually painless, occurs. The color varies from deep red to purple or blue, and there is variation in color with changes in temperature. The patients usually present in the fifth decade, but the tumor has been reported at all ages. The pain associated with the lesion is the most prominent symptom and may occur either spontaneously, with pressure, or in association with trauma. The pain, which is described as stabbing, lancinating, and radiating from the tumor, may be intermittent in character or may occur only when the lesion is touched. The glomus tumor is radioresistant. Encapsulated tumors may be

shelled out, but when an obvious capsule is not seen, wide excision is indicated.

LYMPHATIC MALFORMATIONS

Lymphatic malformations are congenital in origin. The most common type is deep and cavernous, consisting of lymph-filled spaces with thin-walled septums and some areas of fibrosis. A superficial variant presents as circumscribed lesions that appear as small blisters and slightly elevated skin patches. When deep lesions are present in the neck, mediastinum, and axilla, they are referred to as *cystic hygroma* (see Chap. 39) (Fig. 14-11). The treatment is surgical excision which, although frequently incomplete, is rarely associated with recurrence. As with arteriovenous malformations, if the lymphatic malformation invades deep to the subcutaneous tissue, complete excision is virtually impossible. Truly massive lymphangiomas may be impossible to cure.

Dermatofibroma

This is actually a subepidermal nodular fibrosis that occurs chiefly on the extremities and may be related to trauma. Most patients, however, are unable to remember any specific episode of trauma. The tumor presents as a small nonpainful nodule, and the overlying epidermis may be pigmented in such a manner that the lesion is often mistaken for malignant melanoma (Fig. 14-12). The treatment is surgical excision.

Fat Tumors

LIPOMA

This is an extremely common subcutaneous lesion composed of fat and at times difficult to distinguish from the normal subcutaneous adipose tissue. Usually, how-

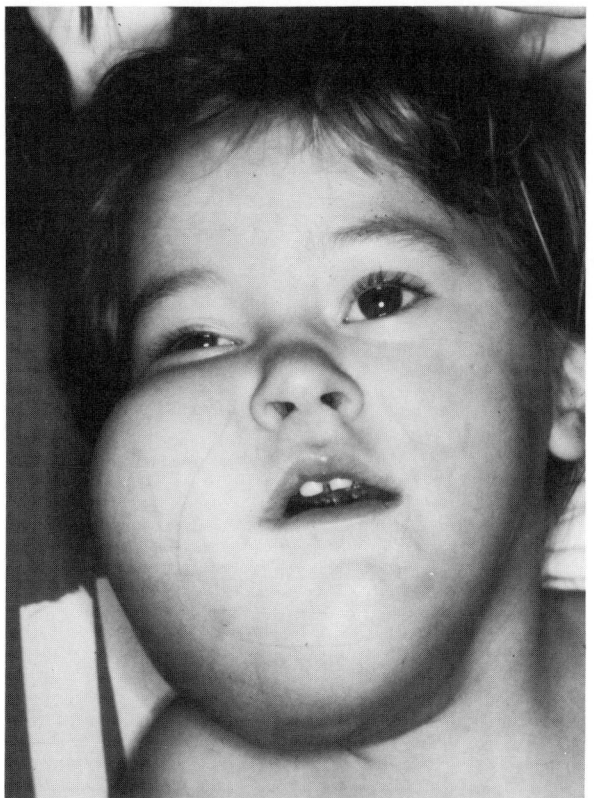

Fig. 14-11. Lymphangioma, diffuse enlargement of inferior one half of right cheek and upper neck.

ever, there is a thin, fibrous capsule, and the lesion can be enucleated from surrounding normal fat. Benign lipomas occur more frequently over the back, between the shoulders, and on the back of the neck, and liposarcomatous transformation is extremely uncommon. Treatment is surgical excision.

Fig. 14-12. Dermatofibroma—darkly pigmented intradermal mass.

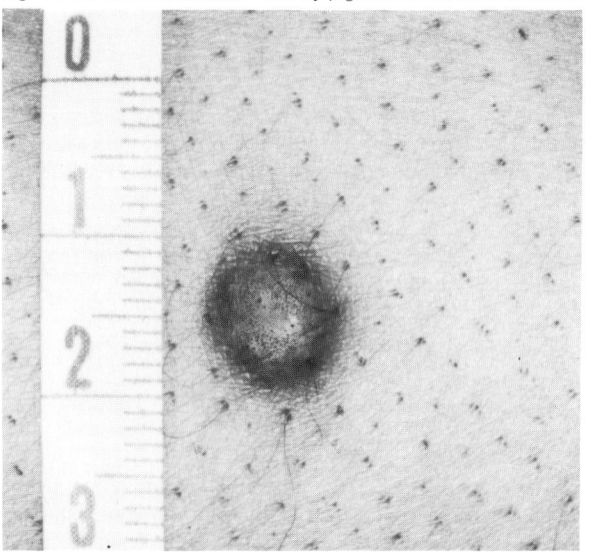

WEBER-CHRISTIAN DISEASE

This is an uncommon inflammatory lesion of the subcutaneous fat characterized by painful reddened areas involving the panniculus. The diagnosis is made by biopsy and is based on the presence of inflammatory cells in the adipose tissue. Many lesions so classified represented facticial dermatitis or skin manifestations of fat necrosis associated with pancreatitis.

Neural Tumors

Neurilemmoma and neurofibroma are the two benign tumors of neural origin. Neurilemmomas arise from the sheath cell of Schwann. Neurofibromas contain the element of peripheral nerves, neurons, Schwann cells, fibroblasts, and perineural cells. Neurilemmomas frequently arise from relatively small nerves and do not produce much pain. Treatment is surgical excision. Neurofibromas may be multiple and may be associated with von Recklinghausen's disease, including café au lait spots and scoliosis. Patients with neurofibromatosis are prone to develop meningiomas, gliomas, and pheochromocytomas; eventual sarcomatous degeneration occurs in approximately 10 percent.

MALIGNANT TUMORS

Carcinoma of the skin occurs predominantly in exposed areas, most frequently in weather-beaten skin. Factors indicted as causes of skin cancer are ultraviolet light, ionizing radiation, chemicals such as tars and pitch, and immunologic and genetic defects. It is generally a low-grade malignant tumor that may metastasize late, in which case the metastasis is usually to regional lymph nodes, so that curability is high compared with that of other tumors.

Basal Cell Carcinoma

This is a localized malignancy that grows slowly, at times taking 1 or more years to double in area. Basal cell carcinoma is more common than the squamous cell tumor, accounting for at least three-fourths of all cases in most clinical series. Lesions may be found over most areas of the body and are waxy, grayish yellow, pink, or translucent, often with telangiectasia below the surface (Fig. 14-13A and B). About 75 percent of basal cell carcinomas are located on the head and neck, 10 percent on the trunk, and 15 percent on the limbs. In some instances, the tumors are darkly pigmented and difficult to distinguish from melanoma (Fig. 14-13B). Basal cell carcinoma may extend deeper subcutaneously than is initially apparent, and extensive ulceration into the deep tissue without marked induration or infiltration has been referred to as rodent ulcer. If the tumor is not treated, it may erode into the deep structures including the skull, orbit, or brain. Less commonly, basal cell carcinoma may appear fungoid and grow large externally.

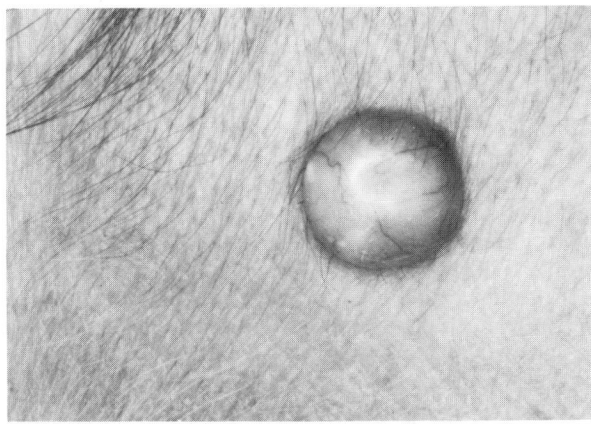

A

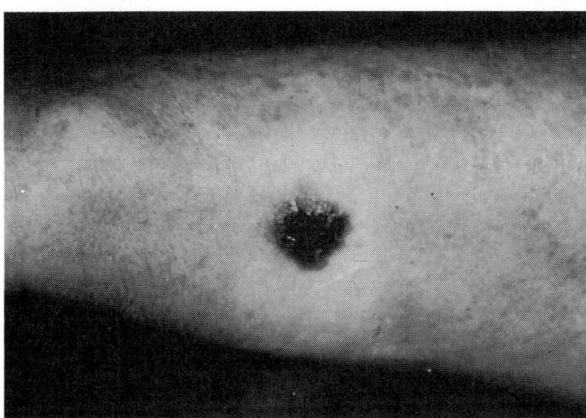

B

Fig. 14-13. *A.* Basal cell carcinoma of cheek—even more typical is a depressed center. *B.* Pigmented basal cell carcinoma. Note characteristics of melanotic tumor.

Squamous Cell Carcinoma

Squamous cell carcinoma presents in a fashion quite similar to basal cell carcinoma. Either may present as a nodule with a translucent surface and telangiectasia. Ulceration may occur in both lesions. Squamous cell carcinoma tends to grow more rapidly, and if an accurate history can be obtained, this may allow differentiation on a clinical basis. Biopsy is necessary for accurate differentiation. Squamous cell carcinoma is both relatively and absolutely less common on the head and neck than is basal cell carcinoma. About 65 percent of squamous cell carcinoma occurs on the head and neck, 30 percent on the limbs, and 5 percent on the trunk (Fig. 14-14).

The primary lesion of the squamous cell carcinoma is occasionally surrounded by satellite nodules, and central ulceration may occur. The degree of induration around the lesion is significant. The center gradually deepens into a crater with an irregular base that is covered by crust. Small pearls may be expressed from the ulcer, and rolled margins surrounding the ulcer contribute to the lesion's resembling a small volcanic crater. Growth may be superficial, or the lesion may burrow into deeper tissue with

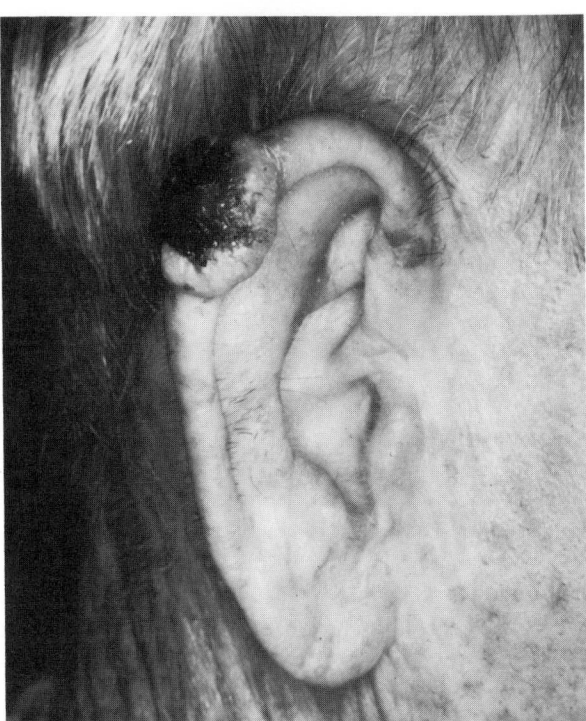

Fig. 14-14. Typical squamous cell carcinoma of ear with raised rolled edges and evidence of recent hemorrhage.

minimal effect on the cutaneous surface. Squamous cell carcinoma is more malignant than the basal cell variety and will metastasize to regional glands more rapidly.

Squamous cell carcinoma is particularly common in the lip at the vermillion border and in the folds of the paranasal area or in the axilla. Lesions occur more frequently in blond individuals with thin, dry skin that is subjected to frequent irritation by rubbing or shaving. Squamous cell carcinoma is also particularly likely to originate in actinic keratosis, atrophonic epidermis, xeroderma pigmentosa, or cutaneous horns, and it develops at the site of postradiation dermatitis and ulcerations in old burn scars (Marjolin's ulcer). The incidence is also higher in people exposed to arsenicals, nitrates, and hydrocarbons.

At times the appearance of *keratoacanthoma* mimics that of both squamous and basal cell carcinoma. Keratoacanthoma presents as a papule with a central keratinous plug and raised rolled edges (Fig. 14-15). Keratoacanthomas are probably derived from hair follicles and are most commonly located on the head and neck. Keratoacanthomas straddle the boundary between benignity and malignancy. The base of a classic-appearing keratoacanthoma may show changes of squamous cell carcinoma. Lacking such changes, local recurrence is possible but not distant metastasis. Although spontaneous resolution will occur in a small percentage of keratoacanthomas, owing to the possibility of malignant changes, surgical excision is the treatment of choice.

Bowen's disease is slowly growing squamous cell carcinoma in situ for which excision is recommended (Fig. 14-16). Adenoacanthoma, which frequently develops on

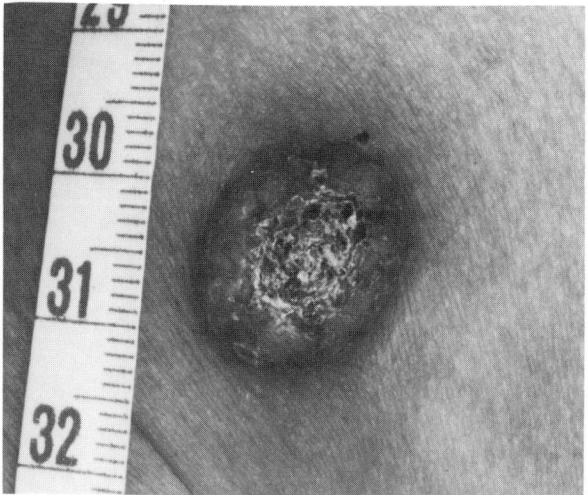

Fig. 14-15. Keratoacanthoma—typical lesion of trunk with keratinous plug surrounded by viable tissue.

the face or ear, is characterized grossly by a verrucous appearance and microscopically by desquamated cells. Local excision only is indicated, since it rarely metastasizes.

Sweat Gland Carcinoma

This rare tumor usually occurs in the sixth and seventh decades of life, but it has been reported in adolescents. Characteristically, a soft tissue mass has been present for

Fig. 14-16. Bowen's disease—erythematous plaque on ventral aspect of penile shaft.

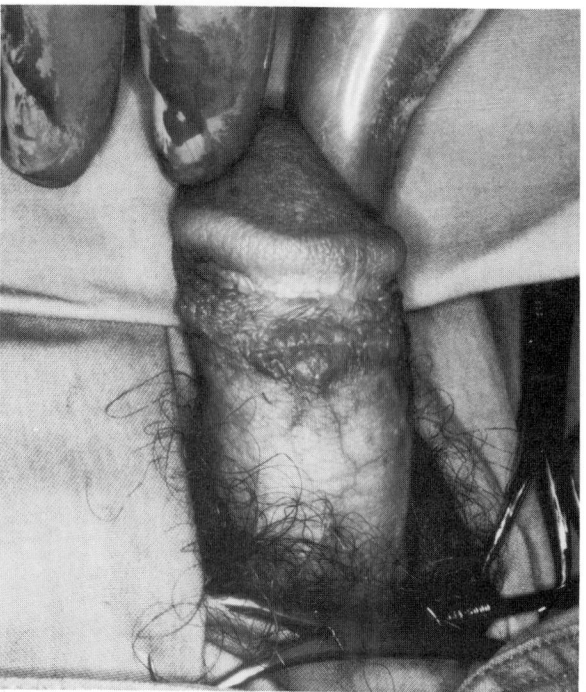

many years. Therapy consists of wide local excision with consideration of lymphadenectomy, since regional lymph nodes are involved in about half the cases. Following treatment, the reported 5-year survival is 38 percent for all patients and 24 percent for those with lymph node involvement.

TREATMENT. Electrodesiccation and Curettage. Electrodesiccation and curettage are applicable for superficial nonrecurrent basal cell carcinomas. Such treatment is not appropriate for squamous and other skin carcinomas. Electrodesiccation and curettage are performed under local anesthesia and consist of treating the surface of the lesion with electrocautery followed by scraping. Traditionally, this sequence is repeated three times at the same sitting. Healing is by secondary intention, and a hypopigmented scar results.

Cryosurgery. After a biopsy to provide diagnosis, cryosurgery, to cure the tumor, is applicable to those lesions treatable by curettage; for palliation it is also applicable to lesions that recur after radiation therapy or curettage. Anesthesia is usually not necessary because the liquid nitrogen freezes the nerve endings. The area treated should extend 2 to 3 mm beyond the margins of the lesion.

Chemosurgery. Mohs originally described a technique of serial excision using zinc chloride paste. His original technique has largely been abandoned and replaced by a fresh-frozen technique. In this technique the lesion is excised under local anesthesia and frozen sections are taken of the entire surface of resection. This is unlike conventional frozen section where only portions of the margin of resection are sampled. For recurrent carcinoma, four to five resections combined with examination of the margin of resection are usually necessary to obtain complete excision. The procedure is repeated until the margins show only healthy tissue. The advantage of this method is the possibility of eradicating small extensions of the central lesion with certainty. The granulation tissue below the lesion heals rapidly and becomes epithelialized. Mohs has achieved 93 percent cures for carcinoma of the skin in all locations on the surface of the body and 87.5 percent cures for carcinoma of the lip. Similar cure rates have been reported following radiation therapy or surgical excision of basal cell and squamous cell carcinoma. The results in *recurrent* basal cell or squamous cell carcinomas reported by Mohs are the best ever reported.

Radiation Therapy. Both basal and squamous cell carcinomas of the skin can be cured by this modality. The site of the lesion may constitute an indication for radiation therapy in that it may provide a better cosmetic result with less effort. It is less appropriate than surgical excision for cancers arising in burn scars or in previously irradiated regions and for tumors invading underlying cartilage or bone.

Surgical Therapy. The advantage of this approach is that the lesion can be completely removed and the extent of the tumor can be assessed. Surgical treatment for carcinoma of the skin should include complete excision of all malignant tissue and a sufficient margin of normal tissue. The acceptable margin of normal tissue to be removed at the margin of the cancer is controversial. Classic recommendations have been 0.5 cm about basal cell carcinomas, and 1 cm about squamous cell carcinomas. More recent evidence indicates that a margin of 3 mm around primary basal cell carcinomas and a margin of 0.5 cm about primary squamous cell carcinomas is sufficient. These margins must extend both laterally and in depth beyond the lesion. For recurrent lesions, the margins of 0.5 cm for basal cell carcinoma and 1 cm for squamous cell carcinoma are indicated. In recurrent lesions, frozen section or permanent section determination of tumor-free margins should precede definitive reconstruction. Primary closure is the treatment of choice. If the dimensions of the lesion physically prevent primary closure or if primary closure distorts normal features (particularly on the head and neck) additional reconstructive technique is useful. Local flaps are the first choice; additional reconstructive technique, at times full-thickness skin grafts, distant flaps, or free flaps may be necessary. Regional lymph-node dissection is performed only for clinical evidence of node involvement.

Treatment of patients with positive margins at the time of resection of basal cell carcinoma is controversial. Only about one-third of patients with positive margins after resection of basal cell carcinoma will ever develop recurrent tumor. If the patient is reliable in returning for follow-up, simple observation may be all that is indicated. If the patient is unreliable, resection of recurrent basal cell carcinoma or any squamous cell carcinoma demands treatment. Repeat surgical excision is usually the best treatment, but at times radiation therapy is indicated.

PROGNOSIS. This is difficult to evaluate, but recurrence rates are very low. A cure rate of about 99 percent for primary basal cell carcinoma should follow either surgical excision, radiation therapy, or electrodesiccation and curettage. About 80 percent of squamous cell carcinomas are cured by surgical excision and a somewhat lower percentage by radiation therapy. About 90 percent of recurrent basal cell carcinoma and 70 percent of recurrent squamous cell carcinoma can be cured by a repeat surgical excision. Mohs has reported about a 95 percent cure rate for recurrent basal cell carcinoma and a 75 percent cure rate for recurrent squamous cell carcinoma.

Other Tumors

Since the dermis has a mesodermal origin, it is logical that sarcomas should develop, and the skin represents the site of origin of 6 percent of all cases of sarcoma. Primary sarcomas vary in degree of malignancy and in histologic characteristics. Excision is associated with an overall incidence of recurrence of 61 percent.

FIBROSARCOMA

This occurs most commonly in women in the buttocks, thigh, and inguinal regions and it occurs particularly frequently in scars. The tumors are usually of relatively low-grade malignancy and are radioresistant. Wide surgical excision is the treatment of choice, but it is followed by a high incidence of recurrence. In one series, 56 percent survived 10 years without recurrence. Distant spread occurs in 25 percent.

HEMANGIOPERICYTOMA

This is a malignant tumor of angioplastic origin and is considered a malignant variant of the glomus tumor. The lesions are extremely malignant, and the prognosis is poor, with only 27 percent surviving 5 years without evidence of disease. Surgical excision has proved unsatisfactory for larger tumors, and x-ray therapy is considered the treatment of choice.

KAPOSI'S SARCOMA

The etiology and pathogenesis of this lesion have not been resolved. It occurs more commonly in men. In Western countries there is a predilection for Jews, Italians, and Prussians. The tumor is prevalent in equatorial Africa. A markedly increased incidence has been noted in homosexuals. Acquired immunodeficiency syndrome (AIDS) is not infrequently associated with Kaposi's sarcoma. Currently the majority of patients with Kaposi's sarcoma also have AIDS. The tumor usually starts in the hands or feet as multiple plaques that are reddish-to-purple and may be flat, ulcerated, or polypoid. The lymph nodes may be involved, and obstruction of the lymph nodes may result in lymphedema.

X-ray may retard the growth of the lesion, but wide surgical excision is also useful. A more extensive operation, such as amputation, is probably not warranted because the skin lesion is merely the manifestation of a systemic disease. Total body radiation followed by bone marrow transplantation is an occasionally successful experimental approach. Patients with florid lesions respond well to actinomycin D (dactinomycin). The prognosis is poor, although some cases have survived for prolonged periods of time. In the terminal stages, the tumor extends to the mucous membranes and portions of the gastrointestinal tract.

OTHER SARCOMAS

A wide variety of other tumors having origin in different cells has been described. Dermatofibrosarcoma protuberans represents one tumor with relatively low-grade malignancy that generally occurs on the trunk. The tumors are radioresistant but respond to surgical excision, and 70 percent have been reported to be free of the disease for at least 5 years. Widespread dissemination is rare, but local recurrence may occur repeatedly.

Lymphangiosarcoma is almost always associated with chronic lymphedema. A review included 186 cases; 162 cases occurred postmastectomy an average of 10 years after operation, with a range of 1 to 26 years. All patients had had radical mastectomy, and the overwhelming majority had received postoperative irradiation. Only 9 percent of the patients survived 5 or more years, and only 2 of 24 patients with nonpostmastectomy lymphangiosarcoma were alive at 5-year follow-up. Amputation gave significantly better results than radiation therapy.

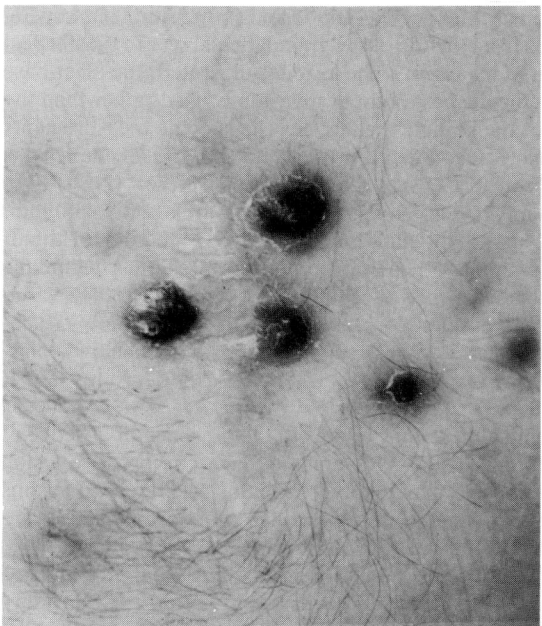

Fig. 14-20. Recurrent satellite nodules. These followed inadequate excision of a malignant melanoma that was thought to be a simple nevus. Note the characteristic deep-black color and emergence of lesions from the subcutaneous tissues to and through the skin.

may occur in the palms, soles, and subungual areas and has a histology similar to the lentigo maligna melanoma. Superficial spreading melanoma is characterized by intradermal spreading that may be present from 1 to 5 years before vertical dermal invasion occurs. It accounts for 60 to 70 percent of all cutaneous melanomas, and has an equal distribution in both sexes. Nodular melanoma, by contrast, has little radial growth, and the size of the lesion is smaller than that of the superficial spreading melanoma. It occurs most commonly on the back, the head, and the neck, and has a predilection for men; it accounts for about 12 percent of all melanomas. Lentigo maligna melanoma constitutes about 10 percent of all cutaneous melanomas, occurs in older age groups, and has the most indolent course. This lesion is twice as common in women. The histologic description of melanoma in the four categories given above has largely been supplanted by Breslow's measurement of tumor thickness. There is some cross correlation, however, and a nodular melanoma and superficial spreading melanoma of equal thickness do have different prognoses. The prognosis of nodular melanoma is significantly worse.

SURGICAL TREATMENT. Surgical excision represents the primary therapeutic modality in the treatment of skin lesions and metastases to regional lymph nodes. Surgical biopsy provides the definitive diagnosis, and permits evaluation of the depth of involvement. Excisional biopsy, with a margin of 2 to 5 mm, is indicated for most pigmented lesions. Incisional biopsy may be required for lesions that are extremely large, and there is no evidence to suggest that this increases the incidence of dissemination.

When all tumor cells are above the basement membrane level and the lesion can be categorized as Clark's Level I excisional biopsy with a very small margin of normal skin is all that is required. The ideal limits of excision of normal tissue about the melanoma have not been defined. Recent evidence indicates that for tumors less than 0.75 mm in thickness, a margin of 2 cm is certainly adequate; data currently being gathered may eventually demonstrate that a 0.5-cm margin is adequate. For lesions 0.76 to 1.5 mm in thickness, a 2-cm margin is probably adequate. For thicker lesions, a 4-cm margin is adequate. The need to remove the underlying fascia has not been resolved. To meet the requirements for wide excision, amputation of a digit is indicated when the lesion is located in the distal part of the finger or toe. When the lesion is located in the proximal half of the digit, disarticulation is performed at the level of the corresponding tarsometatarsal or carpometacarpal joint. The rate of local recurrence for clinical Stage I (Fig. 14-20) malignant melanomas of the limb is approximately 2 percent.

One of the points of contention about the treatment of melanoma relates to the removal of regional lymph nodes. There is no controversy regarding the need to dissect obviously involved nodal areas when other signs of dissemination are not present. There is a question whether lymph-node dissection should be performed in continuity with resection of primary melanoma, particularly in the distal part of the extremities. Some authors have reported an increased incidence of in-transit metastasis after discontinuous lymph-node dissection; other authors have not been able to confirm these findings.

The major problem regarding the surgical treatment of lymph nodes focuses on the uninvolved regional lymph nodes; the problem is whether the surgeon should perform an immediate elective node dissection as soon as the diagnosis of malignant melanoma is made or wait for clinical evidence of node involvement. The chance of having lymph node containing tumor correlates well with tumor thickness. Tumors less than 0.76 mm thick or between 0.77 and 1.5 mm have about a 15 percent association with positive lymph nodes. Lesions between 1.6 and 3.7 mm in thickness have about a 35 percent association with positive lymph nodes. About half the patients with tumors thicker than 3.7 mm have positive lymph nodes. A prospective randomized study by the World Health Organization showed no survival improvement for patients who had undergone elective node dissection. A number of other studies have failed to show any improved survival for prophylactic lymph-node dissection when the melanoma is located on the trunk or limbs. One study has demonstrated a slightly improved survival if prophylactic lymph-node dissection is done for head and neck melanomas. Prophylactic lymph-node dissection does give valuable prognostic information regardless of the location of the melanoma. Veronesi and Cascinelli have suggested that elective regional lymph node dissection be confined to those patients for whom follow-up is a problem. It should also be used when the melanoma originates in the skin covering a lymph node basin, since the postoperative changes following excision of the primary melanoma may

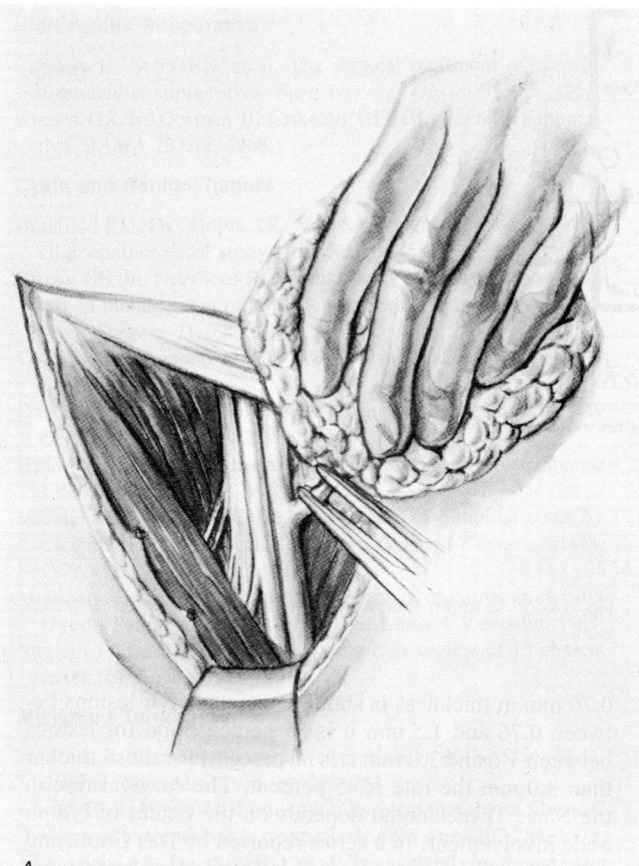

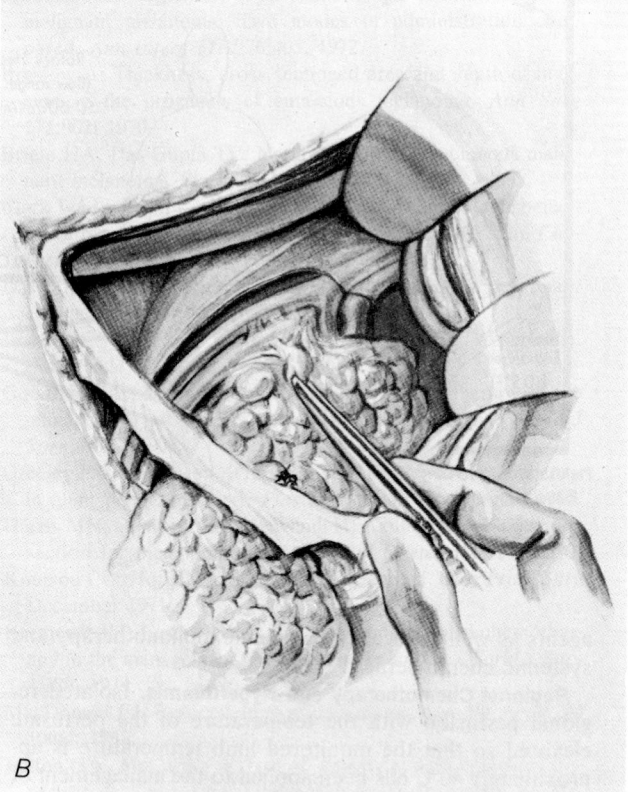

B

A

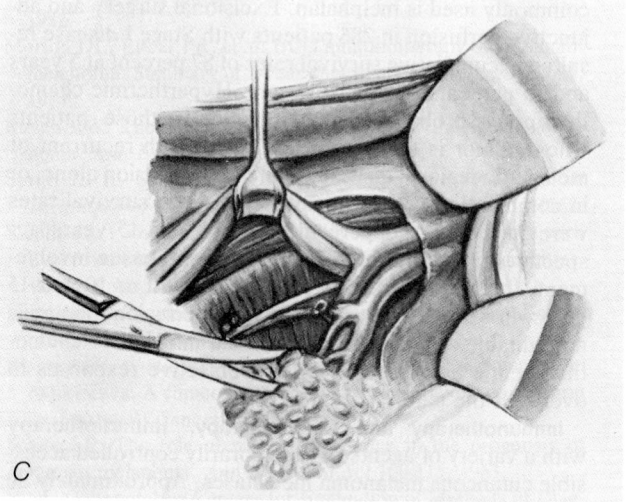

C

Fig. 14-21. Groin dissection. *A.* Dissection of upper thigh and sheath of femoral triangle. *B.* Dissection of inguinal region including excision of endopelvic fascia. Note exposure of iliac vessels. *C.* Dissection of obturator fossa containing medial chain of obturatory lymph nodes. Note that external iliac vein is elevated and obturator nerve is isolated from the fascia.

complicate the clinical evaluation of lymph nodes. They also feel that if the primary melanoma is classified Level V, prophylactic resection of regional lymph nodes seems to increase the chance of cure.

Groin Dissection (Fig. 14-21). Groin dissection is performed preferably through a vertical incision centered over the inguinal lymph nodes. All lymph node bearing tissue in the area of the saphenous vein is removed as well as the subcutaneous tissue extending superiorly on the lower abdominal wall. The saphenous vein is transected. All the fatty tissue about the femoral artery and vein is removed.

Iliac node dissection for melanoma was formerly popular, but recent evidence indicates there is little therapeutic benefit to adding complete iliac node dissection to the groin dissection. Morbidity (lower limb lymphedema) is considerably increased by adding the iliac node dissection. Sampling of the most inferior iliac node is performed by separating the attachment of the transversalis fascia to the inguinal ligament, division of the inferior epigastric

artery and vein, and reflection of the peritoneum. If the most inferior iliac node contains tumor on frozen section, iliac node dissection may be beneficial. The transversalis fascia is reattached to minimize hernia formation. The origin of the sartorius muscle is transected and reflected mediad to cover the femoral artery and vein. The wound is closed over suction catheters.

ADJUNCTIVE TREATMENT. Adjunctive therapy includes regional perfusion with hyperthermic chemotherapeutic

Breast

Benjamin F. Rush, Jr.

The breast is a human being's insignia of membership in the class Mammalia. It is somewhat humbling to reflect that this badge of status had its origin as a modified sweat gland. In the male the breast is, with few exceptions, a dormant structure. In the female, from puberty to death, the breast is subjected to a constant dynamic role of physical changes related to the menstrual cycle, pregnancy, lactation, and the menopause. Associated with this active role are numerous malfunctions and dysfunctions that make diseases of the breast common clinical problems.

EMBRYOLOGY

The human breast makes its first appearance in the sixth week of embryonic development as an ectodermal thickening extending from the axilla to the groin, a distinct linear elevation called the *mammary ridge,* or *milk line.* Lens-shaped thickenings appear along the milk line, presaging the sites of developing breasts. In human beings the caudal two-thirds of the line disappears rapidly,

and the pectoral thickening progresses with the ultimate formation of a breast primordium. Human beings share this pectoral location of the breasts with other primates and with the elephant and sea cow, in contrast to the multiple breasts of the dog and pig and the inguinal location in the cow, goat, and whale.

In the fifth month of embryonic development the human primordial breast develops 15 to 20 solid cords that fan out beneath the skin in the underlying connective tissue. These primary milk ducts branch, and the ends develop club-shaped dilatations. During the seventh or eighth month the ducts hollow to develop lumina. During this same period the point in the skin corresponding to the nipple develops a small depression. At birth the breast is represented by a slight pit pierced by 15 to 20 openings into the primary milk ducts. The areola is a slight thickening in the skin that contains a few glands (of Montgomery). Shortly after birth the nipples become everted, and the areola is distinguished by a slight increase in pigmentation.

A few days after birth, bilateral or unilateral enlargement of the breast occurs in 70 percent of infants. In half the infants the swelling is accompanied by the secretion of a cloudy fluid similar to colostrum, the "witch's milk" of folklore. Histologically, these changes are associated with hypertrophy of the duct system, the appearance of acini, and an increased vascularity of the stroma. These alternatives are considered an indirect effect of the high level of maternal estrogens in the infant's circulating blood. Following birth the falling estrogen level stimulates the hypophysis to produce prolactin, resulting in the mammary changes. These changes occur equally in male and female infants and regress spontaneously by the second or third week of life. Attempts to strip the breasts of their milk, as advocated by some superstitions, provoke the breasts to remain in the secretory state. Hyperplasia of the infant breast persisting over many months with persistent secretions has resulted from such manipulations.

CLINICAL CORRELATIONS. A number of developmental errors of the breast are of clinical importance. Most often observed is the persistence of one or more of the additional nipples in the milk line. These are commonly mis-

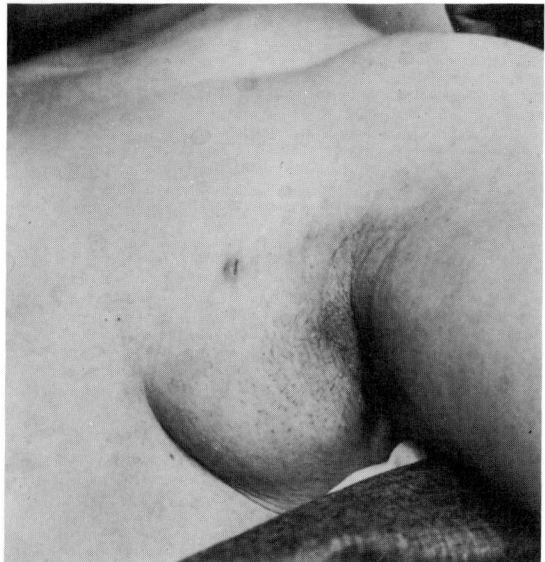

Fig. 15-1. Supernumerary breast.

taken for moles. A rare anomaly is the occurrence of extramammary breast tissue, usually seen in the axilla or over the upper abdomen (Fig. 15-1), often not appearing until the tissue is stimulated by pregnancy and lactation. Excision of these supernumerary structures is the treatment of choice. Absence of one or both nipples or of one or both breasts occurs, though rarely. While these conditions are serious cosmetic and functional defects, a more important functional deficiency is the often associated absence of the underlying pectoralis muscles and chest wall.

Occasionally the nipple fails to evert following birth and remains retracted or inverted throughout life. This is a serious functional problem when the patient attempts to nurse a child.

In some infants the collecting ducts fail to open onto the apex of the nipple, opening onto the areola instead. In a few instances collecting ducts are observed to empty onto the skin of the breast, failing entirely to traverse the nipple. These nippleless collecting ducts recapitulate the normal anatomy of the nippleless breast of the duckbill platypus.

ANATOMY AND DEVELOPMENT

Except for the neonatal period of hypertrophy and a period of slight hypertrophy occurring at puberty, the male breast undergoes little change throughout life. The female breast shows little change through infancy and childhood, but in the prepubertal period and throughout the remainder of life the breasts undergo numerous gross and microscopic changes (Fig. 15-2).

ADOLESCENCE. During the prepubertal period (from eleven to fifteen years) growth of the breast begins with the development of the prepubertal ''bud.'' The areola becomes elevated and forms with the nipple a small coni-

cal protuberance. Histologically, the rudimentary primary ducts begin a rapid process of elongation and terminal branching, pushing down through the subcutaneous tissue toward the pectoral fascia and carrying with them sheaths of periductal connective tissue. A firm plaque of fibrous breast tissue forms as the lobes of the breasts develop, crowding out the subcutaneous fat. Radiographs of the breast at this period show a featureless, fibrous mass without trabeculae. Lobules do not form, however, until ovulation begins. Following ovulation at age fourteen to fifteen the breasts mature into their normal nulliparous form.

THE YOUNG ADULT. Anatomic Limits. The breast is suspended from the anterior chest wall, extending from the second to the sixth rib. The medial boundary is at the lateral border of the sternum, and the lateral border stretches to the anterior axillary line (Fig. 15-3).

Areola and Nipple. The areola in the young female is convex and lens-shaped, surmounted at its center by the nipple. The areola gains a slight amount of pigmentation during adolescence, and although its surface is hairless, a few hairs may appear at the skin of the periphery. Both

Fig. 15-2. Gross and microscopic appearance of breast at different stages of development. Central pictures show three-dimensional projection of microscopic structure. *A.* Adolescence. *B.* Pregnancy. *C.* Lactation. *D.* Postmenopausal period.

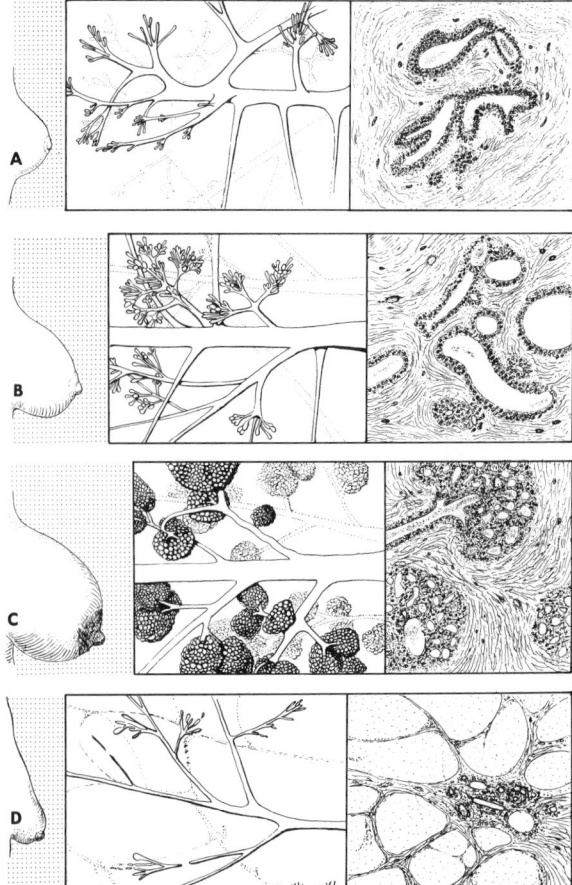

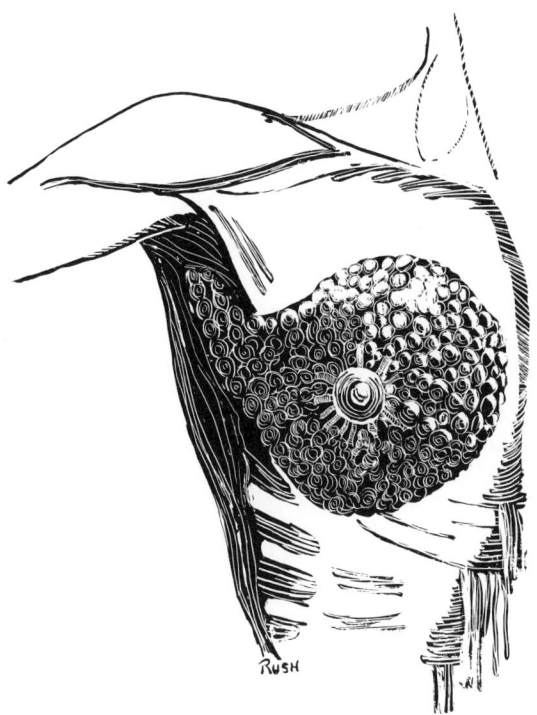

Fig. 15-3. Normal distribution of mammary tissue of adult female breast. Note long tail of Spence extending into axilla.

the subareolar area and the nipple contain much smooth muscle. The fibers of the areola are arranged in concentric rings as well as radially and are inserted into the base of the dermis. They function to contract the areola and to compress the base of the nipple. The bulk of the nipple is made up of smooth muscle fibers arranged both circularly and longitudinally. The nipple is made erect, smaller, and firmer by contraction of these fibers, and this involuntary action serves to aid in emptying the intrapapillary ducts. This response is evoked by sucking or by tactile stimuli. Sir Astley Cooper, a pioneer in describing the anatomy and diseases of the breast, first pointed out that the nipple lies to the lateral side of the center line of the breast and that its axis points upward and outward. The teleologic assumption is that this arrangement is for the convenience of the suckling child.

Glandular Tissue. The functional portion of the breast is a modified cutaneous gland, an appendage of the skin. It is enclosed between the superficial and deep layers of the superficial fascia. The glandular portion of the breast spreads out widely as a layer over the chest wall beneath the integument. It is roughly circular in outline except at the upper outer quadrant, where the axillary tail of Spence extends toward the axilla (Fig. 15-3). The tip of the axillary tail intrudes through an opening in the deep fascia of the axilla, Langer's foramen, to lie well up within the axilla. Neoplasms or deformities in this tail are sometimes mistaken for enlarged axillary nodes.

Portions of the fibrous tissue of the breast parenchyma extend from the surface of the glandular breast anteriorly to intermingle with the superficial layer of the superficial

fascia. Similar processes arise from the deep surface of the gland to cross the retromammary space and fuse with the pectoral fascia. The anterior ligaments were described by Cooper, who noted, "The breast is slung upon the fore part of the chest, for [the ligaments] form a movable but very firm connection with the skin so that the breast has sufficient motion."

Blood Supply and Venous Drainage. Three major arteries generously supply the breast with blood. The perforating branches of the internal mammary artery pass through the first, second, third, and fourth intercostal spaces just lateral to the sternum to penetrate and pass through the origin of the pectoralis major muscle and enter the medial edge of the breast, supplying more than 50 percent of the blood to this organ. The lateral thoracic artery arises from the axillary artery and courses down along the lateral border of the pectoralis minor muscle. Its external mammary branches provide the second largest source of blood to the breast. The third artery of importance is the pectoral branch of the acromiothoracic artery, also a branch of the axillary artery. The pectoral artery is given off by the acromiothoracic at the medial edge of the pectoralis minor muscle. In its course between the pectoralis major and minor muscles, the pectoralis artery gives off branches to the posterior surface of the breast. The superior branch of the axillary artery, the lateral perforating branches of the intercostal arteries, and branches of the subscapular artery also contribute minor amounts to the blood supply.

The mammary glands have a rich, anastomosing network of superficial subcutaneous veins. These veins become markedly dilated during pregnancy and may sometimes become quite prominent over an area of underlying neoplasm. The majority of the superficial veins drain to the internal mammary vein. In some individuals these veins drain into the superficial veins of the lower neck.

The deep veins of the mammary gland drain along routes roughly corresponding to the arterial blood supply. Thus one major route is through the anterior intercostal perforating veins to the internal mammary veins. Another is by way of multiple branches to the axillary vein. A third route is by way of posterior branches anastomosing with the intercostal veins. This last route has special significance, since the intercostal veins communicate with the vertebral veins. This anastomosis with the vertebral veins is offered by Batson as the explanation for the often capricious metastasis of mammary cancer to the vertebral bodies or even the sacrum or pelvis without the presence of metastatic deposits in the lung. He holds that the wide variation in pressure within the thoracic cavity induced by straining or coughing may change the flow patterns within the valveless anastomosing veins so that blood from the breast draining through the lateral perforators to the intercostal vessels is forced down along the vertebral plexus.

The Lymphatics. A generous lymphatic plexus drains the skin and glandular tissues of the breast (Fig. 15-4). The lymphatic vessels empty into two main depots represented by the axillary and the internal mammary lymph nodes. There are an average of 53 lymph nodes in the

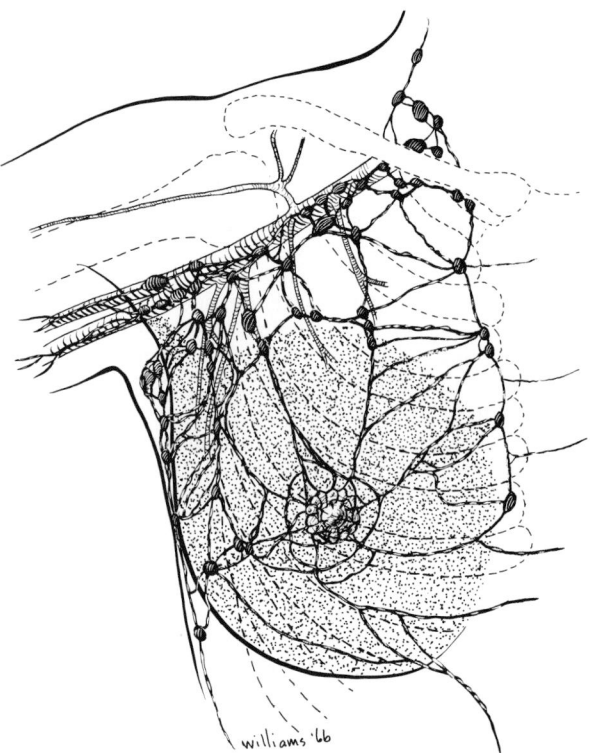

Fig. 15-4. Lymphatic drainage of breast. Nipple drains both laterally and medially. Medial side of breast drains to small internal mammary lymph nodes.

Histology of the Resting Mammary Gland. Each lobe of the mammary gland is an independent compound alveolar gland. The mammary gland is a conglomeration of a variable number of such independent glands, each with its own excretory duct that has its separate opening on the surface of the nipple. The excretory ducts measure from 0.4 to 0.7 mm in diameter at the nipple surface and run perpendicularly through the nipple to turn and radiate out toward the periphery of the breast. Beneath the areola they dilate into a short fusiform area called the *milk sinus*. Beyond the milk sinus the excretory ducts begin to subdivide into smaller and smaller branches forming the lobules of the lobe. Within the lobules the ducts subdivide further, forming terminal, elongated tubes, the alveolar ducts, which are covered by round evaginations, the alveolae. Lobules are peripheral and scanty in the nulliparous breast (Fig. 15-2A).

There is mild controversy as to whether alveolae are present in the resting mammary gland. Some claim that the resting gland is entirely a tubular structure and becomes tuboalveolar only during pregnancy. The majority opinion is that a few alveolae are scattered through the lobules in the resting state.

The walls of the alveolae and the alveolar ducts consist of a prominent basement membrane surrounding a layer of myoepithelial cells, which in turn lie beneath a layer of low columnar glandular cells. The myoepithelial layer is thin and difficult to identify in the acini and the alveolar ducts but becomes more prominent in the more major lobular ducts. These cells take a spiral course about the larger ducts and probably play a role in propelling milk from the acini to the nipple during lactation.

The collecting ducts are lined with a double layer of cuboidal to columnar epithelium until the milk sinus is reached. Here the lining changes to squamous epithelium. This continues through the milk sinus to the surface of the nipple.

Each lobule is surrounded by a coating of dense, firm, interlobular connective tissue, which is an intimate part of the breast parenchyma. The lobules are separated by a looser coating of less dense fibrous tissue, the interlobular connective tissue. This layer represents the supporting stroma of the breast. These layers are easily recognized histologically, but grossly the various lobules are intimately and firmly bound together and cannot be dissected apart.

Cyclic Changes of the Breast. Beginning about the eighth day of the menstrual cycle the female breast gradually increases in size, the volume often increasing by 50 percent by the immediate premenstrual period. At this point the breast is tense and may be somewhat tender. Part of the increase in size is due to interlobular edema and increasing congestion of the vasculature. Ingleby and Gershon-Cohen state that there is also a proliferation of the parenchyma, with the appearance of new lobules. These lobules then regress and fibrose during menstruation. Congestion and edema subside, and the breast again reaches its smallest size on about the eighth day after the onset of menstruation.

axillary fossa, arranged along the course of the arteries and veins. Lymph from the lower outer quadrant of the breast drains to the lateral and inferior axillary nodes, while lymph from the areola, the upper outer quadrant of the breast, and the axillary tail drains to the medial superior axillary nodes. Within the axilla, lymph passes from the lateral inferior to the medial superior nodes at the apex of the axilla. Lymph then courses through lymphatic channels under the clavicle to the supraclavicular lymph nodes and by major lymphatic trunks to the junction of the subclavian and jugular veins. On the right, lymph enters the blood directly through these lymphatic trunks as they join the veins. On the left these trunks may first join with the thoracic duct, which shortly communicates with the venous system.

The internal mammary lymph nodes are much fewer in number than the axillary nodes, averaging but three or four nodes on each side lying along the internal mammary vessels, usually in the first, second, and third interspaces. Despite the scarcity and tiny size of these lymph nodes, most of the lymph from the upper and lower inner quadrants of the breast drains by this channel. Lymph from the nipple and areola may drain to both the internal mammary and the axillary nodes. The internal mammary lymphatic trunks eventually empty into the great veins of the neck, usually by way of the thoracic duct or of the right lymphatic duct.

PREGNANCY AND LACTATION. Implantation of the ovum initiates a profound change in the gross and histologic structures of the breast. Grossly there is a pronounced enlargement of the breast, progressing throughout pregnancy. The normal size may be increased as much as two or three times. The nipple and areola become more prominent and more deeply pigmented. The openings of Montgomery's glands on the areola become prominent and are called *Montgomery's tubercles.* Pigmentation may spread beyond the areola onto the skin, forming a "secondary areola." The veins are engorged, and striae are frequently visible in the skin.

Histologically, the epithelium of the lobular ducts and alveolar ducts proliferates, and new ducts covered with multiple alveolar outpouchings are generated. The total number of lobules increases greatly. By the end of the sixth month the glandular cells of the acini produce small amounts of secretion, colostrum, which increases toward the end of pregnancy (Fig. 15-2C).

Two or three days after delivery, globules appear in the supranuclear cytoplasm of the acinar cells. These push toward the cell lumen, increasing in size. The cell becomes tall and more columnar. Finally the globule is extruded into the lumen, and the cell shrinks to a cuboidal form, to begin the process again. The acini become distended with milk, which is propelled to the nipple during nursing. This process continues as long as suckling continues. When lactation ends, the extralobular tissue involutes, leaving small areas of fibrosis, and the breast gradually returns to the resting state. It never returns to the nulliparous form, however, but has the contour of maturity. The areola recedes into the breast tissue, with only the nipple projecting. Some of the darker pigmentation of the nipple and areola and residual skin striae persist.

MENOPAUSAL CHANGES. Following menopause the mammary gland gradually involutes (Fig. 15-2D). This change is slow and progressive, with gradual disappearance of lobules. Senile involution does not lead to complete extinction of mammary tissue; some lobules always remain, but they are scattered and small. In many areas only the larger lobular and collecting ducts may be found. The parenchyma and stromal fibrous tissue gradually blend together into a homogeneous mass, and the original lobular structure is almost completely lost. As the glandular tissues recede, there is a gradual invasion of fat, which aids in maintaining the breast outline, although in very thin women the breasts may become quite flabby as glandular tissue is lost.

CLINICAL CORRELATION. Both breasts of the adolescent girl usually develop at the same pace. Occasionally development is out of phase, and one breast will develop much more rapidly than the other, leading to distressing asymmetry (Fig. 15-5). The difference in size is usually repaired with time but occasionally persists. Patients complaining of asymmetric breasts during the adolescent period are advised to wait until maturation is complete. If asymmetry persists, a plastic surgical procedure may be required to adjust the difference.

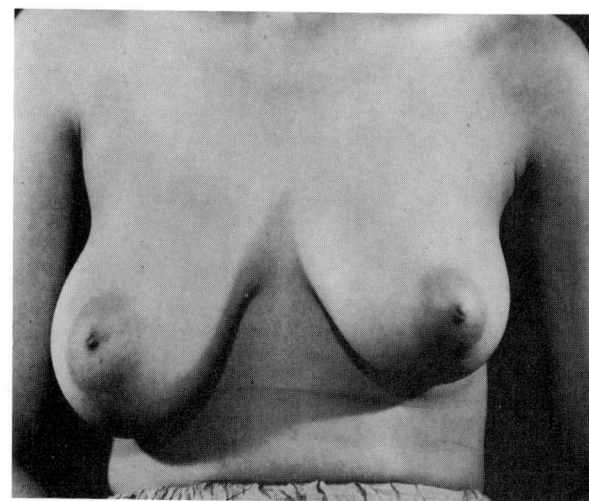
Fig. 15-5. Asymmetric breasts.

A slight swelling of the breasts is often seen in adolescent boys. This is called *gynecomastia* and is a physiologic response to the change in the hormonal milieu in the pubertal male (Fig. 15-6). This slight hypertrophy normally subsides spontaneously but occasionally persists, either unilaterally or bilaterally. Persisting gynecomastia in young manhood requires an evaluation to exclude the possibility of abnormal endocrine secretion. If no abnormalities are found, the small button of hypertrophied breast tissue may be removed surgically to repair an embarrassing cosmetic defect in a young man.

Occasionally the growth of the female breast at puberty fails to cease and the breasts become huge—so-called virginal hypertrophy (Fig. 15-7). Breasts weighing 40 to 50 lb and descending to the level of the genitalia are described.

Fig. 15-6. Gynecomastia.
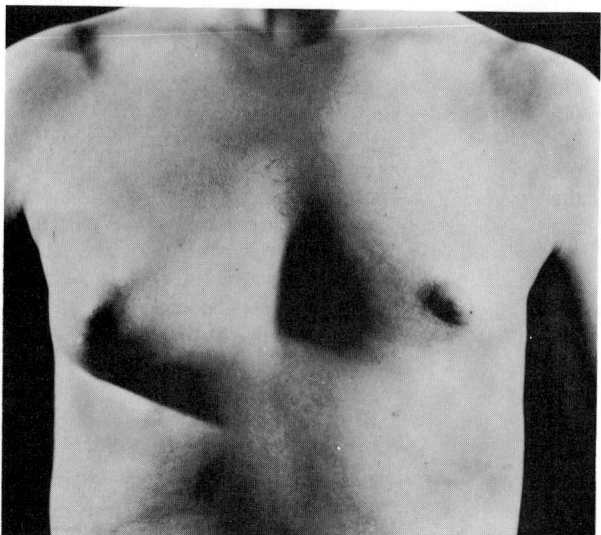

dose of radiation would incite breast cancer in some women. Rapid development of new radiological techniques reduced the absorbed dose of radiation to as little as 0.1 rad at midbreast, and cumulative dose became so small that today the radiation risk is considered negligible.

With the end of the pilot screening program in 1978, a vigorous follow-up program was inaugurated; it was concluded in 1985. Initial reports from this project indicate that screening of breast cancers in women under fifty years of age allows earlier diagnosis and treatment of breast cancer. Disease-free 5-year survival in this group was as high as 93.5 percent.

The American Cancer Society currently recommends that all women begin breast self-examination after the age of twenty, that they obtain a "base-line" mammographic examination some time between thirty-five and forty, that they consult their doctor about the need for regular mammographic screening between forty and fifty, and that they have annual mammographic screening thereafter. This fairly cautious recommendation may be extended even further for examinations in the forty- to fifty-year age group in the light of new findings that radiation exposure involves a risk of cancer induction in women under thirty but that the risk is virtually zero in the cancer age group. Prospective randomized studies of routine mammographic screening have shown 40 percent reduction of Stage II and greater cancers in the screened group and a 30 percent increase in survival in those patients found to have cancer.

Xeroradiography of the breast is basically a radiographic technique that is carried out in exactly the same way as mammography, except that the image is recorded on a xerographic plate instead of the conventional x-ray transparency. The image is positive rather than negative and appears easier to read to the untrained eye. Unfortunately, a badly exposed xeroradiograph, too poor for proper interpretation, is harder to recognize than a poor radiomammograph and may fool the unwary physician.

THERMOGRAPHY. The skin over malignant tumors of the breast is usually warmer than the surrounding areas. Using special heat scanners it is possible to delineate these "hot spots" on film. This method may help to differentiate malignant and benign tumors. Infection may be associated with a false positive, and, conversely, not all cancers are "hot" and so false negatives may occur. The BCDDP abandoned the use of thermography after 3 years because the incidence of false positives and negatives was too high. Research continues to improve the technique, but it is still investigational and not considered a reliable screening method.

ULTRASONOGRAPHY. Ultrasound used in diagnosis of breast lesions is highly effective in differentiating a cystic from a solid mass. It is unsatisfactory for detecting early breast cancers owing to the inability to visualize microcalcification. It is also unlikely to discriminate lesions smaller than 5 mm. While ultrasonography is an excellent method for diagnosing a cyst, needle aspiration as described on page 562 is usually just as effective and a much simpler and less expensive office procedure.

OTHER METHODS. The explosion in technology that has occurred in the past few years has introduced computed tomography (CT), magnetic resonance imaging (MRI), and digital subtraction angiography to the differentiation of breast lesions. In a recent report all of 20 carcinomas of the breast showed an enhanced image when examined with MRI whereas dysplastic or scar tissue enhanced slightly or not at all. This technique has the advantage of avoiding any exposure to radiation. Further experience will be required to determine the incidence of false negative and positive rates for these procedures.

DISEASES OF THE BREAST

Neoplasms

From the standpoint of morbidity and mortality, cancer is by far the most important clinical problem that concerns the breast today. Most benign neoplasms of the breast would have little clinical importance if it were not for the difficulty in differentiating them from cancer. To emphasize this relationship, benign neoplasms are discussed in the section on differential diagnosis of cancer.

In recent years four major controversies have surfaced concerning breast cancer: (1) the relation of treatment to the natural history of the disease; (2) the role of mammography in diagnosis, and especially in screening programs; (3) the appropriate operation for treatment; and (4) the use of postoperative chemotherapy as an adjuvant to primary therapy.

INCIDENCE

Cancer of the breast is the commonest form of cancer in females. The American Cancer Society estimates that 130,000 women in the United States will develop breast cancer in 1987. According to the excellent cancer registry systems in Connecticut and upper New York State, the age-adjusted incidence of new cases has been increasing steadily since the middle 1940s. In the 1970s the chance of developing breast cancer among United States women was estimated at 1 in 13; in 1980 it was 1 in 11, and now it is 1 in 10.

Worldwide figures show that 541,000 cases were diagnosed in 1975 and that the number may approach one million by the year 2000. The Dutch have the highest national mortality of cancer of the breast, with 24.19 patients per 100,000 population. The United States ranks ninth, with 21.38 cases per 100,000 population. The Japanese rank lowest among all nations with reliable statistics, with an incidence of 3.76 per 100,000 population. The factors leading to this wide range of incidence are unknown, although studies seeking an answer are in progress.

ETIOLOGY

Sex is certainly an important contributing factor in this disease, since it is very rare in males. Maleness is not a complete protection, however; there is 1 carcinoma of the breast in men for every 100 carcinomas of the breast in women.

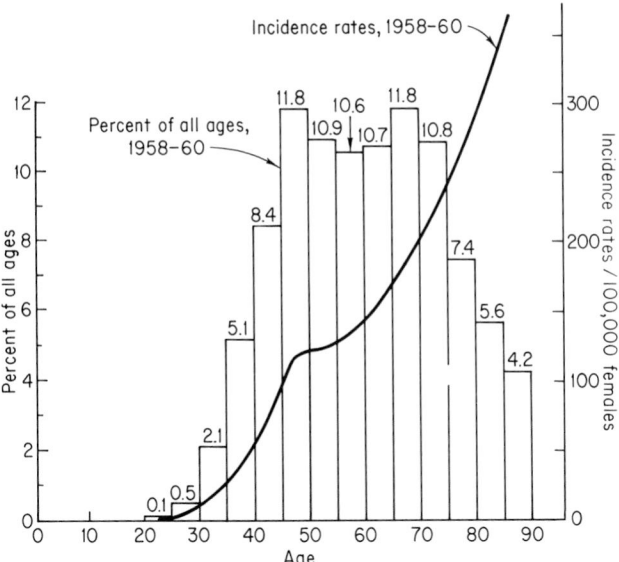

Fig. 15-10. Newly diagnosed breast cancer among women, 1958–1960: percentage distribution and incidence rates by age. Note plateau in incidence between ages forty-five and fifty-five.

The age of the patient is also important (Fig. 15-10). Breast cancer is almost unknown in the prepubertal female and is very rare under the age of twenty. From the age of twenty onward there is a gradually increasing incidence, which reaches a plateau between the ages of forty-five and fifty-five at about 125 new cases each year for every 100,000 females of the age range. After fifty-five the incidence begins to rise again quite sharply, so that the annual risk of developing breast cancer for women eighty to eighty-five is twice as high as for women sixty to sixty-five (312 versus 153 new cases per 100,000 women per year). Some suggest that the plateau of incidence during the menopausal age period reflects the effects of a changing hormonal pattern in women at this time.

Genetic factors play a role in the development of this cancer, though the genetic effect does not seem to be strong and more than one allelic gene must be involved. When the mother has had a breast cancer, the chance of cancer of the breast developing in the daughter is two to three times greater than would be expected in the general population, but no specific pattern of inheritance is evident. Some hypothesize that there is a genotype that has a predisposition to the formation of cancer but that must interact with some nongenetic agent before cancer develops.

Patients in whom breast cancer develops and who have positive family histories for the disease are generally younger and have a higher frequency of bilaterality than breast cancer patients with negative family histories. Blood type O, benign breast disease, and ovarian cysts and tumors also tend to be more common in patients with early diagnosis of breast cancer. Blood type A, diabetes, hypertension, and uterine disorders are more common in those who are older at the time of diagnosis.

Interlinked with factors of age, sex, national origin, and

inheritance in the development of breast cancer is the important role played by hormonal environment. Some breast cancers are highly susceptible to changes in the patient's hormonal pattern and will regress for a time when hormones of various types are given. Mammary cancer can be induced in the mouse and rat by repeated injections of estrogens and in the rat by a combination of estrogen and progesterone. There is a vast literature concerning both experimental and clinical induction and extinction of tumors with hormonal agents. The exact role of hormones in human cancer still remains elusive. It is not known whether hormonal maladjustment is responsible for human breast cancer or what predisposing causes may be required to produce a susceptibility to hormonal change.

Breast cancer may well be multifactorial. Other interesting correlations with breast cancer include the incidence of coronary artery disease, which has a positive correlation with breast cancer death rates in 24 parts of the world. Hems has concluded that "early" breast cancer (age group forty to forty-four) appears to be genetically influenced, while "late" breast cancer (age group sixty-five to sixty-nine) is more closely associated with environmental factors, such as diet. Among younger women, higher risk is associated with late first pregnancy, while among women over fifty years of age the risk appears to increase with weight and the relation of weight to height. Zippin and Petrakis have reported an association between wet cerumen, or earwax, and breast cancer rates in diverse population groups, and breast cancer mortality is closely associated with wet cerumen. Such an association is plausible since the mammary and ceruminous glands are histologically of the apocrine type and have many similarities in their secretions. Cerumen exists in two phenotypic forms, wet and dry, which are controlled by a pair of genes in which the allele for the wet type is dominant over that of the dry type. The dry is homozygous recessive and is highly prevalent in the mongoloid population of Asia and in American Indians. The wet type predominates in Western Europeans, Caucasian Americans, and Negro Americans. These findings support the hypothesis that genetic variations in the apocrine system may influence susceptibility to breast cancer.

Diet in terms of the consumption of animal fat is strongly correlated with breast cancer incidence. Rose and associates plotted correlation of animal fat consumption in 32 countries with incidence of breast cancer and found a highly significant direct relationship (R = 0.74).

It has long been known that breast cancer in mice is related to a viral factor transmitted in the milk. Considerable excitement has attended the discovery of particles in human milk with the same morphologic characteristics as those found to be associated with breast cancer in mice. Antigens to these viral particles have been identified in human plasma. These particles have been found in the milk from the breasts of 60 percent of American women with family histories of breast cancer compared with 5 percent of women without positive family histories. The milk of 39 percent of Parsi women in India also was found to contain these particles. The group of Parsi women is of particular interest because of their endogamous history over the centuries, resulting in an inbred population. Breast cancer accounts for approximately half of the cancers among Parsi women in contrast with Connecticut women, for example, in whom breast cancer represents one-fourth of all cancers.

NATURAL HISTORY

A typical carcinoma of the breast is a scirrhous adenocarcinoma beginning in the ducts and invading the parenchyma (80 percent). Beginning in the upper outer quadrant (40 to 50 percent), it grows slowly, doubling its volume every 2 to 9 months in 70 percent of patients. Starting from a single cell, it takes 30 doubling times for a tumor to attain a size of 1 cm—the smallest tumor of the breast normally found on physical diagnosis. Thus even the fastest-growing tumor of the more common type may require 5 years before it becomes clinically palpable. The use of doubling times to calculate the preclinical course of tumors of the breast is subject to many errors, the most obvious being that growth rates are not always constant, varying with areas of necrosis within the tumor and hormonal changes in the patient. Laboratory and clinical observations indicate, however, that growth rates are more consistent than is usually appreciated, especially during the first 30 doublings. The concept of the origin of these tumors in a single cell with increase in size by doubling is a useful model and suggests the long occult period that probably is present in many tumors before they are diagnosed and treated. Cancers of the breast are often multicentric (15 to 40 percent), but each tumor is assumed to have started from its own individual cell.

A characteristic of malignant cells is the lack of adhesion to adjacent tissue. As the small mass of tumor increases in size, increasing numbers of tumor cells shed into the intercellular spaces to be taken up by the lymphatics. At about the twentieth doubling, the still tiny tumor mass acquires its own blood supply as a network of new capillaries forms. Tumor cells can now be shed directly into the bloodstream. Fisher notes that the cells entering the lymphatic network can cross over into the bloodstream by lymphaticovenous communications. Successful implantation of shed cells is another matter, however, and depends on the number of cells shed, special characteristics of the shed cells, and the resistance of the host. Empiric clinical data indicate that successful implantation of metastatic cells from breast cancer rarely occurs until the primary lesion is larger than 0.5 cm in diameter, or about the twenty-seventh doubling.

Fisher has also introduced the important concept that the appearance of gross tumor in the axillary nodes is an index of the failure of host resistance and that such nodal involvement indicates a probability of disseminated malignant disease. The chance of dissemination is roughly correlated with the number of nodes involved.

As the tumor increases in size and invades the surrounding glandular tissue, the accompanying fibrosis tends to shorten Cooper's ligaments, producing the characteristic dimpling in the skin (Fig. 15-11). Cords of tumor

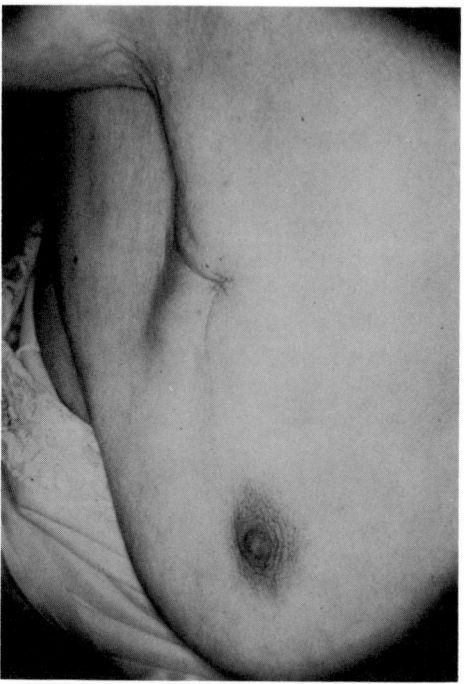

Fig. 15-11. Dimpling of skin over primary carcinoma of breast in upper outer quadrant. Slowly growing lesion in seventy-year-old patient; dimpling had been present for 2 years.

cells grow out along lymphatics, ultimately invading the skin itself. This invasion is preceded by localized edema of the skin as many lymphatic avenues are blocked and drainage of fluid from the skin is impeded. Eventually tumor cells replace the skin, which breaks down to form an ulcer. The tumor increases in size, and new areas of skin invasion may occur, indicated by small satellite nodules adjacent to the ulcer crater. Blood vessels are invaded, and additional tumor cells seed into the circulation, passing into axillary or intercostal veins to be scattered through the pulmonary circuit into the lungs or by way of the vertebral veins up and down the vertebral column.

As the breast tumor extends toward the skin, tumor cells simultaneously pass along the lymphatic vessels from the upper outer quadrant to the axillary nodes, where they implant and grow. As the axillary nodes enlarge, they are at first shotty and fairly soft, then firm and hard as they are increasingly replaced by tumor. Eventually the nodes adhere to one another in a large conglomerate mass, and as the tumor breaks out of the lymphatic capsule the mass of nodes becomes fixed to the medial wall of the axilla. As the axillary nodes become choked with tumor, cells are passed along the chain to the supraclavicular nodes, which also enlarge. Other cancer cells pass by way of the right lymphatic trunk or the thoracic duct into the bloodstream, heart, and lungs. Systemic spread is the rule, and 95 percent of patients who die of uncontrolled breast cancer have distant metastases. Lung (65 percent), liver (56 percent), and bones (56 percent) are the commonest sites for these deposits.

Patients today are rarely allowed to proceed through all stages of carcinoma without some therapeutic intervention. Data are available, however, from the latter half of the 1800s and the first few years of this century indicating the normal course of events in untreated tumors. The excellent report in 1962 by Bloom and associates summarizes much of the data. They cite the experience of the Middlesex Hospital in London, where in 1791 a cancer charity was founded to which patients were admitted to ''remain an unlimited time, until either relieved by art or released by death.'' From the well-preserved records of this charity it was possible to collect a series of 250 advanced cases of untreated breast cancer seen between 1805 and 1933 (Fig. 15-12). All the patients reported died in the hospital, and in every case an autopsy was performed. In the last 86 cases, histologic sections were available. The mean survival in this series and for over 1000 untreated cases collected from the literature was 38.7 months, with a range from 30.2 to 39.8 months. It must be noted that in all reports of untreated patients survival is calculated from the onset of the first symptom. Fifty percent of the patients died in 2.7 years (median survival); 18 percent survived 5 years, 3.6 percent 10 years, and 0.8 percent 15 years. The longest survivor in the group died in the nineteenth year after onset of symptoms. Histologic grading indicated that for 23 patients with grade 1 tumors the mean survival was 47 months. Autopsies indicated that 95 percent of the women died of their carcinoma, only 5 percent of intercurrent disease. Nearly three-fourths of the patients had ulceration of the breast at death, and in 21 percent this was very extensive, sometimes destroying the entire breast and excavating the chest wall. Bloom concluded that treatment of patients with breast cancer appeared to increase the length and improve the quality of survival.

DIAGNOSIS AND STAGING

The normal breast is a nodular structure by virtue of its lobular architecture, and this lobularity may be accentuated during the later portion of the menstrual cycle, pregnancy, or lactation. To the inexperienced examiner the normal nodularity may feel faintly suspicious throughout, although no obvious lesion can be felt. Palpation of the typical carcinoma of the breast normally leaves little doubt in the examiner's mind: the lesion is hard, almost cartilaginous; the edges are distinct, serrated, and irregular. This is true for the 75 to 80 percent of breast tumors associated with productive fibrosis. It is the remaining 20 to 25 percent of tumors, those associated with little fibrosis and those with a medullary or a colloid element or other less typical lesions, which form the spectrum of neoplasms most difficult to distinguish from benign lesions.

Physicians would prefer to have only the clues provided by the local mass to make the physical diagnosis of carcinoma, for it is only when the mass is localized to the breast that one can assume an ''early'' lesion and expect the best possible chance of long survival. Too often the later signs of breast cancer are present to confirm the di-

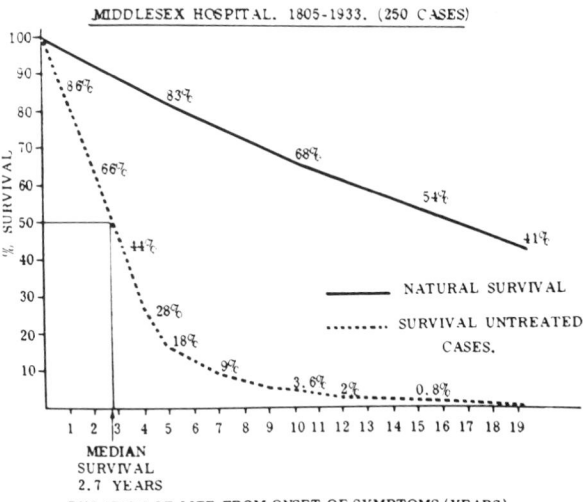

Fig. 15-12. Survival of patients with untreated cancer of breast compared with natural survival. (From: *Bloom HJG, Richardson WW, Harries EJ: Br Med J 5299:213, 1962, with permission.*)

agnosis. As indicated previously, these are skin dimpling or nipple retraction, satellite skin lesions, edema or ulceration, and ipsilateral enlarged axillary or supraclavicular nodes. Signs of even wider spread may be present such as a history of back or leg pain, an enlarged and nodular liver, or perhaps a complaint of dyspnea associated with physical findings of fluid in the chest.

The physical examination of a patient with breast cancer should include an attempt on the part of the examiner to classify and record the stage of the patient's disease specifically. Only consistent classification can make possible clear conclusions concerning prognosis and type of treatment. The problem of comparing the results of treatment from institution to institution and among different operators has been impaired for years by a lack of adequate classification or by varying standards of classification. At present the only acceptable method of classification is a standard system devised by the American Joint Committee on Cancer Staging and End Results Reporting, based on a system proposed by the International Union against Cancer in 1958. This system of classification is called the TNM Classification, the T standing for ''tumor,'' the N for ''nodes,'' and the M for ''metastasis.'' The system is very precise but also complex. If a patient's cancer is staged, it is best to use a staging form as shown in Table 15-1.

DIFFERENTIAL DIAGNOSIS (BENIGN LESIONS)

CHRONIC CYSTIC MASTITIS. Chronic cystic mastitis was first described in the medical literature in the last two decades of the nineteenth century, by Reclus (1883), Brisaud (1884), Schimmelbusch (1890), and König (1893). For a time the disease was known as either Reclus' or Schimmelbusch's disease, but use of these eponyms dwindled following the introduction of the term *chronic cystic mastitis* by König. He chose this term to describe a

Table 15-1. STAGING OF BREAST CARCINOMA

Definitions for all time periods

Primary tumor (T)
- ☐ TX   Tumor cannot be assessed.
- ☐ T0   No evidence of primary tumor.
- ☐ TIS   Paget's disease of the nipple with no demonstrable tumor.

NOTE: Paget's disease with a demonstrable tumor is classified according to the size of the tumor.

T1*   Tumor 2 cm or less in greatest dimension.
- ☐ T1a   No fixation to underlying pectoral fascia or muscle.
- ☐ T1b   Fixation to underlying pectoral fascia and/or muscle.
  (Check below in addition to T1a or T1b)
  - ☐   I   tumor ≤ 0.5 cm.
  - ☐   II tumor > 0.5 ≤ 1.0 cm.
  - ☐   III tumor > 1.0 ≤ 2.0 cm.

T2*   Tumor more than 2 cm but not more than 5 cm in its greatest dimension.
- ☐ T2a   No fixation to underlying pectoral fascia or muscle.
- ☐ T2b   Fixation to underlying pectoral fascia and/or muscle.

T3*   Tumor more than 5 cm in its greatest dimension.
- ☐ T3a   No fixation to underlying pectoral fascia or muscle.
- ☐ T3b   Fixation to underlying pectoral fascia and/or muscle.

T4   Tumor of any size with direct extension to chest wall or skin.

NOTE: Chest wall includes ribs, intercostal muscles, and serratus anterior muscle, but not pectoral muscle.
- ☐ T4a   Fixation to chest wall.
- ☐ T4b   Edema (including peau d'orange), ulceration of the skin of the breast, or satellite skin nodules confined to the same breast.
- ☐ T4c   Both of the above.

Lymph nodes (N)
Definitions for clinical-diagnostic stage
- ☐ NX   Regional lymph nodes cannot be assessed clinically.
- ☐ N0   Homolateral axillary lymph nodes not considered to contain growth.
- ☐ N1   Movable homolateral axillary nodes considered to contain growth.
- ☐ N2   Homolateral axillary nodes considered to contain growth and fixed to one another or to other structures.
- ☐ N3   Homolateral supraclavicular or infraclavicular nodes considered to contain growth, or edema of the arm.†

Lymph nodes (N)
Definitions for surgical evaluative and postsurgical treatment-pathologic
- ☐ NX   Regional lymph nodes cannot be assessed (not removed for study or previously removed).
- ☐ N0   No evidence of homolateral axillary lymph node metastasis.
- ☐ N1   Metastasis to movable homolateral axillary nodes not fixed to one another or to other structure.
  - ☐ N1a   Micrometastasis ≤ 0.2 cm in lymph node(s).
  - ☐ N1b   Gross metastasis in lymph node(s).
    - ☐   I   Metastasis more than 0.2 cm, but less than 2.0 cm in one to three lymph nodes.
    - ☐   II   Metastasis more than 0.2 cm, but less than 2.0 cm in four or more lymph nodes.
    - ☐   III Extension of metastasis beyond the lymph node capsule (less than 2.0 cm in dimension).
    - ☐   IV   Metastasis in lymph node 2.0 cm or more in dimension.
- ☐ N2   Metastasis to homolateral axillary lymph nodes that are fixed to one another or to other structures.
- ☐ N3   Metastasis to homolateral supraclavicular or infraclavicular lymph node(s).

Distant metastases (M)—All time periods
- ☐ MX   Not assessed.
- ☐ M0   No (known) distant metastasis.
- ☐ M1   Distant metastasis present.
  Specify: _____

Tumor size: _____ × _____ × _____ cm.
Predominate lesion
  Measured on: ☐ Patient   ☐ Mammogram
                 ☐ Pathological specimen
Location   ☐ OUQ   ☐ Nipple/areola
(Multiple when   ☐ OLQ   ☐ IUQ   ☐ ILQ
 necessary)

Lymph nodes: Total No. _____   No. with met. _____

Performance status _____ (see reverse side.)

Examination by _____ M.D.

Date _____

STAGE:

☐ Clinical-diagnostic				☐ Postsurgical treatment-pathologic
☐ Stage TIS—In situ				Stage TIS ☐
☐ Stage X—Cannot stage (unstageable)				Stage X ☐
☐ Stage I	☐ T1ai	N0	M0 ☐	Stage I ☐
	☐ T1aii	N0	M0 ☐	
	☐ T1aiii	N0	M0 ☐	
	☐ T1bi	N0	M0 ☐	
	☐ T1bii	N0	M0 ☐	
	☐ T1biii	N0	M0 ☐	
☐ Stage II	☐ T0	N1a or 1b	M0 ☐	Stage II ☐
	☐ T1a or T1b	N1a or 1b	M0 ☐	
	☐ T2a or T2b	N0	M0 ☐	
	☐ T2a or T2b	N1a or 1b	M0 ☐	
☐ Stage IIIa	☐ T0	N2	M0 ☐	Stage IIIa ☐
	☐ T1a or T1b	N2	M0 ☐	
	☐ T2a or T2b	N2	M0 ☐	
	☐ T3a or T3b	N0	M0 ☐	
	☐ T3a or T3b	N1	M0 ☐	
	☐ T3a or T3b	N2	M0 ☐	
☐ Stage IIIb	☐ Any T	N3	M0 ☐	Stage IIIb ☐
	☐ Any T4	Any N	M0 ☐	
☐ Stage IV	☐ Any T	Any N	M1 ☐	Stage IV ☐

* Dimpling of the skin, nipple retraction, or any other skin changes except those in T4b may occur in T1, T2, or T3 without affecting the classification.

NOTE: Cases of inflammatory carcinoma should be reported separately.

† Edema of the arm may be caused by lymphatic obstruction and lymph nodes may not then be palpable.

SOURCE: American Joint Committee on Cancer—1982.

group of pathologic lesions found in the breast because he thought they were due to a "vicious cycle of secretion and irritation." While the disease is indeed chronic, it may not be cystic and is certainly not inflammatory, so this old name is at least two-thirds in error. Nonetheless, attempts to introduce more accurate or at least other nomenclatures have failed. Fibrocystic disease, fibroadenosis, mastopathy, nodular hyperplasia, cyclomastopathy, adenofibromatosis, mazoplasia, cystiphorous epithelial hyperplasia, adenocystic disease, and mammary dysplasia have all been offered, but chronic cystic mastitis is still the most widely used designation.

The term chronic cystic mastitis describes a family of lesions found in the breast. Pathologists disagree as to which lesions are legitimate family relations, so the morphology of the disease, like the terminology, appears rather fuzzy to the casual observer. Foote and Stewart have named 10 lesions often described as members of this group: cysts, papillomatosis, blunt duct adenosis, sclerosing adenosis, apocrine metaplasia, stasis and distention of ducts, periductal mastitis, fat necrosis, hyperplasia of duct epithelium, and fibroadenoma. These writers accept, however, only the first five of this group as being related lesions and forming part of chronic cystic mastitis; the others are held to represent different disease entities. They refer to the first five as the cystic and proliferative group, assuming that the proliferative lesions are responsible for the subsequent formation of cysts. A majority of pathologists accept this list, though some have argued for the inclusion of fibroadenoma. In addition, epithelial hyperplasia is usually accepted as part of the complex, with papillomas representing an advanced manifestation of hyperplasia.

The lesions of chronic cystic mastitis begin to appear in the breasts of a few women in their late twenties. The incidence is greater in the thirties and forties. Originally it was thought that the incidence of these lesions decreased after the menopause, but careful autopsy studies indicate that the lesions are common in the older age groups and may continue to increase in frequency with age. Frantz et al. found a 71 percent incidence of cystic and proliferative lesions in women over seventy years of age. Sandison noted epithelial hyperplasia of the ducts in 7 percent of women in their twenties and in 33 percent of women in their eighties. Rush and Kramer in 1963 reviewed step sections from the breasts of 20 women over seventy years of age. Approximately 100 sections were reviewed per patient, and with this close scrutiny two or more lesions of cystic mastitis were found in all the patients. Moderately severe epithelial hyperplasia was found in 14 of the 20 (Fig. 15-13). A case may be made for considering the lesions of cystic mastitis somewhat as one considers arteriosclerosis: a pathologic process that varies in degree and in time of onset but that is found to some degree in all adult females as they age.

Most of the lesions making up the complex of chronic cystic mastitis are proliferative, and almost from the first recognition of this disease there has been a suspicion that these lesions may represent a premalignant condition. Follow-up studies of patients shown by biopsy to have

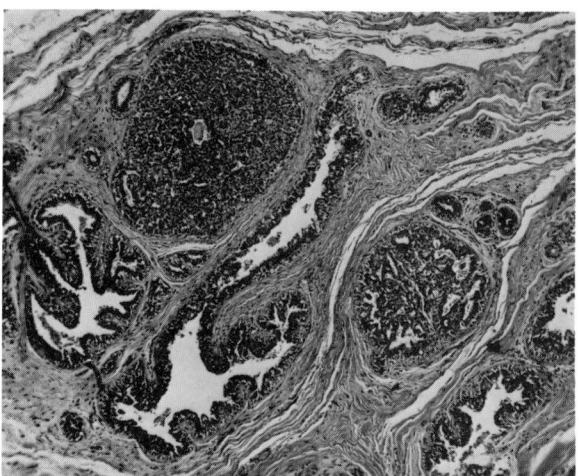

Fig. 15-13. Benign marked intraductal hyperplasia in eighty-eight-year-old female. (Hematoxylin and eosin; ×32.) (From: *Rush BF Jr, Kramer WM: Surg Gynecol Obstet 117:425, 1963, with permission.*)

chronic cystic mastitis uniformly indicate that cancer subsequently occurs three to five times more often in these patients than in the general population.

If one assumes that all women eventually develop some degree of chronic cystic mastitis, how can one conclude that the finding of chronic cystic mastitis on biopsy is associated with an increase in the incidence of cancer of the female breast compared with patients in the general population? Recent studies clearly show that only a small subgroup of lesions, those with severe hyperplasia or atypism, are associated with an increased risk of cancer. All other lesions of the complex have no associated increase in risk. The term fibrocystic *condition* has been proposed to avoid any stigma of premalignancy. This has practical importance, since some insurance companies attempted to raise their rates when the diagnosis of fibrocystic disease was made.

The lesions of chronic cystic mastitis that are most likely to present a problem in differential diagnosis and to require biopsy are cysts, fibroadenoma, ductal papilloma, and sclerosing adenosis.

Treatment. The most important aspect of this condition is the differentiation of the diffuse nodularity of the breast from carcinoma. However, many women suffer associated symptoms of tenderness and swelling of the nodules that occur most commonly during menstruation. Some claim that abstaining from coffee and other xanthine-containing substances will ameliorate the syndrome. Benefits are also claimed for high doses of vitamin E. Neither of these treatments is established as clearly effective. Danazol, a synthetic androgen analog that suppresses follicle-stimulating hormone and luteinizing hormone, is highly effective although expensive. From 100 to 400 mg, given in two divided doses daily, will usually abolish pain and tenderness within a month. Nodularity will diminish and disappear in 2 to 6 months. About half of the patients will show evidence of recurrence of symptoms within a year following the end of therapy. Treatment may be re-

of the nipple in a postmenopausal female that persists for more than a few weeks should be biopsied to exclude the possibility of Paget's disease. Adequate histologic studies of surgical specimens almost always reveal underlying carcinomas of the mammary ducts. Invasion of the skin by these cells produces the interesting Paget's cell, a large cell with clear cytoplasm and commonly with binucleation. This is associated with evidence of chronic inflammation and a surface crust. Robbins and Berg's study of 89 cases indicated that one-third of the patients showed noninfiltrating carcinoma, and in this group the survival rate was 100 percent at 5 years. The remaining patients had infiltrating carcinoma. The overall survival rate for the group was 64 percent, indicating a better prognosis for this lesion than for the average carcinoma of the breast.

NONINFILTRATING CARCINOMAS OF THE MAMMARY DUCTS. These constitute 1 percent of carcinomas of the breast. It is unfortunate that more cancers are not seen at the noninfiltrating stage, since these lesions are carcinomas in situ and operation should result in 100 percent 5-year survival. That this is not the case, 5-year survival being about 90 percent, reflects the fact that the breast is a large organ and that lesions that appear to be noninfiltrating may in fact be infiltrating at some area that the pathologist has not examined. Foote and Stewart report that they have traced progression of intraductal carcinoma from benign papillary hyperplasia through atypism to noninfiltrating intraductal carcinoma and ultimately to infiltrating carcinoma throughout a breast specimen. They state that while this may be one route for the development of cancer of the breast, cancer may arise from normal intraductal cells directly. The differentiation of a noninfiltrating intraductal carcinoma from a benign hyperplasia may be difficult; areas of atypism can blend gradually from one state into the other. Histologically, the duct epithelium is usually seen to be thrown up into papillae that show a loss of cohesiveness and disorientation of cells, with pleomorphism and occasionally mitotic figures but without evidence of invasion of the basement membrane. A more dramatic form is the noninfiltrating comedocarcinoma, in which hyperplasia is more extreme, choking the entire duct for long distances with masses of cells. These lesions commonly develop central necrosis of the cells. A gross section of such a lesion will extrude small cores of tissue from the ducts very much as the core is extruded from a comedo when it is squeezed, thus giving rise to the term comedocarcinoma.

INFILTRATING PAPILLARY CARCINOMA. Presumably a later stage or a more aggressive form of the noninfiltrating papillary lesion, these carcinomas still tend to evolve slowly and have a better 5-year survival rate than the average carcinoma of the breast. They produce a mass rather soft to palpation compared with the typical hard, fibrous lesion usually associated with breast cancer. They may reach large size before metastasizing to the axilla. Dimpling and skin edema are less commonly seen, another index of the late infiltration of the lymphatics and of the failure to stimulate a fibrous response. Noninfiltrating papillary carcinomas are often seen in association with the infiltrating form.

Infiltrating comedocarcinomas comprise approxi-

mately 5 percent of all breast cancers. They are often found in association with other forms of adenocarcinoma that result in productive fibrosis, and the presence of comedocarcinoma together with other elements of carcinoma of the breast does not significantly alter the prognosis from the average.

INFILTRATING DUCT CARCINOMA WITH PRODUCTIVE FIBROSIS. This is the commonest form of breast cancer, constituting 78 percent of the specimens seen. There is a tremendous variation in the amount of fibrosis. The lesion has been termed *scirrhous carcinoma, fibrocarcinoma,* and *sclerosing carcinoma.* The desmoplastic response to the invading cancer cells accounts for the remarkable hardness of the average breast cancer. Grossly the lesions have uneven serrated edges. They cut with great resistance and often with a rather gritty feeling as the knife edge passes through them. Histologically the lesions may vary from scattered, well-differentiated adenomatous clusters and a massive amount of fibrostroma to dense cellular aggregates with only minor amounts of fibroplasia (Fig. 15-16). Electron microscopic examination of these tumors indicates that they originate in the myoepithelial cells of the mammary duct.

MEDULLARY CARCINOMAS. Five percent of carcinomas of the breast assume this pattern, and the diagnosis indicates a favorable prognosis for the patient. Even in the presence of metastatic disease the prognosis remains favorable; the 5-year overall survival rate for the lesion is 85 to 90 percent. These lesions are soft, bulky, and often large. Necrotic areas of varying size are usually present. Occasionally one finds a lesion that is almost totally infarcted. On physical examination these tumors are freely movable, and smaller tumors are likely to be diagnosed clinically as cysts or fibroadenomas. Histologically the tumors are made up of large rounded or polygonal cells with an abundant cytoplasm arranged in broad or narrow plexiform masses anastomosing with one another. Electron microscopic and histochemical evidence suggests that these cells originate in the ductal epithelium. There is

Fig. 15-16. Intraductal carcinoma with stromal invasion in eighty-three-year-old female. Field shows almost entire extent of this very early lesion. (Hematoxylin and eosin; ×32.)

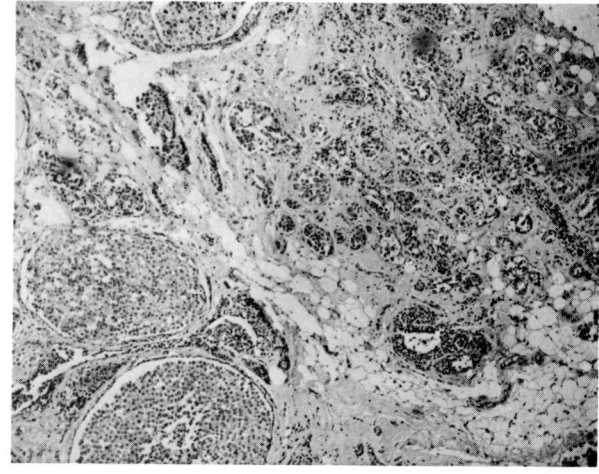

an abundant lymphoid infiltrate. Plasma cells are often seen and are sometimes very prominent. Axillary metastases occur less frequently than in the ordinary carcinoma of the breast but are not uncommon, occurring in about 40 percent. Metastasis frequently involves only a single node.

COLLOID CARCINOMA. This is an infrequent mammary cancer constituting about 1 percent of all breast cancers. The lesions contain a much greater amount of mucin than the usual adenocarcinoma and may be frankly gelatinous on cut section. Clinically these lesions are soft and ill defined and, like the medullary lesions, may be quite bulky before detection. Histologically the predominant picture is of large mucinous lakes in which epithelial aggregates float. Patients with these lesions have a better-than-average survival rate.

TUBULAR CARCINOMA. Also known as "well-differentiated" or "orderly" carcinoma, this lesion has only recently received attention. It may mimic sclerosing or blunt duct adenosis and is made up of tubular structures, typically lined by a single layer of well-differentiated epithelium. It occurs in pure form in only 1.2 percent of cases but may be combined frequently with other histological forms. If a breast carcinoma contains 90 percent or more of the tubular lesion, long-term survival approaches 100 percent.

CARCINOMA OF THE MAMMARY LOBULES. This lesion arises in the mammary lobules from the cells of the acini and the terminal ducts. Most of the acini of a lobule are involved. Lobules may be of normal size or enlarged, with an unsystematic hyperplasia of the lining cells until the lumen is plugged. At the in situ stage of development these are the only changes, and simple mastectomy at this point should produce cure. The lesion subsequently becomes infiltrative and ultimately may give rise to regular scirrhous carcinoma.

Multicentricity and bilaterality are important features of lobular carcinoma. Eighty-eight percent of breast specimens removed for in situ lobular carcinoma show other in situ lesions scattered throughout the specimen. Examination of the contralateral breast has demonstrated in situ lesions in from 35 to 59 percent of specimens.

SARCOMA OF THE BREAST. Sarcomas of the breast are very rare. The commonest sarcoma seen is cystosarcoma phylloides, but only one in ten of these is truly malignant, the great majority being a benign variant of fibroadenoma. Great confusion is created because both the benign and malignant form are called "cystosarcoma." When Müller first described and named the lesion in 1838 he was aware of its predominantly benign nature. At that time "sarcoma" meant simply a fleshy tumor and did not carry the meaning of malignancy that it does today. Modern synonyms for the benign lesion are *giant intracanalicular or pericanalicular fibroadenoma* and *intracanalicular myxoma*. The malignant variant has been called *adenocarcinoma*.

Cystosarcoma phylloides occurs at an older average age (forty), is larger, and has a more cellular stroma than fibroadenoma. When first seen clinically these tumors average 5 to 10 cm, have a firm and rubbery consistency, and may have a bosselated surface. In cut section the tumors have a discrete capsule. Small lesions present leaflike intracanalicular protrusions, and larger lesions have cystic spaces into which project densely packed polypoid masses.

The malignant variant metastasizes most commonly to the lungs, bones, and subcutaneous tissues. Axillary metastasis is so uncommon that simple mastectomy is an adequate procedure for both the benign and the malignant forms.

PRIMARY TREATMENT

The first historical reference to cancer of the breast appears in the Edwin Smith Surgical Papyrus (3000 to 2500 B.C.). The patient described is a man, but the description suggests most of the clinical features of breast cancer. The author concludes that "there is no treatment." References to cancer of the breast are scattered and brief over the following 2500 years. Even in that large body of writings concerning Greek and Roman medicine, the Corpus Hippocraticum, direct reference to the treatment of breast cancer is absent, although it is clear that the condition was recognized.

Celsus, a Roman of the first century, spoke of operation and advised limiting it to early lesions: "None of these can be removed but the cacoethes [early lesion], the rest are irritated by every method of cure. The more violent the operations are, the more angry they grow." Galen, in the second century, inscribed one of the classic clinical observations:

We have often seen in the breast a tumor exactly resembling the animal the crab. Just as the crab has legs on both sides of his body, so in this disease the veins extending out from the unnatural growth take the shape of a crab's legs. We have often cured this disease in its early stages, but after it has reached a large size no one has cured it without operation. In all operations we attempt to excise a pathological tumor in a circle in the region where it borders on the healthy tissue.

Although Galen spoke of operations for tumors, his system of medicine ascribed the disease to an excess of black bile, and logically excision of a local outbreak could not cure the systemic imbalance. The Galenic theories dominated medicine until the Renaissance. Most established physicians looked down on attempts at operative treatment as misdirected and futile. Only when it was again established that a cancer could arise in a part as a local disorder quite separate from a systemic imbalance could excision of the tumor be recognized as rational therapy. Morgagni's definitive study of gross pathology, appropriately entitled *The Seats and Causes of Disease,* supplied this new rationale. Radical mastectomy until recently was the standard treatment for operable cancer of the breast in the United States. This operation involves the removal of the entire breast with a generous portion of overlying skin, all the underlying pectoralis major and minor muscles, and the entire lymphatic and fibrofatty contents of the axilla.

This procedure evolved slowly from simple amputation of the breast. LeDran in the eighteenth century repudiated Galen's humoral theory and stated that cancer of the breast was a local disease that spread by way of the lymphatics to the regional nodes. He removed enlarged axillary nodes in his operations on patients with breast cancer. In the nineteenth century, Moore of Middlesex Hospital, England, emphasized wide removal of the breast and felt that when there was neoplasm in the axilla, the axillary contents should be removed in one block together with the breast. In a presentation before the British Medical Association in 1877, Banks supported Moore's concepts and advocated that axillary nodes should always be removed in one block with the breast tissue whether there were palpable nodes present or not, since occult involvement of the axillary nodes was so often present.

As Lewison notes, it remained for Halsted, the new professor of surgery at a young school called The Johns Hopkins Medical School, to "culminate the operation and germinate the present modern method." Halsted proposed a standard procedure, removing all the structures in one block. His first operation was performed about 1882, and he reported 13 cases in 1890. The procedure was almost exactly as it is today except that the pectoralis minor muscle was not removed. In 1894 he reported more than 50 cases over the preceding 12 years. In the same year Herbert Willy Meyer of New York reported six patients operated upon by a technique he had evolved independently. This procedure, almost a duplicate of the Halsted mastectomy, added the removal of the pectoralis minor muscle. Halsted subsequently accepted this addition, and the modern radical mastectomy is often attributed to both these men. This procedure and the wide-block excision that it incorporated was soon adopted widely and for the following 60 years was the only operation used by the well-trained surgeon for treatment of breast cancer.

Halsted's operation proved so successful because it provided highly reliable locoregional control of breast cancer in an era when almost all patients presenting for treatment had neglected, far-advanced cancer (Stage III or IV) by modern standards. Every one of Halsted's first 50 patients had involved axillary nodes, and he considered a 6-cm mass to be "small." By the middle of this century the situation changed markedly. The average size of lesions when first seen was much smaller, and these were patients with axillary nodal metastasis. As we shall explore in the section on selection of the operation, this greatly expanded the possible procedures available and markedly diminished the role of radical mastectomy.

SELECTION OF PATIENTS. When radical mastectomy was the only treatment available, surgeons attempted to exclude from the operation those patients who would almost certainly develop distant metastasis at a later date. The generally accepted "criteria of inoperability" include fixation of the local breast lesion to the chest wall, fixation of the involved lymph nodes in the axilla, and inflammatory carcinoma of the breast. Haagensen compiled the following detailed list of criteria:

1. Extensive edema of the skin over the breast (Fig. 15-17)
2. Satellite nodules in the skin over the breast
3. Carcinoma of the inflammatory type (Fig. 15-18)
4. Parasternal tumor nodules
5. Proved supraclavicular metastases

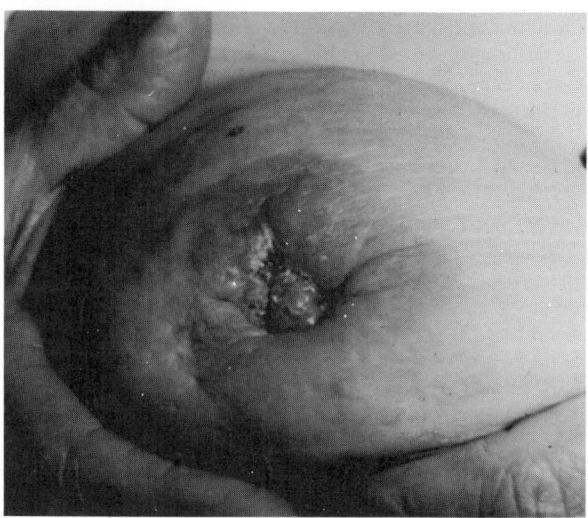

Fig. 15-17. Large cancer of breast with retraction of nipple, skin edema, and several satellite skin nodules.

6. Edema of the arm
7. Distant metastases
8. Any two or more of the following grave signs of locally advanced carcinoma:
   a. Ulceration of the skin
   b. Edema of the skin of limited extent (less than one-third of breast skin involved)
   c. Solid fixation of tumor to the chest wall
   d. Axillary lymph nodes measuring 2.5 cm or more in transverse diameter
   e. Fixation of the axillary nodes to the skin or deep structures of the axilla

At one time these criteria excluded more than 25 percent of patients from surgical treatment. In the average

Fig. 15-18. Inflammatory carcinoma of breast. Bright pink to red suffuses area of skin involvement, reflecting inflammatory response to extensive scattering of tumor cells in subcutaneous tissues. Large skin lesion above nipple is congenital pigmented nevus unrelated to the cancer.

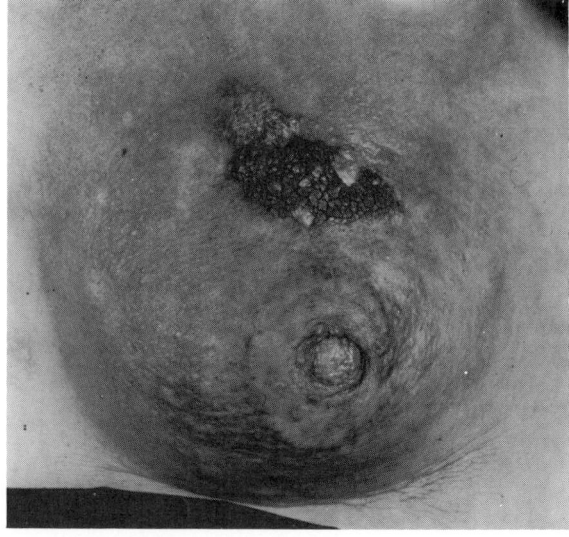

community hospital today less than 15 percent of patients would be found with such advanced tumors. In addition, the successful use of adjuvant chemotherapy has greatly changed our attitude toward patients with a high likelihood of disseminated disease, and if no clinical metastasis is found on initial clinical work-up, most patients will have an operation designed to eradicate the locoregional disease.

Every effort should be made to identify patients with distant metastasis. Search for metastatic lesions preoperatively should include a chest film and liver chemistries. If liver chemistries are altered, a liver scintiscan should be done. If the patient has symptoms of bone pain, a bone scintiscan is indicated. A large number of serum markers for breast carcinomas, both primary and metastatic, are currently under investigation but have yet to emerge into clinical practice.

SELECTION OF THE OPERATION. For the past 20 years a controversy has been raging about the appropriate operation for patients with operable breast cancer. The debate was initially between radical mastectomy and total ("simple") mastectomy plus radiation therapy; then between radical mastectomy and total mastectomy alone; and finally between radical mastectomy alone and partial mastectomy or "lumpectomy" with or without radiation therapy. While these have been the major themes, some minor variations of radical mastectomy also were proposed, either a little less than the radical mastectomy, sparing the pectoralis major (Patey's operation) or both pectoral muscles (Madden's operation), or a little more than the radical mastectomy, taking the internal mammary lymph nodes and adjacent chest wall (Urban's operation). Even more minimal operations include local excision of the breast mass with complete or partial resection of axillary nodes and finally incisional or needle biopsy of the primary lesion with subsequent radiation therapy to the breast and axilla.

The arguments for the various procedures have been remarkably bitter at times, with charges of bias, the citing of incomplete data, and irrationality being hurled not only in the scientific but in the lay press as well. Carter notes that "some women's groups have viewed the discussions about various treatment options in terms of feminist issues. The radical and modified radical mastectomy have been portrayed as procedures devised by male surgeons insensitive to the mutilating effects on women." He compares this with the debate about radical prostatectomy versus radiation for local control of primary prostate cancer "which is not tinged with anything like the emotionalism that similar options evoke for primary breast cancer."

American surgeons have remained reasonably levelheaded during this period, most influenced by maturing data from large, prospective, randomized trials. At first they adhered to the traditional radical mastectomy. After all, the advantages of doing lesser operations were functional and cosmetic, while the penalty of being wrong was the life of a patient. A survey of New Jersey surgeons in 1971 showed that 75 percent would do a radical breast dissection and 15 percent a modified radical operation for a 2-cm lesion in the upper outer quadrant of a fifty-year-old woman. In 1977, surgeons in the same state indicated that approximately 40 percent would do a radical mastectomy, 40 percent a modified radical mastectomy, 15 percent a total mastectomy, and 5 percent some other procedure. By 1982, 90 percent of these surgeons had adopted modified radical mastectomy (Fig. 15-19) for Stage I breast cancers but very few were doing lesser procedures.

Operations for Early Breast Cancer. Stages I and II breast cancers make up 80 to 85 percent of cases now seen in most hospitals in this country. The general consensus until recently was that modified radical mastectomy was the procedure of choice for these lesions, and Maddox reported that a randomized trial showed no significant difference in survival when this procedure was compared with the classic radical mastectomy.

In 1980 Veronesi reported the results of a large, randomized, prospective trial in Italy in which breast tumors 2 cm or less with palpable axillary nodes were randomized to treatment either with radical mastectomy or with "quadrantectomy" (the quadrant of breast in the area of the tumor was removed) plus total axillary node dissection and radiotherapy. Local recurrence rates and survival were the same in both groups. In 1985 Fisher reported the results of the National Surgical Adjuvant Breast Project (NSABP) study that compared three arms of therapy for lesions 4 cm or smaller in diameter with or without palpable axillary lymph nodes. The treatment modalities were modified radical mastectomy, removal of the tumor with a rim of normal tissue, plus removal of lower axillary nodes, plus postoperative radiotherapy; the third group was like the second except that radiation was omitted. Survival and local recurrence were statistically the same in both the first and second arm. In the third arm, patients with local excision and removal of the lower axillary nodes, but without radiation therapy, had a very high local recurrence rate of 24 percent in lymph node negative patients and 36 percent in node positive patients (Fig. 15-20). This finding seems to support the multicentric nature of breast cancer and to indicate that the entire breast on the involved side should be treated. The choice of such treatment may have to be left to bias of the surgeon and the wishes of the patient. The conclusions of the NSABP study are based on 5-year actuarial results and will be firmer if they hold up over time. Past experience from other series suggests that the results will continue to be valid (Fig. 15-21).

The great advantage of sparing the breast by using local excision is the encouragement it gives patients to approach diagnosis and treatment early enough to be eligible for such treatment.

In addition to excision of the local breast mass, the axillary lymph nodes should be removed. The value of removing axillary contents has been defended in the past on the claim of improved survival. The results of controlled cooperative clinical trials indicate that treatment of the axilla does not change survival in patients with clinical Stage I tumors. On the other hand, the added information gained by knowing whether or not axillary nodes are his-

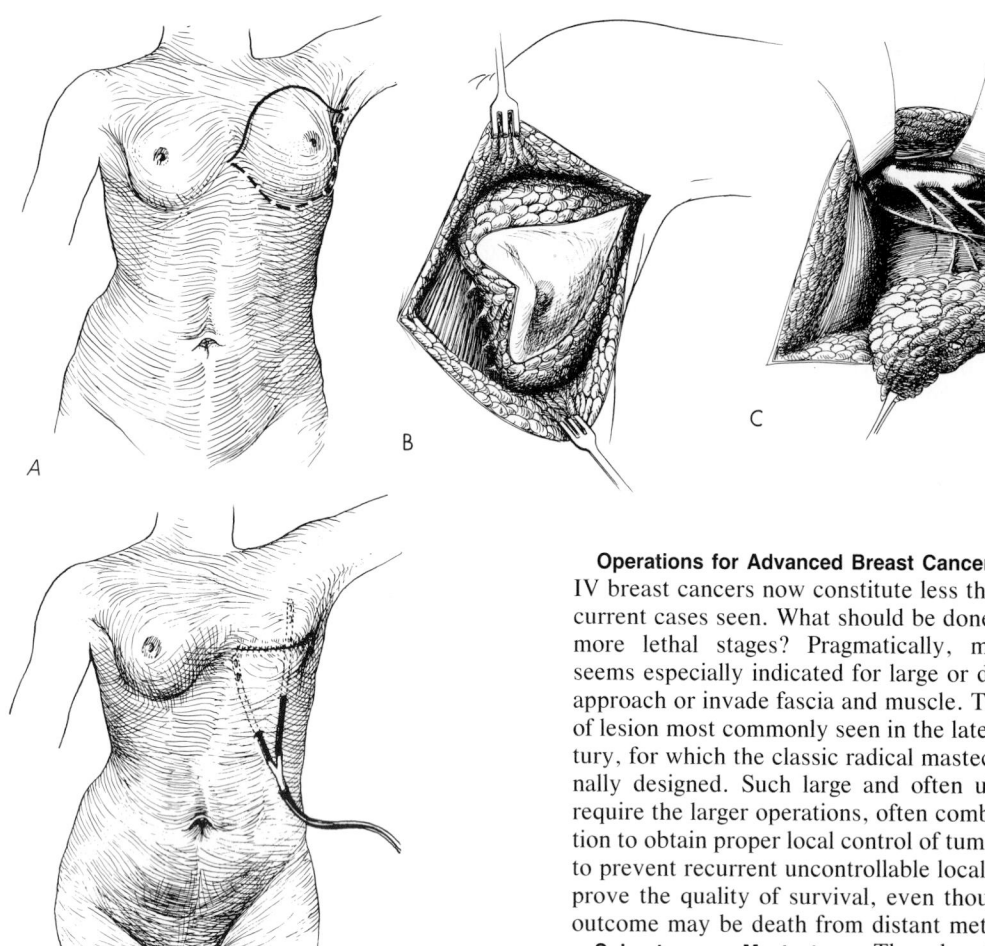

Fig. 15-19. Technique of total mastectomy and axillary dissection (modified radical mastectomy). *A.* Transverse elliptical incision facilitates subsequent reconstruction. *B.* Development of skin flaps. *C.* Clearing of the axillary vein and axilla en bloc with breast. This provides optimal sampling of lymph nodes. The pectoralis major and minor muscles are retracted medially. *D.* Suction drainage obviates accumulation of fluid beneath flaps and allows a small dressing.

tologically involved by malignancy is of enormous value to surgeons and patients, both in rendering an accurate prognosis and in influencing the trend of future therapy. The addition of axillary dissection to breast resection adds very little in risk or morbidity, and the dividend in "staging" the extent of the disease is well worth the price whether survival is improved or not. While "sampling" the lower axilla has been suggested as adequate, several studies indicate that accurate staging is correlated with the completeness of the axillary dissection. In patients treated by local excision and radiation, complete removal of the axillary nodes obviates the need for axillary, supraclavicular radiation, greatly simplifying the radiotherapeutic approach.

Operations for Advanced Breast Cancer. Stages III and IV breast cancers now constitute less than 20 percent of current cases seen. What should be done for these much more lethal stages? Pragmatically, muscle resection seems especially indicated for large or deep tumors that approach or invade fascia and muscle. This was the type of lesion most commonly seen in the late nineteenth century, for which the classic radical mastectomy was originally designed. Such large and often ulcerated tumors require the larger operations, often combined with radiation to obtain proper local control of tumor. The object is to prevent recurrent uncontrollable local disease and improve the quality of survival, even though the eventual outcome may be death from distant metastasis.

Subcutaneous Mastectomy. The advent of mammography has led to an increasing diagnosis of in situ (TIS) and very small microinvasive cancers (T1a). This has coincided with the introduction of subcutaneous mastectomy, a technique in which most of the mammary tissue is removed but the skin of the breast is preserved. Contour is restored by inserting a silastic prosthesis into the subcutaneous pocket left by the excision of breast tissue or now, more commonly, under the pectoralis major muscle. It is impossible to remove all breast tissue by this method, and 1 or 2 percent remains in the subcutaneous layer near the skin even if the nipple is sacrificed. Development of cancer in this residual mammary tissue has been reported, and in view of the multifocal nature of breast cancer, it is expected that some of the foci may be left behind. The risk benefit ratio of this approach remains to be established, and while it is a very attractive alternative for women with in situ cancer of the breast, the accepted procedure for such lesions in the United States is still total mastectomy or possibly radiation therapy.

The Problem of Bilateral Mastectomy. Foote and Stewart have observed that "the most frequent precancerous lesion of the breast is a cancer of the opposite breast." Berg and Robbins noted that the incidence of occurrence of cancer in the contralateral breast following radical mastectomy was approximately 1 percent per year, so that

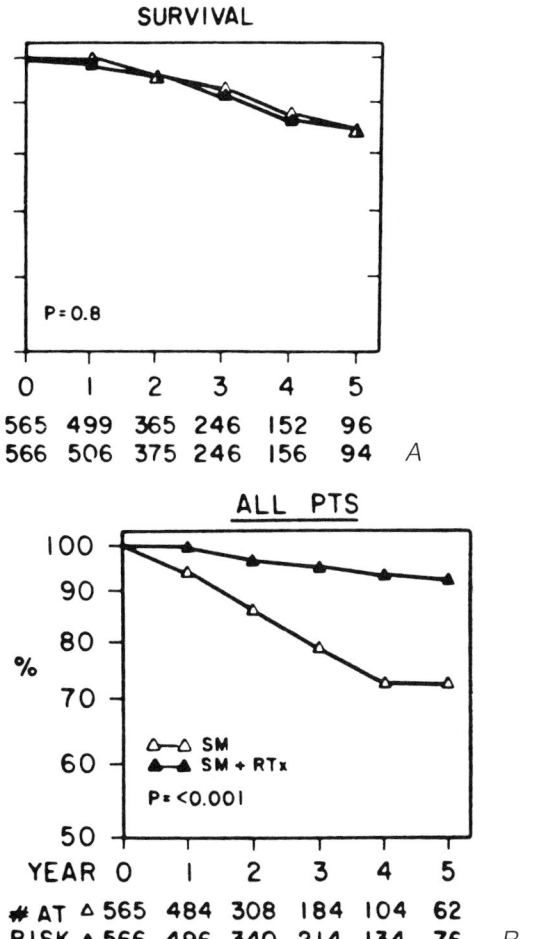

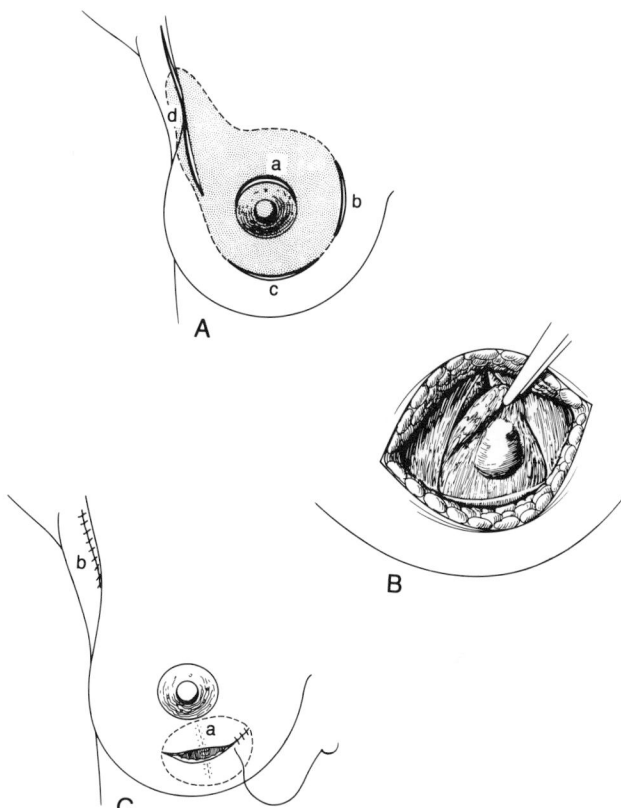

Fig. 15-20. *A.* Survival in patients with segmental mastectomy compared with segmental resection plus radiation. The curves are virtually identical. *B.* Disease-free survival in patients with segmental mastectomy alone, compared with patients with segmental mastectomy plus radiation. (From: *Fisher B et al: N Engl J Med 312:655, 1985, with permission.*)

Fig. 15-21. Technique of segmental mastectomy. *A.* Because of the circumferential skin lines of the breast a circumferential incision gives the best cosmetic results. If the tumor is relatively small and close to the nipple, a periareolar incision, as shown in Aa, is chosen; otherwise circumferential incisions directly over the main body of the tumor as shown in Ab and c should be used. Tumors in the upper outer quadrant, especially close to the axillae, can best be approached through an incision that lies along the tail of the breast and extends into the axillae, parallel to the fibers of the pectoralis major muscle. This incision gives the best access to the outer quadrant, tail of the breast, and axillary contents simultaneously. *B.* This illustrates the approach to a breast tumor through a circumferential incision. Dissection is carried down through the fat until the breast tissue is revealed. Skin and fat are undermined in a radial direction, both away and toward the nipple. A wedge-shaped excision of the full thickness of breast tissue containing the tumor with a 1- to 2-cm margin of normal tissue is removed. *C.* Closure of the incision. The excision of breast tissue has left a wedge-shaped defect in the disclike breast. Rotating the two cut edges of the breast toward each other will result in a nice anatomical closure along a radial line. (a) The skin and fat must have been undermined sufficiently so that the breast tissue will slide together without distorting the skin. The skin is then closed in a circumferential direction using subcuticular sutures. Note that the axillary dissection is not done in continuity except for lesions of the upper outer quadrant. An incision slightly posterior and parallel with the upper lateral border of the pectoralis major muscle (b) provides the best cosmetic approach since it is totally hidden from view and also provides the best exposure to all levels of the axillae.

the cumulative risk of cancer in the remaining breast among patients surviving radical mastectomy for 20 years was as high as 20 percent. As long ago as 1951, Pack published a plea for routine simple mastectomy of the remaining breast at the time of mastectomy for cancer. Presumably because of the psychologic blow to a woman who is asked to lose both her breasts, this approach has rarely been advocated by surgeons, and the usual routine after mastectomy has been to follow the contralateral breast with special care in the ensuing years. The recognition of the high risk of contralateral cancer in patients with in situ lobular carcinoma has caused a change in attitude toward this particular form of the disease. Currently recommended treatment for patients with either in situ or invasive lobular cancer of the breast is total mastectomy of the contralateral breast. Treatment of the other breast with radiation therapy instead may be effective since the

NSABP study seems to establish the effectiveness of radiation therapy for microscopic disease. This inference has not been established by any clinical trials. Should this recommendation be refused, the patient is requested at least to permit a biopsy of the remaining breast. If this biopsy reveals in situ lobular cancer, a total mastectomy is carried out. If invasive lobular cancer is found, modified radical mastectomy is done. If the biopsy is negative, a very careful follow-up is recommended, with mammography and careful breast examination at least twice yearly.

A minority of physicians recommend a "watch" policy for in situ lobular carcinoma. They reason that only one-third of these lesions ultimately become invasive, and that even the invasive lesions of this tumor have a better prognosis than the usual invasive ductal lesion. Close follow-up would thus preserve a substantial number of women from what might be an unnecessary mastectomy. This view of therapy has not proved popular among patients and surgeons. Most women are uneasy about harboring a malignant breast lesion even if it is preinvasive, and most surgeons share this feeling. Moreover, the transition from preinvasive to invasive may go undetected for long periods, since it is not necessarily accompanied by any clinical signs.

OPERATIVE MORTALITY. This is very low for all the various types of mastectomy. Kennedy and Miller reported no deaths following 212 simple mastectomies; Handley and Thackray reported no deaths following 143 modified radical mastectomies; Butcher reported 0.7 percent mortality in 425 radical mastectomies; and Haagensen and his associates had no deaths in 556 radical mastectomies. In all these series any death of a patient up to 3 months after operation was considered an operative death. Even among patients with extended mastectomy, mortality is low. Sugarbaker reported 1 postoperative death in 250 patients with this procedure.

ADJUVANT THERAPY FOLLOWING OPERATIONS FOR BREAST CANCER. The most rewarding event in breast cancer therapy in recent years is the demonstration that adjuvant chemotherapy in high-risk patients contributes substantially to relapse-free long-term survival. This has served as a model for trials of adjuvant therapy in other cancers as well. Fisher deserves the chief credit for first recognizing that early trials of a very brief course of triethylene ethiophosphonamide (Thiotepa) given during and immediately after operation produced a decrease in recurrence rate in long-term follow-up of a small subset of younger patients. As principal investigator of the National Surgical Adjuvant Breast Project (NSABP), he conducted extensive adjuvant studies of a single drug L-PAM (L-phenylalanine mustard), which confirmed his early observation. Bonadonna and his group at the Milan Tumor Institute then found that a three-drug combination of methotrexate, cytoxan, and 5-fluorouracil (CMF) was also effective, and Fisher confirmed in comparative trials that a two-drug combination of L-PAM and 5-FU was superior to L-PAM alone for adjuvant therapy. When several drugs are used in adequate dosages, it also appears that patients in all age groups benefit, rather than only the younger patients who responded to the older one-drug protocols (Fig. 15-22). Bonadonna and others have reported that 6 months of postoperative adjuvant therapy with CMF is as effective as 12 months. The impressive benefit of adjuvant therapy is demonstrated by a report from the South Western Oncology Group (SWOG) in which multidrug adjuvant therapy consisting of CMF plus vincristine and prednisone produced a 5-year relapse-free survival rate of 88 percent in women with one to three positive axillary nodes compared with the 50 percent relapse-free survival rate that occurs in this group without adjuvant treatment. Currently the most frequently used adjuvant therapy following operations for breast cancer is CMF. While this was originally recommended only for women with three or more positive axillary nodes, the present trend has been to use it in any patient with one or more grossly positive axillary nodes. Adjuvant chemotherapy of patients with low-risk Stage I lesions is not recommended, since the mortality due to cancer in this group is less than 10 percent at 5 and 10 years, and long-term hazards of chemotherapeutic drugs, especially the alkylating agents, have not been fully determined. There is some evidence that these are carcinogenic and may themselves induce some cancers. However, considerable effort is being expended to identify subsets of patients at high risk for recurrence. Even when the lesion is Stage I, such patients would be likely candidates for adjuvant therapy.

If a postmenopausal patient has an estrogen-receptor positive tumor, the adjuvant treatment of choice is the antiestrogen, tamoxifen, which will confer a survival advantage at least as good as and probably better than chemotherapy in such patients. Current recommendations of a consensus panel at the NIH for adjuvant therapy for women not on a clinical trial are: for premenopausal node positive women, chemotherapy; for premenopausal node negative women, no adjuvant therapy; for node positive, ER positive, postmenopausal women, tamoxifen; for postmenopausal node negative or node positive, ER negative women, no therapy.

For many decades radiotherapy was the conventional adjuvant therapy used in all patients following radical mastectomy when axillary nodes were found to contain tumor. Multiple randomized clinical trials carried out in the 1950s and 1960s revealed that such radiotherapy had no effect on relapse-free survival or on mortality. Local recurrence rates were favorably affected, with reductions of as much as 50 percent. Most recently the trend has been to advise radiotherapy following operation only in patients at high risk for local recurrence. Even this practice is now debated because a randomized trial indicates that multiple-drug chemotherapy given postoperatively is a substantially superior adjuvant treatment compared with the same drugs given after radiotherapy.

PROGNOSIS

The arguments for and against different forms of therapy in breast cancer are mainly statistical and are chiefly based on survival figures. Before an observer can appreciate this debate, a clear understanding of the data is required. The accurate comparison of results in different series demands that there be a common denominator.

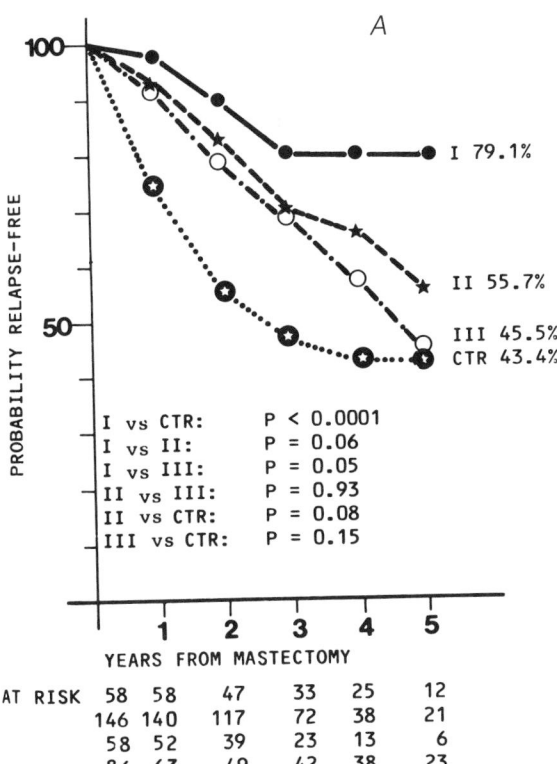

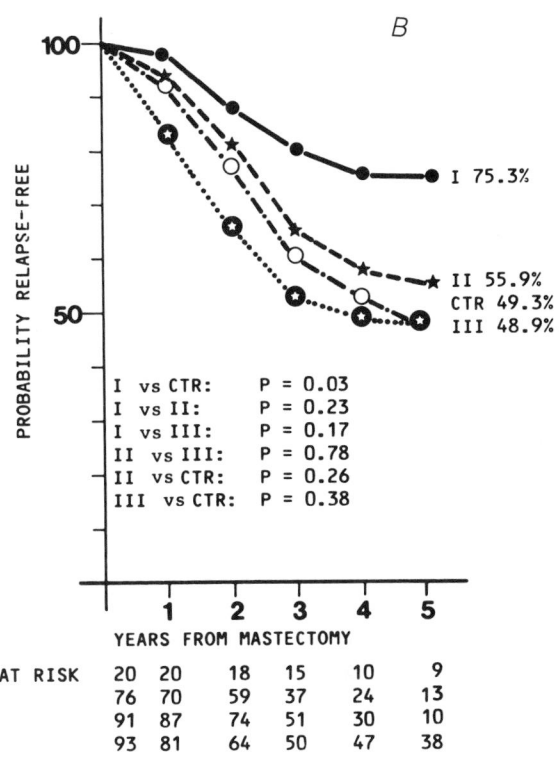

Fig. 15-22. *A.* Relationship of relapse-free survival to dose level in 348 premenopausal patients. The dose levels are indicated by I (>85 percent of the optimal calculated dose), II (65 to 84 percent), and III (<65 percent); CTR denotes controls. The percentages beside the dose levels show the proportion of patients who did not have relapses during the 5 years. *B.* Relationship of relapse-free survival to dose levels in 280 postmenopausal patients; abbreviations are the same as in *A.* Significantly superior and comparable survival occurred in both premenopausal and postmenopausal patients when adequate dosages of CMF were used. (From: *Bonadonna G et al: Cancer Treat Rep 65:61, 1981, with permission.*)

There is great variation in the base line of many published series, and astute investigation is often necessary to determine whether two sets of figures are truly comparable.

An older method of standard reporting required that all patients seen at an institution be reported in the final results, whether they were treated or not. This was called the "absolute," or "crude," survival figure. It had the advantage of indicating the effect of patient selection on the surgical, or "definitive," survival figures. Its disadvantage was that the total experience at different institutions varied greatly. Private hospitals and clinics have a much greater number of early and operable cases compared with cancer hospitals and charity institutions.

Favorable attention has been given to methods of clinical evaluation of the stage of the tumor. By this method the results in patients at an equal stage of disease can be compared among institutions. An advantage of this approach is that since the evaluation is based on pretreatment clinical findings, it is possible to compare the results in patients treated by radiation, radical mastectomy, simple mastectomy, or extended radical mastectomy even though microscopic evaluation of lymph node involvement is available with some forms of treatment and not with others. Disadvantages are that judgment of the extent of involvement is subjective and classification depends greatly on the skill and consistency of the examiner. The system of staging recommended by the American Joint Committee on Cancer Staging and End Results Reporting is most widely accepted (Table 15-1). Other systems include the Columbia classification, the Manchester classification, and the Steinthal classification; these are now obsolete.

New diagnostic methods, especially mammography, have provided a new group of lesions not previously considered by any of the staging methods. Termed by some "minimal breast cancer," these are in situ and microinvasive lesions so small that they are not detectable by conventional palpation of the breast. Current data indicate that 5-year survivals in this group exceed 90 percent.

The best way to evaluate methods of treatment is by cooperative programs among many institutions in which all factors are governed by the same rules and in which random selection of patients for the different methods of therapy is used. Even these trials are not an easy solution to the problem. Such trials tend to be biased toward false-negative results. Only in the largest of the cooperative trials is the chance of error in a negative result reduced to under 10 percent.

NO TREATMENT. In 1951 Park and Lees in a statistical analysis of 5-year survival figures for breast carcinoma tried to show that the course of the disease was not affected by operation. They regarded the improvement in 5-year survival seen following operation as an artifact introduced by operating upon patients earlier in the natural course of the disease. There are now available a number of studies of large groups of patients with untreated breast cancer. Survival computed from the onset of symptoms averages 19 percent at 5 years, 2.5 percent at 10 years. If one computes survival from onset of diagnosis, a figure more comparable with the situation in surgical series, the 5- and 10-year survivals average 8.6 percent and 1.2 percent, respectively. Bloom et al. found that untreated patients with histologically low-grade (grade 1 of 3) neoplasms had survivals of 22 percent, 9 percent, and 0 at 5, 10, and 15 years, respectively. They compared these with survivals of 82, 56, and 37 percent at the same time intervals for lesions of comparable histologic grade in their own treated series (Fig. 15-12).

OPERATIVE THERAPY. If survival data following operative therapy from the introduction of the radical mastectomy to the present are examined, one may wonder why there has been argument and confusion (Fig. 15-23). Dean Lewis and William Reinhoff reported in 1942 that the overall 5-year survival of 393 patients treated at the Johns Hopkins Hospital between 1889 and 1931 was 18 percent, little better than Bloom et al.'s untreated patients. In 1973 the American Joint Committee on Cancer Staging reported in a collected series of 2424 patients treated from 1950 to 1957 an overall survival of 61 percent. Haid and Zuckerman examined the results in 560 patients between

1973 and 1977 and found the 5-year survival was 81 percent. In the first two series the standard operation was radical mastectomy; in the last group most patients underwent modified radical mastectomy. Early diagnosis appears a major factor influencing the change in mortality. The Joint Committee patients had Stage I lesions in 17 percent, while the Haid and Zuckerman patients were classified Stage I in 51 percent. Only 19 percent of their patients were Stage III or IV. Even in this last group there was an improvement in survival, probably because 78 of 288 Stages II and III patients received multidrug therapy following operation. The end result is that the National Cancer Institute and a number of state tumor registries have reported small but steady increases in 5-year survivals in patients with both regional and localized disease since about 1950. Epidemiologic reports from Connecticut and Saskatchewan, Canada, establish a significant increase in the incidence of breast cancer in the last several decades accompanied by a decrease in mortality, thus implying an increase in survival (Fig. 15-24). This trend has continued to the present.

Survival for 5 years following radical mastectomy does not provide the same assurance against recurrence that it does for some other cancers. The risk of death continues higher than for the general population for at least 25 years after the operation, although this risk gradually diminishes with time. According to Berg and Robbins, change in risk over the postoperative period follows a log-normal curve. From this model it can be predicted that after operation the risk of recurrence and death will continue to decrease but will always be present, being about 1 percent in the decade from 30 to 40 years after operation and 0.5 percent from 40 to 50 years after operation.

Our attitudes concerning survival and prognosis continue to be conditioned by our beliefs concerning the natural history of the disease. Mueller has reported data indicating that survival following treatment of breast cancer follows an exponential curve, that is, that the annual risk of recurrence and death remains constant and if patients lived long enough all would eventually die of their tumor. If true, this would imply that all tumors have disseminated and metastasized before clinical detection and treatment. In this circumstance treatment is effective only by altering the slope of the curve and delaying the ultimate death due to the cancer, long enough, it may be hoped, so that the patient dies of other "more natural" causes. This hypothesis is in conflict with the data of Berg and Robbins cited above and those of Blackwood and Rush, who indicated that the hazard function or risk of annual recurrence decreases significantly over time, following a well-known survival curve called the Weibull distribution. Duncan and Kerr have examined a large series of patients treated in the 1940s with a follow-up of 20 or more years. Their data indicate that the "curability" of Stages I and II patients in their era was 30.5 percent (Fig. 15-25). If only lesions of 1 cm were considered without positive nodes clinically, 20-year survival was 90 percent.

Koscielny and his coauthors suggest that there is a critical volume or threshold for each tumor at which the first

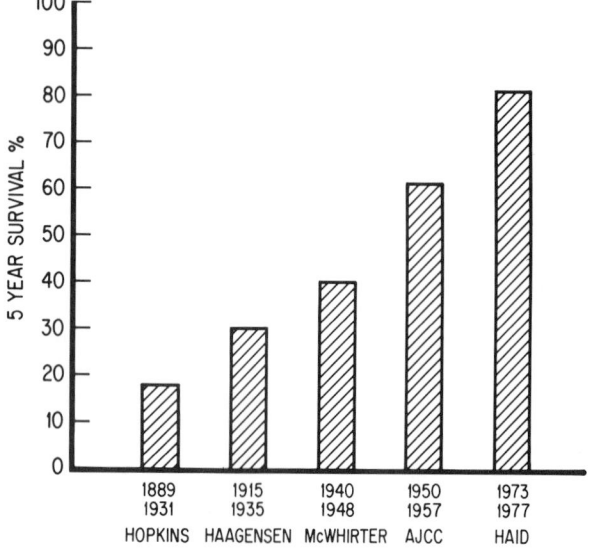

Fig. 15-23. This graph illustrates the startling increase in 5-year survival in patients with "operable" (i.e., Stages I, II, and III) breast cancer in the past century regardless of the mode of therapy. The Hopkins series, the Haagensen series, and the American Joint Committee on Cancer series were treated by radical mastectomy; McWhirter's patients were treated with total mastectomy and radiation therapy; and those in the Haid series were treated with modified radical mastectomy, and in some patients adjuvant chemotherapy was used.

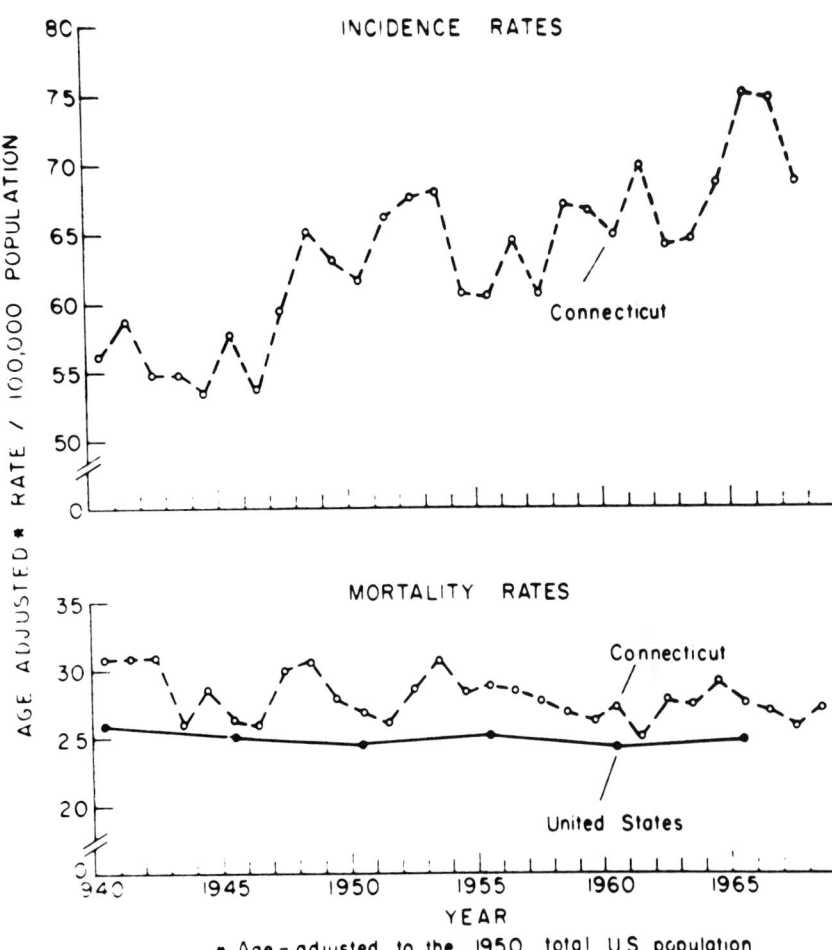

Fig. 15-24. Contrary to past reports data from large population groups now indicate an increasing incidence and a decreasing mortality rate for breast cancer. (From: *Cutler SJ, Christine B, Barcley THC: Cancer 28:1376, 1971, with permission.*)

Fig. 15-25. "Curability" of breast cancer as determined in a group of patients treated 20 or more years. Survival rate in Stages I and II patients parallels the normal population at 20 years, and projection to the base line indicates that 30.5 percent of such patients are curable. (From: *Brinkley D, Haybittle JL: World J Surg 1:287, 1977, with permission.*)

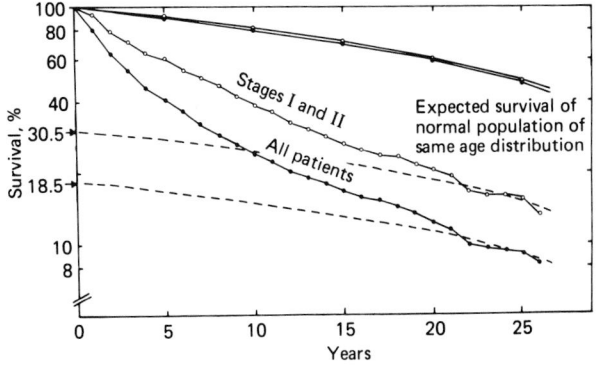

remote metastasis is initiated. The smaller and more well differentiated a tumor is the less likely it is that distant spread will have occurred and the more likely that locoregional methods will cure the lesion.

Radical mastectomy is no longer the routine treatment for all patients with cancer of the breast, and most agree that there is a group of smaller cancers that can be treated by lesser procedures. It is still, however, the reference procedure, the operation with which we have the most experience over the greatest period of time. Comparisons between institutional series have little or no statistical validity at this level of discrimination, and one must turn to the rapidly accumulating data from controlled cooperative clinical trials.

Prognosis for Early Breast Cancer. The current outlook for patients with Stage I breast cancer treated by radical or modified radical mastectomy is remarkably good. Haid and Zuckerman found a 5-year survival of 95 percent in patients with Stage I lesions and 80 percent in patients with Stage II lesions; modified radical mastectomy was the treatment in both groups. The availability of effective adjuvant chemotherapy has provoked an intense search for subsets of patients with early breast cancer who have a poorer prognosis than expected and who would be candidates for adjuvant therapy. Nealon et al. used four histologic criteria to define such high-risk patients: poor cytologic differentiation, lymphatic permeation, blood vessel invasion, and poor circumscription (invasion of tumor into surrounding soft tissues). Using these criteria in a retrospective analysis of patients with negative axillary nodes and tumors 2 cm or less in diameter, they found that all 83 patients classed as low risk survived 10 years and only one had recurrence of disease. Of those with one or more risk criteria, 50 percent had recurrence of tumor within 10 years.

Other criteria of high risk and a poor prognosis not included in the TMN clinical system are rapid growth rate either by history or by evidence of a high thymidine labeling index (indicating an increased number of dividing cells); youth of the patients (the younger the patient the higher the risk); and estrogen receptor negativity.

There are only a few randomized trials that compare the results of different forms of purely *surgical* treatment. Of these the most convincing were those of the NSABP-05 trial in which total mastectomy was compared with radical mastectomy in clinical Stage I patients. Results were identical in both groups up to 10 years after operation. Forrest et al. reported the same outcome in a similar study that differed only in that patients were staged by a partial excision of axillary nodes. Helman's study from South Africa was negated because the project was stopped after 3 years. This was the only study in which clinically positive axillary nodes were *not* treated by either operation or radiation. Subsequent growth of nodes in Stage II patients caused the investigators to abandon the protocol.

Until recently the operation of choice for early cancer of the breast in this country was modified radical mastectomy. A randomized trial comparing this procedure with radical mastectomy has shown that radical and modified radical operations produce the same results.

The psychologic effects of operation would be reduced and early treatment encouraged if sacrifice of the breast were not required. This can be achieved by confining operation to partial mastectomy alone or by combining local excision or simple biopsy of breast cancer with radiation therapy.

A randomized trial of the NSABP compared two surgical arms, lumpectomy and axillary dissection, and total mastectomy with axillary dissection with a combination of lumpectomy and axillary dissection plus irradiation. Omission of treatment of the whole breast by either operation or radiation resulted in a high rate of local recurrence at 5 years, 24 percent for Stage I lesions and 38 percent for Stage II. When radiation of the breast was added to lumpectomy and axillary resection, the local recurrence was 6 percent. In addition, survival rates were slightly but significantly better in the lumpectomy and irradiation treatment arm compared with the other two. This report, together with Veronese's data from Italy, seem to support the use of lumpectomy, axillary resection, and irradiation for breast cancer tumors equal to or smaller than 4 cm in size.

Prognosis in Advanced Breast Cancer. Advanced breast cancers now constitute less than 20 percent of cases and are the lesions that fall into the Joint Committee Stages III and IV. In the recent past prognosis for these patients was bleak, averaging 15 to 20 percent survival at 5 years, little different from the survival of untreated patients. Most of these patients satisfy Haagensen's criteria of inoperability and would previously have been referred for radiation with or without a preceding total mastectomy. The use of adjuvant chemotherapy has cast a new and more hopeful light on this group. Excluding patients with overt distant metastasis (Stage IV), the prognosis for 5-year survival may be doubled in this group. Some of these patients may benefit from radical mastectomy, especially those with large local cancers but few or no axillary nodes. The possibility of controlling disseminated micrometastasis makes a strenuous effort to eliminate gross locoregional disease a rational component of therapy.

The new experiences with control of inflammatory carcinoma of the breast in premenopausal women, the most lethal of all breast cancers, may be an example of the advantages of combining numerous forms of local and systemic therapy. In a sequential series of patients at the MD Anderson Hospital, all 10 patients with inflammatory breast cancer treated by radiotherapy alone suffered relapse by 19 months (median relapse-free survival 9 months). All nine patients treated by chemotherapy and radiation relapsed by 25 months (median relapse-free survival 17 months). Seven patients were treated with chemotherapy followed by extended total mastectomy followed by immunotherapy, maintenance chemotherapy and radiation therapy. After an average follow-up of 21 months, only two patients had relapsed. A more recent report indicates a 5-year survival rate of 74 percent.

Advice to Patients. Carter has observed that controversies about the treatment of primary breast cancer have become so visible to the public that state governments are now entering the picture. In California a new law requires that breast cancer patients be informed by their physicians of the "alternative and effective methods of treatment with an explanation of their risks, advantages and disadvantages." The failure of a physician to so inform a patient would be grounds for a charge of unprofessional conduct. Massachusetts has passed a similar law, and other states are considering like measures.

Medical, surgical, and radiation oncologists are likely to deliver the message concerning breast treatment somewhat differently. In addition there are at least 90 different options for the therapy of Stage I cancer alone. In any case, my advice to patients is to accept those therapies tested by randomized clinical trials as proved effective and regard those therapies not so tested as still experimental. By these standards, total mastectomy or modified radical mastectomy are proved treatments for clinical Stage I cancer, equal in effectiveness to radical mastectomy. Partial mastectomy or lumpectomy is proved effective for tumors 4 cm or less when combined with axillary node dissection and postoperative radiation. Every pa-

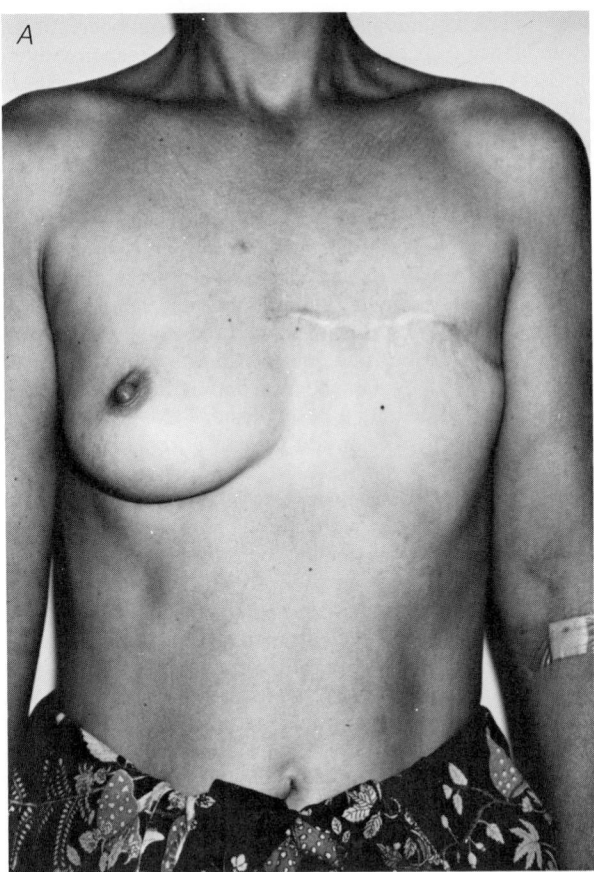 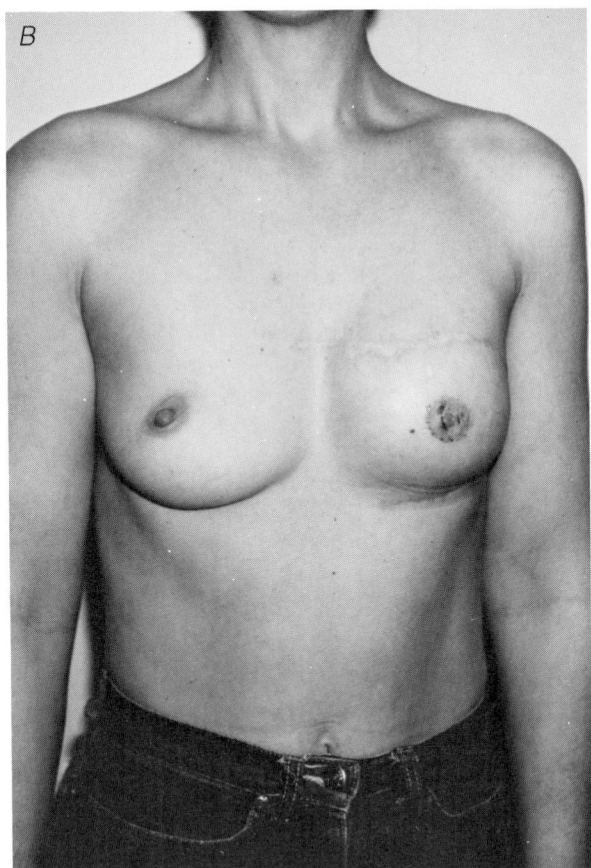

Fig. 15-26. *A.* Postoperative result following modified radical mastectomy with transverse incision. *B.* Reconstruction of the breast with subpectoral silastic implant and of the nipple using skin from the inner thigh. *(Provided by Carl G. Quillen, M.D.)*

tient with clinical Stages I and II breast cancer should have a total removal of axillary lymph nodes, not because it is a proved treatment, but because it is a proved method for effectively staging breast cancer and bringing into the treatment regimen suitably selected adjuvant therapy.

REHABILITATION. Most women require instruction in exercising the arm on the side of operation following radical mastectomy. Proper physical therapy in the immediate postoperative period should ensure complete return to normal function. Following operations that spare the pectoral muscles, full function of the arm usually returns promptly with little or no special help. Psychologic support is also important in restoring the patient's self-image and her confidence that she is still desirable to a present or future companion, or, if the breast has been preserved, that her chances of long survival are good. The Reach to Recovery program of the American Cancer Society has been most successful in providing advisors to the recent mastectomy patient from the ranks of women who have previously had the same operation.

Many women are interested in the possibility of subsequent reconstruction of the excised breast. If the previous operation was radical mastectomy, reconstruction is complex, but good restoration can be accomplished using a myocutaneous latissimus dorsi graft. In patients who have had modified radical or total mastectomy, especially if the operation was performed through a transverse incision, reconstruction with a silastic implant placed under the pectoralis major muscle is a relatively simple and feasible technique (Fig. 15-26). The result is never a perfect match for the remaining breast, and decisions about which patients will find these reconstructions worthwhile must be individualized.

TREATMENT OF RECURRENT CANCER

Prior to the 1950s recurrent cancer of the breast was treated either with radiation or operation or not at all. Radiation remains an extremely useful agent for painful osseous metastases and small subcutaneous lesions. Operation also may be useful for small local lesions. The basic problem in the patient with recurrent cancer is most often wide dissemination, and systemic agents, hormone therapy, and chemotherapy are the treatments of choice.

Selection of hormonal therapy or chemotherapy as the initial treatment of recurrent disease depends on whether the patient's tumor is hormonally sensitive. For decades the only index of hormonal sensitivity was the patient's

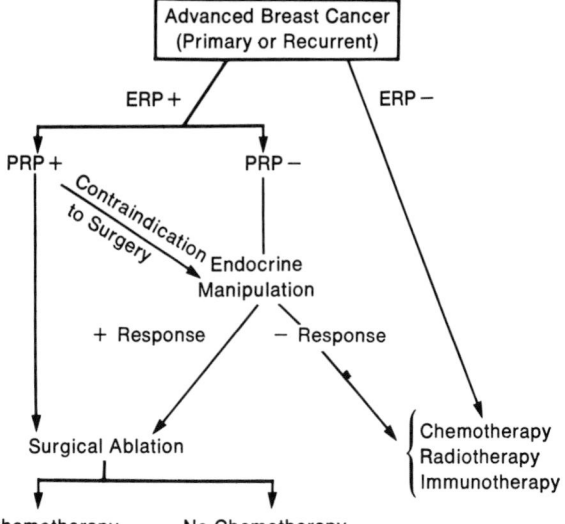

Fig. 15-27. Schema for the treatment of patients with recurrent breast cancer when determinations to estrogen receptors and progesterone receptors are available. Patients who are estrogen receptor–positive (ERP) and progesterone receptor–positive (PRP) have an 80 percent response rate to surgical ablation. (From: *Degenshein GA et al: Breast 3:29, 1977, with permission.*)

response to a trial of hormonal treatment. We now know that the response of breast cancers to hormones is dependent on the presence of hormone receptors in the substance of cancer cells. Hormonal receptors for estrogens, prolactin, progesterone, and corticosteroids have been identified. Dependable clinical tests for estrogen receptors (ER) are now widely available, and all primary cancers should be submitted for testing when first removed; 50 percent of these tumors will prove to be ER-positive. Progesterone receptors (PR) also appear to have a predictive value. Eighty percent of patients with breast cancers that have both ER and PR will respond to hormonal manipulation. Breast cancers that are ER-positive but PR-negative respond in 27 percent, those that are ER-negative and PR-positive (rare) respond in 45 percent, and those that are ER-negative and PR-negative respond in less than 10 percent. A schema for treatment of patients tested for both ER and PR is shown in Fig. 15-27. The presence of hormone receptors is a marker indicating a more differentiated tumor. Such tumors respond to all forms of therapy better than receptor-negative breast cancers.

TREATMENT OF ESTROGEN RECEPTOR–POSITIVE RECURRENT TUMORS. The choices of hormone manipulation are (1) ablation, the removal of estrogen-generating tissue by operation; (2) additive (paradoxically treatment with high doses of estrogens or progesterone is also effective); and (3) antiestrogens. All these techniques produce the same approximate result, regression in about 60 percent of ER-positive patients. Many still consider oophorectomy the therapy of choice for the menstruating pa-

tients; risk is minimal, and there is no concern about compliance over the long term. Favorable response averages 1 year in duration and predicts probable responses to further endocrine maneuvers.

For postmenopausal patients, either naturally or surgically induced, the choice is between additive and antiestrogen therapy. Of these, tamoxifen, an antiestrogen that acts by blocking estrogen receptor sites, is the current favorite. Side effects are minimal, consisting of hot flashes and a mild cytopenia in 10 to 15 percent of patients that does not become clinically important. Diethylstilbesterol, the previous drug of choice, is cheaper but produces nausea in 50 percent of patients, vomiting in 25 percent, and edema in 50 percent. Aminoglutethimide blocks the conversions of cholesterol to pregnenolone and thus inhibits the production of adrenal steroids. It also inhibits the aromatization of androsteredione to estrone in peripheral tissues. When compared with tamoxifen in randomized trials, response rates and durations of survival are similar. Toxicity, consisting of lethargy and a morbilliform rash in about 8 percent, is greater than for tamoxifen. However, patients failing tamoxifen may respond to aminoglutethimide, and it is probably useful as a secondary hormonal treatment. If aminoglutethimide is used, the patients must also receive replacement hydrocortisone or dexamethasone. The effect of aminoglutethimide is often referred to as "medical adrenalectomy," and it seems to eliminate the need for operative adrenalectomy.

TREATMENT OF ESTROGEN RECEPTOR–NEGATIVE RECURRENT TUMORS. Patients who have tumors that are estrogen receptor–negative rarely respond to estrogen ablative therapy (10 percent or less). Such patients, together with the 40 percent who fail to respond to a therapeutic trial of estrogen ablation or antiestrogens, are candidates for cancer chemotherapy. Multiple-drug regimens spaced at much longer intervals than the older single-drug programs are the current mode and have produced a doubling and even tripling of the improvement in the old results with single drugs. Arrest of tumor growth, partial remission, and even complete remissions can be expected in 65 percent of patients so treated. Because of the rapid improvement in the results of chemotherapy, there is now some controversy as to whether hormonal therapy should precede or follow chemotherapy. Wilson and Moore, among several clinicians, have combined total operative estrogen ablation with almost simultaneous cancer chemotherapy in patients with recurrent breast cancer. They suggest that the two forms of therapy work synergistically, with a better response for combination than for sequential use of these techniques when compared with historical controls. No controlled clinical trials are available to confirm this observation, and hormonal therapy remains the first treatment of recurrence at the present. Both therapies are palliative and not curative measures, and most patients will eventually receive most or all of the agents currently available. The aim of therapy is to improve the quality of life and the length of survival, but not as yet to provide cure.

Infection

ACUTE INFECTION

Bacterial infections almost always occur in the lactating breast in the first month or two following delivery. The portal of entry is an abrasion or fissure in the nipple. The best treatment is prevention, with the nursing mother carefully cleaning and drying her nipples after nursing. In general, cleanliness is important. Infections are also seasonal, being more common in the hot summer months.

The milk-containing ducts and acini of the lactating breast are a perfect culture medium, and infection, having gained access, often progresses rapidly through inflammation to suppuration. This is accompanied by extreme pain in the breast, and a good diagnostic sign of abscess is the patient's rapid withdrawal when the physician attempts to palpate the involved breast. The breast is red and the area of abscess indurated and firm. The tendency is to underestimate the size of the abscess on physical examination.

An abscess may be aborted by the use of systemic antibiotics given in the presuppurative period. Treatment of abscess, once it forms, is by surgical drainage. Antibiotics will suppress the process for a time, but it will flare up again when they are discontinued. A curvilinear transverse incision is made in the dependent portion of the breast and the gloved finger or a clamp is used to break up the many septa that separate the cavity into loculations. A rubber drain is left in the wound. Culture of the pus usually demonstrates *Staphylococcus aureus*. Pain is relieved promptly by drainage, and the surrounding inflammation subsides rapidly.

CHRONIC INFECTION

Chronic infection of the breast is now rare. Tuberculosis is the major cause, and as the incidence of this disease has decreased, so have breast lesions caused by it. The index of suspicion for this lesion should still be high in patients with AIDS or those from third world countries. The genesis of breast tuberculosis is either pleural or, more commonly, the breaking down of a mediastinal node to involve one of the costal cartilages. Infection simmers in the cartilage for long periods, giving rise to lesions in the breast, which eventually form one or several fistulas to the skin. Antituberculosis drugs are now the primary treatment for this disease, but care of the breast lesion usually requires excision of the affected costal cartilage.

Bibliography

General

Haagensen CD: *Diseases of the Breast,* 2d ed. Philadelphia, Saunders, 1971.
McKenna R, Murphy G: *Fundamentals of Surgical Oncology.* New York, Macmillan, 1986.
Nealon T: *Problems in General Surgery: Controversies in Cancer of the Breast and Colon.* Philadelphia, Lippincott, 1985.

Anatomy and Development

Batson OV: The function of the vertebral veins and their role in the spread of metastasis. *Ann Surg* 112:138, 1940.
Cooper Sir AP: *The Anatomy and Diseases of the Breast.* Philadelphia, Lea and Blanchard, 1845.
Ingleby H, Gershon-Cohen J: *Cooperative Anatomy: Pathology and Roentgenology of the Breast.* Philadelphia, University of Pennsylvania Press, 1960.
Taylor GT: Anatomy of the breast with particular reference to lymphatic drainage, in Parson WH: *Cancer of the Breast.* Springfield, IL, Charles C Thomas, 1959.

Examination

Clark RL, Copeland MM, et al: Reproducibility of the technic of mammography (Egan) for cancer of the breast. *Am J Surg* 109:127, 1965.
Fagerberg G, Baldetorp L., et al: Effects of repeated mammographic screening on breast cancer stage distribution. Results from a randomized study of 92,934 women in a Swedish county. *Acta Radiol (Oncol)* 24:465, 1985.
Gershon-Cohen J, Berger SM: Detection of breast cancer by periodic x-ray examinations: A five-year survey. *JAMA,* 176:1114, 1961.
Gershon-Cohen J, Berger SM, Klickstein HS: Roentgenography of breast cancer moderating concept of "biologic predeterminism." *Cancer* 16:961, 1963.
Gershon-Cohen J, Ingleby H: Roentgenography of unsuspected carcinoma of breast. *JAMA* 166:869, 1958.
Heywang S, Hahn D, et al: MR imaging of the breast using godolinium DTPA. *J Comput Assist Tomogr* 10:199, 1986.
Horwitz R, Lamas A, Peck D: Mammographic parenchymal patterns and risk of breast cancer in postmenopausal women. *Am J Med* 77:621, 1984.
Ingleby H, Moore L, Gershon-Cohen J: A roentgenographic study of the growth rate of six "early" cancers of the breast. *Cancer* 11:726, 1958.
Snyder RE: Mammography and lobular carcinoma in situ. *Surg Gynecol Obstet* 122:255, 1966.
Treves N, Holleb AI: Cancer of the male breast: a report of 146 cases. *Cancer* 8:1239, 1955.
Watt C, Ackerman L, et al: Differentiation between benign and malignant diseases of the breast using digital subtraction angiography of the breast. *Cancer* 56:1287, 1985.

Neoplasms

Abramson DJ: Delayed mastectomy after outpatient breast biopsy. *Am J Surg* 132:596, 1976.
Adair F, Berg J, et al: Long-term follow-up of breast cancer patients: The 30-year report. *Cancer* 33:1145, 1974.
Baclesse F: Five-year results in 431 breast cancers treated solely by roentgen rays. *Ann Surg* 161:103, 1965.
Baker LH: Breast cancer detection demonstration project: Five-year summary report. *CA* 32:194, 1982.
Barrows G, Anderson T, et al: Fine needle aspiration of breast cancer: Relationship of clinical factors to cytology results in 689 malignancies. *Cancer* 58:1493, 1986.
Berg JW, Robbins GF: Factors influencing short and long-term survival of breast cancer patients. *Surg Gynecol Obstet* 122:1311, 1966.
Blackwood JM, Seelig RF, et al: Survival distribution in breast cancer. *Surgery* 82:443, 1977.

HISTORICAL BACKGROUND

The head and neck are such public regions of the anatomy that one would expect ancient medical manuscripts to give considerable attention to tumors affecting these parts. Strangely, the ancient writers rarely mention such lesions. The Smith Papyrus (2300 B.C.) mentions wounds of the head frequently, but not a single tumor of the area is discussed. The Ebers Papyrus (1500 B.C.) contains references to "eating ulcer" of the gums and "illness of the tongue," but the descriptions are too brief to be adequately interpreted. Celsus (A.D. 178) is often credited with devising an operation for cancer of the lower lip. Martin notes that Celsus recognized and described cancer of the skin or the face, but his operation on the lower lip was for repair of a "mutilation," probably a war wound.

A perusal of *The Surgery of Theodoric* (A.D. 1267) in the translation of Campbell and Colton gives an interesting perspective of the personal experiences of a master surgeon of the era who had a profound knowledge of the writings of preceding centuries. Theodoric describes numerous lesions about the head and neck, mostly of minor significance, i.e., wens, "white pustules or spots which appear by the nose and over the cheeks," "lumps or swellings occurring on the head called horns," "nodes or wens which are formed on the eyelids," lipoma, pustules on the face, freckles, brown patches, wrinkles, and black and blue spots on the face. There is a lengthy section on "the scrofula." He had a much clearer concept of cancer than most of his contemporaries, but in his entire writing he does not mention the treatment of a single lesion of the lip or intraoral area.

This frequent failure to single out cancerous lesions in this area reflects the inability of our medical ancestors to differentiate grossly between chronic infections and cancer. Certainly some miraculous cures were achieved by ointments and spells applied to hard, round ulcers which, in fact, were chronic infections. An early, operable lesion was certain to be treated at length with salves and potions, and when it was evident beyond doubt that the treatment had failed, it was too late to do anything else.

Galen had established firmly the concept that cancer was a systemic disease, an oversupply of black bile. It made more sense by this concept to treat the systemic cause of the affliction by "proper balancing of the constitution" with bleeding or purging or hot and cold baths than it did to attack directly a symptom of the internal problem that happened to occur on the face or in the mouth. The beginnings of rational operations for cancer awaited the discovery of cancer's primary origin in the various organs and the ability to differentiate cancer grossly and microscopically from other confusingly similar diseases.

In addition to the problems of diagnosis, extensive cancer operations were impossible without anesthesia. Even minor operations about the head and neck were few when the patient had to be conscious to witness them. The gruesome habit of excising the tongue for torture and punishment is as old as man, but the first such excision for cancer is attributed to Marchette in 1664. Avicenna (980–1037) described excision of tumors of the lip, the wound being left open to heal by secondary intention, but the classic V excision for cancer of the lip was not described until the first part of the nineteenth century. Tracheotomy to relieve laryngeal obstruction was described by Galen and through the ages was occasionally used to prolong somewhat the lives of those with carcinoma of the larynx, but laryngectomy was not accomplished until the late nineteenth century.

With the advent of anesthesia and microscopic pathology in the mid-1800s, operative attack upon cancer in all areas moved swiftly forward. This was especially true of tumors of the head and neck, since they involved easily seen structures and were so readily diagnosed and the suffering of the untreated patients was so apparent. Surgeons of the German school introduced an array of new techniques for operations upon the tongue, gingiva, mandible, maxilla, and larynx. Partial laryngectomy was introduced by Gurdon Buck in 1853, and total laryngectomy for cancer was first accomplished by Billroth in 1873.

In general, the results of these new procedures were more horrifying than gratifying. Operations in a septic field and without antibiotics produced a postoperative complication rate close to 100 percent with cellulitis, sepsis, abscess, pneumonia, and death the common results. Mortality rates exceeded 50 percent. Moreover, the results of many of the early and unsophisticated operations were not much better than if the cancer had not been treated. Billroth's famous first laryngectomy left the patient with an open pharyngostome and esophagostome, so that he constantly drooled saliva over his neck and had to feed himself with a rubber tube during the entire 8 months that he survived operation.

Operative excision was usually confined to the primary lesion, and in many of the patients fortunate enough to survive the initial operation metastatic disease subsequently developed in cervical nodes. Kocher and Butlin recognized this problem early and recommended excision of the lymphatic contents of the anterior triangle of the neck together with the removal of the primary lesion in the mouth.

At the turn on the century Crile devised radical neck dissection, removing all lymphatic tissue in both the anterior and posterior triangles of the neck together with the jugular vein and the sternocleidomastoid muscle. The basic elements of his classic procedure remain valid to the present.

Patients were willing to risk the high morbidity and mortality of operations in this region because the relentless progress of untreated disease offered a slow death by asphyxia, malnutrition, and eventual hemorrhage. Even the slimmest chance of avoiding this terrible triad seemed worthwhile.

As Crile was developing his operation for treating the cervical lymph nodes, radiation therapy for cancer was introduced. This, it was quickly apparent, offered a preferable alternative to operation, especially for primary lesions of the skin and oral cavity. Until the end of the 1930s most radical operations for cancers of the head and neck were abandoned, and the primary therapy was radiation. Techniques of radiation therapy became more refined and more successful. External radiation replaced radium as the treatment of choice, and fractionated therapy replaced the use of single applications of radium or a single dose of external therapy. With each refinement the percentage of patients who were cured increased. It was soon found that metastatic deposits in the neck did not respond as well to radiation as to operation, and radical neck dissection remained in use. Occasionally, patients who failed to respond to radiation or who had recurrent cancers were submitted to one or another of the old radical procedures. But when these operations were performed in a heavily irradiated fibrotic field, wound breakdown and complications often resembled the results of surgical treatment of the prior century.

In the 1940s, the introduction of endotracheal anesthesia, liberal use of blood transfusions, and antibiotics markedly changed the ability of surgeons to operate in and about the oral cavity. Postoperative morbidity and mortality dropped to a reasonable level. Radiation therapy, so long dominant in the treatment of oral lesions, seemed at a plateau with much dissatisfaction concerning the morbidity of overtreatment. These factors led to a reevaluation of operation. Grant Ward of The Johns Hopkins Hospital and Hayes Martin of the Memorial Center for Cancer led in devising combined operations whereby the primary lesions and the cervical contents were removed in a single block.

Application of this principle improved substantially the prognosis of patients with head and neck carcinomas, especially large lesions involving the oral cavity, hypopharynx, and larynx. In some institutions the pendulum swung from almost exclusive use of radiotherapy to almost exclusive use of operation. Increasing application of these combined operations during the 1950s made possible an evaluation of their mortality, morbidity, and effectiveness. By the end of the decade the place for surgical control of head and neck lesions was much more clearly defined and accepted.

Because of the late development of operative therapy after the long period of dormancy during the radiation era, this field of surgery is still something of a frontier with rapid developments of new techniques and the evolution of new ideas and approaches.

In the meantime, radiation therapy also acquired new techniques. Supervoltage radiation, originally with cobalt 60 and later with linear accelerators, delivered higher doses of therapy with a decreased morbidity, especially sparing the patient's skin and leaving a field more suitable for operation when this was required. Radiotherapists and surgeons who previously tended to disparage the results of each other's methods and to advance their own techniques as the primary treatment for tumors suddenly found that there was considerable common ground for the two methods and that there were patients who frequently could benefit from both operation and radiation as a planned course of integrated treatment.

Detection of most lesions of the head and neck is relatively easy, since the majority are readily available to the eye and the examining finger. Even so, it is tragic to find how often malignant lesions of this area are overlooked, not only lesions more difficult to diagnose, as in the maxillary sinuses and hypopharynx, but lesions readily visualized, such as tumors or the floor of the mouth, tongue, and tonsil.

DIAGNOSIS

Physical Examination

SKIN. The skin (see Chap. 14) of the face and neck should be closely scrutinized, keeping in mind that basal and squamous carcinomas of the skin are the most common of all cancers and that the most common site for such lesions is the area of the head and neck. Seborrheic keratosis, senile keratosis, and patches of atrophic skin often appear side by side with skin neoplasms. Differential diagnosis may be difficult, and biopsy is often required. Pigmented lesions must be examined closely to determine the presence of bleeding ulceration or satellitosis indicating melanoma. All lumps should be palpated to observe their firmness, whether they have a cystic or solid quality, and whether they are fixed to the underlying tissues.

ORAL CAVITY. The oral cavity is often neglected in the course of a complete physical examination. It is said that the internist looks at the top of the tongue depressor, the otolaryngologist looks at the tonsils, and the general surgeon may not look at all. There is no excuse for this neglect, since the oral cavity is a rich source of pathologic processes, not only of local lesions, but often of lesions reflecting pathologic conditions elsewhere in the body.

Proper examination requires the use of a tongue depressor, finger cot or glove, and good lighting. If the examiner is skilled with the use of a head mirror, this will provide ideal illumination. However, there are numerous electric headlights that work equally well and that can be used at different points in the office or at the bedside without requiring an elaborate setup.

With the patient's mouth open, the light is directed into the oral cavity. If the patient has dentures of any sort, they should be removed. The examiner begins by looking at the anterior floor of the mouth and the openings of Wharton's ducts. Then the floor of the mouth is observed, progressing posteriorly along the gingivolingual gutter to the tonsillar pillars on either side. The undersurface of the anterior and lateral tongue can also be observed. This is a good place to detect early jaundice.

The lower gingiva and teeth are examined next. The condition of the teeth and the presence or absence of sepsis are considered. The gingivobuccal gutters are often the hiding place of small malignant lesions and should be inspected thoroughly.

The buccal mucosa can be examined next. Patches of hyperkeratosis are often seen here. The examiner looks for the nipple indicating the opening of Stensen's duct. Pressure on the parotid should express saliva from the orifice. The position and mobility of the tongue are observed. A deviated tongue may indicate injury to the hy-

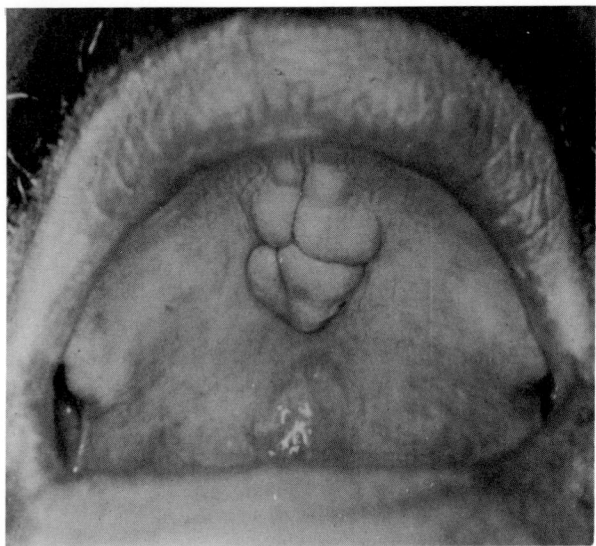

Fig. 16-1. Torus, a congenital lesion formed along the median raphe where the palatine processes of the maxilla join. These protuberances are normally smooth; the lobulation seen here is unusual.

poglossal nerve or a previous stroke. Numerous longitudinal fissures reflect previous syphilis, a condition now rarely seen. Malignant lesions are normally found on the edges or at the tip of the tongue.

Occasionally, a patch of dirty fibers will occupy the surface of the tongue. This condition, called "hairy tongue," often occurs in a dry mouth with impaired salivary secretion. Vitamin deficiencies are reflected by an atrophy of the taste buds with a flat, smooth, erythematous mucosa.

The tonsils and soft palate are considered next. The presence or absence of the tonsils or tonsillar tags should be noted. If the patient gags, the posterior tonsillar pillars rotate toward the midline, better exposing the tonsillar fossa itself. The anterior tonsillar pillar is a common site for patches of hyperkeratosis, or sometimes for very early carcinomas. Inappropriate hypertrophy of one tonsil may reflect a lymphoma. Paralysis of one side of the soft palate is often seen in patients who have had a cerebrovascular accident. Large tumors in the nasopharynx may push the soft palate forward and down.

The examiner can complete the observation with inspection of the hard palate. A smooth or occasionally lobular elevation running down the midline of the palate is usually a torus, a harmless, congenital deformity (Fig. 16-1). Tori of the mandible also occur, projecting into the mouth bilaterally at the level of the canine tooth. They have no particular importance except to the frightened patient who may notice them for the first time in adulthood and mistake them for new growths. Occasionally, patients with atrophied lower alveoli following total loss of the lower teeth will have a spur that projects backward from the midline into the floor of the mouth. This represents a prominence of the symphysis made detectable by the absorption of the surrounding bone.

Palpation is equal in importance to inspection. Many early lesions of the oral cavity cannot be detected except by the sense of touch. This is especially true of lesions buried within the substance of the tongue or in the salivary glands. The gloved finger is passed over the tongue, the floor of the mouth, and the gingivobuccal gutters. Any mass encountered can be made more prominent by bimanual or bidigital palpation, pressing the mass inward from the cheek or submental area toward the oral cavity. If the patient can tolerate it, palpation of the lateral pharyngeal wall may reveal masses in the deep lobe of the parotid. If the index of suspicion is high concerning lesions in the nasopharynx or base of tongue, these areas should be palpated as well.

NECK. Inspection and palpation of the cervical area are done methodically, keeping in mind a distinct list of structures to be felt. These should include the larynx, thyroid, trachea, sternocleidomastoid muscle, lymph node–bearing areas, and salivary glands. The submental area is examined for the presence of enlarged lymph nodes and the size and consistency of the submaxillary glands. In the older patient they may hang low in the anterior cervical triangle as the enveloping fascia becomes lax with age. In this location they often are mistaken initially for enlarged lymph nodes. The presence of any enlarged or firm lymph nodes incorporated within the substance of the submaxillary gland should be noted. Bimanual palpation through the floor of the mouth helps greatly.

The angle of the jaw is a common site for enlarged lymph nodes or not infrequently of a tumor in the tail of the parotid gland. The anterior border of the sternocleidomastoid may overlap a cystic mass representing a branchial cleft cyst. Cystic or fluctuant masses in the posterior cervical triangle may represent a lipoma or a cystic lymphangioma.

The most important consideration in the adult is the presence of enlarged lymph nodes. A number of structures in the neck deceive the novice and at first appear to be enlarged lymph nodes when in fact they are normal structures. The carotid bulb is commonly so mistaken, especially in older patients in whom arteriosclerosis has diminished or obliterated the pulse at the bulb. The tip of the hyoid bone adjacent to the carotid bulb sometimes fools the unwary, unless they are clever enough to palpate for this structure bilaterally. The posterior belly of the omohyoid muscle as it crosses the posterior triangle in the thin patient can mimic a fusiform node until the examiner realizes that the ends of the apparent node cannot be felt. Also in thin patients the tips of the transverse process of the second cervical vertebra are felt posterior to the ascending ramus of the mandible and may seem like a lymph node until it is realized that the structures are bony in consistency and bilateral.

Masses in the thyroid are best felt if the examiner stands behind the patient and palpates the lobes of the gland between thumb and forefinger. A midline mass just above the isthmus of the thyroid may represent an enlarged lymph node, a pyramidal lobe of thyroid, or a thyroglossal duct cyst.

PARANASAL SINUSES. The paranasal sinuses are relatively inaccessible to physical examination. Neoplastic

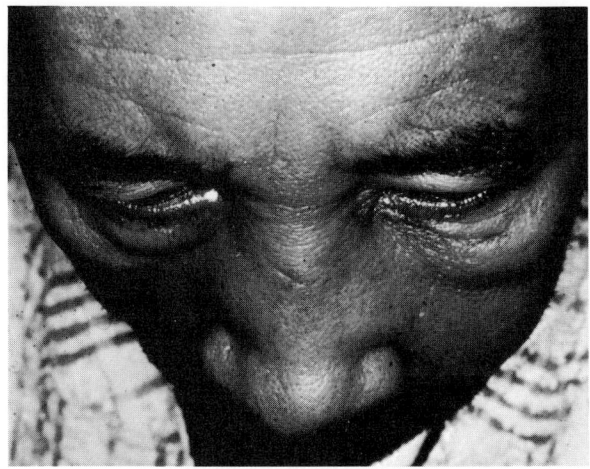

Fig. 16-2. Early swelling of the maxilla, seen best from above, as shown here. The patient had a space-occupying lesion within the sinus that was not as well appreciated in the frontal view.

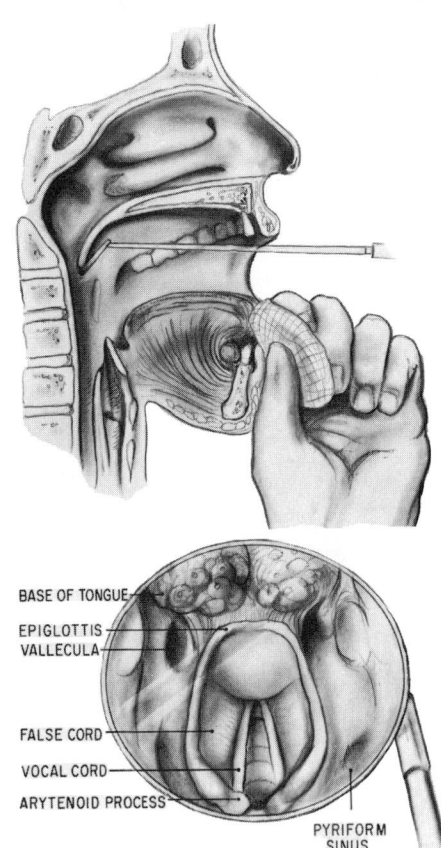

Fig. 16-3. Laryngeal mirror examination of the larynx. Cross section of the oral cavity illustrates the relation of the mirror to the larynx. Insert: View seen by the examiner. Note the epiglottis hiding the anterior portion of the cords.

lesions often hide within these recesses and are not manifest until quite late. Bulging, particularly asymmetric bulging of one maxillary sinus, can best be appreciated by observing the cheeks from above either by having the patient lean toward the examiner or by standing above the patient and looking down (Fig. 16-2). Palpation of the maxillary, ethmoid, or temporal areas may elicit tenderness or a sense of fullness. Transillumination of the sinuses by a bright light placed within the oral cavity of a patient in a dark room may reveal opacification of one or more of the sinuses. This is a relatively crude method of examination compared with x-ray examination.

INDIRECT LARYNGOSCOPY. There is a common misconception that indirect laryngoscopy is an examination to be performed only by specialists. Hoarseness and throat pain are such common symptoms and cancer of the pharynx and larynx so frequent that indirect laryngoscopy should be part of the armamentarium of any physician and part of the routine general physical examination.

The patient is seated in a chair slightly higher than the chair or stool of the examiner. The examiner sits opposite him with his right thigh and knee parallel and immediately adjacent to the right thigh and knee of the patient. The patient should extend his neck, thrusting his chin straight forward, as though he had just finished sneezing. The patient's tongue is wrapped in a gauze sponge, and the examiner, if he is right-handed, grasps the tip of the tongue between the thumb and second finger of the left hand, using the first finger to elevate the patient's upper lip. The tongue is drawn forward, and the patient is instructed to breathe rapidly in short, quick breaths, to "pant like a dog." As long as the patient continues to breathe in this fashion, gagging is inhibited. The examiner inserts a medium to large laryngeal mirror, previously flamed to keep it from fogging, into the oropharynx and shines the headlight on the mirror, reflecting a spot of light down into the hypopharynx (Fig. 16-3).

If one is a novice with the head mirror, an electric head lamp should be used. With the mirror in the oropharynx and directed downward, the posterior third of the tongue, the lateral pharyngeal wall, the posterior pharyngeal wall, the epiglottis, the valleculae, and the pyriform sinuses can all be examined thoroughly. The epiglottis will usually hide most of the glottic opening, and only the posterior portions of the arytenoids may be seen at first. The patient is told to breathe deeply several times. This often throws the uvula forward until more of the glottic opening and a little of the subglottic space is seen. The patient is asked to attempt to enunciate an "ee" sound. This throws the epiglottis even farther forward and usually brings the entire glottis, including the anterior commissure, into view.

The false cords, aryepiglottic folds, and posterior epiglottis can now be examined. The movement of the cords is considered, to determine whether both are moving adequately and whether they meet in the midline. Paralysis of one cord may indicate a malignant lesion in the mediastinum or cervical area or may be related to previous operation or cerebrovascular accident. If nodules in the pharynx or posterior tongue are noted, they should subsequently be palpated. As the examiner acquires skill in this procedure, most of these examinations can be accomplished without local anesthesia. Topical anesthesia

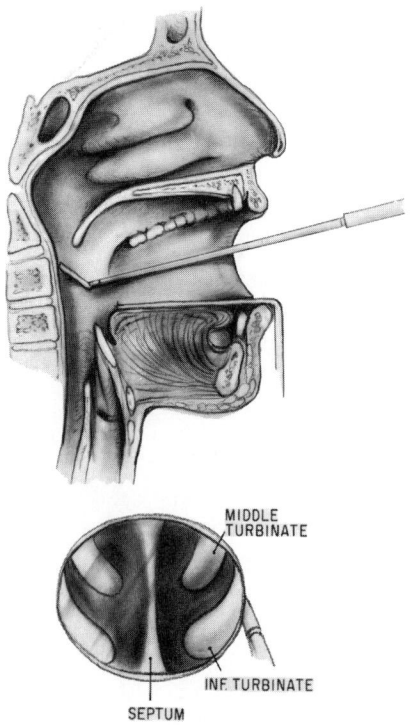

MIDDLE
TURBINATE

INF. TURBINATE

SEPTUM

Fig. 16-4. Mirror view of the nasopharynx. Soft palate is drawn forward, and the mirror in the oropharynx is directed upward. Insert: View seen in the mirror.

with lidocaine 1% should be used by the beginner. Although expensive and somewhat fragile, the flexible fiberoptic nasopharyngoscope is a very handy office instrument and may give novice examiners a better view of the larynx than indirect laryngoscopy.

In one or two patients out of every twenty, examination is incomplete or impossible because of a hypersensitive gag reflex or an acquired or congenital malformation of the epiglottis that makes visualization of the glottis impossible. In such instances, direct laryngoscopy must be used. While direct laryngoscopy is the more sophisticated and complex procedure, indirect laryngoscopy actually gives a better overall picture of the larynx and pharynx. The chief reason for resorting to direct laryngoscopy other than the above is the necessity of biopsy of lesions deep in the larynx. Direct laryngoscopy is sometimes performed using a *suspension laryngoscope,* which, once the cords are visualized, can be fixed in place so that operators do not have to use their hands to hold the laryngoscope. This technique can be combined with the use of an optical device that greatly magnifies the cords so that small irregularities and tiny lesions may be examined. Occasionally in patients with unexplained hoarseness this approach will reveal early localized benign and malignant changes.

NASOPHARYNGOSCOPY. The mirror used for indirect laryngoscopy may be turned over and directed upward. The examiner, standing at the patient's shoulder and depressing the tongue with a tongue blade, may shine the headlight on the mirror and gain a fairly spacious view of the nasopharynx. In most instances the space between the soft palate and posterior pharyngeal wall is too small for the nasopharynx to be adequately visualized in this fashion. If physical findings or the history so indicate, complete examination of the nasopharynx is done by inserting a soft rubber #10 French catheter through either nasal passage, drawing its tip out through the mouth and retracting the soft palate forward, revealing the entire nasopharynx for indirect examination by the mirror (Fig. 16-4). The torus tubarius, the openings of the eustachian tubes, the posterior surface of the soft palate, the posterior aspect of the nasal septum arching back toward the sphenoid sinus, and the posterior tips of the turbinates are seen. The normal lymphatic tissue of the adenoids may lend a granular appearance to some of the posterior and superior mucosal surfaces.

The direct nasopharyngoscope is an instrument that can be used in the office. It is a small instrument like a miniature cystoscope and has a Foroblique or right-angled lens. The diameter of the tube is 5 to 8 mm, and the visual field is quite small and easily obscured by mucus or blood. Use of this instrument is a valuable adjunct to indirect inspection of the nasopharynx and is particularly helpful in searching for small neoplasms.

Introduction of the fiberoptic laryngoscope has made it possible to examine both the nasopharynx and larynx with the same instrument. This thin, flexible instrument is inserted through the nostril and is easily tolerated by the patient. In many offices it is supplanting indirect laryngoscopy.

Diagnostic Studies

RADIOGRAPHY. Most of the bones of the face and neck are adjacent to air-filled cavities or are air-containing, creating an excellent situation for diagnostic radiographs. Lesions of the paranasal sinuses, nasal cavity, orbit, mandible, and larynx are readily revealed.

Arteriography. Injection of contrast medium into the vessels is a useful maneuver for evaluating tumors within the cranium or evaluation of tumors in this region. The rare carotid body tumor can be nicely outlined by the use of radiopaque medium injected into the appropriate common carotid artery, and its appearance when examined in this fashion is pathognomonic. At times, arteriography is useful to outline the extent of a hemangioma of the face or oral cavity (Fig. 16-5).

Laminography. This technique is of great usefulness in examinations of the head and neck, especially for minute examination of the bony walls of the paranasal sinuses. Usually, the clouding of a paranasal sinus by tumor and by infection cannot be differentiated by x-ray unless obvious evidence of bone erosion is seen. Early detection of such erosions is best seen in laminograms. Tumors of the larynx are easily seen from above by indirect laryngoscopy, but their inferior extent is hidden from view unless the lesion is very small. Laminograms and lateral soft tissue views of the larynx play a useful role in revealing the extent of subglottic extension and often the degree of involvement of the pyriform sinuses, which may not other-

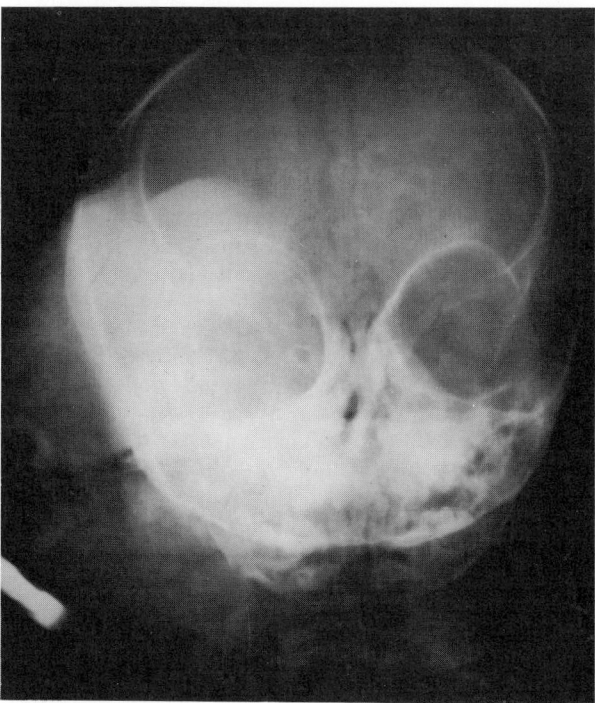

Fig. 16-5. Arteriographic demonstration of hemangioma of the oral cavity. On physical examination, only the cheek appeared involved. In the x-ray view, involvement of the lateral pharyngeal wall and oral cavity is noted. (From: *Rush BF Jr: Ann Surg 164:921, 1966, with permission.*)

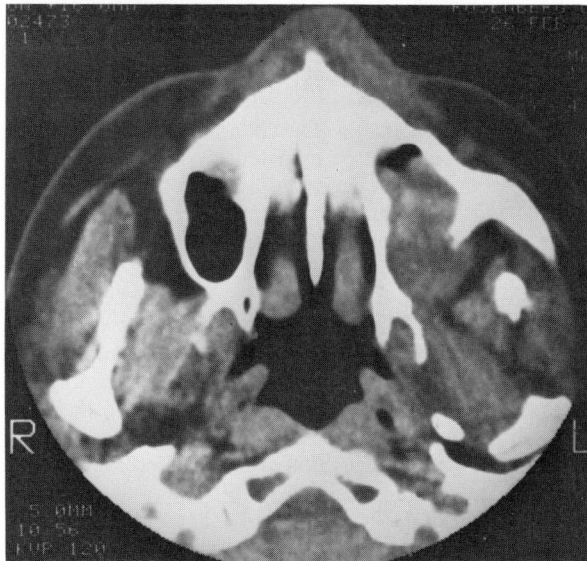

Fig. 16-6. Computer tomography of a squamous cell carcinoma in the left maxillary sinus. Posterior extent of this lesion with perforation of the maxillary wall and proximity to surrounding structures is clearly shown by this technique.

wise be detectable. Details of retropharyngeal and esophageal tumor spread can be seen on the lateral soft tissue view. Laryngograms are performed by the application of barium to the back of the tongue, cords, epiglottis, and all of the intrinsic larynx. A very clear examination of laryngeal structures can be obtained that offers excellent correlation with other diagnostic methods available.

Computer Tomography. This intriguing technique has found applications throughout the body and is especially useful in the head and neck. The true extent of large tumors of this area is best defined by the multisectional studies offered by computer tomography. This is especially true of tumors in the nasopharynx, paranasal sinuses, and the larynx. In these areas the new technique is superior to and is supplanting laminography (Fig. 16-6); when it is used with vascular contrast, enlarged cervical lymph nodes can be detected before they are palpable.

Magnetic Resonance Imaging. Images in the head and neck area provided by this method demonstrate the most detail in soft tissues of any technique available. There is superior differentiation of abnormal from normal tissue. In addition, vascular structures are revealed without having to inject contrast material. Since MRI does not require the use of radiation, it may eventually take the place of arteriography, laminography, and even computer tomography except for very special applications.

BIOPSY. The vast majority of head and neck lesions can be easily biopsied in the office or clinic. The tools required are simple, and the procedure is short and uncom-

plicated. Lesions of the lip, skin, gingiva, floor of the mouth, tongue, and buccal mucosa can quickly be biopsied with a 4-mm dermatologist's skin punch. The area to be biopsied is cleansed with an antiseptic agent infiltrated with a small amount of local anesthesia, and the skin punch is pressed into the lesion to a depth of 4 to 6 mm, cutting a small disc of the tumor, and is withdrawn. The core of tissue that is still connected at its base is grasped with forceps, pulled up until the base is flush with the surface tissues, and cut off with a small pair of scissors. A silver nitrate stick thrust into the depth of the remaining cavity and mild pressure for a minute or two control bleeding in almost all instances. Lesions of the soft palate, tonsillar pillar, or posterior tongue that cannot be reached with a skin punch can often be biopsied easily and quickly with a cervical biopsy forcep; the techniques of anesthesia and hemostasis are essentially the same as described above.

If skill is obtained with indirect laryngoscopy, lesions of the lateral pharyngeal wall, pyriform sinus, epiglottis, and aryepiglottic folds can often be quickly biopsied in the office. While similar biopsies of the true and false cords sometimes can be achieved with skillful manipulation of the indirect mirror, such procedures are best carried out under direct laryngoscopy. Manipulation of biopsy forceps immediately above the cords is much more difficult for the patient to tolerate and may stimulate laryngeal spasm and bleeding at a site where aspiration of blood into the trachea is likely.

Biopsy of the primary lesion is always preferable, but sometimes although cervical nodes are enlarged, no primary tumor can be found. If so, needle biopsy of cervical nodes is indicated and is a rewarding procedure when the node contains metastatic squamous carcinoma. This neoplasm is easily diagnosed even with the smallest fragments of tissue. Nodes involved by lymphoma, on the other hand, are virtually impossible to diagnose by needle biopsy. Positive results of needle biopsy are useful and timesaving; the negative result of a needle biopsy has no significance and must be followed by open biopsy.

Needle biopsy has been rediscovered several times in the 50 years since it was first described. In the last decade there has been considerable excitement over "skinny needly biopsy," biopsy with needles of 20 to 24 gauge. This is a cytologic method, and the fine needles remove cells and tissue fluid rather than any bits of organized tissue. Because tumor cells are less adherent than normal cells, the small needle will often harvest many more abnormal than normal cells, an advantage over the core biopsies taken with larger needles.

There has been much controversy concerning the tendency to spread tumor cells with the use of needle biopsies, and certainly it seems likely that tumor cells are spread into the needle tract by this manipulation. However, this is of greater theoretical than practical importance. Long experience with this technique at a number of major centers has not produced any gross difference in survival rates on long-term follow-up either in the head and neck or elsewhere. Open biopsy of a lymph node seems just as likely to scatter tumor cells, and even more widely.

VITAL DYES. Many cancers of the oral mucosa in their early stages are soft and superficial. They may have an erythematous appearance rather than a white color as usually thought and can easily escape detection even in a careful examination. If suspicion is aroused by a vaguely erythematous patch, the application of toluidine blue will aid in making the diagnosis. This technique will distinguish areas of dysplasia and carcinoma in situ as well as frank carcinoma of the mucosa. The method has its chief use in mapping out the full extent of dysplastic areas or areas of intraepithelial carcinoma.

CYTOLOGY. As used in the oral cavity, exfoliative cytology is a superficial biopsy, since it does not reflect collection of fluid from the entire oral cavity but involves scraping a specific lesion with a spatula and spreading this scraping on a slide. Such cytologic examinations, therefore, require a specific area of suspicion compared with sampling of an entire anatomic area such as in the cervix or bronchial tree. If a specific lesion is present, it is best evaluated by an actual biopsy. The chief virture of oral cytology is that physicians who cannot bring themselves to use office biopsy techniques or who feel they are beyond their competence can still have the opportunity to obtain a histologic specimen from the lesion in question. Unlike biopsy, cytology has no significance when it is negative. Thus, cytology will establish the presence of a lesion but cannot be relied on to rule that a questionable lesion is not malignant.

Tumor Markers. Substances produced by tumor or antigens to these substances sometimes appear in the serum. Few of these appear at an early enough stage in the growth of tumors to be much use in diagnosis, but if they are elevated when the tumor is found, increase or decrease in the marker usually is correlated with increase or decrease in tumor mass. Some head and neck tumors secrete a parahormone-like substance that is associated with an elevated calcium in about 10 percent of Stages III and IV tumors. This finding usually reflects a grim prognosis. Reduction of tumor mass by operation, chemotherapy, or radiation will return the calcium level to normal. Carcinoembryonic antigen (CEA) is sometimes elevated in head and neck tumors and can be used to follow therapy. Squamous cell carcinoma–associated antigen (SCCA) is elevated in 60 to 70 percent of Stages III and IV cancers of the head and neck. Its usefulness as a monitor for therapeutic response is currently under investigation.

CANCER STAGING. An important facet of diagnosis is staging the clinical extent of the tumor. The efforts of the American Joint Commission for Cancer Staging have introduced the now widely accepted TNM system of staging in which T stands for tumor, N for regional lymph nodes, and M for metastasis. In 1987 this system was brought into agreement with the system of the Union Internationale Contre Cancrum (UICC), so there is now a single worldwide staging system. Proper description of each aspect of a malignant lesion permits more precise comparison between series of patients and better evaluation for prognosis. The committee has a book available in which all the major areas for staging in the head and neck are covered. The system has great value but is complex enough that patients should never be staged from memory but only with the staging reference available. Staging may be either clinical, based entirely on the physical examination, or pathologic, based on gross and microscopic examination of the specimen. Recent studies show that thickness of an oral lesion is more important than the area covered when predicting subsequent involvement of cervical nodes and survival.

LIP

Squamous cell carcinomas of the lip are one of the common malignant tumors of the oral cavity, constituting 15 percent of all such lesions and 2.2 percent of all cancers. Basal cell carcinoma is much less frequent; only about 3 are seen for every 100 squamous cell carcinomas of the lip. Benign lesions that are occasionally seen in the lips include mucous cysts, tumors of the minor salivary glands, hemangiomas, lymphangiomas, venous lakes, fibromas, fissures, and hyperkeratosis.

ETIOLOGY. Like tumors of the skin, there is an important relationship between tumors of the lip and exposure to sunlight. About one-third of patients have a history of working outdoors, and the incidence of malignant squamous cancers of the lip increases progressively the farther south the latitude of the patient population being considered. Thus, in the United States the highest incidence is in Florida and Texas. Actinic rays are stronger at higher altitudes and in dryer air, and in areas having these features the incidence of lip (and skin) cancer is increased. Fishermen, sailors, and farmers are among the occupational groups with an increased incidence.

Complexion also plays a role. Susceptible types are fair-skinned, light, blond or ginger-haired, and blue-eyed, with the kind of complexion that freckles and burns rather than tans on exposure to the sun. Resistant people have the opposite characteristics: they are brunet and dark-skinned; blacks are rarely affected.

While there is a relation between lip cancer and tobacco, the exact cause for this is less apparent than in patients with lesions of the intraoral area, larynx, or lungs. The average cigarette smoker receives almost no carcinogen from tobacco directly to the lips, since the smoke is drawn into the oral cavity and tracheobronchial tree without passing over the mucosa of the lips themselves. Some feel that the inmates of nursing homes and institutions are more prone to have carcinoma of the lip from cigarette smoking. Smokers in this population usually treasure their cigarettes, smoking them down to the smallest possible butt. Macerated, moist tobacco and heat are directly applied to the lips.

Reports in the literature implicating pipe smoking as a cause of lip cancer have been appearing since 1795, and the Advisory Committee to the Surgeon General on Smoking and Health has accepted the causal relationship as established. Pipestems of wood and clay that soak up tobacco tars directly and apply a "tar poultice" to the lips have been viewed with special suspicion. In any case, such stems are little used now, and indeed the incidence of cancer of the lip in the United States has been gradually decreasing over the past 30 years. One may speculate whether this reflects the decrease in pipe smoking, outdoor work, use of wood and clay pipestems, or a combination of these and other factors.

Cancer of the lip in women is very rare, occurring in only 1 woman for every 20 to 30 men.

Benign Tumors

The mucosa of the inner surface of the upper and lower lips is subject to the same benign lesions as those throughout the mucosa of the oral cavity. These are discussed in greater detail in the following section, Oral Cavity, and include such lesions as mucous cysts, hemangiomas, tumors of the minor salivary glands, hyperkeratosis, and inflammatory hyperplasia. Specific benign lesions that involve the exposed borders of the lips include venous lakes, pigmented spots, hemangiomas, and very rarely neuromas. Venous lakes are a telangiectasis, usually of the lower lip, occurring in older individuals as a small bluish spot. They appear to have no pathologic significance. The other three lesions all have interesting systemic correlations. Multiple pigmented spots of the lips may be associated with Peutz-Jeghers syndrome and denote the presence of multiple small intestinal polyps, which sometimes lead to bleeding and intussusception but are rarely malignant. Scattered small hemangiomas of the lip may be associated with similar lesions elsewhere in the

oral cavity and gastrointestinal tract, those of Rendu-Osler-Weber disease. Neuromas of the lips, particularly at the commissures, suggest a neuroendocrine dysplasia, a fascinating syndrome associated with pheochromocytomas, medullary carcinoma of the thyroid, hyperparathyroidism, and hypertrophy of the gastrointestinal myenteric plexus.

Hyperkeratosis

This is a premalignant condition of the lips, usually associated with long exposure to sunlight. It typically occurs in fair-skinned individuals in their sixties or seventies who have long histories of outdoor employment. The normal distinct line marking the mucocutaneous border becomes indistinct and gradually retreats, indicating a metaplasia of the outer portion of the mucosa to a keratosquamous epithelium. The mucosa of the lip becomes paler, thinner, and more fragile. There may be perpendicular cracks and fissures. On this base, a white film indicative of early hyperkeratosis appears. This may grow gradually thicker and more exophytic as the condition progresses (Fig. 16-7) or may remain stationary for many years. Gradually, a small area of scabbing and ulceration occurs. This breakdown within the hyperkeratotic tissue represents a failure of the less resistant areas of hyperkeratosis to tolerate normal wear and tear. When such areas of ulceration appear, they continue to break down and heal and often give rise to carcinoma in situ and eventually invasive carcinoma. Persistent hyperkeratosis is a distinct premalignant lesion, and 35 to 40 percent of all carcinomas of the lip are preceded by this condition. Cancers arising on such a base can be prevented by excising the entire exposed mucosa of the lip, elevating the protected mucosa of the inner lip, and advancing it over the bed of the excised mucosa to form a new lining for the

Fig. 16-7. Hyperkeratosis of lower lip. This degree of hyperkeratosis merits serious concern. The entire lower lip is involved and should be treated by excision (lip stripping) and advancement of the mucosa of the inner lip to cover the defect.

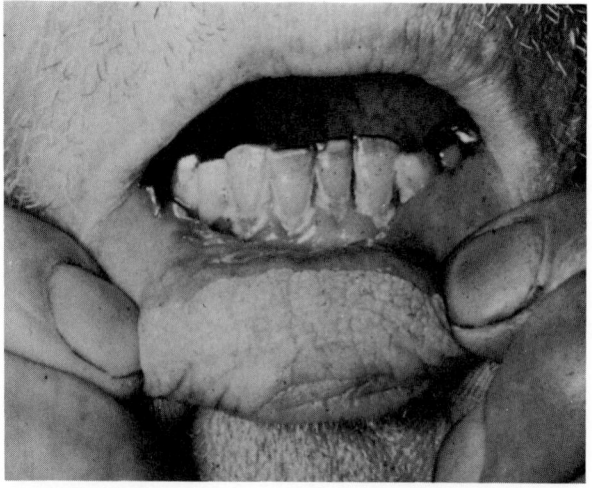

lip. This procedure is called a *lip stripping and resurfacing*.

Carcinoma of the Lip

Most cancers of the lip are squamous carcinomas. When basal cell carcinomas appear, they usually involve the skin of the lip beyond the vermilion border and probably should be considered with the cancers of the skin of the face. Ninety-three percent of the squamous cancers occur on the lower lip. These are usually low-grade, well-differentiated lesions, 80 percent being grade 1 or grade 2. The lesions most frequently start on the outer edge of the mucosa at the vermilion border and seem to favor the middle two-thirds of the lip somewhat more frequently than the commissures (Fig. 16-8).

The natural history of these lesions is of slow but relentless growth. Some grow to great size, destroying the entire lip without ever metastasizing, but the incidence of metastasis gradually increases with the increasing size of the tumors (Fig. 16-9). About 5 to 10 percent of all patients with lip cancer have cervical lymph node metastasis, and in half of these patients only one lymph node is involved. The normal spread of cancer from the lower lip is by way of lymphatics to the submental node on the side of the lesion. Metastases do not involve the opposite submental node unless the primary lesion crosses the midline. Lesions of the upper lip drain to lymph nodes in the anterior portion of the submaxillary gland.

An ulcer of the lip that fails to heal is soon detected by patients or their friends, and in most urban populations such lesions quickly come to the attention of physicians. In rural populations it is surprising how long patients will carry these ulcerations before seeking medical aid.

Treatment for carcinoma of the lip has remained a topic of controversy between radiotherapists and surgeons for many decades. Recent controlled series comparing treatment by both modalities in randomly selected patients

Fig. 16-8. Squamous carcinoma of lip. Any patient with a chronic ulcer of this sort should seek medical advice. The chance of cure at this early stage approaches 100 percent.

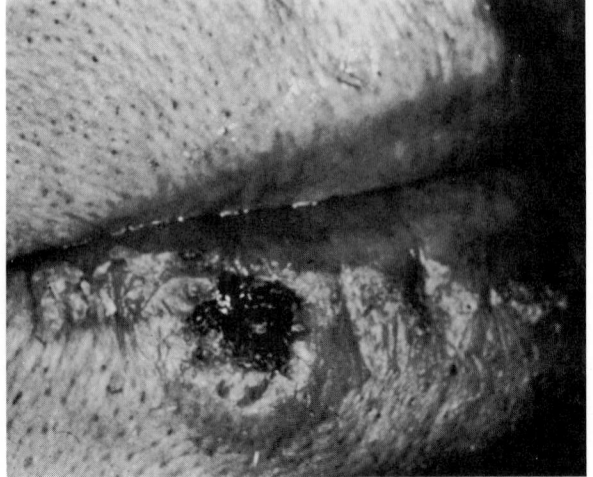

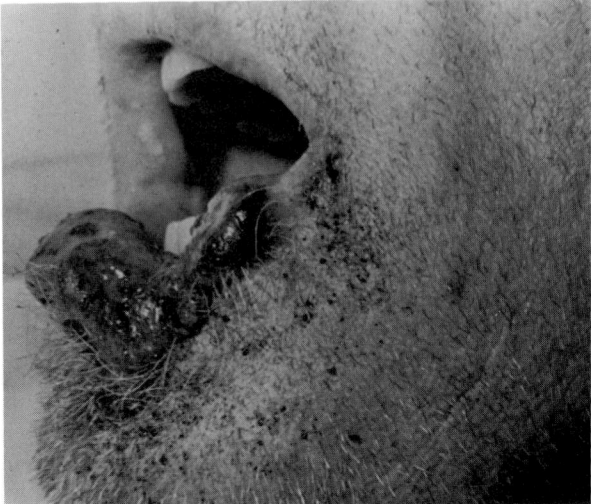

Fig. 16-9. Neglected carcinoma of the lip. A metastatic node is present along the line of the mandible. The chance of cure for this type of lesion is 50 percent or less.

indicate that there is no statistical difference between the two methods in terms of cure rate. The choice for therapy must be made on other grounds. Small lesions of the lip can usually be excised under local anesthesia with little or no hospitalization time. Good radiation therapy producing maximal regression with minimal residual scarring requires 2 to 4 weeks of outpatient therapy. Medium-sized lesions require the use of flaps from the upper lip or elsewhere for closure, and for these lesions radiotherapy often requires the same or less time and less morbidity. For very large lesions that have destroyed most of the lip and are associated with metastasis to the neck, subsequent repair of the lip will be required under any circumstance as well as probable radical neck dissection for removal of cervical nodes; for these major lesions an integration of radiation and surgical therapy may be used to improve cure rates, which are relatively low for either radiation or operation alone. A final consideration is that most carcinomas of the lip are related to solar radiation. Since radiotherapy increases the sensitivity of tissues to such exposure, it is best to avoid radiotherapy in patients who expect to return to outdoor occupations.

Prognosis for lip cancers of 1 cm or less is excellent, ranging from an 87 to 95 percent 5-year survival rate without recurrence. Neglected lesions, especially with associated cervical metastasis, do much more poorly, with a 5-year survival of 50 percent.

ORAL CAVITY

The oral cavity includes the buccal mucosa, upper and lower gingivae, anterior two-thirds of the tongue (that portion anterior to the circumvallate papillae), floor of the mouth, and hard palate.

INCIDENCE. Eight percent of all malignant tumors occur in this area, 95 percent of such tumors being squamous carcinomas. The risk of carcinomas developing here in a male is approximately 1 percent in a lifetime. The risk in females is far less: oral cancer develops in about 1 woman for every 10 males. Benign tumors of the oral cavity are common in both sexes.

ETIOLOGY. Some benign lesions have a specific cause, which will be discussed with the descriptions of the lesions below. Contributing causes to squamous carcinoma are smoking, a heavy intake of alcohol, poor oral hygiene, and syphilis. While cancer often occurs without the presence of any of these factors, they are associated with a majority of the lesions seen.

The *Report on Smoking and Health* by the Advisory Committee to the Surgeon General notes a suggestive relationship between smoking and oral carcinoma. This is especially true in pipe and cigar smokers, where oral cancer has the highest mortality ratio, 3.3,* of all causes of death compared with the nonsmoking population. There are a number of exotic cancers of the oral cavity that serve to indicate the relationship of tobacco to cancer. In Andhra Pradesh, a state in India, the habit of smoking a cigar (i.e., *chutta*) with the burning end inside the mouth is widespread. Carcinoma of the palate, called *chutta cancer,* is common. Presumably, repeated thermal trauma and/or tobacco smoke provide the carcinogenic agents.

In Uttar Pradesh and Bihar, a mixture of tobacco and slaked lime is habitually sucked by men of the districts. The quid is kept in the lower gingivolabial fornix for many hours during the day; a high incidence of carcinoma is found at this site. This has come to be called *khaini cancer,* from the name of the tobacco-lime mixture.

Betel-nut chewing is a common habit among the Indians, Javanese, and Malayans. The chew is made of a mixture of ground betel nut, slaked lime, and spices, such as ginger or pepper. These are wrapped in a betel leaf and chewed. The Indians add tobacco to their betel preparations and have a high incidence of oral cancer, whereas the incidence is low among the Javanese and Malayans, who consume their betel nut without benefit of the tobacco additive. Among betel nut–tobacco chewers, oral cancer comprises 36 percent of all cancers.

Alcoholism has a highly suggestive role in oral cancer. As many as 42 percent of all patients so afflicted have a history of alcoholism. As a corollary, cirrhosis of the liver is a common finding in patients with oral cancer, 20 percent having cirrhosis as compared with 9 percent in a control population. It has been proposed that alcohol acts as an adjuvant to the use of tobacco in producing oral cancer. This is a difficult point to prove, since finding a control population of patients who drink heavily but do not smoke is virtually impossible.

The roles of poor oral hygiene and oral sepsis, mentioned for decades as etiologic agents for oral cancers, are also difficult to evaluate. These conditions are seen most

* That is, 3.3 times as many pipe and cigar smokers died of oral cancer as did nonsmokers in the same age group. The mortality ratio for cancer of the lung in pipe smokers was 1:1, no different from that of the nonsmokers.

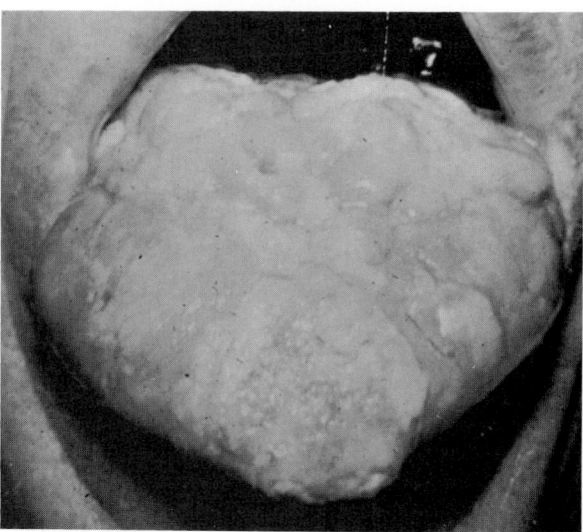

Fig. 16-10. Syphilis of the tongue. The dense, white patches are sometimes mistaken for "geographic tongue." Cancers of the dorsal surface often follow this condition.

commonly in patients at the lower end of the social scale and in the ward population rather than in private practice. Oral hygiene is poor in this group, but it cannot be said whether poor hygiene or social level or other correlated factors are responsible.

Syphilis has a direct relation to cancer of one specific site in the oral cavity, the tongue. When syphilitic glossitis, a lesion of late syphilis, heals, it often leaves the tongue fibrotic and scarred with longitudinal fissures and thick hyperkeratotic plaques. It is on this base that lingual cancer develops (Fig. 16-10). In the days of Bloodgood (1921), 21 percent of American men with lingual cancer had syphilis. Willis still calls this condition "the most clearly established causative factor in European males."

Benign Lesions

Common benign tumors of the oral cavity are inflammatory hyperplasias and cysts. Less commonly seen are giant cell granulomas, salivary tumors, granular cell myoblastomas, dermoids, and hemangiomas.

INFLAMMATORY HYPERPLASIA

The oral mucosa is subject to a number of irritating conditions producing tumorlike projections that are not true neoplasms. Patients develop the nervous habit of sucking a portion of mucosa from the cheek, tongue, or lip between the teeth or through an interdental or edentulous space. The traumatized mucosa becomes edematous and prominent, and the irritation may be compounded by the patient who bites as well as sucks on the offending mucosal fold. Initially, the overlying mucosa is swollen, and eventually this undergoes metaplasia to squamous epithelium. The tissue underlying the elevated mucosa changes from edematous connective tissue to a denser and more fibrotic collection of collagen. At this stage the

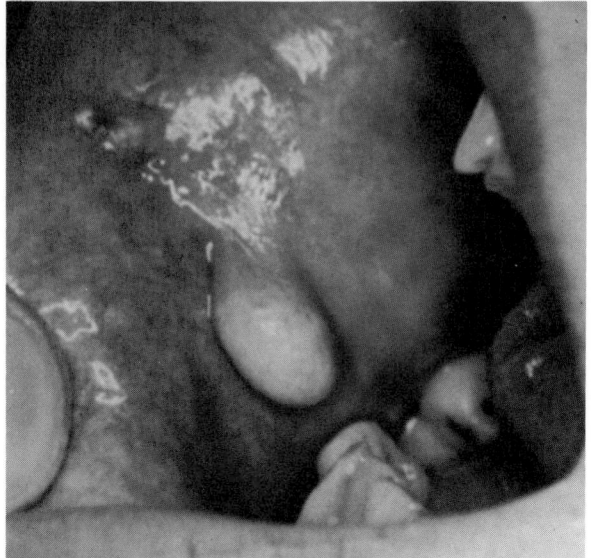

Fig. 16-11. Irritation fibroma. The lesion seen here was caused by persistent sucking and irritation of mucosa through the edentulous space, which can be seen adjacent to this polyp. *(Courtesy of Sheldon Rovin, D.D.S.)*

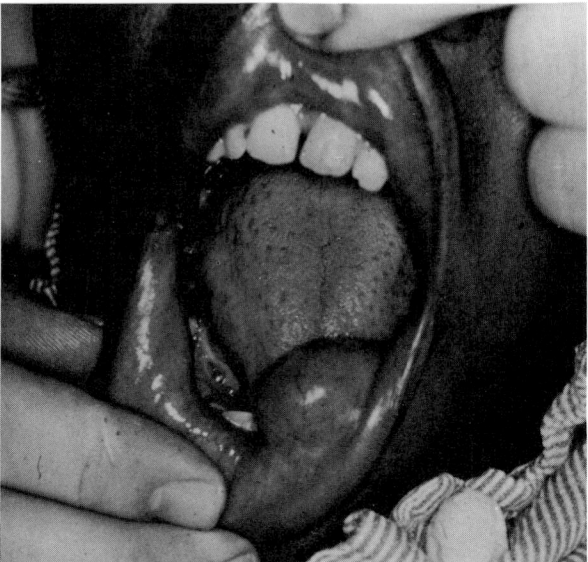

Fig. 16-12. Mucous cyst of the lip, the most common location for this lesion. This mucocele has resulted from rupture of a minor salivary gland duct with spillage of mucus into the surrounding tissue.

lesion may be termed a *fibroepithelial polyp* (Fig. 16-11). Similar lesions are often seen in the gingivobuccal gutter and on the palate in patients with ill-fitting dentures. Those lesions that occur along the vestibular mucosa next to the gingiva in this relation are sometimes called *epulis fissurata*. Another appropriate term, more descriptive of the later stages of these lesions when the fibrosis and scarring has advanced, is *irritation fibroma*. In the early inflammatory phase of these lesions, the overlying mucosa is friable and bleeds easily.

The chief responsibility of the examiner who has recognized the lesion is to reassure the patient that it is not malignant. Although these lesions are usually not ulcerated and are easily recognized, diagnosis should be confirmed by biopsy. Treatment is by correction of the causative factor, either by the design of new dentures or by discouraging the patient from manipulating and traumatizing the area involved. Excision may be necessary, but if the basic problem is not abolished, recurrence is prompt.

CYSTS

Mucous cysts are a common oral lesion occurring on the posterior surface of the lip, floor of the mouth, tongue, and buccal mucosa. These cysts arise from the salivary gland–bearing areas of the oral mucosa and were thought to be due to obstruction of the excretory duct of minor salivary glands. It has been found, however, that these cysts have no epithelial lining and that they result from a rupture of the excretory duct. Saliva spills from the defect in the duct and begins to collect in the tissues. At first it forms a diffuse lesion, but soon a circumscribed cyst with a wall of granulation tissue develops. These mucoceles measure from 1 or 2 mm to 1 or 2 cm in diameter and appear as elevated, translucent, bluish lesions of the mucosa (Fig. 16-12). They frequently rupture, discharging sticky mucoid material, and then recur as the laceration in the overlying mucosa heals. Treatment consists of wide surgical unroofing of the lesion.

A somewhat larger and more dramatic mucocele may result from obstruction and rupture of the major excretory ducts in the floor of the mouth, ducts of the lingual or submaxillary glands. Except for size, these lesions resemble in every way the lesions that result from obstruction of the minor salivary glands but have received the special name of *ranula*.

Dermoids may develop in the floor of the mouth and the base of the tongue along the midline. If neglected, these lesions grow slowly as they accumulate the sloughed-off cells, secretion, and hair of the epidermal lining. They present as both a swelling in the submental triangle and an elevation of the floor of the mouth (Fig. 16-13). They will eventually elevate the floor of the mouth and tongue until it touches the palate and interferes with speech. Treatment consists of operative excision of the cyst, which may be done either intraorally or extraorally. The lesion has a definite, thick capsule and can be shelled out with ease from its relatively avascular midline location.

PERIPHERAL GIANT CELL REPARATIVE GRANULOMA

These benign tumors occur on the gingivae, affecting the maxillary or mandibular gingiva with equal frequency. Grossly, they appear as a slow-growing, reddish, smooth sessile tumor that bleeds easily. They often occur at an area of an interdental papilla (Fig. 16-14) but may also arise in edentulous patients. Histologically, the lesion is covered by stratified squamous epithelium. Endothelial

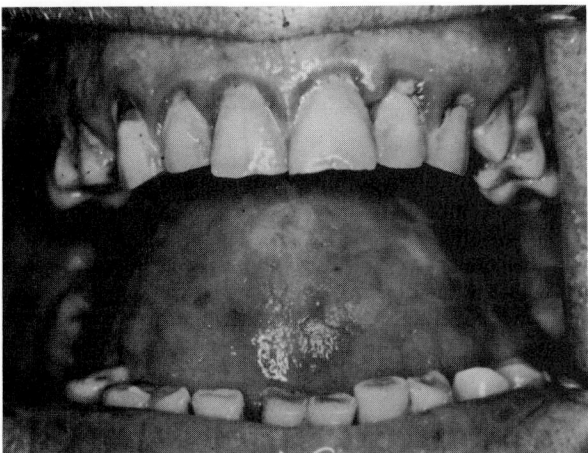

Fig. 16-13. Dermoid of the mouth. This huge dermoid has elevated the floor of the mouth until the tongue is forced against the hard palate and in this illustration is out of sight behind the cyst.

and fibroplastic proliferations, multinucleated giant cells, and extracellular and intracellular hemosiderin are diagnostic microscopic criteria. Multinucleated giant cells are distributed unevenly throughout an area of rich fibroblastic proliferation. Some lesions show spicules of bone tissue. In general, the lesion closely resembles the giant cell tumor of bone seen in hyperparathyroidism. The descriptive term *peripheral* indicates that the lesion is of soft tissue, while the so-called central giant cell reparative granuloma is an intraosseous form found in the mandible or maxilla.

When these lesions arise in the mandible or maxilla, they may be confused with the giant cell tumors of long bones. The distinction between the two lesions must be made, since the oral lesions have no propensity for malignant transformation, as have the lesions seen elsewhere.

Fig. 16-14. Peripheral giant cell tumor. These often arise in interdental spaces, as seen in photograph.

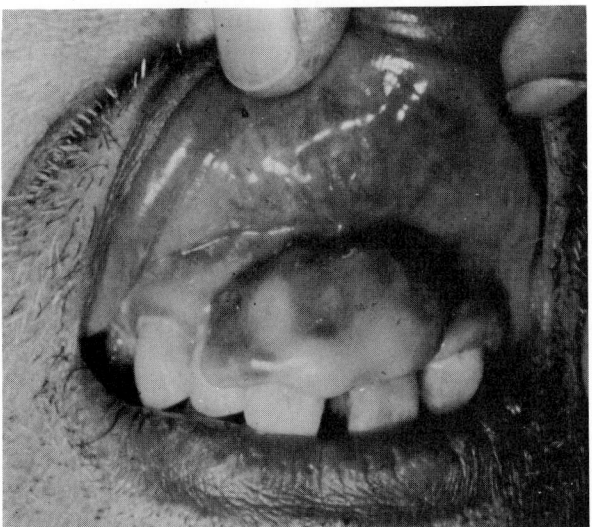

Treatment of the soft tissue lesions is by complete excision. Inadequate removal may result in recurrence.

PERIPHERAL FIBROMA

These are also lesions of the gingiva and are in many respects similar grossly to the giant cell granuloma. They are usually firmer and under the microscope are made up of dense connective tissue. They may also contain bone spicules and may be calcified. One can speculate as to the relation of these lesions to the giant cell granuloma. They may represent a later stage of this lesion or may be a late stage of inflammatory hyperplasia. Excision is usually curative.

GRANULOMA PYOGENICUM

This is an elevated pedunculated or sessile lesion that may occur on the lips, tongue, buccal mucosa, or gingiva. It bleeds readily on being traumatized. Histologically it is made up of edematous, fibrous connective tissue with a prominent endothelial component arranged in lobules of varying sizes separated by bands of collagen. Numerous blood vessels are scattered throughout the tumor. No cause is known for the lesions of the lips, buccal mucosa, and tongue, but lesions of the gingiva are often associated with pregnancy. Thirty to forty percent of pregnant women show some degree of gingival enlargement. Of these, about 1 percent will have an isolated "tumor." These lesions in the pregnant female have been called "granuloma gravidarum." They appear about the third month of pregnancy and increase in size throughout the growth of the child in utero. They usually diminish in size and disappear following delivery, although with a subsequent pregnancy they may appear again in the same location. Lesions unassociated with pregnancy may be treated by excision. It is usually advisable to wait until the end of pregnancy to treat granuloma gravidarum.

SALIVARY TUMORS

Pleomorphic adenomas (mixed tumors) occasionally arise from any of the 400 to 700 minor salivary glands. Occurring most commonly on the lips, tongue, and palate, they can be found anywhere in the oral cavity where minor salivary glands are found. They are usually slow-growing, round masses of a rather rubbery consistency (Fig. 16-15). They have the potential of becoming malignant and if simply enucleated without adequate excision have a marked propensity for local recurrence. Treatment, therefore, is by wide local excision.

HEMANGIOMA

Capillary hemangiomas, not unlike the strawberry hemangioma of the skin, are sometimes seen in the mucous membranes of the oral cavity in infants. Like the lesions of the skin these lesions regress spontaneously, and unless they are so large that they interfere with function, they should be left to regress at their own pace. In most instances they will undergo involution by the end of the fifth year. Unlike the skin lesions they do not disap-

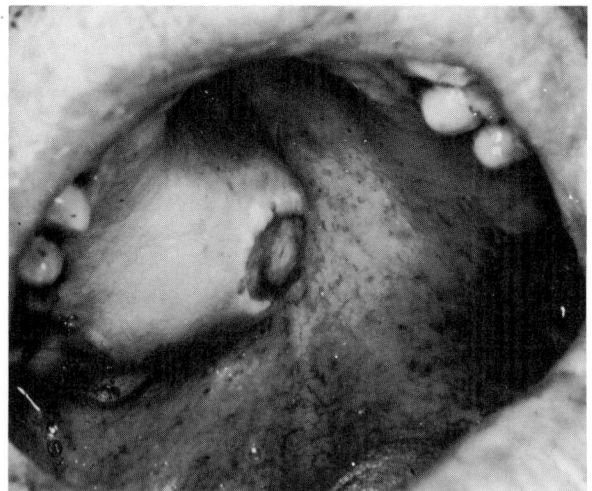

Fig. 16-15. Mixed tumor of palate. This is a benign lesion. Adequate removal to ensure prevention of recurrences includes resection of the underlying hard palate and gingiva.

pear completely and may still be seen as a small, dark lesion underneath the mucosa (Fig. 16-16). It is likely that the transparent nature of the mucosa reveals the sclerosed remnant in a manner that is not seen if the lesion is under the more opaque skin. The sclerosed hemangioma will remain visible throughout life but has no significance and does not require treatment. Rarely, large regional vascular malformations will involve the entire side of the mouth, including the tongue, gingiva, and buccal mucosa. Such lesions do not regress spontaneously. Their treatment is difficult, often requiring multiple plastic procedures to excise the hemangiomatous tissue and to return the contours of the mouth and oral cavity to normal.

GRANULAR CELL MYOBLASTOMA

This is a rare and interesting lesion that occurs most commonly within the muscle of the tongue, presenting as a small, firm spheroid mass detected best by manual palpation. These lesions have no malignant potential but may gradually increase in size with functional impairment. Treatment is by simple excision.

Hyperkeratosis and Erythroplasia

The gross finding of white patches on the oral mucosa elicits the diagnosis of leukoplakia from the clinician. "Leukoplakia" roughly translated means "white patches," so physicians need not feel too proud of their accomplishment; they have only managed to translate English into Latin. To some "leukoplakia" means a specific premalignant lesion. This meaning is not inherent in the original use of this term. Most pathologists adhere to a more rigid description of such lesions and describe the underlying microscopic changes: hyperplasia, keratosis, and dyskeratosis. White patches in the oral cavity may be associated with any or all of these basic changes (Fig. 16-17). Inflammation in this area often stimulates marked hyperplasia of cells, sometimes to the point where they resemble epidermoid tumors and are spoken of as *pseudoepitheliomatous hyperplasia*. Keratosis is a common response of the buccal mucosa and may appear in the presence of lichen planus, chronic dyscoid lupus, and Darier's disease, as well as be a possible accompaniment of malignant change.

Dyskeratosis, the loss of normal stratification or orientation of cells together with irregularity in the size and shape of cells and abnormal staining characteristics, is a much more predictable lesion and much more likely to announce malignant disease. A reddened area in the mucosa or erythroplasia is the earliest indication of dysplasia

Fig. 16-16. Fibrosing hemangioma. Lesions in the mucosal area remain visible under the buccal mucosa, whereas similar lesions may not be discernible under the skin.

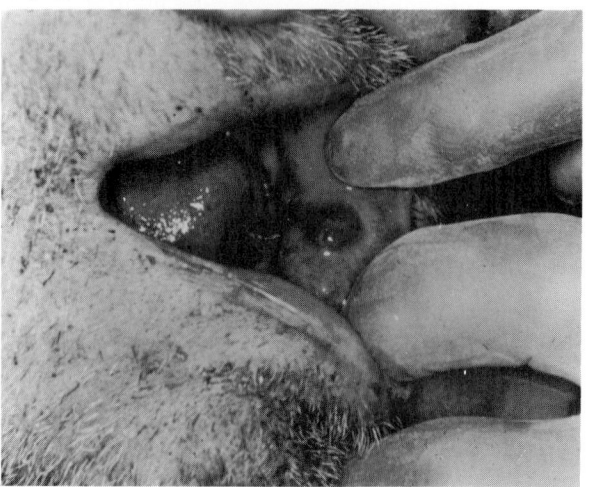

Fig. 16-17. Hyperkeratosis of mucosa. The white mucosa in the gingivobuccal gutter of the patient is due to an ill-fitting denture causing hyperkeratosis, a normal response of the oral mucosa to irritation. *(Courtesy of Sheldon Rovin, D.D.S.)*

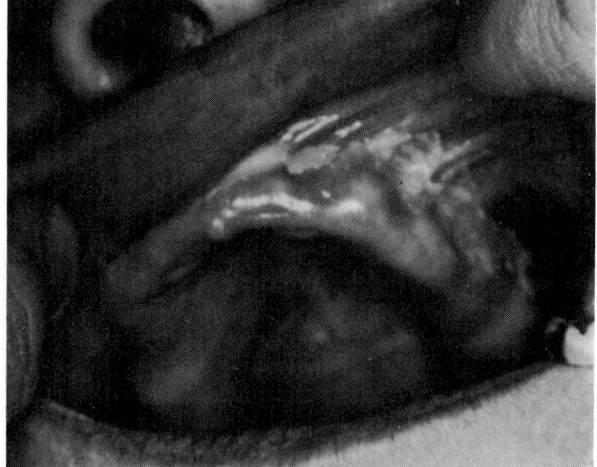

and is the earliest indicator of a malignant or premalignant lesion in the oral cavity. An overproduction of keratin, hyperkeratosis, is a much less common companion (4 percent) of dyskeratosis than it is on the lips, where hyperkeratosis often accompanies dyskeratosis, probably because the squamous cells of the vermilion border normally produce more keratin than the cells of the oral mucosa. Erythroplasia of the oral cavity occurs most commonly in the floor of the mouth, the lingual border, and the anterior tonsillar pillars and may signal not only dysplasia but frank carcinoma in situ and even microinvasive carcinoma. Since erythroplasia is such a definite sign of premalignant or malignant change, all such lesions should be excised promptly. Multiple lesions are common and patients are subject to the appearance of other lesions in the oral cavity and for that matter in the entire aerodigestive tract. Sometimes the dysplastic process will cover a major area such as the entire soft palate or floor of the mouth. Excision, in this case, is futile and radiation of the oral cavity is required after appropriate biopsy.

Malignant Tumors

PATHOLOGY. Low-grade epidermoid carcinomas make up the overwhelming majority of all carcinomas of the oral cavity, varying from highly differentiated tumors, difficult to tell histologically from inflammatory hyperplasia, to less well-organized but still obvious epidermoid tumors usually with associated squamous pearls. Highly undifferentiated and anaplastic lesions are rare. The few adenocarcinomas found are derived from minor salivary glands. The occasional adenoid cystic carcinomas and mucoepidermoid carcinomas seen also arise from salivary tissues.

In the southern United States a very low-grade cancer, verrucous carcinoma, is occasionally seen. This is an exophytic, shaggy white lesion usually found in the gingivobuccal gutter of patients who are tobacco chewers or "snuff dippers." Unless treated by radiation, the lesion never metastasizes, although it frequently invades surrounding tissues, including the mandible.

In general, lesions of the oral cavity are better differentiated and less malignant than lesions occurring in the oropharynx.

TONGUE

Carcinoma of the tongue commonly begins at the tip or along the free borders. It often starts in an area of hyperkeratosis and gradually develops as an ulcerated lesion with a moderately exophytic undermined border. The area of ulceration is related to the rest of the tumor as the tip of an iceberg is to its main mass, and palpation of the tongue may indicate that invasion has occurred deeply throughout underlying muscle (Fig. 16-18). Carcinomas beginning in an area of syphilitic glossitis are exceptions to the normal pattern and occur on the dorsal glossal surface.

Cancer of the tip of the tongue (Fig. 16-19) metastasizes to submental nodes, often bilaterally, while lesions along

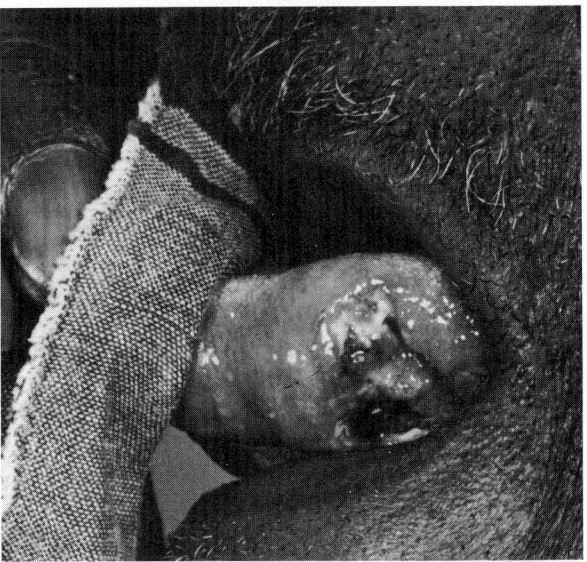

Fig. 16-18. Squamous carcinoma of the lateral border of the middle third of the tongue. The lesion is deeply invasive and much larger than the area of ulceration would indicate. The curled raised border is characteristic.

the borders of the tongue metastasize to ipsilateral submandibular nodes and occasionally to nodes at the angle of the mandible.

These lesions are quick to metastasize, and 40 percent of patients have nodes in the neck when first seen. In another 40 percent nodes develop at some point during therapy or during follow-up. For this reason therapy is designed to attack not only the primary lesion but also the nodes of the ipsilateral neck, as well. Combined operation including wide resection of the oral lesion together with radical neck dissection has been our treatment of choice in the past. More recently we have added either pre- or

Fig. 16-19. Squamous carcinoma of the tip of the tongue. An exophytic, fairly superficial lesion that histologically shows a well-differentiated structure. The prognosis for such a lesion is excellent.

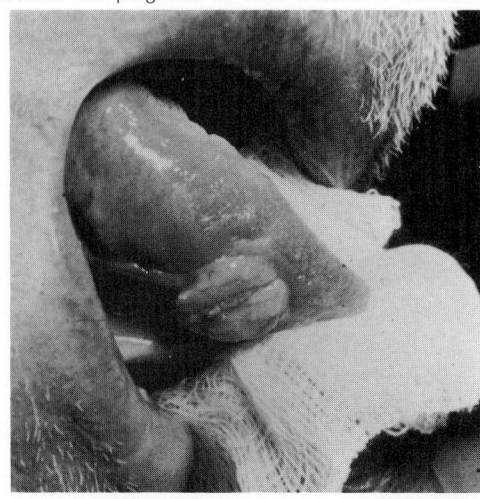

postoperative radiation therapy. The horizontal ramus of the mandible must be resected together with the tumor if the oral cancer has come in contact with the periosteum of the mandible at any point. Such contact seeds the periosteal lymphatics with tumor cells and makes resection of bone mandatory. The determinate 5-year survival for cancer of the tongue is 32 to 40 percent. If no palpable lymph nodes are present, the 5-year survival rate is 53 percent.

FLOOR OF THE MOUTH

The floor of the mouth is that portion of the oral cavity between the tongue and the inner surface of the mandible. This crescentic area of the mucosa lies over the sublingual and submaxillary salivary glands and contains their excretory ducts. It is divided into two halves by the frenulum, a fold of mucosa lying in the midline and extending to the tongue.

Squamous carcinomas developing in this area tend to develop a "run-around" extending anteriorly and posteriorly around the rim of the mandible, and if they are neglected long enough, the entire floor of the mouth becomes involved. This pattern of growth results in common bilateral involvement at the anterior floor of the mouth (Fig. 16-20) with frequent bilateral cervical metastases. These lesions tend to be less well differentiated than lesions of the tongue or gingiva and rapidly invade the surrounding structures, especially the periosteum of the adjacent mandible and the tissues of the submaxillary space. Metastases occur first to the submaxillary lymph nodes and are frequent. Taylor and Nathanson observed that 60 percent of these patients had palpable cervical metastases on admission, and in 90 percent cervical lymph node involvement had developed within a year of diagnosis.

The primary symptoms of these neoplasms are often neglected for some time, since they are quite minimal. Eventually the patient complains of pain, swelling of the tongue, and difficulty in eating and speaking. Early lesions are usually discovered by patients themselves while inspecting the mouth or have been noticed by an alert dentist or physician. Rarely, very early lesions may be seen involving only the superficial mucosa.

Large lesions of the floor of the mouth require wide excision in continuity with resection of a portion of the mandible and radical neck dissection. The neck dissection is done whether lymph nodes are palpable or not, in view of the high incidence of positive cervical nodes. Operative therapy may be integrated with pre- or postoperative radiation in the larger lesions. The much less common superficial and in situ lesions can be treated by local excision only. The 5-year survival rates for cancers in this site are comparable with those for cancer of the tongue. James reports an average determinate survival of 37 percent, and the Tumor Registry of the Memorial Center for Cancer reports a 5-year survival rate of 39 percent.

GINGIVAE

Cancer of the gums is better differentiated and slower in its pattern of growth than lesions of the tongue and floor of the mouth. Patients first note a mass (Fig. 16-21) of slight tenderness of the gum, sometimes with loosening of teeth in the area of the tumor. This often leads them to consult their dentist, who, if not alert to the problem, may extract the teeth under the mistaken impression that the patient has an underlying abscess or cyst. As the lesion progresses, it ulcerates, bleeds, and interferes with mastication. As a neoplasm invades the underlying bone, it can involve the mandibular nerve with the appearance of numbness in the mental and submental areas. Extraction of a tooth often accelerates the invasion of the mandible.

Treatment of cancer of the lower gingiva requires resecton of the involved mandible and overlying gum together with a radical neck dissection. Metastases from cancers at this site are usually to the submaxillary lymph nodes and are present in about half the patients at their first visit. Epidermoid cancers of the upper gingiva are less common and better differentiated than cancers of the

Fig. 16-20. Squamous carcinoma of the floor of the mouth. This lesion is in a typical location in the midline with spread in both directions around the curve of the mandible. It has invaded deeply into underlying structures.

Fig. 16-21. Carcinoma of the gingiva. The adjacent teeth are loose and easily removed. The underlying mandible is already invaded.

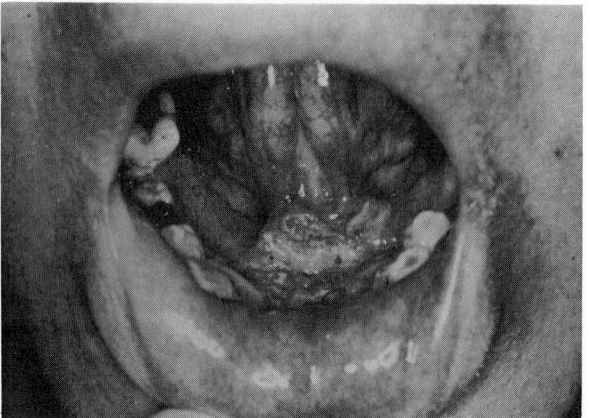

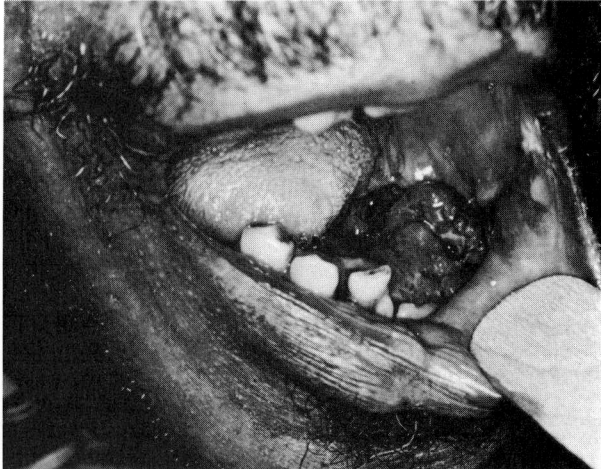

lower gingiva. Metastases to cervical nodes are much less common. Therefore, treatment is restricted to local excision. Radical neck dissection is deferred until there is evidence of palpable cervical node involvement.

The definitive 5-year survival rate following treatment for carcinoma of the gingiva averages 45 percent.

HARD PALATE

The hard palate is the U-shaped area enclosed by the upper gingiva and bounded posteriorly by the attachments of the soft palate. It consists of the palatine processes of the maxillary bones in its anterior two-thirds and of the horizontal portions of the palatine bones in its posterior third.

The most common malignant lesions of the hard palate are tumors of the minor salivary glands. Adenoid cystic carcinomas (Fig. 16-22) and adenocarcinomas occur in almost equal number; malignant mixed tumors are somewhat less frequent. Epidermoid carcinomas primary in the hard palate are rare, although carcinomas primary in the maxillary sinus will occasionally invade the hard palate and perforate into the oral cavity.

The primary symptom is a mass usually noted first by the patient. There is no tenderness or other associated symptom until fairly late in the course of the tumor. As in most salivary malignant tumors, growth is very slow and metastases occur quite late, so that involved cervical lymph nodes are not found initially. Salivary neoplasms respond poorly to radiation therapy, and primary treatment is excision. The chief fault in treatment is underestimation of the extent and potential of these lesions. They are usually fixed to the underlying periosteum, and adequate excision must include resection of the hard palate together with the tumor mass. An attempt to enucleate

the tumor from the underlying bone almost ensures a local recurrence. Excision with a wide margin including the bony palate leaves a substantial palatal defect requiring repair by either surgical reconstruction or the use of an upper plate constructed by a prosthodontist with an obturator that will plug the defect.

Despite the phlegmatic nature of these tumors, complete excision and complete eradication of the lesions are often elusive. The lesions tend to be of a higher grade than malignant lesions of the major salivary glands. Five-year survival rates between 30 and 40 percent are reported, but the incidence of new disease between the fifth and fifteenth year is frequent.

BUCCAL MUCOSA

The lateral walls of the oral cavity are formed by the cheeks, which consist of the buccinator muscle covered on its inner surface by a layer of mucosa extending from the upper to the lower gingivobuccal gutters and from the lateral commissure of the lips anteriorly to the ascending ramus of the mandible posteriorly. Lymphatics from this area pass through the buccinator muscle and follow the facial vein to end in the submaxillary and upper cervical lymph nodes.

The natural evolution of epidermoid carcinoma of the buccal mucosa varies according to the grade of the tumor. About half of the lesions are rather undifferentiated and associated with ulceration, rapid invasion of the cheek, and sometimes even perforation of the skin and formation of an orocutaneous salivary fistula (Fig. 16-23). The majority of such lesions are accompanied by enlarged submaxillary lymph nodes when first seen.

A less aggressive form of buccal cancer is also encountered, especially in patients who are tobacco chewers and "snuff dippers." This is the so-called verrucous carcinoma, which tends to occur in the gingivobuccal gutter and progresses very slowly, sometimes over a period of

Fig. 16-22. Adenoid cystic carcinoma of the hard palate. Although this lesion is much smaller than the mixed tumor in Fig. 16-15, it is malignant. Treatment is by wide excision, including the underlying bone.

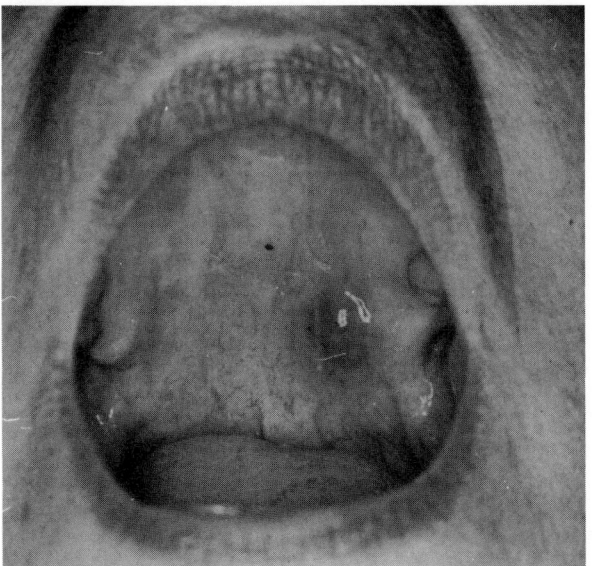

Fig. 16-23. Carcinoma of buccal mucosa. A well-differentiated and slowly growing lesion that was neglected and mismanaged for many years. (From: *Rush BF Jr: Curr Probl Surg May 1966, with permission.*)

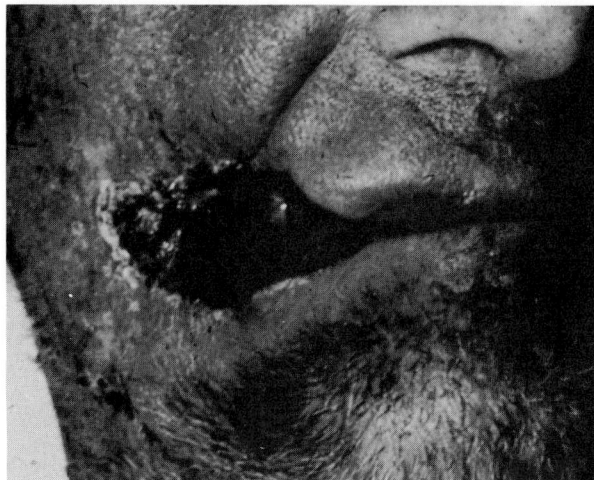

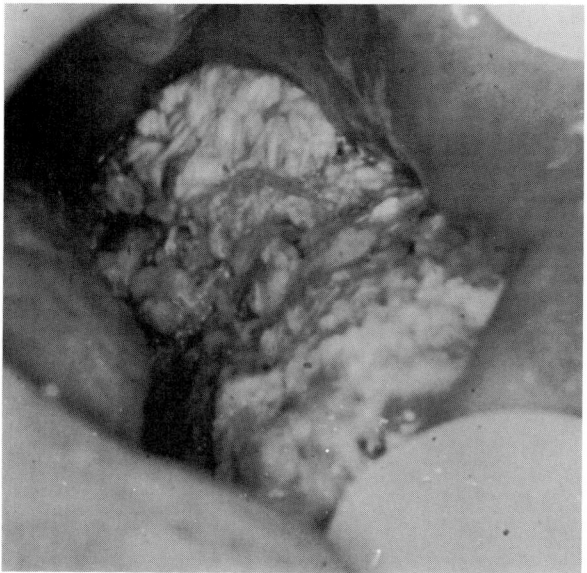

Fig. 16-24. Verrucous carcinoma. The shaggy white plaque along the gingivobuccal gutter is typical. The patient is seventy-five years old and has chewed tobacco for over 50 years.

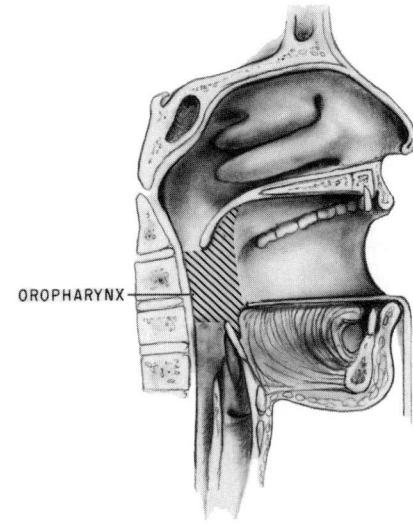

Fig. 16-25. Oropharynx. The shaded area delineates the oropharynx. The nasopharynx is located above, and the hypopharynx and larynx are located below.

years. The tumor is locally invasive, but metastases have never been reported except in patients who have received previous irradiation. Verrucous lesions are easily recognized by their exophytic form and shaggy white appearance (Fig. 16-24). They may cover a wide area, sometimes the entire buccal surface, and have a propensity for bony invasion, often involving a large portion of the mandible or occasionally the maxilla.

Treatment of buccal carcinoma is dictated by the type of lesion encountered. External radiation therapy alone does not eradicate the less well-differentiated lesions, although it has been combined with interstitial therapy with some success. The highly differentiated verrucous carcinomas are fairly radiosensitive but have a marked tendency to recur following an early gratifying regression. In addition, the distressing propensity of these lesions for developing a higher grade of malignancy with metastases after being exposed to radiation is a unique characteristic that has discouraged many from using radiation in treatment. Therefore, the initial therapy for verrucous lesions is wide excision. Since cervical metastases are not ordinarily found, an accompanying radical neck dissection is not done.

For the high-grade lesions, block dissection of the cheek with radical neck resection is the operative treatment of choice. Additional benefit may be derived from combining this with preoperative radiotherapy; this type of combined treatment is still undergoing evaluation. James reported 5-year survival rates in 181 patients with carcinoma of the buccal mucosa of all types as 54.4 percent. The prognosis for the well-differentiated lesions, such as the verrucous carcinoma, should be much better than this.

OROPHARYNX

The oropharynx is the region of the mouth posterior to the anterior tonsillar pillars and the circumvallate papillae of the tongue (Fig. 16-25). It contains the soft palate, tonsil and tonsillar fossa, posterior third of the tongue, anterior surface of the epiglottis, and surrounding pharyngeal walls. The most common site for malignant tumors in this area is the tonsil.

TONSIL

The most common benign lesion of the tonsil is, as every layman knows, inflammatory swelling. This can lead to confusion in diagnosing nonulcerated tumors of these organs. Common malignant lesions are high-grade epidermoid carcinomas (78 percent) and lymphosarcomas (16 percent). A large group of miscellaneous tumors are found, including hemangiomas, neurofibromas, and salivary gland tumors. High-grade epidermoid carcinomas in this area are often described as lymphoepitheliomas and transitional cell carcinomas. It is our feeling that these are simply microscopic variants of highly undifferentiated epidermoid carcinomas.

The frequent first symptom of carcinoma of the tonsil is a slight feeling of tenderness in the area, a typical sore throat. This is easily ignored by the patient for long periods until its persistence finally forces a consultation with the physician. Even then the evidence of a growing tumor may be overlooked and the patient treated for some time with mouthwashes and antibiotics. The lesion will appear grossly as a swelling of the tonsil with a central ulcer. Palpation reveals firmness and induration spreading well beyond the area of ulceration. Trismus and pain in the ear are common complaints. The metastatic spread from this area is to the tonsillar node at the angle of the mandible,

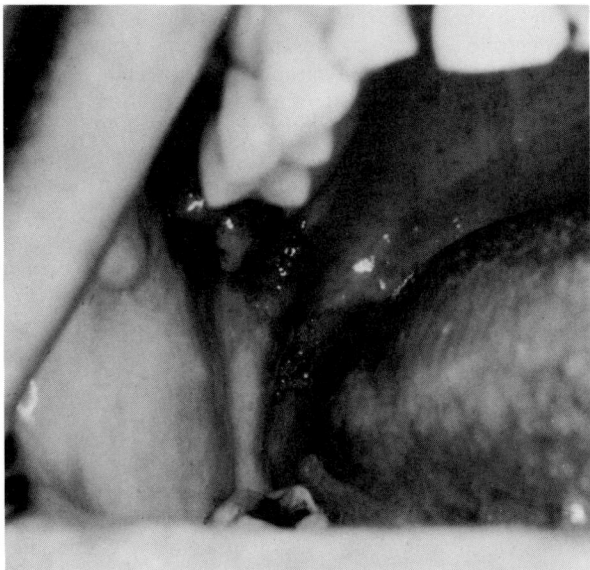

Fig. 16-26. Carcinoma of the anterior tonsillar pillar. These tiny lesions are invasive areas of carcinoma. Despite their size, the patient already had metastatic disease in the ipsilateral neck.

so often enlarged in children who have tonsillitis. The tonsil is a common site for very tiny "occult" carcinomas, which lead to large cervical masses and must be inspected minutely when one is searching for a primary site for cervical metastases (Fig. 16-26). Lymphosarcomas of the tonsil usually present with a more bulky primary lesion and are not as inclined to ulceration. The primary lesions may be bilateral with involvement of both tonsils.

Treatment of tonsillar carcinoma by either radiation or operation has never been very satisfactory. Lymphosarcomas are quite radiosensitive and, if localized, should be treated primarily by radiation. Carcinoma, on the other hand, yields poorly to either form of therapy. Integrated therapy with pre- or postoperative radiation to the tonsil with resection in continuity with a radical neck dissection seems to produce the best results. The definitive 5-year survival following treatment of cancer of the tonsil is 25 percent.

POSTERIOR THIRD OF THE TONGUE

Tumors in the posterior third of the tongue differ markedly in their natural history from those in the anterior two-thirds. Whereas the anterior lesions tend to be well differentiated, remain confined to the primary site, or involve only high cervical nodes for long periods, lesions in the posterior third are of much higher grade, often being classified as *lymphoepitheliomas,* or *transitional cell tumors.* They spread rapidly to the cervical nodes and often beyond to distant sites. A frequent initial symptom of carcinoma of the posterior third of the tongue is a large cervical lymph node accompanied by the complaint of pain on swallowing. Unfortunately, this is a fairly silent area, and lesions may attain considerable size before

causing pain or dysfunction. Wide ulceration causes a malodorous breath and dysphasia. Weight loss is prominent. Treatment has been highly unsatisfactory in the past. Radiation therapy infrequently controls the primary lesion. Operation often results in total loss of the tongue, an overwhelming psychologic and functional deficit. Since these lesions are often across the midline, bilateral neck dissection must be combined with resection of the tongue. Initial experience with combined radiation and operation indicated that occasionally the lesions can be reduced in size sufficiently by preoperative radiation to permit a more conservative resection of the posterior tongue, leaving a functional anterior tongue behind.

SOFT PALATE

Malignant tumors of the soft palate are almost always epidermoid carcinomas. These tend to be well differentiated, slow-growing, and late to metastasize. They are generally superficial lesions spreading over the anterior surface of the soft palate and down the tonsillar pillars. Often it is difficult to determine whether the lesions arose in the tonsil or in the soft palate. Spread may be extensive, covering much of the soft palate, the tonsillar fossa, and the tongue. Pain and dysphagia are the usual first symptoms. Diagnosis by inspection and palpation is a simple matter, and biopsy is easily accomplished.

Response to radiation therapy is only fair. Resection is more likely to produce a cure but often leads to a difficult functional defect, since the patient is unable to close the nasopharynx and will tend to regurgitate food through the nose on swallowing. This is a situation where the clever prosthodontist can help greatly by installing an adequate extension on an upper plate that extends backward into the pharynx to seal the palatal defect. An even more convenient method of closing the palatal defect is to raise a flap from the posterior pharynx and swing it forward to close the defect at the time of the original operation. Prognosis is difficult to determine, since these tumors are usually classed in the literature with tumors of the tonsil or of the hard palate.

EPIGLOTTIS

Malignant tumors of the anterior surface of the epiglottis are usually exophytic and well differentiated and have a slow, natural evolution. Dysphagia and aspiration are early symptoms. Treatment by radiation therapy is quite successful. Hemilaryngectomy of the upper larynx above the cords has also produced good results. Patients who have had resection of the epiglottis must relearn swallowing, and this requires a reasonable level of intelligence. Senile patients or those with poor learning ability should be treated by either radiation or total laryngectomy.

LARYNX

When describing the site of tumors of the larynx, the terminology can be confusing and frustrating. According to current usage, the larynx is made up of those structures lying both above and below the true vocal cords. Thus, the mucosa of the larynx extends along the posterior surface of the epiglottis including its tip, along the aryepiglottic folds, and over the arytenoid cartilages posteriorly. It covers the inner surface of the aryepiglottic folds, the false vocal cords, and the ventricles. All of the larynx thus far described constitutes the supraglottic larynx, i.e., that which is above the true vocal cords. The glottic portion of the larynx is that portion made up of the true cords themselves. The mucosa lining the area underneath the true cords down to the lower border of the cricoid cartilage covers the infraglottic portion of the larynx.

In the past the area just described was called the "endolarynx," or the "intrinsic larynx," although the latter term gradually came to mean the true cords alone. Tumors taking their origin on the outside of the larynx for many years were designated as arising from the "extrinsic larynx." However, this term came to be used for supraglottic lesions as well, so this usage has now been abandoned. Lesions involving any portion of the exterior of the larynx are now spoken of as "hypopharyngeal" or, by some, "laryngopharyngeal."

INCIDENCE AND ETIOLOGY. Cancer of the larynx accounts for 1.62 percent of all cancers in men and only 0.14 percent of all cancers in woman; thus the ratio of incidence favors the male sex over 11:1. The report of the Advisory Committee to the Surgeon General on Smoking and Health reviewed 10 retrospective studies and 7 prospective studies on the relationship of smoking to carcinoma of the larynx. There was a statistically positive relationship in every study. In the prospective studies the mortality ratios for smokers averaged 5.4 times greater for cigarette smokers than for nonsmokers and 2.8 times greater for cigar and pipe smokers than for nonsmokers. Laryngeal cancer mortality has increased somewhat over the past three decades, but the increase has been much less than that for lung cancer. It appears that the induction of carcinoma of the larynx cannot occur solely as a result of tobacco tars but that a further agent, or cocarcinogen, is needed. One such agent may be alcohol, since a high percentage (30 to 40 percent) of patients with carcinoma of the larynx are alcoholics and come from population groups where the risk of alcoholism is great, such as bartenders and entertainers. Cirrhosis of the liver is a common complaint among patients with carcinoma of the larynx; this may be a secondary relationship due to the frequency of alcoholism in this group.

CLASSIFICATION. As it has for other cancers, the American Joint Committee on Cancer Staging and End Results Reporting has developed a TNM system for carcinomas of the larynx. Because of differences in prognosis at different sites the committee has divided the larynx into its three major areas: the supraglottic (posterior surface of the epiglottis, aryepiglottic folds, arytenoids, false cords, ventricles); the glottic (right and left vocal cords and anterior glottic commissure); and the subglottic (subglottic region exclusive of the undersurface of the true cords and down to the lower margin of the cricoid cartilage). About 56 percent of squamous epidermoid cancers of the larynx

occur in the glottic region, 42 percent occur in the supraglottic region, and the remaining 2 percent are subglottic. The combination of topographic spread (T), nodal involvement (N), and distant metastasis (M) in a description of three separate anatomic sites results in a complex system, yet it is the most precise method whereby lesions can be classified and comparisons between institutions adequately made as to the results of treatment.

PATHOLOGY. Polyps, papillomas, granulomas, cysts, and areas of hyperkeratosis make up the common benign lesions of the cords. Rarely hemangiomas and chondromas of the laryngeal cartilages are seen. Ninety-nine percent of the malignant lesions of the larynx are epidermoid carcinomas, and most of these are of the ordinary cornifying (squamous cell) type. These lesions arise from the squamous epithelium of the cords themselves or from areas of metaplasia in the mucosa of the endolarynx. On the cord, carcinoma may be preceded by hyperkeratosis and stages of transition from hyperkeratosis to dyskeratosis, carcinoma in situ, and microinvasive carcinoma. Glottic cancers are usually very well differentiated, slow-growing, and late to metastasize. Supraglottic and infraglottic cancers are less well differentiated and more likely to have spread to lymph nodes when first seen.

DIAGNOSIS. Space-occupying lesions of the larynx produce initial symptoms through interference with phonation and respiration. Hoarseness, the usual first symptom, may be slight and intermittent but gradually becomes constant. What begins as a slight huskiness gradually progresses, until sounds are produced with difficulty. Respiratory obstruction is a later sign, although small lesions on the true cords will produce a greater degree of obstruction than somewhat larger lesions in the supraglottic or infraglottic area. Obstruction progresses in severity until the patient may respire with visible effort, using accessory muscles to force air through the cords, sometimes with audible stridor. At this point the patient's life is in jeopardy. At any moment the slightest additional swelling or edema can cut off breathing completely. The use of sedatives in patients at this phase of obstruction is fraught with danger. Under sedation the patient's tired muscles may fail, with a rapid shallowing of respiration, progressive anoxia, and cardiac arrest. The finding of a tumor on the cord associated with stridor, retraction, or the use of accessory muscles to breathe indicates immediate tracheostomy. It is far better to elect a tracheostomy done in the operating room than to be forced into an emergency tracheostomy in the ward or in the emergency room under much less favorable circumstances.

Late signs of malignant lesions of the larynx are a malodorous breath, pain on swallowing, weight loss, and hemoptysis.

Any patient who has persistent hoarseness for more than 3 or 4 weeks should have a careful inspection of the vocal cords by indirect laryngoscopy. If this reveals no pathologic condition but hoarseness persists, direct laryngoscopy should be used to examine the cords even more closely.

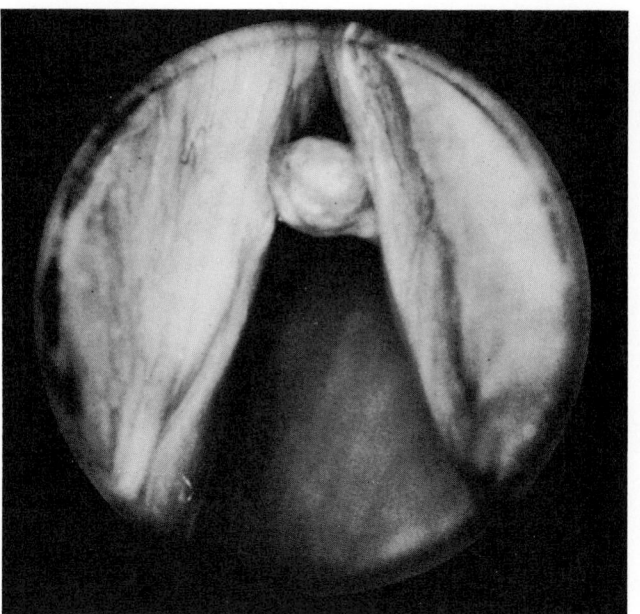

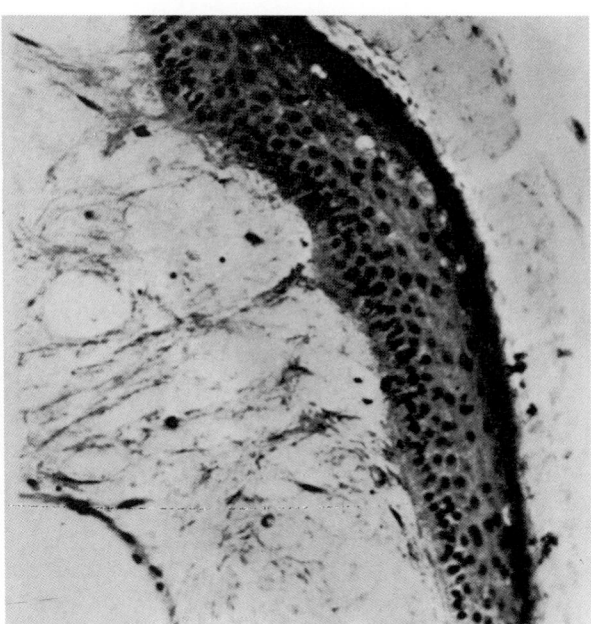

Fig. 16-27. Pedunculated polyp of the right vocal cord arising at the junction of the anterior and middle thirds. (From: *Holinger PH et al: Ann Otol Rhinol Laryngol 56:583, 1947, with permission.*)

Benign Tumors

POLYPS

According to Holinger, 43 percent of all benign lesions of the larynx are simple polyps. These arise on the phonating edge of the cord at the junction between the anterior one-third and the posterior two-thirds (Fig. 16-27). Their cause is obscure. Treatment is by removal with a cupped forceps at direct laryngoscopy.

VOCAL NODULES

The second most common benign tumor of the larynx, these are usually bilateral and, like polyps, occur at the junction of the anterior one-third with the posterior two-thirds of the cords. They are often called "singer's nodules" but certainly are not confined to singers and can occur in any occupational group. Treatment is by removal with the biopsy forceps.

RETENTION CYSTS

About half of these occur on the vocal cords, the remainder being found in the aryepiglottic folds, arytenoids, or epiglottis. They appear to occur as a result of the obstruction of small mucous glands. These lesions can reach considerable size and offer marked embarrassment to respiration.

HYPERKERATOSIS

Hyperkeratosis can affect the vocal cords as it does any of the mucosal areas of the lips, oral cavity, or pharynx.

These lesions are evidence of a premalignant change and should be stripped off the cord with the use of the biopsy forceps. Patients who have developed hyperkeratosis should be followed at twice yearly intervals to guard against recurrence or the appearance of a frank carcinoma.

PAPILLOMAS

These multiple lesions are found most often on the true cords but may appear on any portion of the larynx or pharynx and even on the soft palate. While they are most commonly reported in children prior to adolescence, some adults are also affected. Like warts, these tumors appear to be caused by viruses. Frequently the growths cover the mucosa of the cords in great profusion, causing severe respiratory embarrassment and requiring tracheostomy. They can persist for many years; during this period the patient often must continue to wear a tracheostomy tube while papillomas are cleared from the airway by frequent excisions through the laryngoscope. Repeated excision is the only effective treatment to date. The large number of other forms of therapy attempted indicates the generally unsatisfactory state of therapy. Eventually, after a period of months or years of repeated excisions, the lesions gradually disappear.

Malignant Lesions

Carcinoma of the true cords (Fig. 16-28) is a lesion that should be easily detected. It gives warning of its presence at an early stage through hoarseness and grows slowly enough so that early therapy should be rewarded by a 90 percent or better 5-year survival rate. In many urban areas over half of the lesions of the true cords are stage 1

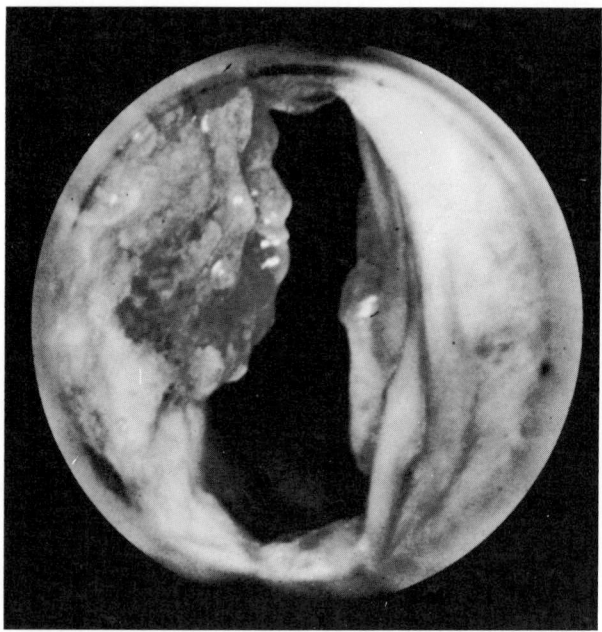

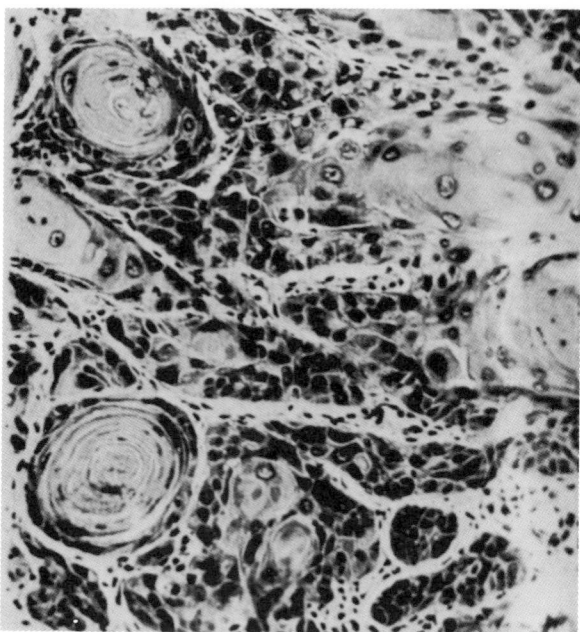

Fig. 16-28. Carcinoma involving the left side of the larynx and anterior commissure. (From: *Holinger PH et al: Ann Otol Rhinol Laryngol 56:583, 1947, with permission.*)

lesions confined entirely to the cord. In contrast, some rural areas report that in only 5 percent of patients reaching the physician the lesions are still in Stage I. As the tumor grows, it extends off the cord, either up into the supraglottic area or less commonly inferiorly into the infraglottic region. Invasion occurs slowly but relentlessly, eventually with perforation of the thyroid cartilage and direct invasion of the soft tissues of the thyroid gland and of the neck.

If cancer remains confined to the true cords, a high percentage of 5-year survivals can be obtained following treatment by radiotherapy alone. Holinger noted that in a series of 102 patients with cordal lesions treated with cobalt irradiation, only 9 patients had residual or recurrent cancer that required subsequent laryngectomy. None of the patients in this series died of carcinoma. Loss of the larynx is such a major functional and psychologic disability that if excellent results can be obtained by irradiation, this should be the treatment of choice.

Cancers that have invaded areas beyond the cord have a much different outlook. Involvement of cervical nodes becomes an important problem, and the ability to eradicate the disease by radiation alone is greatly decreased. For Stages II, III, and IV cancers, partial or total laryngectomy is mandatory. In addition, a radical or modified radical neck dissection on the side of the lesion is often performed, even though palpable nodes are not present. Using this approach, Norris has reported a 70 to 75 percent 5-year survival rate for Stages II and III lesions of glottic and supraglottic origin. Some feel that if no nodes are palpable prophylatic radiation to the neck will suffice. The very large Stage IV lesions do very poorly with surgery alone, with a 5-year survival rate of only 21 percent. Combined radiation therapy and operation in treatment of advanced cancers of the larynx improves the long-term

survival rate. Our recent experience with adding chemotherapy to the integrated treatment of Stage IV lesions indicates a further improvement in survival to as high as 50 percent.

The major problem for the patient after laryngectomy is to regain a useful voice. About half of all such patients will learn to use effective esophageal speech, meaning they can communicate understandably with strangers and casual acquaintances. An additional 25 percent can make themselves understood to members of their family but find that their esophageal speech is too distorted to be useful in the general community. The remaining 25 percent of patients will be unable to conquer the technical problems of learning this method of conversation.

Esophageal speech is by far the most useful technique for speaking after laryngectomy, since it requires no additional paraphernalia and can be refined to the point where it very closely resembles the tone and expression of ordinary speech. It is produced by swallowing air and regurgitating it, creating a vibration in the pharynx—probably at the level of the cricothyroid muscle. The oral cavity modulates this tone just as it would a tone from the larynx.

For the 50 percent of patients who are partly or completely unable to learn esophageal speech, electric vibrating devices can be used to provide a tone in the oral cavity that is modulated by the patient's oral structures, giving a fairly reasonable method of communication.

The realization that any fistula between the trachea and pharynx that permits passage of air from the lungs to the mouth will produce easily understood and controlled speech has led to the development of the Singer-Blom prosthesis. This is a silicone valve that is placed in a passage connecting trachea and pharynx and allows air to

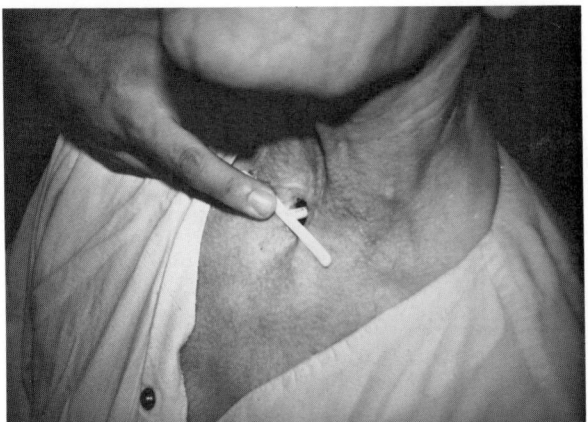

Fig. 16-29. A Singer-Blom prosthesis placed in the fistula between the trachea and pharynx in a laryngectomized patient. The patient will speak by occluding the trachea with a finger, redirecting air from the lungs through the prosthesis into the pharynx. Vibrations induced by pharyngeal structures produce sound that is modulated by the oral cavity to produce excellent speech in most instances.

pass into the pharynx and mouth but prevents saliva from passing into the trachea. With this device successful speech has been reported in from 60 to 90 percent of patients (Fig. 16-29). The principle employed by the Blum-Singer prosthesis has been recognized for many years and operative attempts to create a valved fistula between trachea and pharynx have appeared sporadically for many decades and with increasing frequency in the last 10 years. The major problem has been in establishing a competent valve that prevents aspiration of saliva. Figure 16-30 shows an example of one such operation developed in our clinic that has had some success but requires further development.

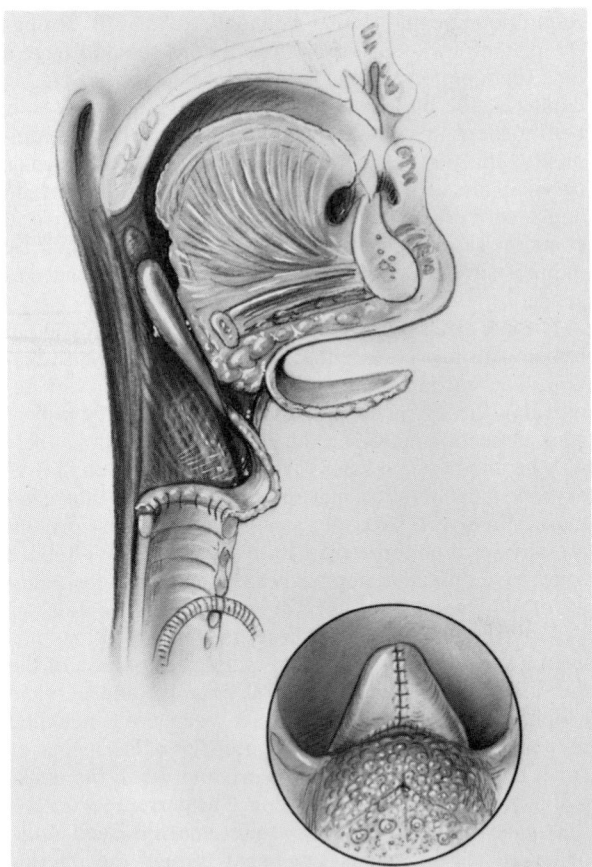

Fig. 16-30. A valved tracheopharyngeal fistula that is formed by a flap turned in from the neck following laryngectomy. Part of the flap forms a "neoepiglottis" (inset) that serves as the valve to close the newly formed glottis when the patient swallows and prevents aspiration. To speak, the patient occludes the tracheostomy, directing air into the pharynx and opening the valve.

HYPOPHARYNX

The hypopharynx is that area of the throat which surrounds the larynx. It is made up of the piriform sinuses on either side, the exterior portions of the aryepiglottic fold, and the lateral and posterior pharyngeal walls. It includes the mucosa overlying the posterior portions of the cricoid cartilage.

INCIDENCE. Cancer of the hypopharynx is three to four times as common as cancer of the larynx and constitutes 4.05 percent of all cancers in males. It is three times more common in men than in women. These tumors appear to be related to smoking. The correlation is stronger with pipe and cigar smoking than with cigarette smoking. Another etiologic factor is the Plummer-Vinson syndrome, found most commonly in Scandinavian women. This deficiency syndrome, now gradually disappearing, is clearly related to carcinoma of the hypopharynx and posterior tongue. At the Radiumhemmet in Stockholm carcinomas of the hypopharynx are seen more frequently in women than in men, and most of these cases are associated with a Plummer-Vinson syndrome.

PATHOLOGY. The great majority of these tumors are epidermoid carcinomas and compared with the oral cavity and endolarynx tend to be of a higher grade with a preponderance of grades 3 and 4 lesions. Better-differentiated forms are seen, however, most commonly on the exterior portions of the aryepiglottic folds and in the postcricoid area. Spread of the tumor occurs promptly and usually by way of the lymphatic channels that drain the hypopharynx, exiting between the lateral portion of the hyoid bone and the upper edge of the thyroid cartilage to travel with the superior thyroid artery to the midjugular chain of lymph nodes. Unlike most head and neck cancers, distant metastases are more common with involvement of mediastinal nodes, lung, liver, and other distant viscera.

DIAGNOSIS. Since these lesions arise outside the endolarynx away from major paths of respiration and speech, hoarseness or dyspnea are uncommon findings until late in the growth of the tumor. Interference with swallowing, on the other hand, is the most common early symptom and is associated with choking and aspiration.

Aspiration pneumonia may be the illness that first brings the patient to the physician. The lesions seem to have a long silent period and can grow to considerable size in the depths of the piriform sinus or on the pharyngeal walls before the first definite symptoms appear. Not uncommonly, the first sign is the appearance of a midjugular cervical node. The better-differentiated lesions invade and ulcerate widely, so that a malodorous breath is a common associated finding. Diagnosis is confirmed by indirect laryngoscopy and biopsy through a laryngoscope.

TREATMENT. Until recent years this was a highly lethal tumor with few cures either by operation or by irradiation. The introduction of wide radical excision with removal of the larynx and hypopharynx and en bloc radical neck dissection increased the cure rate perceptibly. This may be another area where judicious combination of irradiation and operation can improve the cure rate even more. Five-year survival rates with the older form of therapy were no more than 10 to 15 percent. With more aggressive operative approaches, cure rates in the vicinity of 30 percent have been reported.

Rehabilitation following these massive resections has been a very difficult problem requiring restoration of the digestive tract between the oral pharynx and cervical esophagus. Many techniques have been tried including myocutaneous skin flaps, free transfer of segments of small bowel with arterial microanastomosis in the neck, and transfer of a loop of the colon. The current favorite is the "gastric pull-up" whereby the stomach is freed in the abdomen and the fundus is pulled up through the anterior or posterior mediastinum and attached at the base of the tongue. The blood supply is excellent, anastomosis is very reliable, and fistula formation is rare. This procedure is done immediately following resection of the hypopharynx and larynx so that when the patient awakes all continuity has been restored.

NASOPHARYNX

The nasopharynx is at the top of the pharynx, just underneath the base of the skull. The body of the sphenoid bone forms a roof for this cavity, while its floor is formed by the soft palate. There is no anterior wall as such except for the posterior openings of the nasal passage together with the posterior aspects of the nasal septum and the turbinates. The roof of the cavity slopes into the posterior wall made up of the basiocciput and the atlas and the overlying covering of muscle and mucosa. Each lateral wall contains the opening of a eustachian tube guarded by a small prominence, the torus tubarius. The only structure lying within the nasopharynx is the lymphoid tissue of the adenoids scattered on the posterior and superior walls.

INCIDENCE. These tumors are uncommon but not rare, constituting about $\frac{1}{2}$ percent of all cancers. They are somewhat more common in males than in females (2.4:1). There is an interesting relation to race. This is a frequent tumor in the Near East, among the Filipinos, Malays, and

Dayaks, and especially among the Chinese. This cancer accounts for 30.4 percent of all cancers in males in Taiwan. The incidence among the Chinese born in the Far East is more than thirty times greater than in this country, while the incidence among American-born Chinese is about six times as common as the incidence among the other racial groups here. This shift in pattern would suggest that both genetic and environmental causative factors are operating.

Benign Lesions

These include hypertrophied lymphatic tissue, juvenile nasopharyngeal hemangiofibroma, Rathke's pouch cyst, dermoids, and mixed tumors. Of these, hypertrophied adenoids occur commonly, and hemangiofibroma and Rathke's pouch cyst have a special predilection for this site.

Any enlarging, space-occupying lesion of the nasopharynx calls attention to itself by respiratory obstruction and nasal stuffiness. Obstruction to the eustachian tubes provokes earaches and often chronic ear infection. As the lesion encroaches on the soft palate, deglutition is disturbed with pain on swallowing or regurgitation of food and fluids into the nasopharynx and out of the nose.

HYPERTROPHIED ADENOIDS

The adenoids represent a portion of the large circle of lymphatic tissue surrounding the oral respiratory passageway at the level of the posterior tongue and tonsils. Chronic upper respiratory tract infections in infants and children often cause marked and persistent hypertrophy of some of this rim of tissue. In past decades resection of the adenoids and tonsils was one of the most common of operations in children. With the advent of the antibiotics the need for these procedures has diminished markedly. Nonetheless, in an occasional child a persistent hypertrophy of the adenoids will develop that disturbs the breathing pattern, causing mouth breathing, or more importantly will obstruct the eustachian tubes, leading to chronic ear infections with a threat to the child's hearing. These symptoms are adequate indication for operative excision.

JUVENILE NASOPHARYNGEAL HEMANGIOFIBROMA

Made up of a hard stroma of fibrous tissue, richly interlaced with capillaries and cavernous sinuses, this rare and interesting tumor appears to originate on the roof of the nasopharynx perhaps from the periosteum of the sphenoid bone (Fig. 16-31). It increases in size slowly but relentlessly and eventually begins to erode the anterior structures, obstruct the nasal passages, and enter the maxillary sinus on one or both sides. The first symptom may be nasal obstruction but is usually epistaxis, which can be very profuse and even life-threatening.

This lesion is found exclusively in males, usually in the preadolescent or adolescent age groups. In some instances as the boy matures, the lesion appears to regress spontaneously. Just as often it persists, and heman-

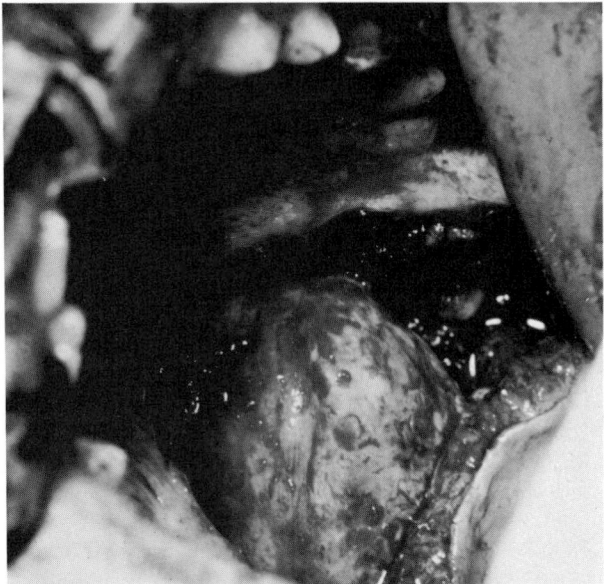

Fig. 16-31. Juvenile nasopharyngeal hemangiofibroma. A fibrous, highly vascular lesion on the posterior wall of the nasopharynx. This was first noted because of epistaxis. Exposure was obtained by an incision between the hard and soft palate with retraction of the soft palate downward.

giofibromas of the nasopharynx have been described in males in their twenties and thirties, either persisting from childhood or appearing for the first time.

The progressive destruction of surrounding bone by pressure and the continuing threat of major hemorrhage require prompt treatment, preferably before the lesions grow too large. Radiation therapy is ineffective, and operative excision appears the only mode of treatment. There is a tendency toward local recurrence following excision, and these patients must be followed carefully for some years after operation.

Malignant Lesions

These are epidermoid carcinoma, lymphosarcoma, adenoid cystic carcinoma, cervical chordoma, sarcoma, and myeloma. The only lesions occurring with any frequency are epidermoid carcinoma and lymphosarcoma.

EPIDERMOID CARCINOMA

These develop from areas of metaplasia in the respiratory epithelium of the nasopharynx and are moderately to highly undifferentiated. There is a liberal amount of lymphoid tissue in the nasopharynx, and frequently malignant epithelial cells are seen mixed with a prominent lymphoid stroma. This mixture of epidermoid and lymphoid cells gave rise to the term "lymphoepithelioma" introduced by Regaud and Schmincke. Many pathologists feel there is no place for this special term, since these tumors are probably highly anaplastic epidermoid carcinomas and the lymphoid element may not constitute an actual malignant part of the growth. Some feel that a large

percentage of lymphoid intermixing indicates a more radiosensitive and more radiocurable tumor.

In addition to the obstructive symptoms described for benign tumors, the invasive qualities of malignant lesions produce a number of characteristic signs and symptoms. These lesions invade the roof of the nasopharynx entering the cavernous sinus with paralysis of the IIId, IVth, Vth, and VIth cranial nerves. The VIth nerve is usually paralyzed first; this is frequently accompanied by pain in the distribution of the supraorbital and infraorbital branches of the Vth nerve. The tumor reaches these nerves by spreading along the eustachian tube into the space between the pharynx and the maxilla, then extending upward through the suture line between the petrous portion of the temporal bone and the lateral wing of the sphenoid. Thus, the symptom complex is called the *petrosphenoidal syndrome*. Metastatic nodes in the retropharyngeal space tend to spread into the area along the base of the skull medial to the parotid gland, where they compress the IXth, Xth, XIth, and XIIth cranial nerves. This causes difficulties with deglutition from hemiparesis of the superior constrictor muscle, a perversion of the sense of taste in the posterior third of the tongue, and hypesthesia of the mucous membranes of the soft palate, pharynx, and larynx. Paralysis of the trapezius muscle, the sternocleidomastoid, the soft palate, and one side of the tongue may also occur. These signs may be associated with Horner's syndrome from compression of the cervical sympathetic chain. Invasion of the orbit and displacement of the globe will cause double vision and proptosis.

Unfortunately, the nasopharynx is a silent area, and tumors here can reach considerable size before any symptoms are evident. The early signs of nasal obstruction or brief episodes of epistaxis are easily ignored. In two-thirds of the patients, by the time diagnosis is made, invasion of the sphenoid bone and base of the skull or nerve paralysis is present. Not infrequently, the primary growth will remain small, even microscopic, and is announced by its cervical metastases. These occur in a characteristic location, high in the neck behind the lower portion of the ear with additional involved nodes scattered along the path of the spinal accessory nerve as it courses down the trapezius muscle (Fig. 16-32). Cervical metastases are found in 50 percent of patients when first seen and are the presenting symptom in one-third.

There is no acceptable way of obtaining an adequate margin of resection when operating upon lesions of the nasopharynx, and the only operative procedure used is biopsy. Treatment of the primary lesion and usually of the metastases is by radiation therapy. Considering the advanced state of most of these lesions when first seen, the 5-year survival rate as a result of therapy is remarkably good, with an overall absolute survival of 28 percent. For the occasional patient who does not have evidence of cervical node metastasis at the beginning of treatment the 5-year survival rate is 55 percent.

LYMPHOSARCOMA

Lymphosarcomas of the nasopharynx tend to occur at the extremes of age in childhood and in the seventh and

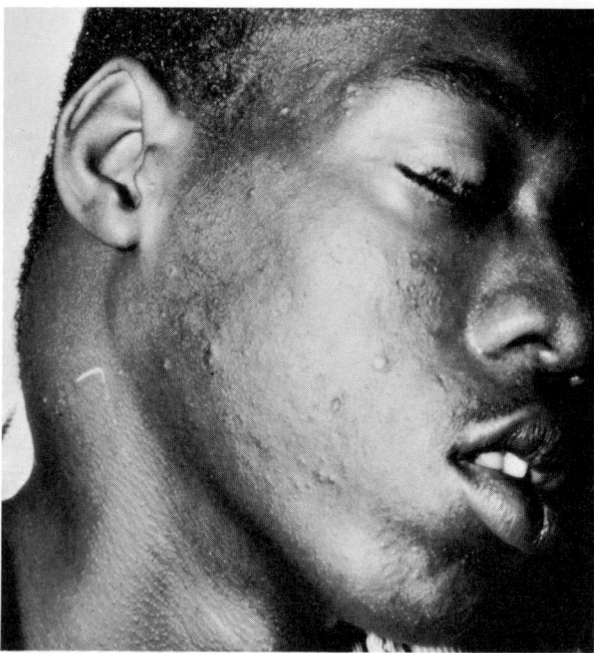

Fig. 16-32. Metastatic lymph nodes in the neck from lymphosarcoma of the nasopharynx. Note the characteristic location behind and inferior to the ear.

eighth decades. These are nearly always non-Hodgkin's lymphomas. The majority of these lesions announce their presence by the occurrence of cervical node metastases, which are usually bulky with a rubbery consistency; the nodes mat together but are less inclined to be invasive and fixed than nodes involved by carcinoma. While lymphosarcoma may mimic all the symptoms produced by epidermoid carcinomas, they invade bone infrequently, and paralysis of nerves is much less common. If there is no evidence of spread beyond the area of the head and neck, the radiotherapist usually administers a high level of therapy in the vicinity of 6000 rad of high-energy (cobalt or linear accelerator) radiation to both the nasopharynx and the cervical lymphatic tissues bilaterally. If the lesions have spread beyond the head and neck or if systemic symptoms are present, chemotherapy is the treatment of choice. Five-year survival in these highly radiosensitive tumors is slightly better than for epidermoid carcinoma, averaging 35 to 40 percent.

NASAL CAVITY AND PARANASAL SINUSES

The position of the eight nasal sinuses surrounding the nasal cavity is often poorly appreciated. The maxillary sinuses lateral to the nasal cavities and beneath the orbits are the largest and most important of the sinus structures. The ethmoid air cells occupying the space between the orbit and the upper nasal cavity are much smaller and are less commonly involved by tumors. The frontal sinuses bilaterally above the orbits are the second largest set of sinuses. The paired sphenoid sinuses divided by a thin septum just below the pituitary and over the roof of the nasopharynx are the most remote of the sinuses. The frontal and sphenoid sinuses are rare primary sites for tumors.

INCIDENCE. Tumors of the nasal cavity and paranasal sinuses represent about 1 percent of all cancer seen. Malignant lesions are found here three times as commonly in men as in women. With the exception of the esthesioneuroblastoma no specific cause is known for lesions arising here.

Benign Tumors

Polyps of the nasal cavity and maxillary sinus are the most common growths seen. These are usually associated with chronic inflammation or, occasionally, allergy. Sometimes the underlying infection may be due to a tumor, so that the discovery of polyps should not be considered an adequate diagnosis until the possibility of an underlying tumor has been ruled out. While polyps can be eradicated by simple excision, they will usually re-form unless the basic pathologic condition leading to their growth has been determined and corrected. This may be allergy, septal deviation, or other factors that obstruct adequate drainage and promote infection.

Malignant Tumors

Of 293 patients with neoplasms of the nasal cavity and paranasal sinus examined at the Mayo Clinic approximately 50 percent had epidermoid carcinomas, 10 percent had lymphomas, and 20 percent had tumors that probably arose from minor salivary tissue. The remaining 20 percent had various soft tissue sarcomas such as fibrosarcoma, chondrosarcoma, neurofibrosarcoma, and osteogenic sarcoma. Among 648 patients seen in Sweden with epidermoid carcinomas arising from the paranasal sinuses, the average age ranged from fifty to seventy years, and the vast majority of the lesions arose in the maxillary sinus (Fig. 16-33). None of these tumors occurred in the sphenoid sinus and only one in the frontal sinus.

Tumors, whether benign or malignant, are announced by pain, nasal obstruction, and persistent nasal secretion. Fifty percent of the patients present with one or more of these three symptoms. Unfortunately, these are also the presenting symptoms of sinusitis; patients may be treated with antibiotics and other measures for long periods before the more serious nature of the disease is realized. Repeated epistaxis is more likely to suggest the presence of tumor but occurs in only 10 percent as a presenting symptom. Swelling or ulceration of the hard palate or gingiva, swelling of the cheek, or ocular symptoms are evidences of a much more advanced stage of tumor growth yet constitute the presenting symptom in 25 to 30 percent of patients (Fig. 16-34). Bone destruction seen on radiographic examination is almost certain evidence of a tumor and unfortunately is also a late sign. Absence of bone destruction does not rule out a malignant tumor. All tissue removed when polyps of the nose or maxillary sinus are treated or when the maxillary sinus is drained should

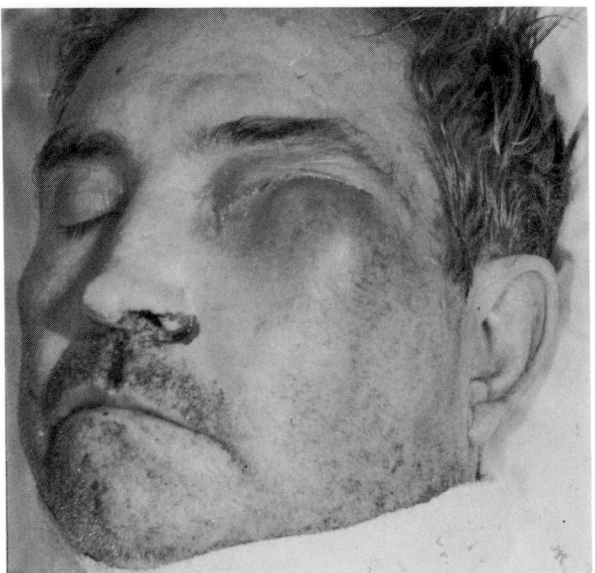

Fig. 16-33. Squamous carcinoma of the maxilla. The lesion had its origin in the upper portion of the maxillary sinus and invaded the floor of the orbit.

Fig. 16-34. Squamous carcinoma of the ethmoid sinuses. This lesion began in the left ethmoid and invaded the nasal cavity and right ethmoid sinus.

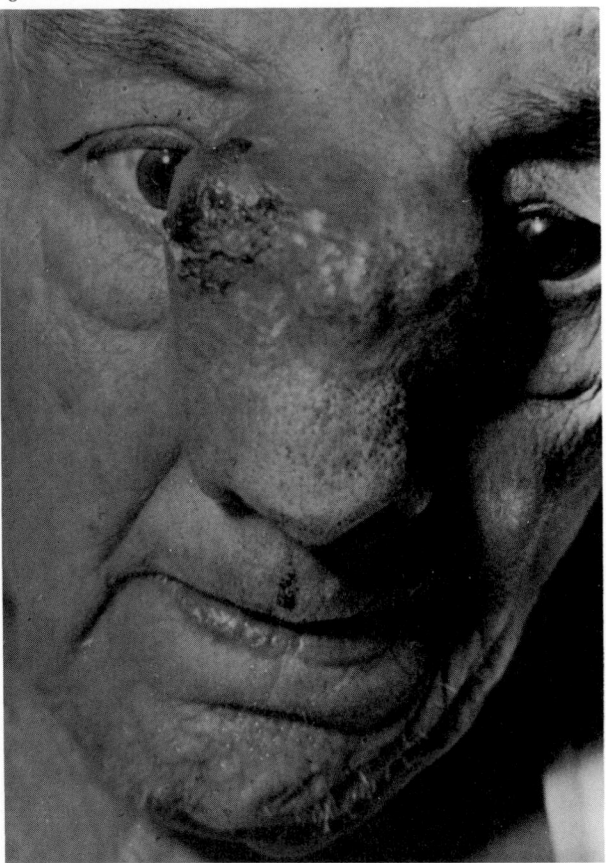

be submitted for histologic examination. Not infrequently this is the first evidence of the presence of an underlying carcinoma and may be the only opportunity for diagnosis of such lesions at an early state.

TREATMENT. Electrosurgical therapy, radiation therapy, and operative excision have all been used to treat these tumors. Lymphomas are ordinarily treated by radiation alone or, depending on type, with appropriate chemotherapy. Epidermoid carcinomas of this site are refractory to either irradiation or operation. Integration of irradiation preoperatively with operative excision has been used for many years and has gained wide acceptance. This approach yields a 5-year survival rate of 30 to 35 percent for lesions of the maxillary sinuses. Cervical lymph nodes are involved late, and radical neck dissections are not done unless palpable nodes are present.

MANDIBLE

Tumors of the mandible arise from two main sources, from the tooth-forming (odontogenic) tissue and from bone.

Odontogenic Tumors

These neoplasms arise from ectodermal odontogenic tissue, mesodermal odontogenic tissue, or a mixture of both. They are invariably benign. The lesions most commonly seen are ectodermal odontogenic cysts: the follicular and radicular cysts. A rare and intriguing tumor is the ameloblastoma. Other odontogenic tumors are too rare to merit consideration here.

FOLLICULAR CYST

Some cysts are derived from the dental lamina and outer enamel epithelium of developing teeth. Remnants of this tissue sequestered during development may undergo proliferation and cystic change. Microscopically, they have fibrous walls usually lined by squamous epithelium. Occasionally remnants of odontogenic epithelium are present from which ameloblastomas may develop. Often the cyst envelops an unerupted tooth. A pathognomonic x-ray finding is the appearance of a smooth symmetric cyst in the mandible containing an unerupted tooth in its cavity. Clinically the tumor is found as a mass causing enlargement of the ramus of the mandible or the rim of the gingiva. Treatment is by intraoral excision, removing the top of the cyst and excising its entire lining membrane.

RADICULAR CYST

Infection of the dental pulp is the most common cause of this frequent cyst. A dental granuloma forms when epithelial remnants of the sheath about the tooth root are entrapped. Nests of epithelial tissue proliferate to line a central lumen usually at the apex of the infected tooth (Fig. 16-35). Cysts may vary in size from 1 to several centimeters. Microscopically, there is a dense, fibrous connective tissue lining covered internally by squamous epi-

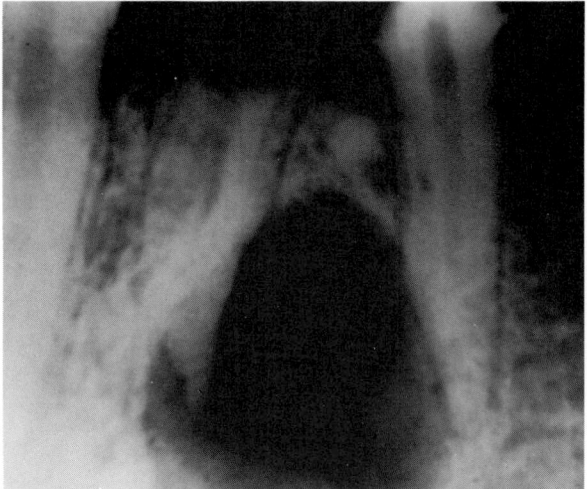

Fig. 16-35. Radiograph of a radicular cyst. Note the root of the tooth from which the cyst took origin. *(Courtesy of Sheldon Rovin, D.D.S.)*

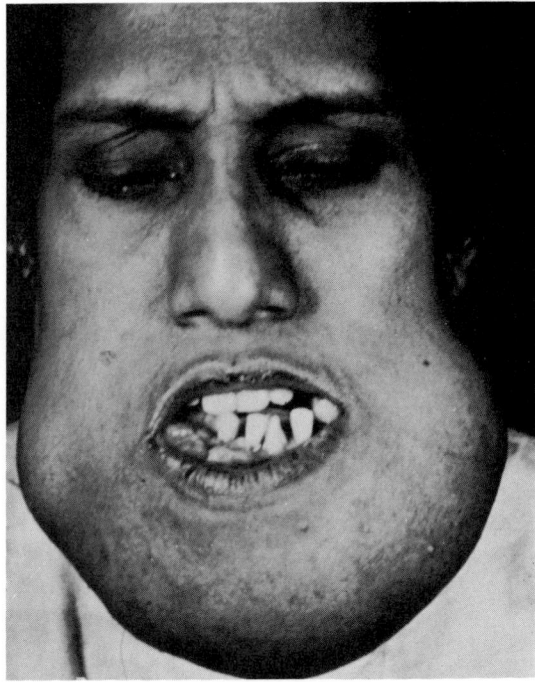

Fig. 16-36. Ameloblastoma. These lesions can grow to fantastic size, as shown here. Aside from the mass and functional disability, they are painless and never become malignant. *(Courtesy of Sheldon Rovin, D.D.S.)*

thelium. Frequently, a generalized inflammatory reaction in the cyst wall is seen. Treatment is by extraction of the tooth involved and excision of the cyst with its lining.

AMELOBLASTOMA

Although very uncommon, this is the most frequent solid tumor of the mandible. It usually appears in the body of the mandible at its junction with the ramus. Growth is slow, and the lesion is relatively asymptomatic, although it may expand the bone about it and eventually attain enormous size, encroaching on soft tissues of the face and neck (Fig. 16-36). Microscopically, the tumor presents interlacing strands and nests of odontogenic epithelium enmeshed in a connective tissue stroma with numerous areas of cystic degeneration. Treatment is by segmental resection of the portion of the mandible affected by the tumor including a centimeter or two of normal bone on either side. Unless the wide excision is accomplished, recurrence is common. The adjacent soft tissues need not be resected, and a good bed is usually left for reconstruction of the mandible.

Osteogenic Tumors

The mandible is affected by the same group of benign and malignant tumors that affect other bones in the body. Benign lesions include exostosis (torus mandibularis), fibrous dysplasia, Paget's disease, and giant cell tumor. Primary malignant lesions are multiple myeloma, Ewing's sarcoma, osteogenic sarcoma, chondrosarcoma (Fig. 16-37), and periosteal fibrosarcoma.

Giant cell tumors of the mandible are often referred to as *central* reparative giant cell tumors and are equivalent to the peripheral giant cell tumors of the gingiva. Although this lesion grows slowly and expands the surrounding bone, it never appears to have the malignant potential of giant cell tumors seen elsewhere in the skeleton and may have a different histogenesis. Microscopically, no distinction can be made between mandibular giant cell tumors and giant cell lesions of other bones. Treatment is usually by unroofing the tumor and curetting its tissue from the bony cavity.

Fig. 16-37. Chondrosarcoma of the mandible. This is a slowly developing lesion and was present in this patient for 9 years before medical aid was sought. The pressure of the upper gingiva has caused the groove that is seen in the dorsal surface of the tumor. Even at this late date, the tumor had not metastasized, and the patient was still alive and well 5 years after resection. (From: *Rush BF Jr, Trinkle K: South Med J 60:714, 1967, with permission.*)

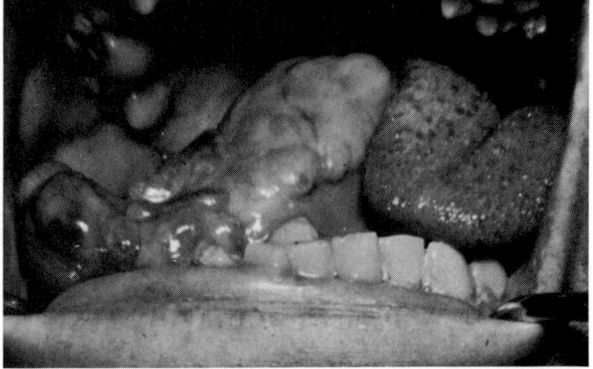

SALIVARY GLANDS

Salivary tissue is found in the parotid gland, the submaxillary gland, the lingual gland, and the numerous salivary glands. The parotid gland is a unilobular structure that is bent in a U shape about the posterior portion of the mandible in such a way that the larger external portion of the gland is often called the *superficial lobe* and the smaller internal portion lying on the internal surface of the ascending ramus is called the *deep lobe*. The VIIth nerve exiting from the skull by way of the stylohyoid foramen crosses the space between the mastoid and the ascending ramus of the mandible and plunges into the parotid gland at the point where it turns the corner around the posterior edge of the ascending ramus. The VIIth nerve usually bifurcates within the substance of the parotid. Each bifurcation further subdivides, and the branches eventually lie between the parotid gland and the underlying masseter muscle. The relationship of the VIIth nerve to the parotid gland is of clinical importance, since tumors of the parotid lie most commonly in the external portion of the gland; on excising such tumors great care must be taken not to cut the branches or the main trunk of this nerve.

The submaxillary gland is an ovoid structure lying in the submaxillary fossa beneath the horizontal ramus of the mandible. It is bounded by the anterior and posterior portions of the digastric muscle, thus occupying most of the digastric triangle in the neck. The important relationships of this gland are to the ramus mandibularis, the lowest branch of the VIIth nerve that courses over the upper portion of the gland. Injury to this nerve blocks innervation of the inferior quarter of the orbicularis oris on the side of the nerve and deprives patients of the ability to pucker their lips normally. The lingual nerve, deep to the upper inferior surface of the submaxillary gland, provides the gland with some small branches. In addition, the lingual nerve parallels the course of Wharton's duct, which conducts saliva from the submaxillary gland to the mouth. When the gland is removed, injury to the lingual nerve can occur either when Wharton's duct is clamped or when the gland is pulled down into the neck dragging the lingual nerve along by its nerve attachments.

The lingual gland is the smallest of the three major salivary glands. It lies beneath the mucosa of the anterior floor of the mouth.

The minor salivary glands are small deposits of salivary tissue that are scattered throughout the mucosa of the oral cavity, maxilla, and nasopharynx. The term *ectopic salivary tissue* is sometimes used but carries an incorrect connotation, since this salivary tissue is a normal finding in all individuals and is not the result of an error in development.

INCIDENCE. About $\frac{1}{3}$ percent of all malignant tumors occurs in the salivary tissues. These tumors are equally common in men and women. About 60 percent of these lesions occur in the parotid glands, which is not surprising, since this is the largest single collection of salivary tissues. The second largest concentration of tumors is found in the submaxillary gland and the third largest in the minor salivary glands. Tumors of the lingual glands are rare. No specific cause is known for any of the benign or malignant tumors of the salivary glands other than the occasional congenital or obstructive cyst. Women with malignant tumors of the salivary glands are known to have a higher incidence of cancer of the breast.

Benign Lesions. A variety of lesions may arise in salivary tissue.

Mixed Tumors. The most common lesion of the salivary glands is the mixed tumor (pleomorphic adenoma). Fifty percent of all tumors of the salivary glands and over 80 percent of all benign tumors are mixed tumors. These probably originate from adult glandular epithelium and, as their name implies, have an extremely diverse structural pattern. In 90 percent of the tumors one finds areas where the tumor grows in a network of strands made up of spindle and stellate cells not always connecting and sometimes lying entirely detached. In about a third of all cases this loose myxoid pattern predominates but is by no means the sole structural component. Half the tumors have pseudocartilaginous structures. Twenty percent show tissue closely resembling hyaline cartilage. Well-formed tubular structures are common and present a wide variety of patterns. The lining epithelium may be single-layered, conspicuously double-layered, stratified, or pseudostratified. Some areas of metaplasia into squamous epithelium may be seen, and well-differentiated squamous epithelium can be found in about a fourth of the cases.

Papillary Cystadenoma Lymphomatosum (Warthin's Tumor). These curious lesions occur only in parotid salivary tissue and almost exclusively (95 percent) in males. About 10 percent of them are bilateral. Characteristically they are made up of a papillary epithelial component intermingled with well-developed lymphoid tissue commonly containing germinal centers. Their histogenesis is uncertain, but many feel they represent parotid duct tissue sequestered in lymph nodes within the parotid gland. They represent the second most common benign tumor of salivary tissue but are a poor second to mixed tumors, which are at least eight times more common.

Mikulicz's Disease. This disease is characterized by a dense infiltration of lymphocytes occasionally arranged in follicles throughout the salivary tissues. This is accompanied by atrophy and disappearance of acinar tissue. Scattered throughout the lymphoid tissue are foci of epithelial and myloepithelial cells in close relationship to distal structures. The more popular modern term for this lesion is *benign lymphoepithelial lesion,* and many feel it represents a phase of the larger disease complex *Sjögren's syndrome.* The diffuse lymphocytic infiltrate, much as one sees in lymphomatous thyroiditis, suggests the possibility of an autoimmune disease. While several of or all the major salivary glands may be involved, a single parotid gland is the most frequent site (80 percent). The highest incidence of the disease is in patients between thirty-one and forty years of age.

Asymptomatic Enlargement of Salivary Tissue. This affection is usually observed in both parotid glands but may involve all the major salivary glands. The characteristic

cinomas, and even an occasional adenocarcinoma will demonstrate considerable sensitivity to x-ray therapy.

PROGNOSIS. Benign mixed tumors will recur in 40 to 50 percent of patients if improperly excised. If excision is by superficial lobectomy, the recurrence rate should be 5 percent or less. Five-year survival rates tend to be misleading, particularly in the chronic, slow-growing tumors. Adenoid cystic carcinoma has an 86 percent 5-year survival rate but a 57 percent 10-year survival. Malignant mixed tumors may have a 5-year survival of 87 to 90 percent and a 10-year survival of 60 to 70 percent.

AIDS-RELATED TUMORS

The epidemic of acquired immunodeficiency syndrome (AIDS) arose through the introduction of human T-cell lymphotrophic virus III (HTLV-III) into the homosexual and drug cultures of this country little more than half a decade ago. It now appears to be spreading through heterosexual contact as well and the case load is believed to be doubling each 6 months. Although patients may have suffered for some time with systemic symptoms of the AIDS-related complex, they may come for initial treatment because of the appearance of tumors, often first noted in the head and neck. The purple-black lesions of Kaposi's sarcoma often appear in the oral cavity where the half palate is the most common site. This tumor may also present on the tonsillar pillars, buccal mucosa, and tongue.

Cervical lymphadenopathy may reflect the persistent generalized adenopathy of the complex or may announce the appearance of a lymphoma. These are usually either B-cell immunoblastic lymphoma or small cell, noncleaved lymphoma (either Burkitt's or Burkitt's-like). Biopsy of the lesions establishes the diagnosis. Treatment with radiation and/or chemotherapy is palliative since the tumors and the syndrome are uniformly fatal.

Patients with AIDS or AIDS-related complex who have malignancies normally unassociated with AIDS may find the course of their tumors greatly altered. In a recent report a patient with AIDS-related complex and a basal cell carcinoma of the chin exhibited diffuse skeletal metastasis.

TUMORS OF THE NECK

Palpable or visible cervical swellings are a common complaint. Two to three percent of all admissions to hospital surgical services are for this condition. About half of these lesions occur in the thyroid gland; the remainder are due to a wide range of malignant, congenital, or inflammatory swellings.

Inflammation

Inflammatory swelling in the adult neck is now a rare hospital problem. Skandalakis and coworkers, in reviewing 1616 nonthyroid masses of the neck, found that only 3.2 percent were inflammatory, whereas 84 percent were neoplastic and 12 percent congenital or miscellaneous. The inflammatory lesions requiring hospitalization of adults are largely acute, often resulting from drainage from infection elsewhere. A common source is an infected tooth draining to the nodes in the submandibular area and causing an abscess. Only two patients in Skandalakis' entire series had tuberculous adenitis (scrofula). This was once the most common cause of neck masses, but with the tuberculin testing of cows and the pasteurization of milk, bovine tuberculosis has virtually disappeared in this country.

Malignant Tumors

The vast majority of cervical masses in adults are due to neoplasms. About 80 percent of these are metastatic from some other site, while the remainder occur from primary lesions in the neck. Primary cervical neoplasms either occur in the major salivary glands (40 percent) or are lymphomas primary in the cervical lymph nodes (60 percent). At one time it was proposed the squamous carcinomas arose primarily in the neck from the lining of branchial cleft cysts. This diagnosis was often made only to discover at a later date that the lesion was actually a metastasis from the oral cavity, nasopharynx, or laryngeal area. While there is some evidence that branchiogenic cysts become malignant, the reported, provable cases number only a handful.

A knowledge of the statistics quickly indicates that a clinician's first suspicion concerning any nonthyroid, cervical mass in adults is of a malignant tumor. He may also suspect that it is metastatic and from a site at some point above the clavicle, since 85 percent of all metastatic cervical lesions come from a supraclavicular site.

When a firm to hard cervical node that suggests malignancy is found, the first responsibility of clinicians is a thorough exploration of possible sites of origin. Cervical tumors appearing below and behind the ear and along the cervical chain are more likely to come from the nasopharynx or lateral pharyngeal walls. Swollen lymph nodes at the angle of the mandible or in the area of the submaxillary gland are most commonly from lesions in the tonsillar area, buccal mucosa, floor of the mouth, and gingiva. Swelling of the lymph nodes in the submental area should provoke a thorough examination of the tip of the tongue, lower lip, and anterior gingivobuccal gutter. Lymph nodes involved by neoplasms that appear in the middle third of the neck should cast suspicion first on the hypopharynx, piriform sinus, larynx, or thyroid.

Only when enlarged lymph nodes appear in the supraclavicular area does metastasis from below the clavicle become a major possibility. These may stem from carcinoma of the upper lobes of the lung or mediastinum or, in women, from carcinoma of the breast. The left supraclavicular nodes are frequently involved by malignant tumors metastatic from the abdomen (Virchow's node). Advanced adenocarcinoma of the stomach, pancreas, biliary tree, and even large bowel metastasize to this site.

If a thorough search of all sites reveals no possible

source of a primary lesion, biopsy of the cervical node is usually carried out. If this confirms the clinical impression of malignancy, further attempts to find the primary lesion are indicated. This can include surgical exploration of the maxillary sinuses. If all avenues have been searched thoroughly and no primary lesion has been found, the problem of local treatment still remains. The best course is to treat the lesion to achieve cure. If operation is chosen, it should be a radical neck dissection; if radiation therapy is used, it should be a full course of therapy. Since lymph nodes involved by metastatic disease respond poorly to radiation, the treatment of choice is normally operation. In the presence of advanced lesions a combination of radiation and operation may be used.

If a group of these patients treated without a known primary lesion is followed for 5 years, 80 percent of the patients will ultimately manifest the primary lesion. In some instances this may subsequently be resected for cure. A few patients may die over this period without ever demonstrating the source for the metastatic lesion, and even at postmortem examination it may not be found. Even more interesting, about 20 percent of the patients survive 5 or more years with apparent "cure" of their metastatic lesion even though the presumed primary lesion has not been found or treated. In those patients who received radiation therapy, either together with operation or alone, it may be that the port included the primary lesion as well. In those patients who are treated by operation alone, the fate of the primary lesion remains a mystery. A few of these patients may represent true branchiogenic carcinoma, or possibly the primary lesion regresses spontaneously.

Other Lesions

A host of other tumors, found infrequently in the area of the neck, present problems in differential diagnosis. Dermoids occur in the midline, most commonly in the submental area and sometimes along the line of the clavicle. Sebaceous cysts are common, especially in men, and probably are related to the trauma of shaving.

Carotid body tumors (chemodectomas) are rare tumors of the paraganglionic tissue found at the carotid bifurcation. Another lesion with a slow evolution, it gradually increases in size over many years, enveloping the bifurcation and slowly compressing the adjacent nerves including the hypoglossal, vagus, and sympathetic chain. For many periods, the only symptom is the mass in the neck. Eventually nerve paralysis, dysphagia, and pain appear. Malignant transformation is rare, but early removal is indicated to avoid the late symptoms. Small lesions can be removed easily (Fig. 16-40), but advanced large tumors require resection of the carotid artery with the risk of subsequent hemiparesis.

TUMORS OF THE NECK IN CHILDREN

The order of frequency of masses in the neck in children differs markedly from that found in adults. Inflam-

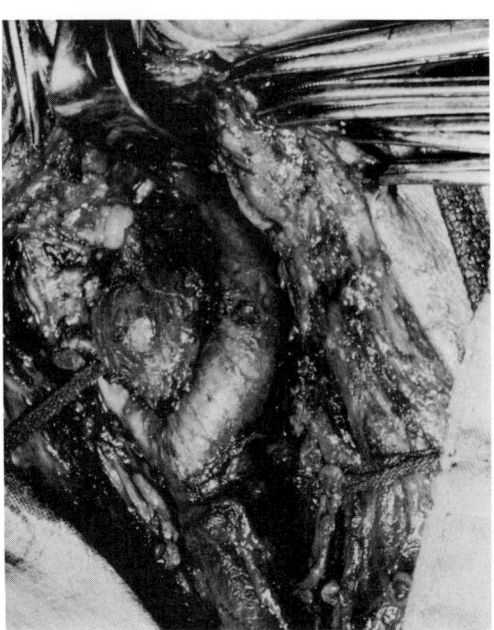

Fig. 16-40. Carotid body tumor of moderate size. The lesion lies between the internal and external branches of the carotid arteries; the adventitial layer binding it to the carotid bulb has been removed. (From: *Rush BF Jr: Ann Surg 157:633, 1963, with permission.*)

matory lesions are by far the most common, often coming from related infections of the tonsils. The most common malignant lesion is the lymphoma, and the second most common is carcinoma of the thyroid. Congenital lesions, of course, are much more common in children than in adults.

CHEMOTHERAPY AND IMMUNOTHERAPY

In the past decade it has been discovered that certain types of neoplasms commonly found in the head and neck area can be cured by chemotherapy. Burkitt's lymphoma, a rare neoplasm in the United States but common in some parts of Africa, was the first such cancer. It became apparent that a predictable and consistent percentage of patients with this disease could be cured by the use of *systemic* chemotherapy alone. Recently we have also learned that squamous cancer of facial skin and of the lips, while in the in situ microinvasive and superficial stages, can be cured by the topical application of 5-fluorouracil used as a cream or paste. These lesions are multiple and often tedious to eradicate by operation or radiation. A third head and neck lesion in which chemotherapy has become important is embryonal rhabdomyosarcoma, an uncommon lesion found in infants and children. Cure of this lesion occasionally has been obtained by combining radiation, chemotherapy, and operation.

Epidermoid cancers of the head and neck respond transiently to a number of single agents. Methotrexate has been the most extensively used. Response rates range from 15 to 57 percent. Bleomycin has also been found to have significant activity, comparable with methotrexate, with reported responses ranging from 15 to 50 percent. Other, less effective, single agents are cyclophosphamide (36 percent), vinblastine (29 percent), hydroxyurea (39 percent), 5-fluorouracil (15 percent), and procarbazine (10 percent). Reports of many of these latter drugs are based on small series and represent, at best, rough estimates. The most recent drug to excite interest in treatment of these tumors is *cis*-dichlorodiamine platinum (II) (DDP or cisplatin), which appears to match or exceed methotrexate and bleomycin in activity, especially when used in high doses with mannitol-induced diuresis to avoid renal injury.

Arterial infusion for the treatment of cancer in the head and neck area has received much attention. This involves the introduction of chemotherapy, usually methotrexate or 5-fluorouracil, into the external carotid artery via a catheter. The agents are administered either continuously or intermittently over 1 to several weeks. At present, this technique is known to produce a substantial to complete regression of the lesions in a large percentage of patients— as high as 50 percent in some series. Unfortunately, the response is usually transient, and the cancers return to continued growth within 2 to 3 months after treatment is discontinued. Long-term regression is uncommonly seen, and the period of regression obtained is rarely worth the morbidity and complications of the treatment itself. Nonetheless, these observations continue to tantalize clinical investigators seeking a clue that will lead to longer or even permanent remissions.

The recent introduction of an implantable, subcutaneous, long-term infusion pump may reduce morbidity, increase convenience, and make this technique more practicable.

The growing body of knowledge concerning the interrelationships between cancer and the body's immune system has touched the field of head and neck cancer through the work of Chretian and others. Squamous carcinoma of the tongue has been found in young men with acquired immune deficiency syndrome. At least half the patients with epidermoid cancer of the oral cavity, hypopharynx, and larynx show some degree of immune incompetence. Moreover, this incompetence is correlated with treatment failure following either radiation or operation. Immune competence can be restored in a number of these patients by improving nutrition, by the use of immunostimulant agents such as BCG or c-Parvum, and by

"reconstitution" agents such as levamisole, thymosin, and transfer factor. Trials to determine the effectiveness of manipulations of the immune system in the immune-incompetent patient have so far shown either no or only marginal benefit.

The rapid expansion in our knowledge of the immune system has introduced a new generation of immunogenic agents that are much more specific in their effects. These include interferon, leukocyte-activated natural killer cells, and monoclonal antibodies to specific tumor antigens. The role of these new modalities and how they should be combined with other therapeutic agents remains to be developed.

Combined forms of treatment for head and neck cancers, which include chemotherapy and immunotherapy as well as radiation and operation, have enjoyed marked clinical and investigative interest in the past several years. The more our knowledge of the natural history of tumor growth develops, the more rational and logical it appears to combine available treatment methods.

Multinodal systemic chemotherapy will double or triple the partial and complete regression rates when the drugs are given as the first part of a therapeutic regimen to patients with previously untreated tumors (Table 16-1). Our current experience suggests that far-advanced (Stage IV) head and neck tumors have double the 2-year disease-free survival if chemotherapy precedes preoperative radiation and operation as compared with preoperative radiation and operation alone (66 vs. 35 percent). This is especially impressive when one realizes that Stage IV tumors ordinarily have a 5-year survival rate of 0 to 15 percent depending upon site (Fig. 16-41).

The practice of using chemotherapy as the first step in the course of multimodal treatment has been called "neoadjuvant" therapy. Several uncontrolled studies have claimed improved survival for late tumors with this technique. On the other hand, several prospective randomized studies report significant early tumor regression but no overall benefit in terms of survival. Since this approach appears to rescue some patients who are otherwise untreatable for cure, it is still under intensive study.

OPERATIONS OF THE HEAD AND NECK

The most commonly performed major operation for cancer of the head and neck is radical neck dissection.

Table 16-1. MULTIDRUG CHEMOTHERAPY FOR UNTREATED HEAD AND NECK CANCER

Drugs	Cycles	No. of pts.	50% Responses	Complete responses	Total responses	Author
DDP, VB, Bleo	3	106	44	22	66	Perry
DDP, MTX	4	82	62	4	66	Tejada
DDP, 5FU	2	26	69	19	88	Kish
DDP, Adra, Bleo, CTX	2	18	33	67	100	Feldman
VCR, Bleo, MTX, 5FU, HYD	2	200	61.5	6.5	67	Price

Abbreviations: DDP = cisplatin; MTX = methotrexate; VCR = vincristine; CTX = cytophosphamide; 5FU = 5-fluorouracil; Bleo = bleomycin; HYD = hydrocortisone; VB = vinblastine; Adra = Adriamycin.

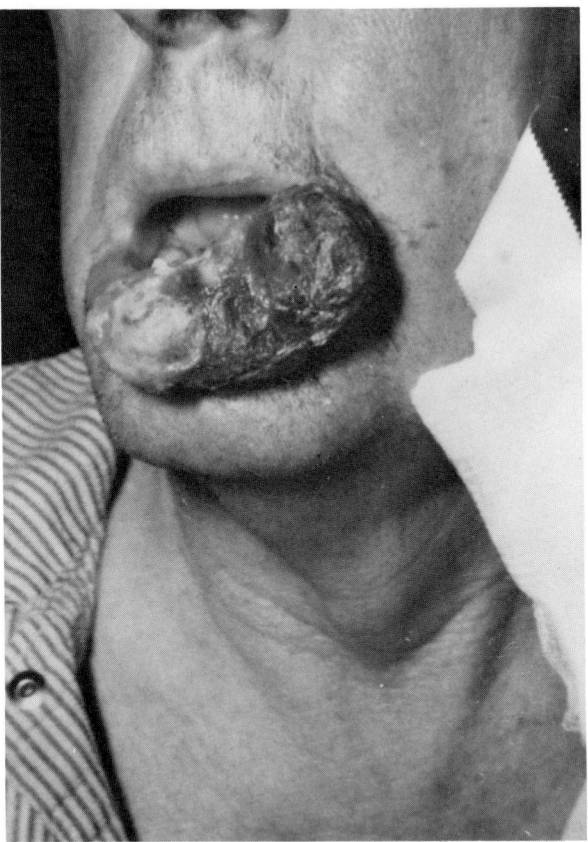

A

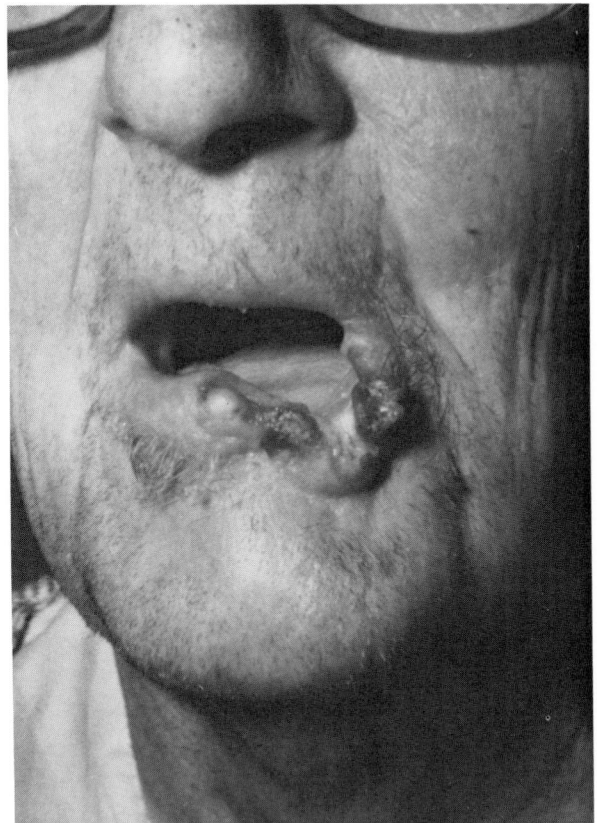

B

Fig. 16-41. Effect of chemotherapy upon squamous carcinoma of the lip. *A.* Lesion prior to treatment. *B.* Lesion following 2d cycle (approximately 4 weeks of treatment) of cisplatin, methotrexate, and bleomycin, 95+ percent regression. Patient had complete regression in another 4 weeks and continued treatment with radiotherapy, operative excision, and reconstruction.

This procedure was originally designed by Crile to eradicate the cervical lymphatic network, thereby eliminating sites of metastasis from cancer of the oral cavity, pharynx, paranasal sinuses, or other areas of the head and neck. In the early days of head and neck surgery radical neck dissections were usually performed after the primary lesion had been controlled through the use of radiation therapy. Today, we are more inclined to combine radical neck dissection with a simultaneous resection of the primary lesion. This is sometimes preceded by a course of radiation therapy to the primary area as part of a planned program of tumor treatment. Combined operations have been called by a number of terms including *composite resections* and *commando operations*. Other common operations in this area are superficial resection of the parotid gland, V excision of carcinoma of the lip, and resection of the maxillary antrum.

Radical Neck Dissection

Incisions for radical neck dissection are numerous and include a T-shaped incision originally used by Crile, a Y

incision described by Ward, and a double Y incision described by Martin (Fig. 16-42). We prefer a hockey-stick shaped incision with the ascending limb along the posterior border of the sternocleidomastoid muscle and the horizontal portion crossing the neck about 2 or 3 cm above the clavicle (Fig. 16-43). This last approach has the advantage of being outside areas of radiation when the neck has had previous exposure to radiation therapy and of being a simple linear incision avoiding small triangular-shaped flaps, which have a tendency to slough. The skin flap is reflected mediad, including the underlying platysma muscle, and dissection of neck structures begins in the posterior triangle, dissecting the fibroareolar tissue of this space away from the trapezius muscle and the underlying brachial plexus and scalene fibers. The portion of the dissection is carried mediad until the phrenic nerve lying on the anterior scalene muscle is identified.

The lower end of the sternocleidomastoid muscle is transected and the jugular vein identified and ligated. The accompanying vagus nerve next to the jugular vein in the carotid sheath is identified and spared. Dissection is then carried up the neck, gradually dissecting the lymph node chain free from underlying fascia and beneath the carotid artery. Just above the level of the carotid bulb the hypoglossal nerve is identified. In the upper portion of the neck the sternocleidomastoid muscle is again transected at the level of the mastoid together with the tip of the

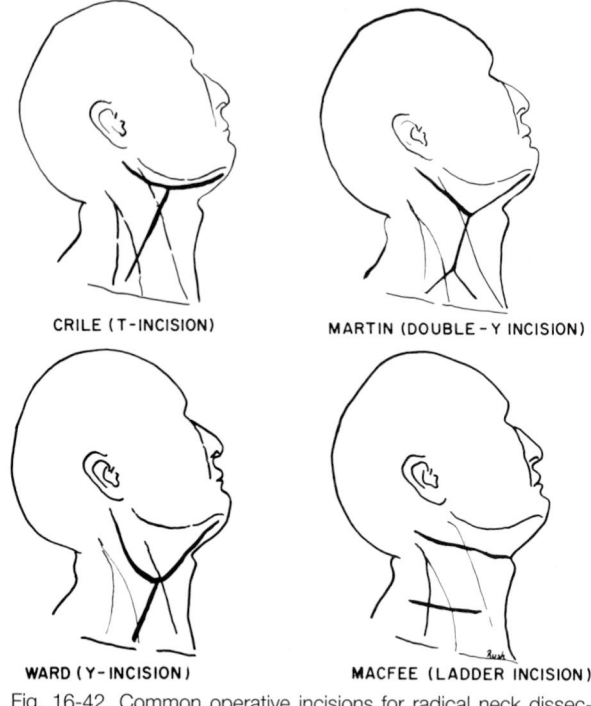

CRILE (T-INCISION)　　　MARTIN (DOUBLE-Y INCISION)

WARD (Y-INCISION)　　　MACFEE (LADDER INCISION)

Fig. 16-42. Common operative incisions for radical neck dissections. (From: *Rush BF Jr: Curr Probl Surg May 1966, with permission.*)

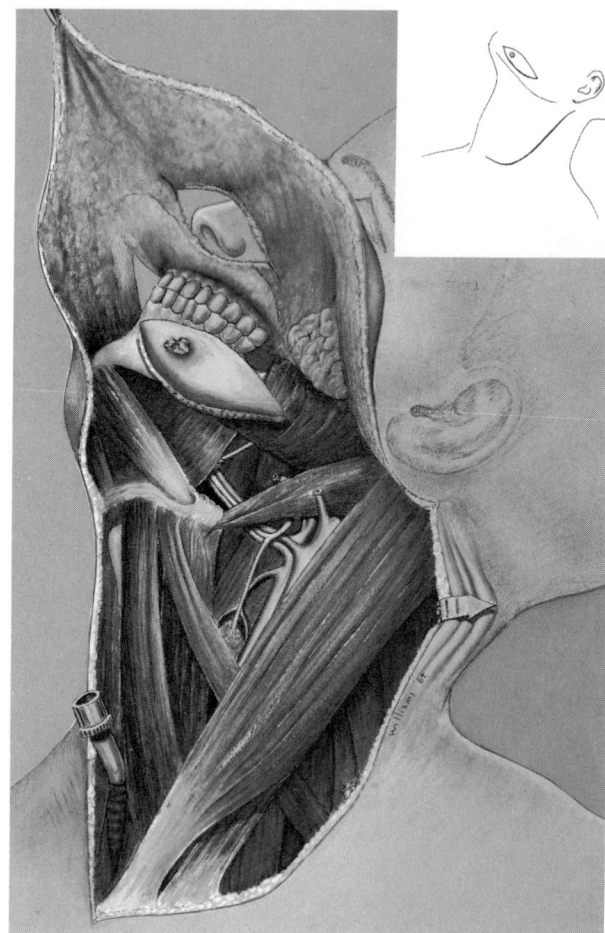

Fig. 16-43. Radical neck dissection through a hockey-stick incision (shown in insert) combined with an exposure of the mandible. The tumor has grown through the mandible and presented on the cheek so that a portion of the skin of the cheek has been left on the specimen. Structures of the neck are shown exposed and intact prior to the start of radical neck dissection. (From: *Rush BF Jr: Surg Gynecol Obstet 121:353, 1965, with permission.*)

parotid gland. The submaxillary gland is dissected free from the digastric fossa and included with the specimen. The lingual nerve and artery in the depths of the submaxillary fossa are visualized and left intact. Care is taken to identify the ramus mandibularis, the tiny fiber of the VIIth nerve that innervates the lower lip, and to reflect this above the submaxillary gland so that its continuity is maintained. The spinal accessory nerve is usually sacrificed, being cut in the lower neck where it enters the trapezius muscle and in the upper neck where it enters the sternocleidomastoid muscle. The operation is completed with the transection of the jugular vein at the point where it leaves the base of the skull (Fig. 16-44). If a radical neck dissection alone is performed, the operation is ended at this point by closing the skin flaps. Multiperforated catheters are left underneath the flaps and are connected to suction. This helps to draw the flap firmly to the structures of the neck and eliminates the problem of fluid collecting under the flap.

MODIFIED RADICAL NECK DISSECTION

This operation is still ill-defined. To some it means preserving the spinal accessory nerve but otherwise doing a complete radical neck. At the other extreme some surgeons spare all the "functional" structures in the neck including the sternocleidomastoid muscle, the spinal accessory nerve, and the jugular vein, removing mainly the lymphoareolar tissue of the anterior and posterior triangle and the submaxillary gland. Our preference is to spare the sternocleidomastoid muscle and the XIth nerve but to remove the jugular vein. There is little morbidity incurred by removing the vein, and the lymphatic tissues of the neck are closely associated with the vein. The indication for limiting radical neck dissection to a modified operation is a negative neck without clinically positive nodes in the presence of a primary lesion with a high risk of occult nodal metastasis.

COMBINED OPERATION

If a radical neck dissection is to be combined with the removal of structures within the oral cavity or tonsillar area, the contents of the neck dissection are left attached to the horizontal ramus of the mandible. The mandible is frequently divided. If the lesion is in the floor of the mouth or tongue, the horizontal ramus of the mandible may be resected. If the lesion is in the tonsillar fossa, the ascending ramus of the mandible is removed. If the lesion

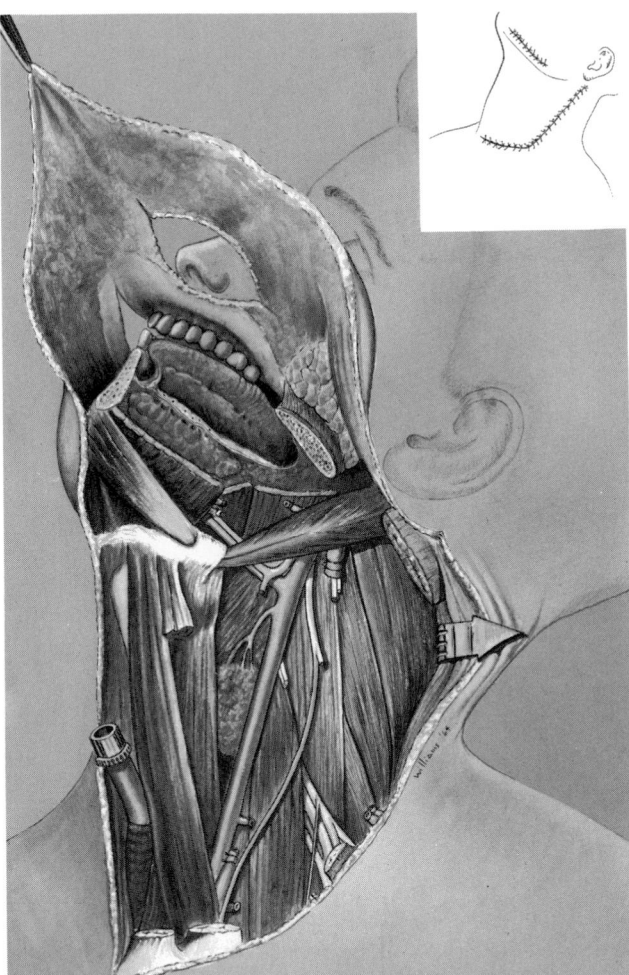

Fig. 16-44. Radical neck dissection completed, combined with excision of the horizontal ramus of the mandible. The jugular vein and sternocleidomastoid muscle have been removed. The phrenic nerve and the common carotid artery are seen coursing across the operative field. The closure of the neck incision is seen in the insert. (From: *Rush BF Jr: Surg Gynecol Obstet 121:353, 1965, with permission.*)

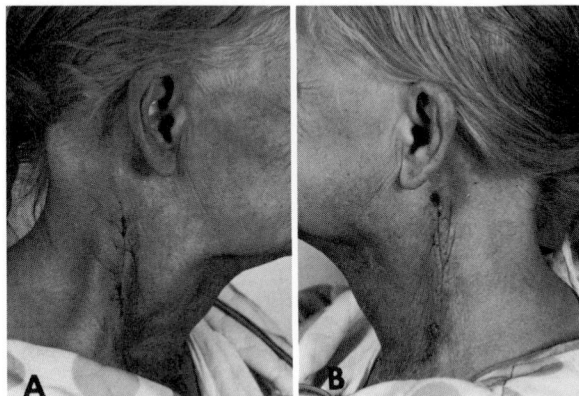

Fig. 16-45. Mandibular resection, 8 days after bilateral neck dissection and partial mandibulectomy on the left, with resection of a portion of the floor of the mouth and the anterior half of the tongue for carcinoma of the tongue. The portion of the jaw was replaced with a Steinmann pin. At 3 years postoperatively there still was no recurrence. Note that it is difficult to determine on which side the mandible was resected. (From: *Rush BF Jr: Curr Probl Surg May 1966, with permission.*)

BILATERAL RADICAL NECK DISSECTION

Lesions that are in the midline of the oral cavity often spread bilaterally, and it is necessary to remove lymph nodes on both sides of the neck. Simultaneous bilateral neck dissections are feasible with an acceptable mortality; however, the postoperative course is likely to be prolonged, since there is a period of marked facial edema following this extensive resection that can persist for several weeks. Some operators will spare the jugular vein on one side when a bilateral neck dissection is done in order to decrease the amount of postoperative edema. Others stage the dissection, allowing a delay of several weeks before operating on the second side.

Parotidectomy

Most lesions in the superficial lobe of the parotid gland are removed by superficial parotidectomy. This operation is designed to give maximal safety in operating about the branches of the VIIth nerve (Fig. 16-46). The VIIth nerve pierces the parotid gland at its posterior margin and lies underneath the gland on the muscles of the face. A Y-shaped incision is made with the lower limb lying behind the angle of the mandible and the arms of the Y on either side of the lobe of the ear. Dissection is carried down to identify the main trunk of the VIIth nerve, which lies in the space between the mandible and the mastoid bone approximately one fingerbreadth below the external auditory meatus. Once the main trunk is identified, dissection is carried along the external surface of the nerve and its branches, gradually separating away the overlying portion of the parotid gland. Stensen's duct is identified at the most medial portion of the midpoint of the parotid gland and is ligated. This technique sometimes causes temporary weakness in the fibers of the VIIth nerve but prevents transecting any of the major trunks of the nerve.

in the oral cavity is quite large, total removal of the hemimandible on the side of the lesion may be necessary. Resection of the mandible is done to remove bone involved by tumor and sometimes to obtain a closure of the oral cavity that would not be feasible without removing a portion of the bony framework. Mandibular resection can be done with the acceptable cosmetic and functional result, especially when the anterior portion of the mandible is preserved (Fig. 16-45). The more anteriorly the mandible is resected, the more likely there is to be facial deformity. If the primary site of the tumor is in the larynx or thyroid, then these structures may also be removed with the radical neck dissection. The mortality for radical neck dissection alone is less than 1 percent. If neck dissection is combined with en bloc excision of a primary lesion, then mortality rates range from 2 to 5 percent.

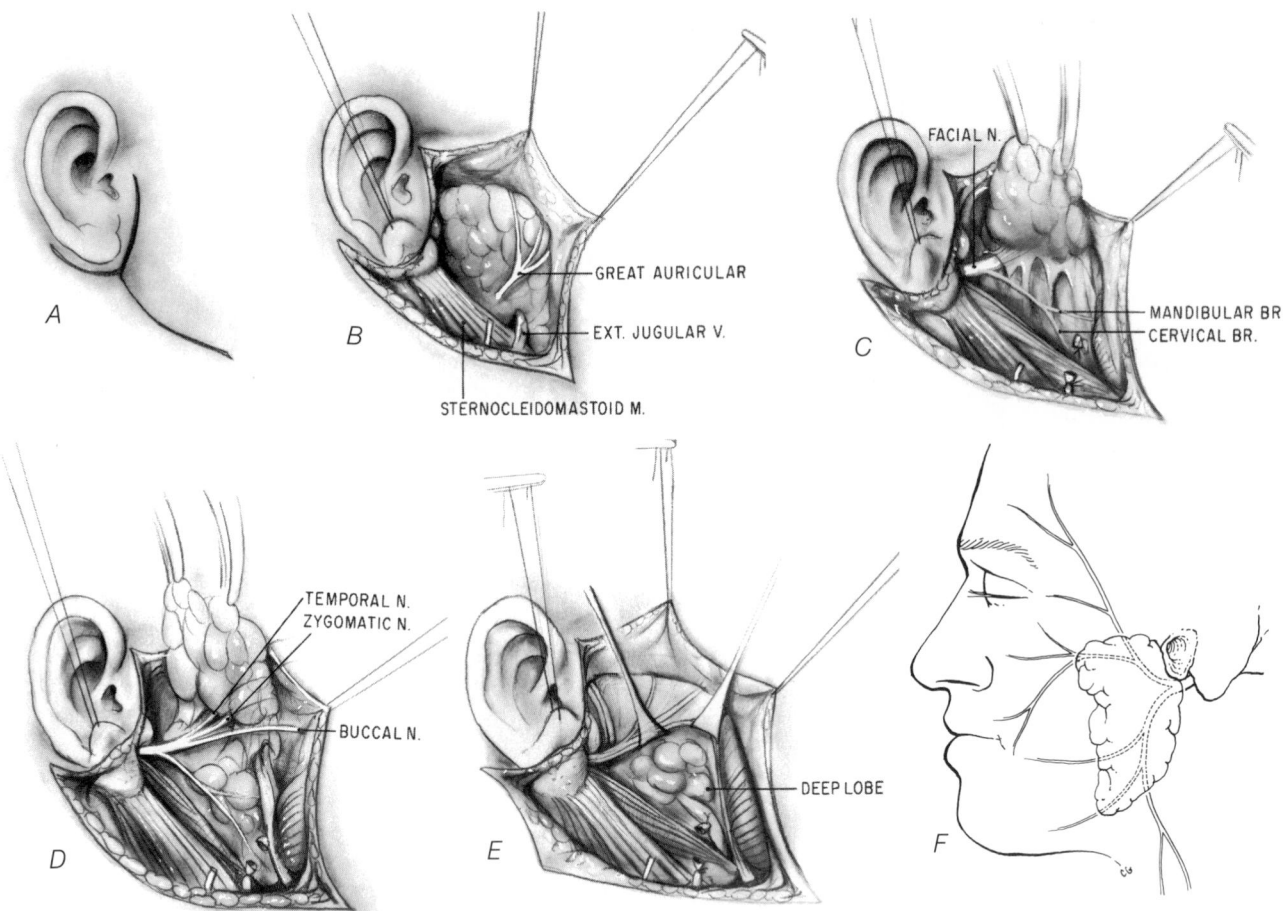

Fig. 16-46. Superficial parotidectomy. *A.* Incision. *B.* Skin flaps established and fascia incised; greater auricular nerve transected and external jugular vein identified. *C.* External jugular vein transected; superficial lobe is being reflected anteriorly, and facial nerve with its mandibular and cervical branches are shown. *D.* Dissection continued anteriorly, demonstrating temporal, zygomatic, and buccal branches. *E.* Superficial lobe removed; if excision of the deep lobe is indicated, the facial nerve can be retracted craniad and the remaining parotid removed. *F.* Relationship of facial nerve and parotid gland. The nerve branches lie between the deep and superficial lobes of the parotid. *(Courtesy of Robert Chase, M.D.)*

Recovery of function in all branches is ensured by the knowledge that they are intact and usually occurs within a week or two following completion of the operation.

V Excision of the Lip

Most cancers of the lower lip are removed with the use of V excision. Between one-fourth and one-third of the lower lip can be easily resected by simple excision without resulting in residual deformity or interference with function. While we refer to this excision as a V. a much better cosmetic result is obtained if the outline of the incision resembles that of a shield. A true V excision results in some flattening of the lower lip with a loss of normal eversion. If a shield-shaped incision is used, the lip will evert normally.

If the tumor involves more area than can be excised with a V excision, a flap is migrated from the upper lip. This involves outlining a V-shaped flap in the upper lip that is left attached at its lower medial corner and is then rotated into the defect in the lower lip. Using this type of closure excision of up to two-thirds of the lower lip can be accomplished without difficulty.

Maxillectomy

Cancer of the hard palate or the lower maxilla requires subtotal excision of the maxillary sinus. Cancer in the upper maxilla involving the orbital plate requires total excision of the maxillary sinus together with an exenteration of the orbital contents. While these excisions are basically mutilating, they can be accomplished with little visible external deformity. The Weber-Fergusson incision is used. This begins at the midpoint of the upper lip, extends to the columella of the nose, and is carried around the edge of the nose and up to the corner of the eye. A horizontal portion continues laterally from the inner canthus to a point just beyond the outer canthus and about 2 or 3 mm below the palpebral fissure. The skin and muscles of the cheek are undermined laterally, so that the entire cheek is turned outward, opening a door to the maxillary sinus. The bony attachments of the maxillary sinus are divided, including the midline of the hard palate, the zygoma, the pterygoid plates; if the orbital plate is to be removed, the bony walls of the medial and lateral orbit are also transected. When this is accomplished, the entire maxillary sinus can be lifted like a small box from its normal position. The inner surface of the Weber-Fergusson flap is covered with a split-thickness skin graft, and the incision is closed. Because it falls in the normal skin lines and about the normal structures of the face, this incision is often difficult to detect after it has healed as long as the structures have been replaced precisely and in good apposition. This operation leaves a large defect in the hard palate on the side of the procedure. This is occasionally closed by subsequent operations, but more commonly a dental prosthesis with a large obturator that fits into the defect is constructed by the prosthodontist. This restores normal speech and relatively normal mastication for the patient.

Total Laryngectomy

Total laryngectomy is traditionally accomplished through a midline longitudinal incision. We have found definite advantages in accomplishing this procedure through a transverse incision in the lower neck very much like the typical thyroidectomy incision. The incision is made 4 cm above the clavicles and approximately 4 cm beyond the edge of the sternocleidomastoid muscles on either side; it is carried down through the platysma muscle, and the upper flap is then developed. The upper limit of dissection is approximately 1 cm above the hyoid, and at this point the entire group of strap muscles and the midportion of the hyoid are exposed. In cancer operations for glottic tumors of any size, all the anterior strap muscles are removed. Occasionally at the election of the operator in the presence of somewhat smaller lesions, the strap muscles on the side contralateral to the lesion may be preserved, or, rarely, the larynx is skeletonized with the preservation of strap muscles on both sides. In the ordinary instance, however, the sternothyroid and sternohyoid muscles are transected at the level of the cricoid, the digastric and mylohyoid muscles are separated from the hyoid above, and the body of the hyoid bone is cut at the junction of the attachments to the lateral wings on either side. The larynx is rocked laterally exposing the pharyngeal constrictors, which are cut at the lateral edge of the thyroid cartilages bilaterally. One can now enter the pharynx laterally, usually on the side opposite the tumor, so that proper visualization of the area can be obtained, and an adequate margin of excision of pharyngeal mucosa will be developed around the tumor. Once the pharynx is entered, it is possible for the surgeon to operate both outside and inside the pharynx. The remaining muscles of the tongue are severed from the hyoid, and the larynx is pulled forward. The vascular pedicles containing the laryngeal arteries and the superior laryngeal nerves are ligated bilaterally. An incision is made in the pharyngeal mucosa just posterior to the arytenoids, entirely circumscribing the point at which the larynx projects into the pharynx. As all pharyngeal mucosa is now separated from the larynx, the larynx is pulled forward, and a plane of dissection is developed between the larynx and the anterior esophageal wall. This dissection is carried inferiorly until the only remaining structure holding the larynx in place is the trachea. This is then divided obliquely around the site of the tracheostomy (if one has been done previous to the operation), or if an endotracheal tube has been used in anesthesia, this is now removed, and a tube is placed in the severed trachea so that anesthesia can be continued. After the larynx has been removed, the defect in the pharynx is closed transversely with an inverting Connell stitch. This is reinforced by interrupted sutures of 4-0 silk which are used to imbricate the constrictor muscles up and around the pharyngeal closure. This closure may further be reinforced by stitches that catch the platysma muscle and draw it down snugly along with the overlying skin. A generous circular portion of skin is removed in the lower midline; this measures about 3 to 4 cm in diameter with three-quarters of the circle lying above the transverse skin incision and one-quarter of the circle lying below. The beveled end of the trachea is then drawn up to the skin by interrupted sutures of nylon. Every attempt is made to obtain a delicate mucosa to skin closure, since the smaller the size of the scar at the junction between mucosa and skin, the less likely there is to be subsequent stenosis of the tracheal opening. The generous amount of skin excised tends to evert the trachea in a slighty "trumpet-like" manner, and this too ensures against subsequent stenosis. This type of trachea skin closure can be maintained without the use of an indwelling tracheostomy tube except for the first 24 h or so postoperatively. The remainder of the wound is closed with interrupted sutures to the platysma muscle and skin. Two suction catheters are left in place on either side of the neck and are usually removed in 24 to 36 h. The patient is maintained on postoperative feeding through a nasal tube made up of a #18 whistle-tip red rubber catheter inserted at the time of operation through the nose and into the esophagus before the pharyngeal defect is closed. This tube is sutured to the nasal columella. The patient is maintained on nasal tube feedings for about 10 days. A liquid diet is usually begun on the fifth or sixth day, and the patient may take solid food on the ninth or tenth day. The nasal tube is removed as soon as it is apparent that patients can well maintain their own nutrition.

Partial Laryngectomy and the Neolarynx

In the past all lesions extending beyond the true cords have been treated by the total laryngectomy. The functional importance of the voice and the great benefit of preserving it for the patient has led to an evaluation of cancer operations that do not remove the entire larynx. Ogura and Biller have led this effort and have proposed a number of new operations that involve removal of most or all of the larynx above the cords (supraglottic laryngectomy) or excision of most of one side of the larynx (hemilaryngectomy) for lesions that are confined enough in their growth to be suitable for this technique. This approach requires careful selection of patients who are young and flexible enough to overcome some of the swallowing and aspiration difficulties that often arise postoperatively. Since the resected margin around the tumor may be very limited, careful diagnostic techniques must be used to identify the outer margins. This technique is almost always combined with preoperative radiation therapy to ensure a lesser threat from residual cells at the periphery of the tumor that may be left by the surgeon. Using these techniques in patients with tumors advanced enough to cause fixation of the cord, Ogura and Biller have reported a 77 percent 3-year survival.

An alternative method for preserving the voice, especially in patients with lesions not amenable to partial laryngectomy, is creation of a pseudolarynx. The most popular method for this procedure is that of Staffieri, in which the open stump of the trachea is covered by a flap of pharyngeal mucosa and a very small mucosa-lined fistula is created connecting the trachea to the pharynx. The patient speaks by occluding a lateral tracheostoma with a finger and diverting air from the lungs into the pharynx and mouth. Aspiration is avoided by the very small size of the fistula but may be a problem in a substantial number of these patients. Attempts at developing a valve of tissue to cover the fistula are in progress, as previously mentioned (Fig. 16-30).

POSTOPERATIVE CARE FOLLOWING HEAD AND NECK OPERATIONS

Tracheostomy is performed at the time of operation in any patient in whom a portion of the mandible is removed or when there is extensive removal of oral structures. Postoperative edema plus the tendency for the larynx to shift position following sacrifice of many of its suspensory muscles predispose to aspiration and obstruction. Catastrophic anoxia may supervene rapidly, with little apparent warning. The tracheostomy tube must be aspirated frequently. This requires the presence of well-trained nursing personnel. If a patient appears to be accumulating unusual amounts of tracheal secretions, it is probable that saliva is being aspirated through an incompetent larynx. This can be controlled by diligent suctioning. In extreme instances, a cuffed tracheostomy may be required temporarily.

The patient with a tracheostomy has lost the usual humidifying effects of the nasal and pharyngeal passageways. The best way to provide humidity for the patient's trachea is to tie an umbilical tape about the neck above the tracheostomy and to hang a moistened 4 by 4 sponge over this tape very much in the manner that a towel is hung over a rail. The sponge must frequently be moistened, and after the first day or two patients can be taught to moisten their own sponges and arrange them for themselves.

There is no need to leave the tracheostomy in place for prolonged periods. As soon as the patient is found to be maintaining a dry, unobstructed airway and the skin flaps are sealed, the tracheostomy tube is covered with a piece of adhesive tape. This is done about 5 days postoperatively. If the patient tolerates the covering of the tracheostomy tube for 24 h, it can be removed. This tube should always be removed in the morning, so that the patient can be observed during the daylight hours following removal.

Patients who have undergone combined resections have had extensive superficial operation, but the body cavities have been undisturbed, and the normal function of the gastrointestinal tract resumes almost immediately. A nasoesophageal tube consisting of a #16 French urethral catheter is left in place at the end of the operative procedure. The tip of the standard urethral catheter reaches to the lower third of the esophagus but does not traverse the esophagocardiac junction. Such tubes can be left in place for long periods without the risk of acid regurgitation and peptic esophagitis. The patient receives fluids intravenously on the day of operation, but on the first postoperative day nasal feedings of half-strength milk are given. On the second postoperative day a nasal formula consisting of a blenderized regular diet diluted with milk is begun. This is continued until the fifth or sixth postoperative day or until patients show evidence that they can tolerate an adequate diet by mouth.

Except for the different flora encountered, there is little difference in the principles of operating on the mouth and other areas in the gastrointestinal tract. This is a contaminated area, and numerous tissue planes are open to this contamination. All patients should be placed on appropriate antibiotics postoperatively. Ketcham et al. demonstrated in a controlled study the advantages of prophylactic antibiotics in these patients.

The mental stress in patients undergoing an oral operation of any magnitude is considerable. They awaken unable to speak because of the tracheostomy. They are unable to control their saliva and find that they are constantly aspirating small amounts of mucus. Their necks and shoulders are completely numb and boardlike because of the section of all cervical sensory nerves on the side of the lesion, and while they have little or no sharp pain, they have a pounding and persistent headache due to the ligation of the jugular vein and concomitant rise of spinal fluid pressure. In a day or two they look into the mirror and may not recognize the swollen, edematous, and possibly deformed face that stares back. It would be abnormal if they were not depressed under these circumstances. Support for the patient depends on good preoperative preparation. The patient must understand clearly what to expect in the postoperative period. Patients do not panic if they understand their problems and realize that most of their deficiencies are reversible as edema subsides and the tracheostomy tube is removed.

REHABILITATION

As Shedd has pointed out, progress in medicine often brings new problems. In head and neck oncology the suc-

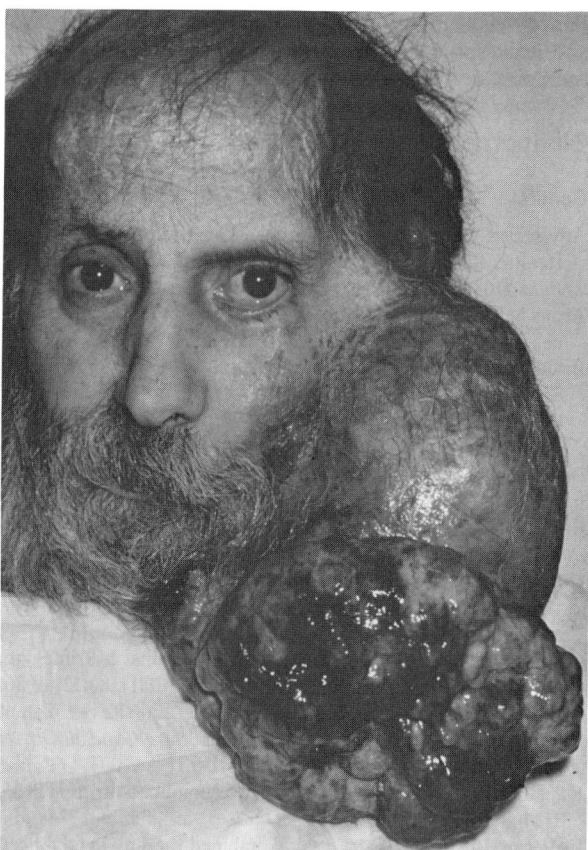

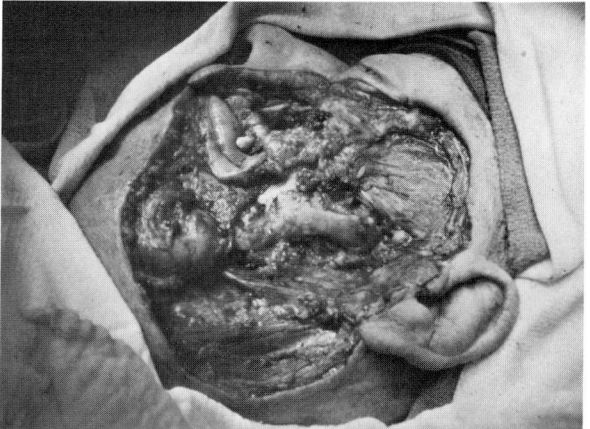

B

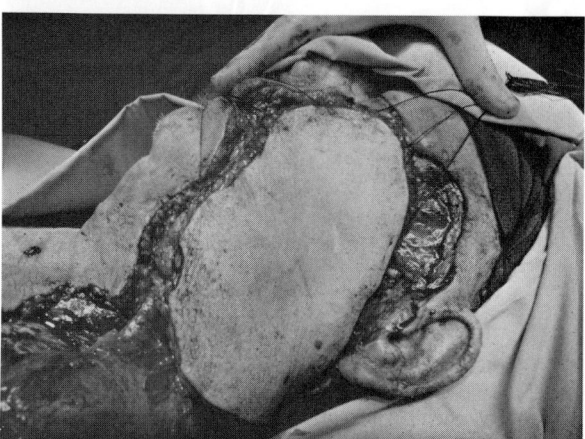

C

A

Fig. 16-47. Pectoralis myocutaneous flap in repair of a facial defect: *A.* Large neglected malignant mixed tumor of parotid with necrosis and ulceration of lower pole. *B.* Operative field after removal of tumor. Ascending ramus of mandible with anterior half removed is in center of field. Tongue is visible at 11 o'clock following removal of entire left cheek and buccal mucosa. Anterior wall of maxillary sinus has been removed. *C.* Pectoralis myocutaneous flap brought up to fill defect. *D.* Seven days after operation, myocutaneous flap in place, slight bulge in lower neck indicates site of muscle pedicle providing blood supply to the flap.

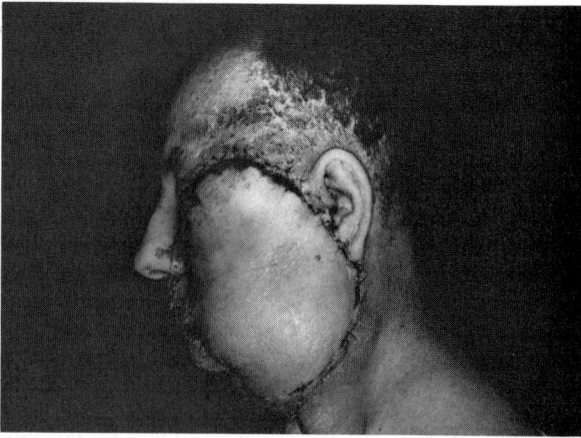

D

cessful control of major cancers may leave a considerable number of patients whose posttreatment life involves a significant degree of disability. Major impairment in appearance, swallowing, taste, and speech all reduce the quality of life and the effectiveness of treatment. While the field of rehabilitation of these patients is too broad to detail here, the major thrust of recent years has been to accomplish as much of the rehabilitation as possible on the operating table at the primary procedure.

The development of free flaps and myocutaneous flaps is a major advance in the reconstruction of head and neck defects. For the first time an adequate source of soft tissue and even bone is immediately available for rapid one-stage reconstruction of operative defects. Myocutaneous flaps are constructed by freeing up one end of a muscle and leaving the blood supply to the other end intact. All or any part of the overlying skin can be brought up with the muscle pedicle to fill the operative defect. The skin obtains its blood supply from the underlying muscle. While there are many muscles that can be used in head and neck reconstructions including the trapezius, sterno-cleidomastoid, and latissimus dorsi, the favorite has become the pectoralis major, which can reach any part of the face and can be fashioned to fill large and small defects (Fig. 16-47*A, B, C,* and *D*).

Rush BF Jr: New voices for old: Attempts to create a new larynx. *Surg Rounds* 4:16, 1981.

Rush BF Jr, Swaminathan AP, et al: Construction of a neolarynx after radiation and laryngectomy. *Am J Surg* 138:619, 1979.

Shahrokh DK, Devine KD, Harrison EG Jr: Statistical evaluation of 115 cases of carcinoma of the epiglottis (1943 to 1952). *Am J Surg* 102:781, 1961.

Shedd DP: Role of surgical measures in voice restoration after laryngectomy, in *Symposium on Malignancies of The Head and Neck*. St Louis, Mosby, 1975.

Spalt L, Greenlaw R, Rush BF Jr: Integrated therapy for carcinoma of the larynx, in Rush BF Jr, Greenlaw RH (eds): *Integrated Radiation and Operation in Cancer Therapy: A Symposium*. Springfield, IL, Charles C Thomas, 1968.

Vuyk H, Tiwara R, Snow GB: Staffier's procedure revisited. *Head Neck Surg* 8:21, 1985.

Nasopharynx

Jesse RH: Preoperative versus postoperative radiation in the treatment of squamous carcinoma of the paranasal sinuses. *Am J Surg* 110:552, 1965.

Moench HC, Phillips TL: Carcinoma of the nasopharynx: Review of 146 patients with emphasis on radiation dose and time factors. *Am J Surg* 124:515, 1971.

Thomas JE, Waltz AG: Neurological manifestations of nasopharyngeal malignant tumors. *JAMA* 192:103, 1965.

Nasal Cavity and Paranasal Sinuses

Kurohara SS, Ellis F, et al: Role of radiation therapy and of surgery in the management of localized epidermoid carcinoma of the maxillary sinus. *Am J Roentgenol Radium Ther Nucl Med* 114:35, 1972.

Moseley HS, et al: Advanced squamous cell carcinoma of the maxillary sinus. Results of combined regional infusion chemotherapy, radiation therapy and surgery. *Am J Surg* 141:522, 1981.

Rush BF Jr, Knightly JJ, Jewell W: Transoral and transverse incision for excision of the maxillary sinus. *J Surg Oncol* 3:53, 1971.

Tabah EJ: Cancer of the paranasal sinuses: A study of the results of various methods of treatment in fifty-four patients. *Am J Surg* 104:741, 1962.

Mandible

Bernier JL: *Tumors of the Odontogenic Apparatus and Jaws*. Washington, Armed Forces Institute of Pathology, 1960.

Cramer LM, Culf NK, et al: Reconstruction management of the mandible in the treatment of head and neck, in *Symposium on Malignancies of The Head and Neck*. St Louis, Mosby, 1975.

Khanna S, Khanna NN, et al: Primary tumors and tumor-like conditions of the mandible. *J Surg Oncol* 16:365, 1981.

Salivary Glands

Beahrs OH, Woolner LB, et al: Surgical management of parotid lesions. *Arch Surg* 80:890, 1960.

Bhaskar SN, Bernier JL: Mikulicz's disease. *Oral Surg* 13:1387, 1960.

Connell HC, Evans JC: Mucoepidermoid carcinoma of the salivary glands. *Am J Surg* 124:519, 1972.

Foote FW, Frazell EL: *Tumors of the Major Salivary Glands*. Washington, Armed Forces Institute of Pathology, 1954.

Gates GA: Current concepts in otolaryngology. Malignant neoplasms of the minor salivary glands. *N Engl J Med* 306:718, 1982.

Grage TB, Lober PH: Benign lymphoepithelial lesion of the salivary glands. *Am J Surg* 108:495, 1964.

Grage TB, Lober PH, Shahon DB: Benign tumors of the major salivary glands. *Surgery* 50:625, 1961.

Katsilambros L: Asymptomatic enlargement of the parotid glands. *JAMA* 178:513, 1961.

Reynolds CT, McAuley RL, Rogers WP Jr: Experience with tumors of minor salivary glands. *Am J Surg* 111:168, 1966.

Rosenfeld L, Sessions DG, et al: Malignant tumors of salivary gland origin: 37-year review of 184 cases. *Ann Surg* 163:726, 1966.

Stewart FW, Foote FW, Becker WF: Mucoepidermoid tumors of salivary glands. *Ann Surg* 122:820, 1945.

Stuteville OH, Corley RD: Surgical management of tumors of intraoral minor salivary glands: Report of eighty cases. *Cancer* 20:1578, 1967.

Suen JY, Johns ME: Chemotherapy for salivary gland cancer. *Laryngoscope* 92:235, 1982.

Winsten J, Ward GE: The parotid gland: An anatomic study. *Surgery* 40:585, 1956.

Tumors of the Neck

Albers GD: Branchial anomalies. *JAMA* 183:399, 1963.

Hoffman E: Branchial cysts within the parotid gland. *Ann Surg* 152:290, 1960.

Jesse RH, Neff LE: Metastatic carcinoma in cervical nodes with an unknown primary lesion. *Am J Surg* 112:547, 1966.

MacComb WS: Diagnosis and treatment of metastatic cervical cancerous nodes from an unknown primary site. *Am J Surg* 124:441, 1972.

Marchetta FC, Murphy WT, Kovaric JJ: Carcinoma of the neck. *Am J Surg* 106:974, 1963.

Mohit-Tabatabai MA, Dasmahapatra KS, et al: Management of squamous cell carcinoma of unknown origin in cervical lymph nodes. *Am Surg* 52, 1986.

Mooney CS, Jewell W, et al: Simultaneous bilateral radical neck dissection following high level radiation therapy. *J Surg Oncol* 1:335, 1969.

Razack MS, Sako K: Carotid artery hemorrhage and ligation in head and neck cancer. *J Surg Oncol* 19:189, 1982.

Roseman JM, James AG: Metastatic cancers to the neck from undermined primary sites long-term follow-up. *J Surg Oncol* 19:247, 1982.

Rush BF Jr: Current concepts in the treatment of carotid body tumors. *Surgery* 52:679, 1962.

Rush BF Jr: Familial bilateral carotid body tumors. *Ann Surg* 157:633, 1963.

Skandalakis JE, Gray SW, et al: Tumors of the neck. *Surgery* 48:375, 1960.

Suarez Nieto D, Estevan Solano JM, et al: Invasion of the carotid artery in tumors of the head and neck. *Clin Otolaryngol* 6:29, 1981.

Chemotherapy and Immunotherapy

Adams GL, Berlinger NT, et al: Immunologic assessment of regional lymph node histology in relation to survival in head and neck carcinoma. *Cancer* 37:697, 1976.

Alexander JC Jr, Chretien PB, et al: Viral-specific humoral immunity to herpes simplex-induced antigens in patients with squamous carcinoma of the head and neck. *Am J Surg* 132:541, 1976.

Blackshear PJ, et al: An implantable pump for long-term intravascular drug infusion. *Med Instrum* 15:226, 1981.

Connors JM, Andiman WA, et al: Treatment of nasopharyngeal carcinoma with human leukocyte interferon. *J Clin Oncol* 3:6, 1985.

Couture J, Deschenes L: Intra-arterial infusion: An adjuvant to the treatment of oral carcinoma. *Cancer* 29:1632, 1972.

Cvitkovic E, Gerold FP, et al: cis-Dichlorodiamineplatinum (II) in the treatment of epidermoid carcinoma of the head and neck. *Cancer Treat Rep* 61:359, 1977.

Dasmahapatra KS, Citrin P, et al: A prospective evaluation of 5-fluorouracil plus cisplatin in advanced squamous-cell cancer of the head and neck. *J Clin Oncol* 3:11, 1985.

Decker DA, et al: Adjuvant chemotherapy with high-dose bolus cis-diamminodichloroplatinum II (CDD) and 120-hour-infusion 5-fluorouracil (5-FU) in stage III and IV squamous cell carcinoma of the head and neck. *Proc Am Soc Clin Oncol* 1:195, 1982.

Ervin TJ, Clark JR, et al: An analysis of induction and adjuvant chemotherapy in the multidisciplinary treatment of squamous-cell carcinoma of the head and neck. *J Clin Oncol* 5:1, 1987.

Feldman J, et al: Up front bleo-cap chemotherapy produces a 100% rate (33%) complete response in previously untreated advanced head and neck cancer. *Proc Am Soc Clin Oncol* 1:193, 1982.

Freckman HA: Results in 169 patients with cancer of the head and neck treated by intra-arterial infusion therapy. *Am J Surg* 124:501, 1972.

Frei Emil II: The national cancer chemotherapy program. *Science* 217:600, 1982.

Holden C: New disease baffles medical community. *Science* 217:618, 1982.

Horn Y, et al: Long-term remission of an advanced head and neck tumor following intra-arterial infusion with *cis*-dichlorodiammineplatinum. *J Surg Oncol* 18:189, 1981.

Kish J, et al: Clinical trial of cisplatin and 5-FU infusion as initial treatment for advanced squamous cell carcinoma of the head and neck. *Cancer Treat Rep* 66:471, 1982.

Milazzo J, Mohit-Tabatabai MA, et al: Preoperative intra-arterial infusion chemotherapy for advanced squamous cell carcinoma of the mouth and oropharynx. *Cancer* 56:1014, 1985.

Perry DJ, Davis RK, Weiss RB: Combined modality treatment with combination chemotherapy for advanced squamous cell carcinoma of the head and neck. *Proc Am Soc Clin Oncol* 1:193, 1982.

Price LA, Hill BT: Safe and effective combination chemotherapy without *cis*-platinum for squamous cell carcinomas of the head and neck. *Cancer Treat Rep* 65 (suppl. 1):149, 1981.

Richman SP, et al: Chemotherapy versus chemoimmunotherapy of head and neck cancer: Report of a randomized study. *Cancer Treat Rep* 60:535, 1976.

Tannock IF, Browman G: Lack of evidence for a role of chemotherapy in the routine management of locally advanced head and neck cancer. *J Clin Oncol* 4:7, 1986.

Tejada F, Chandler JR: Combined therapy for stage III & IV head and neck cancer (H&N). *Proc Am Soc Clin Oncol* 1:199, 1982.

Williams AC: Topical 5 FU: A new approach to skin cancer. *Ann Surg* 173:864, 1971.

Woods JE: The influence of immunologic responsiveness on head and neck cancer. *Plast Reconstr Surg* 56:77, 1975.

Operations of the Head and Neck

Achauer BM, Salibian AH, Furnas DS: Free flaps to the head and neck. *Head Neck Surg* 4:315, 1982.

Frazell EL, Moore OS: Bilateral radical neck dissection performed in stages: Experience with 467 patients. *Am J Surg* 102:809, 1961.

Pradhan SA: Gastric pull-up for cancers of the hypopharynx and cervical esophagus: Our experience. *J Surg Oncol* 26:149, 1984.

Smith PG, Sharkey DE, et al: The infratemporal fossa approach to neoplastic and arterial lesions of the lateral skull base. *Surg Rounds* 9:63, 1986.

Wilson JS, Yiacoumettis AM, O'Neill T: Some observations on 112 pectoralis major myocutaneous flaps. *Am J Surg* 147:273, 1984.

INTRODUCTION

Life depends on a delicate sequence of events that moves air to blood and blood to tissues. The cardiorespiratory system functions to assure those events occur dependably; the margin of error is extremely small. The analysis and management of surgical concerns involving the chest and its contents, whether relating to tumors, trauma, or infection, all focus on the mechanical transport of oxygen to the vital organs and the necessary exchange of gases. Air with adequate oxygen content must pass through the upper airway, the trachea, and the bronchi to reach the alveoli properly warmed and humidified for movement across alveolar membranes. Those membranes must be in condition to allow efficient diffusion of oxygen and carbon dioxide. Blood with sufficient oxygen-carrying capacity must be circulating through the alveolar capillaries in adequate volumes and at the proper speed to allow pickup of oxygen and discharge of carbon dioxide; it must also be at the proper pH and temperature and must have the proper biochemical characteristics for optimum exchange. The vascular system must have the appropriate integrity, pressure gradients, volume, and flow dynamics to traverse the pumps and conduits from alveolar capillaries to vital organ capillaries and back. At the vital organ interface, the characteristics for release from the blood to the tissues of oxygen, and recapture of carbon dioxide must be present. Irreparable damage to vital organs may occur in minutes if any part of the system fails.

Near normal physiologic cardiopulmonary function must continue during surgical procedures involving the chest. Preexisting impairment of pulmonary function, operative removal of tissue from the chest wall or lungs, and postoperative pain are routine hazards to the patient's ability to continue adequate respiratory exchange following operation. The development of thoracic surgery has followed the development of anesthesiology: techniques for tracheal intubation and positive-pressure ventilation. Prior to this recent development, surgeons' efforts were largely limited to the management of trauma, and the history of the field is closely linked to the history of weaponry. Management of chest wounds received in battle was recorded in very ancient writings, including the *Iliad* (ca. 950 B.C.). Galen described a patient who recovered after partial excision of the sternum and pericardium for recurrent abscess due to an injury. Writing about chest wounds in the thirteenth century, Theodoric noted that "the stitches should be placed . . . so that the natural heat cannot escape in any way nor the air outside be able to enter."

The introduction of firearms in the fourteenth century complicated the management of chest wounds because of uncertainty about the intrathoracic damage, and the proper care of the open pneumothorax. Many felt the wound should be kept open for drainage of blood. Consistent with many of his other revolutionary insights, Napoleon's surgeon, Baron Larrey, confirmed the sporadic observations of other surgeons about the lifesaving value of closing an open wound of the thorax. His description of the cardiopulmonary effects of an open chest wound can hardly be improved upon:

> A soldier was brought to the hospital of the Fortress of Ibrahyn Bey, immediately after a wound penetrated the thorax, between the fifth and sixth true ribs. It was about 8 cm in extent. A large quantity of frothy and vermilion blood escaped from it with a hissing noise at each inspiration. His extremities were cold, pulse scarcely perceptible, countenance discolored, and respiration short and laborious; in short, he was every moment threatened with a fatal suffocation. After having examined the wound, the divided edges of the part, I immediately approximated the two lips of the wound, and retained them by means of adhesive plaster and a suitable bandage around the body. In adopting this plan, I intended only to hide from the sight of the patient and his comrades, the distressing spectacle of a hemorrhage, which would soon prove fatal; and I, therefore, thought that the effusion of blood into the cavity of the thorax, could not increase the danger. But the wound was scarcely closed, when he breathed more freely, and felt easier. The heat of the body soon returned, and the pulse rose. In a few hours he became quite calm, and to my great surprise grew better. He was cured in a very few days, and without difficulty.

The history of elective thoracic surgery is the history of airway management. By the late nineteenth century, open thoracic procedures on large animals were successfully performed along with experimentation on mechanical maintenance of ventilation. In 1904, Sauerbruch developed a negative-pressure chamber in which the operating team and the patient could be housed during operation. Under these conditions, the lung would not collapse when the chest was open. Though animal experiments gave some success, operations on patients were not rewarding. Positive-pressure systems with endotracheal intubation were also actively evolving during this fertile period of development. Orotracheal intubation with metal tubes for the treatment of croup and for the prevention of aspiration during oral surgical procedures provided the early experience that led to endotracheal anesthesia for thoracic surgery. An artificial respiration device consisting of a hand bellows and a tracheostomy tube were introduced by Fell in 1893, and modified by O'Dwyer in 1896. The latter substituted an orotracheal tube and a foot bellows with a greater volume capacity. Rudolph Matas in New Orleans advocated the use of the Fell–O'Dwyer apparatus to allow a more general availability of thoracic surgical techniques, and he introduced his own modification of the equipment in 1900. These early techniques to ventilate during thoracotomy were associated with hazards of their own. Consequently, individual surgeons were devising and reporting makeshift techniques to control the open pneumothorax associated with chest wall resections through the first third of this century. These included various packing techniques, preoperative pneumothorax for "conditioning," and suturing the lung to the parietal pleura. Improvements in laryngotracheal intubation techniques, in design and materials of tracheal tubes, and in anesthesia gradually displaced these local improvi-

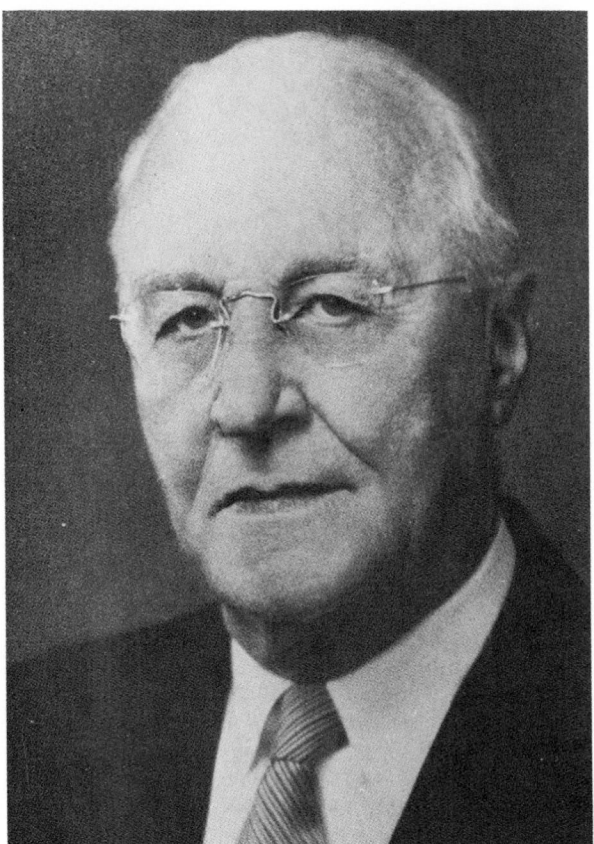

Fig. 17-1. Evarts Ambrose Graham (1883–1957). A dominant figure in the development of the field of thoracic surgery. He performed the first successful pneumonectomy (for bronchogenic carcinoma) on April 5, 1933.

dominate clinical practice as the long-predicted increase in cancers among smoking women has finally succeeded in making lung cancer the most common cancer killer of women as well as men. There is increasing evidence implicating side-stream smoke in health problems of non-smokers, particularly children. New developments in imaging techniques, particularly involving computer-assisted tomography and nuclear-magnetic resonance are making important improvements in the accuracy of diagnosis and staging of intrathoracic diseases. Our evolving skills in fiberoptic endoscopy have opened new diagnostic and therapeutic opportunities in airway, esophageal, and pleural disorders. These techniques are resulting in early detection and surgical resection of some tumors in a preclinical stage and yielding "cure" rates previously considered to be unobtainable. Some unanticipatedly encouraging results are appearing following multimodal therapy with chemotherapy and radiation therapy as pre- or postoperative adjuvant therapy for patients with lung cancer. The diagnostic and/or therapeutic role of immunohistochemical techniques, including monoclonal antibodies, remains uncertain, though recent research in the field presents some exciting theoretic potential for important future contributions. Several centers are now reporting success with heart-lung transplantation applied to the management of young patients with a variety of end-stage cardiopulmonary diseases.

ANATOMY OF THE THORAX AND PLEURA

Anatomic correlation with clinical diagnosis in chest disease is improved because many of the bony parts of the thoracic cage are palpable and cardiac and breath sounds are transmitted through the chest wall. There are a number of anatomic factors, however, that can be quite misleading and lead to errors of analysis and judgment. The "squaring off" effect of the shoulder girdle gives the chest the physical appearance of a rectangle, tempting the examiner to forget that the skeletal chest wall is conical in shape, tapering quite sharply in the upper chest. The diaphragm rises as high as the level of the nipple; the upper part of the abdomen is overlapped by six of the ten anterior ribs and the lower four posterior ribs. The lung apices rise well above the level of the clavicles anteriorly and the scapular posteriorly. These easily overlooked anatomical facts can lead to serious errors, especially in patients with blunt trauma (Fig. 17-2). The lower ribs and costal margin overlap the liver, spleen, stomach, the upper pole of both kidneys, and the distal part of the pancreas.

The framework of the thoracic cage consists of the sternum, twelve thoracic vertebrae, ten pairs of ribs that end anteriorly in segments of cartilage, and two pairs of floating ribs (Fig. 17-3). The thoracic inlet is characterized by having a rigid structural ring formed by the sternal manubrium, the short, semicircular first ribs, and the vertebral column. As a result of its articulation with the manubrium and the attachment of the costoclavicular ligament, the clavicle participates in providing protection for the underlying vascular and neural structures that traverse the tho-

sations. A pivotal figure in most of this evolution of the field of thoracic surgery was Evarts Graham (Fig. 17-1). While a captain in the Army in 1918, he served as chairman of the Empyema Commission and made fundamental observations and recommendations about the cause and care of intrapleural infections, a major cause of death following the disastrous worldwide influenza epidemic at that time. In 1933, he performed the first successful pneumonectomy. The patient was a long-term survivor of lung cancer. Shortly following that dramatic success, the majority of thoracic surgical techniques in use today for noncardiac disease were developed, refined, and widely implemented. He was also among the first to clearly recognize the central role tobacco addiction played in the etiology of most pulmonary diseases and tumors. It is ironic that he died of the consequence of his tobacco addiction (lung cancer) even though he had quit smoking as soon as he recognized the correlation between smoking habits and lung cancer.

Though somewhat overshadowed by the dramatic developments in cardiac surgery, significant recent diagnostic, technical, and therapeutic progress has been occurring in other areas of thoracic surgery. The terrible public health consequences of tobacco addiction continue to

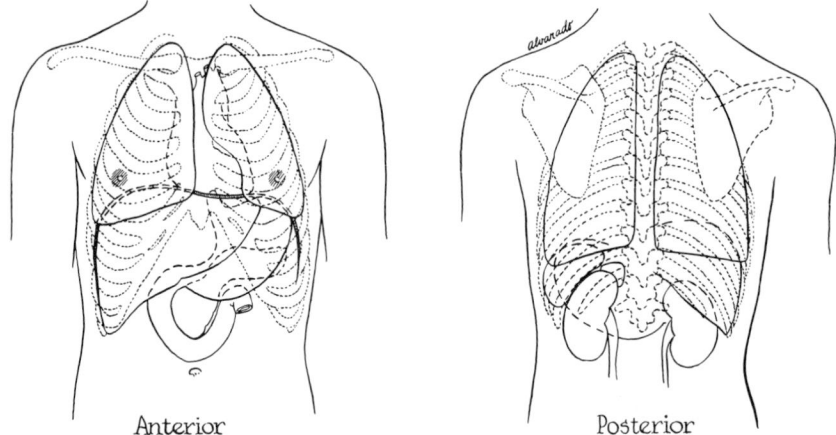

Anterior

Posterior

Fig. 17-2. The relationship of the thoracic cage to the upper abdominal viscera must be remembered to avoid overlooking concomitant abdominal injuries in patients with thoracic trauma.

racic inlet. The same rigidity that provides protection from trauma, however, leaves little room for pathologic swelling, enlarging masses, or postural adjustments with age.

The cartilages of the first six ribs have separate articulations with the sternum; the cartilages of the seventh through the tenth ribs fuse to form the costal margin before attaching to the lower margin of the sternum. As there is significant flexibility of the chest wall in children, serious trauma can be transmitted to the intrathoracic structures with little injury to the bony framework. Even though this flexibility decreases progressively with age, surprising damage can occasionally occur in the chest of adults without evidence of skeletal injury.

The pectoralis major and minor muscles constitute the principal muscular covering of the anterior thorax, and the lower margin of the pectoralis major forms the anterior axillary fold. Auscultation of the chest in the axilla often allows the best determination of breath sounds,

Fig. 17-3. The radiolucent costal cartilages and the poor projection of the sternum on anteroposterior chest x-rays make it difficult to demonstrate major injuries or abnormalities of the anterior part of the chest wall.

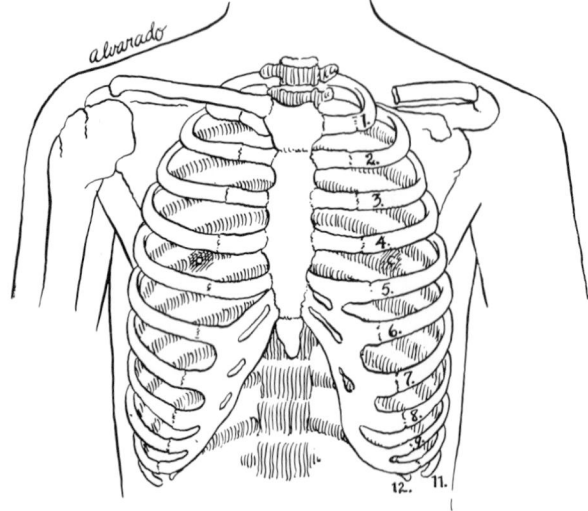

because the thoracic cage is covered only by the origins of the serratus anterior muscle in that location. The long thoracic nerve passes vertically on the axillary surface of that muscle—a point to be remembered when doing a thoracentesis or tube thoracostomy. A convergence of the latissimus dorsi and teres major muscles forms the posterior axillary fold on each side. The triangle of auscultation can often be palpated near the inferior medial border of the scapula, but the latissimus, trapezius, rhomboid, and other shoulder girdle muscles form a strong muscular coat for the posterior thorax. A disadvantage of the heavy muscle coat is the difficulty in accurately identifying specific ribs by palpation of the posterior chest wall.

The sternal angle is almost always palpable, and this allows quick identification of the second rib because of its articulation with the sternum at this location. A plane that is parallel to the floor and passes through the sternal angle of an upright patient will also pass through the fourth or fifth thoracic vertebra. The tracheal bifurcation lies in this same plane, while the apex of the aortic arch is located slightly higher. There is a gradual increase in the length of ribs from the first to the seventh and a progressive lateral displacement of the rib–costal cartilage junctions. Because of the radiolucency of the cartilages, standard anteroposterior chest x-rays may fail to document injury to the thoracic cage even though a severe blunt injury to the chest has disarticulated and fractured multiple costal cartilages.

The pleura is a serous membrane of flat mesothelial cells overlying a thin layer of connective tissue in which a vascular and lymphatic network is distributed. That part covering the lungs is referred to as the visceral pleura, and it is continuous over the pulmonary hilus and the mediastinum with the parietal pleura, which covers the inside of the chest wall and the diaphragm. While it is convenient to consider the pleura as a closed sac around the pleural cavity, that model encourages a static model that misrepresents a highly dynamic structure. The pleural surfaces behave more like a flowing syncytium across which fluids actively move (from visceral pleura to parietal pleura), actively phagocytosing cells and debris and sealing air leaks and capillary leaks. It is this physiologically active membrane that contributes to the general resistance of the pleural space to infection and the lung's remarkable ability to tolerate the trauma of surgery or injury with such a low frequency of persisting air-leak problems. With normal lung expansion the pleural cavity is completely filled and only a potential space exists. As shown in Fig. 17-4, the line of pleural reflection extends slightly beyond the lung border in each direction. This is expected because of the dynamic process of respiration and the need for the pleural sac to accommodate maximum lung expansion with deep inspiration. Conversely, with acute decreases in lung volume, such as that with lobar atelectasis, there is a limit to the pleural accommodation and fluid may be drawn into the pleural cavity to replace partially the lost lung volume.

There is no communication between the pleural cavities, but the anteromedial borders of the two pleural sacs come nearly into apposition behind the sternum. The interior border of each pleural cavity is located at the ninth rib in the midaxillary line, and the borders continue posteriorly in the eleventh intercostal space. Occasionally the pleural sac extends as low as the twelfth rib. Posteriorly, the margins of the two pleural sacs lie on the anterolateral surfaces of the vertebrae, separated by the esophagus. A retroesophageal recess is occasionally formed when the pleural margins are in near apposition, and pulmonary lesions arising in the recess are easily mistaken for mediastinal tumors or cysts. At the inferior margin of the lung hilus on each side, a double layer of mediastinal pleura is formed, the inferior pulmonary ligament.

The structures that occupy the intercostal spaces have considerable significance in relation to thoracic function,

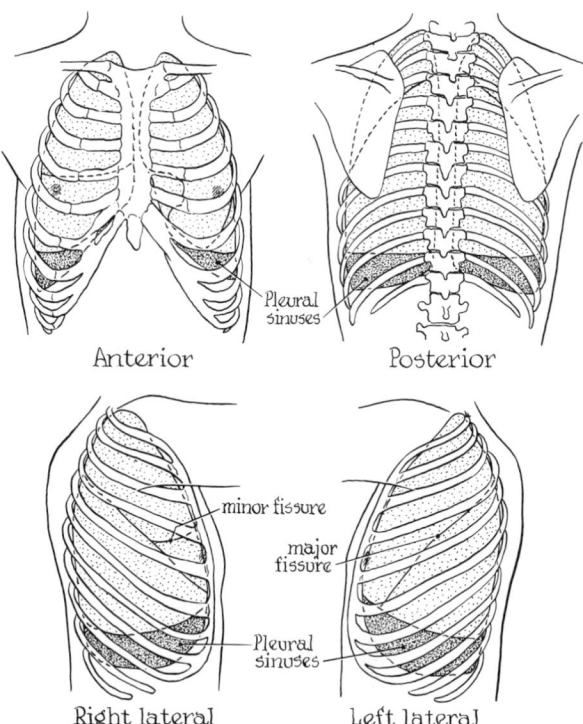

Anterior   Posterior

Right lateral   Left lateral

Fig. 17-4. The relation of the pulmonary lobes and pleural sinuses to the chest wall.

disease, and diagnostic procedures. The parietal pleura, for example, is well supplied with nerve endings for pain, while the visceral pleura is insensitive. Only when pulmonary disease extends to involve the parietal pleura or chest wall is pain produced. Figure 17-5 shows the structures in an intercostal space and emphasizes the layering effect of the muscles and fascia. Three layers of intercostal muscles are present in a major part of the thoracic wall, but some anatomists consider the innermost and the

Fig. 17-5. An illustration of the structures within an intercostal space. (Modified from: *Blevins CE: Anatomy of the thorax and pleura, in Shields TW (ed): General Thoracic Surgery, 2d ed. Philadelphia, Lea & Febiger, 1983, with permission.*)

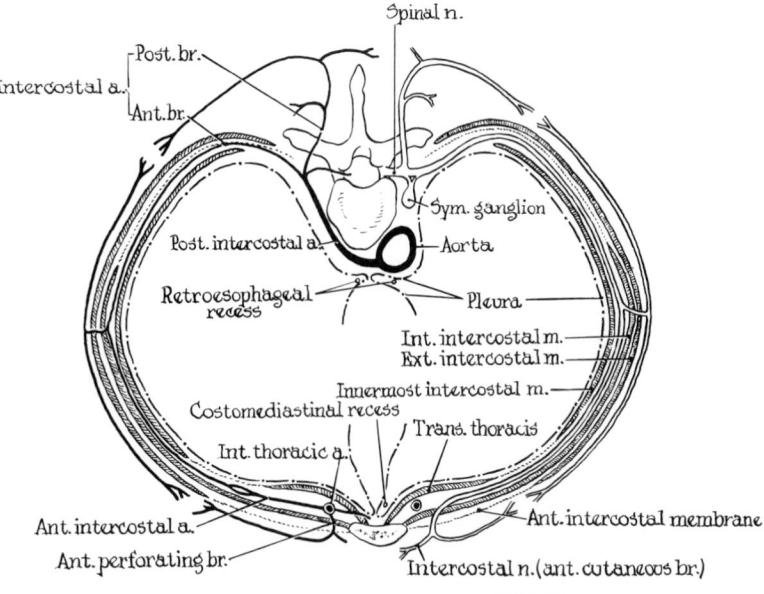

internal intercostals to be a single muscle entity. With quiet respiration the ribs are elevated by synchronous contraction of the intercostal muscles. Because the ribs of each side move as a unit in respiration, a localized painful lesion may eliminate effective function of the entire side. During quiet respiration, however, movements of the diaphragm provide approximately 75 percent of pulmonary ventilation, and temporary loss of unilateral intercostal muscle function is not a threat to breathing. With labored breathing, the muscles of the upper extremity and those cervical muscles that attach to the chest wall assist in elevation and expansion of the thorax.

The endothoracic fascia is a layer of light areolar tissue subjacent to the parietal pleura. At the apex of each hemithorax it is thickened into a more substantial layer referred to as Sibson's fascia.

The vein, artery, and nerve of each interspace are located deep to the external and internal intercostal muscles and lie just behind the lower margin of the rib. For most interspaces a smaller collateral artery runs along the top border of the rib below. There is significant overlap of neural supply by adjacent nerves, and complete anesthesia in an interspace will generally not occur unless the intercostal nerve of the adjacent space above and below and the space in question are anesthetized. To minimize the risk of lacerating the intercostal artery, a thoracentesis needle or a clamp used to perforate the pleura for insertion of a catheter should be passed across the top of the lower rib of the selected interspace.

The lymphatic drainage of the chest wall extends in both anterior and posterior directions. Lymph draining from the anterior region of the first four or five intercostal spaces passes to lymph nodes along the internal thoracic arteries. These nodes may be connected by cross anastomoses before draining into a single or double trunk that joins the thoracic duct, a right lymphatic duct, or a bronchomediastinal trunk. Lymphatics that drain the posterior and lateral regions of the intercostal spaces are tributary to lymph nodes that lie near the vertebral ends of each interspace. In the lower part of the thorax these nodes join the drainage from the posterior mediastinum to contribute to the cisterna chyli. The posterior lymph nodes of the upper thorax drain into the thoracic duct or a right lymphatic duct.

A musculofibrous floor is provided for the thorax by the diaphragm. The peripheral muscular portions of the diaphragm arise from the lower six ribs and costal cartilages, from the lumbar vertebrae (right and left crus), and from the lumbocostal arches. Additional fibers arise from the xiphoid cartilages, and all the muscular elements converge into the central tendon. The central part of the tendon underlies the pericardium, while the right and left divisions extend posteriorly. Some of the lower intercostal nerves are thought to contribute to the sensory innervation of the diaphragm, but motor innervation is supplied by the phrenic nerve on each side.

Of the three major openings in the diaphragm the aortic hiatus is most posterior. The aorta, azygos vein, and thoracic duct pass through this opening. The esophageal hiatus transmits the esophagus and vagus nerves, and only

the inferior vena cava goes through the foramen of that name.

Contemporary imaging techniques (including computer-analyzed tomographic and nuclear-magnetic resonance scanning) have increased the clinician's ability to identify anatomic relationships and their clinical significance. They have dramatically altered the preoperative assessment of both pulmonary and mediastinal lesions.

Figure 17-6 shows the cross-sectional anatomy at four different levels in the thorax associated with identifiable topographical landmarks. These studies provide considerable anatomic clarification of intrathoracic problems.

THORACIC INCISIONS

A basic knowledge of the incisions used to perform thoracic operations is helpful in understanding the postoperative course of patients and the management of complications. Because of the rigidity of the thoracic cage, most incisions for major procedures are relatively large and disrupt the integrity of muscles and bone, or cartilage, though contemporary anesthetic intubation techniques allowing single-lung anesthesia are making less destructive incisions feasible in selected cases. The extensive division of tissues and the distortion or stretching associated with the use of strong mechanical retractors often result in severe postoperative pain.

There are two principal incisions: (1) lateral thoracotomy, performed as either an anterolateral, midlateral (modified transaxillary), or posterolateral incision, and (2) median sternotomy, performed as a vertical, sternal splitting incision. Other incisions are infrequently used, either because experience has shown them to be inferior, or because they are used in unusual circumstances. The thoracoabdominal incision combines an upper abdominal incision with an incision in a lower intercostal space (sixth, seventh, or eighth) that may be carried as far posteriorly as the posterior axillary line. The costal margin and diaphragm are divided to provide an extensive exposure of the upper part of the abdomen and the retroperitoneal and posterior thoracic structures. Prolonged pain associated with incomplete healing of the costal margin, as well as complicated wound management involving two body cavities if infection occurs, has reduced the enthusiasm for this incision. Though elective use of this disabling incision is becoming less common, it is still useful for certain operations involving retroperitoneal structures (kidney, thoracoabdominal aorta), and it may be appropriate for hepatic or thoracoabdominal trauma under emergency conditions.

A bilateral transverse thoracotomy incision with transection of the sternum is rarely used at present but was employed for routine operative approach to the heart and mediastinum before confidence was gained in the median sternotomy incision. The incision generally extends from one anterior axillary line to the other, in either the third or the fourth intercostal space. For reduced exposure needs the incision may be started on the side where the principal dissection will be done and extended only a short distance

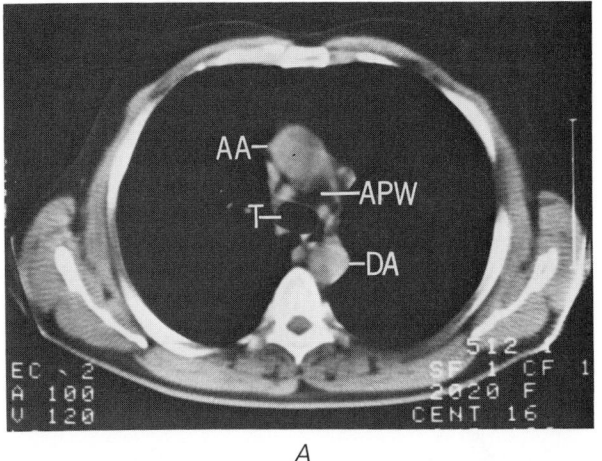

A

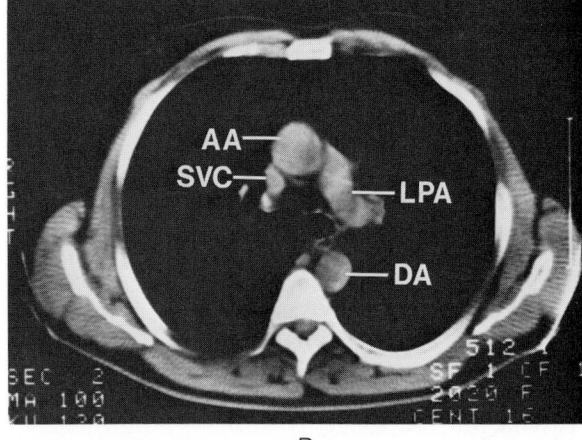

B

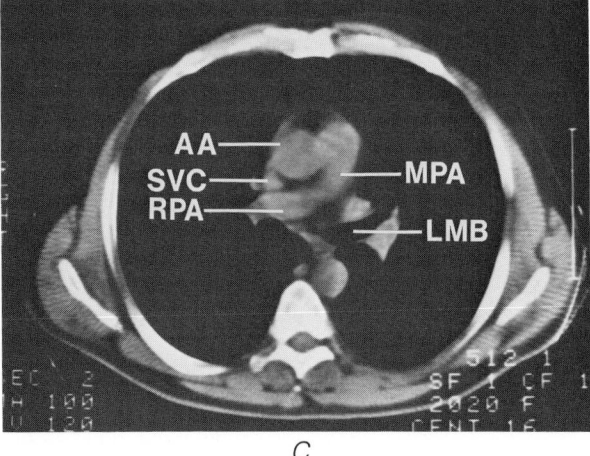

C

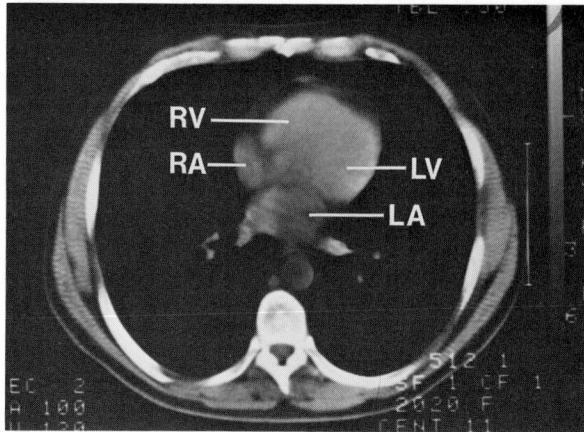

D

Fig. 17-6. Transverse sectional anatomy at four levels as shown by a CT scan of the thorax in a normal person. *A.* A transverse section at the level of the tracheal bifurcation outlines the aortico-pulmonary window, a frequent site of mediastinal lymph-node metastases in patients with bronchogenic carcinoma arising in the left lung. *B.* A section 1 cm inferior to *A* shows the origin of the left pulmonary artery and an air bubble in the esophagus as it lies immediately posterior to the origin of the left main-stem bronchus. *C.* The origin and course of the right pulmonary artery are shown at this level, and the left-upper-lobe bronchus is seen at its origin from the left main bronchus. *D.* At a lower level in the thorax the more complex mediastinal anatomy gives way to the cardiac chambers and pulmonary veins. AA = ascending aorta, DA = descending aorta, APW = aortico-pulmonary window, T = trachea, SVC = superior vena cava, LPA = left pulmonary artery, MPA = main pulmonary artery, RPA = right pulmonary artery, LMB = left main bronchus, RA = right atrium, RV = right ventricle, LA = left ventricle.

into the opposite hemithorax after transection of the sternum. The disadvantages of this incision include the longer time required to make the incision and to close the chest, compared with the median sternotomy incision. Both pleural cavities are usually entered with the transverse incision, but this may be avoided with the median sternotomy approach. In unusual circumstances, where the instruments necessary to perform median sternotomy are not available and there is urgent need to have access to

both sides of the mediastinum, this incision may still be quite useful. It also provides some cosmetic advantage in young women where bilateral submammary incisions leave much less disfiguring scars than the median sternotomy. The sternotomy can be carried out through a submammary incision with large skin flaps, though an anesthetic nipple is a relatively frequent complication of this approach.

The anterolateral and posterolateral thoracotomy incisions are used most frequently for general thoracic operations. Each one requires division of one or more major shoulder-girdle muscles, and this results in voluntary restriction of shoulder motion in the early postoperative period. Because they function as accessory muscles of respiration, it is possible that the selection and placement of the incision to minimize muscle injury could be important in an occasional patient with need for maximal muscle preservation. All patients must be encouraged to begin active shoulder and arm motion after operation, but elderly patients are especially likely to develop a restricted range of shoulder motion if not supervised carefully. The distal parts of the transected muscles lose their nerve supply and atrophy to a significant degree postop-

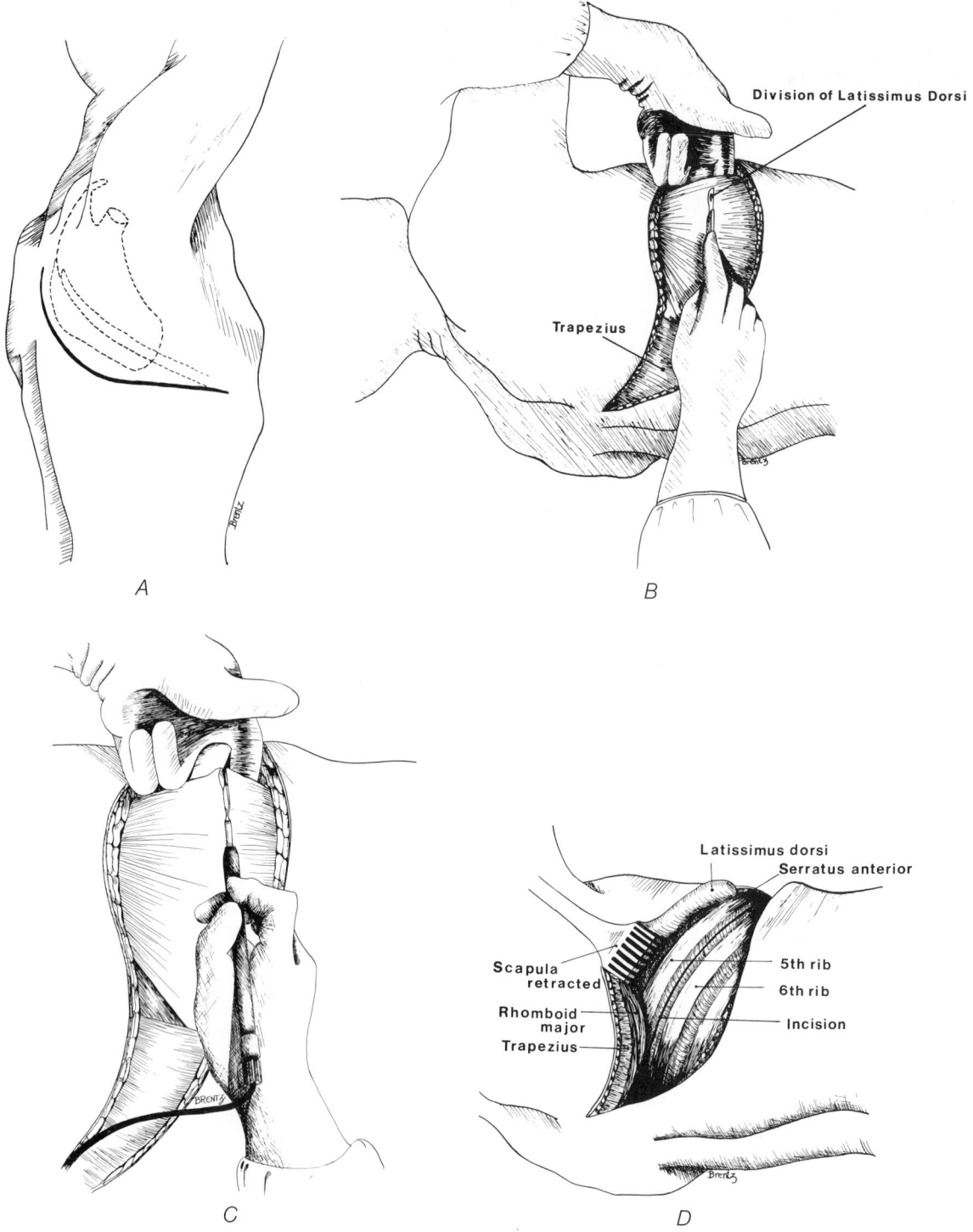

Fig. 17-7. The posterolateral thoracotomy incision. *A.* The skin incision begins near the anterior axillary line and curves posteriorly around the vertebral border of the scapula. *B.* The skin and muscle incisions are located in approximately the same position, whether the pleural cavity is entered in the fourth, fifth, or sixth intercostal space. *C.* Division of the shoulder-girdle muscles with the electrocautery may reduce blood loss and operating time. *D.* The pleural cavity is entered by dividing the intercostal muscles along the lower margin of the interspace.

eratively. Commonly, patients note a zone of reduced sensation in the skin on the caudal side of the incision for months after operation.

The posterolateral thoracotomy is used for the majority of pulmonary resections (except lung biopsy), for esophageal operations, and for the approach to the posterior mediastinum and the vertebral column (Fig. 17-7). When the intent is to enter the pleural cavity in the fifth intercostal space, the most common selection, the skin incision is begun at the anterior axillary line just below the nipple level in the male, and at the corresponding position in the female. The incision extends posteriorly below the tip of the scapula and ascends midway between the vertebral border of the scapula and the spinous processes of the vertebrae. To expose the thoracic cage it is necessary to divide part of the serratus anterior, latissimus dorsi, trapezius, and rhomboid major muscles. The pleural cavity may be entered by dividing the intercostal muscles in the chosen interspace, or by resecting the posterior two-thirds of the corresponding rib. The division of the rib posteriorly before the mechanical rib spreader is put in place may avoid accidental fracture of one or more ribs or a costochondral separation by the instrument. The injury to the rib or cartilage may increase postoperative incisional pain and prolong the restricted motion of the chest cage.

Two advantages of the anterolateral thoracotomy may be important in trauma victims and in patients with an unstable cardiovascular system. The incision can allow rapid entry into the chest, and the patient may be placed in the semisupine position on the operating table. This is tolerated better than the lateral decubitus position, and it gives the anesthesiologist the maximum control over the patient's cardiorespiratory system. The incision may be used for mediastinal operations, for some cardiac procedures, and for wedge resections of the upper and middle lobes of the lung. It is preferable to make a submammary skin incision starting at the sternal border overlying the fourth intercostal space and extending to the midaxillary line. The pectoralis major muscle and part of the pectoralis minor are divided at the level of the fourth or fifth intercostal space, and the incision is extended into the serratus anterior. By extending the chosen intercostal muscle incision posteriorly along the top of the subjacent rib it is possible to obtain a wider opening in the chest than the length of the skin incision would suggest. Still further exposure may be obtained by transecting the sternum.

As most advances in thoracic surgery have followed improvements in techniques of managing the airway, the recent widespread introduction of the double-lumen endotracheal tube has made it possible to utilize a less destructive midlateral thoracotomy incision. This incision is a modification of the transaxillary approach through the bed of the third rib that has been used extensively in some clinics for upper-lobe biopsies, for resection of small apical pulmonary blebs and pleural abrasion in patients with recurrent pneumothorax, for upper thoracic sympathectomy, and for biopsy of upper mediastinal lymph nodes or masses. By moving down the lateral chest wall several ribs, and with the advantage that single-lung anesthesia allows, good exposure can be obtained for most pulmonary resections and hilar dissections. The incision has the advantage that it requires cutting no major muscles, can be rapidly made and closed, and results in significantly less postoperative discomfort. An important requirement for adequate exposure in the incision is proper positioning of the patient. The patient is placed in a straight lateral

position with the arm at right angles (in order to facilitate mobility of the scapula). The skin incision parallels the course of the fifth rib extending from a few centimeters anterior to the middle of the lateral border of the scapula forward toward the submammary fold. The latissimus dorsi is elevated along its entire anterior border, as is the pectoralis major along its axillary border. The serratus is separated from its insertion into the fifth rib, which is removed after the periosteum is stripped. Two Tuffier retractors are placed at right angles to one another, one retracting the two muscle groups anteriorly and posteriorly and one retracting the ribs caudad and cephalad. The upper lung is allowed to collapse as dissection proceeds. Depending on the exposure desired, the skin incision parallels the course of the third, fourth, or fifth rib extending from the middle of the anterior border of the scapula at the posterior axillary fold to the anterior axillary fold (Fig. 17-8).

A hazard that is common to all the lateral thoracotomy incisions is the potential for injury to the brachial plexus and the axillary neurovascular structures from excessive displacement of the shoulder in positioning the patient on the operating table after anesthesia has been induced. By preventing posterior displacement of the shoulder this complication can be minimized.

The median sternotomy incision provides optimum exposure for anterior mediastinal lesions, and it is the principal incision used for cardiac operations. Either pleural cavity may be entered, or incision into the pleural cavity may be avoided if it is unnecessary. Disadvantages of the incision include an increased risk of infection if it is necessary to do a tracheostomy within a few days after operation, and the protracted course that occurs with infection because of involvement of the sternal fragments. An occasional patient who develops an acute wound infection also develops a severe mediastinitis associated with dehiscence of the sternal wound. The mortality rate for this complication is high but has decreased with the evolution of effective treatment.

The skin incision extends from just below the suprasternal notch to a point several centimeters below the xiphoid process (Fig. 17-9). Either an oscillating saw or a Lebsche knife and mallet may be used to split the sternum. A mechanical retractor is used to spread the incision, but the retractor blades may fracture the sternal halves with excessive pressure. Less commonly, there may be injury to the C_8–T_1 component of the brachial plexus, thought to be due to excessive spreading of the sternal halves and high placement of the retractor blades. In some instances a posterior fracture of the first rib can be demonstrated with special rib radiographs. After operation, patients who have had a sternotomy have less pain and less interference with pulmonary function than those who have had a lateral thoracotomy.

The pleural cavity is usually drained with one or two chest tubes connected to an underwater seal system at the conclusion of the intrathoracic portion of the operation. Each chest tube should be brought through a separate stab wound in the chest wall at least two interspaces away from the incision. If the pleural cavity is not entered in operations through a median sternotomy, it is advisable

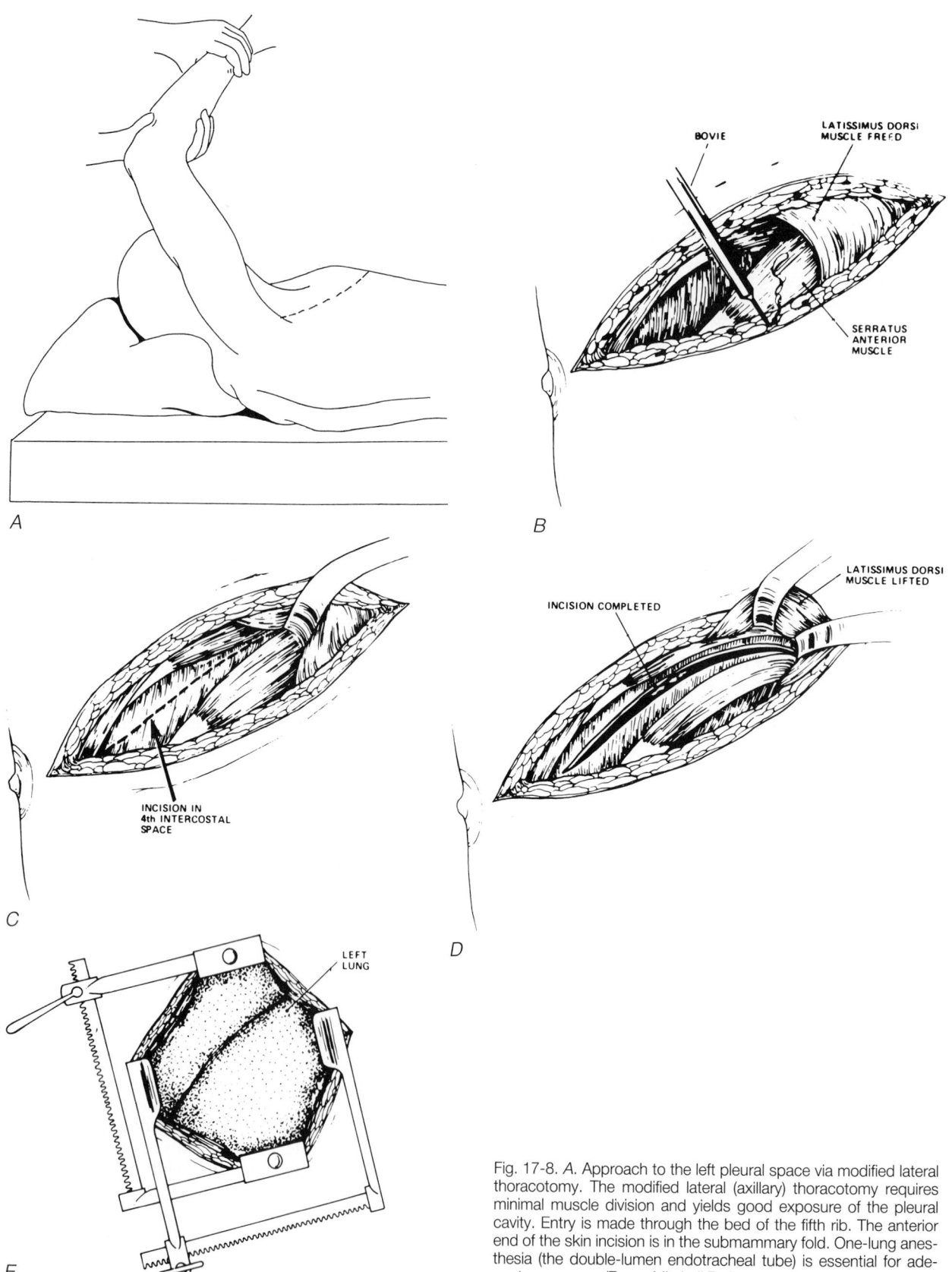

A

B

LATISSIMUS DORSI
MUSCLE FREED

BOVIE

SERRATUS
ANTERIOR
MUSCLE

C

INCISION IN
4th INTERCOSTAL
SPACE

D

INCISION COMPLETED

LATISSIMUS DORSI
MUSCLE LIFTED

E

LEFT
LUNG

Fig. 17-8. *A.* Approach to the left pleural space via modified lateral thoracotomy. The modified lateral (axillary) thoracotomy requires minimal muscle division and yields good exposure of the pleural cavity. Entry is made through the bed of the fifth rib. The anterior end of the skin incision is in the submammary fold. One-lung anesthesia (the double-lumen endotracheal tube) is essential for adequate exposure. (From: *Mitchell R, Angell W, et al, with permission.*)

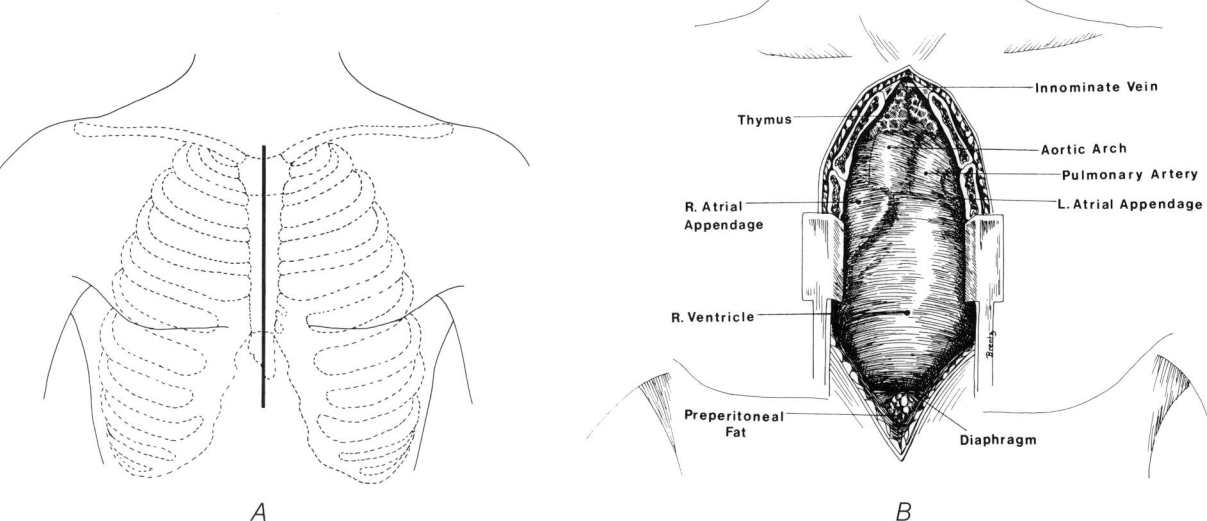

Fig. 17-9. *A*. A median sternotomy incision is outlined. *B*. Exposure of a pleural space would be made optimum by placement of mechanical retractor, rotating the patient slightly, and the use of single-lung anesthesia.

to drain the retrosternal space for 24 h with an intercostal tube that is brought out through a stab wound in the epigastrium.

PATIENT EVALUATION

As diagnostic procedures are being completed in the patient with a thoracic lesion, it is important to assess the ability of the patient to undergo operative treatment. The surgical lesion should be evaluated sufficiently to plan the soundest and most effective operative procedure. Since all operations on the chest result in some short-term respiratory disability, and many require removal or permanent alterations in function of intrathoracic organs, the surgeon must make a careful assessment of the patient's ability to withstand the contemplated procedure. This assessment includes most components of the patient's overall state of health.

The surgeon must make a preliminary decision based on an evaluation of the patient's health, the operation that would be required, the patient's age, and the complications or disability that may occur postoperatively; the potential benefit from operation must be weighed against the involved risk.

The history and physical examination, with the consequence of thoracotomy in mind, constitute the foundation of each patient's evaluation. If the patient is found to be in good health, is young, and has normal values for the hospital admission blood tests and urinalysis, little further evaluation may be necessary. Most candidates for operation, however, have a pulmonary or esophageal neoplasm, or are cigarette smokers with symptoms of chronic bronchitis, and are at least middle-aged. If the patient is a satisfactory candidate for operation, a procedure will be

required that will interfere with cardiopulmonary function, at least temporarily. During an operation, one lung will be either retracted or displaced and will contribute little, if any, to respiratory gas exchange. Further, it may be necessary to retract intermittently against the pericardium interfering with venous return to the atria or precipitating brief arrhythmias. Therefore, the functional status of the contralateral lung and the presence of preexisting cardiac disease are major determinants of the safety of the operation.

MALNUTRITION. Malnutrition increases the morbidity and mortality rate of any major surgical procedure, and an assessment of the preoperative nutritional state is important. While most emphasis has been placed on preexisting protein deficits, both fat and carbohydrate can spare protein and therefore have an effect on nitrogen balance. In clinical practice it may be difficult to separate the effects of total calorie deficit from a deficiency of protein alone. Even so, much of the data relating nutritional deficiency to postoperative complications are based on experimental or clinical effects of hypoproteinemia. There is a reduced blood volume and reduced tolerance for intraoperative bleeding in hypoproteinemic patients. Impaired antibody production, decreased lymphocyte proliferative response, and depression of the delayed skin reactivity to antigens are associated with weight loss and hypoalbuminemia and reduced host resistance to infection.

Particularly important in thoracic surgical patients are the adverse effects of protein depletion on pulmonary functions and ventilatory capacity. As skeletal muscle is catabolized during starvation, the muscle groups in the thorax, abdomen, shoulder, and diaphragm that are involved in respiration and coughing share in the unselective loss of strength that is seen in all muscles. Coupled with the increased tendency for interstitial edema associated with hypoproteinemia, the effects of protein depletion can significantly increase the risk of a major thoracic operation.

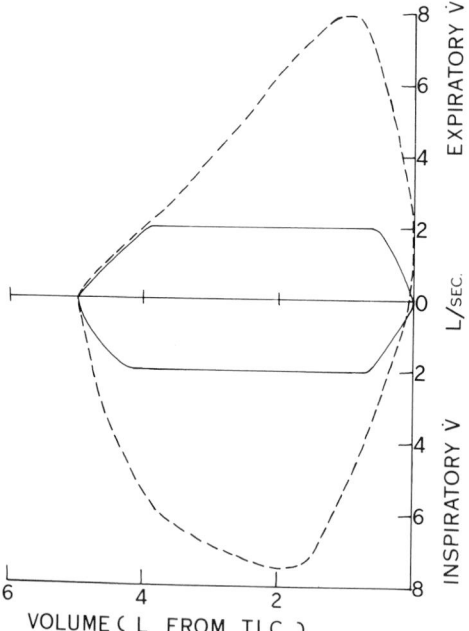

Fig. 17-11. A fixed obstruction in the trachea markedly alters the maximum expiratory flow-volume curve (MEFV). The normal MEFV is shown by the interrupted line. (Reproduced from: *Hyatt RE: Evaluation of major airway lesions using the flow-volume loop. Ann Otol Rhinol Laryngol 84:635, 1975, with permission.*)

significant. Moderate or severe obstructive airway disease invariably decreases the MVV, but patients with pure restrictive lung disease may have normal values for this test. The MVV usually correlates well with the FEV_1, and the expected relationship is $FEV_1 \times 34$ for males, $FEV_1 \times 40$ for females. If the actual measured value fails to correlate with the calculated value, it suggests a poor effort or a fatigued patient. In most laboratories the patient is given an aerosol of a sympathomimetic amine bronchodilator and the spirometry is repeated. An improvement, sometimes significant, in flow rates and in VC may occur. A failure of severely decreased function values to improve does not mean that the patient has irreversible pulmonary disease. Aggressive therapy with the patient's cooperation can often improve pulmonary function, a benefit both to the patient's comfort and to the operative procedure.

The significance of early small-airway disease that is not demonstrated by standard spirometry has not been defined for thoracic surgical patients. Nevertheless, there is interest in two tests that provide data useful in the understanding of pulmonary function. The maximal expiratory flow-volumes curve (MEFV) is inscribed from a plot of airflow against the volume of vital capacity. This relationship of the data may provide information not given by a spirogram. Major airway lesions may distort the MEFV curve; Fig. 17-11 shows the abnormality seen with fixed obstruction of the trachea. The closing volume (CV) depends on the fact that gravity results in a greater negative pressure at the apex of the lung than at the base in an upright person. That lung volume at which lung units in

the dependent regions of the lung cease to ventilate, presumably because of airway closure, is referred to as the CV. The measurement can be made by monitoring the concentration of nitrogen in the exhaled gas during a vital-capacity maneuver after inspiration of a bolus of 100% oxygen. [133]Xe or another gas may be used as the marker. An abrupt increase in the marker concentration in the terminal portion of the vital-capacity curve is the CV, and the value is expressed as a percentage of the vital capacity. Normally, VC is above the RV and below the end-tidal point. The CV increases with age, and it is increased in smokers, in peripheral obstructive airway disease, and in congestive heart failure.

The pulmonary-function values obtained with spirometry in the individual patient must be compared with those obtained from other individuals of the same sex, age, and height who are known to be free of pulmonary disease. Data obtained from the spirometric studies in hundreds of normal males and females form the basis for prediction nomograms that facilitate that comparison. Figure 17-12 shows a prediction nomogram developed from studies of 422 normal adult males in a Veterans Administration–Army Cooperative Study of Pulmonary Function. To demonstrate the considerable information about the individual patient's pulmonary function that may be accumulated, Table 17-3 lists the values for a healthy young male breathing air at sea level. In addition to the studies shown, patients with marginal pulmonary function may require measurements of diffusing capacity, regional lung function with radionuclides, and exercise testing.

Blood-Gas Determination. A measurement of the arterial blood gases and pH should be routine in the preoperative evaluation of a candidate for thoracic surgery. It would be an unusual situation in which the decision to advise operation depended solely on a single measurement of arterial oxygen or carbon dioxide tension. Even so, an occasional patient is discovered to have hypoxemia or CO_2 retention that was not suspected on the basis of clinical examination or spirometry. A measurement of the Pa_{CO_2} provides an immediate indication of the patient's alveolar ventilation; any value above 46 torr means that there is hypoventilation. There are multiple causes for this, and the specific reason should be sought in each patient. The ability of the lungs to excrete CO_2 is remarkable, and any persistent elevation of Pa_{CO_2} in a patient who might other-

Fig. 17-12. A prediction nomogram for pulmonary function in men. FRC, functional residual capacity; TLC, total lung capacity; RV, residual volume; $FEV_{0.5}$, 0.5-s forced expiratory volume; MVV_F, maximal voluntary ventilation (free); FEV_1, 1-s forced expiratory volume; FVC, forced vital capacity. The predicted values for FRC and TLC can be read directly from the left-hand scale, based on the patient's height. The scale at the bottom is for convenience in converting centimeters to inches. RV/TLC (%) may be used directly from the age scale. For the other predicted values, lay a straightedge between patient height and age. Predicted normal values can be read directly from the joints where the straightedge crosses the RV, $FEV_{0.5}$, MVV_F, FEV_1, and FVC scales. (Reproduced from: *Boren HC, Kory RC, Syner JC: The Veterans Administration–Army Cooperative Study of Pulmonary Function: II. The lung volume and its subdivisions in normal men. Am J Med 41:96, 1986, with permission.*)

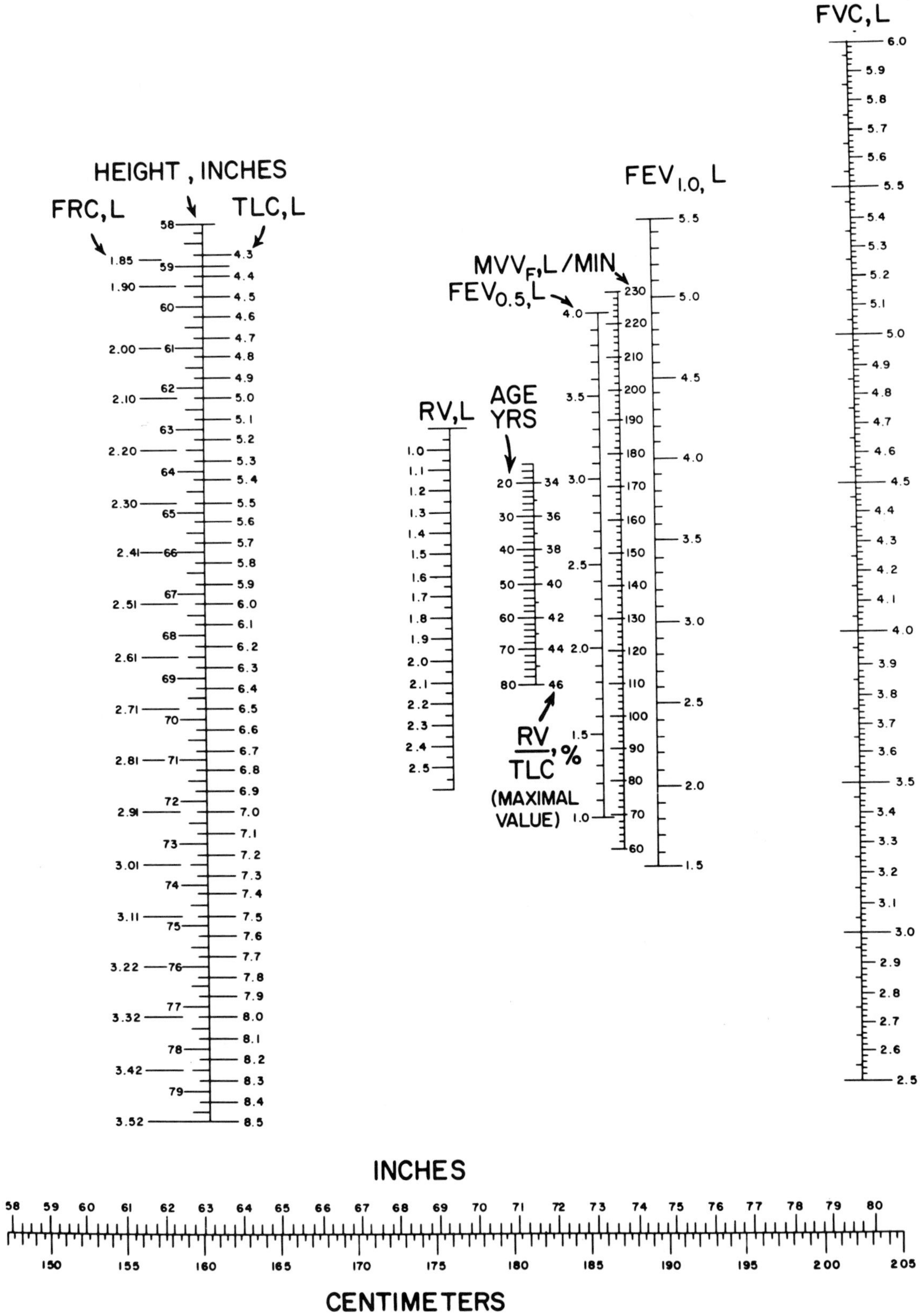

FVC, L

HEIGHT , INCHES

FRC, L   TLC, L

$FEV_{1.0}$, L

MVV_F, L /MIN
$FEV_{0.5}$, L

RV, L   AGE
          YRS

$\dfrac{RV}{TLC}$, %

(MAXIMAL
VALUE)

INCHES

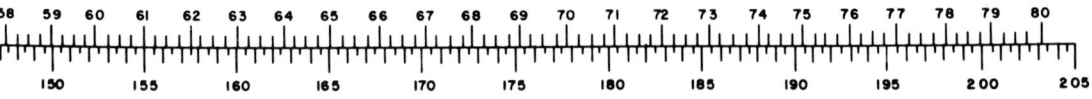

CENTIMETERS

Table 17-3. TYPICAL VALUES IN PULMONARY
FUNCTION TESTS*

Lung volumes:	
Inspiratory capacity, mL	3600
Expiratory reserve volume, mL	1200
Vital capacity, mL	4800
Residual volume (RV), mL	1200
Functional residual capacity, mL	2400
Thoracic gas volume, mL	2400
Total lung capacity (TLC), mL	6000
RV/TLC ×100, %	20
Ventilation:	
Tidal volume, mL	500
Respiratory dead space, mL	150
Respirations/min	12
Minute volume, mL/min	6000
Alveolar ventilation, mL	4200
Mechanics of breathing:	
Maximal voluntary ventilation, L/min	125–170
Forced expiratory volume, % in 1 s	83
Forced expiratory volume, % in 3 s	97
Maximal expiratory flow rate (for 1 L), L/min	400
Maximal inspiration flow rate (for 1 L), L/min	300
Compliance of lungs and thoracic cage, L/cmH$_2$O	0.1
Compliance of lungs, L/cmH$_2$O	0.2
Airway resistance, cmH$_2$O/L/s	1.6
Alveolar ventilation/pulmonary capillary blood flow:	
Alveolar ventilation, L/min/blood flow, L/min	0.8
Physiologic shunt/cardiac output ×100, %	<7
Physiologic dead space/tidal volume ×100, %	<30
Arterial blood:	
Oxygen tension, torr	100
Carbon dioxide tension, torr	40
Oxygen tension (100% inhaled oxygen), torr	640
Alveolar-arterial P_{O_2} difference (100% inhaled oxygen), torr	33
Oxygen saturation (% saturation of hemoglobin)	97.1
pH	7.4

* The values shown are those of a resting young male, 1.7 m^2
body surface area, breathing room air at sea level, except where
specified otherwise.
SOURCE: Modified from Comroe JH Jr: *The Lung,* 2d ed. Year
Book Medical Publishers, Chicago, 1962, with permission.

wise be considered a candidate for a major thoracotomy
suggests serious abnormalities in distribution of ventilation and perfusion. Most operations will temporarily increase the ventilation-perfusion abnormality. A mild elevation of the Pa_{CO_2} in a patient with chronic lung disease
may be treated aggressively to improve pulmonary function and allow the patient to be considered for operation.
If pulmonary resection is contemplated in such an individual, the risk of postoperative respiratory failure is high

and the decision to operate may depend on whether functioning pulmonary tissue would be removed.

The measurement of arterial Pa_{O_2} is valuable in the preoperative assessment of pulmonary function, but the
number reported must be viewed with a consideration of
the possibilities for error in its measurement. At sea level
the normal Pa_{O_2} is above 85 torr. It is remarkable, however, how seldom one sees a patient with even minimal
pulmonary disease who has an arterial oxygen tension in
the normal range. The majority of patients considered by
a thoracic surgeon have a Pa_{O_2} of 80 torr or below, and
values in the range of 70 to 80 torr do not suggest unusual
risk in the absence of other signals of caution. If the Pa_{O_2}
is below 70 torr, an attempt should be made to determine
the cause and to improve the patient's respiratory exchange. The possibilities include right-to-left shunting as
a result of the thoracic disease for which the patient is
being considered, uneven distribution of ventilation and
perfusion, or diffusion barrier. More sophisticated pulmonary function tests may be indicated, including determination of alveolar-arterial oxygen difference, calculation of right-to-left shunt fraction, and split pulmonary
function.

Other Specialized Tests. A specialized test of lung function that has been especially helpful for patients with
compromised pulmonary reserve determined by spirometry is radionuclide perfusion scanning for regional lung
function. This technique has replaced bronchospirometry
for measuring the separate contributions of the right and
left lungs to overall pulmonary function, and the method
is often referred to as a "split-function" study. The data
can be obtained by comparing the counts over each lung
during 99 mTc perfusion scanning, or more detailed information may be utilized if both ventilation and perfusion
scanning are performed.

The practical value of the split-function studies is that
postoperative VC and FEV$_1$ can be predicted for the patient who may require pneumonectomy for adequate resection of a bronchial neoplasm (predicted postoperative
FEV$_1$ = preoperative FEV$_1$ × percent perfusion in noninvolved lung). Even though a patient may require only a
lobectomy for resection of a pulmonary neoplasm, the
effects of a major thoracotomy can be likened to a "functional pneumonectomy" in the early postoperative period
and can be expected to reduce pulmonary function by
approximately 50 percent. This is particularly true if there
is significant preoperative reduction in pulmonary function.

In an important prospective study Boysen and associates demonstrated the validity of the split-function concept in a group of patients with impaired ventilatory function (preoperative FEV$_1$ <2.0 L). If the predicted
postoperative FEV$_1$ exceeded 800 mL, they considered
the patients to be acceptable candidates for pulmonary
resection up to and including a pneumonectomy. The perioperative mortality in their series was 15 percent, a figure
considered acceptable for major pulmonary resections in
extremely high-risk patients. Other investigators have
corroborated their data and have shown the measured
values for FEV$_1$ after a pneumonectomy correlated

closely with the predicted values. Figure 17-13 illustrates the use of a split-function study to decide that a patient with severely decreased pulmonary function is a reasonable risk for pneumonectomy.

In recent years there has been increasing interest in exercise testing for patients who are candidates for pulmonary resection but have impaired pulmonary function. It is particularly indicated for those patients who have reasonable exercise capability despite severe obstructive airway disease. It may be performed as a simple graded exercise test using a treadmill, or it may be done as progressive incremental exercise on a bicycle ergometer with simultaneous respiratory gas analysis. With the treadmill test, the speed is increased every 2 min until 3 mi/h is reached. The elevation is raised in increments to 10°, and patients who complete the test are good risks to tolerate pneumonectomy even with significant impairment on spirometry. By combining respiratory gas analysis with ergometer testing, more sophisticated data can be obtained for correlation of oxygen consumption with work capacity.

Unilateral balloon occlusion of the pulmonary artery with right-heart catheterization is only rarely indicated in the preoperative evaluation of patients who require a major pulmonary resection. Normally, pulmonary vascular resistance decreases with exercise and with pneumonectomy the remaining lung accepts the entire pulmonary blood flow without development of pulmonary hypertension. In a very occasional patient, occlusion of one pulmonary artery results in pulmonary hypertension to levels above 30 torr, and this has been correlated with excessive mortality after pneumonectomy. This test is only done in circumstances where there is conflicting information from the other tests of pulmonary function.

Years of experience and numerous studies have shown that there is no data-analysis technique that will absolutely separate the operable patient from the inoperable. Instead, the goal of preoperative evaluation is to separate patients into low- and high-risk groups. Of the standard function tests, surgeons have come to place the greatest reliance on the expiratory flow rates and MVV as the critical determinants of operability for the patient with reduced function from respiratory disease, advanced age, or chronic illness. Mittman reported a 9 percent cardiopulmonary mortality rate in patients with a maximum breathing capacity (MBC—now called the maximal voluntary ventilation) greater than 50 percent of the predicted value. Those patients whose MBC was less than 50 percent had a 45 percent cardiopulmonary mortality rate after thoracotomy. Miller reported similar results for patients who underwent pneumonectomy, with a slightly lower mortality for those who had a lobectomy.

Other studies have failed to support a precise correlation between a given level of reduced pulmonary function and an expected mortality risk. The continuing improvements in facilities and technology for postoperative care have influenced surgeons to become more aggressive in advising thoracotomy for patients with compromised pulmonary function. In a recent report, Peters and associates presented their results with pulmonary resection in a

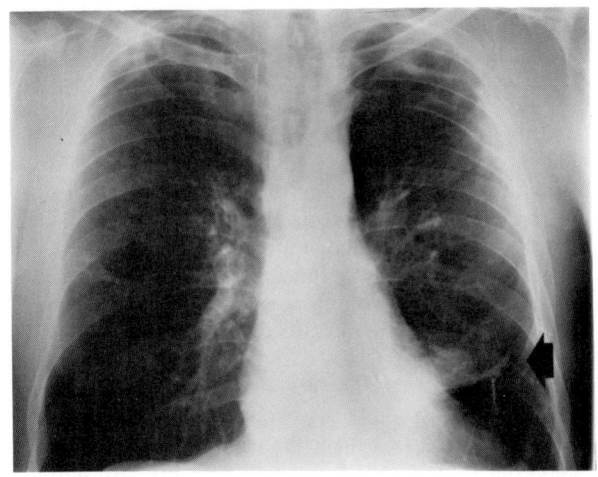

A

Patient - 58 y.o. white male

Spirometry	Measured	Predicted	% Predicted
FEV$_1$	1.72 liters	3.14 liters	55
FVC	2.47	4.37	57
Peak Flow	2.90 liters/s	8.63 liters/s	34
MVV	66.0 liters/min	130.0 liters/min	49

B

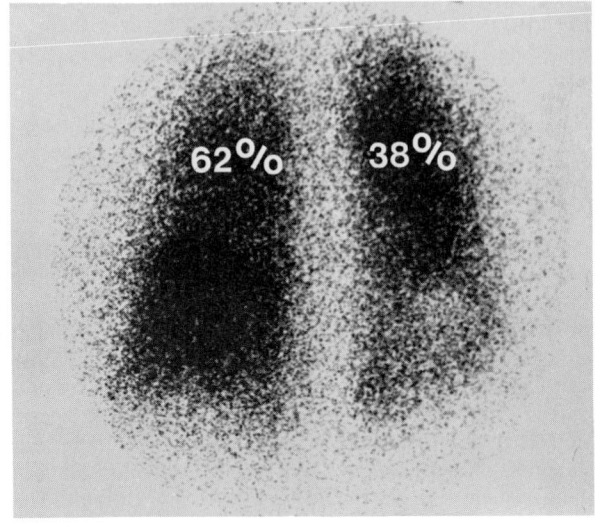

C

Fig. 17-13. An example of the use of radioisotope lung scanning for the prediction of postpneumonectomy pulmonary function. *A.* The P-A chest x-ray of a fifty-eight-year-old man with a recurrent bronchiolo-alveolar cell carcinoma in the left lower lobe. *B.* The results of preoperative spirometry show marked reduction in measured values for expiratory flow rates, vital capacity, and maximum voluntary ventilation. *C.* A lung perfusion scan with macroaggregated radioalbumin shows that approximately 62 percent of pulmonary blood flow is directed to the right lung. Therefore, the predicted values for postoperative vital capacity and FEV$_1$ after left pneumonectomy would be 1.5 and 1.0 L, respectively. These values were marginal but acceptable, and the patient underwent successful pneumonectomy. The actual measured FEV$_1$ 2 weeks after operation was 1.02 L.

group of 22 patients with impaired pulmonary function (FEV_{25-75} less than 1 L/s and FEV_1 less than 70 percent) and recorded only two postoperative deaths. Neither was caused by pulmonary insufficiency. The authors speculated that the low mortality rate was due to the fact that vital capacity was preserved in these patients despite major obstructive disease of the airways. An earlier report by Bryant also suggested a critical relationship between vital capacity and operative results in patients with compromised pulmonary function.

The interest in providing a satisfactory evaluation of the patient before thoracic operation must not obscure the ultimate purpose of the evaluation—to provide the patient with whatever physical and mental preparation is needed. Many patients are smokers, and every effort should be made to persuade them to stop smoking before operation, preferably for 2 weeks or more. All authors agree that the character and amount of bronchial secretions have major impact on postoperative morbidity. Aggressive attention to reducing the amount and tenacity of the secretions must be made before the operation. The etiology of pulmonary infection should be identified and treated intensively, using respiratory therapy, physical therapy, or appropriate techniques. Thoracic operations often are associated with prolonged stays in intensive care units, with multiple chest tubes, with invasive catheters of several types, and with considerable pain. All patients deserve a full explanation of what to expect from the operation, presented in a way that assures them of excellence in their medical care and concern for their well-being.

POSTTHORACOTOMY CONSIDERATIONS (See Also Chapter 12)

PULMONARY FUNCTION CHANGES. Significant pathophysiologic changes in pulmonary function follow major thoracic and abdominal operations. Upper abdominal procedures and thoracic operations produce similar changes in pulmonary function and have similar complications. The magnitude of the changes is affected by preexisting bronchopulmonary disease, length of the operation, postoperative analgesics, and immobilization in bed. Patients without pulmonary disease develop similar changes and are subject to similar complications. The pulmonary changes seen relate to: (1) lung volumes, (2) ventilatory patterns, (3) respiratory gas exchange, and (4) defense mechanisms.

Lung Volume. Total lung capacity and each of its subdivisions are significantly reduced after abdominal or thoracic operations. Vital capacity is reduced by 25 to 50 percent or more, with the maximum reduction occurring during the first 4 days after operation. Similarly, functional residual capacity and expiratory reserve volume are decreased, with a gradual return toward normal beginning in the second week after operation. If a pulmonary resection has been performed, the magnitude of change is even greater and is proportional to the amount of functioning lung that was removed. The reduction in

lung volumes is often accompanied by an increase in the closing volume to potentiate the development of atelectasis.

Ventilatory Pattern. The sedative effect of the anesthetic agent and the postoperative analgesics, combined with the severe pain of the thoracotomy incision, produces sharp reductions in tidal volume after operation. The expected response is an increase in respiratory rate sufficient to maintain minute ventilation. Unfortunately, the parenteral narcotics ordinarily used to manage postoperative pain all depress the respiratory center, inhibiting the rate increase and leading to carbon dioxide retention and hypoxemia.

An equally important effect of the changes in ventilatory pattern is the sharp reduction or elimination of the normal periodic hyperinflations (sighs). Normal adults sigh at the rate of nine or ten times per hour under quiet conditions. With loss of periodic hyperinflations, there is closure of lung units and a reduction in compliance.

Gas Exchange. Decreases in Pa_{O_2} and mild elevations of Pa_{CO_2} are frequent as patients recover from anesthesia. However, Pa_{CO_2} generally returns to normal or below normal in the early postoperative period, while Pa_{O_2} remains depressed during the first week. The factors responsible for reduction in the Pa_{O_2} include abnormal ventilation-perfusion relationships and intrapulmonary shunting associated with closure of terminal lung units.

Pulmonary Defense Mechanisms. The lung is normally protected against inhaled particulate matter and microbes by several mechanisms. The cough reflex defends the upper airways against inhaled or aspirated material in the tracheobronchial tree. Clearance of inhaled particles and microbes from the lower airways is dependent on the mucociliary system, and the alveoli are defended by mucociliary transport, lymphatic drainage, and the alveolar macrophages. Since coughing is inhibited by several mechanisms in the postoperative period, there is significant impairment of that defense mechanism. Ciliary function is decreased, and multiple factors, including arterial hypoxemia, depress the activity of alveolar macrophages. Finally, the composition and physical properties of mucus are altered in a way that reduces the effectiveness of the mucociliary transport system.

COMPLICATIONS. Pulmonary complications of thoracic operations have their origins in these changes and usually begin in the operating room or soon thereafter. The principal pulmonary complications consist of obstructive atelectasis and respiratory infections, and it is possible to consider each of these problems in terms of the complex of factors that contribute to their development.

Atelectasis means closure of lung units, and it exists as microatelectasis, a diffuse sublobular form not visible on chest x-rays, and macroatelectasis, the collapse of a segment, lobe, or entire lung. The three mechanisms that are considered responsible for atelectasis are accentuations of the postoperative pathophysiologic changes described earlier: (1) retained bronchopulmonary secretions, (2) decreased sighing, and (3) decreased expiratory reserve volume.

Retention of secretions is a major cause of atelectasis in

patients with chronic bronchitis. It is more subtle in patients with normal lungs though they also develop either microatelectasis or macroatelectasis. Decreased sighing and reduced tidal volume contribute to the reduced compliance in the postoperative period. Unless reversed by voluntary efforts at deep breathing, induced coughing, or attentive respiratory care techniques, these changes will contribute to the development of both forms of atelectasis. Similarly, the postoperative reductions in lung volumes are related to airway closure that is associated with the changes in ventilatory pattern. The critical relationship may be between the reduced expiratory reserve volume (ERV) and CV. Normally, CV is above residual volume but below the end-tidal point. In the postoperative state with the expected reduction in ERV, the CV may exceed the ERV and be located above the end-tidal point. Under these circumstances, the peripheral airways are subjected to compression and closure during tidal breathing. For some patients the risk of atelectasis is greater because of preexisting abnormalities in ERV and CV. For example, elderly patients and smokers have an increased CV and patients with obstructive airway disease have an increased CV and a decreased ERV. These circumstances potentiate the opportunity for airway closure and significant atelectasis.

Postoperative bronchopulmonary infectious complications consist of tracheobronchitis and pneumonitis. While these complications occur in normal persons, their incidence is higher in patients with preexisting chronic airway disease. Decreased cough, atelectasis, reduced mucociliary clearance of inhaled particles and bacteria, pain, and analgesic drugs all contribute to these infectious complications. Interference with the mucociliary clearance mechanism leads to rapid bacterial proliferation distal to obstruction in an area of atelectasis. Of equal importance has been the demonstration that the respiratory tract becomes colonized with gram-negative bacilli, particularly in the presence of tracheal intubation, coma, hypotension, hypoxia, acidosis, and azotemia. Many of these conditions exist in the postoperative period of patients subjected to major thoracic procedures.

PAIN CONTROL. In the first few postoperative days effective management of incisional pain is of central importance in the maintenance of adequate ventilation. The pain that accompanies the thoracotomy is severe and disabling. Unless well managed, it will cause hypoventilation, retention of secretions, atelectasis, hypoxia, hypoxemia, shallow and ineffective respiratory effort, and pneumonia. It is a constant challenge to find the delicate balance between giving patients enough pain medication so that they are able to cough, without giving them so much that they lose their drive to do so.

In most centers, pain is managed by parenteral narcotics administered intramuscularly or intravenously, on a fixed schedule (by-the-clock) or on-demand (p.r.n.). Particularly when given p.r.n., these techniques are associated with the likelihood of swings in levels from obtundation with respiratory depression and suppression of cough to frightened and agitated patients who hurt too much to move. If parenteral narcotics are to be the primary means

for postthoracotomy pain control, they should probably be given by I.V. drip in a dose carefully regulated by observation to provide adequate continuous pain relief without allowing undue somnolence. Success with this approach requires careful preoperative education of the patient and close nursing care. Nausea and vomiting are frequent side effects.

Some surgeons have reported success with intraoperative intercostal blocks. Either short-acting (lidocaine) or long-acting (bupivacaine) agents can be given but great care must be taken to avoid inadvertent intravascular or subdural injection. Severe vasomotor hypotension has occasionally been reported following this technique, and the patient should be monitored closely whenever it is used. More recently, several investigators have advocated intercostal nerve cryoanalgesia and have reported excellent incisional pain relief by this nerve-freezing approach. Maiwand et al. have reviewed their experience in 600 consecutive cases; the technique is now routine in their unit. Just before the chest is closed, each appropriate nerve receives one 30-s exposure to the probe. While pulmonary function and gas exchange were not uniformly improved over that expected from more conventional management, patients were more comfortable and active, and analgesic medication usage was reduced.

In the mid-1970s opiate receptors were identified in the spinal cord and their specific mediators, endorphins and enkephalin, were characterized. Since that time, active investigation on both sides of the Atlantic has resulted in many highly encouraging reports advocating the use of continuous epidural infusion of preservative-free morphine in doses near 0.1 mg/h. The narcotics can be administered through either a thoracic or a lumbar epidural catheter. While early reports suggested that the obviously more comfortable patients had improved postoperative ventilation characteristics, in a recent controlled, comparative study, Larsen and his group failed to confirm that expectation. Analog pain scores were ordinarily greatly improved, but the profound postoperative decrease in the forced vital capacity and other pulmonary function parameters and the drop in arterial oxygen tension occurred equally in all groups.

Advances in anesthesia techniques, particularly improvements in the design of the various double-lumen endotracheal tubes used with or without high-frequency jet ventilation, have offered the surgeon new options for reducing postthoracotomy pain. The need for wide exposure for delicate hilar dissection was clear when the dissection was carried out around a retracted but filled, moving lung. The ability to work in the chest with a fully deflated lung is encouraging surgeons to seek less traumatic means for entry into the chest. Urschel has reported a large series of lobar resections in both chest cavities through a median sternotomy. The extensive experience with this incision in the open-heart surgery population has demonstrated that it is much less painful and much better tolerated physiologically. Others have worked to improve the straight lateral, or modified axillary incision to allow major resections without the necessity of dividing the muscles to the shoulder girdle. In that

TENSION PNEUMOTHORAX. When an injury to the lung parenchyma has occurred that allows air to enter the pleural space with each respiratory effort, and when the flap-valve effect of the injury prevents that air from reentering the bronchial tree for egress through the trachea during expiration, tension develops within the pleural space until equilibration with the negative pressures the patient is able to generate is reached; at that time effective ventilation ceases and venous blood can no longer enter the chest. The mechanics of a developing tension pneumothorax may not be obvious when the patient is first seen. Pain may be the primary complaint, with no evidence of respiratory distress. But if the lung wound is behaving as a check valve, some air will escape into the pleural cavity with each inspiration or with each cough. Gradually, intrapleural pressure will build up, the lung collapses, and tension pneumothorax may develop. A shift of the mediastinum and compression of the large veins result in a decreased cardiac output that may lead to sudden death.

The diagnosis should be instantly made by the observation of a patient with dilated neck veins making respiratory effort but not respiratory motions, and unable to move air. It is immediately confirmed by the hyperresonant percussion note over the injured hemithorax and absent or distant breath sounds. The immediate release of the tension by placement of a large-bore needle followed immediately by insertion of a thoracostomy tube is lifesaving.

OPEN PNEUMOTHORAX. The sucking chest wound is one in which a segment of the chest wall has been destroyed such that negative intrapleural pressure sucks air directly through the chest wall defect rather than through the trachea into the alveoli. Whenever the cross-sectional area of the defect exceeds that of the trachea, the undesirable preferential air movement takes place. It occurs most commonly after shotgun blasts, explosions with flying debris, or impalement injuries. It may or may not be associated with underlying parenchymal damage.

The diagnosis can be made by noting a patient with normal or collapsed neck veins who is making respiratory motions but not moving air. Confirmation is immediate on inspection of the patient's chest and observation of the wound. The patient is stabilized by any mechanical covering over the open wound. As soon as convenient, a watertight dressing should be placed and an intercostal catheter inserted into the pleural cavity. Early debridement and closure of the wound should then be scheduled.

MASSIVE FLAIL CHEST. Whenever severe blunt injury results in two-point fractures of four or more ribs, a large segment of the chest wall becomes flail. On inspiratory effort, the negative pressure in the chest pulls the unstable segment of the wall inward in a paradoxical motion. The patient may be unable to develop sufficient intratracheal negative pressure to maintain adequate ventilation, and atelectasis, hypoxia, and hypercapnia occur. A patient who is conscious may splint the segment sufficiently to make it inapparent to cursory examination, but the continuing extra effort in the attempt to move air soon leads to tiring and may result in sudden respiratory de-

compensation. The progressing failure is aggravated by the developing pulmonary contusion that accompanies blunt trauma sufficient to break that many ribs. In the unconscious patient, the lesion may be less dangerous, because it is more readily recognized and more apt to be treated early.

In the massive flail chest, the diagnosis may be difficult unless the chest wall is visualized during the respiratory effort. If unconscious, the patient is ordinarily making vigorous respiratory motions, but moving little air; the paradoxical segment should be obvious. The patient who is awake may exhibit a very rapid shallow breathing pattern at or above 40 breaths per minute. Other aspects of the management of lesser flail injuries are discussed below, but when massive flail is diagnosed, endotracheal intubation and positive-pressure controlled ventilation is mandatory.

MASSIVE HEMOTHORAX. When 1500 mL or more of blood is acutely removed from the pleural space as a thoracostomy tube is placed, Rene has shown that urgent thoracotomy will find a surgically correctable lesion in a high proportion of the cases. If a patient with penetrating injury or multiple rib fractures is found to have a complete hemithorax dull to percussion in association with hypotension, a chest tube should be inserted. If massive hemothorax is found, the patient should be taken directly to the operating room as blood volume resuscitation is taking place.

Conditions Requiring Urgent Thoracotomy

CONTINUED INTRAPLEURAL BLEEDING. If bleeding continues from a thoracostomy tube after initial placement at a rate exceeding 100 mL/h for 6 h or more, most surgeons would now agree that a surgically correctable lesion is present. Ordinarily it will be a bleeding intercostal vessel, since bleeding from the lower-pressure pulmonary system will almost always stop when the lung is reexpanded after the pleural space is evacuated. The rate and pattern of bleeding are more important than the amount in deciding to explore.

MASSIVE AIR LEAK. This is an increasingly commonly recognized injury resulting from steering wheel compression of the trachea against the vertebral bodies following high-speed head-on collisions. Complete disruption of the trachea or a major bronchus may occur. The injury is often fatal but may be surprisingly well tolerated for a brief period. All levels of the trachea and all major bronchi have been involved; however, greater than 80 percent of these injuries are within 2.5 cm of the carina. Patients with intrathoracic tracheal or central bronchial disruption may exhibit a variety of signs and symptoms depending on whether there is free communication between the site of injury and the pleural cavity. A particularly important diagnostic finding is complete unilateral atelectasis in the face of a large air leak, or the symmetrical downward displacement of the bilateral hila. Distal injuries often result in pneumothorax, which is manageable by tube thoracostomy alone since the air leak is small. Lazar and King have reported a case in which a complete tracheal disruption just above the carina with 6 cm of discontinuity was tolerated in a young athlete for 24 h before accurate diagnosis and repair. Extreme care must be taken in the evaluation of patients with massive air leaks, since overly aggressive diagnostic bronchoscopy or endotracheal intubation and positive-pressure ventilation before accurate location of the defect and careful operative preparation for approaching it have been made could result in rapid death. Occasionally, as in other tracheobronchial injuries discussed below, an injury may seal itself off and fail to be recognized until severe stenosis develops.

OTHER INDICATIONS. Several other important causes are listed here, but discussed elsewhere.

Acute or rapidly recurring pericardial tamponade
Acute heart failure secondary to valve or septal injury
Widened or widening mediastinum
Perforation of the intrathoracic esophagus

Dangerous but Less Compelling Injuries

DIAPHRAGM RUPTURE. Urgent repair of massive diaphragmatic rupture is sometimes necessary if high-volume herniation of abdominal contents into the chest prevents adequate ventilation. Ordinarily, however, the acute problems associated with diaphragm rupture are related to the associated injuries to abdominal viscera resulting from the force necessary to rupture the diaphragm. Penetrating trauma to the lower chest or upper abdomen and crush injuries, most often secondary to automobile accidents, are the usual causes of traumatic rupture of the diaphragm. The left hemidiaphragm is ruptured more frequently by blunt trauma than the right, the ratio being about 9:1. The right hemidiaphragm is said to be protected by two mechanisms: the liver on the right and the heart in the center have a buffering effect that diffuses the sudden increase in intraabdominal pressure; and cadaver studies have shown an inherent weakness in the posterior lateral aspect of the left diaphragm. When rupture of the right side does occur, the liver is usually the only abdominal structure that herniates into the chest early, though gradual aspiration of the stomach into the right chest through the diaphragmatic defect can occur over time. With rupture of the left hemidiaphragm, the stomach, spleen, left transverse colon, and omentum in any combination may enter the left pleural cavity. When the diagnosis is delayed for several days or longer, there is often a progressive displacement of the abdominal viscera into the chest or progressive gaseous distention of the herniated stomach. The latter may occur despite an indwelling nasogastric tube, and it may precipitate respiratory distress (Fig. 17-15).

Patients with diaphragmatic rupture due to blunt trauma usually have associated injuries that demand first attention and prevent a detailed initial evaluation. The first chest x-ray after rupture of either hemidiaphragm may show nothing more than a blurring of the diaphragm with or without evidence of a small hemothorax. In some patients the diagnosis is made very early because the nasogastric tube is seen to lie within the confines of the left pleural cavity. Injection of air through the nasogastric

tube during auscultation of the left side of the chest may add support to the diagnosis.

Penetrating diaphragmatic injuries rarely produce early symptoms except those related to other structures that may be injured. After several months or years, gastrointestinal obstruction may develop and lead to strangulation of herniated viscera. The hole in the diaphragm is small, and herniation occurs slowly. Early transabdominal operation is indicated when the diagnosis is confirmed, and associated intraabdominal injuries may be repaired at the same time. The wound in the hemidiaphragm may vary from a simple radial tear to an extensive and complex laceration. Repair can usually be accomplished by direct suture, but a prosthetic patch is occasionally required. If the diagnosis is delayed, a transthoracic approach may be preferred. It provides better exposure to (1) reduce the hernia, (2) free adhesions between the abdominal viscera and intrathoracic structures, and (3) repair the defect in the diaphragm.

PNEUMOTHORAX. Pneumothorax is usually the result of injury to the lung or the tracheobronchial tree. Esophageal perforation may be followed by a pneumomediastinum that ruptures into the pleural cavity. Whether the pneumothorax is associated with blunt injury and fractured ribs or is due to a penetrating wound, there is a variable amount of bleeding into the pleural cavity. The decision to use the term hemopneumothorax depends on the amount of blood in the pleural cavity and the likely consequences. If sufficient blood is present to require a concerted effort to assure its removal, or if its loss from the circulating volume requires transfusion replacement, it seems proper to use the double term.

Pneumothorax varies from that which is so slight that it may be missed on the initial x-ray examination to a massive, continuing air leak that displaces the mediastinum, depresses the diaphragm, and compresses the opposite lung, the tension pneumothorax discussed previously (Fig. 17-16). A pneumothorax due to a parenchymal lung injury tends to be self-limited because the developing lung collapse combines with blood clotting in the wound for a sealing effect. For some patients extensive adhesions already present between the visceral and parietal pleura may localize the pleural air and prevent a collapse of the lung (Fig. 17-17).

With any chest injury it is wisest to presume that a pneumothorax is present until proved otherwise. Because of pain and limited chest motion on the injured side, physical examination may be inadequate for diagnosis of a minimal pneumothorax. Since attention may be diverted to the management of other injuries, and because of the risks of tension developing should a general anesthetic with positive-pressure ventilation be given, prophylactic thoracostomy catheters should usually be placed whenever there is significant chest injury. The catheter is usually best placed in the lateral axillary line, just above the fifth rib, after finger exploration has induced a temporary pneumothorax or otherwise assured the pleural space to be free at the site of insertion.

Treatment of the more usual pneumothorax depends on symptoms of respiratory insufficiency, the extent of the

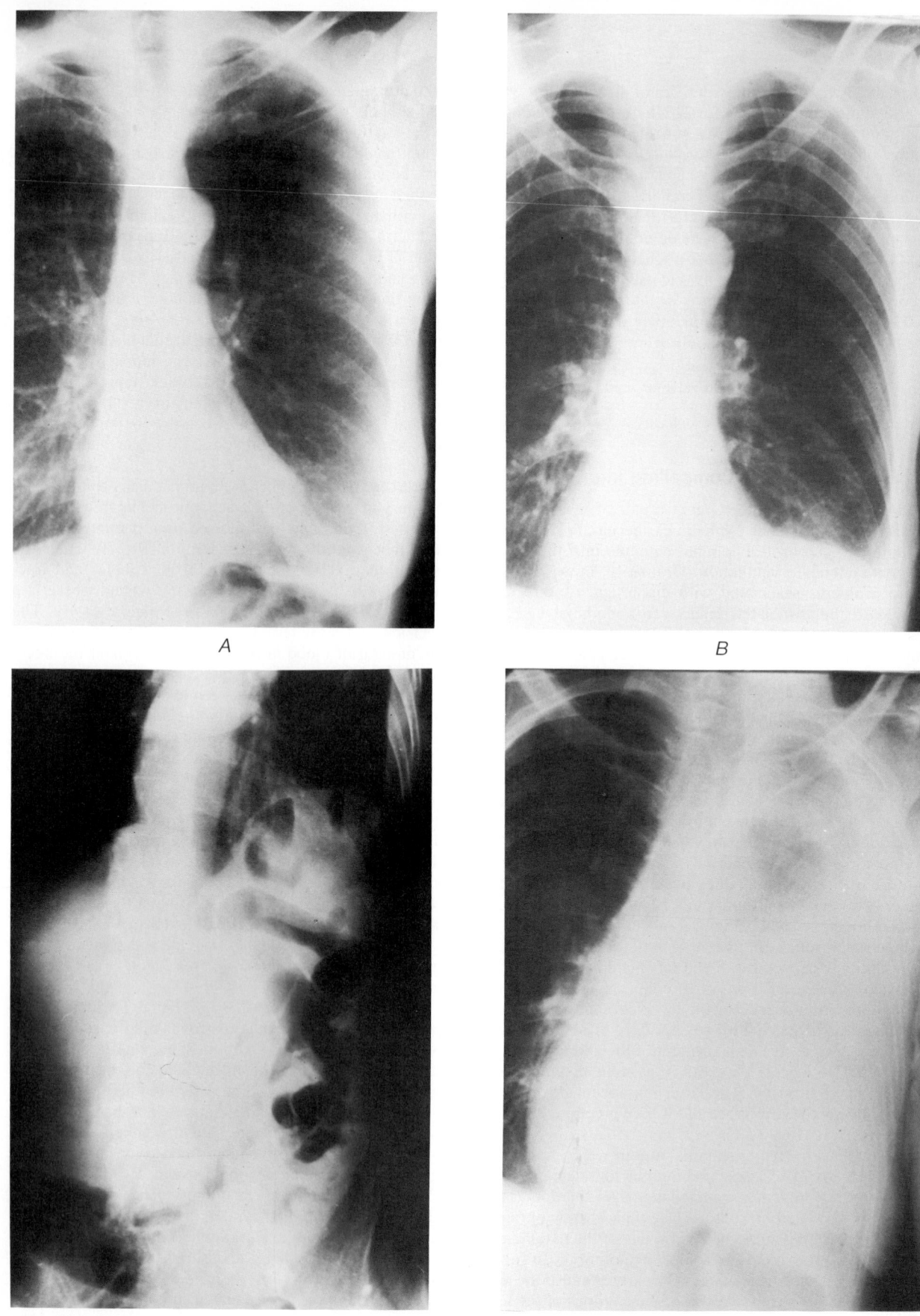

A

B

C

D

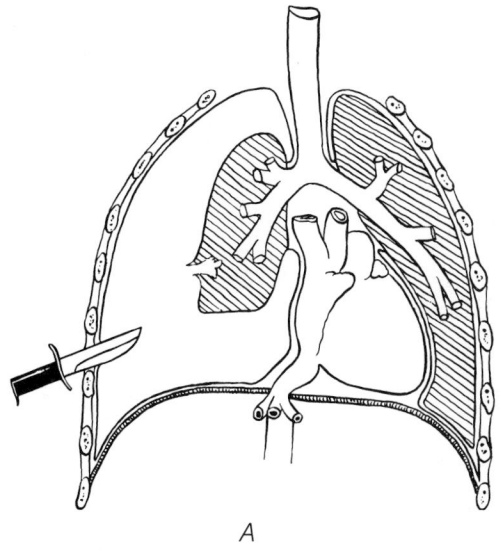

A

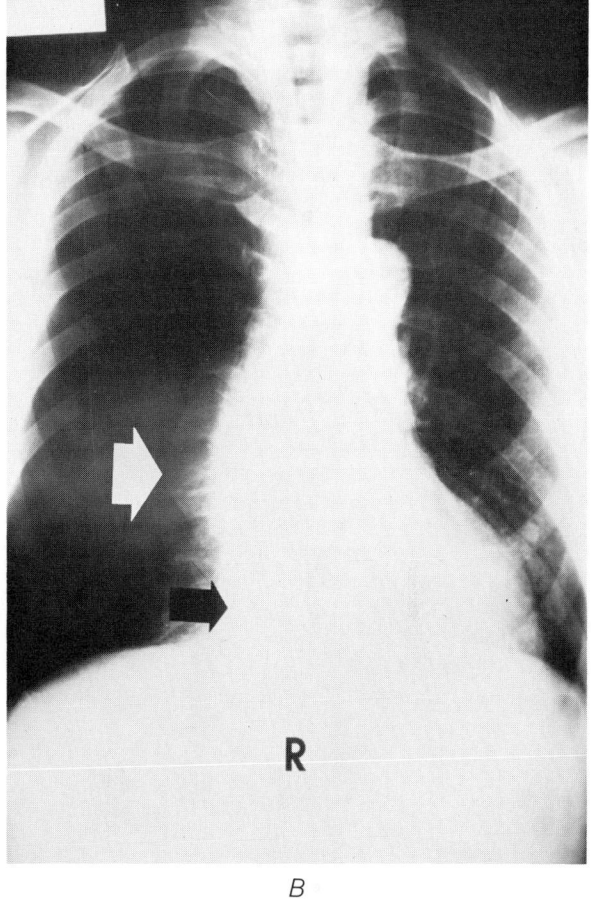

B

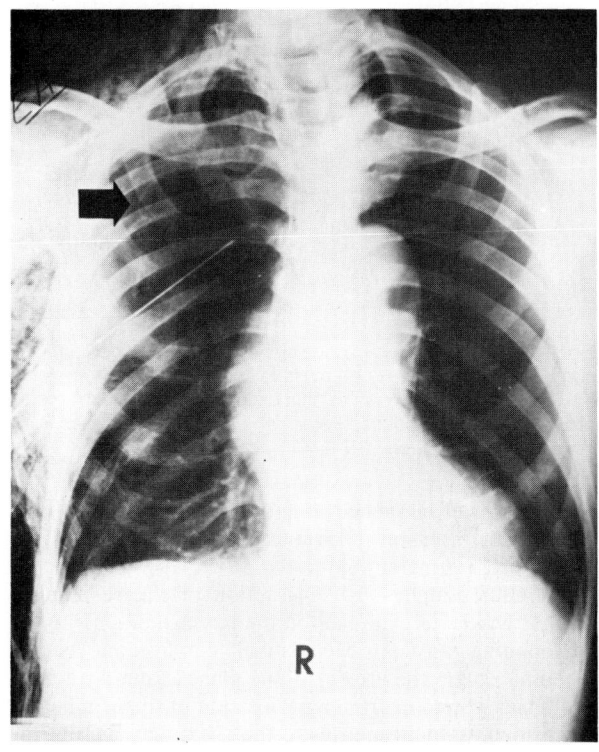

C

Fig. 17-16. *A.* In a tension pneumothorax there is compression of the contralateral lung and a displacement of the mediastinum that may sharply reduce venous return to the atria. *B.* If the diagnosis is strongly suspected, needle aspiration of the pleural space should be done without waiting for the chest x-ray. In this patient, the tension pneumothorax developed slowly and became symptomatic shortly after this film was taken. The lower arrow points to the displacement of the right heart border, and the lung is completely collapsed *(upper arrow)*. *C.* Following needle aspiration a large intercostal tube was put in place, but a major air leak continued for several days and eventually required insertion of an additional chest catheter. The arrow points to the visceral pleura, showing incomplete expansion of the lung.

Fig. 17-15. *A–D.* Traumatic rupture of the diaphragm can present rapidly progressive and life-threatening complications early or late after injury. The patient whose films are pictured here developed increasing herniation of abdominal contents into the left chest over a 3-day period before findings led to urgent thoracotomy for removal of infarcted small intestine. *(Courtesy of Dr. John H.M. Austin.)*

pneumothorax, and the presence of significant hemothorax. There is a tendency to think of pneumothorax in terms of a two-dimensional concept that is conveyed by the anteroposterior chest x-ray. Instead, the hemithorax must be considered a modified cone, and when the lung surface is separated from the chest wall by 3 cm or more, the patient may have a 50 percent lung collapse (by volume) rather than the 25 or 30 percent collapse that the chest x-ray suggests. With a pneumothorax that is less

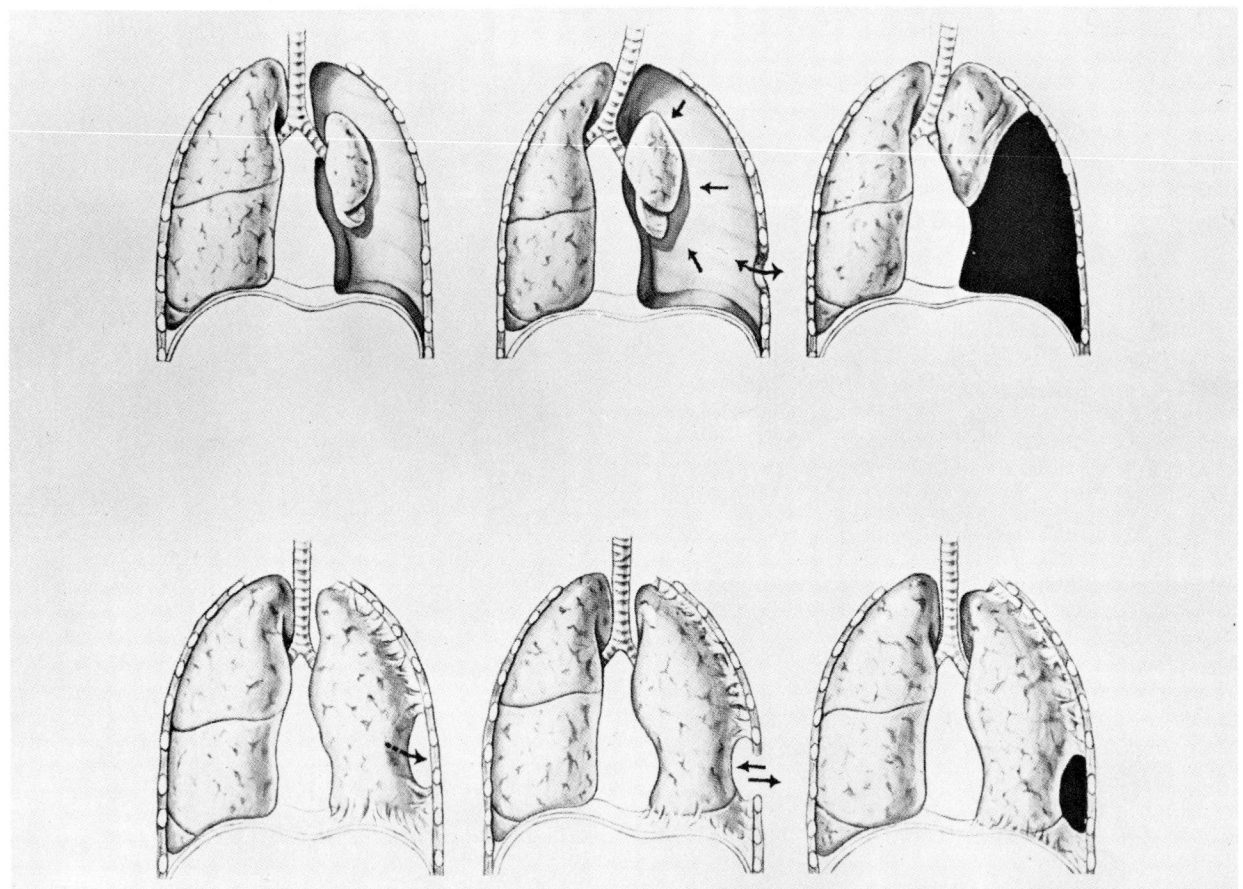

Fig. 17-17. A free pleural space will allow the development of a complete pneumothorax or a massive hemothorax. These potentially fatal complications cannot occur in patients with an obliterated pleural space. (Reproduced from: *Naciero EA: Chest Injuries. New York, Grune & Stratton, 1971, with permission.*)

than this amount, due to a nonpenetrating injury (theoretically, no contamination of the pleural space), and not accompanied by significant blood or fluid in the pleural cavity, treatment may not be required. A decision not to remove the pleural air implies that the patient has had a simple injury and that conditions for observation are ideal. Approximately 1.25 percent of the air will be absorbed each day, with full expansion expected in 3 to 6 weeks.

Aspiration of the air with a needle and insertion of an intercostal catheter only if lung collapse recurs is a reasonable method of treatment advocated by some physicians even when the pneumothorax amounts to as much as 50 percent. In all cases with greater than 50 percent collapse, in those with hemopneumothorax, and in patients whose pneumothorax is the result of penetrating trauma, an intercostal catheter should be inserted and attached to a water seal with 10 to 25 cmH$_2$O negative pressure. In the majority of patients, lung reexpansion and cessation of the air leak will occur within a few hours or a few days. If not, a major bronchial injury may be present, and a thoracotomy may be required after appropriate diagnostic procedures.

The use of prophylactic systemic antibiotics in patients with chest trauma is a subject of current debate, but their use in cases of nonpenetrating trauma seems unjustified. The simple insertion of an intercostal catheter does not justify prescribing antibiotics.

Interstitial Emphysema. Disruption of the respiratory tract at any level will result in the passage of air into the surrounding tissues. Mediastinal emphysema occurs when air enters the areolar tissue planes from a tracheobronchial wound or from a perforation of the esophagus. Occasionally, blunt injuries to the chest may disrupt the integrity of a group of bronchioles or alveolar units without disrupting the visceral pleura. As air escapes into the pulmonary interstitium, it dissects centrally along the bronchi and pulmonary vessels to reach the mediastinum. When the mediastinal pleura remains intact, progressive loss of air into the tissue carries the dissection into the neck, where the air escapes the deep tissue planes and spreads in the subcutaneous tissue. The development of subcutaneous emphysema may cause marked distortion of the patient's appearance, but there is no reason to ''treat'' the condition, except to take whatever steps are appropriate to stop the air leak. The source of the leak must be found, since some potential causes (esophageal perforation or major bronchial injury) require early intervention.

RIB FRACTURES AND LESSER FLAIL INJURIES. The most common injury of the chest is a fracture of one or more ribs, including fracture at the costochondral junction ("separation"). Children seem less liable to rib fractures, but chest x-rays are made less frequently in those young age groups with minor trauma. Fractures occur most commonly in the middle and lower ribs with blunt trama, but the distribution with penetrating wounds varies with the distribution of the penetrating objects.

First Rib Fractures. First rib fractures have historically been associated with high probability of associated upper rib fractures and major vessel injuries. Recent reports by many authors, however, have demonstrated isolated first rib fractures without other significant injuries in the thoracic outlet in a wide variety of patients. Because of the relative high frequency in association with cranial and maxillofacial injuries, and in the "surfer's" rib (an injury occurring in surfers performing the so-called lay-back maneuver), it seems probable that isolated first rib injuries are secondary to avulsion of the first rib by its muscular attachments rather than direct trauma to the relatively protected first rib. There is inconclusive evidence that a direct relationship exists between first and second rib fractures and trauma to major vessels at the apex of the hemithorax (Fig. 17-18). Lazroni et al. recommend arteriography in stable patients with first rib fracture who have (1) absent or decreased upper extremity pulses, (2) hemorrhage, especially large extrapleural hematoma or hemothorax, and (3) brachial plexus injury. Additional criteria for angiography include displacement of fragments and multiple thoracic injuries.

Multiple Fractures. The problem of massive flail chest has been briefly discussed previously. Lesser degrees of flail occur whenever there are multiple fractures of the chest wall skeletal structure. Flail chest is appropriately diagnosed whenever there is paradoxical respiratory movement in a segment of the chest wall. This generally requires at least two segmental fractures in each of three adjacent ribs or costal cartilages or other multiple combinations of rib or sternal fractures with costochrondral or chondrosternal separations. Posterior flail segments, in the absence of disrupted intrathoracic structures, are easier to manage because of the strong muscular and scapular support, and because of patients' natural tendency to lie with their backs against the mattress.

Chest wall stabilization and reduction of respiratory dead space are major goals of treatment. Improvements in respiratory therapy, including bedside measurements of pulmonary mechanics and the widespread availability of arterial blood-gas determinations, have allowed greater individualization in the treatment of patients with flail-chest injuries. For many years endotracheal intubation or early tracheostomy has been recommended for the management of patients with flail chest, because it allows easy access for tracheobronchial suctioning, it reduces dead space, and it facilitates internal stabilization of the chest wall through mechanical ventilation. Intubation is often delayed now until evidence of a need for ventilatory

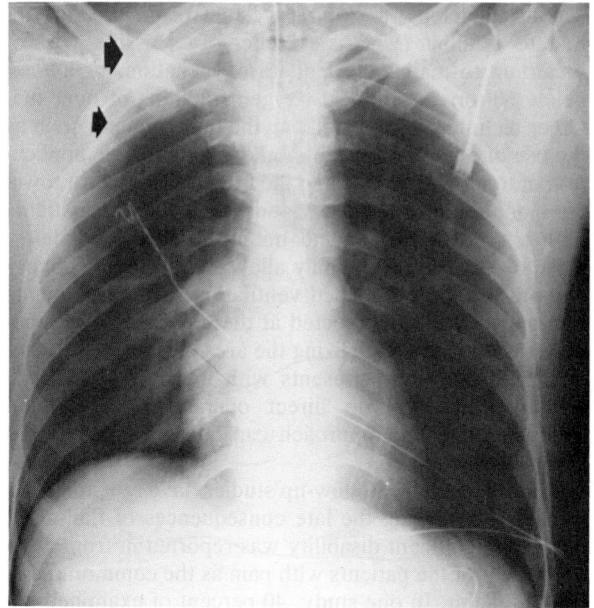

A

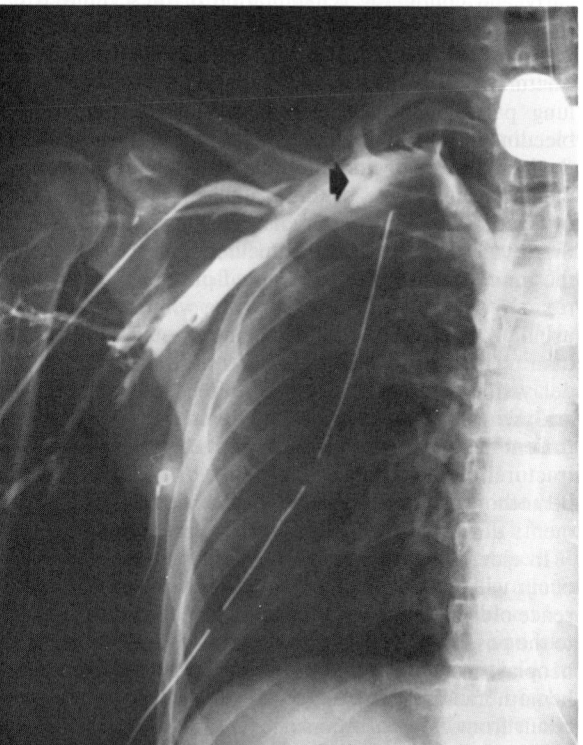

B

Fig. 17-18. *A.* The first chest x-ray of a twenty-five-year-old man who was injured in a motorcycle accident shows a fracture of the right first rib (upper arrow) and a small extrapleural hematoma at the right apex (lower arrow). *B.* A subclavian arteriogram and venogram were done 3 days after admission because of the sudden development of a massive hemothorax (2000 mL blood) on the right side. Bleeding stopped spontaneously, and the venogram shows a tear in the subclavian vein at the rib fracture site.

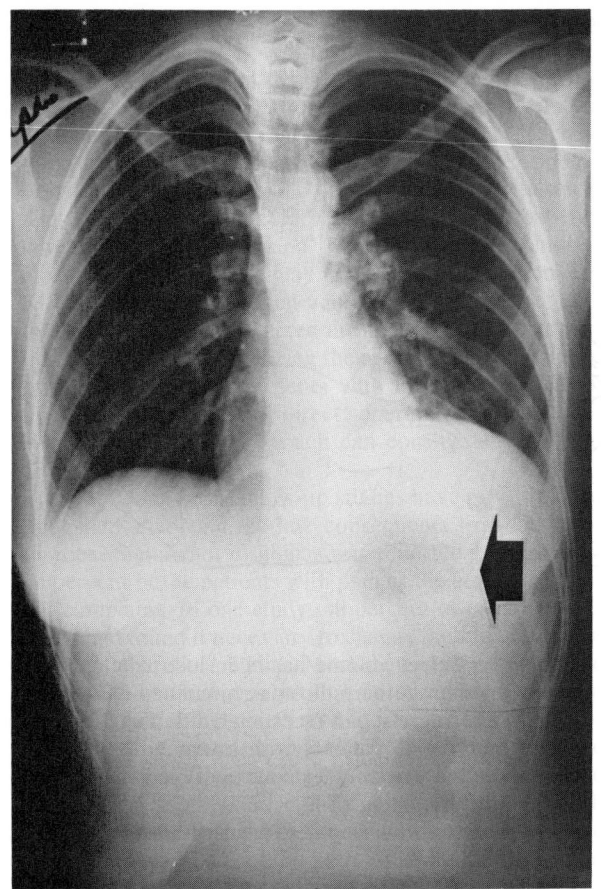

A

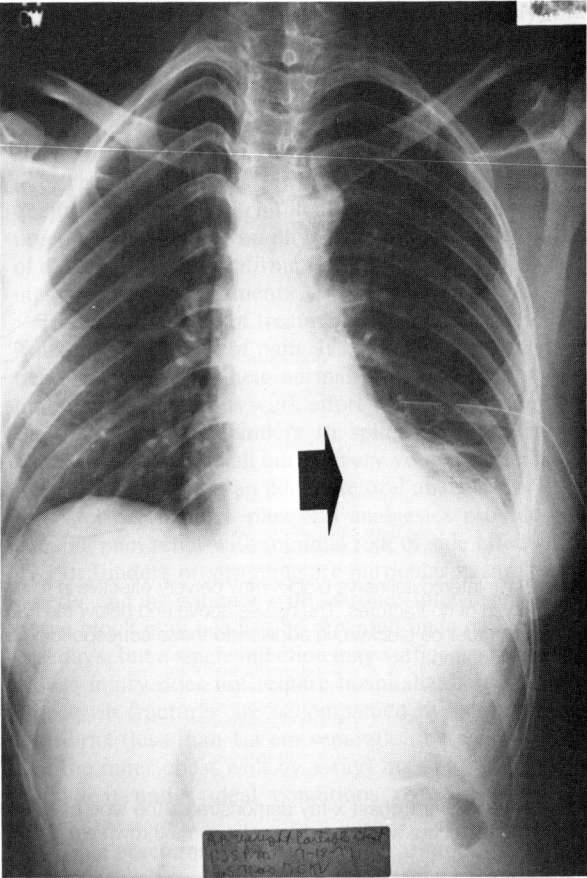

C

B

Fig. 17-21. Traumatic hemothorax due to a stab wound of the left chest in a thirty-two-year-old woman. *A*. The first chest x-ray suggests an elevation of the left diaphragm, and the emergency-room physician did not suspect a hemothorax. The surgical consultant was suspicious of subpulmonary trapping of a hemothorax because of the distance between the top of the apparent diaphragm and the gastric air bubble *(arrow)*. *B*. A lateral decubitis x-ray shows a large collection of blood in the left hemithorax. *C*. Insertion of an intercostal tube resulted in drainage of 600 mL of blood. However, the chest x-ray suggests the presence of residual blood and clots in the pleural cavity *(arrow)*.

not require initial treatment; follow-up x-rays at appropriate intervals will assist with the decision to drain the pleural cavity if there is a progressive accumulation. When the hemothorax exceeds an amount that fills the costophrenic sulcus, or when there is associated pneumothorax, one or more large catheters should be placed in the pleural cavity through the seventh, eighth, or ninth intercostal space in the posterior-axillary line. Underwater drainage alone may be sufficient, but low suction applied to the catheters is often helpful when combined with active efforts at stripping the tubes of blood clot. If the initial drainage of blood is followed by continued bleeding in the absence of a clotting defect, a decision to operate must be made, with a broad consideration of the possible sources of the bleeding.

With a major hemothorax the success of tube drainage is often frustrated by extensive clot that obstructs the tubes. An attitude should be adopted that a nonfunctioning chest tube represents a liability to the patient because of discomfort and the risk of carrying infection from the skin wound into the pleural clot. Especially with penetrating trauma, a hemothorax that fails to drain adequately through intercostal catheters may develop into empyema. An additional hazard is the organization of residual clot to form a fibrothorax. Coselli and his colleagues in Houston have recently reviewed their experience with clotted hemothorax and have found early thoracotomy substantially reduces hospitalization time and empyema rates.

TRACHEOBRONCHIAL INJURY. The management of massive tracheobronchial injuries is discussed above. For small penetrating injuries of the intrathoracic trachea and major bronchi, tracheostomy and effective pleural decompression may provide satisfactory definitive treatment. Those injuries which are associated with an actual defect in the tracheobronchial wall, including partial disruption, require operative exploration and repair. Tracheostomy may be necessary to prevent high intratracheal pressures and to allow tracheal care postoperatively, but positive-pressure assisted ventilation should be avoided.

Penetrating injuries of lobar or segmental bronchi may produce a similar clinical picture to proximal tracheobronchial injuries. Bilateral pneumothorax is rare, and the principal immediate problem is to begin management of the major air leak and confirm the presence of a major bronchial injury. The bronchial air leak often stops soon after an intercostal catheter is put in place. The definitive diagnosis may be delayed if the bronchus becomes obstructed by blood clot or mucus and the air leak ceases. Under these conditions the pulmonary lobe or segment becomes atelectatic and resists conservative methods to produce reexpansion. If infection does not occur, the injured bronchus may heal with significant distortion and obstruction, or the atelectasis may persist and lead subsequently to a correct diagnosis. Operative repair of the disrupted bronchus can be achieved even years after injury. If infection occurs at the site of the bronchial injury, the patient may develop pneumonia, distal bronchiectasis, and empyema. Resection of the bronchus and the involved pulmonary lobe is then required.

PULMONARY INJURY. The lungs have a remarkable ability to tolerate penetrating injuries and blunt trauma without long-term residual effects. Civilian gunshot wounds of the chest penetrate a lung more frequently than any other structure, but the majority of patients with no other significant injury can be treated without a thoracotomy. Any penetrating object produces an air leak with a variable degree of pneumothorax. The disruption of tissue along the missile track causes bleeding, which usually ceases as the damaged parenchyma becomes swollen and filled with blood clot. With small-caliber and low-velocity bullet wounds that pass through the lung periphery, the amount of tissue damage produced may be sufficiently small that late follow-up chest x-rays fail to demonstrate the area of injury. With high-velocity bullets, the tissue destruction extends more widely, and even a peripheral bullet pathway may result in irreversible damage to a lobar or lung hilus.

The immediate management of the patient with a penetrating injury is the insertion of at least one intercostal catheter for evacuation of the associated hemopneumothorax. Serial arterial blood gases and frequent evaluation of the patient's ventilatory ability allow an overall estimate of the effect of the injury on respiratory exchange. Civilian penetrating wounds rarely require ventilatory assistance. Only rarely is there a need for thoracotomy to control bleeding or to perform pulmonary resection for an irreversibly injured lung.

PULMONARY CONTUSION. Pulmonary contusion is the consequence of blunt trauma to the lung. The frequent causes of contusion include rapid deceleration of the chest against an automobile steering wheel, falls from a height, and blast injuries. Particularly in young persons, severe pulmonary contusion can occur by transmission of force through the chest wall with minimal fractures of the ribs or sternum. In middle-aged or elderly persons significant pulmonary contusion is usually accompanied by multiple fractures of the thoracic cage.

The contused lung is characterized by capillary disruption that results in intraalveolar and interstitial hemorrhage, edema, protein and fluid obstruction of small airways, and leukocyte infiltration. Serial chest x-rays begun right after injury show a fluffy infiltrate that progresses in extent and in density over a period of 24 to 48 h. Although the maximum lung injury is directly related to that region of the chest wall that receives the trauma, a "countrecoup" effect may be responsible for a wider distribution of the pulmonary damage. Unless the contusion involves only a small region of one lung, it may result in serious loss of respiratory function. The associated injury to the chest wall is aggravated by the loss of pulmonary compliance, increasing the work of breathing. Small areas of atelectasis become confluent, and progressive hypoxia further diminishes the patient's ability to compensate for the loss of function.

Pulmonary contusion is often part of a major chest injury that includes one or more fractures of the thoracic cage, pneumothorax, and hemothorax. If not present initially, a pneumothorax may subsequently develop from actual disruption of the contused pulmonary parenchyma.

Although it is infrequent in patients who survive to reach the hospital, a major pulmonary laceration may represent the maximum extent of pulmonary contusion. In some instances the tissue disruption is the result of extensive penetration by rib fragments, but in others the causative factor is probably a severe shearing force. The clinical and x-ray findings suggest a serious chest injury but do not differentiate the patient with a major lung laceration from those with pulmonary contusion and associated hemopneumothorax. Continued or uncontrolled hemorrhage and massive air leak generally mandate an early thoracotomy. A major pulmonary resection is often necessary, and the mortality rate is high.

Treatment of pulmonary contusion must include an accurate clinical assessment of the patient's respiratory exchange and careful monitoring by serial measurements of the arterial blood gases. Steroids probably have no role in the management of pulmonary contusion.

A high percentage of patients require temporary assisted ventilation, and it may be evident at the time of admission that endotracheal or nasotracheal intubation should be performed. Without question, aggressive respiratory therapy, including ventilatory support, should be initiated before cardiopulmonary decompensation requires treatment measures that add additional risks. Criteria for instituting assisted ventilation are shown in Table 17-4. For most patients the need for assisted ventilation does not extend beyond 48 to 72 h unless there is major injury to the chest wall or to other body regions.

POSTTRAUMATIC PULMONARY INSUFFICIENCY. The development of acute respiratory failure can be expected in a high percentage of patients who suffer major thoracic trauma. Preexisting pulmonary status will influence the severity of respiratory insufficiency, and the extent of actual pulmonary damage will determine whether the patient survives. An initial evaluation of respiratory exchange and ventilatory ability, confirmed by measurement of pulmonary mechanics and arterial blood gases, should be followed by serial reevaluations.

Especially in patients who have suffered multiple trauma, a respiratory-distress syndrome may develop that is out of proportion to the extent of thoracic injury. A series of terms has evolved over the years to designate several forms of respiratory insufficiency that follow trauma and may be associated with a constellation of causative factors. Such terms as "wet lung," "shock lung," "congestive atelectasis," and "adult respiratory-distress syndrome" reflect some principal features that seemed to be characteristic of the cases that came to the attention of those who coined the terms. There is certainly some overlap in the causation of the several forms of respiratory failure that follow major trauma, and it is important to determine the specific causes in individual patients. Blaisdell and Lewis have presented a thorough discussion of posttraumatic pulmonary insufficiency, choosing the term respiratory-distress syndrome of shock and trauma for those cases not due to a specific cause. They suggest that eight different explanations for respiratory failure other than the respiratory-distress syndrome occur with reasonable frequency in patients who suffer major injury. These include aspiration, simple atelectasis, lung contusion, fat embolism, pneumonia, pneumothorax, pulmonary edema, and pulmonary embolism.

On the basis of their experience with a large number of cases, Blaisdell and Lewis have concluded that the respiratory-distress syndrome (RDS) is one and the same as the fat-embolism syndrome. Originally thought to result from fat embolism from fracture of long bones, the syndrome consists of pulmonary, neurologic, and systemic manifestations. The pulmonary manifestations appear first, generally within 24 to 36 h after injury, and consist of dyspnea, tachycardia, fever, and cyanosis. Documentation that much of the fat that appears in the blood following injury represents a mobilization of free fatty acids from body neutral fat as a result of shock and increased levels of catecholamines has helped in understanding the mechanism of this condition. Because some degree of intravascular coagulation can be demonstrated in all cases, this is almost certainly a factor in development of the syndrome.

For patients who suffer major chest injury it may be impossible to define what part of their respiratory failure is a result of direct trauma and how much is a consequence of the RDS. Treatment must be based on correction of the direct results of injury and on the anticipation or early recognition of respiratory insufficiency. The radiologic changes of RDS, consisting of diffuse lung infiltrates that progress to become confluent, may be super-

Table 17-4. CRITERIA FOR ASSISTED VENTILATION

Function	Normal values	Ventilate
Pulmonary mechanics:		
Respiratory rate	12–20	>35
Vital capacity, mL/kg	65–75	<15
Maximum inspiratory force, cmH$_2$O		
(negative values)	75–100	<25–35
Gas exchange		
Pa_{O_2}, torr	76–100 (room air)	<65–70 (added oxygen)
Alveolar-arterial oxygen difference, torr		
(100% oxygen)	30–70	>350
Pa_{CO_2}, torr	35–45	>50
Dead space/tidal volume ratio	0.25–0.40	>0.6

imposed on the effects of pulmonary contusion and atelectasis. Changes observed on serial chest x-rays lag behind the changes in pulmonary function, and a patient may be in critical respiratory failure before the films suggest a progressive pulmonary lesion.

Management of the RDS requires maintenance of good cardiovascular function and prompt institution of ventilatory support. An adequate volume replacement for external fluid and blood losses is complicated by the internal fluid losses due to increased capillary permeability in the lung, in all areas of direct tissue trauma, and to a varying degree throughout the body. Monitoring central venous pressures is the minimum for guidance of fluid and diuretic therapy in these patients, but placement of a Swan–Ganz catheter to allow left atrial and pulmonary artery pressures is superior. The need for inotropic myocardial support can be detected earlier by this access to left-sided heart pressures.

Ventilatory support techniques have advanced to allow a wider selection of ventilators and methods of assisted respiration. Attention to detail can offer the patient a maximum chance of survival with a minimum risk of complications. An unanswered question is the place of steroid therapy. The experience with these agents has been variable, and their employment is generally delayed until the patient appears to be nearing an irreversible state of progressive respiratory failure. This is probably too late for a reasonable drug effect. Sladen has described an approach that probably justifies a clinical trial. He used pharmacologic doses of methylprednisolone (30 mg/kg) intravenously every 6 h for 48 h in combination with ventilatory support and reported a significant reduction in mortality rate when compared with historical controls.

CHEST WALL

Congenital Deformities

PECTUS EXCAVATUM

The most common congenital deformity of the chest wall is pectus excavatum, in which the body of the sternum is displaced posteriorly to produce a funnel-shaped depression (Fig. 17-22). The etiology is not certain, but most authors ascribe to the notion that overgrowth of the lower costal cartilages and ribs is responsible. The defect varies widely in expression. The depression is most often centered at the xiphisternal junction but may extend to the manubrium in rare cases. In lateral extent the presentation varies from a narrow central cleft to a broad dish-shaped defect extending from nipple to nipple. The depth of the depression is equally variable, with the sternum reaching or even overlapping the spine in extreme forms. Asymmetry is common, and always involves greater depression of the right costal cartilages with rotation of the sternum to the right. Several authors have attempted to classify the severity of defects based on radiographic findings. One method uses the sternovertebral distance measured on a lateral chest x-ray to classify the defects

as slight (>7 cm), moderate (5 to 7 cm), and severe (<5 cm), and others use a ratio of sternovertebral distance to transthoracic diameter. Computed tomography (CT) scanning may allow better quantitative volumetric analysis but has not been widely applied.

Pectus excavatum is present at birth and progresses at a variable and unpredictable rate through childhood. Infants and young children often have a protuberant abdomen that accentuates the deformity. Later in childhood a characteristic posture has been described, with rounded and forward-sloping shoulders, forward angulation of the head and neck, and dorsal kyphosis of the spine. Breast development in young women is frequently asymmetric, with a smaller breast on the right.

Although most cases appear in isolation, a familial tendency has been noted, and the defect is frequently seen in more than one sibling. The anomaly is about three times more frequent in males. Pectus excavatum is frequently seen in Marfan's syndrome and is one of a variety of chest wall deformities seen with increased frequency in patients with congenital heart disease.

That pectus excavatum produces a cosmetic deformity is not a matter of debate. Thirty to seventy percent of patients are reported to be symptomatic, with a broad range of presentations including exercise intolerance, atypical chest pain, dyspnea, bronchospasm, poor feeding, and arrhythmias. In all reported series, symptoms are almost always relieved by operative correction. Systolic ejection murmurs are frequently reported, and are thought to reflect compression of the right ventricular outflow tract. Electrocardiographic abnormalities are frequent and usually resolve after repair, but are thought to reflect changes in axis due to rotation and displacement rather than any fundamental electrophysiologic disturbance.

Whether or not a physiologic defect is responsible for the characteristic symptomatology is still quite controversial. Although most studies of cardiorespiratory function in pectus excavatum have placed patients in the normal or low-normal range, there have been notable exceptions. Weg found a decrease in forced expiratory flow and maximum voluntary ventilation in 25 young men with pectus excavatum. Blickman et al. recently demonstrated abnormal xenon ventilation scintigraphy in 12 of 17 patients before repair, which resolved in 7 of the 12 postoperatively. Perfusion and ventilation-perfusion ratios were abnormal preoperatively in 10 of 17 patients and normalized postoperatively in 6 of the 10. Not surprisingly, the defects were in the lower left lung. The authors did not address the clinical significance of the findings. Cahill et al. recently reported a small improvement in total lung capacity, a significant improvement in maximal voluntary ventilation, and an improvement in exercise performance after repair of pectus excavatum in 14 patients, supporting their belief that a dynamic restrictive pulmonary defect exists in symptomatic pectus excavatum that is reversible with repair.

Indices specific for cardiac performance have also been studied. A diastolic dip-and-plateau configuration in the right ventricular pressure tracing has been occasionally

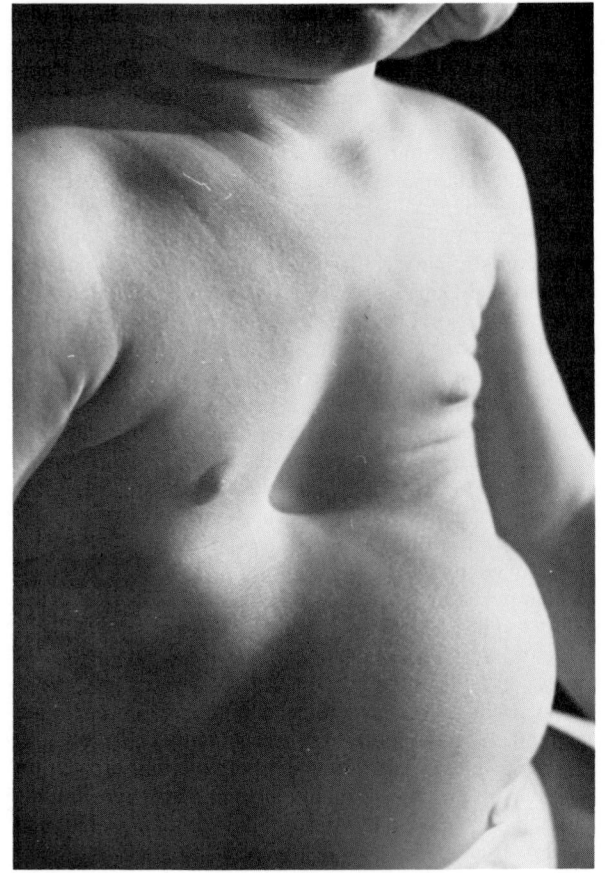

A

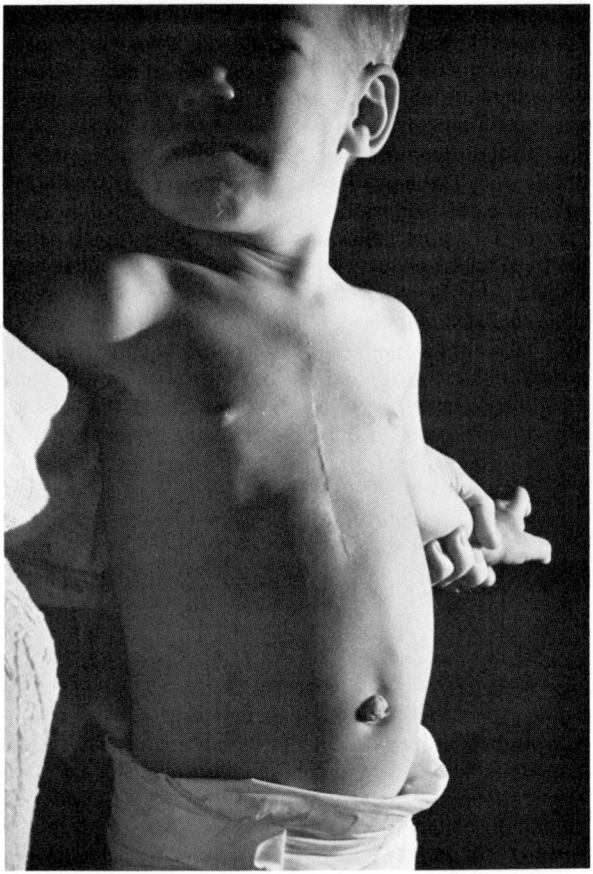

C

B

reported, suggesting a constrictive effect on the right ventricle. Beiser et al. reported normal exercise cardiac index in six supine patients with pectus excavatum that decreased significantly during upright exercise, although the cardiac index during upright exercise was within the reported normal limits in four patients. Of only three patients studied postoperatively, only two had an abnormal exercise cardiac index preoperatively, one of whom continued to be abnormal. In spite of the somewhat confusing findings in a small number of patients, this report has been frequently cited as evidence of abnormal cardiac exercise performance in pectus excavatum.

The largest group of patients (13) with pectus excavatum in whom cardiac performance has been studied was reported in 1985 by Peterson et al. First-pass radionuclide studies during upright rest and bicycle exercise were performed before and at least 6 months after pectus repair. Eighty-five percent of the patients were symptomatic, and all demonstrated striking subjective improvement after repair, correlating with a marked decrease in symptoms during a regulated exercise protocol. Objectively, however, left ventricular ejection fraction and cardiac index were normal before and after repair. Left ventricular end-diastolic volume index and stroke volume index increased at rest after operation, and resting right ventricular end-diastolic volume increased markedly, associated with a decrease in right ventricular ejection fraction. Although the data showed no impairment in exercise cardiac function before or after pectus repair, the increase in ventricular volumes suggested that some degree of cardiac compression was relieved by repair.

Two conclusions are possible. One is that no significant functional disturbance is associated with pectus excavatum. Another is that the methods available to study functional performance are too insensitive to detect the abnormalities that account for the pervasive symptomatology. Underlying the entire controversy is the fact that the anatomic spectrum is very broad and the number of patients available for study comparatively small. Objective study may be further confounded by psychological factors associated with an obvious cosmetic defect.

OPERATIVE TREATMENT. Most authors recommend operative correction during the preschool years (before five years of age) but not before 18 months. Operation at that age is thought to prevent the secondary postural and psychological consequences of the defect. Correction in adolescence or early adulthood is just as frequently performed, and with equal justification based on the desire to wait until evolution of the defect with growth is complete.

◀ Fig. 17-22. A two-year-old child with moderate pectus excavatum. *A.* The posterior displacement of the sternum appears to start at the level of the third chondrosternal junction. *B.* The potbelly that accompanies pectus excavatum in the young child is accentuated in the sitting position. *C.* The postoperative photograph shows an excellent cosmetic result. Either a vertical incision (shown) or a bilateral submammary transverse incision can be used for the repair. *(Photographs courtesy of Dr. Harold A. Albert.)*

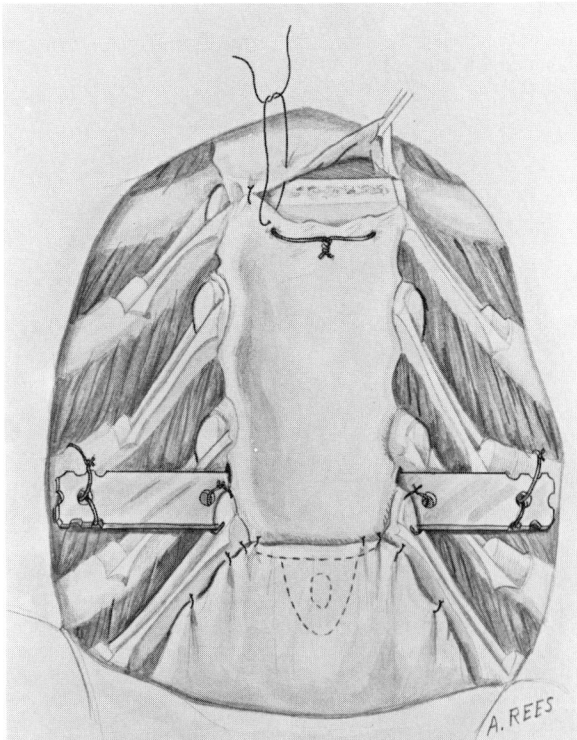

Fig. 17-23. Operative correction of pectus excavatum. The distorted medial portions of the costal cartilages have been resected and a steel bar has been placed behind the lower end of the sternum to decrease the possibility of late posterior sagging of the bone. From 9 to 12 months after operation the steel bar is removed through a small incision at the lateral ends. (From: *Holcomb GW Jr: Surgical correction of pectus excavatum. J Pediatr Surg 12:295, 1977, with permission.*)

The technique most widely used is that described by Ravitch. All the deformed costal cartilages are excised, the xiphisternal joint is disarticulated, and intercostal muscle bundles are separated from the sternum, and transverse posterior osteotomy of the sternum is performed above the point of depression. The osteotomy is combined with a forward fracture of the sternum and insertion of a bone wedge in the osteotomy site to provide an overcorrection of the deformity. Early results are 80 to 90 percent satisfactory.

The few long-term (20-year) results available suggest a disappointing tendency for the defect to slowly recur, and a number of modifications have been developed to counteract this tendency. Holcomb has described such a modification using a metal strut that is removed several months after the repair (Fig. 17-23). Wesselhoeft and Deluca have described a simplified procedure in which the deformed costal cartilages are resected subperichondrially through individual incisions in the pectoral muscles, without mobilizing the sternum from the intercostal muscles. A malleable metal strut is passed transsternally and placed beneath the pectoral muscles laterally. The strut is removed in 4 to 6 months, frequently under local anesthesia. Seventy of seventy-five children followed more than 5 years had an excellent cosmetic result.

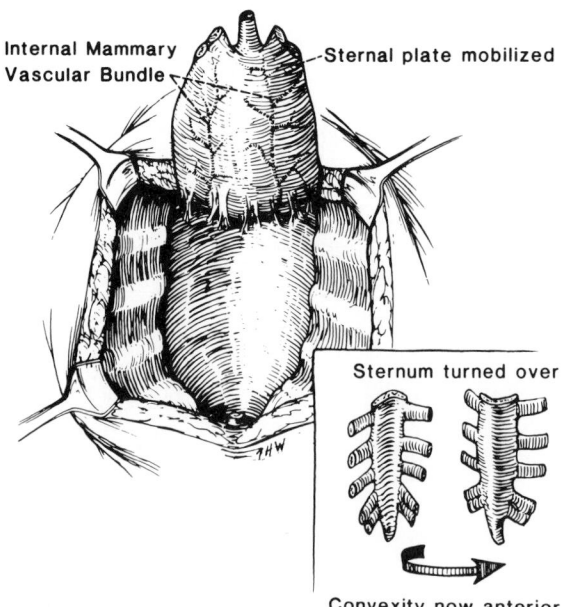

Internal Mammary
Vascular Bundle

Sternal plate mobilized

Sternum turned over

Convexity now anterior

Fig. 17-24. Sternal eversion technique for repair of pectus excavatum. *A.* The sternum is divided transversely just above the beginning of the deformity. The costal cartilages are divided vertically, just lateral to the beginning of the cartilaginous deformity. *B.* The sternal plastron is elevated and rotated so that the convexity is now anterior. The authors prefer to preserve one mammary pedicle. (From: *Hawkins JA, Ehrenhaft JL, et al: 1984, with permission.*)

Kirschner wires, autologous rib struts, Marlex mesh, and other devices have also been described, without reported results that would convincingly favor the use of any particular method.

Sternal eversion is a method that has been widely used in Japan by Wada, who reported satisfactory results in 97 percent of 199 patients over a 15-year experience. A smaller series from Iowa with similar results was reported by Hawkins et al. in 1984. The technique involves transverse division of the sternum, division of the costal cartilages, 180° axial rotation of the sternum (sternal eversion), and suture reattachment. In essence, the concave deformity is made convex. The sternal plastron can be rotated on a mammary artery vascular pedicle or as a free graft (Fig. 17-24).

Surgeons who prefer to focus on the cosmetic defect have used silicone implants to remodel the external appearance of the chest wall, with cosmetically satisfying results. Such a method is not applicable until growth has ceased, and would seem inappropriate in patients whose symptoms or findings suggest a physiologic impairment.

PECTUS CARINATUM

The protrusion deformities of the sternum are much less common than pectus excavatum, accounting for less than 10 percent of patients presenting for repair. Two principal types have been distinguished by Ravitch, although there is considerable variation from patient to patient. The most common type has been called the "chicken breast" type by Ravitch and is characterized by a deep depression of the costal cartilages along each side of the sternum, accentuating mild protrusion of the sternum by creating an illusion of greater anterior projection relative to the ribs. The deformity is usually developed maximally below the nipple level, involving the fourth through the seventh or eighth costal cartilages. As with pectus excavatum, asymmetry is common, most often producing mild rotation of the sternum to the right.

The second type Ravitch has called the "pouter pigeon" variety, characterized by a double angle in the sternum. The manubrium and upper costal cartilages project forward, while the body of the sternum first angulates posteriorly for a variable distance, then sharply reverses to project anteriorly. A depression is created in the lower part of the sternum that resembles pectus excavatum.

Although symptoms reminiscent of pectus excavatum have been associated with the protrusion defects, it appears that most are asymptomatic, and the condition has seldom been studied physiologically. Operative correction is done through a curved submammary incision that allows broad exposure of the deformed cartilages and costochondral junctions (Fig. 17-25). Subperichondral and subperiosteal resection of all deformed cartilages and ribs is performed throughout the length of their deformity. The excessive length of each perichondral bed is obliterated with reefing sutures, and the sternal contour is adjusted with a transverse osteotomy if necessary. Correction of the "pouter-pigeon" variety requires less lateral dissection but does require osteotomy at each of the two sternal angulations.

STERNAL FISSURES

The sternum is formed when two lateral plates of mesoderm fuse in the midline during the tenth week of embryonic development. The clavicular heads also contribute primordia to the manubrium. Failure of fusion can be complete, or it can be confined to the superior end or the inferior end of the sternum.

SUPERIOR STERNAL CLEFT. In this type of defect the cleft is broad and U- or V-shaped, usually extending down to about the fourth costal cartilage (Fig. 17-26). The prominent pulsations of the heart, which is covered only by thoracic fascia and skin, create the illusion of cardiac displacement into the neck. In fact, the heart usually lies in approximately normal position, and the two separate halves of the sternum can be located at the periphery of the defect and reapproximated. Osteotomies in each half, or distal transection of each half is usually necessary to

Fig. 17-25. A fourteen-year-old boy with pectus carinatum. *A.* The preoperative lateral chest x-ray shows remarkable anterior projection of the sternum. *B.* A line drawing demonstrates the forward projection of the sternum that is accentuated by the prominence of the knoblike costal cartilages. *C.* The postoperative photograph of the patient demonstrates a very satisfactory result. *D.* The postoperative lateral chest x-ray contrasts sharply with the preoperative film.

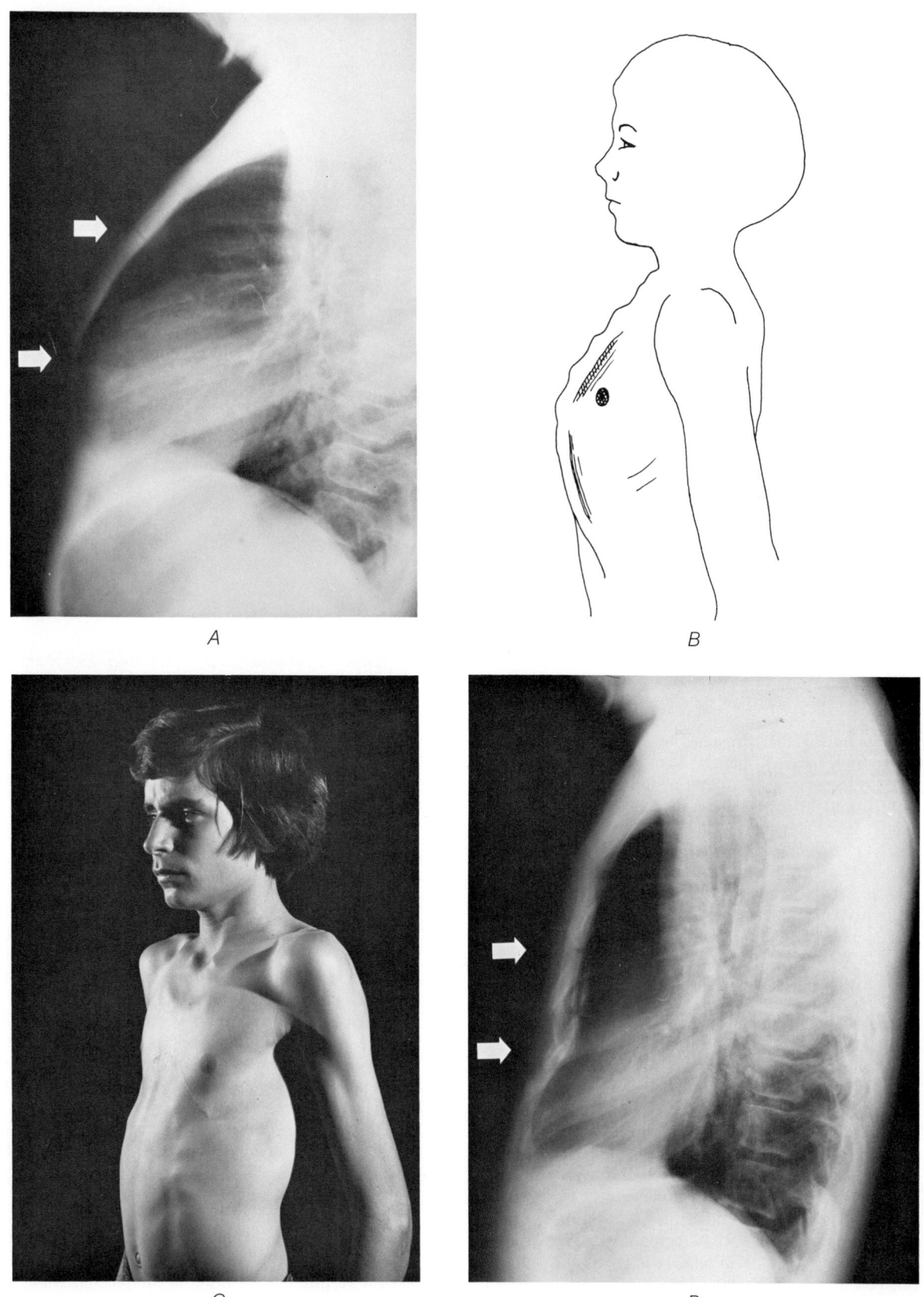

A

B

C

D

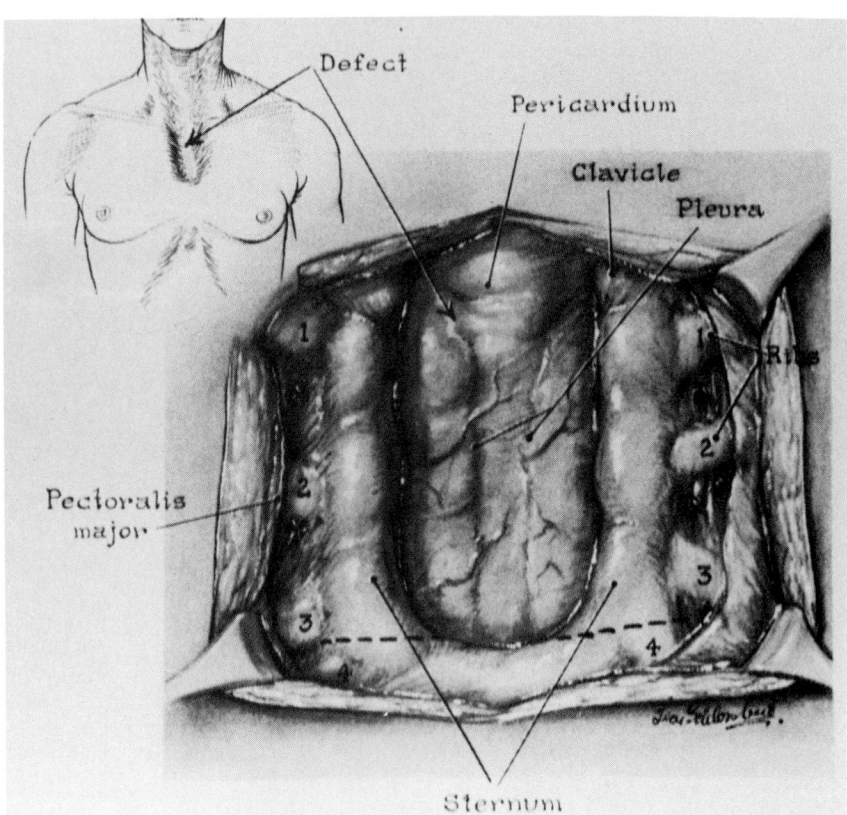

Fig. 17-26. A superior sternal cleft, presenting clinically with striking pulsation at the base of the neck, where the pericardium bulges out through the defect. It is frequently possible to pull the two sternal halves together by transecting the inferior end of the defect (dotted lines), combined with oblique chondrotomies of the costal cartilages. In the case illustrated, an eleven-year-old girl, reduction was not possible, and the defect was successfully repaired with a steel wire mesh covering. (From: *Ravitch MM, with permission.*)

bring them together. In some cases, especially those repaired after infancy, there will not be room for the heart, and coverage with prosthetic material is required.

DISTAL STERNAL CLEFT. A defect in the distal sternal is almost invariably part of a syndrome called Cantrell's pentalogy, which consists of the following five components: (1) a cleft distal sternum, (2) a ventral abdominal wall defect that may be a true omphalocele, (3) an anterior crescentic deficiency of the diaphragm, (4) communication between the parietal and peritoneal cavities through the diaphragm, and (5) congenital heart disease, usually with a ventricular septal defect and a left ventricular diverticulum.

Operative correction requires a staged approach taking into account the priorities of each defect. The omphalocele is usually repaired first. As with other forms of sternal cleft, early reconstruction offers the best chance for primary closure.

COMPLETE STERNAL CLEFT. In this rarest form of sternal cleft, failure of midline fusion is complete, leaving the mediastinal contents bulging through a thin covering of skin and fascia. In the few cases described, an associated failure of midline abdominal fusion has been frequent, and communication between the peritoneum and pericardium common. Repair in infancy is highly desirable and can be quite satisfactory.

MISCELLANEOUS ANOMALIES OF RIB AND COSTAL CARTILAGE

The simplest anomalies consist of deformed, deficient, or enlarged cartilage or rib presenting as an isolated finding in an asymptomatic patient. More complex anomalies include absence or wide divergence of one or more lower ribs and are commonly associated with hemivertebrae, fused bony paravertebral bars, and progressive scoliosis. The chest wall defect can manifest obvious paradoxic respiratory motion and even true lung herniation, but the spinal anomalies are usually more functionally significant and demand more therapeutic attention.

Poland's syndrome consists of absence or hypoplasia of the pectoralis major and minor muscles, breast hypoplasia, and partial absence of the upper costal cartilages (Fig. 17-27). Brachysyndactyly, ectrodactyly, and ectromelia are frequently described associations. It is invariably unilateral. Depending on the extent of cartilage deficiency there may be an impressive lung hernia, paradoxical respiratory motion, or simple flattening of the

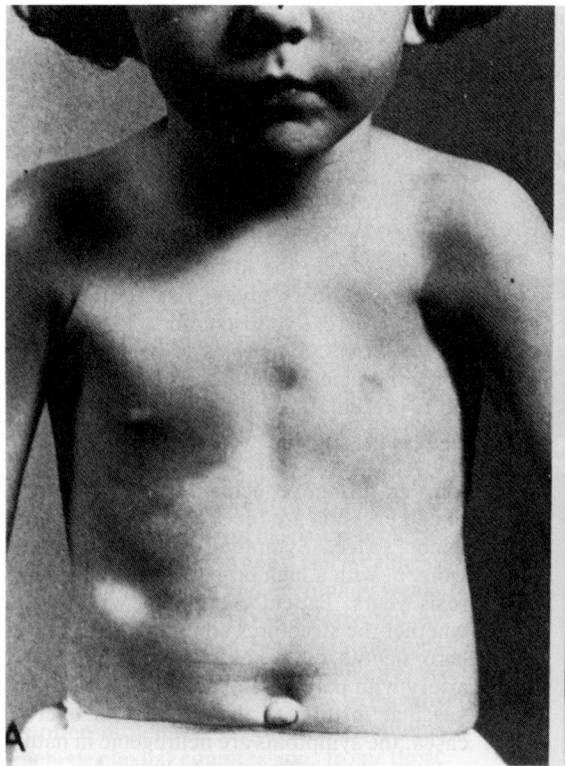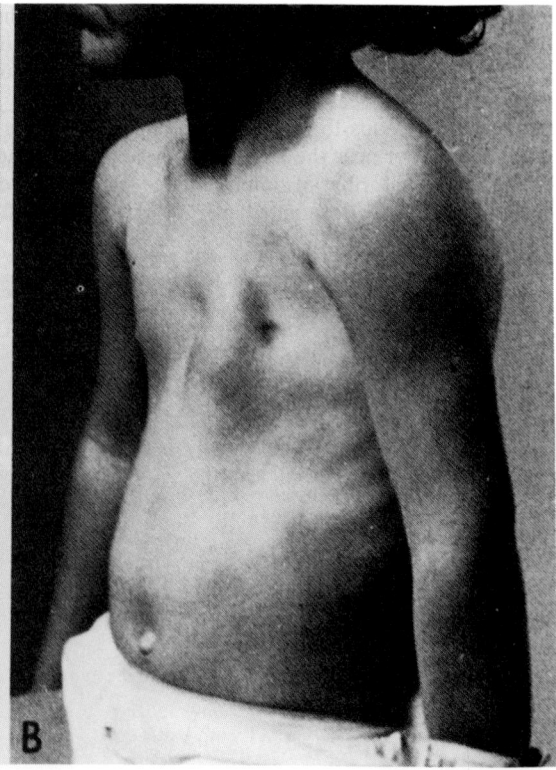

Fig. 17-27. Poland's syndrome in a child. The sternocostal portion of the pectoralis major, the pectoralis minor, and cartilages 2 to 4 are absent on the left side. The nipple, breast, and subcutaneous tissue are hypoplastic. (From: *Ravitch MM, with permission.*)

anterolateral chest wall. When the anomaly is on the left side, the underlying heart and lung are significantly vulnerable, since they are covered only by skin, fascia, and pleura. As the child grows, the concavity tends to become more severe on either side.

Operative reconstruction is recommended for cosmetic reasons, to eliminate paradoxical motion, and to protect intrathoracic structures. Staged procedures involving split rib grafts from the contralateral side combined with Teflon felt or Marlex mesh have been advocated in the past. A logical outgrowth of the increasing popularity of pedicled myocutaneous flaps has been their application in the reconstruction of this anomaly. Urschel et al. described successful single-stage reconstruction in two patients using a lattisimus dorsi flap and simultaneous augmentation mammoplasty.

Thoracic Outlet Syndrome

The thoracic outlet is a tight anatomic space with rigid delimiters and much crowding of the important neurovascular components that must traverse the space. These structural components are subject to a variety of congenital, traumatic, and degenerative abnormalities that may impinge on the vessels and nerve trunks that have low tolerance for compression without symptoms. Osteopo-

rotic or arthritic degenerative changes in cervicothoracic vertebra, callus-rich healing of first rib or clavicular fractures, developmental or fibrotic variations in the course or insertion of the scalene family of muscles, the skeletal anomalies that occur in the first thoracic rib, and the relatively frequent finding of one or more cervical ribs all may contribute to symptomatic neurovascular compression syndromes. Over the past few decades, the several more specific anatomic structures believed to be causing the compression have been labeled ''syndromes'' embracing the symptoms, but currently the cervical rib, scalenus anticus, hyperabduction, costoclavicular, pectoralis minor, and first rib syndromes have all been subsumed under the more general concept of the thoracic outlet syndrome.

Cervical Ribs

Perhaps because they are anatomically easy to demonstrate, the cervical rib anomalies have received a disproportionate attention in symptomatic patients. Cervical ribs occur in about 1 percent of the population, but only a small minority of those (less than 10 percent) have symptoms attributable to the extra ribs. Bilateral in 80 percent of cases, the anomaly is characterized by significant anatomic variation, including variation between the two sides in the same person (Fig. 17-28) and the symptoms may be unilateral, correlating poorly with the extent of anatomic abnormality. In most large series of patients with thoracic outlet syndrome, less than 15 percent are found to have a

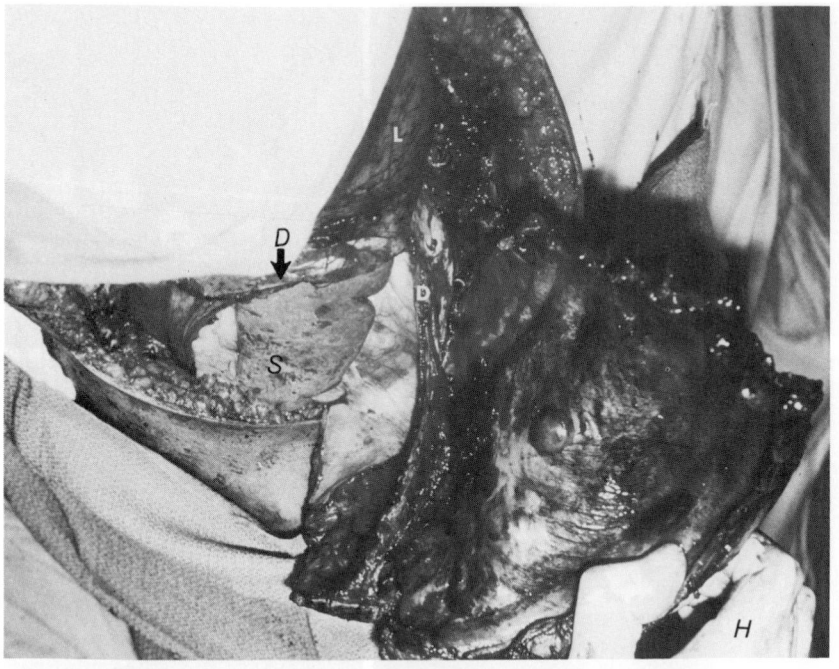

A

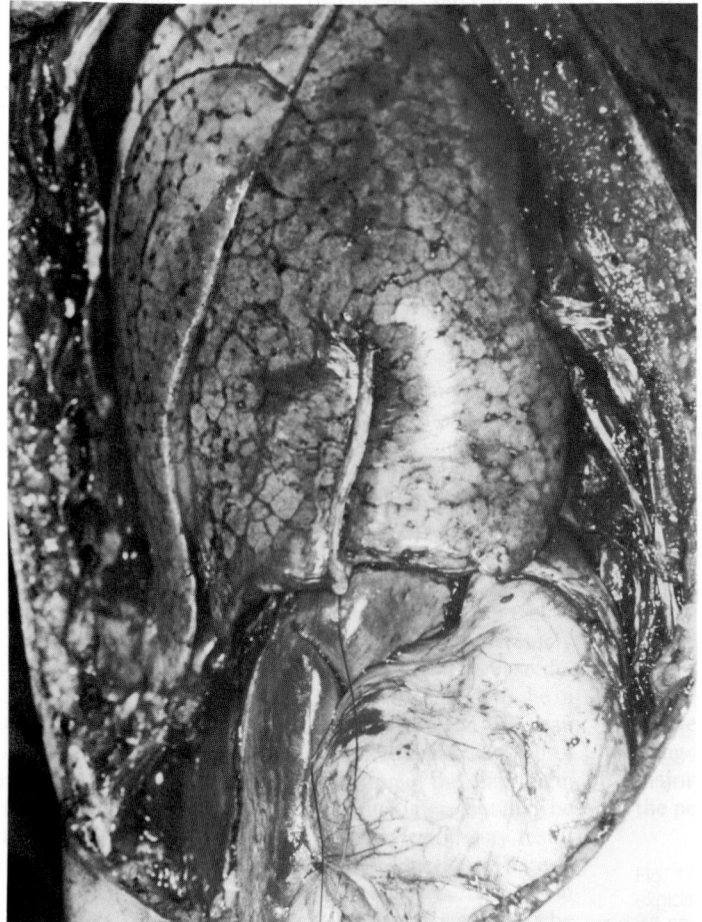

B

Fig. 17-30. Photographs taken in the operating room from the case noted in Fig. 17-29. *A.* The tumor is being resected with two grossly normal ribs above and below the lesion. This required removal of most or all of ribs 3 through 10. H indicates the surgeon's hand retracting the lesion; D marks the cut edge of the diaphragm on both specimen and patient side; S indicates the spleen; L is the lung. *B.* A wedge of lung was removed where pleural adhesions attached to the tumor. The large defect included the lateral third of the diaphragm. This operative view reveals the spleen and abdominal viscera and huge chest wall defect that existed after resection. *C.* The resected specimen. *D.* The prosthesis has been sewed in place. The line of reattachment of the diaphragm is seen in the lower third of the prosthesis. A myocutaneous flap from the left rectus muscle was used to close the skin defect.

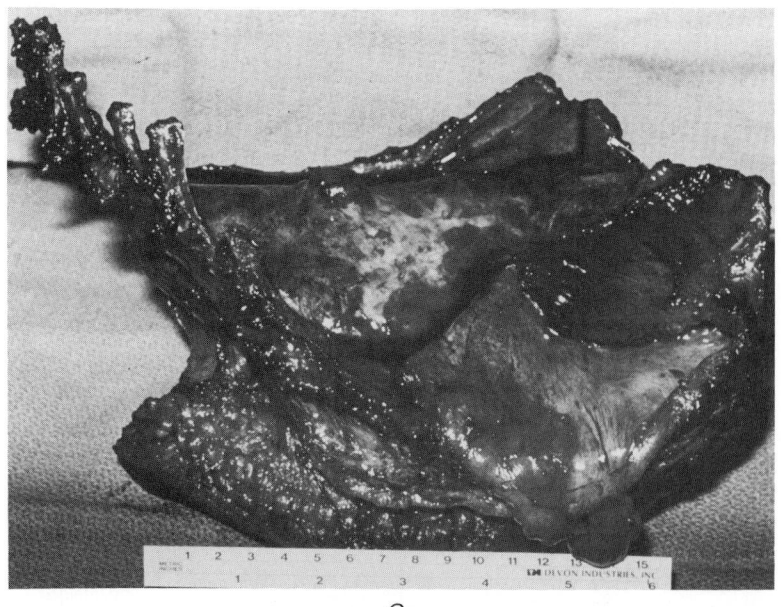

C

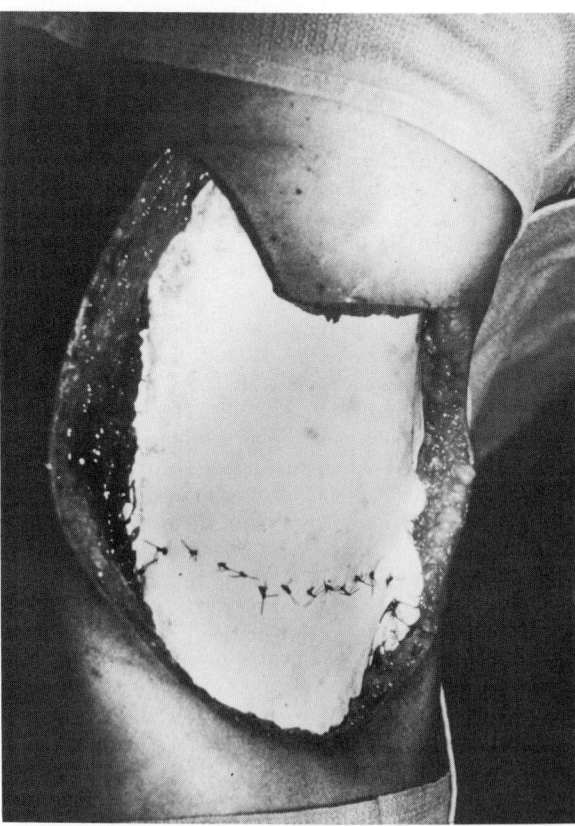

Fig. 17-30 *C,D.* Continued.

D

is appropriate to resect the adjacent part of the pulmonary lobe in continuity (Fig. 17-30*C*). Involvement of the sternum by a malignant tumor requires a total resection of the sternum with the adjacent cartilages. Techniques for postoperative respiratory support are sufficiently good

that resection should not be compromised because of a concern about the patient's ability to ventilate adequately in the early postoperative period.

Reconstruction of a large defect in the chest wall requires the use of some type of material to prevent lung herniation and to provide stability for the chest wall (Fig. 17-30*D*). Mild degrees of paradoxical motion are often well tolerated if the area of instability is relatively small. Pairolero and Arnold have recently reported an extensive experience at the Mayo Clinic of over 200 chest wall reconstructions following removal of significant portions of the bony thorax. They emphasize that both adequate resection and dependable reconstruction are essential ingredients to a successful operation and express the strong belief that a thoracic surgeon–plastic surgeon team is an important collaboration if these complicated problems are to be undertaken. While a wide variety of materials has been used to reestablish chest wall stability including rib autografts, steel struts, acrylic plates, and various synthetic meshes, their current preference is to use a 2-mm-thick polytetrafluoroethylene (Gore–Tex) soft tissue patch with rotation or myocutaneous flaps for coverage.

DISEASES OF THE PLEURA AND PLEURAL SPACE

The inner surface of each hemithorax has a mesothelial lining, the parietal pleura, which is invaginated at each pulmonary hilum to form the visceral pleura. The two surfaces are normally in apposition, lubricated by a thin layer of serous fluid secreted by the mesothelium, so that the steady motion of normal respiration is accomplished without friction. Therefore, the pleural "space" is normally only a potential space lying between the visceral pleura investing the lung and the parietal pleura of the chest wall. The elastic recoil of the lung and the rapid continuous absorption of fluid from the pleural space create a balance of opposing forces that favor apposition of the visceral pleura to the parietal pleura. The introduction of fluid or air breaks this dynamic coupling and converts the potential space to a real space. Normal respiratory mechanics are impaired in proportion to the size of the space created and the pressure within it. Many of the processes affecting the pleural space are essentially mechanical, such as spontaneous pneumothorax or congestive heart failure, and are not associated with any pathologic alteration in either pleural surface. However, virtually any chronic form of pleural space disturbance is associated with pathologic changes that produce thickening and adherence of the visceral and parietal surfaces. The end results vary from a few filmy adhesions of no consequence to a dense fibrous and calcific obliteration of the pleural space with a permanent restrictive defect in pulmonary function.

Pleural Effusion

A pleural effusion is an accumulation of fluid in the pleural space. It is not a disease entity but signals the effect of pleural or systemic disease on the normal daily passage of fluid through the pleural space. Normally, the balance of hydrostatic and colloid osmotic forces favors movement of fluid from systemic capillaries in the parietal pleura to pulmonary capillaries. It is estimated that

Table 17-6. CAUSES OF TRANSUDATIVE EFFUSION

Congestive heart failure
Nephrotic syndrome
Cirrhosis
Hypoproteinemia
Myxedema
Peritoneal dialysis

between 5 and 10 L of protein-free fluid traverses the pleural space in 24 h. Simultaneously, lymphatics drain smaller volumes of fluid containing protein, which would otherwise remain in the pleural space as a source of colloid osmotic pressure favoring retention of fluid. Alterations in systemic hydrostatic or colloid osmotic pressure that disturb the balance of forces across normal pleural surfaces produce an effusion consisting of a protein-poor ultrafiltrate of plasma classified as a transudate. Changes in capillary permeability caused by inflammation or infiltration of the pleura produce a protein-rich effusion classified as an exudate. Common causes of transudates and exudates are listed in Table 17-6 and Table 17-7. The distinction between transudate and exudate has diagnostic relevance, as noted in one series in which effusions were malignant in 42 percent of patients with an exudate and were caused by congestive heart failure in 83 percent of patients with a transudate.

Characteristics of fluid obtained by diagnostic thoracentesis that can help to make the distinction between transudative and exudative effusions are summarized in Table 17-8. Few findings are independently diagnostic, with the exception of positive cultures (empyema) and positive cytology (malignancy). Certain gross findings can be nearly diagnostic, such as the milky white fluid of chylothorax or the foul purulence of an empyema. Other findings can narrow the possibilities considerably. For example, grossly bloody fluid (red cell count >100,000 per mm^3) is almost always caused by trauma, pulmonary infarction, or malignancy. Markedly elevated amylase can be found in sympathetic effusions associated with pancreatitis, pancreatic pseudocyst, and esophageal perforation. Pleural fluid pH <7.20 (with an arterial pH >7.35) strongly suggests bacterial infection, and may appear before culture and Gram's stain are positive in some cases. Low pH has also been reported in some malignant effusions, and in effusions associated with connective tissue disease.

Table 17-7. CAUSES OF EXUDATIVE PLEURAL EFFUSION

Malignancy (primary and metastatic)
Infection
Infarction
Sympathetic (pancreatitis, subphrenic abscess, etc.)
Traumatic
Collagen vascular diseases (rheumatoid arthritis, lupus)

Table 17-8. SOME DISTINGUISHING
CHARACTERISTICS OF TRANSUDATE AND
EXUDATE

	Transudate	*Exudate*
Color	Clear, serous	Cloudy, tan
WBC count	<1000/mm³	>10,000/mm³
RBC count	<10,000/mm³	>10,000/mm³—blood tinged >100,000/mm³—grossly bloody
Glucose	Normal	Low in certain conditions
Protein	<3.0 g/dL	>3.0 g/dL
Protein ratio*	<0.5	>0.5‡
Specific gravity	<1.016	>1.016
LDH	Normal	>67% of upper limit of normal‡
LDH ratio†	<0.6	>0.6‡
pH	Same as arterial	<7.20 suggests empyema
Culture	Negative	May be positive (empyema)
Cytology	Negative	May be positive (malignant)

* Pleural fluid protein divided by serum protein.
† Pleural fluid LDH divided by serum LDH.
‡ From Light RW, MacGregor MI, et al.

There can be considerable overlap in the findings ostensibly separating exudate from transudate, and any chronic effusion tends to develop "exudative" characteristics. Too much can be made of laboratory distinctions, and it is rare for pleural effusion to be the sole manifestation of disease such that diagnosis hinges exclusively on pleural fluid analysis. The etiology of most effusions is best recognized by simply looking carefully at the rest of the patient.

A concave meniscus in the costophrenic angle on an upright chest x-ray suggests the presence of at least 250 mL of pleural fluid. A lateral decubitus view can detect a smaller volume, and confirms that the fluid is free in the pleural space if it is shown to layer out along a dependent surface. In some cases an effusion is completely contained between the base of the lung and the diaphragm (a subpulmonic effusion), and can be difficult to distinguish from an elevated hemidiaphragm or a subdiaphragmatic process. When this occurs on the left side the position of the stomach bubble can provide a useful clue. On a supine film a small to moderate effusion will be completely inapparent, and a large effusion only produces a uniform hazy appearance of the affected hemithorax that can be difficult to detect unless the process is unilateral. A very large effusion can produce complete opacification of one hemithorax that does not change in appearance with changes in position (Fig. 17-31). Adhesions can compartmentalize an effusion into loculations that assume a wide variety of radiographic configurations, frequently requiring multiple views or CT scanning for definition. Presence of an air-fluid level has specific connotations, since the air can only come from the tracheobronchial tree, from the esophagus, or directly through the chest wall.

Thoracentesis is the mainstay of diagnosis. Needle biopsy of the pleura can provide diagnostic tissue but has a

Fig. 17-31. A massive pleural effusion due to metastases from breast carcinoma. *A.* The arrow shows the tracheal displacement to the opposite side. *B.* The malignant effusion has been completely evacuated with a thoracostomy tube, and the mediastinum has shifted back to the midline. The left hemidiaphragm is elevated because of phrenic nerve invasion by pleural metastases.

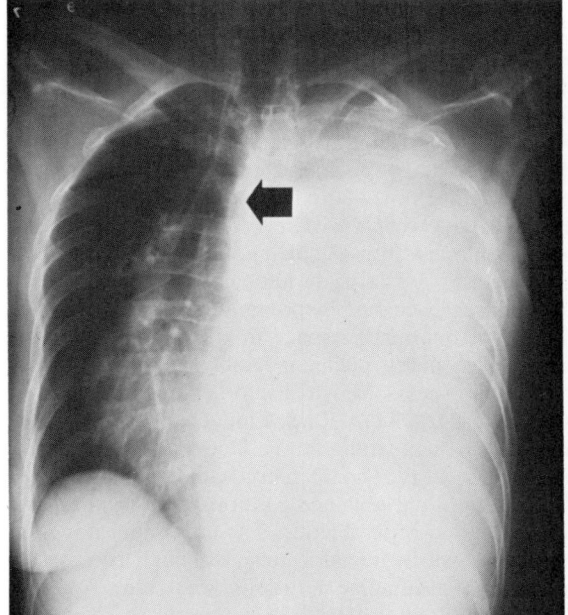

A

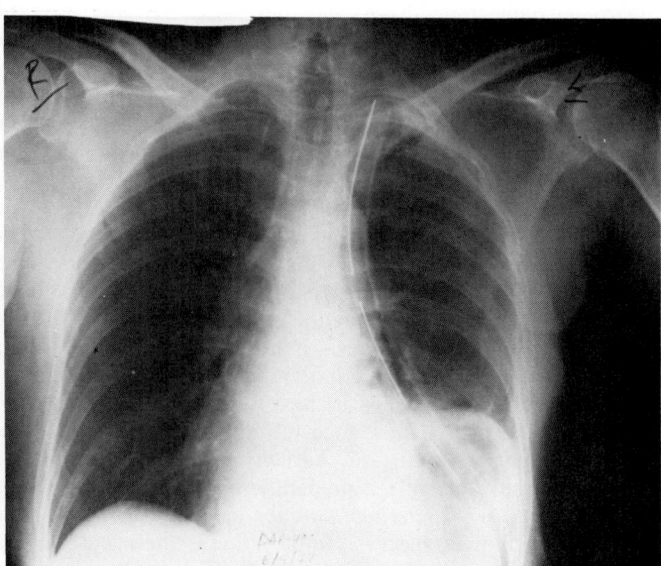

B

high frequency of false negative results because of sampling difficulties in diseases that do not involve the pleura uniformly. Thoracoscopy can increase the specificity of pleural biopsies in selected cases.

Pleural effusions can produce dyspnea but can also be surprisingly asymptomatic at rest. Therapeutic drainage is rarely indicated for transudative effusions since the fluid will rapidly reaccumulate until the underlying condition is improved. Most exudative effusions warrant a more aggressive approach. The treatment of hemothorax is considered elsewhere, and empyema, malignant effusion, and chylothorax are considered separately below. A variety of nonmalignant, uninfected exudative effusions are frequently treated as if they were transudative; examples include collagen vascular disease, pulmonary infarction, and sympathetic effusion secondary to abdominal pathology.

MALIGNANT PLEURAL EFFUSION

More than half of all patients with malignancy will have a pleural effusion at some time in their course. The effusion is frequently massive and symptomatic. The pathophysiology is thought to be interference with venous and lymphatic drainage by direct tumor invasion. Although pleural biopsy is most often normal, the fluid contains malignant cells in at least 80 percent of the patients. Lung carcinoma is the most common primary, with breast and gastrointestinal malignancies close behind. The fluid is exudative in character, and often bloody. Grossly bloody fluid (red cell count >100,000/mL) has a 90 percent probability of being malignant, once trauma and pulmonary infarction are excluded. The presence of a malignant effusion is a poor prognostic sign, with mean survival after diagnosis of 3 to 11 months in most series.

TREATMENT. Treatment is palliative. Repeated thoracentesis has a high failure rate. Chest wall radiation, thoracotomy with decortication and pleurectomy, and even pleuropneumonectomy have been described but carry unacceptable mortality and morbidity to be considered standard treatment. At present the standard therapy is tube thoracostomy and pleurodesis.

Pleurodesis creates an inflammatory fusion between visceral and parietal pleura that eliminates the potential pleural space. An essential first step is complete evacuation of the fluid and reexpansion of the lung (Fig. 17-31), accomplished by inserting a chest tube connected to a water seal drainage system (Fig. 17-32). If loculations or inaccurate tube placement prevent complete fluid removal and lung expansion, pleural symphysis will not occur uniformly and pleurodesis is much less likely to succeed; this is probably more important than the choice of the chemical agent used in the next step. Innumerable agents have been used to induce the inflammation, including talc, nitrogen mustard, Adriamycin, quinacrine, and tetracycline. Recently a preparation of heat-killed, freeze-dried *Corynebacterium parvum* has been tried, reportedly with great success. Tetracycline is the agent most commonly used in the United States. The agent selected is usually administered through the chest tube,

which is removed shortly thereafter. Although each agent has its staunch advocates, reported results suggest that the effusion will not recur in 60 to 90 percent of patients, regardless of which agent is used.

Use of an indwelling shunt connecting the pleural cavity to the peritoneum through a one-way valve has received attention recently. The system is analogous to a LaVeen or Denver shunt, except that the normal pressure gradient between the abdomen and chest is overcome with a subcutaneous squeeze bulb pump. The method has the theoretical disadvantage of continuously circulating malignant cells but does appear capable of producing satisfactory palliation in refractory cases.

EMPYEMA

Empyema is a suppurative infection confined to a natural anatomical space by normal epithelial boundaries; in the thoracic cavity this is the potential space existing between visceral and parietal pleura. Empyema was carefully studied 2400 years ago by Hippocrates, who first described open drainage with rib resection. In the early 1900s empyema complicated pneumonia in 5 to 10 percent of cases, and Sir William Osler required open drainage and rib resection in 1919 for a postpneumonic empyema.

In the postantibiotic era, empyema has become a less frequent complication of pneumonia, now occurring in about 1 percent of cases, and the bacteriologic spectrum has shifted from *Pneumococcus* and *Streptococcus* to *Staphylococcus, Streptococcus,* and gram-negative organisms. Although pneumonia is the most frequent association with empyema, it can also occur following trauma, pulmonary infarction, or pulmonary resection, and can be caused by spread from an intraabdominal source.

Infection of the pleural space initially produces a large, exudative effusion with a high concentration of leukocytes. In hours to days fibrinous adhesions succeed in limiting involvement to one or more loculated compartments. The ability of the lung to expand and obliterate potential space becomes very important in confining the infection, and prevents formation of a fibrous ''peel'' over the visceral pleura that can permanently restrain the lung in a partially collapsed configuration (''trapped lung''). The pleura actually has remarkable ability to resolve infection when assisted by an expanded lung. A persistent air leak (bronchopleural fistula) potentiates infection both by providing a route for constant inoculation of the pleural space, and by promoting lung collapse. The difficulty of obliterating space following pulmonary resection, particularly pneumonectomy, accounts in part for the seriousness of postresection empyema.

CLINICAL MANIFESTATIONS. Empyema should be suspected in a patient with a febrile illness and pleural effusion on chest x-ray. Thoracentesis with Gram's stain and culture of the fluid obtained confirms the diagnosis and guides selection of antibiotics. The gross appearance of the fluid is usually unambiguous, although some seropurulent parapneumonic effusions are sterile. In such cases pleural fluid of pH <7.20 is considered suggestive of empyema. Radiographic findings of loculated fluid or

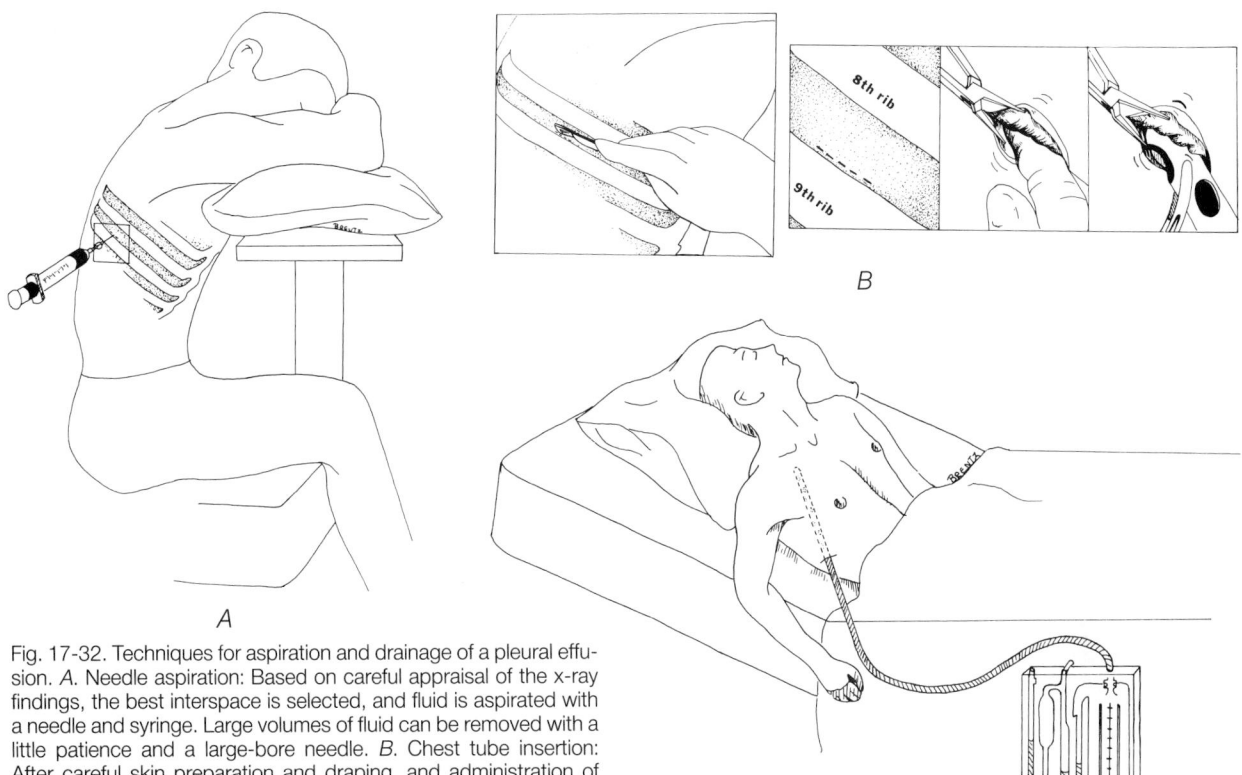

Fig. 17-32. Techniques for aspiration and drainage of a pleural effusion. *A.* Needle aspiration: Based on careful appraisal of the x-ray findings, the best interspace is selected, and fluid is aspirated with a needle and syringe. Large volumes of fluid can be removed with a little patience and a large-bore needle. *B.* Chest tube insertion: After careful skin preparation and draping, and administration of local anesthesia, a short skin incision is made over the correct interspace. The incision is deepened into the intercostal muscles, and the pleura is penetrated, usually with a clamp. When any doubt exists about the status of the pleural space at the site of puncture, the wound is enlarged bluntly to admit a finger, which can be swept around the immediately adjacent pleural space to assess the situation and break down any adhesions. The tube is inserted, with the tip directed toward the optimum position suggested by the chest x-rays. In general, a high anterior tube is best for air (pneumothorax) and a low posterior tube is best for fluid. A 28 to 32F tube is adequate for most situations. A 36F tube is preferred for hemothorax or for a viscous empyema. Many surgeons prefer a very small tube (16 to 20F) for drainage of simple pneumothorax. *C.* The tube is connected to a water seal drainage system. Suction is added if necessary to expand the lung, and will usually be required in a patient with a substantial air leak (bronchopleural fistula).

presence of an air-fluid level also suggest empyema in a clinical setting otherwise consistent with infection but can be difficult to distinguish from a lung abscess, an infected congenital cyst, or an infected bulla (pyocyst). A chest CT scan can be very helpful in avoiding inadvertent tube drainage of parenchyma.

TREATMENT. Successful treatment depends upon early recognition of the problem, selection of appropriate antibacterial therapy based on identification of the organism, and complete obliteration of the emypema space (Table 17-9). Thoracentesis alone has provided adequate treatment in only 9 to 12 percent of two large recent series, and success with this method depends on early treatment of relatively mild infections. Thoracentesis along had a 10 percent success rate even in the preantibiotic era.

A more aggressive form of drainage than thoracentesis is usually required. The first step is insertion of a chest tube connected to a closed drainage system. Suction is applied as necessary to obliterate the cavity and promote lung expansion, which is especially important in the presence of a bronchopleural fistula. Chest tube drainage of most early, moderate infections will result in rapid cessation of drainage and air leak, and obliteration of the cavity within several days. In such cases it is usually possible to simply remove the tube(s).

If early resolution does not occur, drainage of purulent material will continue, usually associated with radiographic evidence of a persistent cavity. It is a simple matter to convert closed-tube drainage to open-tube drainage by cutting the tubes off near the skin and allowing drainage to continue into dressings. With any form of open drainage, suction cannot be applied to the space, so that dependent position of the tube(s) becomes very important. Over a period of weeks to months, the cavity will shrink and eventually obliterate, slowly extruding the tubes, which are progressively shortened.

Conversion to open drainage cannot be done before pleural symphysis at the margins of the cavity has developed enough to prevent pneumothorax when the tube is disconnected from water seal, a process that requires at least 10 to 14 days. If this rule is violated and the lung is allowed to collapse, breaking down the immature symphysis, the empyema can spread rapidly to become a much more serious infection of the entire pleural space. A simple test is to disconnect the tubes and repeat a chest

Table 17-9. TREATMENT OPTIONS FOR
EMPYEMA

1. Antibiotic alone
2. Thoracentesis
3. Closed-tube thoracostomy (drainage to water seal, +/− suction)
4. Closed-tube/catheter drainage with antibiotic irrigation
5. Closed-tube thoracostomy converted to open drainage (no water seal, tubes cut off at the skin and slowly extruded)
6. Formal open drainage with rib resection
7. Thoracotomy and decortication
8. Thoracotomy, decortication, pulmonary resection, thoracoplasty, intrathoracic rotation of pedicled muscle flaps

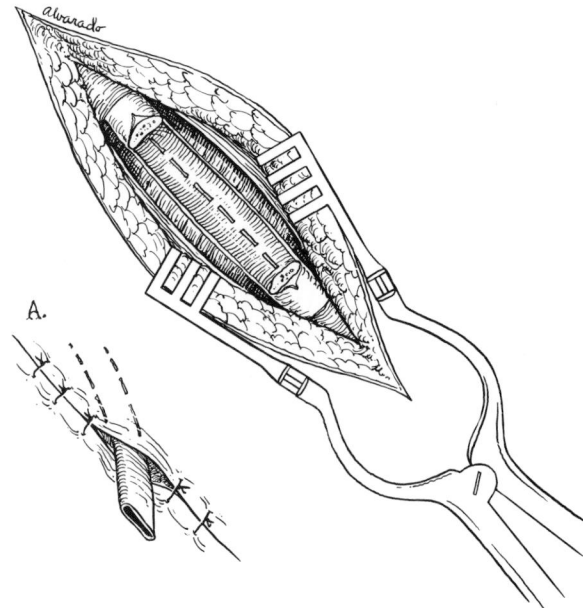

Fig. 17-33. Open drainage through the bed of a resected rib. For an empyema dependent drainage is important and the site is selected accordingly. A tube can be left in place as shown to prevent closure of the skin opening, or the skin edges can be sewed to the parietal pleura to create an epithelialized tract (a modification of an Eloesser flap). Progress can be gauged by periodically measuring the volume of the cavity, which can be done simply by measuring the volume of saline required to overflow it.

x-ray. If the space is ready for conversion to open drainage, the x-ray will be unchanged. Conversion to open drainage is also less attractive in the presence of an air leak, because the bronchopleural fistula is converted to a more chronic bronchopleurocutaneous fistula. In correctly selected patients, a combination of closed- and open-tube drainage is successful in at least 60 percent of cases.

Formal open drainage with rib resection (Fig. 17-33) was done more frequently in the preantibiotic era but is still useful today in the treatment of chronic, mature empyemas with a thick fibrous capsule (Fig. 17-34). Drainage is assured by marsupialization of the empyema cavity. The same cautions important in conversion of closed-tube to open-tube drainage still apply—the cavity must be mature, the drainage site should be dependent, and production of a bronchopleurocutaneous fistula is best avoided. The larger wound allows easier access to the cavity, and drainage can be augmented with irrigation.

A method that appears to be gaining in popularity combines closed-tube drainage with antibiotic irrigation. Results with this method were quite good in two series reported recently from England. Hutter et al. emphasized

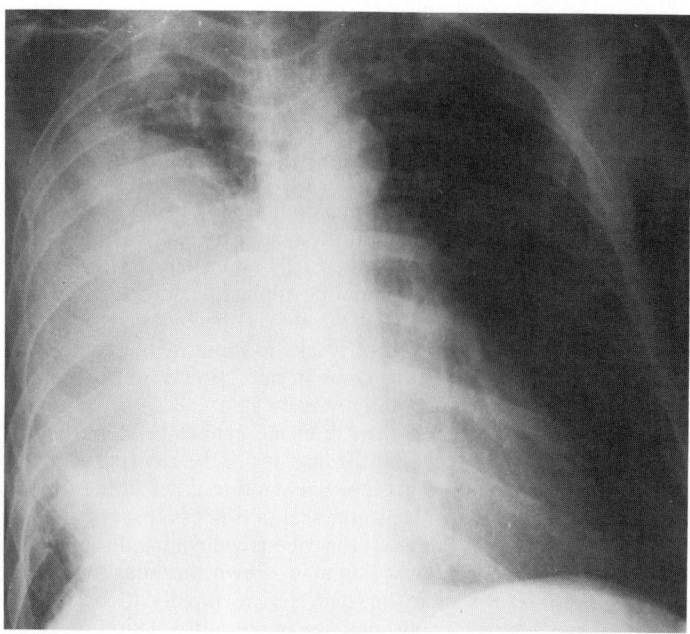

A

Fig. 17-34. *A.* This fifty-four-year-old homeless man presented to the emergency room with a massive consolidation of the right lung. *B.* On antibiotics the radiographic picture slowly evolved into a large cavity with an air-fluid level. *C.* Uncertainty about whether the cavity might be a large lung abscess or infected bulla was largely relieved by the CT scan, which shows a plate of consolidated lung compressed medially by a large empyema cavity. Note the degree of pleural thickening, which contributed to the difficulty encountered obtaining adequate drainage with thoracostomy tubes. Formal open drainage with rib resection was ultimately performed, with gradual resolution of the cavity over several months. At operation the fibrous wall of the cavity was 2 to 3 cm in thickness, precluding any thought of decortication.

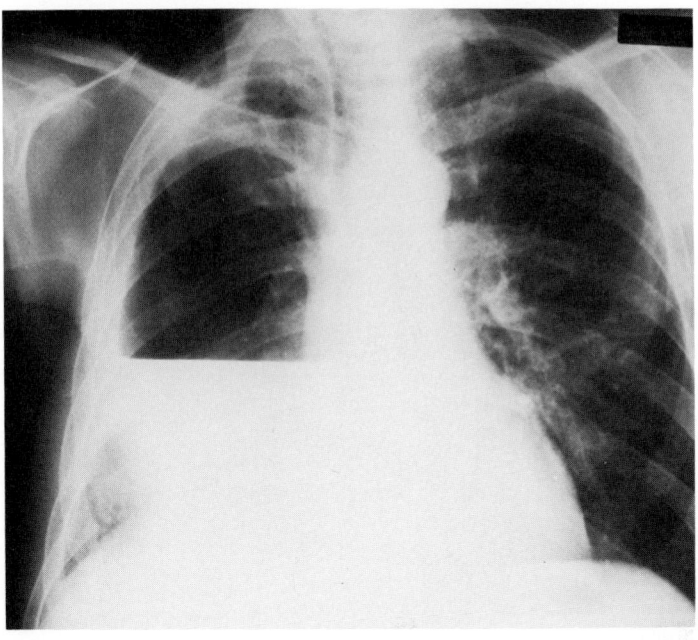

B

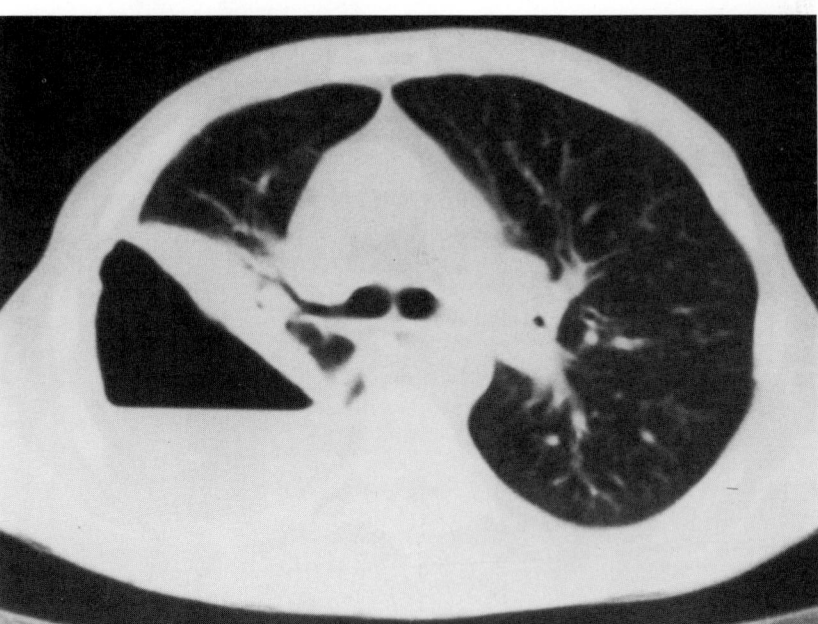

Fig. 17-34 *B,C.* Continued.   *C*

the role of thoracoscopy in this technique, which they feel is an important aid in achieving optimal tube position and lysis of intracavitary loculations.

If drainage fails to expand the lung, a permanent restrictive defect in ventilation on the affected side is likely to result as the inflammatory membrane heals and contracts over the surface of the lung. Failure of expansion is frequent with a bronchopleural fistula. Four to seven days of high-suction drainage is generally considered an

adequate trial, after which thoracotomy and decortication should be performed (Fig. 17-35). The empyema space is completely evacuated under direct vision, and drainage tubes are accurately placed in the most dependent position. The inflammatory "peel" is tightly adherent to the visceral pleura and should be entirely removed, a tedious process that must be done carefully to prevent development of new air leaks from tears in the lung. When an intraparenchymal abscess coexists with a large air leak,

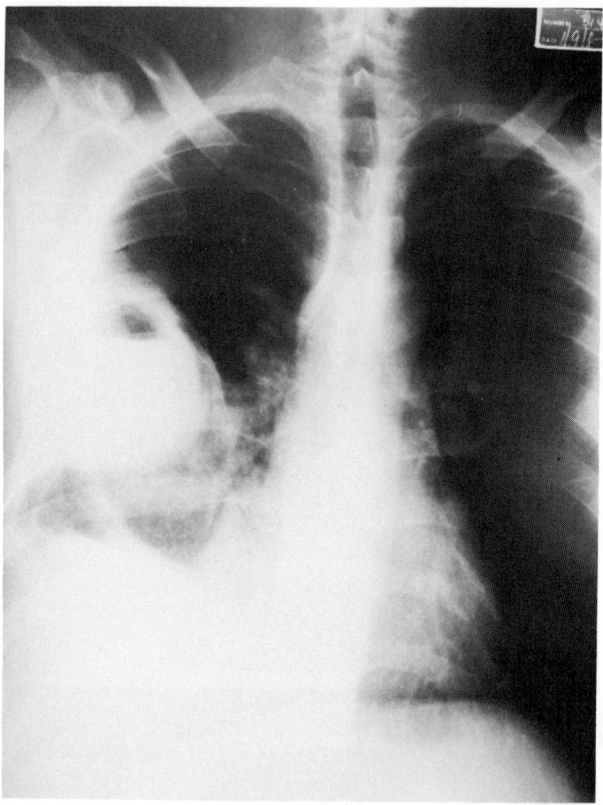

A

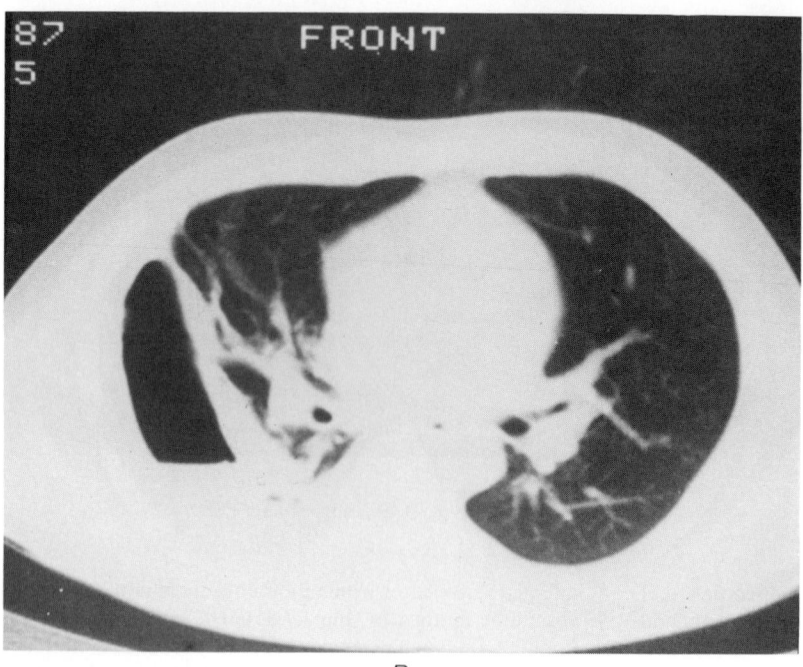

B

Fig. 17-35. *A.* This thirty-seven-year-old intravenous drug abuser presented with pneumonia that evolved into a cavitary process in the right lung, thought to be a lung abscess. *B.* The CT scan showed consolidated right lung compressed medially by a large, thick-walled empyema cavity with an air-fluid level. A decortication was performed through a right posterolateral thoracotomy with excellent results.

pulmonary resection is necessary. Thoracoplasty and intrathoracic rotation of muscle flaps can be added to help obliterate the remaining space.

Decortication has been successful in 80 to 100 percent of cases in reported series, and often shortens hospitalization. It has the disadvantage of requiring general anesthesia and a thoracotomy in patients who frequently have limited ventilatory reserve and are suffering the systemic consequences of chronic infection. Even so, with good anesthesia and aggressive postoperative care, thoracotomy is often better tolerated in the long run than a chronic, draining infection, even one that is slowly improving.

PLEURAL PLAQUES AND CALCIFICATION

Pleural plaques are idiopathic thickenings of parietal pleura, usually smooth and white, and frequently calcified. Most are small (1 to 5 mm) and irregular densities that are frequently bilateral and symmetric and do not occur at the apex or on the visceral pleura. They have no documented relationship to mesothelioma or other neoplasms. Localized inflammatory or traumatic events can heal with production of calcified plaquelike lesions, but they are usually larger and unilateral.

Chronic pleuritis can result in diffuse, remarkably uniform thickening and calcification of parietal pleura. The original pleuritis may result from an unresolved hemothorax, from tuberculous or nontuberculous empyema, and from viral or bacterial pleuritis or pleuropneumonitis. When the wall of a chronic but active empyema becomes calcified, resolution by drainage alone will never occur, and resection, decortication, pleurectomy, and thoracoplasty are likely to be required.

CHYLOTHORAX

Leakage of lymphatic fluid (chyle) from the thoracic duct produces a characteristic milky effusion called a chylothorax. The most common cause is surgical trauma to the thoracic duct, most frequently seen following procedures that involve dissection in the vicinity of the proximal descending thoracic aorta and left subclavian artery (Fig. 17-36), such as ligation of patent ductus or Blalock-Taussig shunt. However, the complication has also been described following a wide range of thoracic, cervical, and even abdominal procedures. Noniatrogenic trauma to the duct is a less common cause of chylothorax, thought to result from hyperextension of the spine producing stretch and rupture of the cysterna chyli over the vertebral bodies. Nontraumatic chylothorax is least common, is associated with malignancy or systemic pathology, and is frequently accompanied by chylous ascites. In nontraumatic cases the pathophysiology is more obscure but is thought to be related to obstruction or erosion of lymphatic channels.

Aspiration of milky-white, odorless fluid from the pleural space is virtually diagnostic. Pseudochyle, which has a similar appearance, is a rare source of confusion seen in certain malignancies, infections, and connective tissue diseases. In comparison with chyle, pseudochyle has a lower fat content and lymphocyte count, and its opalescent appearance is caused by the presence of lecithin-globulin complexes. If the patient is not eating, or if a coexisting problem could significantly dilute the chylous drainage, the gross appearance of the fluid may not be distinguishable from many other effusions. Table 17-10 summarizes characteristics of chyle that can be diagnostically helpful when gross appearance is ambiguous. The

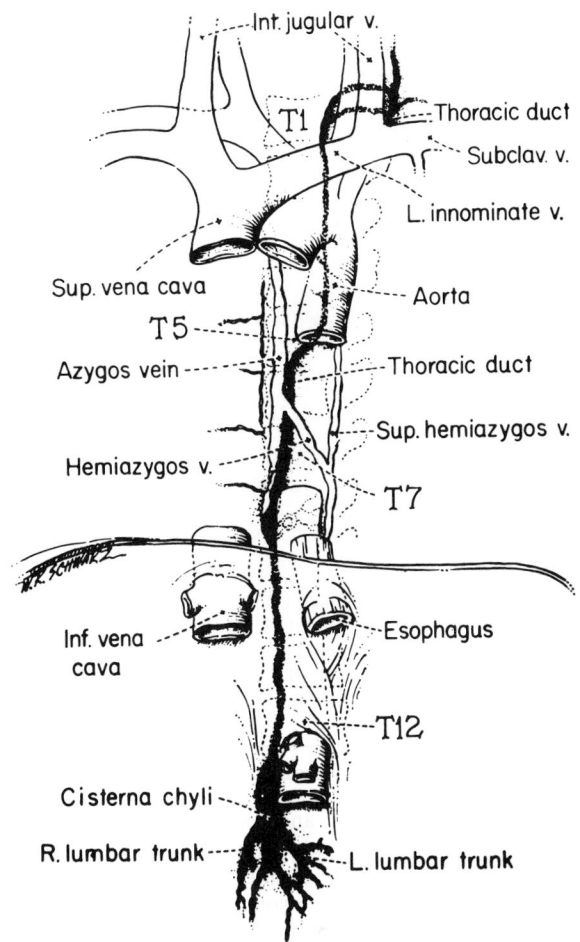

Fig. 17-36. The most common anatomy of the thoracic duct is shown. Anomalous patterns are frequently encountered. After passing through the diaphragm at the aortic hiatus, the duct lies between the aorta and the azygous vein on the anterior surface of the vertebral column, behind the esophagus. Ligation of the duct is most easily performed just above the diaphragm on the right. Although it can be ligated from the left side, the aorta must be mobilized for exposure. At about T_5 the duct crosses to the left side and ascends in the posterior mediastinum, where it is vulnerable to injury during any procedure involving dissection behind the distal transverse aorta. (From: *Bessone LN, Ferguson TB, et al, with permission.*)

lymphocyte count and triglyceride level are most useful. Lymphangiography will occasionally define the site of leak with precision, and is most useful in cases of nontraumatic chylothorax. It is rarely indicated in the traumatic variety.

Normal chyle flow ranges between 1.5 and 2.5 L/day but can vary much more widely depending on diet and on the fat content of the diet. During starvation or intravenous feeding flow falls to about 250 mL/day of clear fluid. Chylothorax is frequently massive (Fig. 17-37) and symptomatic, and significant volume losses can occur through thoracentesis or chest tube drainage. In one recent series, the average amount of fluid lost per day was 756 mL, ranging up to 1720 mL in one nine-year-old patient. Dehy-

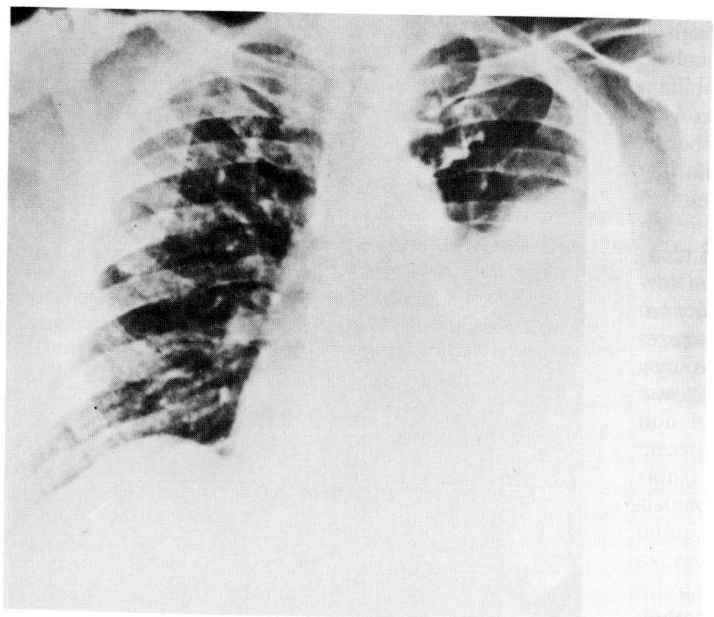

A

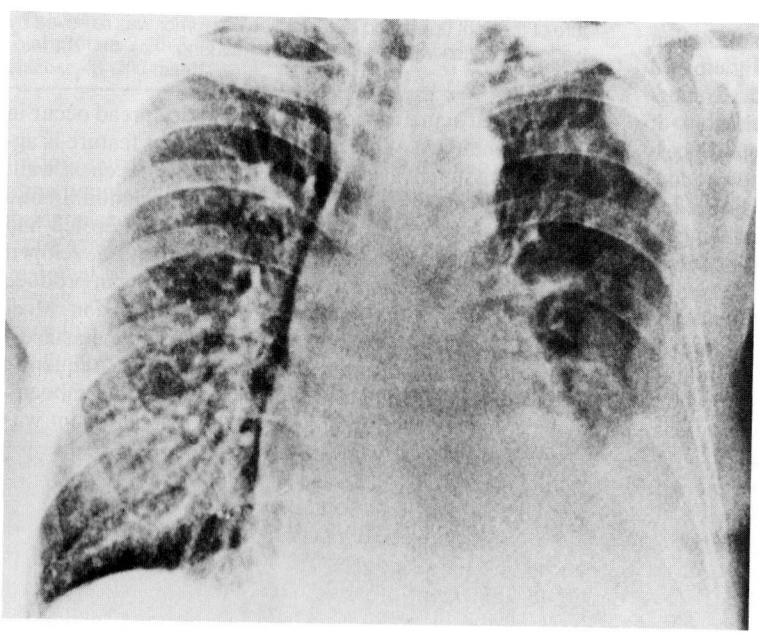

B

Fig. 17-39. Three common radiographic presentations of malignant mesothelioma. *A.* Large pleural effusion without a discrete mass. *B.* Multiple pleural-based masses without an effusion. While the appearance of the left lower lung field is consistent with effusion or mass, the two can be distinguished on the basis of lateral decubitus views and CT scan. *C.* Large pleural-based mass with pleural effusion and thickening. (From: *Martini N, McCormack PM, et al: Ann Thorac Surg 43:113, 1987, Fig 3A–C, p 116, with permission.*)

adequate size is obtained, the epithelial cell type in particular can be easily confused with adenocarcinoma.

TREATMENT. For benign mesothelioma, resection is the treatment of choice and is generally curative. For diffuse malignant mesothelioma treatment is controversial. Since thoracotomy is likely to be required for accurate diagnosis, careful preoperative clinical staging (Table 17-11) should be done to help estimate prognosis. Stages II to IV have a dismal prognosis regardless of treatment, with median survival measured in months. In such cases radiotherapy and chemotherapy are usually given, but proto-

cols with significant benefit have not been established. Even in Stage I disease, a 1986 retrospective analysis of 328 Canadian patients demonstrated median survival of only 17 months regardless of treatment.

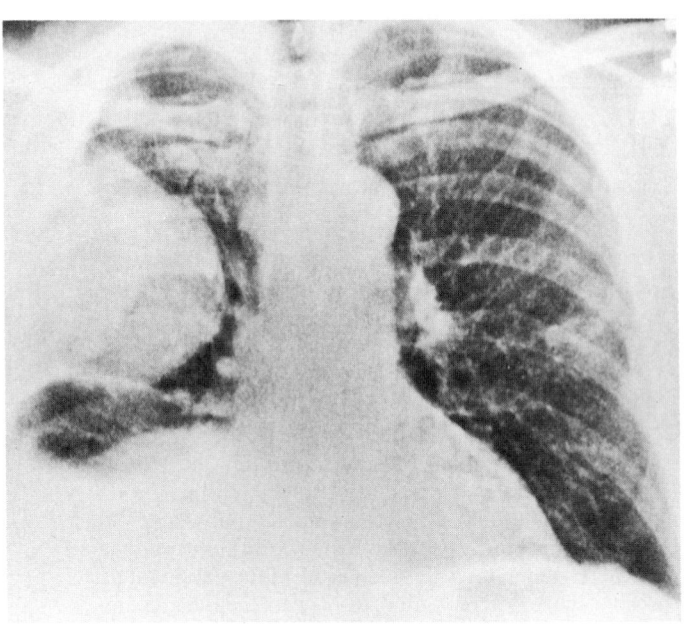

Fig. 17-39 *C.* Continued.   *C*

Radical surgery in Stage I disease is favored by some authors, who feel that meaningful palliation and an occasional long-term survival can be achieved with acceptable mortality and morbidity. At the most radical extreme, DaValle et al. recently reported their experience with 33 patients treated with extrapleural pneumonectomy, including resection of pericardium and diaphragm; 8 patients (24 percent) survived more than 24 months, and 5

Fig. 17-40. CT scan of a diffuse pleural mesothelioma encasing the lung and extending into the major fissure, but without evidence of mediastinal involvement. (From: *Martini N, McCormack PM, et al: Ann Thorac Surg 43:113, 1987, Fig 3A–C, p 116, with permission.*)

survived more than 36 months. Operative mortality was 9 percent, and serious complications occurred in 24 percent. A less radical approach is favored at Memorial Sloan-Kettering Cancer Center in New York, where pleuropneumonectomy has been abandoned in favor of radical pleurectomy, preserving the lung but resecting diaphragm and pericardium when necessary. They emphasize the importance of combined treatment with systemic chemotherapy and radiation, administered as a combination of intraoperative implantation of radioactive material and postoperative external beam. In 94 patients there was no operative mortality, 40 percent survived more than 2 years, and median survival was 21 months.

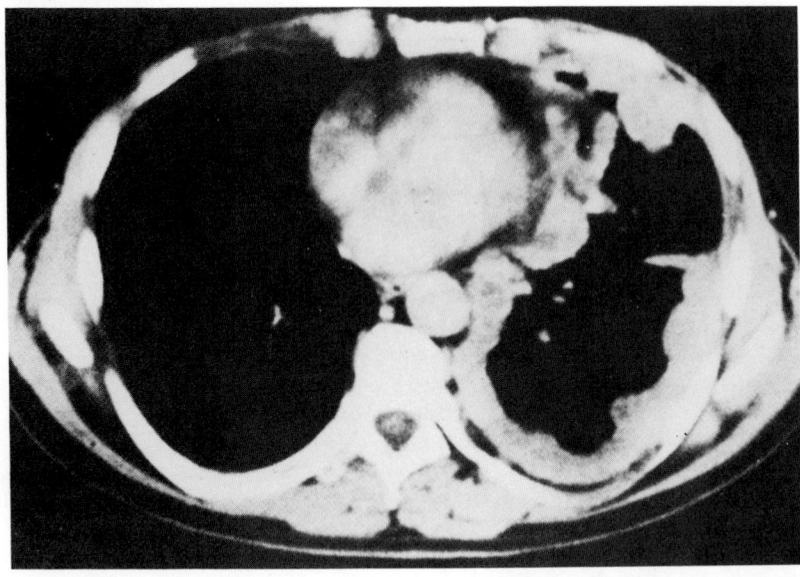

Table 17-11. CLINICAL STAGING OF MALIGNANT MESOTHELIOMA

Stage I:	Tumor confined to ipsilateral pleura or lung
Stage II:	Tumor involving chest wall, mediastinum, pericardium, or contralateral pleura
Stage III:	Tumor on both sides of the diaphragm, or in lymph nodes outside the thorax
Stage IV:	Hematogenous metastases outside the thorax

All authors agree that long-term survival in malignant mesothelioma remains a rare occurrence.

METASTATIC PLEURAL TUMORS

Over 90 percent of pleural tumors are metastatic. Lung and breast carcinoma are the most common primaries. In more than half of all cases, gross tumor is not visible but produces a malignant pleural effusion, which is discussed elsewhere. When multiple nodules or diffuse obliterative spread occur, differentiation from mesothelioma is impossible without biopsy.

Spontaneous Pneumothorax

Nontraumatic pneumothorax most commonly results from rupture of a pulmonary bleb or bulla. Negative intrathoracic pressure throughout the respiratory cycle favors movement of air into the pleural space, with egress prevented by the ball-valve effect of collapsing tissue during expiration. The pneumothorax will continue to progress until the leak seals with fibrin, at a rate directly related to the size of the bleb. Large leaks can produce life-threatening tension pneumothorax. Spontaneous resolution can occur once the leak stops, but the gas in the space is mostly nitrogen and is very slowly reabsorbed by the pleural surfaces.

Up to 80 percent of patients with spontaneous pneumothorax are young adults, usually male, without clinically significant pulmonary disease. A tall, asthenic habitus is common. In 85 percent of cases blebs or bullae of varying size are found in the lung apices (Fig. 17-41), and it is not known whether their origin is congenital or acquired. After the first episode the chance of ipsilateral recurrence is 50 percent, and the risk rises with each recurrence to 62 percent after a second episode and 80 percent after a third episode. The risk of a contralateral pneumothorax after the first episode is about 10 percent.

In patients over age forty, significant pulmonary disease is usually present, most frequently emphysema in a tobacco addict. Catamenial pneumothorax is a rare condition in which pneumothorax occurs predictably within a few days of menses, usually in women over thirty, and almost always on the right side. The mechanism is not known. The two most frequently cited possibilities are pleural endometriosis and small perforations of the diaphragm.

CLINICAL MANIFESTATIONS. Chest pain is the most common presenting symptom, followed by dyspnea. If the lung is more than about 25 percent collapsed, a decrease in breath sounds will be evident to auscultation, and the affected side will be hyperresonant to percussion. Young patients without underlying lung disease can be asymptomatic at rest with nearly complete collapse of one lung, and arterial blood gases will be nearly normal. A more dramatic presentation, including tachypnea, cyanosis, and hypoxia, is seen in patients with underlying lung disease and limited ventilatory reserve. An occasional patient with extensive lung disease and a pleural space obliterated with adhesions will present with massive subcutaneous emphysema and pneumomediastinum, because air escaping from the ruptured bleb follows the path of least resistance retrograde through the peribronchial soft tissue.

Fig. 17-41. An operative photograph showing a giant bulla arising from the upper lobe of an eighteen-year-old man with no symptoms of obstructive airway disease.

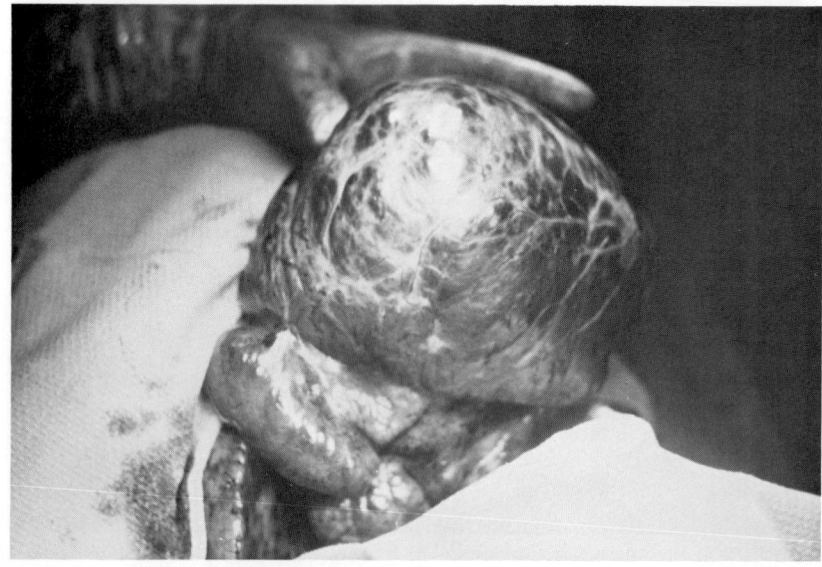

The characteristic radiographic finding is absence of lung markings and a faint visible line defining the edge of the lung. When the lung collapses almost completely, it is visible as an irregular density attached to the hilum (Fig. 17-42). Presence of a small amount of fluid with an air-fluid level is common. The fluid is usually serosanguinous and insignificant. On occasion bleeding from a torn pleural adhesion will produce a large and increasing hemothorax that can require urgent exploration. The lung fields must be closely examined for evidence of gross abnormalities, such as apical blebs or bullae. Although blebs and bullae are frequently obvious at thoracotomy, only about 15 percent are visible radiographically.

An asymptomatic or mildly symptomatic pneumothorax with less than 30 percent collapse that is shown not to increase in size over 6 to 8 h can safely be observed. Simple needle aspiration of the air space can nearly eliminate the space in a stable pneumothorax and will greatly reduce the amount of time required for spontaneous resolution. Needle aspiration of a tension pneumothorax can be a lifesaving temporizing manuever.

Thoracostomy tube drainage is the most common treatment. The tube is inserted either anteriorly (second interspace, midclavicular line) or laterally in a lower interspace (mid to anterior axillary line), with the tip directed toward the apex. The tube is connected to water seal, to which suction can be added to increase the gradient favoring removal of air from the pleural space. Water seal alone will suffice in many cases. As the lung reexpands, the patient will feel pain as the visceral and parietal surfaces reoppose. The pain gradually subsides but is usually much more acute and severe when suction is applied initially. Some authors favor attaching the tube to a one-way flutter valve (Heimlich valve) that permits outpatient treatment of a pneumothorax in a reliable patient with a small leak.

Serial check x-rays are followed to assess reexpansion, and the size of the air leak is monitored by observing the rate of bubbling in the water seal chamber. Air will cross the water seal only with cough or valsalva in a pneumothorax caused by a leak that has already sealed, and the bubbling will usually cease altogether within 24 h. At the opposite extreme, continuous bubbling occurring through both phases of respiration reflects a large active leak that may take days to seal, if it will seal at all. With large air leaks a single tube may be inadequate. If two tubes connected to suction still fail to expand the lung, thoracotomy is required. Even a large leak can seal if the lung can be fully expanded, which promotes adhesion formation between parietal pleura and the site of the leak in the visceral pleura.

Operation is indicated for a massive air leak with failure of lung reexpansion or for a smaller leak that has persisted for more than a week. Because of the frequency of recurrence after one episode, operation is recommended after any second episode and in any patient with a previous contralateral pneumothorax. Operation might be recommended after a first episode to anyone with large apical bullae visible on chest x-ray, to persons likely to be exposed to dangerous changes in atmospheric pressure (airline pilots, scuba divers), or to persons living in re-

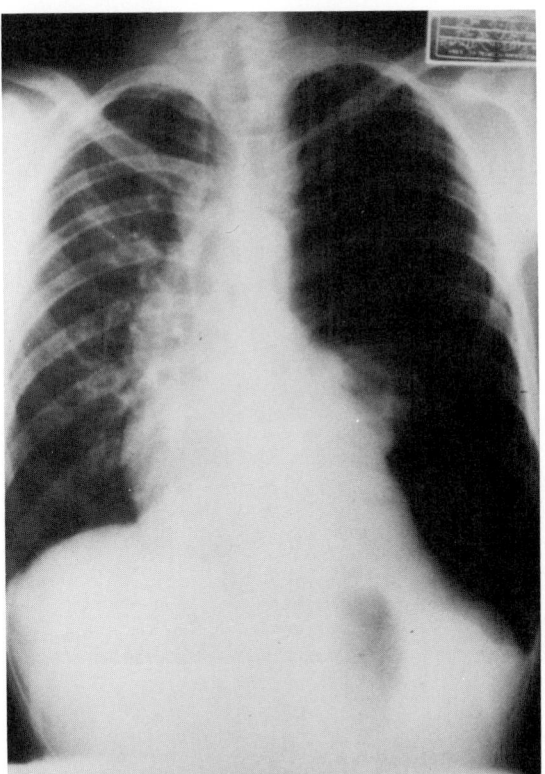

Fig. 17-42. Spontaneous pneumothorax in a young male. The lung is visible as a density collapsed against the mediastinum. The mediastinum is shifted to the right, the diaphragm is pushed down, and the intercostal spaces are wider on the left than on the right—findings that suggest an element of tension pneumothorax. In fact, the patient was hemodynamically stable and only mildly symptomatic.

mote areas. Complications such as empyema or hemothorax occasionally develop and mandate operation. In general, conservative treatment is continued as long as possible in older patients with underlying lung disease because of their limited ventilatory reserve.

At thoracotomy the site of the leak can almost always be identified (Fig. 17-43) and resected, oversewn, or closed with staples. Pleural abrasion should also be performed to promote formation of adhesions between visceral and parietal pleura, an especially important manuever if no leak site can be identified. Pleurectomy, accomplished by stripping all of the parietal pleura off the underlying ribs and intercostal muscles, is undeniably effective but has substantially greater morbidity and is reserved for extreme cases. Either method is 90 to 95 percent effective.

LUNG

Development and Anatomy

In the 4-mm (3-week) embryo, an outpouching from the primitive foregut appears caudad to the paired pharyngeal pouches and bifurcates into the right and left primitive

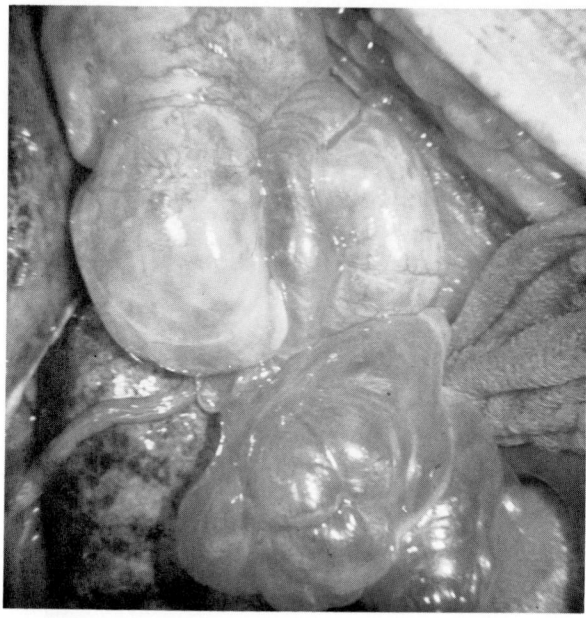

A

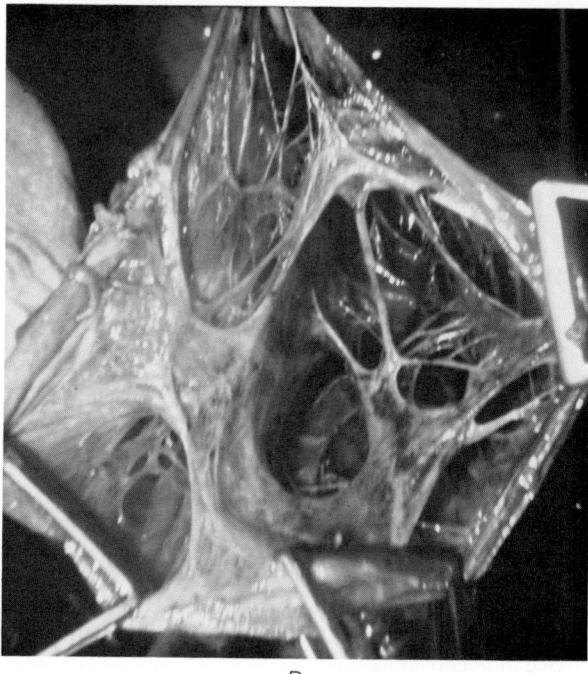

B

Fig. 17-43. This thirty-one-year-old salesman had three episodes of spontaneous pneumothorax over a 2-year period. *A.* At operation multiple bullae were found at the apex of the right upper lobe. *B.* The open bullae reveal a typical cavernous interior trabeculated by bands of fibrous tissue. The involved areas were removed with a wedge resection.

bronchial buds. Over the next two weeks, further branching occurs with 10 segmental tubes on the right and 8 on the left, providing an early indication of the lobar development that will continue in each lung. Progressive branching of epithelial tubes results in a rich arborization of bronchioles, and alveolar ducts and sacs. It is estimated that 300 million alveolar sacs eventually develop. As the structural maturation is taking place, histologic differentiation progresses from the cuboidal epithelium that lines the terminal buds during the first four fetal months to the flattened epithelium present at birth. Boyden and Tomsett have identified 23 to 27 branching generations in infants, adolescents, and adults, supporting the concept that the basic architecture of the lungs is completely developed at birth. As the lungs grow, they bulge into the lateral pleural cavities, leaving a dorsal mesentery to encase the developing mediastinal structures. The most caudal pair of aortic arches (the sixth) gives rise to the pulmonary arteries, with the remnant of the left sixth arch persisting as the ductus arteriosus. Vascular sprouts from the unilocular atrium fuse with the developing capillary vasculature in the lung mesenchyme to become the pulmonary veins.

Although the number of respiratory units may not increase after birth, it does seem apparent that the newborn's lung is structurally immature. In place of alveoli, the lungs are made up of primitive air sacs that differentiate into alveolar ducts and sacs. Alveoli develop by outpouching and compartmentalization, and maturation continues throughout the first eight years of life. The fully developed alveoli give a surface area of 70 to 80 m^2 at three-fourths maximal inflation of the adult lung.

SEGMENTAL ANATOMY. The segmental anatomy of the lungs and bronchial tree is illustrated in Fig. 17-44. Although there is continuity of the pulmonary parenchyma between adjacent segments of each lobe, the separation of the bronchial and vascular stalks allows subsegmental and segmental resections whenever the clinical situation requires or allows preserving lung tissue. This may be particularly important in patients with impaired pulmonary function or in those with disease processes that are apt to be or to become multifocal, requiring multiple resective procedures. Less-than-lobar resections are desirable when dealing with localized inflammatory diseases such as tuberculosis and bronchiectasis that characteristically involve segmental units of the upper and lower lobes, respectively, but often do so in a way that leaves one or more segments of the same lobe unaffected. Both these diseases, as well as metastatic pulmonary neoplasms, may involve more than one pulmonary lobe, either synchronously or metachronously. For many years, Jensik and others have raised questions regarding the necessity of extending the resection of primary lung neoplasms beyond the field necessary for adequate margins around the tumor. The advantages of a segmental concept of surgical treatment are important in all these circumstances.

LYMPHATIC DRAINAGE. Abundant lymphatic vessels are located beneath the visceral pleura of each lung, in the interlobular septums, in the submucosa of the bronchi, and in the perivascular and peribronchial connective tis-

RIGHT LUNG AND BRONCHI

LEFT LUNG AND BRONCHI

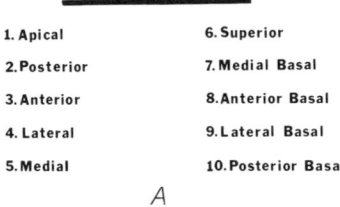
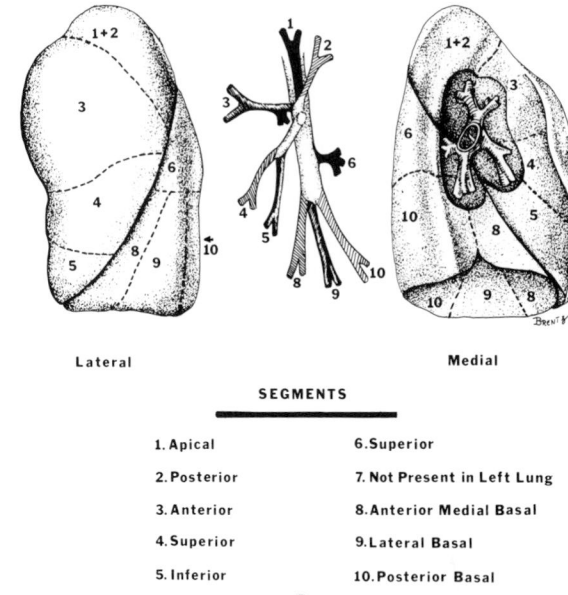

Lateral   Medial

SEGMENTS

1. Apical	6. Superior
2. Posterior	7. Medial Basal
3. Anterior	8. Anterior Basal
4. Lateral	9. Lateral Basal
5. Medial	10. Posterior Basal

A

Lateral   Medial

SEGMENTS

1. Apical	6. Superior
2. Posterior	7. Not Present in Left Lung
3. Anterior	8. Anterior Medial Basal
4. Superior	9. Lateral Basal
5. Inferior	10. Posterior Basal

B

Fig. 17-44. *A* and *B*. The segmental anatomy of the lungs. An appreciation of these anatomic divisions often makes it possible to preserve pulmonary tissue by performing segmental resections for localized disease.

sue. The lymph nodes that drain the lungs are divided into two large groups, the pulmonary lymph nodes and the mediastinal nodes, referred to as N1 and N2 nodes, respectively, in the American Joint Committee Tumor-Nodal Involvement-Metastasis (TNM) system of staging of lung cancer (Fig. 17-45). In turn, the pulmonary lymph nodes consist of (1) intrapulmonary, or segmental, nodes that lie at points of division of segmental bronchi or in the bifurcations of the pulmonary artery, (2) lobar nodes that lie along the upper-, middle, and lower-lobe bronchi, (3) interlobar nodes, situated in the angles formed by the bifurcation of the main bronchi into lobar bronchi, and (4) hilar nodes located along the main bronchi.

The interlobar lymph nodes lie in the depths of the interlobar fissure on each side and have special surgical significance because they constitute a lymphatic sump for each lung, referred to as the lymphatic sump of Borrie (Fig. 17-46). This designation results from the fact that all the pulmonary lobes of the corresponding lung drain into that group of nodes. On the right side the nodes of the lymphatic sump lie around the bronchus intermedius, bounded above by the right-upper-lobe bronchus, and below by the middle lobe and superior-segmental bronchi. The lymphatic sump on the left side is confined to the interlobar fissure, with the lymph nodes disposed in the angle between the lingular and lower-lobe bronchi, and in apposition to the pulmonary artery branches.

The mediastinal lymph nodes consist of four principal groups: (1) anterior mediastinal, (2) posterior mediastinal, (3) tracheobronchial, and (4) paratracheal. The anterior mediastinal nodes are located in association with the

upper surface of the pericardium, the phrenic nerves, the ligamentum arteriosum, and the left innominate vein. Within the inferior pulmonary ligament on each side are found the paraesophageal lymph nodes that constitute a major part of the posterior mediastinal group. Additional paraesophageal nodes may be located more superiorly between the esophagus and trachea in the region of the arch of the azygos vein.

The tracheobronchial lymph nodes are made up of three subgroups that are located about the bifurcation of the trachea. Included are the subcarinal nodes, the lymph nodes lying in the obtuse angle between the trachea and each main-stem bronchus, and a few nodes that lie anterior to the lower end of the trachea. The paratracheal lymph nodes are located in proximity to the trachea in the superior mediastinum. Those on the right side form a chain with the tracheobronchial nodes inferiorly and with some of the deep cervical nodes above. A few of the latter are referred to as the scalene lymph nodes because they lie on the anterior scalene muscle. Lymphatic drainage of the right lung is ipsilateral except for an occasional incidence in which drainage to the superior mediastinum is bilateral. Drainage from the left lung to the superior mediastinum is as frequently ipsilateral as it is to the opposite side.

Diagnostic Evaluation

Two factors make diagnostic evaluation of disorders of the lung more logical than is often the case in other anatomic regions. There is direct communication between the oropharynx and the respiratory system, and the contrasting densities of the contents of the thorax provide exceptional opportunities for a variety of imaging tech-

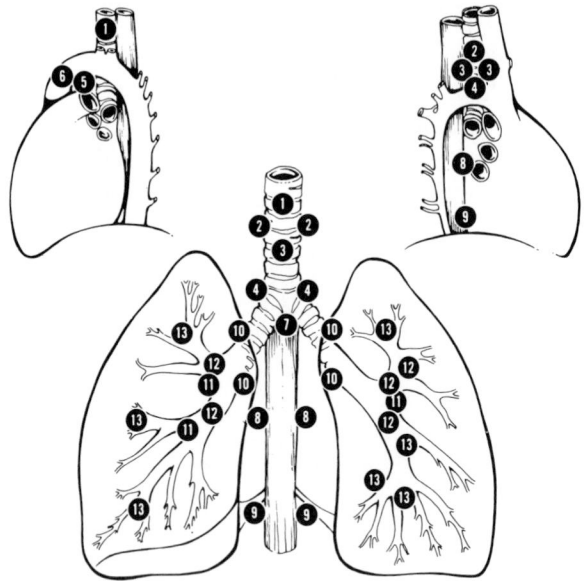

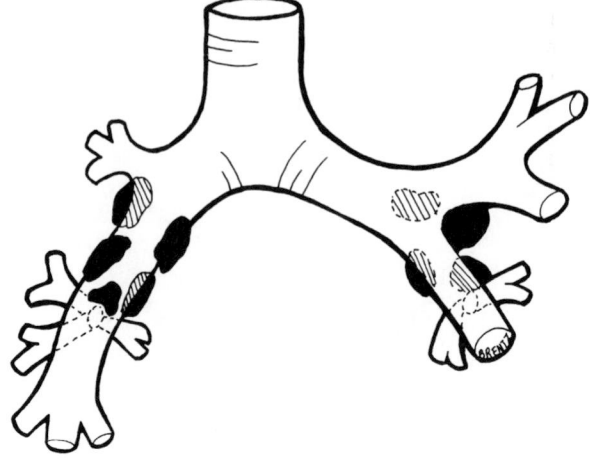

Fig. 17-46. The lymphatic sump of Borrie represents those lymph nodes on each side that receive lymphatic drainage from all lobes of the corresponding lung.

N2 Nodes

- Superior Mediastinal Nodes
  1. Highest Mediastinal
  2. Upper Paratracheal
  3. Pre- and Retrotracheal
  4. Lower Paratracheal
     (including Azygos Nodes)

- Aortic Nodes
  5. Subaortic (aortic window)
  6. Para-aortic (ascending aorta or phrenic)

- Inferior Mediastinal Nodes
  7. Subcarinal
  8. Paraesophageal (below carina)
  9. Pulmonary Ligament

N1 Nodes

10. Hilar
11. Interlobar
12. Lobar
13. Segmental

Fig. 17-45. The American Joint Committee classification of regional lymph nodes. (From: *Staging of Lung Cancer, American Joint Committee for Cancer Staging and End-Results Reporting, Task Force on Lung Cancer, Chicago, 1979,* with permission.)

niques. The first factor allows collection of secretions, abnormal drainage or purulent material, and desquamated cells that may provide a definitive diagnosis. It also allows an orderly sequence of progressively more invasive diagnostic endoscopic procedures for visualization, culture, or biopsy. The ''window'' into the thoracic cavity provided by fluoroscopy, conventional radiography, computed tomography (CT), and magnetic resonance imaging (MRI) allows remarkably clear anatomical definition, opportunities for serial observations, and precise guidance of biopsy needles and forceps.

AIRWAY INVESTIGATION. In most acquired pulmonary diseases sputum collection and examination are indicated as an initial diagnostic procedure. The specific etiologic agent of infections is sought by examination of smears and by culture techniques. The flora of the upper part of the respiratory tract stops abruptly at the level of the larynx, and the tracheobronchial tree is normally sterile. Not frequently, either the patient's sputum is scant, or because it is mixed with saliva and an oral bacterial flora,

its diagnostic usefulness is reduced. To bypass these problems, percutaneous transtracheal aspiration may be performed through the cricothyroid membrane. A 16- or 14-gauge intracatheter needle is used for the procedure after preparation of the skin with soap or iodine solution and local infiltration anesthesia with lidocaine. Coughing may be induced by injecting 5 to 10 mL sterile saline solution without preservative into the trachea. Aspiration of the diluted secretions into a 10- or 20-mL syringe should be followed by immediate delivery of the material to the laboratory.

Bronchoscopy. Whenever malignancy is a diagnostic consideration, or when the preceding studies have failed to yield adequate information, direct visual examination of the tracheobronchial tree is indicated. Information can be gained from this procedure that is available from no other source: cell type of bronchial neoplasms by direct biopsy, mobility of surrounding structures, extent of endobronchial involvement in neoplasms and inflammatory disease, and on occasion, source of bleeding. In addition, the therapeutic aspects of bronchoscopy should not be overlooked. The removal of thick, inspissated secretions from the postoperative patient can be lifesaving. The benefit of foreign body extraction by endoscopic means is obvious.

While the vast majority of endotracheal endoscopic examinations are now made with the flexible bronchoscope, there are still some important uses for the rigid scope, particularly for the removal of certain foreign bodies and the performance of endobronchial resections. The rigid scope provides a large, controlled airway with superb suction capabilities, and room for limited use of snares, scissors, and forceps. In small children, the restricted caliber of the airway may require use of the rigid scope.

The introduction of the flexible bronchoscope in 1967 by Ikeda has greatly extended indications for this procedure. Optically enhanced visualization of tracheobronchial tree to the subsegmental level is now possible and

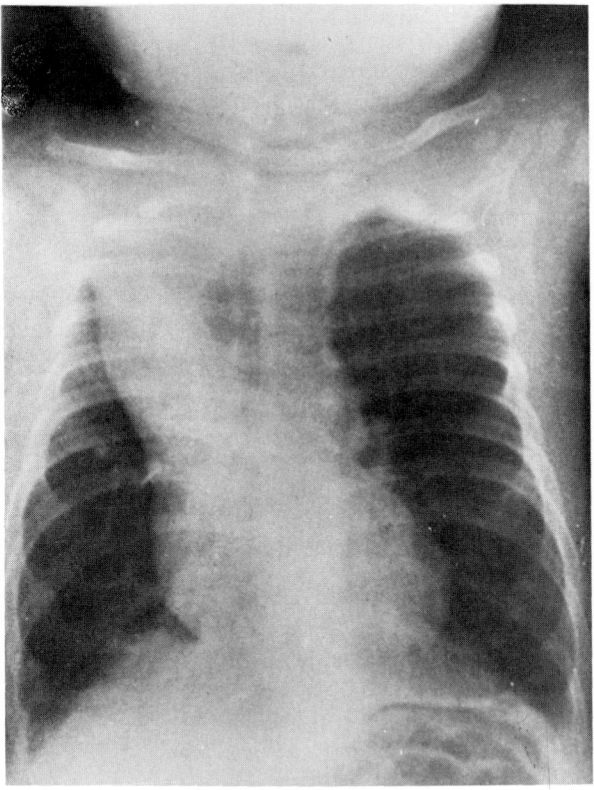

A

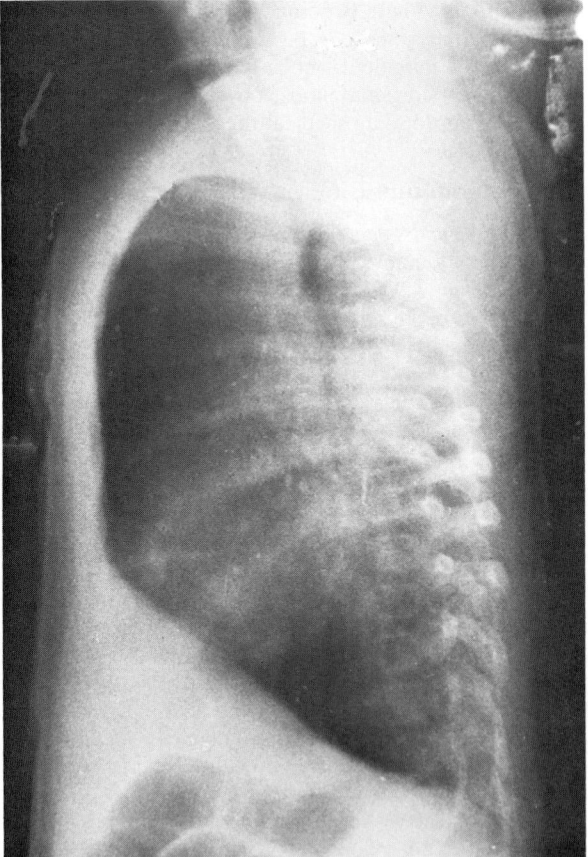

B

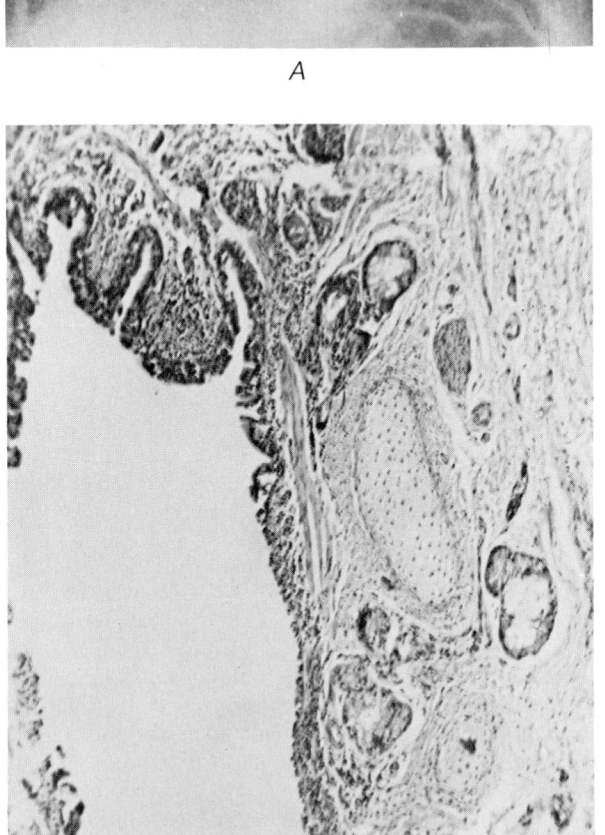

C

Fig. 17-57. Infantile lobar emphysema. *A.* The anteroposterior chest x-ray shows marked overinflation of the left upper lobe, with mediastinal shift to the right and compression of the right upper lobe. *B.* The lateral x-ray shows that most of the hyperinflation is anterior. *C.* Histologic examination of the resected left-upper-lobe bronchus shows incomplete cartilage development. (From: *Michelson E: Clinical spectrum of infantile lobar emphysema. Ann Thorac Surg, 24:182, 1977, with permission.*)

pneumothorax, which is a dangerous misapprehension if it leads to impulsive chest tube insertion. The chest x-ray can also mimic pneumothorax because the distended lung is very hyperlucent. Another common misinterpretation occurs when the compressed normal lung is thought to be atelectatic and the distended lung compensatory. An important radiographic clue is that the diaphragm is usually depressed on both sides with lobar emphysema but is normal or elevated on the side of primary atelectasis (Fig. 17-57).

In an infant with florid, progressive respiratory distress and a characteristic chest x-ray, emergency thoracotomy and lobectomy is indicated without further study. In such circumstances the mortality without operation approaches 50 percent. Involvement of an upper lobe or the right middle lobe is the most frequent finding. Lower lobe involvement is rare. Resection is ordinarily straightforward anatomically and completely curative. When the clinical presentation is less fulminant, the decision is more difficult. There is no question that varying degrees of lobar emphysema can be produced by aspiration of mucus or amniotic fluid, or by acute bronchiolitis. In such cases the emphysema almost always resolves in a few days with appropriate medical therapy.

Emphysematous Blebs and Bullae

Emphysema is characterized by enlarged air spaces produced by a complex process of elastic tissue destruction, alveolar wall breakdown, and coalescence of damaged alveoli, resulting in impaired alveolar ventilation and gas exchange. The disease represents one characteristic expression of advanced chronic obstructive pulmonary disease, overlapping considerably with the secretory, fibrotic bronchiolar obstructive pattern of chronic bronchitis, and with the reactive, atopic pattern of asthma. Pathogenetic differences promoting a predominant pattern of alveolar breakdown are difficult to isolate, and the response to a common mechanism of injury such as cigarette smoking is not predictable. An exception is the emphysematous pattern produced by the loss of normal restraints on tissue destruction seen in alpha$_1$-antitrypsin deficiency.

The surgeon has the luxury of ignoring the confusion of pathogenesis in this complex disorder to concentrate on the parts of the spectrum that have surgical significance. Emphysema is usually not truly diffuse, and involved areas may be quite localized into collections of small cysts (blebs) or very large ones (bullae). Blebs are usually subpleural, do not extend deeply into more central parenchyma, and consequently may have little effect on gas exchange or overall pulmonary function, even when multiple discrete collections of considerable size are present. Their chief significance relates to their potential for rupture with production of pneumothorax. The localized collection of blebs frequently encountered in the apices of otherwise normal lungs in healthy young individuals with spontaneous pneumothorax bear an uncertain pathogenic relationship to emphysema and may be in some way congenital. Although most blebs are apical, the blebs encountered in typical chronic pulmonary disease are more likely to be multiple and in other parts of the lung.

Bullae result from a much larger coalescence of destroyed alveolar septae and tend to develop deep within the lung parenchyma, compressing and distorting adjacent normal lung. They may assume the form of a single large cyst, or remnants of interstitium may remain to form a multiloculated space. Many bullae will remain stable or will increase in size slowly over many years, but they have the potential for rapid expansion, producing acute respiratory distress. An enormous single bulla may be very difficult to distinguish from a tension pneumothorax clinically or radiographically.

Diffuse emphysema is characterized by a uniform destructive process producing profound effects on pulmonary function and gas exchange. The full-blown clinical presentation includes extreme dyspnea, with a barrel chest and attenuation of intercostal and diaphragmatic musculature. Lungs with diffuse emphysema frequently contain areas of bleb or bullous disease as well.

SURGICAL CONSIDERATIONS. The surgeon confronts emphysema in two principal situations: in operations performed on patients with emphysema, and in operations performed for emphysema. In the former category, patients with emphysema undergoing procedures with general anesthesia have an increased operative risk due to their abnormal gas exchange and are at higher risk for barotrauma during mechanical ventilation. Postoperative pulmonary toilet can be a major challenge in a patient with greatly reduced expiratory forces whose ability to cough is further compromised by postoperative pain. Every surgeon has seen patients with marginally compensated emphysema become ventilator-dependent, with a tracheostomy and bilateral chest tubes, following routine abdominal surgery. Elective operation in such patients requires cautious assessment of risks and careful attention to preoperative pulmonary physiotherapy.

Thoracic operations designed to correct specific manifestations of emphysema carry similar risks but also offer the expectation of improvement. The history of operations for emphysema illustrates the danger of allowing surgical intuition to precede an understanding of pathophysiology. Some of the earliest procedures were designed to "make room" for the hyperinflated lung by further enlarging the barrel chest with sternotomy or chondrectomy. Upon observation that such procedures were ineffective at best, attempts were made to decrease lung volume by phrenic nerve destruction or thoracoplasty, with counterproductive results that would be considered predictable today.

Selection for operation is directed toward identifying patients in whom resection of localized bullous disease is likely to improve pulmonary function. Ventilation-perfusion scans and pulmonary angiography can help define areas of normal lung adjacent to large bullae that are compressed and nonventilated but normally perfused (Fig. 17-58). The most favorable patients are young (under age fifty-five years), with unilateral disease and marked asymmetry of function, recently progressive symptoms, well-defined bullae, and evidence of crowded vessels in adjacent parenchyma. Large bullae displacing more than half the hemithorax are more likely to produce symptomatic improvement after resection than smaller bullae.

In all patients every effort is made preoperatively to maximize pulmonary function and eliminate chronic bronchial infection. The disease is usually approached through a posterolateral thoracotomy, although some authors have favored median sternotomy for anterior and superior bullae, claiming that postoperative morbidity is reduced. The resection is carefully tailored to preserve all adjacent vascularized parenchyma. Mechanical stapling devices are extremely helpful. Planes of division through emphysematous lung are friable and prone to air leak. Elimination of any residual pleural space by careful placement of chest tubes and judicious use of pleural tents or thoracoplasty can be essential to success.

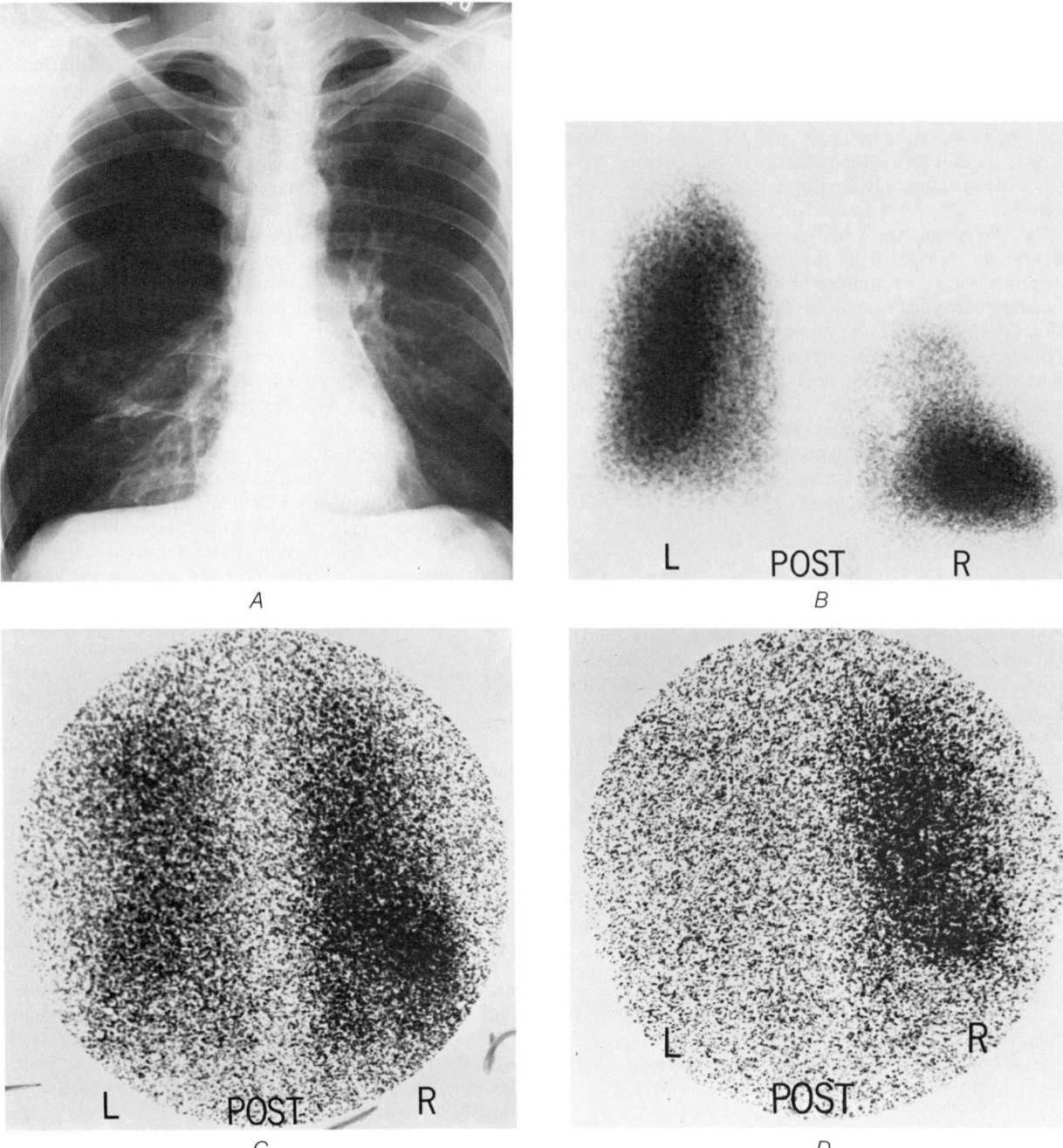

Fig. 17-58. A forty-nine-year-old man with obstructive airway disease (FEV_1 = 50% of predicted) and dyspnea with minimal exertion. *A.* The chest x-ray shows marked radiolucency in the upper half of the right hemithorax, due to giant bullae compressing the remaining normal parenchyma into the lower part of the hemithorax. *B.* A lung perfusion scan with ^{99m}Tc macroaggregated albumin shows loss of perfusion in the right upper and middle lobe regions. *C.* The ventilation scan with ^{33}Xe shows early delay in washout of the radioisotope from the right lung after equilibration. *D.* After 3 min of the washout phase of the ventilation scan, there is marked trapping of the radioisotope in the giant bullae of the right lung. The patient underwent successful resection of the bullae with considerable subjective improvement in symptoms.

Pulmonary Infections

As recently as the early 1960s, thousands of patients each year in the United States required pulmonary resection for lung abscess, bronchiectasis, and chronic granulomatous disease. Since that time effective antibiotics, aggressive methods for accurate early diagnosis, an increased standard of living, and public health programs are among the factors that have diminished the surgeon's role dramatically. Fifteen or twenty years ago it seemed reasonable to hope that suppurative pulmonary infections would remain a common surgical problem only in areas of the world with limited medical technology and limited access to antibiotics. Ironically such problems are becoming increasingly frequent at the high-technology frontiers—patients immunosuppressed following transplant or as part of cancer chemotherapy, and patients with AIDS all too commonly develop serious pulmonary infections.

The pathologic spectrum of pulmonary infections is very broad, ranging from the indolent bronchiolar and peribronchial suppuration of bronchiectasis, to the contained parenchymal necrosis of lung abscess, to the pleural space infection of empyema. The clinical expression of pulmonary infection is determined by the route of inoculation, the competence of host defenses, and the specific organism(s) involved, which can include aerobic and anaerobic bacteria, viruses, and fungi, often in synergistic combinations. This broad spectrum of pathology has an equally broad spectrum of treatment in which surgical management remains important.

LUNG ABSCESS

SPECTRUM OF DISEASE. Lung abscess may be defined as a focus of infection with parenchymal necrosis, usually with cavitation. Distinction between a lung abscess and a consolidated pneumonia is made as areas of cavitation appear on the chest x-ray, and as the peripheral margins of the infection develop sharper definition. Lung abscess and empyema can coexist as confluent or separate processes. Causes of lung abscess are outlined in Table 17-12.

Lung abscess is most commonly a complication of necrotizing pneumonia. Aspiration of gastric contents or sa-

Table 17-12. CAUSES OF LUNG ABSCESS

I. Primary necrotizing pneumonia
    A. Aerobic infection
        1. *Staphylococcus aureus*
        2. *Klebsiella, Pseudomonas,* other gram negatives
        3. *Mycobacteria (M. tuberculosis* and atypical *Myobacteria)*
    B. Anaerobic infection
        1. *Bacteroides (B. fragilis, B. melaninogenicus)*
        2. *Fusobacterium* species
        3. *Actinomyces*
    C. Parasitic infection
        1. *Entameba histolytica*
        2. *Echinococcus (E. granulosus, E. multilocularis)*
II. Aspiration pneumonia
III. Bronchial obstruction
    A. Neoplasm
    B. Foreign body
IV. Complication of systemic sepsis
    A. Septic pulmonary emboli
    B. Seeding of pulmonary infarct
V. Complication of pulmonary trauma
    A. Infection of hematoma or contusion
    B. Contaminated foreign body or penetrating injury
VI. Direct extension from extraparenchymal infection
    A. Pleural empyema
    B. Mediastinal, hepatic, subphrenic abscess

liva produces an infectious focus with enzymatic tissue degradation, mixed aerobic and anaerobic bacterial contamination, and frequently particulate matter that combine to promote abscess formation. Aspiration remains the most common single cause of lung abscess, and has a well-recognized association with altered states of consciousness (Fig. 17-59). Alcoholic stupor is most frequently cited, but drug overdosage, head trauma, cardiopulmonary resuscitation, and general anesthesia can also set the stage for aspiration leading to lung abscess. Because most episodes of aspiration occur with the person supine, the abscess is characteristically located in the lung segments that are dependent in the supine position—the posterior segments of the upper lobes, and the superior segments of both lower lobes. Bacteriologically the infection is usually mixed, with anaerobic mouth organisms such as *Bacterioides* species frequently predominating.

The tissue necrosis that is the hallmark of "necrotizing" pneumonia is a function of the specific organism involved, and is most prominent with *Klebsiella, Pseudomonas,* and other gram-negative organisms. Tissue necrosis is rare with Group B streptococcal pneumonia (*Pneumococcus*), whereas necrosis and abscess formation are frequent with *Staphylococcus aureus* and Group A streptococci. Staphylococcal lung abscess is most common in the first year of life and has characteristic pathology, most frequently with pyopneumothorax and pneumatoceles. The latter are large cystic spaces, typically not containing true pus, that are thought to result from air trapping distal to bronchiolar obstruction. Staphylococcal lung abscess in infancy is also characterized clinically by a remarkable tendency to resolve completely with antibiotics alone, even when temporary drainage of the pleural space has been required.

Establishment of a gram-negative pneumonia begins with major alteration in the bacteriologic composition of upper respiratory flora. The mechanisms that reduce gram negatives to transient visitors in normal individuals are seriously impaired in many hospitalized patients. For example, experiments in mice suggest that an *Escherichia coli* peritonitis interferes with recruitment of polymorphonuclear leukocytes in the lung, increasing susceptibility to gram-negative (*Pseudomonas*) but not to gram-positive infections. Over half the pneumonias seen in seriously ill hospitalized patients are gram-negative, and a significant proportion of such patients manifest a necrotizing infection leading to lung-abscess formation.

Systemic sepsis can produce multiple bilateral foci of parenchymal infection that are radiographically quite discrete, and are most frequently caused by *Staphylococcus* and other gram-positive organisms. One or more of the foci can become an abscess, although most resolve without a trace. Unlike staphylococcal pneumonia of tracheobronchial origin, hematogenous infection does not tend to form pneumatoceles and can be seen in septic patients of any age. Lung abscess developing in a pulmonary infarction following pulmonary embolus is most frequently a special case of hematogenous infection seeding an area of devitalized or injured tissue.

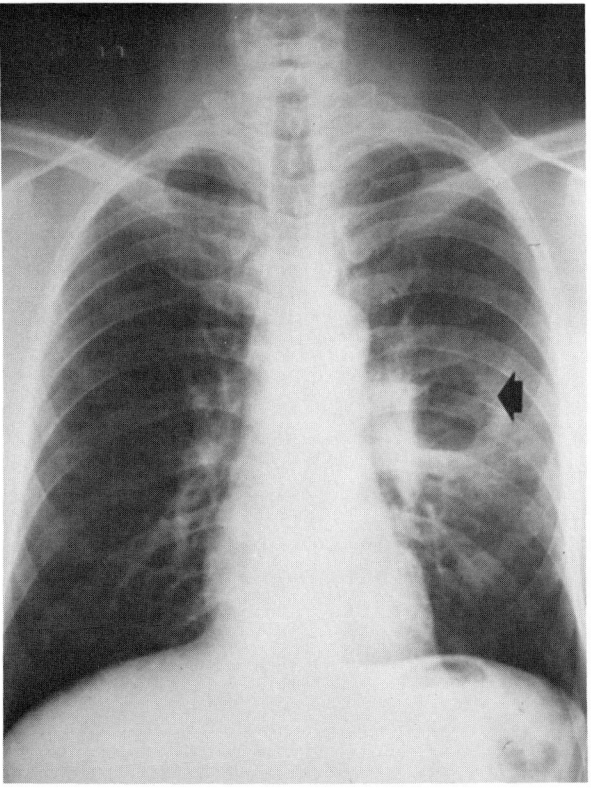

A

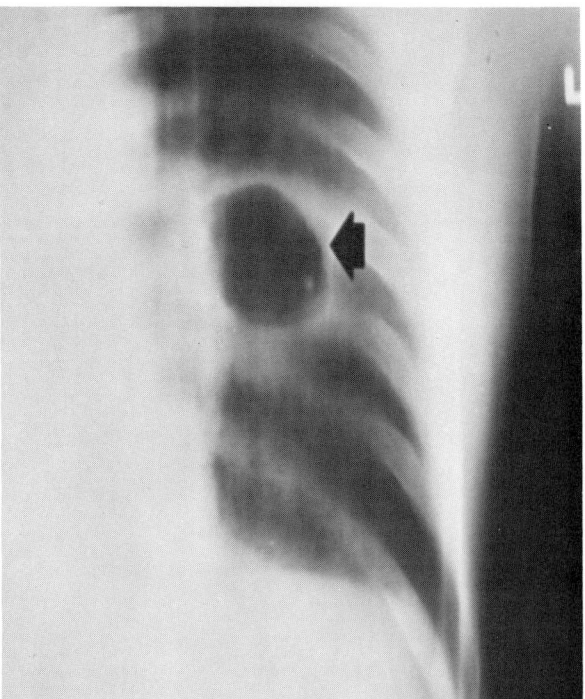

B

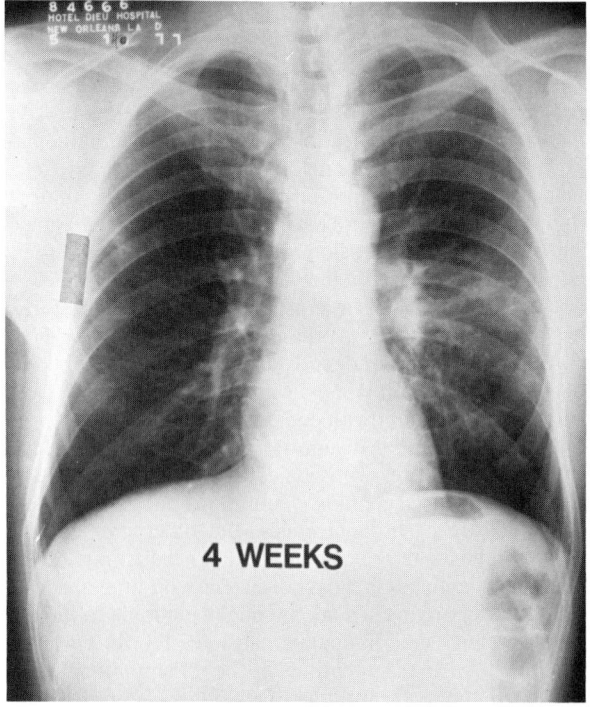

C

Fig. 17-59. Lung abscess due to vomiting and aspiration after an alcoholic binge. *A.* The chest x-ray shows an abscess cavity in the superior segment of the left upper lobe. *B.* A tomogram confirms the thin wall of the abscess, reducing the probability that the lesion could be a cavitated carcinoma. *C.* After 4 weeks of antibiotic therapy and postural drainage the abscess cavity appears to be healing.

A cavitary necrotizing infection can also form distal to an obstructive lung carcinoma or intrabronchial foreign body (Fig. 17-60), a reminder that bronchoscopy is an important diagnostic manuever. Not infrequently a carcinoma becomes visible as the distal infection responds to antibiotic treatment.

In certain parts of the world parasitic infection is a common cause of lung abscess. *Entameba histolytica* can produce lung abscess by hematogenous spread or by direct extension from the liver, in which case it is almost always associated with empyema. Metronidazole is usually effective treatment, and operative intervention is rarely required. Hydatid infection (*Echinococcus* species) is associated with lung abscess in some cases (Fig. 17-61). Intraabdominal pathology is much more prominent. Treatment with oral mebendazole has been moderately successful, but resection has frequently been required. Albendazole is currently in clinical trial and appears to offer the possibility of better results without operation.

CLINICAL MANIFESTATIONS. Regardless of etiology, the clinical presentation is relatively uniform. The patient appears chronically ill, is likely to be febrile, and will often describe recent onset of copious foul sputum pro-

duction, reflecting decompression of the abscess into the airway. Whether the initial infection originated from the airway or the bloodstream, the necrotizing process tends to find its way into the tracheobronchial tree, a develop-

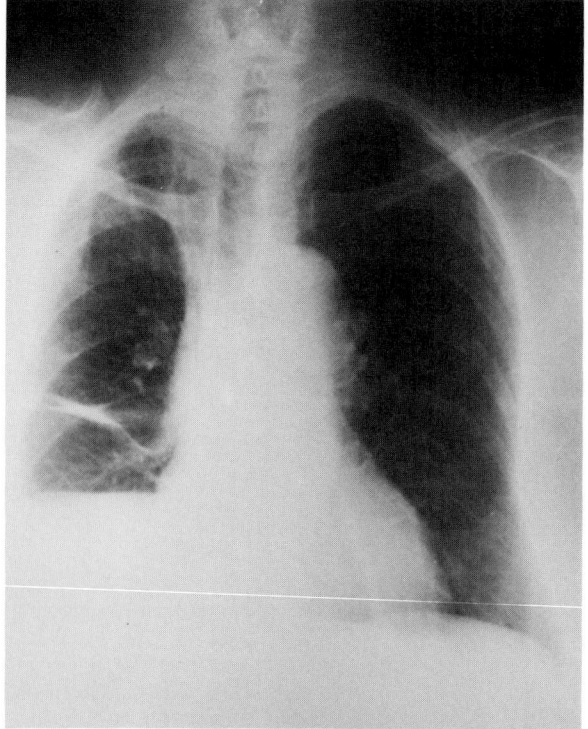

A

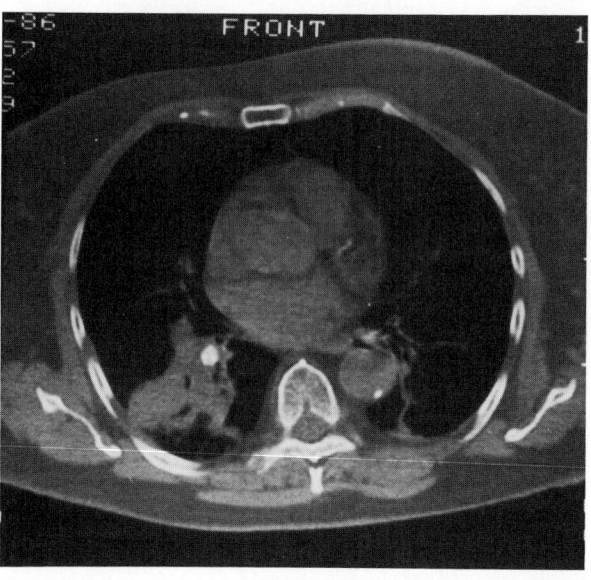

B

Fig. 17-60. *A*. This seventy-two-year-old woman presented with a clinical picture of slowly progressing pneumonia, and chest x-ray revealed right lower lobe consolidation with a pleural effusion. *B*. CT scan demonstrated a large area of consolidation and early abscess formation in the right lower lobe, and a small bone-density mass lying medially within. An obstructing chicken bone was identified by bronchoscopy but could not be removed. A successful right lower lobectomy was performed.

ment heralded radiographically by the appearance of cavitation on chest x-ray. Because of the necrotizing, erosive nature of the communication with the airways, hemoptysis can occur and can be massive. In contrast to pneumonia, dyspnea is not a prominent symptom. Auscultatory findings, if any, are more likely to be attributable to coexistence of a pleural effusion or empyema than to the presence of lung abscess. In the acute phase of abscess development, constitutional symptoms will overlap with those of acute pneumonia. As the process becomes more chronic symptoms frequently ameliorate as the abscess becomes walled off.

In a febrile patient with copious production of foul sputum, the differential diagnosis can be reduced to three entities: lung abscess, bronchiectasis, and cavitating carcinoma. Chronic copious sputum production is most characteristic of bronchiectasis; the other two entities tend to have acute or episodic sputum production. A dramatic febrile illness is most consistent with lung abscess, reflecting its origins in a necrotizing pneumonia, although bronchiectasis and carcinoma can have febrile episodes associated with exacerbations of the inflammatory process surrounding the primary pathology. A chest x-ray showing a well-delineated cavity is against bronchiectasis alone, but the chest x-ray is usually of little help in distinguishing carcinoma from lung abscess, for which bronchoscopy and biopsy are essential. Bronchiectasis is confirmed by bronchography.

TREATMENT. The options for treatment of lung abscess are outlined in Table 17-13. Primary treatment consists of antibiotics and drainage. Antibiotics are administered intravenously in high doses and should be selected based on the sensitivities of the infecting organism. In the most fortunate cases, spontaneous drainage by expectoration is adequate. More commonly, drainage must be achieved by other means, the least invasive of which is bronchoscopic aspiration. Proponents of nonoperative treatment favor at least 8 weeks of antibiotics and "internal" (cough and bronchoscopy) drainage before proceeding to external drainage or resection. Such methods are successful in more than 75 percent of all patients with lung abscess (Fig. 17-59), although convalescence can be prolonged. In one representative nonoperative series the average duration of therapy was 4 months. Numerous surgical series have demonstrated that convalescence can be shortened dramatically in properly selected patients.

The guiding principle governing operative treatment of lung abscess is the establishment of drainage. When internal drainage has been ineffective, external drainage can be established in one of two ways. (1) Tube pneumonostomy is percutaneous insertion of a drainage tube into the abscess cavity, connecting the tube to a water-seal drainage system. The alternative is (2) pneumonotomy, an open drainage procedure that opens the abscess cavity

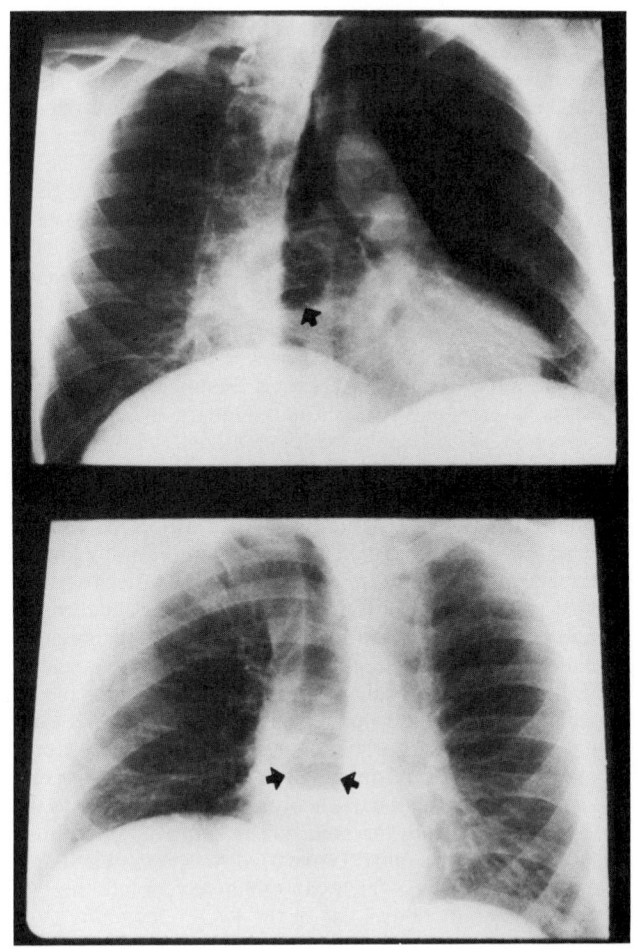

A

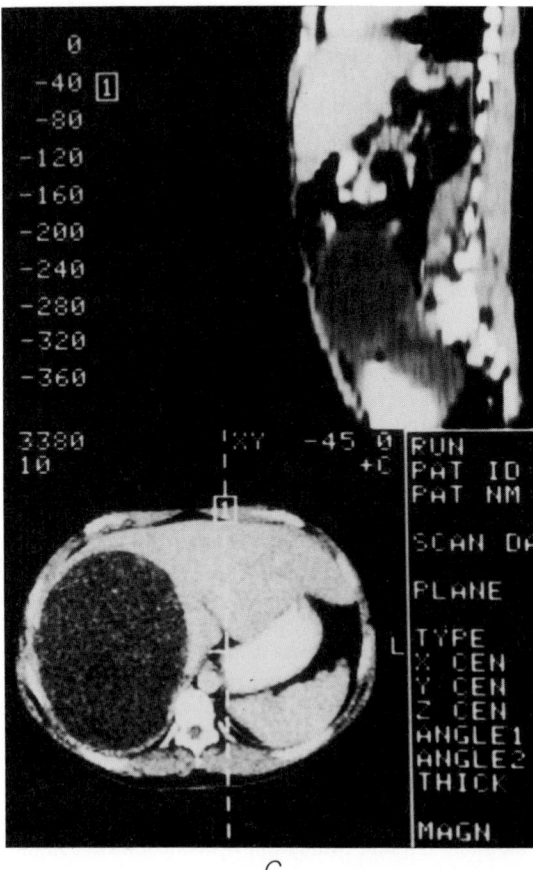

C

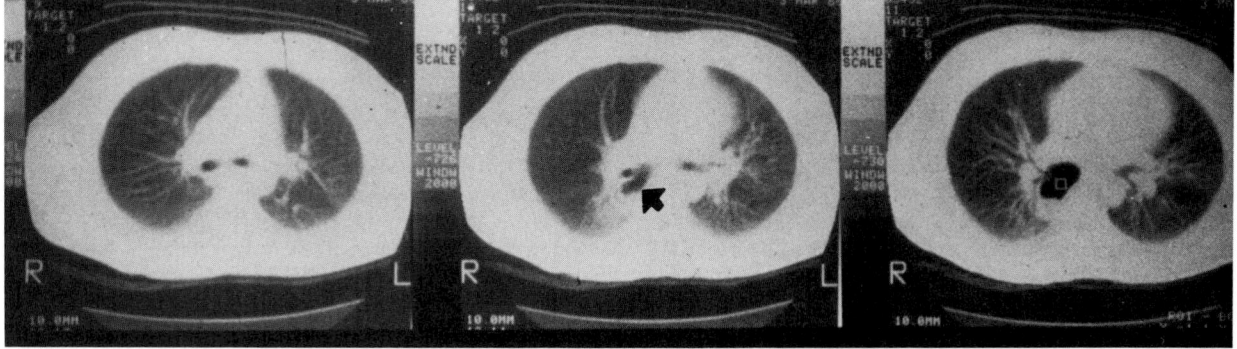

B

Fig. 17-61. *A*. This forty-eight-year-old Yugoslavian immigrant was completely asymptomatic until he presented with a transient episode of copious, foul productive cough. A mediastinal cavity is visible in the oblique views shown *(see arrows)*. *B*. A CT scan of the chest shows the cavity lying just below the right main stem bronchus, and showed that the mediastinal cavity did not communicate with the abdomen. *C*. A CT scan of the abdomen shows further evidence of widespread infection with *Echinococcus granulosus*. The sagittal view shows a large pelvic mass, and the transverse section shows a huge mass in the right lobe of the liver, containing several daughter cysts.

directly to the outside through a generous incision and short rib resection.

Both methods bear obvious superficial resemblance to procedures performed for treatment of empyema. However, there are important differences that are crucial to success and safety. Most fundamentally, both procedures depend on pleural symphysis occurring between the parietal pleura and the visceral pleural surface closest to the

Table 17-13. OPTIONS FOR TREATMENT OF
LUNG ABSCESS

1. Antibiotics and internal drainage (cough, bronchoscopy)
2. External drainage
   a. Pneumonostomy
   b. Pneumonotomy
3. Pulmonary resection

abscess cavity. This commonly occurs in association with infection, and allows drainage to the outside without contamination of the free pleural space. After the body has succeeded in localizing a serious necrotizing infection to an abscess in the lung parenchyma, spilling the contents into the free pleural space can be catastrophic. In addition, the center of an abscess cavity in the lung can communicate directly with large-caliber bronchioles and vascular structures capable of producing major hemorrhage and/or a large bronchopleurocutaneous fistula (a large air leak), especially if the tube penetrates the soft inner surface of the abscess cavity. Therefore, it is critical to accurately localize the abscess in relationship to the chest wall and identify the site where pleural symphysis is likely to have occurred. Unlike drainage of empyema, dependency is not important. Abscess cavities close to the lung periphery are most likely to stimulate an aggressive pleural reaction, are least likely to be lined with major structures, and will be the ones most suitable for external drainage. Fortunately, most abscesses are more peripheral than central; this is particularly true of the common variety caused by aspiration.

Accurate localization of the abscess is obviously critical, and complete evaluation with chest x-rays in multiple views is the minimum required. Chest CT scan should be obtained if possible, it allows placement of skin markers over what appears to be the best drainage site. Ultrasound can be equally helpful and can be used during tube insertion. An essential preliminary step in any method of external drainage is location of the cavity with an aspirating needle inserted along the path proposed for drainage.

If the external drainage procedurre accidentally contaminates the free pleural space, separate drainage of the pleural space is established with a separate tube and drainage system. In performing a pneumonotomy, if inspection through the incision suggests that adequate symphysis has not occurred, the wound can be packed open down to the level of the external surface of the parietal pleura. After several days this usually results in an exuberant pleural reaction and symphysis allowing safe access to the abscess cavity

Choosing between pneumonotomy and pneumonostomy is a purely clinical judgment. Closed-tube drainage (pneumonostomy) is generally adequate and is enjoying a resurgence of popularity in the 1980s (Fig. 17-62), especially in children, based on the impressive results reported in several small series. Tube drainage is theoretically limited by the viscosity and particulate content of the pus. Even so, percutaneous drainage through small-caliber pigtail catheters inserted by invasive radiologists

has had some reported success as well, and seems likely to become a more common practice. On the other hand, the presence of a foreign body in the abscess cavity is thought to increase the risk of erosion and hemorrhage. Pneumonotomy unquestionably provides the swiftest and most reliable drainage, and for that reason might be favored for cavities containing large volumes of especially viscid pus mixed with a large amount of necrotic debris, but open drainage also leaves the patient with a large wound that must eventually heal. It is important to recognize that either method can be complicated by major hemorrhage or the development of a chronic bronchopleurocutaneous fistula.

The most definitive operative treatment for lung abscess is pulmonary resection. Standard indications for resection are chronicity with symptoms, serious hemorrhage, and suspicion of associated carcinoma. Lobectomy is ordinarily preferred to simplify dissection and preserve protective tissue planes. Resection has the advantage of removing the entire infection promptly, and is less hazardous than external drainage when the abscess is very large or centrally located. On the other hand, resection does not eliminate the risk of pleural space contamination. It can be technically difficult to remove a thin-walled abscess presenting close to the visceral pleura without spillage, and empyema following lobectomy is far more serious than primary empyema. Anesthetic technique and patient positioning are critical to prevent spillage of pus through the tracheobronchial tree across to the dependent lung. In the past, the patient was often positioned prone or supine. Currently use of a double-lumen endotracheal tube, which can effectively isolate the two sides, generally allows use of the lateral decubitus position. Safety can be further augmented by frequent intraoperative bronchosopy performed from the head of the table through the endotracheal tube, providing accurate irrigation and aspiration of the airways.

Life-threatening hemorrhage requires prompt resection once the bleeding site is unequivocally localized by bronchoscopy. Unfortunately, this complication most frequently arises in patients least able to tolerate thoracotomy, who are often bleeding because of coagulopathy secondary to sepsis and multiple organ failure. Acceptable temporizing measures designed primarily to protect the uninvolved lung include insertion of a double-lumen endotracheal tube, placement of a bronchial blocker on the affected side, and aggressive toilet of the unaffected side with rigid or flexible bronchoscopy. Bronchial artery embolization is worth consideration but is limited by the rich collateral circulation of the lung.

ACQUIRED IMMUNE DEFICIENCY SYNDROME (AIDS)

Cancer chemotherapy and organ transplantation are creating a steadily increasing population of immunologically compromised individuals who would not have been alive 20 years ago. Patients nursed through major trauma or complications of surgery exhibit a characteristic spectrum of immunologic compromise. As if the increasing numbers put at risk iatrogenically were not enough, pa-

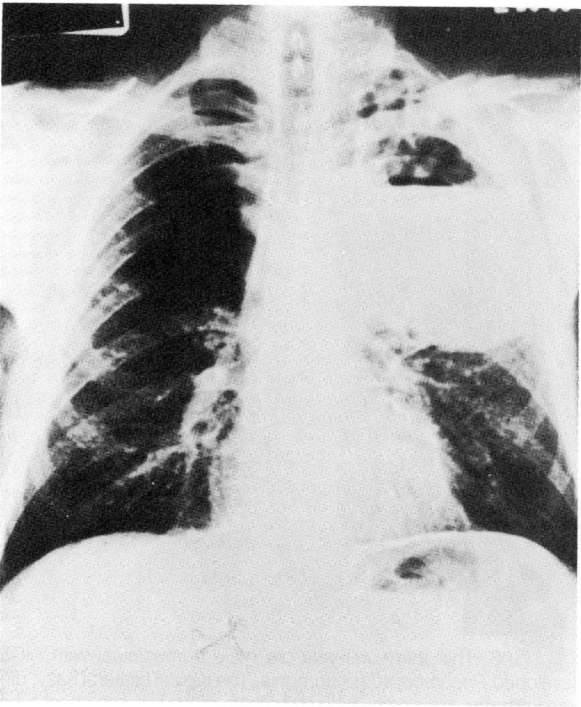

A

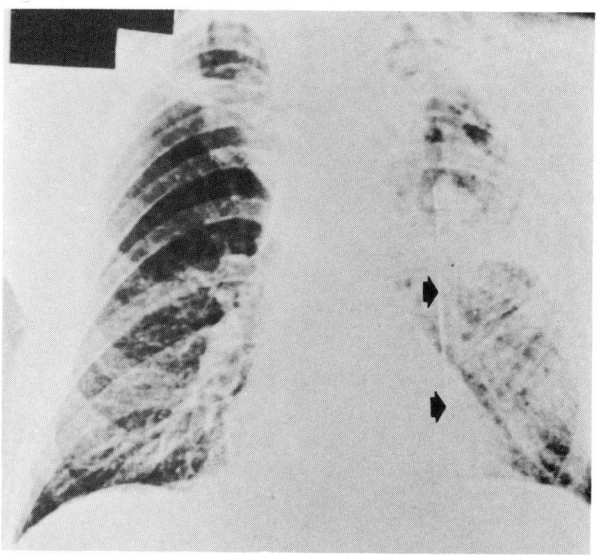

B

Fig. 17-62. *A.* Chest x-ray shows a large abscess cavity in the left upper lobe. The abscess appeared very anterior and adherent to the parietal pleura in lateral views (not shown), making it ideal for percutaneous drainage. *B.* At the bedside, a chest tube *(see arrows)* was inserted in the abscess cavity, and drained 900 mL of thick pus in the first 48 h. After 1 week the tube was amputated, leaving a short segment in the cavity as a straight drain. The patient was discharged on oral antibiotics, and the tube was removed 4 weeks later. *C.* A chest x-ray done 3 months after discharge showed mild residual scarring and a vague outline of the cavity in the left upper lobe. (From: *Mengoli L: J Thorac Cardiovasc Surg 90:189, 1985, Figs 8, 9, 10, with permission.*)

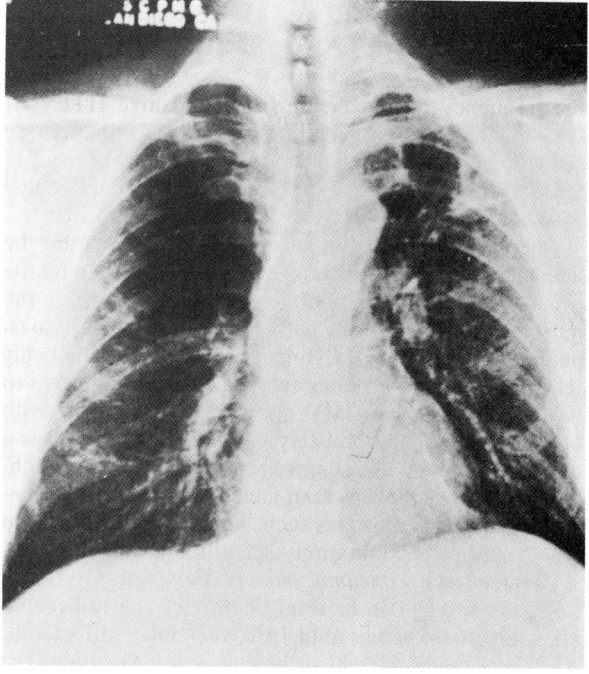

C

tients with the acquired immune deficiency syndrome (AIDS) are beginning to crowd wards in New York City, San Francisco, and elsewhere. All these kinds of susceptible patients share a predilection for pulmonary infections caused by some familiar agents, but even more so by organisms rarely seen in healthy individuals. Perhaps reflecting the fact the lung is the only organ capable of presenting pathogens to a delicate nonsquamous epithelium many times each minute, pulmonary infections are the most common infections seen in immunocompromised patients.

AIDS was defined in 1981 in a group of previously healthy homosexual men with *Pneumocystic carinii* pneumonia and mucosal candidiasis. The causative agent, a retrovirus named the ''human T-lymphotrophic virus type III (HTLV-III),'' was identified in 1983. By early 1986 over 17,000 cases had been reported with 9000 deaths, and it has been predicted that there will be at least 50,000 cases with 31,000 deaths by the end of 1987, and 270,000 cases with over 160,000 deaths by 1991. There are few examples of infectious disease with a higher case fa-

tality rate in previously healthy individuals. At present the average survival from the time of diagnosis is about 12 months, and the mortality for the disease appears to be virtually 100 percent. The syndrome appeared initially to be confined to highly specific groups (73 percent are homosexual males and 17 percent are intravenous drug abusers), but persons outside those groups are legitimately alarmed by the increasing evidence of the disease in the general population. Transmission by heterosexual contact and by blood transfusion has been especially disquieting. Adding to the anxiety is uncertainty concerning

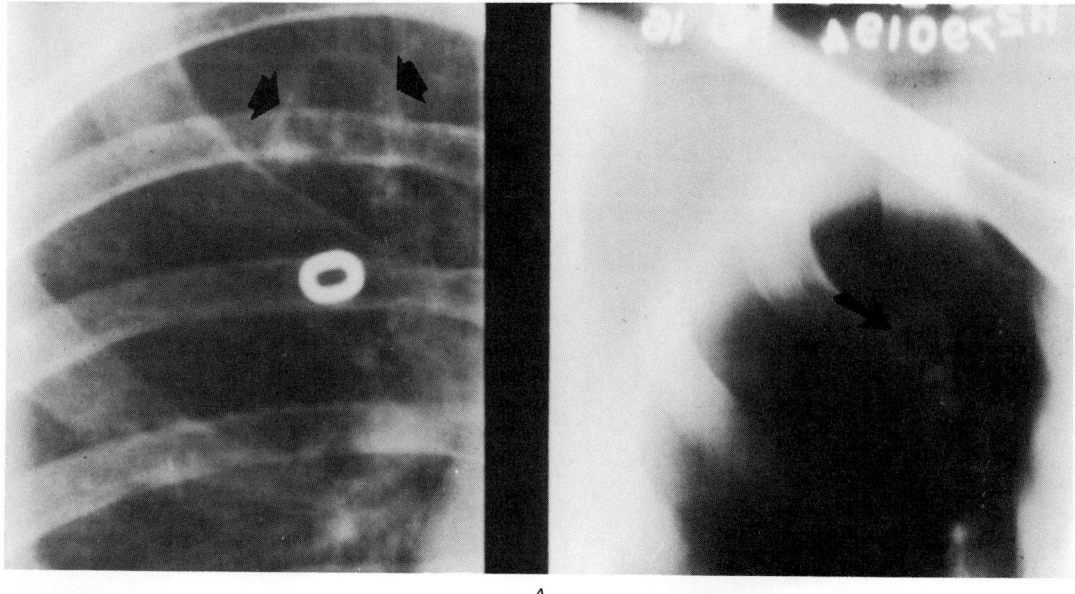

A

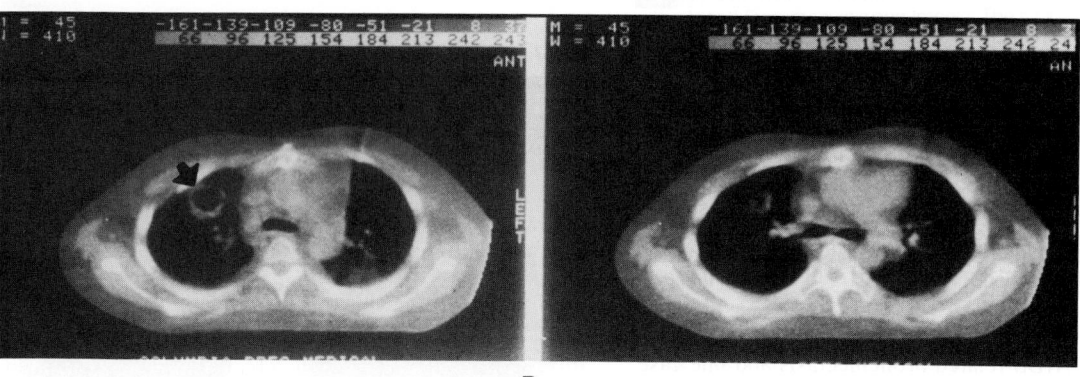

B

Fig. 17-65. *A*. Eight months following cardiac transplant this nineteen-year-old man developed a thin-walled cavity in the right upper lobe, seen (see arrows) in a magnified view of the right apex on the left, and in a tomogram on the right. *B*. CT scan of the lesion (see arrows). The cavity began to grow rapidly, and a right upper lobectomy was performed. The lesion proved to be an aspergilloma. *C*. A thoracoplasty was eventually required for control of a persistent air leak and pneumothorax. A late postoperative chest x-ray is shown. The infection never recurred and the patient was able to resume near-normal activity.

proached aggressively using indications for operation that are the same as those applied to normal hosts with similar infections. Although mortality and morbidity has generally been higher in immunosuppressed patients, it has been possible to perform major pulmonary resection, thoracoplasty, and decortication with excellent long-term results (Fig. 17-65).

BRONCHIECTASIS

Bronchiectasis is characterized by bronchial dilatation, a chronic course, and variable involvement of surrounding parenchyma. Second- to fourth-order segmental bronchi in the basal segments of the lower lobes, the right middle lobe, and the lingula are most frequently involved. Isolated upper-lobe involvement is very rare and is usually associated with tuberculosis or bronchial obstruc-

tion. Approximately one-third of bronchiectasis is unilobar, one-third is unilateral bilobar, and one-third is bilateral. Although the bronchial mucosa usually remains intact and lined with pseudostratified columnar epithelium, the bronchi are filled with mucus, pus, and an occasional broncholith. The changes vary in degree from mild tubular dilation to cystic or saccular changes with almost unrecognizable gross architecture (Fig. 17-66). Collateral

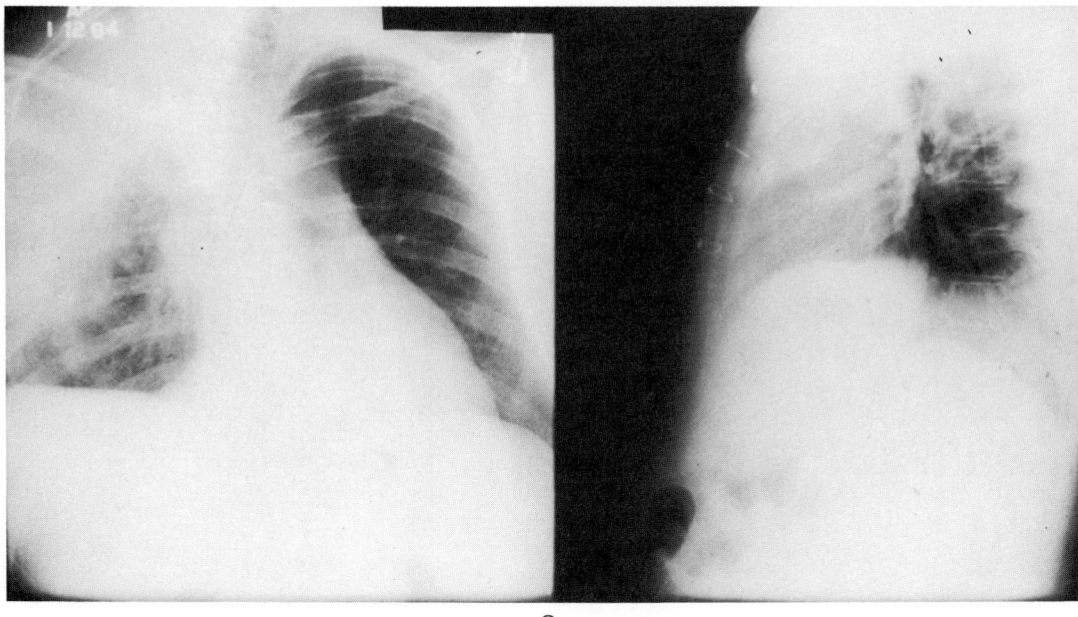

C

Fig. 17-65 *C*. Continued.

air circulation is only partially effective in maintaining expansion of alveoli distal to chronically obstructed segments, and a resected lobe will usually be shrunken and fibrotic. Hypertrophy of bronchial arteries occurs as part of the inflammatory process, producing a locally extensive precapillary left to right shunt into the pulmonary venous system, and laying the substrate for erosive hemorrhage and hemoptysis.

In most cases the disease has to be considered idiopathic. It is occasionally associated with chronic bronchial obstruction by tumor, foreign body, or bronchostenosis. Immune deficiency states have been implicated in certain instances. Kartagener's syndrome (situs inversus, pansinusitis, bronchiectasis) is a rare congenital disorder possibly related to a defect in ciliary function. In many patients afflicted during childhood a history of recurrent bronchitis and bronchopneumonia, presumed to be viral, is present. Bronchiectasis frequently develops during the course of cystic fibrosis.

Fig. 17-66. The cut section of this right lower lobe shows one of several cystic bronchiectatic cavities with surrounding localized pneumonia.

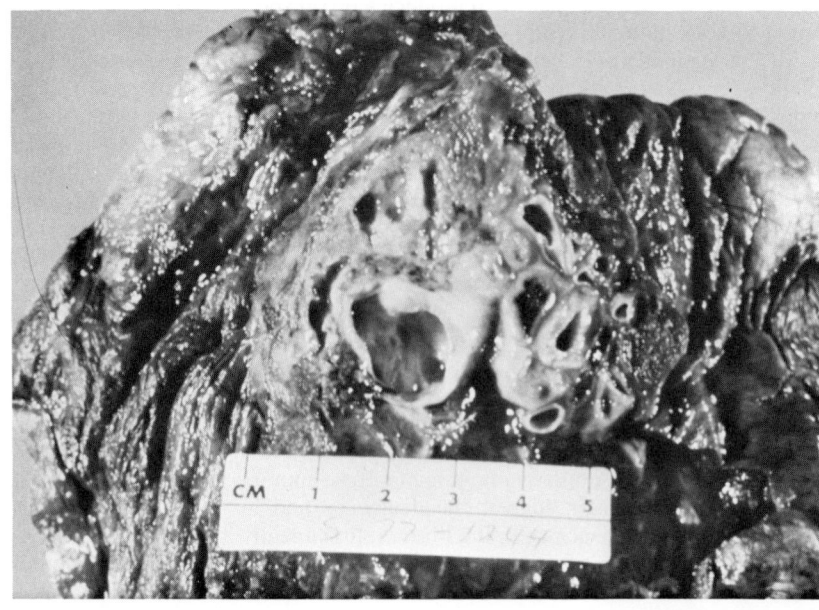

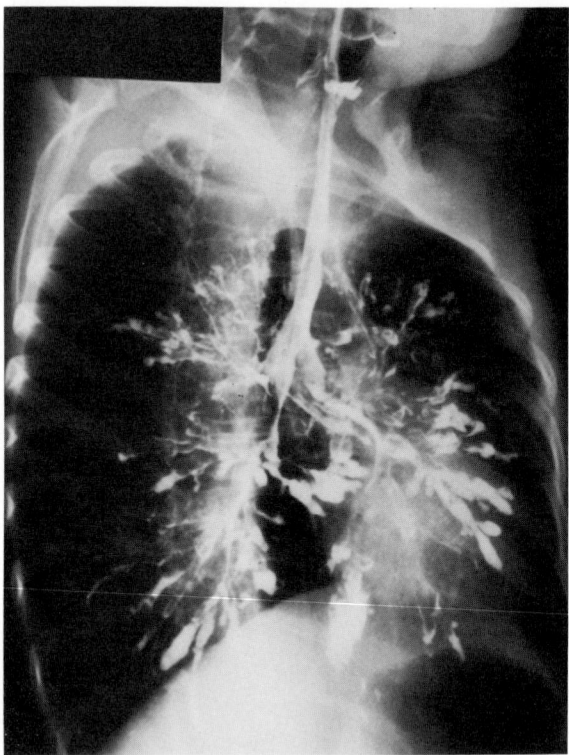

Fig. 17-67. Bronchogram obtained in an eight-year-old Alaskan native, demonstrating widespread saccular and cystic bronchiectasis. This otherwise normal child had a history of repeated respiratory infections, presumed to be viral, during infancy and early childhood. *(Courtesy of JP Wilson.)*

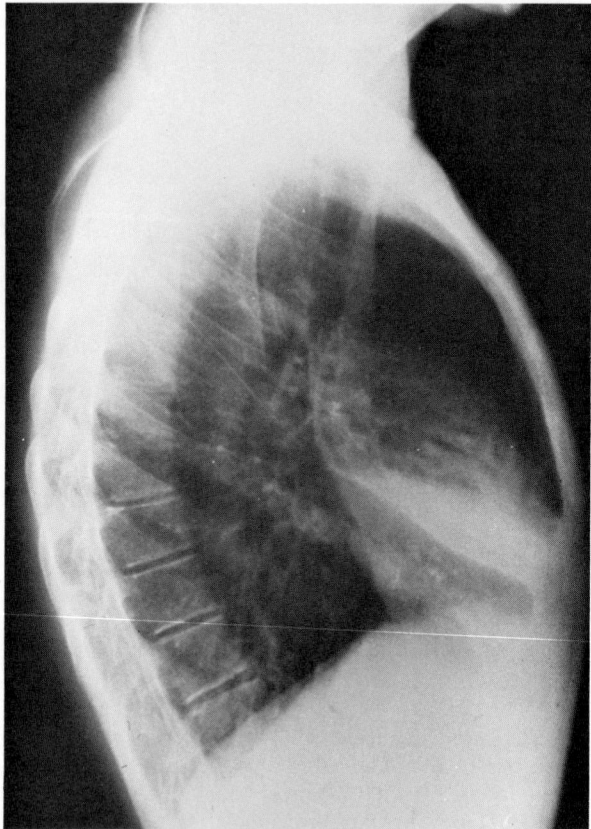

Fig. 17-68. This lateral chest x-ray shows a wedge-shaped density overlying the cardiac shadow and corresponding to a collapsed middle lobe. Resection of the fibrotic lobe showed marked bronchiectasis of the segmental bronchi (middle-lobe syndrome).

CLINICAL MANIFESTATIONS. The clinical picture is dominated by cough and production of mucopurulent sputum, varying in volume from scant to as much as 500 to 1000 mL/day. Fever is usually low-grade with acute exacerbations. The systemic effects of chronic infectious illness can dominate the picture to produce a broad spectrum of constitutional symptoms, weight loss, and retarded development. The disease can occur at any age and is seen equally in both sexes. In the United States an unusually high incidence has been identified in Alaskan Native children, many of whom have required aggressive surgical treatment (Fig. 17-67). Dyspnea is not common except in diffuse disease or in late disease with cor pulmonale. Hemoptysis occurs in about 50 percent of patients, usually late in the disease, and is only major in about 10 percent. Serious hemoptysis is more frequent in association with lung abscess than with bronchiectasis.

Physical findings are dominated by stigmata of chronic disease, and can include digital clubbing and pulmonary osteoarthropathy, even though cyanosis is rare. Auscultatory findings are primarily related to presence or absence of associated pneumonitis and to the effectiveness of pulmonary toilet. A history of chronic profuse sputum production will strongly suggest the diagnosis, and in children associations such as cystic fibrosis, immune deficiency, and alpha₁ antitrypsin deficiency should be ruled out. Chest x-rays tend to be nonspecific but may show linear streaking and volume loss in the affected areas. Bronchiectasis is one possible explanation for the "middle-lobe syndrome," which is isolated middle-lobe atelectasis (Fig. 17-68). Bronchoscopy should be done to exclude the rare case of correctable bronchial obstruction or carcinoma, to obtain accurate cultures, and to aspirate the tracheobronchial tree. Careful bronchoscopic pulmonary toilet can achieve surprisingly durable symptomatic benefit. Complete bronchography remains the definitive test, and is essential to define the anatomy if resection is contemplated (Fig. 17-67). Even bilateral bronchography is usually well tolerated but can produce a febrile response due to chemical and bacterial pneumonitis. It should not be done within about 3 months of an acute episode of pneumonia to reduce this risk, and to avoid overinterpretation of changes that may be reversible.

TREATMENT. The majority of patients with bronchiectasis do not require operative treatment. Postural drainage and chest physical therapy (Fig. 17-69) minimize retention of purulent sputum, and antibiotic treatment of all episodes of pneumonitis should be pursued indefinitely. When debilitating effects of chronic infection become prominent, the anatomy should be carefully defined with

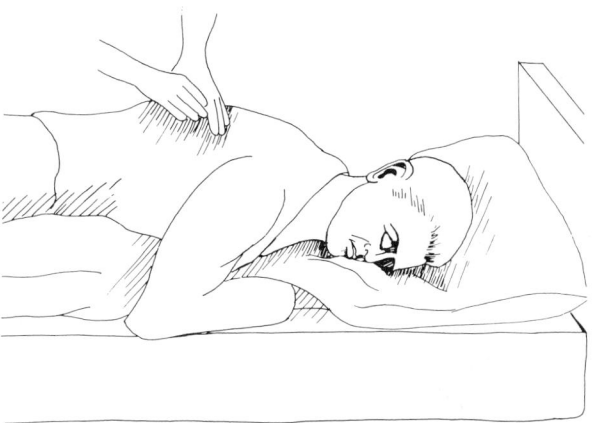

Fig. 17-69. Postural drainage combined with chest physical therapy is important in the medical management of bronchiectasis and in the preoperative care of patients who require pulmonary resection.

bronchography, and resection planned. When extensive saccular disease is confined to one lobe or segment in a sufficiently symptomatic patient, resection is a clear choice. In children, interference with growth should suggest resection. Frequent hemoptysis associated with localized disease deserves operation. Patients with diffuse bilateral disease, of which cystic fibrosis is usually a good example, should be approached cautiously by the surgeon.

All patients should receive a maximal preoperative effort to reduce sputum volume and infection. Care must be taken during anesthesia to prevent spillage of infected secretions into uninvolved segments. A double-lumen endotracheal tube can be used to protect the contralateral lung, and intraoperative flexible fiberoptic bronchoscopy can be used to aspirate uninvolved segments in the ipsilateral lung. As with operation for lung abscess, the risk of postoperative empyema is higher than for clean surgery, and considerable effort must be expended in postoperative pulmonary toilet to assure that residual infected secretions are not allowed to pool in the bronchial stump. The operative strategy is to remove as little normal lung as possible without entering the central focus of infection. This usually requires segmentectomy or lobectomy. Disease so localized as to be treatable with wedge resection probably should not come to operation. Pneumonectomy is almost never indicated for bronchiectasis.

As with many clinical situations in which choice of therapy is based largely on quality of life decisions, there are no prospective controlled series to compare relative benefits of medical versus surgical treatment. In one recent series of 40 patients, the 24 patients resected had an 80 percent chance of becoming nearly or totally asymptomatic. Viewing the group as a whole, the authors estimated that 70 percent of patients with symptomatic bronchiectasis will develop persistent or progressive symptoms on medical therapy. Similar conclusions have been reached in a number of series reported by surgeons, and it is probably fair to say that operation offers the greatest chance for achieving normal or near normal life, if the analysis is confined to the kinds of patients who tend to come to the attention of surgeons with an interest in bronchiectasis.

TUBERCULOSIS

Sanskrit written in 6000 B.C. refers to tuberculosis as the "King of Diseases." Tuberculosis, then called "phthisis," was well known to Hippocrates. A generation beginning to face an uncertain battle with the AIDS complex would do well to recall that pulmonary tuberculosis was epidemic in Europe during the eighteenth and nineteenth centuries and took an extraordinary toll on young adults in the prime of life. In the United States in the 1940s pulmonary resection for tuberculosis carried a mortality rate of about 25 percent, and effective chemotherapy did not exist until streptomycin was discovered in 1944. Tuberculosis remained epidemic in part of the United States (Alaska) as recently as the early 1960s. Yet in a little over 20 years the treatment of tuberculosis has largely been reduced to a straightforward recipe of medical therapy. In spite of such astounding progress, however, about 30,000 new cases are diagnosed each year, and a fraction of these will continue to present operative challenges that are characteristic of the disease.

PATHOPHYSIOLOGY AND CLINICAL MANIFESTATIONS. In broad outline a pulmonary infection with *Mycobacterium tuberculosis* behaves like a lung abscess, with notable differences based primarily on the peculiar growth characteristics of the organism and the nature of the host response. The disease usually becomes clinically apparent when a previously acquired and quiescent infection is reactivated, usually in the apical or posterior segments of an upper lobe or in the superior segment of a lower lobe. In an immunocompetent host the characteristic cycle of caseous necrosis and scar formation will eventually produce what amounts to a tuberculous lung abscess. Just as with pyogenic lung abscess, the smouldering central focus of infection tends to find communication with the tracheobronchial tree, providing a route for drainage and expectoration of purulent sputum loaded with tubercle bacilli, and allowing ingress of air to produce cavitation. The ultimate extent of infection is determined by the size of the inoculum, the immune competence of the host, and the success of antituberculous drugs. Rapid progression can produce a tuberculous empyema surrounding a destroyed lung. If growth of the bacillus is controlled, the cavity may collapse and obliterate or may remain open indefinitely. Such cavities ("open negative") are no longer sites of tuberculous infection but remain potential sites for secondary infection, the classic example of which is an *Aspergillus* "fungus ball" (mycetoma).

As with lung abscess and bronchiectasis, the intense inflammatory process in the periphery of a cavity tends to promote hypertrophy of bronchial arterial and pulmonary arterial branches. These may be eroded by the necrotizing process in the center of the cavity to produce hemoptysis, which can be life-threatening. The vessel responsi-

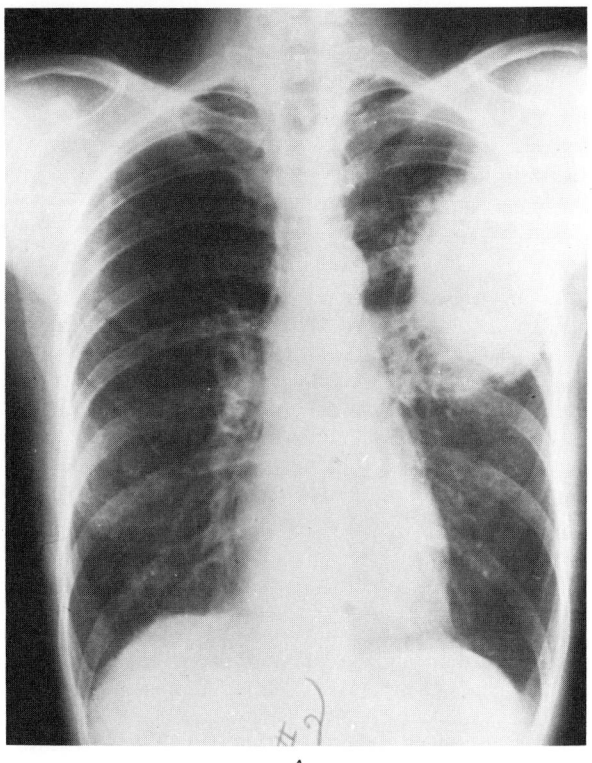

A

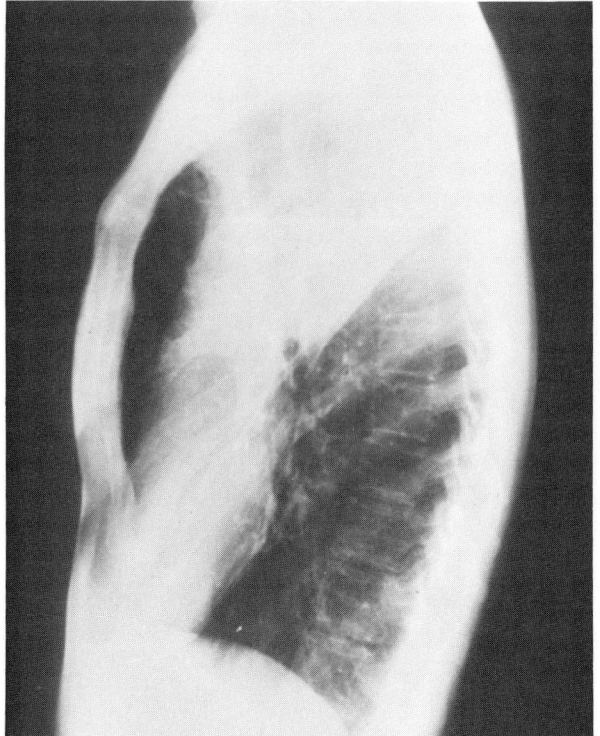

B

Fig. 17-70. Pulmonary tuberculosis, active. *A* and *B*. A large mass in the left upper lobe that was associated with marked atypia of cells obtained by bronchoscopy, and negative sputum smears for acid-fast bacilli. The resected lobe showed active tuberculosis without cavitation.

ble is most frequently a dilated pulmonary arterial branch, referred to as a Rasmussen aneurysm. The management of massive tracheobronchial hemorrhage has been discussed in connection with lung abscess. Because a tuberculous cavity is likely to be more chronic, when major hemoptysis occurs the vessel involved is likely to be larger than that seen in a pyogenic lung abscess, and emergency pulmonary resection is often necessary.

On occasion the most intense inflammatory process is confined to regional lymph nodes, which can enlarge enough to produce bronchial stenosis and distal atelectasis—one cause of the middle-lobe syndrome. If this occurs distal to an evolving cavity, rapid expansion can occur due to air trapping, to produce a "tension cavity." The responsible nodes are choked with caseating granulomata. Discrete bronchial stenosis can also be seen without evidence of extrinsic compression, in which case it is usually ascribed to an intense tuberculous bronchitis occurring in a segment draining an active parenchymal infection.

In a typical case of pulmonary tuberculosis the diagnosis is easily made on the basis of characteristic cavitary changes in an upper lobe on chest x-ray, occurring in a patient with a positive PPD whose sputum has grown *Mycobacterium tuberculosis*. A suggestive x-ray without positive cultures does not confirm the diagnosis, and a negative PPD does not rule out active tuberculosis. Definitive diagnosis rests on growth of the organism in culture (Fig. 17-70). A positive acid-fast stain provides a highly suggestive provisional diagnosis but cannot dis-

criminate completely between *Nocardia* and *M. tuberculosis*.

Culture also allows identification of "atypical" *Mycobacteria,* which deserve special mention. Clinically and pathologically, infection with an atypical *Mycobacterium* can be indistinguishable from infection with *M. tuberculosis*. Resistance to multiple antituberculous drugs is common among the atypical *Mycobacteria*, and chances for a nonoperative cure depend on accurate assessment of appropriate medical therapy. Culture becomes important for identification of a specific species, and for characterization of its drug sensitivities. Even with successful medical treatment the use of three or four drugs for 2 to 4 years can be anticipated. Because of drug resistance, a higher proportion of atypical than of typical mycobacterial pulmonary infections will require operation. *Mycobacterium kansasii* and *M. intracellulare-avium* are the species most often associated with pulmonary disease (Table 17-14).

TREATMENT. Operative treatment of tuberculosis is ordinarily an elective procedure performed after a period of treatment with antituberculous drugs. Emergency operation is only required for life-threatening hemorrhage or massive air leak with tension pneumothorax. The procedure of choice is almost always lobectomy or segmentectomy. The technical precautions necessary to minimize

Table 17-14. CLASSIFICATION OF ATYPICAL MYCOBACTERIA

Group	Example	Principal lesion
I. Photochromogens	*Mycobacterium kansasii*	Pulmonary disease
II. Scotochromogens	*Mycobacterium scrofulaceum*	Cervical lymphadenitis
III. Nonchromogenic	*Mycobacterium intracellulare* (Battey bacillus)	Pulmonary disease
IV. Rapid growers	*Mycobacterium marinum*	Swimming pool skin granuloma

the risk of tracheobronchial or pleural spread of infection are the same as those discussed with regard to resection for lung abscess. Noncontroversial indications for resection include (1) extensive pulmonary destruction with bronchopleural fistula and empyema, (2) persistently active disease with drug-resistant organisms, (3) inability to rule out coexisting bronchogenic carcinoma, (4) pulmonary hemorrhage, and (5) posttuberculous bronchostenosis with recurrent nontuberculous infection. There has always been some controversy regarding resection of an "open negative" cavity. In these patients with negative sputum, the goal of treatment is to ensure that the cavity itself is made truly negative. There is considerable evidence that well-managed long-term medical therapy can produce results at least as good as those following resection. Partial adherence to a drug regimen can encourage emergence of resistant strains, so that noncompliant patients are poor candidates for medical treatment of large residual cavities and should have a resection. This discussion applies equally to typical and atypical Mycobacterial infections.

An occasional patient will have persistent active infection but such limited ventilatory reserve that resection would not be tolerated. Under these circumstances thoracoplasty remains a valid alternative. Thoracoplasty is designed to collapse the affected lung, which can be remarkably effective. Collapse is achieved without entering the pleural space by performing an extrapleural resection of the first five ribs, followed in 10 to 14 days by resection of the sixth and seventh ribs. Although this procedure has its origins in the treatment of tuberculosis, the principle of chest wall collapse is occasionally used to obliterate pleural space following pulmonary resection as well.

FUNGAL INFECTIONS

By about 1900 all the major fungal pathogens had been isolated and named, but recognition of their role in disease underwent a very characteristic evolution. They were initially thought to be rare and fatal infections, but as diagnostic acumen increased, it became clear that mild asymptomatic infection was far more common. Now the pendulum is beginning to swing back somewhat, as fungal infections find their way into our enlarging reservoir of iatrogenically immunocompromised patients. Features common to all fungal infections include protean manifestations in compromised hosts, sensitivity to amphotericin B, and mimicry of carcinoma and tuberculosis. Amphotericin B is a very important drug that has rendered most

fungal infections medically treatable, but it is also a highly toxic drug that cannot be administered as casually as antituberculous drugs are given.

ACTINOMYCOSIS. For many years the actinomycetes were misclassified as fungi because they form branching hyphae and spores. Only in the past 20 years has it been recognized that the actinomycetes are bacteria. This taxonomic distinction has therapeutic relevance, because the pathogens in this group are sensitive to penicillin and sulfonamides but not to amphotericin B.

Actinomycosis is caused by *Actinomyces israelii,* an anaerobic filamentous bacillus that is not found in nature but is a normal commensal inhabitant of the oral cavity and tonsillar crypts. It is not known what causes this organism to become an invasive pathogen, but in about three-fourths of cases some kind of predisposing factor can be identified, such as immunosuppression or breakdown of local tissue barriers (i.e., tooth extraction). About 60 percent of cases are cervicofacial, and only 15 percent are thoracic. Thoracic infection is presumed to result from aspiration of infected secretions. Classically the disease is characterized by suppuration, abscess and sinus tract formation, and relentless invasion with complete disregard for tissue planes. Multiple sinus tracts are observed today in only one-third of cases, and the lesion is more commonly seen as a parenchymal process mimicking bronchogenic carcinoma. Nonetheless, when involvement of ribs or extension into mediastinal structures is seen, actinomycosis must be high on the list of possible causes (Fig. 17-71).

Expectorated sputum, material from a sinus tract, and biopsy material can demonstrate sulfur granules, which are yellow-brown clusters of microcolonies. This finding is highly suggestive, but since *Nocardia,* certain fungi, and *Staphylococcus aureus* are also capable of producing clumps of material resembling sulfur granules, diagnostic confirmation rests on identification of the bacillus within the granules, for which special stains are required. Cultures are positive in only about one-fourth of cases.

The organism is sensitive to penicillin, although large doses are required to penetrate the dense colonies, and medical treatment is most often quite successful. Therefore, the surgical strategy is to make an accurate diagnosis at an early stage of disease. Because the disease can have gross resemblance to fungal infections and to carcinoma, and because tissue stains are essential to the diagnosis, operation is frequently required to obtain adequate biopsy material. Successful diagnosis is followed by high-dose intravenous penicillin and a long subsequent course of oral administration. Resection should rarely be neces-

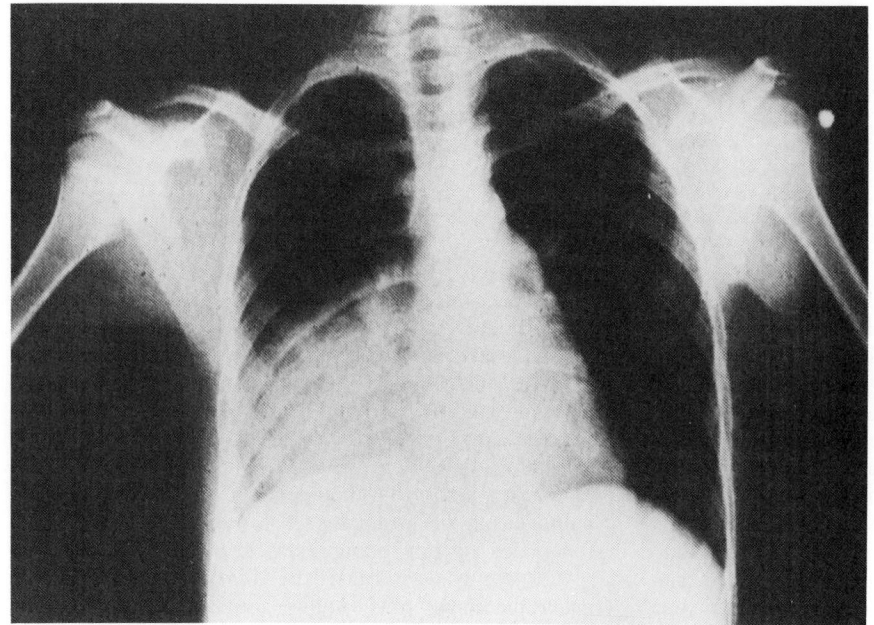

A

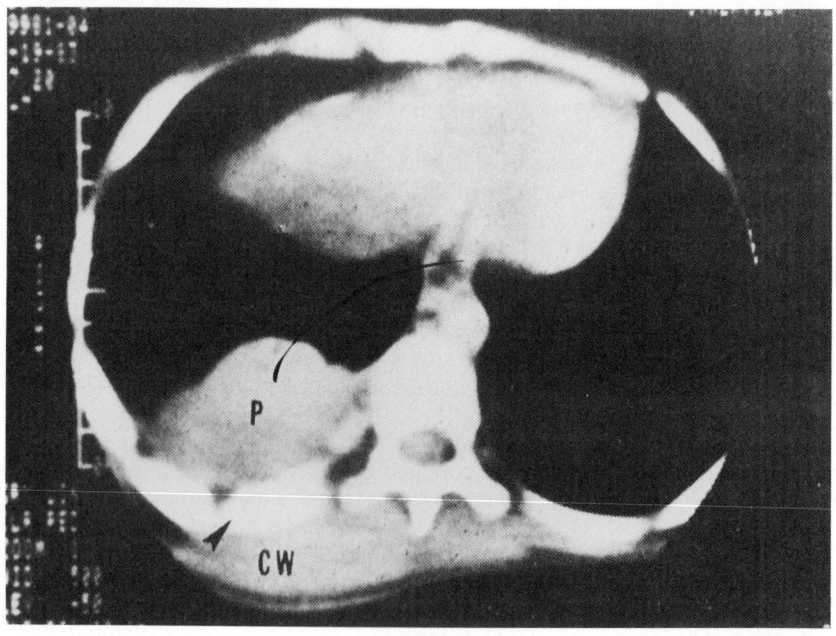

B

sary except in unusually advanced presentations with an inadequate response to penicillin.

Nocardiosis. Nocardiosis is caused by *Nocardia asteroides,* an aerobic acid-fast filamentous bacillus widely distributed in nature as a saprophyte in soil and domestic animals. It is a rare pathogen except in an immunocompromised host and is most often thoracic, beginning as a pneumonic process difficult to distinguish grossly from tuberculosis, fungal infections, and carcinoma. It can also closely mimic actinomycosis, with chest wall involve-

Fig. 17-71. A fourteen-year-old boy presented to his local hospital complaining of a "lump" on his back that had been growing for about 1 month. He recalled an episode of right lung pneumonia 10 months previously. *A.* Chest x-ray on admission showed a density in the right lower lung field and mild levoscoliosis. *B.* A CT scan of the lower thoracic region revealed a mass involving the pleura (P) and the chest wall (CW) with thickening of the eighth rib (arrow). CT sections of the first lumbar vertebra showed lucent bony lesions (not shown). *C.* Biopsy of the mass revealed the characteristic clumped colonies of *Actinomyces.* The patient was treated with 6 weeks of intravenous and 12 months of oral penicillin. The chest x-ray was normal in 3 months. (From: *Golden N, Cohen H, et al: Clin Pediatr 24:646, 1985, Figs 2, 3, 5, with permission.*)

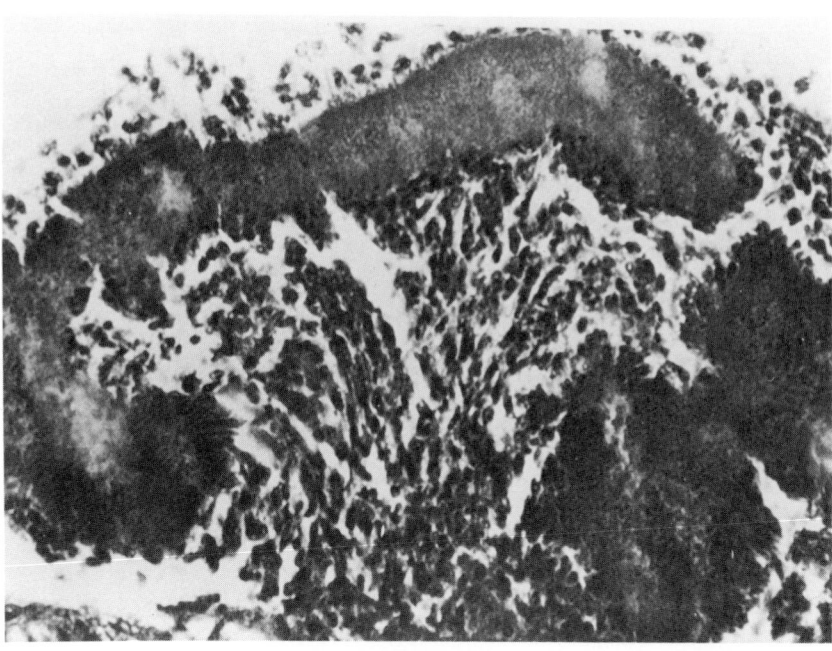

Fig. 17-71 *C*. Continued.   *C*

ment, sinus tract formation, and production of sulfur granules. The acute infection is often much more aggressive than actinomycosis, with extensive pulmonic necrosis and abscess formation, and metastatic dissemination to the central nervous system and elsewhere.

Nocardia is relatively easy to culture and to identify with standard stains, so that the diagnosis can frequently be made by brush or needle biopsy, and even from expectorated sputum. The organism is sensitive to sulfonamides, which usually provide successful therapy. Other drugs can be added in poorly responsive cases (trimethoprim-sulfamethoxasole, minocycline) with good results, and surgery remains purely adjunctive in the majority of cases. Pulmonary resection, drainage of empyema, and similar procedures can be performed safely when necessary.

Histoplasmosis. Histoplasmosis is the most common systemic fungal infection in the United States. *Histoplasma capsulatum* is a dimorphic fungus common in the great river valleys of the midwest, where it lives in mycelial form in soil, decaying organic material, and guano. It assumes yeast form in the cytoplasm of pulmonary alveoli after inhalation. It is extremely common in endemic areas as an asymptomatic infection; the severity of disease is determined by the size of the inoculum and the immune competence of the host. Release of a large inoculum can produce outbreaks of acute pneumonic illness in normal hosts, and usually occurs following an environmental disruption such as excavation or demolition. Such infections ordinarily resolve without specific treatment, but not before widespread lymphatic and hematogenous dissemination has occurred, apparent later as scattered calcific nodules in lungs, mediastinum, spleen, and liver. In symptomatic patients the disease can take many forms and is often distinguishable from tuberculosis only by culture. Skin testing reagents are available but are not as reliable as PPD. Serologic diagnosis is also available but is no more reliable and can be misleading if obtained following skin testing. As with tuberculosis, definitive diagnosis requires growth of the organism from pathologic specimens.

Amphotericin B is effective treatment in the majority of cases and is always the treatment of choice in a serious illness once the diagnosis is made. Most infections are asymptomatic or moderately symptomatic and self-limited, and chemotherapy is not recommended for skin test conversion as it is in tuberculosis. Operation is applied much as it is in tuberculosis. Cavitary disease is quite common, and in a recent large series from an endemic area (Tennessee) this was the most frequent indication for resection. Large, thick-walled cavities that have failed to improve after a course of amphotericin B are likely to progress and can be resected with low morbidity and mortality. Another frequent indication for operative intervention is inability to establish a definitive diagnosis, especially when the lesion presents as a solitary pulmonary nodule grossly consistent with carcinoma (Fig. 17-72). As in tuberculosis, hemoptysis can require operation, and bronchostenosis produced by extrinsic nodal compression can require resection. The lymphogenous phase of *Histoplasma* dissemination leads to remarkable nodal enlargement in some patients, producing symptoms related to compression of mediastinal structures, and a radiographic appearance resembling mediastinal malignancies. Mediastinal involvement can also produce a sclerosing mediastinitis with obstruction of the superior vena cava, pulmonary arteries or veins, esophagus, or tracheobronchial tree. The pathophysiology of

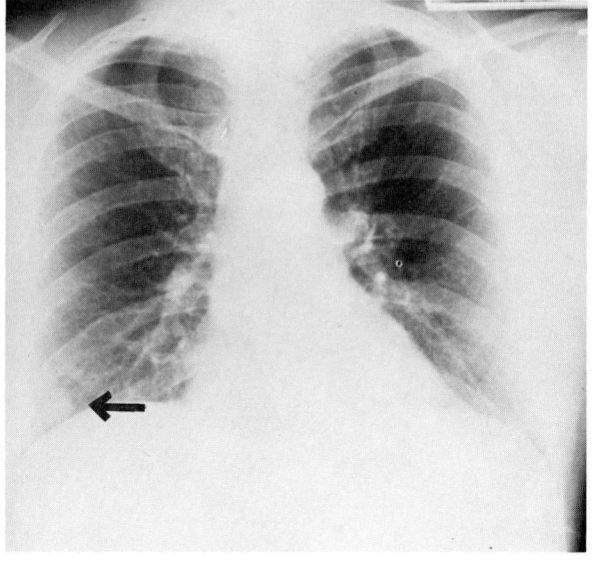

A

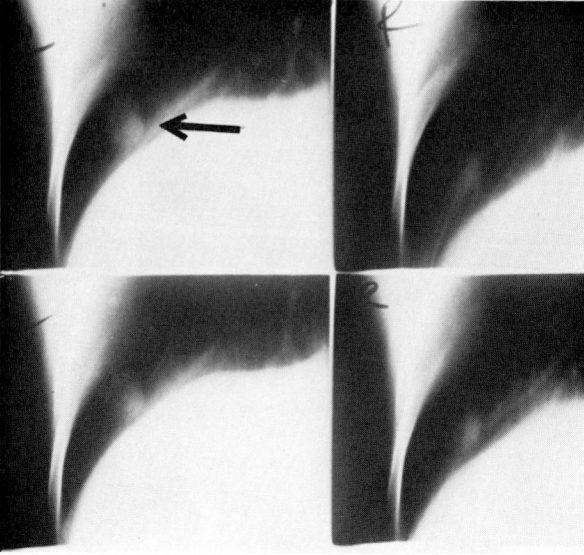

B

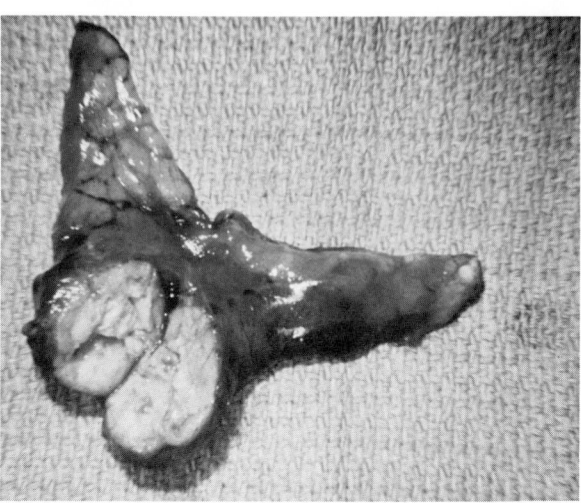

C

Fig. 17-72. Histoplasmosis. *A.* The chest x-ray shows a faint round lesion in the right lower lung field (arrow). *B.* Conventional tomography demonstrates the lesion clearly and shows that it has sharp borders. *C.* The lesion was removed by wedge resection; the cut surface shows a histoplasmoma.

this desmoplastic response to infection is not completely understood but appears to be an idiosyncratic reaction.

Coccidiomycosis. Coccidiomycosis is the second most common fungal infection encountered in the United States. *Coccidioides immitis* is a dimorphic fungus found in mycelial form as a saprophyte in the arid soil of the American Southwest. Arthrospores released by the hyphae are inhaled and initiate the parasitic phase by becoming spherules that release infective endospores. In the normal host most infections are asymptomatic, but some will manifest "valley fever," essentially a mild pneumonic form of the illness. The organism is not difficult to recover from sputum or pathologic specimens. The skin test and serologic titers are almost always positive in active disease but are more ambiguous in the more chronic and indolent forms of infection. Except for a propensity to form thin-walled cavities, the spectrum of

gross and microscopic pathology is similar to that seen in histoplasmosis, tuberculosis, and other fungal infections.

For patients with symptomatic illness requiring treatment, amphotericin B is the primary therapy. As with histoplasmosis, the lungs provide an effective barrier against serious systemic illness in most patients, and specific treatment is frequently not required. Aggressive necrotizing pulmonary infection and disseminated disease are usually seen in immunocompromised hosts, and require early and aggressive medical treatment.

Indications for operation are virtually identical to those applied to histoplasmosis. Resection of cavitary disease and resection for definitive diagnosis of a solitary pulmonary nodule are most frequently performed. Specific indications in cavitary disease include progressive enlargement, hemoptysis, rupture, and secondary infection.

Blastomycosis. Blastomycosis is caused by *Blastomy-*

ces dermatitidis, a round, single budding yeast endemic in the southeastern United States and other scattered areas. Although there is a common cutaneous form, the disease is always acquired through aspiration of spores into the lungs, where it can assume a variety of appearances— pneumonic infiltrates, cavitation, solitary granulomatous nodules, and disseminated disease. The cutaneous form is characterized by crusty, ulcerative lesions from the margins of which the organism can readily be cultured. Cutaneous and pulmonary infection can occur together, and the cutaneous form has a better prognosis. Diagnosis rests on identification of the organism, which can be done with a sputum Papanicolaou stain.

Although it can mimic tuberculosis and other fungal infections, in endemic areas it most frequently mimics bronchogenic carcinoma, and resection will frequently be required if a definitive diagnosis cannot be established (Fig. 17-73). Aggressive infection is treated with amphotericin B. Cutaneous infection and mild pulmonary infection also respond well to 2-hydroxystilbamadine. As with other fungal infections, treatment with amphotericin B can often be avoided in mild presentations of illness, especially in normal hosts during outbreaks in endemic areas.

Aspergillosis. *Aspergillus* is a filamentous fungus with septate hyphae that is ubiquitous in nature. Inhalation of spores from *A. fumigatus, A. niger,* and other species initiates infection in susceptible individuals. Aspergillosis presents in three forms: allergic bronchopulmonary, saprophytic, and invasive. The first is characterized by asthmatic symptoms resulting from host response to fungus in the airways and is of no surgical importance. The invasive form is usually seen in the immunocompromised host, can involve any organ system, and is almost always fatal. Surgical attention focuses on the saprophytic form, produced by colonization of a preexisting pulmonary cavity (an aspergilloma, mycetoma, or "fungus ball"). On chest x-ray the aspergilloma appears as a solid, rounded mass within a cavity, surrounded by a crescent of air between the fungus and the cavity wall (Fig. 17-74). *Aspergillus precipitins* are almost always detectable in patients with aspergilloma. Skin testing is available but is positive in only 30 to 75 percent of cases. The value of sputum cultures has been debated, but recent evidence suggests that two or more positive cultures carry excellent specificity and sensitivity.

For disseminated disease amphotericin B is the mainstay of therapy. Penetration of the drug into a cavity containing an aspergilloma is very poor, so that resection is considered the treatment of choice for a significant aspergilloma. Operative treatment most frequently requires lobectomy, segmentectomy, or pneumonectomy. Cavernostomy (open drainage through the chest wall) is occasionally performed in patients with poor ventilatory reserve and can be augmented by intracavitary instillation of antifungal agents. Operation is most often justified as prevention for hemoptysis, which occurs in 50 to 83 percent of cases and can be life-threatening in a fraction of that total. Even so, operation remains somewhat controversial because it is associated with considerable mortal-

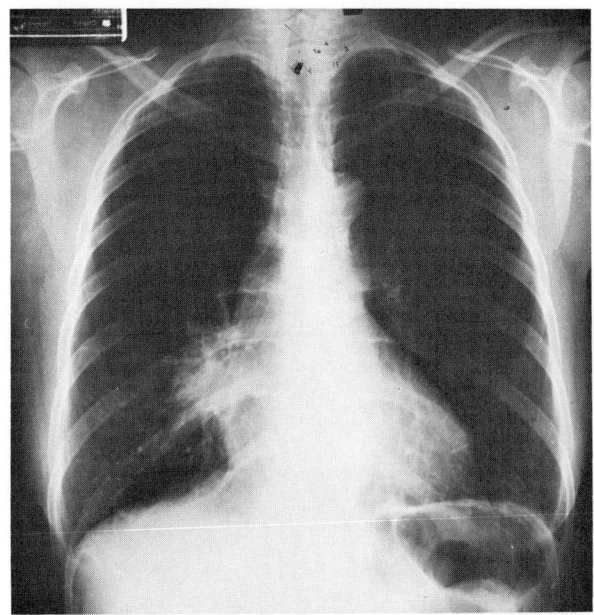

A

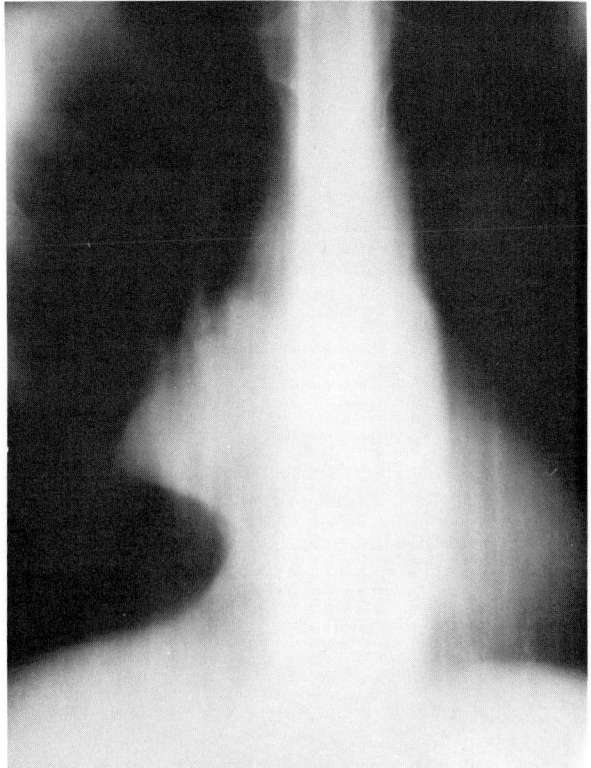

B

Fig. 17-73. North American blastomycosis. *A.* Chest x-ray shows a mass in the right lung field adjacent to the heart border. *B.* Conventional tomography defines the mass more clearly, but neoplasm cannot be excluded. A pulmonary resection revealed active blastomycosis in the right middle lobe.

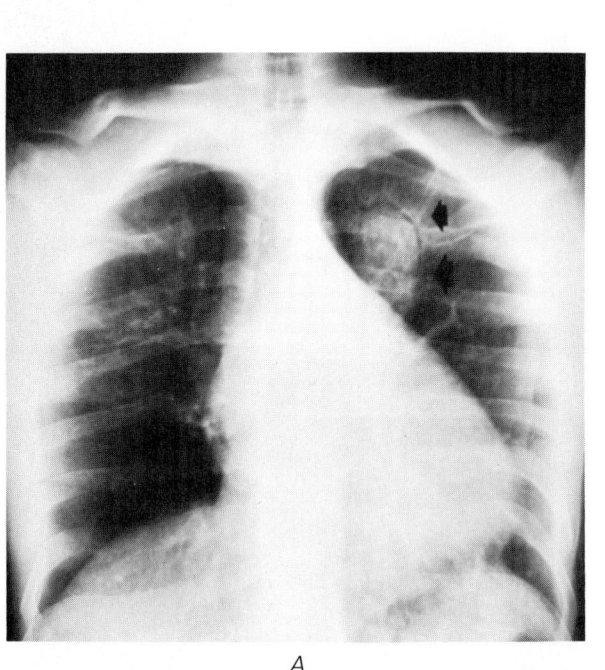

A

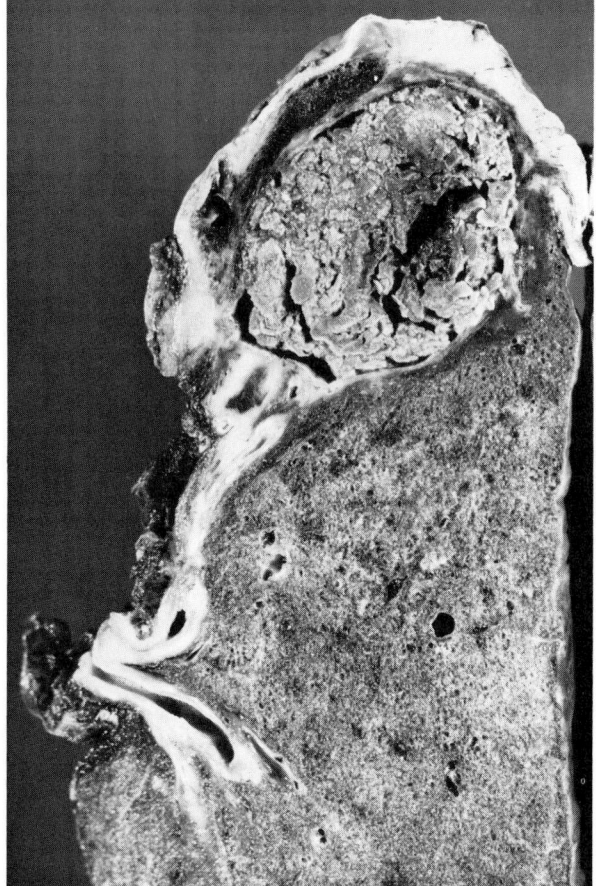

B

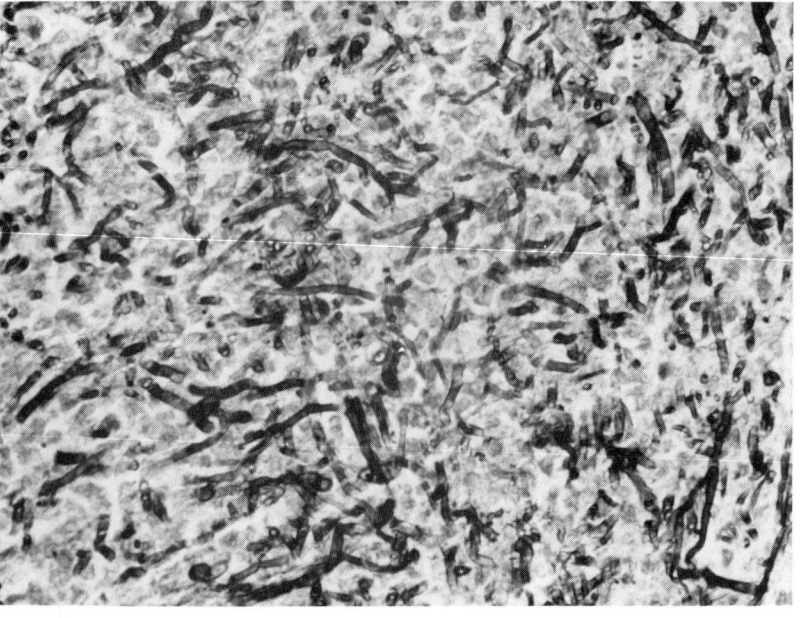

C

Fig. 17-74. A *Aspergillus fumigatus* ''fungus ball.'' *A.* In a patient presenting with recurrent hemoptysis, a lordotic chest x-ray shows a solid mass within a cavity surrounded by a rim of air between the mass and the cavity wall *(arrows),* a finding highly suggestive of an aspergilloma. *B.* After resection of the left upper lobe, cut section reveals the fungus ball filling an old fibrotic cavity. *C.* The histopathology with special stains for fungus demonstrates mycelia infiltrating the tissue in the wall of the cavity.

ity and morbidity. This is related to the poor health of most susceptible hosts and the technical difficulty of resection through dense inflammatory tissue. In a recent series from the Mayo Clinic, for example, either underlying lung disease or immunologic risk factors were present in 92 percent of patients, and complications occurred in 78 percent of patients with complex aspergillomas. In this series and others, operative mortality has been 5 to 10 percent, and complications in "simple" aspergilloma resection have ranged from 25 to 34 percent. Nonetheless, in the Mayo Clinic series the late results were excellent in about 75 percent of cases. In conclusion it is probably prudent to observe small asymptomatic aspergillomas, but in most cases resection should be performed, accepting increased risk in favor of potential benefits (Fig. 17-65).

Cryptococcosis. Cryptococcosis is caused by *Cryptococcus neoformans,* a round, budding yeast found in soil and pigeon droppings. Infection occurs through inhalation of the organism and in most individuals produces a comparatively benign bronchopulmonary illness. The chief radiologic finding is a granulomatous complex with hilar node involvement, indistinguishable from the Ghon complex of tuberculosis. It is rarely of surgical significance except in the compromised host, when the entire spectrum of fungal pulmonary pathology seen in more inherently virulent infections can be seen on occasion (Fig. 17-75). The best-known disseminated manifestation is meningitis. Infection can be controlled in many cases with amphotericin B and 5-fluorocytosine, even with meningeal involvement.

Innumerable other fungi can be associated with pulmonary disease in human beings, but as the list diverges further and further from the recognized pathogens, it becomes increasingly confined to immunocompromised hosts. *Candida,* mucormycosis, sporotrichosis, monospirosis, *Torulopsis,* even *Penicillium*—all have been described. Surgical treatment is rarely indicated and seldom definitive.

Tumors

PRIMARY CARCINOMA

Tobacco addiction (cigarette smoking) is the predominant factor in the etiology of lung cancer. It must puzzle any logical person to observe the paradoxes in the way our society deals with its addiction problems. On the one hand are several substances that, though distressing in individual cases, pose a modest public health problem but are aggressively discouraged with heavy criminal sanctions against production, distribution, or use. On the other hand, we have long subsidized by tax dollars the production and distribution of an addicting drug that is by far this nation's most serious public health problem. How do we rationalize our bizarre tolerance of the "pushers" of this most costly and destructive of all addictive drugs? They spend $1.5 billion dollars each year (more than is spent to advertise any other product) to entice our children to become addicted in their teens to the drug that

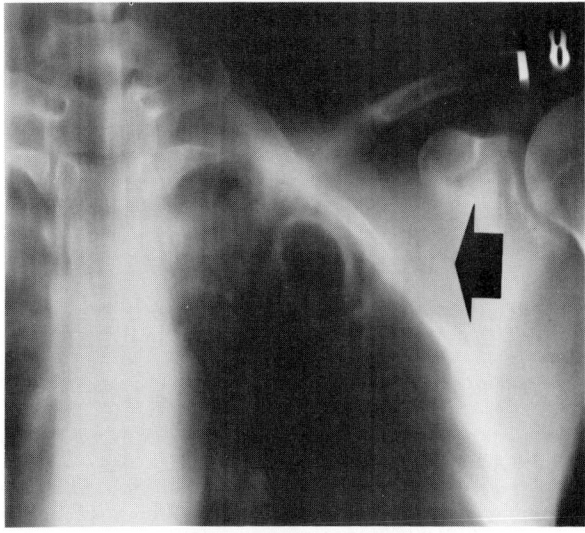

A

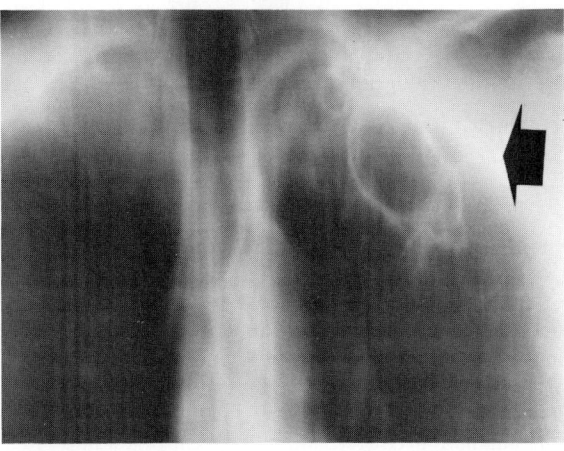

B

Fig. 17-75. *A.* Conventional tomography in a fifty-one-year-old man with hemoptysis showed cavitation within a pulmonary infiltrate in the left upper lobe. Bronchial washings returned a culture diagnosis of cryptococcosis. *B.* Despite two courses of amphotericin B and one course of ketoconazole, tomograms repeated 2 years later demonstrated progressive cavitation. A left upper lobectomy was performed for recurrent hemoptysis and failure of drug therapy.

now is responsible for killing more Americans annually than have been killed in all the wars of this century. Each year in the United States there are 350,000 excess and preventable deaths, and $65 billion in costs attributable to the use of tobacco. For smoker and nonsmoker alike, that represents $200 per person in extra taxes and health insurance premiums, $2.17 for each pack of cigarettes sold. The data from the Framingham study reveal that tobacco addicts are 9 to 10 times more likely to die before age seventy than are nonsmokers. There is no longer any reasonable doubt that those who live or work with tobacco addicts are forced to share a substantial health risk. Physicians must speak clearly on the importance of educating patients and public regarding the consequences of to-

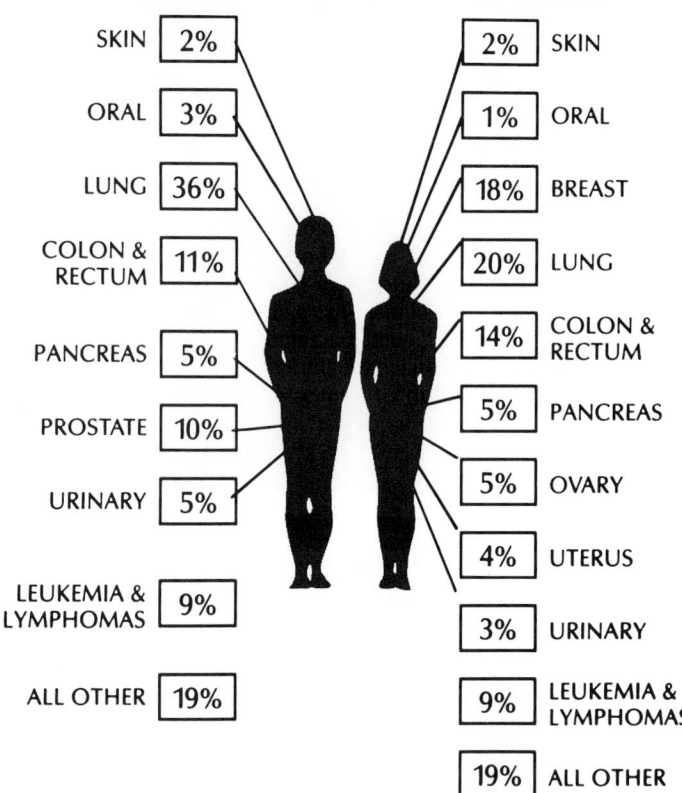

CANCER DEATHS BY SITE AND SEX

	Men		Women	
SKIN	2%		2%	SKIN
ORAL	3%		1%	ORAL
LUNG	36%		18%	BREAST
COLON & RECTUM	11%		20%	LUNG
PANCREAS	5%		14%	COLON & RECTUM
PROSTATE	10%		5%	PANCREAS
URINARY	5%		5%	OVARY
LEUKEMIA & LYMPHOMAS	9%		4%	UTERUS
ALL OTHER	19%		3%	URINARY
			9%	LEUKEMIA & LYMPHOMAS
			19%	ALL OTHER

Fig. 17-76. Lung cancer has long been the leading cancer killer among men; by 1986 it had become the leading killer of women as well. (From: *American Cancer Society, with permission.*)

bacco addiction and on the importance of establishing a smoke-free environment in public and work places for the nonsmoking 70 percent of the population who must not be subjected to this unnecessary health hazard. Reports from Japan and Greece, along with Garfinkel and Auerbach's case control study of 134 cases of lung cancer in nonsmoking women, establish the association between those cancers and the smoking habits of spouses. Even with the best available air-moving and ventilating equipment, Environmental Protection Agency engineers demonstrated that it was not possible to reduce carcinogenic air contamination to an acceptable level for a nonsmoker sharing work space with a tobacco addict. Physical isolation of the addict while engaging in the habit is essential.

In a challenging recent editorial, William Pollin of the National Institute on Drug Abuse in reviewing U.S. statistics reminded us that tobacco addiction causes more excess deaths each year than all other drug and alcohol abuse deaths combined, seven times more than all automobile fatalities per year, more than a hundred times all deaths recorded through the end of 1986 caused by the acquired immunodeficiency syndrome, and more than all American military fatalities in this century put together.

From a trivial health problem at the beginning of this century, and a minor one by 1930 (a death rate of 5 per 100,000), lung cancer has now become the main cancer killer in both men and women (Figs. 17-76 and 17-77). With a death rate of 72 per 100,000 and over 130,000

deaths anticipated in 1986, nearly twice as many will die from lung cancer as will die from all accidents (63,000). A high proportion of those cancers will be in smokers or spouses and coworkers of smokers. Auerbach and his colleagues amplified the long-recognized statistical correlation of smoking and lung cancer by making a detailed analysis of histological changes in the bronchial mucosa of 117 autopsied males. They were able to accurately identify the premorbid smoking habits of the subjects by observing progressive mucosal changes from hyperplasia of the basal cells through stratification, squamous metaplasia, and finally carcinoma in situ. Several groups have closed the loop by producing invasive and metastatic bronchogenic cancers in animal models subjected to forced exposure to tobacco smoke over extended periods. The long exposure required for the development of malignancy provides important and reassuring information for the addict; those who stop smoking will sharply reduce their risk.

Along with tobacco, several other co-carcinogens have been incriminated. There is a potentiation of the cancer risk in tobacco addicts who work in environments contaminated by chromium, nickel, asbestos, mustard gas, arsenic, radioactive minerals, and polycyclic hydrocarbons. Some of the small proportion of lung cancers seen in reported nonsmokers occur in those subjected to these

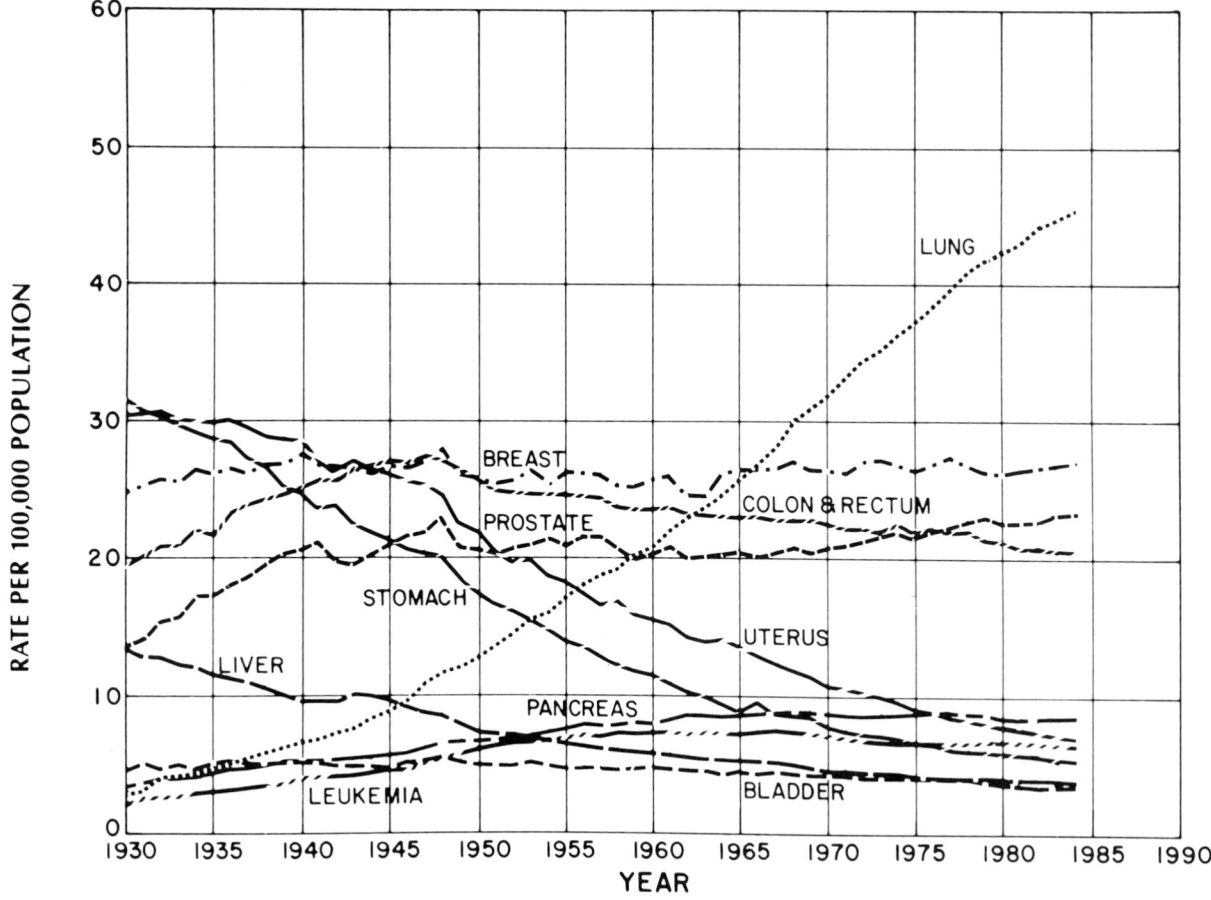

Fig. 17-77. Cancer death rates by site, United States, 1934–1984. Alarming rise in rate of death from lung cancer continues as all other causes of cancer deaths have stabilized or are falling. Rate for the population standardized for age on the 1970 U.S. population. Sources of data: National Center for Health Statistics and Bureau of the Census, United States. Rates for both sexes combined except breast and uterus female population only and prostate male population only. (From: *American Cancer Society, with permission.*)

workplace hazards, but most occur in wives or coworkers of heavily smoking addicts.

PATHOLOGICAL CLASSIFICATION. Several classification systems have been proposed for simplifying analysis and discussion of the various tumors that occur in the lung. Because of distinct differences in approach and management, the most rudimentary division is generally between non-small-cell lung cancer (NSCLC) and small-cell lung cancer (SCLC). Because they have a potential for cure by resection, the NSCLC group have more therapeutic interest to the surgeon. That group of tumors includes squamous cell (or epidermoid) carcinoma, adenocarcinoma, mixed adenosquamous, bronchoalveolar, and large-cell carcinoma.

The traditional histological classification of lung cancers has been based on morphological characteristics visualized by light microscopy. Benfield and Yellin have recently introduced a clinically useful, unifying nomenclature based on more sophisticated modern pathological

techniques, the electron microscope (EM), and immunohistochemistry (Fig. 17-78). These methods prove an interesting overlap among squamous cell carcinomas, adenocarcinomas, and small-cell undifferentiated carcinomas. These observations also clarify the recent reports that show a rising frequency of mixed adenosquamous carcinomas, previously representing under 4 percent of tumors but up to 46 percent in some current reviews. Accurate classification by a pathologist experienced in lung cancer and utilizing modern diagnostic tools is highly desirable.

Most primary bronchogenic carcinomas arise from basal or mucous cells in the surface epithelium of the bronchial tree. Tumors may also arise from the neurosecretory cells or the Clara cells of the distal bronchioles. Atypical epithelial proliferation may precede pulmonary neoplasms. The identification of these changes may provide the early diagnostic clues. Carcinoma in situ is probably a step in the chain of development from squamous metaplasia and dysplasia to invasive carcinoma. An atypical proliferation of Kultchitsky cells is associated with development of the carcinoid tumors.

Non-Small-Cell Lung Cancers (NSCLC). There is frequently a high degree of overlap in the histopathology of most of the various primary lung cancers. Particularly as they become less differentiated, many mixed elements

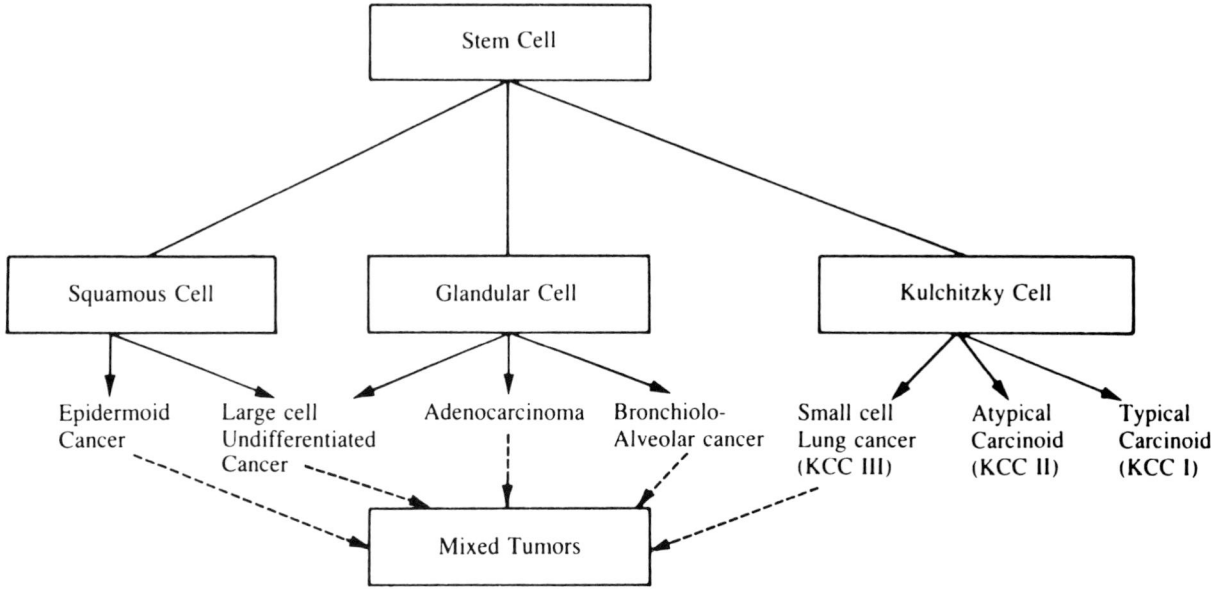

Fig. 17-78. Benfield and Yellin have presented a simplifying scheme for relating the patterns of histopathology seen in lung cancers. There is an increasing frequency of tumors with mixed elements in most current series. (From: *Benfield JR, Yellin A, with permission.*)

may appear that are suggestive of any of the NSCLCs. Except in the most typical situation, the classifications should not be overinterpreted. The therapeutic decisions are largely made on the basis of nodal metastases and other aspects of the clinical behavior of the tumor rather than the specific label assigned.

Squamous Cell Carcinomas. Though more common in upper lobes, bronchogenic carcinomas develop in all parts of the lung. In view of the long exposure to carcinogens in smoke that is required and the progressive mucosal abnormalities that occur, it is likely these cancers are very slow-growing and are present for several years before symptoms occur. It has been estimated that a tumor nodule must go through approximately 30 doublings to become 1 cm in diameter, a size that is large enough to be seen on the routine chest x-ray. This could mean pulmonary tumors may have been present for as long as 8 years before discovery. This slow growth is often a characteristic of squamous cell carcinoma, a tumor that seems to arise after a preliminary squamous metaplasia has replaced the normal respiratory pseudostratified epithelium. The degree of differentiation in squamous neoplasms varies widely. It is occasionally so highly anaplastic that its designation as a squamous tumor is speculative. Until recently, squamous cell carcinoma was the most prevalent type of lung cancer in the United States. Most recent reports documented a progressive increase in the incidence of adenocarcinoma. In many reports, it has now replaced squamous carcinoma as the leading pulmonary neoplasm. The reasons for this apparent change in pattern are unclear, though they may include modification of criteria for determining the histopathology of lung cancer.

Frequently slow-growing and late to metastasize, these tumors may present as central bulky masses obstructing bronchi or as expanding peripheral lesions with cavita-

tion. The centrally located tumors may invade the peribronchial and hilar lymph nodes by direct extension rather than by lymphatic permeation. Evidence of metastases may be absent even with tumors of very large size. When peripheral, the slow growth rate and late metastasis characteristic of these tumors may lead to extensive local chest wall invasion before metastases occur. The surgeons at several large cancer hospitals have recently reported 43 to 54 percent 5-year survival in $T_3N_0M_0$ lesions requiring extensive chest wall resection in continuity with the primary. The Pancoast syndrome represents a specific example of this circumstance wherein a tumor in the superior pulmonary sulcus may invade the brachial plexus, the upper two ribs or transverse processes, and the vascular structures at the thoracic apex.

Adenocarcinoma. These tumors generally arise in the subsegmental bronchi away from the pulmonary hilus. Growth is apt to be more rapid than in squamous tumors, and early metastasis by the vascular route is more common, particularly to the brain and adrenal. Since they are often anaplastic, the pathologist may have difficulty with clear-cut classification, and multiple sections from separate areas of the same neoplasm may suggest a different classification for each area, leading to the designation of adenosquamous carcinoma.

Bronchoalveolar Carcinoma. This variant of lung cancer has some interesting clinical and histopathological characteristics that may distinguish it from the other types. It also often has a more encouraging biologic behavior. It sometimes remains localized, developing as a well-differentiated peripheral tumor. Electron microscopy has been reported to show cellular features suggestive of alveolar origin in some instances, while other tumors have contained atypical Clara cells suggestive of an origin in bronchioles. Resection of the solitary or localized tumor has given a 5-year cure rate from 50 to 75 percent. This contrasts remarkably with the diffuse form of bronchioloalveolar cell carcinoma, in which there is rapid dissemination of the neoplasm in one or both lungs, with no possible consideration of operative treatment. The diffuse form of the neoplasm may be the result of aerogenic dissemination through the tracheobronchial tree from an initial single focus of tumor. In both forms of the disease, it may be possible to demonstrate the typical cells of the neoplasm distributed in alveoli of the surrounding lung parenchyma. Up to one-third of the patients with this relatively rare form of lung cancer may have no significant smoking history.

Scar Carcinoma. The term "scar carcinoma" has been used increasingly in recent years to refer to tumors that seem to arise at the site of previous pulmonary disease (Fig. 17-79). When a patient with previous pulmonary tuberculosis develops a neoplasm in the same area that was scarred by the tuberculosis process, there is generally a speculation about the cause-and-effect relationship. These lesions may be adenocarcinoma or bronchiolar cell carcinoma, and often are of mixed cellular appearance. There is a predominance of upper-lobe location.

Small-Cell Lung Cancer (SCLS). The small-cell anaplastic carcinoma, sometimes referred to as "oat cell carcinoma," is a highly malignant, rapidly growing neoplasm that is most often central in location because of origin from a proximal bronchus. In addition to early spread by hilar and mediastinal lymph-node involvement, this tumor aggressively invades local structures and is disseminated by early vascular invasion. Because of its rapid growth and spread, many consider the oat cell carcinoma to have no place among the bronchogenic tumors that are treated by surgical resection. It has become apparent that certain histologic subtypes of small-cell undifferentiated carcinoma have a better prognosis after curative resection (Fig. 17-80). A number of encouraging multimodal therapy investigative protocols are underway that provide some hope that short-term outlook might be better than has been believed. Surgical resection may still have an important role in the intermediate- (polygonal, fusiform) cell type of small-cell carcinoma, particularly when peripherally located without evidence of lymph-node spread. It is important for the pathologist to distinguish the variants of small-cell carcinoma, because the treatment may depend on the specific subtype.

STAGING. To share information and to standardize evaluation of protocols, the recommendations of the American Joint Committee on Cancer (AJCC) and the International Union Against Cancer (IUCC) have had their systems reconciled with Mountain's staging and the American Joint Committee Task Force on Lung Staging Revision. Recommended variations from the previous AJCC scheme include several modifications of the TNM descriptors. A T_4 category denoting local mediastinal, visceral, great vessel, or bony invasion, or the presence of cytologically malignant pleural effusion has been added and N_3 has been redefined to include contralateral mediastinal, contralateral hilar, or scalene-supraclavicular nodal involvement. Stage III has been subclassified as a and b (b meaning T_4 or N_3 disease). Stage IV has been added to include all M_1 tumors.

Since this classification deviates from the more usually reported earlier AJCC classification, it is worth emphasizing several of the modifications from that version. Stage I no longer includes any patients with any nodal metastases. Stage III has been divided into one group with large locally invasive tumors but with nodes confined to the ipsilateral chest (IIIa) and a second group including contralateral nodal involvement or invasion of mediastinal viscera (IIIb). All tumors metastasizing beyond the thoracic and low cervical lymph nodes are now designated as Stage IV. Using the grading system, patients with NSCLC can be divided clinically into logical treatment groups, whatever the cell type. According to the NCI's current prognosis and treatment recommendations, Stages I and II tumors are usually surgically respectable. The prognosis in this group is 30 to 80 percent 5-year survival, with the range depending on a variety of tumor and host factors. If the patients in these groups have medical conditions that preclude an attempt at curative surgery, radiation therapy can be expected to result in a 20 percent survival at 5 years. A second group of patients with locally advanced cancers (T_3) or certain patterns of regional extension (N_2 or M_1 involving only the supraclavicular area) may respond favorably to extended local resection (the T_3 lesions) combined with radiation and/or chemotherapy, or curative radiation doses directed at the involved nodal areas. Though the overall 5-year survival for this group is 10 percent or less and the median survival is less than a year, as previously noted, several centers have achieved much better results in selected subsets of this group. In Stage IV patients (those with distant metastases at the time of diagnosis), radiation for palliation of symptoms from the primary tumor may be useful. Though progress is being made in the oncology field, at present chemotherapy has not produced much survival benefit. Patients with lung cancer who have extrathoracic disease rarely survive for any significant period. The median survival is less than 6 months.

CLINICAL MANIFESTATIONS. Bronchogenic carcinoma is seen predominantly in men of forty-five to sixty-five years of age, with a peak incidence at fifty-five to sixty years. It is not rare in men less than forty-five years old, and the diagnosis is being made with increasing frequency in women who are in their fifth decade. In a few cases, the disease is discovered incidentally in asymptomatic patients. Such discovery is by means of chest x-ray for the greatest number of patients, but sputum cytology occasionally leads to the eventual identification of an otherwise occult tumor.

Because intermittent or chronic cough is so common among tobacco addicts, it may be difficult to establish an onset of symptoms. Nevertheless, about three-fourths of patients with bronchogenic carcinoma must be said to

THE REVISED (1986) AJCC STAGING SYSTEM

Primary tumor (T)

TX	Tumor proved by the presence of malignant cells in bronchopulmonary secretions but not visualized roentgenographically or bronchoscopically, or any tumor that cannot be assessed as in a retreatment staging
T_0	No evidence of primary tumor
T_{is}	Carcinoma in situ
T_1	A tumor that is 3.0 cm or less in greatest dimension, surrounded by lung or visceral pleura, and without evidence of invasion proximal to a lobar bronchus at bronchoscopy
T_2	A tumor more than 3.0 cm in greatest dimension, or a tumor of any size that either invades the visceral pleura or has associated atelectasis or obstructive pneumonitis extending to the hilar region. At bronchoscopy, the proximal extent of demonstrable tumor must be within a lobar bronchus or at least 2.0 cm distal to the carina. Any associated atelectasis or obstructive pneumonitis must involve less than an entire lung.
T_3	A tumor of any size with direct extension into the chest wall (including superior sulcus tumors), diaphragm, or the mediastinal pleura or pericardium without involving the heart, great vessels, trachea, esophagus or vertebral body, or a tumor in the main bronchus within 2.0 cm of the carina without involving the carina
T_4	A tumor of any size with invasion of the mediastinum or involving heart, great vessels, trachea, esophagus, vertebral body, or carina, or presence of malignant pleural effusion

Nodal involvement (N)

NX	Minimum requirements to access the regional nodes cannot be met
N_0	No demonstrable metastasis to regional lymph nodes
N_1	Metastasis to lymph nodes in the peribronchial or the ipsilateral hilar region, or both, including direct extension
N_2	Metastasis to ipsilateral mediastinal lymph nodes and subcarinal lymph nodes
N_3	Metastasis to contralateral mediastinal lymph nodes, contralateral hilar lymph nodes, ipsilateral or contralateral scalene, or supraclavicular lymph nodes

Distant metastasis (M)

MX	Minimum requirements to assess the presence of distant metastasis cannot be met
M_0	No (known) distant metastasis
M_1	Distant metastasis present

Stage grouping

Occult stage	TX	N_0	M_0
Stage 0	T_{is}	N_0	M_0 (in situ)
Stage I	T_1	N_0	M_0
	T_2	N_0	M_0
Stage II	T_1	N_1	M_0
	T_2	N_1	M_0
Stage IIIa	T_3	N_0	M_0
	T_3	N_1	M_0
	T_{1-3}	N_2	M_0
Stage IIIb	Any T	N_3	M_0
	T_4	Any N	M_0
Stage IV	Any T	Any N	M_1

SUMMARY OF STAGING DEFINITIONS

Occult stage	Microscopically identified cancer cells in lung secretions on multiple occasions (or multiple daily collections); no discernible primary cancer in the lung
Stage 0	Carcinoma in situ
Stage I	Tumor surrounded by lung or visceral pleura arising more than 2 cm distal to the carina (T_{1-2}, N_0)
Stage II	Tumor not extending to adjacent organs, pleura, or chest wall, with hilar lymph-node involvement (T_{1-2}, N_1)
Stage IIIa	Tumor invading chest wall, pleura, or pericardium or within 2 cm but not involving carina; nodes in hilum or ipsilateral mediastinum (T_3, N_{0-1}; T_1, N_2)
Stage IIIb	Direct extension to adjacent organs (pleura, heart, chest wall, diaphragm, or mediastinum); or associated with contralateral mediastinal or supraclavicular lymph-node involvement (T_4 or N_3)
Stage IV	Any tumor with distant metastases (M_1)

have coughing as a principal symptom. Hemoptysis in the form of blood streaking of sputum occurs in about half of all patients, but massive hemoptysis or spitting of blood clots is unusual. Chest pain of dull, nonspecific type is described by some patients whose tumor is subsequently found to be free of chest wall involvement. When there is invasion of the parietal pleura or chest wall, the patient may have mild to severe pain that is either localized or radicular in form. Fever and purulent sputum may mark an increase of symptoms in the patient whose tumor is producing major bronchial obstruction, and wheezing or stridor may also be present.

Involvement of the left recurrent laryngeal nerve (rarely the right nerve), either by direct tumor invasion or by extension from a metastatic lymph node, may result in hoarseness that is often minimized by the patient. Direct tumor extension into the superior vena cava or its compression by the expanding neoplasm produces early symptoms of edema of the eyes and prominence or distension of the superficial veins over the upper part of the body. Dyspnea occurring as a symptom of bronchogenic carcinoma is usually associated with a large pleural effusion, paralysis of a hemidiaphragm due to phrenic nerve invasion, or major bronchial obstruction.

A loss of appetite accompanied by weight loss of more than a few pounds is an ominous sign in the patient with a bronchial neoplasm; such patients usually have either an unresectable tumor or systemic metastases. A deliberate search should be made for evidence of spread by isotope scanning and computed tomography. Because the metastatic spectrum of these tumors is so wide, almost any imaginable symptom can be produced. A rare patient may develop pulmonary hypertrophic osteoarthropathy with clubbing of the digits (Fig. 17-81). Evidence of metastases may be absent, and the process may be dramatically reversed when the tumor is resected.

A small percentage of patients with bronchogenic carcinoma present with extrapulmonary nonmetastatic manifestations that are considered due to elaboration of hormonelike substances by the neoplastic cells. The occurrence of these signs and symptoms does not imply systemic spread of the bronchogenic tumor, and resection of the lesion is generally associated with a regression of the symptoms. Ultrastructural studies have demonstrated the presence of neurosecretory-type granules in the cells of many anaplastic tumors, and the more striking clinical symptoms are associated with oat cell carcinomas. An example is a Cushing-like syndrome that differs from the classic Cushing's syndrome by an older age incidence, a greater frequency in males, and a more rapid clinical course. The ectopic adrenocorticotropic hormone that has been demonstrated in the oat cell tumors appears indistinguishable from the normal hormone. An inappropriate antidiuresis associated with the anaplastic small-cell carcinoma occasionally results in the symptoms of water intoxication with hyponatremia and increasing cerebral symptoms. The carinoid syndrome has been reported in a few patients with oat cell carcinoma, and either 5-hydroxytryptamine or 5-hydroxytryptophan may be secreted.

Hypercalcemia caused by a parathormone-like polypeptide has most often been associated with squamous bronchogenic carcinoma. Tender gynecomastia and ectopic gonadotropin secretion have been identified with large-cell anaplastic carcinoma. Satisfactory resection of the squamous neoplasm reverses the hypercalcemia, but it may return if the tumor recurs. A group of carcinomatous neuromyopathies is included in the nonmetastatic manifestations of lung cancer, and their incidence is thought to be as high as 15 percent. The symptoms may be subtle or somewhat overshadowed by the pulmonary complaints. The patient with bronchogenic carcinoma who mentions weakness along with his cough and chest pain is usually not questioned in detail about the characteristics of the weakness. This is the principal symptom, however, of a myasthenia-like syndrome that is probably due to a defect in neuromuscular conduction. Peripheral and central neuropathies also occur, and their differentiation from the symptoms of metastatic lesions can be im-

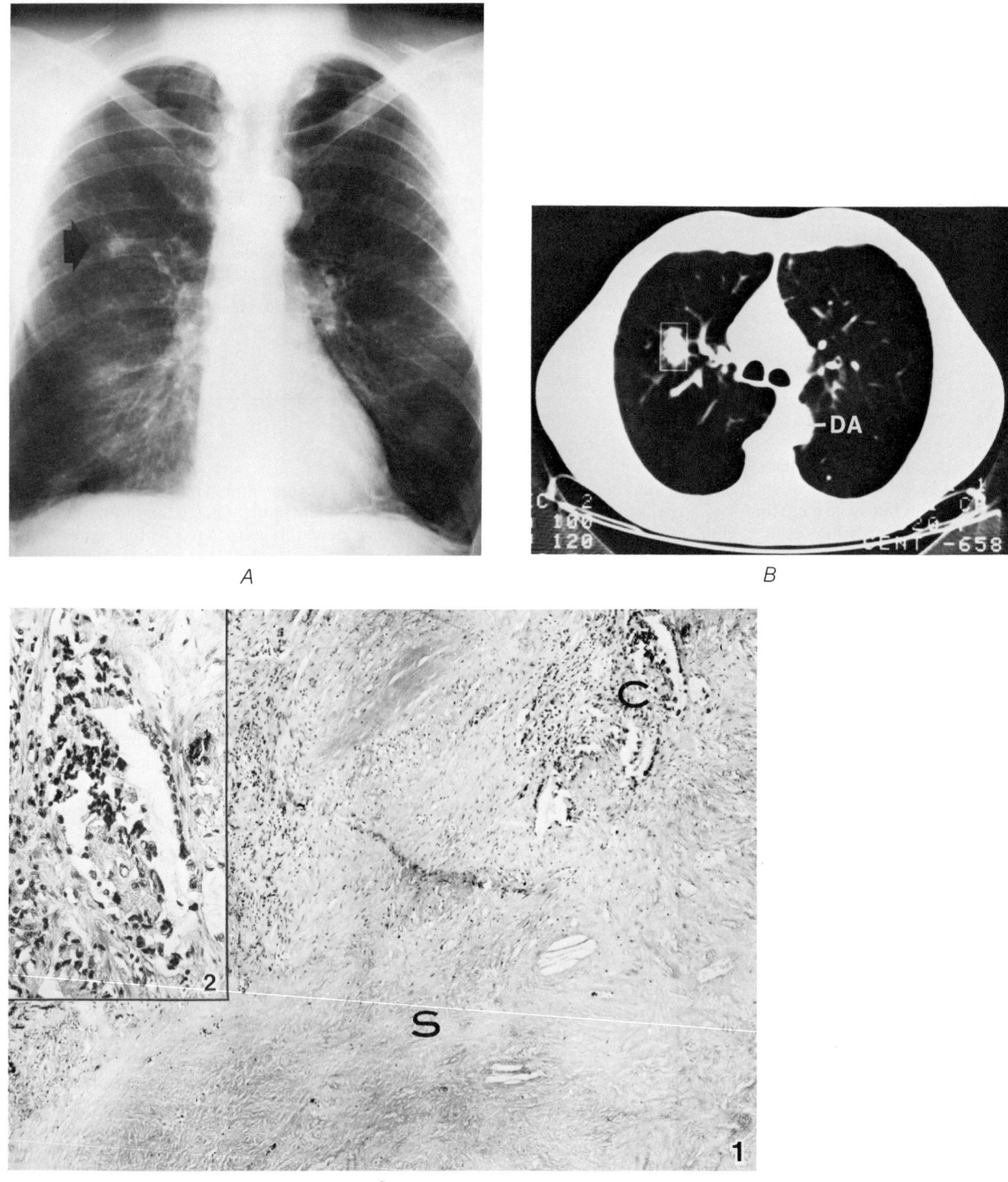

Fig. 17-79. A pulmonary scar carcinoma in a fifty-one-year-old man. *A.* The P-A chest x-ray shows an irregular density in the upper midlung field. *B.* A CT scan at the level of the main-stem bronchi shows a small dense mass in the parenchyma of the right upper lobe. *C.* The photomicrograph made from the resected upper lobe shows the lesion to be a scar carcinoma. The lower portion (S) is ancient hyalinized scar. In the upper right is a focus of adenocarcinoma (C) (×95). The insert is a higher magnification of the adenocarcinoma (×265).

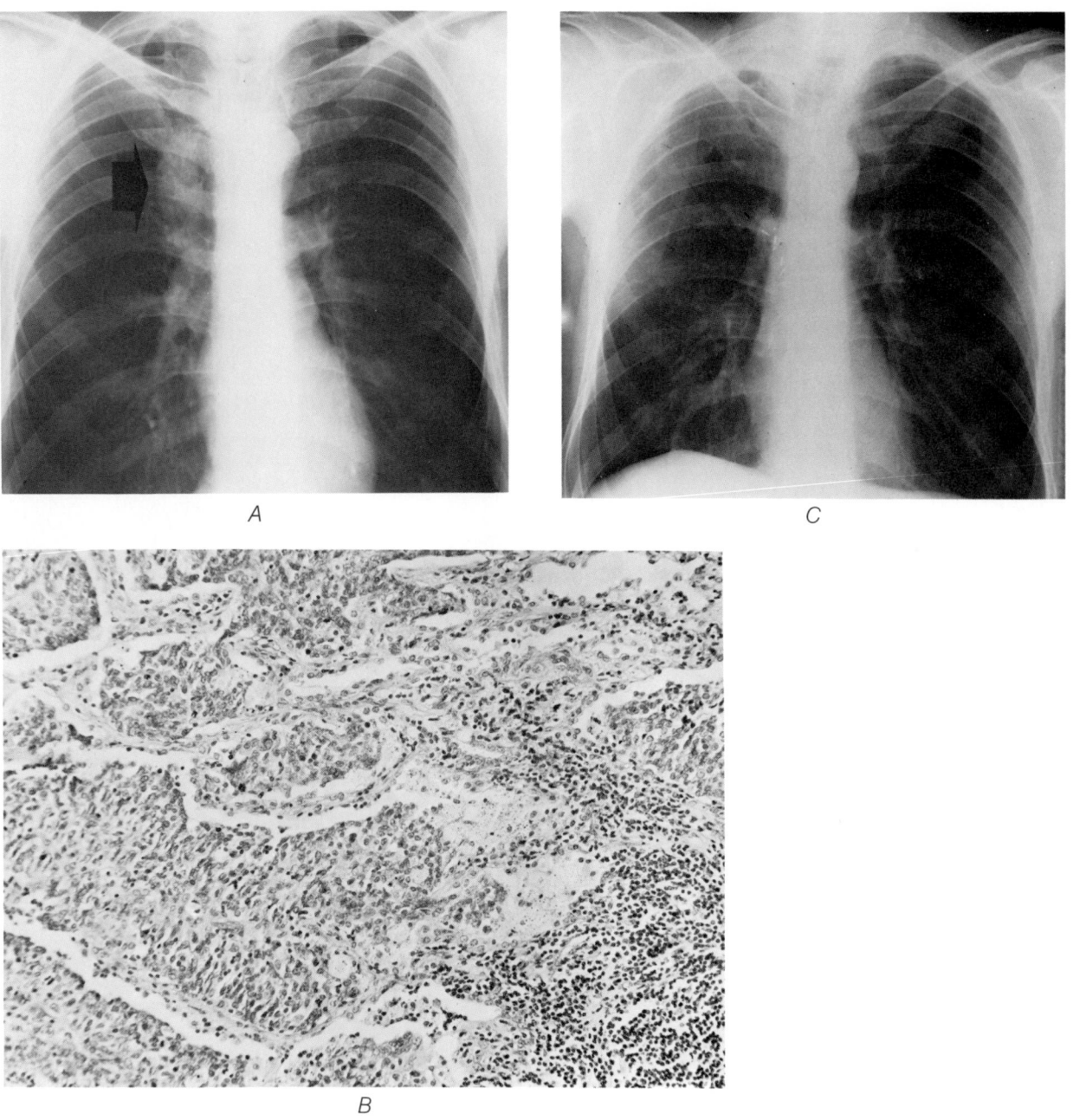

Fig. 17-80. Undifferentiated small-cell carcinoma, intermediate-cell type, in a fifty-five-year-old man. *A.* The preoperative chest x-ray shows a mass above the right hilus. Mediastinoscopy failed to show evidence of mediastinal lymph-node involvement, and the patient underwent right upper lobectomy. *B.* Histological examination of the resected lobe showed an undifferentiated small-cell carcinoma, intermediate-cell type, invading the lung parenchyma. Note the size of tumor cells in comparison with the mature lymphocytes in the lower right corner. (×188.) *C.* A follow-up chest x-ray 4 years after operation shows no evidence of tumor recurrence, and the patient is well.

portant. With the former, pulmonary resection may be possible and may result in disappearance of the symptoms.

DIAGNOSIS AND WORK-UP. Approximately 50 percent of patients with bronchogenic cancer are beyond consideration for operative treatment when the opportunity for definitive diagnosis is first presented. For this reason diagnostic evaluation must include an effort to determine whether localized or metastatic spread has occurred. The key to this effort is a meticulous history. If carefully sought, symptoms can almost always be found that will direct attention to involved organ systems. A thorough

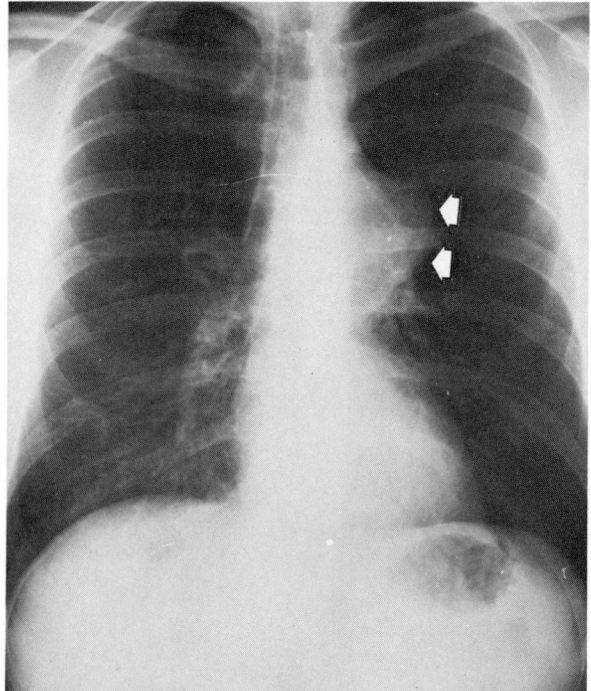

A

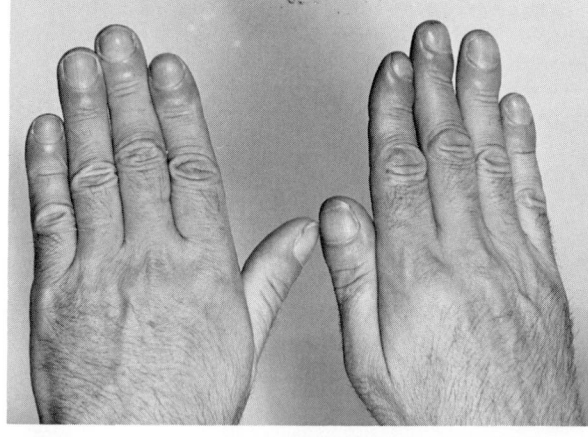

B

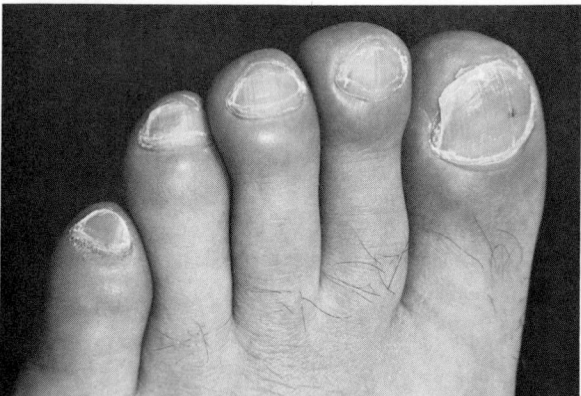

C

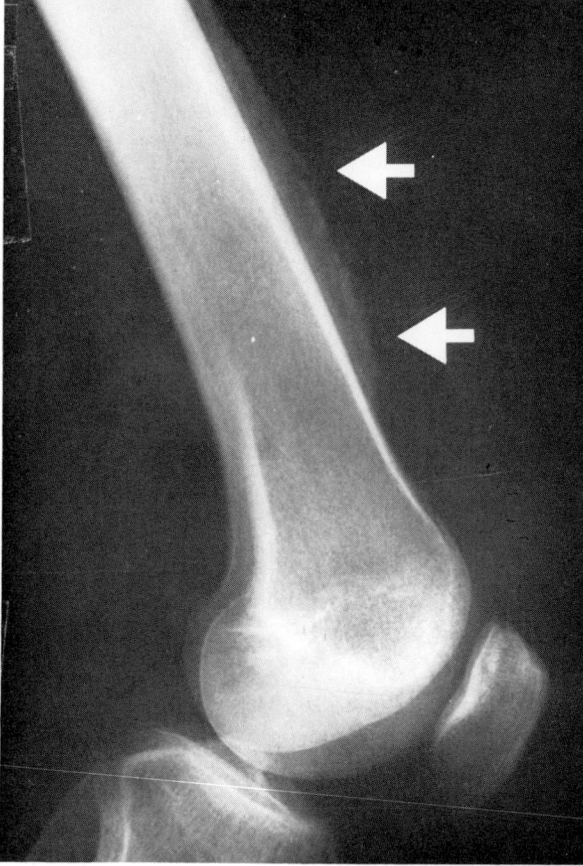

D

examination for suggestive lymph nodes must also be made. Though the yield is low in the absence of symptoms, any or all of the scanning techniques should be used to search for metastatic spread in the presence of suggestive symptoms, or if the patient's general condition suggests systemic spread. With any question of metastasis, an attempt at biopsy should be considered before treatment for the primary neoplasm is planned.

Whenever the differential diagnosis includes lung cancer, aggressive efforts to obtain cytologic or biopsy tissue diagnosis are indicated. Almost any type of pulmonary infiltrate, nodule, mass, or atelectasis should be considered cancer until it can be proved otherwise. This is particularly true if the patient is, has been, or lives with a

Fig. 17-81. Pulmonary hypertrophic osteoarthropathy associated with oat cell carcinoma. *A*. The chest x-ray in a thirty-nine-year-old man shows a left hilar mass that proved to be oat cell carcinoma on bronchial biopsy. *B*. Painful clubbing of the fingers and toes developed during an interval of approximately 3 months. *C*. A close-up of the patient's foot demonstrates clubbing of the toes. *D*. The arrow points to the new bone formation on the femur.

tobacco addict. As previously discussed, there is an orderly and progressively invasive series of investigative studies that can be undertaken to obtain diagnostic tissue. The degree to which a search should be made for extra thoracic disease is a matter of controversy among those who care for lung cancer patients. Radioactive scans of liver, brain, and bones are recommended by many, but evidence is lacking that such searches are fruitful in the absence of symptoms. In one recent analysis of a routine scanning program in patients without symptoms, 16 of 17 positive scans were false positive and 8 of 22 clinically evidence metastases were not detected. Recent reports in the radiology literature have indicated 5 to 20 percent occurrence of demonstrable adrenal metastases in lung cancer patients studied by CT. The demonstrated value of the CT in visualizing the mediastinum has greatly reduced the indication for staging mediastinoscopy, a procedure that had been gaining strong support until recently. Most surgeons now reserve exploration of the mediastinum for those patients with nodes identified on CT as being larger than 1 cm (Fig. 17-82).

Even before the general availability of computed tomography for careful preoperative evaluation of the mediastinum in lung cancer patients, there were differences of opinion about aggressive prethoracotomy staging by mediastinal exploration techniques. For some groups treating lung cancer, the attitude is that positive lymph nodes in the mediastinum preclude thoracotomy because of the very low 5-year survival with resection under these circumstances. Others, however, quoting reasonable survival figures, usually with postoperative adjuvant therapy, have concluded that ipsilateral mediastinal metastases are not a contraindication to pulmonary resection. Therefore, some of the latter surgeons do not feel that routine preoperative staging by mediastinal exploration is warranted.

Along with CT mapping, bronchoscopy is the fundamental diagnostic technique for patients with suspected carcinoma, and the development of the flexible fiberscope has increased the positive diagnosis yield to better than 70 percent in most centers. These results include bronchial brushing and cytologic studies of bronchial washings that may be obtained at the same time. The endoscopist must determine the proximal extent of a visualized neoplasm because the patient's operability may be governed by the closeness of the tumor to the tracheal carina. Murray and colleagues evaluated the relationship between positive bronchoscopy and lymph-node metastases in 42 consecutive patients with tumors of the right lower or middle lobe (Table 17-15). Bronchoscopy was considered positive when a visible endobronchial lesion was identified. When bronchoscopy was negative (21 patients), intraoperative evaluation and pathologic examination of the lymphatic sump of Borrie failed to demonstrate nodal metastases in 18 patients. Hilar nodes were positive in 2 patients, but no patient had mediastinal disease. Pneumonectomy was required in only 3 patients in the negative bronchoscopy group. Of the 20 patients with positive bronchoscopy 9 had metastases to the lymphatic sump and 2 had mediastinal metastases. There was a

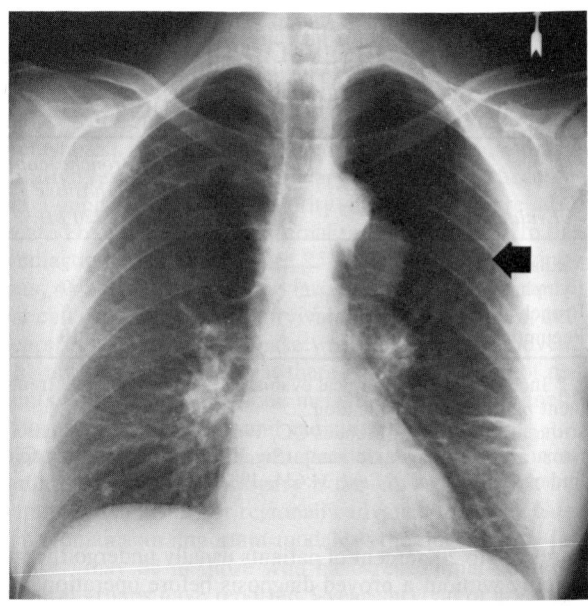

A

B

Fig. 17-82. The use of computed tomography for preoperative staging of bronchogenic carcinoma. *A.* The P-A chest x-ray in a sixty-two-year-old woman shows a mass between the aortic knob and the left hilus. On the lateral chest x-ray the mass was seen to be located in the posterior segment of the left upper lobe. *B.* A CT scan at the level of the tracheal carina shows the tumor in juxtaposition to the descending aorta. The lymph nodes just in front of the carina and posterior to the ascending aorta were interpreted to be at the upper limit of normal size. At operation all lymph nodes were negative for metastases, confirming the CT impression. AA = ascending aorta, LN = lymph nodes, T = tumor, DA = descending aorta.

marked superiority in survival in the negative bronchoscopy group.

A primary goal of the patient's work-up is to confirm the suspected diagnosis of carcinoma by means other than exploratory thoracotomy. Diagnostic procedures should be carried out as techniques for establishing the patient's suitability for operation are completed. Despite a proper application of all reasonable diagnostic proce-

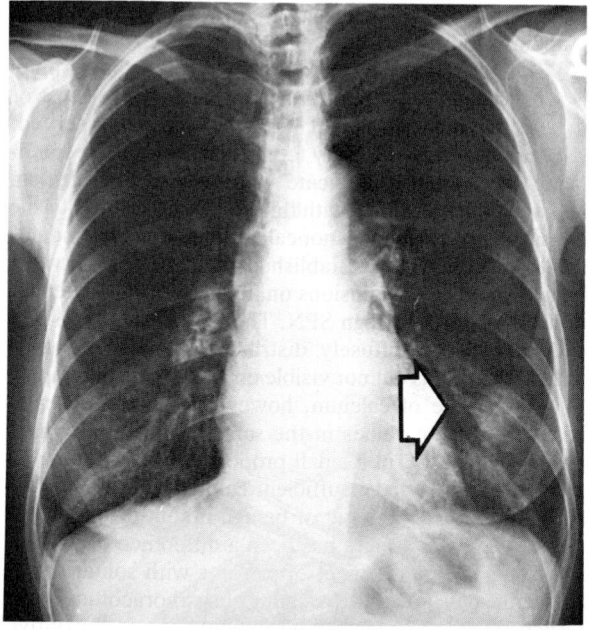

A

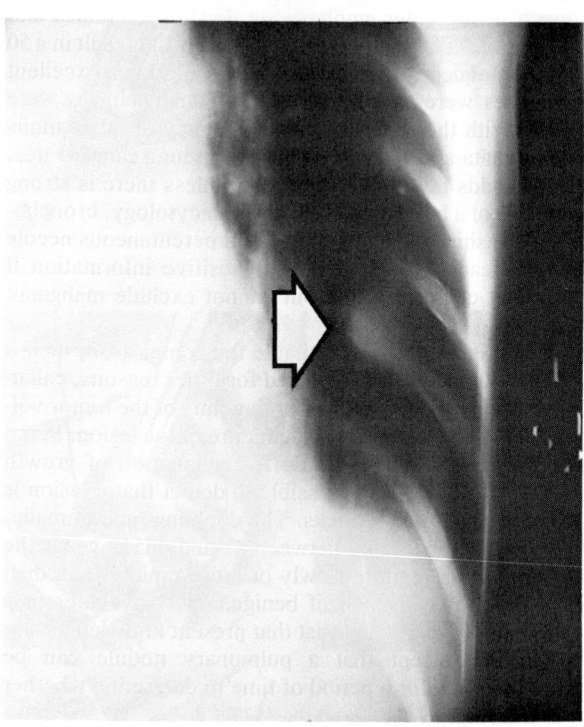

C

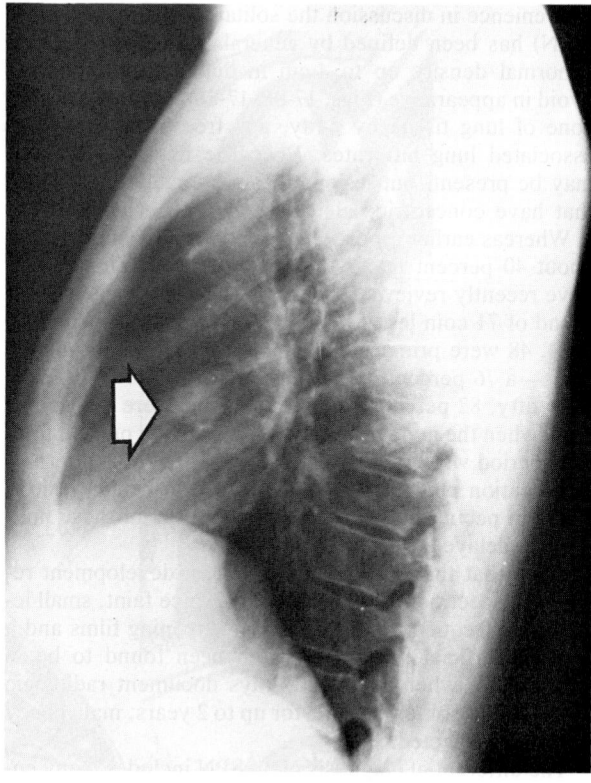

B

Fig. 17-85. A solitary pulmonary nodule. *A* and *B*. The posteroanterior and lateral chest x-rays show a round density in the lingula that had not been present on the patient's previous x-rays. *C*. The lesion is homogeneous, with smooth borders, on tomograms. A wedge resection showed the lesion to be a resolving pulmonary infarct.

bronchial brush biopsy are appropriate, with watchful waiting and close observation for growth or change.

OTHER LUNG TUMORS

BRONCHOPULMONARY NEUROENDOCRINE TUMORS. Both Warren et al. and Benfield's group have recently presented analyses utilizing contemporary electron mi-

croscopic and immunohistochemical techniques to demonstrate the continuum that exists from carcinoids to small-cell undifferentiated lung cancers (SCLC). It now seems clear that this group of tumors are all neuroendocrine neoplasms arising from Kulchitsky cells. At the benign end of the spectrum, the bronchopulmonary carcinoid histologically resembles the carcinoid tumors of the small intestine. Along with cylindroma and mucoepidermoid tumors, the bronchial carcinoid was formerly referred to as a bronchial adenoma. This designation was awkward because the term adenoma implied a fundamental quality of benignancy that was not in keeping with the high incidence of malignant behavior shown by cylindroma and mucoepidermoid tumors. Further, a small proportion of bronchial carcinoids will metastasize to regional lymph nodes, with the result that reference was occasionally made to "metastasizing bronchial adenomas."

Over 80 percent of carcinoids arise in proximal bronchi, but peripheral origin beyond cartilage-containing bronchi does occur. The tumors grow slowly and protrude into the bronchial lumen making signs and symptoms of bronchial obstruction the principal clinical presentation. Unusual vascularity may cause hemoptysis as

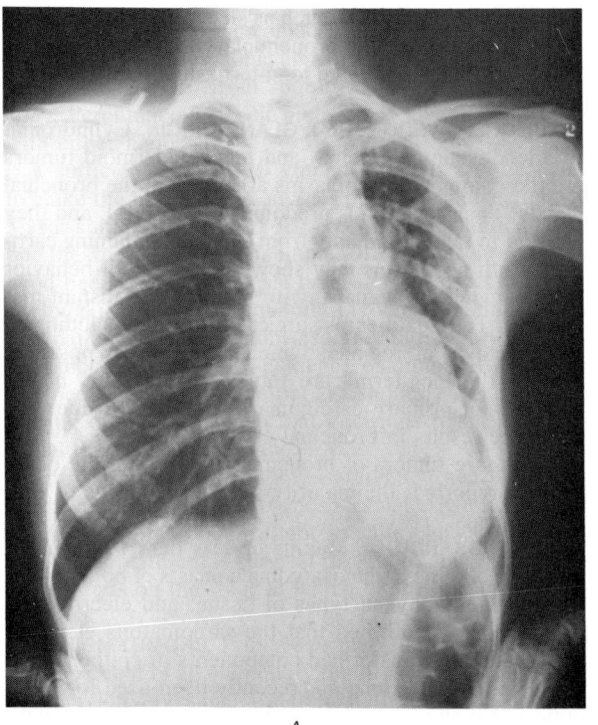

A

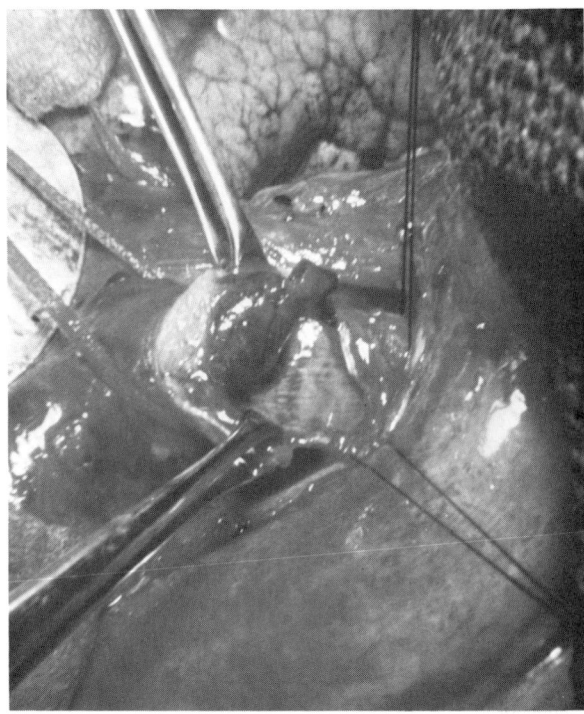

B

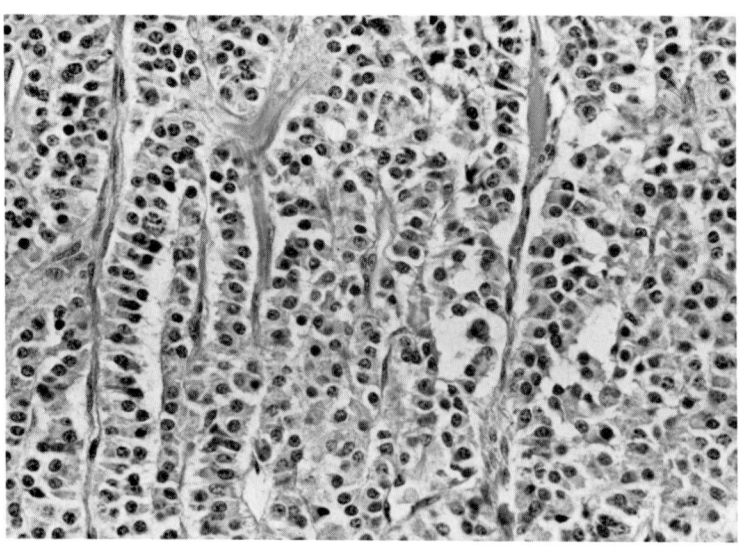

C

Fig. 17-86. A forty-two-year-old woman with a bronchial carcinoid tumor. *A.* The chest x-ray shows collapse of the left lower lobe and shift of the mediastinum to that side. *B.* Bronchotomy of the left stem bronchus confirmed an obstruction of the lower-lobe bronchus by the vascular tumor projecting from the bronchus between the Allis clamps. *C.* Histologic examination of the neoplasm showed it to be a benign carcinoid tumor. (×400.)

a presenting complaint (Fig. 17-86). The vascularity gives the tumor a deep pink or red color when visualized through a bronchoscope.

The extent of bronchial-wall involvement is variable, but there is usually invasion of the underlying cartilages. Rarely, direct extension through the bronchial wall can result in invasion of mediastinal structures. Regional lymph-node deposits are found in approximately 10 percent of patients, liver metastases more rarely. In keeping with the neuroendocrine origin of these tumors, a few

patients with bronchial carcinoid have Cushing-like syndromes that seem attributable to the tumor.

Although the average age of patients with a carcinoid tumor is approximately forty years, the neoplasm does occur in children. Commonly, the clinical presentation is a result of bronchial obstruction with infestation and pulmonary atelectasis. Sputum cytology is negative, but more than 80 percent of the lesions can be visualized by bronchoscopy. The carcinoid syndrome is seen rarely and can occur without extrathoracic metastases. It is wise to

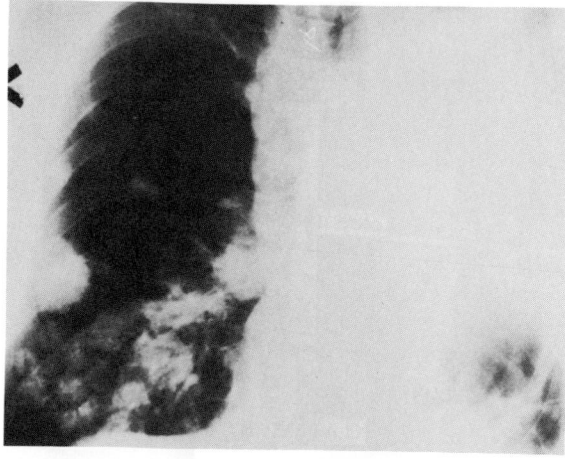

A

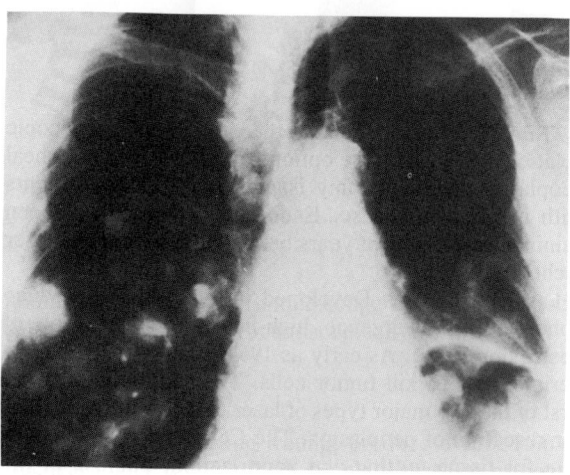

B

Fig. 17-92. *A.* Chest x-ray of a patient with metastatic renal cell carcinoma obstructing the left main-stem bronchus. Note the complete atelectatic opacification of the left lung, and the parenchymal metastases in the right lung. *B.* After Nd-YAG laser ablation of the bronchial lesion the left lung is reexpanded. (From: *Unger M, Atkinson GW: Nd:YAG applications in pulmonary and endotracheal lesions, in Joffe SN, Muckerheide MC, Goldman L (eds): Neodymium-YAG Laser in Medicine and Surgery, chap 9, p 78, Elsevier, 1984, with permission.*)

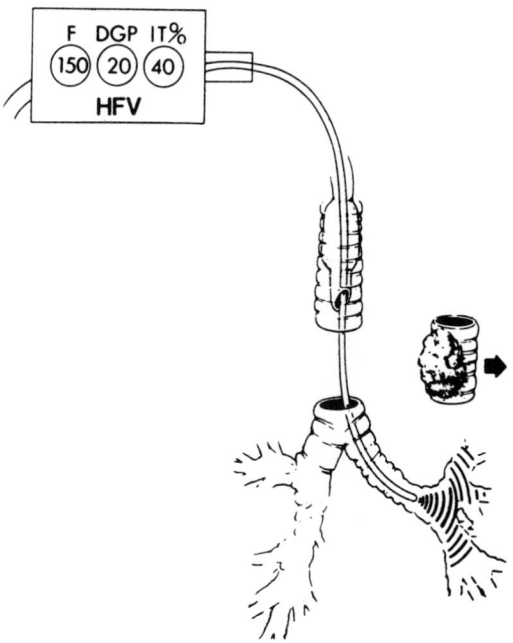

Fig. 17-93. Catheter for high-frequency positive-pressure ventilation ("jet" ventilation) shown passing through the endotracheal tube, across the tracheal lesion, and into the distal left main-stem bronchus. Ventilation is satisfactory with the trachea open, and the field is relatively unobstructed. In the illustration, the high-frequency ventilator (HFV) is set for a frequency of 150 breaths per minute. (From: *El-Baz N, Jensik R, et al: Ann Thorac Surg 34:564, Fig 4, with permission.*)

that four out of five originally inoperable cases became operable and that seven out of ten patients originally thought to require pneumonectomy were treated with lesser resections.

Operative Treatment. Operations on the trachea present both a surgical and an anesthetic challenge. Obstructing lesions make ventilation of the anesthetized patient difficult, and an endotracheal tube offers little advantage because its tip lies above the stenosis. Even when adequate ventilation can be maintained initially, operative manipulation can precipitate complete obstruction and an acute crisis of CO_2 retention, correctable only by the surgeon gaining rapid access to the airway distal to the obstruc-

tion. Furthermore, during reconstruction ventilation must be delivered to the lungs beyond the operative field without interfering with exposure. This has traditionally been accomplished by passing sterile endotracheal tubing off the field that can be placed in the distal airway through the open trachea or bronchus.

The ease of ventilation during tracheal reconstruction has been greatly facilitated by the development of high-frequency "jet" ventilation, which is delivered to the distal airway through a small catheter passed through the endotracheal tube (Fig. 17-93). A small tidal volume is delivered at high frequency (60 to 150 breaths/min), maintaining lung expansion, alveolar ventilation, and oxygenation in the normal range. The catheter is small enough to pass through most stenosis and interferes little with exposure.

The choice of incision for tracheal reconstruction depends on the level of involvement, and somewhat on the age of the patient. In a young patient hyperextension of the neck brings more than half the trachea above the suprasternal notch, accessible through a cervical incision. In older patients, it can be difficult to bring more than the first few tracheal rings above the notch. In general, lesions involving the upper half of the trachea are approached through a cervical collar incision, augmented as necessary with a midline upper sternal extension. Lesions involving the lower half can be approached through a

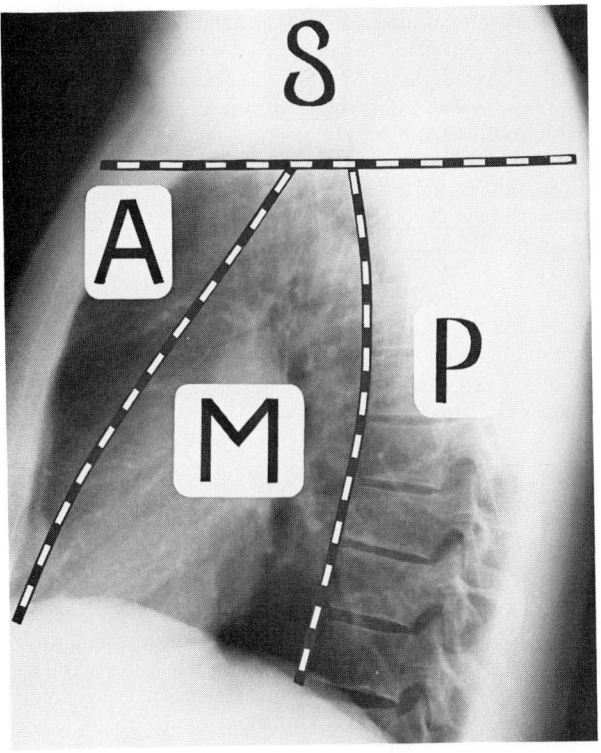

A

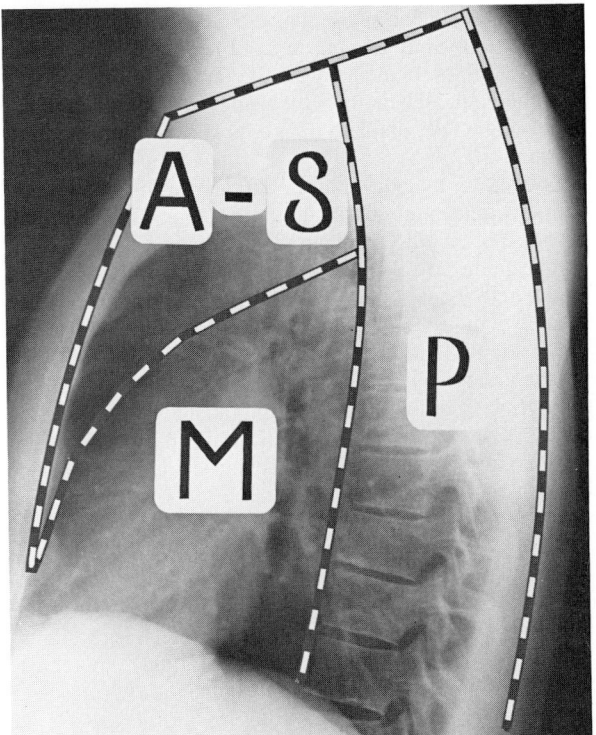

B

Fig. 17-94. The anatomic divisions of the mediastinum. *A.* The traditional classification divides the mediastinum into superior (S), anterior (A), middle (M), and posterior (P) compartments. *B.* A more clinically relevant classification divides the superior compartment between the anterior and posterior compartments. (From: *Burkell CC, Cross JM, et al: Mass lesions of the mediastinum, in Ravitch MM (ed): Current Problems in Surgery. Year Book Medical Publishers, Chicago, 1969, with permission.*)

right posterolateral thoracotomy (Grillo), entering the hemithorax at or above the fifth rib, or through a median sternotomy (Pearson). All cases are preceded by bronchoscopy in the operating room, at which time particularly tight stenoses (lumenal diameter <5 mm) should be dilated to temporarily facilitate anesthesia.

Surprising lengths of trachea can be resected and reconstructed with end-to-end anastomosis. Minimizing tension on the anastomosis is critical and is accomplished by holding the neck in hyperflexion for at least 7 days postoperatively, and by performing a laryngeal release procedure. Care is taken to avoid disturbance of the lateral blood supply, and only 1.5 cm of trachea should be circumferentially dissected on either side of the anastomosis. In most cases, 4.5 to 5 cm of trachea (at least eight rings) should be resectable. A wide variety of complex reconstructions involving the larynx, carina, and both main-stem bronchi have been described in detail by Grillo and others. The use of prosthetic materials for tracheal reconstruction remains anecdotal and experimental. Methods that appeared promising in series reported more than 10 years ago by Neville and by Moghissi have failed to achieve widespread application.

MEDIASTINUM

The mediastinum is the central cavity of the thorax, bounded on either side by the pleural cavities, bounded inferiorly by the diaphragm, and merging superiorly with the thoracic inlet. No compartment of the body carries more physiologic traffic. Many liters of blood pass through the mediastinum each minute, as liters of air, all ingested material and saliva, most autonomic nervous activity, and all of the body's lymphatic fluid pass through the same confined space. Much of the embryologic development of the circulatory, respiratory, and digestive systems takes place within the mediastinum. Congenital, traumatic, inflammatory, and neoplastic processes all find frequent expression in this complex compartment, and produce a broad spectrum of pathology in which anatomic relationships assume paramount importance.

The mediastinum is conveniently divisible along rough anatomic boundaries into subcompartments that contain characteristic lesions. The most traditional classification recognizing four spaces has largely given way to a system recognizing three spaces, which divides the highly overlapping contents of the superior compartment between the more surgically relevant anterior and posterior compartments (Fig. 17-94). In this system the anterior mediastinum lies anterior to the heart and extends cephalad into the anterior half of the thoracic inlet, where it meets the posterior mediastinum. The posterior mediastinum lies behind the heart, extending cephalad into the thoracic inlet where the anterior borders of the upper thoracic vertebrae form its boundary with the anterior mediastinum. The middle mediastinum is the wedge in between, with its base lying on the diaphragm and its apex at the top of the aortic arch.

The anterior mediastinum contains the thymus, along with a variable amount of adipose, areolar, and lymphatic tissue. The middle mediastinum contains the heart and pericardium, aorta, trachea and main-stem bronchi, and associated lymph nodes. The posterior mediastinum contains the descending aorta, the esophagus, autonomic nerve trunks, and the thoracic duct.

The great majority of mediastinal lesions appear as mass lesions radiographically, and most are neoplasms or cysts. A small number of mediastinal mass lesions are inflammatory or infectious. Vascular lesions, such as aneurysms, are considered elsewhere.

Tumors and Cysts

Mediastinal tumors and cysts in adults are distributed by type with similar frequencies in most large series. Neurogenic tumors are most common (about 20 percent), followed closely by thymomas, congenital cysts, and lymphomas. Most series in children from the 1960s and 1970s have reported a predominance of neurogenic tumors as well, followed by lymphoma and cysts, with thymomas rarely seen. In contrast, in a more recent large series of 188 children reported by the Mayo Clinic nearly half of the patients (87) had Hodgkin's or non-Hodgkin's lymphoma, with neurogenic tumors a distant second. Whether this truly reflects a shift in incidence remains to be confirmed. In adult series 25 to 35 percent of all primary tumors of the mediastinum are malignant, and in childhood series the figure is 25 to 45 percent. In either age group the most common malignant tumor is lymphoma, followed in adults in frequency by thymoma and mesenchymal tumors, and in children by neurogenic malignancies.

MANIFESTATIONS AND DIAGNOSIS. Mediastinal masses produce a wide variety of signs and symptoms, and half to one-third of patients are asymptomatic. The most common symptoms are nonspecific (chest pain, cough, dyspnea), and most can be ascribed to compression of adjacent structures, trachea and esophagus in particular. Superior vena caval obstruction, recurrent nerve palsy, and Horner's syndrome are less common examples, but their presence focuses diagnostic attention on the mediastinum. Certain mediastinal tumors are associated with symptomatic endocrine syndromes, such as hypertension (pheochromocytoma), hypercalcemia (parathyroid tumor), thyrotoxicosis (intrathoracic goiter), and gynecomastia (choriocarcinoma). In such cases symptoms have nothing to do with mediastinal location but are systemic consequences of the disease. Pel-Ebstein fevers associated with Hodgkin's disease are a similar example.

The presence of symptoms correlates with malignancy. Ninety-five percent of mediastinal masses that are discovered as incidental radiographic findings are benign, whereas symptomatic lesions are about half benign and half malignant. This correlation is less meaningful in children, whose airways are more vulnerable to compression. In a large series (188 children) from the Mayo Clinic, 78 percent of patients with benign mediastinal masses under age two had symptoms and signs of tracheal compression. Signs and symptoms of nerve compression, such as Horner's syndrome, vocal-cord paralysis, or hemiplegia usually reflect aggressive direct invasion and carry a poor prognosis.

Diagnostic evaluation begins with chest radiography in several views. Simply localizing the mass to one of the three subcompartments of the mediastinum narrows the possibilities (Fig. 17-95) and guides selection of further studies. In most patients the next step is computed tomography (CT), which can sort out the uniform radiographic densities of the mediastinum, identifying normal vascular and soft tissue structures with great cross-sectional clarity. CT of the mediastinum is most diagnostic of benign pathology, such as a cystic mass with an attenuation coefficient close to that of water. The CT appearance of solid malignancies is less definitive, but malignant characteristics such as extension, compression, or invasion are often readily demonstrated. The diagnostic power of CT can be further enhanced by intravascular or intraesophageal injection of contrast. In one series of children with mediastinal abnormalities, CT provided additional diagnostic information in 82 percent of patients, and in 65 percent the CT findings contributed to a change in clinical management.

Magnetic resonance imaging (MRI) is a noninvasive diagnostic modality thought to have great potential for imaging the mediastinum, especially for vascular lesions. Remarkable definition of vascular structures is obtainable in several views, entirely without the need for contrast injection (Fig. 17-96). Early experience has shown somewhat greater difficulty defining soft tissue masses, which tend to appear inhomogeneous or multifocal. The powerful magnetic field employed contraindicates the use of MRI in patients with pacemakers or cerebrovascular metal clips, and complicates examination of critically ill patients on monitors and elaborate life support systems. Fortunately, most metallic hardware likely to occur in the mediastinum (prosthetic valves, vascular clips, sternal wires) does not appear to pose a major hazard.

Plane tomography has been virtually replaced by CT and MRI but can still add useful information, especially in the vicinity of the pulmonary hila. A barium swallow can demonstrate invasion, compression, or displacement of the esophagus, resulting from intrinsic or extrinsic lesions. Arteriography is less frequently necessary with CT and MRI available, but contrast injection of the aorta or pulmonary artery provides information regarding blood supply and anatomic relationship to critical vascular structures that is sometimes not obtainable by any other method. For preoperative evaluation of major vascular disorders (aneurysms), which are discussed elsewhere, angiography is still the diagnostic standard. Venous angiography can provide specific information about the extent of involvement and nature of collateral channels in supe-

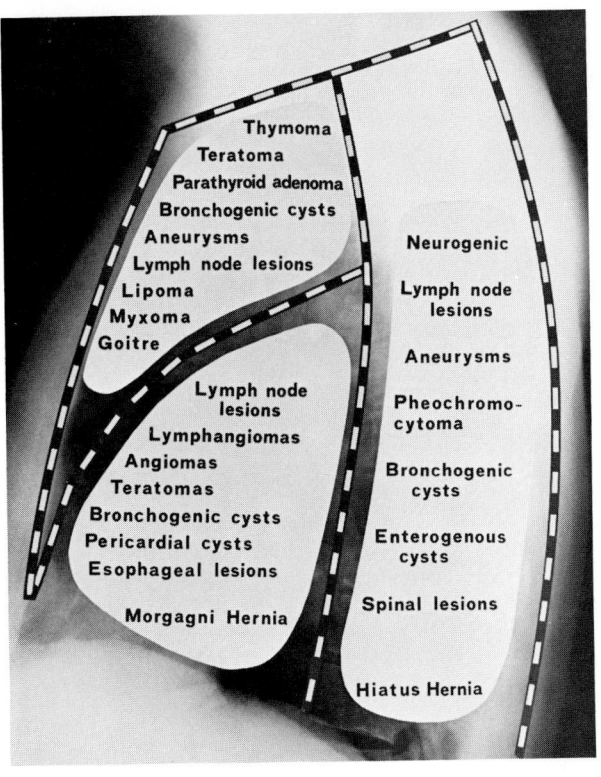

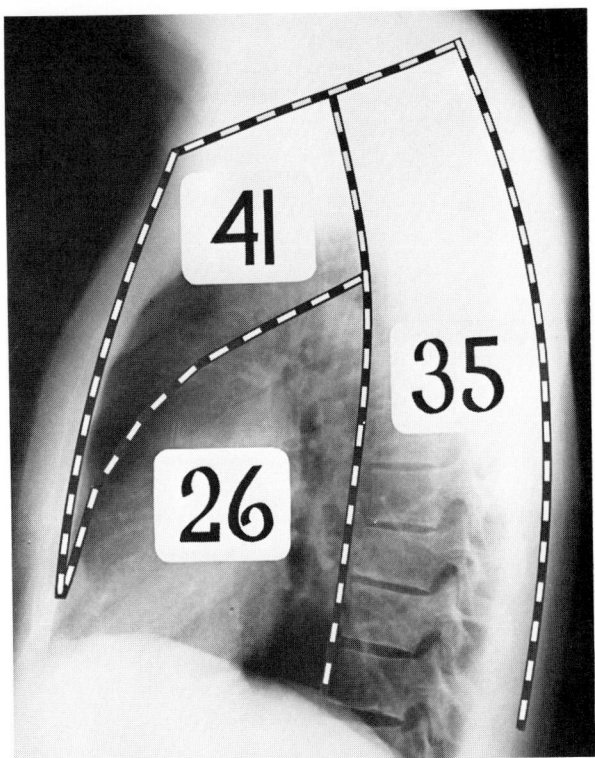

Fig. 17-95. *A.* Mediastinal lesions tend to occur within specific compartments, although some overlap is evident. *B.* The numbers shown indicate the distribution of lesions in 102 patients reported by Burkell and associates. (From: *Burkell CC, Cross JM, et al: Mass lesions of the mediastinum, in Ravitch MM (ed): Current Problems in Surgery. Year Book Medical Publishers, Chicago, 1969, with permission.*)

rior vena caval obstruction but is difficult to justify unless operation and reconstruction are anticipated. Myelography has been considered an essential part of the evaluation of posterior mediastinal tumors lying very close to the vertebral foramina, but this invasive procedure has also been replaced in many cases by CT of the spine.

Radioisotope scanning can provide very specific information when substernal goiter is suspected. Endoscopy of the esophagus or tracheobronchial tree can add observations on gross displacement or erosion by adjacent mass lesions and can occasionally provide biopsy material. Percutaneous needle biopsy, especially with direct fluoroscopic, ultrasonographic, or CT guidance, can be done safely in cases with favorable anatomy. Mediastinoscopy and mediastinotomy can also be employed for diagnosis.

Recitation of the expanding list of potentially applicable diagnostic procedures promotes the impression that operation is being avoided by assiduous diagnosis. On the contrary, there are still few mass lesions that do not come to operation. The operative mortality for resection of mediastinal lesions is quite low, amounting to 1.8 percent in one large series reported by Oldham and Sabiston. Operation provides definitive diagnosis and frequently

simultaneous definitive treatment, and remains an important part of most combined protocols for chemotherapy and radiation. In most cases the diagnostic armamentarium should be viewed as a means to a comprehensive preoperative evaluation.

NEUROGENIC TUMORS

Neurogenic tumors typically arise from sympathetic ganglia or intercostal nerves and are almost always found in the posterior mediastinum lying in the paravertebral gutter. Peak incidence is in adulthood. Since only 10 to 20 percent of adult neurogenic tumors are malignant, presentation as an incidental finding in an asymptomatic young adult is quite common. A higher proportion (20 to 40 percent) of childhood tumors are malignant. Chest wall pain due to nerve compression or bony erosion is the most common symptom. Hemiparesthesia, hemiparesis, and other signs of spinal cord compression can be seen in tumors with "dumbbell" extension through the intervertebral foramina. Hormonally active tumors are most often childhood malignancies, which can produce hypertension, flushing, diarrhea, diaphoresis, anorexia, and fever.

Neurilemmoma. Neurilemmomas (schwannomas) account for 40 to 60 percent of all neurogenic tumors. They arise from mature Schwann cells in intercostal nerves and have a hard, yellowish, well-encapsulated gross appearance consistent with the fact that most are benign. Some form dumbbell extensions through the intervertebral foramina (Fig. 17-97).

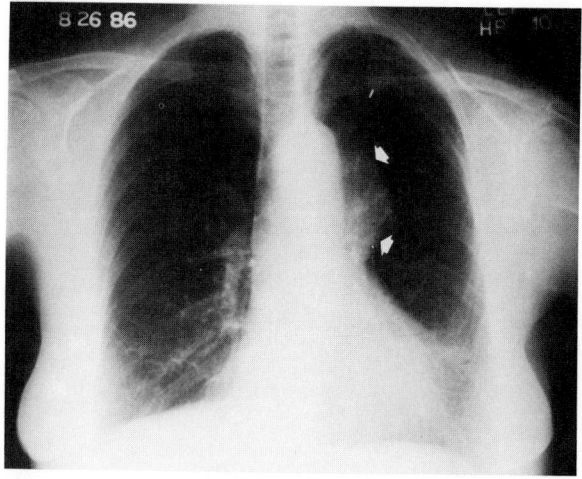
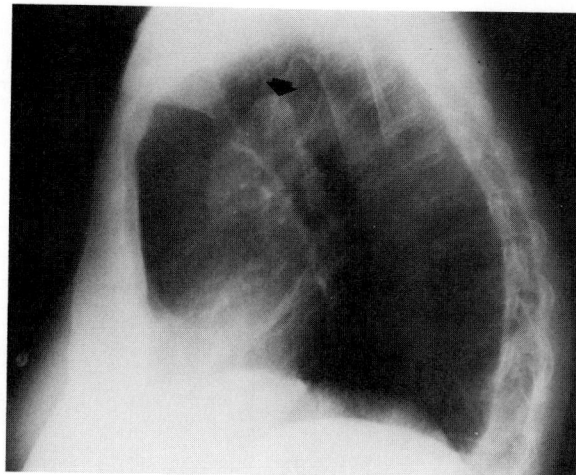

A

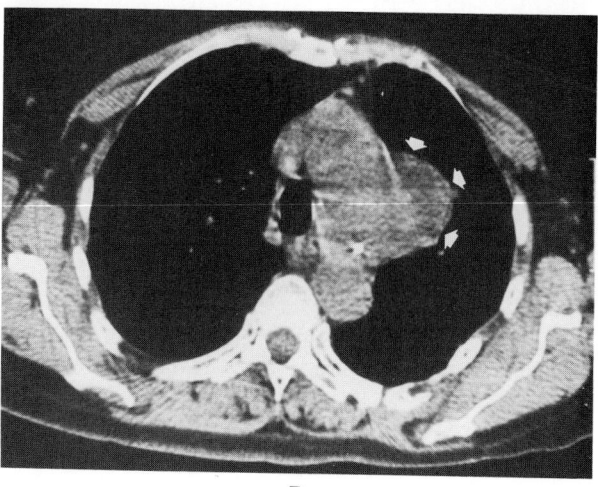

B

Fig. 17-96. *A.* This sixty-four-year-old woman was explored through a left thoracotomy for resection of the mass seen in the middle mediastinum on this chest x-ray *(arrows)*. The gross findings were confusing to the surgeon, and the patient was closed and transferred to another institution. *B.* On CT scan the mass could be seen adjacent to the aorta *(see arrows). C.* An MRI scan demonstrated unequivocally that the mass was an aneurysm of the aortic arch, arising proximal to the left subclavian artery. 1 = ascending aorta, 2 = aneurysm, 3 = descending aorta, 4 = left subclavian artery, P = pulmonary artery, L = left atrium. The patient died suddenly while awaiting reoperation.

Neurofibroma. Neurofibromas contain elements of both nerve sheath and nerve cells, and account for about 10 percent of all neurogenic tumors. They are poorly encapsulated, but radiographically resemble neurilemmomas. Mediastinal neurofibromas can be one feature of generalized neurofibromatosis (von Recklinghausen's disease), in which case the risk of malignant degeneration to neurosarcoma is increased. Advanced age also increases the risk of malignancy. Malignancy is present in 25 to 30 percent of tumors of this type, and carries a poor prognosis because of rapid growth and aggressive local invasion.

Neuroblastoma. Neuroblastomas are the most poorly differentiated tumors arising from the sympathetic nervous system. Only about 10 percent occur as a primary lesion in the mediastinum. More than 75 percent occur in children under four years of age, and many are hormonally active, producing vanillylmandelic acid in sufficient quantity to present with a systemic symptom complex often consisting of hypertension, fever, vomiting, and diarrhea. Bone, liver, and lymph-node metastases, as well as direct spinal cord invasion with neurologic deficits, are not infrequent at the time of diagnosis. Tumors

presenting in such advanced stages are usually unresectable, but the tumors are generally radiosensitive, and debulking followed by radiation therapy can produce long-term survival. Tumors presenting in the mediastinum and those presenting in the first year of life have a more favorable prognosis.

Ganglioneuroma, Ganglioneuroblastoma. Ganglioneuromas arise from mature nerve cells in sympathetic ganglia and are benign tumors that usually present in a younger age group than tumors of neural sheath origin. Radiographically, ganglioneuromas have a triangular configuration, with the base toward the mediastinum, and may be completely obscured by the vertebrae in the lateral projection. They tend to be poorly encapsulated and can be difficult to resect because of adherence to adjacent structures. Ganglioneuroblastomas consist of a mixture of mature and immature cells, and are rare tumors that share features of neuroblastoma. These are usually seen under three years of age, and are rare in adults.

Paraganglionic Tumors. Pheochromocytomas are chromaffin paraganglionic tumors that characteristically secrete catecholamines. Intrathoracic primaries are un-

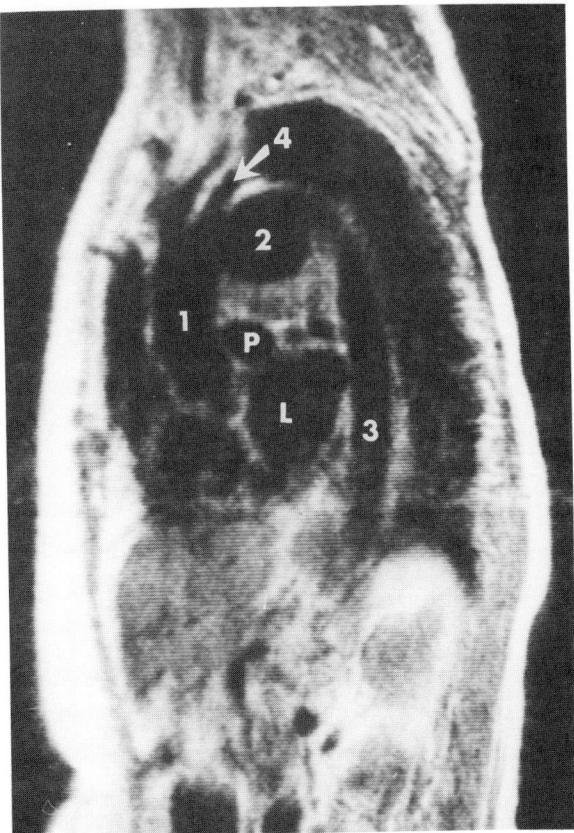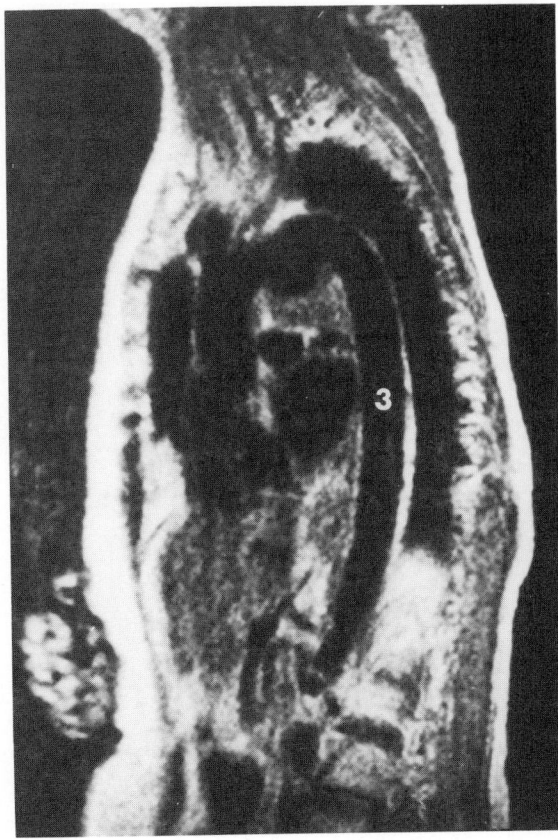

C

Fig. 17-96 *C.* Continued.

usual, occurring in about 1 percent of all pheochromocytomas. As with all extraadrenal locations, intraothoracic tumors are more frequently "silent" (nonsecreting) than their adrenal counterparts but are also more often malignant—about 30 percent of extraadrenal pheochromocytomas are malignant. Chemodectomas are nonchromaffin paraganglionic tumors that rarely secrete catecholamines, and arise from chemoreceptor tissue around the aortic arch, vagus, and aorticosympathetics. They are quite rare, and 15 to 30 percent are malignant.

TREATMENT. Operation is indicated in virtually all posterior mediastinal neurogenic tumors. The region is best approached through a standard posterolateral thoracotomy. Benign tumors should be completely excised. Preoperative evaluation of all posterior mediastinal tumors includes careful evaluation of the intervertebral foramina and vertebral bodies, which is most easily done initially with a CT scan, using magnified views as necessary. Myelography may still be required to confirm intraspinal extension (Fig. 17-97). When intraspinal extension exists, it is best to excise that portion first through a laminectomy, to avoid cord compression from intraspinal hemorrhage during the thoracic excision.

Malignant tumors are excised if possible. Radical operations for neuroblastoma are approached selectively, keeping clearly in mind the age of the patient, the radiosensitivity of the tumor, and the possibility of spontaneous maturation. Resection of an active (secretory) pheochromocytoma requires attention to the perioperative medical management of paroxysmal hypertension.

THYMOMA

In adults thymoma is the most common anterior mediastinal mass, and ranks second in frequency among tumors and cysts of the mediastinum. Thymoma is rare in children and has equal sex distribution, with a peak age incidence between forty and sixty years. About one-third of patients are asymptomatic at the time of diagnosis. Symptomatic patients present either with mass effects on adjacent organs or with systemic effects referable to one of the paraneoplastic syndromes associated with thymoma. Of the former, common examples include cough, chest pain, dyspnea, and superior vena caval obstruction. Of the latter, myasthenia gravis is the most common, although hypogammaglobulinemia and red cell aplasia have been described. It is most often stated that the incidence of myasthenia gravis is 10 to 50 percent in patients with thymoma. Conversely, thymoma is seen in only 8 to 15 percent of patients with myasthenia gravis. Myasthenic patients with thymoma have a poorer prognosis than patients without thymoma, and are less likely to benefit from thymectomy.

Thymoma does not have a characteristic radiographic

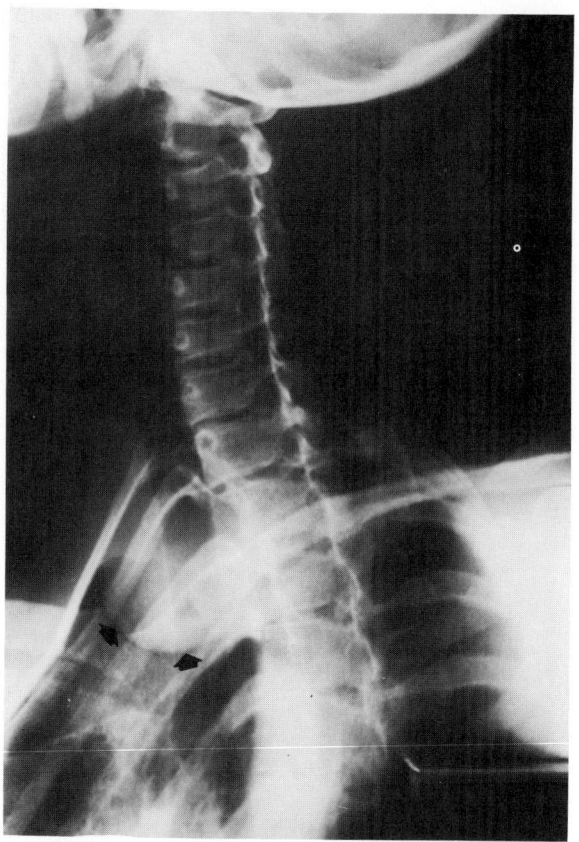

A

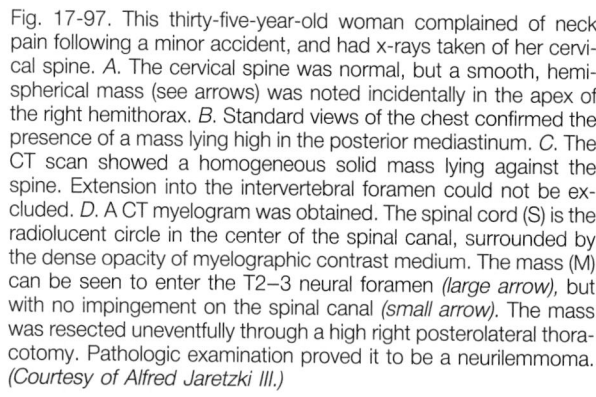

Fig. 17-97. This thirty-five-year-old woman complained of neck pain following a minor accident, and had x-rays taken of her cervical spine. *A.* The cervical spine was normal, but a smooth, hemispherical mass (see arrows) was noted incidentally in the apex of the right hemithorax. *B.* Standard views of the chest confirmed the presence of a mass lying high in the posterior mediastinum. *C.* The CT scan showed a homogeneous solid mass lying against the spine. Extension into the intervertebral foramen could not be excluded. *D.* A CT myelogram was obtained. The spinal cord (S) is the radiolucent circle in the center of the spinal canal, surrounded by the dense opacity of myelographic contrast medium. The mass (M) can be seen to enter the T2–3 neural foramen *(large arrow),* but with no impingement on the spinal canal *(small arrow).* The mass was resected uneventfully through a high right posterolateral thoracotomy. Pathologic examination proved it to be a neurilemmoma. *(Courtesy of Alfred Jaretzki III.)*

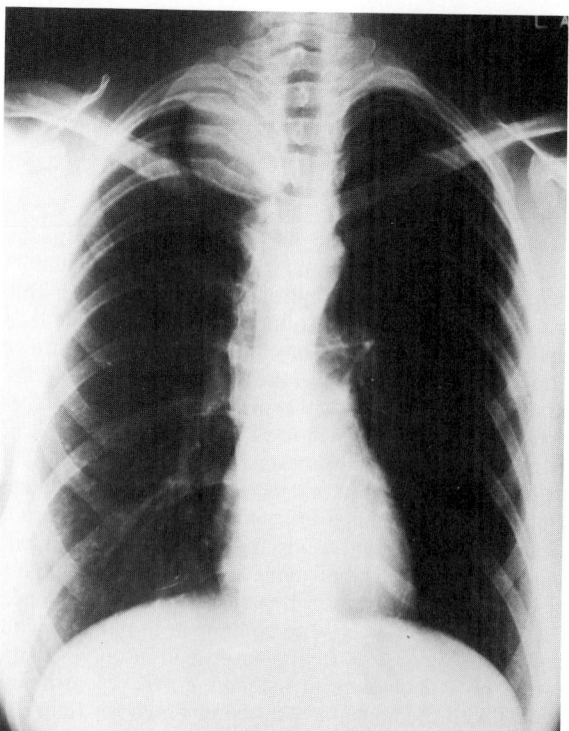

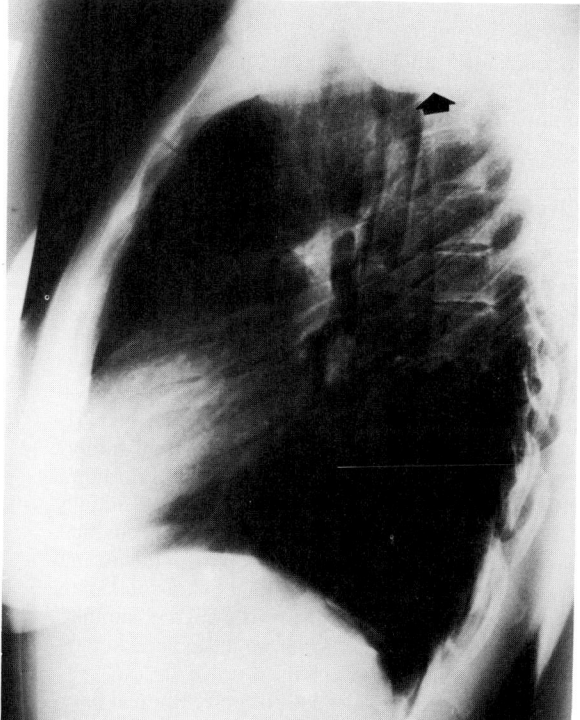

B

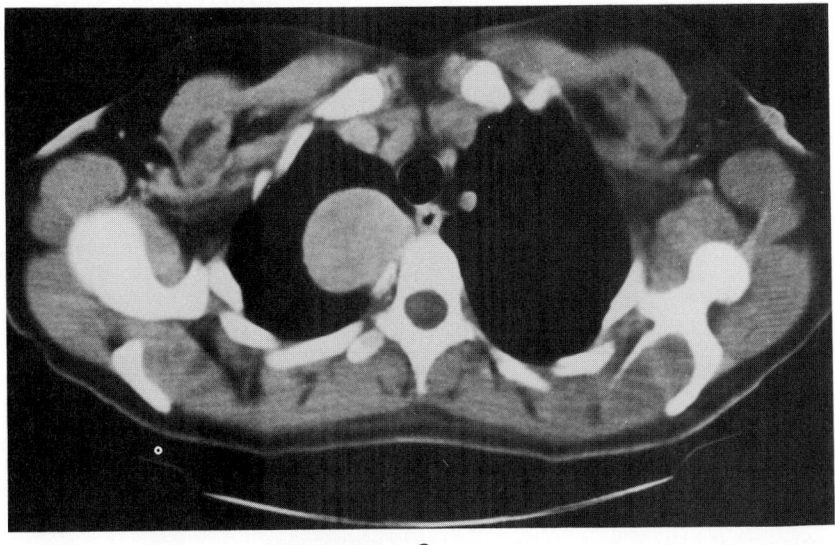

C

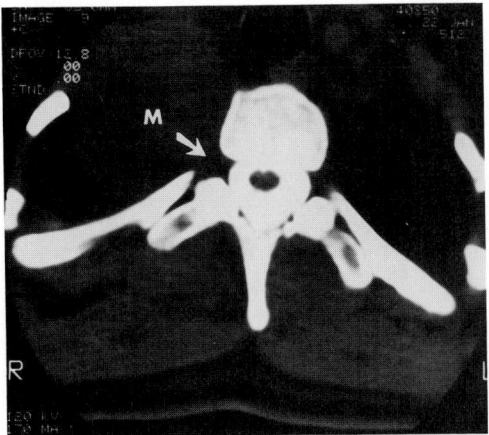

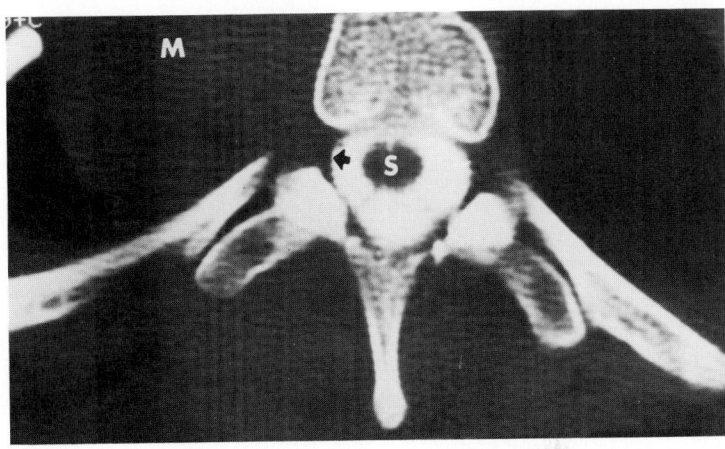

D

Fig. 17-97 *C,D.* Continued.

appearance, and diagnosis is usually made when the mass is excised (Fig. 17-98). The most prevalent histologic classification is based on the relative proportions of lymphocytic and epithelial elements, so that the tumor is described as lymphocytic, epithelial, or mixed. Histology, however, contributes nothing to the distinction between benign and malignant, which is based entirely on invasive gross characteristics. Distant metastases occur but are uncommon. CT scanning can add valuable preoperative radiographic evidence of invasive behavior. Biopsy is not usually recommended because of fear that violation of the capsule might promote invasive behavior, and because almost all such masses deserve an attempt at resection. When the findings suggest that complete resection might be difficult, it is perfectly rational to perform a biopsy followed by radiation or chemotherapy designed to shrink the tumor and simplify later resection.

In most cases resection through a median sternotomy provides the definitive diagnosis. Fifty to sixty-five per-

cent of thymomas are benign and subject to curative resection, which should encompass the entire thymus and all adjacent mediastinal adipose tissue. Truly complete resection is best accomplished with a generous extension into the neck to follow tongues of thymic tissue that commonly extent cephalad. All adjacent nonvital structures invaded by malignant thymoma should also be resected. Postoperative irradiation is of unproved benefit but is generally recommended for patients who have had incomplete resection of a malignant thymoma (Fig. 17-99).

LYMPHOMA

Mediastinal involvement is present in about 50 percent of patients with Hodgkin's and non-Hodgkin's lymphoma, and lymphoma is the most common mediastinal malignancy. Lymphoma is most frequently located in the anterior mediastinum (Fig. 17-100). Hilar nodes in the middle mediastinum are less commonly involved, and

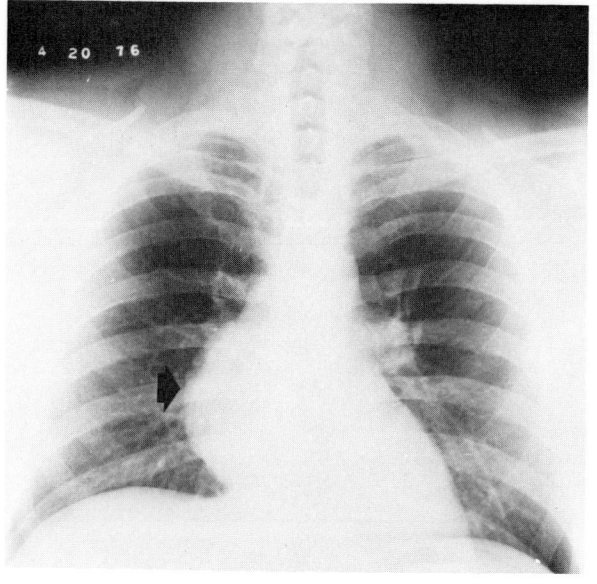

A

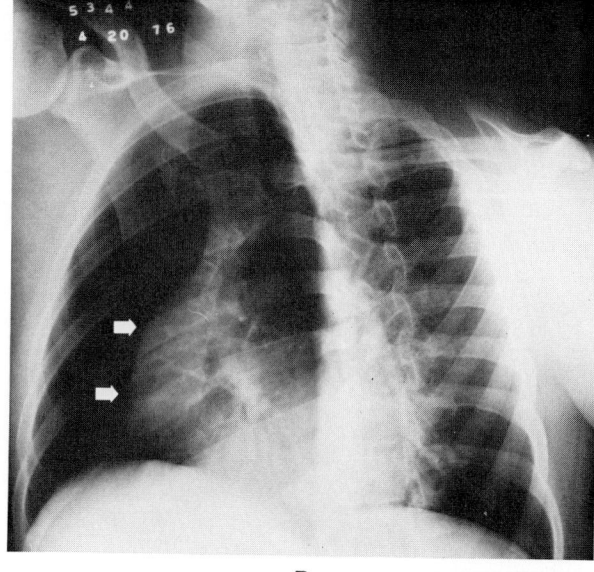

B

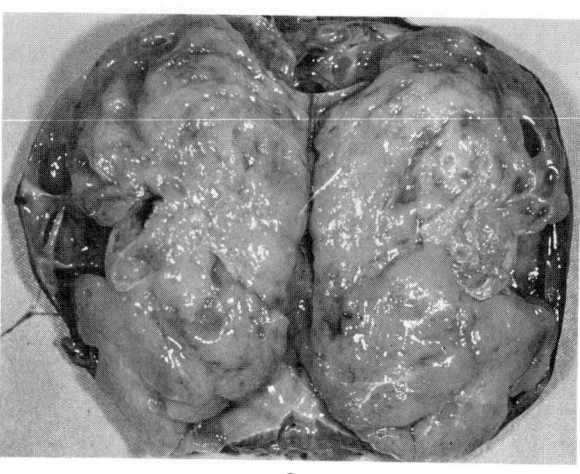

C

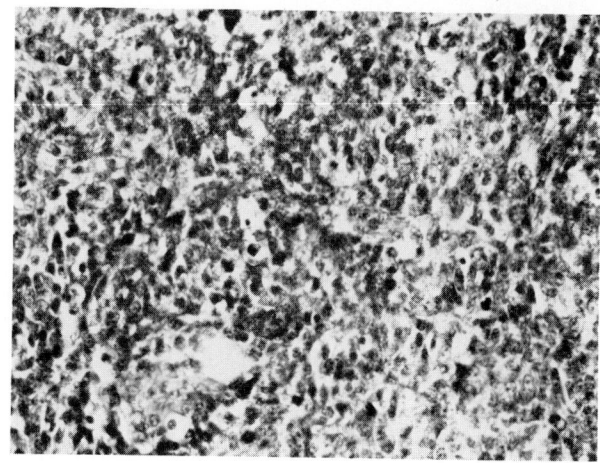

D

Fig. 17-98. A benign thymoma in a thirty-year-old man who presented with a persistent cough. *A.* Chest x-ray shows a large smooth mass contiguous with the right heart border. *B.* An oblique view suggests that the mass is closely related to the pericardium. *C.* The tumor was removed, along with remnants of the thymus, through a high right thoracotomy. This photograph of the bisected tumor shows that it was a well-encapsulated fleshy neoplasm. *D.* Histologic examination of the tumor shows a predominance of lymphocytic elements that justifies its classification as a lympho-cytic type of thymoma.

posterior mediastinal location is rare. Radiation is the standard treatment for most lymphomas, and resection is indicated only for the 5 percent of patients with lymphoma whose disease is confined to the mediastinum, underscoring the importance of a thorough search for involved lymphatic tissue elsewhere.

TERATODERMOID TUMORS

Teratomas account for less than 10 percent of all mediastinal tumors, with almost all found in the anterior mediastinum. By definition teratomas consist of multiple tissue types not normally found at the site of the tumor. They are most often partially cystic and consist primarily of ectodermal elements that can include hair, teeth, and sebaceous glands. Teratomas are thought to arise from branchial cleft and pouch cells associated with the thymus. The mediastinum is second to the gonads as the

most frequent location of teratomas in adults. The sex ratio is roughly equal, and age distribution peaks in early adulthood.

In modern series about two-thirds of patients are asymptomatic at presentation, and the majority of symptoms are nonspecific mass effects such as chest pain, cough, and dyspnea. The classic pathognomonic presentation with cough productive of hair and sebum has become a rarity, as most tumors are detected before eroding

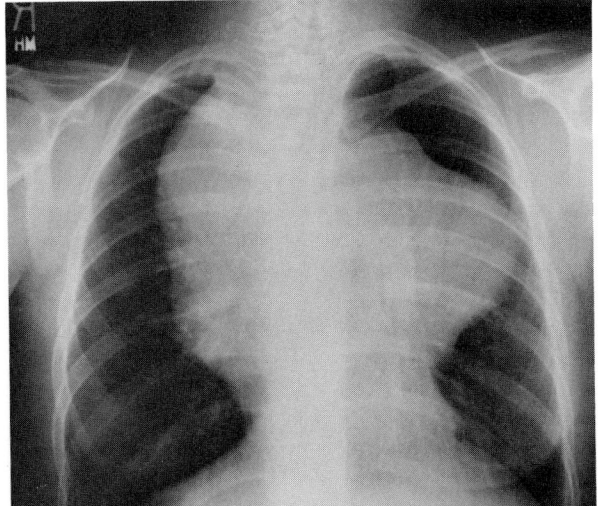

A

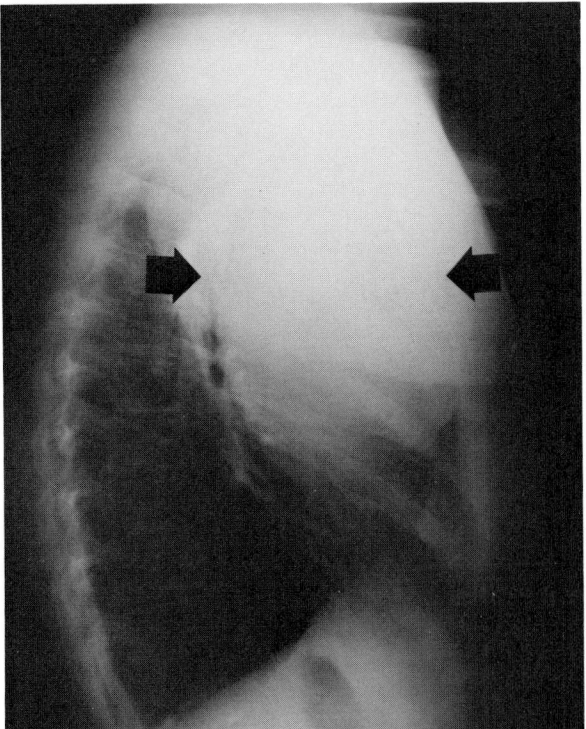

B

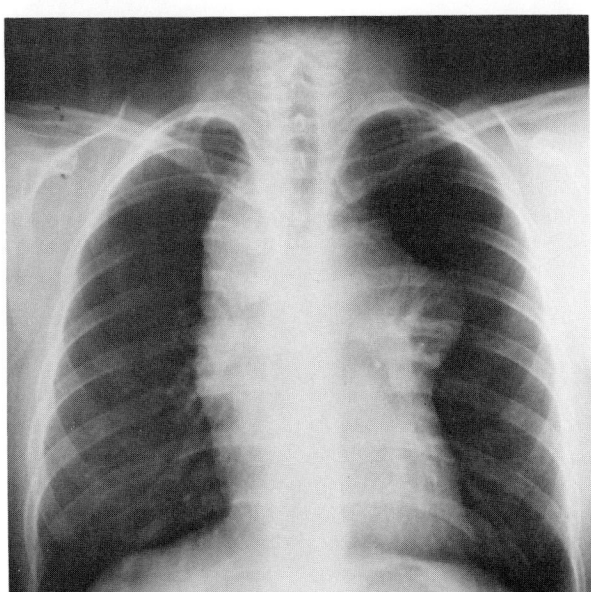

C

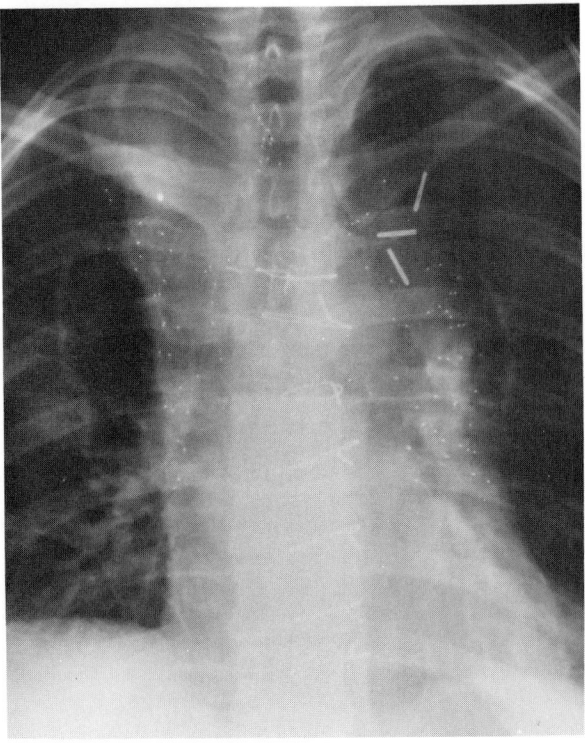

D

Fig. 17-99. A malignant thymoma in a twenty-nine-year-old woman who presented with superior vena caval obstruction and marked tracheal compression. *A.* The initial chest x-ray shows a huge mediastinal mass projecting into both hemithoraces. *B.* In lateral view the mass is seen to lie in the anterior mediastinum, compressing and posteriorly displacing the trachea. A mediastinal biopsy showed thymoma. *C.* After the patient received 2500 rad of external radiation therapy, a repeat chest x-ray shows a significant reduction in the size of the tumor. Symptoms were similarly improved. A subtotal resection was performed through a median sternotomy. The thymoma was found to invade the upper lobes of both lungs, the pericardium, and the areolar tissues of the mediastinum. Residual tumor was implanted with seeds of ^{125}I. *D.* A chest x-ray 1 month after operation shows further reduction in tumor size. The metallic markers of the isotope seeds can be seen throughout the tumor area. The patient has returned to work and is asymptomatic except for a chronic cough.

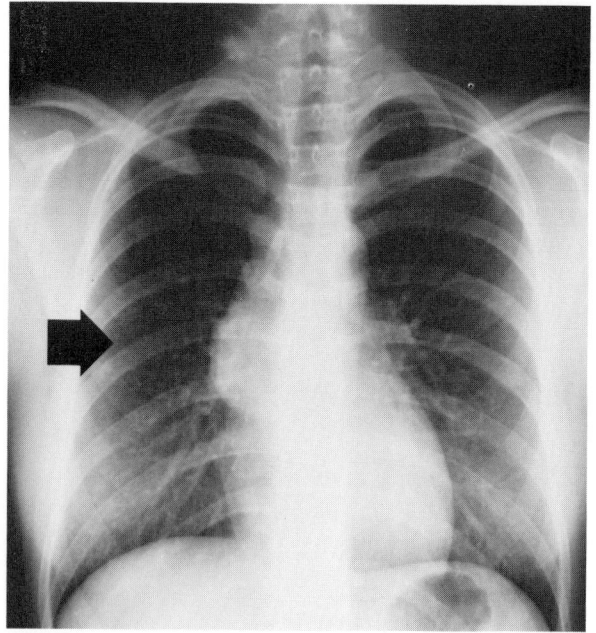

A

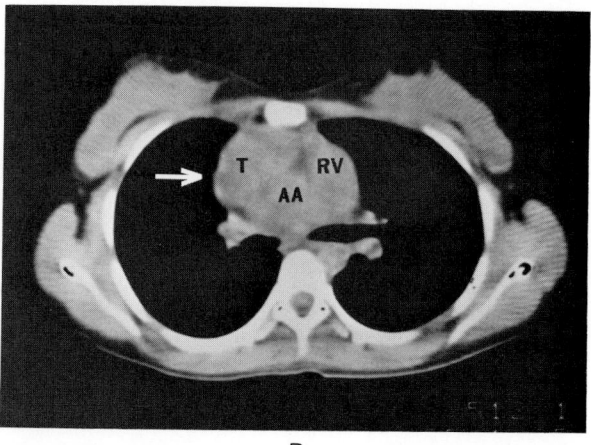

B

Fig. 17-100. Nodular Hodgkin's disease of the mediastinum in an eighteen-year-old woman. *A*. The chest x-ray shows a right mediastinal mass overlying the superior vena cava–right atrial junction. *B*. A CT scan section at the level of the right ventricular outflow tract (RV) shows the intimate relationship of the mass (T) to the ascending aorta (AA).

into the tracheobronchial tree. As with other neoplasms of the region, malignant teratocarcinomas are more likely to present with symptoms related to aggressive invasion of adjacent vital structures.

Typical radiographic appearance is that of a large, well-circumscribed anterior mediastinal mass. Twenty to forty percent of teratomas are calcified, most often appearing as a nonspecific opacity in the cyst wall, although occasionally due to the presence of teeth or bone. CT scanning

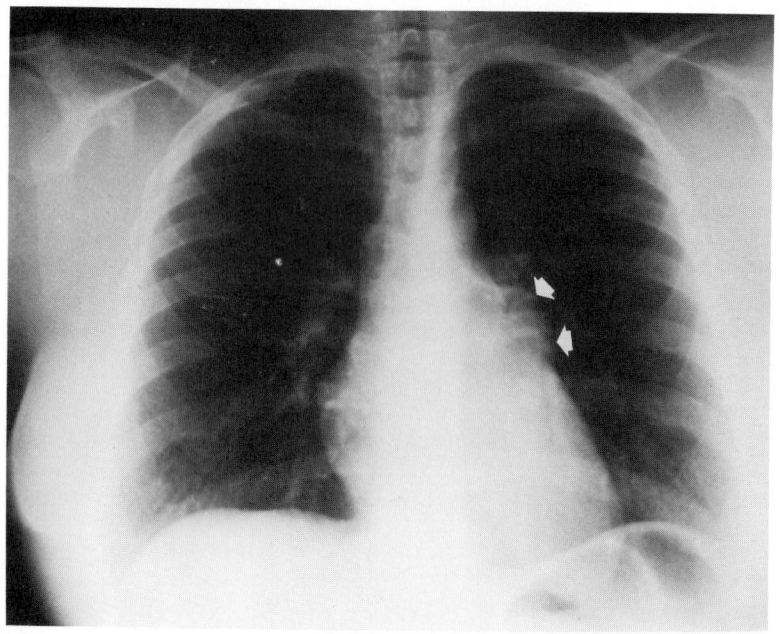

A

Fig. 17-101. *A*. Chest x-ray in an asymptomatic nineteen-year-old woman, demonstrating a mass along the left heart border in the vicinity of the left hilum *(see arrows)*. The lateral (not shown) suggested that the mass was in the anterior mediastinum. *B*. A CT scan without contrast shows a mass with small islands of calcification lying in the anterior mediastinum against the left side of the heart. There is a faint lucency *(see arrows)* suggesting that pericardium separates the mass from the heart. *C*. A CT scan with intravascular contrast injection suggests that the mass (M) is adjacent to but separate from the pulmonary artery (P) and right ventricular outflow tract. Through a median sternotomy a benign teratoma was removed easily along with the left lobe of the thymus. *(Courtesy of Alfred Jaretzki III.)*

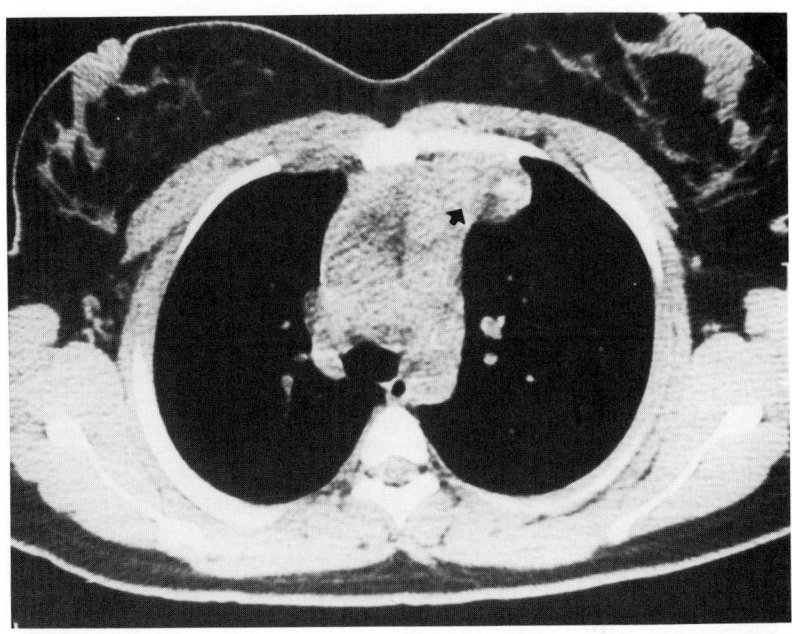

B

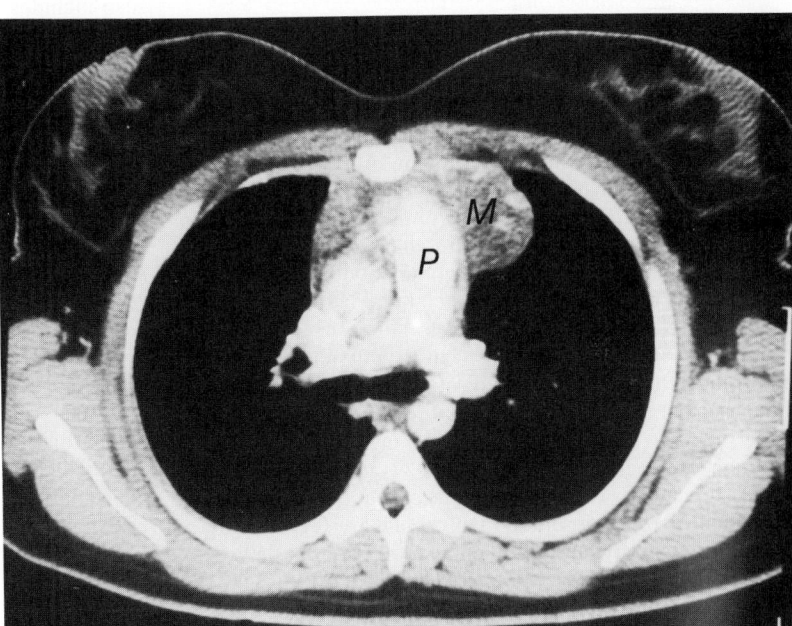

C

Fig. 17-101 *B,C.* Continued.

is very helpful in delineating involvement of adjacent structures, and in confirming fat density in the center of the cystic mass (Fig. 17-101). Elevated serum levels of alpha-fetoprotein and carcinoembryonic antigen suggest malignancy.

Surgical excision through a median sternotomy is the best method of diagnosis and treatment. Eighty percent are benign, and resection is curative. Even with benign forms resection is made more difficult by the tendency for the tumors to be densely adherent to surrounding struc-

tures, most commonly pericardium, lung, great vessels, and thymus, and incomplete resection is occasionally necessary. For benign tumors recurrence is rare even following partial excision. The prognosis for malignant tumors is poor because of local recurrence and distant metastasis.

GERM-CELL TUMORS

Primary extragonadal germ-cell tumors are rare. Although they can be seen in the pineal, sacrococcygeal, and paraaortic regions, they are most often found in the anterior mediastinum, where they comprise less than 1 percent of all mediastinal tumors. The histogenesis of germ-cell tumors outside the gonads is poorly understood, but a theory of origin from pluripotential primordial germ cells in the mediastinum is favored. Mediastinal teratoma should probably be viewed as the end point of benign differentiation in this germ-cell line but is usually considered separately because clinical behavior is quite different.

Five distinct cell types are recognized. Seminoma and embryonal cell carcinoma are most common, followed by choriocarcinoma, malignant teratoma, and endodermal sinus (yolk sac) carcinoma. These tumors are usually seen in young adults, with a male to female ratio of at least 4:1. Since the tumors are highly malignant, it is not surprising that 80 to 90 percent of patients are symptomatic when the diagnosis is made. The most frequent symptoms are nonspecific and result from tumor expansion encroaching on adjacent structures to produce cough, dyspnea, chest pain, or superior vena caval syndrome.

Standard posteroanterior and lateral chest roentgenograms will detect over 90 percent of such tumors. A CT scan can provide very helpful preoperative information regarding anatomic relationships and local invasion but does not substitute for exploration or biopsy. Serum tumor markers, while not specifically diagnostic, are important to obtain prior to treatment as a basis for monitoring relapse and response to treatment. All patients with choriocarcinoma have elevated serum human chorionic gonadotropin (HCG) levels, as will some patients with seminoma and embryonal cell carcinoma. Alpha fetoprotein levels can be elevated, most commonly in embryonal cell tumors, and carcinoembryonic antigen levels are occasionally elevated in all cell types.

The possibility of metastasis from a gonadal tumor must be excluded before a mediastinal germ-cell tumor is declared primary. Primary gonadal tumors rarely metastasize only to the mediastinum, and most often spread through retroperitoneal lymphatics. A gonadal primary can be excluded with reasonable accuracy if there is no evidence of retroperitoneal involvement by CT scan or lymphangiography, and if gonadal nodules are not detectable by palpation or ultrasound examination.

Most patients with mediastinal germ-cell tumors deserve exploration through a median sternotomy and an attempt at complete resection. In a recent large series from the Mayo Clinic, complete resection was achieved in 44 percent of 56 cases. The remainder frequently present with evidence of widespread local invasion or distant metastasis, and are subject to partial resection or to biopsy alone. It is important to separate seminoma from the other tissue types because of its radiosensitivity and generally better prognosis. Five-year survival is about 75 percent for seminoma treated with aggressive resection, followed by irradiation for local disease left behind, and chemotherapy for distant metastases. Prognosis remains poor in the other tissue types, although various protocols of combination chemotherapy have provided increasingly successful palliation.

MESENCHYMAL TUMORS

Tumors of mesenchymal origin constitute about 7 percent of all mediastinal tumors and cysts, with most occurring in the anterior mediastinum. Lipomas are most common and are characteristically soft masses without fixation to surrounding structures that can reach enormous size without producing symptoms. Fibromas are more dense and less common but have similar clinical behavior. The malignant forms (liposarcoma and fibrosarcoma) are seen rarely.

Tumors of lymph-vascular and blood-vascular origin are also classified as mesenchymal neoplasms. Tumors of blood-vascular origin consist of hemangiomas (capillary, cavernous, and venous) and rare malignant hemangiopericytomas. The most common lymph-vascular tumor is a lymphangioma (cystic hygroma). Most vascular tumors present as smooth, often lobulated masses of uniform density on chest x-ray, and will appear as cystic masses on CT scan.

The complete list of mesenchymal mediastinal tumors also includes mesothelioma, hamartoma, myxoma, mesenchymoma, leiomyoma, and leiomyosarcoma, xanthogranuloma, and rhabdomyosarcoma.

ENDOCRINE TUMORS

Thyroid and parathyroid tumors appearing in the mediastinum are most properly considered within the context of their usual cervical manifestations. Less than 10 percent of parathyroid adenomas are located in the mediastinum, and most are approachable through a cervical incision. Because of their embryologic origin from the third branchial cleft they are usually in close association with the upper pole of the thymus gland. Parathyroid tumors rarely present as a mediastinal mass.

Similarly, mediastinal thyroid tissue is usually a direct substernal extension of the cervical gland. Aberrant mediastinal thyroid tissue with agenesis of the cervical gland is exceedingly rare but does provide the rationale for obtaining a radionuclide thyroid scan in any patient with an undiagnosed mass high in the anterior mediastinum.

MEDIASTINAL CYSTS

Congenital cysts constitute approximately 20 percent of all primary mediastinal mass lesions, and account for the vast majority of middle mediastinal primary lesions. On chest x-ray they appear as opaque densities that may be indistinguishable from neoplasms except on the basis of typical location. On CT scan a mass with near water density occurring in a characteristic location is virtually diagnostic, and provides a strong rationale for routine use of CT scanning in mediastinal lesions. In a recent review of experience with mediastinal cysts in 34 children, Snyder et al. found that the accuracy of their preoperative diagnosis increased from 50 percent before the use of CT scanning to 100 percent thereafter.

Pericardial Cysts. These cysts are the most common type occurring in the mediastinum. They are usually detected as an incidental finding in an asymptomatic patient, and very frequently appear at the right costophrenic angle as a smooth-walled cystic mass 3 to 6 cm in diameter. They contain a clear fluid and occasionally communicate with the pericardium. Histologically they are lined with a single layer of mesothelial cells. The location and appearance of pericardial cysts are so characteristic, especially on CT scan, that close observation is becoming a defensible option, although most are still resected for diagnosis.

Bronchogenic Cysts. Bronchogenic cysts are most frequently located just posterior to the carina or main-stem bronchi, although they can be found elsewhere in the mediastinum or more peripherally in the lung (Fig. 17-102). Communication with the tracheobronchial tree can occur to produce an air-fluid level, serving to distinguish them completely from pericardial cysts but allowing for confusion with lung or mediastinal abscess in certain cases. Chest x-ray and CT scan will usually demonstrate a cystic mass in the characteristic location, although bronchogenic cysts can contain a viscid fluid difficult to distinguish from a solid mass by CT scan alone. A contrast esophagram may show compression of the esophagus by an anterior mass. Histologically they are lined with ciliated respiratory epithelium, and contain varying amounts of cartilage, smooth muscle, and mucous glands. They are most frequently symptomatic in children, producing cough, dyspnea, and stridor in more than half. All bronchogenic cysts should be resected, and are usually approached through a posterolateral thoracotomy. Especially when they have formed a communication with the tracheobronchial tree, the chronic infection that frequently results can make resection through dense inflammatory adhesions very difficult.

Enteric Cysts. Enteric cysts are located in the posterior mediastinum adjacent to the esophagus. They are occasionally embedded in the muscularis of the esophagus but rarely communicate with the esophageal lumen. The cysts have a smooth wall with a muscular coat and a lining recognizable as intestinal mucosa, although it may be ciliated, and they contain a clear, colorless mucoid fluid. When lined with an aberrant gastric mucosa, peptic ulceration can lead to perforation of adjacent bronchus or esophagus, producing hemoptysis or hematemesis, and erosion into adjacent lung can produce a lung abscess. A rare association with vertebral anomalies has been described in which the enteric cyst is attached to the spinal cord of meninges, and a patent tract may exist that can be demonstrated by myelography.

Approximately 60 percent of enteric cysts are recognized under one year of age, when symptoms of tracheal and esophageal compression are prominent. Less than one-third of children with enteric cysts are asymptomatic. Complete evaluation of children with a suggestive presentation includes chest x-ray and esophagram followed by a CT scan with contrast in the esophagus. Resection is always indicated. The lesions are approached through a posterolateral thoracotomy with the choice of side determined by the level of involvement and the appearance of projection into either hemithorax.

Mediastinitis

ACUTE MEDIASTINITIS

Acute mediastinitis is a fulminant infectious process with high morbidity and mortality characterized by rapid spread through the areolar planes of the mediastinum. The mediastinal pleura confines the process to the mediastinum only temporarily, with a breach occurring into one or both pleural cavities early in the course of the infection in most cases, after which the negative pressure of the pleural space helps to rapidly spread the infection throughout. The rapid spread of infection is promoted by several factors. One is the separation of tissue planes produced by air forced into soft tissues adjacent to a perforated hollow viscus, most often the esophagus, further promoted by the digestive action of salivary and gastric enzymes. Another is the pressure gradient established from the atmosphere to the negative pressure of the pleural space once the pleura is penetrated, which tends to pull the infection through the mediastinum from its source and into the pleural space. A third factor is the presence of naturally continuous fascial planes connecting the deep cervical compartments with the mediastinum, along which oropharyngeal infection can spread.

The infection is initiated most frequently by esophageal perforation, resulting from instrumentation, trauma, foreign body, suture line leak, or spontaneous postemetic rupture (Boerhaave's syndrome). Tracheal rupture or perforation is a less common cause in which dissemination of air through the soft tissues is massive, and infection is likely to be a secondary development. Direct necrotizing spread of infection without violation of an intrathoracic viscus is seen most commonly with aggressive oropharyngeal infections involving the deep cervical space but has also been described in association with infections of ribs, sternum, and vertebrae.

Chest pain, dysphagia, respiratory distress, and cervical–upper thoracic subcutaneous crepitus are the chief hallmarks of the process during the earliest stages of infection, when it is most important to diagnose the problem and begin treatment. Evidence of fulminant systemic infection is certain to appear within 24 h, and florid sepsis with hemodynamic instability supervenes rapidly in untreated cases.

The chest x-ray may be normal very early in the process, although mediastinal and subcutaneous air becomes apparent in most cases. The mediastinal contour is usually wide, and pleural effusion with or without pneumothorax appears very frequently. A contrast esophagram, for which water-soluble contrast is usually recommended, is essential when esophageal perforation is known or suspected. Esophagoscopy is rarely indicated in acute perforation. Specific diagnostic and therapeutic

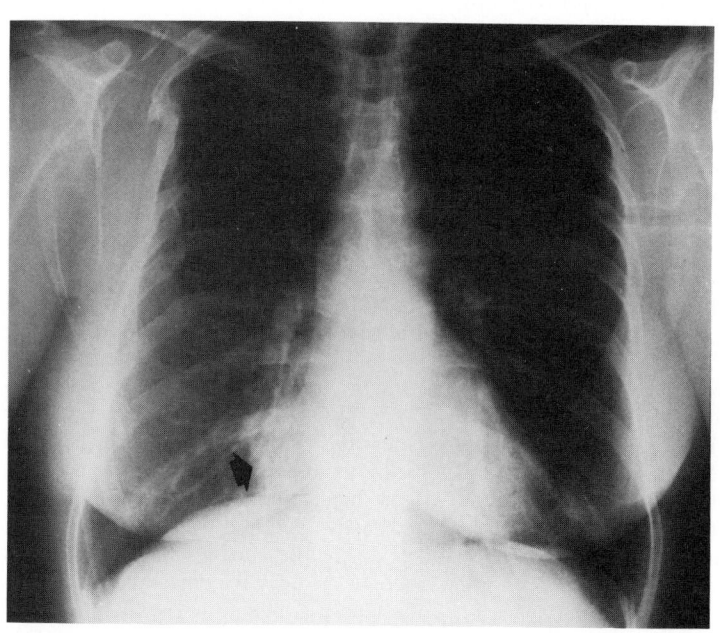
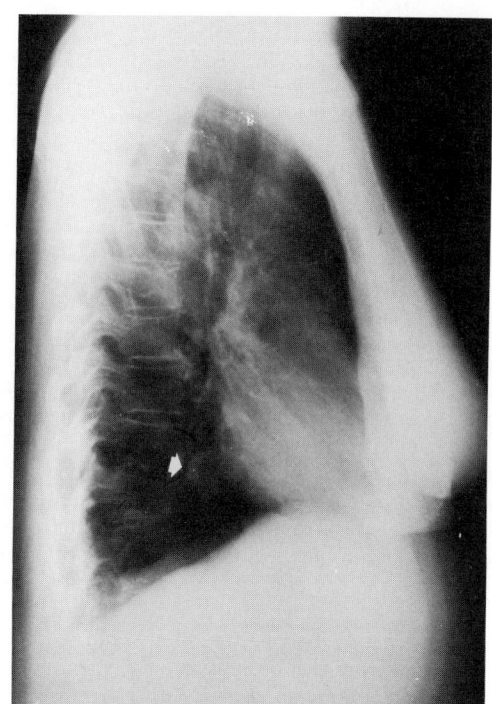

A

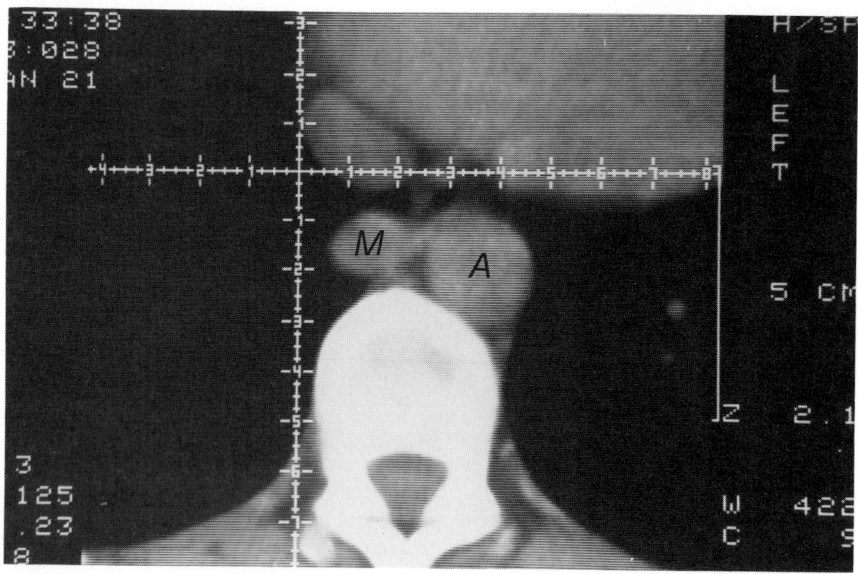

B

approaches to esophageal perforation are dealt with else-where.

Infections resulting from esophageal perforation and those descending from a perioral source are usually caused by a mixture of gram-positive and gram-negative aerobic and anaerobic organisms representing the spec-trum of oral flora. Initial antibiotic coverage should be broad enough to cover all possibilities until cultures are available.

Fig. 17-102. This forty-one-year-old woman had chest x-rays ob-tained during a mild respiratory illness. She was otherwise asymp-tomatic. *A.* A smoothly circumscribed mass is visible along the right heart border near the pericardiophrenic angle, and is seen in the middle mediastinum on the lateral view *(see arrows). B.* A magnified view from the CT scan shows a mass (M) of intermediate density lying just anterior to the spine, and just to the right of the aorta (A). The mass was resected through a right posterolateral thoracotomy, and was found to be a bronchogenic cyst, lined with respiratory epithelium. *(Courtesy of DM Carberry.)*

Treatment must be early and aggressive. Antibiotics and fluid resuscitation are begun immediately. Chest tubes are placed for pneumothorax or effusion. The primary problem, such as esophageal perforation, is treated according to accepted principles, either separately or in combination with drainage procedures. Direct drainage of the neck is occasionally required, entering the deep cervical space through an incision parallel to the sternocleidomastoid muscle and retracting the muscle laterally to expose the carotid sheath and pretracheal and retrovisceral spaces. Unilateral and often bilateral thoracotomy is frequently necessary for direct mediastinal drainage, debridement, and accurate placement of drainage tubes. In rare instances, especially in chronic contained posterior mediastinal infection, drainage is established by approaching the mediastinum extrapleurally through the bed of the posterior end of an overlying rib.

Mediastinitis is seen in 1 to 4 percent of patients following open heart surgery and has accounted for an increasingly large proportion of all cases of mediastinitis as open heart procedures have increased in frequency. It follows a more indolent course than the entities discussed above, is rarely associated with crepitus and mediastinal air on x-ray, and has the bacteriologic spectrum of other wound infections, with *Staphylococcus aureus* and *S. epidermidis* predominating. In recent years the use of muscle flaps rotated into the sternal defect has greatly improved the treatment of this complication, which is discussed more properly in detail as a specific complication of open heart surgery.

CHRONIC MEDIASTINITIS

Chronic inflammation and fibrosis in the mediastinum (sclerosing mediastinitis, fibrosing mediastinitis) are thought to result most often from granulomatous infection such as tuberculosis or histoplasmosis, although identification of an organism in individual patients is rare. It has been postulated that the process begins as an inflammatory reaction in the tissues surrounding involved lymph nodes. The process is likely to remain clinically silent unless it progresses to produce obstruction of the esophagus, airways, superior vena cava, or other mediastinal vascular structures. The chest x-ray may show mediastinal widening but is often normal. CT scanning combined with angiography may be necessary to define the process. Operative exploration is frequently required just to establish a diagnosis, and can also be undertaken to relieve obstruction.

Superior Vena Caval Obstruction

Superior vena caval obstruction is caused by bronchogenic carcinoma in 85 percent of cases. In the remainder the cause is another mediastinal tumor, fibrosing mediastinitis, thoracic aortic aneurysm, or caval thrombosis secondary to chronic indwelling catheters or instrumentation. At least 40 percent of bronchogenic carcinomas producing superior vena caval obstruction are small-cell tumors. Obstruction can be caused by compression or direct invasion. The clinical syndrome produced is easily recognizable, consisting of venous distention, facial edema, and plethora, often accompanied by headache and respiratory symptoms. In rare cases, associated airway compression or laryngeal edema can be life-threatening, but there is otherwise little evidence to support the commonly held notion that superior vena caval obstruction is inherently dangerous. Seizures, intracranial venous thrombosis, and other nonspecific cerebral consequences are unusual and highly associated with the presence of brain metastases. Survival in patients with obstruction due to carcinoma is usually measured in weeks to months, and it can be difficult to separate the dismal prognosis and aggressive behavior of the primary disease from the effects of superior vena caval obstruction alone. As with venous obstruction elsewhere in the body, compensatory venous collaterals develop promptly and largely ameliorate the condition, a fact that also complicates objective assessment of treatment modalities.

The vascular diagnosis can be confirmed by venography, but CT scanning with venous contrast is equally effective, and provides additional information regarding surrounding structures that can be diagnostically valuable. More invasive diagnostic procedures, such as mediastinoscopy, bronchoscopy, and lymph-node biopsy, have long been considered hazardous because of elevated venous pressure. A recent comprehensive review by Ahmann suggests that virtually all invasive procedures can be done with a low incidence of excessive bleeding. Respiratory complications related to venous engorgement and edema of the tracheobronchial mucosa can occur but are almost always manageable in the hands of a careful anesthesiologist. The very dominant clinical tradition favoring emergency radiation therapy for the clinical syndrome prior to obtaining a tissue diagnosis deserves reappraisal.

Especially since the vast majority of cases are caused by an incurable neoplasm, palliative radiation with or without combination chemotherapy is by far the most common treatment modality. The rare cases of benign etiology have occasionally been treated with venous bypass, but without large numbers of reportable patent conduits. Bypasses from the jugular vein to the atrium or distal superior vena cava have been accomplished with femoral vein and with a spiral graft constructed from excised saphenous vein (Fig. 17-103). Saphenojugular bypass has also been described, in which the saphenous vein is routed to the neck through a subcutaneous tunnel and left attached at the saphenous bulb for outflow. All invasive treatments have in common the difficulty of predicting which patients will be unable to establish sufficient venous collaterals over time without operation.

Bibliography

Introduction

Meade RH: *A History of Thoracic Surgery.* Springfield, IL, Charles C Thomas, 1961.

Ravitch MM: *A Century of Surgery 1880–1980.* Philadelphia, Lippincott, 1981.

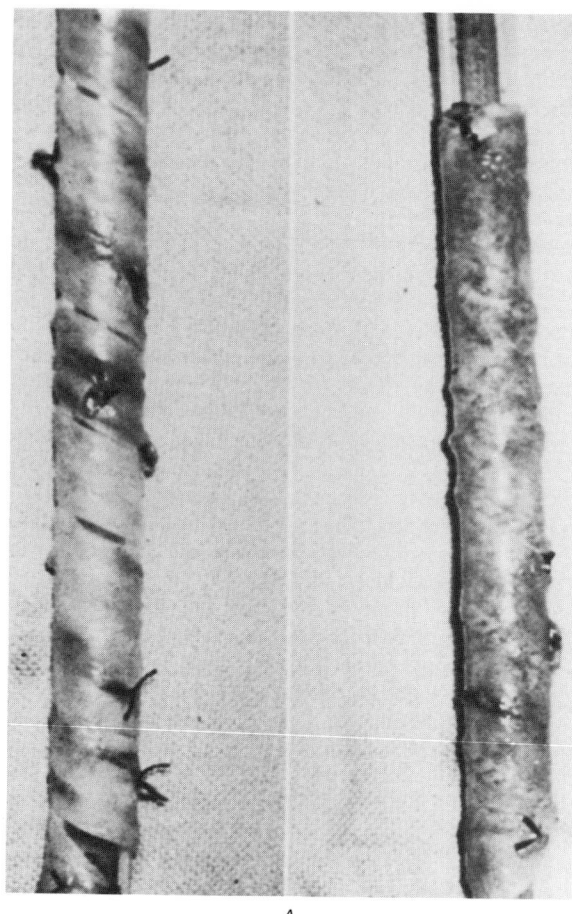

A

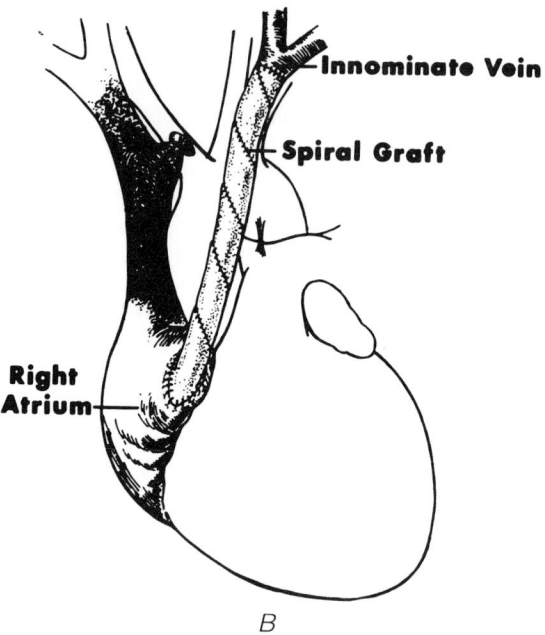

B

Fig. 17-103. Technique of spiral vein graft for bypass of superior vena caval obstruction. *A.* The spiral vein graft is constructed from a saphenous vein that has been opened from one end to the other and wrapped around a tubular stent (left). The opposing edges of vein are sewed together in a continuous spiral with fine monofilament suture (right). *B.* The spiral graft connects the innominate vein to the right atrial appendage. (From: *Doty DB, Baker WH: Bypass of the superior vena cava with spiral vein graft. Ann Thorac Surg 22:492, 1976, with permission.*)

Anatomy of the Thorax

Anderson JE: *Grant's Atlas of Anatomy,* 8th ed. Baltimore, Williams & Wilkins, 1983.

Blevins CE: Anatomy of the thorax and pleura, in Shields TW (ed): *General Thoracic Surgery,* 2d ed. Philadelphia, Lea & Febiger, 1983.

Thoracic Incisions

Asaph JW, Keppel JF: Midline sternotomy for the treatment of primary pulmonary neoplasms. *Am J Surg* 147:589, 1984.

El-Baz NM, Ivankovich AD: One-lung high-frequency ventilation, in Kittle RE (ed): *Current Controversies in Thoracic Surgery.* Philadelphia, Saunders, 1986.

Mitchell R, Angell W, et al: Simplified lateral chest incision for most thoracotomies other than sternotomy. *Ann Thorac Surg* 22:284, 1976.

Noirclerc M, Dor V, et al: Extensive lateral thoracotomy without muscle section. *Ann Chir Thorac Cardiovasc* 12:181, 1973.

Siegel T, Steiger Z: Axillary thoracotomy. *Surg Gynecol Obstet* 155:725, 1982.

Urschel HC Jr, Razzuk MA: Median sternotomy as a standard approach for pulmonary resection. *Ann Thorac Surg* 41:130, 1986.

Evaluation of the Thoracic Surgical Patient

Ali MK, Mountain CF, et al: Predicting loss of pulmonary function after pulmonary resection for bronchogenic carcinoma. *Chest* 77:337, 1980.

Bloomberg AE: Thoracoscopy in perspective. *Surg Gynecol Obstet* 147:433, 1978.

Boren HG, Kory RC, et al: The veterans administration—army cooperative study of pulmonary function: II. The lung volume and its subdivisions in normal men. *Med Clin North Am* 41:96, 1966.

Breyer RH, Karstaedt N, et al: Computed tomography for evaluation of mediastinal lymph nodes in lung cancer: Correlation with surgical staging. *Ann Thorac Surg* 38:215, 1984.

Doyle PT, Weir J, et al: Role of computed tomography in assessing "operability" of bronchial carcinoma. *Br Med J [Clin Res]* 292:231, 1986.

Gamsu G: Magnetic resonance imaging in lung cancer. *Chest* 89:242S, 1986.

Goldman L, Caldera DL, et al: Multifactorial index of cardiac risk in noncardiac surgical procedures. *Arch Surg* 101:140, 1970.

Mittman C: Assessment of operative risk in thoracic surgery. *Am Rev Respir Dis* 84:197, 1961.

Petty TL: *Pulmonary Diagnostic Techniques*. Philadelphia, Lea & Febiger, 1975.

Tisi GM: Preoperative evaluation of pulmonary function. *Am Rev Respir Dis* 119:293, 1979.

von Schulthess GK, McMurdo K, et al: Mediastinal masses: MR imaging. *Radiology* 158:289, 1986.

Postthoracotomy Considerations

Brynitz S, Schroder M: Intraoperative cryolysis of intercostal nerves in thoracic surgery. *Scand J Thorac Cardiovasc Surg* 20:85, 1986.

Conacher ID: Percutaneous cryotherapy for postthoracotomy neuraligia. *Pain* 25:227, 1986.

Cordell RA, Ellison RG: *Complications of Intrathoracic Surgery*. Boston, Little, Brown, 1979.

de la Rocha AG, Chambers K: Pain amelioration after thoracotomy: A prospective, randomized study. *Ann Thorac Surg* 37:239, 1984.

El-Baz NM, Faber LP, et al: Continuous epidural infusion of morphine for treatment of pain after thoracic surgery: A new technique. *Anesth Analg* 63:757, 1984.

Kirsh MM, Rotman H, et al: Complications of pulmonary resection. *Ann Thorac Surg* 20:215, 1975.

Larsen VH, Christensen P, et al: Postoperative pain relief and respiratory performance after thoracotomy: A controlled trial comparing the effect of epidural morphine and subcutaneous nicomorphine. *Dan Med Bull* 33:161, 1986.

Maiwand MO, Makey AR, et al: Cryoanalgesia after thoracotomy. Improvement of technique and review of 600 cases. *J Thorac Cardiovasc Surg* 92:291, 1986.

Mandal AK, Montano J, et al: Prophylactic antibiotics and no antibiotics compared in penetrating chest trauma. *J Trauma* 25:639, 1985.

Middaugh RE, Menk EJ, et al: Epidural block using large volumes of local anesthetic solution for intercostal nerve block. *Anesthesiology* 63:214, 1985.

Peters RM: Pulmonary resection and gas exchange. *J Thorac Cardiovasc Surg* 88:872, 1984.

Restelli L, Movilia P, et al: Management of pain after thoracotomy: A technique of multiple intercostal nerve blocks. *Anesthesiology* 61:353, 1984.

Thoracic Injuries

Albers JE, Rath RK, et al: Severity of intrathoracic injuries associated with first rib fractures. *Ann Thorac Surg* 33:614,1982.

Bailey P: Surfer's rib: Isolated first rib fracture secondary to indirect trauma. *Ann Emerg Med* 14:346, 1985.

Barone JE, Pizzi WF, et al: Indications for intubation in blunt chest trauma. *J Trauma* 26:334, 1986.

Beal SL, Oreskovich MR: Long-term disability associated with flail chest injury. *Am J Surg* 150:324, 1985.

Blaisdell FW, Lewis FR Jr: *Respiratory Distress Syndrome of Shock and Trauma*. Philadelphia, Saunders, 1977.

Chakravarty M: Utilization of angiography in trauma. *Radiol Clin North Am* 24:383, 1986.

Cole FH Jr, Miller MP, et al: Transdiaphragmatic intercostal hernia. *Ann Thorac Surg* 41:565, 1986.

Coselli JS, Mattox KL, et al: Reevaluation of early evacuation of clotted hemothorax. *Am J Surg* 148:786, 1984.

Hoekstra HJ, Kingma LM: Bilateral first rib fractures induced by integral crash helmets. *J Trauma* 25:566, 1985.

Johnson JA, Cogbill TH, et al: Determinants of outcome after pulmonary contusion. *J Trauma* 26:695, 1986.

Kelly JP, Webb WR, et al: Management of airway trauma. I: Tracheobronchial injuries. *Ann Thorac Surg* 40:551, 1985.

Landercasper J, Cogbill TH, et al: Long-term disability after flail chest injury. *J Trauma* 24:410, 1984.

Lazar HL, Thomashow B, King TC: Complete transection of the intrathoracic trachea due to blunt trauma. *Ann Thorac Surg* 37:505, 1984.

Neugebauer MK, Fasburg RG, et al: Routine antibiotic therapy following pleural space intubation. *J Thorac Cardiovasc Surg* 61:882, 1971.

Payne JH, Yellin AE: Traumatic diaphragmatic hernia. *Arch Surg* 117:18, 1982.

Poulton TJ, Haldeman LW, et al: Cardiopulmonary effects of severe thoracic subcutaneous emphysema. *J Trauma* 26:396, 1986.

Ross RM, Cordoba A: Delayed life-threatening hemothorax associated with rib fractures. *J Trauma,* 26:576, 1986.

Sladen A: Methylprednisolone. Pharmacologic doses in shock lung syndrome. *J Thorac Cardiovasc Surg* 71:800, 1976.

Symbas PN, Vlasis SE, et al: Blunt and penetrating diaphragmatic injuries with or without herniation of organs into the chest. *Ann Thorac Surg* 42:158, 1986.

Theriot BA, Gross BD, et al: Isolated fracture of the first rib associated with facial trauma. *J Oral Maxillofac Surg* 42:610, 1984.

Thompson BM, Finger W, et al: Rib radiographs for trauma: Useful or wasteful? *Ann Emerg Med* 15:261, 1986.

Chest Wall—Congenital Deformities

Beiser GC, Epstein SE, et al: Impairment of cardiac function with pectus excavatum with improvement after operative correction. *N Engl J Med* 287:267, 1972.

Blickman JG, Rosen PR, et al: Pectus excavatum in children: Pulmonary scintigraphy before and after corrective surgery. *Radiography* 156:781, 1985.

Cahill JL, Lees GM, et al: A summary of preoperative and postoperative cardiorespiratory performance in patients undergoing pectus excavatum and carinatum repair. *J Pediatr Surg* 19:430, 1984.

Hawkins, JA, Ehrenhaft, JL, et al: Repair of pectus excavatum by sternal eversion. *Ann Thorac Surg* 38:368, 1984.

Holcomb GW Jr: Surgical correction of pectus excavatum. *J Pediatr Surg* 12:295, 1977.

Marks MW, Argenta LC, et al: Silicone implant correction of pectus excavatum: Indications and refinement in technique. *Plast Reconstr Surg* 74:52, 1984.

Peterson RJ, Young WG, et al: Noninvasive assessment of exercise cardiac function before and after pectus excavatum repair. *J Thorac Cardiovasc Surg* 90:251, 1985.

Ravitch MM: Disorders of the sternum and the thoracic wall, in Sabiston DC, Spencer FC (eds): *Gibbon's Surgery of the Chest,* 4th ed. Philadelphia, Saunders, 1983.

Urschel HC Jr, Byrd HS, et al: Poland's syndrome: Improved surgical management. *Ann Thorac Surg* 37:204, 1984.

Wada J, Ikeda K, et al: Results of 271 funnel chest operations. *Ann Thorac Surg* 10:526, 1970.

Weg JG, Krumholz RA, et al: Pulmonary dysfunction in pectus excavatum. *Am Rev Respir Dis* 96:936, 1967.

Wesselhoeft CW Jr, Deluca FG: A simplified approach to the repair of pediatric pectus deformities. *Ann Thorac Surg* 34:640, 1982.

Chest Wall—Tumors and Thoracic-Outlet Syndrome

Blank RH, Connar RG: Arterial complications associated with thoracic outlet compression syndrome. *Ann Thorac Surg* 17:315, 1974.

Capistrant TD: Thoracic outlet syndrome in whiplash injury. *Ann Surg* 185:175, 1977.

Cavanaugh DG, Cabellon S Jr, Peake JB: A logical approach to chest wall neoplasms. *Ann Thorac Surg* 41:436, 1986.

Claggett OT: Presidential address: Research and prosearch. *J Thorac Cardiovasc Surg* 44:153, 1962.

King RM, Pairolero PC, et al: Primary chest wall tumors: Factors affecting survival. *Ann Thorac Surg* 41:597, 1986.

McGough EC, Pearce MB, Byrne JP: Management of thoracic outlet syndrome. *J Thorac Cardiovasc Surg* 77:169, 1979.

Moore M Jr: Thoracic outlet syndrome experience in a metropolitan hospital. *Clin Orthop* 207:29, 1986.

Pairolero PC, Arnold PG: Thoracic wall defects: Surgical management of 205 consecutive patients. *Mayo Clin Proc* 61:557, 1986.

Pairolero PC, Arnold PG: Chest wall tumors. Experience with 100 consecutive patients. *J Thorac Cardiovasc Surg* 90:367, 1985.

Qvarfordt PG, Ehrenfeld WK, et al: Supraclavicular radical scalenectomy and transaxillary first rib resection for the thoracic outlet syndrome. A combined approach. *Am J Surg* 148:111, 1984.

Roos DB: Congenital anomalies associated with thoracic outlet syndrome. Anatomy, symptoms, diagnosis and treatment. *Am J Surg* 132:771, 1976.

Sabanathan S, Salama FD, et al: Primary chest wall tumors. *Ann Thorac Surg* 39:4, 1985.

Sanders RJ, Monsour JW, et al: Scalenectomy versus first rib resection for treatment of the thoracic outlet syndrome. *Surgery,* 85:109, 1979.

Scher LA, Veith FJ, et al: Staging of arterial complications of cervical rib: Guidelines for surgical management. *Surgery* 95:644, 1984.

Diseases of the Pleura

Agostini E: Mechanics of the pleural space. *Physiol Rev* 52:57, 1972.

Azizkhan RG, Canfield J, et al: Pleuroperitoneal shunts in the management of neonatal chylothorax. *J Pediatr Surg* 18:842, 1983.

Bessone LN, Ferguson TB, et al: Chylothorax. *Ann Thorac Surg* 12:527, 1971.

Brenner J, Sordillo PP, et al: Malignant mesothelioma of the pleura. *Cancer* 49:2431, 1982.

Cattaneo SM, Sirak HD, et al: Recurrent spontaneous pneumothorax in the high-risk patient. *J Thorac Cardiovasc Surg* 66:467, 1973.

Chahinian AP, Pajak TF, et al: Diffuse malignant mesothelioma. *Ann Intern Med* 96:746, 1982.

DaValle MJ, Faber LP, et al: Extrapleural pneumonectomy for diffuse, malignant mesothelioma. *Ann Thorac Surg* 42:612, 1986.

de la Rocha AG: Empyema thoracis. *Surg Gynecol Obstet* 155:839, 1982.

DeMeester TR, Lafontaine E: The pleura, in Sabiston DC, Spencer FC (eds): *Gibbon's Surgery of the Chest,* 4th ed. Philadelphia, Saunders, 1983, chap 15.

Ferguson MK, Little AG, et al: Current concepts in the management of postoperative chylothorax. *Ann Thorac Surg* 40:542, 1985.

Fraedrich G, Hofmann D, et al: Instillation of fibrinolytic enzymes in the treatment of pleural empyema. *Thorac Cardiovasc Surg* 30:36, 1982.

Frimodt–Moller PC, Vejlsted H: Early surgical intervention in nonspecific pleural empyema. *Thorac Cardiovasc Surg* 33:41, 1985.

Ginsberg RJ: Diffuse malignant mesothelioma: A therapeutic dilemma. *Ann Thorac Surg* 42:608, 1986.

Hakim M, Milstein BB: Empyema thoracis and infected pneumonectomy space: Case for cyclical irrigation. *Ann Thorac Surg* 41:85, 1986.

Hutter JA, Harari D, et al: The management of empyema thoracis by thoracoscopy and irrigation. *Ann Thorac Surg* 39:517, 1985.

Lampson RS: Traumatic chylothorax. *J Thorac Surg* 17:778, 1948.

Light RW, MacGregor MI, et al: Pleural effusions: The diagnostic separation of transudates and exudates. *Ann Intern Med* 77:507, 1972.

Light RW, MacGregor MI, et al: Diagnostic significance of pleural fluid pH and P_{CO_2}. *Chest* 64:591, 1973.

Martini N, McCormack PM, et al: Pleural mesothelioma. *Ann Thorac Surg* 43:113, 1987.

McCormack PM, Nagasaki F, et al: Surgical treatment of pleural mesothelioma. *J Thorac Cardiovasc Surg* 84:834, 1982.

McLeod DT, Calverley PMA, et al: Further experience of corynebacterium parvum in malignant pleural effusion. *Thorax* 40:515, 1985.

Milsom JW, Kron IL, et al: Chylothorax: An assessment of current surgical management. *J Thorac Cardiovasc Surg* 89:221, 1985.

Reshad K, Inui K, et al: Treatment of malignant pleural effusion. *Chest* 88:393, 1985.

Robinson CLN: The management of chylothorax. *Ann Thorac Surg* 39:90, 1985.

Serementis MG: The management of spontaneous pneumothorax. *Chest* 57:65, 1970.

Strausser JL, Flye MW: Management of nontraumatic chylothorax. *Ann Thorac Surg* 31:520, 1981.

Wehr C, Adkins RB: Empyema thoracis: A ten-year experience. *South Med J* 79:171, 1986.

Lung—Anatomy and Diagnosis

Borrie J: Primary carcinoma of the bronchus: Prognosis following surgical resection. *Ann R Coll Surg Engl* 10:165, 1952.

Boyden EA, Tomsett DH: Congenital absence of the medial basal bronchus in a child: With preliminary observations on postnatal growth of the lungs. *J Thorac Cardiovasc Surg* 43:517, 1962.

Dahlgren S, Nordenstrom B: *Transthoracic Needle Biopsy.* Chicago, Year Book Medical Publishers, 1966.

Garfinkel L, Auerbach O, et al: Involuntary smoking and lung cancer. A case control study. *J Natl Cancer Inst* 75:463, 1985.

Garrison RJ, Castelli WP: Weight and thirty-year mortality of men in the Framingham study. *Ann Intern Med* 103:1006, 1985.

Graves WG, Martinez MJ, et al: The value of computed tomography in staging bronchogenic carcinoma: A changing role for mediastinoscopy. *Ann Thorac Surg* 40:57, 1985.

Hirayama T: Nonsmoking wives of heavy smokers have a high risk of lung cancer: A study from Japan. *Br Med J* 282:183, 1981.

LoCicero J 3d, Frederiksen JW, et al: Experimental air leaks in lung sealed by low-energy carbon dioxide laser irradiation. *Chest* 87:820, 1985.

Martin DH, Newhouse MT: Thoracoscopy: A clinical perspective, in Kittle RE (ed): *Current Controversies in Thoracic Surgery*. Philadelphia, Saunders, 1986.

Martini N, Heelan R, et al: Comparative merits of conventional, computed tomographic, and magnetic resonance imaging in assessing mediastinal involvement in surgically confirmed lung cancer. *J Thorac Cardiovasc Surg* 90:639, 1985.

McKenna RJ Jr, Mountain CF, et al: Open lung biopsy in immunocompromised patients. *Chest* 86:671, 1984.

Mutz N, Baum M, et al: Intraoperative application of high-frequency ventilation. *Crit Care Med* 12:800, 1984.

Oakes DD, Sherck JP, et al: Therapeutic thoracoscopy. *J Thorac Cardiovasc Surg* 87:269, 1984.

Pollin W, Ravenholt RT: Tobacco addiction and tobacco mortality. *JAMA* 252:2849, 1984.

Replace JL, Lowrey AH: An indoor air quality standard for ambient tobacco smoke based on carcinogenic risk. *NY State J Med* 85:381, 1985.

Ross JS, O'Donovan PB, et al: Magnetic resonance of the chest: Initial experience with imaging and in vivo T1 and T2 calculations. *Radiology* 152:95, 1984.

Shields TW: The dilemma of the mediastinal node, in Kittle RE (ed): *Current Controversies in Thoracic Surgery*. Philadelphia, Saunders, 1986.

Sinner WN: Complications of percutaneous transthoracic needle aspiration biopsy. *Acta Radiol (Diagn) (Stockh)* 17:813, 1976.

Todd TR, Weisbrod G, et al: Aspiration needle biopsy of thoracic lesions. *Ann Thorac Surg* 32:154, 1981.

Webb WR, Gamsu G, et al: Magnetic resonance imaging of the normal and abnormal pulmonary hila. *Radiology* 152:89, 1984.

Lung—Congenital Disorders, Emphysema

Brown SE, Wright PW, et al: Staged bilateral thoracotomies for multiple pulmonary arteriovenous malformations complicating hereditary hemorrhagic telangiectasis. *J Thorac Cardiovasc Surg* 83:285, 1982.

Dines DE, Arms RA, et al: Pulmonary arteriovenous fistulas. *Mayo Clin Proc* 49:460, 1974.

Ferguson TB: Congenital lesions of the lungs and emphysema, in Sabiston DC, Spencer FC (eds): *Gibbon's Surgery of the Chest*, 4th ed. Philadelphia, Saunders, 1983.

FitzGerald MX, Keelan PJ, et al: Long-term results of surgery for bullous emphysema. *J Thorac Cardiovasc Surg* 68:566, 1974.

Haller JA Jr, Golladay ES, et al: Surgical management of lung bud anomalies: Lobar emphysema, bronchogenic cyst, cystic adenomatoid malformation, and intralobar pulmonary sequestration. *Ann Thorac Surg* 28:33, 1979.

Iwa T, Watanabe Y, et al: Simultaneous bilateral operations for bullous emphysema by median sternotomy. *J Thorac Cardiovasc Surg* 81:732, 1981.

Michelson E: Clinical spectrum of infantile lobar emphysema. *Ann Thorac Surg* 24:182, 1977.

Tenholder MF, Jones PA, et al: Bullous emphysema: Progressive incremental exercise testing to evaluate candidates for bullectomy. *Chest* 77:802, 1980.

Wesley JR, Heidelberger KP, et al: Diagnosis and management of congenital cystic disease of the lung in children. *J Pediatr Surg* 21:202, 1986.

Lung—Pulmonary Infections

Alexander JC, Wolfe WG: Lung abscess and empyema of the thorax. *Surg Clin North Am* 60:835, 1980.

Amnest LS, Knatz JM, et al: Current results of treatment of bronchiectasis. *J Thorac Cardiovasc Surg* 83:546, 1982.

Battaglini JW, Murray GF, et al: Surgical management of symptomatic pulmonary aspergilloma. *Ann Thorac Surg* 39:512, 1985.

Confronting AIDS: *Directions for Public Health, Health Care, and Research*. Report of the Institute of Medicine, National Academy of Science, National Academic Press, Washington, 1986.

Cooper DKC, Lanza RP, et al: Infectious complication after heart transplantation. *Thorax* 38:822, 1983.

Cunningham RT, Einstein H: Coccidioidal pulmonary cavities with ruptures. *J Thorac Cardiovasc Surg* 84:172, 1982.

Daly RC, Pairolero PC, et al: Pulmonary aspergilloma. *J Thorac Cardiovasc Surg* 92:981, 1986.

Edson RS, Keys TF: Treatment of primary pulmonary blastomycosis. *Mayo Clin Proc* 56:683, 1981.

Elkadi A, Salas R, et al: Surgical treatment of atypical pulmonary tuberculosis. *J Thorac Cardiovasc Surg* 72:435, 1976.

Fuller J, Levinson MM, et al: Legionnaires' disease after heart transplantation. *Ann Thorac Surg* 39:308, 1985.

Golden N, Cohen H, et al: Thoracic actinomycosis in childhood. *Clin Pediatr* 24:646, 1985.

Glimp RA, Bayer AS: Pulmonary aspergilloma. *Arch Intern Med* 143:303, 1983.

Kosloske AM, Ball WS, et al: Drainage of pediatric lung abscess by cough, catheter, or complete resection. *J Pediatr Surg* 21:596, 1986.

Lacey SR, Kosloske AM: Pneumonostomy in the management of pediatric lung abscess. *J Pediatr Surg* 18:625, 1983.

Lemmer JH, Botham MJ, et al: Modern management of adult thoracic empyema. *J Thorac Cardiovasc Surg* 90:849, 1985.

leRoux BT, Mohlala ML, et al: Suppurative diseases of the lung and pleural space. Part I: Empyema. *Curr Probl Surg* 23:1, 1986.

Mammana RB, Eskild AP, et al: Pulmonary infections in cardiac transplant patients: Modes of diagnosis, complications, and effectiveness of therapy. *Ann Thorac Surg* 36:700, 1983.

McKenna RJ, Campbell A, et al: Diagnosis for interstitial lung disease in patients with acquired immunodeficiency syndrome (AIDS): A prospective comparison of bronchial washing, alveolar lavage, transbronchial lung biopsy, and open-lung biopsy. *Ann Thorac Surg* 41:318, 1986.

Mangoli L: Giant lung abscess treated by tube thoracostomy. *J Thorac Cardiovasc Surg* 90:186, 1985.

Miller JI: The thoracic surgical spectrum of acquired immune deficiency syndrome. *J Thorac Cardiovasc Surg* 92:977, 1986.

Newsom BD, Hardy JD: Pulmonary fungal infections. *J Thorac Cardiovasc Surg* 83:218, 1982.

Nonoyama A, Tanaka K, et al: Surgical treatment of pulmonary abscess in children under ten years of age. *Chest* 85:358, 1984.

Pass HI, Potter DA, et al: Thoracic manifestations of the acquired immune deficiency syndrome. *J Thorac Cardiovasc Surg* 88:654, 1984.

Pohlson EC, McNamara JJ, et al: Lung abscess: A changing pattern of the disease. *Am J Surg* 150:97, 1985.

Prager RL, Burney P, et al: Pulmonary, mediastinal, and cardiac presentations of histoplasmosis. *Ann Thorac Surg* 30:385, 1980.

Prober CG, Whyte H, et al: Open lung biopsy in immunocompromised children with pulmonary infiltrates. *Am J Dis Child* 138:60, 1984.

Rao RS, Curzon PGD, et al: Cavernoscopic evacuation of aspergilloma: An alternative method of palliation for haemoptysis in high risk patients. *Thorax* 39:394, 1984.

Rubinstein A, Morecki R, et al: Pulmonary disease in children with acquired immune deficiency syndrome and AIDS-related complex. *J Pediatr* 108:498, 1986.

Shamberger RC, Weinstein HJ, et al: The surgical management of fungal pulmonary infections in children with acute myelogenous leukemia. *J Pediatr Surg* 20:840, 1985.

Solomon NW, Osborne R, et al: Surgical manifestations and results of treatment of pulmonary coccidioidomycosis. *Ann Thorac Surg* 30:433, 1980.

Sterling RP, Bradley BB, et al: Comparison of biopsy-proven *Pneumocystis carinii* pneumonia in acquired immune deficiency syndrome patients and renal allograft recipients. *Ann Thorac Surg* 38:494, 1984.

Tokaro T, Sethi G, et al: Thoracic surgical infections, in Simmons RL, Howard RJ (eds): *Surgical Infectious Diseases.* New York, Appleton Century Crofts, 1982.

Tokara T: Lung infections and diffuse interstitial diseases of the lungs, in Sabiston DC, Spender FC (eds): *Gibbon's Surgery of the Chest.* 4th ed, Philadelphia, Saunders, 1983.

Treger TR, Visscher DW, et al: Diagnosis of pulmonary infection caused by Aspergillus: Usefulness of respiratory cultures. *J Infect Dis* 152:572, 1985.

Weber TR, Grosfeld JL, et al: Surgical implications of endemic histoplasmosis in children. *J Pediatr Surg* 18:486, 1983.

Weiland D, Ferguson RM, et al: Aspergillosis in 25 renal transplant patients. *Ann Surg* 198:622, 1983.

Weissberg D: Percutaneous drainage of lung abscess. *J Thorac Cardiovasc Surg* 87:308, 1984.

White JC, Nelson S, et al: Impairment of antibacterial defense mechanisms of the lung by extrapulmonary infection. *J Infect Dis* 153:202, 1986.

Wilson JF, Decker AM: The surgical management of childhood bronchiectasis: A review of 96 consecutive pulmonary resections in children with non-tuberculous bronchiectasis. *Ann Surg* 195:354, 1982.

Yellin A, Yellin EO, et al: Percutaneous tube drainage: The treatment of choice for refractory lung abscess. *Ann Thorac Surg* 39:266, 1985.

Young WG, Moor GF: The surgical treatment of pulmonary tuberculosis, in Sabiston DC, Spencer FC (eds): *Gibbon's Surgery of the Chest,* 4th ed. Philadelphia, Saunders, 1983.

Lung—Tumors

Aisner J, Whitacre M, et al: Combination chemotherapy for small cell carcinoma of the lung: Continuous versus alternating non-cross-resistant combinations. *Cancer Treat Rep* 66(2):221–230, 1982.

Auerbach O, Garfinkel L, et al: Scar cancer of the lung: Increase over a 21-year period. *Cancer* 43:636, 1979.

Belli L, Meroni A, et al: Bronchoplastic procedures and pulmonary artery reconstruction in the treatment of bronchogenic cancer. *J Thorac Cardiovasc Surg* 90:167, 1985.

Benfield JR, Yellin A: New horizons for lung cancer. *Surg Rounds* April 1985:26–52.

Breyer RH, Jensik RJ: Lung-sparing operations in elderly patients [letter]. *Ann Thorac Surg* 40:636, 1985.

Breyer RH, Zippe C, et al: Thoracotomy in patients over age seventy years. Ten-year experience. *J Thorac Cardiovasc Surg* 81:187, 1981.

Brock L: Long survival after operation for cancer of the lung. *Br J Surg* 62:1, 1975.

Cohen MH, Creaven PJ, et al: Intensive chemotherapy of small cell bronchogenic carcinoma. *Cancer Treat Rep* 61(3):349, 1977.

Cooper JD, Perelman M, et al: Precision cautery excision of pulmonary lesions. *Ann Thorac Surg* 41:51, 1986.

Cortese DA: Endobronchial management of lung cancer. *Chest* 89:234S, 1986.

Cox JD: Non-small cell lung cancer. Role of radiation therapy. *Chest* 89:284S, 1986.

Deslauriers J, Gaulin P, et al: Long-term clinical and functional results of sleeve lobectomy for primary lung cancer. *J Thorac Cardiovasc Surg* 92:871, 1986.

Eagan RT, Frytak S, et al: An evaluation of low-dose cisplatin as part of combined modality therapy of limited small cell lung cancer. *Cancer Clin Trials* 4(3):267, 1981.

Edell ES, Cortese DA: Bronchoscopic phototherapy with hematoporphyrin derivative for treatment of localized bronchogenic carcinoma: A 5-year experience. *Mayo Clin Proc* 62:8, 1987.

Errett LE, Wilson J, et al: Wedge resection as an alternative procedure for peripheral bronchogenic carcinoma in poor-risk patients. *J Thorac Cardiovasc Surg* 90:656, 1985.

Evans WK, Shepherd FA, et al: VP-16 and cisplatin as first-line therapy for small-cell lung cancer. *J Clin Oncol* 3(11):1471, 1985.

Faber LP, Jensik RJ, Kittle CF: Results of sleeve lobectomy for bronchogenic carcinoma in 101 patients. *Ann Thorac Surg* 37:279, 1984.

Feld R, Evans WK, et al: Combined modality induction therapy without maintenance chemotherapy for small cell carcinoma of the lung. *J Clin Oncol* 2(4):294, 1984.

Ferguson MK, Little AG, et al: The role of adjuvant therapy after resection of $T_1N_1M_0$ and $T_2N_1M_0$ non-small cell lung cancer. *J Thorac Cardiovasc Surg* 91:344, 1986.

Firmin RK, Azariades M, et al: Sleeve lobectomy (lobectomy and bronchoplasty) for bronchial carcinoma. *Ann Thorac Surg* 35:442, 1983.

Gail MH, Eagan RT, et al: Prognostic factors in patients with resected stage I non-small cell lung cancer: A report from the Lung Cancer Study Group. *Cancer* 54(9):1802, 1984.

Ginsberg RJ, Hill LD, et al: Modern thirty-day operative mortality for surgical resections in lung cancer. *J Thorac Cardiovasc Surg* 86:654, 1983.

Greco FA, Richardson RL, et al: Small cell lung cancer: Complete remission and improved survival. *Am J Med* 66(4):625, 1979.

Hansen HH, Dombernowsky P, et al: Chemotherapy of advanced small-cell anaplastic carcinoma: Superiority of a four-drug combination to a three-drug combination. *Ann Intern Med* 89(2):177, 1978.

Hardy JD, Ewing HP, et al: Lung carcinoma. Survey of 2286

cases with emphasis on small cell type. *Ann Surg* 193:539, 1981.

Hilaris BS, Gomez J, et al: Combined surgery, intraoperative brachytherapy, and postoperative external radiation in stage III non-small cell lung cancer. *Cancer* 55:1226, 1985.

Homes EC, Gail M: Surgical adjuvant therapy for stage II and stage III adenocarcinoma and large-cell undifferentiated carcinoma. *J Clin Oncol* 4(5):710, 1986.

Holmes EC, Hill LD, et al: A randomized comparsion of the effects of adjuvant therapy on resected stages II and III non-small cell carcinoma of the lung. The Lung Cancer Study Group. *Ann Surg* 202:335, 1985.

Hyman NH, Foster RS Jr, et al: Blood transfusions and survival after lung cancer resection. *Am J Surg* 149:502, 1985.

Ihde DC, Bunn PA, et al: Randomized trial of chemotherapy with or without adjuvant chest irradiation in limited stage small cell lung cancer, in Jones SE, Salmon SE (eds): *Adjuvant Therapy of Cancer IV*. New York, Grune & Stratton, 1984.

Immerman SC, Vanecko RM, et al: Site of recurrence in patients with stages I and II carcinoma of the lung resected for cure. *Ann Thorac Surg* 32:23, 1981.

Jensik RJ, Faber LP, et al: Segmental resection for bronchogenic carcinoma. *Ann Thorac Surg* 28:475, 1979.

Jensik RJ, Faber LP, et al: Survival following resection for second primary bronchogenic carcinoma. *J Thorac Cardiovasc Surg* 82:658, 1981.

Kirsh MM, Rotman H, et al: Carcinoma of the lung: Results of treatment over ten years. *Ann Thorac Surg* 21(5):371, 1976.

Kirsh MM, Tashian J, et al: Carcinoma of the lung in women. *Ann Thorac Surg* 34:34, 1982.

Kittle CF, Faber LP, et al: Pulmonary resection in patients after pneumonectomy. *Ann Thorac Surg* 40:294, 1985.

Komaki R, Cox JD, et al: Characteristics of long-term survivors after treatment for inoperable carcinoma of the lung. *Am J Clin Oncol* 8(5):362, 1985.

Komaki R, Roh J, et al: Superior sulcus tumors: Results of irradiation of 36 patients. *Cancer* 48(7):1563, 1981.

Kreyberg L, Liebow AA, Uehlinger EA: International histologic classification of tumours: No. 1. Histological typing of lung tumours. Geneva, World Health Organization, 2d ed, 1981.

Libshitz HI, McKenna RJ Jr, et al: Patterns of mediastinal metastases in bronchogenic carcinoma. *Chest* 90:229, 1986.

Maassen W, Greschuchna D, Martinez I: The role of surgery in the treatment of small cell carcinoma of the lung. *Recent Results Cancer Res* 97:107, 1985.

Martini N, Beattie EJ: Results of surgical treatment in Stage I lung cancer. *J Thorac Cardiovasc Surg* 74(4):499, 1977.

Martini N, Flehinger BJ, et al: Results of resection in nonoatcell carcinoma of the lung with mediastinal lymph node metastases. *Ann Surg* 198(3):386, 1983.

Martini N, Flehinger BJ, et al: Prospective study of 445 lung carcinomas with mediastinal lymph node metastases. *J Thorac Cardiovasc Surg* 80:390, 1980.

McCaughan BC, Martini N, et al: Chest wall invasion in carcinoma of the lung. Therapeutic and prognostic implications. *J Thorac Cardiovasc Surg* 89:836, 1985.

Meyer JA, Comis RL, et al: Phase II trial of extended indications for resection in small cell carcinoma of the lung. *J Thorac Cardiovasc Surg* 83:12, 1982.

Mountain CF, McMurtrey MJ, et al: Surgery for pulmonary metastasis: A 20-year experience. *Ann Thorac Surg* 38:323, 1984.

Mountain CF: The biological operability of stage III non-small cell lung cancer. *Ann Thorac Surg* 40:60, 1985.

Mountain CF: The new international staging system for lung cancer. *Chest* 89(4 suppl):225S, 1986.

Murray GF, Mendes OC, et al: Bronchial carcinoma and the lymphatic sump: Significance of bronchoscopic findings. *Ann Thorac Surg* 34:634, 1982.

Musset D, Grenier P, et al: Primary lung cancer staging: Prospective comparative study of MR imaging with CT. *Radiology* 160:607, 1986.

Osterlind K, Hansen HH, et al: Mortality and morbidity in long-term surviving patients treated with chemotherapy with or without irradiation for small-cell lung cancer. *J Clin Oncol* 4(7):1044, 1986.

Pairolero PC, Williams DE, et al: Postsurgical stage I bronchogenic carcinoma: Morbid implications of recurrent disease. *Ann Thorac Surg* 38:331, 1984.

Paladugu RR, Benfield JR, et al: Bronchopulmonary Kulchitzky cell carcinomas. A new classification scheme for typical and atypical carcinoids. *Cancer* 55:1303, 1985.

Paulson DL, Reisch JS: Long term survival after resection for bronchogenic carcinoma. *Ann Surg* 184:324, 1976.

Paulson DL: Carcinomas in the superior pulmonary sulcus. *J Thorac Cardiovasc Surg* 70(6):1095, 1975.

Pearson FG, De Larue NC, et al: Significance of positive superior mediastinal nodes identified at mediastinoscopy in patients with resectable cancer of the lung. *Thorac Cardiovasc Surg* 83:1, 1982.

Pearson FG: Lung cancer. The past twenty-five years. *Chest* 98(4 suppl):200S, 1986.

Perloff M, Killen JY, Wittes RE: Small cell bronchogenic carcinoma. *Curr Probl Cancer* 10:169, 1986.

Peters RM, Clausen JL, et al: Extending resectability for carcinoma of the lung in patients with impaired pulmonary function. *Ann Thorac Surg* 26:250, 1978.

Shields TW: The dilemma of the mediastinal node, in Kittle RE (ed): *Current Controversies in Thoracic Surgery*. Philadelphia, Saunders, 1986.

Shields TW, Higgins GA Jr, et al: Surgical resection in the management of small cell carcinoma of the lung. *J Thorac Cardiovasc Surg* 84:481, 1982.

Stair JM, Womble J, et al: Segmental pulmonary resection for cancer. *Am J Surg* 150:659, 1985.

Temeck BK, Flehinger BJ, et al: A retrospective analysis of 10-year survivors from carcinoma of the lung. *Cancer* 53:1405, 1984.

Warren WH, Gould VE, et al: Neuroendocrine neoplasms of the bronchopulmonary tract. A classification of the spectrum of carcinoid to small cell carcinoma and intervening variants. *J Thorac Cardiovasc Surg* 89:819, 1985.

Webb WR, Jensen BG, et al: Bronchogenic carcinoma: Staging with MR compared with staging with CT and surgery. *Radiology* 156:117, 1985.

Yellin A, Hill LR, Benfield JR: Bronchogenic carcinoma associated with upper aerodigestive cancers. *J Thorac Cardiovasc Surg* 91:674, 1986.

Zelen M: Keynote address on biostatistics and data retrieval. *Cancer Chemother Rep* 4(2):31, 1973.

Trachea

Ein SH, Friedberg J, et al: Tracheoplasty—a new operation for complete congenital tracheal stenosis. *J Pediatr Surg* 17:872, 1982.

arch, remaining as the ductus arteriosus. Vascular ring malformations arise from different remnants of these embryonic branchial arches.

The fetal circulation has several distinctive features that may influence association with congenital heart disease. In embryonic life the lungs are collapsed, with a high vascular resistance, and pulmonary blood flow is small. Most of the blood returning through the inferior vena cava to the right atrium goes through the foramen ovale into the left atrium and thence to the left ventricle. Also, most of the blood expelled from the right ventricle into the pulmonary artery is shunted through the ductus arteriosus into the descending thoracic aorta. At birth, with expansion of the lungs, there is a fall in pulmonary vascular resistance, although the vascular resistance does not decrease to that normally found in older individuals for the first 1 to 3 years of life. There is a corresponding persistence during this time of the fetal histologic structure of the pulmonary arteries, characterized principally by an abundance of smooth muscle in the media of the arterial wall. Persistence of the fetal histologic structure of the pulmonary arterioles is associated with pulmonary hypertension.

With expansion of the lungs, the ductus arteriosus normally closes in the first few days after birth. It remains patent in only a small percentage of individuals but is one of the most common forms of congenital heart disease. The foramen ovale is a slitlike channel that is automatically sealed when left atrial pressure becomes higher than right atrial pressure; it normally permits the flow of blood only from the right atrium to the left atrium, not in the reverse direction. Patency of the foramen ovale, usually an innocuous defect, remains throughout adult life in at least 10 to 20 percent of patients. With elevation of right atrial pressure above left atrial pressure from any cause, the foramen ovale may be stretched open and create a right-to-left shunt from the right atrium to the left atrium, resulting in cyanosis from shunting of unoxygenated blood. This characteristically occurs in patients with pulmonic valvular stenosis when right ventricular failure elevates right atrial pressure.

Although a large number of congenital heart defects have been recognized and classified, in a large pediatric cardiac clinic seven malformations will comprise the majority of abnormalities seen. Ventricular septal defect, with or without pulmonic stenosis, is by far the most common, representing 20 percent or more of all patients. The other six malformations, each occurring in 10 to 15 percent of patients, are atrial septal defect, pulmonic valvular stenosis, aortic valvular stenosis, patent ductus arteriosus, coarctation of the aorta, and transposition of the great vessels. The frequency of different defects varies somewhat with the age group evaluated; transposition of the great vessels is more common in the newborn but many do not survive beyond six months of age without an operation.

This gradual evaluation of symptoms is an important consideration in evaluating children with congenital heart disease, for parents are normally apprehensive about consenting to complex diagnostic studies or operative procedures on a child who seems, to the inexperienced eye, to have little disability. Postponing therapy until a child is disabled to a point that is clinically obvious may result in irreversible changes in ventricular muscle, for severe hypertrophy of the right or left ventricle often does not regress completely following surgical correction of the basic cause, such as pulmonic or aortic stenosis. Even more serious is an increase in pulmonary vascular resistance that is usually irreversible.

The three main physiologic disturbances resulting from congenital heart disease are (1) obstruction to emptying of the ventricles, (2) left-to-right shunts with increase in pulmonary blood flow and corresponding decrease in systemic blood flow, and (3) cyanosis. Each of these physiologic disturbances is considered in detail in subsequent sections. With almost all forms of congenital heart disease there is an increased susceptibility to bacterial endocarditis, because the anatomic malformation creates a localized turbulent flow of blood predisposing to local deposition of bacteria during a transient bacteremia.

OBSTRUCTIVE LESIONS. The most common disorders are pulmonic valvular stenosis, aortic valvular stenosis, and coarctation of the aorta. These impede emptying of the involved ventricular chamber, resulting in what has been termed "systolic" overloading and corresponding concentric hypertrophy of the ventricle. As the ventricular response is predominantly concentric hypertrophy, cardiac enlargement cannot be detected by clinical means, and often the chest radiograph is only slightly abnormal. The electrocardiogram and echocardiogram, however, can measure the degree of ventricular hypertrophy that has occurred. With progressive left ventricular hypertrophy angina pectoris may occur, with susceptibility to arrhythmias and even sudden death. Cardiac failure is a late and often preterminal manifestation.

LEFT-TO-RIGHT SHUNTS. As pressures in the left atrium and left ventricle are normally greater than those in the right atrium and right ventricle, a defect in either the atrial or ventricular septum results in a shunt of oxygenated blood from the left side of the heart to the right side. This causes pulmonary congestion from an increase in pulmonary blood flow and often a corresponding decrease in systemic blood flow. Cyanosis, of course, does not occur. With the increase in pulmonary blood flow there is a tendency to develop pulmonary hypertension, varying both with the type of defect and with the individual patient. The most common defects producing left-to-right shunts are atrial septal defects, with or without anomalous pulmonary veins, ventricular septal defects, and patent ductus arteriosus.

Pulmonary Congestion. A shunt becomes physiologically significant when the pulmonary blood flow is 1.5 to 2.0 times as great as the systemic blood flow. Large shunts may produce a pulmonary blood flow three to four times greater than systemic blood flow, with a pulmonary blood flow exceeding 10 to 15 L/min per square meter of body surface. The resulting pulmonary congestion produces a susceptibility to bacterial infection; recurrent bouts of pneumonia may occur in the first few years of life. Beyond early childhood, however, high pulmonary blood flows may produce surprisingly little disability for a period of time. With the increase in pulmonary blood flow there is a corresponding enlargement of the involved ventricle (right ventricle with atrial septal defect, left ventricle with patent ductus arteriosus, both ventricles with ventricular septal defect), resulting in so-called diastolic overloading of the ventricle, with cardiac dilatation rather than hypertrophy. The dilatation can be more easily recognized on clinical examination and on the chest radiograph than its counterpart, concentric hypertrophy. The changes in the electrocardiogram are often less prominent than those seen with concentric hypertrophy. But echocardiography can measure cardiac chamber size precisely. Cardiac failure tends to occur somewhat earlier in the course of the disease than with concentric hypertrophy, and the response to medical therapy is somewhat better than that for predominantly obstructive lesions.

Classification

Congenital heart disease may be classified by the type of anatomic abnormality present, which in turn produces a distinct physiologic disturbance. Four major groups exist: (1) obstructive lesions that restrict the flow of blood, with corresponding increased work loads on the obstructed ventricular chamber; (2) left-to-right shunts that occur through uncomplicated septal defects; (3) right-to-left shunts caused by the combination of a septal defect with obstruction to ventricular emptying; (4) complex malformations. These include abnormal origin or atresia of the aorta or pulmonary artery or hypoplasia or atresia of the right or left ventricle and the corresponding tricuspid and mitral valves.

Pathophysiology

Four degrees of severity of congenital heart disease can be recognized. The mildest form consists only of abnormal physical findings. In some instances, such as trivial pulmonic valvular stenosis, there may never be any sign of heart disease except the characteristic systolic murmur. In the second stage of severity, physiologic abnormalities, such as pressure gradients across stenotic pulmonic or aortic valves, increased blood flow through shunts occurring through atrial or ventricular septal defects, or elevation in pulmonary artery pressure, can be measured by cardiac catheterization. Eventually these physiologic abnormalities produce corresponding anatomic changes (the third stage in severity), manifested principally by cardiac enlargement with hypertrophy of the right or left ventricle, demonstrated by both the electrocardiogram and the radiogram. With the development of pulmonary hypertension, histologic changes occur in the media and intima of the pulmonary arterioles. Cardiac failure, the fourth stage, eventually results from the chronic increased work load on the heart, at times compounded by anoxia.

Increased Pulmonary Vascular Resistance. With the increase in pulmonary blood flow, pulmonary vascular resistance may increase. The mode of development remains incompletely determined. An excellent analysis of the functional pathology of the pulmonary vascular bed was published by Edwards in 1957. Pulmonary hypertension may result from at least three factors: (1) an increase in pulmonary blood flow, (2) histologic changes in the pulmonary vascular bed with corresponding anatomic restriction of distensibility of the pulmonary vessels, or (3) pulmonary venous obstruction. The most important consideration is the pulmonary vascular resistance, not the systolic pulmonary arterial pressure per se. Pulmonary hypertension resulting from an increase in pulmonary blood flow subsides as soon as the cardiac defect producing the increase in blood flow is corrected. Pulmonary hypertension due to increased pulmonary vascular resistance caused by thickening of the media and intima is often irreversible. When severe, surgical therapy is ineffective or contraindicated. Hence, in evaluating pulmonary hypertension, the significant physiologic measurement is the degree of change in the pulmonary vascular resistance, as calculated from the relation between flow and pressure, and not the absolute level of the pulmonary artery pressure per se.

Normally pulmonary arterioles are very distensible and can accommodate an increase in pulmonary blood flow up to three times normal values without any increase in pressure. Further distensibility is limited by the fibrous tissue in the adventitial sheath surrounding the arterioles. In infants and young children with pulmonary hypertension the prominent histologic change in the pulmonary arterioles is hypertrophy of the smooth muscle of the media of the arteriolar wall, which is similar to that normally found in embryonic life. Some consider these histologic changes a failure of involution of the normal fetal pattern. With more severe disease thickening of the intima occurs also. With associated fibrosis this has a serious prognosis, for such histologic changes are usually irreversible, remaining after the underlying cause has been corrected.

More significant than the increase in pulmonary blood flow, however, is the pressure under which blood is expelled into the pulmonary artery. Pulmonary hypertension is much more frequent with ventricular septal defects than with atrial septal defects that produce a similar increase in pulmonary blood flow. The incidence of hypertension with secundum atrial septal defects in children is about 5 percent, while the incidence is about 25 percent in men with ventricular septal defects.

There is also an individual variation in susceptibility to development of pulmonary hypertension. Some children with a large ventricular septal defect and a large increase in pulmonary blood flow will not develop any increase in pulmonary vascular resistance, while others with a smaller septal defect will develop significant pulmonary hypertension at an early age.

Defects such as truncus arteriosus or transposition may produce permanent injury in some infants before six months of age. Most lesions producing an increase in pulmonary vascular resistance, such as ventricular septal defect, patent ductus arteriosus, or atrioventricular canals should be surgically corrected in the first 6 to 12 months of life. The more serious defects, such as transposition or truncus arteriosus, may require operation in the first few weeks or months of life. With simple atrial secundum defect, however, operation at such an early age is virtually never necessary, illustrating the unknown etiologic factors in producing an increase in pulmonary vascular resistance.

Restriction in Systemic Blood Flow. With large left-to-right shunts there is often a decrease in systemic blood flow, frequently associated with a retardation in normal growth and development. This is more prominently seen in children with a patent ductus arteriosus or an atrial septal defect. The appearance of frail, underweight children with atrial septal defect has been termed the *gracile* habitus. Although mental retardation is slightly more common in children with congenital heart disease, beyond this association there is no evidence that congenital heart disease retards mental development. Unfortunately, correction of the cardiac defect does not result in any improvement in mental function. After operation there is often a substantial increase in growth and weight.

RIGHT-TO-LEFT SHUNTS. Right-to-left shunts of venous blood directly into the systemic circulation, producing arterial hypoxemia and cyanosis, result from the combination of an intracardiac septal defect with obstruction to normal flow of blood into the pulmonary artery. The classic example is the tetralogy of Fallot, a combination of ventricular septal defect and pulmonic stenosis. Other cyanotic disorders include the more complex malformations, such as transposition of the great vessels, tricuspid atresia, truncus arteriosus, and total anomalous drainage of the pulmonary veins. Right-to-left shunts produce a large number of physiologic disturbances because of the anoxia resulting from chronic hypoxemia. These are considered in detail in the following paragraphs. It should be emphasized that all these disturbances result from deficient oxygen transport to tissues of the body. With right-to-left shunts there is no increase in cardiac output; the pulmonary blood flow is usually less than normal. Hence cardiac failure is rare with an uncomplicated right-to-left shunt, in contrast to its inevitable eventual occurrence with left-to-right shunts.

Cyanosis. This is the most prominent feature of a right-to-left shunt. The degree of cyanosis depends upon both the degree of anoxia and the blood hemoglobin concentration, for the visible intensity of cyanosis is determined by the number of grams of reduced hemoglobin in the circulation. It has been estimated that about 5 g of reduced hemoglobin is required to produce visible cyanosis. Normally in the capillaries about 2.25 g of reduced hemoglobin is present, so with an average hemoglobin concentration of 15 g/dL of blood, a decrease in arterial oxygen from the normal range of nearly 95 to 75 percent is needed to produce visible cyanosis. In the presence of anemia, however, a more severe degree of anoxia is required to produce visible cyanosis, while with polycythemia and hemoglobin concentrations of 20 g/dL of blood or more, severe cyanosis occurs with lesser degrees of anoxia.

Cyanosis has been conveniently grouped into "central" and "peripheral" types. *Peripheral* cyanosis results simply from a decrease in cardiac output with sluggish regional flow of blood through the capillary circulation, as a result of which more oxygen is extracted and a greater amount of reduced hemoglobin is present. This type of cyanosis occurs with conditions producing a low cardiac output, such as mitral stenosis, and varies with the condition of the patient. It is usually more prominent in certain regions of the body, such as the tips of the fingers, the lips, or the lobes of the ears.

Central cyanosis results either from a defect in oxygenation of blood in the lungs or from an intracardiac shunt. Cyanosis resulting from ventilatory insufficiency can usually be recognized from its prompt improvement when the patient breathes 100% oxygen, increasing the efficiency of pulmonary ventilation. In the catheterization laboratory it can be recognized from the finding that oxygen saturation of blood in the left atrium is less than 95 percent. Pulmonary insufficiency from cardiac disease occurs only with severe pulmonary congestion from cardiac failure or far advanced pulmonary vascular disease.

An intracardiac shunt, permitting direct entry of venous blood into the systemic circulation, is the cause of central cyanosis in most patients. The intensity of the cyanosis is related to the volume of pulmonary blood flow, for ultimately cyanosis depends upon the relative proportions of unoxygenated and oxygenated blood in the arterial circulation. Even though a large intracardiac shunt is present, an increase in pulmonary blood flow to produce a larger amount of oxygenated blood can substantially reduce cyanosis and improve oxygen transport. This was dramatically demonstrated by Blalock with the systemic-pulmonary artery anastomosis for tetralogy of Fallot.

The two distinctive changes that inevitably appear with chronic cyanosis are clubbing of the digits and polycythemia. The triad of cyanosis, clubbing, and polycythemia is a familiar one in children with congenital heart disease. Clubbing of the digits, or hypertrophic osteoarthropathy, is an unusual change in the appearance and structure of the digits, consisting of a rounding of the tips of the fingers and toes, as well as a thickening of the ends, associated with deposition of fibrous tissue. In addition, there may be a pronounced convexity of the fingernails. Histologically, the fingers have increased numbers of capillaries, with a large number of tiny arteriovenous aneurysms. Clubbing is usually not prominent until a cyanotic child is one to two years of age, but in some instances of severe anoxia it may evolve within several weeks. It usually gradually subsides following correction of the intracardiac defect.

Polycythemia is a fortunate physiologic response of the bone marrow to chronic anoxia, as an increase in red cell and hemoglobin concentration increases the ability of the blood to transport oxygen. Hematocrits of 60 to 70 percent are frequent with chronic cyanosis: values exceeding 80 percent are noted in extreme cases. There is a parallel rise in viscosity of the blood, with restriction to the flow of blood as the hematocrit rises. Once the hematocrit exceeds 75 to 80 percent, the increased viscosity constitutes a significant hazard, for transitory dehydration in an infant with a hematocrit above 80 percent may precipitate cerebral venous thrombosis and permanent neurologic injury, apparently from formation of thrombi in the viscous blood.

Limitation of Exercise Tolerance. A decrease in exercise tolerance, with dyspnea on exertion, is characteristic of cyanotic heart disease, for the circulation is unable to increase oxygen transport with exercise. The severity of the disability, or its progression, can be conveniently measured in terms of the patient's ability to walk a measured distance. Associated with exertional dyspnea is squatting, a phenomenon first emphasized by Taussig. The cyanotic child quickly learns that dyspnea on walking can be lessened by assuming a squatting position. Physiologic studies indicate that squatting produces an increase in peripheral vascular resistance, with a corresponding increase in pulmonary blood flow. Squatting is most commonly seen in tetralogy of Fallot, less frequently in other cyanotic conditions.

Neurologic Damage. Periodic episodes of unconsciousness, termed *cyanotic spells,* are grave signs of cerebral anoxia. They often appear in the third to fourth month of life in severely cyanotic children, even in the first few weeks of life with extreme anoxia, but are rare after the fifth to sixth year of life. They characteristically occur at different times, not always associated with exertion, and evolve as episodes of crying, deepening cyanosis, and coma, lasting a few minutes to a few hours. Such episodes are extremely grave, for although recovery may ensue promptly, the spells are recurrent, and any spell may either terminate fatally or result in permanent neurologic injury. Emergency surgical treatment to improve the oxygen content of the arterial blood is strongly indicated.

Another cause of neurologic injury in cyanotic children is brain abscess, for which there is an increased susceptibility especially in children with tetralogy of Fallot. The increased susceptibility is partly related to direct access of bacteria in the venous circulation to the arterial circulation through the right-to-left shunt. This is probably not the entire explanation, however, for a similar increased frequency does not occur in other cyanotic conditions. A localized infarct with subsequent bacterial infection may explain the evolution in some patients.

Another rare cause of cerebral injury is paradoxic embolism through an intracardiac defect, in which a thrombus migrating in the venous circulation, which would normally produce a pulmonary embolus, traverses an intracardiac defect and lodges in the cerebral circulation. Hence permanent neurologic injury, most often seen as hemiplegia, is not uncommon in children with chronic severe cyanosis, constituting a strong indication for early surgical therapy when possible.

Other Changes. In older children with severe cyanosis there is a striking increase in bronchial circulation, apparently a compensatory response to the chronic decrease in pulmonary blood flow. The myriads of collateral vessels, often constituting a mass of varicosities in the mediastinum, are principally of surgical significance because of the risk of bleeding during operation. They may be associated with epistaxis in some children, but hemoptysis is rare because the pulmonary blood flow is usually less than normal, even though the bronchial circulation is greatly increased.

Eventually, with chronic polycythemia in children older than ten to fifteen years of age, multiple defects in blood coagulation occur, with abnormalities in several components of the blood-clotting mechanism. Clinically this may result in mild gastrointestinal bleeding, but the major significance is the increased susceptibility to hemorrhage following surgical procedures.

Clinical Examination

HISTORY. In obtaining the history of a patient with congenital heart disease, the presence of abnormal factors during pregnancy, especially during the first trimester, should be noted. Rubella in the first trimester has been emphasized because of the high incidence of cardiac and other defects. In some disorders, notably hypertrophic muscular aortic stenosis, there is a definite familial history of the disorder. Also, with the majority of patients with congenital heart disease there is about a 2 percent associated occurrence of congenital heart disease in other members of the same family. In most patients, however, no etiologic factors can be found.

The age at which a cardiac murmur was detected for the first time should be carefully noted. Similarly the time of appearance of cyanosis is of significance, whether at birth or subsequently during infancy. Variations in the appearance of cyanosis, as well as its location, are also important. In some patients cyanosis may be recognized at birth, then disappear for months or years, and finally appear again.

A decrease in exercise tolerance, manifested by dyspnea on exertion, is a common symptom and a convenient indication of the severity of the disorder in patients with right-to-left shunts. Squatting can be readily identified by the parents. Symptoms of lesser degrees of restriction in physical capacity, such as undue fatigability or inability to participate in exercise, should be noted, although the ability of many children with large left-to-right shunts to participate vigorously in athletics is impressive. Feeding habits and the pattern of weight are also important features.

Previous neurologic episodes such as cyanotic spells, cerebral embolism, brain abscess, or other signs of cerebral injury should be noted.

An inquiry should be made about infections such as pneumonia, bacterial endocarditis, or rheumatic fever.

PHYSICAL EXAMINATION. Abnormalities in growth and development should be particularly assessed, because these are among the most common signs of cardiac disease. Cyanosis, with clubbing or polycythemia, may be obvious or may require close scrutiny for detection. On examination of the heart, any deformity of the left costal cartilages, indicating long-standing cardiac enlargement, should be noted. A palpable thrill is particularly important, for it almost uniformly indicates significant underlying cardiac disease. Cardiac size should be estimated, although this is difficult in small children and infants and is best determined by the x-ray and echocardiogram. Systolic murmurs are commonly found but often are of little diagnostic significance. Basal systolic murmurs occur with pulmonic stenosis, aortic stenosis, patent ductus in infants, and coarctation of the aorta. A murmur along the left sternal border is particularly prominent with ventricular septal defect. With systolic murmurs the type of murmur, location, and transmission are of particular importance. Diastolic murmurs are infrequent in infants but when present are especially significant. They may occur from aortic insufficiency with prolapse of an aortic cusp, with pulmonic insufficiency from long-standing pulmonary hypertension, or in association with a systolic murmur as the continuous murmur of a patent ductus arteriosus. The cardiac sounds, especially the second sound at the base, may be of importance in certain conditions. The pulmonic second sound is increased with pulmonary hypertension, decreased or absent with pulmonic stenosis or atresia. Variation in splitting of the second sound may be recognized by experienced observers and is of diagnostic importance, especially with atrial septal defect. Disturbances of rhythm are infrequent. The gallop rhythm with its ominous prognosis is seen in terminal forms of cardiac disease.

Examination of the lungs may detect rales from cardiac failure in large left-to-right shunts, but characteristically no abnormalities are found in the lungs with right-to-left shunts producing cyanosis. The hallmark of congestive failure in children is hepatic enlargement, occurring with surprising rapidity and regressing rapidly as failure improves. Hence estimation of the presence and extent of hepatic enlargement is of particular importance. Often hepatic enlargement precedes the detection of audible rales, in contrast to adult forms of cardiac disease. Similarly, edema is usually less prominent clinically than hepatic enlargement.

In the extremities, the presence and quality of the radial, femoral, and pedal pulses should be noted. Faint pulses are characteristic of aortic stenosis. With coarctation, radial pulses are prominent while femoral pulses are weak or absent. Easily palpable, bounding pulses are characteristic of defects producing an abnormal exit of blood from the aorta during diastole, such as patent ductus arteriosus, aortic insufficiency, or a ruptured aneurysm of the sinus of Valsalva. These are associated with an increase in pulse pressure, usually due to a decrease in diastolic pressure. Normally the systolic blood pressure in infants is in the range of 70 to 90 mmHg, rising to about 100 mmHg in the first 5 years of life and subsequently to the normal adult level of 120 mmHg in the next few years. Diastolic pressures are usually in the range of 55 to 60 mmHg.

Examination of the digits is particularly useful with cyanosis, because clubbing is inevitable with chronic severe cyanosis.

LABORATORY STUDIES. The basic noninvasive studies are the chest x-ray, electrocardiogram, and echocardiogram. On the chest x-ray, cardiac size, contour, and vascularity of the lung fields should be noted. Unusual abnormalities include pleural effusion and notching of the ribs, seen in coarctation of the aorta. Cardiac size is best expressed as the cardiothoracic ratio, with a ratio greater than 0.5 indicating cardiac enlargement. In oblique views, enlargement of specific cardiac chambers can be estimated, though this is more precisely done with echocardiography, measuring in centimeters the exact dimensions of the atria and ventricles. Enlargement of the left atrium occurs with mitral insufficiency, ventricular septal defect, patent ductus arteriosus, or any form of left ventricular failures. Left ventricular enlargement is characteristic of aortic disease, mitral insufficiency, coarctation of the aorta, patent ductus arteriosus, and ventricular septal defect. Right atrial enlargement is especially prominent in Ebstein's malformation and also occurs in tricuspid atresia, atrial septal defect, and pulmonic stenosis. Selective enlargement of the right ventricle is frequently seen with pulmonic stenosis, pulmonary hypertension from any cause, atrial septal defect, and ventricular septal defect.

Characteristic changes in contour are seen in certain malformations. The Sabot-shaped heart of tetralogy of Fallot results from hypertrophy of the right ventricle in association with a small pulmonary conus (Fig. 18-1). The egg-shaped heart of transposition of the great vessels (Fig. 18-2) is caused by enlargement of the right ventricle

Fig. 18-1. Chest radiograph of child with tetralogy of Fallot, showing typical cardiac silhouette (sabot-shaped heart). Features include heart of normal size with prominent apex from right ventricular hypertrophy. There is increased concavity at base of heart because pulmonic stenosis produces decrease in size or absence of shadow normally seen from pulmonary artery. Vascularity of lung fields may be normal or decreased. *(Courtesy of Dr. Raymond M. Abrams, Department of Radiology, New York University Medical Center.)*

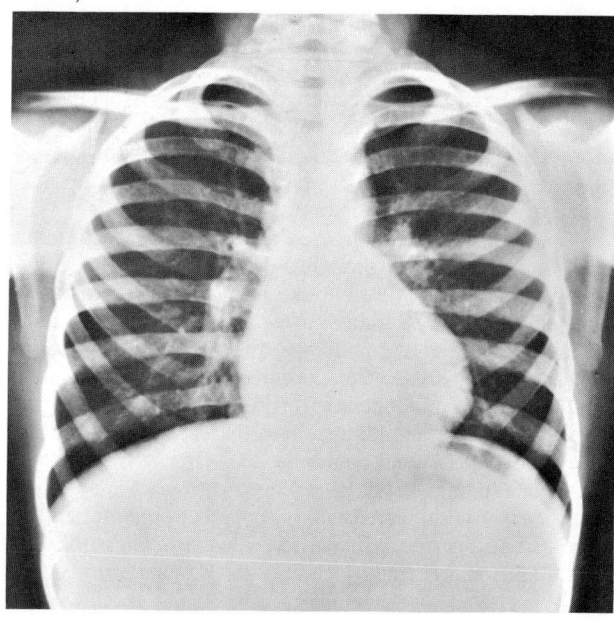

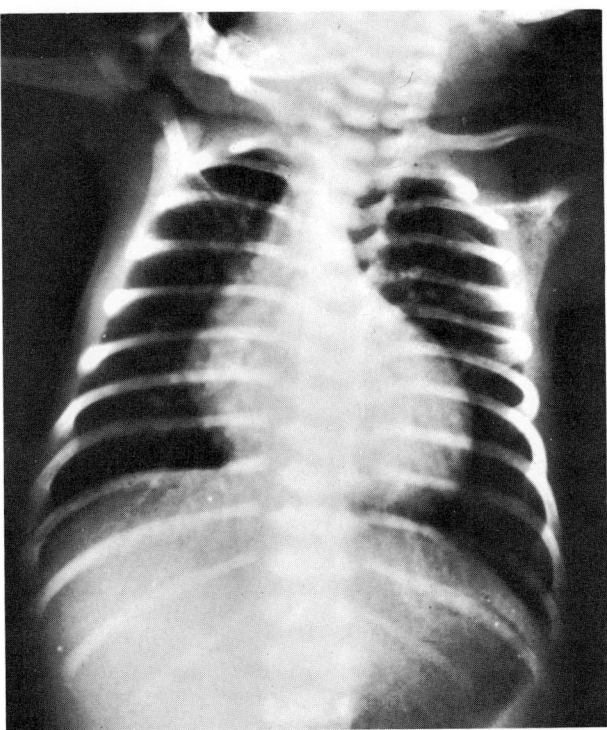

Fig. 18-2. Chest radiograph of child with transposition of great vessels, showing egg-shaped heart with large ventricular silhouette and small "waist," which results from abnormal location of aorta directly anterior to pulmonary artery. *(Courtesy of Dr. Raymond M. Abrams, Department of Radiology, New York University Medical Center.)*

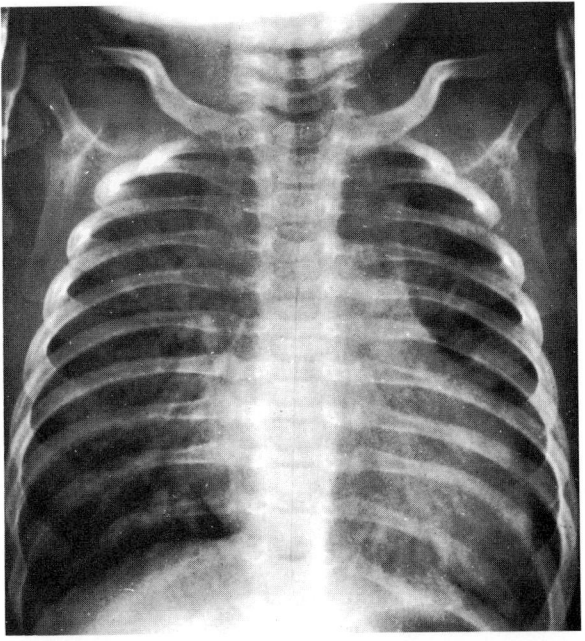

A

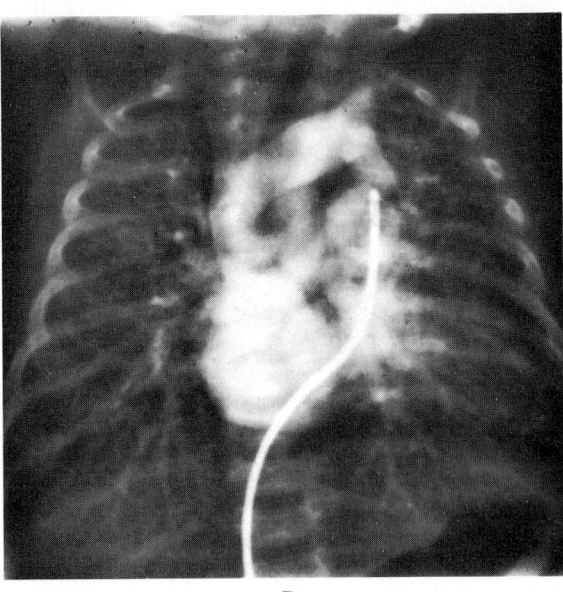

B

Fig. 18-3. *A.* Chest radiograph of child with total anomalous drainage of pulmonary veins through left superior vena cava. Shadow in left upper mediastinum is due to dilated left superior vena cava. *B.* Angiogram demonstrates left superior vena cava emptying into greatly dilated left innominate vein. This x-ray appearance is very suggestive of total anomalous drainage of pulmonary veins into left superior vena cava. *(Courtesy of Dr. Raymond M. Abrams, Department of Radiology, New York University Medical Center.)*

and right atrium, with a narrow shadow at the base from the anterior posterior relation between the aorta and pulmonary arteries. With total anomalous drainage of the pulmonary venous return, a figure of eight abnormality (Fig. 18-3), composed of a large left superior vena cava in the upper mediastinum separate from the cardiac shadow, is characteristic. The size of the pulmonary vessels and the pulmonary vascularity are also important. With left-to-right shunts producing a significant increase in pulmonary flow, the vessels are enlarged with engorgement of the lung fields. The appearance may be strikingly different from conditions with a normal or decreased pulmonary blood flow, as in tetralogy of Fallot.

The electrocardiogram is the best guide to the presence of ventricular hypertrophy. Selective hypertrophy of the left ventricle, as in aortic valvular stenosis, or selective hypertrophy of the right ventricle, as in pulmonic valvular stenosis, can be identified and correlated with the degree of stenosis.

The echocardiogram is often more precise, measuring the wall thickness of the involved chamber in millimeters. Very extensive developments have been made in the field of echocardiography over the past few years, as a result of which classic indications for cardiac catheterization are decreasing. With modern two-dimensional echocardiography, astonishingly clear images can be obtained of the different cardiac chambers. The noninvasive aspects

of echocardiography make it a particularly attractive diagnostic modality for prompt safe evaluation of many conditions, especially in seriously ill newborn infants. For many conditions catheterization with cineangiography is essential for complete evaluation because the measurements of intracardiac blood flow and pressures are far more precise than those that can be obtained by the two-dimensional echocardiogram with Doppler flow studies. With cardiac catheterization the intracardiac pressures can be determined, abnormal shunts of blood recognized, and the ratio between pulmonary and systemic blood flow determined. Mitral and aortic insufficiency are best evaluated by cineangiography.

In the normal heart the right atrial systolic pressure does not exceed 5 mmHg, while left atrial pressure is in the range of 5 to 12 mmHg. In the normal right ventricle systolic pressure ranges from 15 to 30 mmHg, while in the left ventricle pressures average 80 to 120 mmHg systolic and 5 to 12 mmHg diastolic. Continuous pressure recordings as a catheter is withdrawn from one cardiac chamber to another can readily detect the presence of stenosis; pulmonic stenosis can be measured as a catheter is withdrawn from the pulmonary artery to the right ventricle, and aortic stenosis as a catheter is withdrawn from the left ventricle into the aorta. Combined right- and left-heart catheterization is usually done with the introduction of a catheter through a systemic vein into the right side of the heart, combined with introduction of another catheter from a peripheral artery into the aorta and across the aortic valve into the left ventricle to obtain information from both the right and left sides of the heart simultaneously.

All variations from the normal pulmonary and systemic flow of 3 L/min per square meter of body surface may occur with intracardiac shunts. A rise in oxygen saturation of 1 volume percent between cardiac chambers is usually sufficient evidence to diagnose an intracardiac left-to-right shunt. Smaller shunts may be detected with a hydrogen electrode. A pulmonary blood flow one and one-half to two times greater than systemic blood flow is associated with mild physiologic disturbances and is on the borderline of indications for surgical correction. Defects producing greater pulmonary blood flows are usually recommended for operation. From the combination of pulmonary blood flow and pulmonary pressure, pulmonary vascular resistance can be calculated, which in the presence of pulmonary hypertension is one of the most significant physiologic measurements influencing prognosis.

The most precise physiologic evaluation of the degree of valvular stenosis is obtained by calculation of the functional cross-sectional area of the stenotic valve orifice. A normal mitral valve has a functional cross-sectional area of about 5 cm^2; mitral stenosis with an area of less than 1.5 cm^2 is functionally significant. In the aortic valve, normally with a cross-sectional area of 3 to 4 cm^2, a stenosis producing an opening of less than 0.8 cm^2 is functionally significant. Similarly, in the pulmonic valve, with a normal cross-sectional area of 2 to 4 cm^2, a stenosis producing an opening of less than 0.8 cm^2 is functionally significant.

Principles of Operative and Postoperative Care of Infants

Certain principles of management specifically pertain to infants undergoing cardiovascular surgery. For general

principles of operative monitoring, extracorporeal circulation, cardiac massage, and defibrillation, Chap. 19 on acquired heart disease should be consulted.

OPERATIVE MANAGEMENT. Four important aspects of operative care are temperature control, fluid administration, prevention of air emboli, and serial blood-gas monitoring. Temperature control is essential in infants, especially in air-conditioned operating rooms, because body temperature will quickly decrease to below 32°C when the infant is anesthetized and shivering mechanisms are abolished. Constant recording of the temperature with an electric esophageal or rectal probe is mandatory, and some method of warming the infant, preferably a water mattress, should routinely be employed.

Fluids must be administered with unusual precision; a 3-kg infant in cardiac failure should have no more than 20 to 40 mL of fluid in excess of measured losses during an operative procedure.

The danger of air embolism is frequently overlooked in cyanotic infants with right-to-left shunts, in whom air emboli can bypass the heart and lungs to enter the cerebral or the coronary circulation. With intravenous therapy, much care is required to prevent small air emboli, which can easily occur with the usual intravenous therapy during an operation. Only a few small bubbles, if lodged in a coronary artery, can precipitate ventricular fibrillation.

Serial measurement of the pH and the oxygen and carbon dioxide tensions of arterial and central venous blood, usually at 20- to 30-min intervals during an operation, is perhaps the most essential part of monitoring. Using a Swan-Ganz catheter, cardiac output and pulmonary wedge pressure can also be determined. Metabolic and respiratory acidosis are extremely frequent in seriously ill infants and may quickly become intensified with compression of the lung, ineffective cardiac contraction, or hypovolemia. A pH of central venous blood below 7.30 should be promptly corrected by appropriate ventilation, bicarbonate infusion, cessation of anesthesia, or other measures to increase cardiac output. In the author's experience, changes in pH almost always antedate cardiac arrest or ventricular fibrillation. With serial monitoring of blood-gas tensions during operation, desperately ill anoxic children may tolerate procedures that ordinarily would terminate in cardiac arrest or fibrillation.

POSTOPERATIVE CARE. Four important principles in a pediatric intensive care unit are constant observation, monitoring of the electrocardiogram, routine measurement of blood-gas tensions, and respiratory therapy.

Constant observation of the seriously ill infant by experienced staff on a 24-h basis is mandatory. This includes observation of adequacy of ventilation, blood-gas tensions, fluid therapy, and arrhythmias detected on the electrocardiogram. Ventricular fibrillation can appear virtually without warning but can be corrected, usually with electric cardioversion, if therapy can be started within 1 to 3 min. Hence, intensive care unit monitors with electrical alarms are essential.

Serial measurement of blood-gas tensions by analysis of blood samples withdrawn through arterial and central venous catheters is the best measurement of adequacy of ventilation and circulation. Arterial carbon dioxide tensions above 40 mmHg promptly develop with inefficient ventilation, and pH values below 7.30 quickly occur with either metabolic or respiratory acidosis. These changes far antedate any obvious clinical alteration in pulse or blood pressure and accordingly permit more effective therapy. Whether changes in pH and gas tensions are due to metabolic or respiratory causes can be determined by clinical evaluation and by gas analysis of peripheral arterial blood. Periodic measurement of cardiac output is a valuable guide in critically ill patients.

Proper ventilation may be a difficult postoperative problem in an infant following a thoracotomy or sternotomy. Secretions are difficult to remove, the tracheobronchial passages are so small that instrumental manipulation is difficult and can precipitate occlusive edema, and infants quickly develop cardiac arrest with transient anoxia or respiratory acidosis. Many advances in respiratory therapy of infants have been made in the past several years. These include mechanical respirators specifically designed for infants, the continuous positive-pressure breathing system developed by Gregory, and intermittent mandatory ventilation.

The following methods of management have been found useful, but the mode of application varies widely with individual patients. Adequate humidity, with the infant kept in a dense mist following operation, is essential. An endotracheal tube may be left in place for an indeterminate length of time following operation to assist ventilation and removal of secretions. Some have left endotracheal tubes in position for days or weeks, but the author prefers a much shorter period, usually less than 24 to 48 h. When an endotracheal tube is left in position, it may require changing every 6 to 12 h if inspissated secretions occlude the tip of the tube.

Translaryngeal aspiration of the trachea, accomplished with a laryngoscope to permit direct introduction of a soft catheter between the vocal cords into the trachea, is a valuable technique. It must be done by experienced personnel, otherwise trauma and edema of the vocal cords will quickly develop. The flexible bronchoscope is also being used with increasing frequency; it is far less traumatic than the rigid bronchoscope.

Tracheostomy should be avoided if possible but should be done if secretions cannot be adequately removed otherwise. With a precise technique avoiding excision of any tracheal cartilage, complications are far less frequent than in the past. An extensive experience with tracheostomy and mechanical ventilation for several weeks in the treatment of neonatal tetanus has clearly demonstrated the safety of a properly performed tracheostomy in infants.

OBSTRUCTIVE LESIONS

Pulmonic Stenosis

HISTORICAL DATA. In 1947–1948 Brock and Sellors independently performed the first successful valvulotomies for pulmonic valvular stenosis, using a valvulotome through a transventricular approach. A series of 19 patients was reported on by Blalock shortly thereafter. Open cardiotomy, using hypothermia and venous inflow occlusion, was first done in 1954 by Swan and Zeavin. Virtually all operations have been performed with extracorporeal circulation. In critically ill neonates, inflow occlusion and closed valvulotomy are still employed.

Recently, Srinivasan and Subramanian resurrected the concept of closed transventricular valvulotomy and reported survival in 14 of 16 patients less than three months of age. Ten additional infants over three months of age were operated upon using this technique. Late results were excellent in all but one.

INCIDENCE AND ETIOLOGY. Pulmonic stenosis is a common defect, constituting about 10 percent of all patients with congenital heart disease. It was once considered very rare. Taussig, a world-renowned authority, wrote in her classic monograph in 1947 that she had not had an opportunity to study a proven case herself. This astonishing statement indicates the degree to which knowledge of a disease is influenced by the diagnostic and therapeutic methods available. Usually there are no known etiologic factors. Rubella occurring during pregnancy has been implicated.

PATHOLOGIC ANATOMY. Pulmonic stenosis is a spectrum of disorders involving the pulmonary valve cusps, the valve annulus, the pulmonary artery, and the right ventricle. The most common variety results from fusion of the pulmonary valve cusps (Figs. 18-4 and 18-5). The severity varies widely, ranging from mild, clinically insignificant stenosis to "pinhole" stenosis requiring emergency care in neonatal life, to pulmonary atresia. Pulmonary atresia, fortunately, is uncommon, for it is a more severe malformation associated with varying degrees of

Fig. 18-4. Pulmonic valvular stenosis with fused valve cusps creating central stenotic opening. Annulus of pulmonic valve ring is normal. (From: *Cole WH, Zollinger RM: Textbook of Surgery, 8th ed. New York, Appleton-Century-Crofts, 1963, p 935, with permission.*)

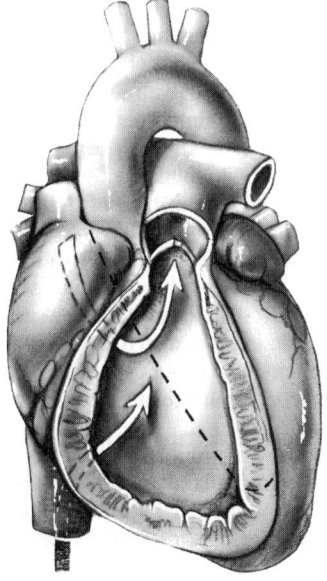

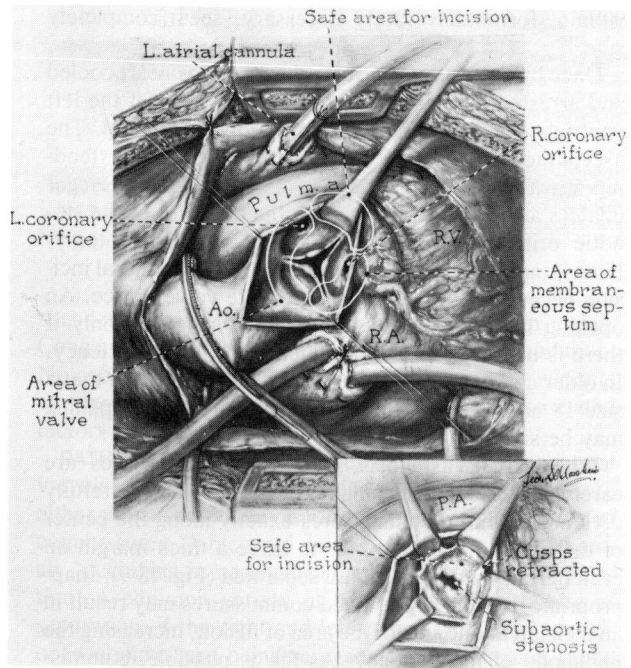

A

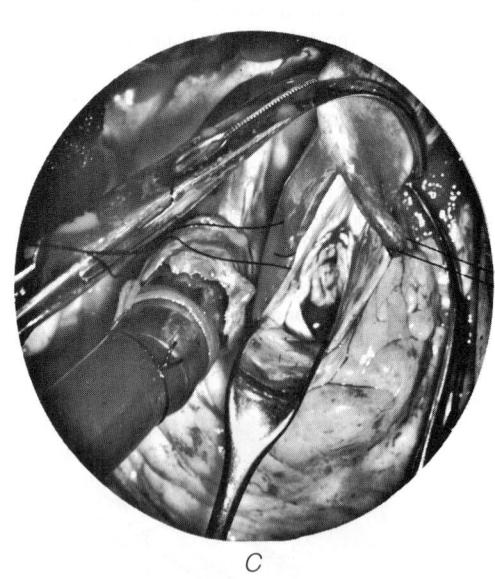

C

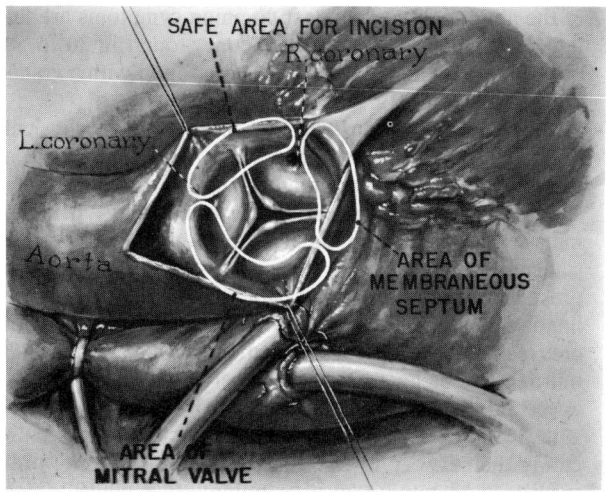

B

Fig. 18-10. *A.* Operative exposure of congenital subaortic stenosis. Valve cusps are normal. Insert shows membranelike subaortic stenosis exposed by retraction of valve cusps. (From: *Am Surg 26:210, 1960, with permission.*) *B.* Diagram of pertinent surgical anatomy with subaortic stenosis. Beneath noncoronary cusps and part of left coronary cusp is aortic leaflet of mitral valve. Beneath part of right coronary cusp is membranous septum. Only in area beneath commissure between right and left coronary cusps is limited zone where underlying ventricular muscle can be safely excised. Failure to observe these landmarks can result in injury to mitral valve or to membranous septum with conduction bundle. *C.* Subaortic stenosis exposed at operation. Aorta has been opened with longitudinal aortotomy and retractor inserted to retract normal aortic cusps. Diaphragmlike subaortic stenosis can be clearly seen with small pinpoint central opening. (From: *Spencer FC, Neill CA, Bahnson HT: The treatment of congenital aortic stenosis with valvulotomy during cardiopulmonary bypass. Surgery 44:117, 1958, with permission of CV Mosby, St Louis.*)

tween the right and left cusps is not well developed. Usually no incision at all is made in this area, leaving the valve as a bicuspid valve. Rarely, a short 2- to 4-mm incision may be cautiously made, but it has the hazard of producing insufficiency. *It is far better to leave some residual stenosis than to produce aortic insufficiency.* Long-term results have been disappointing if significant insufficiency was produced at operation, the patients often requiring aortic valve replacement within a few years because of cardiac failure.

In most patients the stenosis can be adequately relieved without producing significant insufficiency. The technique of commissurotomy has been emphasized in some

detail because most difficulties with aortic insufficiency following aortic valvulotomy have resulted from inept valvulotomies rather than from the pathologic anatomy.

With subvalvular stenosis, the valve cusps can be carefully retracted and the fibrotic ring excised. Excellent visualization is required to prevent injury to the base of the valve cusps. The ring may consist of thin, fibrous tissue, easily removed, or it may be a thick, fibrotic structure requiring excision with a knife and rongeur. Excellent exposure is required because the proximity of the mitral valve and the conduction bundle restricts excision of the ring out to the ventricular muscle to a narrow zone comprising less than 20 percent of the circumference of the ring. This "safe" area corresponds to the area beneath the commissures between the right and left coronary cusps (Fig. 18-10). An adequate rectangular block of hypertrophied muscle must be removed. Radical excision of the fibrotic ring beneath the left coronary cusp may perforate the aortic leaflet of the mitral valve, while radical excision beneath a noncoronary cusp may injure the ventricular septum, creating either a heart block or ventricular septal defect. A right-angled rongeur with a swivel permitting rotation of the instrument to an appropriate angle is particularly useful in small children (Fig. 18-11).

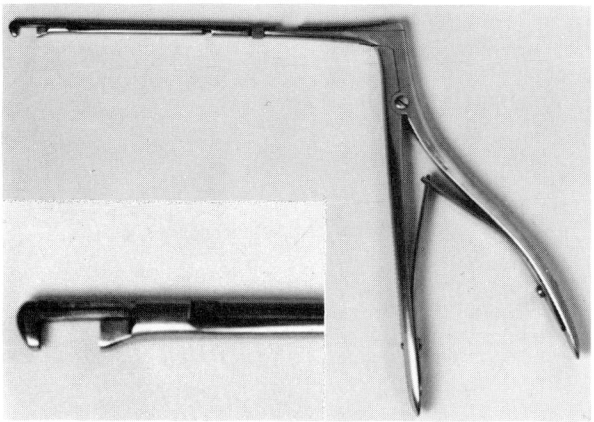

Fig. 18-11. Right-angled sharp rongeur used for excision of suba-ortic stenosis. Swivel mechanism permits rotation of instrument to obtain proper exposure.

With good exposure, an unhurried approach, and appropriate instruments, the area of stenosis can regularly be excised satisfactorily. Optical magnification and focal illumination with a headlight are excellent adjuncts in small children.

Subsequently the aortotomy is closed with a continuous Prolene suture, leaving a small opening for removal of air. Ventricular fibrillation is induced before removal of the clamp on the aorta, permitting the heart to fill with blood and displace air through the aortotomy and the left ventricular vent before the heart is allowed to beat. Following meticulous removal of air from the heart, defibrillation can be done. Following bypass, with a systemic pressure over 100 mmHg, the pressure gradient across the aortic valve should be measured by needle puncture, preferably obtaining a gradient well under 40 mmHg.

The risks of operation are small, about 1 percent, and the results good. Although several reports express pessimism with operations for aortic stenosis, considering them "palliative," our experience has been most favorable. In the past 15 years there have been no deaths following elective operation in patients with uncomplicated valvular or subvalvular stenosis. A satisfactory reduction in systolic gradient has been achieved in almost all patients; only a few had mild aortic insufficiency. Prosthetic replacement of the aortic valve has not been necessary in any patients in the primary operation, and to date has very rarely been necessary as a secondary complication in the 10 to 15 years years after the initial valvulotomy.

In 1986, Hsieh reported long-term results in 59 patients with a mean follow-up of 18 years. Forty-six patients were alive. Sudden death occurred in seven patients, at least four of whom were known to have significant residual disease. Actuarial analysis revealed the probability of reoperation to increase from 2 percent at 5 years to 44 percent at 22 years. Dobell had reported more discouraging results; one-third of the group required a repeat operation within 10 years.

Rarely emergency valvotomy is required in the first few days of life because of pinpoint life-threatening aortic ste-nosis. Usually, such operations have had a high mortality, 30 to 50 percent, but the report by Messina et al. is more encouraging. Eleven newborn infants underwent emergency valvotomy using a short period of cardiopulmonary bypass with only one operative death, and no late deaths.

In patients with severe hypoplasia of the left ventricular outflow tract, the best results follow the Konno procedure. Ebert and associates reported results for 14 patients with no operative deaths and one late death from bacterial endocarditis. This procedure seems to be preferable to the once popular insertion of an apical left ventricular-aortic conduit.

Subsequently the patient should be seen at periodic intervals indefinitely because of the abnormal valve. Long-term prognosis is uncertain, although some patients are now over 20 years since operation without subsequent problems. However, the reports cited in the earlier paragraphs indicate that in some centers 20 to 30 percent of patients have required a subsequent operative procedure within 10 years. In all likelihood, eventually fibrosis and calcification of the thickened aortic cusps will lead to stenosis or insufficiency.

SUPRAVALVULAR AORTIC STENOSIS

Supravalvular aortic stenosis is the rarest form of congenital aortic stenosis. Although the first successfully treated patient was reported by McGoon and Kirklin in 1956, 10 years later Rastelli et al., reporting a personal experience with 16 patients, could only find a total of 88 cases in the medical literature, 51 of which had been treated surgically.

There is considerable variation in the type of aortic obstruction in different patients. Peterson et al., reviewing 68 cases, found three types: hourglass, 45 cases; diffuse hypoplastic, 14 cases; membranous, 9 cases (Fig. 18-12). Associated abnormalities are frequent. In about one-third of the patients abnormalities of the aortic valve cusps are present, frequently consisting of adherence of part of one of the free margins of a cusp to the aortic wall, causing aortic regurgitation. Abnormal coronary arteries are found in over one-half of the patients. Often the right coronary artery is markedly dilated and tortuous. Focal stenotic lesions of branches of the aortic arch and peripheral branches of the pulmonary arteries have also been found.

The usual symptoms, as with other forms of aortic stenosis, are angina and syncope. Supravalvular aortic stenosis may be associated with an unusual "elfin" facies and mental retardation. Multiple peripheral pulmonary artery stenoses are also frequently noted. As physical examination provides no clues to the diagnosis except when the typical facies is present, aortography is required to establish the diagnosis. Sudden death is not uncommon in childhood, probably resulting both from the left ventricular outflow obstruction and from the coronary artery disease. It may be that most untreated patients, especially those with the characteristic facies, die before reaching adult life, because the syndrome is uncommon in adults.

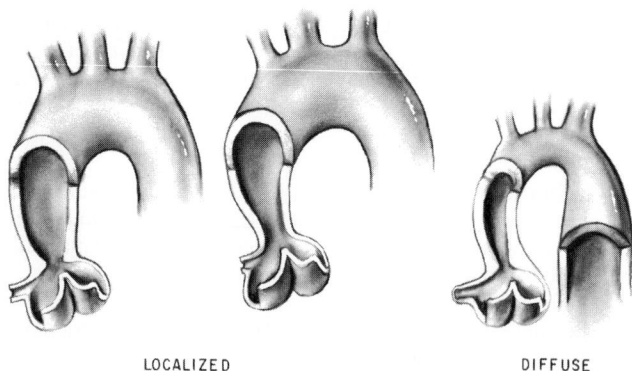

LOCALIZED   DIFFUSE

Fig. 18-12. Different types of supravalvular aortic stenosis, obstruction varying from localized constriction near aortic valve to diffuse hypoplasia of ascending aorta. (From: *Rastelli GC et al: J Thorac Cardiovasc Surg 51:878, 1966, with permission.*)

TREATMENT. With the hourglass type, widening the stenotic area by inserting a patch of Dacron or pericardium is satisfactory. Before the patch is inserted, the intimal ridge lying above the valve cusps should be excised as completely as possible (Figs. 18-13, 18-14). Sudden death has been described in some patients after operation, though the report by Rastelli et al. stated that a follow-up of 15 patients surviving operation found 13 with a good result. All 19 patients in the Kirklin/Barratt-Boyce series have had good short-term results.

Results have been less favorable with the diffuse hypoplastic type of obstruction. Enthusiasm has waned for a left ventricular-aortic conduit because of the high frequency of late complications. Extensive patch grafting of the ascending aorta and transverse aortic arch seems to be the most reasonable approach, though significant data are not available.

When a hypoplastic aortic annulus is present, the ingenious operation reported by Konno in 1975 seems the best approach. This involves extension of the aortotomy down

Fig. 18-13. Operation for localized supravalvular aortic stenosis. Stenotic area is widened by making longitudinal aortotomy and inserting Dacron patch. Partial excision of stenotic membrane is also shown. (From: *Rastelli GC et al: J Thorac Cardiovasc Surg 51:875, 1966, with permission.*)

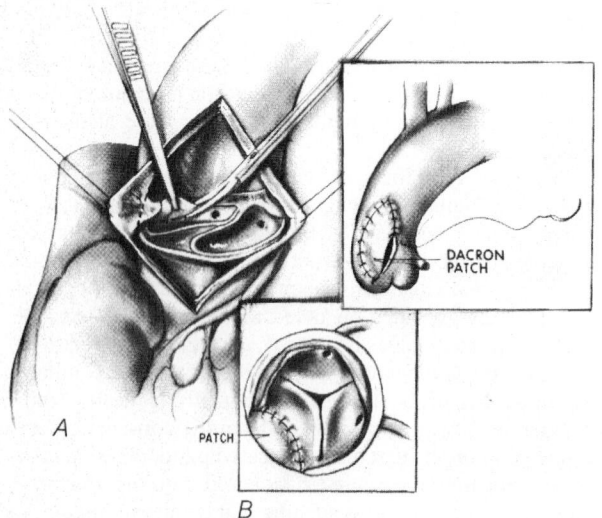

DACRON PATCH

A

PATCH

B

into the upper ventricular septum, with incision of the outflow tract of the right ventricle and the underlying ventricular septum. The complex aortotomy is then repaired with multiple patches after a prosthetic valve has been inserted (Fig. 18-15). Misbach et al. recently reported excellent results in 14 patients. A 23-mm prosthetic valve could be inserted in all patients. There were no operative deaths, one late death from endocarditis, and excellent results in the 13 survivors.

IDIOPATHIC HYPERTROPHIC SUBAORTIC STENOSIS

This disease is a hypertrophic myopathy of the left ventricular muscle, with secondary obstruction of the outflow tract developing from hypertrophy of the septum in about 20 percent of patients. The disease was first characterized in 1960. Diagnosis was greatly facilitated with the development of echocardiography which has recognized asymmetric septal hypertrophy and abnormal systolic anterior motion of the mitral leaflets as characteristic findings. Recognition of patients with few or no symptoms led to confirmation of the fact that the disease is almost always genetic.

Symptoms gradually increase with age, probably as the septal hypertrophy increases. The symptoms are similar to those associated with the more common forms of aortic stenosis and include syncope, angina, and dyspnea. A systolic murmur of medium intensity near the apex, but not prominent at the base of the heart, may be the first clue to the diagnosis. With progressive disease, atrial fibrillation systemic emboli, and sudden death are the most significant events. Sudden death is distressingly common, presumably from an arrhythmia. The chest radiograph and electrocardiogram are not diagnostic, but the 2-D echocardiogram precisely defines the abnormality and establishes the diagnosis. It can be further clarified with catheterization and angiography. On catheterization a gradient varying from 50 to 150 mmHg can be demonstrated in the proximal outflow of the left ventricle. The pressure gradient characteristically increases with the infusion of isoproterenol because of more forceful contraction of the left ventricle.

TREATMENT. Many patients are treated medically, reserving operation for those with symptomatic severe obstruction not improving with medical therapy. Beta

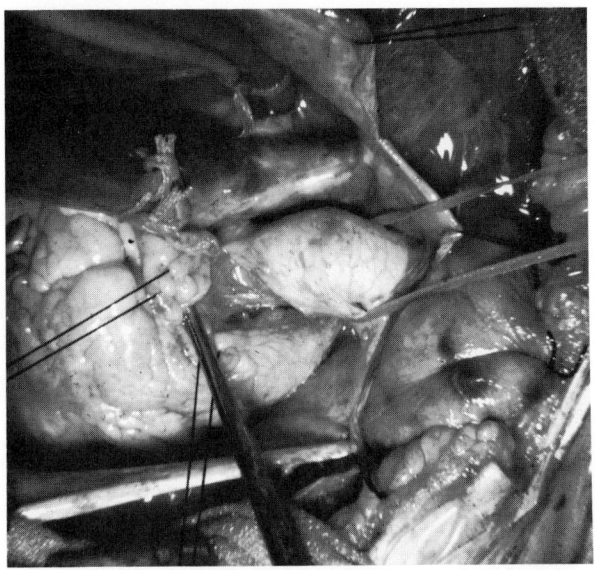

A

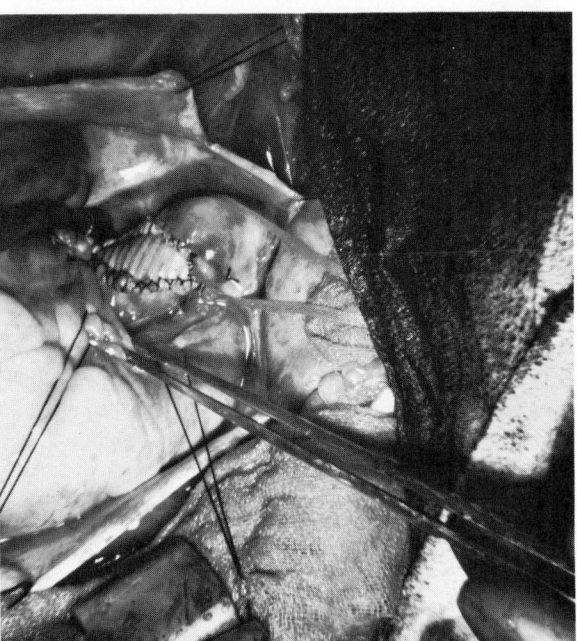

B

Fig. 18-14. *A.* Operative photography of the unusual lesion of supravalvular aortic stenosis. The waistlike narrowing of the ascending aorta just above the aortic valve can be clearly seen. *B.* Operative photograph of correction of supravalvular aortic stenosis by insertion of a Dacron patch to widen the area. The aortic valve gradient was reduced from 80 to near 30 mmHg.

blockade with drugs such as propanolol is usually employed.

Surgical myomectomy, as developed by Morrow, is clearly indicated with symptomatic patients and a gradient of 50 mm or greater. Although Morrow reported excellent results in a series exceeding 200 patients, and others have reported good results in smaller series, the

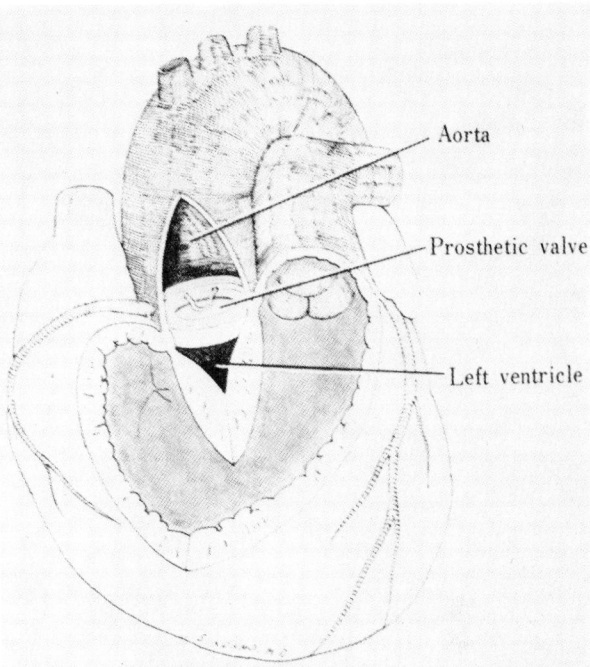

Fig. 18-15. Prosthetic valve is placed in subcoronary position. (From: *Konno S et al: J Thorac Surg 70:909, 1975, with permission.*)

operation is not widely used. Using a transaortic approach, a rectangular block of ventricular muscle is excised from the septum, extending down from the base of the aortic cusp into the ventricular cavity for several centimeters (Fig. 18-16). Late catheterization studies following the radical myomectomy clearly document permanent relief of the outflow tract obstruction.

Kirklin and Barratt-Boyes have reported a combined surgical experience including over 160 patients, with a low operative mortality and excellent long-term results. Symptoms are relieved. Sudden death continues to occur but much less frequently than in nonoperated patients.

Coarctation of the Aorta

HISTORICAL DATA. The characteristic features of coarctation were clearly outlined by Abbott in her classic analysis in 1928. In 1944 and 1945 Blalock and Park, Gross, and Crafoord and Nylin all independently contributed to the first surgical treatment of coarctation by excision and direct anastomosis. Subsequently Gross provided a strong stimulus to the study of vascular grafts by successfully using aortic homografts for patients with coarctation in whom direct anastomosis could not be done.

INCIDENCE AND ETIOLOGY. Coarctation is a common congenital malformation, occurring in 10 to 15 percent of patients with congenital heart disease. It is more common in males (3:1 ratio). Although the cause is unknown, the proximity of the coarctation to the ligamentum arteriosum supports the most plausible theory, that coarctation is an extension of the same fibrotic process that converts the patent ductus into a ligamentum arteriosum.

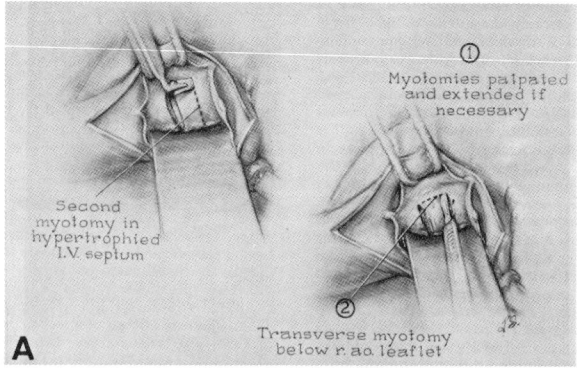

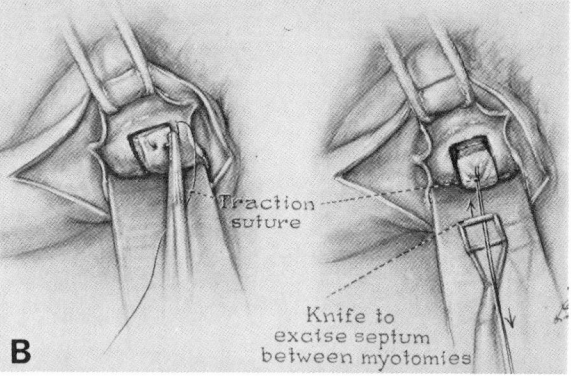

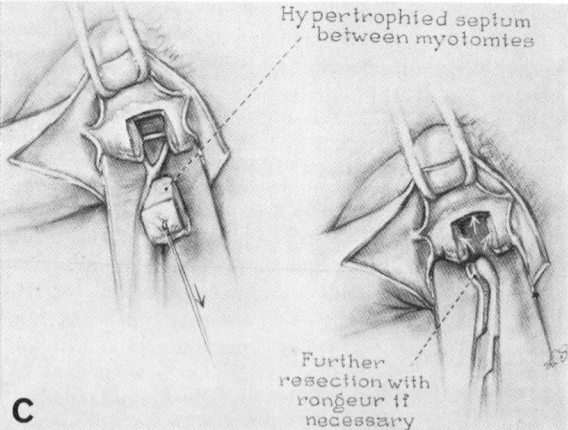

Fig. 18-16. *A.* Second myotomy is made about 1 cm to right (clockwise) of first. Incisions are then deepened if necessary by digital splitting of muscle fibers. Myotomies are usually 12 to 15 mm in depth at most prominent aspect of septum. Transverse incision is then made at base of valve leaflet connecting proximal portions of the myotomies. *B.* Bar of muscle isolated between incisions is held by traction suture as shown or by suitable clamp. Muscle is freed with rectangular knife (devised by Stinson) or with special angled rongeur. *C.* As traction is made on muscle bar, rectangular knife is pushed toward apex, freeing muscle bar from its anterior attachments to septum. Apical portion of resection is often more easily accomplished with rongeur, which may be introduced via aorta or via apical stab wound. In latter case, rongeur is positioned and directed by left index finger passed through valve ring. (From: *Morrow AG et al: Circulation 52:88, 1975, with permission.*)

PATHOLOGIC ANATOMY. In most patients the coarctation consists of a localized stenosis in the first 2 to 4 cm of thoracic aorta beyond the left subclavian artery. Usually there is a 1- to 3-mm lumen, though complete occlusion is present in 20 to 25 percent of patients. The ligamentum arteriosum is attached to the medial surface of the aorta near the site of coarctation. It clearly influences the coarctation, for when surgically divided, the two ends retract sharply, indicating the degree of tension previously exerted.

The stenotic area may have two or three component parts. The most frequent is a localized "shelf," consisting of an infolding of the aortic media into the lumen. This is most visible on the aortic wall opposite the ligamentum arteriosum. In the lumen, a thickened ridge of intima may be present and may increase the severity of the stenosis. In addition, a varying degree of "tubular hypoplasia" consisting of a narrowing of the aorta between the coarctation and the left subclavian artery, often the left common carotid artery, is common.

Distal to the coarctation, the aorta is usually dilated. In adults a true aneurysm forms in a small percentage of patients. Large, dilated intercostal arteries entering the distal aorta, providing collateral circulation around the site of obstruction, are a striking feature. In older patients these large arteries produce "notching" of the ribs. Ultimately they may become aneurysmal and rupture.

Unusual varieties of coarctation include a more proximal site of obstruction, involving the left subclavian artery, or even the left carotid and innominate artery. In some instances there is complete interruption of the aortic arch.

A rare severe anomaly, usually fatal in the first few months of life unless treated, is the so-called preductal coarctation. Usually other severe anomalies coexist. In this condition, a large patent ductus perfuses the distal aorta with blood from the pulmonary artery. The coarctation is located proximal to this. In the few patients who survive infancy without operation, cyanosis may be recognized as localized to the lower half of the body.

PATHOPHYSIOLOGY. In 5 to 10 percent of infants, left ventricular failure may be severe, even fatal, unless operation is performed. After the first year of life, congestive heart failure rarely occurs before the age of twenty.

The hypertension from the coarctation causes rapid degenerative changes in the proximal aorta. Children in their early teens often have obvious fibrosis rigidity in the aortic wall. Without treatment the average life expectancy is only 30 to 40 years. The four most common causes of death in unoperated patients are rupture of the aorta, cardiac failure, rupture of intracranial aneurysms, and bacterial endocarditis.

CLINICAL MANIFESTATIONS. Symptoms. Most children have minimal or no symptoms despite severe hypertension. The diagnosis is often made by a routine school physical examination uncovering hypertension. Headache, epistaxis, and leg fatigue are the most frequent symptoms. Claudication in the lower extremities is uncommon.

Physical Findings. The classic combination of hypertension in the upper extremities with absent or decreased pulses in the lower extremities in a child immediately suggests coarctation. If weak femoral pulsations are present, direct measurement of the blood pressure in the upper and lower extremities may be necessary to confirm the diagnosis. Prominent pulsations from collateral circulation may be visible in the neck and over the muscles of the shoulder girdle. A systolic murmur is usually audible over the left hemithorax.

LABORATORY STUDIES. In older patients the chest radiograph may automatically establish the diagnosis by demonstrating bilateral notching of the ribs posteriorly (Fig. 18-17). Notching is unusual before age six but is almost always present by age fourteen. The electrocardiogram characteristically shows signs of left ventricular hypertrophy, often left ventricular strain. In most patients the diagnosis can be made from the clinical findings in combination with the radiograph and electrocardiogram. 2-D echocardiography may be diagnostic. Cardiac catheterization and aortography should be done routinely to define the location and extent of the obstruction, as well as to detect additional anomalies.

Fig. 18-17. Chest radiograph in patient with coarctation of aorta, demonstrating classic notching of ribs from enlarged intercostal arteries. This x-ray appearance is virtually pathognomonic of coarctation of aorta, as it is rarely produced by any other condition. *(Courtesy of Dr. Raymond M. Abrams, Department of Radiology, New York University Medical Center.)*

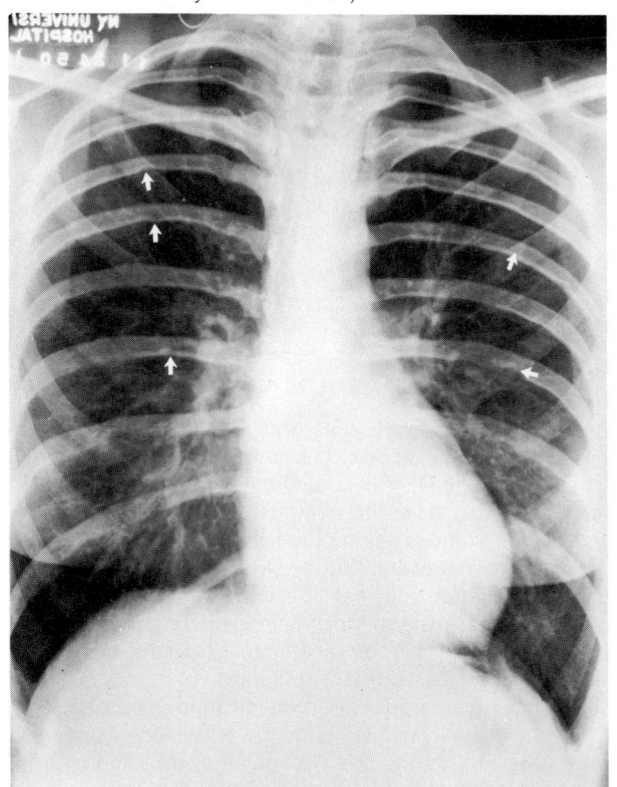

TREATMENT. The ideal age for operation is between three and four years. In infants with congestive failure, operation should be performed urgently, often within the first few weeks of life, because of the high fatality rate. With severe congestive failure, other cardiac anomalies are almost always present. These may require correction during the same hospitalization. When resection and end-to-end anastomosis is performed in infants, the coarctation may recur as the child ages. The subclavian flap technique is the procedure of choice in the first year of life (Fig. 18-18).

Operative Technique. A left posterolateral thoracotomy in the fourth intercostal space is used, dividing the fourth rib posteriorly in older patients (Fig. 18-19). The coarctation is usually readily seen, with the typical medial indentation at the site of insertion of the ligamentum arteriosum, with large, tortuous intercostal arteries entering the distal aorta (Fig. 18-20).

Initially the mediastinal pleura is incised, after which the vagus nerve is retracted medially, noting the course of the recurrent nerve encircling the ligamentum arteriosum. The aorta proximal to the left subclavian artery, the left subclavian, the ligamentum arteriosum, and the distal aorta are serially mobilized and encircled with tapes. Dissection should be kept in the adventitial plane next to the aorta. This minimizes bleeding and also avoids the occasional complication of inadvertent injury to the thoracic duct. Division of the ligamentum arteriosum facilitates dissection, as the aorta is more mobile once the tethering action of the ligamentum is removed.

Dissection of the distal aorta is hazardous in older patients when friable dilated intercostal arteries are present. Intercostal aneurysms, now rare, were found in 45 of 487 patients operated upon by Gross and associates. Usually the aorta can be mobilized sufficiently between the intercostal arteries, individually isolating these and separately occluding them during performance of the anastomosis. The intercostal arteries can also be divided, but this is seldom necessary.

Once the vessels have been adequately mobilized, the proximal aorta, the left subclavian, and the distal aorta are all occluded with vascular clamps, after which the coarctation is excised. The objective, of course, is to obtain an anastomotic lumen as large as the proximal aorta. In children, the widest anastomosis can be obtained by excising the aorta up to the level of the left subclavian. As much as 5 cm of aorta can be excised in a child (Fig. 18-21). In older children, as fibrosis decreases elasticity of the aorta, only 2.5 to 3 cm of aorta can be removed.

An end-to-end anastomosis is usually done with continuous sutures of polypropylene (Prolene) in the posterior row of the anastomosis. Interrupted mattress sutures should be used in small children in the anterior row to permit subsequent growth of the anastomosis.

Following completion of the anastomosis and removal of vascular clamps, the blood pressure should be measured proximal and distal to the anastomosis to confirm that no significant gradient remains. In addition, the circumference of the anastomosis should be measured and

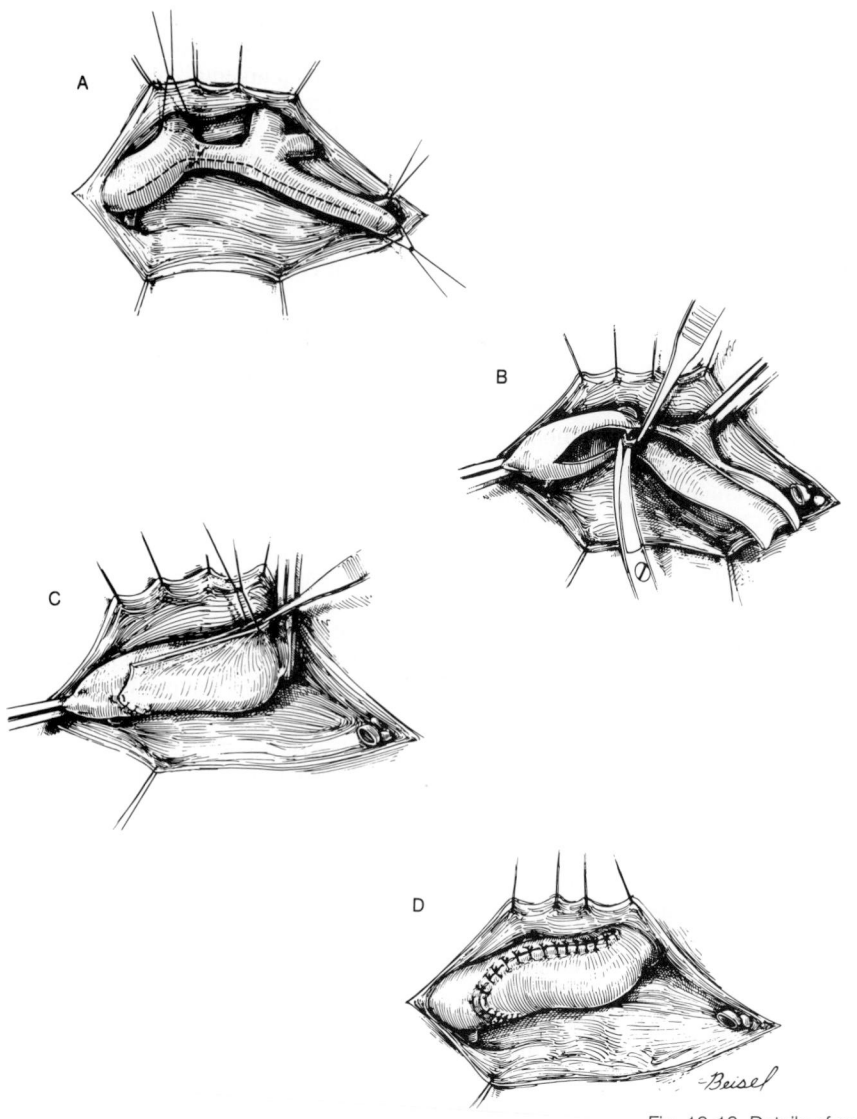

Fig. 18-18. Details of operation. (From: *Campbell DB, Waldhausen JA, et al: Should elective repair of coarctation of the aorta be done in infancy? J Thorac Cardiovasc Surg 88:929, 1984, Fig 2, with permission.*)

compared with that of the proximal aorta. When a gradient greater than 5 to 10 mmHg is present, especially with a circumference smaller than the proximal aorta, clamps should be reapplied after a short period of time, one or two sutures removed from the anterior suture line, and a short anterior arteriotomy made to permit insertion of an appropriate synthetic patch. The dimensions of the patch can be calculated to widen the lumen to the same size as the proximal aorta. This combination of anastomosis and selective patch grafting is a valuable technique, permitting complete correction of the obstruction without insertion of a vascular graft. Fewer than 10 percent of children have an obstruction so diffuse that primary insertion of a graft is necessary. Several reports have described the development of aortic aneurysm in patients 10 to 15 years after extensive patch grafting. We have not noted this development.

In adults, extensive degenerative changes in the aorta from calcification and fibrosis make insertion of a pros-

thetic graft necessary because direct anastomosis cannot be done. A simpler approach in such instances is to insert a bypass graft of Dacron around the obstruction, without attempting to excise the coarctation. This relieves the obstruction without risking the hazards of excision.

Postoperative Course. With present techniques, the risk of operation after one year of age is less than 1 percent. Antibiotics are given routinely during operation and postoperatively for 1 to 3 days. Patients usually recover rapidly and are discharged in 7 to 8 days.

The most feared operative complication is paraplegia. Current data indicate that paraplegia is due to ischemia of the spinal cord during cross-clamping in the majority of instances, and not due to ligation of interiostal arteries or other factors. In a survey of published reports by Brewer

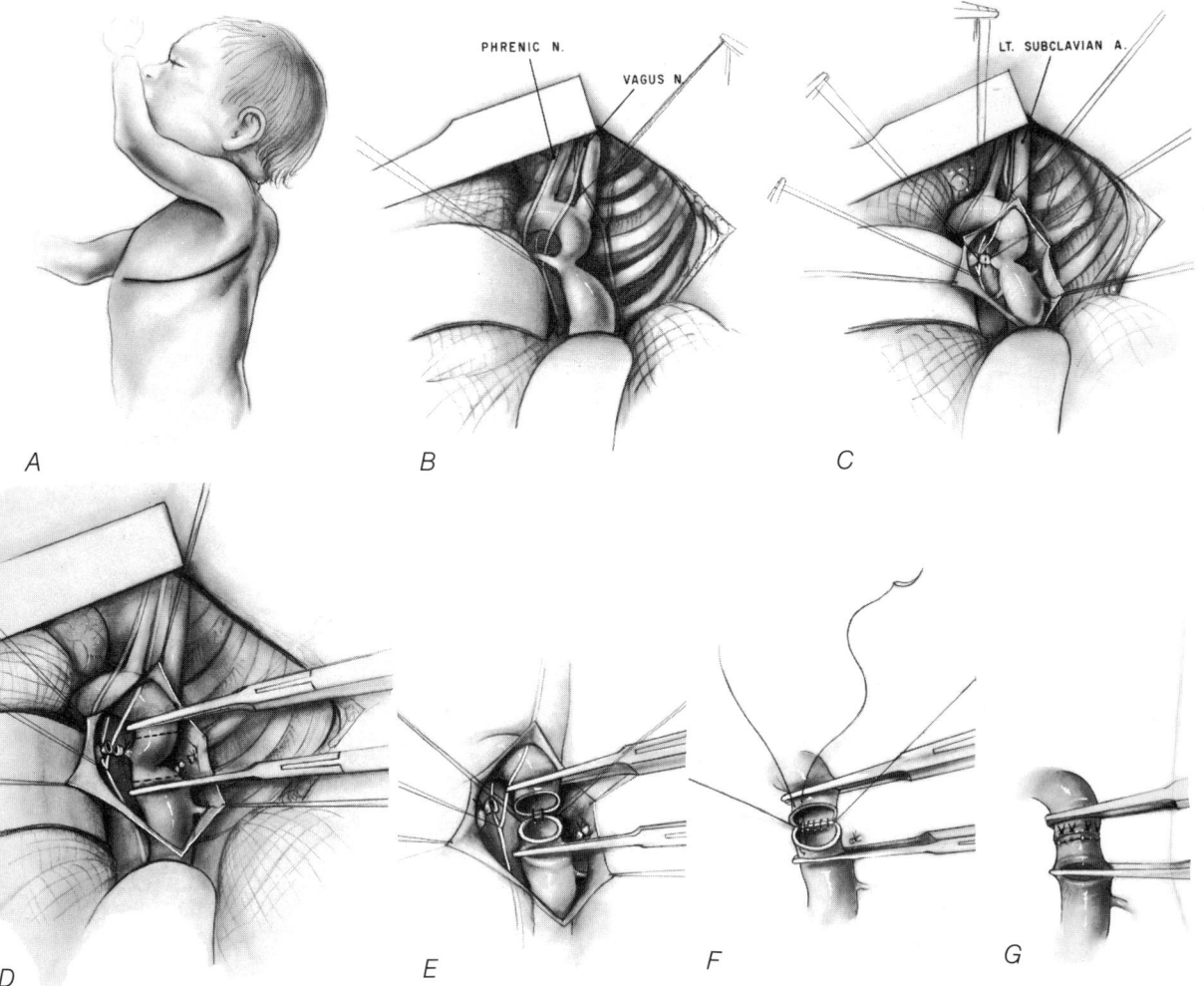

Fig. 18-19. Excision of coarctation of aorta. *A.* Chest is opened with posterolateral incision in fourth intercostal space. *B.* Once chest has been opened and lung retracted, site of coarctation is often visible where aorta is angulated inward toward mediastinum just distal to left subclavian artery. This is site where ligamentum arteriosum is inserted. *C.* After incision of mediastinal pleura overlying coarctation, vessels are isolated proximal and distal to coarctation and ligamentum arteriosum is mobilized and divided. Recurrent laryngeal nerve, often not seen during operative procedure, is displaced mediad with vagus nerve. *D.* After division of ligamentum arteriosum, vascular occlusion clamps are applied to aorta proximal and distal to site of coarctation. Often it is necessary to apply proximal clamp to aorta between left carotid and left subclavian arteries, separately occluding left subclavian artery, in order to excise widely the narrowed segment of aorta. *E.* End-to-end anastomosis is constructed with continuous or interrupted sutures of silk. *F.* After completion of posterior row of anastomosis, interrupted sutures are often used in anterior row in young children to permit growth of anastomosis. *G.* Final view of completed anastomosis.

et al., paraplegia was found to occur in approximately 0.5 percent of patients. The author has personally never had a postoperative neurologic complication following coarctation. For over a decade the pressure in the distal aorta has been continually monitored during excision of the coarctation by inserting a small catheter into the distal aorta before the aorta is clamped. Though it cannot be proved, it seems reasonable that neurologic injury probably should not occur if the distal aortic pressure remains above 60 mmHg. Distal aortic pressure following occlusions of the aorta and the left subclavian artery varies widely, from as low as 30 mmHg to levels greater than 60 mmHg.

Neurologic injury is virtually unknown if the aorta is occluded for less than 20 min. Hence, it seems wise to limit periods of aortic occlusion to less than 20 min if the distal pressure is less than 50 to 60 mmHg. Otherwise a temporary shunt should be used. When 103 patients were treated with those concepts, no neurologic problem occurred.

Often there is a "paradoxical" hypertension in the first 48 to 72 h after operation, occurring to a greater degree in older patients with a severe coarctation. Frequently this is associated with abdominal pain. This syndrome was first described by Sealy. It seemingly is related to an increase in arterial pressure in visceral arteries, previously functioning with a lower mean pressure. Rarely, serious problems such as intestinal necrosis can occur. Prompt treatment with appropriate hypertensive medications,

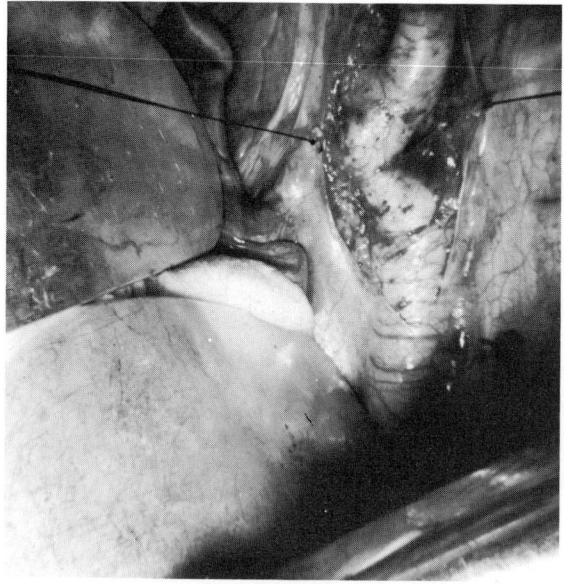

A

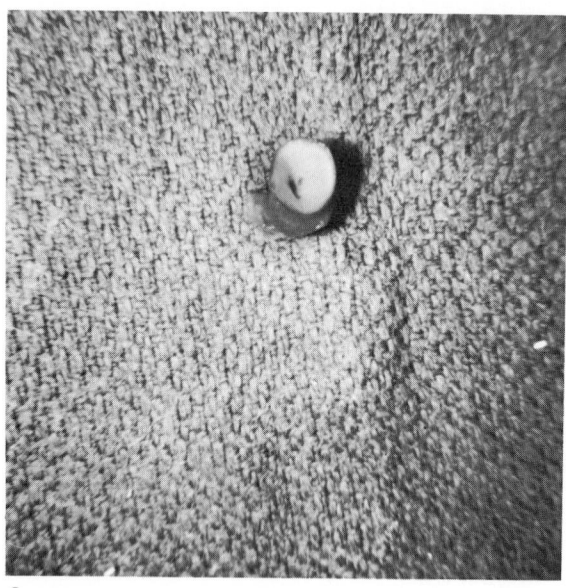

C

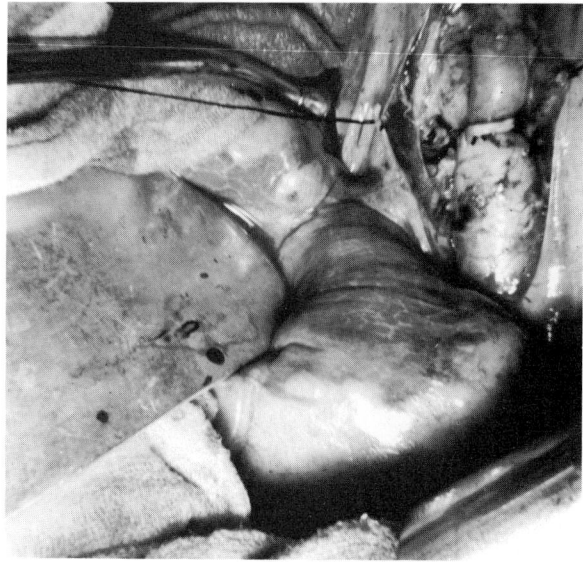

B

Fig. 18-20. *A.* Typical coarctation of aorta in child. Dilated subclavian artery is visible at top of field. At area of coarctation, aorta is angulated into mediastinum, where ligamentum arteriosum is inserted. *B.* Aortic anastomosis performed after excision of coarctation. Anastomosis is made at point of origin of left subclavian artery. *C.* Resected coarctation of aorta, showing narrow lumen that was present.

usually reserpine or nipride, virtually eliminates the problem.

Some residual hypertension is common in patients operated on after five years of age and seems to increase with age. Barratt-Boyes found that 90 percent of patients were normotensive 5 years after operation, but only 50 percent at 20 years and 25 percent at 25 years. A key question is whether residual hypertension will be significantly less in patients operated on at one to four years.

Vascular Rings

HISTORICAL DATA. The clinical significance of vascular rings was recognized by Abbott in her classical survey of congenital heart disease in 1932, but surgical therapy did not develop until 1945 when Gross successfully divided a double aortic arch. Gross subsequently developed most of the basic concepts of vascular rings, classifying and illustrating with clarity and precision the different anomalies found.

INCIDENCE AND ETIOLOGY. Vascular rings are uncommon but are quite significant because surgical therapy is effective with little morbidity or mortality. Embryologically, the vascular rings result from variation in the normal formation of the aorta and pulmonary artery from the six embryonic aortic arches. As six aortic arches exist in the embryo, it is somewhat surprising that such abnormalities are not more frequent. In normal embryonic life, the first two arches disappear, and the fifth never fully develops. The third, fourth, and sixth are significant in normal development. The right common carotid arises from the third arch, the innominate from the right fourth, while the left fourth contributes to the transverse aortic arch. The ductus originates from the sixth.

PATHOLOGIC ANATOMY. Five types of vascular anomalies of clinical significance have been recognized: (1) double aortic arch; (2) right aortic arch with left ligamentum arteriosum; (3) retroesophageal subclavian artery; (4) anomalous origin of innominate artery; and (5) anomalous origin of left common carotid artery. The last two conditions, anomalous origin of the innominate or the left common carotid, are very rare malformations in which the origin of the artery from the aortic arch is such that the trachea is compressed. The recommended method of surgical correction consists of mobilizing the anomalous

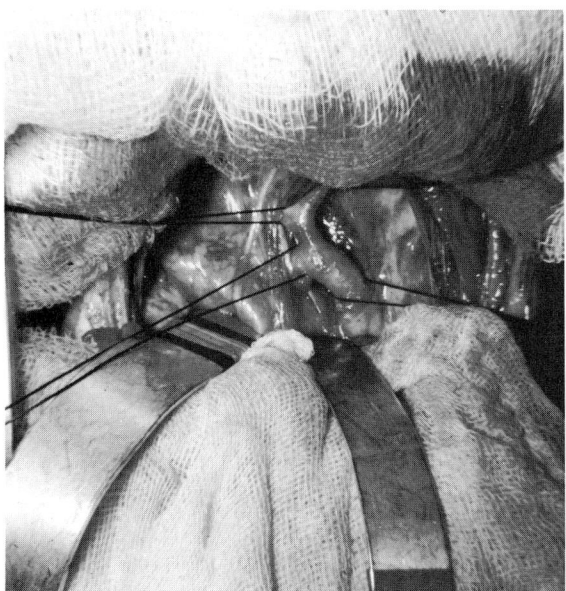

A

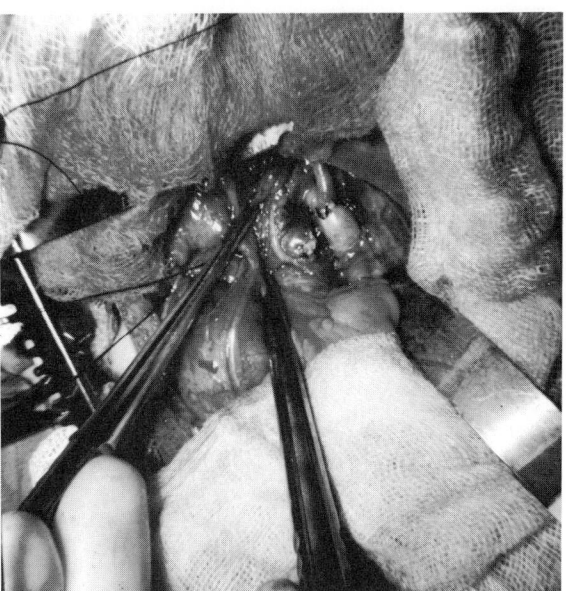

B

Fig. 18-21. *A.* Preductal coarctation exposed at emergency operation on thirteen-day-old infant. Large patent ductus equal in diameter to descending aorta is present. Proximal to patent ductus is coarctation of aorta with narrow proximal aortic segment and narrow subclavian artery. *B.* Appearance after excision of coarctation and suture of patent ductus arteriosus. Anastomosis was conducted proximally at point of origin of left subclavian artery from aorta.

vessel and suturing it into a more normal position. Actually, the mechanism of compression is less precise than in the other three conditions. Its clinical significance is not great.

A double aortic arch with one limb anterior to the trachea and the other limb posterior to the esophagus (Figs. 18-22 and 18-23) is the most severe of these malformations, producing symptoms in early infancy. Usually one limb is smaller than the other. Often the thoracic aorta descends on the right, rather than on the left. A right aortic arch with a retroesophageal ligamentum arteriosum or left subclavian artery is the other most frequent abnormality (Fig. 18-24). A retroesophageal subclavian artery, consisting of a right subclavian artery originating beyond the left subclavian artery and coursing posterior to the esophagus to the right upper extremity, is a common anomaly but usually does not cause symptoms (Fig. 18-25).

CLINICAL MANIFESTATIONS. Almost all symptoms from vascular rings result from compression of the trachea. Rarely is there difficulty in swallowing from compression of the esophagus.

Symptoms. Infants with a double aortic arch often develop difficulty breathing in the first few months of life and become critically ill. Stridor is the most frequent prominent symptom. Periodic episodes of serious respiratory distress, with "crowing" respirations, occur. During these attacks, the infant lies in hyperextension, gasping for breath. Feeding often precipitates such episodes, perhaps from flexion of the neck or aspiration. Infants quickly become underweight and malnourished.

Most patients requiring surgical treatment are seen in infancy. Those with mild symptoms developing after one year of age may spontaneously recover as they grow older. The most common symptoms are intermittent episodes of respiratory compression, at times with a respiratory infection; difficulty in swallowing, which, if present, is mild; and recurrent episodes of pneumonia, perhaps from aspiration. The mildest clinical picture is produced by the retroesophageal subclavian artery, which may cause mild, intermittent dysphagia. Some patients may be

Fig. 18-22. Double aortic arch with small anterior and large posterior limb. *A.* Anterior view of double aortic arch with small anterior limb *B.* Exposure after division of small anterior arch between left carotid and left subclavian artery, followed by displacement of carotid artery anteriorly toward sternum. (From: *Gross RE: The Surgery of Infancy and Childhood. Philadelphia, Saunders, 1953, p 917, with permission.*)

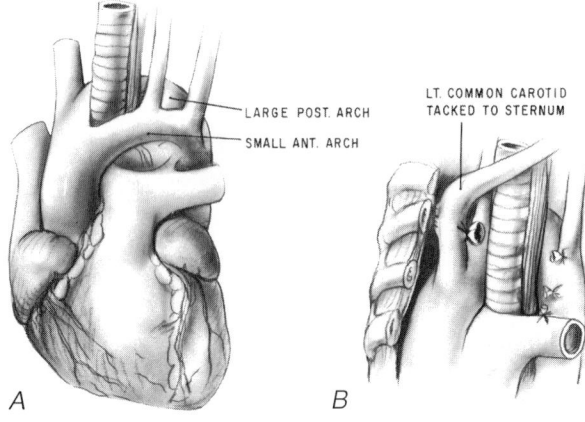

LARGE POST. ARCH
SMALL ANT. ARCH

LT. COMMON CAROTID
TACKED TO STERNUM

A   *B*

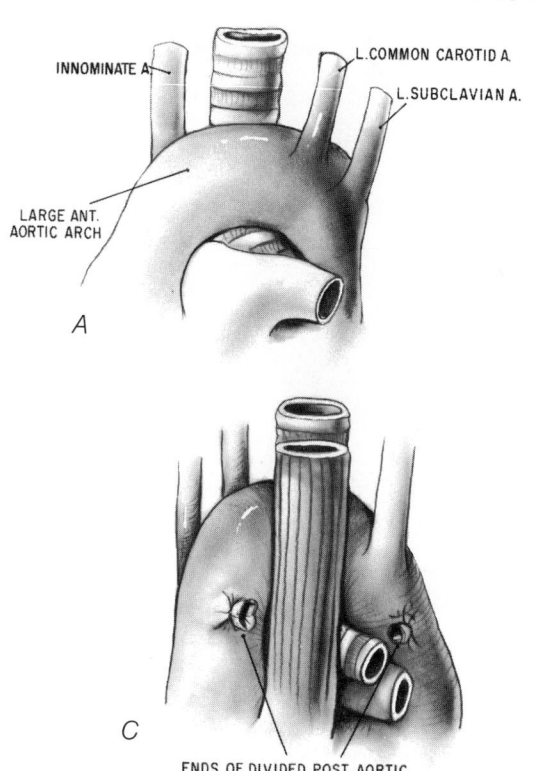

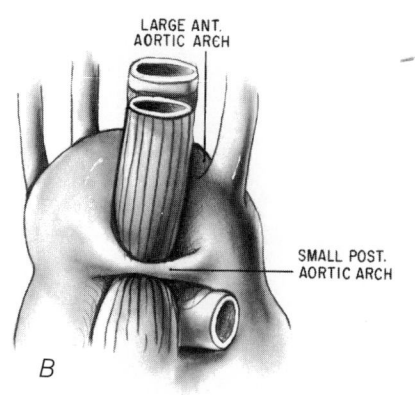

Fig. 18-23. *A.* Double aortic arch with large anterior arch. *B.* Small posterior arch, compressing esophagus. *C.* Appearance after division of small posterior arch. (From: *Gross RE: The Surgery of Infancy and Childhood. Philadelphia, Saunders, 1953, p 918, with permission.*)

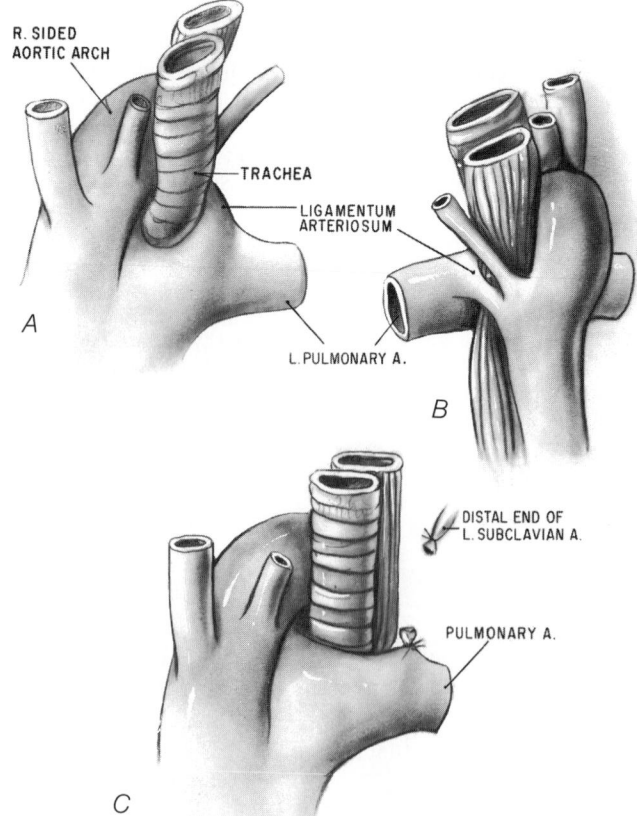

Fig. 18-24. *A.* Right aortic arch with left posterior ligamentum arteriosum. *B.* Posterior view of ligamentum arteriosum extending from right aortic arch to left pulmonary artery, compressing esophagus. Small left subclavian artery arising close to ligamentum arteriosum is also present. *C.* Appearance after division of ligamentum arteriosum and subclavian artery. (From: *Gross RE: The Surgery of Infancy and Childhood. Philadelphia, Saunders, 1953, p 923, with permission.*)

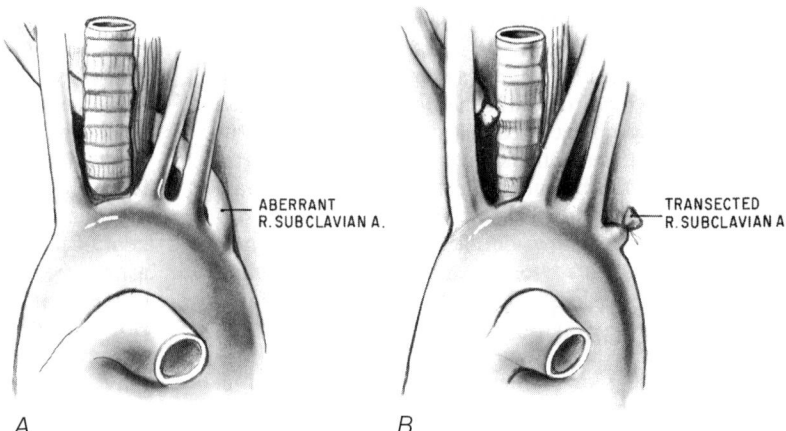

Fig. 18-25. *A.* Retroesophageal right subclavian artery, anomalous vessel arising from aortic arch distal to left subclavian artery. *B.* Appearance after division of anomalous vessel with retraction of distal stump to right of trachea. (From: *Gross RE: The Surgery of Infancy and Childhood. Philadelphia, Saunders, 1953, p 932, with permission.*)

symptomatic in infancy, and spontaneously recover with growth.

Physical Examination. No abnormalities are evident unless respiratory distress is present. If audible stridor is present, the diagnosis should be considered. During episodes of respiratory insufficiency, the infant lies with back arched and neck extended. Attempts to flex the neck may precipitate severe dyspnea and cyanosis.

LABORATORY STUDIES. Both the chest radiograph and electrocardiogram are normal unless aspiration pneumonia is present. Examination of the esophagus with a barium swallow usually establishes the diagnosis, demonstrating a typical area of compression from the retroesophageal artery, usually at the level of the third or fourth thoracic vertebra. This finding virtually confirms the diagnosis.

The precise nature of the obstruction can be defined with further studies. A tracheogram in the lateral view may provide further evidence of a vascular ring, demonstrating anterior compression of the trachea a short distance above the carina combined with posterior compression of the esophagus. Aortography can precisely delineate the abnormal arteries.

TREATMENT. Since a vascular ring has no physiologic significance, no treatment is needed in the absence of symptoms. If symptoms are mild, their origin may be uncertain, and a period of observation may be required to be sure that other difficulties are not responsible. If obvious respiratory compression is present, operation should be performed promptly, however, because death from airway obstruction can easily occur.

Operative Technique. The optimal incision varies with the type of anomaly. Usually an incision through the left four intercostal spaces is selected. An important principle is to dissect the aortic arch completely and identify the innominate artery, the left common carotid artery, and both subclavian arteries. Opening the pericardium facili-

tates identification of these vessels. The vagus nerve should be traced to the recurrent laryngeal nerve and the ligamentum arteriosum divided. Removal of part of the thymus gland will facilitate exposure. It should be emphasized that operative correction is more than simple division of an abnormal ring, because fibrosis surrounding the adventitia of the abnormal vessel may cause continued compression unless the vessels are widely mobilized and all possible compression is relieved.

With a double aortic arch, the smaller of the two arches should be divided. Usually, with a left descending aorta, the anterior arch is smaller and can be divided between the left common carotid and left subclavian artery, after which the mobilized anterior arch can be sutured to the posterior surface of the anterior chest wall to prevent compression of the trachea. If the posterior arch is smaller, it can be divided behind the esophagus. With a right descending thoracic aorta, almost always the posterior arch is the smaller of the two.

With a right aortic arch and a retroesophageal ligamentum arteriosum, division of the ligamentum arteriosum, combined with mobilization of the abnormal vessels, may be all that is necessary. In some patients the left subclavian artery may be in a retroesophageal location and should also be divided. A nubbin of aorta, constituting an aortic diverticulum, has been found in a retroesophageal location in some patients and may require amputation to relieve compression.

With a retroesophageal subclavian artery as an isolated anomaly, simple division of the artery is all that is necessary. Division of this artery through a cervical incision, followed by reimplantation into the right carotid artery, has been reported.

Postoperative Course. Postoperative care consists primarily of careful attention to respiration, with the infant kept in a highly humidified atmosphere and tracheal secretions aspirated. Tracheostomy is rarely necessary. If tracheal compression was present before operation, serious difficulties may develop afterward, probably from dissection around the trachea, creating postoperative edema. Unusually vigilant care for 24 to 72 h may be necessary. After recovery from operation, symptoms soon

TREATMENT. Infants with congestive failure should be operated on promptly. Otherwise, operation can be electively performed between one and two years of age. The operative risk approaches zero, and the results are excellent.

The only contraindication to operation, rarely seen, is cyanosis. Cyanosis may be due to an associated cardiac anomaly such as tetralogy of Fallot, in which case the patent ductus is an important ancillary source of blood flow to the lungs. Cyanosis can also develop with a reversed ductus when pulmonary vascular resistance has increased to exceed systemic vascular resistance, as a result of which blood flows from the pulmonary artery to the aorta and creates cyanosis in the lower half of the body. A reversed ductus cannot be safely closed, for the patent ductus partly decreases the pulmonary hypertension, shunting blood from the pulmonary artery to the aorta. Attempted surgical closure usually results in immediate death. Fortunately, with early operations for patent ductus, such advanced pulmonary vascular disease is almost unknown.

With bacterial endocarditis, intensive antibiotic therapy will effect cure in most patients; operation can then be more safely performed several weeks later. It is rarely necessary to operate in the presence of active infection.

Operative Technique. The operation is preferably done through a posterolateral thoracotomy in the fourth intercostal space, although a left anteriolateral thoracotomy in the third intercostal space has been satisfactorily used in previous years. The author's preferred operative technique is shown in detail in Fig. 18-36.

Patients in the third and fourth decade with pulmonary hypertension and sclerosis or calcification of the ductus constitute a difficult and dangerous technical problem because of friability of the ductus, especially at its junction with the pulmonary artery. Lacerations in this artery may quickly result in fatal hemorrhage. A temporary aortic shunt, either a left atrial–femoral artery bypass or a femoral-femoral bypass, can be employed to permit temporary occlusion of the aorta above and below the ductus, which can then be occluded with a single clamp placed near its junction with the aorta. The ductus can then be divided at its point of origin from the aorta. Alternately, the aorta can be incised and the orifice of the ductus obliterated with a patch applied from within the aorta. Barratt-Boyes has approached some patients through a sternotomy incision, using hypothermia and a brief period of "low flow" to permit opening the pulmonary artery and direct suture of the pulmonary orifice of the ductus.

Ligation of a patent ductus with multiple ligatures was developed and widely used by Blalock. It is now rarely used but is an effective technique in most patients. The original technique included four separate ligatures, with two purse-string sutures at the aortic and pulmonary artery ends of the ductus, followed by two transfixion ligatures.

The author treated a sixty-five-year-old patient with congestive failure and extensive calcification of both the aorta and a large patent ductus. Even simple application of vascular clamps to the calcified vessels seemed unusu-

ally hazardous. Accordingly, the ductus was effectively obliterated with multiple mattress sutures placed through Teflon felt surrounding the ductus. The patient has subsequently remained well.

As illustrated in Fig. 18-36, a valuable technical point for safe division of any patent ductus is the application of a vascular clamp tangentially onto the aorta a few millimeters from the ductus, rather than on the ductus itself. This method of application of the clamp avoids the problem of a short ductus.

Postoperative Course. With an uncomplicated ductus, the operative risk is near zero. As early as 1953 Gross reported experience with 611 patients, with a mortality rate of less than 0.5 percent in those with neither cardiac failure nor infection. Similar figures were described by Jones in a total series of 909 patients. At New York University there has been no mortality or serious complications following division of an uncomplicated patent ductus in the past 15 years.

Convalescence following operation is usually uneventful. A functional systolic murmur may remain audible in a few patients. The electrocardiogram usually returns to normal within a few months. From data now available from over 40 years' experience, it seems certain that cardiac function becomes normal once the ductus has been surgically obliterated.

PATENT DUCTUS IN THE PREMATURE INFANT

In recent years the frequency and significance of the patent ductus in premature infants has become widely recognized. Closure can be significantly hastened by the administration of indomethacin. Apparently, indomethacin acts by blocking the synthesis of prostaglandins, which normally influence contraction of the smooth muscle that obliterates the patent ductus. The frequency of patent ductus in premature infants varies inversely with the birth weight and gestational age, ranging from a frequency of 15 to 80 percent.

Diagnosis may be made from the widened pulse pressure detected through an umbilical arterial catheter. The echocardiogram may be helpful in confirming the diagnosis.

Most patients can be treated with medical therapy, combined with indomethacin when necessary. In the 1983 National Cooperative Study of 3559 patients, this therapy produced ductus closure in 79 percent of the group.

Fig.18-36. Division of patent ductus arteriosus. *A.* Chest is opened ▶ with left posterolateral incision in fourth intercostal space. *B.* Once lung has been retracted, mediastinal pleura is incised longitudinally parallel to vagus nerve. *C.* Initial dissection is along vagus nerve to expose widely the recurrent laryngeal nerve originating from vagus and passing beneath ductus. Wide exposure of recurrent laryngeal nerve is essential part of operative procedure. *D.* After dissection of recurrent laryngeal nerve, lappet of pericardium overlying ductus is freed by sharp dissection proximally to expose pulmonary artery. *E.* Subsequently ductus is encircled, and vascular occlusion clamps are applied. *F.* Ductus is gradually divided and sutured, employing two rows of sutures. *G.* Final view of divided ends of ductus with recurrent laryngeal nerve well exposed.

If the diameter of the main pulmonary artery is less than 2 cm, it is also widened to an appropriate degree with a patch that may be extended when necessary beyond the bifurcation of the artery onto the left pulmonary artery.

Our preference for the prosthetic patch is a section of woven tubular Dacron graft. Pericardium is also a satisfactory material in most patients but has been associated with the subsequent formation of aneurysms in a small number of patients, usually with residual pulmonary hypertension.

Following bypass, intracardiac pressure is measured to confirm that right ventricular obstruction has been corrected. The right ventricular systolic pressure should be reduced to less than 60 to 70 percent of left ventricular systolic pressure. If right ventricular pressure is still elevated above this level, more adequate correction of the ventricular obstruction should be considered, though exact guidelines do not exist. Otherwise fatal depression of cardiac output from right ventricular failure may occur in the early postoperative course. In most patients following bypass a satisfactory result is obtained, with a systolic pressure near 100 mm, a right ventricular systolic pressure between 35 and 50 mm, and a pulmonary artery systolic pressure of 20 to 25 mm.

Fig. 18-41. Right ventricular approach to ventricular septal defect. Ao, aorta; AV, atrioventricular; IVC, inferior vena cava; PA, pulmonary artery; PV, pulmoary valve; RBB, right bundle branch, SVC, superior vena cava; TSM, trabecula septomarginalis; TV, tricuspid valve; VSD, ventricular septal defect. [From: *Kirklin JW, Barratt-Boyes BG: Ventricular septal defect and pulmonary stenosis or atresia, in Kirklin JW, Barratt-Boyes BG (eds): Cardiac Surgery. New York, Wiley, chap 23, pp 732–734, with permission.*]

Postoperative Course. Following operation, particular attention is required in the first 24 h to intrathoracic bleeding, because older cyanotic patients have an increased hemorrhagic tendency from the long-standing polycythemia. Transfusion of fresh frozen plasma, often combined with platelet transfusions, is the best therapy. Close observation is necessary to detect intrathoracic accumulation of blood with cardiac tamponade.

Adequacy of cardiac output is monitored by direct measurement and indirectly by observing blood pressure, blood-gas concentrations in mixed venous blood, and urine output. Blood is transfused in sufficient amounts to keep left atrial pressure in the range of 10 to 15 mmHg if necessary, possibly at higher levels. If cardiac output is inadequate despite these measures, small amounts of inotropic drugs (dobutamine, dopamine, epinephrine, or isoproteronol) are infused. Assisted ventilation may be required for 12 to 24 h but seldom for longer.

The risk of operation varies with the age of the patient and the degree of cyanosis, reflecting the severity of the right ventricular obstruction. The risk is near 2 to 5 percent. Large clinical series showing low operative mortality have also been reported by Kirklin, Malm et al., Shumway et al., and McGoon et al.

Arciniegas et al. reported 209 patients in whom an outflow patch across the pulmonic annulus was employed in nearly 70 percent. Perioperative mortality was 5 percent and delayed mortality was 3 percent. Complete heart block occurred in only one patient. Late results were considered good in 87 percent of the patients.

Following recovery from operation, dramatic improvement is obvious. Cyanosis is, of course, absent, and exer-

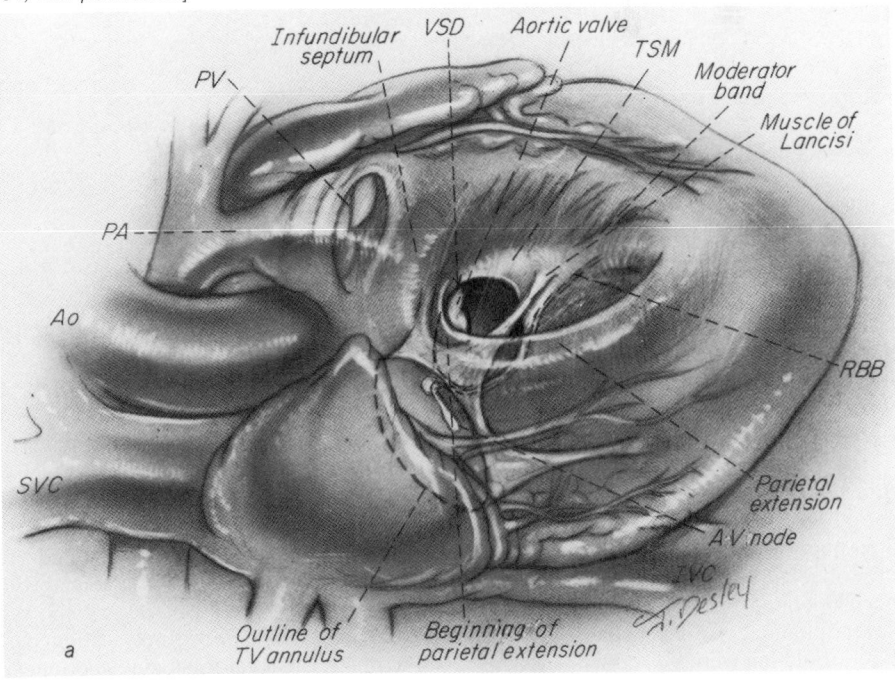

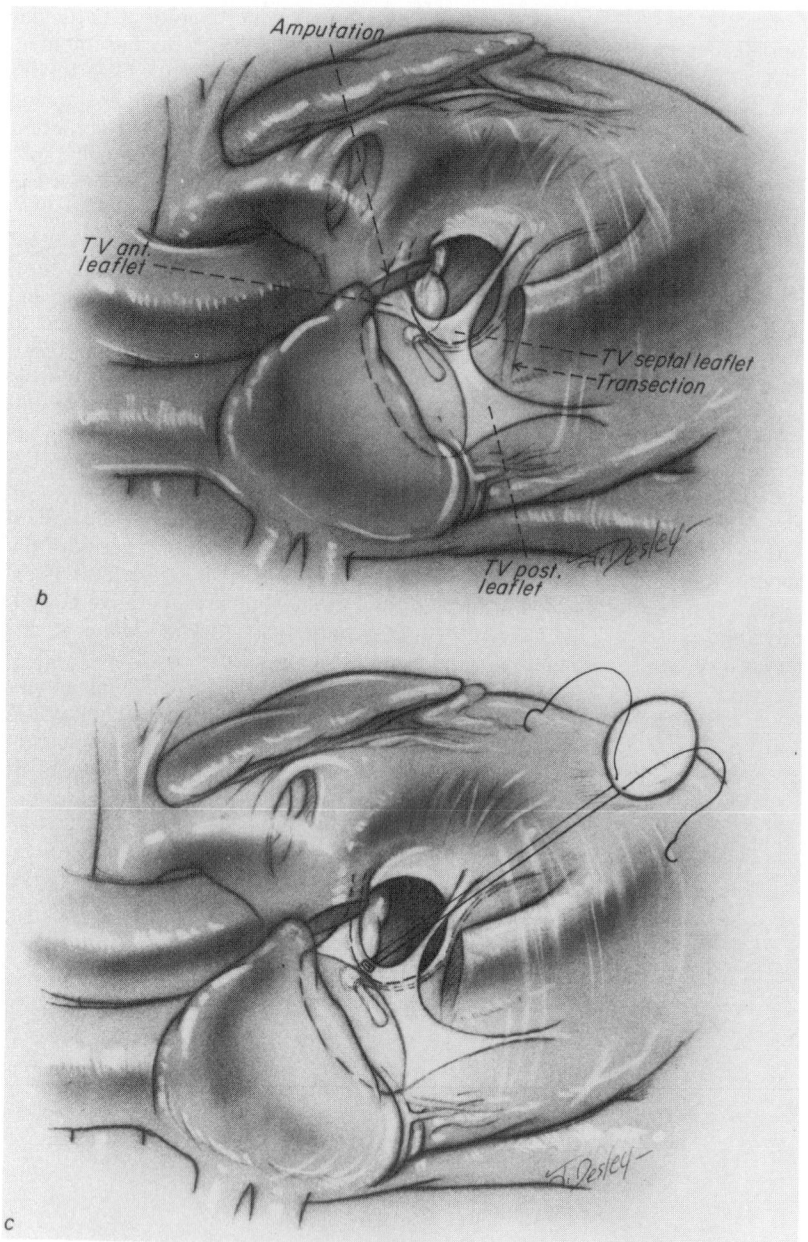

Fig. 18-41. Continued.

cise tolerance within a few months approaches that of a normal individual. If cardiac failure is significant following operation, convalescence may be slow for several weeks. Long-term studies show that most patients have excellent cardiac function.

The tolerance for pulmonic insufficiency after two to three decades is almost unknown, though Lillehei recently reported good long-term results in patients operated upon with a follow-up of more than 30 years. Ebert described repeat operations upon 24 patients who had been operated upon 1 to 21 years earlier. Several with severe pulmonary valve incompetence and right ventricular dysfunction were treated with insertion of a prosthetic valve.

COMPLEX MALFORMATIONS

Transposition of the Great Vessels

HISTORICAL DATA. The clinical syndrome of transposition of the great vessels was clearly described by Taussig in 1938. The first surgical procedure to achieve significant benefit, creation of an atrial septal defect, was reported in 1948 by Blalock and Hanlon. Because of the excellent results now obtained with balloon septostomy, developed by Rashkind in 1969, surgical creation of an atrial septal defect is now seldom performed. Another palliative surgical procedure, no longer used, was developed by Baffes around 1957. He transposed the inferior vena cava and

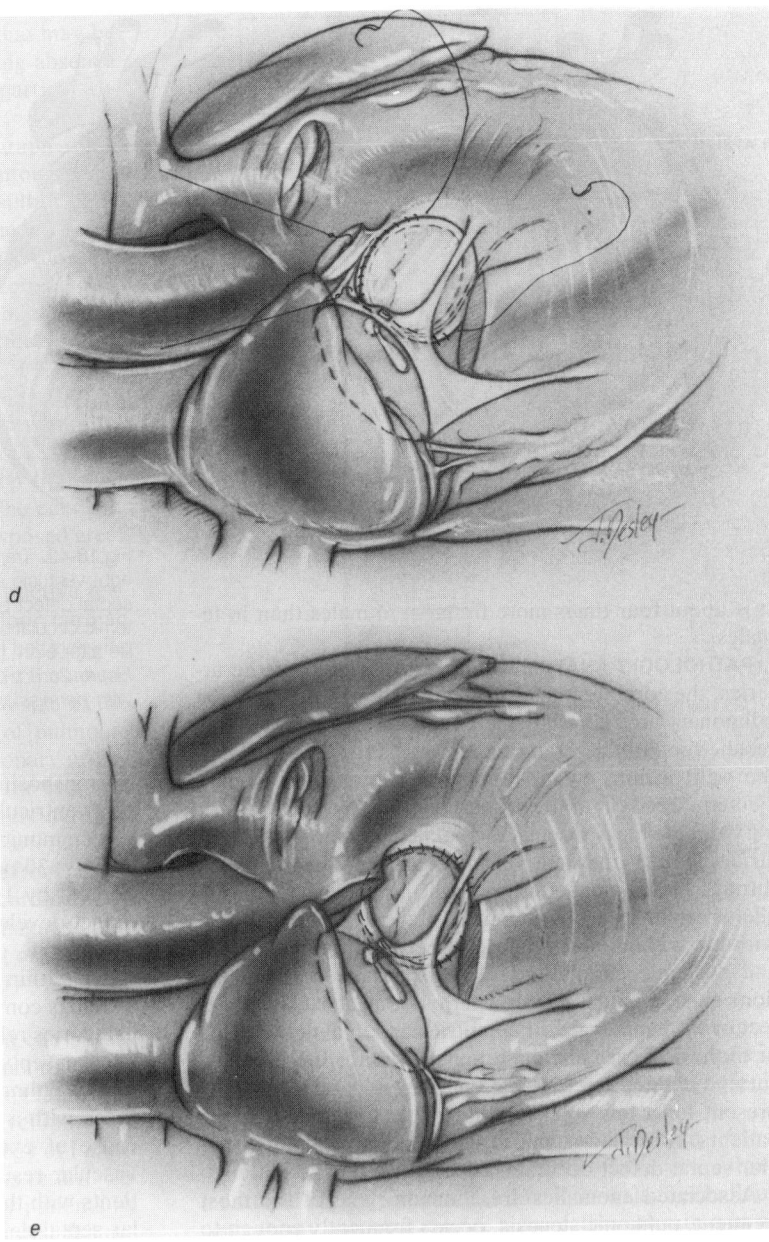

Fig. 18-41. Continued.

the right pulmonary veins. Senning, in 1957, first completely corrected transposition of the great vessels by repositioning the atrial septum, but mortality was prohibitively high. Further experience with a modification of the technique was reported by Senning in 1975. Mustard, in 1964, developed a method of reconstructing the atrial cavity that has produced the best clinical results to date. In the past few years a revised Senning procedure has been adopted by several groups as the procedure of choice.

INCIDENCE AND ETIOLOGY. Successful surgical correction of the transposed aorta and pulmonary artery, the "arterial switch" operation, was first successfully reported by Jatene in 1975. For the first few years, opera-

tive mortality remained excessive, but improved results in the last 3 to 4 years indicate that an arterial switch should be considered the primary operation in many patients. Quaegebeur reported in 1986 experiences with 66 patients with eight operative deaths and *no* late deaths among 33 patients followed for 1 to 8 years.

INCIDENCE AND ETIOLOGY. Transposition of the great vessels is a frequent disorder, representing 5 to 8 percent of all congenital cardiac malformations and accounting for about 25 percent of deaths in the first year of life. It is the most common cause of cardiac failure in the newborn. It results from abnormal division of the bulbar trunk in embryologic development, occurring between the fifth and seventh uterine week. Etiologic factors are unknown.

vascular disease. Either an atrial switch repair, combined with closure of the ventricular septal defect, or an arterial switch can be considered.

In patients with a ventricular septal defect and pulmonic stenosis, hypoxia may require use of a subclavian pulmonary shunt in the first few weeks of life. When older, the Rastelli procedure can be performed if the intracardiac anatomy is satisfactory.

Trusler et al. reported data from the institution in which the Mustard operation was developed. Only two deaths occurred in the last 100 operations. Modification in operative technique has decreased the frequency of pulmonary venous obstruction, caval obstruction, and arrhythmias; 89 percent of patients in the recent group maintained a sinus rhythm. At this time excellent long-term results have been reported with both the Mustard and the Senning methods of atrial correction. Increasingly good results have been reported with the arterial switch procedure.

If an arterial switch operation is performed, it must be done in the first 1 to 2 weeks of life in patients with an intact ventricular septum but may be delayed until about 3 months for those with a ventricular septal defect.

Tricuspid Atresia

HISTORICAL DATA. Systemic-pulmonary arterial shunts for tricuspid atresis were applied soon after their development in 1945–1947. There was significant short-term improvement, but long-term results were disappointing. A significant contribution was made by Glenn in 1958, with the development of the superior vena cava–right pulmonary artery anastomosis. The major advance, however, came in 1968 when Fontan successfully separated the right and left circulations in a patient for the first time, a physiologic concept that had seemed feasible in laboratory studies for over a decade but had never been successfully applied in human beings. In the last 15 years, the Fontan procedure has undergone several modifications but has been established clearly as the procedure of choice for this condition.

PATHOLOGIC ANATOMY. Tricuspid atresia is an important form of congenital heart disease, affecting 3 to 8 percent of children with cyanotic heart disease. The four basic abnormalities are atresia of the tricuspid valve, constituting complete obstruction to the flow of blood; an atrial septal defect; a varying degree of hypoplasia of the right ventricle; and a ventricular septal defect. The mitral valve and the left ventricle are usually normal. Blood enters the rudimentary right ventricle through a ventricular septal defect.

In about 70 percent of patients, the aorta and pulmonary artery are normally located, while in about 30 percent transposition is present. Hence, there are two major types of tricuspid atresia depending upon whether the great vessels are transposed or not. Each of these two major groups has been further subdivided into whether the pulmonary blood flow is normal or increased, decreased, or pulmonary atresia is present (Figs. 18-44, 18-45).

In the patients with normally related great vessels, the majority have a decreased pulmonary blood flow, while about 15 percent have a normal or increased pulmonary blood flow.

When the aorta and pulmonary artery are transposed, about 70 percent of patients have a normal or increased pulmonary blood flow.

Fig. 18-44. Three basic varieties of tricuspid atresia with normally related great arteries. Proximal to the mitral valve, anatomic arrangements are similar, with an interatrial communication providing the right atrium (RA) with its only outlet. Beyond the mitral valve, the anatomic patterns vary (LA–left atrium). *A.* When there is pulmonary atresia, i.e., no interventricular communication, all left ventricular blood enters the aorta (Ao). Pulmonary flow depends on a patent ductus arteriosus or systemic arterial collaterals. *B.* When there is pulmonic stenosis, the zone of obstruction typically consists of a slitlike ventricular septal defect that represents the only communication between the left ventricle (LV) and the small right ventricle (RV). The pulmonary trunk (PT) is normal or hypoplastic, and pulmonic valve stenosis may coexist. *C.* The absence of pulmonic stenosis signifies that there is a large ventricular septal defect with unobstructed flow into the pulmonary circulation. (From: *Perloff JK: The Clinical Recognition of Congenital Heart Disease. Philadelphia, Saunders, chap 25, p 555, with permission.*)

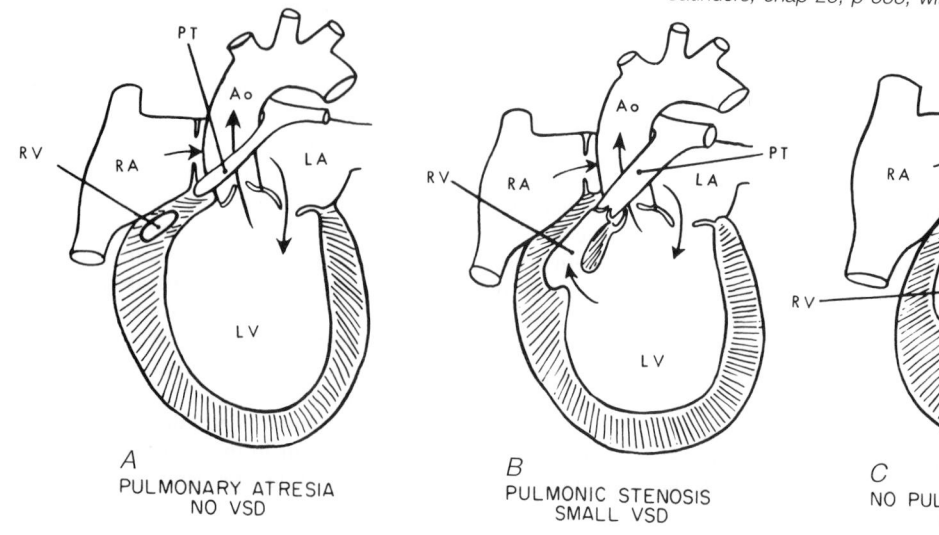

A
PULMONARY ATRESIA
NO VSD

B
PULMONIC STENOSIS
SMALL VSD

C
NO PULMONIC STENOSIS
LARGE VSD

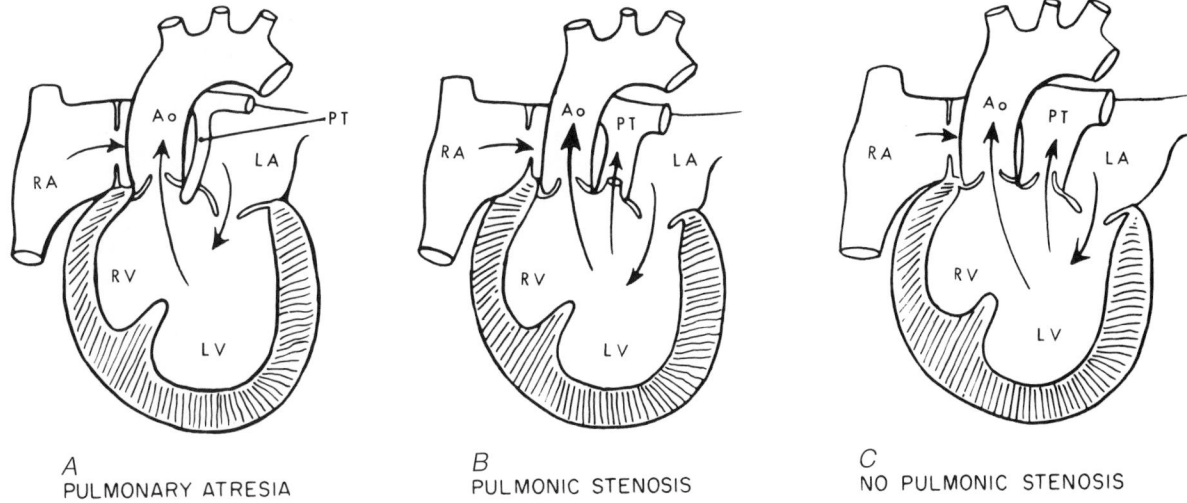

A
PULMONARY ATRESIA

B
PULMONIC STENOSIS

C
NO PULMONIC STENOSIS

Fig. 18-45. Three basic varieties of tricuspid atresia with complete transposition of the great arteries. Proximal to the mitral valve, the anatomic arrangements are similar, with an interatrial communication providing the right atrium (RA) with its only outlet. The ventricular septal defect is characteristically large so there is no obstruction to flow from left ventricle (LV) into the transposed aorta (Ao). Beyond this point the anatomic patterns vary. *A.* When there is pulmonary atresia (imperforate pulmonic valve and hypoplastic pulmonary trunk), all left ventricular blood enters the aorta. Pulmonary flow depends on a patent ductus arteriosus or systemic arterial collaterals. *B.* When pulmonic stenosis is present obstruction is either valvular or subvalvular. *C.* When there is no pulmonic stenosis, the pulmonary vascular resistance determines the amount of blood entering the lungs (RV = right ventricle; PT = pulmonary trunk; LA = left atrium). (From: *Perloff JK: The Clinical Recognition of Congenital Heart Disease. Philadelphia, Saunders, chap 25, p 555, with permission.*)

PATHOPHYSIOLOGY. The disability from hypoxia resulting from inadequate pulmonary blood flow is severe. This is most commonly due to restriction of flow of blood from the left ventricle through the ventricular septal defect and rudimentary right ventricle into the pulmonary artery. The ventricular septal defect usually decreases in size in the first year of life, further decreasing pulmonary blood flow, so over 90 percent of patients die before the first year unless operation is performed.

In the minority of patients with an increase in pulmonary blood flow, with either normal or transposed great arteries, congestive heart failure is present with gradual failure of the left ventricle. Only rarely is the pulmonary blood flow near normal.

CLINICAL MANIFESTATIONS. Disability is severe with cyanosis, usually obvious at birth. Over 50 percent of infants are correctly diagnosed during the first day of life. The clinical manifestations are usually those of severe cyanosis with anoxic spells often terminating in hemiplegia or death. In the few patients with an increased pulmonary blood flow, signs of pulmonary congestion and heart failure may predominate.

The physical examination is usually not diagnostic as the systolic murmur present varies widely, depending upon the size of the ventricular septal defect and the anatomical relationship of the great vessels. The chest roentgenogram shows decreased vascularity if pulmonary blood flow is decreased. Both the electrocardiogram and echocardiogram provide the diagnostic clues that establish the diagnosis. The electrocardiogram is strongly suggestive, showing a typical left axis deviation resulting from the underdevelopment of the right ventricle. The 2-D echocardiogram can often outline the atrial septal defect, the ventricular septal defect, and the relationships of the great arteries. Cardiac catheterization and angiography are required to precisely delineate these abnormalities.

TREATMENT. An emergency shunt is often necessary in the first few days or weeks of life to prevent death from anoxia. A Goretex interposition shunt, as described in the section on Tetralogy, is usually the simplest and most satisfactory.

In some patients, a small atrial septal defect (or foramen ovale) may restrict flow of blood from the right atrium to the left atrium. This can be determined at cardiac catheterization, measuring a gradient between the right and left atrium. If a gradient is present, a balloon septostomy can be performed at that time. Surgical enlargement of the atrial septal defect is almost never required at this time. After six to twelve months of age, a Fontan procedure can be performed, directing the venous blood into the pulmonary circulation.

This landmark procedure was first performed by Fontan in France in 1968 and has subsequently been widely used throughout the world with excellent results. Important modifications of the original Fontan concept were made by Kreutzer and by Bjork. At present, three varieties of connections between the right atrium and the pulmonary artery are performed. The simplest, when feasible, is establishment of a large direct communication between the right atrium and the main pulmonary artery, which is divided at its origin, mobilized, and anastomosed directly to a large circular opening in the right atrium. No valve is inserted (Fig. 18-46).

If the right ventricle is of significant size with a pulmonic valve, a conduit may be established from the right atrium to the right ventricle, either with or without a valve. In all procedures both the atrial and ventricular

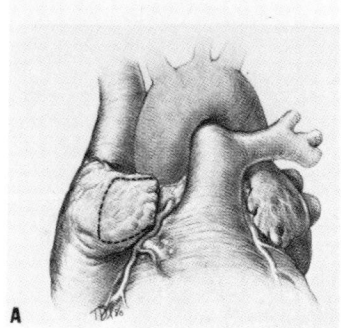
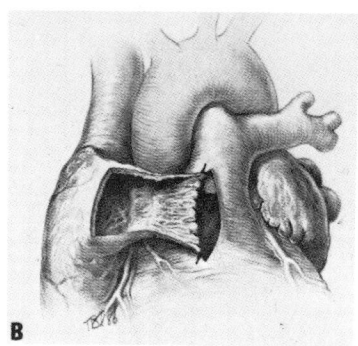
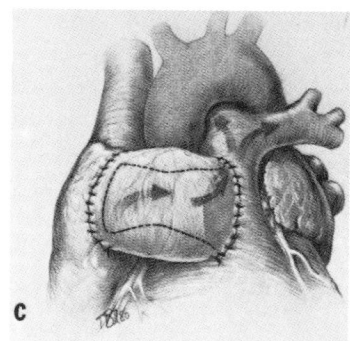

Fig. 18-46. Technique of anastomosing the right atrium to the right ventricle. *A.* An incision is made in the right atrial appendage to form a flap of the anterior wall. *B.* The cut edge of the flap is then sutured to the rightward edge of the longitudinal incision in the right ventricle to form the posterior wall of the tunnel. *C.* The procedure is completed by suturing a pericardial patch from the right atrial appendage to the right ventricle to form the anterior wall of the tunnel. Arrows indicate the flow of blood in the completed conduit. [From: *Stanton RE, Lurie PR, et al: The Fontan procedure for tricuspid atresia. Circulation 64(suppl 2):140, 1981, with permission.*]

septal defects are closed so the two circulations are separated. There are not adequate data at present to determine which of the techniques are preferable.

Operative risk in general is in the range of 5 to 15 percent with reasonably good results for at least 5 to 10 years after operation.

The operation physiologically depends upon using the venous pressure to perfuse the pulmonary vascular bed. This is usually satisfactory if the right atrial pressure remains below 15 mm. Higher levels result in severe problems such as chylothorax and protein-losing enteropathy. Hence, a contraindication to the Fontan procedure is an increase in pulmonary vascular resistance or hypoplasia of the pulmonary arteries.

In the minority of patients who were seen with refractory congestive failure from increased pulmonary blood flow in infancy, banding of the pulmonary artery can be done, followed later by a Fontan procedure and debanding after 1 to 2 years.

The Glenn procedure consists of anastomosis of the superior vena cava to the right pulmonary artery (Fig. 18-47). About 85 percent of patients survive 10 or more years, with generally satisfactory results. Symptoms tend to gradually recur, however, probably related to growth of the patient, development of collateral circulation, and the basic limitation that only part of systemic venous return has been directed into the pulmonary vascular bed.

RARE MALFORMATIONS

Cor Triatriatum

Cor triatriatum is a rare malformation. In 1960 a review by Niwayama found only 36 cases. Excellent embryologic and pathologic studies were reported by Van Praagh, and subsequently by Marin-Garcia.

PATHOLOGIC ANATOMY. The abnormality is best viewed as a variant of total anomalous pulmonary venous

Fig. 18-47. Anastomosis between superior vena cava and right pulmonary artery. *A.* Tangential clamp has been applied to superior vena cava to include origin of azygos vein. Right pulmonary artery has been divided, and end-to-end anastomosis will be constructed. *B.* Posterior row of anastomosis is constructed. *C.* Completed posterior row of anastomosis. *D.* Anterior row of anastomosis is constructed with interrupted sutures to permit growth of anastomosis. After removal of occluding clamps, superior vena cava is doubly ligated at point of juncture with right atrium. (From: *Glenn WWL: N Engl J Med 259:117, 1958, with permission.*)

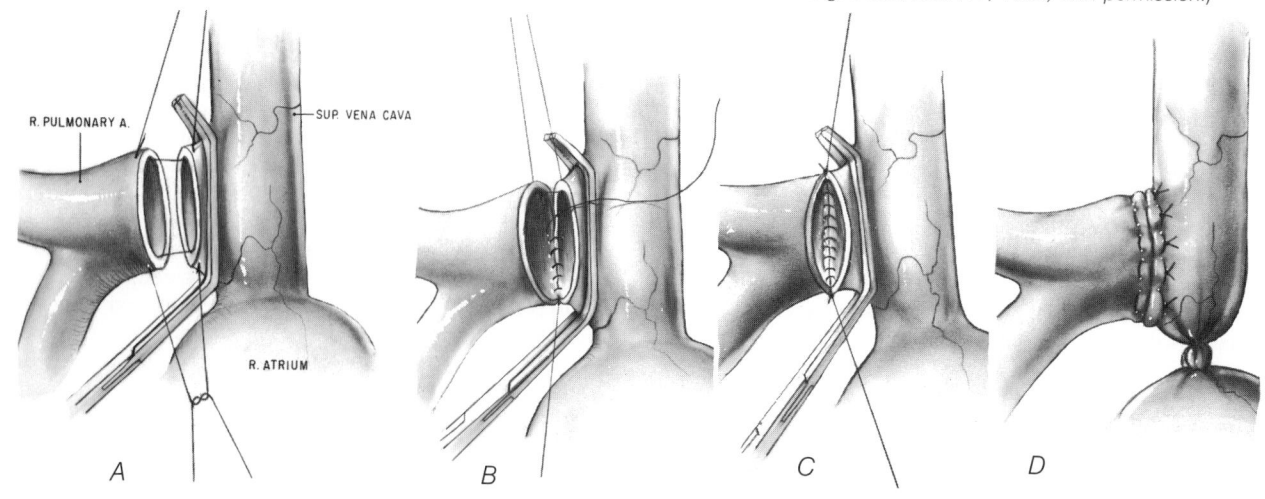

R. PULMONARY A.   SUP. VENA CAVA

R. ATRIUM

A   *B*   *C*   *D*

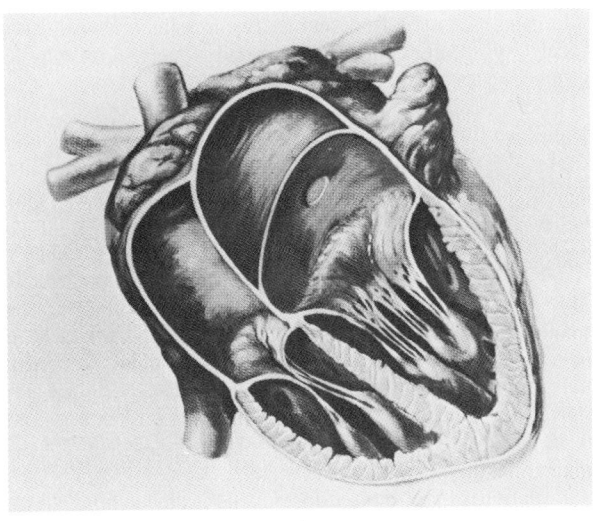

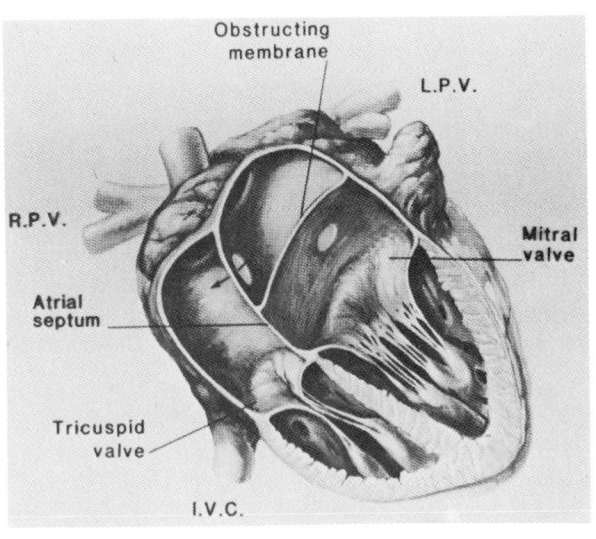

Fig. 18-48. *A.* Cor triatriatum with intact atrial septum (type A). *B.* Cor triatriatum with atrial septal defect between the proximal left atrial chamber and the right atrium (type A₁). (LPV = left pulmonary vein; RPV = right pulmonary vein; IVC = inferior vena cava.) (From: *Arciniegas E, Hakimi M, Green EW: Surgical treatment of cor triatriatum. Ann Thorac Surg 32:571, 1981, with permission.*)

drainage except that the unresorbed common venous sinus empties normally into the left atrium through a restricted aperture, rather than through abnormal channels to the right side of the heart. The common venous chamber is superior and posterior to the normal left atrium with a diaphragm separating this chamber from the true left atrium. The left atrial appendage enters the normal small left atrium. A small opening in a thick muscular diaphragm is the only communication between the two chambers.

This abnormality produces severe pulmonary hypertension, identical to mitral stenosis. Gradients as high as 20 mmHg have been recorded between the venous chamber and normal left atrium.

An atrial septal defect, usually a fossa ovalis, is present in about 70 percent of cases, generally entering the common venous chamber and resulting in a left-to-right shunt.

A classic malformation is shown in Fig. 18-48*A.* The most common variety, with an atrial septal defect between the common venous chamber and the right atrium, is shown in Fig. 18-48*B.*

CLINICAL MANIFESTATIONS. The disability is a severe one from pulmonary congestion, pulmonary hypertension, and heart failure. Without surgical treatment 70 to 75 percent of infants die in the first year of life. The clinical presentation is identical to that of mitral stenosis except that a typical diastolic murmur is often not present.

DIAGNOSTIC CONSIDERATIONS. The x-ray shows pulmonary congestion with right ventricular enlargement. Right ventricular hypertrophy is evident on the electrocardiogram, varying with the degree of pulmonary hypertension. 2-D echocardiography is diagnostic, outlining the abnormal chambers. Some investigators no longer consider cardiac catheterization necessary, although catheterization and angiography permits measurement of pulmonary artery pressure and more precise delineation of other associated anomalies. The classic physiologic abnormalities at catheterization are an elevated pulmonary artery pressure, an increased wedge pressure, and a *normal* pressure in the left atrium. The differential diagnosis includes the two other conditions that can commonly produce pulmonary venous hypertension, mitral stenosis, or stenosis of pulmonary veins.

TREATMENT. Operation should be performed promptly when the diagnosis is recognized in infancy because of the high mortality rate. With proper techniques of extracorporeal circulation, combined with hypothermia and circulatory arrest, operative results are usually excellent. The abnormal septum between the common venous sinus and the left atrium can be readily excised, eliminating the physiologic abnormality. An accompanying atrial septal defect can be closed at the same time. Usually an approach from the right side of the heart is preferable, though this varies with the precise abnormality present. Results in surviving patients are excellent.

Kirklin and Barratt-Boyes reported excellent results in a group of seven patients operated upon over a period of 30 years, emphasizing the rarity of the malformation. Oglietti reported experiences with 25 patients seen over a period of 21 years. The diagnosis was made preoperatively in 14, established at the time of operation for other abnormalities in 10. The anomalous membrane was excised in 18 patients with excellent results in all but one who required reoperation because of incomplete excision of the septum. Arciniegas reported on six patients ranging in age from one and one-half to ninety-three months. There was one postoperative death; the five surviving patients remained in excellent condition 4 years following operation.

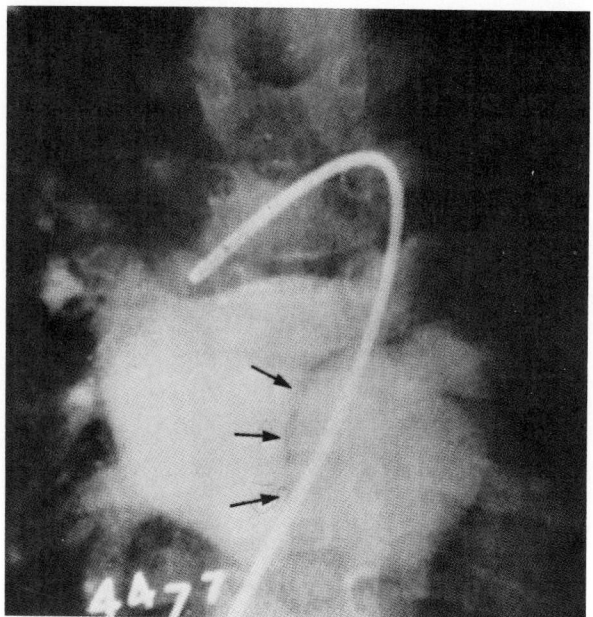

Fig. 18-49. Angiogram shows the subdividing left atrial membrane (arrows). The atrial septum was intact. Contrast material was injected into the pulmonary artery. (From: *Arciniegas E, Hakimi M, Green EW: Surgical treatment of cor triatriatum. Ann Thorac Surg 32:571, 1981, with permission.*)

Congenital Mitral Valve Disease

These abnormalities are rare, about 0.6 percent of all cases of congenital heart disease at autopsy, and about 0.3 percent of clinically diagnosed cases.

In 1967 a review by Tsuji found 131 reported cases, 41 of whom had been operated upon with 21 survivors. One of the most extensive experiences was described by Carpentier, reporting experiences with 47 children, in 14 of whom mitral stenosis was the dominant finding.

PATHOLOGY. Multiple abnormalities in the mitral valve apparatus are usually present. A distinct stenosing *supravalvular* ring has been described in a few patients. The mitral valve annulus is usually small. Usually there are multiple abnormalities in the leaflets with defective commissures. A few patients have a distinct isolated cleft causing insufficiency. The underlying chordae and papillary muscles are often malformed, producing either stenosis or insufficiency. One distinctive malformation, termed a "parachute" mitral valve, consists of a single papillary muscle with all chordae attached to this muscle.

Congenital mitral stenosis exists as an isolated lesion in about 25 percent of patients, in association with a ventricular septal defect in nearly 30 percent. Some form of left ventricular outflow tract obstruction is present in about 40 percent of cases. Van Praagh in 1978 reported an extensive pathologic study of 49 cases.

CLINICAL MANIFESTATIONS. Symptoms of pulmonary venous hypertension often appear in infancy and include dyspnea, orthopnea, and pulmonary edema. It has been estimated that about one-half of patients die within 6 months after symptoms appear. Those with less severe

abnormalities are often seen between ages one and four; rarely symptoms may not become severe until ten to twelve years of age.

Chest x-ray and electrocardiographic abnormalities are similar to those of mitral stenosis. With 2-D echocardiography the diagnosis can usually be made with certainty and the precise abnormalities identified. Additional information can be obtained by subsequent cardiac catheterization and angiography (Fig. 18-49).

TREATMENT. Operation should clearly be postponed as long as possible because of the strong probability of the need for repeat operation as the child grows older. The feasibility of repair versus replacement depends upon the abnormality present. In the extensive experience reported by Carpentier, valve reconstruction was possible in 38 patients; valve replacement was necessary in 9; hospital mortality was 13 percent.

In patients in whom reconstruction was possible, some residual stenosis or insufficiency is usually present. Reasonable long-term results have been reported in the few patients surviving 10 years, with a 63 percent survival and about 80 percent remaining free of reoperation at 10 years.

Aortic-Pulmonary Window

This is a rare abnormality. At the Toronto Children's Hospital, only 23 of 15,000 patients with congenital heart disease who were seen over a period of 20 years had an aortopulmonary window. Synonyms referring to the same lesion include aortopulmonary fistula and aortic septal defect.

One case was treated by ligation by Gross in 1948, another by division and suture by Scott and Sabiston in 1951 (Fig. 18-50). Effective safe correction became possible only with the development of extracorporeal circulation.

PATHOLOGIC ANATOMY. Embryologically, the defect results from incomplete development of the spiral septum dividing the primitive truncus arteriosus into the aorta and pulmonary artery. Persistent truncus arteriosus is a more severe malformation of similar cause. The opening, or "window," between the aorta and pulmonary artery may vary in diameter from 5 to 30 mm. It is usually located proximally near the ostium of the coronary arteries. At least 30 percent of patients have a severe additional cardiac malformation.

PATHOPHYSIOLOGY. The large left-to-right shunt is similar to that of a large patent ductus arteriosus or ventricular septal defect. The course is a malignant one because an increase in pulmonary vascular resistance quickly occurs, similar to a large ventricular septal defect.

CLINICAL MANIFESTATIONS. The clinical findings may be identical to those of patent ductus arteriosus with a continuous murmur and wide pulse pressure. Often, however, only a systolic murmur is present because of the severe pulmonary hypertension. Differential diagnosis includes ventricular septal defect and truncus arteriosus.

LABORATORY FINDINGS. 2-D echocardiography can usually confirm the diagnosis. A CT scan is also usually

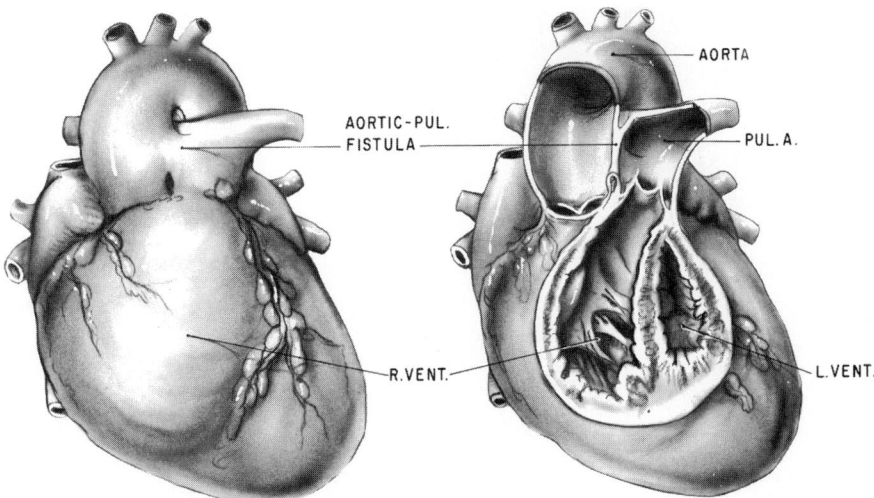

Fig. 18-50. Aortic-pulmonary fistula, showing large communication between aorta and pulmonary artery near base of heart. (From: *Scott HW, Sabiston DC: J Thorac Surg. 25:26 1953, with permission.*)

diagnostic. Cardiac catheterization and aortography should be done to define precisely the relationship to adjacent structures and also confirm that the aortic and pulmonic valve rings are intact. The degree of elevation of pulmonary vascular resistance can also be determined.

TREATMENT. Operation should be performed as soon as the diagnosis has been established because of the rapidity of development of irreversible pulmonary vascular disease. At operation a transaortic approach has usually been employed, closing large defects with a prosthetic patch. Care is taken to avoid injury to the coronary arteries or the pulmonary valve. In patients operated upon in infancy or before the development of severe pulmonary vascular disease, results have been excellent. Little information is available about those surviving with severe elevation in pulmonary vascular resistance.

Doty in 1983 reported 25 patients and reviewed 50 previous reported operative repairs. He concluded that a transaortic approach was preferable with patch closure of the defect. The risk of operation was proportional to the increase in pulmonary vascular resistance.

Ruptured Aneurysm of Sinus of Valsalva

This unusual abnormality produces a distinct syndrome that can be readily diagnosed and effectively treated. Before the development of extracorporeal circulation, it usually caused death from cardiac failure within 1 to 2 years after rupture. The natural history was well described by Sawyer in 1957, reviewing 47 reported patients. Successful operations with extracorporeal circulation were done by Lillehei and by Kirklin in 1956, and other successful care reports soon followed. By 1965 over 90 patients had been operated upon.

PATHOLOGIC ANATOMY. The basic abnormality is a thinning of the aortic media in the wall of the sinus of Valsalva. In embryonic development, the developing ventricular septum inferiorly meets the spiral septum superiorly which separates the aorta and the pulmonary arteries. Incomplete merger of these two structures results in a ventricular septal defect in the membranous septum. An aneurysm of the sinus of Valsalva results from a less severe malformation of a similar type, for the media of the aortic wall does not extend down to the annulus of the aortic valve ring. Hence, there is a spectrum of abnormalities, including ventricular septal defect, aortic valve abnormalities with aortic valve prolapse, and less frequently, pulmonic stenosis.

The right coronary sinus is involved in most patients with rupture into the right ventricle. The noncoronary sinus is involved in about 20 percent of patients, most commonly rupturing into the right atrium. Involvement of the left coronary sinus or rupture into the left atrium or left ventricle is very unusual, probably both because of the differences in anatomy and because of the high pressures in the left ventricle. The typical aneurysm is usually described as a ''windsock'' with a wide base at the aortic origin and a nipplelike apex projecting into a cardiac chamber where rupture eventually occurs.

CLINICAL MANIFESTATIONS. Until rupture occurs, there are no abnormalities unless an enlarging aneurysm distorts the aortic leaflets sufficiently to cause aortic insufficiency. The average age at rupture is 31 years. This is usually without known cause, although a few case reports describe the onset during physical exertion.

About one-third of patients develop acute symptoms at the time of rupture, with chest pain, soon followed by dyspnea and palpitation and the appearance of the characteristic murmur. In nearly one-half of patients, however, the onset is more gradual with progressive dyspnea, while a small percentage have very few symptoms when the cardiac abnormalities are detected. Death seldom occurs from right heart failure shortly following rupture, but over the ensuing weeks and months, cardiac failure relentlessly progresses with few patients tolerating the abnormality for more than 1 to 2 years.

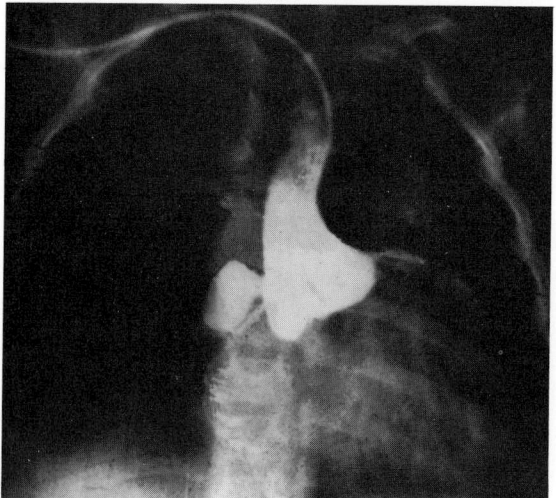

Fig. 18-51. Aortogram confirms diagnosis of ruptured aneurysm of sinus of Valsalva by demonstrating flow of dye from region of aortic sinuses to right atrium. *(Courtesy of Dr. Raymond M. Abrams, Department of Radiology, New York University Medical Center.)*

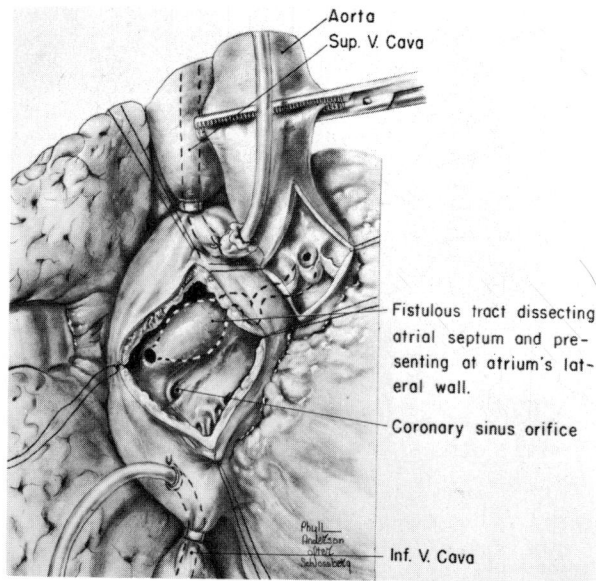

Fig. 18-52. Diagram of unusual type of ruptured aneurysm of sinus of Valsalva. Aneurysm arose from left coronary cusp and developed fistulous tract before rupture into right atrium. Operative closure was performed by opening aorta and closing opening directly. (From: *Ann Surg 152:965, 1960, with permission.*)

On physical examination the classical abnormality is a parasternal murmur, often with a thrill, loudest in the third or fourth interspace. This is often continuous, resembling a patent ductus, but is at a lower location. The usual hemodynamic abnormalities seen with a large patent ductus are present, including a wide pulse pressure, cardiac enlargement, and pulmonary congestion.

The diagnosis can readily be suspected from the history and the physical abnormalities. The chest x-ray shows cardiac enlargement and pulmonary congestion. Cardiac hypertrophy is evident on the electrocardiogram. With 2-D echocardiography the diagnosis can be promptly confirmed. Cardiac catheterization and angiography are usually performed to determine the site of origin, the cardiac chamber involved, and the presence of associated lesions, especially ventricular septal defect or aortic insufficiency (Fig. 18-51).

TREATMENT. Surgical correction, of course, should be performed promptly. The basic objective at operation is to close both the defect and any associated lesions (Fig. 18-52). An approach through both the aorta and the involved cardiac chamber is best, facilitating the correction of associated lesions such as a ventricular septal defect. The aneurysmal sac can be excised back to the aortic origin and closed, preferably with a prosthetic patch. Alternately, the aneurysm can be excised and sutured from within the ventricle, following which a prosthetic patch can be directly sutured over the aortic origin, avoiding any injury to the aortic cusps. The operative risk is small and reported results excellent.

Truncus Arteriosus

Truncus arteriosus is a rare malformation resulting from failure of division of the fetal arterial channel into the aorta and pulmonary arteries and the left and right ventricles. The embryonic origin of the malformation has been analyzed in detail by Rothko.

PATHOLOGIC ANATOMY. In this condition the entire circulation, including the coronary arteries, the pulmonary arteries, and the systemic arteries, arises from a common arterial trunk. There is always a ventricular septal defect. Only one semilunar valve is present, usually with three or four cusps.

In 80 to 85 percent of patients the pulmonary arteries arise from the truncus, either as a common stem or in close apposition. Infrequently, the origin of the two pulmonary arteries is separated a short distance, complicating the anatomic repair. In most patients the ductus arteriosus is absent; if present, it is usually large with corresponding decrease in size of the aortic isthmus (Fig. 18-53).

PATHOPHYSIOLOGY. The disability is a severe one with about 50 percent of patients dying in the first month of life, 90 percent within the first year, usually from congestive heart failure. The severe heart failure results from the large left-to-right shunt through the ventricular septal defect. Severe incompetence of the truncal valve, often from nodular myxomatous degeneration, may contribute significantly.

The blood entering the aorta is a mixture of blood from the systemic and pulmonary circulations, arterial oxygen unsaturation is always present, the degree varying with the volume of pulmonary blood flow. Usually, in infancy, the oxygen saturation is above 80 percent, so cyanosis is minimal. Severe pulmonary vascular disease develops rapidly, often before six months of age. As this progresses, arterial oxygen saturation decreases and cyanosis becomes more prominent.

The majority of infants are obviously seriously ill with congestive heart failure and an overactive heart with a wide pulse pressure. Murmurs are variable, not diagnos-

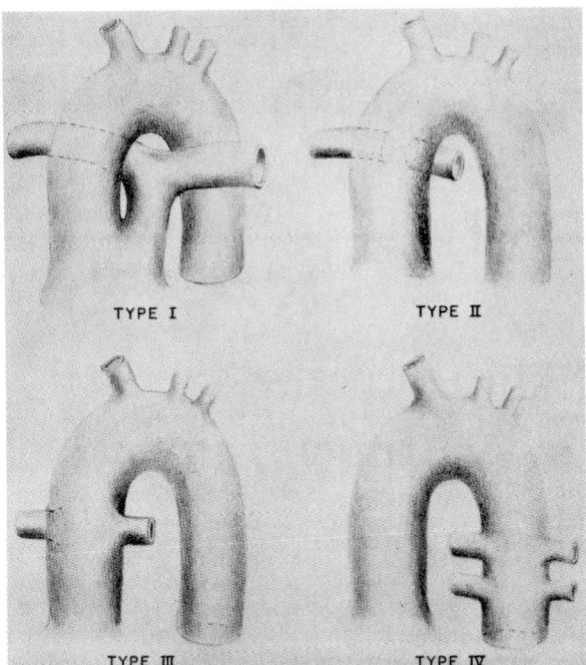

Fig. 18-53. Four anatomic types of truncus arteriosus. (From: *Poirier RA et al: J Thorac Cardiovasc Surg 69:169, 1975, with permission.*)

tic, unless a continuous murmur is audible. The chest x-ray shows cardiomegaly and pulmonary congestion. Both right and left ventricular hypertrophy are evident on the electrocardiogram. 2-D echocardiography is diagnostic, outlining the single vascular trunk originating from the base of the heart. Cardiac catheterization and angiography define the anatomy precisely, including the origin of the pulmonary arteries and the presence of insufficiency of the truncal valve. The pulmonary vascular resistance can be determined, indicating the gravity of the problem, and whether operation can be performed or not.

TREATMENT. Most modern treatment emerged from the excellent work of McGoon, who first successfully used a homograft conduit in 1967. In the procedure developed by McGoon the pulmonary arteries were detached from the truncus, the right ventricle opened, and the ventricular septal defect closed, after which the homograft conduit was inserted between the right ventricle and the distal pulmonary artery.

Most of the early operations were performed upon patients over two years of age, obviously a selective group as only about 10 percent of patients survive beyond the first year of life.

Current experiences at the Mayo Clinic were summarized by DiDonato in 1985, describing experiences with 167 patients over a 17-year period. There were 48 hospital deaths (29 percent mortality). Eighty-four percent of 119 surviving patients were alive at 5 years, 69 percent at 10 years.

In 1985, Sharma reported experiences with 23 patients, 16 of whom were less than one year of age. There were only three operative deaths, two of which occurred in

critically ill infants operated upon under one month of age.

As nearly 50 percent of infants die within 1 month, operation must clearly be performed in the neonatal period if heart failure is severe. Otherwise it may be delayed until three to six months of age, but further delay has the hazard of an irreversible rise in pulmonary vascular resistance.

In 1984, Ebert described experiences with 106 infants. One hundred were corrected by six months of age, with 11 operative deaths. Fifteen of the 86 long-term survivors have returned for change of the conduit because of body growth or pseudo-intimal proliferation in the conduit. There were no mortalities at the time of conduit change. A distinctive feature of the operative technique used by Ebert is minimizing the aortic cross-clamping, performing a significant part of the operation while the heart is beating.

The long-term course of surviving patients is unknown because to date there are few such patients. A progression in pulmonary vascular resistance has occurred in some patients. Another hazard in surviving patients is the development of insufficiency in the abnormal truncal valve.

Operative mortality has been low in the selective group of patients operated upon between five and ten years of age, in whom the pulmonary vascular resistance is less than 0.6 percent of systemic vascular resistance. However, this is a selective group because, as indicated earlier, there is both a high mortality in infancy and also rapid development of irreversible pulmonary vascular disease in many. These considerations were well reviewed in the reports by Poirier in 1975 and by Applebaum in 1976.

Banding of the pulmonary arteries in infancy to protect the pulmonary vascular bed has a surprisingly high mortality, nearly 50 percent from different reports according to Applebaum, and also a significant mortality at the time of attempted correction at a later date. Hence the increasing tendency is to perform corrective surgery with a valve conduit at an earlier age, probably between two and three years, or in the first years of life if symptoms are severe. This has been accomplished in several patients described by Ebert in 1976.

When a conduit is inserted in such small children, it will have to be replaced as the child grows older; Marcelletti and McGoon reported in 1976 that 22 aortic homograft conduits had been successfully replaced with a Dacron conduit, primarily because of deterioration of the aortic homograft.

Single Ventricle

A single ventricle is a severe malformation that fortunately is quite rare. Effective palliative surgery has become possible in a high percentage of cases. The long-term outlook has progressively improved with the effective development of cardiac transplantation.

PATHOLOGIC ANATOMY AND PATHOPHYSIOLOGY. A wide spectrum of abnormalities exists. The basic abnormality is a single functioning ventricle into which both atrioventricular valves empty. The variations include the type of functioning ventricular chamber (morphologically a "left" or a "right" ventricle), the type of hypoplastic ventricular chamber; different abnormalities in the atrioventricular valves; and the origin of the aorta and pulmonary artery from either the large ventricle or the hypoplastic one.

The two physiologic abnormalities are anoxemia from mixture of oxygenated and unoxygenated blood in the single ventricle before entering the aorta, and pulmonary congestion from the high pulmonary blood flow resulting from the origin of the pulmonary artery from the left ventricle. The degree of cyanosis present depends upon the pulmonary blood flow.

CLINICAL MANIFESTATIONS. About one-third of patients do not have significant pulmonic stenosis, so the resulting disability initially resembles that of a large ventricular septal defect with some cyanosis. At the other extreme, severe cyanosis is present from pulmonic stenosis, requiring an emergency shunt procedure in infancy.

In between these two extremes are patients with moderate pulmonic stenosis, often with a pulmonary blood flow about twice normal. Such patients may do reasonably well in the first few years of life.

In most patients the disability is severe, about 40 percent requiring operation in the first year of life, but only about 50 percent of patients alive at four years of age. Excellent morphologic and embryologic studies have been reported by both Van Praagh et al. and by Anderson et al.

CLINICAL MANIFESTATIONS AND DIAGNOSIS. The clinical picture varies with the pulmonary blood flow. Infants with an increased pulmonary blood flow are acyanotic but disabled from pulmonary congestion and cardiac failure. Such infants have been treated previously with pulmonary artery banding, which unfortunately results in subaortic stenosis in a high percentage of patients within the next 1 to 2 years. At the other extreme, with severely decreased pulmonary blood flow, cyanosis is severe so a shunt procedure is often required in infancy. The cardiac murmurs, x-ray, and electrocardiogram are usually diagnostic, but a precise diagnosis can be made by 2-D echocardiography, noting the absence of the normal ventricular septum. Catheterization with selective angiography can further delineate the precise abnormalities present.

TREATMENT. Urgent banding or shunting procedures have been used in infants, depending upon whether the pulmonary blood flow is increased or decreased. In older patients, surgically partitioning the ventricle or separating the two circulations with the Fontan procedure are the two procedures available. Which procedure is selected depends upon the abnormality present and the presence of increased pulmonary vascular resistance. Early experiences with partitioning of the ventricle were reported in four cases by Edie and Malm. In 1977, McGoon et al. reported experiences with 23 patients, obtaining satisfactory results in 61 percent. In 1984, Stefanelli et al. described experiences in 116 patients over a period of 15 years with a 10-year actuarial survival rate of 66 percent. Ventricular septation was performed in 36 patients with 15 deaths. The majority of patients developed com-

plete heart block following septation, requiring a pacemaker.

A total of 73 patients underwent a Fontan-type procedure with a 22 percent mortality and a 10-year actuarial survival rate of 71 percent. Over 95 percent of surviving patients were reported as improving to a functional class I or II status.

A two-stage approach was described in five patients by Ebert, only partly closing the septal defect at the first operation. In this small group, all survived without any rhythm disturbances.

Ebstein's Anomaly

This unusual anomaly was described by Wilhelm Ebstein in 1866. The abnormality is uncommon, about 0.5 percent of all cases of congenital heart disease. There is a nearly 400 times increased frequency of Ebstein's malformation when the mother has taken lithium during the pregnancy.

PATHOLOGIC ANATOMY. The basic abnormality is a malformation of the septal and posterior leaflets of the tricuspid valve. The origin of the leaflets is displaced downward to a variable degree creating a third chamber on the right side of the heart. Both the leaflet tissue and its chordae are also abnormal. The anterior tricuspid leaflet is usually normal and may be unusually large and prominent, described as "sail-like" (Fig. 18-54). The segment of right ventricular wall between the true annulus of the tricuspid valve and the origin of the displaced leaflets becomes functionally part of the right atrium and has been termed the atrialized ventricle. There is a varying degree of hypoplasia of this segment in some patients resembling a true aneurysm that bulges paradoxically. In most patients, the atrialized segment has some muscle fibers with little paradoxical motion. The distal functioning right ventricle is small. Some investigators have felt that there is a true deficiency in the right ventricular fibers as well, contributing to the right ventricular dysfunction in this condition. A foramen ovale or ostium sedundum defect are almost always present. The right atrium is usually dilated, often to a huge size in older patients.

The malformation varies widely in severity, ranging from relatively minor valvular abnormalities to virtual atresia of the valve leaflets.

PATHOPHYSIOLOGY. The main physiologic disturbance is inadequate cardiac output from the right ventricle, a result of both the tricuspid insufficiency and the dysfunction of the right ventricle. A variety of arrhythmias commonly occur in older patients; these are rarely fatal. Massive dilatation of the right atrium gradually develops in some patients. Cyanosis of moderate degree occurs in at least 50 percent of patients because of a right-to-left shunt through the foramen ovale. It gradually becomes more severe in older patients with progressive right ventricular failure.

CLINICAL MANIFESTATIONS. A significant percentage of infants present in the first month of life with tachypnea and cyanosis, probably a manifestation of the elevated pulmonary vascular resistance in the neonatal period. About one-half of patients who are severely symptomatic

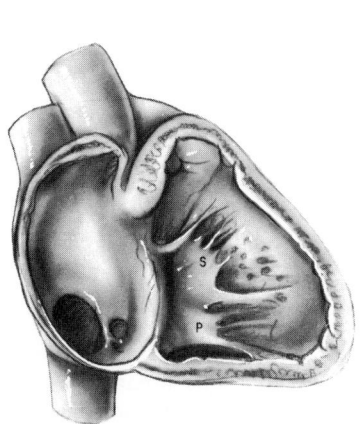
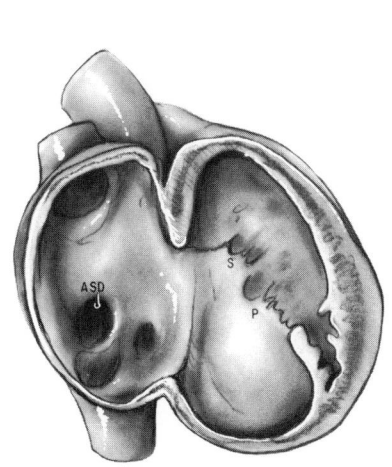
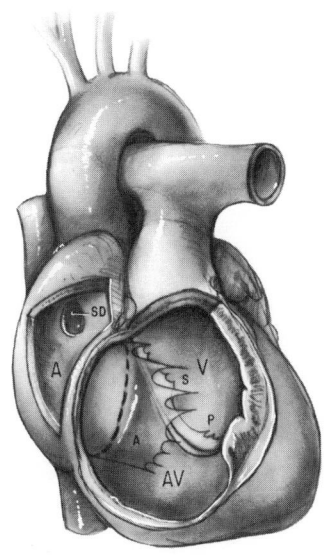

A   *B*   *C*

Fig. 18-54. *A.* Normal heart showing septal and posterior leaflets of tricuspid valve. *B.* Pathologic anatomy in Ebstein's malformation, with displacement of diminutive septal and posterior leaflets down into normal right ventricular cavity. Large anterior leaflet is not shown. *C.* Abnormal pathologic anatomy in Ebstein's malformation. There is large "sail-like" anterior leaflet with hypoplastic septal and posterior leaflets, which are often displaced downward into ventricle, creating third cardiac chamber interposed between right atrium and functioning right ventricle. (From: *Hardy KL et al: J Thorac Cardiovasc Surg 48:931, 1964, with permission.*)

in the first month of life subsequently die. After the first month, disability decreases, often with loss of cyanosis, so disability during childhood is often small. A mortality of about 15 percent has been estimated to occur between ages one and twenty. The course is a gradual one, so that the average age of diagnosis is in the midteens.

Many adults continue to function reasonably well, depending upon the presence of arrhythmias, cyanosis, and cardiac failure. A few patients have lived to beyond seventy years of age, but only about 5 percent of all patients live beyond fifty years.

DIAGNOSTIC CONSIDERATIONS. A variety of systolic and diastolic murmurs are present, though Nadas at one time stated that auscultatory findings were highly suggestive, emphasizing a slow cardiac rate with a triple or quadruple rhythm, a systolic murmur of tricuspid regurgitation, and often a low-pitched diastolic murmur.

The chest x-ray may show grotesque cardiac enlargement because of the huge right atrium and the atrialized right ventricle. Vascularity in the lung fields is usually decreased. Electrocardiographic abnormalities are considered typical with conduction disturbances, a prolonged PR interval, and partial right bundle branch block.

2-D echocardiography is virtually diagnostic, outlining the different abnormalities with surprising precision. Cardiac catheterization should be done carefully, for fatal arrhythmias have occurred. A right-to-left shunt at the atrial level with arterial hypoxemia is found in 25 to 50 percent of patients. The angiocardiogram is usually diagnostic.

TREATMENT. Only limited data are available because surgical treatment has only been used frequently in the past decade. Early corrective operations included prosthetic valve replacement by Barnard, and subsequently by Lillehei. Hardy reported a successful valvuloplasty in 1964, based upon concepts described by Hunter and Lillehei. Bahnson in 1965 reported successful reconstructive operations in two patients.

The best results have been reported by Danielson at the Mayo Clinic, who described in a 1985 report a total experience with 72 patients. Surgical intervention was recommended for all patients at a class III status, or in those with a cardiothoracic ratio enlarging beyond 0.65. In 81 percent of the group reconstruction of the tricuspid valve was possible, converting the valve to a monocusp valve with the functioning anterior leaflet. Prosthetic valve replacement was used in most of the other patients. There were five hospital and three late deaths. The 39 surviving operated patients were 87 percent class I or II at 5 years.

A different approach has been followed by Kirklin and Barratt-Boyes, employing valve replacement in 20 patients operated upon with an overall mortality of 20 percent. The editor feels the data of Danielson are quite convincing and would favor attempted valvuloplasty in the majority of patients operated upon.

At the time of operation the atrial septal defect is closed. Plication of the atrialized ventricle seems unnecessary in the vast majority of patients, employed only when the atrialized segment is clearly extremely thin and contracting paradoxically.

Amomalies of the Coronary Arteries

ANOMALOUS ORIGIN OF THE LEFT CORONARY ARTERY FROM PULMONARY ARTERY

This is a rare malformation, occurring about once in 300,000 live births and representing about 0.25 percent of patients with congenital heart disease. The clinical fea-

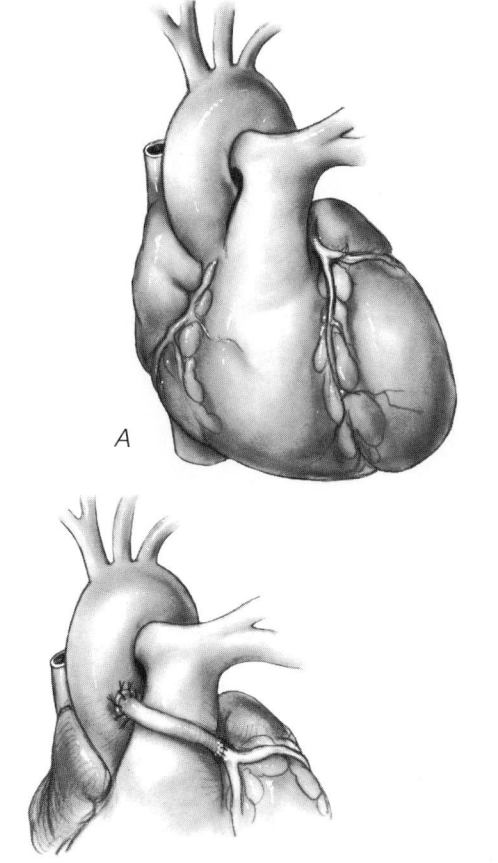

Fig. 18-55. *A.* Anomalous left coronary artery arising from pulmonary artery. *B.* Vein graft used to anastomose coronary artery to aorta. A graft of subclavian artery is preferable. (From: *Cooley DA et al: J Thorac Cardiovasc Surg 52:805, 1966, with permission.*)

tures were well described by Bland and associates in 1933, emphasizing the similarity of the syndrome to myocardial infarction in adults. A particularly significant contribution was made by Sabiston in 1959, conclusively demonstrating that the flow of blood in the anomalous left coronary artery was *retrograde* into the pulmonary artery. Ligation of the anomalous artery was subsequently performed. Reconstruction was first accomplished by Cooley by detaching the coronary artery and connecting it to the aorta with a saphenous vein graft (Fig. 18-55). Unfortunately, the vein graft in a few years became stenotic, so this is no longer considered a satisfactory operation.

PATHOLOGIC ANATOMY AND PHYSIOLOGY. The disability is a severe one, for myocardial infarction and left ventricular failure are commonly present within 3 months after birth. Only about 10 to 20 percent of untreated infants live more than 1 year, apparently because of abundant collateral circulation from the right coronary artery. Symptoms, if present, are usually mild for the first few weeks after birth, probably because of the elevated pulmonary vascular resistance in the neonatal period. Subsequently, symptoms progress with great rapidity. The classic symptom is poor feeding, as attempted feeding produces severe distress. Signs of myocardial infarction or left ventricular failure are soon evident. Initially, only acute episodes occur with feeding, between which the infant may appear normal. During the acute episodes, there is apparently colicky pain, with tachypnea, cyanosis, pallor and sweating, probably angina pectoris, and progressive malnutrition. Subsequently, with chronic congestive failure, tachypnea becomes chronic. On physical examination there may be obvious cardiac enlargement with muffled heart sounds; no characteristic murmurs are found.

The chest x-ray may show extensive enlargement of the left ventricle with pulmonary congestion. Often the electrocardiogram is diagnostic with inverted T waves and prominent Q waves. 2-D echocardiography may confirm the diagnosis, demonstrating absence of the normal origin of the left coronary artery from the aorta, and at times actually demonstrating the anomalous origin from the pulmonary artery. Cardiac catheterization and angiography are diagnostic, demonstrating the abnormal origin of the left coronary artery and a small left-to-right shunt at the level of the pulmonary artery. When coronary angiograms are performed in older children, the right coronary is found dilated and tortous with dye filling the right coronary and subsequently opacifying the left coronary with retrograde flow into the pulmonary artery.

TREATMENT. Operation should be performed in symptomatic infants to prevent progressive myocardial infarction and death. Though reattachment of the coronary artery to the aorta is clearly the ideal operation, data do not clearly indicate better results with reconstruction as compared with simple ligation and interruption of retrograde flow. A mortality near 50 percent unfortunately is common. The ingenious tunnel operation of Takauchi is probably the preferred method of reconstruction, creating an intrapulmonary tunnel to connect the anomalous left coronary ostium to the aorta. If the abnormal anatomy is favorable, the left coronary may be detached from the pulmonary artery and anastomosed directly to the aorta as in the "arterial switch" operation for transposition. In older children a free graft of subclavian artery has been successfully used by several surgeons. A subclavian coronary artery bypass has been successfully performed in a few patients, though simpler techniques of reconstruction are probably preferable in the older patients in whom this type of bypass may be feasible.

In patients operated upon after one year of age, mortality is low and results excellent. The 18 long-term survivors reported by Kirklin were stated to be in excellent condition. Arciniegas reported experiences with 12 patients with only two deaths, but six seriously ill infants were not operated upon, all of whom died. If these six preoperative deaths are included, the total mortality is 40 percent among 20 patients, similar to that reported by other groups.

CORONARY ARTERIOVENOUS FISTULA

Familiarity with this unusual condition grew rapidly with the advent of cardiac angiography and open heart

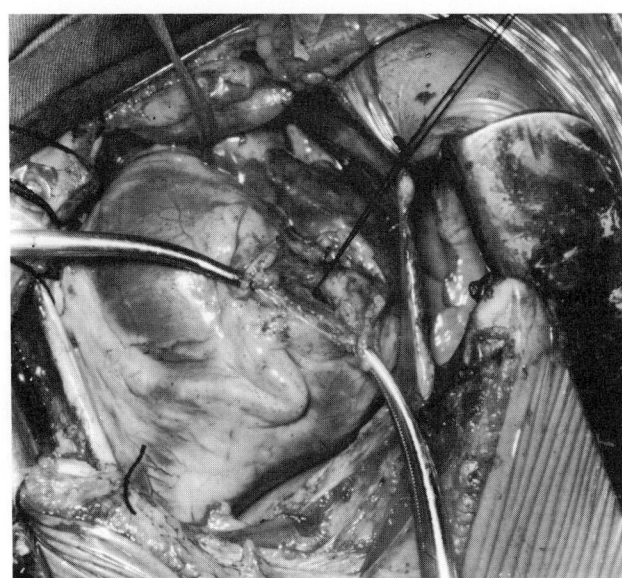

Fig. 18-56. Arteriovenous fistula of right coronary artery. Enlarged, tortuous right coronary artery is clearly visible over surface of right ventricle. Fistulous communication directly into right ventricle was found, as illustrated by ligatures, and ligated.

surgery. In 1960 Gasul found 52 cases in a collective review. At this time well over 300 surgical cases have been reported in the literature; and undoubtedly a much larger number have never been reported.

PATHOLOGIC ANATOMY AND PHYSIOLOGY. The right coronary is involved in about half of the cases, the left coronary in about a third, and both coronaries in only about 5 percent. The artery involved is usually a normal artery with a normal branching pattern. The fistula may be a "side-to-side" one with continuity of the vessel beyond the fistula, or "an end fistula" occurring where the vessel terminates. Over 90 percent of fistulas open into the right heart chambers or its connecting vessels, approximately 25 percent in the right atrium, 40 percent in the right ventricle, 15 to 20 percent in the pulmonary artery, and about 7 percent in the coronary sinus. Fistulas entering the left heart, left ventricle, or left atrium are uncommon. Usually a single fistulous opening is present, in the range of 2 to 5 mm. Rarely there are several openings or a localized angiomatous network. The involved coronary artery is dilated and elongated, at times growing to grotesque serpentine proportions. Actual rupture of an aneurysm, however, is rare (Fig. 18-56).

With fistulas entering the right heart, the resulting shunt is usually small. Only rarely is pulmonary blood flow increased to twice that of systemic flow. As with arteriovenous fistula elsewhere, the usual course is slow but progressive enlargement over decades so the volume of the shunt gradually increases with time.

Bacterial endocarditis may develop in a small percentage of cases, about 5 percent.

CLINICAL FEATURES. The majority of patients are asymptomatic, often evaluated because of the discovery of a continuous murmur. One report found that 80 percent of patients under twenty years of age were asymptomatic, decreasing to less than 50 percent in adults. Rarely, with huge fistulas, symptoms have appeared in the first year of life but are virtually unknown after that during childhood.

In adults the most common symptoms are dyspnea and fatigue from the left-to-right shunt. True angina occurs, probably a "coronary steal," in less than 10 percent. Eventually, congestive heart failure develops in 10 to 15 percent of patients, usually in older life as the shunt gradually enlarges in size.

The distinctive physical finding is a continuous murmur in a location that is unusual for a patent ductus arteriosus. The exact side of maximum intensity of the murmur varies with the cardiac chamber involved, whether it be right atrium, right ventricle, or pulmonary artery. The chest x-ray is either normal or shows slight enlargement with congestion of the lung fields from an increase in pulmonary blood flow. Changes in the electrocardiogram are usually minimal. Echocardiography may outline the dilated tortuous coronary artery. Cardiac catheterization and angiography readily establish the diagnosis and delineate the site of the fistula.

TREATMENT. As most patients are asymptomatic, small fistulas can probably be safely observed. Larger fistulas, however, should certainly be closed because the well-documented course is that of gradual enlargement with increasing disability, similar to that of a small atrial septal defect. The author has treated one patient over fifty years of age with congestive heart failure who subsequently remained in good condition over the next decade.

The present safety of cardiopulmonary bypass indicates that most procedures should either be performed with bypass or with bypass available if the location of the fistula precludes simple treatment without bypass. The fistula may be closed by opening the involved cardiac chamber and suturing the intracardiac communication, or with large fistulas by opening the coronary artery and suturing the opening directly. Preservation of distal coronary flow should be achievable in most patients as opposed to ligation. End fistulas, of course, can simply be treated by ligation.

Fistulas have been treated by placing multiple sutures

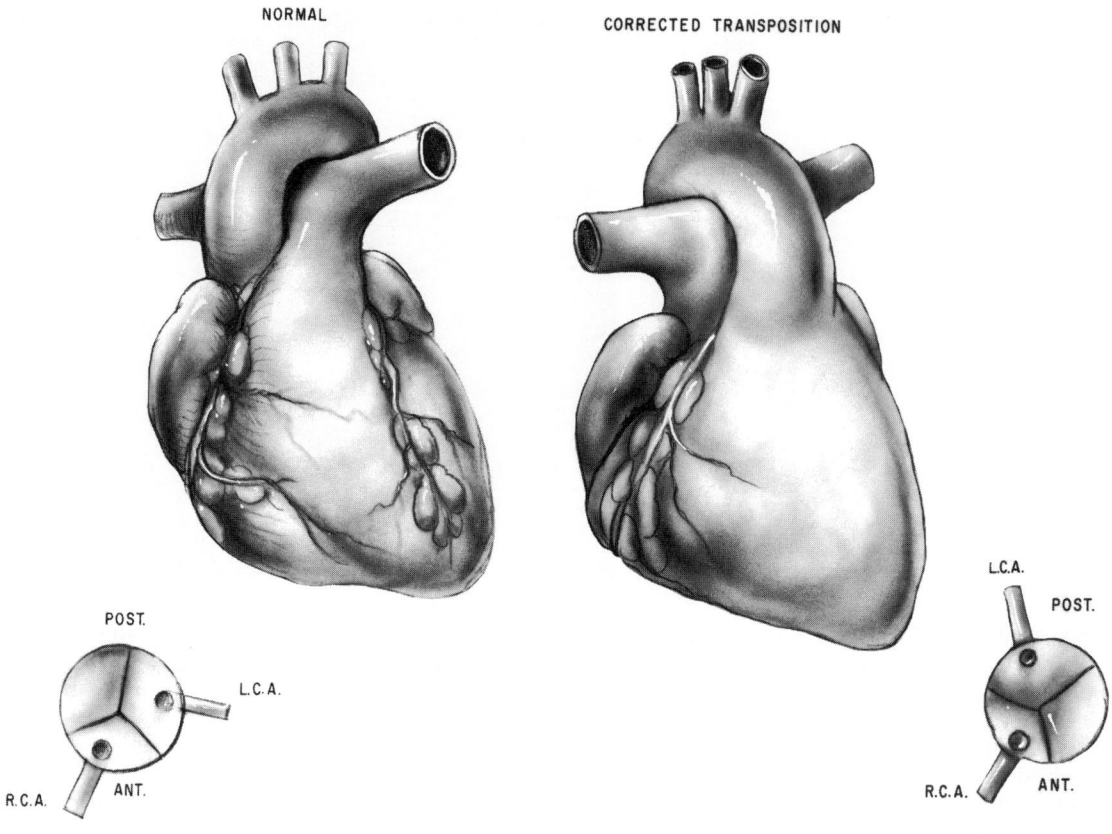

NORMAL   CORRECTED TRANSPOSITION

A   *B*

Fig. 18-57. *A.* Normal cardiac anatomy with pulmonary artery arising from right ventricle and aorta from left ventricle. Comparison
with *B* shows that in corrected transposition, relative positions of
aorta and pulmonary artery are reversed. *B.* In corrected transposition of great vessels, aorta arises anteriorly from ventricle that has
anatomic characteristics of right ventricle. Pulmonary artery arises
posteriorly and to right of aorta—reverse of normal anatomic arrangement. Insert depicts origin of coronary arteries in corrected
transposition. (From: *Nadas AS: Pediatric Cardiology. Philadelphia,
Saunders, 1964, p 714, with permission.*)

beneath the involved artery to obliterate the opening
without precisely identifying it. Recurrences have been
described, however, so this would seem to be a less desirable form of treatment.

In 1981, Lowe reported experiences with 28 patients.
An additional 258 patients were reported by others. Operation was strongly recommended for there were no operative or late deaths and no recurrent fistulas over a period
of 10 years. Urrutia reported experiences with 58 patients
seen. There were no operative deaths in patients with isolated fistulas.

Corrected Transposition

The basic characteristics of this unusual malformation
were described by Anderson in 1957 with additional contributions by Schiebler in 1961.

PATHOLOGIC ANATOMY AND PHYSIOLOGY. In this malformation the aorta and pulmonary artery are transposed
to lie in a position exactly opposite of that normally occurring. The aorta arises from the anterior left border of
the heart and the pulmonary artery from the right posterior area of the heart (Fig. 18-57). The ventricle from
which the aorta arises is the morphologic right ventricle
while that from which the pulmonary artery arises is the
morphologic left ventricle. The atria and ventricle are
also discordant; so blood from a morphologic right atrium
reaches the pulmonary trunk by traversing a mitral valve

and a morphologic left ventricle, while blood from a morphologic left atrium reaches the aorta by traversing a tricuspid valve and a morphologic right ventricle. Hence,
with the "double discordance" the basic circulation is
normal. The anatomic relations of the coronary arteries
are also altered with the right coronary artery arising anteriorly, the left coronary posteriorly, and the noncoronary sinus being located at the anterior left border of the
heart.

The defect apparently arises from a malrotation of the
embryonic heart tube, which bends to the left (L-ventric-
ular loop). The significance of the malformation is primarily from the high incidence of associated abnormalities,
for it has been estimated that only 1 to 2 percent of patients do not have an additional malformation. Four separate malformations commonly occur. The most frequent
is a disturbance in conduction between the atrium and
ventricle, originating from lack of normal continuity from

the AV node to the ventricular septum. Normal AV conduction is present in less than one-half of patients.

A ventricular septal defect is present in the majority of patients, at least 80 percent. Some degree of pulmonic stenosis frequently occurs, which in some patients is of such severity that shunting must be performed in infancy. The fourth malformation, mitral insufficiency, gradually develops in older patients, perhaps a consequence of a tricuspid valve draining into the ventricle from which systemic pressure is generated.

A theoretical question arises from the altered physiology in this condition about whether a morphologic right ventricle can function for a normal lifespan. There are no significant data to indicate that this cannot occur, a particularly important long-term question for patients with transposition surgically corrected by the Senning or Mustard procedures. Most patients die before 50 years of age, usually from complications of the associated anomalies. Only one patient is known to have survived to age seventy-three.

CLINICAL MANIFESTATIONS. Conduction defects may cause problems in infancy as 5 to 10 percent of patients are born with a complete heart block, and subsequently heart block appears in about 2 percent of patients each year, with about 30 percent of patients eventually developing complete block.

Even though a large ventricular septal defect is present, some restriction to pulmonary flow commonly occurs so patients do not develop difficulty as rapidly as those with an uncomplicated large ventricular septal defect. Eventually severe pulmonary vascular disease develops unless significant pulmonic stenosis is present. In about one-third of patients the pulmonic stenosis is of such severity that a shunt must be surgically corrected in infancy or early childhood.

Physical examination is not diagnostic, though such patients have an unusually loud second sound to the left of the sternum, arising from the aortic valve. The chest x-ray characteristically has a narrow "waist" because of the abnormal location of the great arteries.

The electrocardiogram is almost always abnormal, often the first clue to the diagnosis. Characteristic abnormalities include the conduction disturbances and the unusual patterns of ventricular hypertrophy.

Echocardiography is usually diagnostic, but cardiac catheterization and angiography are routinely done to confirm the diagnosis and delineate the severity of associated abnormalities.

TREATMENT. Closure of the ventricular septal defect is technically difficult because a ventriculotomy through the anterior ventricle would injure the ventricle with systemic pressure. The preferred atrial approach is the transvalvular one through the atrium, incising the mitral valve leaflet for exposure if necessary. Heart block frequently occurs after operation, with a frequency of at least 10 to 20 percent. This is partly related to the abnormal location of the conduction bundle, located in the anterior rim of the ventricular septal defect. Pulmonic stenosis, when severe, is best corrected with an extracardiac conduit placed to the pulmonary trunk because the pathologic anatomy precludes an incision across the stenotic pulmonic valve.

The combined series reported in the Kirklin/Barratt-Boyes book total almost 100 patients with an operative mortality between 10 and 15 percent and a 10-year survival between 50 and 75 percent. Less favorable long-term results were reported by Metcalfe. Experiences with 19 patients treated over a decade included a high operative mortality, 37 percent, with only one patient asymptomatic 40 months following operation.

Theoretically, patients could get an excellent result if the ventricular septal defect is corrected before the development of severe pulmonary vascular disease, and conduction problems could be adequately treated with modern pacemakers.

Double Outlet Right Ventricle

This is a congenital malformation in which both great arteries are related to the morphologic right ventricle. It occurs in about 5 percent of all cases of congenital heart disease. Before open heart surgery became possible in 1954–1955, a few cases were reported, but modern knowledge of the condition emerged from surgical observations by Kirklin who, in 1957, first recognized the anatomic problem in the operating room and performed a surgical correction by creation of an intraventricular tunnel, similar to the treatment done today. The term double outlet right ventricle became established as the appropriate designation following a publication by Witham at that time. There are numerous subclassifications of this condition that are beyond the scope of this discussion.

Briefly, four types of relationships of the great arteries at the level of the semilunar valves have been described in this condition, varying with the relationship of the aorta to the pulmonary artery.

In addition, four separate anatomic locations of the ventricular septal defect have been described: subaortic, subpulmonic, beneath both great arteries ("doubly committed"), or beneath neither ("uncommitted"). Theoretically, the existence of two groups of four each creates 16 possible combinations of double outlet right ventricle. At one extreme the condition is that of classic transposition of the great vessels, while at another extreme the condition merges with tetralogy of Fallot. The classic case report by Taussig and Bing in 1949, leading to the eponym Taussig-Bing syndrome, described a double outlet right ventricle with a subpulmonic ventricular septal defect, occurring in about 8 percent of cases.

Clinically, three characteristic types of disability occur. With simply a large ventricular septal defect, the presentation is almost identical to that of a large ventricular septal defect. A high pulmonary vascular resistance develops in infancy with great rapidity. The second familiar clinical syndrome, pulmonic stenosis with a subaortic defect, is virtually identical to that of tetralogy of Fallot. A third variant is the Taussig-Bing, resembling classic transposition with severe disability in infancy from the combination of pulmonary congestion and hypoxemia.

Echocardiography can usually suggest the diagnosis, but precise biplane angiography is necessary for confirmation and delineation of exact details. With modern surgical techniques, most conditions can be corrected satis-

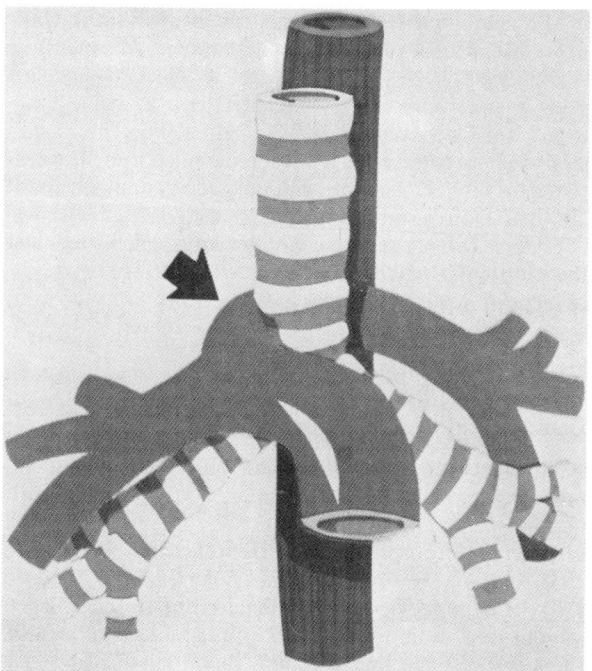

Fig. 18-58. Diagram of anomalous origin of left pulmonary artery from right pulmonary artery. Anatomic relationship of left pulmonary artery to trachea and esophagus is also shown. (From: *Grover FL et al: J Thorac Cardiovasc Surg 69:295, 1975, with permission.*)

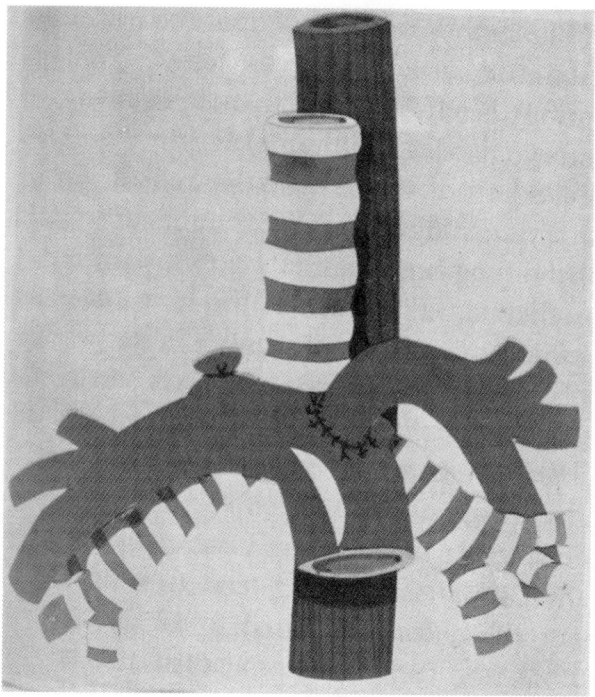

Fig. 18-59. Diagram of anatomy at completion of operation. Note that proximal stump of left pulmonary artery is to right of trachea after having been dissected free. Distal left pulmonary artery has been anastomosed to side of main pulmonary artery. (From: *Grover FL et al: J Thorac Cardiovasc Surg 69:295, 1975, with permission.*)

factorily with a precisely constructed intracardiac tunnel to channel blood from the left ventricle through the defect to the aorta. Excellent illustrations of the technique are present in the recent textbook by Kirklin and Barratt-Boyes.

In the Kirklin/Barratt-Boyes book, the combined experiences by the authors over a period of 15 years include 98 patients with an overall operative mortality of 30 percent. With the common simpler form, that with a subaortic VSD with or without pulmonic stenosis, operative mortality is now less than 10 percent.

Pulmonary Artery Sling

Vascular sling is a rare congenital malformation in which the left pulmonary artery arises from the right pulmonary artery and courses to the left between the trachea and esophagus to reach the left lung hilus, thus forming a sling around the trachea (Fig. 18-58). The term originated from a publication by Contro in 1958. Although the first patient was treated surgically by Potts in 1954, total reported surgical experience remains small. A review of Grover in 1975 described experiences with one patient and found a total of 63 patients reported by others. Twenty of 23 unoperated patients died.

The trachea is often narrowed at the site of compression and, in some patients, significant tracheal stenosis is present with complete cartilagenous rings. Other cardiac anomalies are present in nearly one-half of reported patients.

CLINICAL MANIFESTATIONS. Apparently, most infants develop symptoms in the first few months of life, with wheezing, stridor, and choking. The diagnosis may be suspected from abnormalities visible on the chest x-ray, with a density separating the trachea from the esophagus on the lateral view. An esophageal barium swallow is usually diagnostic, showing anterior indentation of the esophagus just above the carina. A tracheogram and bronchoscopy should routinely be performed to evaluate the severity of associated tracheal malformations, one of the most important determinants of postoperative prognosis. A computerized tomogram will also confirm the diagnosis. Catheterization and angiography are routinely performed to confirm the diagnosis and detect additional anomalies.

The major decision before operation is evaluating the extent of inherent diseases in the trachea. Some infants with tracheal stenoses have ultimately died despite division of the sling and attempted correction of the tracheal malformation. Older patients are occasionally seen with minimal or no symptoms. Such patients often require no specific treatment.

TREATMENT. The operative procedure (Fig. 18-59) is a simple one, dividing the anomalous pulmonary artery at its origin, bringing it from behind the trachea and reanastomosing it to the main pulmonary artery. The ligamentum arteriosum is divided at this time. This has been done through a left lateral thoracotomy and also through a median sternotomy.

The prognosis following operation is determined principally by the inherent disease present in the trachea. Five patients were recorded by Kirklin/Barratt-Boyes, three of whom died after operation while the other two remain asymptomatic. Occlusion of the pulmonary artery has been subsequently found in some patients, probably a reflection of the technique of vascular anastomosis. Campbell, in 1983, reported two patients with good surgical results operating through a median sternotomy and also performing an "aortopexy" to minimize postoperative tracheal compression.

Bibliography

General

Abbott ME: *Atlas of Congenital Cardiac Disease.* New York, The American Heart Association, 1936.

Pulmonic Stenosis

Blalock A, Kiefer RF Jr: Valvulotomy for the relief of congenital valvular pulmonary stenosis with intact ventricular septum. Report of 19 operations by the Rock method. *Ann Surg* 32:496, 1950.

Brock RC: Pulmonary valvulotomy for the relief of congenital stenosis: Report of three cases. *Br Med J* 1:112, 1948.

Coles JG, Freedom RM, et al: Surgical management of critical pulmonary stenosis in the neonate. *Ann Thorac Surg* 38:458, 1984.

Griffith B, Hardesty R, et al: Pulmonary valvulotomy alone for pulmonary stenosis: Results in children with and without muscular infundibular hypertrophy. *J Thorac Cardiovasc Surg* 83:577, 1982.

Jonas RA, Castaneda AR, et al: Pulmonary valvulotomy under normothermic caval inflow occlusion. *Aust NZ J Surg* 55:39, 1985.

Sellors TH: Surgery of pulmonic stenosis. *Lancet* 1:988, 1948.

Srinivasan V, Konyer A, et al: Critical pulmonary stenosis in infants less than three months of age: A reappraisal of closed transventricular pulmonary valvotomy. *Ann Thorac Surg* 34:46, 1982.

Sullivan ID, Robinson PJ, et al: Percutaneous balloon valvuloplasty for pulmonary valve stenosis in infants and children. *Br Heart J* 54:435, 1985.

Congenital Aortic Stenosis

Brown J, Stevens L: Surgery for discrete subvalvular aortic stenosis: Actuarial survival, hemodynamic results, and acquired aortic regurgitation. *Ann Thorac Surg* 40:151, 1985.

Hsieh KS, Keane JF: Long-term follow-up of valvotomy before 1968 for congenital aortic stenosis. *Am J Cardiol* 58:338, 1986.

Hunta JC, Carpenter RJ Jr: Prenatal diagnosis and postnatal management of critical aortic stenosis. *Circulation* 75:573, 1987.

Konno S, Imai Y, et al: New method for prosthetic valve replacement in congenital aortic stenosis associated with hypoplasia of the aortic valve ring. *J Thorac Cardiovasc Surg* 70:909, 1975.

Messina LM, Turley K, et al: Successful aortic valvotomy for severe congenital valvular aortic stenosis in the newborn infant. *J Thorac Cardiovasc Surg* 88:92, 1984.

Misbach G, Turley K, et al: Left ventricular outflow enlargement using the Konno procedure. Paper presented at the American Association for Thoracic Surgery, Phoenix, Arizona, 1982.

Supravalvular Aortic Stenosis

Bernhard WF, Poirier V, LaFarge CG: Relief of congenital obstruction to left ventricular outflow with ventricular-aortic prosthesis. *J Thorac Cardiovasc Surg* 20:136, 1975.

Keane JF, Fellows KE, et al: The surgical management of discrete and diffuse supravalvular aortic stenosis. *Circulation* 54:112, 1976.

Peterson TA, Todd DC, Edwards JE: Supravalvular aortic stenosis. *J Thorac Cardiovasc Surg* 50:734, 1965.

Rastelli GC, McGoon DC, et al: Surgical treatment of supravalvular aortic stenosis: Report of 16 cases and review of literature. *J Thorac Cardiovasc Surg* 51:873, 1966.

Idiopathic Hypertrophic Subaortic Stenosis

Frye RL, Kincaid OW, et al: Results of surgical treatment of patients with diffuse subvalvular aortic stenosis. *Circulation* 32:52, 1965.

Kelly DT, Barratt-Boyes BG, Lowe JB: Results of surgery and hemodynamic observations in muscular subaortic stenosis. *J Thorac Cardiovasc Surg* 51:353, 1966.

Koch J, Maron H, et al: Results of operation for obstructive hypertrophic cardiomyopathy in the elderly. Septal myotomy and myectomy in 20 patients 65 years of age or older. *Am J Cardiol* 46:963, 1980.

Morrow A: Hypertrophic subaortic stenosis. Operative methods utilized to relieve left ventricular outflow obstruction. *J Thorac Cardiovasc Surg* 76:423, 1978.

Coarctation of the Aorta

Abbott ME: Coarctation of the aorta of the adult type: II. A statistical study and historical retrospect of 200 recorded cases, with autopsy, of stenosis or obliteration of the descending arch in subjects above the age of two years. *Am Heart J* 3:392, 1928.

Brewer LA III, Fosburg RG, et al: Spinal cord complications following surgery for coarctation of the aorta: A study of 66 cases. *J Thorac Cardiovasc Surg* 64:368, 1972.

Brom AG: Narrowing of the aortic isthmus and enlargement of the mind. *J Thorac Cardiovasc Surg* 50:166, 1965.

Campbell DB, Waldhausen JA, et al: Should elective repair of coarctation of the aorta be done in infancy? *J Thorac Cardiovasc Surg* 88:929, 1984.

Crafoord C, Nylin G: Congenital coarctation of the aorta and its surgical treatment. *J Thorac Surg* 14:347, 1945.

Fishman NH, Bronstein MH, et al: Surgical management of severe aortic coarctation and interrupted aortic arch in neonates. *J Thorac Cardiovasc Surg* 71:35, 1976.

Hehrlein FW et al: Instance and pathogenesis of late aneurysms after patch graft aortoplasty for coarctation. *J Thorac Cardiovasc Surg* 92:226, 1986.

Kirklin JW, Barratt-Boyes BG: *Cardiac Surgery.* Wiley, New York, 1986.

Krieger KH, Spencer FC: Is paraplegia after repair of coarctation of the aorta due principally to distal hypotension during aortic cross-clamping? *Surgery* 97:2, 1985.

Lerberg D, Hardesty R, et al: Coarctation of the aorta in infants and children: 25 years of experience. *Ann Thorac Surg* 33:159, 1982.

Perloff JK: *The Clinical Recognition of Congenital Heart Disease,* 3d ed. Philadelphia, Saunders, 1987.

Schuster SR, Gross RE: Surgery for coarctation of the aorta: A review of 500 cases. *J Thorac Cardiovasc Surg* 43:54, 1962.

Sealy WC, Harris JS, et al: Paradoxical hypertension following resection of coarctation of the aorta. *Surgery* 42:135, 1957.

Waldhausen J, Nahrwold D: Repair of coarctation of the aorta with a subclavian flap. *J Thorac Cardiovasc Surg* 51:532, 1966.

Yee ES, Soifer SJ, et al: Infant coarctation: A spectrum in clinical presentation and treatment. *Ann Thorac Surg* 42:488, November 1986.

Vascular Rings

Arciniegas E, Hakimi M, et al: Surgical management of congenital vascular rings. *J Thorac Cardiovasc Surg* 77:721, 1979.

Bertrand JM, Chartrand C, et al: Vascular ring: Clinical and physiological assessment of pulmonary function following surgical correction. *Pediatr Pul* 2:378, 1986.

Gross RE: Arterial malformations which cause compression of the trachea or esophagus. *Circulation* 11:124, 1955.

Idbeis B, Levinsky L, et al: Vascular rings: Management and a proposed nomenclature. *Ann Thorac Surg* 31:255, 1981.

Mahoney EB, Manning JA: Congenital abnormalities of the aortic arch. *Surgery* 55:1, 1964.

Roessler M, DeLeval M: Surgical management of vascular ring. *Ann Surg* 197:139, 1983.

Atrial Septal Defects: Secundum Defects

Freed MD, Nasas AS, et al: Is routine preoperative cardiac catheterization necessary before repair of secundum and sinus venosus atrial septal defects? *J Am Coll Cardiol* 4:333, 1984.

Paolillo V, Dawkins KD, Miller GA: Atrial septal defect in patients over the age of fifty. *Int J Cardiol* 9:139, 1985.

Sellers RD, Ferlic RM, et al: Secundum type atrial septal defects: Results with 275 patients. *Surgery* 59:155, 1966.

Sutton M, Tajik A, McGoon D: Atrial septal defect in patients 60 years or older: Operative results and long-term postoperative follow-up. *Circulation* 64:402, 1981.

Trusler G, Kazenelson G, et al: Late results following repair of partial anomalous pulmonary venous connection with sinus venosus atrial septal defect. *J Thorac Cardiovasc Surg* 79:776, 1980.

Anomalous Drainage of Pulmonary Veins

Bahnson HT, Spencer FC, Neill CA: Surgical treatment of 35 cases of drainage of pulmonary veins to the right side of the heart. *J Thorac Cardiovasc Surg* 36:777, 1958.

Blake HA, Hall RC, Manion WC: Anomalous pulmonary venous return. *Circulation* 32:406, 1965.

Brody H: Drainage of the pulmonary veins into the right side of the heart. *Arch Pathol* 33:221, 1942.

Turley K, Wilson J, Ebert P: Atrial repairs of infant complex congenital heart lesions. Emphasis on the first three months of life. *Arch Surg* 115:1335, 1980.

Ostium Primum Defect and Persistent Atrioventricular Canal

Berger T, Blackstone E, et al: Survival and probability of cure without and with operation in complete atrioventricular canal. *Ann Thorac Surg* 27:106, 1979.

Goldfaden D, Jones M, Morrow A: Long-term results of repair of incomplete persistent atrioventricular canal. *J Thorac Cardiovasc Surg* 82:669, 1981.

McGoon D, Puga F: Atrioventricular canal. *Cardiovasc Clin* 11:311, 1981.

McMullan MH, McGoon DC, et al: Surgical treatment of partial atrioventricular canal. *Arch Surg* 107:705, 1973.

Neill CA: Postoperative hemolytic anemia in endocardial cushion defects. *Circulation* 30:801, 1964.

Ventricular Septal Defect

Barratt-Boyes BG, Neutze JM, et al: Repair of ventricular septal defect in the first two years of life using profound hypothermia–circulatory arrest technics. *Ann Surg* 184:376, 1976.

Mattila S, Kostiainen S, et al: Repair of ventricular septal defect in adults. *Scan J Thorac Cardiovasc Surg* 19:29, 1985.

Otterstad JE, Erikssen J, et al: Long term results after operative treatment of isolated ventricular septal defect in adolescents and adults. *Acta Med Scan* 708(suppl):1, 1986.

Richardson J, Schieken R, et al: Repair of large ventricular septal defects in infants and small children. *Ann Surg* 195:318, 1982.

Rizzoli G, Blackstone E, et al: Incremental risk factors in hospital mortality rate after repair of ventricular septal defect. *J Thorac Cardiovasc Surg* 80:494, 1980.

Spencer FC, Doyle EF, et al: Longterm evaluation of aortic valvuloplasty for aortic insufficiency and ventricular septal defect. *J Thorac Cardiovasc Surg* 65:15, 1973.

Walker WJ, Garcia-Gonzalez E, et al: Interventricular septal defect: Analysis of 415 catheterized cases. *Circulation* 31:54, 1965.

Wood P: The Eisenmenger syndrome. *Br Med J* 2:701, 1958.

Yeager SB, Freed MD, et al: Primary surgical closure of ventricular septal defect in the first year of life: Results in 128 infants. *J Am Coll Cardiol* 3:1269, May 1984.

Patent Ductus Arteriosus

Blalock A: Operative closure of the patent ductus arteriosus. *Surg Gynecol Obstet* 82:113, 1946.

Gersony WM, Peckham GJ, et al: Effects of indomethacin in premature infants with patent ductus arteriosus: Results of a national collaborative study. *J Pediatr* 102:895, 1983.

Gold JP, Cohn LH: Operative management of the calcified patent ductus arteriosus. *Ann Thorac Surg* 41:567, 1986.

Gross RE, Hubbard JP: Surgical ligation of a patent ductus arteriosus: Report of first successful case. *JAMA* 112:729, 1939.

Jones JC: Twenty-five years experience with the surgery of patent ductus arteriosus. *J Thorac Cardiovasc Surg* 50:149, 1965.

Kitterman J: Patent ductus arteriosus: Current clinical status. *Arch Dis Child* 55:106, 1980.

Kron IL, Harman PK, et al: The adult ductus surgical results and longterm follow-up. *Am Surg* 49:546, 1983.

Mikhail M, Lee W, et al: Surgical and medical experience with 734 premature infants with patent ductus arteriosus. *J Thorac Cardiovasc Surg* 83:349, 1982.

Tetralogy of Fallot

Ebert PA: Second operation for pulmonary stenosis or insufficiency after repair of tetralogy of Fallot. *Am J Cardiol* 50:637, 1982.

Hammon JW, Henry CL, et al: Tetralogy of Fallot: Selected surgical management can minimize operative mortality. *Ann Thorac Surg* 40:280, 1985.

Kirklin JW, Blackstone E, et al: Risk factors for early and late failure after repair of tetralogy of Fallot and their neutralization. *J Thorac Cardiovasc Surg* 32:208, 1984.

Lillehei CW, Varco RL, et al: The first open heart repairs of ventricular septal defect, atrioventricular communis, and tetralogy of Fallot using extracorporeal circulation by cross-circulation: A 30 year follow-up. *Ann Thorac Surg* 41:421, 1986.

Roh MS, Hardesty R, et al: Blalock shunt: Procedure of choice in infants. *J Cardiovasc Surg* 25:1, 1984.

Transposition of the Great Vessels

Ashraf MM, Cotroneo J, et al: Fate of long-term survivors of Mustard procedure (inflow repair) for simple and complex transposition of the great arteries. *Ann Thorac Surg* 42:385, 1986.

Baffes TG, Riker WL, et al: Surgical correction of transposition of the aorta and the pulmonary artery. *J Thorac Cardiovasc Surg* 34:469, 1957.

Bender H, Graham T, et al: Comparative operative results of the Senning and Mustard procedures for transposition of the great arteries. *Circulation* 62(suppl 1):197, 1980.

Castaneda AR, Norwood WI, et al: Transposition of the great arteries and intact ventricular septum: Anatomical repair in the neonate. *Ann Thorac Surg* 38:438, 1984.

Hanlon CR, Blalock A: Complete transposition of aorta and pulmonary artery: Experimental observations on venous shunts as corrective procedures. *Ann Surg* 127:385, 1948.

Jatene AD, Fontes VF, et al: Successful anatomic correction of transposition of the great vessels: A preliminary report. *Arq Bras Cardiol* 28:461, 1975.

Jatene AD, Fontes VF, et al: Anatomic correction of transposition of the great arteries. *J Thorac Cardiovasc Surg* 83:20, 1982.

Mustard WT, Keith JD, et al: The surgical management of transposition of the great vessels. *J Thorac Cardiovasc Surg* 48:953, 1964.

Piccoli G, Wilkinson J, et al: Appraisal of the Mustard procedure for the physiological correction of "simple" transposition of the great arteries. *J Thorac Cardiovasc Surg* 82:436, 1981.

Quaegebeur JM, Rohmer J, et al: The arterial switch operation. An eight-year experience. *J Thorac Cardiovasc Surg* 92:361, 1986.

Senning A: Surgical correction of transposition of the great vessels. *Surgery* 59:334, 1966.

Stewart S, Alexson C, Manning J: Late results of the Mustard procedure in transposition of the great arteries. *Ann Thorac Surg* 42:419, 1986.

Trusler G, Williams W, et al: Current results with the Mustard operation in isolated transposition of the great arteries. *J Thorac Cardiovasc Surg* 80:381, 1980.

Turley K, Wilson J, Ebert P: Atrial repairs of infant complex congenital heart lesions. *Arch Surg* 115:1335, 1980.

Tricuspid Atresia

Bjork V, Olin C, et al: Right atrial-right ventricular anastomosis for correction of tricuspid atresia. *J Thorac Cardiovasc Surg* 77:452, 1979.

Fontan F, Baudet E: Surgical repair of tricuspid atresia. *Thorax* 26:240, 1971.

Fontan F, Deville C, et al: Repair of tricuspid atresia in 100 patients. *J Thorac Cardiovasc Surg* 85:647, 1983.

Girod DA, Fontan F, et al: Longterm results after the Fontan operation for tricuspid atresia. *Circulation* 75:605, 1987.

Glenn WW: Circulatory bypass with the right side of the heart shunt between superior vena cava and distal right pulmonary artery—Report of clinical application. *N Engl J Med* 259:117, 1958.

Kirklin JK, Blackstone EH, et al: The Fontan operation. *J Thorac Cardiovasc Surg* 92:1049, 1986.

Lee CN, Schaff HB, et al: Comparison of atrial pulmonary vs atrioventricular connections for modified Fontan–Kreutzer repair of tricuspid valve atresia. *J Thorac Cardiovasc Surg* 92:1038, 1986.

Trusler G, Williams G: Long-term results of shunt procedures for tricuspid atresia. *Ann Thorac Surg* 29:312, 1980.

Weinberg P: Anatomy of tricuspid atresia and its relevance to current forms of surgical therapy. *Ann Thorac Surg* 29:306, 1980.

Cor Triatriatum

Arciniegas E, Farooki A, et al: Surgical treatment of cor triatriatum. *Ann Thorac Surg* 32:571, 1981.

Marin-Garcia J, Tandon R, et al: Cor triatriatum: Study of 20 cases. *Am J Cardiol* 35:59, 1975.

Niwayama G: Cor triatriatum. *Am Heart J* 59:291, 1960.

Oglietti J, Cooley DA, et al: Cor triatriatum: Operative results in 25 patients. *Ann Thorac Surg* 35:415, 1983.

Ostman-Smith I, Silverman NH, et al: Cor triatriatum sinistrum: Diagnostic features on cross sectional echocardiography. *Br Heart J* 51:211, 1984.

Van Praagh R, Corsini I: Cor triatriatum: Pathologic anatomy and a consideration of morphogenesis based on 13 postmortem cases and a study of normal development of the pulmonary vein and atrial septum in 83 human embryos. *Am Heart J* 78:379, 1969.

Congenital Mitral Valve Disease

Grenadier E, Sahn DJ, et al: Two-dimensional echo Doppler study of congenital disorders of the mitral valve. *Am Heart J* 107:319, 1984.

Ruckman R, Van Praagh R: Anatomic types of congenital mitral stenosis: Report of 49 autopsy cases with consideration of diagnosis and surgical implications. *Am J Cardiol* 42:592, 1978.

Tsuji HK, Shapiro M, et al: Congenital mitral stenosis: Report of two cases and review of the literature. *J Thorac Cardiovasc Surg* 53:850, 1967.

Vitarelli A, Landolina G, et al: Echocardiographic assessment of congenital mitral stenosis. *Am Heart J* 107:319, 1984.

Aortic-Pulmonary Window

Doty D, Richardson J, et al: Aortopulmonary septal defect: Hemodynamics, angiography, and operation. *Ann Thorac Surg* 32:244, 1981.

Gross RE: Surgical closure of an aortic septal defect. *Circulation* 5:858, 1952.

Jolles PR, Shin MS, Jones WP: Aortopulmonary window lesions: Detection with chest radiography. *Radiology* 159:647, 1986.

Morrow AG, Greenfield LJ, Braunwald E: Congenital aortopulmonary septal defect: Clinical and hemodynamic findings, surgical technique, and results of operative correction. *Circulation* 25:463, 1962.

Scott HW, Sabiston DC: Surgical treatment for congenital aortico-pulmonary fistula. *J Thorac Cardiovasc Surg* 25:26, 1953.

Ruptured Aneurysm of Sinus of Valsalva

Heilman KJ III, Groves BM, et al: Rupture of the left sinus of valsalva aneurysm into the pulmonary artery. *J Am Coll Cardiol* 5:1005, 1985.

Lillehei CW, Stanley P, Varco RL: Surgical treatment of ruptured aneurysms of the sinus of valsalva. *Ann Surg* 146:459, 1957.

Sawyer JL, Adams JE, Scott HW: Surgical treatment for aneurysms of aortic sinuses with aorticoatrial fistula. *Surgery* 41:126, 1957.

Spencer FC, Blake HA, Bahnson HT: Surgical repair of ruptured aneurysm of sinus of valsalva in two patients. *Ann Surg* 162:963, 1960.

Truncus Arteriosus

Ceballos R, Soto B, et al: Truncus arteriosus. An anatomical-angiographic study. *Br Heart J* 49:589, 1983.

DiDonato RM, Fyfe DA, et al: Fifteen-year experience with surgical repair of truncus arteriosus. *J Thorac Cardiovasc Surg* 89:414, 1985.

Ebert PA, Turley K, et al: Surgical treatment of truncus arteriosus in the first 6 months of life. *Ann Surg* 200:451, 1984.

McGoon DC, Wallace RB, Danielson GK: The Rastelli operation: Its indications and results. *J Thorac Cardiovasc Surg* 65:65, 1973.

Rothko K, Moore G, Hutchins G: Truncus arteriosus malformation: A spectrum including fourth and sixth aortic arch interruptions. *Am Heart J* 99:17, 1980.

Sharma AK, Brawn WJ, Mee RB: Truncus arteriosus. Surgical approach. *J Thorac Cardiovasc Surg* 90:45, 1985.

Single Ventricle

Anderson RH, Becker AE, et al: Morphogenesis of univentricular hearts. *Br Heart J* 38:558, 1976.

Anderson RH, Macartney FJ, et al: Univentricular atrioventricular connection: The single ventricle trap unsprung. *Pediatr Cardiol* 4:273, 1983.

Ebert PA: Staged partitioning of single ventricle. *J Thorac Cardiovasc Surg* 88:908, 1984.

Edie RN, Malm JR: Surgical repair of single ventricle. *J Thorac Cardiovasc Surg* 66:350, 1973.

Freedom RM, Benson LN, et al: Subaortic stenosis, the univentricular heart, and banding of the pulmonary artery: An analysis of the courses of 43 patients with univentricular heart palliated by pulmonary artery banding. *Circulation* 73:758, 1986.

McGoon DC, Danielson GK, et al: Correction of the univentricular heart having two atrioventricular valves. *J Thorac Cardiovasc Surg* 74:218, 1977.

Stefanelli G, Kirklin JW, et al: Early and intermediate-term (10 year) results of surgery for univentricular atrioventricular connection ("single ventricle"). *Am J Cardiol* 54:811, 1984.

Van Praagh R, Ongley PA, Swan HJC: Anatomic types of single or common ventricle in man. Morphologic and geometric aspects of 60 necropsied cases. *Am J Cardiol* 13:367, 1964.

Van Praagh R, Van Praagh S, et al: Diagnosis of the anatomic types of single or common ventricle. *Am J Cardiol* 15:345, 1965.

Ebstein's Anomaly

Bahnson HT, Bauersfeld SR, Smith JW: Pathological anatomy and surgical correction of Ebstein's anomaly. *Circulation* 31(suppl 1):3, 1965.

Barbero-Marcial M, Verginelli G, et al: Surgical treatment of Ebstein's anomaly. Early and late results in twenty patients subjected to valve replacement. *J Thorac Cardiovasc Surg* 78:416, 1979.

Hardy, KL, May IA, et al: Ebstein's anomaly: A functional concept and successful definitive repair. *J Thorac Cardiovasc Surg* 48:927, 1964.

Mair DD, Seward JB, et al: Surgical repair of Ebstein's anomaly: Selection of patients and early and late operative results. *Circulation* 72:1170, 1985.

Radford DJ, Graff RF, Neilson GH: Diagnosis and natural history of Ebstein's anomaly. *Br Heart J* 54:517, 1985.

Anomalous Origin of the Left Coronary Artery

Bland EF, White PD, Garland J: Congenital anomalies of the coronary arteries: Report of an unusual case associated with cardiac hypertrophy. *Am Heart J* 787, 1933.

Donaldson RM, Raphael MJ, et al: Hemodynamically significant anomalies of the coronary arteries. Surgical aspects. *Thorac Cardiovasc Surg* 30:7, 1982.

Sabiston DC, Neill CA, Taussig HB: The direction of blood flow in anomalous left coronary artery arising from the pulmonary artery. *Circulation* 22:591, 1960.

Takauchi S, Imamura H, et al: New surgical methods for repair of anomalous left coronary artery from the pulmonary artery. *J Thorac Cardiovasc Surg* 78:7, 1979.

Vesterlund T, Thomsen PE, Hansen OK: Anomalous origin of the left coronary artery from the pulmonary artery in an adult. *Br Heart J* 54:110, 1985.

Coronary Arteriovenous Fistula

Gasul BM, Arcilla RA, et al: Congenital coronary arteriovenous fistula: Clinical, phonocardiographic, angiocardiographic, and hemodynamic studies in five patients. *Pediatrics* 25:531, 1960.

Lowe E, Oldham H, Sabiston D: Surgical management of congenital coronary artery fistulas. *Ann Surg* 194:373, 1981.

Lowe J, Oldham HN Jr, Sabiston DC Jr: Surgical management of congenital coronary artery fistulas. *Ann Surg* 194:373, 1981.

Urrutia SCO, Falaschi G, et al: Surgical management of 56 patients with congenital coronary artery fistulas. *Ann Thorac Surg* 35:300, 1983.

Corrected Transposition

Guit GL, Kroon HM, et al: Congenitally corrected transposition in the adult: Detection by radionuclide angiocardiography. *Radiology* 157:521, 1985.

de Leval M, Bastos P, et al: Surgical technique to reduce the risks of heart block following closure of ventricular septal defect in atrioventricular discordance. *J Thorac Cardiovasc Surg* 78:515, 1979.

Marcelletti C, Maloney J, et al: Corrected transposition and ventricular septal defect. Surgical experience. *Ann Surg* 191:751, 1980.

Metcalfe J, Somerville J: Surgical repair of lesions associated with corrected transposition. Late results. *Br Heart J* 50:476, 1983.

Schiebler GL, Edwards JE, et al: Congenital corrected transposition of the great vessels: A study of 33 cases. *Pediatrics* 27:851, 1961.

Vargas FJ, Kreutzer GO, et al: Repair of corrected transposition associated with ventricular septal defect and pulmonary stenosis. *Ann Thorac Surg* 40:509, 1985.

Waldo AL, Pacifico AD, et al: Electrophysiological delineation of the specialized A-V conduction system in patients with corrected transposition of the great vessels and ventricular septal defect. *Circulation* 52:435, 1975.

Double Outlet Right Ventricle

Anderson RH, Becker AE, et al: Surgical anatomy of double-outlet right ventricle—A reappraisal. *Am J Cardiol* 52:555, 1983.

Judson JP, Danielson GK, et al: Double-outlet right ventricle. *J Thorac Cardiovasc Surg* 85:32, 1983.

Kirklin JW, Pacifico AD, et al: Current risks and protocols for operations for double-outlet right ventricle. Derivation from an 18 year experience. *J Thorac Cardiovasc Surg* 92:913, 1986.

Luber JM, Castaneda AR, et al: Repair of double-outlet right ventricle: Early and late results. *Circulation* 68(2):II 144, 1983.

Pulmonary Artery Sling

Campbell DN, Lilly JR, et al: The surgery of pulmonary artery "sling." *J Pediatr Surg* 18:855, 1983.

Grover FL, Norton JB, et al: Pulmonary sling: Case report and collective review. *J Thorac Cardiovasc Surg* 69:295, 1975.

Gumbiner C, Mullins C, McNamara D: Pulmonary artery sling. *Am J Cardiol* 45:311, 1980.

King HA, Walker D: Pulmonary artery sling. *Thorax* 39:462, 1984.

Marmon LM, Bye MR, et al: Vascular rings and slings: Long-term follow-up of pulmonary function. *J Pediatr Surg* 19:683, 1984.

Chapter 19

Acquired Heart Disease

Frank C. Spencer

CLINICAL MANIFESTATIONS AND DIAGNOSTIC STUDIES

The standard methods for evaluating a patient with heart disease include the history and physical examination; the chest x-ray and electrocardiogram; and special diagnostic studies, especially echocardiography, cardiac catheterization and cineangiography, and special radionuclide studies. Fundamental general considerations are discussed in the following sections. More information is described in the specific section concerning different diseases in this chapter.

HISTORY. The frequent symptoms with cardiac disease include (1) symptoms of left heart failure: dyspnea, other symptoms of pulmonary congestion; (2) symptoms of right heart failure: edema from sodium retention, hepatomegaly and ascites; (3) angina; (4) arrhythmias; (5) syncope; and (6) fatigue. With the exception of angina, symptoms are usually a *late* sign of advanced cardiac disease. The initial change in most cardiac diseases is a rise in intracardiac pressure in the involved cardiac chamber, subsequently followed by cardiac enlargement, usually a combination of dilatation and hypertrophy. This is a manifestation of Starling's law of the heart; an increase in workload can be achieved by an increase in diastolic fiber length. These physiologic and anatomic changes are the early changes from heart disease. Symptoms develop subsequently as different compensatory mechanisms fail. This concept is an important one because abundant data indicate that operation should be considered for many diseases on the basis of physiologic abnormalities, such as reduction of cross-sectional area of an aortic or mitral valve below 1.0 cm^2, rather than the presence of symptoms. Delaying operation until symptoms are severe often results in irreversible ventricular injury, which in turn is a major cause of death in the first few years following operation.

Symptoms of Left Heart Failure. *Dyspnea.* The normal left ventricular end-diastolic pressure is less than 12 mmHg. Pressures in the range of 12 to 20 mmHg represent moderate disease, while pressures of 20 to 30 mmHg represent severe disease. The oncotic pressure of plasma is 30 to 35 mmHg. Hence, as left atrial pressure rises, pulmonary congestion develops as left atrial pressure approaches the colloidal osmotic pressure of plasma. The tolerance for pulmonary congestion depends upon several factors, including the capacity of the pulmonary lymphatics to resorb fluid. *Dyspnea* is one of the cardinal symptoms of left heart failure. It can be graded with the degree of exertion required to initiate dyspnea, as opposed to dyspnea at rest, which represents a severe form of heart disease. With mitral stenosis, dyspnea appears as an early sign because of restriction of flow from the left atrium into the left ventricle. With other forms of heart disease, however, dyspnea is a *late* sign as it develops only after the left ventricle has failed, with the end-diastolic pressure rising above 12 mm. Dyspnea with mitral insufficiency, aortic valvular disease, or coronary disease represents an advanced form of disease, in contrast to mitral stenosis.

A number of other respiratory symptoms represent different degrees of pulmonary congestion. These include orthopnea, paroxysmal nocturnal dyspnea, cough, hemoptysis, and pulmonary edema.

Symptoms of Right Heart Failure. Right atrial pressure is normally less than 5 mmHg. When right ventricular failure results in elevation of right atrial pressure above 5 mmHg, the earliest change is a retention of sodium, a complex homeostatic mechanism initiated by the liver, kidneys, and other organs, which increases blood volume and elevates venous pressure. Retention of more than 7 to 10 lb of fluid results in visible edema of the lower extremities. Hepatomegaly also develops. With chronic severe right heart failure fluid retention is severe, with marked deformities from accumulation of 20, 30, or more pounds of edema fluid, with ascites and massive hepatomegaly.

Angina. Angina is the hallmark of coronary artery disease, a symptom of myocardial anoxia with subsequent anaerobic metabolism. Classic angina is described as a precordial discomfort appearing with exercise, emotion, or eating, relieved by rest or nitroglycerin. This is discussed in more detail in the section on Coronary Artery Disease. It is present in the classic form in 70 to 75 percent of patients with coronary disease. When this history is elicited, the diagnosis of coronary disease can be made with a high degree of certainty. In perhaps 20 to 25 percent of patients, one of the numerous variations of angina occurs, so-called angina equivalents, with symptoms in the shoulders, arms, jaw, epigastrium, or other areas. Also, in a significant number of patients, the exact frequency of which is unknown, angina apparently does not develop, though "silent" ischemia is present.

Angina also is a typical symptom with aortic stenosis, resulting from the combination of decreased cardiac output and left ventricular hypertrophy. It is less common with other forms of heart disease.

With the exception of angina, other forms of pain from heart disease are uncommon; chest pain is usually due to musculoskeletal disorders in the chest wall, pericarditis, or pleural or esophageal disease.

Arrhythmias. Atrial fibrillation is usually one of the first cardiac abnormalities with mitral stenosis, resulting from left atrial hypertrophy evolving from the sustained elevation in left atrial pressure. With other forms of heart disease, arrhythmias are uncommon, occurring sporadically without any predictable consistency. They are more frequent with older patients, probably from intrinsic disease in the atrioventricular conducting mechanism, and in severe cardiac failure, probably a manifestation of generalized cardiac hypoxia.

Syncope. This is an important symptom with aortic stenosis, apparently from a transient decrease in cerebral blood flow. It is of particular importance because it indicates a severity of aortic stenosis that may unpredictably terminate with sudden death. It must be differentiated from syncope from other causes such as bradycardia or heart block.

Fatigue. This is a nonspecific symptom that may arise from many causes. In some patients it probably reflects a generalized decrease in cardiac output. Otherwise, its significance is vague.

PHYSICAL EXAMINATION. Only a few basic physical abnormalities are discussed in this short section, as abnormal physical findings are best discussed with the specific disease causing them. In some cardiac diseases, physical abnormalities are virtually diagnostic of both the disease and the severity of the problem, while in others, such as coronary disease or aortic stenosis, the paucity or absence of *any* physical abnormality can be seriously misleading.

Cardiac Cachexia. The muscular wasting that occurs from chronic congestive failure, reflected in a weight loss of 10 to 40 lb, is due to the long-standing changes of severe congestive failure in combination with a low cardiac output. In some patients, simply inability to eat may be an important cause, resulting in malnutrition from lack of calories and protein. Such patients are especially susceptible to infection following operation because of a generalized decrease in immunity.

Cardiac Size. When a valvular abnormality produces a significant change in intracardiac pressures, the initial physiologic adaptation is enlargement of the involved cardiac chamber, usually from a combination of dilatation and hypertrophy. A fundamental question in evaluation is, "Is there cardiac enlargement?" Accordingly, the finding of a forceful apical impulse in the anterior midaxillary line indicates advanced cardiac disease that usually requires prompt surgical treatment. Less obvious signs of cardiac enlargement may be seen on the chest x-ray, the electrocardiogram, or, most precisely, with the echocardiogram, which can define the exact size of the cardiac chamber and the thickness of the cardiac wall.

Cardiac Murmurs. Diastolic murmurs often establish the diagnosis. The apical diastolic rumble of mitral stenosis is virtually pathognomonic; the parasternal diastolic murmur of aortic insufficiency is also almost equally so.

Systolic murmurs are strongly supportive of the diagnosis of the underlying condition but not to the degree found with diastolic murmurs. These include the basal systolic murmur of aortic stenosis or pulmonic stenosis and the apical systolic murmur of mitral insufficiency.

DIAGNOSTIC STUDIES. Electrocardiography and Radiology. The electrocardiogram and the chest x-ray are the two standard diagnostic studies. The chest x-ray is one of the best guides for answering the basic question, "Is there cardiac enlargement?" Before the development of echocardiography, special oblique views and fluoroscopy provided supplemental information, but echocardiography is far more precise.

Analysis of the pulmonary circulation may show several abnormalities. Pulmonary venous congestion develops when left atrial pressure is chronically elevated above the upper normal limit of 12 mmHg, seen typically with severe mitral stenosis. The signs of pulmonary congestion include engorged pulmonary veins and congestion of pulmonary alveoli. Fluid accumulating in the interlobar planes forms transverse linear opacities perpendicular to the surface of the pleura, termed Kerley "lines." Their presence usually indicates a left atrial pressure exceeding 20 mmHg.

Marked enlargement of the pulmonary arteries may occur from an increase in pulmonary blood flow or an increase in pulmonary vascular resistance with pulmonary hypertension. Normally, the central pulmonary arteries are three to four times larger than the peripheral arteries. With an increase in pulmonary blood flow, as with an atrial septal defect, both central and peripheral arteries are symmetrically enlarged. With pulmonary hypertension, the central pulmonary arteries may become strikingly enlarged while the peripheral arteries are not.

Echocardiography, Cardiac Catheterization, and Cineangiography. Outstanding advances have been made with echocardiography over the past decade. The precise analysis of cardiac chambers, often combined with flow studies and gradient determinations with 2-D Doppler studies, have virtually made cardiac catheterization unnecessary in some conditions. Echocardiography is the most precise method for determining specific chamber enlargement, such as size of the left atrium or left ventricle. This is particularly important in serial evaluation of a patient over months or years, noting an asymptomatic progressive enlargement that could not be detected otherwise. Cardiac catheterization precisely establishes the presence and size of intracardiac shunts or stenoses, as well as the presence of serious physiologic changes of cardiac failure, such as an elevation in end-diastolic pressure or pulmonary hypertension. A sustained rise in left ventricular end-diastolic pressure above the normal upper limit of 12 mmHg is usually the hallmark of serious cardiac disease.

Cineangiography is the fundamental method for evaluation of coronary disease, also for aortic or mitral insufficiency. All three studies are usually performed in the evaluation of a patient with a serious cardiac problem.

PATHOPHYSIOLOGY: GENERAL PRINCIPLES

With valvular heart disease, "When should an operation be performed?" This basic question must be periodically evaluated during the medical therapy of any patient with cardiac valvular disease, because the disease process is usually a progressive one. As a result of several developments, surgical therapy is now being used at a much earlier stage of the disease than in previous years.

At present a decision for operation is best made from physiologic abnormalities found with diagnostic studies, such as cardiac catheterization, angiography, or radionuclide studies, rather than from the severity and disability from symptoms.

Several developments have combined to indicate that operation should be performed earlier. The safety of operative procedures has increased, with the risk of valve replacement now being in the range of 1 to 4 percent in good-risk patients. This is principally due to improvements in myocardial preservation with the widespread adoption of hyperkalemic cold cardiac arrest. The virtually indefinite durability of metallic prosthetic valves is now well established, though anticoagulation with coumadin is required.

Longevity following cardiac valve replacement is strongly influenced by the myocardial function at the time of operation. Patients with early disability (New York Heart Class II or early III) have a 5-year survival near 90 percent, but only 60 to 70 percent of patients with Class IV disability live 5 years. This striking difference is due to irreversible changes in myocardial function that existed before operation, indicating that operation should not be postponed until symptoms are disabling.

Aortic valve replacement should be seriously considered in asymptomatic patients if the orifice cross-sectional area has decreased to near 1.0 cm². An even more liberal indication should be used with mitral stenosis, considering therapy with an orifice cross-sectional area less than 1.5 cm² because a commissurotomy, rather than valve replacement, can usually be performed. The grave hazard always exists of cerebral embolism from thrombi developing in the left atrium, especially when atrial fibrillation has developed. The recent development of balloon valvuloplasty will undoubtedly further change the indications for early treatment.

With aortic and mitral insufficiency, selecting the proper time for operation is more difficult, as this depends upon the left ventricular function. The demonstration of a fall in left ventricular ejection fraction during exercise is probably the best currently available sign that operation should be done. Postponing operation until serious enlargement of the left ventricle develops or a permanent elevation in left ventricular end-diastolic pressure occurs is clearly a mistake because 5-year prognosis following successful operation is greatly decreased.

A patient with cardiac valvular disease is rarely inoperable. If the basic disease process is cardiac valvular disease, an operation, usually prosthetic valve replacement, can almost always be performed with current techniques of myocardial preservation with an operative risk no greater than 5 to 10 percent. Patients are still seen with far advanced Class IV failure and cardiac cachexia who simply have postponed operation for years with the concept that operation was "too dangerous." Some benefit will always result, because if a patient is alive with a malfunctioning valve, that patient will function better with a properly functioning prosthetic valve. The magnitude of benefit often cannot be predicted for some months, depending upon the unmeasurable irreversible loss of ventricular function. Realizing that the degree of improvement in left

Swan-Ganz catheter is almost always inserted in adults to monitor pulmonary artery pressures and cardiac output.

The blood pressure varies widely among different patients during perfusion. It usually decreases sharply with the onset of perfusion, apparently from vasodilatation, and then subsequently rises to above 60 mmHg. The importance of the actual level of mean arterial pressure, as long as flow rate is greater than 2 L/m^2/min, is uncertain. As cerebral autoregulation of blood flow becomes ineffective below a mean pressure of 50 to 60 mmHg, perfusion pressure is usually maintained above 50 mmHg, though with moderate hypothermia (25 to 30°C) an arterial pressure of 40 to 50 mmHg seemingly has no harmful physiologic effects. After 15 to 30 min of perfusion, perfusion pressure may gradually rise from progressive vasoconstriction.

Oxygen and carbon dioxide tensions are periodically measured in the venous blood returned to the oxygenator and the oxygenated blood returned to the patient. Preferably the arterial oxygen tension should be above 100 mmHg and the carbon dioxide tension 30 to 35 mmHg. Venous blood returning to the heart-lung machine with the described flow rate will usually have an oxygen saturation greater than 50 percent. With flow rates and oxygen saturations in this range, metabolic acidosis of significant degree does not occur.

Heparin is gradually metabolized by the body, and so additional heparin is given each hour of perfusion as necessary to keep the ACT above 400 s, usually 1 mg/kg of body weight. During perfusion the lungs are kept stationary in a partially inflated position.

Termination of Perfusion. As perfusion is slowed and stopped, blood is infused from the pump oxygenator to restore normal intracardiac pressures with maintenance of an adequate blood pressure and cardiac output. Left atrial pressure is routinely monitored through an indwelling catheter inserted as bypass is being stopped. Monitoring of left atrial pressure is usually the best guide to monitor infusion of fluids, noting what level of left atrial pressure is needed to maintain an adequate cardiac output.

At NYU an indwelling Swan-Ganz catheter in the pulmonary artery is routinely used to monitor pulmonary artery pressure and cardiac output for 24 to 48 h after operation. In many patients the pulmonary artery diastolic pressure, or wedge pressure, provides a reasonable guide to left atrial pressure.

Heparin is neutralized with protamine, giving sufficient protamine to return the activated clotting time as closely as possible to that existing before bypass. Usually this requires 3 to 4 mg of protamine, given in divided doses. If a coagulopathy is present, the activated clotting time may not return to prebypass levels, indicating the need for infusion of coagulation products, such as fresh frozen plasma, cryoprecipitate, or platelets.

Myocardial Preservation. The development of hyperkalemic hypothermic cardiac arrest for myocardial preservation was a major advance in cardiac surgery. This gradually evolved from laboratories throughout the world after 1975–1976. An unusually large number of substan-

tial contributions came from Buckberg and Maloney at UCLA and from Hirsch and Braimbridge in London. The improved myocardial protection, combined with the increased facility for performing complex cardiac procedures in a dry, quiet field, greatly augmented the safety and effectiveness of virtually all cardiac operations. The results from cardiac operations are now quite different from those obtained in the two decades between 1955 and 1975, when intermittent aortic occlusion was the most widely used technique. Many of the complications of that era were undoubtedly due to myocardial injury and infarction. The status of myocardial preservation in 1980 is well summarized in the Proceedings of the International Symposium on Myocardial Protection held in London that year.

Both crystalloid and blood cardioplegia are widely used, with the exact components of the cardioplegic mixture varying among different institutions. With periods of cardiac arrest for 60 to 90 min, there seems little measurable difference in the two techniques, but with the cold blood technique, regularly used at NYU, the heart can be safely arrested for a surprisingly long period of time, even more than 4 h.

The cardioplegia cold blood solution is that developed by Buckberg et al. with a blood temperature of 7 to 8°C, a potassium concentration near 30 meq/L, and a low calcium concentration.

After the aorta is clamped, blood is infused at a rate sufficient to produce an aortic root pressure initially of 80 to 100 mmHg (200 to 400 mL/min), infusing enough blood to lower myocardial temperature below 15°C, measured in different zones of the myocardium with a needle thermistor. With normal coronary arteries, this can be achieved with 1000 to 1500 mL of cold blood. When diffuse coronary disease produces maldistribution of blood flow, larger amounts may be required, as much as 2000 to 2500 mL. Subsequently, while the aorta is clamped, varying amounts of cold blood are reinfused every 20 to 30 min, usually in the range of 300 to 500 mL. Continuous topical hypothermia, constantly irrigating the pericardium with a 4°C electrolyte solution, is an important part of the procedure to keep the heart from being rewarmed as the temperature of the perfusate in the pump oxygenator is usually 25 to 30°C. With the combination of periodic infusion of cold blood and hypothermia, the myocardial temperature can easily be kept below 15°C.

TRAUMA FROM PERFUSION. Extracorporeal circulation inevitably produces some trauma to the blood, primarily from exposure of blood to gas in the oxygenator and from the use of suction to aspirate intracardiac blood. Minimizing the injury to blood during oxygenation, of course, is the basis for a membrane oxygenator rather than a bubble oxygenator. Trauma to blood from the blood pump itself is surprisingly small. At present, tolerance for long periods of perfusion, even 8 or 10 h, is surprisingly good. The minimal trauma from pump oxygenators is further demonstrated by the selective use of extracorporeal membrane oxygenators (ECMO) for infants with respiratory failure for periods of several days with surprisingly good results.

Studies of capillary microcirculation during perfusion often find a progressive sludging of blood elements, resulting in stasis and maldistribution of capillary blood flow. The clinical significance of these observations is uncertain. Microaggregates can be demonstrated in blood coming from the pump oxygenator, partly removed with filters in the pump circuit. At NYU a filter of 20 to 40 μm capacity is used.

Some derangement of normal clotting mechanisms invariably occurs, reflected by an increased bleeding tendency for 18 to 24 h, even though heparin activity has been neutralized. Such coagulation problems, however, are now far less severe than in previous years with the recognition of the vulnerability of platelets to injury from a wide variety of medications, combined with the availability of platelet transfusions, as well as specific transfusions of fresh frozen plasma or cryoprecipitate for specific coagulation disorders.

Except for the mild coagulation defect, other signs of injury following perfusion are mild. There may be a slight degree of renal insufficiency, manifested by a transient rise in blood urea nitrogen, returning to normal levels within 2 to 3 days. A number of organ systems may sporadically manifest injury with long periods of perfusion, but these are erratic and inconsistent. Respiratory insufficiency has become uncommon. Acute abdominal problems, such as pancreatitis, cholecystitis, or mesenteric infarction, occur in less than 1 percent of patients. With long perfusions, some changes occur in the central nervous system, almost all of which are transitory and of uncertain significance. Reports from England and from Scandinavia found a surprisingly high frequency of transient neurologic abnormalities following perfusion, though the origin and significance of these findings are currently unknown.

Risk of Perfusion. At present the inherent risk from extracorporeal circulation approaches zero, especially if blood transfusion is unnecessary. Large series of coronary bypass procedures have been reported, with an operative risk of less than 1 percent. Also, the risk of aortic valve replacement has decreased to less than 1 percent in several reports. This low risk represents an astonishing achievement, especially when less than four decades ago, 1950–1952, the entire concept of extracorporeal circulation was theoretical and conceived by many to be unachievable. Multiple organ injury was common in the first two decades of extracorporeal perfusion so that perfusion for longer than 1 to 3 h was regularly associated with signs of multiple organ injury. The gradual disappearance of these problems is a tribute to many contributions in the design and manufacture of the pump oxygenators currently used.

Postoperative Care and Complications

GENERAL PROCEDURES. Following a cardiac operation, patients are best kept in a specialized cardiac intensive care unit to permit appropriate monitoring of cardiac functions. With indwelling vascular catheters, the arterial pressure, central venous pressure, intracardiac pressures, and the electrocardiogram are usually displayed on an oscilloscope to permit continuous monitoring. Generally left atrial pressure and pulmonary artery pressures through an indwelling Swan-Ganz catheter are measured.

The key questions in the first 18 to 24 h following an open heart operation are (1) Is there intrathoracic bleeding? (2) Is the cardiac output adequate (near 2.5 L/m²/min)? (3) Is there hypovolemia (manifested by low left atrial or central venous pressure)? (4) Is ventilation adequate? (5) Are any arrhythmias present?

Arterial and venous blood gas measurements (P_{O_2}, P_{CO_2}, and pH) are periodically measured, determining both the adequacy of ventilation and the adequacy of cardiac output. The oxygen tension (P_{O_2}) in mixed venous blood is particularly useful as a P_{O_2} near 30 mmHg indicates both adequate ventilation and adequate cardiac output while one near 25 mmHg or lower indicates that a serious circulatory ventilatory problem may be present.

POSTOPERATIVE COMPLICATIONS. Chest x-rays are periodically made to evaluate hemothorax and pulmonary function. The hematocrit and standard blood chemistries (sodium, potassium, carbon dioxide, chlorides, blood urea nitrogen) are serially measured.

Prophylactic antibiotics are regularly given during the operative procedure and for 24 to 48 h following operation, usually until indwelling intracardiac catheters have been removed. The prophylactic antibiotic used should be chosen on the basis of the most common organism causing infections in the hospital. Cefamandole has been one of the most popular antibiotics for the past few years.

With valvular prostheses, anticoagulant therapy with coumadin is usually begun 2 to 3 days after operation, keeping the prothrombin time slightly above 20 s, about $1\frac{1}{2}$ times normal.

Postoperative Bleeding. Blood coagulation mechanisms are abnormal for at least 18 to 24 h following bypass. With present pump oxygenators, blood loss is small, ranging from a total of 400 to 800 mL with different patients. A blood loss exceeding 1 L usually indicates active intrathoracic hemorrhage that requires return of the patient to the operating room. Unless known coagulation defects are present before operation, such as platelet abnormalities or deficient plasma coagulation factors secondary to liver disease, transfusion of platelets or fresh frozen plasma is seldom necessary.

Cardiac Tamponade. Cardiac tamponade is always a serious hazard in any patients following a cardiac operation. In the first 24 h, it may result from blood clots accumulating in the pericardium, or less commonly simply from myocardial edema with pericardial constriction. In subsequent weeks it may develop from a pericardial effusion; the possibility must be seriously considered with any circulatory problem occurring in a patient for several weeks following a cardiac operation. The classic findings of tamponade include elevated venous pressure, hypotension, and widening of the mediastinal shadow on the chest x-ray. Echocardiography is valuable for detection of pericardial effusions but not of much value for recognition of intrapericardial blood.

A particularly important point is that there is *no certain method* for excluding tamponade short of surgical reexploration. Grave tragedies have occurred from cardiac tamponade progressing to cardiac arrest because subtle findings are easily confused with a low cardiac output from cardiac failure. If a significant decrease in cardiac output is present that does not respond to appropriate treatment with infusion of fluids or inotropic agents, prompt surgical reexploration should be done to exclude cardiac tamponade.

Inadequate Cardiac Output. The adequacy of the cardiac output is the key question in any patient following a cardiac operation. Adequacy of cardiac output, of course, is reflected in the blood pressure and the urine output, but exact measurement of cardiac output is far more precise. This can be simply done with a thermodilution technique if a Swan-Ganz catheter has been inserted. This is the mainstay of treatment in any seriously ill patient. A normal cardiac output, of course, is a cardiac index near 3 L/m^2/min. An output between 2.0 and 2.5 L/m^2 represents moderate cardiac failure, while a decrease below 2 L/min is an ominous finding, often resulting in death from inadequate perfusion of peripheral organs unless cardiac output can be increased. The classic clinical findings of low cardiac output with inadequate oxygen transport are the familiar ones of hypotension, vasoconstriction, oliguria, and metabolic acidosis. Untreated cardiac output is ultimately fatal from either progressive renal failure or arrhythmias.

With treatment of a low cardiac output, the first consideration is to exclude cardiac tamponade or intrathoracic bleeding with hypovolemia. Once these two factors have been excluded, the three forms of therapy may be conveniently grouped as treatment of cardiac *preload, afterload,* and *inotropic agents* to improve cardiac contractility. Preload therapy consists of infusion of sufficient fluids to elevate left atrial pressure to an appropriate level; as defined with the Starling concept, cardiac output rises with a rise in left atrial pressure over a wide range.

Afterload reduction consists of reduction in peripheral vascular resistance with specific drugs to cause vasodilatation. If peripheral vascular resistance is elevated above the normal of 1000 to 1200 units, afterload reduction should be one of the initial forms of therapy. The most popular drugs for intravenous infusion are nipride or nitroglycerin.

A wide variety of inotropic agents have been used to augment myocardial contractility. Our preference is usually for dobutamine or dopamine in most instances, often augmented with small amounts of epinephrine.

If cardiac rhythm is not satisfactory, cardiac pacing should be used to maintain both an adequate rate and rhythm. If a sinus mechanism is not present, atrial-ventricular pacing is valuable.

An intraaortic balloon pump is a valuable form of assisted circulation that can be employed when simpler measures fail, as it augments cardiac output about 700 mL/m^2/min. The need for a balloon pump can easily be determined in the operating room by serial measurements of cardiac output following bypass, using an intraaortic balloon pump if cardiac index remains below 2.0 L/m^2. If this decision is properly made, insertion of an intraaortic balloon pump in the recovery room is seldom necessary. Usually an unexpected fall in cardiac output in the recovery room is due to some specific factor that can be corrected, either in the recovery room or by return of the patient to the operating room. The premature insertion of a balloon pump until all other possible causes of a low cardiac output have been eliminated is a serious error that may have fatal consequences if the basic cause is not recognized.

Cardiac Arrhythmias. An important component of postoperative care is constant, 24 h a day, monitoring of the cardiac rhythm on an oscilloscope for at least 2 to 3 days following operation. In an intensive care unit visual monitoring is satisfactory. Otherwise, some form of telemetry with an appropriate alarm mechanism is needed. Only by *constant* monitoring can serious arrhythmias be detected because such arrhythmias may develop unpredictably despite the presence of a normal cardiac output and without any other signs of circulatory failure. Delayed detection of a significant arrhythmia is a major cause of the rare but tragic unexpected death following cardiac operations. The prevalence of such arrhythmias is the reason that cardiac pacing wires are routinely left in the right ventricle and right atrium for several days following operation.

Ventricular extrasystoles are more serious because their appearance may herald the development of hazardous rhythms such as bigeminy, ventricular tachycardia, or fibrillation. Hypokalemia should always be considered because patients in cardiac failure preoperatively may have significant depletion of body stores of potassium from chronic diuretic therapy. The serum potassium should usually be kept well above 4.0 meq/L.

Intravenous lidocaine, 1 to 3 mg/m, is a valuable form of therapy for temporary control of arrhythmias, as the drug is quickly metabolized. Treatment of more complicated problems should be done in conjunction with a cardiologist. Methods of therapy include the use of digitalis, beta-blocking drugs such as propanolol, a calcium blocking drug such as verapamil, procaine-amide, or quinidine. Unfortunately, virtually all antiarrhythmic agents cause serious side effects in a small percentage of patients; so such patients require careful periodic monitoring. Electric cardioversion is a valuable technique for arrhythmias refractory to simpler forms of therapy.

Renal Failure. In the first 24 h after operation, baseline intravenous fluid therapy is usually in the range of 75 to 100 mL/h, providing a 24-h infusion of near 1500 mL/m^2 of body surface. Usually a limited oral intake of fluids is possible the day following operation; so intravenous therapy is needed for only a short period of time.

There is usually some degree of sodium retention for days or weeks following operation, especially in patients who have had chronic congestive failure beforehand. There is also a normal weight gain of five or more pounds following extracorporeal circulation because of the hemodilution used in the pump oxygenator. Moderate diuretic therapy is usually needed for a few days following operation, noting the change in daily body weight. If preoperative chronic cardiac failure was present, recording daily weight should be continued for weeks or months to permit appropriate adjustment of diuretic therapy.

Renal function is rarely a problem unless there is a persistently low cardiac output or serious preexisting renal disease, with a creatinine clearance less than 30 mL/min. Hourly urine output is carefully measured for 1 to 2 days, usually keeping an average output above 30 mL/h. A transitory elevation of blood urea nitrogen to 30 to 40 mg/dL commonly occurs but apparently is of no clinical significance.

Significant renal failure usually develops as a consequence of a persistent low cardiac output or in patients with minimal renal function before operation. This usually is manifested as a high-output renal failure, with a daily secretion of 1 to 2 L of dilute urine, associated with progressive elevation in blood urea nitrogen. The degree of renal insufficiency may be evaluated simply by performance of a urea clearance test, comparing the urea concentration in the blood and urine. Normally, urea concentration is fifteen to twenty times greater in the urine than in the blood; a urine urea concentration less than ten times that in the blood usually represents severe renal insufficiency.

If renal insufficiency evolves to produce a blood urea nitrogen above 50 to 60 mg/dL, peritoneal dialysis should be started promptly. This is a simple form of therapy that often controls the renal insufficiency until spontaneous recovery of renal function occurs. Permitting the blood urea nitrogen to rise to levels of 90 to 100 mg may precipitate serious cardiac arrhythmias and other metabolic disturbances such as gastrointestinal bleeding.

Oliguric renal failure of severe degree is a more ominous complication. If a short period of peritoneal dialysis is not satisfactory, hemodialysis is often necessary. Renal failure of such severity that hemodialysis is required is a very serious complication, as the mortality rate is at least 50 percent, often greater.

Respiratory Insufficiency. With current pump oxygenators, significant impairment of pulmonary function is uncommon except in patients with severe preexisting pulmonary disease or advanced cardiac failure. The simplest numerical expression of the pulmonary dysfunction is the alveolar-arterial oxygen gradient, representing impaired diffusion of oxygen from the alveoli into the pulmonary venous blood.

Ventilation through an indwelling endotracheal tube for 24 to 72 h is adequate for many patients. If longer periods of ventilation are necessary, a cricothyroidotomy or tracheostomy should be performed, although some patients may tolerate an indwelling endotracheal tube for several days. Removal of pulmonary secretions, however, a major cause of pulmonary infection, is done much better through a tracheostomy or cricothyroidotomy. Ventilatory support for more than a short time is seldom necessary except in chronically ill elderly patients in whom simple physical weakness may significantly impair the effectiveness of breathing and coughing. Such patients may require ventilatory support for days or even weeks.

Fever. A moderate temperature elevation to 100 to 101°F is common for 1 to 2 days following operation, probably reflecting both the operative trauma, impaired pulmonary function, and the products from the pump oxygenator. Fever persisting more than a few days is usu-

ally due to a pleural effusion or the so-called pericardiotomy syndrome. The pericardiotomy syndrome can develop in any patient in whom the pericardium has been opened; it is probably a reaction of a mesothelial lined surface to surgical trauma. The familiar clinical manifestations are fever, often in association with a pericardial friction rub, and pericardial or pleural effusions. The white blood cell count is usually near the normal range of 10,000/mm^3.

Treatment with an anti-inflammatory agent, aspirin, or ibuprofen, is usually satisfactory. With more difficult problems, prednisone therapy may be given for a few days. Investigation should always be done for a bacterial source of infection. Common causes include atelectasis, urinary tract infection, or a wound infection. Blood cultures are usually routinely done to exclude the rare but serious development of endocarditis in patients with prosthetic valves. An infection of the sternotomy incision is a serious complication that requires prompt return to the operating room for treatment with either debridement and antibiotic drainage or debridement and closure with open muscle flaps in refractory cases. Such serious infections are rare, occurring in about 1 percent of all open heart operations.

Central Nervous System Complications. A stroke is perhaps the most serious complication following extracorporeal circulation, occurring with a frequency of 1 to 2 percent following open heart operations. The frequency is greater with older patients, almost surely because of the increasing frequency of atherosclerotic disease of the carotid and vertebral arteries in older patients. Possible causes of stroke that should be routinely investigated include carotid disease, emboli from the heart such as thrombi or calcium fragments from diseased valves, or air emboli from incomplete evacuation of air from the cardiac chambers. In the majority of patients, the cause simply remains unknown; so stroke remains a distressing serious cause of morbidity following any open heart operation. In recent years, at NYU, atherosclerotic disease in the aortic arch has been found by surgical exploration at operation in a significant number of older patients.

Prospective studies of cerebral function have been reported from England and Scandinavian countries in recent years that suggest a significant frequency of transient minor neurologic abnormalities with extracorporeal circulation presumably due to emboli of microaggregates. The significance of these observations is yet unknown.

Gastrointestinal Disturbances. The vast majority of patients recovery uneventfully. An acute abdominal problem has been reported to develop in about 1 percent of all patients following extracorporeal circulation. The specific disease varies widely and unpredictably, including acute cholecystitis, pancreatitis, perforated ulcer, gastrointestinal bleeding, or mesenteric infarction.

CARDIAC ARREST AND VENTRICULAR FIBRILLATION

Cardiac arrest and ventricular fibrillation are considered together because either catastrophe produces immediate cessation of the circulation. An injury causing generalized cardiac depression, such as anoxia, is more likely to lead to cardiac arrest, while agents increasing myocardial irritability, such as digitalis intoxication, are more likely to produce ventricular fibrillation. Diagnosis and treatment of the two conditions are, however, very similar.

HISTORICAL DATA. A successful cardiac resuscitation was performed in 1901 by Igelsrud in Norway, but for many years such experiences were very rare. The first successful case of electrical defibrillation was reported by Beck in 1947. In 1960 the most important advance in cardiac resuscitation occurred when Kouwenhoven, Jude, and Knickerbocker, at the Johns Hopkins Hospital, first introduced the concept of closed-chest massage. This launched the modern era of cardiopulmonary resuscitation, which quickly spread throughout the world. Over the past 10 to 15 years cardiopulmonary resuscitation (CPR) has been successfully taught in organized courses to large numbers of nonmedical personnel with widespread beneficial results. Cobb and associates reported that nearly 300 patients were successfully resuscitated each year. Subsequent studies found that nearly 80 percent had coronary disease but only 25 percent of these had a significant infarction; over 50 percent had no signs of infarction whatsoever, indicating the prevalence and importance of cardiac arrhythmias.

ETIOLOGY. Five frequent causes of cardiac arrest of fibrillation that should be routinely considered in the differential diagnosis are coronary occlusion, anoxia, electrolyte abnormalities, drugs, and arrhythmias.

Coronary Occlusion. Coronary disease is present in the majority of patients. An acute myocardial infarction is a common cause of fibrillation. When chronic coronary disease has produced significant ventricular scarring, cardiac arrhythmias may precipitate ventricular fibrillation in the absence of acute infarction.

Anoxia. Sustained anoxia may lead to ventricular fibrillation or cardiac arrest, both from the low arterial oxygen tension as well as the progressive metabolic acidosis that results. Inadequate ventilation from tracheobroncheal obstruction from aspiration of gastric contents or a foreign body is a frequent cause.

Electrolyte Abnormalities. Either a deficiency or an excess of potassium can cause cardiac arrest or fibrillation. A serum potassium below 4.0 meq or above 6.0 meq can be harmful, though the precise influence is determined by the coexisting concentration of calcium ions and the presence of acidosis or alkalosis.

Drugs. Several drugs may induce ventricular fibrillation or cardiac arrest, either from excessive amounts or from an abnormal sensitivity. Digitalis is one of the most frequent of this group because of its widespread usage. The sensitivity of the myocardium to digitalis varies with a number of factors, one of the most importance of which is the concentration of potassium. Quinidine is a familiar example of a drug that may cause a reaction from abnormal sensitivity, as an occasional patient develops ventricular fibrillation from a very small amount of quinidine.

Arrhythmias. A profound bradycardia, with a heart rate below 60 per minute, may result in ventricular fibrillation or cardiac arrest. This frequently occurs in patients with complete heart block. Ventricular arrhythmias from any cause may progress to bigeminy, ventricular tachycardia, and fibrillation. This well-known sequence is the reason for the fundamental importance of constant visual monitoring of the electrocardiogram on an oscilloscope in a cardiac postoperative unit.

DIAGNOSIS. The cerebral anoxia following circulatory arrest produces brain injury within 3 to 4 min, depending upon the temperature; so diagnosis must be made and treatment begun rapidly to avoid serious brain injury. Periods of anoxia for 6 to 8 min may produce extensive but reversible brain injury whereas longer periods regularly cause irreversible injury. When the diagnosis of cardiac arrest is considered, it should either be excluded within 30 to 60 s or treatment should be begun.

In most patients the diagnosis can be simply made. Loss of consciousness occurs within seconds, as well as absence of respiratory activity except for a few agonal gasps. The rapidity of loss of consciousness is awesome. Abruptly, without a sound or any other warning, the patient simply collapses. This is the reason alarm systems are essential in a busy intensive care unit, for otherwise cardiac arrest may not be recognized unless the patient is under direct visual observation. All peripheral pulses are absent, most easily confirmed by palpation of the femoral or carotid arteries. No cardiac sounds can be heard on auscultation of the chest.

Closed-chest massage should be started promptly, within 1 to 2 min. The electrocardiogram is of little value making a diagnosis of cardiac arrest, for some electrical activity may be visible on the electrocardiogram for a few minutes after effective cardiac contractions have ceased. The main value of the electrocardiogram is to demonstrate ventricular fibrillation, for cardiac arrest can be differentiated from ventricular fibrillation only by the electrocardiogram or by direct inspection of the myocardium.

The most common differential diagnosis from cardiac arrest is extreme bradycardia with hypotension, as in someone who has fainted or developed anaphylactic shock from a hypersensitivity syndrome. In such patients, though unconscious, there is slight respiratory activity and cardiac sounds are usually audible.

TREATMENT. Ventilation. The immediate first step in treatment is to provide adequate oxygenation (Fig. 19-2). Cardiac massage for more than a few seconds without ventilation of the lungs is futile. Ventilation is most quickly accomplished by mouth-to-mouth insufflation of the lungs. This can be begun immediately and continued until equipment for an oral airway or endotracheal intubation is obtained. With a laryngoscope, an endotracheal tube can easily be inserted readily by a physician or other trained personnel. In some patients, as in those with a short, thick neck, the anatomy is such that intubation is difficult, at times almost impossible by highly experienced staff. Unless intubation can be accomplished quickly and with certainty, oral insufflation should be continued until a cricothyroidotomy has been performed. A cricothyroidotomy is far simpler than a tracheostomy and equally satisfactory.

An infrequent but serious error occurs when the endo-

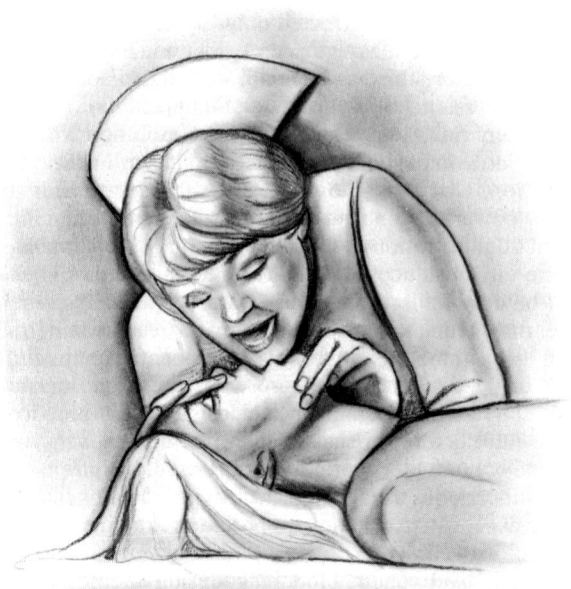

Fig. 19-2. Technique of mouth-to-mouth ventilation. The chin of the patient must be held forward with one hand to prevent obstruction of the nasopharynx by backward displacement of the tongue. The nostrils need to be occluded with the other hand. The head should be extended on the cervical spine to avoid obstruction in the nasopharynx.

tracheal tube is inadvertently placed in the esophagus. Determining whether the endotracheal tube has been placed in the trachea or not can be surprisingly difficult in some patients. If any uncertainty exists after brief auscultation of the lungs, a cricothyroidotomy should be done. A tightly fitting face mask can provide a method of temporary ventilation.

Fig. 19-3. *A*. Closed-chest massage. The heel of the hand should be used to compress intermittently the lower portion of the sternum toward the vertebral column. The effectiveness of the compression should be monitored by palpation of a peripheral pulse by another member of the team. Artificial ventilation must be performed at the same time. *B*. Cross section of chest showing the anatomic basis for closed-chest massage. The heart is seen suspended in the midthorax between the sternum anteriorly and the vertebral column posteriorly. The pericardium must be intact for closed-chest massage to be effective. *C*. Compression of the heart as the sternum is depressed downward toward the vertebral column.

Cardiac Massage. The effectiveness of closed-chest massage probably depends upon intermittent compression of the heart between the sternum and the vertebral column, with lateral motion of the heart limited by the pericardium. The patient must be on a firm surface, usually done by placing a board behind the back. The heel of the hand should be applied over the *lower third* of the sternum with the other hand above it to depress the sternum intermittently for 3 to 4 cm (Fig. 19-3). The sternal compression should be brisk, depress the sternum sharply and then releasing it to permit cardiac filling. Mechanical ventilation must be synchronized with massage.

Compression of the sternum near the xiphoid process may injure the liver; compression over the upper sternum or laterally over the chest wall may produce multiple fractures of the ribs. Massage should be at a rate of about 60/min; more than one person is required since the persons performing massage will fatigue quickly.

The amount of force applied should be judged by palpation of a peripheral pulse, usually the femoral. Caution is required to be certain that a regurgitant pulse in the femoral vein is not confused with a pulse in the femoral artery, for a strong retrograde pulse wave may be propagated down the vena cava during massage.

The influence of technique on effectiveness of massage can be easily judged when intraarterial pressure is visually displayed on an oscilloscope. Small adjustments in the technique of massage may change systolic blood pressure 40 to 60 mmHg.

Weisfeldt and associates proposed that the effectiveness of CPR depended upon the intrathoracic pressure rather than direct compression of the heart between the vertebral column and the sternum. Increasing intrathoracic pressure by inflating the lungs and compressing the abdominal wall with a binder substantially increased the effectiveness of cardiac massage, demonstrated by measuring both flow and pressure in the carotid artery.

If cerebral function is probably intact, massage should be continued as long as significant cardiac activity is present. Cardiac massage is seldom successful after about 15 min.

Retrospective analyses comparing patients who were and were not successfully resuscitated usually find certain basic differences. Patients successfully resuscitated

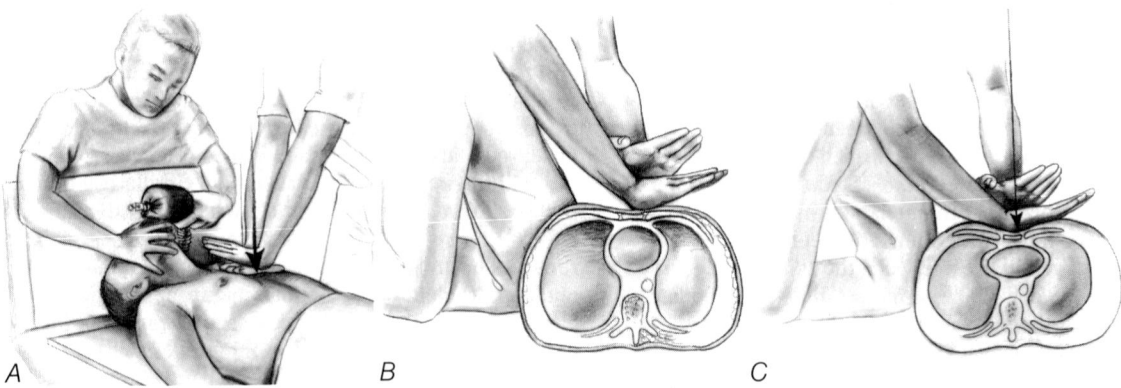

A   *B*   *C*

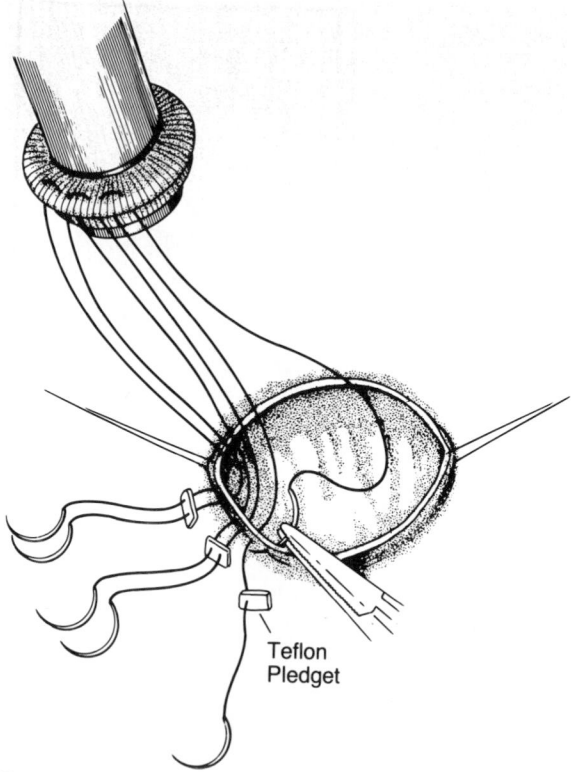

Fig. 19-12. Technique for suturing a mitral valve prosthesis with Dacron pledgets seated above the mitral annulus.

In a report by Halseth et al. only 11 percent of patients required valve replacement at operation. Operative mortality was 1.5 percent; 10-year survival was 81 percent. Only 7 percent of 191 patients required valve replacement in the next several years. In the series reported by Cohn et al. of 120 patients there were no operative deaths and five late deaths from noncardiac causes. Actuarial projections at 10 years found a survival rate near 95 percent, 91 percent freedom from emboli, 84 percent freedom from reoperation.

Fig. 19-13. Bjork-Shiley tilting disc valve.

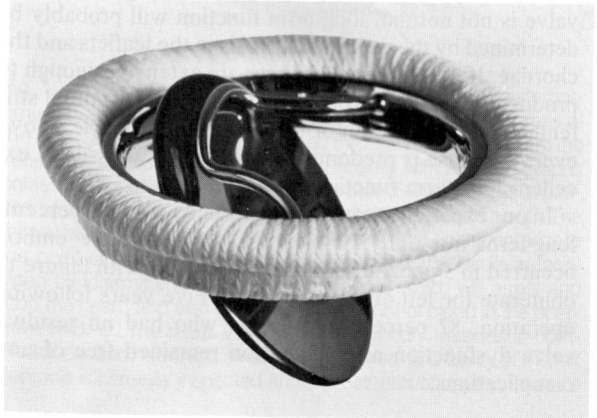

These experiences are particularly significant because during the 1950s and 1960s a recurrence rate as high as 30 to 40 percent within 5 years after operation was reported following commissurotomy, clearly in retrospect owing to an ineffective commissurotomy. Unwarranted pessimism was expressed at that time about the durability of commissurotomy, simply because residual stenosis remained following operation.

These considerations are especially pertinent now because of the recent interest in percutaneous balloon mitral valvuloplasty. The effective mitral valve area has been increased from 0.8 to 1.7 cm^2, but some regurgitation resulted in 43 percent of patients. The noninvasive features make balloon valvuloplasty a serious consideration in patients who are poor candidates for operation because of other diseases such as stroke or advanced age. The data do not support, however, that this procedure is more than a palliative one, with results similar to those obtained with digital commissurotomy in the early 1950s. Far better results can be obtained in good-risk patients with an open operative technique.

Following Valve Replacement. If valve replacement is necessary, long-term results are not nearly as satisfactory as those following commissurotomy. Five-year survival is near 80 percent, 10 years 60 percent. A major factor in determining 5-year survival is the severity of left ventricular failure before operation. Patients in Class II or early Class III have a 5-year survival about 90 percent while those near Class IV are about 60 percent. These data clearly indicate the importance of preoperative irreversible injury to the ventricle and, accordingly, the need for earlier operation. The frequency of emboli has decreased markedly since 1973.

In 1985 Starr summarized his 25 years of experience with over 2000 ball valve prostheses, 34 percent of which were mitral valve replacements. In 1979 Bjork described his experiences with 1800 Bjork-Shiley valves. The 5-year survival after mitral replacement was 66 percent. Frequency of thromboembolism was 4 percent per patient year and frequency of thrombosis of the prosthesis was 1 percent per year.

Edmonds et al. summarized overall reported experiences with thromboembolic complications of different types of valve prostheses. The major problem with tissue prostheses is durability with the estimated failure rate by 10 years of at least 20 percent. Oyer et al. reported a study of over 1400 patients who received Hancock prostheses. The probability of freedom from tissue failure 5 years following operation was 95 percent. At NYU 1643 porcine prostheses in 1492 patients were inserted; 556 patients have isolated mitral replacement. Freedom from late cardiac death was about 85 percent at 5 years.

When either type of prosthetic valve replacement is done, metallic or porcine, there is a small but permanent risk of endocarditis, ranging between 1 and 2 percent per patient per year. Prophylactic antibiotics should be routinely used when episodes of transient bacteremia can be anticipated, such as dental extraction or cystoscopy.

MITRAL INSUFFICIENCY

Prosthetic replacement of the mitral valve is often necessary with rheumatic mitral insufficiency, especially if valvular calcification and fibrosis are severe. If the aortic leaflet of the mitral valve is relatively free of disease, some patients may be treated with annuloplasty. Long-term results following annuloplasty in selected cases have been reported by Reed et al.

Over the past 15 years, Carpentier has serially reported impressive results with a complex mitral valve reconstruction, including excision of part of the diseased mural leaflet and reconstruction of the annulus with a prosthetic ring. Additional technical maneuvers, applicable for specific pathologic problems, include shortening of elongated chordae, attachment of flail chordae to adjacent structures of transposition of chordae. This technique has been used at NYU since 1980 in nearly 200 selected patients with excellent results to date. Long-term data are not available, but in all likelihood the Carpentier technique may be used in the majority of patients with nonrheumatic mitral insufficiency resulting from ruptured chordae tendineae, mitral prolapse, or coronary disease, because inflammatory changes do not destroy the mobility of the leaflets.

ETIOLOGY. In the United States mitral insufficiency from rheumatic fever has steadily decreased in frequency, now representing less than one-half of patients seen. The most common cause is mitral valve prolapse, often complicated by rupture of chordae tendineae. Ischemic papillary muscle disease complicating extensive occlusive disease of the coronary arteries has become an increasingly common cause. Bacterial endocarditis remains an infrequent but important cause.

It is now known that some degree of prolapse of the mitral valve is surprisingly frequent, detectable in as many as 5 percent of the normal population. In the majority of patients, the hemodynamic disturbance is minimal. In chronic cases, however, severe changes evolve with dense extensive calcification, progressive elongation of chordae, and increasing asymmetric dilatation of the annulus of the mitral valve.

PATHOLOGIC ANATOMY. The basic changes with rheumatic fever were described in the preceding section on Mitral Stenosis. Insufficiency develops from fibrosis and contraction of the mitral leaflets, usually combined with calcification restricting mobility. Fibrosis and contraction of chordae tendineae are important contributory factors. These changes are usually gradually progressive because of the turbulent flow of blood.

Carpentier, in a study of over 50 rheumatic hearts, carefully delineated the additional pathologic changes that evolve and augment the insufficiency. These are predominantly progressive elongation of chordae (as much as 5 to 10 mm) and asymmetric dilatation of the mitral annulus, as dilatation predominantly occurs in the posteromedial portion of the annulus of the mural leaflet, not involving the annulus of the aortic leaflet at all, as it is part of the basic fibrous skeleton of the heart.

PATHOPHYSIOLOGY. The basic physiologic change is elevation of left atrial pressure as blood regurgitates through the incompetent mitral valve during ventricular systole. The ventricular pressure spike is commonly to levels of 30 to 40 mmHg, but levels as high as 80 to 90 mmHg have been recorded. In diastole the left atrial pressure drops sharply to approach the left ventricular diastolic pressure, although a small gradient usually remains because of the large blood flow through the mitral valve during diastole. Mean left atrial pressure is usually 15 to 25 mmHg. The mitral regurgitation produces enlargement of the left atrium, although for unknown reasons the degree of left atrial enlargement varies greatly among different patients and is not proportional to the degree of regurgitation. In some patients with significant regurgitation only slight left atrial enlargement is present, while in others giant left atria evolve, enlarging to contact the right chest wall. In contrast to mitral stenosis, pulmonary vascular changes appear rather late in the course of the disease, perhaps as a result of a large left atrium absorbing much of the kinetic energy of the regurgitating blood without sustained elevation of left atrial pressure. Fortunately, the dilated left ventricle with mitral insufficiency may function adequately for surprisingly long periods of time, maintaining the left ventricular diastolic pressure near the normal range of 8 to 12 mmHg until eventually left ventricular failure appears.

As there is little stasis of blood in the left atrium, in contrast to mitral stenosis, left atrial thrombosis and arterial embolism are much less frequent than with mitral stenosis.

Physical Examination. The two characteristic features of mitral insufficiency are the apical systolic murmur and the increased force of the apical impulse. The systolic murmur is heard best at the apex, which is often displaced downward and to the left from enlargement of the left ventricle. It is well transmitted to the axilla. The quality is of a harsh, blowing type. With severe insufficiency, the murmur is pansystolic, appearing immediately after the first sound and continuing until the second sound. The intensity of the murmur does not correlate with the severity of the regurgitation, but the pansystolic characteristic does. Murmurs not extending completely through systole are seen with less serious degrees of regurgitation. The systolic murmur is a highly characteristic feature of mitral insufficiency and is absent only in most unusual circumstances. A diastolic murmur is usually present in addition, resulting from increased flow across the mitral valve as a result of blood regurgitated into the atrium during systole. The absence of an opening snap and the normal quality of the first heart sound both suggest that the diastolic murmur is due to increased flow of blood rather than anatomic mitral stenosis.

CLINICAL MANIFESTATIONS. Symptoms. Patients with mild mitral insufficiency are usually asymptomatic. The diagnosis is usually made after discovery of an apical systolic murmur. In former years, mitral valve prolapse was confused with rheumatic mitral insufficiency. The development of echocardiography has greatly simplified the differential diagnosis.

With significant mitral insufficiency, the most common

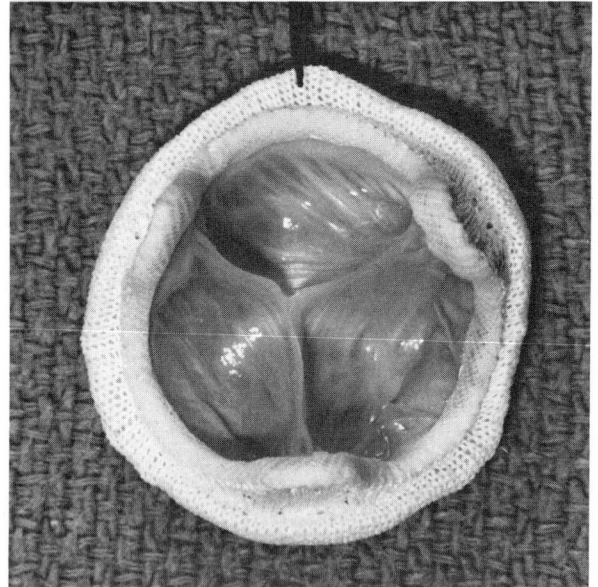

A_1

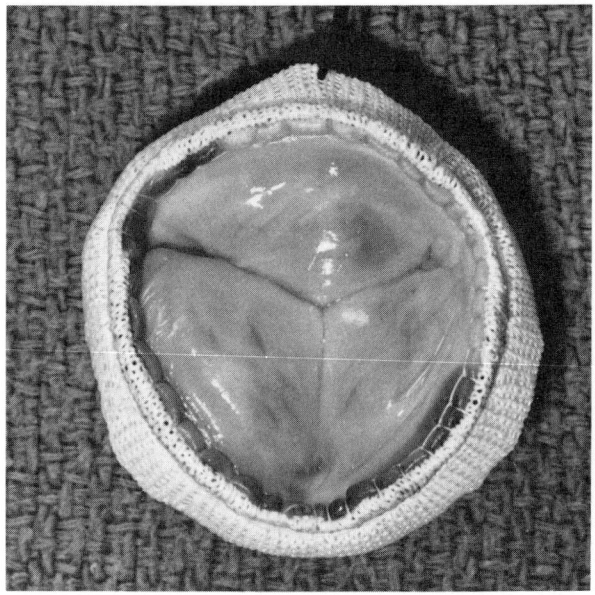

A_2

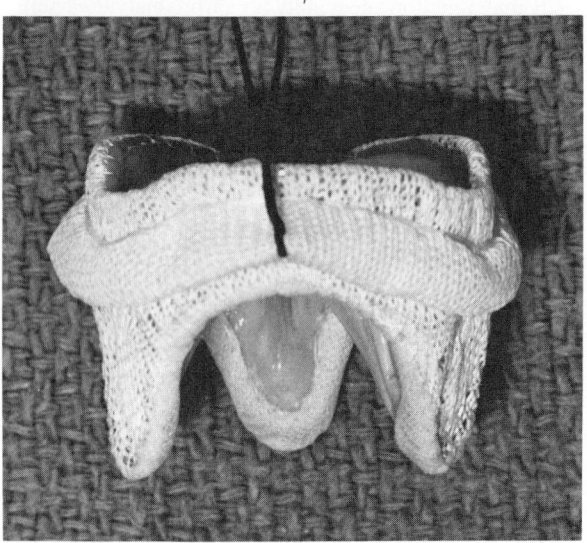

A_3

Fig. 19-14. *A.* Carpentier-Edwards porcine aortic valve prosthesis. A_1. Aortic view; A_2. Ventricular view; A_3. Side view. *B.* Ionescu bovine pericardial prosthesis. B_1. Aortic view; B_2. Ventricular view; B_3. Side view.

symptoms are fatigue, dyspnea on exertion, and palpitation. A most important point is that these symptoms may remain mild despite impressive physical findings of mitral insufficiency with progressive cardiac enlargement. Eventually, left ventricular failure evolves with a rise in end-diastolic pressure and progressive pulmonary congestion. Respiratory symptoms become prominent with exertional dyspnea, cough, and paroxysmal nocturnal dyspnea.

The apical impulse is usually forceful and prolonged, occupying an area of 3 to 4 cm². The first heart sound is usually normal, though it may be confused with the early onset of the systolic murmur.

LABORATORY EXAMINATIONS. The chest x-ray shows enlargement of both the left ventricle and the left atrium

(Fig. 19-15). In some patients, massive enlargement of the left atrium occurs with the wall of the atrium extending to the right chest wall and producing a grotesque deformity. The electrocardiogram does not contribute materially to the diagnosis. It may be normal with significant disease. In about 50 percent of patients, left ventricular hypertrophy can be recognized. 2-D echocardiography combined with Doppler flow studies can reasonably approximate the degree of regurgitation, though the method is far from quantitatively reliable.

The most precise studies are obtained by cardiac catheterization and cineangiography, noting reflux of dye into the left atrium when injected into the left ventricle. With minimal or severe insufficiency the dye studies are quite satisfactory, but with intermediate forms of insufficiency, the method is only reasonably good but thus far the best one available. Left atrial pressure tracings show a prominent V wave from regurgitation of blood during systole.

TREATMENT. Indications for Operation. Symptoms of fatigue and dyspnea may remain only moderately severe for a long time despite progressive deterioration in cardiac function, as evidenced by progressive left ventricular enlargement. Selecting the proper time for operation is best done from laboratory evaluation, not from severity of symptoms. A fall in an ejection fraction with exercise, measured with radionuclide studies, is currently the best measurement of early onset of serious impairment in ventricular function. This change may well antedate visible enlargement of the left ventricle on the chest x-ray. Operation at this earlier stage will avoid the late onset of cardiac failure 3 to 5 years following valve replacement, apparently from preoperative irreversible ventricular dysfunction.

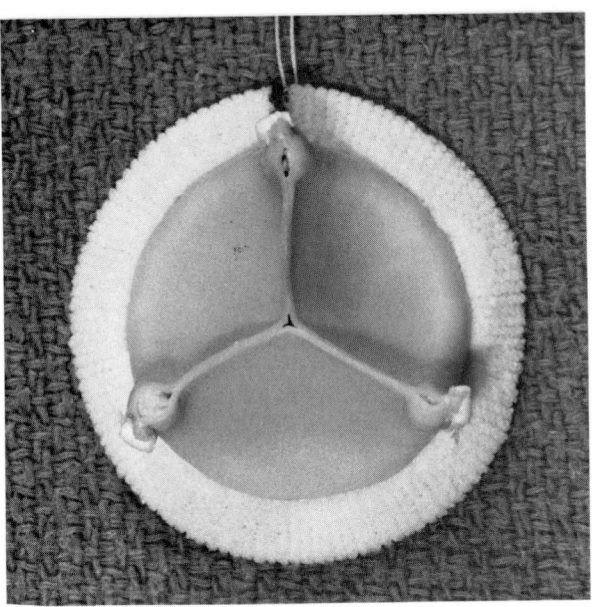

B_1

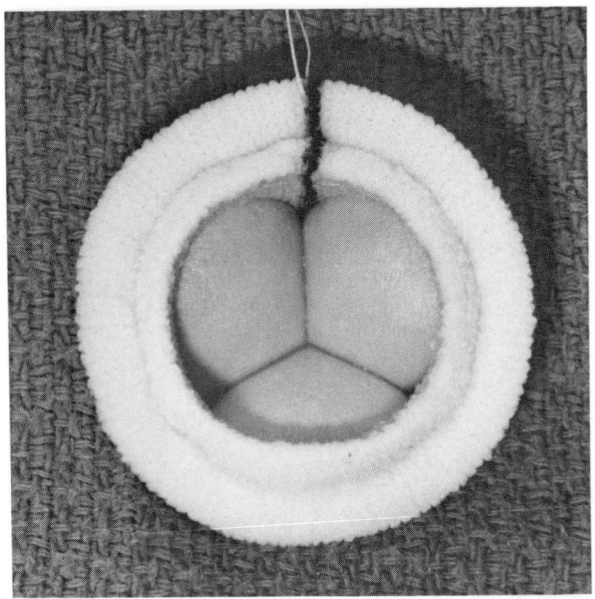

B_2

Fig. 19-14 B_1,B_2,B_3. Continued.

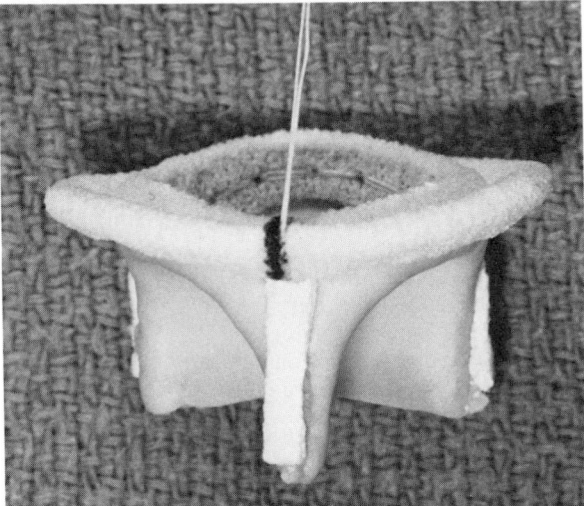

B_3

Replacement versus Reconstruction. Over the past two decades, the majority of patients have been treated with mitral valve replacement. Repair has been employed for some patients with isolated ruptured chordae of the mural leaflet, using the technique developed by McGoon. Reed and Claus successfully used a measured asymmetric annuloplasty for insufficiency in children and adults in whom annular dilatation was prominent. Carpentier, in Paris, France, however, for over 15 years has evaluated methods for mitral valve reconstruction, serially developing several techniques over this time. His overall experiences with over 2000 patients were summarized in 1983. Well over one-half of Carpentier's extensive experience has been with patients with rheumatic valvular disease. A question exists about the applicability of these techniques to nonrheumatic causes of mitral insufficiency, now constituting the majority of cases in this country. Since 1980, we have employed the Carpentier reconstructive techniques, with excellent results to date. The best results have been in patients with prolapse and ruptured chordae, with only one known late recurrence. Similar encouraging results have been reported by Cosgrove et al. If experiences by others in the future are similar, reconstruction, rather than replacement, may become the most commonly performed operation for nonrheumatic mitral insufficiency.

In 1980 Reed summarized experiences with 198 patients. Results were quite good, with a late mortality of only 9 percent, a low frequency of thromboembolism, and only 8 percent of patients requiring repeat operation. This operation is particularly attractive in children, avoiding the use of the Carpentier rigid annuloplasty ring. Chaval et al. described excellent results with reconstruction in 89 children, 84 of whom had rheumatic valve disease. Ten years following operation 90 percent of patients were alive, 98 percent free from thromboemboli, and 78 percent did not require reoperation.

LATE RESULTS. Late results following prosthetic valve replacement were discussed in the preceding section on Mitral Stenosis. Following successful mitral valve reconstruction, significant long-term results are not available from reports in this country except for repair of ruptured chordae. A 1986 study by Orzalak et al. assessed 131 patients who had repair of rupture chordae tendineae of the mitral valve. Mitral valve annuloplasty was performed in addition to leaflet repair in 88 percent of patients. The probability of the patient's requiring a repeat operation was near 10 percent at 5 years, rising to about 25 percent at 10 years. Recurrent rupture of chordae did not occur, a curious phenomenon noted by others.

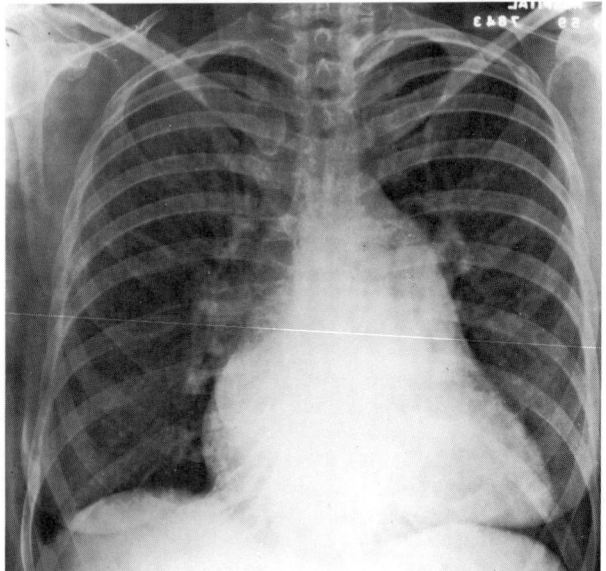

Fig. 19-15. Chest radiograph of a patient with mitral insufficiency. The distinctive features include an enlarged cardiac shadow with a prominent pulmonary artery. The shadow of the left atrium is visible in the right border of the cardiac shadow behind the shadow of the right atrium. The pulmonary vascular markings are prominent.

Carpentier has reported excellent long-term results at both 5 and 10 years following reconstruction. Thromboembolism after the first few months following reconstruction has been gratifyingly low, well under 1 percent per patient year. Recurrent insufficiency requiring repeat operation has occurred in a small percentage of patients each year. The majority of Carpentier's patients had rheumatic mitral insufficiency. Even better long-term results may be obtained when reconstruction has been successfully accomplished in nonrheumatic patients, especially if operation is performed before severe injury to the left ventricle has occurred.

AORTIC STENOSIS

HISTORICAL DATA. Effective surgical treatment of aortic valve disease first became possible in 1960–1961 with the development of satisfactory prosthetic valves by Starr and Edwards and by Harken and associates. Earlier attempts to correct aortic valvular disease by cusp replacement with prosthetic cusps of Teflon cloth or by extensive debridement of calcific material from calcified valve cusps initially gave satisfactory results in some patients, but a high failure rate within 1 to 2 years led to abandonment of these techniques as soon as a satisfactory prosthetic valve became available.

Several modifications of metallic prostheses have been evaluated, but only two basic designs have proved durable, the original ball valve prosthesis and the tilting disc prosthesis. Currently, the durability of these two prostheses is excellent but the major limitation of all metallic prosthetic valves has been thromboembolism, partly controlled with permanent anticoagulation. Despite careful

anticoagulation, some thromboembolic events occur with a frequency of at least 1 to 2 percent per year.

With the significant hazard of thromboembolism, there has been a long and continued investigation of tissue prostheses that often do not require permanent anticoagulation and have a much lower frequency of thromboembolism. One of the most durable has been the homograft aortic valve, first investigated by Barratt-Boyes in 1962 and still used in their institution, using the technique of antibiotic preservation developed in 1968. Currently, about 80 percent of these prostheses are functioning well 10 years following operation.

Several other tissues were evaluated and subsequently discarded because of lack of durability, including autologous fascia lata; allograft dura mater valves; and formaldehyde preserved porcine valves. Subsequently, the gluteraldehyde preserved porcine valve was introduced by Carpentier in 1968 and has subsequently become the most widely used tissue prosthesis. Bovine pericardium, gluteraldehyde treated, was developed by Ionescu but has not been as popular as the porcine valve. At present, 5-year durability with porcine valves is near 95 percent but decreases to about 80 percent at 10 years, with a sharp rise in frequency of failure rate between the eighth and tenth years. Fifteen year data are not available, but the outlook is not encouraging.

ETIOLOGY. About one-half of patients operated upon will be found to have calcification of a congenitally malformed valve, usually a bicuspid valve. Usually, there is a history of negligible disability for decades until calcification has made the valve rigid, with the time interval varying widely from the fourth or even the seventh or eighth decade. In about one-third of patients rheumatic fever is apparently the basic cause.

The third major cause, increasing in frequency with aging of the population, seems to be simply acquired calcific aortic stenosis, a process of diffuse calcification developing in cusps that are neither congenitally malformed nor show any signs of previous inflammation. It is probably similar to calcification that sporadically develops in other soft tissues with aging but is seen more frequently in patients in their seventh and eighth decades.

PATHOLOGY. The pathologic features of diseased aortic valves reviewed at operation in 374 patients were described by Subramanian. A calcified congenital bicuspid valve represented about 46 percent of the cases. The bicuspid valve was fibrosed with deposits of calcium throughout the valve substance as well as on the aortic wall immediately above and the ventricular wall immediately below. Rheumatic aortic stenosis was present in about 35 percent of cases, with the basic findings of fusion of the commissures with supraimposed calcification. In about 10 percent of patients, the disease process was apparently "acquired aortic stenosis," consisting of three leaflets of equal size without significant commissural fusion but dense infiltration of the base of the cusps, rather than the free margins, with calcium.

In older patients coronary atherosclerosis is found in a significant percentage of patients, at least 30 to 50 percent. The frequency is such that routine coronary angiography should be performed upon patients over 40 years of age before operation. With rheumatic aortic disease, mitral stenosis or insufficiency is found in a high percentage of patients. This is as expected, as the aortic valve and the mitral valve are contiguous structures.

A normal aortic valve has a cross-sectional area of 2.5 to 3.5 cm depending upon body size. Moderately severe stenosis is present when the valve orifice has narrowed to about 1.0 cm; 0.8 cm is an approximate area where operation is usually indicated because of pathophysiologic abnormalities. This is a changing field, however, so operation at an earlier time may be recommended in the future because of persistent left ventricular dysfunction following operation in a significant percentage of patients. Cross-sectional areas as low as 0.4 to 0.6 cm^2 may be found in advanced disease, often with a systolic gradient of 100 mm or greater across the valve. Usually, at catheterization a gradient of at least 50 mm is found with significant stenosis.

The increased workload on the myocardium imposed by the stenosis results in progressive concentric ventricular hypertrophy but little dilatation. For this reason heart size may appear almost normal on the chest x-ray. The left ventricular diastolic pressure becomes elevated above the upper limit of normal of 12 mm as the left ventricle gradually fails. Left atrial pressure is not elevated until left ventricular failure develops, explaining the late onset of symptoms.

Myocardial ischemia, manifested as angina pectoris, is a common symptom. This apparently results from the combination of two factors, the increased left ventricular work and myocardial hypertrophy as well as the decreased cardiac output. This factor is apparently responsible for the well-known tendency of aortic stenosis to result in ''sudden death'' with very few premonitory symptoms.

CLINICAL MANIFESTATIONS. Symptoms. Characteristically, there is a long asymptomatic period, sometimes for 10 to 20 years. Classical physical findings may be present with slight dyspnea on exertion as the only symptom. Three symptoms are characteristic, any or all of which may be present: angina pectoris, syncope, or dyspnea. Sudden death, which accounts for 15 to 20 percent of fatalities from aortic stenosis, becomes much more of a threat once these symptoms are present. Syncope develops in about one-third of patients. This apparently is from decreased cerebral blood flow. In some patients, it may result after minimal effort, with little warning. In a small percentage of patients it may result from a conduction abnormality, apparently an intermittent heart block from involvement of the atrioventricular node by calcium spicules arising from the stenotic valve.

Angina pectoris develops in 30 to 40 percent of patients, a manifestation of myocardial ischemia. Probably these episodes are associated with ''silent'' episodes of muscle necrosis because some patients with surprisingly few symptoms are found to have large amounts of myocardium replaced by scar tissue.

The average life expectancy once angina or syncope has appeared is about 3 years.

Left ventricular failure is an even more ominous finding, as the life expectancy is slightly more than a year. Atrial fibrillation, a consequence of prolonged elevation of left atrial pressure, is similarly a grave event, as it indicates an advanced stage of left ventricular failure unless mitral valve disease is present.

The cardiac size is not increased, for the principal change in the left ventricle is concentric hypertrophy, not dilatation. The apical impulse has been described as a ''prolonged heave,'' not a ''forceful thrust,'' as is found with ventricular dilatation from aortic or mitral insufficiency. The peripheral pulse, similarly, is slow and prolonged, well illustrated with a pulse tracing recorded by arterial puncture as a dome-shaped peak in systole, contrasting sharply with the sharp systolic upstroke seen with aortic insufficiency.

LABORATORY STUDIES. The heart size is usually normal on x-ray. Calcification of the aortic valve is usually visible in patients over thirty-five years of age.

The electrocardiogram is not reliable because of the wide variation. In some patients left ventricular hypertrophy is evident, but in some seriously ill patients with severe aortic stenosis the electrocardiogram is virtually normal. The echocardiogram may supply supportive information by noting the increased thickness of the left ventricular wall and also confirming the presence of calcification in the aortic valve. Conduction abnormalities are frequent, apparently from spicules of calcium projecting into the conduction bundle located just beneath the base of the noncoronary sinus. Some patients develop complete heart block.

Cardiac catheterization readily confirms the diagnosis, both measuring the gradient and permitting calculation of the cross-sectional area of the valve. Gradients exceeding 50 mm are usually found with significant stenosis. A cross-sectional area near 0.8 to 1.0 cm^2 is considered the range at which operation should be routinely recommended, though this concept has frequently changed toward more liberal indications for operation as results with aortic valve replacement have improved. With the current interest in balloon valvuloplasty concepts as to what represents critical aortic stenosis will change even further. Probably the best method of following asymptomatic patients and determining the time for operation is evaluation of ventricular function with radionuclide studies once or twice a year, recommending operation when there is a decrease in ejection fraction with exercise, contrary to the normal response.

At catheterization coronary arteriography should be routinely done, for associated coronary disease is found in at least 30 to 50 percent of patients studied, the frequency increasing with the age of the patient studied. Concomitant mitral valve disease and left ventricular function can also be evaluated at catheterization. In some patients with a broad thick chest and distant heart sounds because of emphysematous lungs, the physical findings are deceptively minimal, with a faint unimpressive systolic murmur being the only initial abnormality found on physical examination. In such patients, echocardiography is helpful in deciding whether catheterization should be

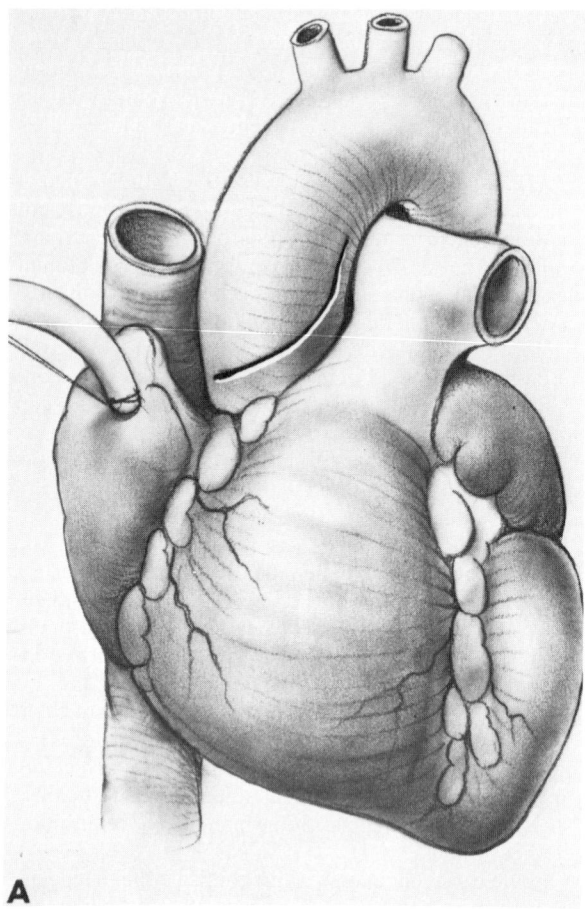

A

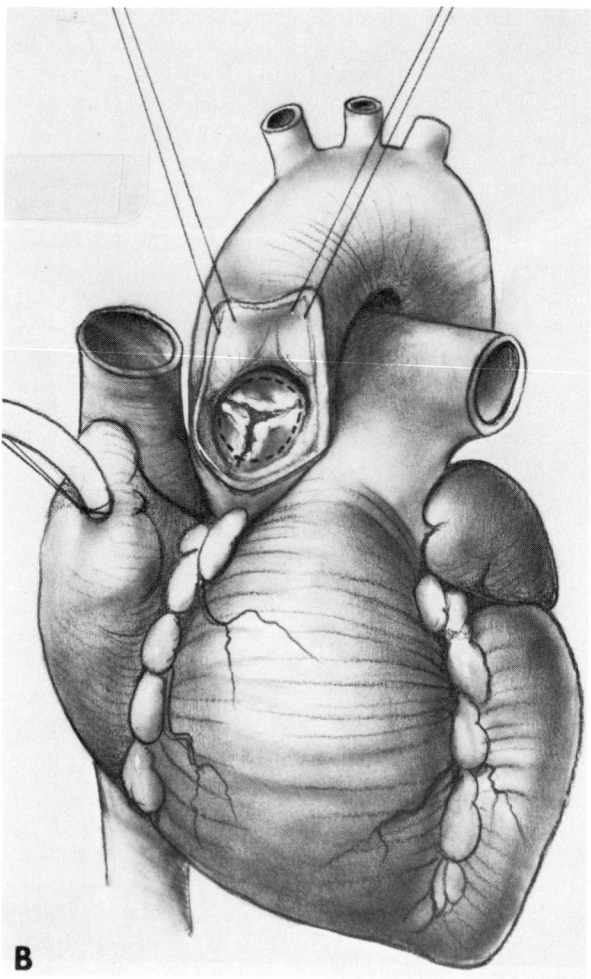

B

done, for a benign aortic systolic murmur becomes increasingly common in older age groups.

TREATMENT. Indications for Operation. In asymptomatic patients, the finding at catheterization of an aortic cross-sectional area of 0.8 cm is clearly an indication for operation. Sudden death remains a small but definite hazard in such patients, so operation should be clearly urged despite the well-being of the patient. In the presence of any of the classic three symptoms, angina, syncope, or dyspnea, operation should similarly be strongly recommended, especially if catheterization demonstrates an aortic valve area near 1.0 cm^2 or less. The frequency of sudden death increases sharply in symptomatic patients.

Technique of Operation (Fig. 19-16). The operative technique is a standard one, using a median sternotomy, cardiopulmonary bypass with hyperkalemic cardioplegia induced with cold blood. If aortic insufficiency is not present, cardiac arrest may be induced by clamping the aorta and infusing cold blood directly into the aortic root. Otherwise, the aorta is clamped and opened, following which cold blood is directly infused into the coronary ostia through a hand-held metallic or silastic coronary cannula. With direct ostial infusion, pressure and flow should be monitored, for excessive flows can induce myocardial edema. Once the heart has arrested, the calculated orifice pressure should be in the range of 50 to

Fig. 19-16. Insertion of aortic valve prosthesis. *A.* Cardiopulmonary bypass is instituted following cannulation of the right atrium with a single large cannula. Usually the ascending aorta is cannulated for arterial return (not shown). The aorta is opened with an oblique incision, initially begun about a centimeter above the right coronary artery. *B.* The heart is arrested with the cold blood potassium technique. Coronary perfusion is no longer employed. The aortic valve is then excised, with care to avoid the loss of any calcific fragments into the ventricle that might subsequently embolize. *C.* The Carpentier porcine prosthesis, which is normally used. *D.* Valve sutured in position. *E.* Final position of the valve. Care is taken, as the valve is tied in position, to seat the valve well below the coronary ostia, actually farther below than is shown here. *F.* The aortotomy is closed with a continuous synthetic suture.

60 mm, usually corresponding with a flow rate near 200 mL/min in a normal left coronary ostium and near 100/min in a right coronary. The flow rates, of course, vary with the size of the coronary arteries. A large amount of cold blood is used, serially monitoring the different areas of the myocardium to be certain that all areas are cooled below 15°C, requiring 1500 to 2000 mL of blood in some patients. Measuring myocardial temperature in at least four zones of the heart with a needle thermistor confirms equal infusion of cold blood. Subsequently, topical hypothermia is routinely employed with

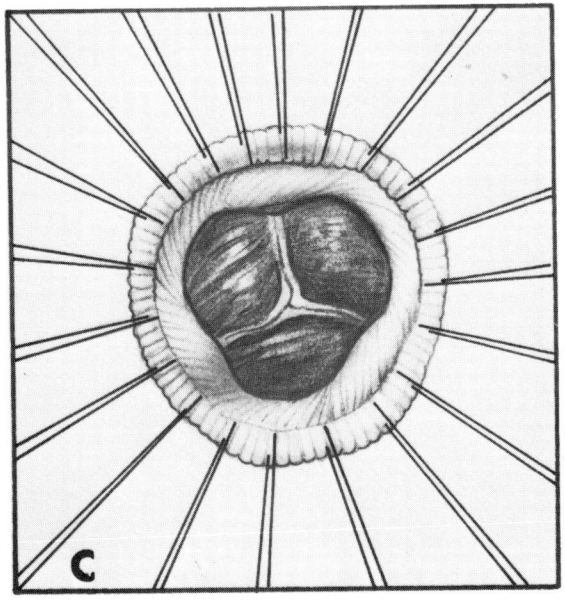

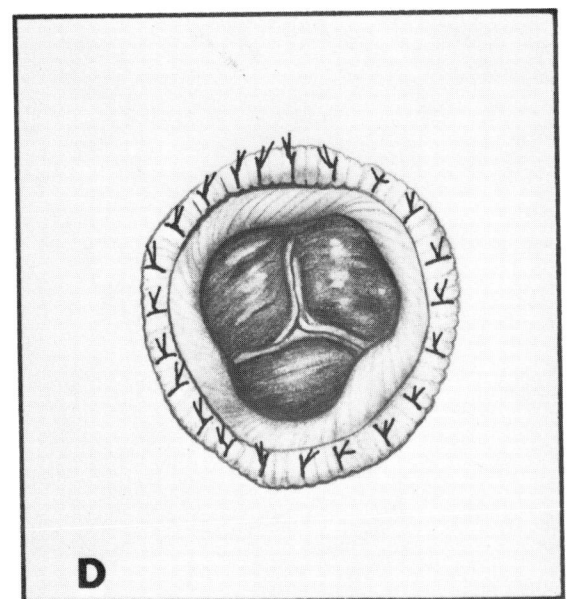

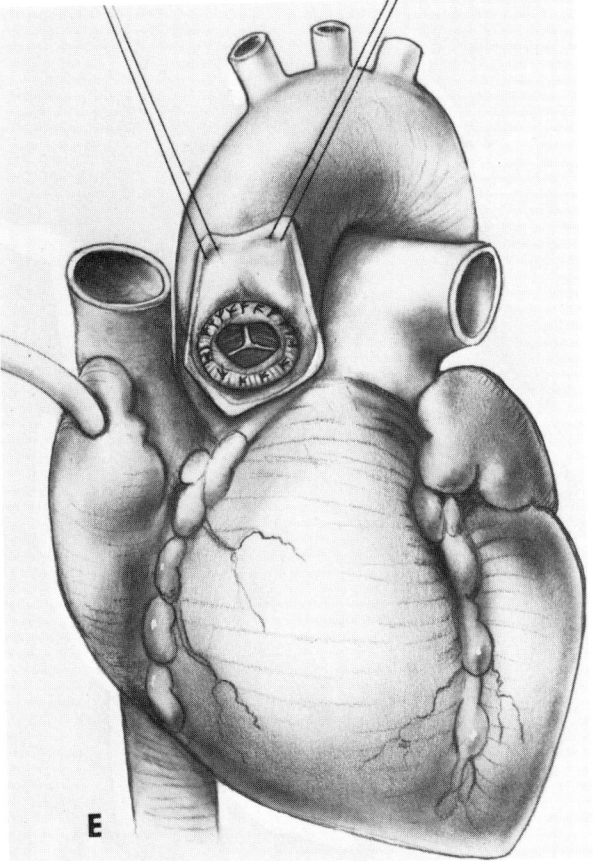

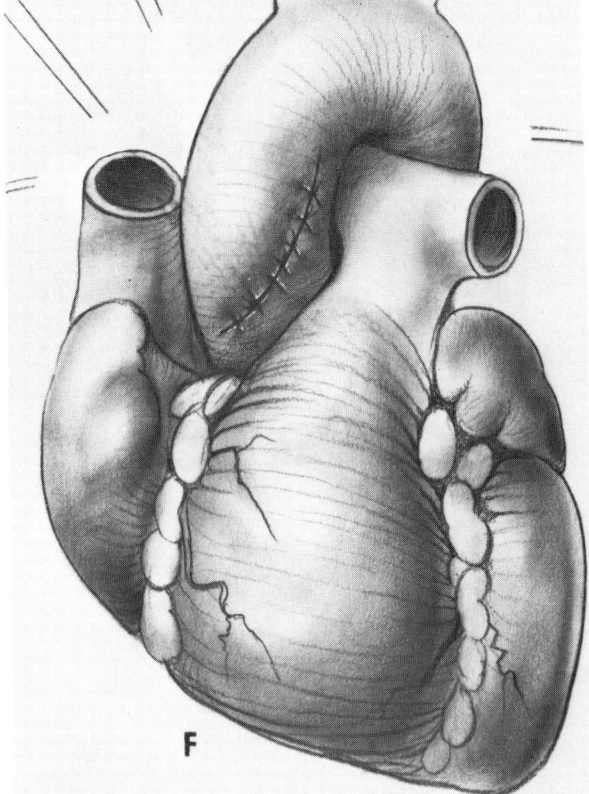

Fig. 19-16 *C,D,E,F.* Continued.

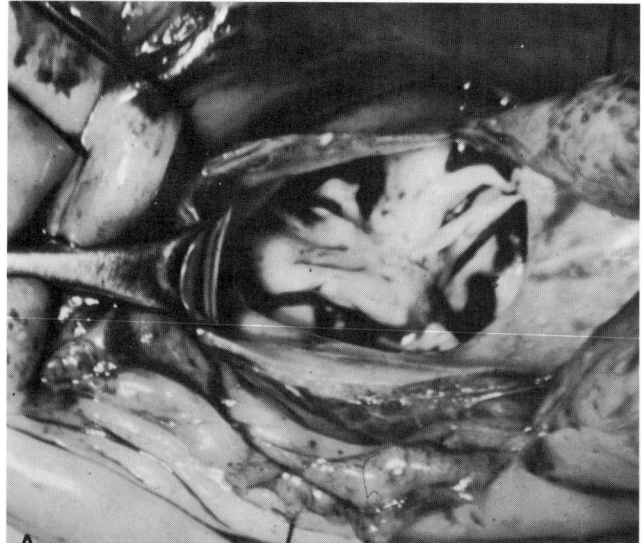 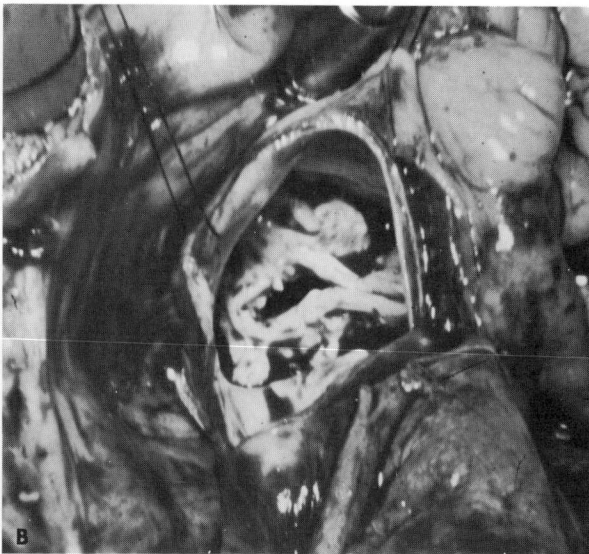

Fig. 19-17. *A.* Stenotic aortic valve exposed during cardiopulmonary bypass through a transverse aortotomy. The valve orifice has been almost obliterated by calcification and apposition of the cusps. *B.* Calcified aortic valve in another patient exposed through a transverse aortotomy. Fusion has produced a small eccentric rigid ostium that is both stenotic and insufficient.

Fig. 19-18. Calcified fragments removed with rongeurs from a patient with severe aortic stenosis. The multiplicity of such fragments emphasizes the grave risk of embolization of calcified material during aortic valve replacement with reduction of severe or fatal neurologic injury. Careful packing of the ventricle with gauze before removal of the calcified valve is essential.

large volumes of a cold electrolyte solution, both filling the pericardium and subsequently wrapping the heart in a laparotomy pad and using a constant infusion of cold fluid. The effectiveness of this method of myocardial preservation is extraordinary because the heart can be safely arrested for 3 h or longer, though this long period of time is seldom necessary.

This form of myocardial preservation provides a dry quiet operative field that has made aortic valve replacement a procedure with a remarkably low mortality and morbidity.

In almost all patients, aortic valve replacement is required (Fig. 19-17). A few elderly patients with a small hypoplastic annulus have been treated by debridement, as long as this does not produce insufficiency. This procedure had a disappointing frequency of recurrence within 3 to 5 years and should be considered a palliative procedure used only when special circumstances indicate prosthetic replacement would be hazardous or unsatisfactory. Great care is taken at operation to avoid losing any calcific fragments detached during removal of the valve that could subsequently be embolized (Fig. 19-18). A gauze pack is routinely placed in the ventricle before removal of the valve is begun. A number of maneuvers during the procedure (frequent removal of the pack, lavage of the ventricle, and keeping the ventricular cavity dry with a vent inserted through the left atrium across the mitral valve) make it possible to avoid emboli in the vast majority of patients.

The choice of a metallic or porcine prosthetic valve was discussed in the section on Mitral Valve Replacement, emphasizing that the surgeon should make a recommendation based upon the specific characteristics of the patient but also emphasizing that the patient should have the final decision. At NYU either the Bjork disc prosthesis or the Starr-Edwards ball valve prosthesis has been used, though recently a small number of the St. Jude metallic

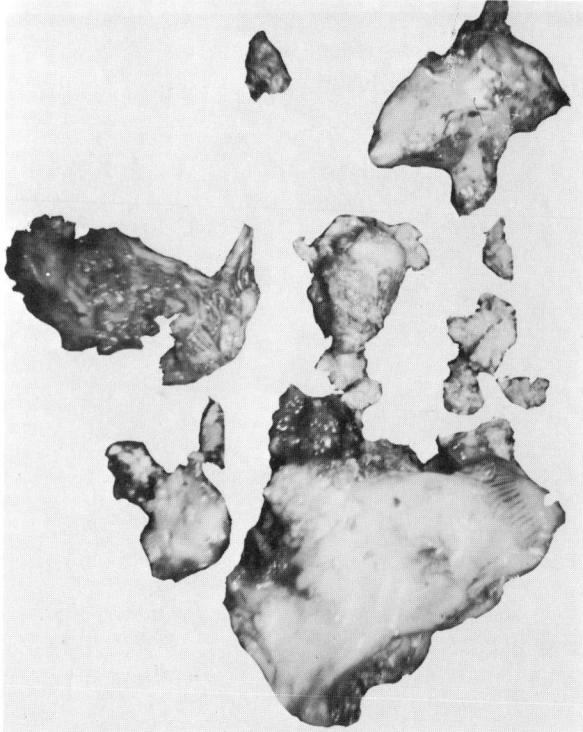

prostheses have been inserted. A larger cross-sectional area with less hemolysis can be obtained with a disc prosthesis than with a ball valve but has the hazard of the rare but catastrophic thrombosis of the prosthesis, virtually unknown with a ball valve prosthesis. A 23-mm Bjork prosthesis, with a cross-sectional area of 250 mm^2, is suitable for the majority of patients, using the 21-mm size for those with a small stature.

With tissue prostheses, the Carpentier porcine prosthesis is currently the most popular. There is less flexibility of valve size with porcine prostheses. A 23-mm valve is satisfactory for most patients under 140 lb, but a larger size is needed otherwise. The 21 mm is too small for all but patients of small stature. A pledgeted mattress suture technique is used routinely, probably unnecessary in many patients, but it clearly virtually eliminates the hazard of periprosthetic leaks (see Fig. 19-12).

The left ventricular-aortic systolic gradient is routinely measured following bypass. Depending upon the cardiac output, a gradient is rarely larger than 10 to 20 mm if a prosthesis of adequate size has been chosen.

Associated coronary disease is present in a large percentage of patients and is usually routinely bypassed at the time of operation.

POSTOPERATIVE CARE. Postoperative care is usually uneventful. Arrhythmias are among the more frequent complications, so 24-h monitoring of the cardiac rhythm with an oscilloscope is routinely done for 2 to 3 days. Pacemaker wires are routinely left in the right ventricle and atrium for 4 to 5 days.

Anticoagulant therapy is started 2 to 3 days following operation, keeping the prothrombin time near 20 s. The anticoagulation program routinely used for tissue valves and metallic valves is discussed under Mitral Valve Replacement.

Except for patients with serious preoperative ventricular dysfunction, patients become asymptomatic with a normal range of physical activity within 2 to 3 months following operation. Permanent periodic medical supervision, however, should be done for all patients because of the problems inherent with any prosthetic valve. Thromboembolism, anticoagulant hemorrhage, and endocarditis are the three principal complications of any patient with a prosthetic valve that requires periodic monitoring. With current prostheses and good anticoagulant therapy, thromboembolism occurs with a frequency of 1 to 2 percent per year in most reports, but fortunately most of these are small. Bloomfield reported an analysis of 540 patients with a disc or a porcine prosthesis inserted, finding no significant difference in the frequency of thromboembolism in patients with different prostheses. Endocarditis remains a grave hazard in any patient if a transient bacteremia occurs, such as a dental extraction or a cystoscopy.

Patients with significant cardiac enlargement and decreased ventricular function following operation should be monitored closely. How carefully this should be done is yet unclear because there remains a significant frequency of sudden death within the first 3 to 5 years following operation. A sobering point is the fact that there is a *greater* risk of death within the first 1 to 2 years following leaving the hospital than from the operation itself.

PROGNOSIS. The operative mortality from aortic valve replacement is at a remarkably low level, usually between 1 and 2 percent for uncomplicated patients, and seldom exceeding 10 percent, even with far advanced complex problems. Christakis et al. reported an analysis of over 40 variables influencing operative results. Operative death was usually a result of operative hemorrhage, or subsequent arrhythmias. Heart block has become uncommon.

Five-year survival in the usual patient is now near 85 to 90 percent. With severe impairment of ventricular function before operation, however, 5-year survival is much smaller, in the range of 60 to 70 percent, emphasizing the need for prompt operation in asymptomatic patients when signs of impaired ventricular function are found with laboratory studies.

Mortality in the first 5 years after operation is due to cardiac causes in at least 50 percent of cases; a significant number of deaths occur suddenly. This fact emphasizes that most patients are currently operated upon after significant permanent ventricular injury has occurred.

In the past 1 to 2 years there has been considerable interest in percutaneous balloon valvuloplasty as a palliative procedure. At present, all physiologic data would indicate that balloon valvuloplasty should be restricted to high-risk elderly patients in whom short-term palliation seems the best immediate goal. Its application to good-risk patients, knowing the excellent results with prosthetic replacement, would seem unwarranted, especially because of the insidious development of permanent injury to the left ventricle in patients who have few symptoms.

AORTIC INSUFFICIENCY

ETIOLOGY AND PATHOLOGY. A variety of diseases can produce aortic insufficiency. Inflammatory disease is a frequent cause. At present, perhaps the most common is bacterial endocarditis that has produced destruction or perforation of a valve cusp. Rheumatic fever was formerly the most common inflammatory disease but is steadily declining in frequency in the United States (Fig. 19-19). Syphilis is now a rarity.

Annular ectasia is an unusual type of collagen disease seen with increasing frequency as the average age of the population increases. This is seen in the most extreme form with the classic Marfan's syndrome with extensive cystic medial necrosis of the aorta, most probably in the ascending aorta. The aortic root gradually enlarges, starting in the sinuses of Valsalva and progressing to a discrete aneurysm in the ascending aorta. The pathology is unusual as the dilatation decreases and almost stops at the level of the innominate artery. The size and shape of the aneurysm is quite characteristic, resembling a truncated cone with the narrow apex near the level of the innominate artery. Aortic insufficiency results from dilatation of the aortic ring.

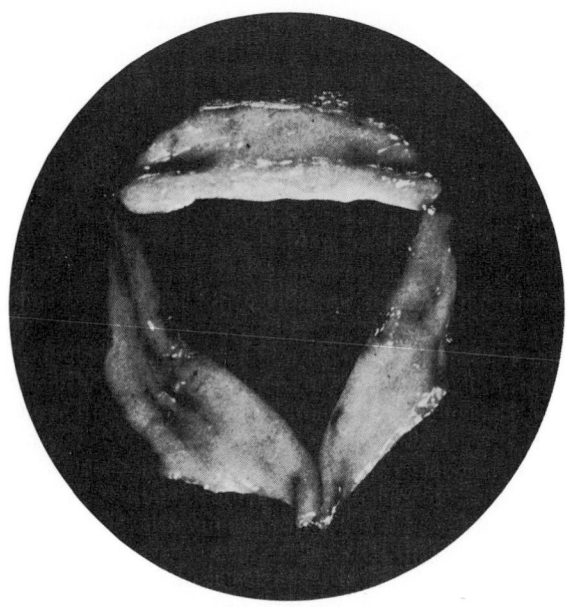

Fig. 19-19. Three aortic valve cusps removed from an eighteen-year-old boy with rheumatic aortic insufficiency. The contracted free margins of each cusp are clearly shown, illustrating the mechanism of production of aortic insufficiency from contracture and retraction of the free margins of the aortic valve cusps.

In less severe forms, there is simply a localized aneurysm in the ascending aorta with or without aortic insufficiency and no other signs of connective tissue disease; histologic examination of the excised aneurysm usually finds the characteristic cystic medial necrosis. Atherosclerotic aneurysms produce insufficiency by dilatation of the ring, though the histologic disease in the aorta is principally in the intima and media, contrasting markedly to that with cystic medial necrosis.

Another variant of collagen disease is the so-called floppy valve, a type of myxomatous degeneration of the valve that becomes elongated and sags into the ventricular lumen, often with no other histologic abnormality. The gross appearance suggests a variant of the more common mitral valve prolapse.

A dissecting aneurysm produces insufficiency by dissection of the aortic wall with detachment and prolapse of the valve cusps, usually the noncoronary. Congenital aortic insufficiency is rarely present at birth but may develop in older patients if stiffening and calcification of the malformed valve produces an insufficient rather than a stenotic valve.

The cardiac response to blood regurgitating into the left ventricle in diastole is an increase in left ventricular stroke volume, accomplished by dilatation of the heart. This results in gradual dilatation of the left ventricle, producing some of the largest hearts seen in clinical cardiology in neglected cases, with an apex of the left ventricle that extends almost to the chest wall and a cardiac weight approaching 1000 g. This cardiac response is quite different from that with aortic stenosis, where concentric muscular hypertrophy with little dilatation is the predominant change.

PATHOPHYSIOLOGY. Surprisingly large volumes of blood regurgitate into the ventricle with severe aortic insufficiency. This may be two or three times greater than the normal stroke volume of 60 to 75 mL. The compensatory ability of the heart is remarkable, as this increased workload may be tolerated for 10 to 15 years or longer. There is little elevation in left ventricular diastolic pressure until cardiac failure develops. There is no increase in left atrial pressure or pulmonary congestion until the onset of cardiac failure, so symptoms of pulmonary congestion appear only with advanced disease, completely contrasting to their early appearance with mitral stenosis. As severe cardiac failure progresses, left ventricular end-diastolic pressure rises to 20 to 30 mm. At this time, the clinical findings of insufficiency may actually decrease because the volume of blood regurgitating during diastole is less.

With marked dilatation of the left ventricle some mitral insufficiency may develop from dilatation of the annulus of the mitral valve. When a rheumatic history is present, it is difficult, or impossible, to determine from angiography whether the mitral insufficiency represents simple dilatation or rheumatic valvulitis. Mitral insufficiency resulting from simple dilatation of the mitral ring usually regresses satisfactorily following replacement of the aortic valve.

CLINICAL MANIFESTATIONS. Symptoms. There is naturally a wide variability in the rate of progression of symptoms, depending upon the degree of insufficiency. A symptom-free period of 8 to 10 years is common, but once symptoms appear, death has usually occurred in the past within 4 to 5 years. In general, citing statistics from the presurgical era, about 40 percent of patients died within 10 years, another 50 percent within 20 years. The terminal illness is usually progressive cardiac failure, as sudden death is much less common than with aortic stenosis.

Palpitation is one of the earliest, nonspecific symptoms, apparently arising from forceful contraction of the dilated left ventricle. Angina pectoris is a common symptom with advanced disease, usually with severe aortic incompetence in which the regurgitant flow is more than 50 percent of forward flow. Dyspnea with exertion appears fairly early during the progression of the disease and gradually increases in severity.

Physical Examination. Palpation readily discloses a prominent cardiac impulse, located downward and to the left of the normal location. The hallmark of aortic insufficiency is a high-pitched decrescendo diastolic murmur along the left sternal border, starting immediately after the second sound. The length of the murmur corresponds somewhat with the severity of the insufficiency. If the murmur is loudest to the right of the sternum, dilatation of the aortic ring, as in Marfan's syndrome, is likely. An ejection systolic murmur of moderate intensity is also frequent.

Examination of the peripheral arterial circulation usually finds several abnormalities. The pulse pressure is increased, partly from an increase in systolic pressure but principally from a decrease in diastolic pressure below the normal range near 80 mm. The diastolic pressure may be as low as 40 mm, but true diastolic pressure, measured by direct arterial puncture, is never less than 30 to 35 mmHg, even though on auscultation a diastolic pressure of 0 may be obtained from dilatation of peripheral arteries. The exact level of diastolic pressure does not closely correlate with the severity of the aortic insufficiency because of the influence of peripheral resistance. With vasodilatation, diastolic pressure may be low without marked regurgitation while conversely, with severe vasoconstriction, diastolic pressure may be elevated but severe regurgitation present.

Peripheral pulses are usually visible, forceful, and bounding. "Pistol shot" sounds are readily heard with the stethoscope over peripheral arteries. A wide variety of other auscultatory phenomena have been described, some over a century ago, all of which indicate vasodilatation and a hyperactive peripheral circulation.

LABORATORY STUDIES AND DIAGNOSIS. The chest x-ray shows enlargement of the left ventricle with the apex displaced downward and to the left. As the normal cardiothoracic ratio is 0.5 or less, asymptomatic patients may be periodically followed with biannual x-rays, as long as the heart size is normal. The size of the left ventricle can be evaluated more precisely with 2-D echocardiography. The electrocardiogram is normal early in the disease, but with cardiac enlargement signs of left ventricular hypertrophy become prominent. The cardiac rhythm usually remains sinus. Atrial fibrillation is uncommon before advanced disease is present and has an ominous prognosis unless it arises from another cause. Its presence from aortic insufficiency indicates an elevation of left ventricular end-diastolic pressure long enough to produce left atrial hypertrophy. Findings on cardiac catheterization are usually normal except for the visible reflux of dye from the aortic root into the ventricle with angiography. With cardiac failure, left ventricular end-diastolic pressure rises above the normal limit of 12 mm. Values of 15 to 20 are common with early cardiac decompensation.

It has long been recognized that postponing operation until symptoms are disabling is not satisfactory, for some patients with early onset of symptoms already have substantial enlargement of the left ventricle and die from cardiac failure in the next 3 to 5 years despite correction of the insufficiency. Hence, clinical investigation for some time has sought a laboratory measurement that would identify the proper time for operation. Simply using changes in the cardiothoracic ratio is also unsatisfactory, for cardiac enlargement to a cardiothoracic ratio of 0.6 or greater indicates advanced disease.

At present, demonstrating a fall in ejection fraction with exercise with radionuclide studies seems one of the best indicators that operation should be performed in asymptomatic patients. The reliability of this "early warning" signs is not yet proved by 5- to 10-year postoperative data because the key question is whether a significant number of patients will continue to die from left ventricular dysfunction in the first 5 years after operation. This has certainly been true in past years when less sensitive criteria were used. Henry assessed echocardiographic findings in this regard, and recommended operation when end-systolic dimension had enlarged to 55 mm.

TREATMENT. The principal decision with treatment is deciding when to operate. In some patients who are still alive despite advanced left ventricular dysfunction, with an end-diastolic pressure of 30 mm or above, uncertainty exists about how much improvement can be expected from aortic valve replacement, as it often appears that the principal symptoms are advanced left ventricular dysfunction (or "myopathy"). Available studies do not permit a precise decision in this regard. In even the most advanced cases, valve replacement can usually be performed with an operative risk less than 10 percent. As death is virtually a certainty unless operation is done, operation is rarely contraindicated on the basis of left ventricular dysfunction, carefully explaining to the patient and the family beforehand that the degree of improvement following operation may be limited and cannot be known with any certainty for at least 6 to 12 months following operation.

The operative technique, choice of valve, postoperative care, and prognosis are very similar to those discussed in the section on Aortic Stenosis.

TRICUSPID STENOSIS AND INSUFFICIENCY

ETIOLOGY. Organic disease of the tricuspid valve is almost always due to rheumatic fever. With the exception of septic endocarditis, usually in drug addicts, it virtually never occurs as an isolated lesion, but only in association with extensive disease of the mitral valve. With mitral disease the frequency of associated tricuspid disease is near 10 to 15 percent, although an incidence as high as 30 percent has been reported. Rarely, blunt trauma produces rupture of a papillary muscle or chordae with resulting tricuspid insufficiency.

Tricuspid insufficiency is the more common lesion encountered; pure stenosis is infrequent, as stenotic lesions usually have concomitant insufficiency. Functional tricuspid insufficiency is much more common than insufficiency from organic disease. It develops from dilatation of the tricuspid annulus and right ventricle as a result of pulmonary hypertension and right ventricular failure. These abnormalities, in turn, result from left ventricular failure and chronic elevation of left atrial pressure.

PATHOLOGY. With tricuspid stenosis the pathologic changes are similar to those found with the more familiar mitral stenosis. There is fusion of the commissures to form a small central opening 1 to 1.5 cm in diameter. As right atrial pressure is normally only 4 to 5 mmHg, significant tricuspid stenosis may be present with a valve orifice considerably larger than that seen with mitral stenosis.

Tricuspid insufficiency results from fibrosis and contraction of the valve leaflets, often in association with shortening and fusion of chordae tendineae. Calcification is rare. With dilation of the tricuspid annulus the valve leaflets appear stretched but otherwise are pliable and seemingly normal even though serious regurgitation is present. Apparently the dilatation and deformity of the annulus are irreversible. Valves with functional tricuspid insufficiency usually do not regain competency, even though the mitral valve disease is corrected and pulmonary artery systolic pressure returns to normal.

PATHOPHYSIOLOGY. With tricuspid stenosis the mean right atrial pressure is elevated to 10 to 20 mmHg. The higher pressures are found with a tricuspid valve orifice smaller than 1.5 cm^2 and a mean diastolic gradient between the atrium and ventricle of 5 to 15 mmHg. A gradient above 5 mm represents significant tricuspid stenosis. When mean right atrial pressure remains above 10 to 15 mmHg, edema and ascites usually appear.

A moderate degree of tricuspid insufficiency may be tolerated, with little adverse influence on the circulation except for a decrease in cardiac output. This is in striking contrast to mitral insufficiency, where the regurgitating blood and elevation of left atrial pressure produces pulmonary congestion. The unusual patient with isolated tricuspid insufficiency produced by a traumatic injury may do well for years, as the only physiologic disturbance is elevation of venous pressure and a decrease in cardiac output. The purest example of the surprising tolerance for tricuspid insufficiency is seen in the drug addict with septic endocarditis who has been treated by total excision of the tricuspid valve. Some, but not all, patients tolerate absence of the tricuspid valve with total tricuspid insufficiency for months or years.

CLINICAL MANIFESTATIONS. The symptoms and signs of tricuspid valve disease are similar to those of right heart failure resulting from mitral valve disease. These all result from chronic elevation of right atrial pressure above 5 to 10 mm. The most familiar ones are edema, ascites, and hepatomegaly. Characteristic murmurs are present and may be associated with hepatic pulsations. As similar findings result from right heart failure without tricuspid disease, the concomitant presence of tricuspid disease in the patient in heart failure with mitral valve disease may be easily overlooked.

Physical Examination. The characteristic murmur of tricuspid stenosis is best heard as a diastolic murmur at the lower end of the sternum. It is a low-pitched murmur of medium intensity and can easily be overlooked, as it is well localized at the lower end of the sternum. During inspiration the intensity of the murmur increases as the volume of blood returning to the heart is temporarily increased by an increase in intrathoracic negative pressure. Tricuspid insufficiency produces a prominent systolic murmur at the lower end of the sternum and also at the cardiac apex, where it may be confused with the systolic murmur of mitral insufficiency. The murmur is often seen in association with an enlarged pulsating liver and prominent engorged peripheral veins. A prominent jugular pulse, especially when the cardiac rhythm is sinus, may be the best clue to unsuspected tricuspid disease.

LABORATORY STUDIES. The x-ray will show enlargement of the right atrium and right ventricle. Prominent P waves may be visible on the electrocardiogram if a sinus rhythm is present. Echocardiography will confirm enlargement of the right atrium and ventricle and may be helpful with Doppler studies in recognizing tricuspid in-

sufficiency. Cardiac catheterization and angiography are required to confirm the diagnosis. Tricuspid stenosis can be confirmed by demonstrating a diastolic gradient between the atrium and ventricle above 4 to 5 mm. As the gradient is small, precise measurements are essential. Cineangiography is the best method for detecting insufficiency but is not always satisfactory because the catheter through which the dye is injected is lying across the tricuspid orifice and may deform the valve leaflets.

Carpentier has cautioned that palpation at the time of operation may be unreliable. If the blood volume and cardiac output are adequate, palpation has been quite reliable in our experience. It should be emphasized that the regurgitant jet is quite different from that present with mitral disease, as the pressures are lower. The jet is of lower volume and much more diffuse.

TREATMENT. Usually the surgical decision about tricuspid insufficiency is a tentative one until the valve is examined at operation. Mild degrees of tricuspid insufficiency are usually left alone, especially in the absence of pulmonary hypertension. The degree of hypertrophy of the right atrial wall is a helpful guide, as the absence of significant right atrial hypertrophy indicates that chronic severe elevation of right atrial pressure has not been present.

With significant tricuspid insufficiency, annuloplasty or tricuspid replacement should usually be done. Precise data confirming the importance of correcting the tricuspid disease in association with mitral valvular disease are virtually impossible to obtain because the hemodynamic changes following correction of the mitral disease far overshadow those of tricuspid disease. However, the significant improvement in cardiac output in the rare patient with isolated tricuspid insufficiency following trauma is the best example of the magnitude of benefit that may be achieved.

In the majority of patients seen clinically, tricuspid disease is due to dilatation of the annulus, as evidenced not only by the large annulus but also by the absence of fibrotic changes in the leaflets. Usually, the leaflets appear entirely normal. Virtually all such patients can be treated by an annuloplasty. For over a decade at NYU a simple posterior leaflet annuloplasty as described by Boyd from our institution in 1974 has been quite satisfactory. The Carpentier ring annuloplasty is a bit more complicated with slight risk of heart block. Excellent results have been reported by Carpentier et al. and by Kirklin et al. The DeVega annuloplasty (a purse-string suture technique) has been widely used, but at least two groups have described a significant late failure rate. In our experience, the posterior leaflet annuloplasty is simpler and safer in the absence of significant leaflet disease or pulmonary hypertension.

In the minority of patients with tricuspid stenosis from commissural fusion, a commissurotomy may be performed. This may often be combined with annuloplasty.

Valve replacement is seldom necessary except in patients with significant pulmonary hypertension and leaflet disease precluding annuloplasty. In a 1986 report of experiences with 151 valve replacements and 63 valve repairs, the prosthetic valve subsequently had to be replaced in 20

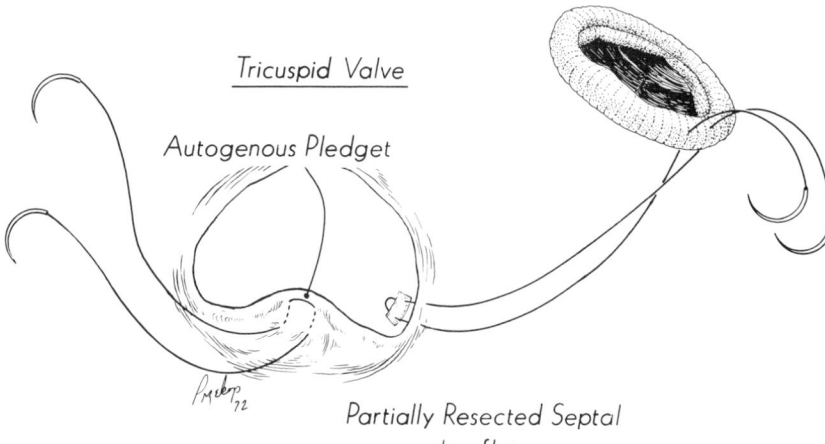

Tricuspid Valve

Autogenous Pledget

Partially Resected Septal Leaflet

Fig. 19-20. Technique for suturing the tricuspid valve prosthesis with Dacron pledgets seated below the tricuspid annulus. The pledgets are used in all areas except the area of the partially resected septal leaflet, which is used as an autogenous pledget to avoid the conduction bundle and the production of heart block.

patients, principally because of progressive thrombosis. These included both ball valves and disc valves. Significant 10-year durability data with porcine prostheses are not yet available, though durability should be higher than the 85 to 90 percent 10-year durability with mitral or aortic porcine prostheses, where higher pressures are present.

Barratt-Boyes et al. preferred an aortic or pulmonary homograft valve, citing experiences with 75 patients, 70 percent of whom were free of valve dysfunction 8 years following operation.

The ball valve prosthesis was initially widely used for tricuspid replacement, but reports of late disastrous thrombotic encapsulation of the cage and ball led to a search for a better prosthesis. The Bjork disc prosthesis has been the preferred mechanical low-profile prosthesis, but the frequency of thrombotic occlusion seems even higher than with the ball valve. At present, any type of prosthesis may ultimately require reoperation, either for thrombosis with a mechanical prosthesis or for biologic deterioration with a porcine prosthesis.

When the prosthetic valve is inserted, particular care is required along the septal leaflet where the conduction bundle is located between the coronary sinus and the ventricular septum. In this area sutures should be placed through the base of the septal leaflet to avoid injury to the conduction bundle (Fig. 19-20). Nevertheless, a heart block may develop sometime after operation, probably a result of an inflammatory reaction stimulated by the prosthetic valve ring.

In the unfortunate patient with septic tricuspid endocarditis, almost always a drug addict, Arbulu demonstrated that total excision of the tricuspid valve *without replacement* could be tolerated. This approach permitted removal of all infected tissue without insertion of a foreign body, increasing the likelihood of cure of the endocarditis with antibiotics. Of the 50 long-term survivors, 11

subsequently required prosthetic replacement. The 15-year survival in this group was near 63 percent, and the majority of late deaths was due to recurrent drug addiction. Stern and Frater questioned this approach, stating that there was little proof that insertion of a prosthetic valve was associated with an immediate high frequency of recurrent endocarditis if the proper antibiotic was given for the infectious organism present.

Operative risk for isolated tricuspid disease is very small, 1 to 2 percent. In previous years, the reported mortality for patients undergoing tricuspid surgery in conjunction with aortic or mitral surgery was high, 25 to 40 percent, primarily because the presence of tricuspid disease represented far advanced cardiac failure. An additional cause of high mortality was probably inadequate myocardial preservation of the hypertrophied right ventricle. With present techniques, however, tricuspid surgery seems to add little increased risk to concomitant aortic or mitral surgery.

PROGNOSIS. Starr reported that 5-year survival was 59 percent, 10-year survival 36 percent with mechanical prostheses, and virtually identical with repair techniques, indicating that long-term prognosis is principally determined by residual myocardial function. Peterffy described hemodynamic findings months or years following tricuspid valve replacement or repair. Higher pressures were found in patients with a tricuspid replacement with a disc prosthesis; postoperative right atrial pressure averaged 11 mm, rising to 17 with exercise. With repair, lower pressures were found, 7 mm at rest, 14 with exercise.

MULTIVALVULAR HEART DISEASE

With rheumatic heart disease, more than one cardiac valve is frequently involved. Prominent signs of disease in one valve can readily mask disease in others. Echocardiography is a valuable noninvasive technique for suggesting that multivalvular disease is present. An important principle at cardiac catheterization with cineangiography is to evaluate all cardiac valves with a combined right and left heart catheterization. With present operative techniques, usually disease in all involved valves can be corrected at operation. Tricuspid disease is one of the most difficult to recognize. This is one of the great advantages of the sternotomy incision, routinely palpating the tricuspid valve with a finger introduced into the right atrial cavity before bypass is started.

MITRAL STENOSIS AND AORTIC STENOSIS. In this type of multivalvular disease the clinical signs of mitral stenosis with pulmonary congestion overshadow those of aortic stenosis because the volume of blood entering the left ventricle is restricted by the stenotic mitral valve. An aortic valve gradient of only 20 to 30 mm may be present if cardiac output is low, but calculation of the cross-sectional area of the aortic valve will precisely diagnose the degree of stenosis. If uncertainty remains, the valve can be examined directly at operation.

MITRAL STENOSIS AND AORTIC INSUFFICIENCY. If aortic insufficiency is prominent, mitral stenosis can easily be overlooked because the classic diastolic rumble of mitral stenosis is overshadowed by the prominent aortic murmurs. Precise cardiac catheterization should make the diagnosis. If there is any uncertainty at operation, the mitral valve should be explored by incising the left atrium.

A difficult clinical problem exists with severe mitral stenosis and minimal to moderate aortic insufficiency. The reduced flow through the mitral valve minimizes the effect of the aortic insufficiency, which may become more troublesome following correction of the mitral stenosis. A final decision must often be made at operation, noting the degree of left ventricular hypertrophy that is present.

MITRAL STENOSIS AND TRICUSPID DISEASE. Tricuspid disease is virtually always associated with severe mitral disease. As physical findings may not be prominent, the *routine palpation of the tricuspid valve* at the time of any mitral valve operation is most important.

AORTIC DISEASE AND FUNCTIONAL MITRAL INSUFFICIENCY. With dilatation of the left ventricle from cardiac failure from aortic insufficiency, dilatation of the mitral annulus can produce functional mitral insufficiency without intrinsic valvular disease. A final decision must usually be made at operation, opening the left atrium and inspecting the mitral valve. Preoperative angiography unfortunately is often indeterminate about the importance of "moderate" mitral insufficiency. With the reliability of the mitral valve reconstructive techniques, especially the annuloplasty ring, significant mitral insufficiency can usually be corrected by reconstruction rather than concomitant mitral valve replacement. Prosthetic valve replacement is probably only necessary in the rare instance of severe leaflet disease, a decision easily made when the valve is inspected at operation.

TRIVALVULAR DISEASE. Severe trivalvular disease is now a rarity because of the decreasing frequency of rheumatic fever. In some patients with advanced heart failure and pulmonary hypertension from aortic and mitral disease, significant tricuspid insufficiency is present from dilatation of the annulus. In such patients tricuspid annuloplasty is usually successful. Replacement of all three

cardiac valves with mechanical prostheses is now seldom necessary.

CARDIAC TRAUMA

Penetrating Trauma

In 1896, Rehn first successfully sutured a stab wound of the heart, but for decades this remained an isolated historic achievement. The hazards of thoracotomy were the principal reason that the 1943 contribution of Blalock and Ravitch, when they introduced pericardial aspiration as a method of treatment for tamponade following penetrating injuries of the heart, was such a significant one. They recognized that many patients survived because the development of tamponade prevented exsanguination. Aspiration remained a definitive and reasonably effective form of therapy for tamponade for over 25 years, but with further advances in therapy has been almost completely replaced for the past two decades with prompt thoracotomy. Aspiration is now used primarily for resuscitation as a lifesaving method of treatment. Removal of as little as 15 to 20 mL of blood by subxyphoid aspiration may abort impending cardiac arrest.

ETIOLOGY AND PATHOLOGY. The two life-threatening problems are tamponade and hemorrhage. Tamponade develops rapidly as the normal pericardium can accommodate only 100 to 250 mL of blood. Small wounds, such as those from an icepick or a knife, often produce tamponade because the laceration in the pericardium is small. Larger wounds, produced by bullets or large knives, threaten immediate death from exsanguination as blood can be expelled through the pericardial laceration into the pleural cavity. The right ventricle, which constitutes most of the anterior portion of the heart, is the cardiac chamber most frequently injured.

TREATMENT. The dominant problem may be hemorrhage, tamponade, or both. The patient should obviously be taken to the operating room as quickly as possible, which will vary with the circumstances and the hospital environment. As stated by Kirklin and Barratt Boyes, "No more than 5 min need elapse between admission and the patient's transfer to the operating table." Rapid transfusion of fluids, intubation, and immediate transportation to the operating room are the key principles in treatment.

Emergency room thoracotomy is frequently done in some institutions, including Bellevue Hospital. It may be lifesaving in some patients with agonal respirations or cardiac arrest but is probably futile with established cardiac arrest and dilated pupils indicating brain injury. After emergency thoracotomy temporary hemostasis may permit restoration of cardiac function long enough for transportation to the operating room. Ivatory reported experiences with emergency room thoracotomy in 22 patients without detectable vital signs. Cardiac function was restored in 16 of these, eight of whom eventually recovered without objective neurologic injury.

An emergency unsterile thoracotomy can be quickly done in less than 1 to 2 min by a trained surgeon. With the patient in a slight left anterolateral position, a curved skin incision is made beneath the left nipple to parallel the intercostal spaces. The fourth or fifth intercostal space should be entered, as the pectoralis major arises from the third to the fifth ribs and causes troublesome bleeding with a higher incision. Once the pleural space is entered, the intercostal incision can be quickly completed with scissors, or the fingers separating the ribs, carrying the incision anteriorly beyond the angle of the rib, almost to the sternum. Unless the incision is long enough, exposure is seriously hampered. Subsequent wound infection following an unsterile thoracotomy is surprisingly rare, less than 5 percent.

The key to cardiac tamponade, the other major life-threatening problem, is simply considering the diagnosis in any patient with hypotension and a penetrating thoracic wound. The classic triad emphasized by Beck decades ago was the combination of hypotension, elevated venous pressure, and a small quiet heart. Only a few conditions, such as cardiac failure or pulmonary embolism, produce the combination of hypotension and elevated venous pressure. When the diagnosis is first suspected, pericardial aspiration, or subxyphoid exploration, should be promptly done. A most dramatic experience is to remove as little as 10 to 15 mL of blood from the pericardium of a moribund patient with an imperceptible blood pressure and be rewarded with a prompt rise in blood pressure to 70 to 80 mm and a return of consciousness. Isaacs demonstrated the exponential rise in intrapericardial pressure as fluid is added. Elevation of intrapericardial pressure above 15 to 17 mm virtually stopped cardiac output unless venous pressure was elevated by infusion of fluids.

In some patients with severe tamponade, an unusual degree of restlessness is present with the patient wildly rolling about. This contrasts strikingly with the usual quiet apathetic state of patients in hemorrhagic shock. This may be due to severe cerebral anoxia, resulting from the combination of arterial hypotension and venous hypertension.

Operative Therapy. In the operating room a median sternotomy is the preferred incision, as it provides ready access to all chambers of the heart. An anterior thoracotomy can be made more rapidly but does not give good exposure of the right heart.

When circumstances permit, a pump oxygenator, or a simpler apparatus for autotransfusion of blood, should be available. This is not often needed, as most cardiac injuries permitting survival long enough to reach the operating room can be controlled by digital pressure and suturing.

Ventricular lacerations can usually be controlled by digital pressure and then sutured with continuous or interrupted mattress sutures. Atrial lacerations may be initially controlled with tangential application of vascular or wide Allis clamps.

Following control of the cardiac laceration, a search should routinely be made for other intrathoracic injuries. Laceration of the internal mammary artery is a common associated injury. Injuries to intracardiac structures, such as a cardiac valve or the ventricular septum, rarely occur but can be treated at a later time.

Following repair of the cardiac laceration and correction of hypovolemia, recovery is uneventful in most patients. Wound infection, pericarditis, or recurrent bleeding are all uncommon.

Blunt Trauma

Blunt cardiac trauma usually results from automobile accidents, such as a "steering wheel" injury or some similar form of severe blunt injury to the chest wall. Probably 900,000 cases of cardiac trauma occur annually in the United States. Many of these are instantaneously fatal. The direct injury may cause an underlying cardiac contusion. Alternately, when the heart is suddenly compressed, intracardiac pressure apparently becomes high enough to rupture different cardiac structures, such as the ventricular septum, the chordae of the mitral or tricuspid valves, or the free cardiac wall. Injuries of this severity are usually fatal. Only rarely is a patient seen with a laceration of a tricuspid valve or the ventricular septum.

The myocardial contusion varies from simple subepicardial hemorrhage to a full-thickness myocardial contusion, which rarely progresses to an infarction.

The clinical picture is that of pericarditis with a pericardial effusion and chest pain. The classic picture of a myocardial infarction or cardiac failure is uncommon.

The electrocardiogram is a nonspecific diagnostic guide, as false-positive and false-negative results are common. The best diagnostic evaluation is done by a combination of serial measurement of myocardial enzymes, combined with 2-D echocardiography. Frazee et al. summarized experiences with 291 patients with thoracic trauma. Twenty percent of the group (58) had elevated cardiac enzymes (CPK-MB) within 24 h. Of this group, 60 percent were classified as simply "cardiac concussion," as the 2-D echocardiogram was normal. The remaining 40 percent were diagnosed as cardiac contusion, as abnormalities were visible on the echocardiogram. Patients with an abnormal echocardiogram were treated like patients with a subendocardial myocardial infarction, as arrhythmias frequently occurred in this group. The majority recovered within a short period of time.

Cardiac injury almost never produces permanent cardiac disability. From a physiologic standpoint, serious cardiac disability does not occur until more than 30 to 50 percent of the myocardium has been lost. An injury severe enough to produce irreversible loss of myocardium of this extent is almost always fatal.

Foreign Bodies

The report by Harken in 1946 is a classic. It describes the successful removal of 56 intramyocardial foreign bodies during World War II without a single death. About two-thirds of the removed foreign bodies had bacteria on culture.

In general, foreign bodies greater than 1 cm usually cause complications, such as pericardial effusion or pericarditis, but smaller foreign bodies are well tolerated. In 1966, Bland and Beebe reported a 20-year follow-up of 40 patients from World War II who had small foreign bodies in the heart. Although major complications did not occur, most patients had a permanent emotional disability, apparently from anxiety associated with the uncertain prognosis of a foreign body in the heart. The difficulty with removing small asymptomatic foreign bodies was emphasized in the report; elective removal was attempted in eight patients, but successfully completed in only three.

Harrison and Sabiston described the intraoperative use of echocardiography with a hand-held probe. After palpation of the heart failed to reveal the location of the bullet, echocardiography identified the fragment, over 1 cm beneath the epicardial surface and about 3 cm from the entrance site. Precise location permitted the performance of a limited ventriculotomy with successful removal of the bullet.

The safety of cardiopulmonary bypass, combined with the use of echocardiography, would suggest that all intramyocardial foreign bodies should be surgically removed. Foreign bodies that are within the cardiac cavities, usually dislodged from a complication of intravascular catheters, can be removed with a percutaneous catheter method. Uflacker et al. reported the successful percutaneous removal of a foreign body in 20 patients.

CARDIAC TUMORS

Metastatic neoplasms are the most common cardiac neoplasms, occurring in 4 to 12 percent of the autopsies performed on patients with neoplastic disease. The most frequent primary cardiac tumor is *myxoma,* comprising 50 to 60 percent of all primary cardiac neoplasms. *Sarcomas* are found in 20 to 25 percent of cases, and *rhabdomyomas* in 10 to 15 percent. Benign but extremely rare neoplasms include fibromas, angiomas, lipomas, teratomas, and cysts.

The clinical significance of cardiac tumors is similar to that of many other cardiac lesions in that accurate diagnosis and successful treatment first became possible with the development of extracorporeal circulation. Before 1950 cardiac tumors were usually first diagnosed at autopsy. Several excellent reviews have previously summarized the pathologic findings and clinical features. A classic analysis was published by Yater in 1931, and a detailed French monograph was published by Mahaim in 1945. In 1949 Whorton described the clinical findings in 100 sarcomas of the heart, and in 1951 Prichard reviewed 150 lesions, most of which were metastatic in origin.

In 1953 Steinberg et al. reported the diagnosis of an atrial myxoma in three patients by angiocardiography. The first successful removal of an atrial myxoma was performed by Crafoord in 1954, using extracorporeal circulation. Other successful reports quickly followed, and in 1967 Thomas et al. stated that there had been 126 attempted excisions of atrial myxomas, either planned or inadvertent, 85 of which had been successful.

The use of echocardiography, first reported in 1968, was a major diagnostic advance. 2-D echocardiography is now the keystone of diagnostic studies. Fyke reported 30 cardiac tumors seen following the introduction of 2-D echocardiography. Twenty-five were operated on based solely on the echocardiographic examination.

Myxoma

Sixty to seventy-five percent of cardiac myxomas develop in the left atrium, almost always from the atrial septum near the fossa ovalis. Most other myxomas develop in the right atrium. Less than 20 have been found in either the right or left ventrile. The curious predilection for a myxoma to develop from the rim of the fossa ovalis in the left atrium has been studied by several observers, but a satisfactory explanation has not been found.

Myxomas are apparently true neoplasms, although their similarity to an organized atrial thrombus led to considerable debate at one time about whether they represented a true neoplasm or not. Their occurrence in the absence of other organic heart disease, histochemical studies demonstrating mucopolysaccharide and glycoprotein, and a distinct histologic appearance all indicate that myxomas are true neoplasms. In 1976 Dang and Hurley reported 19 recurrences of a myxoma following surgical excision in 16 patients, conclusively establishing the low-grade malignant potential of the tumor.

PATHOLOGY. The tumors are usually polypoid, projecting into the atrial cavity from a 1- to 2-cm stalk attached to the atrial septum. The maximum size ranges from 0.5 to greater than 10.0 cm. Only the superficial layer of the septum is involved; invasion of the septum does not occur. Some myxomas grow slowly, for a few patients have had symptoms for many years. There is no tendency to invade other areas of the heart; distant metastases have rarely been reported. The friable consistency of a myxoma is of particular significance, for fatal emboli have occurred following digital manipulation of the tumor at operation.

Histologically, a myxoma is covered with endothelium and composed of a myxomatous stroma with large stellate cells mixed with fusiform or multinucleated cells. Mitoses are infrequent. Lymphocytes and plasmacytes are regularly found. Hemosiderin, a result of hemorrhage into the tumor, is also common.

PATHOPHYSIOLOGY. A myxoma may cause no difficulty until it grows large enough to obstruct the flow of blood through either the mitral or tricuspid valve, or fragments to produce peripheral emboli. The frequency of embolization, estimated to occur in 40 to 50 percent of patients, is not surprising, for an astonishing degree of to-and-fro motion of a myxoma, swinging on a small pedicle with each cardiac contraction, may be seen with echocardiography or angiography. Intermittent acute obstruction of the mitral orifice has been reported to produce syncope or even sudden death. Some myxomas produced generalized symptoms resembling an autoimmune disorder, including fever, weight loss, clubbing, myalgia, and arthralgia. Possibly such patients have an immune reaction to the neoplasm.

CLINICAL MANIFESTATIONS. Symptoms may be those of mitral valve obstruction, resembling mitral stenosis, except for acute exacerbations, presumably due to transient lodging of the myxoma in the mitral orifice; peripheral embolization; or generalized autoimmune symptoms described in the previous section. The diagnosis is made in many patients following an embolic episode, either from histologic examination of the surgically removed embolus or as a result of subsequent diagnostic studies to determine the reason for embolism. The precision and reliability of 2-D echocardiography has greatly simplified diagnosis. Angiography is optional unless additional disease is suspected. Computerized axial tomography has been reported to be helpful with small tumors.

Abnormalities are usually found on examination of the heart and also on the electrocardiogram, but these are not diagnostic.

TREATMENT. Operation should be performed as soon as possible after the diagnosis has been established because a disabling or fatal cerebral embolus is an ever-present hazard.

A sternotomy incision is used. Once extracorporeal circulation has been established, ventricular fibrillation is induced and the aorta clamped to avoid embolism. Palpation is avoided. The right atrium is opened and the fossa ovalis incised to expose the stalk of the myxoma. The left atrium is then opened in the interatrial groove. With the myxoma visualized, the segment of atrial septum from which the tumor arises is excised, after which the myxoma is removed through the incision in the left atrium (Fig. 19-21). The defect in the atrial septum is closed with a small patch. The technique is simple and permits exploration of both atria and ventricles.

A few cases of recurrent myxoma have been reported, some of which have been successfully operated upon. Initially these were thought to represent inadequate excision of the site of origin, but some have recurred at more remote sites in the atrium, indicating the multipotential source of these unusual neoplasms. Hence, it seems prudent to perform periodic echocardiography routinely for 1 to 2 years following operation.

Larrieu et al. described experiences with 18 myxomas in a series of 25 cardiac tumors over a period of 24 years. Fyke et al. treated 21 patients with mitral myxoma in the first 7 years following the introduction of 2-D echocardiography. Kirklin-Barrat Boyce summarized reports of 202 surgically removed myxomas, with 10 operative deaths (5 percent); 160 were in the left atrium, 33 in the right, 2 in both atria, 3 in the right ventricle, and 4 in the left ventricle.

Metastatic Neoplasms

Cardiac metastases have been found in 4 to 12 percent of autopsies performed for neoplastic disease. Although they have occurred from primary neoplasms developing in almost every known site of the body, the most frequent have been carcinoma of the lung or breast, melanoma, and lymphoma. Cardiac metastases involving only the heart are very unusual. Similarly, a solitary cardiac metastasis is infrequent; usually there are multiple areas of

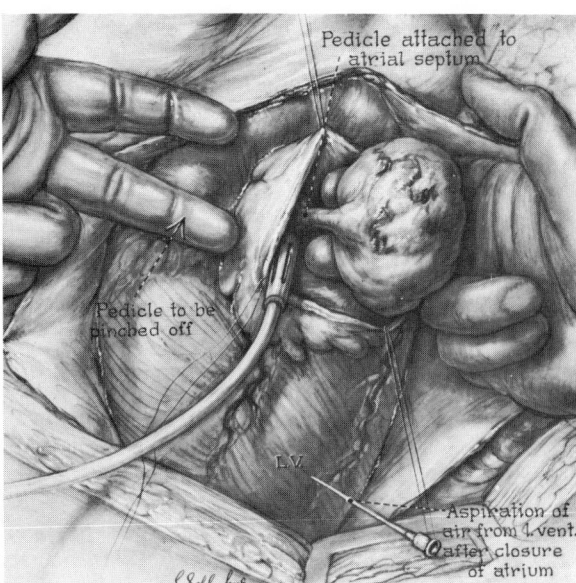

Fig. 19-21. Pedunculated atrial myxoma removed at operation in 1957. The patient has remained free of cardiac symptoms since that time. (From: *Bahnson HT, Spencer FC, Andrus EC: Diagnosis and treatment of intracavitary myxomas of the heart. Ann Surg 145:915, 1957, by permission of Lippincott, Philadelphia.*)

involvement. Cardiac involvement is particularly common with leukemia or lymphoma, developing in 25 to 40 percent of patients. All areas of the heart are involved with equal frequency except the cardiac valves, perhaps as a result of the absence of lymphatics in valves.

The diagnosis of a primary cardiac malignant tumor can be suspected in a patient in whom an unexplained hemorrhagic pericardial effusion develops, especially in association with a bizarre cardiac shadow on the radiograph. Echocardiography should confirm the presence of an abdominal cardiac mass. Thoracotomy is usually required to establish the diagnosis. Only rarely is effective therapy possible.

Rhabdomyoma

A cardiac rhabdomyoma is probably not a true tumor but a hamartoma, representing a focal arrest and maturation of cardiac muscle. The nodules have also been termed *nodular glycogenic degeneration*, being interpreted as a manifestation of glycogen storage disease. About one-half of the patients have tuberous sclerosis of the brain. On histologic examination cells with large vacuoles are found in which the nuclei appear suspended by threads of cytoplasm, giving origin to the term "spider cell."

Although rhabdomyoma is said to be the most common cardiac tumor in children, it is a rare lesion. Reece et al. indicated that only about 110 cases have been reported in the literature prior to 1984.

The cardiac lesions may be solitary or multiple nodules or may present a diffuse infiltration of the cardiac muscle. The lesions do not grow.

Most cases have been recognized in infancy. The average age was 5 months. The disease is apparently fatal, for older children and adults with such tumors are not seen. Whether the death is from the tumor or from associated disease is uncertain.

Symptoms may result from obstruction of a ventricular chamber or from arrhythmias such as recurrent ventricular tachycardia. Complete excision has been accomplished in a few patients. If tuberous sclerosis of the brain is not present, it appears that a rare infant may be successfully operated upon and cured of potentially fatal arrhythmias.

Miscellaneous Tumors

Unusual benign lesions of the heart include fibromas, lipomas, angiomas, teratomas, and cysts. Fewer than 50 examples of each of these types of lesions have been reported. Fibromas have been found most frequently in the left ventricle, often as 2- to 5-cm nodules within the muscle. Sudden death, probably from a cardiac arrhythmia, has been reported with such tumors and may be the reason that only 18 percent of the reported tumors have been found in adults.

Lipomas are usually asymptomatic tumors found projecting from the epicardial or endocardial surface of the heart in older patients. Only about 30 such cases have been reported. Angiomas are commonly small, focal vascular malformations of no clinical significance, except for four that have been found associated with a heart block. Pericardial teratomas and bronchogenic cysts are rare lesions that may cause symptoms from compression of the right atrium and obstruction of venous return. About 30 such patients have been reported in the surgical literature, most of them children. Some of the larger cysts, up to 10 cm in diameter, may produce grotesque deformities from extensive invagination of the right atrial wall. Myxomas are by far the most common benign tumor in adults, but are seldom found in children.

CORONARY ARTERY DISEASE

HISTORICAL DATA. Starting in the late 1930s, different investigators attempted to increase the blood supply of the ischemic heart by developing collateral circulation with vascular adhesions. Beck was the leading investigator, trying different methods for many years, but ultimately all failed. Probably the fundamental biologic reason for failure is the natural tendency for vascular adhesions to progressively fibrose and become more avascular with time.

A separate ingenious concept arose in 1946 when Vineberg developed implantation of the internal mammary artery into a tunnel in the myocardium. This was applied clinically by Vineberg in 1950 and continued for many years. For unknown reasons, the artery remains patent in well over 90 percent of patients, but the amount of flow through the patent artery is distressingly small, often as little as 5 to 10 mL/min. An occasional patient

has been reported in whom the implanted artery was of substantial benefit, carrying as much as 50 mL of blood per minute, but these fortunate results were infrequent. For this reason, the procedure has been virtually abandoned.

Attempts at endarterectomy without bypass grafting have been made sporadically since 1956, but late patency rates were prohibitively low, probably from late cicatrial contractions of collagen in the arterial wall. In recent years some groups have reinvestigated the concept of the combination of endarterectomy with bypass.

In 1986, over 200,000 bypass procedures were performed in the United States. It is estimated that at least 6 million patients in this country have known coronary artery disease.

The development of the bypass operation for coronary occlusive disease between 1967 and 1968 was a dramatic milestone. For the first time it was possible to increase immediately the blood flow to the myocardium. Most of the basic clinical investigations evolved from studies in three centers in the United States during this time. Favalaro et al. from the Cleveland Clinic began using longer and longer segments of saphenous vein to bypass occlusive disease in the right coronary artery, eventually interposing grafts between the aorta proximally and the termination of the right coronary distally. Johnson et al., in 1969, showed that similar grafts could be effectively used for the left coronary artery. This was a quantum achievement. Previously, direct operative procedures upon the left coronary artery had a prohibitive mortality. Green, following extensive experimental studies by others, anastomosed the left internal mammary artery to the anterior descending, using an operative microscope. The internal mammary was not widely used for over a decade but since 1980 has been widely adopted and is now used in the majority of bypass operations. This change resulted from 10-year angiographic studies that found excellent patency rates of internal mammary grafts (>90 percent) but disappointing deterioration in vein grafts between 5 and 10 years after operation with less than 50 percent satisfactory patency.

ETIOLOGY AND PATHOGENESIS. Atherosclerosis is the fundamental cause. It is a common disease in the Caucasian male throughout the world, involving males about four times as frequently as females. The frequency varies widely throughout the world, being less common in populations where the average blood cholesterol is less than 200. The frequency is the lowest in Japan, where the average blood cholesterol is near 160 mg/100 mL. The United States has the second highest frequency in the world.

The basic lesion is a segmental atherosclerotic plaque, often localized within the first 5 cm of the origin of the coronary artery from the aorta. Involvement of small distal vessels is usually less extensive; arterioles and intramyocardial vessels are usually free of disease. This segmental localization makes bypass grafts possible. Among the three major coronary arteries, the proximal anterior descending is often occluded, with the distal half of the artery remaining patent. The right coronary is often occluded throughout its course, but almost always the posterior descending and left atrial-ventricular groove branches are patent. The circumflex is often diseased proximally, but one or more distal marginal branches are patent.

The popular terminology, single, double, or triple vessel disease, refers, of course, to the number of coronary arteries involved. In over 50 percent of patients, "triple" vessel disease is present.

CLINICAL MANIFESTATIONS. The myocardial ischemia produced by coronary disease can produce several serious events: angina pectoris, myocardial infarction, or sudden death. Angina is the most frequent symptom, but unfortunately myocardial infarction or sudden death may appear without warning.

Angina pectoris, the most common manifestation, is demonstrated by periodic discomfort, usually substernal, typically appearing with exertion, after eating, or with extreme emotion. Characteristically these symptoms subside within 3 to 5 min, or may be dramatically relieved by sublingual nitroglycerin. In about 25 percent of patients, the symptoms are not typical and may radiate to bizarre areas, such as the teeth, the shoulder, or the epigastrium. Establishing a diagnosis of angina in these patients is difficult, perhaps impossible without diagnostic studies. Physical examination is usually normal. Differential diagnosis includes anxiety states, musculoskeletal disorders, and reflux esophagitis.

The risk of sudden death varies with the extent of disease and the degree of impairment of ventricular function. It ranges from 2 percent to as high as 10 percent. Death apparently results from ventricular fibrillation, for postmortem examination may not find any acute change.

Myocardial infarction is the most common serious complication. At least 2 million infarcts occur in the United States annually. With modern therapy, mortality is near 10 to 15 percent. Most deaths occur in the first 30 to 60 min after the onset of symptoms, before the patient ever reaches a hospital. With modern treatment in coronary care units, the fatality rate is small.

In a small percentage of patients congestive heart failure eventually develops, resulting from multiple infarctions that ultimately destroy over 40 percent of the left ventricular muscle mass. Often the origin is puzzling. Some patients have had angina for years, with one or more infarctions, but others have been almost asymptomatic for over a decade after a small infarction first established the presence of coronary disease. Despite the paucity of symptoms, ischemic infarction of muscle apparently steadily but "silently" progressed. The frequency, diagnosis, and treatment of so-called silent ischemia is currently one of the most active areas in cardiology (1987). Other patients, by contrast, undergo rapid destruction of ventricular function within 2 to 3 years. Multiple tiny emboli from an ulcerated atherosclerotic plaque may be one possible mechanism.

With chronic congestive failure, manifested by a right atrial pressure above 10 to 15 mmHg, the outlook is ominous, for there is insufficient left ventricular muscle to provide adequate cardiac output. Most patients die within 1 to 2 years. Bypass grafting may be futile in such circumstances unless there is a large ventricular aneurysm present that can be excised. Cardiac transplantation is now being used with increasing frequency in this group of patients with far advanced disease.

LABORATORY STUDIES. The chest x-ray is usually normal, and the electrocardiogram is normal at rest in about 70 percent of patients. The simplest and most widely used study is the stress test with the exercise electrocardiogram, noting electrocardiographic signs of ischemia during graded amounts of exercise. More complex studies include radionuclide imaging with thallium or radionuclide angiography, noting changes in ejection fraction with exercise. A decrease in ejection fraction with exercise is a characteristic finding with significant coronary disease.

Coronary arteriography (Fig. 19-22) remains the cornerstone of evaluation, for it outlines both the location and severity of the disease and the degree of impairment of ventricular function. The number of vessels diseased, the location of proximal stenoses, and the ventricular function as measured by ejection fraction are the three most important prognostic indicators of the severity and prognosis with coronary disease.

"Angiographically significant" stenosis is considered present when the diameter is reduced by more than 70 percent, corresponding to a reduction in cross-sectional area greater than 90 percent; some groups use a more liberal indication, considering a reduction in diameter of 50 percent (equivalent to a 75 percent reduction in cross-sectional area) as significant.

Ventricular function is usually expressed as ejection fraction, considering the range of 0.50 to 0.70 as normal; 0.30 to 0.50 moderately depressed; and below 0.30, especially below 0.20, as severely depressed. An ejection fraction below 0.30 is usually associated with intermittent or chronic congestive heart failure. The long-term course of coronary disease is a balance between two opposing factors, the rate of progression of the atherosclerotic stenoses as balanced by the rate of development of collateral circulation. The ventricular function probably reflects the ability of the heart to develop sufficient collateral circulation to compensate for the arterial stenoses present. This ability to develop collateral circulation varies widely; some patients with extensive triple vessel disease have normal ventricular function while others with less severe disease have marked impairment.

When a ventriculogram is evaluated, the contraction of individual segments of ventricular wall is separately analyzed, i.e., regional wall motion. Segmental wall motion is classified as normal, hypokinetic (impaired), akinetic (little or no visible contraction), or dyskinetic (paradoxical contraction, as with a left ventricular aneurysm).

Although angiography and ventriculography are the most precise methods for evaluating coronary disease, several limitations of the technique should also be emphasized, for erroneous decisions can easily be made.

An angiogram indicates the severity and complexity of the disease but is seldom, if ever, a reliable guide to state that a patient is "inoperable" because of the diffuse dis-

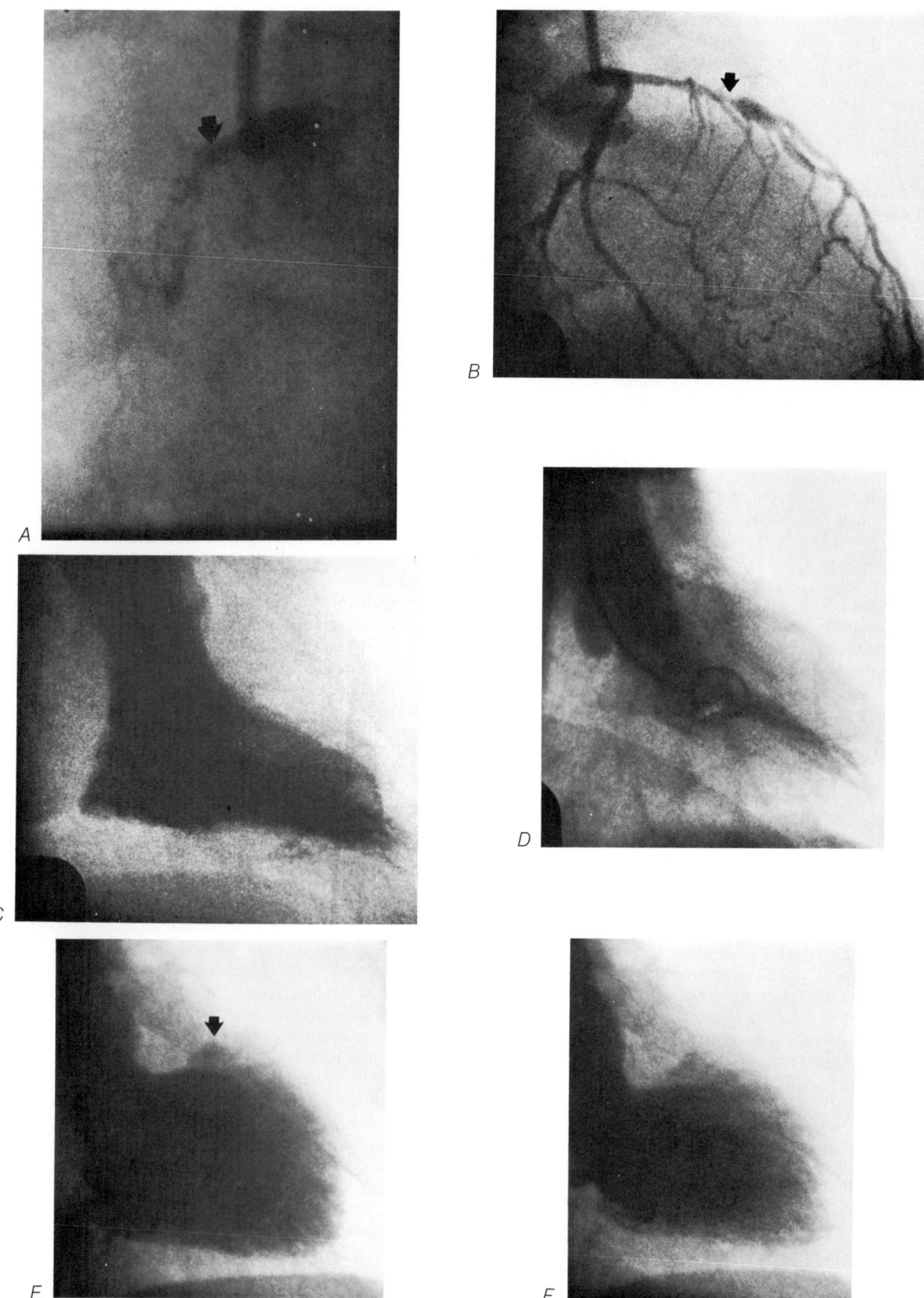

ease present and the small size of the vessels. With the ability to graft vessels as small as 1 mm, combined with endarterectomy when necessary, bypass grafts can virtually always be inserted even though the degree of improvement may be only moderate.

It is also a serious error to conclude from the ventriculogram that a diseased artery supplying an akinetic or dyskinetic area should not be bypassed because that segment of the ventricle is "scar." At operation such areas virtually always contain a significant percentage of viable muscle, estimated to range from 40 to 80 percent. Often improved contractility can be seen following bypass.

The ventriculogram should not be used to conclude that a patient is "inoperable" because of severe impairment of ventricular function, though ejection fraction may be less than 20 percent and end-diastolic pressure above 30 mm. This represents an advanced stage of disease with a grim prognosis, but criteria for operation depend upon the clinical condition of the patient, whether congestive failure is intermittent or chronic, and whether chronic right heart failure is present, reflected by a right atrial pressure near 15 mm or higher, and hepatomegaly.

CORONARY BYPASS. Indications. The clinical status of the patient with coronary disease is usually in one of five groups: asymptomatic, stable angina of varying severity, unstable angina, acute myocardial infarction, and postinfarction angina.

Asymptomatic: Angiographically Significant Coronary Disease with Little or No Angina. This type of patient is the most common clinical problem. The three major types of therapy available are medical (drug) therapy, bypass surgery, or angioplasty. Angioplasty has been applied with steadily increasing frequency for isolated stenotic lesions and by some groups for multiple stenoses. The role of angioplasty will probably not be clearly defined for at least another 5 years. In one series, angioplasty was initially successful in 70 percent of patients, without any deaths, but 33 percent of the successfully dilated patients required either subsequent repeat dilatation or bypass surgery. With significant occlusive disease in the left main coronary, there is virtually uniform agreement that such patients should be operated upon promptly, even if totally asymptomatic.

Stable Angina of Varying Severity. There is uniform agreement that severe angina not responding to drug therapy should be operated upon. The majority of patients have

Fig. 19-22. *A.* Right coronary artery, left anterior oblique projection. There is total obstruction of the vessel immediately distal to its aortic origin *(arrow)*. A network of collateral vessels on the anterior surface of the right atrium and the right ventricle is apparent. *B.* Left coronary artery, right anterior oblique projection. There is severe narrowing of the left anterior descending coronary artery *(arrow)* distal to the origin of the second septal branch. *C.* Left ventricle in right anterior oblique projection in diastole. There is a normal contour of the chamber. *D.* Same ventricle in systole showing excellent contraction of all areas of the ventricle. *E.* Left ventricle in diastole, right anterior oblique projection. There is increased rounding of the ventricle and bulging of the anterolateral wall. A localized bulge on the superior portion of the anterolateral wall is evident *(arrow)*. *F.* The same ventricle in systole. The degree of left ventricular contraction is generally markedly impaired.

extensive disease with little angina. Data increasingly indicate that the presence and severity of angina per se is an unreliable guide for deciding upon operation.

One of the most important studies was done by the European Coronary Surgery Study group in the 1970s. This found that 5-year survival with triple vessel disease was near 90 percent with bypass as compared with near 80 percent with medical therapy. The most extensive study was done by the Coronary Artery Surgery Study (CASS), a multicenter study among 15 institutions between 1974 and 1979, during which over 24,000 patients were entered into the registry. Over 75 percent of patients in the study had a normal ejection fraction (greater than 0.50). Patients with triple vessel disease, good ventricular function, and mild angina did equally well with medical or surgical therapy, as 5-year survival in either group was above 90 percent. These data were initially widely heralded as showing that bypass was "unnecessary," overlooking the disconcerting fact that medical therapy was continued only as long as angina remained stable. In this favorable group, however, 38 percent of patients "crossed over" to surgical therapy within 5 years, indicating the relentless progression of the disease. At present, medical therapy is adequate with good ventricular function only if angina is not progressive.

With triple vessel disease and impaired ventricular function (ejection fraction less than 0.50), results are much better with bypass, as 7-year survival is 84 percent compared with 70 percent with medical therapy.

With single vessel disease, initial treatment with medical therapy or angioplasty is usually satisfactory. However, the outstanding results with internal mammary bypass grafting, an operative risk less than 1 percent, and a 10-year patency rate greater than 90 percent certainly indicate that surgical therapy may be used if either of the other two methods is unsatisfactory. With double vessel disease, intermediate in severity between single and triple vessel disease, bypass is usually not performed in stable patients with satisfactory ventricular function, but multiple factors enter into the decision with individual patients.

Unstable Angina. "Acute coronary insufficiency" exists when angina is persistent and does not respond to therapy with nitroglycerin and other nitrates. It apparently is an acute physiologic state in which the blood flow to a segment of myocardium is seriously jeopardized but necrosis has not yet occurred. It probably arises from a sudden decrease in regional blood flow. Virtually everyone agrees that the condition is a medical emergency. The patient should be promptly hospitalized in a coronary care unit. If collateral blood flow increases and compensates for the ischemia, manifested by subsidence of the angina, recovery is prompt. Otherwise, acute infarction or death can occur.

Most patients respond to acute medical therapy. Those who do not should be operated upon promptly. In patients who recover, coronary angiography should be done soon to decide if elective bypass should be performed, for such patients have a significant frequency of infarction or death within 1 to 2 years after the event.

Acute Infarction. The best therapy for an acute myocardial infarction is one of the most rapidly changing areas in cardiology. Data now are convincing that the infarction is produced by an acute thrombosis in a major artery in the majority of patients. The immediate intravenous administration of a thrombolytic agent, usually streptokinase, is becoming increasingly popular after a study of several thousand uncontrolled patients found a definite decrease in mortality when streptokinase was administered in the first 4 to 6 h after onset of symptoms, with the best results occurring when administration was within 1 to 2 h. In the United States a national study is still evaluating the effectiveness of tissue plasminogen activator (TPA), a far more effective thrombolytic drug.

A more complex form of therapy is the intracoronary administration of the thrombolytic agent in the catheterization laboratory. This may be combined with angioplasty. After thrombolytic therapy has reopened a thrombosed vessel precipitating an acute infarction, the residual stenosis may be treated by angioplasty, bypass, or drug therapy. Thrombolytic therapy, combined with angioplasty, is a simpler and safer procedure than emergency coronary bypass and can be applied more quickly for most patients.

A certain degree of irreversible necrosis develops between 30 and 60 min following occlusion of the coronary artery. Infarction continues to evolve for several hours, probably in the marginal zones of the initial complete infarction. This is probably the basis for the benefit from immediate revascularization, similar to removal of an acute arterial occlusion in other areas of the body. A very short time exists during which therapy may be effective.

When a massive infarction produces cardiogenic shock, mortality remains high, well above 50 percent. Most of these patients have triple vessel disease with a preexisting significant impairment of ventricular function. Probably the best approach for these patients is immediate bypass, perhaps preceded by intraaortic balloon support. Significant data are not yet available.

Postinfarction Angina. Patients recovering from myocardial infarction who develop recurrent angina can be safely operated upon promptly. With present techniques of cardioplegia, the risk of operation seems unrelated to the time lapsing since the initial infarction.

Contraindications. The only absolute contraindication at the author's institution is chronic congestive failure with pulmonary hypertension, a right atrial pressure above 15 mm, and hepatomegaly. The unfortunate patient in this group usually has already necrosed the majority of the left ventricular muscle, so cardiac transplantation is the only therapy likely to be helpful.

Intermittent congestive failure, manifested by intermittent episodes of pulmonary edema, is not a *contraindication* to operation but actually a strong *indication for immediate operation.* This indicates a serious degree of myocardial ischemia that can easily progress to an irreversible stage or death. The intermittent episodes probably evolve from an acute ischemic episode that elevates end-diastolic pressure sufficiently to produce pulmonary edema. Such patients have been regularly operated upon with continuing good long-term results.

A severe depression of ejection fraction to the range of 0.20 to 0.25, or lower, is still erroneously considered a contraindication to bypass, though contrary experiences have been published by several groups. The erroneous concept probably arose from previous experiences with ineffective myocardial preservation that produced some degree of infarction during operation. Jones et al. reported experiences with 188 patients with an ejection fraction below 0.35, about 24 percent of whom had ejection fraction lower than 0.20. Operative mortality was only 2.1 percent.

Pigott and Kouchoukos reported results for 192 patients with an ejection fraction less than 35 percent. Seventy-seven were operated upon; 115 were treated medically. Seven-year actuarial survival was 63 percent in the surgical group, 34 percent in the medical group. Recurrent infarction developed in 19 percent of the medical group as compared with 7 percent of the surgical group.

Operative Technique. At the author's institution all procedures are performed with extracorporeal circulation at a flow rate near 2.3 L/m^2/min and a perfusate temperature of 25 to 30°C. The heart is arrested with the cold blood potassium technique. Cold blood is infused at an aortic root pressure of 80 to 100 mmHg to permit adequate perfusion beyond the occluded vessels. This is confirmed by measuring regional myocardial temperatures in at least four regions of the myocardium, and continuing infusion of cold blood until the "warmest" zone has cooled below 15°C. This can usually be done with 1500 mL but may at times require 2000 or 2500 mL. Topical hypothermia is then employed to prevent rewarming, both by pericardial lavage and by a continuous pericardial infusion of cold electrolyte. Blood is reinfused into the aorta usually after each anastomosis, certainly after every 20 to 30 min. The left heart is decompressed, either by emptying the right heart with a large lumen cannula or with a catheter introduced through a pulmonary vein. Particular attention is given to periodic monitoring of right heart temperatures to be certain that reflux of blood from the cavae does not warm the right ventricle and septum. With this technique, the heart can be arrested for well over 2 h, even though this is rarely necessary. There is ample time for grafting all diseased vessels.

Saphenous veins of appropriate size (greater than 3.5 mm) are removed from the lower extremity, using the lesser saphenous or the cephalic veins if adequate saphenous veins are not available. The left internal mammary artery is routinely used in the vast majority of patients (Fig. 19-23). In recent years, following the lead of others, bilateral mammary grafting has been employed with increasing frequency, usually in healthy patients under fifty-five years of age. With the heart arrested and cooled, bypass grafts are attached to all diseased coronary arteries, making a short arteriotomy and attaching the vein end to side with a continuous suture of 7-0 polypropylene. Three- to four-power optical magnification is routinely used. Internal mammary anastomoses are done with 8-0 polypropylene. Cold blood is routinely infused down each graft after it is constructed. When the aorta is unclamped, warm blood is perfused down the grafts until these are attached to the aorta. This is probably superfluous in

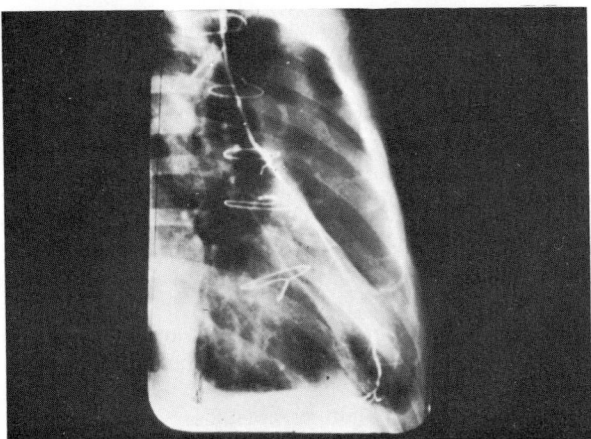

Fig. 19-23. Angiogram performed several months after left internal mammary–left anterior descending coronary bypass, showing a good flow from the internal mammary artery into the anterior descending coronary and its branches.

many patients but seems quite important when serious ischemia is present, especially with left main coronary disease.

An alternative is to attach several grafts to the aorta proximally before bypass is started and then serially construct the distal anastomoses. This is a simpler and more expeditious method, though it requires more judgment about the exact length of grafts and has less freedom of choice once the aorta is clamped and the heart emptied. The usual number of anastomoses constructed varies between three and six. As many as nine to ten anastomoses have been constructed in a few patients with no measurable increase in operative mortality.

Following bypass, flow rates are measured through the grafts with a flowmeter, finding a mean flow between 50 and 80 mL/min in most vessels with an adequate runoff.

Postoperative Management. Postoperative care is usually uncomplicated. The patients remain in a cardiac recovery unit for 12 to 18 h, after which the further care is routine. Initially, adequacy of blood volume and cardiac output are periodically monitored by measurement of left atrial pressure with a catheter inserted at the time of operation and a Swan-Ganz catheter in the pulmonary artery. Minor atrial arrhythmias are fairly common and easily treated with appropriate medication. A mild pericardiotomy syndrome, manifested by fever, a pericardial friction rub, pleural effusion, and a normal white blood cell count, is fairly common and usually responds promptly to therapy with ibuprofen. Prednisone is seldom necessary. Most uncomplicated patients are discharged from the hospital in 7 to 9 days.

Normal sedentary activity is gradually resumed over the next 2 to 3 months. After 3 months have passed, the ejection fraction should probably be routinely measured with exercise before vigorous physical exercise is permitted. If significant arrhythmias were present preoperatively, these must be carefully monitored indefinitely because these are often not improved with bypass and are a fairly common cause of late death. In patients with normal ventricular function beforehand, after 3 months a full return to normal physical activity, with participation in physically active sports, is routinely recommended.

Results. Operative Risk and Major Complications. Operative risk is very small, near 1 percent for the usual patient. Similar low-risk results have been reported by many experienced cardiac surgical groups throughout the world. Moderate impairment of ventricular function does not increase operative risk, though with severe impairment of ventricular function, an ejection fraction less than 0.30, the risk is probably near 3 to 4 percent.

With an uncomplicated operation, electrocardiographic signs of myocardial infarction develop in less than 5 percent of patients. With enzymatic studies, a somewhat higher frequency may be found, though inconsistencies often exist between the electrocardiographic findings and the enzymatic changes. It is rare for enzymatic changes to represent a significant physiologic problem if the patient is asymptomatic without significant changes on the electrocardiogram. A very minimal elevation of myocardial enzymes indicates the absence of any injury, but the significance of a moderate elevation is uncertain.

Operative risk rises somewhat with age, though patients in their seventh or eighth decade are readily operated upon if angina is crippling and cerebral function is satisfactory.

The most serious complication with operation is stroke, a frequency of 1 to 2 percent, more commonly seen in patients in the sixth, seventh, or eighth decades. The exact cause of stroke is usually impossible to determine. The four most common probable causes are atherosclerotic disease in the carotid arteries or the aortic arch, or emboli of thrombotic material or air from the heart. Usually the stroke, fortunately infrequent, is both unexpected and cannot be explained.

We no longer believe that asymptomatic carotid disease is a significant cause of perioperative stroke. Carotid artery disease is surgically treated only in the patient with acute ischemic symptoms such as transient ischemic attacks. Unless acute ischemic symptoms are present, we are not aware of any data that show a benefit from performing carotid endarterectomy either before or concurrently with coronary bypass.

Considerable attention has been focused upon unrecognized atherosclerotic disease in the aortic arch as a source of emboli, especially in older patients. In patients over seventy years of age, a special aortic arch cannula is now routinely used, placing the tip beyond the orifice of the left subclavian artery to avoid dislodgment of atherosclerotic material from the transverse arch by the jet of blood emerging from the perfusion cannula. This cannula is routinely used in all patients with any suspected disease in the transverse aortic arch. In patients with palpable disease of the aortic arch, the aortic arch is also surgically explored, using the technique of circulatory arrest at a perfusate temperature below 18°C. The arch can be readily explored through an appropriately placed 5- to 6-cm aortotomy and any loose atherosclerotic debris removed. This has been done in at least 100 patients, finding intimal ulcerations with loose debris in perhaps 40 to 50 percent of this group. The exploration is clearly safe, with the strong impression that significant protection from stroke results.

Relief of Angina. The immediate relief of angina is the most dramatic aspect of bypass. Angina is either completely relieved or markedly decreased in at least 90 to 95 percent of patients if complete revascularization is done. Persistent angina almost always indicates that either a graft has become occluded or a significant stenosis was not bypassed.

Improvement in Ventricular Function. With former techniques, significant improvement in impaired ventricular function could not be demonstrated. With present techniques of myocardial preservation, the abnormal responses to exercise existing before operation, principally a fall in ejection fraction, are often abolished following complete revascularization. This is also usually associated with an improvement in regional wall motion abnormalities.

Vein Graft Patency. With a proper operative technique, combined with the preoperative use of dipyridamole and aspirin, patency a month following operation should be in the range of 90 to 95 percent. Current data are limited because angiograms are now seldom performed in the immediate postoperative period. In the first 5 years after operation, patency decreases slowly, about 2 to 3 percent per year, so 5-year patency is in the range of 75 to 80 percent. Occlusion of a graft during this time is probably due to the anastomotic technique, trauma to the vein graft at the time of operation, or, rarely, postoperative adhesions.

In the period 5 to 10 years after operation, there is an alarming increase of atherosclerotic disease in the vein grafts, as a result of which vein graft patency at 10 years is probably no better than 50 percent, and significant atherosclerosis is present in many of the grafts remaining patent. For unknown reasons, a small number of grafts, near 20 percent, remain in excellent condition more than 10 years after operation.

For this reason, in the past few years use of the internal mammary artery has increased markedly including the more frequent use of bilateral and sequential mammary grafts.

Progression of Atherosclerosis. All angiographic studies have reported a serious frequency of progressive atherosclerosis in the coronary arteries, ranging from 5 to 10 percent per year. Progressive disease was observed in between 65 and 70 percent of patients treated either medically or surgically.

National studies demonstrated that reduction in total plasma cholesterol and low-density lipoprotein cholesterol, often with an elevation in the high-density lipoprotein, resulted in significant improvement and a 2 percent reduction in coronary risk for each 1 percent reduction in plasma cholesterol levels.

Recurrent Angina. Angina gradually recurs following operation, at a rate of 3 to 5 percent per year. When significant angina recurs, angiography should be promptly done. In the majority of patients, recurrent angina is due to one of two causes, progressive stenosis or occlusion of a bypass graft or progressive stenosis in a previously un-

grafted artery. Either situation can be treated with repeat bypass grafting.

Arrhythmias and Sudden Death. Arrhythmias are usually little improved in patients with significant preoperative myocardial scarring. In some patients with virtually normal ventricular function, arrhythmias may be improved because ischemia was apparently the basic cause. Effective treatment of arrhythmias associated with ventricular scars remains unsatisfactory. The more frequent use of 24-h electrocardiographic monitoring may be helpful in developing more effective antiarrhythmic therapy. Electrophysiologic studies have been of benefit in some patients with recurrent arrhythmias. Patients with recurrent ventricular tachycardia have been effectively treated by electrically locating and then ablating one or more irritable foci.

Sudden death remains a grim possibility in any patient with coronary artery disease. Over 300 patients per year were studied following emergency resuscitation from cardiac arrest on the streets of Seattle. Over 75 percent of the patients had coronary disease, but less than one-half had a significant recent infarction.

The influence of medical and surgical treatment on "sudden death" was reported from results with over 13,000 patients in the CASS. Over a period of 4.6 years, sudden death occurred in 452 patients (3.4 percent of the group). This occurred in 6 percent of the medically treated patients but only 2 percent of the surgically treated patients.

Longevity. The influence of coronary bypass on longevity, of course, depends upon the status of the disease process in the patient operated upon. The CASS data indicate that bypass had little influence on 5-year longevity when performed upon patients with triple vessel disease, little angina, and good ventricular function. Nearly 40 percent of the unusually good risk group developed angina within 5 years and were operated upon. The data were even more convincing for similar patients with single or double vessel disease. For most other categories of patients, which represent a high percentage of all patients with coronary disease, bypass surgery clearly significantly improved longevity. These include patients with left main disease, triple vessel disease with impaired ventricular function, triple vessel disease with severe proximal stenoses or severe angina, and patients with a previous history of severe arrhythmias or "sudden death." In our experiences with 1100 patients operated upon between 1968 and 1975 the 5-year survival rate, including operative deaths, was 88 percent with only 49 cardiac deaths occurring after discharge from the hospital in the entire group. After the patients left the hospital, the average mortality was 1.5 percent per year for the next 5 years, a rate almost identical to that of a matched group of similar age and sex.

The similarity of survival (Fig. 19-24) between the two groups strongly indicated the significant influence of bypass on longevity. This is particularly true because the patients operated upon were usually in a high-risk category with severe angina not responding to medical therapy. Loop et al. noted a 5-year survival among different

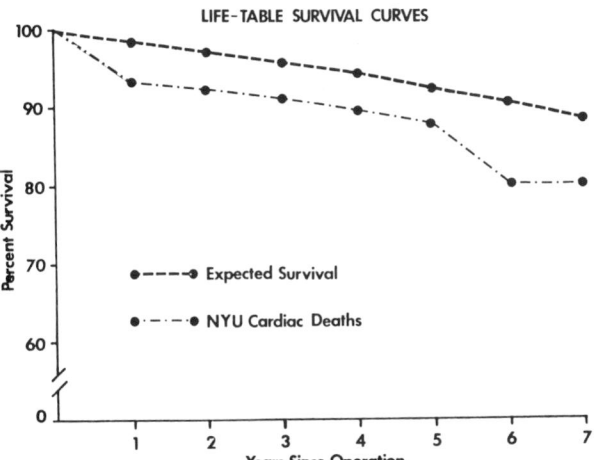

Fig. 19-24. Life table survival curves comparing patients undergoing coronary artery bypass with matched age group.

groups of 90 to 93 percent. Kirklin et al. reported a 5-year survival following triple bypass of 89 percent, and 88 percent following two vessel disease. Most reports show little influence of extent of disease (double or triple vessel disease) on 5-year survival, in marked contrast to that regularly found in medically treated patients.

A 10-year survival of 75 to 88 percent in several thousand patients was reported by Cosgrove et al. for different groups. The 10-year survival varied between 84 percent with a normal ventricle and 54 percent with severe impairment.

Late death, like recurrent angina, is usually found to result from stenosis of a previously inserted bypass graft or progressive disease in an ungrafted vessel. The rare occurrence of death in patients with three functioning grafts, usually from an arrhythmia, also indicates the influence of bypass on longevity. The major factor determining longevity seems to be the adequacy of revascularization of all major coronary arteries.

FUTURE CONSIDERATIONS. Multiple Internal Mammary Anastomoses. Since the 1984 report by Grondin documented the alarming deterioration of vein grafts between 5 and 10 years following operation, while mammary arteries remained patent without change in 90 to 95 percent of patients, a wider application of mammary grafting has been reported by several groups. In brief, certain facts are well established with internal mammary grafting.

1. The 10-year patency rate is near 95 percent, with no signs of deterioration after the first few postoperative months. The mammary artery seems to be relatively immune to atherosclerosis.
2. A patent mammary artery can enlarge substantially over a number of years, perhaps responding to a decrease in peripheral resistance in the coronary vascular bed as atherosclerosis occludes adjacent vessels. This striking ability to enlarge with time indicates the possibilities with multiple anastomoses constructed from a single mammary artery.
3. In retrospect, the concern in the 1970s about the mammary artery was probably due to improper surgical technique, as the vessel is unusually fragile.

4. Data now indicate that bilateral mammary grafts can be performed without significant morbidity. In several significant reports Lytle et al. described experiences with bilateral mammary grafting in 500 patients with little increase in morbidity.

Loop et al. compared longevity in patients who received one mammary graft as compared with those in whom only vein grafts were used. The series included 2306 internal mammary grafts and 3625 vein grafts. There was a statistically significant difference in survival at 10 years, gradually becoming apparent 5 years after operation.

Scanty data are available concerning "free" grafts of mammary artery, in which the artery is divided and reimplanted into the aorta, identical to the method used with a saphenous vein graft. Such "free" grafts no longer function as a pedicle. Loop reported reasonably good results in over 50 such patients operated upon under specific circumstances over a period of years, but no series has yet appeared in which such grafts were used routinely. If excellent results similar to those obtained with mammary pedicle grafts can be obtained with "free" grafts, an even wider use of the mammary artery is possible.

Silent Ischemia. Better therapy is clearly needed to prevent the development of extensive ventricular injury from coronary disease, the so-called "bad" left ventricle with an ejection fraction 0.20 to 0.25 or lower. Such patients are seen too often. The disconcerting fact is that such patients have often had "good" medical management since their coronary disease was first recognized years before, and have had neither recurrent major infarctions nor severe angina. Despite periodic medical observation and therapy, the disease has "silently" progressed. Some method other than severity of angina needs to be used to detect such patients and have bypass performed earlier. Some form of periodic stress testing, perhaps at least annually in patients with known coronary disease, seems to be necessary. One of the most definitive studies at present is a measurement of change in ejection fraction with exercise, especially in comparison with studies done in previous years.

LEFT VENTRICULAR ANEURYSM

HISTORICAL DATA. Safe excision of a ventricular aneurysm was not possible on a routine basis until the development of a pump oxygenator. Cooley, in 1958, is credited with one of the first reports of successful excision of an aneurysm with cardiopulmonary bypass. In the next few years, excision became a standard procedure in most cardiac clinics. Effler reported in 1965 that 61 such patients had been operated upon at the Cleveland Clinic. Series of more than 100 such aneurysms are now frequently reported.

ETIOLOGY, PATHOLOGY, AND PATHOGENESIS. A left ventricular aneurysm develops over a period of 4 to 8 weeks or longer in 10 to 15 percent of patients following a myocardial infarction (Fig. 19-25). It results when a severe transmural infarction destroys virtually all muscular fibers in the area of the infarction, which are subse-

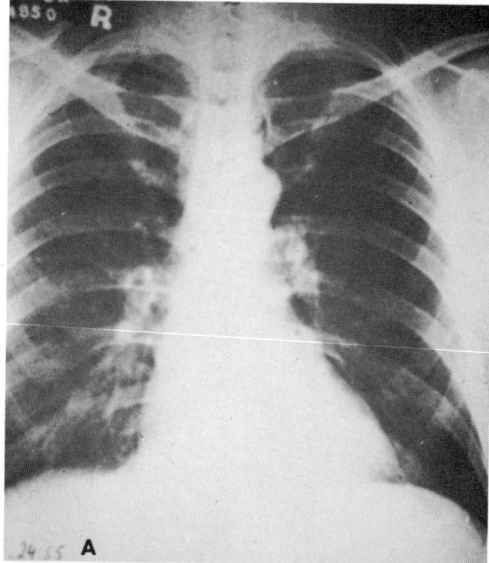

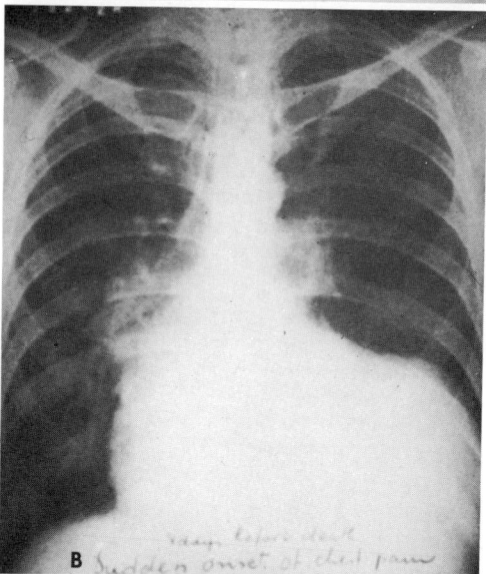

Fig. 19-25. Ventricular aneurysm. *A.* Chest radiograph showing a heart of normal size 2 days following an acute myocardial infarction. *B.* Chest radiograph showing cardiac enlargement from a large left ventricular aneurysm which progressively enlarged before a fatal episode of cardiac arrhythmia.

quently replaced by fibrous tissue. It probably does not occur more frequently following a transmural infarction because collateral circulation is sufficient to maintain viability of a variable number of muscle fibers in the zone of the infarct.

The classic aneurysm is simply an avascular scar 4 to 6 mm thick that bulges outward when the remaining left ventricular muscle contracts in systole. Hence, the term, "paradoxical contraction," more commonly termed "dyskinesis," as opposed to *hypokinesis* (impaired contractility) or *akinesis* (absence of contractility). Mural thrombi are found attached to the ventricular surface of the scar in over one-half of patients, but arterial emboli

are rare. The aneurysm usually enlarges a moderate degree and then becomes stationary; progressive enlargement and rupture, as usually occurs with atherosclerotic aortic aneurysms, is rare. Spotty calcification eventually develops in the aneurysmal wall in chronic cases. Over 80 percent of aneurysms are in the anterolateral portion of the left ventricle, evolving after occlusion of the anterior descending coronary. Lateral or posterior aneurysms are uncommon.

A "false" aneurysm is rare. It is a hematoma that is formed after rupture of a myocardial infarction has been temporarily supported by adjacent fibrous tissue. Excision should be done promptly, for such aneurysms soon expand and rupture.

In 30 to 40 percent of cases, significant coronary disease is limited to the anterior descending coronary, which is either completely occluded or severely stenosed. Multivessel disease is present in the other patients. Small aneurysms (less than 5 cm diameter) have negligible physiologic significance except possibly as a site of arrhythmias. Larger aneurysms decrease ventricular function apparently by dissipating energy of ventricular contraction with the ineffective paradoxical expansion of the wall of the aneurysm during systole. Possibly, the altered geometry of the left ventricular cavity is also significant, though this is difficult to measure. With larger aneurysms, the left ventricular volume is increased and left ventricular hypertrophy develops. The decrease in effective ventricular contraction eventually results in cardiac failure and angina, though angina may be due to the accompanying coronary disease as well. Arrhythmias are prominent in 10 to 15 percent of patients.

As the physiologic burden from an aneurysm is related to its size, the magnitude of improvement following operation is somewhat related to the size of the aneurysm. For this reason, it is doubtful that an aneurysm is ever large enough to be truly "inoperable" simply because of size. If a patient is alive with a large aneurysm, removal of the aneurysm should improve function of the remaining ventricular fibers if these are not harmed at the time of operation from either excessive resection of ventricular wall or inadequate myocardial preservation.

As the development of an aneurysm depends upon almost total destruction of muscle fibers, a true aneurysm, composed of akinetic scar, must be distinguished from a scar that results from an infarction that may be akinetic but whose wall is composed of varying proportions of fibrous tissue and viable muscle fibers. Excision of such akinetic scars has been investigated in some detail in the past but has not been found clinically beneficial.

Because of the wide spectrum between a ventricular "scar" and a true "aneurysm," accurate data to define natural history are almost impossible to obtain. The natural history of a patient with a ventricular aneurysm will, of course, be determined by at least three factors: the size of the aneurysm, the residual coronary disease, and the function of the remaining viable muscle. Five-year survival with an untreated aneurysm has ranged from as low as 10 percent to as high as 70 percent among different reports. Brusche et al. reported that 5-year survival in a patient with an akinetic segment was 70 percent; with a dyskinetic segment and good residual ventricular function, 54 percent; with a dyskinetic segment and poor ventricular function, 36 percent.

CLINICAL MANIFESTATIONS. Dyspnea or angina, either alone or in combination, are the two most common symptoms. Arrhythmias are prominent in a minority of patients. Abnormalities on physical examination are usually not diagnostic. The apical impulse may be forceful and diffuse with a "double impulse."

The chest x-ray may show a localized enlargement in the anteroapical area of the left ventricle. Electrocardiographic changes usually show only the signs of the previous infarction. Most diagnostic information comes from the left ventricular angiogram, outlining an akinetic area bulging paradoxically during systole. Often a clear differentiation cannot be made between an akinetic scar and a true aneurysm, with the final decision being made at the time of operation. If a discrete scar is found at operation, containing few or no muscle fibers, resection is indicated. If a diffuse bulging is present without discrete borders and obviously containing a moderate amount of muscle tissue, resection is probably contraindicated.

TREATMENT. Operation is indicated for symptomatic aneurysms larger than 5 to 6 cm. A moderate asymptomatic aneurysm may be simply observed. The operative procedure includes excision of the aneurysm and bypass grafting of the diseased coronary arteries. Grafting of the diseased anterior descending coronary, which often supplies principally ventricular scar, is of questionable value, though at NYU it has usually been grafted because of the possibility that improved blood supply to the ventricular septum might benefit ventricular arrhythmias.

In general, the aneurysm is not manipulated until the heart has been fibrillated or the aorta clamped to prevent dislodgment of mural thrombi. Once the heart is arrested or fibrillated, the heart is mobilized by freeing the aneurysm from the pericardial adhesions, often by simply incising the wall of the aneurysm and leaving part of the wall attached to the pericardium. After the heart is mobilized completely, a *subtotal* excision of the aneurysm is performed, dividing the wall of the aneurysm about 2 cm from its junction with left ventricular muscle. The *subtotal* concept is a crucial one, as the suture line closing the ventriculotomy is subsequently inserted through scar rather than through viable muscle surrounding the aneurysm. This precaution also avoids any excessive reduction in size of the ventricular cavity (Fig. 19-26). In all likelihood, operative deaths from excision of huge aneurysms probably result from excessive excision of the wall of the aneurysm with injury of the surrounding viable ventricular muscle.

The wall of the aneurysm usually includes the area of the anterior descending coronary, with the scar extending into the ventricular septum. Bypass grafting of the anterior descending in such instances is of uncertain significance, as the muscle supplied by the anterior descending has been infarcted. If significant tributaries to the ventricular septum are patent, the artery should be preserved and a bypass graft attached.

Usually, the extent of the endocardial scar is greater than that of the aneurysm. Because of the hazard of malignant ventricular arrhythmias, a localized excision of the subendocardial scar for one or more centimeters around the periphery of the aneurysm seems worthwhile, as this is easily done without significant injury to functioning ventricular muscle. Electrophysiologic studies have found that trigger zones for arrhythmias are usually located in the scar within 1 to 3 cm of the border of the aneurysm. When preoperative ventricular arrhythmias are prominent, electrophysiologic mapping to locate and excise the irritable foci should be done at the time of operation.

The opening following excision of the aneurysm is closed in an axis that conforms best to that of the residual ventricular fibers. Two or three rows of continuous synthetic sutures are used, occasionally reinforced with Teflon felt if the tissues are friable. Recurrence of an aneurysm is virtually unknown.

Technique of Operation. A sternotomy incision is employed. With huge aneurysms, an additional lateral thoracotomy is occasionally necessary. Pericardial adhesions may be severe. Dissection of these adhesions to mobilize the heart is best postponed until bypass is started. With bypass functioning, the perfusate is cooled, the aorta clamped, and the heart arrested with the cold blood potassium technique.

If concomitant coronary bypass grafting is to be done, the bypass grafts should be attached first to permit intermittent infusion of the cardioplegic solution through the grafts to provide additional myocardial protection. Attachment of all grafts may not be possible until the heart is mobilized and the aneurysm excised.

With the heart arrested and collapsed, pericardial adhesions may be divided and the aneurysm opened. With a huge aneurysm and dense adhesions, after the aneurysm has been opened and the origin from the wall of the left ventricle identified, the aneurysm can simply be divided a short distance from the pericardial adhesions, leaving this part of the aneurysmal wall in situ and thus avoiding troublesome bleeding.

RESULTS. Prognosis is determined principally by the residual ventricular function, which, in turn, is influenced by the size of the aneurysm and the severity of the coronary disease. In general, if angina was the prominent symptom before operation, 5-year survival is 60 percent or better, while if congestive heart failure was the principal indication for operation, 5-year survival is much less, near 30 percent.

Most patients are significantly improved following operation, manifested by relief of angina and improvement in ventricular function. With hemodynamic studies, significant improvement in ventricular function can be demonstrated in some patients, while others show very little change. Improvement in ejection fraction generally occurred when more than 24 cm^2 of aneurysmal wall were resected.

Olearchyk et al. described experiences with 244 cases with a 5-year survival near 70 percent. Dobell et al. in a series of 67 patients found a 5-year survival of 84 percent

ety of arrhythmias, including the "sick sinus syndrome," an alternating bradycardia and tachycardia, and arrhythmias associated with varying degrees of atrioventricular (AV) block.

Approximately 120,000 implants are performed annually in the United States. The chief indications for permanent pacing were sick sinus syndrome (48 percent) and impairment of conduction in the atrioventricular node and HIS-Purkinge system (42 percent).

Heart Block

ETIOLOGY. Acquired heart block in the elderly, now termed "Lev's disease," appears to be a primary disease, a fibrosis of the conduction system without other significant cardiac disease. Another cause is calcification of cardiac valves involving the conduction system. Heart block from myocardial infarction is usually temporary, becoming permanent in only about 5 percent of patients.

Congenital heart block has been reported with increasing frequency. A recent report on 599 infants and children found the greatest risk of death in early infancy. After the first year of life, the outlook was much improved. Children with complete block and additional cardiac disease, however, had a 28 percent mortality. In small premature neonates with congenital complete heart block, permanent pacemakers have been implanted with good long-term results, indicating the refinements in design and size currently available.

Besley et al. reported experiences with implantation of pacemakers in 13 young adults with an average follow-up of 4 years. The authors questioned the concept that congenital heart block in older patients is usually a benign condition.

PATHOLOGY AND PATHOPHYSIOLOGY. In normal cardiac conduction, the cardiac impulse arises in the sinoatrial node near the junction of the superior vena cava with the right atrium. The impulse is propagated through the right atrial wall via internodal pathways to the AV node, lying medial to the ostium of the coronary sinus. From this node it travels along the bundle of HIS near the annulus of the tricuspid valve to pass through the central fibrous body of the ventricular septum near the junction of the muscular and membranous components. Here the bundle divides into right and left bundles, which, in turn, travel to their respective ventricles. The most common surgical trauma producing complete heart block occurs during repair of a ventricular septal defect or an ostium primum defect. It rarely may follow prosthetic replacement of the aortic, mitral, or tricuspid valve, either by direct injury or from traction and subsequent fibrosis. Injuries of the right or left conduction bundle per se are apparently not of great clinical significance.

Heart block seriously impairs cardiac output in several ways. The resulting bradycardia, varying from 25 to 60 beats/min depending upon the idioventricular response, decreases coronary and cerebral circulation. Refractory congestive failure may exist even with rates as high as 45 beats/min. There is intolerance to exercise and even symptoms of cerebral vascular insufficiency with syncope and convulsions.

Clinical symptoms attributed to first-degree heart block (PR interval 0.2 s) are rare. With second-degree heart block (intermittent lack of AV conduction) symptoms become apparent if the bradycardia is severe or persistent. In third-degree heart block (complete lack of AV conduction) bradycardia is persistent and symptoms are quite common.

With complete AV disassociation, there may be periods of transient ventricular asystole with syncope, convulsions, and even death. Equally disastrous in some patients, rather than cardiac arrest, are bouts of ventricular tachycardia or fibrillation, as ventricular "escape" mechanisms result from absence of normal AV conduction. With lesser degrees of heart block, the cardiac rate may be normal most of the time but abruptly change into complete AV disassociation with its attendant complications. Any such episode may be followed by recovery or may result in death. Intermittent attacks of syncope and convulsions with heart block were designated the Stokes-Adams syndrome. Some patients never develop these symptoms but become disabled with cardiac failure.

CLINICAL MANIFESTATIONS. Although some patients may be asymptomatic with a rate as low as 35 beats/min, most have symptoms with a rate less than 45. Episodic Stokes-Adams attacks are the most frequent disability; between attacks the patient feels well. During these episodes, syncope appears abruptly, often with convulsions. The 12-month mortality rate for patients with Stokes-Adams attack who are not paced is 25 to 50 percent.

In milder forms, recurrent syncope may be the only symptom. Differential diagnosis must consider heart block, aortic stenosis, simple syncope, carotid sinus syndrome, epilepsy, or occlusive arterial disease of the cerebral circulation. The diagnosis can be quickly established with the electrocardiogram.

With intermittent heart block, or a "sick sinus syndrome" (tachy-bradyarrhythmia), a 24-h Holter monitoring may be necessary to make the diagnosis. This test is now performed with increasing frequency because certain cardiac arrhythmias can only be recognized by this form of continuous monitoring. Between intermittent episodes, there may be no findings whatever.

Certain electrocardiographic abnormalities suggest the diagnosis. These include trifascicular block, degrees of block less than complete AV disassociation, and the Mobitz type II block. These often signify impending AV disassociation.

As mentioned above, some patients become disabled from progressive heart failure related to inadequate cardiac output. Dramatic improvement, with prompt diuresis, often follows insertion of a pacemaker.

Pacemakers

HISTORICAL DATA. The entire field of pacemakers has expanded to a surprising degree since Bigelow and Callaghan in 1950–1951 developed an electric pacemaker that would increase the rate of the hypothermic heart. In 1952, Zoll convincingly demonstrated clinical possibilities by restarting the hearts of terminal patients with complete heart block, using electrical stimulation through the chest wall with a 60-cycle alternating current–powered Grass stimulator. Surgical interest was heightened with the development of open heart surgery and the unfortunate production of heart block during repair of congenital cardiac lesions. Lillihei demonstrated that direct cardiac pacing could be performed with an electrode implanted in the ventricle, although long-term stimulation with such electrodes ultimately failed, often due to infection. A completely implantable permanent pacemaker was described by Senning in 1959 and by Chardack in 1960. A remarkable clinical discovery was made by Furman and Schwedel in 1959, who found that the heart could be permanently paced with a transvenous catheter wedged into the endocardial surface of the right ventricle. They reported that one could safely leave a catheter in the superior vena cava across the tricuspid valve and permanently positioned in the right ventricle. Once the safety of the technique was established, the transvenous method quickly became the procedure of choice, with far less morbidity and mortality than the previous transthoracic approach.

Other investigators making significant contributions after 1960 include Frank, Kantrowitz, Escher, and Parsonnet. By 1978, Tyers estimated that 100,000 pacemakers were implanted each year for a wide variety of arrhythmias.

Several major technical developments have evolved, rendering pacemaker implantation a safe and predictable form of therapy. Early pacemakers were in epoxy, which permitted some transmission of body fluids. This accounted for the early depletion of the energy cells. Hermetic sealing has gradually been adopted since 1970, virtually avoiding permeation of body fluids. Tyers deserves credit for this important concept. It is estimated that as many as 40,000 early pacemaker recalls were necessary because of the premature power cell failure from penetration of body fluids. Fortunately, this is now almost never seen.

Another major development was the introduction of the lithium-polymer iodine cell in 1968, developed and refined by the Catalyst Research-Wilson Greatbatch Corporation. Over 200,000 of these had been implanted by 1978 without a single proved battery failure. Lithium batteries, a large variety of which have subsequently been developed, have much greater longevity than the zinc–mercuric oxide batteries originally used. Early pacemakers often failed within 2 to 3 years, perhaps sooner, because of permeation of body fluids. With refined lithium-iodine cells, 5 years of pacing is virtually a certainty, and the probability of 10 years of effective pacing is estimated to be greater than 90 percent.

PHYSIOLOGY OF CARDIAC PACEMAKERS. The electrical resistance of the normal heart is 300 to 500 Ω, while the fibrillating threshold to electrical stimulation is at least ten times greater. The efficacy of cardiac pacing depends upon the ability of the heart to respond to short bursts (2 ms) of electric current, ideally less than 1.5 to 2 mA. This amount of current is effective if delivered directly to the heart, but much larger currents are necessary to pace the ventricle through the intact chest wall.

The site of cardiac pacing, the right or left ventricle, apparently is of little significance. The electrode size,

configuration, and material are all important. There is a direct linear relationship between stimulation threshold and electrode surface area, the lowest threshold being associated with the smallest surface area. The optimal surface area for an electrode is about 12 mm^2. The energy capacity of a pacemaker is usually expressed as microjoules. One microjoule is one-millionth of the energy expended by a current of 1 A flowing for 1 s through a resistance of 1 Ω. Energy output in different pacemakers varies from 10 to 150 μJ, depending upon several factors. Other characteristics of the pacemakers include a voltage ranging from 2.5 to 7.5 V, delivering 3.5 to 15 mA, and pulse duration ranging from 0.15 to 1.5 ms.

When a pacemaker is implanted, it is crucial to determine the pacing threshold, measuring this in both milliamperes and volts. Threshold determination is particularly important with intravenous implantations in order to ensure that the catheter in the right ventricle is in the proper position. With satisfactory location of an electrode, a threshold of 0.4 to 0.8 mA at 0.2 to 0.4 V and a pulse width of 1 ms should be obtained.

After implantation, the threshold rises rapidly twofold to threefold in the next 2 to 4 weeks, stabilizing after about 1 month. Hence, the pulse generator output is adjusted in anticipation of this rise in threshold. An excessive rise in threshold may occur from infection or fibrosis, with resultant loss of pacing, termed "exit block." Special high-output pacemaker generators, stimulating up to 10 V, may be used in patients in whom previous pacemakers have failed because of exit block.

Ventricular pacing may be done with unipolar or bipolar leads. In the bipolar system, both the positive and negative electrodes are in contact with the endocardium. With epicardial implantation, both electrodes must be attached. If unipolar pacing, which is the most common, is used, the top of the electrode is the stimulating pole. Most efficient stimulation results from cathodal stimulation. The only particular advantage of bipolar stimulation is that the sensitivity to external magnetic interference is much less.

METHODS OF PACING. Initial pacemakers stimulated the ventricle at a fixed rate. These fixed-rate asynchronous units had numerous disadvantages, including the possible production of ventricular fibrillation by competition with the patient's own rhythm. Fixed-rate pacemakers have been supplanted by demand pacemakers, usually triggered from a ventricular electrode. These are of two types, the R-wave-inhibited type and the R-wave-triggered pacemaker. A more complex type is the atrioventricular pacemaker, requiring an electrode in the right atrium as well as in the ventricle (Fig. 19-27A and B). The resulting pacing may be through the atrium, or it may be atrioventricular synchronous pacing, stimulating first the atrium, then after an appropriate delay, the ventricle (Fig. 19-28). All of these have the advantage of coordinating with the patient's own cardiac rhythm and supplying an "atrial kick" when the atrioventricular sequential pacing is employed. Finally, the development of programmable pacemakers in the last 5 years permits adjustment of rate, pulse amplitude, and duration, which greatly enhances the function of pacemakers in different circum-

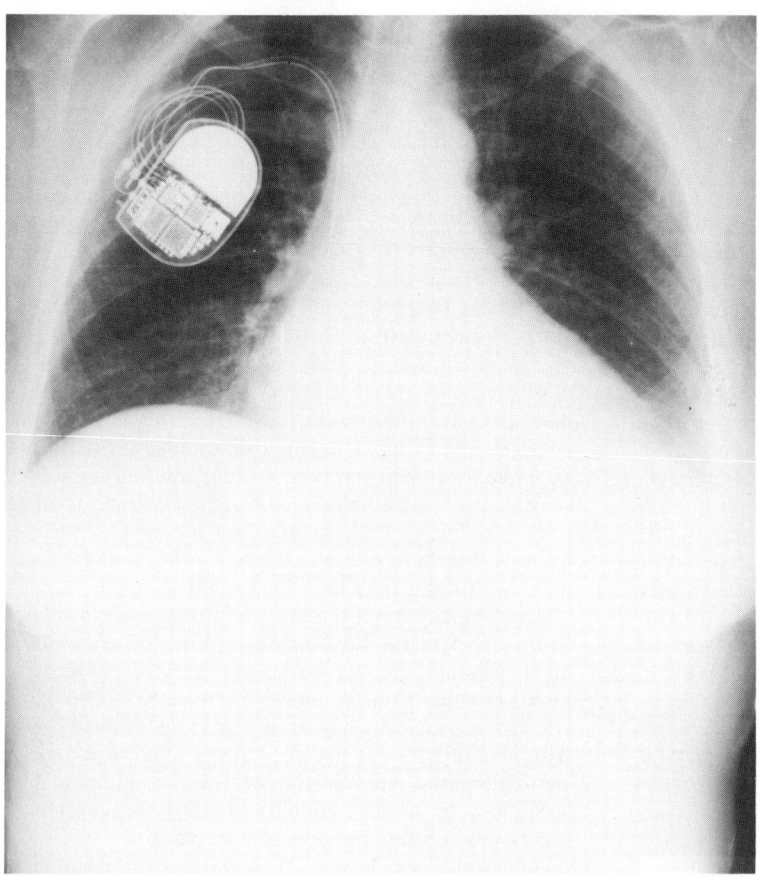

A

Fig. 19-27. *A* and *B*. AP and lateral chest x-ray of patient who developed complete heart block following aortic valve replacement, septal myotomy and myomectomy, ventricular aneurysm resection, and coronary artery bypass grafting. Dual chamber pacing was employed to optimize cardiac output.

stances. Undoubtedly, the entire field will continue to evolve rapidly as new benefits from different types of pacing are found.

With the growing complexity of the mode of pacing, location, and function of cardiac electrodes and with the multiplicity of terms introduced by trade companies, the Pacemaker Study Group of the American Heart Association introduced a simple generic three-letter identification code to identify the chamber paced, the chamber sensed, and the mode of generator function (Table 19-1, Fig. 19-29).

Initial pacemakers were heavy and bulky, a nuisance for adults but a serious problem for children, with the danger of erosion of the overlying skin. Developments in printed electric circuits and semiconductors have led to a progressive decrease in size. In 1978 Culliford et al. reported a technique of implantation in premature infants. In a 1981 review, Young surveyed the status of pacemakers in children, reviewing over 10 reports describing experiences with 448 implantations. The small pacemakers weigh only 50 g with a 20- to 25-mL volume, as compared with older units of 160 to 200 g and 160- to 200-mL volume.

Nuclear Pacemakers. Smyth et al. reported experiences with isotopic pacemakers in 59 patients. Details of nuclear-powered pacemakers are presented in his report.

Tyers and Brownlee raised issues about nuclear pacemakers, which are usually powered by plutonium 238. The basic concern is the long-term effect of radiation on the patient. The amount of radiation is very small in a nuclear pacemaker, but the effects of radiation on the induction of thyroid cancer were not known for over 20 years. Also bone marrow is susceptible to induction of leukemia by radiation. In addition, there is the real risk of environmental contamination. A sobering point is that if one of these units were lost in the ocean, 98 percent of the original 3100 microcuries of plutonium 238 would still be present more than 800 years later. The basic advantage, of course, is that these pacemakers should certainly function for 10 years, possibly indefinitely, and so the probability of battery change is remote. Because of the hazards, however, nuclear pacers are not recommended for younger patients.

IMPLANTATION OF PACEMAKERS. Medical therapy for chronic heart block has virtually disappeared with the development of effective pacemakers. Several years ago, in one group of 100 patients treated before pacemakers were available, 30 percent were dead in 6 months and 75

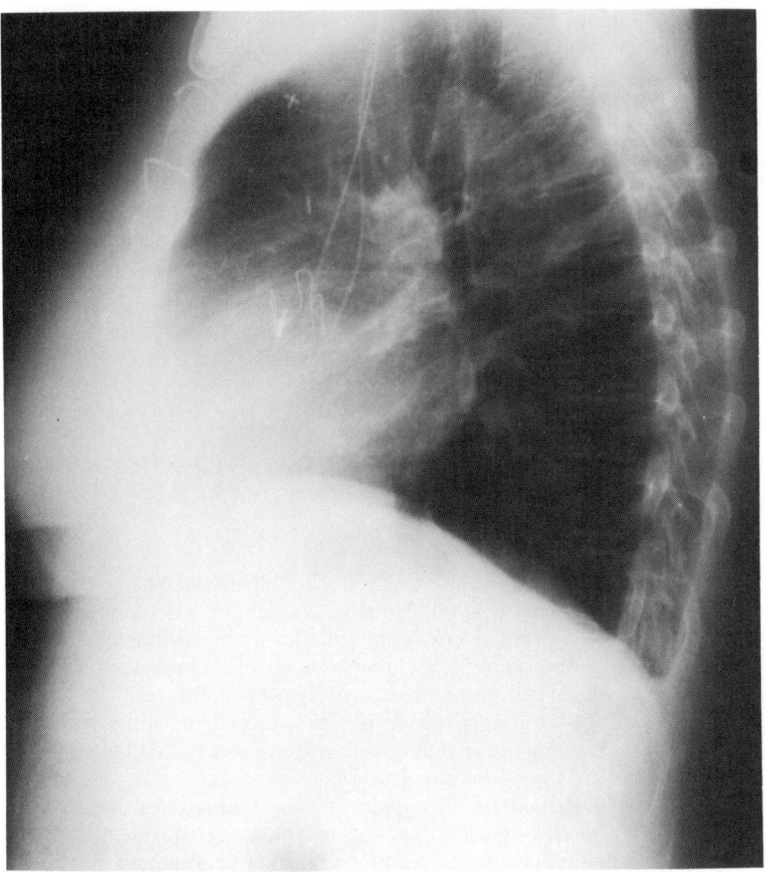

B

Fig. 19-27 *B.* Continued.

percent within 5 years. Hence, pacemakers are now employed promptly for bradycardias, even when they are asymptomatic, and are also widely used for several other arrhythmias. For transitory heart block following myocardial infarction, temporary pacing with a catheter electrode introduced through a peripheral vein and advanced into the right ventricle is usually effective. The block disappears in 90 to 95 percent of patients. Heart block following intracardiac operations is common, almost always subsiding in the next several days. A routine in the majority of cardiac centers is to leave pacing wires in the atrium and ventricle before the chest is closed, removing these several days later. Usually the wires can be used to pace the heart with an external generator for as long as 2 to 3 weeks.

The vast majority of pacemakers are inserted by the transvenous route because of the low morbidity. In order of preference, the cephalic vein, the external jugular vein, or the internal jugular vein may be used. In 1980, Brodman and Furman described a 12-year experience with 1800 patients, in 90 of whom the use of the internal jugular vein was necessary after finding that both the cephalic and external jugular veins were unsatisfactory.

Once the vein has been surgically exposed, the transvenous endocardial electrode can be advanced into the right ventricle, guided under fluoroscopic control, and wedged in an appropriate area. As mentioned earlier, determination of threshold is crucial in securing proper positioning of the catheter. Once the catheter has been positioned, the pacemaker is implanted in a subcutaneous pocket over the chest wall. Morbidity with the transvenous technique is small. Migration of the catheter from improper fixation is the most common complication. Perforation of the ventricle can occur with resultant diaphragmatic pacing or even tamponade. Infection or venous thrombosis is surprisingly rare.

Direct surgical approaches employ one of three routes: short left intercostal, subxiphoid, or left subcostal incision. Morbidity is definitely greater with a direct surgical approach than with a transvenous approach. However, with the development of the sutureless myocardial electrode, a "screw-in" electrode 6 mm in length, morbidity is much less than it used to be. Once the electrode is secured, the frequency of electrode complication is significantly less than with the transvenous approach, though the morbidity from the surgical procedure generally outweighs the advantages. Most would agree that the direct approach should be employed primarily for patients in whom the transvenous route has not been satisfactory because of pulmonary hypertension, dilated right atrium or ventricle, endocardial fibrosis, or tricuspid regurgitation.

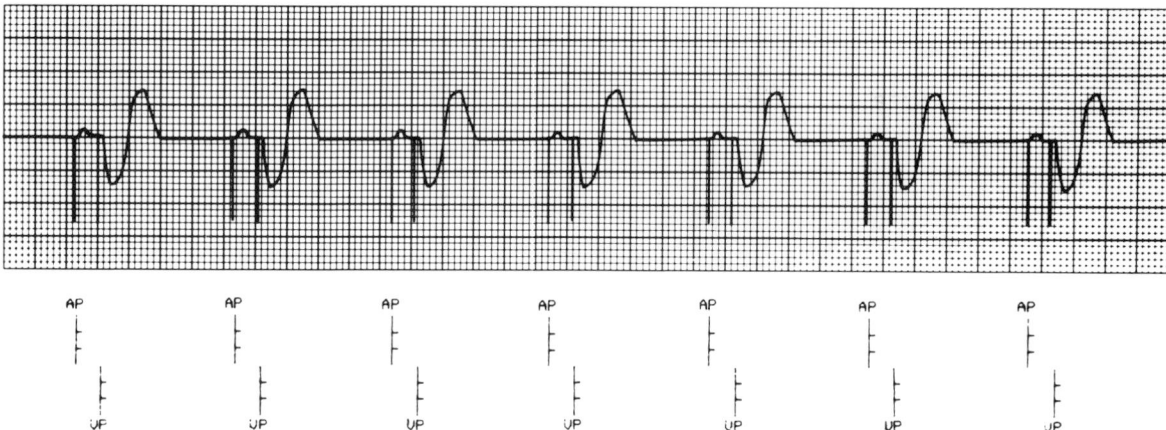

Fig. 19-28. Postoperative electrocardiogram of patient depicted in Fig. 19-27 with AV sequential pacemaker functioning. AP = atrial pace, VP = ventricular pace.

As mentioned earlier, the pacemakers are usually of the "demand" variety, with a basic rate between 70 and 80 beats/min, varying with the patient's own rhythm. The recent development of programmable pacemakers permits the subsequent alteration of pacing rate, pulse width, and amplitude. Also, the mode of pacing can be changed if conditions change.

Recovery following operation is usually uneventful. Antibiotics are given for 3 to 4 days. Difficulties with the subcutaneous implantation of the generator are infrequent, especially with the small generators now available and with meticulous surgical technique at the time of implantation.

Following discharge from the hospital, the patient should be seen in 2 to 3 weeks, because a rise in pacing threshold will occur. After this, the patient should be followed at 3-month intervals indefinitely.

Telephone electrocardiographic surveillance has been a significant advance in periodically evaluating patients over a large geographic distance. Convincing data from several sources indicate that this type of periodic monitoring is mandatory for good care. A typical report from

Rubin et al. described telephonic surveillance over a period of 3 years in 216 patients, finding 82 complications, 60 of which were asymptomatic. They estimated that telephonic surveillance may have decreased the death rate in pacemaker patients by nearly 50 percent.

As the pulse generator fails, there is usually a gradual slowing of the rate, giving ample warning that the generator should be changed.

Patients with permanent pacemakers requiring subsequent surgical procedures in which electrocautery is to be employed are at risk for pacemaker malfunction. Electromagnetic fields as high as 60 V/m are commonly induced with electrocautery, which far exceeds the energy level required to activate the sensing circuit in most pacemakers (usually in the area of 0.1 V/m). As a result, the intense signal may inhibit the pulse generator in a pacemaker-dependent patient or may damage the circuitry or reset programmable units. A variety of arrhythmias have been observed: ventricular asystole, multiple premature ventricular contractions, ventricular tachycardia, and fibrillation. In patients for whom electrocautery cannot be avoided, brief bursts of bipolar cautery should be used because it minimizes the ambient electrical field around the probe. The program for programmable units should be available in the operating room and a thorough preoperative evaluation of the patient may indicate the advisability of a backup temporary transvenous wire in patients who are totally pacemaker-dependent. Awareness of the adverse effects electrocautery may have on paced patients will provide enhanced interoperative and postoperative monitoring. The importance of these potentially serious and lethal complications is reinforced when one considers that many of the over 500,000 individuals in the United States who now have permanent pacemakers will require elective or emergency surgical care in the future.

AUTOMATIC IMPLANTABLE DIFIBRILLATORS. In 1980, Mirowski reported on the successful termination of malignant ventricular arrhythmias with an automatic implantable defibrillator. Although this form of therapy is still in the early stages of development, a 1984 report

Table 19-1. THREE-LETTER IDENTIFICATION CODE

1st letter	2d letter	3d letter
Chamber paced	*Chamber sensed*	*Mode of response*
V—Ventricle		I—Inhibited
A—Atrium		T—Triggered
D—Double chamber		O—Not applicable

First letter: The paced chamber is identified by V for ventricle, A for atrium, or D for double—both atrium and ventricle.
Second letter: The sensed chamber, if either, is again V for ventricle, A for atrium.
Third letter: The mode of response, if any, is either:
  I for inhibited, a pacemaker whose output is blocked by a sensed signal, or
  T for triggered, a unit whose output is discharged by a sensed signal.
  O indicates that a specific comment is not applicable.

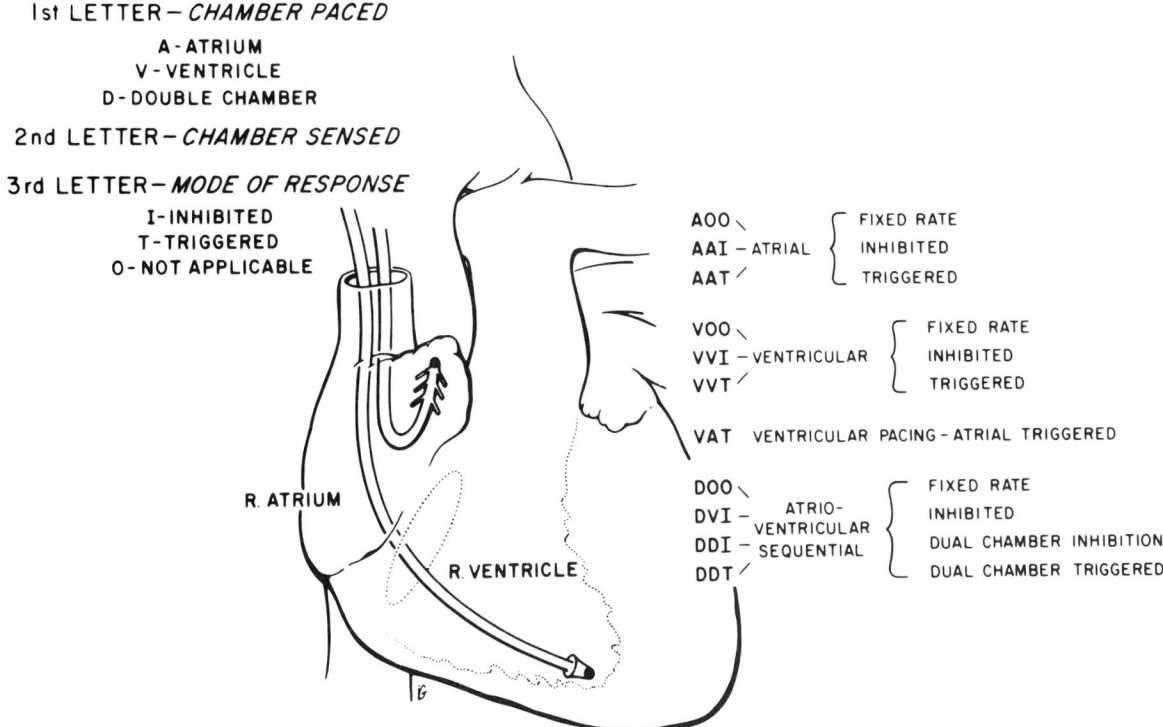

1st LETTER – *CHAMBER PACED*
 A - ATRIUM
 V - VENTRICLE
 D - DOUBLE CHAMBER

2nd LETTER – *CHAMBER SENSED*

3rd LETTER – *MODE OF RESPONSE*
 I - INHIBITED
 T - TRIGGERED
 O - NOT APPLICABLE

R. ATRIUM

R. VENTRICLE

AOO
AAI – ATRIAL
AAT
{ FIXED RATE / INHIBITED / TRIGGERED }

VOO
VVI – VENTRICULAR
VVT
{ FIXED RATE / INHIBITED / TRIGGERED }

VAT VENTRICULAR PACING - ATRIAL TRIGGERED

DOO
DVI – ATRIO-VENTRICULAR
DDI – SEQUENTIAL
DDT
{ FIXED RATE / INHIBITED / DUAL CHAMBER INHIBITION / DUAL CHAMBER TRIGGERED }

Fig. 19-29. Three-letter identification code presently in international use. *(Reprinted courtesy of the American Heart Association.)*

showed apparent early success for 78 consecutive patients with ventricular tachycardia and fibrillation refractory to antiarrhythmic drugs who received implantable automatic internal cardioverter-defibrillator devices.

Others have combined endocardial resection, intraoperative electrophysiologic studies, and implantation of these devices. Twelve such patients were reported by Watkins in 1984. The survival period has been 32 months thus far, with 2 deaths occurring that were not attributable to cardiac causes. The device had been noted to be repetitively successful in terminating fatal ventricular arrhythmias in these patients.

As increasing numbers of patients survive the "sudden cardiac death syndrome" because of prompt treatment and the growing popular awareness of resuscitative techniques, this form of therapy should prove promising for patients failing pharmacologic management of malignant arrhythmias if continued clinical experience and technological advances support the thus far favorable, but limited, clinical observations.

ASSISTED CIRCULATION AND ARTIFICIAL HEARTS

Assisted Circulation

Temporary assisted circulation is a valuable clinical modality when a transient cardiac injury is present, as opposed to a permanent injury such as extensive myocar-

dial infarction. The usual indication for assisted circulation occurs following a cardiac operation when myocardial function is significantly depressed, usually manifested by a cardiac index less than 2.0 $L/m^2/min$. In such instances, assisting the circulation for 24 to 48 h or longer may permit spontaneous improvement in cardiac function, probably from resolution of myocardial edema. The improvement in function is probably accomplished by maintaining adequate perfusion while decreasing the work of the myocardium, hence the term "assisted circulation."

As the concept of temporary assisted circulation is based upon the ability of the heart to spontaneously recover from an existing injury, assisted circulation is seldom effective if required for more than 2 to 3 days, as such patients usually have irreversible myocardial infarction.

Because of the vascular circulation in the heart, the subendocardial area is the most vulnerable, as it is the farthest removed from the coronary arteries on the epicardial surface. With severe myocardial edema from any cause, subendocardial necrosis can result, probably from constriction and compression of terminal coronary arterioles, perhaps analogous to the compartmental syndromes that may occur in the leg after a crush injury, when edema progresses to such an extent that circulation is stopped and tissue necrosis occurs.

The concept of assisting the failing heart by pumping part or all of the circulation through a heart-lung machine has been investigated since the onset of extracorporeal circulation around 1955. It was quickly observed by several groups that a heart unable to maintain circulation after operation with extracorporeal circulation could be supported with a heart-lung machine for 1 to 2 h and then function satisfactorily, apparently recovering from a transient injury. From these observations, the concept of "assisted circulation" was born, supporting the circulation for days, until spontaneous recovery of cardiac function occurred.

If severe myocardial edema is present, the prompt use of assisted circulation may permit full recovery because the edema resolves without the development of extensive necrosis. Delayed use of assisted circulation may permit some patients to spontaneously recover, but others will progress to infarction. Belatedly trying assisted circulation with these patients will inevitably result in a higher mortality because irreversible necrosis is present.

INTRAAORTIC BALLOON PUMPING. Intraaortic balloon pumping is the most effective clinical technique for assisted circulation. This was developed primarily through the efforts of Austen and his associates. A balloon catheter is inserted into a peripheral artery, usually the femoral, and advanced into the thoracic aorta. The safest method for insertion is by direct arteriotomy, but percutaneous insertion of a balloon can be done in urgent problems, initiating balloon pumping much more rapidly. The percutaneous method has more complications, however, especially in females with small femoral arteries.

With electronic synchronization, the balloon is alternately inflated during diastole and deflated during systole. When functioning properly, cardiac index is increased about 0.5 to 0.7 L/min. The pump can be used for several days with minimal morbidity. The blood platelet count usually decreases, probably from trauma from inflation of the balloon. This may be treated with platelet transfusions.

Ischemia of the extremity in which the balloon catheter has been inserted is the most common complication. With large femoral arteries this is unusual. In patients with small or diseased femoral arteries, however, insertion of a balloon may be catastrophic, resulting in either gangrene of the extremity or death. Viability of the extremity must be confirmed by frequent examination of the extremity for the first few hours after the balloon has been inserted. Viability, of course, depends upon continued flow of blood to the extremity around the catheter lying within the artery. If the artery is occluding the lumen, either because of the small size of the artery or because of an atherosclerotic plaque, the same severe ischemia exists as that produced by acute arterial occlusion from an embolus.

At NYU the balloon pump is used promptly if the cardiac index remains below 2 L despite other forms of therapy. It seems lifesaving in postoperative patients, where transient injury may regress after 2 to 4 days. In the last 2 to 3 years, the frequency of use of a balloon has decreased markedly, probably because of the concurrent improvement in the effectiveness of techniques of myocardial preservation.

In one other group, 188 patients were discharged from the hospital following support. The average period of support in these patients was about 60 h. Patients who achieved a cardiac index greater than 2 L were successfully weaned from the pump, while those whose cardiac index remained below the 2.0-L level had a mortality well above 50 percent. In another report only 35 percent of the group ultimately survived hospitalization. Three patients developed the grim complication of paraplegia.

LEFT HEART BYPASS. Dennis demonstrated the benefits of assisted circulation with left heart bypass in experimental studies, withdrawing blood from the atrium and infusing it into a peripheral artery. Difficulties with closed chest cannulation of the left atrium, however, prevented clinical application of the procedure. In the early 1960s Spencer used left heart bypass in a small group of patients by performing a thoracotomy, directly cannulating the left atrium, and employing left heart bypass for 3 to 4 h. Longer periods, however, were impractical.

Clinical use of the technique for patients in cardiogenic shock is under active investigation, though significant data are not yet available. Litwak devised a new type of left heart bypass, to be used in patients who could not be weaned from the heart-lung machine following operation. Silastic cannulae were left in the left atrium and femoral artery and brought through the chest wall before the incision was closed. Pumping was done with a roller pump with silastic tubing, infusing enough heparin to keep the activated clotting time near 150 s. The technique produced significant platelet destruction but otherwise was well tolerated.

With some modifications the Litwak technique was adopted at New York University. Flow rates up to 3500 mL/min could be obtained. Support was used for periods ranging from 16 to 70 h. In 1983 Rose et al. summarized total experiences at NYU with a series of 35 patients. Seventeen patients survived to have the device removed, four of whom died in the next 2 to 4 months. Three of the deaths were from sepsis. Of 13 long-term survivors, five had mild to moderate cardiac symptoms and eight were asymptomatic. The data fully indicate the value of assisted circulation because the device clearly permitted recovery of a heart whose function was temporarily decreased to a near lethal degree.

OTHER FORMS OF LEFT HEART BYPASS. Left heart-aortic bypass with a roller pump has the advantage of ease of applicability and simplicity, but it is moderately traumatic, is nonpulsatile, and is not coordinated with the patient's own cardiac contractions, as is electronically done with intraaortic balloon pumping. Much effort has accordingly been expended to develop physiologically more efficient forms of left heart assist that would effectively support the circulation for weeks or months.

Pierce et al. described experiences with 30 patients over a period of 6 years. Subsequent to 1979, survival increased to about 50 percent, partly because of use of the left atrium rather than the left ventricle for cannulation. Seven patients remained well 5 to 36 months after discharge from the hospital. The Pierce Donachy pump is currently one of the most effective temporary left heart pumps. It is expensive and somewhat difficult to insert but can clearly function satisfactorily for weeks without significant blood trauma. It seems to be a potentially ideal bridge for transplantation. Park and Magovern reported the use of a centrifugal pump in 41 patients, not all of whom required anticoagulation. Schoen et al. reported experiences with diaphragm pumps for temporary circulatory assistance.

Artificial Hearts

Attempts to develop an artificial heart have continued for decades, with a large interdisciplinary program coordinated by the National Heart and Lung Institute. The group headed by Kolff has the longest continued studies of different forms of artificial hearts, with impressive results in calves that survived with an artificial heart for many months. These studies led to the first clinical trial of an artificial heart at Salt Lake City, Utah, in December 1982. The patient survived slightly more than 100 days. Several patients have been successfully operated on, but subsequent thromboembolism was crippling.

The major obstacle is the lack of an artificial substance that resembles a normal intima in the bloodstream. All existing substances result in a surface aggregation of platelets and institution of the thrombotic process. Hence, thromboembolism is a serious or prohibitive risk unless anticoagulation is used, which, in turn, causes problems from bleeding.

Among the several artificial hearts currently under study, the Jarvik-7 model is the most popular. The cumbersome pneumatic-driven pumps, requiring tubes through the chest wall, have been a serious handicap. At present, the best use of heart pumps seems to be as a bridge until clinical transplantation can be done, for results with transplantation are far better. In the future, some type of electrically powered artificial heart seems far preferable to the pneumatic-powered devices.

Griffith et al. in 1987 reported experiences with the Jarvik-7 total artificial heart in six moribund patients, using this as a bridge to transplantation. Four patients were currently well, subsequently having the device removed and a successful transplant performed. In these six patients, total mechanical support was used for a total of 52 days with excellent function of the artificial heart.

Bibliography

Introduction; Clinical Manifestations

Arciniegas E: *Pediatric Cardiac Surgery*. Chicago, Year Book Medical Publishers, 1985.

Gibbon JH Jr, Sabiston DC Jr, Spencer FC: *Surgery of the Chest*, 3d ed. Philadelphia, Saunders, 1976.

Kirklin JW, Barratt-Boyes BG: *Cardiac Surgery*. New York, Wiley, 1986.

Perloff JK: *The Clinical Recognition of Congenital Heart Disease*, 3d ed. Philadelphia, Saunders, 1987.

Smith P: Several consequences of cardiopulmonary bypass. *Lancet* 1:823, 1986.

Sotaniemi KA: Five-year neurological and EEG outcome after open heart surgery. *J Neurol Neurosurg Psychiatry* 48:569, 1985.

Stark J, de Leval M (eds): *Surgery for Congenital Heart Defects*. London, Grune and Stratton, 1983.

Starr A: Presidential address: The thoracic surgical industrial complex. *Ann Thorac Surg* 42:124, 1986.

Extracorporeal Circulation

Bartlett RH, Gazzaniga AB, et al: Extracorporeal membrane oxygenation (ECMO) in neonatal respiratory failure. 100 cases. *Ann Surg* 204(3):236.

Boyd AD, Tremblay RE, et al: Estimation of cardiac output soon after intracardiac surgery with cardiopulmonary bypass. *Ann Surg* 150:613, 1959.

Brantigan CO, Grow JB: Cricothyroidotomy: Elective use in respiratory problems requiring tracheostomy. *J Thorac Cardiovasc Surg* 71:72, 1976.

Buckberg GD: Studies of control reperfusion after ischemia. *J Thorac Cardiovasc Surg* 92(suppl):483, 1986.

DeWall RA, Warden HE, et al: The helix reservoir pump-oxygenator. *Surg Gynecol Obstet* 104:699, 1957.

Esposito R, Culliford A, et al: What is the relationship between plasma heparin concentration and (ACT) activated clotting time? Presented at the 1982 meeting of the American Association for Thoracic Surgery, Phoenix.

Gibbon JH Jr: Application of a mechanical heart and lung apparatus to cardiac surgery. *Minn Med* 37:171, 1954.

Jones RE, Donald DE, et al: Apparatus of the Gibbon type for mechanical bypass of the heart and lungs: Preliminary report. *Proc Staff Meetings Mayo Clin* 30:105, 1955.

Proceedings of Cardioplegia: The First Quarter Century. An International Symposium on Myocardial Protection, London, 1980.

Spencer FC, Benson DW, et al: Use of a mechanical respirator in the management of respiratory insufficiency following trauma or operation for cardiac or pulmonary disease. *J Thorac Cardiovasc Surg* 38:758, 1959.

Stephen Thomas J (ed): *Manual of Cardiac Anesthesia*. New York, Churchill, Livingstone, 1984.

Cardiac Arrest and Ventricular Fibrillation

Cobb LA, Werner JA, Trobaugh GB: Sudden cardiac death. I. A decade's experience with out-of-hospital resuscitation. *Mod Concepts Cardiovasc Dis* 49:31, 1980.

Cobb LA, Werner JA, Trobaugh GB: Sudden cardiac death. II. Outcome of resuscitation; management, and future directions. *Mod Concepts Cardiovasc Dis* 49:37, 1980.

Del Guercio LRM, Feins NR, et al: Comparison of blood flow during external and internal cardiac massage in man. *Circulation* 31(suppl I):I171, 1965.

Dunn HM, McComb JM, et al: Survival to leave hospital from ventricular fibrillation. *Am Heart J* 112:745, 1986.

Geehr EC, Lewis FR, Auerbach PS: Failure of open-heart massage to improve survival after prehospital non-traumatic cardiac arrest. *N Engl J Med* 314:1189, 1986.

Hughes WG, Ruedy JR: Should calcium be used in cardiac arrest? *Am J Med* 81(2):285, 1986.

Joseph WL, Maloney JV Jr: Extracorporeal circulation as an adjunct to resuscitation of the heart. *JAMA* 193:683, 1965.

Jude JR, Elam JO: *Fundamentals of Cardiopulmonary Resuscitation*. Philadelphia, Davis, 1965.

Koehler RC, Chandra N, et al: Augmentation of cerebral perfusion by simultaneous chest compression and lung inflation with abdominal binding after cardiac arrest in dogs. *Circulation* 67(2):266, 1983.

Kouwenhoven WB, Jude JR, Knickerbocker GG: Closed chest cardiac massage. *JAMA* 137:1064, 1960.

Kouwenhoven WB, Milnor WR, et al: Closed chest defibrillation of the heart. *Surgery* 42:550, 1957.

Myerburg RJ, Kessler KM, et al: Long-term survival after pre-hospital cardiac arrest: Analysis of outcome during an eight year study. *Circulation* 70(4):538, 1984.

Roy D, Waxman HL, et al: Clinical characteristics and long-term follow-up in 119 survivors of cardiac arrest: Relation to inducibility at electrophysiologic testing. *Am J Cardiol* 52(8):969, 1983.

Rudikoff MT, Maughan WL, et al: Mechanisms of blood flow during cardiopulmonary resuscitation. *Circulation* 61(2):345, 1980.

Safar P: Cerebral resuscitation after cardiac arrest: A review. *Circulation* 74(6, 2):IV138, 1986.

Sanders AB, Kern KB, et al: Improved resuscitation from cardiac arrest with open-chest massage. *Ann Emerg Med* 13:672, 1984.

Sanders AB, Kern MD, et al: Correspondence: More on open-chest cardiac massage after cardiac arrest. *N Engl J Med* 315:968, 1986.

Spencer FC, Bahnson HT: Treatment of cardiac arrest, in Benson CD, et al (eds): *Pediatric Surgery*. Chicago, Year Book Medical Publishers, 1962, vol I, p 522.

Surawicz B: Ventricular fibrillation. *J Am Coll Cardiol* 5(suppl 6):43B, 1985.

Wilber DJ, Garan H, Ruskin JN: Electrophysiologic testing in survivors of cardiac arrest. *Circulation* 75(suppl III):146, 1987.

Williams GR, Spencer FC: The clinical use of hypothermia following cardiac arrest. *Ann Surg* 148:462, 1958.

Zimmerman JM, Spencer FC: The influence of hypothermia on cerebral injury resulting from circulatory occlusion. *Surg Forum* 9:216, 1958.

Mitral Stenosis and Insufficiency

Chauvaud S, Perier P, et al: Long-term results of valve repair in children with acquired mitral valve incompetence. *Circulation* 74:1104, 1986.

Cobanoglu A, Grunkemeier GL, et al: Mitral replacement: Clinical experience with a ball-valve prosthesis. Twenty-five years later. *Ann Surg* 202:376, 1985.

Cohn LH, Allred EN, et al: Long-term results of open mitral valve reconstruction for mitral stenosis. *Am J Cardiol* 55:731, 1985.

Ferrazzi P, McGiffin DC, et al: Have the results of mitral valve replacement improved? *J Thorac Cardiovasc Surg* 92:186, 1986.

Halseth W, Elliott D, et al: Open mitral commissurotomy: A modern re-evaluation. *J Thorac Cardiovasc Surg* 80:842, 1980.

Hetzer R, Bougioukas G, et al: Mitral valve replacement with preservation of papillary muscles and chordae tendineae—revival of a seemingly forgotten concept. I. Preliminary clinical report. *J Thorac Cardiovasc Surg* 31:291, 1983.

Higgs LM, Glancy DL, et al: Mitral restenosis: An uncommon cause of recurrent symptoms following mitral commissurotomy. *Am J Cardiol* 26:34, 1970.

Isom OW, Spencer FC, et al: Long-term results in 1375 patients undergoing valve replacement with the Starr-Edwards cloth-covered steel ball valve prosthesis. *Ann Surg* 186:310, 1977.

Kirklin JW, Barratt-Boyes BG: *Cardiac Surgery*. New York, Wiley, 1986.

McGoon DC: Repair of mitral insufficiency due to ruptured chordae tendineae. *J Thorac Cardiovasc Surg* 39:357, 1960.

McKay RG, Lock JE, et al: Balloon dilation of mitral stenosis in adult patients: Postmortem and percutaneous mitral valvuloplasty studies. *J Am Coll Cardiol* 9:723, 1987.

Miller DC, Oyer PE, et al: Ten to fifteen year reassessment of the performance characteristics of the Starr Edwards model 6120 mitral valve prosthesis. *J Thorac Cardiovasc Surg* 85:1, 1983.

O'Brien MF, Stafford EG, et al: Aortic valve replacement with cryopreserved homograft valves and with antibiotic 4°C stored valves: A comparative follow-up study. Presented at the 67th Annual Meeting of the American Association for Thoracic Surgery, 1987.

Oyer P, Miller D, et al: Clinical durability of the Hancock porcine bioprosthetic valve. *J Thorac Cardiovasc Surg* 80:824, 1980.

Palacios I, Block PC, et al: Percutaneous balloon valvotomy for patients with severe mitral stenosis. *Circulation* 75:778, 1987.

Reed GE, Pooley R, Moggio R: Durability of measured mitral annuloplasty. Seventeen-year study. *J Thorac Cardiovasc Surg* 79:321, 1980.

Selzer A, Cohn KE: Natural history of mitral stenosis: A review. *Circulation* 45:878, 1972.

Souttar PW: The surgical treatment of mitral stenosis. *Br Med J* 2:603, 1925.

Spencer FC, Colvin SB, et al: Experiences with the Carpentier techniques of mitral valve reconstruction in 103 patients (1980–1985). *J Thorac Cardiovasc Surg* 90:341, 1985.

Spencer FC, Galloway AC, Colvin SB: A clinical evaluation of the hypothesis that rupture of the left ventricle following mitral valve replacement can be prevented by preservation of the chordae of the mural leaflet. *Ann Surg* 202:673, 1985.

Spencer FC, Baumann FG, et al: Experiences with 1643 porcine prosthetic valves in 1492 patients. *Ann Surg* 203:691, 1986.

Starr A, Edwards ML: Mitral replacement: Clinical experience with a ball valve prosthesis. *Ann Surg* 154:726, 1961.

Teply J, Grunkemeier G, et al: The ultimate prognosis after valve replacement: An assessment at twenty years. *Ann Thorac Surg* 32:111, 1981.

Aortic Stenosis and Insufficiency

Arciniegas E: *Pediatric Cardiac Surgery*. Chicago, Year Book Medical Publishers, 1985.

Bloomfield P, Kitchin AH, et al: A prospective evaluation of the Bjork-Shiley, Hancock, and Carpentier-Edwards heart valve prostheses. *Circulation*. 73:1213, 1986.

Christakis GT, Weisel RD, et al: Can the results of contemporary aortic valve replacement be improved? *J Thorac Cardiovasc Surg* 92:37, 1986.

Isner JM, Salem DN, et al: Treatment of calcific aortic stenosis by balloon valvuloplasty. *Am J Cardiol* 59:313, 1987.

Kirklin JW, Barratt-Boyes BG: *Cardiac Surgery*. New York, Wiley, 1986.

Lombard JT, Selzer A: Valvular aortic stenosis. A clinical and hemodynamic profile of patients. *Ann Intern Med* 106:292, 1987.

Meurs AA, Grundemann AM, et al: Early and 8 year results of aortic valve replacement: A clinical study of 232 patients. *Eur Heart J* 6:870, 1985.

O'Brien MF, Stafford EG, et al: Aortic valve replacement with cryopreserved homograft valves and with antibiotic 4°C stored valves: A comparative follow-up study. Presented at the Annual Meeting of the American Association for Thoracic Surgery, April 1987.

Olson LJ, Subramanian R, Edwards WD: Surgical pathology of pure aortic insufficiency: A study of 225 cases. *Mayo Clin Proc* 59:835, 1984.

Perloff JK: *The Clinical Recognition of Congenital Heart Disease*, 3rd ed. Philadelphia, Saunders, 1987.

Schneider JF, Wilson M, Gallant TE: Percutaneous balloon aortic valvuloplasty for aortic stenosis in elderly patients at high risk for surgery. *Ann Intern Med* 106:696, 1987.

Stark J, de Leval M (eds): *Surgery for Congenital Heart Defects*. London, Grune and Stratton, 1983.

Subramanian R, Olson LJ, Edwards WD: Surgical pathology of pure aortic stenosis: A study of 374 cases. *Mayo Clin Proc* 59:683, 1984.

Tricuspid Stenosis and Insufficiency

Arbulu A, Thoms NW, Wilson RF: Valvulectomy without prosthetic replacement: A lifesaving operation for tricuspid *Pseudomonas* endocarditis. *J Thorac Cardiovasc Surg* 64:103, 1972.

Arbulu A, Asfaw I: Tricuspid valvulectomy without prosthetic replacement. Ten years of clinical experience. *J Thorac Cardiovasc Surg* 82:684, 1981.

Boyd AD, Engelman RH, et al: Tricuspid annuloplasty. *J Thorac Cardiovasc Surg* 68:344, 1974.

Carpentier A, Chauvaud S, et al: Reconstructive surgery of mitral valve incompetence. Ten-year appraisal. *J Thorac Cardiovasc Surg* 79:338, 1980.

Cobanoglu A, Starr A: Tricuspid valve surgery: Indications, methods, and results. *Cardiovasc Clin* 16:375, 1986.

Isom OW, Spencer FC, et al: Long-term results in 1375 patients undergoing valve replacement with the Starr-Edwards cloth-covered steel ball valve prosthesis. *Ann Surg* 186:310, 1977.

Peterffy A: Surgical management of tricuspid valvular disease. Ten years' experience of 141 consecutive patients. *Scand J Thorac Cardiovasc Surg* 26(suppl):1, 1980.

Peterffy A, Jonasson R, Henze A: Haemodynamic changes after tricuspid valve surgery. A recatheterization study in forty-five patients. *Scand J Thorac Cardiovasc Surg* 15:161, 1981.

Robin E, Thoms NW, et al: Hemodynamic consequences of total removal of the tricuspid valve without prosthetic replacement. *Am J Cardiol* 35:481, 1981.

Spencer FC, Shabetai R, Adolph R: Successful replacement of the tricuspid valve 10 years after traumatic incompetence. *Am J Cardiol* 18:916, 1966.

Stern HJ, Sisto DA, et al: Immediate tricuspid valve replacement for endocarditis. Indications and results. *J Thorac Cardiovasc Surg* 91:163, 1986.

Thorburn CW, Morgan JJ, et al: Long-term results of tricuspid valve replacement and the problem of prosthetic valve thrombosis. *Am J Cardiol* 51:1128, 1983.

Wellens F, Jacques G: Tricuspid valve replacement. *Cardiovasc Clin* 17:111, 1987.

Multivalvular Heart Disease

Bonchek LI, Starr A: Ball valve prostheses: Current appraisal of late results. *Am J Cardiol* 35:843, 1975.

Kirklin JW, Barratt-Boyes BG: *Cardiac Surgery*. New York, Wiley, 1986.

Spencer FC, Baumann FG, et al: Experiences with 1643 porcine prosthetic valves in 1492 patients. *Ann Surg* 203:691, 1986.

Cardiac Trauma

Blalock A, Ravitch MM: A consideration of the nonoperative treatment of cardiac tamponade resulting from wounds to the heart. *Surgery* 14:157, 1943.

Bland EF, Beebe GW: Missiles in the heart: A 20-year follow-up report of World War II cases. *N Engl J Med* 274:1039, 1966.

Estrera AS, Schreiber JT: Management of acute cardiac trauma. *Cardiol Clin* 2:239, 1984.

Evans J, Gray L, et al: Principles for the management of penetrating cardiac wounds. *Ann Surg* 189:777, 1979.

Frazee RC, Mucha P Jr, et al: Objective evaluation of blunt cardiac trauma. *J Trauma* 26:510, 1986.

Gay W: Blunt trauma to the heart and great vessels. *Surgery* 91:507, 1982.

Harken DE: Foreign bodies in and in relation to the heart and thoracic vessels. *Surg Gynecol Obstet* 83:117, 1946.

Holdeger WF, Lyons C, Edwards WS: Indications for removal of intracardiac foreign bodies. *Ann Surg* 163:249, 1966.

Isaacs JP: Sixty penetrating wounds to the heart: Clinical and experimental observations. *Surgery* 45:696, 1959.

Ivatury R, Shah P, et al: Emergency room thoracotomy for the resuscitation of patients with "fatal" penetrating injuries of the heart. *Ann Thorac Surg* 32:377, 1981.

Marshall WG Jr, Bell JL, Kouchoukos NT: Penetrating cardiac trauma. *J Trauma* 24:147, 1984.

Reid CL, Kawanishi DT, et al: Chest trauma: Evaluation by two-dimensional echocardiography. *Am Heart J* 113:971, 1987.

Spencer FC: Treatment of chest injuries. *Curr Probl Surg* January 1964.

Spencer FC, Kennedy JH: War wounds of the heart. *J Thorac Cardiovasc Surg* 33:361, 1957.

Sugg WL, Ecker RR, et al: Penetrating wounds of the heart: An analysis of 459 cases. *J Thorac Cardiovasc Surg* 56:531, 1968.

Tenzer ML: The spectrum of myocardial contusion: A review. *J Trauma* 25:620, 1985.

Cardiac Tumors

Attar S, Lee Y, et al: Cardiac myxoma. *Ann Thorac Surg* 29:397, 1980.

Bahnson HT, Spencer FC, Andrus EC: Diagnosis and treatment of intracavitary myxomas of the heart. *Ann Surg* 145:915, 1957.

Calhoun T, Terry E, et al: Myocardial fibroma or fibrous hamartoma. *Ann Thorac Surg* 32:406, 1981.

Chan HSL, Sonley MJ, et al: Primary and secondary tumors of childhood involving the heart, pericardium, and great vessels. A report of 75 cases and review of the literature. *Cancer* 56:825, 1985.

Crafoord C: Case report. *Int Symp Cardiovasc Surg Henry Ford Hosp* p 202, 1955.

Fyke FE, Seward JB, et al: Primary cardiac tumors: Experience with 30 consecutive patients since the introduction of two-dimensional echocardiography. *J Am Coll Cardiol* 5(6):1465, 1985.

Gassman HS, Meadows R, Baker LA: Metastatic tumors of the heart. *Am J Med* 19:357, 1955.

Geha AS, Weidman WH, et al: Intramural ventricular cardiac fibroma: Successful removal in two cases and review of the literature. *Circulation* 36:427, 1967.

Hanfling S: Metastatic cancer to the heart. *Circulation* 22:474, 1960.

Larrieu A, Jamieson W, et al: Primary cardiac tumors. Experience with 25 cases. *J Thorac Cardiovasc Surg* 83:339, 1982.

Mahaim I: *Les tumors et les polypes du coeur: Étude anatomoclinique.* Paris, Masson et Cie, 1945.

Prichard RW: Tumors of the heart. *Arch Pathol* 21:98, 1951.

Reece IJ, Cooley DA, et al: Cardiac tumors: Clinical spectrum and prognosis of lesions other than classical benign myxoma in 20 patients. *J Thorac Cardiovasc Surg* 88:439, 1984.

Spencer FC: The heart, in Nealon TF (ed): *Management of the Patient with Cancer.* Philadelphia, Saunders, 1965, p 537.

Whorton CM: Primary malignant tumors of the heart. *Cancer* 2:245, 1949.

Yater WM: Tumors of the heart and pericardium. *Arch Intern Med* 48:627, 1931.

Coronary Artery Disease

Amsterdam EA, Martschinske R, et al: Symptomatic and silent myocardial ischemia during exercise testing in coronary artery disease. *Am J Cardiol* 58:43B, 1986.

Barner HB, Standeven JW, Reese J: Twelve-year experience with internal mammary artery for coronary artery bypass. *J Thorac Cardiovasc Surg* 90:668, 1985.

Cameron A, Kemp HG Jr, Green GE: Bypass surgery with the internal mammary artery graft: 15 year follow-up. *Circulation* 74:III30, 1986.

Catinella FP, Cunningham JN Jr, et al: Cold blood should not be used for vein preparation prior to coronary bypass grafting. *J Thorac Cardiovasc Surg* 82:904, 1981.

Chesebro JH, Clements IP, et al: A platelet-inhibitor-drug trial in coronary-artery bypass operations. *N Engl J Med* 307:73, 1982.

Cobb LA, Werner JA, Trobaugh GB: Sudden cardiac death. I. A decade's experience with out-of-hospital resuscitation. *Mod Concepts Cardiovasc Dis* 49:31, 1980.

Cobb LA, Werner JA, Trobaugh GB: Sudden cardiac death. II. Outcome of resuscitation; management, and future directions. *Mod Concepts Cardiovasc Dis* 49:37, 1980.

Cosgrove DM, Loop FD, et al: Determinants of 10-year survival after primary myocardial revascularization. *Ann Surg* 202:480, 1985.

Culliford AT, Colvin SB, et al: The atherosclerotic ascending aorta and transverse arch: A new technique to prevent cerebral injury during bypass: Experience with 13 patients. *Ann Thorac Surg* 41:27, 1986.

Cunningham JN Jr, Adams PX, et al: Preservation of ATP, ultrastructure, and ventricular function after aortic cross-clamping and reperfusion. Clinical use of blood potassium cardioplegia. *J Thorac Cardiovasc Surg* 78:708, 1979.

Cunningham JN Jr, Catinella FP, Spencer FC: Blood cardioplegia—clinical and experimental results, in Engleman RE, Levitsky S (eds): *A Handbook of Clinical Cardioplegia.* Mt Kisco, NY, Futura, 1982, chap 17.

Dilley RB, Cannon JA, et al: The treatment of coronary occlusive disease by endarterectomy. *J Thorac Cardiovasc Surg* 50:511, 1965.

European Coronary Surgery Study Group: Prospective randomized study of coronary artery bypass surgery in stable angina pectoris. Second interim report. *Lancet* 491, Sept 6, 1980.

Falcone C, deServi S, et al: Clinical significance of exercise-induced silent myocardial ischemia in patients with coronary artery disease. *J Am Coll Cardiol* 9:295, 1987.

Frick MH, Valle M, Harjola PT: Progression of coronary artery disease in randomized medical and surgical patients over a 5-year angiographic follow-up. *Am J Cardiol* 52:681, 1983.

Galbut DL, Traad EA, et al: Twelve-year experience with bilateral internal mammary artery grafts. *Ann Thorac Surg* 40:264, 1985.

Green GE, Spencer FC, et al: Arterial and venous microsurgical bypass grafts for coronary artery disease. *J Thorac Cardiovasc Surg* 60:491, 1970.

Grondin CM, Campeau L, et al: Comparison of late changes in internal mammary artery and saphenous vein grafts in two consecutive series of patients 10 years after operation. *Circulation* 70:1208, 1984.

Holmes DR Jr, Davis KB, et al: The effect of medical and surgical treatment on subsequent sudden cardiac death in patients with coronary artery diease: A report from the coronary artery surgery study. *Circulation* 73:1254, 1986.

Huddleston CB, Stoney WS, et al: Internal mammary artery grafts: Technical factors influencing patency. *Ann Thorac Surg* 42:543, 1986.

Isom OW, Spencer FC, et al: Does coronary bypass increase longevity? *J Thorac Cardiovasc Surg* 75(1):28, 1978.

Isom OW, Spencer FC, et al: Long-term survival following coronary bypass surgery in patients with significant impairment of left ventricular function. *Circulation* 51–52(suppl 1):141, 1975.

Johnson WD, Flemma RJ, et al: Extended treatment of severe coronary artery disease: A total surgical approach. *Ann Surg* 170:460, 1969.

Johnson WD, Brenowitz JB, Gessert R: Long term results of total coronary artery reconstruction. Presented at the American Association for Thoracic Surgery meeting, April 1987.

Kaiser GC: CABG: Lessons for the randomized trials. *Ann Thorac Surg* 43:3, 1986.

Kennedy JW, Killip T, et al: The clinical spectrum of coronary artery disease and its surgical and medical management, 1974–1979. The coronary artery surgery study. *Circulation* 66:III16, 1982.

Levy RI: Cholesterol and coronary artery disease. What do clinicians do now? *Am J Med* 80:18, 1986.

Loop FD, Lytle BW, et al: Free (aorto-coronary) internal mammary artery graft. Late results. *J Thorac Cardiovasc Surg* 92:827, 1986.

Loop FD, Lytle BW, et al: Influence of the internal-mammary-artery graft on 10-year survival and other cardiac events. *N Engl J Med* 314:1, 1986.

Mock M, Ringqvist I, et al: The survival of medically treated patients in the coronary artery surgery study (CASS) registry. *Circulation* 66:562, 1982.

Orszulak TA, Schaff HV, et al: Initial experience with sequential internal mammary artery bypass grafts to the left anterior descending and left anterior descending diagonal coronary arteries. *Mayo Clin Proc* 61:3, 1986.

Pigott JD, Kouchoukos NT, et al: Late results of surgical and medical therapy for patients with coronary artery disease and depressed left ventricular function. *J Am Coll Cardiol* 5:1036, 1985.

Rankin JS, Newman GE, et al: Clinical and angiographic assessment of complex mammary artery bypass grafting. *J Thorac Cardiovasc Surg* 92:832, 1986.

Reeder GS, Vlietstra RE, et al: Comparison of angioplasty and bypass surgery in multivessel coronary artery disease. *Int J Cardiol* 10:213, 1986.

Ringqvist I, Fisher LD, et al: Prognostic values of angiographic indices of coronary artery disease from the coronary artery surgery study (CASS). *J Clin Invest* 71:1854, 1983.

Russo P, Orszulak TA, et al: Use of internal mammary artery

grafts for multiple coronary artery bypasses. *Circulation* 74:III48, 1986.

Sauvage LR, Wu HD, et al: Healing basis and surgical techniques for complete revascularization of the left ventricle using only the internal mammary arteries. *Ann Thorac Surg* 42:449, 1986.

Spencer FC: Binocular loupes (microtelescopes) for coronary artery surgery. *J Thorac Cardiovasc Surg* 62:163, 1971.

Spencer FC: Surgical procedures for coronary atherosclerosis. *Prog Cardiovasc Dis* 14:399, 1972.

Spencer FC: The influence of coronary bypass on ventricular function, consensus meeting on coronary artery bypass surgery, medical and scientific aspects. National Institute of Health, Bethesda, MD, December 1980.

Spencer FC: The internal mammary artery: The ideal coronary bypass graft? *N Engl J Med* 314:50, 1986.

Spencer FC, Green GE, et al: Surgical therapy for coronary artery disease. *Curr Probl Surg* September 1970.

Spencer FC, Green GE, et al: Coronary artery bypass grafts for congestive heart failure. A report of experiences with 40 patients. *J Thorac Cardiovasc Surg* 62:529, 1971.

Spencer FC, Yong NK, Prachuabmoh K: Internal mammary-coronary artery anastomoses performed during cardiopulmonary bypass. *Cardiovasc Surg* 5:292, 1964.

Stoney WS, Alford WC Jr, et al: The fate of arm veins used for aorta-coronary bypass grafts. *J Thorac Cardiovasc Surg* 88:522, 1984.

Tector AJ: Fifteen years' experience with the internal mammary artery graft. *Ann Thorac Surg* 42:S22, 1986.

Vineberg AM: Technical considerations for the combined operation of left internal mammary artery or right and left internal mammary implantations with epicardiectomy and free omental graft. *J Thorac Cardiovasc Surg* 53:837, 1967.

Ventricular Aneurysm

Akins CW: Resection of left ventricular aneurysm during hypothermic fibrillatory arrest without aortic occlusion. *J Thorac Cardiovasc Surg* 91:610, 1986.

Bruschke AV, Proudfit WL, Sones FM: Progress study of 590 consecutive non-surgical cases of coronary disease followed by 5–9 years. Ventriculographic and other correlations. *Circulation* 47:1154, 1973.

Faxon DP, Myers WO, et al: The influence of surgery on the natural history of angiographically documented left ventricular aneurysm: The coronary artery surgery study. *Circulation* 74:110, 1986.

Froehlich RT, Falsetti HL, et al: Prospective study of surgery for left ventricular aneurysm. *Am J Cardiol* 45:923, 1980.

Gay W: Management of ventricular aneurysms following myocardial infarction. *World J Surg* 2:743, 1978.

Jatene AD: Left ventricular aneurysmectomy resection or reconstruction. *J Thorac Cardiovasc Surg* 89:321, 1985.

Josephson M, Harken A, Horowitz L: Long-term results of endocardial resection for sustained ventricular tachycardia in coronary disease patients. *Am Heart J* 104:51, 1982.

Kirklin JW, Barratt-Boyes BG: *Cardiac Surgery.* New York, Wiley, 1986.

Loop F, Cosgrove D: Results of ventricular aneurysmectomy. *Am J Surg* 141:684, 1981.

Novick RJ, Stefaniszyn HJ, et al: Surgery for postinfarction left ventricular aneurysm: Prognosis and long-term follow-up. *Can J Surg* 27:161, 1984.

Olearchyk AS, Lemole GM, Spagna PM: Left ventricular aneurysm. Ten years' experience in surgical treatment of 244 cases. Improved clinical status, hemodynamics, and long-term longevity. *J Thorac Cardiovasc Surg* 88:544, 1986.

Pericarditis

Culliford A, Lipton M, Spencer F: Operation for chronic constrictive pericarditis: Do the surgical approach and degree of pericardial resection influence the outcome significantly? *Ann Thorac Surg* 29:146, 1980.

Hier-Madsen K, Saunamaki KI, et al: Purulent pericarditis in children. Review and case report. *Scand J Thorac Cardiovasc Surg* 19:185, 1985.

Kutcher MA, King SB 3rd, et al: Constrictive pericarditis as a complication of cardiac surgery: Recognition of an entity. *Am J Cardiol* 50:742, 1982.

McCaughan BC, Schaff HV, et al: Early and late results of pericardiectomy for constrictive pericarditis. *J Thorac Cardiovasc Surg* 89:340, 1985.

Miller J, Mansour K, Hatcher C: Pericardiectomy: Current indications, concepts, and results in a university center. *Ann Thorac Surg* 34:40, 1982.

Morgan RJ, Stephenson LW, et al: Surgical treatment of purulent pericarditis in children. *J Thorac Cardiovasc Surg* 85:527, 1983.

Nishimura RA, Connolly DC, et al: Constrictive pericarditis: Assessment of current diagnostic procedures. *Mayo Clin Proc* 60:397, 1985.

Seifert FC, Miller DC, et al: Surgical treatment of constrictive pericarditis: Analysis of outcome and diagnostic error. *Circulation* 72:II264, 1985.

Heart Block and Pacemakers

Besley D, McWilliams G, et al: Long-term follow-up of young adults following permanent pacemaker placement for complete heart block. *Am Heart J* 103:332, 1982.

Brodman R, Furman S: Pacemaker implantation through the internal jugular vein. *Ann Thorac Surg* 29:63, 1980.

Carver J, Spitzer S, Mason D: Current concepts in pacing. *Geriatrics* 36:105, 1981.

Chardack WM, Gage AA, et al: The long-term treatment of heart block. *Prog Cardiovasc Dis* 9:105, 1966.

Culliford A, Isom O, Doyle E: Pacemaker implantation in the extremely young. A safe and cosmetic approach. *J Thorac Cardiovasc Surg* 75:763, 1978.

Furman S, Escher DJ, et al: Implanted transvenous pacemakers: Equipment, technic and clinical experience. *Ann Surg* 164:465, 1966.

Griffin JC, Mason JW, et al: The treatment of ventricular tachycardia using an automatic tachycardia terminating pacemaker. *PACE* 4:582, 1981.

Levine PA, Balady GJ, et al: Electrocautery and pacemakers: Management of the paced patient subject to electrocautery. *Ann Thorac Surg* 41:313, 1986.

Reid PR, Griffith LS, et al: Implantable cardioverter-defibrillator: Patient selection and implantation protocol. *PACE* 7(II):1338, 1984.

Watkins L, Mirowski M, et al: Automatic defibrillation in man: The initial surgical experience, *J Thorac Cardiovasc Surg* 82:492, 1981.

Assisted Circulation and Artificial Hearts

Amsterdam E, Awan N, et al: Intra-aortic balloon counterpulsation: Rationale, application and results, in Rackley C (ed): *Critical Care Cardiology.* Philadelphia, Davis, 1981.

Axelrod HI, Galloway AC, et al: Percutaneous cardiopulmonary bypass with a synchronous pulsatile pump combines effective unloading with ease of application. *J Thorac Cardiovasc Surg* 93:358, 1987.

Bregman D: Mechanical support of the circulation. *Cleveland Clin Q* 48:181, 1981.

Bregman D, Casarella W: Percutaneous intraaortic balloon pumping: Initial clinical experience. *Ann Thorac Surg* 29:133, 1980.

Gaines WE, Pierce WS, et al: The Pennsylvania State University paracorporeal ventricular assist pump: Optimal methods of use. *World J Surg* 9:47, 1985.

Glassman E, Engelman RM, et al: Method of closed-chest cannulation of left atrium for left atrial-femoral artery bypass. *J Thorac Cardiovasc Surg* 69:283, 1975.

Griffith BP, Hardesty RL, et al: Temporary use of the Jarvik-7 total artificial heart before transplantation. *N Engl J Med* 316:130, 1987.

Joyce LD, DeVries WC, et al: Response of the human body to the first permanent implant of the Jarvik-7 total artificial heart. *Trans Am Soc Artif Intern Organs* 29:81, 1983.

Kolff J, Beeb GM: Artificial heart and left ventricular assist devices. *Surg Clin North Am* 65:661, 1985.

Levinson MM, Smith RG, et al: Thromboembolic complications of the Jarvik-7 total artificial heart: Case report. *Artif Organs* 10:236, 1986.

Macoviak J, Stephenson L, et al: The intraaortic balloon pump: An analysis of five years' experience. *Ann Thorac Surg* 29:451, 1980.

Pae WE Jr, Pierce WS, et al: Long-term results of ventricular assist pumping in postcardiotomy cardiogenic shock. *J Thorac Cardiovasc Surg* 93:434, 1987.

Park SB, Liebler GA, et al: Mechanical support of the failing heart. *Ann Thorac Surg* 42:627, 1986.

Pennock JL, Pierce WS, et al: Survival and complications following ventricular assist pumping for cardiogenic shock. *Ann Surg* 198:469, 1983.

Pierce WS: The implantable ventricular assist pump. *J Thorac Cardiovasc Surg* 87:811, 1984.

Pierce WS: The artificial heart—1986: Partial fulfillment of a promise. *ASAIO-Trans* 32:5, 1986.

Pierce W, Myers J, et al: Approaches to the artificial heart. *Surgery* 90:137, 1981.

Rose D, Colvin S, et al: Long-term survival with partial left heart bypass following perioperative myocardial infarction and shock. *J Thorac Cardiovasc Surg* 83:483, 1982.

Rose DM, Colvin SB, et al: Late functional and hemodynamic V status of surviving patients following insertion of the left heart assist device. *J Thorac Cardiovasc Surg* 86:639, 1983.

Schoen FJ, Palmer DC, et al: Clinical temporary ventricular assist. Pathologic findings and their implications in a multi-institutional study of 41 patients. *J Thorac Cardiovasc Surg* 92:1071, 1986.

Spencer FC, Eiseman B, et al: Assisted circulation for cardiac failure following intracardiac surgery with cardiopulmonary bypass. *J Thorac Cardiovasc Surg* 49:56, 1964.

Sturm J, McGee M, et al: Treatment of postoperative low output syndrome with intraaortic balloon pumping: Experience with 419 patients. *Am J Cardiol* 45:1033, 1980.

Van Citters RL, Bauer CB, et al: Artificial heart and assist devices: Directions, needs, costs, societal and ethical issues. *Artif Organs* 9:375, 1985.

Chapter 20

Diseases of Great Vessels

Frank C. Spencer

ANEURYSMS OF THE THORACIC AORTA

Aneurysms of the thoracic aorta may be classified in five groups, varying with the anatomic location: (1) ascending aorta; (2) transverse aortic arch; (3) traumatic, usually occurring distal to the left subclavian artery; (4) descending thoracic aorta; and (5) thoracoabdominal. The etiology, disability, and surgical approach all vary with these different types.

GENERAL CONSIDERATIONS. The most frequent causes of a thoracic aneurysm are atherosclerosis, aortic dissection, or a collagen degenerative disease, the prototype of which is Marfan's syndrome. "Annulo-ectasia" is a popular descriptive term for the common condition of idiopathic dilatation of the aortic annulus, producing aortic insufficiency in association with a localized aneurysm in the ascending aorta. This is probably a localized form of collagen degenerative disease, for it does not develop in other areas of the body. Trauma is an important but infrequent cause of aneurysms in specific locations. Syphilis at one time was a frequent cause but is now very rare. Infrequently, a thoracic aneurysm results from some type of granulomatous disease of unknown etiology.

Dissecting aneurysms are considered in a subsequent section, for the aortic dissection involves a large part or all of the thoracic aorta.

Pathology. The four major types of aneurysm, considered serially in the subsequent sections, are: aneurysms of the ascending aorta, transverse aortic arch, descending thoracic aorta, and thoracoabdominal aneurysms. Aneurysms may be conveniently grouped by their anatomical location, for each type has specific characteristics and requires a form of treatment specific for that anatomical area.

Aneurysms of the ascending aorta are the most frequent, representing over 40 percent of aneurysms in large series. Perhaps this is because the ascending segment is the widest part. The descending thoracic aorta is involved in about 35 percent, the transverse arch and the thoracoabdominal areas in about 10 percent each.

In all areas the natural history is that of progressive enlargement with eventual rupture. Posttraumatic aneurysms are distinctive for their very slow growth, for a few instances of such aneurysms existing for 10 to 20 years before enlarging have been reported. In the vast majority of patients, the aneurysm steadily enlarges until rupture occurs. In a large series reported by Pickerstaff et al., the 1-year survival was about 60 percent, the 5-year survival near 20 percent. McNamara et al. summarized observations with 260 patients with thoracic aneurysms, 126 of whom were treated surgically. Five-year survival in nonsurgically treated patients was only 21 percent. The prognosis for the thoracic aneurysm is somewhat worse than that with an abdominal aneurysm.

Clinical Manifestations. The majority of aneurysms are asymptomatic until significant enlargement has occurred. Pain may infrequently occur, but the majority are accidentally discovered during a routine chest x-ray. Large aneurysms in the transverse aortic arch create symptoms from compression of adjacent structures such as the trachea or superior vena cava. Syphilitic aneurysms were well known for their tendency to invade bone, producing back pain from erosion of the thoracic spine, but this seldom occurs with other aneurysms. Usually, there are no physical abnormalities or any hemodynamic disturbances. Hence, the principal indication for treatment is to prevent death from rupture.

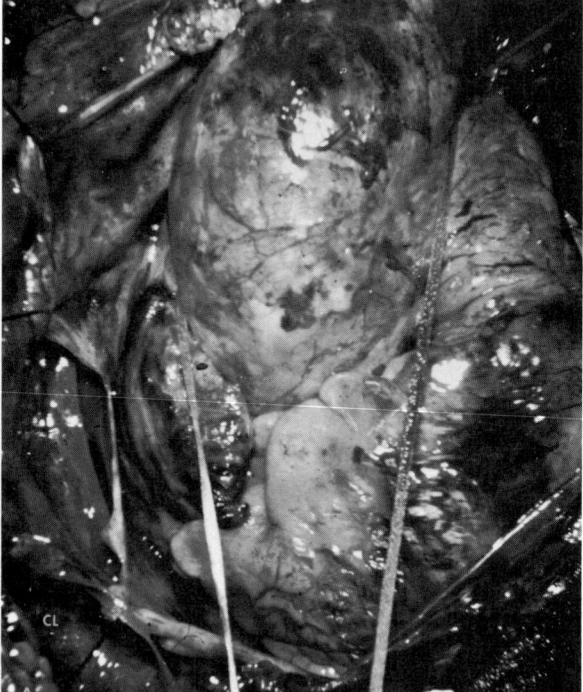

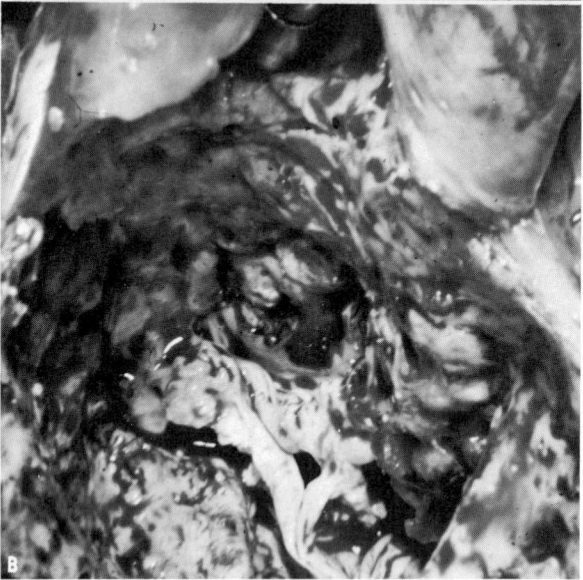

Fig. 20-1. Operative photograph of a patient with a large aneurysm of the ascending aorta. *A.* The aneurysm in the proximal aorta has been isolated and the aorta elevated by encircling umbilical tapes. *B.* Once the aorta has been incised, the incompetent aortic valve is exposed. The aortic insufficiency was produced by dilatation of the aortic annulus.

Once an abnormal shadow has been recognized on the chest x-ray, diagnosis can be readily established with an aortogram or computed tomography (CT). Unless the aneurysm is quite small, all should be treated promptly by excision. If serious complicating diseases, such as age, previous strokes, or heart disease, significantly increase operative risk, they may be observed for a few months or a year, with periodic sonograms or CTs to determine if enlargement is occurring. Once significant enlargement has been demonstrated, operation should be done promptly.

Treatment. The basic steps of treatment are to open the aneurysm, remove the contents and the diseased intima, insert a prosthetic graft (usually Dacron), and then wrap the wall of the aneurysm about the graft. The exact approach varies with different areas and is described in each section. This "inclusion" technique was an important contribution by Rudolf Matas in New Orleans in 1902 but was forgotten until the late 1950s, when it was reinstituted by DeBakey and Cooley and quickly adopted by others.

Aneurysms of the Ascending Aorta

Aneurysms localized to the ascending aorta are often due to a degenerative connective tissue disease of the media of the aortic wall. The origin is usually unknown. This is seen typically as one manifestation of a generalized disorder in Marfan's syndrome or as an isolated disease in Erdheim's cystic medial necrosis. The histologic abnormality described as "cystic medial necrosis" is now recognized as a nonspecific abnormality occurring in several diseases. Atherosclerotic aneurysms are seldom limited to the ascending aorta. Dissecting aneurysms, discussed in the next section, usually begin in the ascending aorta and extend distally. The dissection may stop near the origin of the innominate artery (DeBakey Type II) or may extend throughout the entire thoracic aorta (DeBakey Type I). Syphilis is now an infrequent cause. In the series of 90 patients reported by Miller et al., an unknown degenerative disease of connective tissue was the cause in 60 cases, aortic dissection in 12, syphilis in 10, and atherosclerosis in 8.

PATHOLOGY. As an aneurysm develops in the proximal ascending aorta, dilatation of the annulus of the aortic valve occurs, stretching the cusps of the aortic valve apart and producing aortic insufficiency (Fig. 20-1). Cardiac failure from the resulting aortic insufficiency is often the significant clinical problem rather than enlargement of the aneurysm with compression of adjacent structures or rupture. In the past, saccular syphilitic aneurysms enlarged to massive proportions, eroding through the sternum (Fig. 20-2), but these aneurysms are now rare. Once significant aortic insufficiency has developed, progression is rapid, with death from cardiac failure in 1 to 2 years unless operation is performed. Before surgical therapy was available, most patients with Marfan's syndrome died in the third decade from dissecting aneurysms or aortic insufficiency. Gott et al., based on experience with 50 patients with Marfan's syndrome, concluded that elective operation should be done when the diameter of the aortic root enlarged to 6 cm.

CLINICAL MANIFESTATIONS. Patients are often asymptomatic when the diagnosis is made following recognition of dilatation of the ascending aorta on a chest radiograph performed for other purposes. Frequently, the first symptom is due to congestive heart failure from aortic insuffi-

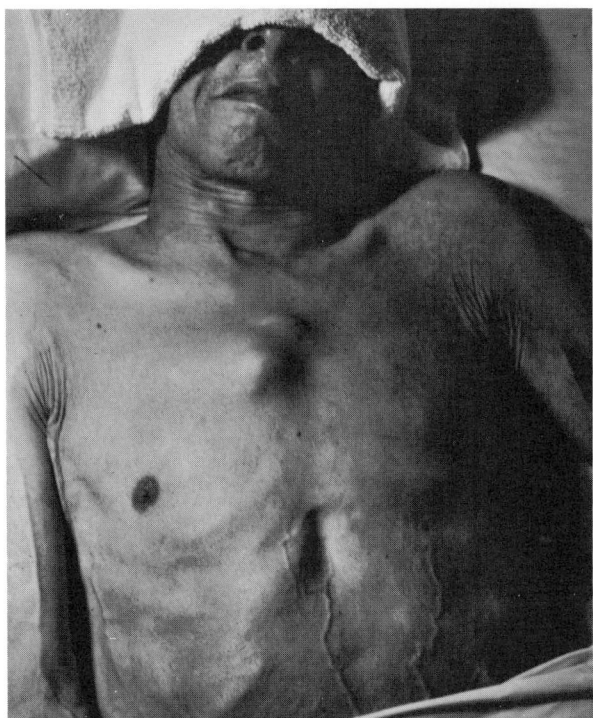

Fig. 20-2. Patient with a large syphilitic aneurysm eroding through the sternum and projecting beneath the skin. Fortunately such lesions are now rare. An attempt at operative extirpation of the lesion was unsuccessful because of hemorrhage.

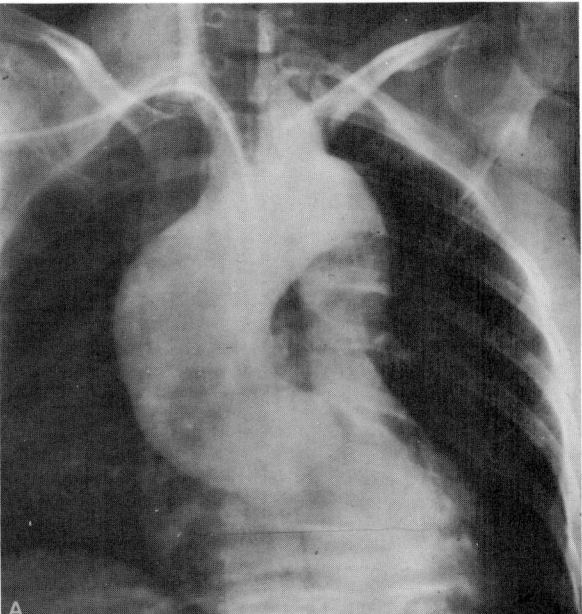

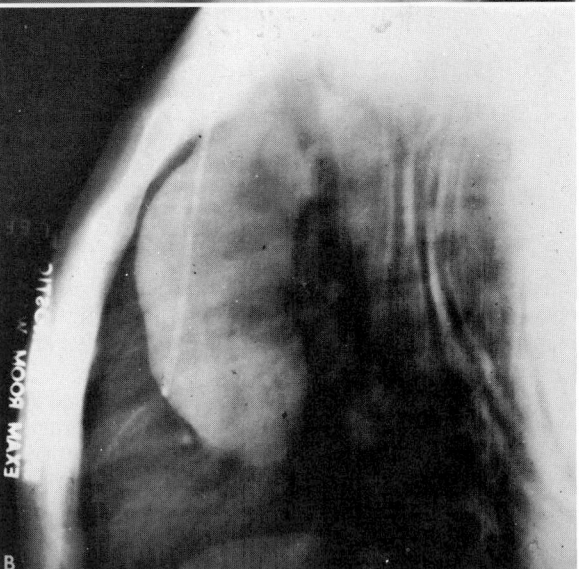

Fig. 20-3. *A.* Posteroanterior view of a thoracic aortogram showing a large aneurysm in the ascending aorta, stopping near the innominate artery. Resection of the aneurysm was successfully performed. The patient was well 15 years following operation. *B.* Lateral view of a thoracic aortogram in the same patient.

ciency. Rarely, expanding saccular aneurysms are seen with symptoms from compression of the superior vena cava or the trachea. Physical examination usually finds no abnormalities except those of aortic insufficiency, the diastolic murmur and the wide pulse pressure.

DIAGNOSTIC FINDINGS. The diagnosis can be suspected from the radiographic findings of dilatation of the ascending aorta. Aortography or a CT scan confirms the diagnosis. The aortographic demonstration of a fusiform aneurysm in the proximal ascending aorta, tapering to an aorta of near-normal diameter at the level of the innominate artery, is virtually diagnostic of cystic medial necrosis (Fig. 20-3).

TREATMENT. Because of the progressive nature of the aortic insufficiency, operation should be performed as soon as possible after the diagnosis is made. As with aortic insufficiency from other causes, postponing operation because of the absence of symptoms while progressive enlargement of the left ventricle occurs is a serious error because the likelihood of sudden death from irreversible ventricular injury is greatly increased in the first few years following operation.

Operation is performed with cardiopulmonary bypass, excising the ascending aorta and replacing it with a woven Dacron graft. Concomitant valve replacement is performed if aortic insufficiency is present.

If aortic valve disease is present but the aortic annulus is not significantly dilated, the aortic valve can be re-

placed and the prosthetic valve inserted a few millimeters above the site of origin of the coronary arteries, leaving the coronary arteries in their normal anatomical location. However, if the aortic annulus is significantly dilated, this should be excised also because of the frequency of recurrent aneurysms in this area. This necessitates replantation of the ostia of the coronary arteries. The decision can usually be readily made at operation, for with significant dilatation of the aortic annulus, the ostia of the coronary arteries are displaced more than 1 cm from the aortic ring.

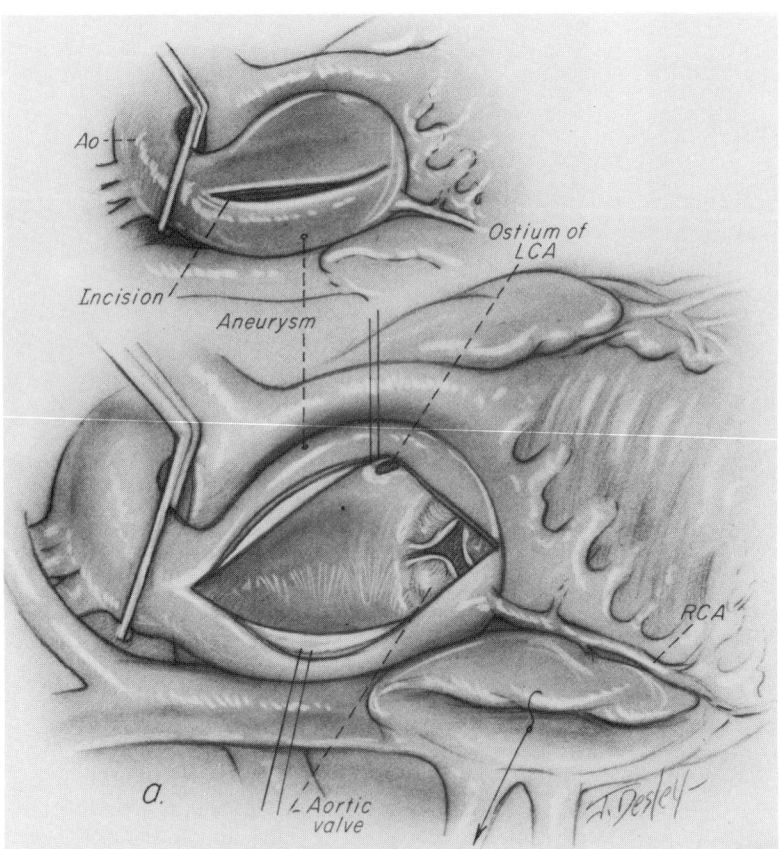

Fig. 20-4. Replacement of aortic valve and ascending aorta using the inclusion technique. *A.* After CPB is established the aortic clamp is placed and the aneurysm is opened longitudinally *(inset)*. The ostia of the left and right coronary arteries are identified, usually displaced somewhat downstream to their normal position. The cold cardioplegic solution is given. *B.* After the aortic valve is excised, the Dacron graft with the attached Bjork-Shiley valve is sutured into place. A hole has been cut in the graft preparatory to suturing this around the ostium of the left coronary artery. *C.* The anastomosis is begun between the graft and the aortic wall around coronary ostium. *D.* Interrupted everting mattress sutures are used, supported by felt strips on the aortic side. *E.* The anastomosis is partially complete. *F.* The anterior row of sutures has been placed. *G.* After felt strips are placed around the aorta, the distal anastomosis is begun with a continuous everting mattress suture. *H.* The distal anastomosis has been completed. The clamp is removed, and the suture lines are inspected for leakage. (From: *Kirklin JW, Barratt-Boyes BG: Cardiac surgery, in Aortic Valve Disease. New York, Wiley, 1986, chap 12, pp 390–392, with permission.)*

This type of reconstruction is termed the "conduit" operation, consisting of replacement of the aortic valve, replantation of the coronary ostia, and replacement of the ascending aorta with prosthetic graft (Fig. 20-4).

The composite operation can be safely performed with excellent results. Kouchoukos et al. reported experiences with 125 patients operated upon over a period of 10 years with an operative mortality of 5 percent. Average follow-up was 55 months with an actuarial survival at 7 years between 65 and 70 percent. In 1985, Cabral et al. reported experiences with 100 patients operated upon over a period of 7 years with an operative mortality of 4 percent and a late mortality of 8 percent during a follow-up period averaging about 3 years. Grey and Cooley described experiences with 140 patients, using the composite repair in 89 of the group and a separate graft-valve repair in 51. In the series reported by Moreno-Cabral et al. 85 percent required concomitant aortic valve replacement.

How often the composite operation should be used as opposed to separate graft-valve replacement varies markedly among different institutions. The long-term durability of the composite operation is yet unknown, for pseudoaneurysms have developed at the site of replantation of the coronary ostia in a few patients.

Aneurysms of the Transverse Aortic Arch

Aneurysms of the transverse aortic arch are almost always due to atherosclerosis. They usually occur in pa-

tients over sixty years of age with associated coronary and cerebral vascular disease. Diagnosis is usually confirmed with aortography and CT to differentiate the aneurysm from a malignant mediastinal tumor. The degree of involvement of the great vessels arising from the aortic arch can also be determined.

TREATMENT. The operative procedure is a complex one involving myocardial protection while the coronary circulation is interrupted, maintenance of blood flow to arteries to the brain, and perfusion of the body distal to the left subclavian artery (Fig. 20-5). Until the concept of

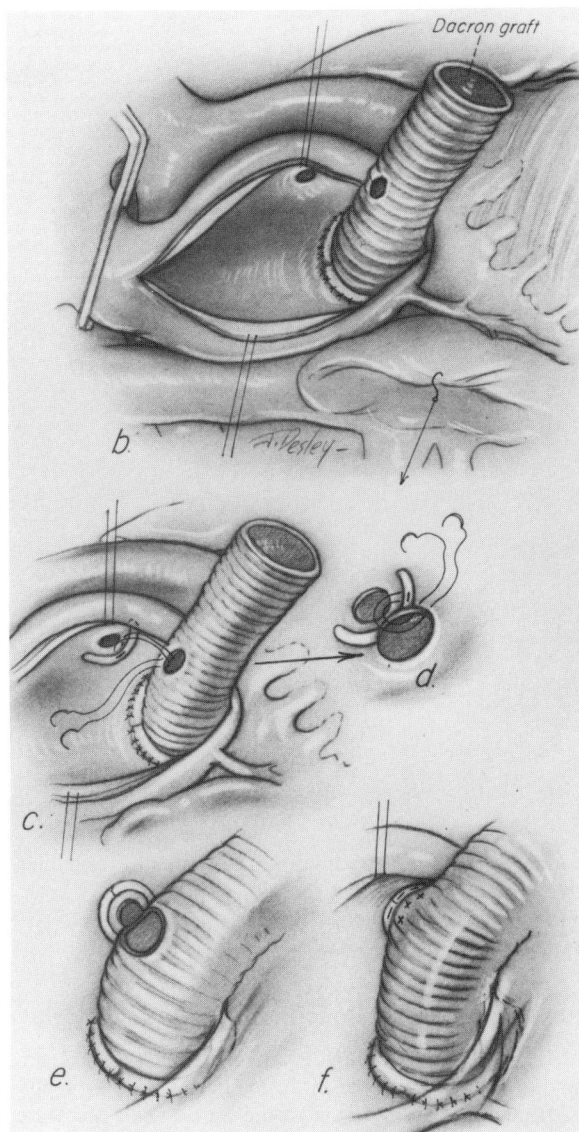

Fig. 20-4 *B,C,D,E,F.* Continued.

combining cardiopulmonary bypass with hypothermia and circulatory arrest was introduced, these aneurysms had the highest operative mortality of any aortic aneurysms, approaching 75 to 80 percent. The demonstration that the brain could tolerate circulatory arrest for 45 min if the brain temperature was carefully lowered to 15 to 17°C formed the basis for the modern approach. Griepp et al. applied the concept for arch aneurysms, reporting a series of 14 patients with an ischemia time near 42 min. Among 10 patients operated upon electively, only one died.

Crawford et al. described experiences with 67 patients, treating aneurysms located in the distal arch by simple proximal and distal clamping, while the hypothermic circulatory arrest technique was used in 27 extensive aneurysms with 26 survivors. Sweeney and Cooley concluded that higher temperatures were safer for short periods and

were accompanied by less bleeding. Most groups, including ourselves, have found a brain temperature near 15°C safer, providing time for a more precise reconstruction.

Aneurysms distal to the innominate artery may be safely treated by a short period of cross-clamping and excision. Cooley et al. described experiences with 32 patients treated with this technique, with an average cross-clamp time of 27 min. The mortality was 6 percent but the occurrence of paraplegia in three patients, all of whom were clamped more than 30 min, is alarming.

More recently Frist et al. proposed reconsidering the old technique of cerebral perfusion, describing experiences with 10 patients with eight survivors and no postoperative strokes. This approach should be considered if a cerebral ischemia time exceeding 45 min is anticipated.

Traumatic Thoracic Aneurysms

ETIOLOGY AND PATHOLOGY. Traumatic aneurysms almost invariably arise from transection of the thoracic aorta due to closed-chest trauma. The majority result from horizontal deceleration injuries, typically steering wheel trauma in an automobile accident. McCollum et al. in 1979 described five different forms of trauma. Out of a group of 50 patients, 35 were injured in an automobile accident, 6 were hurt in crushing injuries, and 4 were injured in falls from a height. Traumatic rupture and traumatic thoracic aneurysms have a common etiology but a different clinical course. Traumatic aneurysms evolve in those few patients fortunate enough not to succumb from exsanguinating hemorrhage in the weeks following injury. If a patient survives longer than 6 to 8 weeks following injury, the risk of acute rupture is small. In a review of the English and French literature between 1950 and 1965, Bennett and Cherry found rupture occurring 9 times in a total of 105 aneurysms. The usual course is one of progressive enlargement with compression of adjacent structures.

Most aneurysms arise just distal to the left subclavian artery, opposite the point of insertion of the ligamentum arteriosum. Fortunately, involvement of the aortic arch or the ascending aorta is rare. Although a huge aneurysm filling most of the hemithorax is occasionally seen, the point of origin is invariably near the ligamentum arteriosum. Reconstruction can usually be done with a short prosthetic graft. Direct anastomosis is seldom possible.

CLINICAL MANIFESTATIONS. Unlike most aneurysms from other causes, traumatic thoracic aneurysms enlarge slowly and in some patients remain stationary for 10 to 20 years; the diagnosis is made in retrospect while evaluating an asymptomatic patient with a history of closed-chest trauma 10 to 20 years before. In the series of McCollum et al., time intervals between trauma and operation varied from 3 months to 32 years, with an average near 12 years for the 50 patients. In 25 patients, the interval was greater than 10 years and in 6 greater than 20 years.

As the aneurysm enlarges, compression of the left recurrent laryngeal nerve, the left main bronchus, and the esophagus occurs. Symptoms usually announce enlargement well before rupture occurs. This small risk of rup-

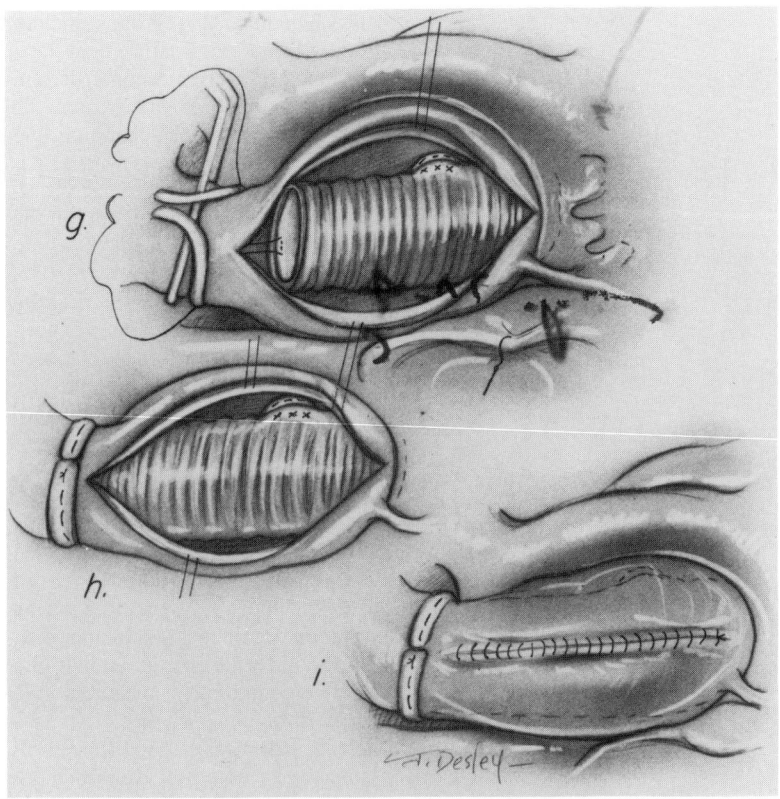

Fig. 20-4 *G,H,I*. Continued.

ture contrasts with the majority of aneurysms from other causes, where the threat of rupture constitutes the major reason for recommending excision before symptoms develop.

In the McCollum series, pain was the most common symptom, occurring in 24 percent of patients. Hoarseness from recurrent laryngeal involvement was present in 14 percent, dyspnea in 8 percent; 28 percent were asymptomatic. Usually there are no abnormalities on physical examination unless compression of the left main bronchus has occurred. No murmurs can be heard.

DIAGNOSTIC FINDINGS. The chest radiograph usually shows an ovoid density near the left subclavian artery. If the aneurysm has been present for several years, calcification is often visible in the wall. Exact dimensions may be outlined by a CT scan. Aortography is needed to confirm the diagnosis as well as the degree of involvement of adjacent structures (Fig. 20-6).

TREATMENT. The problem of management of acute rupture of the thoracic aorta, with the risk of exsanguinating hemorrhage, is discussed in the section Wounds of the Great Vessels. Elective excision is recommended for the majority of patients. An asymptomatic aneurysm first recognized over a decade after injury presents a choice between periodic observation and elective excision. Operative risk is small but not insignificant, and so several factors must be evaluated in making a recommendation for an individual patient. The probability of eventual enlargement requiring operation is the major consideration, as well as the small risk of rupture. I am not aware of an

autopsy report of a traumatic aneurysm that remained asymptomatic throughout the patient's lifetime.

Technique of Operation. (See Descending Thoracic Aneurysm.)

Aneurysms of the Descending Thoracic Aorta

ETIOLOGY AND INCIDENCE. Aneurysms in the descending thoracic aorta may result from atherosclerosis, syphilis, trauma, or a dissection of the aortic wall. Most are due to atherosclerosis and are exceeded only by abdominal aneurysms in frequency of occurrence. They are most common in men in the fifth to the seventh decades. Saccular aneurysms from syphilis, once very common, are now rare. Dissecting aneurysms and traumatic aneurysms are considered in the accompanying sections.

The majority of atherosclerotic aneurysms are located in the proximal part of the descending thoracic aorta, beginning distal to the left subclavian artery. They extend for varying distances and often can involve the entire descending thoracic aorta. They are generally fusiform (Fig. 20-7), rather than saccular.

Thoracic aneurysms enlarge and rupture at a rate greater than abdominal aneurysms. Bickerstaff described the natural history of 72 patients observed over a period of 30 years. The descending aorta was involved in 27. In the overall group, rupture occurred in 53 patients (74 percent). Thirty-seven of these had no prior diagnosis of aneurysms; in 16 others the mean interval between diagnosis and rupture was 2 years. Actuarial 5-year survival for

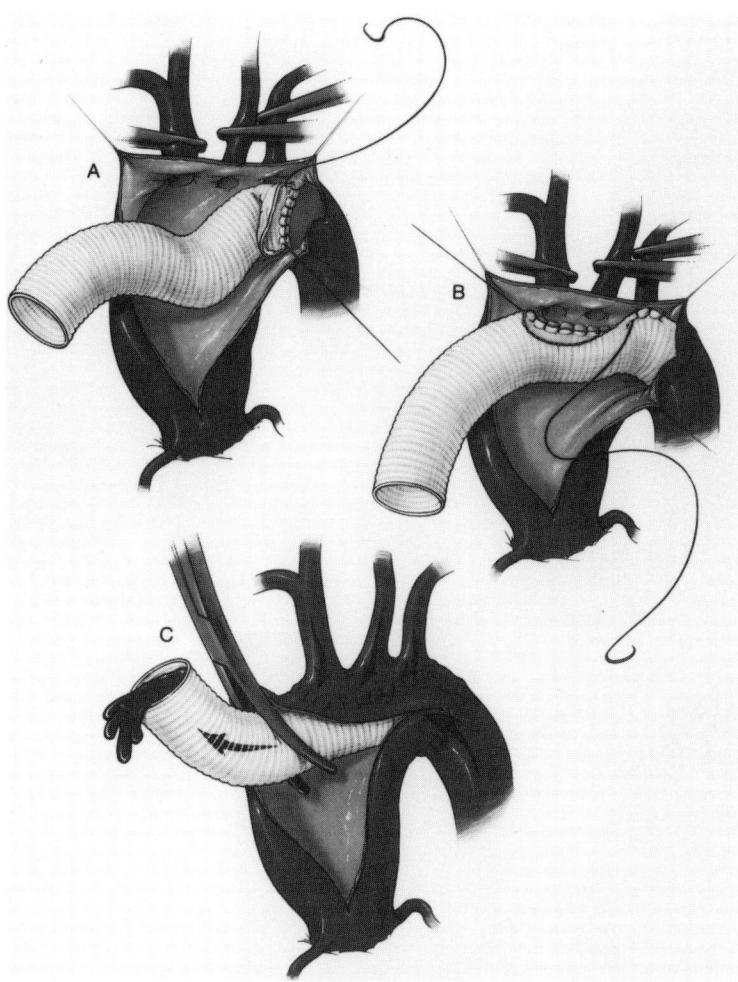

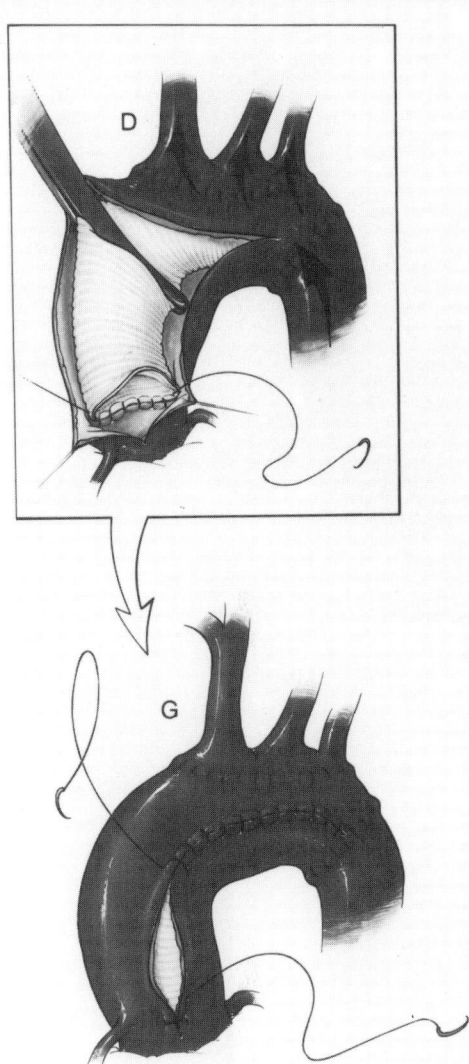

Fig. 20-5. Technique of graft inclusion and direct brachiocephalic arterial reattachment. *A.* With the head of the operating table down, the brachiocephalic arteries are clamped. With perfusion just to fill the aorta, the aneurysm is incised. The distal anastomosis is made between the graft and the normal upper descending thoracic aorta using #000 or #0000 prolene sutures. *B.* Anastomotic leakage is checked by clamping the graft and temporarily increasing perfusion. An oval opening is made with the graft under tension and sutured around the brachiocephalic artery origins. *C.* The head is lowered, the free end of the graft is elevated and filled with blood, and the clamps are removed from the brachiocephalic vessels to expel air. *D.* The graft is clamped proximal to the brachiocephalic arteries, full perfusion is resumed, and rewarming is started. Proximal anastomosis is performed depending on the extent of involvement. When uninvolved, the proximal graft is sutured to the ascending aorta. *G.* In either situation, air is removed by filling the heart and graft with blood as the anastomosis is completed and the aneurysmal wall is sutured around the graft. (From: *Crawford ES, Crawford JL: Diseases of the Aorta. Baltimore, Williams & Wilkins, 1984, pp 24–25, with permission.*)

all patients was 13 percent, for patients without dissection, 20 percent. Similar statistics have been cited by McNamara et al.

CLINICAL MANIFESTATIONS. Most patients are asymptomatic. The diagnosis is made after the accidental finding of an asymptomatic mass on a chest x-ray. In symptomatic patients, most symptoms result from an aneurysm enlarging and compressing the left main bronchus with resulting cough and dyspnea. Erosion into a bronchus or pulmonary parenchyma can produce hemoptysis. Enlarging aneurysms near the left recurrent laryngeal nerve where it encircles the ligamentum arteriosum will paralyze the vocal cord and produce hoarseness.

Physical examination is usually normal. Rarely a bruit is audible in the left paravertebral area. Peripheral pulses are normal unless compression of the origin of the left subclavian artery produces hypotension in the left arm.

DIAGNOSTIC FINDINGS. The diagnosis usually can be suspected from the appearance of a mass in the region of

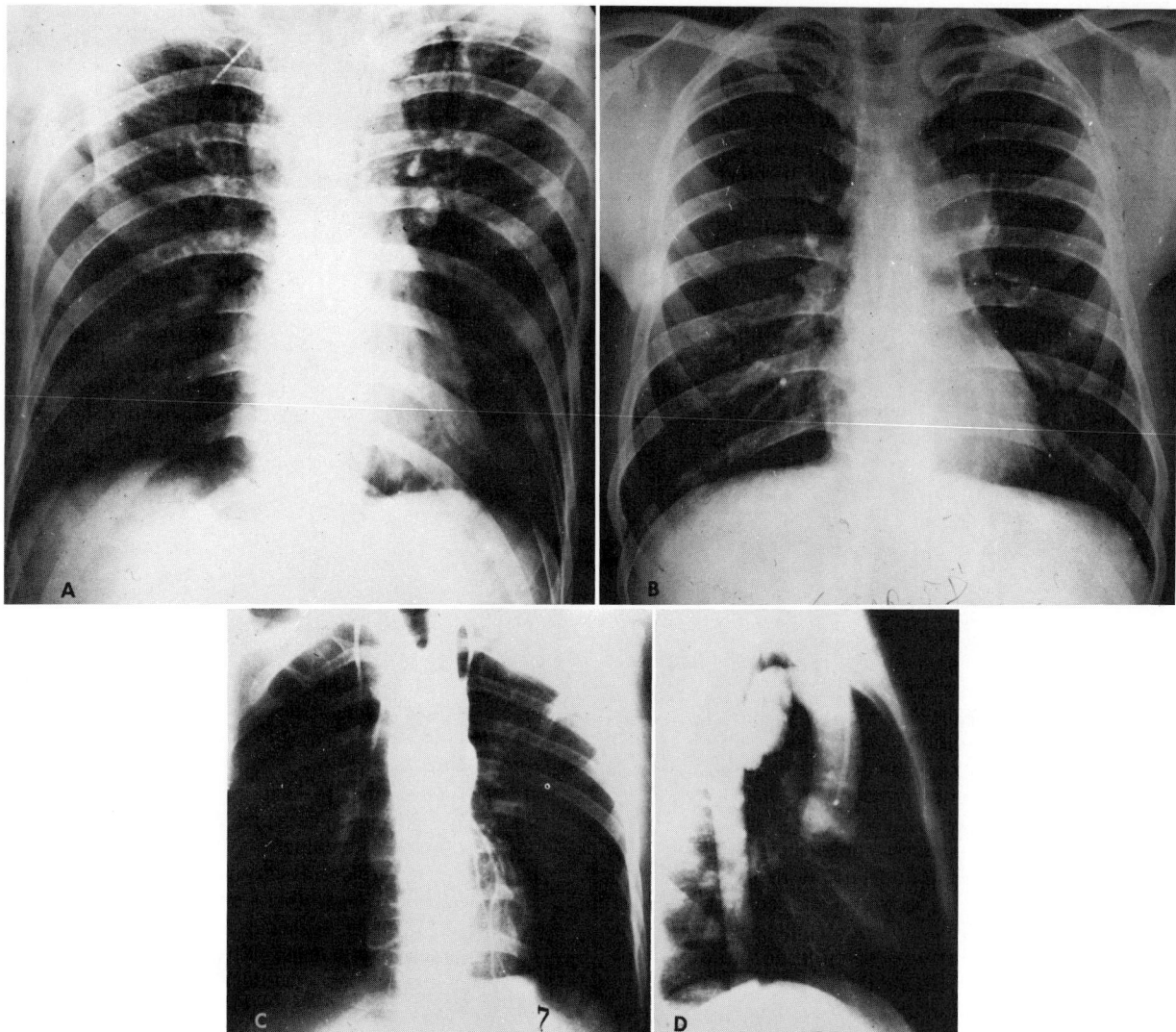

the aorta on the chest radiograph. The differential diagnosis includes bronchogenic carcinoma, metastatic carcinoma, or mediastinal tumors. Laminar calcification may be visible in the wall of the aorta.

CT is a valuable noninvasive technique to determine the size of an aneurysm. It is especially useful to periodically evaluate small aneurysms for enlargement. Aortography may be used to confirm the diagnosis and to delineate the precise extent of the aneurysm. Concomitant atherosclerotic disease in the coronary, renal, and carotid arteries frequently occurs. Hence, preoperative evaluation should carefully investigate these organ systems, often performing coronary arteriography, perhaps carotid arteriography or simpler noninvasive carotid studies.

TREATMENT. In most patients once the diagnosis of a discrete aneurysm has been made, excision should be recommended. Only with small aneurysms associated with significant coronary or cerebral vascular disease is a nonoperative policy of observation with frequent chest radiographs indicated.

Fig. 20-6. *A.* Chest radiograph following an automobile accident, demonstrating widening of the mediastinum with subcutaneous emphysema. Traumatic rupture of the aorta was not recognized at this time. *B.* Chest radiograph 5 months after the injury demonstrated a left upper mediastinal mass. *C.* Posteroanterior view of an aortogram demonstrating a localized thoracic aneurysm. This lesion was excised successfully. *D.* Lateral view of an aortogram in the same patient. *E.* Chest radiograph in a different patient 2 years after an automobile accident demonstrated an asymptomatic mass in the upper mediastinum. *F.* Aortography demonstrated a saccular thoracic aneurysm, which was subsequently resected successfully. *G.* Aortogram in the same patient as in *F.* This film demonstrated the size and extent of the aneurysm as additional contrast material flowed freely within the lesion.

The technique of operation is detailed in Fig. 20-8. A left posterolateral thoracotomy through an appropriate interspace, usually the fourth, fifth, or sixth, is made. Initially, the aorta is mobilized and encircled proximal and distal to the aneurysm. With proximal aneurysms involving the left subclavian artery, the aorta is encircled between the left carotid and left subclavian arteries. This is facilitated by opening the pericardium and dissecting the

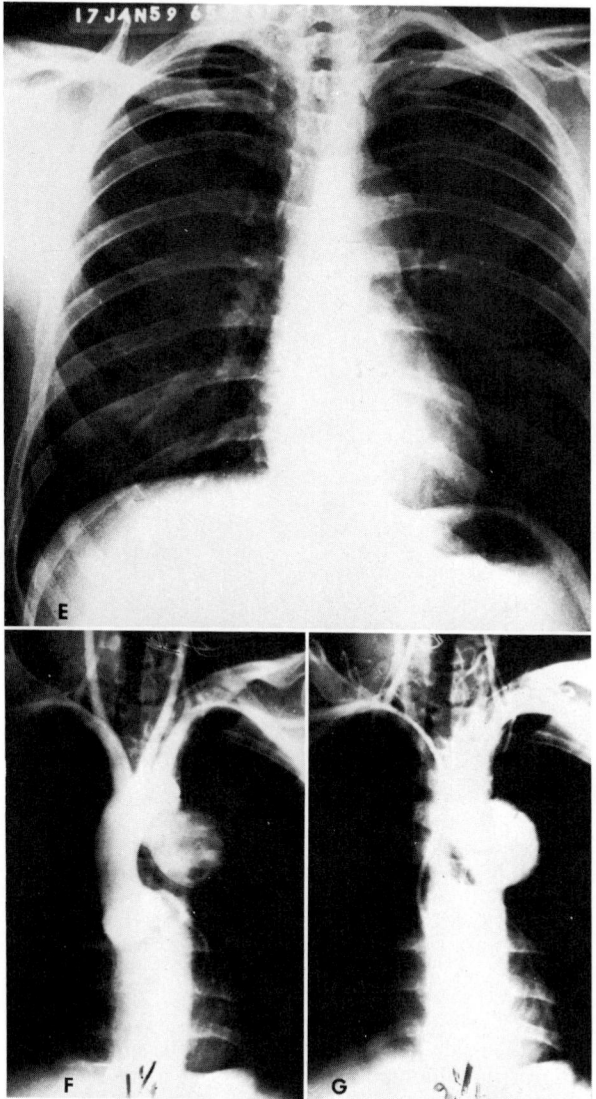

Fig. 20-6 *E,F,G.* Continued.

intrapericardial portion of the aortic arch. The vagus nerve and recurrent laryngeal nerve should be mobilized and protected.

A partial bypass is routinely used at NYU to protect from paraplegia. For the past several years a femoral artery–femoral vein bypass with a pump oxygenator has been used for most patients but with proximal aneurysms, the traditional left atrial–femoral bypass is often used as larger cannulae can be used and a higher flow rate obtained if necessary. A Gott heparinized shunt was used for several years, but this form of shunting is now considered unsatisfactory.

The principal hazards with clamping of the thoracic aorta are paraplegia and renal failure from the distal ischemia produced. Theoretically, this should be preventable by some form of partial bypass, perfusing the distal aorta during this time. Most types of temporary bypass require total body heparinization with subsequent increase in operative hemorrhage.

Somatosensory potential monitoring to evaluate spinal cord function while the aorta was occluded has been routinely used with the majority of operations performed upon the thoracic aorta at our hospital in recent years. Laboratory and clinical data indicate that paraplegia usually results from spinal cord ischemia when thoracic aneurysms do not extend below the diaphragm, while with thoracoabdominal aneurysms, direct interruption of critical blood supply to the spinal cord is a major factor. The inability of temporary bypass to protect from paraplegia over the past two decades has been principally due to an *inadequate flow through the shunt with inadequate distal perfusion pressure*. To date, in aneurysms not extending below the diaphragm, maintaining a distal aortic perfusion pressure above 60 mmHg by providing adequate flow of blood through the temporary bypass has been associated with preservation of sensory potentials during operation and absence of paraplegia, even with occlusion of the thoracic aorta for longer than 60 min. The exact flow rate needed cannot be predicted precisely in advance. Flow rates as high as 4 or more L/min have been needed in some patients. Distal aortic pressure, rather than flow rate, is the key requirement in order to perfuse the spinal cord through collateral circulation. Vascular resistance through collateral circulation is greater than the resistance present when spinal cord blood flow is through normal channels.

Published data do not show a significant reduction in the frequency of paraplegia when conventional temporary bypass is used. Livesay and Cooley reported experiences with 360 thoracic aneurysms employing some form of shunt or bypass in 97 of the group. Paraplegia occurred in 6.5 percent and was not decreased by temporary shunts. Paraplegia occurred principally with extensive aneurysms and with cross-clamp times exceeding 30 min. With thoracoabdominal aneurysms requiring excision of the segment of aorta between T10 and L2, paraplegia occurred in 15 to 20 percent of patients in the series reported by Crawford et al.

The surgical technique is a standard one. Initial dissection is limited to isolating the aorta proximally and distally sufficiently to permit the application of vascular clamps. The aorta is then opened widely, removing the thrombi from the lumen and any gross areas of calcification or degeneration in the intima. Most of the intima and all of the media are carefully preserved. Ostia of bleeding intercostal vessels are directly sutured. A standard woven Dacron graft is then inserted by end-to-end anastomosis (Fig. 20-9), after which the wall of the aneurysmal sac can be sutured around the prosthetic graft to supplement hemostasis.

Operative risk is usually less than 5 percent in elective operations unless serious concomitant coronary artery disease is present. Long-term prognosis is principally determined by the concomitant presence of coronary and cerebral atherosclerosis.

Thoracoabdominal Aneurysms

Thoracoabdominal aneurysms are rare, occurring in older patients with extensive atherosclerosis. Excision is

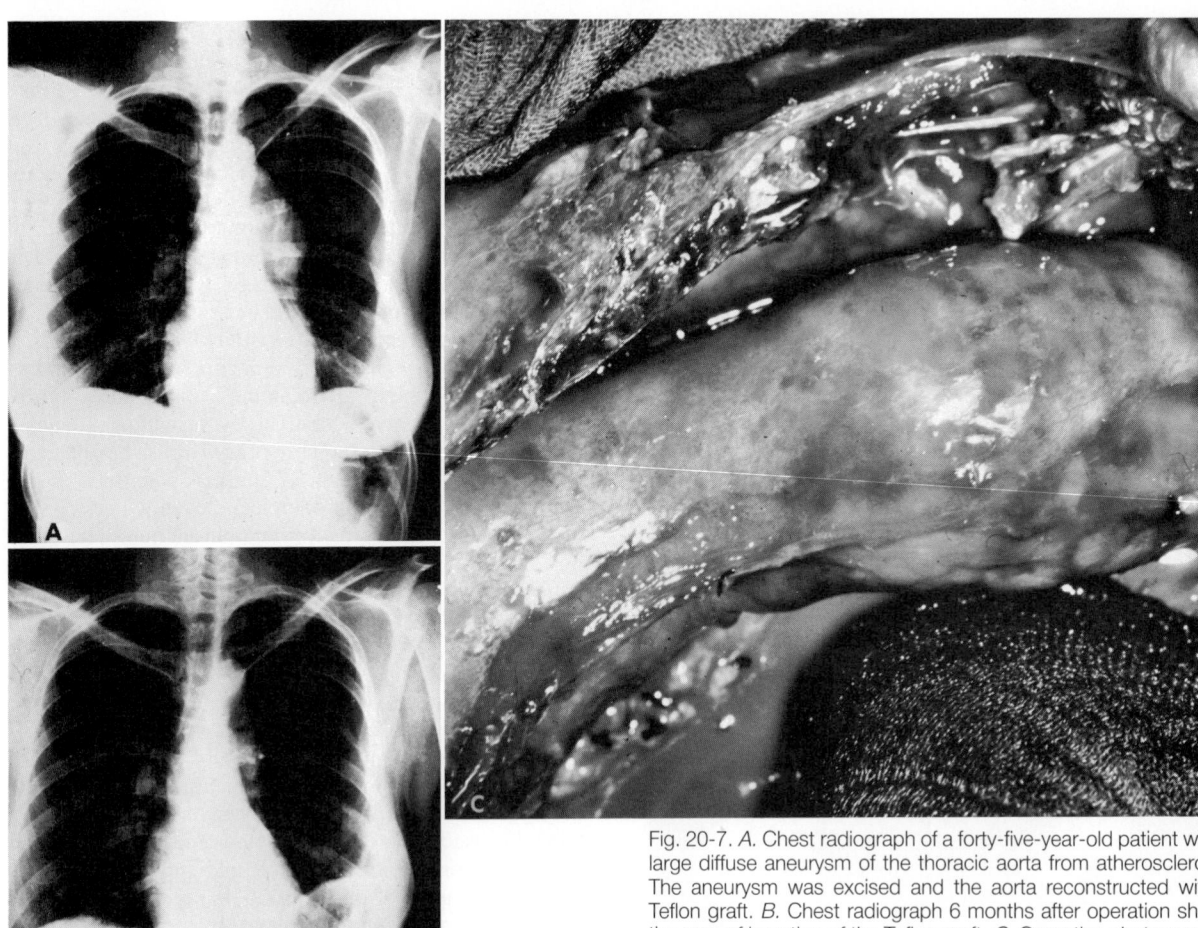

Fig. 20-7. *A.* Chest radiograph of a forty-five-year-old patient with a large diffuse aneurysm of the thoracic aorta from atherosclerosis. The aneurysm was excised and the aorta reconstructed with a Teflon graft. *B.* Chest radiograph 6 months after operation shows the area of insertion of the Teflon graft. *C.* Operative photograph of atherosclerotic aneurysm demonstrated in the chest radiograph seen in *A.*

a complicated surgical procedure, involving restoration of blood flow to the celiac, superior mesenteric, and renal arteries. The diagnosis is often initially made after a chest x-ray shows enlargement of the aorta near the diaphragm. Even with large thoracoabdominal aneurysms, the abdominal component usually cannot be palpated because it is concealed in the upper abdomen by the stomach and pancreas. A diagnosis can be made precisely, however, by aortography and CT.

Early experiences with these complex aneurysms were summarized by DeBakey in 1965. A multiple bypass technique was used, attaching a graft from the thoracic aorta above to the abdominal aorta below (Fig. 20-10). From this initial graft branch grafts were serially attached to the celiac artery, superior mesenteric, and renal arteries. Operative mortality remained at least 50 percent with this complex procedure.

Subsequently, a major advance was developed by Crawford with the intralumenal technique, simply inserting the graft inside the sac of the aneurysm with appropri-

ate side-to-side anastomoses between the graft and the ostia of the different arteries. In 1978, Crawford et al. summarized experiences with 82 patients, 77 of whom survived operation. In 1986, Crawford et al. summarized their very large experience with 605 such operations. About 70 percent of the patients were symptomatic; rupture had occurred in 4 percent of the group. Operative mortality was about 9 percent.

Crawford et al. reported significant observations of the natural history of the disease, describing observations upon 94 patients observed over a period of 25 years in whom operation was not performed for a variety of reasons. Only 24 percent of the group were alive 2 years after a decision was made that operation would not be performed; half of the deaths were due to rupture. By contrast, among 604 patients treated surgically, nearly 60 percent were alive 5 years following operation.

Operations upon the segment of aorta between the tenth thoracic and the second lumbar vertebra have the highest associated frequency of paraplegia, ranging between 20 and 40 percent. Crawford has found that the frequency could be significantly decreased by reattaching large lumbar vessels to the aortic graft at the time of oper-

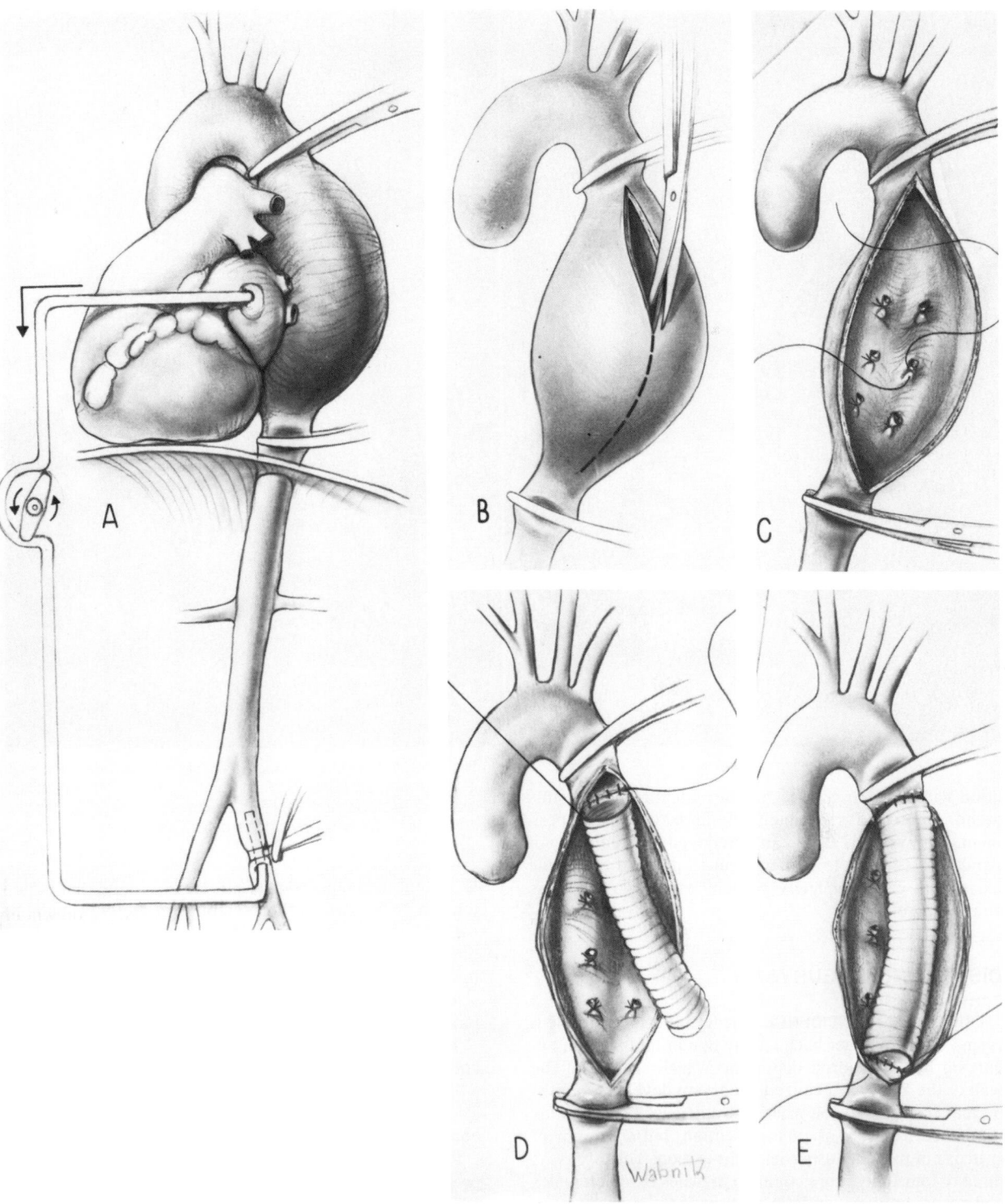

Fig. 20-8. Procedure for excision of an aneurysm of the thoracic aorta. *A.* An aneurysm of the thoracic aorta. Initial dissection is limited to isolation of the aorta proximal and distal to the aneurysm. Left atriofemoral bypass is then instituted at a flow rate near 2 L/min. (See text for other methods of shunting.) Pressures should be monitored in the aorta and also in the femoral artery to ensure adequacy of perfusion of the arterial circulation proximal and distal to the aneurysm. *B.* Aneurysm is widely opened, removing only the inner lining to avoid excessive bleeding where the aneurysm may be adherent to the vertebral column and lung. *C.* Bleeding intercostal arteries may be oversewed from within the lumen of the aneurysm. *D.* A woven Dacron prosthesis is used for reconstruction of the aorta, employing a continuous suture for the anastomosis. *E.* Following completion of the anastomosis the adventitial sac remaining from the aneurysm can be used to surround the graft (not illustrated).

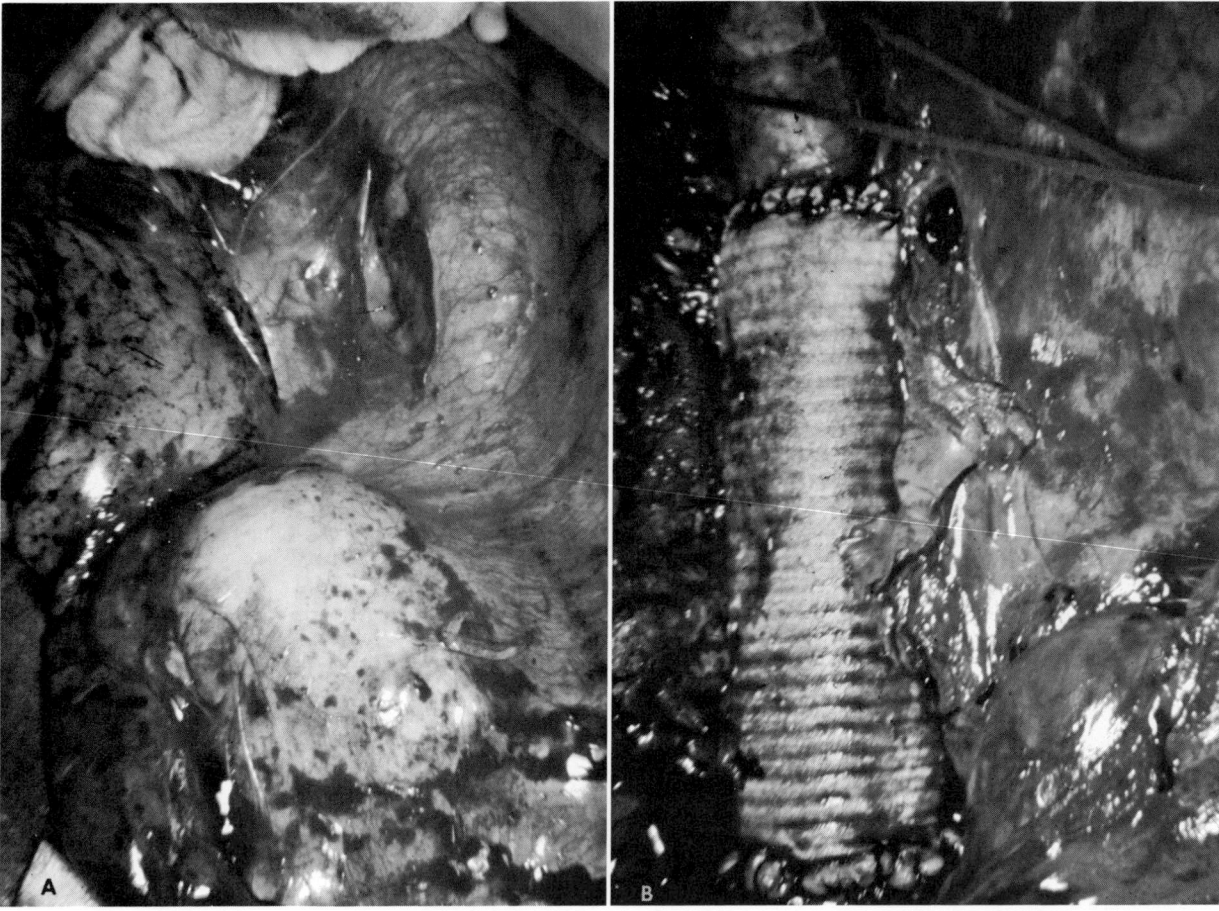

Fig. 20-9. *A.* Operative photograph of saccular syphilitic aneurysm of distal thoracic aorta. *B.* Teflon graft used to restore continuity following excision of a syphilitic aneurysm of the lower thoracic aorta. This graft was used in the patient seen in *A.*

ation with a patch graft technique, a technique that this author described experimentally in laboratory experiments in 1958. This significantly reduced the frequency of paraplegia to near 15 percent, but to date *no technique* exists that can completely prevent paraplegia with this complex problem.

DISSECTING ANEURYSMS

ETIOLOGY AND INCIDENCE. The term "dissecting aneurysm" is a misnomer because the condition is not an aneurysm but an "aortic dissection," a dissection of the wall of the aorta. A localized aneurysm develops months or years later in an area where the aortic wall has become weakened from the original dissection, but a true aneurysm is not present during acute dissection. The disease is three to four times more common in males than in females and occurs predominantly in older patients, those beyond the fifth decade. However, it occurs in every age group, the youngest person being only 14 months of age.

It results from a combination of hypertension and a disease of the media of the aorta of unknown type. Roberts has emphasized that a history of hypertension may be obtainable in only 60 to 75 percent of patients, but hypertrophy of the left ventricle characteristic of hypertension

is present in at least 90 percent. He has found that hypertension is frequently the precipitating factor in patients with Marfan's syndrome who develop dissection, and predicted that proper control of hypertension would virtually eliminate the disease. This prediction well emphasizes the importance of control of hypertension in long-term therapy.

The disease in the media is of unknown type, with no consistent histologic abnormality. Cystic medial necrosis, a histologic abnormality, has been widely described with Marfan's syndrome but is best considered a marker of a connective tissue abnormality, not a disease entity.

Patients with Marfan's syndrome usually develop a progressive fusiform aneurysm in the ascending aorta which eventually ruptures or dissects. There is a greater frequency of dissection in patients with coarctation or congenitally bicuspid aortic valve. Whether this is related to turbulent flow of blood producing these abnormalities or to associated connective tissue defects in the media is uncertain. Disease of the media of the aorta must be a major factor in etiology because there are an estimated 20 million patients with hypertension in the United States,

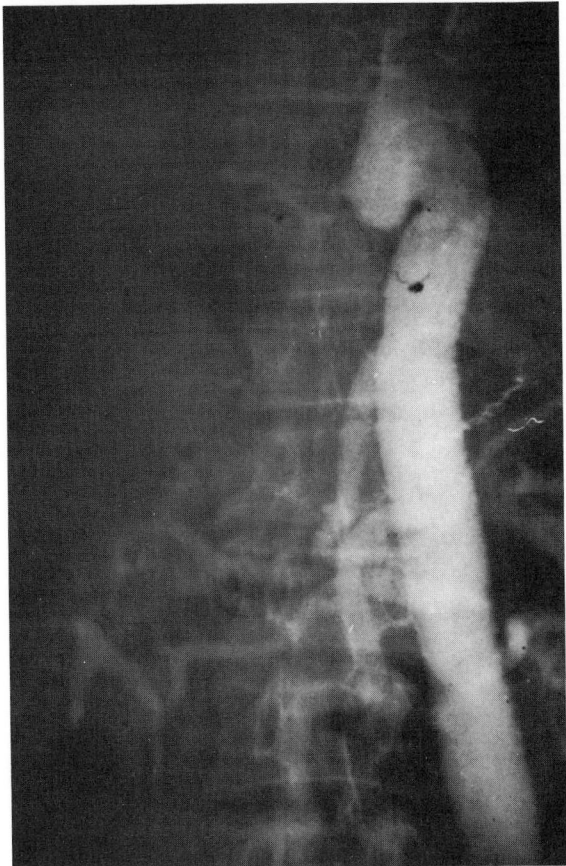

Fig. 20-10. Angiogram of Dacron graft 1 year after excision of thoracoabdominal aneurysm. The graft was inserted between the thoracic aorta, as an end-to-side anastomosis, and the abdominal aorta, not shown in this illustration. Side branches to the superior mesenteric artery, celiac artery, and right and left renal arteries are individually visible.

but only about 2000 dissecting aneurysms are reported each year.

It should be emphasized that the disease is *not due* to atherosclerosis. Atherosclerosis is a disease of the intima, occurring more frequently in the terminal abdominal aorta. Aortic dissection is a disease of the media, almost always occurring in the thoracic aorta. The frequency of occurrence of aortic dissection in older age groups led to confusion with atherosclerosis. The distinction between the two diseases is most important in evaluating prognosis and planning long-term therapy.

Experimentally, a dissecting aneurysm can be produced in young rats with a diet containing 50 percent sweet peas, which causes a distinct abnormality of connective tissue, known as *lathyrism*. The abnormal chemical agent that weakens the cross-linking of collagen is a beta-amino nitrile. To date, this experimental observation has had little clinical significance except to confirm the probable pathogenesis of aortic dissection.

Wilson and Hutchins reviewed 204 patients undergoing autopsy. The most common associated conditions were hypertension, Marfan's syndrome, and inflammatory in-juries of the aortic media. No common pathogenetic mechanism was found.

PATHOLOGY. The two major pathologic abnormalities are a transverse tear of the intima and media, usually involving about half the circumference of the aorta, which permits blood to enter the media. The aortic wall then progressively separates ("dissects") with an inner true lumen and an outer false lumen composed of the outer half of the media and the adventitia. In the detailed analysis published by Roberts, the intimal tear was located in the ascending aorta in about 70 percent of patients, in the aortic arch in 10 percent, in the upper descending thoracic aorta near the ligamentum arteriosum in 20 percent, and in the abdominal aorta in about 2 percent. In the experience of Miller et al. with 125 patients, the intimal tear was in the ascending aorta in 30 percent. In a few patients, no tear in the intima can be found at autopsy, a fact that leads to the theory that dissection of the aorta is the primary process with "rupture of the vasovasorum" and secondary rupture into the aortic lumen. Almost all clinical data make this hypothesis unlikely.

Once the dissection begins, it usually extends rapidly through the thoracic and abdominal aorta into the peripheral arteries. Four types of dissection, proposed by DeBakey as Types A, B, C, and D, depending upon both the site of origin and the extent of distal dissection, are shown in Fig. 20-11. Roberts has estimated that the entire aorta will dissect within minutes unless some structural abnormality that has disrupted continuity of the aortic wall, such as atherosclerosis or coarctation, halts the dissection. In over 50 percent of patients, the dissection process extends into a peripheral artery. If this theory is correct, younger patients with less atherosclerosis would more frequently have dissection of the entire aorta. A "reentry" tear can be identified in about 10 percent of patients, located in the aorta in about half and a peripheral artery in the others.

As dissection progresses, branch vessels are sheared off, either becoming obliterated or establishing a communication with the false lumen occluded by the dissection. Proximally, the coronary arteries may be involved. Frequently one or more aortic valve cusps are detached and prolapse into the lumen, creating aortic insufficiency. Distally, any artery may be involved; carotid artery involvement may produce neurologic injury. Obstruction of the subclavian arteries produces differences in blood pressure between the two arms. Dissection of intercostal arteries may cause spinal cord injury with paraplegia. In one series, 6 of 125 patients had paraplegia on admission. Dissection of renal arteries may produce renal insufficiency. In the extremities, acute obstruction of the iliac or femoral arteries may cause claudication or even gangrene.

The dissection may terminate fatally at any time by rupture of the false lumen with exsanguination. Rupture into the pericardial cavity is the most common, probably because the adventitia is thin over the intrapericardial ascending aorta. Rupture into the left pleural cavity or the retroperitoneal tissues is less common.

The grim mortality is documented in virtually every

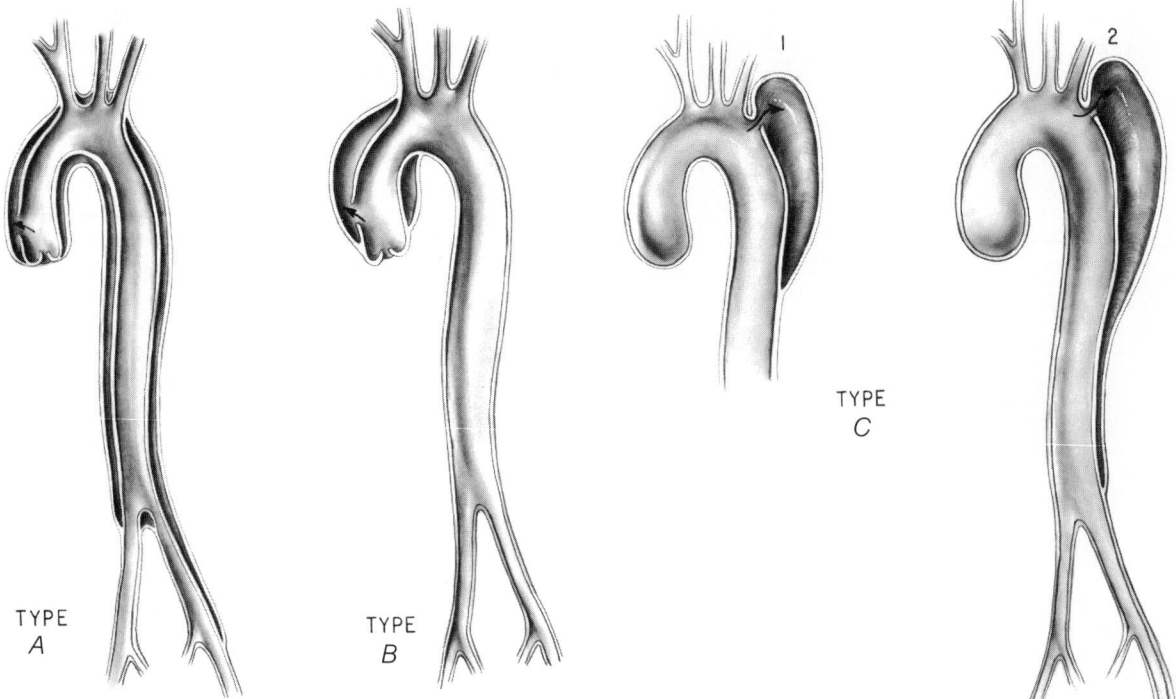

TYPE
A

TYPE
B

TYPE
C

Fig. 20-11. Different types of aortic dissection. *A.* Dissecting aneurysm that begins in the ascending aorta near the aortic valve and extends throughout the aorta down to the external iliac arteries. Unfortunately, this is a common type of dissecting aneurysm. *B.* Dissecting aneurysm limited to the ascending aorta. This is commonly seen in the Marfan syndrome. *C*1. Dissecting aneurysm beginning distal to the left subclavian artery. The localized nature of this aneurysm makes it readily accessible to surgical excision. *C*2. Dissecting aneurysm arising distal to the left subclavian artery but extending into the abdominal aorta. Only partial excision of the area of dissection is possible.

report, with 30 to 50 percent of patients dying within 24 h, 50 to 75 percent within 1 to 2 weeks, and 90 percent of untreated patients within 1 to 3 months. In the classic review of 425 cases by Hirst et al., 74 percent died within 2 weeks and 91 percent within 6 months.

Mortality is much higher with dissection originating in the ascending aorta, almost surely due to the thin adventitia over the intrapericardial aorta. In a group of 62 patients reported by Lindsay and Hurst, almost all of 40 patients whose dissection began in the ascending aorta died within 3 weeks. Only 8 percent of these patients lived 1 month.

This high mortality is the reason emergency operation has been progressively adopted in the last few years for dissections involving the ascending aorta.

In the few patients who survive an aortic dissection, endothelial lining of the false lumen develops, termed a *healed dissecting aneurysm.* This occurs in about 20 percent of patients. Such patients have a so-called double-barreled aorta, with a wide variety of bizarre circulatory patterns. For example, one renal artery may arise from the "false" lumen and the other from the true lumen (Fig. 20-12), or alternatively both renal arteries can arise from the false lumen. In other patients, one iliac artery may originate from the false lumen, the other from the true lumen. In most patients the false lumen gradually becomes aneurysmal and ruptures, especially if significant hypertension is present.

CLINICAL MANIFESTATIONS. The abrupt onset of excruciating pain, almost immediately reaching its peak intensity, is very characteristic of a dissecting aneurysm. A myocardial infarction, by contrast, may gradually develop pain of increasing severity over several minutes.

Sutton et al. reported that chest pain occurred in nearly 80 percent of 113 patients. Usually this was in the anterior chest. Back pain occurred with dissection of the proximal descending aorta in about a third of patients, indicating that absence of back pain did not exclude the dissection of the thoracic aorta. Another significant characteristic of the pain is its tendency to migrate into different areas as dissection extends distally. As might be predicted from the wide variation in the extent of the dissection process, many pain syndromes may occur. Pain may radiate to the neck, the arm, the epigastrium, or the leg. Seldom is pain completely absent, probably in no more than 10 percent of patients.

Syncope occurs in 10 to 20 percent, and some neurologic symptoms are present in 20 to 40 percent. These may result from ischemia of the brain, spinal cord, or a peripheral nerve, depending upon whether a carotid artery, an intercostal artery, or a peripheral artery has been compromised. A stroke develops in about 10 percent of patients, paraplegia in 3 to 5 percent.

Hypertension, often of severe degree, is present in 75 to 85 percent of patients. A frequent clinical picture is that of an acutely ill patient who is hypertensive, pale,

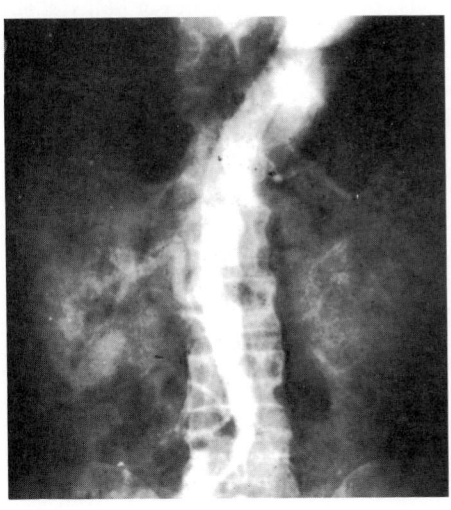
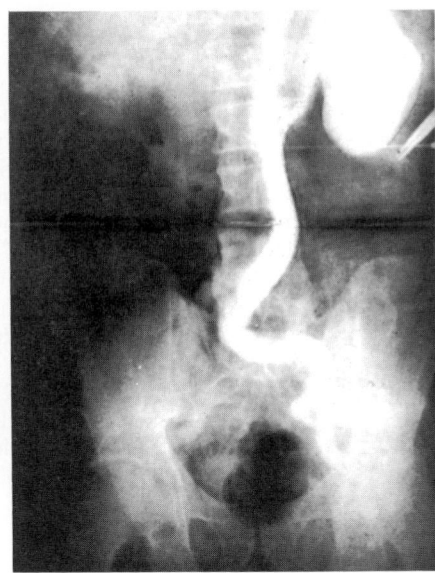
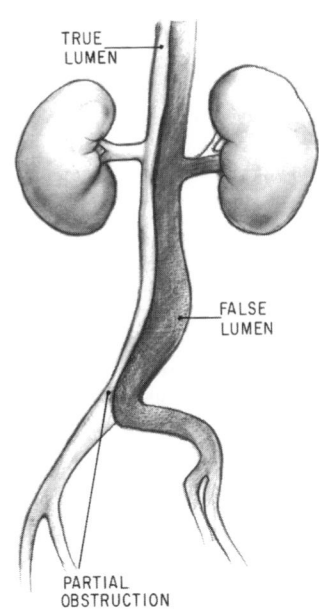

A

B

Fig. 20-12. *A.* Aortogram showing an unusual pattern of aortic dissection in which dissection extended from the thoracic aorta into the abdominal aorta, creating two lumens, with the right renal artery arising from one and the left renal artery from the other. Focal stenosis of the right common iliac artery is seen at the lower part of the field producing intermittent claudication, which was the presenting complaint of the patient. *B.* Aortogram performed by a different root opacifies the left kidney and the left common iliac artery. The condition of the dissected aorta is illustrated in the accompanying drawing. Circulation was reestablished by excising the septum between the two channels at the aortic bifurcation. (From: *Gryboski W, Spencer FC: Intermittent claudication caused by a dissecting aneurysm of the aorta. South Med J 58:593, 1965, with permission.*)

and sweaty from severe vasoconstriction. An aortic diastolic murmur appears in 20 to 30 percent of patients and is of great diagnostic significance, as it originates from detachment of an aortic valve cusp. Unequal carotid or subclavian pulses may be found, caused by unequal compression of these vessels. A variety of neurologic abnormalities may be detected, the most common being either a monoplegia or paraplegia.

DIAGNOSTIC FINDINGS. On the chest radiograph a widened mediastinum or a left pleural effusion from extravasation of blood is frequently seen. In some patients, however, the radiograph may be completely normal. The electrocardiogram is of particular value in distinguishing dissecting aneurysm from myocardial infarction, but there are no characteristic features of aortic dissection. The most common abnormality is left ventricular hypertrophy from the antecedent hypertension.

CT is a valuable noninvasive technique that may establish the diagnosis promptly and quickly in many patients. 2-D echocardiography may also be diagnostic, actually demonstrating the intimal flap. Aortography is the most definitive diagnostic procedure, outlining the double lumen. In some patients, the diagnosis cannot be made by any other technique, as there are no abnormal physical findings and the only symptom is a history of severe back pain.

The importance of immediate aortography or CT in any patient with unexplained sustained severe chest pain cannot be overemphasized. The history of pain may be the *only* abnormality detected. Occasionally a patient is seen a few days or weeks after an acute dissection with no symptoms and no abnormality on physical examination, electrocardiogram, or chest x-ray. Such patients often exsanguinate without any preliminary warning symptoms.

TREATMENT. Modern surgical treatment evolved from the work of DeBakey and Cooley, who reported in 1955 successful excision and grafting of a dissecting aneurysm in the thoracic aorta. Another key concept in treatment, developing from the work of Wheat and colleagues, is the importance of immediate drug therapy both to control the hypertension and to decrease forceful contractility of the left ventricle (dP/dt). Drug therapy should be started as soon as the diagnosis is suspected, preferably in the emergency room, because it may stop the dissection process and prevent exsanguination. Wheat and associates discovered the importance of drug therapy following their ingenious evaluation of observations from the poultry industry that the high fatality rate from spontaneous dissecting aneurysm in certain flocks of turkeys could be dramatically reduced by adding a small amount of reserpine to the turkey food. An intravenous infusion of sodium nitroprusside is usually done, preferably combined with immediate administration of a beta-blocking drug, such as propanolol.

Dissections of the ascending aorta are usually promptly operated upon, generally as an emergency. Both Najafi and Miller have performed emergency operations for over a decade. Ergin and Griepp analyzed 93 publications and recommended immediate operation for both Type A and Type B dissections.

The principal objective at operation is to excise the ascending aorta, as neither excision of the intimal tear nor obliteration of the distal false lumen influences prognosis. In the Miller series of 125 patients, the intimal tear was not excised in 22 percent of patients. Aortic valve replacement was rarely necessary (11 percent); it was sufficient simply to resuspend the aortic cusp, a technique reported by this author in 1962.

With dissections of the descending thoracic aorta many groups use drug therapy initially, as the risk of acute rupture is substantially less. Operation is promptly performed if signs of continued dissection are present, such as continued pain or enlargement of the mediastinal hematoma, or signs of proximal aortic dissection, such as the appearance of an aortic diastolic murmur or a pericardial effusion. With an aggressive policy of emergency operation on all patients the mortality is presently 22 percent with ascending dissections, 14 percent with descending dissections. Wolff et al. reported immediate operation for acute ascending aortic dissection in 48 patients with 6 deaths and overall good results. The incompetent aortic valve was resuspended in 32 of the group; 8 patients required aortic valve replacement as well because of inherent valvular disease. Most patients in recent years with ascending aortic dissections have been operated upon promptly, excising the ascending aorta and restoring continuity with a woven Dacron prosthesis (Figs. 20-13 and 20-14). With descending aortic dissections, drug therapy has been employed initially, reserving operations for patients in whom the dissection process was not controlled.

Several groups, including ours at NYU, have adopted this technique of performance of the distal aortic anastomosis with the "open" technique during a brief period of circulatory arrest. This permits the performance of a more precise anastomosis and also avoids the possible injury of the dissected aorta from application of a vascular clamp. Once the distal anastomosis has been accomplished, the prosthetic graft can be occluded and flow to the brain restored while the proximal anastomosis is performed.

The main cause of operative death is hemorrhage from the suture lines. Performing the distal anastomosis with an "open" technique during circulatory arrest permits precise inclusion of all layers of the dissected aorta with less risk of hemorrhage. At NYU the proximal anastomosis is usually performed with a continuous suture of 4-0 prolene, avoiding undue tension on the suture line which can lacerate the friable intima. An alternative method is to reconstitute the dissected aorta between two strips of Teflon felt, one placed within the lumen and the other around the adventitia, after which the graft is sutured to this reconstructed aorta.

PROGNOSIS. Permanent therapy is necessary because aortic dissection is an acute event in a patient with hypertension and a chronic degenerative disease of the media of the aorta. The false lumen remaining beyond the site of aortic reconstruction may gradually enlarge and become aneurysmal in the first few years following operation. Patients over sixty years of age are also in the age group where atherosclerotic disease of the coronary and cerebral circulations is common. In the series of Miller et al., excluding operative deaths, 5-year survival was 76 percent, 10-year survival 37 percent. Sixty-one percent of late deaths were related to cardiac or cerebral causes.

Control of hypertension is most imortant, as this lessens the frequency of aneurysmal dilatation of the remaining dissected aorta. More than one fatal aortic rupture has resulted from inadvertent cessation of antihypertensive therapy years after recovery from emergent surgical treatment of aortic dissection. These guidelines are especially important in patients with dissections of the descending thoracic aorta, treated initially with drug therapy. They should be carefully observed at 3- to 6-month intervals for development of an aneurysm, as this occurs in at least 25 to 30 percent of such patients. With the present availability of CT and sonography, precise periodic evaluation of the size of the dissected aorta can easily be done.

WOUNDS OF THE GREAT VESSELS

Penetrating Injuries

With penetrating chest wounds, injuries of the heart or great vessels are a frequent cause of death. The two immediate threats to life are cardiac arrest from exsanguination or tamponade. Tamponade is discussed in Chap. 19.

With injuries of the aorta or vena cava, only a few patients are alive when first seen in a hospital emergency room. They are usually in profound shock with signs of massive intrathoracic bleeding. Unless an operating room is immediately available, immediate thoracotomy may offer the only chance for survival. "Slash" thoracotomy with limited aseptic technique has been employed at Bellevue Hospital for several years, occasionally resuscitating a moribund patient. Infection following such a thoracotomy is surprisingly rare. Once hemorrhage has been controlled, the patient can be transferred to the operating room for definitive surgical exploration and repair.

When threatened exsanguination does not mandate immediate thoracotomy, aortography should be seriously considered in any patient with a possible injury of the great vessels from a penetrating wound of the mediastinum. The development of frequent use of aortography is of the major advances in therapy of thoracic trauma of the past decade. Indications should be liberal because some grave injuries may not be recognizable by other methods until serious complications develop.

Aortography helps choose between a sternotomy and a thoracotomy. Median sternotomy, combined with extension into the neck if necessary, provides the best combined exposure of the heart and great vessels. Exposure of the left subclavian artery, however, is limited and may require a lateral thoracotomy, converting the sternotomy to a T incision. This extensive incision in the thoracic cage may require ventilatory support for several days afterward; so it should be avoided if a simpler approach is possible. If aortography indicates that injury of the left

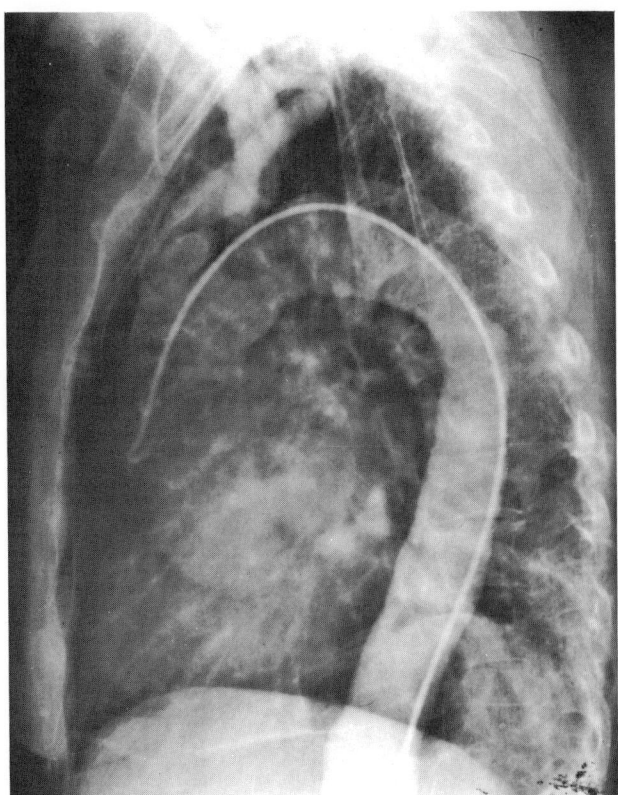

Fig. 20-13. *Opposite.* Thoracic aortogram, performed with a catheter introduced retrograde through the femoral artery, showing a dissecting aneurysm arising distal to the left subclavian artery. The outer channel is faintly visualized as a double density beyond the left subclavian artery. *Lower left.* Operative photograph of dissecting aneurysm arising distal to the left subclavian artery. A clamp is visible on the aorta proximal to the left subclavian artery, which has been encircled with an umbilical tape. The vagus nerve is visible proximally. Laminated clot was found in the lumen of the aneurysm. *Lower right.* Dacron graft inserted to restore aortic continuity following excision of the aneurysm.

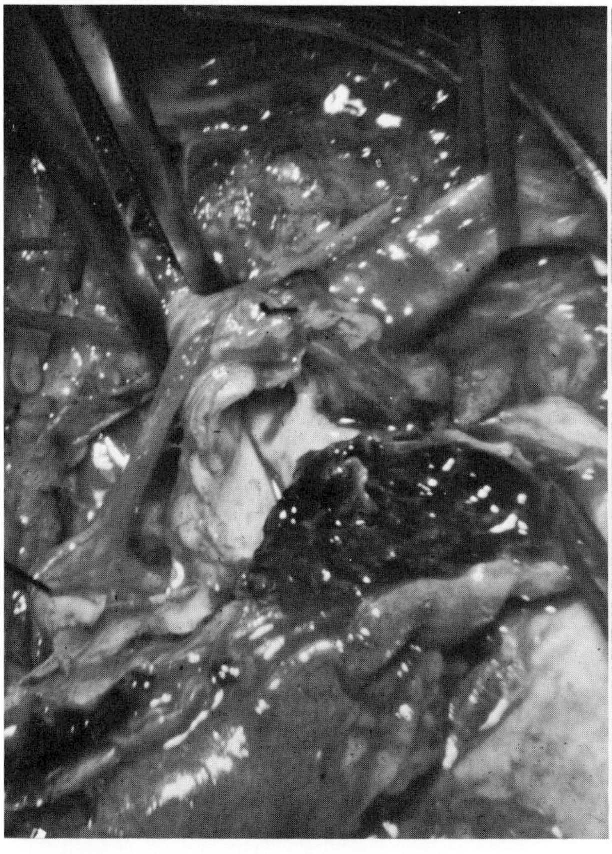

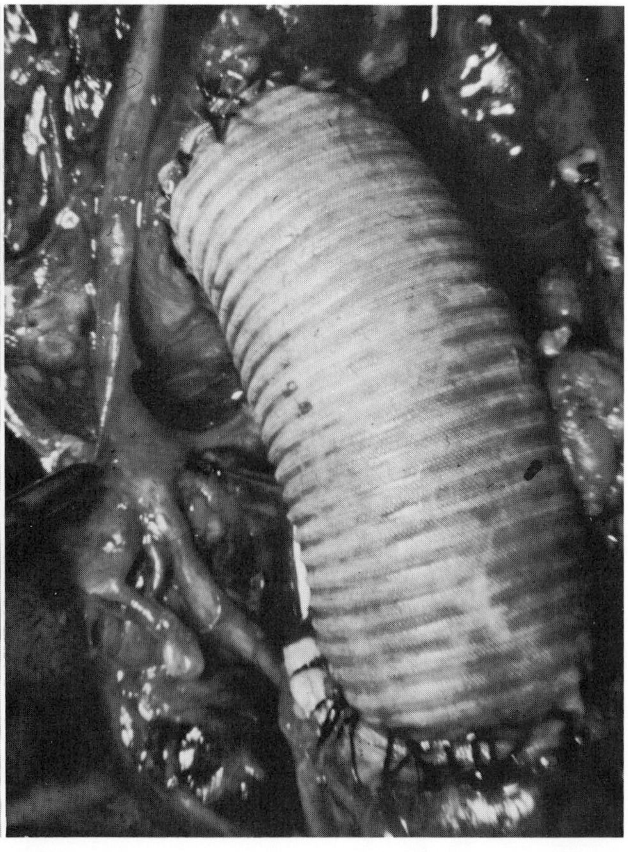

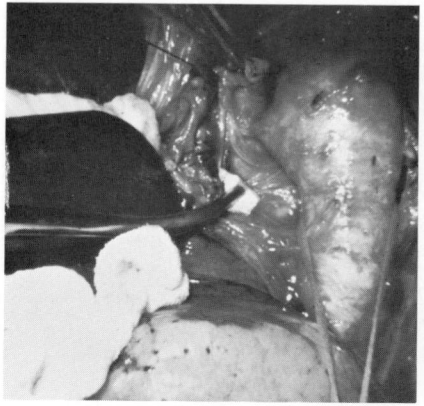 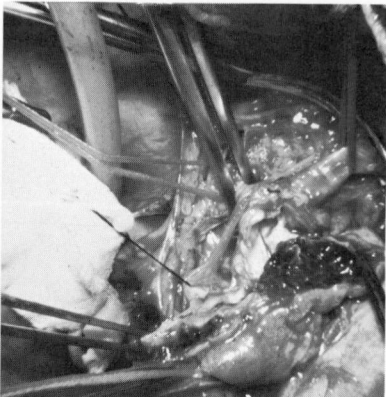 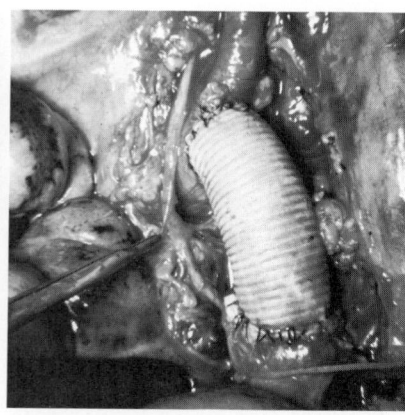

Fig. 20-14. *Left.* Operative photograph of dissecting aneurysm of upper thoracic aorta, starting a few days before operation. The hematoma in the aortic wall is visible. *Center.* With a functioning left atrial bypass, the aorta has been occluded and the aneurysm incised. A tape encircles the left subclavian artery. The vagus nerve with the recurrent nerve encircling the aorta is visible. The aneurysm began in the classic location, just beyond the left subclavian artery. A large thrombus is present in the aortic wall. *Right.* Aortic reconstruction was accomplished with a short woven Dacron graft. The proximal anastomosis is immediately beyond the left subclavian artery.

subclavian artery is the only injury, a left anterior thoracotomy in the third interspace is a better incision.

Richardson described experiences with 76 gunshot wounds of the mediastinum. Immediate operation was performed for 33 patients in *unstable* condition, with 12 deaths. Forty-three patients in *stable* condition had several diagnostic studies, including angiography, after which 27 were operated upon, 11 of whom had injuries to the great vessels. There were three deaths in this group, all from delayed complications (7 percent). In 1985, Zakharia et al. described experiences with nearly 2000 thoracic battle wounds. Over 1400 thoracotomies were performed. Cardiac injuries occurred in 225 patients, great vessel wounds in 54, with an 87 percent survival in those with vessel injuries.

Nonpenetrating Injuries

The possibility of traumatic laceration of the aorta has emerged in the past two decades as one of the most important diagnostic considerations in treating blunt injuries, especially those following an automobile accident. Parmley et al.; they emphasized that between 10 and 20 percent of patients lived longer than 30 min after injury before exsanguination. The frequency of aortic laceration increases with the severity of the trauma; it is a common finding after severe trauma that produces instant death. It is estimated that 10 to 15 percent of patients seen alive following severe blunt trauma will have an aortic laceration. Liberal use of aortography with *all* severe chest injuries is the best diagnostic approach, because *no single* clinical finding can diagnose or exclude significant vascular injuries.

Passaro and Pace in 1959 are credited with the first successful repair of a traumatic aortic laceration. In 1961 the author reported 15 patients with traumatic injuries and reviewed published experiences of others, finding virtually no successful reports of surgical repairs except the one case reported by Passaro.

ETIOLOGY AND PATHOLOGY. Rupture of the aorta usually results from a deceleration-type injury, typically an automobile accident. In the vast majority of patients, the laceration occurs just distal to the left subclavian artery. Apparently the descending thoracic aorta and the aortic arch decelerate at different rates because of differences in anatomic structure, producing a transverse tear near the site of insertion of the ligamentum arteriosum. The tear may involve part or all of the layers of the aortic wall, varying from laceration of the intima to transection of the aorta with retraction of the two ends (Fig. 20-15). Usually the injury is a partial laceration with formation of a localized hematoma. Aortic dissection following trauma is rare.

Fatal hemorrhage is prevented in some patients by the adventitia, which has been reported to constitute 60 percent of the tensile strength of the aortic wall. It is quite astonishing at operation to find the transected edges of the intima retracted for 1 to 2 cm, with exsanguination temporarily prevented by the adventitia.

The extensive 1981 review by Fisher and associates summarized available information. They found that aortic and great vessel laceration constituted the most common site of vascular injury after blunt chest trauma, citing 54 cases of their own and 456 cases previously reported by others. The second most common injury was an innominate artery laceration (26 cases). Injuries of the right carotid or right subclavian are virtually unknown; only 4 cases of laceration of the common carotid artery could be found. There were 13 injuries of the subclavian, virtually all of which involved the left subclavian. Multiple vascular lacerations were found in only 3 percent of cases. Lacerations of the aorta in other areas are very rare, with only isolated reports of injury of the ascending aorta or laceration near the diaphragm.

In surviving patients, a mediastinal hematoma forms and produces widening of the mediastinal shadow, easily recognized on the chest x-ray. This is the *key to the diagnosis.* Several radiographic abnormalities have been de-

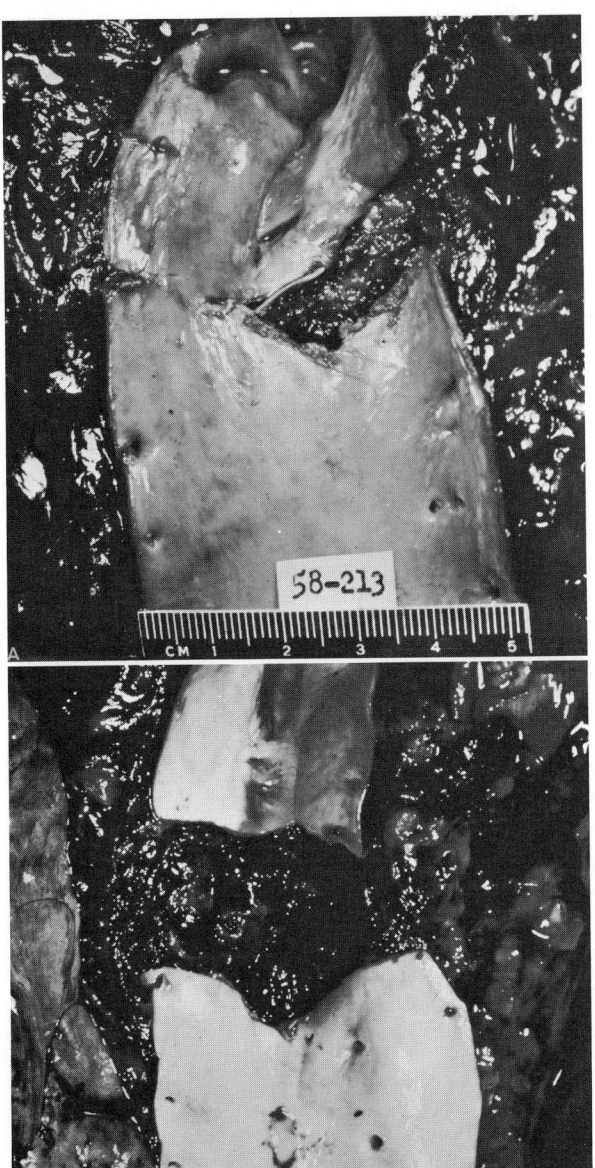

Fig. 20-15. *A.* Translated aorta found at autopsy when the patient was exsanguinated 24 h following injury. The patient had only minor chest pain before the terminal event. The sharp, transverse laceration of the aorta is the usual finding, resulting from the deceleration forces at the time of injury. *B.* Partial transection of the aorta found at autopsy when the patient was suddenly exsanguinated 3 weeks following an automobile accident. An aortic lesion had not been previously suspected.

scribed, but simply recognizing a wide mediastinal shadow is by far the most significant. Several mathematical indices were analyzed, but all were found inferior to the subjective impression of *mediastinal widening.* The critical measurement separating positive from negative cases was a mediastinal width of 8.0 cm.

No single finding either diagnoses or excludes aortic laceration. This can only be done with aortography. A small group of patients, less than 10 percent, have been reported who had aortic laceration but did not have significant mediastinal widening.

In surviving patients first seen in the hospital emergency department, there is a grave risk of imminent rupture, as about 40 percent of such patients exsanguinate within the next 48 h. The statistical risk of fatal rupture within the first 5 days after hospital admission is shown in Fig. 20-16. The risk decreases sharply after 2 weeks. Surviving patients gradually developed a false aneurysm, described earlier in this chapter under Traumatic Thoracic Aneurysms. Although traumatic aneurysms enlarge slowly, there is a small but ever-present hazard of rupture; about 20 percent of patients with false aneurysms seen more than 10 years after injury die from rupture within the next 5 years.

CLINICAL MANIFESTATIONS. Usually there are no symptoms or signs to indicate that an aortic injury is present. Dyspnea and chest pain are usually present, but these result from the almost universally present rib fractures. A hemothorax, with varying degrees of shock, is also common. A murmur has seldom been heard. Rarely, signs of acute obstruction of the aorta, apparently from prolapse of a segment of intima into the lumen, are present.

DIAGNOSTIC FINDINGS. As the history and the physical examination provide virtually no clues to the diagnosis, the chest x-ray is most important. Widening of the mediastinum (Fig. 20-17) is present in 80 to 90 percent of patients. It may result from causes other than rupture of the aorta, hence, aortography is necessary for the definitive diagnosis (Fig. 20-18). As emphasized earlier, an aortogram should be performed in the majority of patients with severe chest trauma, regardless of clinical findings.

TREATMENT. Thoracotomy should be performed as soon as possible after the diagnosis has been established. Akins et al. provide evidence that prompt operation would seem wiser in most instances.

The surgical approach is through a left posterolateral thoracotomy in the fourth intercostal space. At NYU a femoral-femoral bypass with a pump oxygenator and cannulae in a femoral artery and vein is routinely used. The use of a shunt or a bypass during operation, as opposed to the simpler clamp and repair technique, varies widely among different institutions. In a careful survey of published reports by others, Pate found that 8 of 30 patients treated by simply clamping and rapid suture repair developed paraplegia (20 percent). Among 68 patients who had either a shunt or a bypass, only 4 developed papaplegia, a frequency of 6 percent. The key point with femoral-femoral bypass is to use a flow rate high enough to keep the distal aortic pressure above 60 mmHg. Certainly, if the repair could be accomplished predictably within less than 30 min the risk of paraplegia would seem small, but attempting repair of an acute aortic laceration without distal circulation is a serious "gamble."

Once the left chest has been opened, the hematoma overlying the thoracic aorta should not be disturbed until proximal aortic control has been obtained. This is best done by opening the pericardium and encircling the aorta

Mode of Death	No. of Patients
Other subsystem trauma	13
Multiple	8
Head injury	3
Hemorrhagic shock during thoracotomy	2
Acute cardiac failure	4
Diffuse mediastinal and chest wall hemorrhage after repair	2
Total	19

Fig. 20-16. Mode of death after repair of acute traumatic aortic transection (UAB; 1967–July 1984; n = 47, 13 deaths and GLH; 1965–November 1984; n = 32, 6 deaths). (From: *Kirklin JW, Barratt-Boyes BG: Cardiac Surgery. New York, Wiley, chap 53, p 1459, with permission.*)

distal or proximal to the left common carotid artery. Slight manipulation of the mediastinal hematoma may result in abrupt rupture and massive hemorrhage. Surgical repair usually requires the insertion of a short Dacron graft, though some groups have reported repair by direct suture.

Overall mortality with traumatic injuries ranges between 15 and 25 percent, usually because of associated injuries. In the series of 79 patients reported by Kirklin-Barratt-Boyes, mortality was 24 percent and paraplegia developed in 16 percent.

OBSTRUCTION OF THE SUPERIOR VENA CAVA

Obstruction of the superior vena cava produces an unusual but distinctive clinical syndrome that can be easily recognized once the diagnosis is considered. Diagnostic errors are common, primarily because of the infrequent occurrence of the disease and because of lack of familiarity with the distinctive clinical features. The 1981 report by Parish emphasized that the diagnosis can be made on physical examination in most patients.

Fig. 20-17. Chest radiograph of a patient with traumatic rupture of the thoracic aorta, illustrating the characteristic widening of the mediastinum. When this is observed following a chest injury, emergency aortography should be performed to establish the diagnosis of rupture of the thoracic aorta.

Fig. 20-18. Aortogram demonstrating traumatic rupture of the thoracic aorta distal to the left subclavian artery. The point of rupture can be seen as an irregular border of the thoracic aorta, in association with localized bulging. This angiogram represents the *first* instance in which emergency aortography was employed to establish firmly the diagnosis of traumatic rupture of the aorta. (From: *Spencer FC, Guerin PF, et al: A report of 15 patients with traumatic rupture of the thoracic aorta. J Thorac Cardiovasc Surg 41:1, 1961, with permission.*)

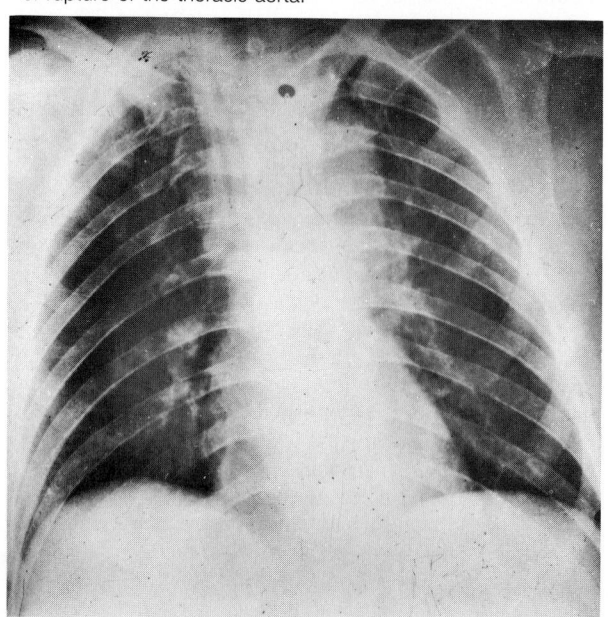

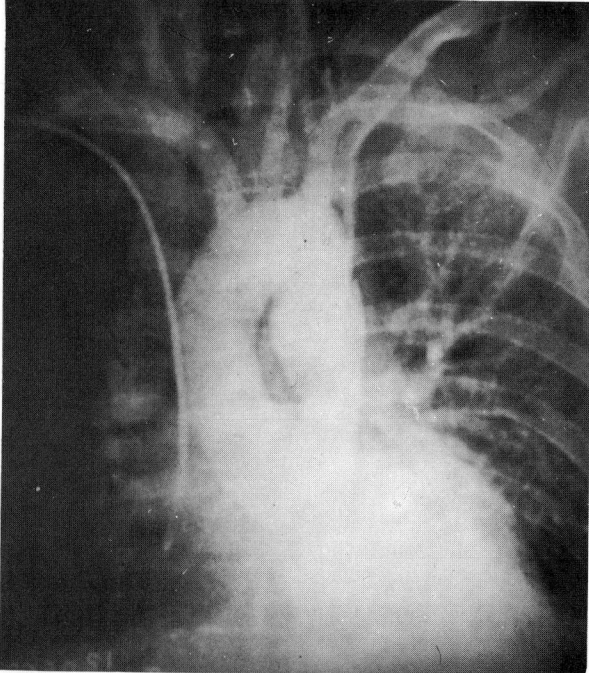

Several excellent reviews of this subject have been published in the last three decades, all finding that a malignant tumor is the most frequent cause. An extensive review made by McIntire and Sykes is a fundamental reference. Effler and Groves reported 64 patients, 48 of whom had a malignant neoplasm. Panker and Maddison summarized reports totaling 438 cases, only 15 percent of which were from benign causes. Mahajan reviewed published reports of benign causes of superior vena cava obstruction, a total of only 16 cases. Lochridge et al. described 66 cases seen in the previous 10 years; 64 were malignant.

ETIOLOGY. Over 90 percent of patients have obstruction from a malignant process. The percentage has apparently risen in recent years, especially since obstruction from expanding aortic aneurysms has decreased. The most common neoplasm is a bronchogenic carcinoma invading the mediastinum. Less frequent lesions are primary mediastinal tumors such as thymoma or lymphoma. Metastatic neoplasms are unusual.

Obstruction from a chronic fibrosing mediastinitis, usually of unknown cause, is infrequent. It is the only condition in which a long-term cure is possible. The etiology in most patients is unknown, although the disorder has been recognized for decades. The Parish report includes three cases resulting from the use of central venous catheters.

PATHOPHYSIOLOGY. With obstruction of the superior vena cava there is an increase in venous pressure to levels between 20 and 50 mmHg. The degree of increase in venous pressure varies with both the rate of development of the obstruction and the site of obstruction. Obstruction between the azygos vein and right atrium is less disabling than at other sites because the azygos vein can provide collateral venous decompression. The usual patient will have obstruction of the vena cava above the level of the azygos. Doty, in a 1982 detailed article, cited a venographic report by Dyet, who found that about 40 percent of patients have displacement but incomplete obstruction by tumor, about 20 percent have obstruction between the azygos vein and the heart, and about 40 percent have obstruction of the superior vena cava above the azygos, the usual finding in patients with disabling symptoms.

Acute obstruction of the vena cava, as during a thoracic operation, can produce fatal cerebral edema within a few minutes. This also occurred with early experiences in infants with the Glenn operation of anastomosis of the superior vena cava to the right pulmonary artery. At the opposite extreme are instances where superior vena cava obstruction develops slowly, permitting time for the development of collateral circulation, as a result of which symptoms are mild.

CLINICAL MANIFESTATIONS. With mild obstruction, frequent symptoms are headache, swelling of the eyelids, puffiness of the face, or enlargement of the neck. The severity is related to posture. Patients quickly find that symptoms increase if they bend over or lie down. With acute obstruction, resulting from hemorrhage into a rapidly growing neoplasm, more serious symptoms of cerebral congestion appear, including drowsiness and blurring of vision. Edema of the vocal cords produces hoarseness

or dyspnea from laryngeal obstruction. As the majority of cases are due to a rapidly growing bronchogenic carcinoma, pulmonary symptoms such as cough and hemoptysis are also often present. In most patients death results within a few months.

In the minority of patients in whom obstruction results from a benign process, usually fibrosing mediastinitis, collateral circulation generally enlarges sufficiently to where little disability is present. Prominent features include dilated veins with edema and cyanosis, the degree varying with the degree of stasis. Venous hypertension is obvious from prominence and distention of veins in the arms and face. Effler and Groves described 16 patients with obstruction from a benign process, all of whom eventually developed sufficient collateral circulation to have minimal symptoms. No fatalities occurred as a result of chronic venous obstruction. We observed one patient over a period of 30 years in whom the superior vena cava became obstructed following an intracardiac operation for correction of anomalous pulmonary veins entering the superior vena cava. Venous hypertension initially was severe, above 35 mmHg, producing a bilateral chylothorax controlled by ligation of the thoracic duct. The child was almost six years of age at this time. Within a few months, however, all symptoms subsided, and the patient, now a young married woman with children, has no limitation of physical activities.

DIAGNOSTIC STUDIES. Although the clinical picture is characteristic when fully developed, early manifestations such as swelling of the eyes or headache may be confused with angioneurotic edema, congestive heart failure, or constrictive pericarditis. Elevation of venous pressure, usually between 20 and 50 mmHg, is diagnostic. Venography readily outlines the location and extent of the obstruction, although the elevated venous pressure may result in bleeding. Often venography is omitted if the diagnosis of a malignant process is obvious. The usual consideration is to determine the type of malignancy present by an appropriate biopsy. Thoracotomy is usually avoided if malignancy is present. Doty has emphasized that morbidity from a thoracic operation is less if a sternotomy is employed, because venous collateral circulation is interrupted to a lesser degree than with a lateral thoracotomy.

TREATMENT. With a malignant process, involvement of the superior vena cava almost precludes surgical resection. Isolated exceptions are rare.

The standard therapy is intensive radiation therapy, often in combination with diuretics and chemotherapy. The degree of improvement in symptoms varies with the type of neoplasm, but the majority improve rapidly, within a few weeks, probably from diminution in edema associated with a growing neoplasm. Death from the neoplasm, however, is virtually inevitable within the next several months, with rare survivors to 2 years.

With benign obstructions, as the report of Effler and Groves indicates, there is no urgency in performing an operation if symptoms are mild. In all likelihood these symptoms will improve, or subside completely, as collateral circulation develops.

pursuing the obliteration too aggressively and precipitating infarction. This is a particularly dangerous complication because not only is tissue lost but also uncontrollable hemorrhage from tissues adjacent to the infant may result. The catheter technique has been successfully applied to malformations of the pelvis and buttock, which were of quite difficult access, as well as to malformations of the head, neck, extremities, and even the brain.

Increasingly favorable experiences with this intraarterial embolization have been reported. Combinations of Gelfoam, pellets, and autologous muscle have been injected by the Seldinger technique. Inoperable lesions may be treated by embolization alone, while extensive lesions may be managed by embolization followed by excision.

ARTERIAL TRAUMA

HISTORICAL DATA. The feasibility of routinely repairing injured limb arteries in military casualties was first demonstrated in the Korean conflict in 1952; earlier attempts in World War II were generally unsuccessful. Several factors contributed to this improvement in results: (1) the prompt evacuation of the wounded by helicopter so that definitive treatment could be started within 2 to 4 h of injury, (2) the realization that extensive debridement of traumatic wounds, together with antibiotic administration and secondary closure controlled infection, and (3) the familiarity of surgeons with new vascular surgical techniques and instruments. Following this war experience, injured extremity arteries encountered in civilians have been almost routinely repaired to avoid the approximately 50 percent incidence of gangrene associated with ligation of major extremity arteries.

PATHOLOGY. Most arterial injuries result from penetrating wounds that partly or completely disrupt the wall of the vessel. Nonpenetrating injuries, usually associated with fractures of adjacent bones, occur less frequently but have a more serious prognosis.

With lacerations or transections, the extent of injury varies with the type of trauma. With clean incised wounds, such as those made by a knife or an icepick, injury to the arterial wall is minimal and repair may require no more than simple suture. By contrast, trauma from high velocity missiles will disrupt the intima and media for a distance beyond the actual laceration and require wider debridement at the time of surgical repair, often necessitating insertion of a conduit to bridge the defect.

Extensive communicated fractures may be associated with either contusion of the artery, leading to thrombosis, or to spasm. Arterial spasm alone, though an infrequent response to injury, may precipitate thrombosis.

Arterial contusion from a blunt injury may result in multiple areas of fragmentation of the arterial wall with intramural hemorrhage or detachment of the intima with prolapse into the lumen. This results in luminal obstruction that can be detected only by arteriotomy and inspection. When contusion is misdiagnosed as spasm, the delay in treatment with persistence of ischemia can result in

gangrene. Volkmann is ischemic contracture of the muscles of the forearm is often due to untreated spasm or contusion of the brachial artery accompanying supracondylar fracture of the humerus.

PATHOPHYSIOLOGY. The consequences of ischemia following an arterial injury vary with the tolerance of different tissues for anoxia. In the extremity the peripheral nerves are the most sensitive. Paralysis and anesthesia quickly develop when arterial blood flow is seriously decreased. Striated muscle is almost equally sensitive and will usually become necrotic if arterial blood flow is decreased to such a degree that anesthesia and paralysis are present. Skin, tendon, and bone all have a greater tolerance for anoxia and may survive an ischemic injury which has produced irreversible extensive muscle necrosis. This is seen in an extremity in which an arterial repair is performed several hours after injury. The skin may appear viable, but the extremity is anesthetic and paralyzed, and after a period of time will be found to have widespread necrosis of the muscles.

Striated muscle will tolerate ischemia 6 to 8 h. Every effort should be made to complete arterial repair within 6 h after injury if anesthesia *or* paralysis is present, indicating a severe degree of ischemia. A definite time limit does not exist, however, beyond which arterial repair is futile, for the importance of the time interval varies with the collateral circulation. The collateral circulation, in turn, varies with the artery injured, with the degree of soft tissue injury which has interrupted collateral circulation, with associated shock, and with ambient temperature. In some patients with little disturbance of collateral circulation, arterial repair may be successfully performed 12 to 15 h after injury.

CLINICAL MANIFESTATIONS. Shock, present in over 50 percent of patients with an arterial injury, is usually due to either hemorrhage from the injured artery or associated injuries. The degree of shock varies with the severity of the blood loss or the severity of other injuries. When profound, the severe associated peripheral vasoconstriction may conceal the presence of an arterial injury until blood pressure has been restored to near normal levels.

With blunt trauma, multiple organ injuries are commonly present. These include skull fractures, rib fractures, or blunt abdominal injuries. Careful assessment of each injury, with subsequent assignment of priorities in therapy, is a critical part of initial evaluation of the patient.

In the injured extremity, fractures and nerve injuries are commonly present either with penetrating wounds or following blunt trauma. The presence of a fracture or extensive soft tissue injury greatly influences the prognosis of an arterial injury. For example, in one series of arterial injuries the presence of a fracture of a femur in association with an injury of the femoral artery raised the incidence of gangrene from 11 to 55 percent.

In the extremity, the arterial injury frequently produces the five abnormal findings associated with acute ischemia, conveniently remembered as five p's: *p*ain, *p*aralysis, *p*aresthesia or anesthesia, loss of *p*ulses, and *p*allor. Of these five, the neurologic findings, paralysis and paresthesia, are the most important, because loss of neurologic function indicates a degree of tissue ischemia that will progress to gangrene unless arterial blood flow is improved. Absence of a pulse in the presence of a normal pulse in the contralateral extremity immediately suggests an arterial injury. In the presence of shock, evaluation of peripheral pulses may be difficult until blood volume is restored. The presence of a peripheral pulse does not exclude an arterial injury since a tangential laceration of the wall of an artery sealed by a blood clot preserves some flow through the arterial lumen.

With penetrating wounds, bright red bleeding, even in small amounts, immediately suggests arterial injury. Contained bleeding may produce a tense hematoma palpable around the wound, without external evidence of bleeding. A systolic bruit or rarely a continuous bruit may indicate that an acute arteriovenous fistula has been produced.

An arterial injury can be present with virtually no abnormalities in the extremity and so a penetrating injury near a major artery should alert to the possibility of an arterial injury that may result in exsanguinating secondary hemorrhage, the occurrence of a false aneurysm, or an arteriovenous fistula in the area where the hematoma formed around the lacerated artery.

With any suspicion of arterial injury, as occurs with diminished or absent pulses or with signs of ischemia, an arteriogram should be performed and is of particular value in determining whether the abnormalities are due to arterial injury or to angulation of the artery at the fracture site.

TREATMENT. Preoperative Considerations. Control of bleeding is the most urgent immediate problem and can usually be accomplished by direct digital pressure on the bleeding site or by tightly packing the wound with gauze and applying a pressure dressing. A large amount of packing may be required, for the efficacy of the packing depends upon compression of the artery between the overlying skin and the underlying bone. Tourniquets are best avoided for most injuries. When used they must be carefully padded to avoid the risk of permanent injury to peripheral nerves.

Shock should be treated by the rapid infusion of fluids (500 mL every 5 to 10 min) until the systolic blood pressure rises to 80 mmHg, after which additional fluids can be infused more gradually. Usually 1000 to 2000 mL of fluid will be required. Blood is preferable, but until the necessary cross-matching has been done, crystalloids, plasma, or dextran may be used.

Antibiotic therapy should be started promptly and appropriate prophylactic therapy for tetanus begun. Sympathetic blocks and systemic anticoagulant therapy have no significant role in preoperative care.

Operative Technique. An important basic tenet regarding arterial trauma is that almost all injuries can be repaired successfully with available surgical techniques. The prognosis then becomes a question of whether the repair was performed before irreversible muscle necrosis developed and how well the bone and associated soft tissue trauma can be managed. The only special instruments required are atraumatic vascular clamps and arterial su-

tures, usually of synthetic fiber (Dacron, polypropylene) fashioned to be monofilamentous, sizes 4-0 to 7-0, with swaged needles. The surgical incisions should be placed to expose the artery proximal and distal to the site of injury, and then the hematoma surrounding the injury can be widely opened and the artery mobilized. When soft tissue trauma is extensive and it is anticipated that arterial anastomosis will be delayed, insertion of a temporary bypass shunt between the proximal and distal ends of the artery to maintain distal flow is recommended to maintain tissue viability while other pressing problems are attended to. When there is associated bone trauma with comminuted displaced fracture fragments, stabilization of the fracture either by internal or external fixation may facilitate the arterial repair and prevent its disruption. Most injuries are best treated by excision of 2 to 4 mm of the injured arterial wall followed by end-to-end anastomosis, avoiding tangential repairs that often result in constriction and subsequent thrombosis. With transection of an artery, retraction of the two ends of the vessel may result in the erroneous impression that a segment of artery has been destroyed. In most instances mobilization of the two ends and application of gentle traction on the ends of the artery with vascular clamps will demonstrate that direct anastomosis can be performed, since 1 to 2 cm of a peripheral artery can be excised and the vessel ends still be approximated. In two series of civilian injuries reported by Patman et al. and by Morris et al., primary repair was possible in 85 to 90 percent of patients. Before the anastomosis is performed, the degree of back-bleeding from the distal artery should be noted and any blood clots removed with a catheter. The anastomosis should be performed with 4-0 or 6-0 arterial sutures using a continuous suture interrupted in two or three areas to avoid a purse-string effect. Individual sutures should be 1 to 1.5 mm in depth and a similar distance apart for large arteries such as the aorta or iliac arteries, but considerably closer for smaller vessels. With arteries smaller than the superficial femoral, interrupted or horizontal mattress sutures may be employed. Either a continuous over-and-over suture or an everting suture is satisfactory (Fig. 21-2).

When direct anastomosis cannot be performed because of loss of 2 cm or more of artery, an autogenous vein is the preferable graft, reversing the ends of the vein which is usually the saphenous. If for some reason a vein cannot be utilized, a graft of Goretex is preferable. If a prosthetic graft is used, the diameter rarely should be more than 6 mm.

When all the major venous structures in an extremity have also been interrupted, failure to restore some venous return results in a higher incidence of failure of arterial reconstruction than if vein continuity is established. In some instances the venous repair will undergo thrombosis and subsequent recanalization, thus restoring the effectiveness of the venous repair.

With contaminated wounds, the best protection from infection following adequate debridement and arterial reconstruction is approximation of the adjacent muscles over the arterial repair, leaving the remaining wound

exertion should be investigated. Characteristically, in most cases, the pain is the first and dominant symptom. Initially, it begins as a dull ache which soon becomes severe and is primarily located over the anterior compartment, where palpation may elicit tenderness. Motion of the leg or foot increases the severity of pain. Subsequently, erythema of the skin over the anterior compartment becomes apparent, and there is measurable increase in the size of the calf. As the syndrome progresses, these signs become more apparent. The dorsalis pedis pulse may be normal, diminished, or absent. Actually, its absence is a late sign and occasionally follows the loss of motor power of the muscles of the anterior compartment. The anterior tibial muscle and the extensor hallucis longus usually become paralyzed first, whereas the extensor digitorum longus loses its function later and is usually the first to return after release of pressure. Loss of the extensor digitorum brevis is an ominous sign. Loss of sensation is confined to the area served by the deep peroneal nerve.

The syndrome must be differentiated from a common condition known as ''shin splints.'' The pain in the latter condition is usually over bone and can be relieved by rest, elevation, and application of cold. There is no associated marked swelling and muscle paresis with shin splints. Other conditions to be differentiated include cellulitis, thrombophlebitis, and stress fractures of the tibia.

TREATMENT. This is directed at decompressing the anterior tibial compartment and should be performed early to avoid anoxic necrosis of the muscle mass. Treatment can be effected with fasciotomy. The skin is incised lateral to the tibial crest over the midportion of the anterior tibial muscle, and the incision is carried through subcutaneous tissue and the fascia. Muscle bellies are then allowed to bulge. The skin may be closed over the bulging muscle or can be left open for secondary closure. A variation of the procedure employs two small incisions, one in the craniad and the other in the caudad portion of the anterior compartment. The fascia is then incised blindly between these two small incisions. An additional maneuver is to divide *between the tibia and fibula* the uppermost inch or two of the ligament over which the anterior tibial artery crosses to pass from the popliteal fossa to the anterior tibial compartment.

PROGNOSIS. If decompression is performed before muscle necrosis is present, return of function is complete. Thus, in many instances, fasciotomy is indicated prior to total disappearance of the pedal pulse. If fasciotomy is delayed until muscle necrosis occurs or neurologic findings are advanced, total recovery of function is not to be anticipated, and rehabilitation is required.

Traumatic Arteriovenous Fistulas

HISTORICAL DATA. That an arteriovenous fistula is a communication between an artery and a vein was first recognized by William Hunter in 1764. Previously the lesion had not been distinguished from a traumatic aneurysm. In a careful description of two patients in whom fistulas developed following phlebotomy, he described

the typical clinical findings of a thrill, continuous murmur, dilated artery proximal to the fistula, and dilated pulsating veins. The abnormal physiology of an arteriovenous fistula was carefully analyzed in a scholarly monograph published by Holman in 1937. Attempted therapy by proximal ligation of the involved artery, which was frequently effective for traumatic aneurysms, was often disastrous for arteriovenous fistulas, because gangrene resulted. The gangrene developed because blood flowing through collateral circulation around the ligated artery would flow through the fistula instead of into the distal extremity.

Matas in 1888 established effective therapy with his technique of endoaneurysmorrhaphy. Directly incising the fistulous sac, followed by suture of the communication between the artery and the vein, was more effective than indirect therapy of proximal and distal ligation of the involved artery and vein.

Although the collateral circulation which develops with an arteriovenous fistula made it possible to treat such fistulas by excision without gangrene resulting, intermittent claudication that results from interruption of the artery was frequently permanent. Consequently, after World War II, reconstruction of the injured artery became the preferable form of treatment.

ETIOLOGY AND PATHOLOGY. An arteriovenous fistula usually results from a penetrating injury that simultaneously injures an artery and an adjacent vein, permitting blood to flow directly from the injured artery into the vein. A fistula may be established immediately at the time of operation, in which case there is little external loss of blood, or it may become apparent days or weeks following injury as clot surrounding the lacerated artery and vein is liquefied.

Unusual forms of arteriovenous fistulas have been reported following different surgical operations. Injury of the iliac artery and vein is a well-recognized, fortunately rare complication of removal of an intervertebral disc. Arteriovenous fistulas have been reported following thyroidectomy, nephrectomy, or even thoracentesis, in all instances representing a concomitant injury of an artery and a vein, sometimes due to simultaneous ligation of artery and vein by the same ligature.

PATHOPHYSIOLOGY. A series of anatomic and physiologic changes begins to evolve when an arteriovenous fistula is produced (Fig. 21-3). The immediate effects are a decrease in blood flow to tissues distal to the lesion and an increase in venous pressure. The peripheral vascular resistance is lowered to that of the venous system as a result of blood bypassing the arteriolar vascular bed resulting in systolic and diastolic blood pressure, an increase in heart rate, and an increase in cardiac output.

In the ensuing days, several compensatory events occur as a result of the decrease in peripheral vascular resistance: The blood volume is increased, systolic blood pressure increases with a corresponding widening of pulse pressure, and a decrease in pulse rate occurs. Locally there is the progressive development of extensive collateral circulation around the fistula, within a few weeks the blood flow to the distal extremity may ap-

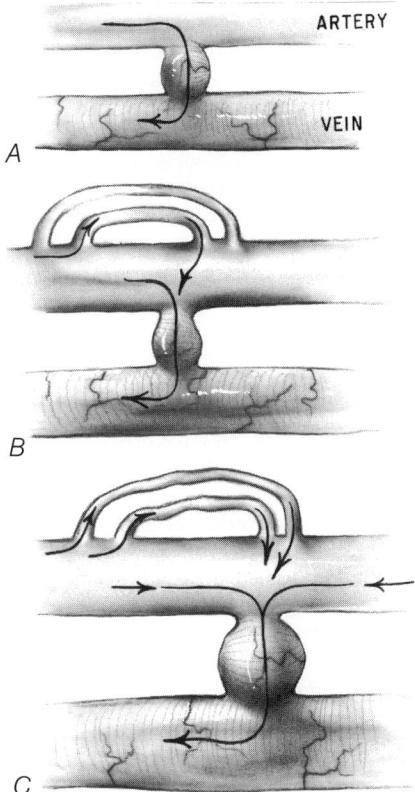

Fig. 21-3. *A.* Immediately following the development of an arteriovenous fistula there is shunting of blood from the artery through the fistula into the vein, from which it returns to the heart. This results in a decrease in peripheral vascular resistance, a fall in diastolic blood pressure, and an increase in heart rate. The venous pressure rises in the involved vein. Peripheral blood flow is decreased in the involved artery distal to the fistula. *B.* After several weeks, collateral circulation enlarges around the fistula because of the decreased vascular resistance at the site of the fistula. As the collateral circulation develops, the involved artery and vein also dilate, increasing the amount of blood flowing through the fistula. *C.* After several years, extensive dilatation may develop about a fistula with marked enlargement of collateral circulation. In addition there is enlargement of the artery immediately distal to the fistula, through which blood flows in a retrograde fashion through the fistula toward the heart. The vein may enlarge to marked proportions, creating varicosities in the extremity. Ultimately such progressive dilatation after a period of years may result in congestive heart failure from the increased cardiac output.

proach normal limits. There is a progressive dilation of the "fistulous circuit," including the heart, the arteries leading to the fistula, the fistula itself, and the venous channels leading from the fistula to the heart.

In subsequent months or years, additional changes evolve. The artery both proximal and distal to the fistula may dilate in response to the marked increase in flow through the fistula. The involved veins progressively dilate with marked tortuosity; external rupture with hemorrhage, however, is very rare. Chronic venous congestion may develop in the extremity, causing skin ulcerations resembling those from varicose veins, and bleeding from the ulcerated areas may become a major problem. In

growing children, there may be hypertrophy of the involved limb from increased growth of the bones and soft tissues. With large fistulas, involving vessels as large as the iliac artery and vein, continued dilation of the heart eventually terminates in heart failure. This, however, is an unusual complication with the majority of arteriovenous fistulas, because the volume of blood shunted is not enough to produce heart failure. Only with large arteries and veins do cardiac symptoms appear.

Two rare complications with arteriovenous fistulas are bacterial endarteritis in the fistula and spontaneous closure. Bacterial endarteritis has been reported in only a few patients and is similar to bacterial endocarditis. Usually with intensive chemotherapy the infection can be controlled or eliminated, after which surgical excision of the fistula should be promptly carried out. A fistula may close spontaneously, occasionally after it has been present for several months. Shumacker reported eight such experiences in 245 patients.

CLINICAL MANIFESTATIONS. A penetrating injury producing an arteriovenous fistula often causes surprisingly few symptoms. External loss of blood can be small, and few disturbances of peripheral circulation develop. Subsequently the patient may be entirely asymptomatic. There is usually awareness of a soft mass in the area of the fistula, which transmits a buzzing sensation when the fingers are placed over it. The patient is rarely totally unaware of the presence of a fistula, the first manifestation of which may be acute congestive heart failure that can be expected to promptly improve with surgical correction of the fistula.

In some patients the venous hypertension produces varices with peripheral pigmentation and ulceration. Surgical mishaps have resulted from unwise attempts to remove such varices without recognizing their origin.

On physical examination, a soft, diffuse mass is usually palpable and often visible. Dilated veins may surround the area. On palpation a thrill is usually felt, maximal in systole. Auscultation reveals a continuous murmur, loudest in systole, which has been described as a "machinery" murmur, emphasizing the rhythmic rise and fall in intensity and pitch during systole and diastole. It is similar to the murmur of a patent ductus arteriosus. Detection of this classic finding establishes the diagnosis and differentiates the lesion from an arterial aneurysm.

Another significant finding is the demonstration of slowing of the pulse when the fistula is obliterated by digital compression, as evidenced by disappearance of the murmur. The slowing of the pulse results from the increase in peripheral vascular resistance when the fistula is digitally occluded causing the blood pressure to rise with reflex slowing of the heart rate. The bradycardia results from a neurogenic reflex mediated through pressure-sensitive receptors in the great vessels and carotid sinuses; it can be blocked by atropine.

Usually there are no signs of arterial insufficiency in the extremity. With large fistulas, the pulse pressure is increased, both from an elevation of systolic pressure and a decrease in diastolic pressure. If cardiac enlargement has occurred, a systolic murmur may be audible at the apex of the heart. Usually cardiac failure is found only with fistulas between large vessels, such as the aorta and the vena cava, or when the fistula has been present for many years, allowing time for progressive enlargement of the fistulous opening. In World War II cardiac failure was rarely seen in a collected series of 593 patients treated surgically.

The physical findings are usually sufficient to establish the diagnosis, but if uncertainty exists, an arteriogram readily demonstrates the rapid opacification of adjacent veins and the greatly increased collateral circulation. As the veins fill rapidly, the exact site of the fistula may be obscured unless serial angiograms are obtained. A common problem in differential diagnosis in the cervical area is with a venous "hum," an auscultatory curiosity resulting from flow of blood in the jugular veins. The murmur of a venous hum promptly disappears when intrathoracic pressure is raised by forced expiration against a closed glottis, as well as by light digital compression of the vein to stop venous flow.

TREATMENT. Formerly treatment of traumatic arteriovenous fistula was delayed for 2 to 4 months to permit the development of collateral circulation in order for the extremity to survive following ligation of the involved artery. Although gangrene virtually never occurred following ligation, claudication frequently resulted, often in as many as 50 percent of patients, despite the abundant collateral circulation. Currently, the majority of patients are treated by division of the fistula and reconstruction of the involved artery, and preferably the injured vein as well. Excision is performed only for fistulas involving small vessels not essential to normal circulation of the extremity, such as the radial or ulnar arteries. Most fistulas are treated at the time of the arterial injury if the proper diagnosis is made. Otherwise operation is performed within 2 or 3 weeks, after the immediate effects of the injury on the soft tissues have subsided and the likelihood of infection occurring from the original injury has decreased significantly. Arteriovenous fistulas have been occluded by glues and coils inserted under radiographic control.

Operative Technique. The incision should be placed so as to permit exposure of the artery and vein proximal and distal to the fistula before the fistula is dissected. Once these vessels are isolated and temporarily occluded, the fistulous sac can be incised and the opening directly isolated. Although a large aneurysmal sac may be present, the basic lesion is usually an incomplete laceration of the arterial wall, involving only a short length of artery. A long segment of artery may be incorporated in the wall of the aneurysmal sac, however, and it must be freed and mobilized to perform arterial repair. Once the involved vessels have been mobilized, most of the remaining sac may be left, for complete excision is difficult and of little benefit.

In many patients the artery can be repaired by direct anastomosis. In a group of 29 aneurysms and arteriovenous fistulas resulting from civilian injuries, all were treated by end-to-end arterial anastomosis. In a series of 134 patients with fistulas, an anastomosis was performed in 61, a vessel graft in 23, a lateral repair in 4, and simple division of the fistula in 10.

Repair of the involved vein is indicated if the vein is a large one, such as an iliac or common femoral vein. Permanent edema has been frequent following ligation of such large veins. Repair can often be done by lateral suture.

PROGNOSIS. Convalescence following operation is usually uneventful, and long-term results are excellent if arterial continuity is preserved. Hughes and Jahnke published a 5-year follow-up of 148 such lesions treated during the Korean conflict with satisfactory results in the majority of patients.

THORACIC OUTLET SYNDROMES

A variety of physical abnormalities have been recognized which constrict or compress the brachial plexus, the subclavian artery, or the subclavian vein near the first rib and clavicle. Several descriptive terms have been employed, indicating the causative mechanism thought to be present. These include cervical rib, scalenus anticus syndrome, costoclavicular syndrome, and hyperabduction syndrome. The disability is dependent upon which of the major neural or vascular structures is compressed. Regardless of the specific mechanism involved, all such abnormalities may be conveniently grouped together as neurovascular compression syndromes occurring near the thoracic outlet.

HISTORICAL DATA. Cervical ribs have been reported as anatomic curiosities for hundreds of years. They occur in about 0.5 percent of the normal population. Murphy in 1905 described a successful operation upon a patient whose subclavian artery was compressed by a cervical rib. By 1916 Halsted was able to find reports of more than 500 cases of symptoms from a cervical rib. Attention was focused on the scalenus anticus muscle in 1927 when Adson and Coffey observed constriction of the subclavian artery by a scalenus anticus muscle and subsequently proposed that compression by an abnormal scalenus anticus muscle created a syndrome identical to that caused by cervical rib. They also emphasized the role of the scalenus anticus muscle in producing symptoms from a cervical rib, the two structures jointly compressing the brachial plexus between them.

Subsequently the frequency of compression between the clavicle and first rib was recognized and the mechanisms well defined in 1943 by the report of Falconer and Weddell, who named this type of compression the *costoclavicular syndrome*. A short time later, in 1945, Wright observed patients in whom vascular symptoms resulted from hyperabduction and introduced the term *hyperabduction syndrome*.

Some degree of compression of the subclavian artery may be demonstrated in a high percentage of normal individuals in whom no symptoms whatever are present, but it formerly was thought that compression syndromes producing significant disability were rare. Since the publication by Roos of a simplified transaxillary approach to relieve compression syndromes at the thoracic outlet and since the introduction of peripheral nerve conduction velocity determinations, the conditions have been recognized with increasing frequency. It has even been suggested that for certain patients who have thoracic outlet syndromes a diagnosis of angina pectoris is erroneously made. Further experience will be needed to determine the exact frequency of these disorders. The aforementioned transaxillary approach to resection of the first rib may help define the frequency of the condition more exactly since this approach permits a clear view of the structures, both normal and abnormal, that produce compression syndromes.

REGIONAL ANATOMY. The subclavian artery leaves the thorax by passing over the first rib between the scalenus anticus muscle anteriorly and the brachial plexus and scalenus medius posteriorly. It then passes under the clavicle and subclavius muscle to enter the axilla beneath the pectoralis minor muscle. The subclavian vein has an almost identical course except that it passes anterior to the scalenus anticus muscle and has an intimate relationship to the head of the clavicle and the most medial portion of the first rib. The route of the brachial plexus nearly parallels that of the subclavian artery in the neck, lying posterolaterally between it and the scalenus posterior muscle.

A potential area of compression exists in the interscalene triangle between the scalenus anticus anteriorly, the scalenus medius posteriorly, and the first rib inferiorly. Only slightly distal to this area, in the narrow space between the clavicle and the first rib, is another potential site of compression. In the axilla, where the pectoralis minor tendon attaches to the coracoid process, an area of potential obstruction of the axillary artery exists where it travels around the coracoid process. During hyperabduction the axillary vessels and brachial plexus are bent at an angle of approximately 90° in this area.

When a cervical rib persists, there may be in addition either a bony or a ligamentous structure, originating on the lowermost cervical vertebra, coursing in, passing under the brachial plexus and subclavian artery, and attaching to the first rib.

ETIOLOGY. Although cervical ribs are found in about 0.5 percent of the normal population, only about 10 percent of these produce symptoms. Asymptomatic anomalies of the first rib are also frequently seen. Thus, additional factors other than the presence of a cervical rib or anomalous first rib must contribute to the compression syndromes. Symptoms are very rare in children and most frequently are seen in thin women in the third and fourth decades. An unusually well-developed musculature seems also to predispose to compression. A congenital variation in the anatomy of the head and neck has been suggested as a predisposing factor, a familiar type of patient being a thin woman with a long, narrow neck. The onset of symptoms in the second and third decade could be due to gradual descent of the shoulder girdle, perhaps from atrophy of the regional musculature.

Local anatomic variations are probably of particular significance. The width of the first rib in individuals in whom we have resected this structure has appeared to be unusually great. The width of the scalene anticus muscle at its insertion into the first rib varies greatly. A wide scalenus anticus muscle, which narrows the space in the interscalene triangle, has often been found at operation in symptomatic patients. Interdigitations of scalene muscles forming slings under the brachial plexus and axillary arteries have been encountered. Cervical ribs vary from short and rudimentary to completely formed and articulating anteriorly with the first rib. Some incomplete ribs are connected by fascial bands to the first rib that compress the brachial plexus. Fractures of the clavicle or first rib may subsequently produce a large bony callus, especially if there is poor alignment of the ends of the fractured bone.

CLINICAL MANIFESTATIONS. Disability from compression may be produced in several ways and depends upon which portions of the neurovascular bundle are involved. Compression of the brachial plexus usually causes pain, paresthesia, and a feeling of numbness. Often these symptoms are greatest in the C_8–T_1 distribution, because the ulnar nerve is derived from this most caudad portion of the plexus which rides over the first rib. Compression of the upper portion of the plexus may also occur, resulting in pain referred to the entire arm and shoulder and occasionally to the neck and cheek. Muscular weakness or paralysis, or atrophy of muscles are less frequent and appear only in far advanced cases. Vascular symptoms may be intermittent from compression or temporary occlusion of the subclavian artery, producing claudication with exercise, pallor, or a sensation of coldness, numbness, or paresthesia. In chronic cases, a different and more serious mechanism evolves, for intermittent compression and trauma of the subclavian arteries produce atheromatous changes in the artery and, rarely, a poststenotic aneurysm. From either arterial abnormality, emboli may be dislodged into the peripheral circulation and produce ischemia in the hand, sometimes with focal areas of gangrene requiring amputation of digits. Thrombosis of the subclavian artery may eventually result.

A third group of vascular symptoms consists of intermittent episodes of vasoconstriction, similar to those seen in Raynaud's disease. Unilateral Raynaud's phenomenon, though rare, almost always suggests a focal disturbance in the blood supply to the involved extremity due to a local lesion such as a cervical rib. A possible explanation for this infrequent occurrence has been proposed by Telford and Mottershead, who, on anatomic dissection, found that in 10 to 15 percent of patients the sympathetic innervation of the extremity traveled in a separate cord not incorporated in the main trunks of the brachial plexus. This isolated filament of fibers presumably would be more prone to direct compression and irritation. Finally, intermittent compression of the subclavian vein may cause signs of venous hypertension in the upper extremity with edema and the development of varicosities. The so-called effort thrombosis, a condition of acute thrombosis of the subclavian vein, may be a result of a thoracic outlet compression syndrome of the axillary vein with intimal damage.

The symptomatology of the thoracic outlet syndrome depends on whether nerves, blood vessels, or both are compressed. Usually compression of one of these dominates the clinical picture. Symptoms of nerve compression manifested by pain and paresthesia are present in almost all patients, the pain usually being of insidious

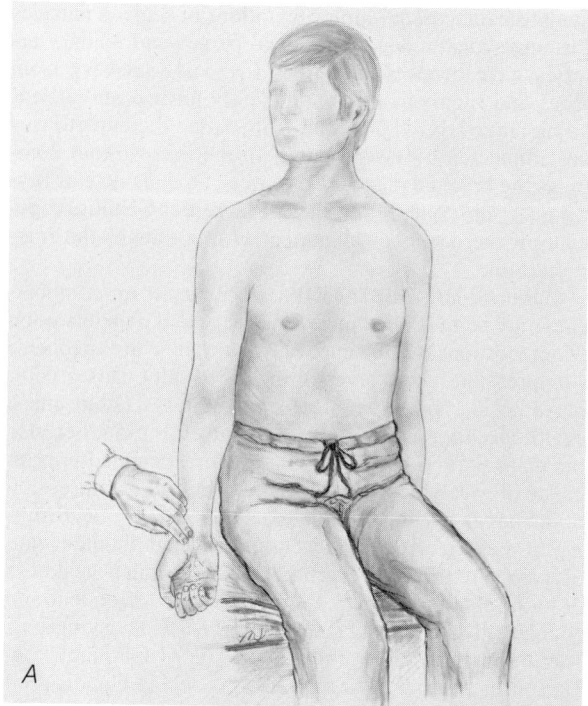

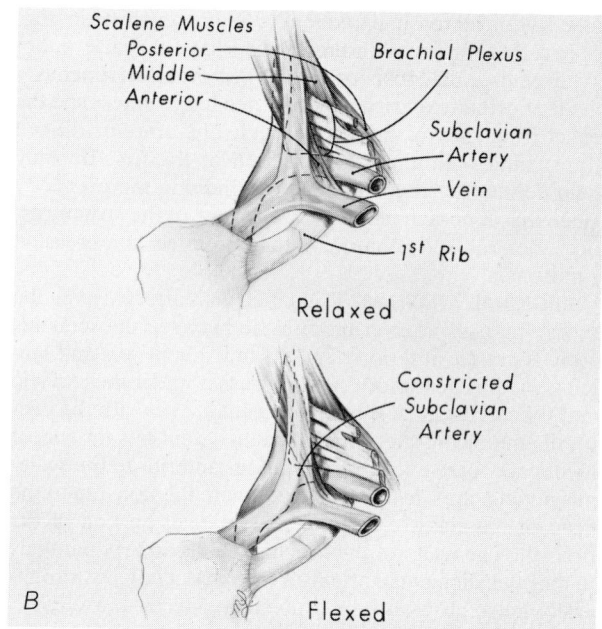

Fig. 21-4. Technique of performance of the Adson maneuver for obstruction of the subclavian artery by the scalenus anticus muscle. *A.* The patient should be seated with his elbows at his sides and his neck extended. During deep inspiration his chin is turned to the affected side, while the intensity of the radial pulse is palpated. All these positions increase the tension on the scalenus anticus muscle. *B.* Course of the brachial plexus and subclavian artery between the scalenus anticus and medius muscles. A localized dilatation of the subclavian artery distal to the scalenus anticus is illustrated. Immediately distal to the scalenus anticus and medius muscles is another potential area of constriction, between the clavicle and the first rib. When the scalenus anticus muscle is relaxed, there is minimal compression of the subclavian artery. With tension on the scalenus anticus muscle, compression of the subclavian artery results in decrease in the radial pulse, in some patients resulting in disappearance of the pulse. A bruit may become audible in the supraclavicular area as the scalenus anticus muscle is progressively stretched to compress the subclavian artery.

onset, commonly involving the neck, shoulder, arm, and hand with occasional radiation to the anterior chest or parascapular area. Paresthesia in a specific nerve distribution occur in most patients, the ulnar nerve being involved in 90 percent.

Symptoms of arterial compression were observed less frequently, in about one-quarter of patients. Raynaud's phenomenon and symptoms of venous compression are even less common.

Physical Examination. Objective physical signs are more common in patients with vascular compression than in those with neural disorders. In only about 20 percent of patients with nerve compression are objective signs of decreased sensation found; some of these show additional muscle weakness or even atrophy. In the presence of neurologic symptoms at least one of the vascular compression signs can be expected, consisting essentially of loss of radial pulse with either Adson's test, hyperabduction, or hyperextension. In Adson's test, the patient sits with his hands on his knees, inspires deeply, extends his head backward, and turns his chin toward the affected side. Deep inspiration, extension of the neck, and turning of the head all tense the scalene anticus muscle and may decrease or obliterate the radial pulse (Fig. 21-4). Simultaneous auscultation of the supraclavicular space for bruit should be performed. In certain patients, a bruit will appear as the head is turned, reach a peak intensity, and cease as compression is increased to the point of obliterating the radial pulse. In other patients turning the head to the opposite side may demonstrate compression more effectively. The possibility of compression of the neurovascular bundle between the first rib and the clavicle also may be tested by displacing the shoulders backward and

downward. The test is considered positive if the radial pulse is obliterated. The hyperabduction maneuver is performed by fully abducting the arm above the head and noting the effect upon the radial pulse.

In evaluating the maneuvers to detect neurovascular compression, it is important to remember that they are positive in a high percentage of normal individuals. This is particularly true of the costoclavicular compression or the hyperabduction test. A positive result, therefore, does not in itself establish a thoracic outlet syndrome; absence of any positive findings, however, suggests some other diagnosis.

The signs of arterial compression may be evident by direct physical examination. There may be differences in the qualities of the pulses between the two arms when the subclavian, brachial, radial, and ulnar arteries are compared. A localized supraclavicular bruit may be present. On occasion a particularly wide pulse, denoting a subclavian or axillary aneurysm, is palpable, usually in the infraclavicular area. With mild forms of ischemia there may be only pallor on elevation while in the more severe forms, especially with embolization, there may be atrophy of the skin, brittle nails, or even focal ulceration. In approximately 5 percent of patients frank Raynaud's phenomenon can be induced by application of cold to the extremity. In the approximately 10 percent of patients, signs of venous obstruction, i.e., edema and venous distention, are apparent.

LABORATORY STUDIES. Chest and cervical spine radiographs may demonstrate bony abnormalities, either as cervical ribs, bifid first ribs, fusion of the first and second ribs, or clavicular deformities either congenital or traumatic.

For diagnosing arterial abnormalities, arteriography may be especially useful in demonstrating intimal irregularities, stenoses, or aneurysms of the subclavian artery. The arteriographic studies are of no value where there is no evidence of arterial compression or occlusion. Venographic studies are useful in patients with signs of venous compression, especially in establishing a differential diagnosis between thoracic outlet compression and other entities which mimic the condition.

The determination of nerve conduction velocities through the thoracic outlet as well as electromyographic determinations have been used to attempt to establish objective criteria for diagnosing neural compression. By applying electrical stimulation to various of the distal components of the brachial plexus and measuring conduction velocities to pinpoint areas of abnormal conduction, it is possible to evaluate sites of involvement of various neural structures. Where atypical thoracic outlet neural compression syndromes are present, other nerves such as the median and the musculocutaneous can be similarly studied. Differential diagnoses between compression at the thoracic outlet, at the carpal tunnel at the wrist, and at the pronator level are possible. When this is combined with carefully performed electromyographic studies, very specific diagnoses are possible.

TREATMENT. The treatment can be divided into that for the arterial, venous, and neurologic compressions. Treatment of the arterial compression depends upon the specific entity produced: embolization, stenosis and thrombosis, aneurysm formation, or intermittent vasospasm (Raynaud's). Occlusion of the subclavian artery, if not associated with severe ischemia, may require no therapy except an exercise program to promote development of collateral circulation. With atherosclerotic plaques or aneurysms of the subclavian artery, frequently associated with embolic episodes, therapy usually involves resection of the first rib, preferably by the transaxillary approach, as well as removing the source of emboli. The presence of a thrombus in an aneurysm or ulceration in an atherosclerotic plaque requires resection of the involved artery through an additional supraclavicular incision that may require resection of the medial half of the clavicle if an aneurysm associated with a cervical rib is present, and replacement, preferably with autologous tissue; composite grafts of saphenous veins have been useful. On occasion direct exposure of the arteries in the arm or forearm is necessary to remove emboli.

The venous occlusions are more difficult to treat, because the compressing mechanism may not be apparent from either physical examination or laboratory studies. It appears clear from results of transaxillary resection of the first rib that the most proximal part of the vein can be decompressed by this procedure, but the roles of the clavicle, the pectoralis minor, and clavipectoral fascia in producing compression cannot be evaluated by this approach. Resection of the medial half of the clavicle may be required for complete decompression of the vein. Those patients with effort thrombosis seen within the first day or two of its occurrence should be considered for combined surgical procedures of venous thrombectomy and relief of the compressing mechanism. Anticoagulation therapy should then be used, perhaps for as long as 1 year.

The management of the neural compression syndromes generally involves a conservative, nonsurgical approach. An exercise program designed to strengthen the muscles of the shoulder girdle and lessen the tendency of the shoulder to droop has been of value in some patients with mild to moderate symptoms. A series of such exercises is carefully described by Allen et al. As an example of this approach, less than half of a group of 300 patients with thoracic outlet syndromes required surgical intervention. The selection of patients for operation should depend upon the severity of the symptoms, failure to respond to a nonsurgical program, and the specificity of the diagnosis.

Operative Technique. It is important to include the entire extremity in the sterile operative field, permitting manipulation of the extremity in order to define the most likely area of compression. Whether or not a cervical rib is present, the transaxillary approach is favored for the decompression for its simplicity, the clarity with which the compression mechanisms can be diagnosed, the excellent cosmetic result, and the ease with which cervical ribs together with the first rib can be excised. If vasomotor symptoms are prominent, sympathectomy can be performed through the same transaxillary approach, exposing the third and second thoracic ganglia as well as the lower third of the stellate ganglion; this includes the first thoracic ganglion but avoids the production of Horner's syndrome. If removal of the second and third intercostal nerves with their ganglia is thought necessary, since 10 to 15 percent of the sympathetic ganglia to the upper extremity are contained in these nerves, it can be carried out.

The transaxillary approach is performed by making an incision in the lowermost portion of the axilla from the pectoralis major anteriorly to the latissimus dorsi posteriorly (Fig. 21-5). The incision is deepened to the muscles of the chest wall, the serratus anterior and the intercostal muscles coming into view. The dissection is continued upward, avoiding the intercostobrachial nerve, with the arm hyperabducted to raise the neurovascular bundle off the first rib. By gentle dissection, it is possible to outline the scalene muscles and identify the attachment of the cervical rib to the first rib if one is present. The scalene muscles are transected and permitted to retract, and the muscles along the inferior border of the first rib are simi-

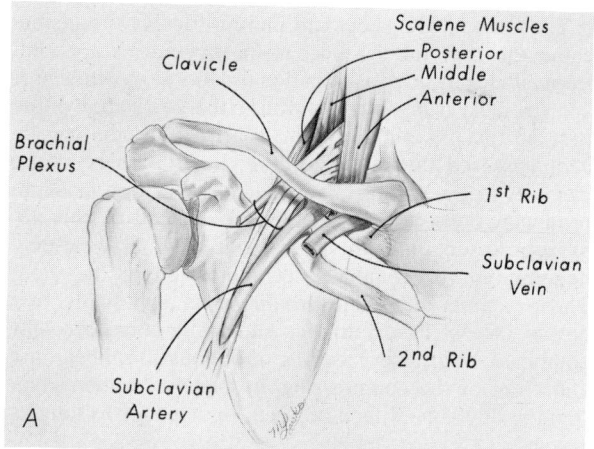

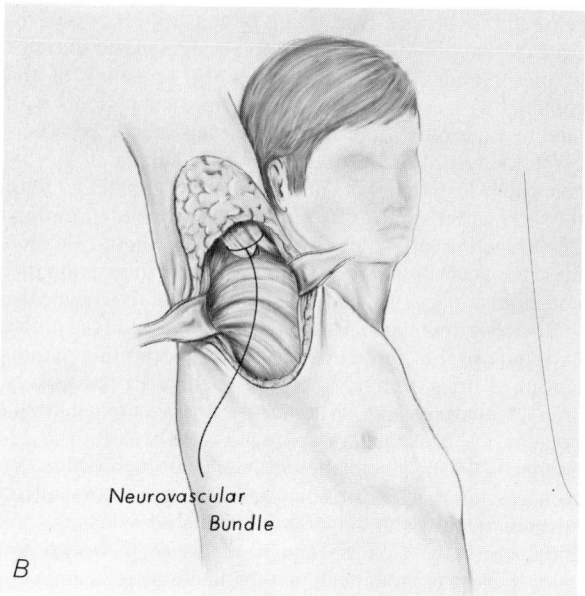

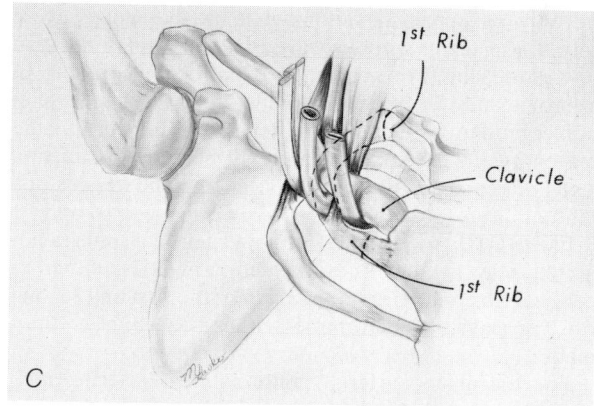

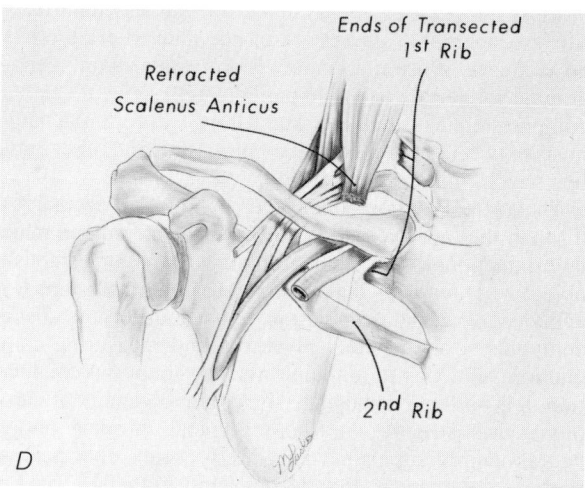

Fig. 21-5. Technique of transaxillary resection of the first rib. *A.* The critical relations of the first rib, clavicle, scalene muscles, and neurovascular structures are shown. The lowermost portion of the brachial plexus, which gives rise to the ulnar nerve, is in contact with the first rib and explains the most characteristic neurologic symptoms usually involving the ulnar aspect of the forearm and fourth and fifth fingers. *B.* Operative incision below the axillary hairline with hyperabduction of the arm which raises the neurovascular bundle out of the operative field. *C.* Effect of hyperabduction in exposing the first rib and scalene muscles, retracting the neurovascular bundle. *D.* Effect of first rib resection, which requires cutting all three scalene muscles, in relieving the compression of artery, vein, and brachial plexus.

larly incised. The first rib and cervical rib usually can be removed in their entirety, including periosteum, from the costochondral junction anteriorly to the posterior angle of the rib. The parietal pleura lies deep to the dissection; care must be taken to avoid puncturing it. If the pleura is punctured, the wound is closed around a catheter in the axilla while the anesthetist expands the lung. This usually suffices to correct the pneumothorax. On occasion it has been necessary to aspirate air from the pleural cavity in the early postoperative period. If resection of the second or third portions of the axillary artery is required due to the presence of an aneurysm associated with a cervical rib or due to marked arterial degeneration posterior to the anterior scalene muscle, a second incision is required, usually in the supraclavicular area, sometimes in association with a resection of the medial half of the clavicle.

If a sympathectomy is indicated, the parietal pleura is stripped from the chest wall attachments and the sympathetic chain exposed, dissected free, and excised.

The postoperative course is usually benign, with the patient ready for discharge by the third postoperative day.

Other approaches have been described for excising the first rib. The posterior approach has been advocated by many but is an operation of greater magnitude. The anterior transthoracic approach has been proposed by others for more extensive exposure. Although most agree that the supraclavicular approach is probably archaic, since it does not permit thorough exploration of the area and easy excision of the first rib (now of paramount importance in treatment), it has been proposed as the first approach to perform scalenectomy, reserving the transaxillary approach for failures of the more simple procedures.

The surgical approach for venous compression is more complex than simply performing transaxillary decompression. With the transaxillary approach it is possible to sever constricting bands which appear to be extensions of the manubrial insertion of the sternocleidomastoid muscles. The head of the clavicle may participate prominently in the compression, so that on occasion it has been necessary to resect the medial half of the clavicle. Upon completion of the external decompression of the vein, an operative venogram is recommended both to confirm the adequacy of the decompression and to detect intrinsic abnormalities of vein, such as webs which may occur at the junction of the subclavian vein with the internal jugular. This latter abnormality may require venotomy and excision of the web with subsequent closure of the subclavian vein.

PROGNOSIS. The prognosis is dependent upon the specific syndrome present. The arterial compression syndromes can be quite satisfactorily relieved and arterial reconstructions performed with a high degree of precision. In our experience it has been possible to stop embolic episodes and restore circulation to the upper extremity by standard arterial reconstructive procedures. Patients with Raynaud's phenomenon and cervical rib in whom associated sympathectomies have been performed have variable results. Although immediate effects of sympathectomy have been excellent, relapses have occurred quite abruptly as early as 6 months following operation.

The venous compression disorders also have given variable results. It is not clear at present whether thrombectomy, with or without relief of the venous compression mechanism, is any better than prolonged anticoagulant therapy. Those patients with chronic venous occlusions of the subclavian and axillary veins who have been followed for years have shown remarkable recovery, with subsidence of edema coincident with the appearance of a prominent venous pattern on the chest wall and little or no resulting disability.

The results of operations performed for neurologic syndromes have been most difficult to evaluate. While some patients have experienced dramatic improvement, others have had no benefit. Still others have had relapses after initial improvement. Roos has reported from a wide experience with transaxillary resection of the first rib that 80 to 90 percent of those with predominantly neurologic symptoms obtained complete relief, while approximately 50 percent of those with predominantly vascular symptoms became free of symptoms.

MANIFESTATIONS OF ARTERIAL OCCLUSIVE DISEASE

Acute Arterial Occlusion

Recognition of acute arterial occlusion is vital, since it may progress to ischemic necrosis within hours. A thrombus propagates distally as well as proximally to the point where it lodges, occluding collateral channels, thereby worsening the ischemia.

Acute occlusion usually appears without specific symptoms. Prompt diagnosis is essential for successful therapy, because within 4 to 8 h after acute occlusion ischemic necrosis in the involved muscles may become irreversible. An additional feature in the pathogenesis of acute arterial occlusion that emphasizes the time factor is the tendency for thrombi to develop in the arteries distal to the point of occlusion where the flow of blood is either decreased or stagnant. This development, superimposed upon the acute obstruction, makes surgical therapy to restore circulation much more difficult. With persisting ischemia, thrombosis finally develops in the venous system as well, making surgical therapy impossible.

The usual causes of acute arterial occlusion are embolism, trauma, or thrombosis. Thrombosis of a previously undiagnosed aneurysm, such as a popliteal aneurysm, is a less frequent cause. Each of these is discussed in subsequent sections. Embolism is noteworthy in that it often appears without any previous signs of underlying disease as an acute catastrophe involving an extremity. In many it is the first symptom of serious underlying heart disease: mitral stenosis, atrial fibrillation, or myocardial infarction. Arterial trauma, when occurring as an isolated injury, may be easily recognized. When complicated with associated fractures or head injuries, the diagnosis may be difficult.

FIVE P's. For emphasis the five prominent features of acute arterial occlusion may be summarized as five p's as discussed above, under Arterial Trauma: *pain*, *paralysis*, *paresthesia*, *pallor*, and absence of *pulses*.

Pain present in 75 to 80 percent of patients with acute arterial occlusion heralds the onset of ischemia. It is absent in some patients, apparently because of the prompt onset of complete anesthesia. In others, when collateral circulation minimizes the degree of ischemia produced, pain may be minimal.

Paralysis and paresthesia (or anesthesia) are most important in evaluating the severity of ischemia. The importance of these features is based on the fact that the peripheral nerve endings are the most sensitive tissues to anoxia in the extremity. A familiar illustration of the sensitivity of sensory nerve endings to anoxia is the common experience of one's foot "going to sleep" while one sits with the extremity flexed in an unusual position. The sensitivity of striated muscles to anoxia is almost as great as that of nerve endings. Hence, an extremity with paralysis and paresthesia will almost surely develop gangrene, while, conversely, if motor and sensory function are intact even though signs of ischemia are present, gangrene probably will not occur. The neurologic findings then are an important clue both to the need for prompt therapy and for the evaluation of the effectiveness of therapy in relieving ischemia. Recognition that a paralyzed anesthetic extremity will develop gangrene in most patients within 6 to 8 h after onset emphasizes the urgency for immediate treatment.

Pallor is also an important sign, representing varying degrees of decreased circulation. Associated with visible pallor may be the sensation of coldness.

Absence of pulses confirms the diagnosis and localizes

the point of occlusion. With uncertainty, as in an edematous extremity, an oscillometer or a Doppler device may be of some value in confirming the absence of pulses. When palpation is indeterminate, the presence of neurologic symptoms indicates the urgency for deciding whether arterial occlusion is present. A frequent example seen is a patient with a swollen extremity with a fracture of the femur in whom swelling of the extremity may make palpation of the pulses difficult. To determine whether an associated injury of the femoral artery is present may require arteriography. If neurologic symptoms are present, angiography should be performed on an emergency basis.

Chronic Arterial Occlusion

The picture of chronic progressive ischemia is typically and most often seen with atherosclerosis involving the abdominal aorta and its branches to the lower extremities, including the iliac, femoral, and popliteal arteries. The course may be gradual and progressive or it may be accelerated with acute episodes due to segmental arterial thrombosis or minor traumatic injuries to the toes resulting in gangrene. Diabetic patients in general tend to have more distal arterial involvement of the popliteal and tibial arteries. Their clinical syndromes are further modified by the not infrequent presence of diabetic neuropathy and by their characteristic susceptibility to necrotizing infections.

Atherosclerotic disease of the arteries to the lower extremities may be divided into three large groups, dependent upon the level of involvement. These are aortoiliac, femoropopliteal, and tibioperoneal. There are distinctive clinical features about each of the categories, although more than one area is involved in at least one-third of patients seen. Aortoiliac disease in the fourth, fifth, and sixth decades is characterized by relatively mild atherosclerosis with aortic occlusion from superimposed thrombosis, while in the seventh and eighth decades atherosclerosis is severe and thrombosis is relatively limited. Isolated femoropopliteal disease is especially frequent in cigarette smokers, while isolated tibioperoneal disease occurs predominantly in diabetics. No matter where the obstruction is located, the physiologic deficit is decreased blood flow to the lower extremities, with symptoms ranging from intermittent claudication to gangrene. Tissue necrosis is more prone to occur with more distal arterial disease because potential for the development of collateral circulation is less.

HISTORY. A detailed history and physical examination are often sufficient to establish the diagnosis of extremity ischemia and to suggest the underlying mechanisms leading to its occurrence. Pain is the key symptom resulting from the ischemia of arterial occlusion. Careful documentation of its mode of onset, its location and distribution, and its character and duration serves as the basis for all additional investigations. When arterial occlusion develops over longer periods of time, ischemia may be subtle and may not become manifest until there are demands for blood beyond basal requirements, such as with exercise.

Pain is experienced during exertion and gradually disappears within minutes upon cessation of activity. This represents the characteristic symptom of *intermittent claudication,* the most common complaint produced by limb ischemia. The areas that are felt to be painful are usually those requiring the largest amount of blood during exertion, e.g., muscle groups. Claudication is a highly specific symptom, virtually diagnostic of chronic arterial insufficiency. For varying periods of time the only measure of progression of arterial insufficiency may be the worsening of claudication with progressively smaller amounts of exercise being required to produce the symptom.

Chronic arterial occlusion may progress, and intermittent pain involving muscle groups may be supplanted by continuous *pain at rest* referred to the sites most distal to the arterial occlusion, viz., toes, feet, fingers, hands. The large muscle groups that are the first to express the ischemic state are almost never the site of rest pain in chronic arterial occlusions. Ischemic rest pain is distinguishable by history from other types of foot or hand pain because pain is worsened by elevation of the extremity, even if only to the supine position, and is relieved by placing the extremity in the dependent position. Patients with pain related to diabetic neuropathy or other painful foot conditions report no such positional dependence.

In the upper extremity, although atherosclerosis that progresses to rest pain and gangrene is unusual, other types of lesions, either embolic or vasospastic, may do so. Claudication of the arm with exercise may be moderately disabling, but more serious symptoms are uncommon. Rest pain and tissue necrosis when present usually denote digital vessel occlusion either due to embolization from proximal lesions or end-stage Raynaud's phenomenon.

Other aspects of history that are critically important in determining treatment and prognosis include smoking, diabetes, cardiac disorders, trauma, familial disease, and occupational history, as well as drug therapy.

PHYSICAL EXAMINATION. Physical examination is of paramount importance in assessing the presence and severity of vascular disease. The color, temperature, and pulse pattern of the extremities involved frequently permits estimation of the level of arterial occlusion, the severity of ischemia, and the abruptness of the onset. Acute arterial occlusion characteristically produces marked color and temperature differences; chronic occlusion may produce no visible changes but only a difference in palpable pulses early in the course of disease. When acute occlusion progresses to gangrene it is manifest frequently as "wet" gangrene, with blebs, bullae, and violaceous discoloration. When chronic occlusion progresses gradually to severe ischemia, characteristic changes associated with atrophy appear and progress to localized tissue necrosis. The final stage is usually the mumification characteristic of dry gangrene, which starts peripherally in the toes and extends proximally to involve the entire foot and leg. Palpation of peripheral pulses is a most important feature of the examination. In the lower extremity, the femoral, popliteal, posterior tibial, and dorsalis pedis pulses should be noted. It is important to remember that the common femoral artery extends only about 5 cm below the inguinal ligament before bifurcating into the profunda femoris and superficial femoral arteries. In the upper extremity the brachial, radial, and ulnar pulses should be noted. In many patients it is possible to feel the digital pulses at the bases of the phalanges. The integrity of the palmar arterial arches can be tested by the performance of the Allen test. This is done by having the patient make a tight fist, then occluding the radial and ulnar arteries at the wrist and having the patient slowly open the hand. With the hand in a relaxed position, the integrity of the radial artery in the hand is determined by releasing radial compression and noting the return of color. The maneuver is repeated releasing the ulnar artery while the radial remains compressed. The ability to determine definitely the presence or absence of a peripheral pulse is one of the most essential features of an adequate evaluation of the peripheral circulation.

With chronic ischemia, characteristic nutritional changes develop in the feet. These include the loss of hair from the toes, the development of brittle, opaque nails, the appearance of atrophy and rubor in the skin, and atrophy of muscles of the feet with increasing prominence of the interosseous spaces. Hence, a simple glance at a foot can determine the presence or absence of serious vascular disease. The importance of this evaluation is emphasized by the fact that gangrene seldom appears in an extremity with chronic vascular disease until these stigmata of chronic ischemia have appeared.

Characteristic color changes also appear with advanced arterial insufficiency, consisting of a purplish rubor in dependency, changing to pallor when the extremity is elevated. The colors are quite different from the chronic congested extremity with venous insufficiency.

The location of ulcerations offers a major clue to cause, for ulceration from venous insufficiency is virtually unknown below the level of the malleolus. By contrast, most ulcers from arterial insufficiency begin over the toes, corresponding to the most distal parts of the arterial tree. Ischemic ulcers on occasion develop on the leg or about the ankle without involvement of the toes, perhaps as a result of local tissue infarction, especially after localized trauma, or from arterioarterial embolization.

Palpation of the extremity for temperature and moisture may provide useful information, especially with vasospastic conditions with increased sympathetic tone, where the cool, sweaty extremity affords an important clue to the diagnosis.

Auscultation is of value for certain disorders, particularly arteriovenous fistulas, where detection of the classic continuous murmur quickly establishes the diagnosis. With localized stenotic lesions in peripheral arteries, usually from atherosclerotic plaques, a systolic bruit may be heard, promptly confirming the presence of arterial stenosis.

Estimation of venous filling time is of some value in the diagnosis of arterial insufficiency, but the test is of no value where incompetent valves are present in the venous system. In the absence of varicosities, the test is performed by elevation of the extremities until collapse of the veins has occurred. The extremities are then quickly lowered, and the time required for the veins to fill, usually on the dorsum of the foot or hand, is noted. Normally venous filling will occur within 10 to 15 s. Prolonged filling frequently denotes arterial insufficiency. Venous filling times of longer than 1 min denote a very high degree of arterial compromise.

The general physical examination is important to determine whether there are any underlying or associated disorders and whether there are additional areas of arterial involvement detectable by finding absent pulses elsewhere or bruits over arteries such as the carotids. It is vital to know about the presence of aneurysms in the abdomen, groin, or thorax. Examination of the heart is essential to determine whether there are valvular lesions, rhythm disorders, or congenital lesions that might serve as the nidus for thromboemboli.

General Laboratory Examinations

In arterial occlusive disease the diagnosis is almost always made by the history and the physical examination. Noninvasive studies using ultrasound, plethysmography, x-ray and magnetic resonance have been useful in confirming the diagnosis and differentiating arterial disease from other clinical syndromes. Angiography continues to be the most important laboratory technique. A high quality study is essential to planning surgical therapy.

Doppler Ultrasound. Doppler ultrasound is based on the shift in ultrasound frequency (called the "Doppler effect") that arises if an ultrasound beam is transmitted to and reflected from moving blood cells. The frequency shift is proportional to the velocity of the blood flow. It may be analyzed audibly by listening to the intensity, pitch, and phasicity of the sound or may be recorded graphically either as a simple wave form or as a complete sound spectrum analysis. A common application of Doppler ultrasound is to determine systolic arterial pressure. The probe is used as a sensitive stethoscope over an artery distal to a pressure cuff. Inflation of the cuff to a suprasystolic level will result in cessation of blood flow and hence, disappearance of the Doppler signal. Pressures obtained by this method are generally compared to the pressure in the arm or unaffected extremity and reported as a ratio of the normal systolic pressure. (If arm pressure is equal to 120 mmHg and dorsalis pedis pressure is equal to 40 mmHg, the ankle/arm index is 0.33.) In patients without arterial disease, the ankle/arm pressure ratio is 1 or higher. In claudication, it is generally between 1 and 0.5 and with more advanced degrees of ischemia is generally less than 0.5. Diabetics may have high indices due to calcification of the arterial wall. When doubt exists about the diagnosis, stress testing is helpful. This may be accomplished by treadmill exercise or by the reactive hyperemia test with a thigh tourniquet. The drop in pressure and the recovery time are proportional to the extent of the arterial occlusive disease. Segmental pressures are obtained by application of cuffs at different levels of the leg. The pressure gradients between the levels provide information about location of the disease.

B-Scan Ultrasound. B-Scan ultrasound can be used for visualization of blood vessels, either as a static or as a real-time echo. The main application is for visualization of aortic aneurysms. The value in the diagnosis of occlusive disease is limited when the vessel wall is extensively calcified. A highly valuable application is in combination with Doppler ultrasound, where the B-Scan is used as a guide for precise placement of the Doppler sample.

Plethysmography. Plethysmography records changes in volume of a limb, digit, or eye to each myocardial contraction. It has applications in peripheral arterial, cerebrovascular, and venous disease. Instrumentation includes strain gauge, photo, impedance, ocular, and air plethysmography. The latter comprises pulse volume recording (PVR) and phleorheography (PRG). Plethysmography can be used for analysis of the pulse waveform and for determination of arterial pressures as well as arterial and venous blood flow.

Arteriography. The most important laboratory examination is selective arteriography to outline the location and extent of arterial obstruction. Selection of the appropriate method of examination varies with the disease present, for virtually every artery in the body can now be successfully outlined by appropriate catheter angiography. Percutaneous introduction of the arterial catheter is the most frequently employed technique. Newer digital subtraction techniques have had some application in special situations. Utilizing a series of radiographic images recorded on a magnetic tape, nonvascular shadows can be subtracted from the image containing the contrast medium. This technique enhances the outline of the artery. Reasonably good views of the arteries can be obtained with less dye and smaller catheters, although resolution may be inferior to conventional arteriography. Also, overlapping images of multiple arteries may interfere with accurate interpretation.

ARTERIAL EMBOLISM

It has been long recognized that the majority of arterial emboli originate in the heart. The embolus originated in the heart in 86 percent of 426 emboli reported by Darling and associates and in 91 percent of 214 emboli reported by Cranley et al. In the past few years there has been increasing recognition of emboli which originate in atherosclerotic arteries, either fragments of a plaque or thrombi adherent to the surface of an ulcerated plaque which subsequently dislodge. For simplicity in presentation, emboli arising from the heart, constituting the majority of emboli seen, are referred to as *cardioarterial embolization*. As a separate entity, the frequency of which is yet unknown, emboli arising from an atherosclerotic artery and lodging in the distal branches are referred to as *arterioarterial emboli*.

Cardioarterial Embolization

HISTORICAL CONSIDERATIONS. Emboli have been long recognized as a cause of acute arterial occlusion resulting in gangrene. Several unsuccessful embolectomies were attempted near the end of the nineteenth century, but the first successful embolectomy is credited to Lahey in 1911. For many years embolectomies performed within 4 to 6 h after lodging of the embolus were successful, while those performed later had a progressively higher failure rate. Less than 15 years ago a serious proposal was made that emboli that had lodged more than 12 h earlier should not be operated upon. It is now well established that such a viewpoint is erroneous. The difficulties with late operation upon still viable extremities have been found due to inadequate removal of distal thrombi. With the combination of operative angiography and the balloon catheter developed by Fogarty et al. in 1963, viability can be preserved in well over 90 percent of patients operated upon if operation is performed before the muscles become necrotic, regardless of whether the embolus lodged 3 h or 3 days beforehand.

INCIDENCE AND ETIOLOGY. In about 90 percent of patients with lower extremity emboli, the embolus originates in the heart from one of three causes: mitral stenosis, atrial fibrillation, or myocardial infarction. In some patients it is the first sign of previously unrecognized heart disease. Hence, an embolus, though a serious or even catastrophic event, is best regarded as a manifestation of serious heart disease that must be treated separately.

With mitral stenosis emboli originate from thrombi that have formed in the left atrium because of restriction of blood flow through the stenotic mitral valve. Most such patients also have atrial fibrillation with impaired contractility of the atrium. Atrial fibrillation from atherosclerosis without mitral stenosis can occur and becomes increasingly frequent in older patients. Emboli have been recognized to occur following the spontaneous or induced conversion of fibrillation to sinus rhythm, probably because the contractions of the atrial appendage expel thrombi that have accumulated during the impaired contractility from fibrillation. Emboli following a myocardial infarction originate from mural thrombi forming over the endocardial surfaces of the infarcts. Their frequency is greatest in the first 2 to 3 weeks following infarction and in some patients are the first sign of myocardial infarction.

An unusual cause of peripheral embolization is the so-called paradoxic embolus, when a thrombus arising in the venous circulation passes through a congenital atrial or ventricular septal defect and lodges in a peripheral artery. Other unusual causes include bacterial endocarditis, mural thrombi in subclavian or popliteal aneurysms, and atrial myxoma. In 4 to 5 percent of patients, despite the most diligent search, the source is never found.

PATHOLOGY. Most emboli ejected from the heart, 70 percent of the 426 emboli reported by Darling, lodge in the arteries of the lower extremities. Unfortunately 20 to 25 percent lodge in the cerebral circulation, usually intracranially, and are surgically inaccessible. Five to ten percent lodge in visceral arteries, the superior mesenteric or renal, and an unknown number lodge in silent areas of the circulation, such as the spleen, for which clinical signs are obscure.

Emboli usually lodge at bifurcations of major arteries where the diameter abruptly narrows. Common sites are the bifurcation of the abdominal aorta, the common iliac artery, the common femoral artery, and the popliteal arteries (Fig. 21-6). In the upper extremities similar patterns are found, including the distal subclavian artery and the bifurcation of the common brachial. The severity of the ischemia produced is due both to the abrupt occlusion and the fact that the site of occlusion involves two major arteries, whereas an occlusion either immediately proximal or distal to a site of bifurcation would permit collateral circulation through the bifurcation.

PATHOPHYSIOLOGY. The result of arterial embolization is the immediate onset of severe ischemia of the tissues normally supplied by the occluded artery. Depending upon the artery involved, if untreated, gangrene occurs in about 50 percent of patients. The prominent early symptoms of pain, paralysis, and paresthesia all result from the great sensitivity of peripheral nerves to oxygen deprivation. Striated muscle is secondary only to peripheral nerves in susceptibility to anoxia. Necrosis may appear within 4 to 6 h after onset of ischemia but varies with a number of factors. These include the size of the artery occluded, the collateral circulation around the site of occlusion, blood pressure, and temperature. If collateral circulation is well developed, necrosis may not appear for 8 to 12 h; occasionally moderate ischemia is present but necrosis does not develop. The fact that muscle necrosis often begins within 4 to 6 h is the reason that surgical embolectomy is successful within 4 to 6 h but considerably less effective after longer periods of time.

Sluggish flow of blood in arteries distal to the embolus results in secondary thrombosis usually in continuity with the original embolism within the distal arterial tree (Fig. 21-7). Secondary thrombi further occlude major collateral channels and intensify the ischemia. Effective therapy becomes more difficult because not only the primary embolus but also the secondary thrombus must be removed. Eventually the progressive circulatory stasis is further complicated by extensive venous thrombosis.

CLINICAL MANIFESTATIONS. The five p's, discussed earlier under Acute Arterial Occlusion, pain, paralysis, paresthesia, absent pulses, and pallor, describe the principal clinical features of arterial embolism. The onset is abrupt in most cases, gradual in a few. In 75 to 80 percent of patients there is severe and unremitting pain, usually referred to the most peripheral portions of the limb. The color may be extreme pallor or mottling from alternate areas of pallor and cyanosis. Sensory disturbances vary from anesthesia to paresthesia. Paralysis may be a feature; complete paralysis and anesthesia mask the true nature of the disorder, diverting the physician into investigations for neurologic disease while muscle necrosis is occurring.

The neurologic symptoms are the crucial prognostic signs. If motor and sensory functions are intact, the extremity will survive even though chronic ischemia may persist.

Physical Examination. The extremity is often pale and cold with collapsed peripheral veins. With less severe

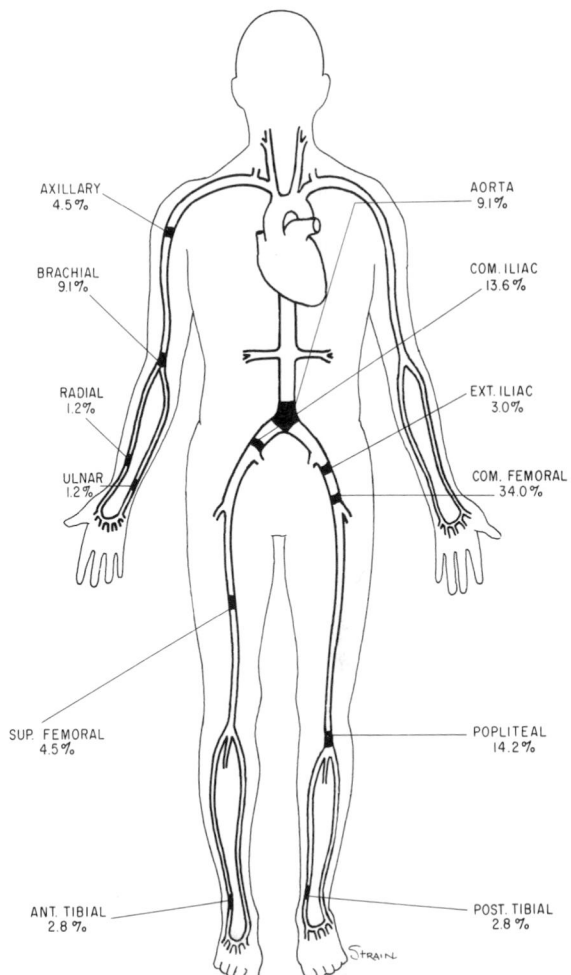

Fig. 21-6. Frequency of involvement of different peripheral arteries by arterial emboli. In the majority of patients arteries in the lower extremity are involved. *(Redrawn from Haimovici H: Peripheral arterial embolism. Angiology 1:20, 1950, with permission.)*

degrees of ischemia there may be cyanosis instead of pallor. A temperature level may be detected that coincides with the level at which the color changes. The arterial pulse is absent at the site of occlusion, frequently with accentuation of the pulse immediately proximal to this point. Sensory impairment varies from hypesthesia to anesthesia, and motor disturbances from weakness to paralysis.

The level of occlusion can often be estimated from the color, temperature level, and pulse findings. Ordinarily acute ischemia develops one joint below the site of occlusion. An iliac embolus produces ischemia at the level of the hip joint, while a common femoral embolus produces ischemia distal to the knee. The extent of ischemia varies with the effectiveness of collateral circulation. Muscle turgor in the ischemic limb is most important. Shortly after the onset of ischemia, the muscles are soft. With continuing ischemia, edema appears, progresses to necrosis, and finally to rigor mortis. Early ischemic edema

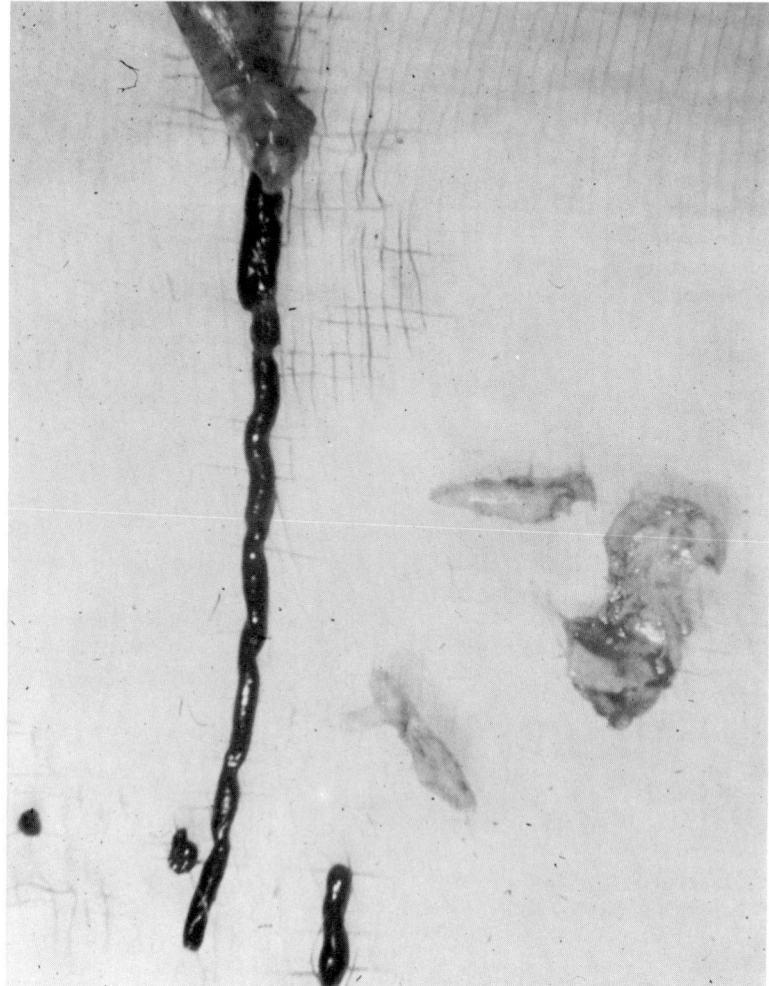

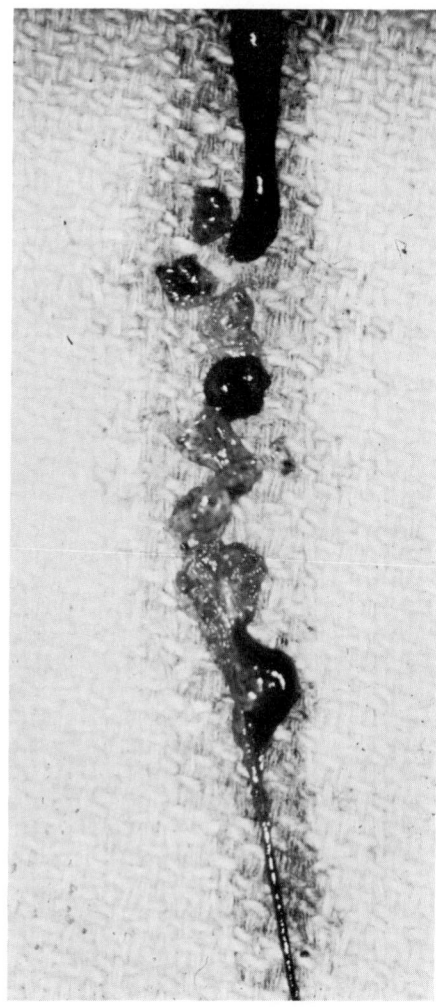

Fig. 21-7. Embolic material and secondary clot. The embolic material that was deposited in the heart chambers during active blood flow is gray to salmon-colored, of firm consistency, and unattached to the arterial wall. It is composed mainly of fibrin and degenerated platelets. The gelatinous clot that appears homogeneous is a secondary stasis clot and was formed when blood flow ceased. It contains all the blood elements and is dark red in color.

creates a "doughy" sensation on palpation. The importance of this physical finding is the fact that as long as the muscles are soft to palpation, the extremity can be salvaged with effective embolectomy and thrombectomy, regardless of how long the embolus has been present. Conversely, the presence of stiff muscles warns that necrosis has occurred. This is most clearly apparent in the leg where the muscle tone of the gastrocnemius and soleus group can be easily evaluated. Some limbs with early muscle necrosis can be salvaged by embolectomy and thrombectomy, combined with extensive fasciotomy and later debridement of localized muscle necrosis, but failure is frequent.

An additional important aspect of physical examination is the cardiac examination for underlying heart disease. The cardiac rhythm, murmurs, or friction rubs may provide clues to atrial fibrillation, mitral stenosis, or acute myocardial infarction. Examination of other peripheral arteries for pulses and bruits provides additional clues to underlying cardiac or arterial disease.

LABORATORY STUDIES. A critical decision to be made when the patient is first encountered is whether an angio-gram should be performed. The diagnosis of acute arterial occlusion can be readily made from the history and physical findings. An electrocardiogram and a chest radiograph should both be done to evaluate the presence of heart disease. If performance of angiography delays surgical therapy beyond the 4- to 6-h "golden period" of therapy, it should be omitted. Intraoperative angiography is one alternative. Angiography is particularly useful where the site of the embolus is uncertain and in distinguishing between arterial embolism and arterial thrombosis superimposed upon an atherosclerotic plaque.

DIAGNOSIS. The condition most easily confused with an arterial embolus is acute thrombosis of an artery previously diseased with atherosclerosis. The importance of differentiating the two conditions is to determine the method of surgical therapy, for a more extensive operative procedure is required with thrombosis. Certain clinical findings suggest thrombosis rather than embolism. Atherosclerosis is usually seen in older age groups, and often symptoms of chronic ischemia, such as claudication, have been present for some time. The involved extremity may show signs of chronic ischemia, such as loss of hair from the toes and atrophy of the skin and nails. The absence of heart disease, which could cause an arterial embolus, further supports the diagnosis of thrombosis. At times differential diagnosis is difficult or even impossible, because an embolus may occur in an older patient with atrial fibrillation who also has claudication from femoral atherosclerosis. In this case, an arteriogram is of great value. With atherosclerosis and secondary arterial thrombosis, diffuse changes of atherosclerosis can be seen throughout the peripheral arteries, often with the development of prominent collateral circulation. By contrast, with embolism, where the distal arteries are usually normal except at the site of occlusion, collateral vessels may not be apparent.

Rarely, acute extensive thrombophlebitis may be confused with acute arterial occlusion. Thrombophlebitis may be associated with extensive vasospasm, causing pain and peripheral vasoconstriction with diminished pulses. A bluish extremity, termed *phlegmasia cerulea dolens,* is also characteristic of venous thrombosis. With arterial embolism, edema appears only after extensive gangrene has developed.

Even more rarely, acute dissecting aneurysm of the thoracic aorta with obliteration of peripheral pulses may suggest multiple peripheral emboli. A dissecting aneurysm can be suspected because of pain in the chest or back, often with a left pleural effusion.

TREATMENT. Indications for Operation. Because patients with arterial emboli usually have serious heart disease, the operative procedure must be planned with regard to the influence of anesthesia and operation on the heart disease. This is particularly critical when the embolus has resulted from a myocardial infarction. With modern vascular techniques, however, embolectomy can be performed in most patients with minimal trauma, often with local anesthesia. Hence, a decision not to operate because of heart disease should be made only if death is imminent. The reason for this is that failure to remove a peripheral embolus, which subsequently produces gangrene, of necessity requires a major amputation, a much greater surgical stress than simple embolectomy.

As emphasized in this chapter, the urgency for performing arterial embolectomy can be simply estimated from the presence of paralysis and anesthesia. When these are present, muscle necrosis often occurs within 4 to 6 h. If they are absent, a more conservative approach may be undertaken. However, their absence does not guarantee that claudication will not subsequently develop in the extremity with resumption of normal physical activity.

An unusual indication for nonsurgical therapy occurs with a migrating embolus. An embolus may lodge in a proximal artery, such as the common femoral, then fragment spontaneously within a few hours and migrate distad. Such patients may on occasion recover completely, but most remain with significant residual occlusion of peripheral arteries. Peripheral pulses should be unequivocally present before simple observation is continued for a long period of time.

Preoperative Therapy. The prompt intravenous administration of heparin to inhibit the development of thrombi distal to the embolus is the most important therapeutic measure in the treatment of an arterial embolus. Heparin, 5000 to 10,000 units, is given intravenously by continuous drip or repeated at 3- to 6-h intervals, depending upon the clotting time, if embolectomy is delayed. Lumbar sympathetic blocks are of dubious value and cannot be safely performed in the presence of systemic anticoagulation. Other measures to influence collateral circulation, such as orally administered vasodilator drugs, are of little value. Intraarterial administration of drugs such as reserpine and tolazoline (Priscoline) sometimes dramatically improves the appearance of acutely ischemic extremities by eliminating functional arterial resistance to flow.

A program for administering extremely large doses of heparin to promote lysis of thrombi and thereby improve the chances of operative success has been proposed by Blaisdell et al., who recommend that 30,000 units of heparin be administered intravenously as a bolus followed by doses of 2000 to 3000 units per hour by continuous I.V. drip. If clinical improvement occurs, operation is deferred. If no clinical improvement is observed, operative intervention is carried out. This requires close observation by highly experienced teams well versed in recognizing the sometimes subtle changes that denote either worsening or improvement of ischemia.

Operative Technique. For operations on the extremities, local anesthesia can be used in seriously ill patients. Frequently the operative incisions are short since the Fogarty balloon catheter has permitted removal of propagated clot both distal and proximal to emboli, making possible performance of the entire operative procedure through limited surgical incisions. Frequently, it is possible to perform the entire embolectomy and thrombectomy through incision in the upper thigh over the common femoral artery. With emboli at the common femoral bifurcation, it is possible to remove thrombi from the arterial tree down to the ankle through the same incision. Rarely is it necessary to enter the peritoneal cavity for aortoiliac embolectomy. This should be avoided when possible, for these patients are usually quite ill from their cardiac disease.

In general, surgical incisions are placed directly over the uppermost level of arterial occlusion unless the aorto-iliac system is involved, in which case incisions are placed over both common femoral arteries. Once the artery has been isolated proximal to distal to the embolus, 5000 units of heparin should be given intravenously. A transverse or a longitudinal arteriotomy is then made in the artery immediately proximal to its bifurcation, where the embolus is usually lodged. The embolus characteristically "pops" out as soon as the lumen is entered and can be recognized by its gray appearance and nonadherence to the arterial wall. Hence, removal is a simple procedure, but removal of thrombi that have formed distad or even proximally may be unusually complex. Fogarty balloon catheters have virtually eliminated the need to make multiple incisions along the course of the arterial tree for the laborious retrograde washing out of thrombi. The preferred technique is to pass the catheter into the distal artery as far as possible, inflate the balloon, and withdraw it in its inflated state. Comparison of the length of the catheter inserted with the length of the extremity indicates how far the catheter has been advanced. Passage of catheters into the aorta for the removal of aortoiliac thrombi is similarly performed. Occasionally it is impossible to pass the balloon catheter into various distal branches, either the anterior and posterior tibial in the calf or the radial and ulnar in the forearm. In such instances separate incisions are made over these vessels, followed by separate introduction of the catheter into each branch. Dale has used polyethylene catheters to aspirate clot. With these techniques, retrograde flushing of the artery through a distal incision is rarely necessary.

As indicated, the most crucial aspect of the operation is determining the completeness of removal of propagated thrombi. Back-bleeding is a notoriously unreliable indicator. Back-bleeding can occur through the nearest arterial branch, while the major artery distad is still occluded. Failure to remove all residual thrombus usually results in reocclusion. The operative procedure should be continued until, by an appropriate combination of techniques, all pulses are restored at the ankle or wrist, or an operative arteriogram has demonstrated that the arteries are patent. On occasion, restoration of a pulse can be misleading, and bounding pulses may be felt in an artery partly reopened but with persisting distal obstruction. For this reason operative angiography is often critical to success.

If severe ischemic injury has been present beforehand, wide fasciotomy of the fascial envelope containing the major muscles may help preserve limb viability, especially if embolectomy has been delayed beyond the golden first 4 to 6 h and increased muscle turgor was palpable before operation.

Postoperative Care. The most important aspect of postoperative care is to be certain that peripheral circulation is adequate. A palpable pulse is the best clinical sign. This should be identified immediately after operation and its presence periodically confirmed by palpation. Pulses which are difficult to feel can be checked with the Doppler instrument, which permits not only auscultation over pedal arteries but also measurement of pressures within those vessels. Disappearance of a previously palpable pulse or a change in Doppler measurements associated with unsatisfactory appearance of the extremity is an indication for either arteriography or immediate reoperation.

The persistence of paralysis and anesthesia following operation is ominous; gangrene is almost a certainty. Conversely, restoration of normal neurologic function indicates adequate circulation for muscle viability. This is particularly reassuring either when pulses cannot be re-

stored or palpation is inconclusive because of edema and swelling.

The mode of heparin administration in the postoperative period is critical, since fresh surgical wounds are subject to hemorrhage, while delay of anticoagulation may predispose to further embolization. Some surgeons give no heparin for 6 h postoperatively and then administer it by intermittent intravenous injection in doses of 5000 units every 4 to 6 h. Oral therapy with coumadin derivatives is begun after 3 to 4 days and continued as long as the patient is at risk. Salzman et al. have reported that continuously administered intravenous heparin, avoiding peak effects which reach infinity during the intermittent administration, is associated with a lesser incidence of hemorrhage. Thrombolysis may accompany heparin administration, especially when porous knitted vascular prostheses are employed. The importance of prompt and continuous anticoagulant therapy cannot be overemphasized, for the arterial embolus is only a symptom of serious heart disease. Recurrence of embolization, each incident associated with a 25 to 30 percent likelihood of lodging in the brain, is distressingly common unless the heart disease is effectively treated. Patients with intractable atrial fibrillation should be maintained on permanent anticoagulant therapy. Those with mitral stenosis should have a mitral valvulotomy performed soon. Those with myocardial infarction should receive anticoagulants for several weeks, by which time the endocardial surface of the infarct will have healed and the likelihood of embolism is small.

Antibiotic therapy generally is started at the time of operation and continued for 2 to 4 days postoperatively.

PROGNOSIS. The most important feature influencing survival of the extremity following embolectomy is the time elapsing between the occurrence of embolization and successful restoration of flow at operation. As mentioned repeatedly, removal within 4 to 6 h after onset is almost always associated with an excellent prognosis, having the two great advantages of avoiding muscle necrosis and limiting secondary thrombus formation beyond the site of embolism. In both of the large series reported by Darling et al. and Cranley et al., excellent results were obtained in 85 to 95 percent of patients. With more than 6 h elapsed between embolization and embolectomy, unsuccessful results were more common. These particularly occur with inexperienced vascular surgeons and limited facilities. The crucial concept is that as long as the calf muscles are "soft" before operation, indicating that muscle necrosis has not occurred, salvage of the extremity should approach 95 percent or higher, regardless of the duration of ischemia. In delayed cases, achieving this goal taxes the resources, skills, and ingenuity of the vascular surgeon to the utmost, for thrombi may have accumulated from the aortic bifurcation to the posterior tibial artery at the ankle and complete removal requires a combination of careful surgical exploration, frequently multiple incisions, and serial operative angiography. If muscle necrosis is present before operation, indicated by a rigid calf muscle, possibilities of limb salvage are small, and the possibility of precipitating fatal myoglobinuria may constitute a contraindication to surgical restoration of flow. Rarely, a functional extremity may be salvaged in which virtually all the calf muscles are lost from necrosis but a viable foot is preserved.

The crucial long-term feature determining prognosis is the ability to prevent further emboli. Without adequate prophylactic anticoagulation, recurrence is dismally inevitable, eventually terminating with fatal or crippling cerebral thrombosis. Vigilance to prevent emboli can be relaxed only when a myocardial infarction has healed or mitral stenosis has been treated by valvulotomy.

In any large series of patients with arterial embolism, death occurs in 25 to 30 percent of patients during that hospitalization. This is almost always due to the underlying heart disease causing the embolus, indicating the gravity of the basic illness. In some instances death is due to either inadequate management of the embolic episode, with the complications of sepsis from gangrene, or to recurrent embolism to the brain or viscera, a result of inadequate anticoagulant therapy.

Arterioarterial Embolization

HISTORICAL CONSIDERATIONS. In the past decade there has been increasing awareness of the existence of arterioarterial embolism and its role in producing previously unexplained ischemic syndromes. With cerebrovascular insufficiency, the ophthalmologic visualization of minute particles of atherosclerotic plaque or platelet fibrin emboli in the retina, in association with an ulcerated atherosclerotic plaque at the bifurcation of the carotid artery, suggested the source of the minute emboli. In the lower extremities, sudden onset of toe and foot ischemia with little or no impairment of peripheral pulses (the "blue toe" syndrome) led to the finding that minute emboli were the mechanism, having originated in aortic or iliac atherosclerotic plaques. The finding of peripheral emboli beyond aneurysms has been described periodically. Miles et al. have cited observations suggesting that small emboli in the coronary circulation could come from ulcerated plaques, producing diffuse myocardial scarring from myriads of tiny emboli.

PATHOGENESIS. The basic process seems to be ulceration of an atherosclerotic plaque with discharge of minute fragments of atherosclerotic debris into the circulation. The ulcerated surface may become covered by platelets and fibrin which in turn are intermittently dislodged. How often these are subsequently resorbed is not known. The embolic may arise from an atherosclerotic artery near the end organ where the emboli lodge or they may originate some distance away, a condition occasionally seen when emboli in the toes apparently originate from plaques in the abdominal or thoracic aorta. Repeated embolic episodes are frequent, at times with almost complete recovery from ischemia between each episode; in other patients progressively greater degrees of ischemia occur, ultimately terminating in necrosis.

CLINICAL FINDINGS. As noted briefly above, a most striking syndrome occurs with emboli from the distal thoracic aorta, the "blue toe" syndrome. There is severe ischemia of the toes and feet, bilaterally, in association with renal failure. Before the pathogenesis was understood, the diagnosis remained an enigma, for pulses often remained palpable even while distal ischemia progressed to gangrene. There is a wide range in severity, from complete clearing of ischemia to progressive occlusion and gangrene. Similar embolization from the infrarenal aorta or iliac arteries also produces blue toes without renal failure.

Similar episodes occur in the cerebrovascular circulation with any combination of neurologic symptoms from the most transient, fleeting symptoms to complete stroke with cerebral infarction. In the upper extremity the subclavian artery is most frequently involved, with repeated attacks simulating Raynaud's phenomenon.

DIAGNOSIS. The diagnosis can be suspected from the combined findings of severe ischemia of a digit with palpable pulses. Determining the source of the emboli is crucial, for many can be corrected surgically, often by simple endarterectomy. Hence, detailed angiographic studies are necessary. The source of the embolus can be estimated by noting the peripheral circulation in other areas, where previous emboli may have lodged. For example, involvement of branches of the profunda femoris artery indicate emboli arising proximal to this level. Concomitant involvement of renal artery branches suggests that the emboli originated in the thoracic aorta. Similarly, in the upper extremity emboli may arise from the subclavian artery or, alternatively, from lesions located far distad, such as small aneurysms in the palm of the hand. These diagnostic possibilities can be resolved only by precise, extensive angiography.

TREATMENT. When the atherosclerotic plaque can be related to the pattern of distal embolization (Fig. 21-8), arterial reconstruction of the atherosclerotic segment by either endarterectomy or replacement with a prosthetic graft has prevented further embolism. In the carotid system, there is now extensive experience with arterial reconstruction to prevent recurrent ischemic episodes, so-called transient ischemic attacks (TIA). The operation is effective and durable. Similar procedures have been performed in the subclavian artery to prevent TIA in the upper extremity. In the lower extremity experience is still limited, but good results in a series of 10 cases operated upon at New York University have confirmed both the validity of the concept and the surgical approach.

In theory, emboli from platelet or fibrin aggregates should be inhibited or prevented by anticoagulants, but their effectiveness is as yet uncertain. Paradoxically, anticoagulant therapy might prevent healing of an ulcerated plaque and thereby increase the tendency to embolization. This may explain the infrequent clinical puzzle of an embolus developing *after* heparin therapy has been started.

ACUTE ARTERIAL THROMBOSIS

ETIOLOGY AND PATHOLOGY. Acute arterial thrombosis usually occurs in an artery previously narrowed by ath-

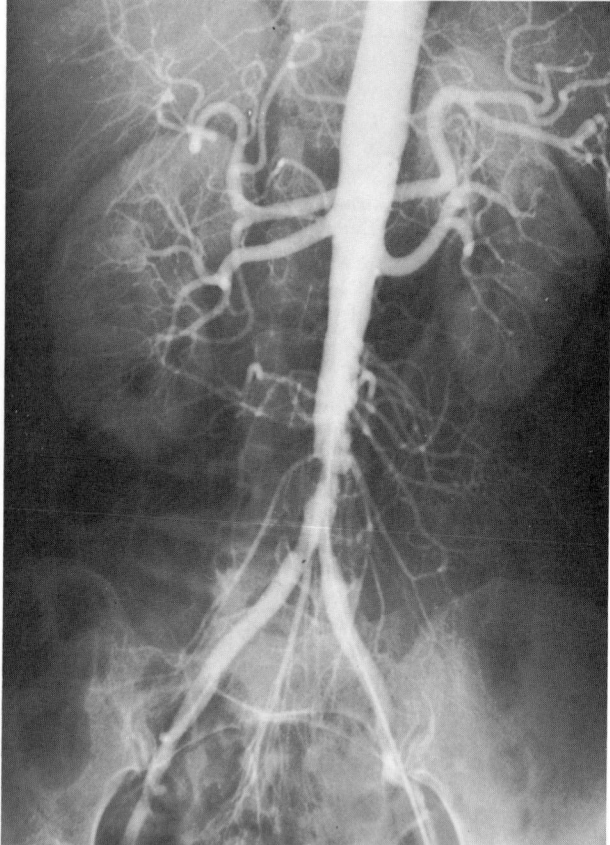

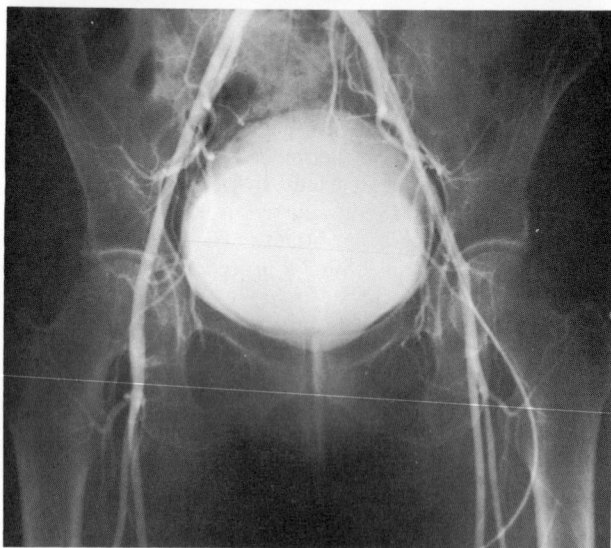

A

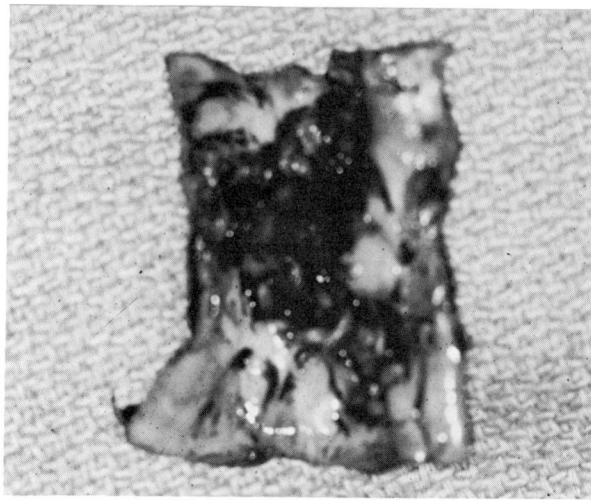

B

Fig. 21-8. Arterioarterial embolization, also known as atheroembolization, in a patient in whom marked ischemia of the toes developed in the presence of palpable pedal pulses. Several attacks occurred with progressive ischemia. *A.* Angiograms showing infrarenal abdominal aortic plaques. Occlusion of small calf arteries without involvement of renal arteries suggested that this infrarenal plaque was the source of emboli. *B.* Aortic plaque removed by endarterectomy. There was no recurrence of embolization at the tenth year follow-up.

erosclerosis. In some patients the process of occlusion is gradual; no acute symptoms appear, but chronic arterial insufficiency slowly becomes more severe. In others, however, sudden thrombosis precipitates acute symptoms, closely mimicking arterial embolization.

Unusual causes of arterial thrombosis are cervical ribs or repeated occupational trauma, such as from operation of pneumatic tools, the vibrations of which locally injure the arterial wall and produce thrombosis. Very rarely arterial thrombosis develops within a normal artery. This can happen with debilitating infections, especially in infants, usually with diarrhea and dehydration. It may also occur with primary hematologic disorders, such as polycythemia vera.

Iatrogenic thrombosis has become much more common due to percutaneous introduction of catheters for cardiac catheterization or selective angiography. Thrombosis develops from detachment of a flap of intima from the arterial wall with subsequent formation of an occluding thrombus. Acute lower extremity arterial thrombosis has also been seen following long periods of immobilization such as long automobile or plane trips. The condition is similar to acute venous thrombosis, which occurs more commonly.

CLINICAL MANIFESTATIONS. When thrombosis occurs suddenly, the findings are similar to those occurring with arterial trauma or embolism: pain, absence of pulses, paresthesia, and paralysis.

A critical differential diagnosis is between arterial embolus and arterial thrombosis, a distinction that cannot always be made with accuracy, although several clues are helpful. A history of claudication in the involved extremity indicates chronic arterial disease. Similarly, examination of the extremity may show the stigmata of chronic arterial insufficiency, including absence of hair and trophic changes in the skin and nails. Significant findings may also be present in the contralateral, asymptomatic extremity. Differentiation between the two conditions is important, because although operation is necessary with either if circulation is impaired to such an extent that gangrene is imminent, the type of operative procedure for each condition varies greatly. Restoration of blood flow in an extremity with chronic occlusive disease, with an arterial thrombosis superimposed upon an artery previously narrowed by atherosclerosis, is much more difficult than the performance of simple embolectomy upon an artery with no intrinsic vascular disease. Additionally, patients with emboli require long-term anticoagulant therapy. Patients with arterial thrombosis should have an arteriogram before operation to assess the extent of occlusive disease and to evaluate the patency of the vascular bed beyond the point of occlusion in order to determine where a bypass graft can be inserted distad.

TREATMENT. Operative correction of the arterial occlusion requires both removal of the thrombus and correction of the atherosclerotic stenosis. The operative techniques are described in detail in the section Chronic Arterial Occlusion. Usually either the atherosclerotic narrowing is removed directly with an endarterectomy or a bypass graft is inserted around the area of obstruction.

ATHEROSCLEROTIC OCCLUSIVE DISEASE

Occlusive Disease of the Lower Extremity

AORTOILIAC DISEASE

Recognition of the ischemic syndrome produced by atherosclerotic disease of the bifurcation of the abdominal aorta is credited to Leriche, who described in the early 1940s the clinical characteristics of occlusion of the abdominal aorta, i.e., claudication, sexual impotence in the male, and absence of gangrene. The development of angiography, pioneered by dos Santos, greatly facilitated diagnosis.

PATHOLOGY. Some degree of atherosclerosis is almost universally seen at autopsy in the abdominal aortas of patients over sixty years of age, but symptoms from decrease in blood flow do not occur unless the cross-sectional area of the aorta has been narrowed by as much as 90 percent. There may be only fibrointimal thickening or typical atherosclerotic plaques with ulceration and superimposed thrombosis or embolization of portions of atherosclerotic plaques. As in other arteries, the disease often begins at bifurcations where flow patterns conducive to intimal thickening occur. Involvement is often greatest at the aortic, the iliac, and the common femoral bifurcations. It may extend proximally in the abdominal aorta up to the level of the renal arteries, but occlusion proximal to the renal arteries is rare.

Patients are occasionally seen in the fifth and sixth decades with thrombosis of the abdominal aorta but only mild atherosclerosis of the common iliac arteries. The thrombus often propagates up to the level of the renal arteries, rarely occluding one renal artery, and extends up to near the superior mesenteric artery. These patients contrast to a curious degree with patients in the seventh and eighth decades who may have unusually severe atherosclerosis but without thrombosis and total occlusion, despite advanced stenosis. This variation with age suggests that some unrecognized factor leading to hypercoagulability in the younger group may precipitate the thrombotic process.

Fortunately clinically significant atherosclerosis of the abdominal aorta is virtually always segmental. Proximally it stops at the level of the renal arteries; distad the profunda femoris artery is almost always patent, though not infrequently involved with correctable stenotic lesions even in the presence of a totally occluded superficial femoral artery (Fig. 21-9). Reconstruction can be done in most of the patients, directing flow distad into the patent profunda femoris artery, which, however, may require either bypass or endarterectomy to serve as a suitable outflow tract. If the superficial femoral artery is also occluded, additional reconstruction is usually not required unless tissue necrosis is present. Otherwise, simple aortoiliac or aortoprofunda femoris reconstruction will suffice to relieve claudication.

A separate therapeutic consideration is the 10 percent of persons with aortoiliac occlusive disease who have small aneurysms as well. This group must be treated by aortic graft replacement of the aneurysmal segment, for aneurysmal dilation may continue following endarterectomy or simple bypass procedures.

Concomitant coronary or cerebral atherosclerosis occurs frequently. This has led to an increased interest in overcoming the effects of aortoiliac occlusions without invading the abdominal cavity, through the performance of so-called extraanatomical bypass grafts, popularized by Blaisdell et al. In these procedures one or both axillary arteries serve as the takeoff vessels for grafts leading to the groin. To overcome unilateral iliac arterial occlusions, cross-femoral grafts also have been used successfully.

In addition, patients with detectable involvement of cerebral or coronary arteries are evaluated for possible angiographic studies of those arteries and for possible cerebrovascular or coronary arterial reconstructive procedures as well.

PATHOPHYSIOLOGY. The slow progression of aortoiliac occlusive disease usually is associated with the development of collateral flow through the lumbar arteries, anastomosing distad with the branches of the gluteal arteries and the profunda femoris arteries sufficient to prevent ischemia at rest, symptoms of claudication appearing only with exercise. Sexual impotence is frequent because of decreased blood flow through the hypogastric arteries. Since blood flow is adequate at rest, the extremities remain well nourished. Only with additional occlusions in the superficial femoral, profunda femoris, or popliteal and tibial arteries do nutritional changes with ulceration and gangrene appear.

Rapidly developing occlusion of the aorta before collateral circulation develops may result in severe ischemic

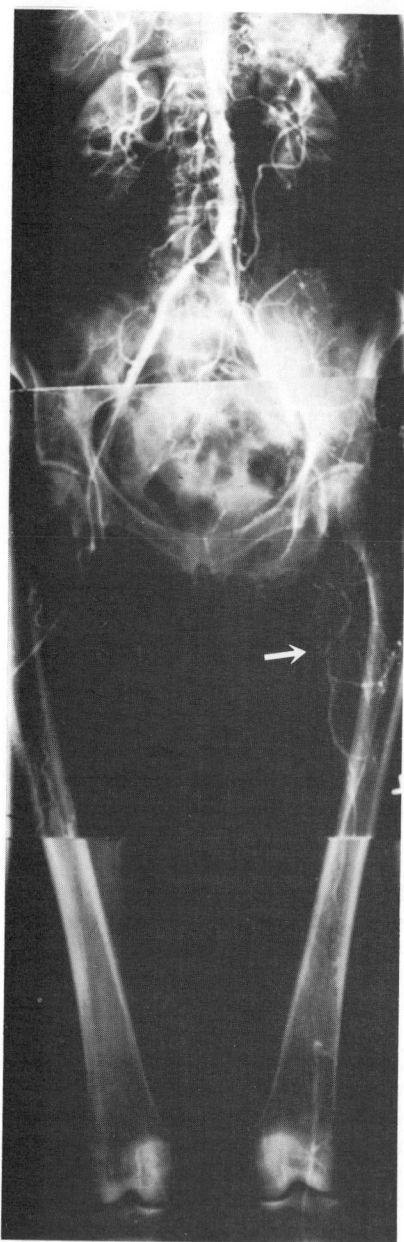

Fig. 21-9. Angiogram illustrating that the profunda femoris artery is usually patent in the presence of aortoiliac occlusive disease. Advanced lesions may be present, however, requiring surgical correction to render the profunda femoris suitable for an outflow tract. Arrow points to patent mid-profunda femoris artery.

changes in the legs, even though no additional disease is present distad. In some extreme cases, thrombosis of an atherosclerotic aorta may propagate up to the level of the renal arteries, rarely occluding one renal artery and extending up to near the superior mesenteric artery.

Yet another manifestation of aortoiliac occlusive disease may be necrotic toe and foot lesions secondary to embolization of minute particles (atheroemboli) from the aorta or iliac arteries. These may occur in the presence of

nonoccluding or even nonstenosing atherosclerotic plaques that give rise to emboli. These emboli may occlude pedal or digital arteries, resulting in the so-called blue or purple toe syndrome (see discussion under Arterioarterial Embolization).

CLINICAL MANIFESTATIONS. The classic symptoms are intermittent claudication involving calf, thigh, and buttock and sexual impotence of varying severity in males. Claudication may be symmetric or asymmetric, depending upon the pattern of involvement of the iliac arteries, and may vary in severity from difficulty after walking three to four blocks to inability to walk, even indoors. Rest pain, ulceration, or gangrene are rare with chronic aortoiliac occlusion, and, when present, almost always indicate additional distal disease, particularly in diabetics where associated occlusions of the tibial arteries are common.

Symptoms may remain stable for years or even improve with exercise as collateral vessels enlarge. Conversely, symptoms may worsen with progression of distal atherosclerosis, sometimes dramatically, with hypotension secondary to myocardial infarction or cardiac arrhythmias, or to administration of drugs that diminish ventricular systolic thrust, such as propanolol. Impotence is a complex syndrome which may arise from multiple causes. Its presence or absence cannot be relied upon to diagnose aortoiliac disease. Although it may improve after successful arterial reconstruction, the outcome in any particular patient is unpredictable.

Physical Examination. The principal finding is diminution or absence of the femoral pulses, combined with absence of popliteal and pedal pulses. Pulsations in the abdominal aorta may be palpable if occlusion is limited to near the aortic bifurcation, but these are absent if the abdominal aorta is occluded up to the renal arteries. A systolic bruit denoting stenosis is often audible over the aorta or iliac arteries. It does not correlate, however, with the degree of stenosis. Nutrition in the extremities is usually normal. With signs of chronic ischemia, such as absence of hair, brittle nails, or rubor, additional atherosclerotic disease in the femoral or popliteal arteries is probably present.

Occasionally patients are seen with aortoiliac disease with acute episodes of severe ischemia of the toes or feet, often with cyanosis and rest pain. The diagnosis may be especially puzzling if the aortoiliac obstruction is not severe. Occasionally pedal pulses are palpable. The syndrome arises from arterioarterial embolization of fragments of atherosclerotic plaques or minute thrombi dislodged from the surface of such plaques. The diagnosis may be suspected if a localized bruit in the abdomen or groin is found.

As multiple areas of atherosclerosis are frequent, particular care should be taken to search for bruits over the carotid or subclavian arteries, as well as to note the adequacy of pulses in the upper extremities.

LABORATORY STUDIES. With the exception of patients experiencing arterioarterial embolization, the diagnosis usually can be established by the history and physical examination. Radiographs often show calcification in the wall of the aorta, but as the calcification is most marked in the media, it does not correlate with the degree of flow obstruction. An unsuspected abdominal aortic aneurysm, however, may be outlined by the calcification within its wall. Noninvasive tests may document reduced blood flow to the lower extremities, confirming the physical findings. These studies are most useful when the vessels are not completely occluded. With stenosis, the patient may have pulses at rest, but after a period of exercise, these values are markedly reduced. Demonstration of this change may be helpful in distinguishing between symptoms due to vascular disease and those due to neurogenic disease. Aortography is performed if surgical reconstruction is being considered. It delineates the proximal extent of the occlusion and, more importantly, may outline the patent arteries beyond the obstruction, especially the profunda femoris vessels that determine the feasibility of revascularization.

MEDICAL MANAGEMENT. The need for surgical reconstruction depends upon the severity of the symptoms and the age of the patient. Intermittent claudication in most instances denotes mild ischemia even in the presence of extensive arterial occlusions and, of itself, is only a relative and weak indication for surgical intervention. In 80 percent of patients affected, the course is relatively benign. Two-thirds of all patients affected can be managed successfully without operative intervention. Few patients fail to improve on a program of active and vigorous leg exercises and cessation of smoking; even in young patients whose livelihood may depend upon walking ability, rarely is operation needed until a 6-month to a 1-year trial of medical therapy has been attempted. By contrast, a retired patient of seventy with angina pectoris and claudication does not require operation. The presence of trophic changes in the feet, rubor, absence of hair, and brittle nails is a useful guide to the risk of gangrene, for gangrene is rare except with acute arterial occlusion as long as trophic changes are absent. Claudicators progress to gangrene at the rate of 2.3 percent per year. These usually are the patients with the most severe claudication and the most marked involvement of the tibial arteries, in whom surgical reconstructions either cannot be done or, if done at higher levels, do not result in control of the necrotizing ischemia. Thus, prophylactic intervention in claudicators probably does not avert the appearance of gangrene at a later date (see Table 21-1).

If operation is not recommended, daily exercise to the point of claudication should be encouraged, for this may enhance collateral circulation, as manifested by gradual increase in walking tolerance. If walking is not feasible, a similar exercise can be performed indoors by having the patient raise himself on his toes and then rock back on his heels, repeating the sequence rapidly until calf cramps occur. Following a rest period the exercise is repeated, as often as twenty or more times daily.

Abstinence from tobacco in any form is mandatory. There is reasonable statistical evidence that claudication improves when smoking is stopped and that the risk of gangrene is greater in patients who smoke. The precise mechanism is unknown, but tobacco is a potent vasocon-

Table 21-1. FATE OF 104 CLAUDICATORS*

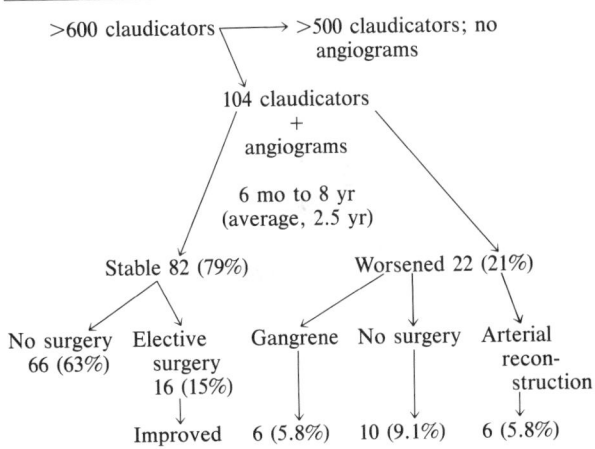

* These patients had arteriograms and were followed for 6 months to 8 years (average, 2.5 years) in an attempt at nonsurgical management.
SOURCE: From Imparato AM, Kim GE, Crowley JG: 1975, with permission.

strictor. Robichek et al. have reported that continued smoking after arterial reconstructions results in premature failures. Drug therapy with vasodilators may be tried, but unfortunately few patients have had any improvement in claudication. Alcohol, orally administered, is employed for its peripheral vasodilator effect.

With severe ischemia, one of the most crucial points in management is educating the patient to protect the feet from any form of trauma, be it thermal, mechanical, or inflicted by trimming of calluses, corns, or toenails. A familiar tragedy is that a trauma that would be minor in a foot with normal circulation will produce gangrene of a toe in a severely ischemic foot that not only fails to heal but may gradually progress upward to result in a low thigh amputation. Infection associated with unguis incarnatus or dermatophytosis similarly may cause decompensation of the circulation with gangrene, probably from an increase in local tissue metabolism.

Therapy directed toward lowering blood lipid concentrations by diet, drugs, or even surgical procedures remains of uncertain benefit. Anticoagulant therapy with heparin or warfarin sodium has not been helpful. The recent exciting discovery that acetylsalicylic acid in small doses strikingly alters platelet aggregation and may thereby prevent intravascular thrombosis is now undergoing clinical evaluation and holds considerable therapeutic promise.

SURGICAL TREATMENT. Operations that have been used to relieve the symptoms of aortoiliac occlusion include (a) direct aortic reconstruction, either by bypass or endarterectomy, (b) indirect revascularization or extraanatomic bypass, or (c) balloon dilatation of stenotic lesions using percutaneous catheters. Occasionally lumbar sympathectomy, either by operation or by phenol injection, has been used to promote peripheral vasodilatation. These will be discussed under the section Femoropopliteal Occlusive Disease.

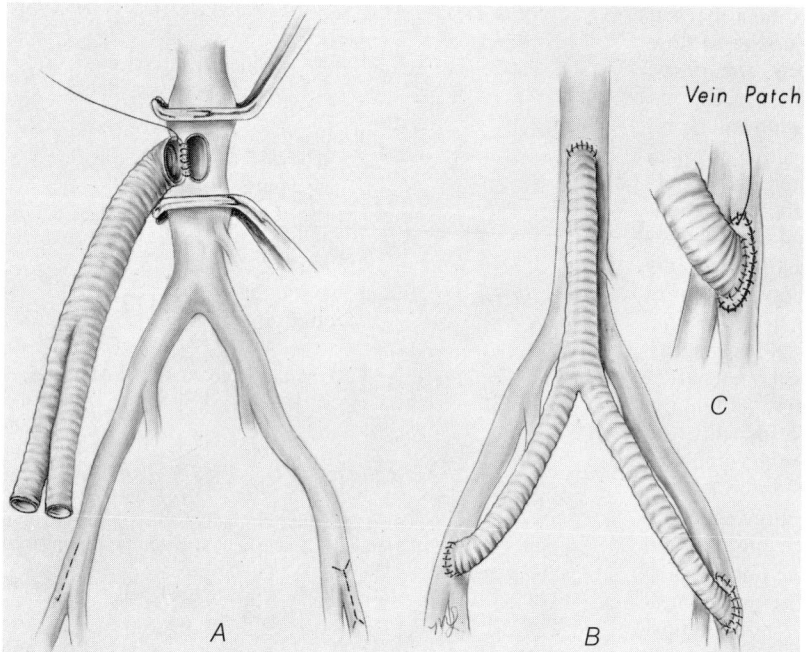

Fig. 21-10. Bypass graft of abdominal aorta. Dissection and exposure are similar to that for endarterectomy procedures. *A.* The proximal anastomosis is performed either end-to-side or end-to-end to the aorta proximal to the point of obstruction. End-to-end aortic anastomosis is preferred by many to lessen the risk of distal embolization. Knitted Dacron is preferred. *B.* The distal anastomoses are performed as end-to-side anastomoses either to the iliac artery proximal to the inguinal ligament or to the common femoral artery at the point of origin of the profunda femoris artery, depending upon the degree of atherosclerotic involvement of the external iliac artery. Anastomoses distal to the inguinal ligament are avoided whenever possible to avoid trauma to the prosthesis passing under the inguinal ligament and to lessen the risk of infection posed by having a plastic prosthesis in the groin. *C.* A vein roof patch may be employed to facilitate suture of the prosthesis to small arteries.

An operation on the abdominal aorta is a major procedure that is associated with a 2 to 10 percent risk of complication depending on the degree of associated medical problems. Complications may stem from associated vascular disease (coronary, carotid, renal, and lower extremity occlusive disease), from failure of other organs (pulmonary and renal), or from perioperative events (bleeding, thrombosis, and infection). Because of these risks, any elective procedure should be carefully planned and discussed with the patient to be certain that the operative risk is matched by the anticipated improvement. Many will refuse operation unless for limb salvage when informed of the risk and reassured about the relatively benign prognosis of intermittent claudication.

Preoperative evaluation should include a thorough history, physical examination, and appropriate diagnostic studies to evaluate the heart, lungs, kidneys, and peripheral vessels. Determination of the left ventricular ejection fraction is particularly useful in evaluating cardiac risk. An angiogram visualizing the aorta from the level of the renal arteries to the arch vessels of the feet is preferred, not only for planning the surgical procedure but also for anticipating possible lower extremity complications. At the time of the operation the blood pressure, cardiac rhythm, urinary output, and intracardiac pressures should be continuously monitored. Careful thought must also be given to the infusion of fluids and blood products.

A number of factors may influence the choice between bypass and endarterectomy for aortic reconstruction. Bypass with a prosthesis is technically less demanding and therefore, for most surgeons, can be performed with less blood loss and operating time. The late complications of infection of the prosthesis, anastomotic aneurysms, and aortoenteric fistulas must be considered because they are all potentially lethal. Endarterectomy leaving only autologous tissue has as good patency rates as bypass, and it is free of the complications associated with plastic prostheses. This operation is especially suited for good risk patients with long life expectancies.

Bypass Grafting (Figs. 21-10 and 21-11). Although bypass may be performed to the iliac vessels, the operation most customarily performed is an aortobifemoral procedure, circumventing occlusive disease in the external iliac and common femoral arteries. Antibiotics are given during the course of the operation. The femoral arteries are exposed from the inguinal ligament distally to the profunda femoris arteries. The latter may require extensive dissection to reach a relatively atherosclerotic free segment. A separate incision is made in the abdomen to expose the infrarenal aorta.

A variety of prosthetic grafts with varying permeabilities is now available. Dacron woven prostheses are less permeable to blood but tend to form a gelatinous neointima that has the potential of embolizing. Knitted grafts are more porous, requiring preclotting, but in time be-

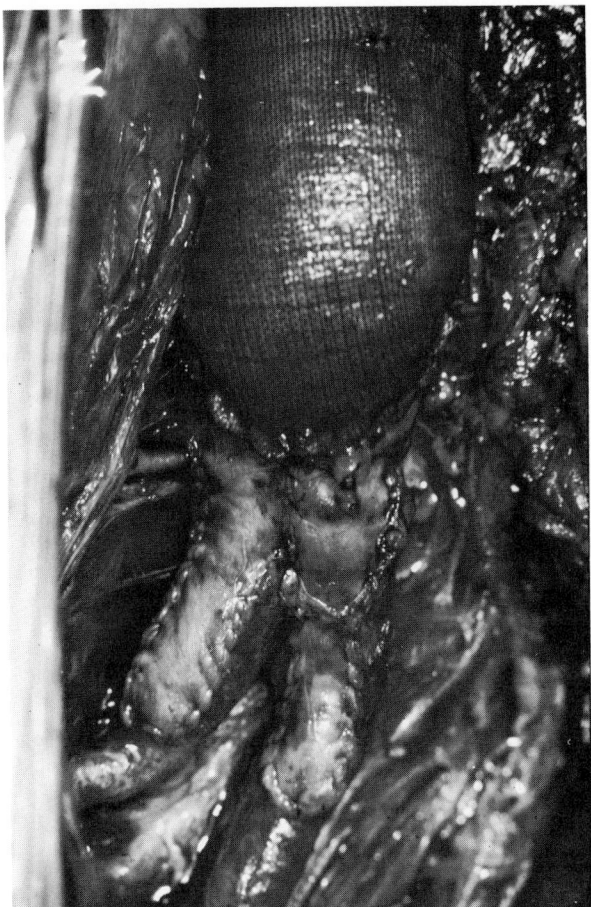

Fig. 21-11. Interposition of vein roof patches over the profunda femoris and superficial femoral arteries facilitates suture of plastic prostheses to the common femoral artery in aortofemoral bypass procedures.

come better incorporated into the surrounding tissues. Over a period of time postoperatively, knitted prostheses have shown a tendency to dilate and collect gelatinous thrombus along the inner wall, losing the original advantage of neointimal incorporation. New woven velous grafts may combine the advantages of both in maintaining diameter and adherent neointima.

After heparinizing the patient, the aorta is clamped and either an end-to-end or an end-to-side anastomosis is constructed using 3-0 or 4-0 nonabsorbable suture. The limbs of the bifurcated graft are then tunneled retroperitoneally, posterior to the ureters and mesosigmoid colon, under the inguinal ligaments to the groin wounds. End-to-side anastomoses are then made to the femoral arteries. A variety of adjunctive techniques, such as local endarterectomy or vein patch angioplasty, may be used if there is extensive atherosclerotic disease of the femoral vessels. After restoring blood flow, intraoperative angiograms are recommended since the potential for technical imperfections, especially at the distal anastomoses, can lead to early and disastrous reocclusions.

Thromboendarterectomy (Fig. 21-12). An alternative procedure that has been used to disobliterate occlusive atherosclerotic disease from the level of the renal arteries to the mid profunda femoris arteries is thromboendarterectomy. It avoids the often precarious complications associated with plastic prostheses and is most useful when the procedure can be limited to the aorta and common iliac arteries. It requires particular skill and expertise for successful performance, is more time consuming when the external iliac and femoral vessels are included in the procedure, but requires later operation for reocclusion, false aneurysm, or infection less frequently than bypass procedures.

A crucial decision about the extent of the endarterectomy performed depends on the distribution of the atherosclerotic process. In some instances termination of significant occlusive atherosclerosis just distal to the bifurcation of the common iliac arteries requires only aortobilateral common iliac endarterectomy. In other cases extensive involvement of the external iliac and common femoral arteries mandates extension to include groin vessels.

The aorta proximally and the external and hypogastric arteries distad are encircled with plastic tapes. The lumbar and inferior mesenteric arteries are similarly exposed. Fifty milligrams of heparin is then given by intravenous injection before occlusive clamps are applied to avoid thrombus formation during the periods of stasis. External iliac clamps are applied before clamping the abdominal aorta to protect from distal embolization. Incisions are made over the distal common iliac arteries, and cleavage planes between the plaques and media are developed. A longitudinal incision is made into the aorta above the level of the inferior mesenteric artery and an appropriate cleavage plane near the junction of the arterial intima and media identified. Using various techniques, including arterial strippers, the core of atherosclerotic material is freed proximally. Usually by blunt dissection the aortic and iliac cores can be mobilized and removed in one piece. A critical aspect of the operative procedure distad is careful inspection of the intima of the proximal external iliac artery to eliminate ledges of thickened intima by suturing. The caliber of the external iliac arteries may be measured with catheters. A diameter smaller than #16 Foley catheter often indicates the necessity of extending the endarterectomy to the common femoral arteries. In the hypogastric arteries, endarterectomy is limited to removal of the occluding material near the ostia, for distal dissection of this artery is usually technically unsatisfactory.

The aortotomy incision is closed with a simple continuous suture of 4-0 or 5-0 monofilament nonabsorbable suture. The iliac arteriotomies may be closed similarly or with a patch graft of either autologous saphenous vein or a prosthetic patch of knitted Dacron. The choice depends upon both the diameter of the artery and the rigidity of the wall. After the incisions are sutured, the occluding clamps are sequentially removed to permit flushing initially into the hypogastric arteries and subsequently into the external iliacs. Strong femoral pulses should be palpa-

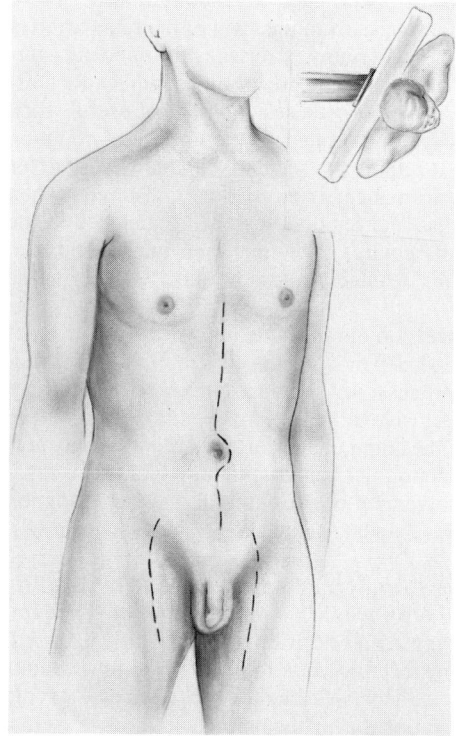

A

Fig. 21-12. Endarterectomy for atherosclerotic obstruction of the aortoiliac segments. *A.* A midline incision from xiphoid process to pubic symphysis is employed. Rotation of the operating table 30 to 40° to the right side facilitates retraction of the intestines. The thighs should be included in the operative field to permit exposure of the bifurcation of the common femoral arteries. *B.* The intestines are either encased in a plastic bag or covered with moist pads. The retroperitoneal tissues are incised exposing the aorta up to the left renal vein. *C.* The arteriotomy incisions are shown placed according to the distribution of the disease. *D.* Endarterectomy strippers may be used to separate the atherosclerotic cores in the iliac arteries. *E.* Following endarterectomy the distal intima is carefully attached to the arterial wall with vertically oriented interrupted sutures to prevent its dissection when circulation is reestablished. *F.* The multiple arteriotomies are either closed by direct suture or with roof patches of autologous vein or Dacron if the vessels are narrow.

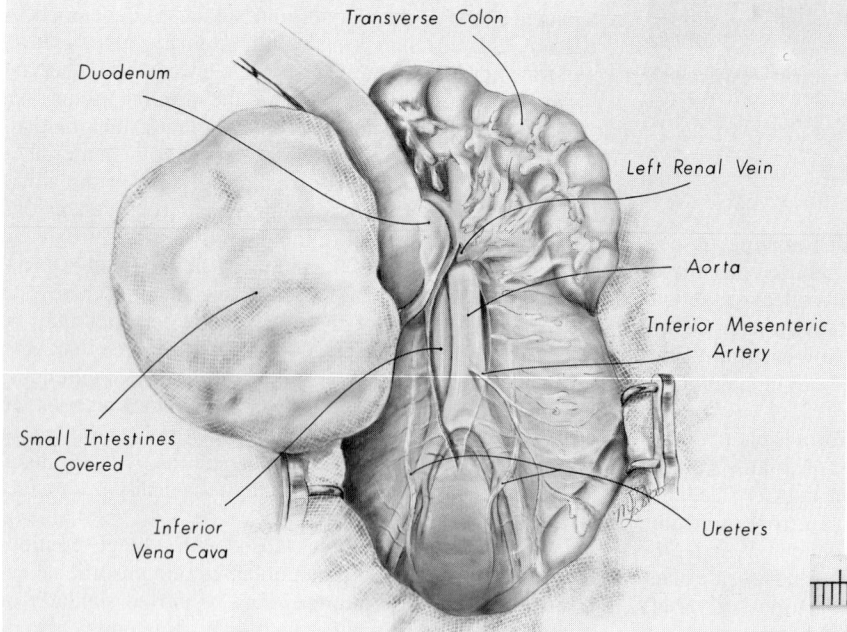

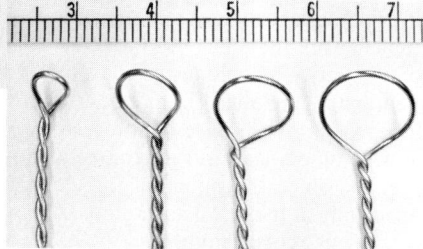

B

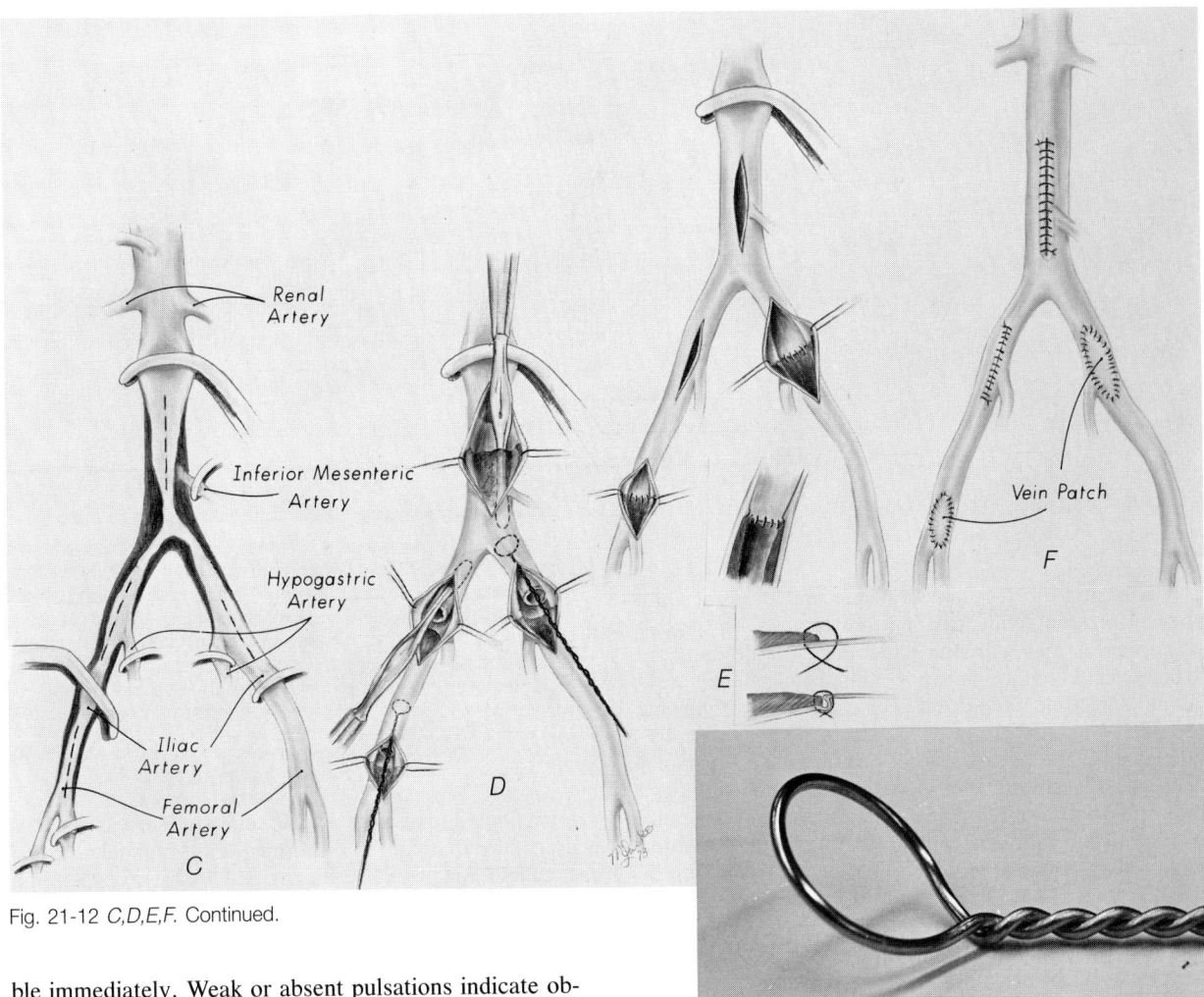

Renal Artery

Inferior Mesenteric Artery

Hypogastric Artery

Iliac Artery

Femoral Artery

C

D

E

Vein Patch

F

Fig. 21-12 *C,D,E,F.* Continued.

ble immediately. Weak or absent pulsations indicate obstruction from either retained plaques or stenotic suture lines, in which case the arteriotomy should be promptly reopened and the obstruction corrected. In such circumstances operative angiography is definitely needed, although completion arteriography is becoming more frequently employed.

Once blood flow is restored, heparin may be neutralized with protamine, giving 1 to 1.5 mg for each milligram of heparin used. Often, unless bleeding appears to be excessive, heparin is not neutralized by protamine administration. The posterior peritoneum is sutured over the reconstructed aorta (Fig. 21-12). A concomitant bilateral lumbar sympathectomy is a simple adjunct to the reconstructive procedure but not clearly beneficial. Many uncontrolled data, attesting to higher patency rates, are available regarding the beneficial effects of sympathectomy performed with arterial reconstruction. In our own series, sympathectomy has been performed on only rare occasions in association with arterial reconstruction, with no apparent effect on patency. When it is performed, the sympathetic chain can be identified by palpation as cordlike nodular structures parallel to the aorta on the left and just under the lateral border of the vena cava on the right.

Results and Prognoses. Immediate results of aortoiliac reconstructions are excellent. Nearly 100 percent patency rates can be achieved by meticulous technique and proper selection of operative procedures. The immediate functional results are predictable from the angiographic patterns of arterial involvement and the preoperative status of the patients (Fig. 21-13). Claudication is almost always relieved. If tissue loss with gangrene is present, however, additional reconstructive procedures in the distal arterial tree are needed in about 50 percent of the patients.

Following aortoiliac reconstruction, long-term patency rates range from 70 to 90 percent. The greatest risk for occlusion of the graft is recurrent stenosis from progressive fibrosis and narrowing of the arterial lumen at the distal anastomoses. Other late complications include false aneurysms at the proximal as well as the distal suture lines. Infection occurs in 1 to 2 percent of patients. The most devastating complication of aortoiliac bypass is aortoenteric fistula. These patients present with gastrointestinal bleeding usually into the third portion of the duodenum from the aortic suture line.

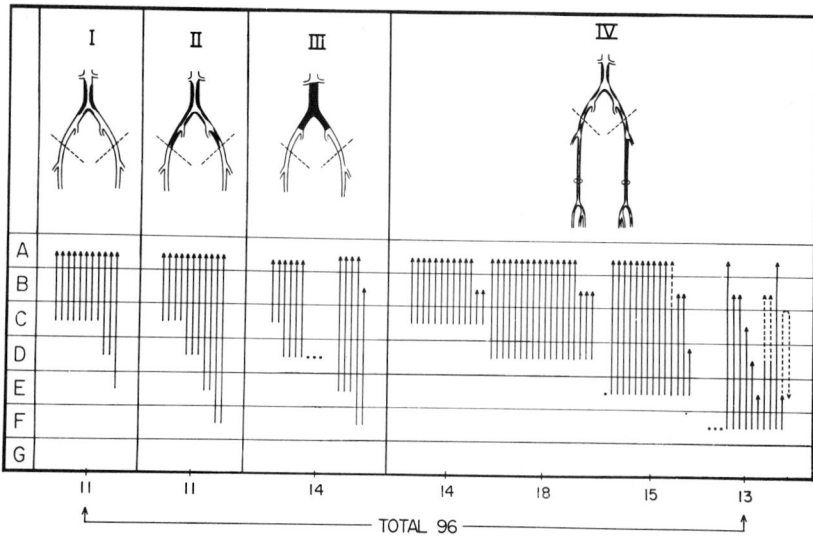

Fig. 21-13. Preoperative angiographic studies provide an excellent index of functional results that can be achieved by aortoiliacfemoral reconstructions. Functional categories *A* to *D* are increasing severities of claudication, while *E* and *F* represent rest pain and gangrene respectively. Even in the presence of disseminated distal occlusive lesions and ischemic lesions, aortoiliac reconstructions to the profunda femoris artery resulted in marked improvement. (From: *Imparato AM et al: Results in 96 aorto-iliac reconstructive procedures. Surgery 68:610, 1970, with permission.*)

It is clear from the data available that the procedure chosen for an individual patient must vary with the disease present and with the experience of the surgeon. Whichever technique is used, immediate patency rates should approach 100 percent. False aneurysms following the use of bypass grafts have greatly decreased in frequency with the use of synthetic sutures and the avoidance of excessive tension on the suture line, although they still occur too frequently. False aneurysms generally do not occur following endarterectomy, and infection with endarterectomy in which autologous tissue only is used, is rare. The principal cause of late death after operation is coronary arterial disease.

It is hoped that with recent advances in diagnosis and treatment of coronary artery disease, perioperative and postoperative deaths from myocardial infarction will be reduced. In recent years we have used the radioactive thallium cardiac function test to identify patients with the most severe coronary disease. Individuals with low left-ventricular ejection fractions are frequently subjected to coronary angiography. With this information, patients may be advised to (a) have coronary bypass surgery prior to undergoing aortic reconstruction, (b) have intensive medical therapy prior to aortic surgery, or (c) not undergo aortic reconstruction.

Extraanatomic Bypass Grafts. A number of factors have led to a growing interest in the use of extraanatomic bypass grafts to overcome the effects of aortoiliac occlusions. The magnitude of the direct aortic operation makes it less suitable for aged, debilitated patients and has led to the development of the axillofemoral and femorofemoral bypass grafts. The early success rate of extraanatomic grafts has made them useful in patients in whom early death from coronary or other vascular disease is quite high. Late graft failure, anastomotic aneurysms, and axillary artery thrombosis have made these procedures less applicable in patients who are good operative risks and have long life expectancies.

When the angiogram has shown the occlusive process

to be limited to a single iliac or common femoral artery, a procedure that can be performed with minimal risk and excellent long-term results is a femoral-cross-femoral bypass. This can be done under regional or even local anesthesia. After exposing both groins, a tunnel is made in the subcutaneous tissue connecting the groin incisions. A Dacron or a PTFE (polytetrafluoroethylene) graft is placed through the tunnel. End-to-side anastomoses are made to each femoral artery. Adjunctive procedures such as endarterectomy or vein patch angioplasty may be necessary depending on the extent of disease in the femoral vessels.

If the aorta and/or both iliac vessels are stenotic, it is necessary to find another inflow vessel for the reconstruction since the pressure will be reduced in both femoral arteries. In this situation, the axillary artery is used as the inflow source.

After suitable outflow tracts have been prepared, either unilaterally or bilaterally as the degree of ischemia of the extremities dictates, the axillary artery is exposed in the infraclavicular region. Care must be taken to select axillary arteries that are fully patent. Comparisons of bilateral upper extremity blood pressures are mandatory, since the relatively high incidence of subclavian arterial lesions, usually on the left side, may lead to graft failure. If a blood pressure differential exists or if supraclavicular bruits are heard, arch aortography is indicated. We now favor the right axillary artery, since the innominate, right subclavian complex seems to be involved less often by advanced atherosclerosis. An incision is made over the coracoid process parallel to the clavicle, exposing the pectoralis major muscle, which is divided in the direction of its fibers, exposing the tendon of the pectoralis minor muscle. This is severed from its attachment to the coracoid process, exposing the axillary artery surrounded by the brachial plexus. The artery is dissected free of these nerves, sometimes producing transient, partial brachial plexus neuropathies. The subscapular artery serves as a useful landmark and is usually though not invariably preserved. A curved tunneler is used to create a subcutaneous tunnel between the infraclavicular incision and the groin incision. When indicated, a suprapubic tunnel is made to connect groin incisions, thereby permitting an additional femorofemoral bypass graft. This latter addition to unilateral axillofemoral grafts is said by some to have a higher late patency rate than the unilateral axillofemoral alone or than bilateral separate axillofemoral grafts.

When doing extraanatomic bypass grafting, it is advisable to check the condition of the entire system with operative angiograms, since there are many pitfalls to the procedure. These include not only the usual problems with operations on atherosclerotic arteries but also accumulations of clot within the prosthesis caused by leakage of tissue thromboplastins and blood from the subcutaneous tunnel into the prosthesis. There are now series that suggest that the immediate and long-term patency rates for axillofemoral grafts are comparable to those for aortofemoral grafts; operative mortality is lower. They are subject to the same complications (such as false aneurysms and infection) as other prostheses anastomosed in the groin.

Balloon Angioplasty. Selected, usually short segmental areas of stenosis or even total occlusion of the common and external iliac arteries lend themselves to percutaneous passage of balloon catheters (Grüntzig) for the purpose of dilating those vessels if stenotic or restoring a lumen if totally occluded. In approximately 10 percent of patients, serious local complications occur and can include rupture of the vessel with retroperitoneal hemorrhage or total occlusion of a previously stenotic vessel, necessitating emergency surgical intervention. In carefully selected patients employing precisely the same indications for other types of surgical intervention, balloon dilation can produce dramatic improvement both radiographically and clinically and therefore is a technique that must be considered in the management of patients with aortoiliac occlusive disease. The technique may be helpful in dealing with multilevel occlusions, especially those in which localized hemodynamically significant lesions of the iliac arteries occur in association with extensive occlusive lesions of the femoral and popliteal in which the aortoiliac inflow lesions can be dilated with a balloon and the occlusive lesions in the thigh and calf are treated by conventional surgical techniques.

FEMOROPOPLITEAL OCCLUSIVE DISEASE

PATHOLOGY. The most common site for atherosclerotic occlusion in the lower extremities is the distal superficial femoral artery within the adductor canal. This may be related to the anatomic relationship between the distal femoral artery and adductor magnus tendon as the artery traverses the adductor foramen to enter the popliteal fossa. Occlusion extends gradually proximally in the superficial femoral artery until it is occluded at its origin from the common femoral. Occlusion of the profunda femoris artery is infrequent, however. Hence, atherosclerotic occlusion of the superficial femoral artery alone usually produces claudication but no more serious circulatory impairment.

The importance of the profunda femoris artery in arterial reconstructions of the aortoiliac system has been realized for many years, and correction of ostial stenoses, incident to femoral popliteal reconstructions, has been routinely performed by some. Recently Martin emphasized its importance as a valuable contributor of blood to the extremity in the presence of superficial femoral arterial occlusions, suggesting that the profunda femoris ostium be enlarged even in the absence of high-grade stenosis. Few direct measurements of flow have been made before and after this reconstruction.

When more extensive occlusive disease develops, usually from occlusion of the popliteal artery or its branches, the anterior and posterior tibial arteries, more serious circulatory insufficiency appears. With occlusion of this extent, ulceration and gangrene are common. Such diffuse patterns of atherosclerosis are particularly common in diabetic patients.

CLINICAL MANIFESTATIONS. Segmental occlusion of the superficial femoral artery produces claudication in the calf with moderate exercise, but no symptoms at rest. Physical examination finds a normal femoral pulse but absent popliteal and pedal pulses. Rarely pedal pulses are present at rest but disappear with exercise. The nutrition of the foot is normal. If additional occlusive disease is present beyond the femoral artery, claudication is more severe, perhaps associated with ischemic rest pain and trophic changes in the foot, and ulceration and gangrene ultimately ensue. Fortunately, the rate of progression of atherosclerotic occlusion is slow in many patients, and the risk of gangrene developing within 5 years in an extremity with claudication as the only symptom is only about 5 percent.

LABORATORY STUDIES. Arteriography is required to determine the segmental nature of the occlusive disease and the consequent possibilities of arterial reconstruction. Adequate visualization of the popliteal artery and its branches is essential (Fig. 21-14). With current techniques, revascularization procedures extended to the popliteal artery are quite satisfactory if the anterior or posterior tibial branches are patent. The peroneal artery, which does not directly contribute to the formation of the pedal arch, is less satisfactory. If all three branches are occluded, under special circumstances, reconstructive procedures may be to blind popliteal segments or extended down to the pedal arches of the foot. This is discussed under Tibioperoneal Arterial Disease. Noninvasive studies of the extremity in patients with localized superficial femoral arterial occlusions are of limited value in planning operative intervention and determining prog-

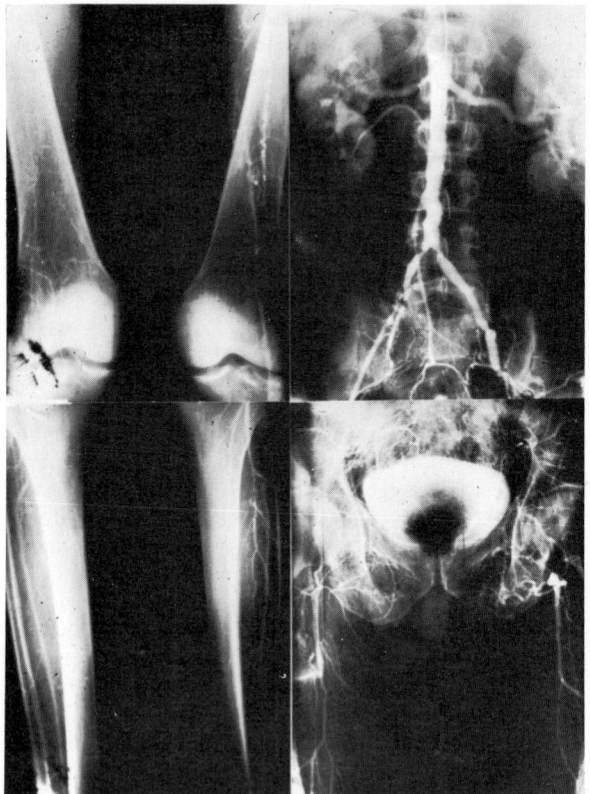

Fig. 21-14. Representative angiographic study required to evaluate patients for arterial reconstruction for claudication. Only in this manner can the inflow and outflow tracts be critically evaluated and arterial reconstructions planned.

nosis, although they are of considerable value in following the postoperative course of such patients and may detect the early signs of threatened graft failure.

TREATMENT. If claudication is the only symptom, operation is an elective decision, determined from the age and occupation of the patient. As the risk of gangrene with claudication alone is small, this alone does not constitute a clear-cut indication for operation. When trophic changes appear in the feet, operation is indicated because of the risk of gangrene. Care to avoid trauma to the foot, described in the section Aortoiliac Disease, is similarly applicable. The patient must avoid even minor trauma or exposure to extremes of heat or cold. Recommendations similar to those made for aortic occlusive disease regarding tobacco, alcohol, exercise, and vasodilatory drugs are applicable. In patients able to walk at least one city block, or 300 feet, a vigorous exercise program of walking at least 1 mile daily has resulted in marked improvement in claudication in at least 50 percent of patients within 6 to 12 months.

Direct Arterial Reconstruction. The basic principle of arterial reconstruction is that there must be both adequate inflow and adequate outflow of blood from the area of reconstruction. Early operative failures are almost always due either to obvious technical faults or to inadequate inflow or outflow.

A variety of techniques and materials have been used to reconstruct the superficial femoral and popliteal arteries. Bypass grafting has been performed using autologous vein (reversed saphenous, nonreversed in situ saphenous, femoral, brachial or cephalic), homograft vein (saphenous or umbilical), bovine arterial grafts, and prosthetic grafts (Dacron and PTFE). Endarterectomy of the superficial femoral and popliteal arteries has also been performed. Autologous reversed saphenous vein bypass has been the most frequently performed operation over the past three decades and remains the standard by which all other operations must be compared. Prosthetic grafts in general have decreased long-term patency rates and therefore are reserved for those situations in which autologous tissue cannot be used. Failure of prosthetic grafts has been related to kinking across joints, fibrointimal proliferation at distal suture lines, and dilatation of the grafts with the development of gelatinous thrombus in the lumen.

Both Wylie and Imparato described similar 5-year results following either endarterectomy or vein bypass. We compared three different techniques—venous bypass, long endarterectomy procedures with a venous roof patch, and endarterectomy performed through multiple arteriotomies with multiple vein roof patches—and found almost identical results 5 to 7 years later. Late failures were due to progressive distal atherosclerosis in one-third, to intimal proliferation in the areas of arterial reconstruction in another third, and to undetermined causes in the remainder.

Bypass Grafting. The technique of bypass grafting is illustrated in Fig. 21-15. It is particularly attractive because of its simplicity and ease of performance. The precision required for obtaining nearly 100 percent immediate patency can best be evaluated by operative angiography. Relatively small imperfections in the anastomotic suture lines or within the body of the graft can lead to deposition of platelet-fibrin aggregates with occlusion within a few hours.

The saphenous vein is carefully removed from the inguinal ligament to the knee, reversed to permit blood to flow in the direction of the venous valves, and then attached with end-to-side anastomoses to the femoral and popliteal arteries proximal and distal to the obstruction. If the vein is small, an alternative technique of leaving the vein in its bed in the nonreversed position has been successfully used. With this in situ method, the valves of the vein are disrupted by passage of an instrument along the course of the vein. Care also must be taken to interrupt the tributaries of the vein, otherwise arteriovenous fistulas will form once the bypass is completed. There are reports of in situ grafts with veins as small as 2 mm in diameter. This technique is particularly useful for long bypasses to the tibial or peroneal arteries since it allows the surgeon to use long, narrow veins and also to have more compatible vessels for suturing at both the proximal and distal anastomoses. The vein should be at least 4 to 5 mm in diameter.

Endarterectomy. Since its introduction over 35 years ago, between 1951 and 1953, endarterectomy has been

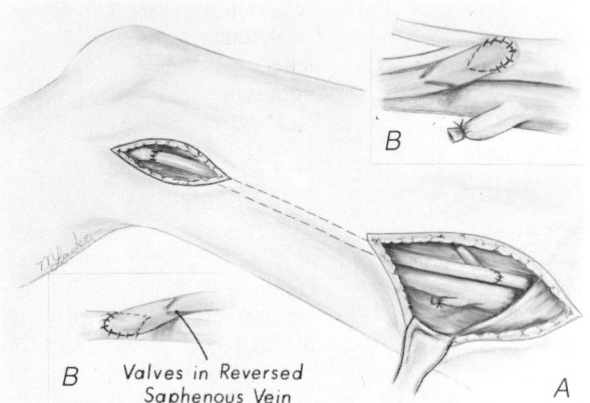

Fig. 21-15. Bypass graft procedure for occlusion of the superficial femoral artery. *A.* Incisions employed for exposure of the major vessels. A proximal incision is made over the saphenous vein from just below the inguinal ligament to the apex of Scarpa's triangle, avoiding undermining of adjacent skin flaps which might result in ischemic necrosis. The distal incision is made on the medial aspect of the popliteal fossa to expose the popliteal artery. The adductor magnus tendon, the site often of most severe superficial femoral arterial involvement, is shown. It is frequently cut to facilitate passing the vein graft from adductor canal to popliteal fossa. *B.* Completed bypass graft of the reversed saphenous vein. The anastomoses are performed end-to-side to the common femoral and popliteal arteries. The vein is brought either subcutaneously or through the subsartorial canal. Inserts show details of the bevel created in the vein bypass and reversal of the valves. An alternative technique is to leave the saphenous vein in its usual location, without reversal, destroying the valves, accomplishing an in situ nonreversed bypass graft.

modified several times. A completely open technique that involved incising the artery throughout its length, removing the atherosclerotic core, and suturing the long arteriotomy had a very high failure rate. Similarly, closed techniques with mechanical strippers often failed, usually due to leaving loose fragments of intima or atherosclerotic plaque in the lumen. Closure of the long arteriotomy with a vein roof patch, developed by Edwards et al., gave significantly better results. A subsequent modification was the use of multiple vein roof patches to close multiple arteriotomies used for semiclosed endarterectomy. This technique is illustrated in Fig. 21-16. Operative angiography is essential to be certain that atherosclerotic debris has been entirely removed from the lumen.

TIBIOPERONEAL ARTERIAL DISEASE

PATHOLOGY. Occlusive disease of the tibial arteries occurs most commonly in patients with diabetes mellitus, in patients with Buerger's disease, and in some instances of arterioarterial embolism.

In the diabetic patient for unknown reasons there are different patterns of disease that can be recognized. All tibial arteries as well as the pedal arches may be occluded. In such instances surgical reconstruction is impossible. In other patients one or more of the tibial arteries may be entirely patent, or there may be proximal occlusion with patent vessels starting at the level of the malleoli. With this pattern of involvement, arterial reconstruction is possible if grafts are extended to the ankles. In some diabetic patients there is additional disease in the aortoiliac or femoral areas that must be dealt with.

CLINICAL MANIFESTATIONS. Tibial arterial occlusions may merely produce claudication of the foot or, more often, advanced ischemia. Diabetic neuropathy may be difficult to differentiate from ischemic rest pain. Characteristically, ischemic pain is relieved by placing the foot in a dependent position, while that of diabetic neuropathy is not. A frequent problem in the diabetic patient is ulceration on the plantar surface of the foot, secondary to pressure associated with diabetic neuropathy. A more serious problem is a spreading necrotizing infection, with absent pedal pulses. Because of associated ischemia the infection is often refractory to both antibiotic therapy and surgical debridement unless revascularization can be done. This type of progressive, refractory infection may lead to amputation before tissue ischemia per se has caused widespread necrosis. Infection undoubtedly increases the metabolic requirements of the tissue and thereby accentuates the degree of ischemia. A third type of terminal event in the ischemic diabetic foot is soft tissue atrophy to a severe degree, terminating with progressive, ischemic dry gangrene of the toes and foot.

LABORATORY STUDIES. Precise angiography is essential to determine the adequacy of the proximal circulation in the aorta and iliac arteries, as well as in the distal arterial tree, especially the small arteries of the ankle and foot. Significant advances in the technique of angiography have permitted excellent delineation of small arterial branches in these areas. Such studies may be done by direct needle puncture of the femoral artery, followed by injection of a large bolus (50 mL) of contrast medium with serial films made over a long period of time (Fig. 21-17). An alternative technique is to produce ischemic vasodilation by temporary arterial occlusion with an inflated blood pressure cuff for 5 min or longer, injecting the dye immediately after deflation of the cuff. This almost invariably produces excellent opacification of distal vessels.

TREATMENT. Unless the extremity is in jeopardy, arterial reconstructions into the tibial arteries are avoided because of the unpredictable outcome in any particular patient. When a reconstruction fails, amputation is usually necessary because the trauma of surgical dissection usually impairs collateral circulation to a significant degree. If operation is not considered indicated, treatment is primarily directed at careful avoidance of foot trauma, as emphasized in the preceding sections.

Surgical reconstruction is most successful if it is to a tibial artery that communicates with a patent pedal arch. Bypasses to peroneal arteries or incomplete tibial vessels are associated with a high incidence of early and late graft failure. In some cases when the pedal arch is thrombosed, even a patent reconstruction may not relieve the ischemia of the distal foot. In these difficult situations, desperate attempts to perform vascular reconstruction may compromise the inevitable amputation. In particular, nonhealing wounds may lead to a below-knee amputation where a transmetatarsal procedure would have suc-

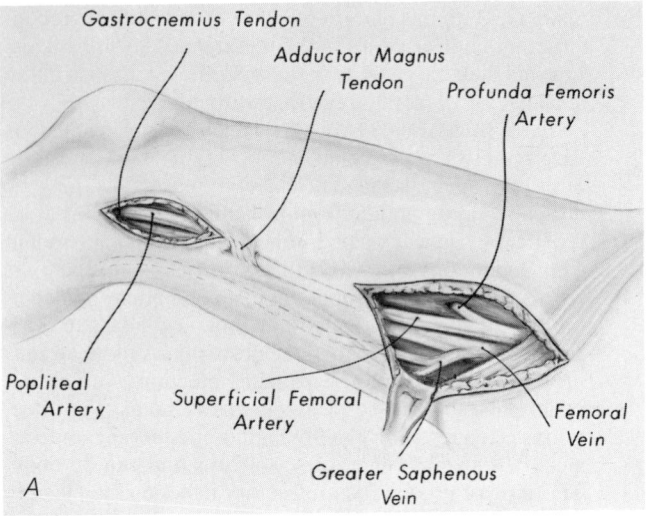

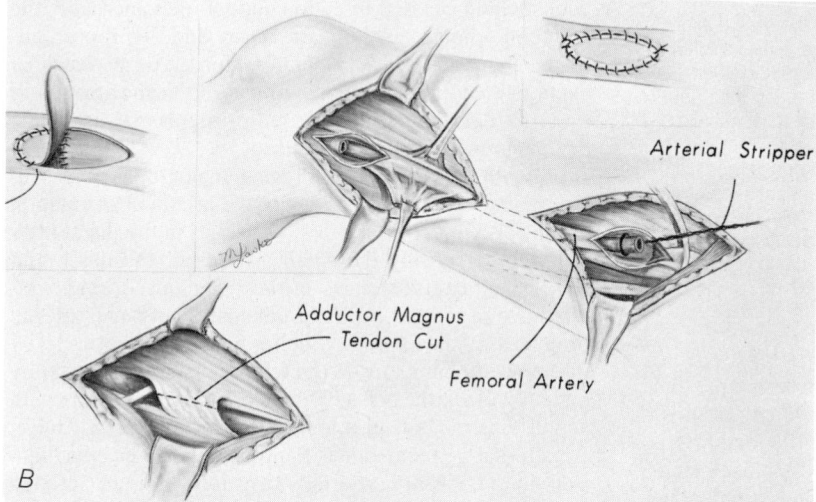

Fig. 21-16. *A.* Femoral popliteal endarterectomy performed by exposing the femoral artery proximally and the popliteal artery distad. *B.* An endarterectomy stripper is used to detach atherosclerotic material via a plane in the media or between media and adventitia. Cutting the adductor magnus tendon facilitates passage of the arterial stripper. The distal intima in the popliteal artery is carefully sutured to prevent detachment and dissection of this free edge when circulation is restored. Arteriotomies are closed with autologous vein roof patches. Angiographic studies are performed to ensure that all debris has been removed, since even minute fragments left behind may result in immediate rethrombosis. Alternative techniques include exposing the entire femoral artery, opening it longitudinally in its entirety and suturing a long roof patch for closure, utilizing CO_2 intramural injection to accomplish endarterectomy, or utilizing a vibrating ring endarterectomy stripper.

ceeded, or an above-knee amputation may become necessary where a below-knee would have succeeded.

When a necrotizing infection is present, characteristically extending as a necrotic phlegmon rather than as an abscess and requiring debridement as opposed to drainage, therapy is almost hopeless without arterial reconstruction. A combined approach of debridement of all infected tissue followed by revascularization into the distal tibial and malleolar vessels has been successful. As a practical guideline, if more than one-half of the sole of the foot has been destroyed, the limb will never be suitable for weight bearing, despite effective arterial reconstruction; so amputation is the primary choice. In all such difficult problems intensive antibiotic therapy for the specific organism involved is essential.

Direct Arterial Reconstruction. Direct arterial reconstructions to the tibial arteries have been successfully performed employing reversed autologous saphenous vein, in situ saphenous vein, and even Goretex. The critical distal anastomoses can be made to accessible portions of the tibial arteries in the calf and ankle to as low as the

level of the malleoli (Fig. 21-18). Combinations of endarterectomy and bypass procedures are possible to the level of the upper third of the calf; in our experience endarterectomy is impossible below that level.

Late results are gratifying when performed for impending limb loss, with limb salvage rates of greater than 50 percent being achieved to as late as the tenth year of

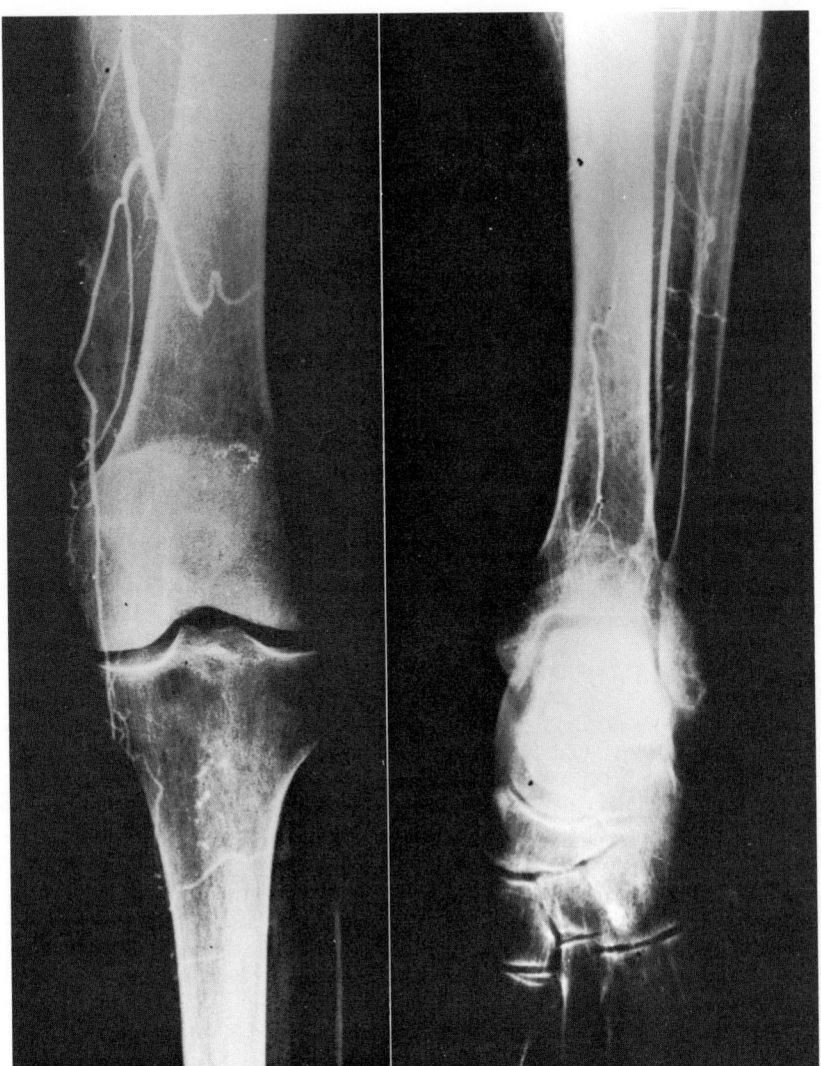
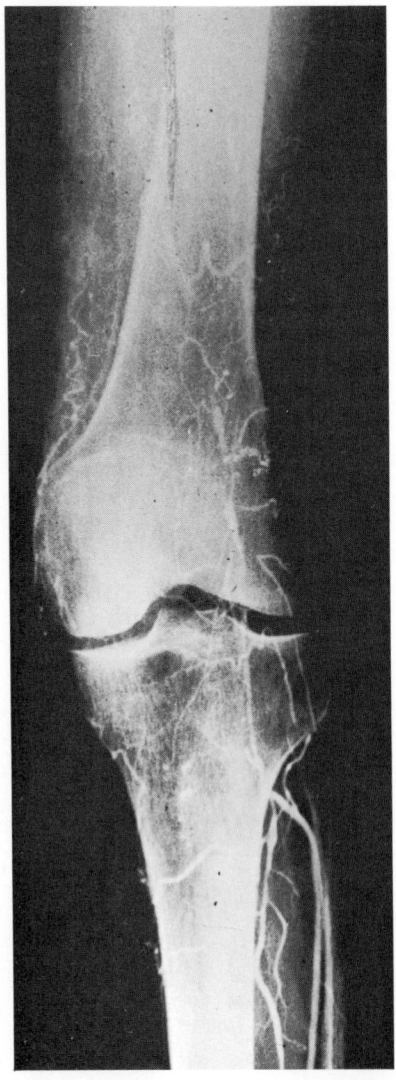

A   *B*

Fig. 21-17. Preoperative angiographic studies in the presence of tibial disease. *A*. Angiographic studies routinely performed showing poor visualization of tibial arteries. *B*. Angiogram in the same patient obtained 6 weeks later, when an ischemic lesion developed in the foot, showing patency of the anterior tibial artery. This degree of opacification was obtained using the ischemic hyperemia technique described in the text.

follow-up, although late patency rates of bypass grafts of tibial arteries may be no more than 10 percent by the tenth year.

The details of surgical technique are critically important and require the use of optical magnification, very fine suture material, and immediate intraoperative angiography upon completion of anastomoses to correct any minor imperfections that result from the surgical manipulations.

Prognosis. As mentioned earlier, arterial reconstructions in this area are performed only when ulceration and gangrene threaten amputation. Arterial reconstruction is initially successful in about 85 percent of patients, both

with reconstruction at the proximal tibioperoneal level and with reconstruction extending down to the malleolus. Immediate failures are almost always due to technical errors or inadequate outflow tracts. Failures occur if the dorsal arch at the ankle is not complete. When the reconstruction is initially successful, limb salvage is excellent, for the necrotic tissue can be debrided and the wound subsequently closed by skin grafting. If the arterial reconstruction fails before complete healing is obtained, however, amputation is usually required.

If healing is complete and the arterial reconstruction subsequently becomes occluded, a significant percentage of patients remain with a viable functional extremity. Some reconstructions into the proximal tibial arteries so far have remained patent for as long as 10 years with limb salvage exceeding 50 percent. Fewer data are available for bypass grafts extending down to the ankle, but the failure rate within 2 years after operation seems to exceed 50 percent, while some reconstructions are still patent up to 7 years.

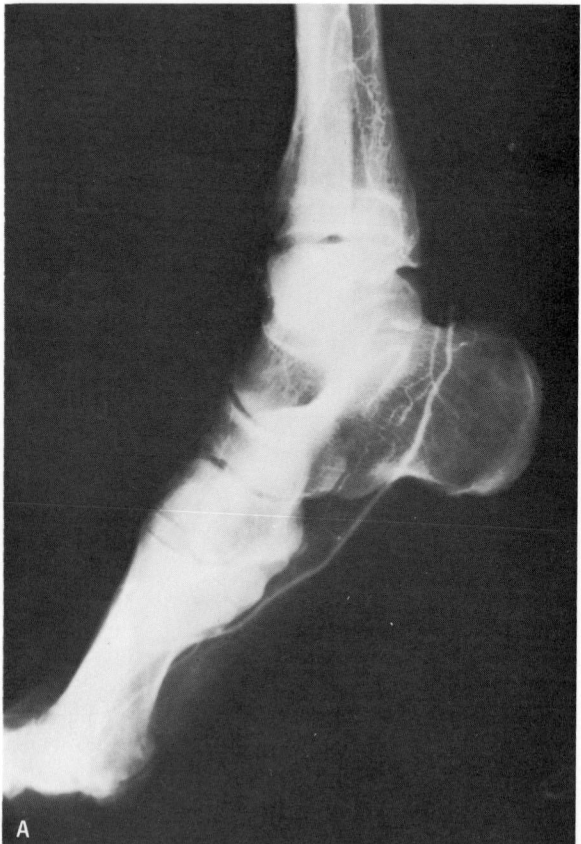

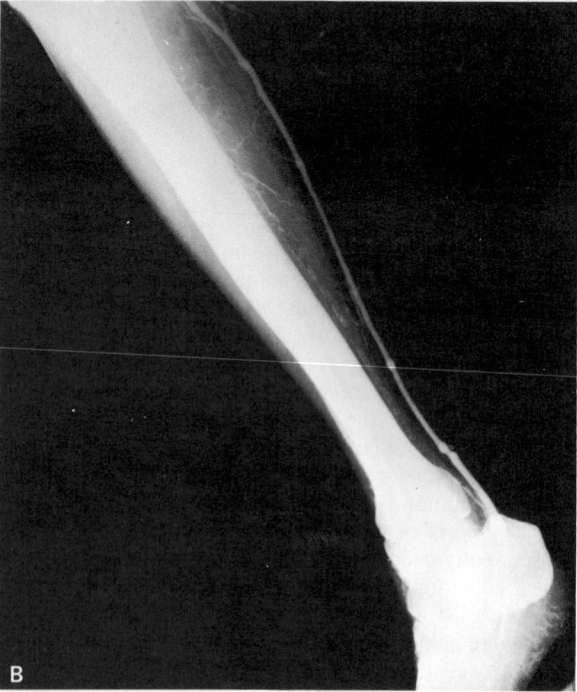

Fig. 21-18. *A.* Operative prereconstruction angiogram showing pedal arch. *B.* Postreconstruction operative angiogram showing reversed autologous saphenous vein bypass graft to the posterior tibial artery at malleolar level.

GENERAL CONSIDERATIONS

COMPLICATIONS OF ARTERIAL RECONSTRUCTIONS.
The most common complication after arterial reconstruction is graft thrombosis. In the early postoperative period, reoperation is usually worthwhile since minor technical errors can result in rapid aggregation of platelets and graft thrombosis. Careful intraoperative analysis using angiography as well as visual inspection of the suture lines often reveals the site of failure. With appropriate corrective action, most grafts can be salvaged. For late graft failures, angiography is essential to planning therapy. Reports of successful treatment with thrombolytic agents and, in some cases, balloon angioplasty have been encouraging. In very late graft failures, decisions to perform reoperation must follow the same criteria used for the original procedure. It has frequently been observed that among patients operated for threatened limb loss, only half go on to require secondary reconstructions if the initial graft fails. Frequently these patients presented initially with a nonhealing ulcer or infections secondary to trauma. If the wounds heal during the period of graft patency, it does not necessarily follow that the wounds will reappear with graft occlusion. Also, in some instances the graft has given the patient time to develop new collateral circulation that then can sustain the limb after the occlusion.

Infected Prosthesis. The large number of patients now alive with artificial, plastic blood vessel replacements has introduced a numerically significant new pathologic entity, viz., the infected plastic prosthesis. Plastic blood vessel substitutes, especially if placed in the groins, are subject to infection that usually cannot be eradicated unless the plastic material is removed from the infected area. Axillofemoral bypass grafts have been employed to permit removal of infected intraabdominal grafts. Infections in the groin, in the presence of noninfected intraabdominal arteries, have been treated by performing iliac to superficial femoral or popliteal bypass grafts, avoiding the infected groin by leading the graft through the obturator foramen to the posteromedial aspect of the thigh or to the medial aspect of the popliteal fossa, thus permitting the radical debridement of infected tissue and grafts from the groins. These have been highly successful when properly planned in association with prolonged antibiotic therapy. These procedures are indicated at a stage when infection may appear relatively innocuous. Injection of a radiopaque contrast medium into the sinuses has been helpful in delineating the true nature and extent of the problem. Aggressive and extensive surgical procedures are required to prevent exsanguinating hemorrhage from breakdown of suture lines secondary to the local infection. Although obturator bypass grafts have been successful in dealing with infections in the groins, removal of aortic prosthesis with end closure of the infrarenal aorta has resulted frequently in subsequent rupture of the aorta.

Lumbar Sympathectomy. Lumbar sympathectomy is often tried in desperation as an alternative to amputation when arterial reconstruction cannot be performed. It also may be combined with reconstruction, although its value in this case cannot be determined. As an isolated procedure, improvement can be significant in 20 to 60 percent of patients in this group. Occasionally a brilliant result occurs, consisting of relief of rest pain and marked increase in temperature of the foot. Unfortunately it has not been possible to predict which patients with impending limb loss would respond favorably. Therefore, in our series all patients, whether diabetic or not, whose conditions were considered inoperable from the point of view of arterial reconstruction on the basis of angiographic studies had lumbar sympathectomies. Some 60 percent responded favorably for longer than 6 months, while 40 percent came to early amputation within 2 months. Extensive gangrene of the forefoot was an unfavorable prognostic sign.

The technique of performing sympathectomy with a percutaneous injection of phenol in the region of the lumbar ganglia has proven to be equally effective and much less hazardous for the patient with lower extremity ischemia. We have used this technique exclusively for the past 5 years when a sympathetic ablation is desired.

Amputation. (See Also Chap. 44.) Some important guidelines should be emphasized when amputation threatens because of progressive ulceration of the foot. First, an arterial reconstructive procedure may be successful if only one major arterial branch is patent, such as a branch of the popliteal artery, the anterior tibial, the posterior tibial, or even the peroneal artery. Second, a foot will remain useful for weight bearing as long as the posterior half, including the heel, is intact. If more than 50 percent of the sole has been lost, however, the foot is probably useless for weight bearing even if arterial reconstruction is successful. With these two guidelines, angiograms should be seriously considered for virtually all patients in whom amputation is being considered. Of 100 patients threatened by amputation, either because of rest pain (38 percent) or ulceration with gangrene (62 percent), arterial reconstructive procedures were performed in 73 and lumbar sympathectomy in 13. The leg was salvaged in 64, and a minor amputation was possible in 10 others.

Both morbidity and mortality are surprisingly high in patients requiring amputation for peripheral vascular disease. Mortality is related to the advanced age in many and to the rate of severe coronary occlusive disease among patients exceeding 50 percent. Morbidity is primarily related to failure of wound healing from improper selection of the site of amputation. In general, as long as gangrene is limited to a toe, the amputation should be delayed and the ischemic toe permitted to mummify and undergo virtual autoamputation. Delay permits growth of collateral circulation in the more proximal tissues so that wound healing may occur if the toe is allowed to gradually separate over a period of weeks; a definite amputation often results in failure and extension of the wound onto the foot. A transmetatarsal amputation may be effective in some diabetic patients when infection superimposed upon a gangrenous toe requires operation. This is successful if pedal pulses are palpable but ineffective if gangrene has extended into the forefoot. Foot amputations proximal to the transmetatarsal level are generally unsatisfactory for weight bearing except for Syme's amputation, which is almost never successful in the presence of peripheral vascular disease.

Below-knee amputations can be successfully performed in a high percentage of patients, even in the absence of a popliteal pulse. Preservation of the knee joint greatly facilitates the wearing of a prosthesis. Guidelines are still being sought to determine the likelihood of wound healing if a below-knee amputation is performed in the absence of a popliteal pulse. The degree of skin bleeding is one of the most useful guidelines, though not infallible, that has yet appeared. Preoperatively, segmental Doppler pressure determinations and radioactive xenon uptake studies have been employed to predict the healing of amputations both at the below-knee level and at the metatarsal level. A below-knee amputation is a significant benefit to the patient if successful but is detrimental if the wound fails to heal and a subsequent above-knee amputation must be performed.

THE DIABETIC FOOT

The foot of the diabetic patient has distinct characteristics and can quickly progress to threaten limb and life. The diabetic has an extraordinary susceptibility to infection. After a seemingly trivial injury, within hours or days a virulent necrotizing infection can appear that rapidly spreads along musculofascial planes. It characteristically begins in an interdigital space, spreads along the plantar fascia, and may continue along tendon sheaths into the muscles of the leg. Frequently the infecting organism is gas producing and may be of the clostridial group. A life-threatening infection quickly evolves. These infections often occur with patent major arteries and seemingly are not closely related to local ischemia.

A second peculiarity of the diabetic is diabetic neuropathy. Characteristically this appears as hypalgesia or true anesthesia of some portion of the sole of the foot, subsequently complicated by trophic ulcers. These also are unrelated to ischemia and often develop with strongly palpable pedal pulses. The trophic ulcer, anesthetic and painless initially, then becomes a portal of entry for necrotizing infection.

In the diabetic foot the arterial occlusive disease typically involves the popliteal artery and its branches down to the pedal arches. The process may be diffuse, or one or more arteries may be spared. Arteries proximal to the popliteal may be normal or may show a typical "nondiabetic" pattern of atherosclerosis. The microangiopathy that is present in diabetics and appears to play a major role in the lesions that develop in the kidney and in the retina of the eye does not appear to play such a role in the ischemic conditions that afflict the foot. If the macroangiopathy can be corrected by revascularization procedures performed to the pedal arteries if necessary, the most severe degrees of ischemia can be reversed. Whether microangiopathy plays a role in the susceptibility to infection is not clear, although radical debridement without correction of the angiopathy in the presence of patent or restored major arteries results in control of the infection.

CLINICAL MANAGEMENT. Infection. In some instances a rampant uncontrolled infection with clostridia may necessitate immediate open amputation through the midcalf or midthigh to prevent death from septic shock. If patients are seen earlier, immediate widespread incision and drainage with debridement of infected tissue may prevent amputation. At an earlier stage, when infection is the dominant process without extensive tissue necrosis, localized debridement combined with intensive antibiotic therapy may be successful. A basic guideline is that all necrotic tissue must be extensively debrided, because simple drainage is hopelessly inadequate in the presence of extensive tissue necrosis, as is radical debridement alone because of the underlying tissue ischemia. In such instances the combination of radical debridement with arterial reconstruction down to the ankle may permit salvage of the extremity.

Gangrene. If gangrene of a toe is present and not complicated by infection, a much more leisurely approach is indicated, quite in contrast to the urgency of therapy if spreading infection is present. Localized dry gangrene of a toe is best treated by postponing operation, often permitting autoamputation over a period of weeks, during which time the development of collateral circulation may permit wound healing to occur. In all likelihood such instances of gangrene of a digit represent occlusion of a critical digital vessel. This may be followed by the development of enough collateral circulation to salvage the foot, but such circulation requires time to develop.

Trophic Ulcers. A trophic ulcer can be readily recognized by several characteristics. It is usually a sharply demarcated, punched out area on the sole of the foot overlying a pressure point, usually the metatarsal heads. A location over the first or third metatarsal head is particularly common. Often the ulcers are completely anesthetic and hence relatively free of pain until secondary infection develops. Similarly, the pedal pulses may be entirely normal.

Treatment in the majority of patients consists of local cleansing, protection from trauma, and most important of all, avoidance of weight bearing. Reconstruction of shoes to distribute weight differently is often effective. Special types of shoes, such as those lined with lamb's wool, are useful. Effective therapy requires long-term careful periodic observation to readjust the weight-bearing characteristics of the foot so that pressure on the area of ulceration is avoided. Any superimposed infection requires antibiotics and local debridement. As most patients do not have any vascular occlusion, arterial reconstruction is not needed.

Occlusive Disease of the Upper Extremity

Upper extremity ischemia can result from a variety of conditions, often complex and difficult to diagnose, unlike lower extremity ischemia where arteriosclerosis and embolic occlusions are the major etiologic conditions. Severe ischemia is more apt to present as focal gangrene of the fingers rather than threatened loss of the entire extremity. The ischemia is less apt to be associated with surgically correctable causes and may require extensive investigation to determine cause and treatment.

PATHOLOGY. The upper extremity is singularly free of occlusive atherosclerotic disease, although atherosclerosis is occasionally encountered in a particularly severe form in young patients with presenile arteriosclerosis. Major arterial occlusions result from emboli originating in the heart, from thoracic outlet compression, from vascular trauma associated with fractures of long bones, and from thrombotic occlusions following the introduction of catheters into upper extremity arteries. These conditions account for most of the surgical interventions required upon upper extremity arteries. Occlusions of aortic arch vessels caused by arteritis or atherosclerosis occasionally warrant intervention to relieve upper extremity ischemia. A host of conditions, including scleroderma, lupus erythematosus, mixed connective tissue diseases, and allergic necrotizing arteritis, affect the small arteries and arterioles of the hands. Occupational injury in workers who use vibrating tools or who inflict trauma upon the hypothenar eminences with the use of hammers, constitutes another group of etiologic factors. Vasospastic disorders presenting with Raynaud's phenomenon constitute a group of disorders peculiar to the upper extremity. A partial listing of conditions that may be associated with upper extremity ischemia is shown in Table 21-2.

PATHOPHYSIOLOGY. Stenosis in major arteries becomes hemodynamically significant only after the cross-sectional area of the artery has been reduced by 75 percent or more, corresponding to a 50 percent or greater reduction in diameter. The compensatory mechanisms in the upper extremity consist of opening and enlargement of collateral channels with dilatation of arterioles. These effectively reduce peripheral resistance distal to a stenotic or occluded artery and are very efficient. Consequently, isolated chronic obstructions and occlusions of the subclavian, axillary, brachial, or even radial or ulnar arteries are well tolerated. Peripheral pulses may be palpable and the extremity may remain symptom-free unless increased metabolic demands are created by exercise, or vasospasm related to the exposure to cold ensues. Acute occlusions of these major arteries may produce more pronounced ischemia because collateral channels may not have time to enlarge, and thrombi may propagate proximal and distal to areas of acute occlusion obstructing collateral channels. Emboli tend to lodge at bifurcations, thereby obstructing main channels as well as collateral channels. Consequently, distal pressures are often reduced, resting flow may be severely diminished, and arterial pulses may disappear. Compensatory mechanisms in the upper extremity are sufficiently active that recovery from even acute arterial occlusions may be quite prompt; improvement in distal flow may occur within relatively few hours as evidenced by the return of palpable pulses.

Vasomotor tone, controlled by the influence of the sympathetic nervous system on the arteriolar bed, can be dramatically affected by exposure to cold, emotional stimuli, and respiratory reflexes. These effects are most impressive in patients afflicted with Raynaud's phenomenon.

Table 21-2. CAUSES OF UPPER EXTREMITY ISCHEMIA

I. Major arterial occlusions
  A. Arteriosclerosis
    1. Atherosclerosis (aortic arch vessels)
    2. Aneurysms (subclavian)
    3. Embolization
      a. Cardiac
      b. Arterioarterial
  B. Trauma
    1. Blunt and penetrating injuries
    2. Iatrogenic
      a. Arteriography, cardiac catheterization, arterial monitoring
      b. Dialysis shunts, occlusions of axillofemoral arterial bypasses
    3. Parenteral drug abuse
  C. Thoracic outlet compression (arterial)
  D. Arteritis
    1. Giant cell arteritis and Takayasu's syndrome
    2. Buerger's disease
II. "Small" vessel occlusions and vasospasm
  A. Autoimmune diseases
    1. Scleroderma
    2. Lupus erythematosus
    3. Rheumatoid arthritis
    4. Mixed connective tissue disorders
    5. Polyarteritis
    6. Allergic
  B. Blood dyscrasias
    1. Cryoglobulinemia
    2. Cold agglutinins
    3. Polycythemia
  C. Trauma
    1. Vibrating tools
    2. Hypothenar hammer syndrome
    3. Frostbite
    4. Radiation injury
    5. Electrical burns
  D. Drug poisoning
    1. Ergot
  E. Uremia
    1. Arteriopathy

CLINICAL MANIFESTATIONS. The clinical manifestations of upper extremity ischemia are determined by the site of arterial occlusion, by the rapidity with which it occurs, and by the mechanism responsible, be it spasm, embolic occlusion, or chronic long-standing or intermittent obstruction. A common clinical entity of acute ischemia is seen in the patient who is subjected to cardiac catheterization through a brachial artery that then becomes occluded. There may be blanching, relatively mild numbness with some easy fatigability of the hand when performing repetitive motions, and absent pulses at the wrist, all of which may appear immediately following occlusion. Within 12 to 24 h there may be a return of a weak radial or ulnar pulse with reappearance of normal color and warm skin. Ischemia may be apparent only when comparing the two extremities raised overhead. Over a period of days or weeks, except under unusual exertion of the hand and forearm or by the use of sophisticated noninvasive testing of segmental pressure or digital pulse volume recordings, all signs of ischemia may have disap-

peared. On the other hand, embolic occlusion may result in progressive ischemia of the entire hand and forearm. In instances of chronic long-standing ischemia, abnormalities may be detected only by careful noninvasive testing or by arteriographic survey, and hand and forearm claudication be minimal.

Occlusion of more distal vessels, as in the hand, due either to microembolization or various types of arteritis, may result in a mottled appearance of the fingertips. This may progress to gangrene with severe pain, even in the presence of palpable pulses at the wrist.

Vasospasm can be quite dramatic; a pink, warm hand may suddenly become ashen or cyanotic and mottled in its entirety, or there may be blanching of single digits that on recovery may pass through a phase of hyperemia before normal color returns.

DIAGNOSIS. The diagnosis of upper extremity ischemia requires a careful history to determine if the ischemia is due primarily to chronic occlusion, to acute occlusion, to intermittent occlusion, or to vasospasm. The circumstances leading to the ischemia must be elicited. An occupational history and a history of drug ingestion must be taken. The physical examination must include a record of the appearance of the extremity and the pulse pattern, including the presence or absence of digital pulses. Palpation of the supraclavicular region may detect the presence of a subclavian artery aneurysm, and palpation of the infraclavicular area may reveal prominent pulsation produced by poststenotic dilatation associated with a cervical rib. Auscultation in this area for bruit must be performed, not only in the neutral resting posture, but also during the shoulder girdle maneuvers. The Allen test is used to determine the patency of the palmar arches. (See the section Thoracic Outlet Syndromes.)

Segmental pressure measurements may define the site of occlusion. Digital pressure measurements or plethysmographic studies combined with physical examination of arm and forearm arteries may help differentiate hand and digital vessel occlusions from vasospastic phenomena and more proximal occlusions. By recording digital pulse volumes and determining digital pulse contours plethysmographically following exposure to heat, cold, or emotional stress, vasomotor tone may be defined. The most definitive examination is angiography. This is done by passing a catheter to the level of the aortic arch through the femoral artery to permit radiographic visualization of the entire upper extremity from the origin of the major vessels to the digital tufts. Complete angiography helps to differentiate between the four major causes of upper extremity ischemia: thrombus, embolus, and vasospastic or arteriopathic disorders. When the occlusive process is predominantly in the arteries of the hand and digits, one must carefully review the angiographic studies for a site from which microemboli might have originated. The major systemic conditions that must be searched for include scleroderma and the CRST syndrome, which includes digital skin binding, telangiectasias, digital calcinosis, and Raynaud's phenomenon. The antinuclear antibody should be measured; Coombs' test coupled with serum complement should be performed; LE cells should be looked for, and SLE antibody against native DNA should be investigated. Mixed connective tissue disease can be detected by an abnormality in circulating antinuclear antibody directed against acid nuclear proteins.

SURGICAL TREATMENT. Severe hand ischemia associated with occlusive lesions of the subclavian, brachial, or antecubital arteries is the prime indication for arterial reconstruction surgery in the upper extremity. Digital arterial occlusions without proximal major arterial occlusions are not amenable to surgical intervention. The specific surgical procedures to be performed on the arterial system depend on the mechanism of occlusion and its site. Proximal reconstructive procedures are best performed using autologous tissue. Vein patches are used to close arteriotomies of arteries that are frequently smaller than those encountered in the lower extremities.

Lesions of the innominate and subclavian arteries are often amenable to bypass procedures with plastic arterial prostheses anastomosing the proximal end to the ascending aorta and the distal end to the most proximal portion of the axillary artery. The brachial and antecubital arteries are best managed either by autologous vein bypass procedures, or, where iatrogenic injury has occurred, by thrombectomy and venous patch angioplasty. Although the forearm arteries are amenable to disobliteration of embolic occlusions, it is unusual for there to be a need to perform direct arterial reconstructions on those vessels. Operations on the palmar arteries, except for small aneurysms that may have been the origin of emboli, are rarely necessary. Digital arterial reconstructions are employed for occlusion induced by acute trauma.

Sympathectomy may be of value in vasospastic disorders and will be discussed under Raynaud's Disease. Combinations of thoracic outlet decompression and arterial reconstruction are discussed under Thoracic Outlet Syndromes.

PROGNOSIS. The prognosis for a patient with a major arterial occlusion of the upper extremity, acute or chronic, is generally excellent. Recovery from an acute occlusion is generally satisfactory even without surgical intervention. When surgical intervention is required, complete or nearly complete restoration of flow is usually achieved. The vasospastic disorders infrequently require surgical intervention on the arterial system, except when small-vessel occlusions are secondary to atheroembolization, as from the subclavian artery at the thoracic outlet or from the innominate or left subclavian arteries at their origins from the aortic arch. Medical therapy is usually satisfactory in the vasospastic disorders unless the underlying metabolic disorder is rapidly progressive, in which case, digital gangrene often leads to multiple amputations. The results of sympathectomy are variable and unpredictable.

Extracranial Occlusive Cerebrovascular Disease

HISTORICAL CONSIDERATIONS. One of the most astonishing historical facts of twentieth century medicine relates to the belated recognition 35 years ago that the majority of ischemic strokes are due to occlusive atherosclerotic disease of the extracranial arteries in the neck, not to intravascular arterial occlusions. The earliest recorded recognition of this possible relationship was made by Wepfer in 1658, rediscovered by Savory in 1856, and again by Hung in 1914. The latter described the postmortem findings of infarction of a cerebral hemisphere in a patient with patent territorial (middle cerebral) arteries but a thrombosed extracranial internal carotid artery. This fact was considered to be a curiosity for almost four more decades, because of both the unavailability of techniques for studying afflicted patients in vivo and the practice of performing incomplete postmortem examinations in order to preserve the cervical carotid arteries for the injection of embalming fluid. The intracranial arteries were examined, as were the origins of the great vessels from the aortic arch, but the critical carotid bifurcation in the neck was left untouched.

The development of safe techniques for cerebral angiography, combined with careful clinical pathologic studies of the type of vascular disease in large numbers of patients with strokes, led to recognition of the frequency with which stroke syndromes were due to extracranial vascular disease. Classic studies were reported by Fischer between 1951 and 1954 and by Hutchinson and Yates in 1956.

The report of Eastcott, Pickering, and Rob documenting the successful operation for carotid bifurcation disease stimulated wide interest in the surgical management of this condition, although three groups, including Carre et al., Stuly et al., and DeBakey, claimed priority in having performed earlier operations. The first significant series in the United States was reported by Lyons and Galbraith in 1957. It was soon established that the operation of endarterectomy for carotid bifurcation atherosclerotic lesions could be performed in large numbers of afflicted individuals with a high degree of safety, in spite of the unmatched sensitivity of the brain to ischemia, and that long-term patency could be expected. The effect of the surgical approach on the natural history of stroke syndromes continues to be the subject of disagreement.

ETIOLOGY AND PATHOLOGY. Although the term *stroke* encompasses a variety of clinical situations in which major neurologic deficits occur because of involvement of the brain, the term *ischemia stroke* refers to cerebral infarction occurring as a result of impairment of regional blood flow. Atherosclerosis is the basis for this in the vast majority of patients. Smaller percentages of ischemic strokes are (1) secondary to cerebral embolization of thrombi that originate in the heart, (2) due to fibromuscular hyperplasia, (3) associated with obliterative ateritis of the great vessels as they originate from the aortic arch (see Aortic Arch Occlusive Disease, in Chap. 20), (4) due to blunt or penetrating trauma, (5) secondary to forceful hyperextension of the neck resulting in dissection and tearing of the carotid intima, and (6) due to dissecting thoracic aortic aneurysms which involve the carotid arteries.

A clinical pathologic correlation between the appearance of surgically removed plaques and the specific syndromes presented by patients operated on at New York University confirmed the early findings of Millard Fisher,

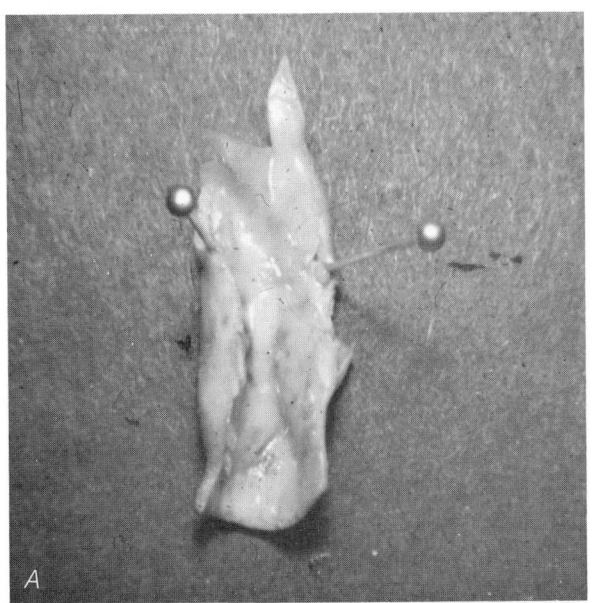

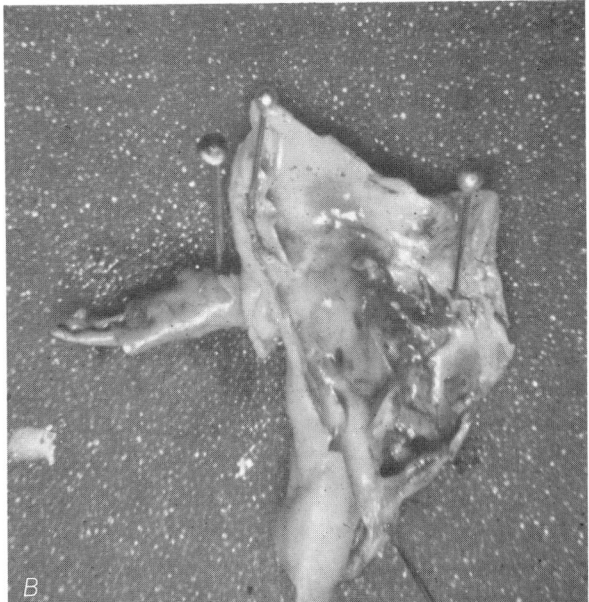

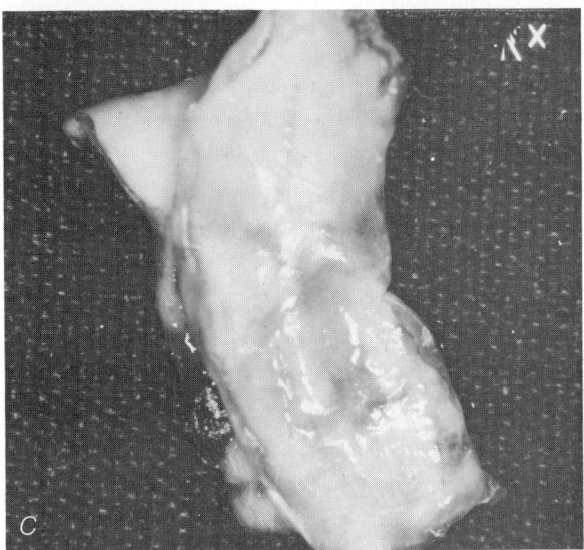

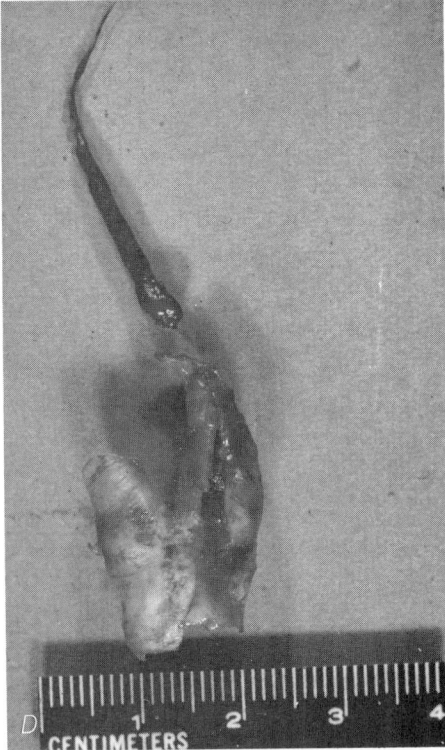

Fig. 21-19. Carotid plaque dynamics in the pathogenesis of stroke syndromes are suggested by the variation in appearance of lesions surgically removed. *A.* Smooth fibrous plaque producing marked stenosis and decreased blood flow. *B.* Ulcerated plaque giving rise to embolization. *C.* Hemorrhage into the wall of a plaque that can result in sudden stenosis or ulceration and subsequent ulceration and embolization. *D.* Total occlusion of an internal carotid artery secondary to thrombosis.

showing that patients with generalized symptoms of cerebral ischemia had major stenotic fibrotic lesions that had smooth surfaces, while those with focal symptoms were found to have plaques with either frank ulcerations or cul de sacs that were thought to be craters created when portions of the plaques broke away as emboli. Intramural hemorrhage was the most common single, pathologic finding and could be responsible for fragmentation of plaques, development of sudden stenosis, breakdown of the plaque, and subsequent thrombosis.

If patients with stroke syndromes are studied with four-vessel angiography, opacifying both carotid and both vertebral arteries from their origins to their points of entry into the skull, significant extracranial occlusive disease will be found in about 75 percent of the group. The segmental localization is impressive. In the carotid artery, almost all plaques are found at the carotid bifurcation, starting in the distal centimeter of the common carotid and involving the proximal external carotid and the proximal 1 to 2 cm of the internal carotid (Fig. 21-19). Fortu-

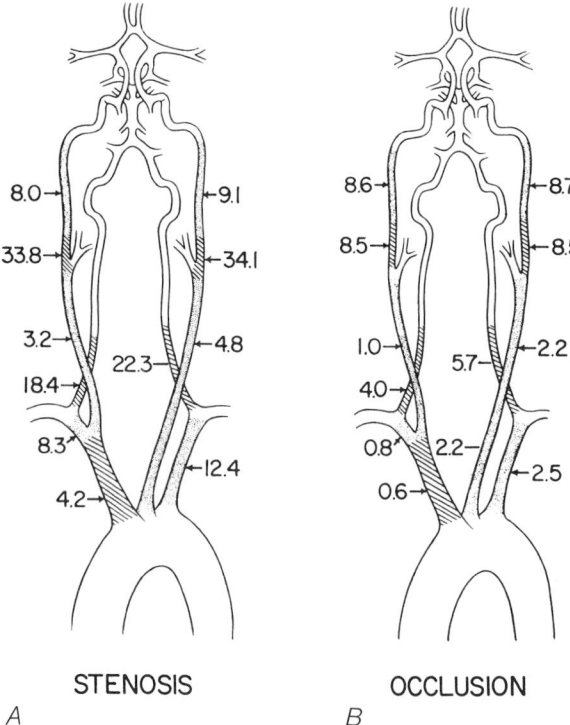

STENOSIS   OCCLUSION

A   *B*

Fig. 21-20. Frequency distribution of lesions according to anatomic locations and stenosis versus occlusion. The predominance of stenotic lesions over occlusions favors embolization as a common mechanism for the production of cerebral ischemia. The predominance of extracranial lesions renders surgical intervention feasible.

nately for surgical reconstruction, and also a striking example of segmental localization of atherosclerosis, the internal carotid beyond the first 1 to 2 cm is usually uninvolved to beyond its point of entry into the skull. The next area of predilection for plaques is at the so-called carotid siphon where the internal carotid artery curves to issue from under the dura. Because of the freedom from involvement of this portion, arterial reconstruction almost always can be done if the internal carotid is not thrombosed. Disease in the middle cerebral artery is rare. In the vertebral-basilar system, plaques are usually at the origin of the vertebrals from the subclavian, and disease of the vertebral beyond its origin is unusual. In the basilar artery localized atherosclerosis is more common. Within the thorax, the great vessels are infrequently diseased. Lesions are multiple in more than 50 percent of patients (Fig. 21-20).

Soon after the recognition of the frequency of extracranial vascular disease, it became apparent that simple reduction in cerebral blood flow from extracranial arterial stenosis and occlusions was not an adequate explanation for many of the neurologic syndromes encountered, and it now seems clear that arterioarterial embolization of fragments of plaque or platelet-fibrin aggregates is probably the most frequent mechanism of neurologic injury (Fig. 21-20). Ophthalmologic visualization of these foreign bodies suddenly appearing in the retina during transient ischemic attacks was one of the first clues to the mechanism of the syndrome. The second method for production

of symptoms is the obvious one of decrease in flow from marked stenosis or occlusion. Because of abundant collateral circulation in the brain through the circle of Willis, major arteries may become narrowed or occluded without any symptoms whatever unless multiple areas are diseased. As with stenotic lesions in the vascular system elsewhere there is little decrease in blood flow until the cross-sectional area of a vessel is narrowed by more than 75 percent. If collateral circulation is adequate, even multiple complete occlusions may be harmless. Routine postmortem studies by Martin and associates of a large group of patients dying from different causes demonstrated that in as many as 40 percent of the patients at least one of the four major extracranial arteries was significantly narrowed or occluded, even though there were no neurologic symptoms before death.

The atherosclerotic plaques removed from the vessels of symptomatic patients have varied greatly in composition and appearance. Some were principally fibrotic, with smooth internal surfaces; others showed advanced degenerative changes, with intramural hemorrhage and little stenosis, but with ulceration of the intimal surface. Plaques with a smooth intimal surface are probably harmless until the cross-sectional area of the artery is reduced to a marked degree. An ulcerated plaque, however, even though the lumen is compromised little, may cause serious or even catastrophic injury from repeated embolization or from thrombosis of the artery.

CLINICAL MANIFESTATIONS. A great variety of clinical syndromes result from the different patterns of occlusive disease in the carotid, vertebral, and subclavian arteries. These will be only briefly summarized here, for they are described in considerable detail in Millikan's excellent paper. The classic stroke from unilateral carotid disease is ipsilateral blindness and contralateral hemiplegia. The presence of aphasia depends upon involvement of the dominant cerebral hemisphere. At the other extreme are the most fleeting focal neurologic defects such as a transient monoplegia, transient hemiplegia, or transient ipsilateral blindness, viz., amaurosis fugax. These episodes, clearing within minutes to hours after an abrupt onset, are termed *transient ischemic attacks* (TIA). Between such episodes the patient may be completely well, but unfortunately such attacks often precede a catastrophic stroke. One retrospective study of patients with severe strokes found that almost 75 percent had such premonitory symptoms in the weeks or months before the stroke appeared.

Between these two extremes, TIA on the one hand and the massive stroke on the other, a wide variety of motor and sensory syndromes of varying severity and duration is seen. Various attempts at simple classification of these syndromes, such as RIND (reversible ischemic neurologic deficit), threatened stroke, stroke in evolution, and completed stroke, have been only partially successful and have led to some confusion, since not all reports use the same criteria for arriving at a classification. Their unilateral localization is strongly suggestive of carotid artery disease. They may be precipitated by hypotension, hypoxia, or changes in position or posture, or they may be unrelated to any known cause.

With disease of the vertebral-basilar system, a number

of brainstem symptoms occur. In contrast to carotid disease, the symptoms are often bilateral, involving either both arms or both legs, but may alternate in severity from one side of the body to the other. Tinnitus, dizziness, vertigo, diplopia, and dysarthria are also common. One type of characteristic syndrome is the so-called drop attack, in which the patient may literally fall to the ground with little or no warning, with or without loss of consciousness, and recover equally rapidly with only residual dizziness or mild ataxia.

Disease of the subclavian artery proximal to the origin of one of the vertebral arteries, more commonly the left, produces the so-called subclavian steal syndrome. The proximal obstruction in the subclavian artery decreases the pressure in that artery at the point of origin of the vertebral artery; this results in an actual reversal of flow in the vertebral artery, with blood draining out of the basilar artery into the arm. Although this phenomenon is seen frequently on angiographic studies, production of symptoms from ischemia of the brainstem by exercising the arm is uncommon.

Physical Examination. Examination is directed primarily at determining the presence of any neurologic deficit as well as the pattern of arterial involvement. Palpation of the carotid pulses is useful only for the rare instance of intrathoracic occlusion of the common carotid artery. Palpation for the internal carotid pulse in the pharynx posterior to the tonsillar pillars is no longer advised. Separate palpation of the external and internal carotid arteries is impossible because of their location next to one another. Hence, the carotid pulses are normal on palpation in almost all patients with occlusive disease at the carotid bifurcation. Auscultation over the carotid bifurcation for a bruit is essential because a bruit is audible just anterior to the sternocleidomastoid muscle near the level of the angle of the mandible in a significant number of patients with stenosis. Auscultation in the supraclavicular fossae may reveal bruits from subclavian-vertebral disease. When bruits are detected, they must be differentiated from murmurs of cardiac valvular lesions, such as aortic stenosis, that are transmitted along the great vessels into the neck. If occlusive disease of a subclavian artery is present, the blood pressures will be significantly different in the two arms.

A number of noninvasive techniques are useful for evaluating the condition of the carotid bifurcations not only in patients with bruits but also as screening techniques in otherwise healthy individuals. The most useful of these are duplex scanning, oculoplethysmography, and B-mode ultrasound imaging.

DIAGNOSIS. The differential diagnosis of cerebrovascular insufficiency syndromes is extremely complex and involves exclusion of a variety of intracranial lesions in addition to generalized conditions that can effect cerebral hypoxia. The latter include myocardial infarction, cardiac arrhythmias, Adams-Stokes-syndrome, Menière's disease, and a number of metabolic disorders, such as diabetic ketosis and hypoglycemia.

The diagnosis of ischemic stroke syndromes ultimately depends upon angiographic delineation of the intra- and extracranial cerebral arteries (Fig. 21-21). The greatest risks related to angiography generally are assumed by the patients most seriously afflicted with arterial disease, particularly those who have already developed serious neurologic deficits. The overall risk of stroke or death incident to cerebral angiography is about 0.5 to 1 percent. Less serious complications, such as hematomas and temporary or permanent loss of arterial pulses distal to puncture sites, occur with greater frequency.

Patients with amaurosis fugax, transient paralysis or weakness of the extremity, weakness of facial muscles, and transient disorders of speech all require more extensive investigation to rule out nonischemic causes, but the ultimate study in these patients is cerebral angiography to delineate the aortic arch and its major branches to their intracranial terminations.

Timing of the angiographic study may be critical. Those patients with transient neurologic deficits may have their studies performed as soon as possible; patients who have suffered profound and extensive neurologic insult, especially if associated with altered consciousness, should have radiographic studies postponed, because if these are performed during the first week of illness, the complication rate is excessive.

The finding of asymptomatic bruits on routine physical examination introduces the need to make difficult decisions. The study by Thompson, in which patients with asymptomatic bruits were shown to have "significant" lesions by angiography and appeared to be protected from future stroke by operative intervention, suggests a more aggressive attitude. A number of other studies, however, suggest that patients with carotid bruits may not be at great risk of stroke during the performance of unrelated operative procedures that are considered to increase stroke risk. Indeed, those who suffered strokes during major operations were those who did not have bruits, raising a number of questions relating to how best to identify stroke-prone individuals and the factors that precipitate cerebral infarction. At the other end of the spectrum are patients with asymptomatic carotid stenoses, discovered either during screening noninvasive studies or investigation of carotid bruits. Computed tomography of the brain has revealed that a number of these patients have suffered silent cerebral infarcts and that this group should have angiographic studies.

The attitude of the authors of this chapter toward asymptomatic bruits, in the face of conflicting data, is to study angiographically those patients who appear to have hemodynamically significant lesions when tested by oculoplethysmography or by duplex scan and who are physiologically fit and thought to have long life expectancies. Operations are offered to patients who have 70 percent stenosis or lesions with irregular contour. Prior to a major intraabdominal or intrathoracic procedure, these patients are studied routinely by duplex scanning of the carotid arteries.

TREATMENT. General Considerations. The Joint Study of Extracranial Arterial Occlusion as a Cause of Stroke clearly shows that to be effective, surgical treatment must be performed before major neurologic deficits are produced from cerebral infarction. Operations are generally performed on patients who have had transient ischemic

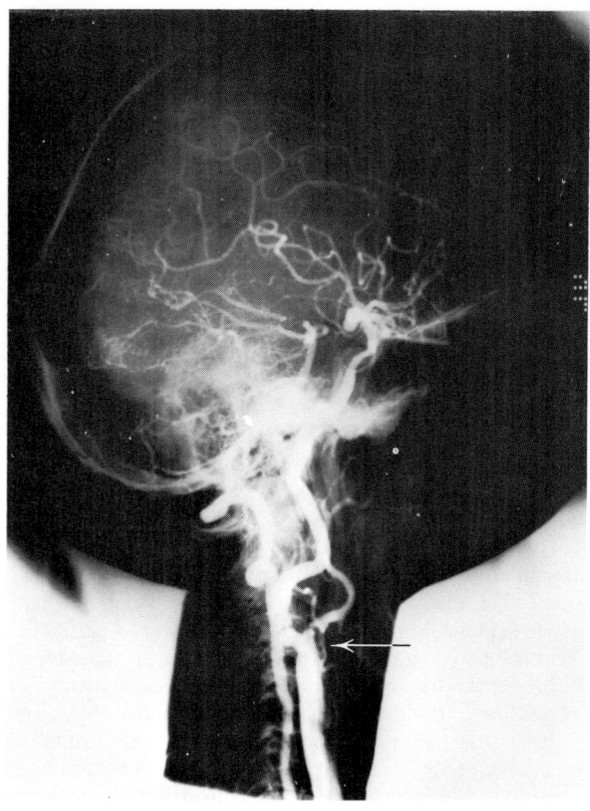

A

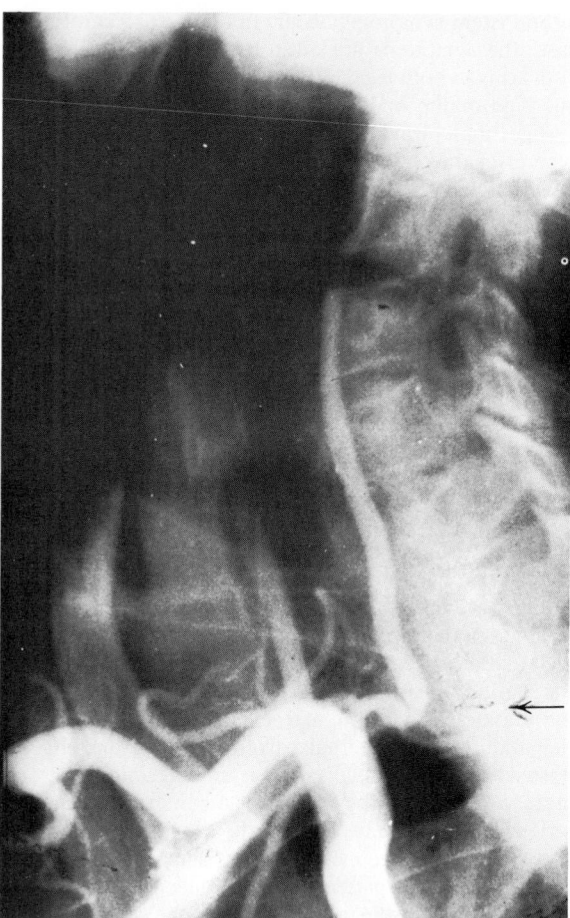

B

Fig. 21-21. Angiographic studies of the cerebral circulation for stroke syndromes should outline the major extracranial as well as the intracranial arteries. This facilitates planning operative procedures and aids in making differential diagnoses of the various causes of stroke syndromes. Cervical carotid and vertebral arteries are outlined by retrograde right brachial arterial injection. *A.* Arrow points to significant lesion in the internal and external carotids. *B.* Arrow points to typical stenotic lesion at the origin of the vertebral with an associated kink.

attacks and carotid lesions that produce 50 to 70 percent stenosis or have irregular contours. Operation upon patients with acute strokes has been associated with a high mortality, considerably higher than that for patients treated medically. Recently, however, this conclusion has been challenged, and certain patients with acute strokes have been successfully operated upon with marked neurologic improvement. Thromboendarterectomy for totally occluded internal carotid arteries in patients with acute neurologic deficits, a procedure previously considered unsafe because of the occurrence of intracerebral hemorrhage resulting from restoration of arterial perfusion through areas of infarcted cerebrum, is now judged feasible by some and has been shown to reverse relatively severe neurologic deficits.

As the prevalence of arterioarterial embolization in the production of stroke syndromes has become clear, there has been renewed interest in altering the coagulability of the blood. Heparin, as therapy for transient cerebral ischemic episodes of increasing frequency, does not appear to decrease the incidence of stroke in patients with high-grade carotid stenoses. Oral anticoagulants may decrease the incidence of TIAs, but not of completed strokes, and are associated with a considerable risk of hemorrhage. The striking finding of the influence of acetylsalicylic acid

on platelet aggregation may be of considerable therapeutic significance. Clinical trials employing aspirin and other antiplatelet drugs have also failed to yield clear-cut results about protection from stroke. One study reported by Bousser, considered definitive, suffers from protocol defects shared by other studies. Angiographic studies to define the presence of extracranial arterial lesions were not performed. The entire spectrum of ischemic cerebral disease was not studied. Only selected and clearly defined clinical categories were included, and patients with tight carotid stenoses were excluded.

An additional question has been raised regarding the universal use of anticoagulant and antiplatelet drugs in patients who exhibit intraplaque hemorrhage resulting in significant stenosis and ulceration. It has been suggested that antithrombotic agents might aggravate such hemorrhages.

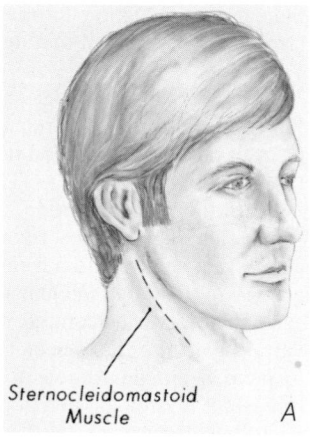

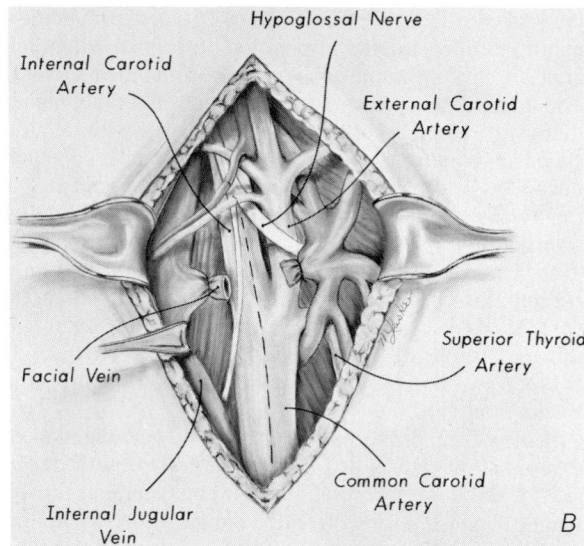

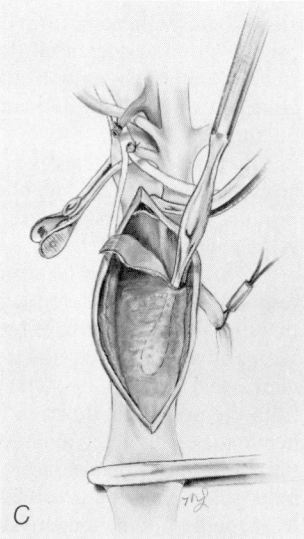

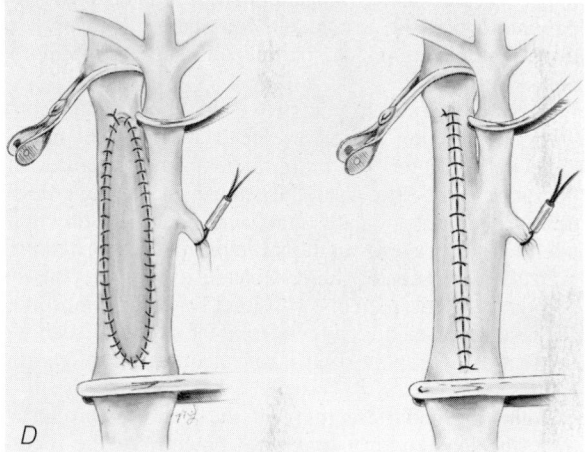

Fig. 21-22. Technique of carotid endarterectomy. *A.* A skin incision is made anterior to the sternocleidomastoid muscle. *B.* The carotid artery branches are widely mobilized. The internal carotid artery is clamped before widely mobilizing the frequently thrombus-containing bulb, thereby protecting the brain from embolization, which may occur during the dissection. The vagus and hypoglossal nerves are carefully protected. Mobilization of the hypoglossal is facilitated by dividing the sternocleidomastoid artery and vein. A longitudinal arteriotomy is made extending above and below the plaque at the carotid bifurcation. *C.* After division of the intima above the plaque, the plaque can be easily dissected from the underlying media or from the adventitia. The distal intima is carefully inspected and sutured if necessary. *D.* The arteriotomy is either closed primarily with 5-0 Tevdek, or a vein roof patch fashioned from autologous saphenous vein is used to avoid producing stenosis. The technique for restoring flow after completion of the closure is crucial to avoid embolization to the brain. The internal carotid clamp is temporarily removed and reapplied. The common and external carotid clamps are removed, and after 1 or 2 min of flushing of the carotid bulb the internal carotid clamp is removed.

Atherosclerotic Disease of the Internal Carotid Artery.
Atherosclerosis of the origin of the internal carotid artery is the most common form of extracranial vascular disease. Involvement is limited to the first 1 to 2 cm of the

origin of the internal carotid and hence is ideal for surgical correction (Fig. 21-21).

When complete occlusion develops in the carotid artery, an organized thrombus develops above the atherosclerotic plaque and extends superiorly into the intracranial internal carotid, making successful operation impossible. In approximately 10 percent of patients with complete occlusion, the thrombus has not propagated more than 2 to 3 cm, and surgical removal is still possible.

The ideal patient for operation is one with TIAs who has been shown to have significant carotid bifurcation disease producing either hemodynamically significant stenosis or marked irregularity of the contour of the arteries at the carotid bulb, without any permanent neurologic abnormality. In such patients operation can be performed with a variety of anesthetic techniques. Mortality and major neurologic complications are in the range of 1 to 4 percent, the risk factors having been defined by a number of authors. Details of the operation are shown in Fig. 21-22.

The hazards of operation are greater and the likelihood of benefit much less when a stroke has occurred. If the internal carotid has become totally occluded, producing a major neurologic deficit, operation performed within 6 h after onset of symptoms may produce dramatic recovery. The operative mortality, however, is considerably higher than with elective operations, especially with altered states of consciousness. If operation is delayed much beyond 6 h after the onset of symptoms, reopening a totally obstructed carotid artery may be followed first by transient improvement, then worsening of symptoms and even death from hemorrhage into the area of infarction precipitated by the restoration of arterial perfusion pressure. It has been suggested by Warren and Triedman that this catastrophe might be prevented by careful avoidance of blood pressure elevation during operation and for some weeks afterward.

If the acute stroke has resulted from embolization of atheromatous debris or platelet aggregates, with occlusion of small intracerebral vessels, emergency operation upon the nonstenosing ulcerated plaque at the carotid bifurcation is not immediately helpful, and carotid clamping might worsen the neurologic deficit. At a later time such patients should be considered for operation to prevent future embolization if the permanent neurologic deficit is not severe.

In patients with chronic strokes in whom acute injury weeks or months earlier produced a permanent neurologic deficit indicative of total hemispheric infarction, operation is of little value. If, however, the neurologic deficit does not indicate total hemispheric dysfunction, operation to prevent additional injury from repeated embolization has been of value. A challenging group consists of asymptomatic patients with loud bruits. Thompson et al. have reported a lowered stroke incidence in such patients if angiographic studies revealed significant carotid lesions.

Following endarterectomy of the stenotic carotid artery, the likelihood of long-term patency of the reconstructed artery is excellent. Early occlusion is due to neointimal hyperplasia; occlusion occurring years postoperatively is due to atherosclerosis.

The effect of prophylactic carotid endarterectomy in altering the incidence of mortality in future stroke has been analyzed in detail by the Joint Study. Although the results of the study were not completely definitive, certain facts emerged. The natural history of the disease definitely can be changed if the operative mortality and stroke rate can be kept at low levels (1 to 5 percent). Those patients with the most severe and extensive involvement, that is to say, those with bilateral carotid lesions or with stenosis opposite complete occlusion, who survive operations enjoy the greatest protection from future stroke and from death from stroke. Strokes in the neurologic area corresponding to the surgically repaired artery are markedly reduced.

In our own series of nearly 2500 carotid operations performed in conscious patients, the perioperative stroke rate has been 2.5 percent, varying from 1.1 percent in patients who were neurologically intact and had bilaterally patent arteries, to 7.7 percent in patients who had contralateral carotid stenosis and failed to tolerate carotid clamping, requiring temporary shunts. Late follow up, indicates a reduction in stroke rate. This reduction in stroke rate is reported to range from 30 to 300 percent for 5 years.

Subclavian-Vertebral Disease. Stenosis involving only the vertebral artery is infrequent. It is physiologically significant only when bilateral or if one vertebral is congenitally hypoplastic or absent. The disease is frequently limited to the site of origin of the vertebral from the subclavian. The atherosclerotic plaques in this area usually have a smooth intimal surface, in contrast to the frequency of ulcerated plaques in the carotid artery. On occasion, however, ulcerated plaques at the origin of the vertebral arteries have been encountered and are thought to have been the source of emboli that produce focal brainstem neurologic deficits. In addition, there are frequently tortuous kinks in the first few centimeters of the vertebral artery that can be shown to result in total occlusion when the head is turned to one side. Symptoms are probably due to decreased flow through the basivertebral system, although embolization cannot be entirely excluded. Concomitant disease in the basilar artery is frequent.

Atherosclerotic stenosis or occlusion of the subclavian artery proximal to the site of origin of the vertebral artery produces the clinical picture termed the *subclavian steal syndrome* and on occasion, embolization to the brainstem arteries. The former abnormality was well defined by Reivich et al. in 1961, following an angiographic description in 1960 by Contorni of retrograde flow in the involved vertebral artery. The reduction in pressure in the subclavian artery beyond the stenosis results in retrograde flow from the brainstem down the vertebral artery to the arm, hence the term "subclavian steal." The clinical picture is that of ischemic neurologic symptoms in association with mild ischemia in the involved arm. Diagnosis can be easily made by finding a decreased pulse and blood pressure in the symptomatic arm, often in association with a localized bruit in the supraclavicular space. Serial angiograms after injection of contrast media into the opposite brachial artery or the ascending aorta will demonstrate reversal of flow in the involved vertebral artery by initially opacifying the opposite vertebral artery in a normal fashion, followed by retrograde opacification of the involved vertebral. Although this phenomenon is not infrequent on angiographic examination, clinical symptoms are not common, perhaps because collateral circulation in the brain can readily compensate for the amount of blood diverted away from the brain by the retrograde vertebral flow.

Operations upon the vertebral artery usually can be performed without thoracotomy. Surgical exposure of the subclavian-vertebral junction is obtained through a transverse supraclavicular incision that divides the clavicular head of the sternocleidomastoid muscle and the underlying scalenus anticus muscle. If the stenosing plaque has a smooth intimal surface, endarterectomy may not be necessary. The artery can be simply widened with a patch angioplasty with autologous saphenous vein. If the vertebral artery is significantly tortuous and redundant, predisposing to kinking, plication can be performed. In 120 arterial reconstructions of vertebral arteries performed by the authors, only 1 postoperative stroke was encountered. Late follow-up, without a comparable control series, reveals a remarkably low stroke rate of about 1 percent per patient follow-up year and normal survival for the age group involved.

Operations for the subclavian steal syndrome are seldom necessary. When done, a transthoracic approach to the subclavian artery can be avoided by employing a bypass graft from the ipsilateral common carotid artery to the distal subclavian artery. This is physiologically possible because the common carotid is large enough to deliver sufficient blood to supply both the brain and the upper extremity. On occasion, when the common carotid or innominate arteries are markedly stenotic and not suitable, axilloaxillary bypass grafting has been useful. Reimplantation of the distal end of the transected subclavian artery to the side of the common carotid is also described.

Aortic Arch Occlusive Disease. Occlusive disease of the major branches of the aortic arch was described as a clinical syndrome by Savory in 1854; it is due to atherosclerosis in this country. In the Orient it occurs in young women, is due to an arteritis, and is known by the eponym "Takayasu's disease," named for the ophthalmologist who described it. Syphilitic arteritis, formerly a common cause, is now most unusual.

Although symptoms are apt to be mild due to the very proximal location of the occlusive process, permitting many pathways for collateral circulation, ischemic symptoms of the upper extremities or the brain can occur. Unless severe ischemic symptoms appear or symptoms that threaten brain function occur, surgical intervention is not indicated. Operative intervention, of necessity, must be via thoracotomy with the use of multiple bypass grafts from the ascending aorta proximally to the carotid or subclavian arteries distally since endarterectomy procedures are usually not possible. Thoracotomy may be avoided in those instances in which one of the arch vessels is spared and a cervical carotid-subclavian bypass can be performed. The theoretic objection that siphoning of blood from a normal artery to a diseased artery may produce a steal syndrome has not been manifest. In one large series, operative mortality was 5 percent, and successful revascularization was achieved in the majority of patients.

ANEURYSMS

Aneurysm can be defined as the inappropriate dilation of an artery. This dilation can involve the entire circumference of the artery and results in a *fusiform* appearance of the artery. It can also be focal, causing a bubblelike projection of the arterial wall and producing a *saccular* appearance. The so-called dissecting aneurysm of the aorta is a misnomer because the primary process is a longitudinal splitting of the layers of the arterial wall, which often results in fusiform and sometimes in saccular dilation of the artery. Fusiform aneurysms are usually secondary to arteriosclerosis and are infrequently due to dis-

section secondary to medial necrosis, as in Marfan's syndrome. Saccular aneurysms may be due to a variety of causes, including trauma, infection, and fibromuscular hyperplasia. Fusiform aneurysms require prosthetic replacement to restore or to maintain arterial continuity; saccular aneurysms may be treated by resection and angioplastic closure of the involved artery.

Aneurysms can further be classified as *true aneurysms* when all the layers of the arterial wall contribute to the dilation and as *false aneurysms* when only a fibrous sac exists. The fibrous sac results from a tangential hole in an artery and the organization of a contained hematoma.

Several milestones in vascular surgery evolved as a consequence of the treatment of aneurysms. In the second century A.D., Antyllus treated an arterial aneurysm by ligature immediately above and below the lesion, followed by incision of the aneurysm, evacuation of the clot, and exteriorization of the cavity. John Hunter, in 1786, electively ligated a femoral artery proximal to a popliteal aneurysm to minimize blood loss during subsequent attempts at extirpation. The anatomic term *Hunter's canal* originated from this surgical episode. In 1888 Rudolph Matas described his operation of endoaneurysmorrhaphy, in which the aneurysm is widely opened and the communications with the parent artery are sutured. This imaginative approach promptly became the standard treatment and was modified little during the next 55 years. Subsequently, as techniques of vascular reconstruction developed and prosthetic conduits became available, modern procedures evolved.

Abdominal Aortic Aneurysms

HISTORICAL DATA. The modern era of treatment of abdominal aneurysms began with the first successful excision of an abdominal aneurysm and replacement with an aortic homograft by Dubost in 1951. Previous therapeutic efforts, such as wiring to promote clotting and wrapping or coating with plastics, and other techniques to include thrombosis, are principally of historic interest. Techniques to promote thrombosis of the aneurysm have been reintroduced, combined with extraanatomic bypass procedures to maintain flow to the lower extremities in poor-risk patients.

INCIDENCE. Abdominal aneurysms, the most common of the arteriosclerotic aneurysms, are increasing in frequency as a consequence of our aging population. Men are affected more frequently than women, in a ratio approximating 10:1.

ETIOLOGY AND PATHOLOGY. The vast majority of abdominal aneurysms are arteriosclerotic in origin, with their pathogenesis probably different from occlusive atherosclerosis. Aneurysms result from degenerative changes in the media, while atherosclerotic occlusion results from a proliferative reaction in the media causing narrowing of the arterial lumen. The distribution of the two processes is different, the atherosclerotic occlusive process involving the aorta at sites of bifurcations, attachments, tapers, and curvatures, while aneurysmal disease has its own characteristic patterns of involvement.

The authors have never seen an abdominal aneurysm arising below the renal arteries from any cause except arteriosclerosis, although they have been reported from syphilis, trauma, Marfan's syndrome, and bacterial endocarditis.

The anatomic location of abdominal aneurysms makes them accessible to surgical therapy, for a graft can be inserted proximally from the abdominal aorta below the renal arteries to the common iliac arteries distad. The size of abdominal aneurysms varies greatly, small ones 2 to 3 cm in diameter being detected accidentally by aortography, sonography, or computed tomography (CT) of the abdomen, while others may enlarge to a diameter of 10 to 15 cm before being discovered accidentally by palpation. The usual course of untreated aneurysms was well documented in the classic report by Estes in 1950. Without treatment there is a 20 percent chance of rupture within 1 year after diagnosis and a 50 percent chance within 4 or 5 years. Complications seldom arise from expanding aneurysms until rupture occurs. Erosion of bone, so common in syphilitic aneurysms, virtually never occurs with arteriosclerotic aneurysms. There is usually no impairment of peripheral circulation unless distal embolization from the shaggy laminated thrombus lining the lumen occurs.

Although aneurysms frequently originate within 1 to 2 cm of the origin of the renal arteries, actual involvement of the origin of the renal arteries in the aneurysm, necessitating reconstruction of the renal arteries during surgical excision, is unusual. In a series of over 170 abdominal aneurysms at the Johns Hopkins Hospital, only 3 aneurysms involving the renal arteries were found.

Adherence to neighboring structures, with the exception of the inferior vena cava and the iliac veins, is unusual unless the lesion is classified as an "inflammatory aneurysm." In this situation there is an intensive adventitial fibroplastic reaction frequently extending from the common iliacs to the origin of the renal arteries. The 3rd and 4th portions of the duodenum and the ureters become firmly attached, making their separation particularly hazardous. Involvement of the renal arteries by this reaction simulates a suprarenal aneurysm when in reality the true aneurysm begins below the level of the renals. Preoperatively the true anatomic involvement is suggested by the CT scan of the abdominal aorta and can be confirmed by aortography to include lateral views.

An abdominal aneurysm is often associated with generalized atherosclerosis. In a series of 1400 patients, some signs of coronary artery disease were present in 30 percent of the patients, and 40 percent of the patients had some increase in systolic blood pressure. Associated occlusive disease of the carotid arteries was found in 7 percent, of the renal arteries in 2 percent, and of the iliac arteries in 16 percent of the patients. Concomitant clinically significant aneurysms were found in the thoracic aorta in 4 percent, in the femoral artery in 3 percent, and in the popliteal artery in 2 percent of the group.

CLINICAL MANIFESTATIONS. Symptoms. Most patients are unaware of their abdominal aneurysms until a mass is discovered by the patient or the physician. The importance of careful deep palpation of the abdomen, outlining

the abdominal aorta when possible, is obvious. Occasionally, low back pain caused by an abdominal aneurysm may be diagnosed erroneously as due to an orthopaedic condition. The pain apparently arises from tension on retroperitoneal tissues from the aneurysm; erosion of bone almost never occurs. Virtually any intraabdominal condition may be simulated by an abdominal aortic aneurysm, including renal colic, acute appendicitis, diverticulitis, peptic ulcer, pancreatitis, or cholecystitis. Rarely, there is gastrointestinal bleeding from erosion into the duodenum as the presenting manifestation. With beginning leakage of the aneurysm or frank rupture momentarily contained retroperitoneally, acute abdominal conditions such as perforated ulcer, hemorrhagic pancreatitis, or generalized peritonitis may be simulated.

Sometimes, sudden vascular collapse with shock is the first indication. Most patients, however, have some premonitory symptoms prior to rupture. The absence of signs preceding fatal rupture is a strong reason for removing most abdominal aneurysms as soon as the diagnosis is made, even though the condition is asymptomatic. Symptoms from an aneurysm are an urgent indication for operation and are sometimes called a *syndrome of impending rupture*.

Physical Examination. An abdominal aneurysm larger than 5 cm in diameter can be diagnosed with reasonable certainty. Once the patient has relaxed the muscles of the abdominal wall, careful deep palpation can usually outline the abdominal aorta near the bifurcation, generally slightly inferior to the umbilicus. The aorta may be traced proximally into the upper abdomen, where it is concealed beneath the pancreas and transverse colon. A normal aorta is seldom over an inch in diameter. Careful palpation can usually distinguish the lateral walls of the aorta and hence provide an estimate of the width. Finding a pulsating mass greater than an inch in diameter should raise the suspicion that an aneurysm is present.

Confusion may arise in thin females with diastasis of the rectus muscles in whom the aortic pulsations are abnormally prominent. This is particularly true if an increased pulse pressure is present. Such patients may come to the physician because of concern over the prominent pulsations, and vague tenderness may be elicited in palpating the aorta. Almost always careful palpation will demonstrate that the aorta is of normal diameter but when palpation is uncertain, an echogram or CT of the abdomen may be required to exclude the presence of a small aneurysm. In the majority of patients palpation either establishes or excludes the diagnosis.

Peripheral pulses should be carefully examined, for associated occlusive vascular disease may be present due to embolization from the aneurysm or occlusive atherosclerosis. The presence of a bruit over the bifurcation of the carotid arteries is particularly significant, because an asymptomatic stenosis of a carotid artery can significantly increase the risk of hypotension occurring during operation.

Laboratory Studies. A radiograph of the abdomen, including anteroposterior and lateral views, will establish the diagnosis in many patients by demonstrating calcifica-

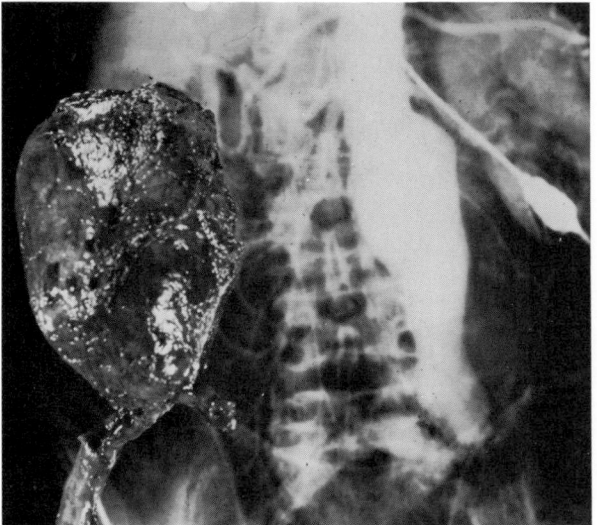

A

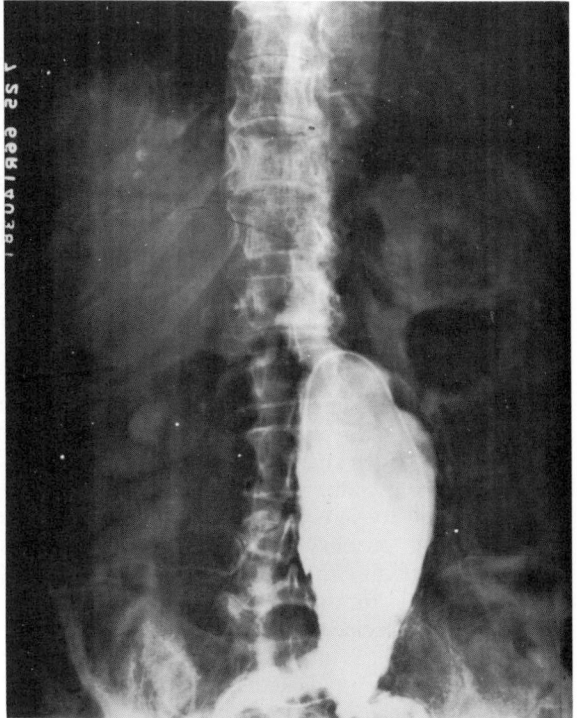

B

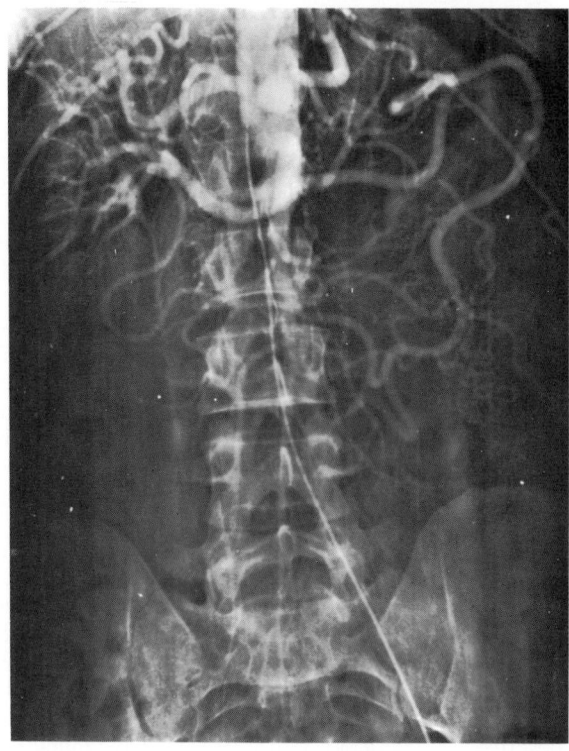

C

Fig. 21-23. *A.* Aortogram showing abdominal aneurysm in the distal aorta. Superimposed on the film is a photograph of a lesion excised at operation, indicating the large laminated clot filling the aneurysm. *(Courtesy of Dr. Henry T. Bahnson, Department of Surgery, University of Pittsburgh.) B.* Anteroposterior lumbar aortogram performed by percutaneous introduction of an arterial catheter, illustrating a large abdominal aneurysm arising in the lower abdominal aorta. Linear calcification of the lower thoracic and upper abdominal aorta is also visible. *C.* Abdominal aortogram in a patient with atherosclerotic occlusion of the abdominal aorta that has extended up to the level of the renal arteries. The superior mesenteric artery is visible as well as the right renal artery. Extensive collateral circulation has developed, particularly in the left flank.

tion in the wall of the aneurysm. The lateral view is particularly helpful, since it permits visualization of the usually thin calcific rim of the aneurysm wall, which may be obscured by the shadows of the vertebral bodies in the frontal projections. An estimate of the size of the aneurysm is obtainable by measuring the distance from the anterior border of the vertebral bodies to the calcium in the anterior wall of the aneurysm and making the appropriate correction for the usual 20 percent magnification produced by the diverging x-rays. The uppermost extent of the aneurysm can often be determined from this view. If combined with left lateral views of the chest it permits recognition of upper abdominal and thoracoabdominal aneurysms. A rapid-sequence excretory urogram may also be useful in detecting renal involvement. The use of ultrasound and especially CT helps to delineate aneurysms more accurately and helps to establish the true size of the aneurysm. This is especially important with aneurysms 4 to 6 cm in diameter where knowledge of true size may be critical in establishing the need for operation.

Aortography (Fig. 21-23) is used infrequently by us because of the small but definite risk it entails and because the diagnosis can usually be established by other means. In addition, a laminated thrombus within the aneurysm may mask the true size of the lesion. Formerly, it was thought that in order to establish relationship of the renal arteries to the aneurysm, aortography was essential, but accumulated experience has found renal artery involvement in only about 1 percent of patients, and CT may provide this information. Nevertheless, some highly experienced vascular groups insist upon performing angiographic studies on all abdominal aortic aneurysm patients to delineate associated vascular lesions. It has not been shown that this has resulted in either increased survival or decreased morbidity, but angiography does result in a higher incidence of incidental operations on the renal and mesenteric arteries.

Our own preference is to perform aortography only for specific indications, avoiding it in the majority of patients. These indications include uncertainty of diagnosis in the presence of small aneurysms (Fig. 21-23), the suspicion of an extensive lesion involving the upper abdominal and thoracic aorta as well, the presence of lower extremity arterial occlusions manifested by absent pulses or to define the extent of the lesion if the existence of an inflammatory aneurysm is suspected. Markedly depressed renal function or uncontrolled hypertension, though somewhat increasing the risk of aortography, are additional indications for this diagnostic procedure.

TREATMENT. Indications for Operation. Aneurysms smaller than 5 cm in diameter can be relatively safely observed unless they expand or become symptomatic. An asymptomatic aneurysm measuring at least 5 to 6 cm in diameter constitutes an indication for operation unless there are other conditions that either markedly increase the operative risk or promise to markedly shorten life expectancy. Asymptomatic aneurysms smaller than 5 to 6 cm are usually considered to carry a very small risk of rupture, while those 5 to 6 cm and larger carry at least a 20 percent yearly risk of rupture. There is very little correlation between the size of the asymptomatic aneurysms beyond 5 to 6 cm, the absence of symptoms, and the tendency to rupture, although the peak incidence of rupture has been reported to occur in 7 cm aneurysms. Operative mortality with a ruptured aneurysm is nearly ten times greater than that for elective excision.

On the other hand, when the aneurysm becomes painful, operation ceases to be elective, for pain often denotes either rupture or impending rupture. The pain may be located in the back, the flank, or the abdominal region and may vary in both intensity and character, simulating many other intraabdominal and musculoskeletal conditions. Abdominal tenderness should increase the suspicion of impending or frank rupture. In such situations the indications for operation are extended to include conditions that might otherwise preclude an elective operation.

Preoperative evaluation to estimate surgical risk, which can then be compared to the risk of rupture of the aneurysm, is critical. Operative mortality for elective aneurysm operations is most often related to acute myocardial infarction. Although many different criteria have been described to determine cardiac risk, we have found estimation of the left ventricular ejection fraction the single most useful parameter. When that fraction is below 35 percent, the risk that the patient will suffer an acute myocardial infarction is 85 percent. Such patients are evaluated with coronary angiography with a view to performing myocardial revascularization prior to or simultaneously with abdominal aortic aneurysm repair. Patients with ejection fractions between 35 and 50 percent, who would experience a 20 percent risk of acute myocardial infarction, are individually evaluated regarding the severity of angina pectoris and the persistence of ischemic ECG changes. This is done to help determine the need for coronary angiography. Those with ejection fractions greater than 50 percent have minimal cardiac risk.

Some surgeons routinely perform coronary angiography prior to abdominal aortic operations and are guided by the distribution and extent of the coronary atherosclerosis in determining which condition should be corrected first. This probably results in too many prophylactic coronary artery operations and has led to aneurysm rupture during the recovery phase from the prophylactic coronary operation.

Excretory urography and especially creatinine clearance studies have been useful. Clearances greater than 30 mL/min usually indicate that there is sufficient renal function for the patient to undergo operation. When lesser levels of clearance are encountered, renal angiography is performed to detect possibly correctable renal lesions.

Duplex scanning of the carotid arteries may be performed to detect flow-impeding lesions that are sometimes corrected prior to the aneurysm operation. Pulmonary function, coagulation, and platelet studies are also valuable in planning operations.

Technique of Operation for Abdominal Aneurysms. The operative procedure for excision of abdominal aneurysms is illustrated in Fig. 21-24. In addition to the obvious risk of hemorrhage, which is avoidable with careful technique, there are several common hazards. These include infection, renal failure, declamping shock, peripheral embolization to lower extremity arteries, and ischemic necrosis of the colon. Infection of a plastic prosthesis is an ever-present and serious complication. It may be prevented by meticulous aseptic technique and by the administration of large doses of antibiotics, preoperatively, during the operation, and for about 5 days postoperatively. Irreversible renal failure has virtually been eliminated (except in the presence of ruptured aneurysm) by careful attention to renal function during the entire operative procedure, especially during the phase of aortic clamping. Normal quarter-hourly urine output is achieved by carefully maintaining normal cardiodynamics and state of hydrations, replacing lost blood promptly, and administering electrolyte solutions to compensate for the known fluid shifts that occur intraoperatively. Diuretics are administered only to evaluate the function of the kidneys if anuria is encountered; fluid boluses or low molecular-weight dextran may be used to expand circulating volume rapidly. An intrapulmonary catheter of the Swan-Ganz type is an invaluable aid in determining normal cardiodynamics and states of hydration.

Declamping hypotension is related to several factors, such as duration of aortic occlusion, adequacy of blood volume, and degree of collateral circulation to the lower extremities. While the aorta is occluded, the lower extremities are relatively ischemic, as a result of which there is pooling of blood in dilated vessels and accumulation of ischemic products of metabolism. If the aorta is unclamped suddenly when ischemia has been severe, profound hypotension, cardiac arrhythmias, and even cardiac arrest can occur. Such problems can be almost completely avoided by different techniques. Hypotension is uncommon if the aorta is occluded for less than 1 h. After longer periods, gradual restoration of the circulation is useful. An effective approach is as follows: Once the proximal aortic anastomosis and one iliac anastomosis have been completed and the system has been flushed antegrade and retrograde to clear clot and atheromatous debris, flow is restored to the ipsilateral hypogastric artery, permitting gradual reopening of the circulation. When adjustment has occurred, the ipsilateral external iliac artery is similarly unclamped while anastomoses are performed on the contralateral side, and the same sequence is repeated. In a series of 750 aortic aneurysm operations reported by Imparato et al., declamping shock did not occur with this technique, vasopressors were not needed, and sodium bicarbonate was not required.

Distal embolization of atherosclerotic or thrombotic debris can be particularly hazardous, varying with the friability of the contents of the aneurysm. The following guidelines are useful: The external and internal iliac arteries are mobilized and occluded before the aorta is clamped proximally. At this time 5000 units of heparin is given intravenously. Subsequently, as the individual iliac anastomoses are completed, retrograde flushing of the iliac arteries is allowed to occur. If this cannot be accomplished, a rubber catheter is passed into the external iliac arteries in order to gently pry apart the walls that may have been deformed by application of arterial clamps. Fogarty catheters are not routinely passed into the distal arteries because, if aneurysmal disease is present in the femoral and popliteal arteries or if there is atherosclerosis, a thrombus or plaque may be dislodged. The selective iliac "flush" technique described above has been very effective. Finally, at the conclusion of the operation, the peripheral pulses are examined to be certain that they are the same as before operation.

Ischemic injury of the colon can be avoided by dissecting within the wall of the aneurysm rather than outside it and ligating the inferior mesenteric artery at its origin, carefully avoiding injury to any collateral vessels in the mesentery of the left colon. The technique of removing only the inner portion of the aneurysm, leaving the adventitial sheath, facilitates dissection, avoids injury to adjacent structures such as the vena cava, and provides a soft-tissue covering of the prosthesis to prevent subsequent erosion of the duodenum or other structures. When the inferior mesenteric artery has been ligated, at least one hypogastric artery must be preserved to maintain collateral circulation to the colon through the middle hemorrhoidal arteries. If one or both hypogastric arteries have been ligated, either transplanting to the aortic prosthesis a button of aneurysm wall containing the inferior mesenteric artery or bypassing from the prosthesis to the infe-

rior mesenteric artery should be performed. With these guidelines, significant ischemic injury of the colon is very rare, occurring probably only when atherosclerosis has compromised the collateral circulation. If ischemic injury is suspected, however, then a "second-look" laparotomy procedure 24 h later is indicated to detect irreversible colon ischemia before bowel perforation and peritonitis occur.

An alternative technique to abdominal aortic aneurysm operation has been a retroperitoneal approach that avoids manipulation of the abdominal viscera. Postoperative recovery is said to be smoother by avoiding the problems of prolonged intestinal atony. For patients who present with apparently prohibitive risks for intraabdominal operations, Leather et al. have described a procedure in which the common iliac arteries are ligated through small groin incisions, thereby promoting thrombosis of the aneurysm. Flow to the lower extremities is maintained by performing axillofemoral, femorofemoral bypasses with plastic prostheses. On occasion it is necessary to occlude lumbar arteries by injecting various types of glues through catheters passed by way of the brachial arteries into the aneurysm itself. It has recently been reported that aneurysms so treated can still rupture unless the infrarenal aorta has also been ligated, thereby decreasing the usefulness of the procedure.

Postoperative Complications. The operative mortality for elective excision of an abdominal aneurysm approaches 2 percent. It varies with the age of the patient and the degree of associated coronary atherosclerosis. Atelectasis, pneumonia, and cardiac arrhythmias are relatively common. Fluid balance must be carefully monitored to avoid congestive heart failure. Nasogastric intubation is required for 4 to 5 days, and if bowel function has not resumed, mechanical intestinal obstruction, which can usually be managed by intestinal intubation, should be suspected. The occurrence of bowel movements during the first 24 to 72 h should raise the suspicion of ischemic colitis, often detectable by the testing of stool for blood. Renal function is estimated from the volume of urinary output and changes in blood chemistry in order to detect the rare instance of progressive renal failure that may be due to a variety of causes, one being embolization to renal arteries during the operative procedure. Lower extremity ischemia associated with loss of previously palpable pedal pulses demands prompt reoperation to remove embolic material originating in the operative site from limb arteries.

With careful management recovery from most elective aneurysm operations is relatively uneventful.

PROGNOSIS. The reported 5-year survival following resection of abdominal aneurysms has varied from 30 to 60 percent. Fatalities are usually due to cardiac or cerebral complications of atherosclerosis. Complications from the prosthetic graft are unusual. The most frequent of these is development of a false aneurysm, often at the proximal suture line, with subsequent rupture or erosion into the duodenum. The possibility of this can be minimized by suturing the prosthesis to the immediate infrarenal aorta that is usually not aneurysmal and covering

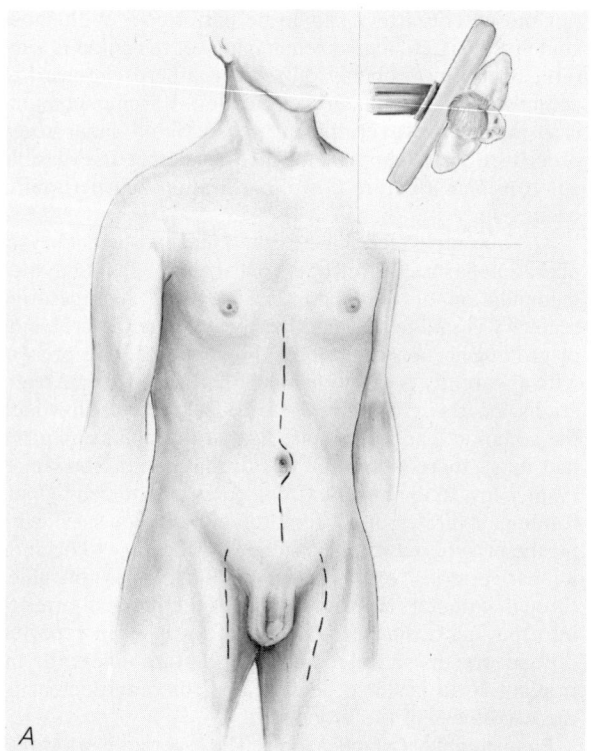

A

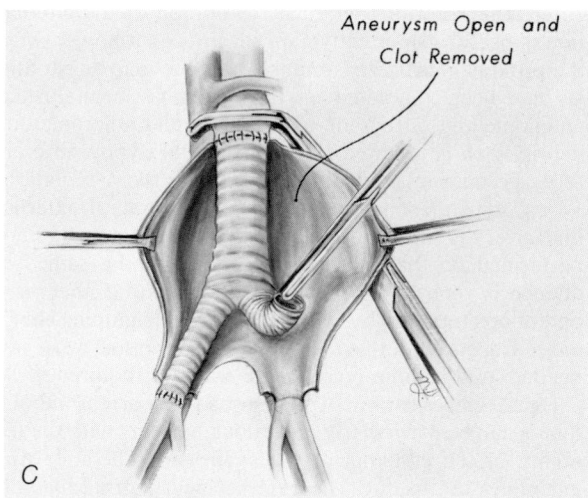

Aneurysm Open and
Clot Removed

C

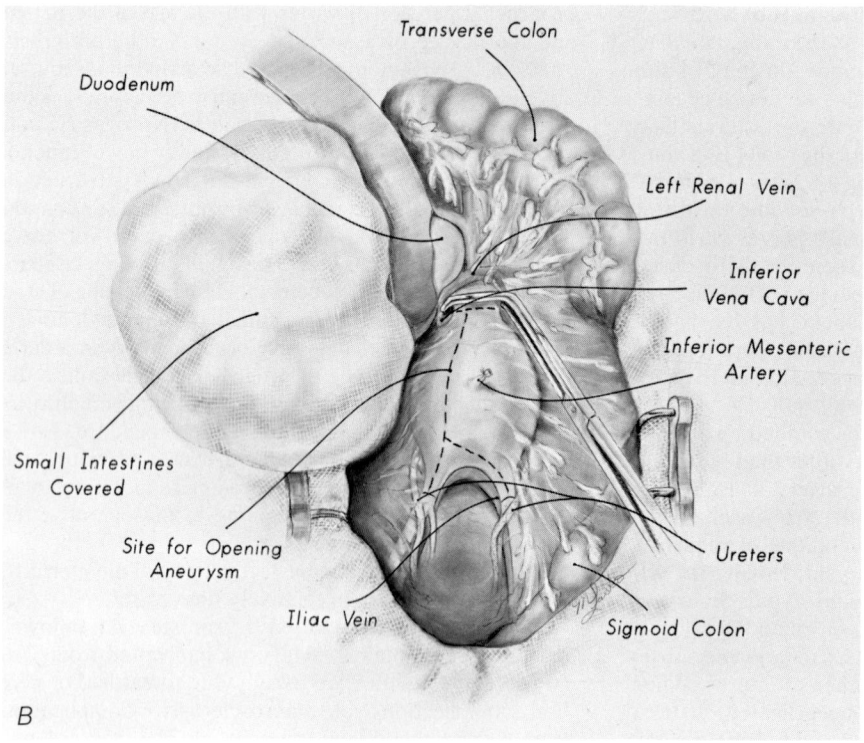

Duodenum

Transverse Colon

Left Renal Vein

Inferior
Vena Cava

Inferior Mesenteric
Artery

Small Intestines
Covered

Site for Opening
Aneurysm

Iliac Vein

Sigmoid Colon

Ureters

B

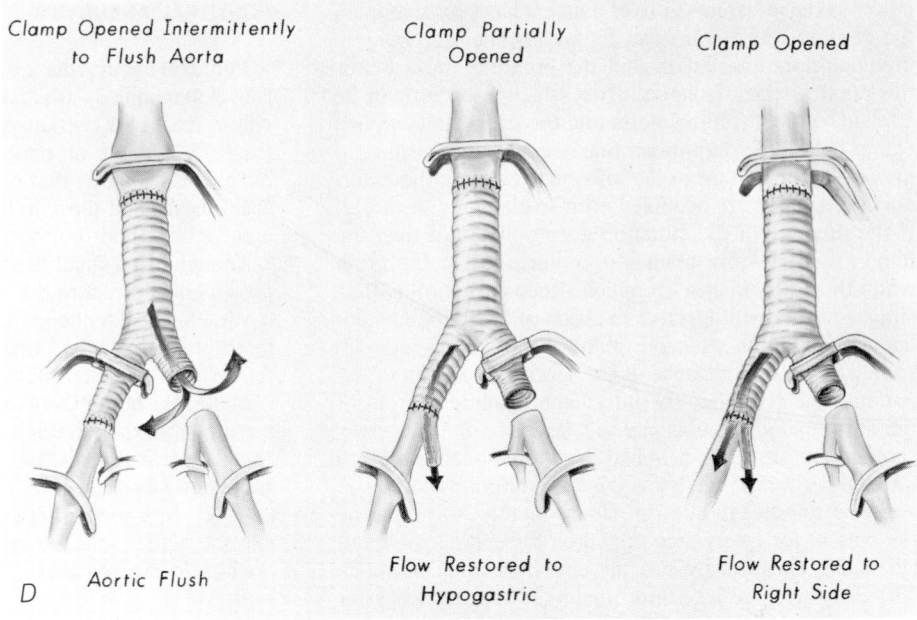

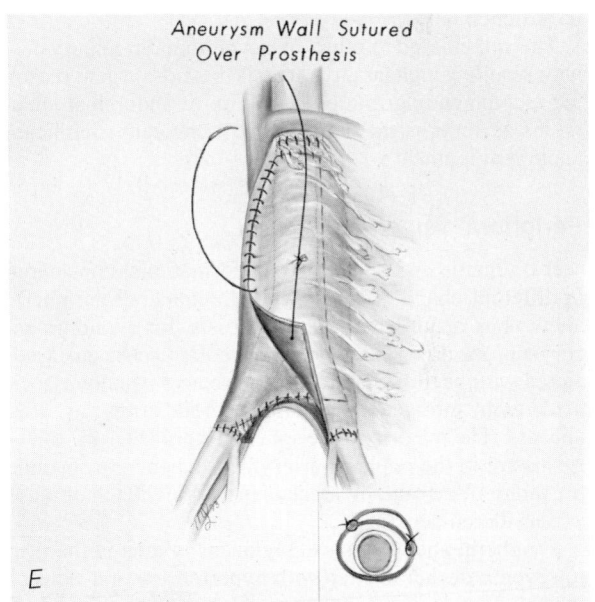

Fig. 21-24. Procedure for substituting aortoiliac bifurcation prosthesis for abdominal aortic aneurysm. *A*. A midline incision extending from xiphoid process to pubic symphysis is usually employed. Insert shows rotation of the table to the patient's right side, which facilitates retraction of the small bowel. *B*. Surgical exposure of vital structures and lines of incision of the aneurysm are shown. *C*. Endarterectomy of the aneurysm wall is performed; the lumbar arteries transfixed with sutures and the prosthesis in place are shown. *D*. Technique for preventing embolization of atherosclerotic debris to the lower extremities and gradually restoring lower extremity circulation to avoid declamping shock. (1) Aorta is flushed through one open limb of the prosthesis. (2) Flow gradually restored to one hypogastric artery and, when the blood pressure has been stabilized, to the ipsilateral external iliac artery. (3) The sequence is repeated on the opposite side. *E*. The remains of the aneurysm wall and the base of the left colon mesentery are carefully sutured over the prosthesis and suture lines to prevent adherence of the bowel and to bolster the suture lines to prevent aorticointestinal fistulas. [From: *Imparato AM et al: Avoidance of shock and peripheral embolism during surgery of the abdominal aorta. Surgery 73(1):68, 1973, with permission.*]

the graft with the adventitia of the aneurysm, thereby separating the prosthetic graft from the intestine. Sexual dysfunction consisting of retrograde ejaculation or impotence occurs in 25 to 50 percent of male patients.

RUPTURED ABDOMINAL ANEURYSM

CLINICAL MANIFESTATIONS. A ruptured abdominal aneurysm is a grave surgical emergency whose onset is characterized by acute vascular collapse, usually with abdominal or flank pain. With collapse, the diagnosis initially may be uncertain, unless a pulsating mass is palpated. A frequent erroneous diagnosis is renal colic or massive myocardial or pulmonary infarction. The diagno-

sis usually can be established by careful, deep palpation of the abdomen that should outline a pulsating, ill-defined mass in the epigastrium or flank.

TREATMENT. Operation should be performed as quickly as possible, infusing 500 to 1000 mL of fluid every few minutes until serious hypotension has been corrected. A midline incision is preferred. Proximal control of the aorta generally can be obtained by isolating the aorta above the stomach just below the diaphragm. This should be done initially, because once the posterior peritoneum is incised and the hematoma surrounding the ruptured aneurysm evacuated, massive hemorrhage can occur with exsanguination. The aorta can be safely clamped below the diaphragm for 20 to 30 min without serious ischemic injury to the intestines or liver. Once it has been clamped, the ruptured aneurysm can be widely incised, intraabdominal clots evacuated, and the proximal aorta below the renal arteries isolated, after which a clamp can be applied to the infrarenal aorta and the previously applied clamp below the diaphragm released. When possible, to prevent embolization to the lower extremities, the external iliac arteries are occluded prior to clamping the aorta. If the urgency of the situation does not permit this, the femoral arteries are manually compressed in the groin while the aortic clamp is applied. Reconstruction is then similar to that with elective excision of an abdominal aneurysm, although excision of the wall of the aneurysm should be limited because of the serious condition of the patient. On occasion, the infradiaphragmatic portion of the aorta cannot be clamped, because of either the massive amount of retroperitoneal hematoma or free rupture into the peritoneal cavity. In this case, left thoracotomy is required to achieve control. Consequently, in preparing the patient for emergency operation for abdominal aneurysm, the chest as well as the abdomen must be made surgically accessible. Unfortunately, despite successful removal of the aneurysm, death results in 30 to 50 percent of patients.

The unheralded rupture of asymptomatic aneurysms, with resulting high fatality rates, is the most urgent reason for recommending routine operation of abdominal aneurysms as soon as the diagnosis of a clinically significant aneurysm is made.

Peripheral Aneurysms

If traumatic and congenital malformations, considered in different chapters, are excluded, almost all peripheral aneurysms result from arteriosclerosis, for syphilitic aneurysms are now seldom seen. Mycotic aneurysms associated with bacterial endocarditis are now usually associated with intravenously administered drugs in drug abusers. The majority of peripheral arteriosclerotic aneurysms are in the popliteal artery. Infrequent sites include the femoral, carotid, or subclavian arteries. Each of these is considered separately.

Peripheral aneurysms usually occur in men in the fifth to seventh decades, often with hypertension and signs of atherosclerosis in other organs. Multiple aneurysms are frequent. In contrast to abdominal or thoracic aneurysms, where rupture is the greatest threat, peripheral aneurysms infrequently rupture but cause disability due to distal embolization or thrombosis, with subsequent ischemia and gangrene of extremities.

Peripheral aneurysms are readily amenable to successful therapy if operated upon electively before embolization with irreversible occlusion of outflow vessels and acute ischemia develop in the extremity. Tortuosity of the involved artery sometimes makes it possible to mobilize the artery proximal and distal to the aneurysm and reestablish continuity following excision by end-to-end anastomosis. Continuity can also be established preferably with saphenous vein, but if this is not possible, a knitted Dacron prosthesis or PTFE is preferred.

POPLITEAL ANEURYSM

Popliteal aneurysms are usually arteriosclerotic, occurring in men in the sixth and seventh decades of life, half of whom may be hyperactive. They occur bilaterally in at least 25 percent of patients afflicted. Their detection raises the suspicion that other arteriosclerotic aneurysms are present, and these must be searched for in the abdomen, groins, and thorax.

Though often small (3 to 4 cm) and asymptomatic, they pose a grave threat to the viability of the affected extremity due to their tendency to embolize to tibial arteries or to thrombose. Once either complication has occurred, retrieval is virtually impossible.

CLINICAL MANIFESTATIONS. Finding of a pulsating mass behind the knee is characteristic enough to permit an accurate diagnosis. Rarely, the aneurysm may enlarge sufficiently to cause local pain and tenderness. Rupture is unusual. In some instances the presenting manifestation may be acute ischemia of the extremity, and the aneurysm is discovered at operation for acute popliteal occlusion.

If the aneurysm is thrombosed, pulsations may be absent, and a mass may or may not be felt. Differential diagnosis must include other cystic tumors about the knee joint, such as Baker's cyst, as well as other causes of tibial arterial occlusion, such as emboli, Buerger's disease, and diabetes mellitus. The presence or absence of pedal pulses should be carefully noted.

Calcification in the wall of the aneurysm is often visible on a radiograph. The diagnosis can be confirmed by CT and by arteriography, although much of the cavity of the aneurysm may be filled with thrombus (Fig. 21-25).

TREATMENT. Because of the hazards of thrombosis, embolization, and gangrene, operation should be performed as soon as possible after the diagnosis is made even though the aneurysm is small, asymptomatic, and seemingly stable. A retrospective study of gangrene and amputation from popliteal aneurysms that have embolized found no warning signs that such a catastrophe was imminent, although the absence or disappearance of one or both pedal pulses in the presence of a pulsating aneurysm usually signifies that distal embolization has occurred and that acute ischemia will occur very shortly.

Operative Technique. With the patient in a prone position, an incision across the popliteal crease readily exposes the artery proximal and distal to the aneurysm. A transverse incision in the line of the popliteal crease, with extension vertically downward on the medial aspect of the upper calf and upward along the posterolateral aspect of the thigh, has also been used. An alternative exposure is particularly useful when the femoral artery needs to be exposed for some distance from the popliteal. With the patient supine, an incision is made on the medial aspect of the lower thigh and extended across the knee joint into the upper calf, transecting the muscles inserting into the upper medial tibial plateau as well as the head of the gastrocnemius tendon. Transection of these muscles provides unusually wide exposure and has not resulted in any late impairment of function of the extremity.

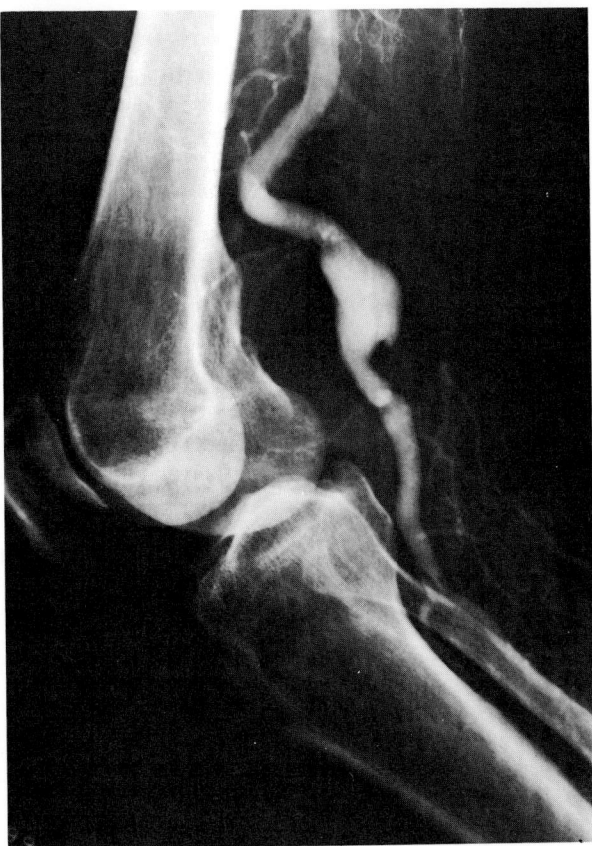

Fig. 21-25. Femoral angiogram indicating the presence of a popliteal aneurysm. Characteristic tortuosity of the involved artery is present. Such tortuosity sometimes makes it possible to establish continuity by direct anastomosis following excision of the aneurysm.

Once the artery has been isolated distal to the aneurysm, vascular clamps are applied and the aneurysm widely opened. Any laminated thrombus is removed, as well as the inner lining of the wall of the aneurysm, preserving the adventitial sheath. The origins of the geniculate branches of the popliteal artery are sutured from within the lumen. This technique preserves branches of the popliteal vein that are usually stretched over the wall of the aneurysm, and also the collateral circulation is less disturbed. A small amount of heparin should be given systemically before the application of clamps.

If the aneurysm is small and the popliteal artery tortuous, an end-to-end anastomosis is sometimes possible. Most patients, however, require a short graft, preferably a reversed autologous saphenous vein. Short grafts of knitted Dacron have also been satisfactory.

Although variations in the suitability of vein grafts in different reports are as low as 43 percent in some, it has been our experience that a vein substitution for the popliteal aneurysm can be achieved in approximately 85 to 90 percent of the patients.

Acute Ischemia. When operation is required because thrombosis has produced severe ischemia with impending gangrene, a different approach is needed, and restoration of flow is difficult and uncertain. Simple excision of the aneurysm, of course, is futile with the obstructed distal circulation. The major consideration is removal of these distal thrombi, which usually have become intimately adherent to the tibial arterial walls, followed by restoration of arterial continuity across the occluded aneurysm, as in elective procedures. Operative incision and exposure should be planned to permit precise cannulation of the anterior and posterior tibial arteries with balloon-tipped catheters to remove propagated thrombus. Retrograde flushing with saline solution from the posterior and anterior tibial arteries is much less satisfactory than the Fogarty catheter technique. Operative angiography should be available to be certain that all thrombi have been removed. In many patients the distal thrombi have become adherent to the arterial wall and resist removal. If thrombi are not completely removed, as confirmed by angiography, rethrombosis terminating in gangrene and amputation is almost a certainty.

FEMORAL ANEURYSM

INCIDENCE AND PATHOLOGY. Although considerably less often encountered than popliteal aneurysms, femoral aneurysms occur in the same population group with the same predisposing factors, exposing patients to the same dangers of embolization, thrombosis, and lower extremity ischemia with a rare incidence of rupture. Their location is in the common femoral or superficial femoral artery, with equal incidence, while approximately half the afflicted patients have involvement of both areas. Involvement of the profunda femoris is extremely rare. The false anastomotic aneurysm associated with aortofemoral artificial prostheses will be discussed under Traumatic Aneurysms.

CLINICAL MANIFESTATIONS. Symptoms usually consist of an awareness of a pulsating mass in the upper thigh until thrombosis or embolization produces ischemic symptoms in the extremity. The diagnosis can often be easily made on physical examination, outlining the pulsating mass in the femoral artery. A radiograph may show calcification in the wall of the aneurysm. Arteriography is useful to delineate the relationship of the aneurysm to the profunda femoris artery, as well as to define the patency of the distal circulation.

TREATMENT. Surgical correction should be performed promptly, unless coexisting cerebral or coronary artery disease makes the risk of operation prohibitive. If operation is postponed because of concomitant disease, such decisions should be made with the full realization that a subsequent amputation because of gangrene may entail an even greater operative risk to the patient.

At operation the arteries can be mobilized proximal and distal to the point of aneurysm and the aneurysm excised. Vascular continuity may be restored with either a saphenous vein graft or an 8-mm knitted Dacron or Goretex prosthesis. Patency of the profunda femoris artery should be maintained by using a Y-bifurcation graft if necessary. Complications following operation are unusual unless peripheral arterial occlusion has already produced severe

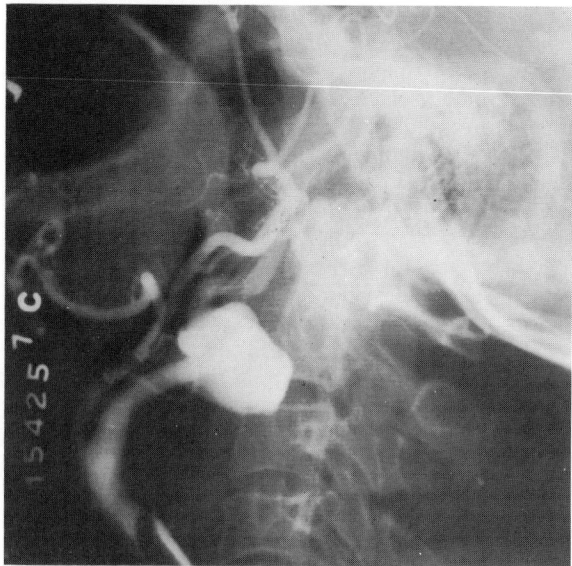

Fig. 21-26. Carotid arteriogram illustrating saccular aneurysm of the internal carotid artery. The internal carotid proximal and distal to the aneurysm is opacified.

ischemic signs. In most patients following operation the prognosis is determined by the coexisting atherosclerotic disease, rather than the femoral aneurysm.

CAROTID ARTERY ANEURYSM

INCIDENCE AND PATHOLOGY. The infrequent occurrence of carotid aneurysms has been documented by several reports. Over a period of time during which 2300 operations for aneurysms had been performed, seven carotid artery aneurysms were noted.

Most carotid aneurysms result from arteriosclerosis and involve either the common carotid artery at the bulb or the extracranial internal carotid artery. Unusual causes include trauma, bacterial infection, or cystic medial necrosis. The main hazard from an aneurysm is embolization of thrombotic material into the cerebral circulation with production of cerebral infarcts. Infrequently, such aneurysms may enlarge and rupture.

CLINICAL MANIFESTATIONS. Patients are usually seen because of a mass in the neck. Pulsations are often prominent and provide an easy clue to the diagnosis. A more difficult problem arises if pulsations are absent, because of laminated thrombus occupying most of the cavity of the aneurysm. Arteriography is the most definitive laboratory technique, establishing the diagnosis and also defining the relationship of the common and internal carotid arteries to the aneurysm (Fig. 21-26). The differential diagnosis should include prominent pulsations from buckling of the carotid artery, a condition seen in hypertensive women, and other solid tumors of the neck, such as a lymph node or a carotid body tumor.

TREATMENT. Because of the constant risk from cerebral infarction, the aneurysm should be excised as soon as possible. The major consideration in planning operation is protection of the brain from ischemic injury while the carotid artery is occluded during excision. In one report, 12 patients were described in whom the aneurysm was excised without any protection of the brain from ischemia. Six of the twelve had a transient neurologic injury, while four developed a permanent neurologic deficit.

The safest surgical technique is excision of the aneurysm under local or regional block anesthesia, keeping the patient awake to assess constantly the tolerance of the brain for temporary occlusion of the carotid artery. If ischemic symptoms develop, an internal shunt may be utilized to maintain cerebral blood flow. Even with a large aneurysm, regional block anesthesia is adequate. On occasion, dislocation of the mandible at the temporomandibular joint is necessary to achieve adequate exposure.

Experiences indicate that in over one-half of the patients there is sufficient tortuosity and elongation of the carotid artery proximal and distal to the site of involvement of the aneurysm to permit mobilization of the ends of the carotid artery and direct anastomosis, although a vein graft may be needed to bridge the gap (Fig. 21-27). Following excision of the aneurysm with reconstruction of the carotid artery, convalescence has usually been uncomplicated, and long-term results are excellent. The most severe complications of the operative procedure are related to proximity of the aneurysm to major cranial nerves VII to XII. Especially with unusually large internal carotid aneurysms, multiple peripheral nerve palsies resulting in marked deviation of the tongue, hoarseness, facial palsies, and difficulty in swallowing should be expected. Even with dislocation of the mandible at the temporomandibular joint, exposure may still be quite limited, and the nerve palsies are to be expected. Recovery from these usually occurs within 6 to 12 months. Even in the absence of transection of these nerves, recovery may be incomplete.

SUBCLAVIAN ANEURYSMS

The majority of subclavian aneurysms develop as secondary complications of a cervical rib and are discussed in the section Thoracic Outlet Syndromes. The extremely rare subclavian aneurysm that results from arteriosclerosis is similar to other peripheral arteriosclerosis aneurysms; it occurs in older men, often with arteriosclerotic aneurysms elsewhere. The diagnosis is usually readily made from physical examination. The most important differential diagnosis is from the frequently seen tortuosity of the innominate and subclavian arteries that occurs in hypertensive patients. Careful examination of the bulge will differentiate a true aneurysm from a tortuous vessel. If aneurysm cannot be excluded, an arteriogram should be done. Excision with reconstruction of the involved artery can be easily performed.

Visceral Aneurysms

SPLENIC ARTERY ANEURYSM

Significant aneurysms of the splenic artery are uncommon. Because of their rarity and unusual manifestations,

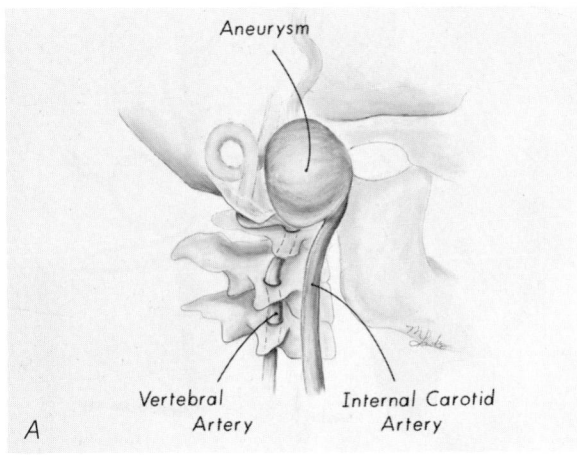

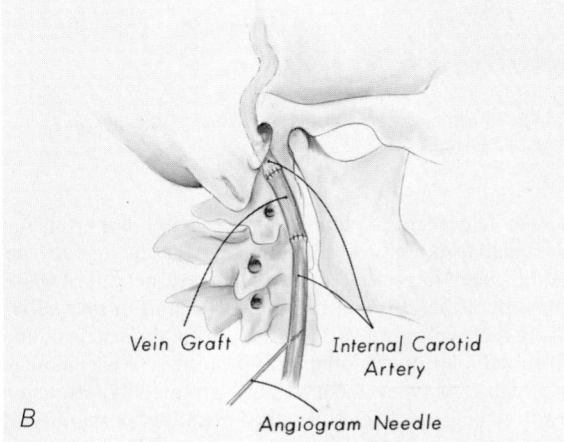

Fig. 21-27. Carotid aneurysmectomy is possible even when the internal carotid artery is involved in its upper extracranial portion, since the artery can be exposed through lateral neck incisions to the base of the skull. *A.* Internal carotid aneurysm. *B.* Replacement with vein graft. (From: *Sanoudos GM et al: Internal carotid aneurysm. Am Surg 39:118, 1973, with permission.*)

several detailed reviews have been published. In 1953 Owens and Coffey reported six patients and found a total of 198 cases in previous reports. Of historical interest is the fact that President Garfield in 1881 died from a traumatic aneurysm of the splenic artery 2 months after being shot by an assassin.

INCIDENCE AND PATHOLOGY. A report of unusual interest is that of Bedford and Lodge in 1960 who published findings from 250 consecutive postmortem examinations in older patients. Routine dissection of the splenic artery found 26 aneurysms, an incidence of nearly 10 percent. All had been asymptomatic. Their size was small, ranging from a few millimeters to as large as 2.5 cm: most were close to 1 cm in diameter. In the 204 cases reviewed by Owens and Coffey, the average diameter was 3 cm. This great discrepancy between the high autopsy incidence and the rarity of clinically symptomatic aneurysms indicates that small aneurysms are probably of no clinical significance and are usually overlooked.

These aneurysms, like other arteriosclerotic aneu-

rysms, occur in older patients with an average age near fifty. Surprisingly, though, the aneurysms are more frequent in women, in contrast to the overwhelming predominance of the usual arteriosclerotic aneurysm in men. In the Owens and Coffey series, 127 patients were women and 63 were men. Bedford and Lodge noted that the aneurysms tended to develop at bifurcations of the splenic artery and suggested that degeneration of the media, as well as atherosclerosis, might be a predisposing factor.

The aneurysms are usually single and in the main trunk of the splenic artery. Rupture is more likely to occur during pregnancy. The actual risk of rupture is uncertain, for many are recognized only after rupture. Rupture is obviously a grave event, for of 131 symptomatic patients reported by Owens and Coffey 94 died from rupture and only 7 from other causes. In 37 female patients, rupture occurred during late pregnancy.

CLINICAL MANIFESTATIONS. Pain in the epigastrium or left flank is the most frequent symptom, occurring in 93 of 131 symptomatic patients in the Owens series. Other symptoms are nonspecific gastrointestinal symptoms, usually interpreted as due to peptic ulcer. These include nausea, vomiting, dyspepsia, and constipation or diarrhea. Gastrointestinal hemorrhage has occurred in about one-third of patients. For unknown reasons gastrointestinal symptoms may exist for months or years before the diagnosis is made. This may be fortuitous.

Often rupture is the first sign of the aneurysm, as it was in 46 percent of the patients in one series. A "double" rupture is a significant clinical sequence, recognized in about one-half of patients. The first rupture is hemorrhage into the lesser omental sac; this ceases temporarily but is followed in 1 to 2 days by secondary hemorrhage and exsanguination.

With the small size of the splenic aneurysms, physical abnormalities are usually not found. For unknown reasons, moderate splenomegaly has been reported in 40 to 50 percent of patients. However, a mass has been palpated in only 20 percent, and pulsations or a bruit in 10 percent. Radiographic identification of a mass with calcium in the walls suggestive of an aneurysm has been reported in 15 percent of the group.

TREATMENT. Obviously symptomatic aneurysms should be excised as soon as the diagnosis is made, usually with concomitant splenectomy. The widespread use of aortography for investigating many abdominal conditions has disclosed aneurysms smaller than 1 cm that are asymptomatic. Their treatment is uncertain because of the rarity of rupture. On the other hand, it is disquieting to note that rupture without preceding symptoms is the first event in one-half of the patients with ruptured splenic aneurysms. From data available, surgical treatment does not seem indicated for asymptomatic aneurysms smaller than 1 cm, but those greater than 3 cm should be excised. Further data are needed to be certain of these guidelines.

RENAL ARTERY ANEURYSM

INCIDENCE AND PATHOLOGY. Aneurysms of the renal artery are similar to aneurysms of the splenic artery in

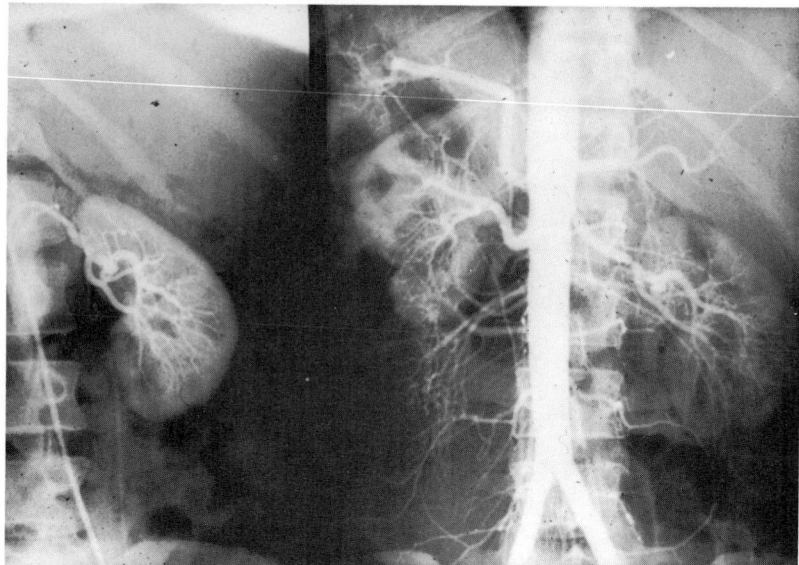

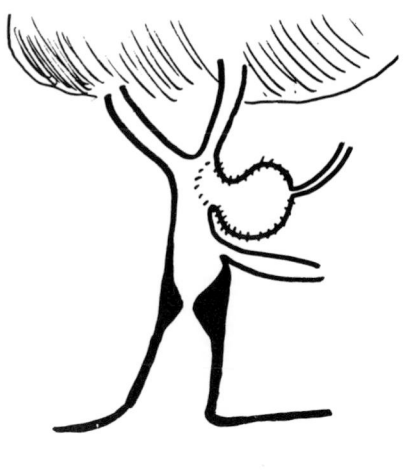

Fig. 21-28. Renal artery aneurysms are frequently saccular, as shown in the angiographic study, and may be associated with arterial hypertension.

that recognition has greatly increased with the use of angiography. The widespread use of renal angiography to investigate patients with hypertension has been chiefly responsible for the increasing recognition of renal aneurysms. Apparently, about 1 percent of hypertensive patients will be found on angiography to have a small aneurysm of one renal artery.

These aneurysms are equally common in males and females, usually in the fifth and sixth decades, but they have been found in all age groups, even in patients as young as nine months. Anatomically they may be saccular or fusiform. Unusual varieties include false aneurysm from trauma, dissecting aneurysm, or arteriovenous fistula. The saccular aneurysm is apparently congenital, arising from a defect in elastic tissue of the wall of the artery, often near a bifurcation. It varies from 1 to 3 cm in size and often develops extensive eccentric calcification, a so-called signet ring on the radiograph. It is infrequently associated with hypertension and rarely ruptures. The fusiform aneurysm develops distal to an area of constriction of the renal artery and is basically a poststenotic aneurysm similar to that seen in other parts of the arterial circulation. Because of the proximal stenosis, it is frequently seen with hypertension.

The aneurysms occur with frequency in either renal artery, usually in the main renal artery or one of its branches. An intrarenal location is uncommon. In one report, 92 aneurysms were in the main renal artery, 44 were in an extrarenal branch, and 15 were intrarenal.

Rupture has been reported in at least 24 patients, with a fatal outcome in 20. Eight of these episodes occurred during pregnancy. Rupture has been recognized rarely in a calcified aneurysm.

CLINICAL MANIFESTATIONS. Abdominal or flank pain has occurred in about 50 percent of the patients but is probably unrelated to the aneurysm. Investigation of the symptom subsequently led to finding the aneurysm. Hematuria, gross or microscopic, has also been reported

in 30 to 40 percent of patients. As expected, hypertension has been frequently seen with poststenotic aneurysms and has been improved or cured in over one-half of these after operation. By contrast, hypertension in one series was present in only 7 of 12 with a saccular aneurysm and improved after operation in only 1 of the 7. A mechanism by which a saccular aneurysm can produce hypertension is not clear except for the rather nebulous possibility of compression or distortion of the renal artery. The association may simply be fortuitous.

There are usually no abnormalities on physical examination. Occasionally a localized bruit is audible. Radiographic examination may show signet ring calcification which must be differentiated from calcification of mesenteric lymph nodes or calcification of other visceral arteries. The intravenous pyelogram is abnormal in about one-half of the patients because of ischemia, infarction, or localized pressure defects. Aortography is essential to establish the diagnosis and define the precise location (Fig. 21-28). As mentioned earlier, most aneurysms have been found during aortography performed for other purposes.

TREATMENT. Prompt operation is indicated whenever an aneurysm is found during investigation of a patient for hypertension. With poststenotic aneurysms the aneurysm can be excised and the renal artery reconstructed, with an excellent likelihood of improving the hypertension. With a saccular aneurysm and hypertension, operation is probably indicated to reconstruct the renal artery, although the prognosis for improving the hypertension is less favorable. In the 17 patients reported by Smith, 5 had successful operations, while 12 with small aneurysms of questionable significance had been followed without operation for an average of 3 years without complications. The "bench" technique, in which the kidney is removed from its bed by transecting the main arteries and veins and leaving the ureter intact, performing microsurgical arterial repair on branch arteries, and then reattaching the main vessels to the iliac vessels, has permitted removal of branch artery aneurysms without sacrifice of kidneys. In a patient with a small calcified aneurysm without symptoms or hypertension, there probably is little indication for operation, for the risk of rupture is almost negligible. With larger aneurysms, certainly with symptoms present, operation should be performed.

ETIOLOGY AND PATHOLOGY. A traumatic aneurysm is produced from a tangential laceration of the wall of an artery. Usually continuity of flow through the lacerated artery is maintained. By contrast, injuries that transect an artery often require immediate treatment because of hemorrhage or ischemia in the affected limb and consequently seldom evolve into an aneurysm.

Following the laceration, blood extravasates into adjacent soft tissues to form a hematoma that compresses and seals the point of injury. If the artery is confined within a small space surrounded by fascia, the hematoma may be small enough to escape recognition. Both the patient and the physician are unaware that an arterial injury has occurred. After days or weeks, the blood clot gradually liquefies; then the firm, immobile mass surrounding the artery begins to pulsate. A descriptive term for these lesions is "pulsating hematoma." With the appearance of pulsation, the aneurysm begins to enlarge. This is ominous, for enlargement is progressive and relentless, destroying nerves, even eroding bone, and eventually terminating in rupture and death.

Traumatic aneurysms are often termed false aneurysms, as distinguished from true aneurysms (see the discussion under Aneurysms, above), for the wall is composed of fibrous tissue rather than components of normal arterial wall, as with arteriosclerotic or syphilitic aneurysms.

As the hematoma enlarges in a recent wound, the tissues are firm, tender, perhaps warm. These findings of redness, tenderness, and heat are, of course, the usual characteristics of an abscess. Occasional vivid reports appear in the surgical literature in which an unsuspecting physician widely incised such a red, tender mass to drain an abscess, with resultant violent hemorrhage.

A similar therapeutic catastrophe occasionally occurs when a traumatic aneurysm stabilizes for years and is subsequently confused with a neoplasm. If the previous history of trauma is not available, the differential diagnosis is difficult, for the aneurysm is partly filled with clot and closely resembles a solid tumor. Attempted biopsy of such lesions, with frightening consequences, has been reported.

Usually there is no disability from a traumatic aneurysm except for the local mass until it enlarges to compress adjacent nerves, causing pain, paresthesia, and eventually paralysis. The peripheral arterial circulation is usually normal. Peripheral embolization of thrombi from the aneurysm is unusual except for the rare aneurysm of the subclavian artery following trauma. Here, intermittent compression by the clavicle may dislodge emboli.

Ischemic symptoms in the arm may dominate the clinical picture, requiring arteriography to disclose small traumatic aneurysms.

CLINICAL MANIFESTATIONS. A localized mass is often the only finding. As it enlarges, there is pain or paralysis from compression of nerves. On physical examination the borders of the mass are ill defined because the hematoma surrounding the aneurysm is beneath the deep fascia. Pulsations may or may not be present, depending upon the amount of thrombus in the lumen. A systolic bruit is frequently audible. Peripheral pulsations are normal.

If the mass pulsates, the diagnosis is reasonably certain from the physical findings. Otherwise arteriography is required to differentiate it from a neoplasm or a cyst. On arteriography the full size is not disclosed, as much of the cavity is filled with thrombus.

TREATMENT. Operation should be performed as soon as the diagnosis has been established because of the inevitable outcome of enlargement and rupture. If neurologic symptoms are present, operation should be done urgently, within hours, to prevent irreversible pressure injury of crucial nerves. At operation the incision should be placed to permit exposure of the uninvolved artery proximal and distal to the aneurysm. With these vessels temporarily occluded, the aneurysm can be widely incised, clots evacuated, and the point of origin from the artery identified. Dissection around the aneurysm before it is opened should be avoided; it is unnecessary, complicated, and often dangerous.

With unusually large aneurysms, it is important to remember that there is only one small opening in the wall of the aneurysm, the tangential laceration of the arterial wall from which the aneurysm began. Hence, if the aneurysm is inadvertently entered, this small opening can be digitally occluded to control bleeding while further exposure is obtained.

Once the aneurysm has been opened and the inner contents removed, the site of communication with the parent artery can be mobilized and the injured area excised. Complete excision of the wall of the aneurysm is unnecessary and should be avoided because of the surrounding dense fibrotic reaction. Once the involved artery has been mobilized, arterial continuity can usually be restored by end-to-end anastomosis or by insertion of a short graft, preferably autologous vein. Ligation should be performed only for small arteries, such as the radial, not essential to normal circulation. Convalescence after operation is usually uneventful and long-term results excellent. Hughes and Jahnke reported continuing good results 5 years after surgical treatment of 67 traumatic aneurysms during the Korean conflict.

ANASTOMOTIC FALSE ANEURYSM

False aneurysm can occur at any arterial suture line but is most frequently encountered where plastic prostheses have been sutured to host arteries, usually in the groin, at the terminal ends of bypass grafts. The longest interval between the original operation and the appearance of false aneurysms in the authors' experience has been 20 years. The incidence was estimated at 2 to 25 percent when suture material such as silk was used. Since the introduction of Prolene and other synthetics, the incidence has decreased.

CLINICAL MANIFESTATIONS. Thrombosis and rupture are the two major complications encountered with false aneurysms. Neighboring structures such as the duodenum may become adherent to an infrarenal aortic suture line and result in an aortoduodenal fistula from rupture, manifest by massive upper gastrointestinal hemorrhage, of a false aneurysm. The clinical presentation depends upon the location of the anastomotic false aneurysm and varies from the presence of a gradually enlarging pulsatile mass to the appearance of acute ischemia of a limb due to thrombosis of, or embolization from, the aneurysm. The patient may present in shock due to the intraabdominal rupture of an iliac or aortic false aneurysm.

TREATMENT. Treatment is surgical and varies according to the location of the aneurysm. The most commonly encountered groin aneurysm can usually be managed by resection of the terminal inch or two of the old prosthesis together with the false aneurysm wall, preserving the posterior wall of the common femoral artery together with the ostia of the profunda femoris artery and the superficial femoral, if it is patent. A segment of new prosthesis is anastomosed to bridge the gap. Immediate results are excellent but recurrences occur.

Mycotic Aneurysm

Mycotic aneurysm is an aneurysm resulting from the introduction of bacteria into the arterial wall. This can be caused by embolization of septic emboli from bacterial endocarditis, from contiguous infection, and from direct trauma to arteries with nonsterile needles, particularly in intravenous drug abusers. The term "infected aneurysm" is preferable for secondary infection of an already existing aneurysm. Since the advent of antibiotics, septic aneurysms resulting from bacterial endocarditis have decreased in incidence and the types of bacteria associated with them has changed from a predominance of *Streptococcus* and *Staphylococcus* to a wider spectrum of bacteria, including enteric organisms and fungi.

CLINICAL MANIFESTATIONS. These vary with the location of the aneurysm, which may remain totally undetected until rupture and shock occur. When a superficial vessel is involved, there may be a tender pulsatile mass with local signs of infection, at times associated with systemic signs of sepsis.

TREATMENT. The underlying condition requires antibiotic therapy. The aneurysm is excised; the involved artery is ligated proximally and distally. Arterial continuity may have to be re-established through extraanatomic routes, preferably with autologous tissue. Many technically complex surgical problems are associated with treatment of mycotic aneurysms. The prognosis for limb survival and patient survival is uncertain. Those mycotic aneurysms encountered in intravenous drug abusers are associated with high rates of recurrence since the original drug addiction is difficult to eliminate and repeated needle trauma persists.

BUERGER'S DISEASE

HISTORICAL DATA. The entity referred to as Buerger's disease was first described by Winiwarter in 1879 and elaborated upon by Buerger in 1908 and again in 1924. The descriptive term *thromboangiitis obliterans* (TAO) emphasizes the inflammatory reaction in the arterial wall, with involvement of the neighboring vein and nerve, terminating in thrombosis of the artery. In 1960 doubt was cast upon the specificity of the pathologic findings when Wessler et al. pointed out that arterial occlusion from any cause, be it atherosclerosis or even embolic occlusion, may result in a similar type of angiitis, indistinguishable from what was usually considered to be specific for TAO. The relatively widespread use of arteriography has shown that many cases of so-called Buerger's disease probably represented presenile atherosclerosis occurring in the third, fourth, and fifth decades of life.

INCIDENCE AND ETIOLOGY. In our experience, we have made the diagnosis in fewer than 0.25 percent of all our patients with occlusive arterial disease of the extremities. The disease is found most frequently in men between twenty and forty years of age, is uncommon in women, who compose only 5 to 10 percent of patients with Buerger's disease, and is also rare in blacks. Initially it was felt that the disease was much more common in the Jewish race; subsequent statistical studies have shown that this frequency has been greatly exaggerated and the incidence is only slightly greater if at all.

Heavy tobacco smoking, usually 20 or more cigarettes per day, has been almost universally associated with this disease. The tobacco habit is firmly entrenched in these individuals in spite of obvious remissions that occur upon cessation of smoking. DeBakey and Cohen analyzed 936 patients and found that only 10 percent successfully stopped smoking over a 10-year period.

Although the correlation between Buerger's disease and smoking is strong, the mechanisms involved are not clear. Either there is a particular response to tobacco (since there are so many more smokers than patients with Buerger's disease), or, as in the Orient, particular brands of cigarettes are associated with the disease. This has never been noted in the West. It has recently been suggested that there is an association with rickettsial disease.

PATHOLOGY. The gross features of Buerger's disease are characteristic of an inflammatory process. The diseased artery is usually surrounded by a dense fibrotic reaction, often incorporating the adjacent vein, less often the neighboring nerve. Although this is usually considered to be characteristic of thromboangiitis obliterans, it also occurs occasionally with atherosclerosis obliterans and very frequently in association with aneurysmal disease.

The distribution of arterial involvement is different from that of atherosclerosis in that smaller, more peripheral arteries, usually in segmental distribution, are involved. In the lower extremities the disease generally occurs beyond the popliteal arteries, starting in tibial vessels extending into the vessels of the foot, in a fashion similar to the typical arterial involvement in the diabetic. In the upper extremities, where atherosclerotic and diabetic involvement are extremely rare, TAO is manifested by arterial involvement usually distal to the forearm in about 30 percent of these patients. The visceral and cardiac circulations can be involved, but this occurs rarely.

Early in the course of Buerger's disease, there is involvement of superficial veins, producing the characteristic migratory, recurrent superficial phlebitis, while the larger and deeper veins (such as femoral and iliac) are rarely affected.

Although some doubt has been raised about the specificity of the histologic findings, most observers consider them to be characteristic. Precise retrospective diagnoses have been made on the basis of histologic examination of amputated extremities.

Microscopic examination of small thrombosed arteries shows extensive proliferation of intimal cells and fibroblasts throughout all segments of the arterial wall, with preservation of the basic architecture of the artery. Lipid deposition and calcification, frequently seen in atherosclerosis, are absent. Inflammatory cells, usually lymphocytes, are observed, while giant cells, whose presence was noted originally by Buerger, generally are absent. Necrosis of the arterial wall is very unusual, as is abscess formation. The thrombus in the arterial wall shows an unusual degree of fibroblastic activity with endothelial proliferation, suggesting the presence of a primary antigen in the blood. Spaces within the thrombus, interpreted as partial though functionally ineffectual recanalization, are common but not particularly characteristic of Buerger's disease, since this is seen with all thrombotic occlusions.

Involvement of the neighboring vein and nerve by the inflammatory and fibrotic reactions completes the histologic appearance of the lesions.

Periods of exacerbation of the acute process may be manifested by acute superficial phlebitis, with eventual progression of arterial occlusions and ischemia counterbalanced by remissions, during which collateral circulation becomes effective in younger patients. The ultimate severity and extent of the extremity ischemia are determined by the frequency and duration of the acute attacks and the length of the quiescent periods. The cycles can usually be broken by cessation of smoking.

DeBakey and Cohen studied this progression in a group of 936 patients followed during a 10-year period after diagnosis and noted a three times higher mortality rate (10 percent), predominantly from cardiovascular disease, than in a control population. Postmortem examination revealed the familiar pattern of atherosclerotic disease in coronary and cerebral vessels, rather than the characteristic histologic pattern of thromboangiitis obliterans found in upper and lower extremity vessels. The limb amputation rate was 20 to 30 percent in 10 years, with an additional 40 percent showing some progression of ischemia but not requiring amputation.

CLINICAL MANIFESTATIONS. There may be a phase of recurrent migratory superficial phlebitis involving superficial veins of the feet, which may occur over a period of years before there is any suspicion of arterial involvement. Invariably the patient is a cigarette smoker, and with continued smoking intermittent claudication appears as the first manifestation of ischemia. Reflecting the peripheral involvement of pedal arteries, pain while walking is usually referred to the arch of the foot, somewhat less often to the calf of the leg, but almost never to the thigh or buttock unless there is associated atherosclerosis obliterans. Upper extremity claudication is rare, probably a reflection of the distribution of arterial involvement, which is usually distal to the wrist. Progression of ischemia is similar to that in all chronic progressive arterial occlusions, in which the initial pain induced by exercise progresses to rest pain, postural color changes, trophic changes, and eventually ulceration and gangrene of one or more digits and finally of an entire foot or hand, necessitating major amputations. Patients with Buerger's disease may eventually require quadruple extremity amputations.

One variant of the typical syndrome is first manifest by painful vesicles of the pulp of fingers with surrounding intensive hyperemia and hypersensitivity, recurring as acute attacks over 2- to 4-year intervals, associated with progressive claudication of the feet and calves. The prognosis appeared to be worsened not only by continued smoking but by smoking certain types of cigarettes.

Pain in Buerger's disease, as in other ischemic conditions of the extremities, is common and may result from phlebitis, ischemic neuritis, or progressive skin and muscle ischemia manifested by the typical ischemic rest pain. This is unremitting and prevents patients from sleeping but is somewhat ameliorated by placing the affected limb in the dependent position. There may be blanching on elevation and rubor on dependence, as well as marked blanching on exposure to cold.

Physical Examination. The most frequent finding is absence of the posterior tibial and dorsalis pedis pulses in the feet. Often the popliteal pulse is palpable, especially in the early stages of the disease. Absence of the posterior tibial pulse is highly suggestive of the diagnosis, especially when bilateral. In the upper extremity, the radial pulse may be congenitally absent in 5 to 10 percent of patients, but absence of both pulses again is very suggestive of the disease. Signs of chronic tissue ischemia include loss of hair from the digits, atrophy of the skin, brittle nails, and rubor on dependency. In more advanced cases there may be ulceration or gangrene in the digits, often beginning near the nail and involving only the distal portion of the digit. With more extensive disease, gangrene extends into the foot. In the upper extremity, fortunately, extension of gangrene beyond the fingers is rare, and amputation of the hand is almost never necessary.

Edema is seen with advanced ischemia, resulting from keeping the extremity in a dependent position to relieve rest pain. Superficial phlebitis involving segments of superficial veins is frequent, but rarely is phlebitis found in the large veins, such as the femoral or iliac. Accordingly, edema on the basis of phlebitis is unusual.

Laboratory Studies. The most significant laboratory examination is arteriography. The arteriographic findings, as emphasized by McKusick et al., are frequently characteristic. Typically, the contours of the large arteries are smooth, without the characteristic irregularities seen in atherosclerosis. In arteries the caliber of the

tibials, there are abrupt areas of occlusion, frequently surrounded by extensive collateral circulation that evolves over many years, is unusually tortuous, and has been termed "tree root" or "spiderlike." A "corkscrew" deformity also has been noted in peripheral arteries, probably representing partial recanalization of arteries previously occluded by thrombi. The combination of extensive occlusive disease in tibial arteries with larger vessels that remain smooth and normal in appearance, especially in association with extensive collateral circulation, is highly characteristic of Buerger's disease and is most useful in differentiating it from atherosclerosis.

DIAGNOSIS. Buerger's disease can be differentiated from atherosclerosis without undue difficulty. Other entities with occlusive disease of tibial arteries, however, closely resemble Buerger's disease. These include diabetes mellitus, popliteal aneurysms, repeated episodes of arterioarterial embolization from proximal atherosclerotic plaques, and different collagen disorders. Patients with any of these may have palpable popliteal pulses, absent pedal pulses, and severe ischemia in the digits. In most of these, however, the upper extremities are not involved. Positive factors supporting the diagnosis of Buerger's disease are its onset in men between the ages of twenty and forty years, a history of migratory phlebitis, strong dependence upon tobacco, usually cigarettes, and associated involvement of the upper extremities. The occurrence of elevated titers to rickettsia has also been suggested as a diagnostic as well as an etiologic factor in the evolution of the disease.

Factors suggesting that the disease is not Buerger's disease include diabetes mellitus, palpable popliteal or abdominal aneurysms, audible bruit over a major artery, high blood cholesterol, calcification of peripheral arteries, and onset after forty years of age.

Usually the diagnosis can be made from the history and physical examination. Angiographic studies are needed for confirmation and to define the possibilities of arterial reconstruction. Final proof of the diagnosis may require gross and microscopic examination of the diseased arteries.

TREATMENT. The most important aspect of treatment is to have the patient forego the use of tobacco in any form. Simply decreasing the frequency of cigarette smoking is ineffective. The great difficulty in getting the patient to stop smoking cannot be overemphasized, for the pernicious addiction to smoking in this disease closely resembles the tenacity of heroin addiction. In most teaching institutions there are one or more pathetic individuals who have undergone amputation of both legs and most of the fingers of each hand but who are trying to get someone to light a cigarette for them.

Sympathectomy may be performed but its benefit is difficult to measure because of the episodic characteristics of Buerger's disease. Perhaps 50 percent of patients significantly benefit from the procedure. Vasodilating drugs may be tried but are of questionable value.

Education regarding foot care similar to that described for the atherosclerotic patient is very important since often gangrene is precipitated by minor trauma to the foot, such as unwise trimming of a callus or wearing tight shoes.

Arteriography should be performed to confirm the diagnosis and exclude other forms of smaller arterial occlusions that may require surgical therapy. If a popliteal pulse is absent, it may indicate the possibility of performing local direct arterial reconstruction.

Occasionally patients with Buerger's disease develop atherosclerotic obstruction of major arteries that are surgically accessible to reconstruction. Such a combination of arterial disease is suggested if the popliteal pulse is absent. In these patients arterial reconstruction may be successfully done upon the atherosclerotic disease, with marked circulatory improvement. Direct surgical approach to the vessels primarily involved by Buerger's disease, however, is usually not possible.

A conservative approach is indicated when amputation is required in these younger patients in the twenty- to forty-year-old age group, since the episodic nature of the disease indicates that conservatism may be rewarded by subsidence of the acute episodes with subsequent partial revascularization by the growth of collateral circulation. As long as gangrene is confined to a toe, amputation should be postponed as long as possible unless rest pain or infection cannot be controlled otherwise.

Once gangrene has involved the foot extensively, there is little point in delaying amputation, because a functional foot can rarely be obtained if the point of amputation is more proximal than the base of the metatarsal bones. Often a below-knee amputation can be performed, rather than an above-knee, because of the lack of involvement of the femoral and popliteal arteries.

Long-term anticoagulant therapy has not been of measurable benefit. Therapy with adrenal steroids, so effective for many inflammatory conditions, has similarly not been of consistent value and may aggravate the intimal changes in the tibial arteries.

PROGNOSIS. The variability of long-term survival data is probably related to the difficulty in establishing the specific diagnosis of Buerger's disease. The risk of amputation within 10 years after onset of symptoms is probably near 20 percent, although this varies with the continued use of tobacco as well as the degree to which the ischemic foot is carefully protected. In the few patients who stop smoking completely, progression of the disease may be greatly restricted. A marked advance in therapy would be the discovery of a method by which abstinence from tobacco could be achieved uniformly in this unfortunate group of individuals.

VASOSPASTIC DISORDERS

Raynaud's Disease

The syndrome described by Maurice Raynaud in 1862, now termed *Raynaud's phenomenon*, consists of recurrent episodes of vasoconstriction in the upper extremities, initiated by exposure to cold or emotional stress. Three sequential phases classically occur: pallor, cyanosis, and rubor. It is now recognized that Raynaud's phenomenon may exist as a primary disorder, termed *Raynaud's disease,* or may be a secondary manifestation of a more serious vascular disease, often not evident for some years after the initial appearance of the recurrent color changes. The more common disorders associated with Raynaud's phenomenon include Buerger's disease (thromboangiitis obliterans), scleroderma, cervical rib or other thoracic outlet syndrome, and atherosclerosis. It occasionally results from recurrent minor trauma, such as from the use of mechanical vibrating tools. Rarely, other collagen diseases, such as periarteritis nodosa or disseminated lupus erythematosus, are found. Hence, in the evaluation of a patient the critical decision is to determine whether the disease is primary Raynaud's disease or a secondary manifestation of a more serious disorder. Some suspect that it is always secondary to some other underlying disorder.

ETIOLOGY. The cause of primary Raynaud's disease is unknown. It is much more frequent in women, with a ratio of about 5:1, and appears in over 90 percent of patients before forty years of age. In men, it is usually much less severe in intensity. DeTakats and Fowler observed abnormal electroencephalograms in some patients, suggesting a primary disease in the midbrain, but the existence of a primary neurologic disease has not been established.

PATHOLOGY. The clinical picture of Raynaud's phenomenon is related to the anatomy and physiology of the arteriolar circulation in the dermis. The arterioles penetrate the dermis at right angles with an irregular reticulate pattern and arborize into a capillary network. Some fluctuation in vasomotor tone, as with pallor or blushing, is a normal physiologic variation. In Raynaud's disease, vasospasm occurs with such severity that dermal circulation momentarily ceases, with the production of severe pallor. If the vasospasm is less severe, with slowing but not cessation of the dermal circulation, cyanosis appears, a result of sluggish flow of blood with an increase in the percentage of reduced hemoglobin in the capillaries. When the vasospasm subsides, a reactive hyperemia with vasodilation develops, probably from the accumulation of tissue metabolites during the anoxic period, producing an unusual redness or rubor.

The basis for the increased tendency of the dermal arterioles to vasoconstriction is unknown. It may be a sensitivity in the arterioles themselves, or possibly may result from hyperactivity of the sympathetic nervous system. Initially the arterioles are normal on histologic examination. With chronic disease, there is progressive hypertrophy of the arteriolar walls and ultimate occlusion. Detailed histologic observation of early phases of Raynaud's disease are not available, because tissue biopsies are seldom performed at this time.

In the majority of patients the episodes of vasoconstriction are precipitated by exposure to cold. In about 25 percent of patients intense emotion, as well as cold, may be the initiating factor. Only rarely is emotion alone the significant stimulus without an abnormal sensitivity to cold.

In most patients the upper extremities are symmetrically involved. Unilateral involvement by Raynaud's phenomenon almost always denotes a proximal mechanical cause, either occlusion of one of the major proximal arteries, recurrent embolization, or neurovascular compression. In 10 to 15 percent of patients the legs are involved as well as the arms.

With repeated episodes of vasoconstriction and ischemia, trophic changes gradually appear. These include atrophy of the skin with loss of elasticity and hair. The term *sclerodactylia* has been applied to this appearance, since it resembles the changes found in scleroderma in other organs. However, long-term studies have demonstrated conclusively that the presence of sclerodactylia in the fingers does not indicate that generalized scleroderma will appear in the future. Focal areas of ulceration develop and leave characteristic scars with healing. Recurrent superficial infections, such as paronychia, may occur. In the more extreme forms of ischemia, gangrene may require amputation of one or more digits, but fortunately gangrene almost never progresses to involve the hands.

CLINICAL MANIFESTATIONS. The patient is usually a young woman who has noted that episodes of cold precipitate vasoconstriction with a repetitive sequence of pallor, cyanosis, and rubor. Several variations in the color phenomena may occur with less severe disease. For example, there may be only cyanosis followed by rubor or only episodes of mild cyanosis.

In addition to the color changes, the patient may have paresthesia and localized pain in the digits. If infection or ulceration is present, pain is more severe. Except for the discomfort in the hands, the patients usually have no other symptoms.

Physical Examination. In the early phases, the extremities may be entirely normal with peripheral pulses of equal volume. The best index to its severity is the extent of trophic changes in the fingers, manifested by atrophy of the skin and nails with loss of hair over the terminal phalanges. In more advanced stages, signs of chronic ischemia are obvious, with punctate scars from healed ulcerations, chronic rubor, and absence of radial or ulnar pulses.

Arteriography is of value in establishing the diagnosis by revealing the absence of occlusive arterial disease and the presence of terminal arterial vasospasm. The most critical examination is demonstration of the vasoconstrictor response to cold. Induction of the characteristic pallor-cyanosis-rubor sequence in both hands following exposure to cold establishes the diagnosis, although it does not differentiate between primary and secondary Raynaud's phenomenon. An electroencephalogram might be obtained to pursue the observation that abnormal electroencephalographic tracings are present in some patients.

Once the presence of Raynaud's phenomenon has been confirmed, the principal question is whether the vasomotor changes are primary or secondary to some other vascular disease. The possibility of early scleroderma can be evaluated by study of the motility of the esophagus and small bowel. Other blood tests to screen for collagen disorders, such as lupus, should be done. The presence of cervical ribs can be easily determined by radiographs of the cervical spine and thorax. Other compression syndromes of the subclavian artery can be detected by performing the maneuvers described under Thoracic Outlet Syndromes. Complete angiographic studies to opacify the arterial circulation from the aortic arch to the small arteries of the hand should be done to exclude the possibility of proximal atherosclerotic plaques producing distal emboli. Occasionally skin and lymph node biopsies are useful.

An important principle in diagnosis is continued observation of the patient over a period of several years. Even after a thorough examination has failed to detect any underlying disease, a disease may appear later. Indeed, patients should be followed indefinitely with this fact in mind.

TREATMENT. In the majority of patients disability is mild. Avoiding cold or other stimuli which precipitate vasoconstriction is adequate. Moving to a warm climate may be considered, but this does not eliminate the attacks. Tobacco certainly should be avoided because of its potent vasoconstrictor action, but this alone does not abolish the syndrome. Various vasodilator drugs have been repeatedly tried, but none has been of consistent benefit. Methyldopa was the earliest effective medication. Intraarterial reserpine often produced dramatic responses of vasodilatation followed by prolonged periods of freedom from recurrent attacks, but its production has been discontinued. Orally administered calcium channel blockers have become the drugs of choice and offer the promise of reasonably good control. Uncontrolled observations show beneficial effects of prostaglandin E, administered intravenously to patients with severe ischemic changes in the fingers and hands. In addition to the healing of ulcerated lesions, improvement in digital blood flow and skin temperature was also reported. The validity of the findings has been questioned, however, because of the failure to observe a control series.

Although cervical dorsal sympathectomy with removal of the first, second, and third thoracic ganglia, preserving the cervical portion of the stellate ganglion to avoid Horner's syndrome, can give excellent immediate results in patients before the advent of the ulceration, relapses are common. DeTakats and Fowler tabulated reports from different groups, including 40 cases of their own, and found that in 424 sympathectomies 55 percent improved. For this reason, sympathectomy is usually employed only when symptoms are severe and other therapy is ineffective. More radical sympathectomies have not given any better results. Proximally all of the stellate ganglion has been removed, producing Horner's syndrome; distad the fourth thoracic ganglion has been included. Another technical modification has been to include the second and third intercostal nerves with the third ganglion because of the demonstration by Skoog that 10 to 15 percent of sympathetic ganglia to the upper extremity are contained in these two intercostal ganglia. Also there has been considerable discussion about differences in preganglionic and postganglionic sympathectomy. None of these variations has been found significant, however, and the conservative sympathectomy involving the first, second, and third

thoracic ganglia is usually performed. Severe trophic changes before operation are unfortunately often associated with a poor result. Patients with scleroderma also obtain little benefit.

Operative Technique. At least four different surgical techniques have been employed at different times for sympathectomy. Originally most were done through a posterior approach, with the patient in a prone position and an incision similar to that for a thoracoplasty. The sympathetic chain was exposed by resecting a short segment of the second or third rib, followed by an extrapleural dissection to isolate the sympathetic chain. In large, muscular individuals this approach is quite difficult and provides only limited exposure. It has been virtually abandoned.

A second technique, a supraclavicular approach, provides excellent exposure in patients of small stature with long thin necks. However, in those with short, thick necks, significant trauma to the brachial plexus, resulting in a painful neuritis, may complicate the postoperative course. An excellent description of the technique was published by Nanson.

Ideal exposure can be obtained by an anterior transthoracic incision, opening the hemithorax in the third or fourth intercostal space. This, of necessity, involves a major thoracotomy, though a simple one. It has been favored by Palumbo, who also emphasized that removal of the lower one-third of the stellate ganglion would adequately sympathectomize the extremity without producing Horner's syndrome.

In recent years the transaxillary approach has become preferred. This is done through a short incision in the axilla, followed by resection of a short segment of the second or third rib and exposure of the sympathetic chain. Good technical descriptions have been published by Roos and by Kirtley et al. The thoracotomy is of much less magnitude than that through the anterior approach, and the incision is in an inconspicuous location.

PROGNOSIS. The prognosis in most patients with primary Raynaud's disease is good, with the exception of the discomfort associated with the abnormal sensitivity to cold. Even in the more advanced forms, tissue loss seldom exceeds the loss of one or more digits. More serious systemic vascular disease does not develop, and although symptoms may continue for many years, there is no known impairment of longevity or health.

On the other hand, patients with secondary Raynaud's phenomenon afflicted with severe collagen disorders frequently progress to loss of tissue, often with amputations of portions of the fingers. This group requires unceasing care of the hands with careful attention to aggressive local treatment of minor injuries and infections.

Uncommon Vasomotor Diseases

Rare, unusual vasomotor diseases include livedo reticularis and acrocyanosis, which primarily result from vasoconstriction, and erythromelalgia, apparently a result of vasodilatation. The disability with these disorders is usually episodic and mild. Their clinical significance lies primarily in differentiating them from more serious underlying disease, such as Buerger's disease, scleroderma, or disseminated lupus erythematosus. Only salient clinical features of these bizarre diseases will be presented here.

LIVEDO RETICULARIS

This unusual vasomotor condition is characterized by a persistent mottled reddish blue discoloration of the skin of the extremities. It is more prominent in the legs and feet than in the hands or arms and only infrequently involves the trunk. Although the severity varies with temperature, becoming worse on exposure to cold, it never entirely disappears spontaneously.

ETIOLOGY AND PATHOLOGY. The cause is unknown, although miscellaneous associated vascular diseases such as hypertension or emotional disorders have been found in different patients.

The pathophysiologic feature apparently is a stenosis of the arterioles that pierce the cutis at right angles and arborize into the peripheral capillaries of the skin. The obstruction of the arterioles, either spastic or organic, therefore affects the peripheral capillary arborizations and accounts for the peculiar reticular nature of the discoloration.

The pathologic change in the arterioles varies from no visible abnormality to proliferation of the intima, in some patients progressing to complete occlusion. With severe organic obstruction, focal ulceration of the skin, usually over the lower legs, may occur.

CLINICAL MANIFESTATIONS. Patients with livedo reticularis complain of the persistent reddish blue mottling over the legs and feet, varying somewhat with temperature. Often the cosmetic appearance is the only concern of the patient. In some there are localized symptoms of coldness, numbness, dull aching, and paresthesia. With severe forms and localized tissue ischemia, there may be pain from local ulceration. These symptoms are more prone to appear during the winter in association with cold temperatures.

The diagnosis is usually made from physical examination, with observation of the persistent blotchy discoloration, and a history of prolonged persistence in association with some variation with environmental temperature. Peripheral pulsations are normal, and trophic changes are not present in the digits. Only with more extreme forms are ischemic ulcers present over the lower legs. These usually heal after a short period of time.

TREATMENT. In most patients no treatment is necessary except reassurance regarding the benign nature of the condition. Gangrene rarely occurs. Avoiding extremes of cold is beneficial in some patients. Vasodilating agents may be tried, but none has been found of consistent benefit. Sympathectomy should be employed if the disability is severe enough to produce local ulceration. After sympathectomy the discoloration may decrease in extent and remain pink rather than blue. In most patients the disorder is a permanent one, remaining as a moderate cosmetic disturbance, but fortunately with no other disability.

ACROCYANOSIS

Acrocyanosis is a disorder characterized by persistent but painless cold and cyanosis of the hands and feet. The cause and the pathologic and pathophysiologic features are virtually unknown, for the disease consists primarily of persistent color changes. Usually it is confused with Raynaud's phenomenon because of the prominent localized cyanosis. Detailed investigation of the pathophysiologic features by Lewis and Landis concluded that the fundamental disorder was a localized abnormality in vasomotor tone in the circulation of the hands and feet. Apparently the basic physiologic condition is a slow rate of blood flow through the skin, the result of chronic arteriolar constriction, which results in a high percentage of reduced hemoglobin in the blood in the capillaries and production of the cyanotic color. Endocrine dysfunction has been found in some patients, but no consistent pattern has been established.

Usually the disorder is found in a young woman who has noted persistent coldness and blueness of the fingers and hands for many years, often with symptoms of less severity in the toes and feet. The abnormalities are more prominent in cold weather, but the extremities are never completely normal. With heat the color may change from deep purple to red, but there are no episodes of blanching, such as occurs with Raynaud's phenomenon. The peripheral pulses are normal, and there are no trophic changes indicative of chronic tissue ischemia, such as atrophy of the skin, sclerosis, or ulceration.

The principal differential diagnosis is from Raynaud's disease because of the prominent color changes in both disorders. The absence of pallor, as well as the absence of signs of chronic ischemia, are the most useful features. Similarly, the constant presence of the color changes in acrocyanosis, as opposed to the intermittent episodic occurrence in Raynaud's disease, is characteristic.

Usually reassurance is the only treatment needed, with the avoidance of cold temperatures when possible. Sympathectomy can be employed with reasonably good results if the disability is more serious. Prognosis is excellent, with tissue loss virtually never occurring. Usually the color changes remain for many years or permanently.

ERYTHROMELALGIA

This rare disorder is characterized by red, warm, painful extremities. The clinical characteristics were described by S. Weir Mitchell in 1872, and the disorder was named by him in 1878. The cause of the primary disease is unknown. Similar phenomena, so-called secondary erythromelalgia, can occur as a result of hypertension or polycythemia vera.

The basic abnormality is an unusual sensitivity to warmth, for skin temperatures of 32 to 36°C, which produce no effects in normal individuals, will regularly induce the painful burning sensation. The exact temperature at which the distress can be produced varies with different patients but may be a precise one for any individual patient. It was termed by Lewis a "critical point." The increase in temperature is usually a result of vasodilatation with increase in blood flow. The exact basis for the spontaneous vasodilatation with the rise in temperature and the burning sensation is not known.

The disease is equally prevalent in men and women, usually of middle age. The distress may be greater in the summer months, but only a general relationship to extremes of heat or cold may be present. The patient soon learns that exposing the extremities to cold, such as by immersing them in ice water, may abort an attack.

Physical examination usually reveals no abnormalities of the peripheral arteries. The diagnosis is usually established by demonstration of a close relationship between the symptoms and skin temperature. This may be induced by direct application of heat, noting the skin temperature at which distress appears. Erythromelalgia should be differentiated from the painful red but cold extremities that occur with Buerger's disease and also with peripheral neuritis.

Aside from the troublesome symptoms, the disorder is a benign one. Avoiding extremes of heat is one of the most useful therapeutic measures. Acetylsalicylic acid, 0.65 g, has been found beneficial in many patients, although the mode of action is uncertain. A trial of therapy with vasoconstrictor drugs, such as ephedrine, should be employed, but consistent value from one drug has not been found. The disorder is usually a permanent one, but no permanent disability results.

FROSTBITE

Several forms of cold injury have been described, usually varying with the environmental conditions under which exposure occurs. These different syndromes include acute pernio (chilblains), chronic pernio, trench foot, immersion foot, and frostbite. Acute and chronic pernio are focal injuries of the skin and subcutaneous tissue resulting from exposure to cold of moderate intensity, representing an increased susceptibility to cold injury in a particular individual. The disorder is seldom a surgical problem, because the lesions are focal, superficial ones that heal readily. Trench foot and immersion foot are primarily military injuries produced by prolonged exposure to cold in damp surroundings, often with temperatures well above freezing, but in circumstances where there is an element of prolonged immobility. Immersion foot is probably simply the seagoing counterpart of trench foot. Such injuries are rarely seen in civilian practice. For practical purposes frostbite is the type of injury usually encountered and will be discussed in detail. The tissue response in the other disorders mentioned, however, is a similar type of response to cold, modified somewhat with the environmental conditions.

ETIOLOGY. Frostbite results when tissues are exposed to cold for varying periods of time. The severity varies both with the temperature and the duration of exposure. It has been demonstrated experimentally that freezing begins in mammalian tissues when the temperature in the deeper parts reaches 10°C and that −5°C is the lowest temperature to which cells may be slowly frozen and still survive. Frostbite injury usually results from exposure

over a period of several hours. In the Korean conflict, 90 percent of the cases occurred at temperatures near −7°C after exposure for 7 to 18 h. A different form of frostbite is produced by acute exposures to below zero temperatures, commonly occurring in airplanes at high altitudes and hence termed "high altitude" frostbite. In such injuries the exposed part is acutely frozen with deposition of ice crystals in the tissues. This unusual form of injury is different from the usual case of frostbite, where a "slow freeze" results.

Several factors influence the injurious effect of cold. Two of the most significant ones are humidity and the presence of wind, both of which accelerate the withdrawal of heat from body tissues. Immobility or occlusive vascular disease also are significant factors, both influencing the rate of peripheral blood flow. Acclimatization has been demonstrated in some persons repeatedly exposed to cold, such as those who live in northern latitudes, and probably is a localized vasomotor adaptation. By contrast, extremities previously injured by cold may remain permanently susceptible to future cold injury, perhaps from an intensified vasoconstrictor response.

PATHOLOGY. The degrees of severity of a frostbite injury have been conventionally grouped into four clinical types analogous to the classification of burn injury. First degree injury consists of edema and redness of the affected part without necrosis; formation of blisters represents a second-degree injury; necrosis of the skin constitutes a third-degree injury; in a fourth-degree injury gangrene of the extremity develops, requiring amputation.

As frostbite occurs, the injured tissue becomes numb and moderately stiff without extensive discomfort. With subsequent rewarming the tissues become reddened, hot, and edematous. At this time blisters erupt and gangrene gradually appears in the more seriously injured tissues. Edema increases to a maximum within 24 to 48 h and then gradually is resorbed as gangrenous tissue begins to demarcate. The extent of gangrene is difficult to estimate initially and requires observations for as long as 30 days or more. Fortunately the degree of gangrene is often much less than that initially feared, because the skin may be gangrenous but the underlying tissue viable. For this reason amputation is delayed until the extent of gangrene is definitely known.

Following recovery of the extremity, there is frequently a permanent increase in vasoconstrictor tone resulting in hyperhidrosis and an abnormal sensitivity to cold. Pain and paresthesia are also common, perhaps as residuals from ischemic neuritis.

It is uncertain whether the fundamental injury from cold results from direct freezing with disruption of cell membranes or whether the injury is primarily an ischemic necrosis from widespread thrombosis of arterioles and capillaries. Certainly vascular occlusion is a prominent feature, whether it is a primary or a secondary event. With exposure to cold, there is severe vasoconstriction, decreasing the rate of blood flow in the chilled extremity, with resulting stasis, sludging of blood, and eventual widespread thrombosis. In clinical experiments, immersion of the arm for 2 h in water at 13°C decreases blood flow to about 3 percent of normal, while immersion of a finger in water at 7°C stops blood flow altogether. In addition to sludging and capillary thrombosis, there is an increase in capillary permeability, resulting in the formation of edema when blood flow is increased after rewarming.

On histologic examination of the injured tissues, edema, infiltration of inflammatory cells, and deposition of fibrin are prominent findings. Widespread thrombosis of small vessels is frequently seen. In addition, focal areas of necrosis may be evident in skin, muscle, and other tissues.

CLINICAL MANIFESTATIONS. Frequently, the patient is unaware that frostbite is occurring. The usual injury occurs with exposure to near freezing temperatures for several hours, often combined with wind, high humidity, damp or wet shoes, or immobility from tightly constricting shoes or confinement in a cramped position. All these factors influence the rate of heat transfer between the extremity and the environment. Initially there may be mild discomfort, but as the extremity becomes numb and somewhat stiff, frequently discomfort is minimal.

When rewarmed, the extremity quickly becomes red, edematous, hot, and painful. This is due to vasodilatation and widespread extravasation of fluid through the walls of capillaries whose permeability has been increased from injury. Edema reaches its peak intensity within 48 h and then gradually subsides over several days. Gangrene gradually becomes evident and slowly demarcates over a period of many days. An ominous sign, indicating that gangrene will develop, is the persistence of coldness and numbness in an area while surrounding tissues become edematous, hot, and painful. The persistent coldness and numbness indicate cessation of all circulation with the certain outcome of ischemic necrosis.

TREATMENT. Frostbite seldom occurs during exposure to cold if proper precautions are taken. This includes wearing dry, insulated, loosely fitting clothing and carefully avoiding long periods of immobility of the exposed extremities. Most cases of clinical frostbite occur in circumstances where exposure to cold inadvertently occurs for long periods of time because of coma from injury, alcohol, or other factors.

Rapid warming of the injured tissue is the most important aspect of treatment. Several studies have clearly demonstrated the advantages of the rapid-rewarming method over any other. The frozen tissue should be placed in warm water, with a temperature in the range of 40 to 44°C. Complete rewarming usually requires about 20 min. Higher temperatures are more injurious than beneficial. A frostbitten part should never be exposed to hot water, an open fire, or excessive dry heat, as in an oven, for the loss of sensitivity in the frozen area makes it especially vulnerable to injury. Warming in water is much more rapid than application of warm blankets, which require three or four times as long as the immersion method.

Following rewarming, the injured extremity should be elevated to minimize formation of edema and carefully protected in a sterile environment. Usually it is left exposed but surrounded by a protective cradle. Blisters are opened only when necessary to remove necrotic skin.

Antibiotic therapy and tetanus antiserum are routinely given to lessen the risk of infection. Demarcation of gangrenous areas should be carefully observed, often for several weeks, before amputation is performed. Often a gangrenous area which initially appears to involve the foot will gradually regress with the separation of superficial areas of gangrenous skin, ultimately with the loss of one or more digits but preservation of the foot.

Angiography of the frostbite patient can define the extent of organic vascular stenosis and the degree of functional vasospasm, thus aiding the choice of therapy. The use of other fast-acting vasodilators such as papaverine might be appropriate.

Both experimental and clinical experiences indicate a beneficial effect from sympathectomy, especially when employed in the first few days after frostbite has occurred. Shumacker and Kilman reported 66 sympathectomies in 38 patients, 24 of which were performed soon after injury. Their experience indicated that sympathectomy should be performed for injuries severe enough to produce necrosis of tissue, both to minimize the extent of necrosis and to prevent the usual late vasomotor sequelae. Golding et al. found in experimental and clinical studies (68 patients) that the proper time for sympathectomy was between 36 and 72 h after injury. Earlier sympathectomies accelerated the rate of edema formation, while sympathectomies performed following the peak intensity of edema seemed to hasten absorption of edema and minimize eventual tissue necrosis. Sympathectomy is also beneficial in alleviating the late sequelae from cold injury, i.e., paresthesia, coldness, and hyperhidrosis.

If vascular injury is the primary event, therapeutic measures to decrease vasoconstriction or blood clotting, such as sympathectomy or the administration of heparin, should be of routine benefit. The theoretic benefit from sympathectomy is the release of vasospasm, which may precipitate thrombosis in injured capillaries and arterioles. Heparin and dextran have also been given in attempts to lessen the degree of small vessel thrombosis that is such a prominent feature on histologic examination of the injured tissues. Although theoretically plausible, consistent benefit has not been demonstrated from the routine use of either heparin or dextran.

PROGNOSIS. Following recovery from injury, all studies have found a significant percentage of residual disability in the extremity. Simeone evaluated 1061 limbs 4 months after frostbite while the patients were still in the hospital and found painful feet and hyperhidrosis the most common complaints. Ervasti described similar sequelae in 812 cases of frostbite 5 to 18 years after injury. Orr and Fainer reported that gangrene occurred in only 6 percent of 1880 cases from the Korean conflict, but some disability remained in 10 to 20 percent of patients.

Bibliography

Occlusive Disease: General

Collins GJ Jr: Vascular occlusive disorders. Medical and surgical management. Mt Kisco, NY, Futura Publishing, 1981.

Dale WA: The beginnings of vascular surgery. *Surgery* 76:849, 1974.

Goldenfarb PB, Cathey MH, Cooper GR: The determination of ADP induced platelet aggregation in normal men. *Atherosclerosis* 12:335, 1970.

Greenhalgh RM, Rosengarten DS, Mervart I: Serum lipids and lipo proteins in peripheral vascular disease. *Lancet* 2:947, 1971.

Hardy JD, Conn JH, Fain WR: Nonatherosclerotic occlusive lesions of small arteries. *Surgery* 57:1, 1965.

Honour AJ, Pickering GW, Sheppard BL: Ultrastructure and behavior of platelet thrombi in injured arteries. *Br J Exp Pathol* 52:482, 1971.

Lassen NA, Holstein P: Use of radioisotopes in assessment of distal blood flow and distal blood pressure in arterial insufficiency. *Surg Clin North Am* 54(1):39, 1974.

Rob CG: *The Classics of Vascular Surgery,* in Reemtsma K (ed): *The Classics of Surgery Library, Classics in Vascular Surgery.* Medford, NJ, Apollo, 1982.

Rutherford RB: *Vascular Surgery.* Philadelphia, Saunders, 1977.

Salzman EW: The limitations of heparin therapy after arterial reconstructions. *Surgery* 57:131, 1965.

Schatz IJ: Classification of primary hyperlipidemia. *JAMA* 210:701, 1969.

Schnetzer GW: Platelets and thrombogenesis: Current concepts. *Am Heart J* 83:552, 1972.

Scott HW Jr: Metabolic surgery for hyperlipidemia and atherosclerosis. *Am J Surg* 123:3, 1972.

Stanley JC, Gewertz BL, et al: Arterial fibrodysplasia: Histopathologic character and current etiologic concepts. *Arch Surg* 110:561, 1975.

Thompson JE, et al: Peripheral-arterial surgery. *N Engl J Med* 302:491, 1980.

Manifestations of Chronic Arterial Occlusion

Bernstein EF: *Noninvasive Diagnostic Techniques in Vascular Disease.* St Louis, Mosby, 1982.

Boyd AM: The natural course of arteriosclerosis of the lower extremities. *Angiology* 11:10, 1960.

Croneweth JL, Warner KG, et al: Intermittent claudication: Current results of nonoperative management. *Arch Surg* 119:430, 1984.

Ekroth R, Dahilof AG, et al: Physical training of patients with intermittent claudication: Indications, methods, and results. *Surgery* 84:640, 1978.

Goldenfarb PB, Cathey MH, Cooper GR: The determination of ADP induced platelet aggregation in normal men. *Atherosclerosis* 12:335, 1970.

Goodreau JJ, Creasy JK, et al: Rational approach to the differentiation of vascular and neurogenic claudication. *Surgery* 84:749, 1978.

Imparato AM, Kim GE, et al: Intermittent claudication: Its natural course. *Surgery* 78:795, 1975.

Karayannacos PE, Yahson D, Vasko JS: Narrow lumbar spine canal with vascular syndromes. *Arch Surg* 111:803, 1976.

Mannick JA: Current concepts in diagnostic methods. Evaluation of chronic lower-extremity ischemia. *N Engl J Med* 309:841, 1983.

Lassen NA, Holstein P: Use of radioisotopes in assessment of distal blood flow and distal blood pressure in arterial insufficiency. *Surg Clin North Am* 54:39, 1974.

Strandness DE: Evaluation of the patient for vascular surgery. *Surg Clin North Am* 54:13, 1974.

Taylor LM Jr, Porter JM: Drug treatment of claudication: Hemorrheologic agents and antiserotonin drugs. *J Vasc Surg* 3:374, 1986.

Yao JST, Bergan JJ: Application of ultrasound to arterial and venous diagnosis. *Surg Clin North Am* 54:25, 1974.

Aortoiliac Occlusive Disease

Brewster DC, Darling RC: Optimal methods of aortoiliac reconstruction. *Surgery* 84:739, 1978.

Flanigan DP, Ryan TJ, et al: Aortofemoral or femoropopliteal revascularization? A prospective evaluation of the papaverine test. *J Vasc Surg* 1:215, 1984.

Garrett HE, Crawford ES, et al: Surgical considerations in the treatment of aorto-iliac occlusive disease. *Surg Clin North Am* 46:949, 1966.

Guida PM, Moore SW: Obturator bypass techniques. *Surg Gynecol Obstet* 128:1307, 1969.

Imparato AM, Sanoudos G, et al: Results in 96 aortoiliac reconstructive procedures: Preoperative angiographic and functional classifications used as prognostic guides. *Surgery* 68:610, 1970.

Inihara T: Endarterectomy for occlusive disease of the aortoiliac and common femoral arteries: Evaluation of results of the eversion technique endarterectomy. *Am J Surg* 124:235, 1972.

Jones AF, Kempezinski RF: Aortofemoral bypass grafting: A reappraisal. *Arch Surg* 116:301, 1981.

Kwaan JHM, Molen RV, et al: Peripheral embolism resulting from unsuspected atheromatous aortic plaques. *Surgery* 78:583, 1975.

LoGerfo FW, Johnson WC, et al: Comparison of the late patency rates of axillobilateral femoral and axillounilateral femoral grafts. *Surgery* 81:33, 1977.

Lorentsen E, Hael BL, Hal R: Evaluation of the functional importance of atherosclerotic obliterations in the aorto-iliac artery by pressure-flow measurements. *Acta Med Scand* 191:399, 1972.

Lowenstein MH, Machleder HI: Sexual function after aortoiliac surgery. *Ann Surg* 191:787, 1975.

Mannick JA, Williams LE, Nabseth DC: The late results of axillofemoral grafts. *Surgery* 68:1038, 1970.

Martinez BD, Hertzer NR, et al: Influence of distal arterial occlusive disease on prognosis following aortobifemoral bypass. *J Vasc Surg* 88:795, 1980.

May AG, Van de Berg L, et al: Critical arterial stenosis. *Surgery* 54:250, 1963.

Nash RL, Menzoian JO, et al: The multidisciplinary approach to vasculogenic impotence. *Surgery* 89:124, 1981.

Ray LI, O'Connor JB, et al: Axillofemoral bypass: A critical reappraisal of its role in the management of aortoiliac occlusive disease. *Am J Surg* 138:117, 1979.

Sethi GK, Scott SM, Takaro T: Multiple-plane angiography for more precise evaluation of aortoiliac disease. *Surgery* 78:15, 1975.

Szilagyi DE, Smith RF, et al: Infection in arterial reconstruction with synthetic grafts. *Ann Surg* 176:321, 1972.

Szilagyi DE, Smith RF, et al: Anastomotic aneurysms after vascular reconstruction: Problems of incidence, etiology, and treatment. *Surgery* 78:800, 1975.

Szilagyi DE, Elliott JP Jr, et al: A thirty-year survey of the reconstructive surgical treatment of aortoiliac occlusive disease. *J Vasc Surg* 3:421, 1986.

Ward RE, Holcroft JW, et al: New concepts in the use of axillofemoral bypass grafts. *Arch Surg* 118:573, 1983.

Transluminal Arterial Balloon Dilatation (Balloon Angioplasty)

Alpert JR, Ring EJ, et al: Balloon dilatation of iliac stenosis with distal arterial surgery. *Arch Surg* 115:715, 1980.

Borozan PG, Schuler JJ, et al: Long-term hemodynamic evaluation of lower extremity percutaneous transluminal angioplasty. *J Vasc Surg* 2:785, 1985.

Colapinto RF, et al: Percutaneous transluminal angioplasty of peripheral vascular disease: A two year experience. *Cardiovasc Intervent Radiol* 3:213, 1980.

Gallino A, Mahler F, et al: Percutaneous transluminal angioplasty of the arteries of the lower limbs. *Circulation* 70:619, 1984.

Gewertz BL, Ball DG, Zareus C: Limb salvage in poor risk patients using transluminal angioplasty. *Arch Surg* 118:1209, 1983.

Kumpe DA, et al: Percutaneous transluminal angioplasty in the selected management of proximal arterial occlusive disease of the lower extremities: A preliminary report. *Surgery* 87:488, 1980.

Martin EC, Fankuchen EL, et al: Angioplasty for femoral artery occlusion: Comparison with surgery. *Am J Rad* 137:915, 1981.

Potter CT, Judkins MP: Transluminal treatment of arteriosclerotic obstruction: Description of a new technique and a preliminary report of its application. *Circulation* 30:654, 1964.

Rush DS, Gewertz BL, Lu C-t: Limb salvage in poor-risk patients using transluminal angioplasty. *Arch Surg* 118:1209, 1983.

Zarins CK, Lu C-t, et al: Limb salvage by percutaneous transluminal recanulization of the occluded superficial femoral artery. *Surgery* 87:701, 1980.

Femoropopliteal Occlusive Disease

Allan JS, Taylor GW: The relationship between blood flow and failure of femoropopliteal reconstructive arterial surgery. *Br J Surg* 59:549, 1972.

Brief DK, Brener BJ, et al: Crossover femoropopliteal grafts followed up five years or more. An analysis. *Arch Surg* 110:1294, 1975.

Cranley JJ, Hafner CD: Newer prosthetic material compared with autogenous saphenous vein for occlusive arterial disease of the lower extremity. *Surgery* 89:2, 1981.

Cutler BS, Thompson JE, et al: Autologous saphenous vein femoropopliteal bypass: Analysis of 298 cases. *Surgery* 79:324, 1976.

Dale WA: Autogenous vein grafts for femoropopliteal arterial repair. *Surg Gynecol Obstet* 123:1282, 1966.

DeWeese JA, Rob CG: Autogenous venous bypass grafts five years later. *Ann Surg* 174:346, 1971.

Evans LE, Webster MW, et al: Expanded polytetrafluoroethylene femoropopliteal grafts: Forty-eight month follow-up. *Surgery* 89:16, 1981.

Imparato AM, Bracco A, Kim GE: Comparisons of three technics for femoral-popliteal arterial reconstructions. *Ann Surg* 177:375, 1973.

Koontz TJ, Stausel HC Jr: Factors influencing patency of the autogenous vein femoropopliteal by-pass graft: An analysis of 74 cases. *Surgery* 71:753, 1972.

Leather RP, Shah DM, et al: Instrumental evolution of the valve incision method of in situ saphenous vein bypass. *J Vasc Surg* 1:113, 1984.

Mannick JA: Femoro-popliteal and femoro-tibial reconstructions. *Surg Clin North Am* 59:581, 1979.

Martin P, Jamieson C: The rationale for and measurement after profundaplasty. *Surg Clin North Am* 54:95, 1974.

Plecha FR, Plecha FM: Femorofemoral bypass grafts: Ten year experience. *J Vasc Surg* 1:555, 1984.

Plecha FR, Pories WJ: Intraoperative angiography in the immediate assessment of arterial reconstruction. *Arch Surg* 105:902, 1972.

Poliwoda H: Treatment of acute and chronic arterial occlusions with streptokinase. *Aust Ann Med* 19(suppl 1):25, 1970.

Reichle FA, Rankin KP, Tyson RR: Long-term results of 474 arterial reconstructions for severely ischemic limbs: A fourteen year follow-up. *Surgery* 85:93, 1979.

Rosenberg N, Thompson JE, et al: The modified bovine arterial graft. *Arch Surg* 111:222, 1976.

Sawyer PN, Kaplitt MJ, et al: Analysis of peripheral gas endarterectomy in 127 patients. *Arch Surg* 97:859, 1968.

Shah DM, Buckbinder D: Modified technique to produce valvular incompetence in in situ saphenous vein arterial bypass. *Arch Surg* 116:356, 1981.

Szilagyi DE, Smith RF, et al: Long-term behavior of a dacron arterial substitute: Clinical, roentgenologic and histologic correlations. *Ann Surg* 162:453, 1965.

Szilagyi DE, Smith RF, et al: Autogenous vein grafting in femoral popliteal atherosclerosis: The limits of its effectiveness. *Surgery* 86:836, 1979.

Towne JB, Bernhard VM, et al: Profundaplasty in perspective: Limitations in the long-term management of limb ischemia. *Surgery* 90:1037, 1981.

Veith FJ, Gupta SK, et al: Six-year prospective multicenter randomized comparison of autologous saphenous vein and expanded polytetrafluoroethylene grafts in infrainguinal arterial reconstructions. *J Vasc Surg* 3:104, 1986.

Vollmar J, Frede M, Laubach K: Principles of reconstructive procedures for chronic femoro-popliteal occlusions: A report of 546 operations. *Ann Surg* 168:215, 1968.

Walker PM, Imparato AM, Riles TS: Long-term results in superficial femoral artery endarterectomy. *Surgery* 89:23, 1981.

Weisel RD, Johnson KW, et al: Comparison of conduits for leg revascularization. *Surgery* 89:8, 1981.

Tibioperoneal Occlusive Disease

Edwards WH, Mucherin JL Jr: The role of graft materials in femorotibial bypass grafts. *Ann Surg* 191:721, 1980.

Flinn WR, Flanigan DP, et al: Sequential femoral-tibial by-pass for severe limb ischemia. *Surgery* 88:357, 1980.

Imparato AM, Kim GE, Chu DS: Surgical exposure for reconstruction of the proximal part of the tibial artery. *Surg Gynecol Obstet* 136:453, 1973.

Imparato AM, Kim GE, et al: Angiographic criteria for successful tibial arterial reconstructions. *Surgery* 74:830, 1973.

Imparato AM, Kim GE, et al: The results of tibial artery reconstruction procedures. *Surg Gynecol Obstet* 138:33, 1974.

Kahn SP, Lindenauer M, et al: Femorotibial vein bypass. *Arch Surg* 107:309, 1973.

Reichle FA, Martinson MW, Kevin PR: Infrapopliteal arterial reconstruction in the severely ischemic lower limb. A comparison of long term results of peroneal and tibial bypasses. *Ann Surg* 191:59, 1980.

Reichle FA, Tyson RR: Comparison of long-term results of 364 femoropopliteal or femorotibial bypasses for revascularization of severely ischemic lower extremities. *Ann Surg* 182:449, 1975.

Occlusive Disease of the Upper Extremity

Machleder HI (ed): *Vascular Disorders of the Upper Extremity.* Mt Kisco, NY, Futura, 1983.

Porter JM, Rivers SP, et al: Evaluation and management of patients with Raynaud's syndrome. *Am J Surg* 142:183, 1981.

Robbs JV, Human RR, Rajaruthnam P: Operative treatment of nonspecific aortoarteritis (Takayusu's arteritis). *J Vasc Surg* 3:605, 1986.

Whitehouse WM Jr, Zelenoc GB, et al: Arterial bypass grafts for upper extremity ischemia. *J Vasc Surg* 3:569, 1986.

Zelenock B, Cronenwett JL, et al: Brachiocephalic arterial occlusions and stenoses. Manifestations and management of complex lesions. *Arch Surg* 120:370, 1985.

Lumbar Sympathectomy

Berardi RS, Siroospour D: Lumbar sympathectomy in the treatment of peripheral vascular occlusive disease: Ten year study. *Am J Surg* 130:309, 1975.

Collins GJ Jr, Rich NM, et al: Clinical results of lumbar sympathectomy. *Ann Surg* 47:31, 1981.

Cross FW, Cotton LT: Chemical lumbar sympathectomy for ischemic rest pain. A randomized, prospective controlled clinical trial. *Am J Surg* 150:341, 1985.

Grover-Johnson N, Baumann FG, et al: Effect of surgical lumbar sympathectomy of innervation of arterioles in the lower limb of patients with diabetes. *Surg Gynecol Obstet* 153:39, 1981.

Kim GE, Ibrahim IM, Imparato AM: Lumbar sympathectomy in end stage arterial occlusive disease. *Ann Surg* 183:157, 1976.

Plecha FR: A new criterion for predicting response to lumbar sympathectomy in patients with severe arteriosclerotic occlusive disease. *Surgery* 88:375, 1980.

Raskin NH, Levinson SA, et al: Post-sympathectomy neuralgia: Amelioration with diphenylhydantoin and carbamazepine. *Am J Surg* 128:75, 1974.

Walker PM, Johnson KW: Predicting the success of a sympathectomy: A prospective study using discriminant function and multiple regression analysis. *Surgery* 87:216, 1980.

Key JA, Mackay IM, Johnson KW: Phenol sympathectomy for vascular occlusive disease. *Surg Gynecol Obstet* 146:741, 1978.

Wright CJ, Cousins MJ: Blood flow distribution in the human leg following epidural sympathetic blockage. *Arch Surg* 105:334, 1972.

Complications of Vascular Reconstructions

Baumann FG, Imparato AM, Kim GE: The evolution of early fibromuscular lesions hemodynamically induced in the dog renal artery: 1. Light and transmission electron microscopy. *Circ Res* 39:809, 1976.

Beebe HG, Clark WF, DeWeese JA: Atherosclerotic change occurring in an autogenous venous arterial graft. *Arch Surg* 101:85, 1970.

Bunt TJ: Synthetic vascular graft infections. I. Graft infections. *Surgery* 93:703, 1984.

Bunt TJ: Synthetic vascular graft infections. II. Graft-enteric erosions and graft-enteric fistulas. *Surgery* 94:1, 1983.

Graor RA, Risius B, et al: Local thrombolysis in the treatment of thrombosed arteries, bypass grafts, and arteriovenous fistulas. *J Vasc Surg* 2:406, 1985.

Hamaker WR, Doyle WF, et al: Subintimal obliterative prolifera-

tion in saphenous vein grafts. A cause of early failure of aorta to coronary artery by-pass grafts. *Ann Thorac Surg* 13:488, 1972.

Imparato AM, Baumann FG, et al: Electron microscopic studies of experimentally produced fibromuscular arterial lesions. *Surg Gynecol Obstet* 68:682, 1976.

Imparato AM, Bracco A, Hammond R: The effect of intimal and neo-intimal fibromuscular fibroplasia on arterial reconstructions. *J Cardiovasc Surg (Torino)* Special Issue, 488, 1975.

Reilly LM, Altman H, et al: Late results following surgical management of vascular graft infection. *J Vasc Surg* 1:36, 1984.

The Diabetic Foot

Barker WF: Peripheral vascular disease in diabetes: Diagnosis and management. *Med Clin North Am* 55:1045, 1971.

Friedman SA, Friedberg P, Colton J: Vasomotor tone in diabetic neuropathy. *Ann Intern Med* 77:353, 1972.

LeFrock JL, Joseph WS: Lower extremity infections in diabetics. *Infect Surg* 135, 1986.

Levin MD, O'Neal LW: *The Diabetic Foot.* St Louis, Mosby, 1973.

Amputations

Barnes RW, Sharick GD, Slaymaker EE: An index of healing in below-knee amputation: Leg blood pressure by Doppler ultrasound. *Surgery* 79:13, 1976.

Beradi RS, Keenin Y: Amputations in peripheral vascular occlusive disease. *Am J Surg* 135:231, 1978.

Bone GE, Pomajzl MJ: Toe blood pressure by photoplethysmography: An index of healing in forefoot amputation. *Surgery* 72:569, 1981.

Cohen SO, Goldman LD, et al: The deleterious effect of immediate postoperative prosthesis in below-knee amputation for ischemic disease. *Surgery* 76:992, 1974.

Delancy JP: The use of radionuclides in the study of limb blood flow, in Bernstein EE (ed): *Noninvasive Diagnostic Techniques in Vascular Surgery.* St Louis, Mosby, 1982, chap 14, p 148.

Denaro JA, Weinstein G, et al: Evaluation of peripheral vascular disease using radioactive xenon. *Rev Surg* 32:65, 1975.

Hicks L, McClelland RN: Below-knee amputations for vascular insufficiency. *Am Surg* 46:239, 1980.

Hunsaker RH, Schwartz JA, et al: Dry ice cryomputation: A twelve-year experience. *J Vasc Surg* 2:812, 1985.

Kelly JP, James JM: Criteria for determining the proper level of amputation in occlusive vascular disease: A review of 323 amputations. *J Bone Joint Surg [Am]* 39A:883, 1957.

Kim GE, Imparato AM, et al: Lower limb amputation for occlusive vascular disease. *Am Surg* 42:598, 1976.

Lim RC, Schecter WP: Transmetatarsal amputation. *Arch Surg* 112:1366, 1977.

McIntyre KE Jr, Bailey SA, et al: Guillotine amputation in the treatment of nonsalvageable lower extremity infections. *Arch Surg* 119:450, 1984.

Moore WS: Amputation level determination using isotope clearance technique, in Bernstein EE (ed): *Noninvasive Diagnostic Techniques in Vascular Surgery.* St Louis, Mosby, 1982, chap 40, p 385.

Pollock SB Jr, Ernst CB: Use of Doppler pressure measurements in predicting success in amputation of the leg. *Am J Surg* 139:303, 1980.

Robinson K: Long posterior flap myoplastic below-knee amputation in ischemic disease. *Lancet* 1:183, 1972.

Rush DS, Huston CC, et al: Operative and late mortality rates of above-knee and below-knee amputations. *Am Surg* 47:36, 1981.

Sizer JS, Wheelock FC Jr: Digital amputations in diabetic patients. *Surgery* 72:980, 1972.

Wagner FW Jr: The syme amputation, in *American Academy of Orthopaedic Surgeons: Atlas of Limb Prosthetics. Surgical and Prosthetic Principles.* St Louis, Mosby, 1981, pp 326–340.

Arterial Embolism

Billig DM, Hallman GL, Cooley DA: Arterial embolism. *Arch Surg* 95:1, 1967.

Blaisdell FW, Graziano CT, Effency DJ: In vivo assessment of anticoagulation. *Surgery* 82:827, 1977.

Blaisdell FW, Steele M, Allen RE: Management of acute lower extremity arterial ischemia due to embolism and thrombosis. *Surgery* 84:822, 1978.

Cranley JJ, Krause RJ, et al: Peripheral arterial embolism: Changing concepts. *Surgery* 55:57, 1964.

Crawford ES, DeBakey ME: The retrograde flush procedure in embolectomy and thrombectomy. *Surgery* 40:737, 1956.

Darling RC, Austen WG, Linton RR: Arterial embolism. *Surg Gynecol Obstet* 124:106, 1967.

Fisher DR Jr, Clagett GP, et al: Dilemmas in dealing with the blue toe syndrome: Aortic versus peripheral source. *Am J Surg* 148:836, 1984.

Fisher ER, Hellstrom HR, Myers JD: Disseminated atheromatous emboli. *Am J Med* 29:176, 1960.

Flory CM: Arterial occlusions produced by emboli from eroded aortic atheromatous plaques. *Am J Pathol* 21:549, 1945.

Fogarty TJ, Cranley JJ, et al: A method for extraction of arterial emboli and thrombi. *Surg Gynecol Obstet* 116:241, 1963.

Haimovici H: Peripheral arterial embolism. *Angiology* 1:20, 1950.

Kassirer JP: Atheroembolic renal disease. *N Engl J Med* 280:817, 1969.

Miles RM, Dale D, Booth JL: The dynamics of peripheral arterial embolism. *Ann Surg* 167:801, 1968.

Spencer FC, Eiseman B: Delayed arterial embolectomy: A new concept. *Surgery* 55:64, 1964.

Tawes RL Jr, Harris EJ, et al: Arterial thromboembolism. A 20-year perspective. *Arch Surg* 120:595, 1985.

Buerger's Disease

Hill GL: A rational basis for management of patients with the Buerger syndrome. *Br J Surg* 61:476, 1974.

Kjeldsen K, Mozes M: Buerger's disease in Israel: Investigations on carboxyhemoglobin and serum cholesterol levels after smoking. *Acta Chir Scand* 135:495, 1969.

McKusick VA, Harris WS, Ottesen OE: The Buerger syndrome in the United States: Arteriographic observations, with special reference to involvement of the upper extremities and the differentiation from atherosclerosis and embolism. *Bull Johns Hopkins Hosp* 110:145, 1962.

McKusick VA, Harris WS, et al: Buerger's disease: A distinct clinical and pathologic entity. *JAMA* 181:5, 1962.

McPherson JR, Guergels JL, Gifford RW Jr: Thromboangiitis obliterans and arteriosclerosis obliterans: Clinical and prognostic differences. *Ann Intern Med* 59:288, 1963.

Silbert S: The etiology of thromboangiitis obliterans. *JAMA* 129:5, 1945.

Walker DH, Mattern WD: Rickettsial vasculitis. *Am Heart J* 100:896, 1980.

Wessler S: Buerger's disease revisited. *Surg Clin North Am* 49:703, 1969.

Wessler S, Si-Chun M, et al: Critical evaluation of thromboangiitis obliterans: Case against Buerger's disease. *N Engl J Med* 262:1149, 1960.

Arterial Trauma

Hughes CW, Cohen A: The repair of injured blood vessels. *Surg Clin North Am* 38:1529, 1958.

Liekweg WG, et al: Management of penetrating carotid arterial injury. *Ann Surg* 188:587, 1978.

Miller HH, Welch CS: Quantitative studies on time factor in arterial injuries. *Ann Surg* 130:428, 1949.

Morris GC Jr, Beall AC Jr, et al: Surgical experience with 220 acute arterial injuries in civilian practice. *Am J Surg* 99:775, 1960.

Mustard WT, Bull CA: A reliable method for relief of traumatic vascular spasm. *Ann Surg* 155:339, 1962.

Patman RD, Poulos E, Shires GT: The management of civilian arterial injuries. *Surg Gynecol Obstet* 118:725, 1964.

Rich NM, Hobson RW, Fedde W: Vascular trauma secondary to diagnostic and therapeutic procedures. *Am J Surg* 128:715, 1974.

Spencer FC: Vascular injury and arteriovenous fistula, in *Lewis-Walters Practice of Surgery*. Hagerstown, MD, WF Prior, 1965, vol XI, chap 8.

Spencer FC, Grewe RV: The management of arterial injuries in battle casualties. *Ann Surg* 141:304, 1955.

Popliteal Artery Entrapment Syndrome

Albertazzi VJ, Elliott TE, Kennedy JA: Popliteal artery entrapment. *Angiology* 20:119, 1969.

Brightmore TGJ, Smellie WAB: Popliteal artery entrapment. *Br J Surg* 58:481, 1971.

Hamming JJ: Intermittent claudication at an early age, due to an anomalous course of the popliteal artery. *Angiology* 10:369, 1959.

Harris JD, Jepson RP: Entrapment of the popliteal artery. *Surgery* 69:246, 1971.

Inshua JA, Young JR, Humphries AW: Popliteal artery entrapment syndrome. *Arch Surg* 101:771, 1970.

Stuart ATP: Note on variation in the course of the popliteal artery. *J Anat Physiol* XIII:162, 1879.

Anterior Compartment Syndrome

Carter AB, Richards RL, Zachary RB: The anterior tibial syndrome. *Lancet* 2:928, 1949.

Getzen LC, Carr JE III: Etiology of anterior tibial compartment syndrome. *Surg Gynecol Obstet* 125:347, 1967.

Hayden JW: Compartment syndromes. Early recognition and treatment. *Postgrad Med* 74:191, 1983.

Mavor GE: The anterior tibial syndrome. *J Bone Joint Surg [Br]* 38B:513, 1956.

Moretz WH: The anterior compartment (anterior tibial) ischemia syndrome. *Ann Surg* 19:728, 1953.

Rollins DL, Bernhard VM, Towne JB: Fasciotomy. An appraisal of controversial issues. *Arch Surg* 116:1747, 1981.

Traumatic Arteriovenous Fistulas

Creech O Jr, Gantt J, Wren H: Traumatic arteriovenous fistula at unusual sites. *Ann Surg* 161:908, 1965.

Hughes CW, Jahnke EJ Jr: The surgery of traumatic arteriovenous fistulas and aneurysms: A five-year follow up study of 215 lesions. *Ann Surg* 148:790, 1958.

Shumacker HB Jr: Arterial aneurysms and arteriovenous fistulas: Report on spontaneous cures, in Elkin DC, DeBakey ME (eds): *Vascular Surgery*. Washington, D.C. Office of the Surgeon General, U.S. Public Health Service, 1955.

Spencer FC: Vascular injury and arteriovenous fistula, in *Lewis-Walters Practice of Surgery*. Hagerstown, MD, WF Prior, 1965, vol XI, chap 8.

Congenital Arteriovenous Fistulas

Cross FS, Glover DM, et al: Congenital arteriovenous aneurysms. *Ann Surg* 148:649, 1958.

Fry WJ: Surgical considerations in congenital arteriovenous fistula. *Surg Clin North Am* 54(1):165, 1974.

Olcott C, Newton TH, et al: Intra-arterial embolization in the management of arteriovenous malformations. *Surgery* 79:3, 1976.

Robertson DJ: Congenital arteriovenous fistulae of the extremities: Hunterian Lecture. *Ann R Coll Surg Engl* 18:73, 1956.

Rosenfeld L: Experiences with vascular abnormalities about the parotid gland and upper neck. *Arch Surg* 79:553, 1959.

Spencer FC: Vascular injury and arteriovenous fistula, in *Lewis-Walters Practice of Surgery*. Hagerstown, MD, WF Prior, 1965, vol XI, chap 8.

Szilagyi ED, Smith RF, et al: Congenital arteriovenous anomalies of the limbs. *Arch Surg* 111:423, 1976.

Tice DA, Clauss RH, et al: Congenital arteriovenous fistulae of the extremities: Observations concerning treatment. *Arch Surg* 86:460, 1963.

Thoracic Outlet Syndromes

Adams JT, DeWeese JA: Effort thrombosis of the axillary and subclavian veins. *J Trauma* 11:923, 1971.

Adson AW: Surgical treatment for symptoms produced by cervical ribs and the scalenus anticus muscle. *Surg Gynecol Obstet* 85:687, 1947.

Beyer JA, Wright IS: The hyperabduction syndrome: With special reference to its relationship to Raynaud's syndrome. *Circulation* 4:161, 1951.

Dale WA: Thoracic outlet compression syndrome. Critique in 1982. *Arch Surg* 117:1437, 1982.

Falconer MA, Weddell G: Costoclavicular compression of the subclavian artery and vein: Relation to the scalenus anticus syndrome. *Lancet* 2:539, 1943.

Jochamisen PR, Hartfall WG: Per axillary upper extremity sympathectomy: Technique reviewed and clinical experience. *Surgery* 71:686, 1972.

Kirtley JA, Riddell DH, et al: Cervico-sympathectomy in neurovascular abnormalities of the upper extremities: Experiences in 76 patients with 104 sympathectomies. *Ann Surg* 165:869, 1967.

Lord JW Jr, Rosati LM: Neurovascular compression syndromes of the upper extremity. *Ciba Found Clin Symp* 10:35, 1958.

Nanson EM: The anterior approach to upper dorsal sympathectomy. *Surg Gynecol Obstet* 104:118, 1957.

Patman RD, Thompson JE, Persson A: Management of post-traumatic pain syndromes: Report of 113 cases. *Ann Surg* 177:780, 1973.

Pollak EW: Surgical anatomy of the thoracic outlet syndrome. *Surg Gynecol Obstet* 150:97, 1980.

Roos DB: Transaxillary first rib resection for thoracic outlet syndrome: Indications and techniques. *Contemp Surg* 26:55, 1985.

Roos DB: The place for scalenectomy and first-rib resection in thoracic outlet syndrome. *Surgery* 92:1077, 1982.

Roos DB: Thoracic outlet and carpal tunnel syndromes, in Rutherford RB (ed): *Vascular Surgery*. Philadelphia, Saunders, 1984, chap 70.

Ross JP: The vascular complications of cervical rib. *Ann Surg* 150:340, 1959.

Sanders RJ, Raymer S: The supraclavicular approach to scalenectomy and first rib resection: Description of a technique. *J Vasc Surg* 2:751, 1985.

Scher LA, Veith FJ, et al: Vascular complications of thoracic outlet syndrome. *J Vasc Surg* 3:565, 1986.

Telford ED, Mottershead S: Pressure at the cervicobrachial junction: An operative and anatomical study. *J Bone Joint Surg [Br]* 30B:249, 1948.

Urschel HD, Paulson DL, McNamara JJ: Thoracic outlet syndrome. *Ann Thorac Surg* 6:1, 1968.

Extracranial Occlusive Cerebrovascular Disease

Baker WH, Littooy FN, et al: Carotid endarterectomy without a shunt: The control series. *J Vasc Surg* 1:50, 1984.

Baker DJ, Gluecklich B, et al: An evaluation of electroencephalographic monitoring for carotid study. *Surgery* 78(6):787, 1975.

Ball JB Jr, Lukin RR, et al: Complications of intravenous digital subtraction angiography. *Arch Neurol* 42:969, 1985.

Barner HB, Kaiser GC, Willman VL: Hemodynamics of carotid-subclavian bypass. *Arch Surg* 103:248, 1971.

Barnes RW, Nix ML, et al: Late outcome of untreated asymptomatic carotid disease following cardiovascular operations. *J Vasc Surg* 2:843, 1985.

Berkoff HA, Tunipseed WD: Patient selection and results of simultaneous coronary and carotid artery procedures. *Ann Thorac Surg* 38:172, 1984.

Bogousslavsky J, Hachiniski SC, et al: Cardiac and arterial lesions in carotid transient ischemic attacks. *Arch Neurol* 43:223, 1986.

Bousser MG, Eschwege E, et al: AICLA controlled trial of aspirin, dipyridamole in secondary prevention of athero-thrombotic cerebral ischemia. *Stroke* 14:5, 1983.

Brewster DC, Moncure AC, et al: Innominate artery lesions: Problems encountered and lessons learned. *J Vasc Surg* 2:99, 1985.

Cebul RD, Ginsberg MD: Noninvasive neurovascular tests for carotid artery disease. *Ann Intern Med* 97:867, 1982.

Cervantes FD, Schneiderman LJ: Anticoagulants in cerebrovascular disease. A critical review of studies. *Arch Intern Med* 135:875, 1975.

Clagett PG, Rabinowitz M, et al: Morphogenesis and clinico-pathologic characteristics of recurrent carotid disease. *J Vasc Surg* 3:10, 1986.

Collins GJ, Rich NM, et al: Fibromuscular dysplasia of the internal carotid arteries. *Ann Surg* 194:89, 1981.

Cote R, Barnett HJ, Taylor DW: Internal carotid occlusion: A prospective study. *Stroke* 14:898, 1983.

Croft RJ, Ellam LD, Harrison MJ: Accuracy of carotid angiography in the assessment of atheroma of the internal carotid artery. *Lancet* 1:997, 1980.

Dent TL, Thompson NW, Fry WJ: Carotid body tumors. *Surgery* 80:365, 1976.

Ehrenfeld WK, Wylie EJ: Spontaneous dissection of the internal carotid artery. *Arch Surg* 111:1294, 1976.

Eikelboom BC, Riles TS, et al: Inaccuracy of angiography in the diagnosis of carotid ulceration. *Stroke* 14:882, 1983.

EC-IC Bypass Study Group: Failure of extracranial-intracranial arterial bypass to reduce the risk of ischemic stroke: Results of an international randomized trial by the EC-IC bypass study group. *N Engl J Med* 313:1191, 1985.

Ferguson GG: Carotid endarterectomy: To shunt or not to shunt. *Arch Neurol* 43:615, 1986.

Fields WM: Selection of stroke patients for arterial reconstructions. *Am J Surg* 125:527, 1973.

Fields WS, Lemak NA, et al: Controlled trial of aspirin in cerebral ischemia. *Stroke* 8:53, 1977.

Fisher DF, Clagett PG, et al: Mandibular subluxation for high carotid exposure. *J Vasc Surg* 1:727, 1984.

Ford JJ, Baker WH, Ehrenhaft JL: Carotid endarterectomy for nonhemispheric transient ischemic attacks. *Arch Surg* 110:1314, 1975.

Giordano JM, Trout HH III, et al: Timing carotid endarterectomy after stroke. *J Vasc Surg* 2:250, 1985.

Glover JL, Bendick PJ, et al: Duplex ultrasonagraphy, digital subtraction angiography and conventional angiography in assessing carotid atherosclerosis. *Arch Surg* 119:664, 1984.

Goldstone J, Effeney DJ: The role of carotid endarterectomy in the treatment of acute neurologic deficits. *Prog Cardiovasc Dis* 22:415, 1980.

Green RM, Messick WJ, et al: Benefits, shortcomings, and costs of EEG monitoring. *Ann Surg* 201:785, 1985.

Halstuk KS, Baker WH, Littoog FN: External carotid endarterectomy. *J Vasc Surg* 1:398, 1984.

Hart R, Hindman B: Mechanisms of perioperative cerebral infarction. *Stroke* 13:766, 1982.

Hays RJ, Levinson SA, Wylie EJ: Intraoperative measurement of carotid back pressure as a guide to operative management for carotid endarterectomy. *Surgery* 72:953, 1972.

Hertzer NR, Beven EG, et al: Early patency of the carotid artery after endarterectomy: Digital subtraction angiography after two hundred sixty-two operations. *Surgery* 92:1049, 1982.

Hirsh J: Progress review: The relationship between dose of aspirin, side effects and antithrombotic effectiveness. *Stroke* 16:1, 1985.

Hugenholz H, Elgie RG: Carotid thrombo-endarterectomy: A reappraisal. Criteria for patient selection. *J Neurosurg* 53:776, 1980.

Humphries AW, Young JR, et al: Relief of vertebrobasilar symptoms by carotid endarterectomy. *Surgery* 57:48, 1965.

Hunter GC, Sieffert G, et al: The accuracy of carotid back pressure as an index for shunt requirements. *Stroke* 13:319, 1982.

Imparato AM: The carotid bifurcation plaque—a model for the study of atherosclerosis. *J Vasc Surg* 3:249, 1986.

Imparato AM: The "major" and "minor" carotid artery in arterial reconstruction. *Stroke* IX:15, 1974.

Imparato AM: Vertebral arterial reconstruction: A nineteen year experience. *J Vasc Surg* 2:626, 1985.

Imparato AM, Baumann G, et al: The significance of gross hemorrhage in carotid plaques. *Ann Surg* 197:195, 1983.

Imparato AM, Bracco A, et al: The hypoglossal nerve in carotid arterial reconstructions. *Stroke* 3:576, 1972.

Imparato AM, Ramirez A, et al: Cerebral protection in carotid surgery. *Arch Surg* 117:1073, 1982.

Imparato AM, Riles TS, Gorstein F: The carotid bifurcation plaque: Pathologic findings associated with cerebral ischemia. *Stroke* 10:238, 1979.

Imparato AM, Riles TS, et al: The management of TIA and acute strokes after carotid endarterectomy, in *Complications in Vascular Surgery.* New York, Grune & Stratton, 1985, chap 43, p 725.

Imparato AM, Riles TS, et al: Controversies in surgery: Anesthetic management in carotid surgery. *Aust NZ J Surg* 55:315, 1985.

Jacobs NM, Grant EG, et al: The role of duplex carotid sonography, digital subtraction angiography, and arteriography in the evaluation of transient ischemic attack and the asymptomatic carotid bruit. *Med Clin North Am* 68:1423, 1984.

Jacobson JH, Mozersky DJ, et al: Axillary-axillary bypass for the subclavian steal syndrome. *Arch Surg* 106:24, 1973.

Joint Study of Extracranial Arterial Occlusion as a Cause of Stroke:

I. Fields WS, North RR, et al: Organization of study and survey of patient population. *JAMA* 203:955, 1968.

II. Hass WK, Fields WS, et al: Arteriography, techniques, sites and complications. *JAMA* 203:961, 1968.

III. Bauer RB, Meyer JS, et al: Progress report of controlled long term survival in patients with and without operation. *JAMA* 208:509, 1969.

IV. Blaisdell WF, Clauss RH, et al: A review of surgical considerations. *JAMA* 209:1889, 1969.

V. Fields WS, Maslenikov V, et al: Progress report of prognosis following surgery or non surgical treatment for transient cerebral ischemic attacks and cervical carotid lesions. *JAMA* 211:1993, 1970.

Killen DA, Foster JH, et al: The subclavian steal syndrome. *J Thorac Cardiovasc Surg* 51:539, 1966.

Kollarits CR, Lubow M, Hissong SL: Retinal strokes: I. Incidence of carotid atheromata. *JAMA* 222:1275, 1972.

Lazar ML, Clark K: Microsurgical cerebral revascularization: Concepts and practice. *Surg Neurol* 1:355, 1973.

Levin SM, Sondheimer FD, Lewis JM: The contralateral diseased but asymptomatic carotid artery: To operate or not? An update. *Am J Surg* 140:203, 1980.

Lusby RJ, Ferrel LD, et al: Carotid plaque hemorrhage: Its role in production of cerebral ischemia. *Arch Surg* 117:1479, 1982.

Meyer FB, Sundt TM, et al: Emergency carotid endarterectomy for patients with acute carotid occlusion and profound neurologic deficits. *Ann Surg* 203:82, 1986.

McCullough JL, Mentzer RM Jr, et al: Carotid endarterectomy after a completed stroke: Reduction in long-term neurologic deterioration. *J Vasc Surg* 2:7, 1985.

Millikan CH: Transient cerebral ischemia: Definition and natural history. *Prog Cardiovasc Dis* 22:303, 1980.

Mohr JP: Lacunes. *Stroke* 13:3, 1982.

Najafi H, Javid H, et al: Emergency carotid thromboendarterectomy: Surgical indication and results. *Arch Surg* 103:610, 1971.

O'Donnel TF, Erdoes L, et al: Correlation of B-mode ultrasound imaging and arteriography with pathologic findings at carotid endarterectomy. *Arch Surg* 120:443, 1985.

Posner MP, Riles TS, et al: Axillo-axillary bypass for symptomatic stenosis of the subclavian artery. *Am J Surg* 145:644, 1983.

Putnam SF, Adams HP Jr: Usefulness of heparin in initial management of patients with recent transient ischemic attacks. *Arch Neurol* 42:960, 1985.

Quinones-Baldrich WJ: Moore WS: Asymptomatic carotid stenosis: Rationale for management. *Arch Neurol* 42:378, 1985.

Reivich M, Holling E, et al: Reversal of blood flow through the vertebral artery and its effect on cerebral circulation. *N Engl J Med* 265:878, 1961.

Rhodes LE, Stanley JC, et al: Aneurysms of extracranial carotid arteries. *Arch Surg* 111:339, 1976.

Riles TS, Imparato AM, Kopelman I: Carotid artery stenosis with contralateral occlusion: Long-term results in fifty-four patients. *Surgery* 87:363, 1980.

Riles TS, Kopelman I, Imparato AM: Myocardial infarction following carotid endarterectomy. *Surgery* 85:249, 1979.

Roederer GO, Langlois YE, et al: The natural history of carotid arterial disease in asymptomatic patients with cervical bruits. *Stroke* 15:605, 1984.

Rosenthal JJ, Gaspar MR, Movius HR: Intraoperative arteriography in carotid thromboendarterectomy. *Arch Surg* 106:806, 1973.

Ross RS, McKusick VA: Aortic arch syndrome. *Arch Intern Med* 92:701, 1953.

Schmidley JW, Caronna JJ: Transient cerebral ischemia: Pathophysiology. *Prog Cardiovasc Dis* 22:325, 1980.

Sobel M, Imparato AM, et al: Contralateral neurologic symptoms after carotid surgery. *J Vasc Surg* 3:623, 1986.

Steed DL, Peitzman AB, et al: Causes of stroke in carotid endarterectomy. *Surg* 92:634, 1982.

Thompson JE: Complications of carotid endarterectomy and their prevention. *World J Surg* 3:155, 1979.

Thompson JE: History of carotid artery surgery. *Surg Clin North Am* 66:225, 1986.

Thompson JE, Patman RD, Persson AV: Management of asymptomatic carotid bruits. *Am Surg* 42:77, 1976.

Thompson JE, et al: Carotid surgery for cerebrovascular insufficiency. *Curr Probl Surg* 15:1, 1981.

Towne JB, Bernhard VM: Neurologic deficit following carotid endarterectomy. *Surg Gynecol Obstet* 154:849, 1982.

Walker PM, Paley D, et al: What determines the symptoms associated with subclavian artery occlusive disease? *J Vasc Surg* 2:154, 1985.

Warlow C: Carotid endarterectomy: Does it work? *Stroke* 15:1068, 1984.

Weinstein GS, Imparato AM: Clinicopathologic correlation in postendarterectomy recurrent stenosis. *J Vasc Surg* 3:657, 1986.

Weksler BB, Lewin M: Anticoagulation in cerebral ischemia. *Stroke* 14:658, 1983.

Wells CE: Role of stroke in dementia. *Stroke* 9:1, 1978.

Whisnant JP, Sandok BA, Sundt TM: Carotid endarterectomy for unilateral carotid system transient cerebral ischemia. *Mayo Clin Proc* 58:171, 1983.

Wylie EJ, Hein MF, Adams JE: Intracranial hemorrhage following surgical revascularization for treatment of acute strokes. *J Neurosurg* 21:212, 1964.

Yatsu FM, Fields WS: Asymptomatic carotid bruit: Stenosis or ulceration. A conservative approach. *Arch Neurol* 42:383, 1985.

Zarins CK, Giddens DP, et al: Carotid bifurcation atherosclerosis: Quantitative correlation of plaque localization with flow velocity profiles and wall shear stress. *Circ Res* 53:502, 1983.

Abdominal Aneurysms

Adar R, Rabbi I, et al: Left renal vein division in abdominal aortic aneurysm operations. Effect of renal function. *Arch Surg* 120:1033, 1985.

Bergan JJ, Yao JST: *Aneurysms, Diagnosis and Treatment.* New York, Grune & Stratton, 1982.

Bernstein EF, Chan EL: Abdominal aortic aneurysm in high risk patients. Outcome of selective management based on size and expansion rate. *Ann Surg* 200:255, 1984.

Bernstein EF, Dilley RB, et al: Growth rates of small abdominal aortic aneurysms. *Surgery* 80:765, 1986.

Boucher CA, Brewster DC, et al: Determination of cardiac risk by dipyridamole-thallium imaging before peripheral vascular surgery. *N Engl J Med* 312:389, 1985.

Brenner DJ, Darling RD, et al: Major venous anomalies complicating abdominal aortic surgery. *Arch Surg* 108:159, 1974.

Brewster DC, Retana A, et al: Angiography in the management of aneurysms of the abdominal aorta: Its value and safety. *N Engl J Med* 292:(16):822, 1975.

Brown OW, Hollier LH, et al: Abdominal aortic aneurysm and coronary artery disease. A reassessment. *Arch Surg* 116:1484, 1981.

Bunt TJ, Wilson TG: Infected abdominal aortic aneurysm. *South Med J* 78:419, 1985.

Bush HL Jr, Huse JB, et al: Prevention of renal insufficiency after abdominal aortic aneurysm resection by optimal volume loading. *Arch Surg* 116:1517, 1981.

Connelly TL, McKinnon W, et al: Abdominal aortic surgery and horseshoe kidney. *Arch Surg* 115:1459, 1980.

Couch NP, O'Mahoney J, et al: The place of abdominal aortography in abdominal aortic aneurysm resection. *Arch Surg* 118:1029, 1983.

Crawford ES, Saleh SA, et al: Infrarenal abdominal aortic aneurysm: Factors influencing survival after operation performed over a 25-year period. *Ann Surg* 193:699, 1981.

Crawford ES, Crawford JL, et al: Thoraco-abdominal aortic aneurysms: Preoperative intraoperative factors determining immediate and long-term results of operation in 605 patients. *J Vasc Surg* 3:389, 1986.

Crawford JL, Stowe CL, et al: Inflammatory aneurysms of the aorta. *J Vasc Surg* 2:113, 1985.

Creech O Jr: Endo-aneurysmorrhaphy and treatment of aortic aneurysm. *Ann Surg* 164:935, 1966.

Darling R, Messina C, et al: Autopsy study of unoperated abdominal aortic aneurysm—the case for early resection. *Circulation* 56 (suppl 2):161, 1977.

Dean RH, Keyser JF III, et al: Aortic and renal disease. Factors affecting the value of combined procedures. *Ann Surg* 200:336, 1984.

DeBakey MR, Crawford ES, et al: Aneurysm of abdominal aorta: Analysis of results of graft replacement therapy one to eleven years after operation. *Ann Surg* 160:622, 1964.

Dent TL, Lindenauer M, et al: Multiple arteriosclerotic arterial aneurysms. *Arch Surg* 105:338, 1972.

Ernst CB: Prevention of intestinal ischemia following abdominal aortic reconstruction. *Surgery* 93:102, 1982.

Estes JE Jr: Abdominal aortic aneurysm: A study of one hundred and two cases. *Circulation* 2:258, 1950.

Flanigan D, Quinn T, Kraft R: Selective management of high risk patients with abdominal aortic aneurysms. *Surg Gynecol Obstet* 150:171, 1980.

Gaspar MR: Role of arteriography in the evaluation of aortic aneurysms: The case against, in Bergan JJ, Yao JST (eds): *Aneurysms, Diagnosis and Treatment.* New York, Grune & Stratton, 1982, p 243.

Gomes AS, Baker JD, et al: Acute renal dysfunction after major arteriography. *AJR* 145:1249, 1985.

Graham LM, Zelenock GB, et al: Clinical significance of arteriosclerotic femoral artery aneurysms. *Arch Surg* 115:502, 1980.

Grindlinger GA, Vegas AM, et al: Volume loading and vasodilators in abdominal aortic aneurysmectomy. *Am J Surg* 139:480, 1980.

Hardy JD, Timmis HH: Abdominal aortic aneurysms: Special problems. *Ann Surg* 173:945, 1971.

Hertzer NR, Beven EG, et al: Coronary artery disease in peripheral vascular patients. A classification of 1000 coronary angiograms and results of surgical management. *Ann Surg* 199:223, 1984.

Hiatt JCG, Wiley FB, et al: Determinants of failure of the treatment of ruptured abdominal aortic aneurysm. *Arch Surg* 118:1264, 1984.

Hicks G, Eastland M, et al: Survival improvement following aortic aneurysm resection. *Ann Surg* 181:863, 1975.

Hollier LH, Stanson AW, et al: Arteriomegaly: Classification and morbid implications of diffuse aneurysmal disease. *Surg* 93:700, 1983.

Imparato AM: Abdominal aortic surgery: Prevention of lower limb ischemia. *Surgery* 93:112, 1983.

Imparato AM, Berman IR, et al: Avoidance of shock and peripheral embolism during surgery of the abdominal aorta. *Surgery* 73:68, 1973.

Inahara T, Geary GL, et al: The contrary position to the nonresective treatment of abdominal aortic aneurysm. *J Vasc Surg* 2:42, 1985.

Jarrett F, Darling CR, et al: Experience with infected aneurysms of the abdominal aorta. *Arch Surg* 110:1381, 1975.

Karmody AM, Leather RP, et al: The current position of nonresective treatment for abdominal aortic aneurysm. *Surgery* 94:591, 1983.

Kim GE, Imparato AM, et al: Dilatation of synthetic grafts and junctional aneurysms. *Arch Surg* 114:1296, 1979.

Knight DG, Lane B, et al: Dynamic preoperative assessment of cardiac reserve in elective aortic surgery. *Br J Surg* 70:362, 1983.

Laetir GM, Crawford ES, et al: Progress in the treatment of ruptured abdominal aortic aneurysm. *World J Surg* 4:653, 1980.

Lawrence RJ, Ferguson MD, et al: Spinal ischemia following abdominal aortic surgery. *Ann Surg* 181:267, 1975.

Leather RP, Shah D, et al: Nonresective treatment of abdominal aortic aneurysm. Use of acute thrombosis and axillo-femoral by-pass. *Arch Surg* 114:1402, 1979.

Lobbato VJ, Rothenberg RE, et al: Coexistence of abdominal aortic aneurysm and carcinoma of the colon: A dilemma. *J Vasc Surg* 2:724, 1985.

McAuley CE, Steed DL, Webster MW: Bacterial presence in aortic thrombus at elective aneurysm resection: Is it clinically significant? *Am J Surg* 147:322, 1984.

Mehrez IO, Nabseth DC, et al: Paraplegia following resection of abdominal aortic aneurysm. *Ann Surg* 156:890, 1962.

Morgan RJ, Abbott WM: Safe management of patients with simultaneously occurring prostatism and abdominal aortic aneurysm. *Am J Surg* 143:319, 1982.

Pairolero PC, Gilmore JC, et al: Isolated iliac artery aneurysms. *Surgery* 93:688, 1983.

Pairolero PC, Walls JT, et al: Subclavian artery aneurysms. *Surgery* 90:757, 1981.

Pasternack PF, Imparato AM, et al: The value of radionuclide angiography as a predictor of perioperative myocardial infarction in patients undergoing abdominal aortic aneurysm resection. *J Vasc Surg* 1:320, 1984.

Pennell RC, Hollier LH, et al: Inflammatory abdominal aortic aneurysms: A 30 year review. *J Vasc Surg* 2:859, 1985.

Porter JM, McGregor F, et al: Renal function following abdominal aortic aneurysmectomy. *Surg Gynecol Obstet* 123:819, 1966.

Rob C: Extraperitoneal approach to the abdominal aorta. *Surgery* 53:87, 1963.

Sethi GK, Hughes RK, Takaro T: Dissecting aortic aneurysms. *Ann Thorac Surg* 18:301, 1974.

Stanley JC, Fry WJ: Pathogenesis and clinical significance of splenic artery aneurysms. *Surgery* 76:898, 1974.

Stanley JC, Thompson NW, Fry WJ: Splanchnic artery aneurysms. *Arch Surg* 101:689, 1970.

Stowe CL, Safi JJ, et al: Inflammatory aneurysms of the aorta. *J Vasc Surg* 2:113, 1985.

String ST: Cholelithiasis and aortic reconstruction. *J Vasc Surg* 1:664, 1985.

Sweeney MS, Gadacz TR: Primary aortoduodenal fistula: Manifestation, diagnosis and treatment. *Surgery* 96:492, 1984.

Szilagyi DE, Elliot JP, Smith RF: Clinical fate of the patient with asymptomatic abdominal aortic aneurysm and unfit for surgical therapy. *Arch Surg* 104:600, 1972.

Szilagyi DE, Hageman JH, et al: Spinal cord damage in surgery of the abdominal aorta. *Surgery* 83:38, 1978.

Szilagyi DE, Smith RF, et al: Contribution of abdominal aortic aneurysmectomy to prolongation of life. *Ann Surg* 164:678, 1966.

Thompson JE, Hollier LH, et al: Surgical management of abdominal aortic aneurysms: Factors influencing mortality and morbidity—a 20 year experience. *Ann Surg* 181:654, 1975.

Trastek VF, Pairolero PC, et al: Splenic artery aneurysms. *Surgery* 91:694, 1982.

Whittemore AD, Clowes AW, et al: Aortic aneurysm repair. Reduced operative mortality associated with maintenance of optimal cardiac performance. *Ann Surg* 192:414, 1980.

Peripheral Aneurysms: General

Howell JF, Crawford ES, et al: Surgical treatment of peripheral arteriosclerotic aneurysm. *Surg Clin North Am* 46:979, 1966.

Popliteal Aneurysm

Alpert J: Aneurysms of the popliteal artery. *J Med Soc NJ* 67:791, 1970.

Anton GE, Hertzer NR, et al: Surgical management of popliteal aneurysms. *J Vasc Surg* 3:125, 1986.

Edmunds LH, Darling RC, Linton RR: Surgical management of popliteal aneurysms. *Circulation* 32:517, 1965.

Gifford RW Jr, Hines EA Jr, Janes JM: Analysis and follow-up study of 100 popliteal aneurysms. *Surgery* 33:284, 1953.

Hunter JA, Julian OC, et al: Arteriosclerotic aneurysms of the popliteal artery. *J Cardiovasc Surg* 2:404, 1961.

Femoral Aneurysm

Crawford ES, Edwards WH, et al: Peripheral arteriosclerotic aneurysm. *J Am Geriatr Soc* 9:1, 1961.

Papas G, Janes JM, et al: Femoral aneurysms: Review of surgical management. *JAMA* 190:489, 1964.

Stoney RJ, Albo RJ, Wylie EJ: False aneurysms occurring after arterial grafting operations. *Am J Surg* 110:153, 1965.

Tolstedt GE, Radke HN, Bell JW: Late sequela of arteriosclerotic femoral aneurysms. *Angiology* 12:601, 1961.

Carotid Artery Aneurysm

Beall AC Jr, Crawford ES, et al: Extracranial aneurysms of the carotid artery: Report of seven cases. *Postgrad Med* 32:93, 1962.

Kianouri M: Extracranial carotid aneurysms. *Ann Surg* 165:152, 1967.

Sanoudos GM, Ramp J, Imparato AM: Internal carotid aneurysm. *Am Surg* 39:118, 1973.

Spencer FC: Aneurysm of the common carotid artery treated by excision and primary anastomosis. *Ann Surg* 145:254, 1957.

Subclavian Aneurysm

Howell JF, Crawford ES, et al: Surgical treatment of peripheral arteriosclerotic aneurysm. *Surg Clin North Am* 46:979, 1966.

Splenic Artery Aneurysm

Bedford PD, Lodge B: Aneurysm of the splenic artery. *Gut* 1:312, 1960.

Owens JC, Coffey RJ: Aneurysm of the splenic artery, including a report of 6 additional cases. *Int Abstr Surg* 97:313, 1953.

Renal Artery Aneurysm

Cerny JC, Chang C, Fry WJ: Renal artery aneurysms. *Arch Surg* 96:653, 1968.

Garritano AP: Aneurysm of the renal artery. *Am J Surg* 94:638, 1957.

Poutasse EF: Renal artery aneurysm: Report of 12 cases, two treated by excision of the aneurysm and repair of renal artery. *J Urol* 77:697, 1957.

Traumatic Aneurysm

Crawford ES, DeBakey ME, Cooley DA: Surgical considerations of peripheral arterial aneurysms. *Arch Surg* 78:226, 1959.

Dickinson EH, Hood RH, Spencer FC: Traumatic aneurysm of the innominate artery. *US Armed Forces Med J* 3:1871, 1952.

Hughes CW, Jahnke EJ Jr: The surgery of traumatic arteriovenous fistulas and aneurysms: A five year follow-up study of lesions. *Ann Surg* 148:790, 1958.

Raynaud's Disease

Burton EE Jr, et al: Raynaud's phenomenon: Treatment with intraarterial reserpine. *Cutis (NY)*, 9:464, 1972.

DeTakats G, Fowler EF: The neurogenic factor in Raynaud's phenomenon. *Surgery* 51:9, 1962.

Farmer RG, Gifford RW Jr, Hines EA Jr: Raynaud's disease with sclerodactylia: A follow-up study of seventy-one patients. *Circulation* 23:13, 1961.

Gifford RW Jr, Hines EA Jr, Craig WMcK: Sympathectomy for Raynaud's phenomenon: Follow-up study of 70 women with Raynaud's disease and 54 women with secondary Raynaud's phenomenon. *Circulation* 17:5, 1958.

Harris RW, Andros G, et al: Large-vessel arterial occlusive disease in symptomatic upper extremity. *Arch Surg* 119:1277, 1984.

Kirtley JA, Riddell DH, et al: Cervicothoracic sympathectomy in neurovascular abnormalities of the upper extremities: Experiences in 76 patients with 104 sympathectomies. *Ann Surg* 165:869, 1967.

Palumbo LT: Anterior transthoracic approach for upper thoracic sympathectomy. *Arch Surg* 72:659, 1956.

Porter JM, Bardana EJ, Baur GM: The clinical significance of Raynaud's syndrome. *Surgery* 80:756, 1976.

Porter JM, et al: Evaluation and management of patients with Raynaud's syndrome. *Am J Surg* 142:183, 1981.

Smith CR, Rodeheffer FJ: Treatment of Raynaud's phenomenon with calcium channel blockers. *Am J Med* 78:(suppl 2B):39, 1985.

Taylor LM Jr, Baur GM, Porter JM: Finger gangrene caused by small artery occlusive disease. *Ann Surg* 193:453, 1981.

Varadi DP, Lawrence AM: Suppression of Raynaud's phenomenon by methyldopa. *Ann Intern Med* 124:13, 1969.

Willerson JT, Decker JL: Raynaud's disease and phenomenon, a medical approach. *Am Heart J* 82:572, 1971.

Uncommon Vasomotor Diseases

Estes JE: Vasoconstrictive and vasodilative syndromes of the extremities. *Mod Concepts Cardiovasc Dis* 25:355, 1956.

Lewis T, Landis EM: Observations upon the vascular mechanism in acrocyanosis. *Heart* 15:229, 1930.

Frostbite

Couch NP, Sullivan J, Crane C: Predictive accuracy of renal vein renin activity in surgery of renovascular hypertension. *Surgery* 79:70, 1976.

Ervasti E: Frostbites of the extremities and their sequelae: A clinical study. *Acta Chir Scand* 299:1, 1962.

Golding MR, Martinez A, et al: The role of sympathectomy in frostbite, with a review of 68 cases. *Surgery* 57:774, 1965.

Mundth ED, Long DM, Brown RB: Treatment of experimental frostbite with low molecular weight dextran. *J Trauma* 4:246, 1964.

Penn I, Schwartz SI: Evaluation of low molecular weight dextran in the treatment of frostbite. *J Trauma* 4:784, 1964.

Shumacker HB Jr, Kilman JW: Sympathectomy in the treatment of frostbite. *Arch Surg* 89:575, 1964.

Simeone FA: A preliminary follow-up report in cases of cold injury from World War II, in Ferrer MI (ed): *Cold Injury. Trans 4th Conf Josiah Macy Jr Found NY* 1956, pp 197–223.

Snider RL, Porter JM: Treatment of experimental frostbite with intra-arterial sympathetic blocking drugs. *Surgery* 77(4):557, 1975.

Chapter 22

Venous and Lymphatic Disease

Lazar J. Greenfield

VENOUS DISEASE

Functional Anatomy of the Veins

Evolution in human beings to an upright position imposed a significant work load on the venous system. Since the systemic veins contain approximately two-thirds of the circulating blood volume under relatively low pressure, movement from the lower extremities must overcome gravity and intraabdominal pressure to return blood to the right ventricle. The left ventricle provides the initial force called *vis a tergo,* which is reduced through the capillary bed to a pressure of about 15 mmHg in the venules. In addition, the calf muscles provide an important pump function as they compress deep veins within an unyielding fascial compartment. Proximal flow is assured by the presence of the delicate but strong venous valves, which prevent reflux distally. Perforating or communicating veins connect the superficial venous system with the deep and direct flow internally from the superficial veins in all areas of the lower extremity except the foot, where the opposite occurs (Fig. 22-1). Each valve is based within a dilated sinus of the vein, which keeps the valve cusps away from the walls and promotes rapid closure when flow ceases. Numbers of valves increase with distance from the heart while the vena cava and common iliac veins are valveless. Valves are the focal point of most of the pathology of venous thrombosis since their sinuses are where the initial thrombus forms and the loss of valvular function after recanalization of a thrombus produces venous insufficiency.

The structure of veins also is related to their functional requirements, with the unsupported superficial vein walls containing more smooth muscle while the deep veins are thin-walled and lacking in significant smooth muscle. In some areas such as the calf, there are spindle-shaped sinusoids that can become sites of venous stasis when the patient is at bed rest, facilitating the development of venous thrombosis.

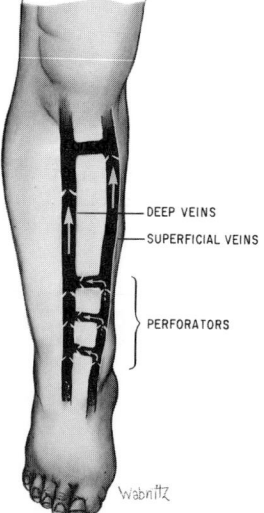

Fig. 22-1. Schematic orientation of venous valves and flow of blood in the superficial, deep, and perforating veins of the lower leg.

The major superficial veins of the lower extremity are the greater and lesser saphenous veins and their tributaries. The deep veins follow the course of the major arteries and share their names. In the lower leg the veins are paired and join at the knee to form the popliteal vein, which continues through the adductor hiatus to become the superficial femoral vein. The latter is joined by the deep femoral vein in the upper thigh to become the common femoral vein, which becomes the external iliac vein as it enters the pelvis beneath the inguinal ligament. The perforating veins are so named because they penetrate the fascia of the lower leg to connect the superficial and deep systems. The perforators adjacent to the medial malleolus are often responsible for the development of stasis ulcers at that level when they become incompetent.

Respiration and exercise have significant effects on normal venous flow. During inspiration, diaphragmatic descent increases intraabdominal pressure, transiently decreasing venous return. During expiration, abdominal pressure falls and the distally trapped blood accelerates flow cephalad. During exercise, the calf muscle pump reduces venous pressure in the deep veins by emptying them and when the muscle relaxes, the superficial veins drain into the deep system rapidly. The ability to move large volumes of blood during the hyperemia of exercise prevents edema formation by maintaining a normal pressure gradient across the capillary bed.

Etiology of Deep Vein Thrombosis

Development of a thrombus within a vein may be considered functionally as an exaggeration of the normal process of hemostasis. When disruption of normal endothelium occurs, subendothelial structures trigger a reaction in platelets, coagulation proteins, and adjacent endothelial cells that results in a hemostatic plug. Soon fibrin is deposited and within 24 h the platelet plug is replaced by fibrin which allows the vessel to heal. The occurrence

of this process in a nontraumatized vein was recognized by Virchow who, in 1856, introduced the term thrombosis and postulated three possible mechanisms: stasis, endothelial damage, and hypercoagulability.

STASIS. In the surgical patient, stasis is the most important factor in the development of deep vein thrombosis (DVT), especially when there is prolonged immobilization in bed. When contrast medium is injected in the veins of the lower extremities of a bedridden patient, it may remain in venous valve sinuses for as long as an hour, confirming the pooling effect in the soleal veins. This is the favored location for the formation of a nidus of thrombus that then promotes successive layering of platelets, fibrin, and leukocytes to produce an organized thrombus. This process can begin under general anesthesia in the operating room but usually requires other contributing factors such as shock, infection, trauma, or congestive heart failure. Aging, obesity, pregnancy, and malignancy are also important added risk factors.

ENDOTHELIAL DAMAGE. Endothelial injury can occur in collapsed vessels when the intimal walls are in contact, and further injury can be demonstrated after hypoxemia that occurs when there is venous stasis. Similarly, leukocyte adherence to endothelial intracellular junctions can be demonstrated in areas of stasis after trauma at a remote site. In spite of these changes, however, routine histological examination of veins containing thrombus usually fails to show an inflammatory response consistent with vessel wall injury.

HYPERCOAGULABILITY. Patients who present at an early age with spontaneous venous thrombosis, who have a strong family history of DVT, or who develop recurrent venous thromboembolism are usually considered "prethrombotic" or "hypercoagulable." They deserve careful study for associated disorders as described by Shattil and listed in Table 22-1.

Idiopathic DVT may also be the first clue to occult malignancy. The association between venous thrombosis and cancer was first suggested by Trousseau and often has been confirmed in postmortem studies. In a recent series reported by Aderka et al., 34 percent of otherwise healthy patients with idiopathic DVT were found to have a malignancy diagnosed an average of 24 months later. Increased likelihood of cancer in these patients was associated with age over sixty-five, anemia, and eosinophilia. The earliest onset malignancies were found within one year and tended to occur in the pelvic organs and breast. Prolonged follow-up is appropriate, however, since some malignancies did not appear until after 5 years, which also suggests coincidence rather than a direct relationship. There is a direct relationship between the use of oral contraceptive anovulatory agents and thrombotic disorders that occur 3 to 6 times more frequently in those women.

The most common transient hypercoagulable states are associated with recent trauma, major surgical procedures and sepsis. In addition to the possible roles of stasis and increased circulating procoagulant factors, the fibrinolytic system is inhibited after surgery and trauma and there is less lytic activity in the veins of the lower extremity than in those of the upper extremity.

Table 22-1. CONDITIONS ASSOCIATED WITH RECURRENT VENOUS THROMBOEMBOLISM

Accelerated or inappropriate hemostatic plug formation

Endothelial cell damage
  Atherosclerosis and hypercholesterolemia
  Homocystinuria
  Vasculitis and the lupus anticoagulant
Inappropriate platelet plug formation
  Essential thrombocythemia
  Paroxysmal nocturnal hemoglobinuria
  Heparin-associated thrombocytopenia
Inappropriate fibrin plug formation
  Disseminated intravascular coagulation
  Infusion of prothrombin complex concentrates

Defects in the mechanism limiting hemostatic plug size

Stasis
  Previous deep vein thrombosis
  Congestive heart failure
  Hyperviscosity syndrome: polycythemia; serum
  hyperviscosity
Antithrombin III deficiency
Protein C deficiency
Defective lysis of fibrin plugs
Dysfibrinogenemia
  Decreased plasminogen activator activity
  Decreased plasminogen activity

SOURCE: Shattil SJ: Diagnosis and treatment of recurrent venous thromboembolism. *Med Clin North Am* 68:577–601, 1984.

Pathophysiology

A propagating thrombus may become attached to the opposite wall, causing interruption of flow, retrograde thrombosis, and signs of venous stasis in the extremity (Fig. 22-2). Subsequent formation of edema within the confines of the deep muscular fascia may produce pain and/or limited dorsiflexion of the foot (Homans's sign). The latter sign as originally described by Homans is only an indication of muscular irritability and its use far exceeds its reliability. More commonly, in about 60 percent of patients the thrombus propagates without interrupting flow and develops a long floating "tail" that is more susceptible to breaking loose from its tenuous anchor within the valvular sinus. It is the latter sequence of events that is the most dangerous aspect of the disorder, because major pulmonary embolism can and does occur without premonitory signs or symptoms at its point of origin.

The site of venous obstruction determines the level at which swelling is observed clinically. Swelling at the thigh level always implies obstruction at the level of the iliofemoral system, whereas swelling of the calf or foot suggests obstruction at the femoropopliteal level (Fig. 22-3). Autopsies suggest that it is more common for thrombi to originate in the veins of the soleus and then propagate proximally, but there is evidence that primary thrombosis of the femoral and iliac venous tributaries occurs as well.

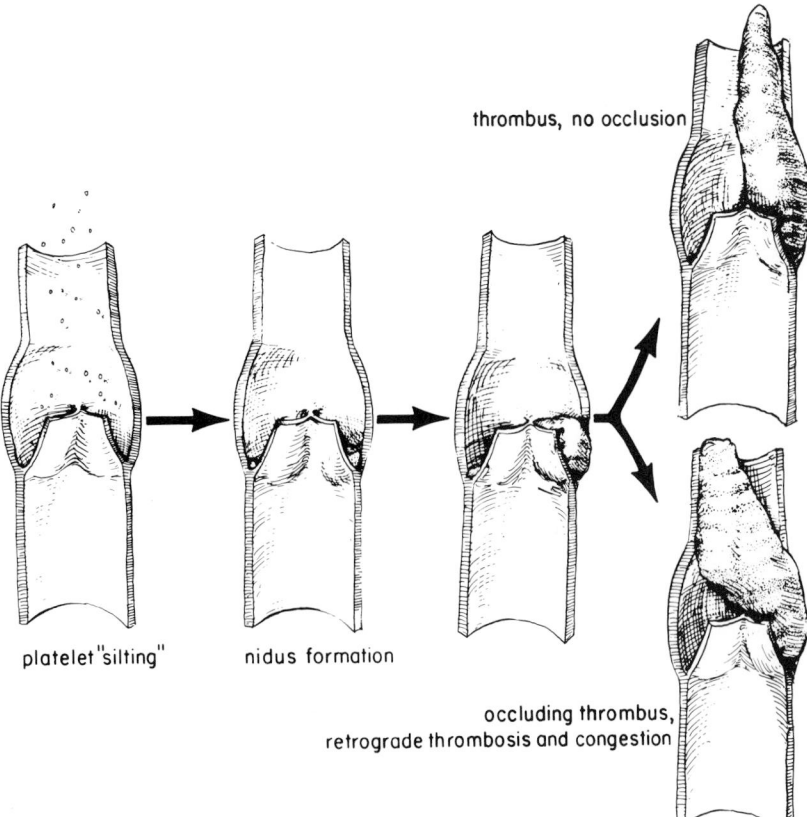

Fig. 22-2. The evolution of venous thrombosis begins with stagnant flow that permits silting of platelets and possibly hypoxemic injury to valvular sinus endothelium. The resulting nidus of thrombus releases thrombin that aggregates more platelets in a cycle of thrombus propagation. As the thrombus grows, it may extend into the lumen without occlusion or may occlude the vein with retrograde thrombosis and venous hypertension. [From: *Greenfield LJ: Acute venous thrombosis and pulmonary embolism, in Hardy JD (ed): Hardy's Textbook of Surgery. Philadelphia, Lippincott, 1983, with permission.*]

thrombus, no occlusion

platelet "silting"

nidus formation

occluding thrombus, retrograde thrombosis and congestion

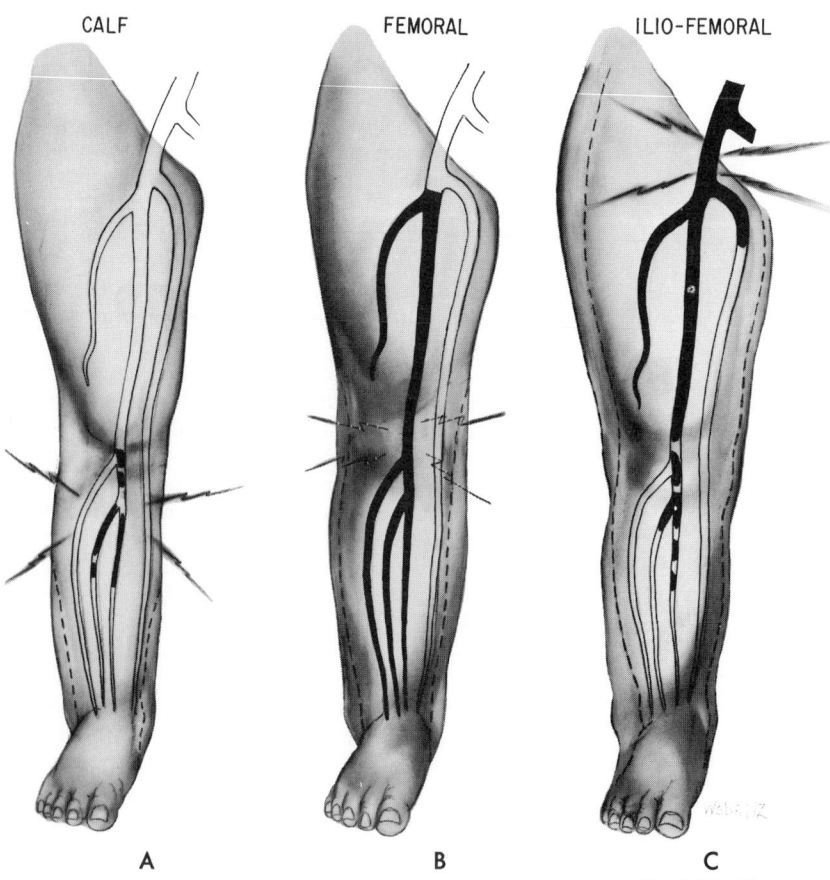

CALF · FEMORAL · ILIO-FEMORAL

A · B · C

Fig. 22-3. Clinical features of venous thrombosis. *A.* When thrombosis is localized to veins of the calf and the popliteal vein, there is minimal swelling at the level of the ankle. Calf pain and tenderness are usually present. *B.* When there is thrombosis of the femoral vein and associated thrombosis of the calf veins, swelling is usually present and extends to just above the level of the knee. Popliteal tenderness and calf tenderness may be present. *C.* In iliofemoral venous thrombosis, there is thrombosis of the iliac and proximal femoral vein, and frequently the calf veins also are involved. Edema is present from the foot to the inguinal ligament. There is usually tenderness in the groin as well as popliteal and calf tenderness.

Resolution of deep vein thrombosis with recanalization will alter the competence of the valves within the veins and can result in the postthrombotic syndrome, which will be discussed.

Diagnosis

CLINICAL MANIFESTATIONS. Major venous thrombosis involving the deep venous system of the thigh and pelvis produces a characteristic clinical picture of pain, extensive pitting edema, and blanching that has been termed *phlegmasia alba dolens* or "milk leg." Association with pregnancy may be related to hormonal effects on blood, relaxation of vessel walls, or mechanical compression of the left iliac vein at the pelvic brim, resulting in the term "milk leg of pregnancy." It was originally believed that the blanching was due to spasm and compromise of arterial flow, but efforts to achieve sympatholysis are ill-advised because it is the subcutaneous edema that is responsible for the blanching. In addition to pregnancy, other mechanical factors that can affect the left iliac vein include compression from the right iliac artery or an overdistended bladder, and congenital webs within the vein. These factors are responsible for the observed 4:1 preponderance of left versus right iliac vein involvement.

As venous thrombosis progresses, impeding most of the venous return from the extremity, there is danger of limb loss from cessation of arterial flow. This clinical picture differs from alba dolens, with more congestion producing *phlegmasia cerulea dolens,* which is characterized by loss of sensory and motor function. Venous gangrene is likely unless an aggressive approach is utilized to remove the thrombus and restore blood flow. A variant of this disorder occurs peripherally in the leg and is associated with concurrent malignant disease and a high mortality rate.

Fortunately, these major complications occur in less than 10 percent of patients with venous thrombosis. Only 40 percent of patients with venous thrombosis have any clinical signs of the disorder. In addition, false-positive clinical signs occur in up to 30 percent of patients studied. Because of this there has been a great deal of interest in the development of screening tests that can reveal thrombi before they become evident clinically. Contrast venography provides direct evidence of both occlusive and nonocclusive thrombi, but it is an invasive procedure and usually requires moving the patient to a radiographic suite. Ideally, the screening test would be accurate, non-invasive, and able to be performed at the bedside. Although the ideal has not yet been achieved, there are a number of tests that have proved useful.

RADIOACTIVE-LABELED FIBRINOGEN. In 1957, Ambrus et al. showed that radioactive thrombi resulted from injection of radiolabeled fibrinogen and thrombin into an occluded vessel, and in 1960, Hobbs and Davies demonstrated preferential uptake of ^{131}I-labeled fibrinogen in formation of a thrombus. Clinical application of this finding required simplification of the test by development of portable scintillation counters for bedside use. After iodine blockage of the thyroid gland, the counts are obtained from marked locations on the lower extremities and expressed as a percentage of the radioactivity measured by counting over the heart. An increase of 20 percent or more in one area indicates the presence of an underlying thrombus. The test permits sequential scanning of the extremities over a period of days and is most sensitive to thrombi forming in the veins of the calves shortly after an operative procedure. It does not permit detection of thrombi in pelvic veins, and it cannot be used in an extremity in which there is a healing wound, fracture, cellulitis, arthritis, edema, ulceration, or superficial thrombophlebitis. It is also contraindicated in patients under thirty years of age and in women of childbearing age. Apart from these conditions it is quite accurate, however, and has a 90 percent positive correlation with contrast venograms. A negative correlation usually is explained by cessation of active thrombosis and failure to incorporate the tagged fibrinogen, making the test most useful clinically in discriminating between old and new venous thrombi.

ULTRASOUND. The Doppler ultrasound probe can be used to advantage to detect major venous thrombi with a high degree of accuracy, but it is a subjective form of testing dependent on the examiner's experience. The principle is based on the change in flow signal produced by intraluminal thrombi. The examination begins at the ankle with identification of the posterior tibial vein signal adjacent to the artery. The flow signal should be altered by distal and proximal compression, producing augmentation and interruption of flow, respectively, which can also be produced by the Valsalva maneuver. The same maneuvers are repeated over the superficial and deep femoral veins and can be done over the popliteal vein as well (Fig. 22-4). Failure of augmentation of flow on compression below the probe or release of interruption of flow above the probe suggests a venous thrombus. The sensitivity of the test exceeds 90 percent, but the specificity is 5 to 10 percent lower because of the possibility of other mechanical problems (e.g., Baker's cyst, hematoma) interfering with venous flow. A negative Doppler ultrasound examination is reassuring, but a positive or equivocal test should be confirmed by contrast venography. A negative test in the leg is not reassuring when thromboembolism is suspected, because the thrombus may have been evacuated from the extremity.

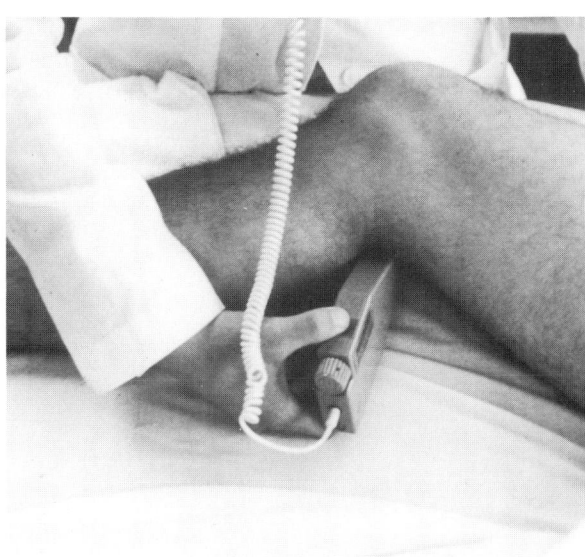

Fig. 22-4. The Doppler probe can be used at the bedside to assess flow in all the venous tributaries of the leg. Distal and proximal compression produce alterations in flow that are attenuated or absent when a thrombus is present.

The addition of real-time B-mode imaging to Doppler measurement in a portable duplex device offers a new approach to detection and characterization of venous thrombi. To date, however, the echographic imaging has been limited to the extremities.

IMPEDANCE PLETHYSMOGRAPHY. The impedance method measures the volume of the extremity to temporary occlusion of the venous system. The diagnosis of venous thrombosis depends on the changes in venous capacitance and rate of emptying after release of the occlusion. A proximal thigh cuff is inflated to 50 mmHg or until maximum filling has occurred by plateau of the electrical signal. The cuff is then rapidly deflated, allowing rapid outflow and reduction of volume in a normal limb (Fig. 22-5). Prolongation of the outflow wave suggests major venous thrombosis with 95 percent accuracy and is much more reliable than any voluntary technique of venous occlusion. The deficiency of this technique, as with all noninvasive methods, is the lack of detection of calf vein thrombosis or old postthrombotic sequelae. The strain gauge plethysmograph can be used in a similar fashion.

VENOGRAPHY. The injection of contrast material for direct visualization of the venous system of the extremity is the most accurate method of confirming the diagnosis of venous thrombosis and the extent of involvement. Injection is usually made into the foot while the superficial veins are occluded by tourniquet, and a supplemental injection into the femoral veins may be required to visualize the iliofemoral system (Fig. 22-6). Potential false-positive examinations may result from external compression of a vein or washout of the contrast material from venous flow from collateral veins. The procedure can also be performed with isotope injection using a gamma scintillation counter to record flow of the isotope. Delayed imaging of

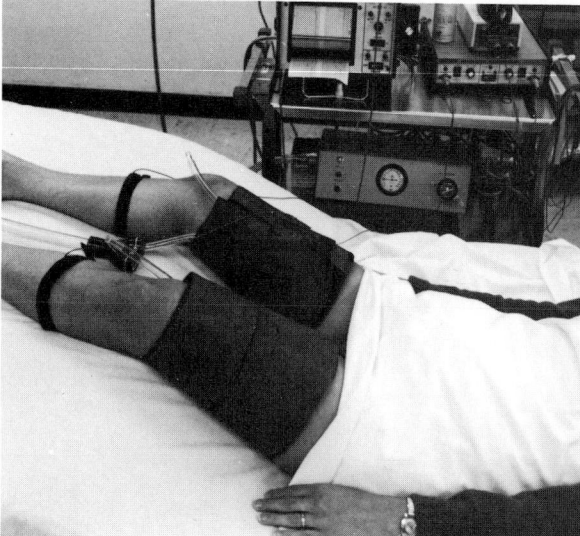

Fig. 22-5. The plethysmograph measures the volume change in the lower extremity following temporary occlusion of venous return by pneumatic cuffs. When the cuff pressure is released, there is rapid outflow of blood and reduction in limb volume unless proximal venous thrombosis is present. Both strain gauge (shown) and impedance sensors may be used for the volume recordings.

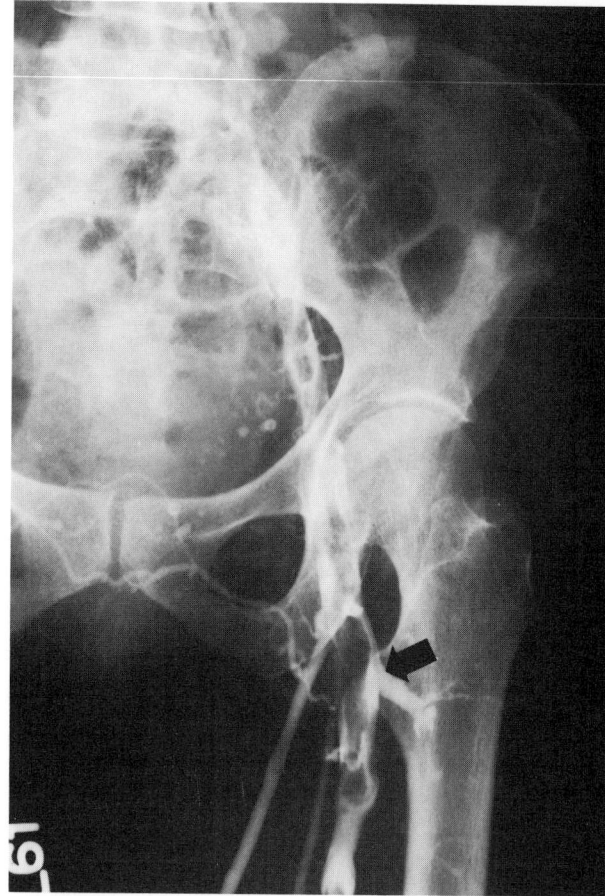

Fig. 22-6. Contrast venogram demonstrating a thrombus within the femoral vein. It is outlined by the contrast material which indicates that it is free-floating at that level. [From: *Greenfield LJ: Complications of venous thrombosis and pulmonary embolism, in Greenfield LJ (ed): Complications in Surgery and Trauma. Philadelphia, Lippincott, 1984, with permission.*]

persistent ''hot spots'' may also reflect isotope retention at the sites of thrombus formation (Fig. 22-7). A perfusion lung scan can also be obtained for baseline comparison and for detection of silent embolism. There is less definition of deep vein thrombi with this technique than with contrast venography, but it is a valuable technique for sequential study of patients and avoids the potential thrombogenesis associated with the injection of contrast medium.

Prophylaxis

Theoretically, it should be possible to prevent formation of venous thrombi either by eliminating or reducing venous stasis or by altering blood coagulability. The belief that early ambulation prevents stasis and reduces the formation of thrombi has been controversial, and studies using tagged fibrinogen have not supported this assumption. One possible explanation for this is that early ambulation often involves having the patient walk to a nearby chair and sit, whereupon the legs are subjected to even more stasis.

There has been more benefit from the prophylactic use of anticoagulant drugs. There are good data to support the use of preoperative oral anticoagulant therapy with warfarin derivatives in high-risk patients. Unfortunately, this procedure increases the risk of hemorrhage, and because of the added difficulties of laboratory control of prothrombin time, there has not been widespread acceptance of this approach. It remains, however, the recommendation of a national task force on prophylaxis for patients undergoing surgery for fractured hips as reported by Hyers, Hull, and Weg. They also recommend adjusted-dose heparin to prolong the APTT to the upper normal

range for patients having elective hip surgery. The administration of dextran, which produces a variety of effects on platelets and clotting factors, has been demonstrated to reduce the incidence of detectable thrombi. However, it too can produce hemorrhagic problems as well as allergic reactions and, in older patients, congestive heart failure.

There has been much wider acceptance of the administration of heparin prior to and following surgery in low (''mini'') doses that do not alter the laboratory clotting profile Generally, a 5000-unit dose is given subcutaneously 2 h preoperatively and then every 12 h postoperatively for 6 days. This provides protection for most high-risk groups with the exception of those undergoing orthopedic or urological procedures. The beneficial effect may be due to the enhancement of heparin cofactor (antithrombin III), a natural inhibitor of activated factor X. Although some studies have failed to show a protective effect, Kakkar et al. in a randomized series of 4121 patients showed that heparin protected against fatal pulmonary embolism as well as deep venous thrombosis.

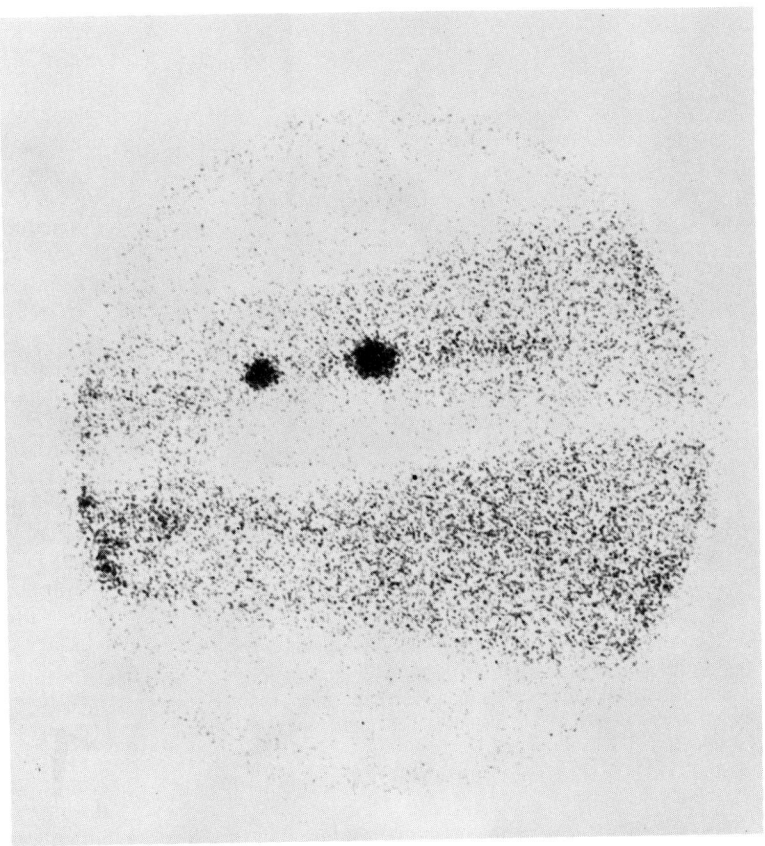

Fig. 22-7. Isotope scan following the injection of macroaggregated albumin ^{131}I showing an acute thrombus in the popliteal vein.

Intermittent pneumatic leg compression prevents stasis and increases fibrinolytic activity with virtually no side effects. The pneumatic boots can be applied in the operating room to minimize the risk of venous thrombosis beginning under general anesthesia. It is recommended for groups in which low-dose heparin is either contraindicated or ineffective, but should not be used in patients with peripheral arterial insufficiency.

Medical Treatment

The approach to management of the patient with deep venous thrombosis is based on three objectives: minimizing the risk of pulmonary embolism, limiting further thrombosis, and facilitating resolution of existing thrombi to avoid the postthrombotic syndrome.

Initially, the patient is anticoagulated and placed at bed rest with the foot of the bed elevated 8 to 10 in. Generally, pain, swelling, and tenderness resolve over a 5- to 7-day period, at which time ambulation can be permitted with elastic stocking support. Standing still and sitting should be prohibited to avoid increased venous pressure and stasis.

ANTICOAGULATION. The foundation of therapy for deep venous thrombosis is adequate anticoagulation, initially with heparin and then with coumarin derivatives for prolonged protection against recurrent thrombosis. Unless there are specific contraindications, heparin should be administered in an initial dose of 100 to 150 units/kg

intravenously. Heparin is an acid mucopolysaccharide that neutralizes thrombin, inhibits thromboplastin, and reduces the platelet release reaction. It may be administered by continuous or intermittent intravenous doses regulated by whole blood clotting time or activated partial thromboplastin time. Bleeding complications can be minimized by doses of heparin that prolong the laboratory clotting determinations by about twice the normal time with no loss of effectiveness. Continuous intravenous infusion regulated by an infusion pump seems to minimize the total dose required for control and is associated with a lower incidence of complications.

Oral administration of anticoagulants is begun shortly after initiation of heparin therapy, because several days are usually required to bring the prothrombin time within the therapeutic range of 1.4 times the control value. The coumarin derivatives block the synthesis of several clotting factors, and prolongation of the prothrombin time beyond the level suggested is associated with a higher incidence of bleeding complications. Fortunately, administration of vitamin K usually can restore the prothrombin time rapidly. After an episode of acute deep venous thrombosis, anticoagulation therapy should be maintained for a minimum of 3 months; some investigators favor 6 months for treatment of thrombi in the larger veins. Many drugs interact with coumarin derivatives (e.g., barbiturates), and therefore it is essential to establish a routine for regular monitoring of prothrombin time after the patient leaves the hospital.

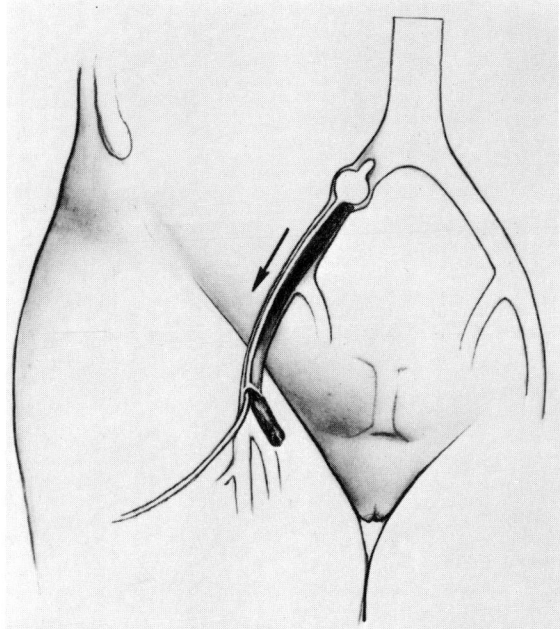

Fig. 22-8. Venous thrombectomy using a Fogarty catheter to extract the proximal thrombus. Increased intraabdominal pressure by the Valsalva maneuver minimizes the risk of embolism. *(Courtesy of C. Rob and R. Smith.)*

FIBRINOLYSIS. There has been great interest in the use of fibrinolytic agents to activate the intrinsic plasmin system. Both streptokinase and urokinase have been used and found to be effective, although they are associated with a relatively high incidence of hemorrhagic complications as reported by Common et al. These agents have no advantage over heparin in the treatment of recurrent venous thrombosis or thrombosis that has existed for over 72 h, and they are contraindicated in postoperative or posttraumatic patients.

In a prospective study of 29 patients with major DVT (thrombosis involving the popliteal veins, with or without calf veins), Kakkar and Lawrence compared hemodynamic and clinical results in patients receiving 5-day treatment with heparin or streptokinase, followed by a 6-month course of coumadin. Overall, at 2-year follow-up they found over half of the limbs with evidence of the postthrombotic syndrome. Clinically, 14 percent of patients had no symptoms, 20 percent had severe symptoms, and the remainder demonstrated mild to moderate changes. No difference was seen between patients receiving heparin or streptokinase. Although a drug to restore venous patency and preserve valve function has not yet been found, other thrombolytic drugs such as tissue plasminogen activator (TPA) are currently under investigation and may provide better alternatives to treatment.

Surgical Approaches

OPERATIVE THROMBECTOMY. The direct surgical approach to remove thrombi from the deep veins of the leg utilizes the common femoral vein and is facilitated by the use of a Fogarty venous balloon catheter and an elastic wrap for milking the extremity (Fig. 22-8). Although the operative results are impressive, venograms obtained prior to discharge from the hospital show iliac occlusion in the majority of patients, and there does not seem to be any lesser incidence of the postthrombotic syndrome. Consequently, the procedure is usually reserved for limb salvage in the presence of phlegmasia cerulea dolens and impending venous gangrene.

In considering the reasons why the procedure has not lived up to expectation, there may be an explanation other than rethrombosis. It is customary to assume that the iliac system has been cleared if there is brisk retrograde blood flow after a proximal thrombus has been removed. This can be misleading if the common iliac vein remains obstructed and the retrograde flow is from the internal iliac vein. Conversely, poor retrograde flow may be seen when an iliac vein valve is intact despite removal of all proximal thrombus. Therefore, intraoperative venography should be performed in all cases. After completion of the thrombectomy, a small catheter may be left in a branch of the saphenous vein for postoperative regional heparin administration and postoperative venography.

In recent reports, an attempt has also been made to prevent rethrombosis after thrombectomy by creation of a peripheral arteriovenous fistula using the saphenous vein or one of its branches. The fistula is either allowed to close or is ligated after 2 to 3 months. Early results in 57 patients reported by Einarsson et al. showed patency of the iliofemoral segment by venography in 61 percent, and 75 percent had a good clinical result. Measurement by venous function, however, using plethysmography and foot volumetry showed normal results in only 29 percent.

VENA CAVAL INTERRUPTION. Adequate anticoagulation is usually effective in managing deep venous thrombosis, but if recurrent pulmonary embolism occurs during anticoagulant therapy or if there is a contraindication to anticoagulation, a surgical approach is necessary. Vena caval interruption is also indicated when a complication of anticoagulation forces is to be discontinued, as prophylaxis against recurrence of embolism after pulmonary embolectomy and in some high-risk patients who could not tolerate even a small embolic recurrence.

Early surgical efforts to prevent recurrence of pulmonary embolism were directed to the common femoral vein, which was ligated bilaterally. This resulted in a high incidence of sequelae due to stasis in the lower extremity and an unacceptable rate of pulmonary embolism. The next approach used was ligation of the inferior vena cava below the renal veins, which added the adverse effect of a sudden reduction in cardiac output under general anesthesia. This effect, coupled with stasis sequelae and recurrent embolism through dilated collateral veins, led to efforts to compartmentalize the vena cava by means of sutures, staples, and external clips in order to provide filtration without occlusion (Fig. 22-9).

Because these procedures required general anesthesia and laparotomy, the next logical step was to devise a transvenous approach that could be performed under local anesthesia. The Mobin–Uddin ''umbrella'' unit was inserted from the jugular vein and positioned under fluoroscopic control below the renal veins, where it usually produced (in 70 percent of cases) thrombosis of the vena cava and occasionally detached, resulting in fatal embolism.

The Greenfield cone-shaped filter was developed to maintain patency after trapping emboli. This is possible because of the unique geometry of the cone that collects emboli in its apex and retains perimeter flow. Preservation of flow avoids stasis and facilitates lysis of the embolus (Fig. 22-10). It can be inserted from either the jugular vein, left axillary vein, or the femoral vein, the latter insertion being reserved for inadequate size or technical problems with the jugular vein, or open wound of the neck. The rate of recurrent embolism with this device has been 5 to 6 percent over 12 years of follow-up. Its long-term patency rate of 95 percent allows it to be placed above the renal veins when necessary for embolism control, such as when there is a thrombus within the renal veins or vena cava. Another device, the Hunter balloon, occludes the vena cava after it is positioned below the renal veins and contributes to stasis sequelae.

The indications for insertion of a vena caval filter are listed in Table 22-2 and will be reviewed in the section on pulmonary thromboembolism.

OTHER TYPES OF VENOUS THROMBOSIS

Superficial Thrombophlebitis

The term thrombophlebitis should be restricted to the disorder of the superficial veins characterized by a local inflammatory process that is usually aseptic (Fig. 22-11). The cause of thrombophlebitis in the upper limb is usually acidic fluid infusion or prolonged cannulation. In the lower extremities it is usually associated with varicose veins and may coexist with deep vein thrombosis. Its association with the injection of contrast material can be

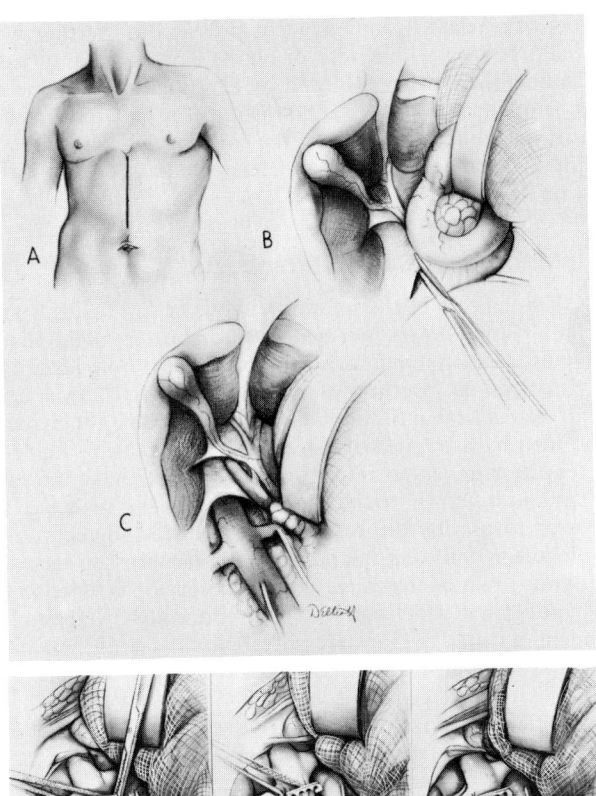

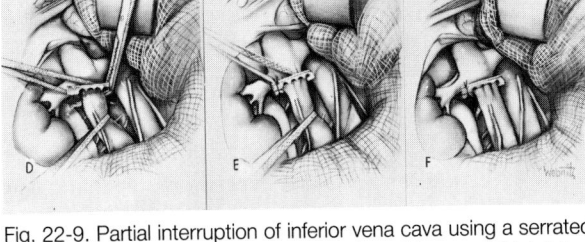

Fig. 22-9. Partial interruption of inferior vena cava using a serrated clip. *A.* Transperitoneal approach is preferred to permit high interruption of vena cava and concomitant ligation of the left spermatic or ovarian veins. *B.* Kocher maneuver. *C.* Vena cava cleared immediately below renal veins. *D.* Clip applied. *E.* Clip closed. *F.* Final position of clip in the immediate infrarenal region to prevent cul-de-sac. (From: *Adams JT, DeWeese JA: Surg Gynecol Obstet 123:1087, 1966, with permission.*)

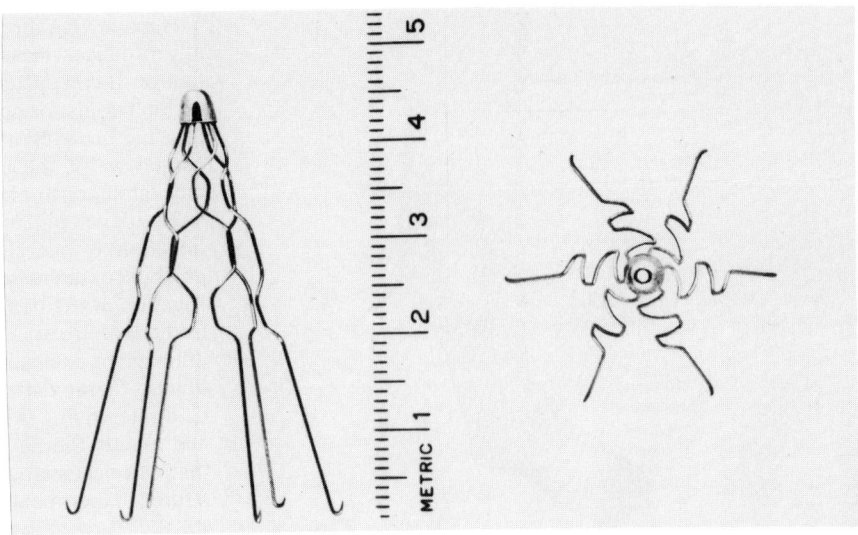

Fig. 22-10. The Greenfield filter is made of stainless steel and shaped in a cone to preserve perimeter flow after an embolus is trapped in its apex. Preservation of flow provides continued filtration, minimizes stasis sequelae, and facilitates lyses of trapped thrombus. The recurved hooks provide secure fixation in the vena cava.

Table 22-2. INDICATIONS FOR INSERTION OF A
VENA CAVAL FILTER

1. Recurrent thromboembolism in spite of adequate anticoagulation
2. Documented thromboembolism in a patient who has a contraindication to anticoagulation
3. Complication of anticoagulation that forces therapy to be discontinued
4. Chronic pulmonary embolism with associated pulmonary hypertension and cor pulmonale (class V)
5. Immediately following pulmonary embolectomy
6. Relative indications—patient with more than 50% of the pulmonary vascular bed occluded (class III) who cannot tolerate any additional embolism; patient with a large free-floating iliofemoral thrombus on venogram

minimized by washout of the contrast material with heparinized saline.

Thrombophlebitis Migrans

Thrombophlebitis migrans, a condition of recurrent episodes of superficial thrombophlebitis, has been associated with visceral malignancy, systemic collagen vascular disease, and blood dyscrasias. Involvement of the deep veins and the visceral veins has also been described.

Subclavian Vein Thrombosis

Thrombosis of the subclavian vein is most likely to be secondary to an indwelling catheter and can occur in the pediatric age group. It may also occur as a primary event in a young athletic person (effort thrombosis), presuma-

bly as a result of injury or compression at the thoracic inlet. If seen within 48 h of onset, it is possible to use thrombolytic drugs followed by a venogram to define a potentially correctable abnormality. If seen later, it usually responds to elevation of the limb and anticoagulation, although some venous insufficiency and discomfort with exercise may persist.

Inferior Vena Caval Thrombosis

Thrombosis of the inferior vena cava can result from tumor invasion or propagating thrombus from the iliac veins. More commonly, however, it results from ligation, plication, or insertion of partially occluding caval devices. Any caval filtration device can become totally occluded by a trapped massive thrombus, causing sudden reduction in venous return and cardiac output. In the patient with known prior pulmonary embolism it is a grave error to ascribe the resulting hypotension to recurrent embolism and treat the patient with vasopressor agents. In this situation the cause of the hypotension is functional hypovolemia which can readily be confirmed by measurement of central venous pressure. Thrombosis of the renal vein can result from extension of vena caval thrombosis but is most likely to occur in association with the nephrotic syndrome. It can be a source of thromboembolism and has been treated successfully by suprarenal placement of the Greenfield filter.

Visceral Venous Thrombosis

Portal vein thrombosis can occur in the neonate, usually secondary to propagating septic thrombophlebitis of the umbilical vein. Collateral development leads to the occurrence of esophageal varices. In the adult, thrombosis of the portal, hepatic, splenic, or superior mesenteric vein can occur spontaneously but usually is associated with hepatic cirrhosis. Thrombosis of mesenteric or omental veins can simulate an acute condition of the abdomen but usually results in prolonged ileus rather than intestinal infarction.

Hepatic vein thrombosis (Budd–Chiari syndrome) usually produces massive hepatomegaly, ascites, and liver failure. It can occur in association with a congenital web, endophlebitis, or polycythemia vera. Although some success has been reported using a direct approach to the congenital webs, the usual treatment is a side-to-side portacaval shunt to allow decompression of the liver.

The development of pelvic sepsis after abortion, tubal infection, or puerperal sepsis can lead to septic thrombophlebitis of the pelvic veins and septic thromboembolism. Ligation of the ovarian vein and vena cava has been the traditional treatment, but the emphasis should be on drainage or excision of the abscesses and appropriate antibiotic therapy. It is also appropriate to use the Greenfield filter in this situation because it is inert stainless steel and avoids the development of an intraluminal abscess that can occur after ligation of the vena cava as demonstrated experimentally by Peyton, Hylemon, et al. in 1983.

Fig. 22-11. Clinical presentation of superficial venous thrombosis. There is usually redness, tenderness, and swelling surrounding a palpable thrombosed superficial vein.

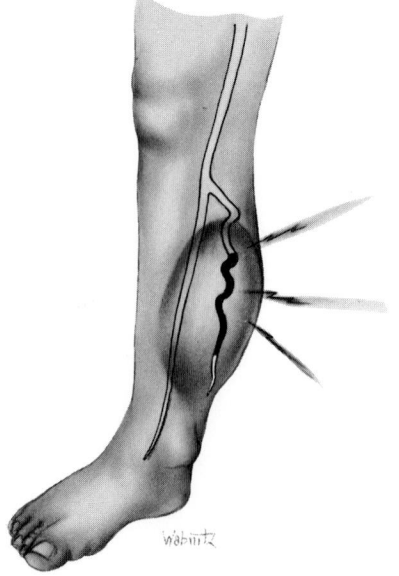

PULMONARY THROMBOEMBOLISM

The clinical significance of major pulmonary embolism can be appreciated by referring to the annual mortality attributed to it, which has been estimated to be 90,000 deaths in the United States alone. It is estimated that 5 of every 1000 adults undergoing major surgery will die from massive pulmonary embolism. Because it represents the most important complication of deep vein thrombosis, it is of particular concern to surgeons whose patients are prone to develop deep vein thrombosis in the immediate postoperative period.

Just as with deep vein thrombosis, our understanding of the pathophysiology of pulmonary embolism dates back to Virchow, who first recognized the association between the two findings. It also became obvious in the early reports by pathologists that pulmonary embolism could be well tolerated by some patients who then died of other causes. In fact, the full spectrum of the disorder ranges from asymptomatic minor embolism to sudden death from massive embolism.

Diagnosis

CLINICAL MANIFESTATIONS. The signs and symptoms of an embolic episode obviously depend primarily on the quantity of embolus involved and, to a lesser extent, on the cardiopulmonary status of the patient. In the classic presentation, the patient suddenly develops chest pain, cough, dyspnea, techypnea, and marked anxiety. Although hemoptysis has traditionally been associated with pulmonary embolism, it is actually an uncommon sign, and when present it usually occurs late in the course of the disease and represents pulmonary infarction. Objectively, the patient with major embolism usually shows tachycardia, an increased pulmonary second sound, cyanosis, prominent jugular veins, and varying degrees of collapse. Less commonly, there may be wheezing, a pleural friction rub, splinting of the chest wall, rales, low-grade fever, ventricular gallop, and wide splitting of the pulmonic second sound. The incidence of these findings found in the Urokinase Pulmonary Embolism Trial is shown in Table 22-3.

The differential diagnosis includes esophageal perforation, pneumonia, septic shock, and myocardial infarction. Since all these entities are life-threatening, it is manda-

Table 22-3. CLINICAL MANIFESTATIONS OF MAJOR PULMONARY EMBOLISM

Symptoms	Incidence, %	Signs	Incidence, %
Dyspnea	80	Tachypnea	88
Apprehension	60	Tachycardia	63
Pleural pain	60	Accentuated P_2	60
Cough	50	Rales	51
Hemoptysis	27	S_3 or S_4	47
Syncope	22	Pleural rub	17

Data from the Urokinase Pulmonary Embolism Trial: A National Cooperative Study. *Circulation* 2(suppl):47, 1973.

tory that an orderly approach be formulated to confirm or reject the working diagnosis. Laboratory studies in general are not very helpful in the differential diagnosis, although a white blood cell count of less than 15,000/mm^3 may be suggestive when a pulmonary infiltrate is present to help rule out pneumonitis. The following examinations are particularly useful in the evaluation of suspected major embolism.

ELECTROCARDIOGRAPHY. The most common electrocardiographic change associated with pulmonary embolism is nonspecific ST and T wave changes (66 percent of patients). More specific signs of right ventricular overload such as the often quoted S_1, Q_3, T_3 pattern are seldom seen. Consequently, the primary value of the electrocardiogram is to exclude the presence of a myocardial infarction. The finding of a myocardial infarction does not exclude the diagnosis of pulmonary embolism, and in some cases a lung scan or pulmonary angiogram may be required to clarify the problem.

CHEST RADIOGRAPHY. Although the chest radiograph may suggest the diagnosis of pulmonary embolism because of central vascular enlargement, asymmetry of the vascular markings with segmental or lobar ischemia (Westermark's sign), or pleural effusion, these signs are nonspecific. The chest radiograph then serves to exclude other diagnostic possibilities such as pneumonia, pneumothorax, esophageal perforation, or congestive heart failure. It is also critical in the interpretation of a lung scan, because any radiographic density or evidence of chronic lung disease makes a perfusion defect less likely to represent pulmonary embolism. Any pulmonary vascular or cardiac disease also reduces the applicability of lung scanning to the diagnosis.

ARTERIAL BLOOD GASES. The widespread availability of blood gas and pH determinations has improved the assessment of all critically ill patients and provides important support for the diagnosis of pulmonary embolism. Hypoxemia with Pa_{O_2} of less than 60 mmHg is found in the majority of patients and is felt to be due to shunting by overperfusion of nonembolized lung and a widened alveolar-arterial oxygen gradient due to reduced cardiac output. The reduction in arterial P_{CO_2} that follows major embolism is the most discriminating finding, because hypoxemia is present in several disorders likely to be misdiagnosed as massive embolism (e.g., septic shock). If hypoxemia and hypocarbia are not present, the diagnosis of major embolism in the severely ill patient is unlikely, and an alternative diagnosis should be sought.

CENTRAL VENOUS PRESSURE. In the patient with systemic hypotension, central venous pressure can supply valuable information, and the line provides access for administration of drugs and fluids as well. Low central venous pressure virtually excludes pulmonary embolism as the primary cause of the hypotension because massive embolism almost always is accompanied by right ventricular overload and elevated right atrial pressures. Elevated right ventricular filling pressures may be transient, however, as hemodynamic accommodation occurs, and in subacute or chronic embolism the central venous pressure may be normal.

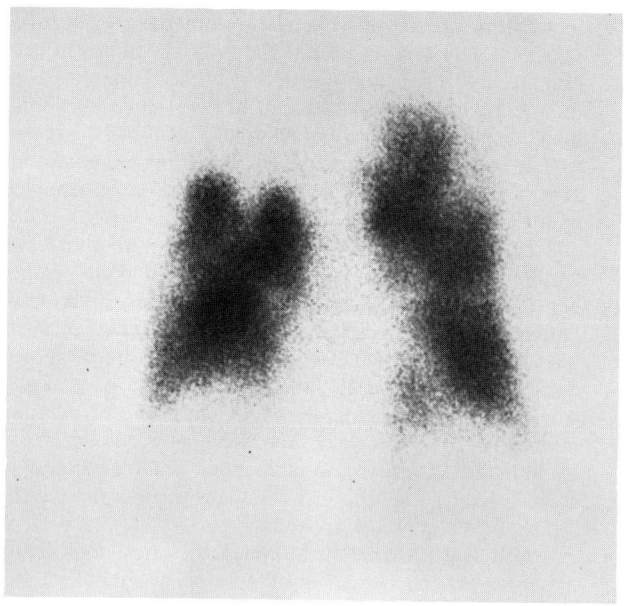

A

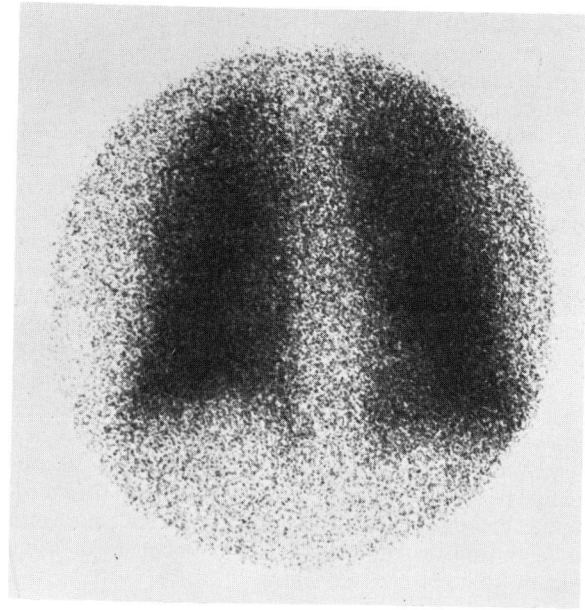

B

Fig. 22-12. *A.* A radionuclide perfusion scan following intravenous injection of macroaggregated albumin tagged ^{99m}Tc showing filling defects in the right lung. *B.* A ventilation scan performed with ^{133}Xe showing normal ventilation. These findings suggest the diagnosis of pulmonary embolism.

LUNG SCAN. The availability and widespread usage of lung photoscanning have led to overemphasis on this test and a tendency to overdiagnose pulmonary embolism. In a nonhypotensive patient with a normal chest radiograph, the lung scan is a valuable screening test that has increasing validity as the size of the perfusion defect approaches lobar distribution (Fig. 22-12). Smaller peripheral perfusion defects are much more difficult to interpret because pneumonitis, atelectasis, or other ventilation abnormalities alter pulmonary perusion. A normal lung scan, on the other hand, usually excludes the diagnosis of pulmonary embolism. Adding a ventilation scan for combined ventilation-perfusion imaging increases the accuracy of the diagnosis of thromboembolism, provided that there are at least two moderate-sized areas or one large area of ventilation-perfusion mismatch. The assumption that the underperfused regions of the lung after embolism will remain normally ventilated, producing the mismatch in the scans, is clouded by the known physiologic effect of bronchoconstriction produced by embolism. When the additional variable of wide variance in scan interpretation among observers is considered, the diagnosis is much more reliable when it is based on arteriography.

PULMONARY ARTERIOGRAPHY. Selective pulmonary arteriography is the most accurate method of confirming the presence, size, and distribution of pulmonary emboli. The procedure is invasive, requiring passage of a cardiac catheter into the pulmonary artery for injection of a bolus of contrast medium. A rapid film changer produces a series of radiographs that outline areas of decreased perfusion and usually show filling defects or the rounded trailing edge of impacted emboli (Fig. 22-13). Straight cutoffs of the smaller pulmonary arteries are more difficult to interpret, particularly if there is associated chronic lung dis-

Fig. 22-13. A selective pulmonary angiogram demonstrating absence of filling of left pulmonary arterial branches due to a large embolus obstructing the left main pulmonary artery.

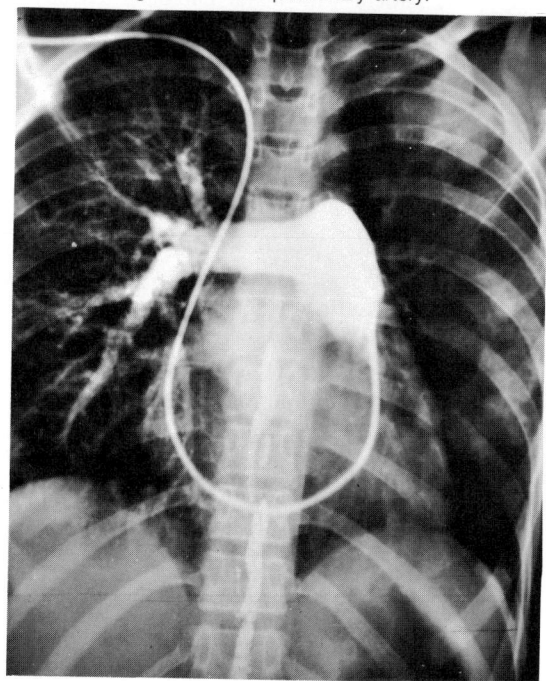

ease that tends to obliterate pulmonary vessels. The procedure can be performed with low risk, although pulmonary hypertensive and cardiac patients are at highest risk for this type of study, which usually carries a 0.3 to 0.5 percent mortality rate. Avoidance of injection of contrast medium into the main pulmonary artery minimizes the complications and mortality rates. Additional useful information is obtained prior to contrast injection by measurement of pulmonary arterial pressures. A normal pulmonary angiogram excludes the diagnosis of pulmonary embolism in acutely ill patients.

Pathophysiology

Although deep vein thrombosis precedes pulmonary embolism, less than 33 percent of patients with documented pulmonary embolism show clinical signs of venous thrombosis. Despite this, it is estimated that 85 to 90 percent of all pulmonary emboli originate from the veins of the lower extremity, and the remainder arise from the right side of the heart or other veins. In addition, the emboli from a recent thrombus tend to be multiple, fragmenting either in the right side of the heart or during impaction into the pulmonary vascular bed. Older thrombi, however, contain laminated fibrin layers that make them more solid and more difficult to lyse.

Once the embolus has lodged and interrupted pulmonary blood flow, the ratio of regional ventilation to perfusion increases, and the lung responds by bronchoconstriction to reduce wasted ventilation. This response is mediated by a local reduction in CO_2 output, since it can be prevented by ventilation with increased concentration of CO_2. Some experimental studies also suggest a generalized neural reflex vasoconstriction, but even if this occurs in human beings, it is not likely to be as significant a factor in survival as the mechanical effect of major vascular occlusion. Similarly, the effects of vasoactive humoral agents can be demonstrated in animals. There is evidence that serotonin is elaborated from platelets adherent to the embolus, which also contributes to the bronchoconstriction. The ability of heparin to inhibit the release of serotonin adds further justification to the early use of this drug. Other vasoactive agents such as histamine and prostaglandins may play a role in human beings, but the net effect is a reduction in size of peripheral airways, reduced lung volume, and reduced static pulmonary compliance.

The hypoxemia that characterizes major embolism is thought to be due to a ventilation-perfusion imbalance secondary to the ventilation changes described above, although the findings in some patients resemble true arteriovenous shunting. Such shunting is anatomically possible if there is an unobliterated foramen ovale that opens in the presence of elevated right atrial pressures. Such an opening can allow passage of a venous embolus into the systemic circulation; it then is termed *paradoxical embolism*. Although there may be some improvement in Pa_{O_2} after supplemental oxygen is administered, the effects usually are minimal. The return of pulmonary blood flow

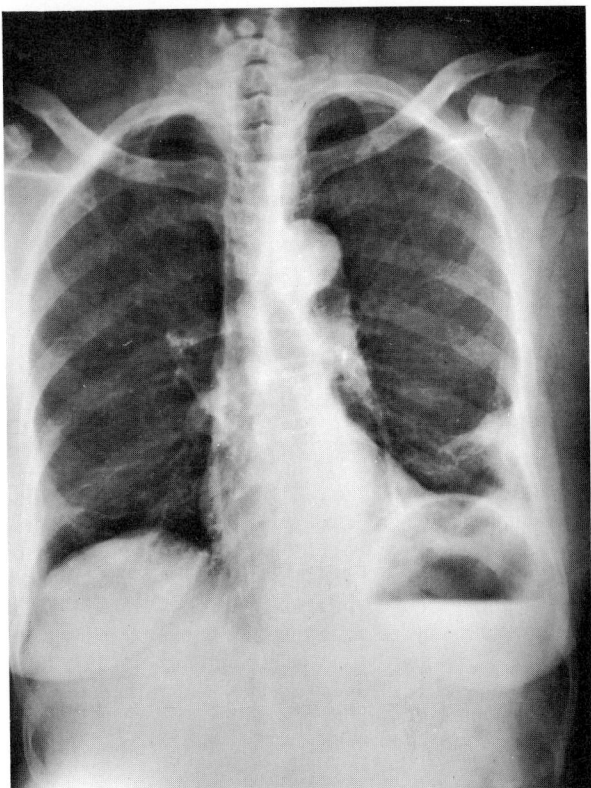

Fig. 22-14. Chest radiograph demonstrating a peripheral wedge-shaped area of infarction on the left side.

effected by embolectomy restores respiratory gas exchange, but the ischemia may result in loss of capillary integrity, causing interstitial pulmonary edema or overt pulmonary hemorrhage.

Pulmonary infarction as a consequence of embolism is relatively rare and is associated clinically with problems of poor systemic perfusion such as shock and congestive heart failure. In these patients the symptoms include pleuritic chest pain, dyspnea, cough, and hemoptysis. The signs include fever, tachycardia, splinting, and occasionally friction rub. There is usually prominent leukocytosis, an elevated lactic dehydrogenase level, and bilirubinemia. A wedge-shaped density usually is seen on chest radiography (Fig. 22-14).

The pulmonary vascular and cardiac effects of embolism are a direct consequence of the degree of filling of the pulmonary vascular bed. Occlusion of more than 30 percent of the vascular tree is required to begin to elevate mean pulmonary artery (PA) pressure, and usually more than 50 percent occlusion is required to reduce systemic pressure. The degree of pulmonary hypertension produced is proportional to the extent of angiographic vascular occlusion, but in a previously normal patient the limit of pressure elevation observed is approximately 40 mmHg mean.

The fate of pulmonary emboli in patients is not easy to predict, although a great deal of experimental work in animals has been reported. Injection of autologous thrombi into the pulmonary circulation of dogs is followed by relatively rapid recovery of pulmonary function and objective evidence of lysis over a period of weeks. Activation of plasminogen to plasmin, which is found in high concentration in the pulmonary circulation, promotes this fibrinolytic effect. The resolution of aged thrombi proceeds more slowly and is hampered further by impaction of the embolus and isolation from pulmonary blood flow. Consequently, resolution after massive embolism in patients is unpredictable and often incomplete. It is not unusual to find residual fibrin strands or webs in the pulmonary arteries at autopsy as remnants of prior embolism.

Management

ANTICOAGULATION. The hemodynamic variables mentioned above provide a means of classification of patients that employs five grades of severity and is a useful guide to therapy and prognosis (Table 22-4). The minor degrees of embolism (classes I and II) can usually be managed by anticoagulants alone with a satisfactory outcome (Fig. 22-15). Heparin is selected for initial treatment in a dose designed to prolong the partial thromboplastin time to at least twice normal. At this dosage of approximately 150 units/kg, there is adequate protection against further attachment of thrombus and platelets to the embolus. Heparin should be administered intravenously by pump-regulated continuous infusion. Conti, Daschbach, and Blaisdell have advocated higher doses of heparin to prolong the activated clotting time to 150 to 190 s with no increase in bleeding complications and improved control of recurrent embolism. However, heparin control of recurrent embolism is imperfect and recurrence was reported in 16 percent of patients by Wilson, Bynum, and Parkay, with a bleeding complication rate of 27 percent. In spite of this, heparin remains the initial treatment of choice and most clinicians also begin oral anticoagulation therapy to allow several days' overlap of the drugs as prothrombin time is extended into the therapeutic range.

THROMBOLYTIC THERAPY. Thrombolytic therapy has been advocated for the treatment of both deep vein thrombosis and pulmonary embolism. Two plasminogen activators, streptokinase and urokinase, are available for this and can be effective as documented in two large clinical trials (Urokinase Pulmonary Embolism Trial). The drugs are administered by intravenous infusion after a loading dose, and beneficial effects in thromboembolism usually can be seen in 12 to 24 h. Present laboratory tests to confirm the presence of a lytic state following streptokinase or urokinase administration have not proved useful in predicting the therapeutic response to these drugs or in preventing hemorrhagic complications. There were hemorrhagic side effects judged to be significant in 30 percent of the patients treated with both drugs, half of whom required transfusion. In addition to bleeding complications, the use of streptokinase for embolism has been associated with allergic reactions, fever, and the adult respiratory distress syndrome as reported by Martin et al. Also, in the first phase of the study, there was no significant difference between urokinase and heparin treatment in terms of the recurrence rate of embolism or mortality rate at 2 weeks.

More recently, recombinant human tissue–type plasminogen activator (rt-PA) has become available as a relatively clot-specific thrombolytic agent. In a series of 36 patients with documented pulmonary embolism by angiography, periopheral infusion of 50 mg over 2 h improved the angiographic score by 21 percent and an additional 40 mg over 6 h improved the average score by 49 percent as reported by Goldhaber et al. Since patients with hypotension were excluded, the initial pulmonary arterial pressure was only moderately evaluated to 22 mmHg and declined to 17 mmHg after infusion. Significant groin hematomas were seen in five patients, hematuria in two patients, and periodontal oozing in three patients. Two patients had major hemorrhage requiring operative treatment that in one case required relief of pericardial tamponade 8 days after coronary artery bypass. One patient had recurrent embolism and died for a mortality rate of 3

Table 22-4. CLASSIFICATION OF PULMONARY THROMBOEMBOLISM

Class	Symptoms	Arterial gases	% PA occlusion	Hemodynamics
I	None	Normal	<20	Normal
II	Anxiety, hyperventilation	Pa_{O_2} <80 mmHg Pa_{CO_2} <35 mmHg	20–30	Tachycardia
III	Dyspnea, collapse	Pa_{O_2} <65 mmHg Pa_{CO_2} <30 mmHg	30–50	CVP elevated, $\overline{PA}$ > 20 mmHg
IV	Shock, dyspnea	Pa_{O_2} <50 mmHg Pa_{CO_2} <30 mmHg	>50	CVP elevated, $\overline{PA}$ > 25 mmHg BP < 100 mmHg
V	Dyspnea, syncope	Pa_{O_2} <50 mmHg Pa_{CO_2} 30–40 mmHg	>50	CVP elevated, $\overline{PA}$ > 40 mmHg CO low, no shock

CVP = central venous pressure
PA = pulmonary artery
$\overline{PA}$ = mean pulmonary artery pressure

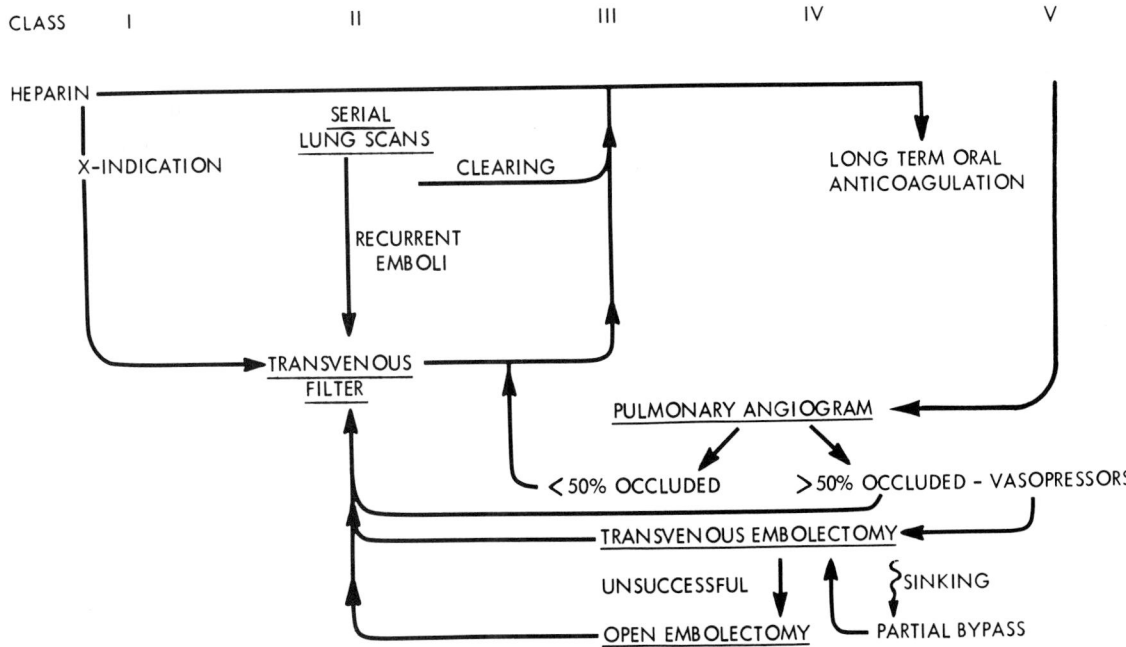

Fig. 22-15. Management algorithm for patients with documented pulmonary embolism stratified by class (see Table 22-4). Treatment is based on anticoagulation as shown for each class. In major embolism (classes III and IV), the findings at angiography and hemodynamic status influence the choice of procedures undertaken. [From: *Greenfield LJ: Acute venous thrombosis and pulmonary embolism, in Hardy JD (ed): Hardy's Textbook of Surgery. Philadelphia, Lippincott, 1983, with permission.*]

percent and a morbidity rate of 33 percent in these patients with submassive embolism. In spite of hope that this agent would be specific for thrombus fibrin, plasma fibrinogen declined 55 percent in patients who received 2-chain rt-PA and 34 percent in those who received 1-chain rt-PA.

The advantage of thrombolytic therapy may well be to improve the ultimate resolution of major thromboembolism as demonstrated by Sharma, Burleson, and Sasakara. Their follow-up studies in patients treated with urokinase or streptokinase showed a better restoration of pulmonary-capillary blood volume and diffusing capacity at 2 weeks than in patients treated with heparin and anticoagulants alone. The reason for the continued improvement that was seen at 1 year was not clear but was felt to be related either to more complete early resolution of the embolic condition, allowing more effective natural lytic processes, or to more complete clearance of peripheral venous thrombi, preventing silent recurrent embolism. Therefore, the patient who is not in shock and who has no clear contraindication to the use of thrombolytic therapy would probably benefit from its use.

VENA CAVAL INTERRUPTION. In some patients, anticoagulants cannot be used because of associated problems (e.g., peptic ulcer disease), and management must be directed toward a mechanical means of protection against recurrent embolism as outlined previously (Table 22-2). Other patients, in whom anticoagulation appears to be

adequate, sustain recurrent embolism and become candidates for surgical intervention. The third indication is when there has been a complication of anticoagulant therapy forcing it to be discontinued and leaving the patient with untreated DVT. Another indication for a vena caval filter is protection against recurrent embolism in a patient who has sustained massive pulmonary embolism requiring open or catheter embolectomy. In these patients, in spite of a satisfactory embolectomy of the pulmonary circulation, the original focus of venous thrombosis remains untreated, and recurrent embolism is likely.

There are two additional relative indications for a vena caval filter in a patient with active or recent deep vein thrombosis. One is the high-risk patient over 40 years of age who is obese and has a serious associated medical illness (e.g., heart disease), malignant disease, or a history of previous embolism and who undergoes a major abdominal or vascular procedure. The final relative indication is the patient in whom 40 to 50 percent of the vascular bed has been occluded (class III) and who would most likely not be able to tolerate additional emboli, particularly if there is associated cardiac or pulmonary disease.

PULMONARY EMBOLECTOMY. In patients who sustain massive embolism (classes III and IV), management must be a coordinated and rapidly responsive effort, since survival may be only a matter of minutes. As indicated earlier, it is critical to document the diagnosis of massive pulmonary embolism by pulmonary arteriography because the clinical diagnosis, regardless of "classic" appearance, often is in error. The initial approach to patients who have either transient collapse (class III) or persistent systemic hypotension (class IV) should include full heparinization and administration of inotropic drugs if necessary to support the circulation while the diagnosis is confirmed. Isoproterenol (4 mg in 1000 mL of 5% dextrose in water) is useful initially because of its bronchodilating and vasodilating effects as well as its positive inotropic cardiac effect. It may provoke arrhythmias, however, and necessitate use of dopamine. In the class II patient who responds to heparin and does not require vasopressors for systemic pressure or urine output, careful monitoring is essential to determine whether anticoagulation alone will control the disorder (Fig. 22-15). In most circumstances the spontaneous lysis of pulmonary emboli will proceed over a period of days and can be documented by serial lung scans performed at weekly intervals. The rate of clearing may be prolonged for weeks, particularly after a sizable embolism, and may be incomplete, as indicated previously. The latter condition has been observed in association with persistent pulmonary hypertension even after additional lytic drugs (e.g., urokinase) were administered. Lytic agents, however, may become a useful adjunct in management in the future.

The direct surgical approach to pulmonary embolism can be traced back to Trendelenburg (1908), who demonstrated the feasibility of pulmonary embolectomy experimentally but had no successes clinically. It remained for his pupil Kirschner (1924) to confirm the possibility of embolectomy by a successful clinical outcome. Because this procedure was attempted without circulatory support using a direct approach to the pulmonary artery at thoracotomy, the number of survivors was very small, and the first successful case in the United States was not reported until 1958 by Steenburg. A modification of this technique using hypothermia to occlude the circulation temporarily was reported by Allison et al. in 1960. The very high mortality rate associated with the Trendelenburg procedure prompted Gibbon to consider the use of extracorporeal circulation to bypass the impacted pulmonary circulation. However, the first successful open embolectomy during cardiopulmonary bypass was not reported by Sharp until 1962. Since then partial bypass support has also been utilized for the patient in shock. Local anesthesia is used, and the femoral artery and vein are cannulated for venoarterial bypass. The equipment is fully portable (Fig. 22-16), and patients can be supported during pulmonary arteriography and then transported to the operating room, where they can tolerate general anesthesia and sternotomy much better while being maintained on partial cardiopulmonary bypass. Once the mediastinum is opened, the partial bypass can be converted to total bypass by insertion of a superior vena caval catheter; the pulmonary emboli are then removed through a pulmonary arteriotomy.

Open pulmonary embolectomy still carries a mortality rate in the range of 50 percent, however, and uncontrollable pulmonary hemorrhage may follow open restoration of pulmonary perfusion. Consequently, an alternative approach utilizing local anesthesia has been suggested by Greenfield et al. for transvenous removal of pulmonary emboli. A cup device attached to a steerable catheter is inserted in either the jugular or the femoral vein, and the cup is positioned under fluoroscopy adjacent to the embolus seen on arteriography (Fig. 22-17). The position is

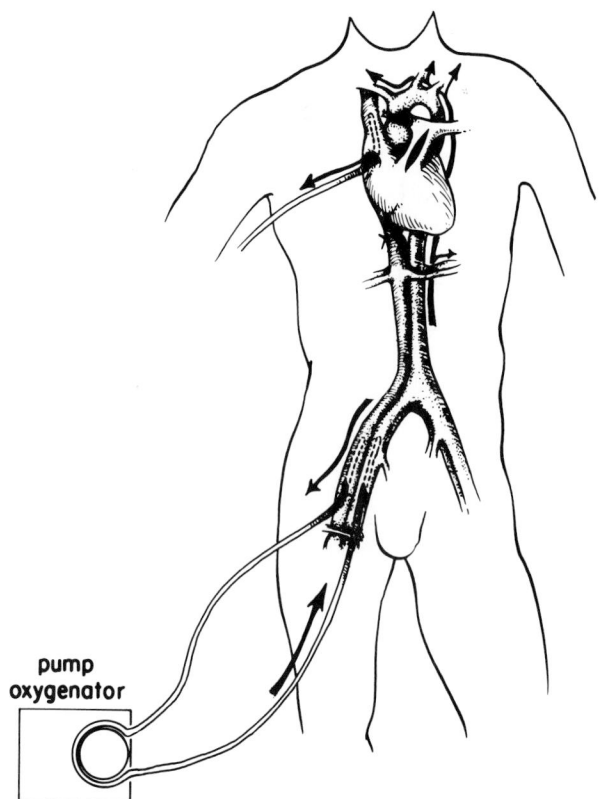

pump oxygenator

Fig. 22-16. The patient who sustains massive pulmonary embolism with shock (class IV) and fails to respond to resuscitation must be supported by partial bypass and considered for open pulmonary embolectomy. The femoral artery and vein can be cannulated under local anesthesia as shown. The patient will then tolerate a general anesthetic and sternotomy, at which time a cannula can be inserted into the superior vena cava for total cardiopulmonary bypass. The main pulmonary artery is opened and the emboli are extracted by forceps and suction. [From: *Greenfield LJ: Complications of venous thrombosis and pulmonary embolism, in Greenfield LJ (ed): Complications in Surgery and Trauma. Philadelphia, Lippincott, 1984, with permission.*]

verified by injection of contrast medium through the catheter. Then syringe suction is applied to aspirate the embolus into the cup, where it is held by suction vacuum as the catheter and captured embolus are withdrawn. Clinical experience with the technique in 29 patients showed that emboli could be extracted in 26 of them (90 percent) with an overall survival of 76 percent. Emboli could not be removed when they had been impacted for more than 72 h or if the patient suffered cardiac arrest at the time of angiography, in which case open embolectomy was required. Placement of a Greenfield vena caval filter after removal of sufficient emboli to produce near normal hemodynamics protected the patients from recurrent embolism.

PULMONARY HYPERTENSION AND THROMBOEMBOLISM

Pulmonary emboli may accumulate gradually over a prolonged period if they fail to undergo lysis and obliter-

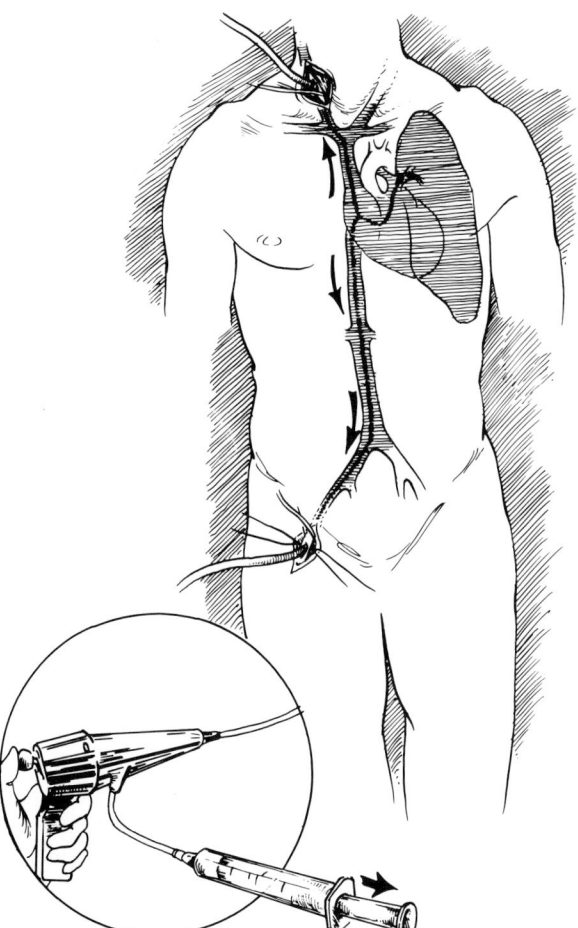

Fig. 22-17. Transvenous pulmonary embolectomy can be performed under local anesthesia via the jugular or femoral vein. The cup-catheter is positioned under fluoroscopy adjacent to the embolus and syringe suction is applied to capture the embolus within the cup. While suction is maintained, the catheter and trailing embolus are withdrawn through the venotomy. Multiple passages allow clearing of the vascular bed and restoration of cardiac output. [From: *Greenfield LJ: Complications of venous thrombosis and pulmonary embolism, in Greenfield LJ (ed): Complications in Surgery and Trauma. Philadelphia, Lippincott, 1984, with permission.*]

ate the pulmonary vascular bed. The clinical picture in this case is one of chronic cor pulmonale because significant pulmonary hypertension results from changes in the pulmonary vascular bed (class V). The presentation may be subtle with only dyspnea or syncope on exertion, but there is a loud P_2 and right-sided strain on the electrocardiogram. The sequence may also occur unaccompanied by significant respiratory symptoms, and this may explain the etiology in some of the patients considered to have primary pulmonary hypertension. When the diagnosis is made, there is very limited life expectancy, but the patient may benefit from a vena caval procedure to prevent further embolism even if the disorder is primary pulmonary hypertension as reported by Greenfield, Scher, and Elkins. The rationale for this is that they will ultimately develop right heart failure, predisposing to pulmonary embolism that is lethal even if small. When acute cardiopulmonary decompensation occurs in these patients after embolism, they are not good candidates for embolectomy because of fixation of the older thrombi to the pulmonary arterial wall. They should be classified separately (class V) and managed by long-term anticoagulation therapy, or in some cases should be considered for heart-lung transplantation.

Recurrent thromboembolism may lead to progressive obliteration of the pulmonary vascular bed if the thrombi fail to undergo lysis. The resultant pulmonary hypertension produces exertional dyspnea and signs of right heart strain with cor pulmonale. With further progression of right heart overload tricuspid insufficiency may develop. This disorder may be difficult to distinguish from primary pulmonary hypertension, although the latter is more likely to be found in women under 20 years of age without a history of deep vein thrombosis. Severe pulmonary hypertension is a serious problem and usually limits the life expectancy to less than 2 years from diagnosis.

Open thrombectomy for chronic occlusion was first performed by Allison et al. in 1958 and remains a possibility for improving pulmonary blood flow. To be eligible for this procedure the occlusion must involve the proximal portion of the pulmonary arterial tree and the distal bed must be patent. The physiologic basis for continued distal patency after proximal occlusion is bronchial arterial collateral flow. The procedure also has a significant mortality, reported at 38 percent by Cabrol et al. in a series of 16 patients. For the majority of patients with severe pulmonary hypertension, however, the outlook is poor unless they receive maximum protection from recurrent embolism, which in our experience has required both anticoagulation therapy and vena caval filter placement.

VARICOSE VEINS

The prevalence of varicose veins in adults increases with age and is generally greater in women. It increases with increasing parity, is directly related to body mass, and has an inconsistent relationship with occupations that require prolonged standing. There is also a striking geographical variation in occurrence that is not well understood, although there appears to be a relationship with low-fiber diets and prolonged sitting as reported by Beaglehole.

Diagnosis

It is important to distinguish between primary varicose veins and the more serious condition of varicosities secondary to underlying deep venous disease. The latter situation is usually associated with stasis dermatitis or ulceration. In primary varicosities there is often a family history and a favorable outcome to medical or surgical treatment. The etiology is unknown, but the more widely accepted hypotheses attribute the disorder to either primary valvular weakness or weakness of the vein walls

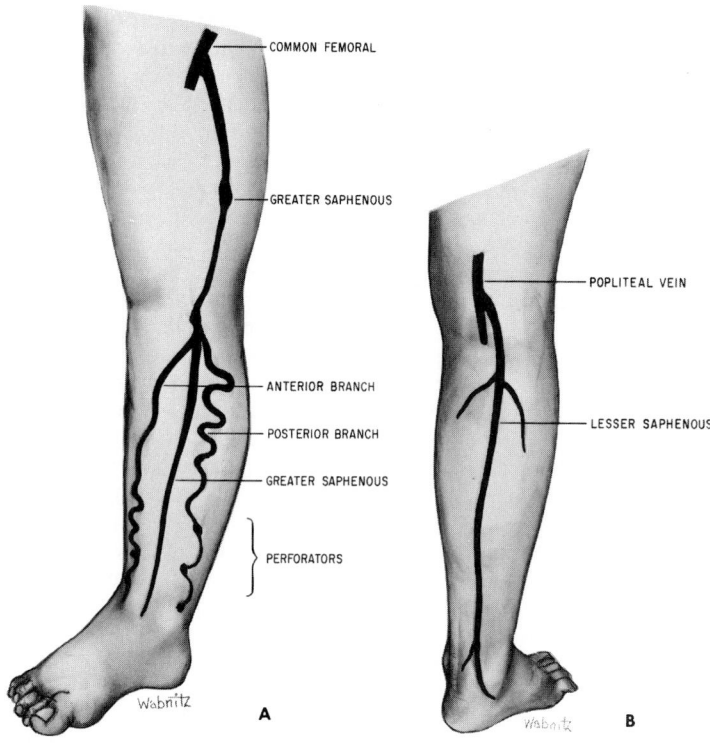

COMMON FEMORAL

GREATER SAPHENOUS

ANTERIOR BRANCH

POSTERIOR BRANCH

GREATER SAPHENOUS

PERFORATORS

A

POPLITEAL VEIN

LESSER SAPHENOUS

B

Fig. 22-18. *A.* The usual course of the greater saphenous vein and its major branches in the lower leg, emphasizing the fact that branch varicosities are the ones usually seen. Perforating veins, posterior and superior to medial malleoli, are indicated. *B.* The usual course of the lesser saphenous vein is shown in the lower leg.

allowing valvular distraction and incompetence. The theory of arteriovenous communication producing high pressure and flow is less well substantiated. There is rarely an association of varicosities with congenital or acquired arteriovenous fistulas. In the Klippel–Trenaunay syndrome, varicose veins develop in the leg in childhood and there is limb hypertrophy. Pelvic visceral varicosities with hemorrhagic complications also may develop. Servelle advises operative treatment in childhood to avoid limb length abnormality and has occasionally found compressive bands over major veins.

Varicose veins are the most common vascular disorder affecting human beings, who are unique among animals in this susceptibility. The term varicose means dilated and the characteristic enlarged and tortuous superficial veins can be diagnosed by inspection of standing patients. The usual distribution of varices is below the knee in branches of the greater saphenous system (Fig. 22-18). In the absence of postthrombotic sequelae, varicose veins are best evaluated by Doppler ultrasound and venous reflux plethysmography. If the abnormalities found are limited to the superficial veins, the condition is probably primary, whereas the finding of deep or perforator venous disease suggests that the varicosities are secondary and no benefit can be expected from their excision. These patients require lifelong elastic stocking support and may require operative treatment for local complications of their venous insufficiency.

The symptoms associated with varicose veins are nonspecific aching and heaviness of the legs that can be attributed to the congestion and pooling of blood in the enlarged superficial venous system. The symptoms are worsened by prolonged sitting and standing and relieved by elevation of the legs above the level of the heart. The use of calf-length elastic stocking support in the range of 20 to 30 mmHg usually suffices to provide relief. Although mild edema may occur from varicosities alone, it usually reflects additional incompetence of the deep or perforating venous system and may require stronger elastic stocking support. Obviously, the differential diagnosis for any patient presenting with bilateral lower-extremity edema also includes cardiac and renal disease, which should be investigated.

Night cramping of the legs is secondary to muscle spasms and is not usually due to venous disease. Arterial insufficiency should be excluded, but it may not be possible to identify a specific etiology. Some patients obtain relief by performing calf-stretching exercises prior to retiring and others may be helped by the administration of quinine sulfate, which reduces muscular irritability.

Treatment

The majority of patients can be managed by conservative methods, but if these fail to control symptoms or if additional complications of venous stasis develop, such as dermatitis, bleeding, thrombosis, or superficial ulceration, the patient may become a candidate for more aggressive management. Cosmetic concern or ill-defined pain patterns are less reliably improved by operation.

The two methods of treatment currently employed are ablative surgery and injection sclerotherapy, the latter being more popular in European countries than in this country. The objective of ablation is to redirect venous

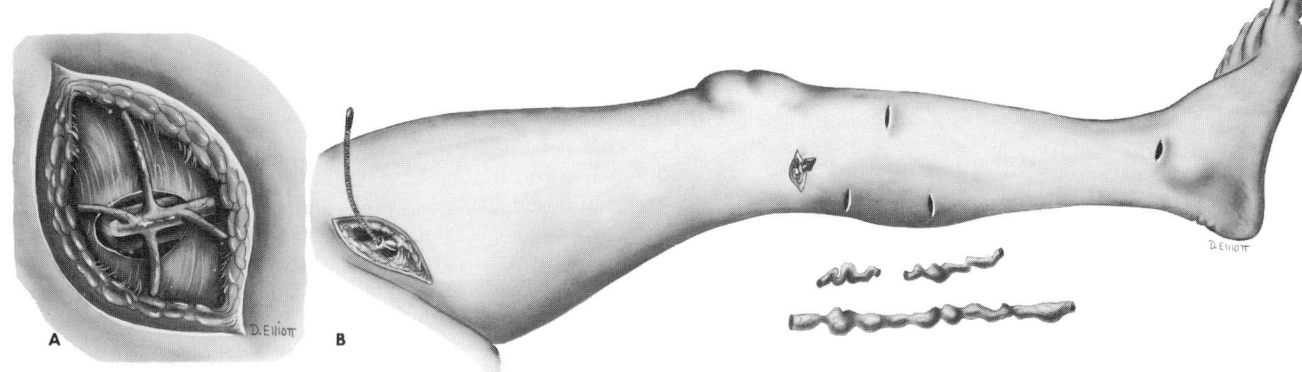

Fig. 22-19. Operative approach for ligation and stripping of the saphenous vein. *A.* The groin incision, showing the junction of the greater saphenous and femoral veins. Note four major branches of the saphenous vein that require ligation and division. *B.* A counterincision at the knee or ankle permits stripping of the saphenous vein. Additional incisions permit removal of branch varicose veins.

return through veins with intact valves and to improve appearance by removal or ligation of the varicosities (Fig. 22-19). The traditional procedure includes stripping of the long saphenous vein from ankle to groin by avulsion from its bed. More recently, Ludbrook and others have pointed out that it is advisable to save the normal portion of the saphenous vein below the knee to avoid the complications of its removal at that level and to allow it to be used for arterial bypass at a future time.

Injection sclerotherapy is designed to destroy the endothelium of the vein and promote its obliteration by scar. If pressure is not applied to the vein after injection of the sclerosant, a thrombus will form and later recanalize, leading not only to recurrence but occasionally to worsening of the problem. The technique for injection involves placement of the needle and syringe with the patient standing followed by elevation of the leg, injection of the agent, and bandage compression of the area for 2 to 3 weeks. Efforts are made to sclerose veins in proximity to perforating veins, which can be palpated as fascial defects, in order to reduce the chances of recurrence. Comparison of these techniques has shown that the results are comparable short-term but that surgical treatment clearly produces the best results after 3 to 5 years of observation as reported by Hobbs. Sclerotherapy also can produce allergic reactions, deep vein thrombosis, and inflammatory reaction with possible skin slough if the sclerosant escapes from the vein. It is useful primarily for management of smaller varicose veins and for recurrent or persistent varicosities after operative treatment.

CHRONIC VENOUS INSUFFICIENCY

In spite of optimal anticoagulation and bed rest for patients with acute deep vein thrombosis, approximately 50 percent will develop the postthrombotic syndrome as a reflection of chronic venous insufficiency. The underlying pathology consists of recanalization of the deep veins

with persistent deformity and incompetence of the valves. The result is a long column of blood unrestrained by valvular support that transmits pressures of over 100 mmHg to the venules, promoting both fluid and protein loss into the tissues. The perivascular fibrinous deposits remain in place because of inadequate fibrinolysis as demonstrated by Browse and interfere with oxygenation and metabolism of the tissues. The result is thickening and liposclerosis of the subcutaneous tissues to produce the characteristic "brawny" edema, which is relatively nonpitting. The loss of red cells results in hemosiderin deposits to produce the characteristic pigmentation. When the distal perforating veins become incompetent there is additional pressure, with skin atrophy leading ultimately to necrosis and chronic stasis ulceration (Fig. 22-20). There is often an associated dermatitis that may be due to various salves and ointments used to treat the condition. Dryness and scaling with pruritus also occur, and with constant scratching, secondary infection and cellulitis may result.

In contrast to normal patients who reduce their distal venous pressure with exercise, patients with the postthrombotic syndrome gain no benefit from their muscle pump (Fig. 22-21). If there has been failure of recanalization with persistent obstruction, the increase in blood flow with exercise may increase venous hypertension to produce ischemic pain referred to as "venous claudica-

Fig. 22-20. Extensive chronic venous ulcers of the lower leg.

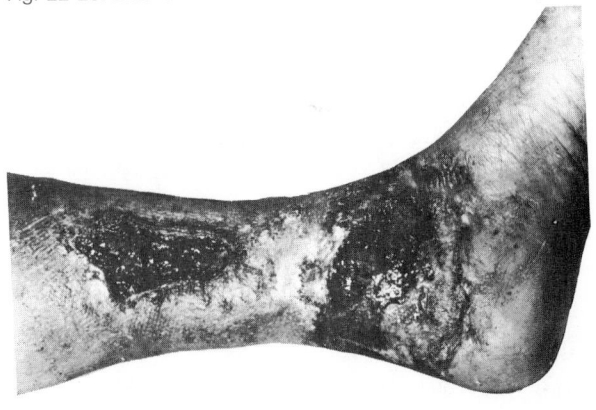

AMBULATORY VENOUS PRESSURE CHANGES

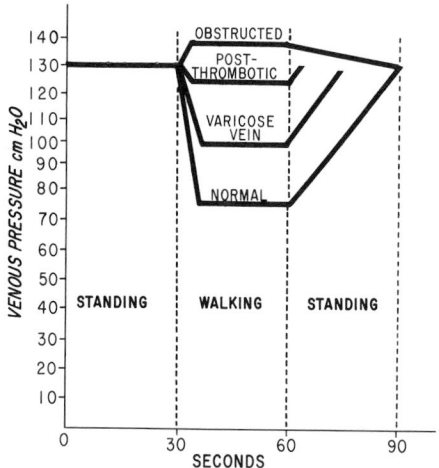

Fig. 22-21. Direct measurement of the responses in venous pressure in the superficial veins at the ankle with exercise. In the standing position, venous pressure is slightly higher than hydrostatic pressure in a column extending from ankle to heart. This pressure is approximately the same for normal persons and for those with venous insufficiency or chronically obstructed veins in which collaterals have formed. With walking, however, normal persons demonstrate a rapid decrease in venous pressure and a slow return to normal when exercise stops; patients with varicose veins show a lesser decrease in pressure with walking but a more prompt return to normal following cessation of exercise; patients with postthrombotic veins demonstrate little if any decrease in venous pressure with walking and a rapid return to normal; patients with obstructed veins show an increase in pressure with walking and a slow return to normal.

tion.'' This may become disabling and lead to consideration of venous bypass procedures to be described.

Diagnosis

Prior to the development of current techniques of noninvasive testing for venous disease, the methods of evaluation depended on physical examination while different sites were compressed. These tests are still useful if a noninvasive vascular laboratory is not available.

CLINICAL COMPRESSION TESTS. In the Trendelenburg test the limb is elevated to evacuate the veins; then pressure by hand or tourniquet is applied to the saphenofemoral junction (Fig. 22-22). With the patient standing, the lower leg is observed for the rate of filling of the varicosities. Gradual filling occurs in normal patients when the perforating veins are competent. Rapid filling occurs if

Fig. 22-22. The four possible results of the Trendelenburg compression test. The patient has been lying down with leg elevated; he then stands up with compression over the saphenofemoral junction. *A.* Negative-negative response in which there is gradual filling of veins from below over a 30-sec period and there is continued slow filling after release of hand. *B.* Negative-positive response. On standing, there is gradual filling of the distal veins; on release of compression there is rapid retrograde filling of the saphenous vein. *C.* Positive-negative response. With the hand in place, filling of superficial varicosities through incompetent perforators occurs; with release of compression there is further slow filling of the veins. *D.* Positive-positive response. On standing with the hand in place, there is filling of varices through incompetent perforators. On release of compression there is additional rapid filling of the saphenous vein.

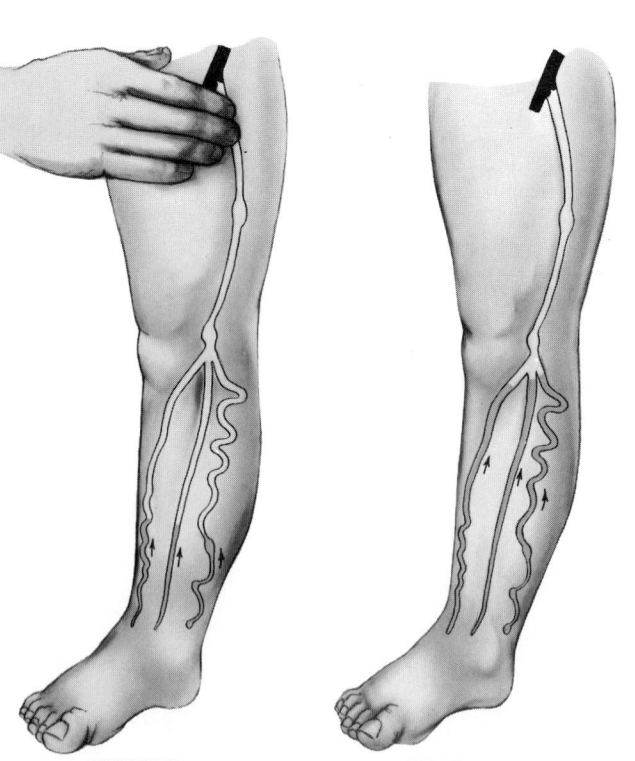

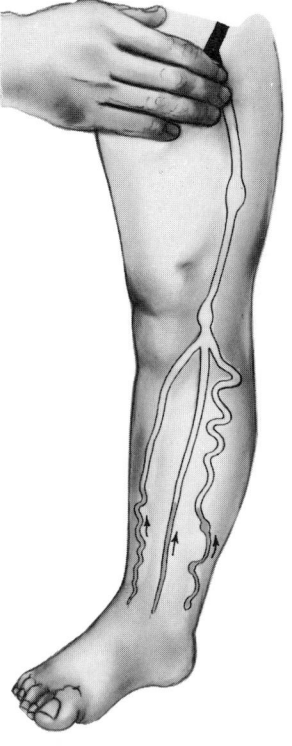

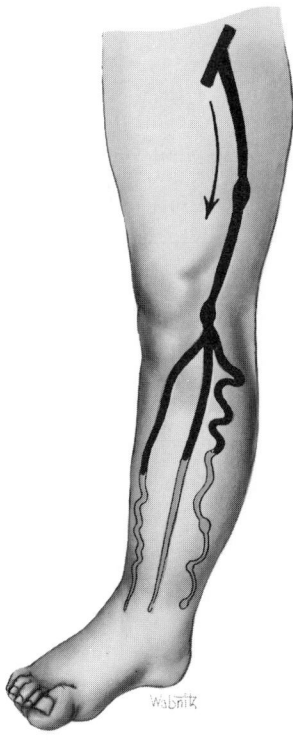

NEGATIVE   **A**   NEGATIVE   NEGATIVE   **B**   POSITIVE

the perforators are incompetent. The second phase of the test consists of release of the pressure to see if the upper thigh varices fill rapidly, indicating incompetence of the saphenofemoral valve.

In the Perthes test a tourniquet is placed around the upper leg and the patient is instructed to walk. If the varicose veins disappear, the deep venous system is patent and the perforating veins are competent. If pain occurs with walking, the deep system is obstructed and the superficial system represents the major source of venous outflow. Obviously, it would be a serious error to excise superficial veins under these circumstances. Sequential tourniquets also may be used to define and isolate areas of incompetent perforating veins (Ochsner–Mahorner test).

LABORATORY MEASUREMENTS. Direct measurement of venous pressure by needle and strain gauge provides the most accurate assessment of venous hemodynamics, but it is invasive and cumbersome to use. It has, however, served to validate the noninvasive tests to be described.

Doppler Examination. A directional Doppler can be used at the bedside to determine venous patency and valvular competence. Reflux retrograde flow can be observed at the femoral level during Valsalva maneuver or at the popliteal level with the patient standing and the calf alternately compressed and released (Fig. 22-4). A similar maneuver should be used when listening over perforating veins.

Plethysmography. The strain gauge plethysmograph measures venous capacity and outflow making it more valuable for acute thrombosis than for chronic changes where it may be normal or indicate persistent obstruction. The photoplethysmograph (PPG) uses infrared light to measure subcutaneous vascular volume and can provide a reliable index of valvular incompetence. The venous refilling time, after calf muscle exercise empties the veins, will be shortened considerably in the presence of valvular incompetence. Although the technique is primarily qualitative, Norris et al. have developed an in vivo calibration technique to provide quantitative information that correlates well with ambulatory venous pressure measured directly.

Duplex Scanning. The most promising of the newer diagnostic techniques is the combination of ultrasound duplex scanning using a B-mode imager with a pulsed Doppler instrument to provide both imaging and flow patterns. Thrombi can be visualized within the veins and flow observed if the vein remains patent. Normal veins can be compressed by the scanner head over the vessel while thrombosed veins are incompressible. Venous valves can also be visualized and their competence assessed under a variety of flow alterations as demonstrated by Kohler and Strandness.

Supportive Therapy

Perhaps the most important aspect of patient management is the education of the patient to emphasize the im-

Fig. 22-22 *C,D.* Continued.

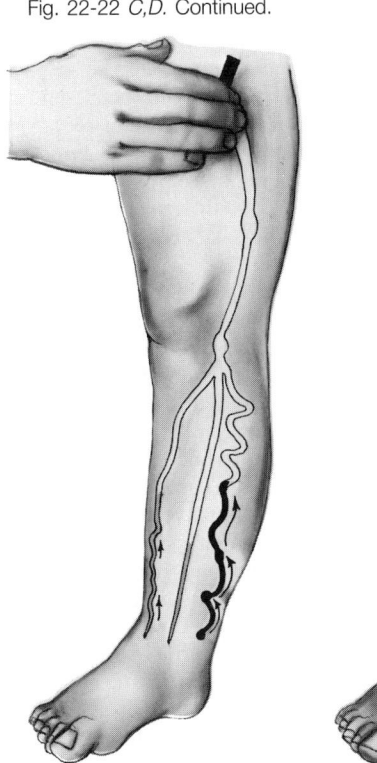
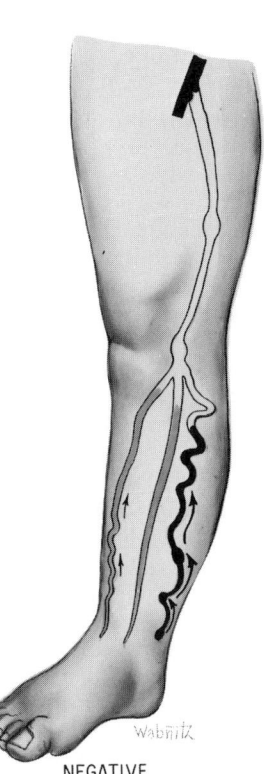
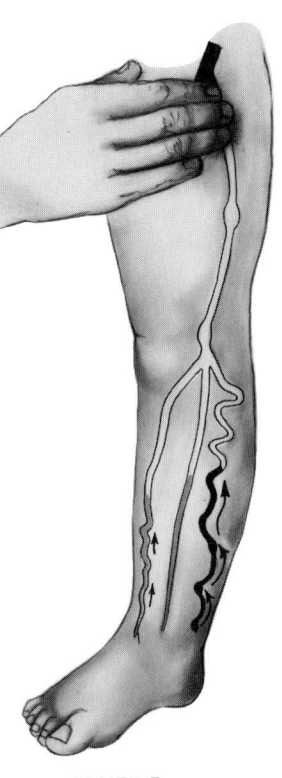
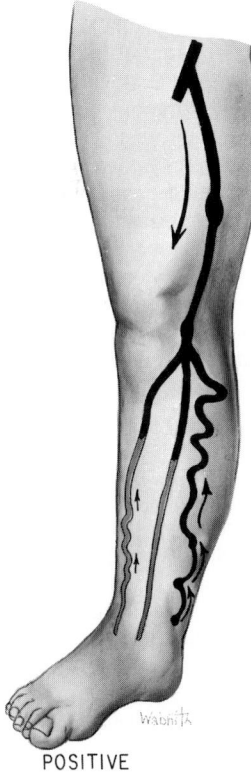

POSITIVE   NEGATIVE
C

POSITIVE   POSITIVE
D

portance of elastic stocking support, frequent elevation of the legs above the level of the heart, and the avoidance of prolonged sitting and standing. Frequent follow-up examinations are essential not only to assess compliance with the prescribed regimen but also to detect early recurrent thrombosis. Patient compliance can be improved by including other family members in the discussion and by the use of calf-length elastic stockings, which are easier to manage than full-length hose and less likely to produce a tourniquet effect at the knee. The patient should acquire two sets of pressure gradient stockings so that a clean pair is always available.

Operative Management

The development of a stasis ulcer requires immediate efforts to promote healing by frequent cleansing, bed rest, foot elevation, and the use of paste boots or elastic sealed dressings. The use of local medications should be avoided to minimize allergic reactions. Patients who fail to heal after prolonged outpatient care will require hospitalization and may need skin grafts for larger ulcers.

PERFORATOR VEIN LIGATION. Permanent healing of chronic stasis ulcers that recur after skin grafting is not likely unless the perforating veins responsible for the ulcer are identified and ligated. The typical location for these is posterior and superior to the medial malleolus as described by Dodd and Cockett. However, ligation of the perforator vessels still leads to recurrent ulceration in 15 percent of patients despite vigorous medical therapy, including support stockings, leg elevation, wound care, and patient education. The patients in whom medical and routine surgical therapy fail may be considered for attempted reconstruction of their venous systems.

VENOUS RECONSTRUCTION. The present attitude of most surgeons toward venous reconstruction is critical and pessimistic as reviewed by Bernstein in 1986. The venous system, unlike the arterial system, tends to recanalize, thus making it more difficult to quantitate the obstruction and identify the patient who may benefit from venous reconstruction. Dale estimated that the percentage of patients with chronic venous insufficiency who could benefit from reconstruction was 1 to 2 percent of that population. Surgical reconstruction can be divided into two categories: bypassing obstructive disease and restoring valvular competence. To evaluate patients, it is necessary to obtain both ascending and descending venograms.

The most widely accepted procedure for venous reconstruction is the saphenous vein cross-over graft, first described by Palma and Esperon in 1958. The procedure consists of isolating the normal contralateral saphenous vein and dividing it distally. The vein is then tunneled suprapubically and anastomosed to the contralateral femoral vein, distal to its obstruction. In 1982, Dale described 59 patients who had the Palma bypass with excellent results in 63 percent, good results in 17 percent, and a failure rate of 20 percent. Husni in 1981 and Smith and Trimble in 1977 had reported similar results. The saphenous

vein cross-over graft has generally been accepted as useful; however, the natural history of iliac vein occlusion is recanalization, and very few patients with iliofemoral thrombosis became candidates for surgery.

Use of the saphenous vein for popliteal-to-femoral vein bypass was described by Warren and Thayer in 1954, with good clinical results in 10 of 14 patients. The saphenous vein is dissected free below the knee and anastomosed to the popliteal vein, which is obstructed proximally. Husni has popularized this procedure and has reported the outcome in 27 patients, with a good result in 63 percent. Dale reported good results in 10 patients (60 percent), and Smith and Trimble, in a collected series of 59 patients, reported good results in 76 percent. However, with rich collateral veins in the thigh, identifying the patient with an obstructed superficial femoral vein who may benefit from the saphenous-to-popliteal vein bypass is difficult. Kistner and Sparkuhl, on the other hand, recognized that patients with superficial femoral vein incompetence and symptoms of thrombotic syndrome could benefit from superficial femoral vein ligation. They ligated the superficial femoral vein of five patients and had good results in four.

Methods of reconstruction for venous incompetence of the iliofemoral system include valvuloplasty as described by Kistner, venous segment transfer as described by Kistner and Sparkuhl, and valve autotransplantation as described by Taheri et al.

Valvuloplasty. In 1980, Kistner, after studying 200 limbs with ascending and descending venography, found 28 that could be treated by valve repair, and 72 percent had an excellent result. In this procedure, floppy incompetent valves are tethered against the vein wall or shortened using interrupted 8-0 monofilament suture (Fig. 22-23). After DVT, most patients have scarred and thickened valves that do not lend themselves to this type of reconstruction. Since Kistner routinely combined valvuloplasty with saphenous vein stripping and perforator ligation, the results have been difficult to interpret, but they have found good to excellent results in 80 percent of cases as reported by Ferris and Kistner.

Vein Segment Transfer. In 1979, Kistner and Sparkuhl described six patients who had vein segment transfer. Of these patients, one had venous occlusion and the other five had good results 1 year postoperatively. In this procedure, competent valves are identified in the saphenous vein, superficial femoral vein, and profundus system. The vessel with the incompetent valve identified by descending venography is divided and anastomosed distal to the portion of the system with a competent valve (Fig. 22-24). This renders the previously incompetent system competent and, when combined with saphenous vein stripping and perforator ligation, improves the clinical and venographic results.

Autologous Vein Transplantation. The third reconstructive procedure for iliofemoral incompetence consists of autologous vein valve transplantation. This was developed by Taheri and coworkers and consists of harvesting a segment of brachial vein with a competent valve from

Valve Repair II

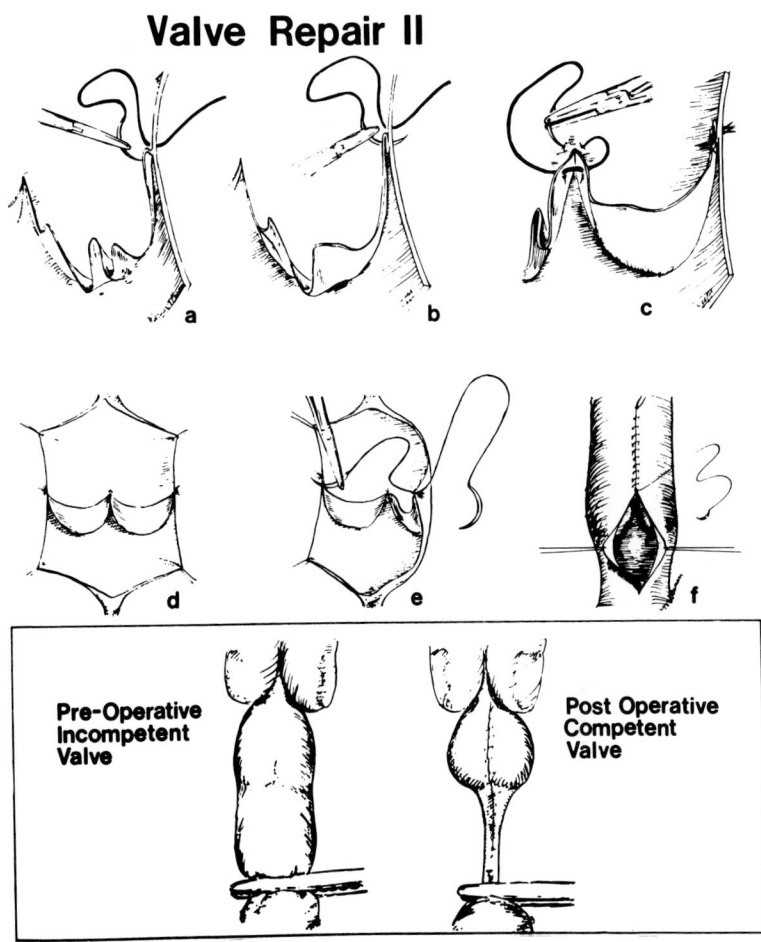

Fig. 22-23. The highest valve in the superficial femoral vein may be eligible for direct repair using the technique proposed by Kistner. A longitudinal venotomy exposes the valve cusps which are repaired by suture plication as shown *(A–E)*. After closure of the vein *(F)*, restored competence of the valve can be demonstrated by milking it proximally. [From: *Bergan J, Yao J (eds): Operative Techniques in Vascular Surgery. Orlando, FL, Grune and Stratton, 1980, with permission.*]

the arm and interposing it into the femoral system just below the origin of the superficial femoral vein or more distally at or above the popliteal vein. In 1986, the investigators described 66 patients, with good results in 78 percent. In this series 31 patients had postoperative venograms, and 28 had valvular competence. This procedure is still considered experimental and is awaiting long-term confirmation. Bergan and colleagues have pointed out that for venous valve surgery to be successful, it usually must be accompanied by saphenous vein stripping and perforator ligation. They reported a series of 12 patients who had only venous valve reconstruction without the more distal stripping and perforator ligation. These patients had good results initially; however, at 1 year, nine of the limbs had reverted to their preoperative condition owing to recurrent symptoms and delayed venous refill time. The difficulty in identifying patients who could

benefit from these procedures was put into perspective by Dale who, after 2 years of investigating, failed to identify a group of patients who would benefit from venous valve transplantation or valvuloplasty.

Husni found that venous reconstruction fails in three situations: when the bypass graft is too small in caliber; when venous hypertension is mild to moderate, that is, less than 80 percent of the standing venous pressure; and when a thrombectomy or endophlebectomy has to be performed before anastomosis. In these patients who are at high risk for failure, he has recommended a distal arteriovenous fistula. The use of arteriovenous fistulas after iliofemoral thrombectomy or reconstruction of the venous system is controversial. Most of the experience has been accumulated in Europe where it is believed to reduce the incidence of early rethrombosis. The two most commonly used sites are the femoral triangle and the ankle. After surgery on the iliofemoral system, an H-shaped fistula can be established easily by anastomosing a branch of the saphenous vein end-to-side to the proximal portion of the superficial femoral artery. At the ankle, the posterior tibial artery may be anastomosed to the posterior tibial vein or the greater saphenous vein. Two problems have led to the reluctance of some surgeons to adopt this procedure:

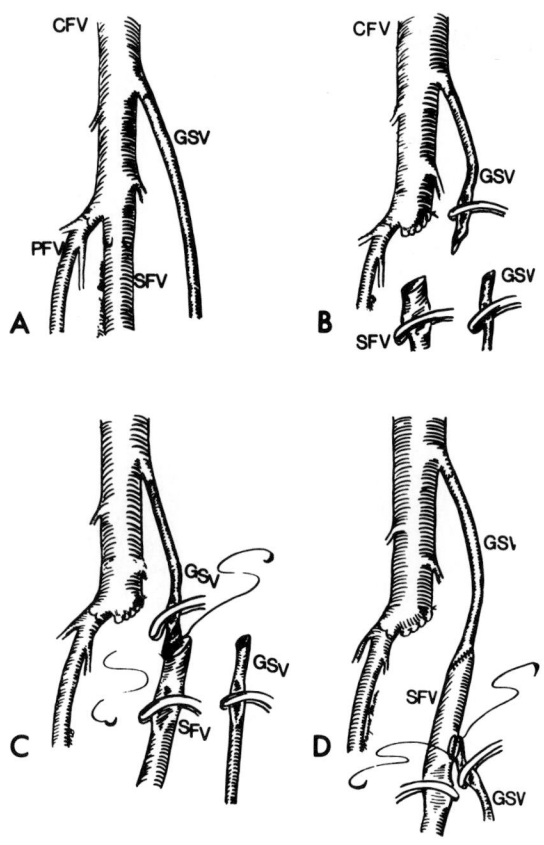

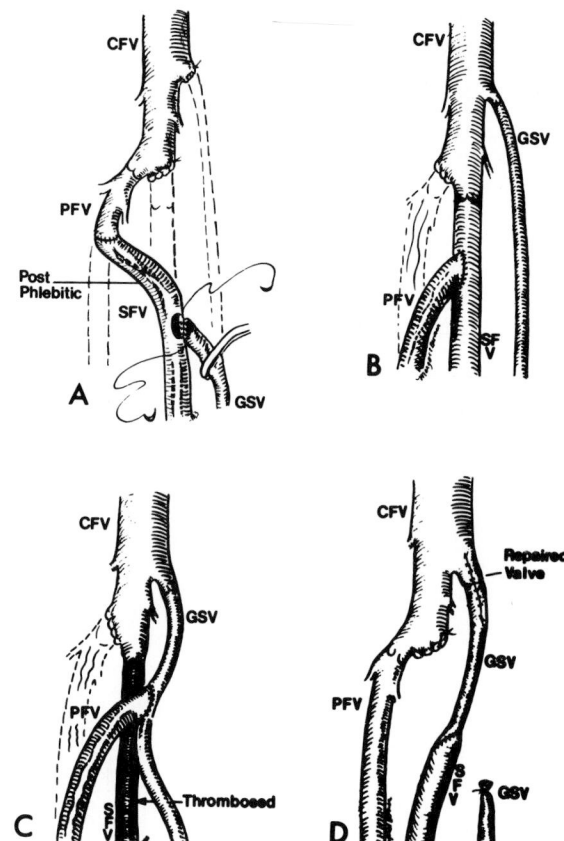

Fig. 22-24. I. An alternative technique for restoring valvular competence is to use the existing competent greater saphenous vein (GSV) as a new conduit for the incompetent superficial femoral vein (SFV) by dividing the veins at the level of the proposed anastomosis (A,B), connecting the SFV to the GSV (C) and then reimplanting the distal GSV into the SFV (D).

II. Where the SFV shows postphlebitic stenosis, it may be preferable to attach it to a competent profunda femoral vein (PFV) and add the inflow from the GSV (A). Where the PFV is incompetent, it can be connected to a competent SFV (B) or to the GSV to bypass an obstructed SFV (C). The transposition procedure can also be used in conjunction with valvuloplasty (D) when both techniques are required for restoring valvular competence. [From: *Bergan J, Yao J (eds): Operative Techniques in Vascular Surgery. Orlando, FL, Grune and Stratton, 1980, with permission.*]

the fear of damaging functioning valves distal to the fistula and the requirement for a second operation to close the fistula. Fistulas are usually closed 3 to 4 months postoperatively, and problems with incompetent valves distal to the fistula have not been reported. In 1981, Kroener and Bernstein reported on the effects of arteriovenous fistulas in dogs. They found a marked increase in the success of venous reconstructive procedures when a fistula was used, and no damage to the venous valves was noted when the fistula was taken down after 5 weeks. Two steps during primary venous reconstruction simplify closing the fistula later. The fistula is made distal to the venous reconstruction, thus avoiding damage to this area at reoperation, and a ligature is wrapped around the fistula and left in the subcutaneous tissue where it can be found under local anesthesia.

It seems reasonable to use the arteriovenous fistula in venous procedures that have been compromised, such as an iliofemoral thrombectomy, when the system has not been effectively cleared, or in a cross-over vein graft where the saphenous vein is of marginal size, since venous dilatation will occur proximal to the fistula. Smith has recommended that the fistula not be used if the ankle-arm index is less than 0.75 to avoid distal arterial problems in the same limb, and that the fistula should not exceed 4 mm in diameter to avoid distal venous hyperten-

sion, valvular damage, and significant effects on cardiac hemodynamics.

It has been noted in the past that the majority of iliofemoral thromboses occur on the left side. This is attributed to the right iliac artery compressing the left iliac vein as it crosses the fifth lumbar vertebra. Various autopsy series and operative studies have documented the presence of left iliac vein webs and scarring in patients who have had iliofemoral thrombosis. There was early interest in this problem by Calnan et al. in 1964 and Cockett and Thomas in 1965 who advocated surgical correction of these lesions. Dale reviewed eight such patients identified by venography and subsequently operated on four, trimming out anterior webs or scar tissue and using a venous

patch for closure. Two of the patients had excellent results, but in one edema developed later, and a fourth patient had a complicated postoperative course, complaining of excruciating pain and postoperative swelling. Dale
currently recommends operations only for the patient
whose symptoms are severe and who will accept the operation knowing that the results are not predictable.
Smith and Trimble have followed 30 patients with this
problem and have operated on 14, with an 85 percent
postoperative improvement rate. Cockett and Thomas,
on the other hand, found the results unsatisfactory, and
after operating on 30 patients using several different
methods, they recommended abandoning the procedure.

VENOUS TRAUMA

Venous injuries of the extremities are usually associated with arterial injuries because of their anatomical
proximity. In this situation, application of a tourniquet
not only renders the limb ischemic but also can increase
blood loss from the venous injury. Since the venous system is under relatively low pressure, direct pressure applied to the wound suffices for control. Direct ligation of
injured superficial veins is appropriate treatment except
when they are the sole remaining venous drainage of the
extremity which mandates their repair.

Treatment of injuries of the deep veins changed dramatically as a result of the military experience in South-
east Asia as reported by Rich et al. It was well demonstrated that ligation of major extremity veins resulted in
higher rates of disability and limb loss than when the
veins were repaired or replaced by autogenous vein segments. The concept of primary repair of venous injuries
by suture vein patch or vein graft interposition has been
extended to civilian injuries by Agarwal et al. with favorable results. These repairs have not been associated with
increased complications such as thrombophlebitis or pulmonary embolism as was originally of concern. Although
injuries to the inferior vena cava are unusual, the morbidity and mortality rates are high, especially for the
retrohepatic vena cava. Kudsk, Bongard, and Lim have
reported their experience in 70 patients with both penetrating and blunt trauma, resulting in 55 percent survivors. They emphasized the importance of adequate resuscitation and the significance of associated injuries. Malt,
Remonsnyder, and Harris showed that venous repair is
also essential for the success of upper extremity replantation after nearly complete or complete traumatic amputation.

Iatrogenic vascular trauma has increased in frequency
with the proliferation of invasive diagnostic and therapeutic puncture and biopsy techniques. The subclavian vein
is particularly vulnerable to injury and thrombosis because of its use for venous access and placement of long-
term catheters. Placement of these catheters also increases the risk of sepsis and the possibility of catheter
breakage with embolization. A technique for retrieval of a
catheter fragment in the subclavian vein by Fogarty catheter was reported by Mathur et al.

Use of a temporary arteriovenous fistula distal to the
repair of a traumatic venous injury of the lower extremity
in eight patients was reported by Richardson et al. in
1986. The posterior tibial artery and vein were utilized
and the external shunt allowed infusion of heparin and
access for postoperative venograms. In six patients the
shunt functioned for an average of 10 days and all patients
with functioning shunts for 72 h or longer had patent venous repairs without subsequent edema.

LYMPHATICS AND LYMPHEDEMA

Developmental Anatomy and Function

The exact origin of lymphatic vessels is a matter of disagreement among embryologists. The original theory of
Sabin traced the origin from the venous system while
Huntington and McClure suggested that lymphatics form
by fusion of mesenchymal spaces or clefts. The latter has
been labeled the centripetal theory. By the sixth week of
gestation, there are paired lymph sacs in the neck and
lumbar areas and at the eighth week, there is a retroperitoneal lymph sac with a developing cisterna chyli. These
systems develop communicating channels that ultimately
form the thoracic duct by merger of the right lymphatic
duct with the left across the fourth to sixth thoracic vertebrae to drain into the left subclavian vein. Smaller lymphatic ducts persist that drain into the right subclavian
vein.

Developmental arrest or abnormalities may result in
primary hypoplasia or absence of ducts and lymph nodes.
Abnormal growth of jugular lymph sacs can produce unilocular or multilocular lymph cysts termed cystic
hygromas. In addition to the neck, these cysts may be
found in the axilla, mediastinum, retroperitoneum, or intestinal mesentery. Hyperplastic changes may also occur
to produce lymphangiomas with or without other vascular
malformations.

The function of the lymphatic system begins with lymphatic capillaries that collect fluid and protein from the
extravascular spaces. In addition to the protein that cannot be reabsorbed by the venules, red cells, bacteria, and
other larger particles can only be evacuated through the
lymphatics. This unique permeability is facilitated by the
absence of a basement membrane beneath the lymphatic
endothelial cells. The lymphatic capillaries are found beneath the epidermis in the superficial dermis. These vessels drain into valved channels in the deep dermis and
subdermal tissues, forming larger channels that follow the
vascular pathways superficial to the deep fascia. Although lymphatics can be found in the intermuscular fascia, they are absent in muscles, tendon, cartilage, brain,
and cornea.

Lymph is transported by afferent vessels to regional
lymph nodes that vary in size according to their function
and activity. Within the medullary sinuses of the node,
circulating lymphocytes are replaced and initial contact of
foreign material with the immune system is made. Efferent lymph leaves the node via hilar channels that are less

numerous than the afferent channels that enter the convex side of the node. In addition to direct thoracic duct drainage into the subclavian vein, there are other lymphovenous communications within nodes and in peripheral vessels. Central lymphatic flow is promoted by the lymphatic valves, muscular contractions in larger ducts, respiration, arterial pulsation, and external massage.

Classification

The original classification of Allen was into two types, one where there was no known cause and one secondary to a known disease or disorder. The primary lymphedemas were called *congenital* when present at birth and *praecox* when there was onset in childhood. When the onset was delayed into later life, Kinmonth added the term *tarda*. With the advent of lymphography it became possible to classify the primary lymphedemas structurally into *hyperplasias* and *hypoplasias*. The present classification as proposed by Kinmonth is as follows:

1. Primary lymphedema
   a. Primary hypoplastic
      (1) Distal hypoplasia or aplasia
      (2) Proximal hypoplasia
      (3) Proximal and distal hypoplasia
   b. Primary hyperplastic
      (1) Bilateral hyperplasia
      (2) Megalymphatic
2. Secondary lymphedema
   a. Malignancy
   b. Radiation
   c. Trauma or surgical excision
   d. Inflammation or parasitic invasion
   e. Paralysis

The primary lymphedemas are hypoplastic in 92 percent of cases. Their subgroups are defined by lymphography and behave differently. Those with distal hypoplasia have a mild, nonprogressive form of the disorder provided that their proximal pathways are normal. Most of these patients are women and notice the onset after puberty. In proximal hypoplasia, the lymphedema is more extensive, involving the entire extremity, and it occurs equally among males and females. The combination of proximal and distal hypoplasia shows features of both groups and tends to be progressive.

The primary hyperplastic lymphedemas are uncommon (8 percent) and those with bilateral hyperplasia can usually be recognized by diffuse capillary angiomata on the lateral sides of the feet. Lymphography shows dilated lymphatics with normal valves in contrast to the findings in the megalymphatic group where no valves can be seen. In this latter group, chylous reflux may produce chylometrorrhea, skin vesicles, or chyluria.

The most common cause of secondary lymphedema in this country is malignant disease metastatic to lymph nodes. Surgical removal of nodes, especially when combined with radiation therapy that produces lymphatic fibrosis, is another common cause. In tropical and subtropical countries, filariasis is the most common cause of secondary lymphedema, producing the typical appearance of elephantiasis. Other infective and chemical agents such as silica can enter the lymphatic system via barefoot walking and cause fibrosis of lymphatics and lymph nodes.

Diagnosis

Lymphedema occurs as the result of an abnormality of the lymphatic system, and the term should be restricted to situations where other causes of edema have been excluded or a specific lymphatic abnormality has been demonstrated. The presence of bilateral dependent "pitting" edema usually indicates a renal or cardiac etiology. Other generalized hypoproteinemias may be seen in malnutrition, cirrhosis, and protein-losing enteropathy, or they may be idiopathic. Allergies or hereditary causes are unusual. In unilateral edema, venous disease is the most likely etiology and can be recognized by the examinations described in the previous section.

CLINICAL MANIFESTATIONS. The patient with lymphedema complains of swelling and fatigue. Limb size increases during the day and decreases at night but is never normal. It is important to determine whether there is a family history of primary lymphedema and whether the patient has visited any countries where filariasis is endemic. The presence of weight loss and diarrhea suggests small bowel lymphangiectasia. On examination, lymphedema is characteristically firm and rubbery but nonpitting. Lymph vesicles may be present containing fluid of high protein concentration. Complications of lymphedema such as infection, cellulitis, erythema, and hyperkeratosis may be present. It is important to document limb size to identify isolated limb gigantism and the Klippel–Trenaunay syndrome which may have hypoplastic lymphatics in addition to venous abnormalities, capillary nevus, and limb elongation. The patient should be examined for upper extremity and genital lymphedema, hydroceles, and amelogenesis imperfecta.

LYMPHATIC VISUALIZATION. Lymphatics can be visualized by dye injection in the extremities and mesentery, and also by ingestion of cream or milk to visualize intestinal lacteals and major ducts.

Dye Infection. A highly diffusible dye such as patent blue as introduced by Hudack and McMaster or sky blue dye as recommended by Butcher and Hoover can be injected in 0.2-mL amounts subcutaneously into each interdigital web. Massage of the skin and movement of the joints will usually define a network of fine intradermal lymphatics (Fig. 22-25). If the collecting vessels are obstructed or inadequate, the dye will diffuse through the dermal lymphatics to produce a marbled appearance called "dermal backflow."

Radiologic Lymphography. The technique of lymphography was developed by Kinmonth, who demonstrated that it was possible to cannulate the lymphatics visualized by dye injection and then inject contrast medium (Lipiodol). This is a meticulous and tedious procedure that may require general anesthesia as originally proposed by Kinmonth. If the lymphatics in the foot are not usable, it is possible either to cannulate lymphatics adjacent to groin nodes or to inject the node directly. With adequate visual-

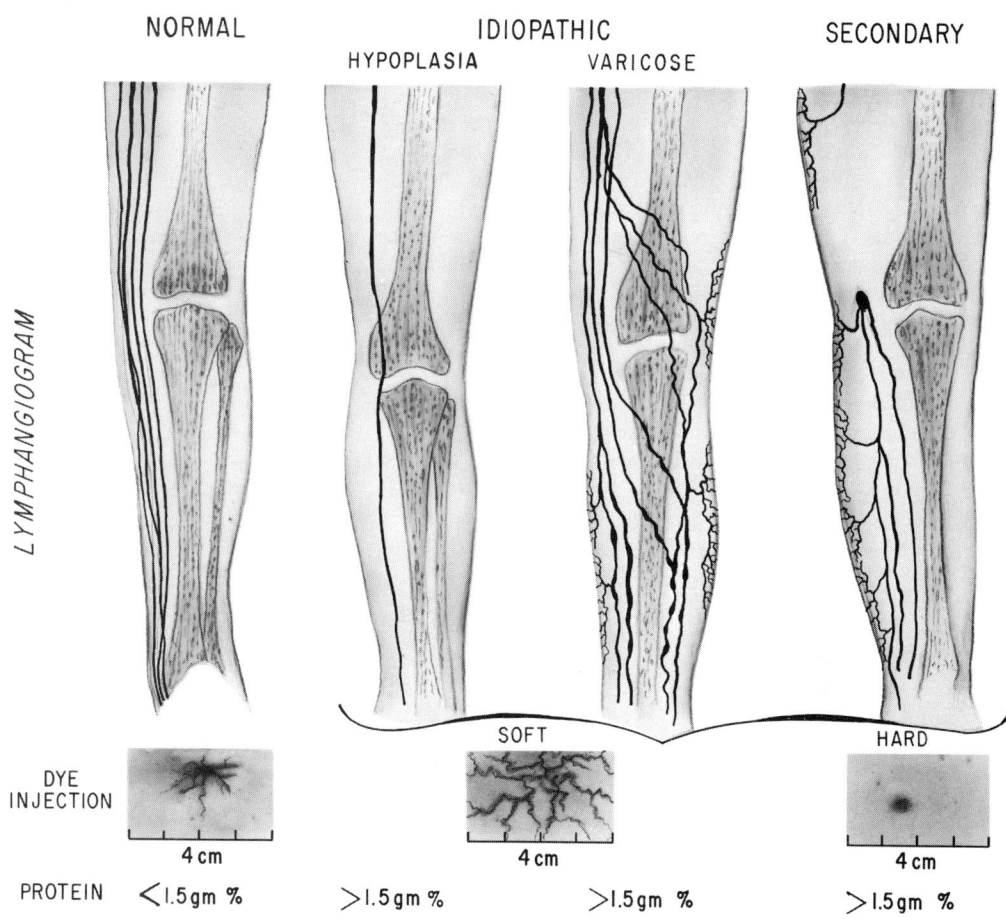

Fig. 22-25. Schematic illustration of the diagnostic procedures for lymphedema: dye injections, lymphangiograms, and protein analysis.

ization, the lymphatics in the extremity will be identified, often as parallel tracks that are of uniform size and bifurcate as they proceed proximally in contrast to the venous system (Fig. 22-25). Normally, there is some dilatation at the level of the valves.

Radionuclide Lymphatic Clearance. Radionuclide scanning using human serum albumin labeled with radioactive iodine or technetium 99m colloid has been used to monitor lymphatic clearance by serial scanning. Although the technique is simpler than standard lymphography, it has major disadvantages due to haziness of the scan, radiation dosage, and distribution of the radionuclide into the extracellular fluid, making calculations of clearance dependent on leg volume.

ANALYSIS OF TISSUE FLUID. Tissue fluid or lymph can be aspirated or collected from a tube in the subcutaneous tissues but contributes little to the diagnosis of lymphedema. Characteristically, lymphedema fluid has a protein content of more than 1.5 g/dL in contrast to edema fluid from venous hypertension, which is usually less. Also, the ratio of albumin to globulin is higher in lymphedema fluid than in plasma, which is helpful in the presence of an inflammatory exudate where the protein content is high but the albumin to globulin ratio is normal.

Management

SUPPORTIVE TREATMENT. There are significant anatomic and physiologic limitations to the treatment of lymphedema. From the standpoint of physiology, the removal of fluid is not as effective as in edema of other causes because of the residual protein in lymphedema. In addition, from an anatomical standpoint, the development of fibrosis produces irreversible changes in the subcutaneous tissues. Therefore, the options are limited and the primary objectives remain for control of edema, maintenance of healthy skin, and avoidance of the complications of cellulitis and lymphangitis.

The initial objective of control of edema can be approached by elevation and the use of sequential pneumatic compression boots to massage the leg. These treatments can be done at home with equipment rented for this purpose. Once the leg has reached optimal size, the patient should be fitted with firm elastic stockings as described earlier for venous insufficiency. The stockings should be removed at night and the foot of the bed elevated to maintain the pressure gradient from leg to right atrium.

The onset of redness, pain, and swelling usually signifies early cellulitis or lymphangitis which can be recognized by red streaking up the leg. The usual causative organism is either staphylococcus or beta-hemolytic streptococcus which must be treated vigorously, usually with intravenous antibiotics. In the absence of treatment, the infection may obliterate more lymphatics and produce constitutional signs of fever, malaise, nausea, and vomiting. Another frequent complication is eczema, which will usually respond to hydrocortisone cream. Antifungal agents may be necessary, both topically and systemically, for chronic infections, particularly between the toes. In contrast to the stasis edema of venous insufficiency, ulceration is unusual, although fissures and lymph fistulas may develop and require surgical excision.

The secondary lymphedemas may lend themselves to treatment of the underlying disorder such as using diethylcarbamazine for filariasis or appropriate antibiotics for tuberculosis or lymphogranuloma venereum. In rare cases of long-standing secondary lymphedema such as in the arm following radical mastectomy, a lymphangiosarcoma may develop appearing as a raised blue or reddish nodule. Satellite tumors and early metastases may develop if it is not recognized and widely excised.

OPERATIVE TREATMENT. Only 15 percent of patients with primary lymphedema become candidates for operative treatment, which usually is directed to reducing leg size. The indications for operation are related to functional rather than cosmetic improvement since the appearance of the extremity even after a successful procedure will still be abnormal and show extensive scarring. The best results are obtained when the bulk of the extremity has severely impaired movement or when there have been recurrent attacks of cellulitis. Although some efforts have been made to develop techniques to improve lymphatic drainage, most of the established procedures consist of excisional operations.

Three of the excisional procedures were based on the incorrect assumption that the deep fascia acted as a barrier to lymphatic drainage, and the efforts of Kondoleon, Sistrunk, and Thompson to excise fascia and/or insert a dermal flap into muscle proved ineffective in improving lymphatic drainage. The original procedure devised by Charles consisting of wide excision of lymphedematous tissue followed by skin grafting is still useful when the overlying skin is in poor condition as in elephantiasis. The procedure used more often, however, is Kinmonth's modification of Homan's procedure where skin flaps are raised to allow excision of the underlying subcutaneous tissues.

The most logical albeit technically demanding approach has been directed to establishing lymphaticovenous anastomoses. Initial efforts in this area were made by Nielubowicz et al. who divided a lymph node, removing the pulp under magnification, and then sutured the node capsule with its afferent lymphatics into a vein. This procedure is more suitable for secondary lymphedema than primary where the disorder lies in the lymphatic channels themselves. Another promising technique of direct lymphovenous connection was developed by Cordeiro and modified by Degni, who used a special needle for insertion of lymphatic vessels directly into veins and fixed them there by a single suture. Using this technique, Fox, Montorsi, and Romagnoli treated 8 secondary and 12 primary lymphedema patients followed for up to 4 years. Good results were obtained in 2 of 4 postmastectomy lymphedemas with poor results in the 2 patients who had postoperative lymphangitis. Nine of 11 patients with primary lymphedemas had good functional results allowing the patients to resume normal activity. The authors recommend long-term preoperative anti-inflammatory and antimicrobial therapy to avoid postoperative lymphangitis.

It is obviously difficult to evaluate the results of such procedures when combined with resectional operations and in the absence of postoperative lymphography to demonstrate patency of the anastomoses. However, the deleterious effects of lymphangiographic contrast on lymphatics were well demonstrated by O'Brien et al., who measured limb volume after lymphangiography in 100 patients and found that 32 percent had a significant increase in leg volume and 19 percent developed lymphangitis. Therefore, it seems advisable to use lymphangiography only for diagnostic studies and not for pre- or postoperative evaluation until safer contrast material becomes available. Further efforts to combine resectional operations with microlymphovenous anastomoses as reported by O'Brien and Shafiroff may offer some brighter prospects for improvement of these debilitating disorders.

Bibliography

Venous Disease

Aderka D, Brown A, et al: Idiopathic deep vein thrombosis in an apparently healthy patient as a premonitory sign of occult cancer. *Cancer* 57:1846, 1986.

Ambrus JS, Ambrus CM, et al: Clinical and experimental studies of fibrinolytic enzymes. *Ann NY Acad Sci* 68:97, 1957.

Common HH, Seaman AJ, et al: Deep vein thrombosis treated with streptokinase or heparin: Follow-up of a randomized study. *Angiology* 27:645, 1976.

Einarsson E, Albrechtsson U, et al: Follow-up evaluation of venous morphologic factors and function after thrombectomy and temporary arteriovenous fistula in thrombosis of iliofemoral vein. *Surg Gynecol Obstet* 163:111, 1986.

Hobbs JT, Davies JWL: Detection of venous thrombosis with ^{131}I-labelled fibrinogen in the rabbit. *Lancet* 2:134, 1960.

Homans J: Diseases of the veins. *N Engl J Med* 231:51, 1944.

Hyers TM, Hull RD, et al: Antithrombotic therapy for venous thromboembolic disease. *Chest* 89(suppl):265, 1986.

Kakkar VV, Carrigan TP, et al: Efficacy of low doses of heparin in prevention of deep vein thrombosis after major surgery: A double blind, randomized trial. *Lancet* 2:101, 1972.

Kakkar VV, Lawrence D: Hemodynamic and clinical assessment after therapy for acute deep vein thrombosis. A prospective study. *Am J Surg* 150:54, 1985.

Peyton JWR, Hylemon MB, et al: Comparison of Greenfield filter and vena caval ligation for experimental septic thromboembolism. *Surgery* 93(4):533, 1983.

Shattil SJ: Diagnosis and treatment of recurrent venous thromboembolism. *Med Clin North Am* 68:577, 1984.

Virchow R: *Gesamelte Abhandlungen zur wissenschaftlichen Medizin.* Frankfurt, Merdinger Sohn, p 219, 1856.

Pulmonary Thromboembolism

Allison PR, Dunhill MS, et al: Pulmonary embolism. *Thorax* 15:273, 1960.

Cabrol C, Cabrol A, et al: Surgical correction of chronic postembolic obstruction of the pulmonary arteries. *J Thorac Cardiovasc Surg* 76:620, 1978.

Conti S, Daschbach M, et al: Comparison of high-dose versus conventional-dose heparin therapy for deep vein thrombosis. *Surgery* 92:972, 1982.

Goldhaber SZ, Vaughan DE, et al: Acute pulmonary embolism treated with tissue plasminogen activator. *Lancet* 2:886, 1986.

Greenfield LJ: Pulmonary embolism: Diagnosis and management. *Curr Probl Surg* 13:1, 1976.

Greenfield LJ: Intraluminal techniques for vena caval interruption and pulmonary embolectomy. *World J Surg* 3:4559, 1978.

Greenfield LJ, Bruce TA, et al: Transvenous pulmonary embolectomy by catheter device. *Ann Surg* 174:881, 1971.

Greenfield LJ, Scher LA, et al: KMA-Greenfield[R] filter placement for chronic pulmonary hypertension. *Ann Surg* 189:560, 1979.

Martin TR, Sandblom RI, et al: Adult respiratory distress syndrome following thrombolytic therapy for pulmonary embolism. *Chest* 1:151, 1973.

Sharma GVRK, Burleson VA, et al: Effect of thrombolytic therapy on pulmonary capillary blood volume in patients with pulmonary embolism. *N Engl J Med* 303:842, 1980.

Steenburg RW, Warren R, et al: A new look at pulmonary embolectomy. *Surg Gynecol Obstet* 107:214, 1958.

Urokinase Pulmonary Embolism Trial: A National Cooperative Study. *Circulation* 2(suppl):47, 1973.

Wilson JE III, Bynum LJ, et al: Heparin therapy in venous thromboembolism. *Am J Med* 70:808, 1981.

Varicose Veins and Chronic Venous Insufficiency

Beaglehole R: Epidemiology of varicose veins. *World J Surg* 10:898, 1986.

Bergan JJ, Flin WR, et al: Venous reconstruction surgery. *Surg Clin North Am* 62:399, 1982.

Bernstein EF: Future prospects in the treatment of venous disease. *World J Surg* 10:959, 1986.

Browse ML, Burnard KG: The postphlebitic syndrome: A new look, in Bergon JJ, Yao JST (eds): *Venous Problems.* Chicago, Year Book Medical Publications, 1978.

Calnan JS, Kountz S, et al: Venous obstruction in the aetiology of lympyoedema praecox. *Br Med J* 2:221, 1964.

Cockett FB, Thomas ML: The iliac compression syndrome. *Br J Surg* 52:816, 1965.

Dale WA: Reconstructive venous surgery. *Arch Surg* 114:1312, 1979.

Dale WA: Venous bypass surgery. *Surg Clin North Am* 62:391, 1982.

Hobbs JT: Surgery and sclerotherapy in the treatment of varicose veins: A random trial. *Arch Surg* 109:793, 1974.

Husni EA: Reconstruction of veins: The need for objectivity. *J Cardiovasc Surg* 24:525, 1983.

Keister HW, Bowers RF: Results obtained by superficial femoral vein ligation. *Surgery* 47:224, 1960.

Kistner RL: Surgical repair of the incompetent femoral vein valve. *Arch Surg* 110:1336, 1975.

Kistner RL: Primary venous valve incompetence of the leg. *Am J Surg* 140:218, 1980.

Kistner RL, Sparkuhl RD: Surgery in acute and chronic venous disease. *Surgery* 85:31, 1979.

Kohler TR, Strandness DE Jr: Noninvasive testing for the evaluation of chronic venous disease. *World J Surg* 10:903, 1986.

Kroener JM, Bernstein EF: Valve competence following experimental venous valve autotransplantation. *Arch Surg* 110:1467, 1981.

Ludbrook J: Primary great saphenous varicose veins revisited. *World J Surg* 10:954, 1986.

Norris CS, Beyran A, et al: Quantitative photoplethysmography in chronic venous insufficiency: A new method of noninvasive estimation of ambulatory venous pressure. *Surgery* 94:758, 1983.

Palma EC, Esperon R: Vein transplants and grafts in the surgical treatment of the postphlebitic syndrome. *J Cardiovasc Surg* 1:94, 1960.

Servelle M: Klippel and Trenaunay's syndrome: 768 operated cases. *Ann Surg* 201:365, 1985.

Smith DE: Surgical management of obstructive venous disease of the lower extremity, in Rutherford RB (ed): *Vascular Surgery.* 2d ed, Philadelphia, Saunders, 1984, pp 1412–1433.

Smith DE, Trimble C: Surgical management of obstructive venous disease of the lower extremity, in Rutherford RB (ed): *Vascular Surgery.* Philadelphia, Saunders, 1977, pp 1247–1268.

Taheri SA, Heffener R, et al: Vein valve transplantation. *Contemp Surg* 22:17, 1983.

Taheri SA, Heffener R, et al: Five years' experience with vein valve transplant. *World J Surg* 10:935, 1986.

Taheri SA, Lazar L, et al: Vein valve transplantation. *Surgery* 1:29, 1982.

Warren R, Thayer TR: Transplantation of the saphenous vein for postphlebitic stasis. *Surgery* 35:867, 1954.

Venous Trauma

Agarwal N, Shah PM, et al: Experience with 115 civilian venous injuries. *J Trauma* 22:827, 1982.

Kudsk KA, Bongard F, et al: Determinants of survival after vena caval injury: Analysis of a 14-year experience. *Arch Surg* 119:1009, 1984.

Malt RA, Remonsnyder JP, et al: Long-term utility of replanted arms. *Ann Surg* 176:334, 1972.

Mathur AP, Pochaczevsky R, et al: Fogarty balloon catheter for removal of catheter fragment in subclavian vein. *JAMA* 217:481, 1971.

Rich NM, Hobson RW II, et al: Repair of lower extremity venous trauma: A more aggressive approach required. *J Trauma* 14:639, 1974.

Richardson JB, Jurkovich GJ, et al: A temporary arteriovenous shunt (Scribner) in the management of traumatic venous injuries of the lower extremity. *J Trauma* 26:503, 1986.

Lymphatics and Lymphedema

Allen EV: Lymphedema of the extremities. Classification, etiology and differential diagnosis: Study of 300 cases. *Arch Intern Med* 54:606, 1934.

Cordeiro AK: Novas tecnias de anastomose linfovenoa para

tratamento cirurgico de linfedma de nembros inferiores e linfedma de membro superior pos mastectomia. *Maternidade
Infuncia* 34:211, 1975.

Degni M: New technique of lymphatic-venous anastomosis for
the treatment of lymphedema. *Vasa* 3:479, 1974.

Huntington GS, McClure CFW: The anatomy and development
of the jugular lymph sacs in the domestic cat. *Am J Anat*
10:177, 1910.

Kinmonth JB: *The Lymphatics. Diseases, Lymphography and
Surgery.* London, Arnold, 1972.

Nielubowicz J, Olszewski W: Surgical lymphaticovenous shunts

in patients with secondary lymphedema. *Br J Surg* 55:440,
1968.

O'Brien BM, Das SK, et al: Effect of lymphangiography on lymphedema. *Plast Reconstr Surg* 68:922, 1981.

O'Brien BM, Shafiroff BB: Microlymphaticovenous and resectional surgery in obstructive lymphedema. *World J Surg* 3:3,
1979.

Sabin FR: On the origin of the lymphatic system from the veins
and the development of lymph hearts and thoracic duct in the
pig. *Am J Anat* 1:367, 1902.

Chapter 23

Surgically Correctable Hypertension

William J. Fry and Richard E. Fry

Elevated blood pressure, especially elevated diastolic pressure, is a too frequent cause of devastating illness and death. In 1981 the American Heart, Lung and Blood Institute released these statistics: One of six Americans, or 35,000,000 people, has definite high blood pressure. Of these individuals, 18,000,000 are aware of their disease; 12,000,000 receive treatment, but only 5,000,000 are adequately treated. Further estimates show that death from myocardial infarction and stroke would be decreased 20 percent if hypertension could be recognized early and appropriately treated.

The ravages of untreated hypertension significantly reduce life expectancy because of secondary involvement of the heart, brain, and kidneys. Insurance tables show that a male with a blood pressure of 150/100 has a risk of death two to three times greater than one with a blood pressure of 110/70. Even modest increase in the diastolic pressure above 82 mmHg can be correlated with a higher mortality, especially of women in the fifteen- to forty year-old age group (Table 23-1). Optimal control of the blood pressure is often difficult. Numerous medications may be necessary, and problems with drug side effects and patient compliance make proper treatment difficult. Palliation is the rule, and the opportunity for cure is seen in those patients with surgically correctable lesions, 5 to 15 percent of the total hypertensive population.

PHYSIOLOGY AND PATHOPHYSIOLOGY

Systolic and diastolic blood pressure are reflections of the peak left ventricular pressure and the static tone of the capacitance vessels during ventricular relaxation. The "normal" values are by age: adults, less than 140/90; adolescents, 100/75; children, 85/55; and infants, 70/45. These values are not absolute, as the aforementioned risk of death with a diastolic pressure greater than 82 attests.

The blood pressure is affected by cardiac output, peripheral resistance, and blood volume. Blood viscosity and vessel compliance have a lesser influence. Increased intravascular volume and red-cell mass as seen in polycythemia rubra vera can cause hypertension, while decreased intravascular volume secondary to hemorrhage will lower the blood pressure. *Cardiac output,* the volume of blood pumped per unit of time by the heart, has great effect on the blood pressure. Hyperdynamic states such as thyrotoxicosis may increase the blood pressure, while ischemic myocardial disease can lead to pump failure and hypotension. *Peripheral vascular resistance,* or the resistance to flow at the arteriolar level, has marked influence on the blood pressure and can vary greatly in response to blood volume changes and circulating vasoactive substances.

Right atrial stretch receptors and carotid and aortic arch baroreceptors modulate the blood pressure through sympathetic and parasympathetic neural signals. These areas are responsible for regulation and maintenance of blood pressure through their influence on cardiac performance and total peripheral resistance. Neural mechanisms may have a role in essential hypertension by the establishment of a higher "set point."

Humoral mechanisms specifically affect the blood pressure. Catecholamines increase small vessel tone; steroids and mineralocorticoids increase total body water and sodium, and potentiate the vasoconstrictive effect of norepinephrine and epinephrine. Angiotensin II, produced by renal ischemia, increases the blood pressure through a combination of its powerful vasoactive properties and its stimulation of aldosterone secretion which expands intravascular volume. Recently, atriopeptides stored in granules within the wall of the atrium have been

Table 23-1. VARIATIONS IN MORTALITY AMONG WOMEN ACCORDING TO SYSTOLIC AND DIASTOLIC PRESSURES. RATIOS OF ACTUAL TO EXPECTED MORTALITY—STANDARD FEMALE RISKS—100 PERCENT

Systolic blood pressure, mmHg	Diastolic blood pressure, mmHg	Mortality ratio %* Issue age		
		15–39	40–69	All ages
128–137	<83	137	93	97
	83–87	147	92	98
	88–92	179	88	93
	93–97	209	92	110
138–147	<83	161	125	128
	83–87	162	150	151
	88–92	150	170	168
	93–97	(394)	168	170
	94–102	(826)	171	220
148–157	<88	—	117	90
	88–92	(301)	219	214
	93–97	—	140	140
	98–102	—	214	183
158–167	<88	—	138	138
	88–92	—	129	127
	93–97	—	179	182
	98–102	—	(246)	(250)

* Where the number of policies terminated by death is 10 to 34, the mortality ratio is enclosed in parentheses. A dash indicates fewer than 10 policies terminated by death.
SOURCE: Lew EA: High blood pressure, other risk factors and longevity: The insurance viewpoint, in JH Laragh (ed): *Hypertension Manual.* New York, Yorke Medical Books, 1974, p 43.

defined. These may contribute to systemic pressure by their natriuretic, diuretic, and antihypertensive effects.

CLINICAL MANIFESTATIONS

Hypertension is an insidious disease. Symptoms such as headache and epistaxis may accompany severe elevation of blood pressure but are nonspecific. Often a patient will realize the presence of hypertension only after hospitalization for myocardial infarction or stroke. Cardiovascular, cerebrovascular, and renovascular disease are the symptoms commonly caused by hypertension. Cardiac effects are secondary to left ventricular hypertrophy. There is an increased distance between the nutrient capillaries in ventricular hypertrophy that effectively compromises nutrient blood flow. The blood supply to the heart may be further compromised by atherosclerotic coronary artery disease. Accelerated atherosclerosis leads to peripheral and splanchnic vascular disease. Cerebrovascular atherosclerosis increases risk of stroke, while chronic hypertension compromises renal function through nephrosclerosis. Malignant hypertension is accompanied by encephalopathy, retinal and cerebral hemorrhage. All of these processes, working in concert or alone, subject the afflicted individual to an increased mortality.

SURGICAL HYPERTENSION AND RATIONALE FOR OPERATIVE THERAPY

Surgically correctable hypertension accounts for 5 to 15 percent of the total spectrum of this disease. A list of

these types may be seen in Table 23-2. All these conditions involve a circulating substance producing increased blood pressure. They differ only in the site of origin and whether the release of the substance is due to a parenchymal disorder such as pheochromocytoma, or due to altered blood flow as in renal artery occlusive disease. The place of surgery in the treatment of "essential" disease is of historical and research interest, but at this time no techniques have been devised that consistently lower blood pressure in those without obvious reasons for operative therapy.

Operative therapy, when appropriate, should be employed rather than instituting or continuing medical therapy. Medical therapy is often ineffective. The myriad medications with their adverse reactions, coupled with poor control of the hypertensive state, are usually not effective. Lowering the blood pressure will do little to ameliorate the ravages of Cushing's disease or to prevent the parenchymal deterioration of renal occlusive disease. Operative therapy offers an opportunity for complete cure rather than palliation.

Table 23-2. SURGICALLY CORRECTABLE FORMS OF HYPERTENSION

Renovascular hypertension
Primary hyperaldosteronism
Hyperadrenocorticism
Pheochromocytoma
Coarctation of the aorta
Unilateral renal parenchymal disease

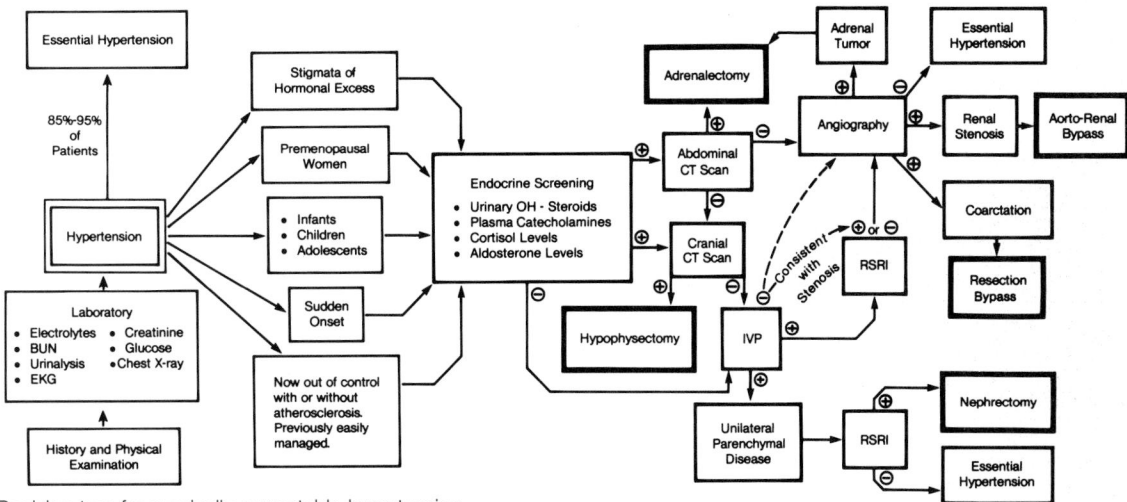

Fig. 23-1. Decision tree for surgically correctable hypertension.

PATIENT EVALUATION AND WORK-UP

Because most patients will have essential hypertension, screening all hypertensives for a surgical lesion may be unproductive and expensive. An algorithm for evaluating the hypertensive patient is shown in Fig. 23-1. A thorough history and physical examination can effectively lead to appropriate evaluation. An operative lesion should be suspected in patients who exhibit (1) sudden onset of severe or malignant hypertension; (2) easily controlled disease, with or without atherosclerosis, that becomes labile or difficult to treat; or (3) signs of hormonal excess. It should also be suspected when hypertension is present in adolescents or children or in premenopausal women. Patients who fall into these categories are more likely to have a surgically correctable lesion. Special attention to the details of the ocular funduscopic examination can help in grading the severity and chronicity of "newly discovered" hypertension. Physical findings such as peripheral edema, pulmonary rales/rhonci, and the presence of a third heart sound may suggest more severe or long-standing hypertension. Basic laboratory studies such as serum electrolytes, blood urea nitrogen (BUN), creatinine, and fasting serum glucose may lead to further endocrine or renal work-up. Electrocardiogram and chest x-ray can document the presence of left ventricular hypertrophy or rib notching. Urinalysis, creatinine clearance, and 24-h protein excretion further evaluate renal function and suggest nephropathy, either hypertensive or inflammatory. These screening examinations should lead to basic endocrine screening and then to the more definitive intravenous pyelogram, CT scanning, and angiographic studies. Information obtained from these tests will direct the clinician to appropriate operative therapy. The specific place and nature of these studies will be discussed later in the chapter.

PHEOCHROMOCYTOMA

Pheochromocytoma is a rare tumor of the adrenal medulla that exhibits a striking variety of presentation, making diagnosis difficult. Afflicted patients can present with a paroxysmal or sustained hypertension associated with sweating, headache, encephalopathy, and cardiac failure, among other symptoms. Pheochromocytomas are found in only 0.1 to 0.6 percent of all patients with hypertension. The severe nature of the disease and the high mortality rate in the untreated dictate early diagnosis and removal of the tumor. Eleven to twenty-three percent of all tumors are found to be malignant; the malignant form of the disease is not easily distinguished from benign, except in locally aggressive or metastatic tumors. The adrenal gland is the site of origin in 87 percent of all cases, the remainder being extraadrenal. Approximately 10 to 15 percent are bilateral and are usually associated with neurofibromatosis, the multiple endocrine adenomatosis (MEA) type II syndrome, and rarely, the von Hippel-Lindau syndrome. Medullary tumors produce both epinephrine and norepinephrine, while extraadrenal sites usually produce nearly pure norepinephrine.

Once a pheochromocytoma is suspected, the screening tests of urinary catecholamine excretion and serum levels should be obtained for normal values (Table 23-3). A recent study has shown increased accuracy of diagnosis using plasma catechol levels rather than urinary levels or levels of catechol metabolites. When chemical evidence is obtained, localization of the tumor may be determined using intravenous pyelogram (IVP), CT scanning, angiography, or venous sampling techniques. Intravenous pyelogram is accurate only 50 percent of the time and has been supplanted by newer methods. CT scanning is a

Table 23-3. NORMAL VALUES FOR URINARY CATECHOLAMINES

Catecholamines	$<100\ \mu g/24$ h
VMA	<6.8 mg/24 h
Metanephrine	<1.3 mg/24 h
Epinephrine	<25 mg/24 h
Norepinephrine	<160 mg/24 h

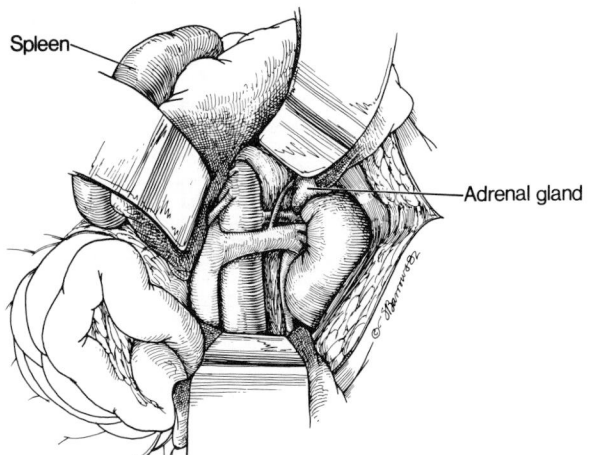

Fig. 23-2. Exposure for left kidney and adrenal gland.

screening procedure of choice and has excellent specificity and sensitivity in identifying adrenal masses. Tumors and normal adrenal glands may be hard to define if there is a paucity of retroperitoneal fat. If a tumor is located and elevated serum catecholamines are present, the diagnosis is complete. Scintigraphic methods using ^{131}I-metaiodobenzylguanidine have been shown to accurately locate pheochromocytomas in 90 percent of patients studied. This method can be useful when a biochemically proved tumor cannot be localized. Angiography and venous sampling techniques should be reserved for those patients with tumors difficult to locate. Transcatheter brush biopsy of inferior vena caval tumor thrombi is a newer technique, but has limited applicability at this time. Transabdominal adrenalectomy with examination of both glands is a preferred surgical approach (Fig. 23-2). The surgeon must also inspect the paraspinous area, bladder, and the organ of Zuckerkandl to rule out the presence of extramedullary tumors. The extent of resection will be dictated by the size of the tumor, the amount of local invasion, and the presence of metastases.

The perioperative treatment plays a major role in the care of the patient with pheochromocytoma. All patients will be relatively hypovolemic, requiring adequate volume replacement. Fluid and cardiac status should be adequately monitored and maintained with pulmonary artery wedge catheterization or at least a central venous line. Use of phenoxybenzamine and nitroprusside can aid in controlling blood pressure during operation, while lidocaine should be available for arrhythmias. After removal of the tumor, hypotension secondary to vasodilatation and hypovolemia are not infrequent. Monitoring of the blood pressure in the intensive care unit with the use of volume replacement and vasopressors, if necessary, is mandatory. Results of benign tumor resection are excellent, with a normal life expectancy. A malignant tumor carries a poor prognosis of 44 percent 5-year survival rate and a 19 percent 5-year disease-free interval. Extra-adrenal lesions have an even poorer outcome because they frequently indicate inoperable tumor and rapid metastases. (See Chap. 37.)

PRIMARY HYPERALDOSTERONISM

Increased primary aldosterone secretion by the zona glomerulosa of the adrenal cortex is associated with hypokalemia, hypernatremia, hypervolemia, and increased blood pressure. Clinically, the patient will exhibit signs of muscle weakness, headache, and malaise. Most patients are women in the thirty- to fifty-year-old age group. Laboratory examination demonstrates increased urinary potassium excretion, increased serum sodium and increased bicarbonate levels. Low plasma renin levels after sodium restriction and furosemide with upright posture is a helpful diagnostic test. The absence of aldosterone suppression after saline loading also aids in diagnosis. The combination of low plasma renins and high serum aldosterone levels gives 95 percent accuracy in diagnosing hyperaldosteronism. CT scanning should be used initially for tumor localization, with angiography and adrenal vein sampling reserved for ambiguous cases. Renal angiography should be strongly considered when the tumor is not easily found. An arterial lesion can be ruled out and a tumor may often be detected. Adrenal venography may be helpful in localizing some tumors when CT scanning and arteriography are not diagnostic.

The decision to employ operative therapy is based on the cause of the increased aldosterone. The anterior abdominal approach is preferred, although flank and posterior approaches are also used (Fig. 23-3). Excision of aldosterone-producing adenomas gives excellent cure rates ranging from 60 to 90 percent. Patients with diffuse cortical hyperplasia do not respond as well to adrenalectomy. If spironolactone can decrease blood pressure effectively preoperatively, the response to operation is generally good. If there is no response, medical treatment may be

Fig. 23-3. Exposure for right kidney and adrenal gland.

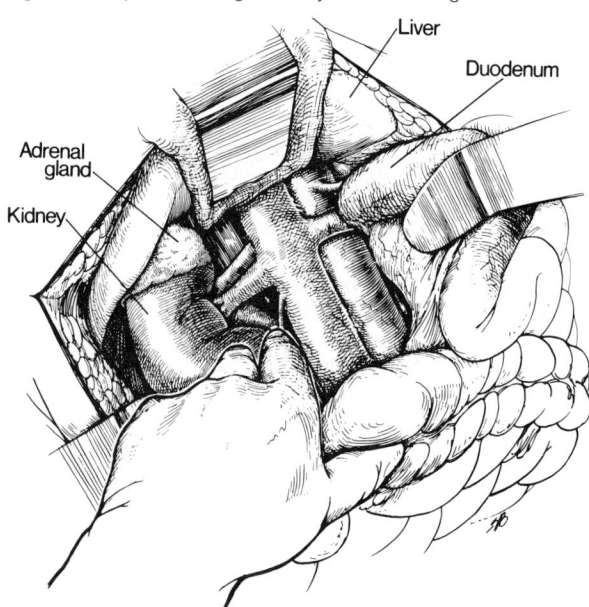

indicated. In cases of adrenal hyperplasia, bilateral adrenalectomy may be considered to alleviate symptoms.

HYPERADRENOCORTICISM

In his book, *The Pituitary Body* (1912), Harvey Cushing described a patient with hypertension, truncal obesity, striae, amenorrhea, and hirsutism. Although the pituitary was thought to be the primary cause of disease, reference was made to planned operative exploration of the adrenal glands. After further investigation, "Cushing's disease" was fully described and more clearly elucidated in 1932. Other causes of adrenal excess are possible, but the classic symptoms are due to an increase in circulating glucocorticoids. Women thirty to fifty years of age are most commonly affected. The cause of the disease may originate in the adrenal gland itself, in the pituitary gland, or from other tumors, the so-called "ectopic ACTH syndrome."

DIAGNOSIS. A more complete explanation of Cushing's disease and its diagnosis is given in Chap. 37. For screening purposes, increased urinary 17-hydroxysteroid levels and loss of diurnal variations in serum cortisol levels are enough to establish a diagnosis of hyperadrenocorticism. Pituitary or adrenal disease can be differentiated by ACTH levels and their response to dexamethasone suppression (see Chap. 37). Abdominal or cranial CT scan and adrenal vein sampling may help in anatomic location. Scintillation scanning of the adrenal with ^{131}I-6 beta-idiomethyl-19-norcholesterol can help localize adrenal or abdominal lesions suspected from biochemical tests. It should be reserved for those patients in whom CT scanning does not localize the lesion. Sella turcica films are not accurate, and the absence of abnormality does not rule out pituitary adenoma.

THERAPY. Surgical therapy should be tailored to the type of lesion, and every effort should be made to locate the tumor before proceeding with adrenal excision. Ectopic and adrenal lesions account for 20 to 25 percent of cases of hyperadrenocorticism and are best treated by excision of the tumor. Bilateral adrenal hyperplasia is usually caused by pituitary tumors. Those patients with moderate symptoms may be effectively treated with pituitary irradiation or transsphenoidal hypophysectomy. If gross sellar enlargement is evident, transsphenoidal ablation may be indicated.

If evaluation of the patient indicates unilateral adrenal enlargement, adenoma or carcinoma is probable. Total or partial adrenalectomy affords excellent cure rates in adenoma. Both glands should be examined at operation, as 10 percent of cases involves both adrenals. Adrenal carcinoma requires extensive dissection with wide excision of the tumor. Cure rates are poor, with most patients surviving only 3 years after diagnosis. Serum cortisol levels should be followed after operation, as these may rise with recurrence. All patients undergoing adrenal surgery for Cushing's disease should be prepared preoperatively with intravenous steroids and followed carefully in the postoperative period for signs of corticosteroid insufficiency.

Ortho para-DDD, a DDT congener, and the agent mitotane have been shown to cause regression in adrenal carcinoma. Use of this drug may provide prolonged remission in patients with metastatic or unresectable tumor.

Ectopic ACTH Syndrome

Several nonadrenal tumors are capable of producing ACTH or ACTH-like substances. Usually this occurs in patients with metastatic malignant tumors. Oat cell tumors of the lung, pancreatic carcinoma, and thymic tumors are the most common cause of this disease. Because of advanced malignancy, classic stigmata are not always present. Tumor removal is preferred; however, extensive tumor growth often makes this impossible. Some palliation may be offered with appropriate chemotherapy.

COARCTATION OF THE AORTA

Congenital narrowing of the aorta, either proximally or distally to the ductus arteriosus, is a frequent cause of hypertension in infants and children. The aortic narrowing and increased resistance to blood flow may contribute to the increased blood pressure, along with decreased renal artery perfusion with secondary hyperreninemia and angiotensin II formation. The entire thoracic and abdominal aorta can be involved, as well as intestinal and renal vessels. Patients with neurofibromatosis and hypertension have an increased incidence of upper thoracic and abdominal coarctation.

Diagnosis is most easily made by comparing blood pressure in the upper and lower extremities. A difference of 20 to 40 mmHg should be seen. Older children and adults may exhibit overdevelopment of the upper body and underdevelopment of the lower limb. Systolic precordial murmurs, left ventricular hypertrophy on ECG, notching of the ribs, and a "3 sign" on chest x-ray are also suggestive of coarctation of the aorta. Arteriographic appearance is diagnostic and helps with operative planning.

Surgical resection with primary anastomosis or graft interposition is the treatment of choice. Use of the left subclavian artery as a "patch graft" is also effective. Untreated patients have a mortality of approximately 60 percent. Most patients should be operated upon between six and sixteen years of age. Early intervention may be necessary if cardiac decompensation supervenes or if medical treatment is not effective. If performed in the optimal age range, a 95 percent cure rate can be seen, with an operative mortality of approximately 1 to 3 percent. When patient age increases, operative mortality increases, since the operation becomes technically more difficult. The cure rate also declines because the hypertension tends to become "fixed" by the long-standing coarctation. (See Chap. 19.)

RENOVASCULAR HYPERTENSION

Renovascular hypertension may be defined as elevation in the diastolic and systolic pressure associated with

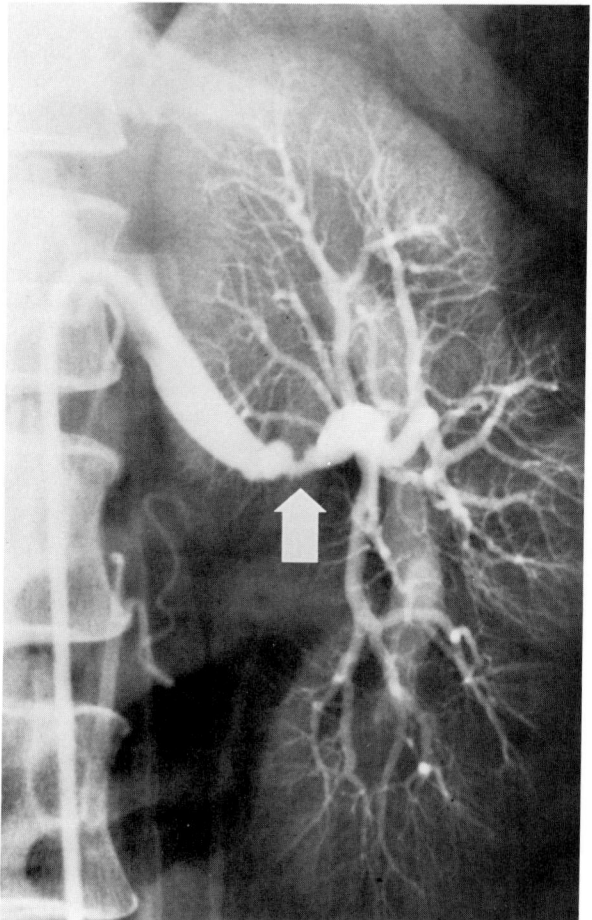

Fig. 23-4. Radiographic appearance of fibromuscular artery disease.

the feasibility of making the correct diagnosis but showed that, with refined techniques in reconstructive vascular surgery, predictable and long-term amelioration of hypertension could be achieved.

ETIOLOGY. Atherosclerosis accounts for over 80 percent of the occluding lesions seen in the renal artery, associated with attendant hypertension (Fig. 23-18A). This is primarily a disease afflicting males between the ages of fifty-five and seventy-five.

Fibrodysplasia accounts for approximately 18 percent of the occluding lesions seen in the renal artery (Fig. 23-4). It is primarily a disease of young people, being the most common etiologic factor in children and young women of the childbearing age group. Fibrodysplasia may take many forms, the most common of which is the medial fibrodysplasia. The classification of this disease process is outlined in Fig. 23-5. Histologically, the vasa vasora are always occluded in this disease, which may account for the overgrowth of collagen tissue. This may lend credence to the theory that this is primarily a disease of trauma or stretching of the renal artery. The right renal artery is affected 85 percent of the time. The right kidney is the most mobile kidney and is stretched repeatedly during pregnancy. Aneurysms are often associated with medial fibrodysplasia, being a secondary consequence of this process. This predisposition in the female may be secondary to the continual stretching of the renal arteries secondary to pregnancy, and/or may be associated with estrogens that are known to cause medial degeneration of the vessel walls. The condition is associated with thrombosis, accounting for the vasa vasora occlusions.

The fibrodysplastic lesions seen in children have so far

renal artery occlusive disease. There must be attendant dampening and reduction in total renal blood flow, causing the juxtaglomerular apparatus to secrete renin. The pathophysiology of renovascular hypertension was clarified by Goldblatt in the 1930s when he produced hypertension in laboratory animals by constriction of the renal artery. Shortly after that, the renoangiotensin system was delineated by Page, Helmer, and Menendez. The first arteriographic demonstration of an occluding lesion to the kidney was demonstrated by John Sid dos Santos. He attempted an endarterectomy of this vessel; it failed and the patient was cured with a nephrectomy. For several years nephrectomy was performed for hypertension in association with small kidneys, and when there was lack of good function on excretory pyelogram. This frequently resulted in failure to relieve hypertension.

It was not until the advent of arteriography and new techniques in vascular surgery that the observations by DeCamp, Morris, DeBakey, and the Cleveland Clinic group spearheaded by Harriet Dustan proved that normal blood pressure could be restored in hypertensive patients with careful technical reconstruction of a stenotic lesion in the renal artery. These pioneers not only demonstrated

Fig. 23-5. Classification of fibromuscular renal artery disease.

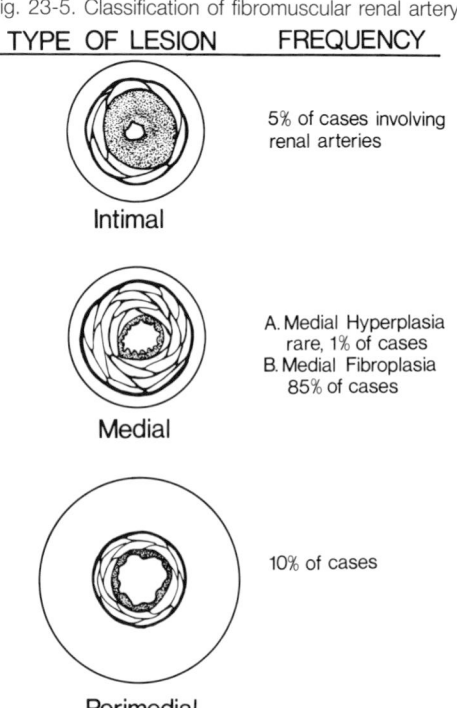

TYPE OF LESION	FREQUENCY
Intimal	5% of cases involving renal arteries
Medial	A. Medial Hyperplasia rare, 1% of cases B. Medial Fibroplasia 85% of cases
Perimedial	10% of cases

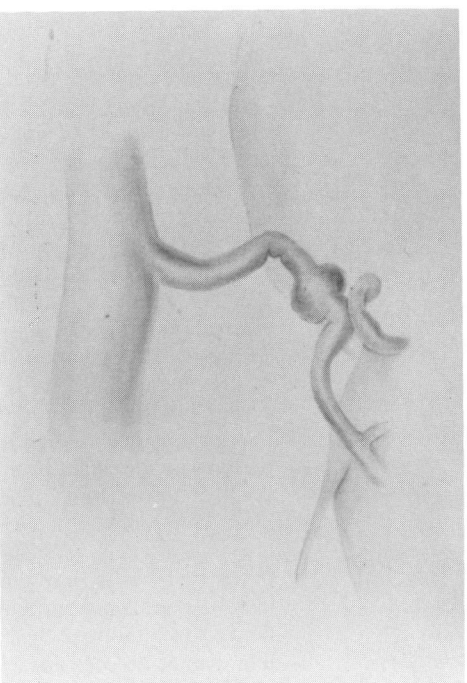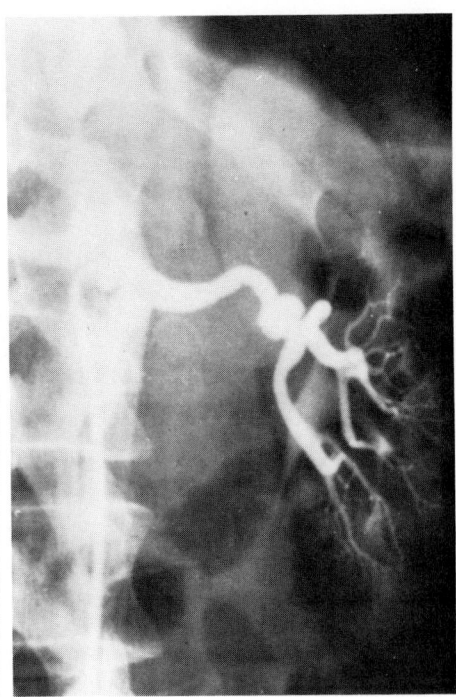

Fig. 23-6. Arteriogram and artist's concept of a solitary renal artery aneurysm.

defied any consistent delineation of etiology. The lesions most commonly seen in children are intimal hyperplasia and medial dysplasia. There is no question that upon occasion this disease progresses, and at least 15 percent of our patients have shown progression or formation of new lesions in 5- and 10-year follow-ups. Medial fibrodysplastic lesions may lend themselves to dilation, either directly or with a Gruntzig catheter. Intimal lesions and perimedial lesions do not lend themselves to dilation.

Trauma is an increasingly common etiologic factor in renovascular occlusive disease. Partial disruption of the renal artery may occur with severe trauma, producing a significant flow pressure gradient. The ability to delineate these problems early is paramount, as the attendant scarring around the renal hilus makes later reconstructive angioplasty exceedingly difficult. Fractures of the kidney may partially devascularize segments of the kidney that, if not recognized, may later produce hypertension.

Aneurysms of the renal arteries in and of themselves do not cause hypertension (Fig. 23-6). They are often associated with medial fibrodysplastic disease or severe atherosclerosis which may cause a secondary narrowing of the renal artery. Upon occasion, renal artery aneurysms will be the source of thrombus which may embolize distally into the renal parenchyma, causing ischemia and secondary hypertension.

Embolus is an uncommon but well-recognized cause of renovascular hypertension, with most emboli originating in the heart, though some originate from atherosclerotic aortic disease.

Dissections of the renal artery may be secondary to trauma, aortic dissections that extend into the renal ar-

tery, or fibrodysplastic disease. Dissections of the renal artery may pose problems in operative repair. With care, in most instances adequate revascularization can be accomplished.

Coarctation of the aorta, either classic or abdominal aortic coarctation, may produce a reduction in flow and pressure to the kidney, activating the release of renin. An abdominal aortic coarctation is depicted in Fig. 23-7.

Other, more obscure causes are vasculitis and collagen disease, rarely cysts or neoplasms of the kidney, and acquired or congenital arteriovenous fistulae within the kidney or the renal vessels.

Renin is produced when there is a reduction in flow and pressure to the renal parenchyma. This activates the juxtaglomerular cells to produce excessive amounts of renin that then sets up the production of angiotensin (Fig. 23-8). The use of angiotensin II antagonists (such as captopril) has been shown to be effective in the diagnosis and treatment of renovascular hypertension. Captopril has renal toxicity and may cause renal artery thrombosis. For these reasons, it should not be used as definitive therapy for renovascular hypertension.

CLINICAL MANIFESTATIONS. The clinical manifestations of renovascular hypertension are not clear. One must have a high index of suspicion in order to make this diagnosis. Renovascular hypertension is one of the most common causes of hypertension in the child. It is usually sustained and severe in nature, not easily controlled by medication. The sudden onset of hypertension in an adult should always alert the clinician to the possibility of renal artery occlusive disease. This is particularly true in women of the childbearing age. In those persons with ath-

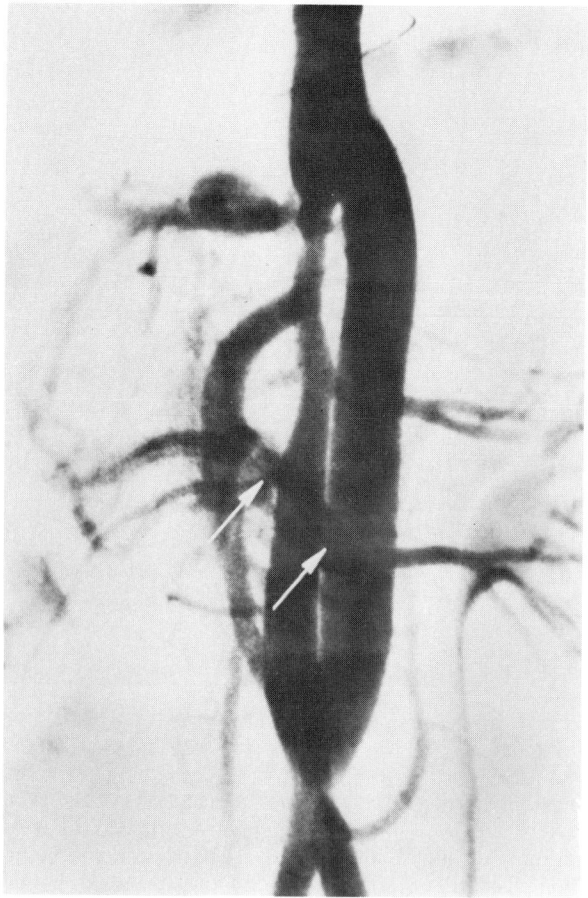

Fig. 23-7. Coarctation of the abdominal aorta after reconstruction. Arrows at repaired renal artery and bypass graft.

erosclerosis, it should likewise be remembered that sudden onset of hypertension may be related to occlusive disease involving the renal artery. The hallmark of renovascular hypertension is a sustained elevation of the diastolic blood pressure that is not readily controlled with

Fig. 23-8. Renin-angiotensin cascade.

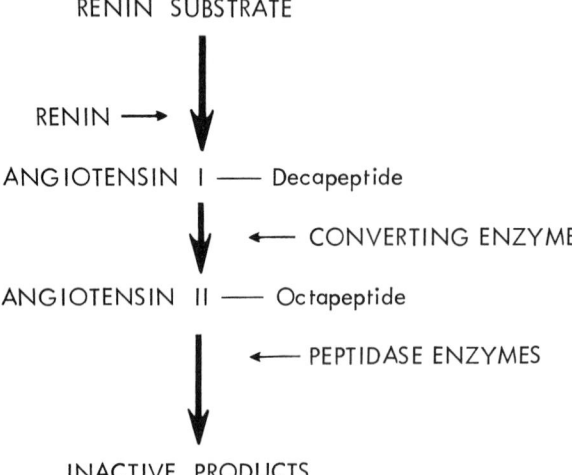

the usual forms of therapy. Easily controlled hypertension is not likely to have occlusive disease of the renal artery as its source. We always hold the child, the adolescent, the young female, and the atherosclerotic male in high suspicion of having occlusive disease of the renal artery when they present with hypertension.

Routine laboratory determinations are mentioned to emphasize the electrolyte derangement as outlined earlier, particularly in aldosterone-producing adenomas of the adrenal gland. An additional emphasis is important, as most hypertensive patients are treated with diuretics and electrolyte imbalance may be common.

Physical examination may or may not be helpful in making the diagnosis of renal artery occlusive disease. It certainly will delineate those patients with coarctation of the aorta as exemplified by reduced femoral pulses, and perhaps an attendant bruit over either the thoracic or abdominal aorta. Bruits over the kidney are common in patients with renovascular occlusive disease, but because of obesity they may be difficult to hear. It must be remembered that bruits may emanate from other vessels and may be confusing, particularly in the atherosclerotic patient. Auscultation of the back in the area of the costovertebral angle on occasion may be helpful in the delineation of a bruit. It is particularly noteworthy that in the atherosclerotic age group there may be other disease, especially of the subclavian vessels, that may not allow the diagnosis of hypertension to be made with one blood pressure determination. Blood pressure taken in both arms is mandatory whenever elevation of the blood pressure is suspected.

LABORATORY EVALUATION. The extent of laboratory evaluation of the hypertensive patient needed to make the diagnosis of renovascular occlusive disease is debated among the experts. There is no question but that in those clinics where an aggressive approach is taken, many more patients with renovascular occlusive disease are seen than in those where little attention is paid to extensive clinical and laboratory evaluation of the hypertensive patient.

Intravenous Pyelography. The intravenous pyelogram is not a good screening procedure for patients with suspected renovascular hypertension. It is least accurate in the child and most accurate in the atherosclerotic adult. There is a 75 percent false-negative rate in children and a 20 to 28 percent false-negative rate in the atherosclerotic adult. Classic findings upon intravenous pyelography—delayed opacification of the collecting system, reduction in size of the affected kidney, and ureteral notching—are the hallmarks of the radiologic diagnosis of renovascular occlusive disease as an etiologic factor in hypertension. We feel very strongly that intravenous pyelography should be done as a screening procedure on those patients suspected of having renovascular hypertension to make sure there are no intrinsic lesions in the kidney, such as ureteropelvic obstructive disease, neoplasm, pyelonephritis, cysts, or other parenchymal lesions associated with hypertension.

Renin Assays. Renin assay studies may be very helpful in the localization and delineation of severity of the renovascular occlusive disease. Before the advent of convert-

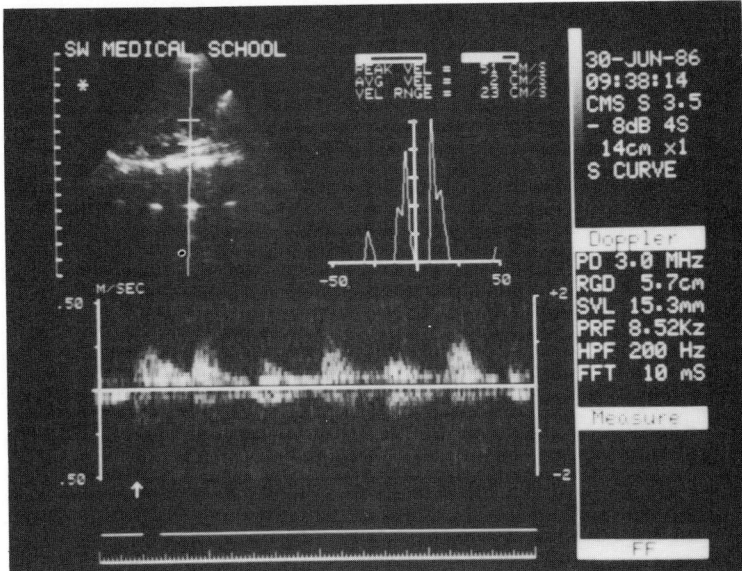

Fig. 23-9. B-mode ultrasonic/coupled Doppler wave-form of stenotic renal artery.

ing enzyme inhibitors (captopril, enalapril), the determination of peripheral venous renin and systemic renins are difficult. Blocking agents such as propranolol depress the output of renin, and to obtain accurate and meaningful renin determinations patients required cessation of medication and a strong natriuresis. This essentially eliminated many patients from study as the risk of hypertensive crisis with cessation of medication was high. It has been shown by several authors that the administration of a converting enzyme inhibitor produces an excess amount of renin in patients with occlusive renovascular disease. This is in spite of the fact that the patient may be on large doses of beta blocking agents such as propranolol. Preliminary work shows that peripheral renin determinations followed by the administration of 25 mg of captopril will produce a marked rise in systemic renin at 1 h. This has made elective renal vein renin determinations more accurate. They now may be done without cessation of therapy and reveal marked differences in the involved kidney vs. the normal kidney. In a study by Thibonnier, 19 patients were shown to have positive differential renin studies after the administration of captopril. All these patients were shown to have renal artery stenosis on arteriography and ultimately underwent successful renal revascularization. The utilization of renal systemic renin indices in conjunction with the captopril test is helpful. This test allows delineation of bilateral disease, comparing one kidney with the other, and demonstrating depression of renin production in the involved kidney. Use of converting enzyme inhibition in the determination of renal systemic index allows accurate prediction of success in operative therapy. The renal systemic renin index (RSRI) is outlined in the formula:

$$RSRI = \frac{\text{individual renal renin activity} - \text{systemic renin activity}}{\text{systemic renin activity}}$$

If the value of the affected kidney is >0.48 with the contralateral kidney ≤0.31, the chance for cure or improvement is high.

Noninvasive Techniques. The advent of the range-gated Doppler ultrasound has enabled accurate visualization and waveform analysis of the renal artery (Fig. 23-9). Strandness and his colleagues have demonstrated the applicability of this technique in the diagnosis of renovascular occlusive disease. These methods are very accurate and can show changes in the flow patterns in the main renal artery and in the kidney itself.

Arteriography. Arteriography remains the only accurate method of diagnosis of occlusive vascular disease involving the kidney. There is real hope that the computer-augmented venous arteriogram may be helpful, as it is much less invasive and may be performed on an outpatient basis. At the present time, 80 percent of the studies done utilizing this technique are accurate and helpful in the diagnosis of occlusive vascular disease of the kidney. Because of various problems with technique, 20 percent of the examinations are not of sufficient quality to make an accurate diagnosis. The drawbacks of digital venous arteriogram are (1) the inability to achieve multiple views of the renal artery, (2) overlap of the renal vessels by the mesenteric vasculature, and (3) poor definition of the intrarenal vessels. Because of these shortcomings, routine use of intravenous digital renal arteriography has been abandoned in our clinic. Use of the duplex scanning techniques coupled with the measurement of systemic renins with converting enzyme inhibition has obviated the need for an invasive screening technique.

The use of intraarterial digital arteriography is helpful because it allows use of small amounts of contrast material and does allow for multiple views of the renal artery. Small-vessel definition is inferior to standard angiography, but it is much better than that seen with the intravenous digital studies. It is also an exceedingly safe tech-

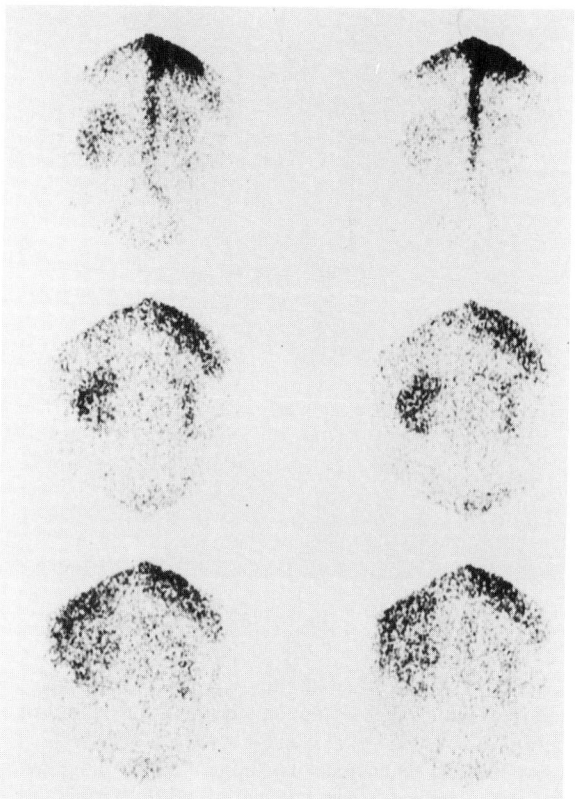

Fig. 23-10. Renal isotope scan showing decreased uptake in the left kidney.

nique, especially when it is combined with the new nonionic contrast material.

The intraarterial injection of contrast material and the selective renal artery injection of contrast material remain the mainstay of the diagnosis of renovascular occlusive disease. This allows for multiple projections to make sure that no lesion is left unrecognized. One may accurately measure the extent of the lesion and the reduction in cross-sectional area, and thus determine the significance of lesions encountered.

We have found that the visualization of collateral vessels around an occluding lesion is an important prognostic sign. This finding reinforces the significance given to an occluding lesion in the renal artery. We, along with others, have noted that there is a relative reduction in renin production as determined by renal vein renin sampling when there are multiple collaterals around a renal artery occluding lesion. It is important to remember this point, as it is one of the main associated factors in false-negative renin determinations.

Split-Renal Function Studies. These are utilized by a small number of clinics throughout the United States. The kidneys seldom vary significantly in their excretive ability to handle water, sodium, or creatinine. The functionally ischemic kidney conserves and reabsorbs sodium and water. This, then, shows a relative concentration of solutes such as creatinine.

These characteristics of the ischemic kidney have led to the description of several function tests that have been utilized in the diagnosis of renovascular hypertension. The Howard test measures urine volume and sodium concentration, as well as creatinine concentration. The involved kidney should have at least a 50 percent reduction in urine volume and 15 percent reduction in serum sodium concentration, with an attendant 15 percent increase in creatinine concentration over the so-called "normal" kidney. The Rappaport test utilizes the sodium-creatinine ratios from each kidney. The tubular rejection fraction ratio is obtained by multiplying the sodium-creatinine ratio on the left by that on the right. A ratio of less than 0.6 indicates significant left renal artery stenosis, and a ratio of more than 1.6 implicates the right renal artery. The test is felt to be negative when the values are between these two levels. The Stamey test utilizes osmotic diuresis or the intravenous infusion of urea. Para-aminohippurate, a solute excreted by the kidney but not reabsorbed by the tubules, is added to the infusion. The Stamey test is positive if there is a two-thirds reduction in urine volume and a 100 percent increase of para-aminohippurate concentration on the affected side. As a side benefit, the Stamey test also determines effective renal plasma flow in each kidney. This adds some credence to the test, as it delineates renal function.

Most clinics do not utilize renal function tests for several reasons. As can be appreciated, ureteral catheters must be placed in each ureter in order to allow individual collections. The introduction of infection and bleeding as a result of the trauma of the inlying catheters imputes a significant morbidity to these procedures. When this fact is combined with the fact that these tests are not as accurate as renal vein renin determinations, and are virtually useless in segmental renal artery lesions and in patients with bilateral disease, the importance of this series of tests is diminished.

Renal Scan. Radioisotope renal scanning allows surgeons to evaluate blood flow to the kidney (Fig. 23-10). Most renal scans depend on renal function. Information obtained by renal scans may be inaccurate if active parenchymal disease exists in conjunction with occlusive vascular disease. The ability to differentiate between primary renal artery occlusive disease and diffuse intraparenchymal disease on a renal scan is difficult. Because of these drawbacks the renal scan is used infrequently as a routine test in patients with renal artery occlusive disease.

Renal Biopsy. Percutaneous renal biopsy may be helpful, on occasion, in the preoperative evaluation of those patients demonstrating significant renal artery occlusive disease. The demonstration of an increased number of granules in the juxtaglomerular cells, with the maintenance of normal glomeruli, may be helpful in predicting the result with revascularization of the kidney. The morbidity associated with percutaneous renal biopsy in the form of bleeding and the production of arteriovenous fistulae has precluded it as a consistently useful modality in the preoperative evaluation of patients for renovascular reconstruction.

TREATMENT. The prognosis in operative therapy after the diagnosis is made depends upon the expertise of the surgeon, the durability of graft material used, and the extent of the secondary ravages of hypertension in the patient.

The refinement of vascular reconstructive techniques has contributed to more effective arterial reconstruction. The morbidity and mortality of the operative procedure are negligible. The utilization of autogenous tissue has assured accurate renal artery anastomoses. There is some excessive growth of scar tissue at the interface between Dacron prostheses and host artery, causing a higher incidence of late failure, but the Dacron prosthesis has proved to be a durable substance in the reconstruction of renal arteries in those adults with suitably sized vessels. PTFE prostheses are also suitable conduits for aortorenal bypass. Their drawback is the same as outlined for Dacron with the exception that these grafts tend to have a higher incidence of intimal proliferation at the graft artery interface. We believe that because of these drawbacks, aspirin therapy should be started the day before operation if one anticipates the use of Dacron or PTFE graft. This may prevent the deposition of platelets at the graft-artery interface, reducing the amount of platelet growth factor and its effect on intimal proliferation at this site. The use of aspirin in the postoperative period appears to be the most effective therapy at this time to reduce intimal proliferation and therefore the chance of recurrent stenosis.

The controversy over medical therapy versus operative therapy continues. Dean has demonstrated that renovascular lesions continue to progress even under optimal therapy, thus contributing to the potential loss of renal function. No accelerated atherosclerosis has been demonstrated in the renal architecture after successful renal artery revascularization. While the Mayo Clinic series was not done by the double-blind method, it would seem to indicate that medical therapy for patients with hypertension secondary to renal artery occlusive disease has a much higher mortality rate than does long-term follow-up of patients treated with operative therapy.

New drug therapy for renovascular hypertension is not without some drawbacks. The advent of the converting enzyme inhibitors such as captopril has brought hope that renovascular hypertension could be treated medically. This is possible in some patients, but there are problems with membranous glomerulopathy associated with long-term drug therapy. Proteinuria and, at times, irreversible renal damage may occur while taking this drug, making it hazardous without careful patient monitoring. In addition, a marked reduction in vascular outflow resistance at the arteriolar level within the kidney can cause stasis and thrombosis distal to a critical renal artery stenosis. This has been reported on many occasions, and we have seen five patients in whom this has occurred with an attendant marked reduction in renal function and mass.

There is no question that renal artery reconstruction in the child is a durable procedure that produces a positive effect, with blood pressure reduction over a long period of time. The same is true with the treatment of fibrodysplastic disease in the young female. There is some debate as to the routine recommendation of operative therapy for the atherosclerotic patient. It would appear that the patient with minimal generalized disease and focal extensive disease involving the ostia of the renal artery benefits most from revascularization of occluding lesions. In the patient with severe generalized atherosclerosis, as manifested by involvement of other organs such as heart and brain, the chance for salutary results is somewhat less; in this group of patients, operation should be reserved for those with uncontrollable hypertension and/or failing renal function secondary to progressive renal artery occlusive disease.

Preoperative Preparation. Past recommendations that most major antihypertensive drugs be stopped at varying times prior to operation are difficult to reconcile. There were isolated reports of death secondary to anesthesia superimposed on a patient taking propranolol. As we have reviewed these incidents, it becomes clear that all these patients were hypovolemic at the time of induction of anesthesia. There is no question but that the beta blockade incurred by the use of propranolol, combined with the alpha blockade induced by anesthesia superimposed on a hypovolemic patient, is dangerous. On the other hand, the authors have observed many problems with uncontrollable hypertension in the preoperative period after important drug therapy is stopped. This is particularly true of the patient with renovascular hypertension where control is often difficult and where sudden changes in blood pressure not only add an extra burden to the heart but place the patient in jeopardy for intracranial bleeding or acute renal failure.

With the recognition that most problems are secondary to hypovolemia and that the correction of this state is critical in the preoperative period, the authors have found it perfectly safe to continue all antihypertensive therapy in the preoperative and perioperative periods.

By definition, the average patient with hypertension is hypovolemic. When drug therapy utilizing a diuretic is superimposed upon this state, patients present themselves in need of volume replacement prior to operation. Cognizance of this fact in treating the young patient with an otherwise normal heart is important. Routinely, these patients are hydrated in the 18 to 24 h preoperatively, with particular attention being paid to potassium replacement. The hypokalemia exhibited by these patients is again usually secondary to the diuretic therapy. Great care must be taken when hydration is accomplished in these patients to prevent excessive elevation of blood pressure. It may be necessary on occasion to control blood pressure during this period of time with vasodilating drugs such as intravenous sodium nitroprusside.

The patient with myocardial disease poses a somewhat different problem than does the young patient with hypertension. Prolonged hypertension causing left ventricular hypertrophy and superimposed coronary artery occlusive disease requires careful monitoring prior to increasing the patient's total blood volume. This requires the placement of a Swan-Ganz catheter, with determination of the patient's cardiac output and total peripheral resistance, as well as of the pulmonary capillary wedge pressure. Most

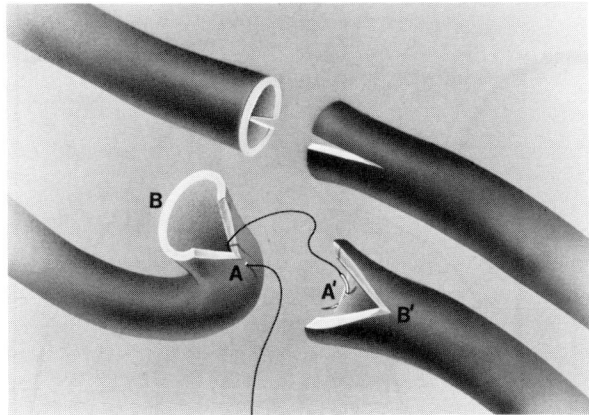

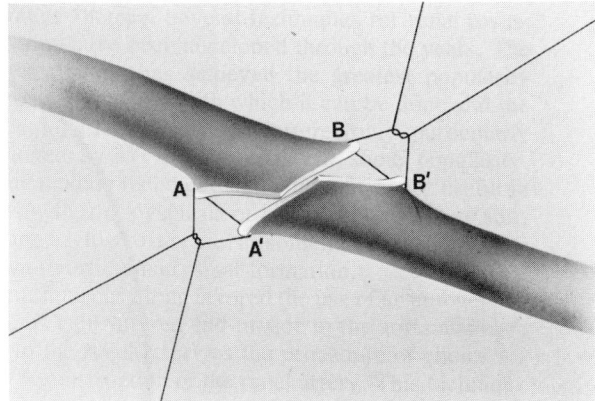

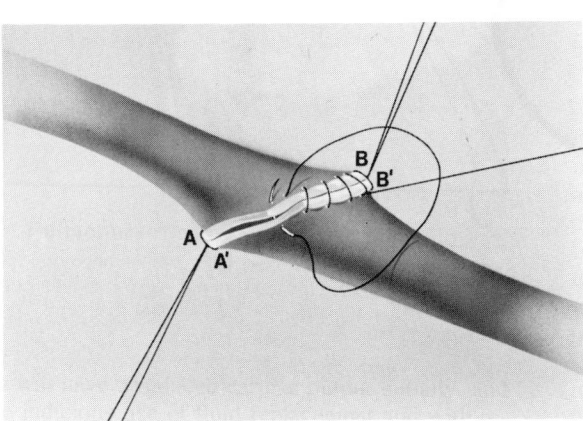

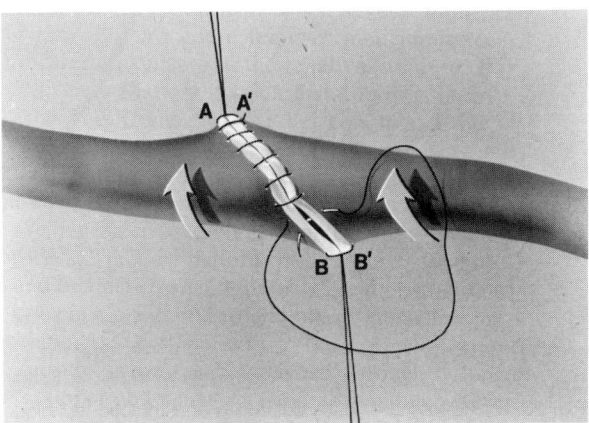

Fig. 23-13. End-to-end spatulated arterial anastomosis using two-point transfixion.

children. Dilatation is seen in approximately 15 percent of the cases. It has not required graft excision; however, these patients must be watched closely. There is some indication that the harvesting and care of the vein are partially responsible for degeneration, but this is not completely substantiated. Because of the incidence of aneurysmal dilation in the autogenous saphenous vein used in children, we would recommend the use of autologous artery whenever possible. Since there have been no aneurysmal changes in vein grafts used in adult patients, we feel that autogenous saphenous vein is the preferable conduit to use in renal arterial reconstruction. Whenever possible the saphenous vein should be harvested at the ankle. This has two advantages. The veins appear thicker; we have seen little in the way of aneurysmal dilatation in veins harvested from this area. In most instances harvesting the vein at the ankle preserves the rest of the saphenous vein for future need.

Transaortic endarterectomy in atheromatous occlusive disease of the renal artery has proved to be a good technique for disobliteration in certain select patients with renal artery occlusive disease. As mentioned before, patients with a soft, ragged aortic intima do not lend themselves well to endarterectomy. This technique is particularly useful in patients who have multiple renal arteries affected by atherosclerosis, allowing a one-stage operative procedure with a relatively short clamp time. Figure

23-14 illustrates five partially occluded renal arteries. Exposure of the aorta is carried out utilizing the same technique as previously described for exposure of the left renal artery. By extending the dissection, the entire abdominal aorta with all its branches may be exposed. Following exposure of the entire upper abdominal aorta, the patient is heparinized, and a clamp is applied to the supraceliac aorta. Following this, the aorta is opened through the midline between the renal arteries, and the incision is carried off to the left superior mesenteric artery (Fig. 23-15).

It is important to note that the renal arteries must be dissected free on both sides prior to opening the aorta. The endarterectomy of the aorta is started superiorly and carried distally to the point of the renal artery ostia. At this point the assistant gently inverts the renal artery so that the entire plaque can be removed; by this technique one can see whether there is feathering of the plaque so that there is no question of a distal intimal flap. Following the removal of the atheromatous material from the aorta and the renal arteries, the endarterectomy is terminated below the renal arteries; the flap may be tacked at this point if necessary (Fig. 23-16). The aortotomy is then closed utilizing a running arterial suture. The clamps are slowly removed, allowing blood flow in the aorta and the

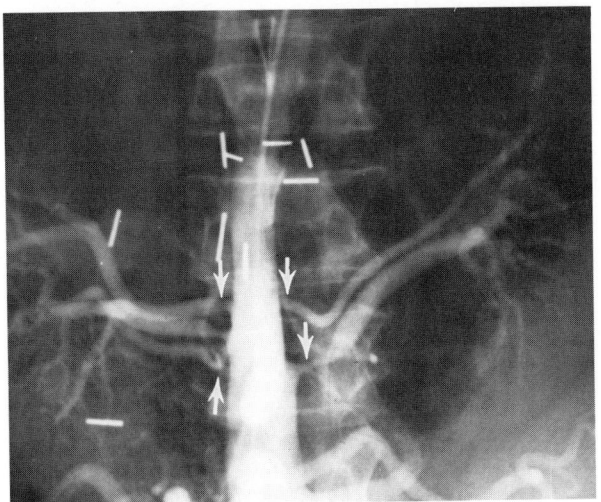

Fig. 23-14. Patient with five renal arteries (see arrows).

visceral and renal arteries. At the completion of the procedure an arteriogram must be done in order to determine good flow to both renal arteries and to rule out any chance for an intimal flap. This is best done by reapplying the clamps and injecting a small amount of contrast material into the aorta in order to visualize both renal arteries. If a small intimal flap is evident it can be dealt with by a separate arteriotomy in the renal artery with or without the utilization of a venous patch graft. When the operative ultrasound is available, it may obviate the need for postoperative angiogram. It has been shown to be exceedingly accurate and when it becomes generally available may replace the need for angiography. Utilizing this technique, Wylie and associates have reported excellent results, substantiated in a limited series by the authors.

The technique of ex vivo repair of renal artery lesions has been championed by Belzer. His reports indicate that, in certain well-selected cases, this technique is very helpful. It should be reserved for lesions that involve mul-

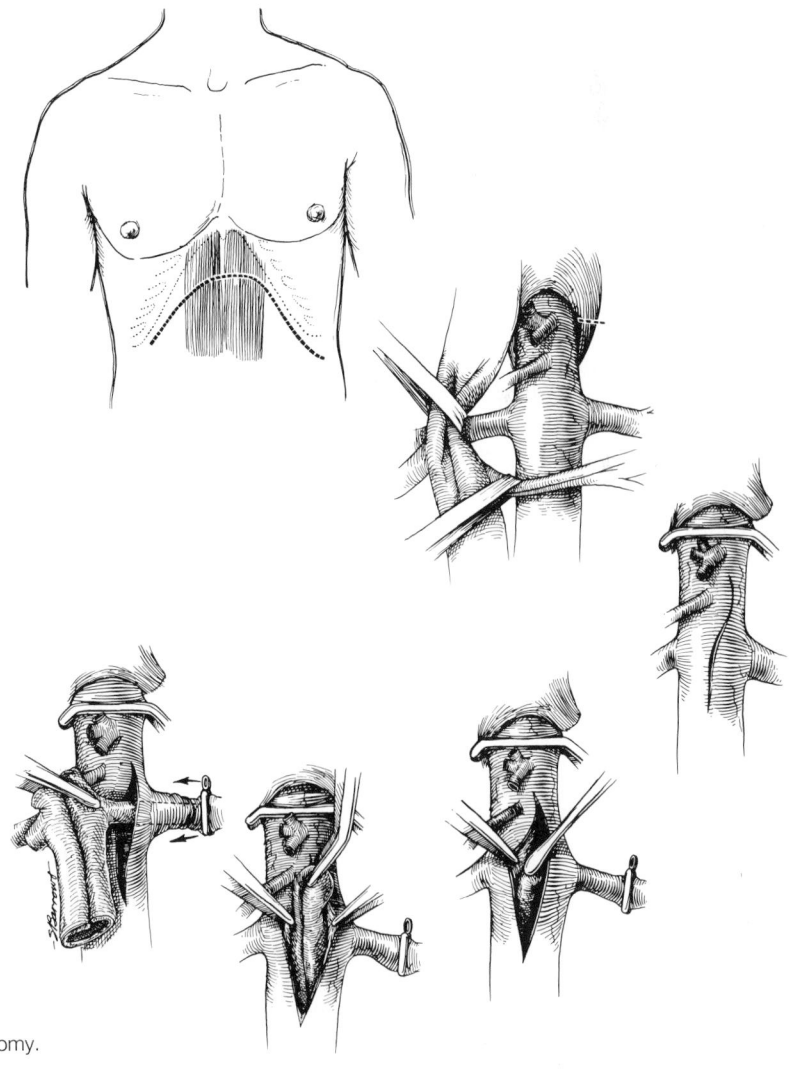

Fig. 23-15. Technique of transaortic endarterectomy.

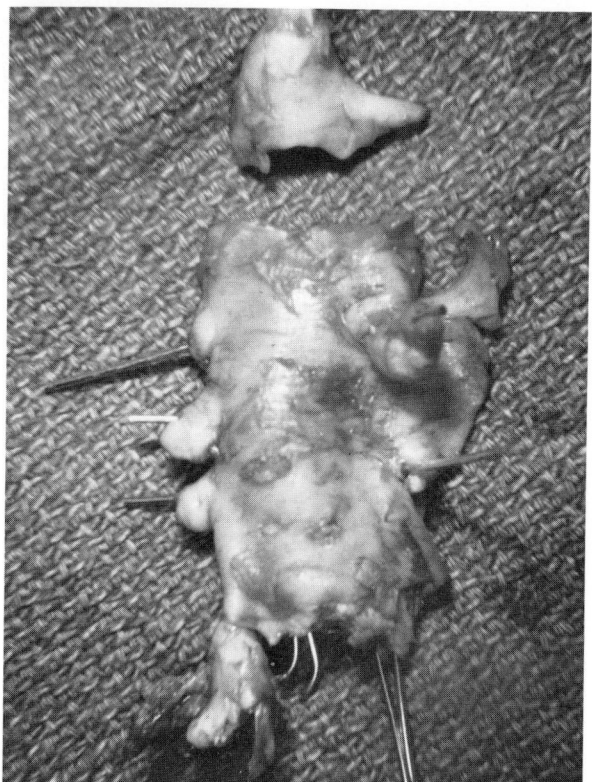

Fig. 23-16. Endarterectomy specimen of lesion seen in Fig. 23-14. Probes are in the renal artery orifices.

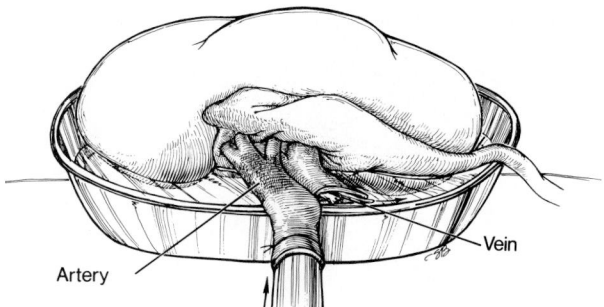

Fig. 23-17. Kidney prepared for ex vivo repair.

tiple branches such as fibrodysplastic disease; aneurysm where multiple branches are involved; renal artery dissections; or those lesions, previously revascularized, with problems such as secondary stenosis. Reoperation on the renal artery is particularly difficult as the renal vein invariably becomes adherent to the renal artery, and it is difficult to dissect free without a great deal of blood loss. The ability to take the kidney out of the abdomen and perfuse it in a bloodless field allows an accurate, safe technique for renal revascularization in the difficult lesion.

The kidney is removed from the abdomen by dividing the renal artery and vein; the renal artery is then perfused with cold Locke's solution at 4°C. This washes all the blood from the renal vasculature and cools the kidney. It allows the surgeon adequate time to carefully dissect out the renal vasculature. Repair can then be instituted (Fig. 23-17). Multiple renal artery lesions can be repaired by utilizing the internal iliac artery or by fashioning multiple branches off an autogenous saphenous vein. Following the completion of the multiple distal anastomoses, the kidney may be implanted back into the original bed or may be moved down into the pelvis, anastomosing the renal artery to the internal iliac artery and renal vein to the iliac vein, a technique similar to that of a renal transplant. If great care is taken in dissecting out the ureter to preserve its blood supply, it is not necessary to reimplant the ureter. We routinely leave the ureter intact and, in

most instances, have reanastomosed the renal vein and utilized the graft, either autogenous saphenous vein or internal iliac graft anastomosis to the side of the aorta. This is feasible and seems to cut down the number of anastomoses and any potential problems with a pelvic kidney.

The problems attendant on the use of this technique are important to recognize. Removal of the kidney from the abdomen completely interrupts all arterial collaterals. Therefore, it is incumbent upon the surgeon to make sure that the anastomoses are technically perfect and that blood flow is reestablished to the kidney at the time of reimplantation. This is best done with a completion arteriogram. If the kidney is placed back in its original bed, it is important to fix it to Gerota's fascia so that it will not rotate on its axis and cause kinking of the renal artery bypass graft.

Belzer has reported outstanding results with this technique; when it is used for the indications outlined, it extends the ability of the vascular surgeon to salvage kidneys with extensive renovascular disease.

Nephrectomy. Nephrectomy is seldom indicated in the treatment of renovascular hypertension because the goal is to preserve renal mass whenever possible. The removal of thrombus from a renal artery where there has been an extensive infarction is contraindicated. This requires a nephrectomy, as the chance for reestablishing significant renal function is negligible (Fig. 23-18*A*, *B*, *C*). Multiple areas of infarction secondary to emboli from a renal artery aneurysm, or from ulcerative aortic disease, are best treated by a nephrectomy unless the contralateral kidney is severely diseased. Severe intraparenchymal occlusive disease, of either an atherosclerotic or a fibrodysplastic nature, does not lend itself to revascularization and is best treated by nephrectomy. This assumes a relatively normal contralateral kidney.

RESULTS. The effectiveness of operative therapy for renal artery occlusive disease is determined by reduction of blood pressure over a long period of time. Over 50 patients in the pediatric age group have been followed by the authors. It has been particularly gratifying to see this group of patients maintain normal pressures through follow-up as long as 18 years. In this series of patients, 85 percent have been cured and are off all medication. Twelve percent are improved, requiring only minimal medication in the form of a diuretic to maintain normal

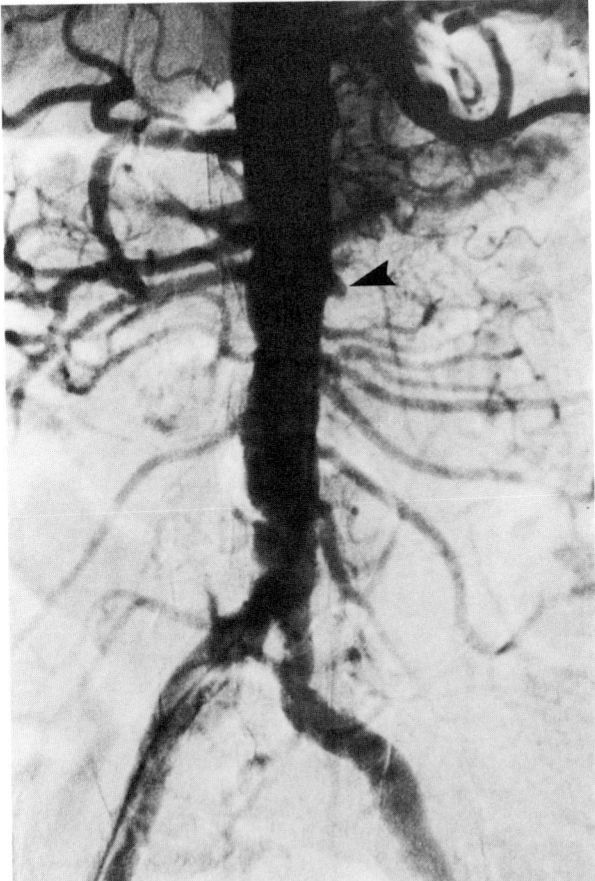

A

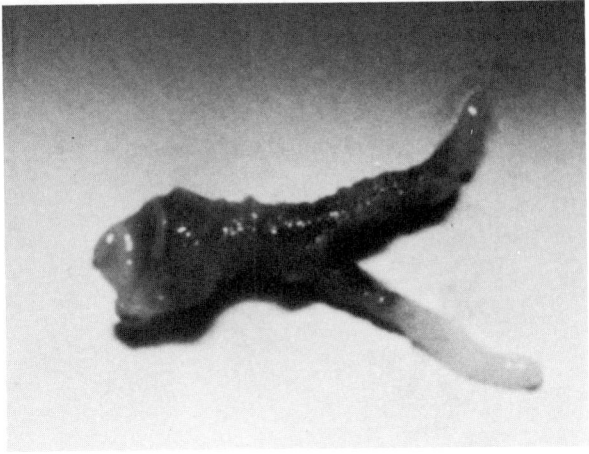

B

440 32 6773

C

Fig. 23-18. *A.* Flush aortogram showing occluded left renal artery with distal vessel reconstitution (arrow). *B.* Extensive thrombus taken from the occluded renal artery seen in the previous arteriogram. *C.* Isotope washout curve of left kidney (bottom curve), showing minimal function after technically successful revascularization.

blood pressure. Of the entire group of children treated, only one patient has had no salutary result from the operative procedure. The latter patient has a diffuse vasculitis involving both renal arteries and the interrenal branches.

Fibrodysplastic disease in the adult, primarily in female patients, has been followed in a series of 144 patients for a minimum of 5 years to a maximum of 21 years. A sustained 55 percent cure rate and a 39 percent improved rate have been noted, giving a total of 94 percent positive results with only a 6 percent failure rate.

Atherosclerosis as a cause of renovascular occlusive disease is difficult to categorize. It is best categorized as *focal* and *diffuse* disease. Focal disease does not have any associated atherosclerotic or aneurysmal involvement of the cerebral, coronary, visceral, or lower extremity vessels. In this group of patients, followed for a minimum of 5 years, the long-term records reveal 91 percent good results with only 9 percent failure. This group generally does well, with a 12 percent attrition rate, secondary to other manifestations of atherosclerosis, over a 5-year period.

Generalized atherosclerosis with overt generalized disease has been a problem in both medical and surgical therapy. The authors have examined a series of 58 patients who fall into this category and were operated upon for renal revascularization. The results were outstanding, with a cure or improved rate of 93 percent. There is a consistent 15 percent renal function improvement rate in this series of patients. The long-term mortality rate of this group is higher than that of any other group because of established generalized atherosclerotic disease. The most common cause of demise is myocardial infarction. In view of these results, the authors have taken a more liberal attitude in recommending operative therapy in this group of patients. Concomitant operative procedures significantly increase the operative mortality of these patients. When aortic grafting for aneurysmal or occlusive disease is performed concomitantly with renal revascularization, great care must be taken in assessing the myocardial reserve of the patient. Extreme care must be taken in monitoring and maintaining optimal cardiac function in the preoperative, perioperative, and postoperative periods.

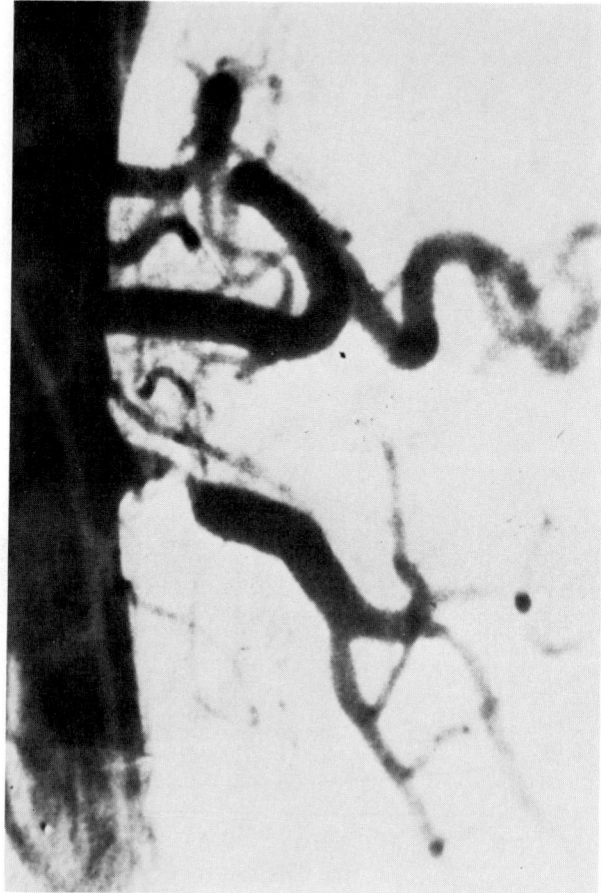

A

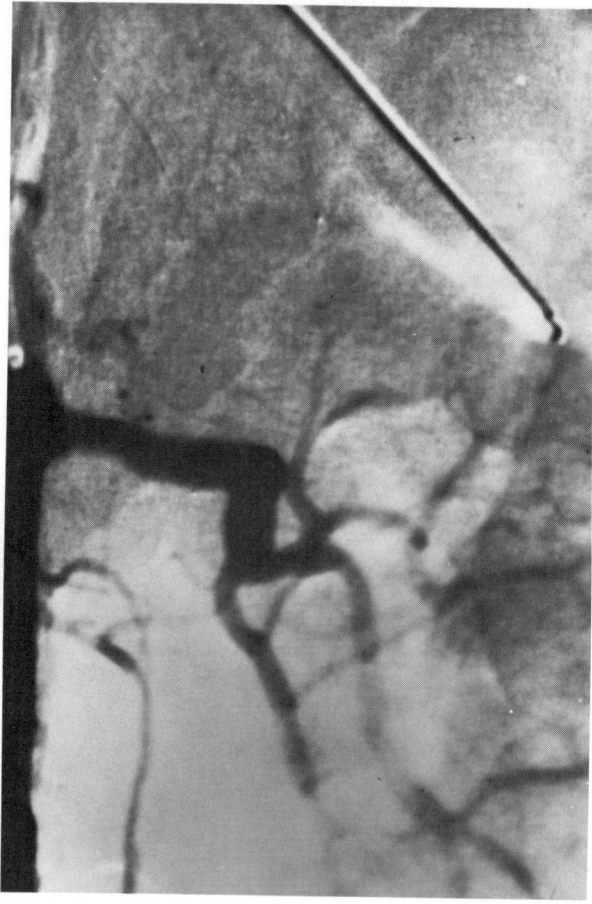

B

Fig. 23-19. *A.* Stenotic atherosclerotic renal artery lesion before balloon angioplasty. *B.* After the procedure.

The utilization of long-term medical therapy for the patient with overt renovascular occlusive disease carries a relatively high mortality, as reported by several authors. Dean has reported a rather alarming progression of atherosclerotic occlusive disease in the renal arteries in those patients treated with a careful medical program. It would seem that this form of therapy is not as good an alternative as arterial reconstruction.

The use of balloon angioplasty to dilate lesions of the renal artery has achieved great popularity (Fig. 23-19*A*, *B*). The longest mean follow-up is approaching 2 years. The cure or improvement rate is generally between 10 and 15 percent lower than that achieved by careful surgical repair. Although the technique has the attractive features of a less invasive procedure and a shorter hospital stay, complications occur. A 5 to 10 percent morbidity rate has been reported, including perforation of the renal artery (Fig. 23-20), thrombosis of the renal artery, distal embolization, disruption of aortic or renal artery atheromata, inability to pass the guidewire through the stenosing lesion, femoral artery thrombosis, and hematoma. It would seem currently that this is an alternative that may supplant surgical therapy in selected fibromuscular or atheromatous lesions involving the midrenal artery. Ostial atheromas and complex fibromuscular lesions are often not suitable for balloon angioplasty.

Bibliography

Endocrine Disease and Hypertension

Bravo EL, Gifford RW: Pheochromocytoma: Diagnosis, localization and management. *N Engl J Med* 311:1298, 1984.

Carpenter PC: Cushing's syndrome: Update of diagnosis and management. *Mayo Clin Proc* 61:49, 1986.

Guerin CK, Wahner HW, et al: Computed tomographic scanning vs. radioisotope imaging in adrenocortical diagnosis. *Am J Med* 75:653, 1983.

Mackett MCT, Crane MG, Smith LL: Surgical treatment of aldosterone-producing adrenal adenomas: A review of 16 patients. *Am J Surg* 142:89, 1981.

Schteingart DE, Motazedi A, et al: Treatment of adrenal carcinomas. *Arch Surg* 117:1142, 1982.

Sisson JC, Shapiro B, et al: Locating pheochromocytomas by scintigraphy using ^{131}I-metaiodobenzylguanidine. *Ca-A* 34:86, 1984.

vanHeerden JA, Scheps SG, et al: Pheochromocytoma: Current status and changing trends. *Surgery* 91:367, 1982.

Coarctation of the Aorta

Dean RH, Scott HW: Subisthmic aortic coarctations, in Dean RH, O'Neill JA (eds): *Vascular Disorders of Childhood*. Philadelphia, Lea & Febiger, 1983.

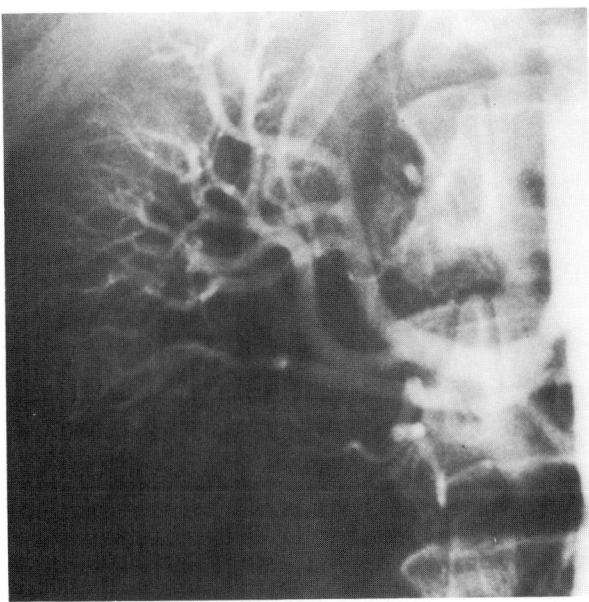

A

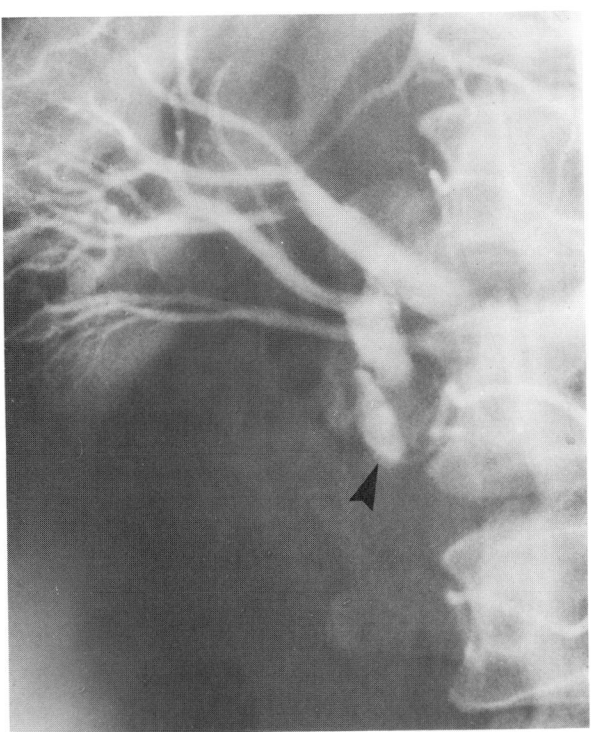

B

Fig. 23-20. *A.* Arteriogram of right renal artery stenosis at ostium. *B.* Perforation of right renal artery after attempted balloon angioplasty (extravasation at arrow).

Marol BJ, Humphries JO, et al: Prognosis of surgically corrected coarctation of the aorta. A twenty-year post-operative appraisal. *Circulation* 47:119, 1973.

Petracek MR, Hammon JW: Thoracic-aortic (isthmic) coarctation, in Dean RH, O'Neill JA (eds): *Vascular Disorders of Childhood.* Philadelphia, Lea & Febiger, 1983.

Schumacker HB Jr, King H, et al: Coarctation of the aorta. *Curr Probl Surg* February 1968.

Renovascular Hypertension

Cohn JN, Franciosa JA: Vasodilator therapy of cardiac failure, part I. *N Engl J Med* 297:27, 1977.

Cohn JN, Franciosa JA: Vasodilator therapy of cardiac failure, part II. *N Engl J Med* 297:254, 1977.

Dean RH, Kiefer RW, et al: Renovascular hypertension: Anatomic and renal function changes during drug therapy. *Arch Surg* 16:1408, 1981.

Dean RH, Krueger TC, et al: Operative management of renovascular hypertension. Results after followup of 15–23 years. *J Vasc Surg* 1:234, 1984.

Dean RH, Lawson JD, et al: Revascularization of the poorly functioning kidney. *Surgery* 85:44, 1979.

Kohler TR, Zierler RE, et al: Noninvasive diagnosis of renal artery stenosis by ultrasonic duplex scanning. *J Vasc Surg* 4:450, 1986.

Kuhlmann U, Greminger P, et al: Long-term experience and percutaneous transluminal dilatation of renal artery stenosis. *Am J Med* 79:692, 1985.

Moncure AC, Brewster DC, Darling RC: Use of splenic and hepatic arteries for renal revascularization. *J Vasc Surg* 3:196, 1986.

Pickering TG, Sos TA, Laragh JH: The role of balloon dilatation in the treatment of renovascular hypertension. *Am J Med* 77 (suppl):61, 1984.

Stanley JC, Ernest CB, Fry WJ: *Renovascular Hypertension.* New York, Saunders, 1984.

Stanley JC, Fry WJ: Pediatric renal artery occlusive disease and renovascular hypertension: Etiology, diagnosis and operative treatment. *Arch Surg* 116:669, 1981.

Stanley JC, Rhodes EL, et al: Renal artery aneurysms: Significance of macroaneurysms exclusive of dissections and fibrodysplastic mural dilations. *Arch Surg* 110:1327, 1975.

Stanley JC, Whitehouse WM, et al: Reoperation for complications of renal artery reconstructive surgery undertaken for treatment of renovascular hypertension. *J Vasc Surg* 2:133, 1985.

Stoney RJ, DeLuccia N, et al: Aorto-renal arterial autographs. Long-term assessment. *Arch Surg* 116:416, 1981.

Stoney RJ, Silane M, Salvatierra O: Ex vivo renal artery reconstruction. *Arch Surg* 113:1272, 1978.

Stuart MT, Smith RB, et al: Concomitant renal revascularization of patients undergoing aortic surgery. *J Vasc Surg* 2:400, 1985.

Textor SC, Gephardt GN, et al: Membranous glomerulopathy associated with captopril therapy. *Am J Med* 74:705, 1983.

Textor SC, Tarazir C, et al: Regulation of renal hemodynamics and glomerular filtration of patients with renovascular hypertension during converting enzyme inhibition with captopril. *Am J Med* 76 (suppl):29, 1984.

Thibonnier M, Joseph A, et al: Improved diagnosis of unilateral renal artery lesions after captopril administration. *JAMA* 251:56, 1984.

Ying CY, Tifft CP, et al: Renal revascularization in the azotemic hypertensive patient resistant to therapy. *N Engl J Med* 311:1070, 1984.

Chapter 24

Manifestations of Gastrointestinal Disease

Seymour I. Schwartz

Symptoms represent subjective manifestations of disturbance in function and are not specific for a disease but rather for a pathophysiologic state. In the gastrointestinal tract, the following changes in physiologic function may be implicated: altered secretion, altered motility, inadequate digestion, inadequate absorption, obstruction. The resultant symptoms of gastrointestinal disease include abdominal pain, dysphagia, anorexia, nausea and vomiting, bloating or distention, constipation, and diarrhea.

Signs of gastrointestinal disease are objective demonstrations of a pathologic process. These include tenderness, abdominal wall rigidity, palpable masses, altered bowel sounds, evidence of gastrointestinal bleeding, poor nutrition, jaundice, and stigmata of hepatic dysfunction.

PAIN

Pain (from the Latin *poena*, penalty, punishment, torment) is the predominant sensory experience by which humans judge the existence of disease within themselves. Most diseases of the abdominal viscera are associated with pain at some time during their course. Indeed, the correct diagnosis of acute abdominal disorders (the "acute abdomen") usually amounts to the correct identification of the cause of the abdominal pain.

Although there is not yet unequivocal proof that each peripheral nerve fiber is devoted to but one type of sensory modality—pain, touch, cold, or warmth—most physiologists now subscribe to the *specificity theory*, which holds that pain is a separate sensory modality with its own specific neural apparatus. In 1965 Melzack and Wall proposed the *gate-control theory*. They disagreed with the proposal that sensation is achieved by a fixed direct-line communication from skin to brain. Their contribution was the suggestion that the amount and quality of perceived pain are determined by many physiologic and psychologic variables. Modulation of nociceptive impulses occurs at the dorsal horn and at various levels of the ascending afferent systems. The gate-control theory has been the basis for methods of pain-inhibiting electrical stimulation. With transcutaneous nerve stimulation (TNS), electrodes are placed on the surface overlying the painful area, and nonpain fibers are activated.

Appropriate stimuli initiate impulses in skin, muscle, or viscera. These sensory impulses are transmitted to the posterior horn of the spinal cord in the primary sensory neuron that has its cell body in the dorsal root ganglion. The secondary sensory neuron in the posterior horn transmits the impulses in the contralateral spinothalamic tract to the posterolateral nucleus of the thalamus. The

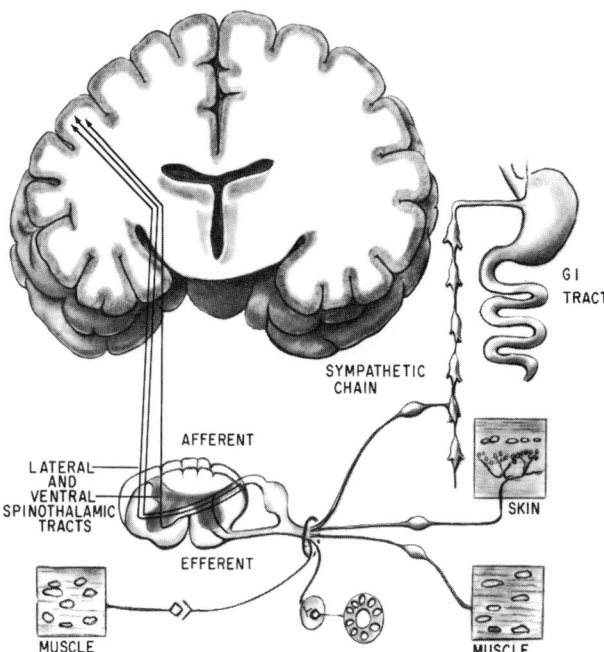

Fig. 24-1. Schematic representation of pathways involved in abdominal pain.

tertiary sensory neuron transmits the impulses from the thalamus to the postcentral gyrus of the cerebral cortex (Fig. 24-1).

Three kinds of pain have been designated: superficial, or cutaneous pain; deep pain from muscles, tendons, joints, and fascia; and visceral pain. The first two may be combined as somatic pain. Knowledge of visceral pain has lagged, in part because of the difficulty of the laboratory investigation.

PAIN PATHWAYS. Until well into the twentieth century, the viscera were thought to be completely insensitive. The first important observer of visceral sensation was William Harvey in the seventeenth century. When the young son of Count Montgomery sustained a chest wound which on healing left the heart exposed, Harvey observed that touching the heart caused not the slightest sensation. After the discovery of local anesthesia, Lennander found that human abdominal viscera are insensitive to cutting, crushing, and even burning. He categorically stated in 1901 that the viscera are wholly insensitive and that only traction or irritation of the parietal peritoneum could cause abdominal pain. The record was set straight in 1911 by Hurst, who demonstrated that distention of any hollow viscus is painful. Ryle amplified this by emphasizing that contraction of smooth muscle of hollow viscera is a physiologic stimulus adequate to cause pain.

The current and preferable terminology uses the term *visceral afferents* to denote all afferent fibers from the viscera including those that give rise to visceral reflexes as well as those that subserve pain. The terms *autonomic, sympathetic,* and *parasympathetic* are reserved for the visceral *efferent* fibers.

Pain impulses from the abdominal cavity reach the central nervous system by three routes: from the viscera via visceral afferents that travel with (1) the sympathetic and (2) the parasympathetic nerves, and from the parietal peritoneum, body wall, diaphragm, and root of mesenteries via somatic afferents that travel in (3) the segmental spinal nerves or phrenic nerves. Primary sensory neurons for pain, both visceral and somatic, are mostly small (1 to 2 μm), unmyelinated fibers but with some small (3 to 4 μm), myelinated fibers (Gasser classes C and A delta, or groups IV and III in Lloyd's terminology).

The route of a typical afferent from an abdominal viscus is as follows: the axons of nerve endings in the wall of the viscus follow the artery to the aorta and then through the collateral sympathetic ganglion without synapsing. They then enter the splanchnic nerve, traverse the paravertebral sympathetic ganglion, again without synapsing, and join the spinal nerve via the white ramus communicans. The cell body of this primary visceral afferent neuron is located in the spinal ganglion from which central processes are sent to the dorsal horn of the spinal cord via the dorsal root.

The central processes of the primary sensory neuron synapse with at least three distinct spinal tracts: (1) secondary pain neurons whose axons ascend for two or three segments and then cross in the anterior commissure to the anterolateral spinothalamic tract, (2) secondary sensory neurons whose processes ascend the posterior columns, and (3) many small neurons in the substantia gelatinosa that contribute to the tract of Lissauer. As the secondary sensory neurons ascend, collaterals are given off to the reticular substance forming the core of the brainstem and to the hypothalamus. The role of these extraspinothalamic pathways is uncertain—they may be alternative pain pathways, may inhibit central pain responses, or may be involved in the affective aspects of pain. Sensory tracts synapse in the thalamus with tertiary neurons that project to the cortex. The cortical areas involved with pain are not completely known. Stimulation of various areas of the postcentral gyrus in the conscious human being produces contralateral paresthesia of small areas of the body, but even total hemispherectomy does not consistently abolish pain, though localization is defective. The functions of the thalamus in human beings, in contrast to animals, are largely expressed through the cortex. But one function that may have been retained in the evolutionary process is the expression of the affective aspects of sensation. Affectivity—pleasantness and unpleasantness—is considered a primitive function that has remained at the thalamic level despite development of the cerebral cortex.

Though the thalamus and frontal cortex are the principal areas of the brain involved with pain, they cannot be considered as *the* brain centers, since the hypothalamus, the limbic system, the brainstem reticular formation, and the parietal cortex are also involved in pain reception. Opiate receptors exist in the brainstem and spinal cord, and naturally occurring opiates are found in the brain and pituitary. These are collectively called *endorphins*. Pain relief from low-frequency electrical stimulation exerts its effect by increasing these endorphin levels, an effect that can be blocked by the opiate antagonist, naloxone.

Abdominal Pain

PATHOPHYSIOLOGY

Three distinct types of pain are involved in the general symptom complex of abdominal pain: visceral pain, (deep) somatic pain, and referred pain.

VISCERAL PAIN. True visceral pain, or splanchnic pain, arises in abdominal organs invested with visceral peritoneum via impulses conducted to the spinal cord over visceral afferent nerve fibers. As noted above, the viscera are normally insensitive to stimuli that produce pain when applied to the skin. Adequate stimuli for visceral pain are those arising from their own environment—pathologic conditions of the viscera. Stimuli that produce pain include increased tension in the wall of hollow viscera from either distention or spastic contraction, stretching of the capsules of solid viscera, ischemia, and certain chemicals. The threshold for pain is lowered by inflammation and by ischemia, so that normal muscular contractions that would ordinarily not be felt may produce pain.

The role of chemical substances in visceral pain is not clear. Experimentally, pain can be produced by the intraarterial injection of acid, alkaline, or hypertonic solutions: lactate, potassium ions, or bradykinin. Potassium that is released from cells by injury or ischemia has long been known as a pain-producing agent, and it has been suggested that the release of intracellular potassium ions may be the actual physiologic stimulus for pain. Some pain receptors have been classified as chemoceptors, and the pain of ischemia has been attributed to increasing concentrations of hydrogen ions. The pain of inflammation is thought to be caused by the accrual of algesic bradykinin peptides that activate pain receptors more or less selectively. The bradykinin effect is facilitated in the presence of prostaglandins, and it is this mechanism that is inhibited by aspirin.

Visceral pain tends to be rather diffuse and poorly localized, has a high threshold, and exhibits an exceedingly slow rate of adaptation. The high threshold and poor localization are probably in part attributable to the relatively sparse distribution of sensory endings in the viscera. The pain is felt by the patient to be "deep" in those cutaneous areas or zones that correspond roughly to the segmental distribution of somatic sensory fibers that take origin from the same segments of the cord as the visceral afferent fibers from the viscus in question.

With severe visceral or deep somatic pain, concomitant responses, presumably due to autonomic reflexes, may be prominent. These include sweating; nausea, sometimes with vomiting; tachycardia or bradycardia; fall in blood pressure; cutaneous hyperalgesia, hyperesthesia, or tenderness; and involuntary spastic contractions of abdominal wall musculature. The muscular rigidity accompanying severe pain is most marked when the body wall is involved by the pain-inciting lesion, e.g., the boardlike rigidity associated with perforated peptic ulcer. The distribution is regional rather than segmental and thus involves sustained reflexes in several segmental nerves. Maintained muscular rigidity may of itself become painful, so that on occasion the deep muscular tenderness outlasts and outweighs the original visceral pain.

SOMATIC PAIN. Pain arising in the abdominal wall, particularly the parietal peritoneum, root of the mesenteries, and respiratory diaphragm, is mediated by somatic afferents in segmental spinal nerves. Pain from parietal structures is for the most part sharper and brighter than visceral pain; it is well localized close to the site of stimulation; and when the source is on one side of the midline, the pain is also lateralized. Acute appendicitis is a common visceral disease that well illustrates typical visceral and somatic abdominal pain. The visceral pain of early appendicitis is perceived diffusely and dully in the periumbilical and lower epigastric regions, and there is little or no rigidity of the abdominal musculature. Later, when parietal peritoneum becomes involved in the inflammatory process, the somatic component of pain is more severe and sharply localized in the right lower quadrant. There is also cutaneous hyperesthesia, tenderness, and muscular rigidity in the right lower quadrant.

REFERRED PAIN. Visceral disease may give rise to pain localized to more superficial areas of the body, often at a considerable distance from the diseased viscus. The reference is usually dermatomic, but on occasion pain may be referred to the scar of a previous surgical operation, trauma, or localized pathologic process. This is called *habit reference* and implies that pain perception is influenced by the individual's prior pain experience.

The currently accepted reasoning for the dermatomic reference of visceral pain is the *convergence-projection* hypothesis. Since the pain fibers in the posterior roots greatly outnumber the fibers in the spinothalamic tracts, several pain fibers must converge on one tract fiber. This same convergence may occur at thalmaic or cortical levels as well. When afferents from the skin and viscera converge on the same neuron at some point in the pain pathway, the resulting impulses, on projection to the brain, are interpreted as coming from the skin, an interpretation learned from previous experiences in which the same tract fiber was stimulated by cutaneous afferents.

CLINICAL CONSIDERATIONS

ETIOLOGY. Abdominal pain may be caused by a great variety of gastrointestinal and intraperitoneal diseases, and, because of overlapping nerve distribution, the pain may be secondary to extraperitoneal disorders. Pain of intraabdominal origin (Table 24-1) may emanate from the peritoneum, hollow intestinal viscera, solid viscera, mesentery, or pelvic organs and may be caused by inflammation, mechanical processes such as obstruction or acute distention, and vascular disturbances.

The extraperitoneal causes of abdominal pain are outlined in Table 24-2. Most of the intrathoracic diseases that

Table 24-1. GASTROINTESTINAL AND INTRAPERITONEAL CAUSES OF ABDOMINAL PAIN

I. Inflammation
  A. Peritoneum
    1. Chemical and nonbacterial peritonitis—perforated peptic ulcer, gallbladder, ruptured ovarian cyst, mittelschmerz
    2. Bacterial peritonitis
      a. Primary peritonitis—pneumococcal, streptococcal, tuberculous
      b. Perforated hollow viscus—stomach, intestine, biliary tract
  B. Hollow intestinal organs
    1. Appendicitis
    2. Cholecystitis
    3. Peptic ulceration
    4. Gastroenteritis
    5. Regional enteritis
    6. Meckel's diverticulitis
    7. Colitis—ulcerative, bacterial, amebic
    8. Diverticulitis
  C. Solid viscera
    1. Pancreatitis
    2. Hepatitis
    3. Hepatic abscess
    4. Splenic abscess
  D. Mesentery
    1. Lymphadenitis
  E. Pelvic organs
    1. Pelvic inflammatory disease
    2. Tuboovarian abscess
    3. Endometritis

II. Mechanical (obstruction, acute distention)
  A. Hollow intestinal organs
    1. Intestinal obstruction—adhesions, hernia, tumor, volvulus, intussusception
    2. Biliary obstruction—calculi, tumor, choledochal cyst, hematobilia
  B. Solid viscera
    1. Acute splenomegaly
    2. Acute hepatomegaly—cardiac failure, Budd-Chiari syndrome
  C. Mesentery
    1. Omental torsion
  D. Pelvic organs
    1. Ovarian cyst
    2. Torsion or degeneration of fibroid
    3. Ectopic pregnancy
III. Vascular
  A. Intraperitoneal bleeding
    1. Ruptured liver
    2. Ruptured spleen
    3. Ruptured mesentery
    4. Ruptured ectopic pregnancy
    5. Ruptured aortic, splenic, or hepatic aneurysm
  B. Ischemia
    1. Mesenteric thrombosis
    2. Hepatic infarction—toxemia, purpura
    3. Splenic infarction
    4. Omental ischemia
IV. Miscellaneous
  A. Endometriosis

cause abdominal pain are confused with upper abdominal disorders, since their segmental distribution is similar. The intraspinal diseases have pain patterns similar to the referred pain from abdominal pathologic conditions, but

Table 24-2. EXTRAPERITONEAL CAUSES OF ABDOMINAL PAIN

Cardiopulmonary	*Vascular*
Pneumonia	Dissection, rupture, or
Empyema	expansion of aortic an-
Myocardial ischemia	eurysm
Active rheumatic heart dis-	Periarteritis
ease	*Metabolic*
Blood	Uremia
Leukemia	Diabetic acidosis
Sickle cell crisis	Porphyria
Neurogenic	Addisonian crisis
Spinal cord tumors	*Toxins*
Osteomyelitis of spine	Bacterial (tetanus)
Tabes dorsalis	Insect bites
Herpes zoster	Venoms
Abdominal epilepsy	Drugs
Genitourinary	Lead poisoning
Nephritis	*Abdominal wall*
Pyelitis	Intramuscular hematoma
Perinephric abscesses	*Psychogenic*
Ureteral obstruction (cal-	
culi, tumors)	
Prostatitis	
Seminal vesiculitis	
Epidydimitis	

they are usually not accompanied by tenderness or muscular rigidity. Inflammation of peripheral nerves, as in the case of herpes zoster, may be accompanied by tenderness and pain before the lesion becomes apparent. The pain usually has a distribution similar to that associated with myocardial infarction or biliary tract disease.

CLINICAL EVALUATION. Since pain is the subjective reaction to a stimulus that initiates transmission along nerve pathways to cortical centers, the patient's response is dependent upon both physical and psychologic factors. Physical requirements for response to pain include the patient's consciousness to permit perception, and integrity of the entire avenue along which impulses are transmitted to the brain. With repeated stimulation, the cortical threshold becomes lowered, and resistance is reduced along nerve pathways, which results in hypersensitivity and "facilitated pain." Hyperthyroidism, hyperadrenalism, and the menopausal syndrome are all associated with increased response to pain, while hypothyroidism is usually accompanied by an increased pain threshold. Sensitivity alters with age, increasing from infancy to adult life and then gradually diminishing in the elderly patient.

The physical responses to painful stimuli are also variable. While superficial pain is frequently associated with diffuse sympathetic nervous system stimulation and outpouring of epinephrine as part of a defense reaction, severe deep pain is more often accompanied by bradycardia, hypotension, nausea and vomiting, sweating, and, at times, syncope. Continued pain may cause a decrease in renal blood flow, renal clearance, and oliguria. Cardiac arrhythmias may also occur, and, in the extreme case, neurogenic shock may result.

History. In eliciting a description of pain, the character, severity, location, timing, and factors that either augment or reduce the pain should all be defined. Certain pathologic states are associated with characteristic pain patterns. Colic—biliary, ureteral, or intestinal—is intermittent, frequently occurring in waves, and is described as cramping, or the patient may use the very term "colicky." Pain of a penetrating ulcer is "burning," while pain accompanying expansion of an abdominal aneurysm is "boring and pounding," and the pain accompanying pleuritis or perforation of a viscus has been described as "knifelike."

The severity of the pain is an expression of the intensity of stimuli plus the patient's physical and emotional response. Colicky pain related to acute distention of the biliary tract, intestine, or ureters, and pain of neurologic origin such as herpes and tabes all have an extremely high intensity. Pain evoked by inflammatory stimuli is less marked. In patients with peritonitis, the degree of pain and muscular rigidity generally parallel each other. Severe pain may be manifested by physical responses, to which previous reference has been made.

In general, abdominal pains that persist for 6 h are caused by conditions of surgical significance. However, it is rare for any pain to be absolutely constant. The pain resulting from distention of hollow viscera is generally intermittent, while the pain of peritonitis is most frequently continuous. Pain that awakens the patient from sleep is usually characteristic of organic disease. Ulcer pain frequently occurs at night or prior to a meal, whereas gallbladder pain may be stimulated by eating. Peptic ulcer pain also has a seasonal variation, occurring more frequently in the spring and fall. In addition to the effect of digestion of food on the pain, the effects of position, motion, and respiration have diagnostic importance.

The location of pain should include a description of original situation, any shifting, and radiation. The initial location may better define the visceral involvement, since once peritonitis occurs, pain becomes diffuse. Because of variation in location of the organs and the pathologic processes, as well as the vagueness of visceral pain, it is difficult to totally exclude diseases on the basis of location, but certain relationships generally pertain (Fig. 24-2). Visceral intestinal pain is usually experienced in the midportion of the abdomen. Duodenal pain is felt in the epigastrium, while the pain of the remainder of the small intestine is characteristically referred to the region of the umbilicus. Pain originating in the large bowel is less well localized and frequently experienced in the hypogastrium. Sigmoid dilatation may result in suprapubic or presacral pain.

The patient's age represents a factor that focuses attention on certain processes. Acute colicky pain in a child under two is suggestive of intussusception, whereas peptic ulcer is extremely uncommon in the young age group. Appendicitis is most frequently a disease of the young adolescent, cholecystitis is more commonly seen in the middle-age group, while diverticulitis rarely occurs before the age of thirty-five.

Vomiting is indicative of severe irritation of the peritoneum, stretching of the mesentery, obstruction, or absorbed toxins. The exact timing of vomiting in relation to the onset of pain is pertinent. Pain almost always precedes vomiting by several hours in patients with appendicitis. Vomiting may also occur early in relation to the onset of pain in patients with peritonitis and biliary or ureteral colic. With intestinal obstruction, the interval between the onset of pain and vomiting provides some indication of the level of obstruction. Frequent vomiting is indicative of intestinal obstruction, while a clear emesis may accompany biliary obstruction or diseases with pyloric obstruction.

An evaluation of bowel habits is particularly pertinent in patients with colonic obstruction, and a menstrual history is imperative in women with lower abdominal or pelvic pain. Past history should be complete and include pertinent medical illnesses, previous surgical treatment, trauma, and drugs.

Physical Examination. Pain itself evokes physical changes which may be manifested on examination. Hyperalgesia may occur at the site of the original stimulus or in the area of referred pain. Muscle contraction may be a consequence of deep pain, or the muscle spasm itself may be responsible for pain. The autonomic responses to pain include pallor, sweating, nausea, vomiting, bradycardia, hypotension, and syncope. Regard for the patient's general appearance includes the attitude in bed, tissue turgor, respiratory rate, and temperature. Restricted motion in bed suggests peritonitis, whereas writhing is more frequently an accompaniment of biliary or ureteral colic.

The abdomen should be examined in a routine manner with inspection, auscultation, percussion, and palpation performed sequentially. On inspection, restricted motion of the abdominal wall during respiration suggests diffuse peritonitis. Maintenance of the hip in a position of flexion is suggestive of a psoas abscess, appendicitis, or a pelvic abscess. Auscultation for bowel sounds may reveal the borborygmi associated with mechanical intestinal obstruction, while an absence of bowel sounds is suggestive of diffuse peritonitis. Percussion is performed for the detection of free peritoneal fluid, distention, and the absence of liver dullness associated with a perforated viscus. Palpation should always begin away from the area of pain and include all possible sites for hernia. Superficial palpation may demonstrate hyperesthesia locally or in a segmental area of referred pain. Deep palpation may detect a mass. Muscle rigidity is a relative term, and its evaluation is dependent on the patient's cooperation. Pelvic and rectal examination are integral procedures for the evaluation of the acute surgical abdomen, as is a thorough examination of the chest for cardiac and pulmonary disease.

Laboratory Procedures. The hemogram with specific interest in the white blood cell count to define the presence of an inflammatory process and a hematocrit reading to determine if there is hemoconcentration or anemia should be routine. Urinalysis is directed toward evaluating dia-

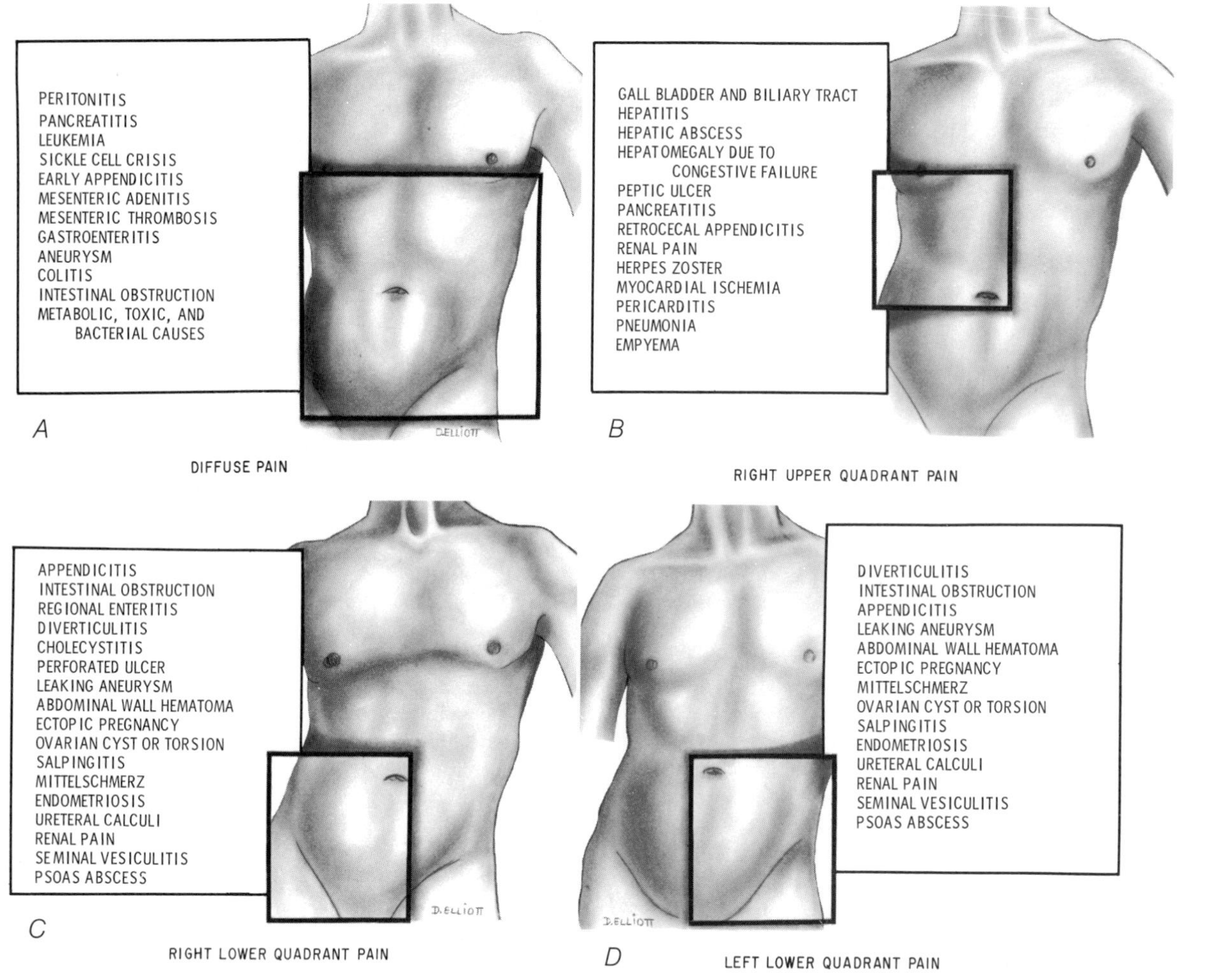

PERITONITIS
PANCREATITIS
LEUKEMIA
SICKLE CELL CRISIS
EARLY APPENDICITIS
MESENTERIC ADENITIS
MESENTERIC THROMBOSIS
GASTROENTERITIS
ANEURYSM
COLITIS
INTESTINAL OBSTRUCTION
METABOLIC, TOXIC, AND
    BACTERIAL CAUSES

A DIFFUSE PAIN

GALL BLADDER AND BILIARY TRACT
HEPATITIS
HEPATIC ABSCESS
HEPATOMEGALY DUE TO
    CONGESTIVE FAILURE
PEPTIC ULCER
PANCREATITIS
RETROCECAL APPENDICITIS
RENAL PAIN
HERPES ZOSTER
MYOCARDIAL ISCHEMIA
PERICARDITIS
PNEUMONIA
EMPYEMA

B RIGHT UPPER QUADRANT PAIN

APPENDICITIS
INTESTINAL OBSTRUCTION
REGIONAL ENTERITIS
DIVERTICULITIS
CHOLECYSTITIS
PERFORATED ULCER
LEAKING ANEURYSM
ABDOMINAL WALL HEMATOMA
ECTOPIC PREGNANCY
OVARIAN CYST OR TORSION
SALPINGITIS
MITTELSCHMERZ
ENDOMETRIOSIS
URETERAL CALCULI
RENAL PAIN
SEMINAL VESICULITIS
PSOAS ABSCESS

C RIGHT LOWER QUADRANT PAIN

DIVERTICULITIS
INTESTINAL OBSTRUCTION
APPENDICITIS
LEAKING ANEURYSM
ABDOMINAL WALL HEMATOMA
ECTOPIC PREGNANCY
MITTELSCHMERZ
OVARIAN CYST OR TORSION
SALPINGITIS
ENDOMETRIOSIS
URETERAL CALCULI
RENAL PAIN
SEMINAL VESICULITIS
PSOAS ABSCESS

D LEFT LOWER QUADRANT PAIN

Fig. 24-2. Characteristic location of abdominal pain associated with various diseases.

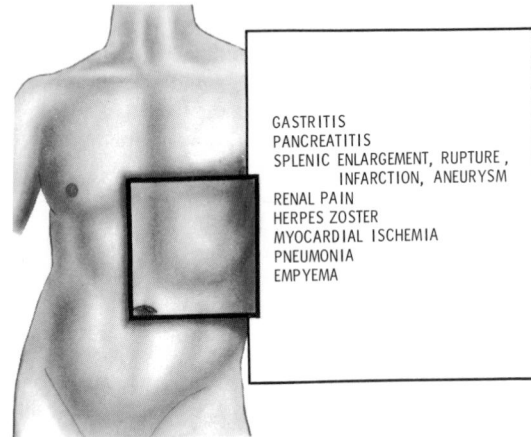

GASTRITIS
PANCREATITIS
SPLENIC ENLARGEMENT, RUPTURE,
    INFARCTION, ANEURYSM
RENAL PAIN
HERPES ZOSTER
MYOCARDIAL ISCHEMIA
PNEUMONIA
EMPYEMA

E LEFT UPPER QUADRANT PAIN

ocholithiasis, and intraabdominal bleeding. A sickle cell preparation may be called for in blacks. Emergency radiographic studies include supine films and upright or lateral decubitus films to determine the presence of air within the intestinal lumen or free within the peritoneal cavity. A chest x-ray is particularly applicable in patients over forty with upper abdominal pain, as is an electrocardiogram to rule out myocardial ischemia, which may mimic cholecystitis. The determination of the presence of free blood or significant amounts of peritoneal fluid may be accomplished by paracentesis with microscopic examination of the specimen or, in the case of lower abdominal or pelvic pain, culdocentesis and culdoscopy. It is to be emphasized that laparotomy may constitute an important tool in the diagnoisis of acute abdominal pain.

INTRACTABLE PAIN

The control of pain associated with diseases that cannot be satisfactorily treated is one of the most challenging and often frustrating problems the clinician has to face. Examples are unresectable carcinoma of the pancreas

betes, porphyria, the presence of infection, or red cells associated with calculi. An elevated serum amylase level is most frequently associated with acute pancreatitis but does occur with a variety of other intraabdominal processes including perforated viscera, cholecystitis, choled-

and chronic pancreatitis. Opiate analgesics if given in sufficient dosage can usually control abdominal pain, but at the risk of addiction and negating the patient's ability to function as an effective person. This is probably the best therapy, however, for a patient with incurable disease and a life expectancy of a few weeks or months. It should not be used in patients with severe pain from nonmalignant causes with an unpredictable life expectancy.

Neurosurgical intervention on the pain pathways, though disappointing at times, is the treatment of choice for intractable pain in properly selected patients. Narcotic addiction prior to surgery usually compromises the result, as an addicted patient continues to be addicted even though pain is relieved by the procedure.

Splanchnicectomy and celiac ganglionectomy can effectively control abdominal pain if somatically innervated structures are not involved in the pain-producing process. When both visceral and somatic pain fibers are involved, posterior rhizotomy or tract interruption is indicated. The spinothalamic tracts are usually interrupted, either by surgical incision or injection of sclerosing chemicals, in the spinal cord a few segments above the segments where the noxious impulses are entering. The interruption has also been done at medullary or mesencephalic levels. After anterolateral chordotomy, pain and temperature sensation are lost, while proprioception and touch are virtually unimpaired. Paresthesia often replaces pain in the anesthetic areas, and in a significant number of patients, after about 1 year, the paresthesia becomes disagreeable and painful. For this reason, root or tract interruption is most useful in patients with intractable pain and a life expectancy of a year or so.

For patients with pain arising from areas too great to be controlled by peripheral interventions, prefrontal lobotomy may be considered. Such lesions do not abolish pain but diminish the reaction to pain. The price paid for such relief, however, includes inability to experience pleasure, as well; i.e., there is a flattening of all affect and the development of a more or less apathetic state.

It is obvious from the above that there is a need for a means to relieve intractable pain that would be nonaddicting, would not affect the patient's personality or mind, and would not destroy normal neural tissue. A dorsal column stimulator is now commercially available. Impulses arising from electrostimulation of descending dorsal column fibers are used to inhibit, in accordance with the gate-control theory, prolonged small-fiber afterdischarge that is uniquely related to pain. Electrodes are implanted four to eight segments above the pain input. The external transmitter is controlled by the patient. There is a buzzing or tingling sensation below the site of the stimulator, but pain is usually controlled without significant alteration of normal sensory function. Transcutaneous electrical stimulation has been used effectively to control postoperative pain.

DYSPHAGIA

Dysphagia refers to a difficulty in swallowing and is related to either a functional alteration in the mechanism of deglutition or physical encroachment upon the lumen of the esophagus. The term *odynophagia* is used when swallowing is painful.

ACT OF SWALLOWING. This is classically divided into three stages. In the first stage the bolus of food or liquid is voluntarily moved into the pharynx by contraction of the mylohyoid muscle. In the second stage, the material is transported through the pharynx by waves of contractions that are involuntary, or reflex. This reflex is initiated by a stimulus from the base of the tongue, soft palate, uvula, and posterior pharyngeal wall and travels up the glossopharyngeal nerve, the second division of the trigeminal nerve, and the superior laryngeal nerve. The impulses terminate in the medulla and initiate a series of efferent stimuli that coordinate contraction of the pharyngeal constrictors. Elevation of the soft palate closes off the nasopharynx, and contraction of the suprahyoid muscles elevates the larynx and trachea. Ventilation is inhibited, and the respiratory tract is completely sealed off by approximation of the vocal cords and posterior displacement of the epiglottis. The terminal phase of the second stage is relaxation of the cricopharyngeus muscles, permitting the bolus to enter the upper esophagus.

The third stage of deglutition transports the bolus through the esophagus into the stomach. Waves of positive pressure sweep down the body of the esophagus in an orderly fashion, and the wave of pressure may reach an intensity of 50 to 100 cmH$_2$O. This wave is effected by a reflex arc, the afferent impulses of which are carried through the glossopharyngeal nerve and the efferent impulses transported by the vagi. Auerbach's plexuses within the wall of the esophagus are also involved. When distention by a solid bolus of food occurs, secondary peristaltic contractions result in that segment. Nonperistaltic tertiary esophageal contractions are seen in the lower esophagus of normal people after the age of forty. They are important considerations in the differential diagnosis of esophageal varices.

Transport of the bolus through the esophagus is dependent upon the pressure gradient produced by the primary peristaltic contraction plus, in the case of liquids, the effect of gravity. The final phase of deglutition is the propulsion of the bolus from the esophagus into the stomach. This is dependent upon relaxation of the inferior esophageal sphincter, which reacts reflexly and autonomously in response to pressure or peristalsis in the lower esophagus.

ETIOLOGY. Dysphagia may be due to oropharyngeal or esophageal causes. The former includes disorders of the mouth, upper respiratory tract, and pharynx. Any painful lesion of the mouth or tongue, including pharyngitis, retropharyngeal abscess, or oral carcinoma, may be implicated. Acute thyroiditis is usually accompanied by pharyngeal dysphagia. Neuromuscular disturbances that may affect deglutition include poliomyelitis, syringomyelia, glossopharyngeal neuritis, and myasthenia. Alteration of the muscle itself, as is seen in amyloidosis and scleroderma, also results in dysphagia, which may be either oropharyngeal or esophageal in location.

Esophageal dysphagia is related to a great variety of

Table 24-3. CAUSES OF ESOPHAGEAL DYSPHAGIA

Cause	Predominant sex	Age incidence		Salient historical and related characteristics
		10–45	45 and over	
Carcinoma	Male	Rare	Common	Duration of symptoms less than 2 years; painful swallowing occurs early, dysphagia later.
Peptic esophagitis	Male	Common	Common	Heartburn for years, often preceding dysphagia; odynophagia later.
Achalasia	Male-female	Common	Common	Liquids, especially cold, cause dysphagia early; regurgitation easy; odynophagia mild and late.
Contractile ring	Male	Rare	Common	Brief, intermittent attacks of dysphagia with no interval symptoms.
Diffuse spasm	Male	Rare	Rare	Affects elderly persons; multiple ringlike contractions along esophageal tube.
Zenker's diverticulum	Male	Rare	Rare	Sticking feeling in neck, gurgling on swallowing; occasional regurgitation of decayed food.
Scleroderma	Female	Common	Rare	Skin changes; Raynaud's disease.
Paraesophageal hiatal hernia	Female	Rare	Rare	Attacks of substernal pressure, pain, dysphagia, and belching during meals.
Extrinsic masses		Common	Rare	Symptoms of primary disorder.

SOURCE: After Ingelfinger, *Med Sci,* Apr. 10, 1960, pp 451–470, with permission.

causes, which are listed in Table 24-3. The level at which the patient localizes a sticking sensation usually corresponds well to the level of the responsible lesion. Dysphagia may be caused by disturbance in esophageal motility with either hypomotility or hypermotility implicated (see Chap. 25). The passage of fluid through the esophagus may also be impaired by encroachment upon the lumen. In the proximal esophagus, Zenker's pharyngoesophageal diverticulum, obstructing bands, and hypertrophic spurs of the anterior cervical vertebrae may be implicated. Dysphagia in the region of the cervical esophagus may also be due to esophageal carcinoma, cervical lymphadenopathy, stenosis secondary to ingestion of a caustic substance, or pressure from an enlarged thyroid. In the middle third of the esophagus, carcinoma, stenosis, esophagitis, and traction diverticulum may all be causes. In addition, a wide variety of mediastinal inflammatory malignant lesions may encroach upon the lumen. Vascular lesions such as enlargement of the left atrium, aneurysm in the arch of the aorta, and anomalous right subclavian artery are rare causes of dysphagia in this region. In the lower third of the esophagus, primary carcinoma and carcinoma of the stomach with craniad extension represent common causes, particularly in the older age group. Other lower esophageal causes of dysphagia include reflux esophagitis, achalasia, contractile rings, and epiphrenic diverticula.

Dysphagia is a relatively common manifestation of emotional diseases. Inability to swallow accompanies anxiety states, conversion hysteria, and anorexia nervosa.

CLINICAL EVALUATION. History should include a precise description of the symptom with particular reference to the duration, location, and timing in relation to ingestion of food. True dysphagia occurs within 15 min of swallowing. The patient can usually pinpoint the site of obstruction. The determination of the amount of weight loss and the presence of associated vomiting are important. Physical examination is directed toward the detection of cervical nodes suggesting mediastinal or esophageal lesions, enlargement of the esophagus, and stigmata of scleroderma. Barium study of the esophagus is frequently diagnostic, and the use of cineradiography and/or manometric motility studies is particularly applicable in determining disorders of motility. In the case of intrinsic esophageal lesions, the ultimate diagnostic study is esophagoscopy with biopsy.

ANOREXIA

Anorexia is the absence of the desire to eat and can be related to a variety of organic and psychologic disturbances. Since appetite is essentially a central phenomenon, anorexia is dependent upon central effects producing a loss of appetite. Animal experiments have demonstrated a feeding center in the lateral hypothalamus and a satiety center in the medial hypothalamus. In most instances, gastric hypofunction, mucosal pallor, and decrease in gastric motility and secretion have been associated with anorexia, but the stomach itself plays a minor role. Anorexia may also occur when both the secretory and motor activity of the stomach and gastrointestinal tract are increased. Visceral stimuli are generally carried to the midbrain via the vagus, pelvic, and sympathetic nerves, but combined sympathetic and parasympathetic denervation may not alter appetite or preclude the possibility of anorexia. The absence of precise pathophysiologic explanation and the protean disorders associated with the symptom of anorexia make it of little diagnostic significance. Among the organic diseases associated with anorexia are inflammatory processes within the intestinal tract; carcinoma of the stomach, pancreas, and liver; hepatitis and alcoholism; advanced renal disease with uremia; congestive heart failure; and certain endocrine disorders such as panhypopituitarism, adrenal cortical insufficiency, and hyperparathyroidism. Many, if not most, drugs can cause anorexia; there is no medication that consistently increases appetite.

NAUSEA AND VOMITING

Nausea and vomiting may occur separately but are closely allied. Nausea usually refers to the feeling of an imminent desire to vomit. Vomiting may be defined as the forceful expulsion of gastrointestinal contents through the mouth. In most instances, nausea precedes vomiting.

In spite of the frequency and great clinical importance of vomiting, the nervous mechanism of the act and the physical and chemical stimuli are not well understood. Most physiologists have agreed to the existence of a vomiting center and to its location in the reticular core of the medulla oblongata. There are actually two medullary centers concerned with emesis: (1) a sensory "chemoreceptive trigger zone" and (2) an integrated center that is concerned directly with the production of vomiting. The former is implicated in drug-induced emesis and also in the vomiting associated with uremia, infections, and radiation sickness.

Afferent pathways to the vomiting center emanate from almost all sites in the body. Impulses from the gastrointestinal system pass through the emetic center by way of afferent fibers in both the vagal and sympathetic nerves. Although neither vagotomy nor sympathectomy alone abolishes the vomiting of peritonitis, the vagus is considered the more important afferent pathway from this stimulus. The vomiting induced by intestinal distention is dependent upon afferent impulses transmitted in the sympathetic nerves, as evidenced by the fact that denervation of the mesenteric pedicle prevents vomiting associated with distention of that segment. Distention of the gallbladder and extrahepatic biliary tract also causes vomiting that may be obviated by a combination of vagotomy and splanchnicectomy. Pyloric pouch distention vomiting is abolished by vagotomy alone. However, it is known that vomiting may be a consequence of surgical vagotomy and that the higher the vagotomy, the more frequent the incidence of vomiting. In this circumstance, the vomiting is related to esophageal stasis with regurgitation of esophageal contents into the pharynx and subsequent pharyngeal irritation.

The act of vomiting is primarily a motor function involving the respiratory and somatic muscular systems in addition to the gastrointestinal tract. Vomiting occurs in the normal fashion following total denervation of the intestine. The efferent neuropathways involve the phrenic nerves to the diaphragm, spinal nerves to the abdominal and intercostal muscles, and efferent visceral fibers along the vagus and sympathetic nerves to the intestine and muscles of the pharynx and larynx. The act of vomiting depends upon the coordinated closure of the glottis, contraction and fixation of the diaphragm in the inspiratory position, closure of the pylorus, and relaxation of the rest of the stomach including the cardia. Relaxation of the upper half of the stomach and the esophageal cardia is followed by peristaltic contractions passing from the midstomach to the incisura angularis. Contraction at the incisura persists and prevents the contents of the stomach from passing into the gastric antrum. This is followed by forceful contraction of the abdominal, diaphragmatic, and intercostal muscles, which transmit a pressure to the stomach and cause regurgitation. Reverse peristalsis in the stomach plays no major role in the mechanism of vomiting. Reverse peristalsis of the small intestine frequently occurs and results in the passage of intestinal contents into the stomach and the presence of bile in the vomitus after repeated retching. This type of intestinal activity, however, has been shown to occur normally in the duodenum and does not contribute to the act of vomiting. Vomiting is frequently associated with autonomic activity, including pallor, sweating, increased salivation, and cardiovascular changes which include irregularity, ectopic beats, heart block, and, rarely, arrest.

All organic diseases of the alimentary tract and its appendages, as well as diseases of almost every organ of the body, have been associated with vomiting. Derangements of the autonomic nervous system, psychogenic disturbances, and the ingestion of noxious materials may also cause vomiting. A broad spectrum of drugs is considered as emetic agents. These include morphine, cardiac glycosides, quinine and quinidine, veratrine alkaloids, pilocarpine, Pituitrin, Pitocin, acetylcholine, ergot alkaloids, atropine, tartar emetic, ipecac, zinc sulfate, and bacterial endotoxins. With each of these causes of vomiting any combination of three major factors may be involved: impulses arising from the gastrointestinal tract, central or cerebral impulses, and chemical materials transported in the blood.

The vomiting associated with shock and severe pain may be related to a reduced blood supply in the cerebral medullary centers or vasoconstriction in the splanchnic areas. Reduction of oxygen supply to the vomiting center has been implicated in the vomiting associated with anemia, vascular occlusion, and increased intracranial pressure. Migraine may also induce vomiting by an effective increase in intracranial pressure with interference of blood supply to the cerebromedullary center. Emetic drugs act in one of two ways, either directly on the cerebrum, hypothalamus, or brainstem or by their irritative effect on the gastric and intestinal mucosa. These two factors may also be involved in vomiting induced by spoiled or contaminated food and the vomiting following the ingestion of alcohol. The vomiting associated with diabetic acidosis, uremia, and Addisonian crisis has been related to changes in electrolytes and, more specifically, acidosis and hyperkalemia affecting the emesis center. An augmented irritability of the emesis center is postulated as playing a significant role in the vomiting of thyrotoxicosis.

The gastrointestinal pathophysiologic processes leading to vomiting are many and varied. Obstruction to passage of food at any level will eventually be accompanied by vomiting. The higher the obstruction, the more rapid the onset of vomiting. The rapidity is also related to the acuteness of onset, since a gradual obstruction is attended by compensation with stretching of muscle fibers and hypertrophy. Inflammatory diseases and malignant tumors of the stomach are frequent causes of vomiting and are usually preceded by anorexia and nausea. In the child under three months of age, vomiting of clear, non-bile-stained materials is highly suggestive of hypertrophic pyloric stenosis. Acute inflammatory diseases of the intestine and pelvic organs are associated with nausea and vomiting through visceral reflexes; the more common disorders include appendicitis, cholecystitis, hepatitis, pancreatitis, and salpingitis.

The pattern of vomiting is of clinical significance. Vomiting without antecedent nausea suggests a central nervous system lesion with increased intracranial pressure, such as hemorrhage or brain tumor. In these cases, vomiting is usually sudden in onset and often projectile. Projectile vomiting is also characteristic of hypertrophic pyloric stenosis. Emesis that follows and relieves epigastric pain is usually associated with intragastric lesions or pyloric spasm. Vomiting that immediately follows eating is noted with toxic causes, such as uremia and hyperemesis gravidarum, gastritis, high intestinal obstruction, and gastric neoplasms. Vomiting of large amounts of digested food at 12- to 48-h intervals is suggestive of chronic pyloric obstruction. Vomiting of feculent material is associated with gastrocolic fistula. Continued retching and vomiting, especially in alcoholics, may lacerate the gastroesophageal mucosa and result in the Mallory-Weiss syndrome with severe bleeding and, at times, exsanguination. An extension of this process is the spontaneous rupture of the esophagus which occurs more frequently in vomiting by the patient with a full stomach (Boerhaave's syndrome).

CONSEQUENCES OF VOMITING. Depending upon its intensity and duration, vomiting may produce hypovolemia, hypokalemia, alteration in the acid-base balance, and the consequences of starvation. Vomitus, without admixture of ingested food, is isoosmotic with the extracellular fluid. The electrolyte composition is extremely variable and dependent upon the extent of hydrogen ion excretion.

When hydrogen ion is excreted into the gastric juice, there is a shift of bicarbonate ion into the plasma, and, to maintain electric neutrality of the blood, chloride is excreted into the gastric juice. Concentration of bicarbonate in the plasma is augmented by the loss of chloride and excessive sodium in the vomitus. In general, an inverse relation exists between the concentration of hydrogen ion and sodium ion in the vomitus. Even in the achlorhydric state, when vomiting results in a depletion of sodium chloride and potassium chloride, chloride is excreted in excess of the physiologic proportions existent in plasma, i.e., 145 meq of sodium and 100 meq of chloride. As the plasma bicarbonate rises, the body compensates by increasing renal excretion of bicarbonate and reducing the rate and depth of respiration to decrease the respiratory loss of $HHCO_3$ to maintain the acid/base ratio. These compensatory features may maintain the normal blood pH, while the urine is alkaline because of excretion of

bicarbonate. Determination of plasma electrolytes is only partly informative, since it is dependent upon the relative loss of electrolytes and water and also upon the solutions ingested.

With continued vomiting, the plasma and extracellular potassium concentration becomes reduced as a result of the increased quantities of potassium excreted in the urine in exchange for sodium, which in turn is related to the lack of availability of hydrogen ions depleted by loss in the vomitus. Adrenal cortical stimulation intensifies the potassium loss and potentiates the absorption of bicarbonate by the renal tubular cell. The extracellular and subsequently intracellular potassium concentrations become reduced, sodium cations shift into the cell, and, in order to conserve sodium, an acid urine is formed in the face of generalized alkalosis. This intensifies the alkalosis and sets up a vicious cycle which includes shift of more potassium out of the cell in exchange for sodium.

The fluid loss results in reduction in the circulating blood volume, and in time the consequences of starvation such as cellular breakdown of protein and increased renal load of nitrogenous waste products cause a rise in the BUN (blood urea nitrogen) level. Fat stores are utilized. Ketone bodies are formed, and since they require sodium for excretion, this further depletes the body stores of sodium.

Therapy should be instituted early, correcting relatively minor defects, since advanced deficiencies are critical and difficult to reverse. Drugs used to treat vomiting include anticholinergics, antihistamines, phenothiazine derivatives, and orthopramides.

CONSTIPATION AND DIARRHEA

Alteration in bowel habits may be related to the type of food ingested, psychologic disorders, or lesions in the gastrointestinal tract.

INTESTINAL TRANSIT. The rate of gastric emptying varies with the amount and quality of food and the emotional state of the individual. Generally, the healthy stomach is emptied within 3 to 4 h, and passage through the duodenum and jejunum is rapid. Digested food usually begins to traverse the ileocolic sphincter in 2 to 3 h and completes its passage into the cecum in 9 h. Some delay occurs almost constantly in the distal ileum, where "segmentation" of a radiopaque bolus can be noted. The contents of the small intestine travel at an average rate of 1 in./min, or 22 ft in 4 h.

The chyme that enters the cecum is semiliquid in consistency. Most of the absorption of water that occurs in the large intestine takes place in the cecum and ascending colon. The intensity and frequency of muscular contractions increase from the duodenum to the rectum. Mass peristalsis carries the bolus from the hepatic flexure onward. These waves occur at varying times but are known to be frequent after meals, the so-called "gastrocolic reflex." Although some food products are evacuated within 24 h of ingestion, the major portion requires several days for disposition.

Normally, the fecal bolus does not pass beyond the sigmoid into the rectum until defecation is about to occur. The passage into the rectum is brought about by powerful peristaltic waves with concomitant relaxation of the smooth musculature at the rectosigmoid junction. Distention of the rectum initiates afferent nervous impulses conducted via hypogastric and pelvic nerves to the sacral cord, whence efferent impulses are discharged. The process of defecation may be entirely involuntary but is usually assisted by voluntary contractions of the muscles of the abdomen and diaphragm and voluntary relaxation of the external anal sphincter. The intraluminal pressure is increased, forcing the stool through the relaxed internal sphincter and the voluntarily relaxed external sphincter. The entire colon, distal to the splenic flexure, is usually emptied at one time.

Although intestinal motility continues after transection of the nerves, under normal conditions the vagi, splanchnics, and pelvic nerves do play a significant role. Parasympathetic efferent supply to the small intestine and proximal colon courses over the vagi, while the remainder of the colon innervation is carried over the lower sacral segment via the pelvic nerves. Splanchnic nerves supply sympathetic innervation. The intrinsic myenteric reflexes are the prime movers, but motility is augmented by parasympathetic stimulation, while sympathetic stimulation results in inhibition of tone. Sympathetic stimulation explains the reflex ileus that is known to accompany retroperitoneal trauma or dissection.

The external anal sphincter, a voluntary muscle, receives nerve fibers from the gray matter of the conus terminalis, where the reflex is located. Transection of the cord in this region does not affect reflex contraction. If the lower segment of the cord is destroyed, the external sphincter becomes relaxed and no longer contracts. If the afferent nerves are destroyed, the fecal bolus may accumulate without sensation. It has been suggested that the medullary center may be implicated in the act of defecation, since a central nervous system influence is capable of causing either diarrhea or constipation.

In addition to neurogenic factors, chemicals also influence defecation. Acetylcholine-like drugs increase the tone and activity of the intestine. Pilocarpine causes smooth muscle contraction, while neostigmine and Mecholyl inhibit the destruction of cholinesterase and produce intestinal activity. Serotonin also alters intestinal motility with resultant increased activity. Guanethidine causes increased motility by its inhibitory effect on the sympathetic nerves, and reserpine acts by its effect on serotonin release. Vasopressin strongly induces motility in the entire intestine. Potassium is implicated in intestinal motility, since the function of the muscle cell is dependent upon its potassium level. Drugs may also delay the passage of intestinal contents. Morphine and codeine decrease the propulsive motility by resulting in a marked increase in tone. Atropine decreases motility by paralyzing the parasympathetic nerve endings.

Constipation

Constipation may be defined as an abnormal retention of fecal matter or undue delay in discharge when compared with the patient's usual bowel habits. The term is used in a variety of ways. It may refer to the fact that the stool occurs with relative infrequency, that the stool is insufficient in quantity, or that it is abnormally hard and dry.

ETIOLOGY. Constipation may be due to psychologic factors, dietary constituents, laxatives and drugs, neurogenic causes, decreased skeletomuscular power, and mechanical factors that are either intrinsic or extrinsic to the gastrointestinal tract.

Psychogenic constipation may be related to improper training, and the symptom frequently dates from early childhood. The end result may be a functional megacolon, which is considered to be more common than Hirschsprung's disease. *Dietary factors* include a lack of bulky foods and the use of laxatives that lead to overstimulation of the bowel with eventual fatigue. Drugs with constipating effects have been referred to in the section Intestinal Transit.

Decreased muscular power in the skeletal muscles of the diaphragm, abdominal wall, and pelvic floor may all cause constipation. Weakness of the diaphragm may be associated with a variety of chronic pulmonary diseases, while weakness of the abdominal wall may occur in pregnancy, in the presence of large, rapidly expanding intraabdominal masses, and in patients with marked ascites. Weakness of the pelvic floor is usually a consequence of pregnancy. The role of *atony of the intestinal muscle* is difficult to evaluate and may be of minimal importance. Hypokalemia results in ileus based on this cause. Collagen and endocrine disorders are thought to be associated with intestinal atony. *Neurogenic causes* include tabes dorsalis, multiple sclerosis, spinal cord tumors, and trauma. These lesions may result in deficient reflex activity or may directly destroy or depress the autonomic innervation of the intestine. In Hirschsprung's disease the neurologic deficit in the myenteric and submucosal plexuses interrupts the peristaltic action to that segment. *Factors intrinsic to the gastrointestinal tract* that contribute to the symptom of constipation include tumors, fecal impactions, intussusception, and volvulus. The mechanical factor is also implicated at the anal sphincter, when spasm and the voluntary avoidance of defecation because of pain occur in patients with hemorrhoids, fissures, or proctitis. *Extrinsic causes* consist of large intraabdominal masses such as ovarian cysts, fibroids, pregnancy, and obstructing adhesions.

ASSOCIATED SYMPTOMS AND EFFECTS. Obstipation, which is defined as the absence of passage of both flatus and feces, is suggestive of mechanical obstruction. Reflex symptoms accompanying constipation include back and hip pain, headache, and, occasionally, tachycardia. So-called intestinal toxemia in patients with chronic constipation remains unproved but probably occurs. Fecal accumulations within the rectum may reach large size and contribute to the formation of anal lesions such as hemorrhoids, fissures, and ulcers. Constipation also has a significant role in the development of colonic diverticula and sigmoid volvulus.

CLINICAL EVALUATION. The history should include complete elaboration of bowel habits and also the patient's dietary intake. Direct questioning concerning the color, consistency, and caliber of the stool, the presence of melena or unaltered blood, mucus, or undigested fats or foods, and the occurrence of tenesmus is indicated. Although abdominal examination may reveal a mass, the rectal is usually the most rewarding aspect of the physical examination. Proctosigmoidoscopy may define the presence of inflammation, tumors, or the melanosis coli of patients who take laxatives chronically. Radiographic examination with a barium enema is indicated in all patients with prolonged constipation.

Diarrhea

Diarrhea refers to an excessively rapid evacuation of excessively fluid stool. It may be acute, in which case it is usually related to dietary, toxic, or infectious causes. When diarrhea is chronic or recurrent, it is more likely a manifestation of gastrointestinal disease.

ETIOLOGY. Even when discussion is limited to chronic diarrhea, classification is at best imperfect. Table 24-4 lists some of the causes of diarrhea that are of interest to surgeons.

PATHOPHYSIOLOGY. The conventional view has been that increased intestinal motor activity producing rapid intestinal transit is responsible for diarrhea. Evidence has now accumulated that the pathophysiologic mechanism for diarrhea is primarily an abnormality of intestinal water and electrolyte transport. Distention of the bowel by this increased fluid stimulates propulsive contractions. Hypermotility then is a secondary phenomenon, not primary, in most types of diarrhea.

There are four principal pathophysiologic mechanisms involved in the production of diarrhea: (1) excessive intestinal secretion ("secretory" diarrhea), (2) the presence in the bowel lumen of increased amounts of poorly absorbable, osmotically active substances ("osmotic" diarrhea), (3) inhibition or absence of a normal active ion transport process, and (4) deranged bowel motility. These mechanisms are by no means mutually exclusive, and more than one mechanism is usually involved in any patient with diarrhea.

Active ion secretion by the small intestine is the most important factor in *secretory diarrhea*. In some syndromes, decreased absorption also plays a role. Cholera has been the most extensively studied of the secretory diarrheas. The toxins of *Vibrio cholerae* activate adenylate cyclase in the basolateral membrane of the mucosal cells, which in turn causes a rise in intracellular cyclic AMP concentration. Cyclic AMP causes chloride and bicarbonate to be actively secreted into the lumen. Water is transported passively in response to osmotic gradients.

Table 24-4. CAUSES OF DIARRHEA

Functional enterocolonic disease	Gastrojejunocolic fistula
Mucous colitis	Inadvertent gastroileostomy
Organic colonic disease	Postvagotomy diarrhea
Ulcerative colitis	Disorders of the solid viscera
Crohn's colitis	Pancreatic insufficiency
Diverticulitis	Biliary fistula
Neoplastic lesions	Watery diarrhea syndrome (VIPoma)
Polyposis	Enteric infections
Villous adenoma	Salmonella
Carcinoma	Shigella
Fecal impaction	Pseudomembranous colitis
Lymphogranuloma venereum	Parasitic infestations
Endometriosis	Amebiasis
Toxic colitis	Leishmaniasis
Arsenic	Ascaris
Mercury	Liver flukes
Alcohol	Schistosomiasis
Small intestinal disease	Trichinella
Crohn's disease	Metabolic disorders
Tuberculous enteritis	Thyroid
Malabsorption due to disease	Thyrotoxicosis
Sprue	Medullary carcinoma—calcitonin
Carcinoid	Hyperparathyroidism
Intestinal lipodystrophy	Uremia
Malabsorption due to mechanical defects	Diabetes mellitus
Short gut syndrome	Addison's disease
Blind loop syndrome	Drugs
Fistulas	Cathartics
Gastric factors	Sympatholytic
Hyperchlorhydria	Propranolol
Zollinger-Ellison syndrome	Parasympathomimetic
Postsurgical problems	Urecholine
Dumping syndrome	Neostigmine
Afferent loop syndrome	Acetylcholine

Characteristic features of secretory diarrhea are (1) the diarrhea is usually voluminous, (2) the osmolality of the stool fluid is isotonic, and (3) the diarrhea usually persists even when the patient fasts.

Osmotic diarrhea results when poorly absorbable solutes accumulate in the bowel lumen. These osmotically active substances result from (1) incomplete digestion of ingested food; (2) failure to absorb a dietary nonelectrolyte that is normally handled by a special transport mechanism, e.g., glucose; and (3) ingestion of poorly absorbable solutes, e.g., the magnesium ion in laxatives. Characteristic features of osmotic diarrhea are (1) the diarrhea stops when the patient fasts or stops ingesting the poorly absorbable solute; (2) the osmolality of fecal fluid is greater than the sum of the concentrations of normal electrolytes.

Malabsorption of a normal ion is an infrequent cause of chronic diarrhea. The best-studied example is congenital chloridorrhea. Passive absorption or secretion down electrochemical gradients is normal, but these patients are unable to actively absorb chloride ion against a gradient. Characteristic features are (1) the diarrhea disappears or is greatly improved on fasting, (2) the osmolality of the fecal fluid is normal; and (3) the ionic composition of the fecal fluid is abnormal, reflecting malabsorption of a specific ion.

Deranged bowel motility is the least understood of the pathophysiologic mechanisms of diarrhea. It is difficult to separate abnormal motility that is secondary to stimulation by distention, as occurs in secretory and osmotic diarrhea, from primary intestinal motility abnormalities. Examples of syndromes in which primary motor abnormalities are thought to play a major role include the diarrheal phase of irritable colon syndrome, diabetic enteropathy, and scleroderma.

CONSEQUENCES OF DIARRHEA. The consequences are dependent upon the intensity and duration of the symptom. Severe or prolonged diarrhea may result in dehydration, electrolyte loss, and acidosis. The fecal sodium and chloride concentrations are usually lower than the plasma levels, whereas the potassium and bicarbonate levels are higher. The villous adenoma excretes a fluid that is particularly high in potassium, with concentrations many times that of plasma.

Acidosis may result because of a high bicarbonate content in the stool or may be related to the production of acid due to starvation or to the dehydration compromising renal function. Dehydration and acidosis accelerate the body depletion of potassium by a shift of the cation out of the cell in exchange for sodium and hydrogen ions. These factors coupled with the large amount of potassium lost in the stool because of excretion into the intestine in exchange for sodium absorption from the lower small intestine and colon may result in significant hypokalemia.

Plasma or electrolyte determinations do not represent a guide to the severity of volume loss, since this reflection is dependent upon the relative tonicity of the stool with respect to extracellular fluid and the amount of fluid lost. In the absence of associated bleeding, the hematocrit is the better index of the severity of dehydration.

CLINICAL EVALUATION. History. Direct questioning should elicit the duration of diarrhea, the time of day during which diarrhea occurs, the patient's description of the stool, the presence of accompanying pain or urge to defecate, and the presence of other manifestations of gastrointestinal disease such as anorexia, nausea, and vomiting. A family or community history of similar episodes suggests an infectious basis. Diarrhea that alternates with constipation occurs with colon lesions such as carcinoma, diverticulitis, partial intestinal obstruction, and chronic constipation treated with laxatives. Recurrent episodes of diarrhea are characteristic of ulcerative colitis, psychogenic causes, and amebic colitis. Ulcerative colitis may be associated with red stools, while the patient may recognize infestation by the presence of the offending organism in the stool. Large, pale, bulky stools suggest pancreatic deficiency. Large amounts of mucus in the stool are seen in patients with mucous colitis, ulcerative colitis, carcinoma of the colon, and villous adenoma.

Pain is frequently present with ulcerative colitis and diverticulitis, and also may be noted when diarrhea is due to carcinoma. Tenesmus commonly accompanies ulcerative colitis, carcinoma of the rectum, and lymphogranuloma venereum. Anorexia, nausea, and/or vomiting are more characteristic symptoms of intestinal malignancy, ulcerative colitis, and severe bacillary or amebic dysentery.

Physical Examination. *Fever* may be present with a variety of inflammatory processes and occurs more rarely as an accompaniment of neoplastic disease, with the exception of lymphoma. Arthritis is particularly common in ulcerative colitis, regional enteritis, and lipodystrophy. This also applies to other hypersensitivity reactions such as iritis and erythema nodosum. A palpable *abdominal mass* should be sought. In the left lower quadrant, this may suggest sigmoid carcinoma or diverticulitis with inflammatory obstruction. Granulomas of regional enteritis, amebic infection, and tuberculosis may all cause palpable masses. *Tenderness* suggests regional enteritis, diverticulitis, or intraabdominal inflammatory processes. *Digital examination* of the rectum may define the presence of lymphogranuloma venereum, carcinoma, granulomas, ulcerative colitis, diffuse polyposis, or a fecal impaction. *Proctosigmoidoscopy* should represent an integral part of the examination of the patient with diarrhea. A friable rectal mucosa may suggest ulcerative colitis or amebiasis. The overwhelming majority of patients with ulcerative colitis have lesions which may be visualized by this technique. Malignant lesions, polyps, and villous adenomas can usually be defined by proctosigmoidoscopy.

Stool. The stool should be evaluated for consistency and the presence of mucus and occult and unaltered blood. Fatty stools suggest pancreatic insufficiency or malabsorption. Carcinoma and diverticulitis may be associated with bloody stools. Microscopic examination for ova and parasites is particularly pertinent to the diagnosis of infestations.

Radiologic Studies. Abdominal films may demonstrate intestinal obstruction, a mass, or calculi associated with chronic pancreatitis. Barium enema is an essential part of the examination and is frequently diagnostic for ulcerative colitis, tumors, and diverticulitis. Reflux into the terminal ileum may define the presence of regional enteritis or tuberculous enteritis. In rare instances, regurgitation of barium into the jejunum or stomach will demonstrate a fistula. The upper gastrointestinal series is also of importance, particularly in determining the presence of gastrocolic fistula, blind loop syndrome, and iatrogenic gastroileostomy. The barium meal may be utilized as a method of determining intestinal transit time in patients with massive resection. Primary malabsorption syndromes may be associated with a small bowel pattern which is quite characteristic. Pancreatography may be indicated.

Laparotomy. In some cases, laparotomy should be considered a diagnostic procedure. Small bowel biopsy is indicated in the differential diagnosis of malabsorption syndrome, regional enteritis, Whipple's disease, lymphomas, and tumors of the small intestine.

INTESTINAL OBSTRUCTION

Intestinal obstruction exists when there is interference with the normal aboral progression of intestinal contents. The term *mechanical intestinal obstruction* is used if an actual physical barrier blocks the intestinal lumen. The term *ileus,* though properly a synonym for intestinal obstruction from whatever cause, by common usage now connotes failure of downward progress of bowel contents because of disordered propulsive motility of the bowel.

Gastric outlet obstruction is discussed in Chap. 26, esophageal obstruction in Chap. 25, and mesenteric vascular obstruction in Chap. 35. Discussion of specific entites causing intestinal obstruction in infancy and childhood will be found in Chap. 39.

Mechanical Obstruction

ETIOLOGY. The causes of mechanical obstruction may be classified according to the manner in which the obstruction is produced: (1) by obturation of the lumen, as in gallstone ileus, (2) by encroachment on the lumen by intrinsic disease of the bowel wall, as in regional enteritis or carcinoma, or (3) by lesions extrinsic to bowel such as an adhesive band (Table 24-5).

Classification of intestinal obstruction on clinical and pathologic grounds is also necessary. In *simple mechanical obstruction* the lumen is obstructed, but the blood supply is intact. If mesenteric vessels are occluded, then *strangulated obstruction* exists. *Closed-loop obstruction* results when both limbs of the loop are obstructed so that neither aboral progression nor regurgitation is possible. Obstruction is further delineated by classification as partial or complete, acute or chronic, high or low, small intestinal or colonic.

INCIDENCE. Probably about 20 percent of surgical admissions for acute abdominal conditions are for intestinal

Table 24-5. MECHANISMS OF INTESTINAL OBSTRUCTION

Mechanical obstruction of the lumen
  Obturation of the lumen
    Meconium
    Intussusception
    Gallstones
    Impactions—fecal, barium, bezoar, worms
  Lesions of bowel
    Congenital
      Atresia and stenosis
      Imperforate anus
      Duplications
      Meckel's diverticulum
    Traumatic
    Inflammatory
      Regional enteritis
      Diverticulitis
      Chronic ulcerative colitis
    Neoplastic
    Miscellaneous
      K^+-induced stricture
      Radiation stricture
      Endometriosis
  Lesions extrinsic to bowel
    Adhesive band constriction or angulation by adhesion
    Hernia and wound dehiscence
    Extrinsic masses
      Annular pancreas
      Anomalous vessels
      Abscesses and hematomas
      Neoplasms
  Volvulus
Inadequate propulsive motility
  Neuromuscular defects
    Megacolon
    Paralytic ileus
      Abdominal causes
        Intestinal distention
        Peritonitis
        Retroperitoneal lesions
      Systemic causes
        Electrolyte imbalance
        Toxemias
    Spastic ileus
  Vascular occlusion
    Arterial
    Venous

obstruction. Adhesive bands are now the most frequent cause of obstruction for all age groups combined. Strangulated groin hernia, formerly the most common cause, is now in second place, with neoplasm of the bowel in third place. In some recently reported series, neoplasm has taken over second place, with hernia now in third. These three etiologic agents account for more than 80 percent of all intestinal obstruction.

The order of frequency differs for different age groups. Hernia is by far the most common cause of obstruction in childhood. Colorectal carcinoma and diverticulitis coli are prominent etiologic agents in the older age group, and these lesions are becoming more prominent in the overall picture as more of the population is living into the geriatric age, where these lesions prevail.

The mortality rate from intestinal obstruction was over 50 percent in the United States in the early part of this century. The mortality rate is now under 10 percent. The factors principally responsible for the reduction are (1) recognition of the role of fluid and electrolyte therapy, (2) gastrointestinal decompression by intubation, and (3) antibiotics.

Though the mortality rate is now but one-fifth of the rate in the early twentieth century, it is still distressingly and needlessly high. This death rate could be appreciably lowered if patients with hernias were urged to have their hernias repaired, since herniorrhaphy can now be done with only about a 0.1 to 0.2 percent mortality even in the presence of other chronic systemic disease. A further lowering of the death rate could be attained if a larger percentage of patients could be operated upon before a simple mechanical obstruction has progressed to strangulated obstruction with its greatly increased morbidity and mortality.

PATHOPHYSIOLOGY. Though simple mechanical obstruction, strangulated obstruction, and ileus have much in common, there are important differences in pathophysiology and management. Also, colon obstruction differs in some aspects from small bowel obstruction.

Simple Mechanical Obstruction of the Small Intestine. The principal physiologic derangements of the mechanically obstructed intestine with intact blood supply are accumulation of fluid and gas above the point of obstruction and altered bowel motility, which lead also to systemic derangements.

Fluid and Electrolyte Losses. Death from intestinal obstruction was for many years attributed to "toxins" that were absorbed from the intestine. In 1912 Hartwell and Hoguet were able to prolong the life of dogs with high intestinal obstruction by the daily parenteral administration of physiologic saline solution. Gamble later demonstrated that the "toxic" factor in simple mechanical obstruction was actually the loss of fluid and electrolytes from the body by vomiting and by sequestering in the obstructed bowel.

Accumulation of large quantities of fluid and gas within the lumen of the bowel above an obstruction is striking and progressive. The net movement of a substance across the intestinal mucosa is equal to the difference between the unidirectional flux from intestinal lumen to blood (absorption) and the opposite flux from blood to lumen (secretion). Accumulation of fluid within the bowel—a negative net flux—will result if the flux from lumen to blood (absorption) is decreased or if the flux from blood to lumen (secretion) is increased. After 48 h of obstruction, the rate of entry of water into the intestinal lumen increases as a consequence of blood to lumen flux. The findings for sodium and potassium are parallel.

Davenport has reported that normal fluxes occurred in the direction of blood to lumen, but fluxes from lumen to blood were depressed or abolished in an obstructed ileal segment. As a result, water, sodium, and chloride (and presumably other ions) moved into the obstructed intestinal segment but not out of it, distending it with fluid having approximately the electrolyte composition of plasma.

Wright et al. studied net flux in patients with mature ileostomies. Closed loops were produced by proximal and distal obstructing balloons inserted through the ileostomy. Absorption of a test solution was found to increase at moderate elevations of pressure, but fell below normal at pressures three or four times normal. Conversely, secretion of fluid into the lumen increased progressively as pressure rose. They concluded that increased secretion is the primary cause of fluid loss and distention in intestinal obstruction, with decreased absorption playing a lesser role. Prostaglandin release in response to bowel distention is thought to be the mechanism by which secretion into obstructed loops is increased.

The bowel immediately above the obstruction is the most affected initially. It becomes distended with fluids and electrolytes, and circulation is impaired. With increasing intraluminal pressure the fluid is dispersed orad until it reaches bowel that is still capable of absorbing. When obstruction has been present for a long time, the proximal portions of the intestine also lose their ability to handle fluid and electrolytes, and the entire bowel proximal to the obstruction becomes distended.

A second route of fluid and electrolyte loss is into the wall of the involved bowel, accounting for the boggy edematous appearance of the bowel often seen at operation. Some of this fluid exudes from the serosal surface of the bowel, resulting in free peritoneal fluid. The extent of fluid and electrolyte loss into the bowel wall and peritoneal cavity depends on the extent of bowel involved in venous congestion and edema, and the length of time before the obstruction is relieved.

The most obvious route of fluid and electrolyte loss is by vomiting—or gastrointestinal tube after treatment is initiated. The aggregate of these losses (1) into the bowel lumen, (2) into the edematous bowel wall, (3) as free peritoneal fluid, and (4) by vomiting or nasogastric suction, rapidly depletes the extracellular fluid space, leading progressively to hemoconcentration, hypovolemia, renal insufficiency, shock, and death unless treatment is prompt and resolute. The blood chemistry values to be expected in intestinal obstruction will be found below under Clinical Manifestations.

Intestinal Gas. Much of the distention of the bowel above a mechanical obstruction can be accounted for by the fluid sequestered within the lumen. Intestinal gas is also responsible for distention.

The approximate composition of small intestine gas (Table 24-6) shows that the basic composition is that of

Table 24-6. INTESTINAL GAS

	Percent
Nitrogen	70
Oxygen	12
Carbon dioxide	8
Hydrogen sulfide	5
Ammonia and amines	4
Hydrogen	1

swallowed air to which small amounts of gases not found in the atmosphere have been added.

Gases are absorbed from the intestine at rates that are directly related to the partial pressure of the particular gas in the intestine, in the plasma, and in the air breathed. Thus with nitrogen there is little diffusion, since the partial pressures of the gas are virtually the same in intestine, plasma, and air. On the other hand carbon dioxide diffuses very rapidly, because the partial pressure of carbon dioxide is high in the intestine, intermediate in plasma, and very low in air. For this reason, though carbon dioxide is produced in large amounts in the intestine, it contributes little to gaseous distention because of its rapid diffusibility.

Bowel Motility. With obstruction of the lumen, peristalsis increases in an "attempt" to overcome the obstruction. After a short time, continuous peristalsis above the obstruction gives way to regularly recurring bursts of peristaltic activity interspersed with quiescent periods. The duration of the quiescent period is related to the level of the obstruction in the gastrointestinal tract—it is 3 to 5 min with high obstruction, 10 to 15 min with lower ileal obstruction. These muscular contractions may be of sufficient magnitude to traumatize the bowel and contribute to the swelling and edema of the bowel wall. As bowel above the obstruction distends, bowel below the obstruction becomes progressively more quiet. This results from an inhibitory reflex initiated by distention of the bowel above.

Strangulated Obstruction. Occlusion of the blood supply to a segment of bowel in addition to obstruction of the lumen is usually referred to as strangulated obstruction. Interference with the mesenteric blood supply is the most serious complication of intestinal obstruction. This frequently occurs secondary to adhesive band obstruction, hernia, and volvulus.

The accumulation of fluid and gas in obstructed loops and the altered motility seen in simple mechanical obstruction are rapidly overshadowed by the consequences of blockage of venous outflow from the strangulated segment—extravasation of bloody fluid into the bowel and bowel wall.

In addition to the loss of blood and plasma-like fluid, the gangrenous bowel leaks toxic materials (not to be confused with the pre-Gamble "toxins") into the peritoneal cavity. These have been variously identified as exotoxins or endotoxins, or toxic hemin breakdown products.

The pathophysiology of the strangulated loop is related to several factors: (1) that the contents of an obstructed bowel are toxic; (2) that bacteria are necessary for the production of this toxin; (3) that neither living tissue nor mucous membrane, nor any of the secretions of the mucous membrane, are necessary for the formation of the toxin; (4) that the toxin does not pass through normal mucosa; (5) that absorption of the toxin is more important than its production, as the toxin is physiologically lost if it exists within a loop and is never absorbed; (6) that circulatory damage aids absorption; and (7) that symptoms may be correlated with the toxin formed in the obstructed intestine.

Closed-Loop Obstruction. When both afferent and efferent limbs of a loop of bowel are obstructed, closed-loop intestinal obstruction exists. This is a clinically dangerous form of obstruction because of the propensity for rapid progression to strangulation of the blood supply before the usual manifestations of intestinal obstruction become obvious. Interference with blood supply may occur either from the same mechanism that produced obstruction of the intestine—twist of the bowel on the mesentery, extrinsic band—or from distention of the obstructed loop. The secretory pressure in the closed loop quite rapidly reaches a level sufficient to interfere with venous return from the loop. Widespread distention of the intestine usually does not occur, and so neither does abdominal distention.

Colon Obstruction. The effects on the patient with colon obstruction are usually less dramatic than the effects of small bowel obstruction. First, colon obstruction, with the exception of volvulus, usually does not strangulate. Second, because the colon is principally a storage organ with relatively minor absorptive and secretory functions, fluid and electrolyte sequestration progresses more slowly. Systemic derangements therefrom are of less magnitude and urgency than in small bowel obstruction.

Progressive distention is the most dangerous aspect of nonstrangulated colon obstruction. If the ileocecal valve is incompetent, then partial decompression of the obstructed colon may occur by reflux into the ileum. But if the ileocecal valve is competent, then the colon becomes essentially a closed loop—closed below by the obstructing lesion and above by the competent valve. If the obstruction is not relieved, distention progressing to rupture of the colon threatens. The cecum is the usual site of rupture, because it is the segment of the colon with the largest diameter. According to the law of Laplace, the pressure required to stretch the walls of a hollow viscus decreases in inverse proportion to the radius of curvature. Applying this law to the colon, given an equal pressure throughout the colon, we find that the greatest distention will occur in the portion of the colon with the largest radius (Fig. 24-3).

CLINICAL MANIFESTATIONS. The initial symptoms of simple mechanical intestinal obstruction are abdominal pain, vomiting, and failure to pass gas or feces by rectum. Abdominal distention is a later symptom.

As the bowel obstructs, severe *cramping pain* is felt synchronously with hyperperistalsis. Initially, the waves of cramps are unremitting, but after a short time attacks of pain alternate with quiescent periods during which the patient may feel quite well. The pain is diffuse, poorly localized, and is felt across the upper abdomen in high obstruction, at the level of the umbilicus in low ileal obstruction, in the lower abdomen in colon obstruction, and in the perineum as well as the abdomen in rectosigmoid obstruction. The period between attacks of pain is short with high intestinal obstruction (4 or 5 min) and is longer the lower the obstruction (15 to 20 min). When obstruction is not relieved, the characteristic colicky pain may cease (as distention becomes extreme) and be replaced by a steady generalized abdominal discomfort. There is no real pain in adynamic ileus, just a steady generalized ab-

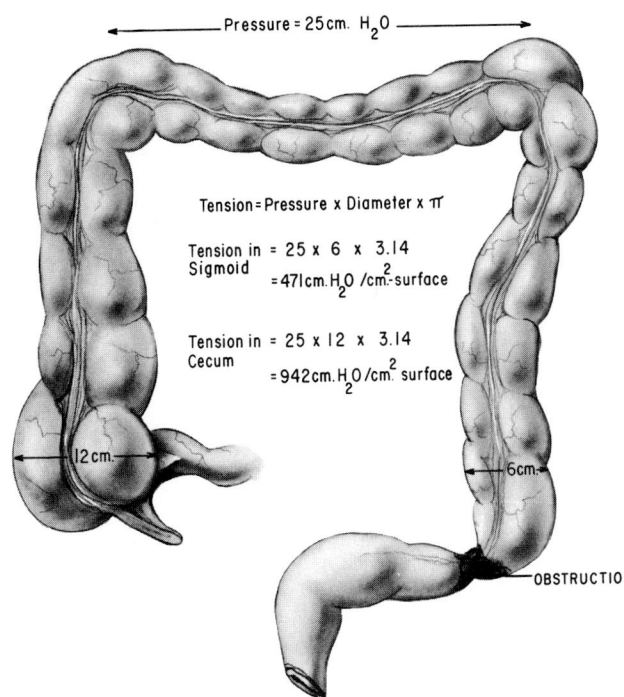

Pressure = 25 cm. H_2O

Tension = Pressure x Diameter x π

Tension in Sigmoid = 25 x 6 x 3.14
= 471 cm. H_2O /cm.^{2}-surface

Tension in Cecum = 25 x 12 x 3.14
= 942 cm. H_2O /cm.^{2} surface

12 cm.

6 cm.

OBSTRUCTION

Fig. 24-3. Physics of cecal rupture in colon obstruction.

dominal discomfort similar to that seen in neglected simple mechanical obstruction. Steady severe pain with no quiescent periods is usually indicative of strangulation.

Vomiting, like pain, usually occurs almost immediately after obstruction of the bowel. This early vomiting is "reflex" vomiting and is followed by a variable quiescent period before vomiting resumes. The quiet interval is short in high obstruction but may even be a day or two with low small bowel obstruction. The vomitus associated with low obstruction frequently becomes thick, dark, and malodorous (i.e., feculent) from stagnation and bacterial action but is not actually regurgitated feces. With high obstruction, vomiting is more frequent and copious and may effectively decompress the obstructed bowel. With low small bowel obstruction, vomiting is less frequent and less productive; little decompression of bowel occurs, because of the excessive length of bowel that the regurgitated material must traverse and because segmentation of the boggy loops prevents regurgitation. Reflex vomiting is unusual in colon obstruction. Thus, vomiting does not occur in most cases until retrograde distention involves the small bowel. When the ileocecal valve is competent, small bowel distention and vomiting may not occur in colonic obstruction.

Failure to pass gas or feces (obstipation) through the rectum is a valuable diagnostic symptom. Gas and feces distal to the obstruction may pass through the rectum after obstruction occurs, however, particularly if the obstruction is high in the jejunum. Cramping pain followed shortly by explosive diarrhea often indicates partial intestinal obstruction.

Abdominal distention is the result of fairly long-standing obstruction. There may be no generalized distention with high small bowel obstruction.

Physical examination of a patient with simple mechanical obstruction within the first 24 h may yield surprisingly few abnormal findings except during periods of colicky pain. Vital signs are essentially normal, and dehydration and distention are not yet marked. Strangulated obstruction is likely if the patient appears seriously ill during this early period. *Palpation* during colic usually demonstrates muscle guarding; between attacks of pain only slight tenderness remains. A mass or localized area of tenderness usually indicates strangulation. *Auscultation* is of great value: in simple mechanical obstruction the abdomen is quiet except during attacks of colic, at which time the sounds become loud, high-pitched, and metallic and occur in bursts or rushes; in paralytic ileus an occasional isolated bowel sound is heard; gangrenous bowel produces complete silence. By the second or third day of obstruction serious illness is obvious. Dehydration and distention are marked, and vital signs are increasingly abnormal, though frank shock does not occur until very late in simple obstruction.

Laboratory Findings. The loss of large amounts of essentially isotonic extracellular fluid into the intestine is principally responsible for the laboratory findings in simple mechanical obstruction. The body responds to this sudden volume decrease by antidiuresis and renal sodium retention. In the early phases, in which the effects are predominantly those of extracellular fluid loss, the hematocrit rises roughly in proportion to the fluid loss. There is little change in the concentration of sodium, potassium, and chloride in the plasma. Acid-base changes, as manifested by the pH and carbon dioxide level, are slight. The markedly reduced urine flow is reflected in a somewhat elevated BUN level. The dehydration and antidiuresis is often so marked that patients may not be able to produce a urine specimen until after intravenous fluid therapy has been started. Urinary specific gravity of 1.025 to 1.030 is the rule; mild proteinuria or acetonuria may also be present.

In the untreated patient, sodium-free water, derived from catabolism of cells and oxidation of fat, tends to restore the acute loss of extracellular fluid volume but at the expense of plasma osmolality. Thus, there is a gradual reduction of the plasma sodium and chloride concentration. Urine volume gradually increases, though not to normal, with excretion of potassium, including the potassium freed by cellular catabolism. The previously noted progressive increase in the hematocrit is halted or actually reversed by the ingress of endogenous water. Acid-base effects are determined by the nature of the fluid lost. Metabolic acidosis due to the combined effects of dehydration, starvation, ketosis, and loss of alkaline secretions is most common. Metabolic alkalosis is infrequent and is principally due to loss of highly acid gastric juice. With great distention of the abdomen, the diaphragm may be sufficiently elevated to embarrass respiration, resulting in carbon dioxide retention and respiratory acidosis.

The white blood cell count is useful in differentiating between different types of obstruction. In general, simple mechanical obstruction calls forth only modest numbers of leukocytes—white blood cell counts often to 15,000/mm^3 with some shift to the left. White blood cell counts of 15,000 to 25,000/mm^3 and marked polymorphonuclear predominance with many immature forms strongly suggest that the obstruction is strangulated, but this is not a sensitive indicator. Very high white cell counts, such as 40,000 to 60,000/mm^3, suggest primary mesenteric vascular occlusion.

Serum amylase level elevations may occur in intestinal obstruction and compromise the differential diagnostic value of the test. Amylase gains entry to the blood by regurgitation from the pancreas because of back pressure in the duodenum, or by peritoneal absorption after leakage from dying bowel. Recently a prospective evaluation of the classic signs of vascular compromise were evaluated. No preoperative clinical parameter, including the presence of continuous abdominal pain, fever, peritoneal signs, leukocytosis, acidosis, hyperamylasemia, or any combination of these were sensitive indicators. The preoperative assessment of the presence or absence of strangulation was correct in only 70 percent of cases.

Radiologic Findings. When properly done, this is the most important diagnostic procedure. The films must be of good technical quality—not the type that are made in the emergency room by a substitute technician with a portable x-ray machine.

X-rays should be made as early in the hospitalization as the patient's condition permits—usually within the first hour. Plain films of the abdomen (without contrast medium) in the supine and upright positions, and posteroanterior and lateral views of the chest are obtained. If the patient is too weak to remain in the sitting position for the 15 min that is necessary to demonstrate air under the diaphragm (best seen on the posteroanterior chest film), then a left lateral decubitus film may be substituted.

The diagnostic features that enable one to distinguish in the majority of cases between simple mechanical obstruction and paralytic ileus are summarized in Table 24-7. Representative films of the three types of obstruction are shown in Fig. 24-4.

Gas-fluid levels are among the important criteria in the x-ray diagnosis of intestinal obstruction. Gas is normally visible in the colon and stomach on plain films of the abdomen in normal adults. Small bowel gas may be visible in infants and occasionally in apparently normal adults. The transit time of swallowed air is normally so rapid that there is an insufficient amount in any one place to show on the x-ray. But if the normal aboral progression of intestinal content is interfered with, then gas collects along with retained fluid and produces gas-fluid levels that are best seen on the upright film of the abdomen. Though gas-fluid levels are highly suggestive of intestinal obstruction (including ileus), they may be seen in other conditions such as extreme aerophagia, gastroenteritis, severe constipation, and sprue.

Barium enema is indicated when the clinical picture and plain films suggest colon obstruction, to give information on the type and location of the obstruction. Barium enema is often helpful also when the distribution of

Table 24-7. RADIOLOGIC SIGNS IN INTESTINAL OBSTRUCTION

Sign	Simple mechanical obstruction (see Fig. 24-4A, B)	Adynamic ileus (see Fig. 24-4C)
Gas in intestine	Large bow-shaped loops in ladder pattern	Copious gas diffusely through intestine
Gas in colon	Less than normal	Increased, scattered through colon
Fluid levels in intestine	Definite	Often very large throughout
Tumor	None	None
Peritoneal exudate	None	Present with peritonitis; otherwise absent
Diaphragm	Somewhat elevated; free motion	Elevated; diminished motion

SOURCE: From Eisenberg RL: *Gastrointestinal Radiology.* Philadelphia, Lippincott, 1983, with permission.

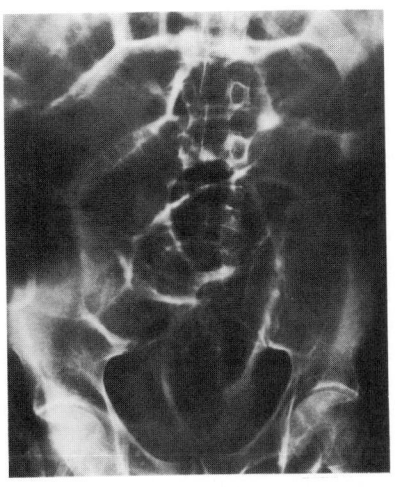
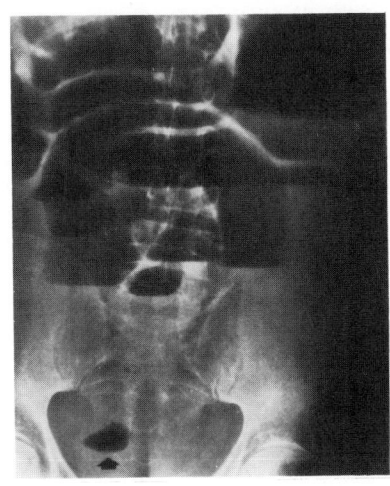
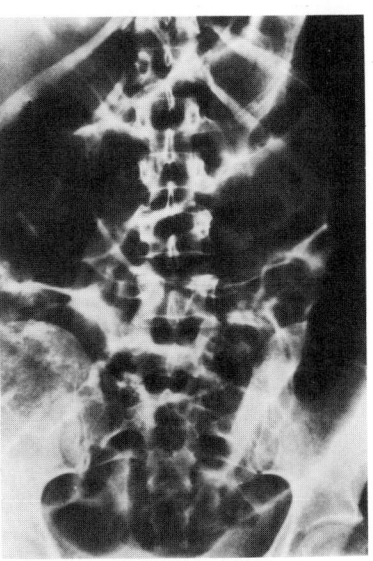

A   *B*

C

Fig. 24-4. *A.* Supine and *B.* upright views demonstrate large amounts of gas in dilated loops of small bowel, but only a single, small collection of gas (arrow) in the colon. *C.* Large amounts of gas and fluid are retained in loops of dilated small and large bowel. The entire small and large bowel appears almost uniformly dilated, with no demonstrable point of obstruction. (From: *Eisenberg RL: Gastrointestinal Radiology. Philadelphia, Lippincott, 1983, p 420, Fig. 33-10, with permission.*)

Fig. 24-5. The antegrade administration of barium demonstrates the precise site of small bowel obstruction. A radiolucent gallstone (arrow) is causing the distal ileal obstruction. (From: *Eisenberg RL: Gastrointestinal Radiology. Philadelphia, Lippincott, 1983, p 420, Fig. 33-13, with permission.*)

gas is not clear on the plain films. Barium enema may be used therapeutically for attempted reduction of nonstrangulated intussusception in children. The dangers of barium enema in obstruction are the possibility of perforating an inflammatory lesion such as diverticulitis or appendicitis and, second, changing a partial colon obstruction to a complete one by forcing barium up past a partially obstructing lesion to form an obstructing concentration of inspissated barium.

Intravenous urography may be indicated to look for ureteral calculi, which often produce marked paralytic ileus.

The principal indication for administration of contrast medium above an obstruction is to differentiate postoperative ileus from mechanical obstruction (Fig. 24-5). The actual point of obstruction rarely can be demonstrated because of dilution of the contrast medium, but if some medium is seen to go through the gastrointestinal tract, the diagnosis of ileus is strengthened. Some surgeons are loath to give barium above an obstruction and prefer to use a liquid medium such as Gastrografin. There is, however, little evidence that small amounts of barium are harmful in small bowel obstruction.

MANAGEMENT. The principles of treatment are fluid and electrolyte therapy, decompression of the bowel, and timed surgical intervention.

Essentially all patients with mechanical intestinal obstruction except those in the immediate postoperative period should be operated upon. The decision to be made is *when* to operate—selection of the optimal time for the individual patient.

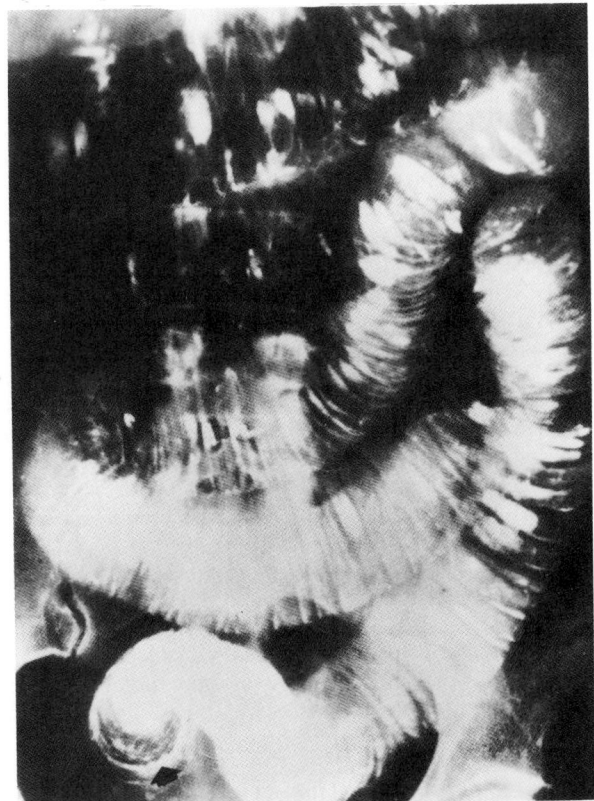

Patients with simple mechanical obstruction who can be operated upon within the first 24 h of the disease do not need extensive preoperative preparation, because water and salt depletion and distention are usually not serious at this stage. After the history and physical examination have established the presumptive diagnosis, laboratory studies should be done, intravenous repletion initiated, decompression started with a nasogastric sump tube in the stomach, and abdominal and chest x-ray films taken on the way to the operating room. This whole process should take less than 2 h. The mortality rate is less than 1 percent for patients with simple mechanical obstruction who are operated upon within the first 24 h.

If the obstruction has been present for more than 24 h when the patient is first seen, depletion and distention may be so severe that if strangulation or closed-loop obstruction seems unlikely, the patient's best interests are served by a period of preparation before the obstruction is surgically relieved. In general, the longer the obstruction has existed, the longer it will take to get the patient ready for surgical treatment. Patients with moderate derangements, particularly hypokalemia, usually require 6 to 12 h; in those with severe problems, up to 24 h may be necessary, mainly because of the hazard of giving intravenous potassium ion faster than it can equilibrate.

With the possible exception of patients with early simple mechanical obstruction, all patients with intestinal obstruction should have a plastic venous catheter threaded into the superior vena cava for frequent measurements of the central venous pressure (CVP), as well as for rapid administration of fluid, and an indwelling catheter inserted into the bladder for accurate continual measurement of the urinary output.

The initial hematocrit reading may be used to estimate the extent of extracellular fluid loss, and thus the volume necessary for restoration of this static debt. For example, if the hematocrit has risen to 55 percent, this indicates a loss of approximately 40 percent of the plasma and extracellular fluid volume.

If acid gastric juice loss is prominent, then normal saline solution is used; otherwise lactated Ringer's solution and 5% dextrose in water in about equal proportions are preferred to replace the lost fluid and to cover maintenance fluid needs. Potassium chloride also will be necessary but should not be given until a good urinary output is established. Antibiotics should also be given in generous dosage and may be added to the intravenous fluids. The choice of antibiotics is a matter of individual preference: the authors currently use ampicillin-gentamycin-clindamycin, or metronidazole with a third-generation cephalosporin.

The rate of fluid administration is best controlled by monitoring the CVP. Fluids may be given rapidly as long as the CVP remains below 10 to 12 cmH$_2$O. The end point of volume replacement is indicated by a sudden rise in the CVP. Other guides are return of skin turgor and the hourly rate of urine production.

The goal in terms of electrolyte concentration and acid-base balance is restoration of these to, or close to, the normal range by the time the volume deficit has been repaired. This is usually possible in patients with reasonably normal renal and pulmonary functions.

When the possibility of strangulation exists, preoperative treatment to fluid-electrolyte normality is not possible or advisable. This is an emergency situation requiring vigorous preparation with fluids and electrolytes, massive antibiotics, nasogastric suction, and an operation at the earliest possible moment to remove the cause of the strangulation and/or nonviable bowel. Despite application of these principles, the mortality rate in strangulated obstruction is still about 25 percent.

Intubation. Tubes for gastrointestinal aspiration, available in bewildering variety, are basically of but two types: "short" tubes for gastric aspiration and "long" tubes for aspiration of the small intestine. The Levin tube, for nasogastric intubation, is preferred by many surgeons for preoperative gastrointestinal decompression in patients with obstruction. Complete decompression of the gastrointestinal tract is not accomplished, since only the intestinal gas and fluid from the upper intestine that regurgitates into the stomach is removed. The stomach is completely emptied, however, which prevents any possible aspiration during anesthesia, and progression of intestinal distention is halted, since all swallowed air is removed. Nasogastric tubes with a double lumen, one for aspiration plus a small second channel to allow ingress of air into the stomach—the sump tube—perform much more efficiently than the old single-lumen tubes.

Long intestinal tubes, of which the Miller-Abbott tube is the prototype, have a lumen for aspiration plus a mercury-containing balloon or small bag at or near the distal end. When inflated in the intestine, the balloon is carried distad by peristalsis. The purpose of the mercury is to aid in getting the tube through the pylorus. After the tube is passed into the stomach, the patient lies on his right side with feet slightly elevated, so that gravity will help pull the tip of the tube through the pylorus.

There is now good evidence that the use of suction as definitive therapy (except as noted below) should be condemned—temporizing may lead to death from strangulated obstruction. The principal indications now for primary intubation therapy are obstruction in the immediate postoperative period, partial small bowel obstruction, or obstruction due to inflammation that is expected to subside under conservative therapy. Some surgeons prefer to use a long intestinal tube for preoperative gastrointestinal decompression in patients with obstruction, feeling that decompression of the intestine per se is sufficiently important to warrant the extra time and trouble necessary to pass an intestinal tube as compared to the Levin nasogastric tube. Emptying of the stomach is inadequate with the long tube, however, and a second short tube is required for this purpose.

Operation. Proper timing of the operation for intestinal obstruction is essential. There are four types of obstruction in which the operation should be done as an emergency as soon as possible after admission: strangulation, closed-loop obstruction, colon obstruction, and early simple mechanical obstruction.

The principal hazard to life in strangulation is septic

shock from transperitoneal absorption of toxins spilled from dying bowel. In closed-loop obstruction, which cannot be decompressed by intubation, the hazard is that the loop will strangulate, and it must be treated with the same urgency as strangulation.

In colon obstruction, which also cannot be decompressed by tube, a competent ileocecal valve preventing regurgitation into the ileum converts the colon into a closed loop. Since fluid and electrolyte abnormalities progress slowly in colon obstruction, a brief period of hydration while laboratory studies are being done is all that is necessary before operation. And, as noted above, when patients with simple mechanical obstruction get to the surgeon early in the course of their disease, immediate surgical procedures may be carried out with essentially no mortality. Thus only in *late* simple mechanical obstruction of the small intestine does extensive preparation for operation take priority over immediate operation.

Anesthesia. General anesthesia is safest for the patient and the method of choice from the point of view of both surgeon and anesthesiologist. Endotracheal intubation, at times performed initially under local anesthesia, is particularly indicated to prevent aspiration of regurgitated gastric content. The surgeon should not be tempted to use local anesthesia for abdominal exploration on the assumption that local anesthesia is easier on the poor-risk patient than general anesthesia—it is not. Local anesthesia should be used only when the surgeon knows the cause of the obstruction and plans a limited procedure only, such as cecostomy.

Surgical Procedures. Surgical procedures for the relief of intestinal obstruction may be divided into five categories:

1. Procedures not requiring opening of bowel—lysis of adhesions, manipulation-reduction of intussusception, reduction of incarcerated hernia
2. Enterotomy for removal of obturation obstruction—gallstone, bezoars
3. Resection of the obstructing lesion or strangulated bowel with primary anastomosis
4. Short-circuiting anastomosis around an obstruction
5. Formation of a cutaneous stoma proximal to the obstruction—cecostomy, transverse colostomy (Figs. 24-6 and 24-7).

On opening the peritoneum, the presence or absence of free peritoneal fluid should be noted, as well as the appearance of the fluid. Bloody fluid denotes strangulation, whereas clear straw-colored fluid is found with simple obstruction. The point of obstruction is usually best found by starting in the right lower quadrant. If the cecum is grossly distended, the obstruction is in the colon. If collapsed small bowel is found, then this is followed back to the point of obstruction, thus avoiding evisceration of the proximal distended loops.

The surgeon is sometimes faced with the difficult decision of whether to resect or to replace in the abdomen a loop of intestine of questionable viability. Before release the strangulated loop of viable bowel has a dull purple-red appearance and is devoid of motion. After release there is a dramatic color change to bright red in the obviously viable loop as well as a return of peristalsis. Conversely, in obviously dead bowel there is no color change and no motion after release of the strangulating obstruction. The loop that only partially pinks up and has little or no motion is the problem. It is usually best to wrap the questionable segment in moist laparotomy pads and leave it completely undisturbed for 10 min by the clock. If the circulation is obviously better at the end of this time, the loop is replaced in the abdomen. If the viability of the segment is still in doubt, resection should be done. Fluorescein staining and Doppler evaluations have been used to distinguish between viable and dead bowel, but results are not consistent. If a very long segment of bowel is involved, requiring a very extensive resection, then an attempt should be made to restore flow in the larger vessels supplying the segment. Even if this is unsuccessful, one should probably accept the risk of replacing nonviable bowel rather than make an intestinal cripple. The patient is observed very closely; if evidence of progressive toxicity develops, reoperation and resection are done. In any event, reexploration and reevaluation of the status of the bowel about 24 h later may be advisable.

Decompression of grossly distended intestine during the operative procedure is sometimes necessary, particularly in late simple mechanical obstruction. Operative decompression is still a contentious point. There is no doubt that the operation is facilitated: the site of obstruction is more easily found, the uncontrolled eventration of distended loops through the incision is avoided, the bowel can be returned to the peritoneal cavity without the kinks that may cause segmentation and postoperative obstruction, and closure of the incision is possible without a struggle. Relief of distention also improves the blood supply to the intestine, and peristalsis returns sooner. It is also probable that removal of toxic bowel content is worthwhile. Whereas the normal mucosa is impermeable to these toxins, permeability is affected by impairment of the blood supply, and absorption may occur in compromised bowel.

Operative aspiration can be done in a variety of ways. Multiple needle aspirations are ineffective and definitely increase the morbidity: studies have shown a wound infection rate of 20 percent versus a rate of 4 percent in a comparable group of patients without needle aspiration. Decompression with an ordinary suction tip through multiple enterotomies, though effective, is similarly attended by an increased infection rate, plus the risk of small bowel fistula. An effective, safe method of decompression is by passage of a tube from above downward, so that the entire gastrointestinal tract proximal to the obstruction is decompressed. A firm tube with generous lumen (Baker tube) is introduced through a proximal jejunostomy. It may be preferable to pass the tube transnasally or through a gastrostomy and thread it into the small intestine. The tube is advanced by manipulation through the intact bowel until the entire length of involved bowel down to the obstructed segment is pleated on the long tube. The tube is secured in that position for postoperative decompression.

Postoperative Care. The principles of postoperative care are the same as for the preoperative preparation of the

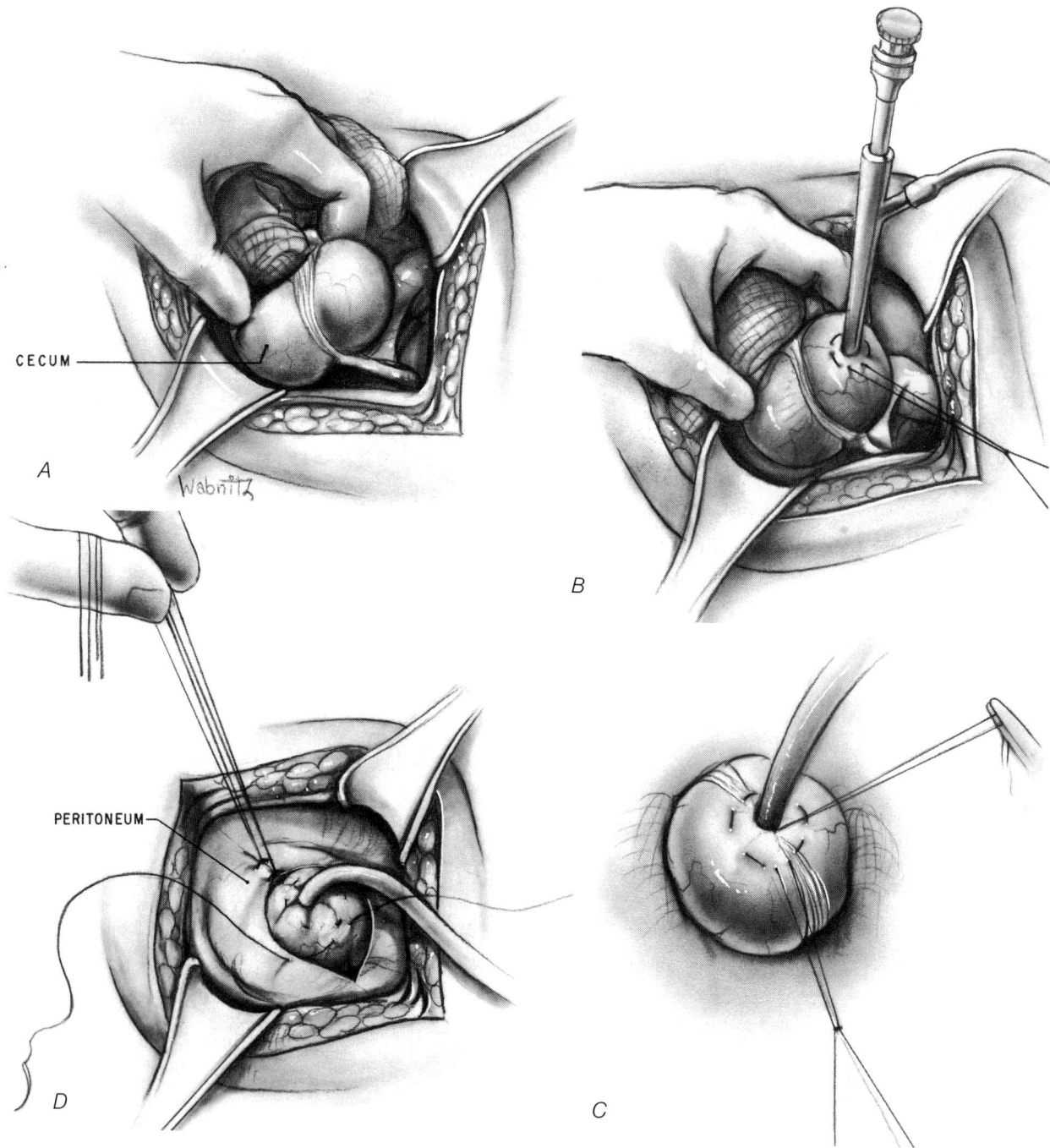

CECUM

Wabnitz

A

B

PERITONEUM

D

C

Fig. 24-6. Tube cecostomy. *A.* A McBurney incision is made in the right lower quadrant, the lateral peritoneal attachment of the cecum is divided, and the cecum is delivered into the wound, using a dry sponge. *B.* The distended cecum is held by the assistant, using gauze sponges, while the surgeon decompresses the cecum with a large trocar connected to suction. If distention is not great, this step may be omitted. *C.* A large rubber tube is then placed in the cecum by enlarging the opening made by the trocar, and the tube is secured in place with two concentric purse-string sutures. *D.* The peritoneum is sutured circumferentially to the cecum. Fascia is approximated; skin and subcutaneous tissues are packed open. The tube is connected to straight drainage.

patient with obstruction—fluids and electrolytes, antibiotics, and gastrointestinal decompression.

Fluid and electrolyte management is more difficult in the postoperative intestinal obstruction patient than in the usual postoperative abdominal surgical patient because of the large third space of sequestered, isotonic fluid. There is continued loss in the immediate postoperative period into the sequestered fluid space. This loss slows in rate, however, and is reversed in direction after a variable pe-

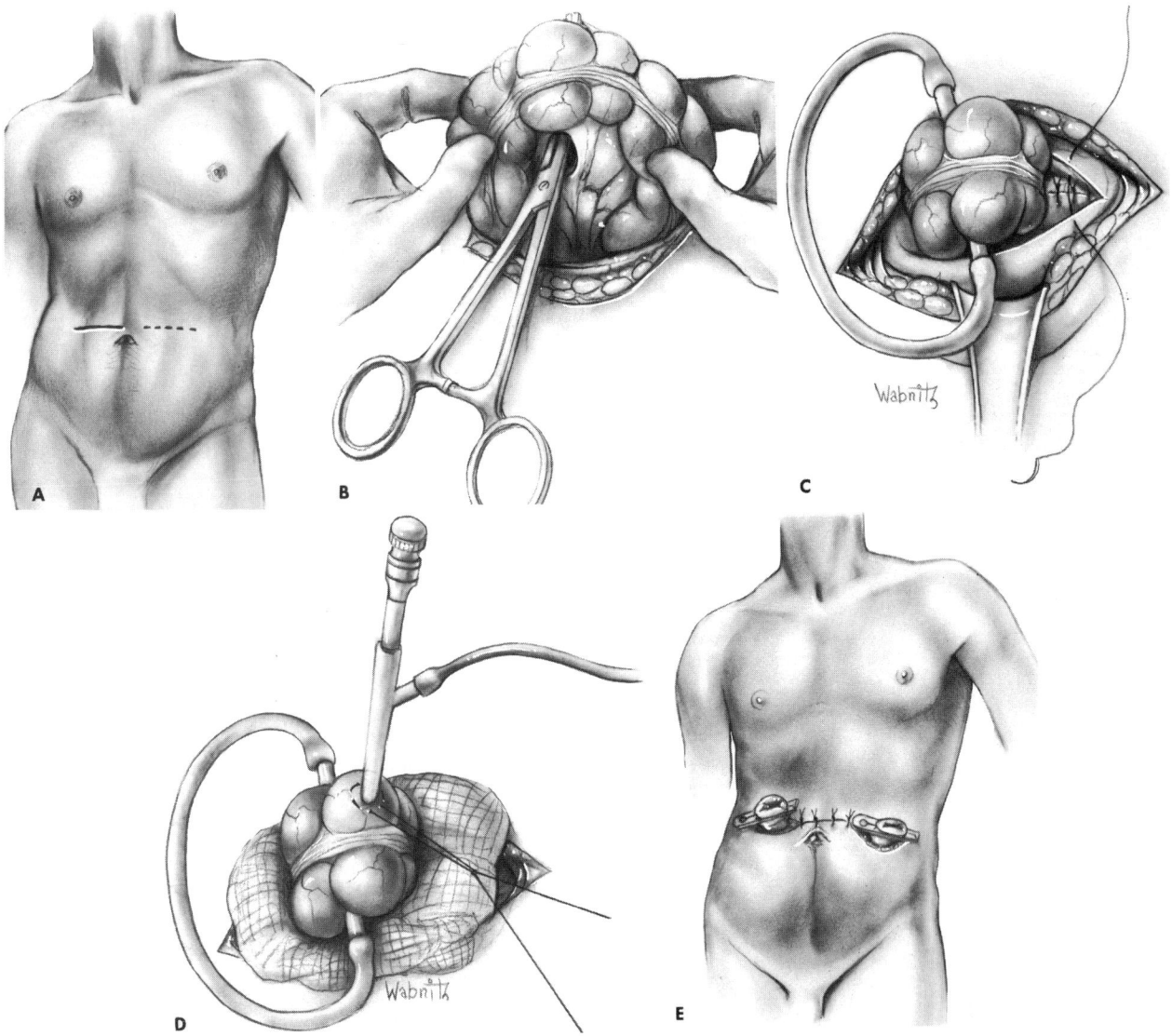

Fig. 24-7. Transverse loop colostomy. *A.* A short transverse incision is made about midway between costal margin and umbilicus. Choice of right or left depends on the type of definitive surgical treatment planned for the future. *B.* After freeing the omentum, an opening is made in an avascular area of the transverse mesocolon close to the bowel. *The middle colic artery must be avoided. C.* A glass rod is inserted through the mesentery and secured in place by rubber tubing. The incision is closed in layers about the colon loop. No sutures are placed in the colon. *D.* If colon distention is extreme, trocar decompression may be done immediately after closing the incision. Otherwise the colostomy is opened with cautery about 24 to 36 h after operation. *E.* Double-barrel colostomy may be performed initially using deMartel's clamps. A small catheter can be inserted into the proximal limb to achieve immediate decompression.

riod, usually about the third postoperative day. This large autoinfusion, as fluid is picked up by the vascular compartment from the sequestered fluid, must be allowed for in planning the daily ration of intravenous fluid therapy, lest the patient be watered into congestive failure. Serum sodium and potassium levels must be watched very closely and kept in the normal range. A deficit of either or both of these ions is associated with prolonged paralysis of the gastrointestinal tract.

Decompression of the gastrointestinal tract is also harder to handle than in the usual postoperative patient, because restoration of normal propulsive intestinal motility is usually significantly delayed after release of intestinal obstruction. Whereas bowel function usually resumes on about the third day after abdominal operation, after intestinal obstruction it is often 5 or 6 days before gastrointestinal decompression can be discontinued. After 2 or 3 days of suction drainage it is often advisable to discontinue the suction and vent the intestinal tube to straight drainage only, to minimize fluid and electrolyte losses. This also obviates the problem of bleeding from ''tube ulcers'' that form when the mucosa is suctioned into the side vents.

Ileus

Ileus may be divided into three groups: *adynamic, or inhibition, ileus,* in which there is diminished or absent motility because of inhibition of the neuromuscular apparatus; *spastic ileus,* in which the bowel musculature remains tightly contracted without coordinated propulsive motility; and the *ileus of vascular occlusion,* in which the bowel wall is incapable of coordinated motility, because it is dying from ischemia.

Spastic ileus, an uncommon form caused by uncoordinated hyperactivity of the intestine, is seen in heavy-metal poisoning, in porphyria, and sometimes in uremia. Therapy of the intestinal manifestations is usually not indicated—therapy should be aimed at the underlying disorder.

Adynamic ileus of some degree is extremely common, since it occurs after every abdominal operation. The rate of recovery of motor function is different in different segments of the gastrointestinal tract: small bowel motility returns within 24 h and gastric motility within 48 h, but colonic inertia persists for 3 to 5 days. Oral intake usually can be resumed on the third or fourth postoperative day. Only when postoperative ileus persists does it become a clinical problem. Common causes of serious degrees of inhibition ileus are many and varied and include intraperitoneal inflammations such as acute appendicitis or acute pancreatitis; retroperitoneal pathologic conditions such as ureteral colic, retroperitoneal hematoma, or fracture of the spine; thoracic lesions such as basal pneumonia or fractured ribs; and systemic causes such as severe toxemia, hyponatremia, hypokalemia, or hypomagnesemia. Several drugs have also been implicated. These include: morphine, propantheline, antacids, anticoagulants, phenothiazines, and ganglionic blocking agents.

Overactivity of the sympathetic system appears to be the common denominator in inhibition ileus associated with many of the lesions listed above; alterations in the composition of the internal environment also play an important role.

Centrally induced inhibition of motility is virtually exclusively dependent on the hormonal component of the sympathoadrenal system. Pseudoobstruction of the colon may develop as a result of inhibition of the sacral parasympathetic nerves.

CLINICAL MANIFESTATIONS. The primary disease causing the ileus may predominate in the clinical picture, or conversely, in some cases, abdominal findings may so predominate that the primary process is overlooked. In postoperative ileus, the division between physiologic ileus and the undue abnormal prolongation of bowel hypofunction is blurred. Instead of passing flatus and becoming hungry on about the third day, as expected following abdominal operation, the patient is noted to be distended and disinterested in food and surroundings. Examination confirms that there is generalized abdominal distention with tympany and scattered, occasional bowel sounds.

Assistance from the laboratory is needed mainly in evaluating some of the causes of ileus, such as acute anemia, sepsis, hyponatremia, hypokalemia, and hypoosmolarity.

As outlined above (Table 24-7 and Fig. 24-4), x-ray can often help in the differential diagnosis between postoperative adynamic ileus and postoperative mechanical obstruction. If the plain films are inconclusive, contrast medium is given by mouth or through a gastrointestinal tube. In inhibition ileus, some medium should reach the cecum in about 4 h, whereas a stationary column of medium for 3 or 4 h indicates complete obstruction of the small intestine.

Adynamic ileus characteristically involves both the small and large bowel to a greater or lesser degree. Occasionally, there is marked distention confined largely to the colon without evidence of mechanical obstruction of the bowel itself or interference with its blood supply—this is known as pseudoobstruction of the colon or Ogilvie's syndrome. Barium enema is indicated to rule out organic obstruction. Cecal perforation may occur even though mechanical intestinal obstruction is absent.

TREATMENT. The treatment of ileus is essentially the treatment of the primary lesion. Postoperative ileus is caused in the vast majority of patients either by focal inflammation—leaking anastomosis, abscess following contamination—or by gross fluid-electrolyte derangements. When these problems are promptly eradicated, the ileus will take care of itself.

Treatment of the distention is best done by passage of a long tube. Unfortunately it is much more difficult to pass than in mechanical obstruction because of the difference in motility of the intestine. If the long tube will not pass the pylorus, then gastric suction should be used and will prevent further distention.

Nonoperative methods of increasing gastrointestinal motility continue to be evaluated. Gastrointestinal pacing by means of an electrode in the tip of the nasogastric tube through which physiologic electric currents are delivered appears to be of little value. Similarly, injections of D-pantothenyl alcohol (a component of coenzyme A that is necessary for the production of acetylcholine) have been shown to be ineffective in postoperative ileus.

Vasopressin, which causes contraction of smooth muscle, and parasympathomimetic drugs such as neostigmine or Urecholine will often increase intestinal motility but are not safe to use, because perforation of the bowel can result if there is mechanical obstruction. Metoclopramide, a dopamine antagonist derived from procainamide, enhances gastrointestinal motility without causing spasm, and has been used extensively in Europe for postoperative ileus. No convincing advantage over placebo can be shown in double-blind studies, however.

Rarely, paralytic ileus does not respond to conservative measures—the obstruction does not relent, and operation must be considered. In most such cases, mechanical obstruction will be found. If no mechanical factors are found, a long tube should be manipulated by the surgeon well down into the small bowel. If the ileocecal valve is competent and marked colon distention is present, then cecostomy should be added. The ileus will be made worse by the operation but can now be managed with adequate decompression. Nonobstructive colon dilation is best managed by colonoscopy.

Pseudoobstruction

Recently a group of patients has been identified that has manifestations of bowel obstruction but no organic lesion. Although the entire gastrointestinal tract is involved, the disorder usually presents with symptoms and signs related to the small intestine. The symptoms are generally intermittent and extend over years. Vomiting that relieves the abdominal pain is characteristic. Distention may be marked. The pseudoobstruction may be caused by an hereditary hollow visceral myopathy. Diabetes mellitus, hypothyroidism, pheochromocytosis, hypoparathyroidism, dermatomyositis, lupus erythematosus, myotonic dystrophy, parkinsonism, multiple sclerosis, and amyloidosis have been associated causes. Esophageal manometry is useful for screening and the mecholyl test is positive for patients who have pseudoobstruction. Treatment of underlying diabetes, collagen vascular disease, or amyloidosis does not relieve the pseudoobstruction.

GASTROINTESTINAL BLEEDING: HEMATEMESIS, MELENA, AND RECTAL BLEEDING

Bleeding may be a manifestation of a variety of diseases along the entire length of the gastrointestinal tract from the oropharynx to the anus. Bleeding represents the initial symptom of gastrointestinal disease in more than one-third of these patients, and in 70 percent there is no history of a previous bleeding episode.

DEFINITIONS. *Hematemesis* refers to the vomiting of blood that is either fresh and unaltered or digested by gastric secretion. It is a manifestation of a bleeding site located between the oropharynx and the ligament of Treitz and may be accompanied by simultaneous melena. The character of the specimen depends on the site of bleeding, the rate of hemorrhage, and the rate of gastric emptying. The presence of blood clots reflects massive bleeding, while a coffee-ground vomitus usually indicates a slower bleeding rate with retention in the stomach and alteration of the blood to form acid hematin.

Melena is usually defined as the passage of a black, tarry stool. Only 50 mL of blood is necessary to produce this sign, and, following the cessation of a bleeding of 1000 mL, the finding may persist for as long as 5 days. A guaiac-positive stool, indicative of occult blood, may persist for 3 weeks following hematemesis or melena. In general, blood from the distal colon is red and not thoroughly mixed with the stool, whereas blood from the upper gastrointestinal tract produces a tarry stool. However, massive bleeding from the upper gastrointestinal tract may be associated with red or currant jelly clots if the bleeding is rapid and gastrointestinal motility is increased. Red or black stools may also result from the ingestion of food dye substances and iron. The tarry color, which accom-

panies upper gastrointestinal bleeding, is attributable to the production of acid hematin by action of gastric acid on the hemoglobin or the production of sulfide from heme by the action of hydrogen sulfide on the iron in the heme molecule. Melena without hematemesis generally indicates a lesion distal to the pylorus but has been associated with bleeding varices and gastritis.

CONSEQUENCES OF GASTROINTESTINAL BLEEDING. Hypotension and shock are dependent upon the rate of the bleeding and the patient's response to the blood loss. It is difficult to estimate the amount of blood loss in either the vomitus or stool, because both specimens contain a mixture of multiple components. The hematocrit and hemoglobin levels are unreliable until equilibration occurs, i.e., 6 to 48 h subsequent to the bleeding, and estimations of blood volume have also proved unreliable, since the error associated with the technique is great and the range of normals for a given physical state is wide. Shortly after bleeding has begun, a vasovagal reaction is associated with bradycardia, whereas with the passage of time the heart rate increases and the cardiac output decreases. The clinical picture of shock may reflect a coronary occlusion or myocardial ischemia precipitated by hemorrhage rather than the consequences of massive blood loss per se. Another consequence of hypotension is reduced renal blood flow, resulting in either oliguria or anuria.

Azotemia, which is characteristically associated with bleeding esophagogastric varices, also occurs in patients with other types of massive hemorrhage. BUN levels of 30 mg/dL or more occur in two-thirds of patients with bleeding varices, and an elevation of 50 mg/dL or more occurs in one-fifth of the cases. Following cessation of the bleeding, normal levels are usually achieved within 3 days. Azotemia usually does not occur with hemorrhage originating in the colon, and since it is dependent upon bacterial action, normal BUN levels may be associated with upper gastrointestinal tract bleeding in patients on antibiotics that sterilize the intestinal flora. The level to which the BUN rises parallels the extent of gastrointestinal bleeding, but it may be potentiated by shock, impairment of renal function, and increased catabolism. In the presence of blood in the intestinal tract renal function can be evaluated by clearance studies.

Upper Gastrointestinal Tract Bleeding

ETIOLOGY. Although a great variety of lesions above the ligament of Treitz have been implicated in the cause of upper gastrointestinal tract hemorrhage, in the vast majority it is due to peptic ulceration, acute mucosal lesions—gastritis and erosions—esophagogastric varices, reflux esophagitis, or gastric neoplasms (Table 24-8).

Peptic ulceration represents the most common cause and accounts for one-half to two-thirds of the cases. Hemorrhage from a duodenal ulcer occurs four times more frequently than from a gastric ulcer, but since this represents the relative incidence of the two lesions, the two types have an equal tendency to bleed. Massive bleeding occurs in 10 to 15 percent of ulcer patients with

Table 24-8. ETIOLOGY OF UPPER GASTROINTESTINAL TRACT BLEEDING IN 14,265 CASES

Author	Year	Number of cases	Peptic ulcer, %	Acute mucosal lesions, %	Esophageal varices, %	Reflex esophagitis, %	Gastric cancer, %	Other, %	Undetermined, %
Ferguson	1962	1124	62	4	7	1	4	1	20
Hirschowitz	1963	216	58	22	1	1	1	5	12
Dorsey	1965	405	68	2	2	3	1	5	20
Jones	1970	4131	58	26	3	2	3	6	3
Katz	1970	800	24	33	17			10	16
Palmer	1970	1400	45	12	19	8		11	7
Schiff	1970	640	53	1	13		2	11	21
Halmagyi	1970	199	65	1	7	6	1	15	5
Preston	1970	535	50	2	30				17
Schiller	1970	2149	45	3	2		2	22	26
Foster	1971	296	67	13	9		3	4	4
Crook	1972	880	50	19	11	3	2	5	4
Himal	1978	964	62	16	7		2	5	11
Dronfield	1982	526	49	5	2	6	3	8	27
Average			52	14	8	2	2	8	14

hemorrhage and is the first symptom in 16 percent of the patients who bleed. The bleeding is generally caused by the inflammatory process eroding into the regional artery. In the case of duodenal ulcers, the gastroduodenal artery is involved, while the left and right gastric arteries and their branches are most frequently involved with gastric ulcers. Most bleeding ulcers are chronic lesions, and the adjacent arteries suffer from local inflammatory changes. Since hemostasis is dependent upon the retraction of the walls of the vessel, persistent bleeding is more likely to occur with chronic lesions and in older patients with atherosclerotic vessels.

Peptic ulceration of the stomal mucosa at the site of a gastroenterostomy is to be considered in any patient who has had previous gastric surgical treatment. It is a more frequent occurrence when less than two-thirds of the stomach has been removed and an accompanying vagotomy has not been performed, especially if there is retained antrum.

The next most common cause of gross upper gastrointestinal tract hemorrhage after peptic ulcer is a diverse group of lesions that can best be collectively termed *acute mucosal lesions* until they are clearly delineated and separated into entities. The reported incidence (Table 24-8) ranges from 1 to 33 percent. The true incidence will not be known until endoscopy is universally applied early in the course of upper gastrointestinal tract hemorrhage. Pathologically, these lesions are sometimes single but more often multiple, or the mucosa may be diffusely involved in hemorrhagic necrosis. The process usually does not extend through the muscularis mucosae, and therefore the lesions are technically *erosions,* not true ulcers. In contradistinction to chronic benign ulcers, which are characteristically located in the antrum or on the lesser curvature, acute erosive lesions are found in the body and fundus of the stomach, sparing the antrum, and on the greater curvature as often as on the lesser curvature. "Tube ulcers," related to suction-drawing mucosa into the apertures of the nasogastric tube, may cause bleeding.

"Stress ulceration" is a much abused term, which, if used at all, should be confined to the acute gastroduodenal lesions that occur secondary to shock and sepsis following operation, trauma, or burns. McClelland et al. have shown in patients with trauma and hemorrhagic shock that gastric secretion is not increased but that splanchnic blood flow is significantly decreased. They conclude that "ischemic damage to the superficial gastric mucosa may induce stress ulceration." Sepsis also plays a prominent role. Upper gastrointestinal tract bleeding has been noted in approximately one-third of surgical patients with septicemia; coagulation abnormalities that attend sepsis have been implicated.

Probably closely related to stress erosion is the acute ulceration or erosion of the stomach and duodenum that occurs in burn patients. Such lesions are usually referred to as *Curling's ulcers,* after the man who described them in 1842. Curling's ulcers occur in about 12 percent of patients hospitalized for burns. The incidence increases with burn size—up to a 40 percent incidence in burns of 70 percent or more of the body surface. Sepsis is an additive stress. In two-thirds of patients with Curling's ulcer the presenting clinical sign is bleeding, and in 45 percent such bleeding is massive. Though there are many similarities between stress erosions and Curling's ulcers, their distribution is somewhat different: Curling's ulcers are about evenly divided between single and multiple, and between stomach and duodenum.

Another eponymic ulcer that is probably closely related to stress erosion is the *Cushing ulcer.* In 1932, Harvey Cushing described a variety of esophagogastroduodenal lesions in nine patients following craniotomy. Since then the belief has persisted that dysfunction in specific areas of the brain leads to gastrointestinal ulceration. In many of these patients, the etiologic factors are probably the same as for patients after any major operation, but there is some evidence that significant gastric hypersecretion may occur after certain intracranial operations or trauma.

Adrenal corticosteroids, given in large doses for prolonged periods, frequently lead to gastroduodenal erosions or ulcers, or to activation of preexisting quiescent peptic ulcers. Patients receiving steroids for rheumatoid arthritis or lupus erythematosus are more prone to this complication than patients with asthma or inflammatory bowel disease. Despite the fact that steroids do not increase the gastric acid output, antacid therapy is often efficacious. The distribution of "steroid ulcers" is much the same as that of postoperative "stress ulcers."

Aspirin and alcohol are the major offenders in a large group of ingested agents that may produce erosive, hemorrhagic gastritis and duodenitis. The incidence with which this lesion is diagnosed is directly related to the degree to which early endoscopic examination is employed. Alcohol is a known gastric secretagogue, but aspirin and similar agents are not; the latter presumably act by increasing back-diffusion of HCl through the gastric mucosa. The hemorrhage is generally mild to moderate but is sometimes massive. Since the gastric mucosa normally renews itself every 48 to 72 h, the process is self-limited if symptoms can be controlled until mucosal regeneration occurs. Emergency operation for exsanguinating hemorrhage is sometimes necessary.

Esophagogastric varices constitute the most common cause of bleeding in patients with cirrhosis or extrahepatic obstruction of the portal vein. These account for approximately 10 percent of all cases of upper gastrointestinal tract bleeding, but the incidence varies widely, being significantly higher in hospitals with a large indigent population. Bleeding varices constitute 95 percent of the cases of massive hematemesis in the child, and they are usually associated with extrahepatic obstruction of the portal vein. In cirrhotic patients, varices are the cause of bleeding in 53 percent of the cases, while gastritis is implicated in 22 percent and duodenal and gastric ulcers in 20 percent. Correlation of the lesions and severity of bleeding reveals that in the majority of cases (70 percent) patients with bleeding from varices have severe hemorrhage while 84 percent of patients with bleeding from gastritis demonstrate mild to moderate blood loss. The precipitation of the bleeding episode has been ascribed to two major factors: increased pressure within the varix and ulceration secondary to esophagitis. Although esophagogastric varices are almost always associated with portal hypertension, the diagnosis has been established in occasional patients with normal portal pressures. The veins responsible for the bleeding are usually opened laterally by transmural erosion, and any hemostasis that occurs is dependent upon occlusion of the opening by a thrombus. The bleeding is nearly always associated with hematemesis and is generally very profuse.

Hiatal hernia frequently may be associated with occult bleeding but is usually not a cause of gross upper gastrointestinal tract hemorrhage, accounting for approximately 2 percent of the cases. The bleeding in the sliding hernia is related to *reflux peptic esophagitis*. Bleeding is more commonly seen with paraesophageal hernias and is thought to be caused by the retention of acid contents within the incarcerated gastric pouch or congestion of the vascular supply of the herniated portion of the stomach.

A variety of miscellaneous lesions account for up to 8 percent of occasional upper gastrointestinal tract bleeding, while in 16 percent the diagnosis is never determined. Neoplasms are not commonly implicated, and there is evidence that the incidence of carcinoma of the stomach is decreasing in the United States. Bleeding associated with *gastric carcinoma* is caused by erosion of the tumor into underlying vessels. It is usually mild to moderate, but if a large vessel is involved, massive bleeding can occur. Massive hemorrhage may be the initial symptom in a patient with gastric carcinoma. Other tumors occur less frequently. Leiomyoma and leiomyosarcoma of the stomach or esophagus may be manifested by profuse bleeding, usually in men in the third decade of life. Leukemia with intestinal infiltrates may cause significant gastrointestinal bleeding. Also, polyps, either single, familial, or associated with the Peutz-Jeghers syndrome, are included as neoplastic lesions with a bleeding potential.

Vascular lesions, including angiomas, hereditary hemorrhagic telangiectasia (Rendu-Osler-Weber syndrome), and vasculitis, have all been reported as etiologic factors in upper gastrointestinal tract bleeding. Spontaneous rupture of aortic, hepatic arterial, and splenic arterial aneurysms into the gastrointestinal tract may produce alarming bleeding. Characteristically, aortoenteric fistula is manifested by moderate bleeding that stops for a variable period of time only to recur as massive bleeding.

Inflammation of the mucosa with erosion of small or large vessels may accompany prolapsing gastric mucosa and duodenal diverticula. Prolapsing gastric mucosa, which is usually not considered a common source of bleeding, may be accompanied by moderate blood loss. Similarly, although duodenal diverticula are generally considered to be asymptomatic, massive hemorrhage has accompanied ulceration of this lesion. Hepatic trauma with development of a central or subcapsular hematoma that discharges into the biliary tree is responsible for the development of the syndrome known as *hematobilia,* which can represent a cause of moderate or massive bleeding. Hematobilia can also occur with cholecystitis, cholelithiasis, and passage of stones. The interval between trauma and the bleeding manifestation is variable. Another traumatic cause of upper gastrointestinal tract bleeding is the Mallory-Weiss syndrome, which consists of linear tears of the esophagogastric junction induced by severe vomiting, usually in alcoholic patients.

DIAGNOSIS. History and Physical Examination. The patient's own account of the amount of bleeding is frequently misleading. Vomiting of large amounts of blood is most suggestive of bleeding ulcer or esophagogastric varices. A history of active ulcer symptoms preceding the hemorrhage with cessation of the pain at the onset of bleeding suggests that the bleeding is originating from a peptic ulcer. Twenty percent of patients with bleeding have no previous history of ulcer. Although there is an increased incidence of the ulcer diathesis in cirrhotic patients, esophagogastric varices represent the most common cause of bleeding in these patients and account for over 50 percent of the bleeding episodes. Violent retching and vomiting in alcoholics or pregnant women is characteristic of Mallory-Weiss syndrome. The history should include questions directed toward the recent ingestion of drugs implicated as causes of gastrointestinal bleeding, particularly salicylates, phenylbutazone (Butazolidin), alcohol, anticoagulants, and steroids. A history regarding the bleeding tendency during childhood, in early adulthood, and in other members of the family focuses on the possibility of hematologic disorders. Previous gastric surgical treatment such as gastroenterostomy or partial gastrectomy directs one's thinking toward the possibility of a marginal ulcer. Heartburn, epigastric substernal pain accentuated by the recumbent position and the ingestion of large meals, suggests the presence of a hiatal hernia. A recent history of upper abdominal or chest trauma is most compatible with a diagnosis of hematobilia, particularly when the bleeding is accompanied by jaundice and intermittent colicky pain.

Examination of the patient with upper gastrointestinal tract bleeding is directed at uncovering stigmata of the various diseases considered in the etiology. The skin and mucous membranes should be examined for icterus, spider angiomas, liver palms, and decreased hair over the extremities, all suggestive of hepatic disease. The mucous membrane should be investigated for melanin spots of the Peutz-Jeghers syndrome. Hereditary telangiectasia lesions are most common on the lips, tongue, and ears. Lymphadenopathy, particularly in the left supraclavicular region, may suggest a malignant intraabdominal process. Abdominal palpation more commonly reveals tenderness when the bleeding is related to ulcer or gastritis, whereas a palpable liver, particularly when accompanied by splenomegaly and abdominal veins that fill in a centrifugal pattern from the umbilicus, is more indicative of bleeding varices. Examination should always include aspiration via nasogastric tube in order to determine presence of blood at this level and the extent of bleeding at the time of examination.

Special Diagnostic Procedures. The extent of anemia may be assessed by the hematocrit level. It should be appreciated that, with acute blood loss, the initial level may be normal, since the hematocrit reduction does not occur for 4 to 6 h, during which time equilibration occurs. Repeat hematocrit readings taken at 4- to 6-h intervals are more meaningful. Leukocytosis, with levels of 25,000/mm^3, may accompany acute hemorrhage, but more marked increases are suggestive of leukemia. Both the neutrophils and platelets may be reduced in the case of hypersplenism secondary to primary hepatic disease, suggesting bleeding from esophagogastric varices.

Clinical chemistries are directed toward evaluating the extent of bleeding and, particularly, determining the presence of hepatocellular dysfunction. None of the tests define the site of bleeding. A rise in the BUN level parallels the extent of hemorrhage and is related to the absorption of blood products from the gastrointestinal tract, possible associated reduction in renal flow secondary to shock or dehydration, and, at times, the presence of preexisting renal disease. In the presence of marked hepatic dysfunction, the BUN level may not be elevated, since the liver is unable to synthesize urea. In this circumstance, the blood

ammonia level is frequently elevated with bleeding varices, since it is related to the extent of portal collateralization and reduced hepatic function. The validity of this test, however, is not uniform. Normal values may be present in patients with variceal bleeding.

Determination of the blood clotting factors is of great importance, particularly in patients bleeding from stress ulceration. Reduced platelet adhesiveness, thrombocytopenia, prolonged prothrombin time, and other clotting defects are common in such patients. The bleeding often stops, obviating emergency operation, following the administration of fresh platelet infusions, vitamin K, and fresh-frozen plasma.

Rarely, bleeding is so rapid that immediate operation without preoperative diagnostic procedures is necessary to save life. More commonly, transfusions can easily allow time for diagnosis and preparation; further, many patients stop bleeding soon after admission. As the above tests are being done, the patient should be rapidly transfused to circulatory normality, with vital signs, central venous pressure, and urinary output as guides. The stomach should be completely evacuated using iced Ringer's lavage through a nasogastric tube; an Ewald tube may be advisable initially if many large clots are present.

Endoscopy is the first special diagnostic procedure to be considered; it is virtually mandatory if the bleeding is thought to be from esophagogastric varices or from an acute mucosal lesion. Esophagoscopy defines the bleeding point in the case of varices, since liver function tests, manometry, barium x-ray, and isotopic studies merely indicate the presence of portal hypertension or varices but do not determine if these lesions are actually bleeding. The reported esophagoscopic accident rate is 0.25 percent, and an experienced endoscopist is required. A 33 percent disagreement rate between two experienced endoscopists evaluating a given group of patients is reported. This is related to the difficulty in differentiating varices from mucosal folds. Gastroduodenoscopy with fiberoptic instruments is particularly valuable in revealing acute gastritis, erosions, and small superficial ulcers that are not demonstrable on upper gastrointestinal tract x-ray.

Radiologic Studies. Radionuclide imaging is emerging as an accurate, safe, minimally invasive method of detecting gastrointestinal bleeding (Fig. 24-8). ^{99m}Tc sulfur colloid has been widely used but has the disadvantages that the intense uptake by the liver and spleen compromises its value in upper gastrointestinal bleeding, and the rapid clearance of the colloid from the blood limits its use to those patients who are bleeding at the time of the injection. ^{99m}Tc-labeled erythrocytes have the advantage that imaging can be continued for up to 24 h. This is a significant advantage since most gastrointestinal bleeders do not bleed continuously. In accuracy and sensitivity the method is at least as good as, and perhaps better than, selective angiography. A disadvantage is that it cannot pinpoint the bleeding site as well as angiography. Radionuclide imaging should be utilized (if available) prior to angiography. Angiography will be unproductive if the technetium scan is negative.

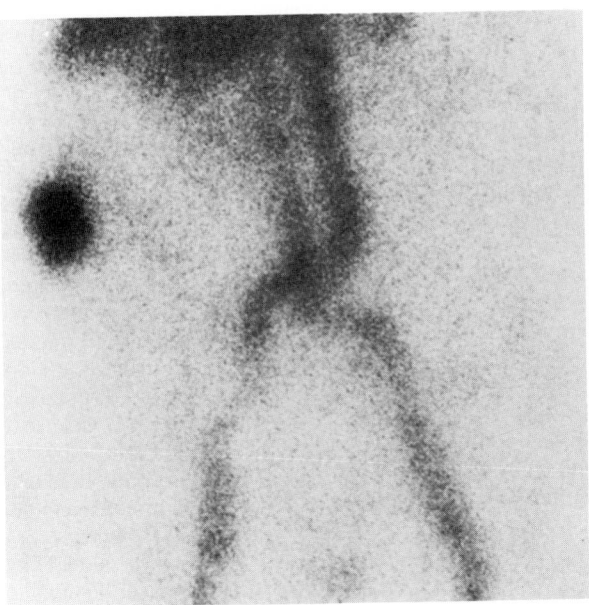

Fig. 24-8. ^{99m}Tc-labeled erythrocyte scan. Fifteen-minute film demonstrating a bleeding site in the right upper quadrant. The diagnosis of bleeding duodenal ulcer was established.

Selective arteriography of the celiac and superior mesenteric arteries and their branches is a relatively safe and accurate method of identifying active bleeding points in the upper gastrointestinal tract (Fig. 24-9). Angiography is usually done after endoscopy and radionuclide imaging. In any event, it must come before the upper gastrointestinal barium x-rays, which will obscure the field. Although bleeding at the rate of 1 to 2 mL/min can be detected experimentally, bleeding must be at the rate of 3 to 5 mL/min for accurate clinical angiographic diagnosis. The diagnostic accuracy of angiography in visualizing actively bleeding arterial lesions is about 90 percent; the accuracy in variceal bleeding, using the venous phase of the angiogram, is only about 20 percent.

In addition to diagnosis, selective arterial catheterization can be used for therapy of gastrointestinal bleeding. After the bleeding point is identified, a small therapeutic catheter is guided into the artery supplying the bleeding area, and vasoconstrictive agents, usually vasopressin at the rate of 0.1 to 0.2 units/min, are infused. Several comparative studies of systemic intravenous vasopressin versus regional arterial vasopressin have not shown any advantage for the more difficult and dangerous arterial route. The selective angiographic catheter may also be used to decrease the blood flow to a vascular bed by transcatheter embolization. Gelfoam soaked in contrast medium is the most frequently used material, but a great variety of materials can be used, including bits of autologous muscle, tiny detachable balloons, mini-coiled springs, and liquid acrylic monomers that instantly solidify on contacting blood. The occlusion is sometimes compromised by the opening up of collateral flow. The principal risk is that the blood supply will be so reduced that infarction occurs.

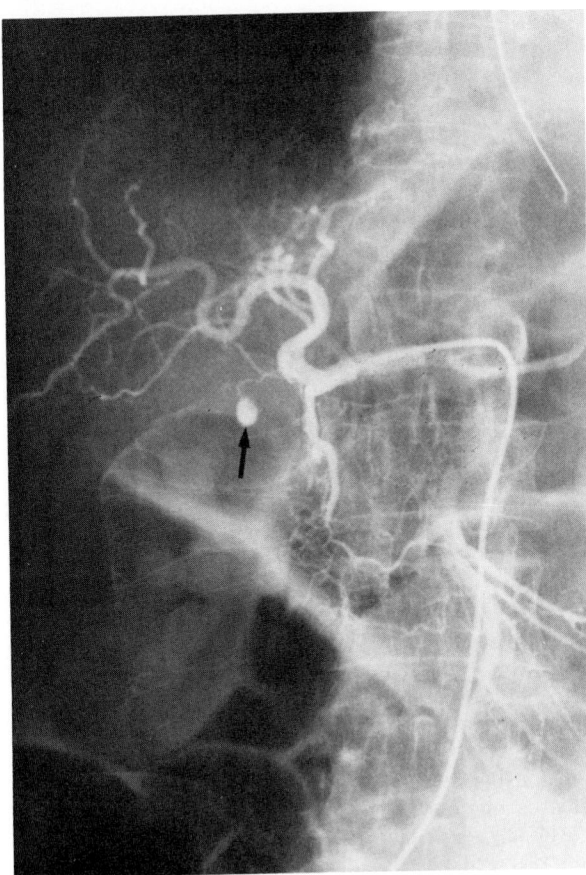

Fig. 24-9. Selective angiography in upper gastrointestinal bleeding. Dye injection into the common hepatic artery has outlined a bleeding duodenal ulcer (arrow). Later films showed a persistent puddling of contrast medium in the duodenum after all intravascular contrast had disappeared.

An upper gastrointestinal tract series, the cornerstone of morphologic radiographic diagnosis, should be done next, if endoscopy and arteriography have not revealed the bleeding site. As with endoscopy, the stomach should be evacuated of clots prior to the examination. In the case of bleeding ulcer, delaying for several days after hemorrhage has ceased does not increase the accuracy of diagnosis. The question of safety in the patient with bleeding has been raised, since the routine gastrointestinal series involves compression that may be attended by increasing hemorrhage. The Hampton technique for demonstration of bleeding ulcers obviates the use of palpation or compression and is attended by a diagnostic accuracy of 86 percent for demonstration of ulcers. The diagnostic accuracy in the case of bleeding varices is approximately 50 percent. Both the Valsalva and Müller maneuvers may occasionally show varices when other methods fail. Radiographs have proved of little value in the diagnosis of gastritis, with a yield of approximately 25 percent.

Percutaneous splenoportography affords a high yield for the diagnosis of esophageal varices but is rarely performed on an emergency basis. Before carrying out this procedure, a platelet count greater than 50,000/mm^3 and a prothrombin time greater than 35 percent of normal should be demonstrated. Splenic pulp manometry has been applied as an emergency test in the differential diagnosis of upper gastrointestinal tract bleeding. A 90 percent accuracy has been reported, but there is a zone of splenic pulp pressures that cannot differentiate variceal bleeding from other causes.

Balloon tamponade has been used as a diagnostic-therapeutic measure. However, varices are controlled even temporarily in only 65 to 75 percent of patients, and a peptic ulcer may coincidentally stop bleeding after a gastric balloon is inflated.

In some instances, an operation is performed on a patient with massive upper gastrointestinal tract bleeding in whom a diagnosis has not been established preoperatively. Laparotomy is to be considered as an important diagnostic tool. Once the peritoneal cavity has been opened, inspection of the liver may reveal cirrhosis, and distention of the omental vessels may suggest portal hypertension. In most cases, however, a determination of the source of bleeding requires a long gastrotomy that permits visualization of the gastric mucosa and the proximal portions of the duodenum. An attempt should be made to identify duodenal ulcer or a gastric lesion, and if these are not apparent, traction on the lower end of the nasogastric tube that is brought out through the gastrotomy will often expose the cardiac end of the stomach and distal esophagus to inspection. Intraoperative esophagogastroscopy by the usual route also may be helpful. Occasionally, in the absence of a preoperative diagnosis, no site of bleeding will be found at operation. In this situation, some surgeons do a vagotomy and drainage procedure; others simply close and hope that if bleeding recurs, the diagnosis can be made at that time and specific therapy instituted. The "blind" gastric resection that was formerly done in this situation has fallen into disfavor.

Lower Gastrointestinal Tract Bleeding

Bleeding distal to the ligament of Treitz is manifested by the passage of tarry stools or unaltered blood (hemochezia) and is characteristically unaccompanied by hematemesis. It is usually moderate or mild but may be massive.

ETIOLOGY. A great variety of lesions extending from the ligament of Treitz to the anus may be implicated as causes of lower gastrointestinal tract bleeding (Table 24-9).

Jejunal and Ileal Bleeding. Meckel's diverticulitis, intussusception, and regional enteritis represent the most common causes. Meckel's diverticulitis with associated bleeding occurs most frequently in children, and the bleeding episode is related to gastric mucosa within the diverticulum stimulating ulceration of the adjacent ileum. Ileocecal intussusception is also a lesion of childhood, occurring most commonly before the age of two and attended by a characteristic currant jelly stool. The cause of this mechanical process in childhood is usually undetermined, while ileocecal intussusception in the adult is usually secondary to an intestinal polyp or tumor. Regional enteritis is accompanied by severe melena in approximately 5 percent of the cases, while some rectal bleeding is a common symptom in about 20 percent of the patients with this disease. Although tumors of the small intestine are rare, approximately half are accompanied by bleeding. The neoplasms include leiomyomas, polyps, either single or multiple (familial polyposis), and the polyps of the Peutz-Jegher syndrome. Carcinomas, sarcomas, and leukemias have all been reported to be associated with bleeding, whereas bleeding is an uncommon manifestation of a carcinoid tumor. Hemangiomas, hereditary telangiectasis, microaneurysms of blood vessels within the wall of the intestine, mesenteric thrombosis, drug reactions, and blood dyscrasias all represent rare causes of small intestinal bleeding.

Colonic Bleeding. The common causes include carcinoma, diverticula, vascular ectasias, colitis, and polyps (Table 24-9). Although carcinoma represents the most common cause of rectal bleeding, the bleeding associated with this lesion is rarely massive. Carcinoma of the right colon, particularly of the cecum, is usually accompanied by melena that may be so subtle that it is not considered until anemia has become established. Diverticulosis presents the most common cause of *massive* rectal bleeding.

Table 24-9. CAUSES OF LOWER GASTROINTESTINAL BLEEDING BY AGE GROUP, IN ORDER OF FREQUENCY*

Infants and children	Adolescents and young adults	Adults to 60 years	Adults over 60 years
Meckel's diverticulum	Meckel's diverticulum	Diverticulosis	Vascular ectasias
Polyps	Inflammatory bowel	Inflammatory bowel	Diverticulosis
Ulcerative colitis	disease	disease	Malignancy
Duplications	Polyps	Polyps	Polyps
		Malignancy	
		Congenital arteriovenous malformations	

* Less frequent causes not specific for any age group. Infectious diarrheas (amebiasis, shigellosis), ischemic colitis, drug-induced cecal ulceration (e.g., vincristine), vascular lesions, vascular tumors, varices, coagulopathies.
SOURCE: From Boley SJ, Brandt LS, Frank MS: 1981, with permission.

This is related to erosion of vessels within the neck of the diverticulum. In contrast, the bleeding that accompanies diverticulitis is mild to moderate and is caused by a superficial erosion of smaller vessels on the surface of the mucosa. Although the bleeding that accompanies ulcerative colitis is usually mild to moderate, massive hemorrhage may occur. Polyps that may be single or multiple and may be located in any segment of the colon represent a relatively frequent source of rectal bleeding. Rarer causes include cecal ulceration, sarcomas, lymphomas, leukemia, hematologic disorders, and impairment of the vascular supply due to mesenteric thrombosis, ischemic colitis, or secondary to aortic resection with interruption of a functionally important inferior mesenteric artery.

Prior to angiography, bleeding lesions of the right colon were thought to be rare, but in the past decade many reports have emphasized that the right colon is a common site of bleeding. Diverticula were thought to be the responsible lesion. Boley and associates have shown that vascular ectasias are probably responsible for much of the right colon bleeding; they suggest that ectasias may be the commonest cause of major lower intestinal bleeding in the elderly. They present evidence that these vascular ectasias (1) are degenerative lesions of aging and are not congenital or neoplastic; (2) occur in patients over sixty years of age; (3) are not associated with angiomatous lesions of the skin or other viscera; (4) occur in the cecum and proximal ascending colon; (5) are small, usually less than 5 mm in diameter; (6) can be diagnosed only by angiography; and (7) usually cannot be identified by the surgeon at operation or by the pathologist using standard techniques—injecting-clearing techniques must be used.

Rectal and Anal Bleeding. This is usually manifested by unaltered blood on the surface of the stool. The causes include hemorrhoids, fissures, and proctitis. It is to be emphasized that the presence of hemorrhoids in a patient with rectal bleeding should not preclude investigation of other possible sources, particularly carcinoma.

DIAGNOSIS. A precise description of the bleeding episode and the nature of the stool is indicated. The question of familial polyposis and drug ingestion should be investigated. Physical examination includes a search for skin and mucosal lesions of hemorrhagic telangiectasia (Rendu-Osler-Weber syndrome) or the Peutz-Jegher syndrome. Abdominal palpation may reveal a mass, tumor, or intussusception, the last frequently accompanied by absence of bowel sounds in the right lower quadrant. Rectal examination may be diagnostic for tumor, polyps, or anal lesions. Proctosigmoidoscopy should be done early in the hospital course. Colonoscopy may be helpful if the patient is not bleeding actively at the time of the examination. With active massive bleeding, colonoscopy is useless.

As with upper gastrointestinal bleeding, radionuclide imaging using ^{99m}Tc-labeled erythrocytes is supplanting angiography as the procedure that follows endoscopy. Bleeding at a rate of 1 mL/min can be detected by this technique.

Selective angiography is still the most accurate method of diagnosis, provided there is active bleeding at the rate of at least 2 or 3 mL/min at the time of the examination. The small intestine and right half of the colon are examined by catheterization of branches of the superior mesenteric artery. Examination of the left colon is sometimes more difficult, since the inferior mesenteric artery may be more difficult to catheterize. As with upper gastrointestinal tract bleeding, regional infusion of vasoconstrictive agents via a catheter in the artery supplying the bleeding site is often an effective method of controlling bleeding.

Barium contrast studies, if needed, should follow angiography so that the contrast material does not obscure the angiographer's field. Barium enema studies, including air contrast, represent a reliable, accurate method of diagnosing colon lesions but yield no information as to whether or not the lesions visualized are responsible for the bleeding. Gastrointestinal series with small bowel follow-through is less productive in the case of lesions of the small intestine. Every effort should be made to demonstrate the bleeding site prior to operation, since diagnosis at the operating table is often not possible.

JAUNDICE

The term *jaundice* is derived from the French word meaning "yellow" and refers to the presence of an excess of bile pigments in the tissues and the serum. It is the presenting sign of a number of hepatic and nonhepatic diseases. The differential diagnosis and management are dependent upon an appreciation of the normal and abnormal variants of bile pigment metabolism. A flow sheet analysis of hyperbilirubinemia is presented in Table 24-10.

NORMAL BILE PIGMENT METABOLISM. The bile pigment bilirubin (Fig. 24-10) is a tetrapyrrole which is formed to the greatest extent from hemoglobin and, to a lesser extent, from myoglobin breakdown and hepatic synthesis itself. When the red blood cell is destroyed by the reticuloendothelial system, either at the end of its natural life span or prematurely, the iron and globin are removed, and the heme ring is opened and transformed into biliverdin, which is green. The latter is reduced to become bilirubin, which is yellow. The bilirubin combines with albumin to form a relatively stable protein-pigment complex and is transported as such to the hepatic parenchymal cell. This complex, which is referred to as *indirect-reacting* bilirubin, since it gives the van den Bergh diazo reaction only after treatment with alcohol and other substances that split the protein bond, is poorly soluble in water and is not excreted in the urine.

In the hepatic parenchymal cell the albumin is removed, and the bilirubin is conjugated with glucuronic acid to form a diglucuronide, which is water-soluble and is excreted into the bile canaliculi. This substance gives an immediate diazo reaction, is therefore termed *direct-reacting,* and is readily passed into the urine. Normally there is less than 1.2 mg of direct-reacting serum bilirubin and less than 0.3 mg of indirect-reacting serum bilirubin per dL of serum.

The conjugated bilirubin, which is excreted via the bile

Table 24-10. ANALYSIS OF A CASE OF HYPERBILIRUBINEMIA

Fractionate serum bilirubin and measure urine bilirubin and urobilinogen to determine whether:

I. Unconjugated hyperbilirubinemia

Determine mechanism on basis of age, clinical features, and laboratory findings:

A. Production of bilirubin beyond excretory capacity. Evidence of:

    1. Hemolysis

        a. Extracorpuscular

            (1) Immune body reactions
                (*a*) Transfusion reactions
                (*b*) Erythroblastosis
            (2) Infections and chemicals
            (3) Physical agents
            (4) Secondary hemolysis in pregnancy

        b. Intracorpuscular

            (1) Congenital hemolytic jaundice
            (2) Sickle cell anemia
            (3) Mediterranean anemia

    2. No hemolysis

        a. Pulmonary infarction
        b. Transfusion of aged red blood cells
        c. Hematomas
        d. "Shunt" hyperbilirubinemia

B. Deficient hepatic uptake of bilirubin:

    1. ? Gilbert's disease (normal biopsy, low-grade hyperbilirubinemia)
    2. ? Acquired liver disease

C. Deficient conjugation of bilirubin:

    1. Physiologic jaundice of newborn

        a. Inadequate bilirubin glucuronide synthesis

    2. Crigler-Najjar syndrome (transferase deficiency)

    3. Inhibition of glucuronyl transferase

        a. Large doses of vitamin K analogs in premature infants
        b. Increase level of pregnanediol
        c. Breast milk containing pregnane-3-(*a*), 20-(*β*)-diol
        d. Novobiocin

    4. Competitive inhibition

        a. Drugs detoxified as glucuronides

II. Conjugated hyperbilirubinemia
Determine mechanism on basis of age, clinical features, and laboratory findings:

A. Defect in bilirubin excretion
Confirm with serum alkaline phosphatase (elevated), cephalin flocculation (normal). In absence of rapid subsidence, exploratory surgery is desirable to differentiate:

1. Extrahepatic biliary obstruction
Identify by radiologic means and/or direct inspection during surgical intervention.
   a. Calculus
   b. Stricture
   c. Neoplasm

2. Intrahepatic biliary obstruction
Confirm absence of extrahepatic biliary obstruction with operative or T-tube cholangiography. Identify localization of lesion by surgical biopsy.
   a. Lesion of bile canaliculi — (1) Drugs (2) Viruses
   b. Lesion of bile ductules — (1) Drugs (2) Viruses
   c. Lesion of bile ducts — (1) Drugs (2) Viruses

B. Deficient liver cell secretion of bilirubin
May need to differentiate from excretory defect by surgical exploration, cholangiography, or biopsy:

1. Persistence of excretory defect in immature liver after development of adequate glucuronide-synthesizing capacity
2. Dubin-Johnson syndrome (biopsy showing characteristic pigment)
3. Rotor syndrome (absence of characteristic pigment)

III. Combined unconjugated and conjugated hyperbilirubinemia
Determine mechanism on basis of clinical features and laboratory findings:

A. Familial defect or immature liver reflected in partial deficiency of glucuronide formation or excretion

B. Acquired liver cell damage
Confirm with liver function tests and determine primary abnormality:

1. Deficient hepatic uptake of bilirubin
2. Deficient conjugation of bilirubin
3. Deficient secretion or excretion of conjugated bilirubin

C. Hemolysis with secondary liver damage.
Demonstrate presence of hemolysis:

1. Hepatic damage secondary to shock
2. Hepatic damage secondary to hemolysis

D. Biliary obstruction with secondary liver damage:

1. Bile stasis with secondary injury
2. Ascending cholangitis

SOURCE: Leevy CM: *Evaluation of Liver Function in Clinical Practice.* Indianapolis, The Lilly Research Laboratories, 1965, with permission.

1093

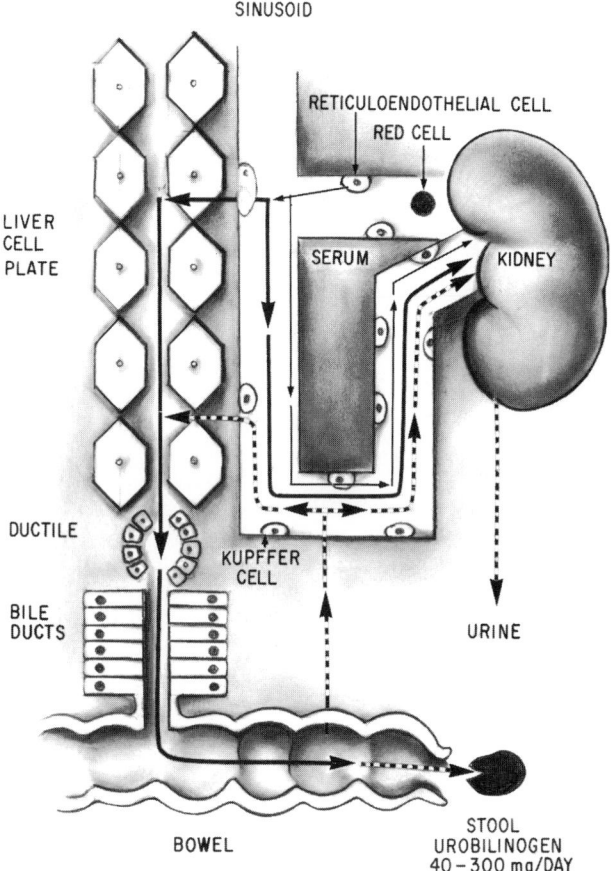

Fig. 24-10. Normal bile pigment metabolism.

into the intestine, is acted upon by bacteria and undergoes a series of reductive reactions leading to the formation of two groups of compounds, the colorless urobilinogens and the colored urobilin. The normal daily fecal excretion ranges between 40 and 300 mg with an average of 100 to 200 mg. In children the values are lower, and in newborn infants, because of the absence of bacterial flora, urobilinogen may be absent. A reduction in enteric bacteria is also responsible for the reduced pigment excretion that accompanies the use of intestinal antibiotics. Some of the urobilinogen is resorbed by way of the portal venous system and returns to the liver, where it is either removed or, to a small extent, excreted in the urine.

ABNORMAL BILE PIGMENT METABOLISM. No classification of jaundice is totally satisfactory. The classification most widely used distinguishes between hemolytic, obstructive, and hepatocellular jaundice. However, it is more reasonable to categorize (1) those disease states in which the bile flow is unimpeded and (2) those types that are associated with an impairment of the bile flow (Fig. 24-11).

Normal Bile Excretion. The overproduction of bile pigment from excessive hemolysis creates a situation in which the normal liver is confronted with more pigment than it is able to remove. This occurs in the physiologic

jaundice of infancy and all pathologic hemolytic states. However, the reserve capacity of the liver is great, and even when the bilirubin production is increased six times, there is only a 2- to 3-mg rise in the serum bilirubin level per dL. In this situation, the increase in serum bilirubin is in the unconjugated indirect-reacting pigment. No bilirubin appears in the urine, but there is an increase in the fecal and urinary urobilinogen. An excess of bilirubin production also occurs in *shunt hyperbilirubinemia,* in which indirect-reacting bilirubin accumulates in the absence of any reduction in red cell life span.

Constitutional defects of liver function may also cause hyperbilirubinemia without impairment of bile flow. In Gilbert's disease, there is a defect in the bilirubin transport into the liver cell, while in the Crigler-Najjar syndrome the defect is an inability of the liver to conjugate the bilirubin with glucuronic acid. In these states, the elevation of bile pigment is in the indirect-reacting fraction. All other hepatic function tests are normal, and no histologic abnormalities are noted. With all of the above-mentioned diseases, the bilirubin pigment is attached to the albumin and cannot be excreted by the kidney, thus prompting the term *acholuric jaundice.*

Impaired Bile Excretion. All other lesions are associated with an accumulation of conjugated bilirubin in the blood and impaired excretion. The bilirubin pigment, which is water-soluble, is readily excreted into the urine, which becomes brown. Obstructive jaundice may be intrahepatic or extrahepatic.

Intrahepatic Obstructive Jaundice. In the Dubin-Johnson syndrome, which is associated with the appearance of iron-free pigment in the hepatic cells and normal liver function, the hepatic excretion of the conjugated bilirubin is impaired. Intrahepatic cholestasis has also been related to a variety of drugs and hepatocellular diseases. Methyltestosterone and norethandrolone damage the microvilli of the bile canaliculi and may cause jaundice. The phenothiazine drugs, such as chlorpromazine, may evoke a hypersensitivity reaction in a small percentage of patients and result in cholangiolitic hepatitis and intrahepatic cholestasis. A lesion along the excretory path within the liver is believed to cause the obstructive jaundice associated with primary biliary cirrhosis.

The jaundice from hepatocellular degeneration, such as occurs in hepatitis and cirrhosis, is associated with morphologic changes in the parenchymal cells and abnormal liver function tests. With these diseases, a Kupffer cell liver block has been proposed to result in regurgitation of bilirubin from the bile canaliculi into the tissue spaces. This defect, coupled with the reduction in the ability of the liver cell to convert the bilirubin protein to the bilirubin glucuronide, causes a rise in both bilirubin and its conjugates. In contrast to the pure obstructive jaundice, urinary urobilinogen may be increased, since the parenchyma is no longer capable of clearing the serum urobilinogen entering from the intestinal tract. However, the excretion of bile may be so suppressed that virtually no bilirubin reaches the intestine; under these conditions the stools are clay-colored, and the production and resorption of the bilirubin from the intestine is diminished, in

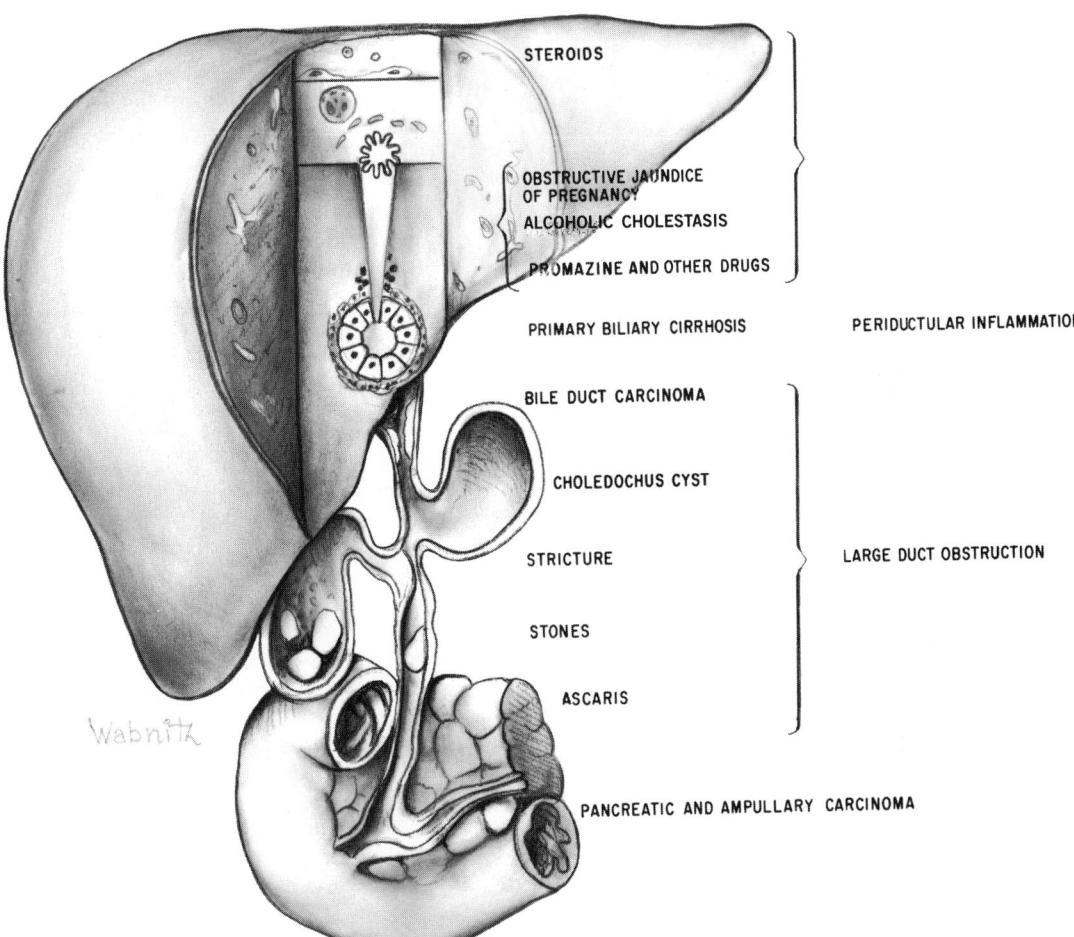

CAUSE OF JAUNDICE	POSTULATED DEFECT
HEMOLYSIS	EXCESS BILIRUBIN PRODUCTION
SHUNT HYPERBILIRUBINEMIA	BILIRUBIN TRANSPORT
GILBERT	BILIRUBIN CONJUGATION
NEONATE, CRIGLER-NAJJAR	CONJUGATION TRANSPORT
DUBIN-JOHNSON HYPERBILIRUBINEMIA	
	CANALICULAR DAMAGE
STEROIDS	
OBSTRUCTIVE JAUNDICE OF PREGNANCY	
ALCOHOLIC CHOLESTASIS	
PROMAZINE AND OTHER DRUGS	
PRIMARY BILIARY CIRRHOSIS	PERIDUCTULAR INFLAMMATION
BILE DUCT CARCINOMA	
CHOLEDOCHUS CYST	
STRICTURE	LARGE DUCT OBSTRUCTION
STONES	
ASCARIS	
PANCREATIC AND AMPULLARY CARCINOMA	

Wabnitz

Fig. 24-11. Abnormal bile pigment metabolism.

which case the urine urobilinogen falls to a low level. In rare instances of intrahepatic bile duct atresia absolute obstruction of the bile conduits within the liver results in jaundice.

Extrahepatic Cholestasis. This is caused by an anatomic obstacle to the flow of bile from the liver to the intestine. The obstacle may be situated anywhere from the junction of the right and left hepatic ducts to the termination of the common bile duct in the duodenum. Atresia, stricture, choledocholithiasis, tumors of the bile duct and pancreas, choledochal cysts, and parasites have all been implicated.

Obstruction of the extrahepatic ducts results in an increase in the serum bilirubin, particularly the direct-reacting type, the appearance of bile in the urine, and the passage of clay-colored stools. When the total bilirubin level is above 3 mg/dL, the increases in both the direct- and indirect-reacting fractions parallel one another. With complete and persistent obstruction, the serum bilirubin may plateau. If the obstruction is fluctuating, the levels will change.

EVALUATION AND MANAGEMENT OF THE PATIENT WITH JAUNDICE. For a discussion of neonatal jaundice and biliary atresia see Chap. 31.

Jaundice is apparent when the serum bilirubin level exceeds 2 mg/dL. Tissues rich in elastic fibers have a particular affinity for bilirubin, thus accounting for the earlier appearance and greater intensity in the sclerae and in the skin of the face and upper trunk. Jaundice is not a mere reflection of yellow light through the skin from underlying interstitial fluid but rather a deposition in the tissue fibers and cells. Tissues stain more readily with direct bilirubin than with the indirect-reacting fraction. There is a failure to stain in areas of marked edema and vitiligo.

The diagnosis of jaundice attempts to define the precise cause and is also directed toward the division into surgically correctable lesions, on the one hand, and other types in which surgical intervention is not indicated.

History. Jaundice secondary to obstruction of the extrahepatic ducts usually starts insidiously and becomes progressively more pronounced. Gastrointestinal disturbances are uncommon, with the exception of those related to biliary calculi. Although, classically, carcinoma of the head of the pancreas is painless, some 20 to 30 percent of these patients do complain of deep epigastric distress or backache. Extrahepatic obstruction associated with ascending cholangitis is accompanied by spiking fevers and abdominal pain. A history of pruritus preceding the onset of jaundice occurs frequently with both extrahepatic biliary obstruction and intrahepatic obstruction secondary to primary cholangiolitis or primary biliary cirrhosis. A detailed family history and history of drug ingestion are imperative before subjecting a patient to surgical treatment, since both constitutional deficiencies and drug-induced jaundice result in a defect in excretion of bile. Loss of appetite, fever, and change of smoking habits are particularly suggestive of hepatitis, and history should be taken of possible contact with persons with known cases and of injections in the previous 6 months. Inquiry into chronic alcohol ingestion is important to rule out jaundice associated with cirrhosis.

Physical Examination. Physical examination also contributes to the diagnosis. Inspection of the skin may reveal a rash, typical of drug reactions, spider angiomas of cirrhosis, or excoriations suggestive of pruritus. Anemia and splenomegaly may be present with hemolytic jaundice. Hepatomegaly and hepatic tenderness are predominant findings with viral hepatitis. A palpable gallbladder in a patient with extrahepatic obstruction occurs more frequently when the obstruction is related to malignancy distal to the cystic duct entrance into the common duct, and less commonly when obstruction is due to biliary calculi. This axiom, known as Courvoisier's law, however, is not universal. Careful search for extrahepatic neoplasm should be made, and the stigmata of portal hypertension including prominent abdominal wall veins and ascites should be investigated.

Laboratory Studies. Hemolytic jaundice is accompanied by anemia and an increased reticulocyte count. Smears for sickle cells, spherocytes, and target cells should be made. The white blood cell count is usually not elevated in viral hepatitis, while it is frequently markedly increased with extrahepatic obstruction and accompanying ascending cholangitis. Stools should be studied for pigment and the presence or absence of guaiac, indicative of

bleeding. With carcinoma of the pancreas, approximately one-third of the patients have guaiac-positive stools; this occurs more frequently in patients with obstructive jaundice secondary to carcinoma of the ampulla of Vater.

The so-called liver function tests are directed toward assessing the degree of functional impairment of the liver and differentiating between "medical" and "surgical" jaundice. The extreme functional reserve of the liver occasionally produces normal results in the face of significant lesions, and none of the tests provides a pathologic diagnosis. Tests should be performed to determine exposure to hepatitis.

Serum bilirubin is normally present in concentrations up to 1.5 mg/dL and, as previously mentioned, appears both in water-insoluble unconjugated form, which gives the indirect van den Bergh reaction, and the water-soluble conjugated form, which reacts directly. Up to 1.2 mg/dL of unconjugated bilirubin is present in the normal serum. Increases in this fraction accompany hemolytic processes such as physiologic jaundice of the newborn, erythroblastosis, and hereditary and acquired hemolytic crises. This fraction is also elevated in the Crigler-Najjar syndrome and in Gilbert's disease. In patients with jaundice secondary to obstruction of the flow of bile or hepatocellular degeneration, the determination of the direct fraction is a more sensitive index of impairment than the total serum bilirubin.

Normally no bilirubin is present in the urine, and bilirubinuria does not accompany hemolytic jaundice or jaundice related to deficiency in the glucuronal transferase system, since the unconjugated fraction, which is increased in these situations, cannot be excreted by the kidney. An elevation in the direct-reacting bilirubin level is associated with bilirubinuria. The production of foam by shaking the urine suggests the elevation. Increased direct-reacting serum bilirubin may not appear in the urine of patients with severe renal failure.

Enzyme studies are also applicable to the differential diagnosis of jaundice. A markedly elevated serum alkaline phosphatase level is usually associated with obstructive jaundice of either extrahepatic or intrahepatic origin. Elevations in SGOT and SGPT are indicative of hepatocellular disease. Gamma glutamyl transpeptidase (GGTP) is elevated in alcoholic liver disease but more markedly increased in patients with extrahepatic cholestasis.

Other laboratory findings, such as a reduction in serum albumin and a reduction in the esterified fraction of the cholesterol, and abnormal turbidity studies are altered with hepatocellular disease. Removal of foreign dye from the liver is dependent upon hepatic blood flow, hepatocellular function, and biliary excretion. The response of prothrombin time to injection of parenteral vitamin K is helpful in establishing a differential diagnosis between hepatocellular and obstructive jaundice. An increase in the prothrombin time within 48 h of parenteral administration suggests the diagnosis of obstructive jaundice, while a lack of response is more compatible with hepatocellular disease.

Other Diagnostic Procedures. *Radiologic Studies.* An x-ray of the abdomen is indicated, since 20 percent of gallstones are radiopaque (see Chap. 31). Oral cholecys-

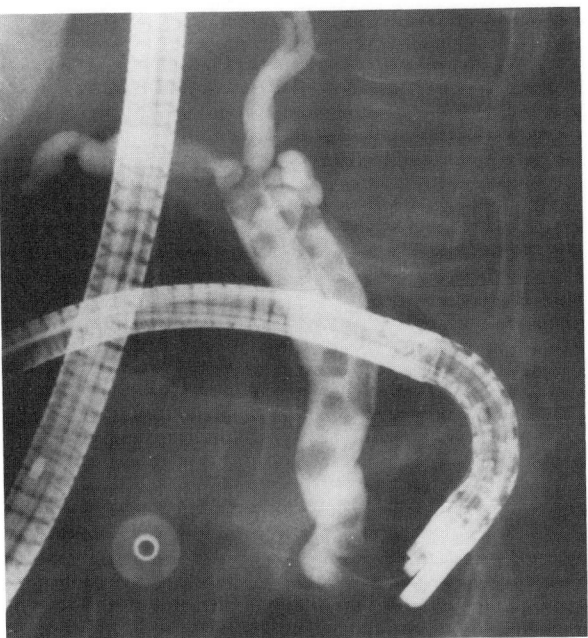

Fig. 24-12. Endoscopic retrograde cholangiopancreatogram (ERCP) showing multiple stones in a dilated common bile duct and in the cystic duct remnant.

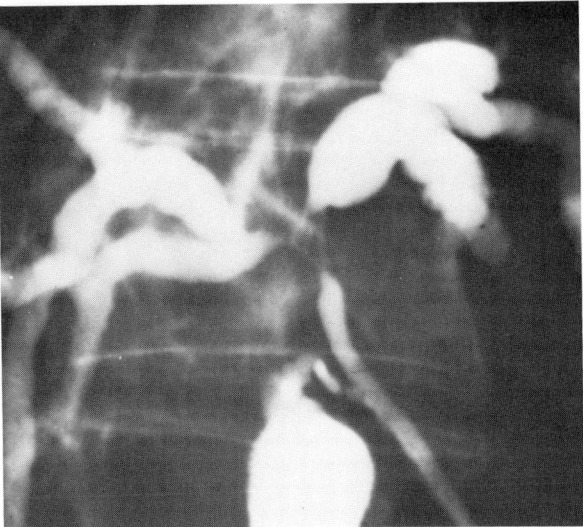

Fig. 24-13. Percutaneous transhepatic cholangiogram defining intrahepatic ductal dilatation. There is almost complete obstruction at the confluence of the right and left hepatic ducts due to carcinoma (Klatskin tumor). Note that there is radiopaque substance in the common duct and gallbladder.

tography is rarely effective if the serum bilirubin level is above 1.8 mg/dL, while the intravenous studies are unrewarding if the serum bilirubin level exceeds 3.5 mg/dL. The upper gastrointestinal series may define a widened ''C loop,'' suggestive of carcinoma of the pancreas.

Recent advances that have contributed significantly in the differential diagnosis of jaundice include endoscopic retrograde cholangiopancreatography (ERCP), percutaneous transhepatic cholangiography (PTC) with the skinny Chiba needle, ultrasonography, computed tomography (CT), and radionuclide scanning. In experienced hands 90 to 95 percent success rates for ERCP (Fig. 24-12) definition of the extrahepatic biliary system have been reported, but in most institutions the yield is less than 65 percent. Cholangitis and pancreatitis are uncommon complications. The technique is uniquely suited to the evaluation of sclerosing cholangitis and carcinoma of the ampulla of Vater, in which case biopsy can establish the diagnosis. In a randomized trial comparing PTC with ERCP for bile duct visualization in deeply jaundiced patients, PTC (see Fig. 24-13) was demonstrated to be the procedure of choice when cholestasis had a surgical cause. PTC was successful in 95 percent of cases with extrahepatic cholestasis and in 25 percent of patients with intrahepatic cholestasis, while ERCP was successful in 62 percent of patients with extrahepatic and 76 percent with intrahepatic cholestasis. In the patient with extrahepatic obstructive jaundice, provision for early operation should be made if bile peritonitis, an uncommon complication, occurs. ERCP is preferred when coagulation defects preclude PTC.

Compound B scanning provides echographic patterns in patients who are deeply jaundiced and whose ducts cannot be visualized with contrast media. Dilated ducts,

calculi, and tumors can be defined by serial laminographic scans. Equipment capable of defining gray scale has increased the sensitivity of this technique (Fig. 24-14). CT employing the body scanner also will demonstrate dilatation of intrahepatic and/or extrahepatic portions of the biliary tract (Fig. 24-15). The ^{99m}Tc-pyridoxylideneglutamate biliary scan is a safe, noninvasive means of distinguishing between jaundice due to hepatobiliary disease and that due to partial or complete extrahepatic biliary duct obstruction. It is applicable even if the bilirubin is elevated to the 20 mg/dL level.

Liver Biopsy. Percutaneous needle biopsy of the liver may, on one hand, prevent procrastination of surgical intervention and progressive parenchymal damage in patients with extrahepatic biliary obstruction; on the other hand, it may preclude laparotomy in patients with severe hepatocellular disease. Patients should be screened for deficiency in the clotting mechanism, and the risk is small. Characteristic lesions of viral hepatitis, cholangiolitic hepatitis, and bile laking suggestive of extrahepatic biliary obstruction can be defined by this technique.

Laparotomy. This is considered an important tool in the diagnostic armamentarium. Laparotomy for obstructive jaundice is never urgent unless there is an acute suppurative cholangitis. Surgical intervention is indicated when other diagnostic procedures have raised a suspicion of extrahepatic obstruction and when the danger of operating on a patient with possible hepatocellular jaundice is considered minimal. An approach to the diagnosis of jaundice in a patient potentially requiring surgical management is shown in Fig. 24-16.

Algorithm for Diagnosis (Fig. 24-16). Given a patient in whom there is a high index of suspicion that jaundice is related to extrahepatic ductal obstruction, the initial investigative procedure, based on yield and cost effectiveness, should be ultrasonography. This will determine if

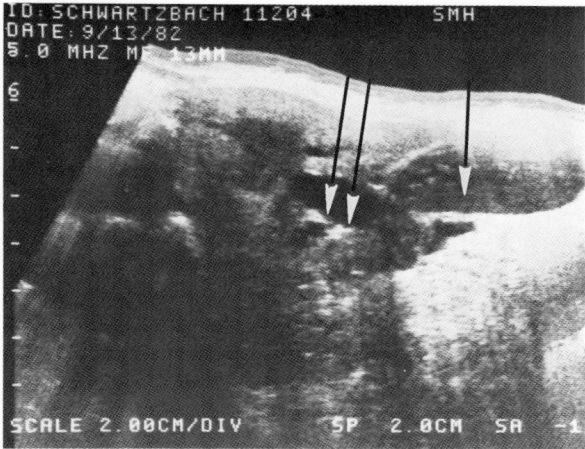

A

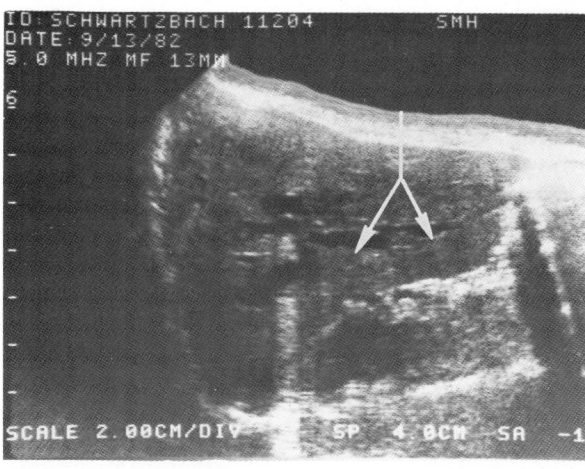

B

Fig. 24-14. Ultrasound of patient with carcinoma of the pancreas causing obstruction of the common bile duct and dilatation of the gallbladder and intrahepatic ducts. *A.* Single arrow points to dilated gallbladder, double arrow to dilated common duct. *B.* Arrow points to dilated intrahepatic duct.

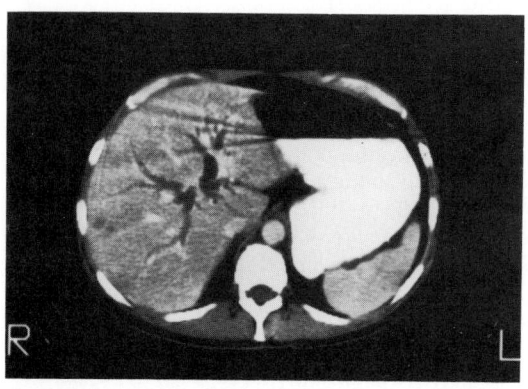

A

B

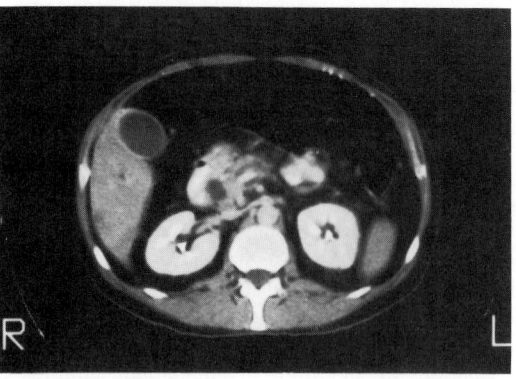

C

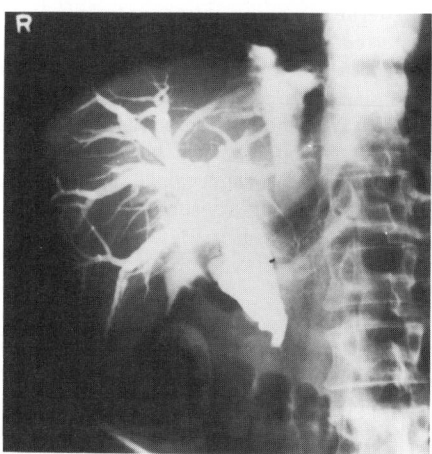

D

Fig. 24-15. Patient with obstructive jaundice due to carcinoma of the head of the pancreas. *A.* CT cut demonstrating intrahepatic ductal dilatation. *B.* CT cut demonstrating dilatation of the gallbladder, common bile duct, and proximal pancreatic duct. *C.* CT cut demonstrating mass in the head of the pancreas. *D.* Percutaneous transhepatic cholangiogram (PTC) demonstrating dilatation of the intrahepatic and extrahepatic bile ducts and the absence of radiopaque material in the duodenum..

Determine Presence or Absence of Intra-and / or Extrahepatic Ductal Obstruction

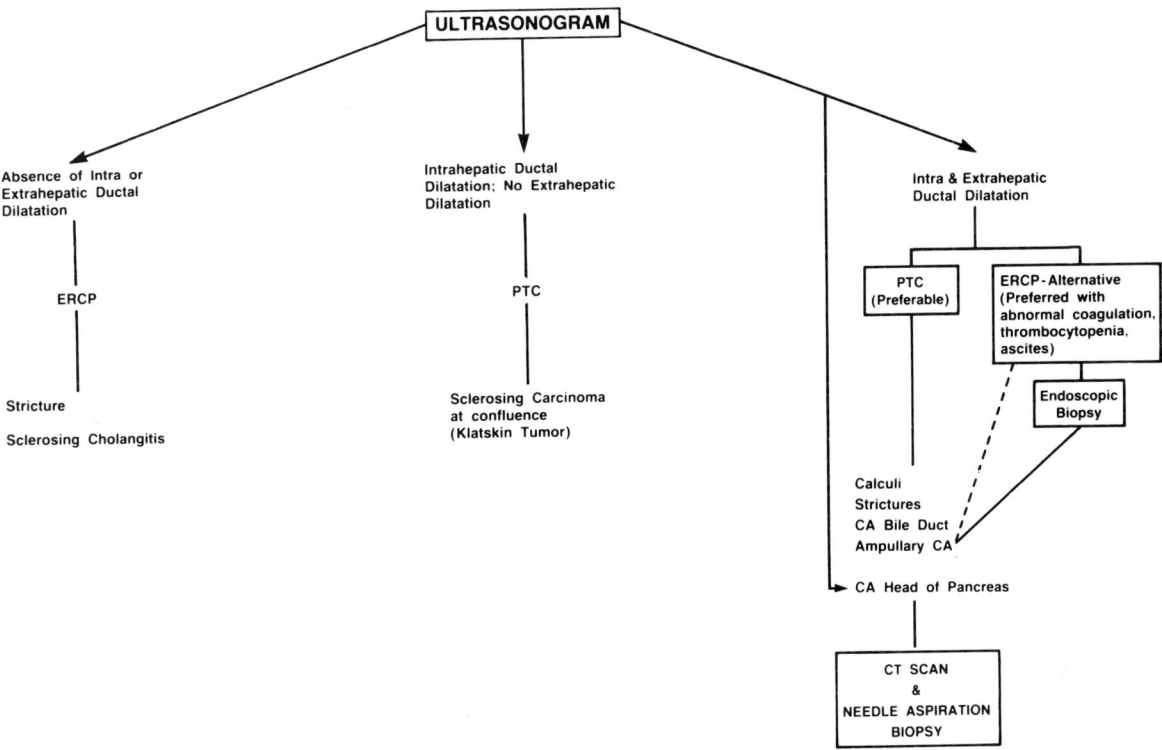

Fig. 24-16. Algorithm for the diagnosis of obstructive jaundice.

intrahepatic ductal dilatation and/or dilatation of the extrahepatic ducts and gallbladder is present. Once ductal dilatation is defined, a PTC should be performed to localize the level of obstruction. If obstruction is present at the confluence of the hepatic ducts, the common hepatic duct, or proximal common duct, no further diagnostic procedure is necessary. If the obstruction is located at the distal common duct, a CT scan may be indicated to define the presence of a mass in the head of the pancreas and the resectability of such a lesion. If no mass is present, ERCP can be performed to determine if an ampullary lesion is present. In most instances upper gastrointestinal series adds little to the diagnosis. This also applies to the liver spleen scan.

Bibliography

Pain

Carlsson CA, Pellettieri L: A clinical view on pain physiology. *Acta Chir Scand* 148:305, 1982.

Cope Z: *The Early Diagnosis of Acute Abdomen,* 15th ed. London, Oxford University Press, 1979.

Long DM: Electrical stimulation for the control of pain. *Arch Surg* 112:884, 1977.

Melzack R, Wall PD: Pain mechanisms: A new theory. *Science* 150:971, 1965.

Nathan PW: Pain. *Br Med Bull* 33:149, 1977.

Pflug AE, Bonica JJ: Physiopathology and control of postoperative pain. *Arch Surg* 112:773, 1977.

Sherman JE, Liebeskind JC: An endorphrinergic, centrifugal substrate of pain modulation. Recent findings, current concepts and complexities, in Bonica JJ (ed): *Pain.* New York, Raven, 1980, p 191.

White JC, Smithwick RH, Simeone FA: *The Autonomic Nervous System: Anatomy, Physiology, Surgical Application,* 3d ed. New York, Macmillan, 1952.

Zimmermann M: Peripheral and central nervous mechanisms of nociception, pain and pain therapy: Facts and hypotheses, in Bonica JJ, Liebeskind JC, Albe-Fessard DG (eds): *Advances in Pain Research and Therapy.* New York, Raven, 1979, vol 3, p 3.

Dysphagia

Davenport HW: *Physiology of the Digestive Tract,* 4th ed. Chicago, Year Book Medical Publishers, 1977.

Grant AK, Skyring A (eds): *Clinical Diagnosis of Gastrointestinal Disease.* Oxford, Blackwell Scientific Publications, 1981.

Greenberger NJ: *Gastrointestinal Disorders: A Pathophysiological Approach,* 2d ed. Chicago, Year Book Medical Publishers, 1981.

Sleisenger MH, Fortran JS: *Gastrointestinal Disease,* 2d ed. Philadelphia, Saunders, 1978.

Anorexia, Nausea, and Vomiting

Davenport HW: *Physiology of the Digestive Tract,* 4th ed. Chicago, Year Book Medical Publishers, 1977.

Grant AK, Skyring A (eds): *Clinical Diagnosis of Gastrointestinal Disease.* Oxford, Blackwell Scientific Publications, 1981.

Greenberger NJ: *Gastrointestinal Disorders: A Pathophysiological Approach,* 2d ed. Chicago, Year Book Medical Publishers, 1981.

Hawkins C: Anorexia and loss of weight. *Br Med J* 2:1373, 1976.

McGuigan JE: Anorexia, nausea and vomiting, in MacBryde CM, Blacklow RS (eds): *Signs and Symptoms,* 5th ed. Philadelphia, Lippincott, 1970.

Constipation and Diarrhea

Davenport HW: *Physiology of the Digestive Tract,* 4th ed. Chicago, Year Book Medical Publishers, 1977.

Dobbins JW, Binder HJ: Pathophysiology of diarrhea: Alterations in fluid and electrolyte transport. *Clin Gastroenterol* 10:605, 1981.

Fingl E, Preston JW: Antidiarrheal agents and laxatives: Changing concepts. *Clin Gastroenterol* 8:161, 1979.

Jaffe BM, Condon S: Prostaglandins E and F in endocrine diarrheagenic syndromes. *Ann Surg* 184:516, 1976.

McJunkin B, Fromm H, et al: Factors in the Mechanism of diarrhea in bile acid malabsorption: Fecal pH—a key determinant. *Gastroenterology* 80:1454, 1981.

Summers RW: Role of motility in infectious diarrhea. *Gastroenterology* 80:1070, 1981.

Intestinal Obstruction

Adams JT: Adynamic ileus of the colon; An indication for cecostomy. *Arch Surg* 109:503, 1974.

Baker JW: Selective usage of the original and modified Baker intestinal tube. *Surg Gynecol Obstet* 149:577, 1979.

Barnett WO, Petro AB, Williamson JW: A current appraisal of problems with gangrenous bowel. *Ann Surg* 183:653, 1976.

Berardi RS: Collective review: Anomalies of midgut rotation in the adult. *Surg Gynecol Obstet* 151:131, 1980.

Berardi RS: Collective review: Paraduodenal hernias. *Surg Gynecol Obstet* 152:99, 1981.

Bizer LS, Liebling RW, et al: Small bowel obstruction: The role of nonoperative treatment in simple intestinal obstruction and predictive criteria for strangulation obstruction. *Surgery* 89:407, 1981.

Boley SJ, Agrawal GP, et al: Pathophysiologic effects of bowel distention on intestinal blood flow. *Am J Surg* 117:228, 1969.

Boley SJ, Sprayregan S, et al: Initial results from an aggressive roentgenological and surgical approach to acute mesenteric ischemia. *Surgery* 82:848, 1977.

Bulkley GB, Zuidema GD, et al: Intraoperative determination of small intestinal viability following ischemic injury. A prospective, controlled trial of two adjuvant methods (Doppler and fluorescein) compared with standard clinical judgment. *Ann Surg* 193:628, 1981.

Davidson ED, Hersh T, et al: The effects of metoclopramide on postoperative ileus. *Ann Surg* 190:27, 1979.

Frimann-Dahl J: *Roentgen Examinations in Acute Abdominal Disease,* 3d ed. Springfield, Ill, Charles C Thomas, 1974.

Gammill SL, Nice CM Jr: Air fluid levels: Their occurrence in normal patients and their role in the analysis of ileus. *Surgery* 71:771, 1972.

Graber JN, Schultz WJ, et al: Relationship of duration of postoperative ileus to extent and site of operative dissection. *Surgery* 92:87, 1982.

Hofstetter SR: Acute adhesive obstruction of the small intestine. *Surg Gynecol Obstet* 152:141, 1981.

Kvist E: Gallstone ileus; a retrospective study. *Acta Chir Scand* 145:101, 1979.

Landman MD, Longmire WP Jr: Neural and hormonal influences of peritonitis on paralytic ileus. *Am Surg* 33:756, 1967.

Levitt MD: Intestinal gas production—recent advances in flatology. *N Engl J Med* 302:1474, 1980.

Levitt MD, Bond JH, Levitt DG: Gastrointestinal gas, in Johnson LR (ed): *Physiology of the Gastrointestinal Tract.* New York, Raven, 1981.

Miller RE, Brahme F: Large amounts of orally administered barium for obstruction of the small intestine. *Surg Gynecol Obstet* 129:1185, 1969.

Nachlas MM, Younis MT, et al: Gastrointestinal motility studies as a guide to postoperative management. *Ann Surg* 175:510, 1972.

Nadrowski L: Paralytic ileus: Recent advances in pathophysiology and treatment. *Curr Surg* 40:260, 1983.

Öhman U: Studies on small intestinal obstruction, I-VI. *Acta Chir Scand* 141:413, 417, 536, 545, 763, 771, 1975.

Osteen RT, Guyton S, et al: Malignant intestinal obstruction. *Surgery* 87:611, 1980.

Politzer J-P, Devroede G, et al: The genesis of bowel sounds: Influence of viscus and gastrointestinal content. *Gastroenterology* 71:282, 1976.

Quatromoni JC, Rosoff L Sr, et al: Early postoperative small bowel obstruction. *Ann Surg* 191:72, 1980.

Sarr MG, Bulkley GB, Zuidema GD: Preoperative recognition of intestinal strangulation obstruction. *Am J Surg* 145:176, 1983.

Shields R: The absorption and secretion of fluid and electrolytes by the obstructed bowel. *Br J Surg* 52:774, 1965.

Smith J, Kelly KA, Weinshilboum RM: Pathophysiology of postoperative ileus. *Arch Surg* 112:203, 1977.

Smith JA, Forward AD, et al: Metronidazole and tobramycin in intra-abdominal sepsis. *Surg Gynecol Obstet* 155:235, 1982.

Snape WJ Jr: Pseudo-obstruction and other obstructive disorders. *Clin Gastroenterol* 11:593, 1982.

Stewardson RH, Bombeck CT, Nyhus LM: Critical operative management of small bowel obstruction. *Ann Surg* 187:189, 1978.

Sykes PA, Boulter KH, Schofield PF: The microflora of the obstructed bowel. *Br J Surg* 63:721, 1976.

Tinker MA, Teicher I, Burdman D: Cellulose granulomas and their relationship to intestinal obstruction. *Am J Surg* 133:134, 1977.

Villar HV, Norton LW: Massive cecal dilation: Pseudoobstruction versus cecal volvulus. *Am J Surg* 137:170: 1979.

Wangensteen OH: Understanding the bowel obstruction problem. *Am J Surg* 135:131, 1978.

Weigelt JA, Snyder WH III, Norman JL: Complications and results of 160 Baker tube plications. *Am J Surg* 140:810, 1980.

Wickstrom P, Haglin JJ, Hitchcock CR: Intraoperative decompression of the obstructed small bowel. *Surgery* 73:212, 1973.

Wolff LH, Wolff WA, Wolff LH Jr: A re-evaluation of tube cecostomy. *Surg Gynecol Obstet* 151:257, 1980.

Wright HK, O'Brien JJ, Tilson MD: Water absorption in experimental closed segment obstruction of the ileum in man. *Am J Surg* 121:96, 1971.

Gastrointestinal Bleeding

Athanasoulis CA: Therapeutic applications of angiography. *N Engl J Med* 302:1117, 1174, 1980.

Atkenson RJ, Nyhus LM: Gastric lavage for hemorrhage in the upper part of the gastrointestinal tract. *Surg Gynecol Obstet* 146:797, 1978.

Boley SJ, Brandt LJ, Frank MS: Severe lower intestinal bleeding: Diagnosis and treatment. *Clin Gastroenterol.* 10:65, 1981.

Boley SJ, Sammartano R, et al: On the nature and etiology of vascular ectasias of the colon: Degenerative lesions of aging. *Gastroenterology* 72:650, 1977.

Bounous G: Acute necrosis of the intestinal mucosa. *Gastroenterology* 82:1457, 1982.

Bowden TA Jr, Hooks VH III, Mansberger AR Jr: Intraoperative gastrointestinal endoscopy. *Ann Surg* 191:680, 1980.

Colacchio TA, Forde KA, et al: Impact of modern diagnostic methods on the management of active rectal bleeding. *Am J Surg* 143:607, 1982.

Dent TL: Collective review: Evaluation of the bleeding patient. *Surg Gynecol Obstet* 151:817, 1980.

Donaldson RM Jr: Assessing the usefulness of diagnostic procedures. *Gastroenterology* 72:762, 1977.

Dronfield MW, Langman MJS, et al: Outcome of endoscopy and barium radiography for acute upper gastrointestinal bleeding: Controlled trial in 1037 patients. *Br Med J* 284:545, 1982.

Dykes PW, Keighley MRB (eds): *Gastrointestinal Hemorrhage.* Bristol, Wright, PSG, 1981.

Eisenberg RL: *Diagnostic Imaging in Internal Medicine.* New York, McGraw-Hill, 1985.

Eisenberg RL: *Diagnostic Imaging in Surgery.* New York, McGraw-Hill, 1987.

Giacchino JL, Geis WP, et al: Changing perspectives in massive lower intestinal hemorrhage. *Surgery* 86:368, 1979.

Hastings PR, Skillman JJ, et al: Antacid titration in the prevention of acute gastrointestinal bleeding: A controlled, randomized trial in 100 critically ill patients. *N Engl J Med* 298:1041, 1978.

Himal HS, Perrault C, Mzabi R: Upper gastrointestinal hemorrhage: Aggressive management decreases mortality. *Surgery* 84:448, 1978.

Johnson WC, Nabseth DC, et al: Bleeding esophageal varices. Treatment with vasopressin, transhepatic embolization and selective splenorenal shunting. *Ann Surg* 195:393, 1982.

Kivilaakso E, Silen W: Pathogenesis of experimental gastric-mucosal injury. *N Engl J Med* 301:364, 1979.

McKusick KA, Froelich J, et al: ^{99m}Tc red blood cells for detection of gastrointestinal bleeding: Experience with 80 patients. *Am J Roentgen* 137:1113, 1981.

Meyers MA, Alonso DR, et al: Pathogenesis of bleeding colonic diverticulosis. *Gastroenterology* 71:577, 1976.

Michel L, Serrano A, Malt RA: Mallory-Weiss syndrome. Evolution of diagnostic and therapeutic patterns over two decades. *Ann Surg* 192:716, 1980.

Milliser RV, Greenberg SR, Neiman BH: Exsanguinating stercoral ulceration. *Am J Dig Dis* 15:485, 1970.

Nance FC, Kaufman HJ, Batson RC: The role of the microbial flora in acute gastric stress ulceration. *Surgery* 72:68, 1972.

Nath RL, Sequeira JC, et al: Lower gastrointestinal bleeding: Diagnostic approach and management conclusions. *Am J Surg* 141:478, 1981.

Odonkor P, Mowat C, Himal HS: Prevention of sepsis-induced gastric lesions in dogs by cimetidine via inhibition of gastric secretion and by prostaglandin via cytoprotection. *Gastroenterology* 80:375, 1981.

O'Donnell TF Jr, Gembarowitz RM, et al: The economic impact of acute variceal bleeding: Cost-effectiveness implications for medical and surgical therapy. *Surgery* 88:693, 1980.

Orloff MJ, Bell RH Jr, et al: Long-term results of emergency portacaval shunt for bleeding esophageal varices in unselected patients with alcoholic cirrhosis. *Ann Surg* 192:325, 1980.

Peterson WL, Barnett CC, et al: Routine early endoscopy in upper-gastrointestinal-tract bleeding. A randomized, controlled trial. *N Engl J Med* 304:925, 1981.

Pruitt BA, Foley FD, Moncrief JA: Curling's ulcer: A clinical-pathological study of 323 cases. *Ann Surg* 172:523, 1970.

Robert A: Cytoprotection by prostaglandins. *Gastroenterology* 77:761, 1979.

Schiff L: Hematemesis and melena, in MacBryde CM (ed): *Signs and Symptoms,* 5th ed. Philadelphia, Lippincott, 1970.

Smith JL, Graham DY: Variceal hemorrhage: A critical evaluation of survival analysis. *Gastroenterology* 82:968, 1982.

Storey DW, Bown SG, et al: Endoscopic prediction of recurrent bleeding in peptic ulcers. *N Engl J Med* 305:915, 1981.

Stothert JC Jr, Simonowitz DA, et al: Randomized prospective evaluation of cimetidine and antacid control of gastric pH in the critically ill. *Ann Surg* 192:169, 1980.

Sutherland D, Frech RS, et al: The bleeding cecal ulcer: Pathogenesis, angiographic diagnosis, and nonoperative control. *Surgery* 71:290, 1972.

Villar HV, Fender HR, et al: Emergency diagnosis of upper gastrointestinal bleedings by fiberoptic endoscopy. *Ann Surg* 185:367, 1977.

Webb WA, McDaniel L, et al: Endoscopic evaluation of 125 cases of upper gastrointestinal bleeding. *Ann Surg* 193:624, 1981.

Winzelberg GG, Froelich JW, et al: Radionuclide localization of lower gastrointestinal hemorrhage. *Radiology* 139:465, 1981.

Zinner MJ, Zuidema GD, et al: The prevention of upper gastrointestinal tract bleeding in patients in an intensive care unit. *Surg Gynecol Obstet* 153:214, 1981.

Jaundice

Boucher IAD: Diagnosis of jaundice. *Br Med J* 283:1281, 1981.

Cooperberg P, Golding RH: Advances in ultrasonography of the gallbladder and biliary tract. *Radiol Clin North Am* 20:611, 1982.

Elias E, Hamlyn AN, et al: A randomized trial of percutaneous transhepatic cholangiography with the Chiba needle versus endoscopic retrograde cholangiography for bile duct visualization in jaundice. *Gastroenterology* 71:439, 1976.

Havrilla TR, Hagga JR, et al: Computed tomography and obstructive biliary disease. *Am J Roentgen* 128:765, 1977.

Jander HP, Galbraith J, Aldrete JS: Percutaneous transhepatic cholangiography using the Chiba needle: Comparison with retrograde pancreatocholecystography. *South Med J* 73:415, 1980.

Levitt RG, Sagel SS, et al: Accuracy of computed tomography of the liver and biliary tract. *Radiology* 124:123, 1977.

Popper H, Schaffner F: *Liver: Structure and Function.* New York, McGraw-Hill, 1957.

Schwartz SI: *Surgical Diseases of the Liver.* New York, McGraw-Hill, 1964.

Sivaprasad R, Gopalaswamy N: Jaundice: An internist's perspective. *Radiol Clin North Am* 18:179, 1980.

Vennes JA, Bond JH: Approach to the jaundiced patient. *Gastroenterol* 84:1615, 1983.

Williams JAR, Baker RJ, et al: Role of biliary scanning in the investigation of the surgically jaundiced patient. *Surg Gynecol Obstet* 144:525, 1977.

PHYSIOLOGY AND PHYSIOLOGIC TESTS

The esophagus provides a channel by which ingested material is conveyed from the pharynx to the stomach. At either end of the tube are regulatory mechanisms that assist in this function. Current knowledge of the physiology of the esophagus has been gained by the use of special recording techniques to detect and record intraesophageal pressures. In routine tests, three or four pressure-detecting units (fine water-filled and perfused polyvinylchloride tubes attached to strain-gauge manometers) are positioned at various points in the esophagus. Some prefer to use a terminal balloon-covered transducer in addition to the tubes with lateral openings at 5-cm intervals (Fig. 25-3). The infusion of distilled water at a constant rate through the open-tipped tubes provides accurate pressure recordings while the balloon-covered transducer provides higher sensitivity in study of sphincter function. Measurements are made with the esophagus at rest and after swallowing, the resting pressures being measured while the units are being withdrawn in stepwise fashion from the stomach into the esophagus prior to the recording of deglutition pressures (Fig. 25-4).

At the upper end of the esophagus there is a zone, about 3 cm long, of increased pressure that relaxes promptly with swallowing and contracts thereafter as a wave of high pressure passes through it (Fig. 25-4). Contractions of this *upper esophageal sphincter* (UES) are in peristaltic sequence with those of the pharynx above and the esophagus below, and the primary peristaltic wave of

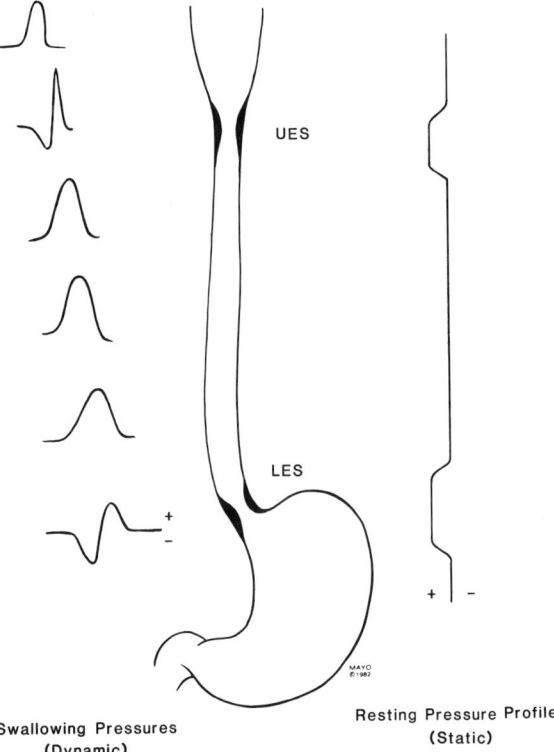

Swallowing Pressures
(Dynamic)

Resting Pressure Profile
(Static)

Fig. 25-4. Simplified representation demonstrating normal physiologic manometric pressures in pharynx, upper esophageal sphincter (UES) esophagus, and lower esophageal sphincter (LES). On right, static or resting high-pressure zones of LES and UES are defined, as pressure-sensing catheter is withdrawn from stomach below to pharynx above. On left are shown normal sequential swallowing pressure events from pharynx downward. Note that these dynamic events are peristaltic, with both upper and lower sphincters showing relaxation prior to contraction and return to resting tone.

Fig. 25-3. Balloon-covered differential transformer and cluster of three polyvinylchloride tubes used in measurement of esophageal and sphincteric pressures. Each tube has side opening (arrow) 5 cm from opening in next tube, is infused with water at rate of 1.4 mL/min by individual pump, and is attached to pressure-sensitive recording device. At Mayo Clinic, balloon-covered pressure transformer is routinely included as highly sensitive additional means of studying sphincter function. (From: *Code CF, Kelley ML Jr, et al: Gastroenterology 43:521, 1962, with permission.*)

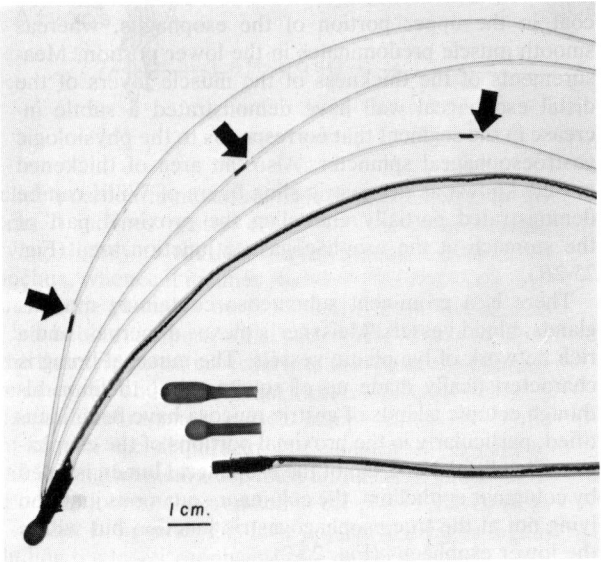

1 cm.

the esophagus is thus initiated. The sphincter relaxes to allow the wave to pass and then closes more tightly before returning to a lower, but elevated, resting tone. This wave of positive pressure sweeps in an orderly peristaltic fashion down the body of the esophagus, reaching an intensity of 50 to 100 cmH$_2$O and being somewhat more forceful in the lower esophagus than above. The resting pressures in the body of the esophagus are normally less than atmospheric, because of negative intrathoracic pressure.

There is also a *lower esophageal sphincter* (LES)—a zone of increased pressure at the lower end of the esophagus, somewhat longer (3 to 5 cm long) than that at the upper end, which can be detected by withdrawing the recording units from the stomach into the esophagus (Fig. 25-4). It is located in the region of the hiatus; and in response to a swallowing effort, relaxation of this zone of increased pressure can be identified, along with the immediately following sphincteric contraction in sequence with the peristaltic wave from the esophagus above (Fig. 25-4).

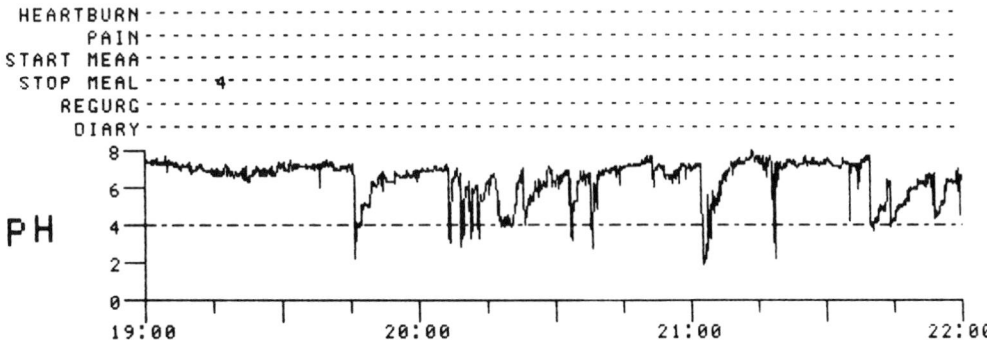

Fig. 25-5. Portion of 24-h pH monitor demonstrating frequent episodes of lower esophageal pH below 4 in a young patient with severe gastroesophageal reflux symptoms.

Measurements of the adaptive response of the LES to graded increases in intragastric pressure provide information pertinent to LES function. This sphincteric response is reflex in nature and is eliminated by vagotomy or atropine. In such a study, with the distal perfused pressure-sensing catheter in the stomach and the next in the higher-pressure zone of the sphincter, intragastric pressure is raised by either abdominal compression or the Valsalva maneuver. The ratio of simultaneous pressure recordings of the two sites provides an index to sphincter function. A ratio of increased sphincter pressure to increased intragastric pressure is usually 1.5, and a ratio less than 1 is considered abnormal. The placement of a third pressure-sensing catheter above the sphincter provides additional information regarding competence. If there is little or no rise in sphincter pressure, there is free transmission of intragastric pressure into the esophagus—the so-called common cavity effect.

The most sensitive objective test of gastroesophageal reflux is the *acid (pH) reflux test,* introduced by Tuttle and Grossman. The acid reflux test is performed by placing 300 mL of $0.1N$ HCl in the stomach. A pH electrode is placed 5 cm proximal to the manometrically defined LES. While a variety of maneuvers to increase intragastric pressure are performed, esophageal pH is monitored. A decrease in pH to less than 4 is considered positive evidence of gastroesophageal reflux. Johnson and DeMeester have further modified the technique by recording pH changes and correlating these with the patient's symptoms over a 24-h period (Fig. 25-5). The final record is analyzed in terms of the percent of time that pH is less than 4 while the patient is upright and recumbent. Additionally, the number of single reflux episodes and of those greater than 5 min duration are scored. Although not widely utilized clinically, this test provides detailed information not otherwise obtainable.

The *acid-clearing test* is used in patients with documented evidence of gastroesophageal reflux to measure the efficiency of the esophagus to clear instilled HCl by dry swallowing. Essentially, it provides an indirect index of the time refluxed gastric secretions are in contact with esophageal mucosa. A close correlation exists between evidence of esophagitis and a positive result on the clearing test. It is performed by placing a pH probe 5 cm above the LES and instilling 15 mL of $0.1N$ HCl 10 cm above the electrode. Normally, the esophagus is able to clear the acid from the distal esophagus with 10 dry swallows.

The *acid perfusion test* was developed by Bernstein and Baker as a provocative test for symptomatic reflux esophagitis, and as a means of reproducing esophageal pain to differentiate it from pain of other causes. The test is performed by introducing, via a tube placed at mid-esophagus, a continuous infusion of saline solution, which is alternated at 15- to 20-min intervals with a solution of $0.1N$ HCl. The results are negative if HCl produces no symptoms and saline reproduces symptoms, or if the pain elicited by infusion is different from spontaneous symptoms. The test is of limited use because of a high incidence of both false-negative and false-positive results.

Helm and associates noted a *galvanometric difference* in the electrical potential of gastric and esophageal mucosa and used this to identify the squamocolumnar junction. An electrode drawn from the stomach through the esophagus will show a 25-mV decrease in potential difference (PD) as it passes from gastric onto esophageal mucosa. While not a critical piece of information, it can be useful in orienting mucosa to manometric events.

Despite extensive knowledge regarding the effects of various hormones, drugs, foods, and other chemicals on lower-esophageal sphincter pressure, there has been only one *pharmacologic test* of esophageal function, and it has largely fallen into disuse. Kramer and Ingelfinger described the increased sensitivity and marked contractile response of the achalasic esophagus to parasympathomimetic drugs, a reaction indicative of denervation as defined by Cannon's law. The test is subjectively unpleasant, and it has been largely replaced by standard manometric studies.

Various safe, noninvasive *radioactive scanning techniques* for studying not only reflux, but the events of esophageal and gastric emptying after the ingestion of labeled liquids or solids, are in the developmental stage.

Although *radiography and endoscopy* are essential in the study of esophageal disease, except possibly for cine radiography, they provide no direct assessment of esophageal function. In addition to the usually ingested liquid radiopaque media, the mixture of barium with solid foods (the so-called barium sandwich) for fluoroscopic examination can provide functional information not defined by other tests and thereby lend objective credence to otherwise unexplained esophageal symptoms.

The details of esophageal innervation remain to be clarified, but esophageal peristalsis seems to be under vagal control, because division of these nerves produces simultaneous low pressures in the body of the esophagus after deglutition. The inferior esophageal sphincter, however, continues to relax with swallowing even after complete denervation, suggesting a certain degree of autonomy.

In spite of the clear demonstration of a physiologic sphincter at the lower end of the esophagus, there remains considerable controversy concerning the exact mechanism by which gastroesophageal reflux is prevented under normal circumstances. Factors that have been suggested as important include the diaphragm, a valve-flap mechanism, the gastric sling fibers and oblique angle of entry, and the mucosal rosette. There is substantial evidence to suggest that the first three are not involved in gastroesophageal competence and that the main antireflux mechanisms, acting together, are the musculature of the intrinsic sphincter and the prominent folds of epithelial gastric lining at the cardia. Studies by Goyal indicate that the LES is controlled by neural, hormonal, myogenic, and mechanical influences.

In the past some observers believed that the basal sphincter pressure was maintained by continuous vagal tone and that sphincter relaxation was a result of a decrease of tonic vagal activity. However, it is now held that both relaxation and contraction of the LES are due to the vagal transmission of active inhibitory or excitatory impulses but that neither acts as the major determinant of basal LES pressure. The role of sympathetic innervation on the LES is less well understood. Stimulation of alpha-adrenergic receptors causes the LES to contract, and stimulation of beta-adrenergic receptors causes it to relax. It is further hypothesized that sympathetic nerves act to modulate vagal activity on the LES. The fact that complete pharmacologic denervation of the LES does not influence basal sphincter pressure suggests that basal sphincter pressure is not due to tonic autonomic neural activity but that it may be due to tonic myogenic activity of the LES muscle itself. Many hormones, drugs, and various chemicals have been known to modify basal pressure of the LES (Table 25-1). It has been held that circulating gastrin is the major determinant of basal LES pressure and that this effect is modulated by interaction of secretin. However, recent studies do not support these views but suggest that the changes previously observed were obtainable only in response to unphysiologically high levels of these hormones. Other hormones such as prostaglandins, histamine, and serotonin produce less clear or more variable effects on LES pressure, depending on experimental conditions.

Thus, at this time it appears that the basal LES pressure is due to background basal tone provided by intrinsic myogenic activity of the sphincter muscle itself and that this tone is modulated by a variety of excitatory and inhibitory neurohormonal influences. The sphincter relaxation is chiefly due to neural activity mediated by inhibitory vagal and extravagal pathways.

Table 25-1. REGULATION OF LES PRESSURE

	Increase	Decrease

Hormones	Gastrin
	Motilin
	Substance P
	Vasopressin
	Glucagon
		Secretin
		Cholecystokinin
		Gastric inhibitory
		  polypeptides
		Vasoactive
		  intestinal
		  polypeptides
		Progestational
		  agents

Drugs	α-Adrenergic
	  agonist
	    Norepinephrine
	    Phenylephrine
	Cholinergic
	    Bethanechol
	    Methacholine
	Anticholinesterase
	    Edrophonium
	Betazole
	Metoclopramide
		α-Adrenergic
		  antagonist
		    Phentolamine
		β-Adrenergic
		  agonist
		    Isoproterenol
		Anticholinergic
		    Atropine
		Theophylline

Miscellaneous	Prostaglandin F$_{2\alpha}$
	Protein meal
	Gastric
	  alkalinization
		Prostaglandins E$_1$,
		  E$_2$, A$_2$
		Nicotine
		Ethanol
		Fat meal
		Chocolate
		Gastric
		  acidification

SOURCE: Data from Castell DO: The lower esophageal sphincter: Physiologic and clinical aspects. *Ann Intern Med* 83:390, 1975.

Loss of the LES basal tone can occur as a consequence of pregnancy (because of elevated levels of progesterone and estrogen), excessive ingestion of alcohol, smoking, and use of drugs that especially inhibit the LES (atropine, nitrites, beta-adrenergic agents, etc.). The LES basal tone can be enhanced by neutralization of gastric acid and by administration of drugs such as bethanecol or metoclopramide.

When the LES is challenged by an increase in intragastric pressure, its resting tone increases. This response is due to a vagus-mediated neural reflex that can be blocked by atropine or vagotomy, as shown by Cohen and Lipshutz. The ability to increase the LES pressure so that it is greater than the rise in intragastric pressure is one of the essential features of the competent LES and the basis of the test alluded to above.

FUNCTIONAL DISTURBANCES OF THE ESOPHAGUS

The development of techniques for physiologic evaluation of esophageal function has permitted the classification of esophageal motor disorders in two main categories: (1) those characterized by disturbances of the esophagus and lower sphincter, such as esophageal achalasia and diffuse spasm of the esophagus; and (2) those characterized by failure of the normal gastroesophageal competence mechanism, which leads to gastro-esophageal reflux and its complications. Although the causes of these conditions remain in doubt, their clinical and physiologic manifestations are well known, so surgical treatment can be undertaken on sound grounds in properly selected patients.

Motility Disturbances

ACHALASIA

Achalasia of the esophagus, or "cardiospasm," as it is more commonly but inaccurately known, has been recognized by the medical profession for more than 300 years. As early as 1674, Thomas Willis in his *Pharmaceutice Rationalis* described the symptoms of this condition and advised forceful dilation as treatment. It is a condition in which peristalsis is absent from the body of the esophagus and the inferior esophageal sphincter fails to relax in response to swallowing.

The causes of the condition are unknown, although a variety have been suggested, including inherent weakness of the esophagus, spasm of the esophagus, mechanical factors such as external compression or trauma, and congenital factors. Most students of the subject now agree that the disease has a neurogenic basis, and pathologic evidence supporting this belief is provided by degeneration or absence of the ganglion cells of Auerbach's plexus in the esophagus of many patients with the disease, a finding first reported by Rake in 1926. Subsequent studies have shown that the changes occur throughout the thoracic esophagus, particularly in the body of the organ, but one-third of the patients are unaffected.

Fig. 25-6. Achalasia of esophagus, radiographs illustrating varying degrees of esophageal dilatation and tortuosity. Effects are absent or mild in 20 percent of patients, moderate in 45 percent, and marked or advanced in 35 percent. All have absent peristalsis and nonrelaxing lower esophageal sphincter.

The reason for these nerve-cell changes remains obscure; infections due to bacteria or viruses, infestations by parasites, and vitamin deficiencies all have been incriminated. That the primary site of the disorder may be in the extraesophageal nerve supply—either the vagus nerve itself or its central nuclei—has been suggested by pathologic studies of biopsy and autopsy material and by experiments involving the selective destruction of the motor nuclei of the vagus nerve in the medulla of the cat and the dog.

CLINICAL MANIFESTATIONS. Whatever the cause of the disease, its clinical manifestations are now well recognized. It occurs with equal frequency in men and in women, and although it may appear at any age, it is more frequently seen in persons between the ages of thirty and fifty years. The earliest and most constant symptom is obstruction to swallowing, which at first may be intermittent. However, as the condition progresses, difficulty is experienced with all efforts to swallow. As a rule, the patient experiences more difficulty with cold than with warm foods, and solids may at first seem to pass more easily than liquids. Pain is rare and is more likely to occur in the early stages of the disease than later; it becomes less noticeable as the esophagus dilates. Regurgitation of ingested food and liquids is a common symptom and may occur particularly at night when the patient is recumbent, leading to aspiration and the development of pulmonary complications. Carcinoma of the esophagus occurs approximately seven times as often in patients with esophageal achalasia as in the general population.

Radiographic studies are helpful in the diagnosis of the disease, because even in its early stages evidence of obstruction at the cardia and slight dilatation of the esophagus may be noted. As the disease progresses, the classic radiographic signs develop (Fig. 25-6), the esophagus becoming dilated and its lower portion projecting beak-like into the distal narrowed segment with very little, if

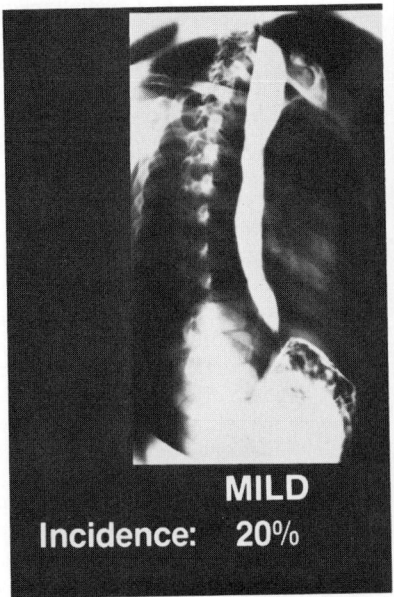
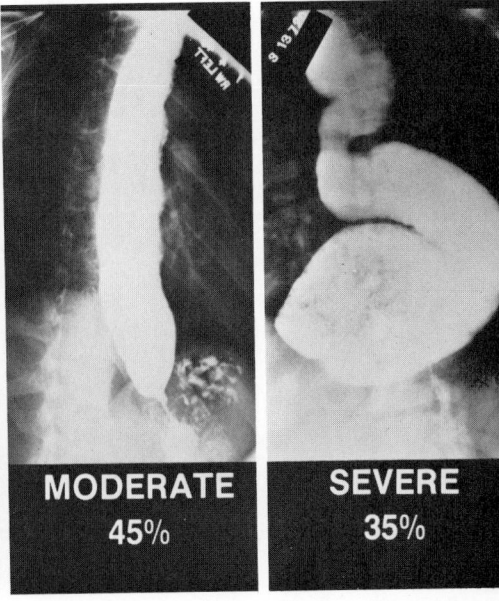

MILD Incidence: 20%   MODERATE 45%   SEVERE 35%

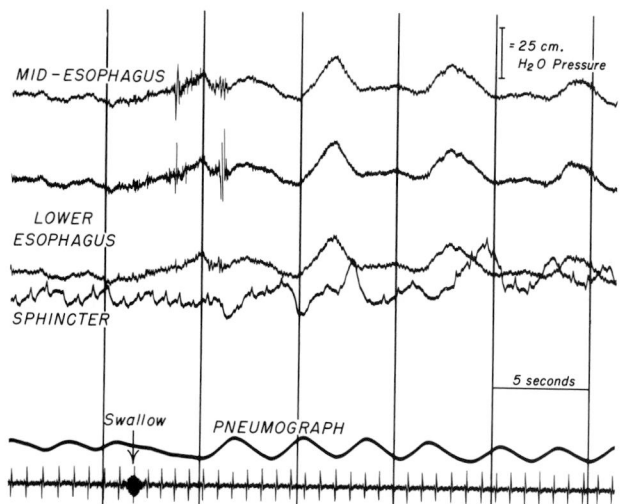

Fig. 25-7. Achalasia of esophagus: response to deglutition. In response to swallowing, feeble simultaneous contractions occur in body of esophagus, with failure of sphincteric relaxation. (From: *Ellis FH Jr, Payne WS: Adv Surg 1:179, 1965. Copyright 1965 by Year Book Medical Publishers, Inc. Used by permission.*)

any, barium present in the stomach. In some cases, the esophagus may reach huge proportions, so that it may be seen on the ordinary thoracic radiograph. Differentiation between early stages of esophageal achalasia and benign stricture or carcinoma of the cardia may be difficult, and esophagoscopy may be required for diagnosis.

Fig. 25-8. Method of performing hydrostatic dilation. *A.* Passage of #41 French olive-tipped bougie into stomach. *B.* Passage of #50 to #60 French sound guided by flexible wire spiral. *C.* Passage of hydrostatic dilator into esophagogastric junction. *D.* Distention of dilator. (From: *Olsen AM, Harrington SW, et al: J Thorac Surg 22:164, 1951, with permission.*)

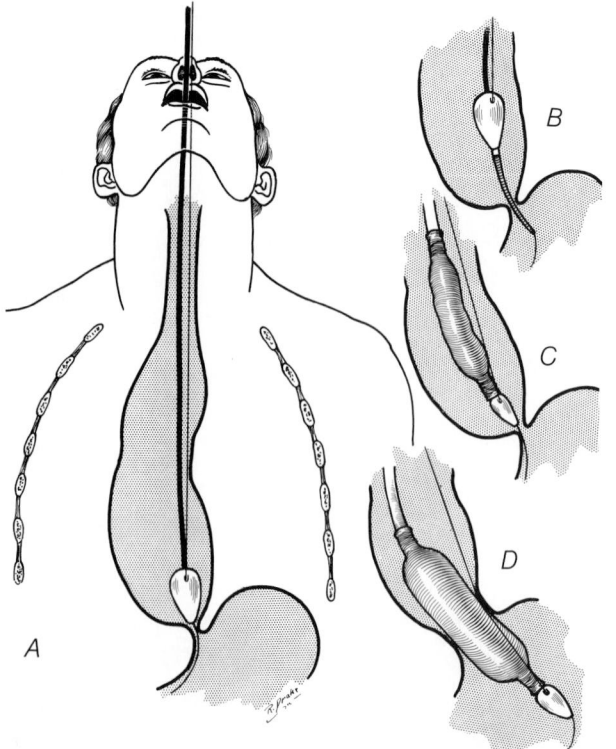

PHYSIOLOGIC STUDIES. Confirmation of the clinical diagnosis can be provided by studies of esophageal motility. Such studies demonstrate that the pressure in the body of the esophagus is higher than normal, often equaling atmospheric pressure, presumably because of esophageal dilatation with retention of food and fluid. In response to a swallowing effort, feeble, simultaneous, repetitive contractions occur throughout the esophagus, but there is no coordinated peristaltic wave (Fig. 25-7). Although relaxation of the UES occurs normally, in the majority of cases the lower sphincter fails to relax after swallowing. Cohen and Lipshutz, using perfused catheters, demonstrated that the LES pressure at rest is increased in patients with achalasia to approximately twice that seen in normal subjects. Furthermore, when the sphincter occasionally does relax during swallowing, the relaxation is incomplete. In some patients with achalasia, contractions of the esophagus and the sphincter may be vigorous and simultaneous, and the term *vigorous achalasia* has been applied to this subgroup.

TREATMENT. Current knowledge does not permit restoration of the disordered esophageal motility to normal. Effective therapy, therefore, can be directed only to relief of the distal esophageal obstruction. Because diet and drugs are ineffective, this must be accomplished either by forceful dilation of the esophagus or by surgical means.

Mechanical, pneumatic, and hydrostatic dilation have been used with success. At the Mayo Clinic, hydrostatic dilation (Fig. 25-8) has been used extensively in the past and has been found to be a useful technique. Okike and associates reported good to excellent results in 65 percent of patients observed for an average of $9\frac{1}{2}$ years (Table 25-2). The method is not without risk; an esophageal perforation occurred in about 2 percent of cases. Forceful dilatation has been done with a pneumatic balloon catheter, inflating the balloon to a 35-mm diameter at approximately 300 torr. This has been performed at the Mayo Clinic in approximately 50 patients; three perforations have occurred. Currently pneumatic dilatation seems most appropriate for those patients who are poor surgical

Table 25-2. COMPARISON OF TWO METHODS USED IN TREATING ACHALASIA AT THE MAYO CLINIC, 1949 THROUGH 1975

Factors	Dilation (N = 431)	Esophagomyotomy (N = 468)
Result, %		
Excellent	28 ⎫ 65*	50 ⎫ 85*
Good	37 ⎭	35 ⎭
Fair	16	9
Poor	19	6
Follow-up, years	1–18	1–17
No. patients	311	456
Percent	72	97
Age, years	1–85	4–81

* Significantly different ($p < 0.001$)
SOURCE: Okike N, Payne WS, et al: *Ann Thorac Surg* 28:119, 1979.

risks or who have recurrent achalasia following a modified Heller myotomy.

Limitations of medical therapy, including the use of forceful dilation, have led to surgical efforts to relieve the symptoms of esophageal achalasia. The techniques have included excisional or bypassing procedures and denervation procedures. The latter were ineffective, and the uniform development of severe reflux esophagitis after any procedure that destroys or bypasses the inferior esophageal sphincter has rightly led to their abandonment.

Current surgical therapy stems historically from the double cardiomyotomy first proposed by Heller in 1913. It has been modified by a number of surgeons in subsequent years. The simplest and most effective modification involves an incision through the muscle layers of the distal esophagus, through a thoracic approach. The mucosa is exposed to free completely the narrowed distal esophageal segment of its circular musculature, but the incision is extended onto the stomach only far enough to ensure completeness of this portion of the procedure (Fig. 25-9). Generally, 1 cm onto the stomach is adequate. The most proximal portion of the stomach can be recognized by multiple transverse mucosal veins. Damage to the vagus nerves and the supporting structures about the hiatus is avoided. An operation carried out in the manner described, without ancillary procedures, should relieve the distal esophageal obstruction in almost every patient and should rarely lead to esophageal reflux. Okike and associates, reviewing the Mayo Clinic experience from 1949 to 1976, reported that 94 percent of 468 patients treated in this fashion were benefited by the operation, and approximately 85 percent had excellent or good results (Table 25-2). More recent reviews of other series confirm our favorable experience with surgical treatment of achalasia.

Because of the superior results obtainable by a properly performed esophagomyotomy, operation is replacing all other forms of treatment for achalasia. Forceful dilation should be used only for selected patients whose general condition precludes a major operation or for patients

who decline to undergo operation. Thus, myotomy should be offered to all but extremely high-risk patients.

The late results of a properly performed esophagomyotomy are so satisfactory that it is neither necessary nor advisable to consider the performance of ancillary esophageal procedures at the time of myotomy. Indeed, Peyton et al., Mansour et al., Menguy, and others have reported the performance of an antireflux procedure at operation on all achalasia patients without a pre-existent sliding esophageal hiatal hernia. Not only does this unnecessarily complicate the surgical approach, it is an overreaction to the 3 percent incidence of incompetence after myotomy alone. Further, the failure rate of antireflux procedures exceeds the failure rate they are designed to prevent. Fewer than 6 percent of patients have poor results requiring reoperation for any cause. Indeed, the majority of patients requiring reoperation for achalasia require treatment for persistent obstruction at the distal esophagus because of persistent achalasia, not because of stricture or esophagitis. In the majority of patients requiring reoperation, the previous myotomy is found to have healed; and the patients respond rather well to performance of a properly designed remyotomy with attention to the details outlined. Only rarely is it necessary to perform esophagogastrectomy. If esophagogastrectomy is required, an antireflux procedure is generally necessary; care, however, must be taken to avoid a 360° fundoplication as this will almost certainly obstruct the amotile esophagus.

DIFFUSE SPASM

The causes of the hypermotility disorders are also unknown, although they too may be related to abnormalities affecting the vagus supply to the organ. Diffuse spasm of the esophagus, hypertensive gastroesophageal sphincter, and the hypercontracting lower esophageal sphincter are the conditions under discussion, and there is little evidence that they may be precursors of esophageal achalasia.

MANIFESTATIONS. Differentiation of these conditions from esophageal achalasia can usually be made on clinical grounds. Pain and dysphagia are the predominant symptoms, pain being more pronounced and dysphagia occurring intermittently or not at all. The pain may manifest only as a sensation of discomfort under the lower half of the sternum, or it may be severe and colicky, with extension through to the back or into the neck, shoulders, or arms, resembling cardiac pain. It may be provoked by eating, or it may come on spontaneously, even awakening the patient at night. Patients so afflicted tend to be high-strung and nervous, and the diagnosis of psychoneurosis may be entertained. The symptoms are intermittent and are more likely to be troublesome than incapacitating; even during an attack, the patient seldom appears to be seriously ill.

Radiologic abnormalities of the esophagus occur in fewer than half the cases. When present, however, they may be striking, with a range from simple narrowing to segmental spasm finally to extreme changes, including

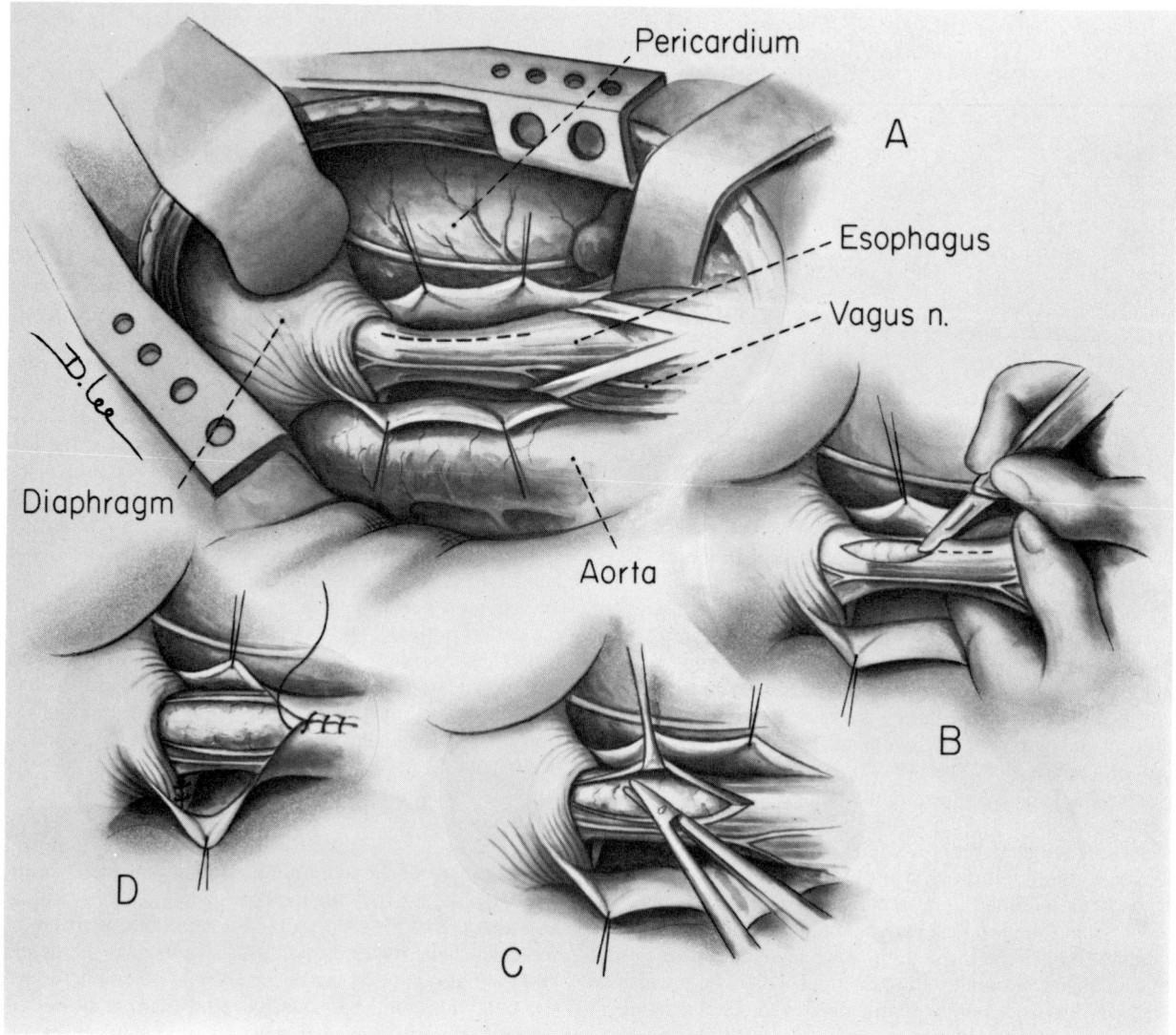

Fig. 25-9. Modified Heller esophagomyotomy for achalasia of esophagus. *A.* Transthoracic exposure of distal esophagus for esophagomyotomy. Esophagus has been mobilized and elevated from its bed by Penrose drain. Intended incision is indicated by dashed line. *B.* Beginning incision. *C.* Dissection of mucosa from muscularis. *D.* Restoration of esophagogastric junction to intraabdominal position, with suture narrowing of esophageal hiatus if necessary. (From: *Ellis FH Jr, Kiser JC, et al: Ann Surg 166:640, 1967, with permission.*)

pseudodiverticulosis (Fig. 25-10). A small diaphragmatic hernia is frequently present, and an epiphrenic diverticulum commonly coexists. A localized area of obstruction may be detectable in patients with hypertensive gastroesophageal sphincter as well as in those with hypercontracting LES.

DIAGNOSIS. Because esophageal radiographs may appear normal in patients with these disorders, and clinical history may be rather nonspecific, the diagnosis usually rests on the results of esophageal-motility studies. In patients with diffuse spasm, there is a specific abnormal pattern of the deglutitive pressures. A primary peristaltic wave can be recognized over the upper half of the esophagus, but in the lower third to two-thirds it is replaced by simultaneous, repetitive, and occasionally prolonged pressure increases of considerable magnitude (Fig. 25-11). Evidence of hiatal herniation is common. In most patients, however, there is no evidence of abnormality of the two sphincters unless there is a hypertension or hy-

percontraction of the LES, in which case resting pressures in that region are excessive and relaxation may be poor or pressures excessive as the swallowing peristalsis passes through the sphincter. Occasionally these sphincteric changes are the only manifestations of disease.

TREATMENT. The use of an extended esophagomyotomy for the treatment of patients with "diffuse nodular myomatosis of the esophagus" was suggested in 1950 by Lortat-Jacob. Although physiologic studies were not made in his patients, many probably had forms of esophageal hypermotility disturbances. A similar approach was

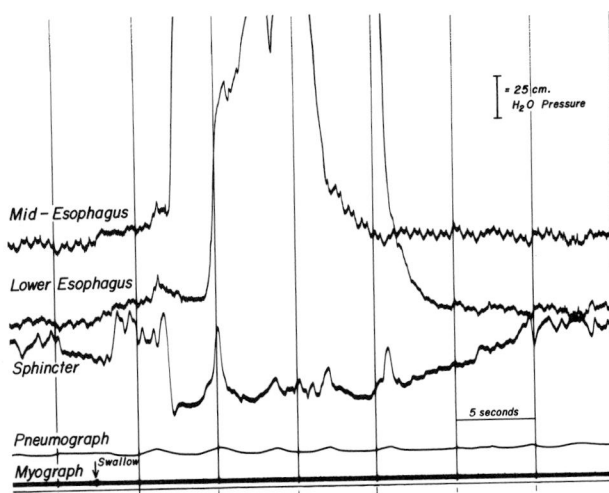

Fig. 25-11. Diffuse spasm: motility in esophagus and sphincter. Note giant repetitive contractions. Sphincter relaxes normally. Peristalsis, although usually absent, is present in this case. (From: *Ellis FH Jr, Code CF, Olsen AM: Surgery 48:155, 1960, with permission.*)

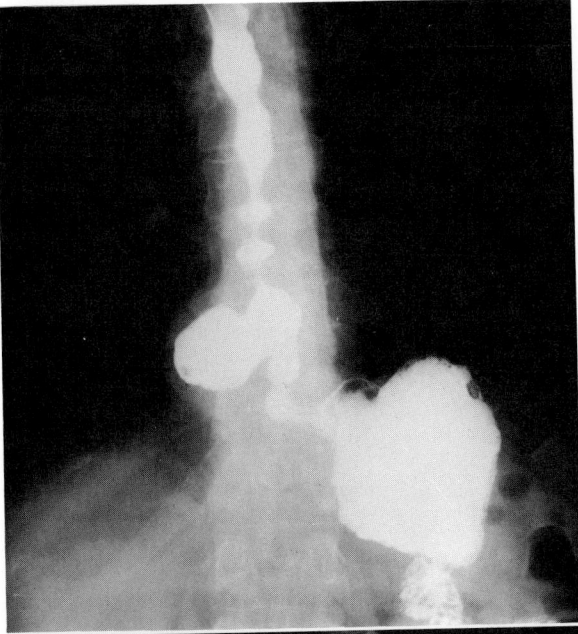

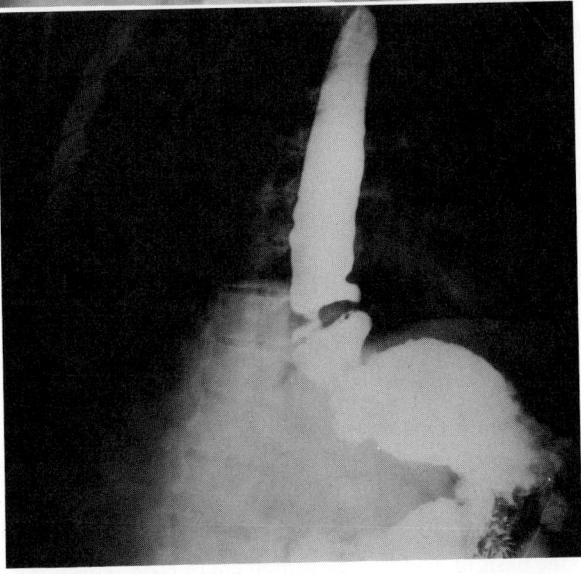

Fig. 25-10. Hypermotility disturbances: esophageal radiographs from two cases. *Top:* Diffuse spasm of esophagus with epiphrenic diverticulum and small hiatal hernia. *Bottom:* Hypertensive gastroesophageal sphincter with small hiatal hernia. (From: *Ellis FH Jr, Payne WS: Adv Surg 1:179, 1965. Copyright 1965 by Year Book Medical Publishers, Inc. Used by permission.*)

initiated independently at the Mayo Clinic in 1956 in order to control the severe symptoms of hypermotility disturbance of the esophagus in carefully selected patients.

In many respects, the technique of the operation resembles that used for achalasia of the esophagus. However, the proximal limit of the esophageal muscular incision varies, depending on the preoperative estimate of the extent of the disease as defined by esophageal motility studies. It may occasionally extend as high as the aortic arch or above (Fig. 25-12). If esophageal motility demon-

strates a hypertensive LES, the myotomy must be carried down onto the stomach as it is for achalasia. If the LES is normal, the myotomy can stop on the distal esophagus. Surgical repair of an associated diaphragmatic hernia is essential. Henderson and associates have stressed the need for an antireflux procedure at operation on all patients with diffuse spasm, and extension of the myotomy from the stomach to 10 cm above the aortic end. Flye and Sealy have reported similar good results with long esophagomyotomy, reserving antireflux operations for patients with manifest hernia or incompetence. Surgical treatment is less effective than for achalasia; only 78 percent of these patients so treated are benefited. Leonardi and associates reported a 91 percent improvement rate in 11 patients when a more proximal myotomy was done to save a sphincter that was not manometrically affected as shown in Fig. 25-12.

Patients therefore should be selected carefully for this operation, the ideal candidate being an emotionally stable person with serious disability from the disease but without evidence of associated gastrointestinal problems. There should be demonstrable evidence of the severity of the disease in the form of a markedly abnormal esophageal motility pattern, ideally associated with radiographic evidence of esophageal spasm.

Disturbances of Gastroesophageal Competence (Gastroesophageal Reflux and Its Complications)

While it is clear that the loss of gastroesophageal competence is the cause for gastroesophageal reflux and its complications, the precise mechanism of competence is still debated. It is generally conceded that there is normally a high-pressure zone (HPZ) 3 to 5 cm long, of 10 to 20 mmHg, which is largely responsible for maintaining a

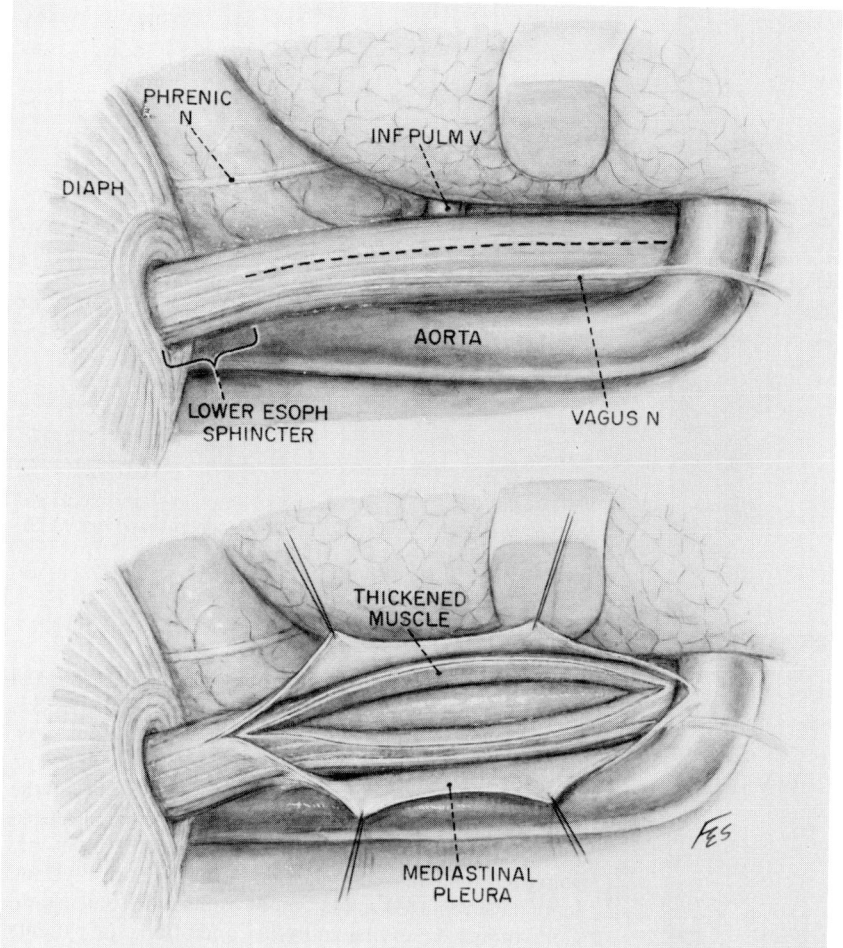

Fig. 25-12. Long esophagomyotomy for diffuse spasm of esophagus. Note that incision extends to aortic arch and spares lower esophageal sphincter. This technique is applicable in diffuse spasm when lower esophageal sphincter is demonstrated manometrically to be normal and only the body of esophagus is affected by motility disturbances.

protective pressure barrier between the stomach and the esophagus to prevent reflux. This barrier relaxes with swallowing to provide unimpeded transport of a bolus, and promptly returns to its resting tone. By mechanisms poorly understood, the intensity of this HPZ increases with intraabdominal and intragastric pressure, effecting an antireflux barrier responsive to changing conditions. Physiologists classically have held that the HPZ is equivalent to LES, but more recently this has been challenged by DeMeester and associates. They conceived that the HPZ was entirely an artifact of esophageal environment and not entirely a result of active motor tone of the sphincter (Fig. 25-13). In brief, they held that the HPZ resulted from exposure of a segment of distal esophagus to intraabdominal positive pressure. Regardless of the merit of these controversies, Cohen and Harris succeeded, by study of the length and magnitude of this HPZ among patients with and without hiatal hernias, in distinguishing those with reflux from those without. Subsequently Olsen and Harrington, Schlegel, and Payne, by the criterion of a hypotensive LES, were able to select a group of patients without hiatal hernia who had significant reflux. In clinical practice, however, it has generally not been possible to select patients for treatment of reflux

on the basis of objective measurement of HPZ. This is not only because there is considerable pressure overlap between refluxers and nonrefluxers in many cases, but mainly because the decision to treat is not whether a given patient is refluxing, but what and how severe are the subjective and objective complications attributable to reflux.

While the majority of patients with clinically significant gastroesophageal reflux have an associated sliding esophageal hiatal hernia, the converse is not true. Indeed, the vast majority of patients with hiatal hernia do not have significant reflux, and the hernia per se does not present a clinical problem.

Sometimes systemic collagen disease involves the esophagus. Scleroderma is probably the most common disease that gives rise to motor failure of the distal esophagus. On manometric study there is a loss of both esophageal peristalsis and sphincter tone. This permits free re-

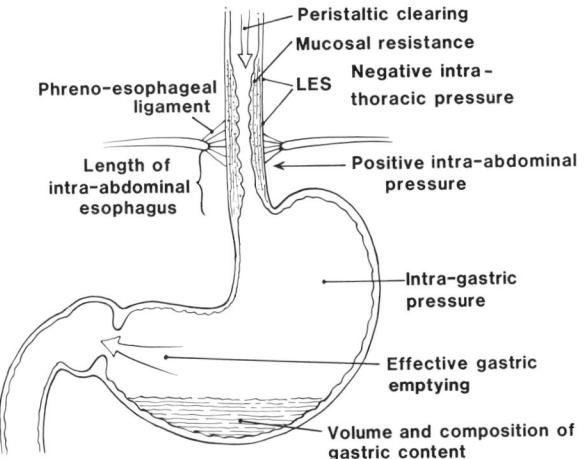

Fig. 25-13. Factors that affect gastroesophageal competence or permit gastroesophageal reflux and its complications. These include esophageal peristalsis with its clearing action, intrinsic lower-esophageal-sphincter tone, intraabdominal position of part of esophagus, site of phrenoesophageal ligament insertions, intraabdominal and intrathoracic pressures, intragastric pressure, effective gastric emptying, and concentration and composition of digestive secretions (acid-bile-pancreatic) present in stomach and available for reflux into esophagus.

flux of gastric contents without a clearing mechanism and results in a particularly virulent form of reflux esophagitis.

Other causes of gastroesophageal reflux include operations that destroy or bypass the normal lower esophageal competence mechanism. These include poorly executed myotomies, resections of the esophagogastric junction, and various types of cardioplasties.

Gastroesophageal reflux may also occur in the presence of a normal competence mechanism, when gastric emptying is impaired by gastric-outlet obstruction or failure of gastric motility.

Almost all of the subjective and objective complications of gastroesophageal reflux (Table 25-3) result from the acute sensitivity of esophageal mucosa to a variety of digestive secretions. While acid peptic secretions are generally implicated, bile and pancreatic secretions, irrespective of pH, are equally irritating and corrosive. The

Table 25-3. COMPLICATIONS OF GASTROESOPHAGEAL REFLUX

Intractable subjective distress
Esophagitis
Bleeding
Stenosis of esophagus
    Reversible
    Irreversible
Shortening of esophagus
    Reversible
    Irreversible
Esophageal-ulcer penetration or perforation
Columnar epithelial-lined lower esophagus (Barrett esophagus)
Motility disturbances of esophagus

severity of complications is related to the type and concentration of secretions refluxed and their contact time with esophageal mucosa.

SYMPTOMS. Heartburn is the classic symptom of gastroesophageal reflux. It is described as a burning retrosternal distress beginning in the epigastrum and extending for varying distances toward the neck. There may be, at times, actual regurgitation of bitter, sour liquid into the mouth, which may cause gagging or retching. Reflux symptoms are usually precipitated by a full stomach or by postural changes such as leaning over, lifting, or recumbency. Nocturnal distress is common, the patients awakening one or more times during sleep with heartburn, regurgitation, or actual respiratory aspiration with cough and choking. Often it is possible to control such symptoms with topical antacids, weight reduction, slant bed, cimetidine, and metoclopramide. When symptoms become intractable to medical management and the patient's ability to function is seriously impaired by symptoms of reflux, surgical restoration of competence is indicated, irrespective of the degree of objective esophagitis or other complications of reflux.

ESOPHAGITIS AND BLEEDING

Esophagitis is an objective finding and not a symptom. It can be suspected from history or esophageal x-rays, but endoscopy is required for diagnosis. It is defined as an objective change in the esophageal mucosa as a consequence of corrosive injury. Objective esophagitis does not necessarily correlate with either the duration or severity of its symptoms, though there is a general parallel. In some patients with intractable subjective distress, no objective endoscopic mucosal change is evident, but mucosal biopsy will demonstrate occult histologic changes. Diffuse distal esophageal erythema is one of the earliest gross signs of esophagitis. This may progress to linear rows of discrete superficial ulcers and subsequently to their coalescence, giving the appearance of linear streaks of ulceration and friable mucosa. Eventually this can lead to an extensive loss of normal epithelium in the distal esophagus or a deep solitary ulcer. When esophagitis becomes severe, patients often complain of painful swallowing *(odynophagia)*. With deep penetrating ulceration, there is often an intractable constant pain radiating to the thoracic spine. Although the esophagus may have a hemorrhagic appearance and there may be chronic blood loss from ulcerative esophagitis, massive upper gastroesophageal bleeding is uncommon. Bleeding, when present, is probably more often attributable to an associated hiatal hernia with gastric erosions in the intrathoracic loculus of the stomach or where the stomach is impinged upon by the hiatus. Severe esophagitis is not often reversible by medical means and usually requires an antireflux operation for its control.

STENOSIS OF THE ESOPHAGUS

As consequences of chronic recurrent corrosive injury, varying degrees of transmural inflammation, muscle contracture, and collagen deposition can occur in the wall of

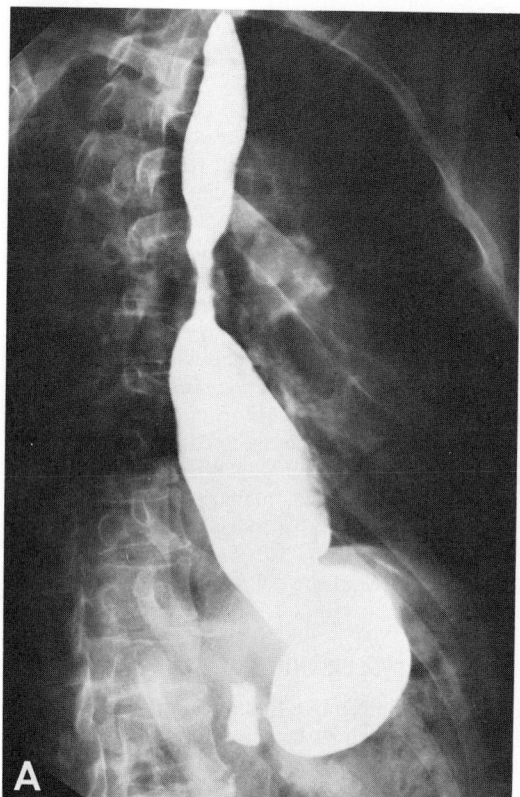 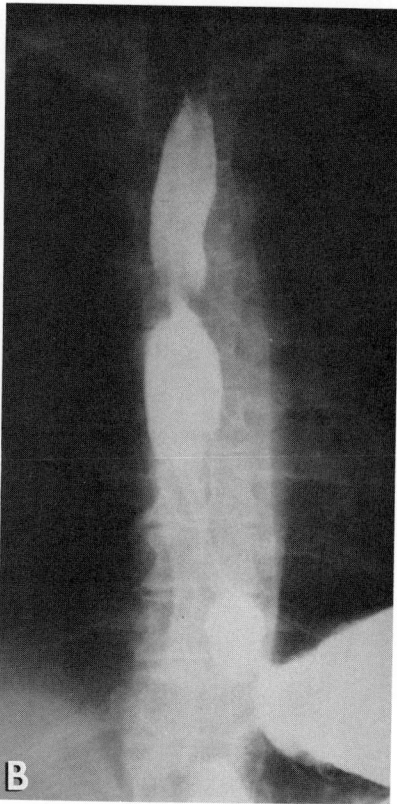

the esophagus. Classically this occurs in the lower few centimeters of the esophagus at the esophagogastric junction. In patients with protracted emesis or with protracted nasogastric intubation, long-tapered stenoses affecting the lower half of the esophagus are seen. These stenoses represent a tissue response to corrosive injury. The vast majority of stenotic lesions are amenable to simple dilation therapy, and symptoms of dysphagia are relieved thereby. Stenosis of the esophagus is an important complication of gastroesophageal reflux; and if it recurs or if symptoms of reflux persist after dilation, an antireflux operation is indicated. Surgical treatment is the most definitive means of preventing progressive and irreversible esophageal injury.

On rare occasions, reflux esophagitis and stenosis progress to such a severe panmural stage that an actual irreversible stricture is formed. If such a stricture cannot be dilated to a #50 French size with use of a swallowed thread or an endoscopically placed wire as a guide, stricture resection is the only method for restoring unobstructed swallowing. This rare late manifestation of reflux esophagitis poses special problems in surgical management to ensure that reflux, esophagitis, and stenosis do not recur after surgical relief of the stricture.

SHORTENED ESOPHAGUS

Just as stenosis of the esophagus is the result of annular contraction of the esophagus due to corrosive injury, so

Fig. 25-14. *A.* Esophagus of patient who had esophageal hiatal hernia with reflux esophagitis, shortened esophagus, and stricture. Esophagogastric junction is at midthoracic level, with stricture (several centimeters long) above. Typical esophageal peristalsis extended up to, but not beyond, midthoracic esophagogastric junction. Most of stomach had been pulled up into chest as consequence of acquired shortening of esophagus. *B.* Barrett esophagus. Small diaphragmatic hernia (sliding type) and midesophageal stricture. Tubular structure between stricture and stomach is columnar epithelial-lined esophagus with typical esophageal motility. (From: *Burgess JN, Payne WS, et al: Mayo Clin Proc, 46:728, 1971, with permission.*)

shortening occurs as the result of linear contracture (Fig. 25-14*A*). Whereas stenosis often accompanies shortening, shortened esophagus is occasionally seen without significant stenosis; and, of course, stenosis is usually seen without shortened esophagus. The vast majority of patients in whom a shortened esophagus is suspected on the basis of x-rays or endoscopic findings do not prove to have the condition when surgically explored. In such cases surgical mobilization usually permits the esophagogastric junction to be reduced below the diaphragm for the performance of one of the antireflux procedures. Under rare circumstances, however, the esophagus is so permanently fibrosed and shortened that one must consider a Collis gastroplasty to effectively lengthen the esophagus so that an antireflux procedure can be done below the diaphragm. In rare cases shortening is so marked that even this cannot be accomplished, and more complex surgical maneuvers are required.

While shortening is an important complication to be aware of in surgical management of gastroesophageal reflux, the symptoms in some patients have ceased entirely or are controllable medically. Thus, as an isolated finding without symptoms, shortening is not an indication for surgical treatment.

COLUMNAR EPITHELIAL-LINED LOWER ESOPHAGUS (BARRETT ESOPHAGUS)

As a consequence of the corrosive injury and destruction when the squamous epithelial lining of the lower esophagus has been damaged or destroyed by the corrosive effect of gastroesophageal reflux, replacement of normal epithelium with columnar epithelium occurs in some patients. It is as yet uncertain whether this is the result of metaplasia or cephalad growth of columnar epithelium from the gastric cardia. The abnormal esophageal lining may extend to the level of the aortic arch or higher (Fig. 25-14*B*). There is often a stenosis of the esophagus at the new squamocolumnar junction and evidence of esophagitis in the squamous epithelial-lined portion above the stricture. The columnar epithelium is largely mucus-producing, with only sparse parietal cells. Rarely, there is a deep, solitary, benign ulcer in the columnar epithelial-lined portion of the lower esophagus. This is referred to as a Barrett ulcer.

The risk of an adenocarcinoma developing in patients with Barrett esophagus is greater than in the general population, but the critical study of a large group of patients with Barrett esophagus to determine the incidence of subsequent malignancy has not been done. At the present time, prophylactic resection is not indicated. Correction of reflux does not prevent subsequent malignant transformation and does not usually cause regression of the abnormal columnar epithelial lining.

Operation is recommended to control intractable symptomatic reflux and stenosis. Standard antireflux procedures usually suffice. Most stenoses are readily dilatable prior to repair. Resection is generally indicated only when cancer is diagnosed or suspected. Many patients with Barrett esophagus are largely asymptomatic at diagnosis. In the absence of other reflux complications, these fortunates do not require specific treatment but do need careful follow-up for early detection of esophageal malignancy.

ESOPHAGEAL-ULCER PENETRATION AND PERFORATION

Esophageal perforation is a rare spontaneous complication of gastroesophageal reflux and esophagitis, yet among patients with postemetic rupture of the distal esophagus a high percentage have preexisting diaphragmatic hernia, esophagitis, and ulceration. The majority of instrumental perforations occur during attempts to dilate benign stenoses of the distal esophagus or to biopsy blindly beyond a stenotic lesion. Penetrating ulcers rarely produce a spontaneous rupture into the mediastinum or pleural spaces. They are more prone to produce intractable penetrating back pain, odynophagia, and bleeding.

MOTILITY DISTURBANCES

Various nonspecific motility disturbances may accompany reflux esophagitis. These may range from increased irritability, with occasional episodes of simultaneous nonperistaltic contraction, to diminution or even complete loss of lower-sphincter tone and contractility of the body of the esophagus. High-amplitude peristaltic contractions may be seen with distal stenotic obstruction, and with time these may give way to fatigue with complete loss of motor activity. Generally, the motility disorders of reflux esophagitis and its complications are reversible by surgical correction of reflux or obstruction.

CONTRACTION RINGS OF LOWER ESOPHAGUS

A ringlike constriction at the squamocolumnar junction, demonstrated radiographically by Schatzki and Gary in patients with diaphragmatic hernia, is now generally recognized as a minor complication of gastroesophageal reflux. It is an organic lesion consisting of a dense annular connective band in the submucosa at the squamocolumnar junction. The degree of impingement of the esophageal lumen varies greatly, and some patients are totally asymptomatic. The symptoms of esophageal obstruction *(dysphagia)* begin to occur with increasing frequency as ring diameter becomes less than 15 mm. Antecedent history of heartburn is frequent, and some patients experience recurrence of gastroesophageal reflux symptoms after the ring is dilated. In the majority, dilation relieves dysphagia, and reflux symptoms are mild and controllable. On rare occasions the mucosal ring will require surgical excision or disruption at the time of hiatal hernia repair and performance of an antireflux procedure.

RESPIRATORY ASPIRATION

Contamination of the upper and lower respiratory tracts by spontaneous gastroesophageal reflux of stomach contents is a generally accepted complication of gastroesophageal incompetence. Upper respiratory infections, sore throat, hoarseness, cough, choking, asthma, fever, pneumonitis, bronchiectasis, and lung abscess are recognized results of aspiration. What is unclear and difficult to document is the incidence of these complications. Some patients give a clear sequential clinical history of recurrent heartburn followed immediately by choking and coughing with recurrent episodes of fever, asthma, or pneumonitis. Others present with a respiratory problem, and the esophageal aspect is otherwise minor or asymptomatic. The 24-h acid-reflux test has the potential of sorting and relating respiratory events objectively to episodes of gastroesophageal reflux and directing therapy appropriately toward antireflux measures. In most cases, however, respiratory aspiration is just one of several well-defined subjective and objective complications of gastroesophageal reflux, and surgical indications are clear.

INDICATIONS FOR SURGICAL TREATMENT

The indications for surgical treatment of gastroesophageal reflux depend on objective assessment of severity and intractability of complications listed in Table 25-3. Although it is essential to correlate the occurrence of complications with that of gastroesophageal reflux as effect and cause, surgery is not indicated for gastroesophageal incompetence alone. Finally, before resorting to operation, it should be established that symptoms and complications cannot be controlled by simpler means.

Since the anatomic repair of esophageal hiatal hernia is an integral part of restoration of gastroesophageal competence and an essential feature of most of the antireflux operations, the details of surgical techniques appear in the succeeding section on esophageal hiatal hernia.

DIAPHRAGMATIC HERNIAS

A variety of acquired and congenital herniations occur through the diaphragm. All are associated with protrusion of abdominal viscera from the high-pressure abdomen into the low-pressure thorax. Like most abdominal hernias, diaphragmatic hernias carry a high risk of volvulus, obstruction, and strangulation of herniated hollow viscera. An exception is the pure sliding esophageal hernia, wherein the only clinical implication is that associated with gastroesophageal reflux and its complications. Another exception is the congenital posterolateral or Bochdalek hernia, in which the threat is not just herniation of viscera, but more importantly the high incidence of associated congenital anomalies, especially a life-threatening congenital dysfunction of the lungs. With these two ex-

ceptions, all the hernias of the diaphragm carry the pure risk of any abdominal hernia and require simple reduction and anatomic repair for management.

Development Anatomy

The diaphragm has a highly complex origin. The classic concept of formation was suggested in 1905 by Broman, who demonstrated that the diaphragm receives contributions from the septum transversum, the mesentery of the esophagus, the pleuroperitoneal membranes, and the musculature of the chest wall. There are two paired (pleuroperitoneal membranes, chest wall musculature) and two unpaired (septum transversum, mesentery) components (Fig. 25-15).

The septum transversum develops during the fourth week of gestation and initially appears as a thick, incomplete partition between the pericardial and peritoneal cavities. Originally, the septum is located opposite the anlage of the cervical vertebrae, but with growth, the septum

Fig. 25-15. Development of diaphragm as viewed from below. *A.* Lateral view of embryo at end of fifth week of gestation (dotted line indicates the level of section B). *B.* Transverse section showing unfused pleuroperitoneal membranes. *C.* Similar section at end of eighth week, showing fusion of pleuroperitoneal membranes. *D.* Transverse section through a 12-week-old embryo, demonstrating ingrowth of chest wall musculature into diaphragm. *E.* View of diaphragm of newborn, indicating probable embryologic origin of its components. (From: *Moore KL: The Developing Human: Clinically Oriented Embryology,* 2d ed. Philadelphia, Saunders, 1977, with permission.)

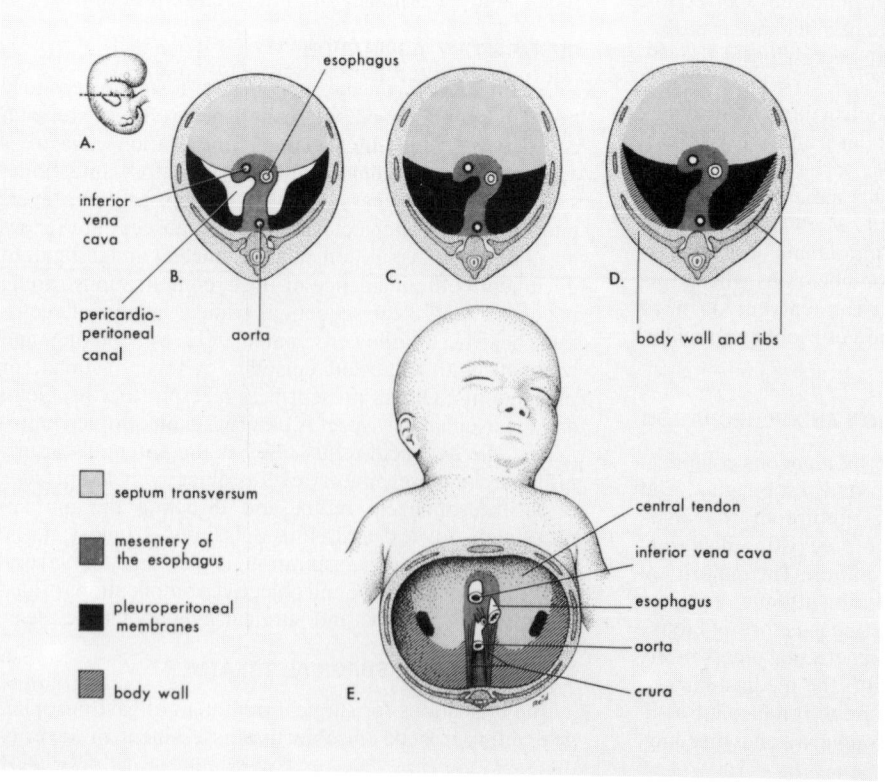

becomes displaced caudally to reach the level of the first lumbar vertebra. Eventually, it fuses dorsally with the ventral mesentery to the esophagus and with the pleuroperitoneal membranes. In the adult, the septum transversum forms the central tendon of the diaphragm. The dorsal mesentery of the esophagus also appears during the fourth week of gestation and constitutes the median portion of the diaphragm dorsal to the septum transversum. In the adult, this mesentery forms the crura of the diaphragm, including the esophageal hiatus and aortic hiatus. During the fifth week of gestation, the pleuroperitoneal membranes first appear along the lateral body wall and extend medially, where they fuse with the dorsal mesentery of the esophagus and the dorsal portion of the septum transversum, thereby completing the partition between the thoracic and abdominal cavities by the eighth week of gestation. Although the pleuroperitoneal membranes may form large portions of the primitive diaphragm, they represent relatively small, intermediate portions of the adult diaphragm. Finally, with further development of the lung, the pleural cavities enlarge and burrow into the lateral body walls where chest wall musculature is split off, forming the peripheral muscular portion of the diaphragm. Failure of any component to develop or to fuse with adjacent structures may result in congenital continuity of the pleural and peritoneal cavities.

Because the diaphragm is formed from the fusion of several components, a number of developmental defects occur, resulting in herniation of abdominal structures into the thorax. A hernial sac may or may not be present. Two fundamental types of defects may occur:

1. Complete or partial absence of the diaphragm. Failure of one or more of the diaphragmatic components to develop or failure of the components to join one another results in a communication between the thorax and the abdomen. No hernial sac is present because the diaphragm never formed. To this group of defects belong absence of the diaphragm, hernia into the pericardium, and herniation through the foramen of Bochdalek.
2. Failure of complete muscularization. In this group of defects, normal fusion of the diaphragmatic components occurs, but the muscular tissue fails to spread over the entire diaphragm. The portion of the diaphragm unsupported by muscle eventually bulges into the thoracic cavity, forming a hernial sac. This thin, bulging membrane may or may not rupture. To this group of defects belong all hernias of the foramen of Morgagni, eventration, and herniation through the foramen of Bochdalek.

Classifying diaphragmatic defects embryologically is not convenient clinically because the hernial sac is not easily detected. Moreover, absence of the sac is not necessarily mean that one was not present initially. A more practical classification incorporates morphology and anatomic location (Table 25-4).

Esophageal Hiatal Hernia

Esophageal hiatal hernias are not only the most common hernias of the diaphragm but also are among the more common abnormalities affecting the upper gastrointestinal tract.

Table 25-4. CLASSIFICATION OF CONGENITAL DIAPHRAGMATIC DEFECTS

Absent diaphragm
Diaphragmatic hernia
   Posterolateral (Bochdalek)
   Anterior (Morgagni)
   Paraesophageal
Eventration

There are two main types of esophageal hiatal hernias: the sliding hernia and the paraesophageal hernia (Fig. 25-16). A third type might well be described as a combination of these two pure types and carries the potential risks of both (Fig. 25-17).

The most common is the *sliding hernia,* in which there is axial displacement of the esophagogastric junction through the esophageal hiatus into the chest. Although such hernias are known to move in and out of the thorax with changes in intrathoracic and intraabdominal pressures, the term "sliding" is applied not because of this behavior but because the hernia has a partial parietal peritoneal sac, whose posterior wall is formed by the stomach.

In the *paraesophageal hiatal hernia,* the esophagogastric junction keeps to its normal position below the diaphragm, but the fundus and successively greater portions of the greater curvature of the stomach roll into the thorax through the esophageal hiatus alongside the esophagus. In its ultimate form the paraesophageal hiatal hernia presents with totally intrathoracic upside-down stomach (Fig. 25-18).

Esophageal hiatal hernia is relatively common, occurring in five individuals per 1000 population. Less than 5 percent ever develop any symptom or complication requiring surgical intervention.

SLIDING ESOPHAGEAL HIATAL HERNIA

This hernia accounts for 90 percent of the esophageal hiatal hernias. It is of clinical significance only because of its very high coincidence with gastroesophageal reflux. A causal relationship has long been sought but has been largely elusive. DeMeester and associates believed that the presence or absence of reflux with hiatal hernia is largely explainable by the absence or presence of a segment of distal esophagus exposed to normal positive intraabdominal pressure. Thus, vagaries in the level of phrenoesophageal ligamentous insertion into the esophagus may explain why some patients with hiatal hernia have competence and others do not. Other investigators have speculated on which comes first, reflux or hernia, or whether there is such a thing as primary sphincter failure in some individuals. Irrespective of the theoretical aspects, current operations for the control of gastroesophageal reflux depend on anatomic repair of the sliding esophageal hernia and reduction by 2 cm or more of the tubular distal esophagus below the diaphragm, as well as an anatomic valvuloplasty.

BASIC SURGICAL PROCEDURES. The primary goal of surgical treatment for sliding esophageal hernia is restora-

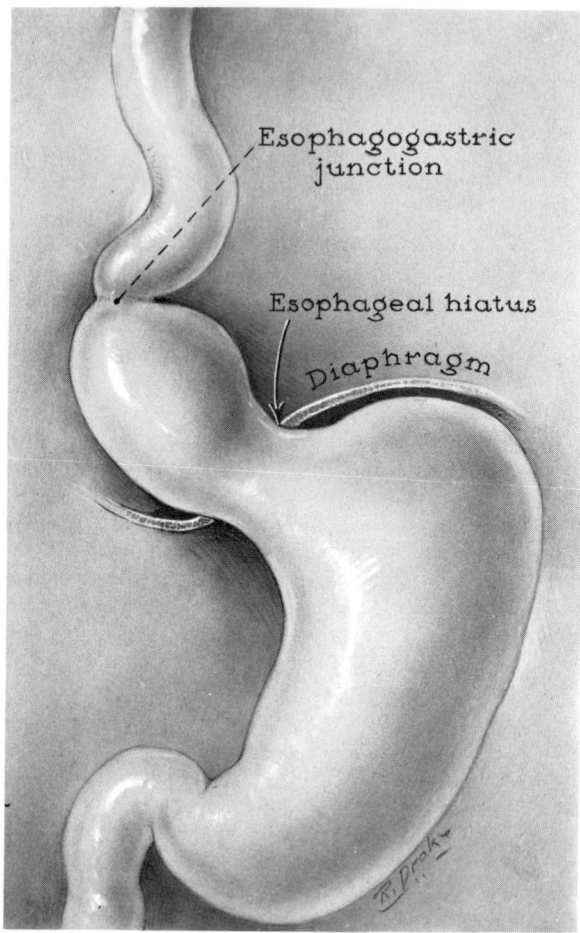

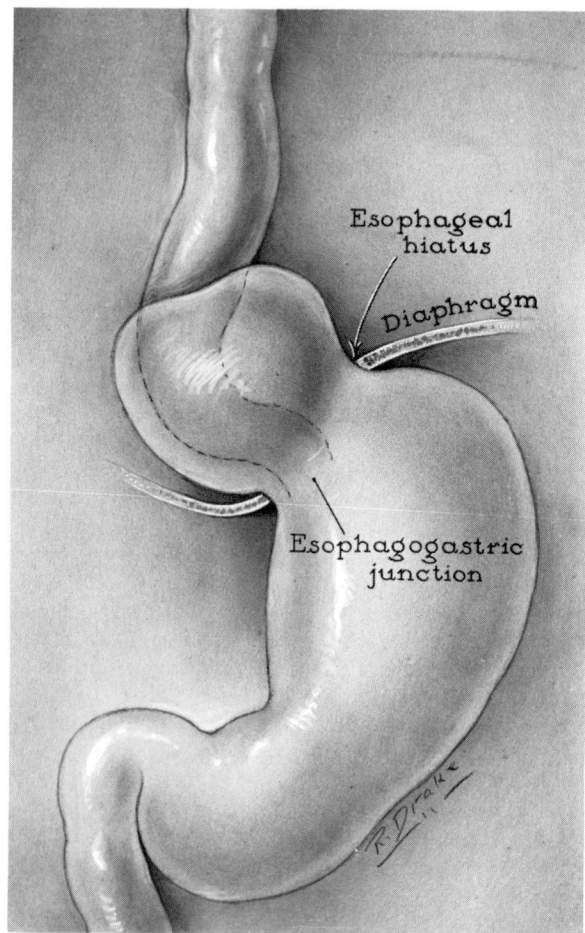

Fig. 25-16. Two chief varieties of esophageal hiatal hernia. *Left:* Sliding esophageal hiatal hernia. *Right:* Paraesophageal hiatal hernia. (From: *Mobley JE, Christensen NA: Gastroenterology 30:1, 1956. By permission of Williams & Wilkins Company.*)

tion of gastroesophageal competence. Because restoration of normal anatomy has been found to be inadequate for restoration of normal pressures to the hypotensive sphincter, "antireflux" operations have been devised to accomplish this end more effectively. Typical of these are the operations associated with the names Belsey, Nissen, and Hill. All are variations of a basic "wrap-around" procedure, and their success in preventing reflux makes it unnecessary, if not irrational, to perform concomitant vagotomy and pyloroplasty unless there is an active duodenal ulcer. The routine use of these additional procedures is also discouraged because of their disagreeable side effects.

Belsey's operation (Fig. 25-19) is a transthoracic procedure that creates a segment of intraabdominal esophagus held in place by a buttress of plicated stomach that surrounds approximately 280° of the distal esophagus. Long-term results indicate that the procedure is successful in relieving symptoms in 85 percent of patients and that the recurrence rate varies between 10 and 15 percent, depending on the length of follow-up.

Nissen's fundoplication can be performed either transabdominally or transthoracically (Fig. 25-20). This operation, which totally surrounds the distal esophagus with the adjacent gastric fundus, also produces good clinical results and a low recurrence rate. A worldwide survey of the results of the Nissen operation indicated an overall success rate of 96 percent, failures being usually the result of either recurrent hernia or postoperative reflux. Some dissatisfaction with this procedure has been expressed by Woodward and associates, who found an unacceptably high rate of dysphagia and the so-called "gas-bloat syndrome"—complications that should be minimal or absent if, during operation, one uses an indwelling nasogastric tube of ample caliber to prevent excessive narrowing of the distal esophagus. Long-term follow-up, furthermore, has shown that these symptoms, when they do occur, become less severe as time goes on. Some believe that the gas-bloat syndrome is due to accidental injury to vagus nerves and note relief with gastric drainage procedures such as pyloroplasty.

Hill's operation (Fig. 25-21) is basically a posterior gastropexy performed transabdominally, but incorporating plicating sutures to narrow the esophagogastric junction.

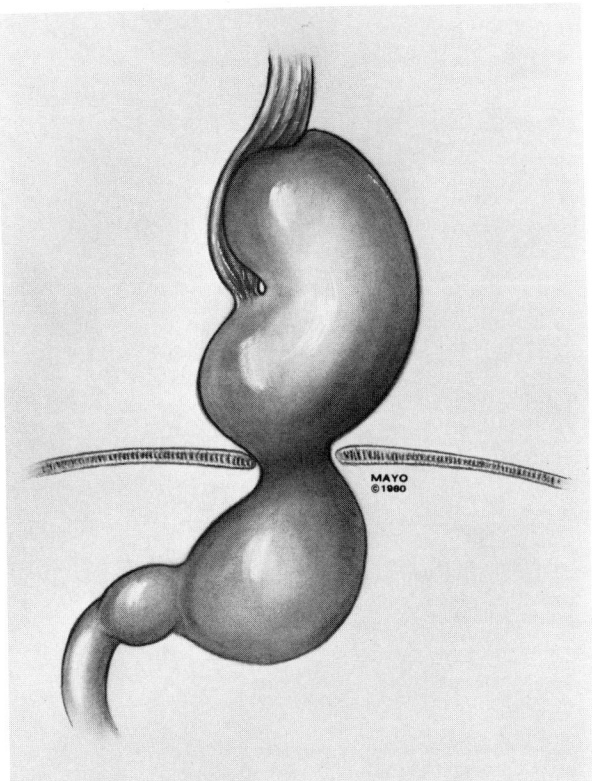

Fig. 25-17. Combined sliding and paraesophageal hiatal hernia. Esophagogastric junction is displaced above diaphragm (sliding component), and greater curvature of stomach has rolled into chest through esophageal hiatus. Hiatus impinges on stomach, producing hour-glass deformity. [From: *Payne WS, in Nyhus LM, Baker RJ (eds): Mastery of Surgery. Boston, Little, Brown, 1984, with permission.*]

He reported 149 cases in which this technique was employed during an 8-year period. There were no deaths and no anatomic recurrences in the follow-up period, and 97 percent of the patients were improved.

In addition to these gratifying clinical and radiologic results, physiologic studies of postoperative sphincteric function are encouraging. Not only is the amplitude of the lower esophageal sphincteric pressure more than doubled, but also the high-pressure zone is lengthened and the normal neural and hormonal response at the sphincter is restored. Now both experimental and clinical evidence suggest that the 360° wrap afforded by the Nissen fundoplication is the most effective of the three antireflux procedures in restoring lower esophageal sphincter pressure and preventing reflux.

Not all surgeons have obtained satisfactory results with these basic antireflux procedures. Therefore, Pearson and his colleagues have encouraged the use of a Collis gastroplasty with a Belsey-type 280° fundoplication. Henderson and Marryatt and Orringer and associates favored the Collis gastroplasty with a 360° Nissen-type fundoplication. Payne utilized an uncut Collis gastroplasty with either Nissen fundoplication if esophageal peristalsis is

present or Belsey-type fundoplication if it is not. Csendes and Larrain favor the performance of a parietal cell vagotomy as a technical aid in effecting a Hill-type repair. Obviously there is not universal agreement on the type of repair to be used.

Technique. The surgical technique of left transthoracic modified (uncut) Collis gastroplasty with Nissen fundoplication performed at the Mayo Clinic is illustrated in Fig. 25-22.

Intraoperative esophageal manometry before and after repair has shown that the procedure restores a high-pressure zone 20 to 40 mmHg in magnitude and 3 to 4 cm in length that corresponds with the region of the fundoplication below the level of the diaphragm.

Piehler and associates recently reported the Mayo Clinic's experience with the uncut Collis–Nissen fundoplication. In a review of 136 patients, there was no operative mortality. Over 90 percent of these patients were improved at 3 years, and 84 percent had good to excellent results. These data support the continued use of the uncut Collis–Nissen operation. Obviously, the perfect operation for gastroesophageal reflux has yet to be devised and continued small modification will no doubt be required in the future. Periodic objective assessment of results is essential in guiding intelligent and rational changes.

MANAGEMENT OF UNUSUAL REFLUX PROBLEMS. A shortened esophagus poses a special problem for surgical correction of gastroesophageal reflux, since it makes reduction of the herniated stomach below the diaphragm infeasible. When the shortening is no greater than 5 to 6 cm, the cut Collis gastroplasty has been an effective means of creating a tubular extension of esophagus made up of lesser curvature of the stomach (Fig. 25-23). One of the standard antireflux procedures, Nissen or Belsey, may then be applied to the distal end below the diaphragm. When shortening is more extensive and the esophagogastric junction is fixed at the carinal or aortic level, one may elect vagotomy, antrectomy, and a long limb (45-cm) Roux en Y gastric drainage procedure (Fig. 25-24); alternatively, bowel interposition or modified Ivor-Lewis resection may be considered.

Esophageal strictures that cannot be dilated are rare, but they too pose a special problem. Whereas resection and reanastomosis is a simple technical feat, recurrence is almost certain. "Inkwelling" of the anastomosis is not reliable in preventing reflux. Intrathoracic Nissen fundoplication is hazardous. Antrectomy with the Roux en Y gastric drainage procedure is a reliable alternative, and bowel interposition another. Woodward and associates have championed the Thal procedure, but this has been met with less than universal enthusiasm by others. The stomach is increasingly being employed as the favored organ for esophageal replacement. When it is placed totally in the thorax and anastomosed high to the esophagus without redundancy—and this disposition is accompanied by pyloroplasty or pyloromyotomy—it usually provides comfortable digestion without reflux problems. This modification of the Ivor-Lewis procedure awaits long-term follow-up in patients with benign disease.

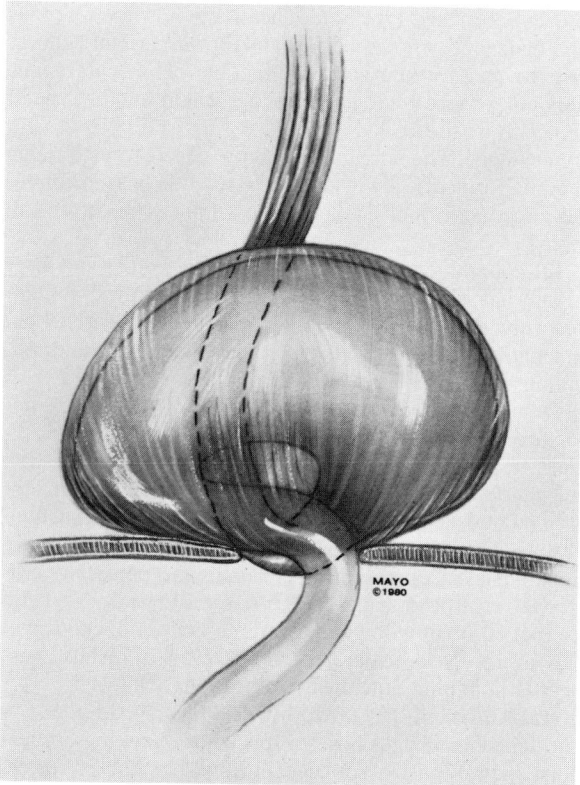

A

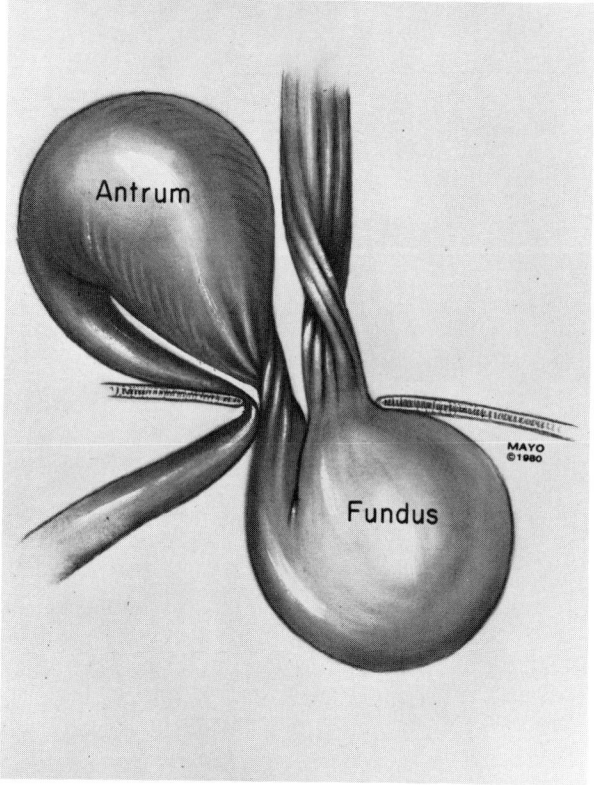

B

Fig. 25-18. *A.* Totally intrathoracic upside-down stomach, or advanced paraesophageal hiatal hernia. *B.* Gastric volvulus is a major complication of totally intrathoracic upside-down stomach. Note that fundus of stomach has fallen below diaphragm, with antrum remaining above diaphragm. This produces twisted obstruction at midstomach and lower esophagus. [From: *Payne WS, in Nyhus LM, Baker RJ (eds): Mastery of Surgery. Boston, Little, Brown, 1984, with permission.*]

PARAESOPHAGEAL HIATAL HERNIA

The pure paraesophageal hiatal hernia is a rare entity. It usually presents as a combined sliding and paraesophageal hernia. Even when the paraesophageal hiatal hernia has advanced to the stage of total intrathoracic upside-down stomach (Fig. 25-18), it has a sliding component as well in most cases. By this, it is implied that the distal esophagus and esophagogastric junction are not well tethered below the diaphragm and that the esophagogastric junction is displaced along with the rolling paraesophageal herniation of the stomach. The observation that most paraesophageal hernias are combined hernias has special implications in treatment to be discussed.

When a paraesophageal hernia of any size presents in pure form, the symptoms and complications result from the anatomic defect and not from any physiologic derangement of gastroesophageal competence. The most common complication—irrespective of the size of the paraesophageal hernia—is chronic, recurrent, asymptomatic occult gastrointestinal blood-loss anemia. Collis has alluded to the occurrence of anemia with hiatal hernia, but more recent studies clearly implicate the paraesophageal component in the genesis of most. A riding ulcer or gastritis where the hiatus impinges on herniated stomach can be demonstrated in some patients. Others appear to bleed from transient erosions secondary to stasis within the suprahiatal loculus of stomach. Classically,

such stasis is evident on chest x-ray as a globular shadow with an air-fluid level superimposed on the cardiac silhouette. When blood-loss anemia occurs in patients with pure or combined paraesophageal hernia and more usual causes for gastrointestinal blood loss can be excluded, surgical correction of the anatomic hernia is usually curative.

The second most frequent complication of paraesophageal hernia is gastric volvulus (Fig. 25-18*B*). This is seen almost exclusively with massive paraesophageal hernia, wherein most or all of the stomach comes to reside in a huge parietal peritoneal sac in the chest behind the heart. Various mechanisms and twisting deformities have been described, the most common being that in which the fundus of the totally intrathoracic stomach descends through the hiatus to the abdomen, leaving the antrum in the chest. This produces complete angulation obstruction of the distal esophagus, and two closed-loop segments of the stomach: the fundus below the diaphragm and antrum above, with duodenum obstructed as it passes through the crowded hiatus. Although detorsion and return of the

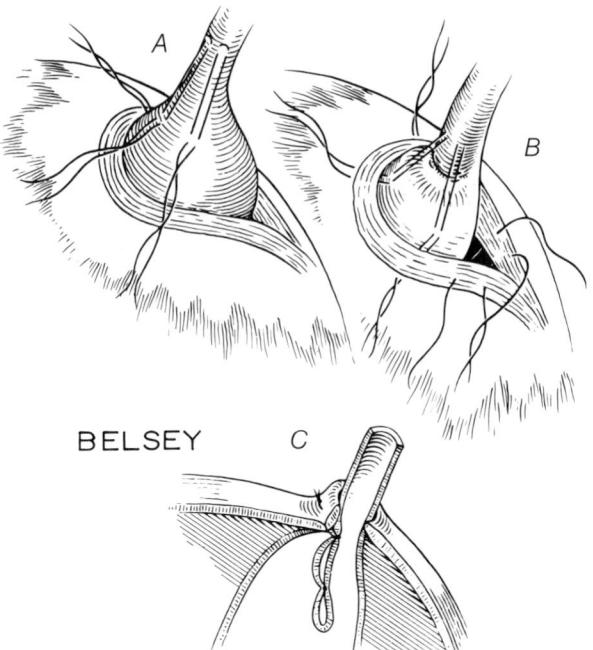

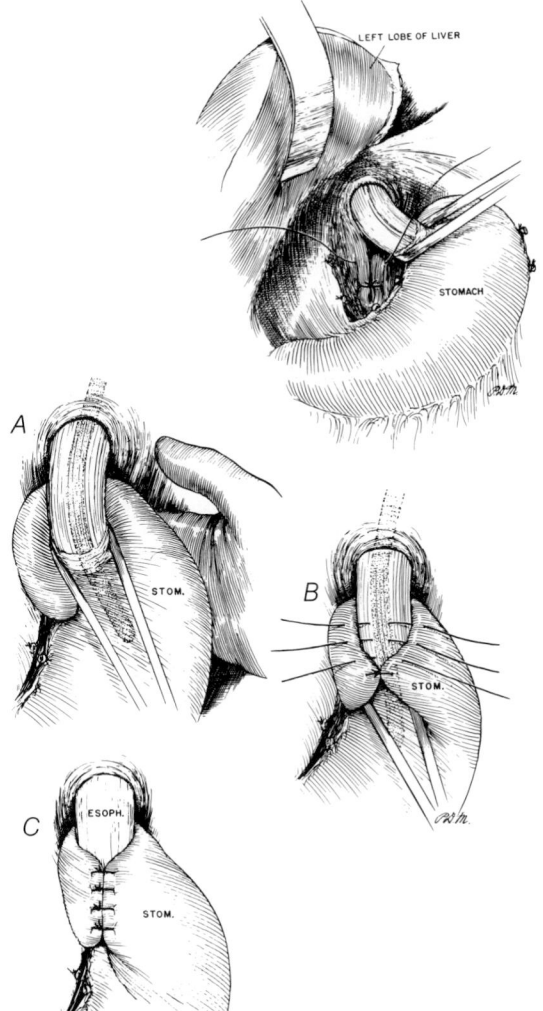

Fig. 25-19. Belsey Mark IV transthoracic repair of sliding esophageal hiatal hernia. Exposure is gained through left thoracotomy incision. After complete mobilization of cardia, lower 4 cm of esophagus is cleared of connective tissue. *A.* Mattress sutures are placed between gastric fundus and muscular layers of esophagus, 1 to 2 cm above and below esophagogastric junction. *B.* After these mattress sutures are tied, a second row of mattress sutures is placed to imbricate additional fundus onto lower esophagus. Note that these sutures pass through hiatus and out through the tendinous portion of diaphragm. Before these sutures are tied, crural sutures are placed to narrow esophageal hiatus. *C.* Completed repair after reduction of hernia and tying of sutures to maintain reconstruction. Previously placed crural sutures have been tied behind esophagus to narrow hiatus (not shown).

Fig. 25-20. Transabdominal Nissen fundoplication. *Above:* Abdominal exposure and mobilization of distal esophagus and upper stomach in preparation for carrying out fundoplication. *A.* Mobilized fundus is displaced behind esophagus by surgeon's right hand. *B.* Placement of sutures to encircle distal esophagus with generous portion of fundus. Note indwelling #40 French gastric tube. *C.* Completed procedure. (From: *Ellis FH Jr: Surg Clin North Am, 51: 575, 1971, with permission.*)

entire stomach to the chest may occur spontaneously, or be effected by nasogastric tube decompression, unrelieved volvulus can progress to gastric strangulation infarction. Gastric volvulus thus is a life-threatening complication of the large paraesophageal hernia. Volvulus may be a chronic recurring problem, alone or in combination with chronic blood-loss anemia.

Because of the high incidence of both bleeding and volvulus in the massive paraesophageal hernias, surgical repair is generally indicated even in the absence of symptoms or complications. The smaller paraesophageal hernias and lesser combined sliding and paraesophageal hernias are repaired only when complicated or symptomatic.

The classic method for repair of pure paraesophageal hiatal hernia differs from that described for sliding esophageal hernia. Since the lower esophageal sphincter functions normally, the esophagogastric junction is not disturbed. Rather, the herniated stomach is reduced, the hernia sac is excised, and the widened hiatus is narrowed by placing sutures in the crura, anterior to the esophagus, as in the technique described by Hill and Tobias.

Recent reviews, however, suggest that the problem is more complex. Simple anatomic repair is followed by a significant incidence of recurrence of anatomic hernia and by organoaxial and other gastric volvuluses, as well as by late occurrence of gastroesophageal reflux. Both the Toronto and Mayo groups have espoused the addition of antireflux measures to anatomic repair, and Geha has suggested gastropexy by temporary gastrostomy tube placement following anatomic repair. Whatever the final answer to this vexing problem, it probably will take into account the extreme rarity of pure paraesophageal hiatal hernia and will always include, in repair of the combined hernias, antireflux features that also fix the mobile stomach so it cannot undergo volvulus.

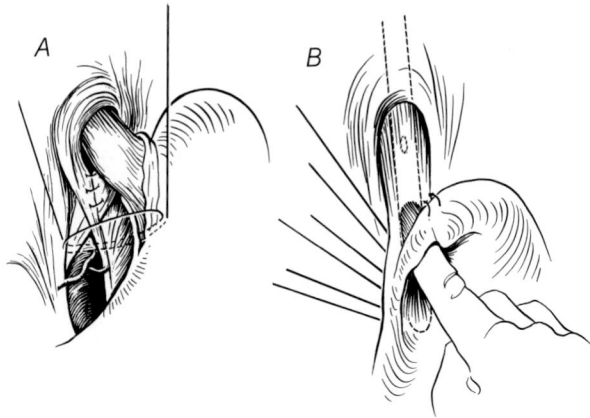

Fig. 25-21. Hill's transabdominal repair of sliding esophageal hiatal hernia. *A.* Reduced esophagogastric junction; crural sutures narrowing hiatus are in place behind esophagus. Single suture is shown incorporating gastrohepatic omentum along lesser curvature of stomach and preaortic fascia. Care is taken in placing sutures to avoid injury to adjacent vagal nerve trunks. Two or three additional sutures are similarly placed on lesser curvature, anchoring stomach posteriorly (posterior gastropexy). *B.* When these sutures are tied, gastric sling fibers should be sufficiently shortened to permit distal phalanx of index finger to invaginate snugly into terminal esophageal lumen alongside Levin tube. Angle of His is further accentuated by placement of sutures between gastric fundus and terminal esophagus. [From: *Payne WS, Ellis FH Jr, in Ellis FH Jr (ed): Lewis-Walters' Practice of Surgery, vol 5, Thoracic Surgery, chap 15, p 1. New York, Harper & Row, 1971, with permission.*]

Posterolateral (Foramen of Bochdalek) Hernia (See also Chapter 39)

Congenital hernias through the posterolateral aspect of the diaphragm are the most frequent diaphragmatic hernias in infants. This hernia was first described by Bochdalek in 1848. These hernias often present as a respiratory emergency at or shortly after birth, depending on the amount of herniated abdominal viscera present in the thorax. Rarely, such defects remain undetected until later childhood (Fig. 25-25) or adult life.

Gastrointestinal rather than respiratory symptoms predominate in older children and adults. Abdominal pain is present in approximately half of these patients. Vomiting, dyspnea, and chest pain occur occasionally. Obstruction is rare.

Foramen of Morgagni Hernias

Although it has been called *anterior diaphragmatic parasternal,* or *retrosternal hernia,* this type is best known by the eponym, foramen of Morgagni hernia (Fig. 25-26). A foramen of Morgagni hernia occurs through the sternocostal hiatus, which is a small triangular area of the diaphragm located on either side of the xyphoid process. Embryologically, the hiatus represents the junction of the septum transversus and the components of the chest wall. Although the hiatus normally permits passage of only vessels, it is a potential site for herniation of abdominal contents. Actual herniation may be the result of trauma

and is almost exclusively seen in adults. Seventy percent of patients are females with ages ranging from 3 months to 78 years. Ninety percent of the hernias occur through a diaphragmatic defect in the right parasternal area. Eight percent are bilateral, and 2 percent occur on the left. A hernial sac is always formed. The abdominal organs found in these hernias in their order of decreasing frequency are omentum, colon, stomach, liver, and small bowel.

Most patients with hernias of the foramen of Morgagni are asymptomatic. Only about one-third have symptoms that could be related to the hernia. These are predominantly gastrointestinal symptoms, with upper abdominal or subcostal discomfort, fullness, cramping, and occasionally vomiting. A few patients have histories suggestive of partial obstruction of the large bowel. Serious complications are rarely encountered, and emergency operations are rarely required. When these hernias occur in infancy and childhood, they may manifest with severe cardiorespiratory symptoms, similar to those associated with hernia of the foramen of Bochdalek. Occasionally, an adult patient with a large hernia of the foramen of Morgagni will present with respiratory distress related to the hernia.

The diagnosis of hernia of the foramen of Morgagni is often obvious on standard x-rays of the thorax, especially when gas-containing bowel is present in the hernial mass. The x-ray reveals a rounded shadow of variable size in the right cardiophrenic angle (Fig. 25-27A and B). Lateral views of the thorax show the lesion anteriorly very near the anterior chest wall (Fig. 25-27B). The demonstration of colon (Fig. 25-27C) within this mass or of angulation of the transverse colon toward the defect after a barium enema provides evidence for diagnosis. Radiographic examination of the upper gastrointestinal tract is usually diagnostically less rewarding. A CT scan may be diagnostic (Fig. 25-27D).

Occasionally, a definitive diagnosis cannot be established before surgical exploration, and other conditions, such as pleuropericardial cyst, pleural or pulmonary neoplasms, and mediastinal and diaphragmatic tumors, are considered in the differential diagnosis.

TREATMENT. Surgical repair is mandatory for all hernias of the foramen of Morgagni. Although a transabdominal approach provides the advantages of greater ease of exposure and repair of the defect, its use should be restricted to those instances in which a preoperative diagnosis is established. An upper abdominal incision provides easy access to either a right- or left-sided hernia or to bilateral hernias. When a definite preoperative diagnosis cannot be established and operation is performed for an indeterminate thoracic mass, a transthoracic operation is indicated. This approach, although technically more difficult for repairing the hernia, affords a better opportunity to diagnose and treat an intrathoracic lesion.

The hernia is reduced, the sac is excised, and the defect is closed. Repair is effected by approximating the posterior margin of the defect to the musculoskeletal chest wall anteriorly with interrupted nonabsorbable suture material. Operative morbidity and mortality rates are negligible.

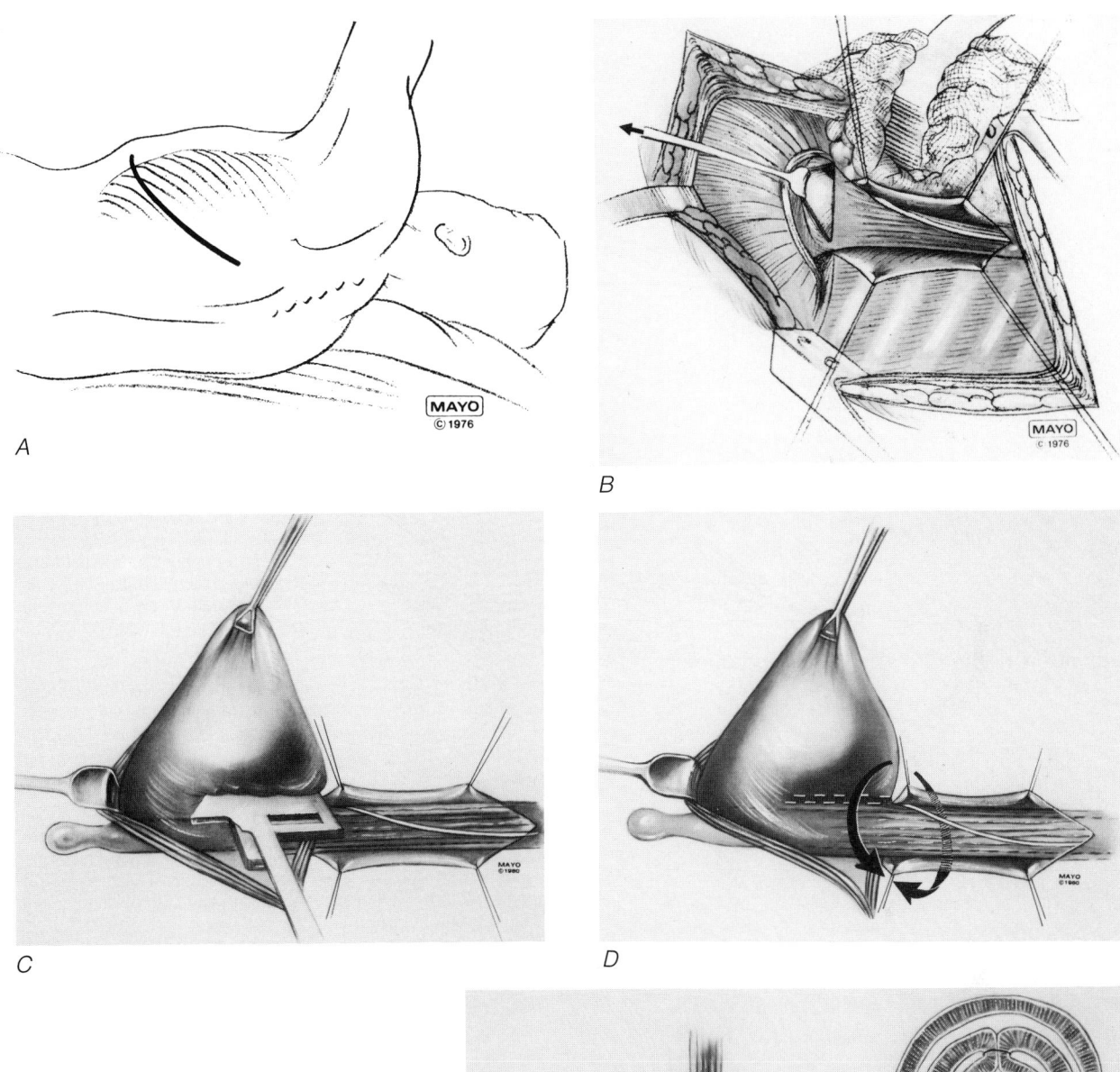

Fig. 25-22. *A*. Placement of incision. *B*. Ventral application of traction through hiatus. *C*. Placement of stapling device. *D*. Tubular extension of esophagus created by stapling. *E*. Completed fundoplication. [From: *Piehler JM, Payne WS, et al: The uncut Collis–Nissen procedure for esophageal hiatal hernia and its complications, in Farnell MB, McIlrath DC (eds): Problems in General Surgery. New Approaches to Old Problems. Philadelphia, Lippincott, vol 1, pp 1–14, 1984, with permission.*]

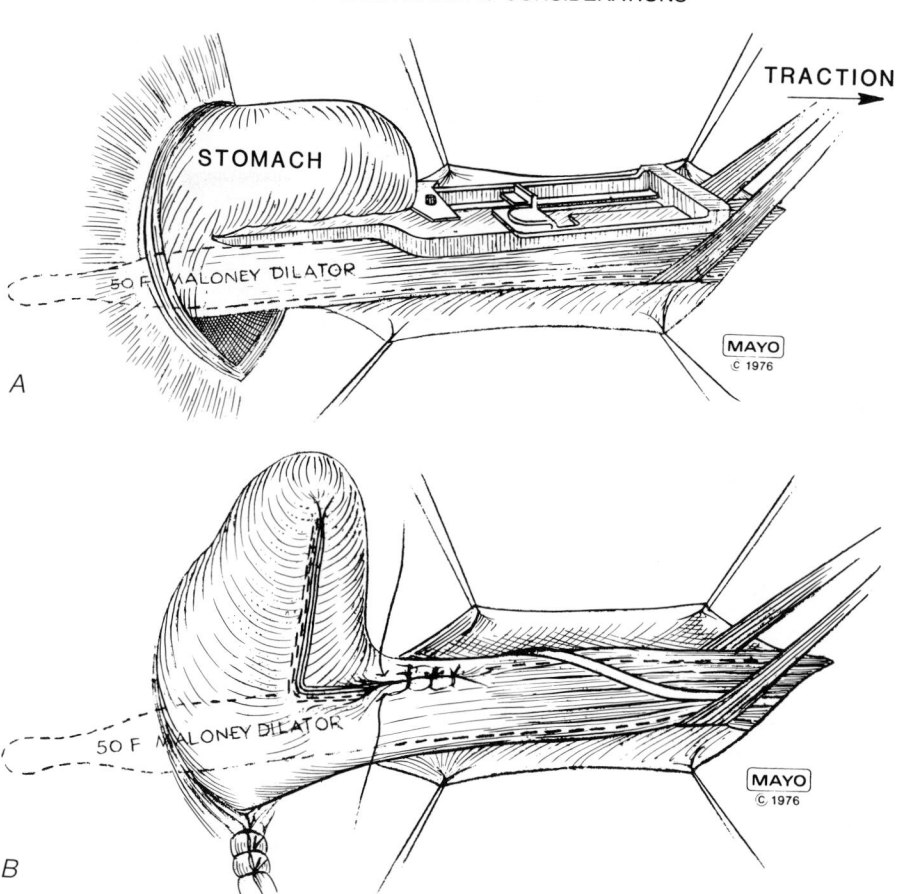

Fig. 25-23. Collis gastroplasty for shortened esophagus. After left thoracotomy, phrenoesophageal attachments have been taken down and multiple short gastric vessels have been interrupted through hiatus. *A.* With #50 French Maloney dilator in place, GIA stapling device is applied to stomach at angle of His, parallel to lesser curvature and Maloney dilator. Activation of instrument creates stapled cut-tubular extension of esophagus made up of lesser curvature of stomach. *B.* Staples are buried beneath a row of sutures. Either 280 or 360° fundoplication can be effected (not shown). Esophageal lengthening procedure permits reduction of valvuloplasty below diaphragm. [From: *Payne WS, in Jackson JW (ed): Operative Surgery: Cardiothoracic Surgery, 3d ed. London, Butterworth, 1978, p 438, with permission.*]

Fig. 25-24. Operative procedures for management of short-esophagus diaphragmatic hernia with stricture. *Left:* Esophagogastrectomy with Roux en Y esophagojejunostomy. *Center:* Esophagogastrectomy with colon interposition and pyloroplasty. *Right:* Gastric tube of Gavriliu.

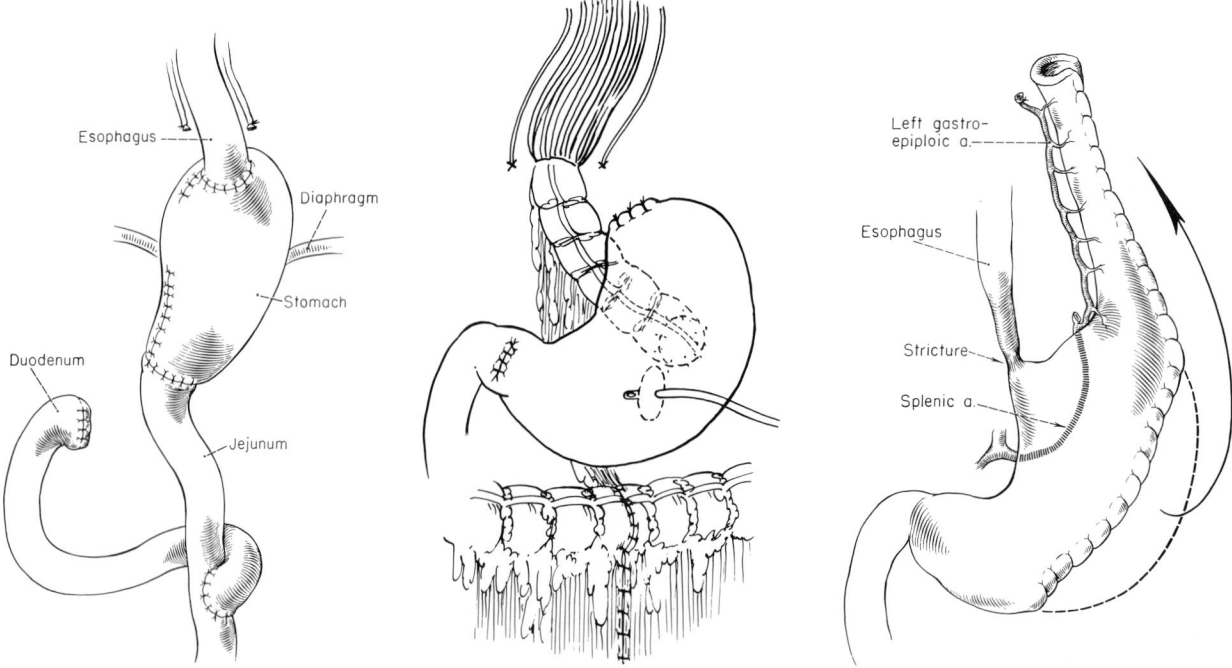

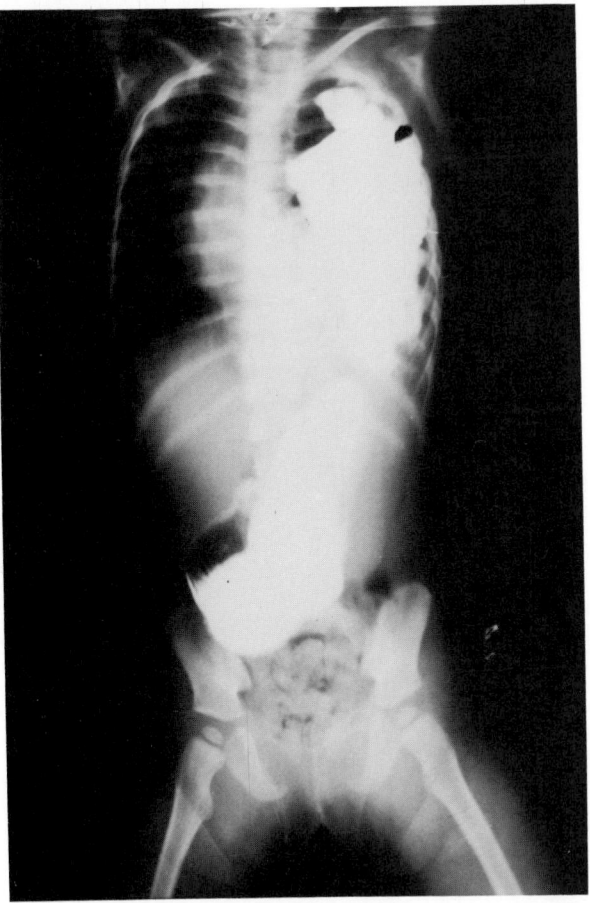

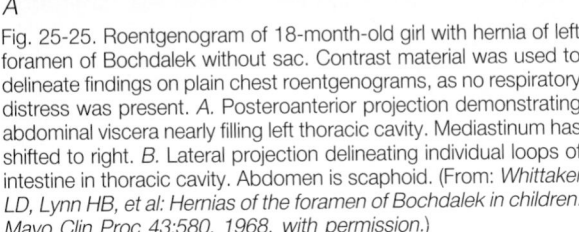

A

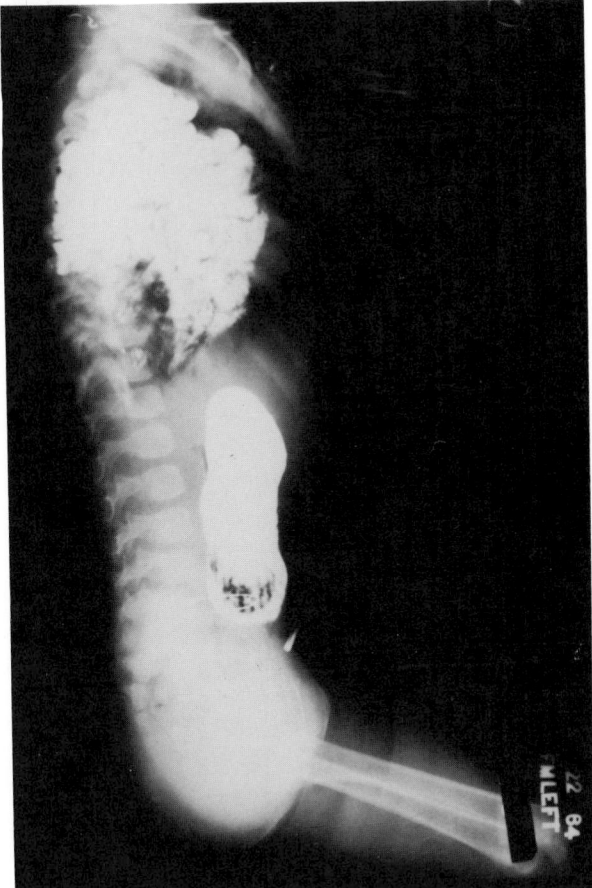

B

Fig. 25-25. Roentgenogram of 18-month-old girl with hernia of left foramen of Bochdalek without sac. Contrast material was used to delineate findings on plain chest roentgenograms, as no respiratory distress was present. A. Posteroanterior projection demonstrating abdominal viscera nearly filling left thoracic cavity. Mediastinum has shifted to right. B. Lateral projection delineating individual loops of intestine in thoracic cavity. Abdomen is scaphoid. (From: *Whittaker LD, Lynn HB, et al: Hernias of the foramen of Bochdalek in children. Mayo Clin Proc 43:580, 1968, with permission.*)

Fig. 25-26. Bilateral foramen of Morgagni hernia as seen at operation from abdominal approach. (From: *Comer TP, Clagett OT: J Thorac Surg 52:461, 1966, with permission.*)

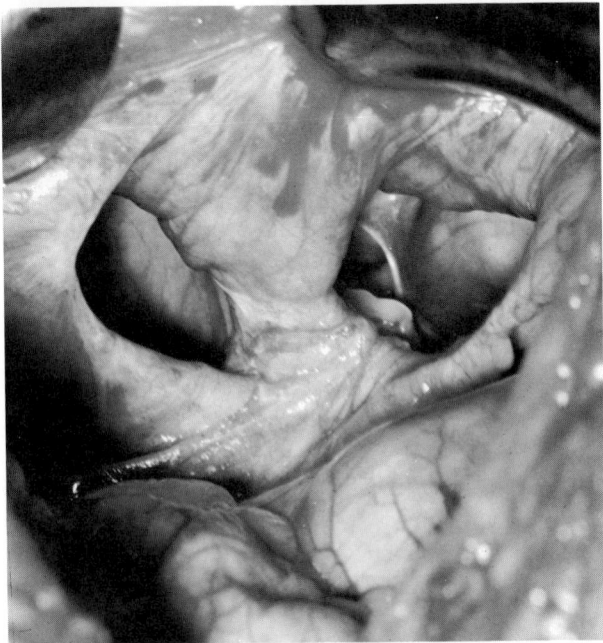

Eventration of the Diaphragm

Complete or partial unilateral elevation of the diaphragm is commonly referred to as eventration. Eventration differs from true diaphragmatic hernias in that there is no localized diaphragmatic defect with discrete margins through which abdominal contents may protrude. Instead, there is a diffuse or localized bulging of the diaphragm itself (Fig. 25-28). In eventration there must be a third layer representing the diaphragm interposed between the pleural and peritoneal layers; this middle layer may consist of only a thin fibrous sheet with scattered atrophic muscle cells. It may be impossible, without resorting to histologic examination, to distinguish eventration from hernias of the foramen of Bochdalek.

Both acquired and congenital factors have been implicated in the genesis of eventration. Acquired eventration implies paralysis of the phrenic nerve subsequent to dis-

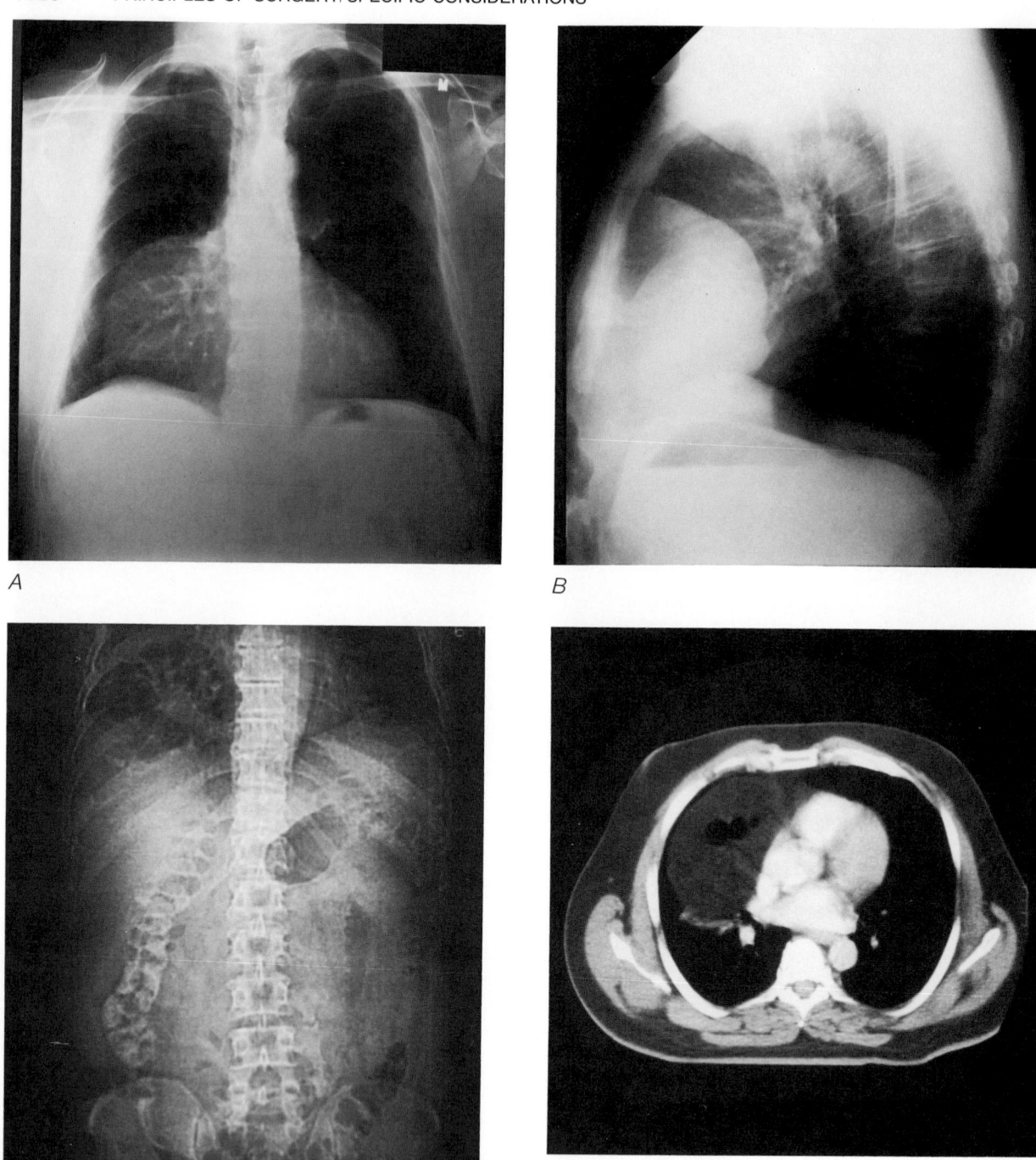

Fig. 25-27. Typical right-sided hernia of foramen of Morgagni. *A.* Anteroposterior projection. *B.* Lateral projection. *C.* Anteroposterior projection demonstrates loop of transverse colon in right-sided foraminal hernia. *D.* Computed tomogram demonstrating omentum and colon in chest.

ease or injury. Infections, neoplasms, poisons, surgical and accidental trauma, including injury to the phrenic nerve at the time of birth, are frequently implicated and may result in either temporary or permanent nerve paral-ysis, followed by elevation of the hemidiaphragm. Con-genital eventration, however, implies anomalous devel-opment of the diaphragm in that there is a failure of normal ingrowth of striated muscle into part or all of the

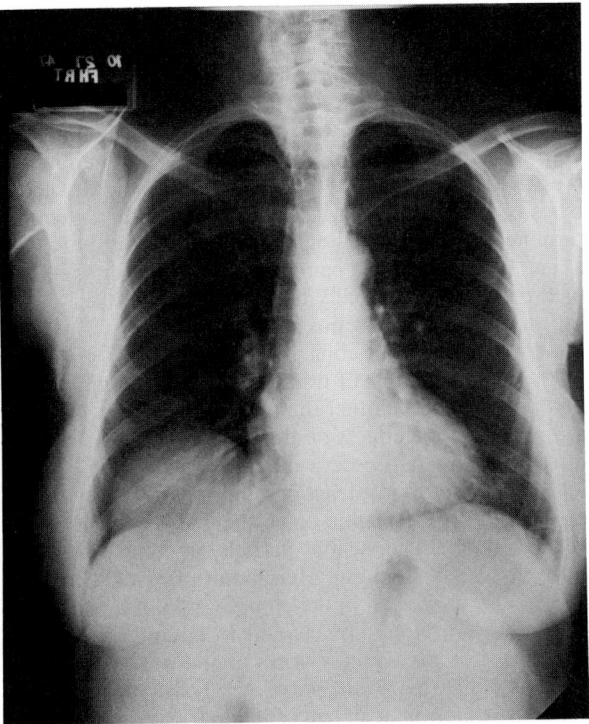
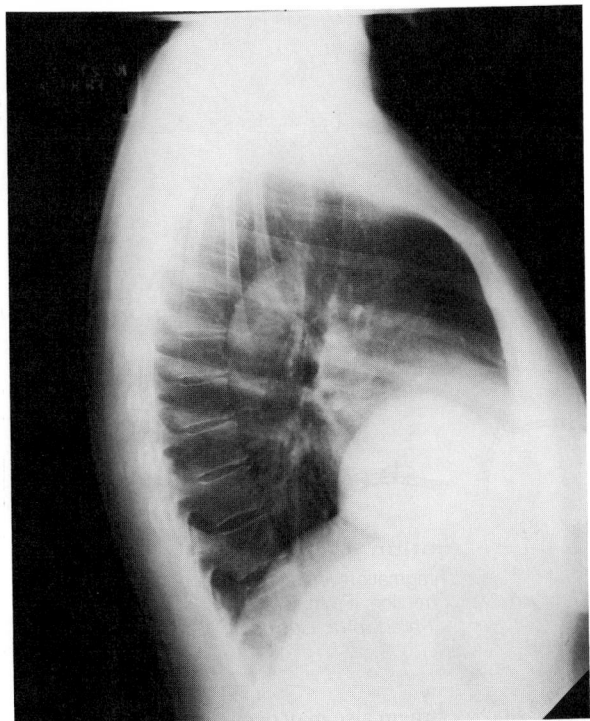

A

B

Fig. 25-28. *A.* Posteroanterior chest roentgenogram demonstrating localized eventration of right diaphragm. *B.* Lateral projection. (From: *Neuman HW, Ellis FH Jr, Andersen HS: Eventration of the diaphragm. Proc Staff Meet Mayo Clin 30:310, 1955, with permission.*)

diaphragm. Congenital eventration is associated with an intact phrenic nerve that may or may not result in diaphragmatic contraction in response to nerve stimulation, depending on the amount of muscle present. Partial or complete inversion of the stomach and intestinal malrotation usually accompanies congenital eventration. Transposition of abdominal organs, megacolon, and hypospadias also have been reported.

Eventration occurs at any age, most commonly on the left, with a male to female ratio of approximately 2:1. Most patients with eventration are asymptomatic, the condition being detected on routine chest x-ray. In the newborn, serious respiratory difficulties are frequently encountered, similar to those of massive congenital diaphragmatic hernias already described. In the adult patient, when decreased cardiopulmonary reserve develops in combination with intraabdominal pressure secondary to obesity, digestive and respiratory symptoms related to eventration may appear for the first time. Digestive symptoms often are vague. Occasionally, palpitations or arrhythmias are encountered. Hemodynamics rarely are affected by mediastinal shift and vascular angulation.

Radiography of the chest is necessary for diagnosis. Ideally, the elevated hemidiaphragm will be visualized high in the thorax. This is in distinction to the picture seen in diaphragmatic hernia in which the diaphragm is located normally with intestines above.

TREATMENT. Prompt emergency surgical repair is indicated in the newborn who is dyspneic and cyanotic. In older children and adults in whom symptoms are disabling, elective surgical repair is indicated. Surgical treatment is directed toward restoration of the diaphragm to its normal position. Such procedures help stabilize the mediastinum and permit more normal pulmonary ventilation. The procedure most frequently used is diaphragmatic plication (Fig. 25-29). In the infant, the transabdominal approach is preferred for the same reasons indicated for the repair of hernias of the foramen of Bochdalek. In adults, the thoracic approach gives better exposure and greater ease of repair. When viscera are adherent to the undersurface of the diaphragm, a thoracoabdominal incision may be advantageous. Because of possible injury to the phrenic nerve, especially in congenital eventration, excision of the diaphragm is rarely performed.

In patients of any age, and particularly in those in whom surgical treatment is contraindicated, symptomatic palliation is indicated. These measures include restriction of activities, weight reduction, and avoidance of abdominal distention, lifting, or straining.

Rupture of the Diaphragm

Loss of continuity of the diaphragm with herniation of the abdominal viscera into the thorax may result from major trauma. Both blunt and penetrating injuries to chest or abdomen have been implicated. Rupture rarely follows disruption of surgical incisions in the diaphragm. Disrup-

ber and severity of associated injuries and the delay both in the recognition of the diaphragmatic injury and in the treatment before the development of related complications.

OROPHARYNGEAL DYSPHAGIA

Swallowing begins in the mouth and ends at the esophagogastric junction. Normally it progresses rapidly as an uninterrupted sequential event from oral to pharyngeal to esophageal phases. Poorly definable dysfunctions of the oral and pharyngeal phases occur as the consequences of primary motor and sensory neurologic deficits and certain neuromuscular and muscular diseases. Although paralysis of the tongue, palate, or vocal cords often is demonstrable on examination, subtle defects in airway closure or impairments of laryngeal excursion and of pharyngeal function with swallowing often escape definition. Of major importance in this group of patients with oropharyngeal dysphagia are those whose condition is largely or exclusively due to cricopharyngeal dysfunction and is potentially reversible (Table 25-5).

Although medical management has succeeded in certain cases of neuromuscular disease, by and large it has been disappointing; so cricopharyngeal myotomy has been tried in refractory cases. The results of myotomy in many of these conditions have been quite variable. The chief problem (alluded to above) appears to be proper selection of patients—presumably just those in whom the problem is largely or exclusively cricopharyngeal. Manometry has been largely disappointing in selection of patients for operation. While incomplete relaxation, hypertension, and premature contractions of the UES have been described, study findings are more often normal or show only weak pharyngeal contractions. Hurwitz and Duranceau, in a collective review, found good results in only 64 percent of patients treated by cricopharyngeal myotomy. Until better selection becomes possible, treatment should be restricted to those in whom voluntary tongue, laryngeal, and pharyngeal movement is intact and pharyngeal sensation is present.

Table 25-5. ETIOLOGY OF OROPHARYNGEAL DYSPHAGIA ASSOCIATED WITH DYSFUNCTION OF THE UPPER ESOPHAGEAL SPHINCTER

CNS disease
  Cerebrovascular accident
  Parkinson's disease
  Bulbar poliomyelitis
  Multiple sclerosis
  Amyotrophic lateral sclerosis
Muscular disease
  Muscular dystrophy (motonic, oculopharyngeal)
  Inflammatory (dermatomyositis, polymyositis)
  Metabolic myopathy (thyrotoxicosis, hypothyroidism)
  Myasthenia gravis
Miscellaneous
  Radical oropharyngeal surgery
  Cricopharyngeal "spasm" (globus)
  Premature contraction (pharyngoesophageal diverticulum)

It is important to appreciate that the above comments apply only to patients with cricopharyngeal dysphagia secondary to neuromuscular disorders or radical surgery. Patients with pharyngoesophageal diverticulum do not have demonstrable etiologic neuromuscular disease; and though UES dysfunction is implicated, the late results of treatment are infinitely superior. The technique for cricopharyngeal myotomy is described under Diverticula.

DIVERTICULA

Diverticula of the esophagus are among the more common lesions that cause esophageal dysfunction. They may have serious consequences if neglected, but current techniques of management offer a particularly rewarding opportunity for effective surgical treatment.

Typical diverticula of the esophagus are thought to be acquired lesions, resulting either from protrusion of mucosa through a defect in the esophageal musculature (*pulsion diverticula*) or from the traction effect of adjacent, chronically inflamed, granulomatous parabronchial lymph nodes (*traction diverticula*). Such acquired lesions should be clearly differentiated from the rare congenital diverticulum of the esophagus and the occasional duplication, enterogenous cyst, or neoplasm that may have a fistulous communication with the esophageal lumen.

Pharyngoesophageal Diverticulum

NATURE AND PRESENTATION. The most common diverticulum of the esophagus arises at the pharyngoesophageal junction. Typically, it is located posteriorly in the midline, protruding between the oblique fibers of the inferior pharyngeal constrictors just above the transverse fibers of the cricopharyngeus. Although the lesion was first described in 1769 by the English surgeon Ludlow, Zenker's name has become intimately associated with it as a result of his studies on 27 collected cases in 1874.

Pharyngoesophageal diverticulum is definitely an acquired abnormality, since it rarely is encountered before thirty years of age and usually occurs after fifty. Esophageal motility studies in patients with pharyngoesophageal diverticulum have demonstrated premature contraction of the cricopharyngeus muscle during swallowing. This occurs frequently enough so that its partial obstructive effects are implicated in the development of the diverticulum. Because of the recurrent pressures involved and the effect of gravity and peristalsis, a globular dependent sac filled with ingested material gradually develops, insinuating itself posteriorly between the esophagus and the cervical vertebrae. In more advanced stages it may descend into the mediastinum. There has been a high association with esophageal conditions, particularly hiatal hernia. Gastroesophageal reflux symptoms, however, are extremely rare.

Since the mouth of the diverticulum is located above the upper esophageal sphincter, there is no barrier to prevent spontaneous pharyngeal reflux and aspiration. Particularly in the sleeping or obtunded patient, this may result in recurrent episodes of airway contamination and aspiration pneumonitis.

A sensation of high cervical obstruction to swallowing is the most common symptom. The patients complain of a noisy, gurgling sound in their throats with drinking and the regurgitation of portions of recent meals into the mouth. This food is undigested, but it may have an offensive odor due to decomposition. Frequently such regurgitation is associated with paroxysms of coughing, which may occur either immediately after meals or on reclining and may even awaken the patient from sleep.

The patient with a neglected pharyngoesophageal diverticulum may find eating to be a slow and laborious process, with dysphagia and interruptions by episodes of regurgitation and cough. In the extreme case, fatigue, malnutrition, hoarseness, and suppurative lung disease may further complicate the clinical course. Occasionally, patients with pharyngoesophageal diverticula are unaware of the abnormality until they experience some complication. An infrequent complication of a chronically neglected diverticulum is the development of squamous cell carcinoma. In a recent review of 1249 patients seen at the Mayo Clinic during a 50-year period, squamous cell carcinoma occurred in 0.4 percent of the patients.

The diagnosis may be strongly suspected from the patient's history, but it can be firmly established only by radiographic examination of the esophagus with contrast medium (Fig. 25-31). Esophagoscopy usually is not necessary. Esophageal motility studies and pH reflux testing are of more theoretical interest than aid in making the diagnosis unless other distal esophageal or gastric abnormalities are suspected.

TREATMENT. In general, any diverticulum arising in the pharyngoesophageal region and producing symptoms warrants surgical treatment. In a given patient, the minimal surgical risks of intervention must be weighed against the severity of symptoms and the risk of present or potential complications arising from the diverticulum or in consequence of associated hypoxic episodes from aspiration.

Currently, most patients with pharyngoesophageal diverticulum seek medical assistance before complications become severe, and little or no preoperative preparation is required. If dehydration is present, it should be corrected prior to operation. When aspiration pneumonitis or lung abscess has complicated a diverticulum, attempts should be made to resolve acute sepsis before proceeding with operation. Usually, however, it is necessary to correct the esophageal problem before the pulmonary process will improve. We also feel that malnutrition should not delay operation, since treatment restores swallowing within 24 h, and oral intake can be supplemented parenterally if necessary. Perforation of the diverticulum is a surgical emergency.

Preoperatively, a liquid diet is provided the evening prior to operation. Endotracheal anesthesia is routinely employed; prior to tracheal intubation, the reverse Trendelenburg position minimizes the risk of aspiration from the diverticulum. After intubation, rapid sealing of the airway with a cuffed balloon prevents intraoperative respiratory contamination by diverticular contents.

One-Stage Diverticulectomy with Myotomy. Although a wide variety of ingenious surgical procedures have been devised and may continue to be used in the treatment of

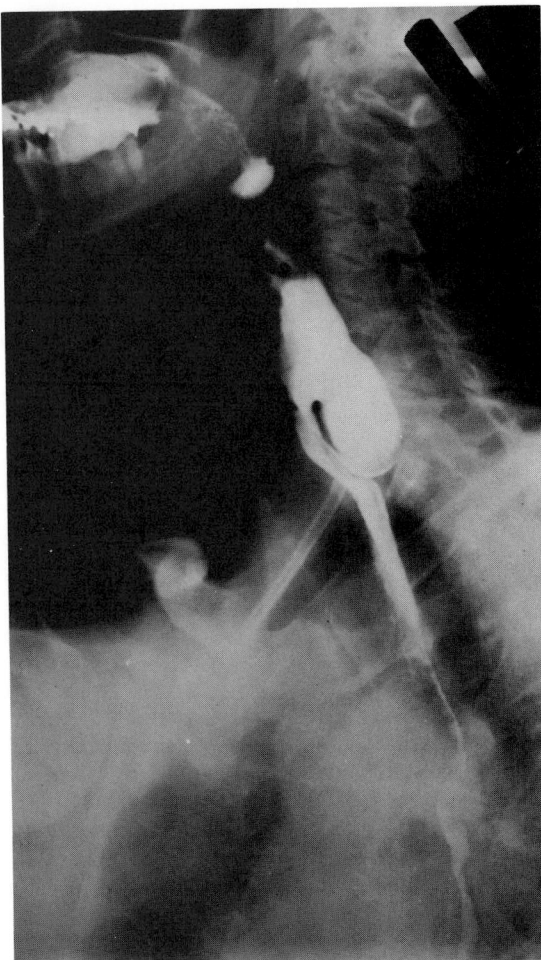

Fig. 25-31. Pharyngoesophageal diverticulum demonstrated radiographically. Note that main lumen is angulated and compressed by this moderate-sized diverticulum. (From: *Payne WS, Clagett OT: Curr Probl Surg April 1965, p 1. Copyright 1965 by Year Book Medical Publishers, Inc. Used by permission.*)

this condition, one-stage diverticulectomy with concomitant esophageal myotomy is the most definitive method of treatment. In our experience, dependable results with myotomy alone are confined to cases of small diverticula, which are less amenable to surgical excision. Therefore, we prefer diverticulectomy with myotomy for the larger diverticula (Fig. 25-32) and myotomy for the smaller diverticula (Fig. 25-33).

The right-handed surgeon will find a left cervical incision provides excellent exposure. Both the horizontal and oblique lower cervical incision have been used. After the incision has been deepened, exposure of the retropharyngeal space and the diverticulum is obtained by retracting the sternocleidomastoid muscle and the carotid sheath and its contents laterally, the thyroid gland and larynx medially, and the omohyoid muscle inferiorly. The apex of the diverticulum is grasped with an Allis forceps and elevated into the wound. The diverticulum must be thoroughly dissected, so that the neck of the mucosal sac and the surrounding ring of the muscular defect are clearly defined.

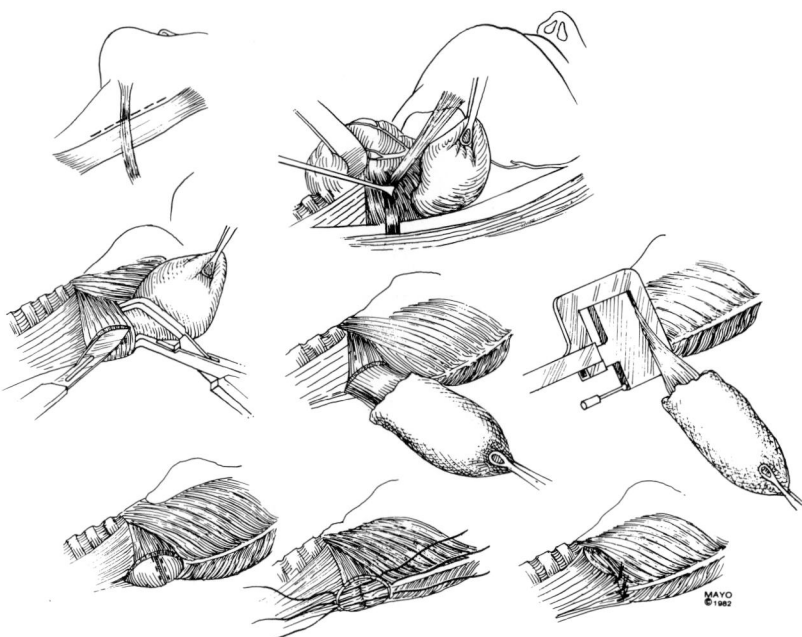

Once the diverticulum is free circumferentially, it is retracted in a cephalad direction. A plane is developed between the cricopharyngeus muscle and the esophageal mucosa at the neck of the diverticulum. The myotomy is carried out for a distance of 3 cm onto the esophagus in the posterior vertical midline. Although the sac can be amputated using a "clamp and sew" technique, we currently prefer a stapling device for transection and closure. The stapling device is applied to the neck of the sac at right angles to the long axis of the pharynx and esophagus. With a #28 French esophageal stethoscope in the lumen of the esophagus, the staples are fired and amputation of the sac is completed, taking care not to encroach on the lumen of the esophagus. When the diverticulum is completely excised and the mucosa satisfactorily approximated, the muscular and fascial layers of the hypopharynx are closed over the repair in a transverse direction. Two small Penrose rubber drains or a suction type of catheter are placed near the site of repair in the prevertebral space and brought to the outside through the lower end of the incision prior to closure.

In Welsh and Payne's 1973 review of 809 consecutive one-stage diverticulotomy operations performed during a 27-year period, the surgical mortality was 1.4 percent. Esophagocutaneous fistulas developed postoperatively in 2.5 percent, but all closed spontaneously in a matter of days. There were no instances of serious mediastinal infection. Unilateral paralysis of the vocal cords was noted postoperatively in 2.8 percent of patients; in only three was this paralysis permanent. Late symptoms or radiologic evidence of recurrence of the diverticulum developed in 7 percent of patients; 93 percent of those followed 5 to 14 years had highly satisfactory results. Addition of cricopharyngeal myotomy to diverticulectomy, a development of the past decade, has not brought significant

Fig. 25-32. The technique of transcervical pharyngoesophageal diverticulectomy with cricopharyngeal myotomy. Steps shown from top left to bottom right. Top row: The approximate location of the oblique skin incision (dotted line) is along the anterior border of the left sternocleidomastoid muscle. The location of the neck of the diverticulum is just cephalad to the omohyoid muscle. Middle row: After the connective tissue has been freed circumferentially from the neck of the diverticulum, the diverticulum is retracted in a cephalad direction and the plane between the cricopharyngeus muscle in the mucosa is developed with right-angle forceps. This myotomy is carried in the vertical posterior plane for 3 cm, completely dividing the cricopharyngeal muscle. With a #28 French esophageal stethoscope in the lumen of the esophagus, the sac is gently retracted and the TA 30 stapling device is applied across the neck of the diverticulum at right angles to the long axis of the pharynx and esophagus. Staples are fired and the amputation of the sac is completed, being careful not to encroach on the lumen. Bottom row: The completed myotomy and closure of the diverticulectomy. Sutures are placed in a transverse fashion of the muscularis layer covering the mucosal staple line. Penrose or suction-type drains are brought out from the retropharyngeal space below the incision. The incision is closed in the usual fashion with absorbable subcuticular suture. [From: *Payne WS, Reynolds RR: Surgical treatment of pharyngoesophageal diverticulum (Zenker's diverticulum). Surg Rounds 5:18, 1982, with permission.*]

improvement in overall results, though postoperative leak has been obviated and symptoms from recurrent diverticula minimized. In the Mayo Clinic's recent experience, radiographic evidence of recurrent phrenoesophageal diverticulum occurred in 2.6 percent of the cases. Symptoms of recurrence were usually high cervical esophageal obstruction with retention and regurgitation of undigested food. A third of the patients had aspiration. Reoperation with diverticulectomy and myotomy was usually curative.

Cricopharyngeal Myotomy Alone (Fig. 25-33). Cross and associates suggested the use of a myotomy as an adjunct to one-stage diverticulectomy to prevent recurrence. Belsey used myotomy with diverticulopexy. Sutherland re-

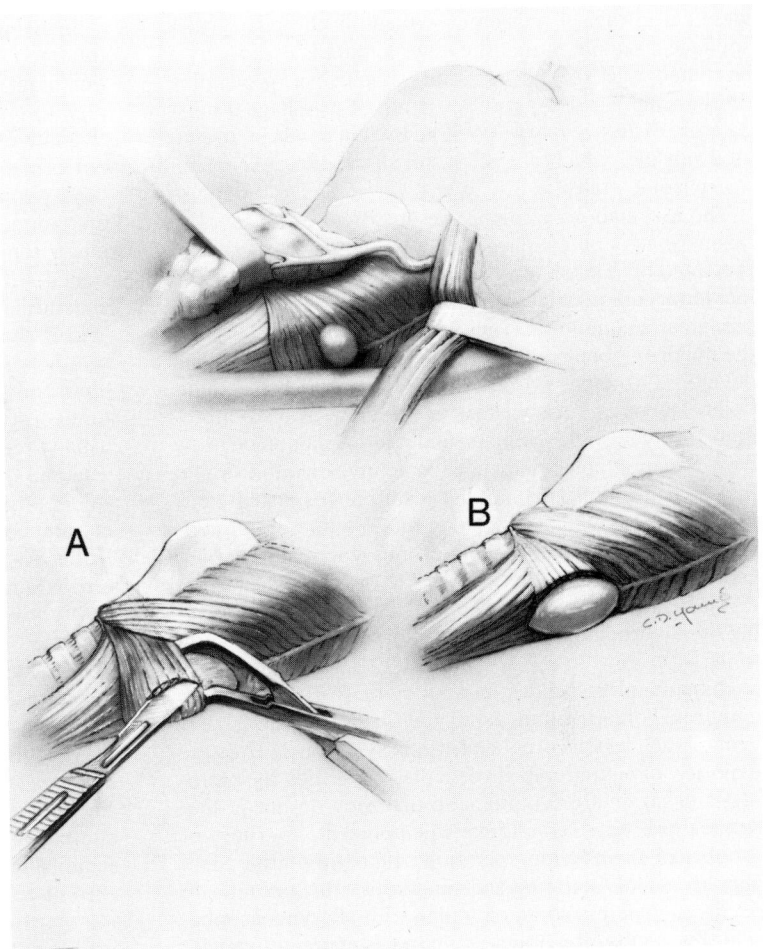

Fig. 25-33. Cricopharyngeal myotomy. This is indicated for smaller diverticula not amenable to diverticulectomy. Surgical exposure of small diverticulum and cricopharyngeus is best obtained below omohyoid. *A.* Right-angled forceps is used to develop a dissection plane below neck of small diverticulum between esophageal mucosa and muscle. *B.* Vertical extramucosal myotomy, 3 to 4 cm long, is effected; and mucosa is allowed to pout through incision. Drainage and closure are provided as with diverticulectomy. [From: *Payne WS, in Shields TW (ed): General Thoracic Surgery, 2d ed. Philadelphia, Lea & Febiger, 1983, p 864, with permission.*]

ported use of cricopharyngeal myotomy as the sole means of treating pharyngoesophageal diverticulum.

Myotomy alone is certainly an effective means of dealing with smaller diverticula, not only because it reduces the tone of the partially obstructing sphincter, but also because it eliminates the distal support of the diverticular neck and obliterates the septating spur. Dohlman and Mattsson have accomplished this same reentry effect by an endoscopic diathermic division of the spur formed by the diverticular esophageal wall.

In regard to the technique of cricopharyngeal myotomy, surgical exposure is accomplished as described for diverticulectomy (Fig. 25-33). After the diverticulum is freed to its neck, the transverse fibers of the cricopharyngeal muscle bordering the inferior margin of the neck of the diverticulum are easily identified and incised verti-

cally. The incision is carried down to mucosa and is extended caudad onto the esophagus in the posterior midline with the length of the incision averaging about 3 cm. After the myotomy, the esophageal and cricopharyngeal muscles are dissected for half the circumference of the mucosal tube to allow the mucosa to protrude freely through the incision. The cervical wound is then closed, with drainage.

Epiphrenic Diverticulum

Probably no other benign lesion affecting the esophagus has been so poorly understood for so long as the epiphrenic diverticulum. Unfortunately, lack of basic knowledge concerning pathogenesis has all too often resulted in poor surgical results. Current surgical methods can provide a safe and rational management in most cases.

NATURE AND PRESENTATION. This diverticulum also is an acquired abnormality, occurring chiefly in adult patients. As its name implies, the epiphrenic diverticulum usually occurs in the lower thoracic esophagus—typically within 10 cm of the cardia—but it may be at higher levels in the thoracic zone. Its pathologic anatomy is almost identical to that of pulsion diverticula in the pharyngoesophageal region, in that the diverticulum is essentially a herniated sac of mucosa and submucosa protruding through the usual supporting sheath of esophageal musculature. The sac may be covered by thin bands of attenuated muscle, which are often not discernible except on microscopic study.

The association of epiphrenic diverticula with motility disturbances and esophageal hiatial hernia was first appreciated by Vinson in 1934. Others since have noted the incidence of associated abnormal esophageal and diaphragmatic conditions. These and other data suggest that the majority of pulsion diverticula of the lower esophagus develop as the result of a variety of esophageal conditions. Debas and associates, in a review of 65 symptomatic Mayo Clinic patients undergoing manometric as well as radiographic and endoscopic investigation, found that 50 had esophageal motility disturbances, usually diffuse spasm or achalasia. Among the 15 with normal peristalsis, it was usual to find esophageal hiatal hernia, esophagitis, or stricture. In only 2 of these 65 cases were no associated esophageal abnormalities detectable, leaving the diverticulum probably the sole cause of the symptoms.

Habein and associates, in a study of 149 patients with epiphrenic diverticulum, estimated that only 15 to 20 percent of such lesions produce definite symptoms. Thus the majority of epiphrenic diverticula are either asymptomatic or so mildly symptomatic that they do not pose a surgical problem. Symptoms, when present, are those of esophageal obstruction, retention, and regurgitation. Tracheobronchial aspiration and suppurative pneumonitis do occur, though less commonly than with pharyngoesophageal diverticula. Regurgitated matter is characteristically bland, containing undigested food and saliva. In some situations it may be difficult to differentiate these symptoms from those caused by related underlying esophageal motor disorders.

The symptoms of epiphrenic diverticulum are often less definite than those of pharyngoesophageal diverticulum and may be only suggestive of the diagnosis. Radiographic examination of the esophagus with contrast medium is the best way to determine the presence and location of this pulsion diverticulum and associated conditions (Fig. 25-10, *top*). Esophagoscopy is not required to establish a diagnosis but should be performed to seek out and define associated esophageal disease, especially stenoses or filling defects. Studies of esophageal motility are essential in planning surgical management of epiphrenic diverticulum.

TREATMENT. The management of epiphrenic diverticulum is surgical, and an operation is indicated in patients with progressive symptoms. Progressive enlargement of an epiphrenic diverticulum is a relative indication for surgical intervention. Diverticulectomy should also be considered when an operation is indicated for an associated esophageal condition. A diverticulum causing few or no symptoms does not warrant surgical intervention if more serious associated conditions can be excluded.

Technique. The chief preoperative considerations in treatment for epiphrenic diverticulum are precise definition of all associated esophageal conditions and a specific plan to deal with each in a definitive manner. Preoperative attempts to empty the esophagus or diverticulum are not ordinarily required or indicated; a liquid diet a few days prior to operation usually suffices. At the time of operation, tracheal intubation with the patient awake under topical anesthesia is prudent. After the airway is sealed with a balloon-cuffed endotracheal tube, general anesthesia is induced.

Left thoracotomy (Fig. 25-34) should be used almost routinely in the surgical treatment of epiphrenic diverticulum, since this incision provides the necessary exposure for excision of the diverticulum and, more importantly, is usually required to correct frequently associated esophageal and diaphragmatic conditions. Furthermore, the results of diverticulectomy are more satisfactory if a long, extramucosal esophagomyotomy is performed routinely. If there is an associated diaphragmatic hernia that needs repair following diverticulectomy and myotomy, a nonobstructive antireflux procedure such as the Belsey Mark IV is advised.

RESULTS. The significance of the present concept of the surgical treatment of pulsion diverticula of the lower esophageal region is clearly apparent on review of the Mayo Clinic experience from 1944 through 1976. Early in this experience, diverticulectomy and correction of associated diaphragmatic hernia were done without concomitant esophagomyotomy. Of 29 patients so treated, 7 had significant postoperative complications—including 4 recurrent epiphrenic diverticula. Later, esophagomyotomy was performed routinely with diverticulectomy; and of the 29 patients so treated, only 1 had a postoperative complication.

Parabronchial or Midesophageal Diverticulum

Granulomatous infections of mediastinal lymph nodes may cause traction diverticula. Although they occur typically in relation to subcarinal and parabronchial lymph nodes in the middle third of the esophagus, they can be at any level. Generally these minute triangular esophageal deformities are of little or no clinical significance except as indications of a previous, often healed infection; they produce no esophageal symptoms and require no treatment. When symptoms are present, they are usually attributable to some other, unrelated process.

If symptoms occur, the usual studies should be carried out to determine the cause and rule out other conditions. These include radiographic examination, endoscopy, and motility studies. When active infection is suspected, appropriate skin tests and microbiologic studies are indicated.

Interest in traction diverticula thus is focused chiefly on distinguishing them from more serious conditions. Rarely, however, such a diverticulum may be the site of serious complications. These include obstruction to swallowing, esophagitis, hemorrhage, perforation, empyema,

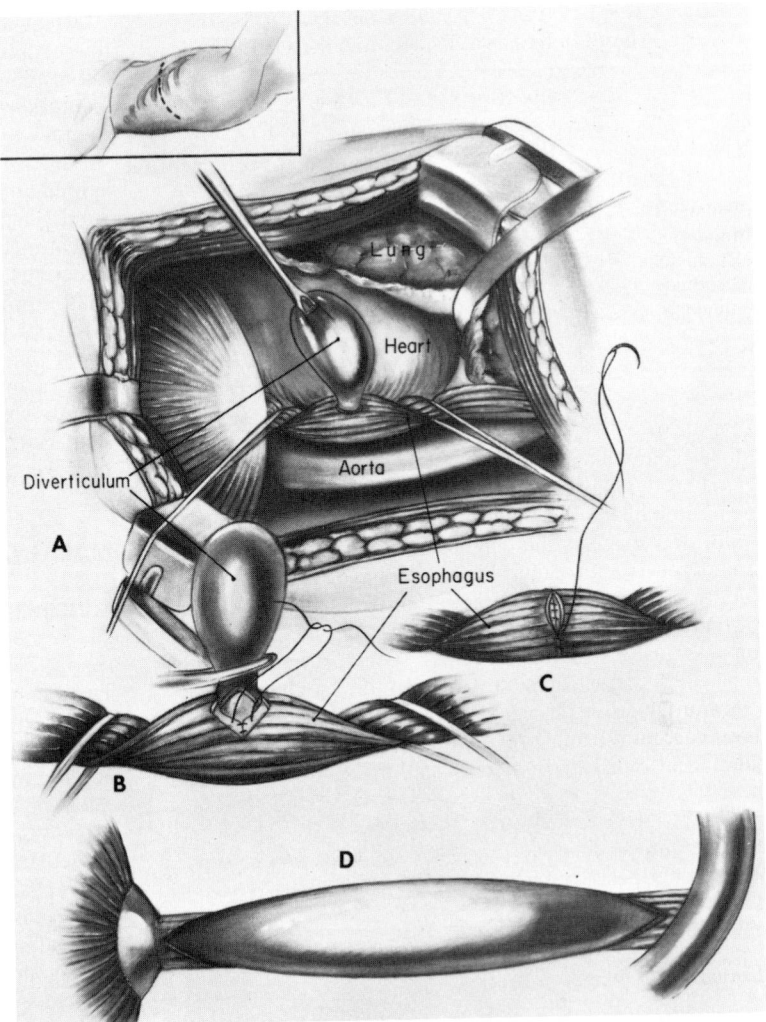

Fig. 25-34. Surgical management of pulsion diverticula of lower esophagus. *Inset:* Placement of left posterolateral thoracotomy incision. *A.* Exposure of diverticulum obtained when chest is entered through bed of left eighth rib. Esophagus has been delivered from its mediastinal bed, tapes have been passed around esophagus, and esophagus has been rotated to bring diverticulum into view. Neck of mucosal diverticulum has been dissected, exposing defect in esophageal muscular wall. *B.* "Cut-and-sew" technique of diverticulectomy. Amputation and closure are effected in transverse axis. Mucosal sutures are tied with knots within esophageal lumen. *C.* Closure of esophageal musculature over mucosal suture line. *D.* Site of diverticular incision has been rotated back to right and is not visible. A long esophagomyotomy, extending from esophagogastric junction to aortic arch, has been performed. Musculature of esophagus has been freed from approximately 50 percent of circumference of esophageal mucosal tube to allow mucosa to bulge through muscular incision. Frequently associated sliding esophageal hiatal hernia is shown. When present, it too should be repaired at time of operation. (From: *Payne WS, Olsen AM: The Esophagus. Philadelphia, Lea & Febiger, 1974, p 220, with permission.*)

pericarditis, or fistula formation with the tracheobronchial tree.

Usually the symptomatic traction diverticulum can be managed by simple excision. Fistulas between the esophagus and lower respiratory tract respond to excision and closure of the communication with interposition of normal tissues to prevent recurrence. Perforation with empyema or pericarditis often requires specific antibiotic treatment as well as surgical drainage and temporary diversion of the esophagus.

BENIGN CYSTS AND TUMORS

Benign cysts and tumors of the esophagus are uncommon and amount to less than 10 percent of esophageal neoplasms. They are of clinical concern, not only because they must be distinguished from more serious conditions but also because on occasion they can produce significant clinical symptoms and even threaten life. More than half of the 246 benign esophageal tumors and cysts seen at the Mayo Clinic were surgically or endoscopically removed; the rest were encountered at autopsy (Table 25-6).

Leiomyomas are the most common benign tumors. Those less than 5 cm in diameter are rarely symptomatic.

Table 25-6. BENIGN TUMORS AND CYSTS OF ESOPHAGUS SEEN AT THE MAYO CLINIC

Type	Total	Type	Total
Leiomyoma	145	Myxofibroma	2
Cyst	55	Fibrolipoma	2
Polyp	12	Neurofibroma	2
Papilloma	5	Fibroma	1
Lipoma	5	Lymphangioma	1
Hemangioma	4	Mucocele	1
Adenoma	3	Duplication	1
Granular cell		Chondroma	1
myoblastoma	3		
Indeterminate	3		

Most leiomyomas occur in the lower half of the esophagus, and the majority of these are extramucosal and can be treated by simple enucleation. Radiographic examination often suggests the diagnosis (Fig. 25-35). Those encountered in the region of the esophagogastric junction tend to be large, circumferential, obstructive lesions and often require esophagogastrectomy for successful removal. Reconstruction requires special attention with regard to unobstructed restoration of esophagogastric continuity, provision against consequences of concomitant vagotomy, and prevention of subsequent gastroesophageal reflux and its complications.

Fig. 25-35. Radiograph of esophagus, demonstrating extramucosal filling defect that proved to be a leiomyoma that could be treated by simple enucleation.

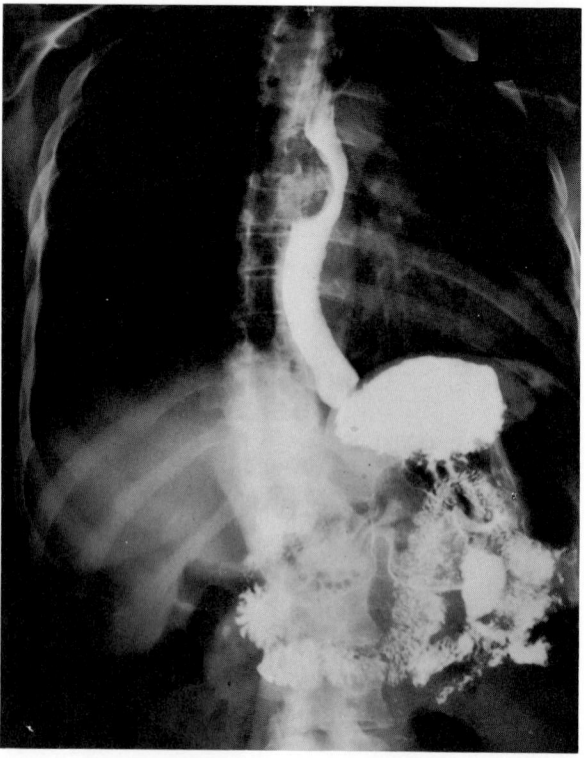

Cysts are the second most common benign lesions of the esophagus. In infants and children they more commonly cause symptoms through compression of the adjacent esophagus or tracheobronchial tree. Most can be removed successfully by enucleation. Complete reduplication is extremely rare; but it is seen, and often features a lining of esophageal, gastric, or small-intestinal epithelium.

Various polypoid intraesophageal tumors have been described, including mucosal polyps, chondromas, lipomas, fibrolipomas, and myxofibromas. Some pedunculated polypoid benign tumors have produced huge esophageal filling defects. Others are more cigar-shaped and have actually been long enough to protrude from the mouth when regurgitated. The smaller lesions can be managed by endoscopic snare; others require esophagotomy for removal.

MALIGNANT TUMORS

INCIDENCE AND ETIOLOGY. Carcinoma of the esophagus is predominantly a disease of males (male-to-female ratio, 3:1) between the ages of fifty and seventy years. The incidence varies widely throughout the world, being notably high in China, Japan, Scotland, Russia, and the Scandinavian countries. In South Africa incidence is especially high among the native Bantu. Although the basic cause of the disease is unknown, dietary and alcoholic habits, as well as tobacco use, have been implicated. A particularly high incidence has been noted among patients with achalasia and corrosive esophagitis. Joske and Benedict found an unusually high incidence of cancer of the cervical esophagus in patients with Plummer–Vinson (Paterson–Kelly) syndrome. Other conditions and disorders associated with a high incidence of esophageal carcinoma include lye burns, diverticula of the esophagus, the columnar epithelial-lined lower esophagus of Barrett, and the syndrome known as *tylosis palmaris et plantaris.*

PATHOLOGY. Although nearly all malignant tumors arising in the body of the esophagus are squamous-cell carcinomas, most of those involving the esophagogastric junction are adenocarcinomas of gastric origin. Figure 25-36 shows the approximate anatomic location and distribution by histopathologic type of the usual esophageal cancers. It should be noted that almost as many tumors affected the cardia as affected the entire cervical and thoracic zones of the esophagus combined.

The remainder of the malignant tumors of the esophagus are rare sarcomas, mostly leiomyosarcomas. These are predominantly extramucosal; but in contrast to the benign leiomyomas, they tend to ulcerate and calcify. Carcinosarcoma, adenoid cystic carcinoma, and small cell carcinoma have been reported. There have also been rare reports of primary malignant melanomas of the esophagus. Nearly all these malignant melanomas were associated with melanosis and had a poor prognosis.

Some carcinomas develop as bulky, fungating, obstructive growths and others as superficially ulcerated, surface-spreading tumors producing little obstruction. All

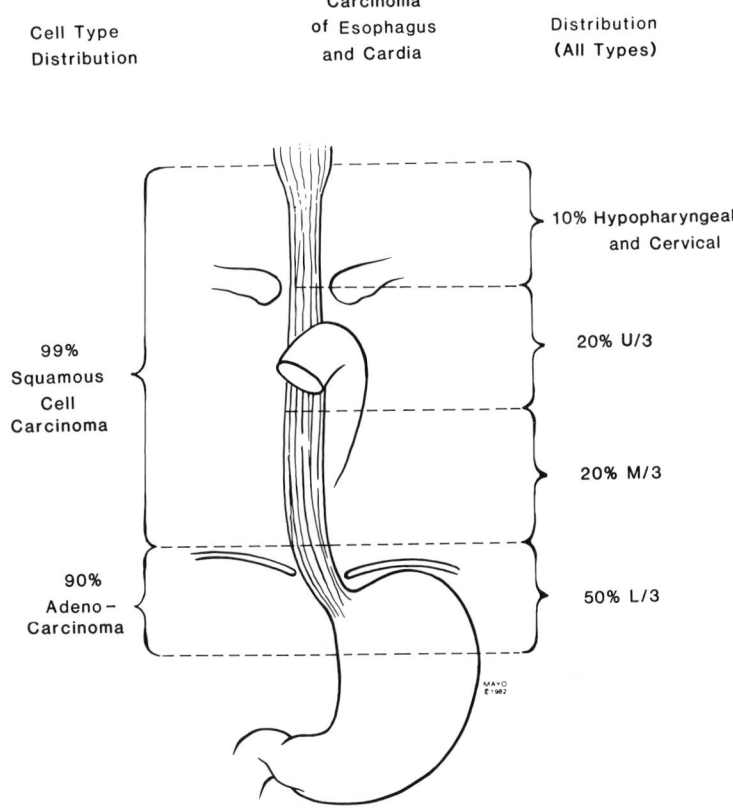

Fig. 25-36. Approximate anatomic distribution of primary carcinomas of esophagus and cardia is shown on right. On left is distribution of the two most common cell types of primary carcinoma. Note that nearly half of carcinomas occur in lower third (L/3) or cardia, and that these are predominantly adenocarcinomas of gastric epithelial origin.

these tumors spread via lymphatic vessels, by direct extension from the esophagus, and by vascular invasion. Tumors of the cervical esophagus disseminate through the lymphatic vessels to cervical nodes, particularly the anterior jugular and supraclavicular nodes. Those arising in the thoracic esophagus spread early to local mediastinal (peritracheal and esophageal) glands as well as supraclavicular and, occasionally, subdiaphragmatic nodes. In contrast, lesions of the gastroesophageal junction spread most frequently to the celiac axis and superior gastric lesser curvature lymph nodes. Occasionally, they may involve middle and superior mediastinal lymph nodes. Neoplasms in any location can metastasize through the bloodstream to the liver, lung, or bone. Reports from China clearly define premalignant esophageal epithelial changes, with atypia progressing to in situ, early invasive, and more massive squamous cell cancers. Evolution from asymptomatic abnormal cytology to dysphagia has been estimated to take about 3 years. Dysphagia usually occurs when about half to two-thirds of the circumference of the esophagus is involved by gross tumor.

MANIFESTATIONS AND DIAGNOSIS. The earliest and almost constant feature of carcinoma of the esophagus is progressive dysphagia. Initially, it is noted with ingestion of solid foods, but ultimately the swallowing of even liquids and saliva becomes difficult. The inevitable consequence is inanition. As obstructive symptoms progress, aspiration pneumonitis is not infrequent. Painful swallowing is especially suggestive of malignancy. Occult mild anemia is common, but massive bleeding is not.

The diagnosis of carcinoma of the esophagus can be made with a high degree of accuracy by the usual radiographic examination of the esophagus and stomach. This usually demonstrates an irregular, ragged mucosal pattern with annular luminal narrowing. Unlike the more chronic benign obstructive lesions, carcinoma usually is not associated with marked proximal dilatation of the esophagus.

Esophagoscopy should be performed in all instances of suspected esophageal cancer—regardless of the interpretation of the radiograph—both to establish a tissue diagnosis and to determine accurately the upper limit of the lesion. When a lesion involves the mid or upper esophagus, it is usually desirable to perform bronchoscopy to detect malignant involvement of the adjacent tracheobronchial tree. Cytologic study of smears made from suggestive lesions is a valuable diagnostic adjunct. Occasionally, study of esophageal motility may suggest malignant involvement, but this technique is of greater assistance in defining one of the more common motility disturbances as a cause for dysphagia. The role of routine computerized tomography (CT) is controversial. Although helpful if distant metastasis to the liver or lung is suspected, the ability of CT to accurately determine the extent of local invasion or metastatic involvement of lymph nodes is less precise and most often the resectability of a tumor can only be

Table 25-7. POSTSURGICAL TNM
CLASSIFICATION FOR ESOPHAGEAL
CARCINOMA

T Classification
    T0 = no evidence of tumor
    T1 = tumor invasion of the mucosa or
           submucosa but not the muscle wall
    T2 = tumor invasion of the muscle wall
    T3 = tumor invasion beyond the muscle wall

N Classification
    N0 = no lymph-node metastasis
    N1 = unilateral regional lymph-node metastasis
    N2 = bilateral regional lymph-node metastasis
    N3 = extensive multiple regional lymph-node metastasis

M Classification
    M0 = no evidence of distant metastasis
    M1 = distant metastasis present

determined at the time of operation. The role of magnetic resonance (MR) scanning is being evaluated. Occasionally surgical exploration is required to establish the presence or absence of malignant growth when clinical manifestations are suggestive but results of diagnostic studies are not definitive.

A report from the Honan province of China indicates that the application of special cytologic screening techniques to a high-risk population permits detection of carcinoma of the esophagus before symptoms develop and at a stage when nearly all cases are resectable, with more than a 90 percent chance of 5-year survival.

TREATMENT. There are only two methods of treatment proved to benefit patients with carcinoma of the esophagus: surgical resection and irradiation. Neither of these methods is new; hence it is not surprising that there has been no recent notable improvement in survival statistics among patients with esophageal cancer in the stage usually encountered. Survival is clearly stage-dependent. Most patients present with advanced disease (Stage III) including full-thickness wall invasion and lymph-node metastases. The TNM staging system (Tables 25-7, 25-8) is currently the only accurate way to predict the survival of subgroups of patients with esophageal carcinoma. Staging also allows more meaningful comparison of the different forms of treatment.

Table 25-8. POSTSURGICAL STAGING FOR
ESOPHAGEAL CARCINOMA

Stage I
    T1 N0 M0

Stage II
    T2 N0 M0

Stage III
    T3 N0 M0
    Any T, any N, M0

Stage IV
    Any T, any N, M1

Irradiation. Squamous cell carcinoma of the esophagus is a radiosensitive and theoretically radiocurable tumor. In contrast, radiation therapy for adenocarcinoma of the gastroesophageal junction is much less effective. Unfortunately, although the primary lesion may be controlled, failures result from the presence of tumor outside the irradiated field, and few permanent cures are obtainable. Pearson, the strongest proponent, reported 17 percent 5-year survival in patients who completed radiation therapy of 5000 to 6000 rad; but nearly half of his patients were unable to complete therapy. Extensive review of reports published in a recent 25-year period suggests 6 percent overall 5-year survival after radiotherapy alone.

Radical radiation therapy is not without risk. Radiation pneumonitis, local tumor recurrence, postradiation stricture, functional dysphagia, tracheoesophageal fistula, perforation, spinal-cord injury, pericardial effusion, and constrictive pericarditis are among the more serious complications—any one of which is likely to occur in half of those treated.

Preoperative radiation in lesser doses of 2000 to 5000 rad and surgical resection at varying intervals after its completion have produced favorable results reported by the originators of these techniques, but not duplicated by others. At best, preoperative radiation appears to improve the resectability rate modestly without affecting survival.

Palliative low-dose radiotherapy (2000 to 3000 rad), judiciously applied, may alleviate distressing symptoms such as pain, dysphagia, and bleeding with minimal risk of morbidity.

Chemotherapy. Chemotherapy alone has had little demonstrable effect in palliating patients with either squamous cell carcinoma or adenocarcinoma of the esophagus. Because of the belief that this disease is often systemic at the time of diagnosis, combined modality treatment using chemotherapy, radiation therapy, and resection in a staged regimen has gained popularity. Recent studies have been encouraging but it is too early to make any long-term predictions.

Surgery. Surgical treatment, too, suffers from being a local form of therapy, but it is more effective in controlling local disease and restoring function. Although it is not without risk (mortality is currently reported at 2 to 6 percent), more than 90 percent of those surviving resection experience unobstructed swallowing throughout their subsequent course. In a recent review of 100 patients with carcinoma of the esophagus and cardia who underwent Ivor Lewis esophagogastrectomy at the Mayo Clinic, 5-year survival for patients with Stage 1 neoplasm was 85.7 percent; Stage II neoplasm 34.1 percent; and Stage III neoplasm 15.2 percent. Overall 5-year survival for the entire 100 patients including operative mortality (3 percent) and death from all causes was 22.7 percent (Fig. 25-37). Cell type, sex, and location of primary tumor did not have an effect on survival. Metastatic lymph-node involvement uniformly adversely influenced survival.

In the past, a large number of ingenious surgical procedures were developed to effect tumor ablation and esophageal reconstruction. Some were elaborate multistaged

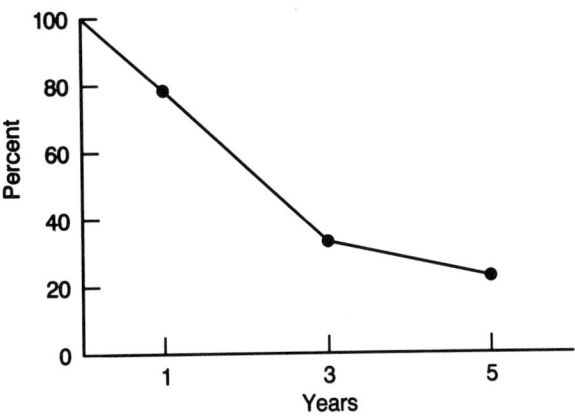

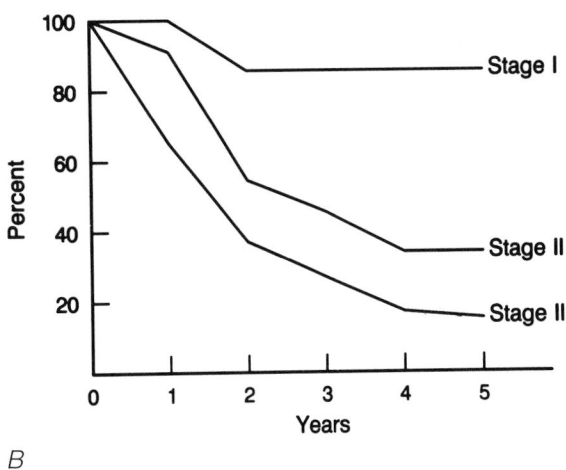

A

B

Fig. 25-37. Survival following resection of esophageal carcinoma. *A.* Overall probability of survival (death from all causes of 100 patients with carcinoma of the esophagus after Ivor Lewis esophagogastrectomy). Zero time on abscissa represents day of operation. *B.* Probability of survival (death from all causes of 100 patients with carcinoma of the esophagus by postsurgical TNM classification). Zero time on abscissa represents day of operation. (From: *King RM, Pairolero PC, et al: Ivor Lewis esophagogastrectomy for carcinoma of the esophagus: Early and late functional results. Ann Thorac Surg 44:119, 1987, with permission.*)

operations and many interfered seriously with eating and digestive comfort, even if the tumor was permanently eradicated. Today every effort is made to minimize the duration of the treatment period, utilizing one-stage pro-

cedures that provide restoration of function with minimal permanent disability.

In most cases—whether the primary lesion is high in the cervical esophagus, at the esophagogastric junction, or in between—the stomach can be effectively mobilized and advanced cephalad at one operation to replace the resected esophagus (Fig. 25-38). Indeed, stomach perfused by right gastric and right gastroepiploic vessels can be made to reach and serve reliably as high as the hyoid bone when placed in the posterior mediastinal bed of the resected esophagus, or as high as the cricoid when passed substernally. Since vagotomy necessarily accompanies

Fig. 25-38. Esophageal reconstruction utilizing stomach. *Above:* Mobilized stomach nourished by distal vascular pedicles of right gastric and right gastroepiploic vessels. Left gastric and short gastric vessels have been interrupted and esophagogastric junction has been divided and closed. Since vagotomy has been effected, a pyloroplasty (or pyloromyotomy) has been performed. *Below left:* Posterior mediastinal passage of vascularized stomach through esophageal hiatus to neck for anastomosis to pharynx or cervical esophagus. *Right:* Substernal or anterior mediastinal tunnel permits passage of stomach to neck for anastomosis to cervical esophagus. Either route can be utilized when colon is interposed between neck and stomach to replace or bypass entire thoracic esophagus.

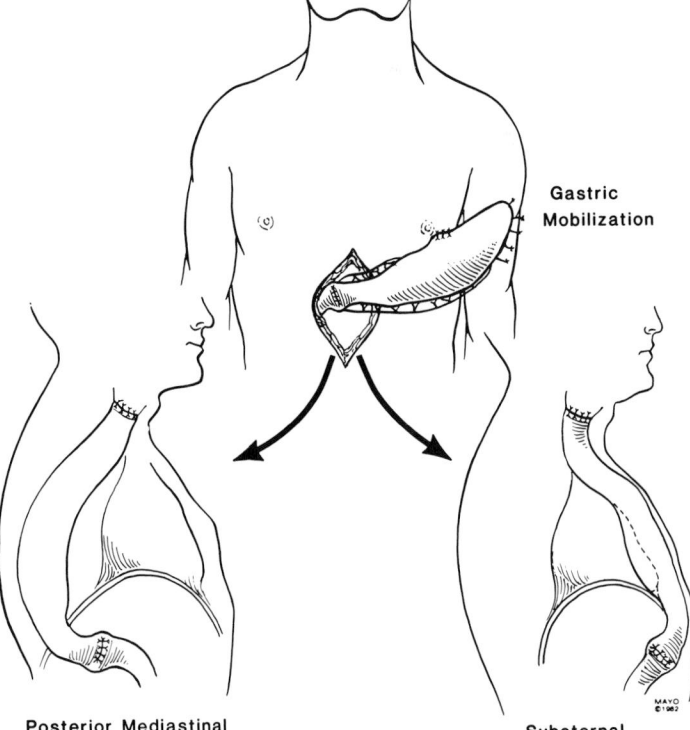

Posterior Mediastinal

Substernal

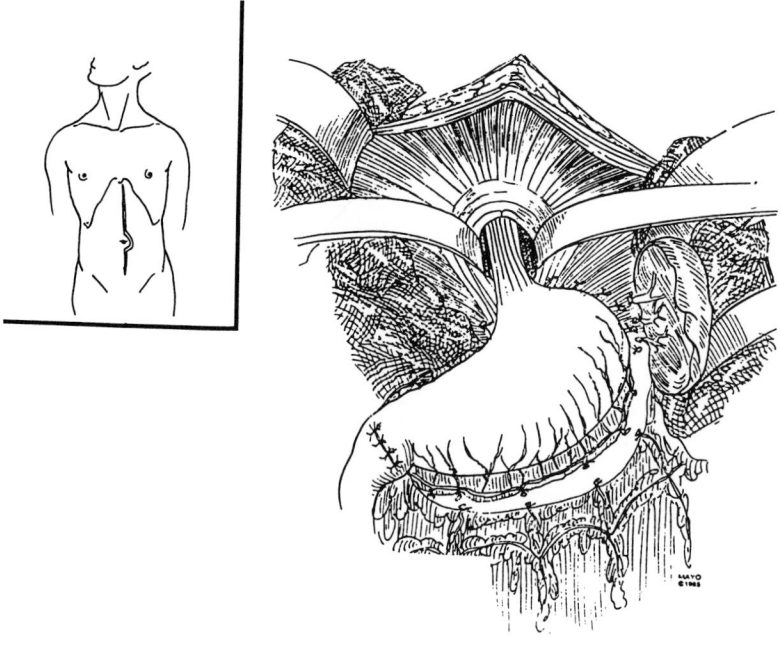

Fig. 25-39. Ivor Lewis esophagogastrectomy-laparotomy. Stomach is prepared for transposition into the chest by preserving right gastric and right gastroepiploic vessels. Pyloromyotomy or pyloroplasty is routinely performed. *Insert:* Upper midline incision from xiphoid to just below umbilicus. (From: *Payne WS, Trastek VF, et al: Current techniques for the surgical management of malignant lesions of the thoracic esophagus and cardia. Mayo Clin Proc 61:564, July 1986, with permission.*)

esophageal resection, pyloroplasty or pyloromyotomy should routinely accompany this use of stomach in esophageal reconstruction.

Generally, both gastroesophageal reflux and gastric dumping are infrequent sequelae of esophagogastrostomy when anastomosis is effected at the carinal level or above, provided the entire stomach lies intrathoracically without redundancy.

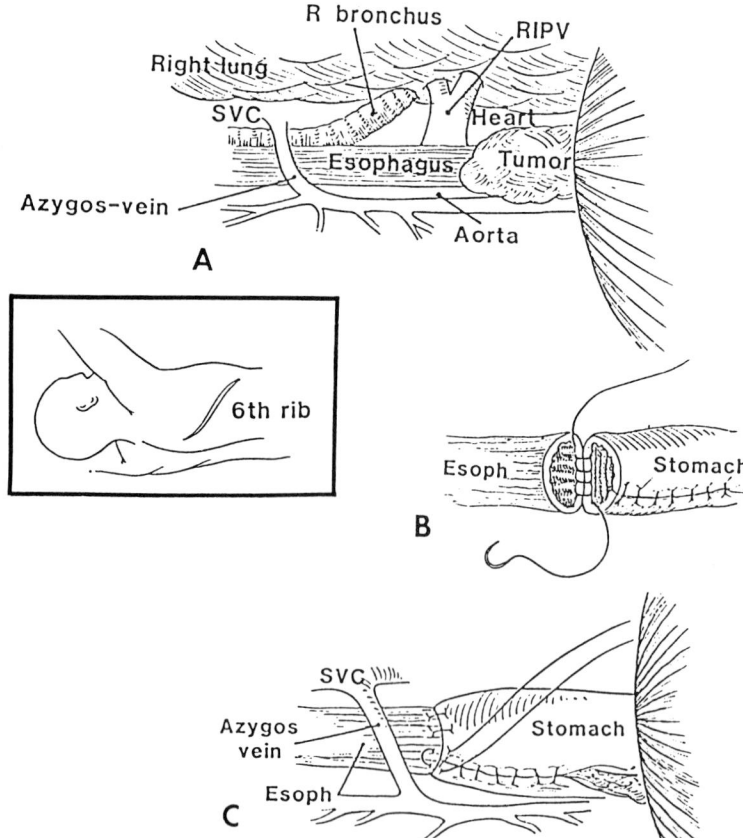

Fig. 25-40. Ivor Lewis esophagogastrectomy-right thoracotomy. *A.* Tumor and esophagus are freed to a level above the azygos vein. *B.* An end-to-end anastomosis is performed over #50 French dilator. *C.* Completed anastomosis. *Insert:* Chest is entered through fifth interspace. (From: *Payne WS, Trastek VF, et al: Current techniques for the surgical management of malignant lesions of the thoracic esophagus and cardia. Mayo Clin Proc 61:564, July 1986, with permission.*)

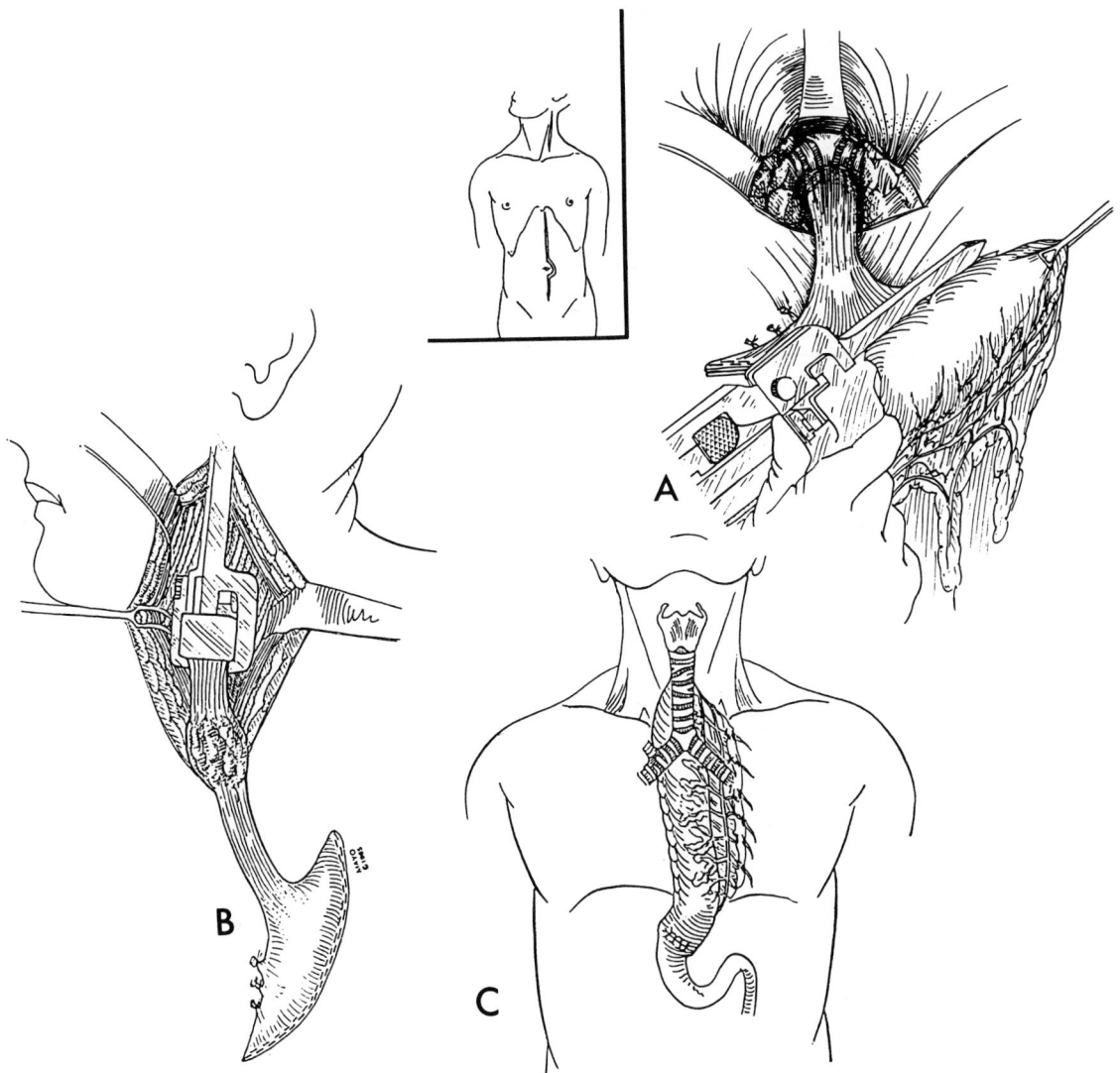

Fig. 25-41. Transhiatal esophagectomy. *Insert:* The neck and abdomen are prepared simultaneously. The midline incision and preparation of the stomach are the same as for the Ivor Lewis esophagogastrectomy (Fig. 25-39). *A.* The stomach is transected just distal to the gastroesophageal junction using the stapling device. *B.* The esophagus is mobilized bluntly from the mediastinum and transposed into the neck, carefully preserving the recurrent nerve. The cervical esophagus is divided using the stapling device. *C.* The stomach is passed through the posterior mediastinal bed, and the anastomosis is constructed at the cervical region over a #50 French dilator. (From: *Payne WS, Trastek VF, et al: Current techniques for the surgical management of malignant lesions of the thoracic esophagus and cardia. Mayo Clin Proc 61:564, July 1986, with permission.*)

Technical Options. The details of the resection and reconstruction vary with individual lesions, surgeons, and surgical intent. Currently the two most commonly performed procedures at the Mayo Clinic are the Ivor Lewis esophagogastrectomy for cardiac and intrathoracic locations (Figs. 25-39, 25-40) and the transhiatal esophagogastrectomy with cervical anastomosis without thoracotomy for a variety of esophageal lesions (Fig. 25-41). Total

gastrectomy with Roux en Y reconstruction is reserved for the gastric lesions that extend up to but are not actually invading the distal esophagus. The left transthoracic esophagogastrectomy with esophagogastrostomy in the left chest for more distal esophageal and gastroesophageal lesions is used only in selected cases. Functional results are enhanced by an anastomotic stoma that accepts a #50 French bougie coupled with invagination into the stomach.

In current practice, colon interposition is largely reserved for those patients in whom disease or previous surgery makes the stomach unsuitable for esophageal replacement (Fig. 25-42). Both the right and left colon and iso- and antiperistaltic segments of the colon have been employed to reach as high as the pharynx. The colon can be passed either substernally or through the posterior mediastinal bed of the resected esophagus. Either the middle colic or inferior mesenteric vessels can serve as blood supply. To improve survival of the colon transposed into the neck, a second blood supply can be con-

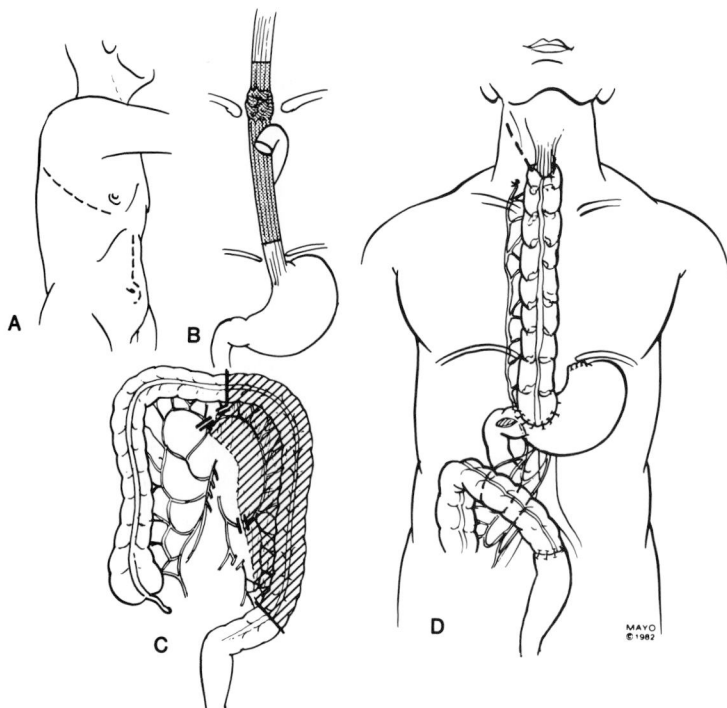

Fig. 25-42. Substernal colon interposition following total esophagectomy for carcinoma. *A* and *B*. At initial operation, esophagus is removed through right thoracotomy and a feeding gastrostomy tube inserted with establishment of proximal cervical esophageal stoma. *C* and *D*. At second operation, left colon is mobilized on vascular pedicle and brought through gastrohepatic omentum. Colon is advanced cephalad through substernal tunnel to neck for anastomosis to cervical esophagus. End-to-side cologastrostomy is effected in abdomen with pyloroplasty or pyloromyotomy. Colonic continuity is restored by colocolostomy.

structed by attaching a colic artery and vein to neck vessels using microvascular techniques.

With colon interposition it is essential that a generous tunnel be provided to minimize vascular compression. If the colon is placed in a substernal position, resection of a portion of the manubrium, clavicle, and first or second costochondral arch is frequently required. The colon must also be straight from proximal anastomosis to

cologastrostomy. When the entire stomach needs to be removed with the esophagus, a long-limb Roux en Y is attached to the abdominal end of the colon interposition to prevent severe bile reflux up to the colon into the mouth (Fig. 25-43).

Decision to Operate and Selection of Techniques. Surgery provides such satisfactory local control of disease, with restoration of swallowing, that many surgeons feel

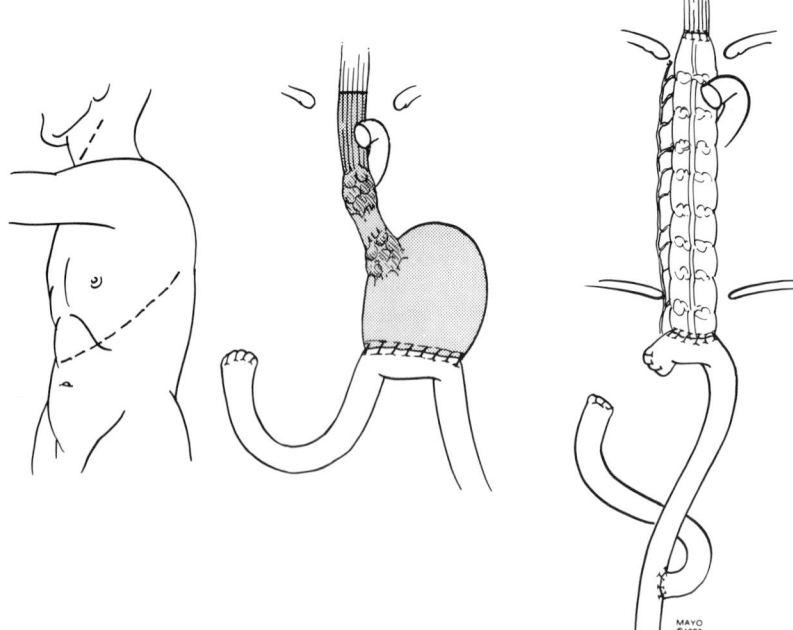

Fig. 25-43. Interposition of colon for esophagus and stomach (latter being unsuitable for interposition because of previous surgery), with long-limb Roux en Y required to prevent bile reflux.

that it should be employed whenever technically feasible. Others cite a median survival of 2 months in patients with known unresectable disease or liver metastases and favor a less aggressive approach. The ability of endoscopic laser therapy to open an obstructed esophagus with minimal morbidity and mortality has made it a primary approach in the palliation of many of these patients. A Celestin or similar palliative tube inserted at the time of abdominal exploration provides a reasonable lumen for unobstructed swallowing in most patients. There is also renewed interest in the palliative transoral endoscopic placement of plastic tubes for inoperable carcinomas. With either method of placement, palliative intubation is restricted to lesions below the cervical esophagus. It may provide satisfactory palliation in cases of acquired malignant tracheoesophageal fistula. Although substernal gastric bypass was initially suggested as a palliative method of management for this type of fistula, a recent review by Orringer has shown a high complication rate, and he no longer recommends this procedure as a palliative maneuver.

Feeding gastrostomy provides no palliation for esophageal obstruction and should be employed only in maintaining nutrition during outpatient radiotherapy, as a temporary measure between stages of esophageal reconstruction, or as an expedient when esophageal obstruction cannot be palliated and parenteral support is impractical. Transendoscopic placement of a gastrostomy tube has been an attractive alternative to surgical placement in selected patients, permitting them to leave the hospital. For others, repeated esophageal dilation treatment can provide reasonable palliation of dysphagia, if they live near the care center.

Unresolved is the management of cervical esophageal and hypopharyngeal cancers. Radiotherapy has surpassed surgery in effecting cure and has the added virtue of preserving voice and laryngeal function if the tumor is locally controlled. Unfortunately, cure and control are not often achieved by this means, and neither esophageal nor laryngeal function is ultimately preserved: the surgeon is often required to perform laryngopharyngoesophagectomy for recurrent or persistent cancer in a heavily radiated field. Reconstruction poses special considerations to restore function (Fig. 25-44).

DeSanto and Carpenter have reviewed the Mayo experience with various reconstructions, which include cervical flaps of the Wookey type, Bakamjian deltopectoral flaps, colon tissue, and gastric interposition of Akiyama. More recently, free transfer of a segment of jejunum has been employed with microvascular anastomosis to cervical vessels. The major problem of hypopharyngeal and cervical esophageal cancer rests not so much with the reconstruction techniques, but with the primary disease and its advanced stage at diagnosis. This, of course, is true for all esophageal cancers.

That cure of early cancer can be achieved frequently with currently available treatment modalities is evident from the Chinese reports of the results in early cancer detected by cytologic screening of a high-risk population. The resectability rate of 170 early esophageal cancers was 100 percent and the 5-year survival was 90 percent.

Postoperative Care. Care following any of the surgical procedures for esophageal cancer is similar to that following any major gastrointestinal and thoracic procedure. Fluid and electrolyte balance, chest physiotherapy, nasogastric intubation, and early ambulation are essential features. Chest tubes, placed at operation, can be removed when drainage ceases. Oral feeding is resumed with the clinical return of gastrointestinal activity, provided contrast radiography demonstrates the absence of anastomotic leak. In nutritionally depleted patients, parenteral alimentation is begun the day after surgery and continued until oral intake is well established. Total hospitalization averages 10 to 12 days.

ESOPHAGEAL PERFORATION

Irrespective of cause, esophageal perforation or rupture may initiate a virulent periesophageal infection. Prompt recognition and proper treatment may avert death or obviate a prolonged and difficult convalescence. In spite of all efforts, esophageal perforation continues to be associated with high mortality and morbidity.

INCIDENCE. Most esophageal perforations today occur after some form of esophageal instrumentation. The number of such perforations appears to have increased over the past 40 years as a result of the greater use of esophagoscopy, gastroscopy, esophageal dilation, and even simple esophageal intubation for diagnosis or treatment.

Of equal interest are those less frequently encountered instances of noninstrumental perforation, which occur as the result of accidental ingestion of foreign bodies or as a consequence of the strain of emesis with or without predisposing esophageal disease. Various other conditions also have been implicated in the noninstrumental perforation of the esophagus, including "stress" associated with neurologic disease or following operations or burns remote from the esophagus. Infrequently, the esophagus may be perforated as the result of either penetrating or nonpenetrating external trauma.

ETIOLOGY. The wall of the esophagus can be breached in a number of ways by either an instrument or a foreign body: (1) simple penetration of the entire wall, (2) simple splitting or rupture of it by strain exceeding its circumferential tensile strength, (3) breaking down of the wall by a localized inflammatory process resulting from mucosal tears, and (4) perforation developing from pressure necrosis or devascularization.

Perforation by instrument or foreign body can occur at any level of the esophagus; however, the sites of normal narrowing are the ones most frequently involved. The greatest narrowing is at the esophageal introitus, and it accounts for the high incidence of perforations seen in this region. Impingement of the rigid scope on bodies of hyperextended cervical vertebrae may crush the mucosa, particularly in the presence of hypertrophic bony spurs.

The second most common site for instrumental or foreign-body perforations has been the lower esophagus, immediately above the point where the organ narrows to pass through the diaphragmatic hiatus. The increased occurrence of disease and frequent need for endoscopic

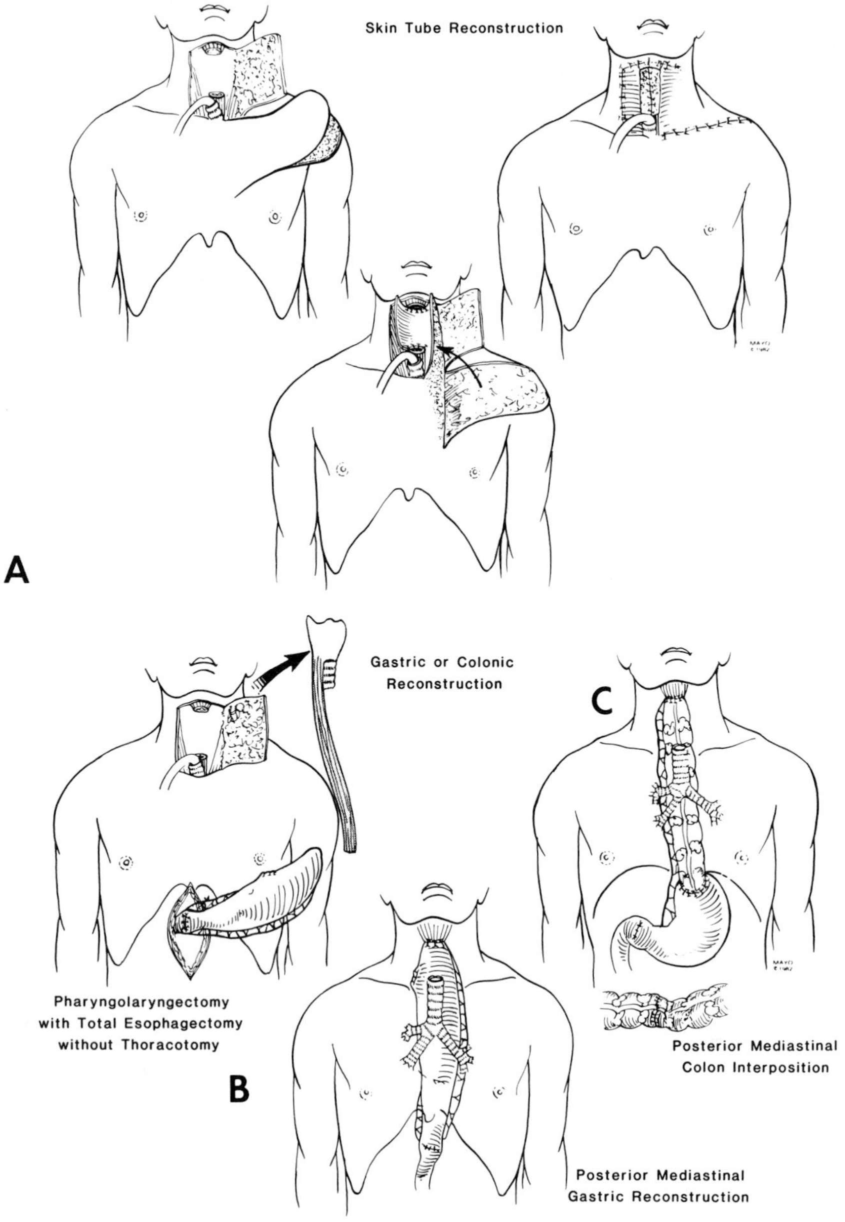

Skin Tube Reconstruction

A

Gastric or Colonic
Reconstruction

C

Pharyngolaryngectomy
with Total Esophagectomy
without Thoracotomy

B

Posterior Mediastinal
Colon Interposition

Posterior Mediastinal
Gastric Reconstruction

Free Segment of Jejunum
(with Microvascular Anastomosis)

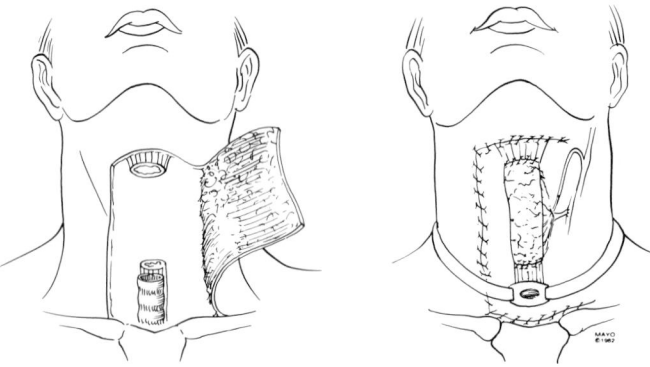

Fig. 25-44. Hypopharyngeal and cervical esophageal cancers pose special reconstruction problems following cervical laryngopharyngoesophagectomy and tracheostomy. Four methods are currently available to effect this reconstruction: *A.* Bakamjian deltopectoral skin-tube reconstruction of pharyngoesophageal continuity. *B.* Posterior mediastinal passage of vascularized pedicle of stomach to neck for anastomosis to pharynx after total esophagectomy. *C.* Posterior mediastinal passage of vascularized colon for interposition between pharynx and stomach. *D.* Free transfer of short segment of jejunum between pharynx and low cortical esophagus with microvascular anastomosis of jejunal vessels to external carotid artery branch and jugular vein.

manipulations in this region contribute further to the incidence of perforation at this level. Perforations of the middle third and abdominal part of the esophagus occur infrequently.

The mechanism of postemetic perforation of the lower esophagus has attracted considerable interest. Mackler showed that inflation of the fresh human cadaveric esophagus resulted in simple longitudinal splitting when the pressure exceeded its circumferential tensile strength. In 95 percent of the 65 specimens studied, such tears occurred in the distal portion of the esophagus. Duval, as reported by Kinsella and coworkers, demonstrated that the rapidity of the increase in pressure rather than the amount of pressure per se may be a critical factor in such injuries. The fact that most postemetic perforations occur in adults rather than in children may be explainable by the higher incidence of predisposing factors in adults and especially by the fact that the strength of the esophagus is thirteen times greater in infants (less than one year old) and four times greater in children (less than twelve years old) than it is in adults.

PATHOPHYSIOLOGY. The consequences of esophageal perforation are due to contamination of periesophageal spaces by corrosive digestive fluids, foods, and bacteria, which leads to a diffuse cellulitis with localized or extensive suppuration.

Anatomic considerations are important, both in the evolution of signs and symptoms and in treatment. The majority of cervical esophageal perforations are posterior and result in suppuration first in the retrovesical space and then extending along fascial planes into the mediastinum.

Perforations of the anterior wall of the cervical esophagus and those involving the lateral pharyngeal spaces and pyriform fossae enter the pretracheal space. The pretracheal space communicates with the mediastinum via the fascial attachment to the pericardium. The manifestations of perforation depend on the relation of the esophagus to the contiguous spaces. The upper two-thirds of the thoracic esophagus is in proximity to the right pleural cavity. The lowest third of the esophagus lies adjacent to the left pleural space. In rare cases, the intraabdominal or subphrenic esophagus may be perforated, leading to peritonitis and intraabdominal abscess.

Although the perforation need not be extensive or impressive to produce marked local or systemic reaction, the consequent sequestration of body fluids in the adjacent spaces may add hypovolemia to bacteremic shock. In addition, the accumulation of fluid and leakage of free air from the perforated hollow viscus may significantly interfere with normal cardiorespiratory dynamics.

MANIFESTATIONS AND DIAGNOSIS. The diagnosis of esophageal perforation depends on suspicious awareness of the possibility as well as on knowledge of the circumstances in which it may occur, the patient's symptoms, the presence of physical signs, and demonstration of the perforation and its secondary manifestations by radiography.

Although the symptoms of perforation depend to a large degree on its site and the extent of inflammatory

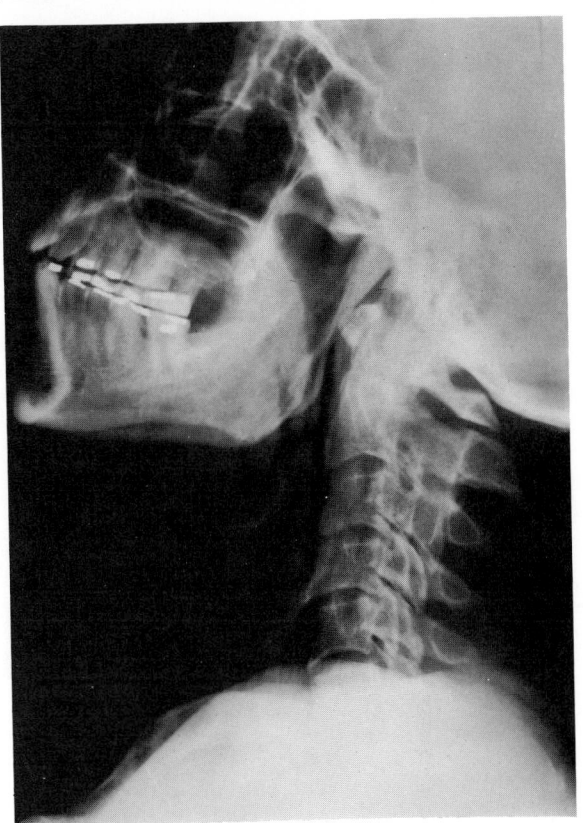

Fig. 25-45. Lateral radiograph of cervical part of spinal column 2 h after instrumental perforation of cervical part of esophagus. Note anterior displacement of trachea by anterior bulging of retrovisceral space, emphysema in tissue planes, and hypertrophic bony spurs on lower cervical vertebrae. [From: *Ellis FH Jr, Payne WS, in Artz CP, Hardy JD (eds): Complications in Surgery and Their Management, 2d ed. Philadelphia, Saunders, 1967, with permission.*]

reaction, the most frequent early complaints are pain, fever, and dysphagia. Dyspnea is usually related to pleural-space involvement, with or without pneumothorax. Cervical tenderness is an early and constant feature of cervical esophageal perforation. Cervical crepitation may be minimal but is an almost constant finding.

The physical findings with thoracic esophageal perforation are usually limited to the thorax. Cervical crepitation may be a feature, but there is usually no cervical tenderness. Auscultation over the heart may elicit signs of mediastinal emphysema (Hamman's sign). With thoracic and subphrenic esophageal perforations, cardiorespiratory embarrassment attended by shock and cyanosis is more commonly seen early, but it may develop at a late stage.

Radiographic studies are of great assistance in diagnosis. Anteroposterior and lateral views of the cervical part of the spinal column often demonstrate pathognomonic signs of cervical perforation (Fig. 25-45). Anterior displacement of the trachea, widening of the retrovisceral space, air in tissue spaces, and occasionally widening of the superior mediastinum are seen. Widening of the superior mediastinum is a common sign in perforation of the cervical or upper thoracic part of the esophagus. Media-

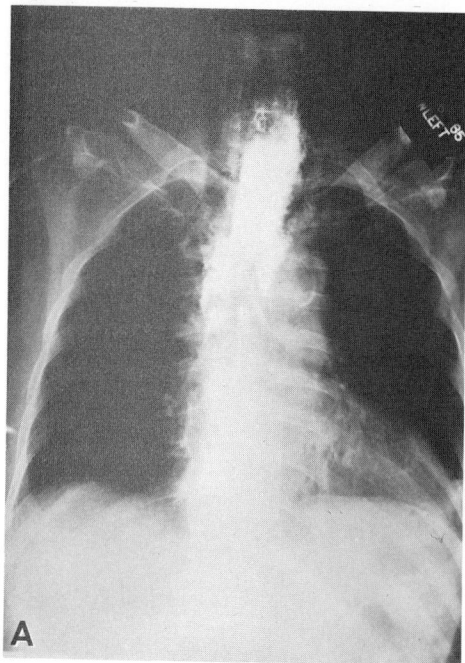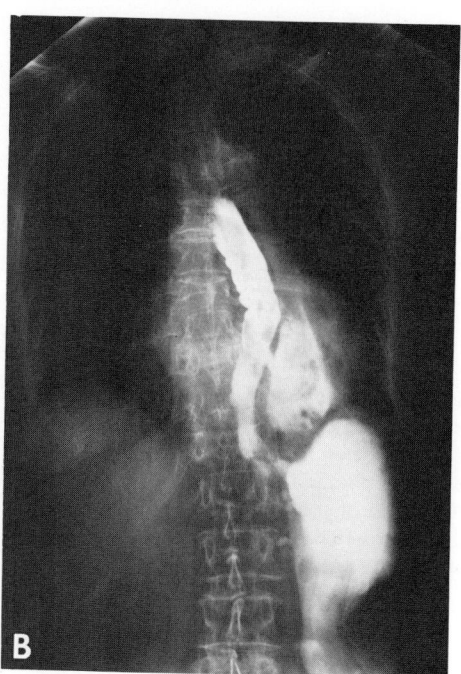

Fig. 25-46. Esophageal perforation. *A.* Extravasation of ingested contrast medium into neck and superior mediastinum, pathognomonic of cervical esophageal perforation. Note failure of distal part of esophagus to fill. [From: *Ellis FH Jr, Payne WS, in Artz CP, Hardy JD (eds): Complications in Surgery and Their Management, 2d ed. Philadelphia, Saunders, 1967, with permission.*] *B.* Postemetic perforation of distal esophagus. Note extravasation of contrast medium into left chest.

stinal emphysema and pleural effusion, with or without pneumothorax, may be present with thoracic or subphrenic esophageal injuries. Studies with opaque medium are indicated to localize the site or sites of perforation and to detect associated abnormalities (Fig. 25-46). The medium should be nonirritating and, preferably, absorbable. Endoscopic procedures are rarely indicated in diagnosis of esophageal perforations, except when a foreign body is present.

TREATMENT. Although there is wide agreement that most perforations of the esophagus are best treated by immediate surgical exploration, repair, and drainage, this is not universally accepted or always feasible. Parenteral antibiotic therapy plus parenteral fluid and electrolyte correction and cardiorespiratory support are appropriate for all patients with esophageal injury.

Confined thoracic esophageal leaks—those demonstrable as local extravasation of contrast media confined to the mediastinum, without pleural contamination and with little or no associated systemic evidence of sepsis—usually will resolve with antibiotics and parenteral alimentation and nothing by mouth.

Surgical Exploration and Management. Simple surgical exploration and drainage of the retrovisceral space—or, on rare occasions, of the pretracheal space—is the treatment of choice for cervical esophageal perforations (Fig. 25-47). Suppuration extending as low as the fourth thoracic vertebra can be evacuated effectively by this route. The usually encountered early cervical perforation may be small, and the inflammatory reaction may be slight; but major lacerations, when present, require suture closure, with drainage of considerable retrovisceral and mediastinal collections.

Instrumental and other perforations of the thoracic and subphrenic parts of the esophagus are often large and require surgical exploration, repair, and drainage. The upper two-thirds of the esophagus is best approached transpleurally by a right midthoracotomy and the lower third by a lower left thoracotomy. The rare subphrenic lacerations are best explored transabdominally. Gastric decompression, either by nasogastric tube or by gastrostomy, is indicated. On occasion, resection of the perforated region and associated esophageal lesion is required.

Late localized cervical and mediastinal abscesses are uncommon complications after adequate early surgical treatment of perforations. When present, they can be drained either by cervical mediastinotomy or transthoracically. As a rule, the late development of empyema after thoracic esophageal perforation can be prevented by early and adequate closed intercostal-tube drainage of the pleural space. When empyema occurs, it usually responds to appropriate open or closed drainage; if it does not, thoracotomy may be required for pulmonary decortication.

Esophagopleural or esophagocutaneous fistulas may occur as a complication of any esophageal perforation. If the esophagus is not obstructed distad and good drainage is provided, such fistulas invariably close with time, provided that there is no undrained local infection, foreign body, malignant change, or epithelialization of the tract. In management of an esophageal fistula, it is best to seek

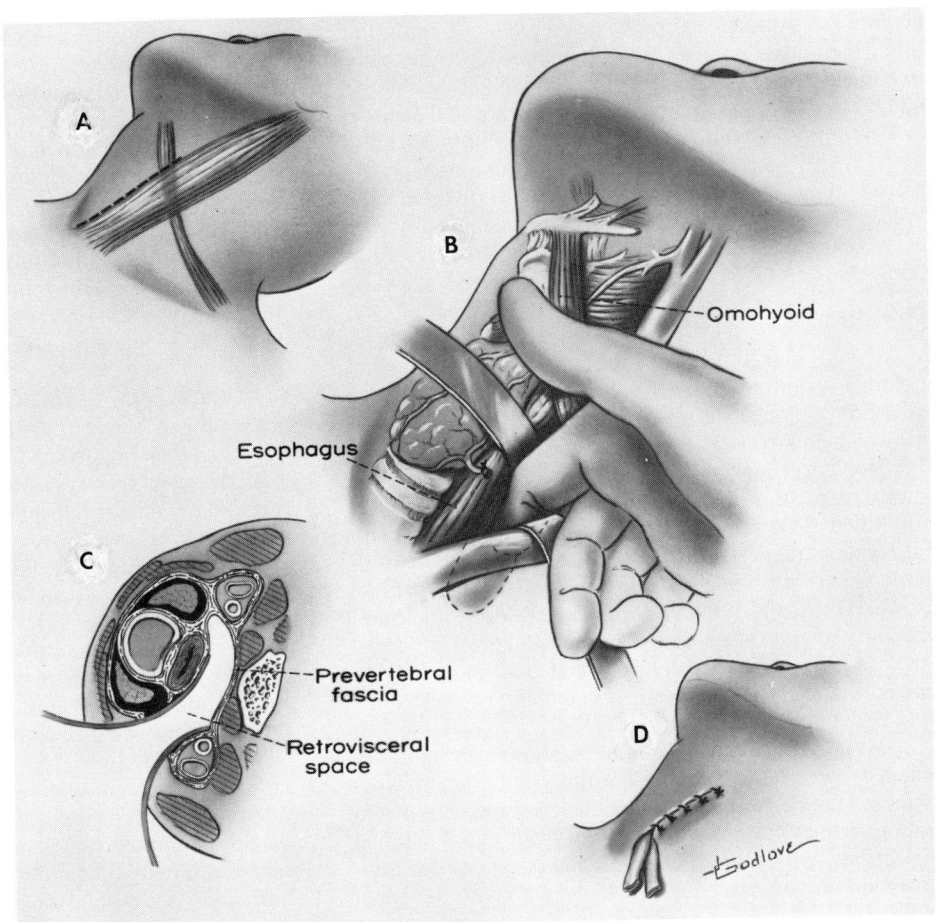

Fig. 25-47. Cervical mediastinotomy. *A.* Access to retrovisceral-prevertebral space is gained through low cervical incision. *B.* Retraction of sternomastoid muscle and cephalic vessels laterally and trachea and thyroid medially gives access to prevertebral (retrovisceral) space. *C.* Gross section of space to be opened in neck. *D.* Posterior collections as low as fourth thoracic vertebra are adequately drained via small rubber drains through this incision. (From: *Payne WS, Larson RH: Surg Clin North Am 49:999, 1969, with permission of Saunders.*)

out and treat for any factors that may contribute to chronicity. Generally it is wise during the healing stage of chronic fistulas to carry out repeated esophageal dilation over a previously swallowed thread, even if no obstruction is demonstrated. With healing, cicatricial narrowing may occur after any perforation; but it is uncommon.

Nutrition is extremely important in the healing of perforations and closure of fistulas. Parenteral alimentation today provides complete nutritional support, which can be maintained indefinitely; but it is usually not required for periods greater than 3 to 4 weeks. If a chronic cutaneous fistula is well drained, oral feedings usually can be resumed despite some nutritional loss through the tract.

RESULTS. The results of the surgical treatment of esophageal perforation depend not only on the cause, site, and severity of the reaction but also, to a large extent, on the lapse of time between perforation and treatment and on the type of treatment.

For perforation of the cervical esophagus, regardless of cause, the results of treatment have been excellent with early cervical exploration and drainage. Even in major cervical injury with marked contamination and delayed treatment, the results of surgical management have been generally satisfactory. However, the incidence of complications, secondary procedures, prolonged hospitalization, and late sequelae has been greater in the group treated initially by medical means only. Mortality from cervical perforation is confined almost exclusively to that subgroup, which further emphasizes the wisdom of early surgical treatment of cervical esophageal perforation.

The results of treatment for perforations of the thoracic and subphrenic esophagus have been less satisfactory. Delay of diagnosis and treatment beyond 18 h appears to be a major factor contributing to morbidity and mortality. Recent reports of series of thoracic esophageal perforations mention mortality in excess of 60 percent with the usual surgical methods in late perforation and between 10 and 30 percent with early treatment.

Differing Opinions

Not all surgeons agree with the operative management outlined. There are instances of cervical and of thoracic esophageal perforation (usually instrumental) in which—

given a late and benign course or the patient's refusal of other methods—success may be obtained by nonoperative management (parenteral alimentation and antibiotics and intercostal tube drainage, etc.). Neuhof and Jemerin in 1943 reported 60 percent survival after surgical drainage alone, but 16 percent after conservative nonsurgical management. A decade later, Seybold and coworkers and Weisel and Raine reported greatly reduced mortality with early suture closure and drainage of esophageal perforation.

Other Methods

The high mortality associated with late diagnosis and treatment of intrathoracic esophageal perforations has led to the development of several other methods of management, which are applicable under various circumstances.

There has been great enthusiasm for reinforcing the suture repair of esophageal tears. Thal has employed gastric fundus as a reinforcing buttress patch; others, pedicles of diaphragm (Rao and associates), pericardium (Millard), intercostal muscle (Dooling and Zick), parietal pleura (Grillo and Wilkins), or latissimus dorsi and other muscle pedicles (Pairolero). Variations on the esophageal exclusion described by Johnson and associates include the partial exclusion and diversion techniques of Urschel and coworkers and of Menguy.

Most current reviews continue to show high mortality when esophageal resective procedures and primary anastomoses are performed in the presence of a recent perforation. It may be preferable to carry out initial surgical resection—with esophageal diversion or one of the complete or partial diversions described above—and deal with reconstruction at a later date.

CONCLUSION. It is impossible, of course, to prescribe a technique applicable to all thoracic esophageal perforations or even those of a given variety. It is essential, however, to have a clear understanding of the clinical problems and the multiple techniques available for rational management of individual patients.

CORROSIVE ESOPHAGITIS (See also Chapter 39)

The ingestion of strong acid or alkali causes a severe inflammatory reaction of the affected mucosa, known as *corrosive esophagitis.* Lye, a strong cleaning agent containing sodium hydroxide and sodium carbonate, is most commonly responsible for such injuries, although various other fluids, including mineral acids, strong bases, phenol, and organic solvents, can produce similar effects. The nature and concentration of the agent ingested determine the degree and extent of the injury, which may involve limited areas of the mouth or esophagus, the entire esophagus, or even the stomach.

PATHOLOGY. The pathologic changes after ingestion of lye are classified in much the same way as thermal burns of the skin. They have been shown experimentally to consist of edema and congestion of the submucosal layer, with associated inflammation and thrombosis of its vessels. Sloughing of the superficial layers occurs, with varying degrees of liquefaction necrosis of the muscularis, followed by fibrosis and delayed reepithelialization. In severe cases the entire mucous membrane of the upper portion of the alimentary tract may slough, and subsequent development of an esophageal stricture is inevitable. Kirsh and Ritter have noted that lye of extremely high concentration in liquid form has become widely available for home use in the past decade. This has markedly altered the extent and severity of injuries following ingestion. Indeed, full-thickness esophageal and gastric necrosis is being seen with increasing frequency. Some of the ingested nonviscous strong acids may miraculously spare the esophagus on their way to causing severe gastric antral burns.

CLINICAL MANIFESTATIONS. During the acute phase of the reaction, burns of the lips, tongue, mouth, and pharynx are apparent. Hoarseness, stridor, and aphonia suggest laryngeal edema or actual epiglottic or laryngeal destruction. Pain in the involved region is common, and there may be associated vomiting. Painful dysphagia is prominent during the acute phase, which lasts from several days to several weeks. As the chronic phase develops, dysphagia due to stricture formation may become the predominant symptom. Gastric injury may be manifested by bleeding or antral obstruction. Clinical signs of perforation of esophagus or stomach, or both, may be apparent and should be sought.

TREATMENT. In view of the instantaneous nature of corrosive injury, it is not reasonable to attempt dilution or neutralization. The immediate effort should be directed to detection and management of attendant airway obstruction and blood-volume depletion. Intravenous fluids and antibiotics are administered promptly, and oral intake is prohibited. The severity of oral burns may be marked, and not necessarily proportional to the severity of esophageal or gastric injury. Early endoscopy and water-soluble contrast radiography of the esophagus and stomach should be performed. The esophagoscope is passed to the first burned area, not beyond. Kirsh and Ritter emphasized the importance of defining, early, the type of corrosive ingested; and they have provided criteria for diagnosing the full-thickness injuries that are more commonly incurred with the liquid corrosives. For injuries of that nature, successful management requires early esophagectomy or total esophagogastrectomy.

Under usual circumstances, however, injury is confined to the mucosa. As soon as patients can swallow their saliva, they are instructed to swallow a thread as a guide for subsequent endoscopy and dilation therapy. Steroids are of questionable efficacy in preventing stricture formation, and they may mask more serious mediastinal, peritoneal, or pulmonary complications. Bouginage, performed early, increases the risk of perforation; so it is not started until acute inflammation has largely subsided, as determined by repeated endoscopy.

Stricture formation is rare if the treatment outlined is initiated promptly. However, should esophagoscopy reveal evidence of stricture formation, dilation of the strictured zone by bouginage over the swallowed thread may be begun within a few weeks of the injury. Some patients may need dilation periodically for a long while, even a year or more. When patients are seen in the chronic phase of the disease and a string has not been ingested previously, it may be necessary to perform gastrostomy for feeding purposes and also for retrograde dilation of the esophageal stricture.

In a small percentage of cases it may become apparent that repeated dilation cannot maintain a satisfactory esophageal lumen. Then extensive reconstructive operative procedures are required to establish a satisfactory, functioning esophageal substitute. Many procedures have been devised, including use of skin-lined tubes and segments of intestine or stomach, as reported by Yudin; the Russian surgeons have had extensive experience with these. Currently preferred is total bypass of the strictured esophagus by a segment of right or left colon interposed substernally between the pharynx and stomach. For lesser degrees of stricture, the lesion may be approached transthoracically and either resected or bypassed with a segment of jejunum or colon. Reconstruction by free transfer of autogenous jejunum with microvascular anastomosis is becoming an important addition to the management of some of these more localized strictures.

MISCELLANEOUS ESOPHAGEAL LESIONS

Plummer–Vinson (Paterson–Kelly) Syndrome

In 1919, Paterson and Kelly independently described a clinical state with which the names of Plummer and Vinson later became associated in the United States. The typical patient is a middle-aged, edentulous woman with atrophic oral mucosa, spoon-shaped fingers and brittle nails, and a long-standing history of anemia and dysphagia. Because of the common finding of iron-deficiency anemia, the term *sideropenic dysphagia* has been used by some to describe the condition, which is more common in the Scandinavian countries than in the United States.

The dysphagia is explained by endoscopic and radiographic demonstration of a fibrous web partially obstructing the esophageal lumen in an eccentric fashion a few millimeters below the cricopharyngeus muscle. A dietary deficiency has been established as the cause, and the condition responds well to iron therapy and forceful dilation of the web.

In approximately 10 percent of cases, a malignant lesion of the oral cavity, hypopharynx, or esophagus develops. The syndrome covers a broad range of clinical entities, and not all patients exhibit hypochromic anemia, nor do they necessarily show evidence of malnutrition. Conversely, not all patients with the other clinical features of the Plummer–Vinson syndrome are found to have esophageal webs. And furthermore, some upper-esophageal webs in younger patients who lack the clinical stigmata of the classic syndrome may have a congenital basis.

Mallory–Weiss Syndrome

In 1929, Mallory and Weiss reported 15 cases of gastrointestinal bleeding after repeated emesis. Linear tears in the mucosa of the esophagogastric junction were demonstrated at postmortem examination in some of these patients. In subsequent years the condition has been noted more commonly, and it should be considered in differential diagnosis of unexplained hematemesis.

The mechanism of the development of the lacerations is similar to that involved in the development of spontaneous rupture of the esophagus—namely, an explosive vomiting effort against a closed cardia or esophagus. A history of prolonged retching or vomiting, often but not always associated with alcoholism, is characteristic. Early diagnosis can be facilitated by radiographic studies to exclude the possibility of other lesions and by endoscopy to identify the site of bleeding.

Bleeding may cease with conservative management, but surgical exploration may be required if it persists. The upper end of the stomach should be exposed through a long gastrotomy, and after manual evacuation of clots and insertion of proper retractors for exposure, the lacerated areas should be repaired with sutures. Prompt arrest of bleeding by this technique can be expected.

Acquired Fistula

Occasionally, a fistulous communication requiring treatment may develop between the esophagus and the lower part of the respiratory tract. Other potential sites of fistulous communication include the aorta, the vena cava, and the heart. The commonest cause of acquired fistula is malignancy, and in the course of incurable carcinoma of the esophagus, the lungs, or the neck structures, such fistula usually is a preterminal event.

Typically, a fistula between the esophagus and the tracheobronchial tree produces cough on eating or drinking, although it may present more subtly, with pulmonary symptoms alone. The basic features of surgical treatment include division of the fistulous tract and suture closure of the defect in the esophagus and respiratory tree, with interposition of viable tissue to prevent recurrence. Additionally, distal esophageal obstruction should be corrected.

The management of congenital tracheoesophageal fistula with and without atresia is discussed in the chapter dealing with pediatric surgery.

Bibliography

General Texts

Brewer LA III: History of surgery of the esophagus. *Am J Surg* 139:730, 1980.

Payne WS, Olsen AM: *The Esophagus*. Philadelphia, Lea & Febiger, 1974.

Postlethwait RW: *Surgery of the Esophagus*. New York, Appleton-Century-Crofts, 1979.

Smith RA, Smith RE: *Surgery of the Oesophagus*. London, Butterworth, 1972.

Anatomy

Carey JM, Hollinshead WH: An anatomic study of the esophageal hiatus. *Surg Gynecol Obstet* 100:196, 1955.

Hayward J: Phreno-oesophageal ligament in hiatal hernia repair. *Thorax* 16:41, 1961.

Higgs B, Shorter RG, Ellis FH Jr: A study of the anatomy of the human esophagus with special reference to the gastroesophageal sphincter. *J Surg Res* 5:503, 1965.

Payne WS: The role of esophageal blood supply, in *Cancer of the Esophagus in 1984: 135 Questions*. Compiled by Giuli R, First Polydisciplinary International Congress of the International Organization for Statistical Studies on Diseases of the Esophagus. Paris, edited and published by Maloine SA, 1984, pp 222–225.

Pera C, Suñer M, Capdevila J: Anatomical demonstration of the lower oesophageal sphincter: A biometrical analysis of 300 specimens (abstract). *Bull Soc Int Chir* 34:285, 1975.

Thomas DM, Langford RM, et al: The anatomical basis for gastric mobilization in total oesophagectomy. *Br J Surg* 66:230, 1979.

Physiology and Physiologic Tests

Bernstein LM, Baker LA: A clinical test for esophagitis. *Gastroenterology* 34:760, 1958.

Bombeck CT, Dillard DH, Nyhus LM: Muscular anatomy of the gastroesophageal junction and role of phrenoesophageal ligament: Autopsy study of sphincter mechanism. *Ann Surg* 164:643, 1966.

Castell DO, Harris LD: Hormonal control of gastroesophageal-sphincter strength. *N Engl J Med* 282:886, 1970.

Castell DO, Levine SM: Lower esophageal sphincter response to gastric alkalinization: A new mechanism for treatment of heartburn with antacids. *Ann Intern Med* 74:223, 1971.

Code CF, Creamer B, et al: *An Atlas of Esophageal Motility in Health and Disease*. Springfield, IL, Charles C Thomas, 1958.

Cohen S, Lipshutz W: Hormonal regulation of human lower esophageal sphincter competence: Interaction of gastrin and secretin. *J Clin Invest* 50:449, 1971.

Earlam R: *Clinical Tests for Oesophageal Function*. New York, Grune & Stratton, 1975.

Henderson RD: *Motor Disorders of the Esophagus*. Baltimore, Williams & Wilkins, 1976.

Ingelfinger FJ: Esophageal motility. *Physiol Rev* 38:533, 1958.

Jahadi MR, Chandler JP: Detecting gastroesophageal reflux by pH recording and acid reflux test. *Am Surg* 38:281, 1972.

Johnson LF, DeMeester TR: Twenty-four-hour pH monitoring of the distal esophagus: A quantitative measure of gastroesophageal reflux. *Am J Gastroenterol* 62:325, 1974.

O'Sullivan GC, DeMeester TR, et al: Interaction of lower esophageal sphincter pressure and length of sphincter in the abdomen as determinants of gastroesophageal competence. *Am J Surg* 143:40, 1982.

Sarna SK, Daniel EE, Waterfall WE: Myogenic and neural control systems for esophageal motility. *Gastroenterology* 73:1345, 1977.

Skinner DB, Belsey RHR, et al (eds): *Gastroesophageal Reflux and Hiatal Hernia*. Boston, Little, Brown, 1972.

Skinner DB, Booth DJ: Assessment of distal esophageal function in patients with hiatal hernia and/or gastroesophageal reflux. *Ann Surg* 172:627, 1970.

Snape WJ Jr, Cohen S: Hormonal control of esophageal function. *Arch Intern Med* 136:538, 1976.

Functional Disturbances of the Esophagus

Motility Disturbances

Arvanitakis C: Achalasia of the esophagus: A reappraisal of esophagomyotomy vs forceful pneumatic dilation. *Am J Dig Dis* 20:841, 1975.

Barker JR, Franklin RH: Heller's operation for achalasia of the cardia: A study of the early and late results. *Br J Surg* 58:466, 1971.

Cohen S, Lipshutz W: Lower esophageal sphincter dysfunction in achalasia. *Gastroenterology* 61:814, 1971.

Creamer B, Donoghue FE, Code CF: Pattern of esophageal motility in diffuse spasm. *Gastroenterology* 34:787, 1958.

Csendes A, Velasco N, et al: A prospective randomized study comparing forceful dilatation and esophagomyotomy in patients with achalasia of the esophagus. *Gastroenterology* 80:789, 1981.

Ellis FH Jr: Surgical management of esophageal motility disturbances. *Am J Surg* 139:752, 1980.

Flye MW, Sealy WC: Diffuse spasm of the esophagus. *Ann Thorac Surg* 19:677, 1975.

Heller E: Extramuköse Cardioplastik beim chronischen Cardiospasmus mit Dilatation des Oesophagus. *Mitt Grengeb Med Chir* 27:141, 1913.

Henderson RD, Ho CS, Davidson JW: Primary disordered motor activity of the esophagus (diffuse spasm): Diagnosis and treatment. *Ann Thorac Surg* 18:327, 1974.

Leonardi HK, Crozier RE, Ellis FH Jr: Reoperation for complications of the Nissen fundoplication. *J Thorac Cardiovasc Surg* 81:50, 1981.

Mansour KA, Symbas PN, et al: A combined surgical approach in the management of achalasia of the esophagus. *Am Surg* 42:192, 1976.

Menguy R: Management of achalasia by transabdominal cardiomyotomy and fundoplication. *Surg Gynecol Obstet* 133:482, 1971.

Nelems JMB, Cooper JD, Pearson FG: Treatment of achalasia: Esophagomyotomy with antireflux procedure. *Can J Surg* 23:588, 1980.

Okike N, Payne WS, et al: Esophagomyotomy versus forceful dilation for achalasia of the esophagus: Results in 899 patients. *Ann Thorac Surg* 28:119, 1979.

Patrick DL, Payne WS, et al: Reoperation for achalasia of the esophagus. *Arch Surg* 103:122, 1971.

Peyton MD, Greenfield LJ, Elkins RC: Combined myotomy and hiatal herniorrhaphy: A new approach to achalasia. *Am J Surg* 128:786, 1974.

Vantrappen G, Hellemans J: Treatment of achalasia and related motor disorders. *Gastroenterology* 79:144, 1980.

Disturbances of Gastroesophageal Competence

Barrett NR: Chronic peptic ulcer of the oesophagus and "oesophagitis." *Br J Surg* 38:175, 1950.

Behar J, Biancani P, Sheahan DG: Evaluation of esophageal tests in the diagnosis of reflux esophagitis. *Gastroenterology* 71:9, 1976.

Borrie J, Goldwater L: Columnar cell-lined esophagus: Assessment of etiology and treatment; A 22-year experience. *J Thorac Cardiovasc Surg* 71:825, 1976.

Brand DL, Ylvisaker JT, et al: Regression of columnar esophageal (Barrett's) epithelium after anti-reflux surgery. *N Engl J Med* 302:844, 1980.

Burgess JN, Payne WS, et al: Barrett esophagus: The columnar-epithelial-lined lower esophagus. *Mayo Clin Proc* 46:728, 1971.

Cameron AJ, Ott BJ, Payne WS: The incidence of adenocarcinoma in columnar-lined (Barrett's) esophagus. *N Engl J Med* 313:857, 1985.

Henderson RD, Pearson FG: Surgical management of esophageal scleroderma. *J Thorac Cardiovasc Surg* 66:686, 1973.

Lam CR, Taber RE, Arciniegas E: The nature and surgical treatment of lower esophageal ring (Schatzki's ring). *J Thorac Cardiovasc Surg* 63:34, 1972.

Orringer MB: Respiratory symptoms and esophageal reflux. *Chest* 76:618, 1979. (Editorial.)

Orringer MB, Dabich L, et al: Gastroesophageal reflux in esophageal schleroderma: Diagnosis and implications. *Ann Thorac Surg* 22:120, 1976.

Ottinger LW, Wilkins EW Jr: Late results in patients with Schatzki rings undergoing destruction of the ring and hiatus herniorrhaphy. *Am J Surg* 139:591, 1980.

Payne WS, McAfee MK, et al: Adenocarcinoma of the columnar epithelial-lined lower esophagus of Barrett, in Delarue NC, Wilkins EW, Wong J (eds): *International Trends in General Thoracic Surgery,* vol V, *Esophageal Carcinoma.* St. Louis, Mosby. (In press.)

Schatzki R, Gary JE: Dysphagia due to a diaphragm-like localized narrowing in the lower esophagus ("lower esophageal ring"). *Am J Roentgen* 70:911, 1953.

Diaphragmatic Hernias

Esophageal Hiatal Hernia

Behar J, Sheahan DG, et al: Medical and surgical management of reflux esophagitis: A 38-month report on a prospective clinical trial. *N Engl J Med* 293:263, 1975.

Belsey R: Reconstruction of the esophagus with left colon. *J Thorac Cardiovasc Surg* 49:33, 1965.

Bushkin FL, Neustein CL, et al: Nissen fundoplication for reflux peptic esophagitis. *Ann Surg* 185:672, 1977.

DeMeester TR, Johnson LF, Kent AH: Evaluation of current operations for the prevention of gastroesophageal reflux. *Ann Surg* 180:511, 1974.

Demos NJ: A simplified, improved technique for the Collis gastroplasty for dilatable esophageal strictures. *Surg Gynecol Obstet* 142:591, 1976.

Demos NJ: Correction of paraesophageal hiatal hernia. *NY State J Med* 77:1281, 1977.

Ellis FH Jr: Controversies regarding the management of hiatus hernia. *Am J Surg* 139:782, 1980.

Fonkalsrud EW, Ament ME, et al: Gastroesophageal fundoplication for the management of reflux in infants and children. *J Thorac Cardiovasc Surg* 76:655, 1978.

Gavriliu D: État actuel du procédé de reconstruction de l'oesophage par tube gastrique (138 malades opérés). *Ann Chir* 19:219, 1965.

Glasgow JC, Cannon JP, Elkins RC: Colon interposition for benign esophageal disease. *Am J Surg* 137:175, 1979.

Hawe A, Payne WS, et al: Adenocarcinoma in the columnar epithelial lined lower (Barrett) oesophagus. *Thorax* 28:511, 1973.

Hiebert CA, O'Mara CS: The Belsey operation for hiatal hernia: A twenty year experience. *Am J Surg* 137:532, 1979.

Hill LD: An effective operation for hiatal hernia: An eight year appraisal. *Ann Surg* 166:681, 1967.

Hill LD: Incarcerated paraesophageal hernia: A surgical emergency. *Am J Surg* 126:286, 1973.

Jolley SG, Herbst JJ, et al: Surgery in children with gastroesophageal reflux and respiratory symptoms. *J Pediatr* 96:194, 1980.

Leonardi HK, Crozier RE, Ellis FH Jr: Reoperation for complications of the Nissen fundoplication. *J Thorac Cardiovasc Surg* 81:50, 1981.

Mansour KA, Burton HG, et al: Complications of intrathoracic Nissen fundoplication. *Ann Thorac Surg* 32:173, 1981.

Nissen R: Eine Einfache Operation zur Beeinflussung der Refluxoesophagitis. *Schweiz Med Wochenschr* 86:590, 1956.

Orringer MB, Orringer JS, et al: Combined Collis gastroplasty—fundoplication operations for scleroderma reflux esophagitis. *Surgery* 90:624, 1981.

Orringer MB, Skinner DB, Belsey RHR: Long-term results of the Mark IV operation for hiatal hernia and analyses of recurrences and their treatment. *J Thorac Cardiovasc Surg* 63:25, 1972.

Orringer MB, Sloan H: Complications and failings of the combined Collis-Belsey operation. *J Thorac Cardiovasc Surg* 74:726, 1977.

Payne WS: Surgical treatment of paraesophageal hiatal hernia, in Nyhus LM, Baker RJ (eds): *Mastery of Surgery.* Boston, Little, Brown, 1984.

Payne WS: Prevention and treatment of biliary-pancreatic reflux esophagitis. *Surg Clin North Am* 63:851, August 1983.

Payne WS: Surgical management of reflux-induced oesophageal stenoses: Results in 101 patients. *Br J Surg* 71:971, December 1984.

Payne WS: Paraesophageal hiatal hernia, in Nyhus LM, Baker RJ (eds): *Mastery of Surgery.* Boston, Little, Brown, 1984, pp 329–337.

Payne WS: Reflux oesophagitis with stricture: Alternative methods of management, in Dudley H, Carter DC, Jackson JW, Cooper DKC (eds): *Operative Surgery.* London, Butterworth, 1986, pp 314–325.

Payne WS, Andersen HA, Ellis FH Jr: Reappraisal of esophagogastrectomy and antral excision in the treatment of short esophagus. *Surgery* 55:344, 1964.

Pearson FG, Langer B, Henderson RD: Gastroplasty and Belsey hiatus hernia repair: An operation for the management of peptic stricture with acquired short esophagus. *J Thorac Cardiovasc Surg* 61:50, 1971.

Piehler JM, Payne WS, et al: The uncut Collis-Nissen procedure for esophageal hiatal hernia and its complications. *Probl Gen Surg* 1:1, 1984.

Pridie RB: Incidence and coincidence of hiatus hernia. *Gut* 7:188, 1966.

Richardson JD, Larson GM, Polk HC Jr: Intrathoracic fundoplication for shortened esophagus: Treacherous solution to a challenging problem. *Am J Surg* 143:29, 1982.

Skinner DB: Esophageal reconstruction. *Am J Surg* 139:810, 1980.

Urschel HC Jr, Razzuk MA: "Collis-Belsey" fundoplication for uncomplicated hiatal hernia and gastroesophageal reflux. *Ann Thorac Surg* 27:564, 1979.

Miscellaneous Diaphragmatic Conditions

Beck WC, Motsay DS: Eventration of diaphragm. *Arch Surg* 65:557, 1952.

Bekassy SM, Dave KS, et al: "Spontaneous" and traumatic rupture of the diaphragm: Long-term results. *Ann Surg* 177:320, 1973.

Broman I: Über die Entwickelung und Bedeutung der Mesenterien und der Korperhohlen bei den Wirbeltieren. *Ergeb Anat Entwicklngsgesch* 15:332, 1905.

Carter R, Brewer LA III: Strangulating diaphragmatic hernia. *Ann Thorac Surg* 12:281, 1971.

Chin EF, Duchesne ER: The parasternal defect. *Thorax* 10:214, 1955.

Comer TP, Clagett OT: Surgical treatment of hernia of the foramen of Morgagni. *J Thorac Cardiovasc Surg* 52:461, 1966.

Drews JA, et al: Acute diaphragmatic injuries. *Ann Thorac Surg* 16:67, 1973.

Hill LD: Injuries of the diaphragm following blunt trauma. *Surg Clin North Am* 52:611, 1972.

Pairolero PC, Payne WS: Diaphragm, in Goldsmith HS: *Practice of Surgery*. Hagerstown, Harper & Row, 1980.

Shoemaker R, Palmer G, et al: Aggressive treatment of acquired phrenic nerve paralysis in infants and small children. *Ann Thorac Surg* 32:251, 1981.

Wilson RF: Discussion. *Ann Thorac Surg* 16:77, 1973.

Oropharyngeal Dysphagia

Black RJ: Cricopharyngeal myotomy. *J Otolaryng* 10:145, 1981.

Duranceau A, Forand MD, Fauteux JP: Surgery in oculopharyngeal muscular dystrophy. *Am J Surg* 139:33, 1980.

Ellis FH Jr, Crozier RE: Cervical esophageal dysphagia: Indications for and results of cricopharyngeal myotomy. *Ann Surg* 194:279, 1981.

Orringer MB: Extended cervical esophagomyotomy for cricopharyngeal dysfunction. *J Thorac Cardiovasc Surg* 80:669, 1980.

Palmer ED: Disorders of the cricopharyngeus muscle: A review. *Gastroenterology* 71:510, 1976.

Diverticula

Allen TH, Clagett OT: Changing concepts in the surgical treatment of pulsion diverticula of the lower esophagus. *J Thorac Cardiovasc Surg* 50:455, 1965.

Debas HT, Payne WS, et al: Physiopathology of lower esophageal diverticulum and its implications for treatment. *Surg Gynecol Obstet* 151:593, 1980.

Habein HC Jr, Moersch HJ, Kirklin JW: Diverticula of the lower part of the esophagus: A clinical study of 149 nonsurgical cases. *Arch Intern Med* 97:768, 1956.

Huang B, Payne WS, Cameron AJ: Surgical management for recurrent pharyngoesophageal (Zenker's) diverticulum. *Ann Thorac Surg* 37:189, March 1984.

Huang BS, Unni KK, Payne WS: Long-term survival following diverticulectomy for cancer in pharyngoesophageal (Zenker's) diverticulum. *Ann Thorac Surg* 38(3):207, September 1984.

Payne WS, Pairolero PC, Piehler JM: The management of Zenker's diverticulum: Diverticulectomy, in Kittle CF (ed): *Current Controversies in Thoracic Surgery*. Philadelphia, Saunders, 1986, pp 3–9.

Payne WS, Reynolds RR: Surgical treatment of pharyngoesophageal diverticulum (Zenker's diverticulum). *Surg Rounds* 5(6):18, June 1982.

Payne WS, Trastek VF: The role of stapling devices in the treatment of pharyngoesophageal (Zenker's) diverticulum, in Ravitch MM, Steichen FM (eds): *Principles and Practices of Surgical Stapling*. Chicago, Year Book Medical Publishers, 1987, pp 79–98.

Welsh GF, Payne WS: The present status of one-stage pharyngoesophageal diverticulectomy. *Surg Clin North Am* 53:953, 1973.

Benign Cysts and Tumors

Bernatz PE, Smith JL, et al: Benign, pedunculated intraluminal tumors of the esophagus. *J Thorac Surg* 35:503, 1958.

Schmidt HW, Clagett OT, Harrison EG Jr: Benign tumors and cysts of the esophagus. *J Thorac Cardiovasc Surg* 41:717, 1961.

Malignant Tumors

Akiyama H, Hiyama M, Miyazono H: Total esophageal reconstruction after extraction of the esophagus. *Ann Surg* 182:547, 1975.

Akiyama H, Tsurumaru M, et al: Principles of surgical treatment for carcinoma of the esophagus: Analysis of lymph node involvement. *Ann Surg* 194(4):438, 1981.

Bakamjian VY: Total reconstruction of pharynx with medially based deltopectoral skin flap. *NY State J Med* 68:2771, 1968.

Beahrs OH, Myers MA (eds): *Manual for Staging of Cancer*. American Joint Committee on Cancer Staging. Lippincott Medical, 1983.

Belsey RHR: Palliative management of esophageal carcinoma. *Am J Surg* 139:789, 1980.

Cameron AJ, Ott BJ, Payne WS: The incidence of adenocarcinoma in columnar-lined (Barrett's) esophagus. *N Engl J Med* 313:857, 1985.

Chang TS, Hwang OL, Wang-Wei: Reconstruction of esophageal defects with microsurgically revascularized jejunal segments: A report of 13 cases. *J Microsurg* 2:83, 1980.

Cooper JD, Jamieson WRE, et al: The palliative value of surgical resection for carcinoma of the esophagus. *Can J Surg* 24:145, 1981.

DeSanto LW, Carpenter RJ: Reconstruction of the pharynx and upper esophagus after resection for cancer. *Head Neck Surg* 2:369, 1980.

DiCostanzo DP, Urmacher C: Primary malignant melanoma of the esophagus. *Am J Surg Pathol* 11(1):46, 1987.

Drucker MH, Mansour KA, et al: Esophageal carcinoma: An aggressive approach. *Ann Thorac Surg* 28:133, 1979.

Earlam R, Cunha-Melo JR: Oesophageal squamous cell carcinoma: I. A critical review of surgery. *Br J Surg* 67:381, 1980.

Ellis FH Jr: Esophagogastrectomy for carcinoma: Technical considerations based on anatomic location of lesion. *Surg Clin North Am* 60:265, April 1980.

Ellis FH Jr, Gibb P, Watkins E Jr: Esophagogastrectomy: A safe, widely applicable, and expeditious form of palliation for patients with carcinoma of the esophagus and cardia. *Ann Surg* 198(4):531, 1983.

Ellis FH Jr, Salzman FA: Carcinoma of the esophagus: Surgery versus radiotherapy. *Postgrad Med* 61:167, 1977.

Gatzinsky P, Berglin E, et al: Resectional operations and long-term results in carcinoma of the esophagus. *J Thorac Cardiovasc Surg* 89:71, 1985.

Gluckman JL, McDonough J, et al: The free jejunal graft in head and neck reconstruction. *Laryngoscope* 91:1887, 1981.

Goldberg SJ, King KH: Endoscopic Nd:YAG laser coagulation as palliative therapy for obstructing esophageal carcinoma. *Am J Gastroenterol* 81(8):629, 1986.

Goldfaden D, Orringer MB, et al: Adenocarcinoma of the distal esophagus and gastric cardia: Comparison of results of transhiatal esophagectomy and thoracoabdominal esophagogastrectomy. *J Thorac Cardiovasc Surg* 91:242, 1986.

Guojun H, Lingfang S, et al: Diagnosis and surgical treatment of early esophageal carcinoma. *Chin Med J* 94:229, April 1981.

Harrison DFN: Surgical repair in hypopharyngeal and cervical esophageal cancer: Analysis of 162 patients. *Ann Otol Rhinol Laryng* 90:372, 1981.

Harrison DFN, Thompson AE, Buchanan G: Radical resection for cancer of the hypopharynx and cervical oesophagus with repair by stomach transposition. *Br J Surg* 68:781, 1981.

Hawe A, Payne WS, et al: Adenocarcinoma in the columnar epithelial lined lower (Barrett) oesophagus. *Thorax* 28:511, 1973.

Keagy BA, Murray GF, et al: Esophagogastrectomy as palliative treatment for esophageal carcinoma: Results obtained in the setting of a thoracic surgery residency program. *Ann Thorac Surg* 38(6):611, 1984.

King RM, Pairolero PC, et al: Ivor Lewis esophagogastrectomy for carcinoma of the esophagus: Early and late functional results. *Ann Thorac Surg.* (In press.)

Kiviranta UK: Corrosion carcinoma of the esophagus: 381 cases of corrosion and nine cases of corrosion carcinoma. *Acta Otolaryng (Stockh)* 42:89, 1952.

Lea JW, Prager RL, Bender HW Jr: The questionable role of computed tomography in preoperative staging of esophageal cancer. *Ann Thorac Surg* 38(5):479, 1984.

Lewis I: The surgical treatment of carcinoma of the oesophagus: With special reference to a new operation for growths of the middle third. *Br J Surg* 34:18, 1946.

Marcial–Rojas RA, Valleciool LA: Primary adenoidcystic carcinoma of the esophagus: Report of one case and review of the literature. *Arch Otolaryng* 70:197, 1959.

Marks RD Jr, Scruggs HJ, Wallace KM: Preoperative radiation therapy for carcinoma of the esophagus. *Cancer* 38:84, 1976.

Meyers WC, Seigler HF, et al: Postoperative function of "free" jejunal transplants for replacement of the cervical esophagus. *Ann Surg* 192:439, 1980.

Miller JI, McIntyre B, Hatcher CR: Combined treatment approach in surgical management of carcinoma of the esophagus: A preliminary report. *Ann Thorac Surg* 40(3):289, 1985.

Molina JE, Lawton BR, et al: Esophagogastrectomy for adenocarcinoma of the cardia: Ten years' experience and current approach. *Ann Surg* 195:146, 1982.

Nakamura T, Nagamachi Y: Long loop Roux–Y esophagojejunostomy following total gastrectomy. *Gastroenterol Jpn* 13:415, 1978.

Ong GB: Resection and reconstruction of the oesophagus in oesophageal cancer. *J Jpn Assoc Thorac Surg* 22:769, 1974.

Orringer MB: Substernal gastric bypass of the excluded esophagus—results of an ill-advised operation. *Surgery* 96:(3):467, 1984.

Orringer MB: Transhiatal esophagectomy without thoracotomy for carcinoma of the thoracic esophagus. *Ann Surg* 200(3): 282, 1984.

Payne WS, Bernatz PE: One-stage resection and reconstruction for carcinoma of the esophagogastric junction, in Varco RL, Delaney JP (eds): *Controversy in Surgery.* Philadelphia, Saunders, 1976.

Payne WS, Fisher J: Esophageal reconstruction: Free jejunal transfer or circulatory augmentation of pedicled intestinal interpositions using microvascular surgery. *International Trends in General Thoracic Surgery,* vol 5, 1986.

Payne WS, Trastek VF, et al: Current techniques for the surgical management of malignant lesions of the thoracic esophagus and cardia. *Mayo Clin Proc* 61:564–572, 1986.

Shields TW, Rosen ST, et al: Multimodality approach to treatment of carcinoma of the esophagus. *Arch Surg* 119:558, 1984.

Skinner DB: En bloc resection for neoplasms of the esophagus and cardia. *J Thorac Cardiovasc Surg* 85:59, 1983.

Skinner DB, DeMeester TR: Permanent extracorporeal esophagogastric tube for esophageal replacement. *Ann Thorac Surg* 22:107, 1976.

Steiger Z, Franklin R, et al: Eradication and palliation of squamous cell carcinoma of the esophagus with chemotherapy,
radiotherapy, and surgical therapy. *J Thorac Cardiovasc Surg* 82:713, 1981.

Talbert JL, Cantrell JR: Clinical and pathologic characteristics of carcinosarcoma of the esophagus. *J Thorac Cardiovasc Surg* 45:1, 1963.

West PN, Marbarger JP, et al: Esophagogastrostomy with the EEA stapler. *Ann Surg* 193:76, 1981.

Wilkins EW Jr: Long-segment colon substitution for the esophagus. *Ann Surg* 192:722, 1980.

Wookey H: Cited by Bakamjian VY, Total reconstruction of pharynx with medially based deltopectoral skin flap. *NY State J Med* 68:2771, 1968.

Wychulis AR, Gunnlaugsson GH, Clagett OT: Carcinoma occurring in pharyngoesophageal diverticulum: Report of three cases. *Surgery* 66:979, 1969.

Esophageal Perforation

Bradley SL, Pairolero PC, et al: Spontaneous rupture of the esophagus. *Arch Surg* 116:755, 1981.

Cameron JL, Kieffer RF, et al: Selective nonoperative management of contained intrathoracic esophageal disruptions. *Ann Thorac Surg* 27:404, 1979.

Finley RJ, Pearson FG, et al: The management of nonmalignant intrathoracic esophageal perforations. *Ann Thorac Surg* 30:575, 1980.

Grillo HC, Wilkins EW Jr: Esophageal repair following late diagnosis of intrathoracic perforation. *Ann Thorac Surg* 20:387, 1975.

Michel L, Grillo HC, Malt RA: Operative and nonoperative management of esophageal perforations. *Ann Surg* 194:57, 1981.

Michel L, Grillo HC, Malt RA: Esophageal perforation. *Ann Thorac Surg* 33:203, 1982.

Pairolero PC, Payne WS: Esophageal perforation, in English GM (ed): *Otolaryngology.* Hagerstown, Harper & Row, 1981.

Payne WS, Larson RH: Acute mediastinitis. *Surg Clin North Am* 49:999, 1969.

Sarr MG, Pemberton JH, Payne WS: Management of instrumental perforations of the esophagus. *J Thorac Cardiovasc Surg* 84:211, August 1982.

Schwartz ML, McQuarrie DG: Surgical management of esophageal perforation. *Surg Gynecol Obstet* 151:668, 1980.

Skinner DB, Little AG, DeMeester TR: Management of esophageal perforation. *Am J Surg* 139:760, 1980.

Worman LW, Hurley JD, et al: Rupture of the esophagus from external blunt trauma. *Arch Surg* 85:333, 1962.

Wychulis AR, Fontana RS, Payne WS: Instrumental perforations of the esophagus. *Dis Chest* 55:184, 1969.

Wychulis AR, Fontana RS, Payne WS: Noninstrumental perforations of the esophagus. *Dis Chest* 55:190, 1969.

Corrosive Esophagitis

Buntain WL, Payne WS, Lynn HB: Esophageal reconstruction for benign disease: A long-term appraisal. *Am Surg* 46:67, 1980.

Campbell GS, Burnett HF, et al: Treatment of corrosive burns of the esophagus. *Arch Surg* 112:495, 1977.

Kirsh MM, Ritter F: Caustic ingestion and subsequent damage to the oropharyngeal and digestive passages. *Ann Thorac Surg* 21:74, 1976.

Yudin SS: The surgical construction of 80 cases of artificial esophagus. *Surg Gynecol Obstet* 78:561, 1944.

Miscellaneous Esophageal Lesions

Adler RH: Congenital esophageal webs. *J Thorac Cardiovasc Surg* 45:175, 1963.

Hastings PR, Peters KW, Cohn I Jr: Mallory-Weiss syndrome: Review of 69 cases. *Am J Surg* 142:560, 1981.

Mallory GK, Weiss S: Hemorrhages from lacerations of the cardiac orifice of the stomach due to vomiting. *Am J Med Sci* 178:506, 1929.

Chapter 26

Stomach

Frank G. Moody, James M. McGreevy, and Thomas A. Miller

ANATOMY

FUNCTIONAL RELATIONSHIPS. The stomach is an expanded segment of the foregut responsible for the initial breakdown and predigestion of a meal. Its location in the upper abdomen beneath the left hemidiaphragm allows for free expansion of its thin-walled distensible fundus, which receives and stores solid foods that pass into it from the esophagus above. The thicker-walled, more muscular distal portion of the stomach, the antrum, grinds and mixes the food and then forces it back into the fundus for further reduction in size and predigestion. Small particles move forward into the duodenum where they are further processed by intestinal secretions. The distal stomach is delineated by a thick band of circular smooth muscle, the pyloric sphincter. This sphincter prevents duodenogastric reflux and assists in gastric emptying by relaxing during antral propulsive contractions.

The fundus is lined by a highly specialized epithelium that secretes hydrochloric acid, pepsin, and intrinsic factor. The mucosa of the antrum participates in the process of gastric acid secretion by releasing the secretagogue, gastrin, into the circulation. This event is mediated by vagal release of acetylcholine and is modulated by the pH of the antral lumen. The stomach, therefore, can be considered as two organs: its proximal portion is designed for storage and digestion, and its distal part is adapted to the role of mixing and evacuation.

Of importance to the functional activity of the stomach in disease is its relationship to other intraabdominal organs. The most important adjacent organs are the pancreas and the liver, which lie dorsad and ventrad, respectively, and the spleen, which lies directly to the left of the stomach's greater curve (Fig. 26-1). Inflammation of the pancreas may delay gastric emptying, while enlargement by neoplasm may cause a sense of fullness or even obstruction to the gastric outlet. Liver or splenic enlargement may also interfere with the storage capacity of the stomach by infringing on its lumen. The transverse colon, which lies caudad, may also interfere with gastric function by direct neoplastic extension. More commonly, however, the stomach affects adjacent organs by penetration from peptic ulceration of either the stomach or duodenum. Another closely related structure is the biliary tree. It runs posterior to the first part of the duodenum only a few centimeters from the gastric outlet and is vulnerable to injury not only from peptic ulcer of the duodenum but from attempts at treatment by gastrectomy.

BLOOD SUPPLY AND LYMPHATICS. The stomach has a blood supply so extensive and interconnected that three of its four major nutrient arteries can be ablated without incurring necrosis or even significant dysfunction. A submucosal plexus of arterioles provides for rapid healing of wounds and a low incidence of anastomotic disruption after operative manipulation. Because of this vascular anatomy, mucosal lesions may bleed extensively, even when small or superficial. The major arterial supply to the

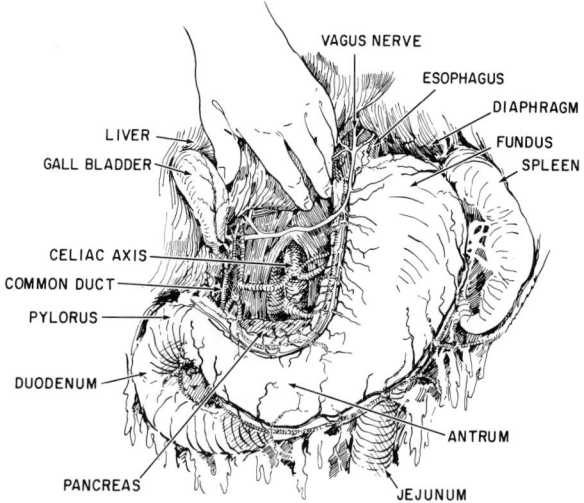

Fig. 26-1. Position of the stomach relative to the other principal organs of the upper abdomen.

stomach is shown in Fig. 26-2. The lesser curve of the stomach is supplied primarily by the left gastric artery, which arises from the celiac axis. The right gastric artery, arising from the ascending hepatic artery, is usually a small vessel that provides branches to the first part of the

Fig. 26-2. Blood supply to the stomach. Legend: F—fundus; C—cardia; P—pylorus; S—spleen; A—aorta; E—esophageal arteries; SP—splenic artery; LG—left gastric artery; CH—common hepatic artery; RG—right gastric artery; GD—gastroduodenal artery; PD—pancreaticoduodenal artery; RGE—right gastroepiploic artery; LGE—left gastroepiploic artery; SG—short gastric arteries. *(Courtesy of KR Larsen, PhD.)*

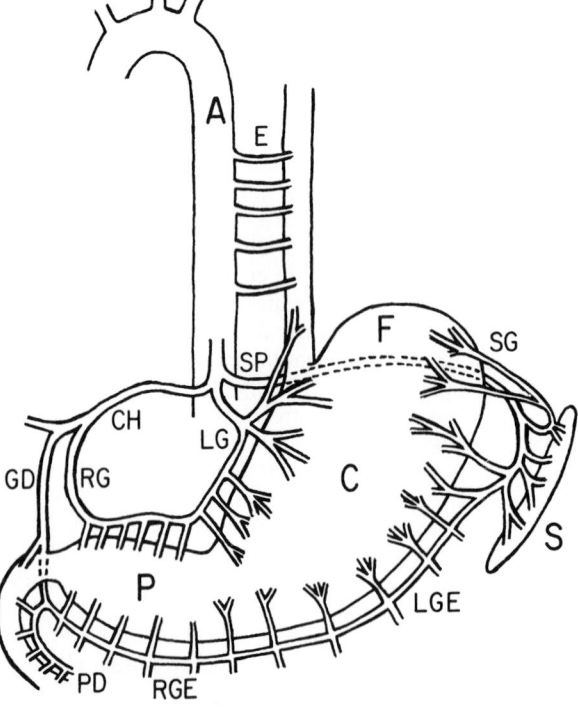

duodenum and the pylorus. Right and left gastroepiploic arteries arise from the gastroduodenal and splenic arteries, respectively. They form an arcade along the greater curve, the right providing blood to the antrum and the left supplying the lower portion of the fundus. The short gastric arteries arising from the splenic artery are small and relatively insignificant in terms of the amount of blood that they deliver to the most proximal portion of the body of the stomach.

The lymphatic drainage of the stomach follows the distribution of the blood supply. An understanding of lymphatic channels and their nodal communications is important to the assessment of tumor spread from gastric cancer. These routes of flow are shown schematically in Fig. 26-3. Lymph from the upper lesser curvature of the stomach drains into the left gastric and paracardial nodes (Region I). The antral segment on the lesser curve (Region II) drains into the right suprapancreatic nodes. Lymph from Region III, high on the greater curvature, flows into the left gastroepiploic and splenic nodes, while the distribution of flow along the right gastroepiploic enters nodes at the base of the vascular pedicle serving this area (Region IV). Knowledge of these areas is of practical importance when operating for cure of gastric cancer. Unfortunately, the routes of metastatic spread in this disease are unpredictable. Therefore, removal of lymph nodes is more important for ascertaining prognosis than for gaining a cure.

INNERVATION. Motor aspects as well as secretory aspects of gastric function are controlled by the autonomic nervous system. The vagus nerves provide a predominant part of this innervation. The major branches of the vagi are shown schematically in Fig. 26-4. Each vagus has a single branch within the abdomen: the hepatic arising from the left anterior vagus, and the celiac from the right posterior vagus. The axial orientation of the vagi relates to the rotation of the stomach to the left as the lengthened foregut returns to the celomic cavity from the yolk sac during gestation. Each vagus terminates in the anterior and posterior nerves of Laterjet, respectively. Small branches course along the smaller blood vessels as they enter the gastric wall along its lesser curve. Knowledge of the anatomy of these nerves has resulted in a new technique, highly selective vagotomy, for treatment of peptic ulcer. In this procedure, the antral branches called the "crow's-foot" are preserved, while the more proximal branches are divided as they enter the stomach. The left anterior vagus will often divide into two or three branches before passing through the esophageal hiatus. The right posterior vagus may occasionally give off a small branch that courses to the left behind the esophagus to join the cardia. This branch has been termed the "criminal nerve of Grassi" in recognition of its important role in the etiology of recurrent ulcer when it is left undivided.

The splanchnic innervation to the stomach is less distinct than that of vagal origin. It has been demonstrated that some of the vagal fibers are adrenergic as well as cholinergic. The majority of sympathetic innervations, however, appear to be adrenergic. They accompany the gastrosplenic artery and its branches, which is appropriate for their function of control of blood flow and muscu-

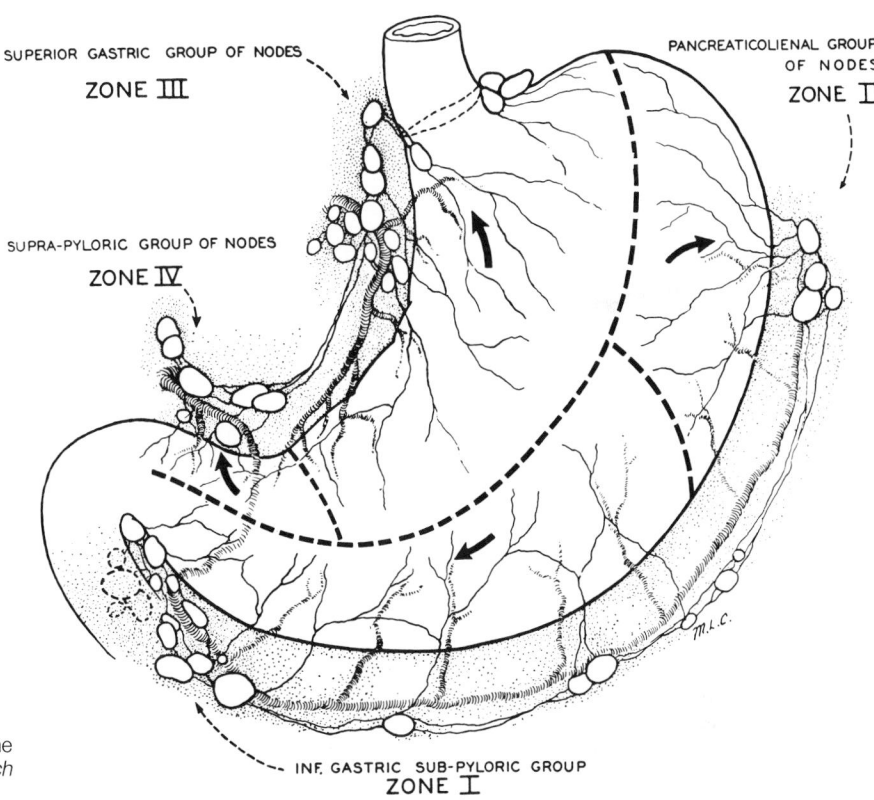

SUPERIOR GASTRIC GROUP OF NODES
ZONE III

PANCREATICOLIENAL GROUP OF NODES
ZONE II

SUPRA-PYLORIC GROUP OF NODES
ZONE IV

INF. GASTRIC SUB-PYLORIC GROUP
ZONE I

Fig. 26-3. Lymphatic drainage of the stomach. (From: *Coller FA, et al: Arch Surg 43:751, 1941, with permission.*)

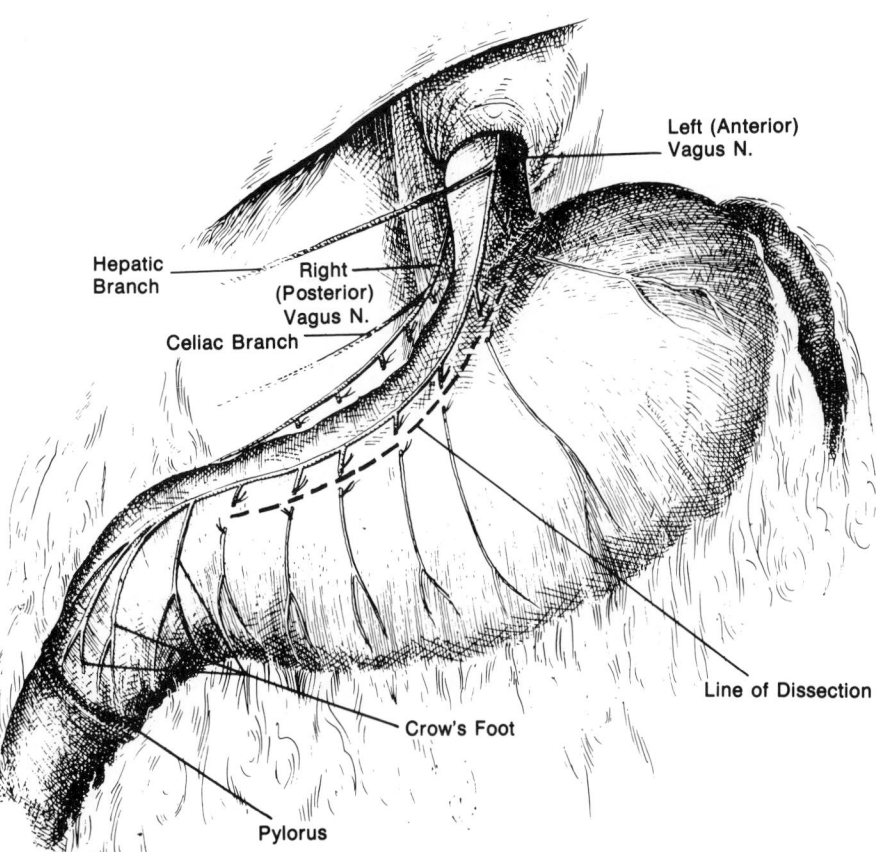

Left (Anterior) Vagus N.

Hepatic Branch

Right (Posterior) Vagus N.

Celiac Branch

Line of Dissection

Crow's Foot

Pylorus

Fig. 26-4. Diagram of the distribution of the vagus nerve within the abdomen. It also shows where the branches of the nerve of Laterjet are divided for a parietal cell vagotomy. (From: *Moody FG: Mt Kisco, NY: Futura, 1:1–15, 1980.*)

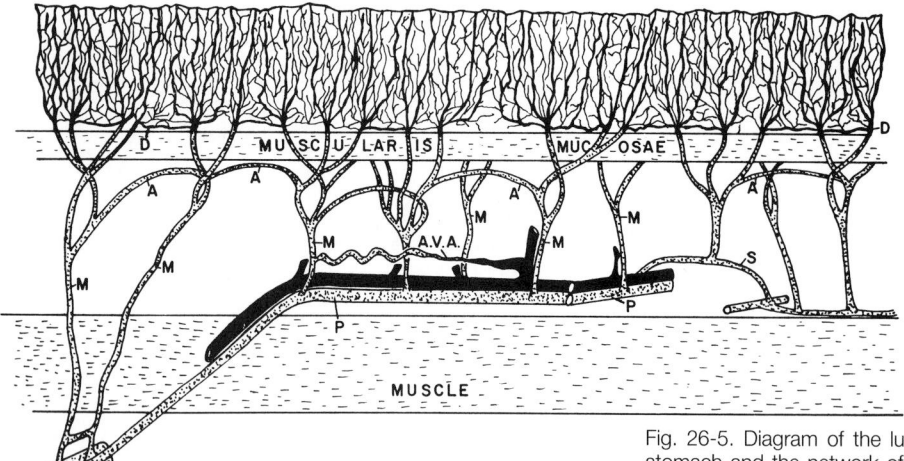

Fig. 26-5. Diagram of the lush mucosal capillary network of the stomach and the network of relatively large caliber arterioles that exist in the submucosa. Legend: D—anastomosing channels; A—anastomosis; M—mucosal arteries; AVA—arteriovenous anastomosis; P—submucous plexus; S—subsidiary anastomosing channels. (From: *Barlow TE, et al: Surg Gynecol Obstet 93:668, 1951, with permission.*)

lar function rather than secretory events within the mucosa. There is, in general, a paucity of knowledge about the precise role that local sympathetic nerves play in gastric function.

MORPHOLOGY. The gastric wall consists of an external serosa that covers an inner oblique, a middle circular, and an outer longitudinal layer of smooth muscle. The submucosa and mucosa provide a continuous inner integument that is separated by a thin sheet of smooth muscle, the muscularis mucosa (Fig. 26-5). A prominent characteristic of the mucosa is a rich mucosal capillary network that

Fig. 26-6. Fundic gastric mucosa illustrating multiple gastric pits (P), some of which are filled with secretion (S). "Cobblestone" appearance of the epithelium is suggested *(arrows)* (×400). *(Courtesy of CA Zalewsky, PhD.)*

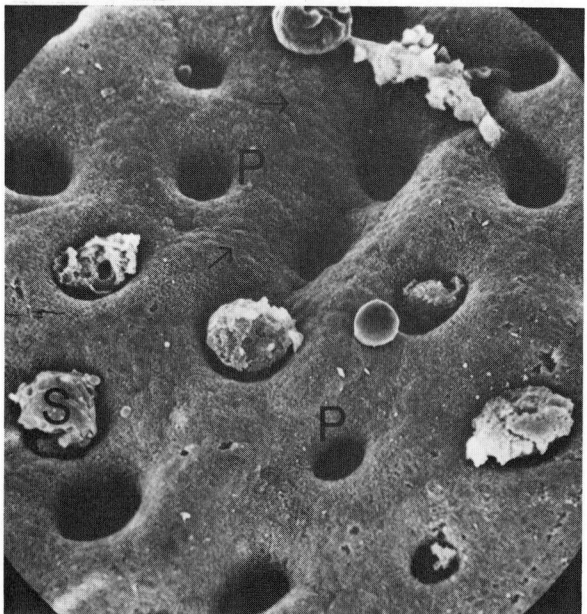

is derived from small arteries that originate in the submucosa. Arteriovenous shunts are rarely seen within the gastric wall.

The mucosal lining of the gastric antrum (distal one-third) is distinctly different from that of the gastric fundus (proximal two-thirds). The latter has an elaborate network of deep glands, four or five of which join an indentation within the mucosal surface called a *pit* or *foveolus.* Individual pits are seen along with the cells that line the interfoveolar area in a scanning electron micrograph in Fig. 26-6. The gastric glands consist of six major cell types: surface, mucous neck, progenitor, chief, parietal, and endocrine cells (Fig. 26-7). The surface epithelial cells are distinguished by abundant mucous granules within their apical surface. These cells are designed to protect the epithelium from ingestants and the injurious effects of gastric acid. They are also the likely source of a sodium-rich alkaline secretion. The mucous neck cells line the entrance to gastric glands. They may serve the purpose of partially buffering nascent acid as it enters the gastric pits. Cells at the base of the gastric pits serve as stem or progenitor cells for the development of new surface cells and also the cells of the gastric glands. Knowledge of the function of the parietal cells distributed within the gastric glands is more secure than that of surface cells, for it has been proved that they are the site of secretion of hydrochloric acid. The characteristics of a resting and secreting cell are shown in Fig. 26-8A and B. Chief cells are the source of pepsinogen, a proteolytic enzyme that is converted to its active form, pepsin, at a pH below 2.5. A variety of endocrine cells exist within the gastric gland. Some secrete gastrin or serotonin, while the function of the others has not as yet been elucidated.

The antral mucosa is less specialized than that within the fundic area. In fact, by light microscopy, one can only identify surface epithelial cells and mucous neck cells. There are no parietal or chief cells. Gastrin-producing

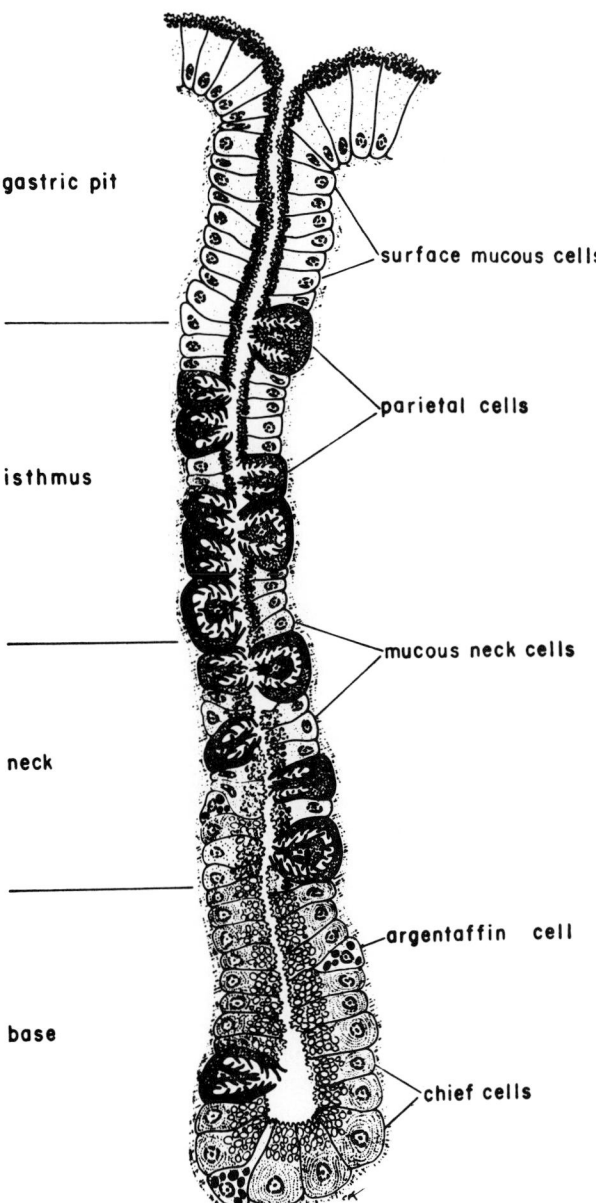

gastric pit

surface mucous cells

parietal cells

isthmus

mucous neck cells

neck

argentaffin cell

base

chief cells

Fig. 26-7. Diagram of a single gastric gland of the bat. Between five and seven of these units open into the base of a single gastric pit (foveolus). (From: *Ito S, et al: J Cell Biol 16:543, 1963, with permission.*)

cells (G-cells), however, can be identified by radioimmunofluorescence.

SPHINCTERS. The entrance of ingestants into the stomach is controlled by a highly specialized 5-cm area of smooth muscle, termed the *lower esophageal sphincter.* This sphincter, which presents a high-pressure zone between the esophagus and stomach, relaxes to allow the passage of foodstuffs. It then contracts to prevent the regurgitation of gastric contents into the esophagus. This sphincter is important because it protects the esophageal mucosa from corrosion by gastric acid.

The lower esophageal sphincter does not have a physical correlate, i.e., an identifiable mound of smooth muscle that can be easily felt and even seen when cut in cross section. By contrast, the pyloric sphincter, which prevents (or minimizes) duodenogastric reflux, is both anatomic and physiologic. It also serves as a metering point for the movement of food particles into the duodenum. Particles that are more than 2 mm in size are rejected and forced back into the body of the stomach for further trituration and preliminary digestion.

PHYSIOLOGY

STORAGE. The major function of the stomach is to prepare ingested food for digestion and absorption as it descends through the small intestine. The process of early digestion requires that solid foodstuffs be stored for a prolonged period of time (4 hours) as they undergo reduction in size and preliminary breakdown into basic metabolic constituents. Once the meal has been processed to an appropriate particulate size and chemical composition, it is delivered intermittently to the duodenum for further digestion.

The storage function of the stomach is greatly enhanced by the process of receptive relaxation. This is an event whereby the upper portion of the stomach relaxes as the intake of food is anticipated. Solid food settles and layers within the greater curvature of the fundic area of the stomach. Liquids pass rapidly from the stomach along its lesser curve (the magenstrasse), thereby leaving the solid mass quite undisturbed. Processing of the food mass is initiated by a skimming from the outermost layers of the gastric bolus. Salivary digestion occurs within its middle and gastric digestion at its periphery. Food particles are reduced in size by a grinding action of the antrum as well as digestion and dilution by the gastric secretions. The storage function of the stomach is enhanced by the antrum and pylorus, which constantly return material to the proximal stomach until it is ready for delivery to the duodenum. A surprising aspect of this very active mechanical process is that it proceeds for several hours after a solid meal without sensation of its occurrence.

Satiety is a feeling of gratification after eating. Morbidly obese individuals do not experience this feeling until they have consumed more food (calories) than they need. Appetite control is based upon genetic, cultural, psychological, environmental, and physical factors, all of which play a role in how much one eats. The pathophysiologic consequence of abnormalities of this appetite control mechanism is obesity more often than malnutrition.

DIGESTION. Gastric digestion involves the breakdown of foodstuffs into fine particles. Starches undergo enzymatic breakdown as long as the pH within the center of the gastric bolus remains favorable for the activity of salivary alpha-amylase (pH > 5). Peptic digestion within the stomach is primarily designed to reduce the size of meat particles and initiate the dispersion of fats, proteins, and carbohydrates by breaking down cell walls. The gastric mucosa also secretes a lipase that assists in the early

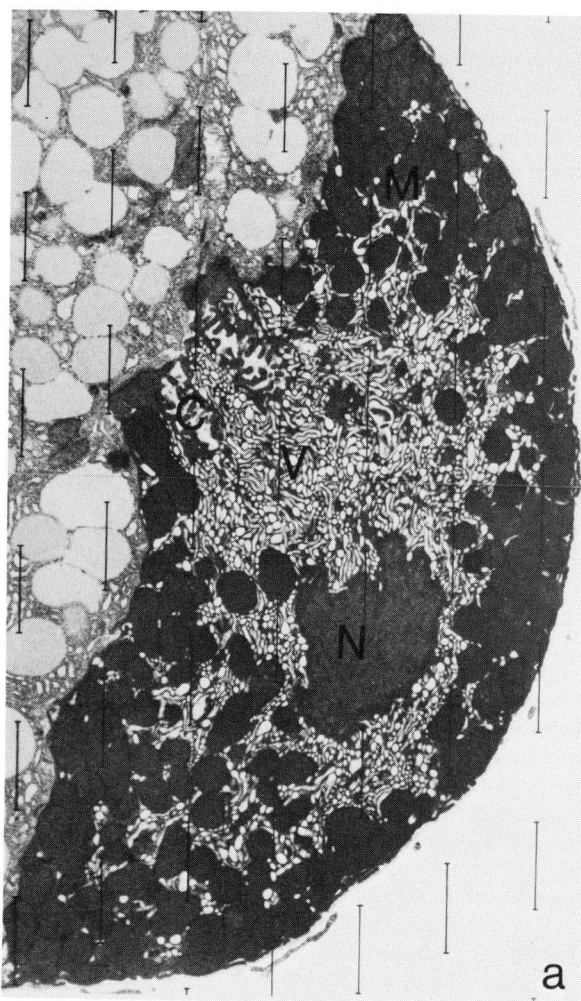

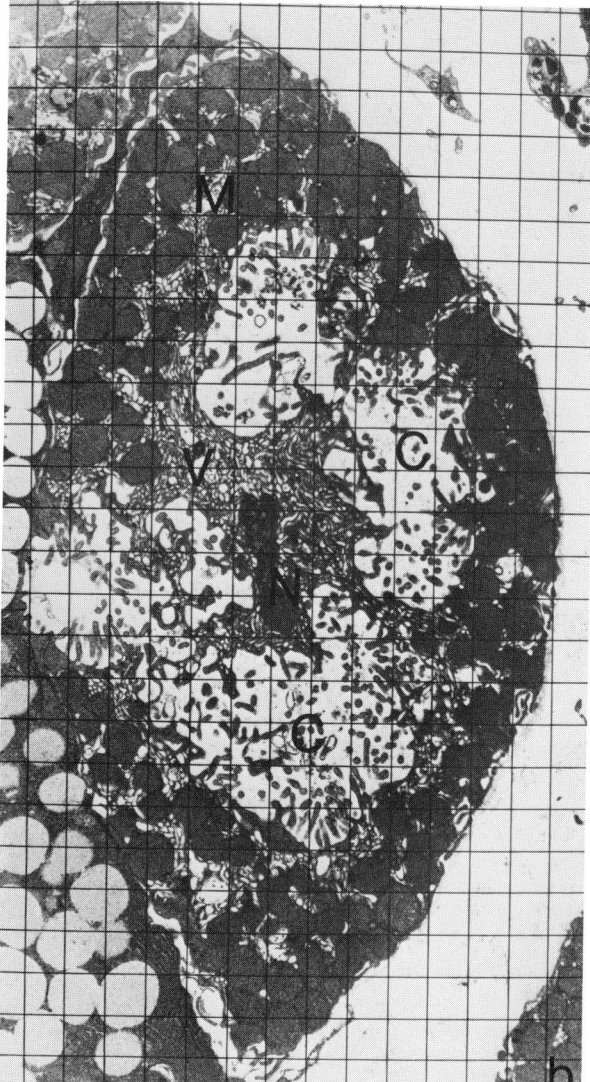

Fig. 26-8. *A.* Resting, unstimulated parietal cell in which the cytoplasm is occupied primarily by tubulovesicles (V) and peripheral mitochondria (M). Apical canaliculi (C) and nucleus (N) are present. A stereometric grid to measure membrane density covers the cell (×9500). *B.* Histamine-stimulated parietal cell with extensive development of canaliculi (C). Remaining tubulovesicles (V) surround the nucleus (N), and mitochondria (M) occupy the periphery. A stereometric grid to measure membrane density covers the cell (×9000). *(Courtesy of CA Zalewsky PhD.)*

phase of fat digestion. The majority of digestion occurs within the duodenum and upper small bowel. The stomach is merely responsible for improving the efficiency of the process.

Gastric Acid Secretion. Acid-peptic disease of the esophagus, stomach, and duodenum represents one of the most common pathologic entities of the foregut. While gastric acid is usually not the single or even the predominant causative factor in peptic diseases, it is a critical component in their genesis. The dictum "no acid, no ulcer" has gained general support since the discovery by Beaumont (1833) that the stomach could secrete hydrochloric acid. Furthermore, all therapies for gastric and duodenal ulcer are based on control of intraluminal pH by either neutralization or inhibition of acid secretion.

It is convenient to consider the secretion of gastric acid in terms of its neurohumoral control. There is only a low rate of acid secretion during the interdigestive period when the stomach is at rest (2 to 3 meq/h). The sight and

smell of food and its ingestion lead to a brisk secretion of hydrochloric acid. This activity is initiated by stimuli that pass from the cerebral cortex to the vagal centers within the hypothalamus. Action potentials descend the vagi and release acetylcholine within the enteric plexuses and their nerve endings in the gastric wall. Acetylcholine in turn leads to the release of gastrin from the antral mucosa and the secretion of acid and pepsinogen from the fundic mucosa. Gastrin is also a stimulant of acid secretion, and its action is greatly enhanced by the vagal release of acetylcholine. Histamine also participates in the acid secretory event and may, in fact, be a critical modulator of the process.

The gastrointestinal hormone, gastrin, is a polypeptide that has been well studied during the past decade since its isolation and purification by Gregory and Tracy. Numerous clinicians and scientists have made important contributions to our understanding of how this hormone might carry out its important activities within the gastrointestinal tract. Foremost among these is the late Morton Grossman who, over a 30-year period, stimulated numerous collaborators to find out how gastrin might contribute to acid secretion in the normal state and in disease. Unfortunately, the answer is still not known. It is to the credit of Yalow and Berson, and their collaborators, that the technique of radioimmunoassay has allowed a reasonably full description of its biologic function.

The vagal release of gastrin is enhanced by antral distension and contact of its mucosa with proteins. The ingestion of a meal is associated with a cumulative release of gastrin that provides for a constant flow of acid secretion during gastric digestion. This gastrin release is facilitated as long as the intraluminal pH is high. Conversely, gastrin release is attenuated by a low pH on the antral mucosal surface. This negative feedback mechanism provides the principal control for the rate of acid secretion. Furthermore, it offers a check on the indiscriminate secretion of acid during the interdigestive period. The process described above is called the "cephalogastric" phase of acid secretion.

The duodenum and intestines also play a role in controlling acid secretion. Acidification of the duodenum leads to the release of secretin. Secretin inhibits both gastrin release and the secretion of gastric acid. Gastrin, which is also present within the mucosa of the duodenum and upper intestine, may be the source of the small stimulus for acid secretion that occurs as the products of a meal move through the intestinal tract. The intestinal phase of gastric secretion accounts for about 5 percent of the cumulative acid secretory response during the ingestion of a meal.

Parietal Cell Function. The parietal cell (Fig. 26-8A and B) is the putative site of hydrochloric acid secretion. In the resting state, its cytoplasm consists of numerous mitochondria and tubulovesicles. With stimulation, there is a remarkable elaboration of membrane into an intracellular canaliculus. This is the presumed site of the transfer of hydrogen ions (H^+) to the luminal side of the plasma membrane into the tubule of the gastric gland. How this occurs is not completely known. A current scheme involves the translocation of a proton (H^+) at some site on the membrane in exchange for a potassium ion (K^+). This H^+ for K^+ exchange requires energy provided by oxidative phosphorylation. The hydrolysis of ATP derived from this process is facilitated by a specific enzyme, adenosine triphosphatase (ATPase). There is speculation that the Cl^- in this process is provided by its own translocation process. The extraordinary aspect of gastric acid secretion is that it moves H^+ against a millionfold chemical gradient (10^{-7} in the blood to 10^{-1} in gastric juice).

The parietal cell will secrete acid in response to acetylcholine, gastrin, and histamine. Acid secretion can be inhibited by a class of agents (cimetidine) that block histamine receptors on the parietal cell (H_2, as opposed to the heart and lung histamine receptors called H_1). Recently, an inhibitor (omeprazole) of the hydrogen-potassium ATPase has been discovered that may have clinical value because of its specificity. Prostaglandins are also potent inhibitors of acid secretion that are being evaluated for their clinical usefulness. Anticholinergics in high doses are partial antagonists of the secretory process, but their pronounced effects on delaying gastric emptying preclude their value as antisecretory agents. Vagotomy profoundly diminishes the response of the parietal cell to gastrin and histamine, an effect that has contributed to its effectiveness as a therapy for peptic ulcer.

Surface Cell Function. The surface epithelial cells line the outermost layer of the gastric epithelium and thereby are exposed to the contents of the gastric lumen. They are relatively impervious to H^+ ions and are protected from mechanical injury by a thin layer of mucus. This mucus layer is renewed constantly by a large number of mucus granules stored beneath the apical plasma membrane. Surface cells also produce a sodium-rich alkaline (bicarbonate) secretion that may play an important role in reducing the pH at the apical surface. This is a new concept that has not yet assumed clinical relevance because of the low rate of alkaline secretion. It is important to recognize that a break in the barrier to H^+ ions may render the epithelium of the stomach susceptible to acute erosive gastritis.

Gastric Analysis. There are a variety of ways to assess the acid secretory capacity of the stomach. The most accurate is to aspirate gastric contents under controlled conditions through a nasogastric tube. It is best to have the patient lying in a semirecumbent position on the left side. The study is commenced by aspirating the stomach of its contents and then instilling and immediately recovering 50 mL of normal saline. Complete recovery reveals appropriate tube placement. Aspirations are then done by hand syringe every 5 min for 1 h. The aspirates are pooled in 15-min aliquots. At the end of the final aspirate, the stomach is stimulated to secrete by the intravenous administration of histalog in a dose of 2 μg/kg, or pentagastrin in a dose of 6 μg/kg. Aspiration is continued as described above, with four 15-min collections obtained over a 1-h period. The volume of the collections is measured, and an aliquot is titrated electrometrically to determine its content of H^+. The rate of secretion is then expressed as the number of milliequivalents produced per hour during the basal or prestimulatory phase and during maximal and peak output. Maximal acid output (MAO) is obtained by averaging the output of the two final 15-min periods. Peak output is the highest rate of secretion obtained during a 15-min period after stimulation. Basal acid output (BAO) is normally 2 to 3 meq/h; secretory output (MAO) is in the range of 10 to 15 meq/h. Patients with duodenal ulcer have higher values, while those with gastric ulcer may have lower values. However, there is remarkable overlap between either condition and the normal. Another role for gastric analysis is its use as a screen for the Zollinger-Ellison (ZE) syndrome. In this illness characterized by flagrant ulcer disease, basal acid outputs may be in excess of 50 meq/h.

Pepsinogen. The role of pepsinogen in gastroduodenal disease has not been well defined. Pepsinogen, a proenzyme, does not assume its proteolytic activity until activated by a pH below 2.5. Pepsin, the activated enzyme, can digest food and devitalized tissue but has virtually no effect on healthy, well-nourished cells. Its role, therefore, in the pathogenesis of peptic ulcer is obscure. The well-circumscribed, clean nature of a peptic ulcer bed, however, is likely a consequence of its activity. Pepsinogen is stored within chief cells in the form of granules whose release is under vagal control. It is interesting that so little is known about a substance that assumes illusionary importance by the terms "peptic ulcer" and "dyspepsia."

GASTRIC EMPTYING. Control Mechanisms. Gastric emptying is modulated by a highly integrated process that includes mechanical, chemical, and neurohumoral mechanisms. Solids are preprocessed in the stomach over a period of hours during which they are reduced in size and dispersed within the gastric juice for efficient digestion. In addition, the osmolality of the chyme is reduced by dilution. The latter function is important in the prevention of the dumping syndrome. Dumping occurs when an osmotic load is delivered to the intestine, causing an influx of water, intestinal distention, and rapid transit of the predigested meal. This leads to light-headedness, sweating, tachycardia, crampy abdominal pain, and diarrhea. It is, therefore, logical that one of the important control mechanisms should include osmoreceptors within the duodenum.

An understanding of the neurohumoral control of gastric emptying is currently incomplete. The observation that truncal vagotomy does not predictably lead to delayed gastric emptying has lead to ambiguity about the role of the autonomic nervous system. In fact, vagotomy may hasten the transit of liquids when a pyloroplasty or gastroenterostomy has been performed. The antrum appears to be the key component in propulsion from the stomach, and its activity is clearly under vagal control. Apparently the myenteric plexuses that are a component of the enteric nervous system can continue to function in response to intraluminal stimulation of food even in the absence of central vagal innervation. Furthermore, denervation causes an increase in serum gastrin as a consequence of loss of antral acidification. Possibly the law of Cannon, in which denervated receptors become more sensitive to chemical stimuli, is at work in this situation, whereby the gastrin receptors that stimulate gastric smooth muscle contractions may be rendered supersensitive to a point of compensating for the loss of centrally mediated vagal release of acetylcholine.

What is known is as follows: Anticipation of a meal leads to vagally mediated gastrin release, gastric acid secretion, receptive relaxation of the proximal stomach, rhythmic antral contractions, and coordinated relaxation of the pyloric sphincter. Ingestion of the meal accentuates all these responses. Emptying of liquids is continuous and relatively rapid, depending on the osmolarity. Solids must

be reduced to a few millimeters in diameter before antral discharge occurs.

Gastric motor function is related in some way to the electromyographic activity within its smooth muscle. The stomach has a pacemaker high on the greater curve that likely initiates contractions in the area by phasic spike potentials that entrain a series of action potentials toward the pylorus (Fig. 26-9). The precise role of the myoelectric entrainment is not understood, nor is it a critical phenomenon since division of the stomach does not interfere with aboral electrical activity or gastric emptying.

Fats delay gastric emptying by an unknown mechanism. Gastric lipase may be responsible in that it is slow to reduce the droplet size of fats. It is also possible that the antral or duodenal mucosa may have a chemical sensor for specific fatty acids. Finally, lipid-related cholecystokinin release may affect gastric emptying by retarding emptying.

Gastric Emptying Studies. There are a variety of ways to assess gastric emptying. The simplest is to instill a known volume of saline into the stomach and attempt to recover it at a fixed time. Lewis recommends instillation at 750 mL into the unoperated stomach. Gastric aspiration at 30 min with returns of less than 200 mL indicates normal pyloric function. Pyloric dysfunction or obstruction usually yields greater than 400 mL. This saline load test can provide a qualitative view of the stomach's capacity to empty a liquid meal. A barium radiograph can also provide some information on adequacy of emptying and may reveal pathology that might contribute to a delay such as pyloric obstruction. Computerized radionuclide scans have provided a quantitative way to measure the emptying rate of liquids as well as solids. Radiolabeled technetium is used to monitor the rate of liquid emptying. The solid phase is measured with radioactive chicken livers. An example of the appearance of such a study is shown in Fig. 26-10. These studies are particularly helpful in patients who have gastric atony from vagal denervation, diabetes, or other associated illness.

OTHER GASTRIC FUNCTIONS. The stomach plays an important role in hematopoiesis through its production of intrinsic factor by the parietal cell. Intrinsic factor is essential for the ileal absorption of vitamin B_{12}. Of added, but not critical, importance is a relationship between acid secretion and iron absorption by the duodenum, a relationship that involves the important role of acid in proteolysis and breakdown of animal cells.

Gastric acidification is also important in maintaining sterility of the foregut. Only a few unusual fusiform bacillae can withstand the challenges of a low gastric pH. It is known that the upper gastrointestinal tract is rapidly colonized by enteric bacteria when the stomach is rendered achlorhydric by medical or surgical means.

Immunologic Sensing. It is reasonable to assume that the gastric mucosa is involved in the detection of harmful ingestants. It is well suited for this purpose with its ability to protect its surface by rapid mucus release, creating an unstirred layer that may form a first line of defense against harmful macromolecules. If potentially dangerous substances (with chemical or oncological portend) should

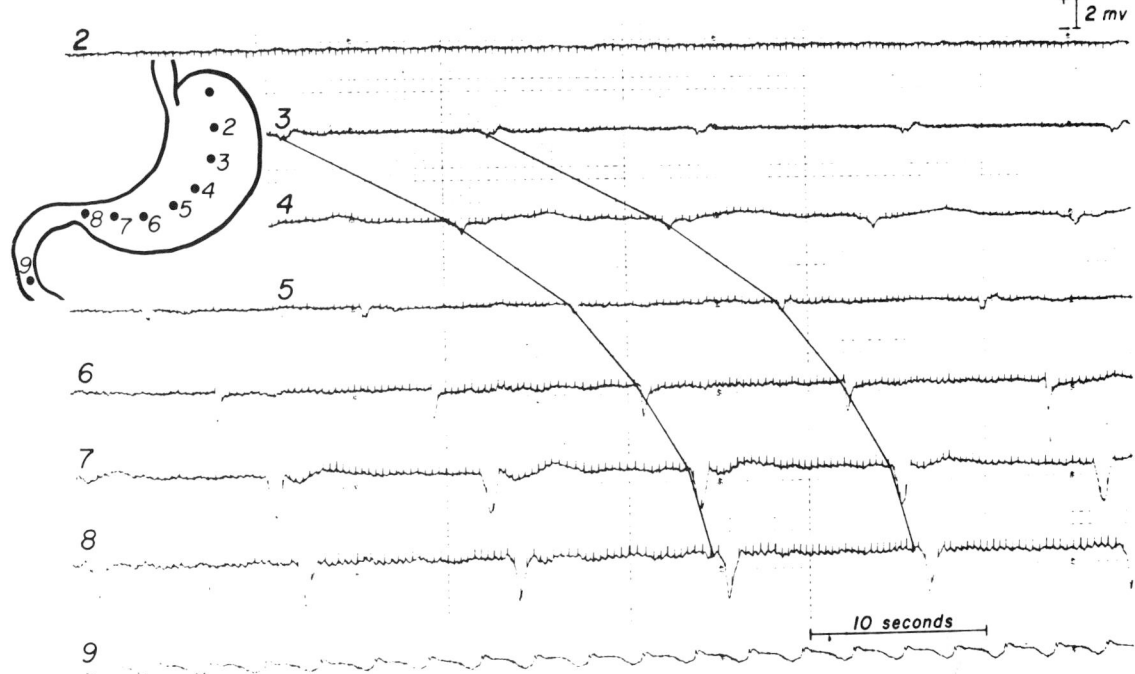

Fig. 26-9. Illustration of electrical activity measured at different sites on the stomach. The recordings demonstrate the distal migration of myoelectric complexes from the gastric pacemaker. (From: *Kelly KA, et al: Am J Physiol 217:465, 1969, with permission.*)

permeate the mucosa, they immediately encounter the lamina propria and its army of mast cells and free-floating macrophages and lymphocytes. The role of the gastric mucosa in immunosurveillance has not yet been elucidated.

Heat Exchange. The stomach with its lush mucosal microcirculation is an excellent heat exchanger. This is an important function, for it ensures the intraluminal contents a relatively stable thermal environment for their

Fig. 26-10. A normal solid-phase gastric emptying study using 100 μC technetium sulfur colloid. Gamma camera images were made at *A*, immediately after ingestion of the radioactive meal; *B*, after 15 min; *C*, after 30 min; *D*, after 45 min; *E*, after 60 min; and *F*, after 90 min. The sequential pictures show more activity in the small bowel and less in the stomach. *(Courtesy of P Christian.)*

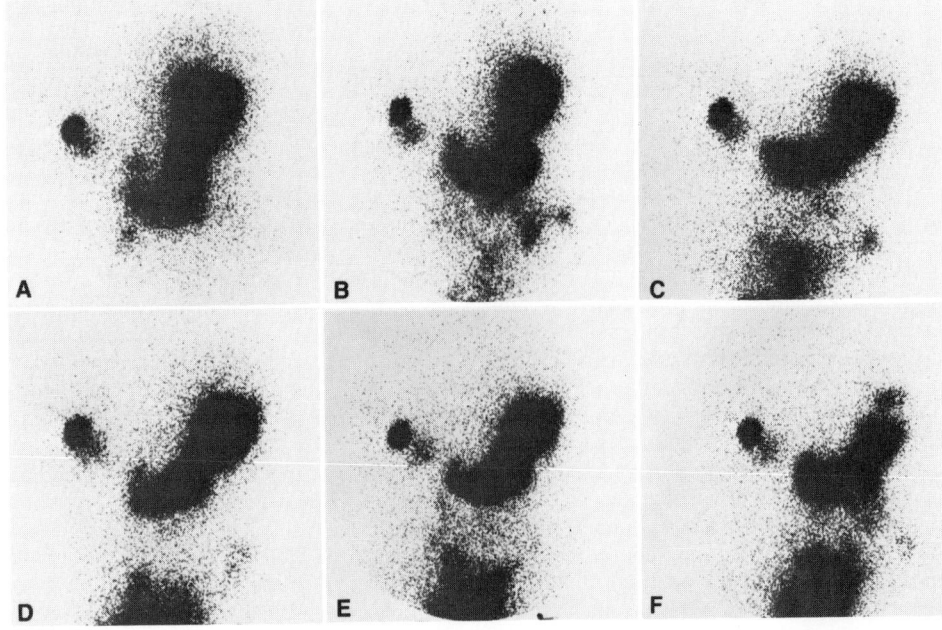

enzymatic digestion. Furthermore, the mechanism offers protection against cooling of adjacent viscera or significant changes in core temperature.

GASTRIC DYSFUNCTION

SYMPTOMS. Anorexia. Lack of appetite, or anorexia, is a common symptom that everyone has from time to time, especially during a viral illness. In fact, it is so frequently associated with psychologic stress that it may initially be overlooked as an early sign of a serious illness. For example, most patients with cancer of the gastrointestinal tract will recall that they were anorectic during the early phase of their illness. Anorexia is usually the reason for weight loss in neoplastic as well as other diseases within the gastrointestinal tract.

Nausea and Vomiting. The gastrointestinal tract is capable of protecting itself from harmful ingestants by a forceful evacuation of its contents through the mouth. Vomiting is a complex process. After a deep breath, the glottis is closed. The stomach then evacuates its contents by retropulsion. The reversed movement of gastrointestinal contents is assisted by a tightening of the muscles of the abdomen and thorax, a decrease in acid secretion, and an autonomic response that includes sweating, pallor, and tachycardia. Nausea is a sensation of impending emesis and may be of central or peripheral origin. It is not always accompanied by vomiting. In fact, many patients with vaguely defined gastrointestinal disease will complain of nausea. It is a symptom that accompanies low-grade visceral pain such as might occur in gallstone disease, mild pancreatitis, peptic ulcer, or the early phase of acute appendicitis.

The vomiting of "intestinal origin" is often associated with other signs such as abdominal distention or emesis of blood (varices, gastritis, or peptic ulcer) or intestinal contents. The character of the vomitus may be helpful in establishing a diagnosis. Lack of bile suggests a point of obstruction above the papilla of Vater. Feculent vomiting is associated with low small bowel obstruction, its brown color and foul odor being a result of bacterial overgrowth by enteric organisms. Obstruction at this level is usually accompanied by generalized abdominal distention, in contrast to chronic pyloric obstruction in which there is distention of the mid and left upper abdomen from a fluid- and air-filled stomach.

Pain. The mucosa of the stomach is devoid of pain endings. This explains in part the relatively painless nature of erosive gastritis, gastric cancer, and even peptic ulcer disease of the stomach. Acute gastric distention may also be a relatively pain-free event, especially in the postoperative period. Acid-peptic disease of the duodenum, however, has a very characteristic pain pattern depending upon the depth of ulceration. Early superficial ulceration is usually associated with a gnawing sensation within the midepigastrium. When acid is unbuffered, such as might occur in the early morning hours, the pain is sharp and more intense. A characteristic of duodenal ulcer pain is that it disappears as soon as an antacid or other neutralizing substance is ingested. Gastric ulcer pain is more

subtle and diffuse in nature, often coming on during or after eating, rather than before. The sudden onset of severe, unrelenting, generalized abdominal pain is a sign of ulcer perforation. This, of course, is a catastrophic event that requires immediate surgical attention.

Regurgitation. The reflux of gastric contents into the esophagus may be associated with three complaints: (1) heartburn, (2) expectoration of gastric chyme, and (3) cough from aspiration. Heartburn is a sensation of mild to moderate substernal discomfort. It is an annoying, diffuse, burning pain that is usually well tolerated by the patient. Not only acid but also alkaline regurgitation can cause this symptom, which may be associated with inflammation within the esophageal mucosa. A severe subxiphoid or substernal pain exacerbated by feeding (odynophagia) is a sign of esophageal ulceration. Difficulty in swallowing (dysphagia) accompanies esophageal obstruction from peptic stricture, esophagogastric cancer, or a primary motor disturbance such as achalasia or esophageal spasm.

Regurgitation is a sign of loss of the high-pressure zone that normally exists between the stomach and esophagus. Recall that the pressure within the body of the esophagus reflects intrathoracic pressure, and therefore is subatmospheric (-5 to -10 mmHg). Gastric pressures are positive, 5 to 10 mmHg. The pressures within the lower esophageal segment (LES) must, therefore, be in excess of 15 mmHg in order to prevent reflux. Factors that control the pressure within the LES are not completely known, but they include vagal release of acetylcholine, intraabdominal pressure, intragastric pressure, and ill-defined humoral mechanisms, which may include cyclic nucleotides and prostaglandins. Pharmacologic doses of acetylcholine, metoclopromide, gastrin, and calcium blocking agents can reconstitute low esophageal sphincter pressures. The LES can also be repaired operatively by wrapping the upper part of the stomach around the lower end of the esophagus (Nissen fundoplication).

SIGNS. Bleeding. Upper gastrointestinal bleeding demands a thorough evaluation of the alimentary tract. Hematemesis (vomiting of blood) may be a dramatic, exsanguinating event, or it may be a manifestation of a minor bleed from gastritis or peptic ulcer. The nature of the vomitus may provide a clue to the rate and site of bleeding. Coffee-ground emesis (acid-hematin) is usually a sign of peptic ulcer. Bright-red emesis may be from an esophageal varix, a gastric mucosal tear, gastritis, or a peptic ulcer. Gastric or duodenal bleeding can occur without hematemesis. In this instance the stool is usually black. More rapid bleeding, however, can result in bright-red stools. Newer technology now permits rapid identification and control of the offending lesion. This is accomplished by upper gastrointestinal endoscopy whereby the esophagus, stomach, and duodenum can be safely and quickly inspected. Bleeding sites can be controlled by electrocoagulation or photocoagulation, and biopsies of suspicious lesions can be obtained for histologic examination.

Weight Loss. Gastric disease, especially neoplasia, is usually accompanied by gradual loss of weight. Benign gastric ulcer is associated with weight loss as a consequence of the avoidance of food which might induce abdominal pain. Duodenal ulcer is usually accompanied by weight gain in response to pain control by the ingestion of milk and other alkalinizing foods.

Gastric Distention. Acute gastric dilatation provokes an intense autonomic response that includes pallor, rapid respirations, bradycardia, and hypotension. This is a dramatic and serious complication that may follow any operation within the abdomen. It can easily be diagnosed by inspection and percussion of the abdomen which reveals a markedly distended stomach. Once recognized, the problem is easily remedied, by the passage of a nasogastric tube and gastric aspiration.

Abdominal Tenderness. Peptic ulcer disease may be accompanied by tenderness on deep palpation within the midepigastrium. This is a common sign when an active ulcer is present within the duodenum; gastric ulcers, except when they penetrate through the gastric wall, are usually nontender. Gastric neoplasms are also not associated with discomfort on palpation. Perforated ulcers are usually accompanied by marked, generalized tenderness in response to the intense chemical peritonitis that accompanies the leak of gastric acid into the abdominal cavity.

Palpable Tumor. Gastric neoplasms of the distal stomach may present as a palpable mass within the epigastrium or left upper abdomen. Gastric tumors can usually be distinguished from mass lesions that arise within the pancreas, since they are more anterior and often movable. Liver tumors are even more superficial and usually will descend with deep inspiration. Neoplasms of the proximal stomach are hidden from detection by physical examination by the left hemithorax.

DIAGNOSIS. Radiography. Visualization of the upper gastrointestinal tract by barium radiography has provided a safe, convenient, reliable way to detect gastric and duodenal disease. Unfortunately, over half of the acute lesions of the duodenum and almost all superficial erosions of the stomach go undetected by this type of examination. It still remains, however, a starting point for patients with chronic symptoms of upper gastrointestinal disease. A normal upper gastrointestinal barium series is shown in Fig. 26-11. Multiple views are required to gain a full view of the stomach and duodenal bulb.

Endoscopy. Patients who present with the signs and symptoms of upper gastrointestinal hemorrhage are usually subjected to endoscopy early in their hospital course, especially when the bleeding is massive or persistent. Endoscopy for chronic symptoms is also a routine procedure that can be done on an ambulatory basis with high yield and little risk or discomfort to the patient. Most gastroenterologists, and an increasing number of general surgeons, are proficient at the technique of upper gastrointestinal endoscopy. An advantage of the technique is the opportunity it provides to obtain photographs and biopsies of suspicious lesions.

POSTGASTRECTOMY SYNDROMES. Operations upon the stomach that include resection, pyloric ablation (pyloroplasty) or bypass (gastroenterostomy), and total gastric vagotomy may be accompanied by unpleasant side effects. For convenience, they have been termed

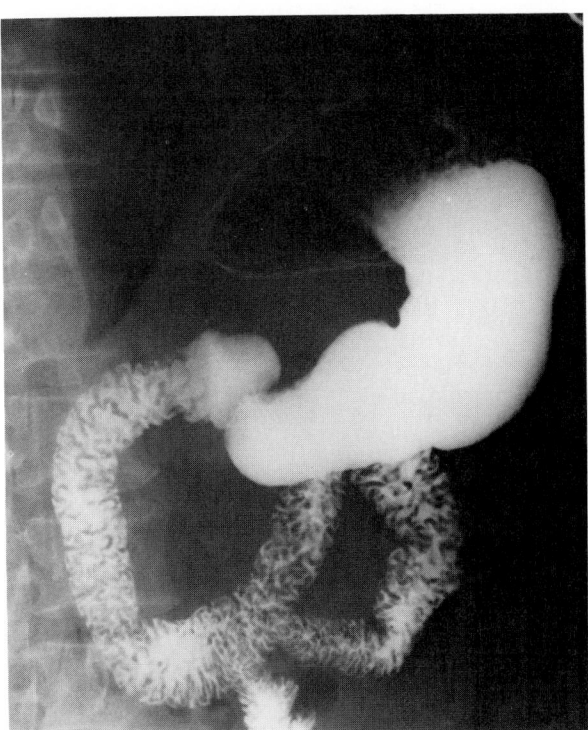

Fig. 26-11. Normal upper gastrointestinal barium radiograph.

"postgastrectomy syndromes" (Table 26-1). They occur to varying degrees in about 20 percent of patients in the early months after stomach surgery. With time and attention to diet, the symptoms disappear in the majority of patients. About 5 percent of patients, however, remain symptomatic for the remainder of their lives, and 1 percent become permanently disabled to a point of being considered "gastric cripples." It is for this reason that lesser procedures such as proximal gastric vagotomy without drainage have replaced the more extensive 75 percent gastric resection or pyloroplasty and truncal vagotomy for the treatment of acid-peptic disease of the duodenum.

Surprisingly, total gastrectomy with esophagojejunal reconstruction is fairly well tolerated by patients who require it for gastric cancer or the Zollinger-Ellison syndrome. They usually remain on the slender side but have few gastrointestinal complaints if they eat several small meals a day. It is essential that they receive injections of vitamin B_{12} on a monthly basis, since they cannot absorb

Table 26-1. POSTGASTRECTOMY SYNDROMES

Small capacity
Dumping
Bile gastritis
Afferent loop
Efferent loop
Postvagotomy diarrhea
Anemia
Metabolic bone disease

it from the gut in the absence of intrinsic factor that formerly came from the parietal cells.

The dumping syndrome, characterized by light-headedness, diaphoresis, palpitations, crampy abdominal pain, and diarrhea, is a consequence of the rapid movement of gastric contents into the upper intestinal tract. It usually is related to the ingestion of a high-carbohydrate meal. Pyloric bypass or ablation appears to be the main contributor to this syndrome. Vagotomy and the type of gastric reconstruction do not appear to be important variables in its frequency. The mystery is why it occurs as a chronic symptom so infrequently.

Extensive gastrectomy is accompanied by early satiety, a symptom called the *small-capacity syndrome*. This is a serious problem, since it can lead to profound weight loss and malnutrition.

Truncal vagotomy requires an accompanying drainage procedure (pyloroplasty or gastroenterostomy); otherwise gastric stasis may lead to nausea, vomiting, or gastric ulceration. The extragastric vagal denervation associated with this procedure may also contribute to gallstone formation and incapacitating, explosive diarrhea.

Bile gastritis has been recognized as a consequence of gastrectomy in recent years. It is an entity that is characterized by vague symptoms of low-grade epigastric pain, chronic nausea, and bilious vomiting. Barium examination of the stomach is usually nonrevealing. Erosive gastritis may be seen during endoscopic examination of the gastric mucosa. Biopsy often reveals round cell infiltration and edema, especially at the site of mucosal lesions. Unfortunately, patients without gastrointestinal complaints may have similar findings. The strongest evidence that bile may be involved in the syndrome relates to the observation that approximately half of individuals who undergo biliary diversion by Roux en Y gastrojejunostomy will gain symptomatic relief.

The afferent loop syndrome is a clearly defined entity that is characterized by bilious vomiting after distal gastric resection and gastrojejunal anastomosis (Billroth II). The patient will complain of a severe midepigastric pain after eating which is relieved by the emesis of a large volume of bile. Its pathogenesis relates to an obstruction at the junction of the afferent limb coming from the duodenum to the gastric remnant. Food usually has already passed from the stomach into the efferent limb; therefore, it is not mixed with the emesis, as is the case when the efferent loop is obstructed. These conditions are mechanical in nature, as a consequence of either recurrent ulcer or a technical error at the time of reconstruction. Their correction requires reoperation.

Acid-reducing procedures of all types can be accompanied by an iron deficiency or even macrocytic anemia. Bile gastritis and duodenal bypass may increase the frequency and severity of hematologic disturbances. Also of concern is an increased incidence of cancer in the gastric remnant after acid reduction procedures for duodenal ulcer. Little attention has been given to the pathogenesis of this unusual but serious complication.

Diarrhea is one of the most common and distressing complaints after gastric surgery. In a small number of patients it contributes to profound, life-threatening malnutrition. In most patients, however, avoidance of foods that contribute to dumping provides a return to a normal bowel habit. Postvagotomy diarrhea is explosive and unpredictable, a most undesirable sequela that has no therapy except antimotility drug control. Occasionally, gastric surgery will unmask nontropical sprue or a lactase deficiency. These conditions can be diagnosed by small bowel mucosal biopsy, with specific histochemical staining for the presence or absence of lactase.

Recurrent ulcer is a disappointing postgastrectomy sequela. Some patients may present with multiple symptoms including dumping, bilious vomiting, and pain from recurrent ulcer. This presents a quandary in diagnosis and management. Most students of the postgastrectomy syndromes are ultraconservative in offering patients further reconstructive surgery, since the results are modest even in the hands of those skilled in the management of such complex problems.

GASTRIC DISEASE

Peptic Ulcer—Duodenum

Peptic ulcer disease of the duodenum is one of the most common illnesses of the foregut. The stomach's complicity relates to the presumed role of gastric acid secretion in ulcerogenesis. While it is true that achlorhydric patients rarely develop peptic ulcers and that most patients with hyperchlorhydria from gastrinoma (Zollinger-Ellison syndrome) have severe ulcer disease, patients with more common forms of duodenal ulcer may not have hypersecretion of acid. It is for this reason that the role of acid in ulcerogenesis is ambiguous and to this day subject to challenge.

PATHOPHYSIOLOGY. Chronic duodenal ulceration is almost never of neoplastic origin except in rare instances of duodenal cancer. Acute ulcers may occur in a setting of extreme psychological or physical stress. The etiology of acute and chronic ulceration is multivariate. It involves aggressive factors, such as gastric acid and pepsin, and protective factors, which include the alkaline duodenal secretions (bile, pancreatic juice, and duodenal secretion from Brunner's glands) and the duodenal epithelium (hydrogen for sodium exchange, bicarbonate secretion, blood flow, and release of antisecretory hormones such as secretin).

Several observations suggest that duodenal ulcer disease in many patients is a consequence of the secretion of acid in excess of the amount that can be efficiently disposed of by the duodenum. Such patients have an increased basal and stimulated acid secretory output. In addition, they have an augmented cumulative gastrin response to an ingested meal. They also have acidification of the duodenum for prolonged periods (pH < 2), an event rarely seen in normal patients. That hypersecretion of acid can cause duodenal ulceration has been well established in experimental animal models. Furthermore, as mentioned above, patients with hypersecretion of acid on the basis of hypergastrinemia from a pancreatic tumor have a severe ulcer diathesis that subsides when acid secretion is controlled by antisecretory agents. The usual forms of duodenal ulcer also heal when gastric acid is either neutralized by ingestion of antacids or inhibited by antisecretory agents.

There is abundant evidence that reduction of duodenal buffers contributes to ulceration. An example is the removal of bile from the duodenum by biliary diversion into a limb of jejunum. Another is the reduction in the flow of pancreatic juice in chronic pancreatitis or following extensive pancreatic resection. Transposition of the bile and pancreatic secretions into the small intestine at a point where they cannot reflux into the duodenum in experimental animals uniformly leads to chronic duodenal ulceration.

The surgical treatment of peptic ulcer has as its rationale the reduction of acid secretory output to a point that will provide permanent cure for peptic ulcer. There has been a gradual evolution of how this can best be accomplished. Initial efforts were directed toward diversion of acid from the duodenum (gastroenterostomy) and reduction of the acid secretory mass by extensive resection. Knowledge that acid secretion is under vagal control has led to vagotomy as a simpler operative approach with less immediate and late morbidity.

CLINICAL MANIFESTATIONS. Chronic duodenal ulcer disease can present in a number of ways. It usually has its onset in early or midadult life and occurs more frequently in males than in females (4 to 1). The clinical stereotype of an intense, compulsive, cigarette-smoking, alcohol-drinking executive has not been well established in careful epidemiologic studies, but such individuals do represent a high-risk group. There may also be genetic factors other than those that relate to families with gastrinoma or hyperparathyroidism as a component of a multiple endocrine neoplasia syndrome (MEN).

Abdominal Pain. The most common feature of duodenal ulcer is a gnawing, sometimes sharp, well-localized midepigastric pain. The pain is tolerable and usually relieved by alkali or milk. It is for this reason that many patients do not seek medical advice until they have had the disease for many years. In addition, the pain is episodic, coming and going over periods of months for unknown reasons. There appears to be a spring and fall seasonal occurrence and a relapse during periods of extreme stress. The development of constant pain is a sign of deep penetration. Referral of pain to the back is often associated with penetration into the pancreas. Generalized severe abdominal pain is a sign of free perforation.

Bleeding. Gastrointestinal bleeding is a common manifestation of duodenal ulcer. This is not surprising, since the duodenal wall has an abundant blood supply, and there are several large blood vessels posterior to the duodenal bulb. In fact, most cases of massive upper gastrointestinal hemorrhage are secondary to a posterior ulcer that has penetrated into the gastroduodenal artery or one of its branches. Most ulcers are more superficial or are located on the duodenal wall that is not adjacent to large blood vessels. This is the reason why most duodenal ul-

cers present with only minor bleeding episodes, usually detected by melenic (black) or guaiac positive feces.

Obstruction. Duodenal ulcer during a period of activity is often associated with delayed gastric emptying characterized by anorexia, or nausea, or vomiting. These symptoms may be a consequence of pylorospasm or obstruction to the gastric outlet by an inflammatory mass. In cases of protracted vomiting, patients may become dehydrated and develop a hypokalemic, hypochlorhydric alkalosis from the loss of large amounts of gastric juice that is rich in hydrogen, chloride, and potassium ions. Therapy, therefore, includes intravenous restitution of these losses and nasogastric suction for control and assessment of replacement needs. Until the chloride and potassium deficits have been replaced, the kidney is unable to correct the metabolic alkalosis.

Long-standing duodenal ulcer, with recurrent episodes of healing and repair, may lead to cicatricial stenosis of the lumen of the duodenum. Patients with pyloric obstruction on this basis usually have painless vomiting of large volumes of undigested food once or twice a day. The stomach in this condition is usually massively dilated and has lost its muscular tone. This form of obstruction may be associated with marked weight loss and malnutrition. Treatment is always surgical after appropriate metabolic and nutritional preparation that may include a period of parenteral hyperalimentation.

Perforation. Penetration of an ulcer through the duodenal wall is usually accompanied by an effort at containment by the greater omentum or adjacent viscera. Occasionally (about 5 percent of the time), a penetrating ulcer will perforate into the free peritoneal cavity. This is a dramatic clinical event, characterized by severe generalized abdominal pain, fever, tachycardia, dehydration, and ileus. This complication represents a surgical emergency. The diagnosis is easily made by palpation of the abdomen, which almost always reveals exquisite tenderness, rigidity, and rebound. Percussion demonstrates loss of liver dullness. An upright radiograph of the chest will usually demonstrate free air beneath the diaphragm. Operation to close the perforation and clean the peritoneal cavity should be carried out within a few hours after the patient enters the emergency department. Operation should be delayed only for appropriate fluid resuscitation. Early intervention will usually reveal sterile exudate within the abdomen; delay will most certainly be associated with a subsequent septic complication. A prompt operation may also provide an opportunity for performing an acid-reducing procedure if indicated.

Zollinger-Ellison Syndrome. The description of an association between a pancreatic tumor and severe ulcer disease by Zollinger and Ellison in 1955 initiated a new era in the study and treatment of acid-peptic disease of the duodenum. Their observation was made before the isolation and characterization of gastrin and the ability to measure its presence in the bloodstream by radioimmunoassay. Gastrointestinal endoscopy was in its early phase of development, and medical treatment for ulcer disease centered on antacids. A great deal of knowledge about peptic ulcer has derived from the study of the Zollinger-Ellison

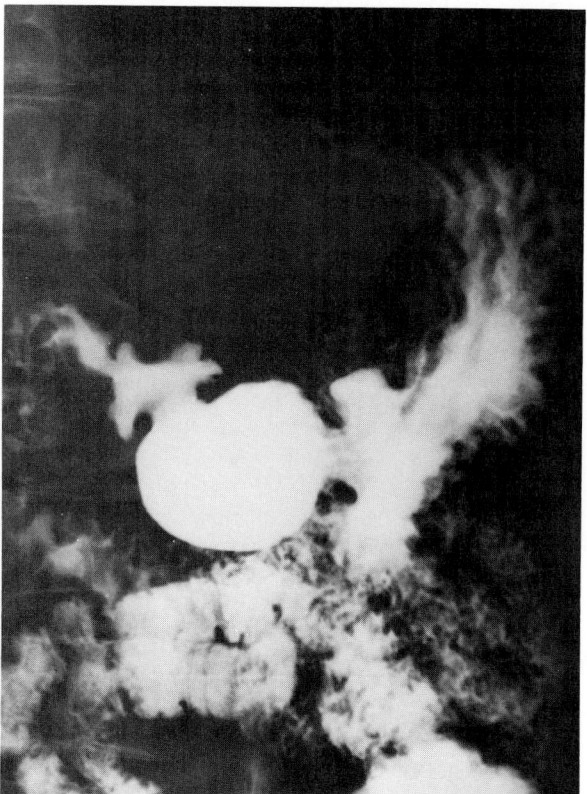

Fig. 26-12. Barium radiograph demonstrating the classic cloverleaf appearance of a deformed duodenal bulb due to the scarring of chronic ulcer disease. *(Courtesy of FA Mann, MD.)*

syndrome, a disease characterized clinically by flagrant duodenal ulcer disease, high basal acid secretory outputs, and a pancreatic tumor. Serum gastrin levels are usually in excess of 1000 pg/mL, but in some cases, the serum gastrin may be only mildly elevated for reasons not yet known. In the latter cases, serum gastrin levels can be increased by provocation with the intravenous administration of calcium or secretin. Increase in serum gastrin to above 350 pg/mL when calcium is infused at a rate of 4 μg/(kg · h) is indicative of a gastrinoma. An increase of serum gastrin in excess of 150 pg/mL in response to a bolus dose of 2 μg/kg of secretin is also considered to be a positive response. The true value of these tests is still being studied.

The pancreatic tumor of Zollinger-Ellison disease is a true neoplasm. In fact, approximately half of the patients have metastases to adjacent pancreatic nodes or the liver at the time of the discovery of the disease. Fortunately, the neoplasm has a slow growth pattern, and survival, even with proved metastases, is in the range of decades rather than months or years, as is true of most gastrointestinal malignancies.

DIAGNOSIS. Active ulcer disease of the duodenum can usually be detected by a directed history and careful physical examination. When epigastric pain and tenderness are the only findings, a clinical trial of antacid or antisecretory therapy may be sufficient to provide symp-

tomatic relief, healing, and in some instances a cure. This is especially true when symptoms are of an acute nature and related to environmental stress. In most cases, however, there is a history of chronic dyspepsia, and activity is manifested by bleeding or incapacitating pain. These symptoms require endoscopic examination of the duodenum to determine the precise nature of the lesion. Examination of the upper gastrointestinal tract by barium radiography is also a useful study to determine the location and depth of penetration of the ulcer, as well as the extent of deformation from chronic fibrosis (Fig. 26-12). Unfortunately, superficial ulceration will not be detected by this technique. False negatives in the range of 50 percent have been documented by follow-up endoscopy when ulcer symptoms are present and barium radiographs are negative. Pyloric obstruction is easily diagnosed by an upright radiograph of the abdomen; perforation is best detected by a chest x-ray also performed in the upright position (Fig. 26-13A and B).

TREATMENT. Medical. The medical therapy of duodenal ulcer is based upon the premise that it is a chronic, incurable disease. Treatment, therefore, is directed toward symptomatic relief during periods of acute exacerbation. This is best accomplished by a 6-week course of the H_2 blocker, cimetidine, in a dose of 300 mg four times a day. The frequent (every-hour) ingestion of antacids is as effective as antisecretory therapy for symptomatic relief, but the H_2 blockers shorten the period of complete healing. Furthermore, patient compliance appears to be higher on H_2 blockers in view of the ease of taking a pill and the avoidance of the undesirable intestinal symptoms (diarrhea or constipation) associated with antacid ingestion. Tranquilizers and diets have not proved to be efficacious, although both are employed on an empiric basis by most clinicians. A six-feeding bland diet may help to reduce the gastric phase of acid secretion. Tranquilizers themselves have a modest antisecretory effect. A new generation of H_2 blockers (ranitidine) are now available that are more potent and associated with even fewer side effects than cimetidine. A highly specific inhibitor of the hydrogen-potassium ATPase is also undergoing human trials (omeprazole). These advances will offer not only the possibility of providing symptomatic relief during activity but also the possibility of protection against recurrences. Knowledge derived from their mechanisms of action may also lead to an understanding of the pathogenesis of the disease and its ultimate prevention. There is no question that acid antisecretory agents have made a profound impact on the treatment of this common disease.

Surgical. Surgical therapy for chronic duodenal ulcer has two purposes: (1) to salvage patients from the life-threatening complications of perforation, massive hemorrhage, and gastric outlet obstruction and (2) to provide cure for the disease in the form of protection from recurrence. The indications for surgery, therefore, include perforation, obstruction, massive bleeding, and intractable abdominal pain.

The objective of therapy for perforation is early recognition of the complication and prompt closure of the opening in the duodenum. This procedure, termed "plica-

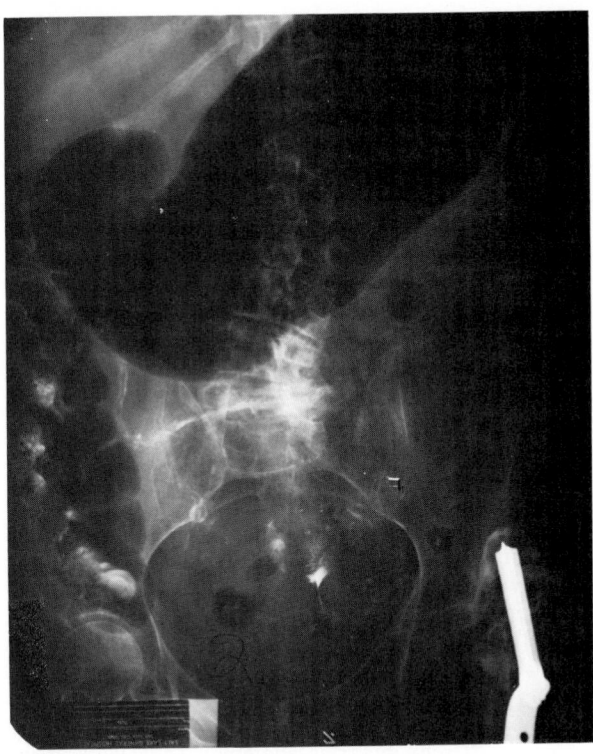

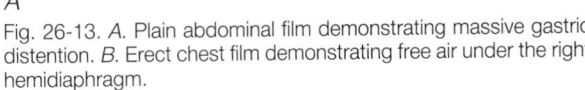

A

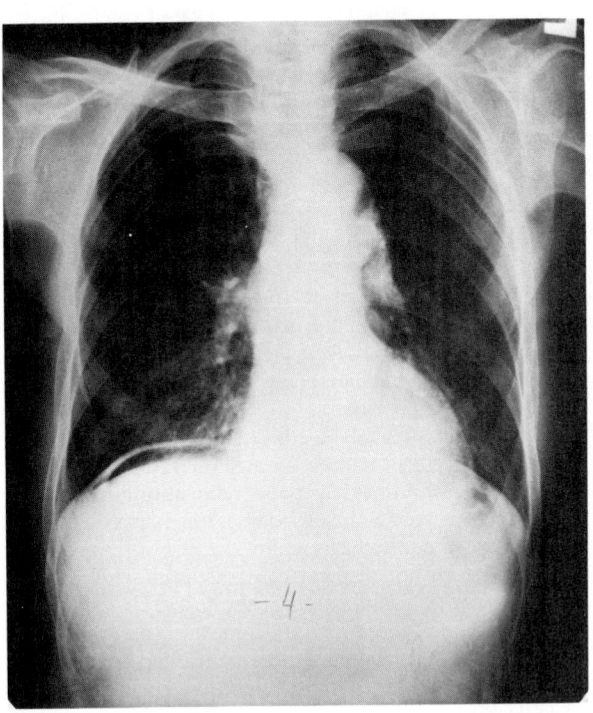

B

Fig. 26-13. *A*. Plain abdominal film demonstrating massive gastric distention. *B*. Erect chest film demonstrating free air under the right hemidiaphragm.

tion,'' is accomplished through an upper midline incision. Usually three or four silk (00) sutures placed in seromuscular fashion across the site of perforation is sufficient for secure closure. It is customary to tie in a tag of omentum with these sutures to provide a biologic buttress, a procedure termed a ''Graham patch.'' Thorough cleansing of the peritoneal cavity by irrigation is an essential part of the operation. A major decision relates to whether an acid-reducing procedure should be performed as part of the therapy. The criteria for this approach include longstanding ulcer symptoms, a perforation of less than 6 h duration, and a patient whose condition is conducive to a longer operation than is associated with simple plication. The procedure of choice is a truncal vagotomy and Heineke-Mikulicz pyloroplasty (Fig. 26-14) with excision of the ulcer that is almost always on the anterior surface of the first part of the duodenum.

Pyloric obstruction can be treated by either a partial gastrectomy or vagotomy and drainage procedure. The former is preferred when the stomach is massively dilated. By this approach, the potentially deleterious effects of vagotomy on gastric emptying are avoided. Truncal vagotomy with pyloroplasty or gastroenterostomy, however, conserves the gastric reservoir and can be done with a lower risk in these patients who may have incompletely corrected fluid and electrolyte imbalance or malnutrition. A newer and more rational approach is the per-

Fig. 26-14. Diagram of the most frequently used drainage procedures: *A*. Heineke-Mikulicz pyloroplasty. *B*. Finney pyloroplasty. *C*. Jaboulay pyloroplasty. *D*. Gastroenterostomy.

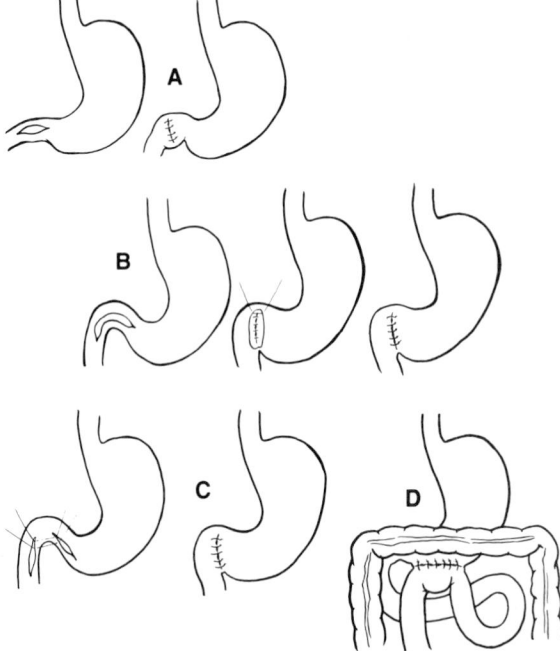

Table 26-2. RESULTS OF OPERATIONS FOR
DUODENAL ULCER

	Mortality	Morbidity	Recurrence
Partial gastrectomy	3%	10%	5%
Vagotomy and antrectomy	2%	12%	1%
Vagotomy and drainage	1%	15%	10%
Proximal gastric vagotomy	0.5%	5%	15%

formance of a proximal gastric vagotomy with either a pyloroplasty or gastroenterostomy (Fig. 26-14). This operation allows for preservation of the antral pump, thereby reducing the incidence of dumping, gastric stasis, and bile reflux gastritis.

Rapid, uncontrolled bleeding from a duodenal ulcer (usually posterior) requires surgical intervention once the intravascular volume has been reconstituted. Immediately upon entering the abdomen, the surgeon incises through the midanterior aspect of the distal 3 cm of stomach and the proximal 2 cm of duodenum. This incision provides direct visualization of the posterior wall of the duodenum, the ulcer crater, and the spurting vessel within its base. Bleeding can be controlled by compression with the left index finger, and the open vessel can then be easily secured by undersewing the finger with 00 silk on a stout needle. Sutures should be placed above and below this point in order to ensure complete encirclement of the gastroduodenal artery in this area. It may be necessary to place sutures deep at all four quadrants of the lesion. Some surgeons prefer a horizontal mattress stitch to encompass the bleeding vessel. Careful suture ligature of the vessel is essential if rebleeding is to be avoided. The operation is completed by a truncal vagotomy and pyloroplasty. A gastric resection should not be attempted because of the possibilities of pancreatic injury, anastomotic leak, or blown duodenal stump, complications that account for the majority of deaths in ulcer surgery.

The management of a medically controlled major bleed, or recurrent minor bleed, is controversial. Availability of effective antisecretory agents has introduced an element of uncertainty in these complications that were considered to be indications for operation in the recent past. Proximal gastric vagotomy is the preferred approach for reasons that will be discussed below.

Intractable pain is no longer a common indication for ulcer surgery. It has been reasonably well demonstrated that patients with intractable pain are usually poorly compliant in their antacid therapy. Antisecretory therapy has improved compliance of medical therapy and may account for the remarkable decrease in the number of cases of intractable pain referred for surgical therapy during the past 5 to 10 years. An operative approach is necessary in truly noncompliant patients or in those who cannot bear the expense or inconvenience of prolonged or repeated courses of H_2 blockage. These individuals should have a proximal gastric vagotomy as the next step in the treatment of their disease.

The relative advantages of the various operations for duodenal ulcer are shown in Table 26-2. Notice that proximal gastric vagotomy has a remarkably low morbidity and mortality but has a recurrence rate that is comparable with or even higher than truncal vagotomy and drainage. Antrectomy and vagotomy provide the best assurance of a low recurrence rate but at a mortality and morbidity that would be unacceptable for patients with easily controllable ulcer symptoms, which represents the majority. Candidates for vagotomy and antrectomy include patients who are to undergo an elective operation for a major complication of their ulcer and who are at high risk for recurrence. These would include individuals in high-stress situations, heavy smokers, chronic alcoholics, and patients who have known high acid secretory rates unrelated to hypergastrinemia. Such patients are usually middle-aged, heavy-set, aggressive, reasonably successful males.

There is some evidence that females do not tolerate truncal vagotomy as well as males. The availability of proximal gastric vagotomy offers an excellent alternative to partial gastrectomy for use in females needing surgery for peptic ulcer. The surgical therapy for duodenal ulcer, other than Zollinger-Ellison syndrome and the exceptions listed above, is based upon the reduction of the acid secretory response by vagotomy. This can be accomplished by division of the vagi above their major abdominal branches, thereby incurring a complete vagal denervation of the intraabdominal viscera. Selective vagotomy, whereby the major trunks are divided below the hepatic and celiac branches to include transection of the nerves of Laterjet, provides for total gastric denervation. Proximal gastric vagotomy, wherein the small branches of the nerves of Laterjet to the fundus are divided close to the gastric wall, leaves the vagal innervation undisturbed to the antrum and other intraabdominal viscera. Truncal vagotomy is currently the most popular method of gastric denervation because of its simplicity. Selective vagotomy is the best way to denervate the gastric remnant following antrectomy, but it does not reduce the incidence of postgastrectomy sequelae. Because of its low early and late morbidity, proximal gastric vagotomy has emerged as the preferred operation for duodenal ulcer when drainage is not required.

Truncal and selective vagotomy may lead to gastric stasis and therefore must be accompanied by a drainage procedure. Three types of pyloroplasty (Heineke-Mikulicz, Finney, and Jaboulay) are recommended for this purpose. They differ in the way in which the pylorus is reconstructed or bypassed, as shown in Fig. 26-14. A gastroenterostomy is also an acceptable way to prevent stasis following truncal gastric vagotomy, but it is more complex than pyloroplasty and therefore used when the latter cannot be easily performed.

Gastric resections are described by the amount of stomach removed: antrectomy (one-third), hemigastrectomy (one-half), partial gastrectomy (two-thirds), subtotal gastrectomy (three-fourths), and total gastrectomy. Except as described below for gastric cancer and the Zollinger-Ellison syndrome, attempts are made to preserve antral function and the gastric reservoir. When resection

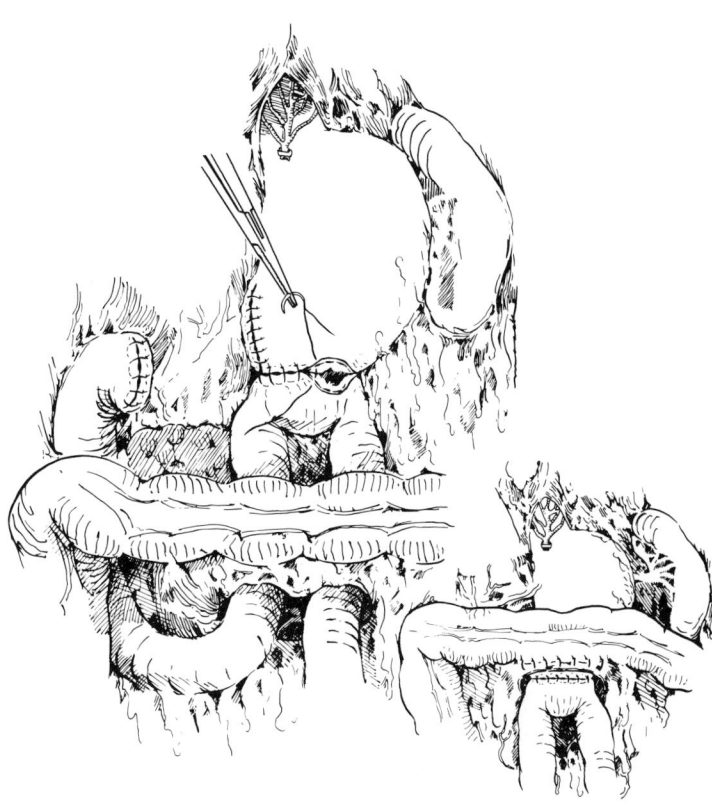

Fig. 26-15. Diagram of a Billroth II gastrojejunostomy placed behind the transverse colon. For cancer, the anastomosis is usually done in front of the colon away from areas of possible recurrence.

is required for benign ulcer of the duodenum or stomach, the gastric remnant is usually anastomosed to the duodenum (Billroth I), whereas resection for neoplasm is usually followed by a gastrojejunostomy (Billroth II) in order to avoid obstruction from tumor recurrence at the anastomosis (Fig. 26-15).

The surgical treatment of the Zollinger-Ellison syndrome has undergone dramatic change in recent years since the introduction of the H₂ blocker, cimetidine. Patients who are refractory to cimetidine or ranitidine usually respond to omeprazole. Dosages of cimetidine in the range of 600 mg four times a day have been effective in controlling the severe ulcer diathesis associated with the syndrome. Unfortunately, medical control precludes staging of the extent of the neoplastic process within the pancreas and adjacent lymph nodes and viscera. In addition, there are increasing numbers of reports documenting that many patients with a gastrinoma gradually become refractory to cimetidine and require total gastrectomy for control of ulcer disease. More recently it has been observed that proximal gastric vagotomy serves as a useful adjunct to cimetidine therapy by rendering the acid secretory cells more sensitive to lower doses of the drug. Another advantage to utilizing proximal gastric vagotomy as a component of initial pharmacologic therapy is the opportunity that it provides for assessing the extent of tumor. Occasionally (<5 percent of the time), the gastrinoma consists of a single tumor mass located within the distal pancreas that is readily accessible to excision and permanent cure. It is generally agreed that Zollinger-

Ellison patients should not have partial gastric resections, since recurrences in this situation can be catastrophic. Total gastrectomy with esophagojejunostomy in Roux en Y fashion (Fig. 26-16) is a safe operation that is well tolerated in the Zollinger-Ellison patient.

Peptic Ulcer—Stomach

ACUTE EROSIVE GASTRITIS

The gastric epithelium is constantly at risk of injury from ingestants in combination with its own secretions. Acute mucosal injury, called *erosive gastritis,* is the most common cause of upper gastrointestinal bleeding and by far the most frequent pathologic process within the stomach. The clinical problem is compounded by its relatively frequent occurrence in the setting of severe illness, or following physical or thermal injury, sepsis, or shock. Stress erosive gastritis has been of particular interest to the surgeon since it may require a surgical intervention in an already critically ill patient. Fortunately, advances in the understanding of the pathogenesis of the disease have led to a variety of ways to prevent its occurrence or progression.

MECHANISMS. The pathogenesis of erosive gastritis involves five variables: (1) acid secretion, (2) rate of back-diffusion of H⁺ ions (the gastric barrier), (3) gastric mucosal blood flow, (4) mucus and alkaline secretion, and (5) submucosal buffers. Obviously, many other factors are involved in maintaining normal epithelial function,

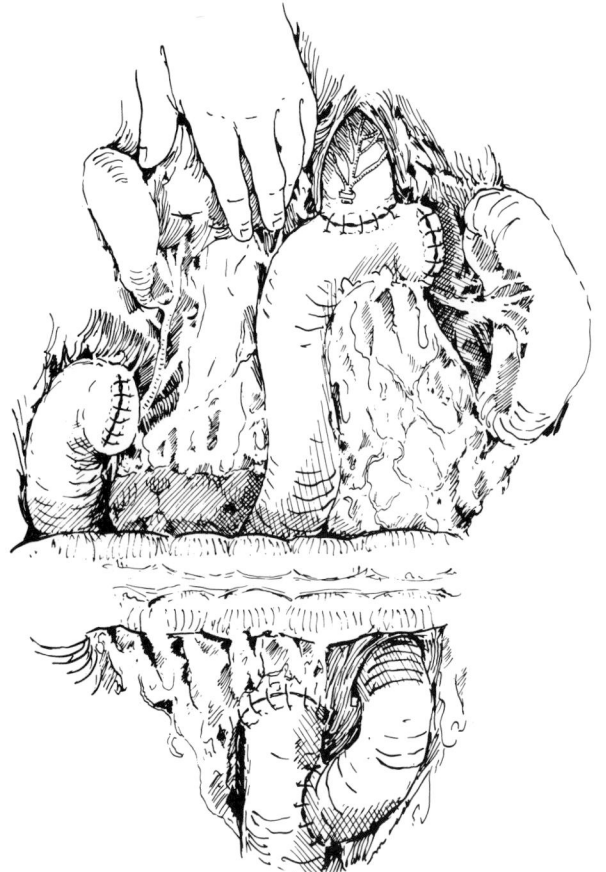

Fig. 26-16. Roux en Y reconstruction after total gastrectomy.

but their role in the pathogenesis of erosive gastritis has not yet been identified.

The dictum "no acid, no ulcer" clearly applies to erosive gastritis. This has been well established in experimental models and in the clinical situation. In fact, it represents the basis for modern therapy of the disease.

The precise role of H$^+$ ions in ulcerogenesis is not known. It has been well established, however, that the gastric epithelium is relatively impervious to H$^+$ ions, thereby accounting for their millionfold gradient from blood to gastric lumen. A disruption of this cation barrier leads to an influx of H$^+$ ions and an efflux of Na$^+$ ions, bicarbonate, and water. Breaking of the barrier by noxious agents such as aspirin, alcohol, or bile salts may lead to acute erosions within the superficial layers of the gastric epithelium. A variety of protective mechanisms attempt to counteract this possibility. Mucus and an alkaline secretion are produced by the surface epithelial cells in an attempt to wash away and neutralize the effects of the barrier breaker and H$^+$ ions by dilution and alkalinization. These functions of the surface cell represent the first line of defense against external injury.

Gastric mucosal blood flow maintains the epithelial integrity by delivery of buffers and nutrients to the gastric cells. Substrates for oxidative metabolism such as oxygen

play a key role in this regard. Curiously, even prolonged intervals of hypoxia or hypoperfusion do not induce injury in the absence of H$^+$ ions and chemical disruption of the barrier. A critical relationship exists between the rate of hydrogen ion back diffusion, gastric mucosal blood flow, and extent of mucosal injury.

The role of mucus and buffer secretion by surface cells is only now being studied in a comprehensive way. Knowledge of these events is much too new to make a clear statement of their importance in the pathogenesis of acute lesions. It is possible that thickening of the mucus coat on the luminal side of the surface cell may provide an unstirred layer that allows entrapment and a titration sink for H$^+$ ions. This theory is currently under study in several laboratories.

Another area of intense inquiry relates to the fate of H$^+$ ions once they permeate the surface cell layer. It has been well established that acidification of the lamina propria can lead to surface cell injury, and that neutralization of this process by parenteral alkalinization can prevent cell loss. For example, the secreting stomach is less prone to experimental injury, possibly as a consequence of the delivery of alkali to the lamina propria following its discharge into the gastric venous effluent after the secretion of an H$^+$ ion into the stomach. The importance of this concept to the clinical problem has yet to be defined.

DIAGNOSIS. Painless upper gastrointestinal bleeding is the clinical hallmark of erosive gastritis. It may be characterized by hematemesis, bloody nasogastric aspirate, melena, or anemia associated with the detection of occult blood in the stool. Pain is uncommon and, when present, is a sign of a penetrating ulcer. Small amounts of blood in the nasogastric aspirate of patients in a critical care setting are so common that they provide enough evidence for making a presumptive working diagnosis without further work-up. Massive hematemesis requires gastric lavage for cleansing and endoscopic examination to determine the anatomic lesion. Superficial erosions rarely bleed rapidly; vomiting of large volumes of blood is an indication of penetration of an erosion into a large blood vessel within the submucosa or the presence of a chronic gastric or duodenal ulcer. Barium studies are not useful in this disease.

TREATMENT. The therapy of erosive gastritis is directed toward intravascular volume replacement and early control of hemorrhage by nonsurgical means. Gastric lavage with room temperature solutions such as water or saline is an important first step in therapy. The stomach must be completely evacuated of its blood contents in order to reduce fibrinolysis at bleeding sites. In addition, the stomach will be stimulated to secrete acid if the antrum is distended by clots. More than 80 percent of patients stop bleeding with this simple maneuver.

The third step in management is to provide for intragastric neutralization. This may be accomplished by inhibiting acid secretion with cimetidine (300 mg I.V. every 6 h) or the instillation of antacids (30 to 60 mL/h) into the stomach, checking its effectiveness by assessing gastric neutrality (pH > 5) by pH-sensitive paper at the end of each hour. The latter process must be pursued diligently if further penetration of erosions with rebleeding is to be avoided. Furthermore, antacid therapy must be included when cimetidine is used in the treatment of erosive gastritis.

If bleeding persists or recurs, the patient should be treated by transendoscopic bipolar electrocautery or by laser photocoagulation. Pharmacologic control by the selective infusion of pitressin into the left gastric artery is also effective, since it induces spasm and thrombosis of the bleeding artery. The associated decrease in mucosal perfusion does not lead to further ulceration if the gastric contents are carefully alkalinized during therapy. Transluminal occlusion of the left gastric artery by a gel forms a clot, or a coil is also an effective way to control bleeding from a branch of this vessel.

Bleeding that recurs or persists, requiring more than 6 units of blood (3000 mL), is an indication for operation. Since most erosions occur in the fundus of the stomach, a long anterior gastrotomy is made in this area. The gastric lumen is cleared of blood, and the mucosal surface is inspected for bleeding points in deeply penetrating lesions. These are secured with silk (00) by a figure-of-eight stitch taken deep within the gastric wall. Each actively bleeding site should be secured in this way. The majority of superficial erosions will not be actively bleeding and do not require ligature unless a blood vessel can be felt or seen at its base. The operation is completed by closure of the anterior gastrotomy and the performance of a truncal vagotomy and pyloroplasty. The incidence of rebleeding is less than 5 percent if bleeding points are carefully looked for and secured.

Some surgeons prefer a liberal partial gastrectomy and vagotomy. In fact, near-total gastrectomy even has its advocates because of concern over the possibilities of rebleeding. This radical surgical approach has no justification except in the rare instance in which suture ligature with vagotomy and pyloroplasty fails.

PREVENTION. An understanding of the importance of intragastric neutralization in erosive gastritis has provided a rationale for the prevention of the disease in critically ill patients. The efficacy of alkalinization has been established by randomized controlled trials. Inhibition of acid secretion by cimetidine has emerged as a useful adjunct to antacid therapy, since it reduces the need for instillation of large volumes of buffer that can lead to undesirable side effects. Cimetidine alone, however, does not provide adequate protection.

Prostaglandins of the E series have emerged as a potentially important group of compounds that may in themselves offer protection to the gastric epithelium. Their mechanism of action is not precisely known, but they may work through stimulation of mucus and alkaline secretion, enhancement of mucosal blood flow, or inhibition of acid secretion. The importance of the latter biologic property of prostaglandins has been challenged, since prostaglandins provide cytoprotection at dosages below those that inhibit acid secretion, and noninhibitory prostaglandins can also prevent experimentally induced gastritis. Prostaglandins have not yet been made available for clinical use because of undesirable side effects.

CHRONIC GASTRIC ULCER

DIFFERENTIAL DIAGNOSIS. Chronic gastric ulceration presents a unique challenge in diagnosis since malignant and benign lesions share many clinical and pathologic features. The advent of endoscopic biopsy and brush cytology has reduced uncertainty in this area, but a significant false-negative rate (5 to 10 percent), i.e., the lesion is neoplastic but the biopsies are benign, still exists. It is for this reason that patients with gastric ulcer require careful follow-up by radiographs and repeat endoscopy with biopsy if the ulcer persists. Gastric analysis can also be helpful since achlorhydria to maximal histamine stimulation excludes the possibility of a peptic ulcer.

The pathogenesis of a benign gastric ulcer remains unknown. Several prominent contributing factors are age (>forty), sex (female/male, 2/1), ingestion of barrier-breaking drugs such as aspirin, and malnutrition. Numerous attempts have been made to implicate chronic gastric ischemia, but with little success. The occurrence of the lesions on the lesser curvature at the junction of the antral and fundic mucosa suggests the possibility of a breakdown of mucosal protective factors at that site, but there is no evidence to support this speculation. It has been well demonstrated, however, that patients with gastric ulcer have an epithelium that is ''leaky'' to H^+ ions. This observation has suggested that regurgitation of bile acids and other barrier breakers within the duodenal succus may play an important role in the disease. Against this possibility is the fact that the experimental rerouting of bile through the stomach by a cholecystogastrostomy does not cause ulceration. Furthermore, chronic gastric ulceration is uncommon in patients with a gastroenterostomy, a situation in which bile is constantly bathing the mucosa of the gastric antrum. The most compelling evidence that the disease is acid-peptic in origin relates to the rapid healing that follows antacid therapy or vagotomy, even when the lesion-bearing portion of the stomach is left intact.

Ulceration within a gastric cancer is somewhat easier to explain. This lesion is most likely a consequence of local ischemia and malnourishment of the tissues within the center of the neoplastic process. It is easy to visualize how this might occur as the younger cells at the advancing edge of the penetrating neoplasm deprive the older cells within its center of nutrients and oxygen. The bulk lesion and infiltration of the gastric wall as revealed by barium radiographs provide the major diagnostic clues of the neoplastic nature of malignant ulcers. Furthermore, achlorhydria precludes peptic digestion of devitalized cells within the ulcer bed, resulting in an irregular, shaggy appearance in contrast to the clean, well-demarcated base of a benign peptic ulcer.

SYMPTOMS. Lack of appetite with vague upper abdominal distress following a meal is a common presenting complaint of patients with a benign gastric ulcer. This form of dyspepsia usually is accompanied by a gradual loss of weight as a consequence of a decrease in the intake of food. Severe pain is an unusual manifestation of the disease, except when the ulcer is located within the distal stomach or pyloric channel. Ulcers in this location assume the characteristics of a duodenal ulcer in that they are associated with increased rates of acid secretion, epigastric pain during the interdigestive period, and prompt relief with antacid ingestion. Gastric ulcers in the proximal stomach have less dramatic symptomatology and consequently may assume a large size and extensive depth of penetration before their detection.

Massive hemorrhage is an unusual event in chronic gastric ulceration; melena, or the detection of occult blood in the stool, is common. Gastric outlet obstruction as manifested by nausea and vomiting is also a rare finding, while delayed gastric emptying is frequent and the likely source of the vague "indigestion" experienced by this patient population.

DIAGNOSIS. Radiography. The upper gastrointestinal barium radiograph is the first step in diagnosis after a careful history and physical examination have focused attention on the stomach as the likely source of the patient's complaints. This is a simple, safe, convenient study that provides a great deal of diagnostic information in the hands of a well-trained radiologist. The radiographic characteristics of a benign gastric ulcer are shown in Fig. 26-17. A common mistake in the diagnostic approach is the utilization of endoscopic visualization of the lesion without obtaining a barium study. The two procedures complement each other. Their order of performance is obvious; barium examination performed first serves to identify the presence and location of a lesion

Fig. 26-17. This air contrast barium radiograph shows an ulcer with smooth margins. The rugal folds radiate toward the ulcer crater. This is the typical appearance of a benign ulcer. *(Courtesy of FA Mann, MD.)*

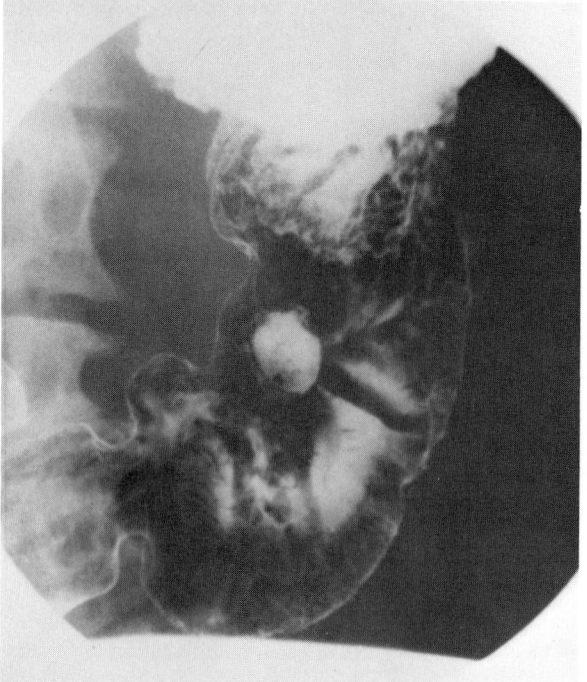

and the probability of its benign or malignant nature; subsequent endoscopy with biopsy provides a histologic diagnosis.

Endoscopy. The endoscopic appearance of a gastric ulcer offers information about its pathologic identity. Benign lesions usually have a well-demarcated, "punched-out" appearance, with a smooth base and a sharp, flat margin. Malignant ulcers usually have an irregular, "heaped-up" margin and a rough, necrotic-appearing base. Unfortunately, there is overlap, especially between benign ulcers and ulcerating cancers early in their genesis. This is why careful endoscopic biopsy at multiple sites at the margin of all gastric ulcers is a mandatory diagnostic procedure. It should not be omitted even when the radiograph and the eye suggest that the lesion is benign in appearance.

TREATMENT. Medical. The initial therapy for a benign gastric ulcer is a so-called medical trial. Unfortunately, there is no specific therapy for a gastric ulcer, since its etiology is unknown. The empiric use of antacid therapy appears to hasten the rate of ulcer healing. H_2 blockers such as cimetidine may also be a useful adjunct, but they were not found to be more effective than antacid therapy in ulcer healing. There has been a great deal of interest in diet manipulation that includes abstention from alcohol, spicy foods, and large meals that might aggravate symptoms associated with delayed gastric emptying. A six-feeding bland gastric diet is usually recommended for this reason. Aspirin and other barrier-breaking drugs (nonsteroidal, anti-inflammatory agents) must be stopped during the period of therapy. Sulfated glycoproteins (sucralfate), a new generation of antiulcer agents, appear to hasten the healing rate of gastric ulcer by binding to the devitalized tissues within the ulcer bed and thereby protecting it from further peptic digestion. Cytoprotective agents such as the prostaglandins of the E series may also play a role in the future of patients who must take barrier-threatening drugs on a chronic basis. This is currently an active area of investigation.

Unfortunately, some gastric ulcers, even when benign, fail to heal at a satisfactory rate (6 weeks) to provide symptomatic relief or assurance that they are not neoplastic. This situation requires a period of hospitalization for further evaluation and careful supervision of medical therapy. Since gastric ulcers are notorious for their tendency to recur even after a successful course of medical therapy, an operative approach should be considered early in patients with recalcitrant or recurrent benign gastric ulcers or when malignancy is even a remote possibility.

Surgical. The indications for surgical management of benign gastric ulcer are fairly clear-cut and include persistent bleeding, perforation, obstruction, failure to heal, recurrence, and suspicion of malignancy. Combined gastric and duodenal ulcer is also best treated by an acid-reducing procedure such as truncal vagotomy and antrectomy to include resection of the gastric ulcer. In fact, it is important to keep in mind that the surgical treatment of gastric ulcer must include a consideration of the presence of duodenal ulcer disease, since the rate of anastomotic ulcer is high (50 percent) if only a distal gastrectomy is used for this purpose.

The most popular operation for a benign lesser curvature gastric ulcer is a distal gastrectomy (antrectomy) to include the ulcer. Gastroduodenostomy is preferred since it reduces the risk of bile gastritis, iron deficiency, and afferent loop syndrome. The recurrence rate and incidence of undesirable side effects are low with this approach in the absence of duodenal ulcer disease or an overlooked cancer.

High-lying gastric ulcers near the esophagogastric junction present a special challenge in management. These can be locally excised or left in place in conjunction with a truncal vagotomy and pyloroplasty. Giant (>4 cm) benign ulcers are also a problem, since they may require an extensive gastric resection. Usually they occur in a malnourished, elderly patient who may have an underlying chronic disease. These patients are best managed by a period of hospitalization, parenteral hyperalimentation, and interval surgery (4 to 6 weeks) if inability to eat persists. Usually the ulcer reduces to a small size or heals during this period. Distal gastric and pyloric channel ulcers should be treated as a duodenal ulcer, since they usually are similar in their clinical presentation and relationship to acid hypersecretion.

Gastric Neoplasia

MALIGNANT TUMORS

The vast majority of gastric tumors are malignant, and of these, adenocarcinoma of the stomach is by far the most common (95 percent). Lymphomas (4 percent) and leiomyosarcomas (1 percent) constitute the rest, except for rare lesions such as squamous cell carcinoma, angiosarcoma, carcinosarcoma, and metastasis from adjacent or distant primary sites.

Cancer

Epidemiology. Gastric cancer is a biologically aggressive disease that is virtually incurable when discovered in its symptomatic phase. While it is worldwide in occurrence, its frequency varies greatly. Chile, Japan, and Iceland have the highest incidence. The disease is rarely encountered in Malaysia. The United States has experienced a rapid decline in stomach cancer deaths from a rate of 30 per 100,000 in 1930 to 8 per 100,000 today. The reason for this favorable trend is not known. Nor is the high incidence in some geographic areas understood, although a high consumption of smoked fish appears to be a characteristic common to these high-risk populations. Patients with pernicious anemia and blood group A also have an increased incidence of the disease, suggesting that genetic as well as environmental factors play a role. An important clue to pathogenesis is the high incidence of gastric cancer observed in the gastric remnant following operation for duodenal ulcer. This lesion is presumed to have its origins within the bile-induced gastritis so commonly found in this patient population.

Symptoms and Signs. Anorexia with weight loss is the most common sign of gastric cancer (>95 percent). Unfortunately, patients are relatively asymptomatic until there is extensive involvement of the gastric wall and adjacent viscera, or widespread metastases. Massive hematemesis occurs in less than 5 percent of patients, although the finding of occult blood in the stool is common. Nausea and vomiting may occur when distal lesions encroach upon the pylorus. Dysphagia is a dominant symptom when cancer arises within the cardia of the stomach. Pain is a late and uncommon complaint. While abdominal tenderness is a rare finding, a palpable abdominal mass is common (50 percent). Hepatomegaly is also a frequent finding and must arouse suspicion of liver metastases. Peritoneal seeding may cause massive ascites or involvement of the ovaries (Krukenberg tumor) or pelvic cul-de-sac (Bloomer's shelf) by gravitational metastases. These manifestations of advanced gastric cancer may lead to pelvic pain and constipation. A palpable lymph node in the left supraclavicular space (Virchow's node) is also a sign of advanced malignancy.

Pathologic Features. Gastric cancer may involve the stomach in a variety of ways (Table 26-3), even though each type usually originates from the progenitor cells at the base of the gastric pits. The most favorable form of the disease is superficial spreading carcinoma. In that condition, the neoplastic process does not penetrate through the muscularis mucosa, nor is it associated with a breakdown of the epithelium and chronic ulceration. Early detection by endoscopic biopsy and gastrectomy is associated with a good prognosis (75 percent with 10-year survival). Lesions of this type are usually detected by mass screening of high-risk populations by endoscopic visualization or photography.

Most symptomatic gastric cancers are infiltrating lesions that penetrate deep into the gastric wall. The luminal portion of the neoplastic process may be represented by a bulky tumor mass, a polypoid excrescence, or a flat, ulcerating lesion. Large cancers of this type are easily detected by radiography or endoscopy. Linitis plastica is an extensive infiltration of the gastric wall without tumor or ulceration. This form of gastric cancer produces a peculiar "leather-bottle" appearance to the gastric radiograph because of the rigid, nondistensible stomach.

Gastric cancer may spread in four ways: (1) lymphatics, (2) bloodstream, (3) peritoneal seeding, and (4) direct extension. More than half of the patients already have tumor spread at the time they seek medical therapy. It, therefore, is important to recognize high-risk groups. A family history of gastric cancer, detection of pernicious anemia, unexplained weight loss, and gastric symptoms that have their onset many years after gastrectomy re-

Table 26-3. TYPES OF GASTRIC CANCER

Superficial spreading
Polypoid
Ulcerative
Scirrhous-linitus plastica

quire careful medical evaluation. There is concern that chronic hypochlorhydria, even when obtained by H_2 blockers, may present a high-risk situation since bacterial overgrowth within the stomach may allow a buildup of oncogenic substances such as nitrosoureas.

Natural History. The tendency for gastric cancer to be advanced at the time of its detection has led to considerable therapeutic nihilism. This is not entirely justified, since gastric resection can provide excellent palliation in most patients and an occasional cure when the cancer is confined to the gastric epithelium. The latter form of the disease mimics chronic gastric ulcer. Even when such neoplastic ulcers are neglected, patients with them may survive for prolonged periods of time.

Chronic wasting and progressive weakness and cachexia constitute the usual mode of death. Liver and pulmonary metastases are common. Metastases to bone are uncommon; therefore, pain is usually not a major problem in management. Nutrition becomes the rate-limiting step in maintaining function due to mechanical or functional gastric obstruction caused by the cancer.

Therapeutic Alternatives. The therapy of gastric cancer is primarily surgical. Radiation and chemotherapy have little to offer even in the way of palliation. Except in advanced cases of carcinomatosis, a palliative subtotal gastrectomy should be done to provide a route for oral alimentation. When there is no evidence of distal spread, a radical subtotal gastrectomy should be performed for cure. This operation includes resection of the gastrocolic omentum and ligation of the right gastric, right gastroepiploic, and left gastric arteries at their origin. Approximately 4 cm of the proximal duodenum is included in the resection. More than 85 percent of the stomach is removed, and gastrointestinal continuity is reestablished by a gastrojejunostomy. Splenectomy and even total gastrectomy may be required when the lesion is large or within the proximal portion of the stomach.

Gastric resection usually provides a symptom-free interval of 1 or 2 years. Recurrences may respond to chemotherapy, although such responses are usually of short duration. The reported 5-year survival rate when gastric resection is performed for cure is less than 10 percent. Clearly, efforts must be directed toward early detection and prevention if survival statistics are to be improved. Mass screening in Japan by gastroscopy has established the validity of an aggressive public health approach. Cure rates are reported in the range of 85 percent at 5 years when gastric cancer is discovered in an early stage, when it is still confined to the epithelial surface of the stomach.

Lymphoma (Lymphosarcoma)

Gastric lymphoma may occur as an isolated neoplasm confined to the stomach, or it may be a manifestation of widespread infiltrative disease. The lesion may present as a tumor mass or, more commonly, as a thickening of the rugal epithelial folds secondary to lymphocytic infiltration within the submucosa. Anorexia and weight loss are the most common presenting complaints. Early satiety may also be a prominent symptom as the gastric wall becomes thickened, and the lumen is progressively compromised by the neoplastic infiltrate. Bleeding is uncommon.

Definitive diagnosis is made by endoscopic biopsy. Bulky lesions, with associated gastric outlet obstruction, are best treated by subtotal gastric resection and postoperative irradiation. Radiation therapy alone, however, provides a long-standing remission that is equal to that obtained by gastric resection in most cases. Radiation, in fact, has emerged as the treatment of choice because of its low morbidity. A combined approach is associated with an 85 percent, 5-year survival when the process is limited to the stomach. Involvement of the stomach by generalized lymphosarcoma is usually treated by radiation or chemotherapy. Gastrectomy in such cases is undertaken only when complications ensue or when the stomach is the major source of disabling symptoms, e.g., obstruction.

Leiomyosarcoma

This tumor of smooth muscle origin is the least common of gastric malignancies. Unfortunately, it usually grows to a very large size before detection because of its outward growth away from the gastric lumen. Distal spread, however, is late, and even massive tumors that become adherent to the liver or pancreas can be resected with prolonged survival. Leiomyosarcomas are not responsive to radiation or chemotherapy. They usually are detected following a gastrointestinal hemorrhage from a breakdown of overlying epithelium or as a consequence of malnutrition secondary to compromise of gastric storage capacity. They often are palpable on abdominal examination when they present in this way. Preoperative assessment can be enhanced by visceral angiography in order to determine mesenteric or hepatic vascular interrelationships to the tumor. Cleansing and chemical preparation of the large intestine are also useful, since resection of its transverse portion or splenic flexure may be required in order to encompass the tumor. Resection is the preferred treatment, even when all the tumor cannot be safely removed, since long-term survival is usual even in this incurable situation.

BENIGN TUMORS

Polyps

Papillary excrescences of the gastric epithelium (polyps) are the most common benign tumors of the stomach of clinical significance. They are of two types—inflammatory and adenomatous. While the latter are less common, they represent the more important lesion, since they are true neoplasms and may have a malignant potential. They can be distinguished from inflammatory polyps because of their long stalk and tendency to occur in the atrophic mucosa of patients with pernicious anemia. Occasionally, adenomatous polyps will arise in the stomach in conjunction with the multiple small bowel polyposis of the Peutz-Jeghers syndrome or the familial polyposis of Gardner's syndrome.

Inflammatory polyps are usually sessile excrescences within the antrum or fundus of the stomach. They are asymptomatic, except when they are adjacent to and prolapse through the pylorus. Hypertrophic gastritis

(Menetrier's disease) may also be associated with multiple inflammatory polypoid lesions within the fundic area of the stomach. These lesions can be distinguished from multiple gastric adenomatous polyposis by biopsy and histologic examination. They do not require surgical extirpation.

Gastric polyps should be biopsied and excised by ensnarement through the endoscope when their adenomatous nature has been determined. Malignant polyps should be treated as a gastric cancer by a partial gastrectomy. Patients with pernicious anemia require careful monitoring by gastric barium radiograph or endoscopy in order to detect neoplastic polyps early in their genesis.

Leiomyoma

Small, benign leiomyomas are commonly found within the smooth muscle of the gastric wall at autopsy or during palpation of the stomach at laparotomy. They are of little clinical significance until they enlarge to greater than 4 cm in diameter. At this point, they begin to compromise the blood supply to the overlying gastric epithelium. This leads to ulceration and proteolytic digestion of the core of the neoplasm that itself may have undergone central necrosis. This process culminates in a massive upper gastrointestinal hemorrhage that may require emergency gastric resection for control. Such lesions when large cannot be distinguished from their malignant counterparts and therefore should be treated by distal gastrectomy with a liberal margin (4 cm) proximally. Smaller lesions (<4 cm) can be shelled out of the gastric wall or removed by a wedge resection.

Lipoma

Lipomas of the stomach are asymptomatic submucosal lesions that are a radiographic curiosity, distinguished by their smooth contour. Endoscopy will reveal their submucosal position. They need not be biopsied or excised.

Ectopic Pancreas

Rarely, a pancreatic rest will reside within the antrum of the stomach. While this lesion is usually submucosal, it often will present within the gastric lumen as an umbilicated dimple. It may require excision if there is a question about its nature or when patients present with unremitting dyspeptic symptoms that are refractory to antiulcer therapy.

Other Gastric Lesions

HYPERTROPHIC GASTRITIS (MENETRIER'S DISEASE)

Menetrier's disease is a rare inflammatory disease of the gastric epithelium that is characterized by massive gastric folds within the proximal stomach. In advanced stages, the epithelium assumes the appearance of large multiple polypoid excrescences as shown in Fig. 26-18. Histologic examination reveals that the thickened folds consist of a hypertrophy of the gastric glandular epithelium as well as a remarkable increase in the size of the submucosa that is edematous and contains a large number of small round cells. The latter finding has suggested that the disease may have an autoimmune component.

Menetrier's disease is characterized clinically by the massive amount of plasma proteins that can be lost through an epithelium that ordinarily is extremely tight to large molecules. The reason for this extraordinary event

Fig. 26-18. Gross appearance of hypertrophic gastritis (Menetrier's disease).

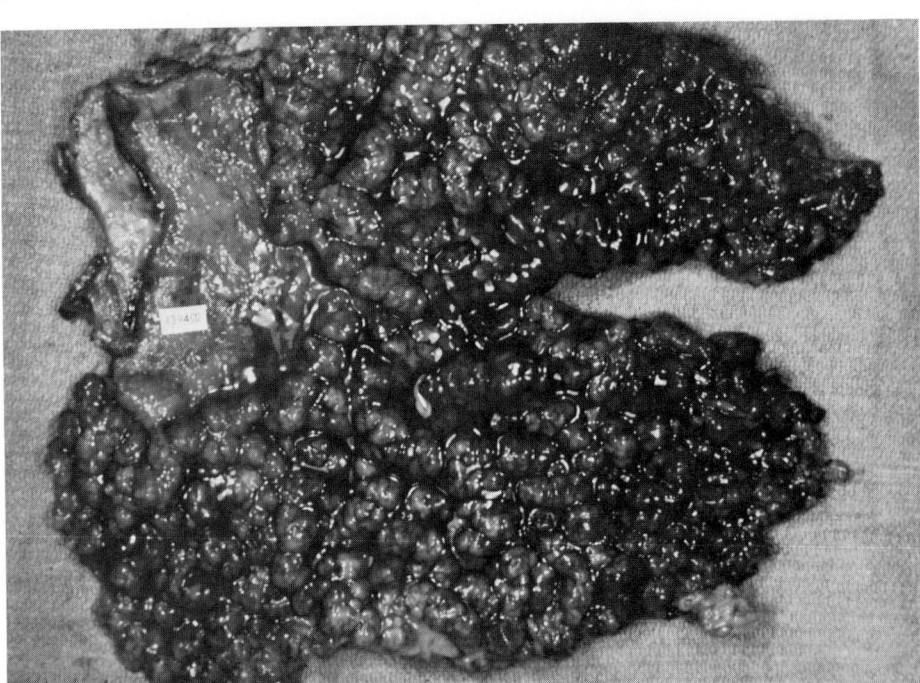

is not known. The immunologic aspects of the disease have not yet been studied.

Most cases of hypertrophic gastritis can be managed nonoperatively with treatment directed toward maintaining good nutrition and symptomatic relief of the vague gastric complaints offered by these patients. Rarely, loss of plasma proteins is so persistent and rapid that hypoproteinemia ensues. If left unrecognized, a state of severe protein deprivation may develop (kwashiorkor), with its attendant hepatic dysfunction, ascites, and peripheral edema. Cases with massive protein loss should have a total gastrectomy following a period of parenteral hyperalimentation. Individuals with less severe forms of the disease should be followed carefully by barium or endoscopic examination in view of the high incidence of gastric cancer reported in some series.

MALLORY-WEISS TEAR

Violent retching can lead to a disruption of the gastric mucosa high on its lesser curve at the esophagogastric junction. The usual story is that of retching after ingestion of solid food, which is followed shortly thereafter by bright red hematemesis. The mucosal tear often extends deep into the submucosa where a large arteriole is encountered as the source of bleeding. However, this lesion is associated with massive upper gastrointestinal bleeding in only 10 percent of cases. Alcoholics with portal hypertension may have as their source of bleeding a submucosal gastric or esophageal varix.

The diagnosis is suspected by history and confirmed by esophagogastroscopy. Rapidly bleeding lesions require immediate operation following reconstitution of intravascular volume. Nonactively bleeding tears can be safely observed and usually proceed to complete healing without symptoms or further evidence of bleeding.

The operation for persistent bleeding from a Mallory-Weiss tear is carried out through an upper midline incision. The lesion at the esophagogastric junction is approached through a long anterior gastrotomy. This provides a full view of the bleeding site which is secured by several deep 2-0 silk ligatures placed in such a way that the mucosal edges are reapproximated in an anatomic fashion. A supplemental antisecretory operation is not necessary. Extension of the tear into the lower end of the esophagus may require mobilization of the esophagogastric junction in order to approximate the margins of the esophageal component of tear. The operation is completed by a fundoplication whereby the upper part of the stomach is wrapped around the lower end of the esophagus. This provides protection to the closure. Furthermore, lesions of this type often occur in association with reflux esophagitis and direct hiatal hernia.

GASTRIC MUCOSAL PROLAPSE

There is uncertainty about whether the prolapse of antral gastric mucosa through the pylorus can lead to gastrointestinal symptoms. Unfortunately, it is observed as a radiologic finding in some patients with symptoms of acid-peptic disease who otherwise have no other findings to explain them. It is unlikely that the nonspecific complaints offered by such patients are a consequence of this radiographic curiosity.

ACUTE GASTRIC DILATATION

Sudden rapid distention of the stomach is associated with a vagovagal response characterized by pallor, sweating, bradycardia, hypotension, and abdominal pain in the nonsedated patient. Unfortunately, many patients develop this problem early after an operative procedure when they are under the influence of anesthetics and analgesics. If left unrecognized, gastric dilatation may lead to vomiting with aspiration, tissue decompensation from hypoxia, or bleeding from stress erosive gastritis. Treatment consists of nasogastric aspiration which can be dramatic in providing relief of associated symptoms. The stomach often requires a period of 24 to 48 h to regain normal emptying. Nasogastric aspiration should be maintained throughout this period of recovery.

GASTRIC VOLVULUS

Torsion of the stomach is an uncommon, serious complication that occurs in association with a paraesophageal hiatal hernia. In this condition, the stomach, which is located within the mediastinum in an orad-caudad reversal (upside-down stomach), can rotate in a clockwise manner, thereby entrapping ingestants, air, and gastric juice. The associated distention and venous obstruction lead to ischemic gangrene of the gastric wall and subsequent perforation. It is for this reason that patients with the otherwise relatively asymptomatic condition of paraesophageal hiatal hernia are advised to have an operative repair. The procedure usually involves returning the stomach to the abdominal cavity and closure of the large opening within the diaphragm adjacent to the right crus.

FOREIGN BODIES AND BEZOARS

The stomach becomes a repository for objects other than food that are taken into the mouth. Infants and those who are mentally deranged represent those most vulnerable to this complication. Children most commonly swallow coins, small parts of toys, or their diaper pins when they are very young. As a rule of thumb, blunt objects that enter the stomach will usually pass on through the intestinal tract. Sharp objects should be retrieved by endoscopy. If this cannot be easily accomplished, the progress of the object should be followed radiographically while carefully observing the patient for signs of perforation. Adults may ingest numerous large objects that make endoscopic retrieval both time-consuming and difficult. These cases usually require operative evacuation. Bulky, solid, nondigestible objects, retained for prolonged periods of time, may, even when single, require operative extraction.

Bezoars are conglomerates of nondigestible materials usually of vegetable origin. Persimmon peels or pits, orange or grapefruit pulp, or fruit pits are the usual offenders, especially in the postgastrectomy stomach. Patients of this type must be advised to avoid foodstuffs that have a great deal of cellulose or other vegetable fiber. Bezoars are associated with vague upper abdominal discomfort, nausea, and vomiting. A barium radiograph will reveal a mass lesion within the lumen of the stomach. Treatment consists of dissolution of the undigested bolus by ingestion of proteolytic enzymes such as papain or by mechanical fragmentation via the endoscope. Recurrence can be prevented by dietary management.

ATROPHIC GASTRITIS

Pernicious anemia is associated with a gradual thinning of the gastric epithelium of the proximal stomach and a complete loss of parietal cells. This results in achlorhydria and a loss of the secretion of intrinsic factor which is responsible for the absorption of vitamin B$_{12}$. A deficiency of this vitamin will develop within 3 or 4 years if it is not provided by monthly replacement (1000 μg I.M.). Atrophic gastritis itself does not produce symptoms. Its major significance is a high risk for gastric malignancy.

EOSINOPHILIC ANTRITIS

Rarely, eosinophils may infiltrate beneath the submucosa of the antrum, producing a nodular deformity. Patients with this lesion usually present with ill-defined complaints. The diagnosis can be confirmed by endoscopic biopsy. The pathogenesis and natural history of these lesions are unknown. Careful follow-up and observation are therefore essential if for no other reason than to learn what the clinical significance of this lesion might be.

CORROSIVE GASTRITIS

The ingestion of strong alkali or acid may lead to gastric as well as esophageal injury. Lye remains a principal cause of this problem even though alterations in packaging of caustic materials have decreased the frequency of accidental ingestion. Suicide attempts by ingestion of large volumes of liquid lye lead to severe erosive esophagitis and gastritis. The subsequent healing process may be associated with gastric outlet obstruction as well as esophageal stricture. Gastric perforation, however, is unusual.

The ingestion of strong acid (sulfuric or hydrochloric) may lead to a full-thickness perforation of the stomach. History of this form of caustic injury requires endoscopic visualization of the gastric epithelium. The identification of large areas of epithelial necrosis should lead to immediate exploration and resection of the involved stomach.

GASTRIC PROCEDURES FOR MORBID OBESITY

RATIONALE. Morbid obesity is a condition wherein people exceed twice their ideal weight. This physical state is not associated with symptoms or disease in early life. By midlife, however, the morbidly obese may develop hypertension, carbohydrate intolerance (adult-onset diabetes), degenerative arthritis, cardiopulmonary dysfunction, or gallstones. Possibly of equal importance is the fact that afflicted individuals are forced to live a suboptimum life since our culture is designed for slim people.

The pathogenesis of morbid obesity is poorly understood. Of the many factors involved, probably the most dominant is a combination of a genetic predisposition and an affluent society where there is an abundance of food. Childhood or teenage onset obesity appears to have this background. However, obesity that starts in midlife does not usually reach massive proportions. Obesity has been presumed to be an inequality of energy intake versus expenditure. Recent results from both animal and human studies suggest that body weight is not always directly related to the amount of food one eats. Some obesity may result from an inability to burn off excess calories as heat, leading to storage of these calories as fat. It is speculated that this disturbance in thermogenesis is due to a decreased amount of brown adipose tissue.

It is generally agreed that morbid obesity is refractory to medical therapy. Jejuno-ileal bypass, wherein the length of the small bowel is shortened, has been an effective way to induce weight loss in the morbidly obese. Its efficacy has been based upon the malabsorption of excess food. Diarrhea associated with overeating also contributes to a reduction in food intake. Unfortunately, the operation which involves anastomosis of the jejunum 14 in. beyond the ligament of Treitz to the ileum, 4 in. from the ileocecal valve, requires bypass of the majority of the small bowel. The bypassed segment in some way contributes to the development of liver disease in 5 to 10 percent of patients. Malabsorption is associated with fluid and electrolyte abnormalities in an additional 5 percent. Over 50 percent of jejuno-ileal bypass patients develop oxalate kidney stones. Bloating with crampy abdominal pain is also a common complaint. These side effects have led to an abandonment of the procedure.

OPERATIONS. Gastric operations for morbid obesity are designed to reduce the daily intake of food to less than 800 cal until weight reduction has been achieved. A variety of such operations have been developed and evaluated by Edward Mason and his colleagues at the University of Iowa. These procedures are depicted in Fig. 26-19. Gastric bypass, which consists of constructing a small proximal pouch that is drained into a loop or Roux en Y limb of jejunum, is the oldest and still the most popular procedure. Its disadvantages include a high operative morbidity, a 5 percent incidence of stomal ulcer, and uncertainties as to the future problems associated with bypass of the lower stomach and duodenum.

Attempts to gain and maintain weight loss by gastroplasty (gastric partition) have been less successful even though perioperative mortality and complications have been less. This procedure is accomplished by placing staples across the upper portion of the stomach. The size of the proximal pouch and stoma is usually similar to that employed in gastric bypass. Stomas have been placed on

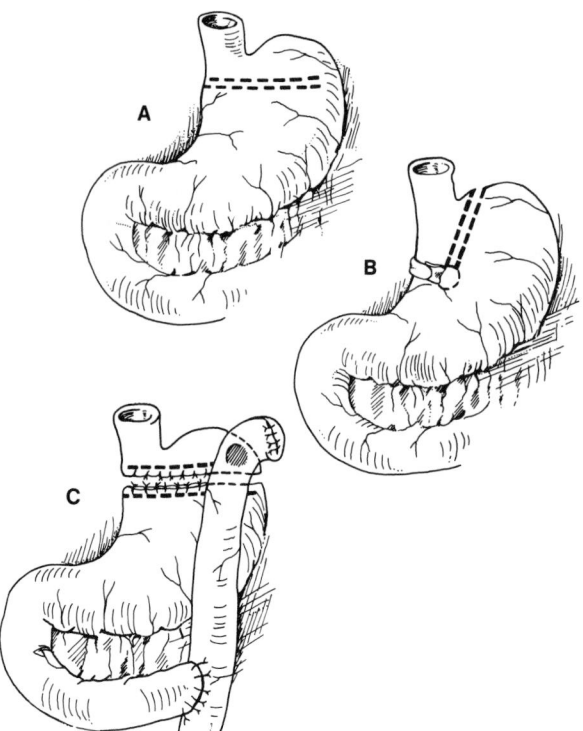

Fig. 26-19. Most common procedures designed to reduce gastric capacity and induce weight loss. *A.* Horizontal gastric partition. *B.* Vertical banded gastroplasty. *C.* Gastric emptying.

<table>
<tr><td colspan="2">*Table 26-4.* MAJOR COMPLICATIONS OF GASTRIC BYPASS*</td></tr>
</table>

Wound infection	14%
Wound hernia	6%
Splenectomy	2%
Subphrenic abscess	2%
Gastric leak	5%
Pouch ulcer	3%
Pouch obstruction	5%
Bile gastritis	1%
Pneumonia	2%
Atelectasis	3%
Embolism	1%
Early reoperation	7%
Readmission for vomiting	5%
Postoperative death	
Pulmonary embolus	0.6%
Peritonitis	2%

* Adapted from Mason EE: Surgical treatment of obesity, in Ebert PA (ed): *Major Problems in Clinical Surgery*. Philadelphia, Saunders, 1981, vol XXVI, p 154.

either curvature of the stomach or its middle with comparable results. This procedure, called *gastric partition* or *stapling,* has a low morbidity and allows for subsequent visualization of the lower stomach and duodenum by radiography or endoscopy. In addition, the potential harmful side effects of antral and duodenal bypass can be avoided. Unfortunately, many patients ultimately lose the feeling of early satiety that they experienced in the early postoperative period (12 to 18 months). As they increase their intake, they stretch the pouch and the stoma. Ultimately, they are able to eat larger meals and slowly regain weight. Attempts to overcome this problem include use of a circumferential suture to prevent stomal dilatation, vertical rather than horizontal stapling to utilize the lesser curve as a nonelastic or less stretchable portion of the stomach, and gastric wrapping whereby the lumen is compromised by infolding of the gastric wall. These variations are currently under investigation.

RESULTS. There is no ideal operation for chronic morbid obesity. In fact, it may be an incurable disease at this stage because of our lack of understanding of its origins. For this reason safety and avoidance of long-term side effects must take precedence over efficacy as it might relate to a long-term cure. While gastric partition provides the best chance for safe palliation and retention of the integrity of the upper gastrointestinal tract, it does not provide for the rapid, extensive weight reduction that accompanies gastric bypass. However, gastric partition is still in the early phase of perfection and evaluation.

Mason and his colleagues have reported the largest and best studied series of patients undergoing gastric bypass. Their mortality and morbidity are shown in Table 26-4. More recently, they have abandoned gastric bypass in favor of gastric partitioning, currently performed by fashioning a 30-mL pouch along the proximal lesser curvature that communicates with the main stomach by a 1-cm conduit that is encircled by a Teflon ring. This is called a *vertical banded gastroplasty* since staples are placed in a vertical manner from the angle of His caudad in order to fashion the proximal pouch. Mason feels that this is the ultimate in gastric procedures for morbid obesity. However, the follow-up is too short for his results to support this contention. The need for performing an operation so deforming to the gastric outlet to gain dietary compliance is further testimony to the complex nature of the disease for which it is designed. The development of a multidisciplinary team approach has strengthened the follow-up and improved the results in most series. Dietary counseling, motivational support, exercise instruction, and social rehabilitation through a self-help group have greatly enhanced the effectiveness of the surgical approach.

Mason has pointed out that all forms of gastric capacity reduction will provide a 50 percent loss of excess weight in 75 percent of patients so treated. The remaining problem is that of long-term weight containment, which can be achieved only by a lifetime of dieting. For most patients with morbid obesity, this means 1000 cal or less each day for the rest of their lives.

Bibliography

History

Beaumont W: *Experiments and Observations on the Gastric Juice and the Physiology of Digestion.* New York, Dover, 1959.

Blalock JB Jr: History and evolution of peptic ulcer surgery. *Am J Surg* 141:317, 1981.

Jordan PH Jr: Duodenal ulcers and their surgical treatment: Where did they come from? *Am J Surg* 149:2, 1985.

Wagensteen OH, Wagensteen SD: Gastric surgery, in *The Rise of Surgery*. Minneapolis, University of Minnesota Press, 1978.

Zollinger RM: Reflections on gastric surgery. *Am J Surg,* 139:10, 1980.

Anatomy

Griffith CA: Anatomy, in Harkins HN, Nyhus LM (eds): *Surgery of the Stomach and Duodenum*. Boston, Little, Brown, 1969, p 25.

Lillibridge CB: The fine structure of normal human gastric mucosa. *Gastroenterology* 47:269, 1964.

McGuigan JE: Gastric mucosal intracellular localization of gastrin by immunofluorescence. *Gastroenterology,* 55:315, 1968.

Michels NA: Blood supply of the stomach and the esophagus, in *Blood Supply and Anatomy of the Upper Abdominal Organs*. Philadelphia, Lippincott, 1955, p 248.

Schofield GC: Anatomy of muscular and neural tissues in the alimentary canal, in Code CF (ed): *Handbook of Physiology*. Washington, DC, American Physiological Society, 1968, sec 6, p 1579.

Physiology

Card WI, Marks IN: The relationship between the acid output of the stomach following "maximal" histamine stimulation and the parietal cell mass. *Clin Sci* 19:147, 1960.

Cooke AR: Control of gastric emptying and motility. *Gastroenterology* 68:804, 1975.

Davenport HW: Gastric secretion, in *Physiology of the Digestive Tract*. Chicago, Year Book Medical Publishers, 1971, p 95.

Davenport HW: Why the stomach does not digest itself. *Sci Am* 226:86, 1972.

Davenport HW, et al: Functional significance of gastric mucosal barrier to sodium. *Gastroenterology* 57:142, 1964.

Debas HT, Hollinshead J, et al: Vagal control of gastrin release in the dog: Pathways for stimulation and inhibition. *Surgery* 95:34, 1984.

Dragstedt LR: The physiology of the gastric antrum. *Arch Surg* 75:552, 1957.

Edkins JS: The chemical mechanism of gastric secretion. *J Physiol* 34:183, 1906.

Flemstrom G: Gastroduodenal mucosal secretion of bicarbonate and mucus. Physiologic control and stimulation by prostaglandins. *Am J Med* 81:18, 1986.

Fordtran JS, Walsh JH: Gastric acid secretion rate and buffer control of the stomach after eating: Results in normal subjects and in patients with duodenal ulcer. *J Clin Invest* 52:645, 1973.

Gregory RA: Memorial lecture: The isolation and chemistry of gastrin. *Gastroenterology* 51:953, 1966.

Gregory RA, Tracy HJ: The constitution and properties of two gastrins extracted from hog antral mucosa. *Gut* 5:103, 1964.

Grossman MI: Neural and hormonal stimulation of gastric secretion of acid, in Code CF (ed): *Handbook of Physiology*. Washington, DC, American Physiological Society, 1967, sec 6, vol II, p 835.

Grossman MI, et al: Candidate hormones of the gut. *Gastroenterology* 67:730, 1974.

Heading RC, et al: Gastric emptying rate measurement in man. A double isotope scanning technique for simultaneous study of liquid and solid components of a meal. *Gastroenterology* 71:45, 1976.

Hunt JN, Knox MT: Regulation of gastric emptying, in Code CF (ed): *Handbook of Physiology*. Washington, DC, American Physiological Society, 1968, sec 6, vol IV, p 1917.

Hunt JN, Stubbs DF: The volume and energy content of meals as determinants of gastric emptying. *J Physiol (London)* 245:209, 1975.

Ippoliti AF, et al: Demonstration of the intestinal phase of gastric acid secretion in man. *Gastroenterology* 70:896, 1976.

Jeffries GH: Gastric secretion in intrinsic factor, in Code CF (ed): *Handbook of Physiology*. Washington, DC, American Physiological Society, 1967, sec 6, vol II, p 919.

Johnson LR: Progress in gastroenterology: The trophic action of gastrointestinal hormones. *Gastroenterology* 70:278, 1976.

Kelly KA, Code CF: Canine gastric pacemaker. *Am J Physiol* 220:112, 1971.

Kleibeuker JH, Eysselein VE, et al: Role of endogenous secretin in acid-induced inhibition of human gastric function. *J Clin Invest* 73:526, 1984.

Makhlouf GM, et al: A quantitative statement of the two component hypothesis of gastric secretion. *Gastroenterology* 51:149, 1966.

Malagelada JR, et al: Measurement of gastric function during digestion of ordinary solid meals in man. *Gastroenterology* 70:203, 1976.

Meyer JH, Mayer EA, et al: Gastric processing and emptying of fat. *Gastroenterology* 90:1176, 1986.

Nyhus LM, et al: The control of gastric release: An experimental study illustrating a new concept. *Gastroenterology* 39:582, 1960.

Richardson CT, et al: Studies on the role of cephalic-vagal stimulation in the acid secretory response to eating in normal human subjects. *J Clin Invest* 60:435, 1977.

Samloff IM: Pepsinogens, pepsins and pepsin inhibitors. *Gastroenterology* 69:586, 1971.

Sircus W: The intestinal phase of gastric secretion. *Q J Exp Physiol* 38:91, 1953.

Thompson JC: Gastrointestinal hormones—introduction to symposium on gastrointestinal hormones. *World J Surg* 3:389, 1979.

Uvnas B: Role of duodenum in inhibition of gastric acid secretion. *Scand J Gastroent* 6:113, 1971.

Walsh JH, Grossman MI: Gastrin. *N Engl J Med* 292:1324, 1975.

White CM, Poxon V, et al: The importance of the distal stomach in gastric emptying of liquids in man. *Surg Gastroenterol* 3:13, 1984.

Wolf S, Wolff HG: *Human Gastric Function*. London, Oxford University Press, 1943.

Woodward ER: The role of the gastric antrum in the regulation of gastric secretion. *Gastroenterology* 38:7, 1960.

Gastric Dysfunction

Alexander-Williams J: Alkaline reflux gastritis: A myth or a disease? *Am J Surg* 143:17, 1982.

Barnes AD, Cox AG: Diarrhea, in Williams JA, Cox AG (eds): *After Vagotomy*. London, Butterworth, 1969, p 211.

Baron JH: The clinical use of gastric function tests. *Scand J Gastroent Suppl* 6:9, 1970.

Becker JM, Sava P, et al: Intestinal pacing for canine postgastrectomy dumping. *Gastroenterology* 84:383, 1983.

Condon JR, et al: The cause and treatment of postvagotomy diarrhea. *Br J Surg* 62:309, 1975.

Fiore AC, et al: Surgical management of alkaline reflux gastritis. *Arch Surg* 117:689, 1982.

Goldberg J, et al: A clinical evaluation of the maximal histalog test. *Am J Dig Dis* 12:468, 1967.

Gustavsson S, et al: Scintigraphic assessment of biliary reflux into the residual stomach after subtotal gastrectomy and gastrojejunostomy. *Acta Radiol [Diagn] (Stockh)* 21:639, 1980.

Halpern NB, et al: Failure to achieve success with remedial gastric surgery. *Am J Surg* 125:108, 1973.

Herrington JL Jr, Sawyers JL: Surgical management of alkaline reflux gastritis and esophagitis. *Surg Annu* 13:341, 1981.

Herrington JL Jr, et al: Surgical management of reflux gastritis. *Ann Surg* 180:526, 1974.

Hirschowitz BI, et al: Demonstration of a new gastroscope, the "Fiberscope." *Gastroenterology* 35:50, 1958.

Isenberg JI, et al: Pentagastrin vs betazole as stimulant of gastric secretion. *JAMA* 206:2897, 1968.

Johnstone FR, et al: Postgastrectomy problems in patients with personality defects: The "albatross" syndrome. *Can Med Assoc J* 96:1559, 1967.

Jordon GL: Surgical management of postgastrectomy problems. *Arch Surg* 102:251, 1971.

Kelly KA: Gastric motility in health and after gastric surgery. *Viewpoints, Dig Dis* 8:1, 1976.

Kennedy T: The failures of gastric surgery. *Br J Surg* 68:677, 1981.

Laufer I: A simple method for routine double constrast study of the upper gastrointestinal tract. *Radiology* 117:513, 1975.

Laufer I, et al: The diagnostic accuracy of barium studies of the stomach and duodenum—correlation with endoscopy. *Radiology* 115:569, 1975.

LeQuesne LP, et al: The dumping syndrome—1. Factors responsible for the symptoms. *Br Med J* 1:141, 1960.

Lundh G: Intestinal digestion and absorption after gastrectomy. *Acta Chir Scand Suppl* 231:1, 1958.

Martin LF, Larson GM, et al: Bleeding from stress gastritis. Has prophylactic pH control made a difference? *Am Surg* 5:189, 1985.

Mathias JR, Fernandez A, et al: Nausea, vomiting, and abdominal pain after Roux en Y anastomosis: Motility of the jejunal limb. *Gastroenterology* 88:101–107.

Metzger WH, et al: Effect of metoclopramide in chronic gastric retention after gastric surgery. *Gastroenterology* 71:30, 1976.

Phillips JC, et al: Gastric leiomyosarcoma; Roentgenologic and clinical findings. *Am J Dig Dis* 15:239, 1970.

Reasbeck PG, Van Rij AM: The effect of somatostatin on dumping after gastric surgery: A preliminary report. *Surgery* 99:462, 1986.

Reber HA, Way LW: Surgical treatment of late postgastrectomy syndromes. *Am J Surg* 129:71, 1975.

Sakita T, Oguro Y: Endoscopic diagnosis of early gastric cancer, in Berry LH (ed): *Gastrointestinal Pan-Endoscopy*. Springfield, IL, Charles C Thomas, 1974, p 278.

Sawyers JL, et al: Remedial operation for alkaline reflux gastritis and associated postgastrectomy syndromes. *Arch Surg* 115:519, 1980.

Seaman WB: Non-neoplastic diseases of the stomach, in Mar-gulis AR, Burhenne HJ (eds): *Alimentary Tract Roentgenology*. St Louis, CV Mosby, 1973, vol 1, p 607.

Shaffer EA: The effect of vagotomy on gallbladder function and bile composition in man. *Ann Surg* 195:413, 1982.

Sheiner HJ, et al: Gastric motility and emptying in normal and post-vagotomy subjects. *Gut* 21:753, 1980.

Shirakabe H, et al: *Atlas of X-ray Diagnosis of Early Gastric Cancer*. Philadelphia, Lippincott, 1966.

Tovey FI, Clark CG: Anaemia after partial gastrectomy: A neglected curable condition. *Lancet* 1:956, 1980.

van Heerden JA, et al: Postoperative reflux gastritis. *Am J Surg* 129:82, 1975.

Vogel SB, Vair DB, et al: Alterations in gastrointestinal emptying of 99m-technetium-labeled solids following sequential antrectomy, truncal vagotomy and Roux Y gastroenterostomy. *Ann Surg* 198:506, 1983.

Wormsley KG, Grossman MI: Maximal histalog test in control subjects and patients with peptic ulcer. *Gut* 6:427, 1965.

Yalow RS, Berson SA: Radioimmunoassay of gastrin. *Gastroenterology* 58:1, 1970.

Zboralske FF: Gastric ulcer, in Margulis AR, Burhenne HJ (eds): *Alimentary Tract Roentgenology*. St Louis, CV Mosby, 1967, vol 1, p 475.

Gastric and Duodenal Disease

Adami H, Enander L, et al: Recurrences one to ten years after highly selective vagotomy in prepyloric and duodenal ulcer. *Ann Surg* 199:393, 1984.

Adkins RB Jr, DeLozier JB III, et al: The management of gastric ulcers: A current review. *Ann Surg* 201:741, 1985.

Amdrup E: Recurrent ulcer. *Br J Surg* 68:679, 1981.

Amdrup E, Jensen HE: Selective vagotomy of the parietal cell mass preserving innervation of the undrained antrum. *Gastroenterology* 59:522, 1970.

Amdrup E, et al: Clinical results of parietal cell vagotomy (highly selective vagotomy) two to four years after operation. *Ann Surg* 180:279, 1974.

Amdrup E, et al: Parietal cell (highly selective or proximal gastric) vagotomy for peptic ulcer disease. *World J Surg* 1:19, 1977.

Anderson JR, et al: Cholelithiasis following peptic ulcer surgery: A prospective controlled study. *Br J Surg* 67:618, 1980.

Asbaugh D, et al: Gastroscopy in corrosive burn of the stomach. *JAMA* 216:1638, 1971.

Bader JP: The surgical treatment of peptic ulcer disease. A physician's view. *Dig Dis Sci* 30(11 suppl):52S, 1985.

Bardhan DD: Refractory duodenal ulcer. *Gut* 25:711–717, 1984.

Barragry TP, Blatchford JW, et al: Giant gastric ulcers, a review of 49 cases. *Ann Surg* 203:255, 1986.

Bergegardh S, et al: Gastric acid responses to graded I.V. infusion of pentagastrin and histalog in peptic ulcer patients before and after antrum-bulb resection. *Scand J Gastroent* 11:337, 1976.

Berne CJ, Rosoff L: Peptic ulcer perforation of the gastroduodenal artery complex. *Ann Surg* 169:141, 1969.

Binder HJ, et al: Cimetidine in the treatment of duodenal ulcer: A multicenter double-blind study. *Gastroenterology* 74:380, 1978.

Bittner R, Schirrow H, et al: Total gastrectomy: A 15-year experience with particular reference to the patient over 70 years of age. *Arch Surg* 120:1120, 1985.

Blumenthal IS: Digestive disease as a national problem. III. Social cost of peptic ulcer. *Gastroenterology* 54:86, 1968.

Bonfils S, et al: Cimetidine treatment of acute and chronic Zollinger-Ellison syndrome. *World J Surg* 3:597, 1979.

Bringaze WL III, Chappuis CW, et al: Early gastric cancer. *Ann Surg* 204:103, 1986.

Burgess JN, et al: Sarcomatous lesions of the stomach. *Ann Surg* 173:758, 1971.

Burhenne HJ: The postoperative stomach, in Margulis AR, Burhenne HJ (eds): *Alimentary Tract Roentgenology*. St Louis, CV Mosby, 1973, vol 1, p 740.

Castrini G, Pappalardo G: Carcinoma of the cardia: Tactical problem. *J Thorac Cardiovasc Surg* 82:190, 1981.

Cathcart PM, et al: Tumors of gastric smooth muscle. *South Med J* 73:18, 1980.

Cello JP, Grendell JH: Endoscopic laser treatment for gastrointestinal vascular ectasias. *Ann Intern Med* 104:352, 1986.

Christiansen J, et al: Prospective controlled vagotomy trial for duodenal ulcer: Primary results, sequelae, acid secretion, and recurrence rates two to five years after operation. *Ann Surg* 193:49, 1981.

Chung R, DenBesten L: Fiberoptic endoscopy in treatment of corrosive injury of the stomach. *Arch Surg* 110:725, 1975.

Collen MJ, Howard JM, et al: Comparison of ranitidine and cimetidine in the treatment of gastric hypersecretion. *Ann Intern Med* 100:52, 1984.

Conn HO, et al: Intra-arterial vasopressin in the treatment of upper gastrointestinal hemorrhage. A prospective, controlled clinical trial. *Gastroenterology* 68:211, 1975.

Cooke AR: The role of the mucosal barrier in drug-induced gastric ulceration and erosions. *Am J Dig Dis* 21:155, 1976.

Cooperative Study Group: Omeprazole in duodenal ulceration: Acid inhibition, symptom relief, endoscopic healing, and recurrence. *Br Med J* 289:525, September 1984.

Cowley DJ, et al: Acid secretion in relation to recurrence of duodenal ulcer after vagotomy and drainage. *Br J Surg* 60:517, 1973.

Cox AJ Jr: Pathology, in Harkins HN, Nyhus LM (eds): *Surgery of the Stomach and Duodenum*, 2d ed. Boston, Little, Brown, 1969.

Cross S, et al: Carbenoxolone: Its protective action on gastric mucosa, in *Biologie et Gastroenterologie*. 9th International Congress of Gastroenterology, Paris, 5:568C, 1972.

Csendes A, Braghetto L, et al: Surgical treatment of high gastric ulcer. *Am J Surg* 149:765, 1985.

Czaja AJ, et al: Gastric acid secretion and acute gastroduodenal disease after burns. *Arch Surg* 111:243, 1976.

DeBakey M, Ochsner A: Bezoars and concretions. *Surgery* 4:934, 1938.

Diggory RT, Cuschieri A: R2/3 gastrectomy for gastric carcinoma: An audited experience of a consecutive series. *Br J Surg* 72:146, 1985.

Donovan AJ, et al: Selective treatment of duodenal ulcer with perforation. *Ann Surg* 189:627, 1979.

Dougherty SH, et al: Stomach cancer following gastric surgery for benign disease. *Arch Surg* 117:294, 1982.

Dragstedt LR, Owens FM Jr: Supradiaphragmatic secretion of vagus nerves in treatment of duodenal ulcer. *Proc Soc Exp Biol Med* 53:152, 1943.

DuPlessis DJ: Pathogenesis of gastric ulceration. *Lancet* 1:974, 1965.

Duthie HL, et al: Surgical treatment of gastric ulcers. Controlled comparison of billroth-I gastrectomy and vagotomy and pyloroplasty. *Br J Surg* 57:784, 1970.

Elashoff JD, Van Deventer G, et al: Long-term follow-up of duodenal ulcer patients. *J Clin Gastroenterol* 5:509, 1983.

Ellis FH Jr: Esophagogastrectomy for carcinoma: Technical considerations based on anatomic location of lesion. *Surg Clin North Am* 60:265, 1980.

Emas S, Aly A: Acid and pepsin responses to graded doses of pentagastrin in duodenal and corporeal gastric ulcer patients before and after selective proximal vagotomy. *Am J Surg* 150:543, 1985.

Emas S, Fernstrom M: Prospective, randomized trial of selective vagotomy with pyloroplasty and selective proximal vagotomy with and without pyloroplasty in the treatment of duodenal, pyloric, and prepyloric ulcers. *Am J Surg* 149:236, 1985.

Engstrom PF, Lavin PT, et al: Postoperative adjuvant 5-fluorouracil plus methyl-CCNU therapy for gastric cancer patients: Eastern Cooperative Oncology Group Study (EST 3275). *Cancer* 55:1863, 1985.

Fakhry SM, Herbst CA Jr, et al: Complications requiring intervention after gastric bariatric surgery. *South Med J* 78:536, 1985.

Farris JM, Smith GK: Vagotomy and pyloroplasty: A solution to the management of bleeding duodenal ulcer. *Ann Surg* 152:416, 1960.

Feczko PJ, Halpert RD: Gastric polyps: Radiological evaluation and clinical significance. *Radiology* 155:581, 1985.

Finsberg HV, Pearlman LA: Surgical treatment of peptic ulcer in the United States. Trends before and after the introduction of cimetidine. *Lancet* 1:1305, 1981.

Fleischer D: Endoscopic laser therapy for gastrointestinal neoplasms. *Surg Clin North Am* 64:947, 1984.

Fleming ID, et al: The role of surgery in the management of gastric lymphoma. *Cancer* 49:1135, 1982.

Fordtran JS, et al: In vivo and in vitro evaluation of liquid antacids. *N Engl J Med* 288:293, 1973.

Foster JH, et al: Factors influencing mortality following emergency operation for massive upper gastrointestinal hemorrhage. *Surg Gynecol Obstet* 117:257, 1963.

Fraser AG, Brunt PW, et al: Comparison of highly selective vagotomy with truncal vagotomy and pyloroplasty: One surgeon's results after 5 years. *Br J Surg* 70:485, 1983.

Fraser GM, Earnshaw PM: Double-contrast barium meal: Correlation with endoscopy. *Clin Radiol* 34:121, 1983.

Friedman GD, et al: Cigarettes, alcohol, coffee and peptic ulcer. *N Engl J Med* 290:469, 1974.

Gall FP, Hermanek P: New aspects in the surgical treatment of gastric carcinoma—a comparative study of 1636 patients operated on between 1969 and 1982. *Eur J Surg Oncol* 11:19, 1985.

Gentsch HH, et al: Results of surgical treatment of early gastric cancer in 113 patients. *World J Surg* 5:103, 1981.

Gilbert DA, Surawicz CM, et al: Prevention of acute aspirin-induced gastric mucosal injury by 15-R-15 methyl prostaglandin E_2: Endoscopic study. *Gastroenterology* 86:339, 1984.

Gledhill T, Buck M, et al: Cimetidine or vagotomy? Comparison of the effects of proximal gastric vagotomy, cimetidine, and placebo on nocturnal intragastric acidity and acid secretion in patients with cimetidine-resistant duodenal ulcer. *Br J Surg* 70:7043, 1983.

Goldstein F, Kline TS, et al: Early gastric cancer in a United States hospital. *Am J Gastroenterol* 78:715, 1983.

Goligher JC: A technique for highly selective (parietal cell or proximal gastric) vagotomy for duodenal ulcer. *Br J Surg* 61:337, 1974.

Goligher JC, et al: Controlled trial of vagotomy and gastroenterostomy, vagotomy and antrectomy and subtotal gastrectomy in elective treatment of duodenal ulcer: Interim report. *Br Med J* 1:455, 1964.

Goligher JC, et al: Five to eight year results of truncal vagotomy and pyloroplasty for duodenal ulcer. *Br Med J* 1:7, 1972.

Gough KR, Korman MG, et al: Rantidine and cimetidine in prevention of duodenal ulcer relapse: Double-blind, randomized, multicenter, comparative trial. *Lancet* 2:659, 1984.

Graffner HO, Liedberg GF, et al: Parietal cell vagotomy in the surgical treatment of chronic duodenal, pyloric and prepyloric ulcer disease. *Int Surg* 70:139, 1985.

Graffner HO, Liedberg GF, et al: Recurrence after parietal cell vagotomy for peptic ulcer disease. *Am J Surg* 150:336, 1985.

Greenall MJ, Lehnert T: Vagotomy or gastrectomy for elective treatment of benign gastric ulceration? *Dig Dis Sci* 30:353, 1985.

Greenall MJ, et al: Long term effect of highly selective vagotomy on basal and maximal acid output in man. *Gastroenterology* 68:1421, 1975.

Gregory RA, et al: Extraction of gastrin-like substance from pancreatic tumor in case of Zollinger-Ellison syndrome. *Lancet* 1:1045, 1960.

Griffith CA, Harkins HN: Partial gastric vagotomy. An experimental study. *Gastroenterology* 32:96, 1957.

Grossman MI: Some minor heresies about vagotomy. *Gastroenterology* 67:1016, 1974.

Grossman MI, et al: A new look at peptic ulcer. *Ann Intern Med* 84:57, 1976.

Grossman MI, et al: Peptic ulcer: New therapies, new diseases. *Ann Intern Med* 95:609, 1981.

Hallenbeck GA, et al: Proximal gastric vagotomy: Effects of two operative techniques on clinical and gastric secretory results. *Ann Surg* 184:435, 1976.

Hastings PR, et al: Mallory-Weiss syndrome, review of 69 cases. *Am J Surg* 142:560, 1981.

Herrington JL, et al: A twenty-five year experience with vagotomy-antrectomy. *Arch Surg* 106:469, 1973.

Hirschowitz BI, Luketic GC: Endoscopy in the post-gastrectomy patient: An analysis of 580 patients. *Gastrointest Endosc* 18:27, 1971.

Hunt PS: Surgical management of bleeding chronic peptic ulcer: A 10-year prospective study. *Ann Surg* 199:44, 1984.

Hunt PS, et al: The management of bleeding gastric ulcer: A prospective study. *Aust NZ J Surg* 50:41, 1980.

Iishi H, Tatsuta M, et al: Enoscopic diagnosis of minute gastric cancer of less than 5 mm in diameter. *Cancer* 56:655, 1985.

Inberg MV, et al: Total and proximal gastrectomy in the treatment of gastric carcinoma: A series of 305 cases. *World J Surg* 5:249, 1981.

Ippoliti AF, et al: Cimetidine versus intensive antacid therapy for duodenal ulcer: A multicenter trial. *Gastroenterology* 74:393, 1978.

Isenberg JI, Peterson WL, et al: Healing of benign gastric ulcer with low-dose antacid or cimetidine: A double-blind randomized, placebo-controlled trial. *N Engl J Med* 308:1319, 1983.

Ivy AC, et al: *Peptic Ulcer*. Philadelphia, Blakiston, 1950.

Jaffin BW, Kaye MD: The prognosis of gastric outlet obstruction. *Ann Surg* 201:176, 1985.

Johnston D, Wilkinson AR: Highly selective vagotomy without a drainage procedure in the treatment of duodenal ulcer. *Br J Surg* 57:289, 1970.

Jordan GL Jr, et al: Surgical management of perforated peptic ulcer. *Ann Surg* 179:628, 1974.

Jordan PH Jr, Condon RE: A prospective evaluation of vagotomy-pyloroplasty and vagotomy-antrectomy for treatment of duodenal ulcer. *Ann Surg* 172:547, 1970.

Klein TS, Goldstein F: Malignant lymphoma involving the stomach. *Cancer* 32:961, 1973.

Knauer CM: Mallory-Weiss syndrome. Characterization of 75 Mallory-Weiss lacerations in 528 patients with upper gastrointestinal hemorrhage. *Gastroenterology* 71:5, 1976.

Koga S, et al: Results of total gastrectomy for gastric cancer. *Am J Surg* 140:636, 1980.

Koo J, Lam SK, et al: Proximal gastric vagotomy, truncal vagotomy with drainage, and truncal vagotomy with antrectomy for chronic duodenal ulcer: A propsective, randomized controlled trial. *Ann Surg* 197:265, 1983.

Kuster GGR, et al: Gastric cancer in pernicious anemia and in patients with and without achlorhydria. *Ann Surg* 175:783, 1972.

Lamers, CBHW, Lind T, et al: Omeprazole in Zollinger–Ellison syndrome: Effects of a single dose and of long-term treatment in patients resistant to histamine H_2-receptor antagonists. *N Engl J Med* 310:758, 1984.

Laurence BH, et al: Endoscopic laser photocoagulation for bleeding peptic ulcers. *Lancet* 1:124, 1980.

Lieberman DA, Keller FS, et al: Arterial embolization for massive upper gastrointestinal tract bleeding in poor surgical candidates. *Gastroenterology* 86:376, 1984.

Littman A (ed): The Veterans Administration cooperative study on gastric ulcer. *Gastroenterology* 61:567, 1971.

Longmire WP Jr: Gastric carcinoma: Is radical gastrectomy worthwhile? *Ann R Coll Surg Engl* 62:25, 1980.

Lucas CE, et al: Natural history and surgical dilemma of "stress" gastric bleeding. *Arch Surg* 102:266, 1971.

Lunde OC, Liavag I, et al: Proximal gastric vagotomy and pyloroplasty for duodenal ulcer with pyloric stenosis: A thirteen-year experience. *World J Surg* 9:165, 1985.

Lygidakis NJ: Gastric stump carcinoma after surgery for gastro-duodenal ulcer. *Ann R Coll Surg Engl* 63:203, 1981.

Lygidakis NJ: Total gastrectomy for gastric carcinoma: A retrospective study of different procedures and assessment of a new technique of gastric reconstruction. *Br J Surg* 68:649, 1981.

McCarthy DM: Report of the United States experience with cimetidine in the Zollinger-Ellison syndrome and other hypersecretory states. *Gastroenterology* 74:453, 1978.

McCarthy E, et al: H_2-histamine receptor blocking agents in the Zollinger-Ellison syndrome. *Ann Intern Med* 87:668, 1977.

MacLeod LA, Mills PR, et al: Neodymium-yttrium-aluminum-garnet laser photocoagulation for a major hemorrhage from peptic ulcers and single vessels: A single-blind controlled study. *Br Med J* 286:345, 1983.

Madsen P, Kronborg O: Recurrent ulcer $5\frac{1}{2}$–8 years after highly selective vagotomy without drainage and selective vagotomy with pyloroplasty. *Scand J Gastroenterol* 15:193, 1980.

Malagelada JR: Medical versus surgical therapy for duodenal ulcer: Making the right choices. *Mayo Clin Proc* 55:25, 1980.

Malagelada JR, Ahlquist DA, et al: Defects in prostaglandin synthesis and metabolism in ulcer disease. *Dig Dis Sci* 31(suppl 2):20S, 1986.

Malagelada J, Edis AJ, et al: Medical and surgical options in the management of patients with gastrinoma. *Gastroenterology* 84:1524, 1983.

Malagelada J, Phillips SF, et al: Postoperative reflux gastritis: Pathophysiology and long-term outcome after Roux en Y diversion. *Ann Intern Med* 103:178, 1985.

Mallory GK, Weiss S: Hemorrhages from lacerations of cardiac orifice of the stomach due to vomiting. *Am J Med Sci* 178:506, 1929.

Marshak RH, Lindner AE: The Zollinger-Ellison syndrome, in *Radiology of the Small Intestine.* Philadelphia, Saunders, 1970, p 88.

Mekelvey STD: Gastric incontinence and postvagotomy diarrhea. *Br J Surg* 57:741, 1970.

Mendeloff AI: What has been happening to duodenal ulcer? *Gastroenterology* 67:1020, 1974.

Menetrier P: Des polyadenomes gastriques et de leurs rapports avec le cancer de l'estomac. *Arch Physiol Norm Path* 1:32, 226, 1888.

Menguy R: Pathophysiology of peptic ulcer. *Am J Surg* 120:282, 1970.

Menguy R, et al: Mechanism of stress ulcer: Influence of hypovolemic shock on energy metabolism in the gastric mucosa. *Gastroenterology* 66:46, 1974.

Menguy R, et al: The surgical management of acute gastric mucosal bleeding. Stress ulcer, acute erosive gastritis, and acute hemorrhagic gastritis. *Arch Surg* 99:198, 1969.

Messer J, Reitman D, et al: Association of adrenocorticosteroid therapy and peptic ulcer disease. *N Engl J Med* 309:21, 1983.

Mizuno H, et al: Endoscopic followup of gastric polyps. *Gastrointest Endosc* 21:112, 1975.

Moertel CG, et al: Sequential and combination chemotherapy of advanced gastric cancer. *Cancer* 38:678, 1976.

Monaco AP, et al: Adenomatous polyps of the stomach. A clinical and pathological study of 153 cases. *Cancer* 15:456, 1962.

Moody FG: Role of mucosal blood flow in the pathogenesis of gastric ulcers, in Holton P (ed): *International Encyclopedia of Pharmacology and Therapeutics.* Oxford, Pergamon, 1973, sec 39A, vol 1.

Moody FG, et al: Stress and the acute gastric mucosal lesion. *Am J Dig Dis* 21:148, 1976.

Nicosia J, et al: Surgical management of corrosive gastric injuries. *Ann Surg* 180:139, 1974.

Norton JA, Doppman JL, et al: Aggressive resection of metastatic disease in selected patients with malignant gastrinoma. *Ann Surg* 203:352, 1986.

Nyhus LM: Gastric ulcer, in Harkins HN, Nyhus LM (eds): *Surgery of the Stomach and Duodenum,* 2d ed. Boston, Little, Brown, 1969, p 203.

O'Brien JJ, Burakoff R, et al: Early gastric cancer: Clinicopathologic study. *Am J Med* 78:195, 1985.

Ochsner A, et al: Cancer of the stomach. *Am J Surg* 141:10, 1981.

Oi M, et al: The location of gastric ulcer. *Gastroenterology* 36:45, 1959.

O'Neill JA, et al: Studies related to the pathogenesis of Curling's ulcer. *J Trauma* 7:275, 1967.

Orlando R III, Welch JP: Carcinoma of the stomach after gastric operation. *Am J Surg* 141:487, 1981.

O'Rourke IC: Elective surgery for peptic ulcer: A five-year review. *Med J Aust* 143:13, 1985.

Overholt BF, Jeffries GH: Hypertrophic, hypersecretory protein-losing gastropathy. *Gastroenterology* 58:80, 1970.

Palmer ED: The vigorous diagnostic approach to upper gastrointestinal tract hemorrhage. *JAMA* 207:1477, 1969.

Pellegrini CA, Patti MG, et al: Alkaline reflux gastritis and the effect of biliary diversion on gastric emptying of solid food. *Am J Surg* 150:166, 1985.

Primrose JN, Ratcliffe JG, et al: Differences between peptic ulcer and control patients on the basis of the response to secretion. *Digestion* 32:249, 1985.

Richardson CT, Peters MN, et al: Treatment of Zollinger–Ellison syndrome with exploratory laparotomy, proximal gastric vagotomy, and H_2-receptor antagonists: A prospective study. *Gastroenterology* 89:357, 1985.

Richardson CT, Walsh JH: The value of a histamine H_2-receptor antagonist in the management of patients with the Zollinger-Ellison syndrome. *N Engl J Med* 294:133, 1976.

Ritchie WP Jr: Alkaline reflux gastritis, late results on a controlled trial of diagnosis and treatment. *Ann Surg* 203:537, 1986.

Romanus ME, Neal JA, et al: Comparison of four provocative tests for the diagnosis of gastrinoma. *Ann Surg* 198:608, 1983.

Rossi RL, et al: Parietal cell vagotomy for intractable and obstructing duodenal ulcer. *Am J Surg* 141:482, 1981.

Rotter JL, et al: Genetics of peptic ulcer disease: Segregation of serum group I pepsinogen concentrations in families with peptic ulcer disease. *Clin Res* 25:114A, 1977.

Sakita T, et al: Observations on the healing of ulcerations in early gastric cancer. The life cycle of the malignant ulcer. *Gastroenterology* 60:835, 1971.

Sawyers JL, Scott HW Jr: Selective gastric vagotomy with antrectomy or pyloroplasty. *Ann Surg* 174:541, 1971.

Schafer LW, Larson DE, et al: Risk of development of gastric carcinoma in patients with pernicious anemia: A population-based study in Rochester, Minnesota. *Mayo Clinic Proc* 60:444, 1985.

Scott, HW Jr, Adkins RB Jr, et al: Results of an aggressive surgical approach to gastric carcinoma during a twenty-three-year period. *Surgery* 97:55, 1985.

Shepherd AF, Allan RN, et al: The surgical treatment of gastroduodenal Crohn's disease. *Ann R Coll Surg Engl* 67:382, 1985.

Shimm DS, Dosoretz DE, et al: Primary gastric lymphoma: An analysis with emphasis on prognostic factors and radiation therapy. *Cancer* 52:2044, 1983.

Sirinek KR, et al: Simple closure of perforated peptic ulcer. Still an effective procedure for patients with delay in treatment. *Arch Surg* 116:591, 1981.

Stabile BE, Passaro E Jr: Recurrent peptic ulcer. *Gastroenterology* 70:124, 1976.

Stanten A, Peters H Jr: Enzymatic dissolution of phytobezoars. *Am J Surg* 130:259, 1975.

Stempien SJ, et al: Hypertrophic hypersecretory gastropathy. *Am J Dig Dis* 9:471, 1964.

Swain CP, Storey DW, et al: Nature of the bleeding vessel in recurrently bleeding gastric ulcers. *Gastroenterology* 90:595, 1986.

Tanphiphat C, Tanprayoon T, et al: Surgical treatment of perforated duodenal ulcer: A prospective trial between simple closure and definitive surgery. *Br J Surg* 72:370, 1985.

Thomas WE, et al: The long-term outcome of billroth I partial gastrectomy for benign gastric ulcer. *Ann Surg* 195:189, 1982.

Thomsen F, et al: Cimetidine treatment of recurrent ulcer after vagotomy. *Acta Chir Scand* 146:35, 1980.

Vallon AG, et al: Randomized trial of endoscopic argon laser photocoagulation in bleeding peptic ulcers. *Gut* 22:228, 1981.

Wara P: Endoscopic management of the bleeding ulcer. *Danish Med Bull* 33:1, 1986.

Wastell C, Ellis H: Volvulus of the stomach. *Br J Surg* 58:557, 1971.

Weaver RM, Temple JG: Proximal gastric vagotomy in patients resistant to cimetidine. *Br J Surg* 72:177, 1985.

Weiland D, et al: Gastric outlet obstruction in peptic ulcer disease: An indication for surgery. *Am J Surg* 143:90, 1982.

Weinberg JA: Treatment of the massively bleeding duodenal ulcer by ligation. Pyloroplasty and vagotomy *Am J Surg* 102:158, 1961.

Wermer P: Multiple endocrine adenomatosis: Multiple hormone producing tumors, a familial syndrome. in Bonfils S (ed): *Endocrine-Secreting Tumours of the Gastrointestinal Tract.* Philadelphia, Saunders, 1974, p 671.

Wilson SD, Ellison EH: Survival in patients with Zollinger-Ellison syndrome treated by total gastrectomy. *Am J Surg* 111:787, 1966.

Wilson WS, et al: Superficial gastric erosions. Response to surgical treatment. *Am J Surg* 126:133, 1973.

Wyllie JH, et al: Effect of cimetidine on surgery for duodenal ulcer. *Lancet* 1:1307, 1981.

Yalow RS, Berson SA: Size and charge distinctions beween endogenous human plasma gastrin in peripheral blood and heptadecapeptide gastrins. *Gastroenterology* 58:609, 1970.

Yan CJ, Brooks JR: Surgical management of gastric adenocarcinoma. *Am J Surg* 149:771, 1985.

Zollinger RM: Gastrinoma: Factors influencing prognosis. *Surgery* 97:49, 1985.

Zollinger RM, Ellison EH: Primary peptic ulcerations of the jejunum associated with islet cell tumors of the pancreas. *Ann Surg* 142:709, 1955.

Gastric Procedures for Morbid Obesity

Agha FP, Eckhauser FE, et al: Mason's vertical banded gastroplasty for morbid obesity: Surgical procedure and radiographic evaluation. *Radiology* 150:825, 1984.

Buckwalter JA: Clinical trial of jejunoileal and gastric bypass for the treatment of morbid obesity: Four-year progress report. *Am Surg* 46:377, 1980.

Flickinger EG, Pories WJ, et al: The Greenville gastric bypass: Progress report at 3 years. *Ann Surg* 199:555, 1984.

Flickinger EG, Sinar DR, et al: The bypassed stomach. *Am J Surg* 149:151, 1985.

Freeman JB, Burchett HJ: A comparison of gastric bypass and gastroplasty for morbid obesity. *Surgery* 88:433, 1980.

Gannon MX, Pears DJ, et al: The effect of gastric partitioning on gastric emptying in morbidly obese patients. *Br J Surg* 72:952, 1985.

Gentry K, Halverson JD, et al: Psychologic assessment of morbidly obese patients undergoing gastrc bypass: A comparison of preoperative and postoperative adjustment. *Surgery* 95:215, 1984.

Gomez CA: Gastroplasty in the surgical treatment of morbid obesity. *Am J Clin Nutr* 33(2 suppl):406, 1980.

Griffen WO Jr, et al: Experiences with conversion of jejunoileal bypass to gastric bypass: Its use for maintenance of weight loss. *Arch Surg* 116:320, 1981.

Halverson JD, et al: Gastric bypass for morbid obesity: A medical-surgical assessment. *Ann Surg* 194:152, 1981.

Halverson JD, Koehler RE: Assessment of patients with failed gastric operations for morbid obesity. *Am J Surg* 145:357, 1983.

Jones KB Jr: Horizontal gastroplasty: A safe, effective alternative to gastric bypsss in the surgical management of morbid obesity. *Ann Surg* 50:128, 1984.

Laws HL, Piantadosi S: Superior gastric reduction procedure for morbid obesity: A prospective, randomized trial. *Ann Surg* 193:334, 1981.

MacLean LD, et al: Gastroplasty for obesity. *Surg Gynecol Obstet* 153:200, 1981.

Makarewicz PA, Freeman JB, et al: Vertical banded gastroplasty: Assessment of efficacy. *Surgery* 98:700, 1985.

Mason EE: Vertical banded gastroplasty for obesity. *Arch Surg* 117:701, 1982.

Mason EE, et al: Gastric bypass in morbid obesity. *Am J Clin Nutr* 33(2 suppl):395, 1980.

O'Leary JP: Partition of the lesser curvature of the stomach in morbid obesity. *Surg Gynecol Obstet* 154:85, 1982.

Sugarman HJ, Fairman RP, et al: Gastric surgery for respiratory insufficiency of obesity. *Chest* 90:81, 1986.

Villar HV, et al: Mechanisms of satiety and gastric emptying after gastric partitioning and bypass. *Surgery* 90:229, 1981.

Chapter 27

Small Intestine

Courtney M. Townsend, Jr., and James C. Thompson

INTRODUCTION

Considered teleologically, the small bowel is the *raison d'être* for the entire gut. The esophagus brings food to the stomach, which prepares it for digestion. The exocrine secretions of the liver and pancreas make digestion possible. Digestion is achieved in the lumen of the small bowel, and food is absorbed through the small bowel mucosa; the colon disposes of whatever is left.

In addition to its vital function in nutrition, the small bowel has other important roles. It is the largest endocrine organ in the body. It has tremendous defenses against infection and is one of the most, if not the most, important organ in immune defense. It is a marvel of efficiency and works so well that, excepting the proximal 3 cm of the duodenum, it is not a common site for disease. We are supplied with a great excess of small bowel and can exist on far less than one-half of the absorptive surface provided.

Until recently, the small intestine had been relatively inaccessible for nonoperative diagnostic procedures compared to the stomach or colon. Several diagnostic techniques are now available for specific diseases of the small bowel. Mucosal biopsies obtained with the peroral biopsy capsule are often diagnostic in diffuse mucosal diseases. Enteroclysis is a more sensitive radiographic technique than the conventional barium follow-through examination of the small bowel. Selective mesenteric angiography is often helpful in cases of discrete lesions with abnormal vascular patterns, such as neoplasms, vascular malformations, or actively bleeding lesions. Scintigraphy may be helpful in localizing sites of bleeding. Fiberoptic endoscopy of the duodenum, proximal jejunum, and distal ileum are routinely employed.

Some diseases affecting the small intestine are discussed in other chapters: intestinal obstruction (Chap.

24), mesenteric vascular disease (Chap. 35), diseases of the intestine in infancy and childhood (Chap. 39), the intestine in trauma (Chap. 6), and duodenal and gastro-jejunal peptic ulcer (Chap. 26).

ANATOMY

The most impressive thing about the small bowel is its immense mucosal surface area, which is responsible for the organ's tremendously efficient digestion of food. Several layers of muscle, combined with actin and myosin components in the microstructures, provide great motility, so that not only is there great surface area, but the interface between the surface and the luminal contents, presented for absorption, is in constant motion as well.

Gross Anatomy

The small bowel extends from the pylorus to the cecum. The length of the small intestine depends entirely upon the state of bowel activity at the time of measurement. Careful estimates provide a duodenal length of 20 cm, a jejunal length of 100 to 110 cm, and an ileal length of 150 to 160 cm. The jejunoileum extends from the peritoneal fold that supports the duodenal-jejunal junction (the ligament of Treitz) downward to the ileocecal valve. The jejunoileum is estimated to comprise 60 percent of the entire length of the gut and to be approximately 160 percent of the body height, so that the small bowel, of couse, is considerably longer in a 7-ft basketball player than it is in a 5-ft jockey.

Generally, the jejunum occupies the upper abdomen, especially on the left, and is in contact with the pancreas, spleen, colon, and left kidney and adrenals. Affliction of these organs may affect the jejunum; pancreatitis, for example, may cause local ileus (the "sentinel loop") of the jejunum.

The jejunum has a larger circumference and is thicker than the ileum, and it may be identified at operation because of this and also because the mesenteric vessels usually form only one or two arcades and send out long straight vasa recta to the mesenteric border of the bowel. By contrast, the blood supply to the ileum may have four or five separate arcades, the vasa recta are shorter, and, most importantly, there is usually much more fat in the mesentery of the ileum than in the jejunum (Fig. 27-1). The jejunal mesentery may be transparent, but mesenteric fat will usually reach all the way to the bowel in the ileum. The ileum occupies the lower abdomen, especially on the right, and the pelvis. It is smaller in diameter and somewhat more mobile.

Except for the duodenum, the small bowel is entirely covered with visceral peritoneum (the serosa) and is tethered only by its attachment to the mesentery, through which course arteries, veins, and lymphatics. The mesentery is obliquely attached to the posterior body wall, beginning superiorly well to the left of the second lumbar vertebra and ending obliquely downward and to the right to overlie the right sacroiliac joint. The mesentery is normally covered with glistening peritoneum, which is nonadherent, but after trauma (external, chemical, septic, or operative), it may become adherent to other surfaces (mesenteric, visceral, or parietal) and greatly limit bowel mobility.

Except for the proximal duodenum, which is supplied by branches of the celiac axis, the blood supply of the small bowel is entirely from the superior mesenteric artery, which is the second major branch of the infradiaphragmatic aorta. The superior mesenteric artery also supplies the appendix, cecum, and ascending and proximal transverse colons. There is an abundant collateral supply to the small bowel, provided by the vascular arcades in the mesentery. In spite of this collateral supply, occlusion of a major branch of the superior mesenteric artery, or of the superior mesenteric artery itself, will lead to bowel death if not quickly corrected. Venous drainage of the segments of the small bowel is in parallel with the arterial supply. The superior mesenteric vein joins the splenic behind the neck of the pancreas to form the portal vein. The relatively high oxygen content of the blood leaving the gut provides a significant portion of the oxygen supply to the liver.

Fig. 27-1. Jejunum contrasted with ileum. Note the larger jejunal diameter, the thicker wall, prominent plicae circulares, one or two arterial arcades, long vasa recta, and translucent (fat-free) areas at the mesenteric border. The ileum is smaller, thinner walled, has few plicae, multiple vascular arcades with short vasa recta, and abundant mesenteric fat.

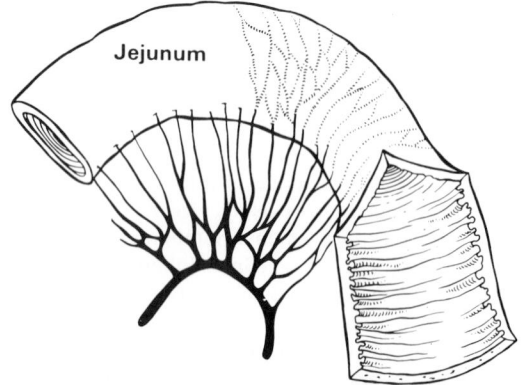

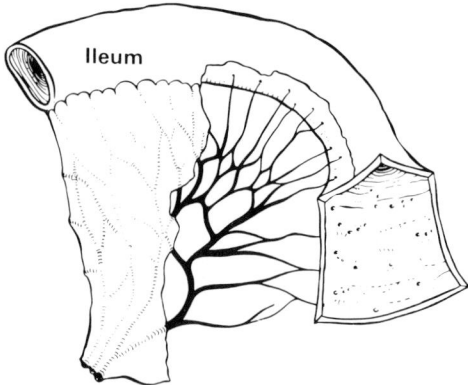

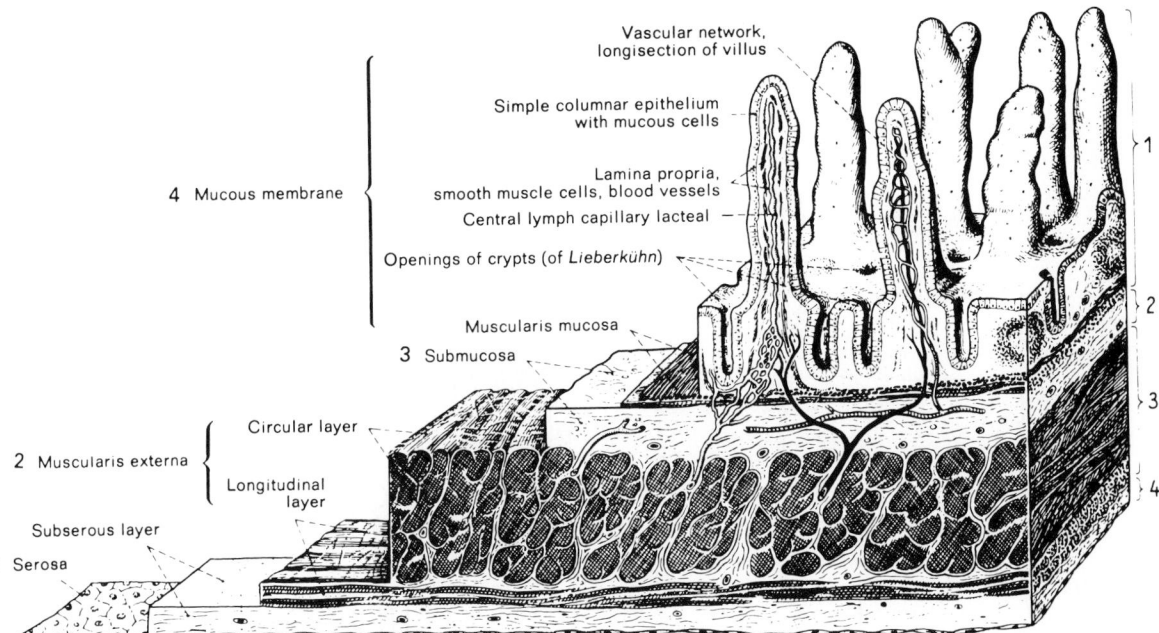

Vascular network,
longisection of villus

Simple columnar epithelium
with mucous cells

Lamina propria,
smooth muscle cells, blood vessels

Central lymph capillary lacteal

Openings of crypts (of *Lieberkühn*)

4 Mucous membrane

Muscularis mucosa

3 Submucosa

Circular layer

2 Muscularis externa

Longitudinal
layer

Subserous layer

1 Serosa

1

2

3

4

Fig. 27-2. Layers of the small intestine: A large surface is provided by villi for the absorption of required nutriments. The solitary lymph follicles in the lamina propria of the mucous membrane (not labeled). In the stroma of both sectioned villi are shown the central chyle vessels (lacteal) or the villous capillaries. (From: *Sabotta/Figge: Atlas of Human Anatomy. New York, Hafner, 1974*, with permission.)

If the mesentery is not greatly infiltrated by fat, and if there are no peritoneal adhesions, the bowel is extraordinarily mobile on its vascular tether, and in some individuals, jejunal segments may be sufficiently mobilized to allow anastomosis in the neck to replace the cervical esophagus.

The small bowel contains major deposits of lymphatic tissue, particularly in the Peyer's patches of the ileum. There is a rich lymphatic drainage of the entire small bowel, and this plays a major role in fat absorption. Lymphatic drainage proceeds from the mucosa through the wall of the bowel to a set of nodes adjacent to the bowel in the mesentery. Drainage continues to a group of regional nodes adjacent to the mesenteric arterial arcades and then to a group at the base of the superior mesenteric vessels. From there, lymph goes to the cisterna chyli and from thence up the thoracic ducts to empty into the venous system in the neck. The lymphatics of the gut play a major role in immune defense and also in the spread of cells arising from neoplasms in the gut.

The small bowel mucosa is characterized by transverse folds (plicae circulares or valves of Kerckring), but actually these are absent in the duodenal bulb and in the distal ileum. They are more prominent in the distal duodenum and jejunum, where they may reach 1 cm in height and form interlocking transverse ridges (Fig. 27-1). The small bowel mucosa has a pink velvet-like appearance with a glistening surface. It is usually thicker in the jejunum than in the ileum, where there may be no folds and the surface

may be entirely smooth, except for small scattered lymphatic nodules.

The innervation of the small bowel comes from both sympathetic and parasympathetic systems. Parasympathetic fibers come from the vagus and traverse the celiac ganglia. They affect secretion and motility and probably all phases of bowel activity. Vagal afferent fibers are present but apparently do not carry pain impulses. The sympathetic fibers come from the three sets of splanchnic nerves and have their ganglion cells usually in a plexus around the base of the superior mesenteric artery. Their motor impulses affect blood vessel motility and probably gut secretion and motility. Pain from the intestine is mediated through general visceral afferent fibers in the sympathetic system.

Histology

The wall of the small bowel has four layers, the serosa, the muscularis, the submucosa, and the mucosa (Fig. 27-2).

SEROSA. The serosa is the outermost layer and consists of visceral peritoneum that encircles the jejunoileum, but that covers the duodenum only anteriorly. It consists of a single layer of flattened mesophelial cells overlying loose connective tissue.

MUSCULARIS. The muscularis consists of a thin outer longitudinal layer and a thicker inner circular layer of smooth muscle. Specialized gaps in the muscle-cell membranes permit cell-to-cell communication, which facilitates the ability of the muscle layer to function as an electrical syncytium. Ganglion cells from the myenteric (Auerbach's) plexus are interposed between the two muscle layers and send fibers into both layers.

SUBMUCOSA. The submucosa is a layer of fibroelastic connective tissue containing blood vessels and nerves. It

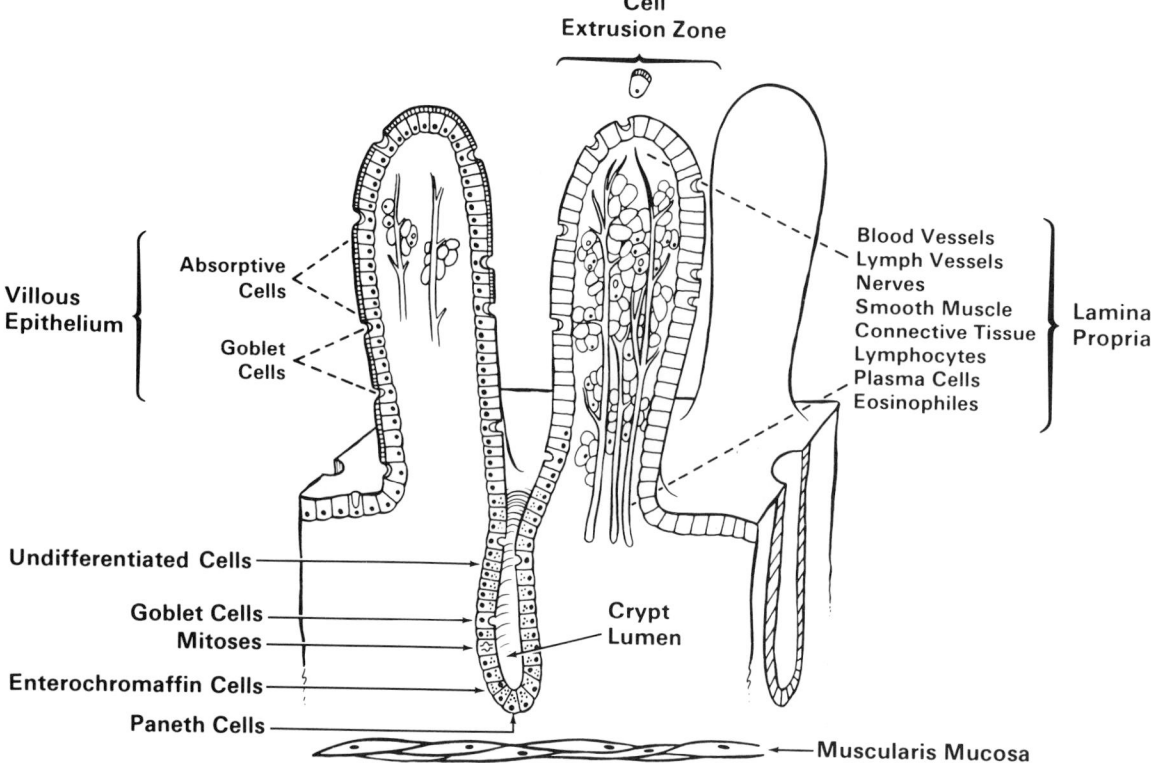

Fig. 27-3. Schematic diagram of two sectioned villi and a crypt of Lieberkühn illustrating the histologic organization of the small intestine mucosa. [Adapted and redrawn from: *Trier JS et al, in Sleisenger MH, Fordtran JS (eds): Gastrointestinal Disease. Pathophysiology, Diagnosis, Management. Philadelphia, Saunders, 1983, chap 48, with permission.*]

is the strongest component of the bowel wall and must, therefore, be included in placing sutures through the bowel. It contains elaborate networks of lymphatics and arterioles and venules and an extensive plexus of nerve fibers and ganglion cells (Meissner's plexus). Although frequently subdivided, the nerves from the mucosa, submucosa, and muscle layers are interconnected by small nerve fibers, and cross-connections between adrenergic and cholinergic elements have been described.

MUCOSA. Looked upon as a device to increase absorptive surface, the small bowel mucosa is an architectural marvel. The gross transverse folds, the finger-like villi protruding into the lumen of the bowel, the microvilli (brush border) covering the cells, and the glycocalyx fuzz covering the microvilli each tremendously increase the surface area exposed to luminal contents. Villi protrude $\frac{1}{2}$ to 1 mm into the lumen, are tallest in the distal duodenum and proximal jejunum, and become progressively shorter towards the terminal ileum.

The mucosa can be divided into three layers, the muscularis mucosae, lamina propria, and the epithelium. The deepest of these, the muscularis mucosae, is a thin sheet of muscle separating mucosa from submucosa. The lamina propria is a continuous layer of connective tissue between the epithelium and the muscularis mucosae. It extends into the villi and around the pitlike crypts of Lieberkühn (Fig. 27-3). The lamina propria contains, additionally, a variety of cells—plasma cells, lymphocytes, mast cells, eosinophils, macrophages, fibroblasts, smooth muscle cells—and noncellular connective tissue. The

lamina propria is the architectural base upon which the epithelium lies, but it also has important functions of its own and apparently serves protectively to combat microorganisms that penetrate the overlying epithelium. The plasma cells are an active site of synthesis of immunoglobulins.

Epithelium. The innermost mucosal layer is a continual sheet, one layer thick, of epithelial cells covering the villi and lining the crypts of Lieberkühn (see Fig. 27-3). The crypts contain four types of cells, goblet cells that secrete mucus, enterochromaffin cells whose endocrine function is unknown, Paneth cells that secrete zymogen granules and whose function is also unknown, and undifferentiated epithelial cells whose function is to provide for cell renewal. The epithelium of the small intestine is rapidly proliferating tissue in which old cells are discarded into the lumen and are replaced by newly-formed cells that appear to march up from the crypt into the villus in orderly sequence. This trip takes 5 to 7 days in the proximal small bowel, but in the ileum, labeled cells may travel from crypt to villous tip in 3 days.

The epithelium covering the villi consists of scattered endocrine cells, goblet cells, and absorptive cells. The major known functions of the villi are digestion and absorption. These functions are carried out by the absorp-

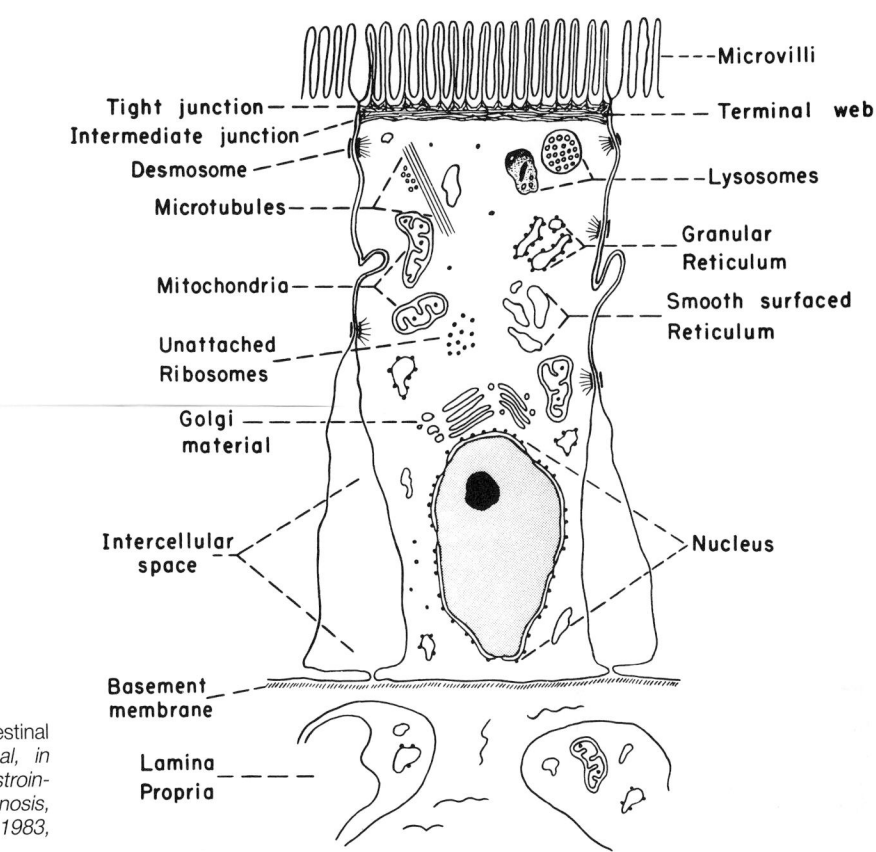

Fig. 27-4. Schematic diagram of an intestinal absorptive cell. [From: *Trier JS et al, in Sleisenger MH, Fordtran JS (eds): Gastrointestinal Disease. Pathophysiology, Diagnosis, Management. Philadelphia, Saunders, 1983, chap 48, with permission.*]

tive cells, tall columnar cells resting on a thin basement membrane that separates them from the lamina propria. Their luminal surface is covered by microvilli that rest on a terminal web (Fig. 27-4). The microvillar projections multiply the cell surface exposed to the lumen 30 times. The microvilli are covered in turn by a fuzzy coat of glycoprotein, the glycocalyx (Fig. 27-5). The microvilli participate actively in absorption and digestion: they contain enzymes for digestion of disaccharides and peptides, and certain cells may contain specific receptors that facilitate absorption (for example, certain ileal cells have receptors for vitamin B_{12} on their microvilli).

The plasma (or cell) membranes of the epithelial cells consist of three layers and are thicker over the microvilli than over the lateral and basal portions of the cell (Fig. 27-5). The lateral portion of the plasma membrane is also specialized. There are tight junctions between epithelial cells that prevent communication between intercellular spaces and the lumen. Immediately underneath the tight junction is a narrow space called an intermediate junction and beneath that is a desmosome, which provides tight attachments of adjacent membrane, by binding adjacent cells together. The depths of the tight junctions are greater between adjacent absorptive cells than between adjacent undifferentiated crypt cells. The permeability of the barrier between the intestinal lumen and the space between cells may vary from one location to another.

Fig. 27-5. Schematic illustration of the specializations of the apical cytoplasm of the plasma membrane of intestinal absorptive cells. [From: *Tier JS et al, in Sleisenger MH, Fordtran JS (eds): Gastrointestinal Disease. Pathophysiology, Diagnosis, Management. Philadelphia, Saunders, 1983, chap 48, with permission.*]

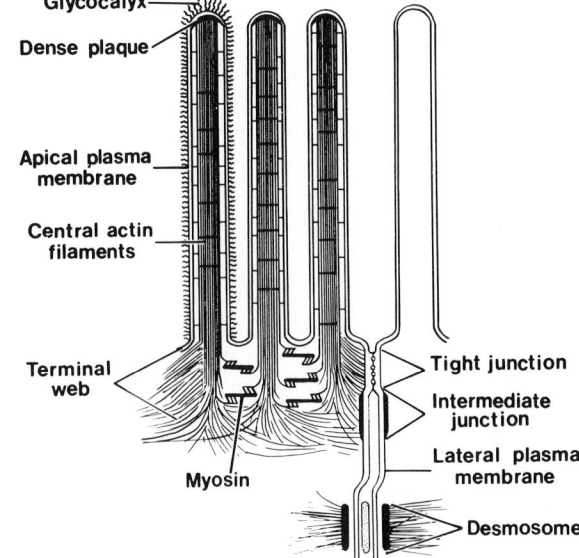

The cytoplasm immediately beneath the microvilli consists of fine filaments, known as the terminal web. This interconnects with filaments forming the core of the microvilli, which contain actin (Fig. 27-5). Myosin may also be present at the base of the microvilli, and these contractile proteins may allow for movement and contraction of the microvilli.

The processes of digestion and absorption within the epithelial cells are carried out by specific organelles (Fig. 27-4). The mitochondria participate in intracellular oxidation and provide energy for metabolism. The lysosomal sacs contain cytotoxic substances and intracellular waste products. The endoplasmic reticulum is the main synthesizing element within the cell and appears to be responsible for at least two major processes in fat absorption, the resynthesis of triglycerides from absorbed fatty acid fragments and the synthesis of the lipoprotein coat for chylomicrons. It is also the major synthetic site for intracellular digestive enzymes. The Golgi apparatus segregates, stores, and chemically modifies material that is absorbed and synthesized by the cell.

It may be useful to follow the path of a food element absorbed from the intestinal lumen. Initial contact is with the glycocalyx coating the microvilli, where some digestion may occur. Products of this digestion may go through the microvillous membrane, traversing the terminal web into the cytoplasm. The absorbed material may then either go laterally into the intracellular spaces or enter the channels of the endoplasmic reticulum, where it may be biochemically modified and transmitted to the Golgi material, where it may be stored. Eventually the material leaves the cell by crossing either the lateral or basal plasma (cell) membrane. It penetrates the basal lamina to enter the lamina propria, where it traverses the lymphatic or capillary endothelial cells to gain access to lymph or blood.

PHYSIOLOGY

Motility

Food is propelled through the small bowel by a complex series of muscular contractions. Motility patterns in the small bowel vary greatly in the fed and fasting state. Pace-setter potentials, probably originating in the duodenum, initiate a series of contractions that propel food through the small bowel. These contractions are of two types, segmentation and peristalsis. Contractions of the circular muscle divide the bowel into segments that are moved to and fro over the column of bowel contents for a short distance. The contents of adjacent segments then combine, and the process is repeated. About 40 percent of contractions are segmental. The circular muscle also initiates peristalsis, circular contractions migrating in an aboral direction propelling intestinal contents onward. The peristaltic reflex may function independently of extrinsic nerves. Abnormal waves of powerful contractions (*peristaltic rushes*) may rapidly traverse the entire segment of small intestine during episodes of enteritis.

During the interdigestive (fasting) period between meals, the bowel is regularly swept by a series of contractions initiated by the migrating myoelectric complex (MMC). The MMC is under neural and humoral control and initiates a triphasic series of contractions, phase I of which is resting, phase II intermittent contractions of moderate amplitude, and phase III the activity front that consists of a brief series of high-pressure waves. The MMC in man is stimulated by some (but not all) fluctuating increases in serum concentrations of motilin.

Small bowel motility is modulated by neural and humoral influences. Extrinsic nerves to the small bowel are vagal and sympathetic. Vagal fibers have two functionally different effects, one is cholinergic and excitatory and the other is peptidergic and probably inhibitory. Sympathetic fibers from the splanchnics appear chiefly to modulate the activity of intrinsic nerves.

Although gut peptides clearly influence bowel motility, their physiologic function is uncertain, except for the role of motilin in initiating MMC activity. Gastrin, cholecystokinin, and motilin are known to stimulate muscle contraction, whereas muscle activity is inhibited by secretin and often by glucagon (Table 27-1). Cholecystokinin may be physiologically important, since ingestion of a fatty meal may stimulate peristaltic contraction.

Digestion and Absorption

Liters of water and hundreds of grams of food move across the intestinal mucosa from the lumen to the blood stream each day. The process is remarkably efficient, nearly all food is absorbed unless protected by indigestible cellulose. There is no apparent governor; food absorption is just as efficient in the corpulent as it is in the starving.

FAT. Most individuals in Western Europe and North America consume 60 to 100 g of fat per day in the form of triglycerides. Fat digestion and absorption occurs in the small intestine, where triglycerides are partially hydrolyzed by pancreatic lipase, which splits off the two exposed fatty acids to leave a single central fatty acid still combined with glycerol (beta monoglyceride) plus two fatty acids (Fig. 27-6). Both are poorly soluble in water but combine with bile salts to form micelles. A mixed micelle is composed of bile salts, fatty acids, and the beta monoglyceride, and may also include phospholipids, cholesterol, and fat-soluble vitamins. The micelle must traverse three diffusion barriers in the passive process of entry into the intestinal epithelial cell. These are the unstirred water layer, the mucous coat overlying the brush border, and finally the lipid bilayer membrane making up the brush border. The micelle may release its fatty acid and monoglyceride component in traversing these barriers. After disaggregation of the micelle, bile salts remain within the intestinal lumen to enter into the formation of other micelles, and the released fatty acids and monoglycerides traverse the plasma membrane into the epithelial cell. The major metabolic pathway within the cell is initiated by reformation of the triglyceride through the interactions of intracellular enzymes (see Fig. 27-6) that are associated with the endoplasmic reticulum.

The triglycerides then combine with cholesterol and

Table 27-1. EFFECTS OF GASTROINTESTINAL HORMONES ON SMALL BOWEL MOTILITY

Gastrin — ↑ [a]
CCK — ↑ [a]
Secretin — ↓ [a]
Vasoactive intestinal peptide (VIP) — ↑↓
Glucagon — ↑↓ [a]
Motilin — ↑ [b,c]
Substance P — ↑

Neurotensin — ↑
Somatostatin — ↑↓ [c]
Bombesin — ↑↓
Enkephalins — ↑↓ [c]
Pancreatic polypeptide — ↑
Peptide YY (PYY) — ↓

↑ Increased
↓ Decreased
[a] Induction of fed pattern of motility from fasting
[b] Possible physiologic role
[c] Induction of migrating motor complexes
SOURCE: Adapted from: Sakamoto T, Guo Y-S, Thompson JC: Motility: gut and biliary, in Thompson JC, Greeley GH Jr, Rayford PL, Townsend CM Jr (eds): *Gastrointestinal Endocrinology.* New York, McGraw-Hill, 1987, pp 123–136.

phospholipids and apoproteins to form chylomicrons. These consist of an inner core containing almost all triglycerides with a membranous outer coat of phospholipids and apoproteins. The chylomicron exits the cell from the basolateral region and preferentially enters the central lacteal of the villus from whence it moves to the thoracic duct. Small fatty acids with chain lengths of C_{10} and less may move directly through the cell into capillaries to flow into the portal vein. The bulk of chylomicron assimilation from the intestinal cell is via lymphatics, but some direct transfer to the portal vein may take place, particularly during periods between meals.

Bile salts are resorbed into the enterohepatic circulation from the distal ileum, in one of the examples of selective sites of resorption (Table 27-2). The total bile salt pool in man is about 5 g, and it recirculates about 6 times every 24 h (the enterohepatic circulation of bile salts). Only about 0.5 g is lost in the stool every day, and this is replaced by resynthesis from cholesterol. All ingested fat

Fig. 27-6. Diagrammatic representation of fat digestion and absorption. Abbreviated structures and names are given. DG = diglyceride; C_{10} and C_{15} = carbon chain length of amino acids. [From: *Gray GM, in Sleisenger MH, Fordtran JS (eds): Gastrointestinal Disease. Pathophysiology, Diagnosis, Management. Philadelphia, Saunders, 1983, chap 51, with permission.*]

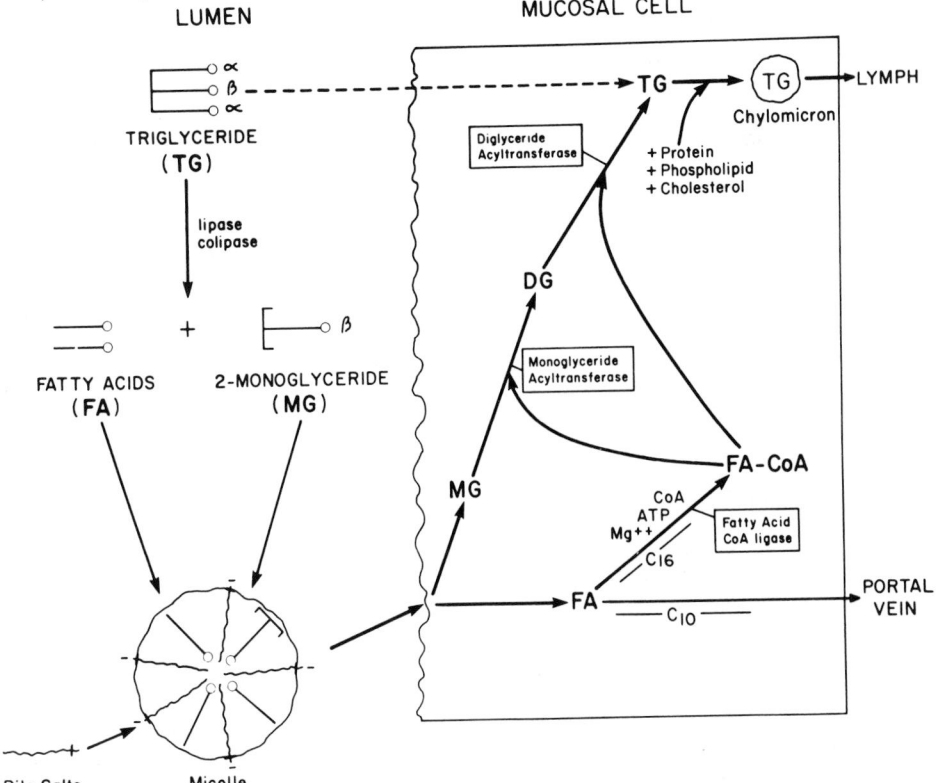

Table 27-2. DIFFERENTIAL SITES OF
ABSORPTION FROM THE JEJUNOILEUM

Proximal	*Distal*
Calcium	Bile salts
Fat (absorbed mainly	Vitamin B_{12}
in jejunum)	
Folate	
Iron	

is usually absorbed, and the small amount appearing in the stool comes from sloughed cells and bacteria.

PROTEIN. Protein digestion is initiated in the stomach, where gastric acid denatures proteins, and proteolysis is initiated by activated pepsin. Little actual digestion takes place, however, until protein enters the duodenum and upper jejunum, when proteins come under the influence of pancreatic proteases. Pancreatic trypsinogen is activated by the duodenal mucosal enzyme, enterokinase, and then activated trypsin further activates all proteases. Endopeptidases (trypsin, elastase, chymotrypsin) act on peptide bonds at the interior of the protein molecule, producing peptides that are substrates for exopeptidases (carboxypeptidases), which serially remove a single amino acid at a time from the carboxy-terminal end of the peptide. The final products are amino acids and peptides of 2–6 amino acid residues. The intraluminal action of pancreatic proteases is efficient and yields 70 percent short-chain peptides and 30 percent amino acids. Short peptides are optimal substrates for the peptide transport mechanism that brings di- and tripeptides into the cell. Of peptides that are assimilated intact, at least 90 percent are hydrolyzed to free amino acids by cytosol peptidases, before delivery to the portal venous system.

CARBOHYDRATE. Western men and women take in about 400 g of carbohydrates a day, 60 percent as starch, 30 percent as sucrose, and 10 percent as lactose. Carbohydrates comprise about half the calories ingested in our society, but in underdeveloped countries they may provide a much higher proportion.

Starch is a polysaccharide consisting of long chains of glucose molecules. Amylose makes up 20 percent of starch in the diet and has an alpha glucose-to-glucose bridge. Amylopectin (80 percent of dietary starch) has branching points every 25 molecules along the straight glucose chains. Both have an $alpha_{1-4}$ glucose-linked chain. Alpha amylase attacks the $alpha_{1-4}$ linkage and converts amylose to maltotriose and maltose. Amylase converts amylopectin to shorter dextrins. Intraluminal digestion of starch in the duodenum is rapid because of the huge amounts of pancreatic amylase, and digestion is often complete by the time the starch enters the jejunum.

The enzyme responsible for final surface digestion is concentrated in the brush border of the luminal surface (Fig. 27-7). After dietary carbohydrate is reduced to monosaccharides by surface digestion, transport of the released hexoses (glucose, galactose, or fructose) is carried out by a specific process. Glucose and galactose are actively transported across the intestinal membrane,

whereas fructose is absorbed by facilitated diffusion. The rate-limiting phenomenon for most carbohydrate absorption occurs during transport through the intestinal cell, but luminal hydrolysis of lactose is slower than its transport capacity, so that surface hydrolysis of lactose is rate-limiting.

WATER AND ELECTROLYTES. In addition to ingested water, salivary, gastric, biliary, pancreatic, and intestinal fluids add up to 8 to 10 L of water per day, of which all but about 0.5 L per day is resorbed proximal to the ileocecal valve. The small bowel secretes and absorbs huge amounts of water. Net absorption is the algebraic sum of two fluxes going in opposite directions. Water may simply diffuse in or out of the cell or may be drawn through by osmotic or hydrostatic pressures. The osmotic pressures result from active transport of sodium glucose or amino acids into cells. Diffusion occurs through pores in plasma cell membranes. Jejunal pores are larger (7 to 9 Å) than those in the ileum (3 to 4 Å). Hypertonic solutions in the duodenum and upper jejunum are rapidly equilibrated to isotonicity by the influx of large amounts of water.

Sodium and chloride are absorbed from the small bowel by active transport, by coupling to organic solutes and cotransport by carriers of neutral sodium chloride. A small portion of sodium absorption in the jejunum is by active transport, but the bulk is by coupling to organic solutes. In the ileum, sodium is absorbed against deep gradients and is not stimulated by glucose, galactose, or bicarbonate. Bicarbonate is absorbed by a sodium-hydrogen exchange, so that one bicarbonate ion is released into interstitial fluid for every hydrogen ion secreted. Calcium is absorbed by active transport, particularly in the duodenum and jejunum. Absorption appears to be facilitated by an acid environment and is enhanced by vitamin D and parathormone. Potassium appears to be absorbed by passive diffusion.

Endocrine Function

The mucosa of the small bowel is the primary source of regulatory peptides of the gut, and the muscle wall of the small bowel is rich in peptidergic nerves containing neuroendocrine peptides. Although we often call these agents hormones, they do not always function in a truly endocrine fashion, that is, the active peptides are not always discharged into blood vessels to act upon some distant site. Sometimes they are discharged and act locally in a paracrine fashion [for example, bombesin (gastrin-releasing peptide) and somatostatin], or they may serve as neurotransmitters, or they may be discharged into blood vessels after nerve stimulation in a true neuroendocrine manner. We will briefly describe some of these agents.

SECRETIN. The discovery of secretin in 1902 gave birth to the entire field of endocrinology. Secretin is a 27-amino acid, helical peptide that is present in specialized cells in the small bowel mucosa and is released by acidification or by contact with bile and perhaps fat. It acts to stimulate release of water and bicarbonate from pancreatic ductal cells, and when this combination flows into the duodenal lumen, the bicarbonate neutralizes gastric acid. The

LUMEN

INTESTINAL CELL

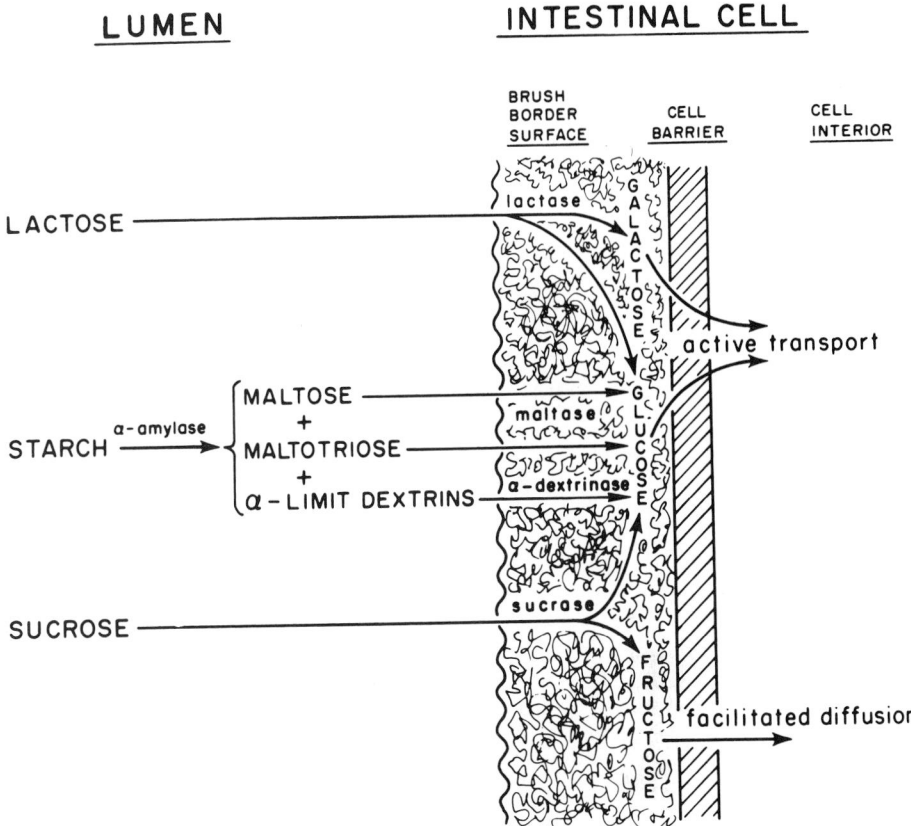

Fig. 27-7. The digestion and absorption of carbohydrate. Note that only starch is digested in the lumen; other dietary saccharides are hydrolyzed by constitutive enzymes of the intestinal surface. The final monosaccharide products are then transported by their specific mechanisms. [From: *Gray GM, in Sleisenger MH, Fordtran JS (eds): Gastrointestinal Disease. Pathophysiology, Diagnosis, Management. Philadelphia, Saunders, 1983, chap 51, with permission.*]

amount of pancreatic bicarbonate released after a meal closely approximates the amount of acid secreted by the stomach. Secretin also acts to stimulate the flow of bile and to inhibit gastrin release, gastric acid secretion, and gastrointestinal motility. Secretin has the unique ability to release gastrin from gastrinomas, and intravenous secretin is used as a diagnostic test in patients with the Zollinger-Ellison syndrome.

CHOLECYSTOKININ. Cholecystokinin (CCK) is released from small bowel mucosa by contact with certain amino acids (especially tryptophan and phenylalanine) and medium- to long-chain fatty acids. It has two major actions, one to stimulate contractions of the gallbladder and relaxation of the sphincter of Oddi and the other to stimulate the secretion of enzymes by pancreatic acinar cells. CCK also stimulates growth of bowel mucosa and pancreas, it stimulates bowel motility, and it releases insulin. CCK exists in multiple molecular forms (CCK-8, CCK-33, CCK-39, among others), and the larger forms contain the smaller ones. CCK and gastrin share the identical C-terminal tetrapeptide (Trp-Met-Asp-Phe-NH₂), which explains many of the similarities in their action.

OTHER PEPTIDES. Largely through the efforts of Viktor Mutt and colleagues at the Karolinska Institute, several active agents have been isolated from the mucosa of the small bowel that greatly influence physiologic activities of the gut. Of these, only *gastric inhibitory polypeptide* (GIP) has satisfied rigid criteria for hormonal status, but others will be discussed as well. GIP is a 43-amino acid peptide member of the secretin-glucagon family that is released by glucose and by fat. Although it was initially studied for its properties of inhibition of gastric secretion, later studies showed that it was a prime incretin candidate because it greatly stimulated insulin release when levels of glucose were elevated. Glucose-stimulated release of intestinal GIP apparently solves the conundrum posed by the fact that oral ingestion of a fixed amount of glucose releases more insulin than the intravenous administration of the same amount. A family of peptides reacting with glucagon antibodies is present in small bowel mucosa, and it has been given a variety of names. *Enteroglucagon* is a term used to designate all such gut peptides. It inhibits bowel motility, and it apparently stimulates mucosal growth. *Vasoactive intestinal peptide* (VIP) is a 28-amino acid basic peptide of the secretin-glucagon family that appears to function chiefly as a neuropeptide. VIP is a potent vasodilator and stimulates pancreatic and intestinal secretion and inhibits gastric acid secretion. It is the chief agent in the watery diarrhea syndrome caused by pancreatic endocrine tumors. *Motilin* is a 22-amino acid

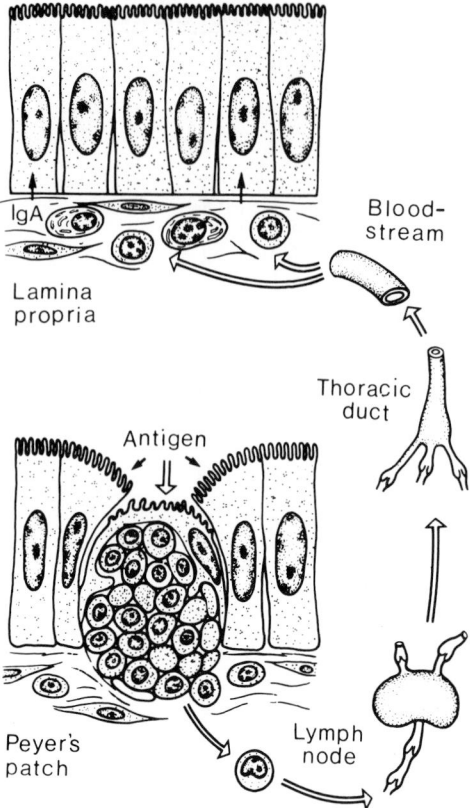

Fig. 27-8. Schematic representation of the pathways involved in the secretory immune system. Lymphocytes in Peyer's patches exposed to antigens from the gut lumen migrate to regional lymph nodes and thence to the bloodstream. Circulating in the blood, they home into the lamina propria of the gut and there develop into plasma cells secreting IgA, which acquires a secretory piece in the epithelium and is released into the gut lumen. (From: *Fawcett DW: A Textbook of Histology. Philadelphia, Saunders, 1986, with permission.*)

peptide widely distributed through the gut. It causes contraction of intestinal smooth muscle, including the gallbladder, and appears to be involved in the interdigestive pattern of gut motility. *Bombesin* is a 14-amino acid peptide first isolated from frog skin. It has the capacity to release probably all gut peptides except secretin. Its mammalian equivalent, gastrin-releasing peptide, is present in small bowel mucosa, where it probably serves as an "on" switch regulating release of gastrointestinal hormones. *Somatostatin* is a 14-amino acid peptide first isolated from the brain that is also widely distributed in the gut, where it probably functions in a paracrine fashion as an "off" switch. *Peptide YY* (PYY) is a 36-amino acid peptide in the distal ileum and colon. It inhibits gastric and pancreatic secretion but has no effect on gallbladder motility. PYY is released by perfusion of the colon with fat and may be involved in the physiologic inhibition of pancreatic secretion.

Immune Function

We ingest thousands of bacteria and parasites and viruses every day. Only a few of these are pathogenic, but the huge surface of the small bowel mucosa represents a massive potential portal of entry. An important component of bowel defense is the secretory immune system that produces a special group of antibodies that resist bacterial proliferation, neutralize virus, and minimize the penetration of enterotoxins.

The small bowel is a major source of immunoglobulin A (IgA). Cells of the lamina propria of the small intestine contain plasma cells that produce IgA. The population of cells producing IgA (the secretory immunoglobulin) is ten times greater than that producing IgG (the antibody mediating general humoral immunity).

Antigens from the intestinal lumen crossing the mucosal barrier contact M cells overlying lymphoid nodules. These cells are specialized for uptake and transport of antigen, which they convey to the underlying lymphoblasts that produce IgA. After interacting with the antigen, the lymphoblasts migrate to the regional lymph nodes from which they enter the systemic circulation. They then are returned to the intestine, where they are widely distributed in the lamina propria (Fig. 27-8). In the lamina propria, they differentiate into plasma cells that produce a specific IgA antibody directed to the absorbed antigen. This IgA antibody traverses the epithelial cell to the lumen by means of a protein carrier (the secretory component) that not only transports the IgA, but also protects it against the intracellular lysosomes. The antibodies at the free surface of the cell collect in the glycocalyx where they are in a strategic position to combat new antigens, preventing their attachment to the cell membrane, achieving immune exclusion.

INFLAMMATORY DISEASES

Crohn's Disease

Crohn's disease is a chronic granulomatous disease of the alimentary tract first described as regional ileitis by Crohn, Ginzburg, and Openheimer in 1932. In the introduction to their landmark paper, they stated

We propose to describe, with pathologic and clinical details, a disease of the terminal ileum affecting mainly young adults, characterized by a subacute or chronic necrotizing and cicatrizing inflammation. The ulceration of the mucosa is accompanied by a disproportionate connective tissue reaction of the remaining walls of the involved intestine, a process which frequently leads to stenosis of the lumen of the intestine, associated with the formation of multiple fistulas.

This disease has never been more elegantly, accurately, or completely described. Many different terms have been used to describe this disease, but because of its multiple clinical appearances and because the disease is not confined to the terminal ileum, Crohn's disease has been universally accepted as its name.

Since 1932, we have learned a great deal about the disease; unfortunately, we still do not know the etiology, and curative treatment has not been devised. We have learned, however, that extensive surgical resection, in an attempt at cure, plays no role in the management of patients with Crohn's disease. Our discussion will be limited to Crohn's disease of the small intestine.

Crohn's disease is a chronic inflammatory disease characterized by spontaneous remissions and acute exacerbations. There is a peak age of onset between the second and fourth decades. The typical patient is a young adult with a long history of chronic abdominal pain, diarrhea, and weight loss. The diagnosis is often delayed; an average of 3 years has elapsed between the onset of symptoms and the time the diagnosis is established. The abdominal pain is usually cramping, and often becomes constant. Diarrhea is intermittent, explosive, associated with meals, and frequently nocturnal. Weight loss usually appears later and is the result of decreased food intake, as well as nutritional abnormalities that develop as a result of defects of digestion and absorption in the diseased bowel.

Crohn's disease is the most common surgical disease of the small intestine. The incidence of Crohn's disease is greatest in North America and Northern Europe and is still increasing. For example, the incidence increased from 1.8 to 3.7 per 100,000 from 1963 to 1973 in the United States. There is a familial association with Crohn's disease, but no specific pattern of inheritance has been described. The risk for Crohn's disease is increased 30 times in siblings of patients with the disease and 13 times for all first-degree relatives. Although surgical resection is not curative, 75 percent of patients studied in the National Cooperative Crohn's Disease Study (NCCDS) required one or more surgical procedures within 20 years of onset of the disease. Operations are used only to treat complications. Recurrence rates after operation are high; surgical cure is not possible.

PATHOLOGY. The usual sequence in discussion of a disease is etiology, pathogenesis, and pathology. This sequence is here reversed in order to relate pathologic findings, which are well known, to hypotheses concerning pathogenic and etiologic factors, which are not known.

Microscopic features of Crohn's disease vary, but some histologic features occur with sufficient consistency to create a pattern that, while not specific, is at least characteristic of the disease. Some understanding of pathogenesis may be gained by observing the progression of changes from early to late phases of regional enteritis.

Intense mucosal and submucosal edema may be seen microscopically before any gross changes are apparent. The earliest gross pathologic lesion is a superficial aphthous ulcer. As the disease progresses, the ulceration becomes more pronounced and complete transmural inflammation results. The inflammatory reaction is characterized by extensive edema, hyperemia, lymphangiectasia, an intense infiltration of mononuclear cells, and hyperplasia of lymphoid follicles. The ulcers are characteristically linear. As the disease progresses, linear ulcers may coalesce to produce transverse clefts and sinuses that result in the characteristic cobblestone appearance of the mucosa. There is thickening and hypertrophy of the submucosa and the muscularis, which results in narrowing of the gut lumen; obliterative lymphangitis occurs; the bowel wall becomes thickened and edematous and quite rigid. Granulomas appear later and are found in the bowel wall and in regional lymph nodes. These are noncaseating granulomas with Langhans' giant cells. As the transmural inflammation progresses, the mesentery becomes involved in the inflammatory reaction and becomes thickened and shortened. At operation, one observes thickened, grayish pink or dull purple-red loops of bowel with areas of thick, gray-white exudate or fibrosis of the serosa. Areas of diseased bowel separated by areas of grossly normal bowel, called skip areas, are commonly encountered. A striking finding of Crohn's disease at operation is extensive fat-wrapping, caused by circumferential growth of the mesenteric fat around the wall of the bowel. The thickened bowel wall is very firm, rubbery, and virtually incompressible. The uninvolved proximal bowel is often dilated because of the considerable degree of obstruction present in the diseased segment. Involved segments are often adherent to adjacent loops or other viscera, or several loops may be matted together into a bulky conglomerate mass. Internal fistulas are common in such adherent areas. The mesentery of the segment is characteristically greatly thickened, dull, and rubbery, and contains masses of lymph nodes up to 3 or 4 cm in size.

Crohn's disease is a chronic granulomatous disease of unknown etiology. Despite years of trials, no animal model has been developed for Crohn's disease. Theories that have been put forth to suggest causative factors in the development of the disease have included immunologic abnormalities or the presence of transmissible agents.

Immunologic abnormalities that have been found in patients have included both humoral and cell-mediated immune reactions directed against gut cells, suggesting autoimmunity. However, there has been no direct correlation between these abnormalities, immunologic reactivity, and the development of Crohn's disease; they are probably epiphenomena.

A transmissible agent was first suggested in 1970 by Mitchell and Rees who inoculated the foot pads of mice with extracts of diseased bowel from patients; granulomatous lesions were produced in the footpads. These lesions were proposed as evidence of transmissable agents causing Crohn's disease. Other workers have failed to confirm these findings. Cytotrophic agents, or viruses, have been found by some investigators in diseased human tissue; however, there is controversy as to whether their findings represent true viruses. Electron microscopic analysis of large numbers of specimens has failed to reveal any viruses. Mycobacteria (*Mycobacterium kansasii*) have also been implicated, but presently, no etiologic agent has been found.

CLINICAL MANIFESTATIONS. A typical patient is a young adult with a long history of recurring and persistent abdominal pain, diarrhea, and weight loss. About one-third of patients have fever. There are three patterns of involvement: the small bowel is involved alone in 30 percent of patients; ileocolitis is present in 55 percent of patients; and 15 percent of patients have involvement of only the colon. These findings from the NCCDS differ from some British and Australian series in which as many as 50 percent of patients have only colonic involvement. The site of involvement is an indicator of prognosis; ileocolitis has the highest incidence of recurrence after resection.

Perianal disease (fissure, fistula, stricture, or abscess) is common, occurring in 25 percent of patients with small intestinal disease, 41 percent of patients with ileocolitis, and 48 percent of patients with exclusively colonic involvement. Perianal disease may be the sole presenting feature in 5 percent of patients and may precede the onset of intestinal disease by months to years. Any patient with multiple, chronic, recurrent perianal fistulas should be suspected of Crohn's disease. Extraintestinal manifestations of Crohn's disease include arthritis and arthralgia, uveitis and iritis, hepatitis and pericholangitis, and erythema nodosum and pyoderma gangrenosum.

In the majority of patients, the onset of disease is insidious, with a slow, protracted course. There are symptomatic periods of abdominal pain and diarrhea interspersed with varying intervals of remission; but over time, symptomatic periods gradually become more frequent and more severe and long-lasting. Pain (the most common symptom) is usually intermittent and cramping early in the course of the disease, but may develop into persistent, dull aching abdominal pain, most prominent in the lower abdomen.

Diarrhea is the next most frequent symptom and is present, at least intermittently, in 85 percent of patients. The frequency of stools is not great compared with ulcerative colitis, numbering two to five daily, and, unlike ulcerative colitis, the stools rarely contain mucus, pus, or blood.

Fever is present in about one-third of these patients; moderate weight loss, loss of strength, and easy fatigability, in over one-half. Frank nutritional disorders and steatorrhea are uncommon before surgical treatment.

DIAGNOSIS. Patients with chronic, recurring episodes (often of long duration) of abdominal pain, diarrhea, and weight loss should be suspected of having Crohn's disease. Diagnosis is confirmed by barium radiographic studies of the small bowel. The most accurate technique of examination is radiographic enteroclysis. Although numerous findings have been described for Crohn's disease, the most common findings noted in the NCCDS survey were a nodular contour, diffuse narrowing of the lumen, sinuses, clefts, and linear ulcers, separation of bowel loops, and asymmetrical involvement of the bowel wall. One-half of patients had a cobblestone mucosal pattern composed of linear ulcers and transverse sinuses and clefts. This study showed that the radiographic features of Crohn's disease of the small bowel did not correlate with clinical symptoms or response to drug therapy. Therefore, there is no need for ritual, periodic radiographic examination of the small bowel in patients with established Crohn's disease, except in one of the following situations: (1) evaluating the appearance of Crohn's disease in a patient with severe clinical exacerbation, looking particularly for evidence of stricture with obstruction or fistula; (2) preoperative evaluation of patients undergoing planned resection; or (3) evaluation of post-operative patients who develop clinical symptoms of recurrence.

TREATMENT. Patients presenting with signs and symptoms of acute intestinal obstruction are common; however, complete obstruction is unusual. Most patients with these findings will improve on a conservative program of intravenous fluids, nasogastric suction, and medications. Complete obstruction is uncommon compared to partial obstruction. The acute obstruction is produced by intense edema and inflammation of the bowel wall. Emergency operation for obstruction per se is usually not necessary, since most patients respond rather quickly to nonoperative measures. Elective operative treatment for high-grade partial obstruction (characterized by Kantor's string sign on barium radiographic studies, (Fig. 27-9) is usually indicated, however, as soon as the patient can be prepared.

Medical treatment of Crohn's disease is largely symptomatic and empiric and is usually followed by remissions and exacerbations until a complication that requires surgical intervention supervenes. Goals of medical therapy are relieving abdominal pain, controlling diarrhea, treating infection, and correcting any nutritional deficiencies.

Intraluminal antibiotics, particularly sulfasalazine (Azulfidine), do have significant beneficial effects in certain patients. Corticosteroids are also useful in effecting re-

Fig. 27-9. This radiograph demonstrates Kantor's string sign (arrows). The string sign is the result of narrowing of the lumen due to mucosal ulceration, extensive thickening, and rigidity of the bowel wall.

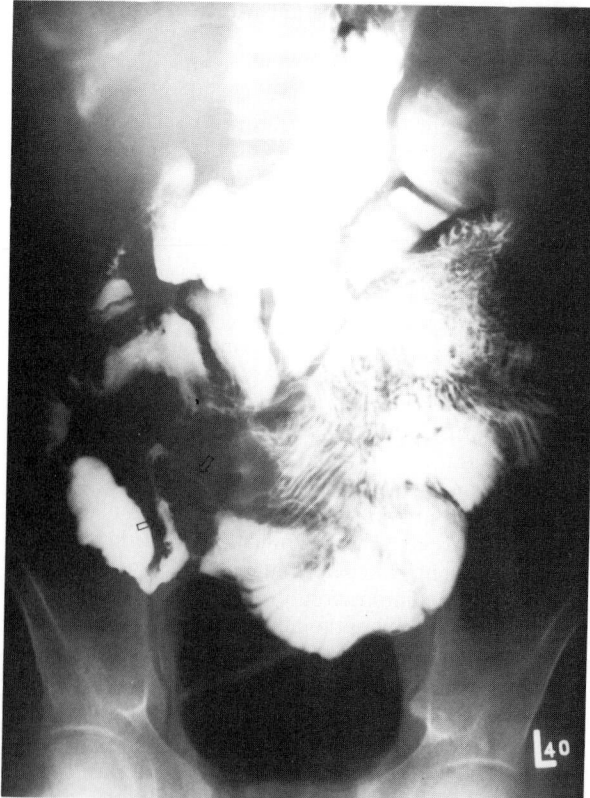

mission of symptoms during acute exacerbations of ileitis, and a combination of sulfasalazine and steroids may be used to maintain patients for a short period of time after resolution of an acute inflammatory episode. Long-term maintenance therapy, with either agent alone or in combination, however, has not been shown to be of benefit in preventing recurrence of the disease. Although there have been implications of immunologic abnormality in Crohn's disease, immunosuppressive treatment with azathioprine and 6-mercaptopurine have not been conclusively shown to be of advantage when compared to placebo. Systemic antibiotics are valuable in the management of infectious complications, but have no effect on the primary disease process and should not be considered to be therapeutic.

Elemental diets and total parenteral nutrition have been touted as being beneficial, even curative, in patients with acute Crohn's disease or in patients with complications such as enterocutaneous fistulas. There is no specific therapeutic benefit in any dietary measure. The provision of adequate nutrition is much more important in preparing patients for operation than it is for cure.

There is a subgroup of patients with acute abdominal signs and symptoms in whom the usual preoperative diagnosis is acute appendicitis. At operation, the appendix is found to be normal, but the terminal ileum is edematous and beefy red, having a thickened mesentery with enlarged lymph nodes. The condition is acute ileitis, a self-limiting disease, which does not lead to subsequent development of Crohn's disease. The precise etiology of acute ileitis is unknown; however, some patients have been found to have *Yersinia* or *Campylobacter* infections.

Although in the past, performance of appendectomy has been controversial in this setting, the place of appendectomy now seems clear. In the absence of acute inflammatory involvement of the appendix or the cecum, appendectomy should be performed. This removes the possibility of acute appendicitis in the differential diagnosis of any subsequent abdominal complaints in these patients. In the few patients who have developed enterocutaneous fistulas after appendectomy, the fistulas have all originated from the ileum.

Although medical management is certainly indicated during acute exacerbations of disease, the majority of patients with chronic Crohn's disease will require operation sometime during the course of their illness. In patients with more than 20 years of disease, the NCCDS reported that the cumulative probability of operation was 78 percent.

Cure of patients with Crohn's disease is not possible by either medical or surgical therapy. Indications for operation are limited to complications, including: obstruction, abscess, fistula, free perforation, urologic complications, hemorrhage, cancer, perianal disease, and growth retardation.

Patients with Crohn's disease who have had a previous abdominal operation and who develop signs of mechanical bowel obstruction pose a difficult problem. The most likely cause is progressive disease, but the obstruction may be caused by postoperative adhesions. In this set-

ting, the historical sequence of symptoms becomes most important. A history of increasing pain, diarrhea, and fever over days to weeks points toward a recrudescence of Crohn's disease. A short history (hours) of the acute onset and rapid progression of cramping abdominal pain, nausea, and vomiting, without an antecedent history of increasing disease activity, usually means adhesions.

At operation, only the segment of the bowel involved in the obstructive process should be resected. Even if adjacent areas of bowel are clearly diseased, they should be ignored unless also obstructed. Early in the history of surgical treatment of Crohn's disease, many surgeons tended towards wide resection in an attempt to effect cure. Repeated wide resections lead to the short bowel syndrome, a devastating surgical complication. In the past, the most common cause of the short bowel syndrome was repeated resections for Crohn's disease. We and most other surgeons have, for at least the past two decades, concluded that it is extremely difficult surgically to eradicate this disease, and we have, for example, given up frozen-section study of the resected margin because we generally limit our resection to areas that are grossly involved adjacent to sites of obstruction or fistulization. We ignore microscopic evidence of involvement.

Fistulas in patients with Crohn's disease are usually enteroenteral or enterocutaneous. The presence of a radiographically demonstrable enteroenteral fistula without any signs of sepsis or other complication is not in itself an indication for operation. However, the vast majority of patients who have radiographic demonstration of enteroenteral fistulas will develop later complications, most commonly sepsis, and will require resection of the fistula. Enterocutaneous fistulas are rarely spontaneous, but follow resections or external drainage of intraabdominal abscesses. All enterocutaneous fistulas associated with active Crohn's disease must be treated by resection of the involved segment of the bowel, in addition to closure of the fistula. The formation of enteroenteric or enterovesicle fistulas usually involves either a previous intestinal perforation with formation of a walled-off abscess that finally perforates or the adherence of one diseased loop of bowel to another diseased loop of bowel or an adjacent normal organ. If the fistula forms between two or more adjacent loops of diseased bowel, the entire involved segment should be excised. On the other hand, if the fistula involves an adjacent normal organ, such as the bladder or the colon, only the segment of the diseased small bowel and fistulous track should be resected, and the defect that is left in the normal organ is simply closed. Block and Schraut have shown that the majority of patients with ileosigmoid fistulas do not require resection of the sigmoid because the disease is confined to the small bowel. If the segment of sigmoid involved in an ileosigmoid fistula is found to have Crohn's disease, it should be resected, along with the segment of diseased small bowel.

Perforation into the free peritoneal cavity is not common, but occurs occasionally. Free perforation usually occurs in a diseased segment of bowel but can also occur in bowel proximal to an obstruction. The segment should be resected back to relatively good bowel on each side of the perforation, and no attempt should be made to eradicate all diseased bowel. If generalized peritonitis is present, an anastomosis should not be done because of the high rate of anastomotic dehiscence; an ileostomy should be performed until intraabdominal sepsis is controlled. Later restoration of intestinal continuity can be carried out safely.

The most common urologic complication is ureteral obstruction, which is usually due to ileocolic disease with retroperitoneal abscess. Periureteric fibrosis may be present and may require extensive ureteral lysis.

Although anemia from chronic blood loss is common, life-threatening hemorrhage is rare. When it occurs, the segment involved should be resected and intestinal continuity restored. Up to one-fourth of children with Crohn's disease may have significant growth retardation that may precede the appearance of active bowel disease. In these children, bowel resection, in the absence of other common indications, is indicated and will often result in restoration of normal growth.

Treatment of perianal disease should be conservative, and wide excisions of abscesses or fistulas are not indicated. Definitive fistulotomy is indicated in the majority of patients, although one must recognize that some degree of anal stenosis may occur as a result of the chronic inflammation. Fissures are usually lateral, relatively painless, large and indolent, and will usually respond to conservative management. Abscesses should be drained, but large excisions of tissue should not be carried out.

The optimum treatment of complications of Crohn's disease is surgical resection of the involved segment with restoration of intestinal continuity. Current evidence indicates that results are not improved by increasing the margins of normal tissue proximal and distal to the diseased intestine. Thus, the proximal margin should be through soft, pliable bowel—dilatation does not necessarily indicate disease—and microscopic control of margins with frozen sections is not helpful and is often confusing. With disease in the terminal ileum, the distal line of resection should be in the ascending colon, although the standard right colectomy is technically easier. No attempt should be made to remove all enlarged mesenteric lymph nodes, since this does not change the rate of recurrence and may endanger the blood supply to otherwise normal intestine. In selected patients with obstruction caused by strictures (either single or multiple), many surgeons utilize strictureplasty as an alternative to resection. The technique involves longitudinal incision of the stricture, including one centimeter of bowel on either side of the stricture. The incision is then closed transversely. This technique is said to be associated with no increased incidence of leaks or recurrence of disease compared to resection. We do not use this method. No one should be confused; the standard surgical treatment is limited resection and anastomosis of diseased bowel.

In the past, bypass procedures were commonly used, but today, bypass with exclusion is now only used in elderly, poor-risk patients; in patients who have had several prior resections and can ill afford to lose any more bowel; and in patients in whom resection would necessitate entering an abscess or endangering normal structures. The reasons for this are twofold: the disease often persists in the bypassed segment with development of intraabdominal sepsis, and cancer may occur in the bypassed segment.

PROGNOSIS. The occurrence of cancer in Crohn's disease has been well documented. Cancer is reported to be 60 to 300 times more frequent in patients with Crohn's ileitis than in patients the same age without Crohn's disease. Cancer arising in the small bowel afflicted with Crohn's disease is different than small bowel cancer in patients without Crohn's disease. The cancers occur more commonly in the ileum, they occur more often in men, they have a worse prognosis, and Crohn's disease patients are younger.

There is no surgical cure for Crohn's disease. It is now clear that a substantial proportion of patients who have had one operation will require another operation for complications of Crohn's disease. In one study, the cumulative recurrence rates were reported to be 29 percent at 5 years, 52 percent at 10 years, 64 percent at 15 years, and 84 percent at 25 years. No important differences were noted between disease location and the type of operation. One cannot predict which patients will develop recurrent disease. Sex, age, duration of disease, granulomas, enteral or perirectal fistulas, the length of resection, the length of diseased gut, and the proximal resection margin had no significant influence on the rate of recurrent disease or functional outcome. The most common site of recurrence is the small bowel proximal to the site of previous resection. Recurrence is five times more likely to involve the adjacent or remote colon in patients with ileocolitis compared to ileitis. Few patients with ileitis eventually require ileostomy, whereas one-third of patients with ileocolitis or colitis often may require permanent ileostomy.

Crohn's disease gradually burns out with advancing age. Active disease is unusual between the ages of 50 and 55, but gradual cicatrization with healing may cause bowel obstruction in old patients.

Tuberculous Enteritis

Tuberculosis of the gut is now rare in Western countries, but is still a significant problem in India and developing countries. Tuberculosis of the gastrointestinal tract occurs in two forms. Primary infection is usually due to the bovine strain of *Mycobacterium tuberculosis* and results from ingesting infected milk. This now accounts for less than 10 percent of reported cases. Secondary infection, due to the human strain, results from the swallowing of bacilli by patients with active pulmonary tuberculosis. Chemotherapy has greatly decreased the incidence of secondary tuberculous enteritis, so that it now occurs in only about 1 percent of patients with pulmonary tuberculosis.

The ileocecal region is the site of involvement in about 85 percent of patients with tuberculous enteritis, presumably because of the abundance of lymphoid tissue in this area. Three patterns of involvement are seen: hypertrophic, ulcerative, or ulcerohypertrophic.

Occasionally, a hypertrophic reaction produces contracture and stenosis of the lumen of distal ileum, which requires resection. The diagnosis is not often made preoperatively; only 50 percent of patients have evidence of active pulmonary tuberculosis; 45 percent of patients have negative skin tests. If the diagnosis is suspected preoperatively, chemotherapy, best given as a combination of isoniazid, 100 mg three times a day, with either rifampin (600 mg daily) or ethanibutol (15 mg/kg daily), should be administered for about 2 weeks before operation. If unsuspected tuberculosis is found at operation, chemotherapy should be started, and in both instances, drugs should be continued for 1 year after the patient has become asymptomatic. Surgical therapy of hypertrophic tuberculous enteritis is usually inadvisable unless bowel obstruction due to high-grade stenosis requires relief. Resection and anastomosis should be performed unless extensive disease is present, otherwise ileocolic bypass is the safer procedure.

Symptoms of the more common ulcerative form of tuberculous enteritis include alternating constipation and diarrhea associated with crampy lower abdominal pain. At times, the diagnosis may only be made by radiographic intestinal examination of patients with pulmonary tuberculosis. In severe cases, diarrhea is persistent, and anemia and inanition are progressive. Clinical confirmation of a presumptive diagnosis may be obtained by a prompt response to antituberculous chemotherapy. Surgical therapy is contraindicated except for the rare complications of perforation, obstruction, or hemorrhage.

Typhoid Enteritis

Typhoid enteritis is an acute, systemic infection of several weeks' duration, caused by *Salmonella typhosa*. There is hyperplasia and ulceration of Peyer's patches of the intestine, mesenteric lymphadenopathy, splenomegaly, and parenchymatous changes in the liver. Confirmation of diagnosis is obtained by culturing *S. typhosa* from blood or feces or by finding a high titer of agglutinins against the O and H antigens.

Typhoid fever is still a major disease in areas of the world that have not yet attained high public health standards, but it is now rare in the West. The death rate, formerly about 10 percent, is now about 2 percent, in large part because of the specific antimicrobial chloramphenicol, introduced in 1948.

There is some disagreement as to whether chloramphenicol remains the drug of choice, however, because of the emergence of resistant strains, high relapse rate, and risk of marrow toxicity. Trimethoprim-sulfamethoxazole has emerged as the best successor to chloramphenicol. Trimethoprim-160 mg and sulfamethoxazole-800 mg are given, either orally or parenterally, twice daily for 2 weeks. Amoxycillin is also effective and should be given intravenously or intramuscularly in doses of 1 g every 6 h for 2 weeks.

Gross hemorrhage occurs in 10 to 20 percent of hospitalized patients, even while on adequate therapy. Transfusion is indicated and usually suffices. Every effort should be made to avoid operation, since the bleeding is often from multiple ulcers and the bowel is exceedingly friable. Rarely, laparotomy must be done for uncontrollable, life-threatening hemorrhage.

Perforation, through ulcerated Peyer's patches, is usually single and found in the terminal ileum, and occurs in about 2 percent of cases. Operative treatment is indicated unless the patient is moribund, since localization or walling-off of the perforation is uncommon. Simple closure of the perforation is successful in the majority of patients. With multiple perforations, which occur in about one-fourth of patients, resection with primary anastomosis or a temporary ileostomy is preferred. The mortality rate of those with free perforation is about 10 percent.

NEOPLASMS

General Considerations

Primary neoplasms of the small bowel are extremely rare, despite the much greater mucosal surface area and rapidity of cell turnover of the small bowel compared to the stomach and colon; neoplasms are 40 times more common in the colon; the reasons for this difference are not clear. Several theories have been proposed as possible explanations: rapid transit time decreases the time for contact of carcinogens with the mucosa; the local immune system of the small bowel mucosa; the alkaline pH of the *succus entericus*; the absence of bacteria that might convert certain ingested products to carcinogens; and the presence of mucosal enzymes that destroy certain carcinogens.

Primary small bowel neoplasms are either benign or malignant and may arise from any of the cells of the small bowel. The frequency of benign and malignant neoplasms is reported to be equal in surgical series, whereas benign neoplasms far exceed malignant neoplasms in autopsy series. Malignant neoplasms (75 to 80 percent) more often produce symptoms than benign neoplasms.

Symptoms associated with small bowel neoplasms are often vague; they include epigastric discomfort, nausea, vomiting, abdominal pain (often intermittent and colicky), diarrhea, and bleeding (often manifest as symptoms of anemia). Symptoms may be present for months to years prior to operation. Bleeding is usually occult; hematochezia or hematemesis may occur, although life-threatening hemorrhage is not common. The most common indications for operation in patients with neoplasms of the small bowel are obstruction, bleeding, and pain. The mechanism of obstruction differs, depending upon whether it is caused by a benign or malignant neoplasm. Benign neoplasms are the most common cause of intussusception in the adult; whereas malignant neoplasms commonly cause obstruction by circumferential growth or kinking of the bowel due to longitudinal, intramural growth.

Because of their relative infrequency and the vague symptoms they produce, the diagnosis of small bowel neoplasms requires informed suspicion. Endoscopy is useful in evaluating the duodenum and possibly the most proximal jejunum, just beyond the ligament of Treitz. The

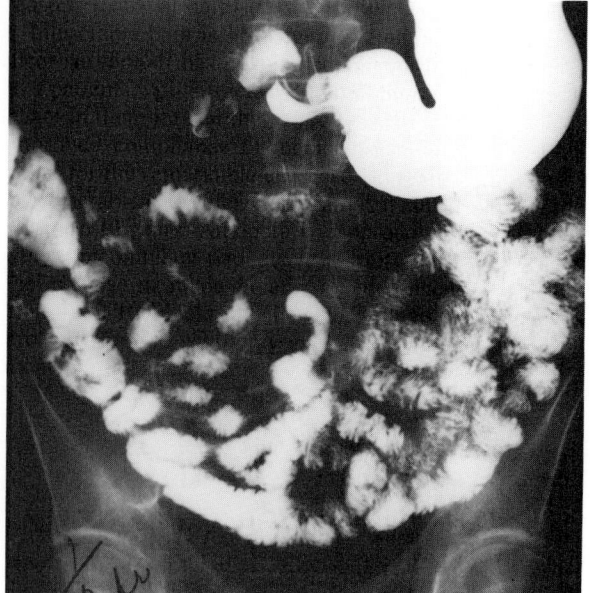

A

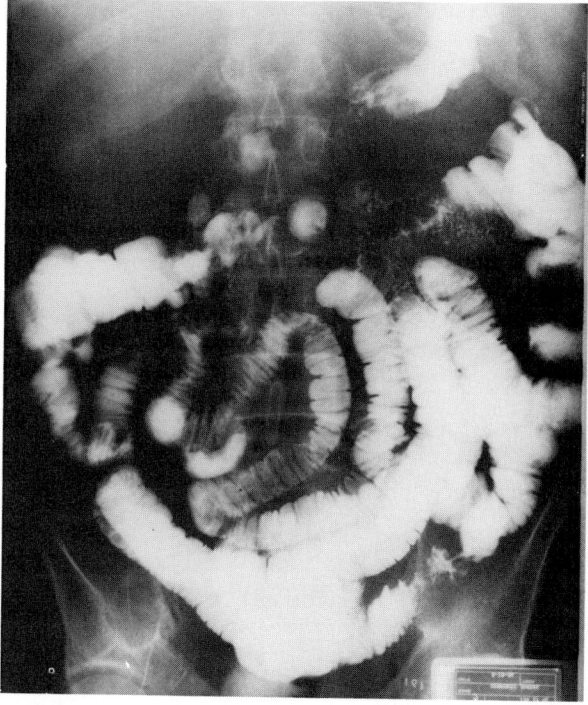

B

Fig. 27-10. Enteroclysis compared to small bowel follow-through. *A.* An overhead view obtained one-half hour after administration of barium in a small bowel follow-through examination. Note the incomplete filling and poor distention of bowel loops. The lesion in the ileum was not found. *B.* An overhead view from an enteroclysis examination in the same patient. The entire small bowel is nicely distended, except for ileal loops in the right abdomen. Each loop is individually examined by compression. *C.* This is a compression film of the involved ileal loops. These loops exhibit thickened, irregular mucosal folds; the thickening and kinking of the bowel wall are characteristic of an infiltrating carcinoid tumor.

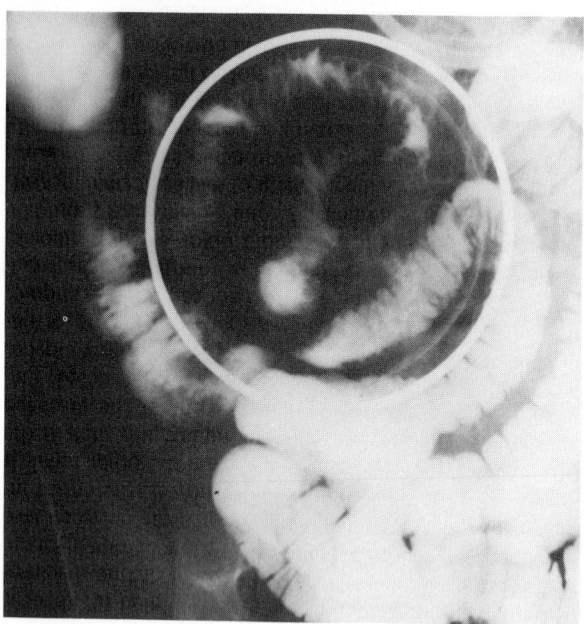

C

great majority of the small bowel is not accessible to endoscopic scrutiny. Barium contrast radiography is therefore required.

Hypotonic duodenography employing glucagon to produce temporary paralysis of the duodenum allows excellent visualization of the duodenal mucosa; exquisite detail can be obtained and accurate diagnoses rendered.

For the small bowel distal to the ligament of Treitz, however, traditionally, the motor meal, or small bowel follow-through, examination was employed. This was accomplished by taking overhead radiographs every 15 to 30 min after ingestion of barium until barium reached the cecum. Compression films of the terminal ileum were also obtained. This method is limited by low diagnostic sensitivity. Intubation infusion for small bowel examination, termed *enteroclysis*, has recently been widely employed. The availability of better intubation techniques, improved mixtures of barium, and improved results have increased its use.

In performing enteroclysis, the tip of a naso-small bowel tube is placed just beyond the ligament of Treitz, and dilute barium sulfate is instilled at a constant flow rate by an electric pump. The examination is complete when the barium reaches the cecum; this usually occurs within 10 to 15 min. Enteroclysis (Fig. 27-10) is superior to small bowel follow-through for detection of small filling defects and for determination of changes in mucosal pattern; the diagnostic accuracy of enteroclysis approaches 90 percent. The sensitivity and accuracy of enteroclysis has led to its acceptance by more gastrointestinal radiologists as the examination of choice for radiographic study of the small bowel.

Benign Neoplasms

PATHOLOGY. Benign tumors of the small bowel may either be of epithelial or of connective tissue origin. The most common lesions are adenomas, leiomyomas, and lipomas. Other benign lesions include hamartomas, fibromas, angiomas, lymphangiomas, neurofibromas, and hemangiomas. Adenomas are the most common benign tumors reported in autopsy series; however, leiomyomas are the most common benign small bowel lesions that produce symptoms.

Histologic types of benign small bowel tumors and their relative incidence are shown in Table 27-3. The incidence of these tumors varies, depending upon whether they are reported from autopsy or clinical series.

CLINICAL MANIFESTATIONS. An appreciable number of small bowel benign tumors apparently cause no serious symptoms during life and are incidental findings at autopsy. The diagnosis is delayed or missed in many patients because symptoms may be absent or vague or nonspecific until significant complications have developed. Physical examination rarely provides any clue unless intestinal obstruction is present, and radiographic studies of the small bowel and selective angiography, the only specific diagnostic aids, may fail to demonstrate an existing tumor, even though it is suspected clinically. In only about one-half of small bowel tumors found at operation has the correct diagnosis been made preoperatively.

The two most common clinical manifestations of small bowel tumors are bleeding and obstruction. Rarely, perforation of the bowel wall occurs, resulting in abscess or internal fistula formation, peritonitis, or pneumatosis cystoides intestinalis. Bleeding occurs in about one-third of patients but is rarely gross hemorrhage. More commonly, bleeding is occult and intermittent, producing guaiac-positive stools and iron-deficiency anemia. Leiomyomas and hemangiomas are the lesions that most often cause bleeding.

TREATMENT. Surgical treatment of benign tumors is nearly always indicated because of the risk of subsequent complications and because the diagnosis of benign disease cannot be made without microscopic evaluation.

Table 27-3. TYPES AND RELATIVE FREQUENCY OF SMALL BOWEL BENIGN NEOPLASMS

Neoplasms	Percent
Leiomyomas	17
Lipomas	16
Adenomas	14
Polyps	14
Polyposis, Peutz-Jeghers	3
Hemangiomas	10
Fibromas	10
Neurogenic tumors	5
Fibromyomas	5
Myxomas	2
Lymphangiomas	2
Fibroadenomas	1
Others	1

Complications of benign neoplasms most often requiring treatment are bleeding and obstruction. Segmental resection and primary reanastomosis is most commonly used except for very small lesions that may be excised by enterotomy. The entire small bowel should be searched for other lesions since they are often multiple.

ADENOMA

Adenomas are of three primary types: true adenomas, villous adenomas, or Brunner's gland adenomas. Twenty percent of adenomas are found in the duodenum, 30 percent in the jejunum, and 50 percent in the ileum. The majority of adenomas are asymptomatic, single, and are most commonly found incidentally at autopsy. If adenomas cause symptoms, they usually are associated with bleeding or obstruction. Villous adenomas of the small bowel are rare but do occur and are most commonly found in the duodenum. Their presence may be suspected by the characteristic "soap bubble" appearance on contrast radiography. They may attain large size (greater than 5 cm in diameter) and are usually found because of pain or bleeding. Obstruction may also occur. There have been no reports of secretory diarrhea associated with villous tumors of the small bowel; however, the malignant potential of these lesions is reportedly between 35 and 55 percent.

Brunner's gland adenomas are hyperplastic proliferations of normal exocrine glands located in the duodenum. Brunner's gland adenomas may produce symptoms that mimic those of peptic ulcer disease or may cause obstruction. Diagnosis can be made by endoscopy and biopsy, and symptomatic lesions in an accessible region should be resected. There is no malignant potential for Brunner's gland adenomas, and a radical resection should not be employed.

LEIOMYOMA

The most common symptomatic benign lesions of the small bowel are leiomyomas. Leiomyomas are benign tumors of smooth muscle that are most common in the jejunum. They are usually single, although multiple tumors may occur. The incidence is equal in men and women. Two growth patterns are noted: (1) the tumor may grow primarily intramurally and cause obstruction; (2) both intramural and extramural growth occurs and produces a dumbbell-shaped mass. These tumors may attain considerable size, outgrowing their blood supply, and tumor necrosis with bleeding may occur. The most common indication for operation on leiomyomas is bleeding. Angiography may provide the correct preoperative diagnosis.

LIPOMA

Lipomas are most common in the ileum and are single intramural lesions, submucosal in location, and usually small. Less than one-third of lipomas are found at operation and, when found, usually are the cause of obstruction, most commonly as the lead point of an intussuscep-

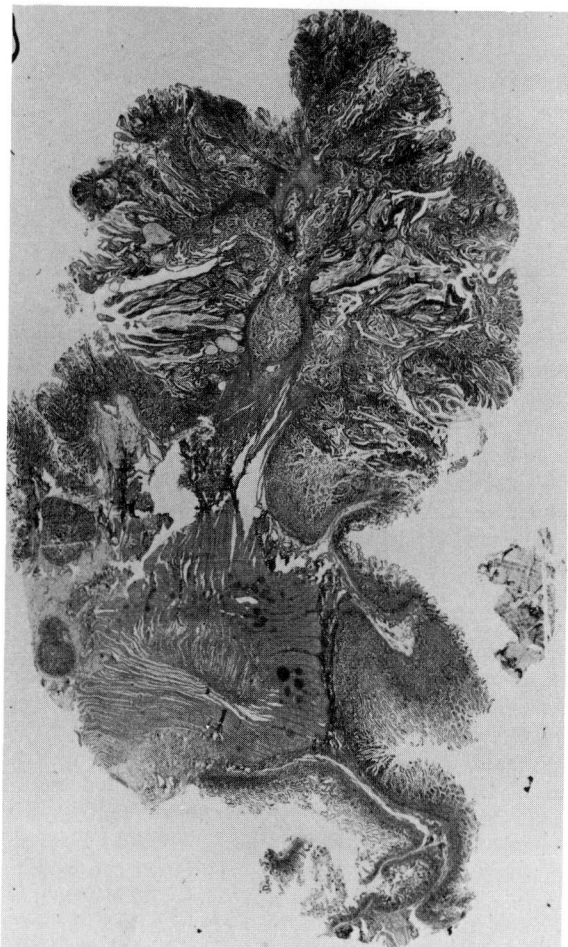

Fig. 27-11. Low-power photomicrograph of a Peutz-Jeghers jejunal polyp. Instead of one predominant cell, as seen in most intestinal polyps, these contain all cells of normal intestinal mucosa interspersed within bands of smooth muscle. They are hamartomas.

tion. Bleeding may occur from ulceration of the overlying mucosa. Lipomas do not possess malignant potential and, therefore, when found incidentally, should be removed only if the resection is simple. Pedunculated lipomas should be excised.

Peutz-Jeghers Syndrome

This is an inherited syndrome of mucocutaneous melanotic pigmentation and gastrointestinal polyps. The pattern of inheritance is simple mendelian dominant, with a high degree of penetrance. A single pleiotropic gene is responsible for both polyps and melanin spots. The classic pigmented lesions are small, 1 to 2 mm brown or black spots, located on the circumoral region of the face, buccal mucosa, forearms, palms of the hands, soles of the feet, the digits, and the perianal area. The syndrome was first reported in 1921 by Peutz. Jeghers et al. redescribed it in 1949. Multiple pigmented lesions may be noted or only a single buccal lesion may be present. Pigmentation appears in childhood. All cutaneous lesions may fade, leaving only buccal lesions. Pigmentation with polyposis and polyposis without pigmentation have been reported. The entire jejunum and ileum are the most frequent portions of the gastrointestinal tract to be involved with multiple polyps. Fifty percent of patients may, in addition, have rectal and colonic polyps, and one-fourth of the patients may have gastric polyps. The chief point to note is that if a patient with multiple rectal, colonic, or gastric polyps is found to have hamartomas rather than adenomas, a search for small bowel polyposis and pigmented lesions should be carried out.

The lesions are not true polyps but are hamartomas and, as such, are not premalignant (Fig. 27-11). However, there have been a few reported cases of malignant tumors of the gastrointestinal tract associated with Peutz-Jeghers syndrome. Some of these adenomatous and carcinomatous changes were noted in the hamartomatous polyps. It is not clear, however, whether this represents a coincidence or a true malignant transformation of this syndrome.

The most common symptom is recurrent colicky abdominal pain, due to intermittent intussusception. Lower abdominal pain associated with palpable mass has been reported to occur in one-third of patients. Hemorrhage occurs less frequently and is most commonly manifested by insidious involvement of anemia. Acute life-threatening hemorrhage is uncommon but may occur.

Surgical therapy is required only for obstruction or persistent bleeding. The resection should be limited to the segment of bowel that is producing complications, that is, polypectomy or limited resection. Because of the widespread nature of intestinal involvement, cure is not possible and extensive resections are not indicated.

Malignant Neoplasms

The most common malignant neoplasms of the small bowel are adenocarcinomas, carcinoids, sarcomas, and lymphomas, in about that order of frequency.

CLINICAL MANIFESTATIONS. Rochlin and Longmire called attention to three distinct clinical presentations of patients with malignant small bowel neoplasms: diarrhea, with large amounts of mucus and tenesmus; obstruction, with nausea, vomiting, and cramping abdominal pain; and chronic blood loss, with anemia, weakness, guaiac-positive stools, and occasionally melena or hematochezia. As with benign neoplasms, symptoms of malignant neoplasms are often present for many months before the diagnosis is made, emphasizing their insidious nature.

TREATMENT. The treatment for malignant neoplasms of the small bowel is wide resection, including regional lymph nodes. This may require a radical pancreatoduodenectomy (Whipple operation) for duodenal lesions. Because of the extent of the disease at the time of operation, curative resection may not be possible. Palliative resection should be performed when possible to prevent further complications of bleeding, obstruction, and perforation. However, if that is not possible, bypass of the involved segment is an alternative that may provide worthwhile relief of symptoms. If this is used, the proximal end of the bypassed segment should be brought out as a mucous fistula to prevent development of a closed loop.

PROGNOSIS. The overall survival of malignant neoplasms of the small bowel is not good. The highest survival rates are reported for duodenal periampullary carcinomas (about 30 to 40 percent), whereas adenocarcinomas occurring elsewhere in the small bowel have a 5-year survival of 20 percent or less. Leiomyosarcomas of the small bowel have a 5-year survival of between 30 to 40 percent. Radiation and chemotherapy play little role in treatment of patients with adenocarcinomas of the small bowel. There may be some improvement in survival when radiation therapy is employed in patients with sarcomas. Determinants of survival for patients with lymphomas is the cell type and extent of disease. Radiation therapy and chemotherapy, combined with surgical excision, provide the best survivals for patients with lymphomas. Five-year survivals have been reported to range between 10 and 50 percent, with an average of about 30 percent.

CARCINOMA

Carcinomas comprise about 50 percent of the malignant tumors of the small bowel in most reported series and are twice as common in men as in women. The average age at diagnosis is 50 years. Adenocarcinomas are more common in the duodenum and proximal jejunum than in the remainder of the small bowel. The reasons for this are unclear. About half of duodenal carcinomas involve the ampulla of Vater.

The location in the small bowel often determines the presenting symptoms. For example, periampullary adenocarcinomas are associated with intermittent jaundice, whereas carcinomas of the jejunum usually produce symptoms of mechanical small bowel obstruction (Fig. 27-12). The presence of jaundice, often intermittent, and a positive stool test for guaiac should immediately call to mind the possibility of a periampullary carcinoma.

As with carcinomas arising in other organs, survival of patients with small bowel carcinomas is related to the stage of disease at the time of diagnosis. Diagnosis is often delayed, and disease is often far advanced at the time of operation. The delay in diagnosis is due to a combination of factors, including lack of suspicion because of the relative rarity of the lesions, vagueness of symptoms, and absence of physical findings.

Fig. 27-12. Malignant tumors. *A.* Adenocarcinomas produce a typical apple core or napkin ring deformity of the small bowel. *B.* The operative specimen illustrates a fungating intraluminal mass that is typical of adenocarcinoma.

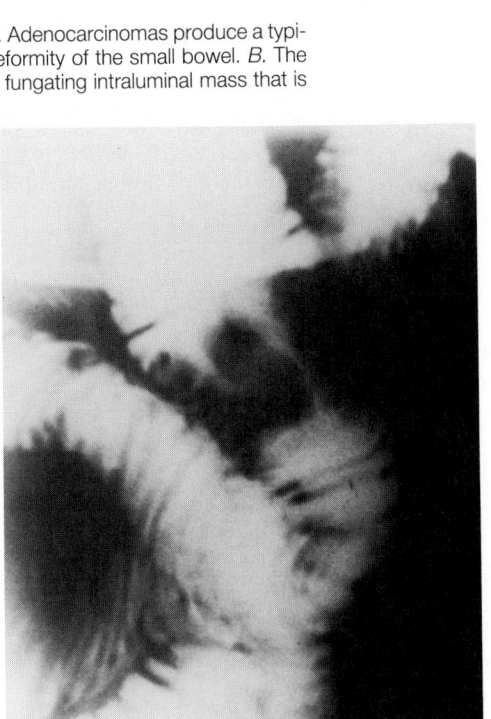

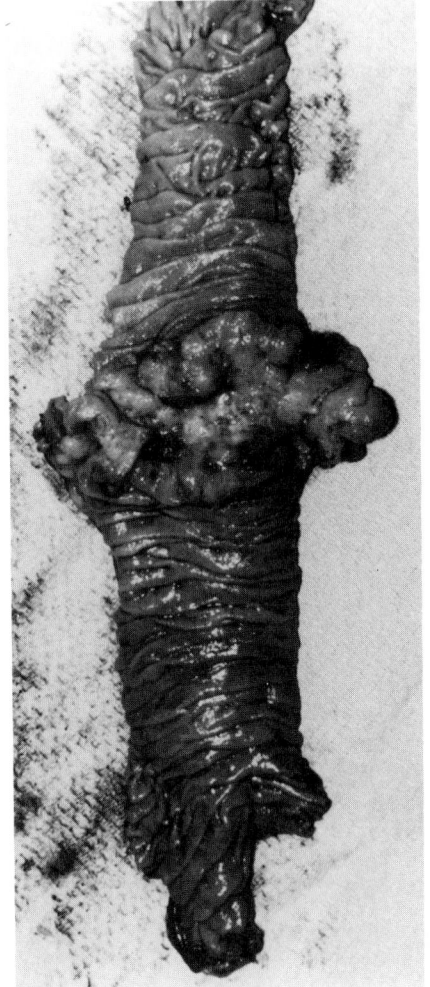

A

B

SARCOMA

Sarcomas comprise about 20 percent of malignant neoplasms of the small bowel, and the most common by far is the leiomyosarcoma. Leiomyosarcomas are evenly distributed throughout the small bowel, the incidence between men and women is equal, and the most common age at diagnosis is the sixth decade. The most common indications for operation are bleeding and obstruction, although free perforation due to hemorrhagic necrosis in large tumor masses may occur. Leiomyosarcomas are spread by direct invasion of adjacent structures, by hematogenous dissemination, or by transperitoneal seeding producing sarcomatosis.

LYMPHOMA

Lymphomas comprise about 10 to 15 percent of small bowel malignant tumors and are most commonly found in the ileum, where the greatest concentration of gut-associated lymphoid tissue is present. Lymphomas may be primary or part of a generalized disease. Dawson and colleagues have devised criteria to determine whether lymphoma of the small bowel is primary. These include: (1) absence of peripheral lymphadenopathy; (2) normal chest x-ray without evidence of mediastinal lymph node enlargement; (3) normal white blood cell count, total and differential; (4) at operation, the bowel lesion must predominate and the only involved nodes are associated with the bowel lesion; and (5) absence of disease in the liver and spleen. Even when these criteria are employed, one-third or more of patients with lymphomatous involvement of the small bowel will be found to have generalized lymphoma.

There are three syndromes of small bowel lymphoma. Western lymphoma is a disease predominantly of adults, typically found in the western hemisphere and associated with severe malabsorption in 5 to 10 percent of patients. Another form, known as "Mediterranean," is a malignant lymphoma first noted in non-Ashkenazi Jews and Arabs in Israel, which has subsequently been reported in other countries and in other ethnic groups, including Hispanic Americans. Since this disease is not confined to the Mediterranean basin, the term *immunoproliferative small intestinal disease* has been used. One-third of the patients may be found to have an abnormal fragment of IgA heavy-chain in their serum, which is produced by plasma cells infiltrating the small bowel. This variant is known as "heavy-chain disease."

The third intestinal manifestation of lymphoma is childhood abdominal lymphoma. This is a group of lymphomas including American (nonendemic) Burkitt's lymphoma, undifferentiated non-Burkitt's lymphoma, and diffuse histiocytic lymphoma.

CARCINOID

Carcinoids of the small bowel arise from the enterochromaffin, or Kulchitsky, cells found in the crypts of Lieberkühn. These cells are also known as argentaffin cells because of their staining by silver compounds. Car-

cinoids of the small bowel occur with almost the same frequency as adenocarcinoma and together they make up the preponderance of malignant neoplasms of the small bowel. Carcinoids have variable malignant potential and are composed of multipotential cells with the ability to secrete numerous humoral agents, the most prominent of which are serotonin and substance P. Although the carcinoid syndrome, characterized by episodic attacks of cutaneous flushing, bronchospasm, diarrhea, and vasomotor collapse occurs in fewer than 5 percent of the patients with malignant carcinoids, it is quite dramatic and has been extensively described and discussed with fascination by many authors.

The primary importance of carcinoid tumors is not, however, the carcinoid syndrome, but the malignant potential of the tumors themselves. Oberndorfer coined the term *karzinoide* to denote that this tumor was carcinomalike, and to emphasize the assumed lack of malignant potential. By 1930, this concept was no longer supported, since many patients with metastatic carcinoid tumors had been reported. In 1953 and 1954, the carcinoid syndrome was described.

PATHOLOGY. Carcinoids may arise in organs derived from the foregut, midgut, and hindgut. In the gastrointestinal tract, the appendix is most frequently involved (46 percent), followed by the ileum (28 percent), and rectum (17 percent). Other locations are shown in Table 27-4. The malignant potential, thus the ability to metastasize, appears to be related to the site of origin and the size of the primary tumor. Only about 3 percent of appendiceal carcinoids metastasize, but about 35 percent of ileal carcinoids are associated with metastasis. Seventy-five percent of gastrointestinal carcinoids are less than 1 cm in diameter; only 2 percent of this group metastasize. About 20 percent of primary tumors are 1 to 2 cm in diameter,

Table 27-4. DISTRIBUTION OF GASTROINTESTINAL CARCINOIDS: INCIDENCE OF METASTASES AND OF CARCINOID SYNDROME

Site	Cases	Average metastasis, %	Cases of carcinoid syndrome
Esophagus	1	—	0
Stomach	93	23	8
Duodenum	135	20	4
Jejunoileum	1032	34	91
Meckel's diverticulum	42	19	3
Appendix	1686	2	6
Colon	91	60	5
Rectum	592	18	1
Ovary	34	6	17
Biliary tract	10	30	0
Pancreas	2	—	1
	3718		136

SOURCE: From Wilson JM, Cheek RC, et al: 1970, with permission.

and 50 percent of this group metastasize. Only about 5 percent are over 2 cm in diameter; 80 to 90 percent of these metastasize. Multiple carcinoids of the small bowel occur in 30 percent of cases but are rare in the appendix. This tendency to multicentricity exceeds that of any other malignant neoplasm of the gastrointestinal tract. An unusual observation that is yet unexplained is the frequent coexistence of a second primary malignant neoplasm of a different histologic type; a second primary neoplasm was reported in 25 percent of patients in one large series.

Carcinoids present grossly as a slightly elevated, smooth, rounded, hard nodule, covered with normal mucosa. On cut section, they have a characteristic yellow-gray or tan appearance. Extensive fibrosis of the mesentery and of the bowel wall, due to an intense desmoplastic reaction, may be present. This fibrosis may produce mechanical bowel obstruction from kinking or matting of loops of small bowel together. Obstruction is rarely due to direct tumor encroachment on the lumen of the bowel. In addition to the desmoplastic reaction apparently produced by humoral agents elaborated by the tumor, metastases to mesenteric nodes also result in kinking and fixation by large, metastatic tumor deposits. An often remarked upon finding is that of a small primary tumor associated with massive mesenteric metastases.

CLINICAL MANIFESTATIONS. In the absence of the malignant carcinoid syndrome, symptoms of patients with carcinoid tumors of the small bowel are similar to those of patients with small bowel tumors of other histologic types. The most common symptoms are abdominal pain, bowel obstruction, diarrhea, and weight loss. In the majority of patients (in the absence of the malignant carcinoid syndrome), the diarrhea is due to partial bowel obstruction, rather than secretory diarrhea. On rare occasions, malignant carcinoid tumors of the ampulla of Vater may be found in patients with disseminated neurofibromatosis (von Recklinghausen's disease).

DIAGNOSTIC FINDINGS. Radiographic studies of the small bowel may exhibit multiple filling defects sometimes due to tumors but more often due to kinking and fibrosis of the bowel, mesenteric calcifications, and fixed rigid loops of intestine. Mesenteric vascular angiography may reveal abnormal arrangement of mesenteric arteries, and narrowing of peripheral branches together with poor accumulation of contrast and poor venous drainage of the tumor area. Tumor staining during angiography may be enhanced by administration of norepinephrine. Angiography is the most sensitive diagnostic test to detect hepatic metastasis, particularly diffuse metastatic disease with fine nodular distribution. Hepatic metastases are hypervascular and intensely stained during arteriography.

TREATMENT. The treatment of patients with small bowel carcinoid tumors is based upon size and site of the tumor and the presence or absence of metastatic disease. For primary tumors less than 1 cm in diameter without evidence of regional lymph node metastasis, a segmental intestinal resection is adequate. For lesions greater than 1 cm, for patients with multiple tumors, and in the presence of regional lymph node metastasis regardless of the size of the primary tumor, wide excision of bowel and mesentery is required. Since the majority of small bowel carcinoids are found in the ileum, wide excision usually entails a right hemicolectomy. Malignant carcinoid tumors of the duodenum may require radical pancreatoduodenectomy.

Treatment of Carcinoid Tumors of the Appendix.

Simple appendectomy is curative for patients with tumors less than 1 cm in diameter without gross evidence of metastasis. Because of the potential for metastasis, right hemicolectomy should be performed for tumors greater than 2 cm. Intramural lymphatic invasion, serosal involvement, or microscopic involvement of the mesoappendix associated with tumors less than 2 cm is not an indication for extensive resection.

PROGNOSIS. Survival for small bowel carcinoid tumors has been reported to be 75 percent for those tumors staged as local, 59 percent for regional tumors, and 19 percent for tumors with distant spread. The overall survival rate is 54 percent. Attempts to relate microscopic growth patterns to prognosis suggests that, as the site of origin of carcinoid tumor is an independent predictor of outcome, the growth pattern is likewise an independent predictor of outcome. Decreasing order of median survival time of the various growth patterns is illustrated: mixed insular plus glandular, 4.4 years; insular, 2.9 years; trabecular, 2.5 years; mixed insular plus trabecular, 2.3 years; glandular growth pattern, 0.9 years; and undifferentiated, 0.5 years.

When widespread metastatic disease precludes cure, extensive resection for palliation is indicated. Since these tumors are often indolent and slow growing, long-term palliation often results. Bypass procedures may be used in poor-risk patients with extensive disease. The overall 5-year survival rate after resection of intestinal carcinoids is about 50 percent. If "curative resection" is done, 70 percent of patients live 5 years. Chemotherapy has not been entirely successful; however, treatment with streptozocin and 5-fluorouracil (5-FU) may provide significant palliation. Up to 25 percent of patients with palliative resections survive 5 years.

MALIGNANT CARCINOID SYNDROME

This rare syndrome is widely described but rarely seen. The infrequent occurrence of this syndrome is emphasized when one considers that 30 to 70 percent of carcinoid tumors of the gut are metastatic at the time of diagnosis, but that only 6 to 9 percent of patients with metastatic disease will develop manifestations of the malignant carcinoid syndrome. By far the most commonly associated primary tumor is located in the small bowel, and massive hepatic replacement by metastatic tumor is usually found.

CLINICAL MANIFESTATIONS. The syndrome is characterized by hepatomegaly, diarrhea, and flushing in 80 percent of patients, right heart valvular disease in 50 percent, and asthma in 25 percent. Malabsorption and pellagra (dementia, dermatitis, and diarrhea) may infrequently be present and are thought to be due to excessive diversion of dietary tryptophan to meet the metabolic requirements of the tumor.

Diarrhea is episodic, often occurring after meals, and is due to elevated circulating levels of serotonin, which stimulates secretion of small bowel fluid and electrolytes, and increases intestinal motility. Some patients may present with acute abdominal symptoms, characterized by severe abdominal cramping without mechanical bowel obstruction. This has been called "carcinoid abdominal crisis." The mechanism of this crisis is thought to be intestinal ischemia, caused by the vasoactive substances elaborated by the tumor, combined with decreased mesenteric blood supply due to perivascular fibrosis.

Flushing is not temporally related to diarrhea, and although both may be present, either may be present without the other. The lack of relationship between flushing and diarrhea suggests that these two manifestations of the syndrome are due to different mediators. Although substance P produces all of the vasomotor phenomena associated with the flush, it has been questioned as the primary mediator. Besides serotonin and substance P, other substances that have been implicated include bradykinin and prostaglandins E and F.

Valvular heart disease is due to irreversible endocardial fibrosis, which is similar in genesis to the fibrosis noted in the gut wall, retroperitoneum, and around the mesenteric blood vessels. It occurs in patients with hepatic metastases and is limited to tricuspid and pulmonary valves. The reason that the right side valvular lesions predominate is that they are exposed to high levels of serotonin. The pulmonary filter deactivates serotonin, thereby preventing left sided valvular lesions.

Asthma is due to bronchoconstriction, which may be produced by serotonin, bradykinin, or substance P. Treatment of asthma associated with carcinoid syndrome must be carried out very carefully, since use of adrenergic drugs may cause release of humoral agents that may cause status asthmaticus.

Although the syndrome is seen in patients with high circulating levels of serotonin and often substance P, these are probably not the only mediators of all components of the syndrome. The malignant enterochromaffin cells produce 5-hydroxytryptamine, also called serotonin (5-HT). Circulating serotonin is metabolized in the liver and in the lung to 5-hydroxyindoleacetic acid (5-HIAA), which is pharmacologically inactive. Elevated levels of 5-HIAA are only seen in patients with metastasis. However, not all patients with metastasis have increased levels of 5-HIAA. The majority of patients who exhibit malignant carcinoid syndrome have massive hepatic replacement by their metastatic disease. Tumors that bypass the hepatic filter, specifically ovarian and retroperitoneal carcinoids, may produce the syndrome in the absence of liver metastasis.

DIAGNOSTIC FINDINGS. The diagnosis is most reliably established by repeated determination of urinary 5-HIAA. A single determination may be normal in the presence of metastatic disease. Provocative testing to reproduce symptoms has employed injection of pentagastrin, calcium, or epinephrine. The pentagastrin test is by far the most reliable and safest provocative test. During times of testing for increased levels of 5-HIAA, the patient must avoid foods rich in serotonin, such as bananas, tomatoes, walnuts, pineapples and certain drugs, including phenothiazines, glycerol guaiacolate, or reserpine.

TREATMENT. Treatment of the carcinoid syndrome would require removal of all tumor; this is rarely possible. Hepatic resection, however, even when known tumor is left behind, may result in significant relief of symptoms due to removal of the mass of tumor. When resection is not possible, hepatic dearterialization or embolization of the hepatic arterial branches may provide some relief. The duration of response after resection was 6 months compared to 4.8 months for hepatic artery ligation.

Drug therapy for prevention or relief of symptoms is directed at blockade of the effects of humoral agents elaborated by the tumor. Interferon has provided some symptomatic improvement in a small group of patients. Somatostatin or the long-acting analogue of somatostatin (SMS 201-995, Sandoz) prevents diarrhea and flushing in the majority of patients with the syndrome. Chemotherapeutic attacks on the tumor itself have been disappointing, although streptozocin, alone or combined with 5-FU, appears to be the most effective.

Treatment of carcinoid tumors remains wide surgical resection of the small bowel and regional lymph nodes. In addition, significant palliation may be achieved with aggressive hepatic resection in patients with malignant carcinoid syndrome.

DIVERTICULAR DISEASE

Diverticula of the small bowel may either be congenital or acquired. A congenital diverticulum is a true diverticulum; it is composed of all layers of the bowel wall. An acquired diverticulum is a false diverticulum; only mucosa and submucosa protrude through a defect in the muscle coat of the bowel wall. Diverticula may occur in any portion of small intestine. Duodenal diverticula are the most common acquired diverticula of the small bowel. Meckel's diverticulum is the most common true diverticulum of the small bowel.

Duodenal Diverticula

The true incidence of duodenal diverticula is unknown and varies depending upon whether they are found clinically (by x-ray, endoscopy, or operation) or at autopsy. It has been reported that between 1 to 5 percent of upper gastrointestinal x-ray examinations will reveal duodenal diverticula; between 9 to 20 percent of upper gastrointestinal endoscopic examinations show them. This is compared to a 10 to 20 percent incidence reported from autopsy series. More than 90 percent of these diverticula are clearly asymptomatic, and less than 5 percent will require operation due to a complication of the diverticulum itself. The ratio of appearance in men to women is about 1:2. Duodenal diverticula are rare in patients under 40 years of age, and the incidence increases with increasing age.

Two-thirds to three-fourths of duodenal diverticula are found in a periampullary region and project from the medial wall of the duodenum (Fig. 27-13). Duodenal diverticula are clinically important for two reasons: they may occasionally produce symptoms related to the diverticulum, including obstruction, perforation, or bleeding, and the presence of the diverticulum may cause recurrent pancreatitis, cholangitis, or recurrent common-duct stones after cholecystectomy.

Only those diverticula associated with the ampulla of Vater have significant relationship to complications of cholangitis, pancreatitis, and stone disease. In patients with these diverticula, the ampulla most often enters the duodenum at the superior margin of the diverticulum, rather than through the diverticulum itself. The mechanism proposed for the increased incidence of complications of the biliary tract is the location of the periavaterian diverticula, which may produce mechanical distortion of the common bile duct as it enters the duodenum, resulting in partial obstruction and stasis. Bile stasis allows proliferation of bacteria and subsequent formation of stones. The incidence of bactibilia is significantly increased in patients with periavaterian diverticula compared to diverticula located in other parts of the duodenum. The bacteria isolated from the bile duct and from the diverticula are identical. There is also evidence that dysfunction of the choledochal sphincter is produced by presence of diverticula. In one study of 101 patients who had undergone cholecystectomy more than 2 years previously, a significantly increased incidence of recurrent calculi was noted in patients with diverticula compared to patients without. A causal relationship of duodenal diverticula and biliary tract stones, however, has not been demonstrated. The great majority of duodenal diverticula cause no trouble and should be left alone unless they can be closely related to disease.

Fewer than 60 patients have been reported with intraluminal duodenal diverticula. These diverticula, which probably originate from incomplete duodenal webs, are lined both inside and out with duodenal mucosa, have a characteristic picture of a barium-filled wind sock on contrast radiography, and most often have required operation because of duodenal obstruction or recurrent pancreatitis. In these diverticula the common bile duct and pancreatic duct usually enter the diverticulum, and a second orifice is present that allows drainage of the biliary-pancreatic secretions into the lumen of the gut.

Symptoms related to duodenal diverticula, in the absence of any other demonstrable disease, are usually nonspecific epigastric complaints. Bleeding, perforation, and diverticulitis are all rare. The morbidity and mortality caused by complications of diverticula are nonetheless high because of delay in diagnosis due to the lack of suspicion of the underlying condition. Diagnosis is seldom made preoperatively.

TREATMENT. Treatment of complications of the diverticulum are directed toward the control of the complication. In those patients who have bleeding or symptoms that are related to the duodenal diverticulum, several operative procedures have been described. The most

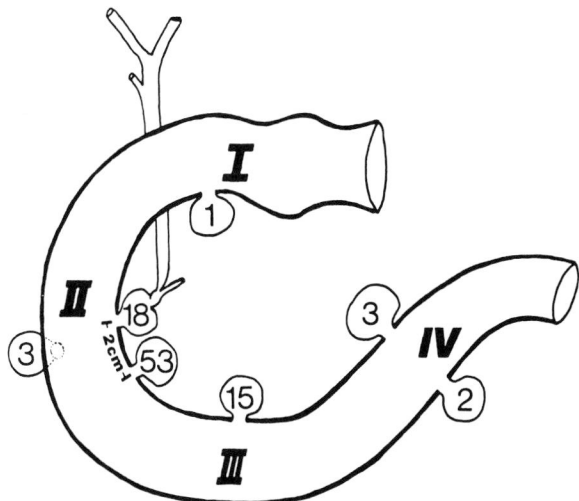

Fig. 27-13. Distribution of 95 duodenal diverticula within the four portions of the duodenum. (From: *Eggert A, Wittmann DH: Surg Gynecol Obstet 154:62, 1982, with permission.*)

common and most effective treatment in this situation is diverticulectomy. This is most easily accomplished by performing a wide Kocher maneuver that exposes the diverticulum. The diverticulum can then be excised, and the duodenum is closed in a transverse or longitudinal manner, whichever technique produces the least amount of luminal obstruction. For those diverticula embedded deep within the head of the pancreas, lateral duodenotomy is performed, and the diverticulum is invaginated into the lumen and excised, and the wall closed. An alternative method that has been described for the duodenal diverticula associated with the ampulla of Vater is an extended sphincteroplasty through the common wall of the ampulla and the diverticulum.

A perforated diverticulum may cause great trouble. When found, the perforated diverticulum should be excised and the duodenum closed with a serosal patch from the jejunal loop. If the inflammation is severe, it may be necessary to divert enteric flow away from the site of the perforation, with either a gastrojejunostomy or, preferably, a duodenojejunostomy if possible. It may be possible to interrupt duodenal countinuity proximal to the perforated diverticulum with a row of staples. Great care should be taken if the perforation is adjacent to the papilla. In one early perforation, we were able simply to invert the diverticulum, close the duodenal wall, and reinforce this with a serosal patch.

Because of the relationship of the common bile duct and pancreatic duct in patients with intraluminal diverticula associated with the ampulla of Vater, subtotal resection of the diverticulum should be carried out to protect the entry of the biliary-pancreatic ducts. If an intraluminal diverticulum arises at a site distant from the ampulla, complete excision may be possible.

Although fascinating, the vast majority of duodenal diverticula are asymptomatic, boringly benign, and, when found incidentally, should not be resected.

Jejunal and Ileal Diverticula

Diverticula of the jejunum and ileum are much less common than duodenal diverticula, with an incidence between 0.5 and 1 percent on small bowel x-ray examination. Jejunal diverticula are more common and are larger than those in the ileum. Multiple diverticula are more common in the jejunum and ileum than in the duodenum. These are false diverticula, usually protrude from the mesenteric border of the bowel, and may be overlooked at operation because they are embedded within the small bowel mesentery. When jejunal and ileal diverticula give trouble, the symptoms are usually due to imcomplete bowel obstruction, acute diverticulitis, hemorrhage, or malabsorption due to bacterial overgrowth within the diverticulum. A specific syndrome of intestinal pseudoobstruction or jejunal dyskinesia is characterized by symptoms of intermittent partial bowel obstruction. On enteroclysis examination, barium may be seen to pass back and forth from the intestinal lumen into the diverticulum, rather than move normally through the bowel. This condition may be associated with hypertrophy and dilatation of the bowel proximal to the diverticulum. A recent study found that the condition may be associated with one of three syndromes: systemic sclerosis, visceral myopathy, or visceral neuropathy. If this condition is the only finding, resection of a large segment of jejunum containing diverticula should be avoided. Treatment of complications of obstruction, bleeding, and perforation is by intestinal resection and end-to-end anastomosis. Patients with malabsorption due to production of the blind loop syndrome by bacterial overgrowth within the diverticulum can usually be treated with antibiotics. Asymptomatic diverticula require no treatment.

Meckel's Diverticulum

The most common true diverticulum of the gastrointestinal tract is Meckel's diverticulum. This is a congenital diverticulum that results from incomplete closure of the omphalomesenteric or vitelline duct. Meckel's diverticula are located usually within 2 to 3 ft of the ileocecal valve and vary in length from 1 to 12 cm. Heterotopic gastric or pancreatic tissue is often found in Meckel's diverticula. The great majority of symptomatic Meckel's diverticula will be found in childhood, and the most common symptom in childhood is bleeding. A 2 percent incidence of Meckel's diverticula in the general population is based upon reports of several autopsy series. In adults, most Meckel's diverticula are found incidentally by radiographic examination of the small bowel. Enteroclysis has a very high incidence of accurate diagnosis. Another technique for detection of Meckel's diverticulum in symptomatic patients is radionuclide scanning, using ^{99m}Tc-pertechnetate. The basis for this is the uptake of radioisotope by the heterotopic gastric mucosa within the diverticulum. The diagnostic accuracy of this scanning technique may be increased by administration of pentagastrin (6 mg/kg subcutaneously) 15 min before the scan, which enhances the uptake of the radioisotope by the gas-

tric mucosa. It has been shown, however, that the parietal cells do not specifically accumulate pertechnetate and are not essential for detection purposes. The scan is not nearly so useful in adults as it is in children.

Complications of Meckel's diverticulum in adults include intestinal obstruction, bleeding, acute diverticulitis, or the presence of a diverticulum in a hernia sac (Littre's hernia). Obstruction may be produced by one of two mechanisms. The most common is volvulus or kinking around a band running from the tip of the diverticulum to the umbilicus, abdominal wall, or mesentery. The diverticulum may also cause obstruction by intussusception. Bleeding is the second most common complication and is usually found only in those patients who have heterotopic gastric mucosa within the diverticulum. The bleeding ulcer is found not in the diverticulum, but in the ileum adjacent to the diverticulum.

Meckel's diverticulitis, which is clinically indistinguishable from appendicitis, is the third most common complication in adults. The incidence of perforation or peritonitis with Meckel's diverticulitis is about 50 percent.

A Meckel's diverticulum should be considered in the differential diagnosis of patients who present with a mechanical bowel obstruction, with low small bowel hemorrhage, or with signs and symptoms of inflammation or peritonitis. Treatment is prompt surgical intervention with resection of the diverticulum or resection of the segment of ileum bearing the diverticulum. Segmental intestinal resection is required for treatment of patients with bleeding, because the bleeding site is usually in the ileum adjacent to the diverticulum.

Removal of an asymptomatic Meckel's diverticulum found incidentally at laparotomy in adults should not be performed. Soltero and Bill have estimated that the likelihood of Meckel's diverticulum becoming symptomatic in an adult is 2 percent or less and that morbidity from incidental removal (reported to be as high as 12 percent) far exceeds the potential for prevention of disease.

MISCELLANEOUS PROBLEMS

Small Bowel Ulcerations

The majority of ulcerations of the small bowel have definable causes, which include the following: drug-induced (enteric-coated potassium chloride tablets or corticosteroids), vascular (occlusion or vasculitis), Crohn's disease, syphillis, typhoid fever, tuberculosis, lymphoma, heterotopic gastric mucosa (Meckel's diverticulum), and ulcers associated with gastrinoma. This discussion is limited to those ulcerations of the small intestine in which no etiologic agent can be identified.

Patients with discrete isolated ulcers of the small bowel, without any identifiable underlying disease, have nonspecific ulcers. Ulcers are more common in the terminal ileum. These appear to be self-limited and do not recur after bowel resection.

These patients usually present with a single ulceration,

although multiple ulcers may be present. Indications for operation are for complications of the ulcers, including perforation, bleeding, or stricture. Recurrence of ulceration in the small bowel distal to the duodenum is rare. A review of 59 patients studied from 1956 to 1979 reports the overall incidence of 4 patients per 100,000 new patients seen at the Mayo Clinic. These investigators noted that the yearly rate fell from 3.6 new cases per year from 1960 to 1969 to 1.2 cases per year from 1970 to 1979. They believe, despite the absence of a documented underlying etiology, that the decrease in incidence was directly related to the removal of enteric-coated potassium chloride tablets.

The ulcers are discrete, vary in size from 0.3 to 5 cm in diameter, are sharply demarcated, and the surrounding mucosa is perfectly normal. They occur more frequently on the antimesenteric border and may be associated with fibrous scar formation, which produces the obstruction. The characteristic microscopic findings include acute granulation tissue and inflammatory cells at the base of the ulcer, local hyperplasia of the muscularis mucosae, and pyloric metaplasia of the adjacent mucosa. Varying degrees of edema and fibrosis, depending upon the chronicity of the ulcer, are noted. There is no evidence of vascular disease associated with the ulcer. With time, the ulcers may increase in size, become annular, and, with healing, may produce fibrous strictures of the intestine, which may produce obstruction.

Diagnosis is rarely if ever made before operation; the majority of patients present with complications. In a Mayo Clinic series, 63 percent of patients had intermittent small bowel obstruction, while 25 percent had bleeding, and 12 percent had symptoms of acute abdominal inflammation caused by perforation. With the increasing use of enteroclysis, the diagnosis of small bowel ulcer may be made more frequently, and an asymptomatic solitary ulcer does not require treatment.

TREATMENT. The treatment of small bowel ulcers depends upon the complications encountered at the time of diagnosis. Mechanical bowel obstruction and bleeding should be treated by segmental resection. Although excision and primary closure of perforated ulcers has been advocated by some, high recurrence rates have been associated with this technique. Resection of the ulcerated segment of bowel should be done.

Ingested Foreign Bodies

A great variety of objects that are capable of penetrating the wall of the gut are swallowed, usually accidentally, but sometimes intentionally by the mentally deranged. These include glass and metal fragments, pins, needles, cocktail toothpicks, fish bones, coins, whistles, toys, and broken razor blades.

Treatment is expectant, since the vast majority pass without difficulty. If the object is radiopaque, progress can be followed by serial plain films. Catharsis is contraindicated.

Sharp, pointed objects such as sewing needles may penetrate the bowel wall. If abdominal pain, tenderness, fever or leukocytosis occur, immediate surgical removal of the offending object is indicated. Abscess or granuloma formation are the usual outcomes without surgical therapy.

Small Bowel Fistulas

The vast majority of small bowel fistulas are due to operation; less than 2 percent are associated with granulomatous disease of the bowel (Crohn's disease) or trauma. In some patients, there are contributing factors, such as preoperative radiotherapy, intestinal obstruction, inflammatory bowel disease, mesenteric vascular disease, and intraabdominal sepsis. But in the majority, surgical misadventures are the primary cause. These include anastomotic leak, injury of bowel or blood supply at operation, laceration of bowel by wire mesh or retention sutures, and retained sponges. We have seen fistulas result from injury by suction catheters and from erosion by abscesses.

The major complications associated with small bowel fistulas include sepsis, fluid and electrolyte depletion, necrosis of the skin at the site of external drainage, and malnutrition. Successful management of patients with small bowel fistulas requires meticulous attention to detail and a logical, stepwise plan of management. One must establish controlled drainage, manage sepsis, prevent fluid and electrolyte depletion, protect the skin, and provide for adequate nutrition.

Mortality for patients with intestinal fistulas remains high, 20 percent or greater, even with the use of total parenteral nutrition (TPN). Although TPN has not been shown to reduce mortality significantly, it is the single most important advance in the management of patients with enterocutaneous fistulas. Fluid, electrolyte, and nutritional status may be maintained from the time the fistula becomes apparent and throughout the time required for control of sepsis. The key to successful management of intestinal fistulas is control of sepsis and prevention of malnutrition.

Diagnosis of small bowel fistula is usually not difficult. When the damaged area of the small bowel breaks down and discharges its contents, dissemination may occur widely in the peritoneal cavity, producing generalized peritonitis. More commonly, however, the process is more or less walled-off to the immediate area of the leak, with formation of an abscess. This usually underlies the operative incision, so that when a few skin sutures are removed to ascertain why the incision is becoming red and tender, contents of the abscess are discharged and the fistula established. The discharge may initially be purulent or bloody, but this is followed, sometimes immediately, sometimes within a day or two, by drainage of obvious small bowel contents. If the diagnosis is in doubt, confirmation can be obtained by oral administration of a nonabsorbable marker such as charcoal or Congo red.

Small bowel fistulas are classified according to their location and volume of daily output, since these factors dictate treatment as well as morbidity and mortality rates. In general, the more proximal the fistula in the intestine, the more serious the problem. Proximal fistulas have a greater fluid and electrolyte loss, the drainage has a greater digestive capacity, and an important (distal) segment is not available for food absorption. High-output fistulas are those which discharge 500 mL or more each 24 h. It is important, therefore, as soon as the patient's condition is stabilized, to identify the site of the fistula, to determine the extent of the associated abscess cavity by fistulogram, and to ascertain whether there is distal obstruction, since fistulas will not close in the presence of distal obstruction. Upper gastrointestinal series with small bowel follow-through and barium enema studies usually provide this information.

TREATMENT. Control of sepsis is aided by sump suction, which provides drainage of the associated intraabdominal abscess cavity and prevents accumulation of intestinal contents. Control of fistula output is most easily accomplished by percutaneous intubation of the fistula track. Protection of the skin around the fistulous opening is important. In the past, frequent applications of zinc oxide, aluminum paste ointment, or karya powder were required; excoriation and destruction of skin still occurred. The advent of stomahesive appliances used for colostomy and ileostomy bags greatly improved and facilitated protection of the skin at the site of fistula. The stomahesive appliance should be cut so that the opening just fits over the fistulous opening and no unprotected skin remains. The suction catheter can be brought out through the end of the bag which is fixed firmly about the tube. This allows for collection of all the drainage and accurate quantitation of the lost volume.

The volume depletion that occurs from a proximal small bowel fistula may present a formidable problem. Patients with volume losses exceeding 5 L/day are not uncommon. Agents that inhibit gut motility (codeine, Lomotil, or loperamide) are not generally helpful. Somatostatin inhibits both intestinal secretion and motility. We have successfully used a long-acting analog of somatostatin (SMS-201995 Sandoz) to stop fistula output in three patients. Somatostatin, however, is a general "off" switch, and ileus can be a problem. In none of our patients was spontaneous healing effected, but the analog ameliorated the problems associated with massive volume loss. Systemic antibiotics should be administered until sepsis is controlled. At the same time, TPN should be instituted because a prolonged course of inability to use the gut for nutrition is likely.

Several factors may prevent spontaneous closure of fistulas. Fistulas will not close spontaneously if there is high output (>500 mL/24 h) or severe disruption of intestinal continuity (>50 percent of the circumference of the bowel involved in the fistula). A fistula will not close spontaneously if it arises from a segment of bowel involved with active granulomatous disease, cancer, or radiation enteritis, if there is distal obstruction, or if there is an undrained abscess cavity. If a foreign body is in the track, if the fistulous track is less than 2.5 cm in length, or if there is epithelialization of the track, spontaneous closure will not occur. Radiographic investigation of the fistula by means of injection of water soluble contrast material through the fistulous track should be carried out early to delineate the presence and extent of any abscess cavities and obtain information about the length of the track and the extent of bowel wall disruption. A diligent search by means of contrast studies for distal obstruction should be performed. CT will often reveal undrained collections of fluid.

When any of the conditions noted above are present, spontaneous closure is unlikely; therefore, management should be directed toward obtaining prompt control of sepsis, maintaining positive nitrogen balance, and early operation.

Conservative treatment for up to 3 months with TPN has been advocated by some to allow spontaneous closure of the fistula. We do not believe that the results support this plan. Fewer than 30 percent of all small bowel fistulas will close spontaneously. In patients with low output fistulas, particularly those located in the distal small bowel without any of the conditions that will prevent spontaneous closure, a wait of up to 6 weeks may be indicated. The patient can usually wait at home. When we reviewed reported series that advocate conservative therapy for longer than 6 weeks, we found that the majority of fistulas that close spontaneously do so within 3 weeks after their appearance. After 3 weeks, if sepsis has been controlled and adequate nutritional status has been achieved, operative control of the fistula should be carried out promptly. Delay only produces delay. TPN simplifies management of patients, but it does not cure fistulas. The single most important determinant in successful treatment of fistulas is sepsis. If sepsis is not controlled, the patient will die. After sepsis has been controlled, one should not wait endlessly for a fistula to spontaneously close simply because malnutrition can be avoided by use of TPN. The proper role of TPN is prevention or treatment of malnutrition prior to operative closure of fistulas.

Operation is most easily accomplished by entering the previous abdominal wound. The wound should be reopened with great care to avoid needless reinjury to the bowel. The fistulous track is excised, the bowel should be completely mobilized, and the portion of bowel involved in the fistula resected. The technique of excision and fistula closure must be precise and accurate, and all rigid or diseased bowel must be resected. Simple closure of the fistula after removing the fistulous track and minimal mobilization of the bowel almost always results in recurrence of the fistula.

If an unexpected abscess is encountered or if the bowel wall is rigid and distended over a large distance, a proximal enterostomy should be performed. Later, resection of the bowel involved in the fistula will be required for successful closure. Side-to-side bypass should not be done.

The overall mortality rate in enterocutaneous fistulas of the small bowel is still greater than 20 percent. It is higher in jejunal fistulas and significantly lower in ileal fistulas. Successful treatment of the majority of patients with small bowel fistulas requires control of sepsis, provision of adequate nutrition, and operative closure.

Pneumatosis Cystoides Intestinalis

This is an uncommon condition manifested by multiple gas-filled cysts of the gastrointestinal tract. The cysts are either submucosal or subserosal and vary in size from microscopic to several centimeters in diameter. The jejunum is most frequently involved, followed by the ileocecal region and colon. Gas cysts are associated with other lesions of the gastrointestinal tract in about 85 percent of cases. Pneumatosis not associated with other lesions (15 percent of cases) is called "primary."

Grossly, the cysts resemble cystic lymphangiomas or hydatid cysts. On section, the involved portion has a honeycomb appearance. The cysts are thin-walled and break easily. Spontaneous rupture gives rise to pneumoperitoneum.

Symptoms are nonspecific and in "secondary" pneumatosis may be those of the associated disease. In primary pneumatosis, symptoms, when present, resemble those of irritable bowel syndrome. The diagnosis is usually made radiographically (Fig. 27-14). No treatment is necessary unless one of the very rare complications supervenes, such as rectal bleeding, cyst-induced volvulus, or tension pneumoperitoneum. Prognosis in most patients is that of the underlying disease. When pneumatosis occurs in infants with necrotizing enterocolitis, it does not make the outlook any worse. The cysts may disappear spontaneously or may persist for prolonged periods without serious symptoms.

Blind Loop Syndrome

This is a rare clinical syndrome manifested by diarrhea, steatorrhea, anemia, weight loss, abdominal pain, multiple vitamin deficiencies, and neurologic disorders. The underlying cause is not a blind loop per se, but bacterial overgrowth in stagnant areas of small bowel produced by stricture, stenosis, fistulas, blind pouch, or diverticula (Table 27-5). The bacterial flora are altered in the stagnant area, both in number and in kind. Bacteria compete successfully for vitamin B_{12}, producing a systemic deficiency of B_{12} and megaloblastic anemia. Steatorrhea also occurs; bacteria in the stagnant area deconjugate bile salts, causing disruption of micellar solubilization of fats. There may also be absorptive defects of other macro- and micronutrients, probably caused by direct injury of the mucosal cells.

The syndrome can be confirmed by a series of laboratory investigations. First, a Schilling test (^{60}Co-labeled B_{12} absorption) is performed; this should reveal a pattern of urinary excretion of vitamin B_{12} resembling pernicious anemia (that is, a urinary loss of 0 to 6 percent of vitamin B_{12}, compared with the normal of 7 to 25 percent). The test is then repeated with the addition of intrinsic factor. In true pernicious anemia, the excretion should rise to normal; in the blind loop syndrome, the addition of intrinsic factor will not increase the excretion of B_{12}. Next, the patient is given a course of tetracycline for 3 to 5 days, and the Schilling test is repeated. With blind loop syn-

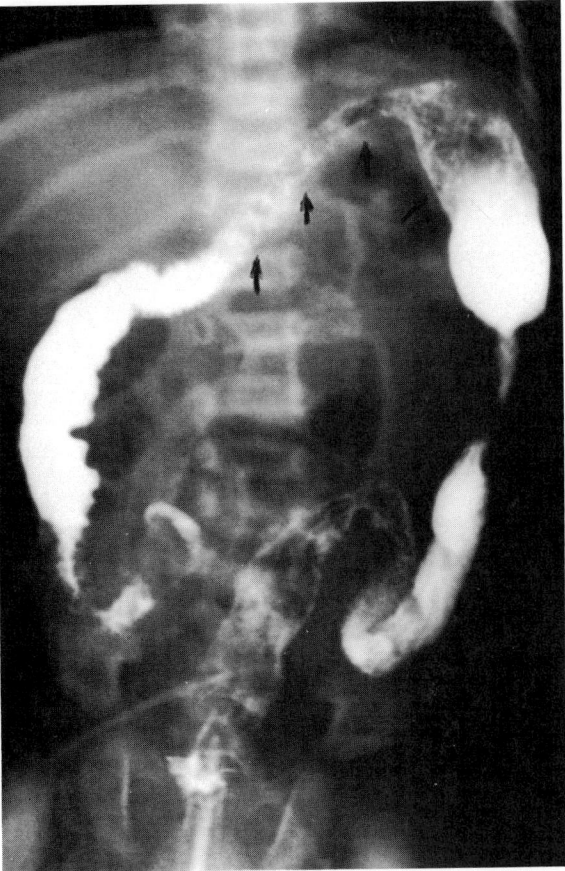

Fig. 27-14. Barium enema radiograph of an infant with pneumatosis cystoides coli. Arrows point to several submucosal gas cysts.

Table 27-5. CLINICAL CONDITIONS PREDISPOSING TO BACTERIAL OVERGROWTH WITHIN THE SMALL BOWEL

Gastric proliferation
    Achlorhydria, especially when combined with motor or anatomic disturbance
Small intestinal stagnation
    Anatomic
    Afferent loop of Billroth II partial gastrectomy
    Duodenal/jejunal diverticulosis
    Surgical blind loop (end-to-side anastomosis)
    Surgical recirculating loop (side-to-side anastomosis)
    Obstruction (stricture, adhesion, inflammation, cancer)
    Motor
    Diabetic autonomic neuropathy
    Scleroderma
    Idiopathic intestinal pseudoobstruction
    Absence of "intestinal housekeeper"
Abnormal communication between proximal and distal gastrointestinal tract
    Gastrocolic or jejunocolic fistula
    Resection of ileocecal valve

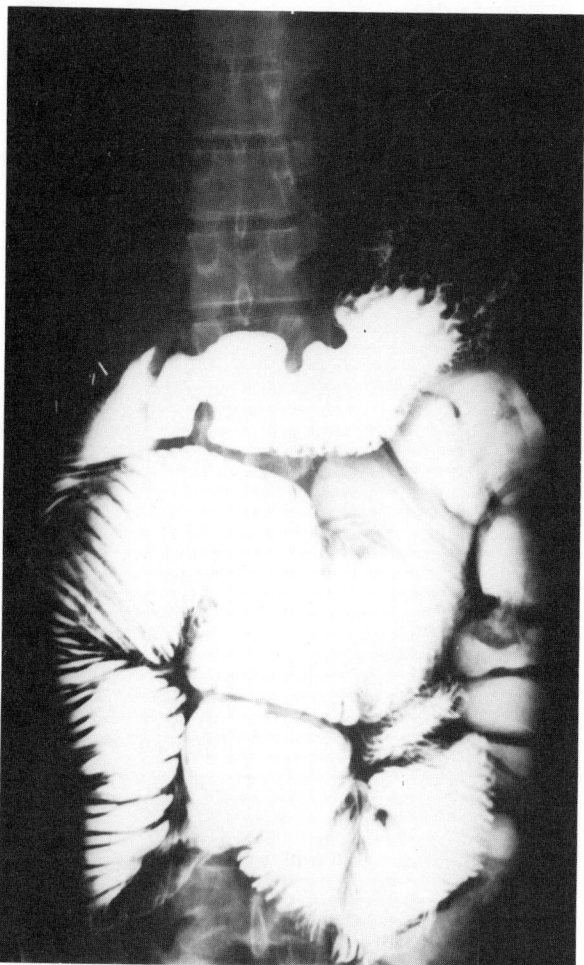

Fig. 27-15. This picture illustrates small intestine adaptation at 18 months after massive bowel resection.

drome, absorption of ^{60}Co-labeled B_{12} returns to normal; this does not occur in the macrocytic anemia due to steatorrhea. Patients with the blind loop syndrome respond to tetracycline and parenteral B_{12} therapy. Medical treatment is not definitive, but should be employed to prepare patients for operation. Surgical correction of the condition producing stagnation and blind loop syndrome effects a permanent cure and is indicated.

Short Bowel Syndrome

Emergency massive resection of the small bowel must sometimes be done when extensive gangrene precludes revascularization. Mesenteric occlusion, midgut volvulus, and traumatic disruption of the superior mesenteric vessels are the most frequent causes. Short bowel syndrome may result from such massive resections; it may also be produced by several bowel resections in patients with severe recurrent Crohn's disease.

The short bowel syndrome is a group of signs and symptoms that result from a length of small bowel that is inadequate to support nutrition. The clinical hallmarks of

the short bowel syndrome include diarrhea, fluid and electrolyte deficiency, and malnutrition. The small bowel has two primary functions, digestion and absorption of nutrients. Problems that result from extensive resection of the small bowel can be divided into two types: (1) those related to the extent of small bowel loss and (2) those related to the specific area of bowel removed.

Although there is considerable individual variation, resection of up to 70 percent of the small bowel can usually be tolerated if the terminal ileum and ileocecal valve are preserved. Length alone, however, is not the only determining factor of complications of small bowel resection. For example, if the distal two-thirds of the ileum, including the ileocecal valve, are resected, significant abnormalities of absorption of bile salts and B_{12} may occur, although only 25 percent of the total length of the small bowel has been removed. Proximal bowel resection is tolerated much better than distal resection.

Digestion and absorption in the small bowel depend upon the presence of brush border enzymes, an adequate number of enterocytes for absorption, and normal intestinal motility. With massive resection of the small bowel, there is reduced absorption of all nutrients, including electrolytes, water, carbohydrates, protein, fat, trace elements, and vitamins. The proximal small bowel is the primary site of absorption of iron, folate, and calcium, whereas the distal small bowel is the site of absorption of bile salts and vitamin B_{12} (Table 27-2).

The bowel has an intrinsic capacity to adapt after small bowel resection, and in many instances, this process of intestinal adaptation effectively prevents severe complications due to the reduced surface area of the small bowel available for absorption and digestion. Any adaptive mechanism can be overwhelmed; maximum adaptation will be inadequate if sufficient small bowel is lost. Intestinal adaptation is characterized by increased absorptive surface due to hyperplasia of the remaining enterocytes. The villi lengthen (but do not increase in number), more cells are produced, and there is increased cell renewal and migration to the villous tip. This allows for a total increase in absorptive surface. Although there are more cells, individual cells do not increase their life span (they must migrate farther) or their capacity to synthesize digestive enzymes or to increase absorptive processes, so the overall net increase in digestive efficacy is not great (Fig. 27-15).

Mechanisms responsible for intestinal adaptation have been studied widely in animals. Multiple factors are responsible and are required for development of successful intestinal adaptation. For reasons that are not known, the ileum exhibits a much greater adaptive response than the jejunum. Luminal nutrients, trophic gut hormones, and pancreatic and biliary secretions are all required for complete adaptation to occur. In animals maintained on TPN after extensive small bowel resection, nutrition may be maintained, but intestinal adaptation does not occur. The trophic gut peptides studied most intensively in small bowel adaptation are gastrin, CCK, secretin, and enteroglucagon. We now know that, although hypergastrinemia is associated with the short bowel syndrome, gastrin does not play a major role in the adaptive response after resection. CCK and secretin may have direct effects on enterocyte replication; however, their primary importance in intestinal adaptation may be in stimulation of pancreaticobiliary secretions rather than in directly stimulating enterocyte proliferation. Enteroglucagon has been recently emphasized as the primary trophic stimulus for intestinal adaptation. This idea is based upon the findings of increased numbers of cells containing enteroglucagon in the intestinal mucosa and measured increases of plasma enteroglucagon after bowel resection. Direct analysis of the effects of enteroglucagon on intestinal growth have not been possible because of the lack of pure peptide for such studies.

In man, the adaptive responses to massive resection have been found to be increased caliber of the remaining small bowel, hypertrophy of the gut wall, increased villous height, and increased numbers of enterocytes. This process often takes weeks to months to complete after small bowel resection. With time, absorptive function increases. This increase is characterized by decreasing stool losses of water and electrolyte and increased absorption of glucose and vitamin B_{12}.

Hypergastrinemia and gastric hypersecretion occur after massive small bowel resection and have been widely studied in experimental animals; some information has come from man. Diarrhea associated with gastric hypersecretion is caused by (1) delivery of a massive volume of fluid and electrolytes to the shortened small bowel, (2) steatorrhea due to failure of lipolysis by pancreatic lipase, which requires an intraluminal pH greater than 5.0 for activity (pancreatic secretion of lipase is not affected), and (3) acid enteritis. Although acid hypersecretion was at one time thought to be of prime importance in producing diarrhea after extensive small bowel resection, both hypergastrinemia and hypersecretion of acid are transient. Acid hypersecretion is now easily managed by H_2-receptor antagonists. Control of acid secretion controls diarrhea to a great extent during the early phase. Several operations, including vagotomy and pyloroplasty, or vagotomy and antrectomy, have been employed with treatment of the short bowel syndrome to control acid hypersecretion. Since the problem is self-limited, however, these procedures are not indicated and should not be done.

Resection of specific segments of the small bowel leads to specific problems. Resection of the distal small bowel results in diarrhea, steatorrhea, and malabsorption. Conjugated bile salts, essential for normal fat absorption, are almost totally absorbed in the distal ileum by active transport mechanisms. Resection of the ileum results in disruption of the enterohepatic circulation of bile salts and may lead to two types of diarrhea. If less than 100 cm of small bowel is resected, excessive amounts of bile salts enter the colon and produce a chemical enteritis; this type of diarrhea has been termed *cholerrheic*. The toxic effects of bile acids on colonic epithelial cells are twofold: bile salts inhibit absorption of water and electrolytes in the colon, and the injured colonic cells secrete excessive amounts of water and electrolytes. The response to de-

creased absorption of bile salts is increased hepatic production of bile salts, and this leads to perpetuation of diarrhea.

When more than 100 cm of ileum has been resected, the loss of bile salts is so great that hepatic synthesis cannot compensate. In addition to the direct toxic effects of bile salts on the colonic epithelium, fat malabsorption (steatorrhea) occurs. Differentiation of the two types of diarrhea associated with distal resection is important because treatment is different. Measurement of stool fat content, vitamin B_{12} absorptive capacity, and fecal bile salt concentrations are important for accurate determination of deficits produced. For those patients who have cholerrheic diarrhea, agents that bind bile acids (cholestyramine) may alleviate diarrhea. If steatorrhea is present, then medium-chain triglycerides that do not require micelle formation for absorption should also be used.

Another factor contributing to diarrhea after ileal resection is loss of the ileocecal valve. The ileocecal valve has two important actions. It prolongs intestinal transit time, and it prevents retrograde passage of colonic bacteria into the small bowel, which, if not prevented, causes bacterial enteritis.

Other complications associated with alteration of enterohepatic circulation of bile acids include gallstones and anemia. The changes in the bile salt pool produce lithogenic bile; the incidence of gallstones in patients with ileal resection is three to four times greater than that of the normal population. The ileum is the specific site for transport mechanisms for intrinsic-factor–mediated vitamin B_{12} absorption, and with total ileal resection, stores of vitamin B_{12} are depleted, and anemia will result.

TREATMENT. The most important principle in treatment of short bowel syndrome is prevention. This means that at operation, when intestinal viability is questionable, the smallest possible resections should be performed, and "second look" operations 24 to 48 h later should be carried out to allow the ischemic bowel to demarcate. Delay may prevent unnecessary, extensive resection of bowel. In patients with Crohn's disease, the devastating complications of the short bowel syndrome have led all students of the disease to recognize that only limited resections should be performed.

After massive small bowel resection, the program for treatment may be properly divided into early and late. Early on, treatment is primarily directed at the control of diarrhea, replacement of fluid and electrolytes, and the prompt institution of total parenteral nutrition. Volume losses may exceed 5 L/day, and vigorous monitoring of intake and output with adequate replacement must be carried out. Depletion of fluid volume caused by diarrhea, especially in the early phase, is often a formidable problem. Judicious use of agents that inhibit gut motility (codeine, Lomotil, loperamide) may be helpful. These drugs may cause profound ileus if used excessively, and you simply trade volume lost through the gut for volume lost through nasogastric suction. In addition, prolonged ileus with dilatation and edema of the bowel wall may result.

As intestinal adaptation progresses, and gut absorption increases, the stool volume gradually decreases. Once patients have completely adapted to an oral diet, semi-formed stools may appear, but these patients will likely never have the normal number or consistency of stools.

As soon as the patient has recovered from the acute phase, he or she should begin enteral nutrition, so that intestinal adaptation may begin early and proceed successfully. The most common types of enteral diets are either elemental diets (Vivonex, Flexical) or polymeric diets (Isocal, Ensure). Each presents problems with increased osmolality and may contain foodstuffs that may not be absorbed due to enzyme deficiency (for example, deficiency of lactase). Milk products should be avoided, and diets should be begun at isoosmolar concentrations and with small volumes (50 mL/h), even though the full nutrient value may not be obtained. As the gut adapts, the osmolality volume and caloric content may be increased.

Reduction of dietary fat has long been considered to be important in the treatment of patients with the short bowel syndrome. High-carbohydrate, high-protein, low-fat diets have been prescribed. Fat has more than twice as many calories per gram as protein and carbohydrate and is important for maintenance of proper nutrition. Supplementation of the diet with 100 g or more of fat should be carried out. Often this requires the use of medium-chain triglycerides, which may be absorbed in the proximal bowel without micelle formation. Vitamins, especially fat-soluble vitamins, as well as calcium, magnesium and zinc supplementation, must also be provided. H_2-receptor antagonists may greatly diminish the diarrhea that is largely caused by the early, transient acid hypersecretion. Measurement of intragastric pH can be used to guide the dose of drugs required. Antacids are not useful because they may aggravate diarrhea or bind essential ions. In no case should gastric resection or vagotomy be used for the treatment of the short bowel syndrome.

Since the dysfunction of massive small bowel resection is caused by decreased absorptive surface and rapid transit time, most attempts at surgical treatment have been directed toward increasing the absorptive surface or slowing the intestinal transit time. These operations have included serosal patches of the colon in order to stimulate neomucosal growth, longitudinal small bowel division and lengthening, construction of valves (artificial sphincters), reversed segments of small bowel or colon, or insertion of isoperistaltic colonic segments. None of these surgical operations has been found effective, and they should not be performed.

The present treatment of the short bowel syndrome is palliative and is directed toward control of diarrhea and prevention of dehydration and malnutrition. Only with the development of successful allotransplantation of the gut will the short bowel syndrome be cured.

Intestinal Bypass

MORBID OBESITY

Surgical procedures to treat morbid obesity (defined as more than 100 lb over ideal weight) have become popular because the long-term success rate of nonsurgical treatment of this condition is only 1 percent. The original procedure designed to create a short-gut malabsorption syndrome, jejunocolostomy, had to be abandoned because of an unacceptable rate of complications. It was succeeded by jejunoileostomy, either end-to-side (Payne procedure) or end-to-end (Scott procedure). Many thousands of these procedures have been done in the United States. These too have been abandoned. An alternative method of operative therapy of obesity is the gastric bypass or partition. This method limits food intake by reducing the reservoir capacity of the stomach to 5 to 10 percent of normal.

Jejunoileal bypass produces very significant weight loss in the majority of patients, with the heaviest patients losing the most weight. Weight loss goes on for 12 to 18 months and then plateaus at a level that is still considerably above the ideal, but well below the preoperative weight. Despite the effectiveness of jejunoileal bypass in producing weight loss, there is widespread disenchantment with the procedure, principally due to very serious long-term complications, and it has been abandoned by most surgeons.

The operative mortality rate of jejunoileostomy is 2 to 5 percent. The morbidity, as always in operations on very obese patients, is appreciable and includes atelectasis, pneumonia, wound infection and dehiscence, and thromboembolism.

The late mortality rate has been about 10 percent, one-half the deaths being from liver failure. Late complications are many and formidable; they include hepatic steatosis, cirrhosis, and failure; hyperoxaluria and calcium oxalate urinary tract calculi; hyperbilirubinemia and gallstones; electrolyte imbalances, including hypocalcemia, hypomagnesemia, and hypokalemia; avitaminoses; psychologic problems and emotional upsets; loss of hair; polyarthropathy; pancreatitis; blind loop syndrome; pneumatosis cystoides intestinalis; colonic pseudo-obstruction; intussusception of bypassed jejunum; and bypass enteritis. Although many morbidly obese (and some not so morbidly obese) patients are eager to submit to these procedures and many surgeons appear eager to comply, these procedures are metabolically unsound.

Fifteen to 25 percent of patients in whom jejunoileal bypass has been performed have had the shunt reversed. The morbidity and mortality of the reanastomosis is not inconsequential in patients who are often nutritionally and metabolically crippled. The principal indications have been hepatic failure, unmanageable electrolyte and metabolic imbalances, persistent uncontrollable diarrhea or associated severe anorectal problems, excessive or excessively rapid weight loss, and inadequate weight loss.

Alpers has pointed out three major problems with operations for morbid obesity: lack of criteria for proper patient selection, lack of clear superiority for any operative procedure, and the lack of any long-term benefit of decreased mortality.

HYPERLIPIDEMIA

Surgical bypass of a portion of the small intestine is a useful method of treating hypercholesterolemia and hypertriglyceridemia. The operation, designed by Buchwald and Varco, short-circuits either the distal 200 cm or one-third of the small intestine length, whichever is greater. This operation, though occasionally associated with diarrhea, does not cause significant weight loss and is not associated with the undesirable side effects of the jejuno-ileal bypass.

This procedure lowers serum cholesterol level through two mechanisms: by interfering with the absorption of cholesterol by short-circuiting the usual site of absorption, and by increasing cholesterol and bile acid excretion, which accelerates cholesterol turnover.

Clinical metabolic studies have demonstrated a 60 percent decrease in cholesterol absorption, a 40 percent reduction in serum cholesterol, and a more than 50 percent reduction in plasma triglycerides. About 70 percent of patients with angina have had improvement or total remission of symptoms after this operation. Thus, partial ileal bypass, when employed for the correction of hyperlipidemia, appears to be an effective method of lipid reduction. It is obligatory in its actions, safe, and is associated with minimal side effects.

Bibliography

Anatomy

Fawcett DW (ed): Intestines, in *A Textbook of Histology*. Philadelphia, Saunders, 1986, pp 641–660.

Grand RJ, Watkins JB, et al: Development of the human gastrointestinal tract. *Gastroenterology* 70:790, 1976.

Hirsch J, Ahrens EH Jr, et al: Measurement of the human intestinal length in vivo and some causes of variation. *Gastroenterology* 31:274, 1956.

Trier JS: Morphology of the epithelium of the small intestine, in Code CF (ed): *Handbook of Physiology*, sect 6. Washington, DC, American Physiological Society, 1968, pp 1125–1175.

Trier JS: Diagnostic value of peroral biopsy of the proximal small intestine. *N Engl J Med* 285:1470, 1971.

Trier JS, Krone CL, et al: Anatomy, embryology, and developmental abnormalities of the small intestine and colon, in Sleisenger MH, Fordtran JS (eds): *Gastrointestinal Disease. Pathophysiology, Diagnosis, Management*. Philadelphia, Saunders, 1983, pp 780–811.

Physiology

Alpers DH: Absorption of water-soluble vitamins, folate, minerals, and vitamin D, in Sleisenger MH, Fordtran JS (eds): *Gastrointestinal Disease. Pathophysiology, Diagnosis, Management*. Philadelphia, Saunders, 1983, pp 830–844.

Becker JM, Duff WM, et al: Myoelectric control of gastrointestinal and biliary motility: A review. *Surgery* 89:466, 1981.

Binder HJ: Absorption and secretion of water and electrolytes by small and large intestine, in Sleisenger MH, Fordtran JS (eds): *Gastrointestinal Disease. Pathophysiology, Diagnosis, Management*. Philadelphia, Saunders, 1983, pp 811–829.

Code CF (ed): *Handbook of Physiology*, sect 6. Washington, DC, American Physiological Society, 1968.

Cohen S, Snape WJ Jr: Movement of the small and large intestines, in Sleisenger MH, Fordtran JS (eds): *Gastrointestinal Disease. Pathophysiology, Diagnosis, Management*. Philadelphia, Saunders, 1983, pp 859–873.

Davenport HW (ed.): Intestinal secretion, in *Physiology of the Digestive Tract*. Chicago, Yearbook Medical Publishers, 1982, pp 174–178.

Hofmann AF: A physicochemical approach to the intraluminal phase of fat absorption. *Gastroenterology* 50:56, 1966.

Gangl A, Ockner RK: Intestinal metabolism of lipids and lipoproteins. *Gastroenterology* 68:167, 1975.

Gray GM: Mechanisms of digestion and absorption of food, in Sleisenger MH, Fordtran JS (eds): *Gastrointestinal Disease. Pathophysiology, Diagnosis, Management*. Philadelphia, Saunders, 1983, pp 844–858.

Scratcherd T, Grundy D: The physiology of intestinal motility and secretion. *Br J Anaesth* 56:3, 1984.

Thompsom JC, Greeley George H Jr, et al (eds): *Gastrointestinal Endocrinology*, New York, McGraw-Hill, 1987.

Thompson JC, Marx M: Gastrointestinal hormones. *Curr Probl Surg* 21:1, 1984.

Inflammatory Diseases

Alexander-Williams J, Haynes IG: Up-to-date management of small-bowel Crohn's disease. *Adv Surg* 20:245, 1987.

Aston NO, de Costa AM: Tuberculous perforation of the small bowel. *Postgrad Med J* 61:251, 1985.

Bartlett JG: *Clostridium difficile* and inflammatory bowel disease. *Gastroenterology* 80:863, 1981.

Beart RW Jr, McIlrath DC, et al: Surgical management of inflammatory bowel disease. *Curr Probl Surg* 17(10):533, 1980.

Block GE, Enker WE, et al: Significance and treatment of occult obstructive uropathy complicating Crohn's disease. *Ann Surg* 178:322, 1973.

Block GE, Schraut WH: The operative treatment of Crohn's enteritis complicated by ileosigmoid fistula. *Ann Surg* 196:356, 1982.

Bluth EI, McVay LV III, et al: Ultrasonic characteristics of ileal tuberculosis. *Dis Colon Rectum* 28:613, 1985.

Broe PJ, Bayless TM, et al: Crohn's disease: Are enteroenteral fistulas an indication for surgery? *Surgery* 91:249, 1982.

Chouhan MK, Pande SK: Typhoid enteric perforation. *Br J Surg* 69:173, 1982.

Collier PE, Turowski P, et al: Small intestinal adenocarcinoma complicating regional enteritis. *Cancer* 55:516, 1985.

Crohn BB, Ginzburg L, et al: Regional enteritis. A pathologic and clinical entity. *JAMA* 99:1323, 1932.

Eggleston FC, Santoshi B, et al: Typhoid perforation of the bowel. *Ann Surg* 190:31, 1979.

Eustache J-M, Kreis DJ Jr: Typhoid perforation of the intestine. *Arch Surg* 118:1269, 1983.

Farmer RG, Hawk WA, et al: Indications for surgery in Crohn's disease: Analysis of 500 cases. *Gastroenterology* 71:245, 1976.

Fresko D, Lazarus SS, et al: Early presentation of carcinoma of the small bowel in Crohn's disease ("Crohn's carcinoma"). *Gastroenterology* 82:783, 1982.

Gilinsky NH, Marks IN, et al: Abdominal tuberculosis. A 10-year review. *SA Med J* 64:849, 1983.

Gitnick G: Is Crohn's disease a mycobacterial disease after all? *Dig Dis Sci* 29:1086, 1984.

Goldberg HI, Caruthers SB Jr, et al: Radiographic findings of the National Cooperative Crohn's Disease Study. *Gastroenterology* 77:925, 1979.

Greenstein AJ, Janowitz HD, et al: The extraintestinal manifestations of Crohn's disease and ulcerative colitis: A study of 700 patients. *Medicine* (Balt) 55:401, 1976.

Greenstein AJ, Meyers S, et al: Surgery and its sequelae in Crohn's colitis and ileocolitis. *Arch Surg* 116:285, 1981.

Greenstein AJ, Sachar D, et al: Cancer in Crohn's disease after diversionary surgery. A report of seven carcinomas occurring in excluded bowel. *Am J Surg* 135:86, 1978.

Greenstein AJ, Sachar DB, et al: Patterns of neoplasia in Crohn's disease and ulcerative colitis. *Cancer* 46:403, 1980.

Gryboski JD, Spiro HM.: Prognosis in children with Crohn's disease. *Gastroenterology* 74:807, 1978.

Hamilton SR, Reese J, et al: The role of resection margin frozen section in the surgical management of Crohn's disease. *Surg Gynecol Obstet* 160:57, 1985.

Hawker PC, Givel JC, et al: Management of enterocutaneous fistulae in Crohn's disease. *Gut* 24:284, 1983.

Heuman R, Boeryd B, et al: The influence of disease at the margin of resection on the outcome of Crohn's disease. *Br J Surg* 70:519, 1983.

Homan WP, Dineen P: Comparison of the results of resection, bypass, and bypass with exclusion for ileocecal Crohn's disease. *Ann Surg* 187:530, 1978.

Homan WP, Tank C-K, et al: Acute massive hemorrhage from intestinal Crohn's disease: Report of seven cases and review of the literature. *Arch Surg* 111:901, 1976.

Janowitz HD: Crohn's disease—50 years later. *N Engl J Med* 304:1600, 1981.

Kakar A, Aranya RC, et al: Acute perforation of small intestine due to tuberculosis. *Aust NZ J Surg* 53:381, 1983.

Kendall GPN, Hawley PR, et al: Strictureplasty. A good operation for small bowel Crohn's disease? *Dis Colon Rectum* 29:312, 1986.

Kewenter J, Hulten L, et al: The relationship and epidemiology of acute terminal ileitis and Crohn's disease. *Gut* 15:801, 1974.

Khanna AK, Misra MK: Typhoid perforation of the gut. *Postgrad Med J* 60:523, 1984.

Kim J-P, Oh S-K, et al: Management of ileal perforation due to typhoid fever. *Ann Surg* 181:88, 1975.

Kirschner BS, Voinchet O, et al: Growth retardation in inflammatory bowel disease. *N Engl J Med* 306:775, 837, 1982.

Knutson L, Arosenius K-E: Tuberculosis of the large bowel. Report of two cases. *Acta Chir Scand* 150:345, 1984.

Korelitz BI, Present DH: Favorable effect of 6-mercaptopurine on fistulae of Crohn's disease. *Dig Dis Sci* 30:58, 1985.

Lennard-Jones JE: Azathioprine and 6-mercaptopurine have a role in the treatment of Crohn's disease. *Dig Dis Sci* 26:364, 1981.

Lennard-Jones JE, Singleton JW: The Azathioprine controversy. *Dig Dis Sci* 26:364, 1981.

Lizarralde AE: Typhoid perforation of the ileum in children. *J Pediatr Surg* 16:1012, 1981.

Lock MR, Farmer RG, et al: Recurrence and reoperation for Crohn's disease: The role of disease location in prognosis. *N Engl J Med* 304:1586, 1981.

Mayberry JF, Rhodes J: Epidemiological aspects of Crohn's disease: A review of the literature. *Gut* 25:886, 1984.

Mekhjian HS, Switz DM, et al: Clinical features and natural history of Crohn's disease. *Gastroenterology* 77:898, 1979.

Mekhjian HS, Switz DM, et al: National Cooperative Crohn's Disease Study: Factors determining recurrence of Crohn's disease after surgery. *Gastroenterology* 77:907, 1979.

Menguy R: Surgical management of free perforation of the small intestine complicating regional enteritis. *Ann Surg* 175:178, 1972.

Meyers S, Walfish JS, et al: Quality of life after surgery for Crohn's disease: A psychosocial survey. *Gastroenterology* 78:1, 1980.

Nugent FW, Richmond M, et al: Crohn's disease of the duodenum. *Gut* 18:115, 1977.

Pennington L, Hamilton SR, et al: Surgical management of Crohn's disease: Influence of disease at margin of resection. *Ann Surg* 192:311, 1980.

Present DH, Korelitz BI, et al: Treatment of Crohn's disease with 6-mercaptopurine: A long-term, randomized, double-blind study. *N Engl J Med* 302:981, 1980.

Prior P, Gyde S, et al: Mortality in Crohn's disease. *Gastroenterology* 80:307, 1981.

Rankin GB, Watts HD, et al: National Cooperative Crohn's Disease Study: Extraintestinal manifestations and perianal complications. *Gastroenterology* 77:914, 1979.

Rombeau JL, Barot LR, et al: Preoperative total parenteral nutrition and surgical outcome in patients with inflammatory bowel disease. *Am J Surg* 143:139, 1982.

Sachar DB, Auslander MO: Missing pieces in the puzzle of Crohn's disease. *Gastroenterology* 75:745, 1978.

Sachar DB, Auslander MO, et al: Aetiological theories of inflammatory bowel disease. *Clin Gastroenterol* 9:231, 1980.

Sachar DB, Wolfson DM, et al: Risk factors for postoperative recurrence of Crohn's disease. *Gastroenterology* 85:917, 1983.

Seashore JH, Hillemeier AC, et al: Total parenteral nutrition in the management of inflammatory bowel disease in children: A limited role. *Am J Surg* 143:504, 1982.

Shorter RG, Huizenga KA, et al: A working hypothesis for the etiology and pathogenesis of nonspecific inflammatory bowel disease. *Am J Dig Dis* 17:1024, 1972.

Simpson S, Traube J, et al: The histologic appearance of dysplasia (precarcinomatous change) in Crohn's disease of the small and large intestines. *Gastroenterology* 81:492, 1981.

Singleton JW: The National Cooperative Crohn's Disease Study. *Gastroenterology* 77:825, 1979.

Singleton JW: Azathioprine has a very limited role in the treatment of Crohn's disease. *Dig Dis Sci* 26:368, 1981.

Sleisenger MH: How should we treat Crohn's disease? *N Engl J Med* 302:1024, 1980.

Stead WW, Dutt AK: Chemotherapy for tuberculosis today. *Am Rev Respir Dis* 125:94, 1982.

Strobel CT, Byrne WJ, et al: Home parenteral nutrition in children with Crohn's disease: An effective management alternative. *Gastroenterology* 77:272, 1979.

Summers RW, Switz DM, et al: National Cooperative Crohn's Disease Study: Results of drug treatment. *Gastroenterology* 77:847, 1979.

Tandon HD, Prakash A: Pathology of intestinal tuberculosis and its distinction from Crohn's disease. *Gut* 13:260, 1972.

Trnka YM, Glotzer DJ, et al: The long-term outcome of restorative operation in Crohn's disease. *Ann Surg* 196:345, 1982.

Vaidya MG, Sodhi JS: Gastrointestinal tract tuberculosis: A study of 102 cases including 55 hemicolectomies. *Clin Radiol* 29:189, 1978.

Vantrappen G, Ponette E, et al: Yersinia enteritis and enterocolitis: Gastroenterological aspects. *Gastroenterology* 72:220, 1977.

Weakley FL, Turnbull FL: Recognition of regional ileitis in the operating room. *Dis Colon Rectum* 14:17, 1971.

Wolff BG, Beart RW Jr, et al: The importance of disease-free margins in resections for Crohn's disease. *Dis Colon Rectum* 26:239, 1983.

Wolfson DM, Sachar DB, et al: Granulomas do not affect postoperative recurrence rates in Crohn's disease. *Gastroenterology* 83:405, 1982.

Neoplasms

Ahlman H, Dahlstrom A, et al: The pentagastrin test in the diagnosis of the carcinoid syndrome. Blockade of gastrointestinal symptoms by Ketanserin. *Ann Surg* 201:81, 1985.

Akwari OE, Dozois RR, et al: Leiomyosarcoma of the small and large bowel. *Cancer* 42:1375, 1978.

Awrich AE, Irish CE, et al: A twenty-five year experience with primary malignant tumors of the small intestine. *Surg Gynecol Obstet* 151:9, 1980.

Bancks NH, Goldstein HM, et al: The roentgenologic spectrum of small intestinal carcinoid tumors. *Am J Roentgenol* 123:274, 1975.

Barclay THC, Schapira DV: Malignant tumors of the small intestine. *Cancer* 51:878, 1983.

Beaton H, Homan W, et al: Gastrointestinal carcinoids and the malignant carcinoid syndrome. *Surg Gynecol Obstet* 152:268, 1981.

Boddie AW Jr, Mullins JD, et al: Extranodal lymphoma: Surgical and other therapeutic alternatives. *Curr Probl Cancer* 6:1, 1982.

Bremer EH, Battaile WG, et al: Villous tumors of the upper gastrointestinal tract. Clinical review and report of a case. *Am J Gastroenterol* 50:135, 1968.

Darling RC, Welch CE: Tumors of the small intestine. *N Engl J Med* 260:397, 1959.

Davis GR, Camp RC, et al: Effect of somatostatin infusion on jejunal water and electrolyte transport in a patient with secretory diarrhea due to malignant carcinoid syndrome. *Gastroenterology* 78:346, 1980.

Davis Z, Moertel CG, et al: The malignant carcinoid syndrome. *Surg Gynecol Obstet* 137:637, 1973.

Dawson IMP, Cornes JS, et al: Primary malignant lymphoid tumours of the intestinal tract. Report of 37 cases with a study of factors influencing prognosis. *Br J Surg* 49:80, 1961.

Emson PC, Gilbert RFT, et al: Elevated concentrations of substance P and 5-HT in plasma in patients with carcinoid tumors. *Cancer* 54:715, 1984.

Godwin JD II: Carcinoid tumors. An analysis of 2837 cases. *Cancer* 36:560, 1975.

Goedert M, Otten U, et al: Dopamine, norepinephrine, and serotonin production by an intestinal carcinoid tumor. *Cancer* 45:104, 1980.

Halpert RD, Feczko PJ, et al: Enteroclysis for the examination of the small bowel. *Henry Ford Hosp Med J* 33:116, 1985.

Herbsman H, Wetstein L, et al: Tumors of the small intestine. *Curr Probl Surg* 17(3):121, 1980.

Jeghers H, McKusick VA, et al: Generalized intestinal polyposis and melanin spots on the oral mucosa, lips and digits. *N Engl J Med* 241:993, 1949.

Johnson LA, Lavin P, et al: Carcinoids: The association of histologic growth pattern and survival. *Cancer* 51:882, 1983.

Kvols LK, Moertel CG, et al: Treatment of the malignant carcinoid syndrome. Evaluation of a long-acting somatostatin analogue. *N Engl J Med* 315:663, 1986.

Long RG, Peters JR, et al: Somatostatin, gastrointestinal peptides, and the carcinoid syndrome. *Gut* 22:549, 1981.

Maglinte DDT, Hall R, et al: Detection of surgical lesions of the small bowel by enteroclysis. *Am J Surg* 147:225, 1984.

Martin JK Jr, Moertel CG, et al: Surgical treatment of functioning metastatic carcinoid tumors. *Arch Surg* 118:537, 1983.

McAllister AJ, Richards KF: Peutz-Jeghers syndrome: Experience with twenty patients in five generations. *Am J Surg* 134:717, 1977.

McDermott WV, Hensle TW: Metastatic carcinoid to the liver treated by hepatic dearterialization. *Ann Surg* 180:305, 1974.

Moertel CG, Dockerty MB, et al: Carcinoid tumors of the vermiform appendix. *Cancer* 21:270, 1968.

Moertel CG, Sauer WG, et al: Life history of the carcinoid tumor of the small intestine. *Cancer* 14:901, 1961.

Nagorney DM, Sarr MG, et al: Surgical management of intussusception in the adult. *Ann Surg* 193:230, 1981.

Oates JA: The carcinoid syndrome. *N Engl J Med* 315:702, 1986.

Pagtalunan RJG, Mayo CW, et al: Primary malignant tumors of the small intestine. *Am J Surg* 108:13, 1964.

Perzin KH, Bridge MF: Adenomatous and carcinomatous changes in hamartomatous polyps of the small intestine (Peutz-Jeghers syndrome): Report of a case and review of the literature. *Cancer* 49:971, 1982.

Rao AR, Kagan AR, et al: Management of gastrointestinal lymphoma. *Am J Clin Oncol* 7:213, 1984.

River L, Silverstein J, et al: Benign neoplasms of the small intestine. A critical comprehensive review with reports of 20 new cases. *Intl Abst Surg* 102:1, 1956.

Rochlin DB, Longmire WP Jr: Primary tumors of the small intestine. *Surgery* 50:586, 1961.

Salem PA, Nassar VH, et al: Mediterranean abdominal lymphoma, or immunoproliferative small intestinal disease. Part I: Clinical aspects. *Cancer* 40:2941, 1977.

Schulten MF Jr, Oyasu R, et al: Villous adenoma of the duodenum. A case report and review of the literature. *Am J Surg* 132:90, 1976.

Starr GF, Dockerty MB: Leiomyomas and leiomyosarcomas of the small intestine. *Cancer* 8:101, 1955.

Stothert JC Jr, Riaz MA, et al: Preoperative angiographic diagnosis of small bowel leiomyomas. *Arch Surg* 113:643, 1978.

Strodel WE, Talpos G, et al: Surgical therapy for small-bowel carcinoid tumors. *Arch Surg* 118:291, 1983.

Stubenbord WT, Thorbjarnarson B: Intussusception in adults. *Ann Surg* 172:306, 1970.

Weingrad DN, DeCosse JJ, et al: Primary gastrointestinal lymphoma: A 30-year review. *Cancer* 49:1258, 1982.

Wilson H, Cheek RC, et al: Carcinoid syndrome. *Curr Probl Surg* 36:41, 1970.

Wilson JM, Melvin DB, et al: Primary malignancies of the small bowel: A report of 96 cases and review of the literature. *Ann Surg* 180:175, 1974.

Wilson JM, Melvin DB, et al: Benign small bowel tumor. *Ann Surg* 181:247, 1975.

Zollinger RM Jr, Sternfeld WC, et al: Primary neoplasms of the small intestine. *Am J Surg* 151:654, 1986.

Diverticular Disease

Adams DB: Management of the intraluminal duodenal diverticulum: Endoscopy or duodenostomy? *Am J Surg* 151:524, 1986.

Brian JE Jr, Stair JM: Noncolonic diverticular disease. *Surg Gynecol Obstet* 161:189, 1985.

Critchlow JF, Shapiro MD, et al: Duodenojejunostomy for the pancreaticobiliary complications of duodenal diverticulum. *Ann Surg* 202:56, 1985.

DeBartolo HM Jr, van Heerden JA: Meckel's diverticulum. *Ann Surg* 183:30, 1976.

Eckhauser FE, Zelenock GB, et al: Acute complications of jejuno-ileal pseudodiverticulosis: Surgical implications and management. *Am J Surg* 138:320, 1979.

Economides NG, McBurney RP, et al: Intraluminal duodenal diverticulum in the adult. *Ann Surg* 185:147, 1977.

Eggert A, Teichmann W, et al: The pathologic implication of duodenal diverticula. *Surg Gynecol Obstet* 154:62, 1982.

Griffin M, Carey WD, et al: Recurrent acute pancreatitis and intussusception complicating an intraluminal duodenal diverticulum. *Gastroenterology* 81:345, 1981.

Haugh DC, McBee MH: Perforation of duodenal diverticula. *Contemp Surg* 25:72, 1984.

Howard JM, Wynn OB, et al: Intraluminal duodenal diverticulum: An unusual cause of acute pancreatitis. *Am J Surg* 151:505, 1986.

Kaminsky HH, Thompson WR, et al: Extended sphincteroplasty for juxtapapillary duodenal diverticulum. *Surg Gynecol Obstet* 162:280, 1986.

Karoll MP, Ghahremani GG, et al: Diagnosis and management of intraluminal duodenal diverticulum. *Dig Dis Sci* 28:411, 1983.

Kellum JM, Boucher JK, et al: Serosal patch repair for benign duodenocolic fistula secondary to duodenal diverticulum. *Am J Surg* 131:607, 1976.

Kilpatrick ZM, Aseron CA: Radioisotope detection of Meckel's diverticulum causing acute rectal hemorrhage. *N Engl J Med* 287:653, 1972.

Krishnamurthy S, Kelly MM, et al: Jejunal diverticulosis. A heterogenous disorder caused by a variety of abnormalities of smooth muscle or myenteric plexus. *Gastroenterology* 85:538, 1983.

Leinkram C, Roberts-Thomson IC, et al: Juxtapapillary duodenal diverticula. Association with gallstones and pancreatitis. *Med J Aust* 1:209, 1980.

Løtveit T, Osnes M: Duodenal diverticula. *Scand J Gastroenterol* 19:579, 1984.

Løtveit T, Osnes M, et al: Studies of the choledocho-duodenal sphincter in patients with and without juxtapapillary duodenal diverticula. *Scand J Gastroenterol* 15:875, 1980.

Løtveit T, Osnes M, et al: Recurrent biliary calculi. Duodenal diverticula as a predisposing factor. *Ann Surg* 196:30, 1982.

Manny J, Muga M, et al: The continuing clinical enigma of duodenal diverticulum. *Am J Surg* 142:596, 1981.

Mendelson RM, Shepherd HA, et al: "Inverted" diverticulum mimicking an ulcerated duodenal tumour. *Br J Radiol* 57:426, 1984.

Scudamore CH, Harrison RC, et al: Management of duodenal diverticula. *Can J Surg* 24:311, 1982.

Soltero MJ, Bill AH: The natural history of Meckel's diverticulum and its relation to incidental removal. A study of 202 cases of diseased Meckel's diverticulum found in King County, Washington, over a fifteen-year period. *Am J Surg* 132:168, 1976.

Williams RA, Davidson DD, et al: Surgical problems of diverticula of the small intestine. *Surg Gynecol Obstet* 152:621, 1981.

Ulcers

Boydstun JS Jr, Gaffey TA, et al: Clinicopathologic study of nonspecific ulcers of the small intestine. *Dig Dis Sci* 26:911, 1981.

Guest JL: Nonspecific ulceration of the intestine: Collective review. *Surg Gynecol Obstet* 117:409, 1963.

McMahon FG, Akdamar K: Gastric ulceration after "slow-K." *N Engl J Med* 295:733, 1976,

Thomas WEG, Williamson RCN: Enteric ulceration and its complications. *World J Surg* 9:876, 1985.

Foreign Bodies

Goldman AL: Foreign bodies of the gastrointestinal tract. *Contemp Surg* 18:45, 1981.

McCanse DE, Kurchin A, et al: Gastrointestinal foreign bodies. *Am J Surg* 142:335, 1981.

Schwartz JT, Graham DY: Toothpick perforation of the intestines. *Ann Surg* 185:64, 1977.

Fistulas

Blackett RL, Hill GL: Postoperative external small bowel fistulas: A study of a consecutive series of patients treated with intravenous hyperalimentation. *Br J Surg* 65:775, 1978.

Chapman R, Foran R, et al: Management of intestinal fistulas. *Am J Surg* 108:157, 1964.

Coutsoftides T, Fazio VW: Small intestine cutaneous fistulas. *Surg Gynecol Obstet* 149:333, 1979.

Edmunds LH, Williams GM, et al: External fistulas arising from the gastrointestinal tract. *Ann Surg* 152:445, 1960.

Hill GL: Operative strategy in the treatment of enterocutaneous fistulas. *World J Surg* 7:495, 1983.

Jones SA, Gazzaniga AB, et al: The serosal patch: A surgical parachute. *Am J Surg* 126:186, 1973.

Kingsnorth AN, Moss JG, et al: Failure of somatostatin to accelerate closure of enterocutaneous fistulas in patients receiving total parenteral nutrition. *Lancet* 1:1271, 1986.

Knighton DR, Burns K, et al: The use of stomahesive in the care of the skin of enterocutaneous fistulas. *Surg Gynecol Obstet* 143:449, 1976.

Malangoni MA, Madura JA, et al: Management of lateral duodenal fistulas: A study of fourteen cases. *Surgery* 90:645, 1981.

McIntyre PB, Ritchie JK, et al: Management of enterocutaneous fistulas: A review of 132 cases. *Br J Surg* 71:293, 1984.

McLean GK, Mackie JA, et al: Enterocutaneous fistulae: Interventional radiologic management. *AJR* 138:615, 1982.

Reber HA, Roberts C, et al: Management of external gastrointestinal fistulas. *Ann Surg* 188:460, 1978.

Soeters PB, Ebeid AM, et al: Review of 404 patients with gastrointestinal fistulas. Impact of parenteral nutrition. *Ann Surg* 190:189, 1979.

Webster MW Jr, Carey LC: Fistulae of the intestinal tract. *Curr Probl Surg* 13(6):1, 1976.

Zera RT, Bubrick MP, et al: Enterocutaneous fistulas. Effects of total parenteral nutrition and surgery. *Dis Colon Rectum* 26:109, 1983.

Enterocutaneous fistulas—Encouraging trends. *Lancet* 2:204, 1984 (Editorial.)

Blind Loop Syndrome

Fromm D: Ileal resection, or disease, and the blind loop syndrome: Current concepts of pathophysiology. *Surgery* 73:639, 1973.

Kern L: Bacterial contamination syndrome of the small bowel. *Clin Gastroenterol* 8:397, 1979.

King CE, Toskes PP: Small intestine bacterial overgrowth. *Gastroenterology* 76:1035, 1979.

Short Bowel Syndrome

Boeckman CR, Traylor R: Bowel lengthening for short gut syndrome. *J Pediatr Surg* 16:996, 1981.

Bristol JB, Williamson RCN: Postoperative adaptation of the small intestine. *World J Surg* 9:825, 1985.

Cortot A, Fleming CR, et al: Improved nutrient absorption after cimetidine in short-bowel syndrome with gastric hypersecretion. *N Engl J Med* 300:79, 1979.

Fleming CR, Beart RW Jr, et al: Home parenteral nutrition for management of the severely malnourished adult patient. *Gastroenterology* 79:11, 1980.

Gladen HE, Kelly KA: Electrical pacing for short bowel syndrome. *Surg Gynecol Obstet* 153:697, 1981.

Grosfeld JL, Rescorla FJ, et al: Short bowel syndrome in infancy and childhood. Analysis of survival in 60 patients. *Am J Surg* 151:41, 1986.

Hyman PE, Everett SL, et al: Gastric acid hypersecretion in short bowel syndrome in infants: Association with extent of resection and enteral feeding. *J Pediatr Gastroenterol Nutr* 5:191, 1986.

Koretz RL, Meyer JH: Elemental diets—facts and fantasies. *Gastroenterology* 78:393, 1980.

Krejs GJ: Intestinal resection. *Clin Gastroenterol* 8:373, 1979.

McIntyre PB: The short bowel. *Br J Surg* 72:592, 1985.

Mitchell A, Watkins RM, et al: Surgical treatment of the short bowel syndrome. *Br J Surg* 71:329, 1984.

Murphy JP Jr, King DR, et al: Treatment of gastric hypersecretion with cimetidine in the short-bowel syndrome. *N Engl J Med* 300:80, 1979.

Postuma R, Moroz S, et al: Extreme short-bowel syndrome in an infant. *J Pediatr Surg* 18:264, 1983.

Ricotta J, Zuidema GD, et al: Construction of an ileocecal valve and its role in massive resection of the small intestine. *Surg Gynecol Obstet* 152:310, 1981.

Ricour C, Duhamel JF, et al: Enteral and parenteral nutrition in the short bowel syndrome in children. *World J Surg* 9:310, 1985.

Russell RI: Intestinal adaptation to an elemental diet. *Proc Nutr Soc* 44:87, 1985.

Sheldon GF: Role of parenteral nutrition in patients with short bowel syndrome. *Am J Med* 67:1021, 1979.

Tepas JJ III, MacLean WC Jr, et al: Total management of short gut secondary to midgut volvulus without prolonged total parenteral alimentation. *J Pediatr Surg* 13:622, 1978.

Thompson JS: Surgical therapy for the short bowel syndrome. *J Surg Res* 39:81, 1985.

Weser E: Short bowel syndrome. *Gastroenterology* 77:572, 1979.

Williams RCN: Medical progress: Intestinal adaptation. Part 1, Structural, functional and cytokinetic changes. Part 2, Mechanisms of control. *N Engl J Med* 298:1393, 1444, 1978.

Williams NS, Evans P, et al: Gastric acid secretion and gastrin production in the short bowel syndrome. *Gut* 26:914, 1985.

Winchester DP, Dorsey JM: Intestinal segments and pouches in gastrointestinal surgery. *Surg Gynecol Obstet* 132:131, 1971.

Ziegler MM: Short bowel syndrome in infancy: Etiology and management. *Clin Perinatol* 13:163, 1986.

Intestinal Bypass

Alpers DH: Surgical therapy for obesity. *N Engl J Med* 308:1026, 1983.

Buchwald H, Moore RB, et al: Ten years clinical experience with partial ileal bypass in management of the hyperlipidemias. *Ann Surg* 180:384, 1974.

Griffen WO Jr, Young VL, et al: A prospective comparison of gastric and jejunoileal bypass for morbid obesity. *Ann Surg* 186:500, 1977.

Halverson JD: Obesity surgery in perspective. *Surgery* 87:119, 1980.

Ravitch MM, Brolin RE: The price of weight loss by jejunoileal shunt. *Ann Surg* 190:382, 1979.

Terry BE: Surgical management of morbid obesity. *Bull Am Col Surg* 67:3, 1982.

Chapter 28

Colon, Rectum, and Anus

Stanley M. Goldberg, Santhat Nivatvongs, and David A. Rothenberger

ANATOMY

The large intestine extends from the ileocecal valve to the anus. It consists of the colon, rectum, and anal canal. The colon is divided into several parts according to location: cecum, ascending colon, hepatic flexure, transverse colon, splenic flexure, descending colon, and sigmoid colon.

Colon

The colon starts from the end of the ileum and arbitrarily ends at the promontory of the sacrum where the teniae coli disappear as distinct bands. The *teniae coli* are the three strips of longitudinal muscle distributed at 120° intervals around the circumference of the colon. Thus, the outer longitudinal muscle layer of the gut is incomplete in the colon. The three bands converge proximally on the appendix and may be used as a means of locating it in difficult cases. The *haustra* are sacculations about the bowel and are the result of the outpouchings of bowel wall between the teniae. The haustra are separated by the *plicae semilunares*, or crescentic folds of bowel wall, which give the colon its characteristic x-ray appearance when filled with either barium or air. The *appendices epiploicae,* or fatty appendages along the bowel, have no anatomic function but are often useful in helping to protect a suture line or closure of a perforation in the colon.

The length of the colon varies between 3 and 5 ft and is approximately one-fifth the length of the entire gastrointestinal tract. The fixation of the colon is related to the retroperitoneal location of the ascending and descending portions of the bowel. The intraperitoneal transverse colon is comparatively free, but it is marked by a relatively constant location and by the attachment of the omentum to its anterior superior edge. The fixation of the ascending and descending colon in the lateral peritoneal gutters eliminates these areas from the problem of volvulus, which occurs most commonly in the mobile sigmoid and less commonly in the cecum or transverse colon. Since the colon comes into contact with almost every organ in the peritoneal and retroperitoneal spaces, its diseases may be made manifest by symptoms related to any of these organs or areas.

The internal diameter of the colon is greatest in the cecum, where it averages from 7.5 to 8.5 cm; it diminishes in size progressively to an averge of 2.5 cm in the sigmoid. The narrow lumen of the sigmoid, with its bulky and more solid fecal contents, explains how relatively small lesions can create significant obstruction, while lesions of the same size in the cecum, with its large diameter and liquid contents, often produce no symptoms. The large size of the cecum also explains why it is the first part of the bowel to rupture in the presence of unrelieved distal obstruction, since Laplace's law relates tension *(T)* in the wall of the bowel to the radius *(R)* of the tube and its internal pressure *(P)* *(T = PR)*.

ARTERAL SUPPLY. Although the blood supply of the colon varies from person to person, there is generally a distinct main artery to each segment of the colon arising either from the superior mesenteric artery (ileocolic artery, right colic artery, and middle colic artery) or from the inferior mesenteric artery (left colic artery, sigmoid arteries, and superior rectal artery) (Fig. 28-1). The marginal artery generally known as the artery of Drummond is a series of arcades of arteries along the mesenteric border of the entire colon. It is the branch connecting the superior and the inferior mesenteric arteries.

Fig. 28-1. Arterial supply of the colon. (From: *Nivatvongs S, Becker ER, 1987, with permission.*)

Mid Col	**Middle Colic A.**	**Lt Col**	**Left Colic A.**
Rt Col	**Right Colic A.**	**Sig**	**Sigmoidal A.**
Ic	**Ileocolic A.**	**Sup Rec**	**Superior Rectal A.**
Sup mes	**Superior Mesenteric A.**		
Inf mes	**Inferior Mesenteric A.**		

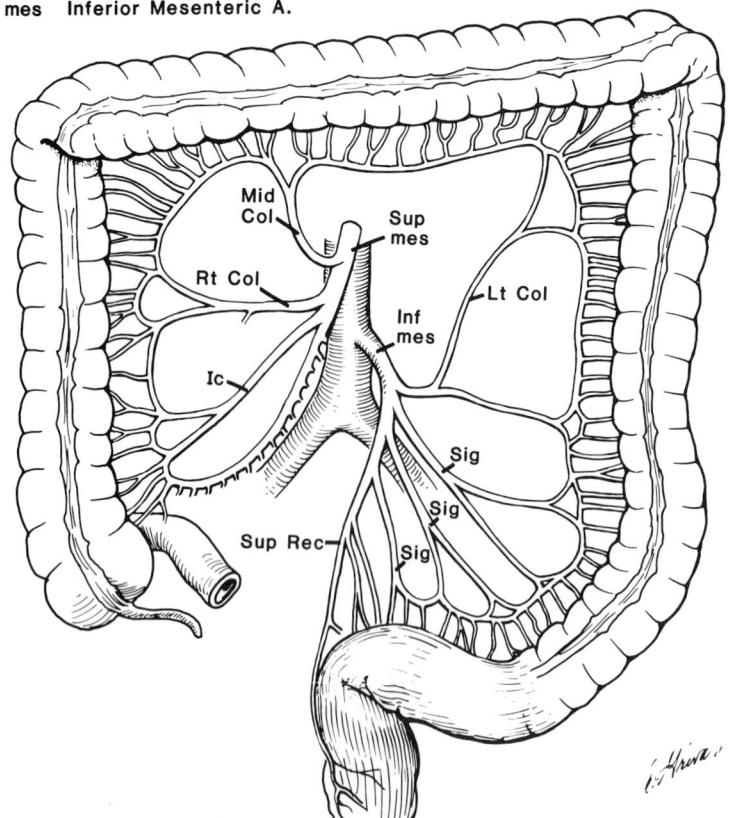

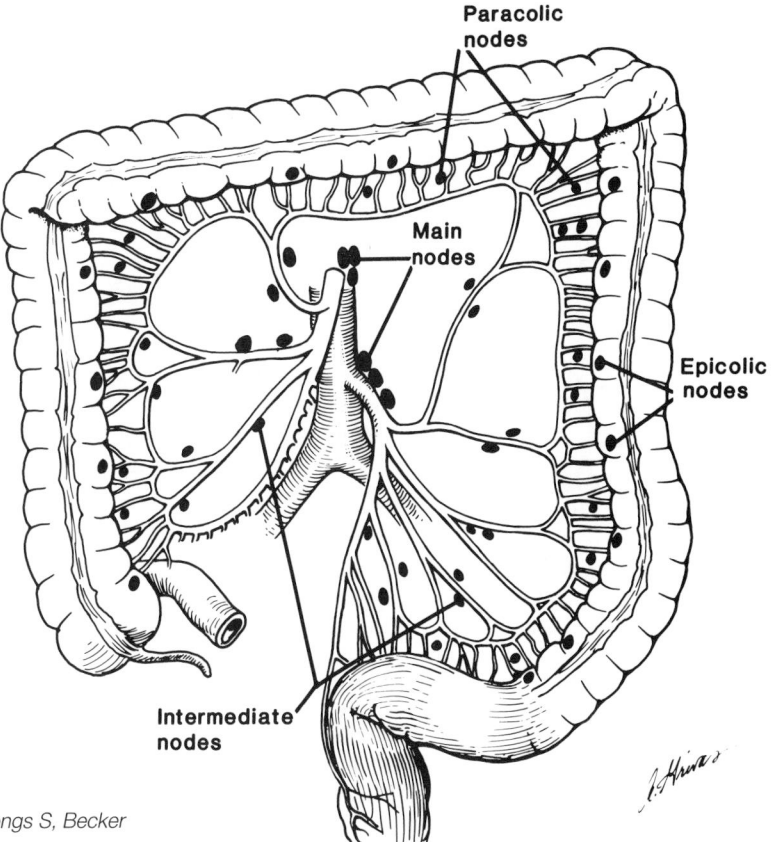

Fig. 28-2. Lymph nodes of the colon. (From: *Nivatvongs S, Becker ER, 1987, with permission.*)

VENOUS DRAINAGE. Except for the inferior mesenteric vein, the veins of the colon follow their corresponding arteries and bear the same terminology. At the level of the left colic artery, the inferior mesenteric vein follows its own course and ascends in the retroperitoneal plane over the psoas muscle to the left of the ligament of Treitz. It continues behind the body of the pancreas and enters the splenic vein.

LYMPHATIC DRAINAGE. The lymphatic drainage of the colon starts with an intramural network of lymphatic vessels and lymph follicles in the muscularis mucosa. The extramural lymphatic vessels and lymph nodes follow the regional arteries and consist of four groups: (1) Epicolic nodes lie on the bowel wall. (2) The paracolic nodes lie along the inner margin of the bowel, mainly between the intestine and the arterial arcades. (3) The intermediate nodes lie around the stem of the arteries before they divide. (4) The main nodes lie along the origin of the superior and inferor mesenteric arteries (Fig. 28-2).

NERVE SUPPLY. The nerve supply of the colon consists of both sympathetic and parsympathetic fibers that follow the course of the arteries. The sympathetic nerves inhibit and the parasympathetic nerves stimulate peristalsis of the colon and rectum. The sympathetic nerves supplying the colon originate from the lower thoracic and upper lumbar segments of the spinal cord. The parasympathetic nerve of the right colon is the vagus nerve. The vagus fibers are probably distributed as far as the splenic flexure. The parasympathetic nerve supply to the left colon is

from the sacral nerves, where the fibers from the pelvic plexus ascend.

Rectum and Anal Canal

The rectum starts at the level of the promontory of the sacrum where the three teniae spread out to form a complete layer of longitudinal smooth muscle. The rectum extends inferiorly to the level of the levator ani muscles and varies from 12 to 15 cm in length. It has two or three lateral curves forming the submucosal folds in the lumen known as *valves of Houston.* Peritoneum covers the upper two-thirds of the rectum anteriorly; the anterior peritoneal reflection is about 6 to 8 cm from the anal verge. Laterally, only the upper third of the rectum is covered with peritoneum, while the lower third of the rectum is entirely devoid of peritoneum. The posterior peritoneal reflection is usually 12 to 15 cm from the anal verge.

The extraperitoneal rectum is covered with endopelvic fascia. Posteriorly, this is called the *fascia propria* of the rectum. The presacral fascia is a strong endopelvic fascia covering the entire anterior surface of the sacrum and the underlying vessels and nerves. At about the level of S4, the presacral fascia also runs forward and downward and attaches to the rectum. This is referred to as the Waldeyer's fascia or the *rectosacral fascia.* The endopelvic fascia covering the anterior extraperitoneal rectum is called *Denonvilliers' fascia.* The lateral endopelvic fascia

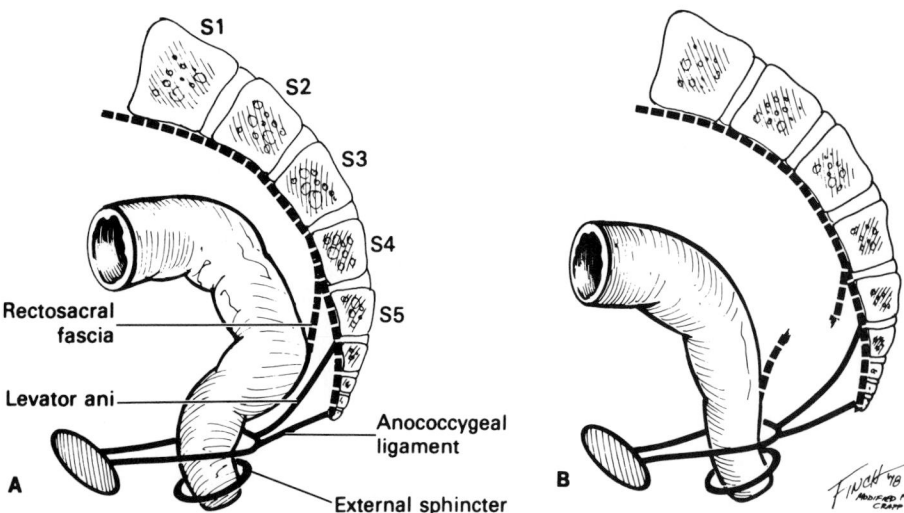

Fig. 28-3. The rectosacral fascia *(A)* and division of the rectosacral fascia for full mobilization of the rectum *(B)*. (From: *Goldberg SM, Gordon PH, Santhat N, 1980,* with permission.)

is thicker and is called the *lateral stalks*. Full mobilization of the rectum requires division of the lateral stalks, Denonvilliers' fascia, and Waldeyer's fascia (Fig. 28-3).

The surgical anal canal, about 4 cm in length, is the terminal portion of the large bowel that passes through the levator ani muscles and opens to the anal verge. It differs from the anatomic anal canal that is measured from the dentate line to the anal verge. The inner muscular wall of the anal canal is the continuation of the circular smooth muscle layer of the rectum that has become thickened and is called the *internal sphincter*. It is innervated by the autonomic nervous system. This is surrounded by

Fig. 28-4. U-shaped anal sphincters.

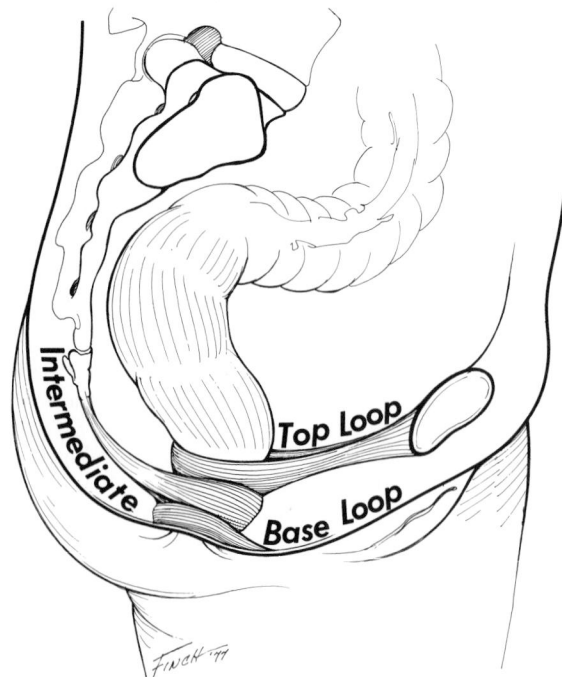

an outer, funnel-shaped tube of skeletal muscle with somatic innervation, arranged in three U-shaped loops. The top loop is the *puborectalis;* it is the deep portion of the external sphincter muscle that arises from the pubis and loops around the upper part of the anal canal with a downward inclination. The intermediate loop is the *superficial external sphincter muscle* that surrounds the anal canal and is attached via the anococcygeal ligament to the coccyx. The base loop is the *subcutaneous* portion of the external sphincter muscle (Fig. 28-4).

The "anorectal ring" is the upper portion of the anal canal where there is a thickening as the puborectalis wraps around it. This can be felt on digital examination in the lateral and posterior quadrants. From the level of the anorectal ring distally and between the internal and external sphincter muscles, the longitudinal muscle coat of the rectum is joined by fibers of the levator ani and puborectalis muscles to form the *conjoined longitudinal muscle*. In its distal part, many muscle fibers cover the lower portion of the external sphincter to insert on the perianal skin, causing wrinkling of the anal verge. These fibers are referred to as the *corrugator cutis ani*.

The anal canal is lined by different kinds of epithelium. At about the midpoint of the anal canal, there is an undulating demarcation called the *dentate* or *pectinate line,* which is about 2 cm from the anal verge. There are 6 to 14 longitudinal folds of the mucosal lining above the dentate line known as *columns of Morgagni*. Between these, at the lower end, there are small crypts through which the ducts of the anal glands empty. For a distance of about 1 cm at the dentate line, the epithelial lining may be columnar, transitional, or stratified squamous epithelium. This is referred to as the *transitional* or *cloacogenic zone*. This is also the area where the internal hemorrhoidal plexus lies. The area above the transitional zone is lined by columnar epithelium while below the dentate line, squamous epithelium is found (Fig. 28-5).

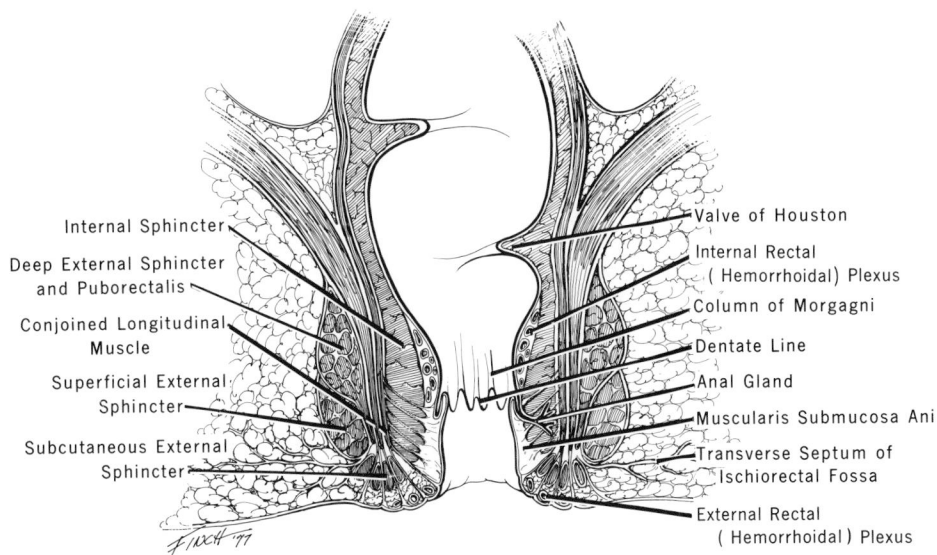

Fig. 28-5. Coronal section of the rectum and anal canal, showing sphincter muscles and the lining of anal canal.

PELVIC FLOOR. The *levator ani muscle* is a broad, thin muscle plate that forms the floor of the pelvic cavity and is innervated by the fourth sacral nerve. This muscle consists of the iliococcygeus and pubococcygeus. It has become evident that the receptors of a fullness sensation in the rectum are in the pelvic floor muscles rather than in the rectal wall itself.

The *iliococcygeus* arises from the ischial spine and posterior part of the obturator fossa, passes downward, backward, and medially, and becomes inserted on the last two segments of the sacrum and the anococcygeal raphe.

The *pubococcygeus* arises from the anterior half of the obturator fossa and back of the pubis. Its fibers are directed backward, downward, and medially, where they decussate with fibers of the opposite side. This line of decussation is called the *anococcygeal raphe* (Fig. 28-6). Some fibers, which lie more posteriorly, are attached directly to the tip of the coccyx and the last segment of the sacrum. This muscle also sends fibers to share in the formation of the conjoined longitudinal muscle.

The muscle fibers of the pubococcygeus, while proceeding backward, downward, and medially, form an elliptical space called the *levator hiatus* (Fig. 28-6) through which pass the lower part of the rectum, prostatic urethra, and dorsal vein of the penis in men or vagina and urethra in women. The intrahiatal viscera are bound together by part of the pelvic fascia that is more condensed at the level of the anorectal junction and has been called the *hiatal ligament* (Fig. 28-7). It is believed that the func-

Fig. 28-6. The levator ani muscle. (From: *Goldberg SM, Gordon PH, Santhat N, 1980, with permission.*)

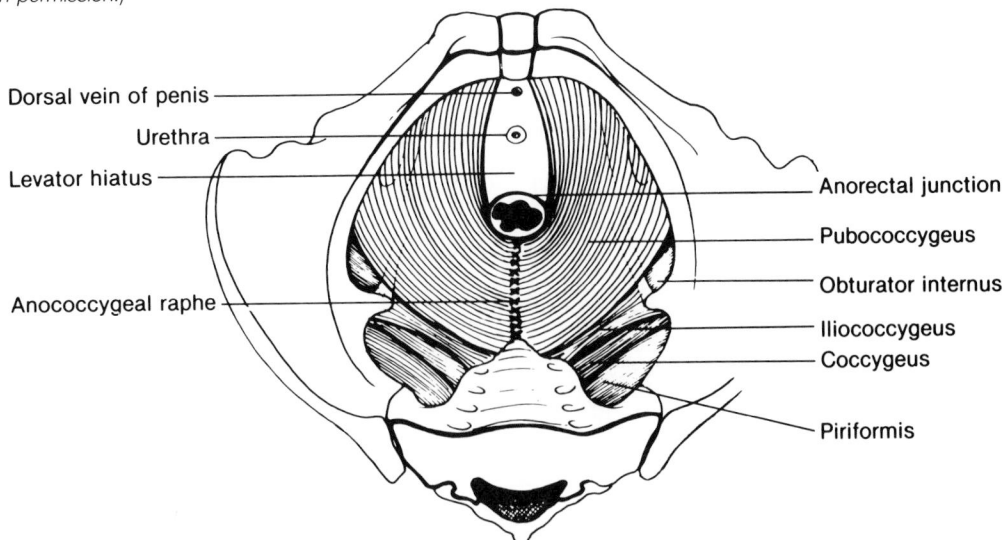

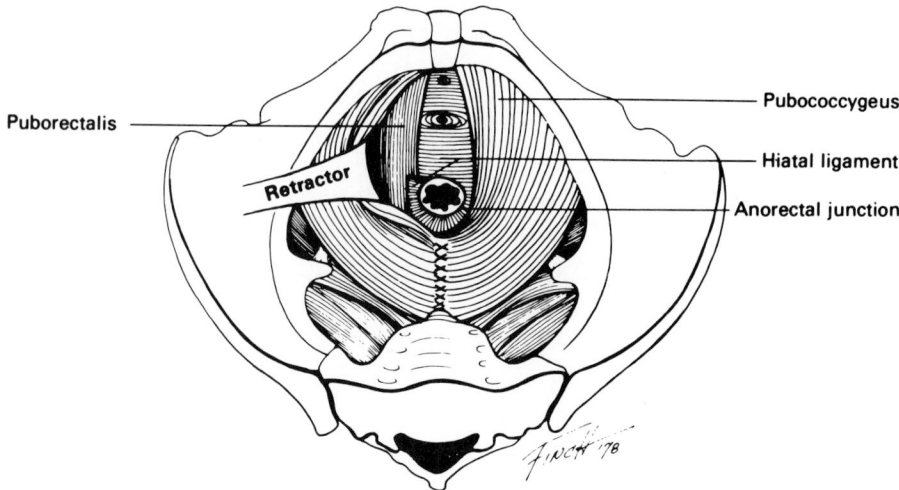

Fig. 28-7. Structures related to the levator ani muscle. (From: *Goldberg SM, Gordon PH, Santhat N, 1980, with permission.*)

tion of this ligament is to keep the movement of the intrahiatal structures in harmony with the levator ani muscle. The crisscross arrangement of the anococcygeal raphe prevents the constrictor effect on the intrahiatal structures during levator ani contraction and causes a dilator effect. The puborectalis and levator ani muscles have a reciprocal action: as one contracts, the other relaxes. During defecation, there is puborectalis relaxation accompanied by levator ani contraction, which widens the hiatus and elevates the lower rectum and anal canal. In an upright position, the levator ani muscle supports the viscera.

ARTERIAL SUPPLY (Fig. 28-8). The superior rectal (hemorrhoidal) artery is the continuation of the inferior

mesenteric artery and descends posteriorly to the rectum, where it bifurcates to supply the rectum and the upper portion of the anal canal.

The middle rectal (hemorrhoidal) arteries arise from the internal iliac artery on each side and enter the lower portion of the rectum anterolaterally at the level of the levator ani muscle; they do not enter the lateral stalks, as previously believed. These arteries anastomose with the branches of the superior rectal artery.

The inferior rectal arteries arise on each side from the internal pudendal artery, a branch of the internal iliac ar-

Fig. 28-8. Arterial supply of the rectum and anal canal.

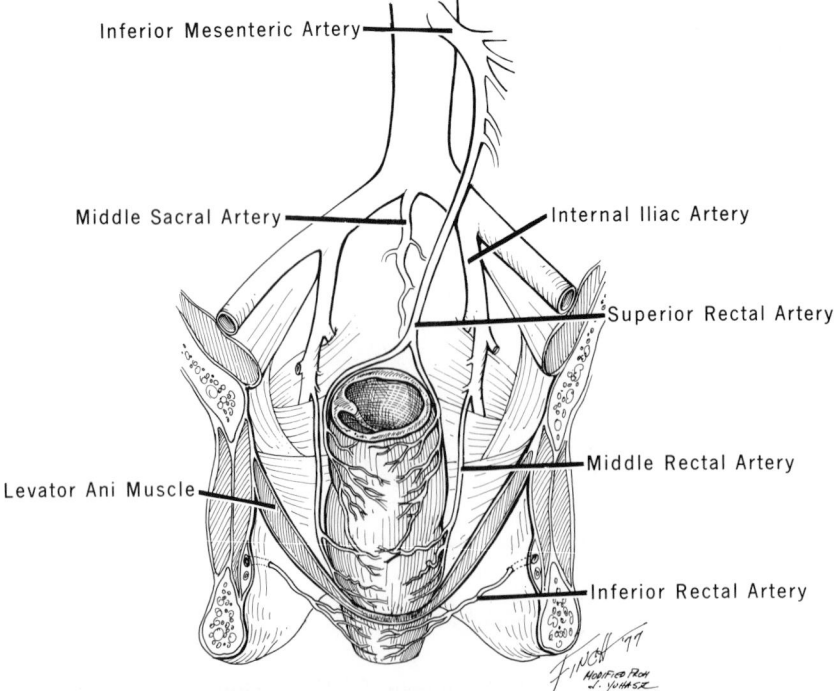

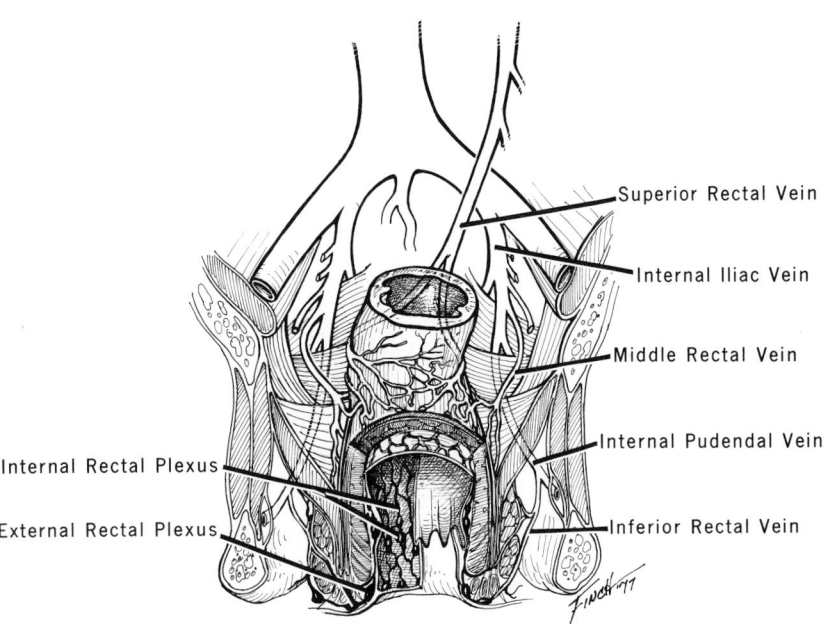

Superior Rectal Vein

Internal Iliac Vein

Middle Rectal Vein

Internal Pudendal Vein

Inferior Rectal Vein

Internal Rectal Plexus

External Rectal Plexus

Fig. 28-9. Venous drainage of the rectum and anal canal.

tery, and traverse the ischiorectal fossa on each side to supply the anal sphincter muscles. There is no evidence of direct anastomosis between the superior and inferior rectal arteries.

The middle sacral artery provides an insignificant amount of the blood supply to the rectum. It arises posteriorly, just above the bifurcation of the aorta, descends over the lumbar vertebrae, sacrum, and coccyx, and gives only small branches to the posterior wall of the lower portion of the rectum.

VENOUS DRAINAGE (Fig. 28-9). Return of blood from the rectum and the anal canal is via two systems: portal and systemic. The superior rectal (hemorrhoidal) veins drain the rectum and upper part of the anal canal into the portal system via the inferior mesenteric vein. The middle rectal veins drain the lower part of the rectum and the upper part of the anal canal. They accompany the middle rectal arteries and terminate in the internal iliac veins. The inferior rectal veins, following the corresponding arteries, drain the lower part of the anal canal via the internal pudendal veins, which empty into the internal iliac veins. Dilatation of the inferior rectal veins leads to external hemorrhoids.

The superior, middle, and inferior rectal veins converge to form the internal rectal (hemorrhoidal) plexus in the submucosa of the columns of Morgagni. Dilatation of this plexus gives rise to internal hemorrhoids.

LYMPHATIC DRAINAGE. Lymph from the upper and middle parts of the rectum ascends along the superior rectal artery and subsequently to the inferior mesenteric lymph nodes. The lower part of the rectum drains cephalad via the superior rectal lymphatics to the inferior mesenteric nodes and laterally via the middle rectal lymphatics to the internal iliac nodes (Fig. 28-10).

Lymphatics from the anal canal above the dentate line drain cephalad via the superior rectal lymphatics to the inferior mesenteric nodes and laterally along both the middle rectal vessels and inferior rectal vessels through the ischiorectal fossa to the internal iliac nodes. Lymph from the anal canal below the dentate line usually drains to the inguinal nodes. It can also drain to the superior rectal lymph nodes or along the inferior rectal lymphatics to the ischiorectal fossa, if obstruction occurs in the primary drainage (Fig. 28-11).

Studies of the lymphatic drainage of the anorectum in women have shown that when dye is injected 5 cm above the anal verge, spread of dye occurs to the posterior vaginal wall, uterus, cervix, broad ligament, fallopian tubes, ovaries, and cul-de-sac. When dye is injected at 10 cm above the anal verge, the spread occurs only to the broad ligament and the cul-de-sac; whereas injection at the 15 cm level shows no spread to the genital organs. It has been generally known that retrograde lymphatic spread in carcinoma of the rectum and anal canal occurs only after there has been extensive involvement of perirectal structures, serosal surfaces, veins, perineural lymphatic and proximal lymphatic channels. This information is obviously helpful in planning a curative operation for a patient with a malignant tumor of the rectal or anal canal.

NERVE SUPPLY OF THE RECTUM AND UROGENITAL ORGANS. Sympathetic and parasympathetic nerves of the autonomic nervous system not only supply the anorectum but also send branches to the adjacent urogenital organs. These nerves are very close to the rectum and are prone to injury during mobilization of the rectum. Sexual dysfunction, especially in males, and, to a lesser degree, urinary dysfunction, can easily occur unless specific precautions are taken.

Sympathetic nerve fibers to the rectum are derived from the first three lumbar segments of the spinal cord. They pass through the ganglionated sympathetic chains and leave as a lumbar sympathetic nerve that joins the

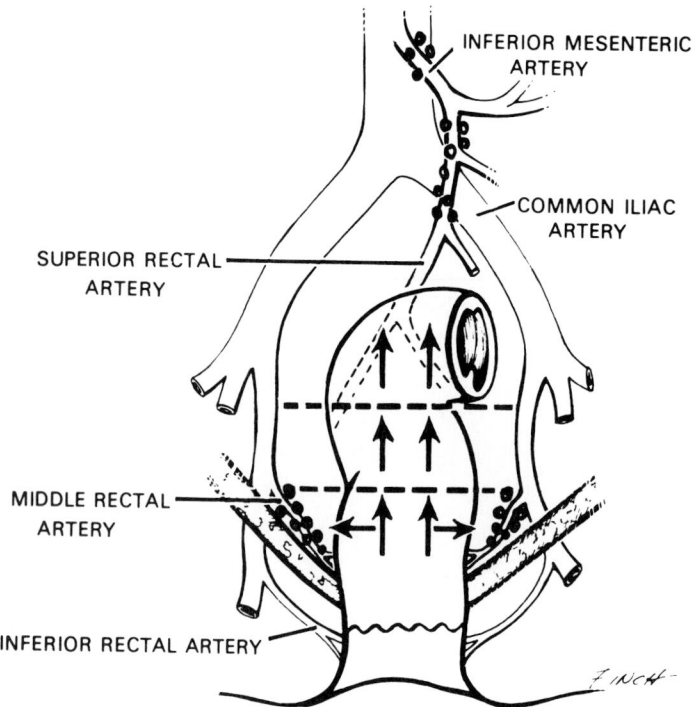

Fig. 28-10. Lymphatic drainage of the rectum. (From: *Goldberg SM, Gordon PH, Santhat N, 1980, with permission.*)

preaortic plexus. The preaortic fibers extend below the bifurcation of the aorta to form the superior *hypogastric plexus,* or presacral nerve (Fig. 28-12). The plexus thus formed divides into left and right branches on each side of the pelvis where they join the branches of the parasympathetic nerve fibers to create the pelvic plexuses.

The sacral parasympathetic nerves or *nervi erigentes* originate from the second, third, and fourth sacral nerves.

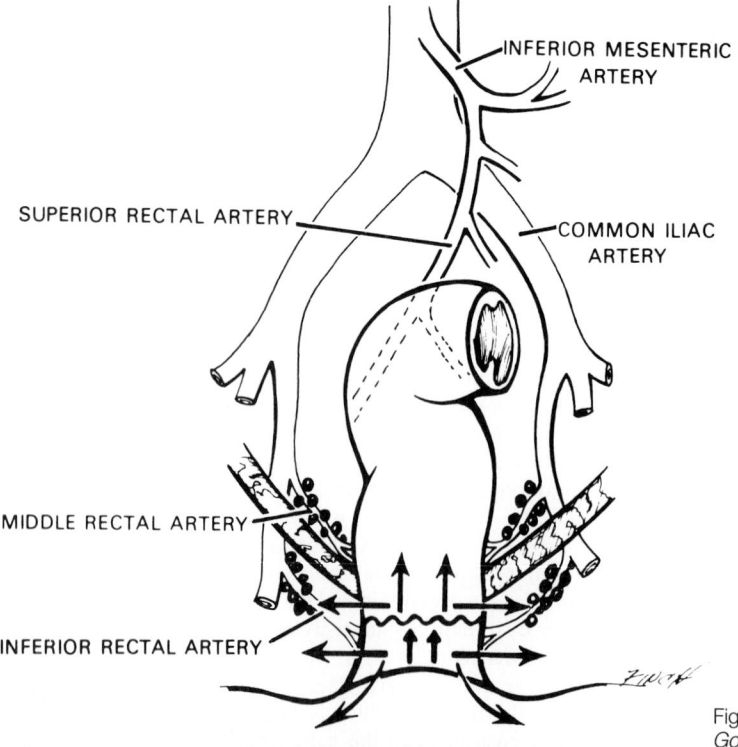

Fig. 28-11. Lymphatic drainage of the anal canal. (From: *Goldberg SM, Gordon PH, Santhat N, 1980, with permission.*)

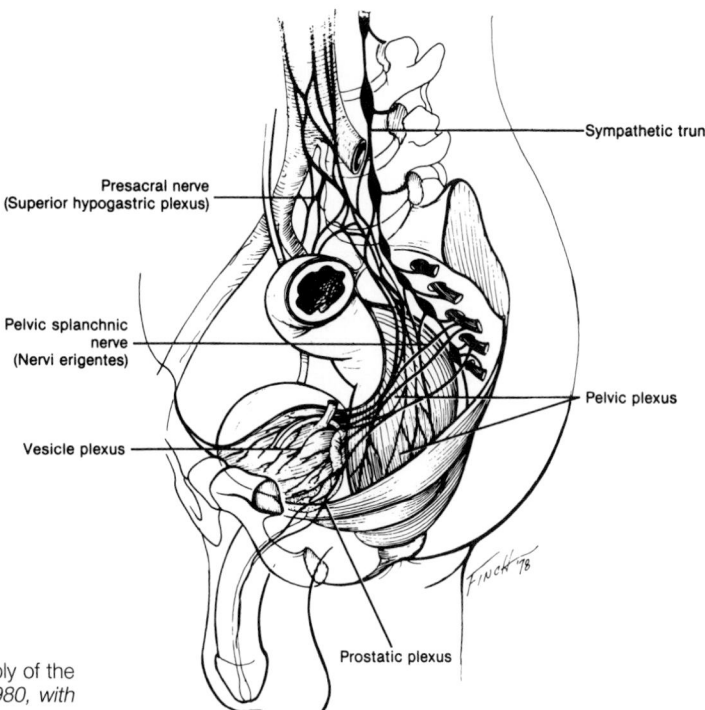

Fig. 28-12. Sympathetic and parasympathetic nerve supply of the rectum. (From: *Goldberg SM, Gordon PH, Santhat N, 1980, with permission.*)

The fibers pass inward and forward to join the sympathetic nerve fibers to form the *pelvic plexuses* (Fig. 28-12). From here the two types of nerve fibers are distributed to the urinary and sexual organs and to the lower rectum and anal canal.

In women, the sympathetic nerve fibers from the hypogastric plexus pass toward the uterosacral ligament close to the rectum. In men, the nerve fibers from the hypogastric plexus pass immediately adjacent to the anterolateral wall of the rectum in the retroperitoneal tissue.

The pelvic plexuses give rise to the periprostatic plexus, an important subdivision that is essential to sexual function in men. The periprostatic plexus distributes fibers to the prostate, seminal vesicles, corpora cavernosum, terminal part of the vas deferens, prostatic and membranous urethra, ejaculatory ducts, and the bulbourethral glands.

Both parasympathetic and sympathetic nervous systems are involved in erection. The nerve impulses from the parasympathetic nerves that lead to erection produce arteriolar vasodilation and they increase blood in the cavernous spaces of the penis. Activity of the sympathetic system inhibits vasoconstriction of the penile vessels, thereby adding to vascular engorgement and sustained erection. Sympathetic activity also causes contraction of the ejaculatory ducts, seminal vesicles, and prostate with subsequent expulsion of semen into the posterior urethra. Depending on which nerves have been damaged, certain deficiencies may occur, including incomplete erection, lack of ejaculation, retrograde ejaculation, or total impotence.

Prevention of Injury. Unlike the technique of proctectomy for cancer, the dissection of the rectum for be-

nign diseases such as inflammatory bowel diseases and familial polyposis coli should be done close to the rectal wall. Precautions can be exercised to avoid nerve injuries: (1) Stay close to the bowel wall posteriorly when mobilizing the rectosigmoid and to avoid injury of the hypogastric plexus do not disturb the retroperitoneal tissue. (2) Cut the peritoneum on each side close to the rectum and brush off the retroperitoneal tissue laterally to avoid injury to the left and right branches of the hypogastric plexus. (3) Divide the lateral stalks close to the rectum to avoid injury to the nervi erigentes and the pelvic plexus. (4) Stay in the proper plane when separating the anterior wall of the rectum from the Denonvillier's fascia in order to avoid injury to the seminal vesicles and prostate.

The *pudendal nerve* arises from the sacral plexus (S2, 3, 4). It leaves the pelvis through the greater sciatic foramen, crosses the ischial spine, and then continues in the pudendal canal (Alcock's canal) toward the ischial tuberosity in the lateral wall of the ischiorectal fossa on each side. Three of its important branches are the *inferior rectal, perineal,* and *dorsal nerve of penis* or *clitoris*. The pudendal nerve is anatomically protected from injury during mobilization of the rectum. Sensory stimuli from the penis and clitoris are mediated by the pudendal nerve and are preserved after proctectomy.

NERVE SUPPLY OF THE ANAL CANAL. Motor Innervation. The internal sphincter is supplied by both sumpathetics and parasympathetics, which presumably reach the muscle by the same route as that followed to the lower rectum. Contrary to the previously held belief that sympathetic nerve is stimulant and parasympathetic nerve inhibitory to the internal sphincter, it has been found that both the sympathetic and parasympathetic nerves are inhibitory to the anal sphincter. The external sphincter and puborectalis are supplied by the inferior rectal branch of the internal pudendal and the perineal branch of the fourth sacral nerve. The levator ani is supplied not only by the pudendal but also by the direct branch of the third, fourth, and frequently fifth sacral nerves which lies above the pelvic floor.

Sensory Innervation. The sensory nerve supply of the anal canal is the inferior rectal nerve, a branch of the pudendal nerve. The epithelium of the anal canal is profusely innervated with sensory nerve endings, especially in the vicinity of the dentate line. Pain sensation in the anal canal can be felt up to 1.5 cm proximal to the dentate line.

PHYSIOLOGY

Colon

The colon is much more than a storage organ. In health, the colon absorbs water, sodium and chloride, short-chain fatty acids, and nitrogen substances, while secreting potassium and bicarbonate. The colon can respond to body requirements and has an important role in fluid and electrolyte balance.

ABSORPTION AND SECRETION. In a normal person, each day about 1500 to 2000 mL of fluid from the gastrointestinal tract enters the large bowel, but only 100 to 200 mL of water is contained in the feces. Thus, over 90 percent of the water is absorbed in the large bowel. The rectum has little or no ability to absorb water or electrolytes. It is estimated that the human colon is capable of absorbing at least 2500 mL of water each day and as much as 5700 mL by using slow perfusion technique. The capacity is reduced if the fluid enters the cecum rapidly. Unlike the gallbladder, the small intestine, and the renal proximal tubules which all absorb isotonic fluid, the colon appears capable of absorbing hypertonic solution. The main forces influencing water movement across the colon seem to be osmotic gradients and sodium transport. Water can be absorbed against a lumen-to-blood osmotic gradient of 50 mO/kg. Net movement of water into the colon increases when the osmotic gradient between the lumen and blood rises.

Sodium. Sodium is absorbed against an electrochemical potential by an active transport system. Its absorption is related to the lumenal concentration of sodium. No sodium absorption occurs when the lumenal concentration is below 25 meq/L. In contrast to the small bowel, sodium and water absorption in the colon are not enhanced by addition of glucose, and the glucose is not absorbed from the colon. The colon is the main source of sodium absorption and has the capacity to absorb up to 400 meq/day if there is a slow and constant rate of perfusion. A patient without a colon, such as one with an ileostomy, cannot tolerate a low sodium intake.

Chloride and Bicarbonate. Chloride is actively absorbed against concentration gradients, and this capacity for absorption is greater than that of sodium. While chloride is absorbed, bicarbonate is secreted, and the presence of chloride in the lumen facilitates secretions of bicarbonate. There is an ion exchange between chloride and bicarbonate. Chloride and bicarbonate exchange can account for only about one-fourth of the chloride that is absorbed during perfusion of physiologic solution. There is a large fraction of chloride absorption that is independent of an ion exchange. Hyperchloremia in patients with a ureterocolic anastomosis results from absorption of urinary chloride by the colon.

Potassium. In contrast, potassium transport is related to the concentration of potassium in the large bowel lumen. Potassium is absorbed by passive diffusion. The normal colon has a capacity to secrete about 32 meq/L of potassium a day. In diseased states, abnormal permeability of an active potassium secretion might play a role in losing a large amount of potassium through the colon.

Short-Chain Fatty Acids (SCFA). Short-chain fatty acids are produced from dietary carbohydrates and dietary fibers by anaerobic bacterial fermentation. When lumenal formation of SCFA exceeds its absorption, diarrhea results. The transport process is accompanied by increased sodium, potassium, and water absorption, by lumenal alkalinization due to secretion of bicarbonate and by a fall in lumenal PCO_2.

Ammonia and Urea. The colon is an important site for the production and absorption of ammonia. The most important source of ammonia in the colon is urea. At least one-fourth of urea synthesized by the liver is continuously hydrolyzed by intestinal bacteria. Only a small amount of urea enters the colon from the ileum, and very little urea and ammonia are found in the feces. Most of the urea metabolized in the colon is secreted into the colon, and the product of its metabolism (ammonia) is almost completely absorbed. A smaller source of ammonia in the colon is derived from nitrogen in diet, desquamated epithelial and bacterial debris. The absorbed ammonia is delivered to the liver through the portal circulation, where it enters the ornithine-citrulline-arginine cycle to form urea, which is excreted by the kidney. The rate of ammonia absorption is dependent on the pH of the colonic lumen. As the lumenal pH falls, the rate of absorption decreases. This provides the rationale for giving lactulose in patients with portal-systemic encephalopathy. Lactulose is metabolized by bacteria into lactic and acidic acids that lower the pH of the colon and retard the absorption of ammonia. Another possible explanation is that lactulose may stimulate the incorporation of ammonia into bacterial protein.

MOTILITY. Two motility patterns are observed in the colon. Agitating or segmenting contractions knead and mix the fecal mass primarily in the right and transverse colon. These movements appear to aid water absorption. A second type of contraction, "mass movement," propels the colonic contents distad. These contraction waves are not true peristalsis, since there is a simultaneous constriction of long segments of colon. The mass movements empty the contents of the right colon into the sigmoid and upper rectum.

Colonic motility may be altered by a number of stimuli. Morphine and codeine markedly increase muscle tone of the large bowel and reduce propulsive action. Anticholinergics and glucagon are potent inhibitors of colonic motility, while parasympathomimetic drugs such as neostigmine increase colonic motor activity.

LARGE BOWEL GAS. The sources of intestinal gases are swallowed air, diffusion from the blood into the lumen, liberation of carbon dioxide from reaction of hydrogen and bicarbonate, and production of gas within the lumen from bacterial metabolism and fermentation. Normally the gastrointestinal tract contains 100 to 200 mL of gas at a given time. But between 400 and 1200 mL of gas is normally expelled per day as flatus, depending on amount and type of food ingested. Flatus is composed mainly of carbon dioxide, hydrogen, methane, nitrogen, and a small amount of oxygen. Flatus carbon dioxide and hydrogen are derived almost entirely in the colon. Methane (CH_4) is produced only in the colon. Approximately two-thirds of adults do not harbor methane-producing bacteria, while one-third do. The tendency to produce large quantities of methane appears to be familial.

Hydrogen and methane are the two potentially explosive gases in the gastrointestinal tract. The explosive concentration of H_2 ranges from 4 to 74% and of CH_4 from 5 to 15%. Human flatus may contain concentrations as high as 44% for H_2 and 30% for CH_4. Explosion can occur during polypectomy or electrocoagulation of a large bowel polyp. Bowel preparation with laxatives, enemas, polyethylene glycol solutions, clear liquids and overnight fasting has been shown to decrease H_2 and CH_4 to negligible levels. This makes it safe to use electrocoagulation without CO_2 insufflation. Bowel preparation with mannitol, an unabsorbable carbohydrate, must be avoided if electrocautery is to be used. In a situation when a thorough large bowel preparation cleansing is not achieved, the risk of explosion can be minimized by a thorough exchange of the intraluminal gas with suction and insufflation of air, or by a continuous infusion of the bowel lumen with an inert gas such as CO_2.

Rectum and Anal Canal

DEFECATION. Defecation is an act of evacuating fecal material from the rectum. It is a complex process that involves both a reflex response and a voluntary performance.

When a fecal bolus enters the rectum, the receptors, believed to be outside the rectal wall and most likely in the pelvic floor, will register a sensation and a feeling of an urge to defecate. Distention of the rectum causes a reflex relaxation of the internal sphincter that allows the content to make contact with the anal canal while the external sphincter and puborectalis contract. This "sampling response" allows the sensory epithelium of the anal canal to sense and discriminate the content. If the rectal distention is maintained for a long period of time, the rectal musculature adapts to decrease the rectal pressure. This is known as *accommodation response*. Urgent defecation arises if the stimulus from the rectum increases

rapidly to overcome the accommodation response, as when a large amount of liquid stool enters the rectum. The act of defecation proceeds with the subject assuming the squatting or sitting position and with the relaxation of the puborectalis to flatten out the angle between the rectum and the anal canal. Expulsion of the feces is accomplished by contracting the rectum and increasing intraabdominal pressure by the Valsalva maneuver. Although any rise in abdominal pressure causes an immediate increase in the reflex tone of the pelvic floor muscle, defecation straining abolishes the reflex tone of the pelvic floor muscle and the anal sphincter muscles. After defecation is completed, the voluntary sphincters contract actively and the normal postural tone is restored.

CONTINENCE. Normal anorectal continence is controlled by the interaction of the visceral internal anal sphincter and the somatic external anal sphincter and puborectalis. The internal and external sphincters are both tonically active at rest and surround the anal canal. The internal anal sphincter provides most of the resting sphincter tone. Injury or degeneration is associated with minor impairment of continence exhibited by soiling and by incontinence of liquid stool. The external anal sphincter contributes about 20 percent of the high pressure zone at rest and is responsible for the squeeze contraction. Degeneration or injury may be associated with varying degrees of incontinence. It is sometimes possible to divide the whole of the internal and external sphincters and retain normal continence as long as the puborectalis sling is intact. Children, following operations for congenital anorectal anomalies in which the anal canal is only surrounded by the puborectalis, suffer no loss of gross continence. It is generally agreed that the puborectalis is the most important muscle of continence and responsible for maintaining the normal anorectal rectal angle of approximately 90 to 100°. A flutter valve theory of continence in which the lower rectum is occluded by raised intraabdominal pressure acting on an area of rectum above the pelvic floor has been suggested. Continence is further augmented by the surface tension adherence of the anteroposterior slitlike aperture of the anal canal.

CLINICAL EVALUATION

A careful and complete history and physical examination is the starting point for evaluation of any patient with suspected disease of the colon or rectum. Visual examination of the anus and a careful digital rectal examination are essential parts of any complete physical examination.

OCCULT BLOOD. *Hemoccult* is a commercial guaiac-impregnated filter paper used to detect blood in the stool. It does so with good sensitivity, although specificity is not high. The test can be done by the individual at home by smearing some stool on the paper slides provided. These are then sent back to the physician for determination of blood. Basically, the test is to detect peroxidase in the hemoglobin molecule, which will turn a blue color in the filter paper with a reagent. The Hemoccult test is not specific since many foods also contain peroxidase, e.g. raw meat, pheasant, salmon, sardines, turnip, radish, cherry, tomato, and many other fruits and vegetables. These may give a false-positive test. Vitamin C is known to give false-positive tests. During the test, all these substances must be avoided. A restricted diet is recommended for two or three days before the test and should be continued during the test. In addition, roughage should be obtained by taking bran or psyllium seed. The stool is smeared on the filter paper slides; two slides each day from three consecutive stools are examined. A complete colon and rectal examination is indicated if any of the slides is positive. The tests can easily be done once a year in persons fifty years or older. Although the results may be negative in the presence of polyps or carcinoma, a controlled study using Hemoccult testing conducted at the University of Minnesota led to a diagnosis of colorectal carcinoma in 4 percent and polyps in 20 percent of the positive slides. The detected cancers by Hemoccult had favorable staging: Dukes' A, 57 percent; Dukes' B, 21 percent; Dukes' C, 19 percent; and Dukes' D, 3 percent. Whether this is translatable into a better long-term survival remains to be seen.

The newer HemoQuant, a qualitative assay of fecal blood based on the fluorescence of heme-derived porphyrin, is more sensitive and specific than the Hemoccult and may be more useful.

LABORATORY TESTS. Laboratory tests that should be performed in a patient with known or suspected disease of the colon will be determined by the specifics of the case. In a patient who is being prepared for major colonic surgery, some information about the hematologic, cardiac, respiratory, and renal status should be part of the general information obtained preoperatively. For the patient with severe diarrhea, or marked obstruction, knowledge of the electrolyte status is important. In the patient who has metastatic disease, knowledge of the functional capacity of the organ with metastases may be desirable. Liver function tests may be helpful, but it is recognized that there can be extensive malignant involvement of the liver with little or no alteration in any of the commonly available biochemical tests of liver function. An elevated alkaline phosphatase level is a suggestive sign of liver metastases. The carcinoembryonic antigen (CEA) was originally proposed as a screening test for occult colon cancer, but the lack of specificity and sensitivity of the examination has led to a reappraisal of its use for this purpose. It has proved useful for detecting recurrence in patients following resection of colon cancers. A repeatedly rising CEA level may be an indication for a second-look procedure and also may have preoperative predictive value for postoperative recurrence.

ENDOSCOPY. Anoscopy, rigid proctoscopy, and flexible sigmoidoscopy are the most important screening diagnostic studies for patients with colonic or anorectal disease. The standard rigid proctoscope is a 25-cm tube with a light source, a magnifying eyepiece, and provisions for aspiration, biopsy, electrodesiccation, and swabbing of the mucosa. The anoscope is shorter (8 cm) and larger in diameter. It is useful for diagnosis and treatment of lesions at or near the anal verge, such as hemorrhoids and fissures. Flexible sigmoidoscopes utilize fiberoptic light

sources and are available in a variety of lengths up to 60 cm.

Normally, the distal colon is cleansed by administration of two packaged enemas. The examination is conducted with the patient in the prone jackknife, knee-chest, or left lateral position. Careful visual inspection of the anus and digital rectal examination should precede the introduction of the instrument. For rigid proctoscopy, the instrument with the obturator in place is gently inserted into the rectum. The obturator is removed and the proctoscope is then passed under direct vision the maximum comfortable distance. Introduction of the first 15 cm will cause little discomfort, but at this point angulation of the bowel occurs and further insertion of the proctoscope must be done carefully and gently, aided by occasional air insufflation. Often, it is impossible to insert the proctoscope to 25 cm. Lesions seen during insertion of the proctoscope are noted, but careful examination is performed during its withdrawal. The instrument is withdrawn slowly and rotated so that every inch of mucosa is seen. Small lesions may successfully hide on a valve of Houston or in the posterior rectal vault. The location of all abnormalities should be carefully described in anatomic terms.

Polypoid lesions less than 1 cm usually can be removed for pathologic examination. For benign lesions this is also therapeutic. The possibility of synchronous lesions must be excluded, usually by colonoscopy, and at times it may be best to defer polypectomy or biopsy until full colonic evaluation is performed. If one plans an immediate barium enema, rectal polypectomy or biopsy should not be done since perforation at the biopsy site during the barium enema could occur. Diffuse disease, such as radiation colitis, ulcerative colitis, or large lesions, may be identified grossly and by biopsy. If infectious disease, such as amebic colitis, is suspected, mucosal swab for trophozoites and culture may be obtained.

Fiberoptic sigmoidoscopy may be used in place of rigid proctoscopy. This has the advantages of usually being a more comfortable examination while allowing a more complete study of the upper rectum, sigmoid, and sometimes the descending colon. Lesions beyond the reach of the conventional proctoscope can be identified during routine screening examinations.

Colonoscopes are flexible instruments up to 200 cm in length that utilize fiberoptic light sources. Indications for colonoscopy include: (1) abnormalities on barium x-ray (filling defects, segmental colonic narrowing, and polyps), (2) chronic gastrointestinal bleeding, (3) anatomic abnormalities following colonic surgery, (4) chronic inflammatory bowel disease in carefully selected patients, and (5) rectal lesions including polyps to rule out synchronous colonic lesions. Acute inflammatory bowel disease is a relative contraindication to colonoscopy because of the danger of perforation. Intraoperative colonoscopy is sometimes useful. The management of polyps of the colon has changed drastically since the introduction of these fiberoptic instruments. In the hands of an experienced, well-trained colonoscopist, the risk of colonoscopy is minimal, and the accuracy of the procedure is high.

RADIOLOGIC STUDIES. Plain flat and upright films of the abdomen may reveal a closed-loop obstruction of the colon due to a competent ileocecal valve, a volvulus with its tremendous dilatation and characteristic distribution of air, or the presence of free air. Contrast examinations with water-soluble agents may establish the presence of a fistulous tract and its location or the site and extent of colon obstruction. Barium enema remains a valuable examination for identifying colonic disease. Digital examination of the rectum and proctoscopy or flexible sigmoidoscopy should be done first in almost all cases to rule out distal disease. The radiologist should be forewarned if the patient is thought to have obstruction, perforation, or any inflammatory disease of the colon in order to minimize the dangers of perforation. While barium enema is helpful, it is not infallible. Colonoscopy appears more accurate than barium enema in detecting neoplasms. Air contrast barium enema appears more accurate than single column barium enema in detecting neoplasms, especially if sessile or small. Even an expert radiologist will have difficulty on occasion distinguishing between a carcinoma and an area of constriction resulting from diverticulitis.

Selective angiography has been useful in locating sites of bleeding within the colon and in identifying vascular lesions of the bowel. The technique requires selective catheterization of the superior or inferior mesenteric arteries. In some cases, infusion of vasopressin or epinephrine has stopped bleeding in patients who might otherwise have required emergency operation for massive colonic hemorrhage. Radioisotope scanning, ultrasound, computed tomography, or nuclear magnetic resonance imaging may provide additional information regarding metastatic involvement of the liver or extent of pelvic recurrence.

Interest in the preoperative staging of rectal cancer has

Fig. 28-13. Granular appearance of mucosa in chronic ulcerative colitis. (From: *Nivatvongs S, Becker ER, 1987, with permission.*)

been rekindled because of alternative forms of therapy that are less morbid than radical operations but are of value only in certain circumstances. Computed tomography scanning and more recently endoluminal ultrasound have provided more objective, reproducible staging. The high resolution of the images may allow accurate assessment of the depth of tumor invasion in the rectal wall. The advantage of this degree of accuracy in staging may have important implications for the management of rectal cancer, enabling the more precise planning of surgical treatment and, in particular, defining those patients suitable for local excision and restorative surgery. The key issue in these patients is whether the tumor is confined to the rectal wall or whether it has extended into the perirectal fat. It may also play an important role in trials of preoperative and postoperative radiotherapy.

INFLAMMATORY BOWEL DISEASE

Ulcerative Colitis

Ulcerative colitis is a nonspecific inflammatory bowel disease of the large bowel that affects both sexes and occurs at all ages, with maximum onset between the second and fourth decades. The cause is unknown, and no epidemiologic data to date suggest that a transmissible causative agent is responsible.

PATHOLOGY. Gross Appearance. The bowel is foreshortened in long-standing cases, but the bowel wall on the outside is not thickened or inflamed. The appearance of the mucosa varies according to severity of the disease. The inflammation in ulcerative colitis is confined to the mucosa and submucosa. Typically, the mucosa is granular, swollen, and friable (Fig. 28-13). In severe cases, there are patchy full-thickness ulcerations of the mucosa. In long-standing ulcerative colitis, most of the mucosa

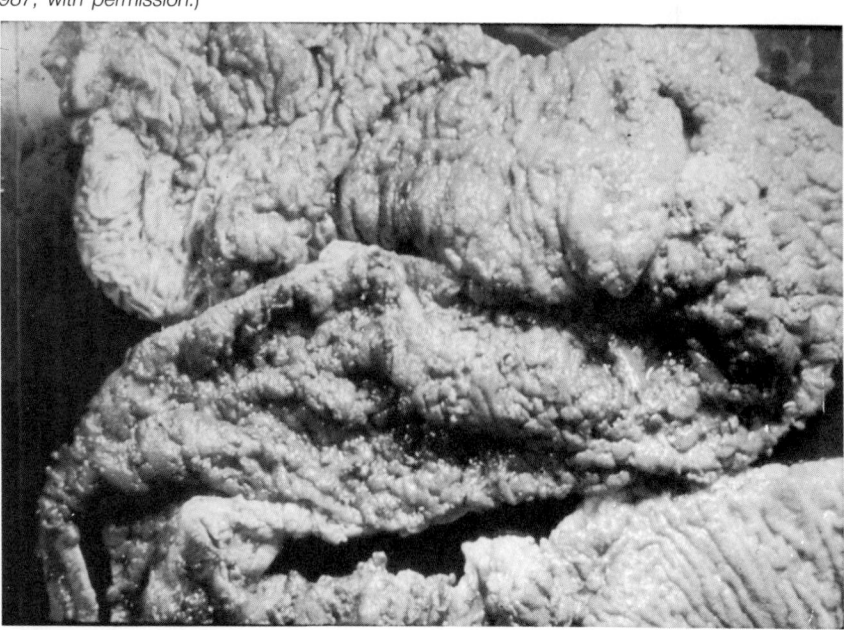

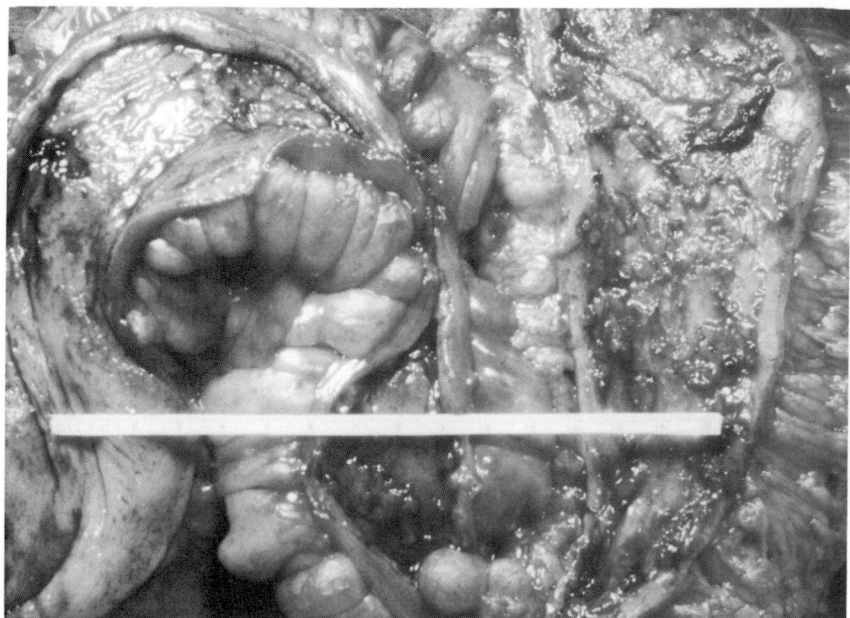

Fig. 28-14. "Burned out" mucosa in long-standing ulcerative colitis. (From: *Nivatvongs S, Becker ER, 1987, with permission.*)

may be lost or "burned out" (Fig. 28-14). The mucosa sometimes shows multiple pseudopolyps. These inflammatory polyps result from regeneration of inflamed mucosa accompanying previous ulcerations.

Microscopy. There are infiltrations of acute and chronic inflammatory cells in the mucosa and submucosa (Fig. 28-15). The muscularis propria and the serosa are normal. The mucosa is atrophic, with a decrease in goblet cells. Multiple crypt abscesses may be present, but this is not pathognomonic for ulcertive colitis since it may also be

Fig. 28-15. Infiltrations of acute and chronic inflammatory cells in the mucosa and submucosa. (From: *Nivatvongs S, Becker ER, 1987, with permission.*)

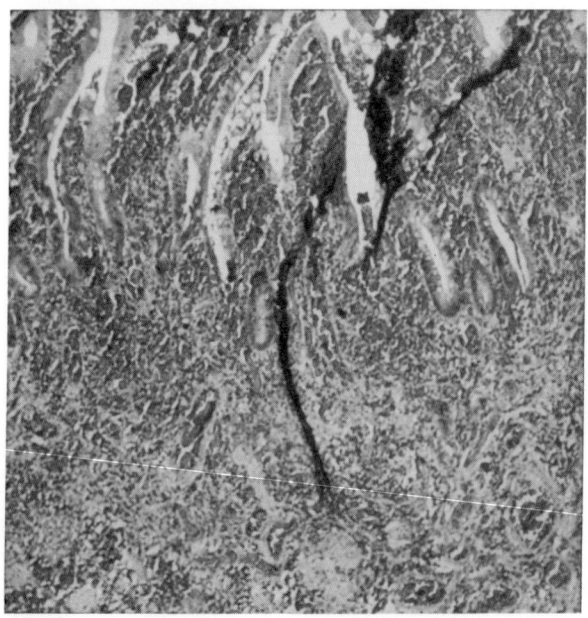

present in Crohn's colitis. In quiescent ulcerative colitis, the acute inflammatory cells are absent. Mucosal atrophy with distortion of crypts and thinning of the distance between the muscularis mucosa and the surface of the epithelium are evident.

CLINICAL MANIFESTATIONS. Ulcerative colitis is a dynamic disease characterized by remissions and exacerbations. The clinical spectrum ranges from an inactive or quiescent phase to low-grade active disease and to fulminant disease. The rectum is invariably involved. The disease may involve just the rectum (proctitis) or the rectum and sigmoid (proctosigmoiditis) or the rectum and left colon (left-sided colitis) or the entire colon and rectum (pancolitis). Ulcerative colitis does not involve the small bowel, but frequently the distal few inches of the terminal ileum are inflamed. This is called "backwash ileitis," a reversible process. It must not be confused with ileocolitis on Crohn's disease.

The onset of ulcerative colitis can be insidious, with minimal bloody stools and/or diarrhea, or the onset can be abrupt, with explosive severe diarrhea with bleeding, tenesmus, crampy abdominal pain, and fever.

The basic symptoms of ulcerative colitis are bleeding per rectum and diarrhea. The severity of diffuse oozing of blood from the diseased mucosa is directly related to the stage, extent, and intensity of the inflammatory process. Massive hemorrhage is infrequent, occuring in about 2 to 3 percent of patients. Diarrhea may be as often as once every 1 to 2 h. Nocturnal diarrhea is a reliable sign of an organic problem. The stool is usually a small amount, often only blood and mucus.

The physical findings are nonspecific and depend on the severity of the disease. Abdominal pain and tenderness may be present. Abdominal distention in association with toxic signs of fever, tachycardia, and an elevated white blood count is an ominous sign of toxic megacolon.

Endoscopy. Diagnosis of ulcerative colitis must be made by endoscopy. Since the rectum is almost invariably involved, proctoscopy may be adequate to establish the diagnosis. A complete evaluation with total colonoscopy or barium enema is contraindicated during an acute attack because of the risk of perforation. The mucosa in ulcerative colitis ranges from granular with minimal edema and friability in the mild stage, to frank ulceration with marked edema and bleeding from the mucosa in the acute stage. The most sensitive sign is loss of the normal vascular pattern as a result of mucosal edema; with more severe inflammation, mucosal erythema, contact bleeding, ulceration, and pus or mucus in the lumen are seen. Fine granularity indicates acute inflammation, while coarse granularity is a manifestation of chronic disease in which previous repair and mucosal regeneration have occurred. Biopsy of the mucosa is unnecessary in the acute stage. The report is usually a nonspecific inflammation and is not worth the risk of possible complication.

After the patient has recovered from an acute attack, a total colonoscopy should be performed to determine the extent of the disease. Multiple random biopsies of the mucosa can be done to check for mucosal dysplasia, particularly when the disease has been present for longer than 10 years. Photographs can be obtained to serve as a base line for future reference.

Radiologic Findings. Barium enema examination can be performed to establish the diagnosis of ulcerative colitis, to determine the extent of the disease, and to serve as a base-line study for follow-up of the progress of the disease. Barium enema, however, is less sensitive in detecting early disease. In long-standing ulcerative colitis, the colon is foreshortened and has lost normal haustration (Fig. 28-16). Tiny ulcers are seen as fine marginal irregularities (Fig. 28-17). Deep ulcers are seen as "collar buttons" (Fig. 28-18) or as a linear collection of barium parallel to the bowel lumen (Fig. 28-19). Benign stricture of the colon in long-standing ulcerative colitis is uncommon and is usually from spasm or hypertrophy of the muscularis mucosa. Stricture in ulcerative colitis must be presumed to be malignant until proved otherwise.

DIFFERENTIAL DIAGNOSIS. Continuous disease starting in the upper anal canal and spreading proximally suggests ulcerative colitis, whereas patchy disease with intervening areas of normal mucosa is more likely to be found in Crohn's disease. A small bowel gastrointestinal study may be helpful in patients with suspected Crohn's disease. Besides Crohn's colitis, many infectious diarrheal diseases have signs and symptoms similar to ulcerative colitis. Infective colitis caused by *Campylobacter* or *Entamoeba histolytica* may be indistinguishable from ulcerative colitis. Stool culture for enteric pathogens should be done in all cases of ulcerative colitis, particularly shigella, salmonella, campylobacter, and *Clostridium difficile.* Fresh stool should be examined for ova and parasites, particularly to exclude amebic colitis. Gonoccoccal proctitis is characterized by the presence of a purulent exudate adherent to the mucosa with little mucosal erythema

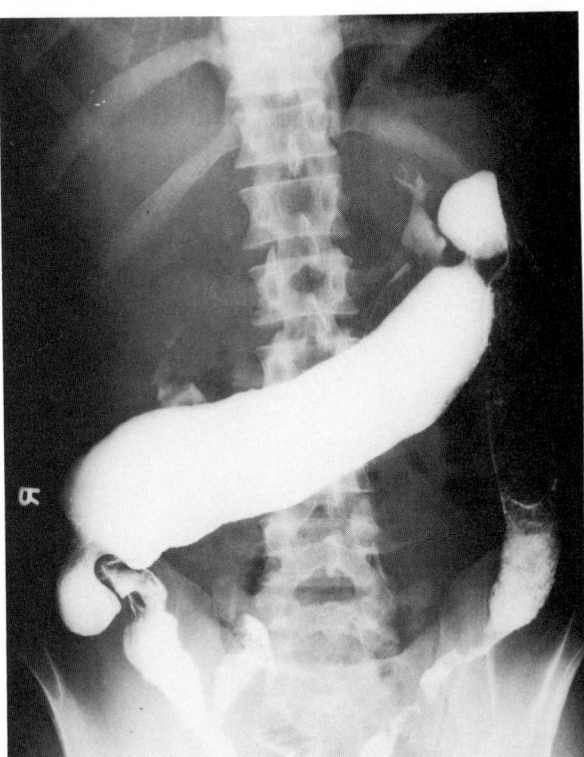

Fig. 28-16. Foreshortened colon from long-standing ulcerative colitis. Note stricture of sigmoid colon due to carcinoma. (From: *Nivatvongs S, Becker ER, 1987, with permission.*)

or bleeding. Inflammation rarely extends beyond the lower rectum. In suspected gonococcal proctitis, rectal, urethral and high vaginal cultures should be taken.

EXTRAINTESTINAL MANIFESTATIONS OF INFLAMMATORY BOWEL DISEASE. Fatty infiltration of the liver is present in up to 40 to 50 percent and cirrhosis is found in 2 to 5 percent of patients with inflammatory bowel disease. Control of the primary disease medically or surgically will reverse or improve the fatty infiltration of the liver, but once cirrhosis has developed, it is irreversible.

Primary sclerosing cholangitis is a progressive disease causing obstruction and jaundice. It is best diagnosed by endoscopic retrograde cholangiopancreatogram, which will show characteristic beadlike extra- and intrahepatic bile ducts. The condition is not reversible.

Pericholangitis frequently occurs in association with inflammatory bowel disease. It may not be clinically apparent, but liver function tests can reveal an elevated AST or SGOT. The diagnosis is confirmed by liver biopsy that shows intensive infiltration of the portal triads.

Bile duct carcinoma is a rare complication of long-standing inflammatory bowel disease. Patients who develop bile duct carcinoma secondary to inflammatory bowel disease are on average 20 or more years younger than other patients with bile duct carcinoma.

The incidence of arthritis in inflammatory bowel disease is 20 times greater than in the general population. The knees, ankles, and wrists are most commonly af-

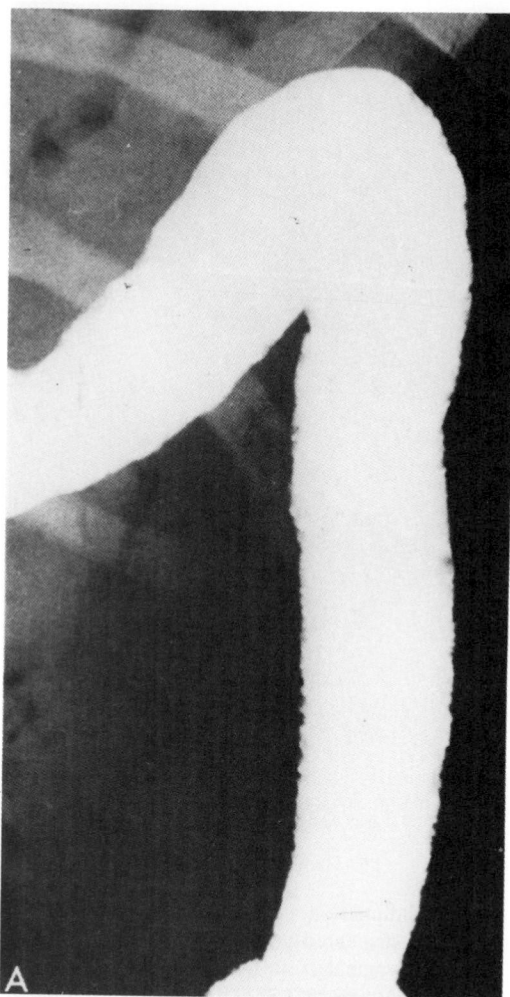

Fig. 28-17. Tiny ulcers are seen as fine marginal irregularities. [From: *Stein GN, Sabri PJ: Roentgen features, in JE Berk (ed): Bockus Gastroenterology, 4th ed. Philadelphia, Saunders, 1985, Fig 126-23, p 2169, with permission.*]

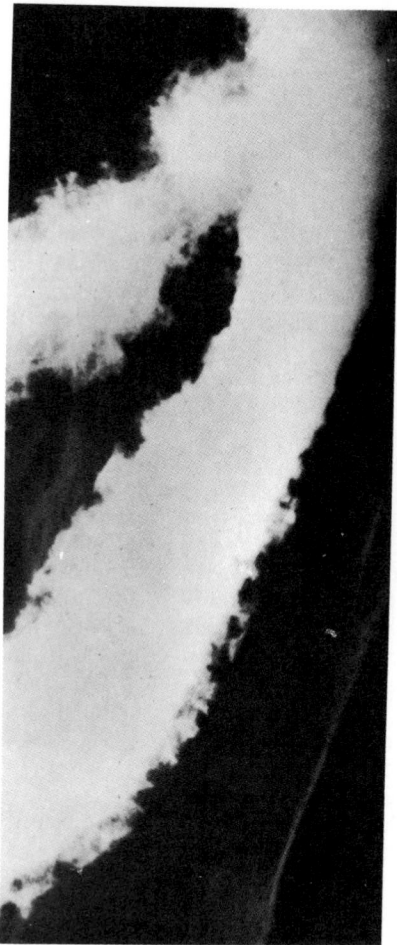

Fig. 28-18. Deep ulcers are seen as "collar buttons." [From: *Stein GN, Sabri PJ: Roentgen features, in JE Berk (ed): Bockus Gastroenterology, 4th ed. Philadelphia, Saunders, 1985, Fig 126-25, p 2170, with permission.*]

fected, but any joint may be involved. Arthritis from inflammatory bowel disease can be differentiated from rheumatoid arthritis in that there are no subcutaneous nodules, tendinitis, or residual deformities. The arthritis usually improves when the bowel disease improves.

The relationship between sacroiliitis and ankylosing spondylitis to inflammatory bowel disease is not well understood, since these conditions also occur in other types of intestinal disease, including Whipple's disease and other acute enteric bacterial infections. Spondylitis may be detected before the intestinal disease is recognized. There is little or no correlation between the spondylitis and the extent, duration, or severity of the colitis. Symptomatic relief is all that can be offered to the patient. Medical or surgical treatment directed at the underlying colitis has little or no effect on the sacroiliitis and spondylitis.

Erythema nodosum is seen in 5 to 15 percent of patients and usually coincides with clinical disease activity but

may precede an acute exacerbation. Females are affected three to four times more frequently than males. The characteristic lesions are raised, red, and predominantly on the lower legs. Some of the lesions ulcerate but they do not become chronic. Erythema nodosum is thought to be due to hypersensitivity, but specific antigens have not been identified.

Pyoderma gangrenosum is an uncommon but serious condition that occurs almost exclusively in patients with inflammatory bowel disease. The lesion begins as an erythematous plaque, papule or bleb, usually situated on the pretibial region of the lower leg, but occasionally elsewhere. The lesions soon progress into an ulcerated, necrotizing, and painful wound with ragged purple-red margins. There appears to be two subgroups of patients with pyoderma gangrenosum. In one group, the skin lesions seem related to bowel activity. In this group of patients, surgical resection of all diseased bowel is followed by prompt skin healing. The second group of patients has pyoderma gangrenosum with quiescent bowel disease.

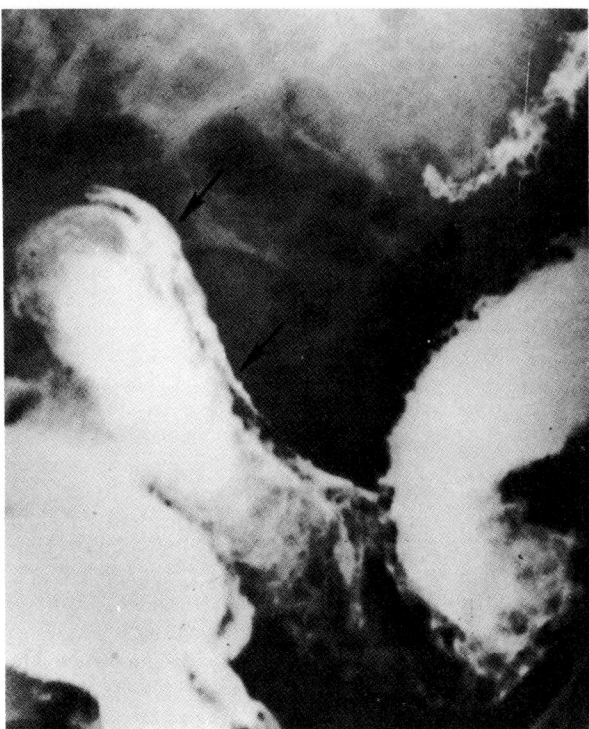

Fig. 28-19. A linear collection of barium parallel to the bowel lumen (arrows). [From: *Stein GN, Sabri PJ: Roentgen features, in JE Berk (ed): Bockus Gastroenterology, 4th ed. Philadelphia, Saunders, 1985, Fig 126-26, p 2170, with permission.*]

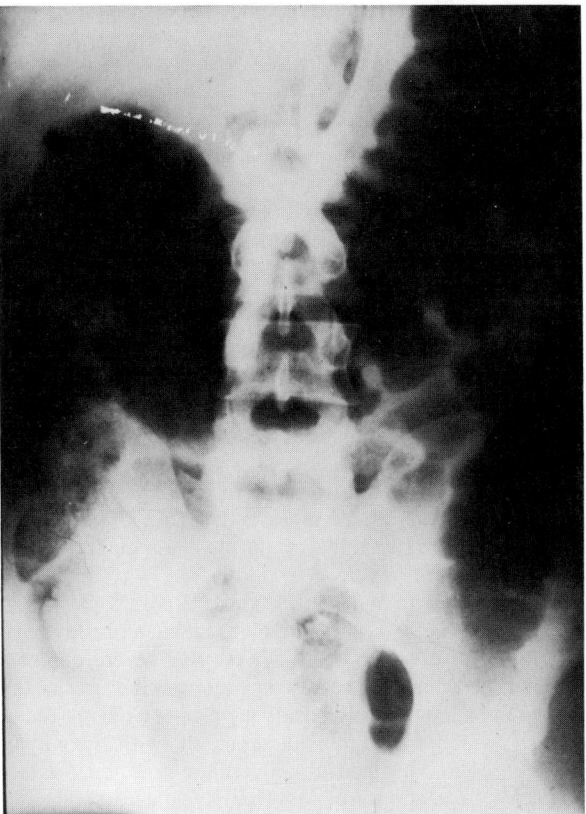

Fig. 28-20. Dilated transverse colon with air in toxic megacolon. (From: *Nivatvongs S, Becker ER, 1987, with permission.*)

Colectomy in this group does not heal the skin lesions promptly.

Aphthous ulcerations of the buccal mucosa, soft palate, gums, lips, tongue, and uvula are frequent complications of inflammatory bowel disease. Treatment is symptomatic. Control of the active bowel disease helps resolve these oral lesions.

Up to 10 percent of patients with inflammatory bowel disease develop ocular lesions. These include uveitis, iritis, episcleritis, and conjunctivitis. They usually develop in conjunction with an acute exacerbation of the bowel disease and subside as the bowel disease improves. The cause of these eye lesions is not known.

Toxic Megacolon. Toxic megacolon is an emergency, life-threatening complication of both ulcerative colitis and Crohn's colitis. It may occur as an acute exacerbation of chronic disease but more frequently develops during the initial presentation. In recent years, it has become a rare complication, probably because of better medical management and earlier referral of the patient for operation. Toxic megacolon is a clinical term for an acute colitis with segmental or total dilatation of the colon associated with signs of toxicity (Fig. 28-20). Usually these patients are very ill with high fever, abdominal pain and tenderness, tachycardia, and leukocytosis. Patients may develop toxicity without megacolon or megacolon without severe toxic signs. The etiology of megacolon is unclear but known factors that precipitate the condition are antidiar-

rheal agents, opiates, belladonna alkaloids, and barium enema.

Medical Management. These patients are very ill and require vigorous resuscitation to maintain homeostasis. Antibiotics to cover colonic bacterial flora are given as soon as possible. Intravenous corticosteroids are mandatory for those patients receiving or recently treated with corticosteroids to prevent adrenal insufficiency. Intravenous corticosteroids are the mainstay of medical therapy, but if the patient has never been on corticosteroids before and the decision has been made to operate, hydrocortisone should not be started. Properly managed, more than half of the patients respond to medical treatment and operation can be postponed. Ultimately, most of these patients will require resection.

Surgical Therapy. An operation is indicated if the patient's condition is not clearly improved within 24 h. This approach minimizes the incidence of colonic perforation, which is associated with an 80 percent mortality rate compared with less than 10 percent if there is no perforation.

Controversy exists regarding the best operation in this setting. Total proctocolectomy has the advantage that the entire disease is eliminated. On the other hand, subtotal colectomy without removal of the rectum is significantly less of an operation for the very ill patient. The disadvantage is that the diseased rectum remains, risking continued complications. Since the introduction of the ileal pouch anal pull-through procedure, the trend at the present time is to save the rectum if feasible, particularly in young patients, hoping that the restorative procedure can be performed at a later date. About 50 percent of patients with Crohn's colitis have minimal involvement of the rectum. This makes it logical not to remove the rectum at this critical time. In selected patients, an ileorectal anastomosis can be done as a second stage.

CANCER SURVEILLANCE. One of the most serious complications of ulcerative colitis is the development of colon and rectal carcinoma. The exact incidence of carcinoma in ulcerative colitis is not known. The known factors that increase the risk are onset in childhood, total large bowel involvement, duration of the disease longer than 10 years, and persistent inflammation.

Carcinoma in ulcerative colitis is difficult to diagnose since in most instances it develops as a flat lesion. Frequently, multiple lesions are found. About 20 percent of the patients are incurable by the time the diagnosis has been made.

In 1967 Morson and Fang studied 23 colectomy specimens removed for colitis in which one or more invasive carcinomas were found. They found that severe mucosal dysplasia was present near and away from the sites of the carcinomas in all specimens. They proposed using rectal biopsy to identify the individual patients with chronic ulcerative colitis destined to get carcinoma. Their original work has been supported by other investigators. The development of colonoscopy has enabled biopsies to be obtained from all parts of the colon and rectum and has further increased its accuracy. Since carcinoma is unusual in chronic ulcerative colitis of less than 10 years duration, it is recommended that patients with ulcerative colitis for more than 10 years should have colonoscopy and multiple biopsies every 6 to 12 months. If severe dysplasia is present on repeat biopsies, operation should be strongly considered.

Cancer surveillance using mucosal biopsies is suitable only in patients with chronic or quiescent colitis. In acute and active colitis, it is usually impossible for the pathologist to differentiate between true dysplasia and reactive dysplasia. Although attractive in concept, the practical application of this screening technique has been difficult. Pathologists cannot uniformly agree on the diagnosis of severe dysplasia.

MEDICAL MANAGEMENT. In long-standing active ulcerative colitis, the patient may have had bleeding and diarrhea for a long period of time, leading to anemia, hypoproteinemia, weight loss, and vitamin deficiency. The degree of abnormality is directly related to severity and duration of the disease. Some patients may require admission for intensive therapy. Parental hyperalimentation has not been shown to be beneficial as a primary therapy. It is valuable and is used as a preoperative adjunctive treatment for patients who are severely malnourished.

Cortisone enemas are frequently used empirically in patients with symptomatic ulcerative proctitis and proctosigmoiditis with good results, although there has been no controlled study to evaluate their efficacy. Cortisone enema has limited value in total proctocolitis. Recently, 5-aminosalicylic acid enema has also been shown to help.

Sulfasalazine (Azulfidine) is part of the standard treatment for ulcerative colitis. Sulfasalazine is a conjugate of 5-aminosalicylic acid and sulfapiridine linked by an azo bond. Most of the ingested drug is absorbed from the small intestine. The remainder is returned to the bowel unchanged by way of bile. On reaching the colon, sulfasalazine is split by colonic bacteria into 5-aminosalicylic acid and sulfapiridine. The 5-aminosalicylic acid remains in the colon and is excreted in the stool. It has been shown that 5-aminosalicylate acts topically in the lumen of the colon and inhibits the inflammatory process. The usual dose is 1 g orally twice daily, increasing to 4 g/day. Improvement and therapeutic response may take up to 3 to 4 weeks. About 10 to 15 percent of patients develop side effects, which include nausea, vomiting, stomach upset, rash, and headache. 5-ASA alone is being used orally in the hope of minimizing side effects to sulfasalazine. Sulfasalazine is usually used as a long-term therapy with a maintenance dose of 2 g/day. Its main benefit is to prolong the remission time. Oral sulfasalazine 2 to 3 g/day is commonly used to treat refractory proctosigmoiditis.

Corticosteroids are the primary drugs used for the acute stage of ulcerative colitis. In a fulminant colitis, intravenous hydrocortisone 100 mg every 8 h or its equivalent is used. In a less severe form, prednisone 40 to 60 mg/day with a gradual tapering for a period of weeks to 20 mg or less is the usual treatment. Response should be evident within one week. Long-term use of prednisone has not been shown to prevent the relapse. Side effects of long-term use of corticosteroids are multiple and potentially serious. Corticosteroids are therefore used only on a short-term basis.

Many patients with acute ulcerative colitis have diarrhea almost every hour. Antidiarrheal drugs are helpful to decrease the frequency of bowel movements and help to relieve abdominal cramps. Diphenoxylate (Lomotil) and loperamine (Imodium) are the drugs of choice. Codeine and morphine should be avoided, especially in the acute state since they may precipitate toxic megacolon. Antispasmodic drugs are of limited value.

Antibiotics are rarely indicated in the management of ulcerative colitis. While infectious colitis is being excluded with appropriate cultures, antibiotics may be used empirically. Anecdotal reports of response of colitis or proctitis to a variety of antibiotics are difficult to interpret.

SURGICAL THERAPY. The indications for operation include disease that has been present for over 15 years, intractability, severe mucosal dysplasia, carcinoma, and cutaneous or systemic manifestations. An urgent procedure may be required for massive hemorrhage, fulminant colitis, or toxic megacolon. A variety of operations have been employed.

Total Proctocolectomy and Ileostomy

This operation removes the entire disease and is considered the "gold standard" treatment. Most patients adjust well physically and psychologically to the permanent ileostomy, although some will never adapt to it or accept it psychologically.

Colectomy with Ileorectal Anastomosis

In properly selected patients, particularly young patients with good anal continence and good compliance, in the presence of mild or moderately inflamed mucosa, colectomy with ileorectal anastomosis works well. The advantage to preserving the rectum is obvious. The patient continues to have bowel movement naturally. Since the rectum is not disturbed, the possibility of causing impotence from mobilization of the rectum during surgery does not exist. This is particularly important in young male patients. The disadvantages are the frequency of bowel movement, which may be up to 6 to 10 times per day but is more commonly 2 to 3 times per day, and the risk of incontinence if the patients are not properly selected. The disease remaining in the rectum may exacerbate, and the rectum continues to be at risk to develop cancer. The risk of cancer is directly related to the duration of the disease, about 2 percent at 15 years and 15 percent at 30 years. It is important that patients return for periodic biopsy to check for mucosal dysplasia every 6 to 12 months. The patients should also understand that approximately 50 percent will ultimately require another operation to remove the rectum because of bowel symptoms, severe dysplasia, or cancer.

Total Proctocolectomy with Continent Ileostomy (Kock's Pouch) (Fig. 28-21). In 1969 Kock et al. pioneered an ileal reservoir that was subsequently improved to build a nipple valve to maintain continence of the ileostomy. The ileal content in the reservoir is evacuated via intubation with a catheter 4 to 6 times a day. The primary advantage of this procedure is the elimination of the disease without having to wear an ileostomy bag. The disadvantage is that the patients still have an ileostomy. The operation is rather extensive, with a relatively high rate of complications, especially extrusion of the valve, which causes incontinence. This operation has never become widely used because of its unpredictable success in maintaining continence.

Total Colectomy, Rectal Mucosectomy, Ileal Pouch-Anal Anastomosis (Fig. 28-22). The concept of an ileal reservoir that could be pulled through the anal sphincter mechanism to maintain natural continence has great appeal, since it would not only rid the patient of the disease but preserve bowel continuity and anal continence. The operation consists of colectomy to the level just above the levator ani muscles. The diseased mucosa in the remaining short rectum is then stripped off its underlying muscle. An ileal reservoir is created and then brought through the anorectal muscle tube and anastomosed to the dentate line. A temporary ileostomy is usually constructed about $1\frac{1}{2}$ to 2 ft proximal to the reservoir. The functional results of this operation are good to excellent in the majority of patients. Some patients have significant seepage of mucus and even stool, especially at night. Patients have an average of six bowel movements per 24 h period, but the range is highly variable. Common early postoperative complications are pelvic abscess and small bowel obstruction. The common late postoperative complications are pouchitis (inflammation of the reservoir) and anastomotic stricture.

In patients with ulcerative colitis the ileal pouch-anal anastomosis is contraindicated if there is perianal sepsis, anal stenosis, fecal incontinence, or if the patient is in poor general health, unreliable, and over 50 years of age. A previous small bowel resection may preclude the procedure. If an operation is being performed, such a complex procedure usually should not be performed as an

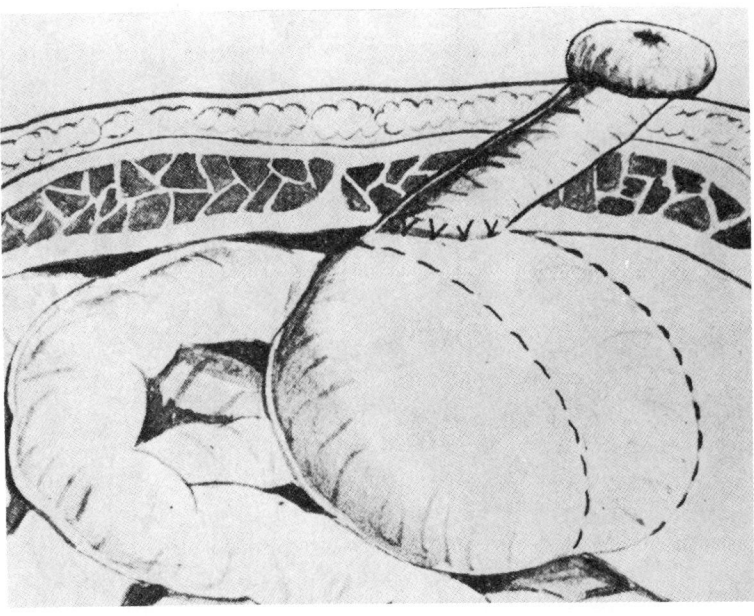

Fig. 28-21. Continent ileostomy (Kock's pouch).

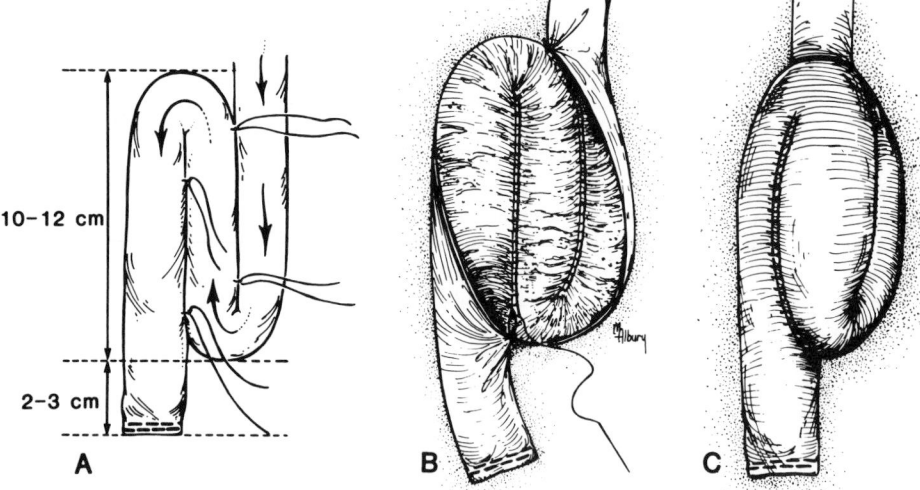

A   B   C

Fig. 28-22. The S-pouch (Parks' pouch). *A.* Terminal ileum is aligned in S shape with 2 to 3 cm projection. *B.* Creation of the pouch by joining the limbs together. *C.* The completed pouch. The projection of the pouch is anastomosed to the anal canal at the dentate line.

emergency procedure. The operation is not applicable to patients with Crohn's colitis.

Crohn's Colitis

In 1932 Crohn et al. presented the classic description of this nonspecific inflammatory bowel disease; at that time it was thought to be limited to the terminal ileum and was called regional enteritis. Crohn's disease of the colon was not recognized as an entity until 1960, when a report by Lockhart-Mummery and Morson appeared. It has now been realized that Crohn's disease can occur anywhere in the gastrointestinal tract from mouth to anus. Extraintestinal disease may precede the intestinal manifestations by many years.

PATHOLOGY. Crohn's disease is a transmural, predominantly submucosal inflammation with cobblestone ap-

pearance (Fig. 28-23). Typically, there is submucosal edema, lymphoid aggregation (Fig. 28-24), and, ultimately, fibrosis. In severe and chronic disease, the bowel wall becomes thickened and rigid, with creeping of fat from the mesentery to the bowel wall. The histologic hallmark of the disease is the sarcoid-like epithelioid granuloma (Fig. 28-25). This is found in roughly 50 to 75 percent of cases, and provides the alternative nomenclature *granulomatous bowel disease.*

Complications include obstruction, enterocutaneous fistula, internal fistula, free perforation, anal complica-

Fig. 28-23. Cobblestone appearance of Crohn's colitis. (From: *Nivatvongs S, Becker ER, 1987, with permission.*)

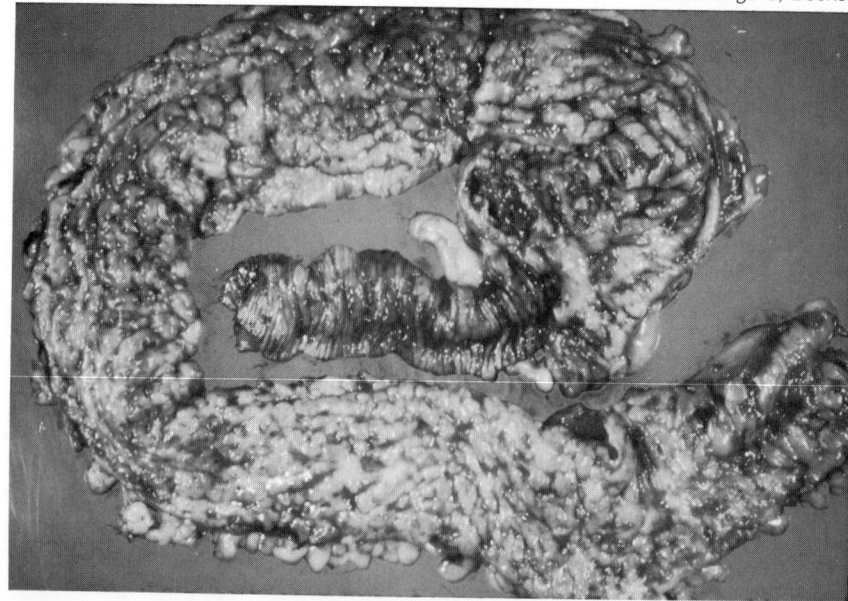

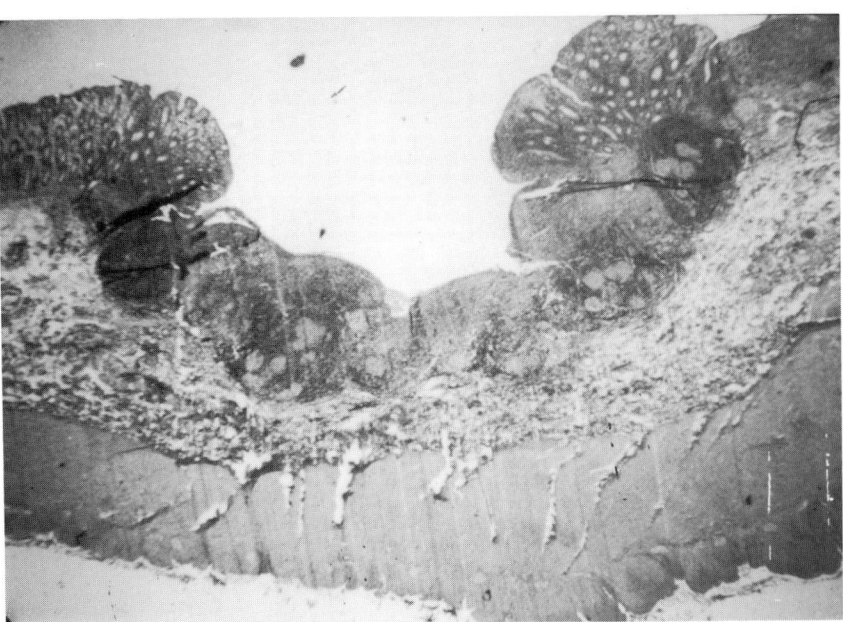

Fig. 28-24. Mucosal ulceration with submucosal edema and lymphoid aggregations. (From: *Nivatvongs S, Becker ER, 1987, with permission.*)

tions, massive hemorrhage, toxic megacolon, carcinoma, and cutaneous and systemic complications.

CLINICAL MANIFESTATIONS. The course of the disease is characterized by remissions and exacerbations like ulcerative colitis, but Crohn's disease tends to be a slowly progressive disease with eventual development of complications that require an operation. Unlike ulcerative colitis, Crohn's disease can involve both the small and large bowel, with its characteristic segmental involvement.

In a study of clinical patterns in Crohn's disease involving a series of 615 consecutive patients seen at the Cleveland Clinic, four clinical patterns were noted: ileocolic involvement of ileum and right colon 41 percent; colonic involvement without small intestinal involvement 28 percent; small intestinal involvement without colonic disease 27 percent; and anorectal involvement only 3 percent.

The onset of Crohn's disease is insidious. The symptoms are subtle and the manifestations are protean, depending on whether another part of the small bowel is also involved. Most patients have diarrhea that is usually not bloody. Abdominal pain is a typical symptom of

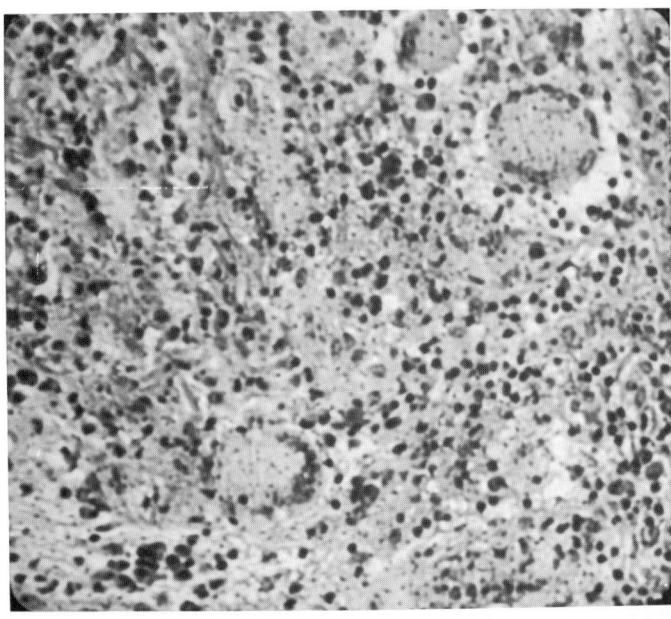

Fig. 28-25. Sarcoid-type epithelioid granulomas. (From: *Nivatvongs S, Becker ER, 1987, with permission.*)

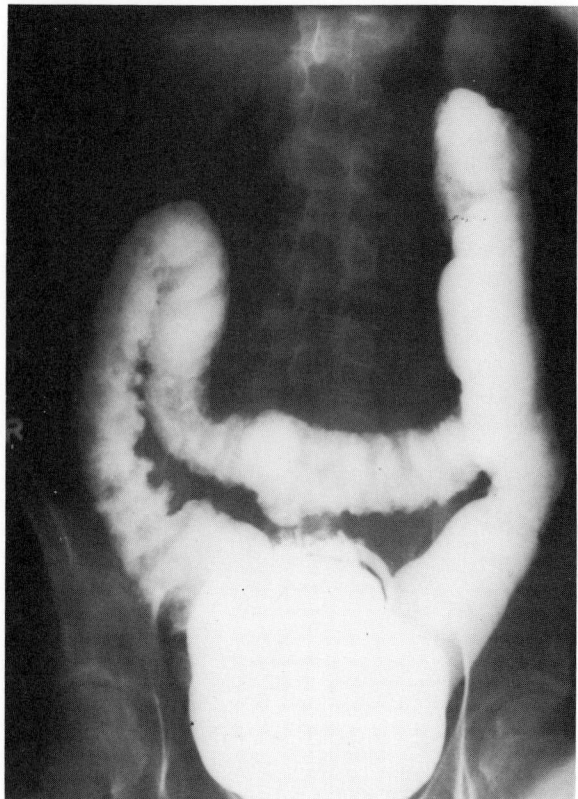

Fig. 28-26. Irregular nodular defect of Crohn's colitis or barium enema. (From: *Nivatvongs S, Becker ER, 1987, with permission.*)

Table 28-1. ULCERATIVE COLITIS AND CROHN'S COLITIS: CONTRASTING AND SIMILAR FEATURES

	Ulcerative colitis	*Crohn's colitis*
Manifestation		
Bleeding per rectum	3+	1+
Diarrhea	3+	3+
Abdominal pain	1+	3+ especially with involvement of ileum
Fever	R	2+
Palpable abdominal mass	R	2+
Internal fistula	R	4+
Intestinal obstruction (stricture or infection)	0	4+
Rectal involvement	4+	1+
Small bowel involvement	0	4+
Anal and perianal involvement	R	4+
Thumbprinting sign on barium enema	R	1+
Risk of cancer	2+	1+
Clinical course	Remission and relapse	Slowly progressive
Gross appearance		
Thickened bowel wall	0	4+
Shortening of bowel	2+	R
Fat-creeping onto serosa	0	4+
Segmental involvement	0	4+
Aphthous ulcer	0	4+
Linear ulcer	0	4+
Microscopic picture		
Depth of involvement	Mucosa and submucosa	Full thickness
Lymphoid aggregation	0	4+
Sarcoid-type granuloma	0	4+
Fissuring	0	2+
Surgical treatment		
Total proctocolectomy	"Gold standard"	Indicated in total large bowel involvement
Segmental resection	Infrequent	Frequent
Ileal pouch procedure	Excellent option in selected patients	Contraindicated
Prognosis		
Recurrence after surgery	0	3+

NOTE: R = rare; 0 = not found; 1+ = may be present; 2+ = common; 3+ = usual finding; 4+ = characteristic (not necessarily common).

ileocolitis. Weight loss associated with anemia and hypoproteinemia is common.

Endoscopy. Only half the patients with Crohn's colitis have rectal involvement; therefore, proctoscopy is not an adequate examination. Colonoscopy is the most sensitive tool for diagnosis, particularly in mild and early disease. Typically, the disease is patchy in distribution. Mucosal edema and aphthous ulcers are a feature of early Crohn's disease. Deep linear ulcers and fibrotic strictures are typical for more chronic Crohn's disease. Some patients have granular and friable mucosa with continuous involvement of the entire colon and rectum. In this situation, it is impossible to differentiate it from ulcerative colitis. Biopsies of the mucosa are rarely helpful unless a sarcoid-type giant cell granuloma is seen.

Radiologic Findings. Upper intestinal and small bowel follow-through barium studies may aid in the diagnosis. One of the striking features of Crohn's disease of the colon is the frequency of concomitant involvement of the small bowel. The characteristic roentgen features of Crohn's colitis are skip lesions, contour defects, longitudinal and transverse ulcers, cobblestone-like mucosal pattern, narrowing or stricture, thickening of the haustral margin, irregular nodular defects, and involvement of the terminal ileum (Fig. 28-26).

DIFFERENTIATION BETWEEN ULCERATIVE COLITIS AND CROHN'S COLITIS (Table 28-1). Ulcerative colitis and Crohn's colitis are grouped together as nonspecific inflammatory bowel diseases because of their similarity in many clinical aspects. Yet they also have many contrasting features. Most of the time they can be differentiated from each other without much difficulty. In 10 to 15 percent of cases, it is impossible to tell one from the other even in the hands of an experienced pathologist.

With the introduction of the ileal pouch-anal procedure, it has become more important to know the preoperative diagnosis as accurately as possible. The ileoanal pouch procedure is contraindicated in Crohn's colitis because of the high risk of recurrent Crohn's disease within the pouch.

MEDICAL MANAGEMENT. Contrary to previous belief, epidemiologic studies have shown that Crohn's colitis has a four- to twentyfold increased risk of development of carcinoma compared with the general population. Colorectal carcinoma in Crohn's disease is rarely seen probably because most Crohn's colitis requires surgery before it has time to develop carcinoma. The anatomic sites of the cancers are not significantly different from those of usual colorectal carcinomas. Mucosal dysplasia is also identified in patients with Crohn's disease similar to patients with ulcerative colitis. Some have advised periodic mucosal biopsies as part of the surveillance for cancer in long-standing Crohn's colitis.

There is no specific medical therapy for Crohn's colitis. The aims of treatment are to reduce the bowel inflammation, promote symptomatic relief for the intestinal and extraintestinal manifestations, and correct nutritional disturbances. Control rather than cure of the disease is the expectation of treatment.

Mild and moderately severe disease can be treated on an outpatient basis. In severe disease, the patient should be admitted to the hospital for bowel rest and institution of vigorous nutritional and medical supportive therapy.

Sulfasalazine should be initiated in all patients with mild to moderate Crohn's colitis. The usual oral dose is 1 g twice a day, increasing to a total of 4 g daily. The therapy is continued for as long as the patient remains symptomatic. Once clinical remission is achieved, the dosage is gradually reduced and the drug discontinued. Unlike ulcerative colitis, long-term maintenance of sulfasalazine has not been shown to prolong the remission time.

In a double-blind trial conducted in Sweden comparing metronidazole with sulfasalazine, there was no difference in efficacy between the two drugs. Low doses of metronidazole are well tolerated by patients and may be a valuable therapeutic option. The drug would seem especially useful for those patients who cannot tolerate or who are unresponsive to sulfasalazine.

Corticosteroids are widely used for the treatment of active, severe, symptomatic Crohn's colitis. Good initial symptomatic response can be expected in 75 to 90 percent of the patients, although not necessarily associated with concomitant improvement of radiologic abnormalities. Prednisone 60 mg orally, given in 3 or 4 divided doses is maintained for 10 to 14 days. Prednisone is then tapered at the rate of 5 mg every week, preferably from the evening dose. The dose of the prednisone is increased if there is any sign of relapse in the disease activity. Sulfasalazine can be added. In very ill patients, intravenous hydrocortisone 100 mg every 8 h or its equivalent should be given until the patient can start on oral prednisone. There has been no good evidence to support the use of prophylactic steroid therapy in both quiescent disease and after surgical therapy.

There has been controversy regarding the use of the immunosuppressive agents azathioprine and 6-mercaptopurine in the treatment of Crohn's colitis. Recently it has been shown that when properly used, the response rate is high (60 to 70 percent), though prolonged treatment is necessary. The indications are steroid toxicity, steroid dependence, fistulization (perianal, enterocutaneous, internal fistula), and recurrent Crohn's disease with previous multiple small bowel resections. The drugs have had many known side effects: gastrointestinal complaints, headache, leukopenia, and bone marrow depression. Of most concern is the risk of malignancy, particularly non-Hodgkin's lymphoma, which occurs among patients after a renal transplantation. The dosage used for Crohn's colitis is low and the risk of this potential complication is not known.

SURGICAL THERAPY. Indications for operation include intractability, obstruction, internal fistula, colo- or enterocutaneous fistula, intraabdominal abscess, massive hemorrhage, fulminating colitis, toxic megacolon, free perforation, cutaneous and systemic complications, severe anal and perianal involvement, severe mucosal dysplasia, and carcinoma. A variety of procedures may be used.

In patients with limited colonic involvement, a segmental resection to grossly normal margins is advisable. With more extensive disease of the colon, the status of the rectum should determine the choice of the procedure: subtotal colectomy if the rectum is relatively spared or total proctocolectomy if rectal and/or severe perianal disease is present. An abdominal perineal resection and sigmoid colostomy seems an appropriate procedure for the rare patient with severe rectal and/or perineal disease but an otherwise apparently normal colon.

Segmental Resection. Segmental resection is utilized for patients with isolated ileocolic Crohn's disease. The involved terminal ileum and the right colon are resected and a primary anastomosis is done. Segmental resection can also be performed if the disease is confined to a small segment of the colon. This is an uncommon situation.

Colectomy and Ileorectal Anastomosis. In Crohn's colitis in which the rectum and sigmoid colon are spared or have minimal involvement, a total colectomy with ileorectal or ileosigmoid anastomosis is a viable option. Although the recurrence is frequent, the advantage of avoiding a stoma is significant.

Total Proctocolectomy and Ileostomy. This procedure is the standard treatment of Crohn's disease that involves the entire colon and rectum. Unlike in ulcerative colitis, the patient can still develop recurrent disease anywhere in the small bowel. Most commonly this occurs in the ileum just proximal to the ileostomy.

Abdominoperineal Resection and Colostomy. If the disease is confined to the rectum or anal canal and surgical treatment becomes necessary, an abdominoperineal resection with sigmoid colostomy can be done. Such a localized distal involvement of the disease is uncommon and recurrence in the colon is likely. Some would thus favor a total proctocolectomy and ileostomy in this setting.

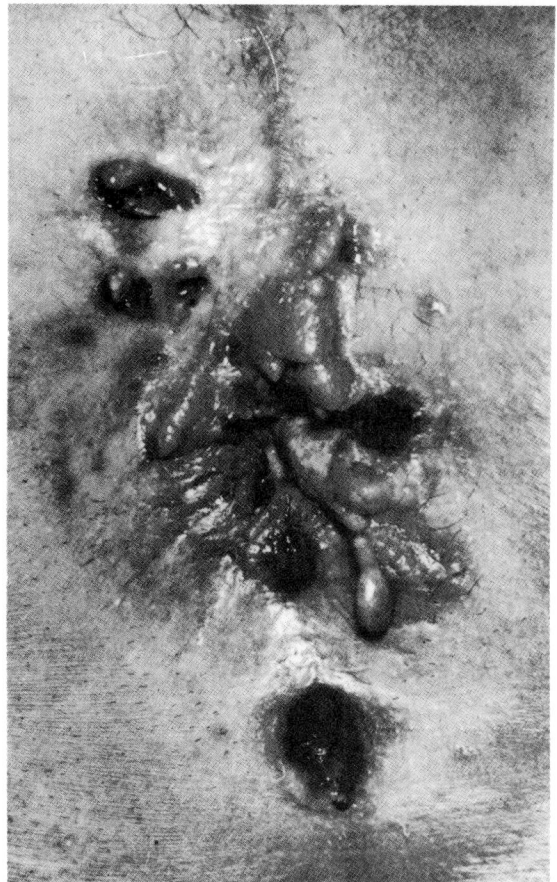

Fig. 28-27. Anal involvement in Crohn's disease. Multiple fistulas and edematous skin tags are present. [From: *Hamilton SR, Borson BC: Crohn's disease: Pathology, in JE Berk (ed): Bockus Gastroenterology, 4th ed. Philadelphia, Saunders, 1985, Fig 127-5, p 2229, with permission.*]

Management of Ileosigmoid Fistula

The finding of an ileosigmoid fistula in a patient with ileal Crohn's disease poses a dilemma, i.e., should a segment of sigmoid colon be resected en bloc with the involved ileum or should the fistula's opening into the sigmoid simply be closed. Concern over anastomotic leak and late sigmoidocutaneous fistula must be balanced against the risks of an unnecessary colon resection. Simple excision of the fistula and closure of the sigmoid defect is safe as long as the sigmoid colon has not been involved with obvious Crohn's disease or a severe inflammatory reaction.

Recurrence after Surgical Treatment

Unlike in ulcerative colitis, even complete resection of the diseased bowel does not cure the patient of Crohn's disease. The recurrence rate is directly related to the type of operation, duration of the follow-up, and the definition of recurrence. The highest rate of recurrence is seen in

those patients who underwent resection and anastomosis (up to 80 percent after 20 years), while the lowest rate is seen in patients who underwent total proctocolectomy and ileostomy for isolated Crohn's colitis. Not all recurrences, however, require reoperation. Some patients with known recurrence continue to lead a normal life. Most patients will need multiple operations during their lifetime.

ANAL AND PERIANAL CROHN'S DISEASE

Anal and perianal manifestations of Crohn's disease are very common. Anal lesions are the first manifestation of large bowel Crohn's disease in 25 percent of cases and occur in 50 to 70 percent of patients with colonic or rectal involvement. Their incidence in small bowel or ileocecal Crohn's disease without apparent colonic disease is 10 to 30 percent. Up to 90 percent of patients will have some anal or perianal involvement, but they usually have only mild symptoms. Anal and perianal Crohn's disease as the primary site occurs in about 3 percent of patients. It may precede the more proximal involvement of Crohn's disease by many years. When anal Crohn's disease is suspected, a complete gastrointestinal workup is indicated.

CLINICAL MANIFESTATIONS. Presentation may be acute or chronic depending on the lesion, and anal disease may be the most troublesome aspect or it may be overshadowed by symptoms from other sites of involvement. The most common anal finding is the edematous *skin tags* that usually cause minimal symptoms (Fig. 28-27). *Fissures* are common. They are usually deep and indolent looking, but as a rule are not as painful as they appear. Severe pain in anal fissures of Crohn's disease may be a sign of an abscess formation that should be carefully drained. *Hemorrhoids* are not a common feature of anal Crohn's disease. What are usually regarded by patients or inexperienced physicians as hemorrhoids are actually skin irritations, anal fissues, or ulcerations. *Stricture* or *stenosis* is a common complication of long-standing anal disease or occurs as a result of anorectal surgery. *Perianal abscesses* in Crohn's disease can be single, multiple, simple, or complicated. They may develop from underlying active disease in the anal canal, rectum, or even colon or small bowel. *Anal incontinence* usually occurs because of diarrhea and overflow rather than from an involvement of the anal sphincter muscle with Crohn's disease. Destruction of the anal sphincter muscle is usually the result of aggressive surgery for perianal problems.

Granulomata are found in about 75 percent of the rectal biopsy specimens, although they occur much less frequently in tissue taken from anal lesions (33 percent).

MANAGEMENT. The basic principle is to provide conservative management for symptomatic disease. In many cases, anal hygiene and control of diarrhea will be sufficient therapy. Medical treatment of underlying symptomatic bowel disease with corticosteroids, sulfasalazine, bowel rest with hyperalimentation or elemental diet, and sometimes immunosuppressants like 6-mercaptopurine will often result in control of the perianal and anal symptoms. Metronidazole has been used for anal and perianal Crohn's disease with variable success.

Skin tags may be excised if they become painful or interfere with anal hygiene. Hemorrhoidectomy in patients with Crohn's disease may leave the patient with chronic unhealing anal wounds or fistula in ano. In one study 67 percent of the patients needed an excision of their rectum following hemorrhoidectomy. Formal hemorrhoidectomy is therefore contraindicated in Crohn's disease but highly symptomatic hemorrhoidal thromboses or prolapse may be treated by excision or banding.

Fissures associated with Crohn's disease are usually not in the typical position in the midline posterior and the midline anterior. If they are troublesome, however, the fissures can be "cleaned up" by excising overhanging edges and flattening the wound. Examination for underlying fistula or abscess should be carried out under anesthesia. Occasionally, a highly symptomatic typical fissure in ano is seen in a patient with Crohn's disease. Sphincterotomy may be necessary if it does not heal with conservative management. A sphincterotomy runs the risk of creating a perianal wound that may fail to heal and that may lead to incontinence. Symptomatic anal stricture or stenosis is best treated by repeated dilatation to one finger's breadth.

Abscesses must be adequately drained. Simple fistulas can be left alone, or if necessary can be laid open like ordinary fistulas. Conventional laying open of low fistulas in Crohn's disease results in healing in 90 percent of cases. Some patients may be helped by treatment with metronidazole, which often reduces discharge although it rarely produces permanent healing.

High fistulas should be considered for treatment with a silastic seton rather than by transecting a large amount of sphincter and risking incontinence. The patient will tolerate a persistent small discharge of purulent material better than incontinence. A silastic tube is loosely tied around the involved sphincter muscle overlying the fistula. In many cases, the seton can be removed a few weeks later without dividing the muscle. In other cases, the seton can be left in place indefinitely to prevent recurrent abscesses. Severe anorectal sepsis uncontrolled by a local procedure is indication for proctectomy. In practice this is necessary only in a small proportion of patients with fistula (10 to 15 percent), most of whom also have severe rectal disease as a contributing factor. The majority of patients can be successfully managed by local operation which may, however, need to be repeated.

In well-selected cases, a rectovaginal fistula can be repaired if there is no active anorectal disease. The same principle is applied to anal incontinence. In severe anal and perianal disease, particularly when there is active anorectal disease, proctectomy may be necessary. Most of the time this is done because of intolerable anal incontinence or pain.

There is no convincing evidence that temporary diversion or resection of the proximal bowel with active Crohn's disease will cure anal or perianal Crohn's disease.

Ischemic Colitis

Mesenteric vascular occlusion without major vessel involvement may produce localized ischemia. In the past decade, ischemic colitis has emerged as a clearly defined clinicopathologic entity. Ischemic colitis presents as three quite different clinical syndromes depending on (1) the extent of the vascular occlusion, (2) the duration of the occlusion, (3) the efficiency of the collateral circulation, and (4) the extent of secondary bacterial invasion. With transitory impairment of arterial supply, which is soon compensated by collateral flow, there is a partial mucosal slough that is healed by mucosal regeneration within 2 or 3 days—*reversible* or *transient ischemic colitis* (Table 28-2). Gross impairment of arterial supply results in hemorrhagic infarction of the mucosa, which ulcerates, allowing invasion of bowel bacteria. Healing is by fibrosis, which often produces stenosis—*stricturing ischemic colitis*. With complete loss of arterial flow, there is full-thickness infarction, gangrene, and, if untreated, perforation with peritonitis and death—*gangrenous ischemic colitis*.

Early reports stressed that the splenic flexure is the most vulnerable segment, presumably because this is the area at the periphery of both superior and inferior mesenteric artery supply and because in this area the marginal artery of Drummond is at its greatest distance from the bowel wall. It is now clear, however, that ischemic colitis can affect any segment from the cecum to the rectosigmoid. Major vascular occlusion does not correlate with ischemic colitis; many patients, particularly those with abdominal aneurysms, have occlusion of the inferior mesenteric artery without bowel symptoms. Conversely, some patients with frank ischemic colitis have demonstrably patent major mesenteric arteries. Experimentally, ligation of the inferior mesenteric artery in the dog has no deleterious effect on the colon; it is only when the small vessels between the mesenteric arcade and the bowel are ligated that colonic ischemia is produced.

Most patients with ischemic colitis are in the older age group; it is rarely seen under age forty-five. The majority also have associated medical problems such as cardiovascular disease, rheumatoid arthritis, or diabetes. The onset of ischemic colitis is characteristically acute with mild to moderate generalized or lower abdominal cramping pain followed by passage of blood per rectum. Vomiting is uncommon. Further symptoms depend on which of the three types of ischemic colitis is developing. With the gangrenous type, the abdominal pain becomes more severe until it is constant. Systemic symptoms of an abdominal catastrophe ensue. On physical examination, abdominal tenderness is usually generalized but is often most marked over the ischemic segment. Voluntary guarding and involuntary spasm are present but are not marked. Bowel sounds, which are hyperactive early, gradually cease. Later, with progression of infarction to gangrene, necrosis, and perforation, the findings are those of spreading bacterial peritonitis and septic shock. Diagnosis can usually be made from the clinical picture alone.

Table 28-2. ISCHEMIC COLON DISEASE

	Form 1	Form 2	Form 3
Synonyms	Nonspecific colitis; ulcerative colitis of aged; reversible ischemia of colon	Ischemic stricture	Colonic infarction; necrotizing colitis; gangrene of colon; irreversible ischemia
Symptoms	Cramping abdominal pain; bloody diarrhea	Cramping abdominal pain; abdominal distention; decreased bowel movements	Diffuse abdominal pain; obtundation; bloody diarrhea
Signs	Localized tenderness; hyperactive intestinal sounds; mild pyrexia; leukocytosis	Abdominal distention, hyperactive intestinal sounds; normal temperature; normal white blood cell count	Diffuse-direct and rebound tenderness; rigid abdomen; hypoactive or absent intestinal sounds; abdominal distention; pyrexia, leukocytosis, tachycardia, hypotension
Barium enema	Mucosal irregularity; thumbprinting; local narrowing	Stricture; intestinal obstruction	Mucosal irregularity; dilatation of colon; thickening of intestinal wall; perforation
Treatment	Medical	Resection of involved intestine	Correction of predisposing factors; immediate operation
Results	Resolution	Correction of symptoms	High mortality rate due to associated diseases or complications of colonic gangrene

SOURCE: From O'Connell, Kadell, and Tompkins, 1976, with permission.

Proctoscopy reveals only a normal distal segment with blood coming from above. If the rectosigmoid is the segment involved, a blue-black, sloughing mucosa oozing blood is seen. Flexible sigmoidoscopy or even colonoscopy can more specifically identify the sites of ischemia, but perforation is a risk that must be avoided.

Barium enema is contraindicated in gangrenous colitis, and arteriography is unnecessary and delays proper treatment. Plain abdominal radiographs are often confirmatory and reveal adynamic ileus with the gaseous distention stopping at the involved segment. Occasionally small bubbles of gas may be detected in the wall of the infarcted bowel. Treatment is emergency operation as soon as the patient's condition is stabilized by vigorous preparatory therapy. Under favorable circumstances, the involved segment is resected and primary anastomosis performed. More frequently, however, this disease in this age group dictates exteriorization of the involved segment.

With impairment but not complete loss of blood supply, the patient's symptoms do not progress, but neither do they disappear promptly. Mild to moderate abdominal pain continues, as does rectal bleeding, which, however, is usually not massive. There may also be symptoms and signs of partial intestinal obstruction. Barium enema radiography is diagnostic. Marginal "thumbprinting," or "pseudotumors," due to submucosal hemorrhage and pericolic fat inflammation is seen. Spasm and ulceration also may be present. Conservation therapy is indicated at this point since the process may be self-limited and reversible. Anticoagulants should not be used. After sev-

eral days the barium enema findings revert toward normality, but repeat barium enema in a few weeks often reveals stricture formation at the ischemic site. The strictured colon should be electively resected with primary anastomosis.

In the transient or reversible form of ischemic colitis, symptoms are mild and last only 2 to 4 days. Barium enema, if done promptly, usually reveals thumbprinting or superficial ulceration but promptly reverts to normal. Follow-up barium enema is also within normal limits. No specific therapy is necessary.

Radiation Enterocolitis

That x-rays have deleterious effects on the intestine has been known since 1897, 2 years after their discovery, when Walsh described a self-limited instance of diarrhea and cramps which was resolved by placing a metal shield between the observer and the source of radiation. Radiation enterocolitis has become a major problem in recent years because of the higher radiation doses employed in the therapy of uterine, bladder, and prostatic malignancies, and, perhaps, because the newer external radiation sources deliver large visceral doses with little or no skin reaction to alert the therapist.

The incidence of radiation injury to the bowel is very roughly dose-dependent. At tissue doses below 4000 rad, significant bowel injury is quite uncommon. With 5000 rad, essentially all patients will have some demonstrable damage; in 5 to 10 percent the damage will be significant and ongoing. Other factors that increase the likelihood of problems include asthenia, advanced age, hypertension, arteriosclerotic vascular disease, diabetes, and previous abdominal surgery with resulting adhesions that fix the bowel.

The rapidly proliferating intestinal epithelium is most sensitive to ionizing radiation and shows changes early in the course. These are mucosal hyperemia and edema, an extensive inflammatory cell infiltrate, and crypt abscesses. With higher doses there are areas of ulceration because of failure of epithelial regeneration. After cessation of therapy, reepithelialization is the rule but with a thin mucosa with shortened villi. Of more serious import is the long-term effect of radiation on blood vessels. Beginning several weeks after radiation exposure and continuing for years is a progressive vasculitis, affecting principally the small arterioles in the submucosa with marked thickening of the vessel wall and leading to luminal occlusion and thrombosis. Large foam cells seen beneath the intima are said to be pathognomonic of radiation vasculitis. The progressive ischemia is accompanied by progressive thickening and fibrosis, principally of the submucosa. As ischemia progresses, ulceration supervenes. This in turn leads to abscess and fistula formation, also on an ischemic basis.

At least 75 percent of patients undergoing radiotherapy with exposure of the gastrointestinal tract will have nausea and vomiting, and often diarrhea with cramping. With high doses of radiation there may also be rectal bleeding and tenesmus. Most patients can be managed symptomatically, but in some the reaction is so severe that the therapy has to be stopped for a time or prolonged. These acute symptoms subside fairly promptly after completion of therapy.

Late symptoms of radiation damage to the intestines appear from several months to many years after exposure. The clinical presentation is determined by the segment of bowel involved as well as by the type of lesion: atrophic mucosa, ulcer, stricture, abscess, fistula, or perforation. The rectum is by far the most common site of involvement because of its proximity to the cervix and its fixed position. Rectal ulcers are most commonly seen on the anterior wall at 4 to 6 cm above the dentate line and cause the passage of bloody mucus and tenesmus. Symptomatic rectal strictures are usually found at the 8- to 12-cm level and produce the picture of partial colonic obstruction. A particularly distressing complication is a postradiation fistula from rectum into bladder or vagina producing feculent vaginal discharge or pneumaturia.

Radiation-induced rectovaginal fistula is most commonly seen in patients who received radiation for carcinoma of the cervix. The development of the fistula usually is preceded by bleeding and ulceration in the rectum or vagina 6 to 18 months after completion of radiation therapy. Once the fistula has occurred, vaginal discharge of feces begins. In occasional patients, vesicovaginal fistula may develop to add to their discomfort. Virtually all the lesions are located 4 to 10 cm from the anus. Diagnosis may be difficult because of the difficulty in distinguishing between radiation changes and recurrent tumor.

Barium contrast radiographic studies usually demonstrate rather characteristic changes, but these are not specific. Angiography also usually demonstrates changes that are characteristic of, but not specific for, radiation damage. Endoscopy with biopsy yields a specific diagnosis in some cases but not in all. If a positive histologic diagnosis is not possible prior to treatment, the patient should be given the benefit of the doubt and not denied maximal therapy, since the lesion may be recurrent cancer. Diverting colostomy is necessary. In patients with biopsy-proved recurrent tumors, this palliative procedure may be sufficient. In patients without recurrent tumor, an attempt should be made at repair of the fistula. Under protection of the colostomy, local excision of the fistula is feasible. If the lesion is high enough, anterior resection or a coloanal pull-through can be attempted.

Management of radiation injuries is difficult and often unsatisfactory. Conservative measures should be used as long as they are effective. Ischemic fibrotic tissues make for poor wound healing, anastomotic disruption, infection, and occult perforation. Morgenstern and associates have well summarized several caveats for the surgeon: (1) Avoid entry into the abdomen for radiation injury unless absolutely forced to operate. (2) Avoid extensive resections and multiple anastomoses. Short isolated segments are best resected, but long segments are most safely treated by side-to-side bypass. (3) Avoid extensive adhesiolysis. Lysis of adhesions in damaged intestine produces minute openings into the intestine that lead to postoperative perforation or fistulas. (4) Use frozen-section control of the intestinal ends to be anastomosed to rule out unsuspected radiation changes. (5) Protect anastomoses. Colon anastomoses should be protected with a proximal colostomy; small bowel anastomoses, with a long tube.

The outlook in radiation enterocolitis is grim. Many patients are spared this travail because they die of their primary diseases before radiation damage supervenes. But many more will die as a result of the treatment that cured their cancer. DeCosse and associates followed 90 patients with radiation enterocolitis. Of these, 27 were living, 28 died from cancer, 13 died from other causes, and 22 died from complications of radiation enterocolitis.

Pseudomembranous Colitis

Pseudomembranous colitis is an acute, severe diarrheal syndrome, characterized by plaques and pseudomembranes on the colonic mucosa, that follows administration of antimicrobials. An enterotoxin secreted by *C. difficile* organisms has been implicated as the etiologic agent.

Since first described by Billroth in 1867, pseudomembranous colitis, or *enterocolitis,* has been linked to major operations, debilitating medical diseases, and immunosuppression. The syndrome was reported with increased frequency in the 1950s and 1960s, associated with many different antibiotics, and thought to be caused by overgrowth of resistant *Staphylococcus aureus* in the gastrointestinal tract. The terms *staphylococcal enterocolitis* and *antibiotic-induced enterocolitis* were commonly used

of hyperemic edge. In some patients, the mucosa is red and granular without gross ulceration, mimicking a localized proctitis. A full-thickness rectal prolapse may be present.

DIAGNOSIS. A biopsy is essential to exclude carcinoma. The most characteristic histologic features are (1) obliteration of the lamina propria of the mucosal layer in the region of the ulcer by fibroblasts and muscle fibers derived from the muscularis mucosa, (2) a muscularis mucosa that is thicker than normal with fibers extending into the lamina propria, (3) few inflammatory cells in the lamina propria, and (4) tubules sometimes showing cystic dilatation, which may be displaced into the submucosa. Most of the time, the diagnosis can be made by the gross appearance of the lesions. Differential diagnosis of solitary ulcer of the rectum includes carcinoma, Crohn's disease, proctitis, and lymphogranuloma venereum.

Anal-rectal manometric studies do not contribute to the diagnosis but may be helpful in assessing the sphincter mechanism in cases of incontinence.

TREATMENT. Treatment of this condition is directed at correcting the associated problems, particularly the full-thickness rectal prolapse (procidentia) and rectal mucosal prolapse. Neither medical treatment nor local excision of the lesion achieves relief of symptoms or healing of the ulcer. Adjustment of diet to avoid straining at stool may be helpful.

Abdominal rectopexy is indicated in patients with simultaneous complete rectal prolapse. Healing rates after this procedure of over 80 percent have been reported. In cases without prolapse, the management is less straightforward. Conservative management consists of trying to prevent straining at stool. Surgical excision of the ulcerated area is followed by recurrence. The ulcer has been observed to heal following a colostomy, only to recur after subsequent closure.

DIVERTICULAR DISEASE

GENERAL CONSIDERATIONS. Two types of diverticula of the colon are recognized. One is a very common, acquired disease that consists of multiple false diverticula, principally in the left colon. A false colonic diverticulum is a herniation of the mucosa, including the muscularis mucosa, through the colonic muscle wall. These are pulsion-type protrusions. The other type of diverticula is very uncommon, is probably a congenital disease, and consists of a single true diverticulum of the cecum or ascending colon.

Diverticulosis implies the presence of a diverticulum or diverticula without inflammation. The term *diverticular disease* is used to describe the clinical spectrum of the disease with or without complications. Diverticulosis is the most common clinically encountered colonic condition. It is rare below the age of thirty but increases in incidence thereafter, with one-third of people studied over the age of sixty having diverticula on barium enema examination. In patients under fifty years of age, it is more common in males. This subgroup is more likely to

have symptoms and to develop complications, with about 50 percent requiring an operation. In elderly people it is more common in females and operation is rarely required.

ETIOLOGY. Although diverticulosis can occur in any segment of the colon, the sigmoid colon is the most common site. In a study by Parks, the sigmoid colon alone accounted for 66 percent, the sigmoid colon combined with other segments was present in 96 percent, and total colonic involvement was seen in 7 percent of cases. The rectum is rarely affected.

Colonic diverticula occur between the teniae coli, at points of weakness where the main blood vessels pass to supply the colonic mucosa (Fig. 28-28). Most diverticula develop between the mesenteric and antimesenteric teniae coli. Smaller and fewer diverticula are found between the two antimesenteric teniae.

The cause of diverticulosis is unknown. There is some evidence that points to large bowel muscle wall abnormalities. The most striking change in the sigmoid colon affected by diverticulosis is thickening of the muscle wall. The greatly thickened circular muscle gives rise to corrugation inside the bowel lumen (Fig. 28-29). These muscle clefts are responsible for the sawtooth signs on barium enema studies. Histologic examination of the colonic muscle in diverticulosis reveals thickening but shows no evidence of either hyperplasia or hypertrophy of muscle cells. Simple diverticulosis without muscle thickening of the bowel wall is commonly seen by radiologists and surgeons, particularly in older persons (Fig. 28-30). There is no good explanation for this.

Painter et al. studied the colons of patients by means of simultaneous cineradiography and intraluminal pressure recordings. Contraction rings form in the sigmoid colon. These close the lumen, creating a series of "bladders," each of which has its outflow obstructed at either end. With contraction of the colonic muscle forming the wall of the segments, intraluminal pressures up to at least 90 mmHg are generated. Contraction of these closed segments creates a pulsion force that was observed to distend existing diverticula. This mechanism may well be responsible for the initial mucosal herniation.

Depletion of dietary fibers has been postulated to be responsible for the genesis of colonic diverticular disease. Painter theorizes that a narrow colon results from a diet low in fiber content and that a narrow colon can segment more efficiently than a colon of large bore and hence build up high localized pressures that may lead to diverticulosis. The higher incidence of diverticulosis in the older age group is probably due to deteriorating integrity of the bowel wall. Although collagen, elastin, and reticular tissues of the colonic wall increase with age, mechanical tests on postmortem colons show a decline in tensile strength with age. The tensile strength is lowest in the distal colon. Diverticulosis coli has been produced in the rat and rabbit by feeding them a low-residue diet, a diet similar to that of industrial societies.

Some workers have attempted to compare colonic motility on the basis of an index derived from measurements of colonic activity at rest, during stimulation with neostigmine (Prostigmin) or morphine, and after eating. Reports

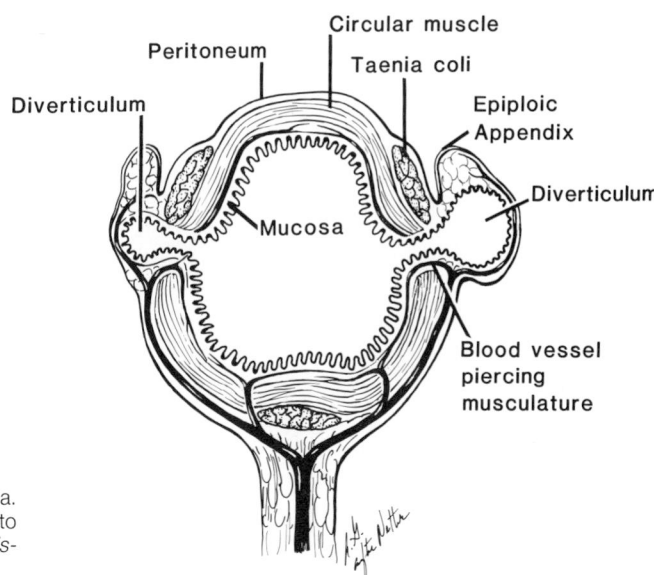

Fig. 28-28. Diverticulosis. Herniation of mucosa between two tenia. Note the point of weakness where main blood vessel passes into the mucosa. (From: *Nivatvongs S, Becker ER, 1987, with permission.*)

have varied from no difference in motility index to an increased motility index in patients with symptomatic diverticular disease. Bile salts stimulate colonic motility, and some workers have reported higher daily output in patients with diverticular disease compared with controls.

CLINICAL MANIFESTATIONS. Most patients with diverticula are asymptomatic and are only identified by barium enema or endoscopic examination. Although specific treatment is not indicated, it is reasonable to encourage these patients to be on a high-roughage diet, or a supple-

ment of bulk-producing agents such as raw wheat, bran, or psyllium seed.

Patients with symptoms can be divided into those with uncomplicated and those with complicated diverticular disease. This last group is a minority. Most symptoms and signs are the result of inflammation around diverticula, leading to acute diverticulitis, perforation, abscess and fistula formation, or stenosis. Diverticular hemorrhage is uncommon but it can cause massive colonic bleeding.

Painful Diverticular Disease

Many patients who have sigmoid diverticulosis with muscle abnormality develop left lower abdominal pain,

Fig. 28-29. Greatly thickened circular muscle causing corrugation inside the colonic lumen. (From: *Gallagher D, Russell TK: Surgical management of diverticular disease. Surg Clin North Am 58:563, 1987, with permission.*)

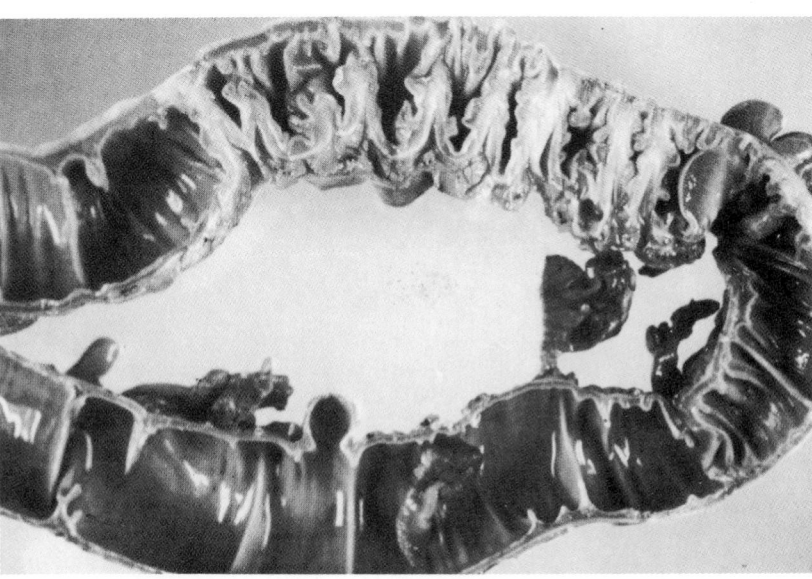

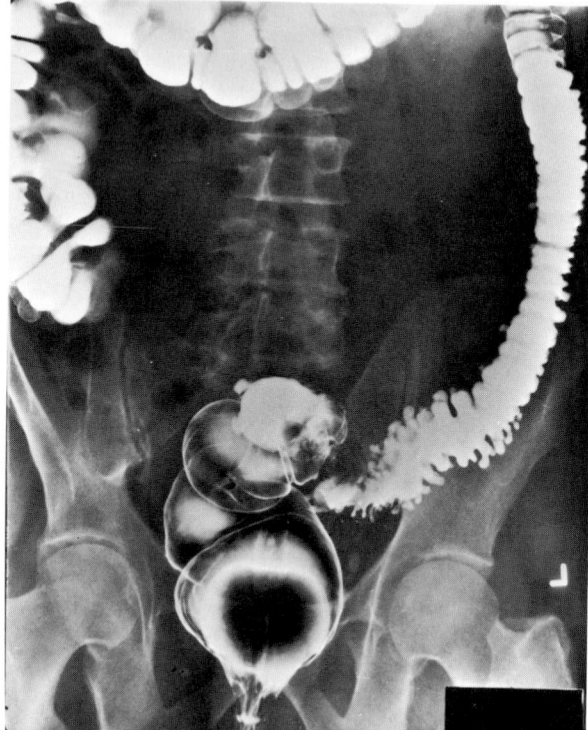

Fig. 28-30. Simple diverticulosis without muscle thickening. (From: *Nivatvongs S, Becker ER, 1987, with permission.*)

sometimes with palpable tenderness in the left lower quadrant. The symptoms may mimic diverticulitis except that there is no rebound tenderness, fever, or elevated white blood cell count. Unlike diverticulitis, the symptoms are chronic and often insidious. Change in bowel habits such as constipation and diarrhea can be experienced during attacks. The symptoms are believed to be from hyperactivity and hypersegmentation of the colon. Diagnosis depends on radiographic confirmation of spastic diverticulosis without features of acute inflammation. The symptoms of diverticular disease may be the same as the symptoms in irritable bowel syndrome.

Treatment is symptomatic. Morphine and codeine are avoided. In the acute situation, low-residue feedings are useful to decrease pain and spasm. In the nonacute phase, basic treatment is a bulk-producing agent in the form of psyllium seed or raw wheat bran. Occasionally, resection is necessary for chronic symptoms.

Diverticulitis

PATHOGENESIS. Diverticula readily fill with colonic contents, as evidenced by barium enema examination, but emptying is often slow because of the narrow neck and the lack of musculature of the diverticulum. If an inspissated fecal plug obstructs the neck of the diverticulum, continued mucus secretion and proliferation of ever-present bacteria distend the flask-shaped diverticulum and produce inflammation at the apex. This focal diverticulitis often resolves by discharge of the contents into the colonic lumen, but if the obstructing plug remains in place, inflammation spreads to peridiverticular tissues. Initial spread is to the pericolic fat between the muscularis propria and serosa. Extension is usually longitudinal in this plane, giving rise to intramural fistulas, which are one of the diagnostic signs of diverticulitis on barium enema (Fig. 28-31). Diverticulitis is thought to start as inflammation of a single diverticulum; other diverticula may become secondarily involved as edema from the initial diverticulitis narrows their necks, preventing emptying and thus initiating another inflammatory focus. Berman and associates have presented evidence that actual perforation of a single diverticulum is the initiating event, followed by an inflammatory focus in the pericolic fat.

DIAGNOSIS. Although diverticulosis can involve the entire colon, infection of a diverticulum is usually in the sigmoid colon, and more than one diverticulum is rarely involved. The diagnosis of acute diverticulitis is aided by a history of previous demonstration of diverticulosis with barium enema radiography. The clinical picture of sigmoid diverticulitis so resembles appendicitis that it is often called "left-sided appendicitis." The patient presents with sudden onset of left-sided abdominal pain, fever, and an elevated white blood cell count. The diagnosis is made entirely on clinical grounds. Flat plate abdominal films and/or a gentle limited Gastrografin enema should be done if perforation is suspected. Enemas, barium studies, laxatives, and colonoscopy should be postponed until the acute symptoms have subsided for fear of perforation.

TREATMENT. The patient should be admitted to the hospital. Nonoperative therapy should be instituted for the first attack of uncomplicated diverticulitis. A clear liquid diet is allowed unless there are signs of ileus or bowel obstruction. A single agent broad spectrum antibiotic or combination therapy with an aminoglycoside and a drug effective against anaerobes is given intravenously. Morphine and codeine should be avoided. Meperidine is used as needed. As soon as the fever has subsided, a contrast x-ray may be obtained. Gastrografin enema shows segmental spasm with serrations (sawtoothing) of the bowel in the area of the disease. Mucosal edema, fixation of the bowel, and narrowing of the lumen may be present. On x-ray, diverticulitis may be difficult to differentiate from cancer, but the following features are suggestive of diverticulitis: (1) involvement of a long segment of bowel, (2) spasm, (3) presence of diverticula elsewhere in the bowel, and (4) tapered or conical ends in the bowel segment involved. Occasionally the contrast enema will show a leak into an abscess cavity or a fistula into an adjacent organ. As soon as the fever is gone and there is no evidence of bowel obstruction, regular diet and a bulk-producing agent such as psyllium seed or raw wheat bran should be started to prevent hypersegmentation of the sigmoid colon. Endoscopic examination at a later time when all inflammation has subsided should be considered to exclude carcinoma.

Surgical therapy of diverticulitis is reserved for complications, for those patients who fail to respond to medical therapy, for recurrent episodes of acute diverticulitis, and

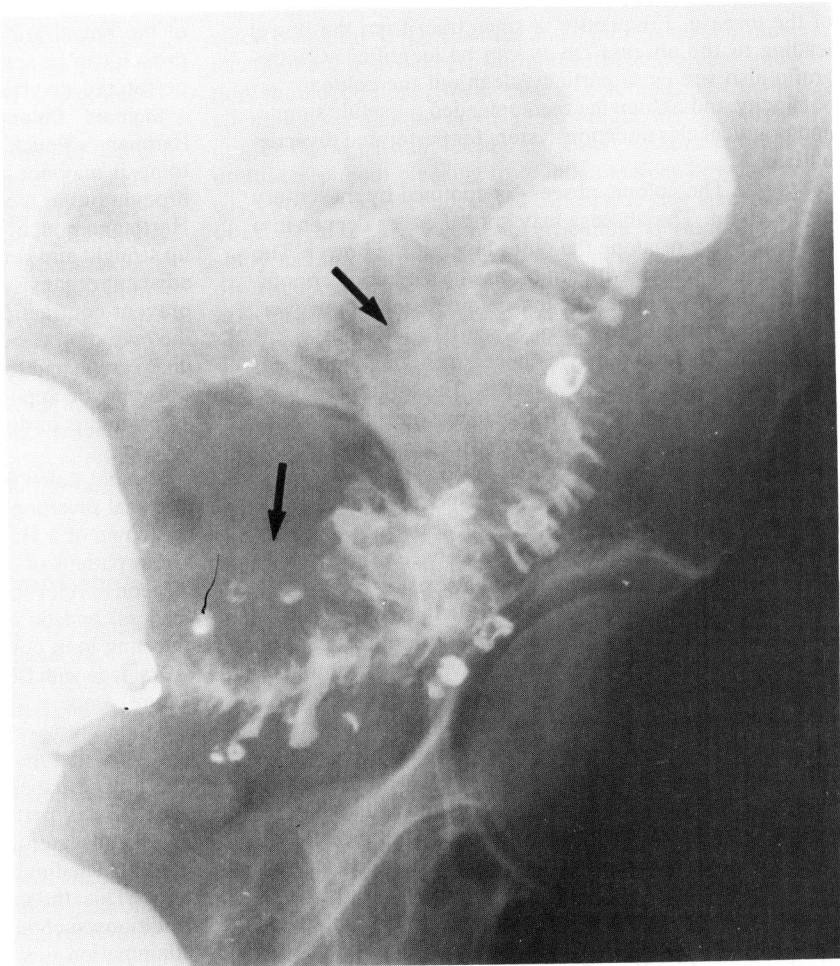

Fig. 28-31. Barium radiograph of diverticulitis of sigmoid colon. Note long length of involvement. Arrows point to intramural abscesses.

if carcinoma cannot be excluded. Of patients who require operation, half do so due to repeated attacks that do not respond to medical therapy. These patients may undergo elective resection of the involved segment of colon with very low operative risk. The remaining 50 to 60 percent of patients who require surgical intervention undergo an emergency procedure for one of the complications: perforation (30 to 35 percent), fistula (10 to 15 percent), obstruction (10 percent), and bleeding (6 to 10 percent).

The difference in mortality between elective and emergency surgery in patients with diverticulitis has led many surgeons to urge earlier elective resection in patients who have repeated episodes of local tenderness in the left lower quadrant, a persistent mass, marked narrowing on roentgenologic examination, or lesions difficult to differentiate from cancer.

Elective colectomy is curative and may be carried out with minimal risk to the patient. The operative technique differs from resections for cancer in that only the involved segment of colon need be removed and extensive mesenteric dissection is unnecessary. Resection should be extended to the nonperitonealized rectum distally. Proximal resection should include all thickened muscle. Anastomotic complications are somewhat more common than after operations for cancer because edema and thickening of the bowel may be present. A one-stage resection is the usual procedure. Recurrence rates of 11 percent have been reported, especially when the resection did not extend distally to the extraperitoneal rectum.

PERFORATED DIVERTICULITIS

DIAGNOSIS. Symptoms of perforated diverticulitis vary depending on severity of the infection. The usual presentation is a rather sudden onset of left lower quadrant pain associated with tenderness, fever, leukocytosis, and, frequently, dehydration and tachycardia.

Abdominal x-ray is not specific, unless there is a free perforation, which is uncommon. Differential diagnosis includes perforated appendicitis, perforated viscus, bowel obstruction, mesenteric vascular insufficiency, and ruptured abdominal aortic aneurysm. During the attack, barium enema studies and colonoscopy are contraindicated. Gastrografin enema without using pressure is very helpful to confirm the diagnosis and to evaluate the extent

Cystoscopy is the most important and the most accurate procedure to diagnose colovesical fistula. Fistulogram via the cystoscope is highly successful in demonstrating the fistula to the colon. Biopsy can also be taken if carcinoma is suspected. Cystogram rarely demonstrates the fistula. Barium enema studies should be done to evaluate the extent of the sigmoid diverticular disease but define the fistula in only 25 percent of the cases. After gastrointestinal barium studies the urine may be collected and centrifuged and examined for barium sediment by x-ray. Proctoscopy, flexible sigmoidoscopy, or colonoscopy is performed to rule out associated colonic lesions but rarely demonstrates the fistula. Intravenous pyelogram is not helpful in the diagnosis of the fistula but may be useful to rule out abnormalities of the urinary tract. Charcoal ingestion with subsequent examination of the urine may be helpful, but false-positive results from perineal contamination in females have been reported. Methylene blue enemas have been used with success but must be interpreted with caution. The positive urine examination for methylene blue could be a result of the absorption of the dye from the rectum subsequently excreted into the urine. CT is not useful to document the fistula.

TREATMENT. Colovesical fistula, as a rule, does not present as an acute abdomen. Sepsis, if present, is usually due to an underlying urinary tract infection. This must be adequately treated immediately. Occasionally, a pelvic abscess is also present and responsible for sepsis. Percutaneous drainage via CT guidance is usually possible. Once sepsis is under control, the operation can be scheduled on a more elective basis.

Rectosigmoid and sigmoid colon resection is the definitive treatment for most cases of diverticular disease complicated by a fistula. Bowel preparation is usually possible and thus a primary anastomosis can be safely done with little morbidity. A potential complication during operation is injury of the ureter. If difficulty is anticipated, particularly when a mass is palpable, ureteral catheters should be inserted via cystoscopy before the laparotomy begins. Usually, one can "pinch off" the fistula site and separate the involved segment of colon from the organ secondarily involved by the fistula. If dealing with a coloenteric fistula, the small bowel site can be oversewn or the edges of the inflammation excised and a primary repair performed. Resection of the small bowel is rarely necessary.

For colovaginal or colouterine fistulas, nothing need be done to the secondary opening. Similarly, for colovesical fistulas, the opening in the bladder usually need not be closed since it will spontaneously heal after the sigmoid diverticular disease is resected, provided that a Foley catheter is left in the bladder for at least one week. Closure of the bladder fistula in the presence of significant inflammation often is insecure and risks injury to the ureteral orifices. If the circumstance dictates, such as an unprepared bowel or marked inflammation of the colonic wall, a sigmoid colon resection is carried out, exteriorizing the proximal end as a colostomy and closing the distal end as a Hartmann pouch. In rare instances, when the inflammatory mass is so severe that resection cannot be safely done, a transverse colostomy is performed and the inflammatory mass adequately drained. A few months later, the inflamed colon is resected. The final stage is to close the colostomy.

In selected patients, especially elderly or high-risk patients, with minimal or no urinary tract sepsis and no evidence of distal colon obstruction in whom carcinoma has been excluded, nonoperative treatment using antibiotics to suppress urinary tract infection is a viable option.

Diverticulum of the Right Colon

The cecum and ascending colon infrequently are involved in diverticulosis coli. Even more uncommon is a solitary true diverticulum, usually called *cecal diverticulitis,* that is found only in the cecum or ascending colon. In contrast to the false diverticula of diverticulosis coli, solitary cecal diverticula contain all layers of the bowel wall and are, therefore, true diverticula. Because of this and because these lesions are found in younger individuals, they are considered to be congenital in origin. The condition is more common among the native Hawaiian population.

Symptoms are produced in the same manner as in diverticulitis coli or acute appendicitis. The ostium of the diverticulum becomes obstructed by a plug of feces or fecalith, creating a miniature closed loop. Inflammation ensues from continued secretion within the diverticulum and infection by resident bacteria.

DIAGNOSIS. Clinical manifestations of acture cecal diverticulitis are essentially identical to those of acute appendicitis. The true nature of the lesion may be suspected if there is a history of numerous frequent episodes of similar attacks. The correct diagnosis is made preoperatively in only about 5 percent of patients, nearly always by barium enema demonstration of the diverticulum. The preoperative diagnosis is acute appendicitis in about 80 percent, tumor in about 5 percent.

TREATMENT. The operative procedure is determined by the findings. If inflammation is limited to the diverticulum, then simple diverticulectomy with inversion of the stump is done as for appendicitis. Ruptured diverticulum with abscess is treated by drainage and removal of the diverticulum if it can easily be done; otherwise only drainage is performed, and interval diverticulectomy is carried out later. When inflammation involves the cecum also, resection of diverticulum and adjacent cecum is indicated if the cecal closure is through healthy tissue, and the ileocecal valve is not encroached upon. When the cecum is extensively involved, terminal ileum and cecum are resected with ileo-ascending colon anastomosis. If frank peritonitis is present, ileo-ascending colectomy, cutaneous ileostomy, and creation of a transverse colon mucous fistula should be done because of the risk of primary anastomosis in this situation. Chronic diverticular disease with extensive productive inflammation and fibrosis may be indistinguishable from neoplasm at the operating table. Right colectomy with ileo-transverse colostomy as for cancer is indicated.

No treatment is indicated for asymptomatic cecal diverticula that are an incidental finding on barium enema. Diverticula found incidentally at operation should be removed if their removal does not add significantly to the risk of the primary procedure.

MEGACOLON

The term *megacolon,* meaning large colon, also implies chronic dilation, elongation, and hypertrophy of the colon. Megacolon may be congenital or acquired. Acquired megacolon may be due to organic causes or may be idiopathic. The common denominator in megacolon is chronic partial colon obstruction with associated chronic constipation. In general, the degree of megacolon is proportional to the duration of the partial obstruction. Megacolon is of interest to surgeons not only because many patients require surgical correction but also because of their propensity for volvulus.

Congenital Megacolon (Hirschsprung's Disease) (See Chap. 39)

This disease is due to congenital absence of ganglion cells in the myenteric plexus of the bowel. The rectosigmoid is frequently involved, but the aganglionosis is sometimes more extensive, even involving the entire colon. The functional defect is the inability of the aganglionic segment to relax to allow a peristaltic wave to pass, thus producing a functional partial obstruction with proximal retention of feces, which in turn causes megacolon above the aganglionic segment. This is primarily a disease of infants and children but occasionally may not become manifest until later in life. It is therefore advisable, whenever performing operations for megacolon or volvulus, to have a frozen section of colon examined for ganglion cells.

A different form of megacolon that may be congenital has been reported to occur in certain areas of the world, such as Eastern Europe and Okinawa, where the vegetable diets are high in roughage and residue. It is not clear whether the unusually large, long colon is acquired by the individual as an adaptation to the high-residue diet or whether this is a hereditary characteristic that was selected in the evolutionary process because of its adaptive significance.

Acquired Megacolon

Chagas' disease is caused by infection with a protozoan, *Trypanosoma cruzi,* and is endemic in South and Central America. Megacolon, one of the complications of the chronic form of the disease, is attributable to widespread destruction of the intramural nervous system. Surgical therapy is sometimes necessary for severe constipation, recurring fecal impaction, or volvulus. Subtotal colectomy with ileoproctostomy is probably the procedure of choice, though some surgeons prefer abdominoendoanal rectosigmoidectomy.

Acquired organic megacolon results also from partial mechanical obstruction of the lower colon, rectum, or anus. More common causes are postoperative anorectal stricture; lymphogranuloma venereum (lymphopathia venereum); endometriosis; radiation proctitis; and anorectal injury, either accidental or from sexual perversion. Treatment is aimed at the offending stricture. The secondary megacolon regresses toward, but not to, normal when the primary cause is removed.

Megacolon is also seen in association with neurologic disorders such as paraplegia or poliomyelitis. Constipation is a problem because the contribution of the voluntary muscles to the defecatory act is lost. If constipation is avoided by the use of enemas and stool softeners, megacolon is avoided.

Acute dilatation of the colon, as seen in fulminating colitis, septic shock, prolonged adynamic ileus, or diabetes, has no relationship to chronic megacolon.

Megacolon is frequent in institutionalized psychotic patients. No organic cause has been found, and it is referred to as psychogenic or idiopathic megacolon. Severe constipation, because of extreme inactivity and perhaps voluntary inhibition of defecation, is presumed to be the principal cause. Psychogenic megacolon has also been seen in young children, presumably as an extension of problems with bowel training. Colectomy for megacolon is occasionally justified in these patients. If sigmoid volvulus occurs in patients with megacolon, subtotal colectomy to "straighten out" the colon is preferable to sigmoid segmental colectomy.

FECAL IMPACTION

Impaction is the arrest and accumulation of feces in the rectum or colon. Feces are progressively dehydrated by the colonic mucosa the longer they remain in the colon. When normal progression of feces does not occur, the hard dry fecal mass is increased in size as more feces are pushed downward from above. Retained barium after radiographic studies and calcium carbonate used as ulcer therapy frequently contribute to fecal impactions. With dehydration these substances attain a consistency resembling concrete.

Many of the patients with chronic constipation (discussed under Acquired Megacolon) frequently have impactions. A common cause in otherwise healthy persons is an acute painful lesion of the anus—fissures, fistulas, thrombosed external hemorrhoids, or recent anorectal surgical therapy.

CLINICAL MANIFESTATIONS. The most common symptom of a rectal impaction is the passage of frequent loose stools without relief of the sense of rectal urgency and fullness. This is "overflow" evacuation around a partial obstruction. Marked rectal urgency but inability to defecate is also common. In patients who have lost rectal sensation, as occurs in paraplegia or spina bifida, or in psychotics, there may be no symptoms of fecal impactions until a complication supervenes.

Infrequently, full-blown mechanical obstruction of the colon is the presenting picture. A rare but serious complication may occur when the fecal impaction does not obstruct completely and allows overflow evacuation to occur. The unmoving hard mass eventually erodes the mucosa with production of a stercoral ulcer. If the ulcer is in the rectum, serious bleeding may ensue; if in the abdominal colon, perforation with spreading fecal peritonitis may develop. Management of this complication is the same as for perforated diverticulitis.

Diagnosis is usually easily made by digital rectal examination. If the impaction is higher, large, hard fecal masses can be palpated in the colon. These masses can also be seen on plain radiographs of the abdomen.

TREATMENT. Unless a complication is present, fecal impaction is treated by instillation of tap water enema. This will usually soften the stool sufficiently that it can be passed. If defecation still does not occur, impaction must be broken up and delivered digitally. It is helpful in female patients to exert gentle digital pressure on the rectal mass through the rectovaginal septum with two fingers in the vagina while the mass is delivered through the anus with the other hand. If a painful anal condition is present, hot sitz baths and an anesthetic ointment often relieve the spasm and permit defecation.

VOLVULUS

Volvulus of the colon is a twisting of a segment of the colon about its mesentery (Fig. 28-32). It requires a redundant colon with a narrow mesentery at its base, and

Fig. 28-32. Sigmoid volvulus. (From: *Nivatvongs S, Becker ER, 1987, with permission.*)

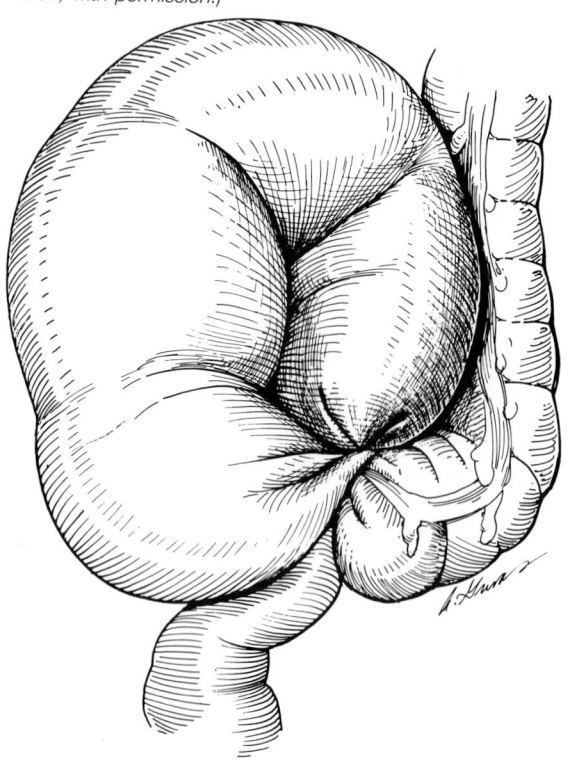

distention with air. Volvulus almost never occurs when the colon is filled with solid stool. Volvulus of the colon may spontaneously reduce and recur as a chronic problem, but more frequently the colon becomes acutely obstructed, which may lead to strangulation and gangrene if not treated. Although a common cause of bowel obstruction in Asia and Africa, volvulus of the colon is uncommon in the United States, accounting for only 3 percent of the cases of large bowel obstruction.

Sigmoid Volvulus

This is the most common type in the United States, accounting for about 90 percent of the cases of volvulus of the colon. In this country, most patients are the elderly from institutions or nursing homes. Colonic dysfunction associated with chronic constipation probably predisposes to volvulus.

DIAGNOSIS. The patients present with acute abdominal pain and distention. The symptoms rapidly progress to generalized abdominal pain and tenderness. If gangrene is present, fever and high white blood cell count will be apparent. Another group of patients, usually older, have had a long previous history of intermittent abdominal pain and distention and intermittent chronic volvulus.

Plain x-ray films of the abdomen reveal markedly dilated loops of large bowel forming the so-called bent inner tube or omega loop sign, with the convexity of the loop lying away from the site of obstruction. Pointing toward the obstruction is the so-called bird's beak, a narrowing of the air-filled colon.

Two air-fluid levels are almost always seen within the sigmoid loop. Gastrografin enema characteristically shows a narrowing at the site of torsion with "spiraling" of the mucosal folds and the pathognomonic "bird's beak" (Fig. 28-33) or "ace of spades" deformity. Barium enema is contraindicated when gangrene is suspected, because of the danger of perforation of the necrotic segment.

MANAGEMENT. Unless there are obvious signs of gangrene or perforation, the initial management after the appropriate resuscitation is proctoscopic decompression with a rectal tube. If frank mucosal ulceration, slough, or dark blood is seen, strangulated obstruction is probable, and emergency operative intervention is indicated. If no signs of strangulation are seen, a well-lubricated long rectal tube is gently advanced via the sigmoidoscope through the obstructing twist into the distended sigmoid loop. Dramatic deflation usually results. The tube may be secured in place in the loop and left in place for two or three days, until bowel function resumes. Patients must be closely watched for signs of gangrenous bowel, which is present occasionally but unrecognized at the time of tube deflation. The success rate is about 70 percent. More recently the colonoscope has been used with success to reduce the volvulus.

If proctoscopic reduction is successful, further treatment should be considered because of the extremely high recurrence rate (33 to 60 percent). Elective resection with primary anastomosis should be done as soon as the pa-

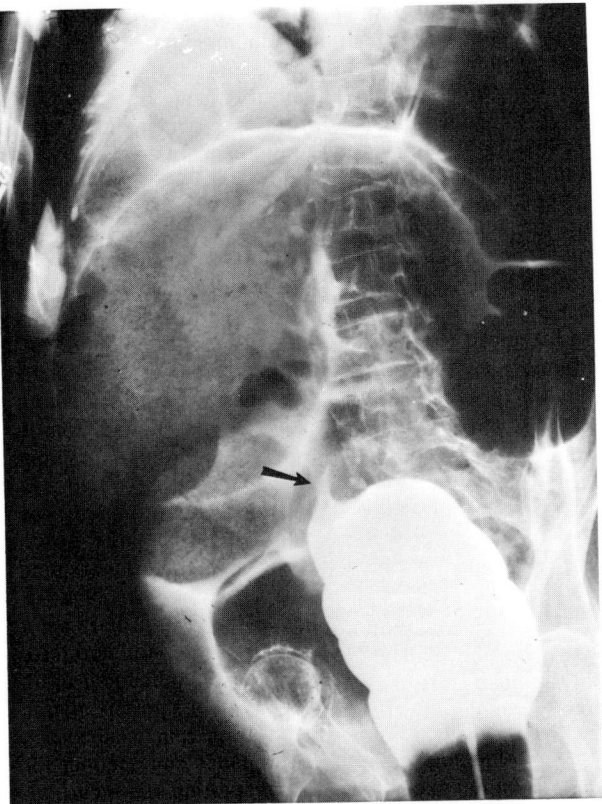

Fig. 28-33. ''Bird-beak'' sign (arrow) on Gastrografin enema in sigmoid volvulus. (From: *Nivatvongs S, Becker ER, 1987, with permission.*)

tient can be properly prepared, preferably within a week or so, because the risk of recurrent volvulus is so great. Not infrequently, the volvulus recurs while the patient is being prepared for elective resection.

Unsuccessful detorsion of sigmoid volvulus by rectal tube or colonoscopy may indicate strangulation or gangrene and an immediate exploratory celiotomy is indicated. Nonviable colon must be resected. The proximal end is brought out as a colostomy and the distal end closed as a Hartmann pouch. If the sigmoid colon is viable, resection with or without anastomosis is considered based on the condition of the colon and the patient.

The mortality rate for elective sigmoid colon resection is less than 10 percent. Emergency sigmoid colon resection for nongangrenous sigmoid colon is associated with a mortality of about 12 percent. When the colon is gangrenous, a 50 percent mortality is reported.

Cecal Volvulus

In cadaver studies, about 10 to 20 percent of people have a freely mobile right colon and are possible candidates to develop cecal volvulus. This is much less frequent than sigmoid volvulus. Rotation of the hypermobile cecum, usually 360° or up to 720° around the mesenteric pedicle of the ileocolic artery, produces a closed-loop obstruction. Circulatory impairment of the loop is fre-

quent and occurs early in the course. Cecal volvulus can occur simultaneously with sigmoid volvulus.

DIAGNOSIS. The clinical picture of cecal volvulus is that of a small bowel obstruction. If gangrene develops, an acute abdomen is apparent. Abdominal x-ray examination reveals a dilated large bowel filled with gas, and the cecum can be seen anywhere in the abdomen. The findings can be confused with ileus or acute pseudo-obstruction of the colum. The small bowel is usually dilated with gas to a variable degree. Characteristically a large midabdominal ovoid dilated segment is seen, with distended small bowel loops and a relatively empty large bowel. The diagnosis should be confirmed by Gastrografin enema, which has the benefit of cleaning out the colon as well.

MANAGEMENT. Once diagnosed, exploratory celiotomy should be done. There have been sporadic reports of colonoscopic detorsion of cecal volvulus.

For gangrenous bowel, a right hemicolectomy is indicated, with or without primary anastomosis. If the bowel is viable, there is controversy as to the choice of operation. Many authors recommend simple detorsion with cecopexy and/or cecostomy. The definitive treatment is a right hemicolectomy and, in the majority of patients, a primary anastomosis can be done. The mortality in cecal volvulus with gangrenous bowel is about 30 to 40 percent, compared with about 10 to 15 percent if the bowel is viable.

Transverse colon volvulus is unusual, and radiograms are suggestive of sigmoid volvulus. The point of obstruction is defined by barium enema. Resection is preferred to detorsion because of the high recurrence rate. Colonoscopy is technically difficult, but it can detorse the bowel. The operative mortality is as high as 33 percent.

MISCELLANEOUS BENIGN LESIONS

Angiodysplasia

Angiodysplasia was recognized only after the introduction of selective angiography. The lesions are not visible on macroscopic examination of resected specimens but can be demonstrated on histologic examination after injection of the specimen with silicone rubber and barium paste compounds. They are usually only a few millimeters in size and consist of dilated submucosal vascular spaces. Mucosal involvement may occur, and arteriovenous shunts have been described. The lesions almost always are located in the cecum and ascending colon.

Angiodysplasia is thought to be an acquired condition, possibly due to degeneration of blood vessel walls. The disease is usually seen in older individuals, although young adults may be affected. It has been suggested that venous congestion due to increased intramural muscle tension may lead to dilatation of submucosal veins, and it may be that the association between right-sided diverticular disease and bleeding is due to coexisting angiodysplasia.

DIAGNOSIS. Patients often give a history of previous gastrointestinal bleeding. When bleeding is minor and intermittent, the diagnosis should be considered in any patient with a normal barium enema examination. Colonoscopy may reveal a small area of tortuous dilated submucosal vessels or of nonulcerated reddening.

Persistent minor bleeding with a normal colonoscopy is an indication for gastroscopy and small bowel contrast radiography. If these are normal, selective angiography should be carried out to demonstrate a lesion in the area of distribution of the blood vessels to the right colon.

In patients who present with major bleeding, emergency colonoscopy has been advocated by some endoscopists, but others have not found it helpful since vision is often obscured by blood. When aspiration of gastric contents reveals no blood, selective angiography is the investigation of choice. Preliminary barium studies are contraindicated since residual barium will mask any features on the angiogram. The site of an actively bleeding lesion may be seen as a blush of extravasated contrast if the rate of blood loss is over about 1 mL/min. Radiolabeled red cell scintigraphy has been used to localize the site.

TREATMENT. Treatment is by surgical resection. In the elective case, right hemicolectomy will satisfactorily remove the lesion. A total colectomy is the operation of choice in cases of acute hemorrhage that has failed to stop spontaneously and in which a specific lesion has not been defined.

Endometriosis

Progressive involvement of the colonic or rectal wall with endometriosis may initiate luminal obstruction that may be partial or complete. In the colon, especially the sigmoid, endometrial nodules may implant and proliferate to initiate complete obstruction. Ectopic endometrium in the cul-de-sac of Douglas may cause dense adherence of the anterior rectal wall to the posterior uterus. Colonic obstructive symptoms are rare, as the rectal diameter is large enough to obviate these symptoms. Dyspareunia, tenesmus, or bowel irritability symptoms may be present. Hematochezia is uncommon. Typically, this presentation occurs in the reproductive age group and is rare in the postmenopausal patient.

DIAGNOSIS. Diagnosis is usually established by history and the symptoms of menstrual irregularity and exaggerated cyclic menstrual pain. The finding in bimanual pelvic examination of tender endometrial nodules in the rectovaginal septum or the cul-de-sac is classic. The presence of a solitary mass in the rectosigmoid and the absence of disease in the cul-de-sac makes the diagnosis of endometriosis dubious. Palpation of the mass initiates pain, characteristically absent in carcinomatous lesions. Submucosal biopsy should be attempted but may not be diagnostic when the endometrial implant occupies a deep submucosal or submuscularis position in the bowel wall. Laparoscopic examination is of value if uterine, pelvic, or peritoneal implants can be visualized and biopsied. An intramural submucosal lesion may be noted on air contrast barium enema study.

TREATMENT. Treatment aimed at medical control of the estrogen-sensitive endometrial implants may initiate complete regression of the colorectal symptoms. The antigonadotropin compound danazol (Danocrine) has effectively controlled the pelvic and abdominal symptoms via feedback inhibition of the pituitary-ovarian stimuli common with cyclic proliferation of the endometriomas. The side effects of this drug in the moderately high doses (400 to 800 mg twice daily for 3 to 6 months) that are necessary to control the symptoms represent a detracting feature. As patients approach menopause, endometrial symptoms commonly begin to regress. Resolution of the pelvic and colonic symptoms may be complete following surgical castration. For individuals who fail hormonal medical therapy, or in whom previous surgical excision has been unsuccessful, limited surgical resection of the involved colorectal segment is indicated, with restoration of intestinal continuity.

Lipoma

Lipomas are benign neoplasms that commonly present in the colon. Most often their origin is near the ileocecal valve, but they can be distributed throughout the colorectal submucosa. Lipomas may initiate symptoms of bleeding, incomplete obstruction, and intussusception. These lesions may be resected endoscopically; however, sleeve (segmental) resections are indicated for large lesions not amenable to endoscopic removal.

POLYPS

Polyp is a nonspecific clinical term that describes any projection from the surface of the intestinal mucosa regardless of its histologic nature. Polyps can be conveniently classified according to their histologic appearance:

1. Neoplastic: tubular adenoma, villous adenoma, and tubulovillous adenoma
2. Hamartomatous: juvenile, Peutz-Jeghers, Cronkhite-Canada
3. Inflammatory: inflammatory or pseudopolyp, benign lymphoid polyp
4. Unclassified: hyperplastic (metaplastic)

Neoplastic Polyps

Tubular adenomas (Fig. 28-34) account for 75 percent of all neoplastic polyps, villous adenomas (Fig. 28-35) account for 10 percent, and tubulovillous adenomas (Fig. 28-36) 15 percent. The malignant potential of neoplastic polyps is related to the type and size of the polyp. The malignant rate for tubular adenomas is 5 percent, compared with 40 percent for villous adenomas and 22 percent for tubulovillous adenomas. Invasive carcinomas are uncommon in polyps smaller than 1 cm in diameter and the incidence increases with the increase in size.

Some benign neoplastic polyps will transform into cancers. This theory can be supported by findings of benign

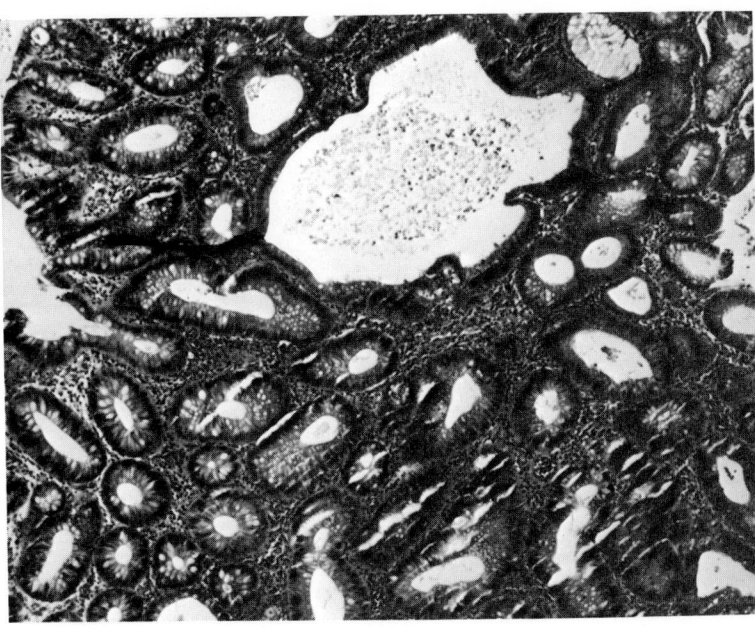

Fig. 28-34. Tubular adenoma.

adenomatous tissues in continuity with a cancer. In early cancers invading the submucosa, benign adenomatous tissues can be found in 57 percent of the cases. With the spread of cancers into the muscle wall, benign adenomatous tissues can be seen in 18 percent, and when the invasion is through the bowel wall they can be seen in 8 percent. It is likely that as carcinomas spread through the bowel wall, they tend to destroy the surviving benign tumor. The concept that most cancers of the large bowel evolved from isolated adenomas is called the *polyp-cancer* or the *adenoma-carcinoma sequence*. Polypectomy is thus prophylactic for the development of large bowel cancers and in some instances, therapeutic as well. It has been shown by Gilbertsen that removal of rectal polyps in patients under surveillance results in a lower than expected incidence of rectal cancer.

DIAGNOSIS. Adenomas of the large bowel are usually asymptomatic and are frequently discovered on routine barium enema studies or endoscopic examinations. Bleeding per rectum is the most common symptom if the polyp is situated in the rectum or sigmoid colon. A large pedunculated polyp in the lower part of the rectum may prolapse through the anus. A large villous adenoma may manifest as watery diarrhea, and in rare instances cause fluid and electrolyte imbalance. Intermittent abdominal pain from recurrent intussusception or spasm with a large colonic polyp may occur but is unusual. Mild anemia may follow chronic bleeding from an ulcerative polyp.

Proctosigmoidoscopy examination is an incomplete surveillance. Neoplastic polyps are often multiple, and associated cancers are found in a small percentage of patients. Once a polyp is detected, a complete examination of the large bowel is indicated. This can be done with proctoscopy or flexible sigmoidoscopy followed by air contrast barium enema or total colonoscopy.

The risk of cancer is significant in polyps larger than 1 cm in diameter, and polypectomy should be performed. Carcinoma in polyps smaller than 1 cm in diameter is uncommon but does occur. Questions often arise whether these lesions should be removed. It is recommended that all large-bowel polyps be removed unless difficulty or risk is anticipated. The rationale for their removal is to eliminate the small risk that cancer exists in these small polyps and to eliminate the potential future development of cancer in such polyps.

Fig. 28-35. Villous adenoma.

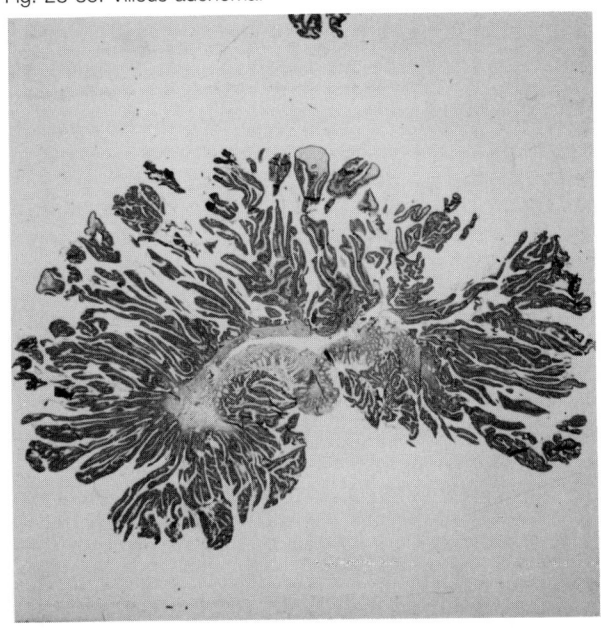

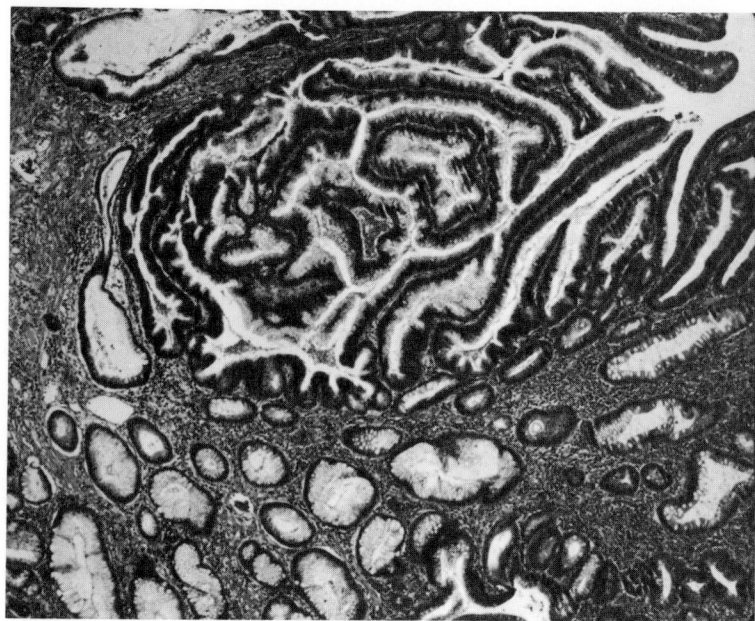

Fig. 28-36. Tubulovillous adenoma, mixture of tubular and villous glands.

MANAGEMENT. Fiberoptic colonoscopy has revolutionized the management of large bowel polyps. Most benign polyps throughout the entire colon and rectum can be excised via the colonoscope with minimal morbidity. Colon resection is reserved for cases in which colonoscopic polypectomy cannot be done, such as lesions that are too large or too flat or when the colonoscope cannot be passed to the site of the polyp.

Most pedunculated polyps can be snared in one piece since the size of the pedicles is rarely larger than 2 cm in diameter. Sessile polyps smaller than 2 cm can usually be snared in one piece. Large sessile polyps should be snared piecemeal and, at times, in more than one session.

It is important that excised polyps are properly prepared and sectioned so that all the layers can be examined microscopically.

Management of Polyps with Invasive Carcinoma

The term invasive carcinoma is applied only when the cancer cells have invaded through the muscularis mucosa of the polyp (Fig. 28-37.) Carcinoma of the mucosa is called *carcinoma in situ* or *superficial carcinoma*. For this type of lesion, complete excision is all that is necessary since it does not metastasize.

Polyps with invasive carcinoma metastasize to lymph

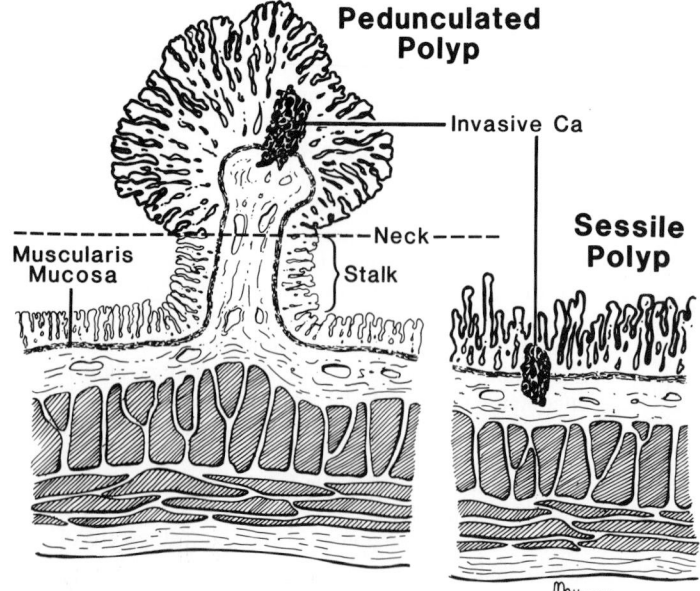

Fig. 28-37. Anatomic landmarks of colon and rectal polyps. Definition of invasive carcinoma. Cancer cells have invaded the muscularis mucosal layer. [From: *Nivatvongs S: Management of polyps containing invasive carcinoma, in IJ Kodner, RD Fry, JP Roe (eds): Colon, Rectal, and Anal Surgery: Current Technique and Controversies. St Louis, Mosby, 1985, chap 15, Fig 15-1, p 174, with permission.*]

nodes in 9 percent of cases. The risk varies according to the type of lesion. In sessile polyps with invasive carcinoma, the incidence of lymph node metastasis is 15 percent and the incidence of residual tumor after snaring is 6 percent, a failure rate of 21 percent. Bowel resection is indicated in these lesions unless the patient is a high operative risk.

In pedunculated polyps with invasive carcinoma, the incidence of lymph node metastasis and residual tumor are 7.8 and 2.3 percent respectively, a failure rate of 10 percent. If these lesions are further divided into those in which carcinomas are limited to the head of the polyps and those in which carcinoma has invaded to the neck of the stalk, it becomes apparent that the risk is much higher in the latter group. In pedunculated polyps with invasive carcinoma into the neck of the stalk, the incidence of lymph node metastasis is 20 percent, and bowel resection is usually indicated. If the invasion is limited to only the head of the polyps, the risk of lymph node metastasis is only 3 percent.

Hamartomatous Polyps

Juvenile polyp is the characteristic polyp of children but may present at any age. This lesion is a hamartoma and is not precancerous. The cut section shows a characteristic "Swiss cheese" appearance from dilated cystic spaces. Dilated glands are filled with mucus, and the lamina propria has a mesenchymal appearance (Fig. 28-38). The muscularis mucosa does not participate in the structure of the polyp. Bleeding per rectum is a common finding. A moderate amount of bleeding can occur if the polyp is autoamputated, a phenomenon not seen in other types of polyps. Intussusception of the colon occasionally occurs if the polyp is large. Treatment is by excision or snaring via colonoscope or sigmoidoscope.

Familial juvenile polyposis coli is a recognized entity in which there are hundreds or even thousands of polyps distributed throughout the entire colon and rectum and with occasional involvement of the stomach and small bowel. It has an autosomal dominant inheritance. Rectal bleeding is the most common symptom. Prolapse or protrusion of rectal mass, intestinal or colonic intussusception, abdominal pain, diarrhea, and protein loss can also be present. Unlike solitary juvenile polyps, which are not premalignant, diffuse juvenile polyposis can degenerate into adenomas and, eventually, carcinoma. Sometimes adenomatous polyps coexist in the same patient. The treatment is subtotal colectomy with ileorectal anastomosis. If the rectum is carpeted with the polyps, total proctocolectomy and ileostomy or an ileal pouch and pull-through procedure is indicated.

Peutz-Jeghers syndrome was originally described by Peutz in 1921, but it was not clearly identified until Jeghers in 1949 brought it to attention. The syndrome consists of melanin spots on the buccal mucosa and lips—the face and digits may be involved to a variable extent, but the mouth pigmentation is the sine qua non of this portion of the syndrome; the presence of polyps in the small bowel is the constant finding of this syndrome, but

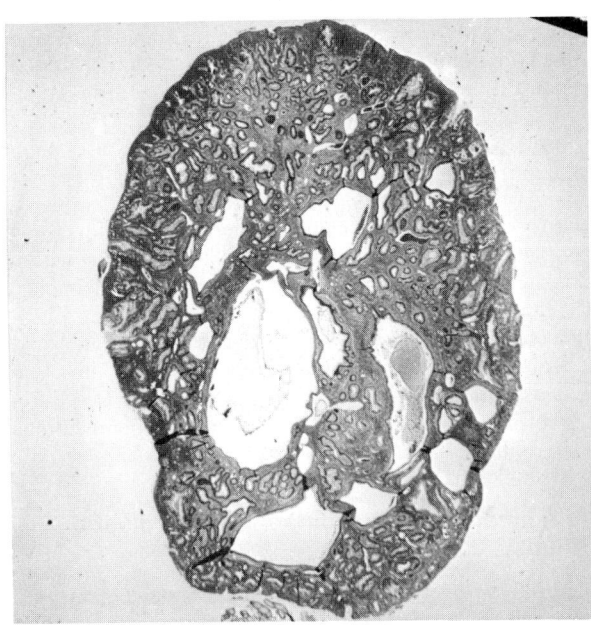

Fig. 28-38. Juvenile of retention polyp. Note Swiss-cheese appearance from dilated glands.

the stomach, colon, and rectum may also be involved. The characteristic picture of Peutz-Jeghers polyps is an abnormal muscularis branching into the lamina propria, giving the appearance of a Christmas tree (Fig. 28-39). It is considered a hamartoma, which, in general, should not degenerate into malignancy. In the past several years, however, there have been a few documented cases of Peutz-Jeghers polyps that have become invasive adenocarcinomas.

Fig. 28-39. Peutz-Jeghers polyp. Note Christmas tree appearance from branching of muscularis mucosa.

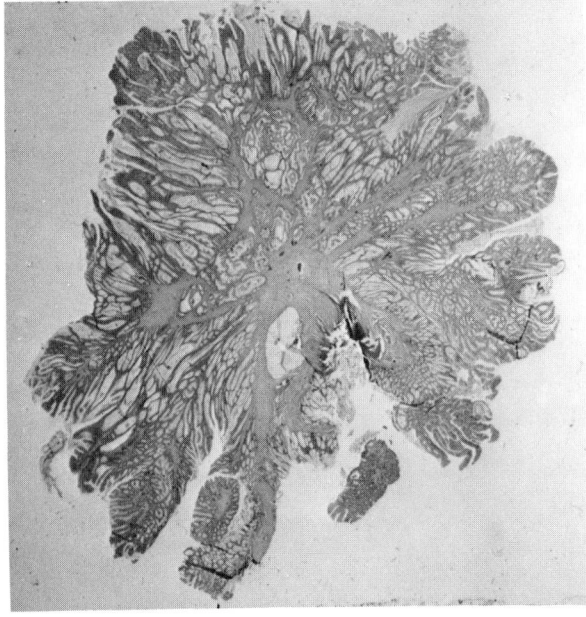

Cronkhite-Canada syndrome is characterized by generalized gastrointestinal polyposis in association with alopecia, cutaneous pigmentation, and atrophy of fingernails and toenails. Diarrhea is prominent. Vomiting, malabsorption, and protein-losing enteropathy are also common clinical manifestations. The polyps consist of cystic dilatation of the epithelial tubules as with juvenile polyps, but the lesions are usually smaller and do not show marked excess of lamina propria. Most patients die within a relatively short period of time following the diagnosis, but there have been a few reports of spontaneous remission. The cause of Cronkhite-Canada syndrome is not clear but may be related to fat, protein, and carbohydrate malabsorption. The treatment is symptomatic. Bowel resection is reserved for cases that develop complications such as bowel obstruction.

Inflammatory, Lymphoid, and Hyperplastic Polyps

Inflammatory polyps or *pseudopolyps* may look grossly like adenomatous polyps. Microscopic examination shows islands of normal mucosa with or without slight inflammation. They are caused by previous attacks of severe colitis (ulcerative colitis, Crohn's colitis, amebic colitis, ischemic colitis, and schistosomal colitis) resulting in partial loss of mucosa, leaving remnants or islands of relatively normal mucosa.

Benign lymphoid polyps are an enlargement of lymphoid follicles and are commonly seen in the rectum. They may be solitary or diffuse. The cause is unknown. Lymphoid polyps must not be confused with familial adenomatous polyposis.

Hyperplastic polyps are nonneoplastic polyps, commonly found in the rectum as small, pale, and glassy mucosal nodules. Most of them are 3 to 5 mm in diameter, although larger ones can be seen in the more proximal part of the colon. The majority of small polyps, particularly those in the more proximal colon, are adenomatous polyps, in contrast to the previous clinical impression that most small polyps are hyperplastic. Although gross differentiation is unreliable, histologic differentiation from neoplastic polyps presents no problem. The characteristic picture is a sawtooth appearance of the lining of epithelial cells producing a papillary outline (Fig. 28-40). There is no nuclear dysplasia. Hyperplastic polyps have no malignant potential.

Familial Adenomatous Polyposis Coli

Familial adenomatous polyposis coli is an inherited non-sex-linked autosomal dominant disease in which there are at least 100 adenomatous polyps throughout the entire large bowel. The rectum is invariably involved. This disease has high penetrance, with 50 percent chance of developing the disease in the affected family. Approximately one out of three patients with polyposis coli has no family history, and in this case the disorder represents spontaneous mutation. No means has been found of indicating which children of a polyposis parent will develop the disease. Screening of all offspring is mandatory.

CLINICAL MANIFESTATIONS. Normally symptoms do not develop until there is a full-blown development of polyposis. Bleeding per rectum and diarrhea are the most common symptoms. The diagnosis is made by endoscopic examination of the colon and rectum or by barium enema studies. Diagnosis must be confirmed by histologic findings of an adenomatous polyp.

The average age at which the disease is diagnosed is 36 years. The adenomas actually appear much earlier, as is

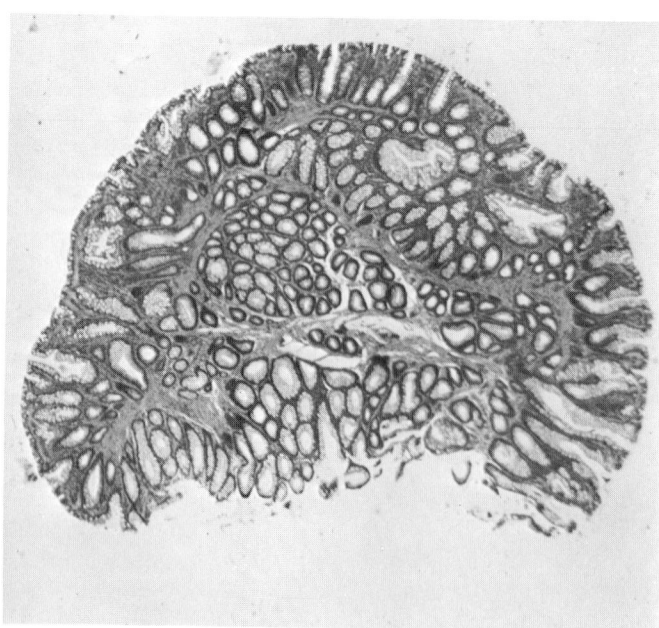

Fig. 28-40. Hyperplastic polyp. Note the typical sawtooth appearance of the surface epithelium with a papillary appearance.

seen by comparing the age at which the family members called up for examination are diagnosed. In this group of patients the average age is twenty-four years.

Nearly two out of three patients who present because of symptoms already have cancer. The average age at the time of diagnosis of colorectal cancer in these patients is thirty-nine years, compared with sixty-five years in the normal population.

Extracolonic Expression

In 1952 Gardner reported findings of osteomatosis, epidermoid cyst, and fibromas of the skin, a triad in familial polyposis known as *Gardner's syndrome*. Since then these extracolonic expressions of familial adenomatous polyposis coli have been expanded to include other lesions: gastric and small bowel polyps, desmoid tumor, impacted supernumerary teeth, lipoma, lymphoid hyperplasia, periampullary carcinoma, carcinoma of small intestine, carcinoma of thyroid, carcinoma of renal gland, carcinoma of gallbladder, pancreatitis, ovarian cyst, renal cyst, and uterine myoma. Gardner's syndrome should be considered as a variant of familial adenomatous polyposis coli rather than a separate entity.

The most important extracolonic expression of familial polyposis is desmoid tumor. About 15 percent of patients develop a desmoid tumor or fibromatosis, usually after colonic resection. Intraabdominal desmoid tumors are the most common, and they are life threatening. An intraabdominal desmoid tumor can grow to a very large size and can cause nutritional crippling after massive bowel resection.

MANAGEMENT. Pathologic verification of adenoma is essential so that confusion with familial juvenile polyposis, hyperplastic polyposis, pseudopolyposis, and lymphoid polyposis is avoided. Total colonoscopy and biopsy is the best method. Upper intestinal tract workup is also essential. This should include gastroduodenoscopy and small bowel follow-through barium studies to rule out any polyps. About 40 to 50 percent of patients have polyps of the upper intestinal tract although most of them are small and do not require treatment. Cancers of the duodenum and other parts of the small bowel in association with familial adenomatous polyposis coli are rare.

All patients with familial adenomatous polyposis coli should have prophylactic colectomy because development of carcinoma is inevitable. At the present time, there are several options.

Total Proctocolectomy with Ileostomy. This should be considered the "gold standard" treatment. It removes all the disease, but an obvious disadvantage is a permanent ileostomy, a procedure not well accepted by many patients, particularly young people.

Colectomy with Ileorectal Anastomosis. This procedure is the most popular option. It reduces the risk of development of cancer to only the last 15 to 20 cm of the rectum or rectosigmoid colon. The patients require a close follow-up at least twice a year for the rest of their lives, with electrocoagulation of the polyps as indicated. This

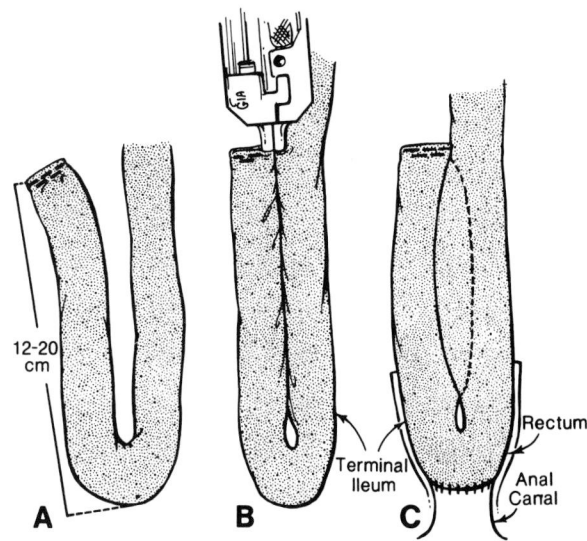

Fig. 28-41. The J pouch. *A.* Terminal ileum is aligned in a J shape. The length of the limb varies so that maximum length to pull it down to the anus can be achieved. *B.* Side-to-side anastomosis is made by GIA stapler. *C.* Anastomosis of the J pouch to the anal canal at the dentate line. [From: *Rolfmeyer E, Rothenberger DA, et al: Ileoanal pull-through, in IJ Kodner, RD Fry, JP Roe (eds): Colon, Rectal, and Anal Surgery: Current Techniques and Controversies. St Louis, Mosby, 1985, chap 26, Fig 28-8, p 322, with permission.*]

procedure should be selected for patients in whom the rectum is not carpeted with polyps and in patients who are reliable and willing to return for follow-up. The data from the Mayo Clinic show that in spite of periodic electrocoagulation of rectal polyps, the risk of development of cancer in the remaining rectum is still very high—59 percent at twenty-three years. Data from St. Mark's Hospital in London place this risk of carcinoma at 5 percent. This procedure should now be considered a temporary measure in most patients.

Total Proctocolectomy with Ileal Reservoir-Anal Anastomosis. This relatively new operation cures the patient by eliminating the disease while the patient maintains bowel continuity and continence. A reservoir using the terminal ileum is created, then anastomosed to the anal canal at the dentate line (Fig. 28-41), and a total colectomy and rectal mucosectomy is performed. The average number of bowel movements is six a day. The operation is complicated, with potential for major morbidity, especially sepsis, bowel obstruction, and pouchitis. It is ideal for young patients who are not obese. Patient satisfaction and functional results have been good.

Total Proctocolectomy with Continent Ileostomy. The procedure was a popular option in the 1970s. After total proctocolectomy, an ileal reservoir with a nipple valve is created from the terminal ileum and brought out as an ileostomy. The advantage over the conventional ileostomy is that an ileostomy bag is not required. The pouch has to be evacuated 4 to 6 times a day with a catheter. Because of the frequent extrusion of the nipple valve, which results in incontinence, the procedure is now limited to a small number of patients. The ileal reservoir-anal anastomosis has largely replaced this procedure.

Follow-up after Prophylactic Colectomy. In patients who still have the rectum preserved, proctoscopy or flexible sigmoidoscopy should be performed at least every six months. If present, as many polyps as possible should be electrocoagulated. In patients whose entire colon and rectum have been removed, upper gastrointestinal tract with small bowel follow-through barium studies should be done periodically. Routine physical examination to detect abnormality of other organs should also be performed on a regular basis.

Examination of the Family. The management of familiar adenomatous polyposis coli cannot be complete without examination of the other members of the family to prevent bowel cancer. The experience at St. Marks Hospital in London showed that cancer develops in only 8 percent of the called-up group compared with 65 percent in the propositus group. There is no fixed rule when to start examining members of the affected family. Since polyps in familiar polyposis rarely develop before fourteen years, it is reasonable to start flexible sigmoidoscopy or colonoscopy at this age.

CARCINOMA

INCIDENCE. Cancer of the colon and rectum continues to be the most common cancer of the gastrointestinal tract. In men, colon and rectal cancer is the third most common cancer, preceded only by cancer of the lung and prostate. In women, it is outnumbered only by cancer of the breast.

Each year, 140,000 new cases of large bowel cancer develop in the United States; about 60,000 patients will die as a result of the cancer, despite treatment. Colon and rectal cancer has maintained a steady frequency of occurrence in both men and women since 1940. The ratio of large bowel cancer in men to large bowel cancer in women is about equal.

Cancer of the large bowel affects mostly the older age group, with the incidence rising steadily from fifty years of age to peak at eighty years of age and an average age of sixty-seven at the time of diagnosis. About 6 to 8 percent of colorectal cancers are diagnosed before age forty.

ETIOLOGY. The etiology of colorectal carcinoma is unknown. Hereditary factors have been implicated in some patients, but the overwhelming majority of cases appear to be related to extragenetic factors. The observation that the incidence of carcinoma of the large bowel is low in Japan but increases among Japanese immigrants to the United States when they adopt a Western diet suggests that dietary factors are of etiological significance in the development of this disease. North Americans and Western Europeans, who generally consume a mixed Western diet high in animal fat and low in fiber, have a high incidence of colorectal cancer. It is postulated that a high-fiber diet may decrease the colonic transit time and thus decrease the contact time of carcinogens with the large bowel mucosa. Because of the increased bulk of the stools, the concentration of carcinogens is diluted. These factors may explain how a high-fiber diet could lower the incidence of carcinoma of the large bowel. High-fiber, bran diets significantly lower the incidence of neoplastic changes in colons of mice receiving 1,2-dimethyl hydrazine, a drug known for its specificity of causing cancer of the colon in mice.

Persons on a conventional American mixed diet excrete about three times as much bile acids and neutral sterols in the feces as do vegetarians. A high-fat diet also changes the composition of the intestinal flora, with an increase in the bacterial species known to chemically alter primary bile acids and sterols. These cholesterol and bile acid metabolites are thought to be carcinogenic. The diet therefore controls both the supply of substrate and the flora acting on it, and this perhaps explains the correlation between diet and colonic cancer.

A corollary of the bile acid-intestinal flora hypothesis of colonic cancer is the observation that there is a twofold increased risk of developing cancer of the right colon after cholecystectomy. Absence of a gallbladder results in a continuous circulation of the bile salt pool that prolongs the exposure of the bile salts to intestinal bacteria. The conjugated bile acids are hydrolyzed and subsequently transformed into secondary bile acids, a step in the formation of known carcinogens.

PATHOLOGY. Distribution. Carcinoma of the colon and rectum occurs with different frequency in the various segments of the colon. During the past three decades, there has been a gradual shift of the cancers toward the right colon, so that now cancer of the rectum constitutes 15 to 35 percent. The most striking findings were reported by Morgenstern and Lee. In 1009 consecutive cases of colorectal cancers diagnosed by conventional methods, fifteen percent occurred in the rectum compared with a 40 to 50 percent incidence in older studies. Right colon cancers increased in incidence to 24 percent compared with 12 to 15 percent previously. These figures are in accordance with the study of Nivatvongs et al. in asymptomatic patients between fifty and eighty years of age diagnosed by Hemoccult and colonoscopy. The reasons for this shifting are unclear. It is speculated that the decreasing incidence of rectal cancers could be the result of eradication of benign rectal polyps, a widespread practice during the past thirty years.

Macroscopy. The two most common macroscopic forms are the ulcerating type and the polypoid or fungating type (Fig. 28-42). About 10 to 15 percent display a bulky growth with a gelatinous appearance and are referred to as colloid carcinomas. An uncommon form is the intracellular mucinous or signet-ring cell carcinomas. In rare instances there is thickening of the rectal wall extending submucosally for at least 5 to 7 cm. This is the infiltrating carcinoma similar to linitis plastica of the stomach. The gross appearance of carcinoma may be of clinical importance. Greaney showed that ulcerated lesions regardless of size and polypoid lesions larger than 5 cm are associated with a 50 percent incidence of lymph node metastasis. For polypoid carcinomas smaller than 5 cm, lymph node involvement is much less common.

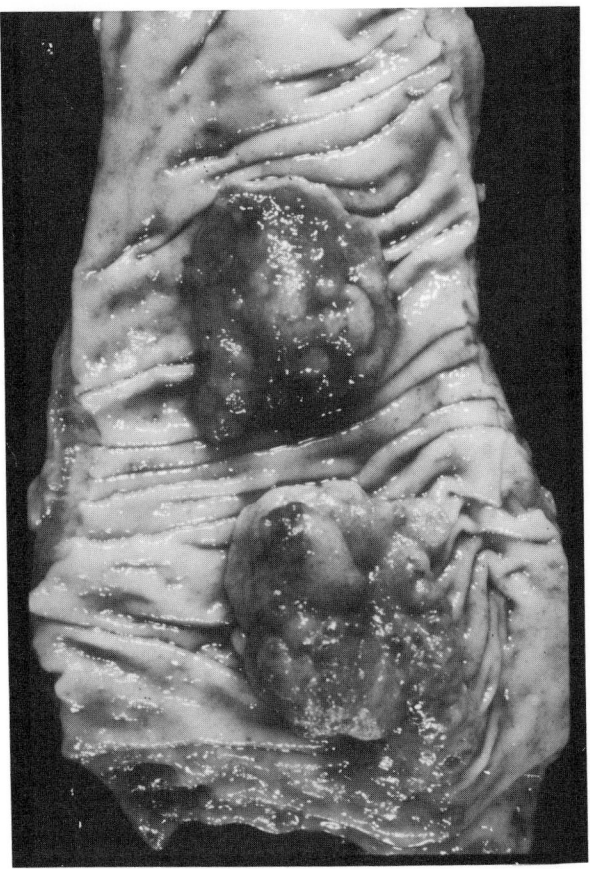

Fig. 28-42. Polypoid carcinomas of the rectum. (From: *Nivatvongs S, Becker ER, 1987, with permission.*)

Fig. 28-43. Grade I, or well-differentiated, adenocarcinoma. (From: *Goldberg SM, Gordon PH, Nivatvongs S, 1980, with permission.*)

Microscopy. Almost all carcinomas of the rectum are adenocarcinomas, but their histologic appearance differs considerably. In 1925 Broders divided the microscopic features of carcinoma of the rectum into four grades according to the degree of differentiation. While trying to apply this grading to prognosis, Grinnell found it more practical to grade large bowel carcinoma in relation to invasive tendency, glandular arrangement, nuclear polarity, and frequency of mitosis. This grading system is used worldwide at the present time.

Grade I. This variety displays a well-differentiated and compact glandular structure. The acini are lined with two or three layers of cells whose nuclei tend to remain close to the basal layer of the gland leaving a clear zone near the lumen. There is little tendency for individual cells or small groups of cells to extend into surrounding tissue. Mitoses are infrequent (Fig. 28-43).

Grade II. The glandular arrangement is still preserved, but some glands appear to be loosely and irregularly arranged. The walls are thicker and composed of cells in three or more layers with their nuclei scattered throughout the wall of the gland. The central zone in the cytoplasm of cells around the lumen is largely lost. A tendency of the cells to stray off into adjacent tissue can be seen, especially at the deep, advanced edge of the lesion. Mitosis are more numerous (Fig. 28-44).

Grade III. The glandular structure may be completely or nearly completely lost. At lease parts of the growth may show neoplastic cells growing in solid masses, or cords with little or no tendency to arrange themselves around a central lumen. Nearly all the polarity of the cells is lost. Mitoses are frequent (Fig. 28-45).

This grading system has been modified and adopted by others as *well differentiated* (low grade), *moderately differentiated* (average grade), and *poorly differentiated* (high grade). In addition, about 10 to 15 percent of colo-

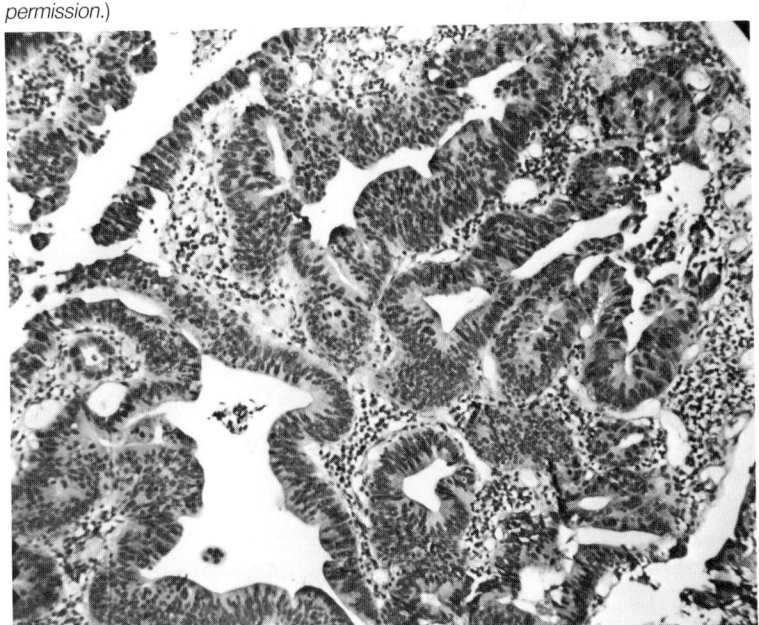

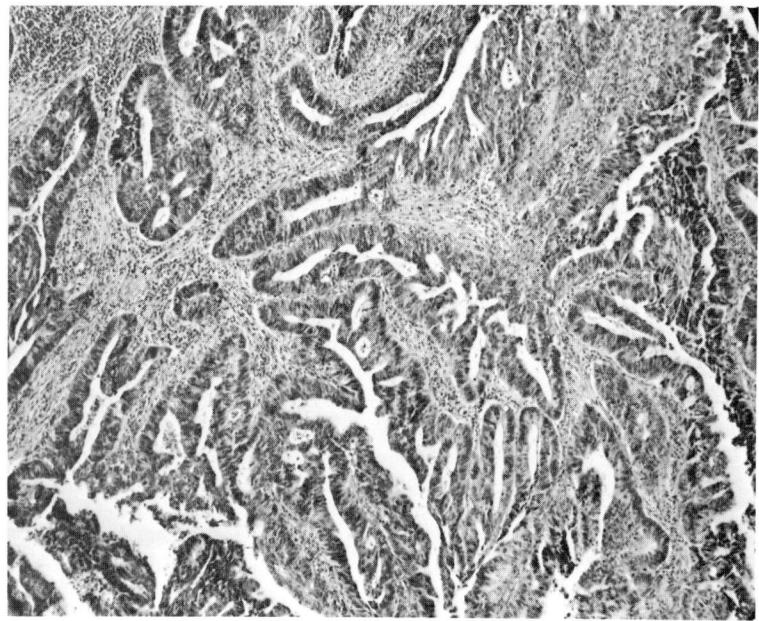

Fig. 28-44. Grade II, or moderately differentiated, adenocarcinoma, (From: *Goldberg SM, Gordon PH, Nivatvongs S, 1980, with permission.*)

rectal carcinomas produce mucin and are called mucinous carcinomas (Fig. 28-46). This type of cancer has more tendency to spread locally and distantly and carries a poor prognosis. The signet-ring cell carcinoma, a rare intracellular mucinous carcinoma, has also been found to have poor prognosis (Fig. 28-47).

STAGING SYSTEMS. Prognosis is related not only to dissemination but to the local extent of the carcinoma and to the presence or absence of lymphatic and venous invasion. This can be determined accurately only by histological examination of the resected specimen. Assessment by the pathologist involves dissection of the specimen to identify nodes, veins, and section of the primary tumor through the area of greatest penetration. The accuracy of the report depends on how carefully this has been done. Dukes' pathologic staging system has been modified in various ways so that, unfortunately, there is now no uniform standard worldwide. Although the majority of pathologists in Europe apply Dukes' system, those in the

Fig. 28-45. Grade III, or poorly differentiated, adenocarcinoma. (From: *Goldberg SM, Gordon PH, Nivatvongs S, 1980, with permission.*)

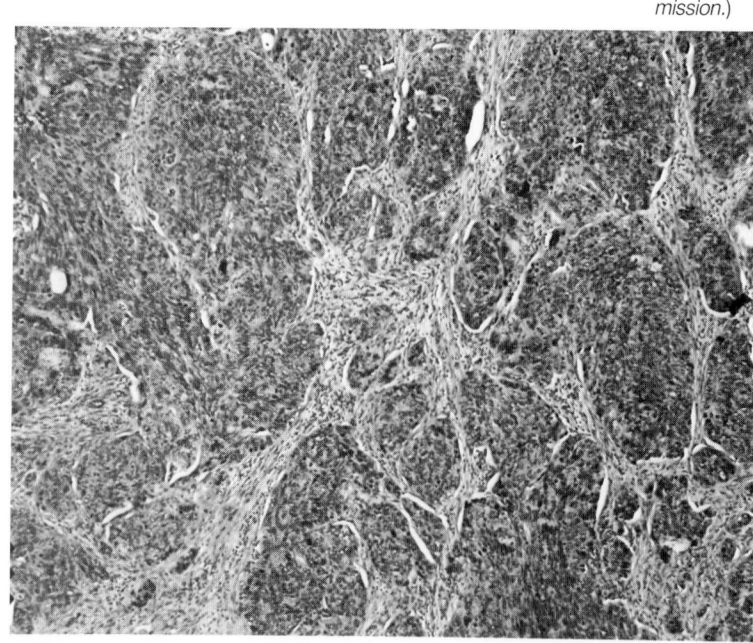

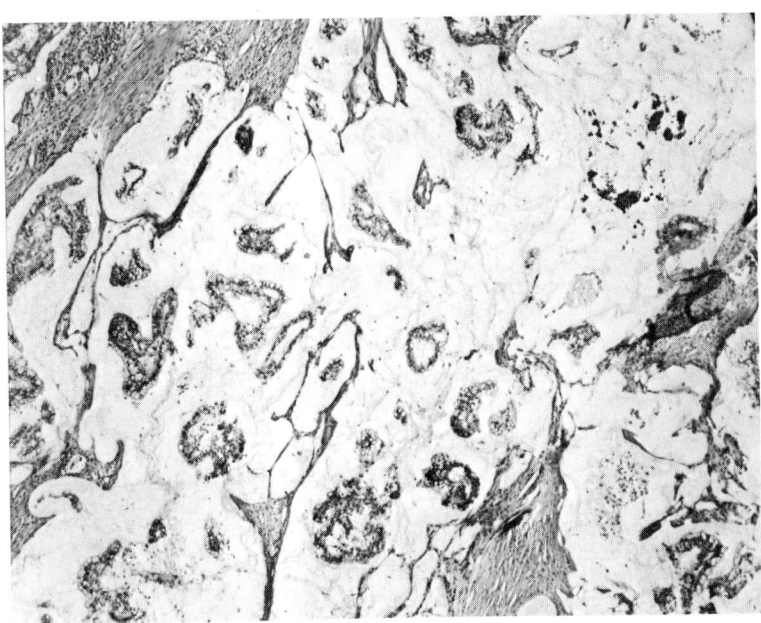

Fig. 28-46. Mucinous adenocarcinoma. (From: *Goldberg SM, Gordon PH, Nivatvongs S, 1980, with permission.*)

United States mostly use the modification of Astler and Coller. Both have adopted an ABC notation, but despite this confusion there is a clear relationship between stage and five-year survival using either method.

Pathologic staging systems are really an attempt to combine two pathologic features of a tumor (depth of the bowel wall involvement and the presence or absence of lymph node metastases) into a simplified scale of indices. All systems have failed, however, to include two other features, namely the presence or absence of venous invasion and the extent of direct local spread within the tissues outside the bowel.

Dukes' Staging (Figure 28-48)

Prognosis of colorectal carcinoma varies according to many factors. Some factors are impossible to measure, others are not practical. In 1932, Dukes developed a staging system to predict the prognosis of cancer of the rectum. This was later applied to carcinoma of the colon as well. His classification proved to be simple, practical, and easily remembered and understood. At the present time,

Fig. 28-47. Signet-ring cell carcinoma in a pool of mucin. (From: *Nivatvongs S, Becker ER, 1987, with permission.*)

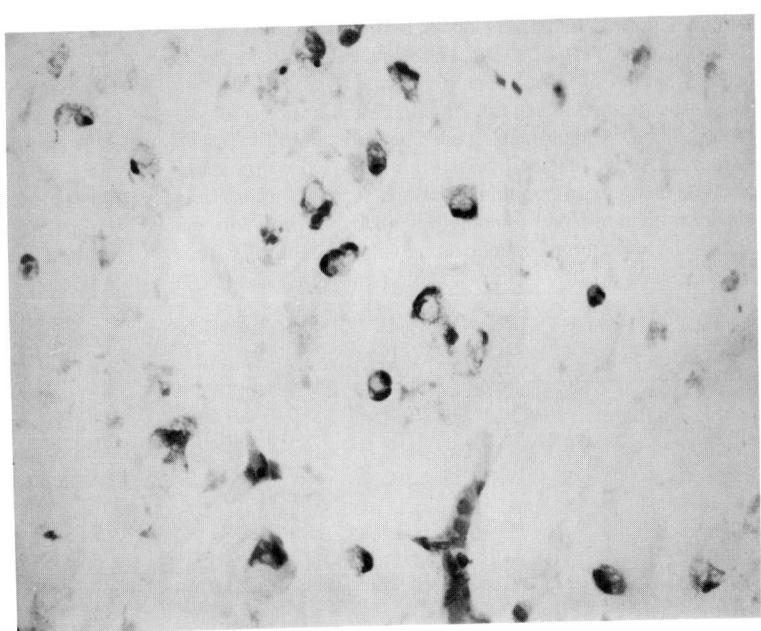

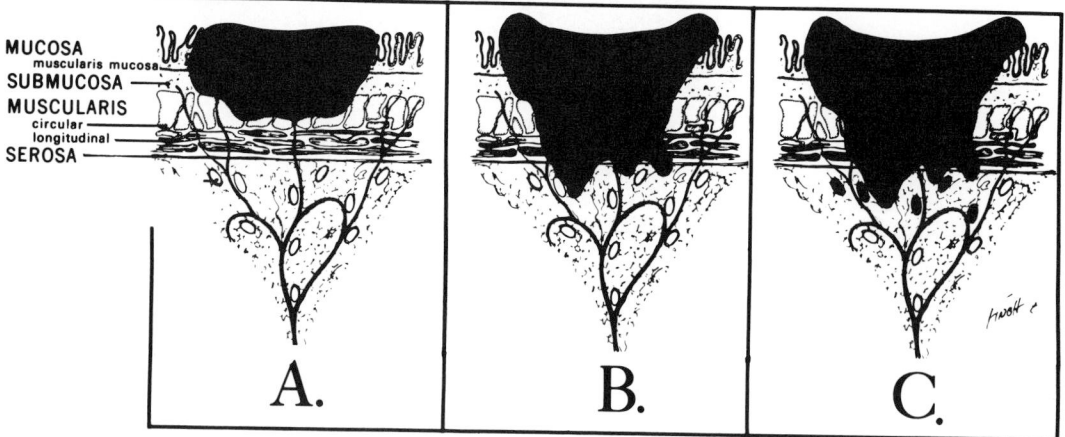

Fig. 28-48. The Dukes' staging system (A, B, and C). (From: *Goldberg SM, Gordon PH, Nivatvongs S, 1980, with permission.*)

this staging system is the most practical prognostic indicator.

Stage A connotes invasion at least through the muscularis mucosa to, but not through, the muscularis propria; the lymph nodes are free from metastasis.

Stage B connotes invasion through the full thickness of the bowel but lymph nodes free from metastasis.

Stage C connotes lymph node metastasis regardless of the depth of the invasion. When the depth of invasion is limited to the muscularis propria, the risk of lymph node metastasis is about 12 percent, whereas when invasion is full thickness, the risk of lymph node metastasis is 50 percent. Dukes' original report was strengthened by a comprehensive analysis of the system in 1958. Dukes and Bussey analyzed the 5 year survivals of Stages A, B, and C carcinomas of the rectum (Table 28-3).

Dukes subsequently subdivided Stage C into C-1 and C-2. Stage C-1 is when only adjacent regional lymph nodes contain metastasis, whereas C-2 is when lymphatic spread involves the nodes of the point of ligature of the blood vessels (Fig. 28-49). The survival rates in these cases are also different (Table 28-4).

In most large series, the staging distribution is as follows: Dukes' Stage A, 15 percent; Dukes' Stage B, 35 percent; Dukes' Stage C, 50 percent. About two-thirds of Stage C cases correspond to the definition of Dukes' C-1, and one-third to that of Dukes' C-2. This distribution has not changed during the past thirty years except in studies

emphasizing early detection by aggressive screening techniques.

The Dukes classification is based entirely on pathologic findings of the resected specimen. Problems do occur with this system when the clinical findings reveal local invasion to adjacent organs or distant metastasis to the liver or lung. It has been generally understood that a "Stage D" is added for the cancer with distant metastasis or with adjacent organ involvement, although Dukes never used such a term. Other modifications of the Dukes system have been suggested, but most of these have added more to the confusion regarding staging than to improved accuracy.

Aster-Coller Modification. In this classification *A* refers to lesions limited to the mucosa, *B-1* to lesions limited to the muscularis propria with negative nodes, *B-2* to lesions penetrating the muscularis propria with negative nodes, *C-1* to lesions limited to the wall with positive nodes, and *C-2* refers to lesions that have extended through the wall with positive nodes. The 5-year survival rate has been correlated with the class (Table 28-5).

A new system, the Australian Clinical-Pathological Staging (ACPS) system, has also been proposed. This system requires the accurate use of precise definitions, cooperation between surgeons and pathologists, and a complete pathology report. Under it, all the information available—clinical, radiologic, operative, pathologic—is considered before a stage is allotted. Whether this more exhaustive system can be put into practice worldwide remains to be seen.

In order to obtain some uniformity in staging, it has been suggested that a TNM classification should be introduced, similar to that used for breast carcinoma. This has not been universally adopted. To investigate the significance of the number of lymph node metastases, cases with lymphatic spread have been further subdivided into one metastasis, two to five metastases, six to nine metastases, and ten or more metastases. Using this criterion, the 5 year survival is shown in Table 28-6.

Table 28-3. RELATIONSHIP OF DUKES' STAGING TO SURVIVAL

Stage	Number of patients	Corrected 5-year survival rate, %
A	308	98
B	692	78
C	1037	32
Total	2037	57.4

SOURCE: Dukes CE, Bussey HJR: 1958, with permission.

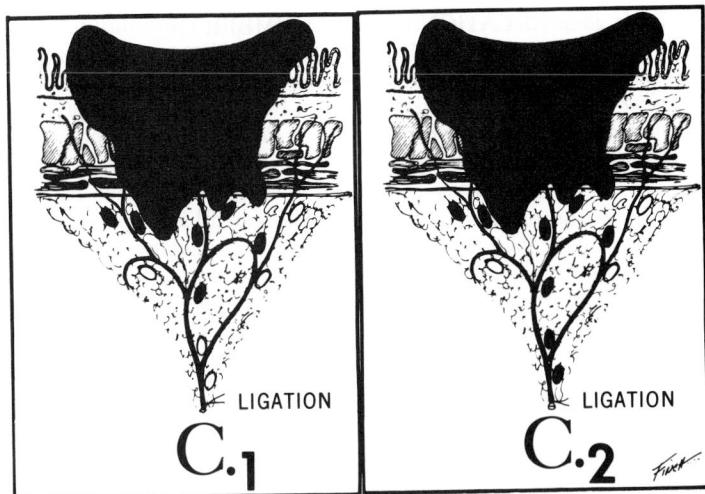

Fig. 28-49. The Dukes' staging system (C$_1$ and C$_2$). (From: *Goldberg SM, Gordon PH, Nivatvongs S, 1980, with permission.*)

MECHANISM OF SPREAD. Direct Spread. Carcinoma of the colon and rectum originates in the mucosa. It subsequently penetrates the thickness of the bowel wall rather than just growing in the longitudinal axis. Untreated, it finally involves the full thickness of the bowel and eventually invades the adjacent tissues. It is unusual to find direct upward or downward microscopic spread greater than 2.5 cm beyond the visible borders of the lesion.

Transperitoneal Spread. Peritoneal involvement of carcinoma of the large bowel probably starts from local extension, which continues through the peritoneum, and, subsequently, is disseminated within the peritoneal cavity. Once this occurs, it is beyond hope of surgical cure.

Implantation. It has been postulated that desquamated colorectal cancer cells may implant on anal wounds after hemorrhoidectomy, fistulectomy, fissurectomy, and on the cut ends of bowel. Although this hypothesis has gained widespread acceptance, evidence is contradictory. A study by Rothenberger and colleagues failed to show the viability of exfoliated cells. Recent data by Umpledy et al. demonstrated viable exfoliated tumor cells in 70 percent of the specimens. Their presence in large numbers at the site of bowel anastomosis may play a role in the etiology of suture-line recurrence. Most suture-line recurrences of the colon and rectum, however, are caused by extension of local recurrences at the previously removed tumor bed, extending into the lumen of the bowel.

Lymphatic Spread. Regional lymph node involvement is the most common form of metastasis in colorectal carcinoma. When carcinoma has extended through the bowel wall, the chance of lymph node metastasis is 50 percent, compared with 15 percent if the cancer has not penetrated through the muscularis layer. In about 85 percent of lymph node metastases, the lymph node most proximal to the tumor will be the first one involved. Fifteen percent of the time, the metastasis may skip to the ones closer to the aorta.

Lymphatic spread in the rectum is different from that in the colon. Basically, the lymphatic drainage of the rectum ascends along the superior rectal vessels to the inferior mesenteric nodes. Lymphatic drainage of the lower third of the rectum may secondarily drain laterally along the middle rectal vessels. Retrograde metastasis to pararectal nodes rarely occurs and usually is the result of proximal lymphatic blockage from metastasis.

Hematogenous Spread. The development of distant metastasis from primary carcinoma can only result from dissemination of malignant cells into the bloodstream. Circulating malignant cells are found infrequently in the

Table 28-4. PROGNOSIS OF DUKES' C-1 AND C-2 STAGES

Stage	Number of patients	Corrected 5-year survival rate, %
C-1	680	41
C-2	282	14
Unclassified	75	20
Total	1037	32

SOURCE: Dukes CE, Bussey HJR: 1958, with permission.

Table 28-5. CLASSIFICATION OF COLORECTAL CANCER

Class	Extent	5-year survival rate, %
A	Lesions limited to mucosa	100.0
B-1	To muscularis propria with negative nodes	66.4
B-2	Penetrating muscularis Proptid with negative nodes	53.9
C-1	Limited to wall with positive nodes	42.8
C-2	Through the wall with positive nodes	22.4

SOURCE: Holyoke ED, Mittleman A: Cancer of the colon and rectum, in Pilch YH (ed): *Surgical Oncology.* New York, McGraw-Hill, 1984, Chap 28, p 602, with permission.

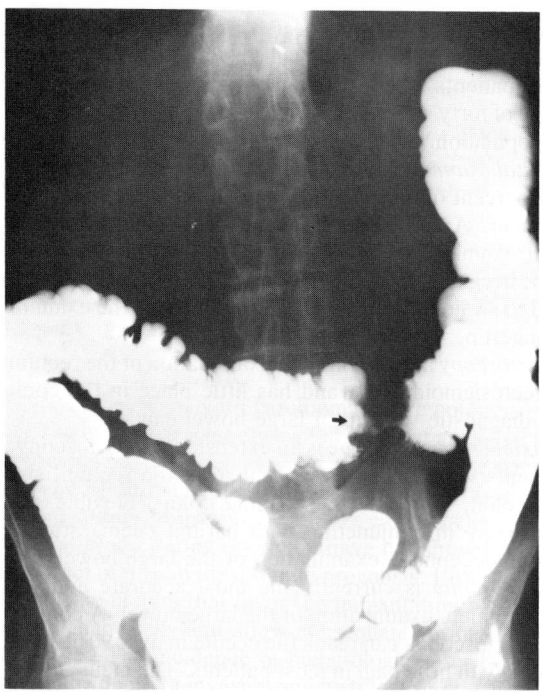

Fig. 28-50. An apple-core lesion on barium enema (arrow). (From: *Nivatvongs S, Becker ER, 1987, with permission.*)

These include cancers of the stomach, breast, and lung, liver disease, history of excessive smoking, pancreatitis, and ulcerative colitis. CEA has no value in screening for large bowel cancer, but it has been shown to have prognostic value. When preoperative CEA is abnormal, the chance of subsequent recurrence or metastasis is higher than when the preoperative CEA is normal. Some surgeons advocate a routine CEA determination in colorectal carcinoma preoperatively as a base-line study. Its main usefulness is for postoperative follow-up.

Early Detection

Symptoms of large bowel cancer often do not manifest until the tumor is large enough to cause some partial obstruction. Bleeding from large bowel cancers can occur at any stage but as a rule is intermittent. The amount of bleeding ranges from occult blood to a moderate amount of bright red blood. The only way to diagnose large bowel cancer before any symptoms develop is to have a complete colonic examination, particularly colonoscopy. This obviously is impracticable, costly, and the yield is low for the general population. For practical purposes, the workup should be divided into two groups of people.

High-Risk Group. This group consists of individuals with a family history of cancers, particularly colorectal cancer, cancers of the prostate and bladder in men, and cancers of the cervix, uterus, ovary, and breast in women. Preexisting conditions have been known to have a higher risk of large bowel cancer—colorectal polyp, endometrial carcinoma, cancer of the breast, cancer of the head and neck, lymphoma, and prior colorectal cancer. In the high-risk

group, colonic workup should be done before the age of forty years and every 3 to 5 years thereafter.

Low-Risk Group. This is the population at large in which there are no known risk factors or signs and symptoms to suggest colorectal cancer. At the present time, the mass screening test for occult blood in the stool is the most practical method of early detection.

TREATMENT. Standard therapy for carcinoma of the colon and rectum consists of surgical excision. Distinct operative procedures are performed for intraperitoneal colon carcinomas as compared to carcinoma of the rectum. There is general agreement regarding the appropriate operation for carcinoma of the intraperitoneal colon. Controversy exists concerning the particulars of resection for rectal carcinoma. Local therapy, either electrocoagulation or radiation, has been used as an alternative to resection in patients with rectal carcinoma. Radiation therapy and/or chemotherapy has been used in combination with surgical excision to improve the cure rate and also as palliation.

Preoperative Bowel Preparation

Wound infection and intraabdominal abscess used to be common problems after colorectal surgery. The primary source of infection is the endogenous bacteria in the bowel lumen. Although the colon and rectum cannot be sterilized completely, a complete mechanical clearance of its contents is the most important method to decrease the bacterial count. The conventional regimen of 3-day course of purgatives, enemas, and dietary restriction has now often been replaced by whole-gut lavage with polyethylene glycol-electrolyte solution (Golytely or Colyte). With this method of cleansing, the patient is allowed a light solid meal up to lunch time of the day prior to the operation. Metoclopramide (Reglan), 10 mg, may be given orally or intramuscularly half an hour to an hour prior to starting bowel preparation to reduce nausea. The patient drinks the solution or the solution is given via a small nasogastric tube at the rate of 250 mL every 10 min, until the diarrheal effluent is clear. It may take from 3 to 10 h to complete the process. It is convenient to start at 4:00 or 5:00 P.M. the evening before colon surgery.

Preoperative prophylactic antibiotics have been shown to markedly reduce the infection rate. The choice of antibiotics is a matter of personal preference, but in general the potent broad spectrum antibiotics should be reserved for therapeutic use. A long-acting first generation cephalosporin along with metronidazole given prior to abdominal incision is an effective regimen. Another is to give a second generation cephalosorin only. In uncomplicated cases the antibiotics may be continued for two more doses. There is no benefit to prolonging the administration of prophylactic antibiotics; it may be dangerous by aiding in the production of antibiotic-resistant bacteria.

Operative Treatment: Intraperitoneal Colon Carcinoma. The objective in the treatment of carcinoma of the colon is to remove the primary tumor along with the surrounding soft tissues and lymphatics draining the tumor. Since lymphatics of the colon accompany the main arterial supply, the length of the bowel resected is dependent on which vessels are supplying the segment involved with cancer. If the tumor is adherent to or invading adjacent organs such as the small bowel, ovaries, uterus, or kidney, an en bloc resection should be performed if technically feasible. Adhesions between the tumor and the contiguous organ are often inflammatory, but this cannot usually be determined prior to resection. If all tumor cannot be removed, a palliative colon resection is generally performed to relieve symptoms. In the rare situation of a nonresectable tumor, a bypass operation should be considered to relieve or prevent bowel obstruction. In multiple colon carcinomas, or in colon carcinoma associated with multiple neoplastic polyps, a subtotal colectomy with ileorectosigmoid colon anastomosis should be considered.

For carcinoma of the right colon, right hemicolectomy should include ligation of the ileocolic artery, right colic artery, and right branch of the middle colic artery. About 10 to 12 cm of the terminal ileum is included, and the ileum is anastomosed to the left transverse colon (Fig. 28-51). The anastomosis can be performed by either hand sewn or stapling technique.

For carcinoma of the hepatic flexure and the right transverse colon, a right hemicolectomy is extended to include the middle colic artery along with its left branch (Fig. 21-51*B*).

For carcinoma of the mid-transverse colon, the middle colic artery is taken near its base (Fig. 28-51*C*). Another option is to do an extended right hemicolectomy taking the ileocolic, right colic, and middle colic arteries. The anastomosis is made between the terminal ileum and upper descending colon.

For carcinoma of the splenic flexure, the left transverse colon, or the descending colon, the left branch of the middle colic artery, the left colic artery, and the first branch of the sigmoid artery should be taken (Fig. 28-51*D*).

For carcinoma of the descending colon, the left branch of the middle colic artery along with the left colic artery and an upper branch of the sigmoid artery are taken. (Fig. 28-51*E*).

For carcinoma of the sigmoid and rectosigmoid colon, all the sigmoid arterial branches are taken (Fig. 28-51*E*).

Emergency Operations. When surgical treatment must be carried out on unprepared bowel because of obstruction, perforation, or hemorrhage, or when a colorectal cancer is encountered unexpectedly, most surgeons prefer to proceed with the definitive resection and anastomosis if the lesion is in the right half of the colon. Although a few surgeons also perform emergency primary anastomosis after resection of left colon lesions, most prefer to resect the lesion and bring both cut ends of the colon out—proximally as an end colostomy, distally as a mucous fistula. If the distal end is too short to exteriorize, the Hartmann procedure is used.

While preliminary decompressive procedures continue to have a role in select situations of obstruction of the distal colon due to carcinoma, the current trend is toward primary resection with or without immediate anastomosis. The various primary resective procedures that can be

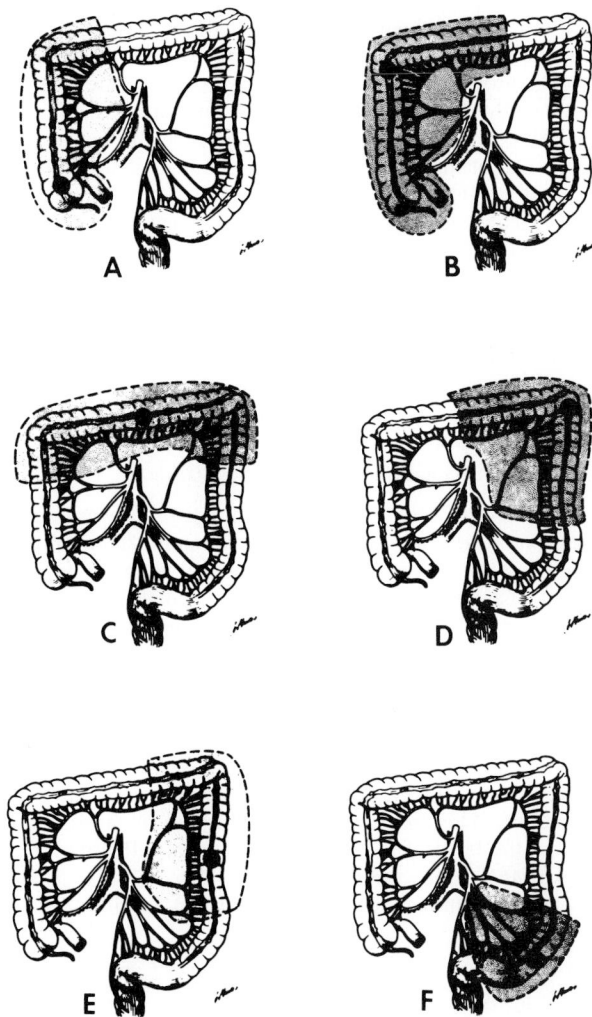

Fig. 28-51. Extent of resection in carcinoma of the colon. *A.* Carcinoma of cecum. *B.* Carcinoma of hepatic flexure. *C.* Carcinoma of transverse colon. *D.* Carcinoma of splenic flexure. *E.* Carcinoma of descending colon. *F.* Carcinoma of sigmoid colon. (From: *Nivatvongs S, Becker ER, 1987, with permission.*)

utilized in this setting include: (1) primary resection with anastomosis, (2) primary resection without anastomosis, (3) primary resection with anastomosis and proximal protective colostomy, and (4) subtotal colectomy with ileosigmoidostomy.

Primary resection with immediate anastomosis carries an average mortality of 37 percent and probably should be used only in isolated situations by surgeons thoroughly familiar with the details of patient selection and operative technique. In most cases, primary resection with end colostomy and mucous fistula or the Hartmann procedure is preferred, especially if there is an associated perforation.

Proximal decompressive colostomy probably offers little protection in the setting of emergency left colon resection and primary anastomosis. Therefore, this procedure has limited application. Several recent reports have demonstrated that emergency subtotal colectomy with immediate ileosigmoidostomy can be used very effectively in this setting. This procedure removes the septic or neoplastic process, and the anastomosis is constructed utilizing healthy ileum and collapsed distal colon.

Primary anastomosis should not be performed in the presence of markedly edematous colon or ileum loaded with stool. If the tumor cannot be safely removed, a proximal fecal diversion such as ileostomy or transverse colostomy should be done as the first stage. Later, after the bowel is appropriately prepared, the colon is resected and anastomosis performed. The ileostomy or transverse colostomy is closed at the third stage. The 5-year survival rate is low in patients with perforating cancers in any segment and in those with obstructing cancers of the right colon.

Operations: Rectal Carcinoma

An *anterior resection* is the term used to describe resection of the colorectum with partial mobilization of the rectum. The inferior mesenteric artery is taken at the point just distal to takeoff of the left colic artery (Fig. 28-52) or at the aorta. The anastomosis is made above the anterior peritoneal reflection.

In a *low anterior resection,* the rectum is fully mobilized to the level of the levator ani muscle. The lateral stalks on each side are cut and ligated. Anterior mobilization is done to the level of the pubis. The inferior mesenteric artery is taken at the same area as it is in anterior resection. The anastomosis is performed in the rectum below the level of the anterior peritoneal reflection.

An *abdominoperineal resection* (Figs. 28-53–28-55) means the removal of the colorectum in a fashion similar

Fig. 28-52. Extent of resection in carcinoma of upper rectum. (From: *Nivatvongs S, Becker ER, 1987, with permission.*)

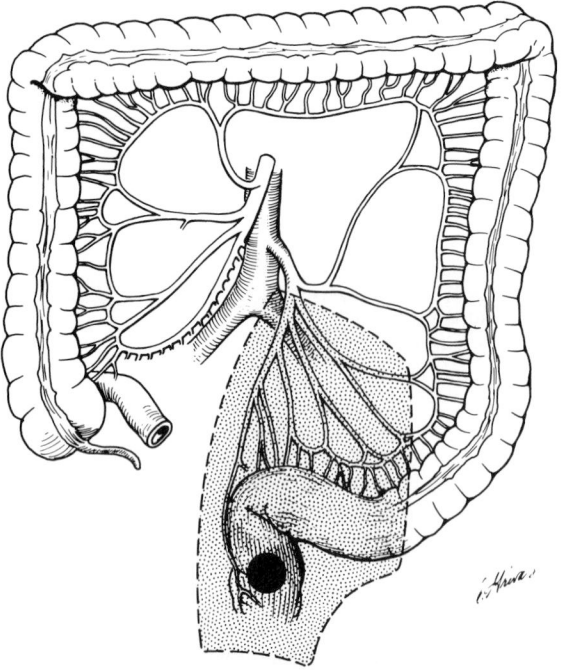

to the technique for low anterior resection, along with the anal canal. The anal canal below the level of the levator ani muscle is excised via a perineal approach. The proximal blood vessels are taken at the same area as for anterior resection. The sigmoid colon is brought out as a permanent colostomy.

For carcinoma of the upper rectum, an anterior resection is the standard treatment. The anastomosis can be performed with hand-sewn sutures without much difficulty (Fig. 28-56).

Most carcinomas of the midrectum are amenable to a low anterior resection. In most hands, a low anastomosis using an intraluminal stapling device is more secure than a handsewn anatomosis at the same level (Fig. 28-57). Mobilization of the splenic flexure may be necessary to bring the ends together without tension. A temporary proximal colostomy or ileostomy is advisable when there is any question about a low anastomosis. If anastomosis is technically impossible, such as in patients with a very narrow pelvis or in obese patients, then an abdominoperineal 7 cm resection is necessary. Carcinomas in the distal rectum, i.e., within 7 cm of the anal verge, are generally removed by abdominoperineal resection.

Evolution of Operations (Fig. 28-58). In 1885, Kraske described his technique of sacral excision of the rectum. Lockhart-Mummery popularized the extended perineal excision which became the most common operation for rectal cancer in the early 1900s in England. These two operations were associated with an operative mortality of about 12 percent but yielded a 5-year survival rate among the survivors of 30 and 40 percent, respectively.

In 1908, following investigation of the lymphatic spread of rectal cancer, Miles described his technique of combined abdominoperineal excision. This was the first widely accepted procedure primarily to approach rectal carcinoma by the abdomen. In 1923, Hartmann reported his anterior resection without anastomosis leaving the inverted rectal stump in situ. This was associated with less morbidity and mortality than abdominoperineal resection. As operations became safer, however, it was the abdominoperineal resection that became widely accepted as standard therapy for rectal cancer. It remains the "gold standard" to which the results of all other operations for rectal carcinoma are compared.

Increased knowledge of the routes of spread of rectal cancer and of the physiology of anal continence and the increased safety of gastrointestinal anastomoses promoted the development of restorative procedures as alternatives to abdominoperineal resection. In the 1930s and 1940s, Dixon and Wangesteen promoted an anterior approach to rectosigmoid and intraperitoneal rectal tumors through the abdominal cavity with sutured anastomosis. It soon was demonstrated that anterior resection of upper rectal tumors resulted in cure rates equal to those achieved by abdominoperineal excision. Not surprisingly, anterior resection was applied to midrectal cancers. Because of the technical difficulties often encountered with a low handsewn anastomosis, a variety of operations were revived and modified to facilitate reestablishment of intestinal continuity. Abdominosacral re-

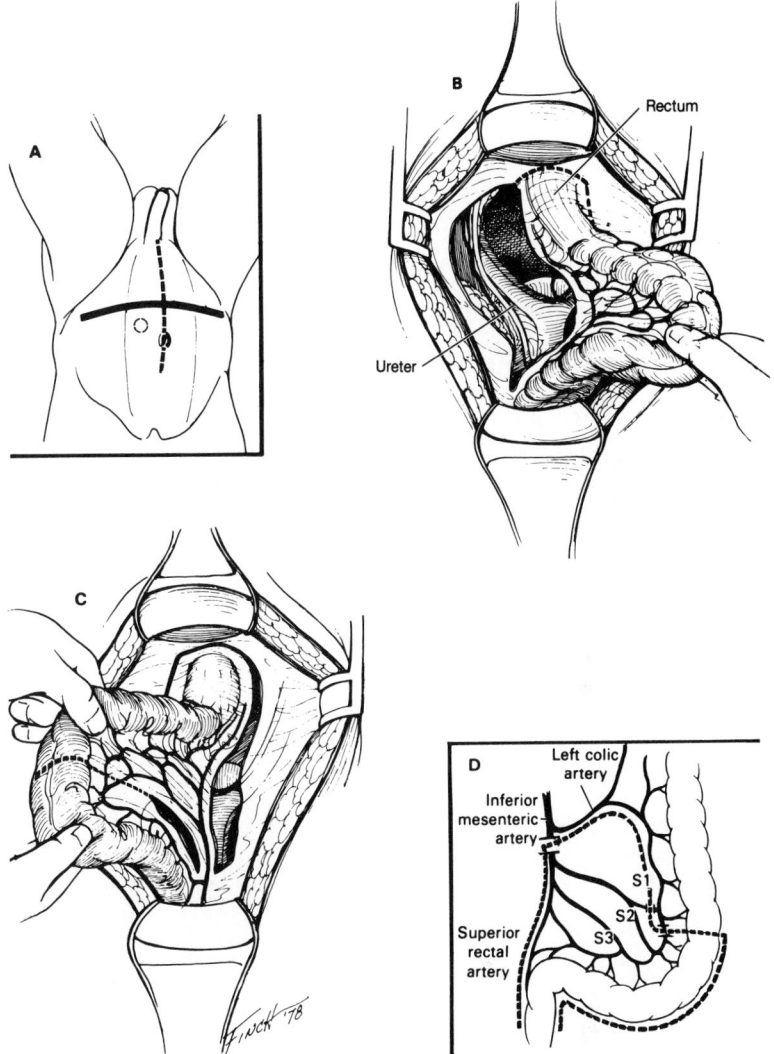

Fig. 28-53. Technique of abdominoperineal resection: abdominal phase. *A.* Infraumbilical, transverse, or midline incision can be used. *B.* Mobilization of sigmoid colon medially. Left ureter is identified. *C.* Extent of proximal resection. *D.* Inferior mesenteric artery is taken below the take-off of left colic artery. *E.* The rectum is pulling up taut. Posterior mobilization should be done by sharp dissection. *F.* Rectosacral fascia is divided by scissors to enter the supralevator space. *G.* Anteriorly, the rectum is dissected free from the bladder, to just below seminal vesicles in male and to the upper part of vagina in female. *H.* Lateral stalk on each side is divided and tied with absorbable sutures. *I.* Excess rectosigmoid colon transected. The rectal stump along with the cancer is left in place, to be removed in the perineal phase. *J.* Extraperitoneal tunnel is created in the left flank. *K.* The colon is brought through the extraperitoneal tunnel for the extraperitoneal colostomy. *L.* Pelvic peritoneum closed. *M.* Maturation of colostomy. Note generous protrusion. (From: *Nivatvongs S, Becker ER, 1987, with permission.*)

section, a variety of pull-through operations, Parks' abdominal transanal resection with coloanal anastomosis, and the abdominal transsphincteric resection promoted by York Mason are examples of such operations.

The introduction of the circular intraluminal stapling devices in 1978 has for most surgeons provided a techni-

cally more acceptable means of restoring continuity than the alternatives just discussed. Low anterior resection is now extended to even more distal lesions by more complete mobilization of the rectum. Anastomosis is accomplished by transanal placement of the circular stapling device.

Local surgical therapy for rectal cancer was advocated in the form of local excision by Bevan in 1917 and by electrocoagulation as first described by Strauss and associates in 1935. Though interest in local measures subsequently waned as resectional procedures became the accepted standard, a recent resurgence of application has been led by Madden and Kandalaft and others.

Controversies (Fig. 28-59). There are several current controversies regarding the techniques for excision of rectal carcinomas. One relates to the question of high versus low ligation of the inferior mesenteric artery pedicle. The authors feel that high ligation is of no value in treating Dukes' A and B lesions, nor does it have any value if distant spread has occurred. There is a potential benefit

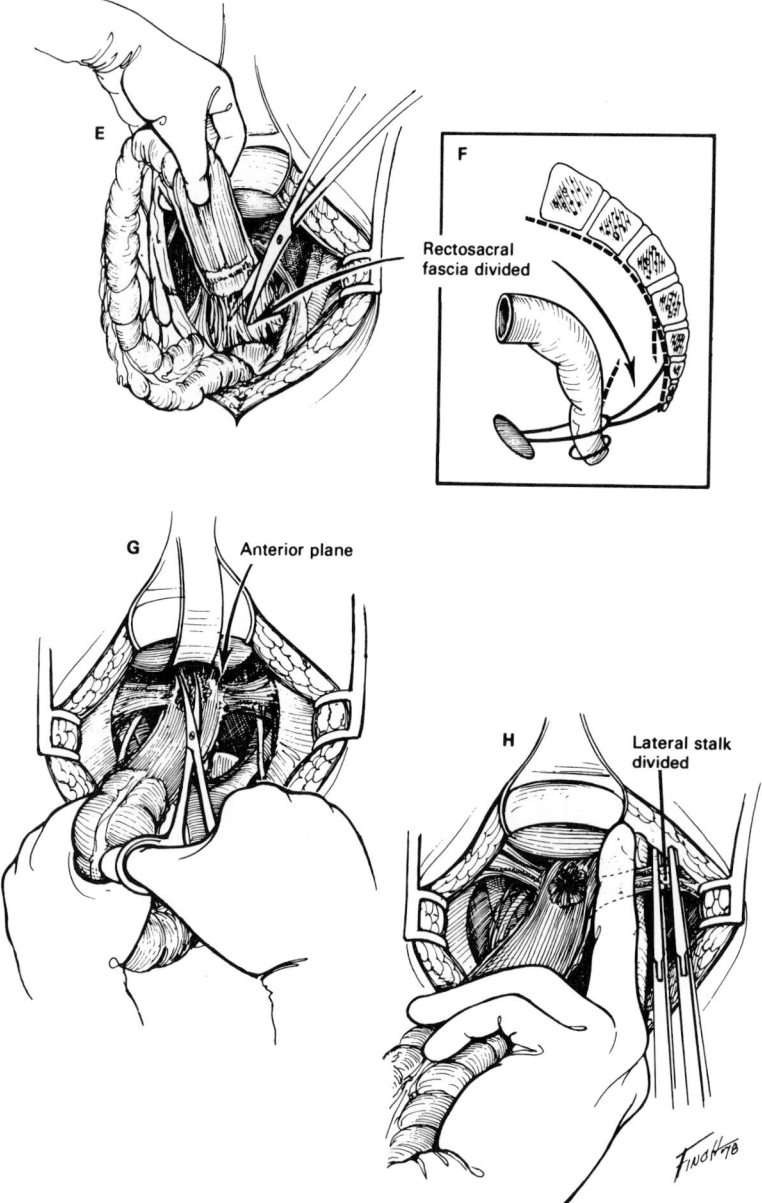

Fig. 28-53 *E,F,G,H.* Continued.

associated with high ligation in patients with Dukes' C lesions when modal metastases have spread to a level proximal to the left colic artery but have not spread beyond the origin of the inferior mesenteric artery. It is, therefore, reasonable to selectively utilize high ligation in good-risk patients in whom the dissection is easily accomplished.

There is a difference in opinion regarding the extent of lateral dissection and pelvic lymphadenectomy that should be employed during the course of excising lesions of the distal two-thirds of the rectum. There is no firm data to suggest that survival rate is enhanced by removing lateral hypogastric nodes, while the morbidity in terms of genitourinary complications is increased. The question as to whether such a dissection would effect reduction of local recurrences has not been resolved.

Another controversy relates to the extent of distal margin required so that cure is not compromised. This is particularly pertinent because it impacts on the trend toward sphincter-preserving operations. The authors feel that at least a 2-cm margin distal to gross evidence of tumor is mandatory. When feasible without jeopardizing restoration, a margin up to 5 cm should be obtained. To some extent the margin should be related to the type of tumor, in that a smaller margin might be acceptable for more differentiated carcinomas because more poorly differentiated tumors have been noted to have more extensive intramural spread.

Another controversy relates to the issue of concomitant organ resection. In the absence of distant metastasis, organs adherent to the primary carcinoma are treated as though the tumor had spread directly and are removed by

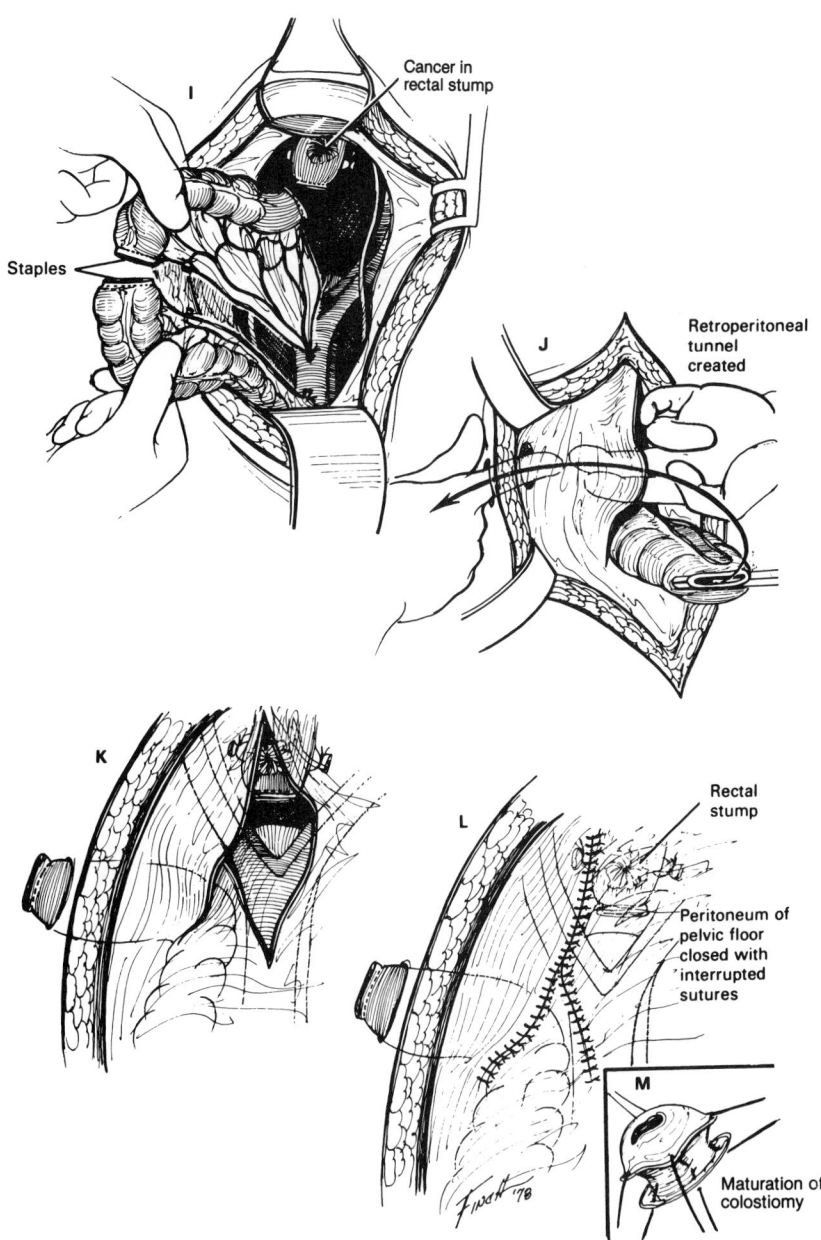

Fig. 28-53 *I,J,K,L,M.* Continued.

means of an en bloc resection. The authors perform oo-phorectomy in all postmenopausal females at the time of primary resection and in premenopausal women if there is any gross abnormality or if peritoneal implants are detected.

Resection Results. The operative mortality for both abdominoperineal resection and restorative resection varies between 0.6 and 12 percent. It averages about 5 percent. The morbidity is significant. The incidence of bladder dysfunction, impotence, injury to adjacent viscera, and major cardiopulmonary complications has been reported to be as high as 41 percent for low anterior resection and 53 percent for abdominoperineal resection. Whereas abdominoperineal resection may have problems related to the stoma and the perineal wound, the primary risk of

restorative procedures is anastomotic disruption and sepsis. Goligher and associates demonstrated a subclinical leak in 70 percent and 40 percent of cases after low and high handsewn anastomoses, respectively. An initial clinical leak rate for low anterior resection of 20 percent has been reported. A more recent series has reported a low incidence of fecal fistula and abscess associated with circular intraluminal stapling devices.

The functional results after abdominoperineal resection depend on the ability of the individual patient to adjust to a permanent stoma. In most instances this is not a major problem. Some patients find that an irrigation regimen affords sufficient control that an appliance is not required.

Although anal continence can be preserved with only a

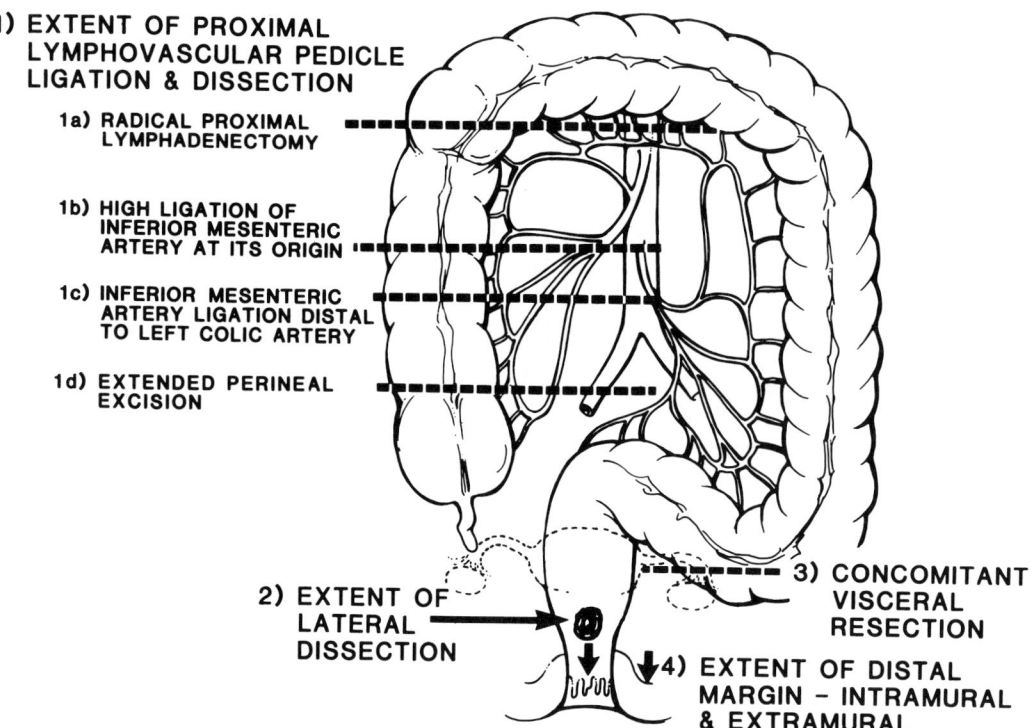

1) EXTENT OF PROXIMAL LYMPHOVASCULAR PEDICLE LIGATION & DISSECTION

1a) RADICAL PROXIMAL LYMPHADENECTOMY

1b) HIGH LIGATION OF INFERIOR MESENTERIC ARTERY AT ITS ORIGIN

1c) INFERIOR MESENTERIC ARTERY LIGATION DISTAL TO LEFT COLIC ARTERY

1d) EXTENDED PERINEAL EXCISION

2) EXTENT OF LATERAL DISSECTION

3) CONCOMITANT VISCERAL RESECTION

4) EXTENT OF DISTAL MARGIN – INTRAMURAL & EXTRAMURAL

Fig. 28-59. The four major areas of controversy regarding the ideal extent of major resections for carcinoma of the rectum. Lockhart-Mummery's extended perineal excision ligated the superior rectal vessels 5 to 7.5 cm below the sacral promontory (1d). Miles' abdominoperineal resection improved survival rates of patients with Dukes' C lesions by extending the proximal dissection to the level of the inferior mesenteric artery just distal to the left colic (1c). More proximal ligation at the level of the origin of the inferior mesenteric artery (1b) may be of value. More proximal dissection along the aorta and vena cava (1a) is of unproved value. Whether the lateral dissection should include hypogastric lymphadenectomy is debated (2). The ideal distal margin remains controversial (3). The efficacy of concomitant visceral resection of grossly uninvolved viscera remains open to question (4). (From: *Rothenberger DA, Wong WD: Rectal cancer. Surg Annu 17:318, 1985, with permission.*)

because they are submucosal, rarely can be seen on barium enema. If found incidentally, they may safely be removed by wedge excision. Most carcinoids larger than 1 cm that produce symptoms are malignant, and more than half have nodal metastases at the time of diagnosis. Clinical and radiographic manifestations of symptomatic carcinoids are essentially the same as in adenocarcinomas of the colon. A definitive cancer resection is done if liver metastases are not demonstrable. Worthwhile palliation is often attained in patients with unresectable disease by resection of the primary tumor. Some patients have lived in relative comfort for many years with residual disease.

Most rectal carcinoids are small, asymptomatic, yellow-gray submucosal nodules found incidentally at proctosigmoidoscopy. Larger lesions may bleed and cause rectal pain. Rectal lesions, unless frankly malignant clinically, should be completely excised transanally with the deep margin extending into the muscularis propria. The diagnosis of malignancy is based on invasion; cytologic criteria are unreliable. If invasive malignancy is found, anterior resection or abdominoperineal resection is indicated.

Leiomyosarcoma

Leiomyosarcoma of the large bowel arises from smooth muscle of the bowel wall and projects either as a submucosal mass into the bowel lumen or on the external surface of the bowel. The degree of differentiation varies and

the pathologist may have difficulty in distinguishing between benign and malignant tumors. Malignant tumors spread by direct extension or by bloodstream. Lymphatic spread occurs rarely.

Symptoms of leiomyosarcoma are indistinguishable from those of other tumors although massive bleeding can occasionally occur. Local excision is reserved for small lesions since the recurrence is high. Larger lesions require bowel resection or abdominoperineal resection if they occur in the lower rectum.

Lymphoma

Malignant lymphoma of the colon and rectum is rare but accounts for about 10 percent of all gastrointestinal lymphomas. The cecum is involved more commonly than the left colon or the rectum, but this distribution is probably due to spread into the cecum from a lymphoma arising in the terminal ileum. Clinical presentation is usually indistinguishable from that of an adenocarcinoma. Bowel resection is the treatment of choice. Postoperative irradiation and chemotherapy are given according to the stage of the disease. The prognosis depends on the extent of the disease: whether it is confined to the bowel wall, has spread to regional lymph nodes or para-aortic lymph nodes, or has direct extension to adjacent organs. Overall, the 5-year survival following curative resection is about 60 percent.

ANAL NEOPLASMS

Malignancies of the anal canal are uncommon. They account for about 2 percent of large bowel cancers. Neoplasms of the anal canal should be divided into two categories as designated by the World Health Organization (WHO). In this classification, the anal canal is arbitrarily divided into the area above the dentate line as "anal canal" and the area below the dentate line as "anal margin."

Anal Margin Neoplasms

SQUAMOUS CELL CARCINOMA (Fig. 28-60). Squamous cell carcinoma of the anal margin grows slowly and typically has rolled, everted edges with central ulceration. Any chronic unhealed and indurated ulceration in the anal area should be considered a potential squamous cell carcinoma until proved otherwise by biopsy. It is usually well differentiated histologically with well-developed patterns of keratination. These tumors have a greater tendency to spread to inguinal nodes than anal canal squamous cell carcinoma. Despite the surface location, the lesions are usually diagnosed late, with 50 percent of cases detected more than 24 months following onset of symptoms.

Treatment is by radiotherapy or surgical excision. Since carcinoma of the anal margin is late to metastasize, adequate local excision can be carried out in many cases. If the carcinoma has invaded the underlying sphincter muscles, an abdominoperineal resection is indicated. In selected cases, radium implantation also gives good results. A radical groin dissection should be carried out only if there are metastases to the inguinal nodes. The overall 5-year survival of squamous cell carcinoma of the anal margin is about 60 percent.

BASAL CELL CARCINOMA. Basal cell carcinoma of the anal margin is rare. It occurs three times as frequently in men as in women. The lesion is characterized by a central ulceration with irregular and raised edges. It remains superficial, mobile, and rarely metastasizes, although frequently inguinal lymphadenopathy develops from reactive inflammation. The patients present with complaints of mild discomfort, itching, or bleeding.

Treatment is by local excision or radiotherapy, which is equally effective. The inguinal nodes are rarely involved, and the prognosis is excellent.

BOWEN'S DISEASE (Fig. 28-61). Bowen's disease of the perianal skin is a rare, slow-growing, intraepidermal squamous cell carcinoma (carcinoma in situ). The lesion appears as discrete, scaly, or crusted plaques, sometimes exhibiting a moist surface. It produces a chronic dermatosis not unlike Paget's disease and can also be mistaken for psoriasis, excoriation in pruritus ani, or eczema. The patients may complain of itching, burning, or spotty bleeding.

Fig. 28-60. Squamous cell carcinoma. (From: *Goldberg SM, Gordon PH, Nivatvongs S, 1980, with permission.*)

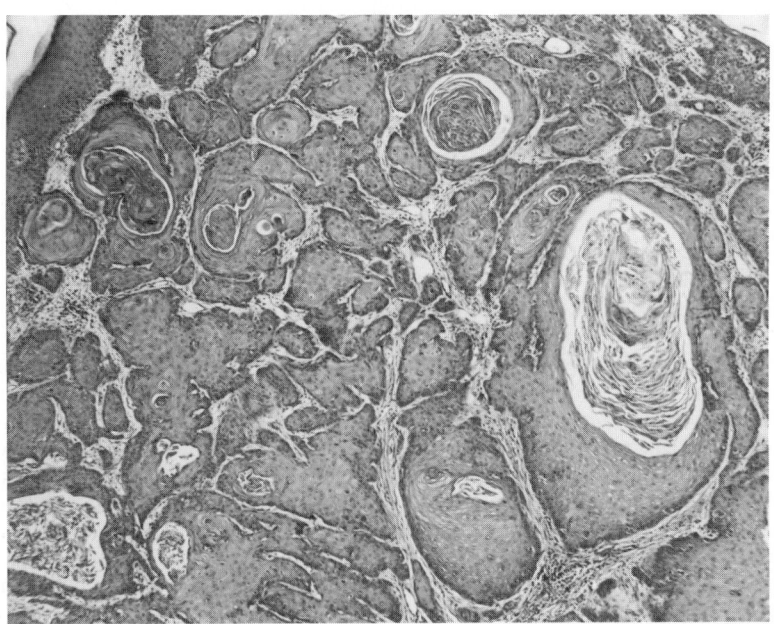

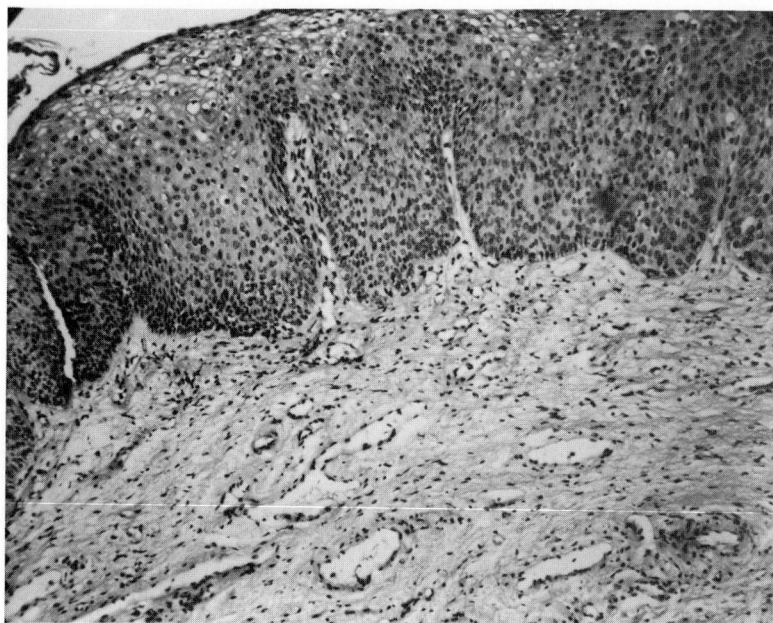

Fig. 28-61. Bowen's disease. Atypical epithelial cells involve full thickness of the epidermis (carcinoma in situ). (From: *Goldberg SM, Gordon PH, Nivatvongs S, 1980, with permission.*)

Only a biopsy will confirm the diagnosis. An important feature of this type of tumor is that up to 70 to 80 percent of these patients have one or more primary internal malignancy or a primary cancer of the skin with metastasis. It is essential to rule out other primary malignancies. Wide local excision is the treatment of choice. Because excision may need to be extensive, skin grafting, rotation flaps, or advancement flaps may be necessary. The prognosis is good, and if local recurrence develops, further local excision is sufficient.

PERIANAL PAGET'S DISEASE. Sir James Paget first described this disease in relation to the nipple of the breast in females. Extramammary Paget's disease may be found in the axilla and anogenital region (labia majora, penis, scrotum, groin, pubic area, perineum, perianal region, thigh, and buttock). Paget's disease of the perianal area is a malignant neoplasm of the intraepidermal portion of the apocrine glands with or without associated dermal involvement. It has a long preinvasive phase, but if the patient lives long enough, an adenocarcinoma of the apocrine-gland will develop. It is more common in women than men, with the highest incidence in the seventh decade. As in Bowen's disease, up to 80 percent of the patients with Paget's disease are found to have or develop a coexisting carcinoma.

Intractable anal itching is usually present for many months. Macroscopically, the lesion appears as an erythematous, scaly, or eczematoid plaque-like lesion similar to other cutaneous lesions, making clinical diagnosis difficult. Diagnosis is made by biopsy, which shows characteristic Paget cells: large, pale, vacuolated cells with hyperchromatic eccentric nuclei (Fig. 28-62). They invariably contain acid mucosubstances, an important feature in the differential diagnosis with melanoma and Bowen's disease.

Wide local excision is the treatment of choice for the localized lesion. Because of the high incidence of local recurrence due to residual tumor, it is of vital importance to obtain an adequate margin. Grossly, the extent of involvement is ill-defined. Multiple punch biopsies may be required to determine the extent of the involvement. For more advanced lesions with an underlying carcinoma, an abdominoperineal resection is indicated. Inguinal lymph node dissection is performed only if the groin lymph nodes are positive for metastasis. Because diagnosis is often delayed (on average 4 years), about 25 percent of patients with perianal Paget's disease have metastases. The sites of metastasis, in order of frequency, are inguinal and pelvic lymph nodes, liver, bone, lung, brain, bladder, prostate, and adrenal gland. The prognosis is poor once metastasis has occurred.

Anal Canal Neoplasms

SQUAMOUS CELL CARCINOMA. This type of carcinoma arises from the cloacogenic area. It is a flat, ulcerating, nonkeratinizing neoplasm that occurs more frequently in women. Minor perianal problems such as bleeding occur in about half of the patients. Other symptoms include pain and an anal mass. Almost one-third of the patients in most series had a mistaken initial diagnosis of benign or inflammatory disease. At the time of treatment, squamous cell carcinomas of the anal canal have been found to metastasize to the superior rectal lymph nodes in about 40 percent and to the inguinal nodes is about 30 percent of the cases. The overall corrected 5-year survival is about 50 percent.

BASALOID CARCINOMA (CLOACOGENIC CARCINOMA). These are a variant of squamous cell carcinomas that in

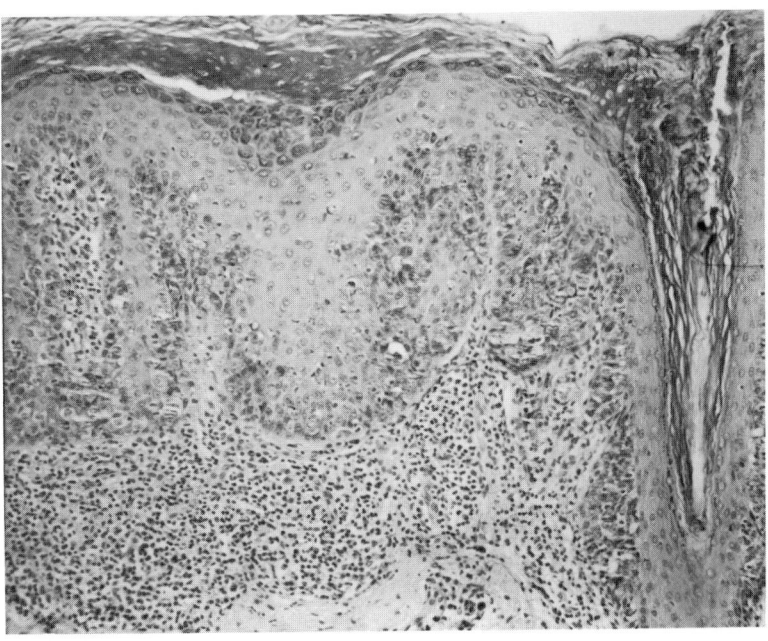

Fig. 28-62. Perianal Paget's disease. Paget cells are present just above the basal layer.

some degree resemble basal cell carcinomas of the skin. *Basaloid* refers to the histologic appearance of palisading nuclei seen in the periphery of the clumps of cells which characterize this malignancy (Fig. 28-63). Histologically they are unlike basal cell carcinoma in that there are areas of eosinophilic necrosis within clumps of the neoplastic cells. There is nuclear irregularity and the presence of giant cells, especially in the anaplastic variety. There is

female preponderance, and the average age of onset is sixty years with a range from forty to eighty years.

This type of carcinoma arises from the transitional zone about the dentate line, and, therefore, the term *transitional cloacogenic carcinoma* is also used. Because of their similar behavior, some authors group them together with squamous cell carcinomas as *epidermoid carcinomas of the anal canal*. The clinical features are similar to squamous cell carcinomas of the anal canal.

As in squamous cell carcinomas of the anal canal, about 50 percent of patients already have regional lymph node involvement at the time of operation. The prognosis

Fig. 28-63. Basaloid (cloacogenic) carcinoma. (From: *Goldberg SM, Gordon PH, Nivatvongs S, 1980, with permission.*)

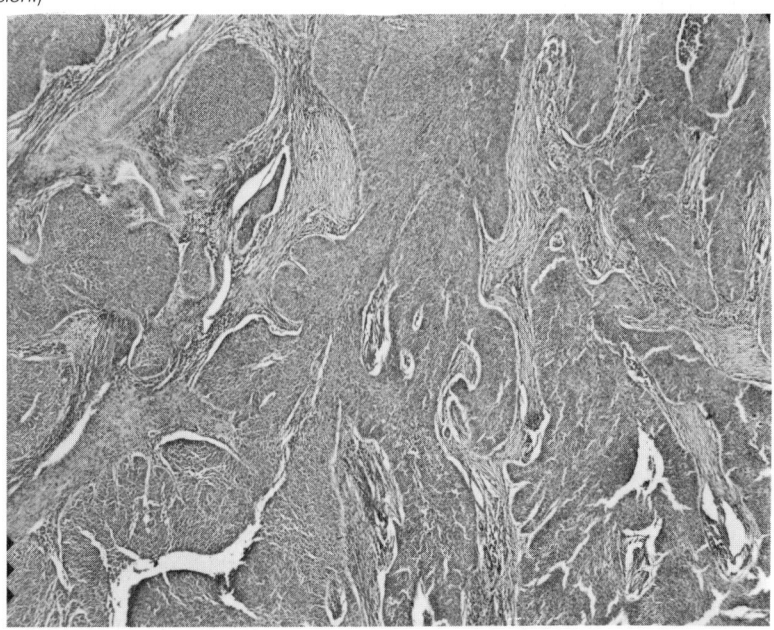

is related to the grading of the carcinoma. The 5-year survival for patients with well-differentiated lesions is 90 percent, with moderately differentiated lesion 60 percent, and for those with anaplastic lesions there is almost no 5-year survival. The overall 5-year survival is about 50 percent.

MUCOEPIDERMOID CARCINOMA. This is another variant of squamous cell carcinoma and has the same basic histologic pattern except for the addition of mucin, which varies in amount from lesion to lesion, and even within different areas of the same lesion. There is slight female preponderance. The behavior and prognosis of this lesion is similar to squamous cell or basaloid carcinoma.

Treatment of Epidermoid Carcinoma of the Anal Canal (Squamous Cell Carcinoma, Basaloid or Cloacogenic Carcinoma, and Mucoepidermoid Carcinoma)

Local Excision. This form of therapy should be reserved only for early lesions or well-differentiated lesions that are confined to the submucosa. It may also be considered for individuals who are a poor risk for an extensive operation.

Combined Therapy. In 1972 Nigro et al. instituted a protocol consisting of preoperative irradiation and chemotherapy with the intent of reducing the extent of the disease to permit more effective removal by radical operation. The addition of chemotherapy, particularly mitomycin C, which is a radiosensitizer, was directed at decreasing the radiation dose so that its effect would not delay wound healing. The regimen of treatment is as follows:

External irradiation 3000 rads (30 cGy) to the primary tumor, pelvic and inguinal nods
Day one to day 21 (200 rads/day)
Systemic chemotherapy
5-FU: 1000 mg/m^2/24 h as a continuous infusion for 4 days. Starts on day one.
Mitomycin C: 15 mg/m^2/IV bolus on day one
5-FU: repeated day 28 to day 31

Operation is performed 4 to 6 weeks after completion of the irradiation. If the lesion disappears, as proved by adequate excision and biopsy, no further treatment is necessary. If residual cancer is present, and if there is no evidence of disseminated disease, abdominoperineal resection should follow.

Of 104 patients evaluated for the effect of chemoradiation therapy, 97 patients had no gross tumor remaining in the anal canal, while in seven patients gross tumor was present, although reduced in size. Eighty-two patients were alive and apparently free of disease from 2 to 11 years. It appears that this combined regimen is at least as effective as the previous standard treatment with abdominoperineal resection.

MELANOMA. Melanoma, a rare malignant tumor of the anal canal, accounts for 0.5 to 1 percent of anal canal malignancies. The anal canal represents the third most common site for melanomas, preceded only by the skin and eyes. Almost all the tumors arise from the epidermoid lining of the anal canal. Most melanomas occur adjacent

to the dentate line, although there are a few reports of these tumors arising in the rectum.

Rectal bleeding is the most common symptom. Melanoma is suspected when a deeply pigmented lesion is noted, but this can be confused with thrombosed hemorrhoids. The majority of tumors are lightly pigmented or are nonpigmented, and they often are misdiagnosed as polyps or epidermoid carcinomas.

Anal canal melanomas have a marked tendency to spread submucosally into the rectum, but they rarely invade adjacent organs. Lymphatic spread to the mesenteric nodes occurs in about one-third of the patients; spread to the inguinal nodes is less common. Hematogenous spread to the liver and lung is early and rapid, accounting for most of the deaths.

Melanomas are radioresistant and do not respond well to chemotherapy. The only chance for cure, therefore, is early diagnosis followed by radical operation. Abdominoperineal resection represents the approach of choice, but the prognosis remains extremely poor. Survival after total rectal excision or local excision appears to be similar, with mean values ranging from 12 to 18 months. Because of this poor prognosis, in many cases only a local excision should be considered.

ADENOCARCINOMAS OF THE ANAL CANAL. Carcinomas of the lower rectum occasionally extend downward to involve the anal canal; therefore, it may be impossible to determine the origin of the lesion. The ducts of the anal glands are lined primarily by squamous epithelium, but close to their opening in the crypts they are lined by transitional epithelium, and in the depth of the gland by mucin-secreting columnar epithelium.

Patients usually present with complaints of pain and swelling in the anal area but no mass in the anal canal. They may also present with a perianal or ischiorectal abscess or a fistula-in-ano. Occasionally these are incidental findings in hemorrhoidectomy specimens. The diagnosis is usually made late, and the disease has frequently spread beyond hope for cure.

Adenocarcinomas developing in long-standing fistulas-in-ano have occasionally been reported. It has been suggested that these carcinomas are due to chronic irritation of the epithelium around either the internal or the external openings of fistulas over a period of years. Some authors, however, believe that carcinomas in fistulas are ductal in origin.

The treatment of adenocarcinoma of the anal canal is the same as for adenocarcinoma of the rectum.

RECTAL PROLAPSE

Prolapse of the rectum (procidentia) is an uncommon condition in which the full thickness of the rectal wall turns inside out, into or through the anal canal. Typically, the extruded rectum is seen as concentric rings of mucosa (Fig. 28-64). This should not be confused with rectal mucosal prolapse (Table 28-7) or prolapsed hemorrhoids, in which the radial folds of mucosa extrude through the anus. Although prolapse of the rectum can occur at any

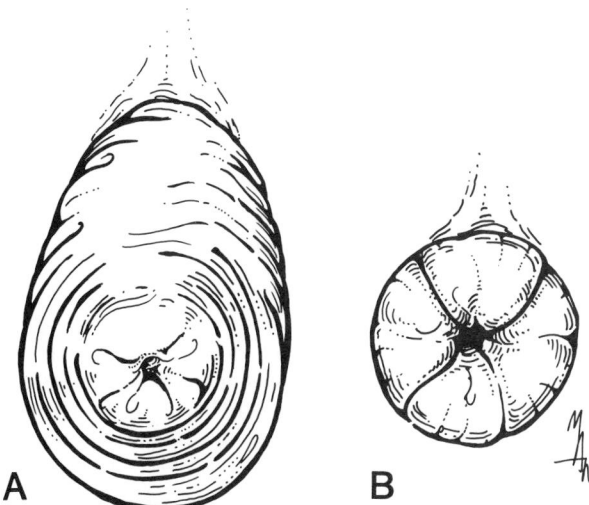

Fig. 28-64. Differential diagnosis of true rectal prolapse vs. mucosal prolapse. In true rectal prolapse *(A)*, note the circumferential folds. In mucosal prolapse *(B)*, folds are in the radial configurations. (From: *Wassef R, Rothenberger DA, Goldberg SM: Rectal prolapse. Curr Probl Surg 23:402, 1986, with permission.*)

age, the peak incidence is between sixty and seventy years in women. In men the age distribution is constant. Female to male ratio is between 5 and 10:1.

Cineradiography has demonstrated that procidentia begins as an intussusception that occurs circumferentially at 6 to 7 cm from the anal verge. Certain anatomic defects that are in some way related but not necessarily the cause of the prolapse are well known. The levator muscles are diastased. The endopelvic fascia is loose. The normal horizontal position of the rectum is lost. The anterior rectovaginal or rectovesical pouch is unusually deep. The anal sphincter muscle is commonly weak. Surgical treatment of rectal prolapse focuses on correction of one or several or these anatomic changes. Because these are not the cause of the prolapse, surgical correction is not universally successful, and there is a high incidence of recurrence.

CLINICAL MANIFESTATION. The early symptoms are minor, including anorectal pain or discomfort during defecation. Difficulty to initiate bowel movement and the feeling of incomplete evacuation are also common.

In the advanced stage, fecal and urinary incontinence

Table 28-7. DIAGNOSTIC CHARACTERISTICS OF PROCIDENTIA AND RECTAL MUCOSAL PROLAPSE

Procidentia	*Mucosal prolapse*
Concentric furrows	Longitudinal furrows
Anus in normal anatomic position	Anus everted
Sulcus between anus and protruding bowel	No sulcus present

SOURCE: From Carter HG: *South Med J* 64:1238, 1971, with permission.

are common. Parks et al. have shown that the incontinence is the consequence of entrapment or stretching of the pudendal or perineal nerve resulting in neuromuscular dysfunction. It is therefore essential to repair the prolapse before this mishap occurs. The diagnosis is easy if the prolapse comes through the anus. When the prolapse remains in the upper anal canal (''hidden prolapse''), the diagnosis can be difficult. Redness of the rectal mucosa, especially anteriorly at the 6 to 7 cm level, gives a clue. Straining of the anorectum with an anoscope or with a flexible sigmoidoscope in place can confirm the diagnosis of hidden prolapse.

DIAGNOSTIC STUDIES. Although a barium enema is usually performed for completeness, it is often unrewarding. Patients with rectal prolapse have difficulty retaining the contrast material, and abundant fecal residue often obscures the study. Cinedefecography may be useful in demonstrating internal intussusception that has not yet exteriorized through the anal canal. Balloon proctography is another means of documenting some of the anatomic features typical of these patients (loss of the anorectal angle, lax squeeze pressures, etc.). Transit time studies can be helpful in identifying the subgroup of patients with marked colonic inertia. Along with conventional manometry, these tests have documented in a reproducible and quantifiable manner the clinically obvious anatomic or functional defects encountered in these patients.

These investigations may prove useful in establishing an individual treatment plan for each patient. Perhaps their greatest role will be in predicting the functional prognosis or in assessing the need for additional surgery (such as postanal or sphincter repair for incontinence or subtotal colectomy for chronic constipation).

TREATMENT. Surgical therapy for rectal prolapse is based on narrowing of anal orifice; obliteration of peritoneal pouch of Douglas; restoration of pelvic floor; resection of redundant bowel; suspension or fixation of rectum; and combinations of the above. A wide diversity of surgical repairs exist for patients with rectal prolapse.

Rectal Sling. Several variations on a main theme exist with this procedure (Fig. 28-65). An abdominal approach is required, whereby the rectum with its mesentery is mobilized for varying degrees posteriorly. The partially or completely mobilized rectum is anchored to the front of the sacrum, utilizing a sling of Teflon or Marlex mesh or other foreign material. If this type of technique is used, it is important to ensure that the sling is loose enough to allow easy passage of two fingers between it and the rectum. If made too snug, fecal impaction above the level of the sling may occur.

Ivalon Sponge Wrap. This technique involves no abdominal approach (Fig. 28-66). Although not popular in this country, it has been widely utilized in the United Kingdom and Europe. The rectum with its mesentery is completely mobilized posteriorly. Polyvinyl alcohol sponge material is wrapped around the back of the rectum and then is attached to the presacral fascia and periosteum on the sacrum. In some instances Marlex or Teflon mesh is used in preference to the polyvinyl alcohol sponge.

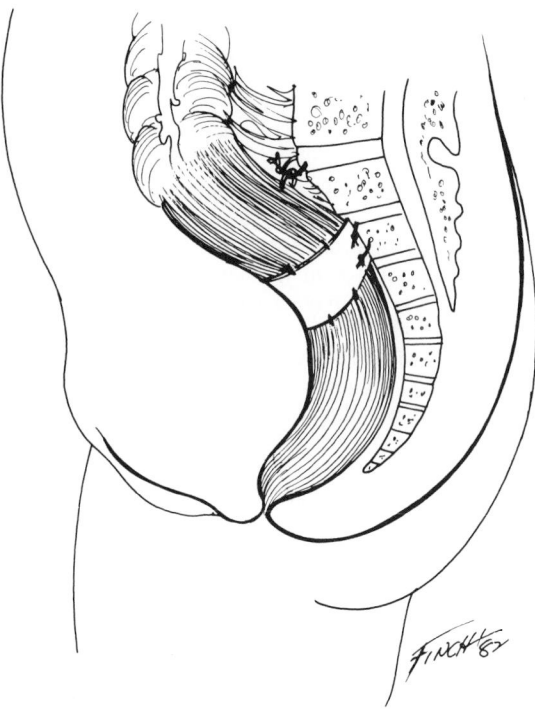

Fig. 28-65. Rectal sling operation. A 5-cm band of Teflon or Marlex mesh is placed around the fully mobilized rectum and sutured to the presacral fascia.

Fig. 28-66. Ivalon sponge wrap operation. A sheet of Ivalon sponge is sutured to the presacral fascia, then wrapped over and sutured to the rectum.

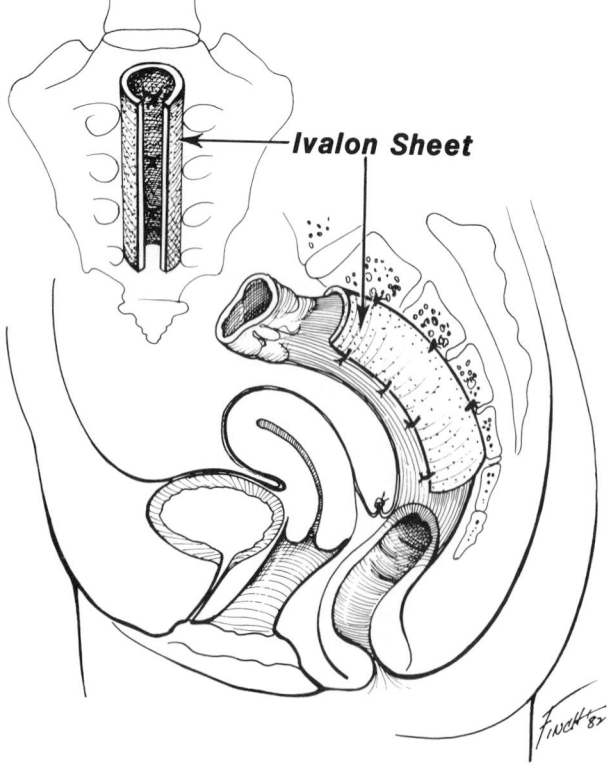

Anterior Resection. An abdominal approach is required, with the operative technique being similar to that for low anterior resection of the rectum. Dissection close to the rectal wall minimizes the chance of injury to the pelvic autonomic nerves. The rectum at or just above the anterior peritoneal reflection, which is the starting point of the intussusception, is resected. The proximal line of resection should be at a convenient level in the rectosigmoid or sigmoid colon so that any redundancy is removed without tension on the anastomosis.

Transabdominal Proctopexy and Sigmoid Resection. This is an abdominal procedure whereby the rectum is fixed to the front of the sacrum without the necessity of using a foreign material (Fig. 28-67). This operation is our procedure of choice. Our preference is to use a low transverse abdominal incision. The rectum is fully mobilized posteriorly and laterally down to the pelvic floor. The lateral ligaments of the rectum are not divided. The mobilized rectum is drawn up toward the sacrum, and the peritoneum, including the endopelvic fascia of the lateral ligament on each side of the rectum, is sutured to the presacral fascia and periosteum just below the promontory of the sacrum. One to three sutures of 2-0 silk on each side are all that is necessary. No attempt is made to obliterate the anterior cul-de-sac or to approximate the levator hiatus. In most instances rectosigmoid colon resection with a high end-to-end anastomosis is performed because of the concurrent presence of marked redundancy, predisposing to sigmoid volvulus.

Perineal Rectosigmoidectomy. This procedure is well tolerated by all patients, especially the elderly or frail, and general, regional, or even local anesthesia can be used. The procedure may be performed in the lithotomy or prone jackknife positions. The prolapse is exteriorized and a circular incision is made at 2 cm proximal to the dentate line. This is deepened so that the intussusception along with the redundant rectosigmoid and sigmoid colon can be resected and an end-to-end anastomosis performed perineally (Fig. 28-68).

Delorme Procedure. This is a perineal operation. The technique is based on a submucosal resection, with reefing and plication of the lower rectal musculature to produce in effect an encirclement of the anal sphincters. It has the advantage, like the perineal rectosigmoidectomy, of avoiding an abdominal approach.

Transsacral Approaches. This type of surgical approach to the treatment of complete rectal prolapse has remained unpopular despite obvious theoretical advantages and good clinical results (Fig. 28-69). This approach entails removal of the coccyx, as well as the lowermost two segments of the sacrum. The fascia of Waldeyer is incised and the levator ani muscle separated to expose the rectum, which is then mobilized and freed from the adjacent structures. The peritoneal layer is identified anterior to the rectum and incised. If redundancy of the sigmoid is encountered, a resection can be performed by withdrawing a loop of sigmoid colon through the peritoneal incision. Following the resection, an end-to-end anastomosis if performed. The medial borders of the levator ani muscles and the puborectalis are identified and approximated anterior to the rectum.

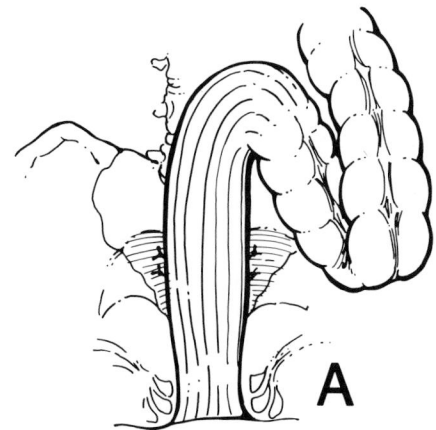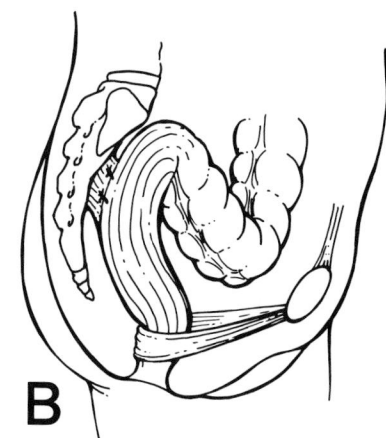

Fig. 28-67. Transabdominal proctopexy. The fully mobilized rectum is fixed to the presacral fascia with 00 silk.

Fig. 28-68. Perineal rectosigmoidectomy (the patient in lithotomy position). *A.* A circular incision is made 2 cm proximal to the dentate line. *B.* The anterior peritoneal reflection is opened. *C.* The mesentery is divided. *D.* The previously opened peritoneum is resutured to the bowel wall. *E.* The prolapse along with the redundant bowel is resected. *F.* Anastomosis is made, using one layer interrupted 4-0 Vicryl or Dexon.

Davidian and Thomas reported on 30 such patients followed for 1 to 11 years. There was no mortality. Morbidity was minimal when no resection was performed. There was no recurrence. Hagihara et al. have also advocated this approach, claiming that it offers the following advantages: it is simple and safe even for the elderly; it avoids an abdominal incision with its concomitant postoperative complications; it allows complete correction of all associated abnormalities; and it has been performed with a low recurrence rate.

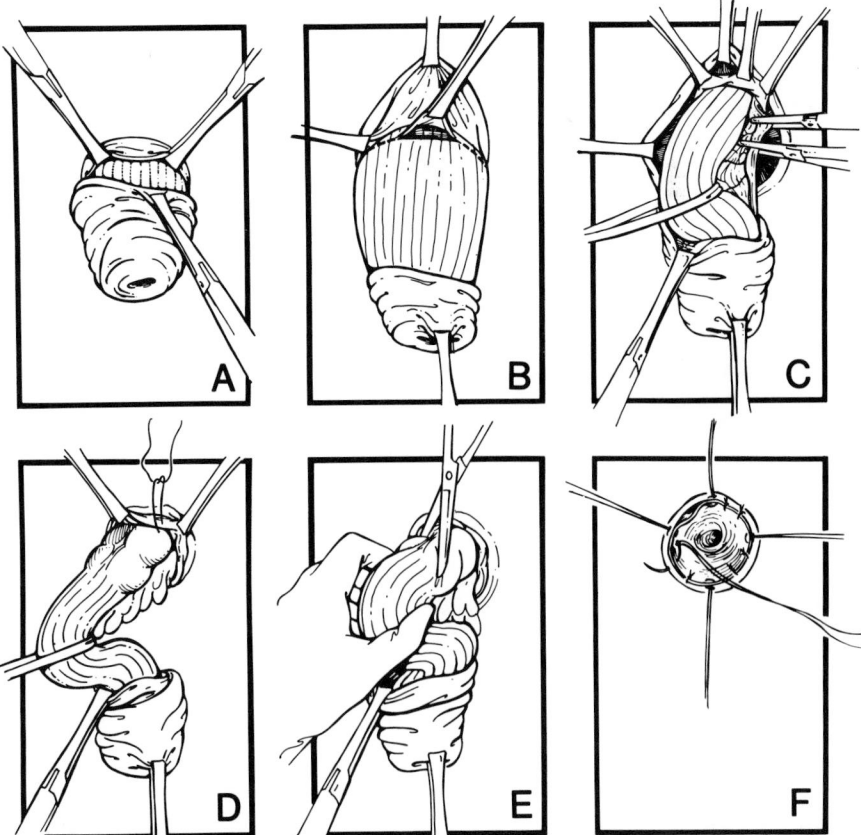

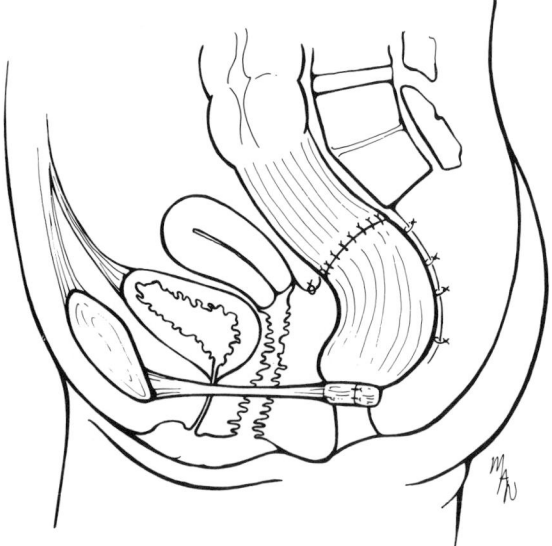

Fig. 28-69. Through a transsacral approach the rectum is mobilized and any rectosigmoid redundancy resected. Following the completion of the anastomosis, plication of the levator ani muscles is carried out as well as an excision of the deep pouch of Douglas. The rectum is then fixed to the periosteum of the anterior surface of the sacrum with a few stitches on each side. (From: *Wassef R, Rothenberger DA, Goldberg SM: Rectal prolapse. Curr Probl Surg 23:402, 1986, with permission.*)

This approach has not been reported extensively and seems to remain unpopular. The main disadvantage of this procedure, as pointed out by Goligher, is that surgeons in general are very familiar with the abdominal approach from their experience in the treatment of malignant disease of the rectum, whereas very few are acquainted with the sacral approach.

Anal incontinence accompanies complete rectal prolapse in approximately 50 percent of the cases. Definitive surgical repair of the prolapsing rectum results in resolution of or improvement in the continence problems in a large percentage of patients. In those patients in whom incontinence persists despite a successful repair of the prolapse, further operative intervention may become necessary. Under such circumstances extensive denervation of the sphincter muscle often exists, precluding direct sphincteric repair. Decreasing the anorectal angle by performing a postanal repair through the intersphincteric plane has been successful in some individuals with this problem (Fig. 28-70).

Our choice of procedure has been the transabdominal proctopexy for all good-risk patients. For patients who are considered not suitable for a safe intraabdominal procedure but who can withstand general or regional anesthesia, perineal rectosigmoidectomy is the method of choice. In the elderly and in those whose general medical condition preclude a definitive repair, a perineal rectosigmoidectomy can be performed using local anesthesia. The Thiersch wire encirclement procedures are not rec-

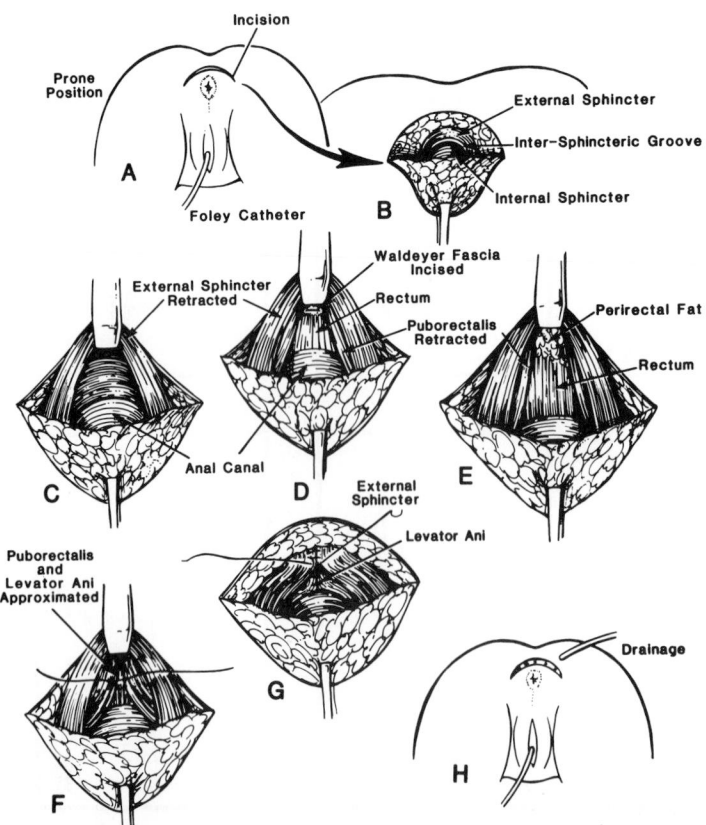

Fig. 28-70. Techniques of postanal intersphincteric sphincteroplasty and pelvic floor repair.

ommended even in the poor-risk patient. Such procedures, although simple, produce an alarmingly high incidence of fecal impaction, which makes nursing more difficult. Under such circumstances it is probably better not to offer any surgical therapy at all.

RECTAL, ANAL, PERIRECTAL, AND PERIANAL INFECTIONS

GONOCOCCAL PROCTITIS. Gonococcal proctitis is found most commonly among homosexual males. In the female, the rectum may be infected by the spread of discharge from gonococcal cervicitis or urethritis. Patients are generally asymptomatic but may have mild anal burning, pain, or discharge in the acute phase. Proctoscopic examination reveals hyperemic and edematous rectal mucosa with purulent discharge in the anal crypts. In the chronic phase, examination of the anal canal and rectum may show them to be normal. Diagnosis is confirmed by Gram smears of the discharge and culture in the appropriate medium, either Thayer-Martin or Stuart.

Penicillin remains the antibiotic of choice. When penicillin is contraindicated or fails to effect a response, oral tetracycline or intramuscular injection of spectinomycin hydrochloride may be used. Cure is determined by smears and cultures taken at regular intervals after treatment.

CHLAMYDIA PROCTITIS (LYMPHOGRANULOMA VENEREUM). *Chlamydia trachomatis* is an obligate human intracellular parasite that causes, among other conditions, urogenital and anorectal infections. *C. trachomatis* will cause various degrees of clinical and subclinical proctitis.

The proctitis is mainly a condition of tropical and subtropical climates. In females it tends to involve the rectum late in the course of the disease by spreading via the lymphatics in the rectovaginal septum. In most men proctitis arises from the practice of anal intercourse, it may present early.

Diagnosis of chlamydial infections of the anorectum is by tissue culture and, in the case of lymphogranuloma venereum (LGV), by serological tests with additional information from biopsy. Treatment is with tetracyclines or, as a second choice, erythromycin.

Lymphogranuloma venereum is either an acute or a chronic venereal disease caused by *C. trachomatis*. Transmission of the disease is by intercourse or contact with contaminated exudate from active lesions. In the male, the most common sites for the primary lesion are the coronal sulcus, prepuce, glans penis, and urethra. In the female, the primary lesion may appear on any part of the external genitalia, but the most common site is the posterior vaginal wall. The lesion usually is single, consisting of a small erosion, blister, or ulcer, without induration or infiltration. The primary focus is painless and so transient that few patients with LGV are aware of it. Adenitis develops in the lymphatic drainage area soon after the primary lesion disappears, although, at times, several months elapse.

Rectal stricture is a sequel of perirectal lymphatic involvement or direct anorectal mucosal infection. The stricture usually is several centimeters above the anal orifice and is 4 to 10 cm in length. Involvement of the perirectal tissues causes perirectal abscess or chronic anal fistulas. Diagnosis is confirmed by the Frei intradermal test and the LGV complement fixation test. A cross-reaction with organisms of psittacosis and other chlamydiae may take place. Once positive, the test remains positive for life, and a persistent negative result in the presence of the disease is rare.

Tetracycline or chloramphenicol is the drug of choice. In early stricture, dilatation by finger of dilator is recommended. Colostomy is indicated for complete obstruction. Biopsy for possible malignancy is mandatory.

ANORECTAL HERPES. Anorectal herpes is caused by *Herpesvirus hominis* type II, the same organism that is implicated in genital herpes. Anorectal herpes is less common than gonorrhea but more common than syphilis. The clinical presentation usually begins with itching and soreness in or around the anus, followed by severe anorectal pain. The pain may be so intense that the patient is reluctant to have a bowel movement, leading to constipation and fecal impaction. Examination reveals erythematous, red areas with small groups of vesicles that rupture and become ulcerated. The diagnosis is confirmed by viral culture of the vesicular fluid. There is no effective cure for herpes. The lesions should be kept clean by frequent sitz baths. Symptomatic relief is obtained by the use of analgesic drugs and the local application of soothing agents.

ACQUIRED IMMUNODEFICIENCY SYNDROME (AIDS). Rectal infections seen in AIDS can be caused directly by human insufficiency virus (HIV) or by one of the concomitant opportunistic infections. HIV can involve the bowel wall, causing malabsorption and resultant diarrhea.

Mycobacterium avium intracellulare (MAI) is a frequent AIDS-related opportunistic infection. Involvement of the bowel wall results in diarrhea and occasionally superficial ulcers. The diagnosis is made by appropriate staining of stool or rectal biopsy. Treatment remains extremely difficult even with multiple agents. *Cytomegalovirus colitis* can also cause diarrhea and superficial ulceration. Reports of inflammatory bowel disease and perforation have been noted. Although the virus primarily affects the cecum, rectal involvement has been noted. Antiviral therapy has been ineffective.

Chronic perianal *herpes simplex* is frequently seen as a complication of AIDS. Severe tenesmus, rectal pain, and hematochezia are characteristic and often disabling symptoms. The lesion is readily recognizable and appropriate culture confirms the diagnosis. Acyclovir can be effective in controlling symptoms. *Salmonella enterocolitis* is seen occasionally in AIDS with frequent resultant bacteremia. Other enteric organisms such as *Shigella, Campylobacter, Entamoeba,* and *Giardia* are often seen in sexually active individuals who practice anal intercourse, and the consequences may be profound in the immunocompromised host.

Anorectal AIDS-related malignancies may be seen as the primary presenting complaint or as a manifestation of

AIDS elsewhere in the body. Kaposi's sarcoma is the most common AIDS-related malignancy. The characteristic raised violet- to purple-appearing lesions can be seen throughout the gastrointestinal tract, including the rectum and anus. Symptoms of diarrhea, melena, hematochezia, or rectal discomfort are noted. Biopsies will show the characteristic histopathologic features. Chemotherapy with vincristine and vinblastine is highly effective in inducing remission. Localized radiation is sometimes undertaken.

Squamous cell carinoma of the rectum and cloacogenic carcinoma of the rectum had been described in anally receptive sexually active individuals prior to the era of AIDS. The cause of these carcinomas has been related to trauma and chemicals such as lubricants. Exposure to sexually transmitted viruses, and especially to condyloma acuminata, has also been felt to play a role in these entities.

CONDYLOMA ACUMINATA. Anal condylomata acuminata, or warts, are caused by a papilloma virus. Condylomata occur in the perianal area or the squamous epithelium of the anal canal. Occasionally, the mucosa of the upper part of the anal canal or the lower part of the rectum is involved. The extent of the disease varies from a few small warts to an extensive mass, occluding the anal canal. Bleeding, itching, and irritation are common symptoms. The diagnosis is based on the characteristically soft, papillary appearance. Since most cases are transmitted by sexual contact, other coexisting venereal diseases, especially syphilis and gonorrhea, should be excluded. Multiple biopsies and histologic examination should be done in the case of extensive warts, since a few cases of squamous cell carcinoma arising from condylomata acuminata have been reported.

Small perianal warts may be destroyed by applying bichloracetic acid or 25 percent podophyllin solution. Extensive warts in the perianal area or in the anal canal require excision and/or fulguration under anesthesia. Frequent postoperative follow-up is necessary, since recurrence is as high as 65 percent. Immunotherapy, using autogenous wart-tissue vaccine, in conjunction with excision of the lesions, has been found to be effective and has reduced the recurrence rate to within 10 percent. Immunotherapy should be used with caution, since the vaccine contains an oncogenic virus. Counseling regarding the sexual transmission of the virus should be part of any treatment plan.

ANORECTAL ABSCESS. Anatomy of Perianal Spaces. Around the anorectum, there are several potential spaces that are normally filled with areolar tissues or fat. These spaces can become infected and abscesses can form (Figs. 28-71 and 28-72).

The *perianal space* is in the immediate area of the anus. Laterally, it becomes continuous with the subcutaneous fat of the buttocks. Medially, it is bound by the anoderm up to the level of the dentate line.

The *ischiorectal space* is a triangular-shaped space below the levator ani muscle. It is bound medially by the external sphincter muscle, laterally by the ischium, and inferiorly by the transverse septum. The space on each side is filled with fat and contains the inferior rectal vessels and lymphatics.

The *deep postanal space* connects the ischiorectal space on each side posteriorly. It lies between the levator ani muscle above and the anococcygeal ligament below. The deep postanal space is an important pathway in the formation of an abscess that can spread to one ischiorectal fossa or both, resulting in the so-called horseshoe abscess.

The *intersphincteric space* lies between the internal and external sphincter muscles. It is continuous below with the perianal space and extends above into the wall of the rectum.

The *supralevator space* is situated on each side of the rectum above the levator ani muscle. The two supralevator spaces communicate with each other posteriorly.

Fig. 28-71. Anatomy of perianorectal spaces (A-P view). (From: *Goldberg SM, Gordon PH, Nivatvongs S, 1980, with permission.*)

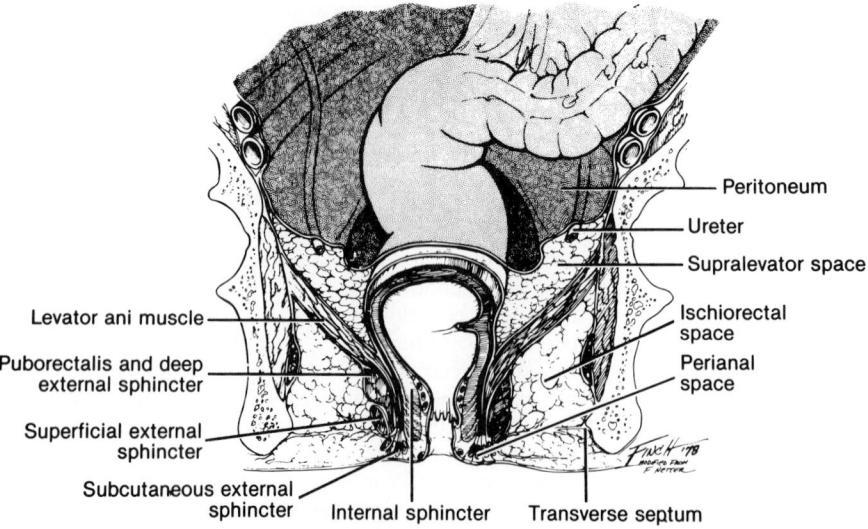

Labels: Peritoneum / Ureter / Supralevator space / Ischiorectal space / Perianal space / Levator ani muscle / Puborectalis and deep external sphincter / Superficial external sphincter / Subcutaneous external sphincter / Internal sphincter / Transverse septum

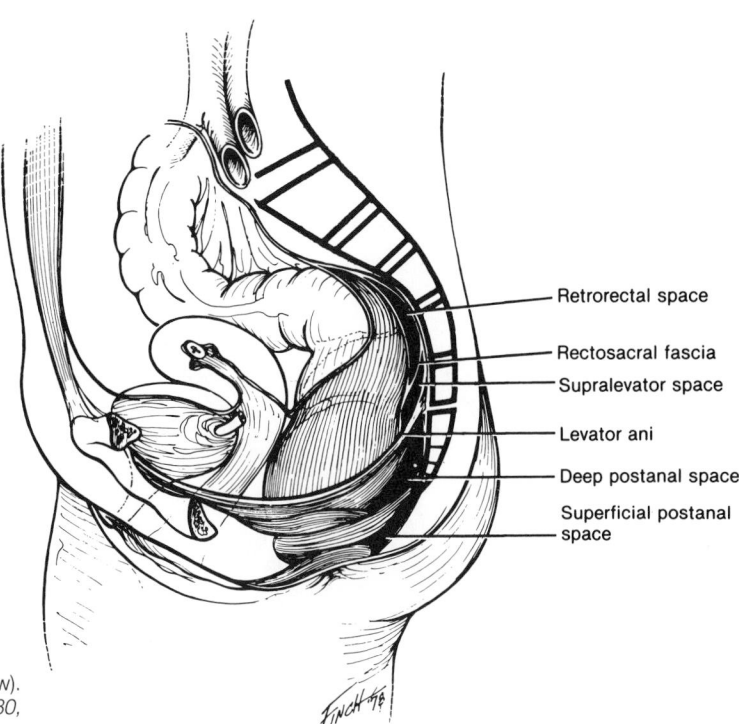

Fig. 28-72. Anatomy of perianorectal spaces (lateral view). (From: *Goldberg SM, Gordon PH, Nivatvongs S, 1980, with permission.*)

Etiology

In the wall of the anal canal, there are a variable number of anal glands (4 to 10) lined by stratified columnar epithelium that have direct openings into the anal crypts in the dentate line. Current evidence suggests that infection of the anal glands is probably the most common origin of perianal abscesses. Because the anal glands lie between the internal and external sphincter muscles, an intersphincteric abscess is formed. The infection may then spread to different spaces (Fig. 28-73). The locations of abscesses in order of frequency are perianal, ischiorectal, intersphincteric, and supralevator.

As a rule, bacteria in perianal abscesses are a mixture of fecal flora and cutaneous flora. The common organisms are *E. coli, Bacteroides, Peptostreptococcus, Streptococcus, Clostridium, Peptococcus, Staphylococcus,* and other gram-negative rods.

CLINICAL MANIFESTATIONS. The initial symptom of most anorectal abscesses is severe pain in the anal region. The pain is throbbing or dully aching in character, aggravated by walking, straining, coughing, and sneezing. Depending on the location of the abscess, a swollen mass may or may not be felt by the patient. Fever or even septicemia may be present. In some patients urinary retention occurs.

Treatment

Like an abscess in any other part of the body, an anorectal abscess must be drained as soon as possible. When properly treated, it results in an uncomplicated recovery with minimal morbidity, although many will progress to a fistula-in-ano. Delayed treatment or inadequate treatment may occasionally cause extensive and life-threatening suppuration associated with massive tissue necrosis and

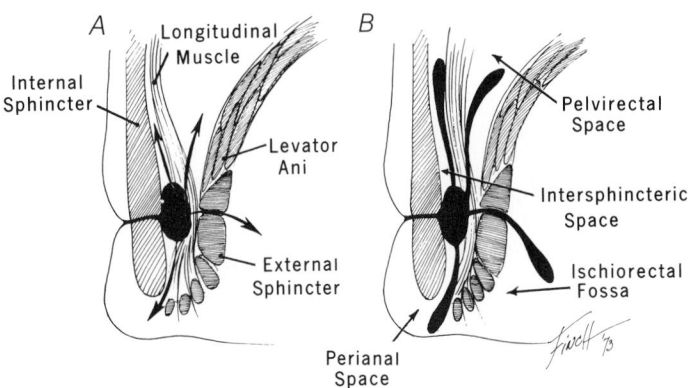

Fig. 28-73. Pathways of infection in perianal spaces.

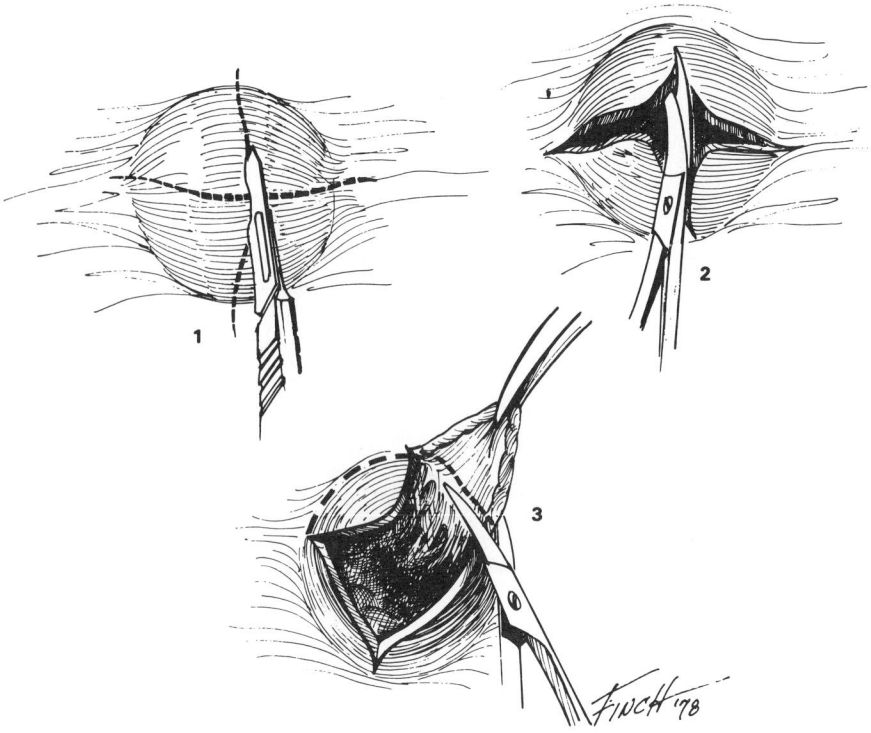

Fig. 28-74. Technique of drainage of perianal abscess. (From: *Goldberg SM, Gordon PH, Nivatvongs S, 1980, with permission.*)

septicemia, with risk of high mortality. In general, an antibiotic is not necessary after the abscess is adequately drained but may be essential in a certain group of patients. In patients who have septicemia and in patients who have immune deficiency, severe diabetes mellitus, and agranulocytosis, broad-spectrum antibiotics should be initiated, pending the results of culture and sensitivity

Fig. 28-75. Drainage of horseshoe abscess. The deep postanal space is entered, incising the anococcygeal ligament. A counter drainage is made of each limb of the ischiorectal space.

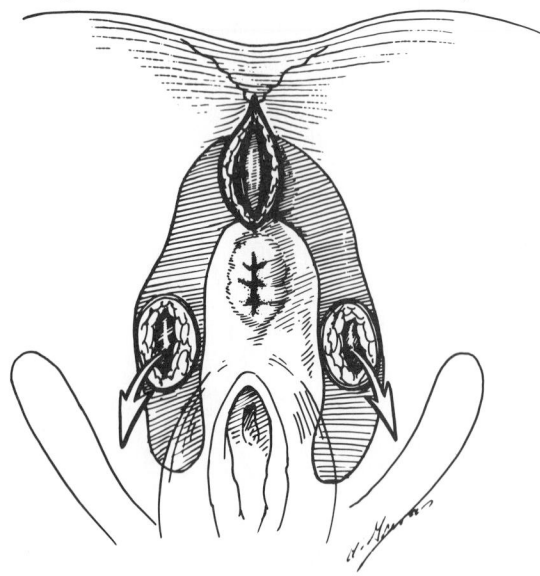

tests. Patients who have heart valve abnormalities and patients with a prosthesis should also receive antibiotic coverage.

Perianal Abscess. This type is the most superficial and the easiest to treat. The abscess is usually small and can be drained under local anesthesia in the office, clinic, or emergency room. A cruciate incision is made in the most prominent part of the skin and subcutaneous tissue overlying the abscess cavity (Fig. 28-74). The dog ears are excised to prevent premature closure of the abscess. No packing is necessary. Sitz baths are started the next day.

Ischiorectal Abscess. The ischiorectal abscess causes a diffuse swelling of the ischiorectal fossa. It may involve one side or both sides, forming a horseshoe abscess. The origin of this type of ischiorectal abscess is in the deep postanal space, then it spreads to the ischiorectal space, which has the capacity to hold a large amount of pus.

A horseshoe abscess should be drained through the deep postanal space. Ideally the procedure should be done under general or regional anesthesia, but local anesthesia can be used. A longitudinal incision is made on the skin between the tip of the coccyx and the anus to expose the anococcygeal ligament. The anococcygeal ligament is incised along its fibers entering the deep postanal space. The abscess cavity is drained and irrigated with normal saline solution. A counter-drainage incision is made on one or both limbs of the ischiorectal space (Fig. 28-75). No packing is used. Sitz baths are started the next day.

Intersphincteric Abscess. Unlike perianal and ischiorectal abscesses, there are no apparent signs of swelling or induration in the perianal area in intersphincteric abscesses. The diagnosis is made by a high index of suspicion, particularly when the anorectal pain is so severe that rectal examination is impossible. One clue to an intersphincteric abscess is a deep-seated tenderness when circumanal pressure is applied. A proper examination should be done under general or regional anesthesia in the operating room. Most intersphincteric abscesses are located in the posterior quadrant, but they can also develop anywhere around the anal canal. An indurated or bulging mass can be felt in the anal wall above the dentate line and can extend into the rectum for a variable distance.

The intersphincteric abscess is drained by incising the anal canal lining and incising through the internal sphincter muscle. The abscess cavity is curetted and irrigated with saline solution until clean. No packing is placed. Postoperative care consists of warm sitz baths for comfort. A bulk-producing agent such as bran or psyllium seed is started the next day.

Supralevator Abscess. This type of abscess is uncommon and can be difficult to diagnose. Because of its proximity to the abdominal cavity, a supralevator abscess can mimic acute intraabdominal conditions. Digital examination reveals an indurated or bulging tender mass on either side of the lower rectum or, posteriorly, above the level of the anorectal ring.

The supralevator abscess may develop in one of three ways. It may be due to the upward extension of an intersphincteric abscess, the upward extension of an ischiorectal abscess, or from intraabdominal diseases such as diverticular abscess, appendiceal abscess, or abscess from Crohn's disease.

It is essential to determine the origin of the abscess prior to treatment. If the abscess is secondary to an upward extension of an intersphincteric abscess, it should be drained into the rectum. If it is drained through the ischiorectal fossa, a complicated suprasphincteric fistula can be formed. If a supralevator abscess arises from the upward extension of an ischiorectal abscess, it should be drained through the ischiorectal fossa. Attempts at draining this kind of abscess into the rectum may result in an extrasphincteric fistula (Fig. 28-76). If the abscess is secondary to intraabdominal disease, the primary disease is removed, and the supralevator abscess is drained into the rectum, through the ischiorectal fossa, or through the abdominal wall.

NECROTIZING PERIANAL AND PERINEAL INFECTIONS.
This is the most lethal form of infection in the anorectal area. The routes of infection are most commonly from progression of anorectal abscesses, less commonly from urinary tract infection particularly periurethral gland infection) or from trauma to the anorectal area. Occasionally no apparent source of infection can be found.

Clinical Manifestations

As a rule, necrotizing perianal and perineal infections are the result of neglected or delayed treatment of the primary anorectal infection. Patients with diabetes mellitus are more prone to this type of infection. Pain, ten-

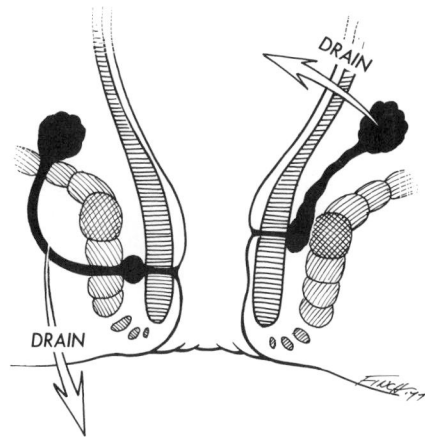

Fig. 28-76. Proper route of drainage in supralevator abscess.

derness, and swelling with crepitation of the perianal area, perineum, scrotum, or labia, are characteristic. The swelling and crepitation may spread to the back, abdominal wall, and thigh. A distinct "black spot" on the skin is indicative of underlying tissue necrosis. Fever and high white blood cell count are consistent findings.

Management

The infections are mixed synergistic gram-negative rods and anaerobic or microaerophilic bacteria flora that result in considerable gas formation. Although *C. perfringens* is usually isolated, it is not the major offending microorganism. Multiple antibiotics are started as soon as possible. These include penicillin or cephalosporin for gram-positive cocci, an aminoglycoside to cover gram-negative rods, and metronidazole or clindamycin for anaerobes. They should be adjusted when the results of culture and sensitivity tests return.

The most important aspect of treatment is an immediate excision under general anesthesia. All dead tissue must be excised irrespective of the size or site of the residual defect. Typically the underlying subcutaneous tissue necrosis is more extensive than initially appreciated. Hyperbaric oxygen treatment is not indicated unless the infection is proved to be myonecrosis caused by *C. perfringens*.

During the postoperative period, it is important to examine the patient several times a day. If the necrosis or infection spreads further, reoperation is indicated and has to be done as many times as necessary. Once the infection has arrested, whirlpool treatment is helpful. The patient should also be evaluated for consideration of hyperalimentation, diverting colostomy, or cystostomy. Because of the extensive wound, skin grafting is usually necessary at a later date.

PRURITUS ANI.
Pruritus ani is a common problem. The perianal area is sensitive, and any condition causing soiling or moisture to the area can produce itching. The surgically correctable conditions contributing to this condition are prolapsing hemorrhoids, ectropion, anal fissure, fistula-in-ano, condylomata acuminata, and neoplasm of the

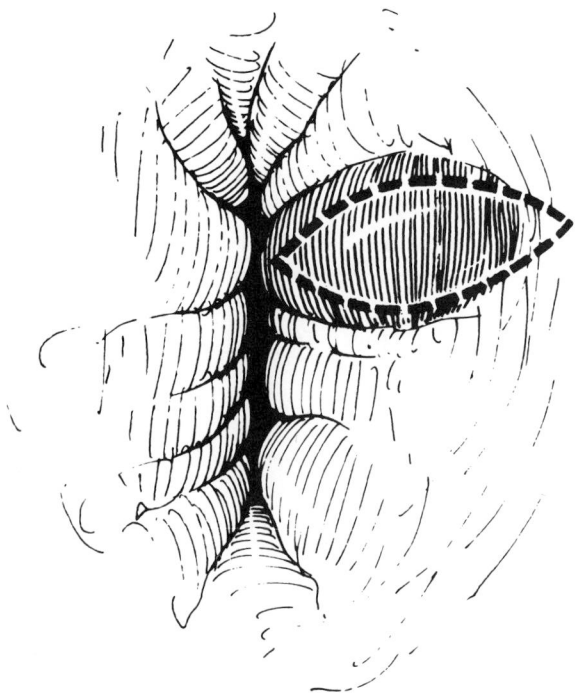

Fig. 28-77. Elliptical excision of thrombosed external hemorrhoid. (From: *Goldberg SM, Gordon PH, Nivatvongs S, 1980, with permission.*)

anal canal and perineum. Other conditions include diabetes mellitus, dermatitis, jaundice, diarrhea, and leukorrhea. Fungus infections, most commonly due to *Monilia* and *Epidermophyton* organisms, are mainly secondary invaders. In children, *Enterobius vermicularis* (pinworm) is a common cause. When no specific causes are found, the pruritus is called "idiopathic" and can be very difficult to treat.

There is no specific treatment for idiopathic pruritus ani. Anal hygiene, consisting of gentle cleansing of the anal canal with moist tissue or water, is the cornerstone of successful control. Bowel habit regulation to prevent incomplete evacuation and soiling must be emphasized. All other possible causes (e.g., sensitivity to toilet paper or to various dyes in underclothing, allergy to soap, cream, and ointment) should be excluded. Hydrocortisone, 0.5 percent preparation, applied locally, gives temporary symptomatic relief. Topical fungicides have also been used successfully for symptomatic control of pruritus ani.

The undercutting operation described for idiopathic pruritus ani is to be condemned, since it provides only temporary relief. Similarly, the subcutaneous injection of alcohol, tattooing with mercury sulfate, and topical irradiation have been abandoned, since they are ineffective or achieve only transient relief.

HEMORRHOIDS. Hemorrhoids are cushions of submucosal tissue located in the anal canal. They are composed of connective tissue containing venules, arterioles, and smooth muscle fibers. Usually there are three cushions— left lateral, right anterior, and right posterior. This ana-

tomic arrangement is remarkably constant and bears no relationship, as previously thought, to the terminal branches of the superior rectal vessels, which are quite inconstant. The function of these cushions is a matter of speculation. By their bulk, they aid in anal continence, and during the act of defecation when they become engorged with blood, they cushion the anal canal and support the lining.

An *external skin tag* is redundant fibrotic skin at the anal verge. It is usually the result of a previously thrombosed external hemorrhoid or past anal operation. Excision is indicated only if it causes pain, irritation, or interferes with anal hygiene.

External hemorrhoids are dilated venules of the inferior hemorrhoidal plexus located distal to the pectinate, or dentate, line. A *thrombosed external hemorrhoid* is an external hemorrhoid containing intravascular clots in these vessels. It may cause extreme pain during the first 48 h. Excision is the treatment of choice and is usually done under local anesthesia as an office or outpatient procedure (Fig. 28-77). Incision should be discouraged since the clots are multiloculated. If the pair is subsiding, excision is unnecessary. Warm sitz baths will speed up resolution.

Internal hemorrhoids most commonly are manifested by painless, bright-red rectal bleeding associated with a bowel movement and by symptoms of prolapse. A feeling of incomplete evacuation is also common. In chronic prolapse, mucus frequently causes perianal irritation. Pain is not a common symptom of internal hemorrhoids unless they are complicated by an anal fissure, stenosis, or thrombosis.

The severity of internal hemorrhoids is graded according to the degree of prolapse. *First degree hemorrhoids:* The anal cushions slide down beyond the dentate line on straining. The most common symptom is painless rectal bleeding. Treatment consists of bulk-forming agents such as bran or psyllium seed. If bleeding persists, rubber band ligation should be done (Fig. 28-78). *Second degree hemorrhoids:* The anal cushions prolapse through the anus on straining but are spontaneously reduced. Rubber band ligation is the treatment of choice, along with bran or psyllium seed. *Third degree hemorrhoids:* The anal cushions prolapse through the anus upon staining or walking and require manual replacement into the anal canal. Hemorrhoidectomy gives the best results, but rubber band ligation is often effective and should usually be tried first. *Fourth degree hemorrhoids:* The prolapse stays out all the time. Hemorrhoidectomy is indicated. The prolapse may become strangulated and requires urgent or emergent hemorrhoidectomy.

Postpartum hemorrhoids usually occur in patients who have had some problems with hemorrhoids before or during pregnancy. Prolonged straining during labor causes thrombosis and/or strangulation. Hemorrhoidectomy is the treatment of choice for most cases. If a thrombosed external hemorrhoid develops, excision is indicated.

Hemorrhoids in portal hypertension do not occur more frequently than in the normal population. Active bleeding usually emanates from ulceration at the external or inter-

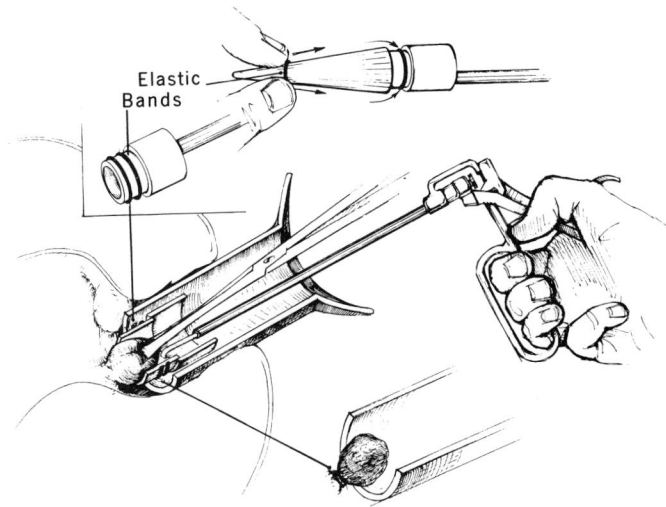

Elastic Bands

Fig. 28-78. Lateral partial internal sphincterotomy (opened technique).

nal hemorrhoid. A "stick-tie" at the bleeding site will solve the problem. In some cases a hemorrhoidectomy at the site of bleeding is necessary.

Hemorrhoidectomy

The technique described here is closed excision of an intraanal hemorrhoid. The patient is placed in prone position with a roll under the pubis. If the operation is done under local anesthesia, a left anterolateral position (Sims' position) will be more comfortable to the patient. The cheeks of the buttock are tapered apart, prepped, and draped. The anal canal and perianal skin are infiltrated with 0.25% bupivacaine (marcaine) containing 1:200,000 epinephrine for local anesthesia and for the purpose of decreasing bleeding.

The anal canal is examined with a Pratt bivalve speculum to determine how many hemorrhoids need to be removed. A Fansler anal speculum is used to expose the operative field. Dissection is started on the perianal skin just distal to the anal verge. A narrow, elliptical excision is made with Metzenbaum scissors removing the skin, external hemorrhoids, and internal hemorrhoids down to the underlying internal sphincter muscle. The redundant mucosa is excised up to the level of the anorectal ring. Excess mucosa and anoderm are trimmed, and the wound is closed with running 3-0 chromic catgut (Fig. 28-79). The same procedure is performed at other quadrants. No packing is placed in the anal canal.

Urinary retention is related in part to the amount of intravenous fluid administered during and after the procedure. Demerol intramuscularly or orally or another nonconstipating analgesic is prescribed. Sitz baths are started 4 h later if the procedure is performed under local anesthesia but should be postponed until the next morning if general or regional anesthesia is used. Bran or psyllium seed bulk laxatives are started the next morning. A mild laxative such as milk of magnesia may be given the following night. The patient is kept in the hospital until the pain is minimal or until the patient can void spontaneously, usually 1 to 3 days.

ANAL FISSURE. An anal fissure is a tear of the skin-lined part of the anal canal, i.e., the area from the pectinate, or dentate, line to the anal verge. It is usually a few millimeters in width and rarely larger than 1 cm. Most anal fissures initiate from passage of a large, hard stool. Due to poor muscular support of the anal canal posteriorly, the majority of the fissures occur in the posterior midline and less frequently in the anterior midline. An anal fissure off the midline posterior or anterior is usually secondary to other conditions, such as Crohn's disease, chronic ulcerative colitis, syphilis, tuberculosis, and leukemia. Anal fissures occur mostly in young and middle-aged adults.

Clinical Manifestations. The characteristic symptom is a sharp burning pain during and after bowel movement. Another common complaint is bright-red blood on the toilet paper upon wiping. Gentle separation of the buttock will usually reveal the fissure. Digital and anoscopic examination may be necessary to establish the diagnosis, provided that the examination does not cause too much pain. Proctoscopic examination should also be done to exclude any associated abnormalities of the anal canal and rectum, especially inflammatory bowel disease.

Treatment. For an acute fissure, conservative treatment consisting of anal hygiene, bulk-producing agents such as bran and psyllium seed, warm sitz baths, and a local anesthetic jelly, is usually therapeutic. Once the fissure progresses into a chronic stage, surgical treatment is usually required. The treatment of choice is usually a lateral internal sphincterotomy (Figs. 28-80 and 28-81). A fissurectomy may occasionally be indicated, particularly if a superficial fistula is present.

FISTULA-IN-ANO. Fistula-in-ano is an inflammatory track with a secondary opening (external opening) in the perianal skin and a primary opening (internal opening) in the anal canal at the dentate line. The fistula originates in an abscess in the intersphincteric space of the anal canal.

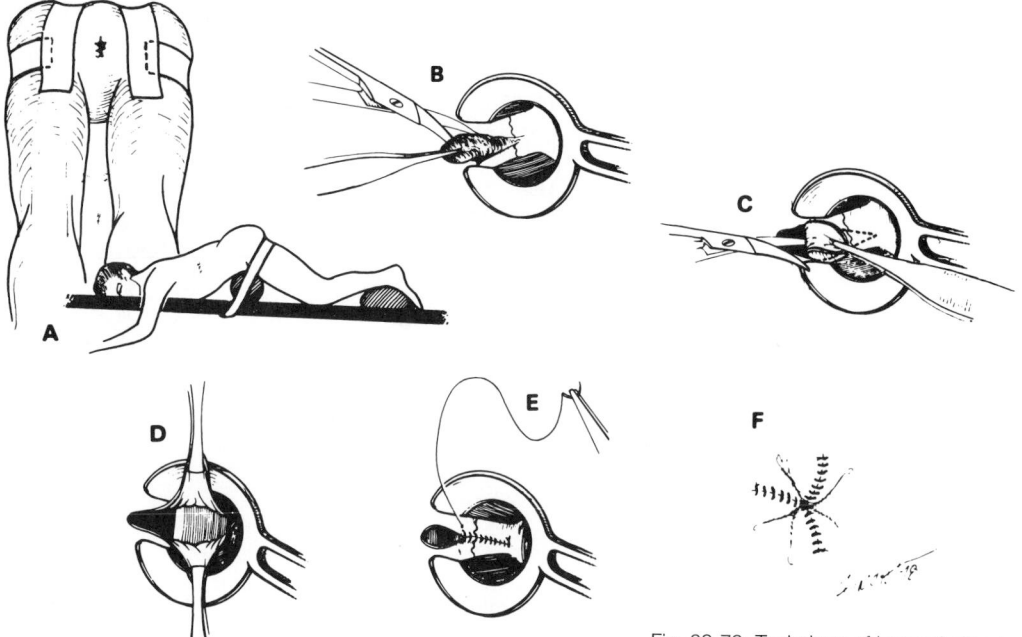

Goodsall's rule relates the location of the internal opening to the location of the external opening (Fig. 28-82). If the external opening is anterior to an imaginary line drawn across the midpoint of the anus, the fistula usually runs directly into the anal canal. If the external opening is pos-

Fig. 28-79. Technique of hemorrhoidectomy. *A.* Positioning of patient in prone. *B.* Exposure of the hemorrhoid using Fansler operative scope. *C.* Elliptical excision starting at the perianal skin to anorectal ring. *D.* Submucosal hemorrhoidal plexuses dissected from the internal sphincter, anoderm, and mucosa. *E.* Wound closed with running absorbable suture. *F.* Completion of procedure. (From: *Goldberg SM, Gordon PH, Nivatvongs S, 1980, with permission.*)

Fig. 28-80. Lateral partial internal sphincterotomy.

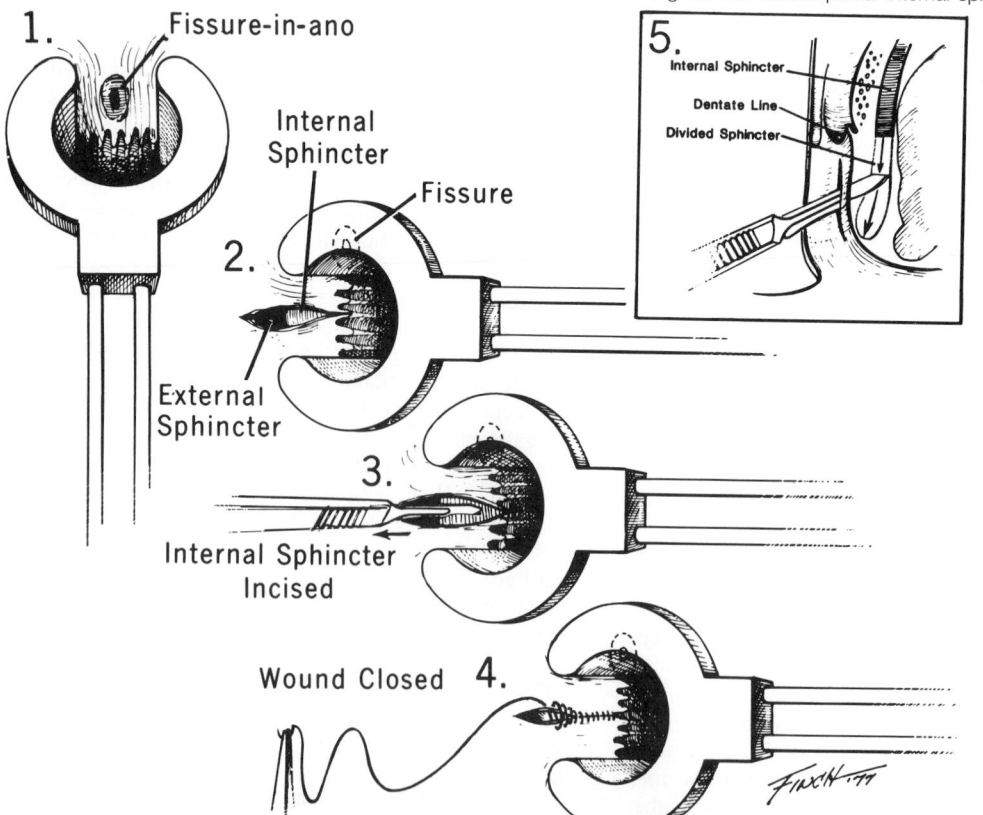

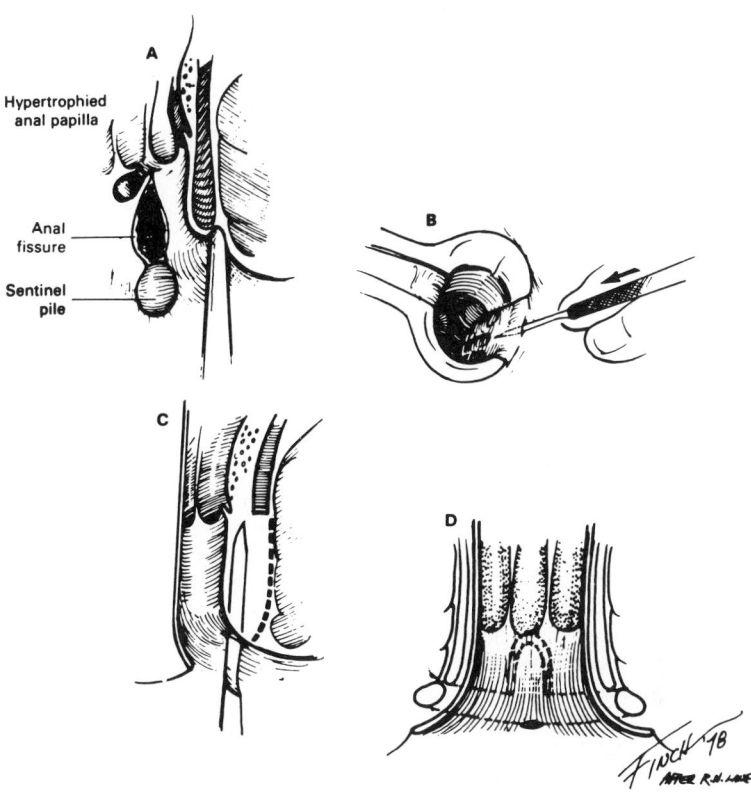

Fig. 28-81. Lateral partial internal sphincterotomy (closed technique). (From: *Goldberg SM, Gordon PH, Nivatvongs S, 1980, with permission.*)

terior to that line, the track usually will curve to the posterior midline of the anal canal. An exception to this rule is an external opening anterior to this imaginary line and greater than 3 cm from the anus, in which case the track may curve posteriorly and end in the posterior midline.

A more precise classification of fistula-in-ano has been proposed by Parks, Gordon, and Hardcastle. It consists of four categories based on the relationship of the fistula to the sphincter muscles: intersphincteric, transsphincteric, suprasphincteric, and extraphincteric (Fig. 28-83).

Clinical Manifestations. Most patients present with previous history of anorectal abscess associated with intermittent drainage. Recurrence of a perianal abscess suggests the presence of a fistula-in-ano. The external opening is usually visible as a red elevation of granulation tissue with purulent or serosanguineous drainage on compression. In the simple or superficial fistula, the track can be palpated as an indurated cord. Deep, high, or horseshoe fistulas usually are not palpable.

It is important to rule out fistulas associated with ulcerative colitis and Crohn's disease; in these cases one may refrain from extensive operative procedures for fistula-in-

Fig. 28-82. Goodsall's rule.

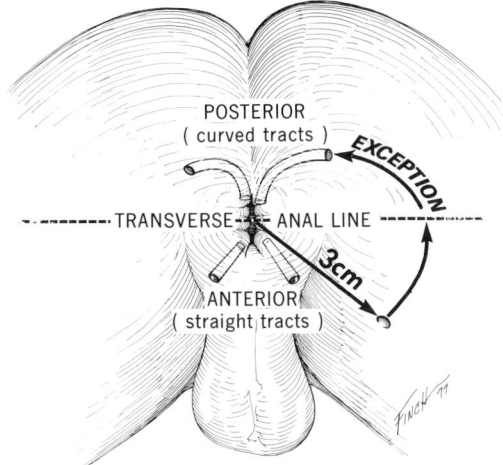

Fig. 28-83. The four main anatomic types of fistula: (1) intersphincteric, (2) transsphincteric, (3) suprasphincteric, and (4) extrasphincteric.

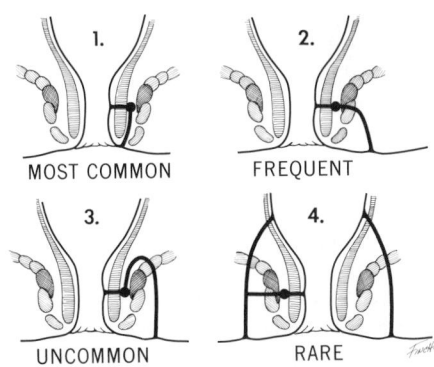

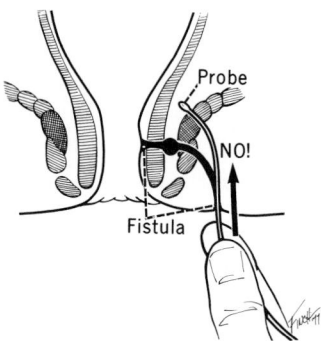

Fig. 28-84. Iatrogenic track created by injudicious probing of a fistula-in-ano.

ano because of poor secondary healing. This differential can be established by proctoscopy, upper gastrointestinal examination with small bowel follow-through, and barium enema. Diverticulitis of the sigmoid colon, with perforation and fistulization to the perineum, occurs rarely. Hidradenitis suppurativa is differentiated by the presence of multiple perianal skin openings. A pilonidal sinus with perianal extension and infected perianal sebaceous cysts must be considered. Low rectal and anal canal carcinomas rarely present as a fistula in the perineum. Carcinomas may sometimes develop in long-standing fistulas.

Treatment. The first step in management is the identification of the primary opening of the fistulous track. About 50 percent of patients do not have clinically detectable openings. Positive identification is best accomplished in the operating room under anesthesia. Bidigital palpation, using the index finger and the thumb, may trace the indurated track to the primary opening. Probing the track from the external opening is successful in 50 percent of cases, but care must be taken to avoid creating an artificial opening and seeding infected material into clean tissue, thus risking iatrogenic extensions above or beyond the original fistula (Fig. 28-84). The injection of diluted methylene blue may be helpful. Fistulography, utilizing a water-soluble contrast solution, is a valuable method of identifying and managing high, complicated fistulas. If definition of the primary opening is impossible at operation, the crypt-bearing area suspected of harboring the infected duct and gland must be excised.

The principles of fistulotomy include unroofing all fistulas, eliminating the primary opening (infective source), and establishing adequate drainage. The tracks are unroofed from the primary source at the dentate line through the secondary opening or openings by incising all overlying tissue, including sphincter (Fig. 28-85). Failure to unroof the entire track and divide the necessary amount of sphincter may lead to recurrence. The wound is allowed to heal by secondary intention. Fistulectomy is the excision of the entire fistulous track and is rarely necessary.

Occasionally, a patient may present with an acute perianal abscess associated with an obvious fistula-in-ano. Incision and drainage of the abscess and primary fistulotomy are indicated. If the fistula is high in relation to

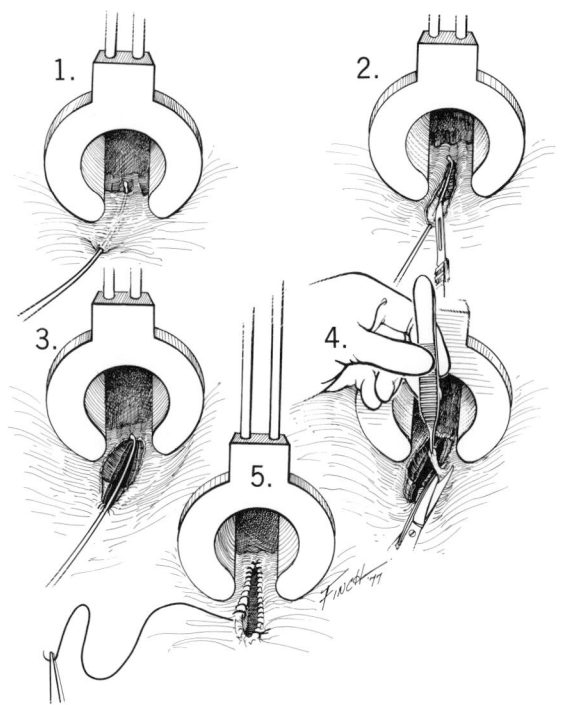

Fig. 28-85. Fistulotomy. 1. The probe is in the fistulous track. 2 and 3. Unroofing of the fistulous track over the probe. 4. Redundant skin is excised. 5. The wound is marsupialized.

the anorectal ring, a two-stage procedure may be indicated. In the first stage, a seton of heavy black silk or a rubber band is placed loosely around the sphincter muscle as a marker (Fig. 28-86). This stimulates fibrosis adjacent to the sphincter muscle so that when the second stage, which involves laying open the transsphincteric portion of the fistulous track, is completed, the sphincter will not separate as widely. Incontinence is the most serious complication of operations for fistula.

Horseshoe fistula, an uncommon form of fistula-in-ano, is a direct extension of an intersphincteric abscess, and usually starts in the deep postanal space. Radical unroofing procedures are seldom necessary. A posterior midline internal sphincterotomy combined with laying open the deep postanal space and coring or excising the lateral tracks as recommended by Hanley has proved effective (Fig. 28-87).

ANAL INCONTINENCE. Anal incontinence results when there is loss of control of the anal sphincter. The term actually covers a broad spectrum of anal function impairment, ranging from simple involuntary passage of formed stool.

The external sphincter and the puborectalis muscles are primarily responsible for voluntary control. The internal sphincter muscle maintains continence at rest. Anal continence has a complex mechanism, made up of multiple factors other than the sphincter muscles. These factors include the ability of the anorectum to perceive sensation from stool and gas. These receptors are in the pelvic wall and anoderm. Structural arrangements are

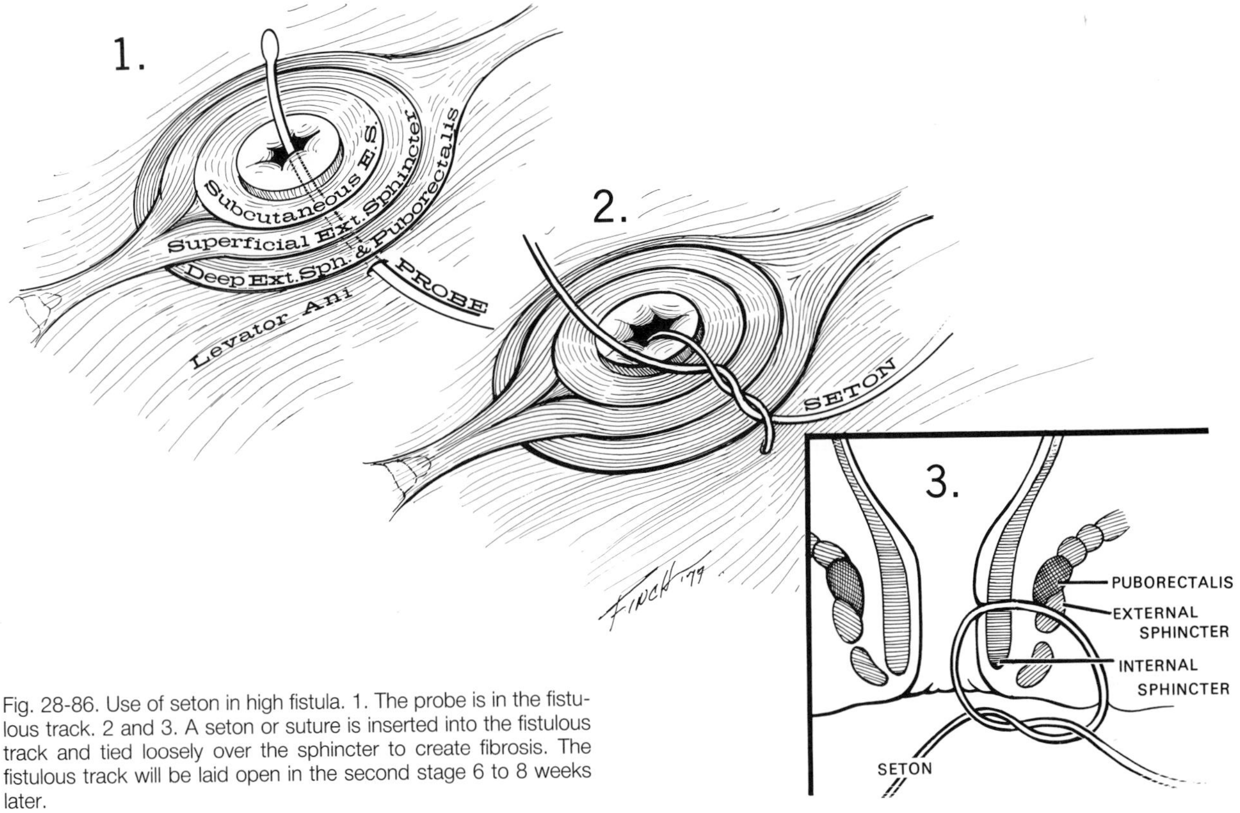

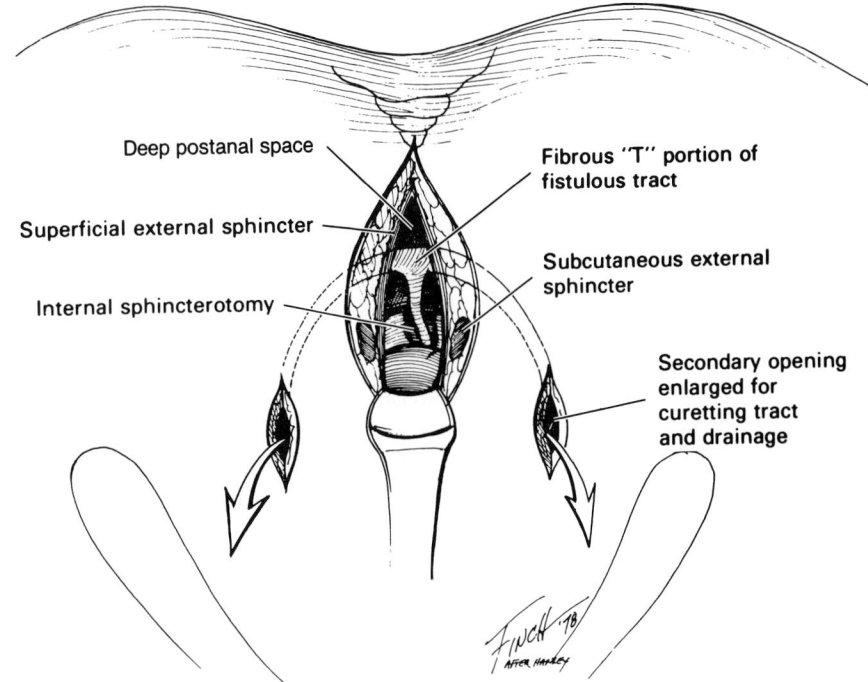

Fig. 28-86. Use of seton in high fistula. 1. The probe is in the fistulous track. 2 and 3. A seton or suture is inserted into the fistulous track and tied loosely over the sphincter to create fibrosis. The fistulous track will be laid open in the second stage 6 to 8 weeks later.

Fig. 28-87. Hanley's fistulectomy: laying open of deep postanal space along with posterior midline internal sphincterotomy. The lateral tracts are excised or cored out.

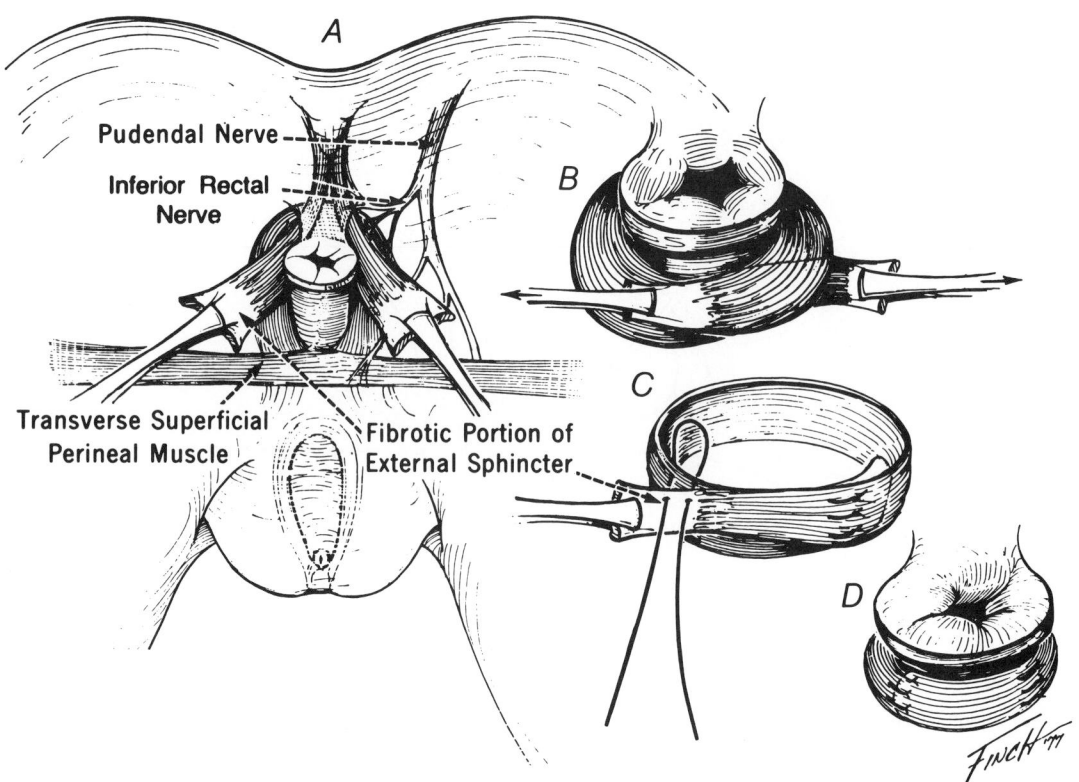

Fig. 28-88. Sphincteroplasty. *A.* The external sphincter muscles is mobilized along with the fibrotic ends. Care should be taken not to injure the inferior rectal nerve. *B.* The well-mobilized external sphincter muscle is wrapped around the anal canal. *C.* Mattress sutures of 2-0 polyglycol inserted into the fibrotic ends. *D.* At completion, the anal canal should admit only an index finger.

also important anatomic aids to continence. These include the curves of the rectum, the anorectal angle (normally 80 to 90°), and the flutter valve created by the pelvic pressure. The anal cushions (internal hemorrhoidal plexus) serve to resist opening of the anus.

There are many and varied causes of incontinence. Acquired anal incontinence secondary to obstetrical tear, previous anorectal surgery (hemorrhoidectomy, fistulectomy), or trauma (e.g., perineal injury) are the most common causes. In recent years, these injuries have been the most amenable to surgical management. Other causes of incontinence such as long-standing rectal prolapse (procidentia) or severe prolapsed hemorrhoids often respond to treatment of the primary disorder alone. On the other hand, neurogenic problems such as myelomeningocele, demyelinating disease or trauma, or neoplasm of the spinal cord are usually impossible to correct.

Preoperative evaluation of the patient with fecal incontinence is important and should include a complete history and physical examination. Differentiation should be made between incontinence and urgency or diarrhea related to diet or bowel habits. Mild forms of incontinence may respond adequately to nonoperative therapy, such as diet control, bowel training, sphincter exercises, and improved hygiene. Endoscopy and barium enema studies should be used to rule out tumors and colitis. Overflow incontinence secondary to fecal impaction is not an uncommon problem in the elderly, particularly nursing home patients. The large bolus of feces distends the rectal ampulla causing relaxation of the internal sphincter and is responsible for loss of the defecation reflex.

Treatment

Warp-around Sphincteroplasty. This is most suitable to incontinence secondary to obstetrical trauma or injury secondary to anorectal surgery. The procedure involves mobilization of the divided sphincter muscle and reapproximation without tension (Fig. 28-88).

Postanal Intersphincteric Sphincteroplasty. This relatively new method of repair was pioneered by Parks. It works well for incontinence caused by prolapse of the rectum and certain cases of idiopathic incontinence where there is loss of anorectal angle. The approach is via the intersphincteric plane posteriorly. The levator ani muscle is then approximated to restore the anorectal angle to normal. The puborectalis and the external sphincter muscles are also tightened with sutures. The procedure also lengthens the anal canal to a significant degree (Fig. 28-70).

Gracilis Muscle Transposition. It is suitable in cases where there is significant loss of the anosphincter muscle mass, or in cases in which other techniques have failed. The gracilis muscle from the thigh is mobilized and detached from its insertion at the tibial tuberosity. It is then tunneled through the perineum and encircled around the anal canal to replace the anosphincter muscle (Fig. 28-89).

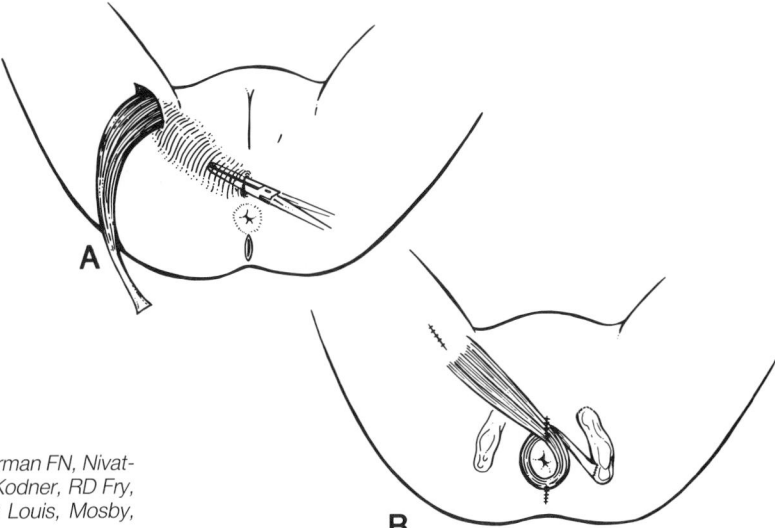

Fig. 28-89. Gracilis muscle transposition. [From: *Herman FN, Nivatvongs S, et al: Anal sphincter reconstruction, in IJ Kodner, RD Fry, JP Roe (eds): Colon, Rectal and Anal Surgery, St Louis, Mosby, chap 4, 1985, p 37, with permission.*]

Sigmoid Colostomy. Not all patients with severe anal incontinence are suitable for repair. In such situations, if the patient cannot live with it, a permanent sigmoid colostomy is an excellent alternative.

PROCTALGIA FUGAX AND LEVATOR ANI SYNDROME. Proctalgia fugax is a severe, spasmodic rectal pain lasting a few minutes or longer. The exact cause is unknown, but the condition may be due to levator ani muscle spasm. The symptom generally occurs in patients who are anxious and overworked. The characteristic history is that of severe pain awakening the patient. The pain usually is located in the midrectum and disappears spontaneously without residual symptoms. Complete proctosigmoidoscopic examination should be performed to rule out anorectal disease. Treatment to relieve the spasm during an acute attack consist of warm baths or a heating pad applied to the perineum. Since many of these patients are anxious and have cancer phobia, reassurance is an important aspect of therapy.

Another group of patients has chronic vague pain in the anorectum. Examination reveals tenderness of the levator ani muscle, more often on the left side. This is termed *levator ani syndrome*. Digital massage of the tender muscle at weekly intervals may provide an effective relief. Care must be taken to ensure that patients with these symptom-complexes do not undergo an unnecessary rectal operation.

Bibliography

General Considerations

Goldberg SM, Gordon PH, Nivatvongs S: *Essentials of Anorectal Surgery.* Philadelphia, Lippincott, 1980.

Goligher JC: The functional results after sphincter-saving resections of the rectum. *Ann R Coll Surg Engl* 8:421, 1951.

Morson BC: Adenomas and adenoma-carcinoma sequence, in Morson BC, Dawson IMP (eds): *Gastrointestinal Pathology,* 2d ed. Oxford, England, Blackwell Scientific Publications, 1979.

Nivatvongs S, Becker ER: Colon, rectum and anal canal, in James EC, Corry RJ, Perry JCF Jr (eds): *Basic Surgical Practice.* Philadelphia, Hanley & Belfus, 1987.

Anatomy, Physiology, and Clinical Evaluation

Bartolo DCC, Roe AM, et al: Flap-valve theory of anorectal continence. *Br J Surg* 73:1012, 1986.

Beynon J, Mortensen McC, et al: Preoperative assessment of local invasion in rectal cancer: Digital examination, endoluminal sonography or computed tomography? *Br J Surg* 73:1015, 1986.

Bigard MA, Gaucher P, Lassalle C: Fatal colonic explosion during colonoscopic polypectomy. *Gastroenterology* 77:1307, 1979.

Block IR, Enquist IF: Lymphatic studies pertaining to local spread of carcinoma of the rectum in females. *Surg Gynecol Obstet* 112:41, 1961.

Bond JH, Levitt MD: Colonic gas explosion—is a fire extinguisher necessary? *Gastroenterology* 77:1349, 1979.

Boxall TA, Smart PJG, Griffiths JD: The blood supply of the distal segment of the rectum in anterior resection. *Br J Surg* 50:399, 1962.

Crapp AR, Cuthbertson AM: William Waldeyer and the rectosacral fascia. *Surg Gynecol Obstet* 138:252, 1974.

Devroede G, Phillips SF: Conservation of sodium chloride and water by human colon. *Gastroenterology* 56:101, 1969.

Debongnie JC, Phillips SF: Capacity of the human colon to absorb fluid. *Gastroenterology* 74:698, 1978.

Duthie HL: Dynamics of the rectum and anus. *Clin Gastroenterol* 4:467, 1975.

Duthie HL, Gairns FW: Sensory nerve-endings and sensation in the anal canal region of man. *Br J Surg* 47:585, 1960.

Gaston EA: Physiologic basis for preservation of fecal continence after resection of rectum. *JAMA* 146:1486, 1951.

Goldberg SM, Gordon PH, Nivatvongs S: *Essentials of Anorectal Surgery.* Philadelphia, Lippincott, 1980.

Levitt MD, Bond JR Jr: Volume, composition, and source of intestinal gas. *Gastroenterology* 59:921, 1970.

Levitt MD: Intestinal gas production—recent advances in flatology. *N Engl J Med* 302:1474, 1980.

Nivatvongs S, Stern HS, Fryd DS: The length of the anal canal. *Dis Colon Rectum* 24:600, 1982.

Nivatvongs S, Becker ER: Colon, rectum and anal canal, in James EC, Corry RJ, Perry JF Jr (eds): *Basic Surgical Practice*. Philadelphia, Hanley & Belfus, 1987.

Oh C, Kark AE: Anatomy of the external sphincter. *Br J Surg* 59:717, 1972.

Phillips SF, Edwards DAW: Some aspects of anal continence and defaecation. *Gut* 6:396, 1965.

Shafik A: A new concept of anatomy of the anal sphincter mechanism and the physiology of defecation. The external anal sphincter: A triple-loop system. *Invest Urol* 12:412, 1975.

Shafik A: A new concept of the anatomy of the anal sphincter mechanism and the physiology of defecation. II. Anatomy of the levator ani muscle with special reference to puborectalis. *Invest Urol* 13:175, 1975.

Sonneland J, Anson BJ, Benton LE: Surgical anatomy of the arterial supply to the colon from the superior mesenteric artery based upon a study of 600 specimens. *Surg Gynecol Obstet* 106:385, 1958.

Turnberg LA: Electrolyte absorption from the colon. *Gut* 11:1049, 1970.

Varma KK, Stephens FD: Neuro-muscular reflexes of anal continence. *Austr NZ J Surg* 41:263, 1972.

Wunderlich M, Parks AG: Physiology and pathophysiology of the anal sphincters. *Int Surg* 67:291, 1983.

Inflammatory Bowel Disease

Buchmann P, Waterman IT, et al: The prognosis of ileorectal anastomosis in Crohn's disease. *Br J Surg* 68:7, 1981.

Dissanayake AS, Truelove SC: A controlled therapeutic trail of long-term maintenance treatment of ulcerative colitis and sulfasalazine (salazopyrin). *Gut* 14:923, 1973.

Fauci AS, Macher AM, et al: Acquired immunodeficiency syndrome: Epidemiology, clinical, immunologic and therapeutic considerations. *Ann Internal Med* 100:92, 1984.

Ford MJ Jr, Anderson JR, et al: Clinical spectrum of "solitary ulcer" of the rectum. *Gastroenterology* 84:1533, 1983.

Hamilton SR: Colorectal carcinoma in patients with Crohn's disease. *Gastroenterology* 89:398, 1985.

Henry MM, Parks AG, Swash M: The pelvic floor musculature in the descending perineum syndrome. *Br J Surg* 53:760, 1982.

Keighley MRB, Fielding JL, Alexander-Williams J: Results of abdominal rectopexy using polypropylene (Marlex) mesh in 100 consecutive patients. *Br J Surg* 70:229, 1983.

Kennedy DK, Hughes ESR, Masterton JP: The natural history of benign ulcer of the rectum. *Surg Gynecol Obstet* 144:718, 1979.

Madigan MR, Morson BC: Solitary ulcer of the rectum. *Gut* 10:871, 1969.

Martin CJ, Parks TG, Biggert JD: Solitary rectal ulcer syndrome in Northern Ireland. *Br J Surg* 68:744, 1981.

Mekhjian HS, Switz DM, et al: Clinical features and natural history of Crohn's disease. *Gastroenterology* 77:898, 1979.

Metcalf AM, Dozois RR, et al: Ileal "J" pouch-anal anastomosis. Clinical outcome. *Ann Surg* 202:735, 1985.

Nicholls J, Glass R: *Coloproctology*. New York, Springer-Verlag, 1985.

Present DH, Korelitz BI, et al: Treatment of Crohn's disease with 6-mercaptopurine. A long-term, randomized, double blind study. *N Engl J Med* 302:981, 1980.

Price AB, Morson BC: Inflammatory bowel disease. The surgical pathology of Crohn's disease and ulcerative colitis. *Human Pathol* 6:7, 1975.

Rankin GB, Watts HD, et al: National cooperative Crohn's disease study: Extraintestinal manifestations and perianal complications. *Gastroenterology* 77:914, 1979.

Riddell RH, Goldman H, et al: Dysplasia in inflammatory bowel disease: Standardized classification with provisional clinical applications. *Human Pathol* 14:931, 1983.

Rosenstock E, Farmer RG, et al: Surveillance for colonic carcinoma in ulcerative colitis. *Gastroenterology* 89:1342, 1985.

Singleton JW, Summers RW, et al: A trial of sulfasalazine as adjunctive therapy in Crohn's disease. *Gastroenterology* 77:887, 1979.

Van Heerden JA, Beart RW Jr: Carcinoma of the colon and rectum complicating chronic ulcerative colitis. *Dis Colon Rectum* 23:155, 1980.

Wong WD, Rotherberger DA, Goldbert SM: Ileoanal pouch procedures. *Curr Probl Surg* 22:1, 1985.

Diverticular Disease

Arfwidsson S: Pathogenesis of multiple diverticula of the sigmoid colon in diverticular disease. *Acta Chir Scand Suppl* 342:1, 1964.

Auguste L, Borrero E, Wise L: Surgical management of perforated colonic diverticulitis. *Arch Surg* 120:450, 1985.

Bowden TA Jr, Hooks VH III, Mansberger AR: Intraoperative gastrointestinal endoscopy. *Ann Surg* 191:680, 1980.

Hyland JMP, Taylor I: Does a high fiber diet prevent the complications of diverticular disease? *Br J Surg* 67:77, 1980.

Kadir S, Ernst CB: Current concepts in angiographic management of gastrointestinal bleeding. *Curr Probl Surg* 20:287, 1983.

Killingback M: Management of perforative diverticulitis. *Surg Clin North Am* 63:97, 1983.

Ouriel K, Schwartz SI: Diverticular disease in young patient. *Surg Gynecol Obstet* 156(1): 1, 1983.

Painter NS. Truelove SC, et al: Segmentation and the localization of intraluminal pressures in the human colon, with special reference to the pathogenesis of colonic diverticula. *Gastroenterology* 49:169, 1965.

Painter NS, Burkitt DP: Diverticular disease of the colon: A deficiency disease of western civilization. *Br Med J* 2:450, 1971.

Parks TG: Natural history of diverticular disease of the colon: A review of 521 cases. *Br Med J* 4:639, 1969.

Rodkey GV, Welch CE: Changing patterns in the surgical treatment of diverticular disease. *Ann Surg* 200:466, 1984.

Ryan P: Changing concepts in diverticular disease. *Dis Colon Rectum* 26:12, 1983.

Slack WW: The anatomy, pathology, and some clinical features of diverticulitis of the colon. *Br J Surg* 50:185, 1962.

Wolff BG, Ready RG, et al: Influence of sigmoid resection on progression of diverticular disease of the colon. *Dis Colon Rectum* 27:645, 1984.

Megacolon

Olness K, McParland FA, Piper J: Biofeedback: A new modality in the management of children with fecal soiling. *J Pediatr* 96:505, 1980.

Preston DM, Hawley PR, et al: Results of colectomy for severe idiopathic constipation in women (Arbuthnot Lane's disease). *Br J Surg* 71:547, 1984.

Watkins GL, Oliver GA: Giant megacolon in the insane: Further observation on patients treated by subtotal colectomy. *Gastroenterology* 48:718, 1965.

Volvulus

Ballantyne GH: Review of sigmoid volvulus. History and results of treatment. *Dis Colon Rectum* 25:494, 1982.

Ballantyne GH, Brandner MD, et al: Volvulus of the colon. Incidence and mortality. *Ann Surg* 202:83, 1985.

Brunsgaard C: Volvulus of the sigmoid colon and its treatment. *Surgery* 22:466, 1947.

Jorgensen K, Kronberg O: The colonoscope in volvulus of the transverse colon. *Dis Colon Rectum* 23:357, 1980.

Zinken LD, Katz LD, Rosin JD: Volvulus of the transverse colon: Report of a case and review of the literature. *Dis Colon Rectum* 22:492, 1979.

Miscellaneous Benign Lesions

Bowden TA Jr, Hookes VH III, et al: Occult gastrointestinal bleeding: Locating the cause. *Am Surg* 46:80, 1980.

Bowden TA Jr, Hooks VH III, Mansberger AR Jr: Intestinal vascular ectasias: A new look at an old disease. *S Med J* 75:1310, 1982.

Dmowski WP, Cohen MR: Antigonadotropin (Danazol) in the treatment of endometriosis: Evaluation of posttreatment fertility and three-year follow-up data. *Am J Obstet Gynecol* 130:41, 1978.

Haginara PF, Chauang VP, Griffin WO: Arteriovenous malformations of the colon. *Am J Surg* 133:681, 1977.

Morson BC, Dawson IMP: *Gastrointestinal Pathology*. Oxford, London, Blackwell Scientific Publications, 1972.

Pillay SP, Hardie IR: Intestinal complications of endometriosis. *Br J Surg* 67:677, 1980.

Polyps

Bess MA, Adson MA, et al: Rectal cancer following colectomy for polyposis. *Arch Surg* 115:460, 1960.

Bussey JJR, Veale AMD, Morson BC: Genetics of gastrointestinal polyposis. *Gastroenterology* 74:1325, 1978.

Cooper HS: Surgical pathology of endoscopically removed malignant polyps of the colon and rectum. *Am J Surg Pathol* 7:613, 1983.

Fenoglio-Preiser CM: Colorectal polyps: Pathologic diagnosis and clinical significance. *Cancer* 35:322, 1985.

Haggitt RC, Glotzbach RE, et al: Prognostic factors in colorectal carcinomas arising in adenomas: Implications for lesions removed by endoscopic polypectomy. *Gastroenterology* 89:328, 1985.

Linos DA, Dozois RR, et al: Does Peutz-Jeghers syndrome predispose to gastrointestinal malignancy? A later look. *Arch Surg* 116:1182, 1981.

Lipper S, Kahn LB, Ackerman LV: The significance of microscopic invasive cancer in endoscopically removed polyps of the large bowel. A clinicopathologic study of 51 cases. *Cancer* 52:1691, 1983.

Morson BC, Whiteway JE, et al: Histopathology and prognosis of malignant colorectal polyps treated by endoscopic polypectomy. *Gut* 25:437, 1984.

Reed K, Vose PC: Diffuse juvenile polyposis of the colon: A premalignant condition? *Dis Colon Rectum* 24:205, 1981.

Riddle RH: Hands off "cancerous" large bowel polyps. *Gastroenterology* 89:432, 1985.

Russell DM, Bhathal PS, St John DJB: Complete remission in Cronkhite-Canada syndrome. *Gastroenterology* 85:180, 1983.

Seuer SF, Miller HH, DeCosse JJ: The spectrum of polyposis. *Surg Gynecol Obstet* 159:525, 1984.

Carcinoma

Bacon HE: Major surgery of the colon and rectum: Rehabilitation and survival rate in 2457 patients. *Dis Colon Rectum* 3:393, 1960.

Bacon HE, Khubchandani IT: the rationale of aortoiliopelvic lymphadenectomy and high ligation of the inferior mesenteric artery for carcinoma of the left half of the colon and rectum. *Surg Gynecol Obstet* 119:503, 1964.

Baker AR: Local procedures in the management of rectal cancer. *Semin Oncol* 7:385, 1980.

Beart RW, Jagelman DG, Salvati EP: Symposium: Sphincter saving operations for rectal cancer. *Cont Surg* 21:59, 1982.

Bennett RC, Hughes ESR, Cuthbertson A: Long-term review of function following pull-through operations of the rectum. *Br J Surg* 59:723, 1972.

Birnkrant A, Sampson J, Sugarbaker PH: Ovarian metastasis from colorectal cancer. *Dis Colon Rectum* 29:767, 1986.

Black BM: Combined abdominoperineal resection: Reappraisal of a pull-through procedure. *Surg Clin North Am* 47:977, 1967.

Bland KI, Polk HC: Therapeutic measures applied for the curative and palliative control of colorectal carcinoma. *Surg Annu* 15:123, 1983.

Bown SG, Barr H, et al: Endoscopic treatment of inoperable colorectal cancers with the Nd YAG laser. *Br J Surg* 73:949, 1986.

Cohen AM, Wood WC, et al: Pathological studies in cancer. *Cancer* 45:2965, 1980.

Coutsoftides T, Sival MV Jr, et al: Colonoscopy and the management of polyps containing invasive carcinoma. *Ann Surg* 188:638, 1978.

Davis NC, Evans EB, et al: Staging of colorectal cancer: The Australian clinico-pathological staging (ACPS) system compared with Dukes' system. *Dis Colon Rectum* 27:707, 1984.

Dukes CE, Bussey HJR: The spread of rectal cancer and its effect on prognosis. *Br J Cancer* 12:309, 1958.

Eisenstat TE, Deak ST, et al: Five-year survival in patients with carcinoma of the rectum treated by electrocoagulation. *Am J Surg* 143:127, 1982.

Elliot MS, Todd IP, Nicholls RJ: Radical restorative surgery for poorly differentiated carcinoma of the mid-rectum. *Br J Surg* 69:273, 1982.

Enker WE, Laffer UT, Block GE: Enhanced survival of patients with colon and rectal cancer based upon wide anatomic resection. *Ann Surg* 190:350, 1979.

Gabriel WB, Dukes C, Bussey HJ, cited in Sugarbaker PH: Influence of surgical techniques on survival in patients with colorectal cancer. *Dis Colon Rectum* 25:545, 1982.

Gerard A: Surgical aspect of colo-rectal cancer therapy. *Int J Radiation Oncol Biol Phys* 8:1757, 1982.

Gilbertsen VA, McHugh R, et al: The earlier detection of colorectal cancers: A preliminary report of the results of the occult blood study. *Cancer* 45:2899, 1980.

Gingold BS, Mitty WF, Tadros M: Importance of patient selection in local treatment of carcinoma of the rectum. *Am J Surg* 145:293, 1983.

Goligher JC, Graham NG, DeDombal FT: Anastomotic dehiscence after anterior resection of the rectum and rectosigmoid. *Br J Surg* 57:109, 1970.

Graffner HOL, Alm POA, Oscarson JEA: Prophylactic oophorectomy in colorectal carcinoma. *Am J Surg* 146:233, 1983.

Griffiths JD, McKinna JA, et al: Carcinoma of the colon and rectum: Circulating malignant cells and five-year survival. *Cancer* 31:226, 1973.

Hager TH, Gall FP, Harmanek P: Local excision of cancer of the rectum. *Dis Colon Rectum* 26:149, 1983.

Heald RJ: Chir M, Leigester RJ: The low stapled anastomosis. *Dis Colon Rectum* 24:437, 1981.

Heald RJ, Husband EM, Rydall RD: The mesorectum in rectal cancer surgery: The clue to pelvic recurrence? *Br J Surg* 69:613, 1982.

Heberer G, Denecke H, et al: Anterior and low anterior resection. *World J Surg* 6:517, 1982.

Hermanek P: Evolution and pathology of rectal cancer. *World J Surg* 6:502, 1982.

Hojo K, Koyama Y, Moriya Y: Lymphatic spread and its prognostic value in patients with rectal cancer. *Am J Surg* 144:350, 1982.

Jones PF, Thomson HJ: Long term results of a consistent policy of sphincter preservation in the treatment of carcinoma of the rectum. *Br J Surg* 69:564, 1982.

Keighley MRB, Matheson D: Functional results of rectal excision and endo-anal anastomosis. *Br J Surg* 67:757, 1980.

Kirwan WO, Turnbull RB, et al: Pullthrough operation with delayed anastomosis for rectal cancer. *Br J Surg* 64:695, 1978.

Lambrianides AL, Ghilchik MW: Cryosurgery in the treatment of rectal carcinoma. *Postgrad Med J* 59:244, 1983.

Langevin JM, Nivatvongs S: The true incidence of synchronous cancer of the large bowel. A prospective study. *Am J Surg* 147:330, 1984.

Localio SA, Eng K, Coppa GF: Abdominosacral resection for midrectal cancer: A fifteen year experience. *Ann Surg* 198:320, 1983.

Lock MR, Cairns DW, et al: The treatment of early colorectal cancer by local excision. *Br J Surg* 65:346, 1978.

Lockhart-Mummery HE, Ritchie JK, Hawley PR: The results of surgical treatment for carcinoma of the rectum at St. Mark's Hospital from 1948 to 1972. *Br J Surg* 63:673, 1976.

Lynch HT, Rozen P, Schuelke GS: Hereditary colon cancer: Polyposis and nonpolyposis variants, *CA* 35:95, 1985.

MacKeigan JM, Ferguson JA: Prophylactic oophorectomy and colorectal cancer in premenopausal patients. *Dis Colon Rectum* 22:401, 1979.

Madden JL, Kandalaft SI: Electrocoagulation as a primary curative method in the treatment of carcinoma of the rectum. *Surg Gynecol Obstet* 157:164, 1983.

Manson PN, Corman ML, et al: Anterior resection for adenocarcinoma: Lahey Clinic experience from 1963 through 1969. *Am J Surg* 131:434, 1976.

Mason YA: Transsphincteric exposure for low rectal anastomosis. *Proc R Soc Med* 65:974, 1972.

Mayo W, cited in Breen RE, Garnjobst W: Surgical procedures for carcinoma of the rectum; a historical review. *Dis Colon Rectum* 26:680, 1983.

McDermott FT, Hughes ESR, et al: Changing survival prospects in carcinoma of the rectum. *Br J Surg* 76:775, 1980.

McDermott F, Hughes E, et al: Long term results of restorative resection and total excision for carcinoma of the middle third of the rectum. *Surg Gynecol Obstet* 154:833, 1982.

Mettlin C, Mittelman A, et al: Trends in the United States for the management of adenocarcinoma of the rectum. *Surg Gynecol Obstet* 153:701, 1981.

Morgenstern L, Lee SE: Spatial distribution of colonic carcinoma. *Arch Surg* 113:1142, 1978.

Morson BC, Bussey HJR, Samoorian S: Policy of local excision of early cancer of the colorectum. *Gut* 18:1045, 1977.

Morson BC: Adenomas and adenoma-carcinoma sequence, in Morson BC, Dawson IMP (eds): *Gastrointestinal Pathology*, 2d ed. Oxford, England, Blackwell Scientific Publications, 1979.

Muto T, Kamiya J, et al: Colonoscopic polypectomy in diagnosis and treatment of early carcinoma of the large intestine. *Dis Colon Rectum* 23:68, 1980.

Nicholls RJ, Ritchie JK, et al: Total excision or restorative resection for carcinoma of the middle third of the rectum. *Br J Surg* 66:625, 1979.

Nicholls RJ: Surgery. *Cancer Res* 83:101, 1982.

Nivatvongs S, Gilbertsen VA, et al: Distribution of large-bowel cancers detected by occult blood test in asymptomatic patients. *Dis Colon Rectum* 25:420, 1982.

O'Connell MJ: Chemotherapy for colorectal carcinoma. *CA* 36(6):360, 1986.

Osborne DR, Higgins AF, Hobbs KEF: Cryosurgery in the management of rectal tumours, *Br J Surg* 65:859, 1978.

Papillon J: New prospects in the conservative treatment of rectal cancer. *Dis Colon Rectum* 27:695, 1984.

Parks AG: Transanal technique in low rectal anastomosis. *Proc R Soc Med* 65:975, 1972.

Parks A, Nicholls RJ, cited in DeCosse JJ; Sphincter preserving operations, in *Large Bowel Cancer*. Churchill Livingston, New York, 1981, chap 8, pp 113–117.

Parks AG, Percy JP: Resection and sutured colo-anal anastomosis for rectal carcinoma. *Br J Surg* 69:301, 1982.

Patel SC, Tovee EB, Langer B: Twenty-five years of experience with radical surgical treatment of carcinoma of the extraperitoneal rectum. *Surgery* 82:460, 1977.

Pezim ME, Nicholls RJ: Survival after high or low ligation of the inferior mesenteric artery during curative surgery for rectal cancer. *Ann Surg* 200:729, 1984.

Polk HC: Extended resection for selected adenocarcinomas of the large bowel. *Ann Surg* 175:892, 1972.

Pollett WG, Nicholls RJ: The relationship between the extent of distal clearance and survival and local recurrence rates after curative anterior resection for carcinoma of the rectum. *Ann Surg* 198:159, 1983.

Rosenberg IL, Russell CW, Giles GR: Cell viability studies on the exfoliated colonic cancer cell. *Br J Surg* 65:188, 1978.

Rothenberger DA, Wong WD: Rectal cancer—adequacy of surgical management. *Surg Annu* 17:309, 1985.

Rouviere, cited in Bonfanti F, Doci R, et al: Results of extended surgery for cancer of the rectum and sigmoid. *Br J Surg* 69:305, 1982.

Salvati EP, Rubin RJ: Electrocoagulation as primary therapy for rectal carcinoma. *Am J Surg* 132:583, 1976.

Sanderson ER: Henri Hartmann and the Hartmann operation. *Arch Surg* 115:792, 1980.

Shinya H, Cooperman A, Wolff WI: A rationale for the endoscopic management of colonic polyps. *Surg Clin North Am* 62:861, 1982.

Silverberg BS, Lubera JA: A review of American Cancer Society estimates of cancer cases and deaths. *CA* 33:2, 1983.

Simon JB: Occult blood screening for colorectal carcinoma: A critical review. *Gastroenterology* 88:820, 1985.

Sischy B, Gunderson LL: The evolving role of radiation therapy in the management of colorectal cancer. *CA* 36(6):351, 1986.

Slanetz CA, Herter FP, Grinnell RS: Anterior resection versus abdominoperineal resection for cancer of the rectum and rectosigmoid. *Am J Surg* 123:110, 1972.

Strauss AA, Strauss SF, et al: Surgical diathermy of carcinoma of the rectum: Its clinical results. *JAMA* 104:1480, 1935.

Sugarbaker PH, Corlew S: Influence of surgical techniques on survival in patients with colorectal cancer. *Dis Colon Rectum* 25:545, 1982.

Tonak J, Gall FP, et al: Incidence of local recurrence after curative operations for cancer of the rectum. *Aust NZ J Surg* 52:23, 1982.

Williams NS, Dixon MF, Johnston DP: Reappraisal of the 5 centimetre rule of distal excision for carcinoma of the rectum: A study of distal intramural spread and of patients' survival. *Br J Surg* 70:150, 1983.

Other Neoplasms

Akwari OE, Dozois RR, et al: Leiomyosarcoma of the small and large bowel. *Cancer* 42:1375, 1978.

Godnin JD: Carcinoid tumors—an analysis of 2837 cases. *Cancer* 36:560, 1975.

Orloff MJ: Carcinoid tumors of the rectum. *Cancer* 28:175, 1971.

Anal Canal Neoplasms

Boman BM, Moertel CG, et al: Carcinoma of the anal canal. A clinical and pathologic study of 188 cases. *Cancer* 54:114, 1984.

Clark J, Petrelli N, et al: Epidermoid carcinoma of the anal canal. *Cancer* 57:400, 1986.

Cooper PH, Mills SE, Allen MS: Malignant melanoma of the anus. Report of 12 cases and analysis of 255 additional cases. *Dis Colon Rectum* 25:693, 1982.

Cummings B, Keane T, et al: Results and toxicity of the treatment of anal canal carcinoma by radiation therapy or radiation therapy and chemotherapy. *Cancer* 54:2062, 1984.

Goldberg SM, Gordon PH, Nivatvongs S: *Essentials of Anorectal Surgery*. Philadelphia, Lippincott, 1980.

Greenall MJ, Quan SHQ, DeCosse JJ: Epidermoid cancer of the anus. *Br J Surg* (suppl) Sept:S97, 1985.

Greenall MJ, Quan SHQ, et al: Epidermoid cancer of the anal margin. Pathologic features, treatment, and clinical results. *Am J Surg* 149:95, 1985.

Leichman L, Nigro N, et al: Cancer of the anal canal. Model for preoperative adjuvent combined modality therapy. *Am J Med* 78:211, 1985.

Nicholls J, Glass R: *Coloproctology*. New York, Springer-Verlag, 1985.

Nivatvongs S, Becker ER: Colon, rectum and anal canal, in James EC, Corry RJ, Perry JF Jr (eds): *Basic Surgical Practice*. Philadelphia, Hanley & Belfus, 1987, chap 24.

Nigro ND: An evaluation of combined therapy for squamous cell cancer of the anal canal. *Dis Colon Rectum* 27:763, 1984.

Oster MW, Magun A, et al: Colorectal carcinoma 15 years after the diagnosis of perianal Paget disease. *J Surg Oncol* 12:379, 1979.

Papillon J, Mayer M, et al: A new approach to the management of epidermoid carcinoma of the anal canal. *Cancer* 51:1830, 1983.

Ramos R, Salinas H, Tucker L: Conservative approach to the treatment of Bowen's disease of the anus. *Dis Colon Rectum* 16:712, 1983.

Sischy B, Remington JH, et al: Definitive treatment of anal-canal carcinoma by means of radiation therapy and chemotherapy. *Dis Colon Rectum* 25:685, 1982.

Strauss RJ, Fazio VW: Bowen's disease of the anal and perianal area. A report and analysis of twelve cases. *Am J Surg* 137:231, 1979.

White WB, Schneiderman H, Sayre JT: Basal cell carcinoma of the anus: Clinical and pathological distinction from cloacogenic carcinoma. *J Clin Gastroenterol* 6:441, 1984.

Rectal Prolapse

Altemeier WA, Culbertson WR, et al: Nineteen years experience with one-step perineal repair of rectal prolapse. *Ann Surg* 173:993, 1971.

Broden B, Snellman B: Procidentia of the rectum studied with cineradiography: A contribution to the discussion of causative mechanism. *Dis Colon Rectum* 11:330, 1968.

Davidian UA, Thomas CG: Trans-sacral repair of rectal prolapse. *Am J Surg* 123:231, 1972.

Frykman HM, Goldberg SM: The surgical treatment of rectal procidentia. *Surg Gynecol Obstet* 129:1225, 1969.

Goldberg SM, Gordon PH: Treatment of rectal prolapse. *Clin Gastroenterol* 4:489, 1975.

Hagihara PF, Griffin WD Jr: Transsacral repair of rectal prolapse. *Arch Surg* 110:343, 1975.

Keighley MR, Fielding JW, Alexander-Williams J: Rectopexy for rectal prolapse in 100 consecutive patients. *Br J Surg* 70:229, 1983.

Keighley MR, Matheson DM: Results of treatment of rectal prolapse and fecal incontinence. *Dis Colon Rectum* 24:449, 1981.

Moody FG, Carey LC, Jones RS, Kelly KA, Nahrwold DL, Skinner DB: *Surgical Treatment of Digestive Disease*. Chicago, Year Book Medical 1986.

Parks AG: Anorectal incontinence. *Proc R Soc Med* 68:681, 1975.

Ripstein CB: Surgical care of massive rectal prolapse. *Dis Colon Rectum* 8:34, 1965.

Schlinkert RT, Beart RW Jr, et al: Anterior resection for complete rectal prolapse. *Dis Colon Rectum* 28:409, 1985.

Thomas CG, Jenkins SG: Results of the posterior approach in the repair of rectal prolapse. *Ann Surg* 161:897, 1965.

Uhlig BE, Sullivan ES: The modified Delorme operations: Its place in surgical treatment of massive rectal prolapse. *Dis Colon Rectum* 22:513, 1979.

Vermeulen FD, Nivatvongs S, et al: A technique for perineal rectosigmoidectomy using autosuture devices. *Surg Gynecol Obstet* 156:85, 1983.

Wassef R, Rothenberger DA, Goldberg SM: Rectal prolapse. *Curr Prob Surg* 23(6):402, 1986.

Watts JD, Rothenberger DA, et al: The management of procidentia—30 years experience. *Dis Colon Rectum* 28:96, 1985.

Rectal, Anal, Perirectal, and Perianal Infections

Billingham RP, Lewis FG: Laser versus electrical cautery in the treatment of condyloma accuminata of the anus. *Surg Gynecol Obstet* 155:865, 1982.

Bubrick MP, Hitchcock CR: Necrotizing anorectal and perineal infections. *Surgery* 86:655, 1979.

Clay CC: Sexually transmitted diseases, in Bouchier IAD, Allan RN, Hodgson HJF, Keighley MRB (eds): *Textbook of Gastroenterology*. London, England, Bailliere Tindall, 1984.

Cone LA, Woodard DR, et al: An update on the acquired immunodeficiency syndrome (AIDS) associated disorders of the alimentary tract. *Dis Colon Rectum* 2:60, 1986.

Cooper HS, Patchefsky AS, Marks G: Cloacogenic carcinoma of the anorectum in homosexual men: An observation of four cases. *Dis Colon Rectum* 22:557, 1979.

Croxson T, Chabon AB, et al: Intraepithelial carcinoma of the anus in homosexual men. *Dis Colon Rectum* 27:325, 1984.

Douglas JM, Critchlow C, et al: A double-blind study of oral acyclovir for suppression of recurrences of genital herpes simplex virus infection. *N Engl J Med* 310:1551, 1984.

Ejeckam GC, Idikio HA, et al: Malignant transformation in an anal condyloma acuminatum. *Can J Surg* 26:170, 1983.

Ferenczy A, Mitao M, et al: Latent papillomavirus and recurring genital warts. *N Engl J Med* 313:784, 1985.

Friedberg MJ, Serlin O: Condyloma acuminatum: Its association with malignancy. *Dis Colon Rectum* 6:352, 1963.

Goodell SE, Quinn TC, et al: Herpes simplex virus proctitis in homosexual men. Clinical, sigmoidoscopic, and histopathological features. *N Engl J Med* 308:868, 1983.

Hanley PH: Reflections on anorectal abscess fistula: 1984. *Dis Colon Rectum* 28:528, 1985.

Holmes K: The chlamydia epidemic. *JAMA* 245:1718, 1981.

Kram HB, Hino ST, et al: Spontaneous colonic perforation secondary to cytomegalovirus in a patient with acquired immune deficiency syndrome. *Crit Care Med* 12:469, 1984.

Lee MH, Waxman M, Gillooley JF: Primary malignant lymphoma of the anorectum in homosexual men. *Dis Colon Rectum* 29:413, 1986.

Marks G, Chase WV, Mervine TB: The fatal potential of fistula-in-ano with abscess: Analysis of 11 deaths. *Dis Colon Rectum* 16:224, 1973.

Read DR, Abcarian H: A prospective survey of 474 patients with anorectal abscess. *Dis Colon Rectum* 22:566, 1979.

Sands M: Treatment of anorectal gonorrhea infections in men. *JAMA* 243:1143, 1980.

Scoma JA, Salvati EP, Rubin RJ: Incidence of fistulas subsequent to anal abscesses. *Dis Colon Rectum* 17:357, 1974.

Wolke A, Myers S, et al: Mycobacterium avium-intracellulare-associated colitis in a patient with the acquired immunodeficiency syndrome. *J Clin Gastroenterol* 6:225, 1984.

Miscellaneous Anal Disorders

Abcarian H: Surgical correction of chronic anal fissure. Results of lateral internal sphincterotomy vs fissurectomy—midline sphincterotomy. *Dis Colon Rectum* 23:31, 1980.

Blaisdell PC: Plastic repair of the incontinent sphincter. *Am J Surg* 79:174, 1950.

Buls JG, Goldberg SM: Modern management of hemorrhoids. *Surg Clin North Am* 58:469, 1978.

Corman ML: Anal incontinence following obstetric injury. *Dis Colon Rectum* 28:86, 1985.

Corman ML: Gracilis muscle transposition for anal incontinence: Late results. *Br J Surg* 72:S21, 1985.

Fang DT, Nivatvongs S, et al: Overlapping sphincteroplasty for acquired anal incontinence. *Dis Colon Rectum* 27:720, 1984.

Grant SR, Salvati EP, Rubin RJ: Levator syndrome: An analysis of 316 cases. *Dis Colon Rectum* 18:161, 1975.

Hanley PH, Ray JE, et al: Fistula-in-ano: A ten-year follow-up study of horseshoe-abscess fistula-in-ano. *Dis Colon Rectum* 19:507, 1976.

Hagihara PF, Griffin WO Jr: Delayed correction of anorectal incontinence due to anal sphincteric injury. *Arch Surg* 111:63, 1976.

Henry MM, Simson JNL: Results of postanal repair: A retrospective study. *Br J Surg* 72:S17, 1986.

Horn HR, Schoetz DJ Jr, et al: Sphincter repair with a silastic sling for anal incontinence and rectal procidentia. *Dis Colon Rectum* 28(11):868, 1985.

Iwai W, Kaneda H, et al: Objective assessment of anorectal function after sphincter reconstruction using the gluteus maximum muscle. *Dis Colon Rectum* 28:973, 1985.

Keighley MRB: Postanal repair for faecal incontinence. *J R Soc Med* 77:285, 1984.

Labow S, Rubin RJ, et al: Perineal repair of rectal procidentia with an elastic fabric sling. *Dis Colon Rectum* 23:467, 1980.

Leguit P, VanBaal JF, Brummelkamp WH: Gracilis muscle transposition in the treatment of fecal incontinence: Long-term follow-up and evaluation of anal pressure recordings. *Dis Colon Rectum* 28(1):1, 1985.

Lomas MI, Cooperman H: Correction of rectal procidentia by use of polypropylene mesh (Marlex). *Dis Colon Rectum* 15:416, 1972.

Marks CG, Ritchie JK: Anal fistulas at St. Mark's Hospital. *Br J Surg* 64:84, 1977.

Mazier WP: Emergency hemorrhoidectomy—a worthwhile procedure. *Dis Colon Rectum* 16:200, 1973.

Motson RW: Sphincter indications for and results of sphincter repair. *Br J Surg* 72:S19, 1985.

Nicosia JF, Abcarian H: Levator syndrome. A treatment that works. *Dis Colon Rectum* 28:406, 1985.

Notaras MJ: The treatment of anal fissure by lateral subcutaneous internal sphincterotomy—a technique and results. *Br J Surg* 59:96, 1971.

Parks AG: Anorectal incontinence. *Proc R Soc Med* 68:681, 1975.

Parks AG: Etiology and surgical treatment of fistula-in-ano. *Dis Colon Rectum* 61:17, 1963.

Parks AG, Gordon PH, Hardcastle JD: A classification of fistula-in-ano. *Br J Surg* 63:1, 1976.

Pickrell KL: Gracilis muscle transplant for the correction of neurogenic rectal incontinence. *Surg Clin North Am* 39:1405, 1959.

Rothenberger DA, Goldberg SM: The management of rectovaginal fistula. *Surg Clin North Am* 62:61, 1983.

Russell TR, Donohue JH: Hemorrhoidal banding. A warning. *Dis Colon Rectum* 28:291, 1985.

Schoetz DJ Jr: Operative therapy for anal incontinence. *Surg Clin North Am* 65:35, 1985.

Schottler JL, Balcos EG, Goldberg SM: Postpartum hemorrhoidectomy. *Dis Colon Rectum* 16:395, 1973.

Slade MS, Goldberg SM, et al: Sphincteroplasty for acquired anal incontinence. *Dis Colon Rectum* 20:33, 1977.

Smith LE, Henrichs D, McCullah RD: Prospective studies on the etiology and treatment of pruritus ani. *Dis Colon Rectum* 25:358, 1982.

Thomson WHF: The nature of hemorrhoids. *Br J Surg* 62:542, 1975.

Vasilevsky CA, Gordon PH: Results of treatment of fistula-in-ano. *Dis Colon Rectum* 28:225, 1984.

Vasilevsky CA, Gordon PH: The incidence of recurrent abscesses or fistula-in-ano following anorectal suppuration. *Dis Colon Rectum* 27:126, 1984.

Walker WA, Rothenberger DA, Goldberg SM: Morbidity of internal sphincterotomy for anal fissure and stenosis. *Dis Colon Rectum* 28(11):832, 1985.

Wrobleski DE, Corman ML, et al: Long-term evaluation of rubber ring ligation in hemorrhoidal disease. *Dis Colon Rectum* 23:478, 1980.

Chapter 29

Appendix

Seymour I. Schwartz

FUNCTION AND DEVELOPMENT

The human vermiform appendix is usually referred to as "a vestigial organ with no known function." This implies a more fully developed organ in an earlier stage of the individual or in earlier stages in the evolution of the species. There is little evidence that this is the case. On the contrary, currently available evidence suggests that the appendix is a highly specialized part of the alimentary tract.

Lymphoid tissue first appears in the human appendix about 2 weeks after birth. The number of lymph follicles gradually increases to a peak of about 200 between the ages of twelve and twenty. After thirty there is an abrupt reduction to less than half and then to a trace or total absence of lymphoid tissue after sixty. Concurrent with lymphoid atrophy is fibrosis, which partially or totally obliterates the lumen in many older persons.

In the 1960s, it was proposed that the lymphoepithelial tissues of Peyer's patches and the appendix in the human are probably the equivalent of the avian bursa of Fabricius in terms of processing and maturation of thymus independent lymphocytes. It has since been shown that sites outside the gut also function as central organs for the maturation of B lymphocytes.

The appendix also participates in the secretory immune system in the gut. Secretory immunoglobins produced by the gut-associated lymphoid tissues (GALT) function as a very effective barrier that protects the milieu intérieur against the hostile milieu extérieur. Though the appendix is an integral part of the GALT-mediated secretory globulin immune mechanism, it is not indispensable. Removal of the appendix produces no detectable defect in the functioning of the immunoglobulin system. Thus, the human appendix is a useful, though not indispensable, immunologic organ.

Another possible role for the appendix in human disease was suggested in the 1960s by several retrospective studies of necropsy data. The incidence of previous appendectomy in patients dying of carcinoma of the colon was found to be higher than in comparable control groups. The widespread practice of incidental appendectomy in the course of another operation began to be questioned. But subsequent retrospective studies could not confirm the relationship. And in a prospective study designed to answer the question "In how many patients who have undergone appendectomy will cancer develop?" Moertel and associates could find no evidence that appendectomy predisposes to cancer. Thus, on the basis of currently available evidence, the practice of incidental appendectomy seems advisable since acute appendicitis and its complications continue to be significant sources of morbidity and mortality which removal of the appendix effectively prevents.

At birth the cecum and appendix have the so-called infantile contour—the appendix arising from the inferior tip of the cecum, which is shaped like an inverted pyramid. The cecum becomes bilaterally sacculated in early childhood but with the appendix still at the inferior tip. Further growth of the cecum is unequal, rapid growth of the right side and anterior aspects rotating the appendix to its adult position on the posteromedial aspect, below the ileocecal valve. The relation of the base of the appendix to the cecum is essentially constant, whereas the free end is found in a variety of locations—pelvic, retrocecal, retroileal, left lower quadrant, as well as right lower quadrant. The three taeniae coli meet at the junction of cecum with appendix and form the outer longitudinal muscle layer of the appendix. Thus the taeniae, particularly the anterior taenia, may be used as a landmark to identify an elusive appendix.

INFLAMMATION OF THE APPENDIX

Congenital defects of the appendix such as diverticula, duplication, or congenital absence are rare and of little clinical importance. The appendix occasionally gives rise to tumors, such as carcinoid or adenocarcinoma, and may be involved in inflammatory diseases of the cecum and ileum, such as tuberculosis, typhoid fever, or regional enteritis. However, by far the most important disease of the appendix is acute inflammation.

Acute Appendicitis

HISTORICAL BACKGROUND. There are isolated reports of appendectomy from 1736 on, when Amyand successfully removed from a hernial sac an appendix that had been perforated by a pin. There are also many reports, from 1581 on, of fatal suppurative disease of the cecal region, usually referred to, however, as "perityphlitis." The recognition of appendicitis as a clinical and pathologic entity for which surgical therapy is essential dates from 1886 when Reginald Fitz, Professor of Pathologic Anatomy at Harvard, gave a paper at the first meeting of the Association of American Physicians entitled "Perforating Inflammation of the Vermiform Appendix: With Special Reference to Its Early Diagnosis and Treatment." Soon thereafter McBurney described the clinical manifestations of early acute appendicitis prior to rupture, including the point of maximal abdominal tenderness, and an incision "made in the abdominal wall in cases of appendicitis."

INCIDENCE. Acute appendicitis is the most common acute surgical condition of the abdomen. The disease occurs at all ages but is most frequent in the second and third decades of life. It is quite rare in the very young, probably because the configuration of the appendix at this age makes obstruction of the lumen unlikely. There is a rough parallel between the amount of lymphoid tissue in the appendix and the incidence of acute appendicitis, the peak for both occurring in the middle teens.

The sex ratio in acute appendicitis is about 1:1 prior to puberty. At puberty the frequency in males increases, so that the male-to-female ratio is about 2:1 between the ages of fifteen and twenty-five, after which the male incidence gradually declines until the sex-related incidences are again equal.

The incidence of acute appendicitis requiring appendectomy has significantly decreased over the past 3 or 4 decades, and the trend appears to be continuing. The decline has been noted in many countries, particularly the United States, Great Britain, and Scandinavia. Some of the decrease in the number of primary appendectomies is attributable to better diagnosis (and perhaps the advent of tissue committees): acute appendicitis is being reported in 80 to 85 percent of primary appendectomies in the 1960s, as opposed to 50 to 60 percent in the 1940s. But the declining incidence is much greater than can be accounted for by better diagnosis alone. No reason for the declining incidence of appendicitis has been established. Specula-

tion has included changing dietary habits, changing intestinal flora, better nutrition, higher vitamin intake, antibiotics, and many other reasons.

ETIOLOGY AND PATHOGENESIS. Obstruction of the lumen is the dominant factor in the production of acute appendicitis. Fecaliths are the usual cause of appendiceal obstruction. Less common are hypertrophy of lymphoid tissue; inspissated barium from previous x-ray studies; vegetable and fruit seeds; and intestinal worms, particularly ascarids.

The frequency with which appendiceal obstruction is found is proportional to the diligence with which it is looked for. The frequency of obstruction also rises with the severity of the inflammatory process. Fecaliths are found in about 40 percent in simple acute appendicitis, in about 65 percent in gangrenous appendicitis without rupture, and in about 90 percent in gangrenous appendicitis with rupture.

The sequence of events following occlusion of the lumen is probably as follows: A closed-loop obstruction (Chap. 24) is produced by the proximal block, and continuing normal secretion of the appendiceal mucosa very rapidly produces distention. The luminal capacity of the normal appendix is only about 0.1 mL—there is no real lumen. Secretion of as little as 0.5 mL distal to a block raises the intraluminal pressure to about 60 cmH$_2$O. The human being is one of the few animals with an appendix capable of secreting at pressures high enough to lead to gangrene and perforation. Distention stimulates nerve endings of visceral afferent pain fibers, producing vague, dull, diffuse pain in the midabdomen or lower epigastrium. Peristalsis is also stimulated by the rather sudden distention, so that some cramping may be superimposed on the visceral pain early in the course of appendicitis.

Distention continues, not only from continued mucosal secretion, but also from rapid multiplication of the resident bacteria of the appendix. As pressure in the organ increases, venous pressure is exceeded. Capillaries and venules are occluded, but arteriolar inflow continues, resulting in engorgement and vascular congestion. Distention of this magnitude usually causes reflex nausea and vomiting, and the diffuse visceral pain becomes more severe. The inflammatory process soon involves the serosa of the appendix and in turn parietal peritoneum in the region, producing the characteristic shift in pain to the right lower quadrant.

The mucosa of the gastrointestinal tract, including the appendix, is very susceptible to impairment of blood supply. Thus its integrity is compromised early in the process, allowing bacterial invasion of the deeper coats. Fever, tachycardia, and leukocytosis develop as a consequence of absorption of dead tissue products and bacterial toxins. As progressive distention encroaches on the arteriolar pressure, the area with the poorest blood supply suffers most—ellipsoidal infarcts develop in the antimesenteric border. As distention, bacterial invasion, compromise of vascular supply, and infarction progress, perforation occurs, usually through one of the infarcted areas on the antimesenteric border.

This sequence is not inevitable—some episodes of acute appendicitis apparently subside spontaneously. Many patients who are found at operation to have acute appendicitis give a history of previous similar but less severe attacks of right lower quadrant pain. Pathologic examination of the appendices removed from these patients often reveals thickening and scarring, suggesting old healed acute inflammation. Presumably obstruction of the lumen when due to lymphoid hypertrophy or soft fecalith can be spontaneously relieved, allowing subsidence of appendiceal inflammation and attendant symptoms.

CLINICAL MANIFESTATIONS. Symptoms. Abdominal pain is the prime symptom of acute appendicitis. Classically the pain initially is diffusely centered in the lower epigastrium or umbilical area, is moderately severe, and is steady—sometimes with intermittent cramping superimposed. After a period varying from 1 to 12 h, but usually within 4 to 6 h, the pain localizes in the right lower quadrant. This classic pain sequence, though usual, is not invariable. In some patients the pain of appendicitis begins in the right lower quadrant and remains there. Variations in the anatomic location of the appendix account for many of the variations in the principal locus of the somatic phase of the pain. For example, a long appendix with the inflamed tip in the left lower quadrant causes pain in that area; a rectrocecal appendix may cause principally flank or back pain; a pelvic appendix, principally suprapubic pain; and a retroileal appendix may cause testicular pain, presumably from irritation of the spermatic artery and ureter. Malrotation is also responsible for puzzling pain patterns. The visceral component is in the normal location, but the somatic component is felt in that part of the abdomen where the cecum has been arrested in rotation.

Anorexia nearly always accompanies appendicitis. It is so constant that the diagnosis should be questioned if the patient is not anorectic. Vomiting occurs in about 75 percent of patients, but is not prominent or prolonged, most patients vomiting only once or twice.

Most patients give a history of obstipation from before the onset of abdominal pain, and many feel that defecation would relieve their abdominal pain. Diarrhea occurs in some patients, however, particularly children, so that the pattern of bowel function is of little differential diagnostic value.

The sequence of symptom appearance has great differential diagnostic significance. In over 95 percent of patients with acute appendicitis, anorexia is the first symptom, followed by abdominal pain, which is followed in turn by vomiting (if vomiting occurs). If vomiting precedes the onset of pain, the diagnosis should be questioned.

Signs. Physical findings are determined principally by the anatomic position of the inflamed appendix as well as by whether the organ has already ruptured when the patient is first examined.

Vital signs are not changed very much by uncomplicated appendicitis. Temperature elevation is rarely more than 1°C; the pulse rate is normal or slightly elevated. Changes of greater magnitude usually mean that a complication has occurred or that another diagnosis should be considered.

Patients with appendicitis usually prefer to lie supine with the thighs, particularly the right, drawn up, because any motion increases pain. If asked to move, they do so slowly and gingerly.

The classic right lower quadrant physical signs are present when the inflamed appendix lies in the anterior position. Tenderness is often maximal at or near the point described by McBurney as being "located exactly between an inch and a half and two inches from the anterior spinous process of the ileum on a straight line drawn from that process to the umbilicus." Direct rebound tenderness usually, and referred or indirect rebound tenderness frequently, is present and is also felt maximally in the right lower quadrant, indicating peritoneal irritation. Rovsing's sign—pain in the right lower quadrant when palpatory pressure is exerted in the left lower quadrant—also indicates the site of peritoneal irritation. Cutaneous hyperesthesia in the area supplied by the spinal nerves on the right at T_{10}, T_{11}, and T_{12} is a frequent but not a constant accompaniment of acute appendicitis. In patients with obvious appendicitis, this sign is superfluous, but in some early cases it may be the first positive sign. It is elicited either by needle prick or, better, by gently picking up the skin between the forefinger and thumb. This ordinarily is not unpleasant but is painful in areas of cutaneous hyperesthesia.

Muscular resistance to palpation of the abdominal wall roughly parallels the severity of the inflammatory process. Early in the disease, resistance, if present, consists mainly of voluntary guarding. As peritoneal irritation progresses, muscle spasm increases and becomes largely involuntary—true reflex rigidity as opposed to voluntary guarding.

Variations in the position of the inflamed appendix produce variations from the usual in physical findings. With a retrocecal appendix, the anterior abdominal findings are less striking, and tenderness may be most marked in the flank. When the inflamed appendix hangs into the pelvis, abdominal findings may be entirely absent, and the diagnosis may be missed unless the rectum is examined. As the examining finger exerts pressure on the peritoneum of the cul-de-sac of Douglas, pain is felt in the suprapubic area as well as locally. Signs of localized muscle irritation may also be present. The *psoas* sign indicates an irritative focus in proximity to that muscle. The test is performed by having patients lie on their left side; the examiner then slowly extends the right thigh, thus stretching the iliopsoas muscle. The test is positive if extension produces pain. Similarly, a positive *obturator* sign of hypogastric pain on stretching the obturator internus indicates irritation at that locus. The test is performed by passive internal rotation of the flexed right thigh with the patient supine.

LABORATORY FINDINGS. Moderate leukocytosis, ranging from about 10,000 to 18,000/mm³ and accompanied by a moderate polymorphonuclear predominance, is the rule in acute uncomplicated appendicitis. With normal total and differential white blood cell counts, the diagnosis of appendicitis is in question though not ruled out. If the white cell count is greater than about 18,000/mm^3 or if the shift to the left is extreme, perforated appendicitis or an acute inflammatory disease of greater magnitude than appendicitis is probable.

Urinalysis, except for the high specific gravity of dehydration, is normal unless the inflamed appendix lies near the ureter or bladder, in which case white cells and occasionally even red cells may be seen. Bacilluria in a fresh catheterized urine is not seen in appendicitis, however, allowing differentiation from urinary tract infection.

Radiography. The diagnosis of acute appendicitis is usually based on history and clinical findings. X-rays are used, therefore, only in differential diagnosis and to demonstrate complications of appendicitis.

Plain films of the abdomen in acute appendicitis often reveal a distended loop or two of small bowel in the right lower quadrant, less often a distended cecum. Visualization of a gas-filled appendix usually, but not invariably, indicates acute appendicitis with proximal appendiceal obstruction. A radiopaque fecalith when present in the right lower quadrant is nearly always associated with gangrenous appendicitis. Barium enema examination may be helpful in selected patients, particularly children, in whom the diagnosis remains unclear and operation is thought to be hazardous. It is done cautiously and gently, without prior preparation of the colon and without external manipulation or pressure. Complete filling of the appendix and absence of mucosal changes in both the appendix and ileocecal region rule out acute appendicitis. Pathognomonic findings of acute appendicitis on barium enema consist of nonfilling of the appendix, mass effect on the medial and inferior borders of the cecum, and mass effect or mucosal irregularities of the terminal ileum.

Chest films are sometimes necessary to rule out disease in the right lower lung field, since lesions that irritate nerves at T_{10}, T_{11}, and T_{12} may simulate appendicitis.

COMPLICATIONS—APPENDICEAL RUPTURE. Though some patients with acute appendicitis have spontaneous subsidence of the acute process, there is no way of predicting in which patients this will occur. The only safe course of action in uncomplicated acute appendicitis is immediate appendectomy. Ideally, every patient would have the offending organ removed before complications, particularly rupture, supervene. Some progress has been made, but too many patients still are seen first only after rupture has occurred, and some physicians still are needlessly indecisive. The use of antibiotic therapy in an attempt to avoid or postpone operative therapy ignores the obstructive etiology of acute appendicitis, is dangerous, and is ill-advised.

Pathogenesis. Unrelenting obstruction of the appendiceal lumen leads inexorably to gangrene and rupture of the pus-filled organ. Among the sequelae are appendiceal phlegmon, abscesses, spreading peritonitis, suppurative pylephlebitis, and intestinal obstruction.

Rupture of the appendix nearly always is distal to an occluding fecalith. The contents of the distended distal appendix spill through the necrotic rent, but this is rarely more than a few milliliters because of the small capacity of the appendix. Retrograde spill of cecal contents is ordinarily prevented by the occluding fecalith, unless the fecalith becomes dislodged through the rupture site or the necrotic area involves the base of the appendix and contiguous cecum.

During the several hours elapsing between onset of acute appendicitis and rupture, nature's walling-off process is able to quarantine the inflammation in about 95 percent of patients and confine the spill to the periappendiceal area.

A phlegmon is produced consisting of a mass of inflamed, matted intestines and omentum but with little or no discrete collection of pus. This process may slowly resolve spontaneously or may be hastened in resolution by timely surgical intervention. In some patients, however, a progressive suppurative process produces an expanding collection of pus contained by the walling-off process—a periappendiceal abscess.

If the walling-off process has not been completed by the time appendiceal rupture occurs, contamination spreads beyond the right lower quadrant. The two sites of predilection are the pelvic cul-de-sac via gravity drainage, and the right subhepatic space, which is reached via the right gutter (see also Chap. 34). With indiscriminate centrifugal contamination, virulent bacteria thus seeded initiate spreading diffuse peritonitis. An even more lethal form of peritonitis is produced by secondary rupture of intraabdominal abscesses that were produced by ruptured appendicitis. Ascending septic thrombophlebitis of the portal venous system—pylethrombophlebitis—is a very grave but fortunately rare complication of gangrenous appendicitis. It is heralded by chills and spiking fever, followed by right upper quadrant pain and jaundice. Septic clots from the involved mesenteric radicles embolize the liver, producing multiple pyogenic abscesses (Chap. 30).

Incidence. The proportion of patients with acute appendicitis who already have ruptured appendicitis when they are first seen varies with the age of the patients and with the type of hospital reporting. Twenty-five to thirty percent of charity hospital patients have ruptured appendicitis on admission versus about 15 percent in private hospitals. The rupture incidence is also significantly higher in the pediatric and geriatric age groups.

Diagnosis. Diagnosis usually is not difficult after rupture has occurred. The patient is obviously quite ill, prostrated, toxic, dehydrated, and distended. Right lower quadrant pain increases in severity and spreads over a somewhat larger area. Abdominal pain has been said to lessen dramatically at the moment of perforation and to be diminished for a few hours thereafter. This was attributed to sudden relief of the pain-producing distention of the obstructed appendix. Temporary relief of pain is rarely seen, however, occurring in only 4 percent in one series. In the vast majority, pain continues unabated—apparently local peritonitis is as effective in producing pain as distention of the appendix.

Physical findings are also more definite after rupture. With periappendiceal phlegmon or abscess, a tender, boggy mass with ill-defined margins usually can be felt. Tenderness, which is fingerpoint with simple acute appendicitis, now encompasses the whole right lower quadrant. Rebound tenderness and muscular rigidity are usually marked and correspond in extent to the extent of the local peritonitis. As in simple acute peritonitis, however, physical findings depend on the position of the appendix. For example, the only physical finding with a pelvic abscess secondary to a ruptured pelvic appendix may be a boggy tender mass on rectal examination. With spreading peritonitis, the physical signs advance with the spread of the inflammation (see also Chap. 34). Abdominal distention and paralytic ileus roughly parallel the severity and duration of the inflammatory process.

Fever and pulse also parallel the severity of the process. The temperature, which is rarely over 38°C in simple acute appendicitis, rises to about 39°C with localized peritonitis and often spikes over 40°C with diffuse peritonitis. Leukocytosis increases to 20,000 to 30,000 cells/mm^3 with extreme polymorphonuclear predominance and marked shift to immature forms. Hemoconcentration and desalting are variable and reflect the amount of fluid sequestered in the inflamed area as well as loss of oral intake.

DIFFERENTIAL DIAGNOSIS. The differential diagnosis of acute appendicitis is essentially the diagnosis of the "acute abdomen" (see Chap. 24). This is because clinical manifestations are not specific for a given disease but are specific for disturbance of a physiologic function or functions. Thus an essentially identical clinical picture can result from a wide variety of acute processes within or near the peritoneal cavity that produce the same alterations of function as acute appendicitis.

Accuracy of preoperative diagnosis should be about 85 percent. If it is consistently less, some unnecessary operations are probably being done, and a more rigorous preoperative differential diagnosis is in order. On the other hand, an accuracy consistently greater than 90 percent should also cause concern, since this may mean that some patients with atypical but bona fide acute appendicitis are being "observed" when they should have prompt surgical intervention. The Haller group has shown, however, that this is not invariably true. Prior to their study, the perforation rate at the hospital where the study took place was 26.7 percent, and acute appendicitis was found at 80 percent of the operations. By a policy of intensive in-hospital observation when the diagnosis of appendicitis was unclear, the group raised its rate of appendicitis found at operation to 94 percent, while the perforation rate remained unchanged at 27.5 percent.

There are a few conditions in which operation is contraindicated, but in general the disease processes that are confused with appendicitis are also surgical problems or, if not, are not made worse by operation. The more frequent error is to make a preoperative diagnosis of acute appendicitis only to find some other condition (or nothing) at operation; much less frequently, acute appendicitis is found after a preoperative diagnosis of another condi-

tion. Most common erroneous preoperative diagnoses—accounting for more than 75 percent—in descending order of frequency are acute mesenteric lymphadenitis, no organic pathologic condition, acute pelvic inflammatory disease, twisted ovarian cyst or ruptured graafian follicle, and acute gastroenteritis.

Differential diagnosis of appendicitis depends upon three major factors: the anatomic location of the inflamed appendix, the stage of the process—whether simple or ruptured, and the age and sex of the patient.

Acute Mesenteric Adenitis (Chap. 35). This is the disease most often confused with acute appendicitis in children. Almost invariably an upper respiratory infection is present or has recently subsided. The pain is usually less or more diffuse, and tenderness is not as sharply localized as in appendicitis. Voluntary guarding is sometimes present, but true rigidity is rare. Generalized lymphadenopathy may be noted. Laboratory procedures are of little help in differentiating, though a relative lymphocytosis, when present, suggests mesenteric adenitis. Observation for several hours to allow the clinical picture to clarify is in order if the diagnosis of mesenteric adenitis seems likely, since this is a self-limited disease, but if the differentiation remains in doubt, immediate operation is the only safe course.

Acute Gastroenteritis. This is very common in childhood but usually can easily be differentiated from appendicitis. Viral gastroenteritis, an acute self-limited infection of diverse causes, is characterized by profuse watery diarrhea, nausea, and vomiting. Hyperperistaltic abdominal cramps precede the watery stools. The abdomen is relaxed between cramps, and there are no localizing signs. Laboratory values are normal.

Salmonella gastroenteritis results from ingestion of contaminated food. Abdominal findings are usually similar to those in viral gastroenteritis, but in some the abdominal pain is intense, localized, and associated with rebound tenderness. Chills and fever are common. Leukocyte count is usually normal. The causative organisms can be isolated from essentially 100 percent of patients, but this may take too long to help the clinician in differential diagnosis of abdominal pain. Similar attacks in other persons eating the same food as the patient greatly strengthen the presumptive diagnosis of salmonella gastroenteritis.

Typhoid fever is now a rare disease. This probably accounts for the frequency of missed diagnosis—it is rarely seen and rarely thought of. The onset is less acute than appendicitis, with prodrome of several days. Differentiation is usually possible because of the prostration, maculopapular rash, inappropriate bradycardia, and leukopenia. Diagnosis is confirmed by culture of *Salmonella typhosa* from stool or blood. Intestinal perforation, usually in the lower ileum, develops in about 1 percent of cases and requires immediate surgical therapy.

Ruptured Ectopic Pregnancy. This is manifested by lower abdominal pain and symptoms of hypovolemia. A tuboovarian mass is usually palpable on pelvic examination. Culdocentesis yields nonclotting blood.

Disease of the Male. Diseases of males (Chap. 40) must

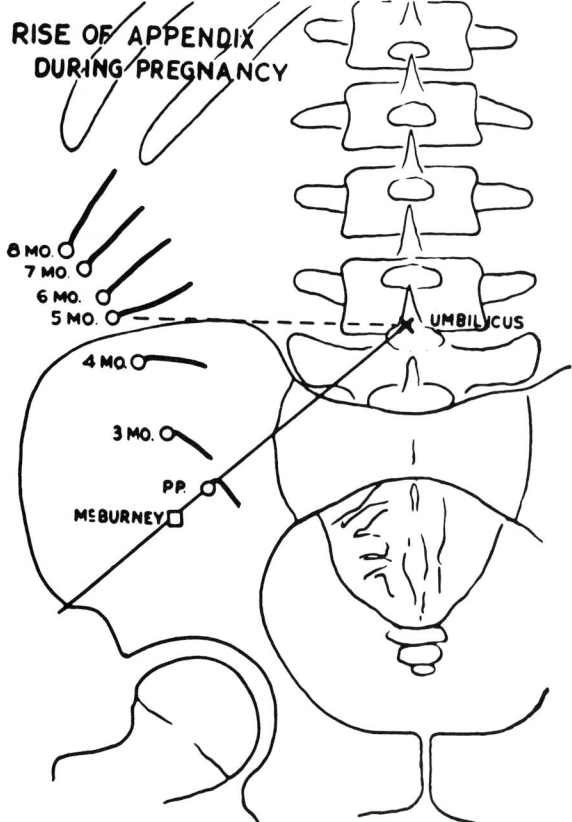

Fig. 29-1. Changes in position and direction of appendix during pregnancy. PP = postpartum. (From: *Baer JL, Reis RA, Arens RA: Appendicitis in pregnancy. JAMA 98:1359, Copyright 1932, American Medical Association, with permission.*)

perforation and generalized peritonitis. Fetal mortality overall is 2 to 8.5 percent, but is about 35 percent in perforation and peritonitis. It is obviously imperative to remove acutely inflamed appendices before they perforate.

TREATMENT. There is but one treatment for acute appendicitis and its complications. To attempt to treat appendicitis with antibiotics is misguided because it ignores the obstructive etiology of appendicitis and is to be condemned. Thus the only question to be resolved is when—the timing of surgical intervention.

Immediate appendectomy is indicated in acute appendicitis without rupture just as soon as the minimal workup compatible with good medical practice is completed. Ruptured appendicitis with local peritonitis or phlegmon formation also should be operated upon early in the hospital course. A brief period of preparation is advisable during which nasogastric suction is instituted and sufficient intravenous fluids, usually Ringer's lactate solution and 5% dextrose in water, are given to correct systemic fluid and electrolyte deficits. Systemic antibiotics in large doses are administered: since bacteroides organisms play such a major role in appendiceal infections, clindamycin should be one of the antibiotics used pending culture-sensitivity data. (See also Chap. 5.)

Patients with ruptured appendicitis producing spreading peritonitis should similarly be prepared with "all deliberate haste" for early surgical intervention. Preparation (Chap. 34) may take somewhat longer than with localized peritonitis because of the greater magnitude of the physiologic derangements caused by the more extensive process but rarely requires more than 3 or 4 h. It is essential to remove the necrotic appendix to prevent continued contamination of the peritoneum.

There is general agreement on the timing of the operation for the three categories of appendicitis mentioned above—acute appendicitis without rupture, ruptured appendix with local peritonitis or phlegmon formation, and ruptured appendix with spreading peritonitis. There has been a difference of opinion, however, concerning the optimal timing of the operation for ruptured appendicitis with frank periappendiceal abscess formation. "Expectant treatment" was advocated by A. J. Ochsner in 1901. As now practiced this consists of intravenous fluids, nasogastric suction, and large doses of antibiotics. Vital signs, leukocytosis, and size of the mass are followed closely. If progression occurs, the abscess is drained. If the patient improves, conservative treatment is continued. With these measures the majority of appendiceal abscesses resolve satisfactorily, although many days of hospital treatment are required. An elective appendectomy 6 weeks to 3 months later is strongly advised, since the recurrence rate is very high.

Most surgeons urge prompt operation for ruptured appendix with abscess as soon as the patient can be prepared. With the supportive measures now available, and particularly with the now widespread availability of well-trained surgeons, prompt operation can be done with a lower mortality and morbidity than with conservative treatment. Prompt operation for all categories of appendicitis is especially important in children since expectant treatment of ruptured appendicitis has been less successful than in adults.

Nonoperative therapy may be appropriate if, when the patient is first seen, symptoms are of several days' duration and are subsiding, and there is a discrete right lower quadrant mass; or if expert surgical care is not available.

Preoperative Antibiotics. Many trials have demonstrated the efficacy of preoperative antibiotics in lowering the infectious complications in appendicitis. It is not yet clear, however, which of many different regimens is best. There are currently three principal practices: (1) antibiotics are started preoperatively only if perforative appendicitis is thought to be present; (2) antibiotics are started preoperatively in all, and if gangrenous or perforative appendicitis is found, antibiotics are continued (author's preference); (3) antibiotics are started preoperatively in all patients with a diagnosis of acute appendicitis; if appendicitis of any stage is found, antibiotics are continued for 3 to 5 days.

The bacterial flora customarily found in acute appendicitis is a mixed colonic flora with both aerobic and anaerobic organisms. But the most important pathogen in appendicitis-related infections is the gram-negative rod *Bacteroides fragilis*. Thus an agent effective against this

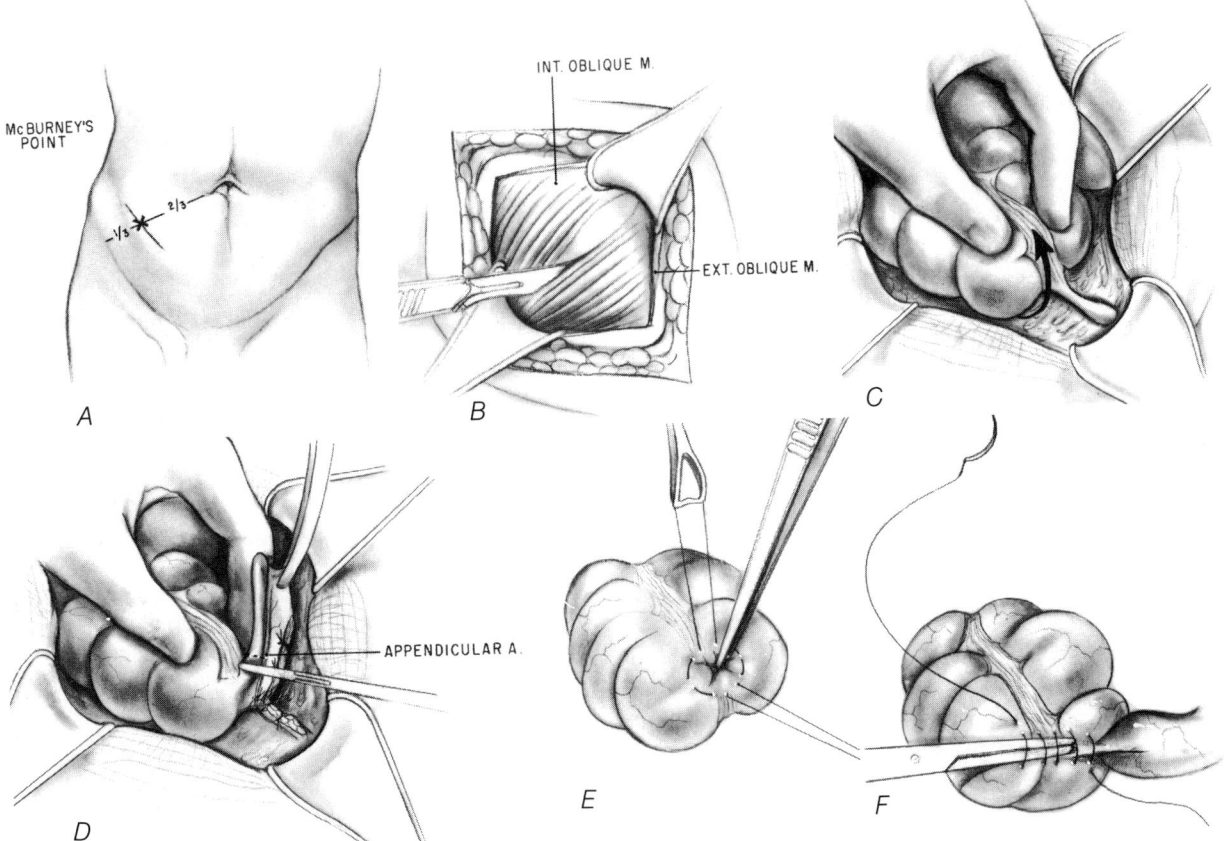

Fig. 29-2. Appendectomy. *A.* McBurney incision passing through McBurney's point, which is located one-third of the distance from the anterior superior iliac spine to the umbilicus. *B.* The incision has been carried through skin and subcutaneous tissue and has divided the aponeurosis of the external oblique muscle in the course of its fibers. The internal oblique muscle is being separated in the direction of its fibers. *C.* The peritoneum has been incised and the peritoneal cavity entered. The appendix is delivered into the wound by rotation of the cecum up and out. *D.* The vessels within the mesoappendix have been doubly ligated and transected with particular attention directed toward the appendicular artery. A crushing clamp is applied to the base of the appendix and then moved distad (to dotted line), so that a ligature may be placed in the resulting groove. *E.* The stump of the appendix may or may not be tied with a ligature. It is customary to invert the stump and place a purse-string suture through the seromuscular layers of the cecum. *F.* An alternative method of inverting the appendiceal stump is demonstrated with a continuous seromuscular suture. A Z suture can also be used to achieve this end.

species should be part of the regimen. Clindamycin plus an aminoglycoside is popular in the United States; the single agent metronidazole is often used in the United Kingdom.

Conduct of the Operation (Fig. 29-2). Many surgeons (including the author) prefer a McBurney (or Rockey-Davis) incision in all patients with suspected appendicitis, while others use a McBurney incision in clear-cut appendicitis but use a right paramedian (or midline) incision if the diagnosis is in doubt, particularly in females. The principal argument against the McBurney incision is that a second incision may be necessary if a procedure other than appendectomy has to be done. The principal argument against the paramedian incision is that if the patient does indeed have appendicitis, the diseased organ can be removed only by traversing the previously unsoiled peritoneal cavity.

When a periappendiceal abscess is suspected, paramedian incision is contraindicated. The abscess is approached from a laterally placed McBurney incision without entering the free peritoneal cavity. The abscess is evacuated, with care to avoid breaking down any of the walling-off process. The appendix should be removed if possible, but if extensive dissection is necessary to expose the organ, appendectomy is hazardous. Interval appendectomy should be done some weeks later.

There are several methods of managing the appendiceal stump. The traditional method of ligation-inversion has the advantage that peritonealization and hemostasis are secured, but the disadvantage of inverting an infected stump into a closed cavity is the risk of an intramural abscess of the cecum. However, if the ligation is done with fine plain catgut this risk is minimal. Inversion without ligation obviates the risk of abscess, but hemostasis of the intramural branch of the appendiceal artery may not be secure. Ligation without inversion avoids burying the stump and secures hemostasis but is unsurgical because there remains free in the peritoneal cavity a contaminated raw surface. Contamination of the peritoneal cavity may result from the ligated stump either from bacteria on the stump or from the slipping of the ligature or necrosis of the stump as a result of the ligation. A recent study demonstrated that invagination of the stump significantly reduced the incidence of bacterial contamination of the peritoneal cavity.

If appendicitis is not found, an orderly investigation for the cause of the symptoms must be done. This should include gross examination and immediate Gram stain of any peritoneal fluid or exudate. With the assistant elevating the anterior abdominal wall by retraction, the pelvic organs are examined. Next the gallbladder and gastroduodenal areas are visualized. The mesentery is examined for nodes. The small intestine is then "run" in a retrograde manner, starting at the cecum, looking particularly for regional enteritis and Meckel's diverticulum. Finally, palpation of the colon and kidneys is done as well as is possible through a McBurney incision. It is axiomatic that if the cause of the acute abdomen is found, exploration is terminated and appropriate therapy for the offending process undertaken.

Drainage of localized collections of pus is indicated and should be done with one or more soft rubber drains to each collection, brought out through the McBurney incision. If a paramedian incision has been used, a separate stab wound is preferred to avoid incisional hernia. A sump drain is more effective in large collections. Drainage of diffuse peritonitis is unwarranted, because it is physically impossible and physiologically undesirable. If an intact though inflamed appendix has been removed, all layers of the incision should be closed without drainage. However, if a ruptured appendix is removed the peritoneum and fascial layers are closed but the subcutaneous tissues and skin are left open because of the risk of wound infection if they are closed. The wound may be allowed to granulate or be closed secondarily in 4 or 5 days.

PROGNOSIS. Mortality. The mortality from appendicitis in the United States has steadily decreased from a rate of 9.9 per 100,000 in 1939 to 0.2 per 100,000 in 1986. Among the factors responsible are the significantly decreasing incidence of appendicitis; better diagnosis and treatment, attributable to the now available antibiotics, intravenous fluids, blood, and plasma, and a higher percentage of patients receiving definitive treatment before rupture.

Principal factors in mortality are whether or not rupture occurs prior to surgical treatment and the age of the patient. The overall mortality rate in unruptured acute appendicitis is little higher than the rate for a general anesthetic (0.06 percent) and is now about 0.1 percent. The overall mortality rate in ruptured acute appendicitis is about 3 percent—a thirtyfold increase. The mortality rate of ruptured appendicitis in the elderly is about 15 percent— a fivefold increase from the overall rate.

Death is usually attributable to uncontrolled sepsis— peritonitis, intraabdominal abscesses, or gram-negative septicemia. Sepsis may impose metabolic demands of such magnitude on the cardiovascular or respiratory systems that they cannot be met, in which case cardiac or respiratory insufficiency is the direct cause of death. Pulmonary embolism continues to account for some deaths. Aspiration producing drowning in the patient's vomitus is a prominent mode of death in the older age group.

Morbidity. Morbidity rates parallel mortality rates, being precipitously increased by rupture of the appendix and to a lesser extent by old age. In one report, complications occurred in 3 percent of patients with nonperforated appendicitis and in 47 percent of patients with perforations. Most of the serious early complications are septic and include abscess (Chap. 34) and wound infection. Wound infection is common but is nearly always confined to the subcutaneous tissues and promptly responds to wound drainage, which is accomplished by reopening the skin incision. Wound infection predisposes to wound dehiscence also. The type of incision is relevant, since complete dehiscence rarely occurs in a McBurney incision. The efficacy of systemic antibiotics in reducing the incidence of wound infections has not been established. But Foster et al. reported a significant reduction in patients receiving metronidazole.

The incidence of intraabdominal abscesses secondary to peritoneal contamination from gangrenous or perforated appendicitis has decreased markedly since the introduction of potent antibiotics. The sites of predilection for abscesses are appendiceal fossa, pouch of Douglas, subhepatic space, and interloop, which are usually multiple. Transrectal drainage is preferred for an abscess that bulges into the rectum.

Fecal fistula is an annoying but not particularly dangerous complication of appendectomy. This may be produced by sloughing of that portion of the cecum inside a constricting purse-string suture, by the ligature's slipping off a tied but not inverted appendiceal stump, or by necrosis from an abscess encroaching on the cecum.

Intestinal obstruction, initially paralytic but sometimes progressing to mechanical, may occur with slowly resolving peritonitis with loculated abscesses and exuberant adhesion formation (Chap. 24).

Late complications are quite uncommon. Adhesive band intestinal obstruction after appendectomy does occur but much less frequently than after pelvic surgical therapy. The incidence of inguinal hernia is three times greater in patients who have had an appendectomy. Incisional hernia is analogous to wound dehiscence— infection predisposes to it, and it rarely occurs in a McBurney incision but is not uncommon in a lower right paramedian incision.

TUMORS

Neoplasms of the appendix are very uncommon and are usually diagnosed at operation or autopsy. Three histologic types of malignant tumors occur: carcinoid, adenocarcinoma, and malignant mucocele. Various benign tumors also occur but are of no clinical significance except as a very rare etiologic agent in the production of acute appendicitis from appendiceal obstruction. In a study of 50,000 appendices the incidence of carcinoid was 0.5 percent, primary adenocarcinoma 0.08 percent, and mucocele 0.2 percent.

Carcinoid

Forty-five percent of all reported carcinoid tumors of the gastrointestinal tract have been found in the appendix. The true incidence probably exceeds 75 percent, since carcinoids of the appendix are not sufficiently unusual to elicit the urge to publish while carcinoids elsewhere more often are. Although cytologic criteria of malignancy are not uncommonly present, biologic malignancy evidenced by metastasis has been demonstrated in only 2.9 percent of appendiceal carcinoids. There are but six reported cases of malignant carcinoid of the appendix producing the malignant carcinoid syndrome (Chap. 27).

Carcinoids of the appendix are typically small, firm, circumscribed, yellow-brown tumors. About three-fourths occur in the distal third of the appendix; less than 10 percent occur at the base. They are nearly always an incidental finding at the time of appendectomy (or autopsy), though rarely they may initiate acute appendicitis. Simple appendectomy with wide excision of the mesoappendix is adequate treatment unless invasion beyond the line of resection and/or nodal metastasis is demonstrated, in which case right colectomy with excision of the node-bearing mesentery is indicated.

Adenocarcinoma

This is often referred to as "colonic" type of carcinoma of the appendix because of the resemblance in behavior and in gross and microscopic appearance to colonic cancer. It also serves to distinguish it from the mucocele. Preoperative diagnosis may be based on the visualization of an extracecal mass on barium enema, but usually the appendiceal tumor is not suspected prior to operation, which is usually an appendectomy. In a few instances the lesion is unrecognized at appendectomy and is detected on pathologic examination of the specimen. Treatment is right colectomy including mesentery. The prognosis is probably about the same as for carcinoma of the cecum.

Mucocele

This is a cystic dilatation of the appendix containing mucoid material. Histologically, mucoceles are divided into a benign type, which results from noninflammatory occlusion of the proximal lumen of the appendix and thus is not a neoplasm, and a malignant type, which is a grade 1 mucous papillary adenocarcinoma. Appendectomy is adequate treatment, but care should be taken to avoid rupture, since pseudomyxoma peritonei has been reported to occur following rupture and peritoneal dissemination of the appendiceal contents.

Bibliography

Function and Development

Buschard K, Kjaeldgaard A: Investigation and analysis of the position, fixation, length and embryology of the vermiform appendix. *Acta Chir Scand* 139:293, 1973.

McVay JR Jr: The appendix in relation to neoplastic disease. *Cancer* 17:929, 1964.

Moertel CG, Nobrega FT, et al: A prospective study of appendectomy and predisposition to cancer. *Surg Gynecol Obstet* 138:549, 1974.

Walker WA, Isselbacher KJ: Intestinal antibodies. *N Engl J Med* 297:767, 1977.

Inflammation of the Appendix

Amyand C: Of an inguinal rupture with a pin in the appendix caeci encrusted with stone: Some observations on wounds in the guts. *Philosoph Trans* 39:329, 1736.

Arnbjornsson E: Invagination of the appendiceal stump for the reduction of peritoneal bacterial contamination. *Curr Surg* 42:184, 1985.

Bailey LE, Finley RK Jr, et al: Acute appendicitis during pregnancy. *Am Surg* 52:218, 1986.

Bongard F, Landers DV, Lewis F: Differential diagnosis of appendicitis and pelvic inflammatory disease. *Am J Surg* 150:90, 1985.

Bower RJ, Bell MJ, Ternberg JL: Controversial aspects of appendicitis management in children. *Arch Surg* 116:885, 1981.

Bower RJ, Bell MJ, Ternberg JL: Diagnostic value of the white blood count and neutrophil percentage in the evaluation of abdominal pain in children. *Surg Gynecol Obstet* 152:424, 1981.

Brook I: Bacterial studies of peritoneal cavity and postoperative surgical wound drainage following perforated appendix in children. *Ann Surg* 192:208, 1980.

Burkitt DP: The aetiology of appendicitis. *Br J Surg* 58:695, 1971.

Busuttil RW, Davidson RK, et al: Effect of prophylactic antibiotics in acute nonperforated appendicitis: A prospective, randomized, double-blind clinical study. *Ann Surg* 194:502, 1981.

Butler C: Surgical pathology of acute appendicitis. *Hum Pathology* 12:870, 1981.

Cooperman M: Complications of appendectomy. *Surg Clin North Am* 63:1233, 1983.

Donovan IA, Ellis D, et al: One-dose antibiotic prophylaxis against wound infection after appendicectomy: A randomized trial of clindamycin, cefazolin sodium and a placebo. *Br J Surg* 66:193, 1979.

Fitz RH: Perforating inflammation of the vermiform appendix: With special reference to its early diagnosis and treatment. *Trans Assoc Am Physicians* 1:107, 1886.

Foster GE, Bolwell J, et al: Clinical and economic consequences of wound sepsis after appendicectomy and their modification by metronidazole or povidone iodine. *Lancet* 1:769, 1981.

Gilbert SR, Emmens RW, Putnam TC: Appendicitis in children. *Surg Gynecol Obstet* 161:261, 1985.

Greenall MJ, Evans M, Pollock AV: Should you drain a perforated appendix? *Br J Surg* 65:880, 1978.

Haller JA Jr, Shaker IH, et al: Peritoneal drainage versus nondrainage for generalized peritonitis from ruptured appendicitis in children. *Ann Surg* 177:595, 1973.

Harrison MW, Lindner DJ, et al: Acute appendicitis in children: Factors affecting morbidity. *Am J Surg* 147:605, 1984.

Jepsen OB, Korner B, et al: *Yersinia enterocolitica* infection in patients with acute surgical abdominal disease. *Scand J Infect Dis* 8:189, 1976.

Jordan JS, Kovalcik PJ, Schwab CW: Appendicitis with a palpable mass. *Ann Surg* 193:227, 1981.

Knight PJ, Vassy LE: Specific diseases mimicking appendicitis in childhood. *Arch Surg* 116:744, 1981.

Koepsell TD, Inui TS, Farewell VT: Factors affecting perforation in acute appendicitis. *Surg Gynecol Obstet* 153:508, 1981.

Lau WY, Fan ST, et al: Acute appendicitis in the elderly. *Surg Gynecol Obstet* 161:157, 1985.

Law D, Law R, Eiseman B: The continuing challenge of acute and perforated appendicitis. *Am J Surg* 131:533, 1976.

Lewis FR, Holcroft JW, et al: Appendicitis. A critical review of diagnosis and treatment in 1000 cases. *Arch Surg* 110:677, 1975.

McBurney C: Experience with early operative interference in cases of disease of the vermiform appendix. *NY State Med J* 50:676, 1889.

McBurney C: The incision made in the abdominal wall in cases of appendicitis. *Ann Surg* 20:38, 1894.

McDonald JC: Nonspecific mesenteric lymphadenitis: Collective review. *Surg Gynecol Obstet* 116:409, 1963.

Masters K, Levine BA, et al: Diagnosing appendicitis during pregnancy. *Am J Surg* 148:768, 1984.

Miranda R, Johnston AD, O'Leary JP: Incidental appendectomy: Frequency of pathologic abnormalities. *Am Surg* 46:355, 1980.

Morrison JD: Yersinia and viruses in acute non-specific abdominal pain and appendicitis. *Br J Surg* 68:284, 1981.

Moss JP: Historical and current perspectives on surgical drainage—collective review. *Surg Gynecol Obstet* 152:517, 1981.

Noer T: Decreasing incidence of acute appendicitis. *Acta Chir Scand* 141:431, 1975.

Pinto DJ, Sanderson PJ: Rational use of antibiotic therapy after appendicectomy. *Br Med J* 280:275, 1980.

Savrin RA, Clausen K, et al: Chronic and recurrent appendicitis. *Am J Surg* 137:355, 1979.

Seal A: Appendicitis: A historical review. *Canad J Surg* 24:427, 1981.

Smith DE, Kirchmer NA, Stewart DR: Use of the barium enema in the diagnosis of acute appendicitis and its complications. *Am J Surg* 138:829, 1979.

Stone HH, Hooper CA, Millikan WJ Jr: Abdominal drainage following appendectomy and cholecystectomy. *Ann Surg* 187:606, 1978.

Verrier ED, Bossart KJ, Heer FW: Reduction of infection rates in abdominal incisions by delayed wound closure techniques. *Am J Surg* 138:22, 1979.

Weingold AB: Appendicitis in pregnancy. *Clin Obstet Gynecol* 26:801, 1983.

White J, Santillana M, Haller JA Jr: Intensive inhospital observation: A safe way to decrease unnecessary appendectomy. *Am Surg* 41:793, 1975.

Williamson WA, Bush RD, Williams LF Jr: Retrocecal appendicitis. *Am J Surg* 141:507, 1981.

Tumors

Aranha GV, Reyes CV: Primary epithelial tumors of the appendix and a reappraisal of the appendiceal "mucocele." *Dis Colon Rectum* 22:472, 1979.

Chang P, Attiyeh FF: Adenocarcinoma of the appendix. *Dis Colon Rectum* 24:176, 1981.

Higa E, Rosai J, et al: Mucosal hyperplasia, mucinous cystadenoma, and mucinous cystadenocarcinoma of the appendix: A re-evaluation of appendiceal "mucocele." *Cancer* 32:1525, 1973.

Syracuse DC, Perzin KH, et al: Carcinoid tumors of the appendix: Mesoappendiceal extension and nodal metastases. *Ann Surg* 190:58, 1979.

Wilson H, Cheek RC, et al: Carcinoid tumors. *Curr Probl Surg* November 1970.

Wolff M, Ahmed N: Epithelial neoplasms of the vermiform appendix (exclusive of carcinoid): I. Adenocarcinoma of the appendix. *Cancer* 37:2493, 1976.

Wolff M, Ahmed N: Epithelial neoplasms of the vermiform appendix (exclusive of carcinoid): II. Cystadenomas, papillary adenomas, and adenomatous polyps of the appendix. *Cancer* 37:2511, 1976.

Liver

Seymour I. Schwartz

ANATOMY

The liver constitutes approximately one-fiftieth of the total body weight. Its size reflects the complexity of its functions. True division into right and left lobes is in line with the fossa for the inferior vena cava posteriorly and the gallbladder fossa anteroinferiorly (Fig. 30-1). A right segmental fissure divides the right lobe into anterior and posterior segments, while the falciform ligament divides the left lobe into medial and lateral segments. True segmental divisions can be observed only in cast specimens in which the glissonian structures, i.e., hepatic artery, portal vein, and bile ducts, have been injected. These casts have produced a "functional" anatomy that permits a description of hepatic segmentation based on the distribution of portal pedicles and the location of hepatic veins. A schematic representation is shown in Fig. 30-2. The liver is divided into two "livers" (lobes) by the portal scissura in which the middle hepatic vein courses. The right lobe is divided into two "sectors" by the right portal scissura containing the right hepatic vein. The right posterolateral "sector" contains segment VI anteriorly and segment VII posteriorly. The right anterolateral "sector" contains segment V anteriorly and segment VIII posteriorly. The left lobe is divided by the left portal scissura containing the left hepatic vein. The left anterior sector is divided by the umbilical fissure into segment IV, the anterior part of which is the quadrate lobe, and segment III, which is the anterior part of the left lobe. The posterior sector is segment II. The dorsal segment I, in regard to its vascularization, is independent of the portal division and the three main hepatic veins (Fig. 30-3).

BILIARY DRAINAGE. Each sector is drained by a major segmental duct formed by the confluence of subsegmental draining structures. The anterior and posterior sectoral ducts in the right lobe join to form the right hepatic duct, while the medial and lateral segmental ducts in the left lobe terminate in the left hepatic duct, which joins the right duct to form a common hepatic duct in the porta hepatis. This lies anteriorly in relation to other structures in the area.

BLOOD SUPPLY. The afferent blood supply to the liver arises from two sources: (1) the hepatic artery, which carries oxygenated blood and accounts for approximately 25 percent of hepatic blood flow and (2) the portal vein, which accounts for approximately 75 percent of hepatic

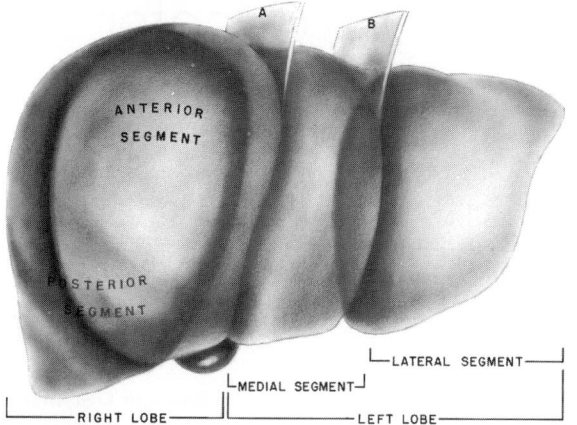

Fig. 30-1. Lobar and segmental divisions of the liver. *A*. Lobar fissure. *B*. Left segmental fissure. A right segmental fissure divides the right lobe into its anterior and posterior segments. (From: *Schwartz SI: Surgical Diseases of the Liver. New York, McGraw-Hill, 1964, with permission.*)

blood flow and drains the splanchnic circulation. The common hepatic artery originates from the celiac axis and, after contributing the gastroduodenal and right gastric artery, ascends in the hepatoduodenal ligament to the left of the common bile duct and anterior to the portal vein. It bifurcates into a right and left branch to the left of the main lobar fissure. The major right hepatic artery originates from the superior mesenteric artery in 17 percent of people. Intrahepatic anastomoses between the right and left hepatic arteries do not occur. The cystic artery is usually an extrahepatic branch of the right hepatic artery.

The portal venous system contains no valves (Fig. 30-4). It returns to the liver the blood that the celiac, superior mesenteric, and inferior mesenteric arteries supply to the gastrointestinal tract, pancreas, and spleen. The vessel is

formed behind the pancreas, at the level of L_1 to L_2, by the confluence of the superior mesenteric and splenic veins and, at times, the inferior mesenteric vein. The portal vein resides posteriorly in relation to the hepatic artery and bile duct in the hepatoduodenal ligament but, in rare instances, is located anterior to the pancreas and first portion of the duodenum, in which circumstance it is frequently associated with a partial or complete situs inversus and is subject to injury during cholecystectomy or gastrectomy. In the porta hepatis the vein divides into two branches, which course to each lobe. The average length of the main portal vein is 6.5 cm, and the average diameter is 0.8 cm. Much has been written concerning the streaming phenomenon within the portal vein accounting for preferential metastases to the right and left lobe depending on the venous drainage of the primary site. Experimental and clinical findings have refuted this concept.

The hepatic venous system (Fig. 30-5) begins as a central vein of the liver lobule and represents the only vessel in human beings into which the sinusoids empty. The central veins unite to form sublobular veins, which in turn fuse to form collecting veins. The collecting veins gradually increase in size by joining other large intrahepatic collecting channels, which coalesce to form the three major hepatic veins. The hepatic venous tributaries occupy the fissures and are intersectoral in position. The major hepatic veins are classified as right, left, and middle. The right hepatic vein drains the entire posterior portion as well as the superior area of the anterior portion of the right lobe. The left hepatic vein drains the entire lateral area to the left of the umbilical fissure. The inferior areas of the medial and anterior portions of the two lobes are drained by the middle vein. In human beings there are no valves in the hepatic venous system. Total hepatic blood flow can be measured by means of hepatic vein catheterization and the use of the Fick principle. The average value is 1500 mL/min per 1.73 m² of body surface.

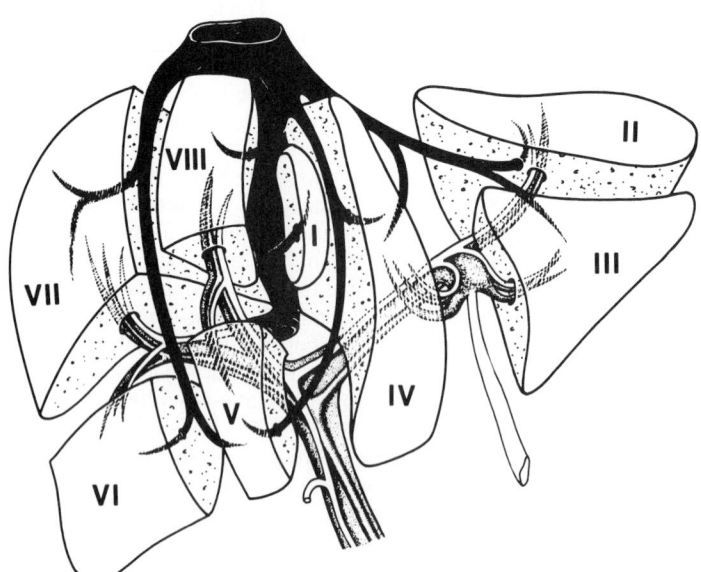

Fig. 30-2. The functional division of the liver and the segments according to Couinaud's nomenclature. (From: *Bismuth H: Surgical anatomy and anatomical surgery of the liver. World J Surg 6:6, 1982, with permission.*)

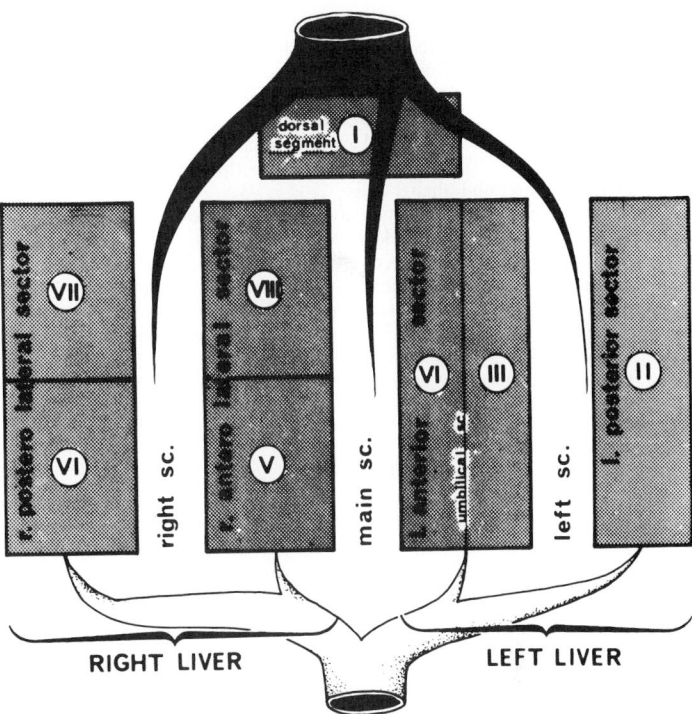

Fig. 30-3. Schematic representation of the functional anatomy of the liver; three main hepatic veins divide the liver into four sectors, each of them receiving a portal pedicle; hepatic veins and portal pedicles are intertwined as the fingers of the two hands. (From: *Bismuth H: Surgical anatomy and anatomical surgery of the liver. World J Surg 6:4, 1982, with permission.*)

Fig. 30-4. Anatomy of the extrahepatic portal venous system, anterior aspect. The termination of each vein is shown as it was encountered most frequently in 92 dissections. The pancreas is represented by the shaded area. *A.P.,* accessory pancreatic vein; *C.,* coronary vein; *Cystic,* cystic vein; *I.,* intestinal veins; *I.C.,* ileocolic vein; *I.M.,* inferior mesenteric vein; *I.P.D.,* inferior pancreaticoduodenal vein; *L.,* liver; *L.B.P.,* left branch of portal vein; *L.C.,* left colic vein; *L.G.E.,* left gastroepiploic vein; *M.C.,* middle colic vein; *O.,* omental vein; *P.,* pancreatic veins; *Pyloric,* pyloric vein; *R.C.,* right colic vein; *R.G.E.,* right gastroepiploic vein; *R.B.P.,* right branch of portal vein; *S.,* splenic vein; *S.G.,* short gastric veins; *S.H.,* superior hemorrhoidal vein; *S.M.,* superior mesenteric vein; *S.P.D.,* superior pancreaticoduodenal vein; *S.T.,* splenic trunks. (From: *Douglass et al: Surg Gynecol Obstet 91:562, 1950, with permission.*)

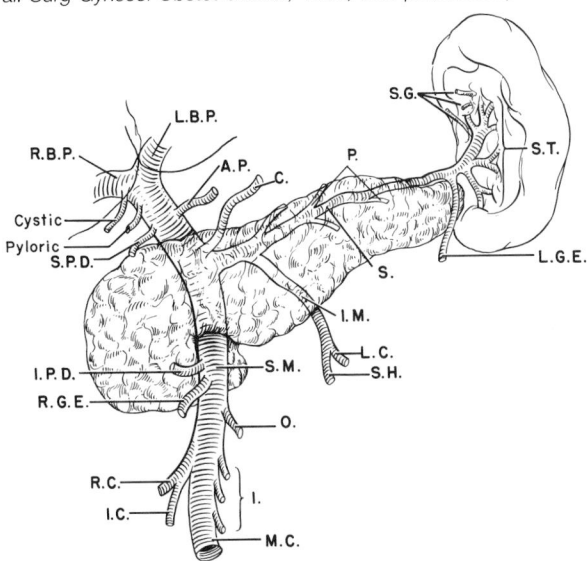

LIVER FUNCTION

The liver consists of four physiologic-anatomic units that are interrelated:

1. The circulatory system. A dual blood supply nourishes the liver and acts as a vehicle for material absorbed from the intestinal tract to be utilized in the metabolic pool. Blood vessels are accompanied by lymphatics and nerve fibers that contribute to the regulation of blood flow and intrasinusoidal pressure.

Fig. 30-5. Prevailing pattern of drainage of hepatic veins in the human liver. (From: *Schwartz SI: Surgical Diseases of the Liver. New York, McGraw-Hill, 1964, with permission.*)

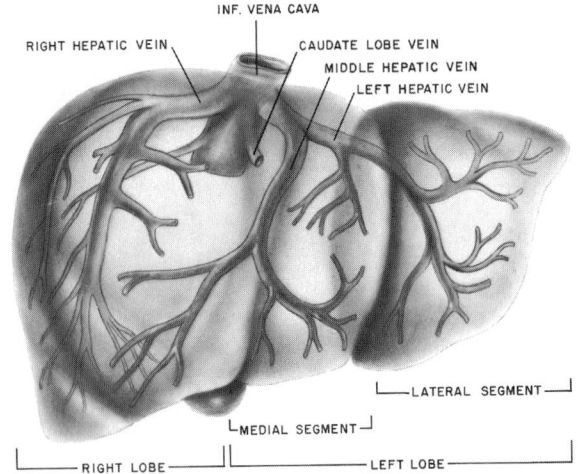

2. Biliary passages. These serve as channels of exit for materials secreted by the liver cells, including bilirubin, cholesterol, and detoxified drugs. This system originates with the Golgi apparatus adjacent to the microvilli of the bile canaliculi and eventually terminates in the common bile duct.
3. The reticuloendothelial system. This system has 60 percent of its cellular elements in the liver and includes the phagocytic Kupffer cells and endothelial cells.
4. The functioning liver cells, which are capable of a wide variation of activity. The metabolic pool in the liver serves the needs of the entire body. The cell performs both anabolic and catabolic activities, secretes, and stores. The large amount of energies required for these transformations result from the conversion of adenosine triphosphate (ATP) to adenosine diphosphate (ADP). A second source is the aerobic oxygenation in the metabolic pool via the tricarboxylic acid cycle of Krebs.

Function Tests (Table 30-1)

The so-called liver "function" tests evaluate liver activity by assessing the degree of functional impairment. They do not provide a pathologic diagnosis, and the extreme functional reserve of the organ occasionally produces normal results in the face of significant lesions. Many of these tests do not measure a specific function of the liver, and other organ systems may be implicated. False positives for each of the tests are found in about 2.5 percent of normal controls and in about 10 percent of hospital controls. False-negative tests also occur in about 10 percent of most tests.

PROTEINS. Hepatic cells are responsible for the synthesis of albumin, fibrinogen, prothrombin, and other factors involved in blood clotting. A reduction of serum albumin is one of the most accurate reflections of the extent of liver disease and the effects of medical therapy. Because the half-life of albumin is 8 to 10 days, impairment of hepatic synthesis must be present for over 2 weeks before abnormalities are noted. The correlation between total protein and disease of the liver is not as close as that between the serum albumin level and liver disease, since albumin is produced only by hepatic cells and a reduction is frequently compensated for by an increase in the level of globulin.

CARBOHYDRATES AND LIPIDS. Glycogenesis, glycogen storage, glycogenolysis, and the conversion of galactose into glucose all represent hepatic functions. Hypoglycemia is a rare accompaniment of extensive hepatic disease, but the amelioration of diabetes in patients with hemochromatosis is considered an indication of neoplastic change. The more common effect of hepatic disease is a deficiency of glycogenesis with resultant hyperglycemia. A hepatic enzyme system is responsible for the conversion of galactose into glucose, and abnormal galactose tolerance tests are seen in hepatitis and active cirrhosis. In rare instances, a familial deficiency in this enzyme system accounts for spontaneous galactosemia accompanied by an obstructive type of jaundice that appears after the first week of life and subsides when lactose is removed from the diet.

Synthesis of both phospholipid and cholesterol takes place in the liver, and the latter serves as a standard for the determination of lipid metabolism. The liver is the major organ involved in the synthesis, esterification, and excretion of cholesterol. In the presence of parenchymal damage, both the total cholesterol and percentage of esterified fraction decrease. Biliary obstruction results in a rise in cholesterol, and the most pronounced elevations are noted with primary biliary cirrhosis and the cholangiolitis accompanying toxic reactions to phenothiazine derivatives.

ENZYMES. The three enzymes that achieve abnormal serum levels in hepatic disease that have been widely studied are alkaline phosphatase, serum glutamic oxalacetic transaminase (SGOT), and serum glutamic pyruvic transaminase (SGPT). The SGOT is present in the liver, myocardium, skeletal muscles, kidney, and pancreas. Cellular damage in any of the above-mentioned tissues results in elevation of the serum level. In reference to the liver, the most marked increases accompany acute cellular damage regardless of cause, and extremely high levels are noted in patients with hepatitis. The SGOT is only moderately increased in cirrhosis and biliary obstruction. The SGPT is more particularly applicable to the evaluation of liver disease, since the hepatic content greatly exceeds myocardial concentration. Elevations accompany acute hepatocellular damage. Lactic acid dehydrogenase (LDH) levels also may be elevated.

A variety of methods of assaying the serum alkaline phosphatase are currently in use, and in all notations of results normal values should be parenthetically indicated. Serum alkaline phosphatase provides an evaluation of the patency of the bile channels at all levels, intrahepatic and extrahepatic. Elevation is demonstrated in 94 percent of patients with obstruction of the extrahepatic biliary tract due to neoplasm and 76 percent of those in whom the

Table 30-1. NORMAL VALUES FOR HEPATIC "FUNCTION" TESTS

Test	Normal value
Serum albumin	3.5–4.6 g/dL
Total protein	6.0–7.4 g/dL
Cholesterol	135–300 mg/dL
Alkaline phosphatase	24–100 I.U./dL
Serum glutamic oxalacetic transaminase (AST)	10–36 units/dL
Serum glutamic pyruvic transaminase (ALT)	10–48 units/dL
Gamma glutamyl transferase (GGT)	0–48 units/dL males
	4–26 units/dL females
Lactic acid dehydrogenase (LD)	180–225 units/dL
Prothrombin time	90–100% of laboratory control
Fibrinogen	200–400 mg/dL
Blood "ammonia"	10–63 μg/dL
Serum bilirubin:	
Total	Less than 1.4 mg/dL
Direct	Less than 0.3 mg/dL
Indirect	Less than 1.1 mg/dL
Urinary bilirubin	0

obstruction is caused by calculi. Intrahepatic biliary obstruction and cholestasis also cause a rise in the enzyme level. In the presence of space-occupying lesions such as metastases, primary hepatic carcinoma, and abscesses, the alkaline phosphatase is also increased. The overall correlation between metastatic carcinoma of the liver and an elevated enzyme level is as high as 92 percent. Sixty percent of patients with primary hepatic carcinoma also demonstrate a significant increase. Granulomatous and infiltrative lesions such as sarcoidosis, tuberculosis, and lymphoma are irregularly associated with mild to moderate increases in the alkaline phosphatase. Elevation of the serum level of this enzyme is also associated with diseases that have as a common denominator increased osteoblastic activity.

5'-Nucleotidase is a phosphatase that catalyzes hydrolysis of nucleotides. Levels are elevated in hepatobiliary disease, and the relative sensitivity and selectivity compared with alkaline phosphatase has not been defined.

DYE EXCRETION. The hepatic removal of dyes from the circulation is dependent upon hepatic blood flow, hepatocellular function, and biliary excretion. Sulfobromophthalein (Bromsulphalein, or BSP) provides an assessment of hepatic function, although 20 percent is removed by an extrahepatic means. The presence of jaundice produces a disproportionate BSP retention, and fever, shock, hemorrhage, and recent surgical treatment may all result in increased levels. An increased retention is associated with acute cellular damage and is also noted in patients with cirrhosis, carcinoma, and chronic passive congestion. Since the rate of disappearance from the blood is constant, hepatic blood flow can be determined by injecting the dye at a rate that will maintain a constant blood level and applying Fick's principle to the blood removed from a catheterized hepatic vein. An intestinal xenon technique has been shown to provide an accurate method of measuring portal vein and total hepatic blood flow.

Indocyanine green now is used more frequently to determine hepatic blood flow. Rose bengal is another phthalein dye that, when labeled with radioactive iodine, has been useful in the evaluation of liver disease. Since all this material is removed by the hepatic parenchymal cell, it provides a more accurate estimate of hepatic blood flow. Determination of the fecal excretion of the radioactive material has been applied to the differential diagnosis of obstructive jaundice, particularly in the establishment of the diagnosis of congenital atresia of the bile ducts.

COAGULATION FACTORS. In liver disease, multiple coagulation defects may occur. Two mechanisms contribute to the deficiency of coagulation factors: (1) in obstructive jaundice, the bile source required for the absorption of the fat-soluble vitamin K results in a decreased synthesis of prothrombin, and (2) hepatocellular dysfunction is accompanied by an inability of the liver to synthesize the prothrombin. Abnormal values for prothrombin time have been noted in a variety of hepatic diseases with parenchymal damage, and determination is particularly applicable in the evaluation of patients undergoing liver biopsy or surgical procedures. An increase in prothrombin time subsequent to the injection of parenteral vitamin K is used as an indication of hepatic function and suggests obstructive jaundice. Decreases in factors V, VII, IX, and fibrinogen have also been noted in hepatic disease. Cirrhosis has also been associated with an increased fibrinolysis due to defective synthesis of fibrinolytic inhibitors and delayed removal of plasminogen activators.

QUANTITATIVE TESTS. Maximal rate of urea synthesis after an oral challenge with casein or an intravenous bolus of amino acids provides an assessment of hepatic function as does the determination of galactose elimination capacity.

BILE PIGMENT METABOLISM. See the section on Jaundice in Chap. 24.

SPECIAL STUDIES

NEEDLE BIOPSY OF THE LIVER. This is the one study that provides a pathologic diagnosis. It is dependent on an area of tissue measuring 1 to 4 cm in length and containing approximately 5 to 20 lobules representing a general anatomic change. Close to 100 percent accuracy has been demonstrated for both posthepatitic and postnecrotic cirrhosis. Intrahepatic cholestasis, hepatitis, and cellular degeneration resulting from toxicity are all diffuse lesions and readily diagnosed. Focal lesions, such as neoplasm, granulomas, and abscess may be missed, but the correlation between needle biopsy and operative and autopsy findings is high. A mortality rate of 0.08 percent has been determined, and pain, pneumothorax, hemorrhage, and bile peritonitis are the complications to be considered.

ULTRASONOGRAPHY, COMPUTER TOMOGRAPHY, AND MAGNETIC RESONANCE IMAGING. These tests define solid and cystic parenchymal lesions and can distinguish one from the other. A diagnosis of hydatid cysts can be made based on either of these studies alone; a hepatic abscess can be localized and drained transhepatically. The distribution of primary and metastatic solid tumors can be ascertained. Hemangiomas may be specifically diagnosed. These studies also can be used to assess the patency of a portacaval shunt. Intraoperative ultrasonography provides a sensitive method of demonstrating parenchymal lesions and the intrahepatic vasculature, thereby contributing to patient evaluation and selection of an appropriate procedure.

SCINTILLATION SCANNING. This technique has been used as a method of evaluating liver size, shape, and position, and also to determine the presence and location of intrahepatic neoplasms or focal lesions. Technetium-sulfur colloid (^{99m}Tc), which is deposited in the reticuloendothelial system, is generally used. For lesions over 1.5 cm, the correlation with autopsy and operative findings is excellent and is over 83 percent for metastatic lesions.

A prospective analysis of laboratory tests and imaging studies has shown greater than 65 percent accuracy in the detection of hepatic lesions. No combination of laboratory tests increased this accuracy. If the laboratory tests were used with one of the imaging studies, the accuracy was increased to 76 percent. The use of all the liver imaging tests and laboratory tests lowers the accuracy and needlessly increases the expense.

ANGIOGRAPHY. Since hepatic tumors, both primary and metastatic, are dependent on an arterial circulation, unusual vascular patterns are also detected by injection of the hepatic artery with the radiopaque material. Unusual arrangements of the arteries and "tumor staining," analogous to that found in cerebral and osseous neoplasms, may be noted. Angiography also demonstrates extrahepatic vascular anatomy and provides a "road map" for the surgeon.

MEASUREMENTS OF PORTAL PRESSURE, AND EVALUATION OF PORTAL CIRCULATION. See Portal Hypertension, later in this chapter.

TRAUMA

INCIDENCE. The liver ranks high on the list of intraabdominal organs involved by injury (Table 30-2). It is only surpassed by the spleen as the most commonly injured intraperitoneal organ. The rapid increase in motor traffic has resulted in an increasing incidence and in a change of pattern from one with a predominance of penetrating wounds to the present higher incidence of blunt traumatic injuries. There is a higher frequency of hepatic trauma in children.

Rupture of the liver also occurs spontaneously in pathologic organs. It occurs in approximately 8 percent of patients with primary carcinoma and has been reported with increasing frequency for benign hepatic adenoma and in association with toxemia of pregnancy. Rupture of the liver in the newborn infant is related to the trauma of birth and is more common in infants who are larger than average and classified as "postmature."

PATHOLOGY. Liver injuries are classified as *transcapsular, subcapsular, or central* (Fig. 30-6). When rupture of the liver extends through Glisson's capsule, extravasated blood and bile are found in the peritoneal cavity. If the capsule remains intact, the collection of blood between the capsule and parenchyma is usually found on the superior surface of the organ. Central rupture consists in interruption of the parenchyma of the liver. Blunt trauma may be associated with hepatic parenchymal emboli to the right heart and lungs, causing death.

Persons with injury about the hilus rarely survive long enough for surgical exploration. Nonpenetrating injuries result in a tear in the anteroposterior portion. The dome of the liver is frequently involved, particularly in older patients. With penetrating lesions of the lower thorax, the dome is also most frequently involved, and the ratio of right lobe to left lobe involvement is 7:1.

CLINICAL MANIFESTATIONS. These are determined by the pathologic types. With rupture of Glisson's capsule, signs and symptoms are related to shock and peritoneal irritation. Shock is present in over three-quarters of the cases, and abdominal pain, spasm, and rigidity are usual accompaniments.

DIAGNOSTIC STUDIES. Shortly after trauma, an increased leukocyte count is more consistent than a reduced hemoglobin. Infrequently mild elevation of the serum bilirubin level occurs on the third or fourth day. X-ray may reveal evidence of fluid in the peritoneum and pelvis or a wide right flank stripe indicating blood accumulated between the ascending colon and the peritoneal line. CT is the most useful study to define the extent of trauma (Fig. 30-7). Ultrasonography may indicate the presence of intraperitoneal fluid. Paracentesis is useful in verifying the presence of hemoperitoneum, but a negative tap does not exclude the diagnosis. Celiac angiography also may identify hepatic rupture.

TREATMENT. Shock is corrected and associated thoracic lesions are treated first. Surgical procedures are directed at the control of bleeding, the removal of necrotic devitalized tissue, and the establishment of external drainage. These should be initiated early, because time has proved to be a definite factor in morbidity and mortality statistics. With penetrating wounds of the liver, particularly knife wounds, the bleeding has usually stopped at the time of exploration and simple drainage is all that is required. Such is usually not the case with blunt trauma and shotgun wounds. Subcapsular hematomas diagnosed by technetium scan may be managed nonoperatively. Also, a few patients with transcapsular trauma and intraperitoneal bleeding defined by CT will not require exploration if vital signs remain stable and transfusion requirements are limited.

Hemorrhages are controlled preferably by occluding the vascular inflow (Pringle maneuver) and with the finger fracture technique exposing individual bleeders within the parenchyma of the liver and ligating these vessels. The technique of placing a row of interlocking through-and-through mattress sutures parallel to the surfaces of the laceration should be avoided, since this adds to the amount of tissue necrosis. In general, hepatic resection is not carried out along precise anatomic lines unless the injury demands it. Most resections are best regarded as sublobar debridements, with as much tissue preserved as possible. All the devitalized tissue and markedly traumatized tissue is removed to avoid subsequent autolysis, abscess formation, and secondary hemorrhage.

Table 30-2. RELATIVE FREQUENCY OF VISCERAL INJURY FROM BLUNT TRAUMA

Viscera involved	Series					
	I	*II*	*III*	*IV*	*V*	*VI*
Spleen	56	20	53	37	20	38
Intestine	14	3	27	13	4	19
Liver	6	9	45	5	14	19
Kidneys	8	25	Not incl.	26	27	91
Bladder	11	9	Not incl.	4		8
Others, including pancreas, the diaphragm, and mesentery	46	8	8	39	7	25
Total	141	74	183	124	72	200

SOURCE: From McCort: *Radiology* 78:49, 1962.

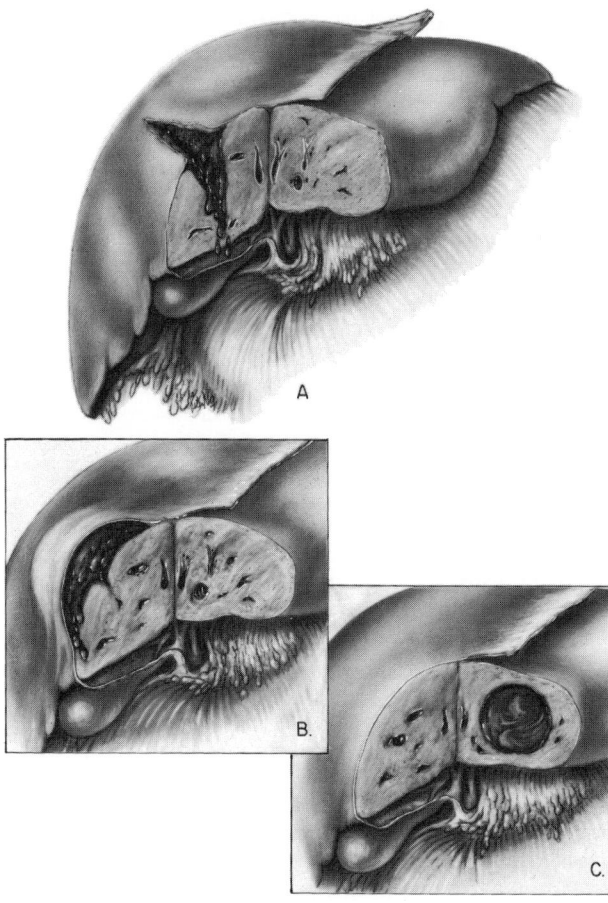

Fig. 30-6. Diagram of three types of liver rupture. *A.* Transcapsular.
B. Subcapsular. *C.* Central. (From: *Schwartz SI: Surgical Diseases
of the Liver. New York, McGraw-Hill, 1964, with permission.*)

Fig. 30-7. CT demonstrating traumatic rupture of the right lobe of
the liver. Patient treated nonoperatively.

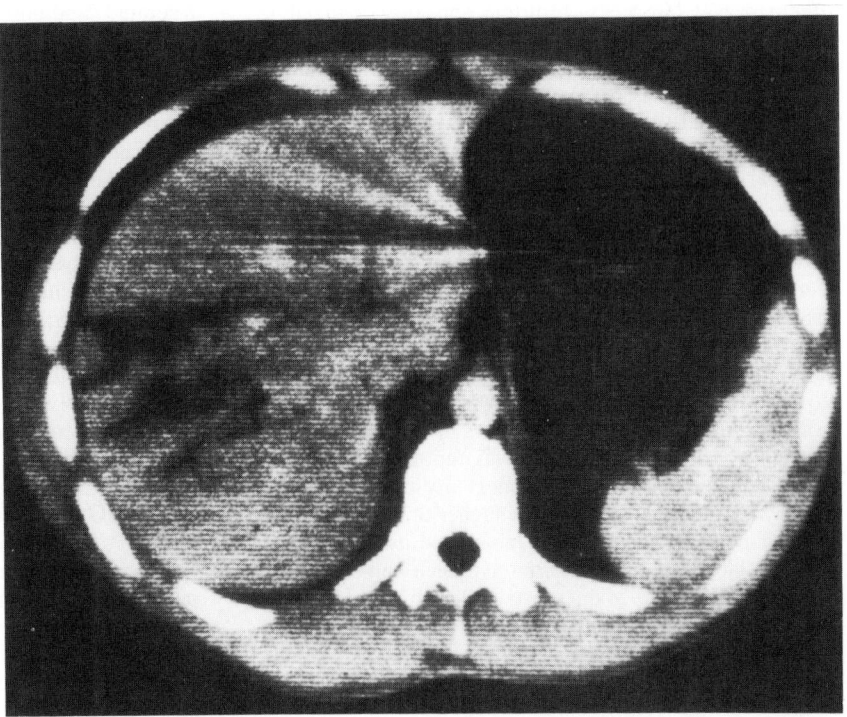

Continued bleeding following attempts at control may be tamponaded with packs. Removal of these usually is not associated with recurrent bleeding. A "second look" operation allows further debridement of nonviable tissue and the insertion of new drains. Hepatic arterial bleeding may be controlled by selective hepatic arterial ligation. This maneuver should not be applied prophylactically to all patients with hepatic trauma; it will not prevent postoperative bleeding or hematobilia, and it is not physiologically innocuous. The most vigorous bleeding associated with hepatic trauma is usually caused by involvement of the hepatic veins. This cannot be controlled by hepatic arterial ligation.

External drainage should be carried out in almost all cases and is directed at the prevention of abscess and bile peritonitis. Routine T-tube drainage of the common duct offers no advantage and has been associated with an increased complication rate.

COMPLICATIONS. The incidence of complications is well over 50 percent and is related to the extent of injury to other organs. Hemorrhage is the most important cause of death, and recurrent bleeding may occur secondarily to necrosis and sequestration of infected tissue.

Hematobilia

The pathologic *sine qua non* for this condition is free communication between a blood vessel and the biliary tree. It is a consequence of central or subcapsular hematomas and also capsular wounds that have been primarily closed or packed. The world literature records only about 75 cases related to trauma. The triad of abdominal injury, subsequent gastrointestinal hemorrhage, and colicky pain should raise a high index of suspicion. This may occur within a few days after injury or, more characteristically, after a period of weeks. Multiple episodes of bleeding with some suggestion of periodicity occur. Melena is more frequent than hematemesis, and jaundice of mild to severe proportion is present in some cases. Diagnosis is established and the lesion located by angiographic techniques; embolization has been effective. Operations have been varied and have included resection of the lesion, which is preferable, debridement and unroofing, or ligation of the contributing hepatic artery.

PROGNOSIS. The improvement in mortality statistics accompanying hepatic injuries is evident from war experience. During World War II with the institution of routine drainage and the elimination of gauze packs, the mortality rate dropped from 30 to 17 percent. During the Korean war, penetrating injuries were associated with a mortality rate of 14 percent, whereas in the Vietnam war a mortality rate of 4.2 percent was reported for United States military personnel. The mortality rate associated with blunt trauma is consistently higher than that accompanying penetrating injuries. Defore and associates' report of a large civilian series noted a declining mortality. Between 1971 and 1974 the mortality for stab wounds was about 1 percent, gunshot wounds 6 percent, and blunt trauma 30 percent, although only 2.5 percent of patients underwent laboratory or segmental debridement. The mortality rate was 59 percent in this group. In all situations mortality rates were proportional to the number of organs injured.

MAJOR VASCULAR INJURIES. The effects of ligation of the major vessels are diagramed in Fig. 30-8. When the common or proper hepatic artery is ligated, collateral supply is apparent radiographically within 4 h, and it is unusual for major dysfunction caused by hepatic ischemia to occur. However, primary repair of a surgically traumatized artery and restoration of flow are indicated.

Hepatic vein injuries represent a significant factor in the high mortality accompanying blunt liver trauma. Fifteen percent of patients with blunt hepatic trauma have sustained injury to the hepatic veins, and most of these patients die from uncontrollable hemorrhage either in the operating room or prior to operation. Because the hepatic veins are multiple, often forming connecting channels, the safe approach is to expose all the veins and the entire retrohepatic inferior vena cava. Control of the bleeding vein or veins may be accomplished by occluding the porta hepatis and inserting a catheter via either the inferior vena cava or the right atrium in such a fashion that umbilical tapes may be placed above and below the area of the hepatic veins. Temporary total inflow and outflow occlusion, with occlusion of the aorta above the celiac artery, the vessels in the hepatoduodenal ligament, and the supra- and infrahepatic vena cava, is more expeditious.

Portal vein injury is rare, and can be managed by end-to-end anastomosis, lateral venorrhaphy, graft interposition, superior mesenteric vein to splenic vein anastomosis, ligation of the portal vein with portal systemic shunt, and ligation of the portal vein alone. Lateral venorrhaphy with primary repair of the portal vein is the procedure of choice when this is feasible. Portal vein ligation can be tolerated, and portal systemic diversion of the initial surgical procedure may be more hazardous than acute ligation alone and carries its own inherent complication. Graft interposition is usually doomed to thrombosis.

Stone and associates reported 83 patients with wounds of the portal and/or superior mesenteric veins who underwent emergency laparotomy. Over 90 percent of the wounds were caused by penetrating trauma. Lateral phleborrhaphy resulted in survival in two-thirds of the patients so treated. End-to-end reanastomosis of the portal vein was successful in only one of three patients, while the single portacaval shunt resulted in metabolic death. In the more recently treated patients, immediate ligation of the portal vein was successful in 17 of 20 patients. There was no survival if both superior mesenteric and portal vein had been injured.

HEPATIC ABSCESSES

Hepatic abscesses are related to two distinct groups of pathogens, pyogenic bacteria and *Entameba histolytica*. Distinctive features in the clinical manifestations and therapy of these two variations necessitate separate consideration.

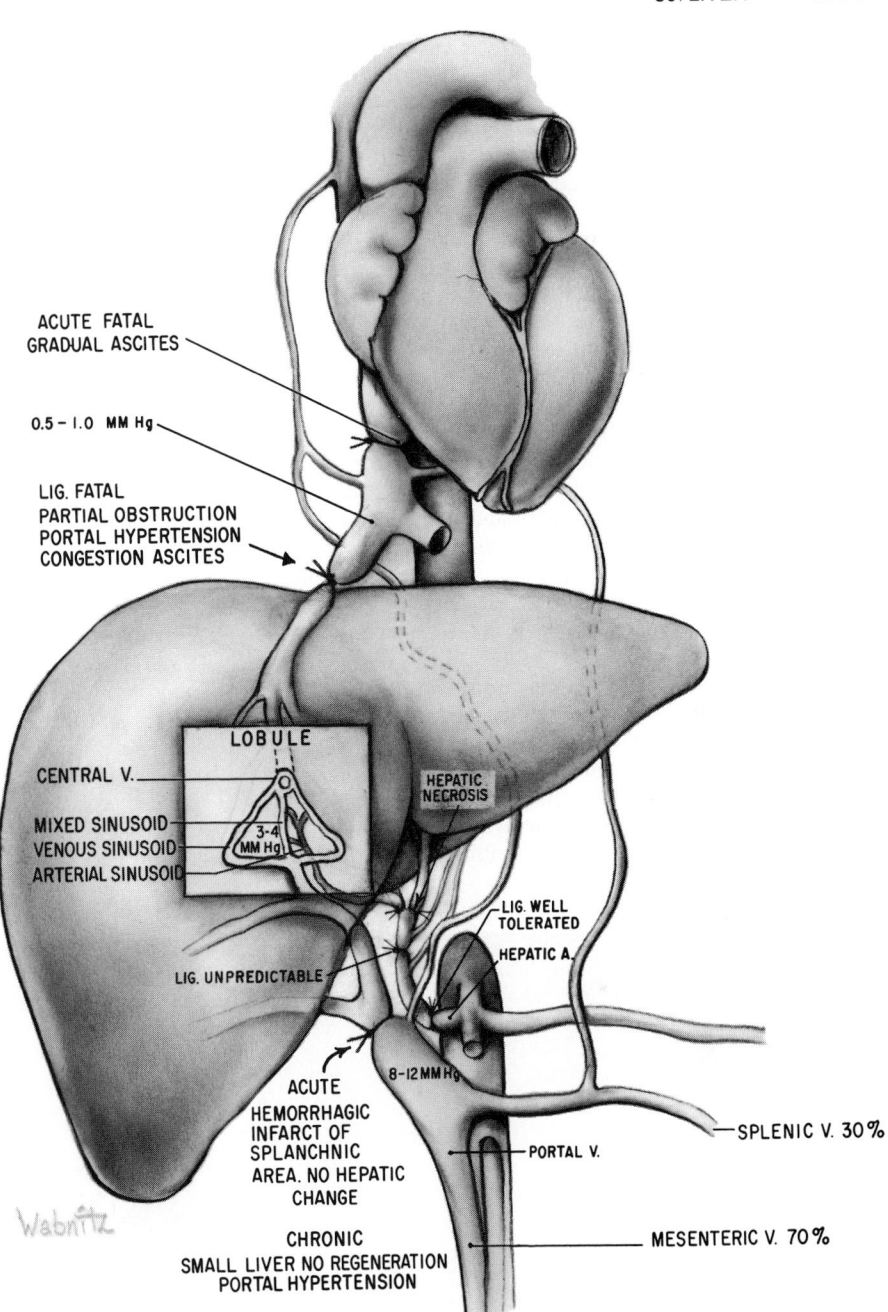

ACUTE FATAL
GRADUAL ASCITES

0.5 - 1.0 MM Hg

LIG. FATAL
PARTIAL OBSTRUCTION
PORTAL HYPERTENSION
CONGESTION ASCITES

LOBULE

CENTRAL V.

MIXED SINUSOID
VENOUS SINUSOID
ARTERIAL SINUSOID

3-4 MM Hg

HEPATIC NECROSIS

LIG. WELL TOLERATED

HEPATIC A.

LIG. UNPREDICTABLE

8-12 MM Hg

SPLENIC V. 30%

PORTAL V.

MESENTERIC V. 70%

ACUTE
HEMORRHAGIC
INFARCT OF
SPLANCHNIC
AREA. NO HEPATIC
CHANGE

CHRONIC
SMALL LIVER NO REGENERATION
PORTAL HYPERTENSION

Wabnitz

Fig. 30-8. Pressures and effects of ligations in the blood vessels of the liver. (From: *Popper H, Schaffner F: Liver: Structure and Function. New York, McGraw-Hill, 1957, with permission.*)

Pyogenic Abscesses

INCIDENCE. The lesion is present in 0.36 percent of autopsies. Prior to the widespread use of antibiotic therapy, this incidence was 0.44 percent as contrasted with 0.28 percent in autopsies since 1945. The highest percentage of cases occur in the sixth and seventh decade, and there is no predilection for either sex.

ETIOLOGY. Pyogenic abscesses of the liver result from (1) ascending biliary infection, (2) hematogenous spread via the portal venous system, (3) generalized septicemia with involvement of the liver by way of the hepatic arterial circulation, (4) direct extension from intraperitoneal infection, (5) other causes, including hepatic trauma. Recently, the most frequent antecedent cause has been cholangitis secondary to calculi or carcinoma in the extrahepatic biliary duct system. The second most common cause is related to generalized septicemia, while the portal venous route of infection has decreased in importance.

Pylephlebitis occurs in 0.05 percent of cases of acute appendicitis and 3 percent of patients with perforated appendicitis. No segment of the intestine drained by the portal venous system can be excluded as a possible cause, and the incidence associated with acute diverticulitis is as high as that of appendicitis. There has been an increase in the percentage in which no cause is apparent. These account for about 20 percent of the cases.

Positive cultures are obtained from pyogenic abscesses in only 50 percent of cases. *Escherichia coli,* which accounts for about one-third of positive cultures, has been the dominant microorganism in abscesses secondary to biliary tract infection and infection along the portal venous route. By contrast, the cocci, particularly *Staphylococcus aureus* and hemolytic streptococcus, are usually isolated from abscesses related to systemic infection. *Proteus* and *Klebsiella* were each indicted in about 10 percent of abscesses. *Bacteroides* and other anaerobes have become increasingly prevalent as a cause.

Pyogenic abscesses may be solitary, multiple, and multilocular. Single and multiple abscesses occur with equal frequency. When a single abscess is present, it is usually located in the right lobe.

CLINICAL MANIFESTATIONS. Since most pyogenic hepatic abscesses are secondary to other significant infections, it is difficult to delineate a pathognomonic symptom. Fever is the most common symptom, and a "picket fence" configuration of the temperature chart generally has been noted. Fever is frequently accompanied by chills, profuse sweating, nausea, vomiting, and anorexia.

Pain is a late symptom and is more common with large solitary abscesses. Liver enlargement was noted in 30 to 60 percent of cases. Hepatic tenderness was absent in one-half of the patients. Jaundice is a relatively uncommon finding.

DIAGNOSTIC STUDIES. Leukocytosis with white blood cell counts ranging between 18,000 and 20,000 is usual. Half of the patients are anemic. Positive blood cultures are demonstrated in approximately 30 percent of patients, the most significant yields accompanying abscesses secondary to systemic septicemia. Liver function tests are not diagnostic but elevation of the alkaline phosphatase level is the most frequent abnormality. Hypoalbuminemia is common. Characteristically, x-rays reveal an elevation and immobility or restriction of motion of the right leaf of the diaphragm. There is also obliteration of the right cardiophrenic angle on the posteroanterior chest film and the anterior costophrenic angle on the lateral film. Abscesses produced by gas-forming microorganisms are associated with air-fluid levels in the liver. Ultrasonography, ^{99m}Tc-sulfur colloid scan, or computed tomography (CT) may suggest the diagnosis (Figs. 30-9 and 30-10).

TREATMENT. This is based on appropriate antibiotic therapy combined with drainage in selected cases. The abscesses may be drained percutaneously under ultrasonographic or CT control. Several series have reported success rates of 80 percent using this technique. The route of surgical access depends on the position of the abscess and may be transthoracic or transabdominal (Figs. 30-11 and

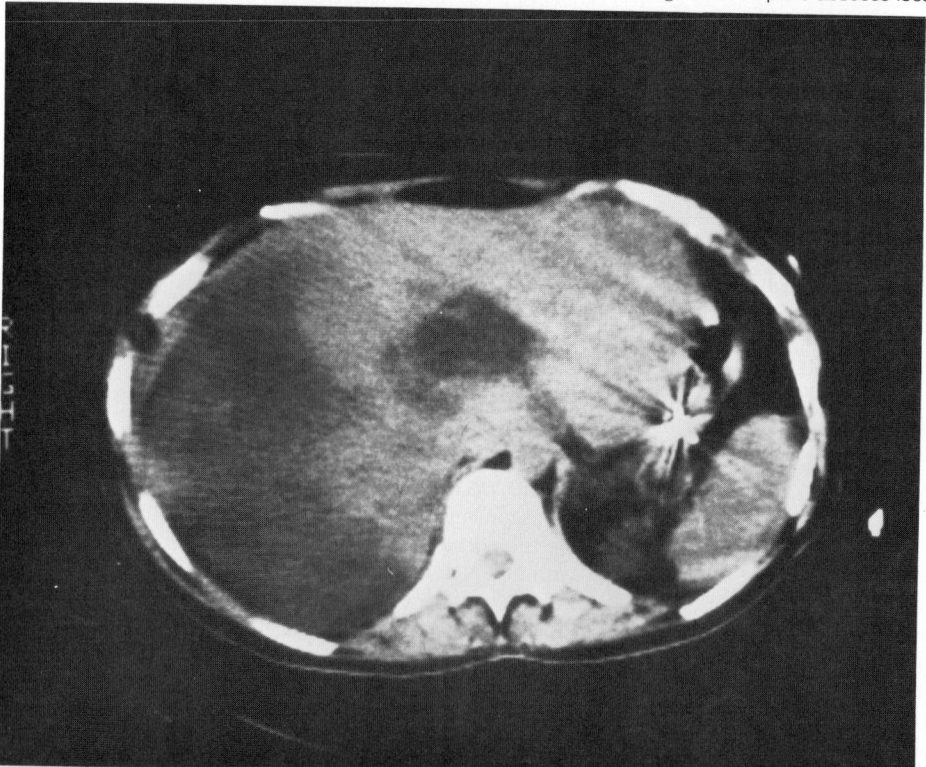

Fig. 30-9. Hepatic abscess located in medial segment of left lobe.

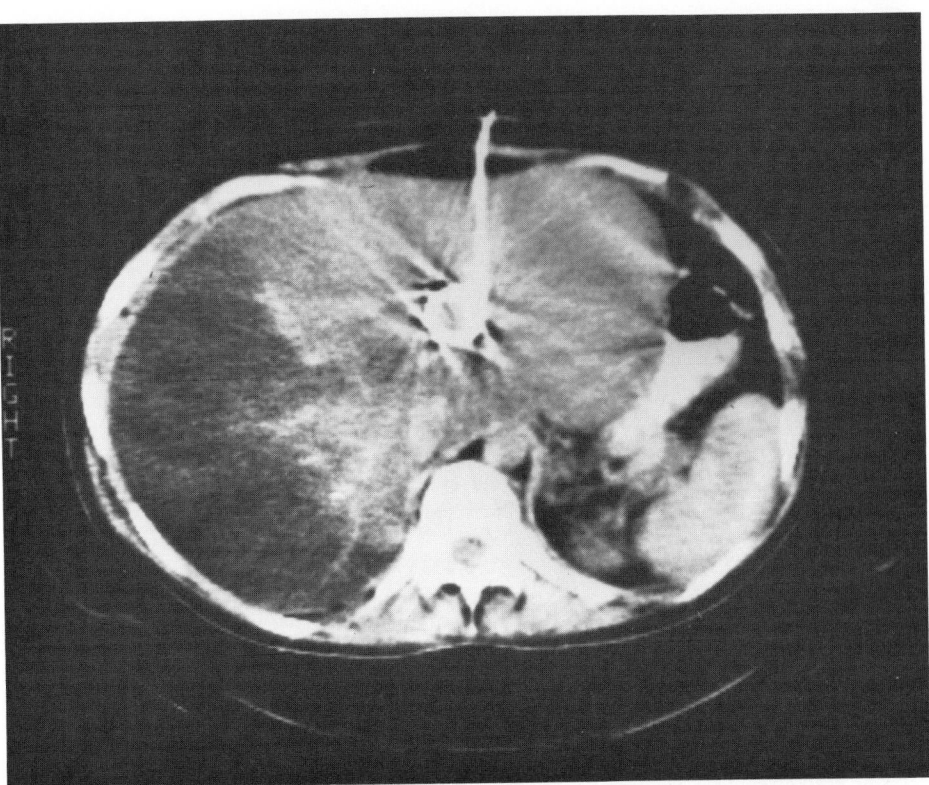

Fig. 30-10. Abscess as pictured in Fig. 30-9, drained extrasonographically with pigtailed catheter.

30-12). Because of the availability of antibacterial agents, transperitoneal drainage is no longer associated with prohibitive morbidity or mortality. In a small group of patients with multiple abscesses confined to a lobe, treatment is best managed by resection.

PROGNOSIS AND COMPLICATIONS. The mortality rate for patients with solitary pyogenic abscesses is less than that for patients with multiple abscesses. The mortality rate for undrained hepatic abscesses approaches 100 percent.

Amebic Abscesses

INCIDENCE. *Entameba histolytica* has been found wherever surveys have been made on the human population from northern Canada to the Straits of Magellan. It has been estimated that at least 10 percent of the population of this country is infected with the parasite. Amebic abscess of the liver is a disease of the middle-aged adult and predominates in the male with a 9:1 ratio. The concept of racial immunity is invalid.

PATHOLOGY. Amebas reach the liver by way of the portal venous system from a focus of ulceration in the bowel wall. Hepatic involvement is usually a large single abscess containing liquefied material with a characteristic reddish brown ''anchovy paste'' fluid. The lesions are usually single and occur in the right lobe of the liver, either near the dome or on the inferior surface in juxtaposition to the hepatic flexure. The wall is only a few millimeters thick and consists of granulation tissue with little or no fibrosis. Microscopically, three zones are recognized: a necrotic center, a middle zone with destruction of parenchymal cells, and an outer zone of relatively normal hepatic tissue in which amebas may be demonstrated. The concept of amebic hepatitis or presuppurative hepatitis has been challenged, since it is not certain that biliary abscesses or even larger central hepatic abscesses do not exist.

CLINICAL MANIFESTATIONS. Abscesses become evident when they cause generalized systemic disturbances coupled with symptoms and signs of hepatic involvement. The chief complaints are fever and liver pain. Pain is present in 88 percent of patients, and the pattern is related to the location of the hepatic abscess. With pain and tenderness over the right lower intercostal spaces, there may be associated bulging and pitting edema of the subcutaneous tissue. Superior surface abscesses result in pain referred to the right shoulder, while abscesses in the bare area, which have no contact with the serosal surface, are latent as far as pain is concerned. Left lobe abscesses present as a painful epigastric swelling.

Fever accompanied by chills and sweating is present in over three-quarters of the patients, but the temperature does not reach the levels resulting from pyogenic abscesses unless there is secondary infection. One-third to one-half of the adults offer a history of antecedent diarrhea, while in children grossly bloody mucous stool occurs more frequently. Tender hepatomegaly is an almost constant feature. Clinical jaundice is relatively rare.

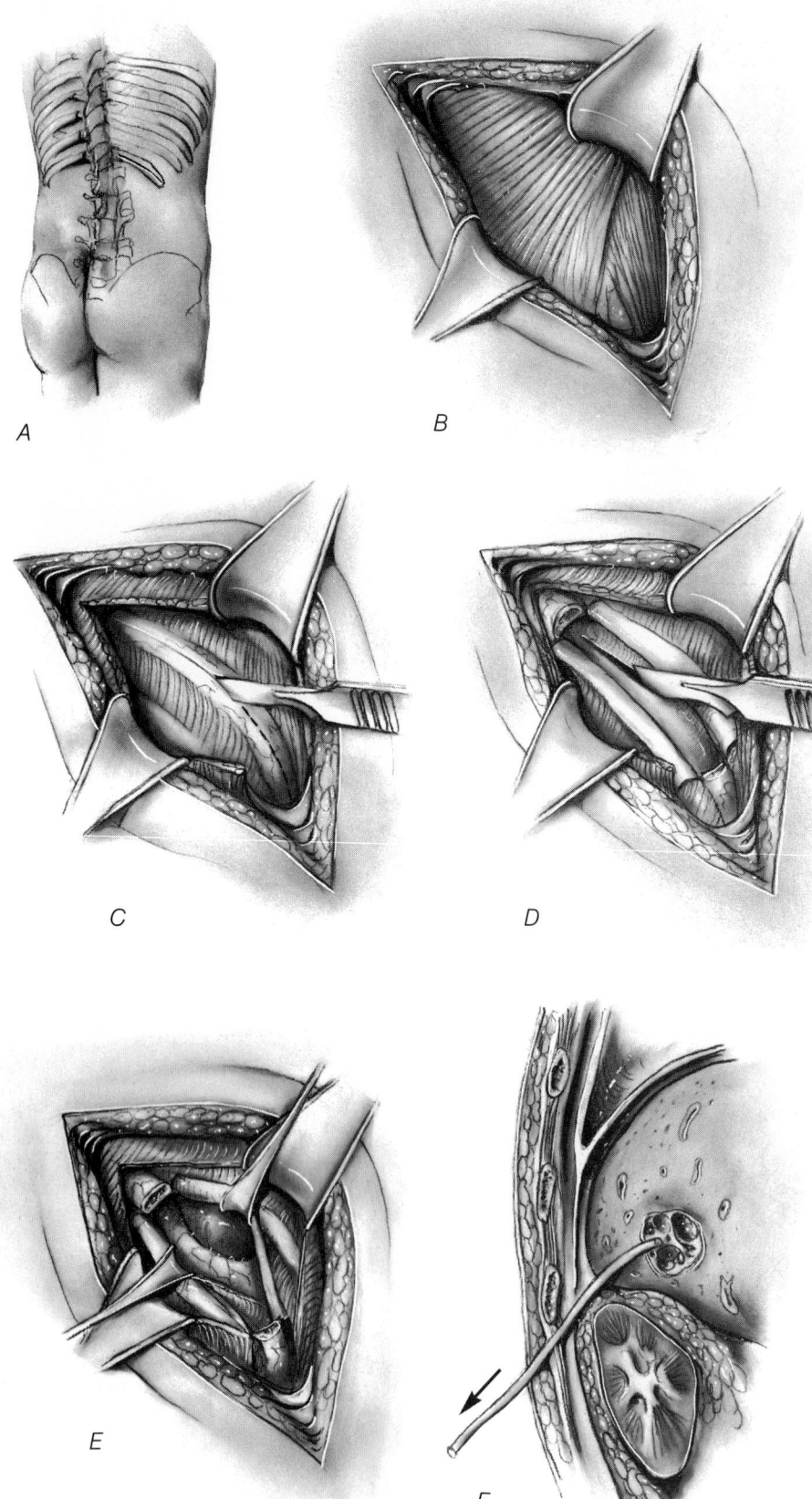

Fig. 30-11. Extraserous transthoracic drainage. *A.* Incision is made posteriorly over right twelfth rib. *B.* Latissimus dorsi muscle exposed. *C.* Periosteum of twelfth rib incised. *D.* Twelfth rib removed subperiosteally and bed incised. *E.* Diaphragm is detached and peritoneum is reflected from the inferior surface of diaphragm. *F.* Schematic drawing of position of drain. (From: *Schwartz SI: Surgical Diseases of the Liver. New York, McGraw-Hill, 1964,* with permission.)

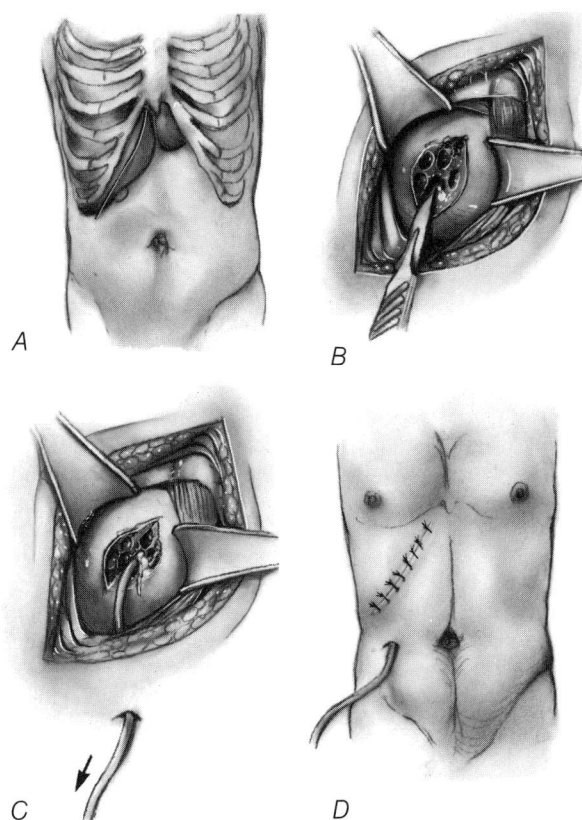

A

B

C

D

Fig. 30-12. Transabdominal drainage. *A.* Subcostal incision. *B.* Peritoneum has been entered and abscess incised. *C.* Drain is positioned in abscess and brought out through the stab wound. *D.* Closure of wound and position of stab wound. (From: *Schwartz SI: Surgical Diseases of the Liver. New York, McGraw-Hill, 1964, with permission.*)

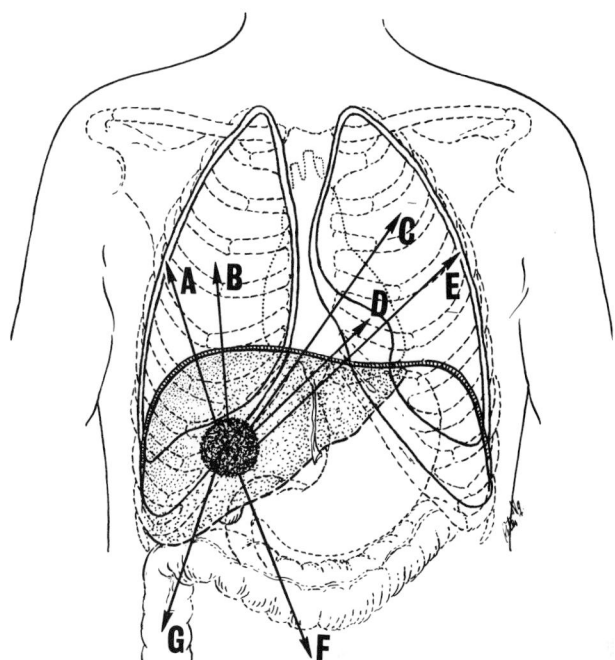

Fig. 30-13. Directions of rupture in 44 cases of amebic liver abscess: *A.* 8 cases, right pleural cavity. *B.* 13 cases, right lung. *C.* 4 cases left lung. *D.* 7 cases, pericardium. *E.* 1 case, left pleural cavity. *F.* 10 cases, peritoneal cavity. *G.* 1 case, colon. (After: *Lamont: Q J Med 27:389, 1958, with permission.*)

DIAGNOSTIC STUDIES. Patients with acute disease show no anemia but an appreciable degree of leukocytosis, whereas those with prolonged illness have anemia with less marked leukocytosis. Examination of the stool does not provide a high diagnostic yield. Amebas are found in the stool of only 15.4 percent of cases collected from the literature. Liver function tests are not helpful in establishing the diagnosis. A specific complement-fixation test has been more reliable than a history of diarrhea, stool examination, and proctoscopy. A negative test does not exclude the diagnosis. Radiographic findings are similar to those described for pyogenic abscesses. Scintillography, ultrasonography, and angiography have also helped to localize the lesion.

Diagnosis is frequently established by aspiration of the abscess cavity, a relatively innocuous procedure. Although the "anchovy paste" aspirate is considered pathognomonic, the abscess content may be creamy white, even though there is no secondary bacterial infection. Amebic trophozoites are demonstrated in the aspirate of fewer than one-third of the patients.

COMPLICATIONS. The most common complication is secondary infection, which occurs in approximately 22 percent of patients. Rupture of the amebic abscess ac-

counts for the next most common group of complications. The direction of rupture is reproduced in Fig. 30-13. Pleuropulmonary complications occur in 20 percent of patients. This is usually the result of direct extension of the hepatic process. The most serious route of rupture is into the pericardial cavity, and this is usually secondary to extension of an abscess in the left lobe. Rupture into the peritoneal cavity or into an intraabdominal viscus occurs in 6 to 9 percent of the patients.

TREATMENT. This consists of administration of amebicidal drugs combined with aspiration or surgical drainage when indicated. The initial approach is usually conservative and directed toward eradicating the parasite from the intestinal tract, liver, and abscess itself. In general, the patient is not considered for surgical treatment until the intestinal phase is controlled. Metronidazole, which acts in both the hepatic and intestinal sites, has replaced emetine and chloroquine. Both the hepatic and intestinal infections have generally been cured by 400 mg three times a day for 4 days combined with closed aspiration. A single dose of 2.5 g combined with aspiration also has had dramatic results. Since both emetine, which may be cardiotoxic, and chloroquine act mainly on the hepatic phase, following completion of therapy with these drugs, intestinal amebicidals such as Diodoquin, chiniofon, and tetracycline must be administered to control the intestinal phase.

Surgical Procedures. The indications for aspiration are (1) the persistence of clinical manifestations following a course of amebicidal drugs, (2) clinical or radiographic evidence of a hepatic abscess, and (3) absence of findings that would suggest secondary infection of a liver abscess. Drug therapy should be instituted several days prior to aspiration. There is no indication for injection of any drug directly into the abscess cavity. In the absence of localizing signs, the preferred route is through the ninth or tenth interspace between the anterior and posterior axillary line. Once an abscess has been demonstrated to be secondarily infected, open drainage is the treatment of choice.

PROGNOSIS. This is dependent upon the relative virulence of the organism and the resistance of the host, the stage of infection, the multiplicity of abscesses, and the presence of complications. In uncomplicated cases, the mortality rate is only 7 percent, whereas with complications a 43 percent mortality has been reported.

CYSTS AND BENIGN TUMORS

Nonparasitic Cysts

These lesions may be single, multiple, diffuse, localized, unilocular, or multilocular. They include (1) blood and degenerative cysts, (2) dermoid cysts, (3) lymphatic cysts, (4) endothelial cysts, (5) retention cysts, consisting of (a) solitary retention cysts and (b) multiple retention cysts (polycystic disease), and (6) proliferative cysts (cystadenomas). Autopsy incidences of approximately 0.15 percent have been reported. The clinically apparent cystic disease and nonparasitic solitary cysts occur more frequently in the fourth, fifth, and sixth decades, at an average age of fifty-two years. Polycystic, hepatic disease also occurs much more frequently in the female.

PATHOLOGY. Solitary nonparasitic cysts are usually located in the right lobe of the liver. The cyst content is a clear, watery material, and characteristically the cysts have a low internal pressure in contrast to the high tension in parasitic cysts. Occasionally the fluid is yellowish-brown, suggesting necrosis of adjacent parenchyma. Polycystic disease of the liver has a honeycomb appearance with multiple cavities, and the lesions are commonly distributed throughout the entire liver, but at times one lobe, more frequently the right, is preferentially involved. Unlike the solitary nonparasitic cyst, polycystic disease of the liver (Fig. 30-14) is frequently associated with cystic involvement of other organs; 51.6 percent of polycystic livers are associated with polycystic kidneys. Conversely, the incidence of hepatic cysts in patients with known polycystic renal disease varies between 19 and 34 percent. Polycystic livers have been implicated as a rare cause of portal hypertension and also have been associated with atresia of the bile ducts, cholangitis, and hemangiomas.

Traumatic cysts are usually single, are filled with bile, and contain no epithelial lining. Cystadenomas are grossly smooth, encapsulated, and lobular, and contain a mucoid material. They are lined by a proliferative columnar epithelium.

CLINICAL MANIFESTATIONS. Both solitary and polycystic lesions grow slowly and are relatively asymptomatic.

A painless right upper quadrant mass is the most frequent complaint, and when symptoms occur, they are usually related to pressure on adjacent viscera. Acute abdominal pain may accompany the complications of torsion, intracystic hemorrhage, or intraperitoneal rupture. Physical examination may reveal the mass, and the kidneys may be palpable. Jaundice is rare. Liver function tests are of little diagnostic aid. Scintillography, CT scan, ultrasonography, and arteriography have been used to define the intrahepatic position of the mass, and peritoneoscopy may be diagnostic (Fig. 30-15).

TREATMENT. With the exceptions of rupture, torsion, and intracystic hemorrhage, the treatment is elective. Asymptomatic nonparasitic cysts should not be treated surgically or by percutaneous drainage. If there is an indication for intervention, complete extirpation is the treatment of choice. Solitary cysts that are superficial should be resected, but resection of a large cyst extending deep into the parenchyma may be hazardous. When the cyst contents are sterile and contain no bile, unroofing the cyst and establishing a free connection with the peritoneal cavity is satisfactory. The presence of purulent contents mandates external drainage or marsupialization. Wide unroofing has been shown to be the treatment of choice even when the cyst fluid is bile stained. The complication rate is less than that attendant upon either marsupialization or Roux en Y drainage. With polycystic disease of the liver and serious renal involvement, excisional therapy for the hepatic cyst is contraindicated. Also, if the patient has been asymptomatic and excision is deemed to be technically difficult, resection should not be carried out. If the patient is in good health and symptomatic related to a mass effect, even partial excision is justifiable.

PROGNOSIS. The prognosis of polycystic disease is essentially that of the accompanying renal disease. Hepatic failure, jaundice, and the manifestations of portal hypertension are rare. The mortality rate for surgically treated nonparasitic cysts of the liver approaches zero.

Hydatid Cysts

Hydatid disease *(echinococcosis)* is characterized by worldwide distribution and frequent hepatic involvement. The incidence among human beings is dependent on the incidence in intermediate hosts including sheep, pigs, and cattle. The southern half of South America, Iceland, Australia, New Zealand, and southern parts of Africa are regarded as intensive endemic areas. Most cases reported in the United States have occurred in immigrants from Greece and Italy.

PATHOLOGY. The most common unilocular hydatid cyst is caused by *Echinococcus granulosus,* while the alveolar type is caused by *Echinococcus multilocularis.* Approximately 70 percent of hydatid cysts are located in the liver, and in one-quarter to one-third of these cases there are multiple cysts. The right lobe is affected in 85 percent of patients. Cysts are usually superficial and are composed of a two-layer laminated wall, an inner germinative membrane, and an outer adventitia. The two membranes are in close contact with each other but are not linked. The fluid in the hydatid cyst has a high pressure of

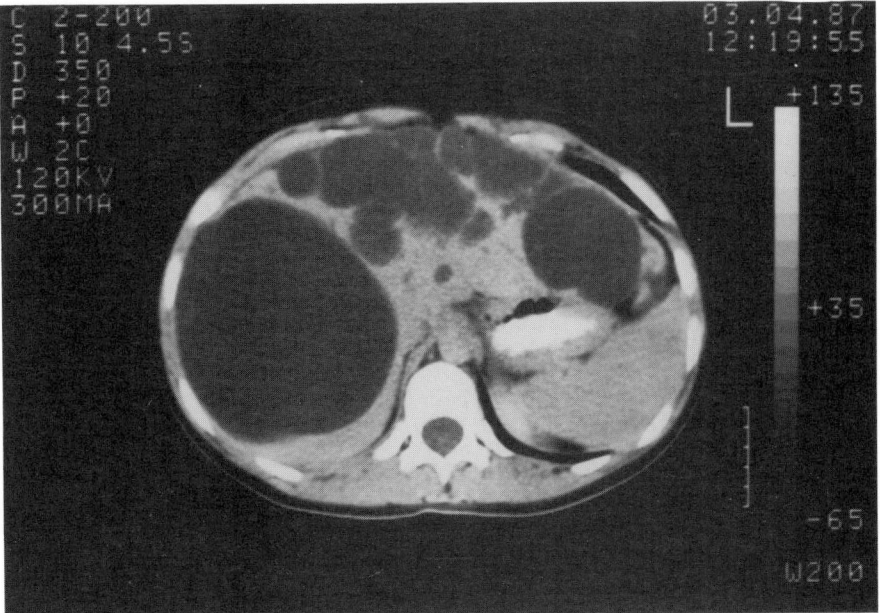

A

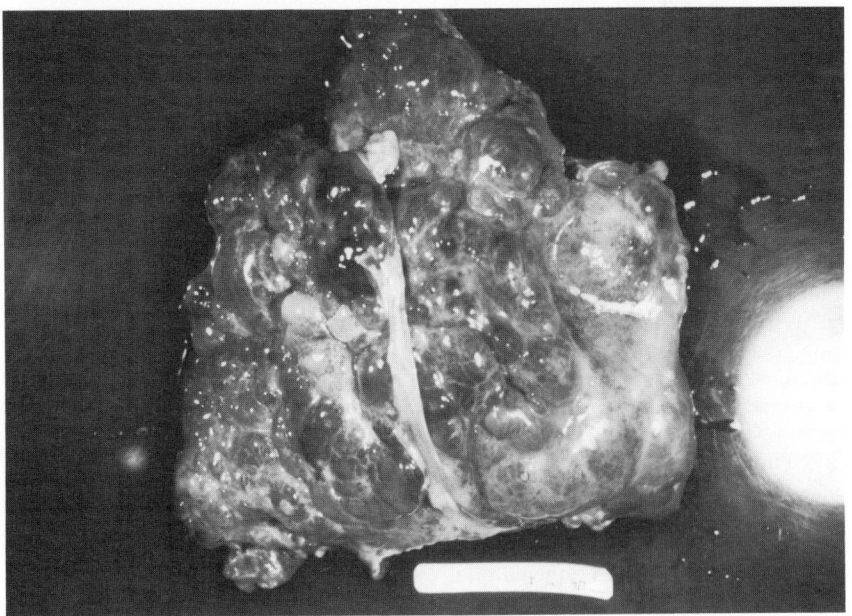

B

Fig. 30-14. *A.* CT scan of polycystic liver demonstrating large cyst in right lobe and multiple cysts throughout the right lobe. *B.* Specimen of resected polycystic left lobe of liver. Right cyst was unroofed.

approximately 300 mL of water and is colorless, opalescent, and slightly alkaline. Inside the main hydatid vesicle daughter cysts are usually found. Extension is commonly into the peritoneal cavity, but progressive intrahepatic expansion may result in the replacement of liver parenchyma.

In contrast to the unilocular hydatid cysts, the alveolar hydatid is a growth without a capsule and with a tendency toward multiple metastases. As growth progresses, the center becomes necrotic, and the peripheral invades the blood vessels and lymph channels. The causative agent of this lesion is found more frequently in the colder regions of Alaska, Russia, and the Alps.

COMPLICATIONS. Intrabiliary rupture represents the most common complication and occurs in 5 to 10 percent of cases. Suppuration, the second most common complication, is caused by bacteria from the biliary tract. The formation of the purulent material results in the death of the parasite and conversion into a pyogenic abscess. Intraperitoneal rupture results in the showering of hydatid

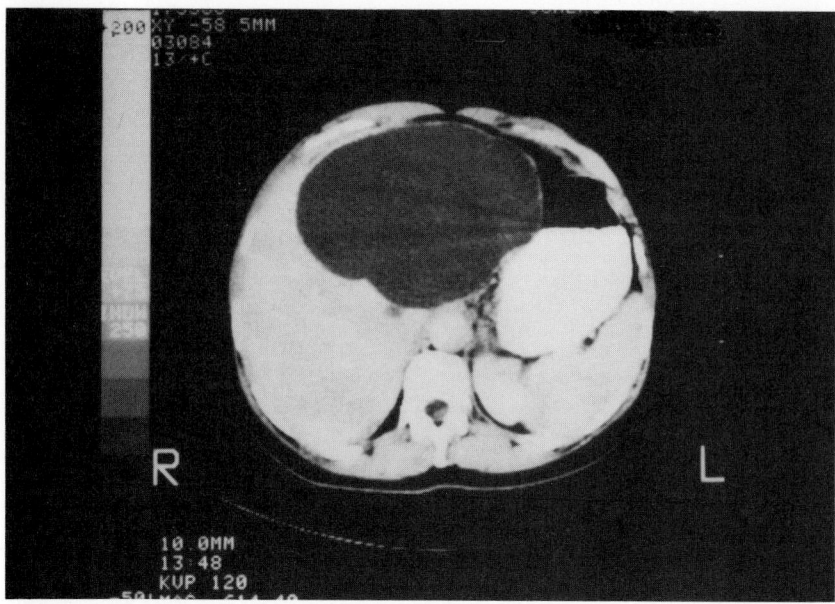

Fig. 30-15. CT scan demonstrating solitary, nonparasitic cyst of left lobe of liver.

fluid, brood capsules, and scolices into the peritoneum, leading to transient peritoneal irritation of varying intensity. Usually, the reproductive elements survive and initiate the formation of new cysts, *secondary echinococcosis of the peritoneum.* Cysts located in the superior portion of the liver tend to grow craniad into the pleural cavity and become intrathoracic. These can be differentiated from primary pulmonary cysts by the presence of daughter cysts and bile pigments. Empyema and bronchopleural fistula must result.

CLINICAL MANIFESTATIONS. Patients with simple or uncomplicated multivesicular cysts are usually asymptomatic. When symptoms occur, they are caused by pressure on adjacent organs. Abdominal pain and tenderness are the most common complaints followed by a palpable mass. A tumor, which is palpable in 70 percent of the patients, or diffuse hepatic enlargement in a patient who has lived in an endemic region is cause for suspicion. The so-called hydatid thrill and fremitus are quite rare. Jaundice and ascites are uncommon. With secondary infection, tender hepatomegaly, chills, and spiking temperatures occur. Urticaria and erythema offer evidence of a generalized anaphylactic reaction. With biliary rupture, the classic triad of biliary colic, jaundice, and urticaria may be noted. Vomiting with passage of hydatid membranes in the emesis *(hydatidemesia)* and passage of membranes in the stool *(hydatidenteria)* may also occur. The complication of intraperitoneal rupture is heralded by abdominal pain and signs of anaphylactic shock. Intrathoracic rupture is associated with shoulder pain and cough initially productive of a frothy blood-stained fluid that subsequently becomes bile-stained. Membranes are intermittently expectorated in 80 percent of these cases.

DIAGNOSTIC STUDIES. Radiographically, an unruptured cyst presents as a round, reticulated calcified shadow in the liver (Fig. 30-16). Secondary infection with gas-producing organisms may demonstrate as daughter cysts. With intrabiliary rupture, gas is noted in the remaining cyst cavity. CT scans furnish useful information and correlate well with operative findings (Fig. 30-17). Eosinophilia is the least reliable of immunologic responses, being present in only 25 percent of all patients. The indirect agglutination test is positive in about 85 percent of cases; the complement fixation test is slightly less sensitive. This reaction becomes negative 2 to 6 months after removal of the cyst. Casoni's skin test is positive in approximately 90 percent of patients, and the reaction

Fig. 30-16. Hydatid cyst of liver, demonstrating calcification. (From: *Schwartz SI: Surgical Diseases of the Liver. New York, McGraw-Hill, 1964, with permission.)*

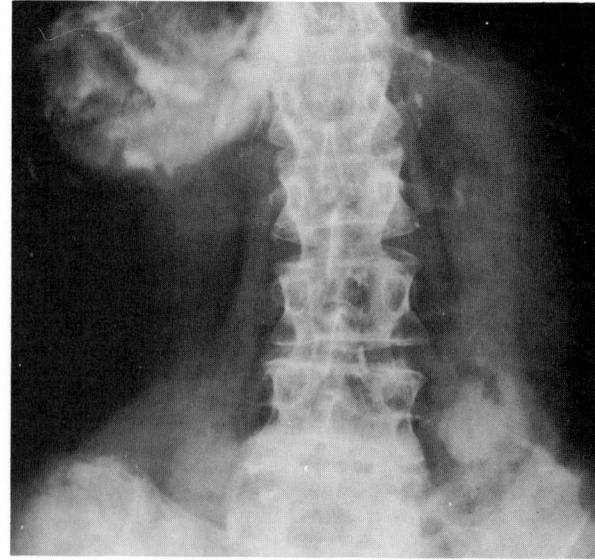

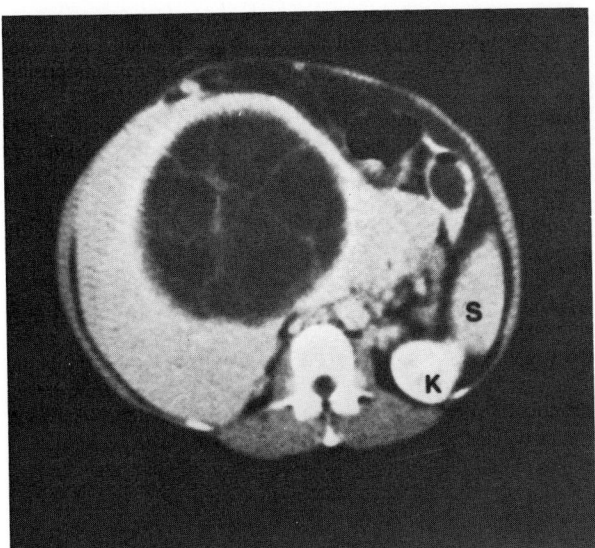

Fig. 30-17. CT scan showing large echinococcus cyst with multiple septa.

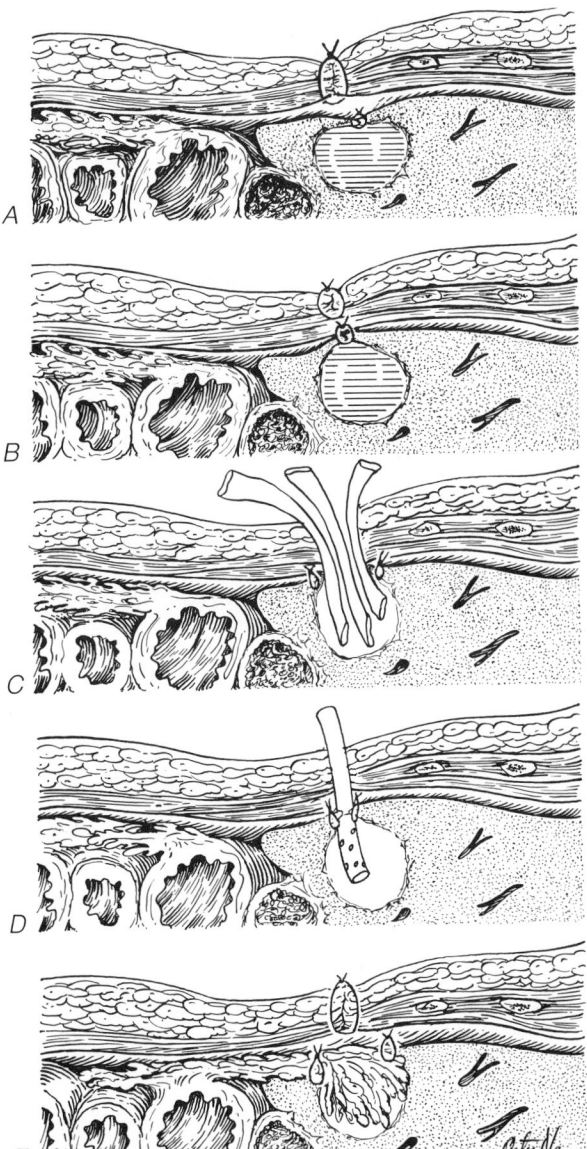

Fig. 30-18. Methods of handling residual hepatic cavity. *A.* Suture without drainage (capsulorraphy). Cavity is filled with sterile saline solution, and adventitia is closed without drainage. *B.* Same as *A* but peripheral peritoneum of anterior abdominal wall is sutured to periphery of capsule to facilitate extraperitoneal drainage of secondary infection, if one arises. *C.* Marsupialization. Edges of cavity are sutured to abdominal wall, and several drains are inserted into depths of wound. *D.* Variant of marsupialization. Catheter is inserted into cavity, and closed drainage is used. *E.* Omentoplasty. Omentum is used to fill remaining cavity and is sutured to periphery of fibrous capsule. Vascular omental pedicle absorbs effusion. (From: *Schwartz SI: Surgical Diseases of the Liver. New York, McGraw-Hill, 1964, with permission.*)

may be obtained years after surgical removal of the cyst or after the parasite has died.

TREATMENT. Small calcified cysts in patients with negative serologic test results need no treatment. Treatment is surgical, since there is no response to drug administration or radiation therapy. Therapy consists of removal of the cyst contents without contaminating the patient, followed by appropriate management of any remaining cavity. Since the hydatid fluid is under high tension, evacuation and sterilization are carried out initially with a scolicidal agent such as hibitane, alcohol, or hypertonic saline. Following evacuation and irrigation, primary closure may effect cure. External drainage or marsupialization are accompanied by high complication rates and prolonged drainage. Removal of the parasite is accomplished by excision of the hydatid vesicle using the natural cleavage plane that exists between the germinative layer and adventitia. Omentoplasty provides a method of successfully managing the cavity (Fig. 30-18). Total removal of the cysts, including the adventitial layer, may also be performed. Partial hepatectomy with controlled hepatic resection has been advised for larger and multiple cysts. Marsupialization or partial hepatectomy are the alternatives for large or infected cysts. In uncomplicated cases, the results of surgical treatment are excellent, and the postoperative mortality is less than 5 percent. With intrabiliary rupture, marsupialization should be accompanied by drainage of the bile duct if there is associated obstruction. Rupture into the peritoneal cavity is treated by laparotomy and thorough cleansing, although it is frequently impossible to prevent secondary contamination. Intrathoracic rupture generally can be controlled by evacuating and draining the hepatic cysts. Alveolar disease of the liver was inevitably fatal, but, more recently, satisfactory results have been obtained with extensive hepatic resection.

Benign Tumors

HAMARTOMA. Hamartomas are composed of tissues normally present in the organ but arranged in a disorderly fashion. The lesions vary from minute nodules to large tumors and are rarely of clinical significance. Large mes-

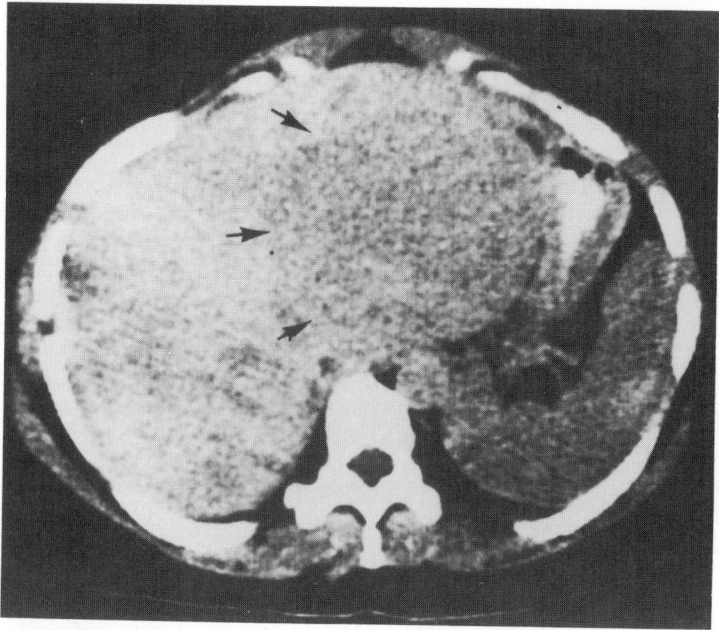

A

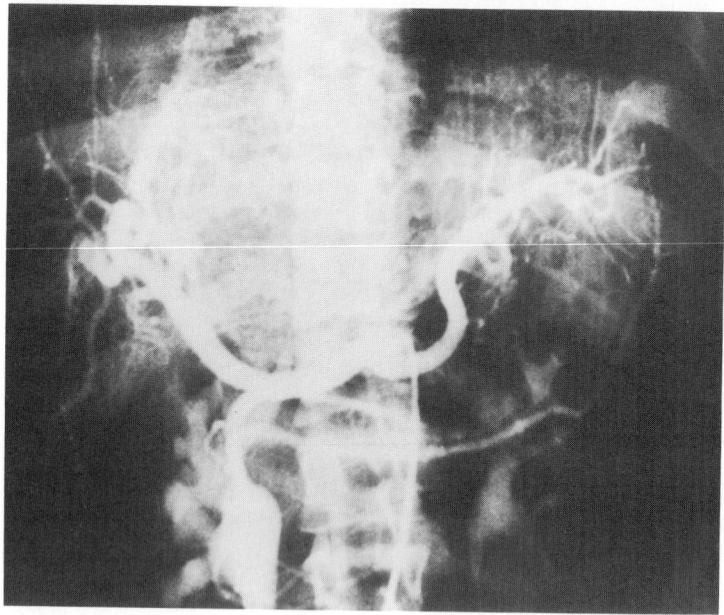

B

Fig. 30-19. *A.* CT scan demonstrates a solid, low-density mass occupying most of the left lobe of the liver *(arrows)*. *B.* Arteriogram shows a large hypervascular mass involving the entire left lobe. Tumor had tortuous, encased, and distorted vessels supplied by branches of the left hepatic artery. A vascular flush was apparent in the capillary phase. (From: *Gutierrez O, Schwartz SI: Atlas of Hepatic Tumors and Focal Lesions. New York, McGraw-Hill, 1984, pp 83–84, with permission.*)

enchymal hamartomas have presented as rapidly growing abdominal masses in children. Grossly, the tumors are firm, nodular, and located immediately beneath the surface of the liver, and may be solitary or multiple. They are generally well encapsulated and often cystic. With lesions of clinical significance, surgical excision is generally indicated. Deeply located lesions should be left alone after histologic diagnosis has been established, since they do not grow rapidly and do not undergo malignant transformation.

ADENOMA. In the past hepatic adenomas were extremely rare. They now appear more common. In 1973, a relationship between intraperitoneal bleeding from these lesions and contraceptive drugs was reported. The relationship between adenoma and estrogen, progesterone, or a combination has not been established. It occurs in men and in women who have never taken contraceptive medication. Most reported patients, however, have been women receiving oral contraceptives. Regression has been documented following cessation of the drug. This is

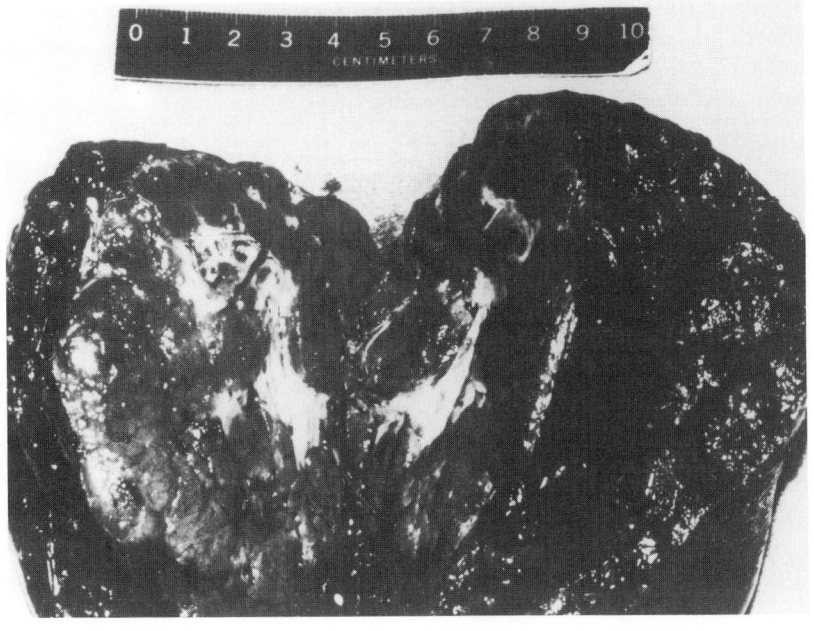

A

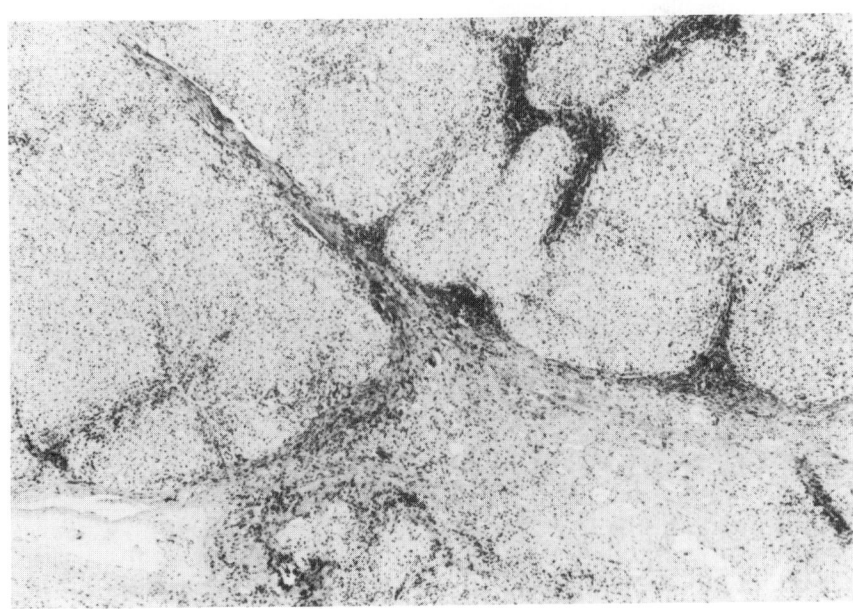

B

Fig. 30-20. *A.* Focal Nodular Hyperplasia gross specimen. *B.* Microscopy demonstrated normal parenchymal cells surrounding large scar. (From: *Gutierrez O, Schwartz SI: Atlas of Hepatic Tumors and Focal Lesions. New York, McGraw-Hill, 1984, p 99, with permission.*)

particularly true of patients who present with intraperitoneal bleeding. CT can usually demonstrate the lesion, shown to be hypervascular on angiogram (Fig. 30-19*A* and *B*). Resection is indicated for lesions that bleed or increase in size. Asymptomatic adenomas should be watched, contraceptives should be discontinued, and the lesion should be followed with sequential scans.

FOCAL NODULAR HYPERPLASIA (FNH). No statistically significant correlation between oral contraceptives and FNH has been established. The lesion may represent response to insult to the liver cells. The tumors are usually solitary and frequently found near the free edge of the liver on cut section. They are tan, usually without a capsule, and have a central stellate scar (Fig. 30-20).

Most FNH produce no symptoms and they rarely rupture. Diagnosis can be made by angiographic demonstration of a stellate lesion. Resection is indicated only for symptoms that can be related to the tumor.

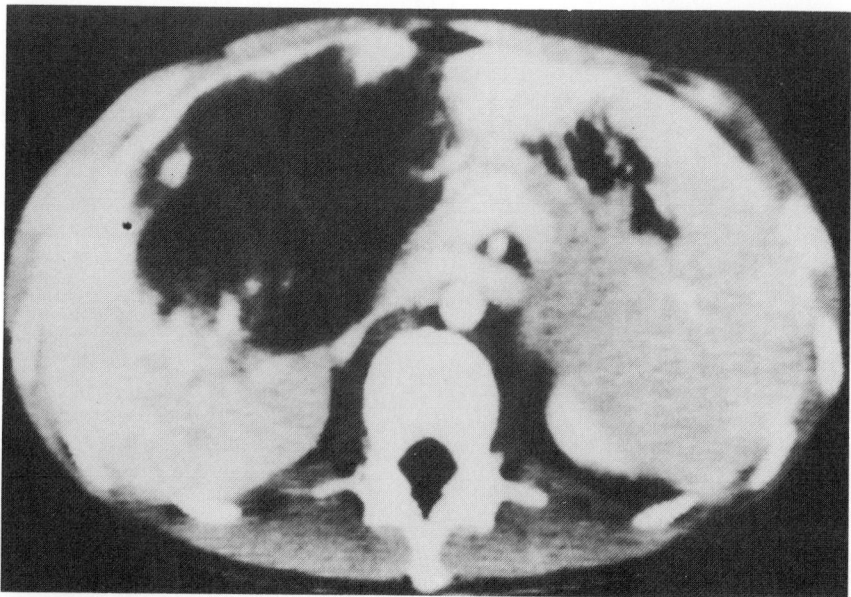

A

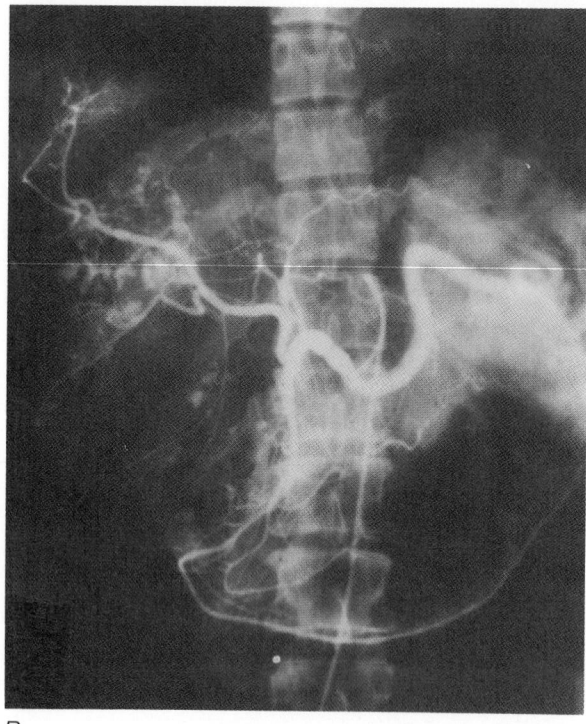

B

Fig. 30-21. *A.* Celiac angiogram demonstrating typical pooling of radiopaque throughout right lobe of liver. *B.* Infusion CT scan showing large, centrally located hemangioma of liver containing several organized clots. (From: *Schwartz SI, Husser WC: Cavernous hemangioma of the liver. Ann Surg 205:456, 1987, with permission.*)

ticentric lesions accompanied by vascular involvement of the skin and occurs in children with clinical manifestations in the first week of life.

A mass is occasionally apparent. Pain may be related to large lesions. The overwhelming majority of patients remains asymptomatic. A bruit is heard only rarely. The major complication is rupture with intraperitoneal hemorrhage, which occurs more commonly in children and in gestational females. Large tumors in infants may be associated with high-output cardiac failure. Selective hepatic arteriography is the most informative diagnostic technique (Fig. 30-21*A*). Ultrasonography, CT (Fig. 30-21*B*), and MRI all provide definition of an intrahepatic hemangioma. Percutaneous needle biopsy, either radiographically or laparoscopically controlled, can be diagnostic but is associated with the complication of bleeding.

In infants with high-output congestive heart failure, supportive therapy, at times with the addition of steroids, is effective and the lesion regresses. In rare cases hepatic artery ligation may be required to reverse cardiac failure. In adults, most hepatic hemangiomas should not be excised. Even large lesions followed for long periods showed no notable increase in size or clinical manifestations. Only anecdotal experiences indict hormonal alteration as a potential stimulus for growth of the tumor. The potential for rupture is minimal and should not constitute an indication for excision. Pain, mass effect, significant growth, and rupture are indications for surgical excision. Few reports have documented reduction in size with radiation therapy. In adults hepatic arterial ligation is ineffective.

HEMANGIOMA. Hemangioma is the most common nodule in the liver, and the liver is the internal organ most frequently affected with this lesion. The tumor occurs five times more frequently in the female than in the male. These are occasionally associated with focal nodular hyperplasia, cysts of the liver and pancreas. Malignant degeneration does not occur, but the hemangioma must be distinguished from a hemangioendothelioma or diffuse hemangiomatosis. The latter consists of widespread mul-

MALIGNANT TUMORS

Primary Carcinoma

INCIDENCE. Although the disease is rare in people of western Europe and North America, it is remarkably common among the aboriginal inhabitants of Africa and certain parts of Asia. Postmortem rates in the United States average 0.27 percent, whereas in Africa the postmortem rate is 1.1 percent, hepatic carcinomas representing 17 to 53 percent of all cancers.

Primary carcinoma of the liver occurs with greater frequency in males. In the Caucasian it is rare before the age of forty, while in the African and Indonesian the affection is primarily one of youth, usually occurring before the age of forty. The American black does not exhibit a predisposition toward the disease. In contrast, a higher incidence is present in Chinese subjects even after they have changed their habitation. In children, the first appearance of the neoplasm is usually before the age of two, and primary carcinoma of the liver represents the most common carcinoma in the first few years of life. Hepatoblastoma usually affects children less than two years old; the male to female ratio is 6:1. This lesion also occurs in adults. Fibrolamellar carcinoma, a variant of hepatocellular carcinoma, has a propensity for adolescents and young adults, with an equal sex incidence.

ETIOLOGY. A variety of etiologic factors have been implicated. Aflatoxins of the mold *Aspergillus flavus* contaminate the diet in African and Asian communities with high incidence of hepatocellular carcinoma. Low protein intake and consequent kwashiorkor also may be factors. Just as almost every type of experimentally induced cirrhosis may be followed by carcinoma of the liver, so a definite association between cirrhosis and primary carcinoma has been noted in the human being. Postnecrotic cirrhosis is the type most commonly preceding hepatocellular carcinoma; cirrhosis is present in 60 percent of cases. Hepatic malignant tumors occur in 4.5 percent of cirrhotic patients, and the incidence is increased in patients with hemochromatosis. Parasitic infestation with the liver fluke *Clonorchis sinensis* has been considered a factor in the development of cholangiocarcinoma, but this is open to question. There is no increased risk for hepatic carcinoma following infectious hepatitis. In the pediatric age group the tumor is rarely related to cirrhosis.

PATHOLOGY. Liver cell carcinoma *(hepatocellular)* is the most common type; the tumor cells resemble the parenchymal cell. Bile duct carcinoma *(cholangiocarcinoma)* is apparently derived from bile duct epithelium. *Hepatoblastoma* represents an immature variant of the hepatic cell carcinoma.

Grossly, each of these types may present as a single large nodule, as extensive nodularity, or as a diffuse permeation throughout the organ. The anatomic distribution of fibrolamellar carcinoma is unusual in that 75 percent present as solitary large left lobe tumors. They have a prominent central scar. The hepatocellular carcinomas have a trabecular structure, and vascularity is a prominent feature. These lesions frequently invade branches of the portal vein and occasionally the hepatic veins. The formation of giant cells is a feature of hepatocellular carcinoma and aids in distinguishing this lesion from the secondary carcinoma of the liver. Fibrolamellar carcinoma is characterized by eosinophilic hepatocytes and abundant fibrous stroma arranged in parallel bands around tumor cells. The cell type of the bile duct carcinoma is columnar, and its microscopic appearance may be impossible to distinguish from that of carcinoma of the gallbladder or extrahepatic biliary duct system. Bile is never seen in the acini or the cells, whereas mucus formation is common.

Hepatic tumors extend by four methods:

1. Centrifugal growth indicates nodular expansion leading to compression of the surrounding hepatic tissue.
2. Parasinusoidal extension refers to tumor invasion into the surrounding parenchyma, either through the parasinusoidal spaces or through the sinusoids themselves.
3. Venous spread is the extension of tumor from small branches of the portal system in a retrograde fashion into larger branches and eventually into the main portal vein. Invasion of hepatic vein tributaries is less common but may extend up to the inferior vena cava or right atrium.
4. Distant metastases are the result of invasion of lymph channels and vascular systems. The most frequently involved locations are regional lymph nodes and the lungs.

Metastases occur in 48 to 73 percent of cases.

CLINICAL MANIFESTATIONS. Weight loss and weakness occur in 80 percent of cases, while abdominal pain is present in half (75 percent in patients with fibrolamellar carcinoma). The pain is usually dull and persistent, but dramatic sudden onset may occur in patients with intraperitoneal hemorrhage secondary to rupture of a necrotic nodule or erosion of a blood vessel. Bleeding varices are infrequent, but foreboding symptoms and delirium have almost always represented a terminal event (Table 30-3).

Table 30-3. PRIMARY EPITHELIAL CANCER IN ADULTS: 1974 LIVER TUMOR SURVEY— SYMPTOMS AND SIGNS OF HOSPITAL ADMISSION

Mass	60
Pain	51
Weight loss	29
Epigastric distress	16
Intraperitoneal hemorrhage	15
Hepatomegaly	14
Fever	9
Incidental at laparotomy for other disease	7
Diarrhea	6
Anorexia	6
Nausea and vomiting	6
Weakness, malaise	5
Misdiagnosis—cholecystitis	5
Endocrine symptoms	3
Pruritus	3
Jaundice	2
Calcification on x-ray	1
Needle biopsy for benign disease	1
Abnormal liver function tests	1
Abnormal scan	1

SOURCE: Foster J, Berman M: *Solid Liver Tumors.* Philadelphia, Saunders, 1977, vol XXII.

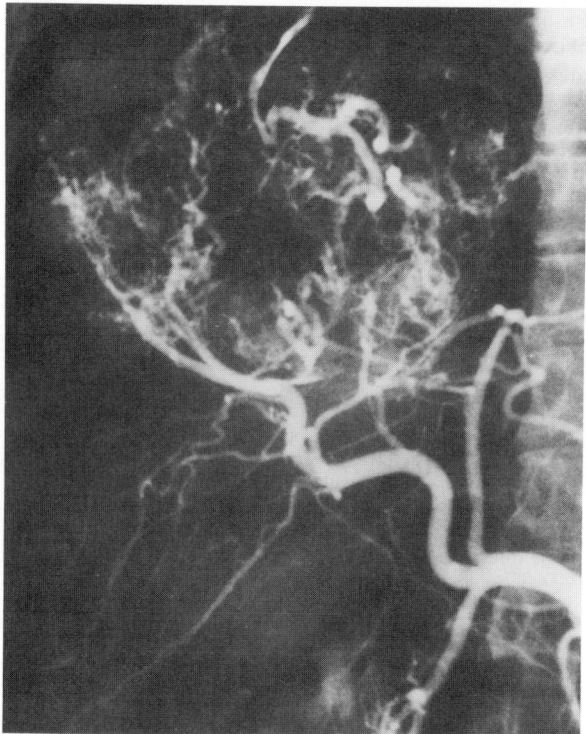

A

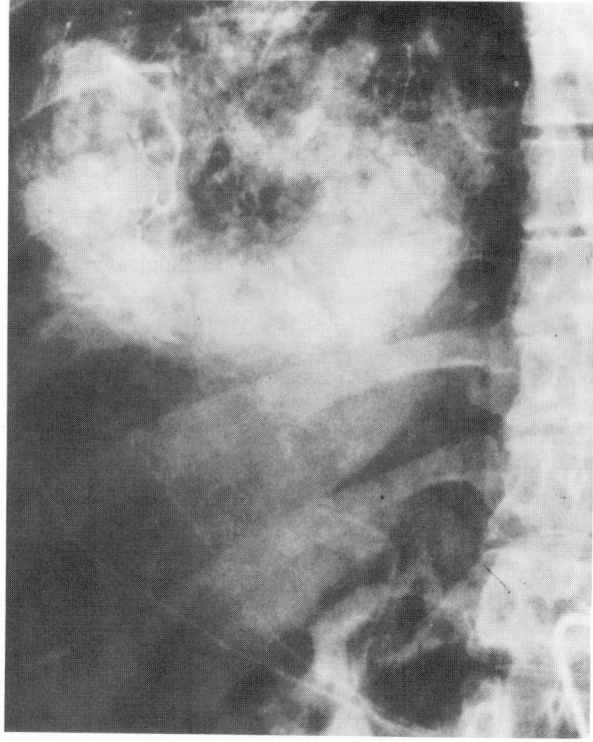

B

Fig. 30-22. *A*. Hepatic arteriogram showing a 13×14 cm hypervascular mass in the superior portion of the right lobe of the liver supplied by vessels from the right and medial branches of the left hepatic artery. *B*. A lucent center within this mass represented either central necrosis or hemorrhage. (From: *Gutierrez O, Schwartz SI: Atlas of Hepatic Tumors and Focal Lesions. New York, McGraw-Hill, 1984, p 19, with permission.*)

The liver is almost always enlarged but not tender. Splenic enlargement is present in one-third of the cases, as are other signs of portal hypertension. The incidence of jaundice varies from 20 to 58 percent. Ascites develops in one-half to three-quarters of patients. A rapid increase in the symptoms and signs associated with cirrhosis or hemachromatosis is highly suggestive of superimposed hepatic carcinoma. In these cases, the amelioration of diabetes and occasional hypoglycemic intervals also indicate neoplastic change.

In over half the pediatric cases the first evidence is an abdominal mass. Hemihypertrophy and sexual precocity occur in an occasional pediatric patient with hepatoblastoma.

DIAGNOSTIC STUDIES. The most consistently altered liver function tests are the BSP and alkaline phosphatase. The serum bilirubin level is usually normal; 5' nucleotidase is usually elevated.

The demonstration of α-fetoprotein (AFP) in the serum by immunodiffusion, immunoelectrophoresis, and immunoassay techniques is useful in differential diagnosis and epidemiologic studies. This protein is normally present in the fetus but disappears a few weeks after birth. Positive AFP tests are noted in about 75 percent of Africans but in only 30 percent of patients in the United States and Europe. False-positive results occur with embryonic tumors of the ovary and testis. Resection of the tumor converts the test to "negative"; recurrence may be detected by the reappearance of AFP in the serum.

Selective hepatic arteriography has been utilized to demonstrate an arterial pattern within the tumor, characterized by pooling and increased vascularity (Fig. 30-22). Scintillation scanning may also identify the space-occupying lesion within the liver, but computed tomography and MRI are more sensitive. Percutaneous needle biopsy can provide a definitive diagnosis. Ultrasonography is particularly helpful in differentiating cystic from solid tumor. Intraoperative ultrasonography has added an important surgical refinement and permitted more limited resections.

TREATMENT. The only curative therapy is surgical excision. In most instances this entails a lobectomy, but with an appreciation of segmental anatomy, lesser "anatomic" resections are being performed more frequently. A major resection is compromised by cirrhosis because of increased vascularity, increased morbidity, and an inability for the cirrhotic liver to regenerate. The use of intraoperative ultrasonography has permitted limited resections particularly in cirrhotic patients.

Neither radiation therapy nor chemotherapy is curative, but a combination of these modalities in children with hepatoblastoma has converted nonresectable lesions into resectable ones, and in some instances cure was achieved. Direct arterial infusion of chemotherapeutic drugs has effected a reduction in tumor size and extension of survival in about 25 percent of cases. Hepatic dearterialization is generally unrewarding.

PROGNOSIS. The outlook for untreated primary carcinoma of the liver is extremely poor, and the duration of the disease is rarely longer than 4 months from the time of onset of symptoms. Death is the result of cachexia, hepatic failure, sequelae of portal vein thrombosis, intraperitoneal hemorrhage, and metastases. In children under age two years with hepatoblastoma, 21 of 27 who survived operation were alive and well with no evidence of disease for a mean of 53 months. In adults, 5- and 10-year survival rates of 36 percent and 33 percent, respectively, have been reported.

Other Primary Neoplasms

The three major lesions are sarcoma, mesenchymoma, and infantile hemangioendothelioma. All hepatic mesenchymal lesions are considered malignant. Angiosarcoma is the most common primary sarcoma of the liver. Exposure to vinyl chloride and thorotrast injection have been implicated as etiologic factors.

Angiosarcoma is characterized by short illness, jaundice, and coma progressing rapidly to death. Infantile hemangioendotheliomas occur in children under the age of five and are associated with skin lesions and cardiac failure secondary to arteriovenous shunts within the tumor. Although most of these pediatric lesions are fatal, spontaneous regression has been recorded, as has success with partial hepatectomy.

Metastatic Neoplasms

These represent the most common malignant tumor of the liver. The relative proportion of primary to secondary neoplasms is estimated to be 1:20, and there is no statistical difference between those with and those without cirrhosis. The liver is second only to regional lymph nodes as a site of metastases for tumors, and 25 to 50 percent of all patients dying of cancer have been found to have hepatic metastases. Fifty percent of patients with gastrointestinal tumors have hepatic metastases when autopsied.

Metastatic neoplasms reach the liver by four routes: (1) portal venous circulation, (2) lymphatic spread, (3) hepatic arterial system, and (4) direct extension.

Metastases appear in the liver at varying times in relation to primary lesions: (1) Precocious metastasis is evident when the primary lesion is not suspected (carcinoid of the ileum). (2) Synchronous metastases occur when the hepatic neoplasm is detected at the same time as the primary lesion. (3) Metachronous metastasis is one in which appearance is delayed following the successful removal of a primary tumor (ocular melanoma). The growth pattern of the metastatic tumor is frequently more rapid than the original lesion, and the mitotic count of the metastatic hepatic neoplasms has been shown to be five times greater than that of the extrahepatic primary lesion.

CLINICAL MANIFESTATIONS. Symptoms referable to the liver are present in 67 percent of patients with proved metastases. These include hepatic pain, ascites, jaundice, anorexia, and weight loss. On examination, hepatic nodularity is apparent in half the cases, and a friction rub is audible in 10 percent. Jaundice, ascites, and the signs of portal hypertension are present in approximately one-quarter to one-third of the patients. With carcinoid tumors, hepatic metastases are of major importance in the pathogenesis of the flushing syndrome.

DIAGNOSTIC STUDIES. The alkaline phosphatase level is increased in over 80 percent of patients. The SGOT level is elevated in approximately two-thirds of the patients, but the serum α-fetoprotein determination is negative. The carcinoembryonic antigen may provide a marker for metastatic colon carcinoma. The combination of computed tomography, MRI, and angiography best defines the presence, location, and operability of lesions. Intraoperative ultrasonography has aided in the definition of resectable lesions.

TREATMENT. Surgical treatment of hepatic metastases should be considered only if (1) control of the primary tumor is accomplished or anticipated, (2) there are no systemic or intraabdominal metastases, (3) the patient's condition will tolerate the major operative procedure, and (4) the extent of hepatic involvement is such that resection and total extirpation of the metastasis is feasible. Resection of segments of the liver containing metastases has effected reasonable long-term survival without recurrence for patients with primaries in the colon and rectum and for Wilms' tumor. Rare survivors have been reported for other primaries. A metastasis noted during a colon resection should be removed at that time if it is readily removable without anticipated blood loss. However, if it appears that a major hepatic resection will be required, the operation is delayed for months and is preceded by CT scan and angiography to assess resectability. Although 20 percent of patients with colorectal cancer have hepatic metastasis, only one-quarter of these are potentially resectable; half of these, in turn, have other metastases that would negate the value of resection.

In one institution there was a 5-year survival rate for approximately 40 percent of 60 patients who had had removal by local excision of small hepatic metastases from colorectal cancer. Almost 30 percent of patients who underwent major hepatic resection for colorectal carcinoma survived 5 years. Long-term survival was not related to the interval between resection of the primary lesion and resection of liver metastases.

In several series patients with multiple metastases, provided there were fewer than four, confined to one lobe, did as well as patients with a single metastasis. Of 13 Wilms' tumor patients who survived resection of liver metastases, nine were alive and well $1\frac{1}{2}$ to 7 years later. Resection of metastases from melanoma, breast, stomach, uterus, cervix, and kidney is occasionally curative.

Palliative surgical measures are indicated for marked pain associated with hepatic neoplasm and for the excision of metastases in patients with the flushing syndrome of carcinoid tumor. Resection of the major portion of hepatic metastases (debulking procedure), even if residual tumor remains, has resulted in significant symptomatic improvement and reduction of the five HIAA levels to normal. These subjective and objective changes have persisted for several years. Dearterialization and radiographically controlled embolization have achieved similar results.

Symptomatic improvement and objective evidence of reduction of size of hepatic metastases from colorectal carcinomas have been achieved with hepatic arterial infusion of Floxuridine (FUDR) and mitomycin C. The infusion can be accomplished by percutaneous placement of the catheter. Recently a percutaneous refillable pump has been well received by patients; it is implanted in the subcutaneous tissue and attached to a catheter surgically positioned in the hepatic artery. This provides a long-term intraarterial infusion of chemotherapy. Improvement of intravenous administration has not been uniformly demonstrated. Intraarterial infusion has been associated with gastrointestinal symptoms, hepatitis, and sclerosing cholangitis.

HEPATIC RESECTION

The present indications for hepatic resection include (1) trauma with resultant necrosis of hepatic tissue, (2) cysts, (3) granulomas, (4) primary neoplasms of the liver, and (5) secondary malignant tumors that involve the liver either by direct extension or as metastatic lesions.

Removal of up to 80 percent of the liver is compatible with life. Following excision of this amount, patients maintain normal blood ammonia levels and normal prothrombin times. Fibrinogen production is insignificantly impaired; clinical jaundice is a transient phenomenon. By the fifth postoperative day, 95 percent of patients show clinical improvement in function, with the bilirubin and alkaline phosphatase returning to normal by the end of the third week. The most profound changes are noted in the serum albumin, which, by the third week, is usually restored to normal. Regeneration results from marked hypertrophy of the remaining tissue. The remaining portion of the liver responds as rapidly and completely after second and third partial hepatectomies as after an initial insult. There is experimental evidence for hepatotropic substances in portal venous blood. Insulin may represent the major anabolic factor and may be counterbalanced by glucagon. It is now felt that portal venous blood flow is an important contributory factor in liver regeneration. Very little restoration occurs after partial hepatectomy of the cirrhotic liver.

MANAGEMENT OF THE PATIENT. Preoperative therapy is directed at maintaining optimal liver function and correcting any defects that may be present. A diet high in calories, proteins, and carbohydrates is utilized, and the administration of albumin may be required to achieve normal levels. Vitamin K is given routinely until a normal prothrombin time results. In the presence of jaundice, other fat-soluble vitamins are added. Fresh-frozen plasma will rapidly replenish coagulation factors. Since many patients have a reduced hematocrit, transfusion with fresh whole blood rich in platelets and coagulation factors

is indicated. Major hepatic resection is attended by a prohibitive mortality rate in the patient with BSP retention greater than 35 percent, a serum albumin level lower than 2.0 g, and an increased prothrombin time that does not respond to parenteral vitamin K.

Postoperatively, infusion of 10% glucose or fructose is continued until the patient maintains an adequate oral intake to obviate severe hypoglycemia, which has been reported. Daily administration of 25 to 50 g of albumin is usually required for 7 to 10 days to maintain the serum level above 3 g/dL. Antibiotics are administered prophylactically. Analgesics and hypnotics that are detoxified by the liver are used only sparingly.

OPERATIVE PROCEDURES. Control of Bleeding. This may be accomplished by (1) ligation or compression of blood vessels within the substance of the remaining liver segment, (2) efforts directed at the raw surface, and (3) control of the main blood vessels entering the porta hepatis. Omental grafts, peritoneal grafts, Gelfoam, micronized collagen, and rapidly polymerizing adhesives have been applied to the raw surface as local hemostatic agents. Compression of the main vessels entering the liver facilitates the demonstration of bleeding sites along the raw surface. The hepatic artery and portal vein may be compressed for over an hour without affecting hepatic structure or function.

Technique of Resection. On the basis of new concepts of segmental anatomy, the following classification of hepatic resection is applicable (Fig. 30-23): (1) *Subsegmental,* or *wedge, resection* is the removal of an area of the liver that is less than a segment and without an anatomic dissection

Fig. 30-23. Nomenclature for hepatic resection.

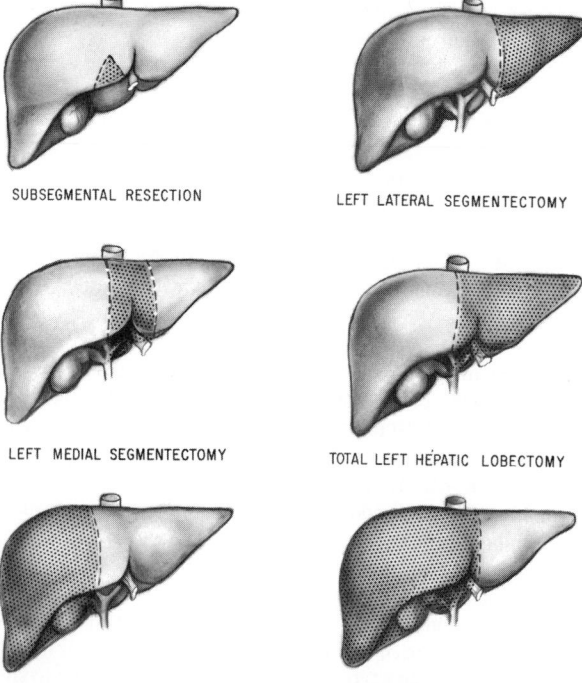

SUBSEGMENTAL RESECTION

LEFT LATERAL SEGMENTECTOMY

LEFT MEDIAL SEGMENTECTOMY

TOTAL LEFT HEPATIC LOBECTOMY

RIGHT LOBECTOMY

EXTENDED RIGHT LOBECTOMY

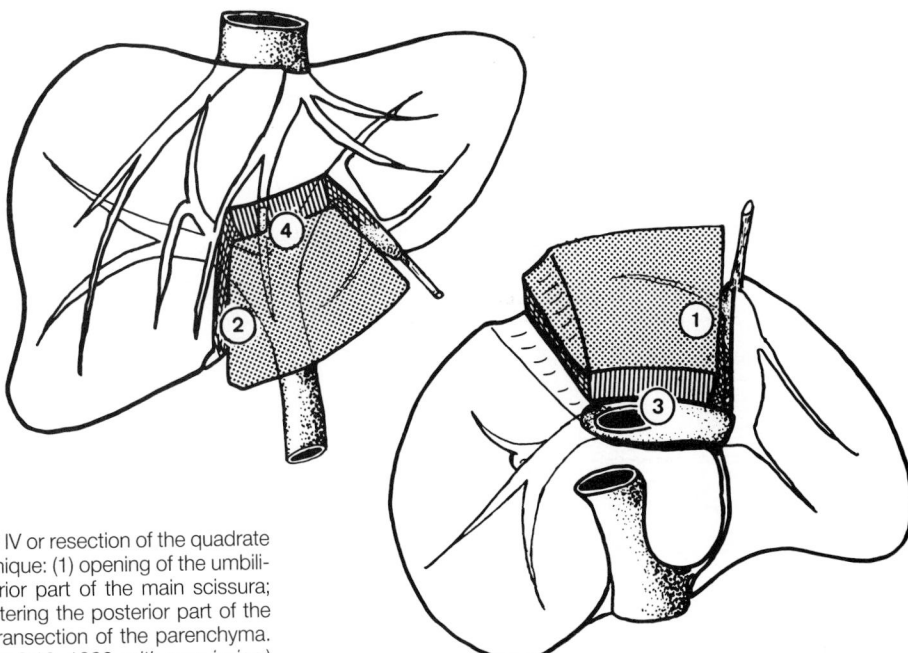

Fig. 30-24. Anterior segmentectomy IV or resection of the quadrate lobe. The different steps of the technique: (1) opening of the umbilical fissure; (2) opening of the anterior part of the main scissura; (3) ligation of the portal pedicles entering the posterior part of the quadrate lobe; and (4) transverse transection of the parenchyma. (From: *Bismuth H et al: World J Surg 6:10, 1982, with permission.*)

plane. (2) *Left lateral segmentectomy* ("left lobectomy" in old nomenclature) is the excision of the liver mass to the left of the left segmental fissure along an anatomic plane. (3) *Left medial segmentectomy* is resection between the main interlobar fissure and the left segmental fissure. (4) *Left lobectomy* is the excision of all hepatic tissue to the left of the main lobar fissure. (5) *Right lobectomy* is the removal of the liver to the right of the main lobar fissure. (6) The *extended right lobectomy* is the excision of the entire right lobe plus the medial segment of the left lobe (*trisegmentectomy*), i.e., excision of all tissue to the right of the umbilical fossa, fossa for the ligamentum venosum, and the ligamentum teres.

Based upon portal distribution, Couinaud has defined eight hepatic segments (see Fig. 30-2). Segmental resections of one or two contiguous segments can be performed by a transparenchymatous approach following the anatomical scissura to the vascular pedicle (Fig. 30-24). These procedures are indicated for (1) benign tumors; (2) some liver trauma; (3) carcinoma of the gallbladder discovered histologically after cholecystectomy; and (4) malignant tumors in patients at risk for liver failure.

The liver is initially mobilized by dividing the appropriate ligamentous attachments, i.e., ligamentum teres and triangular and coronary ligaments (Fig. 30-25). Dissection of the porta hepatis identifies the branches of the hepatic artery, portal vein, and biliary duct system supplying the segment or lobe to be removed (Fig. 30-26). These are individually temporarily occluded. By rotating the liver, the hepatic veins may be isolated at their junctions with the inferior vena cava and ligated (Fig. 30-27). Glisson's capsule is then incised along the surgical plane (Fig. 30-28A), and the cleavage plane of the hepatic parenchyma itself is best established by means of a scalpel handle or

finger to permit exposure of the larger ducts and vessels, which may be individually clamped and ligated as they are encountered. This incision is continued posteriorly until the major hepatic vein or veins are identified (Fig. 30-28B), doubly ligated, and transected. The specimen is removed. The previously occluded structures in the porta hepatis are unclamped and if bleeding or biliary drainage from the raw surface persists, the appropriate structure is ligated. The remaining raw surface may be covered with omentum. The blood flow to and from the remaining segments of the liver must be carefully preserved.

The majority of lobar resections, even right lobe resections, can be carried out transabdominally, and it is not necessary to proceed along the outlined sequence of events for surgical excision. Finger fracture is employed for trauma but is also applied in many instances for tumor. The sequence is summarized in Fig. 30-29. One can reduce the blood flow into the liver by temporarily cross clamping the hepatoduodenal ligament; this procedure can be carried out for 60 min using a vascular clamp intermittently. Glisson's capsule is then incised anteroinferiorly, and the incision is carried down to the region of the porta hepatis. The vessels in the porta hepatis are then picked up in the parenchyma as they enter the liver. The parenchymal dissection is continued along anatomic planes, picking up vessels and ducts as they traverse the liver, until the hepatic venous structures are also picked up in the hepatic parenchyma. An ultrasonic disruption of the parenchyma can be used to isolate vessels as they traverse the resection plane. The operative time is significantly reduced by this technique, and the blood loss is only moderately increased. Trisegmentectomy necessitates anatomic dissection in order to avoid interrupting veins from the remaining segment.

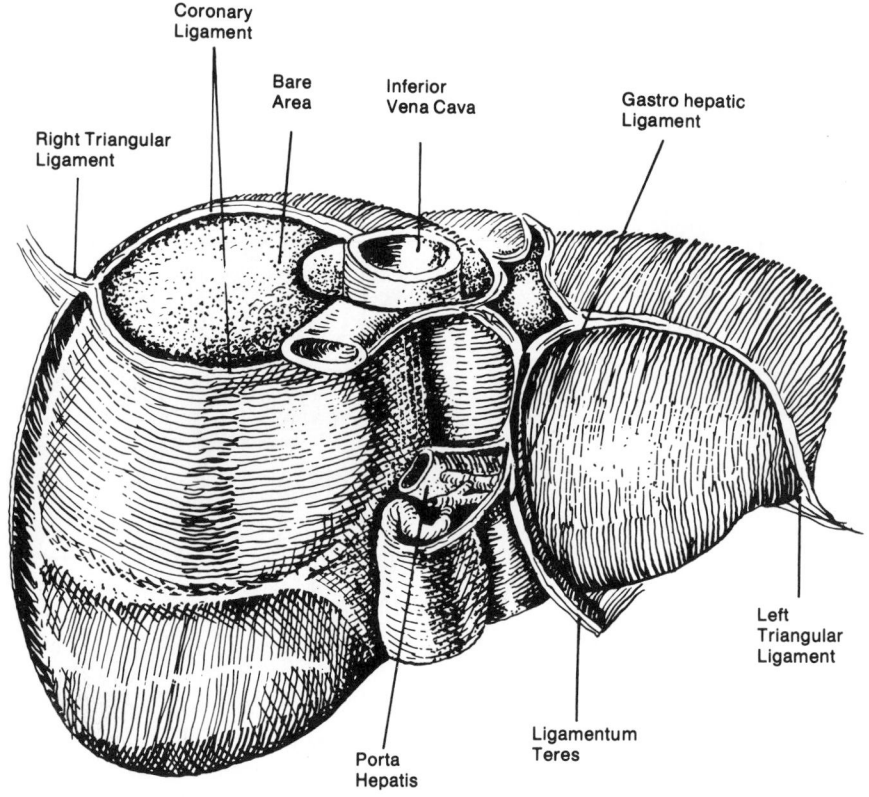

Fig. 30-25. Ligamentous attachments of the liver. (From: *Schwartz SI: Liver resection in Modern Technics in Surgery. Mt Kisco, Futura, 1981, p 10-6, with permission.*)

PORTAL HYPERTENSION

Hypertension within the portal vein and its tributaries may accompany hepatic disease or disturbance in the anatomy of the extrahepatic vascular system. As a consequence of this elevated pressure or in association with it, congestion of collateral pathways is established and may be manifested by esophagogastric varices, ascites, hypersplenism, or encephalopathy.

ETIOLOGY. The etiologic factors implicated in portal hypertension are listed in Table 30-4. Increased hepatopetal flow is an infrequent cause of portal hypertension. Hepatic arterial-portal venous fistula has been reported rarely, and the diagnosis can be established by CT, MRI, or angiography. Successful treatment has been effected by ligation of the hepatic artery or by direct closure of the fistula through an arteriotomy. Splenic arteriovenous fistula is also a relatively uncommon lesion. This has a predilection for females between the ages of twenty and fifty and may become symptomatic during pregnancy. Calcification in the left upper quadrant is suggestive, and aortography may be diagnostic. Resection of the fistula or splenic artery, and splenectomy is therapeutic. An increase in forward blood flow in the portal venous system has also been proposed as the cause of portal hypertension in patients with tropical splenomegaly and myeloid metaplasia. A small group of well-documented cases of bleeding esophageal varices with portal hypertension in the absence of demonstrable intrahepatic or extrahepatic

obstruction may be related to a similar intrasplenic pathology. In patients with increased hepatopetal flow related to splenomegaly, splenectomy alone may be therapeutic.

Since the hepatic veins constitute the sole efferent vascular drainage of the liver, obstruction or increased pressure within these vessels or their radicals results in an increased sinusoidal and portal pressure. This outflow obstruction (Budd-Chiari) syndrome is most frequently associated with an endophlebitis of the hepatic veins, which may be isolated or part of a generalized thrombophlebitis process. A web in the suprahepatic vena cava has been reported to cause the syndrome in Japanese people. The clinical picture depends on the rapidity and degree of venous obstruction. With sudden and complete obstruction, the presentation is that of an abdominal catastrophe with severe abdominal pain, nausea, vomiting, and rapid enlargement of the abdomen by ascites. This rarely occurs. More commonly, obstruction to the hepatic venous system appears to be gradual and is associated with mild to moderate abdominal discomfort and ascites. Treatment demands a side-to-side portal systemic anastomosis, since the portal vein must act as an efferent hepatic conduit. A peritoneovenous shunt has provided relief. If the inferior vena cava is obstructed, a mesenteric-atrial shunt with a conduit may be therapeutic but does not address the intrahepatic congestion. In some

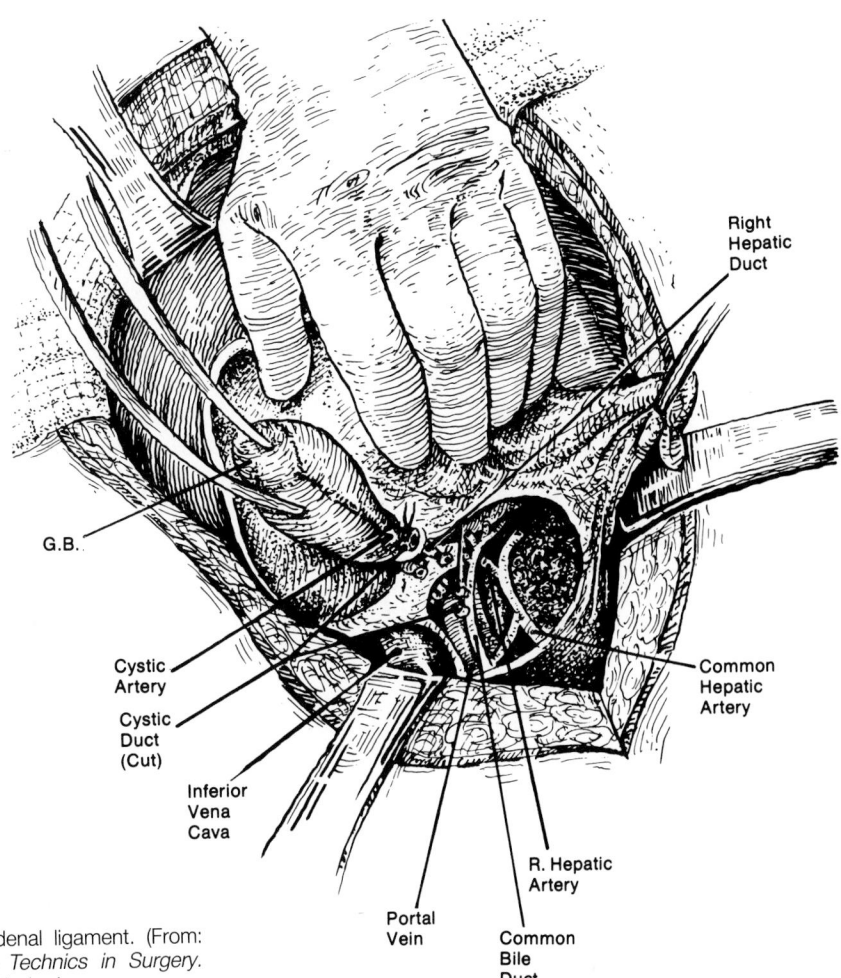

Fig. 30-26. Dissection of the hepatoduodenal ligament. (From: *Schwartz SI: Liver resection, in Modern Technics in Surgery. Mt Kisco, Futura, 1981, p 10-7, with permission.*)

patients the manifestations have disappeared spontaneously.

Portal hypertension secondary to impaired flow in the extrahepatic portal venous system is unique in that the hypertension usually is not complicated by hepatocellular dysfunction. Congenital atresia or hypoplasia, as an extension of the obliterative process of the umbilical vein and ductus venosus, is rare. More commonly, there is a cavernomatous transformation of the portal vein that probably represents organization and recanalization of thrombi within the vessel. The most common etiologic factor in the development of extrahepatic portal venous obstruction in childhood may be some form of infection. Bacteria may be transmitted via a patent umbilical vein, but a history of neonatal omphalitis is rarely obtainable. Extrahepatic obstruction also may be secondary to trauma and extrinsic compression caused by adhesions, inflammatory processes, and tumors. Isolated splenic vein thrombosis, usually a consequence of alcoholic pancreatitis, may cause esophagogastric varices. In this case splenectomy cures the portal hypertension.

The overwhelming majority of cases of portal hypertension is related to an intrahepatic obstruction. This ac-

counts for over 90 percent of patients with portal hypertension in most large series. A variety of hepatic diseases have been implicated, but no single explanation of pathogenesis has proved totally satisfactory. The pathogenic factors include (1) hepatic fibrosis with compression of portal venules, (2) compression by regenerative nodules, (3) increased arterial blood flow, (4) fatty infiltration and acute inflammation, and (5) intrahepatic vascular obstruction. The hepatic diseases associated with portal hypertension include nutritional cirrhosis, postnecrotic cirrhosis, schistosomiasis, biliary cirrhosis, hemochromatosis, Wilson's disease, congenital hepatic fibrosis, and infiltrative lesions.

Nutritional cirrhosis is the most common and has a worldwide distribution. In the western countries, it is frequently associated with chronic alcoholism. As it is true with all intrahepatic lesions, with the exception of congenital hepatic fibrosis and schistosomiasis, the major resistance to the flow of portal blood is located on the hepatic venous side of the sinusoid (postsinusoidal). Postnecrotic cirrhosis accounts for 5 to 12 percent of the cases and represents progression of an acute viral hepatitis or toxic hepatic injury. Frequently a history of viral

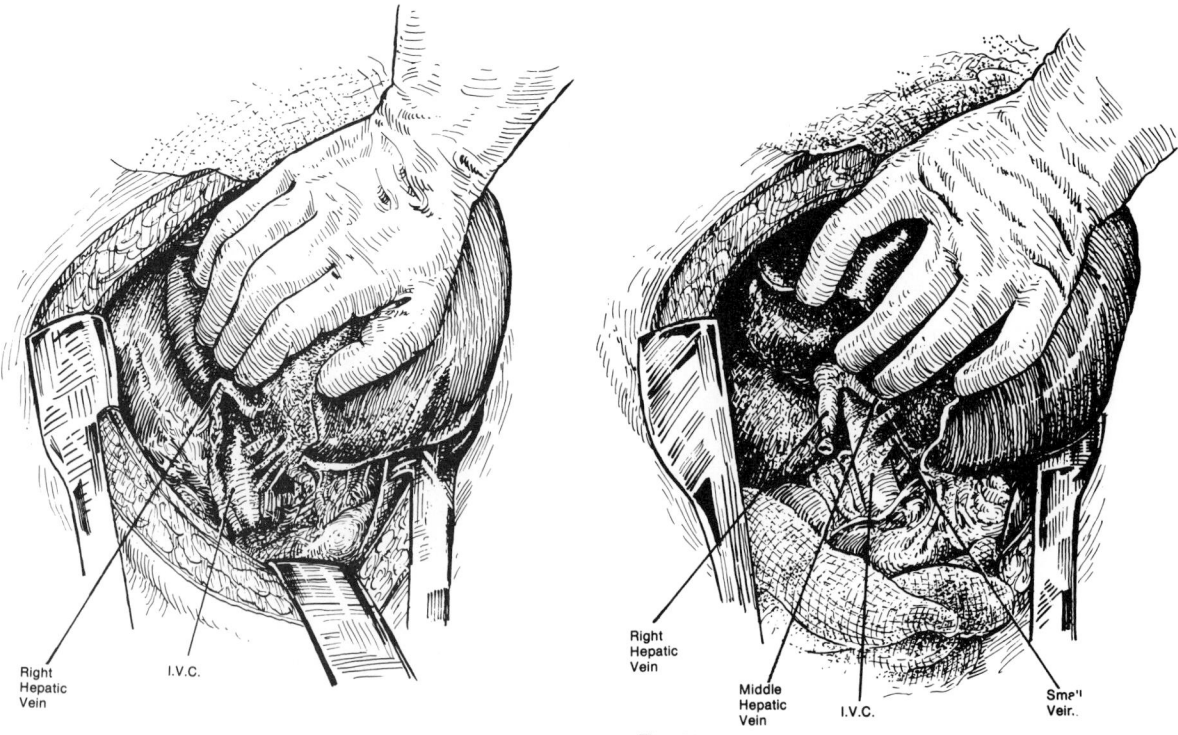

Right
Hepatic
Vein   I.V.C.

Right
Hepatic
Vein

Middle
Hepatic
Vein   I.V.C.   Sme'l
                                   Veir..

Fig. 30-27. Dissection and ligation of hepatic veins draining right lobe of liver. (From: *Schwartz SI: Liver resection, in Modern Technics in Surgery. Mt Kisco, Futura, 1981, p 10-9–10, with permission.*)

infection is not obtainable. Biliary cirrhosis may be due to extrahepatic obstruction and secondary cirrhosis or to a primary hepatic lesion. Advanced portal cirrhosis is an almost invariable feature of hemochromatosis. Wilson's disease (hepatolenticular degeneration) is characterized by alteration of hepatic function and structure and by

Fig. 30-28. *A.* Finger fracture of anteroinferior portion of the liver to isolate portal structures. *B.* Intraparenchymal isolation of hepatic vein. (From: *Schwartz SI: Liver resection, in Modern Technics in Surgery. Mt Kisco, Futura, 1981, pp 10-13–14, with permission.*)

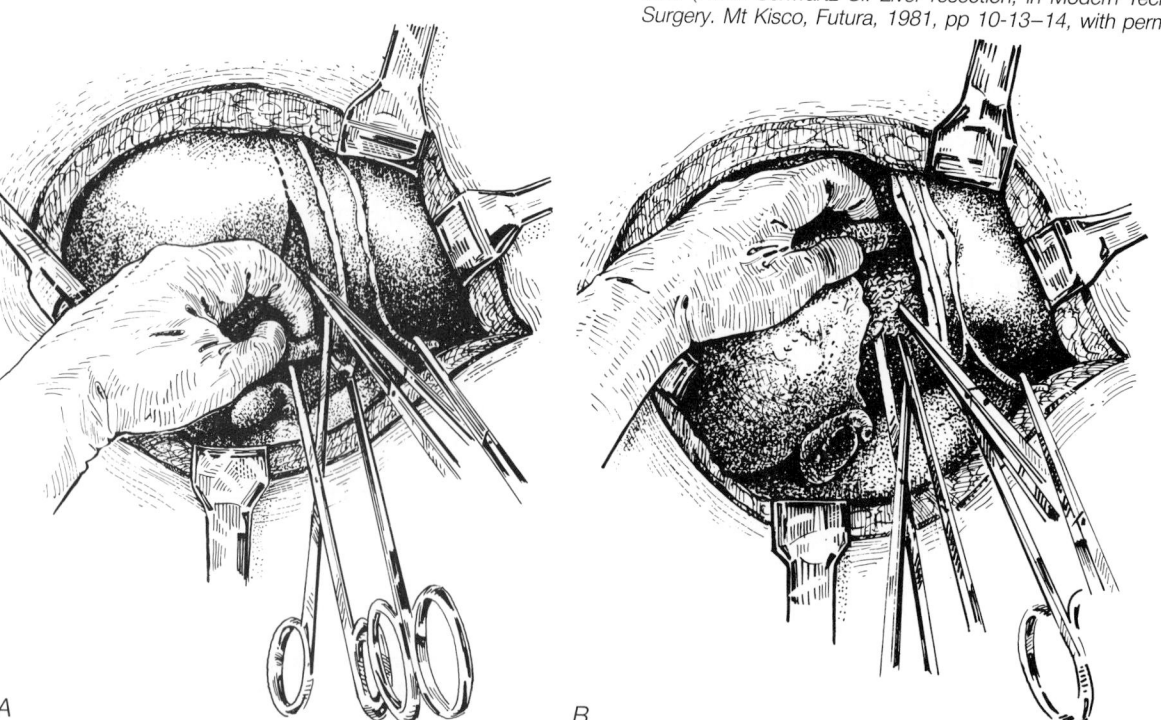

A   *B*

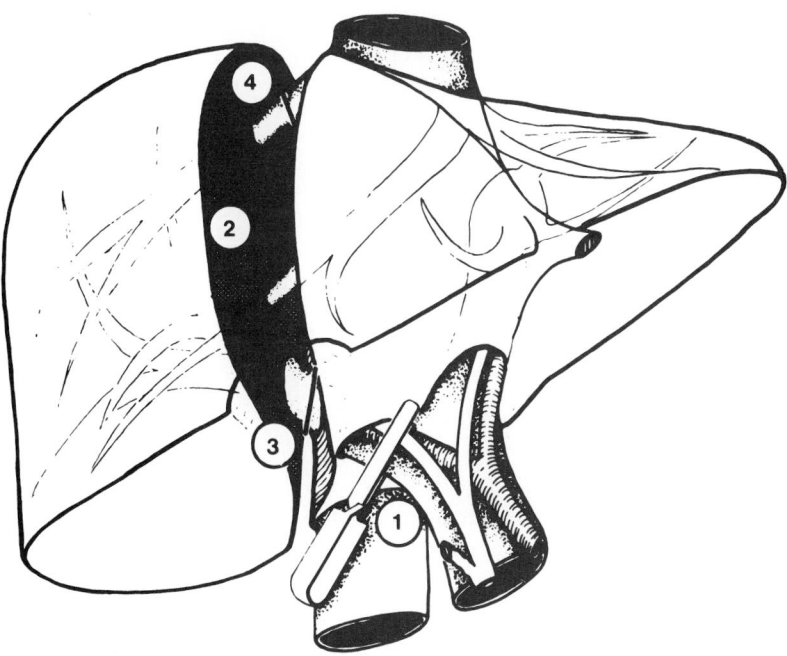

Fig. 30-29. Sequence of events: (1) temporary occlusion of structures in hepatoduodenal ligation; (2) anterior parenchymal dissection; (3) parenchymal dissection of portal structures; and (4) parenchymal dissection of hepatic vein. (From: *Bismuth H: Surgical anatomy and anatomical surgery of the liver. World J Surg 6:3, 1982, with permission.*)

mental deterioration. Congenital hepatic fibrosis may be related to dilatation of the intrahepatic bile ducts. It is usually an autosomal recessive disease. Clinical features include gross enlargement and firm consistency of the liver, accompanied by manifestations of portal hyperten-

Table 30-4. ETIOLOGY OF PORTAL HYPERTENSION

A. Increased hepatopetal flow without obstruction
  1. Hepatic arterial-portal venous fistula
  2. Splenic arteriovenous fistula
  3. Intrasplenic origin
B. Extrahepatic outflow obstruction
  1. Budd-Chiari syndrome
  2. Failure of right side of heart
C. Obstruction of extrahepatic portal venous system
  1. Congenital obstruction
  2. Cavernomatous transformation of portal vein
  3. Infection
  4. Trauma
  5. Extrinsic compression
D. Intrahepatic obstruction
  1. Nutritional cirrhosis
  2. Postnecrotic cirrhosis
  3. Biliary cirrhosis
  4. Other diseases with hepatic fibrosis
    a. Hemochromatosis
    b. Wilson's disease
    c. Congenital hepatic fibrosis
  5. Infiltrative lesions
  6. Venoocclusive diseases
    a. Senecio poisoning
    b. Schistosomiasis

sion and cholangitis. Hepatic function is not disturbed. As hepatic infestation with *Schistosoma mansoni* results in presinusoidal obstruction, there is no impairment of hepatic function until late in the course of the disease.

PATHOPHYSIOLOGY. Portal hypertension refers to an elevated pressure within the portal venous system. This pressure reflects a dynamic, constantly fluctuating force. In addition to diurnal fluctuations, the pressure varies with changes of position, phases of respiration, and intra-abdominal pressure. The normal portal pressure is less than 250 mm of water with a mean value of 215 mm of water. Portal pressure can be assessed by a variety of techniques. During an operative procedure, cannulation of an omental vein or the portal vein itself provides a direct recording. The pressure can also be determined by occlusive catheterization of a hepatic venule (OHVP). This procedure is analogous to determination of pulmonary capillary pressure, in that it is based on the assumption that the occluding catheter creates a static column of blood extending from the hepatic vein to the junction of the hepatic arterial and portal venous streams as they converge in the sinusoidal bed. The procedure is carried out by cardiac catheterization technique and is particularly valuable in the diagnosis of extrahepatic portal obstruction. In this situation, the presinusoidal obstruction is associated with a normal OHVP and an elevated splenic pulp pressure.

In all instances of portal hypertension, splenic pulp pressure is elevated. Intrasplenic pressure is essentially uniform throughout the pulp and is unrelated to the size of the organ. The pressure is usually 2 to 6 mmHg higher than the pressure within the portal vein per se, a function of the direction of venous flow. Splenic pulp manometry is carried out under local anesthesia but is contraindicated in patients with a bleeding tendency, thrombocytopenia, or severe jaundice.

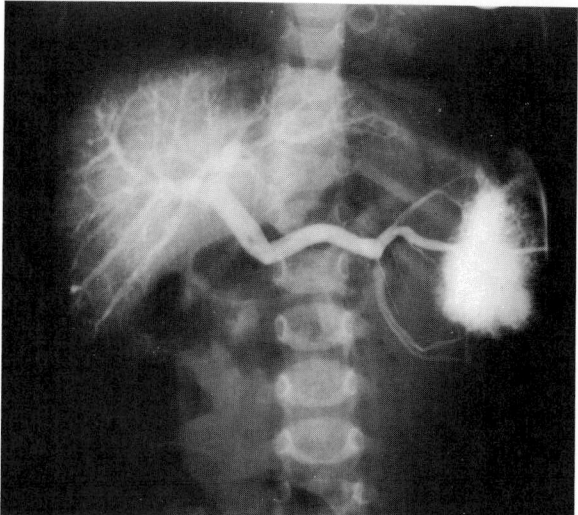

Fig. 30-30. Normal splenoportogram. Note site of injection in spleen and diffusion of radiopaque material through organ. Main splenic vein and two hilar veins are visualized. Portal vein, major branches, and intrahepatic arborization can be seen. No collateral veins are present. Note radiolucency at junction of splenic and superior mesenteric veins. (From: *Schwartz SI: Surgical Diseases of the Liver. New York, McGraw-Hill, 1964, with permission.*)

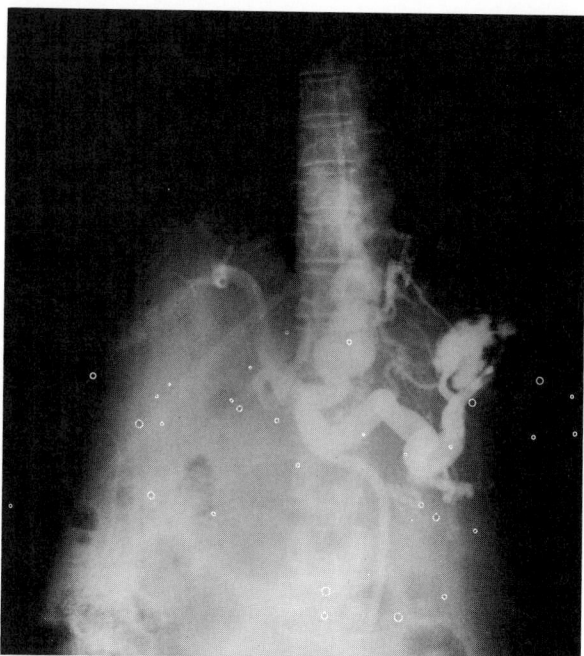

Fig. 30-31. Splenoportogram: portal hypertension secondary to intrahepatic obstruction. Note large tortuous coronary vein and inferior mesenteric vein. Intrahepatic arborization is minimal. (From: *Schwartz SI: Surgical Diseases of the Liver. New York, McGraw-Hill, 1964, with permission.*)

Splenoportography or the venous phase of celiac and superior mesenteric angiography defines the pathologic features of the portal circulation. The studies provide a demonstration of collateral veins, particularly esophagogastric varices. They also provide graphic demonstration of the site of obstruction, i.e., intrahepatic or extrahepatic. Under normal circumstances no collaterals are visualized and a good arborization is noted in the liver (Fig. 30-30). Whenever collaterals are apparent, the diagnosis of portal hypertension is suggested. Usually one can define the coronary vein contributing to esophageal varices by this technique (Fig. 30-31).

The umbilical vein also has been used to outline the portal system. In 80 percent of these cases the obliterated vein can be isolated and dilated to permit passage of a catheter and injection of radiopaque material in the left portal vein. The portal and hepatic veins can also be visualized by percutaneous transhepatic cannulation.

PATHOLOGIC ANATOMY. The collateral vessels (Fig. 30-32) that become functional in cases of portal hypertension are classified in two groups:

1. Hepatopetal circulation occurs only when the intrahepatic vasculature is normal and obstruction is limited to the portal vein. In this situation, the accessory veins of Sappey, the deep cystic veins, the epiploic veins, the hepatocolic and hepatorenal veins, the diaphragmatic veins, and the veins of the suspensory ligaments carry a limited amount of portal venous blood to the liver.
2. Hepatofugal flow is the type most commonly provided by the collateral circulation.

The vessels of the hepatofugal circulation include

1. The coronary vein, which courses to the esophageal veins and thence to the azygos and hemiazygos veins with eventual termination in the superior vena cava.

2. The superior hemorrhoidal veins, which communicate by way of the hemorrhoidal plexus with hemorrhoidal branches of the middle and inferior hemorrhoidal veins and ultimately drain into the inferior vena cava.
3. The umbilical and paraumbilical veins, which communicate with superficial veins of the abdominal wall and anastomose freely with the superior and inferior epigastric veins. Dilatation occurs in 22 percent of patients with portal cirrhosis, and the advanced stage is known as the *caput Medusae*. The cephalad portion of the obliterated umbilical vein may remain patent in adult life or become recanalized, contributing to the Cruveilhier-Baumgarten syndrome.
4. Retroperitoneally, the veins of Retzius, which form an anastomosis between the mesenteric and peritoneal veins and empty directly into the inferior vena cava.

In general, the collateral circulation does not effectively decompress the portal system, and the amount of blood shunted is relatively insignificant. Assuming the cross-sectional diameter of the normal portal vein to be 2 cm, then, according to Poiseuille's law, over 4000 collateral veins $\frac{1}{2}$ cm in diameter will be needed to provide equivalent flow. The highest values of portal pressure are recorded in the group in which collateralization is more marked. In rare instances, spontaneous portal systemic shunts have effectively decompressed the portal system.

Esophagogastric Varices

As the veins become engorged, vessels in the submucosal plexus of the esophagus increase in size and become dilated. In the later stages, the overlying submucosa may disappear and the walls of the vein actually form a lining

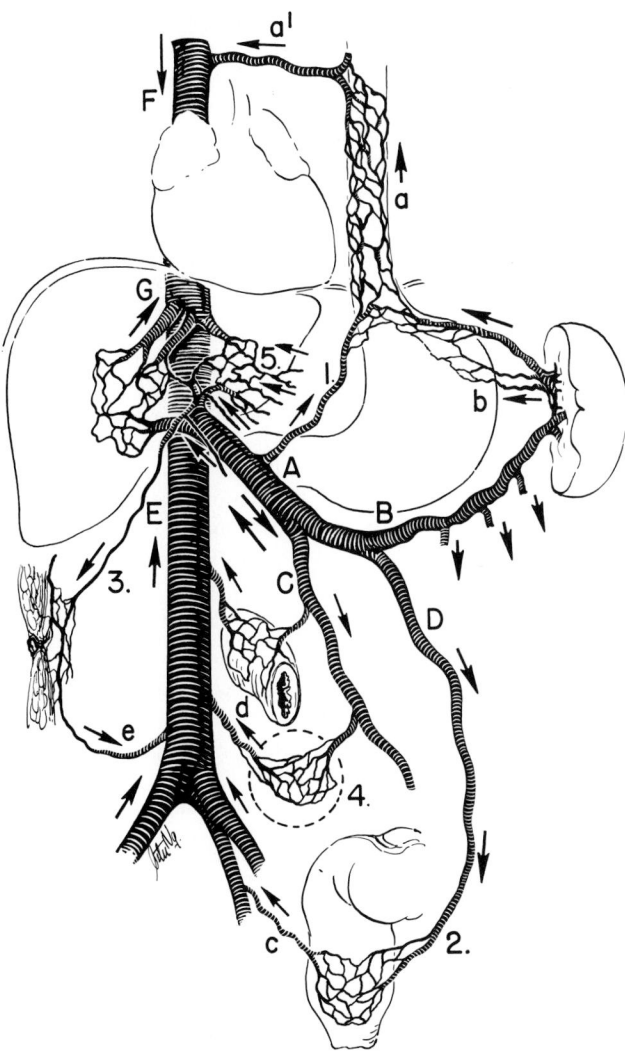

Fig. 30-32. Collateral circulation. 1, Coronary vein; 2, superior hemorrhoidal veins; 3, paraumbilical veins; 4, veins of Retzius; 5, veins of Sappey; A, portal vein; B, splenic vein; C, superior mesenteric vein; D, inferior mesenteric vein; E, inferior vena cava; F, superior vena cava; G, hepatic veins; a, esophageal veins; a¹, azygos system; b, vasa brevia; c, middle and inferior hemorrhoidal veins; d, intestinal; e, epigastric veins. (From: *Schwartz SI: Surgical Diseases of the Liver. New York, McGraw-Hill, 1964, with permission.*)

of the esophagus. The submucosal veins in the fundus and subfundal regions of the stomach also become varicose. Gastric varices occur predominantly in the cardiac end of the stomach but have also been found along the lesser curvature. Varices also have been demonstrated in the duodenum and ileum.

Although the presence of esophagogastric varices is, in itself, of minor consequence, rupture and bleeding from these vessels constitute the most alarming and serious complication of portal hypertension. The varices are almost always associated with portal hypertension but infrequently have occurred in patients with normal pressure. Over 90 percent of adult patients demonstrate intrahepatic disease, whereas in childhood the varices are

usually related to extrahepatic portal obstruction. Precipitation of the bleeding episode has been ascribed to two factors, increased pressure within the varix and ulceration secondary to esophagitis. Regurgitation of gastric juice into the esophagus has been implicated, and ulcers of the esophagus have been demonstrated in 25 percent of nonintubated and 50 percent of intubated patients. The frequency and severity of bleeding also is related to the degree of hepatocellular dysfunction and ingestion of salicylates.

NATURAL COURSE. Bleeding is to be anticipated in approximately 30 percent of cirrhotic patients with demonstrable varices. The elapsed time from the diagnosis of varices to the first hemorrhage varies between 1 and 187 weeks. Almost all hemorrhages occur within 2 years of the initial observation. Etiology is a prime consideration. Varices secondary to extrahepatic portal obstruction must be considered separately, since it is rare for these patients to die of hemorrhage. By contrast, the mortality risk of repeated hemorrhage in patients with esophageal varices secondary to cirrhosis is extremely high. Approximately 70 percent of these patients die within 1 year of the first hemorrhage. Sixty percent of cirrhotic patients who have hemorrhaged once rebleed massively within 1 year.

A prophylactic shunt is not advised for a patient with varices that have not bled, since one cannot predict which patients will bleed; the survival is not improved and encephalopathy may be induced. A cooperative Japanese study group has presented data suggesting that a prophylactic devascularization procedure or selective shunt can prevent bleeding without leading to a significant increase in mortality or morbidity in Child's A and B patients.

ACUTE BLEEDING. In children, massive hematemesis almost always emanates from bleeding varices. Acute hemorrhage is usually the first manifestation of portal hypertension in children. Seventy percent of patients experience their first bleeding episode before the age of seven, and almost 90 percent hemorrhage before the age of ten.

In the adult, bleeding varices comprise one-quarter to one-third of the cases of massive upper gastrointestinal tract bleeding. In cirrhotic patients, varices are the source of bleeding in approximately 50 percent, whereas gastritis is implicated in 30 percent and duodenal ulcers in 9 percent. It is now felt that peptic ulcer does not occur more frequently in cirrhotic patients. Correlation of the lesion with the severity of bleeding reveals that in the majority of cases bleeding from varices is severe hemorrhage, whereas bleeding from gastritis involves only mild to moderate blood loss.

Since the management of bleeding varices differs significantly from that of bleeding due to other causes, it is important to establish a diagnosis on an emergency basis. Physical examination may reveal the stigmata of cirrhosis. Splenomegaly is particularly suggestive of portal hypertension. Tests of hepatic function have been used but do not have uniform reliability. Barium-swallow has a significantly high percentage of false-negative results. In a series of patients with proved varices, radiographic demonstration was present in only half. Celiac or superior mesenteric arteriography will rule out an arterial bleeding site, and the venous phase of the arteriogram will demonstrate collateral venous circulation. Bleeding from a varix is not visualized. A 90 percent correlation has been reported for splenic pulp manometry, but there is a zone of splenic pulp pressures that may be characteristic of patients bleeding from varices or from other causes. Esophageal balloon tamponade has also been used as a diagnostic measure, but varices are controlled in only two-thirds of the patients, and, moreover, peptic ulcer may stop bleeding after the gastric balloon is inflated. Esophagoscopy represents the single most reliable technique, since it alone defines the bleeding point. On the other hand, esophagoscopy may fail to reveal varices because of variations in transvariceal blood flow. In addition, there is a significant observer variation in the endoscopic evaluation of varices.

TREATMENT. The therapeutic regimen is directed at promptly controlling bleeding without further disturbing an already impaired hepatic function. Rapid control is critical in order to avoid the injurious effects of shock on hepatic function and also the toxic effects of absorption of blood from the gastrointestinal tract. The therapeutic approaches may be divided into methods that directly approach the bleeding site and techniques that act indirectly by decreasing portal pressure (Table 30-5).

Balloon tamponade has reduced the mortality and morbidity from bleeding varices in good-risk patients, particularly those in whom the varices were secondary to extrahepatic portal hypertension or compensated cirrhosis. Little change has been noted in the mortality rate for poor-risk patients, and reports have indicated failure to control hemorrhage in 25 to 55 percent of cases. Increasing awareness of the complications associated with this technique, including aspiration, asphyxiation, and ulceration at the site of the tamponade, has reduced its use. Either a four-lumen tube should be used or a small nasogastric tube should be positioned proximal to the esophageal balloon to provide suction and prevent aspiration.

Table 30-5. CONTROL OF ACUTE BLEEDING

A. Nonoperative
   1. Direct: control of bleeding site
      a. Tamponade
      b. Local hypothermia
      c. Esophagoscopic injection of sclerosing solution
      d. Transhepatic sclerosis of coronary vein
   2. Indirect: reduction of portal pressure
      a. Vasopressin
      b. Propranolol
      c. Paracentesis
B. Operative
   1. Direct control of bleeding site
      a. Transesophageal ligation/esophageal transection
      b. Devascularization (Sugiura)
      c. Gastroesophageal resection: colon or jejunum interposition
   2. Indirect: reduction of variceal pressure
      a. Portal-systemic shunt

Endoscopic injection of a sclerosing solution into varices has also successfully controlled bleeding. In a large series, bleeding was controlled in 93 percent of patients. But the results have not been uniformly that successful, and Cello et al. reported that the 30-day mortality was less for a group of Child's C patients who underwent an emergency portacaval shunt than for a matched group treated by sclerotherapy.

Drug therapy to reduce portal hypertension has employed surgical vasopressin, which acts by constricting the splanchnic arterial circulation and consequently reducing portal pressure and flow by approximately 40 percent. The drug is contraindicated in patients with angina, since generalized vasoconstriction results. Effective control has accompanied direct infusion of vasopressin, 0.2 unit/mL per minute, into the superior mesenteric artery. Equal efficacy has been achieved with the same dosage administered into a peripheral vein. Isoproterenol may be given to reduce the hemodynamic hazards of vasopressin related to its potential effect on the cardiac output. Propranolol has been used to prevent recurrent bleeding by reducing cardiac output. Paracentesis in a patient with bleeding varices and tense ascites will immediately reduce portal pressure.

Surgical therapy includes transesophageal ligation and emergency portal-systemic shunt. The results of transesophageal ligation have not been uniformly encouraging, and in cirrhotic patients the procedure has been accompanied by a high incidence of recurrent bleeding. Devascularization procedures such as Sugiura's have had variable success. Success rates from Western nations have not matched the Japanese success.

A more liberal use of emergency portacaval shunts to stop bleeding has been advised for the cirrhotic patients whose bleeding cannot be controlled by tamponade or vasopressin. The base figure that serves as a frame of reference for comparison is the mortality for patients with bleeding varices not subjected to emergency portacaval shunts, and this ranges between 66 and 73 percent. There is little question that an effective portal-systemic decompressive procedure almost always stops bleeding. A review of reported experiences indicates that so-called emergency shunts are associated with survival for immediate hospitalization in 50 to 71 percent of cases, despite a more liberal attitude toward acceptability of patients in reference to their liver profile. Orloff and his associates have reported an operative survival of 48 percent and an actuarial 7-year survival of 42 percent in consecutive, unselected patients with alcoholic cirrhosis and bleeding varices operated on within 8 h of admission to hospital. In regard to selection of patients, reported results could not be correlated with the patient's liver function profile in some series. No significance could be attributed to the presence or absence of jaundice, but ascites, when present, was associated with a marked reduction of survival rate.

In the pediatric age group, despite the fact that the bleeding is often alarming, spontaneous cessation almost always occurs, and esophageal tamponade or vasopressin is rarely necessary. Hospitalization, bed rest, blood replacement, and sedation almost always suffice for patients with bleeding secondary to extrahepatic portal obstruction.

The majority of patients with acute bleeding varices is not in shock at the time of admission to the hospital, although the hematocrit is often reduced and blood replacement may be necessary. Fresh blood or frozen red blood cells and fresh-frozen plasma should be employed for transfusing cirrhotic patients. This provides the clotting factors that are frequently diminished in the presence of hepatic disease and avoids the increased ammonia content and diminished platelet and prothrombin supply characteristic of old blood. There is a linearly progressive daily increment of 35 μg/dL of ammonia nitrogen in banked blood, which can be responsible for exogenous hepatic coma. Therapy directed at preventing hyperammonemia and hepatic coma consists primarily of removing blood from the gastrointestinal tract. Catharsis, gastric lavage, and enemas are employed. If vasopressin has been administered, it will induce intestinal motility and effect a catharsis. A reduction in intestinal bacterial flora also contributes to the prevention of coma, and nonabsorbable antibiotic therapy is used to accomplish this.

PREVENTION OF RECURRENT HEMORRHAGE. The case for surgical intervention is based on the precept that a patient who has bled from esophageal varices is likely to rebleed and that subsequent bleeding episodes are associated with a higher mortality than an elective operative procedure.

A difference of opinion exists regarding the role of decompressive procedures in children with portal hypertension due to extrahepatic portal venous thrombosis. Some children can be treated satisfactorily and safely without operation despite repeated episodes of variceal bleeding. The results of operation in terms of survival are significantly more encouraging in this population than in adults. Therefore, many series have suggested an aggressive approach in children with recurrent bleeding episodes. The central splenorenal shunt or an anastomosis between the inferior vena cava and superior mesenteric vein is applicable to this group of patients. The incidence of postoperative encephalopathy has been negligible.

Presinusoidal obstruction (hepatic fibrosis, extrahepatic portal venous thrombosis, schistosomiasis) is characterized by portal hypertension and may be associated with normal hepatic function. In patients with hepatic fibrosis and extrahepatic portal venous obstruction the results are gratifying; the surgical procedure will generally prevent subsequent bleeding and provide the patient with an essentially normal life expectancy. The patients with schistosomiasis are a unique group in that they are extremely liable to postshunt encephalopathy. A selective splenorenal shunt or devascularization procedure is the preferred operation.

Postsinusoidal portal hypertension is invariably complicated by impaired hepatic function. The role of decompressive procedures is least well defined for this group of cirrhotic patients. Elective procedure should be considered when the presence of an active intrahepatic process such as hyaline necrosis or acute fatty infiltration has

been ruled out. Ascites that fails to respond to medical therapy, a prothrombin time that remains prolonged following parenteral administration of vitamin K, a serum bilirubin above 3 mg/dL, a BSP retention greater than 20 percent, and a serum albumin level less than 2.5 g/dL are all associated with a poor postoperative prognosis. In these patients there is immediate deterioration following portacaval shunting, but this is actually no greater than after other operations of comparable severity. Child's criteria and other assessments of hepatic function are not completely predictive and relate only to the immediate postoperative course.

Two randomized series have been reported. The Cooperative Study of the Veterans Administration randomized cirrhotic patients who had at least one major gastrointestinal hemorrhage and were considered suitable for an operative procedure. Increased survival rate was noted in the group of patients who were operated upon. By contrast, the Boston Interhospital Liver Group's study of patients on whom a therapeutic portacaval shunt had been performed showed that recurrent variceal bleeding could be prevented but that greater longevity could not be expected for these patients. Increased survival following shunting procedures in patients with a single major variceal hemorrhage remained a statistical possibility. It has been shown that better results are to be anticipated in patients with biliary cirrhosis than in those with nutritional, alcoholic, or cryptogenic cirrhosis.

Ascites

ETIOLOGY. The mechanisms contributing to the formation of ascites are complex and incompletely understood. Portal hypertension is regarded as a contributory but minor factor, since there is no correlation between the degree of portal hypertension and the extent of ascites. Ascites is not a usual accompaniment of extrahepatic portal venous obstruction but has been noted occasionally. Impairment of hepatic venous outflow with subsequent congestion of the liver is the experimental method most consistently used to produce ascites. This lesion is accompanied by an increase in the size of lymphatic vessels and increased production of the hepatic lymph that extravasates through the capsule of the liver into the peritoneal cavity. In clinical cirrhosis, there is an increase in the size of hepatic channels and an augmented flow of thoracic duct lymph. Two distinct patterns of intrahepatic vasculature have been correlated with the presence or absence of ascites. With irreversible ascites, there is an absolute decrease in the hepatic venous bed and a concomitant increase in both the portal venous and hepatic arterial beds. By contrast, when cirrhosis is unaccompanied by ascites, there is a deficit in all vascular systems.

Reduced serum osmotic pressure related to hypoalbuminemia does exert some influence. The response of patients to albumin infusion is variable, and the reduced osmotic pressure may represent the result rather than the cause of fluid accumulation. The most profound biochemical change that accompanies the formation of ascites is the retention of sodium and water. There is evidence that the adrenal cortical hormone is a factor in the renal retention of sodium, and higher concentrations of antidiuretic substances have been noted in the urine of patients with cirrhosis and ascites.

TREATMENT. Bed rest reduces the functional demand on the liver. A diet high in calories with an excess of carbohydrates and proteins, supplemented by vitamins, is directed toward improving hepatic function, while low sodium (10 to 20 meq daily) intake is essential. Fluid is usually not restricted, and potassium supplements are routinely provided to treat the potassium depletion that accompanies the formation of ascites.

Chlorothiazide is usually used to initiate diuretic therapy, and approximately two-thirds of patients will respond to this medication. Potassium supplements are required. The aldosterone antagonists are employed for patients with incipient hepatic coma. Abdominal paracentesis as an initial procedure has diagnostic value, but repeated procedures are contraindicated, since they deplete the body of protein and contribute to the development of systemic hyponatremia. Furosemide (Lasix) is the most frequently used drug. In some refractory cases ethacrynic acid will help.

Emphasis on the importance of obstruction of hepatic venous outflow led to the proposal of side-to-side portacaval shunts as a method of therapy. These procedures were based on the hypothesis of providing a second outflow tract with the portal vein acting as a hepatofugal conduit. At present, the operation is limited to patients with Budd-Chiari syndrome and to those patients who cannot be managed on a strict low-sodium diet and diuretic therapy, an unusual circumstance. Peritoneal venous shunts of the Leveen and Denver types have effectively controlled medically intractable ascites. Improvement may be related to increased creatinine clearance and normalization of renin activity and aldosterone levels. Adverse consequences of the procedures include disseminated intravascular coagulopathy and initiation of variceal bleeding.

Umbilical herniorraphy in a cirrhotic patient with marked ascites presents a significant risk, with hazards of leakage of ascitic fluid, infection, necrosis of the abdominal wall, and variceal bleeding due to interruption of collateral veins.

Hypersplenism

Splenomegaly, with engorgement of the vascular spaces, frequently accompanies portal hypertension. There is little correlation between the size of the spleen and the degree of hypertension. When hematologic abnormalities occur, they have been related to sequestration and destruction of the circulating cells by immune mechanisms mediated by the enlarged spleen or secretion by the hyperactive spleen of a substance that inhibits bone marrow activity. The patient may demonstrate reduction of any or all of the cellular elements of blood. The usual criteria are a white blood cell count below 4000 and a platelet count below 100,000/mm³. Schistosomal fibrosis frequently induces hypersplenism, which is best deter-

mined by the size of the spleen. No correlation exists between degree of anemia or leukopenia and the 5-year survival rate in patients. Splenectomy is rarely indicated and does not permanently reduce portal pressure. Removal of the spleen negates the possibility of performing a selective shunt. Decompression of the portal venous system is rarely indicated for treatment of hypersplenism alone. Significant hypersplenism in a patient undergoing elective surgical treatment for bleeding varices favors a splenorenal anastomosis, but both portacaval anastomosis and selective splenorenal shunt have been accompanied by reduction of the spleen and correction of the hypersplenism in about two-thirds of the cases.

Hepatic Coma

The development of neuropsychiatric symptoms and signs is related to natural and surgically created portal-systemic shunts and is identified by the term *portal-systemic encephalopathy*. This rarely occurs in patients with obstruction of the extrahepatic portal venous system without hepatocellular dysfunction. The neuropsychiatric syndrome usually is associated with cirrhosis and occurs in patients with marked hepatic dysfunction. Postshunt encephalopathy rarely occurs in patients with extrahepatic portal obstruction unaccompanied by hepatic dysfunction. Operative procedures that decompress the portal system have also been associated with varying incidences of encephalopathy in cirrhotic patients. With splenorenal anastomoses, the syndrome is demonstrated in 5 to 19 percent, while it has been reported in 11 to 38 percent following a portacaval anastomosis. The Warren distal splenorenal shunt has been associated with a reduced incidence of postoperative encephalopathy, compared with portacaval and mesocaval shunts.

Hepatic coma has been related to hyperammonemia and ammonia intoxication (Fig. 30-33). Both exogenous and endogenous sources contribute to the blood ammonia level. Dietary protein is the usual source of intestinal ammonia. In patients who bleed, blood within the intestinal tract is also converted into ammonia by bacteria. In the patient with hepatic disease, the ammonia formed within the intestine is carried to the liver but because of hepatic dysfunction cannot enter the Krebs-Henseleit (ornithine-citrulline-arginine) cycle. Endogenous urea produced within the gastrointestinal tract also represents an important source of ammonia, and gastric ammonia production from urea is a significant factor in patients with azotemia and cirrhosis. Galambos and associates have reported a randomized trial in which there was less deterioration of maximum urea synthesis following a selective splenorenal shunt than after total shunts.

In the cirrhotic patient with portal hypertension, the two factors implicated in the disturbed ammonia metabolism are impairment of hepatocellular function and portal-systemic collateralization. The blood ammonia level is also raised by increased ammonia production by the kidneys and increased ammonia production by muscles that are actively contracting during delirium tremens. The neuropsychiatric manifestations involve the state of con-

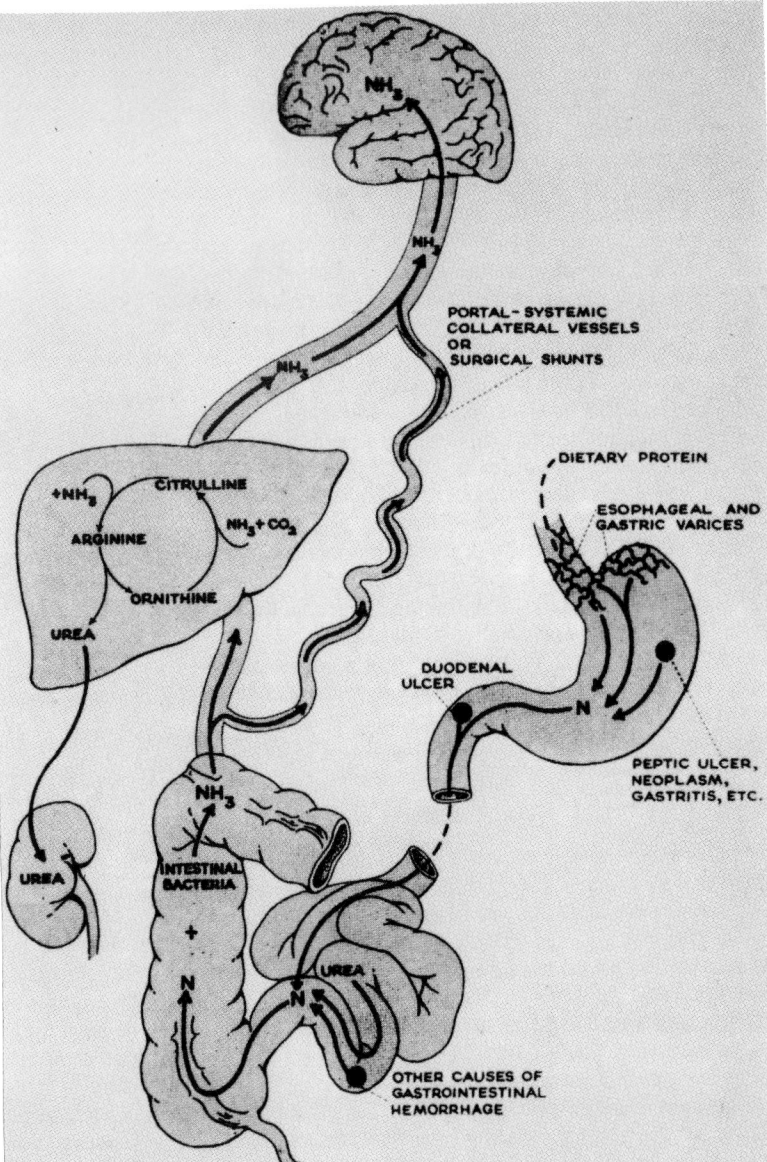

Fig. 30-33. A summary of normal and abnormal aspects of ammonia metabolism. Dietary protein is the normal primary source of intestinal nitrogen However, when gastrointestinal bleeding occurs, the blood that accumulates within the intestine may become an important source of intestinal nitrogen. Urea, which is excreted in part into the gastrointestinal tract, also adds to the intestinal nitrogen pool. All these nitrogen-containing compounds are converted into ammonia by the numerous bacteria within the colon. This ammonia is absorbed into the portal circulation and, under normal conditions, is rapidly removed in the liver by the formation of urea, which is excreted by the kidneys. This mechanism of detoxification of ammonia is so efficient that little or no ammonia can be found in the peripheral blood. Because of the important role of the liver in the detoxification of ammonia, (1) a decrease in hepatic function or (2) a bypass of the liver associated with (a) the development of portal systemic collaterals or (b) surgical shunting procedures will result in an increase in concentrations of ammonia in the peripheral blood, which will exert its toxic effects on the central nervous system. (From: Najarian et al: Am J Surg 96:172, 1958, with permission.)

sciousness, motor activity, and deep tendon reflexes. These have been divided into three stages: delirium, stupor, and coma. In the early stages there is mental confusion and exaggerated reflexes. The characteristic ''liver flap'' may be elicited. In the second stage, there is an accentuation of muscular hypertonicity, to the extent of rigidity, and in the final stage there is complete flaccidity. The electroencephalogram is a sensitive indicator of portal-systemic encephalopathy, and the changes antedate clinical manifestations. Blood ammonia level does not define precisely the nature of material measured by standard tests. In patients with hepatic coma, the concentration of ammonia in the blood has correlated well with the clinical progress in over 90 percent of the cases. An elevated level, over 125 μg/dL, is usually associated with

the clinical features of hepatic coma. Treatment with antibiotics negates the value of the test.

TREATMENT. Treatment is directed at (1) reducing nitrogenous material within the intestinal tract, (2) reducing the production of ammonia from this nitrogenous material, and (3) increasing ammonia metabolism. Since ammonia is an end product of protein metabolism, dietary protein must be drastically reduced to 50 g daily or less. Glucose is included in the diet, since it inhibits ammonia production by bacteria. Gastrointestinal hemorrhage frequently precipitates portal-systemic encephalopathy with blood acting as a source of ammonia. A major factor in the prophylaxis of hepatic coma is prompt control of active bleeding. Potassium supplements are administered, particularly in patients who are receiving thiazide diuretics, since the rise in blood ammonia that accompanies diuresis has been related to hypokalemia.

The protein substrate on which bacteria can act may be initially reduced by using cathartics and enemas to purge the gastrointestinal tract. If active bleeding has occurred, infused vasopressin plays a dual role in temporarily stopping the bleeding as well as stimulating motility and evacuation of the intestine. Bacteria within the bowel are reduced by administering nonabsorbable antibiotics such as neomycin or kanamycin. In the presence of renal disease, kanamycin is preferred since there is less associated renal toxicity. For patients with severe renal impairment, chlortetracycline is more appropriate since it is not excreted primarily by the kidneys. Lactulose acts as a mild cathartic, and the products of its oxidation by bacteria include lactic and acetic acids, which lower the colonic pH and interfere with ammonia transfer across colonic mucosa. This drug has produced encouraging results in the treatment of hepatic encephalopathy.

Since the colon is the site of most ammonia absorption into the portal circulation, partial colectomy has been suggested as treatment of intractable encephalopathy. Resnick and associates studied a matched group of patients, randomly selecting half the group for colon bypass. The longevity figures for the two groups were identical, and the dietary protein tolerance and encephalopathy control only slightly favored the bypass group.

Surgery of Portal Hypertension

The surgical therapy of portal hypertension may be divided into two major categories: (1) procedures that directly attack a manifestation of portal hypertension, such as bleeding varices or ascites; and (2) procedures aimed at decreasing the portal hypertension and/or portal venous flow (Table 30-6).

TRANSESOPHAGEAL LIGATION OF VARICES AND ESOPHAGEAL TRANSECTION. Using either a transthoracic or transabdominal approach, transesophageal ligation of varices and esophageal transection have been directed at controlling bleeding varices. The end-to-end stapler has facilitated the procedure. The procedures do provide temporary control, particularly in children with extrahepatic portal block who are too small to be considered for splenorenal anastomosis. However, control is not prolonged. In patients without cirrhosis, recurrent bleeding has been reported in 28 percent, while among the cirrhotic group approximately 50 percent of survivors have recurrent bleeding. The operative mortality rate associated with this procedure is high, but it must be appreciated that the technique generally is applied to the poorest-risk patients.

Technique. Transthoracic ligation (Fig. 30-34) is performed through the eighth left intercostal space. The lower esophagus is freed, but the esophageal hiatus of the diaphragm is not disturbed. An umbilical tape is tightened around the esophagus just above the hiatus in order to minimize bleeding. A 7-cm longitudinal incision is made through all layers, and three tortuous columns of veins, coursing longitudinally and communicating with one an-

Table 30-6. OPERATIVE PROCEDURES

I. Control of manifestation
  A. Bleeding varices
    1. Ligation of varices
      a. Transthoracic
      b. Transabdominal
    2. Transection procedures
      a. Gastric
      b. Esophageal (stapler)
      c. Esophageal, with paraesophageal devascularization
    3. Resection of varix-bearing area-esophagogastrectomy
      a. Roux en Y
      b. Jejunal interposition
      c. Colonic interposition
      d. Reversed gastric tube
  B. Ascites
    1. Peritoneal cavity–venous shunt
II. Reduction of portal pressure and flow
  1. Splenectomy
  2. Portacaval shunt
    a. End-to-side
      (1) End-to-side shunt with arterialization of the portal vein stump
    b. Side-to-side
    c. H graft
  3. Splenorenal shunt
    a. End-to-end
    b. End-to-side
    c. Distal (selective)
  4. Superior mesenteric–inferior vena cava shunt
    a. Side-to-end
    b. H graft

other, are obliterated with continuous locking sutures of 3-0 chromic catgut. The esophagotomy is closed in two layers with interrupted silk sutures and the edges of the defect in the mediastinal pleura are reapproximated. Direct ligation of varices can be performed transabdominally.

For transection of the esophagus, the peritoneal cavity is entered and the esophagogastric junction is exposed. The lower 3 cm of the esophagus is mobilized, and care is taken to avoid the vagus nerves. The periesophageal veins are ligated. A high, vertical incision is made in the anterior wall of the stomach, and the EEA stapler is inserted, using the largest size cartridge possible. The esophagus is tied over the center rod 2 cm above the gastric junction. The instrument is fired, resulting in simultaneous transection and reanastomosis of the esophagus (Fig. 30-35).

ESOPHAGEAL TRANSECTION WITH PARAESOPHAGEAL DEVASCULARIZATION. The procedure introduced by Sugiura (Fig. 30-36) has been applied to over 3000 cases of bleeding varices. The perioperative mortality was about 7 percent in elective cases and 25 percent in emergency cases. Hepatic function was not compromised, and postoperative encephalopathy did not occur. Unfortunately, American studies have not duplicated these results. The initial and late mortality rates were high, and over half the patients re-bled. The procedure consists of

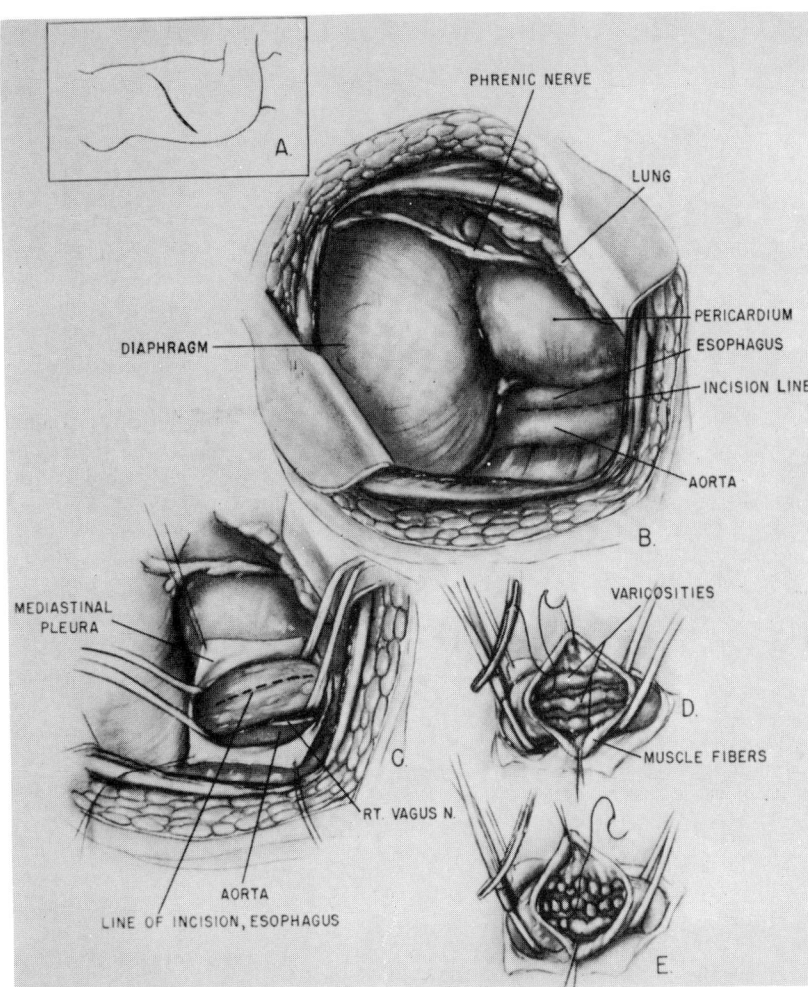

Fig. 30-34. Transthoracic transesophageal ligation. *A.* Left eighth intercostal space incision. Patient in right lateral decubitus position. *B.* Pulmonary ligament has been divided to permit retraction of lung, and line of incision in mediastinal pleura is outlined. *C.* Mediastinal pleura is incised, esophagus is mobilized, and line of incision in esophagus is outlined. *D.* Umbilical tape is tightened around esophagus just above hiatus to minimize bleeding, and edges of esophageal incision are retracted by stay sutures. *E.* The tortuous columns of esophageal veins are obliterated with continuous locked suture of 3-0 chromic catgut swaged on an atraumatic needle. (From: *Schwartz SI: Surgical Diseases of the Liver. New York, McGraw-Hill, 1964, with permission.*)

esophageal transection and paraesophagogastric devascularization, splenectomy, and either selective vagotomy and pyloroplasty or highly selective vagotomy without pyloroplasty.

PROCEDURES FOR REDUCTION OF PORTAL PRESSURE. The operations directed at portal hypertension are based on the consideration that any reduction in portal pressure should decrease the potential for bleeding from varices. Splenectomy is effective only when portal hypertension is due to splenic vein thrombosis or increased flow, as in the massive splenomegaly of myeloproliferative disorders. Reduction of portal pressure by diffuse shunts between a high-pressure portal venous system and low-pressure systemic circulation was attempted. These procedures included omentopexy, posterior mediastinal packing, and transposition of the spleen into the thoracic cavity. Application of Poiseuille's law would suggest that any diffuse shunting would be less effective than a major portal systemic shunt.

Functionally, portal-systemic shunts have been categorized as either totally or partially diverting portal venous flow away from the liver and also as decompressing or failing to decompress intrahepatic venous hypertension

(Fig. 30-37). The end-to-side portacaval shunt prevents blood from reaching the liver by providing complete drainage of the splanchnic venous circulation to the vena cava. The associated alteration of hepatic blood flow is extremely variable, ranging from an increase of 34 percent to a decrease of 53 percent. This shunt also prevents the portal vein from serving as an efferent conduit from the liver. It has been shown that following the end-to-side shunt, the wedged hepatic vein pressure declines. Proponents of the end-to-side shunt have indicated this as the best method of preventing recurrent bleeding from varices, since it most completely decompresses the portal venous system's splanchnic circulation. In refutation, it has been shown that end-to-side and side-to-side portacaval shunts demonstrate equal flow and equivalent reductions of portal pressure.

The concept that the side-to-side portacaval shunt provides the liver with portal venous flow is erroneous in most circumstances. Injection of radioisotope into the distal portal vein results in minimal recovery in the portal vein cephalad to a side-to-side anastomosis. Accumulated evidence indicates that the side-to-side portacaval shunt converts the cephalad portion of the portal vein to an out-

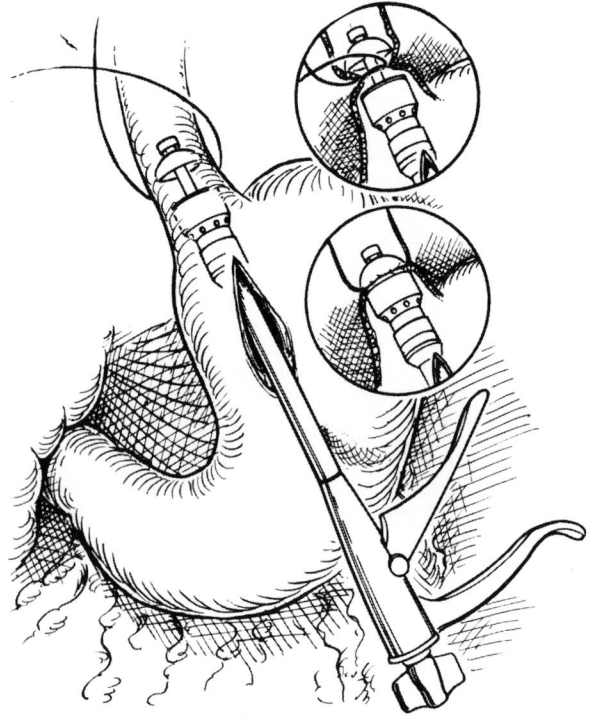

Fig. 30-35. The EEA stapler is introduced and the esophagus securely tied over the center rod 2 cm above the gastric junction. The instrument gap is closed and the trigger fired, completing the simultaneous transection and reanastomosis. (From: *Wexler MJ: Surgery 88:406, 1980, with permission.*)

flow tract from the liver. This is an important feature in patients with Budd-Chiari syndrome. Whether decompression of sinusoidal hypertension is greater with the side-to-side shunt than with the end-to-side shunt has not been defined. There is also concern whether the portal vein is beneficial or harmful as an efferent conduit, because of a possible siphon effect that may reduce the blood available to the hepatic cell.

The classic end-to-side splenorenal shunt using the central end of the splenic vein also prevents the flow of portal venous blood to the liver if it adequately performs its prescribed function of decompressing esophagogastric varices. The other functional side-to-side shunts, including the end-to-side inferior vena cava–superior mesenteric shunt and the interposition of an H graft between these vessels, do not maintain hepatic perfusion with portal venous blood.

The distal splenorenal shunt proposed by Warren and associates is the one procedure that can be classified as truly selective, because it decompresses esophagogastric varices while maintaining portal hypertension within the portal veins and hepatic sinusoids. Portal perfusion has been demonstrated in over 90 percent of patients with selective distal splenorenal shunts; the total hepatic blood flow has been shown to be unchanged, while the splenic venous circulation and esophagogastric veins have been reasonably decompressed. Angiographic and other studies have demonstrated that the distal splenorenal shunt loses its selectivity a few months after the operation. Prospective randomized trials comparing the distal

Fig. 30-36. Illustration of esophageal transection with paraesophagogastric devascularization (Sugiura procedure). (From: *Sugiura M, Futagawa S: Arch Surg 112:1317, 1977. Copyright 1977, American Medical Association.*)

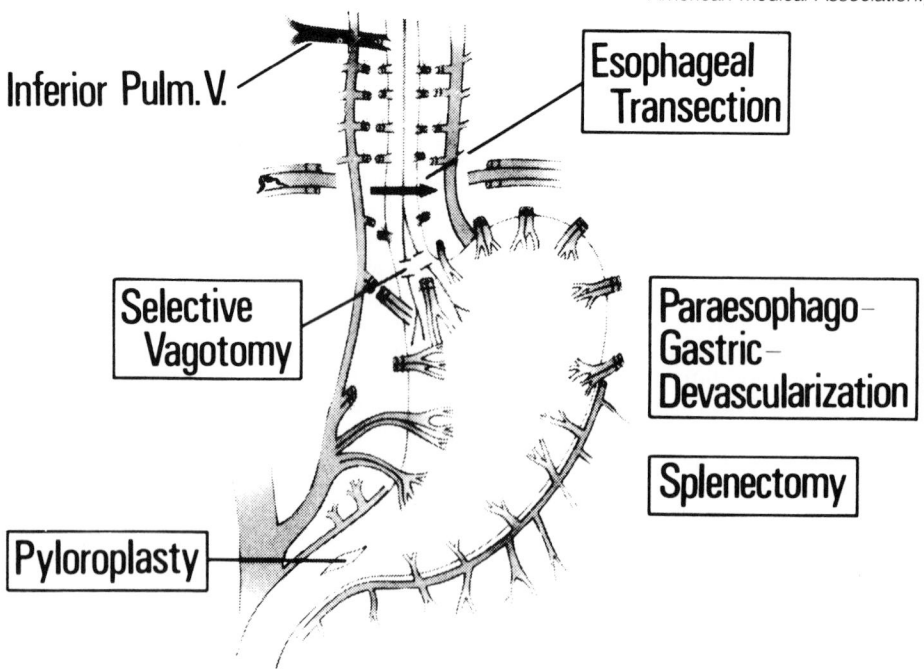

Inferior Pulm. V.

Esophageal Transection

Selective Vagotomy

Paraesophago-Gastric-Devascularization

Splenectomy

Pyloroplasty

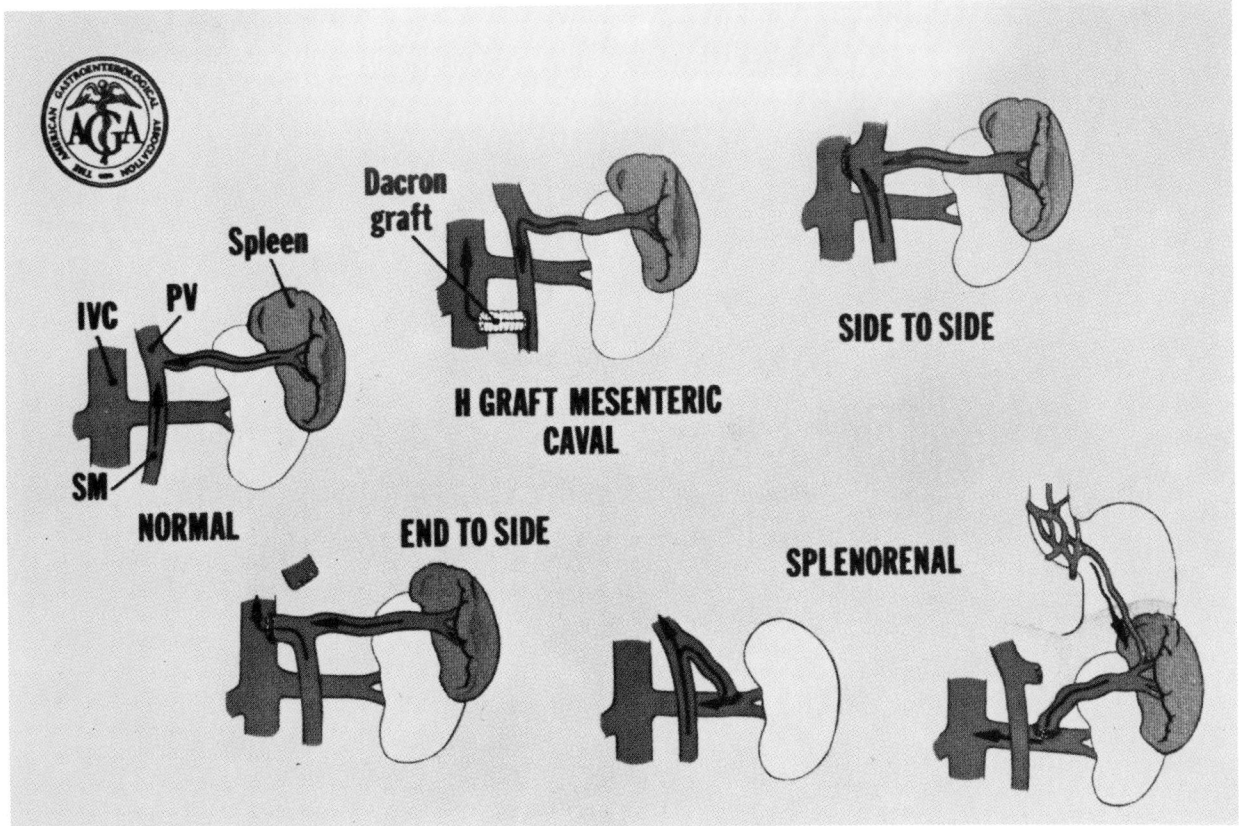

Fig. 30-37. Surgical portacaval shunts.

splenorenal shunt with nonselective (portacaval or mesocaval) shunts demonstrate no difference in survival, postoperative complications, or ascites. It is generally felt that the selective shunt is associated with a lower incidence of encephalopathy.

Selection of Procedure. Before a major shunt is performed, the presence of portal hypertension should be defined manometrically. Infrahepatic venacaval pressure should also be measured to rule out caval hypertension that would interfere with splanchnic venous decompression. A splenoportogram or a selective superior mesenteric arteriogram with a venous phase should be obtained to determine the status of the major veins. Portal vein thrombosis occurs as a complication in approximately 2 percent of the patients with portal cirrhosis. But lack of visualization of the portal vein in and of itself does not establish this diagnosis, and collateral veins of Sappey must be visualized. If a selective or central splenorenal shunt is being considered, the anatomy of the left renal vein and its relation to the splenic vein should be identified. Estimations of hepatic blood flow are fraught with errors in interpretation, particularly in cirrhotic patients. Large series have shown that pressure determinations and differentials within the portal venous system, measurements of the estimated hepatic blood flow, and splenoportographic findings did not approximate true flow and these findings could not be related to the subsequent development of postshunt encephalopathy. The increase in hepatic arterial flow subsequent to the creation of a portacaval shunt has offered a hemodynamic correlate with the patient's prognosis.

The end-to-side portacaval shunt is the procedure most commonly performed, since it is technically easiest and has been associated with the lowest incidence of thrombosis. The presence of a large caudate lobe is less compromising to this procedure than to a side-to-side shunt. For some patients with extensive adhesions from previous operative procedures in the right upper quadrant, the splenorenal and mesocaval shunts are preferred. Thrombosis with or without recanalization of the portal vein (cavernomatous transformation) generally precludes a portacaval anastomosis. The Budd-Chiari syndrome, related to endophlebitis of the hepatic veins, dictates a side-to-side shunt to decompress the liver.

In reference to the factor of ascites as a determinant of the decompressive procedure, in one series 39 percent of patients with end-to-side shunts who had preoperative ascites experienced postoperative relief; in 12 percent, ascites appeared after the shunt, while all patients with side-to-side shunts and ascites had permanent relief. The splenorenal shunt, which is a functional side-to-side shunt, failed to relieve ascites in 12 percent of the cases,

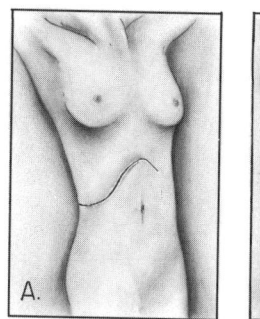

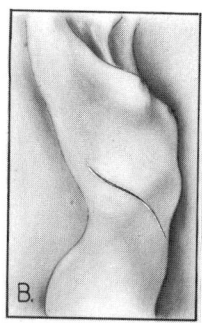

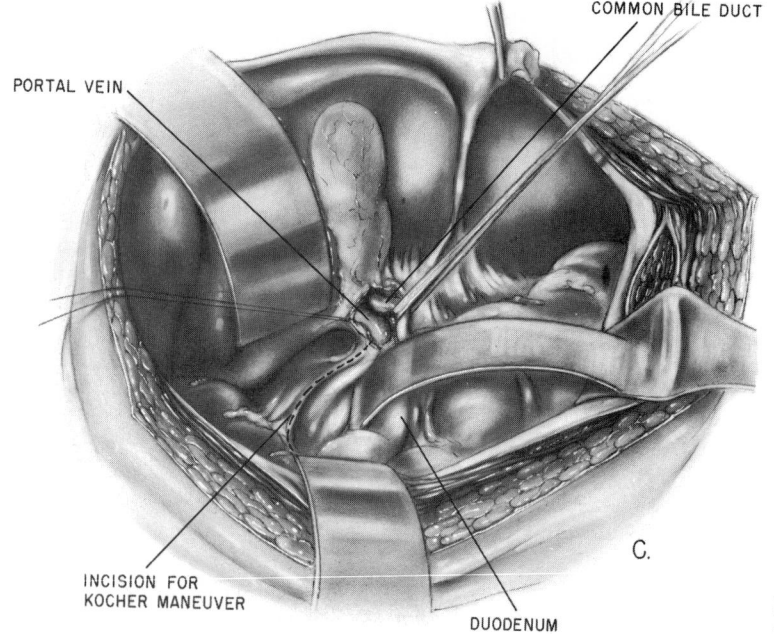

COMMON BILE DUCT

PORTAL VEIN

INCISION FOR
KOCHER MANEUVER

DUODENUM

C.

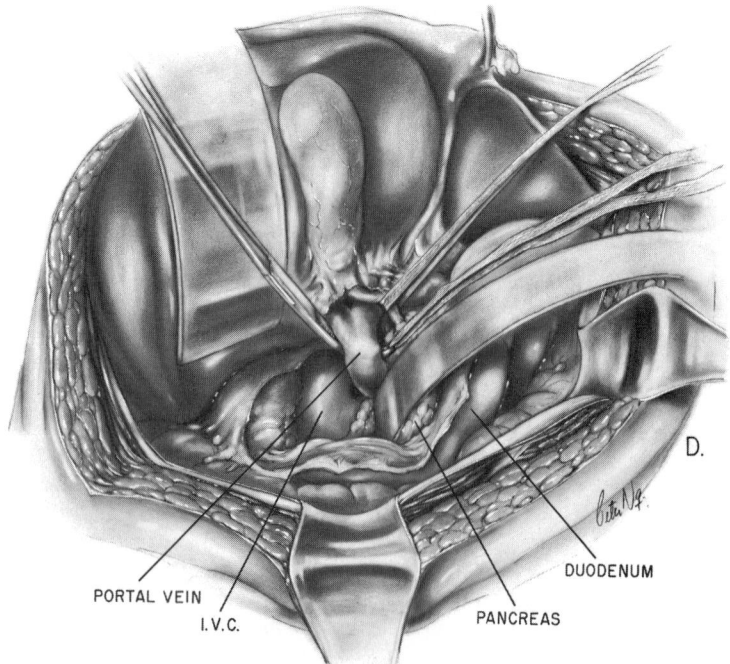

PORTAL VEIN

I.V.C.

DUODENUM

PANCREAS

D.

Fig. 30-38. Three kinds of portacaval shunt. (1) End-to-side portacaval shunt: *A.* Subcostal transabdominal incision. *B.* Thoracoabdominal incision over ninth intercostal space. *C.* Line of incision for Kocher maneuver. Initial dissection of hepatoduodenal ligament, with isolation and retraction of common bile duct and exposure of portal vein. *D.* Completion of dissection of portal vein, with demonstration of bifurcation in porta hepatis. Dissection of retroperitoneum to clear inferior vena cava. *E.* Technique for end-to-side anastomosis. Note partially occluding clamp on anteromedial aspect of inferior vena cava. Atraumatic clamps are applied to proximal and distal portions of portal vein. *F.* An ellipse has been removed from inferior vena cava. This should measure $1\frac{1}{2}$ times diameter of portal vein. Portal vein has been transected. *G.* Distal end of portal vein has been oversewn with continuous silk sutures. (This may be handled by ligature and transfixion ligature.) Portal vein has been approximated to stoma of inferior vena cava. Two stay sutures are initially tied, and posterior layer is in place. *H.* Placement of posterior layer of sutures is facilitated by passing cranial suture into lumen of portal vein and continuing this suture to caudal limb of portal vein, where it is then passed to outside and tied. *I.* Closure of anterior row is accomplished with interrupted horizontal mattress sutures. (A continuous suture may also be employed.) *J.* Completed anastomosis. (2) Side-to-side portacaval shunt. (From: *Schwartz SI: Surgical Diseases of the Liver. New York, McGraw-Hill, 1964, with permission.*)

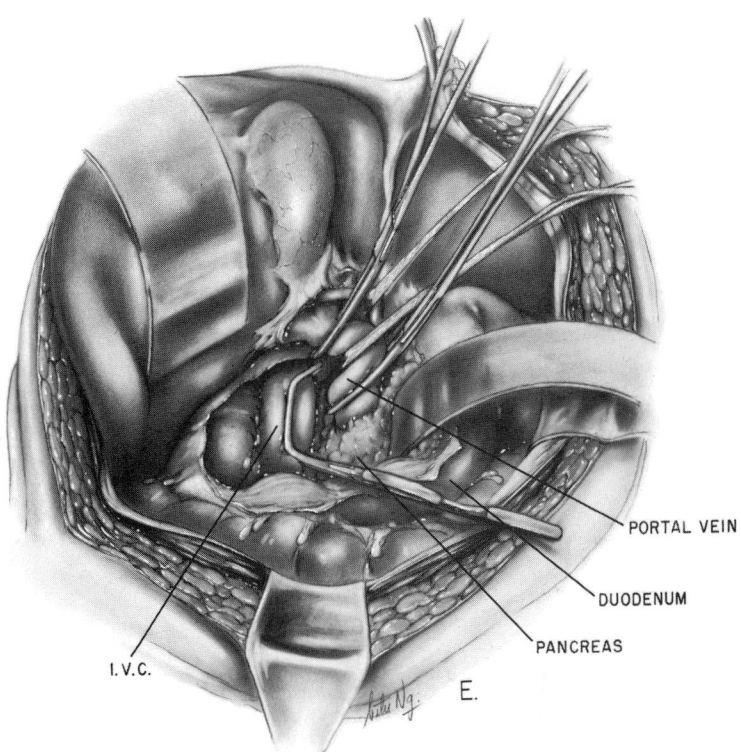

PORTAL VEIN

DUODENUM

PANCREAS

I.V.C.

E.

Fig. 30-38 *E.* Continued.

and ascites appeared after the shunt in 16 percent. It is therefore felt that ascites per se cannot be considered a significant factor in determining the shunt to be performed. Some series have indicated that the selective splenorenal shunt is not acitogenic.

Similarly, whether previous encephalopathy or the presence of asterixis are important determinants of the type of shunt has not been resolved. In general the selective splenorenal shunt is associated with a lower incidence of encephalopathy than other decompressive procedures; devascularization operations rarely cause encephalopathy.

Selection of Patients. Ascites that failed to respond to medical therapy, a prothrombin time that remained prolonged after parenteral administration of vitamin K, serum albumin less than 3, serum bilirubin greater than 1, and BSP retention greater than 10 percent are all associated with poor postoperative prognosis. Child divided patients into three groups including those with good hepatic function (A), those with moderate hepatic function (B), and those with advanced disease and poor reserve (C). In group A are patients with a serum bilirubin below 2, albumin above 3.5, no ascites, no neurologic disorders, and excellent nutrition. Patients in the B group have bilirubin between 2 and 3, albumin between 3 and 3.5, easily controlled ascites, minimum neurologic disorder, and good nutrition. In the C group, bilirubin is above 3, the albumin is below 3, and the ascites is poorly controlled with advanced coma and wasting. Operative mortality following portacaval shunts in the A group was zero, in the B group was 9 percent, and in the C group was 53

percent. There is general agreement that hepatic function is more important than the type of shunt in determining prognosis.

Portacaval Shunt Technique. This shunt (Fig. 30-38) generally is performed through a subcostal incision, but in the presence of extreme hepatomegaly or obesity a thoracoabdominal approach may be used. The liver is retracted craniad and a Kocher maneuver performed to permit mobilization of the duodenum. Dissection is begun in the hepatoduodenal ligament, and the portal vein, which resides posteriorly in relation to the common bile duct, is dissected free along the entire course. Attention is then directed to the dissection of the inferior vena cava. The incision in the retroperitoneum is extended, and the anterior and lateral aspects of the inferior vena cava are exposed from the renal veins to the point where the vessel passes retrohepatically. Atraumatic clamps are applied to the portal vein just above its origin and just below its bifurcation, after which the vein is transected as far craniad as possible. The hepatic end is either ligated or oversewn. A sidearm, nonocclusive clamp is positioned along the anterior aspect of the inferior vena cava and an incision is made in the inferior vena cava wall. This should be approximately $1\frac{1}{2}$ times as long as the diameter of the portal vein. Employing vascular suture techniques, an anastomosis is made between the portal vein and the side of the inferior vena cava, utilizing a continuous suture that is interrupted at the two ends. Following mobilization of the portal vein and inferior vena cava, a side-to-side shunt may be performed. After the anastomosis is completed, the clamp is removed from the inferior vena cava, and

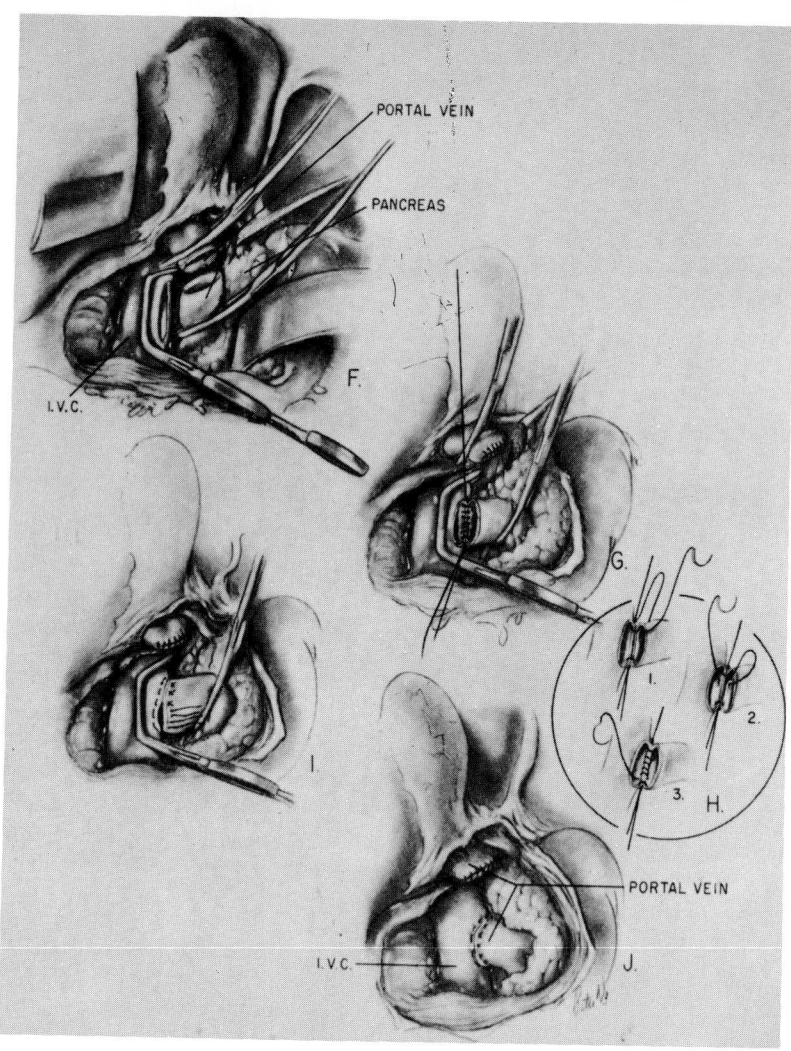

Fig. 30-38 *F,G,H,I,J.* Continued.

then the clamp occluding the portal vein is removed. Pressure should be recorded directly from the portal vein.

Central Splenorenal Shunt. In the cirrhotic patient with postsinusoidal obstruction, the splenorenal anastomosis is not as hemodynamically efficient as the portacaval shunt and is associated with a higher incidence of recurrent bleeding. Proponents of this procedure indicate that in their experience the prevention of recurrent bleeding is similar to that resulting from a portacaval shunt, and the incidence of portal-systemic encephalopathy and persistent hypersplenism is reduced. The operation is generally employed in patients with obstruction of the extrahepatic portal venous system in which the portal vein is not available for shunting. In the pediatric age group, it is preferable to postpone this procedure until the child is ten years old and the splenic vein is large enough to maintain its patency.

Technique (Fig. 30-39). An oblique subcostal incision or thoracoabdominal approach may be used. The transverse colon and splenic flexure are mobilized and re-

tracted caudad, and the short gastric vessels are doubly ligated and transected. The splenophrenic and splenorenal ligaments are then transected and dissection continued in the hilus until an ultimate pedicle of splenic artery and vein remains. The splenic vein is freed as it courses along the pancreas. The posterior peritoneum is incised just medial to the hilus of the kidney and the left renal artery and vein are dissected free. Tapes are passed around the main renal vein and the major branches in the hilus of the kidney. Traction on these tapes establishes control of bleeding and minimizes the number of clamps interfering with the anastomosis. The splenic artery is double ligated and transected, and an atraumatic clamp is applied to the central end of the splenic vein. The splenic vein is then transected as close to the hilus of the spleen as possible and brought down to an appropriate site on the anterosuperior aspect of the renal vein. The renal artery is occluded temporarily with a bulldog clamp, and an incision is made in the renal vein. An end-to-side anastomosis is performed by initially securing two stay sutures

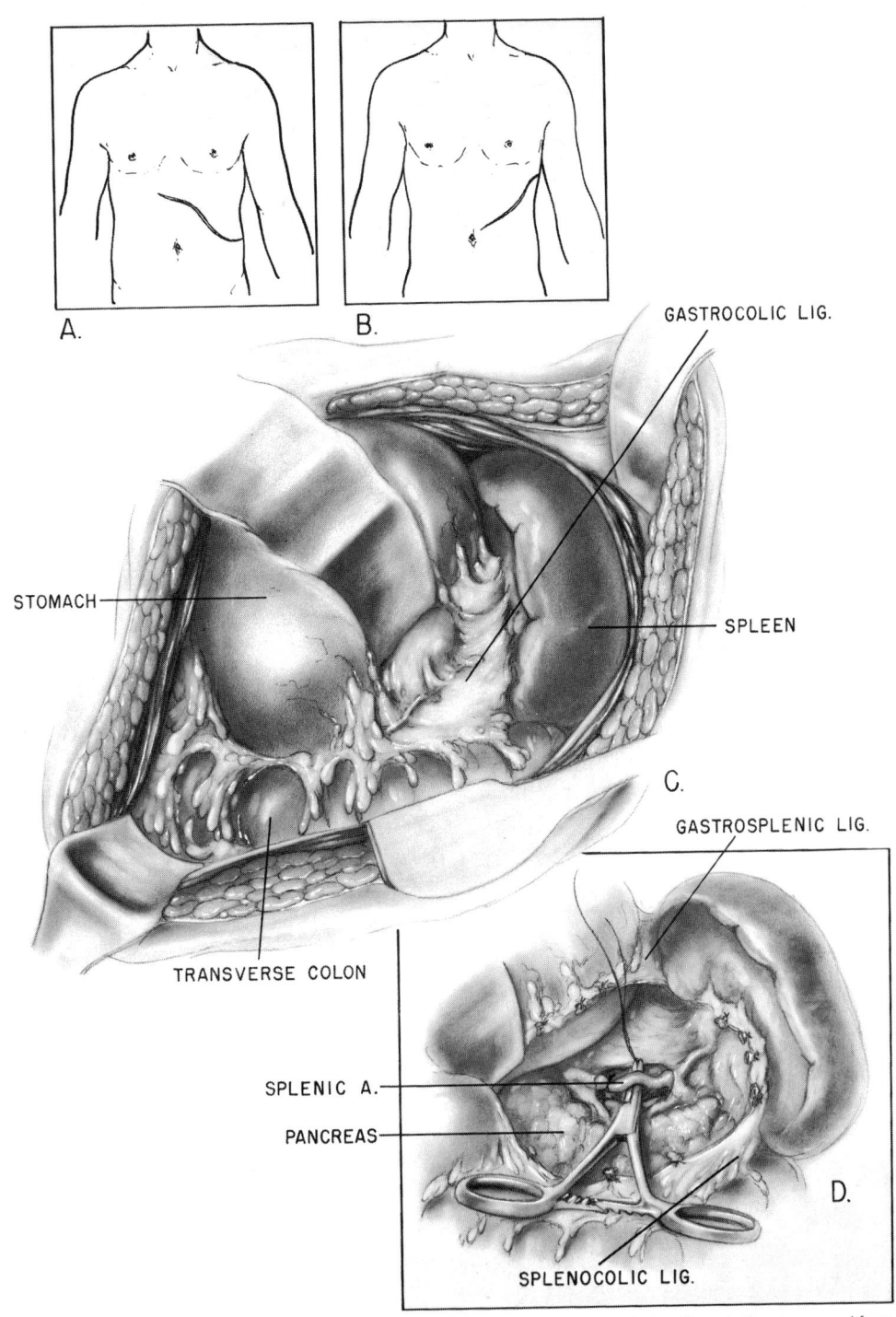

GASTROCOLIC LIG.

STOMACH

SPLEEN

TRANSVERSE COLON

C.

GASTROSPLENIC LIG.

SPLENIC A.

PANCREAS

SPLENOCOLIC LIG.

D.

Fig. 30-39. Splenorenal anastomosis. *A.* Subcostal transabdominal incision. *B.* Thoracoabdominal incision overlying ninth intercostal space. *C.* Retraction of stomach medially. *D.* Vasa brevia have been transected. Splenic artery is ligated. Gastrosplenic and splenocolic ligament are to be transected. *E.* Spleen is mobilized so that an ultimate pedicle of splenic vein remains. *F.* Retroperitoneum has been incised, and tapes are placed around renal artery and renal vein. *G.* Tapes are placed around major tributaries of renal vein within hilus of kidney and around main renal vein. Renal artery is occluded with bulldog clamp, and traction is applied to tapes around renal vein to secure control. An ellipse is then removed from anterosuperior aspect of renal vein. This should be 1½ times diameter of splenic vein. Vascular clamp has been applied to splenic vein, and spleen is removed; as long a segment of splenic vein as possible is retained. *H.* Splenic vein is brought down and anastomosed to stoma that has been created in main renal vein. Occlusive tapes have been removed from splenic vein and renal artery. (From: *Schwartz SI: Surgical Diseases of the Liver. New York, McGraw-Hill, 1964, with permission.*)

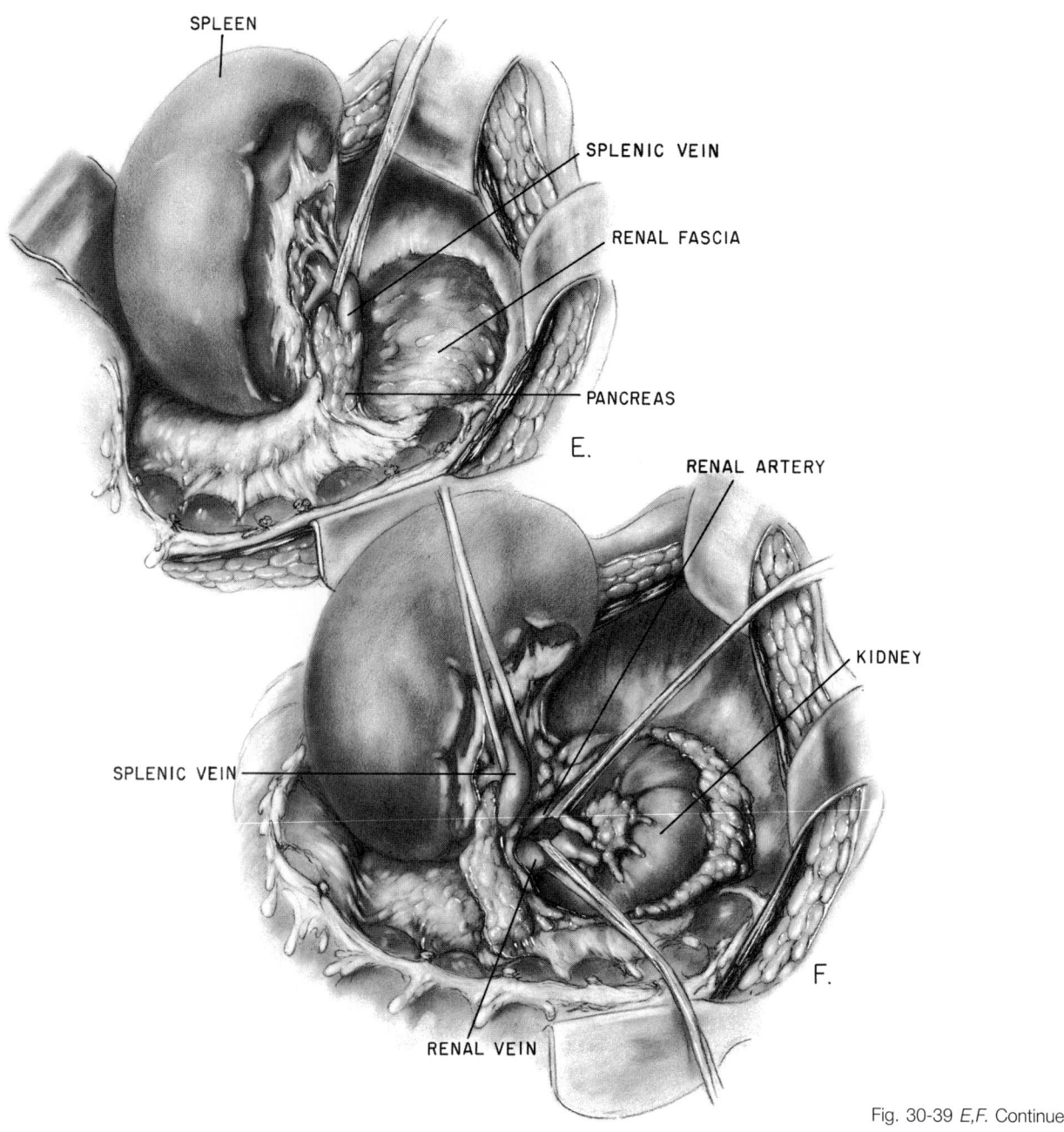

SPLEEN

SPLENIC VEIN

RENAL FASCIA

PANCREAS

E.

RENAL ARTERY

KIDNEY

SPLENIC VEIN

F.

RENAL VEIN

Fig. 30-39 *E,F.* Continued.

and completing the posterior layer as a continuous suture. Anastomosis of the anterior layer is accomplished with either horizontal mattress sutures or a continuous suture.

Superior Mesenteric–Inferior Vena Cava Shunt. This operation is generally employed for patients with extrahepatic vein obstruction and is particularly applicable to the patient in whom a previous splenorenal shunt failed or to a small child in whom a splenorenal anastomosis is doomed to failure because of the size of the splenic vein. The operation is also advised for patients with cirrhosis if there is associated thrombosis of the portal vein or exten-

sive scarring in the right upper quadrant that precludes safe dissection of the portal vein or marked enlargement of the caudate lobe of the liver.

Interruption of the inferior cava, which is required for the end-to-side shunt, results in venous stasis in the lower extremity, and in the immediate postoperative period the foot of the bed must be elevated to reduce potential edema. The procedure is well tolerated by young patients in whom postoperative chronic dependent edema of the legs is uncommon. In older patients, any edema may be readily controlled with elastic stockings.

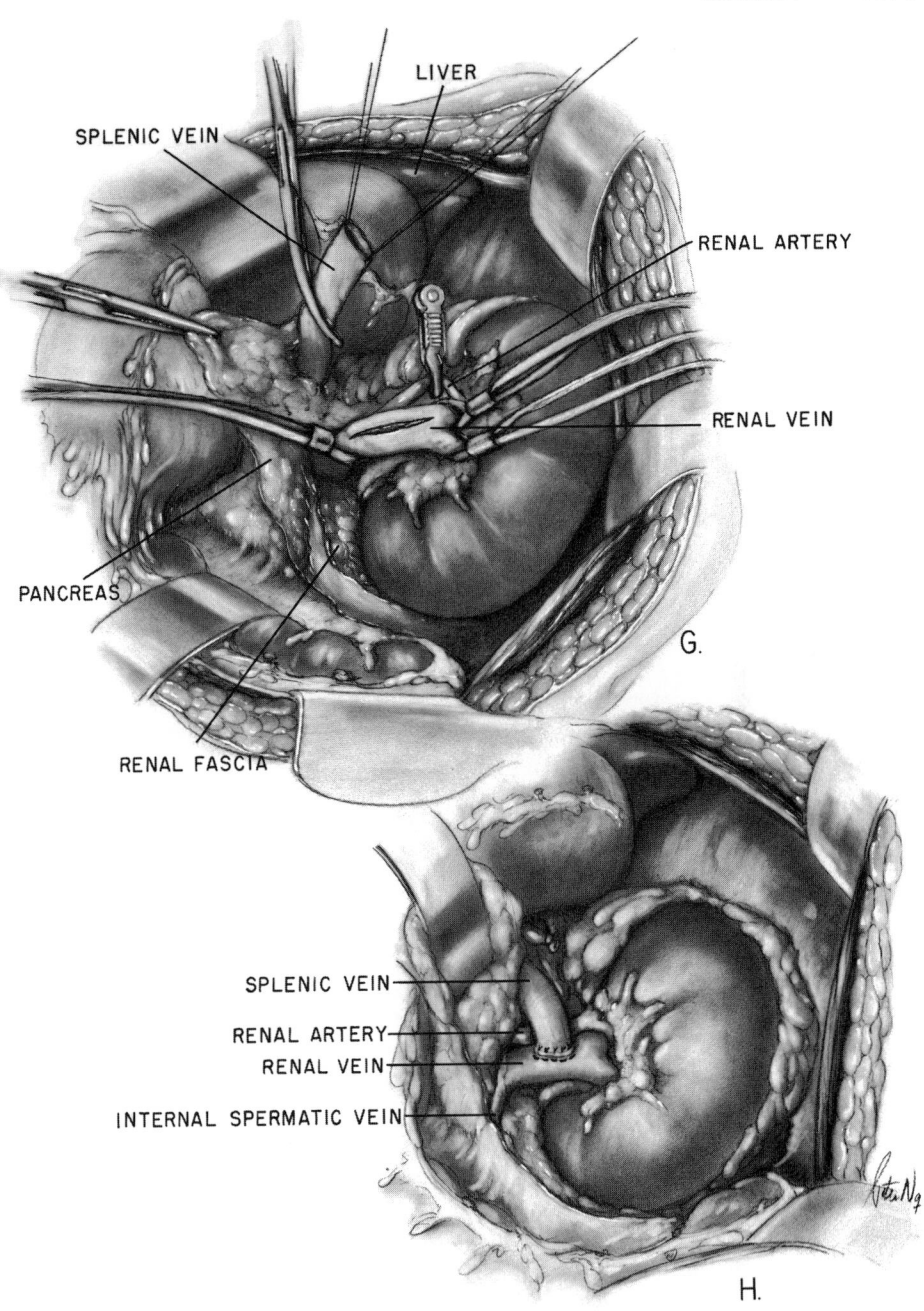

LIVER

SPLENIC VEIN

RENAL ARTERY

RENAL VEIN

PANCREAS

RENAL FASCIA

G.

SPLENIC VEIN
RENAL ARTERY
RENAL VEIN
INTERNAL SPERMATIC VEIN

H.

Fig. 30-39 *G,H.* Continued.

Technique (Fig. 30-40). The peritoneal cavity is entered through a midline or right paramedian incision extending from the xiphoid process to well below the umbilicus. Upward traction on the transverse colon exposes the superior mesenteric vessels. The peritoneum is incised in the region of the superior mesenteric arterial pulse, and the superior mesenteric vein is identified and dissected free. The lateral reflection of the ascending colon is then incised along its entire length to permit medial displacement of the transverse and ascending colons and the medial reflection of the ascending mesocolon. This exposes

the inferior vena cava and the third portion of the duodenum. The inferior vena cava is mobilized from its origin up to the entrance of the right renal vein. The paired lumbar veins are ligated and transected. After the entire inferior vena cava has been freed, vascular clamps are applied immediately below the renal veins and at the junction of the iliac veins. The inferior vena cava is transected as far distad as possible and the caudal stump ligated. The right iliac vein may be left attached to the vena cava to achieve greater length. A window is created in the mesentery of the small intestine between the ileocolic

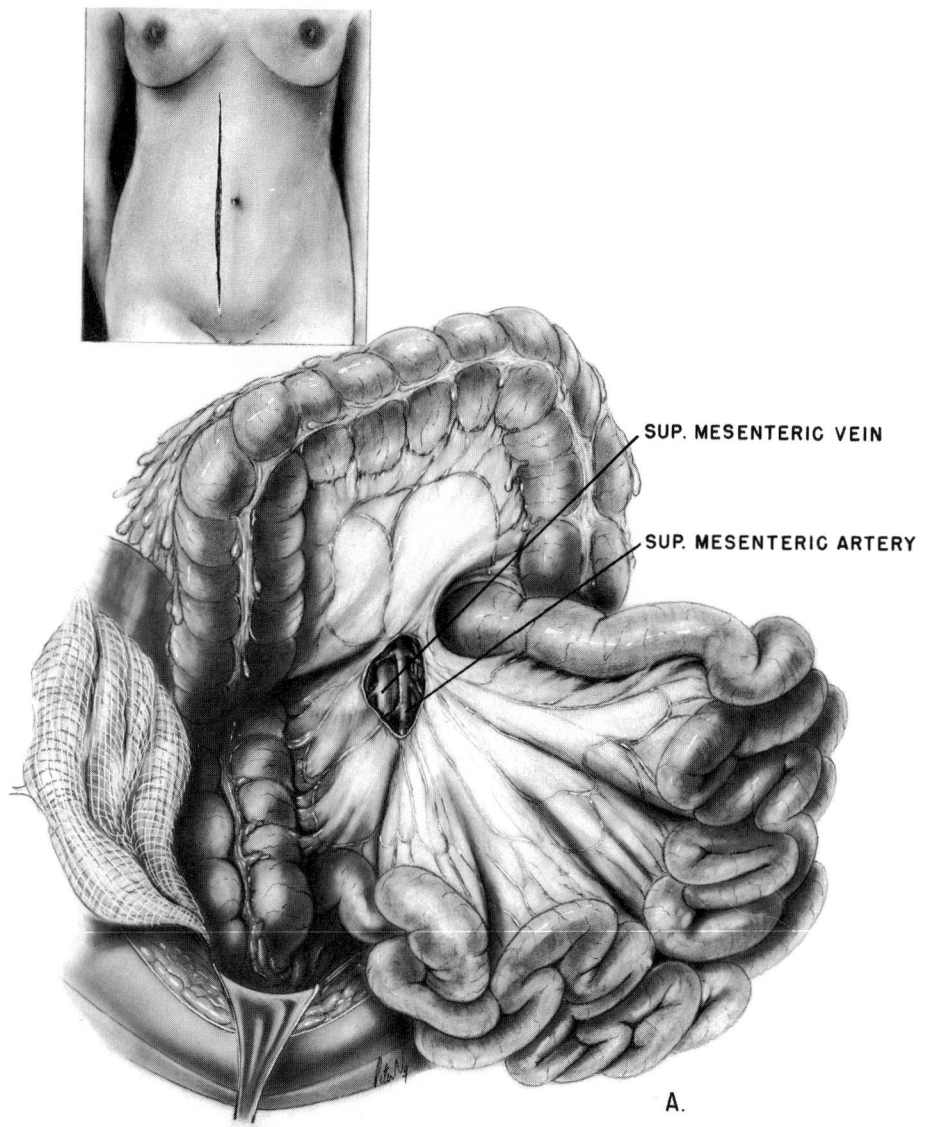

SUP. MESENTERIC VEIN

SUP. MESENTERIC ARTERY

A.

vessels and the origin of the main ileal trunk to permit approximation of the end of the inferior vena cava to the right posterolateral aspect of the superior mesenteric vein. The anastomosis between the inferior vena cava and the superior mesenteric vein is usually performed proximal to the right colic vein, utilizing a continuous arterial suture interrupted at both ends.

Decompression is more commonly accomplished by the construction of an H graft using a 19- to 22-mm prosthesis interposed between the superior mesenteric vein and the inferior vena cava (see Fig. 30-41). A high incidence of immediate and long-term thrombosis of the graft has been reported from some institutions, but this is not uniform.

Selective Splenorenal Shunt. The indications for the selective distal splenorenal shunt include a substantial portal venous flow to the liver, favorable anatomic features

Fig. 30-40. Superior mesenteric-inferior vena cava shunt, right route. *A*. Insert: right paramedian incision. Traction applied to transverse colon exposes superior mesenteric artery and vein. Peritoneum over vessels has been incised. Right side of superior mesenteric vein is dissected carefully to preserve colic branches. *B*. Lateral reflection of ascending colon has been incised, and colon is reflected medially. This has exposed inferior vena cava and third portion of duodenum. Inferior vena cava is mobilized from convergence of two common iliac veins up to entrance of right renal vein. In course of this dissection, paired lumbar veins are ligated in continuity and transected. *C*. Inferior vena cava has been transected. Stay sutures are inserted into adventitia of proximal vena cava, to be used to traction and orientation. Window has been created in small intestinal mesentery between ileocolic vessels and origin of main ileal trunk. *D*. Distal end of inferior vena cava has been oversewn. Proximal inferior vena cava is passed anterior to third portion of duodenum and through window in mesentery. Anastomosis is made between end of inferior vena cava and right posterolateral aspect of superior mesenteric vein. (From: *Schwartz SI: Surgical Diseases of the Liver. New York, McGraw-Hill, 1964, with permission.*)

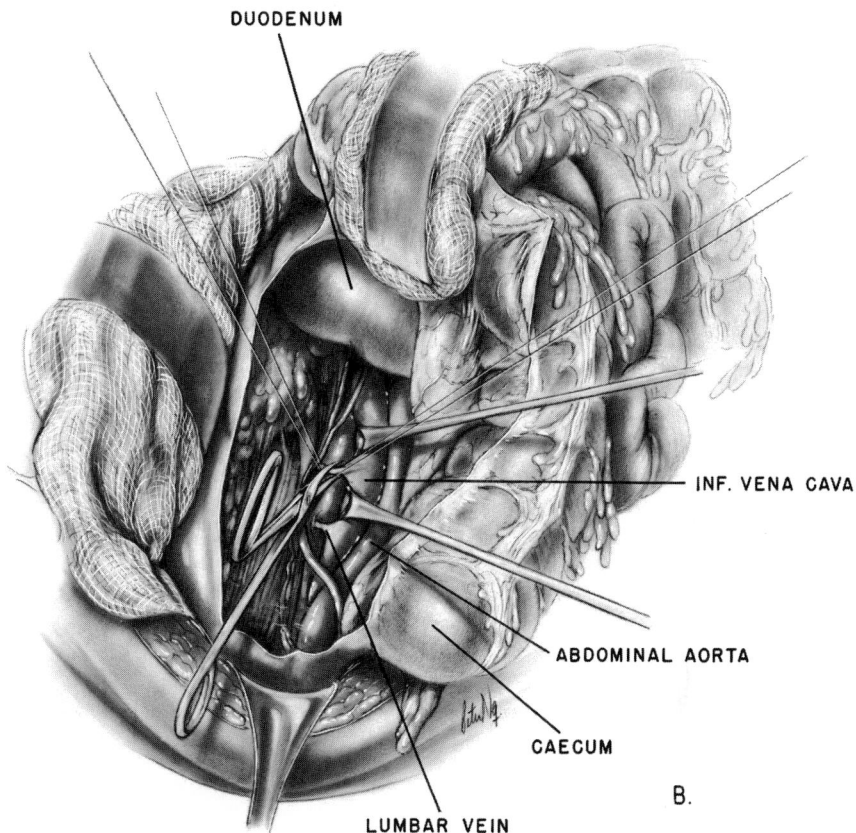

DUODENUM

INF. VENA CAVA

ABDOMINAL AORTA

CAECUM

B.

Fig. 30-40 *B.* Continued.

LUMBAR VEIN

related to the site and patency of the splenic vein and the site and size of the left renal vein, and satisfactory liver function in the absence of marked ascites.

Technique. The operative procedure is shown in schematic fashion in Fig. 30-42. Decompression is effected through the short gastric vessels in the spleen. The spleen is not removed, and the distal or splenic side of the splenic vein is used for an anastomosis to the left renal vein. This technique can be modified by transecting the left renal vein close to the hilus of the kidney, turning and anastomosing the caval side of the renal vein to the side of the splenic vein, and ligating the splenic vein close to the confluence with the superior mesenteric vein. Included in the procedure is ligation of the coronary vein and devascularization of the stomach by ligating of all vessels with the exception of the right gastric artery and the short gastric veins. Both Inokuchi and Warren have devised modifications of splenopancreatic disconnection to prevent future portal malcirculation.

Complications of Portal-Systemic Shunts. The complications uniquely associated with portal-systemic shunting procedures occur intraoperatively or during the postoperative period. The intraoperative complications include bleeding and a nonshuntable situation, while the postoperative complications include rebleeding, hepatic failure, changes in cardiorespiratory dynamics, the hepatorenal

syndrome, plus delayed complications of hemosiderosis, peptic ulcer, and portal-systemic encephalopathy.

The complication of intraoperative bleeding can be reduced by correction of coagulation defects and by continuing the infusion of vasopressin during the operative procedure. A nonshuntable situation may be related to extension of cavernomatous transformation of the portal vein to involve the superior mesenteric vein and the splenic vein. In these patients, the so-called makeshift shunt, using large collaterals, is generally doomed to failure. The circumstance of caval hypertension caused by hypertrophy and nodularity of the caudate lobe encroaching on the infrahepatic vena cava has been referred to previously. Attempts have been made to shunt between the superior mesenteric vein and the atrium.

Early postoperative bleeding is usually related to thrombosis of a reconstructed shunt. This can be defined by splenoportography in the case of a portacaval shunt. The rapid onset of ascites during the early postoperative period may be managed by restriction of sodium intake and the administration of diuretic agents. In this circumstance the early institution of a peritoneal-venous shunt has provided dramatic relief. Renal failure following a portal-systemic shunt is not predictable, and treatment consists of supportive measures. The early postoperative development of hepatic coma is an ominous sign.

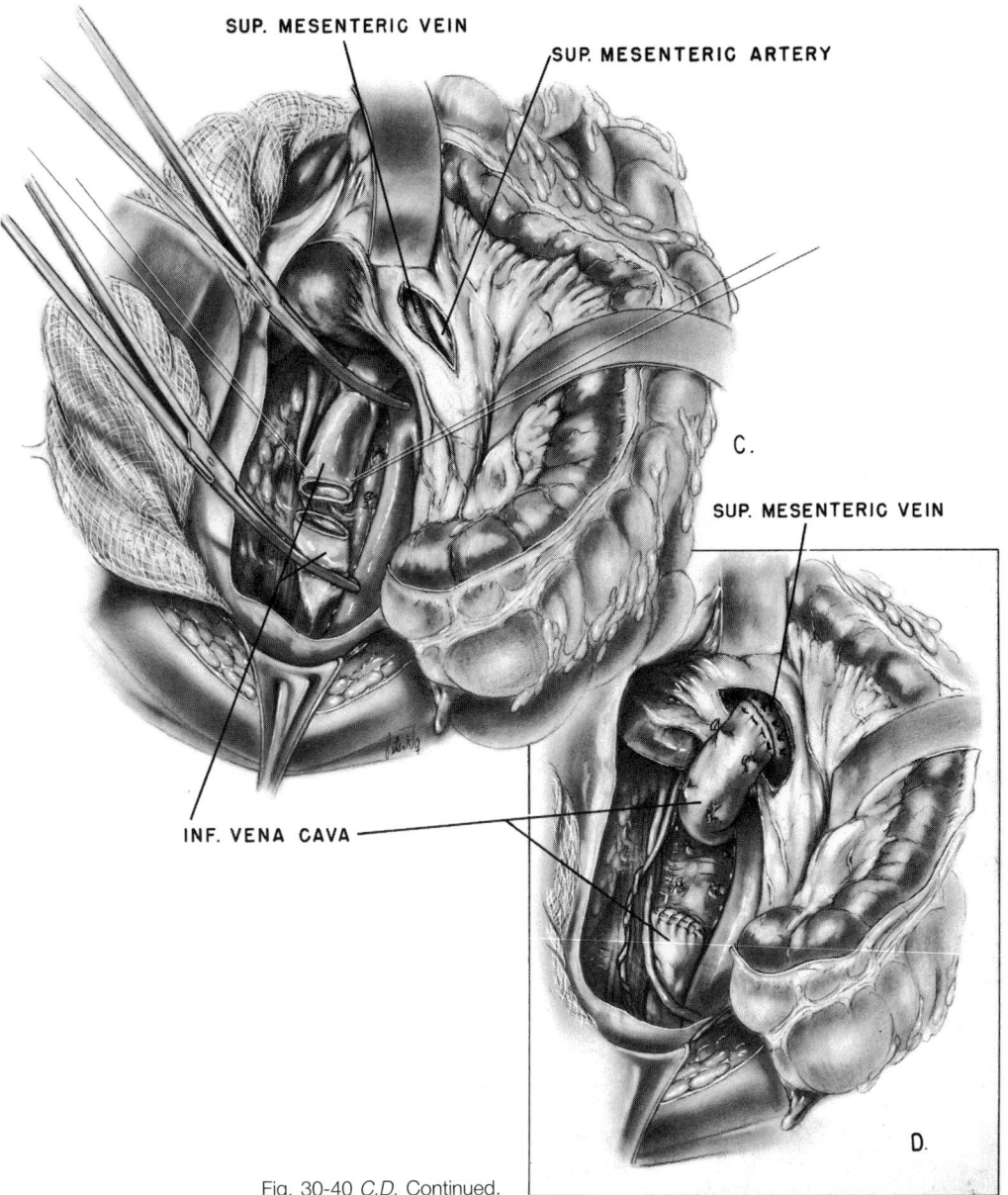

SUP. MESENTERIC VEIN

SUP. MESENTERIC ARTERY

C.

SUP. MESENTERIC VEIN

INF. VENA CAVA

D.

Fig. 30-40 *C,D*. Continued.

Portacaval Shunt for Glycogen Storage Disease and Hypercholesterolemia

In 1963, Starzl and associates performed a portacaval transposition on an eight-year-old child with type III glycogen storage disease, which resulted in resumption of weight gain and growth rate. Since then, several investigators have reported clinical improvement following an end-to-side portacaval shunt in children with type I glycogen storage disease in which the enzyme glucose 6-phosphatase is deficient or absent. Intravenous hyperalimentation for 2 to 3 weeks prior to surgery is advised to reduce the liver size, restore the bleeding time to normal, correct acidosis and hypoglycemia, and promote a favorable outcome of the shunting procedure. Children who

have undergone diversion of portal flow have shown no evidence of encephalopathy. Portacaval shunts also have been applied with success to a few patients with homozygous hypercholesterolemia and to an occasional patient with heterozygous type 2 hypercholesterolemia.

FULMINANT HEPATIC FAILURE

This refers to the clinical syndrome characterized by sudden, severe impairment of hepatic function generally as a consequence of massive necrosis of liver cells. In most instances, the cause is acute hepatitis of viral origin. Massive necrosis and dysfunction have been reported

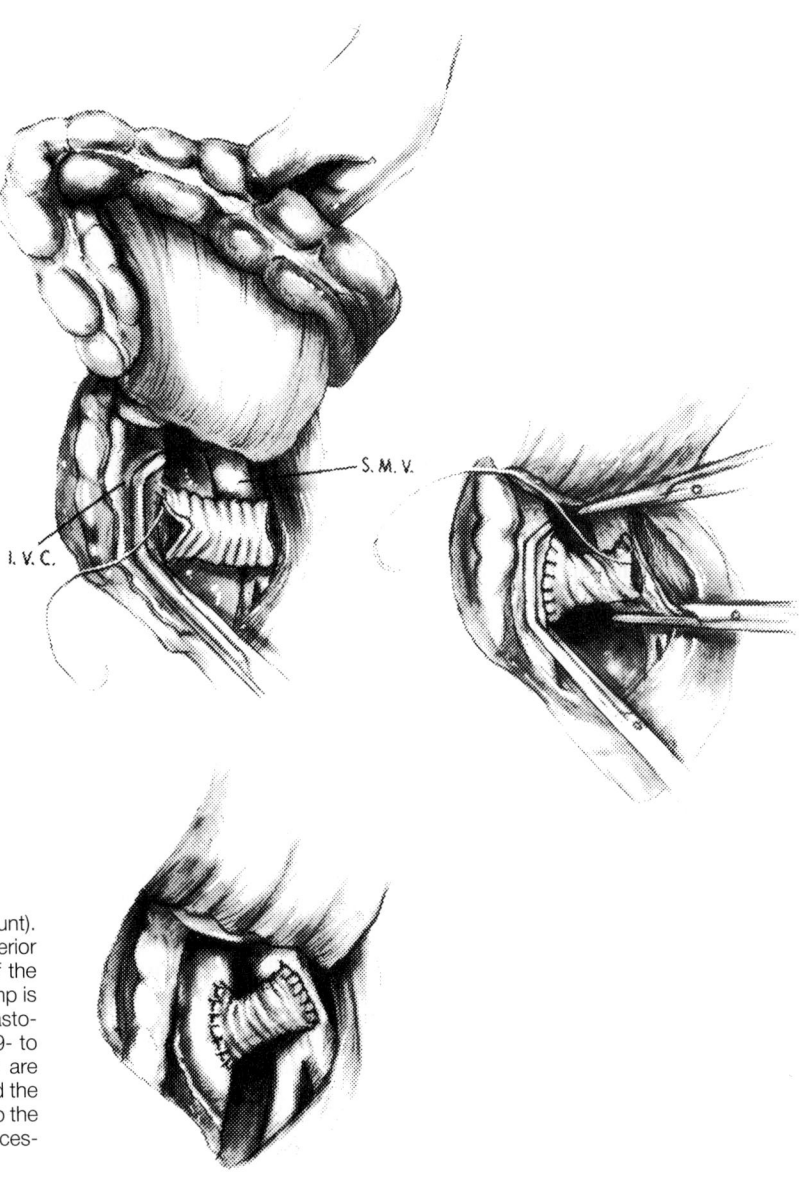

Fig. 30-41. H graft (interposition mesocaval shunt). The transverse colon is elevated, and the superior mesenteric vein is dissected free at the route of the small bowel mesentery. A partially occlusive clamp is applied to the infrarenal vena cava, and an anastomosis is made between the vena cava and a 19- to 22-mm Dacron prosthesis. Occlusive clamps are then placed on the superior mesenteric vein, and the graft is anastomosed in an end-to-side fashion to the superior mesenteric vein. Heparinization is unnecessary.

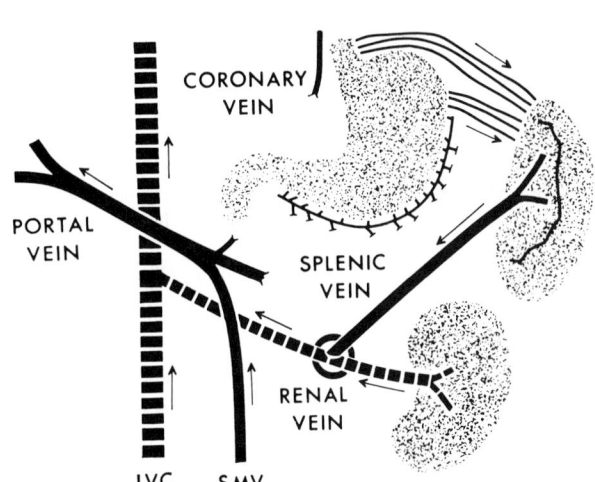

Fig. 30-42. Diagrammatic illustration of the selective distal splenorenal shunt. Note coronary vein ligation and gastric devascularization which protects the vasa brevia and other collateral vessels from esophagus and diaphragm. (From: *Salam AA et al: Ann Surg 173:827, 1971, with permission.*)

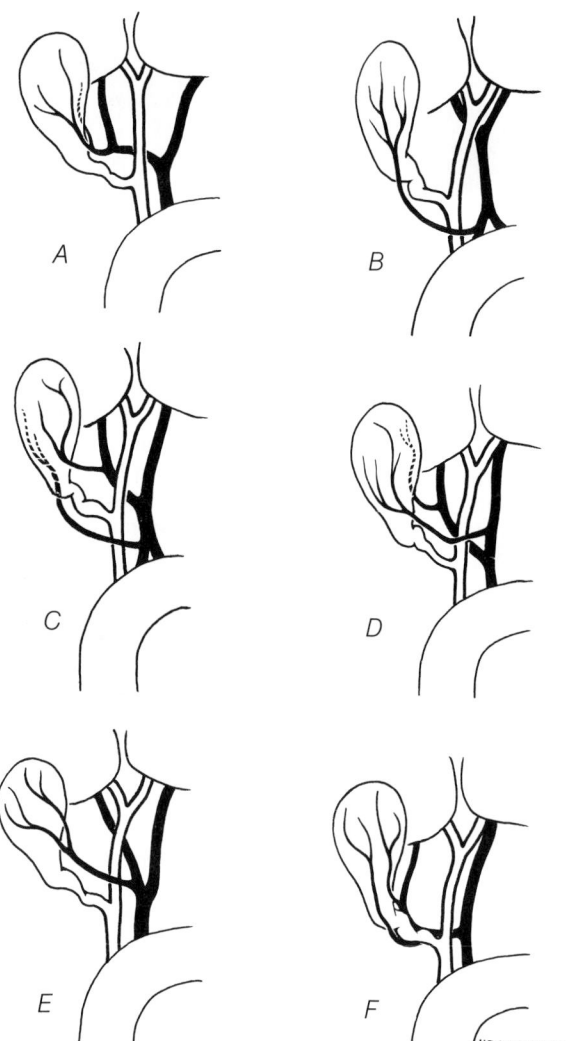

Fig. 31-3. Anomalies of the arteries to the gallbladder. *A.* Cystic artery arises from right hepatic artery in 95 percent of cases. *B.* Cystic artery arises from gastroduodenal artery. *C.* Two cystic arteries, one arising from right hepatic artery and the other from common hepatic artery. *D.* Two cystic arteries. Abnormal one arises from left hepatic artery and crosses common hepatic duct anteriorly. *E.* Cystic artery arises from right hepatic artery but courses anterior to common hepatic duct. *F.* Two cystic arteries arising from right hepatic artery. Right hepatic artery is adherent to cystic duct and neck of gallbladder. Posterior cystic artery is very short (a common finding).

cases there are two hepatic arteries—one originating from the common hepatic and the other from the superior mesenteric artery. The right hepatic artery is vulnerable during surgical procedures, particularly when it parallels the cystic duct and is adherent to it or when it resides in the mesentery of the gallbladder. A "caterpillar hump" right hepatic artery may be mistaken for the cystic artery. The right hepatic artery may course anterior to the common duct. In 10 percent of cases, the cystic artery originates from the left hepatic artery or from the junction of the left or right hepatic arteries with the common hepatic

artery. In about 15 percent of cases, the cystic artery passes in front of the common hepatic duct, rather than to the right of or posterior to this duct. Double cystic arteries occur in about 25 percent of cases, and they may both arise from the right hepatic artery, or one may have an abnormal origin.

CYSTIC DISEASE OF THE EXTRAHEPATIC BILIARY TRACT (CHOLEDOCHAL CYST)

Congenital cystic abnormalities may occur throughout the entire biliary system, i.e., from intrahepatic biliary radicles to the terminal common duct. Intrahepatic cystic dilatation is discussed in Chap. 30, Liver. Choledochal cysts are discussed in Chap. 39. There are three major varieties (Fig. 31-4): cystic dilatation involving the entire common bile duct and common hepatic duct with the cystic duct entering the choledochal cyst; a small cyst usually localized to the distal common bile duct; and diffuse fusiform dilatation of the common bile duct.

CONGENITAL BILIARY ATRESIA (See Chap. 39)

PHYSIOLOGY

BILE SECRETION. The normal adult with an intact hepatic circulation and consuming an average diet secretes from the hepatic cells 250 to 1000 mL bile per day. This is an active process that is dependent upon hepatic blood flow and an oxygen supply available to the hepatic cell. The secretion of bile is responsive to neurogenic, humoral, and chemical control. Vagal stimulation increases secretion, whereas stimulation of the splanchnic nerves results in vasoconstriction and decreased bile flow. The release of secretin from the duodenum following the stimulus of hydrochloric acid, breakdown products of protein, and fatty acids results in an increased bile flow. Bile salts are effective cholerectics, acting directly on the liver to augment secretion.

COMPOSITION OF BILE. The main constituents of bile include electrolytes, bile salts, proteins, cholesterol, fats, and bile pigments. Sodium, potassium, calcium, and chloride have approximately the same concentration in bile as in plasma. There is a direct relation between the rate of secretion and the electrolyte concentration. As the former increases, there is an increase in bicarbonate and pH and a slight increase in chloride. The pH of liver bile, which usually ranges between 5.7 and 8.6, tending to the alkaline side, varies with the diet, an increase in protein ingestion shifting the pH to the acid side.

Bile salts act as anions that are balanced by sodium. The major salts, cholic, deoxycholic, and chenodeoxycholic acids, conjugate with taurine or glycine and are present in the bile in concentrations of 10 to 20 meq/L. The bile salt anion has extremely weak osmotic activity because of its tendency to form large molecular aggregates. Proteins are present in lesser concentrations than in plasma, with the exception of mucoproteins and lipoproteins that are not present in plasma. Liver bile contains unesterified cholesterol, lecithin, and neutral fat,

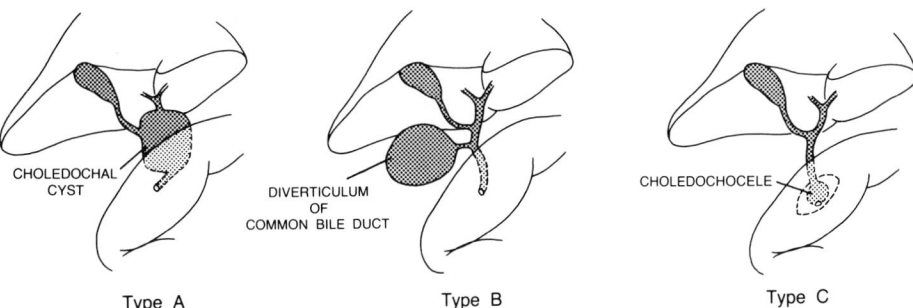

CHOLEDOCHAL
CYST

DIVERTICULUM
OF
COMMON BILE DUCT

CHOLEDOCHOCELE

Type A   Type B   Type C

Fig. 31-4. Choledochal cyst. Three major varieties, Alonso-Lej classification.

which consists of palmitic, oleic, and linoleic acids. The concentrations of both cholesterol and phospholipids are lower in hepatic bile than in plasma.

The color of the bile secreted by the liver is related to the presence of the pigment bilirubin diglucuronide, which is the metabolic product of the breakdown of hemoglobin and is secreted into the bile in concentrations 100 times greater than that present in the plasma. After this pigment has been acted upon by the bacteria in the intestine and converted into urobilinogen, a small fraction of the urobilinogen is absorbed and also secreted into the bile. A variety of dyes foreign to the body, such as sulfobromophthalein (BSP), rose bengal, and indocyanine green, are removed from the blood by the liver, concentrated, and secreted into the bile.

GALLBLADDER FUNCTION. The gallbladder provides storage and effects concentration of bile. Sodium, chloride, and water are selectively absorbed, while the absorption of potassium and calcium is less complete and the concentration of bicarbonate in the gallbladder bile is twice that in plasma. This absorption of water and electrolytes results in a tenfold concentration of bile salts, bile pigments, and cholesterol in relation to levels present in liver bile. The gallbladder mucosa has the greatest absorptive power per unit area of any structure in the body, and this rapid absorption prevents a rise in pressure within the biliary system under normal circumstances.

Secretion of mucus in amounts approximating 20 mL/24 h protects the mucosa from the lytic action of bile and facilitates the passage of bile through the cystic duct. This mucus makes up the colorless "white bile" present in hydrops of the gallbladder resulting from obstruction of the cystic duct. The gallbladder also secretes calcium in the presence of inflammation or obstruction of the cystic duct.

Motor activity is a critical function, since the passage of bile into the duodenum requires the coordinated contraction of the gallbladder and relaxation of the sphincter of Oddi. In addition to rhythmic contractions occurring two to six times per minute and mediating of pressure less than 30 mm water, tonic contractions lasting 5 to 30 min increase the pressure within the gallbladder up to 300 mm water. Since the hepatic secretory pressure is 375 mm water and is greater than the maximal pressure mediated within the gallbladder, the passage of bile is dependent upon the relaxation of the sphincter of Oddi. The gallbladder empties following humoral or nervous stimulation. The main stimulus in human beings is cholecystokinin, which is released from the intestinal mucosa in response to food, particularly fat entering the duodenum. Following the intravenous injection of cholecystokinin, the gallbladder begins to contract in 1 to 2 min and is two-thirds evacuated within 30 min. Cholecystokinin also relaxes the terminal bile duct, the sphincter of Oddi, and the duodenal musculature. Splanchnic sympathetic stimulation is inhibitory to the motor activity of the gallbladder, while the vagus stimulates contraction. Although vagotomy for duodenal ulcer will increase the size and volume of the gallbladder, the rate of emptying is unchanged. A gallbladder that contains calculi should be removed concomitantly with vagotomy, in view of a significant incidence of early postoperative cholecystitis in this circumstance. Parasympathomimetic drugs contract the gallbladder, whereas atropine tends to relax the organ. Magnesium sulfate acts as a potent evacuator of the gallbladder. Hydrochloric acid and bile salts have little direct effect on motor activity.

Evacuation of the gallbladder occurs $\frac{1}{2}$ h after a fatty meal. There is an increased risk of gallbladder disease in patients receiving total parenteral nutrition (TPN) related to consequent stasis of the gallbladder. The incidence of calculous or acalculous cholecystitis in patients receiving long-term TPN is about 45 percent.

The common bile duct was generally regarded as an inert tube until cineradiographic studies demonstrated waves of peristalsis. The sphincter of Oddi is a major factor in the evacuation of bile. During starvation, the sphincter maintains an intraductal pressure approximating the maximal expulsive power of the gallbladder, i.e., 300 mm water, and thus prevents evacuation. Following the ingestion of food, this is reduced to 100 mm water. When pressures within the biliary system are greater than 360 mm water, there is suppression of bile secretion. Following obstruction or occlusion of the common bile duct, the time required to reach this pressure level and to result in jaundice is dependent upon the presence and function of the gallbladder. When the gallbladder is absent, the bilirubin levels are raised within 6 h of total occlusion, while with a functioning gallbladder jaundice may not occur for 46 to 48 h.

Motor Dysfunction. *Biliary dyskinesia,* a term introduced by Westphal in 1923, lacks objective findings. It was originally used to describe functional disturbances of biliary tract motility that occurred in the absence of anatomic changes and were related to alterations in autonomic reflex activity. Subsequently, the term has been applied to both this primary condition and situations secondary to other biliary tract diseases, such as cholecystitis and cholelithiasis, and following biliary tract surgical treatment. The origin of biliary tract pain itself has not been precisely defined. Experiments inducing gallbladder contraction by fatty foods and cholecystokinin in the presence of a closed sphincter of Oddi have demonstrated that pain can result from motor incoordination. The factor of distention remains suspect, but this is difficult to implicate, since above pressures of 300 to 360 mm water bile secretion ceases. Acute distention of the common bile duct produced by inflation of a balloon-tipped catheter results in colicky pain. When identical pressures are used but dilatation is increased gradually, distress rather than colic results. Biliary tract pain has also been related to spasm of the sphincter of Oddi per se. The concept of hyperplastic cholecystoses, characterized by a functional abnormality manifested by hyperconcentrating and excessive emptying of the gallbladder on cholecystogram, is questionable. Cholecystectomy is reported to be curative in symptomatic patients, but results are difficult to evaluate.

DIAGNOSIS OF BILIARY TRACT DISEASE

(See also Jaundice in Chap. 24.)

Radiologic Studies

ROUTINE ABDOMINAL X-RAYS (Fig. 31-5). Plain films of the abdomen prior to the administration of any radiopaque material are indicated, since biliary calculi have

Fig. 31-5. Routine abdominal x-ray demonstrating radiopaque biliary calculi in gallbladder.

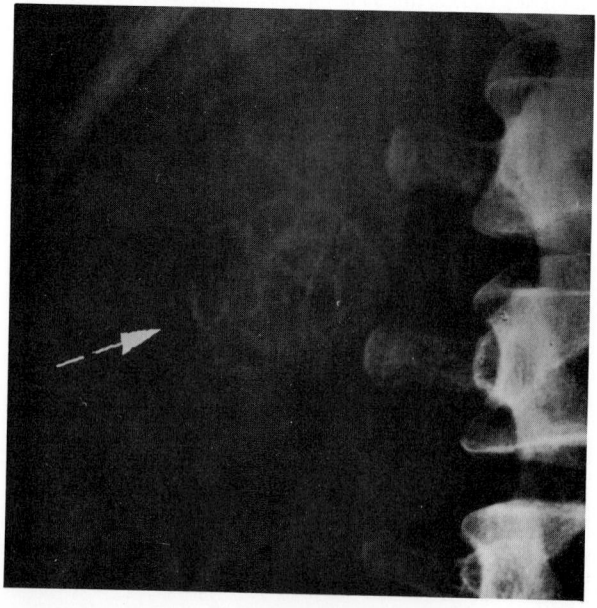

been demonstrated in up to 15 percent of cases, and faintly calcified stones may be rendered invisible when contrast materials surround them. Bile pigment calculi, which are characteristically associated with hemolytic disorders, generally are nonradiopaque, but they may contain sufficient amounts of calcium to be noted on routine x-ray. Similarly, the pure cholesterol calculus is nonradiopaque, whereas calcium carbonate calculi are all visible. Gallstones formed in association with infection or inflammation are generally mixed and contain two or all elements. Their visibility is dependent upon the amount of calcium present.

ORAL CHOLECYSTOGRAPHY. In 1924, Graham and Cole introduced the use of contrast media for visualizing the gallbladder. Successful visualization of the gallbladder by a radiopaque iodine-containing compound is dependent upon blood flow to the liver, functional ability of the liver cell to excrete the dye into the bile, patency of the hepatic and cystic duct system, and water absorption by the gallbladder to concentrate the excreted dye. Most diseases of the gallbladder reduce the absorptive capacity in the mucosa; an exception is cholesterosis, in which the dye may concentrate beyond normal.

This procedure (Fig. 31-6) provides visualization of the normal gallbladder. Subsequent to the ingestion of a fatty meal, contraction begins promptly, and within 40 min the gallbladder should be reduced to at least one-third or one-fourth of its normal size. The abnormal cholecystogram may demonstrate poor visualization or nonvisualization of the gallbladder or may indicate the presence of filling defects such as calculi or tumors. Reliability of the Telepaque examination has been reported as 98 percent accurate when compared with surgical findings. Nonvisualization with the use of the dye may be caused by failure to retain the oral medication, faulty absorption such as with pyloric obstruction, hepatic dysfunction, hepatic or cystic duct obstruction, loss of concentrating ability of the gallbladder mucosa, or faulty x-ray technique. Oral cholecystography is seldom effective if the serum bilirubin is over 1.8 mg/dL. Oral cholecystography is the best method of demonstrating calculi, either by direct visualization of filling defects or by demonstration of a nonopacifying gallbladder, which is associated with a 90 percent incidence of calculi. It remains the standard procedure for establishing the diagnosis of chronic cholecystitis and cholelithiasis in the anicteric patient. Cholecystokinin (CCK) cholecystography has been used to define gallbladder disease in patients with suggestive pain and a normal cholecystogram; 75 Ivy units of CCK are instilled intraduodenally or intravenously. The normal gallbladder will demonstrate a volume reduction greater than 50 percent in 20 min. Cholecystokinin cholecystography is usually combined with aspiration of duodenal contents to determine if there are more than 10 cholesterol monohydrate or calcium bilirubinate crystals per slide. The outcome of cholecystectomy in patients with abnormal findings on either test is equivalent to that obtained in patients with a conventional diagnosis.

PERCUTANEOUS TRANSHEPATIC CHOLANGIOGRAPHY (PTC), ENDOSCOPIC RETROGRADE CHOLANGIOPANCREATOGRAPHY (ERCP) (See Jaundice in Chap. 24).

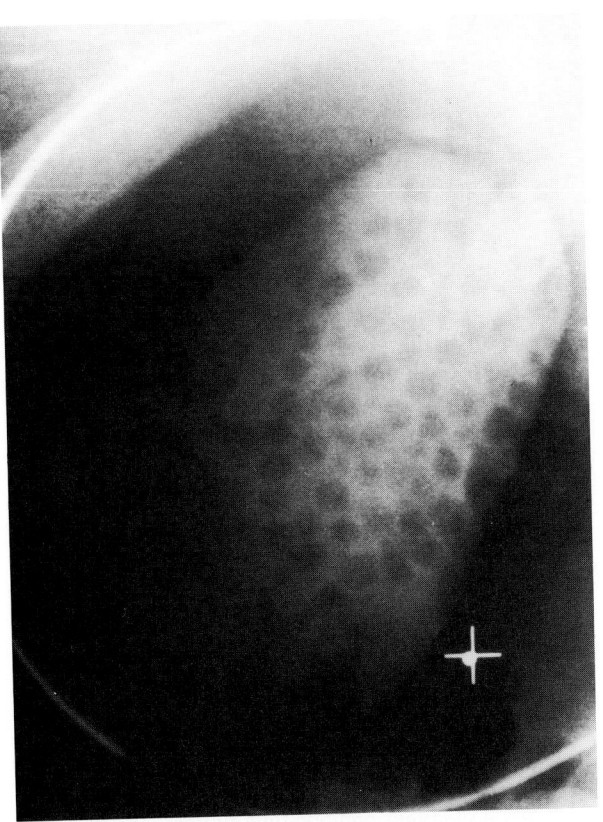

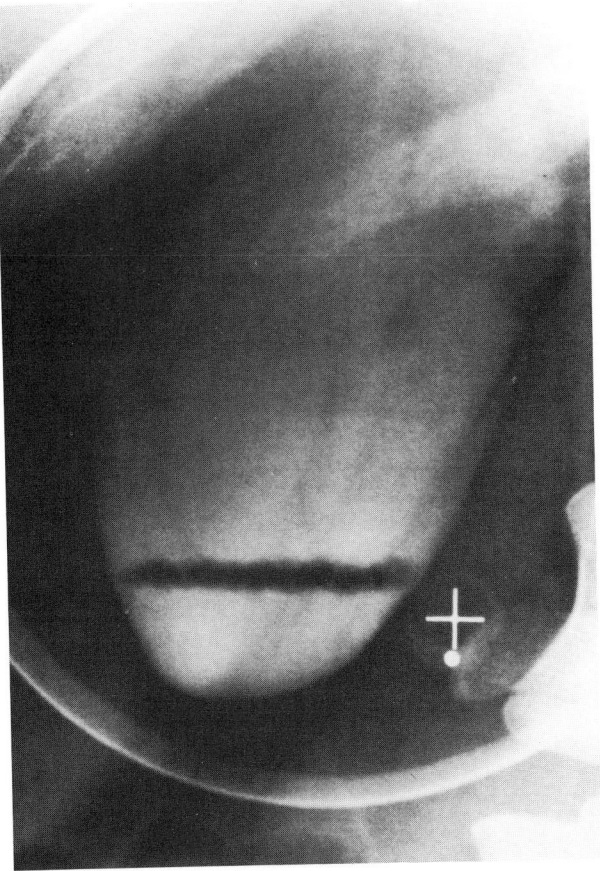

A

B

Fig. 31-6. Multiple gallbladder stones. *A.* With the patient supine, the stones are seen scattered throughout the gallbladder. *B.* With the patient upright and a horizontal x-ray beam, the stones are in a dense layer (arrow) floating in a partially contrast-filled gallbladder. [From: *Skucas J: Diagnostic and interventional radiology, in Schwartz SI, Ellis H (eds): Maingot's Abdominal Operations. Norwalk, CT: Appleton-Century-Crofts, 1985, pp 68–69, with permission.*]

Fig. 31-7. T-tube cholangiogram demonstrating normal caliber of duct with absence of choledocholithiasis. Liver arborization is normal. Tapering at terminal portion of common bile duct is normal, and radiopaque material is noted in duodenum.

Operative Cholangiography (T-Tube Cholangiography). This procedure (Fig. 31-7) is frequently performed in the operating room at the time of exploration of the biliary tract, with injection of radiopaque material either into the cystic duct or into the T tube placed in the common duct. The main application of cystic duct cholangiography is to avoid common bile duct exploration. It is also used to identify calculi that have escaped palpation in order to avoid a subsequent common duct exploration. The technique may contribute to confusion because of failure of the opaque medium to enter the duodenum, despite the fact that there is no abnormality present in the sphincter of Oddi and no obstruction within the common duct. Postoperative cholangiography is usually performed in the x-ray suite prior to removal of a T tube to demonstrate the patency of the common duct, the absence of retained stones, and free passage of bile into the duodenum. The most rewarding technique employs 10 to 15 mL 50% Hypaque diluted to 30 mL with saline solution and administered slowly.

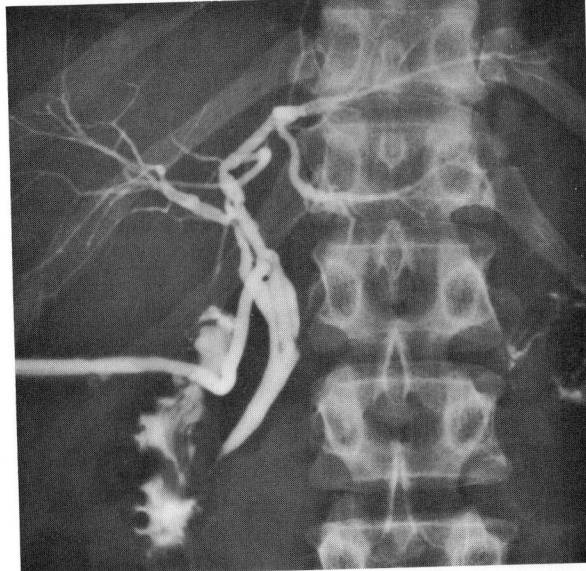

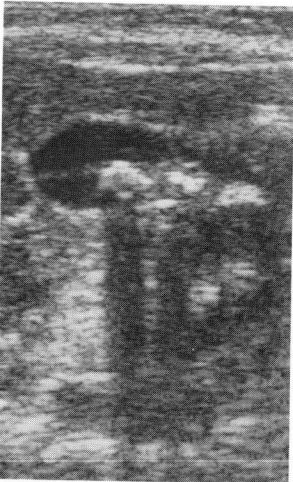

Fig. 31-8. Ultrasound reveals multiple large stones in gallbladder and shadowing effect of stones.

Ultrasonography and Computed Tomography

Gray-scale B-mode ultrasonography (Fig. 31-8) has a diagnostic accuracy of over 90 percent for defining biliary calculi. Diagnostic errors occur with very small calculi and when a single stone is impacted in the cystic duct. A gallbladder packed with stones may not be identified. The technique is particularly pertinent in the evaluation of the patient who is vomiting, or pregnant, and in the emergency assessment of patients with suspected biliary tract disease. It is also applicable in the initial evaluation of the jaundiced patient to define the presence of proximal ductal dilatation and calculi. Computed tomography can be applied for the same situations but provides little advantage and is more expensive.

Isotopic Scans (Fig. 31-9)

A variety of ^{99m}Tc labeled iminodiacetic acid isotopes that are secreted in the bile have been used to define gallbladder function and pathology. These are gamma-emit-

Fig. 31-9. HIDA scan of biliary tract. *Left:* normal, with visualization of the gallbladder, hepatic ducts, and common bile ducts, and also second portion of the duodenum. *Right:* acute cholecystitis with visualization of common bile duct, and second and third portions of the duodenum. The gallbladder failed to visualize.

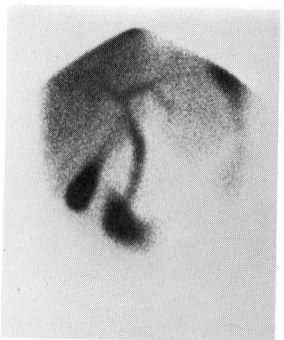 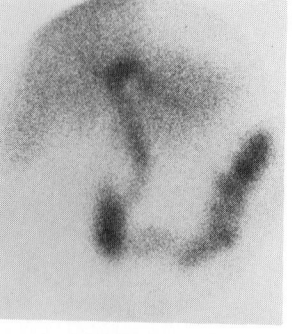

ting agents with a 6-h half-life. Hepatobiliary scanning has become the diagnostic tool of choice for defining acute cholecystitis secondary to cystic duct obstruction. Visualization of the gallbladder rules out this diagnosis. The technique can also define obstruction of the extrahepatic ducts. There is no toxicity and less compromise by hyperbilirubinemia in contrast to intravenous cholangiography, which scanning has almost completely replaced.

Cholangiomanometry

This procedure, which frequently combines determination of bile duct pressure (normal is 12 ± 3 cm) and flow of an infused solution (normal is 23.0 ± 7 mL/min), is widely used by the European surgeon but rarely used in North America. Proponents of the method suggest that the additional 5 min of operative time increases the yield for diagnoses of abnormalities in the common duct, stones in the distal end of the duct, and most particularly organic changes in the sphincter that cause functional changes.

Choledochoscopy

Both rigid and flexible choledochoscopes inserted into the supraduodenal common duct to visualize the lumen of the extrahepatic ducts have been applied to determine the presence or absence of calculi; an accuracy of over 90 percent has been reported. The technique is used as an addendum to operative cholangiography when the common duct is explored. Choledochoscopy can also aid in the removal of stones and bile duct tumors, and stenoses can be inspected and biopsied.

TRAUMA

Penetrating and Nonpenetrating Injuries of the Gallbladder

Injuries of the gallbladder are uncommon, occurring in 1.9 to 8.6 percent of cases with major abdominal trauma. Penetrating injuries are usually due to gunshot wounds or stab wounds and occur rarely during attempted needle biopsy of the liver, particularly in patients with obstructive jaundice. Nonpenetrating injuries are most frequently caused by automobile accidents, kicks, blows, and falls. They are extremely rare; only about 50 cases have been reported. The associated visceral damage with both penetrating and nonpenetrating gallbladder injuries includes involvement of the liver in 72 percent, small bowel in 36 percent, colon in 32 percent, and in only 20 percent of the cases is the trauma isolated to the gallbladder. Although it is very uncommon for the gallbladder to be the only organ involved with nonpenetrating injuries to the abdomen, isolated involvement of the gallbladder due to penetrating injuries is relatively frequent.

The types of injuries include (1) contusion, (2) avulsion, (3) rupture, and (4) traumatic cholecystitis. Contusion is difficult to verify but may be associated with vague or temporary symptoms that require no specific therapy. The contused area may undergo necrosis and perforate. Avulsion of the gallbladder from its liver bed occurs as a result of nonpenetrating injury. When the gallbladder's attachments are torn, the organ usually hangs by its neck but may be attached only by the cystic duct and artery. Volvulus of the gallbladder may result. Traumatic cholecystectomy, in which the cystic duct, cystic artery, and gallbladder attachments are transected, has been reported. An acutely inflamed gallbladder may be avulsed from the liver as a result of minor trauma. Laceration is the most common type of injury following penetrating wounds but also may result from blunt trauma. Cases of delayed rupture of the gallbladder occur days to weeks following injury. Traumatic cholecystitis is an unusual condition that occurs as a result of blunt trauma. Bleeding into the gallbladder, due to injury either of the gallbladder or of the liver, precipitates cholecystitis and, at times, gangrene of the gallbladder. The retained blood may clot and block the cystic duct, and the patient presents with the manifestations of hematobilia, including intermittent jaundice, colicky pain, hematemesis, and melena.

EFFECTS OF INTRAPERITONEAL BILE. Effects of extravasation of bile into the peritoneal cavity depend upon whether or not the bile is infected. When infected bile escapes into the peritoneal cavity, a fulminating and frequently fatal peritonitis results. On the other hand, when bile is sterile, it is well tolerated and results in a chemical peritonitis that may be relatively mild. In the majority of gallbladder injuries, the organ is normal and the bile is sterile. The fact that sterile bile is relatively innocuous is borne out by the very low mortality rate associated with nonpenetrating wounds of the gallbladder. Penetrating wounds are potentially more serious because of the danger of secondary infection. Continuous leakage of noninfected bile, however, is not innocuous. The extravasated bile may produce ascites or become encysted, and extensive chemical peritonitis causes an outpouring of fluid into the peritoneal cavity from the general circulation that may result in shock. There is also some evidence to indicate that absorption of large amounts of bile salts may be toxic.

CLINICAL MANIFESTATIONS. The diagnosis of involvement of the gallbladder or extrahepatic biliary tract is frequently entertained preoperatively in patients with penetrating injuries, in contrast to a low incidence of diagnosis associated with blunt trauma. Bile leakage through the penetrating wound suggests the possibility of damage to the biliary system, but duodenal laceration may have a similar manifestation. With blunt trauma, manifestations may be delayed for 36 h or more. This has been related to the fact that there are other serious injuries that mask injury of the biliary tract and that the sterile bile causes only minimal symptoms. The presence of severe shock and pain in the right upper quadrant or lower part of the right side of the chest should make one suspicious. The manifestations of bacterial peritonitis may ensue, or if the bile leakage is minimal, the patient may recover only to subsequently develop ascites or an intraperitoneal cyst. The finding of bile-stained fluid during diagnostic paracentesis is suggestive, but a negative tap does not exclude gallbladder injury. In most instances, the diagnosis is made at celiotomy, emphasizing the necessity for careful examination of the biliary system following abdominal trauma.

TREATMENT. The injured gallbladder has been successfully treated by simple suture of the laceration, cholecystostomy, and cholecystectomy. In general, it is preferable to remove the traumatized gallbladder. Cholecystectomy is usually quite easy to perform, since the gallbladder is rarely diseased, and must be performed if the gallbladder has been avulsed or the cystic artery torn. In the severely ill patient, cholecystostomy may be used for treatment of the extensive laceration or traumatic cholecystitis in order to reduce the time of operative procedure and avoid injury to the common duct. Prognosis is directly related to the incidence of associated injuries.

Injury of the Extrahepatic Bile Ducts

Rare cases of solitary penetrating wounds involving the bile duct have been reported, but there is usually associated trauma to other viscera. Approximately 100 cases of traumatic rupture of the extrahepatic bile duct have been reported, and in 15 cases complete transection occurred. The clinical manifestations are similar to those described for gallbladder injury, and diagnosis is extremely difficult.

Treatment consists initially of meticulous exploration, particularly if injury to the gallbladder has been excluded and bile has been demonstrated retroperitoneally or within the peritoneal cavity. A Kocher maneuver should be performed to rule out perforation of the common duct behind the duodenum. The presence of hematoma in this region should make one suspicious. Tangential injuries may be treated by primary repair. Complete transection by a knife of either the common hepatic duct or common bile duct may be treated by debridement and an end-to-end anastomosis over a T tube, which should be left in place for several weeks, but in most cases of complete transection or injuries caused by blunt trauma, the proximal end of the duct should be anastomosed to a Roux en Y of jejunum. The patient should be placed on appropriate antibiotics.

Operative Injury of the Bile Ducts

The great majority of injuries of the extrahepatic biliary duct system are iatrogenic, occurring in the course of gallbladder surgical procedures. In over 70 percent of the cases, the cholecystectomy had apparently been carried out without incident. In the remaining 30 percent, a variety of factors were implicated. These included cholecystectomy for contracted gallbladder, intimate association between the ampulla of the gallbladder and the common hepatic duct, massive hemorrhage at the time of operation with attempted "blind control," during which the duct was occluded and traumatized, and excessive tension when ligating a cystic duct. Lack of appreciation of anatomy and possible anomalies in the region increase the incidence of surgical trauma of the common duct.

DIAGNOSIS. In approximately 15 percent of the cases, ductal injuries are recognized and treated at the time of operation. The remaining 85 percent become manifest by either increasing obstructive jaundice or profuse and persistent drainage of bile through a fistula. Jaundice usually becomes manifest in 2 to 3 days but, in some instances, does not develop for weeks. It may be continuous or intermittent; if intermittent, it is frequently accompanied by attacks of chills and fever suggesting ascending cholangitis. Hepatomegaly almost always accompanies jaundice if it has been persistent for a period of time, and splenomegaly may also occur if secondary biliary cirrhosis has evolved. Some patients do not display the signs or symptoms of partial or complete blockage until months or years after surgical treatment. This is related to increasing fibrosis and narrowing of the channel and repeated episodes of cholangitis, which, in turn, leads to fibrosis. Percutaneous transhepatic cholangiography most clearly defines the site of obstruction or leak.

TREATMENT. Patients with jaundice or persistent fistula require a vigorous preoperative regimen including a high-protein, low-fat diet and intravenous administration of fat-soluble vitamins, particularly vitamin K. If there is concomitant portal hypertension with bleeding varices, this preempts repair of the common duct, and the portal hypertension is usually best treated by a splenorenal shunt because of extensive scarring of the right upper quadrant. Sedgwick and associates have described 12 such patients, 5 of whom were salvaged.

Operative Approach. Injury of the bile duct recognized during surgical operation should be corrected with an immediate reconstructive procedure. Restoration of the continuity of the duct with an end-to-end anastomosis over a T tube may be feasible, but following such a procedure stricture develops in about half the cases. Direct anastomosis is usually impractical for acute injuries and chronic strictures where the proximal end of the duct should be anastomosed to a Roux en Y of jejunum. A mucosa-to-mucosa approximation provides the best long-term results. If this is not feasible, a lateral-lateral anastomosis between the left hepatic duct and a Roux en Y limb of jejunum (Hepp-Soupault) is preferable to the Smith transhepatic mucosal pull-through technique. The Longmire operation, with transection of the left lobe of the liver and anastomosis of the jejunum to a large intrahepatic bile duct, has been associated with discouraging results.

The operative mortality of patients with chronic stricture is reported to be 8 percent, and approximately 10 percent of patients die of liver failure or its attendant complications after leaving the hospital. A satisfactory result is obtained in about 70 percent of patients after one or more operative procedures. If the patients are symptom-free 4 years after reconstruction, the cure is almost always permanent.

GALLSTONES

COMPOSITION. The major elements involved in the formation of gallstones are cholesterol, bile pigment, and calcium. Other constituents include iron, phosphorus, carbonates, proteins, carbohydrates, mucus, and cellular debris. In Western cultures, most stones are made up of the three major elements and have a particularly high content of cholesterol, averaging 71 percent. Pure cholesterol stones are uncommon, usually large with smooth surfaces, and solitary. Bilirubin pigment stones are also uncommon, with a characteristic smooth, glistening green or black surface. The pigment stones may be "pure" or consist of calcium bilirubinate. The "pure" pigment stones are usually associated with hemolytic jaundice or situations in which the bile is abnormally concentrated. Increased red blood cell destruction following cardiac valve replacement has resulted in production of gallstones. Calcium bilirubinate stones are prevalent in Asia, where they constitute 30 to 40 percent of all gallstones.

FORMATION. Gallstones form as a result of solids settling out of solution. The solubility of cholesterol depends on the concentrations of conjugated bile salts, phospholipids, and cholesterol in bile. Lecithin is the predominant phospholipid in bile and, although insoluble in aqueous solutions, is dissolved by bile salts in micelles. Cholesterol is also insoluble in aqueous solution but becomes soluble when incorporated into the lecithin–bile salt micelle. By plotting the percentages of cholesterol, lecithin, and bile salts on triangular coordinates (Fig. 31-10), the limits of micellar liquid in which bile is less than saturated with cholesterol may be defined. Above these limits, the bile is either a supersaturated liquid or a two-phase sys-

Fig. 31-10. Three major components of bile (bile salts, lecithin, and cholesterol) plotted on triangular coordinates. Point *P* represents bile consisting of 80 mol percent bile salt, 5 percent cholesterol, and 15 percent lecithin. Line *ABC* represents the maximal solubility of cholesterol in varying mixtures of bile salt and lecithin. Because point *P* falls below line *ABC* and within the zone of a single phase of micellar liquid, this bile is less than saturated with cholesterol. Bile with a composition that would place it above line *ABC* would contain excess cholesterol in supersaturated or precipitated form. (After: *Small DM: Gallstones. N Engl J Med 279:588, 1968,* with permission.)

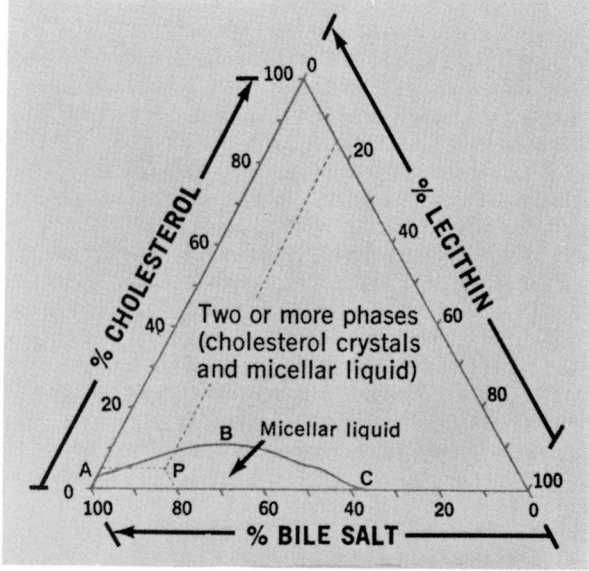

tem of liquid bile and solid crystalline cholesterol. When crystals achieve macroscopic size during a period of entrapment in the gallbladder, gallstones form. The basic secretory defect in nonobese patients is decreased bile salt and phospholipid secretion. Conversely, in obese subjects cholesterol secretion is greatly increased without any reduction in bile salt or phospholipid secretion.

Factors that have been implicated in the formation and precipitation of cholesterol include constitutional elements, bacteria, fungi, reflux of intestinal and pancreatic fluid, hormones, and bile stasis. Constitutional elements are best exemplified in the Pima Indians, of whom 70 percent of females by age 30 and 70 percent of males by age 60 have gallstones. The Masai of Africa, on the other hand, do not have gallstones. Evidence in favor of infection as a cause includes the isolation of such organisms as *Escherichia coli, Bacterium typhosum,* and *Streptococcus* from gallbladder walls and centers of stones in a high percentage of cases, and the demonstration of slow-growing actinomyces recovered from over half the stones examined in one series. The development of gallstones in the absence of infection or inflammation argues against infection as a universal factor. In Oriental people, concretions are known to form about liver flukes and other parasites within the bile ducts.

The reflux factor receives support from the findings of pancreatic enzymes in the gallbladders of patients with cholelithiasis. Trypsin disturbs colloidal balance, and pancreatic phospholipase A can convert lecithin into toxic lysolecithin. Hormones have been implicated in an unproved correlation between calculi and parity, diabetes, hyperthyroidism, and the predominance in females.

Stasis, which includes temporary cessation of bile flow into the intestine and stagnation in the gallbladder, has also been assigned a major role. Temporary bile stasis may be due to functional disorders or to a mechanical blockage in the region of the choledochoduodenal junction or gallbladder. The interruption of bile flow to the intestine is associated with an interruption in enterohepatic circulation, which, in turn, is accompanied by a decrease in the output of bile salts and phospholipids, reducing the solubility of cholesterol. When over 20 percent of bile is diverted, the bile salt pool cannot be maintained. Bile salt secretion is also diminished by reduction of the distal third of the intestine, explaining the development of stones in patients with ileal resection or disease. Cholecystectomy causes a greater fraction of the bile salt pool to cycle around the enterohepatic circulation, thereby increasing bile salt and phospholipid secretion.

Solubility has been investigated as a possible regimen to prevent the development of stones in patients at risk and also to dissolve stones already formed. Chenodeoxycholic acid, which replenishes the bile acid pool and reduces cholesterol synthesis and secretion, administered to potential stone formers may return supersaturated bile to its normal composition, preventing stone formation. In one series the drug was administered for 2 years; complete dissolution of radiolucent stones occurred in 13.5 percent of patients. Partial dissolution occurred in 41 percent. The effects were more frequent in women, thin patients, and in patients with serum cholesterol levels greater than 227 mg/dL. Clinically significant hepatotoxicity was rare. Lithotripsy has successfully fragmented biliary calculi but generally is not regarded as appropriate therapy because a diseased organ remains to form new stones and the flushing effected by normal bile flow is not equivalent to that of urinary flow.

Asymptomatic Gallstones

Asymptomatic cholelithiasis is rare. Of 3012 patients with cholecystitis and cholelithiasis, only 134 had no symptoms attributable to gallbladder disease. The liberal use of cholecystography and ultrasonography has resulted in the diagnosis of calculi in patients without symptoms referable to the biliary tract. In several large series of asymptomatic patients with gallstones who were followed without surgical treatment, symptoms developed in 50 percent, and serious complications occurred in 20 percent. By contrast, McSherry and associates reported that only 10 percent of patients developed symptoms during a mean 5-year follow-up. Similarly, Grace and Ransohoff reported that none of 123 patients with asymptomatic gallstones died of gallbladder disease and the 15-year cumulative probability of developing symptoms was 18 percent. The relationship of cholelithiasis and carcinoma of the gallbladder is also of some significance. A review of several series showed that the incidence of calculi in cancer of the gallbladder varied between 65 and 100 percent, with a mean of 90 percent. Conversely, the incidence of cancer of the gallbladder in patients with symptomatic gallstones ranged between 1 and 15 percent, with a mean of 4.5 percent. Comfort et al. reported no carcinoma among 112 patients with asymptomatic cholelithiasis.

Cystic Duct Obstruction

Calculi, usually of the cholesterol type, may become impacted in the cystic duct or neck of the gallbladder, resulting in a hydrops. The bile is absorbed, and the gallbladder becomes filled and distended with mucinous material. The gallbladder is generally palpable and tender, and the impacted stone with the resulting edema may encroach upon the common duct and cause mild jaundice. Although hydrops may persist with few consequences, early cholecystectomy is generally indicated to avoid the complications of biliary tract infection or perforation of the gallbladder. In questionable cases, isotopic scanning of the gallbladder following intravenous CCK (cholecystokinin) can define cystic obstruction or patency.

Choledocholithiasis

Common duct stones may be single or multiple and are found in approximately 12 percent of cases subjected to cholecystectomy. Most common duct calculi are formed within the gallbladder and migrate down the cystic duct into the common bile duct. Less commonly, stones are thought to form within the ducts. In patients infected with tropical parasites such as *Clonorchis sinensis* and in the Oriental population in Asia, stones may form within the hepatic ducts or the common bile duct itself. Although small stones may pass via the common duct into the duodenum, the distal duct with its narrow lumen (2 to 3 mm) and thick wall frequently obstructs their passage. Edema, spasm, or fibrosis of the distal duct secondary to irritation by the calculi contribute to biliary obstruction. Both extrahepatic and intrahepatic bile ducts become dilated, and there is evidence of laking in the biliary radicles of the liver. There is also thickening of the duct walls and inflammatory cell infiltration. Chronic biliary obstruction may cause secondary biliary cirrhosis with bile thrombi, bile duct proliferation, and fibrosis of the portal tracts. Also associated with chronic obstruction is the development of infection within the bile duct giving rise to ascending cholangitis and occasionally extending up to the liver, resulting in hepatic abscesses. The offending organism is almost always *E. coli*.

CLINICAL MANIFESTATIONS. The manifestations of calculi within the common duct are variable. Stones may be present within the extrahepatic duct system for many years without causing symptoms. Characteristically, the symptom complex consists of colicky pain in the right upper quadrant radiating to the right shoulder with intermittent jaundice accompanied by pale stools and dark urine. Biliary obstruction is usually chronic and incomplete but may be acute or complete. If obstruction is complete, jaundice progresses but is rarely intense. In contrast to patients with neoplastic obstruction of the common bile duct or ampulla of Vater, the gallbladder is usually not distended because of associated inflammation (Courvoisier's law). Liver function tests demonstrate the pattern of obstructive jaundice, and the alkaline phosphatase level usually becomes elevated earlier and remains abnormal for longer periods of time than the serum bilirubin. The prothrombin time is frequently prolonged, because the absorption of vitamin K is dependent upon bile entering the intestine, but a normal level can usually be achieved with parenteral vitamin K. Tests of hepatocellular function are generally normal. In patients with ascending cholangitis, Charcot's intermittent fever accompanied by abdominal pain and jaundice is characteristic. The diagnosis may be established by ERCP or PTC.

TREATMENT. When surgical operation is performed to establish the cause of obstructive jaundice, there is little question whether the duct should be explored, since there is dilatation and thickening of the duct and stones are usually palpable. Criteria for exploration of the common bile duct during cholecystectomy for cholelithiasis have been proposed. The three obvious indications are (1) palpable stones within the common bile duct, (2) dilated common bile duct, and (3) significant jaundice or a definite history of jaundice. Other indications are recurrent chills and fever suggestive of cholangitis, gallstone pancreatitis, multiple small stones within the gallbladder, and inflamed gallbladder that is empty of stones in a patient with biliary tract symptoms.

The optimal time for exploration of the common bile duct is during the initial procedure of cholecystectomy, provided acute inflammation does not obscure the anatomy. One large prospective series showed that exploration of the common bile duct in the presence of acute cholecystitis carried no greater risk than during elective cholecystectomy. The higher the incidence of duct exploration at the time of cholecystectomy, the lower the incidence of residual stones but the higher the incidence of negative exploration. Considering all patients, including those with jaundice, the performance of a concomitant choledochostomy at the time of cholecystectomy increases the operative mortality by 0.2 to 1.2 percent. If one excludes the jaundiced patients, there is little difference in operative mortality between cholecystectomy alone and cholecystectomy plus concomitant choledochostomy. Early operation for choledochal calculi accompanied by hyperamylassemia is not attended by increased mortality. But there is a significant increase in postoperative morbidity and hospital stay. In order to avoid the negative duct explorations, an operative cholangiogram via a catheter inserted into the cystic duct has been used. This study will demonstrate the caliber of the duct, and a duct greater than 12 mm in diameter should be considered pathologic. The technique will also indicate the presence or absence of filling defects, in which case air bubbles within the ductal system must be differentiated before applying a diagnosis of choledocholithiasis. With this technique, the incidence of concomitant exploration of the common bile duct has been reduced while the incidence of positive exploration has been increased.

The treatment for stones within the common bile duct or hepatic ducts is surgical removal. Preoperatively, patients with common duct stones should be prepared with fat-soluble vitamins, particularly vitamin K if the prothrombin time is prolonged, and if there is evidence of ascending cholangitis, antibiotics should be administered. At the time of exploration, all stones and sludge should be removed, and free passage into the duodenum should be demonstrated. Removal of stones from the common and hepatic ducts may be facilitated by the use of balloon-tipped catheters. As instrumentation has been refined, choledochoscopic techniques have been more widely applied. After the common duct is explored, a T tube is inserted prior to closure and drainage is maintained for approximately 1 week, at which time a T-tube cholangiogram is performed in order to demonstrate patency of the duct and absence of retained stones. If these criteria are met, the T tube can then be removed. Intraoperatively if there is obstruction of the distal duct, transduodenal sphincteroplasty and removal of the stone may be performed, or, if the common duct is dilated, choledochoduodenostomy may be carried out. Choledochoduodenostomy has become increasingly popular for patients, particularly the elderly, with enlarged ducts and multiple retained stones. A wide sphincteroplasty is preferred by others, particularly when there is no ductal dilatation and if a stone is impacted at the ampulla of Vater.

RETAINED COMMON DUCT STONES. If stones are noted to be present when a T-tube cholangiogram is performed postoperatively (Fig. 31-11), there are five general approaches that can be entertained. Small stones, particularly those located in the branches of the hepatic duct, may be disregarded since the majority will remain asymp-

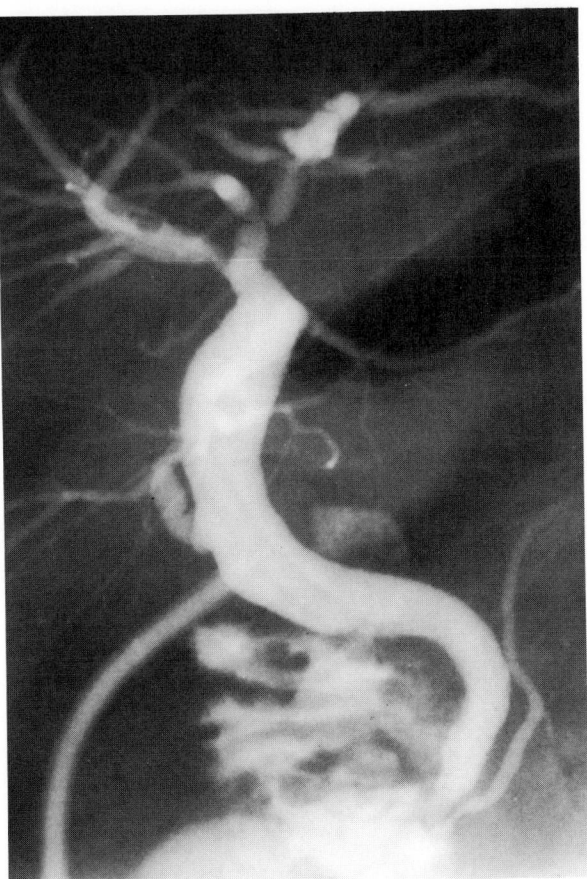

Fig. 31-11. T-tube cholangiogram demonstrating calculus in the right hepatic duct. [From: *Skucas J, Spataro RF: Liver and biliary tract, in Skucas J, Spataro RF (eds): Radiology of the Acute Abdomen. New York, Churchill Livingstone, 1986, Fig 9-30, with permission.*]

tomatic and if symptoms ensue, operative extraction is not associated with significantly increased morbidity. A second approach employs either flushing or chemical dissolution. Capmul 8210, a mono-octanoin, is the agent of choice. Heparin, 250,000 units in a 250-mL solution infused every 8 h for 5 days, has been successful.

The most encouraging approach employs mechanical extraction of the retained stone under radiographic control. Mazzariello achieved success in 96 percent of 1086 cases, while Burhenne and associates, reporting on 612 patients managed at 38 hospitals, reported no deaths and no significant complications, coupled with a 91 percent success rate. The T tube is generally left in place for at least 4 weeks after the operation; it is then extracted and a polyethylene catheter is used to instill radiopaque material into the common duct. A Dormia basket is then advanced through the catheter to entrap the stone (Fig. 31-12).

If the T tube had been removed and a common duct stone demonstrated cholangiographically, transduodenal papillotomy with extraction of the stone under endoscopic visualization may be applied (Fig. 31-13). The suc-

cess rate for extraction or spontaneous passage following this procedure was 86 percent for 731 collected cases. A complication rate of 7 percent was noted, but two-thirds were treated conservatively. The mortality rate related to the technique was 1.25 percent. Operative intervention is indicated in some cases if there is evidence of obstruction and/or cholangitis, or if nonoperative methods fail.

Most calculi in the intrahepatic ducts either pass into distal ducts or are extractable. Some calculi remain within the liver and may cause irreversible damage. The most common location is a left main hepatic duct that forms a cisterna, and treatment is best achieved in this circumstance by hepatic resection of the left lobe of the liver.

Biliary Enteric Fistula and Gallstone Ileus

Biliary enteric fistulas usually develop between the gallbladder and duodenum but 15 percent are cholecystocolic fistulas. Mechanical obstruction of the gastrointestinal tract caused by gallstones is a relatively infrequent occurrence. Gallstone ileus causes 1 to 2 percent of mechanical small intestinal obstructions and was associated with high mortality rates. Currently the mortality rate is less than 10 percent.

Since cholelithiasis occurs three to six times more commonly in the female than in the male, the higher incidence of gallstone ileus in the female is to be anticipated. Preponderance in the female is actually higher than one would expect, and in several series all patients were female. It is characteristically a disease of the aged, with an average age of sixty-four, and is unusual under the age of fifty. Associated diseases are common, diabetes occurring in 50 percent and major cardiovascular disorders in 58 percent.

The process usually begins with formation of the stone within the gallbladder, but cases have been reported in which the gallbladder was not present, having been removed several years prior to the intestinal obstruction. After the gallstone has left the gallbladder, it may obstruct the alimentary tract in one of two ways: rarely, it enters the peritoneal cavity, causing kinking or inflammation and extrinsic obstruction of the intestine; more commonly, the blockage is caused by the entrance of the stone into the gastrointestinal tract, producing an intraluminal type of obstruction. The stone may enter the duodenum via the common duct, but this is unusual, and almost always the offending calculus enters through a cholecystoenteric fistula. The fistulous tract may connect the gallbladder with the stomach, duodenum, jejunum, ileum, or colon. In addition, internal biliary fistulas may communicate with the pleural or pericardial cavities, tracheobronchial tree, pregnant uterus, ovarian cyst, renal pelvis, and urinary bladder. In a series of 176 fistulas caused by gallstones, the duodenum was involved in 101, the colon in 33, the stomach in 7, and multiple sites in 11.

The fistula probably originates with a stone obstructing the cystic duct, acute cholecystitis, empyema, and the formation of adhesions between the gallbladder and adjacent viscera. Perforation then occurs between the inti-

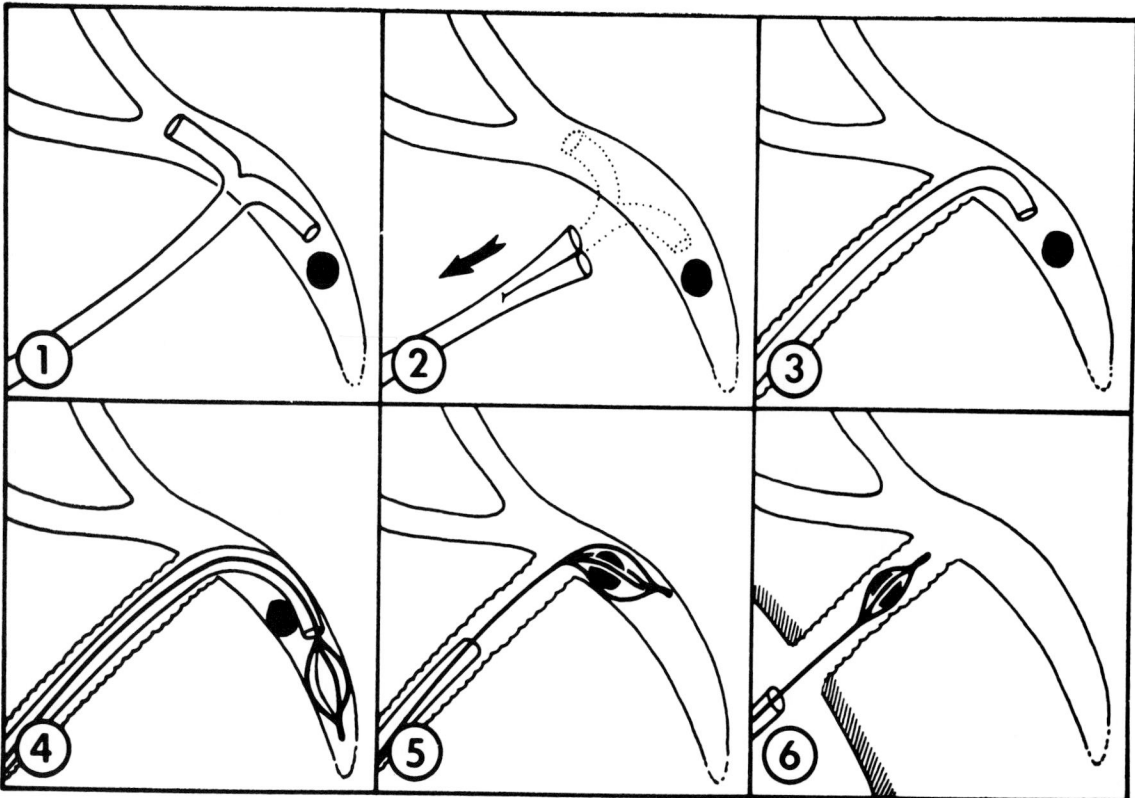

Fig. 31-12. Technical steps for retained common duct stone extraction. 1. Repeat T-tube cholangiogram is obtained on the day of stone extraction 4 to 5 weeks after choledochotomy. 2. After the location of the retained stone has been ascertained, the T tube is withdrawn. 3. Using the sinus tract of the T tube, the steerable catheter is guided into the bile duct, and its movable tip is advanced beyond the retained stone. 4. The basket is inserted through the steerable catheter, the catheter is withdrawn, and the basket is opened. 5. The open basket is withdrawn in order to engage the stone. The basket is only retracted, never advanced, outside the enclosure of the steerable catheter. 6. The stone is extracted through the drain tract. (After: *Burhenne HJ: Radium therapy and nuclear medicine. Am J Roentgenol 117:388, 1973, with permission.*)

Fig. 31-13. Steps in endoscopic sphincterotomy. *A.* Sphincterotome is inserted in closed position into common bile duct. *B.* Proximal part of bent wire appears just outside papilla. *C.* Current is applied for cutting sphincter. *D.* Extraction of stone through opened papilla. (After: *Safrany L: World J Surg, 2:457 1978, with permission.*)

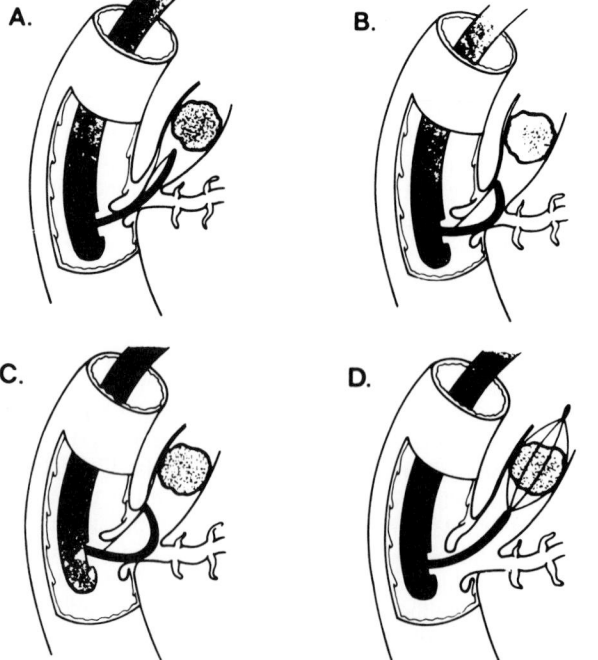

mately adherent organs, and the stone traverses the fistula. The cholecystoenteric fistula then frequently closes, and only a fibrous remnant remains. Having entered the alimentary tract, the gallstone, which is usually single, may be vomited or passed spontaneously per rectum. The size of the stone is important, since stones smaller than 2 to 3 cm usually pass. When obstruction occurs, the site is usually at the terminal ileum, which is the narrowest portion of the small intestine. Of 154 collective cases, the duodenum was obstructed in 6, the jejunum in 14, the proximal ileum in 6, the middle ileum in 31, the terminal ileum in 88, the colon in 3, and the rectum in 2. When a gallstone blocks the small intestine, the morbid anatomic and physiologic effects of a mechanical obstruction pertain. There are extremely large losses of fluid into the intestine. Edema, ulceration, or necrosis of the bowel may occur, and perforation may result.

CLINICAL MANIFESTATIONS. A past history suggestive of cholelithiasis is present in 50 to 75 percent of patients.

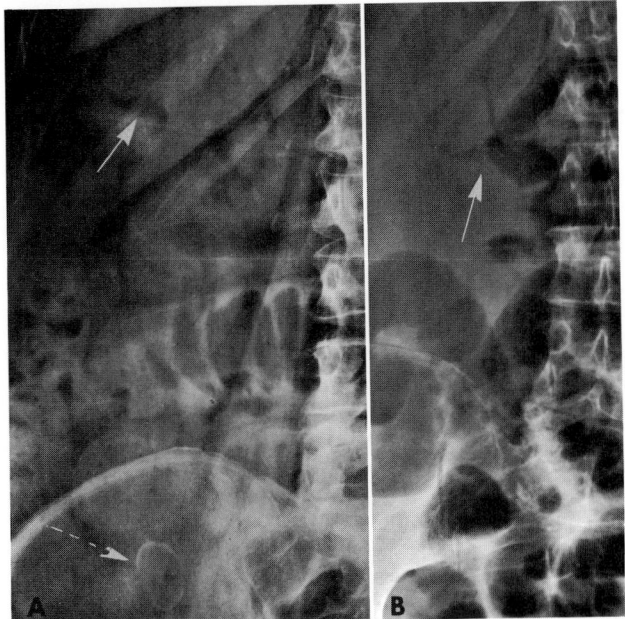

Fig. 31-14. Gallstone ileus. *A.* Radiopaque calculus present in right lower quadrant; suggestion of air in biliary tract within liver. *B.* Demonstration of air in intrahepatic biliary system.

Symptoms of acute cholecystitis immediately preceding the onset of gallstone ileus occur in one-quarter to one-third of the cases. A history of jaundice is present in about 10 percent of the cases. Occasionally, there may be an initial episode of pain suggestive of biliary colic, but major pain is usually not experienced until the intestinal colic results. There is associated cramping, nausea, and vomiting, which may be intermittent. When complete small intestinal obstruction occurs, the vomiting increases and the patient becomes obstipated. Analysis of the incidence of varying symptoms indicates that vomiting is present in almost 100 percent, cramps in 90 percent, distention in 90 percent, obstipation in 78 percent, and feculent vomiting in 67 percent. Serum electrolytes reveal the pattern of lower intestinal obstruction with marked hypochloremia, hyponatremia, hypokalemia, and an elevated carbonate level.

The correct preoperative diagnosis is infrequently made, ranging between 13 and 30 percent in several series. The usual diagnosis is that of intestinal obstruction of unknown cause. Radiologic examination may be diagnostic if air is demonstrated within the biliary tract (Fig. 31-14). Flat, upright, and lateral films plus spot films over the liver are indicated if the diagnosis is considered. The plain x-ray reveals the pattern of small intestinal obstruction, and in less than 20 percent of the cases a stone is visualized. The diagnosis has also been based on the migration of a previously observed radiopaque gallstone.

TREATMENT. Biliary enteric fistulas are managed by cholecystectomy and closure by primary repair of the intestinal opening. The patient with gallstone ileus often requires fluid and electrolyte replacement in order to correct deficiency, and a nasogastric tube is used to decompress the stomach. Definitive therapy consists of locating the stone or stones, enterotomy proximal to the stone, and removing the offending calculi with closure of the

intestine. The recurrence rate of gallstone ileus is 5 to 9 percent, and it is important to palpate the entire small intestine, gallbladder, and common duct for retained stones, particularly if the obstructing stone is faceted. Either concomitant or planned interval cholecystectomy and closure of the fistula, if patent, is indicated, since recurrent symptoms or complications develop in one-third of the patients and in eight cases carcinoma of the gallbladder was either present or developed 5 to 16 years after removal of the obstructing gallstone. Performance of concomitant cholecystectomy is determined by the patient's general condition. Many of these patients are extremely ill and depleted; prolongation of the operative procedure in these patients is contraindicated.

INFLAMMATORY AND OTHER BENIGN LESIONS

Cholecystitis

In 85 to 95 percent of the cases, inflammation of the gallbladder is associated with calculi. Whether the stones represent cause or effect has not been defined, but they are generally implicated as a cause of the acute inflammatory process. Stasis of the gallbladder with consequent maintenance of contact between stagnant bile and the gallbladder wall is also considered a cause of cholecystitis. A bacterial cause of cholecystitis has been proposed, and positive bile cultures have been noted in 60 percent of patients with acute cholecystitis. A variety of organisms have been cultured in both acute and chronically inflamed gallbladders. *E. coli,* streptococci, *Aerobacter aerogenes, Salmonella,* and clostridia have all been implicated, but in many cases of both acute and chronic cholecystitis cultures of the bile are negative. In addition to bile, which in its concentrated or desiccated form is known to cause acute cholecystitis, pancreatic juice with its enzymatic properties is also considered a chemical irritant. Since pressures developed in the pancreatic duct are generally greater than those in the biliary tract, the presence of a common channel permits entrance of pancreatic juice into the gallbladder; the frequent finding of amylase in the bile supports this assumption.

ACUTE CHOLECYSTITIS

In the overwhelming majority of cases, acute cholecystitis is associated with an obstruction of the neck of the gallbladder or cystic duct due to stones impacted in Hartmann's pouch. Direct pressure of the calculus on the mucosa results in ischemia, necrosis, and ulceration with swelling, edema, and impairment of venous return. These processes, in turn, increase and extend the intensity of the inflammation. The ulceration may be so extensive that the mucosa is frequently hard to define on microscopic examination and there are segmented leukocytes infiltrating all layers. The results of necrosis are perforation with pericholecystic abscess formation, fistulization, or bile peritonitis. In the past, acute cholecystitis secondary to systemic infection occurred most commonly with typhoid fever, but this is now rare. Acute cholecystitis, due either to generalized sepsis or to stasis and/or impaction of a calculus, may occur while the patient is recovering from trauma or an operation. Among other causes of acute cholecystitis are the vascular effects of collagen disease, terminal states of hypertensive vascular disease, and thrombosis of the main cystic artery. Less than 1 percent of acutely inflamed gallbladders contain a malignant tumor that may play a role in causing obstruction. The incidence of common duct calculi is similar in acute and chronic cholecystitis, averaging 7 to 15 percent.

CLINICAL MANIFESTATIONS. Most attacks of acute cholecystitis occur in patients who give a past history compatible with chronic cholecystitis and cholelithiasis. Acute cholecystitis can occur at any age, but the greatest incidence is between the fourth and eighth decades, and patients over sixty comprise between one-quarter and one-third of the group. Caucasians are afflicted more frequently than blacks.

The onset of acute symptoms is frequently related to a vigorous attempt of the gallbladder to empty its contents, usually after a heavy, fatty, or fried meal. Moderate to severe pain is experienced in the right upper quadrant or epigastrium and may radiate to the back in the region of the angle of the scapula or in the interscapular area. The patient is often febrile, and vomiting may be severe. Tenderness, usually along the right costal margin, often associated with rebound tenderness and spasm, is characteristic. The gallbladder may be palpable. Mild icterus may be present and can be related to calculi within the ampulla and edema encroaching upon the common duct. Moderate to marked jaundice, particularly with a serum bilirubin greater than 6 mg/dL suggests the presence of associated choledocholithiasis but can occur with isolated cholecystitis.

The differential diagnosis includes perforation or pene-

tration of peptic ulcer, appendicitis, pancreatitis, hepatitis, myocardial ischemia or infarction, pneumonia, pleurisy, and herpes zoster involving an intercostal nerve.

The hemogram usually demonstrates leukocytosis with a shift to the left. Radiograms of the chest and abdomen are indicated to rule out thoracic processes. A radiopaque calculus is noted in less than 20 percent of the cases. The serum bilirubin level may determine the presence of common duct obstruction. Although the elevated amylase level is generally regarded as evidence of acute pancreatitis, levels as high as 1000 Somogyi units have been associated with acute cholecystitis uncomplicated by pancreatitis. To rule out myocardial ischemia, an electrocardiogram should be made on any patient over the age of forty-five being considered for surgical treatment. However, acute cholecystitis may be responsible for some changes. Oral cholecystography is of limited value because of impaired absorption of dye. An ultrasonogram may demonstrate calculi and/or a thickened wall of the gallbladder. Radionuclide scanning with DISIDA or PIPIDA is the most effective diagnostic study in this situation.

TREATMENT. Conflicting opinions concerning the management of acute cholecystitis, with particular reference to the optimal time for surgical intervention, persist. For the purpose of discussion, early operation is defined as one performed within 72 h after the onset of the acute process; intermediate operation is one carried out between 72 h and the cessation of clinical manifestations; delayed operative management permits the acute inflammatory process to subside; and scheduled elective surgery is performed at an interval of 6 weeks to 3 months.

The proponents of the conservative treatment, i.e., delayed operative management, base their thesis on the following premises: (1) Most cases of acute cholecystitis subside on conservative management without significant complications. (2) Operation performed in the presence of inflammation with vascular congestion may be injurious as a result of spreading infection. (3) The acute inflammatory changes obscure the anatomy and lead to technical errors. In the presence of intense inflammatory process, exploration of the common duct for stones is compromised. (4) Many of the patients with acute cholecystitis have associated diseases and do not represent optimal risk for surgical intervention.

Nonoperative management is directed at creating a situation of functional rest for the gallbladder and upper gastrointestinal tract and relaxing spasm of the sphincter of Oddi. The regimen includes restriction of fluid and food intake and continuous nasogastric suction. Anticholinergic drugs are administered in an effort to decrease spasm of the sphincter. Pain is treated with small amounts of Demerol, while morphine is withheld, because it causes more profound sphincteric spasm. Antibiotics are advised by many physicians.

The proponents of nonoperative management of acute cholecystitis argue against the importance of perforation and bile peritonitis. In one series of 679 patients subjected to laparotomy, although perforation was noted in 9 percent of the patients, only 3 percent demonstrated free perforation into the peritoneal cavity. In another series of 441 patients treated surgically, there were only 2 instances of free perforation, while 11 patients had pericholecystic abscesses. In several series, there was no serious morbidity associated with perforation.

The arguments for early or intermediate cholecystectomy point out that about 5 percent of patients fail to respond to medical management and more than half of the patients who respond initially experience an exacerbation. Unless there is a medical contraindication, eventual surgical intervention is indicated for almost all patients with cholecystitis and cholelithiasis. Low mortality rates have been reported for early cholecystectomy, and these rates are quite comparable with those reported for the elective procedure. The risk of operating in an area of inflammation, in the early stages of acute cholecystitis, is refuted. In the first 2 to 3 days after the onset of symptoms, although edema may be significant, there is usually little difficulty in displaying the duct system. If the structures can be safely defined, exploration of the common duct for stones can be carried out without increased risk. If early operation is performed and the inflammatory process has progressed to obscure the structures, cholecystostomy, which can be carried out with a low mortality rate, speeds the patient's recovery. Acute cholecystitis in the diabetic is associated with higher incidences of complications and mortality than in the nondiabetic.

In the United States the majority of surgeons favor early operation, whereas in Great Britain it is more customary to treat the condition conservatively, unless there is specific indication for surgical intervention.

The mortality rate for emergency cholecystectomy ranges from near zero to 5 percent and, in several series, is comparable with the mortality rate for elective cholecystectomy. In one series, the mortality rate for cholecystectomy was 3.9 percent, while the nonoperative patients had a mortality of 5.5 percent. A randomized series shows that early cholecystectomy is as safe as the nonoperative approach and that the period of morbidity and disability is shortened. Cholecystostomy for extremely ill patients was accompanied by a mortality rate of 15 percent in one series, in contrast to the 1.5 percent mortality rate reported by Dunphy and Ross.

Author's Approach. If the diagnosis of acute cholecystitis is relatively unequivocal and the patient presents within 3 days of the onset of symptoms, early operation is performed. The presence of hyperamylasemia per se does not influence the decision. Immediate *emergency* cholecystectomy is rarely indicated, and the patient should be thoroughly investigated and prepared prior to operation. If the patient is extremely ill with a palpable gallbladder, surgical treatment is usually carried out within 24 h of admission. If possible, cholecystectomy is performed. However, if the patient will not tolerate this procedure because of extreme toxicity or otherwise complicating medical illness, a cholecystostomy, under local anesthesia, is carried out. If a cholecystectomy has been planned but the inflammatory process is so marked that it compromises the dissection, cholecystostomy terminates the procedure. Patients whose symptoms continued to progress under medical management are operated upon. With associated cholangitis, a course of antibiotics is initiated, and early operation is performed for relief of obstruction. If the patient presents 72 h after the onset of symptoms and shows signs of improvement during the early periods of hospitalization, surgical intervention is deferred, and an elective operation is planned in approximately 6 weeks in most instances, but there is no hesitation in operating after the "golden" 72 h.

At the time of surgical treatment for acute cholecystitis, the indications for common bile duct exploration are the same as those which pertain during elective cholecystectomy. Patients with obstructive jaundice due to stones or ascending cholangitis require early surgical relief of obstruction and drainage of the common bile duct. Palpable stones and ductal dilatation demonstrated at operation constitute indications for common duct exploration. Pancreatitis is not, in itself, an indication in the presence of acute cholecystitis, since the yield is small, and it is best to perform an operative cholangiogram via the cystic duct to determine if stones are present in the common duct. If indications for exploration of the common duct are present but the inflammatory process compromises dissection, cholecystostomy is performed and the stones are removed from the gallbladder. An attempt may be made to pass a catheter via the cystic duct into the common bile duct.

Emphysematous Cholecystitis. This is a rare form of acute, usually gangrenous, cholecystitis, caused by gas-forming organisms and characterized radiologically by the presence of gas in the gallbladder (Fig. 31-15). Unlike ordinary acute cholecystitis, which is more prevalent among women, emphysematous cholecystitis is more often found in men, with a sex incidence of 75 percent for males and 25 percent for females. Pathogenesis is related to acute inflammation of the gallbladder, which often begins aseptically, complicated by a secondary infection with gas-forming bacilli. These may reach the gallbladder by bile ducts, bloodstream, or lymphatic channels and grow in an anaerobic environment. The clinical manifestations are similar to those present in acute cholecystitis. In approximately half the patients, a history of previous gallbladder attacks can be elicited. Cholelithiasis is also present in half the patients, who are frequently diabetic. The diagnosis is usually made on the basis of radiographic findings that show a globular shadow, distended with gas, in the region of the gallbladder. Later, intramural or submucosal gas may appear, and gas may also appear in the pericholecystic area, denoting extension of the pathologic process outside the confines of the gallbladder. The treatment of choice is early operation, since the incidence of free perforation is reported to be 40 to 60 percent. Cholecystectomy is indicated, but if this is not feasible, cholecystostomy should be performed. In 9 percent of cases, choledocholithiasis is present, and exploration of the common duct may be required. Although positive bile cultures are found in only half the cases, antibiotics directed toward the clostridial and coliform organisms are indicated. The mortality rate is significantly greater than that for nonemphysematous cholecystitis.

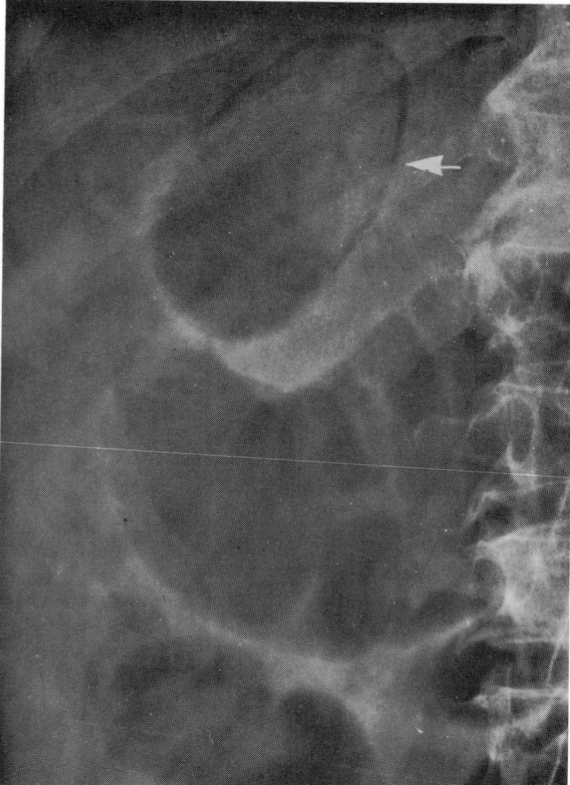

Fig. 31-15. Emphysematous cholecystitis. Gallbladder is shown as gas-filled organ.

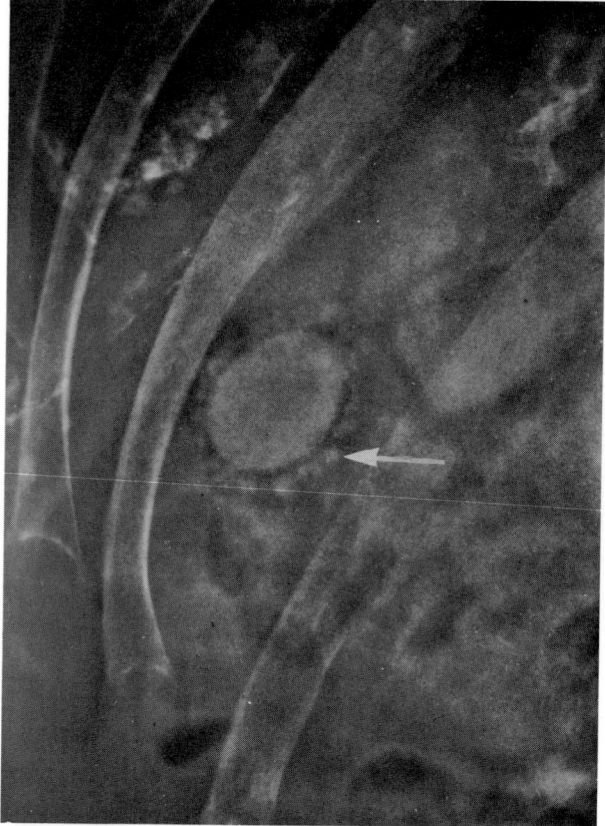

Fig. 31-16. Rokitansky-Aschoff sinuses presenting as a halo effect, a finding present in chronic cholecystitis.

CHRONIC CHOLECYSTITIS

Chronic inflammation of the gallbladder is generally associated with cholelithiasis and consists of round cell infiltration and fibrosis of the wall. Buried crypts of mucosa (Rokitansky-Aschoff sinuses) may be seen dipping into the mucosa (Fig. 31-16). Obstruction by gallstones of the neck of the cystic duct may produce a mucocele of the gallbladder (hydrops). The bile is initially sterile but may be secondarily infected with coliform bacilli, streptococci, and occasionally clostridia or *Salmonella* (typhoid). Secondary effects of cholecystitis include obstruction of the common duct, cholangitis, perforation of the gallbladder with formation of a pericholecystic abscess or a cholecystoenteric fistula, bile peritonitis, and pancreatitis. There may be associated carcinoma of the gallbladder.

CLINICAL MANIFESTATIONS. The patients generally present with moderate intermittent abdominal pain in the right upper quadrant and epigastrium, occasionally radiating to the scapula and intrascapular region. There is usually a history of intolerance of fatty and/or fried foods, and the patient may have noted intermittent nausea and anorexia. If the patient is not experiencing acute pain, there may be no diagnostic findings on physical examination. Occasionally tenderness is elicited over the gallbladder. This is usually maximal during inspiration. The diagnosis is usually established by an oral cholecystogram,

which demonstrates either the absence of filling of the gallbladder or the presence of stones. An ultrasonogram may demonstrate calculi.

TREATMENT. The treatment of chronic cholecystitis and cholelithiasis is cholecystectomy, and the results are usually excellent. Early cholecystectomy is particularly important for the diabetic patient. Operative mortality of less than 1 percent has been reported for large series. Seventy-five percent of patients undergoing cholecystectomy for cholelithiasis are completely relieved of all preoperative symptoms, and the remaining 25 percent have only mild symptoms that are apparently unrelated to the biliary system.

POSTCHOLECYSTECTOMY SYNDROME. This ill-defined syndrome refers to symptoms that either develop subsequent to or continue in spite of cholecystectomy. In patients with abdominal symptoms subsequent to cholecystectomy for chronic cholecystitis and cholelithiasis, these symptoms are usually related to an extrabiliary cause such as hiatal hernia, peptic ulceration, or pancreatitis. Symptoms may also be due to a residual stone in the common bile duct, residual cystic duct stones, or spasm of the sphincter of Oddi. The etiology is best defined by ERCP.

The *cystic duct stump* is rarely responsible for clinical manifestations similar to those of cholecystitis. The residual stump may undergo changes of inflammation and is capable of forming calculi.

ACALCULOUS CHOLECYSTITIS

Acute and chronic inflammatory disease of the gall-bladder can occur without stones. Acute acalculous cholecystitis frequently is a complication of burns, sepsis, multiple system failure, cardiovascular disease, diabetes, prolonged illness, or a major operation.

The incidence of chronic acalculous is difficult to establish. It is present in over 50 percent of children and 35 percent of Nigerians with gallbladder disease, and the accepted incidence for adults in the United States is less than 5 percent. Possible causes include (1) anatomic conditions such as kinking, fibrosis, and obstruction of the cystic duct due to tumor or anomalous vessels; (2) thrombosis of major blood vessels producing ischemia and gangrene; (3) spasm of fibrosis of the sphincter of Oddi in patients with a "common channel" with or without associated pancreatitis; (4) systemic diseases such as diabetes mellitus and collagen diseases; (5) specific infections such as typhoid fever, actinomycoses, and parasitic infestation; and (6) scarlet fever and a wide variety of febrile illnesses in young children. The DISIDA or PIPIDA scan and the ultrasonogram are occasionally normal in these patients.

TREATMENT. Cholecystectomy is preferable, but the patients' condition mandated cholecystostomy in 14 of 16 cases in one series. In children with acute febrile illness, cholecystostomy has been particularly effective, and subsequent cholecystectomy has not been required in many of these patients.

Cholangitis

Infection within the biliary duct system is most frequently associated with choledocholithiasis but has also accompanied choledochal cysts and carcinoma of the bile duct, and has followed sphincteroplasty. Infection and inflammatory changes may extend up the duct system into the liver and give rise to multiple hepatic abscesses. Clinically, the condition is characterized by intermittent fever, upper abdominal pain, exacerbation of jaundice, pruritus, and at times rigor.

In patients with common duct stones in whom there is ascending cholangitis, a broad-spectrum antibiotic directed particularly at *E. coli,* which is the most common offending organism, should be given for several days prior to surgical treatment. Antibiotics usually control the infection, but if the temperature does not fall, surgical intervention should not be delayed. Occasionally, the patient may be so ill as to allow only insertion of a T tube into the common duct, and when cholangitis has subsided, a second operation can be performed to remove the stone.

ACUTE SUPPURATIVE CHOLANGITIS. Suppurative cholangitis, in which there is gross pus within the biliary tract, merits special consideration, since it constitutes one of the most urgent causes for laparotomy in patients with obstructive jaundice. The entity was first described in 1877 by Charcot, who suggested a diagnostic triad of jaundice, chills and fever, and pain in the right upper quadrant. To these, Reynolds and Dargan added shock and central nervous system depression as specific identifying features of the condition.

The disease occurs almost exclusively in patients over seventy years. All patients are febrile, and a majority are jaundiced. Hypotension, confusion, or lethargy occur in about 20 percent of cases. A white blood cell count of less than 12,000 has been reported in over half the patients, probably related to the age and lack of response. Bilirubin, SGOT, and alkaline phosphatase levels are characteristically elevated, but the serum amylase is usually normal. The correct diagnosis has been made in less than a third of the patients.

At operation, all patients demonstrate gross distention of the common bile duct, with frank pus, frequently under considerable pressure, and choledocholithiasis, or a tumor obstructing the distal bile duct. If the gallbladder is present, it is invariably distended and inflamed. Spontaneous perforation of the bile ducts has been reported. Surgical treatment is directed at rapid decompression of the duct system and is combined with large doses of antibiotics, particularly those which achieve high levels in the bile. In a review of the literature, it was reported that all patients who were not operated upon died, while mortality following surgical procedures ranged between zero and 88 percent, averaging 33 percent. A group of patients whose common duct diameter was, in each case, larger than 1.5 cm were managed by choledochoduodenostomy, with results equivalent to T-tube drainage. Some patients have been managed emergently by establishing initial drainage via ERCP or PTC followed by a definitive operation.

Cholangiohepatitis

Cholangiohepatitis, which is also known as "recurrent pyogenic cholangitis," is found almost exclusively among the Chinese, with the largest number of cases seen among Cantonese living in the Pearl River delta in China. In Hong Kong it is the most commonly encountered disease of the biliary passages and is the third most common abdominal emergency after appendicitis and perforated ulcer. It has also been encountered in Great Britian, in Australia, and in the Chinese population in the United States. Cholangiohepatitis occurs most frequently in the third and fourth decades but has been reported at all ages and has an equal sex frequency.

The etiology is summarized in Fig. 31-17. The pyogenic element probably originates from the bowel and is caused by *E. coli* or *Streptococcus faecalis.* In most instances, positive cultures are obtainable from the bile and portal venous blood. The Chinese liver fluke, *C. sinensis,* was thought to be an important contributing factor. Other factors that have been implicated as contributing causes for cholangiohepatitis include ascariasis and hemolysis associated with malaria.

PATHOLOGY. The gallbladder wall is thickened but not grossly inflamed. The common bile duct is also usually grossly distended and contains large stones. The stones are produced by precipitation of bile pigments, desqua-

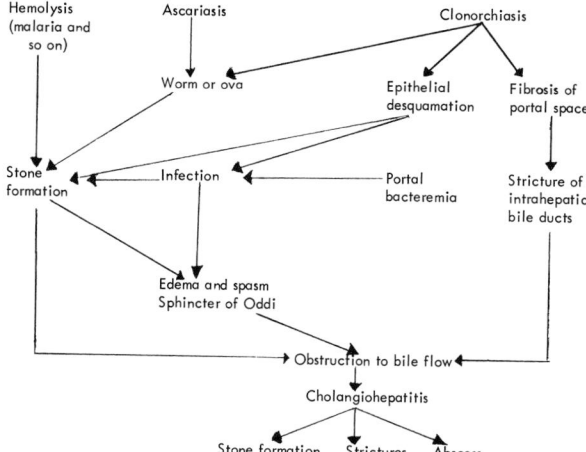

Fig. 31-17. Schema of etiologic factors implicated in cholangiohepatitis. [After: *Stock FE, Fung JHY: Oriental Cholangiohepatitis, in Smith R, Sherlock S (eds): Surgery of the Gall Bladder and Bile Ducts. London, Butterworth, 1964, with permission.*]

mation of epithelium, and products of inflammation, and, not infrequently, the nucleus of the stone may contain an adult *Clonorchis* worm, an ovum, or an ascarid. Acute or hemorrhagic pancreatitis occurs in less than 1 percent of the cases. The most marked changes occur in the liver, where the intrahepatic bile ducts are both dilated and constricted. Inflammatory changes are present in the periductal tissue and may progress to frank abscess formation.

CLINICAL MANIFESTATIONS. In highly endemic areas, cholangiohepatitis is the first consideration in patients with jaundice, pain, and pyrexia. Pain is usually located in the right upper quadrant and epigastrium and may be colicky or constant. In most acute attacks, there is fever accompanied by chills and rigors, and 50 percent of the patients are jaundiced, while the remainder have an elevation of the serum bilirubin level. Recurrence of symptoms is one of the most characteristic features of the disease.

Most patients appear toxic, with temperatures up to 40°C. There is tenderness and guarding in the right upper quadrant. The white blood cell count is usually about 15,000, and the serum bilirubin level is generally above 2 mg/dL with accompanying bilirubinuria. There may be evidence of impairment of hepatocellular function. In the majority of cases calculi are not demonstrable on routine x-rays. An occasional finding of significance is the presence of air in the biliary tree, which may be due to a secondary gas-forming organism or a fistula between the duct and duodenum. Endoscopic retrograde cholangiopancreatography (ERCP) or PTC may establish the diagnosis. Operative cholangiography also is helpful in revealing intrahepatic stones, constrictions of intrahepatic ducts, and small filling defects due to the liver fluke. Manifestations of portal hypertension may be present.

TREATMENT. Patients are generally prepared with antibiotics. Surgical therapy, however, should not be delayed for the patient who is jaundiced and has pain and pyrexia.

Cholecystostomy is reserved for the seriously ill patient showing signs of rupture of the gallbladder. The definitive operative procedure, however, consists of removal of stones and debris from the extrahepatic bile ducts and providing an improved communication between the duct system and the intestine. Transduodenal sphincteroplasty has been performed in cases where the common duct was not grossly dilated, but wide choledochoduodenostomy or Roux en Y choledochojejunostomy is the treatment of choice with ductal dilatation. T-tube drainage represents a temporizing procedure, since obstruction frequently recurs after the tube has been removed. The gallbladder is usually removed, although it is rarely acutely inflamed and never represents the primary site of disease.

If large hepatic abscesses are noted, drainage should be performed. Left hepatic lobectomy has been carried out on occasion, when there has been gross dilatation of the ducts and abscess formation in the left lobe while the right was apparently normal.

The prognosis is generally guarded, since recurrence is not uncommon. Choi et al. reported the operative results in 150 patients with primary intrahepatic stones. Common duct exploration, transhepatic intubation, and hepatotomy were associated with recurrence rates of 24, 37, and 75 percent, respectively. Hepatic resection had a failure rate of only 4 percent, and none of the patients had recurrent stones. In advanced cases, particularly with multiple abscesses, the prognosis is poor, and the patient eventually succumbs to liver failure, septicemia, or cholangiocarcinoma.

Sclerosing Cholangitis

Sclerosing cholangitis is an uncommon disease that involves either all or part of the extrahepatic biliary duct system and, occasionally, affects the intrahepatic biliary radicles. The disease has also been called *obliterative cholangitis* and *stenosing cholangitis,* in reference to a progressive thickening of the bile duct walls encroaching upon the lumen. It may be associated with gallstones, but several series have been presented in which there were no stones in either the gallbladder or the common duct. A significant number of cases have been associated with ulcerative colitis, Crohn's disease, Riedel's struma, retroperitoneal fibrosis, and porphyria cutanea tarda.

Schwartz and Dale reviewed the literature prior to 1958, and only 13 cases satisfied their criteria of generalized extrahepatic bile duct stenosis in the absence of previous biliary surgical treatment and gallstones. More recently institutional series of 19, 29, and 50 cases have been reported.

Most patients present with symptoms during the fourth, fifth, and sixth decades of life, and the disease appears to occur more often in males, in contrast to acute cholecystitis.

The cause of sclerosing cholangitis is unknown. Histologic sections in several cases failed to reveal any granulomatous lesion, metaplasia, or neoplasia. In several series, none of the patients had had previous surgical treatment, and therefore trauma was excluded as an etiologic agent; irritation of the common duct by passage of calculi is refuted by the fact that there are usually no stones present in either the common duct or the gallbladder. It has been suggested that the disease may be caused by local response to viral infection, since a relative lymphocytosis with atypical lymphocytes has been noted. Immune response and collagen disease have also been considered as possible etiologic factors. A positive cellular immune response to biliary antigens has been demonstrated.

PATHOLOGY. Grossly there is diffuse thickening of the wall of the extrahepatic biliary tract and, at times, of the intrahepatic ducts, with a concomitant encroachment upon the lumen, resulting in marked luminal narrowing. The duct system may be completely involved, or the hepatic ducts may be spared and the disease restricted to the entire length of the common duct. The gallbladder is usually not involved, but the lymph nodes in the region of the common duct and foramen of Winslow are usually markedly enlarged and succulent. Microscopic analyses of the affected duct show that the walls are as much as eight times thicker than normal. The areas of inflammation and fibrosis are in the submucosal and subserosal portions with an edematous field between them. The mucosa is intact throughout. Biopsy of the liver may reveal bile stasis or, in long-standing cases, biliary cirrhosis. The histologic evaluation is critical, since it is difficult to differentiate this disease from sclerosing carcinoma of bile ducts.

CLINICAL MANIFESTATIONS. The diagnosis is to be considered in patients, particularly those in middle age, with a clinical and laboratory picture of extrahepatic jaundice. Jaundice is usually associated with intermittent pain in the right upper quadrant, nausea, vomiting, and occasionally chills and fevers. In long-standing cases with biliary cirrhosis, the manifestations of portal hypertension, such as bleeding varices and ascites, may be apparent. The diagnosis has been established by ERCP. At operation a dense inflammatory reaction in the region of the gallbladder and gastrohepatic ligament is noted. Palpation of the duct reveals a cordlike structure that may feel like a thrombosed blood vessel, but the wall of the common duct is obviously thickened and cuts with difficulty. The edges of the incision characteristically pout out. Usually, only a fine probe or small Bâkes dilator can be inserted into the lumen. Cholangiography may vividly demonstrate the extensive narrowing of the lumen (Fig. 31-18).

TREATMENT. The appropriate management of sclerosing cholangitis remains unclear. No drug therapy has achieved consistent, or even usual, success. Operative intervention is no longer required for diagnostic purposes in most patients except to distinguish between sclerosing cholangitis and carcinoma of the bile ducts in some patients. Both the medical regimens and the operative procedures are palliative in nature. These facts, coupled with the variations in clinical course of the patients and the lack of any controlled trials, precludes any sense of assurance in prescribing a particular therapeutic approach.

The asymptomatic anicteric patient is not treated and is not studied with repeated cholangiograms if jaundice or cholangitis does not develop. The pruritic and icteric patient is treated for 4 to 6 weeks with prednisone; if there is no improvement, or if cholangitis is present or develops, an operation is performed with a preoperative cholangiogram as a guide. If there is minimal intrahepatic involvement and dilatation of a segment of the common duct or common hepatic duct proximal to marked stenosis, the stenotic segment is excised as a biopsy section to rule out cholangiocarcinoma and a direct mucosa-to-mucosa anastomosis is effected between the dilated segment of

Fig. 31-18. Operative cholangiogram demonstrating diffuse narrowing of the common bile duct, dilatation of the main hepatic ducts, and beading of the intrahepatic ducts.

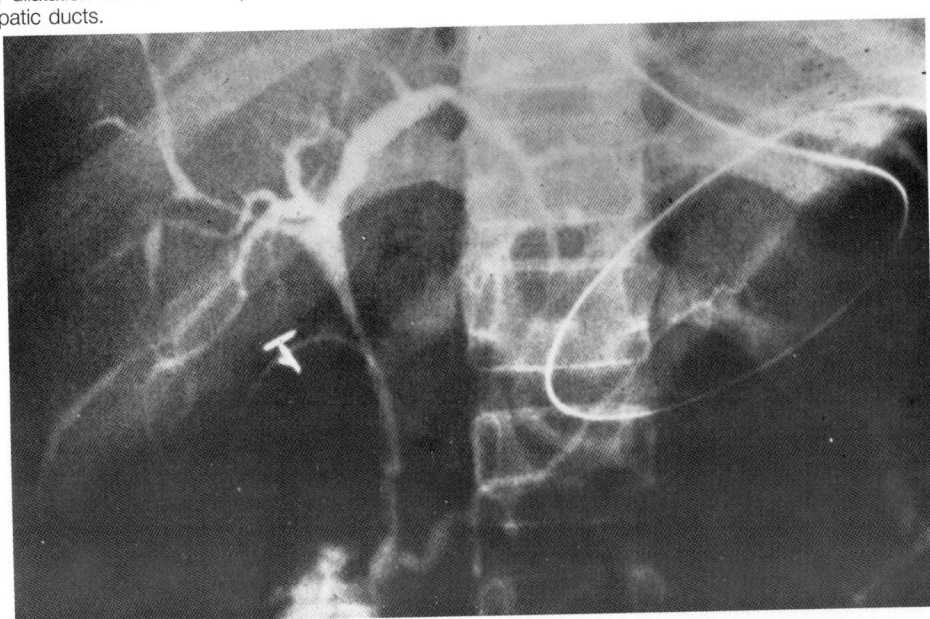

duct and a Roux limb of jejunum, preferably without a stent. Stricture of the confluence of the hepatic ducts is managed by excision of the distal ducts for pathologic evaluation and anastomosis of the hepatic ducts to the Roux limb of jejunum by the mucosa-to-mucosa technique. If the hepatic ducts are sufficiently dilated, no stent is used. If these ducts are small, transhepatic stents are used, but no attempt is made to dilate intrahepatic ducts. If the entire extra- and intrahepatic systems are dominated by areas of marked stenosis and narrowing, with minimal dilatation, a small T tube is inserted, steroid therapy is used, and the patient is followed by sequential T-tube cholangiograms that will define improvement. If the disease has progressed to the stage of marked hyperbilirubinemia and liver failure or cirrhosis, transplantation is advised, avoiding a shunt to decompress portal hypertension even if there has been variceal bleeding.

Fibrosis or Stenosis of the Sphincter of Oddi

In 1884, Langenbuch, only 2 years after reporting the first successful removal of a gallbladder, suggested transduodenal division of the "diverticulum" of Vater in cases of cicatricial stenosis for chronic inflammation. In 1901, Opie called attention to the "common channel" theory as the cause of pancreatitis, and in 1913 Archibald suggested sphincteroplasty as the treatment for pancreatitis.

The pathogenesis of fibrosis or stenosis of the sphincter of Oddi and the papilla of Vater is not fully understood. Long-standing spasm may play an important role, and infection of the biliary tract or pancreas has also been implicated. Irritation from stones within the common duct may also lead to fibrosis. In a series of 50 patients in whom sphincteroplasty was performed because of inability to pass a small Bâkes dilator, biopsies revealed no abnormalities in 18, while 18 showed inflammatory infiltration, 17 had minimal fibrosis, and 2 had diffuse fibrosis. No definite correlation could be found between the various manifestations of biliary tract disease and the histologic changes.

CLINICAL MANIFESTATIONS. The main symptom is abdominal pain, which is usually colicky and frequently associated with nausea and vomiting. The pain begins in the right upper quadrant and radiates to the shoulder, and it may be intermittent in nature. Over half the patients give a history of intermittent jaundice, and many indicate that they have had previous cholecystectomy without relief of symptoms.

TREATMENT. The diagnosis is generally made at operation when there is difficulty in passing a 3-mm Bâkes dilator through the ampulla of Vater into the duodenum. Operative cholangiography and pressure studies on the common bile duct have theoretical application. If a 3-mm dilator cannot be easily passed through the ampulla, a transduodenal exploration should be carried out. Thomas et al. compared the results of transduodenal sphincteroplasty and choledochoduodenostomy in 30 patients with stenosis or stricture of the sphincter. The procedures were equally and highly effective, and neither was associated with a significant incidence of subsequent cholangitis. Sphincteroplasty is preferable if the common duct is small, and a transduodenal approach is indicated if an ampullary tumor is suspected. Endoscopic papillotomy has been used successfully, particularly in Europe where the disorder is more frequently diagnosed. Choledochoduodenostomy appears preferable if the stenosis is long, if it is difficult to identify the sphincter, or if exposure is difficult.

PAPILLITIS

In 1926, DelValle first described a benign inflammatory and fibrous process of the ampulla of Vater and indicated that it was a factor in producing stenosis. It was postulated that acute and subacute inflammatory changes occur and that stenosis is the final and irreversible result of these changes. Acosta and Nardi have presented 61 cases of papillitis, 21 of which were chronic ulcerative papillitis, 20 chronic sclerosing papillitis, 15 chronic granulomatous papillitis, and 5 chronic adenomatous papillitis. The acute stage, which is characterized by edema, papillary dilatation, hemorrhage, and infiltration, may be reversible, while sclerosing papillitis and chronic granulomatous papillitis are considered irreversible in view of their inevitable evolution into scar tissue.

The clinical and pathologic features associated with papillitis include the postcholecystectomy syndrome in 30 percent, dilatation of the common duct in 50 percent, biliary disease without stones in 25 percent, obstructive jaundice in 60 percent, pancreatitis in 70 percent, and liver damage in 25 percent. There has been no correlation between the specific clinical syndromes and the pathologic changes. A pancreatic evocative test, utilizing morphine-prostigmine or secretin-CCK, has been used. Elevation of at least one serum pancreatic enzyme by a factor of 4 over the normal, coupled with reproduction of the patient's pain, is considered a positive test result. The efficacy of this test has been disputed. Since the majority of patients with papillitis have irreversible lesions, sphincteroplasty is generally employed.

TUMORS

Carcinoma of the Gallbladder

Carcinoma of the gallbladder represents the fifth most common type of carcinoma involving the gastrointestinal tract and accounts for 4 percent of all carcinomas. Its occurrence in random autopsy series averages approximately 0.4 percent, while approximately 1 percent of patients undergoing biliary tract operations are noted to have carcinoma. Approximately 80 percent of patients in most series are female. The lesion usually presents after the age of sixty.

PATHOLOGY. The relationship between gallstones and carcinoma has been emphasized for many years. Approximately 90 percent of patients with carcinoma have associated cholelithiasis. Five to ten percent of patients over the age of sixty-five with symptomatic gallstones have carcinoma of the gallbladder. In patients with asymptomatic cholelithiasis the frequency of occurrence is extremely low. Malignant transformation of sessile adenomas of the gallbladder is rare.

Approximately 80 percent of the tumors are adenocarcinomas, while the remainder are either undifferentiated or squamous cell carcinomas. Of the adenocarcinomas, 70 percent are scirrhous, 20 percent are papillary, and 10 percent are mucoid. The routes of metastases include spread along the lymphatics to the choledochal and pancreatic or duodenal nodes, localized involvement of the venules and veins of the gallbladder, and invasion of the liver. In approximately one-third of the cases the disease spreads directly to the liver, an important consideration as far as therapy is concerned. In patients with metastases, the liver is involved in two-thirds of the cases, the regional lymph nodes in about one-half, and the omentum, duodenum, colon, or porta hepatis in about one-fourth. Pulmonary metastases are relatively uncommon.

CLINICAL MANIFESTATIONS. Signs and symptoms of carcinoma of the gallbladder are generally indistinguishable from those associated with cholecystitis and cholelithiasis. Most patients present with abdominal distress, epigastric and right upper quadrant pain, nausea, and vomiting. About half the patients are jaundiced, and in two-thirds there is a palpable right upper quadrant mass. Less than 10 percent present with normal findings on abdominal examination.

Laboratory findings are of little assistance. The liver function tests are diagnostic of obstructive jaundice, and the gallbladder is usually not visualized by cholecystography. In many patients the gallbladder carcinoma is found incidentally during routine cholecystectomy.

TREATMENT. Surgical treatment offers the only, albeit small, hope for cure. Most of the reported long-term survivors are patients who underwent surgical treatment for acute and chronic cholecystitis and in whom an incidental localized microscopic focus of neoplasia was detected in the specimen. Some have recommended removal of an adjacent wedge or the anterior portion of segment V of liver for this lesion. The best results in patients with grossly visable carcinoma have been achieved with cholecystectomy and regional lymphadenectomy. When the lymph nodes are removed, the portal vein, hepatic artery, hepatic duct, and common bile duct should be skeletonized from the pylorus to the porta hepatis. A formal right hepatic lobectomy has been suggested, but the 5-year survival rate has not been improved by this approach. The prognosis for 5-year survival is extremely poor, however, approximating 2 percent. Ninety percent of patients die before the end of 1 year. In patients with tumor confined to the mucosa and submucosa, a survival rate of 64 percent has been reported.

Carcinoma of the Extrahepatic Bile Ducts Exclusive of the Periampullary Region

This lesion has an average autopsy incidence of approximately 0.3 percent. The ratio of incidence of carcinoma of the extrahepatic bile duct exclusive of the periampullary region to that of carcinoma of the gallbladder ranges from 1:2 to 1:5 in various series, while the ratio of this lesion to carcinoma of the ampulla is 3:2. The tumor occurs more frequently in males and has the highest incidence in the sixth and seventh decades.

PATHOLOGY. The primary lesion is often small but so located as to cause symptoms early. Approximately one-third of the cases occur in the common bile duct, and one-fifth are at the junction of the cystic and common hepatic ducts. Almost two-thirds occur above this level. The tumor usually involves the whole thickness of the duct, resulting in complete anatomic obstruction in about one-third of the cases. Grossly, the tumor presents as a firm, circumscribed, grayish tan mass that causes a "napkin ring" obstruction. In rare instances, the growth projects into the lumen of the duct in the form of a polypoid mass. Histologically, all lesions are adenocarcinomas. Metastatic spread has been reported in about three-fourths of autopsy cases, liver and regional lymph nodes being most frequently involved. Spread to adjacent structures accounts for 20 percent of metastases. The incidence of metastases at operation was reported to be approximately 50 percent. Multicentric lesions in the duct have been demonstrated choledochoscopically. In some instances there is severe bile stasis, while in others there are suppurative cholangitis and hepatic abscesses. Cholelithiasis has been implicated as a contributing factor just as in carcinoma of the gallbladder. The incidence of calculi within the bile ducts themselves is extremely low.

CLINICAL MANIFESTATIONS. The symptoms are variable, and the correct preoperative diagnosis is seldom made. Characteristically, there is a rapid onset of jaundice, which is present in almost all patients. This is frequently preceded by pruritus. Nearly always there is weight loss, and abdominal pain occurs in over half the patients. Cholangitis is a frequent consequence. The liver is palpable in about 50 percent of the cases and is usually nontender and rarely nodular. The gallbladder is palpable in about one-third of the patients with distal lesions who have not undergone previous cholecystectomy. The serum bilirubin is usually elevated, often to an extremely high level, and fluctuation of the bilirubin level has been recorded in about 60 percent of the cases. Intravenous cholangiography rarely visualizes the ducts because of the high degree of obstructive jaundice. ERCP may be diagnostic, but transhepatic cholangiography is associated with the highest yield (Fig. 31-19). At the time of surgical treatment, an operative cholangiogram is very helpful in establishing the diagnosis and choledochoscopy should be performed to assess multicentricity.

TREATMENT. The surgical procedure is potentially curative or palliative. Tumors may be resected or bypassed by anastomosing the dilated proximal duct system to a segment of intestine, preferably by a Roux en Y procedure. There is now a more aggressive attitude about these lesions. Distal third tumors in the intrapancreatic part of the common duct are managed by radial pancreaticoduodenectomy. Middle third tumors are most easily resected and biliary drainage is established with a Roux

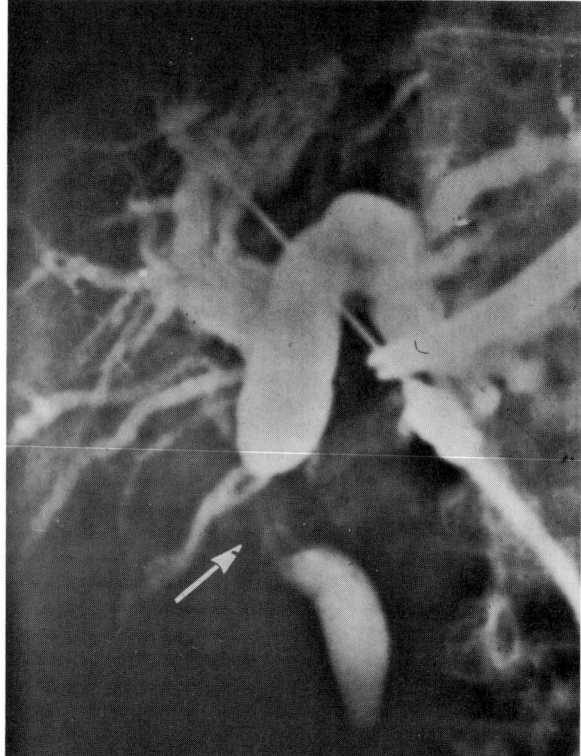

Fig. 31-19. Transhepatic cholangiogram demonstrating a tumor of the common bile duct.

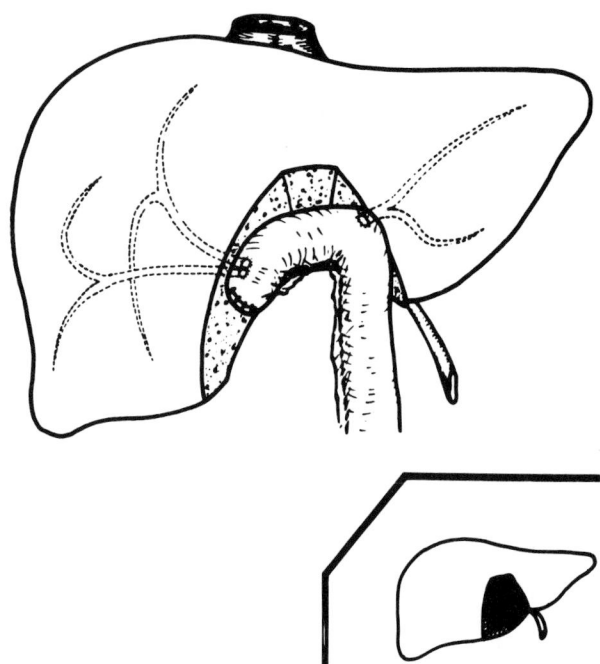

Fig. 31-20. Diagram of resection of main hepatic duct junction and segment IV. After resection of segment IV, performed to obtain adequate exposure of hilus of the liver, en bloc excision of entire major hepatic duct junction, gallbladder, cystic duct, and common bile duct was made and followed by anastomosis of a Roux en Y jejunal loop. The right hepatic ducts, divided proximal to a secondary junction, were inserted into jejunal loop in "double-barreled" manner, the left hepatic duct was inserted into the loop direct. (From: *Launois B, Campion J-P, et al: Carcinoma of the hepatic hilus. Ann Surg 190:151, 1979, with permission.*)

en Y hepaticodochojejunostomy. Removal of upper third tumors may require resection of the hepatic hilus and hepatic parenchyma and anastomosis of the right and/or left hepatic ducts to a Roux en Y limb of jejunum (Fig. 31-20). Although resectability rate of these tumors is only 15 to 20 percent, and the cure rate is low, the 5-year survival and quality of life was better in patients who underwent resection rather than drainage alone.

The addition of adjuvant internal and external radiation has not been consistently effective. In poor-risk patients or when the tumor is not resectable, percutaneous transhepatic catheter drainage can relieve the jaundice and pruritus temporarily and at times for prolonged periods.

Sclerosing carcinoma usually arises from the major hepatic ducts near the hilus of the liver and extends into the intrahepatic ducts, developing slowly and often mimicking a chronic inflammatory process. As the tumor obstructs the bile ducts, progressive jaundice, cholestasis, suppurative cholangitis, and hepatic abscess may result. The average age at diagnosis is about sixty-five, and the ratio of male to female has been reported at 8:1.

The signs and symptoms are variable. There is characteristically insidious and progressive jaundice, and there is usually associated marked weight loss. Fever is noted in over half the patients. The syndrome may progress to hepatic coma, renal failure, or septicemia. An ultrasonogram followed by PTC defines intrahepatic ductal dilatation and the site of obstruction.

OPERATIONS ON THE BILIARY TRACT

ANTIBIOTIC THERAPY. The infectious complications of an operation on the biliary tract are more frequent in patients with infected bile than in those with sterile bile. It has been shown that patients over the age of seventy who have acute cholecystitis, common bile duct stones, jaundice, or diabetes have a significantly higher incidence of positive bile cultures and therefore are at risk for postoperative infection. This group of patients should receive antibiotics preoperatively. In all cases, the gallbladder bile should be cultured at the time of the operative procedure. The selection of antibiotics should be based on appreciation of the fact that most organisms are *E. coli* or *Klebsiella*. Patients undergoing a T-tube cholangiogram or a radiologically controlled extraction of a common duct stone should be protected with prophylactic antibiotics.

CHOLECYSTOSTOMY. The procedure accomplishes decompression and drainage of the distended, hydroptic, or empyematous gallbladder. It is particularly applicable if the patient's general condition is such that it precludes prolonged anesthesia, since the operation may be performed under local anesthesia. It is also performed for the situation in which marked inflammatory reaction obscures the anatomic relation of critical structures. Chole-cystostomy may be a definitive procedure, particularly if a postoperative tube cholangiogram is normal.

Technique (Fig. 31-21). A circumferential purse-string suture is placed in the fundus of the gallbladder, and a small incision is made through the serosa within the suture. A trochar is inserted into the lumen of the gallbladder, which is then decompressed. After the gallbladder has been emptied, a stone forceps may be introduced to the junction of the ampulla and cystic duct, and obstructing calculi may be removed. A mushroom or Foley catheter is inserted into the lumen of the gallbladder, and a second purse-string suture is placed concentrically in relation to the first one. The sutures are tied, inverting the serosa. Unless a small, oblique incision was employed initially, the drainage tube should be brought out through a stab wound.

If the fundus of the gallbladder is necrotic, the gangrenous portion should be excised and the remainder of the gallbladder closed around the catheter, using purse-string sutures as previously described.

CHOLECYSTECTOMY. A principal aim of the technique is to avoid injury to the common duct while transecting the cystic duct close to its junction with the common bile duct to obviate a long cystic duct remnant. A more conservative approach toward elective cholecystectomy is indicated for cirrhotic patients. If an operation is performed, increased bleeding should be anticipated; external intrahepatic dissection should be avoided. Intraoperative infusion of vasopressin and an antifibrinolytic agent should be considered.

Technique (Fig. 31-22). The gallbladder may be approached through an oblique right upper quadrant incision (Kocher or Courvoisier), through a vertical right paramedian incision, or through the upper midline. There are frequently adhesions between the gallbladder, particularly the ampulla, and the duodenum and colon. These should be lysed by sharp dissection. By applying traction laterally to the ampulla and retracting the duodenum medially, the veil of peritoneum running from ampulla to hepatoduodenal ligament may be accentuated and incised. The cystic duct is identified and a silk ligature passed around it. Traction is applied to the ligature to prevent passage of a stone down the cystic duct during dissection of the gallbladder. Dissection is continued craniad in this peritoneal fold, and the cystic artery is identified. The course of this artery to the gallbladder should be demonstrated to avoid ligating the right hepatic artery. The cystic artery should be doubly ligated and transected. If bleeding occurs from the cystic artery, it is best controlled by applying pressure on the hepatic artery within the hepatoduodenal ligament. The artery is compressed between the index finger, which is inserted into the foramen of Winslow posteriorly, and the thumb anteriorly. The peritoneum overlying the gallbladder is then incised close to the liver, and dissection is begun from the fundus of the gallbladder down to an ultimate pedicle of cystic duct. During this dissection, blood vessels coursing from the liver may require ligation, and the gallbladder bed should be inspected for large draining ducts, which

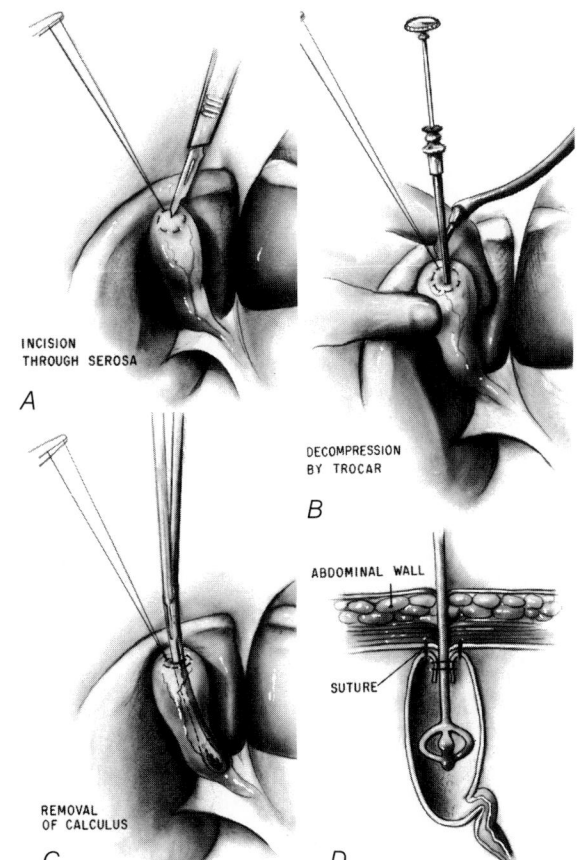

Fig. 31-21. Cholecystostomy. *A.* Placement of purse-string suture in fundus of gallbladder, and incision through serosa. *B.* Trochar decompression. *C.* Removal of calculus from ampulla. *D.* Sagittal section demonstrating two concentric purse-string sutures, intraluminal catheter, and suturing of serosa of gallbladder to peritoneum.

should also be ligated. Attention is then directed toward visualization of the junction of the cystic duct with the common duct. The cystic duct is transected and ligated 3 mm from the common bile duct. It is not necessary to close the bed of the gallbladder. A drain may be brought out from the hepatorenal pouch, which is the most dependent portion of the upper abdomen with the patient in the supine position, via a separate stab wound if there is concern that blood will accumulate or if there is marked pseudocholecystic inflammation and edema. Several series have shown that in the absence of specific indications, drainage is not required.

The above-described method is directed at facilitating demonstration of the junction between the cystic duct and common bile duct. The gallbladder may also be removed in a so-called "retrograde" fashion, in which the cystic duct is ligated close to the junction with the common duct as the initial part of the procedure. Then, after the cystic duct and artery have been transected, dissection is begun from the cystic duct and continued outward toward the fundus (Fig. 31-23).

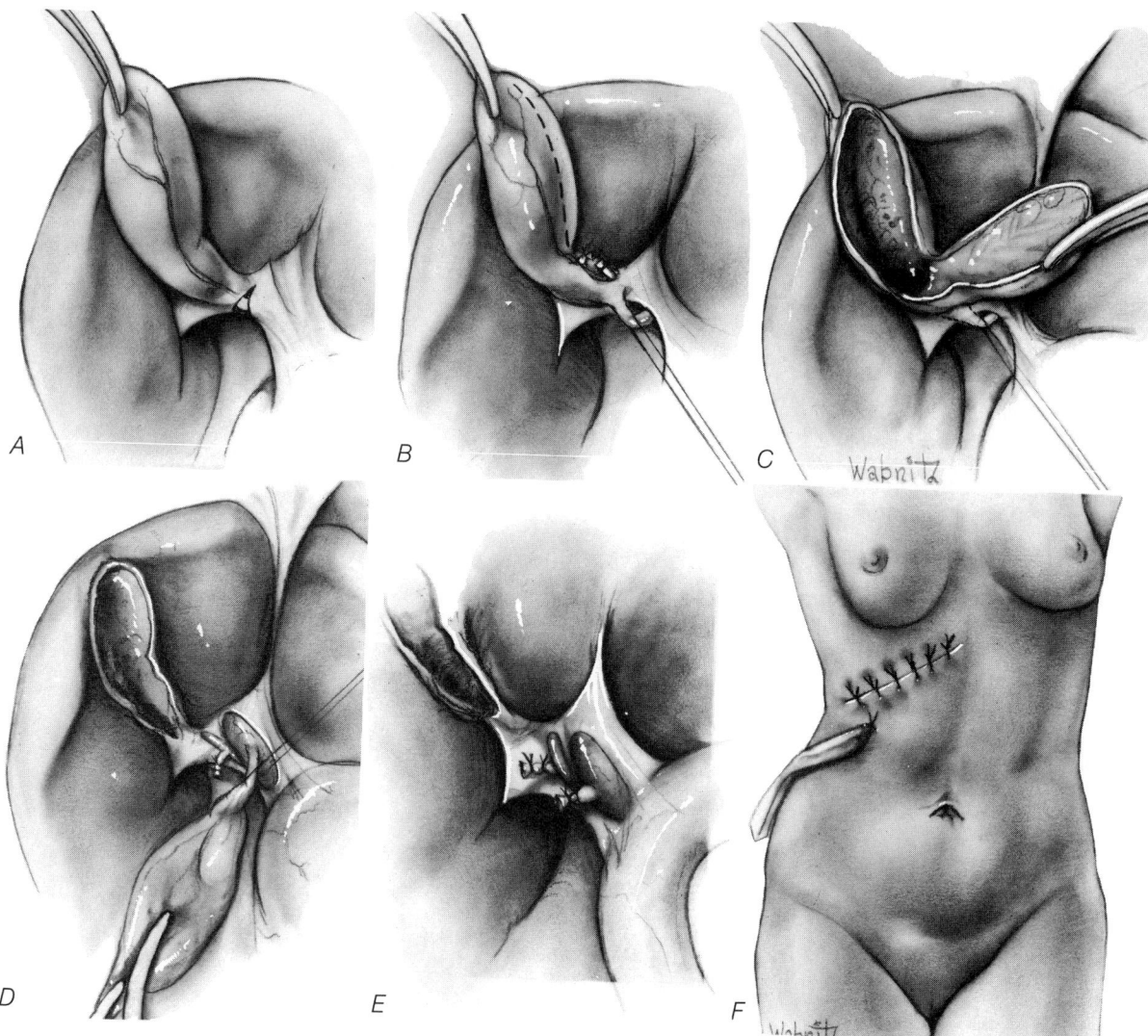

Fig. 31-22. Cholecystectomy (preferred approach.) *A.* Veil of peritoneum coursing from ampulla to hepatoduodenal ligament is transected, and cystic duct is identified. *B.* Ligature is passed around cystic duct and traction applied to prevent passage of calculi from gallbladder into common duct during the course of subsequent dissection. Dissection is continued along same fold of peritoneum, and cystic artery is doubly ligated and transected. Incision is made in peritoneum overlying gallbladder. *C.* Gallbladder is removed from its bed, and if large vessels or bile ducts are encountered, they are ligated. Dissection continues from fundus toward junction between cystic duct and common bile duct. *D.* Ultimate pedicle of cystic duct is established, and junction between cystic duct and common bile duct is defined. *E.* Cystic duct is ligated and transfixed and then transected approximately 3 mm from its junction with the common bile duct. *F.* Drain is brought out via stab wound from the hepatorenal (Morison's) pouch.

OPERATIONS OF THE COMMON BILE DUCT. The situations necessitating operative procedure on the common bile duct include exploration for calculi, repair of a surgically interrupted or injured common duct, stenosis of the sphincter of Oddi, and bypass procedures for obstructive jaundice secondary to trauma, tumors, and atresia. The indications for concomitant exploration of the common bile duct during cholecystectomy have been enumerated in the section on choledocholithiasis.

Initial Exploration for Choledocholithiasis. When the procedure (Fig. 31-24) is being performed at the time of cholecystectomy, the cystic duct should be identified initially. Traction is applied to a ligature passed around this duct to avoid passage of stones from the gallbladder into the common duct. The gallbladder is generally removed after the common duct has been thoroughly explored and distal patency demonstrated. After the common duct has been visualized, aspiration with a fine needle provides confirmation. Two fixation sutures are placed distal to the junction of the cystic and common bile duct, and a vertical incision is made between these through the anterior

wall. Calculi are removed by a combination of stone forceps, scoops, balloon-tipped catheters, and irrigation. These procedures should first be applied to the common bile duct toward the ampulla of Vater and subsequently to each of the main hepatic ducts. After the stones have been removed, a #3 Bâkes dilator should pass readily into the duodenum, and the tip of the dilator should be

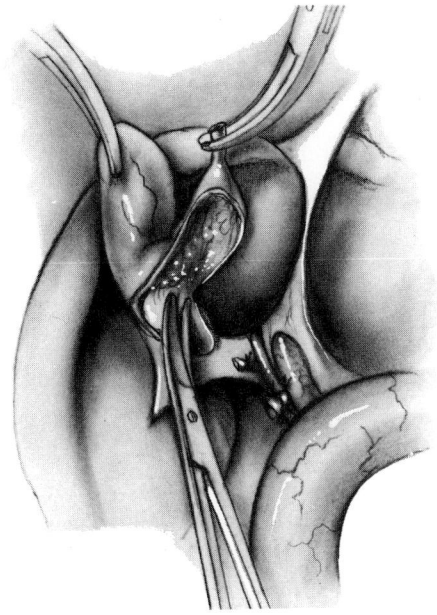

Fig. 31-23. Retrograde dissection of gallbladder. After cystic duct has been identified, its junction with common bile duct is defined, and cystic duct is transected. Cystic artery is also doubly ligated and transected, and gallbladder is removed from its bed with dissection progressing from the cystic duct and ampulla outward toward fundus.

Fig. 31-24. Exploration of the common bile duct. *A.* Ligature has been placed around cystic duct to prevent passage of stones from gallbladder into common duct. After common bile duct has been identified by dissection and aspiration, two stay sutures are placed on either side. A longitudinal incision is made in the common duct. *B.* Duct is explored with stone forceps and scoops, and irrigated in both directions, i.e., toward liver and toward ampulla of Vater. Prior to insertion of a T tube, a #3 Bâkes dilator should pass readily into duodenum. *C.* An ellipse is removed from junction of horizontal and vertical limbs of the T tube, and a T tube is inserted into common duct via choledochotomy. Distal limb of T tube should be short and should not pass through ampulla of Vater. Proximal limb should also be short and positioned so that is does not obstruct either of the hepatic ducts. *D.* Choledochostomy is closed tightly around T tube, which is irrigated to demonstrate absence of leakage.

visualized through the wall of the intestine. After free passage of the dilator has been demonstrated, a T tube, with the ellipse removed from the junction of the horizontal and vertical limbs of the T to facilitate removal of the tube postoperatively, is inserted into the common duct. The limbs of the T should be short, so that the distal limb does not pass through the ampulla of Vater and the proximal limb does not obstruct either of the hepatic ducts. The common duct is then closed with interrupted sutures, and saline solution is injected into the T tube to demonstrate absence of leaks. At this stage an operative cholangiogram should be performed to rule out retained stones and demonstrate free passage of the radiopaque medium into the duodenum. The T tube should be brought out through a stab wound to prevent dislodgment when the major incision is dressed. Postoperative cholangiogram is performed on the seventh to eighth day, and if absence of stones plus clear passage of radiopaque into the duodenum is demonstrated, the tube can be removed.

Transduodenal Choledochotomy: Sphincteroplasty (Fig. 31-25). In the event that a stone is impacted at the ampulla of Vater or that a Bâkes dilator cannot be passed into the duodenum, thus suggesting fibrosis of the sphincter of Oddi, a duodenotomy is performed. The procedure is also applicable to the problem of multiple or recurrent stones. The lateral peritoneal reflection of the second portion of the duodenum is incised (Kocher maneuver) to facilitate exposure. A longitudinal duodenotomy is performed on the anterior aspect of the duodenum and, with the Bâkes dilator in place in the common duct to facilitate demonstration of the sphincter, the sphincter is incised, and the impacted calculus is removed. If there is evidence of fibrosis of the sphincter, a V segment should be removed from the area at "11 o'clock" to avoid injury of the pancreatic duct. Absorbable sutures are used to approximate duodenal mucosa to distal mucosa. Free passage of a #3 Bâkes dilator into the duodenum from the common bile duct should then be demonstrated and a T tube inserted into the common duct. The duodenotomy is preferably

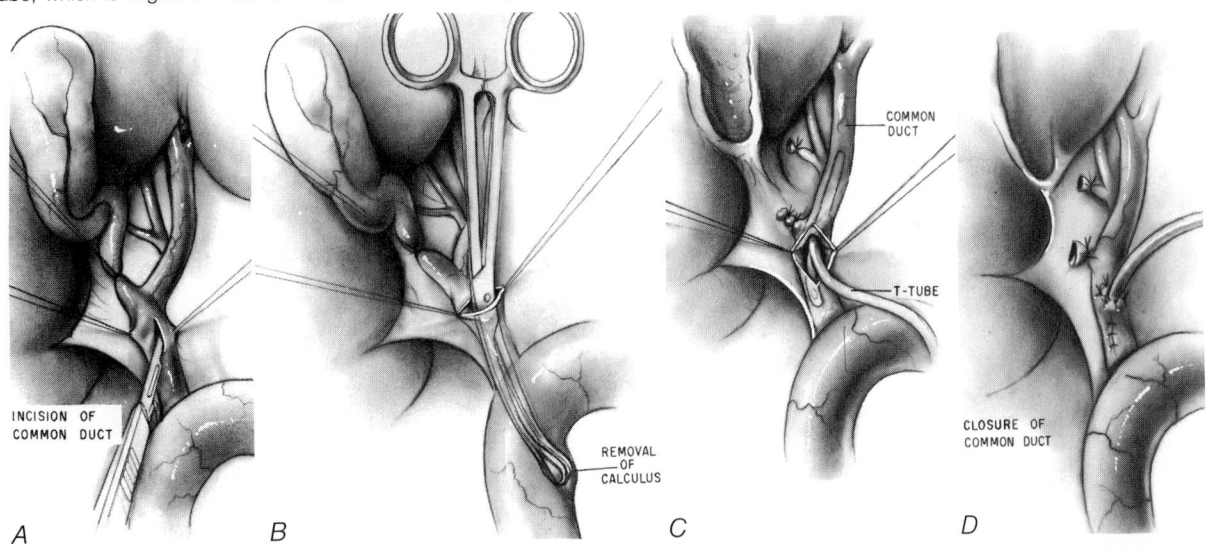

A   INCISION OF COMMON DUCT

B   REMOVAL OF CALCULUS

C   COMMON DUCT   T-TUBE

D   CLOSURE OF COMMON DUCT

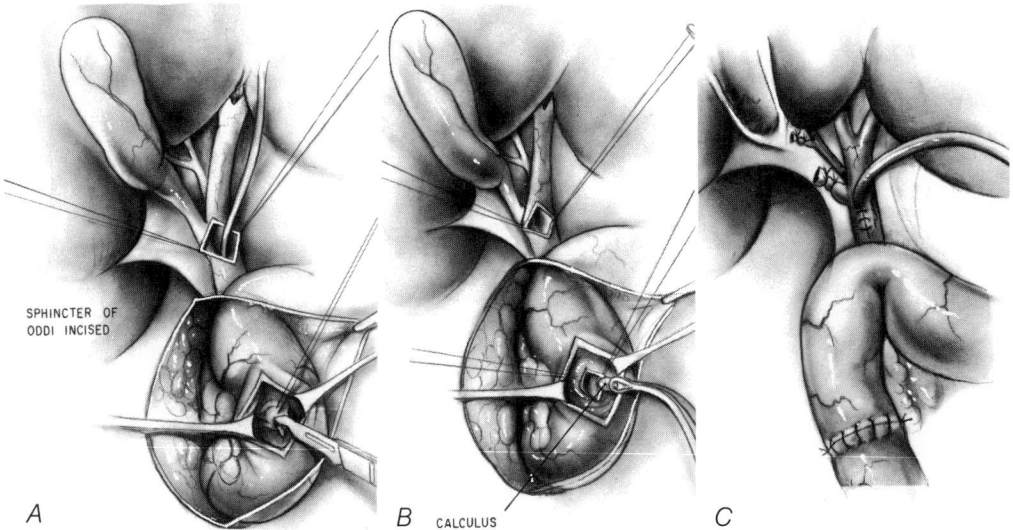

closed in two layers. The longitudinal incision may be converted into a transverse closure to prevent stenosis.

Operative Procedures for Recurrent Choledocholithiasis: Choledochoduodenostomy (Fig. 31-26). Common duct exploration is carried out as described above. If the surgeon is concerned about the possibility of subsequent reexplorations, either because of the patient's age or the fact that the surgeon is not totally satisfied that all stones have been removed, a choledochoduodenostomy may be performed provided that the common duct is dilated. The incision in the common duct should be enlarged, and after all apparent stones have been removed, a Kocher maneuver is performed on the duodenum, and a side-to-side anastomosis between the common duct and the duodenum is carried out. One or two layers may be used for this anastomosis, but it is imperative that the stoma be large enough so that subsequent scarring does not result in spontaneous closure.

Repair of Injured or Strictured Common Duct (Fig. 31-27). If transection of the common bile duct is noted at opera-

Fig. 31-25. Transduodenal choledochotomy: sphincterotomy. *A.* Kocher maneuver is performed on second portion of duodenum, and longitudinal duodenotomy is carried out. With Bâkes dilator inserted in common duct in order to define ampulla of Vater, stay suture is placed in ampulla, which is incised. *B.* Wedge of tissue should be removed from sphincter, and calculus impacted in this region can readily be excised. *C.* T tube is inserted into the common bile duct, and duodenotomy is closed transversely.

tion, an end-to-end anastomosis over a T-tube stent is indicated. A single layer of sutures is sufficient, and the results are usually excellent.

If the stricture has developed subsequent to injury of the common duct, the preferable method of treatment is direct repair of the common bile duct over a T tube. The

Fig. 31-26. Choledochoduodenostomy. *A.* Kocher maneuver is performed on second portion of duodenum, and common bile duct has been isolated. *B.* Seromuscular suture approximates duodenum to common bile duct. Longitudinal incision is made in distal common bile duct and in duodenum. *C.* Anterior row of anastomosis is completed, and wide stoma between duodenum and common bile duct is created.

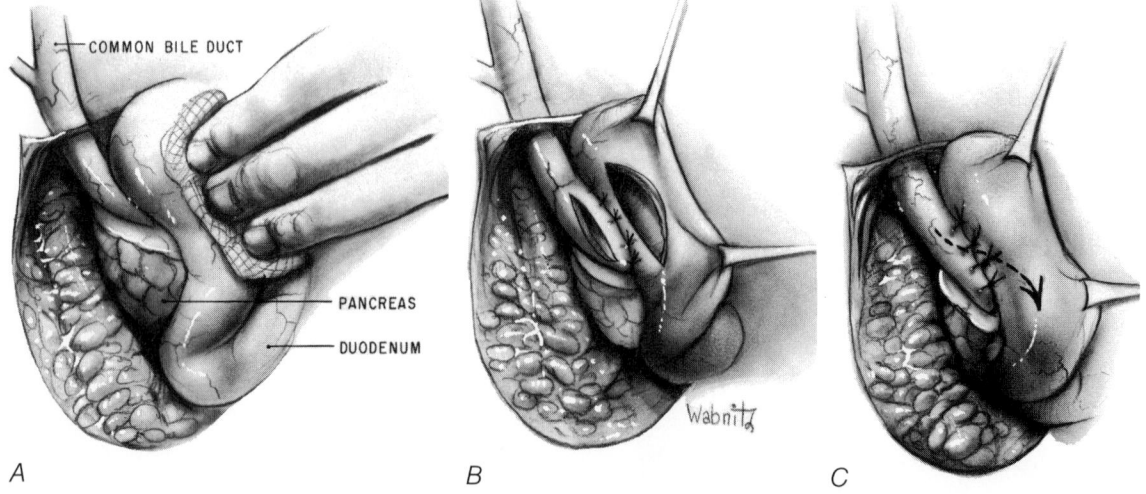

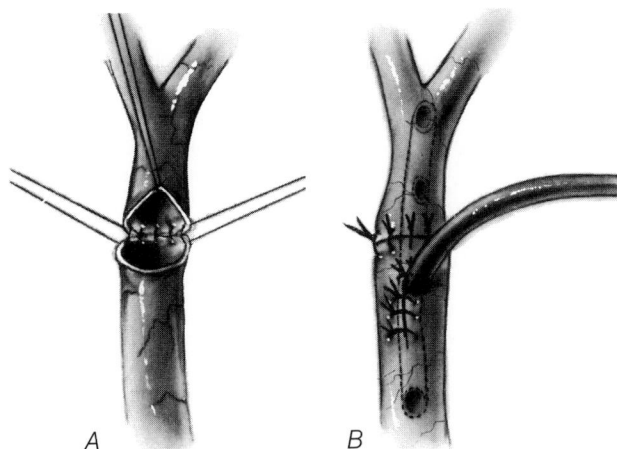

Fig. 31-27. Immediate repair of injured common duct. *A.* End-to-end anastomosis using interrupted suture is effected after cut ends of duct have been debrided. This procedure can also be carried out if there is stricture of common duct and both proximal and distal segments are identifiable. *B.* Anastomosis is complete, and T tube has been inserted as a stent via separate choledochostomy.

strictured area may be excised and the common duct mobilized so that an end-to-end anastomosis is possible. If the area of stricture is extensive and if the distal common bile duct cannot be identified, a proximal decompressive procedure is indicated.

Decompressive Procedures. A great variety of procedures are applicable, and the selection is primarily dependent upon the availability of the gallbladder or proximal ducts. If obstruction is at the level of the distal common duct, an anastomosis between proximal common duct and intestine is indicated. The common duct may be anastomosed to the side of the jejunum or preferably to a Roux en Y jejunal segment 30 cm in length. The latter has the theoretic advantage of decreasing the incidence of ascending cholangitis. With obstruction of the proximal common bile duct, the gallbladder, if present, can be anastomosed to the jejunum, or the common hepatic duct may be anastomosed as a Roux en Y. If obstruction is at the confluence of the hepatic ducts, in the porta hepatis, decompression is more difficult, but a single hepatic duct may be anastomosed to the Roux en Y of the jejunum, or the liver may be split along its anatomic plane and the confluence anastomosed to the intestine. With high ductal obstruction, the mucosal graft of Smith has been applied (Fig. 31-28). Although the procedure is facilitated by this maneuver stricture frequently occurs. A mucosal-to-mucosal suture is associated with a reduced incidence of stricture. In the face of a scarred hilus, the left hepatic duct can be anastomosed side-to-side to a Roux en Y limb of jejunum (Hepp-Couinaud) (Fig. 31-29).

Bibliography

General

Smith R, Sherlock S: *Surgery of the Gall Bladder and Bile Ducts.* London, Butterworth, 1981.

Fig. 31-28. Decompression of intrahepatic ducts by jejunal mucosal graft (Smith). *A.* Jejunal Roux en Y established and elipse of serosa removed. *B.* Catheter passed through liver parenchyma and into jejunal limb, where it is secured with catgut sutures. *C.* Jejunal limb pulled up so that mucosal patch abuts stoma of hepatic duct.

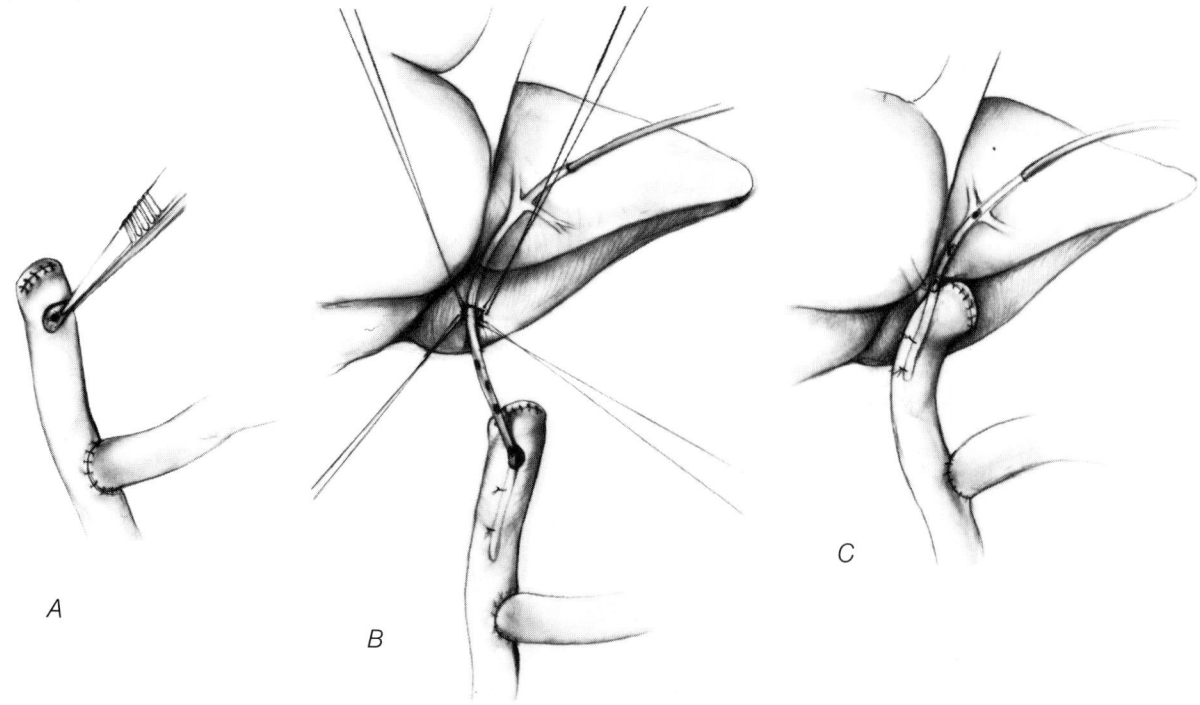

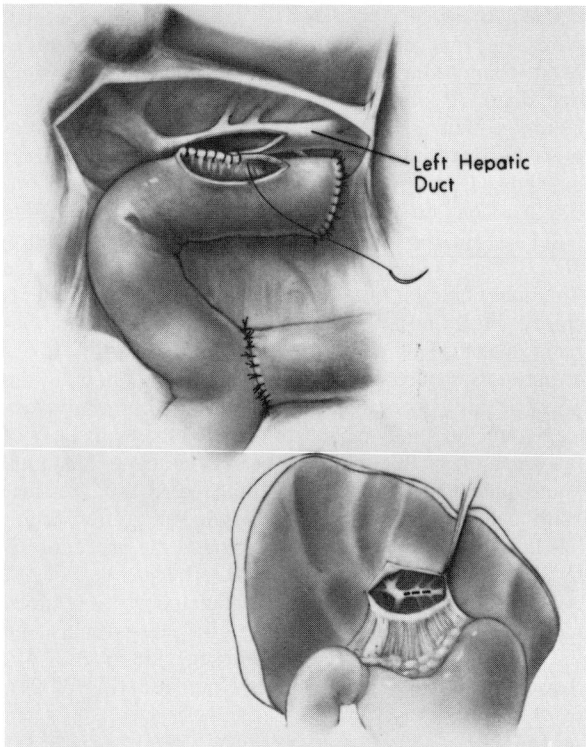

Fig. 31-29. Hepp-Couinaud procedure. Lower illustration demonstrates detachment of tissue in hilus of liver to visualize the left hepatic duct, which is incised longitudinally. Upper illustration demonstrates side-to-side anastomosis between main left hepatic duct and a defunctionalized (Roux en Y) limb of jejunum.

Way LW, Pellegrini CA: *Surgery of the Gallbladder and Bile Ducts*. Philadelphia, Saunders, 1987.

Anatomy

Alonso-Lej F, Rever WB, Pessagno DJ: Congenital choledochal cyst, with a report of 2, and an analysis of 94 cases. *Surg Gynecol Obstet* 108:1, 1958.

Benson EA, Page RE: A practical reappraisal of the anatomy of the extrahepatic bile ducts and arteries. *Br J Surg* 63:853, 1976.

Boyden EA: The anatomy of the choledochoduodenal junction in man. *Surg Gynecol Obstet* 104:641, 1957.

Deziel DJ, Rossi RL, et al: Management of bile duct cysts in adults. *Arch Surg* 121:410, 1986.

Longmire WP Jr, Mandiola SA, Gordon HE: Congenital cystic disease of the liver and biliary system. *Ann Surg* 174:711, 1971.

Mercadier M, Chigot JP, et al: Caroli's disease. *World J Surg* 8:22, 1984.

Michels NA: *Blood Supply and Anatomy of the Upper Abdominal Organs*. Philadelphia, Lippincott, 1955.

Nagorney DM, McIlrath DC, Adson MA: Choledochal cysts in adults: Clinical management. *Surgery* 96:656, 1984.

Sugura K, Miyano T, et al: Study on hepatic portoenterostomy for treatment of atresia of the biliary tract. *Surg Gynecol Obstet* 159:53, 1984.

Physiology

Jacobs LA, DeMeester TR, et al: Hyperplastic cholecystoses. *Arch Surg* 104:193, 1972.

Roslyn JJ, Pitt HA, et al: Gallbladder disease in patients on long-term parenteral nutrition. *Gastroenterology* 84:148, 1983.

Roslyn JJ, Pitt HA, et al: Parenteral nutrition-induced gallbladder disease: Reason for early cholecystectomy. *Am J Surg* 148:63, 1984.

Diagnosis of Biliary Tract Disease

Berci G, Shore JM, et al: Choledochoscopy and operative fluorocholangiography in the prevention of retained bile duct stones. *World J Surg* 2:411, 1978.

Burnstein MJ, Vassal KP, et al: Results of combined biliary drainage and cholecystokinin cholecystography in 81 patients with normal oral cholecystograms. *Ann Surg* 196:627, 1982.

Escat J, Fourtanier G, et al: Choledochoscopy in common bile duct surgery for choleocholithiasis: A must—eight years experience in 441 consecutive patients. *Am Surg* 51:166, 1985.

Freeman JB, Cohen WN, Den Besten L: Cholecystokinin cholangiography and analysis of duodenal bile in investigation of pain in right upper quadrant of the abdomen without gallstones. *Surg Gynecol Obstet* 140:371, 1975.

Frei GJ, Frei VT et al: Biliary pancreatitis: Clinical presentation and surgical management *Am J Surg* 151:170, 1986.

Jakimowicz JJ, Carol EJ, et al: An operative choledochoscopy using the flexible choledochoscope. *Surg Gynecol Obstet* 162:2–5, 1986.

Prian GW, Norton LW, et al: Clinical indications and accuracy of Gray-scale ultrasonography in the patient with suspected biliary tract disease. *Am J Surg* 134:705, 1977.

Rattner DW, Warshaw AL: Impact of choledochoscopy on the management of choledocholithiasis: Experience with 499 common duct explorations at the Massachusetts General Hospital. *Ann Surg* 194:76, 1981.

Suarez CA, Block F, et al: Role of HIDA/PIPIDA scanning in diagnosing cystic duct obstruction. *Ann Surg* 191:391, 1980.

Sugawa C, Clift D, et al: Endoscopic retrograde cholangiopancreatography after cholecystectomy. *Surg Gynecol Obstet* 157:247, 1983.

White TT, Waisman H, et al: Radiomanometry, flow rates, and cholangiography in the evaluation of common bile duct disease. *Am J Surg* 123:73, 1972.

Trauma

Andren-Sandberg A, Johansson S, et al: Accidental lesions of the common bile duct at cholecystectomy: II. Results of treatment. *Ann Surg* 201:452, 1985.

Blumgart LH, Kelley CJ, et al: Benign bile duct stricture following cholecystectomy: Critical factors in management. *Br J Surg* 71:836, 1984.

Diethrich EB, Beall AC Jr, et al: Traumatic injuries to the extrahepatic biliary tract. *Am J Surg* 112:756, 1966.

Ellis H, Cronin K: Bile peritonitis. *Br J Surg* 48:166, 1960.

Ivatury RR, Rohman M, et al: The morbidity of injuries of the extrahepatic biliary system. *J Trauma* 25:967, 1985.

Longmire WP Jr: Early management of injury to the extrahepatic biliary tract. *JAMA* 195:623, 1966.

Schwartz SI, Adams JT, et al: Blunt trauma to the upper abdomen. *Surg Annu* 3:273, 1971.

Sedgwick C, Poulantas J, Kune G: Management of portal hypertension secondary to bile duct strictures: Review of 18 cases with splenorenal shunt. *Ann Surg* 163:949, 1966.

Turney WH, Lee JP, Raju S: Complete transection of common bile duct due to blunt trauma. *Ann Surg* 179:440, 1974.

Gallstones

Adson MA, Nagorney DM: Hepatic resection for intrahepatic ductal stones. *Arch Surg* 117:611, 1982.

Bartlett MK, Waddell WR: Indications for common-duct exploration: Evaluation in 1,000 cases. *N Engl J Med* 258:164, 1958.

Braasch JW, Fender HR, Benneval MM: Refractory primary common bile duct stone disease. *Am J Surg* 139:526, 1980.

Burhenne HJ: Complications of nonoperative extraction of retained common duct stones. *Am J Surg* 131:260, 1976.

Comfort MW, Gray HK, Wilson JM: Silent gallstone: 10 to 20 year follow-up study of 112 cases. *Ann Surg* 128:931, 1948.

Cotton PB, Vallon AG: Duodenoscopic sphincterotomy for removal of bile duct stones in patients with gallbladders. *Surgery* 91:628 1982.

Day EA, Marks C: Gallstone ileus: Review of literature and presentation of 34 new cases. *Am J Surg* 129:552, 1975.

Degenshein GA: Choledochoduodenostomy: An 18-year study of 175 consecutive cases. *Surgery* 76:319, 1974.

Fung J: Liver fluke infestation and cholangio-hepatitis. *Br J Surg* 48:404, 1961.

Glenn F, Reed C, Grafe WR: Biliary enteric fistula. *Surg Gynecol Obstet* 153:527, 1981.

Gracie WA, Ransohoff DF: The natural history of silent gallstones. The innocent gallstone is not a myth. *N Engl J Med* 307:798, 1982.

Large AM: On the formation of gallstones. *Surgery* 54:928, 1963.

Mack E, Patzer EP, et al: Retained biliary tract stones: Nonsurgical treatment with Capmul 8210, a new cholesterol gallstone dissolution agent. *Arch Surg* 116:341, 1981.

Madden JL, Chun JY, et al: Choledochoduodenostomy: An unjustly maligned surgical procedure? *Am J Surg* 119:45, 1970.

Mazzariello RM: A fourteen-year experience with nonoperative instrument extraction of retained bile duct stones. *World J Surg* 2:447, 1978.

McSherry CK, Ferstenberg H, et al: The natural history of diagnosed gallstone disease in symptomatic and asymptomatic patients. *Ann Surg* 202:59, 1985.

Merendino KA, Manhas DR: Man-made gallstones: New entity following cardiac valve replacement. *Ann Surg* 177:694, 1973.

Safrany L: Transduodenal endoscopic sphincterotomy and extraction of bile duct stones. *World J Surg* 2:457, 1978.

Sauerbruch T, Delius M, et al: Fragmentation of gallstones by extracorporeal shock waves. *N Engl J Med* 314:818, 1986.

Schoenfield LJ, Lachin JM, et al: Chenodiol (chenodeoxycholic acid) for dissolution of gallstones: The National Cooperative Gallstone Study. *Ann Intern Med* 95:257, 1981.

Seifert E: Endoscopic papillotomy and removal of gallstones. *Am J Gastroenterol* 69:154, 1978.

Shaffer EA, Small DM: Biliary lipid secretion in cholesterol gallstones disease: Effect of cholecystectomy and obesity. *J Clin Invest* 59:828, 1977.

Small DM: Gallstones: Diagnosis and treatment. *Postgrad Med* 51:187, 1972.

Thistle JL, Schoenfield LJ: Lithogenic bile among young indian women: Lithogenic potential disease with chenodeoxycholic acid. *N Engl J Med* 284:177, 1971.

Vogt DP, Hermann RE: Choledochoduodenostomy, choledochojejunostomy or sphincteroplasty for biliary and pancreatic disease. *Ann Surg* 193:161, 1981.

Warshaw AL, Bartlett MK: Choice of operation for gallstone intestinal obstruction. *Ann Surg* 164:1051, 1966.

Inflammatory and Other Benign Lesions

Acosta J, Nardi GL: Papillitis of the ampulla of Vater. *Arch Surg* 92:354, 1966.

Adams JT, Libertino JA, Schwartz SI: Significance of an elevated serum amylase. *Surgery* 63:877, 1968.

Boey JH, Way LW: Acute cholangitis. *Ann Surg* 191:264, 1980.

Burnett W: The management of acute cholecystitis. *Aust New Zeal J Surg* 41:25, 1971.

Cameron JL, Gayler BW, et al: Sclerosing cholangitis: Biliary reconstruction with silastic transhepatic stents. *Surgery* 94:324, 1983.

Carmona RH, Crass RA: Oriental cholangitis. *Am J Surg* 148:117, 1984.

Cattell RB, Colcock BP: Fibrosis of the sphincter of oddi. *Ann Surg* 137:797, 1953.

Charcot JM: *Leçons sur les maladies du foie des voies filiares et des reins*. Faculté de Médecine de Paris, 1877.

Chetlin SH, Elliott DW: Biliary bacteremia. *Arch Surg* 102:303, 1971.

Choi TK, Wong J, et al: Late results of sphincteroplasty in the treatment of primary cholangitis. *Arch Surg* 116:1173, 1981.

Choi TK, Wong J, Ong GB: The surgical management of primary intrahepatic stones. *Br J Surg* 69:86, 1982.

Dunphy JE, Ross FP: Studies in acute cholecystitis. *Surgery* 26:539, 1949.

Fox MS, Wilk PJ, et al: Acute acalculous cholecystitis. *Surg Gynecol Obstet* 159:13, 1984.

Glenn F: Acute acalculous cholecystitis. *Ann Surg* 195:131, 1982.

Goldstein F, Grunt R, Margulies M: Cholecystokinin cholecystography in differential diagnosis of acalculous gallbladder disease. *Am J Dig Dis* 19:835, 1974.

Haupert AP, Carey LC, et al: Acute suppurative cholangitis: Experience with 15 consecutive cases. *Arch Surg* 94:460, 1967.

Hoerr SO, Hazard JB: Acute cholecystitis without gallbladder stones. *Am J Surg* 111:47, 1966.

Järvinen HJ, Hastbacka J: Early cholecystectomy for acute cholecystitis: Prospective randomized study. *Ann Surg* 191:501, 1980.

Keighley MRB, Lister CM, et al: Hazards of surgical treatment due to microorganisms in bile. *Surgery* 75:578, 1974.

LoGiudice JA, Geenen JE, et al: Efficacy of the morphine-prostigim test for evaluating patients with suspected papillary stenosis. *Dig Dis Sci* 24:455, 1979.

Long TN, Heimbach DM, Carrico CJ: Acalculous cholecystitis in critically ill patients. *Am J Surg* 136:31, 1978.

Lygidakis NJ: Acute suppurative cholangitis: Comparison of internal and external biliary drainage. *Am J Surg* 143:304, 1982.

Mentzer RM Jr, Golden GT, et al: Comparative appraisal of emphysematous cholecystitis. *Am J Surg* 129:10, 1975.

Mercer LC, Saltzstein EC, et al: Early surgery for biliary pancreatitis. *Am J Surg* 148:749, 1984.

Ottinger LW: Acute cholecystitis as a postoperative complication. *Ann Surg* 184:162, 1976.

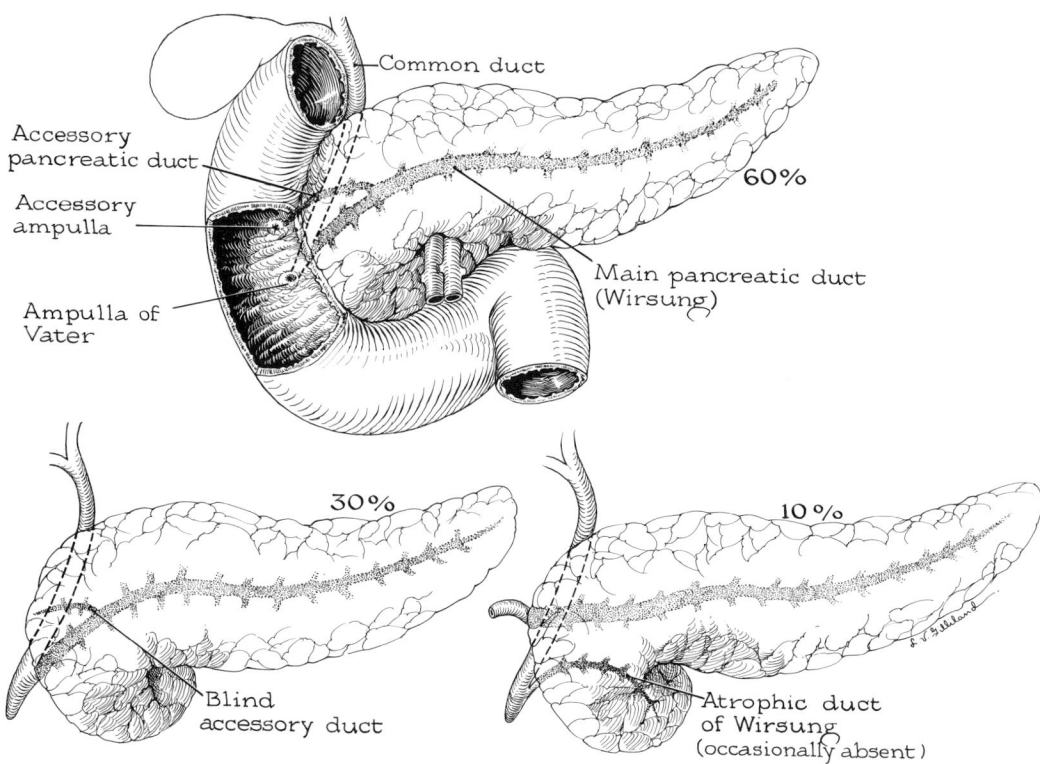

Fig. 32-1. Anatomic configuration of the intrapancreatic ductal system. Note the lack of communication between the two ducts in 10 percent of cases. (From: *Silen W: Surg Clin North Am 44:1253, 1964, with permission.*)

3 to 4 mm in diameter. As aging progresses, the ducts become larger, and in persons over the age of seventy, ducts 5 to 6 mm in diameter are commonly encountered in the normal pancreas.

BLOOD SUPPLY. The arterial supply to the pancreas is remarkably constant (Fig. 32-2). Anterior and posterior arcades supply the head of the pancreas; each arcade derives a superior component from the gastroduodenal artery and an inferior component from the superior mesenteric artery. The anterosuperior pancreaticoduodenal and anteroinferior pancreaticoduodenal arteries join to form the anterior arcade; the posterosuperior pancreaticoduodenal and posteroinferior pancreaticoduodenal arteries form the posterior arcade. This arrangement

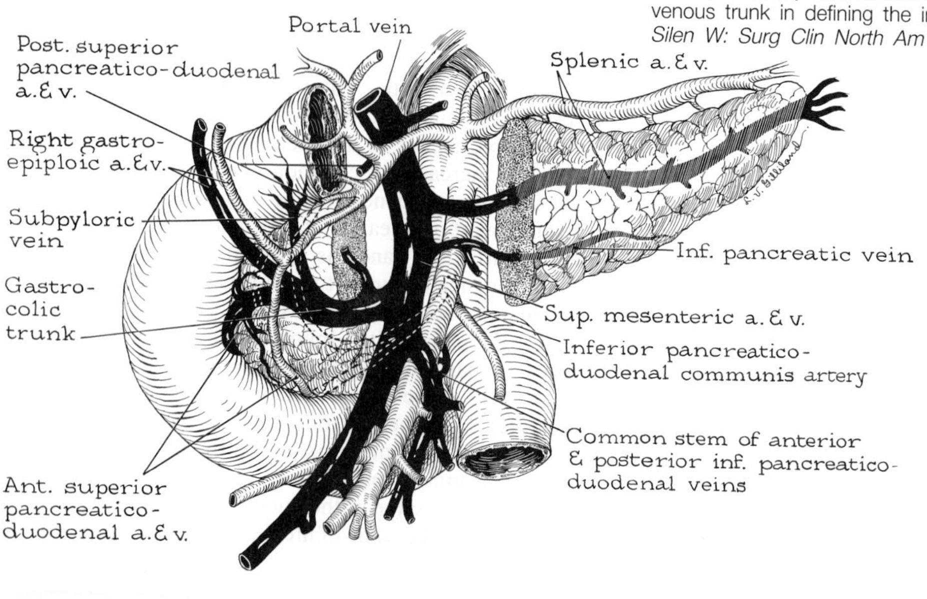

Fig. 32-2. Arterial supply and venous drainage of the pancreas. Note particularly the anatomic importance of the gastrocolic venous trunk in defining the inferior portion of the neck. (From: *Silen W: Surg Clin North Am 44:1253, 1964, with permission.*)

occurs in almost 100 percent of cases. The anterior arcade constitutes virtually the only major group of blood vessels on the anterior surface of the pancreas, an important surgical consideration.

The inferior pancreatic artery, which is nearly always constant, runs along the posteroinferior surface of the pancreas in intimate contact with the organ. Its origin is variable; it may start from the superior mesenteric artery, anterosuperior or anteroinferior pancreaticoduodenal artery, or superior pancreatic artery.

The superior pancreatic artery is present in from 50 to 90 percent of patients and arises from the splenic, hepatic, superior mesenteric, or celiac arteries. It lies along the posterosuperior portion of the neck and body of the pancreas. The body and tail of the pancreas are also supplied by branches from the splenic and left gastroepiploic arteries.

The venous drainage of the pancreas follows the course of the arteries quite closely, but the veins lie superficial to their arterial counterparts. Anterior and posterior venous arcades are always present around the head of the pancreas. The confluence of the right gastroepiploic vein, anterosuperior pancreaticoduodenal vein, and middle colic vein forms the gastrocolic trunk, which empties directly into the superior mesenteric vein at the inferior border of the neck of the pancreas. This provides an important landmark for location of the superior mesenteric vein when the pancreas is mobilized to determine operability of pancreatic tumors.

From the surgical standpoint it is important to remember that occasionally the hepatic artery may arise from the superior mesenteric artery and pass behind the pancreas and common bile duct. An unusually long and tortuous hepatic artery may lie close to the superior border of the head of the pancreas, or in some cases it may be within the pancreas itself. Under these circumstances, the hepatic artery may be injured during resection of the body and tail of the pancreas and may require ligation. Pierson has pointed out that the distal duodenum and proximal jejunum receive their arterial supply from one of the inferior pancreaticoduodenal arteries, so that interruption of these vessels probably will necessitate resection of the proximal 3 to 5 cm of jejunum.

Anatomy textbooks usually state that the anterior surface of the superior mesenteric and portal veins is free of tributaries in the region of the pancreas. However, the superior pancreaticoduodenal vein often joins the portal vein at the anterior surface of the pancreas, and the gastrocolic vein almost always joins the anterior surface of the superior mesenteric vein inferior to the neck. Other small venous tributaries from the pancreas to the portal and superior mesenteric veins are often present, although hidden from view. The posterosuperior pancreaticoduodenal vein may be the source of severe hemorrhage during mobilization of the portal vein for portacaval shunt.

LYMPHATIC DRAINAGE AND NERVE SUPPLY. The lymphatic capillaries from the tail drain into the nodes at the hilus of the spleen. From the right side of the pancreas the lymphatics drain into the pancreaticoduodenal lymph nodes lying in the groove between the duodenum and

pancreas and into the subpyloric nodes. Anteriorly the drainage is to the superior pancreatic, superior gastric, and hepatic nodes along the hepatic artery. Posteriorly the lymphatics pass to the inferior pancreatic, mesocolic, mesenteric, and aortic nodes.

The sympathetic nerve supply to the pancreas is derived from the greater, lesser, and lowest splanchnic nerves via the celiac ganglia and plexus. These fibers conduct the afferent pain fibers from the pancreas. The sympathetic nerves intermingle with branches of the right vagus nerve to form the splenic plexus from which most of the nerve supply to the pancreas emanates. The celiac branch of the right, or posterior, vagus nerve provides parasympathetic supply to the pancreas. This branch can be spared during selective gastric vagotomy for duodenal ulcer.

Annular Pancreas and Heterotopic Pancreas

Annular pancreas is a rare anatomic abnormality that results when two limbs of pancreatic tissue encircle the second portion of the duodenum because of incomplete migration of the ventral anlage of the gland. A variable degree of duodenal obstruction occurs, and associated anomalies, particularly complete atresia of the duodenum, are common. Histologically, the lesion presents as normal pancreatic tissue. Frequently there are no symptoms, and the finding is incidental. When symptoms occur, they are related to acute and recurrent duodenal obstruction and include abdominal pain, nausea, and vomiting. The onset of symptoms appears at all ages, but one-third present under the age of one. The diagnosis is suggested by the radiographic finding of partial or complete duodenal obstruction with notching of the right lateral duodenal wall (Fig. 32-3). A variety of surgical procedures have been proposed, including partial resection of the annular portion of the gland or bypassing the area of obstruction. The former is frequently followed by pancreatic fistula, and it is the consensus that duodenojejunostomy is the least hazardous and most effective way of relieving the obstruction.

Heterotopic (accessory) *pancreas* is most commonly found in the stomach and in a Meckel's diverticulum, but such islands of ectopic tissue have also been reported in the gallbladder and small intestine. Grossly, these are firm yellow nodules from 0.2 to 4.0 cm in size located submucosally with a central umbilication on the mucosal surface. Heterotopic pancreas can be confused with a leiomyoma or gastric or duodenal ulcer. Most gastric lesions are on the greater curvature of the antrum. No special symptom complex can be attributed to this condition.

PHYSIOLOGY

Exocrine Pancreas

FLUID AND ELECTROLYTE SECRETION. The human pancreas daily produces from 1500 to 2500 mL of a colorless, odorless fluid that has a pH of 8.0 to 8.3. Fluid and electrolytes are secreted by the centroacinar and ductal

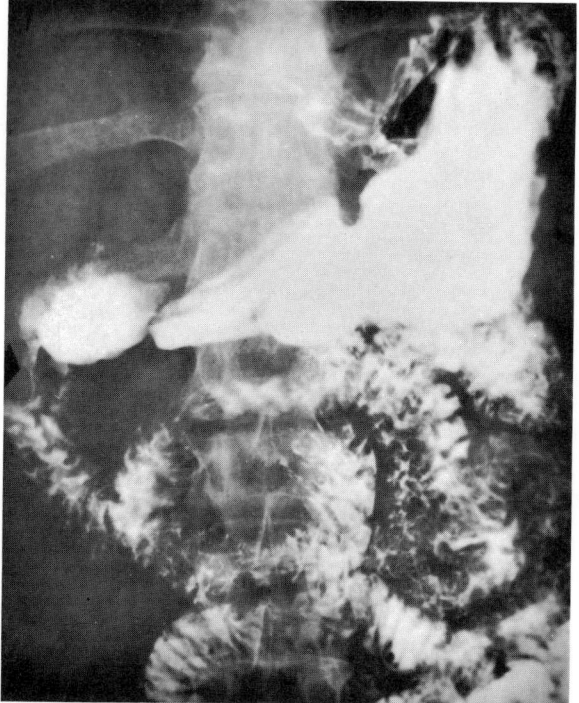

Fig. 32-3. Radiograph demonstrating annular pancreas.

cells in response to secretin stimulation. The secretion is isosmotic with the plasma, and its osmolality is independent of the rate of flow, in both health and disease. The bicarbonate of pancreatic juice is secreted by an active transport mechanism, and as the solution moves down the collecting system, exchange with chloride ion takes place. The sum of the concentrations of bicarbonate and chloride is constant under all conditions of secretion, although bicarbonate concentration rises with increasing rates of secretion. The secretion of bicarbonate is under the catalytic influence of carbonic anhydrase. The concentration of sodium and potassium is only slightly higher than that of plasma, which indicates that these ions are moved passively rather than actively.

Pancreatic juice contains between 1 and 3 percent protein, 90 percent of which is made up of digestive enzymes. Since the metabolic turnover of protein in the acinar cells of the pancreas is the highest of any cells in the body, the pancreas is dependent upon a constant supply of amino acids. It is not surprising, therefore, that protein deficiency may be associated with severe defects in exocrine pancreatic function, as in kwashiorkor. Proteolytic, lipolytic, and amylolytic enzymes are present in the pancreatic juice; the optimal pH for activity of all three enzyme systems is greater than 7.

Digestive enzymes are synthesized on polysomes attached to the endoplasmic reticulum (*rough endoplasmic reticulum,* RER). The nascent polypeptide chains elongate within the cisternae of the RER until a "signal sequence" is reached, at which point the chain is cleaved and the newly synthesized protein achieves its final structure within the cisternal space. From this point, the newly synthesized digestive enzymes migrate through a series of membrane-enclosed spaces (cisternae, Golgi complex, condensing vacuoles, zymogen granules). Eventually fusion and fission of the zymogen granule and plasma membranes allows exocytosis of the digestive enzymes into the luminal space of the ductal system. Some of the digestive enzymes are secreted in their active form (e.g., amylase, lipase) while others, particularly the proteolytic enzymes (trypsin, chymotrypsin, carboxypeptidases A and B), are released as inactive zymogens. The enzymes of the latter group are activated within the duodenum, where enterokinase converts trypsinogen to trypsin and trypsin activates chymotrypsinogen and the procarboxypeptidases. Pancreatic juice also contains elastase, phospholipase, ribonuclease, and deoxyribonuclease as well as colipase, which is a cofactor for lipase. Within the intestine, the pancreatic proteolytic enzymes split proteins into peptides, lipase breaks fats into glycerol and fatty acids, and amylase degrades starches to disaccharides and dextrins.

REGULATION OF PANCREATIC SECRETION (Table 32-1). Pancreatic exocrine secretion is regulated by both neural and humoral mechanisms. Acetylcholine, released from vagal nerve terminals, stimulates digestive enzyme secretion. The circulating hormone cholecystokinin (formerly

Table 32-1. REGULATION OF PANCREATIC EXOCRINE SECRETION

Phase	Stimulus	Mediator	Pancreatic response
Cephalic	Sight and smell of food	Vagus	Enzyme secretion
Gastric	Food in stomach, distention; gastric distention; acid discharged to duodenum	Gastrin release	Enzyme secretion
		Gastrin	Enzyme secretion
		Vagus	Enzyme secretion
		Secretin	HCO_3^- and H_2O secretion
Intestinal	Acid in intestine; amino acids, peptides, fatty acids	Secretin	HCO_3^- and H_2O secretion
		CCK	Enzyme secretion
		Vagus	Enzyme secretion
Postcibal	Fat in distal intestine; intravenous glucose and protein hydrolysate	?	Inhibition of secretion
		?	Inhibition of secretion

called cholecystokinin-pancreozymin) is also a strong stimulant of enzyme secretion and a weak stimulant of water and bicarbonate secretion. In contrast, secretin and vasoactive intestinal peptide (VIP) strongly stimulate water and bicarbonate secretion and are weak stimulants of enzyme secretion. Hormones originating in the islets of Langerhans are also believed to regulate exocrine function. Pancreatic polypeptide, somatostatin, and glucagon inhibit exocrine secretion. Finally, peptidergic nerves, which release agents such as somatostatin, enkephlin, and vasoactive intestinal peptide, may also play a role in the regulation of pancreatic function. A local, paracrine role for these agents has been suggested. Vasoactive intestinal peptide acts like secretin to stimulate fluid and bicarbonate secretion, while somatostatin and enkephlin inhibit exocrine secretion.

The sight and smell of food initiates the *cephalic phase* of pancreatic secretion that is vagally mediated. Direct vagal stimulation results in the secretion of a low-volume, enzyme-rich juice. Vagal stimulation also results in gastrin release from the stomach, and circulating gastrin may also stimulate pancreatic enzyme secretion. During the *gastric phase* of a meal, gastric distention and the presence of protein in the stomach cause the release of gastrin and stimulate gastric vagal afferent nerves (*gastropancreatic reflex*). Both events lead to the stimulation of enzyme secretion by the pancreas as well as acid secretion by the stomach. During the *intestinal phase,* acid in the duodenum stimulates secretin release and, thus, pancreatic fluid and bicarbonate secretion. Peptides and amino acids as well as fatty acids and monoglycerides stimulate release of cholecystokinin. The latter hormone causes a slow but sustained increase in the rate of enzyme secretion by the pancreas. In addition, the products of digestion stimulate intestinal vagal afferent fibers and initiate an enteropancreatic reflex that promotes the rapid, but short-lived, discharge of digestive enzymes from the pancreas. The *postcibal phase* of digestion is characterized by the inhibition of pancreatic secretion. Intravenous infusions of glucose or protein hydrolysate and the presence of fat in the distal intestine can inhibit pancreatic secretion, but the physiologic basis for this response has not been established.

EFFECTS OF LOSS OF PANCREATIC JUICE. Exclusion of pancreatic juice from the gastrointestinal tract by pancreatectomy, by ligation of the pancreatic ducts, or by total external pancreatic fistula results in severe impairment of the digestion and absorption of various foodstuffs, particularly fat. On the other hand, digestion is probably only slightly impaired if only a fraction of normal pancreatic juice enters the duodenum and clinically apparent steatorrhea develops only after loss of more than 90 percent of pancreatic digestive enzyme secretion.

Profound gastric hypersecretion always occurs experimentally whenever pancreatic secretions are diverted from the intestine. It is likely that the absence of pancreatic juice from the intestine prevents normal fat inhibition by enterogastrone and that the nutritional consequences of inadequate digestion cause hepatic damage, which may also enhance gastric hypersecretion. Two conclusions of surgical importance can be reached: (1) if the head of the pancreas is resected, digestion is better, and the chances of marginal ulceration are less if the remaining pancreatic remnant is anastomosed to the gastrointestinal tract rather than being ligated; and (2) pancreatic extracts should be used freely whenever postoperative deficiency of external pancreatic secretion exists. Pancreatic digestive enzymes can be degraded by acid in the stomach, and their pH optima are alkaline. For these reasons, inhibition of gastric acid secretion, by agents such as the H_2-antagonists cimetidine and ranitidine or by neutralization with antacids, improves the therapeutic effectiveness of exogenously administered pancreatic enzymes.

Impaired absorption of vitamin B_{12}, seemingly associated with a low duodenal pH, has been observed in patients with pancreatic insufficiency, and improved absorption of vitamin B_{12} may follow administration of sodium bicarbonate, pancreatic extract, or both. Apparently, normal secretion of pancreatic juice is essential for unimpaired absorption of vitamin B_{12}. Conversely, pancreatic extracts may depress the abnormally high absorption of iron in hemochromatosis or pancreatitis. These findings provide further strong reasons for administering pancreatic extract to patients with pancreatic insufficiency.

PANCREATICOBILIARY PRESSURE RELATIONSHIPS. Studies of intrabiliary pressure in patients in whom T tubes have been placed in the common duct after cholecystectomy indicate that responses are similar to those observed in dogs. Menguy et al. have shown in dogs that resting pancreatic pressures consistently exceed those in the biliary tree, although the pressure in the bile duct rises after cholecystectomy. The pressure in both ductal systems rises after a meal. When the rate of flow of pancreatic juice is increased by injecting secretin, the pressure in the pancreatic ducts does not rise, although intravenous administration of sodium dehydrocholate definitely increases biliary pressure. Acid instilled into the duodenum causes little change in pancreatic intraductal pressure, in contrast to alcohol, which uniformly increases both pancreatic and biliary pressure. Morphine, codeine, and meperidine hydrochloride increase intrapancreatic pressure but raise biliary pressure only in the absence of the gallbladder. Atropine consistently lowers pancreatic intraductal pressure, and pilocarpine increases pressure. Infected bile, probably as a result of bacterial deconjugation of bile salts, causes a marked rise in resistance of the sphincter of Oddi.

Endocrine Pancreas

The internal secretions of the pancreas are formed by the islets of Langerhans, which approximate 1 million in number yet represent only about 1.5 percent of the normal pancreas by weight. The individual islets are 75 to 150 μm in diameter and comprise 75 percent beta (B) cells, 20 percent alpha (A) cells, 5 percent delta (D) cells, and a small number of C cells. The various cell types are arranged in layers with the alpha cells outermost, delta cells intermediate, and beta cells central. Alpha cells are the source of glucagon and beta cells the source of insulin. Delta cells produce somatostatin, gastrin, and pancreatic polypeptide. Recent studies have indicated that all these endocrine hormones can modulate pancreatic exocrine function, and a capillary bed connecting the endocrine and exocrine pancreas has been demonstrated. Parainsular cells that are intermediate in appearance, resembling both endocrine and exocrine pancreatic cells, have been noted in several species, but their function and importance have not been established.

Glucagon is composed of 20 amino acids arranged in a straight chain and has a molecular weight of 3485. It causes glycogenolysis in the liver and release of glucose into the bloodstream. A decreased response to glucagon occurs in diseases of the liver. Purified glucagon, 1 mg given intravenously, will usually raise the blood sugar by 50 to 80 mg/dL and a gradual return to normal follows in about 90 min. Glucagon is also secreted by the intestinal mucosa.

Insulin has a molecular weight of about 6000 and consists of two polypeptide chains. The prime function of insulin is to promote the transfer of glucose and other sugars across certain cell membranes. The transfer of sugars into muscle cells, fibroblasts, and adipose tissue requires insulin, but neurons, erythrocytes, hepatic cells, and intestinal cells can accomplish this process without it. In the absence of glucose, fat is utilized, and ketosis and acidosis occur. Amino acids may be oxidized to provide energy and may cause a negative nitrogen balance when glucose is not being used properly. Insulin may also play a role in the conversion of glucose to glycogen in the liver.

Regulation of insulin secretion does not seem to depend upon trophic support, since neither vagotomy nor ablation of the anterior pituitary gland has an effect upon insulin secretion. The primary stimulus to the secretion of insulin is the blood sugar itself; an increase in blood sugar causes degranulation of the beta cells. Various hormones that increase the blood sugar, such as growth hormone, glucocorticoids, thyroid hormone, and epinephrine, may secondarily increase the secretion of insulin.

It has recently been demonstrated that all three of the major nutrient substrates, namely, glucose, amino acids, and fatty acids, stimulate varying degrees of insulin secretion. Gastrin, secretin, and cholecystokinin all produce a rise in insulin after injection, but the response to gastrin is quantitatively trivial while that to secretin is modest. Cholecystokinin elicits substantial release of both insulin and glucagon and augments the release of these two hormones by amino acids. Leucine and the sulfonureas used in the treatment of diabetes are known to produce their effects by releasing insulin from the beta cell granules.

PANCREATITIS

Acute Pancreatitis

ETIOLOGY. There are two main types of pancreatitis, *acute* and *chronic*. Reference is frequently made in the literature to a form of "chronic relapsing pancreatitis" which is discussed as a third form of the disease. Most of these cases are actually recurrent attacks of acute pancreatitis or are simply acute exacerbations in the course of chronic pancreatitis.

Pancreatitis Associated with Gallstones. Approximately two-thirds of patients with pancreatitis in private hospitals have gallstones, but in charity hospitals only one-third or less prove to have gallstone pancreatitis. For many years, a common channel between the common bile duct and the duct of Wirsung was thought to be of great importance in the pathogenesis, not only of gallstone pancreatitis, but also of pancreatitis due to many other causes. It is true that, on occasion, a calculus impacted at the ampulla of Vater may produce pancreatitis. Yet, even though a clear association exists between gallstones and acute pancreatitis and treatment of the biliary tract disease almost always cures the pancreatitis, the mechanism by which the pancreatitis is produced remains an enigma. Recent studies show that a high proportion of patients with gallstone pancreatitis have recoverable biliary calculi in the stools.

The classic experimental method for production of pancreatitis is injection of bile into the ductal system, but many facts militate against this mechanism in human gallstone pancreatitis. Continuous perfusion of the unobstructed pancreatic ductal system with bile in dogs and goats has not led to acute pancreatitis. In experimental biliary pancreatitis the bile is usually injected with sufficient pressure to rupture the pancreatic acini. The normal secretory pressure relationships argue against reflux, since pancreatic secretory pressure is generally higher than that of the liver. Radiocinemanometric studies have shown that contraction of the sphincter of Oddi often occludes both the biliary and the pancreatic ducts and isolates them from each other rather than producing an open common channel. Furthermore, reflux into the pancreatic duct occurs quite often during operative or T-tube cholangiography without apparent ill effects. Nevertheless, the bile factor cannot be discarded completely. Elliott et al. have shown that resistance to the flow of bile into the pancreatic duct greatly decreases after incubation of bile with pancreatic juice. Two components of bile, deconjugated bile salts and lysolecithins, have recently been found to be extremely toxic to the pancreas during experimental reflux. Deconjugated bile salts may be formed by bacterial action on conjugated bile salts, and lysolecithin results from the conversion of biliary lecithin by phospholipase A of pancreatic juice. It has been demonstrated that bile in the pancreas may cause vascular injury, stasis, and spasm, which may initiate pancreatitis.

Several studies have indicated that choledocholithiasis can lead to the development of acute pancreatitis even in the absence of a common biliary-pancreatic channel and/or reflux of bile into the pancreatic duct. Presumably, the presence of an ampullary stone or edema at the papilla can obstruct pancreatic duct outflow without altering the rate of pancreatic secretion and, thus, can result in the development of ductal hypertension.

Alcoholic Pancreatitis. About two-thirds of patients with pancreatitis in charity hospitals, but only one-third of such patients in private hospitals, have alcoholic pancreatitis. Alcohol is now known to cause an increase in protein concentration in pancreatic juice, precipitation of which may form a nidus upon which subsequent calcification occurs, and intraduodenal instillation of alcohol also causes a profound and sustained rise in pancreatic ductal pressure in dogs. Duodenal inflammation, induced by alcohol, may produce some degree of ductal obstruction in a gland actively secreting in response to the acid-secretin mechanism. Experimental ductal obstruction alone does not cause pancreatitis, but if hypersecretion induced by food, secretin, or vascular injury is also present, severe pancreatitis ensues. Persistent vomiting may cause regurgitation of duodenal contents into the pancreatic ducts. Dietary-induced hypertriglyceridemia has now been shown to produce a clinical syndrome of acute pancreatitis in about half of alcoholic patients who previously exhibited alcoholic pancreatitis. Pancreatic calculi and multiple stenoses within the ductal system late in the course of chronic pancreatitis are probably the sequelae of pancreatitis rather than the cause. As important as the mechanical factors may be, nutritional factors may ultimately prove to be more crucial. Since the turnover of protein by the pancreas is the greatest of any organ, it is not surprising that protein deficiency states have been associated with degeneration, atrophy, and fibrosis of the pancreas.

Postoperative Pancreatitis. Pancreatitis occasionally occurs after intraabdominal operations, especially those on the biliary tract and stomach. Rarely, it may develop after operations remote from the pancreas. It is clear that the pancreatitis that follows biliary operations occurs only when the common bile duct has been explored, especially if a long-armed T tube has been placed through the sphincter of Oddi. Pancreatitis is also likely to follow a gastrectomy in which the region of the head of the pancreas has been dissected. Direct ligation or laceration of the duct of Santorini may provide the insult that triggers the pancreatitis. Vascular injury, together with the damage to the duct, may set the stage for this serious disease. The interaction of obstruction and vascular factors is demonstrated by the development of experimental pancreatitis when the second part of the duodenum is converted into a closed loop. The clinical counterpart of this experiment is the occurrence of pancreatitis in a patient with afferent loop obstruction after a Billroth II gastrectomy. The mortality of postoperative pancreatitis is approximately 50 percent. After splenectomy, postoperative pancreatitis is usually the direct result of operative injury to the tail of the pancreas.

Metabolic Factors. It has been claimed that an association between hyperparathyroidism and pancreatitis exists and that an attack of acute pancreatitis may be the first sign of hyperparathyroidism. Some have suggested that patients with otherwise unexplained pancreatitis should be evaluated for possible hyperparathyroidism. Recently, however, evidence has been presented that indicates that hyperparathyroidism is an unlikely cause of pancreatitis and that most hyperparathyroid patients with pancreatitis have other, more common, processes that are more likely to have led to their pancreatic disease (i.e., gallstone, al-

cohol abuse). Hyperparathyroidism-induced pancreatitis, if it occurs at all, must be a rare event.

A small group of patients with a hereditary type of pancreatitis has been described in whom aminoaciduria is a fairly consistent finding. Lysinuria and cystinuria are frequently observed, but the metabolic defect that produces the pancreatitis is not known. The disease usually begins in childhood, and inheritance follows the pattern of an autosomal gene. Some of these patients have calcification of the pancreas. The prognosis is generally good.

It has been known for many years that *transient* hyperlipemia may occur during the course of clinical and experimental acute pancreatitis. Release of an inhibitor of the "clearing factor," lipoprotein lipase, by the diseased pancreas is the most likely cause of the hyperlipemia. This secondary type of hyperlipemia is to be distinguished from an idiopathic form in which the pancreatitis is probably caused by the hyperlipemia. In the idiopathic form, the neutral fats usually increase immediately before the onset of abdominal symptoms and return to normal when the attack is over. Klatskin and Gordon have suggested that the pancreatitis may be caused by fat emboli. The differentiation between the primary and secondary types of hyperlipemia is extremely important, because the attacks of pancreatitis may be prevented by a low-fat diet in the primary group. Dietary-induced hypertriglyceridemia can also cause attacks of acute pancreatitis in alcoholic patients.

Hemochromatosis has been thought to produce pancreatic fibrosis and atrophy because of the irritating properties of the deposited iron. However, iron absorption often increases after pancreatic damage caused by several diseases, and siderosis may in fact be secondary to the pancreatic disease.

Vascular, Toxic, Allergic, and Other Factors. Vascular stasis is an important factor in experimental pancreatitis. The process may be diffuse, probably at the arteriolar level, since ligation of major vessels to the pancreas alone causes only small infarcts. Occasionally, older patients who have widespread vascular obstruction and patients who have undergone cardiopulmonary bypass are seen with severe hemorrhagic pancreatitis. The role of vascular spasm and obstruction in other forms of pancreatitis is not clear.

Various toxins, such as methyl alcohol, zinc oxide, choline esterase inhibitors, cobaltous chloride, and chlorothiazide, have been known to produce pancreatic injury. Although Thal and others have implicated autoimmune mechanisms in the pathogenesis of pancreatitis, there is little evidence to suggest that these are of any particular importance in human pancreatitis.

Despite frequent reports of pancreatitis during mumps, no fatalities or complications have been recorded. The serum amylase may increase in patients with mumps, but whether this results from the parotitis or pancreatitis is unknown. The coxsackie virus has recently been shown to cause pancreatitis.

CLINICAL MANIFESTATIONS. Acute pancreatitis is sometimes divided into the acute edematous type and a hemorrhagic or necrotic form. This is a purely arbitrary distinction by the clinician that can be made only at operation or autopsy.

Attacks of acute pancreatitis often occur after a heavy meal or an episode of acute alcoholism. The pain usually begins suddenly but may start gradually. The pain is frequently located in the midepigastrium and often radiates to the back. The patient's discomfort is in many instances improved by sitting and aggravated by lying. The character of the pain is extremely variable, ranging from steady, knifelike distress to an agonizing intermittent cramping pain. Pain in the left or right upper quadrants is not uncommon and is caused by particularly severe involvement of the tail or the head of the gland.

Persistent and repeated vomiting without nausea but often to the point of extreme retching is common. The character of the vomitus is unremarkable, and the vomiting occurs with an empty stomach. Physical examination usually shows upper abdominal tenderness and guarding, sometimes far greater than what might be expected for the amount of pain the patient seems to have. About 90 percent of patients with proved pancreatitis have fever, tachycardia, and leukocytosis. Shock may be present, depending upon the amount of fluid and blood lost in the retroperitoneal area and peritoneal cavity, as well as the volume deficit incurred by persistent vomiting. Dissection of irritating exudate from the pancreas into the lower quadrants of the abdomen or even into the chest may produce signs and symptoms in these areas, as well as even greater volume deficits because of the local outpouring of fluid in response to the exudate. Adynamic ileus with intraluminal sequestration of fluid also contributes to extracellular fluid deficit. Lefer, with Wangensteen and others, has demonstrated a myocardial depressant factor (MDF) released from the pancreas during pancreatitis that may also contribute to the shock. Acute renal insufficiency often occurs in these patients. Mild jaundice occurs in 20 to 30 percent of the patients. This is partly due to swelling of the head of the pancreas and perhaps also to hemolysis of red blood cells, which become more fragile in acute pancreatitis. Carpopedal spasm may occur if true hypocalcemia develops. It has been proposed recently that a substantial degree of hypocalcemia may be caused by the hypoalbuminemia found in patients with acute pancreatitis. Other factors that may contribute to the development of hypocalcemia include end-organ unresponsiveness to parathormone and stimulation of thyrocalcitonin secretion. The latter process has been shown in experimental animals to follow administration of glucagon, and hyperglucagonemia is known to occur during pancreatitis.

LABORATORY STUDIES. Acute pancreatitis is largely diagnosed by clinical history and findings rather than by laboratory studies. Disastrous outcomes have occurred when elevated serum amylase values have led the physician or surgeon immediately to eliminate from consideration any diagnosis but acute pancreatitis. Not only is simple elevation of the serum amylase level an inadequate diagnostic test of acute pancreatitis, but there is also ample evidence that serum amylase values of over 1000 units are frequently caused by conditions other than acute pancreatitis. Blood drawn during the course of proved pancreatitis, when the amylase might be expected to be elevated, has indicated that approximately one-third of the patients had values of less than 200 Somogyi units, one-third had levels between 200 and 500 units, and one-third had more than 500 units.

Apart from acute pancreatitis, the most frequent causes of marked elevations of the serum amylase level are acute cholecystitis, common duct stone with or without cholangitis, perforated peptic ulcer, and strangulating obstruction of the small intestine. Other conditions in which the serum amylase level is elevated include acute alcoholism without pancreatitis, afferent loop obstruction after gastrectomy, ectopic pregnancy, perforated duodenal diverticulum, renal failure, carcinoma of the pancreas, and mumps. Although frequently claimed to have more diagnostic value than the serum amylase test, serum lipase not only is a difficult determination to perform but also has proved to be disappointingly inaccurate.

Estimation of the total amount of amylase in a 2-h urine sample is more accurate than is the simple measurement of the concentration of the enzyme in the urine, blood, or the serum lipase. The number of positive diagnoses of pancreatitis is doubled when the amylase output in the urine exceeds 300 units in 1 h. It has been suggested that the renal clearance of amylase in acute pancreatitis is much greater, relative to the creatinine clearance, than in any other condition and that a ratio of amylase/creatinine clearance of >5 is virtually diagnostic. Exceptions to this have been found in burned patients and in diabetic ketoacidosis, and the test has been largely discarded because it has proved to be no more accurate than the serum or urinary amylase. Elevated amylase values in pleural fluid are diagnostic of pancreatitis. Abdominal paracentesis may provide useful information, but increased amylase in abdominal fluid has been reported in other conditions as well. Estimations of trypsin levels in the blood and the separation of various organ-specific isoenzymes of the blood, especially those of amylase, seem to be encouraging but are not yet sufficiently well evaluated to warrant widespread use.

Serum calcium values of less than 7.5 mg/dL generally indicate a poor prognosis and reflect the extensiveness of the disease process. Transient hyperglycemia and glycosuria have formerly been attributed to inadequate production of insulin by the injured pancreas, but recent work has shown that injection of amylase into the bloodstream converts glycogen to glucose in the liver, and that glucagon is released during the course of pancreatitis.

Radiologic examinations have only occasional value. The so-called "sentinel loop" of distended jejunum in the left upper quadrant is extremely nonspecific. Oral cholecystography or nuclear (HIDA) scans during, or immediately following, an episode of acute pancreatitis usually show visualization of the gallbladder, but failure of the gallbladder to visualize occurs in as many as 20 or 30 percent of cases of acute pancreatitis, even when it is completely normal. CT scans early in the course of the disease may show an enlarged pancreas, occasionally with surrounding edema.

The diagnosis of acute pancreatitis is usually made

from clinical findings, although intelligent use of serum and urinary amylase tests and the HIDA scan may provide useful if not clearly diagnostic information. Frequent clinical reassessment of the patient is of the utmost importance. On occasion, laparotomy may be necessary in a carefully prepared patient as a purely diagnostic maneuver in order to avoid missing a strangulating obstruction of the small intestine or another potentially lethal but curable condition.

TREATMENT. Meticulous replacement of losses of colloid, fluid, and electrolytes, and adequate maintenance therapy are of the utmost importance. Constant attention to the urinary output, alterations in the hematocrit, blood volume, and central venous pressure, and estimation of the occult losses into the peritoneum and retroperitoneal area are mandatory. Blood transfusion may be required in hemorrhagic pancreatitis. Small doses of insulin may be necessary if hyperglycemia is marked and diabetic acidosis is imminent. Calcium gluconate should be given intravenously if the serum calcium level is depressed.

In addition to proper metabolic management, continuous aspiration of the stomach and withholding ingestion of food or fluids often relieves discomfort immediately. These maneuvers are designed to put the pancreas to rest by diminishing the acid-secretin mechanism of pancreatic stimulation, by eliminating gastric distention, which in turn invokes the gastropancreatic reflex and the production of antral gastrin, and by preventing the flow of pancreatic juice stimulated by foodstuffs in the duodenum. Adynamic ileus is also favorably affected by intubation. Such therapy is continued until the patient no longer has pain and tenderness. In spite of its apparent rationale, randomized trials suggest that nasogastric drainage does not affect the course of alcoholic pancreatitis. Other treatment modalities such as the administration of glucagon, atropine, and the trypsin inhibitor Trasylol have also been noted not to alter the outcome of acute pancreatitis.

Although many authorities advocate the routine administration of antibiotics to patients with acute pancreatitis, randomized trials have indicated that antibiotic administration does not alter the incidence of septic complications of pancreatitis. In spite of this, we use these agents in the occasional severe fulminating case, since these patients are the ones in whom secondary abscesses are most likely to develop. There is no evidence to support the belief that infection is an important contributing factor in the development of pancreatitis or that antibiotics can actually prevent the development of an abscess.

Meperidine is usually used to relieve pain, because it has less effect on the sphincter of Oddi than morphine and other opiates, although it does not relax the muscle as was formerly believed.

Recent reports have indicated that removal of common duct stones by either choledochotomy or endoscopic papillotomy reduces the severity and mortality of gallstone pancreatitis. The optimal timing of such procedures has not yet been established. Surgical intervention may also be indicated in certain patients who fail to respond to supportive measures. Total or near-total pancreatectomy for severe hemorrhagic pancreatitis has been proposed,

but this operation is associated with an extremely high mortality rate and its value in the treatment of acute pancreatitis has not been established. A recently reported prospective randomized trial has indicated that peritoneal lavage provides no treatment benefit in this disease.

COMPLICATIONS, MORBIDITY, AND MORTALITY. Pseudocyst is the most common complication of acute pancreatitis. Abscesses are rare but mortality is high, approaching 100 percent if clostridial organisms are the cause of the infection. Pseudocysts rarely appear before the second week of the disease and abscesses not usually before the third week. Obstruction of the common bile duct and duodenum is not common in the acute cases. The remaining complications of acute pancreatitis may be grouped together, since they are caused by the necrotizing effects of the process itself. These include rupture or thrombosis of the splenic, mesenteric, or portal vessels, necrosis and perforation of the common bile duct or colon, and perforation of the stomach and duodenum.

Just as important as the early complications of acute pancreatitis and perhaps even more so is the insidious development of sequelae of repeated attacks. Pancreatic calcification, secondary diabetes, and steatorrhea are far more common in alcoholic pancreatitis than in gallstone pancreatitis, in which these phenomena are almost nonexistent. Pseudocysts too are less frequently encountered in the course of gallstone pancreatitis.

The overall mortality rate from acute pancreatitis in the past 10 years has been 10 to 15 percent. Twenty-five years ago most patients died during the first week of the disease, but now the vast majority do not succumb for several weeks after the onset, probably because of better early metabolic management. The mortality rate of alcoholic pancreatitis is approximately three times that of gallstone pancreatitis in most series, but reverse incidences have been recorded in a few reports. It is virtually impossible to determine the true mortality rate of hemorrhagic pancreatitis, since a clinical diagnosis may be impossible without operative or postmortem observation. Operation is generally regarded as detrimental to the outcome of the disease unless specific indications, as outlined above, are present. Paradoxically, operation has not increased the mortality rates in most reports. Secondary hemorrhage from major vessels, fulminating uncontrollable shock without hemorrhage, and infection are the most common causes of death.

Ranson and coworkers, as well as a number of other groups, have retrospectively analyzed large numbers of cases of acute pancreatitis to determine early signs that might identify those patients with severe attacks and those most likely to develop complications or to die from their attack. Ranson's early signs of severity are listed in Table 32-2. Similar criteria have been proposed by others. The mortality rate for those with less than three signs of severe pancreatitis is approximately 1 percent, while for those with three or more signs it is 33 percent. Early recognition of the severity of an attack may allow for a more rational approach to therapy, including the need for admission to an intensive care unit.

One of the most dread complications of acute pancrea-

Table 32-2. SIGNS USED TO CLASSIFY SEVERITY OF ACUTE PANCREATITIS

At admission	
1. Age > 55	4. LDH > 350 I.U./L
2. WBC > 16,000/mm³	5. SGOT > 250 Frankel
3. Glucose > 200 mg/dL	units %
During initial 48 h	
1. Hematocrit fall > 10%	4. Arterial P_{O_2} < 60 mmHg
2. BUN rise > 5% per mg/dL	5. Base deficit > 4 meq/L
3. Ca⁺⁺ < 8 mg/dL	6. Fluid sequestration > 6 L

titis is "pancreatic abscess," a misnomer because the process is not usually pancreatic nor is there a true abscess. Except in instances of infected pseudocysts (see below), there is usually no single collection of purulent material. Rather, the process is characterized by extensive necrosis of retroperitoneal fat, mesentery, and mesocolon while the pancreas remains intact, albeit swollen and inflamed. It is likely that infection is secondary and of intestinal origin because the most common organisms are coliforms, *Streptococcus faecalis,* and clostridia, but the mechanism by which the organisms gain access to the necrotic retroperitoneal material is unclear. Infection is most frequently encountered 2 to 3 weeks after an attack of acute pancreatitis, but earlier instances are not rare. An episode of severe pancreatitis usually precedes a pancreatic abscess. The latter should be suspected in such patients who continue to be ill with fever, leukocytosis, abdominal pain, and adynamic ileus. The diagnosis can be established with certainty only if gas can be detected by plain film or CT scan in the retroperitoneum, or if bacteria are grown from blood cultures. The mortality rate of unoperated pancreatic abscess is 100 percent. Early and wide debridement, often requiring multiple operations, is the only known successful treatment, but even under optimal circumstances the best reported results have still reached survivals of only about 75 percent. Simple drainage without debridement is usually inadequate because it does not eliminate the necrotic foci of tissue. It is not clear whether early debridement of the *uninfected* retroperitoneal phlegmon will prevent the development of abscess with its high attendant mortality.

Chronic Pancreatitis

This diagnosis usually refers to a clinical entity rather than a specific pathologic process. This is especially true during its early stages, when repeated attacks of acute pancreatitis of varying severity are likely to occur, whatever the precipitating factor. As the disease progresses, however, the edges of the pancreas become rounded, and the organ becomes smaller, indurated, and nodular. Histologically, lobules of functional acinar and islet tissue are surrounded by thick bands of fibrous tissue. Alternating areas of stricture and dilatation of the main ductal system may occur late in the disease. In the very last stages calcification occurs. It is almost always intraductal and rarely interstitial. Calcification is usually superimposed upon

precipitates of protein that have been found in increased quantities in the juice of patients with chronic pancreatites. These severe changes are confined largely to patients with alcoholic pancreatitis and are extremely rare in gallstone pancreatitis. Calcification and ductal distortion have also been seen in familial or hereditary pancreatitis. Occasionally in chronic alcoholic pancreatitis, progressive fibrosis of the gland without ductal dilatation or calcification seems to be the primary pathologic process.

CLINICAL MANIFESTATIONS. Typical patients with chronic pancreatitis are in their late thirties or early forties and have a long history of alcoholism and repeated attacks of acute pancreatitis, often with delirium tremens. After approximately 10 years, the pain changes from intermittent to persistent and continuous. It is located in the epigastrium but radiates to the back and is often partially relieved if the patient sits in a hunched position. Anorexia and weight loss are common, and nausea and vomiting occur if an exacerbation has been precipitated by an acute bout of alcoholism. Diabetes and steatorrhea with foul-smelling, bulky, greasy stools are common. At this stage, addiction to narcotics as well as alcohol is extremely common. Pseudocysts are frequently found in these patients.

This picture is in sharp contrast to the patient who has recurrent pancreatitis in association with biliary tract disease. Such persons generally have episodic bouts of acute pancreatitis, sometimes in association with attacks of acute cholecystitis or cholangitis caused by common duct calculi. Severe pancreatic fibrosis and insufficiency almost never occur in association solely with biliary tract disease. Recurrent attacks of acute pancreatitis may also occur in patients who have severe ductal stenosis resulting from major trauma to the pancreas. Occasionally the picture of familial pancreatitis may be similar to that seen in alcoholic chronic pancreatitis, but these cases are rare, and at times severe damage to the pancreas and calcification may be present without any symptoms at all and in the absence of a known cause.

LABORATORY STUDIES. Many psychoneurotic patients with abdominal pains are labeled as having chronic pancreatitis without adequate substantiation for such a serious diagnosis. Documentation is difficult, but in these instances thorough radiologic examinations of the biliary tree and upper gastrointestinal tract are mandatory. The advent of endoscopic retrograde cannulation of the pancreatic duct has proved of great value in these cases, since abnormalities of the ductal system are readily detected. Determination of serum or urinary amylase or serum lipase may not be fruitful, especially if the pancreas has been seriously damaged. The presence of calcification in the pancreas virtually establishes the diagnosis.

TREATMENT. The wide variety of operative procedures devised for chronic pancreatitis are a reflection of the generally unsatisfactory results of treatment. However, some confusion has been created by our own inability, or refusal, to differentiate clearly among the various types of chronic pancreatitis.

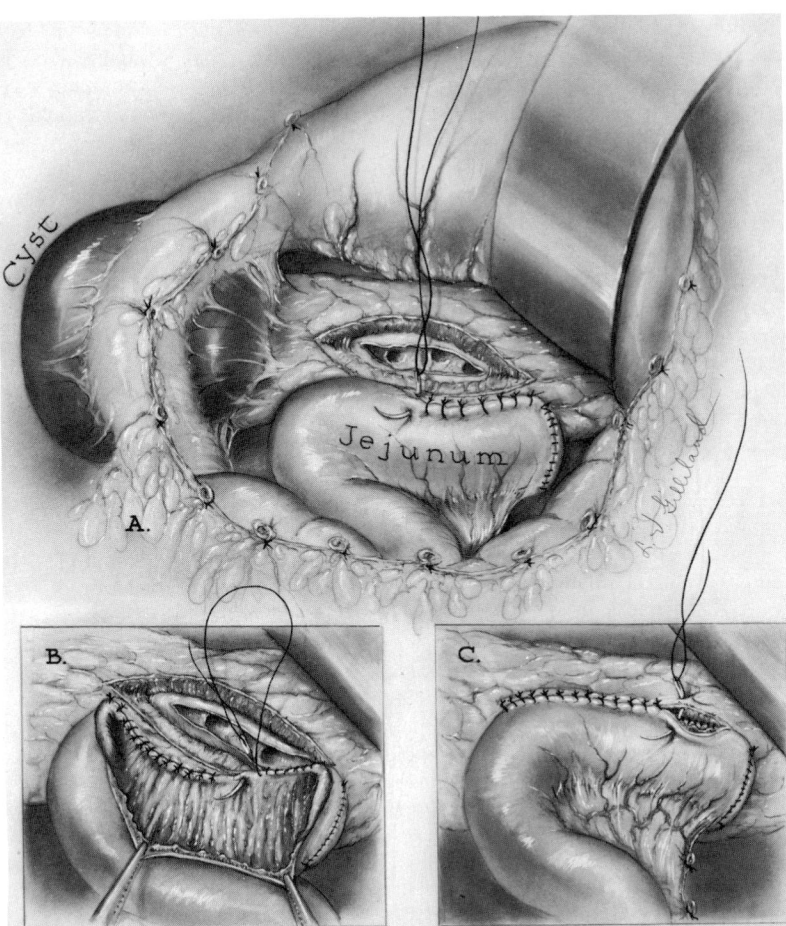

Fig. 32-4. Side-to-side pancreaticojejunostomy with preservation of the tail of the pancreas and spleen. An exploring needle is used to locate the dilated pancreatic duct, which is then incised. The end of the defunctionalized jejunum is closed and brought up for anastomosis with the opened pancreas in side-to-side fashion. *A*. The posterior row of sutures is placed first. *B*. The jejunum is then opened, and an inner layer of continuous sutures is placed, uniting jejunal mucosa and pancreatic duct *C*. An anterior row of interrupted sutures completes the anastomosis. A Roux en Y is then constructed to complete intestinal continuity. (From: *Silen W, Baldwin J, Goldman L: Am J Surg 106:243, 1963, with permission.*)

It is evident that definitive and corrective biliary tract operations are almost always curative in gallstone pancreatitis. Whether this implies simple cholecystectomy or common duct exploration, with or without sphincteroplasty, is dictated by the local and cholangiographic findings at operation. Sporadic initial success with biliary operations led to their widespread, indiscriminate use without due regard for the precipitating cause of the pancreatitis. Large numbers of patients with alcoholic pancreatitis were subjected to cholecystectomy and a variety of other biliary tract procedures, only to find that relief was not obtained. Even when biliary calculi are present in the alcoholic patient, correction of the biliary tract disease will not alter the course of the pancreatic disease, especially if the ingestion of alcohol is continued.

In the case of chronic alcoholic pancreatitis, the only logical and effective therapy is complete abstinence from alcohol before the stage of fibrosis, calcification, steatorrhea, and diabetes is reached, but rarely can this be achieved. Once the severe complications of chronic pancreatitis have developed, consideration should be given to pancreaticojejunostomy, originally advocated by Puestow and Gillesby. Operation is indicated *only* for persistent and unrelenting pain. This procedure is based on the fact that multiple areas of stricture within the pancreatic ductal system often occur in patients with severe chronic pancreatitis, so that simple retrograde drainage of the pancreas via its tail, as originally proposed by DuVal, does not adequately decompress the pancreatic ducts. The limb of jejunum may be anastomosed, side to side, to the pancreas after wide incision of almost the entire pancreatic duct but without removal of the spleen or mobilization of the pancreas (Fig. 32-4). This procedure can be carried out rather simply, with an extremely low mortality and little morbidity. It can be expected that about 75 to 80 percent of patients will have complete relief. The relief of pain is dramatic, particularly if the duct is dilated at operation. The most accurate preoperative indication of a dilated duct is the presence of calcification or the demonstration of dilatation by endoscopic retrograde cholangiopancreatography (ERCP).

Lateral pancreaticojejunostomy also provides for the return of pancreatic juice to the intestine. In addition, the adequacy of ductal exploration, removal of calculi, and drainage is far greater than that which can be accomplished through a transduodenal sphincterotomy, advocated by some. If the pancreatic duct is small, without evidence of stricture, yet severe chronic pancreatitis is present and is causing unremitting pain, the results of operation are less satisfactory than when a dilated duct is present. The choice lies between 95 percent distal pancreatectomy and a new procedure that removes most of the head of the pancreas and totally denervates the remaining tail and body. Experience with the latter procedure is too limited to allow assessment of its efficacy. The 95 percent pancreatectomy is associated with a high incidence of diabetes and exocrine pancreatic insufficiency, both of which may be excessively morbid in the nonresponsible alcoholic patient. Relief of pain occurs in the majority of patients, but the quality of life is poor because of the associated brittle diabetes, pancreatic insufficiency, and on-going alcohol ingestion.

Sphincterotomy, ligation of the pancreatic ducts, and lumbodorsal sympathectomy and splanchnicectomy have all failed to provide lasting relief in patients with chronic pancreatitis. On occasion, the Whipple pancreaticoduoenal resection may be indicated if stricture of the common bile duct or stenosis of the duodenum is the result of chronic pancreatitis localized to the head of the pancreas.

TRAUMA

MECHANISMS OF INJURY. Penetrating trauma, caused by gunshot or stab wounds, is more common than blunt injury to the pancreas and constitutes from 70 to 80 percent of pancreatic injuries, even in civilian practice. Penetrating injuries, especially knife wounds, usually cause less destruction and disruption of the organ than does blunt trauma. In gunshot wounds an area of contusion usually surrounds the track of the missile. Injury to adjacent structures is exceedingly common (70 to 90 percent). The stomach, liver, small intestine, spleen, colon, kidney, and duodenum are the most frequently wounded. These organs are usually the source of the most significant hemorrhage.

The immobility of the pancreas accounts for its vulnerability to blunt trauma, which may fracture it posteriorly across the rigid vertebral column. Usually the disruption occurs at the neck of the pancreas overlying the mesenteric vessels, although occasionally the gland may become completely separated from the duodenum. Associated injury to other organs is not as frequent as in penetrating trauma.

Although frequently referred to as "traumatic pancreatitis," the consequences of these injuries, such as fistula, pseudocyst, or death, are usually the result of disruption of the organ itself or its ductal system rather than pancreatitis per se. Crushing injury to the pancreas in itself does not seem to produce extensive inflammation in the remainder of the gland, but may be followed by fistula or pseudocyst, e.g., following splenectomy in which hemostats applied to the splenic vessels may injure the distal duct of Wirsung.

CLINICAL MANIFESTATIONS. It is significant that the interval between injury and surgical exploration is considerably longer after blunt trauma to the pancreas, often consisting of many days. Adequate awareness of the possibility of this type of injury may shorten delay and reduce morbidity and mortality. Abdominal pain and findings on examination may be surprisingly minimal, which partly explains the frequent procrastination in undertaking laparotomy. Clinical and laboratory evidence of continuing hemorrhage makes the decision of operation an easy one. Continued abdominal pain, tenderness, fever, and ileus should immediately arouse suspicion of pancreatic injury. Standard radiologic examinations, with or without contrast media, are rarely helpful, but CT scans sometimes show the lesion. Paracentesis may provide a clear-cut indication for operation if the fluid is positive for blood or is rich in amylase, but a negative result should not deter the surgeon from exploration. Although frequently forgotten in cases of blunt trauma, serum amylase determination and amylase/creatinine clearance ratio may be of great help. These are elevated in over 80 percent of the patients with pancreatic injuries in whom they are measured. Unfortunately, hyperamylasemia is common in trauma patients who do not have pancreatic injury and, therefore, the specificity of serum amylase measurement is low. Possibly of greater surgical importance is the fact that persistent elevations of the serum amylase usually mean inadequate drainage of the injured pancreas.

TREATMENT. The high incidence of complications and the excessive mortality suggest that the treatment leaves much to be desired. It is generally agreed that early operation is necessary in both penetrating wounds and in blunt injury.

Proper evaluation of the extent of the pancreatic injury is the key to adequate surgical therapy. It is impossible to explore the pancreas without widely exposing it by division of the gastrocolic omentum, as far as is necessary to provide adequate assessment of the major portion of the gland (Fig. 32-5). Care must be taken to protect the middle colic vessels during the procedure. If the injury is in the region of the head of the pancreas, the duodenum must be mobilized by the method of Kocher (Fig. 32-6) so that the full extent of the damage can be ascertained and the duodenum, common bile duct, and adjacent structures can be examined. If a hematoma is found over the pancreas, it should not be treated by drainage alone but must be examined carefully, since it may hide major vascular or ductal injury. Vascular instruments should always be readily available in the operating room when operations of this type are being performed.

During exploration of the hematoma, attention should be first directed toward hemostasis. Blind clamping in the depths of the pancreas or deep, carelessly placed sutures may injure the pancreatic ductal system, leading to pancreatitis or fistula. Damaged tissue should be thoroughly debrided; carefully placed nonabsorbable suture ligatures

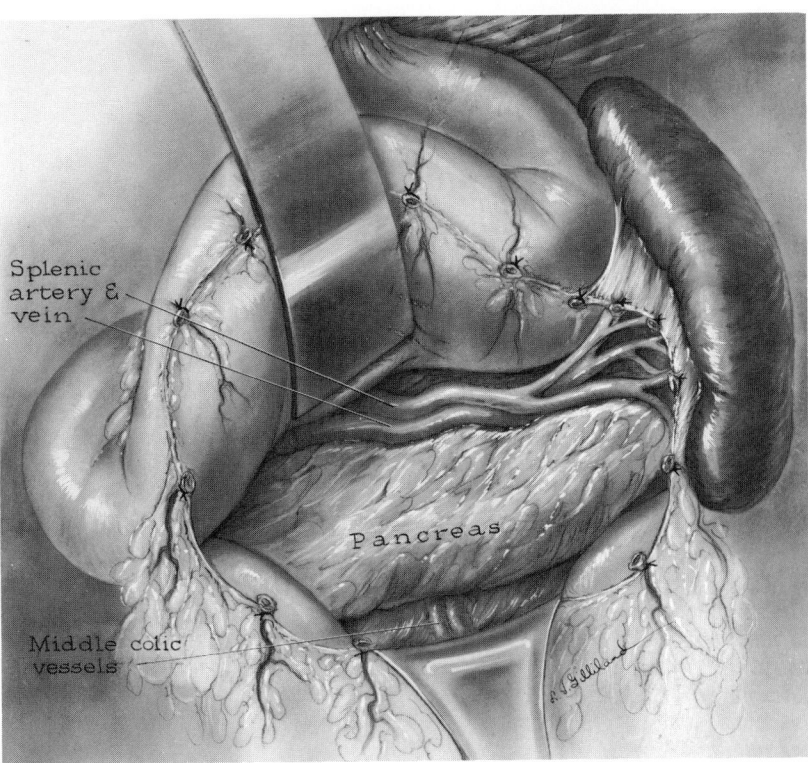

Fig. 32-5. Wide exposure of the pancreas obtained by the gastro-colic omental route. The middle colic vessels must be located and preserved. (From: *Silen W: Surg Clin North Am 44:1253, 1964, with permission.*)

Fig. 32-6. Operative exposure of the head of the pancreas after the Kocher maneuver. Note that portal or superior mesenteric veins are covered posteriorly by the uncinate process, preventing direct vision of these structures inferiorly. (From: *Silen W: Surg Clin North Am 44:1253, 1964, with permission.*)

permit adequate hemostasis. If the ductal system is uninjured, these procedures, together with adequate drainage, may be sufficient to treat small penetrating injuries.

A much more aggressive approach is probably necessary when the pancreas is badly lacerated. Should the severely injured area involve only the tail or distal body

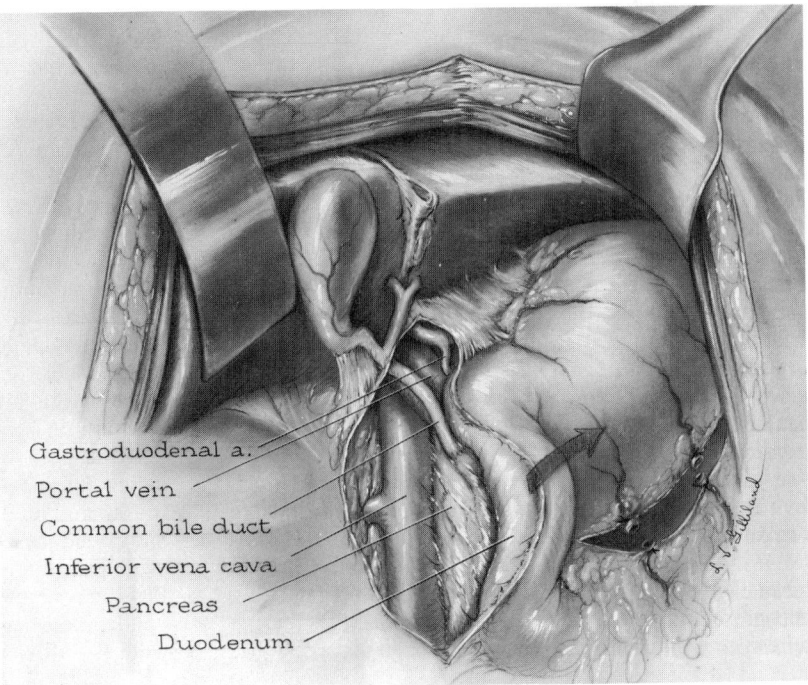

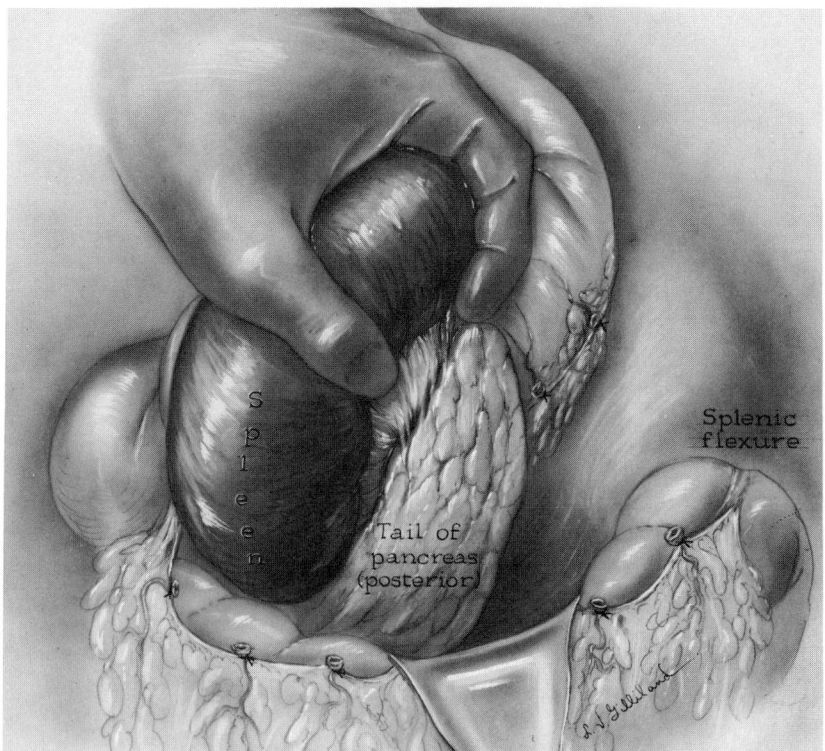

Fig. 32-7. Mobilization of tail and body of pancreas with spleen. (From: *Silen W: Surg Clin North Am 44:1253, 1964, with permission.*)

of the pancreas, the simplest procedure is resection. Mobilization of the spleen and distal pancreas is easily carried out (Fig. 32-7). Since the gastrocolic omentum has already been opened, only a few vasa brevia remain to be ligated and divided; the distal pancreas and spleen can easily be delivered into the wound after division of the lienorenal and splenocolic ligaments and the thin posterosuperior and posteroinferior peritoneal attachments of the pancreas. After the splenic artery and vein are ligated and divided, the injured pancreas may be removed. The distal end of the pancreas remaining in situ should be carefully inspected for adequate hemostasis. If possible, the duct of Wirsung should be ligated with nonabsorbable sutures, and the area is then drained.

If the pancreas is transected near its neck or even farther to the right, preservation of pancreatic tissue may be important. The lacerated proximal segment is managed as outlined above. The distal transected portion of the organ can be anastomosed end to end with a Roux en Y limb of jejunum. Generally, the limb of jejunum is placed in a retrocolic position. The transected proximal pancreas can also be implanted into the same limb of jejunum used for the distal end, but this is unduly complicated and probably is not necessary.

Although these procedures might appear too involved to be used in seriously injured patients, less adequate therapy results in a high incidence of severe complications and death. Furthermore, ductal obstruction and the late development of chronic pancreatitis in inadequately recognized and treated injuries support an aggressive approach to such lesions. Thal and Wilson proposed that

pancreaticoduodenal resection be carried out for severe lesions of the head of the pancreas. Berne advocates distal Billroth II gastrectomy with careful local repair of the badly injured duodenum and pancreas, coupled with adequate drainage, for injuries of this area. The choice between this procedure and the Whipple operation is determined by the extent of the injury. Should the pancreas be sheared away from the duodenum, disrupting pancreatic and biliary ductal continuity, careful reanastomosis to the duodenum may be carried out if the blood supply to the pancreas and duodenum has not been disrupted. The importance of recognizing major ductal injury in any case of pancreatic injury cannot be overemphasized. Cannulation of the pancreatic duct can sometimes be facilitated by intubation through a transduodenal sphincterotomy, as suggested by Doubilet and Mulholland. Although drainage of the ductal system can undoubtedly be achieved in this manner, definitive therapy by splinting of the duct alone by this method will not prevent subsequent ductal stricture and pancreatitis.

MORBIDITY AND MORTALITY. The most serious complications of pancreatic injury are fistulization, pseudocyst formation, infection, and delayed hemorrhage. Fistula and pseudocyst are the result of disruption of a duct of significant size. Doubilet and Mulholland have suggested that the resistance to the flow of pancreatic juice into the duodenum by the duodenal musculature and sphincter of Oddi is sufficiently great so that in cases of injury the juice will preferentially flow into the retroperitoneal area. The incidence of complications in most series averages 30 percent. Pancreatic complications seem to occur much more frequently after blunt trauma than in penetrating injuries.

The overall mortality rate in recent years, like the complication rate, has averaged 20 percent. Usually the death rate after penetrating injuries is higher than that after blunt trauma, probably because adjacent organs are often injured. The most frequent causes of death are shock, renal failure, and sepsis.

CYSTS AND PSEUDOCYSTS

True cysts of the pancreas are filled with fluid and have an epithelial lining. These cysts are to be distinguished from the much more common *pseudocysts,* which have fibrous lining rather than epithelium.

True Cysts

A simple classification of true cysts of the pancreas is presented in Table 32-3.

Congenital cysts of the pancreas are extremely rare, and *parasitic cysts* of the pancreas have not been reported in the United States. *Retention cysts* are cystic dilatations of the pancreatic ducts and are almost always caused by pancreatitis. Although not as rare as the congenital cysts, *neoplastic cysts* of the pancreas are relatively uncommon. Cystadenoma and cystadenocarcinoma are discussed below.

Pseudocysts

More than three-quarters of all cystic lesions of the pancreas are pseudocysts. The fibrous wall of a pseudocyst surrounds a collection of pancreatic juice (with or without blood clot) and necrotic or suppurative pancreatic tissue. Most pseudocysts are unilocular and are located in the lesser sac. However, they occasionally occur within the pancreas (retention cysts), transverse mesocolon, or omentum and even more rarely may be found behind the pancreas or within the mediastinum. Since a pseudocyst usually results from disruption of the ductal system of the pancreas, the ultimate form and location of the lesion are dependent upon the position and the extent of pancreatic injury and the secretory pressure of the pancreas distal to the point of ductal damage. The fluid within a pseudocyst varies from clear and colorless to a brown or green murky material, depending upon the amount of blood or necrotic pancreas present.

Pancreatitis and trauma are the most important causes of pseudocysts, accounting for about 75 and 25 percent of cases, respectively. Neoplasm and parasites are extremely rare causes, and occasionally pseudocysts develop without any demonstrable cause whatever. In patients with pseudocysts caused by pancreatitis, alcoholism is more common than cholelithiasis. For this reason, pseudocysts appear most frequently in the fourth and fifth decades of life and are more common in men.

Table 32-3. CLASSIFICATION OF TRUE CYSTS OF THE PANCREAS

A. Congenital
  1. Single cyst
  2. Multiple (polycystic disease)
  3. Dermoid cyst
  4. Fibrocystic disease
B. Acquired
  1. Retention cysts
  2. Parasitic cysts
  3. Neoplastic cysts
     a. Benign cystadenoma
     b. Cystadenocarcinoma

CLINICAL MANIFESTATIONS. The usual clinical findings in patients with pseudocysts are persistent pain, fever, and ileus, appearing 2 to 3 weeks after an attack of pancreatitis or trauma to the pancreas. Although a pseudocyst may develop after one attack of pancreatitis, the patient often has had several previous attacks. Pain, in the epigastrium or the left upper quadrant with occasional radiation to the back, is the most common symptom. A mass, nausea, vomiting, and anorexia occur in approximately 20 percent of the patients. Rarely, gastrointestinal hemorrhage from gastroesophageal varices occurs if the portal venous system is compressed by the pseudocyst. Narrowing of the common bile duct may cause jaundice.

A mass is found on physical examination in about 75 percent of patients and is usually nontender or only slightly tender. The amount of movement of the mass is variable, depending upon the degree of surrounding inflammatory reaction and fixation to adjacent structures. The mass often changes in size, probably because of partial drainage into the ductal system of the pancreas. The complete and prolonged disappearance of the mass in some patients may be explained by the fact that these masses develop after attacks of acute pancreatitis and may represent small fluid collections, matted omentum, and enlarged pancreas, all of which resolve after the acute attack has subsided. Occasionally the mass may be confused with an aortic aneurysm because of the pulsations transmitted by the aorta immediately posterior to the pancreas. Patients may present with pleural effusion as the sole finding, undoubtedly caused by transdiaphragmatic drainage of pancreatic lymph. Pleural or pulmonary manifestations are common.

The diagnosis of pseudocyst is not particularly difficult. In addition to persistent pain, fever, and ileus during or after an attack of pancreatitis, continued elevation of the serum amylase level should suggest the development of a pseudocyst. The most helpful radiologic examination is the CT scan, which usually shows a mass adjacent to the pancreas displacing the stomach anteriorly and superiorly. Occasionally the lesser curvature of the stomach may be flattened by a high-lying pseudocyst (Figs. 32-8 and 32-9). Ultrasonography is of value in detecting a pseudocyst, especially as a preliminary to the CT scan. Endoscopic retrograde cannulation of the pancreatic duct may show either obstruction of the duct of Wirsung or

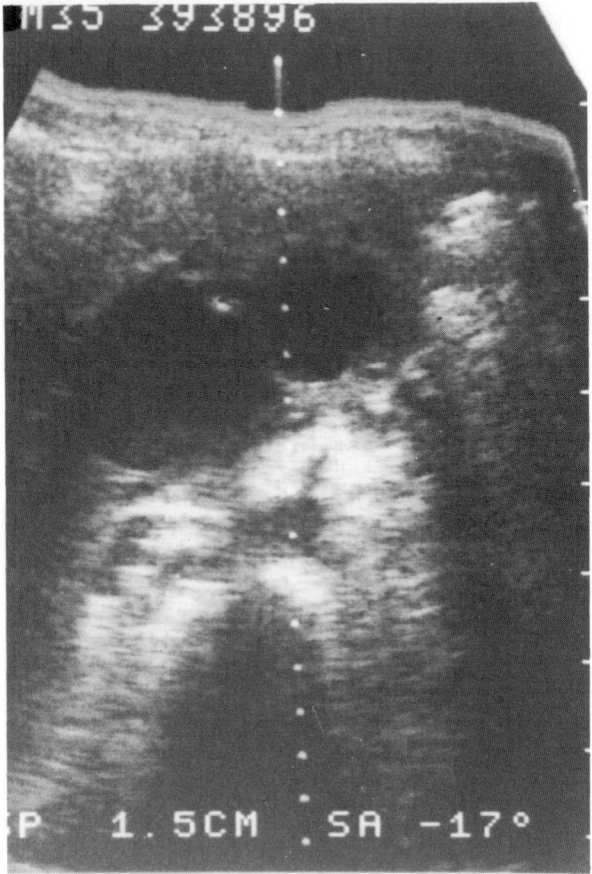

Fig. 32-8. Ultrasound examination of patient with chronic pancreatitis. Note two large pseudocysts that happen to communicate with each other.

extravasation of dye into the pseudocyst but is not usually necessary.

Secondary infection of a pseudocyst is detected by accentuation of fever and toxicity, usually at least 3 weeks after the onset of an attack of acute pancreatitis. The presence of gas bubbles on a plain film of the abdomen or CT scan and bacterial growth in the bloodstream may help establish the diagnosis. The clinician should also be alert to the syndrome of pancreatic ascites, which is caused by leakage of pancreatic juice from a pseudocyst or actual pancreatic ductal disruption. The demonstration of high amylase content of ascitic fluid that also has the characteristics of an exudate serves to differentiate this condition from ascites of hepatic origin.

TREATMENT. Surgical treatment is recommended for pseudocyst of the pancreas for two reasons: first, complications such as secondary infection, severe hemorrhage, or rupture into an adjacent viscus or into the free peritoneal cavity may occur if a pseudocyst remains untreated; second, these lesions rarely resolve once a thick fibrous wall has developed. A patient who develops a mass during an attack of acute pancreatitis and whose condition remains satisfactory should be observed for several weeks. Should the mass enlarge or the patient become more ill during this period, immediate operation is indicated. If physical and radiologic examination show complete disappearance of the mass, operation may be postponed indefinitely, but pseudocysts that persist for 4 to 6 weeks are unlikely to resolve spontaneously and should be treated aggressively. True intrapancreatic pseudocysts often vary greatly in size and frequently disappear completely only to reappear at a later date.

No single operative procedure is appropriate for every pseudocyst of the pancreas. Simple external drainage or

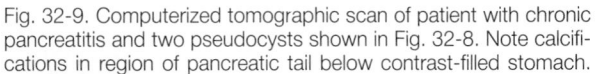

Fig. 32-9. Computerized tomographic scan of patient with chronic pancreatitis and two pseudocysts shown in Fig. 32-8. Note calcifications in region of pancreatic tail below contrast-filled stomach.

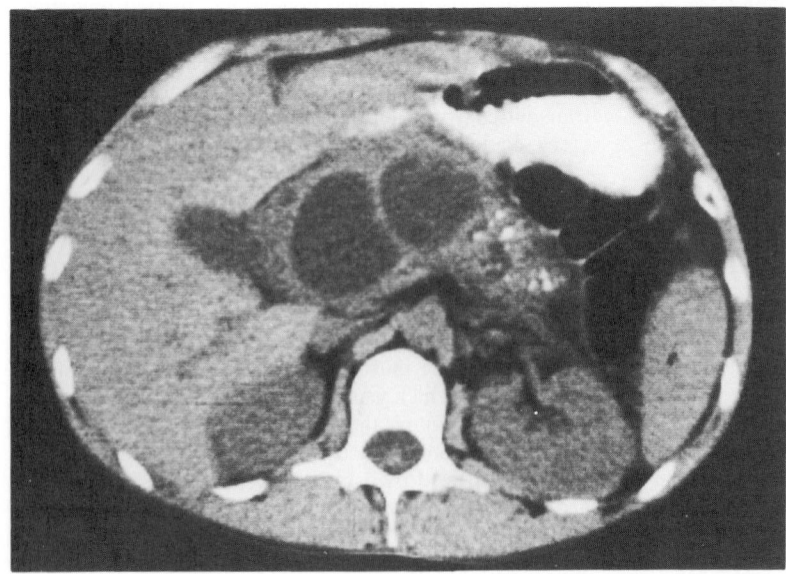

marsupialization should be used in extremely ill patients requiring urgent drainage in whom more extensive procedures might endanger life. If the pseudocyst has a thin flimsy wall, external drainage may be the only means of treatment. The mortality rate of this procedure is low (about 4.5 percent) but the morbidity (prolonged drainage, loss of electrolytes, and a relatively high rate of recurrence) is about 17 percent. Contrary to the radical debridement required for the typical case of pancreatic abscess, infected pseudocysts may be treated by internal or external drainage as for any uninfected pseudocyst. The reported cures of pancreatic abscess by percutaneous drainage in the majority of instances are infected pseudocysts rather than the type of pancreatic abscess described above.

Extirpation theoretically is an ideal method of therapy. Yet only the rare, very small pseudocyst located in the distal pancreas and unattached to vital structures lends itself to excision. Extirpation is not recommended except in these special circumstances, since the mortality is high.

Internal drainage of some type is the best treatment for most pseudocysts. Transgastric cystogastrostomy when the lesion is adherent to the stomach or transduodenal cystoduodenostomy if the cyst is located in the head of the pancreas have produced mortality rates of 2.5 to 5 percent with approximately the same low rate of recurrence. They are almost as easily accomplished as external drainage. Suturing of the edges of the stomach and cyst or excision of a large ellipse of tissue may predispose to regurgitation of gastrointestinal fluids into the cyst. Pancreatic abscesses and gastric ulcer have also been sequelae of cystogastrostomy, and therefore cystojejunostomy to a Roux en Y of jejunum is preferred. A small piece of the wall of the cyst should always be excised and submitted for microscopic examination to exclude the possibility of a neoplastic cyst. Anastomosis of a Roux en Y jejunum to the wall of the pseudocyst requires a thick fibrous wall and results in the same mortality and recurrence rates as cystogastrostomy or cystoduodenostomy.

Drainage through the duct of Wirsung after transduodenal sphincterotomy has been advocated by Doubilet and Mulholland, based on the principle that pseudocysts have major ductal communications. There is little question that drainage of the ductal system will accomplish decompression of most pseudocysts, but the procedures mentioned above would seem to be simpler and more direct in most cases. The primary indication for transphincteric drainage is in patients with gallstone pancreatitis who are undergoing corrective biliary tract operation. In these cases, common duct exploration is frequently performed, making transphincteric drainage a rather simple matter, and recurrence of the pancreatitis is unlikely.

A number of recent reports have suggested that external drainage of pseudocysts, accomplished using catheters placed with CT or ultrasound guidance, provides an effective method of treating pancreatic pseudocysts. Greater experience with this approach will be needed, however, before its value can be determined, as a number of patients treated in this manner have had their pseudocysts recur.

For cases of pancreatic ascites, internal drainage of the offending pseudocyst or resection of the pancreas distal to a ductal disruption is curative.

TUMORS

Carcinoma of the Pancreas and Periampullary Area

The manifestations of carcinoma of the pancreas and other malignant tumors of the periampullary areas (see Chap. 31 for carcinoma of the bile ducts) are so frequently indistinguishable that it seems reasonable to consider these neoplasms as a group. The relative frequency of these lesions in a series of 159 patients is shown in Table 32-4.

The average age of patients with carcinoma of the pancreas, duodenum, and common bile duct is sixty years, but in carcinoma of the ampulla the average age is about five years less. Males are more frequently affected by all these lesions, but there is no special racial predilection. The incidence of carcinoma of the pancreas has risen steadily over the past 10 years, but the reason for this is unknown. Cigarette smoking and consumption of coffee have been implicated as causative factors, but the relationship has not been proved. Biliary lithiasis has been suspected as a cause of carcinoma of the common bile duct, but not all such patients have cholelithiasis.

PATHOLOGY. Although its cell of origin is not known with certainty, carcinoma of the pancreas is believed to arise from the ductal system in 90 percent of the cases and from the acini in the remainder. Adenocarcinoma is the predominant lesion, often accompanied by extreme fibrous connective tissue stromal proliferation. The lesion itself is frequently small, in many instances one-third to one-half of the bulk of the gross lesion, the remainder consisting of a zone of pancreatitis. These tumors are most frequently found within the head of the pancreas and compress the pancreatic and common bile ducts. The pancreatic duct may become extremely dilated and tortuous and is often easily palpable at operation, especially if the surrounding pancreas is somewhat atrophic and

Table 32-4. RELATIVE FREQUENCY OF PERIAMPULLARY NEOPLASMS

	Percent
Pancreas	83
Ampulla of Vater	10
Duodenum	4
Common bile duct	3

SOURCE: Taken with permission from Jordan GL Jr: Benign and malignant tumors of the pancreas and the periampullary region, in Howard JM, Jordan GL Jr (eds): *Surgical Diseases of the Pancreas.* Philadelphia, Lippincott, 1960.

firmer than usual. Other adjacent structures, such as the portal vein, stomach, duodenum, and vena cava, may be invaded by tumor. Regional lymph-node metastasis is present in 90 percent of patients, and perineural invasion is extremely common. About 80 percent of the patients have liver metastases.

Carcinomas of the ampulla of Vater and the duodenum are frequently impossible to differentiate. Grossly and microscopically, they are columnar cell adenocarcinomas. Frequently, a large area of pancreatitis in the head of the pancreas will not only obscure the small primary lesion but may also be erroneously interpreted as the primary neoplasm itself. Some tumors of the ampulla are so small that they are not readily detected at operation, since biliary obstruction may have occurred very early. In both these neoplasms, intermittent jaundice is caused by recurrent sloughing of the central portion of the tumor. The pattern of metastatic spread is similar to that of carcinoma of the pancreas. Carcinomas of the common bile duct occasionally are fleshy fungating growths but more frequently form a hard mass that may be mistaken for a stone or stricture. In the absence of previous operation, a stricture should be considered to be carcinoma even though biopsies may not initially confirm this. Metastases generally follow the same route as other tumors in this region.

Cystadenoma and cystadenocarcinoma of the pancreas are rare lesions with a predilection for females. Their importance lies in the fact that growth is slow and metastasis late even though these neoplasms may become very large. In addition, these lesions should not be confused with pseudocysts and thereby subjected to cystenterostomy. The gross and histologic differentiation between the benign and malignant varieties is difficult and sometimes impossible, but the benign form seems to be much more common. These tumors comprise numerous cystic spaces separated from each other by thick fibrous septae. The extreme vascularity of these lesions may give rise to a bruit and accounts for a characteristic angiographic blush that is not present in the more common adenocarcinomas. Because of a far better prognosis than other pancreatic tumors, resection of cystadenomas and cystadenocarcinomas should be carried out when possible.

CLINICAL MANIFESTATIONS. Weight loss is the single most common symptom in carcinoma of the pancreas, no matter where the lesion is located. Pain is extremely frequent (70 to 80 percent), although it is rarely of the dramatic type caused by biliary colic resulting from a stone in the common bile duct. The pain is usually dull and aching and is most often confined to the midepigastrium. Radiation to the back is frequent, although the pain may extend to both lower quadrants. A helpful diagnostic feature of the pain is that it is relieved by sitting in a hunched position and accentuated by lying supine. Eating may aggravate the pain, which often antedates jaundice by many weeks or months, depending upon the proximity of the primary lesion to the common bile duct. Distention of the common bile duct, and especially of the pancreatic duct, and perineural invasion by tumor are usually re-

sponsible for pain in carcinoma of the pancreas. Cystadenomas and cystadenocarcinomas are frequently asymptomatic.

Progressive jaundice occurs in about 75 percent of patients with carcinoma of the head of the pancreas; the incidence of jaundice decreases as the location of the lesion progresses to the left. Occasionally a tumor may deform the second part of the duodenum without obstructing the common bile duct. Anorexia and weakness are common (about 50 percent of cases). Diarrhea, constipation, nausea, and vomiting are inconstant symptoms. Chills and fever are rare. Pruritus is frequent and may be an extremely trying symptom for the patient. The liver is palpable in 50 to 70 percent of patients with carcinoma of the head of the pancreas, but the gallbladder can be palpated in only one-third to one-fourth of the cases. These findings are obviously much less frequent in lesions of the body and tail of the pancreas. An enlarged palpable gallbladder in a jaundiced patient without chills or fever is most certainly a reliable diagnostic criterion for malignant choledochal obstruction, but no diagnostic inference is justified if the gallbladder cannot be palpated. Tenderness, ascites, the presence of an abdominal mass, a rectal shelf, or Virchow's nodes are all less frequent findings.

Pancreatic malignant tumors occur at least twice as frequently in diabetic as in nondiabetic patients, but diabetes is rarely the first sign of pancreatic cancer. Approximately 10 percent of patients with carcinoma of the pancreas are overtly diabetic, and 20 percent have asymptomatic glycosuria or hyperglycemia. It has often been stated that because of the high incidence of thrombosis in carcinoma of the pancreas, it must be seriously considered in all patients who have a spontaneous onset of venous or arterial thrombosis. In fact, clinically detectable thromboses are quite rare in patients with carcinoma of the pancreas.

The clinical signs of carcinoma of the ampulla of Vater, common bile duct, and duodenum are similar to those of carcinoma of the head of the pancreas. Yet, a few distinguishing features may allow differentiation of these lesions from carcinoma of the pancreas. Pain is somewhat less frequent; when present it is apt to be more colicky in nature than the pain of pancreatic cancer. The jaundice is usually less intense when the patient is admitted to the hospital and is more likely to be intermittent (25 percent). Chills and fever are also somewhat more common. In carcinoma of the duodenum, duodenal obstruction and gastrointestinal hemorrhage are more common than in carcinoma of the pancreas.

LABORATORY AND DIAGNOSTIC STUDIES. The most important laboratory studies in periampullary and pancreatic carcinoma are tests for obstructive jaundice. No great significance can be attached to the relationship between the direct and indirect fractions of bilirubin, since they are nearly equal even in only moderately advanced obstructive jaundice. The serum bilirubin almost never rises above 30 to 35 mg/dL in pancreatic cancer, whereas acute hepatic necrosis may be associated with much higher levels. The alkaline phosphatase is almost always increased, occasionally even before the onset of jaundice. Serum transaminase is of value in ruling out hepatitis, since in this disease the serum transaminase often rises to more than 1000 units. In mechanical biliary obstruction, values below 500 are the rule. Exfoliative cytology and the response of the pancreas to secretin and pancreozymin are time-consuming and rarely of real diagnostic help.

Fifty to sixty percent of patients with pancreaticoduodenal cancer will have some radiologic abnormality, such as distortion and flattening of the gastric antrum or second and third parts of the duodenum, anterior displacement of the stomach, gross distortion of the duodenum and "reverse 3" sign, or widening of the duodenal loop. Definitive radiologic diagnosis by upper gastrointestinal series is usually impossible, however. The recent improvement in ultrasonic techniques and the advent of computed tomography (CT) have revolutionized the diagnosis. Both are advocated when carcinoma of the pancreas is suspected. If the diagnosis is still in doubt, especially in cases of lesions of the body of the pancreas, ERCP is indicated. When obstructive jaundice is present, we prefer transhepatic cholangiography (THC) with a fine needle to ERCP because a better definition of the site of encroachment upon the biliary tree is possible with the former. Carcinoma produces a smooth, tapering obstruction, but calculi cause a typical convex deformity. Since hemorrhage and bile peritonitis may occur, THC should only be done when the patient is thoroughly prepared for operation. Selective angiography may be of value in selected cases more to ascertain operability as determined by absence of encasement of major vessels than to establish the diagnosis of the neoplasm itself. Percutaneous fine needle aspiration biopsy of pancreatic tumors has recently been shown to be safe and accurate in 60 to 70 percent of cases. Since operation is indicated in most cases for biliary decompression and/or gastric bypass, we prefer intraoperative fine needle aspiration to the percutaneous technique.

DIAGNOSIS. In the absence of jaundice, a high index of clinical suspicion should be maintained when a patient has obscure abdominal pain. Many of these patients are thought to be psychoneurotic and are sent from one physician to another, often ending up in the care of a psychiatrist. It is for these cases that ultrasound and CT examinations are of special value. The diagnosis of carcinoma of the head of the pancreas and other periampullary lesions, on the other hand, is easier. Differentiation between the various types of pancreaticoduodenal carcinoma is an interesting intellectual exercise and is to be encouraged, but definitive diagnosis from clinical and laboratory examination may be impossible. Hepatitis can usually be excluded by its tendency to affect younger persons; the 1- to 2-week prodromal period of malaise, anorexia, and fever that precedes the onset of jaundice; the presence of diffuse hepatic tenderness; and a marked increase in serum transaminase. Profound weight loss in a jaundiced patient almost always means carcinoma. Cholestatic jaundice due to viral hepatitis or drugs may be difficult to differen-

tiate from obstruction caused by tumors, because the hepatic function tests show similar abnormalities. In these instances, needle biopsy of the liver should be done and may be invaluable.

TREATMENT AND PROGNOSIS. Once the diagnosis of obstructive jaundice has been established, early operation is advised. Procrastination can only lead to further deterioration of hepatic function and increased operative risk as the patient continues to lose weight. Preliminary transhepatic biliary drainage for 7 to 10 days may be of value in improving hepatic function in deeply jaundiced patients, but controlled trials show that overall outcome of operation is not improved because of an increased incidence of infection. Adequate nutrition and correction of anemia should be accomplished as rapidly as possible. Preoperative evaluation of renal function is essential, since postoperative renal failure is common in severely jaundiced patients. Adequate hydration immediately prior to operation is mandatory for the same reason.

The only definitive and potentially curative therapy for pancreaticoduodenal carcinoma is adequate surgical resection. This implies pancreaticoduodenal resection of the type first successfully performed by Whipple in 1935. During the early years after this formidable operation was first introduced, mortality and morbidity were extremely high, often 40 to 50 percent. Because of these dismal statistics, many surgeons developed a fatalistic attitude toward the therapy of pancreaticoduodenal carcinoma, regarding surgical treatment as merely palliative. Recent improvements in preoperative and postoperative care as well as meticulous attention to technical details have markedly reduced mortality rates, in one instance to 0 percent in 41 consecutive cases, making this operation a feasible therapeutic technique, especially since no other method of cure is now known.

Most surgeons agree that pancreaticoduodenectomy should be performed for localized carcinoma of the ampulla of Vater, duodenum, or common bile duct in good-risk patients. Although many surgeons do not advocate excision of primary carcinoma of the pancreas, if the lesion is relatively confined and there is no evidence of spread to the liver, resection should be carried out. Additional reasons for resection in those cases that are locally removable include the surgeon's inability to differentiate between a primary lesion of the head of the pancreas and a tumor of the ampulla or the lower end of the common bile duct and also a longer, more comfortable survival after resection even for those who ultimately succumb to their disease.

A recent review of the large Mayo Clinic experience over 25 years with carcinoma of the pancreas indicates that potentially curative operation could be done in only 13 percent of 1272 patients. When hospital deaths were excluded, the overall 1-, 2-, and 5-year survival rates in these 162 patients were 54, 29, and 8 percent, respectively. The prognosis was not influenced by the histologic grade of the lesion, its nodal status, or whether the Whipple operation or total pancreatectomy was performed. The decision for or against partial pancreatectomy should, therefore, rest upon the technical ease and safety of anastomosis between the pancreas and jejunum and the frozen-section examination of the margins of resection. The 5-year survival rate for carcinoma of the ampulla of Vater and duodenum is at least twice as high as for carcinoma of the pancreas.

The major problem confronting surgeons at operation is accurate diagnosis, especially before they embark upon a procedure as large as pancreaticoduodenectomy. Carcinoma of the ampulla of Vater and duodenum can usually be diagnosed rather easily by biopsy of the lesion through a duodenotomy. In expert hands intraoperative fine-needle aspiration cytology now offers a diagnostic accuracy as high as 75 percent for lesions of the pancreas. Establishing the existence of carcinoma of the head of the pancreas or lower end of the common bile duct is sometimes impossible, however. The decision for resection in these cases must be made on the basis of the clinical and operative findings of a mass in the region of the head of the pancreas in a patient in the sixth or seventh decade of life, very frequently with dilatation of the duct of Wirsung. If a calculus can be ruled out by exploration of the common bile duct and cholangiography, surgeons can take solace in the fact that they will rarely be wrong in the diagnosis of malignancy. Furthermore, if pancreatitis has progressed to the point of obstructing the common bile duct and if the resection can be performed with a reasonably low mortality rate, successful resection for this benign lesion cannot be too strongly criticized.

Although the resectability rate of carcinoma of the ampulla and duodenum is between 65 and 75 percent, only 10 to 15 percent of patients with carcinoma of the pancreas have resectable lesions. The surgeon's role in palliation is, therefore, an important one even though the average survival after diagnosis in patients with unresectable neoplastic obstructions of the biliary tract is approximately 6 months. Rarely do these patients live longer than 1 year. However, the relief of the jaundice, with its attendant pruritus, and possibly alleviation of obstruction, will often provide significant palliation for these unfortunate patients. A simple cholecystojejunostomy to a loop of jejunum without enteroenterostomy is easily performed and is rarely followed by cholangitis. Choledochojejunostomy may be necessary when the gallbladder is absent or the cystic duct is obstructed by tumor. Anastomosis of the biliary tree to the duodenum has been done successfully but is unwise if duodenal obstruction is likely. Invasion of the duodenum and stomach produces gastrointestinal obstruction in 20 percent of patients with carcinoma of the pancreas, and for this reason gastroenterostomy may be advisable. Intraoperative injection of the celiac plexus with 95% alcohol provides significant relief of pain in many patients. The use of high-dose intraoperative radiotherapy has recently shown some promising results in terms of palliation, but it is too soon to know its true place.

For the occasional debilitated and aged poor-risk patient, long-term internal drainage by the percutaneous transhepatic technique may offer reasonable palliation for the remaining life of the individual. Combined external beam radiation therapy and 5-fluorouracil have recently been shown to significantly prolong comfortable survival of patients with carcinoma of the head of the pancreas and may be of value for some patients who have undergone potentially curative resections.

Pancreaticoduodenal Resection (Fig. 32-10). Pancreaticoduodenectomy is almost always performed in one stage. The two-stage procedure has been replaced by preliminary transhepatic biliary drainage in deeply jaundiced patients with prolonged obstruction and consequent hepatic injury.

A vertical or a transverse abdominal incision may be used, depending upon the habitus of the patient. The duodenum should have been thoroughly mobilized by the maneuver of Kocher, not only in its second part, but also in the third portion to the superior mesenteric vessels. This usually requires prior mobilization of the hepatic flexure. Gentle dissection between the vessels and the neck of the pancreas with a blunt-nosed clamp is performed once the gastrocolic trunk and pancreatic tributaries have been divided and the posterosuperior pancreaticoduodenal vein has been located. At this point, surgeons may still turn back, before they have performed an irrevocable maneuver, but excellent assessment of the entire area is still available.

The gastrocolic omentum may also be divided at this point to allow better evaluation or so that resection can be continued. The right gastric, gastroduodenal, and descending branch of the left gastric arteries are divided and ligated. The stomach is transected, leaving the entire antrum with the specimen. The pancreas is transected, usually at its neck. Large vessels are transfixed with fine nonabsorbable sutures. The uncinate process is mobilized by dividing numerous vessels to it between ligatures. Varying amounts of pancreas, or even the entire organ, may be removed with this procedure, at the discretion of the surgeon. The jejunal mesentery and jejunum are divided to allow removal of a few inches of jejunum distal to the ligament of Treitz; the jejunum is withdrawn from beneath the mesenteric vessels. The entire specimen may now be removed by division of the common bile duct. A concomitant cholecystectomy is not always necessary but is usually performed.

Many methods of reconstruction are available. The end of the jejunum is brought into the upper abdomen in a retrocolic position but anterior to the mesenteric vessels. Of prime importance is the anastomosis of the biliary and pancreatic ducts above, or proximal to, the gastrojejunal anastomosis, to prevent marginal ulceration. Vagotomy is not generally performed, although it has been recommended by some. If the common duct and jejunum are of equal size, they are joined end to end. When the jejunum is larger than the common bile duct, the end of the jejunum is closed, and end-to-side anastomosis is carried out. The pancreaticojejunostomy is performed between the end of the pancreas and the side of the jejunum several inches distal to the choledochojejunostomy, suturing the duct of Wirsung to jejunal mucosa. A gastrojejunostomy

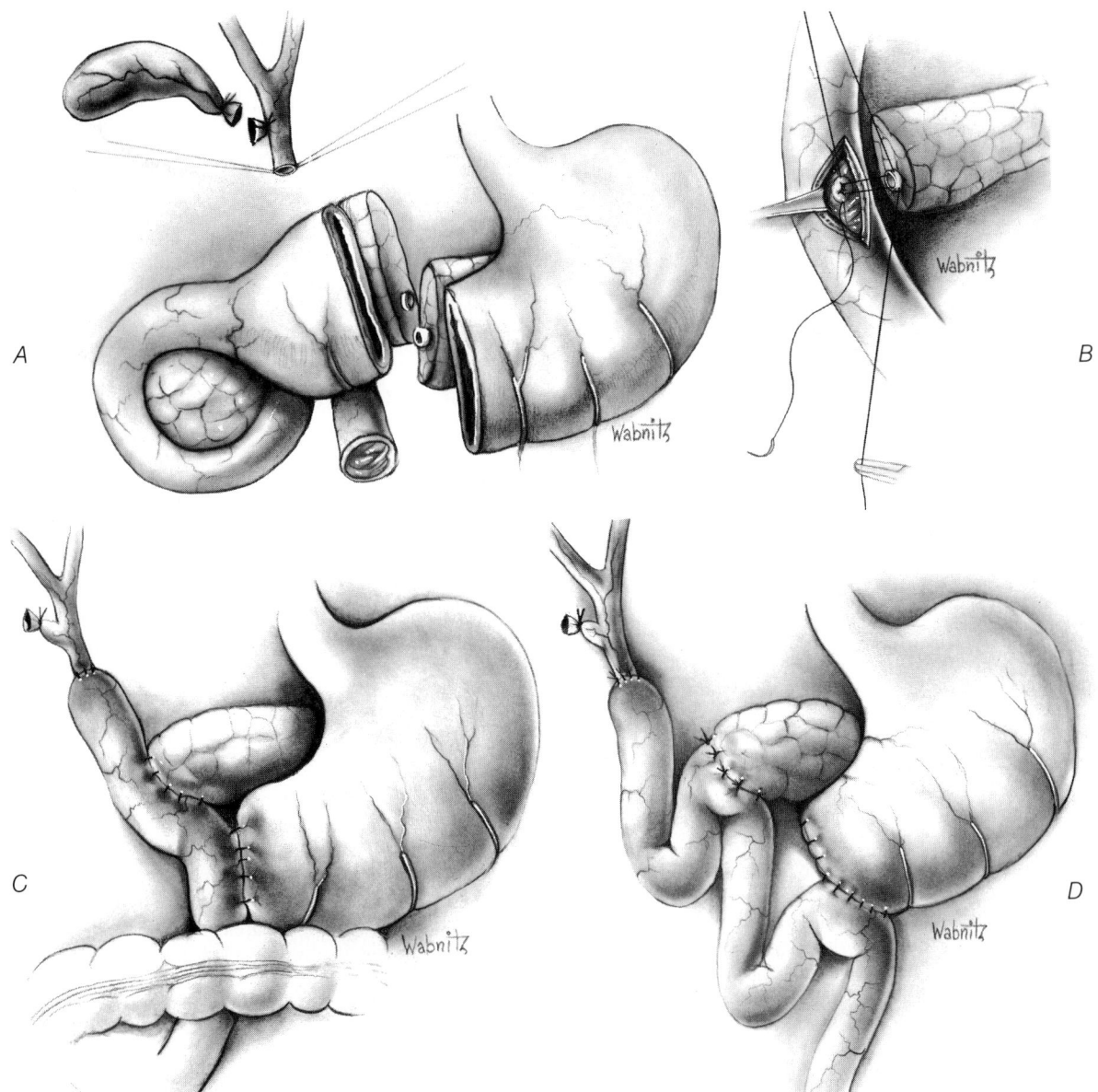

Fig. 32-10. *A.* Pancreaticoduodenectomy. Extent of resection. *B.* Anastomosis of pancreatic duct. *C.* Retrocolic method of reconstitution. *D.* Antecolic method of reconstitution.

completes the operative procedure. A single soft Penrose drain is left in place close to, but not in apposition with, the pancreaticojejunal anastomosis.

Hemorrhage and renal failure are the most common complications in the early postoperative period. Meticulous hemostasis during operation and the administration of vitamin K will generally prevent hemorrhage and later renal failure. The importance of adequate replacement of blood, fluids, and electrolytes cannot be overemphasized. Pancreatic fistula is the third most common complication and is particularly apt to occur if the stump of the pancreas is closed. Careful pancreaticojejunostomy with

anastomosis of the duct of Wirsung to the mucosa of the jejunum over a fine tube or invagination of the cut end of the pancreas into the jejunum has largely obviated this complication. Should a pancreatic fistula occur, sump drainage should be instituted. The fistula will usually close in 2 to 3 weeks if adequate nutrition and electrolyte balance are maintained.

Metabolic Consequences of Pancreaticoduodenectomy. Most patients tolerate pancreaticoduodenectomy relatively well. Although some patients gain weight and thrive, the majority tend to lose some weight and may have varying degrees of malabsorption. The management of these problems is not unlike that in the postgastrectomy patient, but exocrine pancreatic substitution therapy is often necessary. Viokase or pancreatin in divided doses, up to 20 g daily, is preferred. Whether resection of the head, uncinate process, and neck of the pancreas or closure of the pancreaticojejunostomy causes the pancreatic insufficiency often seen after pancreaticoduodenectomy is unknown.

The nutritional and metabolic picture is quite different in the case of total pancreatectomy. The postoperative diabetes, even though mild and rarely requiring more than 30 units of insulin daily, is exceedingly difficult to manage because of the patient's extreme sensitivity to insulin. Diabetic retinopathy and glomerulosclerosis have been reported but are rare. Loss of nitrogen in the stool increases, and fat absorption is severely impaired. Iron absorption is very poor, and negative calcium and phosphorus balance is common. Theoretically, total pancreatectomy should improve the results of surgical therapy for carcinoma of the pancreas, since the tumor may spread via the pancreatic duct; the lesion is often multifocal; and the gross extent of the tumor may be difficult to ascertain at operation. However, the extreme metabolic derangements produced by total pancreatectomy and the absence of data to indicate that this operation increases survival in cancer of the pancreas make its use debatable at the present time.

The APUD Concept

APUD is an acronym taken from the initial letters of the most common cytochemical properties of a series of cells whose apparent common function is the synthesis and secretion of peptide or amine hormones. *A* refers to their content of amines, *P* and *U* to their potential for preferential uptake of the amino acid precursors of dopamine and 5-hydroxytryptamine, and *D* to their decarboxylation of these relevant precursors. These cells exhibit the property of masked metachromasia and argyrophilia, have a high content of nonspecific esterases or cholinesterases, have high levels of mitochondrial α-glycerophosphate dehydrogenase, and demonstrate endocrine-type granules by electron microscopy.

APUD cells of the central division are located in the pituitary, pineal, and hypothalamus. APUD cells in the pituitary are known to secrete ACTH, melanocyte-stimulating hormone, somatotropin, and prolactin. In the hypothalamus, APUD cells produce oxytocin, vasopressin, thyrotropin-releasing factor, somatotropin-releasing hormone, melanotropin-releasing factor, somatotropin-release inhibiting factor (somatostatin), and perhaps others. APUD cells of the peripheral neuroendocrine division are found in the pancreas, stomach, intestine, thyroid (calcitonin), parathyroid (parathormone), carotid body, skin, adrenal, lung, and urogenital system. In the pancreas, APUD cells normally produce insulin, glucagon, somatostatin, and pancreatic polypeptide. Gastrin, glucagon and substance P are secreted by gastric APUD cells. Intestinal APUD cells have been shown to produce motilin, substance P, enteroglucagon, secretin, somatostatin, CCK, GIP, and VIP.

The clinical and pathologic implications of the APUD concept are that the widely distributed APUD cells have a multipotential capacity for the production of peptide hormones. Thus, it would not be surprising to find in the pancreas gastrin- or VIP-producing APUD cell tumors or carcinoid tumors that secrete a variety of peptide hormones normally produced almost anywhere in the gastroenteropancreatic system. The multiple endocrine adenomas (MEA) syndromes are also readily reconciled by the APUD concept. At one time, it was believed that APUD cells shared a common embryology and originated from the neural crest. This belief is no longer commonly held.

Islet-Cell Tumors and Hyperinsulinism

Roscoe Graham achieved the first recorded cure of organic hyperinsulinism by removing an islet-cell adenoma. In a review of the literature published between 1929 and 1958, Moss and Rhoads found 766 cases, of which only 93 were malignant.

PATHOPHYSIOLOGY. The beta cells of the pancreatic islets secrete insulin, and tumors that cause hyperinsulinism arise from these cells. Bioassays of these tumors have usually shown large quantities of insulin, and recent studies of plasma insulin in patients harboring beta cell tumors have indicated markedly elevated levels after islet-cell stimulation by a variety of means.

The excessive circulating insulin causes profound hypoglycemia. Since the brain depends primarily on glucose for its metabolism and cannot store either glucose or glycogen in significant amounts, the hypoglycemia may cause convulsions, severe cerebral depression, and coma, which if allowed to persist for a prolonged period will be followed by death within 3 to 20 days. Mental deterioration, ataxia, hemiparesis, and a wide variety of neurologic sequelae may result from repeated minor hypoglycemic episodes. Early diagnosis and prompt treatment are of importance in the prevention of these irreversible changes.

Administration of glucose promptly reverses the hypoglycemia and relieves the symptoms. The spontaneous recovery that is so frequent in patients with organic hyperinsulinism has not been adequately explained. However, it has been suggested that hypoglycemia stimulates the release of epinephrine and glucagon, which in turn mobilize sufficient glycogen to elevate the blood sugar.

PATHOLOGY. Approximately 75 percent of patients with pancreatic organic hyperinsulinism have benign adenomas; 12.9 percent have suspiciously malignant lesions, and in 12.1 percent the lesions are clearly malignant. About 15 percent of the patients have multiple adenomas, but only a few cases of diffuse adenomatosis involving the entire pancreas have been described. Most of the adenomas measure between 1 and 3 cm, but the size of the tumor seems to have little relationship to the severity of the clinical symptoms. Metastases from malignant beta cell tumors may be functional or nonfunctional. In infants, the entity of nesidioblastosis, a proliferation of beta cells in close apposition to ductal cells, has recently been recognized as a cause of about one-fourth of the cases encountered in this age group.

CLINICAL MANIFESTATIONS. Most of the patients with this syndrome are in the fourth to seventh decades of life. The sex incidence is approximately equal. Insulinomas are occasionally a feature of the multiple endocrine adenomatosis (MEA-I) syndrome (see below under Ulcerogenic Tumors of the Islets). Functioning islet-cell tumors are rare in childhood, but spontaneous hypoglycemia occasionally occurs without tumor or with nesidioblastosis.

The symptoms may take one of two general forms, but between the two extremes many combinations of clinical signs may occur. The absolute level of blood sugar often bears little relationship to the severity or character of the symptoms, even in the same patient on different days. If the blood sugar falls rapidly, the primary symptoms may be referable to the release of epinephrine caused by the hypoglycemia. Sweating, hunger, weakness, tachycardia, and "inward trembling" result from this mechanism. A slower decrease in blood sugar produces "cerebral" symptoms, such as headache, mental confusion, visual disturbances, convulsions, and coma. Symptoms may last for a few weeks or as long as 20 years. Signs and symptoms of progressive muscular atrophy have been reported in these cases. The widest possible variety of bizarre neurologic or psychiatric disorders may be mimicked by organic hyperinsulinism. Fear of attacks leads many patients to consume large quantities of food, especially carbohydrates, and they often become extremely obese.

LABORATORY AND DIAGNOSTIC STUDIES. Whipple's triad consists of (1) attacks precipitated by fasting or exertion, (2) fasting blood sugar concentrations below 50 mg/dL, and (3) symptoms relieved by oral or intravenous administration of glucose. These criteria should always be met before considering operation. Three types of spontaneous hypoglycemia account for about 80 percent of all such cases: (1) functional hyperinsulinism, (2) organic hyperinsulinism due to pancreatic islet-cell tumor, and (3) hepatogenic hypoglycemia. Functional and alimentary hypoglycemia are usually easily ruled out, because they never occur in the fasting state and invariably occur 2 to 4 h after eating. Hepatogenic hypoglycemia may be almost impossible to differentiate from insulinoma. Abnormal hepatic function and a high-plateau type of glucose tolerance curve that does not respond to a high-carbohydrate diet are the keystones to diagnosis of hepatogenic hypoglycemia. Abnormalities of the pituitary, adrenal, and central nervous system may also cause organic hypoglycemia but can usually be ruled out.

Apart from satisfying the conditions of Whipple's triad, prolonged fasting with or without exercise is the single most valuable test in the diagnosis of insulinoma. The blood sugar will invariably decrease to below 50 mg/dL under these circumstances, and fasting for longer than 30 h is almost never necessary. Simultaneous measurement of serum insulin and blood sugar levels with the finding of an insulin level inappropriately high for the level of the blood sugar is diagnostic of insulinoma. The glucose tolerance test has been unduly deprecated because of the wide variation in the responses. However, if care is taken to restore the sensitivity of the islets in the nontumorous portion of the pancreas by feeding carbohydrates for a few days, the typical flat low curve will almost always be seen. Once the diagnosis has been established by biochemical means, pancreatic angiography and pancreatic venous sampling for insulin assay have been advocated for localization of the lesion. Unfortunately, these studies have been helpful in only about 30 percent of cases. Since most of the tumors are small, CT scans are of value in a limited number of cases.

TREATMENT. Although dietary therapy has been attempted, the only permanent cure of organic pancreatic hyperinsulinism is by removal of the offending lesion. Streptozotocin, a potent antibiotic that destroys islets, is useful in treating patients with far-advanced metastatic islet-cell carcinoma but should be reserved for these patients because of the antibiotic's toxic side effects. The preoperative management is concerned mainly with the provision of adequate quantities of glucose, usually in the form of 10% dextrose solutions. ACTH and cortisone have been recommended, presumably to prevent hyperthermia during, or immediately after, operation. However, it is not necessary to use these drugs, and there is no sound physiologic reason for them. Diazoxide inhibits insulin release from beta cells and also stimulates release of epinephrine. It may be of use in control of hypoglycemia preoperatively if other measures fail, but fluid retention, gastric irritation, and agranulocytosis may occur.

Surgically, every portion of the pancreas must be carefully examined. The entire anterior aspect of the body, tail, and a portion of the head of the pancreas should be exposed. Then the entire body and tail of the pancreas with the spleen must be mobilized into the wound by division of the splenocolic and lienorenal ligaments and incision of the parietal peritoneum along the inferior and superior aspects of the pancreas. The entire posterior surface of the organ as far right as the superior mesenteric vessels may then be palpated and visualized. The head of the pancreas must be completely mobilized by the Kocher maneuver. Particular attention should be paid to exposure of the neck of the pancreas by division and ligation of the gastrocolic venous trunk and to the uncinate process. The latter is best seen after meticulous clearing of the superior mesenteric vessels. Adenomas in the stomach, duodenum, jejunum, ileum, mesentery, and omentum are aberrant locations in 1 to 2 percent of cases, and these areas should be carefully searched.

Simple excision of the adenoma is sufficient in most cases, since the majority are benign. If malignancy is suspected, a pancreatic resection should be done. Complete exploration should be performed even if a single tumor is found, since about 14 percent are multiple.

The greatest current controversy concerns proper procedure when the tumor cannot be found after thorough examination. Classically, a distal subtotal pancreatectomy to the left of the mesenteric vessels has been advocated under these circumstances, with the hope that a small adenoma might be present in this tissue (21 percent chance) or that hyperplasia of the islets might be ameliorated. It is doubtful whether there are any authenticated cases of hyperplasia of the islets in adults. Yet Moss and Rhoads have found that 42.6 percent of 129 patients were cured and 10.9 percent were improved after "blind" distal pancreatectomy when no tumor was found. The original diagnosis in those who were improved is questionable. Fonkalsrud et al. have suggested that pancreaticoduodenal resection with preservation of the tail of the pancreas should be done when the pancreatic tumor cannot be found after thorough exploration. These investigators feel that a small tumor is much more easily overlooked in the head and uncinate process than in the tail or body. They believe that distal pancreatectomy would be far easier technically after "blind" pancreaticoduodenectomy when no tumor has been found than the reverse sequence of operations. We are reluctant to advocate "blind" pancreaticoduodenectomy because of the higher morbidity and mortality and would still choose distal resection. The distal pancreatectomy can be extended to a 90 percent resection or more if necessary, more easily and with less morbidity than pancreaticoduodenectomy. However, it cannot be stressed strongly enough that all of the pancreas, and especially the head and uncinate process, must be seen and felt. A marked increase in blood glucose within 30 min of removal of tissue suspected of being responsible for the hyperinsulinism is confirmatory evidence that the disease has been eradicated. Subsequent determination of serum insulin levels on the same blood taken at operation will provide postoperative substantiation of cure.

The child with organic hypoglycemia can usually be managed with diet and ACTH or cortisone. If a response is not evident and if the patient seems to be deteriorating, operation is indicated, even though tumors are exceedingly rare in children. If no tumor is found, distal subtotal pancreatectomy in a child is a much more logical procedure than in adults, since hyperplasia of the islets and nesidioblastosis do occur and are responsive to partial resection.

The overall operative mortality for removal of a localized islet-cell tumor is 8.2 percent, and for partial resection (distal) of the pancreas it is 9.6 percent.

Ulcerogenic Tumors of the Islets

In 1955, Zollinger and Ellison reported two patients with coincidental fulminant peptic ulceration and non-beta cell tumors of the pancreas. Since then, many cases of ulcerogenic tumors of the pancreas have been described.

CLINICAL MANIFESTATIONS. The triad described originally by Zollinger and Ellison remains extremely useful today: (1) fulminant and often complicated peptic ulceration, frequently found in atypical locations, (2) extreme gastric hypersecretion, and (3) non-beta cell tumor of the pancreatic islets. The symptoms are similar to those caused by ordinary peptic ulceration and in recent years, more cases are being uncovered in patients with "garden variety" duodenal ulcer. Some patients with this syndrome have had explosive and unrelenting ulceration from onset; others have had symptoms for several years that suddenly become fulminant. Perforation, hemorrhage, obstruction, internal fistulization, and intractability may occur. The ulceration, although often present in the first portion of the duodenum, occasionally is found in unusual locations, such as the third and fourth parts of the duodenum or the jejunum. Perforation or any other complication of jejunal ulceration should always make one suspect the presence of an ulcerogenic pancreatic tumor, since peptic ulceration of the jejunum rarely occurs when no tumor is present.

Fulminant ulceration often recurs within weeks after ordinarily effective surgical therapy. Subtotal gastrectomy with or without vagotomy, vagotomy with a drainage procedure, radiation therapy, and prodigious doses of alkalinizing and anticholinergic agents have generally been ineffective in controlling the ulcer diatheses. H_2-receptor antagonists have recently proved to be effective in selected patients who may have inoperable situations or as an adjunct to some forms of operation directed at the ulcer diathesis. Many patients have undergone several of these procedures before the true nature of the process was discovered.

The syndrome is slightly more common in males, the ratio being approximately 6:4. Most of the patients are in the third to fourth decade of life, although a few cases have occurred in the first decade and a rare case in the ninth. Even the smallest remnants of gastric mucosa can cause extreme hypersecretion and recurrent ulceration in these patients. Since the secretory rates are already close to their maximum, further stimulation with histamine generally produces very little response. Marks et al. have suggested that a ratio of basal acid output to histamine-stimulated output of greater than 60 percent is virtually diagnostic of the Zollinger-Ellison syndrome, but exceptions are more common than generally recognized.

The extreme gastric hypersecretion is associated with distressing watery diarrhea in about a third of the reported cases. Some patients have excreted between 2 and 8 liters of liquid stool daily, and in many cases profound diarrhea has preceded the onset of peptic ulceration. In some cases in which diarrhea is the sole symptom, the patient has had gastric hypersecretion without peptic ulceration. Steatorrhea may also occur and probably is caused by three mechanisms: (1) inactivation of pancreatic and intestinal lipase by the abnormally acid environment of the upper small intestine, (2) precipitation of bile salts, and (3) irritative and inflammatory action of the acid environment upon the mucosa of the small bowel. Aspiration of the gastric secretion often temporarily relieves the diarrhea.

A sharp distinction should be made between the diarrhea of the Zollinger-Ellison syndrome and another syndrome of watery diarrhea and non-beta cell tumors of the pancreas that is much less common than the former (see below).

In addition to the usual radiologic findings of peptic ulceration, duodenal ileus with enlargement of rugal folds, hypertrophy of the gastric mucosa, and an abnormal feathery pattern of the small bowel are frequently found in patients with the Zollinger-Ellison syndrome.

PATHOLOGY AND PATHOPHYSIOLOGY. The origin of these tumors is from the islets. The typical tumor is composed of rather uniform cuboidal cells arranged mainly in strands and ribbons or occasionally in sheets and clumps. The nucleus is oval and has one or more round nucleoli. The cytoplasm usually contains fine stippling and irregular vacuoles. These tumors often bear a striking resemblance to argentaffin tumors (carcinoids) but do not react to silver stains. The growth pattern of these two tumors is remarkably similar in that both tend to grow slowly, metastasize late, and exhibit little correlation between the microscopic appearance and growth propensities. The patient with an islet-cell tumor often dies from the unremitting peptic ulceration rather than from metastasis, although recent long-term follow-up indicates an increasing and unexpected incidence of death from metastatic disease. Grossly, the tumors are slate gray to red-brown and vary from 2 mm to 10 cm. Most are solid, although a few cystic tumors have been reported.

In 249 collected cases, 61 percent of the patients had malignant tumors, and 44 percent of these had metastases, usually to the regional lymph nodes. The tumors are located with equal frequency in the head and tail of the pancreas. Diffuse microadenomatosis has been observed in 19 percent of the cases. A significant number of patients have had lesions in the duodenal wall. This is of particular interest because removal of the tumor alone in these cases has frequently sufficed to eradicate the disease, in contradistinction to the radical treatment by total gastrectomy usually advocated in this syndrome.

Associated endocrine disease has been found in 21 percent of the patients with the Zollinger-Ellison syndrome. This usually consists of adenomas of other endocrine glands, such as the pituitary, parathyroid, pancreatic islets (beta cells), and adrenal cortex, in that order of frequency. These patients usually do not have family histories of similar disturbances; therefore, most of these cases can be distinguished from the group described by Wermer in 1954. He pointed out that some patients with polyendocrine adenomas and peptic ulceration often have giant gastric rugae (Ménétrier's disease) and that an abnormal gene may be responsible. Ellison and Wilson have found that only 3 percent of the patients with the Zollinger-Ellison syndrome fall into this classification. It is now known that Wermer's syndrome is caused by an autosomal dominant gene that has a high degree of penetrance. The acronym MEA-I (multiple endocrine adenomatosis) has been used for this syndrome, in which 90 percent of patients have hyperparathyroidism, usually caused by hyperplasia of the parathyroids, 50 to 85 percent have gastrinomas of the pancreas indistinguishable from the sporadic type, 30 percent have pituitary adenomas, and 30 to 50 percent have adrenocortical hyperplasia. A few cases of insulinoma have also been reported.

Gastrin is secreted by these tumors, and that extracted from tumors has physiologic effects identical to those of synthesized pure gastrin. Thus, the diagnosis can be substantiated by the detection of high levels of gastrin in the serum, although gastrinomas have been found in some patients with serum gastrin levels as low as 200 pg/mL. Elevation of the serum gastrin is common in patients with pernicious anemia but the absence of basal acid hypersecretion excludes this diagnosis. An exaggerated response of the serum gastrin to the intravenous infusion of calcium and a paradoxical rise of the serum gastrin level after intravenous infusion of secretin serve to elucidate the diagnosis in doubtful cases. These findings, together with the absence of a rise in serum gastrin level after a meal, are helpful in differentiating patients with gastrinoma from those who have the recently described antral G cell hyperplasia. Selective sampling of portal venous blood for determination of localized elevations of gastrin has been advocated by some but has recently been shown to be of extremely limited value.

TREATMENT AND PROGNOSIS. Total gastrectomy was originally the cornerstone of treatment for several years after gastrinomas were first described, because the high incidence of functioning metastases and the multiplicity of the pancreatic lesions often led to the demise of the patient from fulminating ulcer disease when lesser gastric operations were performed or when attempts were made to remove the pancreatic lesion alone. The relatively protracted course of the tumor, even when it had metastasized, justified this seemingly radical approach. Recent follow-up studies indicate, however, that roughly 60 percent of patients with gastrinoma will be dead (40 percent) or dying (20 percent) of metastatic tumor at 20 years. These data, together with some promising results with H_2-receptor antagonists, have prompted a reexamination of the role of total gastrectomy. A few authors have found that with careful adjustment of dosage and timing of H_2-receptor antagonists in cooperative and reliable patients, the ulcer diathesis can be controlled for up to 7 years. In some instances, lesser operations, such as highly selective vagotomy, have made control of the acid hypersecretion with these drugs more readily achieved. Thus, efforts have been directed preliminarily to exploration of the patient with the intent of cure of the tumor by resection, if that seems possible, coupled with highly selective vagotomy to reduce the required dose of H_2-receptor antagonist. Whether this approach will produce longevity equivalent to that achieved by total gastrectomy and an improved quality of life remains to be established. In any case, when H_2-receptor antagonists are used, the response of the basal acid secretion to the drug must be assessed and titrated to reduce basal acid secretion to at least 2 meq/h 6 h after the drug is administered. The H_2-receptor antagonists have found a very real place in the preparation of debilitated gastrinoma patients for operation when complications such as hemorrhage or perforation have required emergency treatment. Persistence of serum gastrin levels above 1500 pg/mL, or the posttherapeutic elevation to such levels, usually indicates the presence of metastatic disease. Streptozotocin has been effective in a few instances of extensive metastatic disease, but the results in general have been disappointing.

Oberhelman et al. have had good results from removal of the tumor alone without total gastrectomy when the tumor has been located in the duodenal wall, and others have had similar results. Whether these tumors differ materially from those in the pancreas is not known, although the microscopic appearance is similar.

Diarrheagenic Islet Tumors, Glucagonoma, and Somatostatinoma

Diarrheagenic tumors are extremely rare, somewhat less than 100 cases having been reported. The clinical syndrome has been called "pancreatic cholera," or the Verner-Morrison syndrome after the authors who first described it. The acronym WDHA has also been used and refers to the watery diarrhea, hypokalemia, and gastric anacidity or hypochlorhydria that are commonly encountered. Middle-aged females are most frequently affected. The diarrhea is usually profuse, averaging 4 to 5 L/day, and contains 200 to 400 meq of potassium daily. Symptoms of severe hypokalemia are common, and peptic ulcers do not occur because acid secretory rates are low. Hypercalcemia occurs in about one-third of cases, but the parathyroid glands are normal. Glucose intolerance is common, and cutaneous flushing has been noted in a few cases. The most likely explanation for the symptoms is the secretion of vasoactive intestinal peptide (VIP) by the tumor, causing a profuse secretory diarrhea. About 40 percent of the patients have had benign islet tumors; 40 percent have malignancies, usually with metastases; and 20 percent have hyperplasia of the islets. The most important differential diagnoses include laxative abuse, villous adenoma, and celiac disease. Resection provides the only effective means for cure or long-lasting remission.

Glucagonomas have recently been reported with increasing frequency, although these tumors are still very rare. A classical syndrome of cutaneous lesions, diabetes, glossitis, anemia, weight loss, severe depression, and venous thrombosis has been found in most of the cases. The cutaneous lesions are characteristically on the lower abdomen and perineum, but the perioral skin and lower limbs are also often affected. The lesions are migratory from one place to another, have a marginated appearance, and destroy the superficial layers of the epithelium while maintaining a background of profound erythema. The cutaneous lesion has been called necrolytic migratory erythema. Many of these patients have attended dermatology and/or diabetes clinics for years. Occasionally, glucagonoma occurs without the cutaneous syndrome, and in these cases severe diabetes is the only manifestation. The most satisfactory treatment is resection, but the majority of patients have metastases when the disease is first discovered. The cutaneous lesions and other manifestations of the syndrome disappear when the tumor can be removed completely. Chemotherapy has been disappointing in advanced cases.

Another potentially surgically curable cause of diabetes is a somatostatin-producing tumor of the islets. In addition to diabetes, the clinical syndrome includes abdominal pain, diarrhea, profound steatorrhea, achlorhydria, and gallstones. All these symptoms can be explained by the well-known inhibitory effect of somatostatin on hormone secretion and motility of the gastrointestinal tract. Only a few cases have been reported.

Bibliography

Anatomy

Kleitsch WP: Anatomy of the pancreas: A study with special reference to the duct system. *Arch Surg* 71:795, 1955.

Payne RL Jr: Annular pancreas. *Ann Surg* 133:754, 1951.

Pierson JM: The arterial blood supply of the pancreas. *Surg Gynecol Obstet* 77:426, 1943.

Physiology

Case RM: Synthesis, intracellular transport and discharge of exportable proteins in the pancreatic acinar cell and other tissues. *Biol Rev* 55:211, 1978.

Gardner JD, Jensen RJ: Regulation of pancreatic enzyme secretion *in vitro*, in Johnson LR (ed): *Physiology of the Gastrointestinal Tract*. New York, Raven, 1981, pp 831–871.

Konturek SJ, Radecki T, et al: Effect of vagotomy on pancreatic secretion evoked by endogenous and exogenous cholecystokinin and caerulein. *Gastroenterology* 63:273, 1972.

Malagelada JR: Gastric, pancreatic and biliary responses to a meal, in Johnson LR (ed): *Physiology of the Gastrointestinal Tract*. New York, Raven, 1981, pp 893–924.

Menguy RB, Hallenbeck GA, et al: Intraductal pressures and sphincteric resistance in canine pancreatic and biliary ducts after various stimuli. *Surg Gynecol Obstet* 106:306, 1958.

Meyer JH: Control of pancreatic exocrine secretion, in Johnson LR (ed): *Physiology of the Gastrointestinal Tract*. New York, Raven, 1981, pp 821–829.

Meyer JH, Spingola LJ, Grossman MI: Endogenous cholecystokinin potentiates exogenous secretin on pancreas of dog. *Am J Physiol* 221:742, 1971.

Meyer JH, Way LW, Grossman MI: Pancreatic response to acidification of varying lengths of proximal intestine in dog. *Am J Physiol* 219:971, 1970.

Moreland HJ, Johnson LR: Effect of vagotomy of pancreatic secretion stimulated by endogenous and exogenous secretin. *Gastroenterology* 60:425, 1971.

Palade GE: Intracellular aspects of the process of protein synthesis. *Science* 189:347, 1975.

Poncelot PR, Thompson AG: Role of infected bile in spasm of sphincter of Oddi. *Am J Surg* 126:387, 1973.

Routley EF, Mann FC, et al: Effects of vagotomy on pancreatic secretion in dogs with chronic pancreatic fistula. *Surg Gynecol Obstet* 95:529, 1952.

Schulz I: Electrolyte and fluid secretion in the exocrine pancreas, in Johnson LR (ed): *Physiology of the Gastrointestinal Tract*. New York, Raven, 1981, pp 795–819.

Thomas JE: Mechanism of action of pancreatic stimuli studied by means of atropine-like drugs. *Am J Physiol* 206:124, 1964.

Unger RH, Eisentraut AM: Enteroinsular axis. *Arch Intern Med* 123:261, 1969.

Unger RH, Ketterer H, et al: The effects of secretin, pancreozymin, and gastrin on insulin and glucagon secretion in anesthetized dogs. *J Clin Invest* 46:630, 1967.

Veeger W, Abels J, et al: Effect of sodium bicarbonate and pancreatin on the absorption of vitamin B_{12} and fat in pancreatic insufficiency. *N Engl J Med* 267:1341, 1962.

Wang CC, Grossman MI: Physiological determination of release of secretin and pancreozymin from intestine of dogs with transplanted pancreas. *Am J Physiol* 164:527, 1951.

Acute Pancreatitis

Acosta JM, Pelligrini CA, et al: Etiology and pathogenesis of acute biliary pancreatitis. *Surgery* 88:118, 1980.

Acosta JM, Rossi R, et al: Early surgery for acute gallstone pancreatitis: Evaluation of a systematic approach. *Surgery* 83:367, 1978.

Adams JT, Libertino JA, et al: Significance of an elevated serum amylase. *Surgery* 63:877, 1968.

Albo RJ, Silen W, et al: A critical clinical analysis of acute pancreatitis. *Arch Surg* 86:1032, 1963.

Beger HG, Bittner R, et al: Bacterial contamination of pancreatic necrosis. A prospective clinical study. *Gastroenterology* 91:433, 1986.

Bernard HR, Criscione JR, et al: The pathologic significance of the serum amylase concentration: An evaluation with special reference to pancreatitis and biliary lithiasis. *Arch Surg* 79:311, 1959.

Bradley EL III, Clements JL Jr, et al: The natural history of pancreatic pseudocysts: A unified concept of management. *Am J Surg* 137:135, 1979.

Cameron JL, Zuidema GD, et al: Pathogenesis for alcoholic pancreatitis. *Surgery* 77:754, 1975.

Delhaye M, Engelholm L, et al: Pancreas divisum: Congenital anatomic variant or anomaly? Contribution of endoscopic retrograde dorsal pancreatography. *Gastroenterology* 89:951, 1985.

Finch WT, Sawyers JL, et al: A prospective study to determine the efficacy of antibiotics in acute pancreatitis. *Ann Surg* 183:667, 1976.

Gross JB, Comfort MW: Hereditary pancreatitis. *Proc Staff Meeting Mayo Clinic* 32:354, 1957.

Gross JB, Ehrlich EW: The etiology of pancreatitis: A review of clinical experience. *Ann Surg* 152:135, 1960.

Kim E, Sheth M: Optimal timing of surgical intervention in patients with acute pancreatitis associated with cholelithiasis. *Surg Gynecol Obstet* 150:499, 1980.

Klatskin G, Gordon M: Relationship between relapsing pancreatitis and essential hyperlipemia. *Am J Med* 12:3, 1952.

Lawson DW, Daggett WM, et al: Surgical treatment of acute necrotizing pancreatitis. *Ann Surg* 172:605, 1970.

Levitt MD, Rapoport M, et al: The renal clearance of amylase in renal insufficiency, acute pancreatitis, and macroamylasemia. *Ann Intern Med* 71:919, 1969.

Mayer AD, McMahon MJ, et al: Controlled clinical trial of peritoneal lavage for the treatment of severe acute pancreatitis. *N Engl J Med* 312:399, 1985.

Medical Research Council Multicentre Trial: Morbidity of acute pancreatitis: The effect of aprotinin and glucagon. *Gut* 21:334, 1980.

Neoptolemos JP, London N, et al: A prospective study of ERCP and endoscopic sphincterotomy in the diagnosis and treatment of gallstone acute pancreatitis. A rational and safe approach to management. *Arch Surg* 121:697, 1986.

Ranson JHC: Surgical treatment of acute pancreatitis. *Dig Dis Sci* 25:453, 1980.

Ranson JHC, Balthazar E, et al: Computed tomography and the prediction of pancreatic abscess in acute pancreatitis. *Ann Surg* 201:656, 1985.

Ranson JHC, Rivkind KM, et al: Prognostic signs and role of operative management in acute pancreatitis. *Surg Gynecol Obstet* 139:69, 1974.

Ranson JHC, Rivkind KM, Turner JW: Diagnostic sepsis and nonoperative peritoneal lavage in acute pancreatitis. *Surg Gynecol Obstet* 176:209, 1976.

Russel RC, Wong NW, et al: Accessory sphincterotomy (endoscopic and surgical) in patients with pancreas divisum. *Br J Surg* 71:954, 1984.

Smith RB III, Warren WD, et al: Pancreatic ascites: Diagnosis and management with particular reference to surgical technics. *Ann Surg* 177:689, 1973.

Sostre CF, Flournoy JG, et al: Pancreatic phlegmon: Clinical features and course. *Dig Dis Sci* 30:918, 1985.

Stone HH, Fabian TC, et al: Gallstone pancreatitis biliary tract pathology in relation to time of operation. *Ann Surg* 194:305, 1981.

Stone HH, Strom PR, et al: Pancreatic abscess management by subtotal resection and packing. *World J Surg* 8:340, 1984.

Stroud WH, Cullom JW, et al: Hemorrhagic complications of severe pancreatitis. *Surgery* 90:657, 1981.

Watts GT: Total pancreatectomy for fulminant pancreatitis. *Lancet* 2:384, 1963.

Chronic Pancreatitis

Arvanitakis C, Cooke AR: Diagnostic tests of exocrine pancreatic function and disease. *Gastroenterology* 74:932, 1978.

Fry CF, Child CG III, et al: Pancreatectomy for chronic pancreatitis. *Ann Surg* 184:403, 1976.

Garcia-Puges AM, Navarro S, et al: Reversibility of exocrine pancreatic failure in chronic pancreatitis. *Gastroenterology* 91:17, 1986.

Joffe BI, Banks S, et al: Insulin reserve in patients with chronic pancreatitis. *Lancet* 2:890, 1968.

Kalser MH, Leite CA, et al: Fat assimilation after massive distal pancreatectomy. *N Engl J Med* 279:570, 1968.

Nagata A, Homma T, et al: A study of chronic pancreatitis by serial endoscopic pancreatography. *Gastroenterology* 81:884, 1981.

Owens JL, Howard JM: Pancreatic calcification: A late sequel in the natural history of chronic alcoholism and alcoholic pancreatitis. *Ann Surg* 147:326, 1958.

Prinz RA, Greenlee HB: Pancreatic duct drainage in 100 patients with pancreatitis. *Ann Surg* 194:313, 1981.

Proctor HJ, Mendez OC, et al: Surgery for chronic pancreatitis: Drainage versus resection. *Ann Surg* 189:664, 1979.

Stone HH, Mullins RJ et al: Vagotomy plus Billroth II gastrectomy for the prevention of recurrent alcohol-induced pancreatitis. *Ann Surg* 201:684, 1985.

White TT, Hart MJ: Pancreaticojejunostomy versus resection in the treatment of chronic pancreatitis. *Am J Surg* 138:129, 1979.

Trauma

Balasegaram M: Surgical management of pancreatic trauma. *Curr Probl Surg* 16:1, 1979.

Berne CJ, Donovan AJ, et al: Duodenal "diverticulization" for duodenal and pancreatic injury. *Am J Surg* 127:503, 1974.

Doubilet H, Mulholland JH: Some observations on the treatment of trauma to the pancreas. *Am J Surg* 105:741, 1963.

Freeark RJ, Kane JM, et al: Traumatic disruption of the head of the pancreas. *Arch Surg* 91:5, 1965.

Jones RC, Shires GT: Pancreatic trauma. *Arch Surg* 102:424, 1971.

Northup WF, Simmons RL: Pancreatic trauma: A review. *Surgery* 71:27, 1972.

Olsen WR: The serum amylase in blunt abdominal trauma. *J Trauma* 13:200, 1973.

Stone HH, Fabian TC, et al: Experiences in the management of pancreatic trauma. *J Trauma* 21:257, 1981.

Thal AP, Wilson RF: A pattern of severe blunt trauma to the region of the pancreas. *Surg Gynecol Obstet* 119:773, 1964.

Cysts and Pseudocysts

Balfour JF: Pancreatic pseudocysts: Complications and their relation to the timing of treatment. *Surg Clin North Am* 50:395, 1970.

Cullen PK Jr, ReMine WH, et al: A clinicopathological study of cystadenocarcinoma of the pancreas. *Surg Gynecol Obstet* 117:189, 1963.

Doubilet H, Mulholland HJ: Pancreatic cysts. *Surg Gynecol Obstet* 96:683, 1953.

Gerzof SG, Johnson WC, et al: Percutaneous drainage of infected pancreatic pseudocysts. *Arch Surg* 119:888, 1984.

Piper CE, ReMine WH, et al: Pancreatic cystadenoma: Report of 20 cases. *JAMA* 180:648, 1962.

Polk HC, Zeppa R, et al: Surgical significance of differentiation between acute and chronic pancreatic collections. *Ann Surg* 169:444, 1969.

Schindler SC, Schaefer JW, et al: Chronic pancreatic ascites. *Gastroenterology* 59:453, 1970.

Varriale P, Bonanno CA, et al: Portal hypertension secondary to pancreatic pseudocysts. *Arch Intern Med* 112:191, 1963.

Carcinoma of the Pancreas and Periampullary Area

Braasch JW, Gongliang J, et al: Pancreatoduodenectomy with preservation of the pylorus. *World J Surg* 8:900, 1984.

Cotton PB: Endoscopic methods for relief of malignant obstructive jaundice. *World J Surg* 8:854, 1984.

Dobelbower RR, Milligan AJ: Treatment of pancreatic cancer by radiation therapy. *World J Surg* 8:919, 1984.

Edis AJ, Kiernan PD, et al: Attempted curative resection of carcinoma of the pancreas: Review of Mayo Clinic experience 1951–1975. *Mayo Clin Proc* 55:531, 1980.

Ellison CE, Van Aman ME, et al: Preoperative transhepatic biliary decompression in pancreatic and periampullary cancer. *World J Surg* 8:862, 1984.

Howard JM: Pancreatico-duodenectomy. Forty-one consecutive Whipple resections without an operative mortality. *Ann Surg* 168:629, 1968.

Ihse I, Isaksson G: Preoperative and operative diagnosis of pancreatic cancer. *World J Surg* 8:846, 1984.

Longmire WP: Cancer of the pancreas: Palliative operation, Whipple procedure, or total pancreatectomy. *World J Surg* 8:872, 1984.

McPherson GA, Benjamin IS, et al: Pre-operative percutaneous transhepatic billary drainage: The results of a controlled trial. *Br J Surg* 71:371, 1984.

Moertel CG, Reitemeier RJ, et al: Combined 5-fluorouracil and supervoltage radiation therapy of locally unresectable gastrointestinal cancer. *Lancet* 2:865, 1969.

Monge JJ, Dockerty MB, et al: Clinicopathologic observations on radical pancreatoduodenal resection for peripapillary carcinoma. *Surg Gynecol Obstet* 118:275, 1964.

Sarr MG, Cameron JL: Surgical palliation of unresectable carcinoma of the pancreas. *World J Surg* 8:906, 1984.

Shipley WU, Tepper JE, et al: Intraoperative radiation therapy for patients with pancreatic carcinoma. *World J Surg* 8:929, 1984.

Shipley WU, Woods WC, et al: Intraoperative electron beam irradiation for patients with unresectable pancreatic carcinoma. *Ann Surg* 200:289, 1984.

Silen W: Surgical anatomy of the pancreas. *Surg Clin North Am* 44:1253, 1964.

Soreide P, Skaarland E, et al: Fine-needle biopsy of the pancreas: Results of 204 routinely performed biopsies in 190 patients. *World J Surg* 9:960, 1985.

Taft DA, Freeny PC: Cystic neoplasms of the pancreas. *Am J Surg* 142:30, 1981.

van Heerden JA: Pancreatic resection for carcinoma of the pancreas: Whipple versus total pancreatectomy—an institutional perspective. *World J Surg* 8:880, 1984.

Wittenberg J, Ferrucci JT Jr, et al: Contribution of computed tomography to patients with pancreatic adenocarcinoma. *World J Surg* 8:831, 1984.

The APUD Concept and Islet-Cell Tumors

Dunn E, Stein S: Percutaneous transhepatic pancreatic vein catheterization in localization of insulinoma. *Arch Surg* 116:232, 1981.

Fonkalsrud EW, Dilley RB, et al: Insulin secreting tumors of the pancreas. *Ann Surg* 159:730, 1964.

Friesen SR, Tomita T: Further experience with pseudo-Zollinger-Ellison syndrome: Its place in the management of neuroendocrine duodenal ulceration. *World J Surg* 8:552, 1984.

Harrison TS, Fajans SS, et al: Prevalence of diffuse pancreatic beta islet cell disease with hyperinsulinism: Problems in recognition and management. *World J Surg* 8:583, 1984.

Hsien-chiu T, Chong-zheng Y, et al: Percutaneous transhepatic portal vein catheterization for localization of insulinoma. *World J Surg* 8:575, 1984.

Ingemansson S, Kuhl C, et al: Localization of insulinomas and islet cell hyperplasias by pancreatic vein catheterization and insulin assay. *Surg Gynecol Obstet* 146:725, 1978.

Krejs GJ, Orci L, et al.: Somatostatinoma syndrome: Biochemical, morphologic and clinical features. *N Engl J Med* 301:285, 1979.

Le Quesne LP, Nabarro JD, et al: The management of insulin tumours of the pancreas. *Br J Surg* 66:373, 1979.

Pearse AGE: The diffuse neuroendocrine system and the APUD concept: Related 'endocrine' peptides in brain, intestine, pituitary, placenta, and anuran cutaneous glands. *Med Biol* 55:115, 1977.

Verner JV, Morrison AB: Islet cell tumor and a syndrome of refractory watery diarrhea and hypokalemia. *Am J Med* 25:734, 1958.

Zollinger RM, Ellison EC, et al: Thirty years' experience with gastrinoma. *World J Surg* 8:427, 1984.

Spleen

Seymour I. Schwartz

ANATOMY

The spleen arises by mesenchymal differentiation along the left side of the dorsal mesogastrium in the 8-mm embryo. The weight of the spleen in the healthy adult ranges between 75 and 100 g, decreasing somewhat with age. The organ is located in the left upper quadrant, having a superior relationship to the under surface of the left leaf of the diaphragm and protected anteriorly, laterally, and posteriorly by the lower portion of the rib cage. Its position is maintained by several suspensory ligaments, the major ones being the splenophrenic, splenorenal, splenocolic, and gastrosplenic ligaments (Fig. 33-1). The gastrosplenic ligament normally contains the short gastric vessels, while the remaining ligaments are generally avascular, except in patients with portal hypertension when collateral veins become apparent. Arterial blood enters the spleen via the splenic artery, a branch of the celiac artery. The major venous drainage courses through the splenic vein, which joins the superior mesenteric vein to form the portal vein.

Accessory spleens have been reported in 14 to 30 percent of patients, with a higher incidence occurring in patients operated on for hematologic disorders. These accessory organs, which receive their vascular supply from the splenic artery, are present, in decreasing order of frequency, in the hilus of the spleen, the gastrosplenic and splenocolic ligaments, the gastrocolic ligament, the splenorenal ligament, and the greater omentum (Fig. 33-2). They also may occur in the pelvis of the female, and functioning splenic tissue has been removed from the scrotum in juxtaposition to the left testicle.

The spleen consists of a capsule that is normally 1 to 2 mm thick and trabeculae that enclose the pulp. The pulp, itself, has conventionally been divided into three zones: white, marginal, and red. Peripheral to the white pulp is the marginal zone that contains end arteries arising from the central artery and from the penicillar arteries. The marginal zone contains lymphocytes, macrophages, and some red cells that have exited the terminal arteries. The marginal zone contains the marginal sinus that filters material from the white pulp. Locally produced immunoglobulins enter this sinus and course to the peripheral circulation. Peripheral to the marginal zone is the red pulp that consists of cords and sinuses that contain cellular elements of blood in transit.

Blood brought to the spleen via the splenic arteries courses through branches, the trabecular arteries, that leave the trabeculae and enter the white pulp as central arteries (Fig. 33-3). These central arteries give off at right angles many arterioles, some of which terminate in the white pulp. The perpendicularity contributes to a skimming effect by which plasma exits while most red cells pass to the red pulp. Other branches cross the white pulp and end in the marginal zone or in the red pulp, itself. The branch of the central artery that terminates in the red pulp, known as the "artery of the pulp," breaks up into many branches. Within the red pulp, the blood is collected in splenic sinuses. These large, thin-walled venous

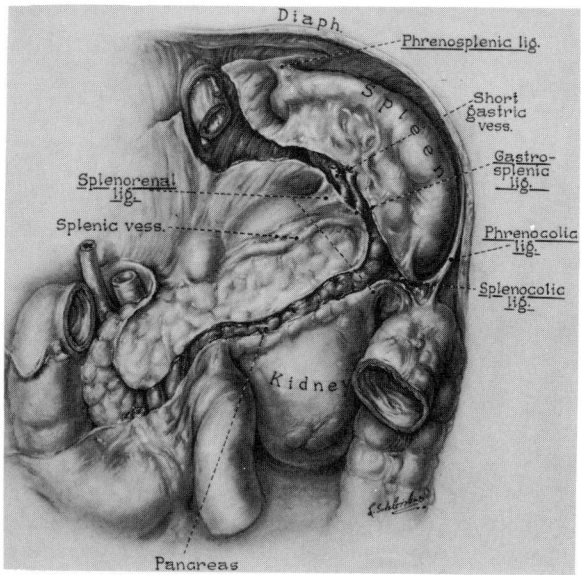

Fig. 33-1. Ligaments of the spleen. (From: *Erslev AJ, Ballinger WF II: Splenectomy. Curr Probl Surg, 1965. Copyright 1965, Chicago, Year Book Medical Publishers. Used by permission.*)

spaces drain into the pulp veins which, in turn, drain into the trabecular veins and then into the main splenic veins to enter the portal circulation. Thus splenic pulp pressure reflects pressure throughout the portal venous system. The tissue between the splenic sinuses is a reticular, connective tissue meshwork that appears as cords on histologic section, hence designated the "splenic cords." At points of passage from cords to sinuses, deformability and flexibility are demanded of the red blood cells so that they can squeeze through. Although these fenestrations are of small diameter (0.5 to 5.0 μm), they are traversed by normal red cells, which easily adjust to these dimensions. Under normal conditions, 10 percent of red cells pass from terminal arterioles through arteriovenous connections; 90 percent of cells course from terminal arterioles into pulp cords and into splenic sinuses after traversing the cordal–sinus wall apertures. The total splenic blood flow averages 300 mL/min.

PHYSIOLOGY AND PATHOPHYSIOLOGY

Galen is credited with the phrase "The spleen is an organ full of mystery"; to date this mystery has been only minimally unraveled. During the fifth to eighth month of fetal life, the spleen contributes actively to the production of both red cells and white cells that enter the circulation. This function does not continue in the normal adult, and both the qualitative and quantitative effects of splenic extramedullary hematopoiesis seen in myeloproliferative disorders have not been consistent. The role of the spleen in the immunologic processes of the body is discussed in Chap. 10. The splenic function that is the focus of surgical attention relates to the organ's reticuloendothelial tissue which contributes to the removal of cellular elements

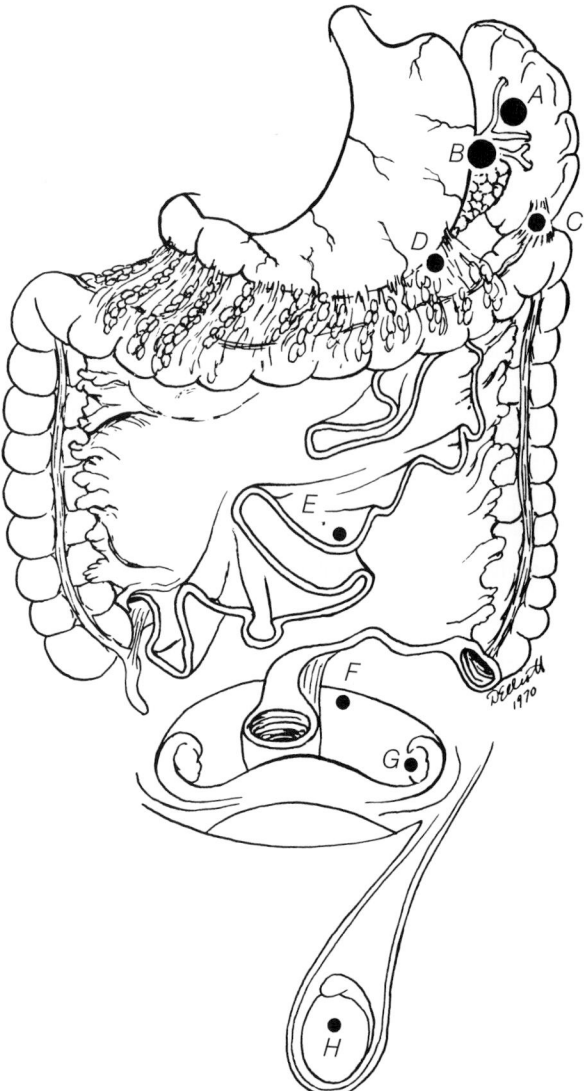

Fig. 33-2. Location of accessory spleens. *A.* Splenic hilus. *B.* Along splenic vessels; tail of pancreas. *C.* Splenocolic ligament. *D.* Greater omentum; perirenal regions. *E.* Mesentery. *F.* Presacral region. *G.* Adnexal region. *H.* Peritesticular region. (From: *Schwartz SI, Adams JT, Bauman AW: Splenectomy for hematologic disorders. Curr Probl Surg May 1971. Copyright 1971, Chicago, Year Book Medical Publishers. Used by permission.*)

from the circulating blood. Normally, cells pass through the spleen rapidly, but in the presence of splenomegaly and other disease states, the flow patterns become circuitous, contain more obstacles, and result in pooling of cells within the cords. ^{51}Cr studies have demonstrated that the slow-circulating component may have a half-life of 30 min.

Abnormal and aged erythrocytes, abnormal granulocytes, normal and abnormal platelets, and cellular debris may be cleared by the spleen, which apparently is capable of discriminating between these and normal cellular components. In the normal adult, the spleen is the most important site of selective erythrocyte sequestration and,

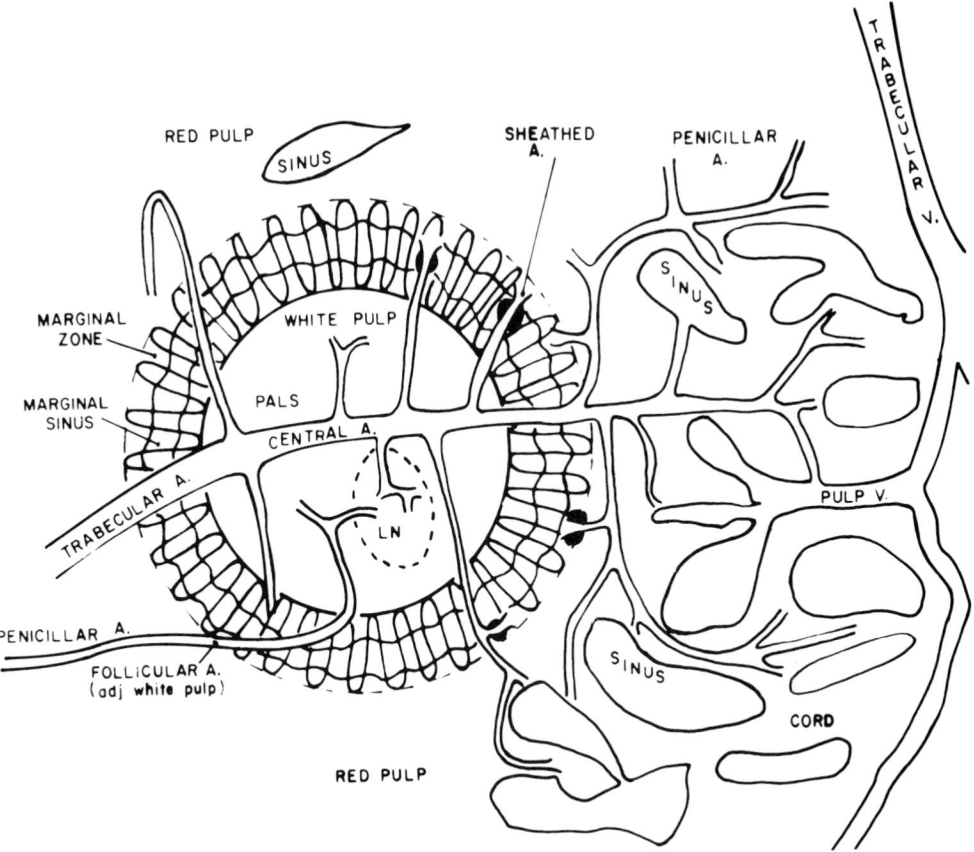

Fig. 33-3. Diagram illustrating splenic compartments and potential vascular supply routes. Symbols: A = artery or arteriole; V = vein; LN = lymphatic nodule that may include germinal center; PALS = periarterial lymphatic sheath. (From: *Barnhart MI, Lusher JM: Structural physiology of the human spleen. Am J Pediatr Hematol Oncol 1:311, 1979, with permission.*)

during its 120-day life cycle, the red cell spends an estimated minimum of 2 days within the spleen.

The action of the spleen that results in the pathological reduction of circulating cellular elements of blood has been attributed to three possible mechanisms: (1) excessive splenic destruction of cellular elements, (2) splenic production of an antibody that results in the destruction of cells within the circulating blood, and (3) splenic inhibition of the bone marrow causing failure of maturation and cell release. The last proposal is not important in most circumstances. The production of antibodies may be important in certain circumstances, but, as this is not an exclusive function of splenic immunocytes, antibody production would continue in the absence of the spleen. Overactivity of splenic function leading to accelerated removal of any or all of the circulating cellular elements of the blood with resultant anemia, leukopenia, or thrombocytopenia, alone or in combination, is referred to as *hypersplenism*.

The normal adult spleen contains about 25 mL of red blood cells, but relatively few of these are removed during a single passage through the organ. The spleen is ca-

pable of removing nuclear remnants from circulating erythrocytes (Howell-Jolly bodies) leaving the intact parent erythrocyte and cytoplasmic siderotic granules. The postsplenectomy blood smear is characterized by the presence of circulating erythrocytes with Howell-Jolly bodies and Pappenheimer bodies (siderotic granules that stain with Wright's stain) as a result of the loss of the pitting function of the spleen.

During the course of a day, approximately 20 mL of aged red blood cells are removed. The alterations in the red cell that make it sensitive to splenic destruction after 105 to 120 days in circulation have not been established with certainty. It appears that aging changes the biophysical properties of the red cell, making splenic entrapment more likely. In parallel, the enzyme activity and, therefore, the metabolic capacity of the red cell wanes with cell aging. Delay in splenic transit of aged or abnormal cells can lead to further cell injury because of the relatively hypoxic, acidotic, and substrate (glucose)-deprived environment that is present in congested splenic red pulp cords. These environmental conditions lead to further physical and chemical deterioration of the erythrocyte, making it more susceptible to phagocytosis by splenic macrophages and reticuloendothelial cells or to intrasinusoidal disintegration. The central event in cytolysis may be the fall in cellular adenosine triphosphate (ATP) to very low levels and the loss of vital cellular functions dependent on ATP, such as sodium and calcium efflux, priming of glycolysis, and maintenance of membrane integrity. To what extent repeated passages through the spleen contribute to normal red cell aging is not certain, but evidence that the red cell loses surface area with aging, combined with the ability of the spleen to remove bits of red cell with surgical precision, raises this possibility. On the other hand, the presence of a normal red cell life span in splenectomized subjects suggests that red cell aging occurs independently of splenic presence and at approximately the normal rate. A variety of erythrocytes altered by intrinsic factors (membrane, hemoglobin, or enzymic abnormalities) or extrinsic factors (antibody and nonantibody injury) may be prematurely removed by the spleen. Severely damaged cells may be removed by the reticuloendothelial system at a variety of sites. Minimally altered erythrocytes may require the specific rigors of the splenic circulation for premature destruction and, therefore, may have normal or near-normal survival after splenic removal. In the dog and cat, unlike man, the spleen may contract significantly in response to hypovolemia or catecholamines, resulting in an autotransfusion; this is an important consideration in studies of experimental shock.

The neutrophil is removed from the circulation with a half-life of about 6.0 h. Although the role of the spleen in the destruction of neutrophils under normal conditions is not well quantified, in some hypersplenic states the spleen's role is augmented, with resulting neutropenia. This augmented removal can occur because of splenic enlargement and accelerated sequestration of granulocytes or because of enhanced splenic removal of altered granulocytes, as seen in immune neutropenias.

The platelet (thrombocyte), under normal circumstances, survives about 10 days in the circulation. One-third of the total platelet pool is normally sequestered in the spleen, but the role of the spleen in the final removal of normal platelets has not been precisely defined. With splenomegaly, a larger proportion of platelets is sequestered in the spleen (up to 80 percent), and this and accelerated platelet destruction in the spleen account for thrombocytopenia. Splenectomy results in an increase in platelets, which at times reach levels greater than 1 million cells per cubic millimeter. Postsplenectomy thrombocytosis is often transient but may persist. This is particularly notable in congenital hemolytic states that do not respond well to splenectomy. In these circumstances, continued hemolysis in the absence of the splenic removal mechanism can lead to persistent, extreme thrombocytosis and intravenous thrombosis.

DIAGNOSTIC CONSIDERATIONS

EVALUATION OF SIZE. Normally the spleen is not palpable on abdominal examination, but the organ may be felt in about 2 percent of healthy adults. In healthy subjects, no significant dullness is elicited by percussion over the spleen either anteriorly or laterally. As the organ enlarges, dullness may be detected at the level of the ninth intercostal space in the left anterior axillary line especially on expiration. Thereafter, it becomes first percussible and then palpable below the left costal margin. With increasing splenomegaly, notching may be palpable on the anteromedial surface, distinguishing the spleen from other abdominal masses.

Routine radiologic examination of the abdomen usually provides an accurate estimate of the size of the spleen. Although splenomegaly may be suggested by medial or caudad displacement of the stomach bubble, frequently accompanied by caudad displacement of air in the splenic flexure, the organ's outline can often be clearly demarcated in the left upper quadrant, corroborating enlargement. Computer tomography and magnetic resonance imaging (MRI) depict the spleen and define abnormalities in size, shape, and parenchymal pathology, i.e., cyst, abscess, tumor (Fig. 33-4). Radioisotopic scanning with ^{99m}Tc-sulfur colloid (Fig. 33-5) also defines the organ;

Fig. 33-4. Splenic abscess. *A.* Coronal sonogram of spleen. Large irregular anechoic area (A) containing a few internal scattered echoes due to debris. *B.* Transverse axial sonogram of spleen demonstrates abscess (A). *C.* CT scan at corresponding level. Abscess (a) is area of diminished attenuation in center of spleen. Lesion was drained percutaneously. (From: *Pawar S, Kay CJ, et al: Sonography of splenic abscess. AJR 138:259, 1982, with permission.*)

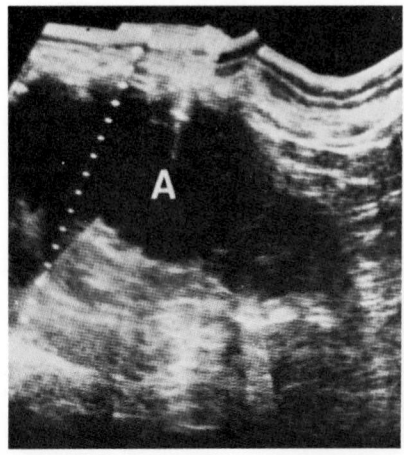
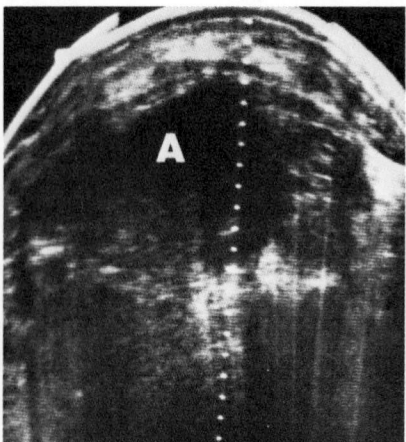
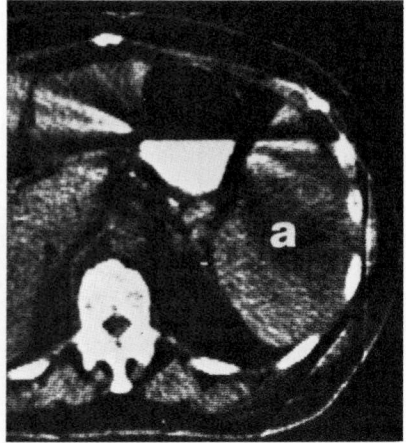

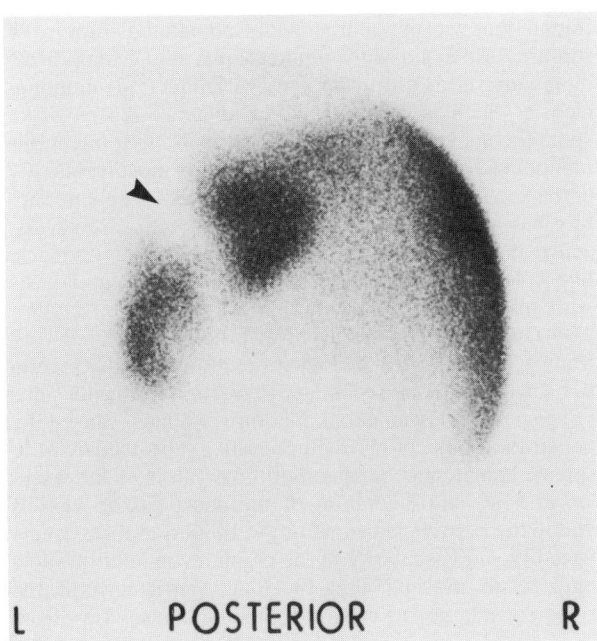

Fig. 33-5. Splenic rupture; patient treated without operative intervention.

Fig. 33-6. ^{51}Cr-labeled red cell determination of hemolytic anemia and splenic sequestration. Top, disappearance of ^{51}Cr-labeled normal autogenous red cells from the bloodstream and accumulation by the tissues in normal subjects and in patients with hemolytic anemia. Bottom, accumulation of radioactivity in liver and spleen of normal subjects and patients with hemolytic anemia and splenic sequestration. (After: *Jandl J et al: J Clin Invest 35:842, 1956.*)

vascular shunts that allow blood to bypass splenic phagocytes interfere with the procedure.

EVALUATION OF FUNCTION. The functional abnormality of hypersplenism may be manifested by a reduction in the number of red cells, neutrophils, or platelets in the peripheral blood. An increase in the rate of red cell destruction will always result in a compensatory rise in the rate of production unless disease of the marrow coexists. The hallmark of increased red cell turnover (hemolysis) is reticulocytosis in the absence of blood loss. Other tests such as the plasma bilirubin, haptoglobin, and hemoglobin are less sensitive, dependent on the rate of hemolysis, the sites of hemolysis, and liver function, and are therefore only of adjunctive value.

Reduced red blood cell survival in patients with hemolytic anemia may be more precisely demonstrated by measuring the disappearance of blood radioactivity after the patient's erythrocytes are labeled with $Na_2{}^{51}CrO_4$ (Fig. 33-6). With this technique, the normal half-life of the red cells is about 30 days, i.e., 50 percent of the cells remain in the circulation at that time. A half-life of 15 days or less indicates significantly increased hemolysis. The spleen's role in a hemolytic anemia may be assessed by determining the relative uptakes of ^{51}Cr-tagged erythrocytes by the spleen and the liver. A spleen-liver ratio greater than 2:1 indicates significant preferential splenic sequestration and anticipates a beneficial effect of splenectomy. Radioisotopic labeling also has been used to evaluate the survival of neutrophils and platelets. Presently there is no clinically practical method of assessing

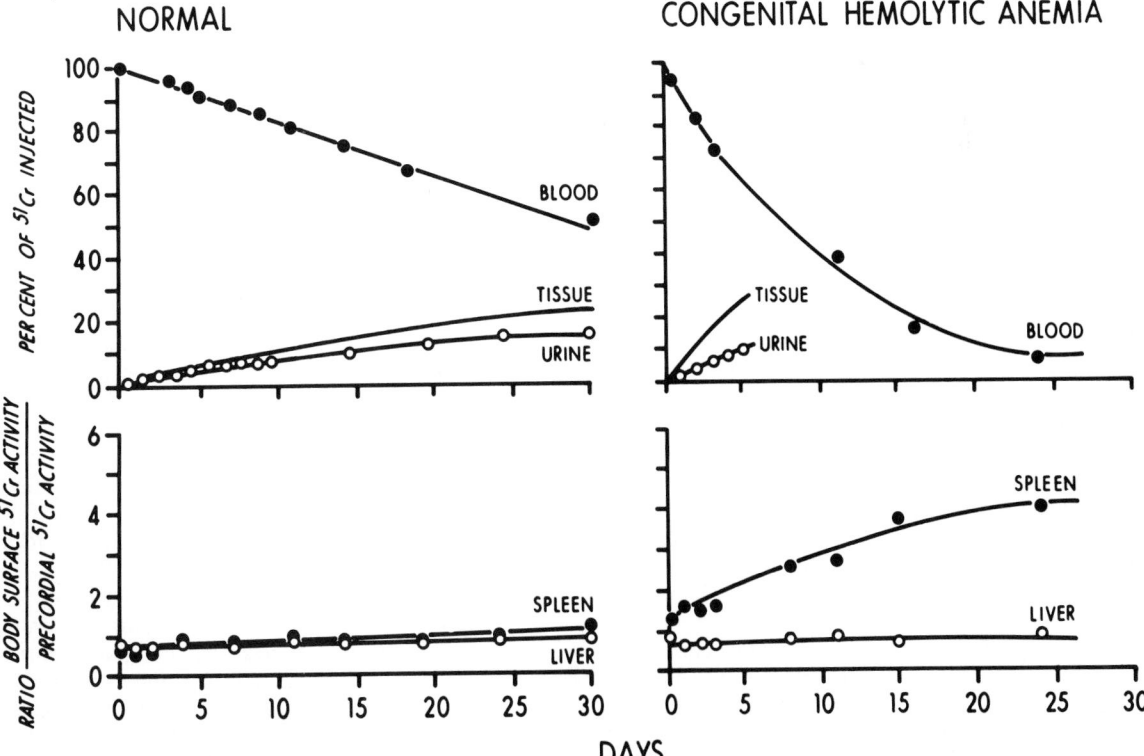

the decreased longevity of neutrophils or of measuring the role of the spleen in the destruction of these cells. The role of the spleen as a major offending organ has been precisely defined in patients with hypersplenism or immune thrombocytopenia. Platelet destruction in the spleen is such a common mechanism in thrombocytopenia that radioisotopic studies are not often done if the bone marrow aspirate indicates an abundance of megakaryocytes, suggesting adequate platelet production.

RUPTURE OF THE SPLEEN

The term "rupture" has been applied to splenic injuries in which there is disruption of the organ's parenchyma, capsule, or blood supply.

ETIOLOGY. The causes of splenic rupture include either transabdominal or transthoracic penetrating trauma, nonpenetrating trauma, operative trauma, and rarely, a spontaneous event.

Penetrating Trauma. Rupture of the spleen may occur as a consequence of large gunshot wounds or small puncture lacerations due to stabbing or missiles. The trajectory of the penetrating wound may pass through the anterior abdominal wall, through the flank, or transthoracically, piercing the pleural space, the lung, and the diaphragm. Isolated splenic injury may be present. With penetrating trauma, the associated organs most frequently injured include the stomach, the left kidney, the pancreas, and vascular structures at the root of the mesentery. Percutaneous splenic puncture to perform splenic pulp manometry and splenoportography may be associated with persistent bleeding, but this is uncommon in patients whose platelet counts are above 70,000 and whose prothrombin times are greater than 20 percent of normal.

Nonpenetrating Trauma. The spleen, alone or in combination with other viscera, is the most frequently injured organ following blunt trauma to the abdomen or the lower thoracic cage. Automobile accidents provide the predominating cause, while falls, sledding and bicycle injuries, and blows incurred during contact sports are frequently implicated in children. Splenic rupture that follows blunt trauma is an isolated event in only 30 percent of patients. The other organs that may be injured, in decreasing order of incidence, include (1) chest (rib fracture), (2) kidney, (3) spinal cord (fracture), (4) liver, (5) lung, (6) craniocerebral structures, (7) small intestine, (8) large intestine, (9) pancreas, and (10) stomach.

Operative Trauma. Operative trauma to the spleen most commonly occurs during operations on adjacent viscera. The spleen has been injured in about 2 percent of patients whose operations involved viscera of the left upper quadrant. Injury usually results from retractors placed against the organ in order to obtain exposure. This injury generally permits repair but may require splenectomy.

Spontaneous Rupture. Although spontaneous rupture of the normal spleen has been reported, it is a much more common event when the spleen is involved with a hematologic disorder. It is likely that the majority of patients classified as experiencing spontaneous rupture had

trauma that was not appreciated. Spontaneous rupture or rupture associated with minor trauma is the most common cause of death for patients with infectious mononucleosis which is second only to malaria as a cause of spontaneous splenic rupture. In patients with infectious mononucleosis, this complication occurs most frequently in the second to fourth weeks of the disease. Splenic rupture has also been reported in patients with sarcoidosis, acute and chronic leukemia, hemolytic anemia, congestive splenomegaly, polycythemia vera, and candidiasis with splenic abscesses.

PATHOLOGY. The spectrum of lesions associated with trauma to the spleen includes linear and stellate lacerations, capsular tears secondary to traction from adhesions or suspensory ligaments, puncture wounds caused by penetrating objects or fractured ribs, subcapsular intrasplenic hematomas, avulsion of the organ from its vascular pedicle, and laceration of the short gastric vessels within the gastrosplenic omentum. In view of the extreme friability and vascularity of the organ, even minor trauma may result in significant bleeding, particularly if the spleen is enlarged or diseased. Splenic injuries vary from simple transverse tears of the parenchyma to transverse cracks of the hilus, longitudinal injuries, subcapsular hematomas, or complete disruption of the organ and its vessels. Most injuries result in transverse ruptures of the parenchyma, the direction of rupture determined by the internal architecture of the organ which is arranged in a transverse plane.

Splenic rupture may be acute, delayed, or occult. *Acute rupture* that is attended by immediate intraperitoneal bleeding occurs in about 90 percent of the cases of blunt trauma to the spleen. *Delayed rupture,* with an interval of days or weeks between the injury and intraperitoneal bleeding, is reported in 10 to 15 percent of the cases of blunt trauma. The quiescent period, referred to as the "latent period of Baudet," persists for less than 7 days in half of these patients and less than 2 weeks in three-quarters of them. This is probably related to a temporary tamponade of a minor laceration or the presence of a slowly enlarging subcapsular hematoma that eventually ruptures. *Occult splenic rupture* is the term applied to traumatic pseudocysts of the spleen when injury to the organ previously has not been diagnosed. These appear in less than 1 percent of patients sustaining trauma and are generally caused by organization of an intrasplenic or parasplenic hematoma. Another pathologic lesion related to splenic trauma is *splenosis,* which is the result of autotransplantation of fragments of the traumatized spleen onto the peritoneal surfaces. Patients with splenosis are generally asymptomatic, but the lesions may stimulate adhesions that, in turn, lead to intestinal obstruction.

CLINICAL MANIFESTATIONS. The signs and symptoms produced by trauma to the spleen vary according to the severity and rapidity of intraabdominal hemorrhage, the presence of other organ injuries, and the interval between the injury and examination. The majority of patients present with some degree of hypovolemia, and tachycardia is almost always present. The latter is particularly evident when the pulse is recorded with the head of the patient elevated. A slight reduction of the blood pressure is characteristic. The patient usually complains of generalized upper abdominal pain, which in one-third of the cases is localized in the left upper quadrant. Pain at the tip of the shoulder (Kehr's sign) is evidence of diaphragmatic irritation but occurs in less than half the patients. If the patient is placed in the Trendelenburg position, left shoulder pain may be produced. Tenderness of the left upper quadrant or left flank is a frequent physical sign. A mass or a percussible area of fixed dullness in this region (Ballance's sign), secondary to subcapsular hematoma or omentum surrounding an extracapsular hemotoma, is rarely detected.

DIAGNOSTIC STUDIES. The hematocrit may be reduced if there is major bleeding, but the initial determination may be normal, emphasizing the fact that serial hematocrits are more meaningful. Increases of the white blood cell count to levels frequently greater than $15,000/mL^3$ are to be anticipated. Routine abdominal radiographs may demonstrate fractured ribs which should arouse suspicion of injury to the spleen. More specific findings that may be noted on abdominal films include: (1) elevated immobile left diaphragm, (2) an enlarged splenic shadow, (3) medial displacement of the gastric shadow with serration of the greater curvature due to dissection of blood into the gastrosplenic omentum, and (4) widening of the space between the splenic flexure and the properitoneal fat pad. Abdominal paracentesis yields a positive tap, i.e., return of blood that does not clot, in about 50 percent of the cases. A CT or radionuclide scan may define the lesion (Fig. 33-5). The diagnosis may be established angiographically by visualization of (1) the disruption, (2) radiopacity in the peritoneal cavity, or (3) early filling of the splenic vein.

TREATMENT. Iatrogenic lacerations that are detected intraoperatively usually can be repaired. Concern with the risk of asplenic sepsis has led to a change in approach to penetrating and blunt splenic trauma. In children many series have observed and avoided operative intervention for the majority of patients in whom scans have defined parenchymal rupture. The patients are observed for 7 to 14 days; delayed rupture rarely occurs. Operation is mandated if there is a suggestion of injury of other intraabdominal organs. The great majority of adult patients require surgical intervention. In children and adults in whom operation is performed, splenic repair can be successfully effected for the majority of parenchymal injuries. Hilar injury and extensive splenic injuries are more safely handled by splenectomy. Splenectomy as a lifesaving procedure is still the standard in many cases. The risk of late overwhelming postsplenectomy infection (OPSI) after splenectomy for trauma is very low in adults. Although some authors have championed reimplantation of splenic tissue in the omentum and have demonstrated its viability, there is consensus that the amount of tissue mass and the blood supply do not provide sufficient phagocytic clearance of the encapsulated bacteria implicated. In a recent series of 326 patients operated on for splenic trauma in whom 51 percent had penetrating wounds,

splenorrhaphy or no repair was performed in 42 percent. No patient required reexploration from the splenorrhaphy site.

An upper midline incision is generally preferred since this may be performed rapidly and can be extended to manage other intraabdominal injuries. The posterior approach to the splenic pedicle, emphasized by Dunphy, offers the most rapid means of controlling hemorrhage. Manual compression of the pedicle usually controls the bleeding and permits transection of the splenic ligaments and mobilization of the spleen forward and medially. Under adequate exposure lacerations may be sutured over omentum, oxidized cellulose, or micronized collagen. A damaged pole or segment may be excised and the raw edges compressed using sutures tied over the same hemostatic materials. The operative mortality for isolated penetrating injuries of the spleen is less than 1 percent. Operative mortality for blunt trauma to the spleen alone ranges between 5 and 15 percent, while the rates are between 15 and 40 percent when other serious concomitant injuries occur. All splenectomized patients should receive Pneumovax *Haemophilus influenzae* vaccine, if available, and children should also be given oral penicillin daily until age eighteen.

HEMATOLOGIC DISORDERS FOR WHICH SPLENECTOMY IS POTENTIALLY THERAPEUTIC

In 1887, Spencer-Wells performed a therapeutic splenectomy in a patient with what subsequently proved to be hereditary spherocytosis. Since then, as a consequence of appreciation of the physiology and pathophysiology of the spleen, the application of splenectomy for hematologic disorders has been extended.

Hemolytic Anemias

This category includes a broad spectrum of disorders in which there is accelerated destruction of mature red blood cells. Hemolytic anemias are generally classified as congenital or acquired. The congenital anemias are due to an intrinsic abnormality of the erythrocytes, and the acquired anemias are related to an extracorpuscular factor acting on an intrinsically normal cell. In both types of disorder, the reduced red blood cell survival may be demonstrated by measuring the disappearance of the patient's radioactive erythrocytes (labeled with ^{51}Cr), and the spleen's role may be evaluated by determining the relative uptakes of this radioactivity by the spleen and liver (Fig. 33-6).

HEREDITARY SPHEROCYTOSIS. Hereditary spherocytosis is transmitted as an autosomal dominant trait and is the most common of the symptomatic familial hemolytic anemias. The fundamental abnormality stems from a defective erythrocyte membrane that causes the cell to be smaller than normal, unusually thick, and almost spherical in shape. These cells also demonstrate increased osmotic fragility, i.e., lysis occurs at a higher concentration of sodium chloride than normal. The role of the spleen in this disorder is related to the inability of the spherocytic cells to pass through the splenic pulp. The cells that escape from the spleen are more susceptible to trapping and disintegration during each successive passage, until cell loss ensues. The precise pathogenesis of the cell injury may relate to a decreased availability of red cell ATP in the environment of the spleen, combined with a cell membrane that has been shown in in vitro studies to be more susceptible to reduction in ATP levels.

The salient clinical features of the disease are anemia, reticulocytosis, jaundice, and splenomegaly. It is unusual for the anemia to be extremely severe, and the jaundice usually parallels the severity of the anemia. Periodic and sudden increases in the intensity of the anemia and jaundice may occur, and rare, fatal crises have been reported. Cholelithiasis with gallstones of the pigmented variety has been reported in 30 to 60 percent of the patients but is rare in children under the age of ten. Leg ulcers are uncommon specific manifestations.

Diagnosis is generally established by the peripheral blood smear, which demonstrates that more than 60 percent of the red blood cells are spherocytic-shaped with a mean diameter less than normal and a thickness greater than normal. Increased osmotic fragility of the red blood cells provides diagnostic confirmation, but this test rarely is performed.

Splenectomy is the sole therapy for hereditary spherocytosis. It is generally recommended that the operation be delayed until the fourth year of life. Intractable leg ulcers indicate early splenectomy, as they heal only after the spleen is removed. The results of splenectomy have been uniformly good. Although an inherent membrane abnormality persists and the spherocytosis and increased osmotic fragility of the cells are not altered, in vivo hemolysis virtually ceases and, following removal of the spleen, the erythrocytes achieve a normal life span and the jaundice, if present, disappears. It is appropriate to perform an oral cholecystogram or ultrasonogram prior to splenectomy, and the gallbladder should always be examined at the time of operation. If gallstones are present, the gallbladder should be removed during the operation.

HEREDITARY ELLIPTOCYTOSIS. Ovalocytosis and stomatocytosis usually exist as harmless traits, but occasionally, when these forms constitute 50 to 90 percent of the red cell population, clinical manifestations indistinguishable from those noted with hereditary spherocytosis may occur. Splenectomy is indicated for all symptomatic patients since removal of the organ often is followed by decreased hemolysis and corrected anemia, although the morphologic abnormality of the red blood cell remains unchanged. Associated cholelithiasis should be managed as in hereditary spherocytosis.

HEREDITARY HEMOLYTIC ANEMIA WITH ENZYME DEFICIENCY. Included in this category are: (1) enzyme deficiencies in anaerobic glycolytic pathways, the prototype of which is the pyruvate-kinase deficiency (PK), and (2) enzyme deficiencies in the hexose monophosphate shunt, the prototype of which is the glucose-6-phosphate deficiency (G-6-PD). These deficiencies render the cells susceptible to increased hemolysis. Splenic enlargement occurs more frequently with PK deficiency, and the spleen is rarely enlarged in patients with G-6-PD deficiency. Specific enzyme assays are employed to define the deficiency.

The majority of patients maintain hemoglobins greater than 8 g/dL, are asymptomatic, and do not require therapy. With significant anemia, blood transfusions are indicated, and the transfused cells survive normally. ^{51}Cr-tagged red cell studies are not predictive of results with a high enough degree of accuracy to be useful. In severe cases of PK deficiency, splenectomy may be worthwhile. In patients with this disorder, postoperative thrombocytosis with consequent hepatic, portal, or inferior vena caval thrombosis may occur if the hemolytic rate is unabated. Splenectomy is not indicated for patients with G-6-PD deficiency.

THALASSEMIA. Thalassemia (Mediterranean anemia) is transmitted as a dominant trait and primarily derives from a defect in hemoglobin synthesis. The development of intracellular precipitates (Heinz bodies) contributes to premature red cell destruction. The disease is classified as alpha, beta, and gamma types, determined by the specific defect in synthesis rate of the peptide chain. In the United States, most patients are of southern European origin and suffer from beta thalassemia, i.e., a quantitative reduction in the rate of beta chain synthesis, resulting in a decrease in hemoglobin A (Hb-A). Thalassemia occurs in two major degrees of severity: homozygous thalassemia (thalassemia major), a severe disorder in which the affected child receives a gene for thalassemia from each parent, and heterozygous thalassemia (thalassemia minor), a mild disorder in which the affected child receives a gene from only one parent. Gradations of thalassemia range from heterozygous thalassemia (minor), often not detected until examination of the blood for an unrelated problem, to homozygous thalassemia, a severe, chronic anemia, with icterus, splenomegaly, and death early in life. In thalassemia minor, Hb-A$_2$ is always increased, and slight increases in Hb-F occur in 50 percent of patients. In both types of thalassemia, the hemoglobin-deficient cells are small, thin, and misshapen. These cells appear washed out and have a characteristic resistance to osmotic lysis.

The clinical manifestations of thalassemia major usually occur in the first year of life and consist of pallor, retarded body growth, and enlargement of the head. Intractable leg ulcers may be noted, intercurrent infections are common, and gallstones are reported in about 24 percent of patients. The manifestations of thalassemia minor may vary. Most patients with thalassemia minor lead normal lives, but some patients have a more severe expression of their disease (referred to as thalassemia intermedia) and generally present with signs and symptoms attributable to mild anemia, chronic mild jaundice, and moderate splenomegaly.

The diagnosis of thalassemia major is established by the smear revealing the hypochromic, microcytic anemia with markedly distorted red cells of various sizes and shapes. Nucleated red cells invariably are present, and the reticulocyte count is elevated, as is the white blood count. The characteristic feature of the disease is the persistence of Hb-F and a reduction in Hb-A, demonstrated by the alkali denaturation study. Importantly, both parents should have evidence of thalassemia minor.

Treatment is directed only at symptomatic patients. Transfusions are usually required at regular intervals, but as most patients accommodate to low hemoglobin levels, the transfusions should be directed at maintaining the hemoglobin level at 10 g/dL. Although splenectomy does not influence the basic hematologic disorder, it may reduce both the hemolytic process and the transfusion requirements. Marked splenomegaly and/or symptomatic repeated splenic infarction also constitute indications for splenectomy. Severe infection generally occurs within 10 years of splenectomy. Because there is little difference in the risk of infection related to removal of the organ, the overall benefit-to-risk ratio favors splenectomy when appropriate indications are present.

SICKLE CELL DISEASE. Sickle cell anemia is a hereditary hemolytic anemia seen predominantly in blacks and characterized by the presence of sickle- and crescent-shaped erythrocytes. In this hereditary hemoglobinopathy, the normal Hb-A is replaced by the abnormal form of hemoglobin, sickle hemoglobin (Hb-S). Hb-F is also usually mildly increased. Combinations of Hb-S with other hemoglobin variants also occur as a result of an abnormal trait inherited from each parent, e.g., Hb-S/Hb-C or Hb-S/thalassemia.

Under conditions of reduced oxygen tension, Hb-S molecules undergo crystallization within the red cell, which elongates and distorts the cell. The sickling phenomenon occurs more readily with higher percentages of Hb-S, with a reduced pH, and under conditions of circulatory stasis that tend to exaggerate hemoglobin deoxygenation. The sickle cells, themselves, contribute to increased blood viscosity and circulatory stasis, thus establishing a vicious cycle. The primary consequence of this stagnation is thrombosis, which leads to ischemia, necrosis, and organ fibrosis.

The role of the spleen in this disorder is not clear. Early in the course of the disease, splenomegaly occurs, but following varying intervals in most patients, the spleen undergoes infarction and marked contraction with eventual autosplenectomy.

Although the sickle cell trait occurs in approximately 9 percent of the black population, the majority of patients are asymptomatic. However, sickle cell anemia has been observed in 0.3 to 1.3 percent of blacks, who often show remarkable adaptation to the state of chronic anemia and jaundice. This adaptive state may be interrupted at intervals by acute symptoms or crises that are related to vascular occlusion. Depending on the vessels involved, the patient may have bone or joint pain, hematuria, priapism, neurologic manifestations, or ulcers over the malleoli. Abdominal pain and cramps due to visceral stasis are frequent, stimulating an acute surgical abdomen. Thrombosis of the splenic vessels may result in an unusual complication of splenic abscess, manifested by splenomegaly, splenic pain, and fever. Most patients with sickle cell

anemia die in the first decade of life, but a few survive to the fifth decade. Death may be the result of intercurrent infections or cardiac or renal failure.

The diagnosis is established by the presence of anemia, characteristic sickle cells on smear, hemoglobin electrophoresis showing 80 percent or more Hb-S, and the presence of the trait in both parents. Leukocytosis is often noted, and the platelets are frequently increased in number. There may be modest elevation of the serum bilirubin, and cholelithiasis is a frequent accompaniment.

For most patients only palliative treatment is possible. Recently, studies have shown that sodium cyanate will prevent sickling of Hb-S. Transfusions may be required to maintain adequate hemoglobin levels. Adequate hydration and partial exchange transfusion may help during a crisis. In the circumstance of splenic abscess, incision and drainage of the abscess cavity within the parenchyma of the spleen may be necessitated, since removal of the organ is hindered by marked inflammatory and adhesive processes. Splenectomy may be of benefit in a very few patients in whom acute splenic sequestration of red cells can be demonstrated, although the operation does not affect the sickling process. A recent report reviewed the data on 46 children who underwent splenectomy for hypersplenism and 14 patients operated on for acute splenic sequestration. The median follow-up was 6 years. Two patients died of overwhelming sepsis; neither received prophylaxis, and neither pneumococcal septicemia nor meningitis was confirmed.

IDIOPATHIC AUTOIMMUNE HEMOLYTIC ANEMIA. This is a disorder in which the life span of a presumably normal erythrocyte is shortened when exposed to an endogenous hemolytic mechanism. The etiology has not been defined, but an autoimmune process appears to be fundamental. In such patients, antibodies reacting with the patient's normal red cells have been defined, and there is evidence that the spleen may serve as a source of antibody. Both "warm" and "cold" antibodies have been described. Some "warm" antibodies have Rh specificity. Most of these antibodies are hemagglutinins rather than hemolysins. It is believed that the reticuloendothelial system traps and destroys the immunologically altered cells. Sequestration occurs primarily in the spleen. By binding the F_c portion of the IgG molecule to the corresponding macrophage surface F_c receptor, the spherocytes become more rigid and more sensitive to destruction in the splenic circulation.

Although autoimmune hemolytic anemia may be encountered at any age, it occurs more frequently after the age of fifty and twice as often in females. Mild jaundice is often present. The spleen is palpably enlarged in half the cases, and gallstones have been demonstrated in a quarter of the cases. The extent of anemia varies, and hemoglobinuria and tubular necrosis have been reported in severe cases. In this circumstance, the prognosis is serious, as the mortality rate is 40 to 50 percent.

The diagnosis of hemolysis is made by demonstrating anemia and reticulocytosis accompanied by the products of red cell destruction in the blood, urine, and stool. The bone marrow is hypercellular with a predominance of

by fragmentation and immature forms and poikilocytosis with numerous teardrop and elongated shapes. Characteristically, the patients have anemia of the normochromic type. The white blood cell count is under 50,000 in the majority of the cases but may reach extremely high levels. Immature myeloid cells are found in the peripheral smear. The platelet counts are normal in about a quarter of the patients, thrombocytopenia is present in about one-third, and marked thrombocytopenia is present in 5 percent. Thrombocytosis over 1 million per cubic millimeter is observed in one-quarter of the patients. The platelets frequently are enlarged and bizarre in appearance. The leukocyte alkaline phosphatase usually is high, and hyperuricemia frequently is present. Radiographs of the bone demonstrate increased density in approximately 50 percent of the patients, particularly in the pelvic region. Marrow biopsy sections show varying degrees of bone marrow replacement by fibrous tissue interposed with small foci of megakaryocytes, erythropoiesis, and myeloid cells.

Treatment is generally directed at the anemia and splenomegaly. It usually consists of transfusions, hormones, chemotherapy, and radiotherapy. Male hormone preparations may be of value in patients with anemia due to marrow failure. Alkylating agents may be effective in reducing splenic size and transfusion requirements as well as for patients whose predominant clinical problem is hypermetabolism. Busulfan is the most commonly used alkylating agent, but cyclophosphamide may also be used in thrombocytopenic subjects since it is less likely to suppress platelet production. Since patients with myelofibrosis are very sensitive to chemotherapy, such agents must be used very cautiously.

Although splenectomy does not alter the general course of the disorder, the procedure is indicated for control of anemia, thrombocytopenia, and for symptoms attributable to splenomegaly. Thrombocytopenia associated with sufficiently reduced megakaryocytes to contraindicate chemotherapy is also a frequent indication for splenectomy, as is the large spleen that causes digestive difficulties or is symptomatic because of multiple infarctions despite chemotherapy and/or local irradiation. In patients with esophagogastric varices portal pressures should be determined before and after splenectomy. In most instances splenectomy alone will effect significant reduction in pressure and obviate the need for a concomitant splenorenal or portacaval shunt.

Splenectomy rarely has a deleterious effect on the hematologic status of the patient, and the old concept that splenectomy resulted in the removal of a significant hemopoietic element does not pertain. The incidence of the mortality and morbidity rates for patients with myeloid metaplasia undergoing splenectomy are higher than those reported for other hematologic disorders. Postoperative thrombocytosis and/or thrombosis of the splenic vein extending into the portal and mesenteric vein occur more commonly in these patients. The incidence of this complication can be reduced by correction of a thrombocytotic state, if present, preoperatively using alkylating agents and the use of drugs to prevent platelet aggregation during the perioperative period.

Hodgkin's Disease, Lymphomas, and Leukemias

Chemotherapy and/or radiation therapy are the standard approaches to treatment of these disorders. Splenectomy may be indicated for patients with symptomatic splenomegaly, with anemia and increasing transfusion requirements, or with cytopenia that limits systemic therapy.

In both Hodgkin's disease and non-Hodgkin's lymphoma splenectomy has improved cytopenia in over 75 percent of cases. In these patients, palliative splenectomy should be performed before the platelet count is excessively low or there are marked clinical abnormalities. In these groups of patients 2- and 5-year survivals after splenectomy of 44 and 26 percent, respectively, have been reported. Equally favorable hematologic responses have also been reported for patients with chronic lymphatic leukemia. Palliative splenectomy may be indicated for symptomatic splenomegaly in these patients and an occasional patient with myelogenous leukemia. It has been reported that survival is extended by splenectomy in patients with blastic crises, but this has not been substantiated.

Hairy cell leukemia, or reticuloendotheliosis, is characterized by malignant cells with filamentous cytoplasmic projections. Patients without symptomatic splenomegaly and few "hairy" cells in the circulating blood do well without any treatment. Patients who live 4 years after the diagnosis has been established have a favorable long-term prognosis. Hairy cell leukemia frequently is accompanied by problems caused by neutropenia, thrombocytopenia, and anemia. Splenectomy is very effective therapy in these situations. A complete response occurs in two-thirds to three-quarters of patients and a partial response is effected in another 20 percent. The 5-year survival has been reported as 61 to 76 percent. The response to splenectomy is unrelated to the weight of the spleen. Failures are managed with steroids and chemotherapeutic agents. Survival is not related to the hematologic response to splenectomy.

STAGING OF HODGKIN'S DISEASE AND NON-HODGKIN'S LYMPHOMA

The diagnosis of Hodgkin's disease is generally established by histologic evaluation of a clinically suspect area of lymphadenopathy or splenomegaly. Demonstration of the typical, large, multinuclear cell, the Sternberg-Reed cell, is regarded as essential for the diagnosis. However, these cells do not form the bulk of the tumor. Four major histologic types have been defined: lymphocyte predominance, nodular sclerosis, mixed cellularity, and lymphocyte depletion. Survival with Hodgkin's disease is related in part to the histologic type and also to the distribution of disease and the presence or absence of specific symptoms. Stage I disease is defined as limited to one anatomic region; Stage II disease is limited to two or more contiguous or noncontiguous regions on the same side of the diaphragm; Stage III disease refers to disease on both sides of the diaphragm with involvement limited to lymph nodes, spleen, and Waldeyer's ring; and Stage IV refers to involvement of the bone marrow, lung, liver, skin, gastrointestinal tract, and any organ or tissue other than the lymph nodes or Waldeyer's ring.

The application of laparotomy, splenectomy, liver biopsy, and retroperitoneal node biopsy as diagnostic tools is based on the following considerations: (1) the lesion generally begins as a single focus and spreads in a predictable manner along adjacent lymph channels, (2) prognosis is related to clinical stage, (3) therapy may be dictated by clinical stage, and (4) previous methods of evaluating the clinical stage, including the physical examination, laboratory studies, and radiographic studies have significant degrees of inaccuracy. The procedure begins with a wedge biopsy of the liver performed before retractors are applied to avoid confusion of white cell migration. Splenectomy is then performed, the entire periaortic chain of lymph nodes is examined, and representative nodes are removed. The sites of lymph node removal are chosen according to preoperative CT, lymphangiography, and surgical evaluation. Examination of the upper aortic chain, facilitated by transecting the ligament of Treitz, has proved most rewarding in regard to positive lymph node findings. Representative mesenteric and hepatoduodenal nodes should also be biopsied. A liberal iliac crest marrow biopsy is generally included.

The spleen is involved with Hodgkin's disease in 39 percent of patients surgically staged. The error for patients with preoperative diagnoses of splenic involvement based on palpability, and/or scintillation scan studies that suggested enlargement is 38 percent, while the error for patients with preoperative diagnoses of normal spleens is 36 percent. Accessory spleens are positive for disease in 7 percent of cases. The liver is suspected of being infiltrated by Hodgkin's disease if there is evidence of hepatomegaly, if liver function tests demonstrate abnormalities, or if liver scans define a space-occupying lesion. Preoperative suspicion of Hodgkin's disease of the liver is incorrect in 45 percent of the cases, whereas clinical judgment that the liver is not involved is incorrect in only 4 percent. Abdominal lymphoangiography has been replaced largely by computer tomographic assessment of lymphatic involvement. Thirty percent of positive lymphangiograms were not confirmed by laparotomy, while 15 percent of patients whose lymphangiograms were considered normal were shown to have Hodgkin's involvement of the retroperitoneal nodes. Summary of the reported cases indicates that surgical staging upgraded the clinical stage in 27 to 36 percent of cases and decreased it in 7 to 15 percent, for a total alteration of about 42 percent.

In staging young women, oophoropexy should be performed to reduce the incidence of radiation-induced menopause and to permit subsequent pregnancies. In the Stanford series of 825 staging laparotomies, 48 women had 70 pregnancies subsequent to the procedure and definite therapy. Restaging laparotomy has been useful in documenting residual or recurrent disease. A laparotomy with negative findings spares the patient added treatment without compromising survival.

The applicability of surgical staging in patients with Hodgkin's disease has not been resolved. It is generally agreed that the procedure is indicated for a patient with Hodgkin's disease who presents evidence or suggestion of disease in the upper part of the abdomen, provided that the patient is not jaundiced and does not have other evidence of significant hepatic dysfunction. Other generally accepted indications include the presence of systemic symptoms in clinical Stages I and II patients, and a mixed cellularity or lymphocyte depletion type of histology. By contrast, in patients with high cervical, lymphocyte-predominant lesions and no evidence of mediastinal involvement, staging is not indicated, since these lesions rarely involve the subdiaphragmatic nodes.

The argument regarding the role of staging centers around patients with clinical Stage I-A or II-A (asymptomatic). Those in favor base their opinion on negligible mortality and morbidity rates coupled with the additional "bonus" that splenectomy has facilitated radiation therapy and reduced the potential radiation pneumonitis and/or nephritis as well as leukopenia and thrombocytopenia that may complicate either radiotherapy or chemotherapy. The objections to routine staging in these patients relate to the facts that (1) some series do include perioperative deaths, and (2) the problem of susceptibility to infection subsequent to splenectomy has not been resolved. It has also been pointed out that ablation of the spleen can be accomplished by radiation therapy; many therapists advocate prophylactically treating all infradiaphragmatic areas in patients with Stages I and II Hodgkin's disease.

In reference to the routine staging for non-Hodgkin's lymphoma, a difference of opinion also pertains. Veronesi and associates conclude that diagnostic laparotomy and staging should be carried out in centers in which the information can be translated into aggressive treatment, but feel that it should not have the wide adoption that Hodgkin's staging has had. Chabner et al. reported that percutaneous and peritoneoscopically directed biopsies were reasonable alternatives to staging for non-Hodgkin's lymphoma and that the presence or absence of subdiaphragmatic disease could be established in over 80 percent of the patients by nonsurgical procedures, including lymphangiography, marrow biopsy, and percutaneous liver biopsy.

Miscellaneous Diseases

FELTY'S SYNDROME. The triad of rheumatoid arthritis, splenomegaly, and neutropenia is referred to as Felty's syndrome. Mild anemia and/or thrombocytopenia have been noted in some cases, and gastric achlorhydria is common. An antibody specifically directed against neutrophil nuclei is nearly always demonstrable by fluorescent stains. Corticosteroids and splenectomy have been used to reverse the neutropenia in order to reduce susceptibility to infection. The response to steroids is usually not long-lasting, but the hematologic effects of splenectomy generally are excellent. Splenectomy in these patients should be reserved for neutropenic patients having serious or recurrent infections, patients requiring transfusions for anemia, patients with profound thrombocytopenia, and for those with intractable leg ulcers. There is a sharp rise in the total number of leukocytes in the first 24 h, reaching a peak at about the third postoperative day. Although relative neutropenia may persist, the neutrophilic response to infection in the postsplenectomy state becomes normal. However, the clinical course of the arthritis is rarely altered.

SARCOIDOSIS. This disease affects young adults. There are few constitutional symptoms, and fever is unusual, although night sweats have been noted. Cough and shortness of breath may attend mediastinal or pulmonary involvement. Skin lesions appear in about 50 percent of patients, and generalized lymphadenopathy is frequent. Involvement of the liver and spleen may produce hepatomegaly and splenomegaly in about 25 percent of the cases. About 20 percent of the patients with splenomegaly develop manifestations of hypersplenism, particularly thrombocytopenic purpura. Hemolytic anemia, neutropenia, pancytopenia, and spontaneous splenic rupture have all been observed.

There is no specific treatment, and spontaneous recovery can be anticipated in the majority of cases. Splenectomy should be considered for patients with splenomegaly when there are complications of hypersplenism, since the operation has been almost uniformly followed by correction of the hematologic abnormality.

GAUCHER'S DISEASE. This is a familial disorder characterized by abnormal storage or retention of glycolipid cerebrosides in reticuloendothelial cells. Proliferation and enlargement of these cells produces enlargement of the spleen, liver, and lymph nodes. The disease is generally discovered in childhood but may become evident either early in infancy or late in adult life.

The sole clinical manifestation may be awareness of a progressively enlarging abdominal mass, primarily due to splenomegaly and, to a lesser extent, to hepatomegaly. The yellowish-brown pigmentation of the head and extremities occurs in about 45 to 75 percent of cases. Bone pain and pathologic fracture may develop in long-standing cases. Many patients develop the hematologic manifestations of hypersplenism as a result of excessive sequestration of formed blood elements. Moderate to severe thrombocytopenia and normocytic anemia are almost always present, and often there is mild leukopenia. In the patients with hypersplenism, splenectomy almost uniformly has been beneficial in correcting the hematologic disorder, but there is no evidence that the operation influences the course of the basic disease. Partial splenectomy has been performed in children for symptomatic splenomegaly and hypersplenism to obviate OPSI; 400 to 3800 g of tissue has been removed without complication. There has been no OPSI and no postoperative increase in accu-

mulation of beta-glucocerebroside in the liver or bones. All children had an improved growth wave and hematologic picture.

PORPHYRIA ERYTHROPOIETICA. This is a congenital disorder of erythrocyte pyrrole metabolism that is transmitted as a recessive trait and characterized by the excessive deposition of porphyrins in the tissues. In the skin this results in pronounced photosensitization and severe bullous dermatitis. Premature red cell destruction within the spleen contributes to severe anemia. When the disease is complicated by hemolysis or splenomegaly, splenectomy is followed by marked improvement in the anemia and decreased concentrations of porphyrins in the red cells, bone marrow, and urine.

MISCELLANEOUS LESIONS

ECTOPIC SPLEEN. This unusual condition is ascribed to lengthening of the splenic ligaments that results in extreme mobility of the organ so that the spleen of normal size may be palpable in the lower abdomen or in the pelvis. In some cases, acute torsion of the pedicle occurs, necessitating surgical intervention.

SPLENIC ARTERY ANEURYSM. The splenic artery is the most common site of intraabdominal aneurysm other than the aorta. The incidence of splenic artery aneurysm ranges between 0.02 and 0.16 percent in autopsy series. The lesions occur more frequently in females, and the most common predisposing factor is atherosclerosis. Splenic artery aneurysms are usually discovered as incidental findings on an abdominal x-ray, and a bruit is rarely heard in the left upper quadrant. The frequency of rupture is generally less than 10 percent, with about 20 percent of ruptures having occurred during pregnancy. Excision of the aneurysm, with or without splenectomy, is recommended for enlarging or symptomatic aneurysms, and in women in the child-bearing age. In many asymptomatic patients close observation is justified.

CYSTS AND TUMORS. Cysts of the spleen are unusual. Parasitic cysts are usually due to echinococcal involvement, while the nonparasitic cysts may be categorized as dermoid, epidermoid, epithelial, and pseudocysts. Pseudocysts occur after occult rupture of the spleen.

Primary and malignant tumors of the spleen are sarcomatous. Recent autopsy series have refuted the concept that metastases to the spleen are rare. However, laparotomy for undiagnosed splenomegaly that reveals unsuspected metastatic deposit in the absence of known generalized metastases is extremely uncommon.

ABSCESSES. Splenic abscess is an uncommon cause of abdominal sepsis. Primary splenic abscesses occur much more often in the tropics, where they are frequently related to thrombosis of the splenic vessels with infarction in patients with sickle cell anemia. Clinical manifestations include fever, chills, splenomegaly, and left upper quadrant tenderness. Diagnosis may be established by ultrasound and CT scan (see Fig. 33-8) or angiography. Removal of the spleen is the operation of choice, but some cases have been treated with splenotomy and drainage

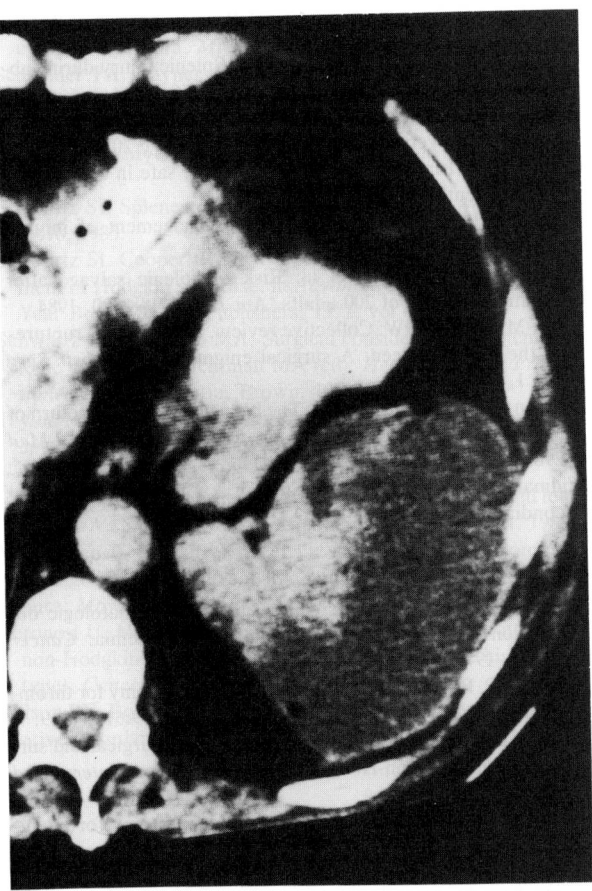

Fig. 33-8. Initial CT scan at the level of the spleen. There is a large low-density area in the spleen containing tiny gas pockets indicative of splenic abscess. (*Courtesy of Robert M. Lerner, Department of Radiology, University of Rochester Medical Center.*)

when there were gross adhesions or the condition of the patient did not permit splenectomy. Splenic fungal abscesses have developed in patients taking steroids and chemotherapeutic agents. Many of these patients have been on systemic antibiotics and intestinal colonization with candida developed. In some cases, the abscesses resolved with antifungal drugs, but more often success has been achieved when the drugs were combined with splenectomy.

SPLENECTOMY

When elective splenectomy is performed for hematologic disorders, specific considerations arise. Patients with malignant lymphoma and leukemia may develop cryoglobulinemia and, therefore, the blood should be administered at room temperature. For patients with thalassemia and, more particularly, acquired hemolytic anemia, typing and cross matching may be difficult, and sufficient time should be allotted during the preoperative period to accumulate the blood that may be required during the operation. For patients with marked immune

thrombocytopenia (ITP), platelet packs are not administered preoperatively since the platelets are rapidly destroyed by the spleen and, therefore, are not very effective. A nasogastric tube is inserted after endotracheal intubation to decompress the stomach and to facilitate handling of the short gastric veins.

TECHNIQUE. Although the midline incision is preferred for exposure of a ruptured spleen, either a left subcostal incision or midline incision may be used for elective resection. The spleen is mobilized initially by dividing the ligamentous attachments, which are usually avascular but may contain large vessels in patients with secondary hypersplenism and myeloid metaplasia. The short gastric vessels then are doubly ligated and transected, taking care not to traumatize the stomach itself. If compromise of blood supply to the fundic portion of the greater curvature of the stomach is a concern, enfolding of this area should be performed to prevent the development of a gastric fistula. This permits ultimate dissection of the splenic hilus with individual ligation and division of the splenic artery and vein. During the course of hilar dissection, care should be taken to avoid injury to the tail of the pancreas in order to obviate pseudocyst formation. The technique of initial ligation of the splenic artery by exposure through the gastrosplenic omentum is applicable to the small spleen but not appropriate when there is marked splenomegaly or when large lymphomatous lymph nodes encircle the splenic vessels. Whenever splenectomy is performed for hematologic disorder, a careful search should be made for accessory spleens. The splenic bed is not drained routinely, but drains are used in patients with myeloid metaplasia if there is a question of continued oozing from distended collateral veins.

POSTOPERATIVE COURSE AND COMPLICATIONS. Following splenectomy, characteristic changes in blood composition occur. Howell-Jolly bodies are present in almost all patients, and siderocytes are common. Generally, leukocytosis and increased platelet counts are observed. In patients with marked thrombocytopenia, the platelet count often returns to normal within 2 days, but peak levels may not be reached for 2 weeks. The white blood cell count usually is elevated the first day and may remain persistently elevated for several months. The most frequent complication is that of left lower lobe atelectasis. Other complications include subphrenic hematoma and abscess, injury to the pancreas causing fistula, or pancreatitis. Excessively elevated platelet counts, particularly in patients with myeloid metaplasia, and increased platelet adhesiveness have been reported. Although these factors have been implicated in the greater incidence of thrombophlebitis following splenectomy, many series can show no good correlation between these complications and the platelet counts. In patients with hereditary hemolytic anemia and associated red cell enzyme deficiency, postoperative thrombocytosis may lead to hepatic, portal, or caval thrombosis particularly if the hemolytic rate is unabated by splenectomy.

There has been increasing concern regarding infection and sepsis in splenectomized patients. In a large review Singer reported that deaths from sepsis in splenectomized

additional responses due to the presence of infection also occur. The general responses, found to some degree whenever peritonitis occurs, are described here; the additional reactions specific to the various clinical forms of peritonitis are described in following sections.

Primary Responses in Peritonitis

MEMBRANE INFLAMMATION. The peritoneum responds to insult with hyperemia followed by transudation. Edema and vascular congestion occur in the subperitoneal tissues immediately external to the peritoneal membrane. Absorption across inflamed peritoneum in early peritonitis is slightly increased. In later stages, and in chronic peritonitis, absorption is decreased. Absorption of macromolecules appears to be more affected than absorption of small molecules. Transudation of fluid with a low protein content from the extracellular interstitial compartment into the abdominal cavity is accompanied by diapedesis of large numbers of polymorphonuclear leukocytes. During the early vascular and transudative phase of engorgement, the peritoneum acts as a "two-way street," so that toxins and other materials that may be present in peritoneal fluid are readily absorbed, enter the lymphatics and bloodstream, and may lead to systemic symptoms.

Transudation of interstitial fluid into the peritoneal cavity across the inflamed peritoneum is shortly followed by exudation of protein-rich fluid. The fluid exudate in the peritoneal cavity contains large amounts of fibrin and other plasma proteins in concentrations sufficient to bring about clotting that, in turn, results in agglutination of loops of bowel, other viscera, and the parietes in the area of peritoneal inflammation. This response helps to confine the source of peritoneal contamination.

The metabolic changes in the inflamed human peritoneum are similar to those of dermal inflammation but occur more quickly. There is increased synthesis of membrane glycoproteins and proteoglycans. The concentration of uronic acid also increases, probably reflecting exudation of plasma proteins in the early stages of peritonitis and, in later stages, increased synthesis of glycoaminoglycans due to the activation of fibroblasts and mesothelial cells.

Changes in noncollagen protein synthesis and in collagen concentration are two other metabolic events that occur in the inflamed peritoneum during peritonitis. In early peritonitis, noncollagen protein synthesis is increased while collagen concentration is decreased. Later, collagen concentration increases owing to increased total protein synthesis. The RNA/DNA ratio, an index of the protein synthesizing capability of tissues, increases during the first week of peritonitis.

Experimental studies of energy metabolism of the peritoneal membrane in peritonitis have shown increased oxygen and glucose consumption and increased lactate production. There is also increased anaerobic metabolism due mainly to glycolysis. Coupled with decreasing oxygen partial pressure and increased oxygen consumption, this leads to a hypoxic environment in the peritoneal cavity that may favor adhesion formation. Though these metabolic changes return to normal with time, removal of the causative agent and the oxygen-consuming peritoneal fluid cells is the cornerstone of treatment of peritonitis.

BOWEL RESPONSE. The initial response of the bowel to peritoneal irritation is transient hypermotility. After a short interval, motility becomes depressed, and nearly complete adynamic ileus soon follows. The bowel distends, and both air and fluid accumulate in the lumen. The source of the accumulating gas is largely swallowed air. Fluid secretion (exsorption) into the bowel lumen is enhanced in ileus, while resorption (insorption) is relatively impaired, promoting sequestration of fluid in the bowel lumen that contributes to the decreased extracellular fluid volume found in peritonitis. In bacterial peritonitis, oxygen consumption of the bowel is decreased possibly owing to absorption of toxic substances through its peritoneal (serosal) surface.

HYPOVOLEMIA. The peritoneum reacts to irritation by vascular dilation and an outpouring of plasmalike fluid from the extracellular, intravascular, and interstitial compartments into the peritoneal space as an exudate. The loose connective tissue beneath the mesothelium of the viscera, the mesenteries, and the parietes traps extracellular fluid as edema. The atonic, dilated bowel also accumulates fluid in its lumen that is derived from the extracellular fluid volume. This translocation of water, electrolytes, and protein into a sequestered "third space" functionally removes this volume temporarily from the body economy. The rate of functional extracellular fluid loss is proportional to the surface area of peritoneum involved in the inflammatory process. With extensive peritonitis, fluid translocation of 4 to 6 L or more in 24 h is not uncommon.

Secondary Responses in Peritonitis

ENDOCRINE RESPONSE. Peritonitis acts as a stimulus to many endocrine organs. There is an almost immediate adrenal medullary response, with outpouring of epinephrine and norepinephrine, producing systemic vasoconstriction, tachycardia, and sweating. The adrenal cortex is stimulated to increased secretion of cortical hormones during the first 2 to 3 days following peritoneal injury. Originally thought to be the cause of the increased nitrogen excretion that persists throughout peritonitis, it has now been shown that the elevation in adrenocortical hormones persists only for about 72 h. Circulating concentrations of these hormones have returned to normal long before nitrogen losses cease to occur.

Secretion of both aldosterone and antidiuretic hormone also is increased as a response to the hypovolemia of peritonitis, resulting in enhanced renal conservation of sodium and water. Water retention may be greater than sodium retention, so that there is dilution of plasma sodium (hyponatremia). Thyroid metabolism probably is unaltered despite increased rates of energy utilization and heat production by the body during peritonitis.

CARDIAC RESPONSE. The effects of peritonitis on cardiac function are a reflection both of the decrease in extracellular fluid volume and of progressing acidosis. The volume deficit results in decreased venous return and diminished cardiac output. The heart rate increases in an attempt to maintain cardiac output, but compensation usually is incomplete. Progressive acidosis brings about secondary dysfunction in cardiac contractility and a further decrease in cardiac output. These alterations are, in part, related to relative failure during acidosis of oxidative membrane transport.

The cardiac response is seen primarily in untreated hypovolemia associated with peritonitis. Animal studies and retrospective clinical observations suggest that expansion of the intravascular volume by rapid infusion of intravenous fluids will augment cardiac output during peritonitis. This would improve oxygen delivery to the tissues, improve oxygen consumption and cellular metabolism, maintain aerobic metabolism, and avert acidosis and its adverse effects on cardiac contractibility.

RESPIRATORY RESPONSE. Abdominal distention, primarily due to adynamic ileus, coupled with restriction of both diaphragmatic and intercostal respiratory movements due to pain, results in a decrease in ventilatory volume and the early appearance of basilar atelectasis. Early in the course of peritonitis, an increase in respiratory rate may be noted, stimulated both by the hypoxia of diminished ventilation and by beginning accumulation of acidic end products of anaerobic tissue metabolism. Ventilation-perfusion imbalance results from continued pulmonary perfusion of underventilated or nonventilated alveoli, producing increased functional intrapulmonary shunting of blood and peripheral hypoxemia.

RENAL RESPONSE. Hypovolemia, reduced cardiac output, and increased secretion of antidiuretic hormone and of aldosterone in peritonitis all act synergistically on the kidney. Renal blood flow is diminished, resulting in a decrease in the volume of glomerular filtrate and in tubular urine flow. Reabsorption of both sodium and water is increased, often in imbalance; potassium is wasted. Urine volume output is diminished, and renal capacity to handle an excess of solute is impaired. The tendency to develop metabolic acidosis is enhanced.

METABOLIC RESPONSE. The metabolic rate generally is increased with a corresponding increase in peripheral oxygen demand. Simultaneously, the capacity of the lungs and the heart to deliver oxygen is diminished. Poor circulation leads to a shift from aerobic to anaerobic metabolism in muscle and other peripheral tissues. As a result, anaerobic end products of carbohydrate metabolism accumulate and lactic acidosis begins to develop.

Under normal circumstances, local tissue perfusion is controlled by regional metabolic requirements. If anaerobic metabolic end products begin to accumulate, local arteriolar dilation occurs. Cardiac output, in the absence of hypovolemia, increases to maintain circulatory homeostasis. Perfusion in the periphery improves, the acidic metabolic end products are cleared, and the tissues return to aerobic metabolism.

This fine balance is easily upset by the circulatory insufficiency due to hypovolemia that accompanies peritonitis. Cardiac output may be inadequate to maintain normal arterial blood pressure and to supply required perfusion of all body tissues. Compensatory vasoconstriction results in increased total peripheral resistance, which, in turn, maintains essential perfusion to the heart and brain. The skin, muscles, splanchnic bed, and, to some degree, kidneys are denied a portion of their normal circulatory volume. As a result of decreased tissue perfusion and oxygenation, anaerobic glycolysis persists and leads to a progressive increase in lactic acid and other acidic metabolic end products. Decreased renal clearance of these acidic solutes, secondary to reduced renal perfusion, contributes to the metabolic acidosis. The body attempts to compensate with increased respiratory effort to excrete carbon dioxide, but the increased respiratory effort, in turn, places on the already inadequate circulation an additional demand to perfuse the muscles of respiration.

The appearance, in some cases of peritonitis, of lactic acidosis before systemic hypotension or hypoxemia suggests the possible existence of a primary cellular insult that makes cells unable to use available oxygen and substrate. This hypothesis was investigated in isolated hepatic mitochondria harvested following induction of peritonitis by cecal ligation. In these experiments, hepatic cellular hypoxia followed the development of peritonitis even while systemic oxygenation was adequate and hypotension had not yet developed. Mitochondrial respiration, however, was unaltered in these experiments, suggesting that primary cellular injury does not occur in peritonitis but that alterations in oxygen delivery are responsible for reduced oxygen consumption and lactic acidosis.

Another contributor to lactic acidosis in peritonitis may be the bacteria causing the peritoneal infection. Both D- and L-isomers of lactate are produced by bacterial metabolism and may be absorbed during peritonitis. Human beings can rapidly metabolize L-lactate but have a relatively limited capacity to handle D-lactate. The dextrorotary isomer then accumulates in body fluids, and contributes to metabolic acidosis.

Hepatic glycogen stores are utilized promptly in peritonitis. Insulin secretion by islet cells increases, but relative insulin resistance to utilization of glucose by muscle is unchanged, and an energy deficit persists. While increased lipolysis also occurs, fat is not utilized efficiently as an energy source in peritonitis.

Protein catabolism begins early in peritonitis and becomes progressively more severe. Only a part of the amino acids made available by catabolism are readily utilized as energy sources since muscle cells can use only branched-chain amino acids directly. However, some data indicate that the rate of synthesis of plasma proteins is increased in terms of both concentration and turnover. Thus, plasma proteins preferentially are synthesized while muscle proteins preferentially are catabolized during peritonitis. Weight loss of 25 to 30 percent of lean body mass can occur if peritonitis persists. Albumin synthesis also is apparently increased during peritonitis, as judged by increased uptake of radioactive label, but the increased synthesis occurs in the face of a decreasing concentration of circulating albumin. One reason for this disparity is that a considerable amount of albumin accumulates in the peritoneal cavity and thus is lost to the general circulation.

Clinical Manifestations

The appearance of a patient with advanced peritonitis was described by Hippocrates: "hollow eyes, collapsed temples; the ears cold, contracted and their lobes turned out; the skin about the forehead being rough, distended, and parched; the color of the whole face being brown, black, livid, or lead-colored." Patients with peritonitis that is so advanced as to present this classic Hippocratic facies are usually in a preterminal state. But even much earlier in the clinical course of peritonitis, patients quite obviously appear gravely ill. Characteristically, they lie quietly in bed, supine, with knees flexed and with frequent limited intercostal respirations since any motion intensifies their abdominal pain.

Abdominal pain almost always is the predominant symptom, unless its perception is masked by the administration of anodynes of the presence of a fresh surgical wound. The pain may have been sudden in onset, associated with rupture of a viscus, or more insidious. When fully developed, pain is steady, unrelenting, burning, and aggravated by any motion. Pain usually is most intense in the area of most advanced peritoneal inflammation. Decreasing intensity and extent of pain with time suggest localization of the inflammatory process, while increasing intensity and extent imply the presence of a spreading peritonitis.

Anorexia almost always is present. Nausea is frequent and may be accompanied by vomiting. The patient usually complains of thirst and of feeling feverish, often with intermittent chills. Body temperature elevation in peritonitis usually is in the range of 38 to 40°C. Fever is usually higher and more spiking in character in younger and healthier patients, while infants and older, debilitated patients may exhibit only a modest febrile response. Hypothermia may occur, instead of fever, in severely ill patients with high cardiac output and peripheral vasodilation.

Tachycardia and a diminished peripheral pulse volume are early signs of hypovolemia. The blood pressure is maintained in the early stages of peritonitis, but as hypovolemia progresses, compensatory vasoconstrictive responses may be overcome with the rapid appearance of hypovolemic shock. Respirations typically are rapid and shallow; rapid because of progressively greater tissue demands for oxygen and a need to correct developing acidosis, and shallow because deep respirations intensify the perception of abdominal pain.

The abdomen is distended, quiet to auscultation, and tender to palpation. Tenderness is present over the entire extent of the peritoneum involved in the inflammatory process. Maximal tenderness usually is noted in the region of the organ in which the process originated, but in some cases, maximal tenderness is found over the advancing edge of the peritoneal inflammation. Direct, percussion, or referred rebound tenderness confirm the presence of peritoneal irritation. Percussion tenderness sometimes is more accurate than direct palpation in locating the point of maximal tenderness as well as in delineating the extent of peritoneal irritation.

Rigidity of the abdominal muscles is produced initially by voluntary guarding and, following involvement of the parietal peritoneum by inflammation, also by reflex muscular spasm. As peritonitis advances, reflex spasm may become so severe that boardlike abdominal rigidity is produced. Hyperresonance due to accumulating gas in the paralyzed, distended intestine usually can be demonstrated easily by percussion. If a pneumoperitoneum has resulted from rupture of a hollow viscus, gas accumulating under the right side of the diaphragm may result in a decrease in the vertical extent of liver dullness to percussion.

Some bowel sounds may be audible on auscultation early in peritonitis, but as inflammation spreads, the nearly silent abdomen of adynamic ileus supervenes. Rectal examination, and vaginal examination of female patients, are important in establishing the diagnosis. The location and extent of tenderness, and the possible presence of a pelvic mass, permit assessment of the degree of involvement of pelvic peritoneum. Vaginal examination of the cervix may provide clues to the origin of an inflammatory process within the female generative organs.

Leukocytosis is usual in acute peritonitis, but the total white cell count, taken alone without a differential count, can be very misleading. Massive peritoneal inflammation may mobilize sufficient numbers of leukocytes into the diseased area so that only 3000 to 4000 white cells/mm^3 remain behind in the circulating blood. The differential count shows a moderate to a marked left shift in peritonitis, and the predominance of polymorphonucleocytes in the differential count provides evidence of the presence of inflammation even when the total leukocyte count is not markedly elevated. Blood chemistry determinations are quite variable but usually will reflect homoconcentration due to dehydration (increased hematocrit) as well as metabolic acidosis.

The radiologic picture of generalized peritonitis is that of paralytic ileus, with distention of both small intestine and colon. Inflammatory exudate and edema of the intestinal wall may produce widening of the spaces between adjacent bowel loops noted on a flat film of the abdomen. Peritoneal fat lines in the flanks and the psoas shadows may be obliterated. Free air may be visible on an upright abdominal or lateral decubitus film if a ruptured viscus is the cause of peritonitis. Air beneath the diaphragm also may be noted on upright x-rays of the chest.

In general, the importance of laboratory work in the diagnosis of peritonitis has been overemphasized, a statement that also holds true for almost every other acute intraabdominal disease. Though laboratory determinations undoubtedly are of occasional help, the major emphasis in both the diagnosis and management of peritonitis should be on clinical examination of the patient. Amelioration of symptoms and restoration of the patient's physical state toward normal are the best indicators of effective treatment. Laboratory and radiologic examinations should be employed only to help exclude other causes of abdominal pain such as pneumonia. In an occasional case that is a difficult diagnostic problem, peritoneal lavage may be useful in patients with diffuse peritonitis. It is of limited value and thought not to be very useful for routine cases.

ACUTE SUPPURATIVE PERITONITIS

The overall incidence of acute suppurative peritonitis is declining but the disorder remains a major clinical concern for surgeons. This process is generally diffuse in nature and may be caused by a number of intraabdominal problems. Diffuse peritoneal contamination may follow penetrating or blunt abdominal trauma, postoperative anastomotic dehiscence, loss of bowel integrity secondary to ischemia, or the occurrence of primary intraabdominal disease associated with an inflammatory process or, less commonly, an obstetric-gynecologic infection.

While no longer the overwhelming clinical problem it once was, postoperative suppurative peritonitis still is a common cause of death directly related to an abdominal operation and is more lethal than other forms of peritonitis. In two recent collected series, the overall mortality of diffuse peritonitis was reported to vary between 16 and 38 percent. In the review by Bohnen and associates, patients with postoperative peritonitis had a mortality of 60 percent while the mortality due to peritonitis related to primary appendicitis and to perforated ulcer was only 10 percent.

Although there is some degree of peritoneal inflammation every time the peritoneal cavity is entered surgically, because of mechanical and desiccation injury of exposed peritoneum as well as intraoperative bacterial contamination from the environment, spillage during manipulation of viscera, or minor breaks in aseptic technique, such contamination usually is not so great that clinically significant peritonitis ensues. Peritonitis following an operation is due most commonly to anastomotic dehiscence. The integrity of an anastomosis is endangered by tension on the suture line, ischemia, hemorrhage, infection, or the presence of a drain in apposition to the suture line, as well as all the systemic factors that interfere with wound healing (see Chap. 8).

Perforated peptic ulcer is the most common cause of peritonitis due to visceral rupture. Appendicitis, formerly the most common cause, is now less frequent because of an overall decline in the incidence of appendicitis and prompt exploration in most cases when the diagnosis is suspected. Gangrene of the bowel from strangulation obstruction, acute mesenteric vascular occlusion, or nonocclusive, low-perfusion states such as cardiac failure also are important causes of peritonitis. Other visceral diseases that may lead to peritonitis due to rupture of an inflamed organ are acute gangrenous cholecystitis and colonic diverticulitis. Pelvic inflammatory disease is a common cause of pelvic peritonitis; in a severe infection, it may progress to generalized peritonitis. Diffuse disease may also be seen with septic abortion and puerperal sepsis.

Trauma to the abdomen may produce peritonitis through contamination of the abdominal cavity with foreign material, such as shotgun wadding or clothing, or through disruption of a hollow abdominal viscus as the result of a stab or gunshot wound, or severe blunt trauma. Blunt abdominal trauma also may disrupt the vascular supply to abdominal viscera, leading to gangrene or rupture of the involved organ.

Interactions of Bacteria and the Peritoneum

The presence of bacteria within the peritoneal cavity by no means invariably results in spreading diffuse peritonitis. On the contrary, peritoneal defense mechanisms clear bacteria from the peritoneal cavity and contain the insult in most instances. Bacterial clearing occurs rapidly by way of the stomata and submesothelial lacunae of the diaphragm that drain into thoracic lymphatics and then into the systemic circulation. Rapid phagocytosis by resident peritoneal macrophages of opsonized bacteria also occurs within the peritoneum. These defense mechanisms often successfully limit the inflammatory process and restore the peritoneum to a relatively normal state.

If peritoneal defenses are successful in localizing the infectious process but the interaction between invading microorganisms and body defense mechanisms does not result in early elimination of the bacteria, confined suppuration and abscess formation ensues. On occasion, however, initial defense reactions are insufficient to localize the infection, and a more diffuse peritonitis ensues. The general responses to peritonitis then follow. They are mediated largely by translocation of extracellular fluid into the peritoneal cavity, with both the local (primary) and systemic (secondary) consequences enumerated above (see Peritonitis, General Responses).

In suppurative peritonitis, in addition, a group of specific responses due to the presence of overwhelming numbers of bacteria is superimposed on the general responses to peritonitis (Fig. 34-2). The magnitude of the specific responses to generalized spreading peritonitis is, in part, determined by (1) the *virulence* of the contaminating bacteria, (2) the *extent and duration* of contamination, (3) the presence or absence of an *adjuvant,* and (4) the *appropriateness of initial therapy.* If initial treatment fails to bring about prompt control of peritoneal infection, endotoxemia and septic shock may ensue.

VIRULENCE OF CONTAMINATING BACTERIA. A mixed, or polymicrobial, bacterial flora usually is present in patients suffering acute suppurative peritonitis secondary to contamination of the abdominal cavity from the gastrointestinal tract. The most common offending organisms include aerobic coliform bacilli, particularly *Escherichia coli,* anaerobic *Bacteroides* species, anaerobic and aerobic streptococci, enterococci, and *Clostridia* (Table 34-1). These bacteria are significant pathogens for human beings.

Experiments of Nichols and colleagues, in which the entire range of peritonitis from overwhelming sepsis to resolution with an abscess was produced, indicate that mortality risk is a bacterial dose-related phenomenon and correlates directly with the total number of pathogenic bacteria present in the peritoneal cavity (Fig. 34-3). Experimental evidence also indicates that the mixed fecal

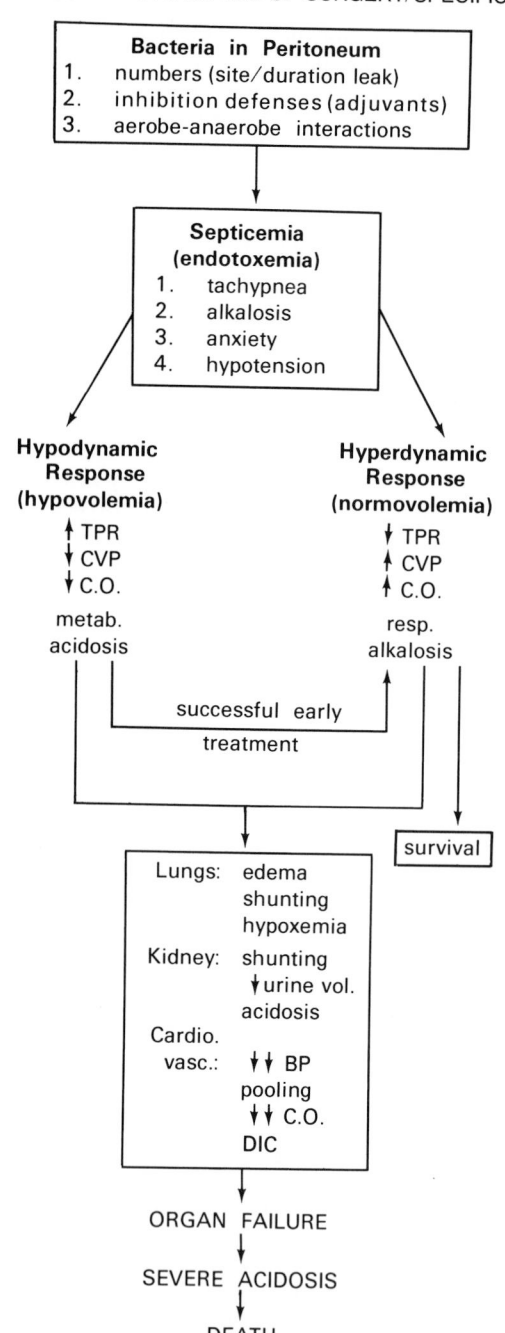

Fig. 34-2. The specific responses to suppurative peritonitis begin with septicemia, which initiates tachypnea, respiratory alkalosis, anxiety, and moderate hypotension in most cases. Continuing responses depend on the status of total body fluid volumes; in most cases of peritonitis, patients are hypovolemic and a hypodynamic response pattern is seen. Successful early fluid resuscitation may convert the hypodynamic response to a hyperdynamic one. If sepsis continues uncontrolled, major functional deficits appear in the vital organ systems that are essential to survival, and death ensues.

flora usually found in peritonitis acts synergistically, so that total virulence is greater than the sum of its parts. Experimentally, injection of massive numbers of single species of fecal pathogens may not produce a fatality.

Mixtures of organisms in the same total numbers, particularly combinations of aerobes and anaerobes, however, can result in overwhelming peritonitis and death. Further, there is evidence that apparently nonpathogenic microorganisms may increase the virulence of pathogenic bacteria with which they are associated.

Years ago, Meleney and Altemeier both emphasized the role of anaerobic bacteria in peritonitis. Although the frequency with which anaerobic bacteria participate in peritoneal infections probably has not changed over the years, modern culture methods have greatly improved the rate at which these organisms are recovered. Thus, the importance of anaerobic bacteria in peritonitis has become more widely recognized, and surgeons now treat patients with fecal peritonitis using antibiotics effective against anaerobes.

Experimental evidence indicates that aerobic organisms enhance the virulence of anaerobes by lowering the redox potential and elaborating essential nutrients, and the anaerobic microorganisms enhance the virulence of aerobic pathogens by elaborating enzymes that destroy antibiotics. Stone and colleagues demonstrated in patients undergoing operation that recoverability of anaerobic organisms from a soiled peritoneal cavity showed a progressive decline with the passage of time. Nichols and associates subsequently demonstrated that the concentration of both aerobic and anaerobic bacteria decline progressively during operative exploration of a contaminated abdomen. Although it has been suggested that in some cases exposure to room air might be sufficient to manage the anaerobic component of peritoneal sepsis, specific antibiotic therapy obviously is more certain.

EXTENT AND DURATION OF CONTAMINATION. Massive sudden contamination, as from a burst carcinoma of the cecum, often spreads bacteria rapidly throughout the peritoneal cavity. Dissemination occurs before defensive localization mechanisms have time to be effective. Experimentally, bacteria or liquid radiopaque media injected intraperitoneally at one locus can be demonstrated to spread throughout the entire peritoneal cavity within 3 to 6 h. Spread is produced by normal intestinal and abdominal movements, by the suction effect of the diaphragm during respiration (which establishes a cyclic negative pressure differential between the subphrenic space and the rest of the peritoneal cavity, promoting upward flow of fluid and particulate matter), and by the effect of gravity related to body position which tends to promote flow into the pelvic cavity. Even though infection spreads diffusely throughout the peritoneal cavity, if the source is controlled by early surgical intervention, peritonitis usually responds to vigorous antibiotic and supportive therapy. On the other hand, if the source of contamination persists, death nearly always results because of continuing peritoneal soiling.

The severity and extent of peritonitis secondary to spontaneous or traumatic perforation of the gastrointestinal tract varies not only with the size of the perforation but also with its location. Spillage of distal ileal or cecal content is associated with greater morbidity than a perforation proximally or distally in the gastrointestinal tract. Proximally there are few bacteria; distally the fecal con-

Table 34-1. BACTERIOLOGY OF SECONDARY PERITONITIS

	No. cultures growing specified organism					Relative frequency, %
	Gorbach 1974	Lorber 1975	Stone 1975	Jones 1987	Total	
Aerobic bacteria:						
E. coli	28	43	164	94	329	31.9
Streptococci	3	28	11	190	232	22.5
Enterococci	2	9	55	—	66	6.4
Staphylococci	16	—	13	35	64	6.2
Enterobacteriaceae/Klebsiella	17	6	78	53	154	14.9
Proteus	10	8	69	18	105	10.1
Pseudomonas	8	2	20	30	60	5.8
Candida	4	—	2	15	21	2.0
Anaerobic bacteria:						
Bacteroides sp.	36	45	136	257	474	39.1
B. fragilis	28	71	54	—	153	12.6
Eubacteria	11	8	75	69	163	13.4
Clostridia	31	7	29	90	157	12.9
Peptostreptococci	14	43	40	60	157	12.9
Proprionobacteria	2	—	34	9	45	3.7
Fusobacteria	6	15	13	30	64	5.3

tent is more solid and tends to be more easily localized. But ileal and cecal content is fluid and contains high concentrations of bacteria as well as residual active enzymes that increase the severity of peritonitis and prevent effective local sequestration.

Fig. 34-3. Experimental (rat) model indicating cumulative percentage mortality with varying inoculum size of human fecal material in the peritoneal cavity. (From: *Nichols et al, 1978, with permission.*)

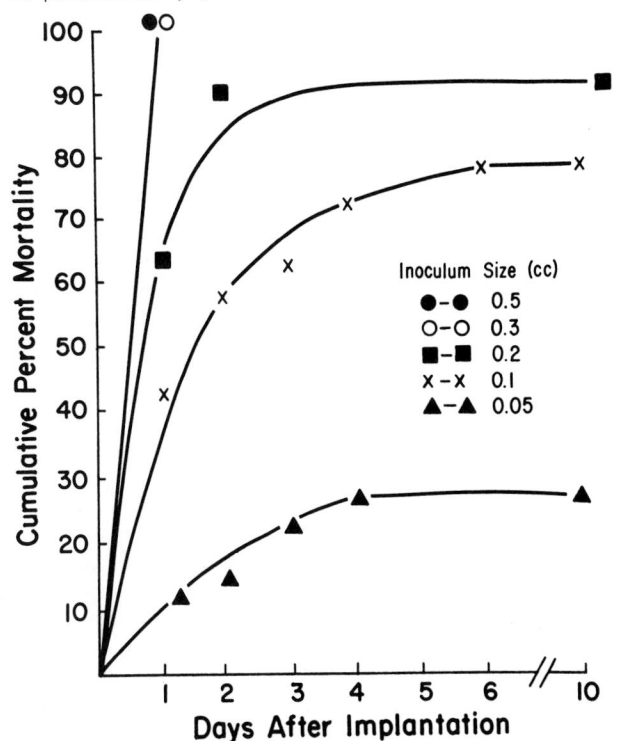

INFLUENCE OF ADJUVANTS. The virulence of peritonitis not only is determined by the nature of the contaminating mixture of bacteria and the duration of peritoneal soiling but also is influenced by the presence of adjuvant substances such as mucus and hemoglobin. Trauma or any foreign body will retard clearance of bacteria from the peritoneal cavity and can act as an adjuvant. Hemoglobin experimentally increases the lethality of *E. coli* peritonitis, but the mechanism of action is not well defined. It has no adverse effect on leukocyte function, as was previously suggested, and no influence on peritoneal clearance of bacteria, as demonstrated experimentally in studies of *E. coli* peritonitis. In other studies of the adjuvant effects of hemoglobin in experimental peritonitis, increased bacterial proliferation was seen. This increase in number of bacteria may account for increased host lethality. It also has been suggested that local host defense mechanisms may be inhibited by a leukotoxin elaborated by bacteria in the presence of hemoglobin. These experimental studies have been conducted with monocontaminated *E. coli* peritonitis.

The presence of an adjuvant nearly always is necessary to produce lethal experimental peritonitis. Intraperitoneal injection of bacteria can be made lethal by the addition of such foreign substances as bile salts, talc, gum tragacanth, gastric mucin, feces, or barium. The enhancement of virulence is attributed to the adverse effect of these adjuvants on the function of phagocytic cells. The body apparently does not differentiate between bacteria and the adjuvant, attacking both with vigor. The presence of the adjuvant dilutes the net effectiveness of phagocytosis, since a proportion of leukocytes is diverted to phagocytosis of the adjuvant, retarding clearance of bacteria from the peritoneal cavity.

An adjuvant role in the lethality of experimental bacterial peritonitis has also been attributed to the presence of a large volume of fluid within the peritoneal cavity. The fluid volume, whether left after irrigation during laparotomy or due to ascites, may delay bacterial clearance, enhance bacterial growth, or diminish phagocytosis by diluting intraperitoneal opsonins.

INAPPROPRIATE THERAPY. Peritonitis may be spread by errors of omission as well as by errors of commission. A frequently fatal error of omission is failure to diagnose the presence of a ruptured viscus and to undertake surgical control of the source of contamination of the peritoneum in timely fashion. Another error of omission occurs in attempting to control a persisting intraabdominal infection by administration of antibiotics without adequate surgical debridement or drainage. Subsequent rupture of an undrained abscess will broadcast highly virulent contents throughout the abdomen, often with fatal consequences. Conversely, an error of commission may occur if laxatives or enemas are administered to patients suffering abdominal pain, thus increasing the risk of rupture of an inflamed portion of the bowel.

Pathophysiology of Sepsis

The presence of bacteria in suppurative peritonitis leads to a number of both local and systemic responses that are related directly to the effects of the microorganisms. These responses are in addition to and superimposed on the general primary and secondary pathophysiologic responses that occur in all cases of peritonitis.

TOXIC ABSORPTION. The inflamed peritoneum acts as a bidirectionally permeable membrane, not only secreting fluid into the peritoneal cavity in the presence of peritonitis, but also permitting ready absorption of both bacteria and bacterial toxins from peritoneal fluid. Endotoxins derived from the cell wall of aerobic gram-negative bacilli, such as E. coli, are most frequently involved and are the most important in generating systemic responses, although absorption of performed exotoxins, elaborated by gram-positive organisms such as Clostridia, are the dominant influence in an occasional case.

Endotoxin is a lipopolysaccharide. It acts primarily on blood vessels, producing arteriolar and venular dilation and loss of endothelial integrity. Capillary leakage, accumulation of fluid in tissues, and intraorgan shunting are some of the consequences of endotoxin action that lead to the clinical features of septic shock. Exotoxins, in contrast, are proteins. They cause hemolysis of red cells or destruction of other body cells, or interfere with metabolic or other cellular processes. Exotoxins may also cause peripheral arteriolar dilation, but exotoxin effects tend to be more cellularly specific compared with the effects of endotoxins.

Gram-negative sepsis of major proportions often begins with chills, rapid elevation of the temperature above 38.5°C, and moderate hypotension. Because of predominant peripheral vasodilation, the clinical picture often is characterized as "warm" shock unless the effects of hypovolemia predominate, in which case the clinical picture is of more typical "cold" shock.

The severity of septic shock varies depending on the amount and duration of exposure of body tissues to circulating gram-negative organisms and their endotoxins. Transient, self-limited bacteremia may produce minimal adverse systemic effects, whereas persisting or repetitive episodes of septicemia overwhelm the vital cardiorespiratory and renal support systems and, obviously, result in a much poorer prognosis. The presence of underlying disease of the cardiac, pulmonary, hepatic, or renal systems renders the patient more susceptible to organ dysfunction and also impairs responses to the septic insult.

There are considerable species differences in responses to septicemia. Though the use of experimental animal models has contributed a great deal to our understanding of this form of shock, direct extrapolation of findings in animals to human septic shock cannot be made. For example, injection of lipopolysaccharide endotoxin in a dog causes splanchnic pooling as a consequence of hepatic venous constriction. Decreased venous return, reduction in cardiac output, and an abrupt fall in blood pressure follow immediately after injection of endotoxin. This pattern is very different from that seen in subhuman primates and in human beings, in whom injection of endotoxin produces chills, fever, transient vasoconstriction, then peripheral vasodilation; cardiac output initially rises and then declines.

There also are differences in response to experimental injection of performed endotoxin as compared with septicemia produced by injection of live bacteria. Hypoglycemia and hypoinsulinemia are regularly observed after live E. coli-induced shock; hyperglycemia is a consistent hallmark in endotoxin-infused models. Renal fibrin thrombi due to disseminated intravascular coagulation (DIC) are present after live E. coli administration, while tubular necrosis is found following both organism and endotoxin infusions. Liver dysfunction is indicated by elevation of blood levels of hepatic enzymes and morphologic alterations in both models. The responses of the live E. coli-injected baboon appear to bear a closer similarity to the clinical entity of human septic shock than do endotoxin-treated animals.

Renal morphologic changes induced during experimental septic shock can be prevented by administration of heparin, although in all other respects, heparin-treated animals are identical to unheparinized animals in their reactions to injection of live organisms or endotoxin and suffer the same mortality risk. In particular, abnormal renal function, as reflected in rising BUN, creatinine, and uric acid levels, is not modified by administration of heparin.

INFLUENCE OF HYPOVOLEMIA. Septic shock in normovolemic patients begins with a hyperdynamic response associated with increased cardiac output, normal or high central venous pressure, low peripheral resistance, warm extremities despite a low blood pressure, hyperventilation, and respiratory alkalosis. Despite the increased cardiac output, effective tissue perfusion in the liver and kidneys may be decreased. Depressed ketogenesis and impaired uptake of amino acids have been observed.

In sepsis secondary to peritonitis, hypovolemia is characteristically present owing to fluid shifts from the intravascular fluid compartment to the interstitial space as a direct result of inflammation of the peritoneal membrane and increased vascular permeability. Hypovolemia is responsible for the decreased cardiac output, decreased central venous pressure, low blood pressure, cold extremities, and vasoconstriction with high peripheral resistance seen in the septic hypodynamic state.

As the fluid deficit is corrected, the hyperdynamic state characteristic of normovolemic septic shock may ensue, and is a favorable prognostic sign. If the hypodynamic state is not treated or is undertreated, low cardiac output and decreased tissue perfusion will persist, resulting in profound metabolic acidosis that may be responsible for further cardiac dysfunction and, possibly, death.

RESPIRATORY RESPONSES. Compromise of vascular endothelial integrity in the lung during sepsis results in increased capillary permeability, leading to leakage of fluid from pulmonary arterioles and capillaries into the interstitial pulmonary space. The accumulating fluid makes the lungs less compliant and causes an increase in pulmonary vascular resistance. This interstitial edema also acts, in effect, as a barrier between pulmonary capillaries and adjacent alveoli, retarding uptake of oxygen and producing mild hypoxemia. Compensatory hyperventilation and respiratory alkalosis result. At this stage there is little clinical or x-ray evidence of pulmonary compromise. The development of mild hyperventilation, respiratory alkalosis, and an altered sensorium may be the earliest signs of gram-negative sepsis; this triad may precede more obvious signs of sepsis or shock by many hours.

As pulmonary edema progresses, protein-rich fluid accumulates in the alveoli. Septicemia not only lowers the hydrostatic pressure threshold at which pulmonary edema begins to accumulate but also leads to a loss of pulmonary surfactant, promoting alveolar collapse and progressive pulmonary consolidation. The chest x-ray at this point shows patchy infiltrates diffusely in the lungs.

Changes in extravascular lung water are not exclusively responsible for the degree of shunting in the lung during sepsis. Maintenance of circulation to areas of the lung that have lost effective capacity for oxygen uptake also produces ventilation-perfusion inequality. In addition, excessive beta-adrenergic stimulation is common in sepsis and causes opening of splanchnic and pulmonary arteriovenous shunts. Pulmonary dysfunction in sepsis also may be related to loss of hypoxic vasoconstrictive responses within the pulmonary capillary bed.

Both functional and actual intrapulmonary shunting results in return of poorly oxygenated blood to the general arterial circulation. This leads to tissue hypoxia, further compensatory hyperventilation, and respiratory alkalosis. *Adult respiratory distress syndrome* (ARDS) is the term used to describe the clinical and radiologic effects of this process. Subsequently, the picture frequently is one of rapid deterioration of pulmonary function, confluence of patchy infiltrates, and severe hypoxemia.

RENAL RESPONSE. The decrease in glomerular perfusion and filtration brought about by hypovolemia in peritonitis is reinforced by endotoxin-induced opening of intrarenal shunts at the corticomedullary level. The blood circulating to the kidneys now preferentially perfuses more central renal tissues, while the cortex receives little blood flow at all. This phenomenon of "corticomedullary disconnection" profoundly decreases glomerular perfusion and results, when fully elaborated, in formation of little glomerular filtrate. As a consequence, urine flow is greatly diminished; this is recognized clinically by oliguria and progressive systemic accumulation of unexcreted acidic end products of metabolism (metabolic acidosis). Recent evidence also indicates that prolonged sepsis in some cases may be accompanied by development of proliferative glomerulonephritis, leading not only to acute renal failure but also to chronic renal insufficiency in survivors.

LEUKOCYTE AND PLATELET FUNCTION. Altered leukocyte responsiveness, particularly neutrophil dysfunction, is seen in patients with septicemia. The neutrophil dysfunction may be manifested by impaired or defective migration, altered phagocytosis or degranulation. Although neutrophil dysfunction is temporally related to the septic state, it is not firmly established that generalized sepsis occurs as a result of altered leukocyte responsiveness. It is also not clear that there is increased susceptibility to remote infections in patients who present initially with intraabdominal sepsis.

The mechanisms of altered leukocyte function are not completely defined. It has been suggested that defective migration may be secondary to inadequate levels of circulating chemotactic factors. There also is evidence indicating that inadequate complement-mediated opsonic activity may be responsible for decreased bacterial phagocytosis, particularly in the presence of abundant numbers of normal-appearing neutrophils. Lymphocyte responsiveness also may be decreased as a result of generalized sepsis. Though the significance of such impairment in early sepsis is unclear, lymphocytes along with macrophages do serve important functions in the immune response.

Thrombocytopenia also commonly occurs in peritonitis. In most instances, the drop in platelet count is not a reflection of disseminated intravascular coagulation or bone marrow suppression, and clinical bleeding usually does not occur. The effect is transient, and platelet transfusion is not needed.

MULTIPLE ORGAN SYSTEM FAILURE. In addition to the morbidity and mortality accountable to peritonitis, per se, there is a tight correlation between mortality and the systemic physiologic and metabolic abnormalities that occur as the result of uncontrolled sepsis, a state called "multiple organ system failure." A number of risk factors have been identified in patients with persisting sepsis who develop multiple organ system failure. Shock (mean blood pressure below 80 mmHg) is the single factor best predicting death. Other important risk factors synergistic with shock in predicting organ dysfunction and death are age over 70 years, alcohol abuse, malnutrition, and bowel infarction.

The initial event in the cascade of multiple organ system failure is often cardiac and circulatory dysfunction, followed by impairment of the pulmonary and renal systems. Metabolic and hepatic failure follow next and are manifest by carbohydrate intolerance and jaundice. Thrombocytopenia may appear at any time. The risk of dying increases sequentially with increasing organ involvement, and ranges from 30 percent with failure of a single organ to 100 percent with impairment of four or more organ systems. The overall mortality of multiple organ system failure is about 70 percent. Prompt and effective control of the underlying peritoneal infection is essential to minimize mortality.

Clinical Manifestations

The patient with suppurative peritonitis presents all the features that characterize peritonitis in general: a distended, tender, abdomen; rapid, shallow respirations; fever, and tachycardia. In addition, disorientation progressing to coma also is frequently present. The acute symptoms are of rapid onset and progression. Occasional patients report a history of symptoms suggesting past subacute episodes.

The history and location of pain in the abdomen may provide clues to the possible organ source of peritonitis. Pain may increase or decrease at the time of viscus rupture. Thereafter, the story is one of progressively worse pain, initially diffuse but tending to localize if peritoneal defense mechanisms can contain the spillage. Tenderness increases, percussion tenderness appears or worsens, bowel sounds diminish and disappear, muscular rigidity replaces guarding, and distention worsens. Leukocytosis with a left shift is usually but may not be marked in elderly or debilitated patients. In patients with advanced peritonitis, trapping of neutrophils in the peritoneal cavity may produce a normal or low total white count in the blood, but the left shift persists. Severe leukopenia is an ominous sign. Abdominal x-ray films may show paralytic ileus, free air, or atelectactic changes in the lung bases.

In some cases of septic peritonitis, fever may be misleading. Subnormal temperatures may occur, particularly later in the course, because body compensatory mechanisms are unable to prevent hypothermia consequent upon peripheral vasodilation. Shock, due to accumulation of fluid in peripheral tissues as well as failure of compensatory vasoconstrictive mechanisms, is out of proportion to the degree of measurable hypovolemia.

In patients with generalized peritonitis, serum bilirubin and alkaline phosphatase levels demonstrate an irregular relationship. Sepsis is known to be associated with jaundice; it has been shown that some endotoxins inhibit mitochondrial respiration in human liver preparations. In patients with peritonitis, the presence of persisting or recurring hyperbilirubinemia is a warning sign of an intraabdominal abscess or of a leaking anastomosis.

Management

Initially, both therapeutic and diagnostic efforts are conducted simultaneously. Therapeutic efforts are directed to restoration of an effective total body fluid volume. Diagnosis is directed to the cause of the peritoneal

sepsis. The objective is to determine the need for and timing of operation.

Nonsurgical conditions simulating peritonitis should be considered and excluded. Pneumonia, particularly in the aged or very young, often is accompanied by abdominal distention and ileus, simulating a slowly progressive peritonitis. Diaphragmatic pleurisy may be associated with abdominal pain suggestive of acute cholecystitis or a perforated ulcer. Uremia commonly is associated with abdominal distention and ileus. A variety of other conditions, including acute gastroenteritis, ureteral calculi, and the various female pelvic disorders including twisted ovarian cyst, ectopic pregnancy, and ruptured ovarian follicle may produce abdominal pain simulating early acute peritonitis.

PREOPERATIVE PREPARATION. The essential features of preoperative treatment of suppurative peritonitis involve (1) fluid resuscitation, (2) antibiotics, (3) oxygen and, if needed, ventilator support, and (4) nasogastric intubation, urinary catheterization, and monitoring of vital signs and biochemical and hemodynamic data. An additional measure that may need to be considered in selected cases is the requirement for vasopressor drugs after fluid volume resuscitation has been completed.

Patients are better served if major metabolic derangements and fluid deficits are corrected prior to operation, although an inordinately long time cannot be taken in this exercise. Certain causes of peritonitis require more urgent intervention than others. For example, intestinal infarction demands nearly immediately intervention, whereas inflammatory perforation of a sigmoid diverticulum with developing fecal peritonitis usually will permit 1 or 2 h of resuscitative effort prior to laparotomy.

Fluid Resuscitation. Extensive inflammation of the peritoneal membrane causes fluid to shift into the peritoneal cavity and the interstitial space. Large volumes of fluid may be necessary to restore intravascular volume and to maintain a satisfactory urine output. Volume losses may be difficult to estimate, sometimes resulting in inadequate or excessive replacement. The functional peritoneal surface area is approximately equal to the body surface area, so fluid replacement in peritonitis may be calculated and administered as though treating a burn to the body surface.

Since it is difficult to estimate the extent of peritonitis, careful monitoring of the response to rapid fluid resuscitation is necessary, particularly if large fluid volumes are required to maintain an adequate circulation. Monitoring usually entails frequent vital signs, hourly urine output, central venous pressure measurement, or, preferably, Swan-Ganz catheter placement for pulmonary capillary wedge and pulmonary artery pressure determinations. Along with the clinical examination, these measurements provide a good assessment of the adequacy of fluid replacement therapy. Whole blood or packed red blood cells are administered, if needed, to correct anemia and to maintain an adequate red cell mass (hematocrit of 30 to 35).

Crystalloid or Colloid. There is agreement that deficits in the interstitial fluid volume in patients with peritonitis should be replaced with a crystalloid solution, preferably Ringer's lactate. But controversy exists about replacement of the deficient plasma volume. Some authorities advocate administration of more crystalloid; others argue for administration of colloid.

The argument turns on the applicability of Starling's law to the pulmonary circulation, the liability to develop interstitial pulmonary edema due to leakage from pulmonary capillaries, and the comparative efficiency of the two forms of therapy. Colloid solutions are theoretically more efficient but also more expensive. Crystalloid solutions are readily available and more economical but require administration of a large excess volume that must later be excreted by the kidneys.

Though it is clear that albumin or other colloids will restore an effective plasma volume efficiently in terms of the total volume administered, the same end can be achieved if one gives three to four times as much crystalloid solution. The theoretical advantages of administering albumin in resuscitation of patients suffering peritonitis are that salt overload, peripheral edema, and weight gain are less likely. Administering crystalloid solutions in excess volume might result in interstitial fluid accumulation in the lung because of a reduction in the colloid oncotic pressure-pulmonary capillary wedge pressure gradient. This hypothesis is based on Starling's law of fluid movement across a semipermeable membrane, which, in essence, indicates that net movement of fluid is governed by the algebraic sum of the hydrostatic and colloid osmotic pressures on the two sides of the membrane.

The strict applicability of the Starling hypothesis to fluid dynamics in the human lung has been questioned. It appears from experimental evidence that the oncotic pressure gradient as it relates to the alveolar-capillary membrane is not an important factor in the development of pulmonary edema. In studies in which pulmonary capillary wedge pressure has been measured, no relationship between colloid oncotic pressure or intrapulmonary pressure gradients and the development of pulmonary edema has been identified.

Liablity to development of pulmonary interstitial edema is related primarily to the degree of endothelial leakiness present in sepsis rather than the type of resuscitation fluid administered. There is extravasation of albumin into interstitial tissues when given to septic primates. Both crystalloid and colloid solutions are equally liable to be associated with pulmonary edema due to leakage from pulmonary capillaries. Exclusive crystalloid resuscitation is more likely to be associated with additional risks of pulmonary edema due to volume overload.

When excessively large doses of albumin are administered to traumatized or septic patients, pulmonary dysfunction is greater than in crystalloid-resuscitated patients. But a definitive clinical trial, utilizing more clinically reasonable volumes of colloid and crystalloid versus crystalloid alone for resuscitation of patients with impaired cardiopulmonary function who are in sepsis, has yet to be reported. We usually rely mainly on crystalloid solutions for resuscitation of most patients with septic peritonitis, but employ partial colloid resuscitation in patients known to have preexisting cardiopulmonary disease.

Antibiotic Therapy. The bacterial flora in suppurative peritonitis is polymicrobic in nature, an observation established by Altemeier in 1938 in a study of appendiceal abscesses, and confirmed by more recent studies of bacterial peritonitis (Table 34-1). In a typical specimen of bacterial peritonitis fluid, an average of five species of bacteria are isolated in cultures—three anaerobes and two aerobes. In more elegant microbiologic studies, an average of 14 different bacterial species are isolated—nine anaerobes and five aerobes. The most common anaerobes are species of *Bacteroides*, *Clostridium*, and *Peptostreptococci*. The most common aerobes are *E. coli* and other enterobacteriaceae and streptococci.

Antibiotics play an important, although adjunctive, role in the treatment of suppurative peritonitis. At the time of initial diagnosis, empiric antimicrobial therapy should be directed against likely aerobic and anaerobic pathogens, considering the probable organ source of bacteria contaminating the peritoneum. In addition to specific activity against contaminating pathogens, the efficacy of antimicrobial agents in peritonitis may be influenced by (1) the degree of bacterial contamination (inoculum size), (2) trauma or nontrauma setting of peritonitis, and (3) the presence of resistant organisms or of opportunistic pathogens, e.g., *Candida*.

To be effective in the treatment of peritonitis, antibiotic therapy must be initiated prior to, and continued during and after, surgical therapy. The specific antibiotics chosen should be effective against all suspected or documented pathogens. Consideration should also be given to the pharmacokinetics of the drug and its ability to penetrate tissues. Agents considered effective in the treatment of peritonitis are the combinations of clindamycin or metronidazole with an aminoglycoside, as well as chloramphenicol, and the second-generation cephalosporins (cefoxitin, cefotetan, moxalactam). Third-generation cephalosporins and the newer broad-spectrum penicillins are being evaluated as single agents for treatment of bacterial peritonitis, but evidence documenting their possible efficacy does not yet permit a recommendation.

Oxygen and Ventilator Support. Oxygen is administered to overcome the mild hypoxemia that is commonly present in peritonitis because of the increased metabolic demands of infection, some degree of intrapulmonary shunting, and the mechanical impairment of pulmonary ventilation by the distended, tender abdomen. Assessment of respiratory function should be made clinically, noting apparent tidal volume and work of breathing. If any impairment is suspected, measurement of ventilatory volume and of arterial blood gases is indicated.

Ventilator support should be initiated whenever any of the following are present: (1) inability to maintain adequate alveolar ventilation as evidenced by a rising Pa_{CO_2} of 50 mmHg or greater; (2) hypoxemia reflected in a Pa_{O_2} less than 55 mmHg on FI_{O_2} of 1.0; (3) evidence of shallow, rapid respirations due to muscular tiring, or the use of accessory muscles of respiration. Positive end-expiratory pressure (PEEP) should be added to ventilator support if adequate oxygenation is not maintained on an F_{IO_2} of 0.4.

Intubation, Catheterization, and Hemodynamic Monitoring. Nasogastric intubation is performed to evacuate the stomach, to prevent further vomiting, and, most importantly, to reduce accumulation of additional air in the paralyzed bowel. Urinary catheterization is utilized to record initial bladder urine volume and to monitor subsequent urinary output.

A central venous catheter should be placed through the subclavian or internal jugular vein to assess current hydration and the ability of the right heart to accommodate intravenous replacement. A chest radiograph is taken after catheter insertion to assure correct placement of the catheter tip and the absence of a pneumothorax or other complication. A Swan-Ganz catheter should be inserted if there is any suspicion of cardiopulmonary dysfunction in order to measure pulmonary capillary wedge pressure and pulmonary artery pressure. In addition, assessment of pulmonary shunting and cardiac output by the thermodilution technique can be obtained. Continuous monitoring of physiologic functions provides objective assessment of the overall adequacy of therapy.

Vital signs (temperature, blood pressure, pulse, and respirations) are recorded at least every 4 h. Preoperative biochemical evaluation should include measurement of serum electrolytes, creatinine, glucose, bilirubin, and alkaline phosphatase, and a urinalysis.

Vasoactive Drugs. Drugs with predominant alpha-adrenergic effects are of limited value in the treatment of sepsis secondary to peritonitis, since artificial attempts to maintain blood pressure by inducing vasoconstriction without thought to its consequences on tissue blood flow are potentially harmful. When adequate volume replacement and other measures have failed to restore the circulation, administration of dopamine or dobutamine may be helpful.

Steroids. Administration of pharmacologic doses of steroids to septic patients has been advocated in the past on the basis of experimental work, but controlled trials of steroids in the treatment of septic patients have failed to show any clear-cut advantage. Recent clinical studies support the idea that large doses of steroids may delay mortality in sepsis, particularly if given before or early after the onset of shock, but do not alter the eventual outcome.

Narcotics. Analgesic drugs should not be administered to patients with suspected peritonitis, or any other acute abdominal process, until a diagnosis has been made or, at least, a decision to operate has been made. The reason is that analgesia may obscure abdominal findings and hamper establishment of a diagnosis of peritonitis. Once a decision to operate has been made, pain should be relieved with potent narcotics. Morphine is preferred to other drugs and should be given in intravenous doses of 1 to 3 mg, repeated every 20 to 30 min or even more frequently, to maintain the patient's comfort. Small intravenous doses are safer than the traditional larger intramuscular doses, particularly in patients whose condition is unstable.

Naloxone, an opiate antagonist, has been suggested as a pharmacologic agent to treat persistent hypotension seen in septic shock. The presence of endorphins in septic patients, and the beneficial effects of naloxone in endotoxic animals has been the basis for the use of naloxone in septic patients. Release of endorphins (endogenous opiates) from central nervous system neurons contributes to sustained hypotension. In early clinical reports on the use of naloxone in septic patients, clinically significant improvement in mean arterial blood pressure was seen. More recent reports have shown no beneficial effect of naloxone in terms of improvement in cardiovascular parameters or survival in patients with septic shock. In the collected reported studies (Table 34-2), very few patients with sepsis secondary to peritonitis can be identified and the outcome related to naloxone therapy determined. Based on these reports, naloxone does not appear to be effective in treating prolonged hypotension associated with septic shock that is not responsive to other supportive therapy.

Fever. A temperature above 38.5°C may be associated with difficulties in administration of anesthesia. Patients with such hyperthemia, and also those with hypothermia, should have their temperature corrected toward normal prior to operation. Administration of salicylates often will be effective in reducing fever. If not, or if the patient is hypothermic, a cooling-warming mattress should be employed.

OPERATIVE MANAGEMENT. The primary therapy in management of generalized suppurative peritonitis is surgical. An operation is usually required since the fundamental objective of treatment is to control the source of peritoneal contamination. This may require closure of a perforation, or resection of bowel with primary anastomosis or exteriorization. The specific procedure performed depends upon the findings at operation. In addition to dealing with the organ responsible for contamination or in the site of perforation, the other aim of operative therapy is to remove adjuvant substances from the peritoneal cavity (fibrin, feces, bile, hemoglobin, gastric mucus) and to irrigate the peritoneal cavity in order to decrease the inoculum size and number of virulent bacteria.

Though there are a number of other factors that affect the outcome in suppurative peritonitis, the timing of operation is an important variable that is often overlooked. A significantly higher mortality occurs in patients whose operation is delayed more than 24 h from onset of peritonitis compared with those operated on more promptly.

Table 34-2. NALOXONE THERAPY IN SEPTIC SHOCK

References	Patients treated	Patients with peritonitis
Peters et al, 1981	13	1
Hughes et al, 1983	8	0
Groegor et al, 1983	10	1
Rock et al, 1985	12	2
DeMaria et al, 1985	10	0
Total	53	4

In adult patients with diffuse suppurative peritonitis, the operative approach is made through a midline vertical incision. This incision allows ready access to all quadrants of the abdominal cavity and is quick to open and close. Exceptions to the vertical midline approach are made in infants less than two years of age, in which a transverse incision is safer, and in the presence of localized peritonitis. In the latter case, an incision may be made directly over the suspected site of inflammation, avoiding spread of contamination to other quadrants of the abdomen.

Odor and Gram's Stain of Peritoneal Pus. Immediately on opening the abdomen, any odor should be noted and a representative sample of peritoneal pus or fluid should be sent for immediate Gram's stain and for aerobic and anaerobic culture. The odor of peritonitis pus is of diagnostic importance. Altemeier studied the ability of *E. coli* to produce a putrid odor when grown on sterile human pus and found that no odor resulted, although good growth of bacteria was obtained. On the other hand, when similar sterile pus was inoculated with anaerobic streptococci and *Bacteroides melaninogenicus,* a marked, penetrating foul odor was produced. In addition to these two organisms, other anaerobic bacteria, particularly members of the *Clostridium* group, recovered from peritonitis pus are capable of producing unpleasant odors.

The general rule is that aerobic infections do not produce a marked odor, whereas infections containing anaerobes do. Combining information provided by the odor of the pus in peritonitis with the staining characteristics of bacteria noted on a Gram's stain of the same material, together with knowledge of the regional differences in the intestinal microflora provides information of the possible organisms present when there is peritonitis due to perforation of the gastrointestinal tract or the biliary system, and permits a presumptive diagnosis of the infecting organisms.

Improvement in techniques for isolation and identification of anaerobic bacteria, particularly the use of selective media and gas-liquid chromatography, have resulted in more accurate early identification of anaerobic organisms in cultures of patients with peritonitis. The contribution of both aerobic and anaerobic microorganisms in the pathogenesis of peritonitis (see Interactions of Bacteria and the Peritoneum, above) dictates that initial antibiotic coverage be provided to combat both groups of organisms. The results of a Gram's stain on a properly submitted fluid specimen, as well as later culture results, helps to decide the choice of antibiotics.

Debridement of Exudate. In the operative management of peritonitis, judicious mechanical debridement is important. The objective is to remove as much debris as possible without stirring up additional bleeding. All peritoneal pus, pseudomembranes, loosely adherent fibrin, and other exudates, as well as the content of any localized collections or abscesses, should be completely excised once the source of the peritonitis has been controlled. Viable bacteria become trapped in fibrin exudate in the early stages of peritonitis. If not removed, they form a focus for later reinfection or for abscess formation. Experimentally, administration of heparin improves the outcome in septic peritonitis; the effect is thought due to prevention of fibrin deposition.

Fibrin may also play a role in intraperitoneal adhesion formation. Gentle dissection of all adhesions of bowel and mesentery should be done together with removal of pus and exudate from the subhepatic, subdiaphragmatic, and pelvic cavities. Moderate debridement that does not induce significant bleeding was associated with no mortality in a group of 92 patients with peritonitis reported by Hudspeth. More radical debridement, however, is not beneficial.

Lavage. Presently, the only widely accepted method of cleaning the peritoneal cavity is irrigation with saline solution of all parts of the peritoneal cavity until the effluent is clear. Washing the contaminated peritoneal cavity with large volumes of irrigant was first advocated by Price in 1905. The next year, Torek reported that large-volume irrigation reduced mortality in generalized peritonitis following appendicitis to 14 percent, an extremely good experience at the time of that report. The procedure later fell into disrepute because of the fear, never clinically documented, that lavage disseminates peritoneal contamination.

Burnett reintroduced peritoneal lavage in the management of suppurative peritonitis, and reported a two-thirds reduction in mortality. The modern concept of peritoneal lavage views the contaminated peritoneum in the same way as a contaminated dermal wound: copious irrigation is a major component of therapy and involves the use of large volumes, up to 10 L and occasionally more, of saline solution with the objective of diluting and removing all contaminated peritoneal contents.

Although peritoneal irrigation is a safe procedure, its efficacy in reducing morbidity and mortality associated with suppurative peritonitis remains controversial. Experimentally, lavage reduces mortality in fecal peritonitis. Further, there is no difference in mortality following local or diffuse peritoneal contamination by feces containing equal numbers of bacteria, so that even if dissemination occurs during lavage the negative effect would be counterbalanced by reduction in numbers of bacteria through dilution. Lavage also has been objected to on the basis that phagocytic macrophages and neutrophils cannot function unless attached to serosa: "phagocytes can't function if they're swimming." But phagocytes dislodged from peritoneal serosa are already either dead or nonfunctional, in which case lavage causes no harm. In more recent experimental reports, systemic antibiotic therapy combined with crystalloid irrigation resulted in improved cure in induced fecal peritonitis. But addition of antibiotics directly to peritoneal lavage fluid has had mixed effects on abscess formation and survival; the bacterial count in the peritoneum, and associated mortality, also is decreased considerably following saline irrigation in controls.

In 1967, Noon and associates reported the first prospective randomized trial of the effectiveness of topically administered antibiotics in peritonitis. They demonstrated decreased mortality and a lower incidence of wound infection using a kanamycin-bacitracin solution as a "final rinse" in patients with purulent peritonitis. The incidence of wound infection was decreased to 12 percent from 24 percent in controls, but there was no benefit of antibiotic lavage in reducing intraabdominal infections.

Jennings and colleagues reported the efficacy of continuous, postoperative peritoneal lavage in the setting of severe peritonitis. A significant benefit was realized with no septic complications and no deaths secondary to sepsis, although the overall mortality in the group of 20 patients was 15 percent. Washington and associates, in a prospective study of 50 patients, added antibiotic and heparin to the peritoneal lavage solution. A decreased incidence of abscess formation was seen in the lavage group. However, a statistically significant difference in mortality was not observed between the lavage and control groups. It appears that an important beneficial effect of lavage is its mechanical action in removing adjuvant substances from the peritoneal cavity.

The effectiveness of antiseptic agents, as contrasted to antibiotics, as irrigation solutions in bacterial peritonitis remains controversial. In an experimental model of suppurative peritonitis, the antiseptics taurolin, noxytiolin, povidine-iodine, and hypochlorite were found to be ineffective in reducing mortality, but chlorhexidine gluconate was efficacious. In a randomized trial, a povidine-iodine solution was effective in decreasing intraabdominal infectious complications compared with saline irrigation. But, when studied in an animal model of bacteria peritonitis, povidine-iodine was both ineffective and deleterious.

A resurgence of enthusiasm for treating widespread intraabdominal infection by leaving the postoperative abdomen completely open has recently occurred. The purported advantage of this method of management is ease in bedside exploration of the abdomen to break up loculi of purulent material that may occur after operation. The major difficulties with this technique are the risk of evisceration, poor efficacy in completely draining intraabdominal infections, need for ventilatory support, and recurrent sepsis. An alternative to the open method is placement of polypropylene mesh with a zipper to allow repetitive access to the abdominal cavity for lavage and exploration of patients with severe suppurative peritonitis. Neither technique has been widely adopted.

Drains. The use of drains, particularly sump-suction drains, is an important feature in the surgical management of an intraabdominal abscess or similarly localized peritoneal fluid collection. Insertion of drains in cases of severe pancreatitis is a common practice, although somewhat controversial. But placement of drains in cases of generalized peritonitis is of no benefit. In fact, the presence of drains in such cases is harmful since they interfere with peritoneal defense mechanisms, provide a route for exogenous bacterial contamination, and promote formation of unwanted adhesions. The failure of drains in management of generalized peritonitis was clearly demonstrated by Yates in 1905; his observations have been confirmed in several more recent studies. Drains should not be used in peritonitis unless there is an abscess or similar space to be drained.

Closure. If a midline wound has been made, the fascia may be closed as a single layer with running monofila-

ment suture (polypropylene or nylon), taking generous bites of tissue on either side. Some surgeons recommend use of interrupted fascial suture technique and also favor placement of additional retention sutures; the reasons advanced for recommending these more tedious suture techniques are a supposed reduction in the incidence of wound dehiscence. However, the occurrence of dehiscence in suppurative peritonitis is primarily due to infection in the wound. Septic wounds are likely to fail to heal whatever suture technique is used for closure; interrupted or retention sutures will not prevent subsequent dehiscence.

The skin and subcutaneous portions of the wound usually should be left open. A few layers of fine gauze soaked in antibiotic irrigating solution are used to cover the subcutaneous tissues, but the wound should not be tightly packed. Dry gauze dressings then lightly cover the wound. All dressings, including those within the wound, are removed in 24 to 48 h and replaced with a simple covering bandage. Delayed primary closure with adhesive strips can be begun 4 or 5 days later if the wound remains healthy.

POSTOPERATIVE MANAGEMENT. The general principles of postoperative care include continued administration of intravenous fluids and antibiotics. Complications of sepsis—particularly respiratory failure, renal failure, and disseminated intravascular coagulation—should be expected and searched for continuously by monitoring ventilatory volume, urine output, blood gases, serum creatinine, and coagulation factors. Abnormalities in the physiologic responses of these organ systems and metabolic abnormalities as evidenced by a rising bilirubin or persisting acidosis are early signs of an intraperitoneal source of continuing sepsis and developing organ failure.

When the results of antibiotic sensitivity studies done on the operative specimen of peritoneal pus are available, consideration should be given to changing antibiotic therapy to the most specific and least toxic of the drugs that appear to be effective (see Chap. 5). If the patient is stable, and clinical evidence of sepsis is subsiding, antibiotics should not necessarily be changed only on the basis of laboratory sensitivity studies. But patients who remain febrile or demonstrate persistent leukocytosis without fever for more than 7 to 10 days have a higher incidence of developing a relapse of intraabdominal infection despite exhibiting an initial favorable clinical response; a change in antibiotic therapy is appropriate in such patients. Antibiotic treatment should not be stopped until the patient is clinically well enough to be consuming a regular diet and other clinical evidence (fever <100°F and WBC <12,000 for 48 h) indicates that residual infection is unlikely.

ASEPTIC (CHEMICAL) PERITONITIS

This form of peritonitis develops whenever irritant materials gain entry to the peritoneal cavity, usually because of rupture of a solid or upper abdominal hollow viscus. The soilage initially is sterile or nearly so, a feature by which chemical peritonitis differs from suppurative peritonitis. The aseptic inflammatory reaction gives rise to the general clinical symptoms and physiologic sequellae discussed under Peritonitis: General Responses. Translocation of plasma volume into the peritoneal cavity with the secondary systemic responses of hypovolemia is the major initial reaction.

Secondary bacterial invasion may occur, sometimes as early as 12 h after the initial peritoneal insult, even when no bacteria enter the peritoneal cavity via a perforated viscus or from the environment through a traumatic wound. Presumably because episodes of transient portal vein bacteremia are relatively common though ordinarily innocuous, an initially aseptic peritonitis cannot be expected to remain sterile. Most of the substances that cause aseptic peritonitis are capable of acting as adjuvants whenever secondary bacterial contamination occurs, promoting proliferation of microorganisms and, later, onset of the systemic effects of suppurative peritonitis.

Symptoms typically are sudden, severe pain, tenderness, and rigidity of the abdominal muscles. Backache occurs if the retroperitoneal area is involved. During the next few hours, peritoneal fluid dilution and neutralization of the irritant may produce a deceptive sense of improvement. Leukocytosis is present. Plain abdominal and chest films are useful in showing bowel distention, intraabdominal fluid accumulation, and specific injuries after trauma. The most helpful diagnostic test in some situations, apart from exploratory laparotomy itself, is a peritoneal tap.

The principles of surgical management in cases of aseptic peritonitis include preoperative resuscitation with fluids and similar measures; control of the source of contamination during laparotomy by suture closure or excision, as appropriate; debridement of foreign substances; copious lavage; and administration of antibiotics to combat the risks of existing infection.

GASTRIC CONTENTS. Gastric juice is highly irritating to the peritoneum, not only because of its hydrochloric acid content but also because of the presence of mucin and digestive enzymes. If gastric juice gains access to the peritoneal cavity through a perforated duodenal ulcer, spilled material initially is sterile in the majority of cases because the normal "acid barrier" of the stomach effectively kills swallowed microorganisms. In patients who have been treated with H_2-blocker drugs, and in cases of perforated gastric ulcer in which a high proportion of patients also have a defective gastric acid barrier to bacteria due to diminished secretion of acid, the spilled gastric juice regularly is contaminated with swallowed aerobic and anaerobic organisms derived from the oral (mouth) flora and from the environment.

In gastroduodenal perforation, the interval between the occurrence of the perforation and its closure is viewed by many surgeons as the primary determinant of postoperative morbidity and mortality. But Hamilton and Harbrecht, in a review of patients with perforated ulcer, found the degree of peritoneal contamination and the incidence of contaminating virulent pathogens greater when

operation was performed 6 h or less after perforation than in operations done after 24 h. The incidence of negative cultures in this study (about 50 percent) was the same whether spillage was light or marked. Postoperative complications (64 percent of which were septic) were related only to the presence of marked spillage. This apparent paradox must be due partially to peritoneal fluid dilution that occurs during the initial inflammatory response to the peritoneal insult and to killing of bacteria in the peritoneum by host defense mechanisms. Unfortunately, the use and duration of antibiotic therapy in these patients was not recorded. The findings in this study are in contrast to the usually accepted surgical wisdom that indicates that the incidence of peritoneal contamination by virulent pathogens is less when the operation is performed within 6 h of perforation compared with later operative times. The important point illustrated by this study is that taking sufficient time preoperatively to complete fluid resuscitation and otherwise prepare the patient for operation is rewarded by a reduction in mortality risk.

PANCREATIC JUICE. Pancreatic secretions enter the peritoneal cavity during episodes of acute pancreatitis or following pancreatic trauma. If the mode of entry is due to rupture of a pancreatic duct or of a pseudocyst, with release of relatively large volumes of activated pancreatic juice, pancreatic ascites ensues. Because the pancreatic juice is diluted in the ascites, the overall peritoneal reaction varies considerably, from mild to relatively severe inflammation. Alternatively, pancreatic juice may transude through the retroperitoneum in acute pancreatitis. In these cases, typically, the volume of accumulating intraperitoneal fluid is less. If the pancreatic exudate is combined with blood and breakdown products of pancreatic necrosis, as is true in cases of hemorrhagic pancreatitis, secondary infection occurs in a higher proportion of instances.

BILE. Most commonly, bile enters the peritoneal cavity as a result of leakage following exploration of the common bile duct or other operation on the biliary system. Rupture of the gallbladder during acute cholecystitis, perforation of a gallbladder carcinoma, or infrequently, rupture of the common duct due to necrosis from a common duct stone also may lead to spill of bile into the peritoneal cavity. Although bile peritonitis follows rupture of an inflamed gallbladder, biliary peritonitis can occur without detectable gallbladder perforation. In such cases, presumably, the mechanism for leakage of bile involves transudation through an ischemic portion of the acutely inflamed gallbladder wall.

Sterile bile is a chemical irritant. Frequently, bacterial contamination, either associated with the cause of the biliary rupture, itself, or having been acquired secondarily, leads to a particularly virulent form of septic biliary peritonitis. Experimental studies of bile peritonitis have shown that both inflammation and lethality in animals are reduced if therapeutic serum levels of antibiotics have been achieved at the time of biliary leakage.

URINE. Intraperitoneal rupture of the bladder usually is a sequela of severe trauma. Sterile urine is an extremely irritating substance, and the chemical insult frequently is followed by secondary infection. Spontaneous intraperitoneal perforation of the urinary bladder also occurs in neurologically handicapped patients. Necrosis of the bladder wall in these patients, secondary to chronic intramural infection, results in spill of infected urine into the peritoneal cavity. In addition to the direct peritoneal irritation caused by hyperosmolar urine, reabsorption of acidic metabolic acid end-products and urea leads to acidosis and uremia.

ACUTE HEMOPERITONEUM (ABDOMINAL APOPLEXY). Intraperitoneal blood is not very irritating. If red cells lyse, the released cell contents act as a mild hyperosmolar irritant. Blood can be transfused intraperitoneally; the rate at which red cells subsequently enter the general circulation is slow, but the fraction of a transfused unit of blood detectable in the circulating blood volume 48 to 96 h after intraperitoneal injection is the same as after an intravenous transfusion. It is not blood, per se, which is of concern in relation to peritonitis, but the fact that blood or, more particularly, hemoglobin and ferrous iron act as adjuvants of a particularly noxious sort should subsequent bacterial infection of the peritoneal cavity occur.

Spontaneous rupture of a visceral artery, most frequently the splenic and less commonly the hepatic or a gastroepiploic artery, or rupture of the spleen, liver, or of a hepatic tumor may produce a massive acute hemoperitoneum. The clinical symptoms are of abdominal pain accompanied by tenderness, absent bowel sounds, and other clinical signs of peritonitis. The leukocyte count may be elevated. Treatment consists of early laparotomy and control of the bleeding source.

MECONIUM. Intrauterine perforation of the bowel with leakage of sterile meconium produces a marked sterile peritonitis, resulting in matted adhesive obliteration of the abdominal cavity. If the bowel perforation remains uncontrolled after birth of the infant, secondary bacterial infection is the rule. Aggressive operative management and the administration of broad-spectrum antibiotics sometimes improve what is otherwise a grim situation.

CHYLE. Chronic chylous effusion into the peritoneal cavity as chylous ascites or into the chest as chylothorax is not rare; acute symptoms are unusual. Acute chylous peritonitis, on the other hand, which results from a sudden outpouring of chyle into the free peritoneal cavity, may produce signs and symptoms suggestive of an acute abdominal catastrophe but is a distinctly rare clinical syndrome. Chylous peritoneal leaks usually are secondary to injuries of the larger lymphatic vessels during operations on retroperitoneal organs.

MUCUS AND SIMILAR SUBSTANCES. Mucus from intestinal secretions released in small-bowel rupture, or the contents from a ruptured ovarian cyst or mucocele of the appendix, induce a sterile inflammatory reaction of the peritoneum. Rupture of a dermoid cyst of the ovary can produce a severe peritonitis, because of the cyst content of cholesterol, hair, and other irritant materials.

ENDOTOXIC PERITONITIS. Under certain circumstances, constriction or occlusion of intestinal vessels produces sufficient ischemia that there is increased permeability of the bowel wall, permitting transudation of preformed endotoxin generated by the intestinal flora within the bowel lumen into the peritoneal cavity. Transperitoneal absorption of endotoxin then produces systemic symptoms of gram-negative sepsis. The degree of peritoneal inflammation, per se, in such instances ordinarily is not great unless bowel wall necrosis or perforation ensues. The vascular obstruction leading to this syndrome can involve either large or small bowel and may be segmental or extensive. A history of symptoms or episodes suggestive of arrhythmia or heart failure should be sought.

Generalized crampy abdominal pain, tenderness, low-grade fever, mental apathy or agitation, abdominal distention, and bowel hypomotility may be accompanied by vomiting, anorexia, and mucoid or bloody diarrhea. Leukocytosis with a left shift is consistently present. The serum amylase level is elevated, since amylase also escapes from the bowel into the peritoneal cavity and is absorbed. Plain films of the abdomen show only ileus. When mesenteric occlusion is suspected, arteriography may establish the diagnosis and also permits intraarterial vasodilator perfusion before and during laparotomy.

Episodes of aseptic endotoxic peritonitis also have been reported among patients undergoing chronic peritoneal dialysis due to contamination of dialysis fluid by preformed coliform endotoxin. Onset of symptoms occurs on the average 7 h after initiation of dialysis with the contaminated fluid. Diffuse abdominal pain and rebound tenderness are the predominant findings; fever is present in only about half the patients. Discontinuation of dialysis usually relieves the pain promptly, and the symptoms rapidly clear.

FOREIGN BODIES. A foreign body may be deposited in the peritoneal cavity during an operative procedure (sponge or instrument inadvertently left behind) or may result from penetrating injuries, with the penetrating missile itself or material carried with it (clothing, earth) acting as a foreign body. Foreign bodies such as fish bones, wood splinters, needles, pins, and glass may perforate the gastrointestinal or genitourinary tracts to enter the peritoneal cavity.

The relative amounts of acute exudation and later fibrosis vary greatly depending on the nature of the foreign body and the degree of bacterial contamination that occurs in conjunction with it. A foreign body may lead to formation of an abscess with an interval course of fever, chills, and toxicity, and the eventual appearance of an intraabdominal mass. On the other hand, small foreign bodies, such as shrapnel, simply may be walled off by fibrous tissue and give rise to few if any significant clinical manifestations.

BARIUM. Barium sulfate may be spilled into the peritoneal cavity during radiologic investigation of the gastrointestinal tract if a perforation is present or occurs during the examination. Spillage of barium causes *barium peritonitis,* a clinical and pathologic sequence of specific events secondary to the association of intraperitoneal barium and enteric contents including bacteria.

Barium is extremely irritating to peritoneal surfaces and, in combination with enteric contents, poses a lethal challenge to a patient. It has been shown experimentally that the association of barium and feces is more deleterious than either alone. The chemical injury to the peritoneal surface by barium causes release of histamine and other permeability factors from peritoneal mast cells. The free barium may activate the clotting system by way of the intrinsic pathway. Also, because of tissue injury, factors are released from injured cells that may then activate the clotting system by way of the extrinsic pathway. Both pathways result in the conversion of prothrombin to thrombin which then converts fibrinogen to fibrin. The end result is a severe *fibrinous peritonitis*.

Zheutlin and colleagues, in a collective review of 53 cases of barium peritonitis secondary to colon perforation, reported in 1952 a mortality of 53 percent for patients with laparotomy and of 58 percent for patients treated nonoperatively. More recent studies, though of smaller groups of patients, indicate a more favorable outcome with early surgical exploration, removal of as much barium as possible, and control of the source of leak. Yamamura and colleagues have suggested that using urokinase solution for irrigation and for wiping the peritoneal surfaces is most effective in removing barium. Other key factors in patient survival are adequate intravenous fluids to replace the large intraperitoneal fluid losses that occur with severe peritonitis and appropriate antibiotic therapy for treatment of bacterial contamination.

GRANULOMATOUS PERITONITIS

This group of diseases is characterized by a peritoneal reaction that includes formation of granulomas and is associated with a markedly increased incidence of adhesion formation compared with other forms of peritonitis.

TUBERCULOUS PERITONITIS. Formerly quite common, the incidence of tuberculous peritonitis has declined as has the incidence of all forms of human tuberculosis over the past several decades. This now is a rare disease; it usually occurs in patients who are malnourished or who have cirrhosis. The primary focus of infection from which secondary involvement of the peritoneal cavity occurs may not be clinically apparent in tuberculous peritonitis. Although nearly all patients dying with tuberculous peritonitis have a primary focus identified at autopsy, in only about a third of cases currently being seen clinically is the primary focus readily diagnosed. In cases in which the primary focus of tuberculous infection remains obscure, it is almost always later demonstrated to be in the lung. Most cases are due to reactivation of latent peritoneal tuberculosis which has been established by hematogenous spread from a pulmonary focus during an earlier episode of acute disease. In the past, the disease has been classified into wet and dry phases. The ''wet'' phase refers to the early, subacute, ascitis stage of the disease, while the ''dry'' phase refers to later resolution, during which dense adhesions are formed.

Clinically, tuberculous peritonitis is insidious, presenting with fever, anorexia, weakness, and weight loss. Some ascites almost always is present, and more than half of affected patients have dull, diffuse abdominal pain. On examination, the abdomen is modestly tender, but the classically described ''doughy abdomen'' is rarely found today. Clinical manifestations of generalized tuberculous infection are seen in about one-third of patients, and include anorexia, weight loss, and night sweats. Tubercle bacilli can be retrieved 80 percent of the time from ascitic fluid if more than 1 L of fluid is cultured. The ascitic fluid has an increased protein concentration, lymphocytic pleocytosis, and a glucose concentration below 30 mg/dL. If these measures do not establish the diagnosis, peritoneoscopy and direct biopsy of the peritoneum are recommended.

The peritoneoscopic appearance of tuberculous peritonitis is characteristic. Typical stalactite-like fibrinous masses hang from the parietal peritoneum in the lower part of the abdomen. A directed, percutaneous needle biopsy of a granulomatous lesion, as well as samples of peritoneal fluid for direct smear examination and injection into a guinea pig, should be obtained. As a last resort, exploratory laparotomy may be undertaken to establish the diagnosis. If laparotomy is carried out, a peritoneal biopsy should be taken; the placement of drains or the exteriorization of bowel should be avoided.

Tuberculous peritonitis, formerly frequently fatal as a manifestation of uncontrolled generalized tuberculosis, now is arrested by chemotherapy in nearly all patients. Triple antituberculous drug therapy, instituted early in the course of the disease, is associated with a good prognosis. Therapy should continue for at least 2 years after the patient becomes asymptomatic. Since tuberculosis peritonitis may heal with formation of dense fibrous adhesions, patients suffering this disease always are liable to the future development of an intestinal obstruction. Treatment with prednisone during the initial few months of antituberculous drug therapy reduces the incidence of adhesion formation and the subsequent development of obstruction.

***CANDIDA* PERITONITIS.** While *Candida* and other yeast organisms are ubiquitous in the lumen of the gastrointestinal tract, only occasionally do these yeasts become pathogenic. Solomkin and coworkers have reviewed 56 episodes of *Candida* peritonitis with an associated mortality of 25 percent. Once *Candida* is cultured from peritoneal fluid, it is important to distinguish whether this is due to colonization or to infection. The presence of *Candida* in the urine or sputum, as well as the appearance of pseudohyphae in tissue biopsies, indicates infection. The presence of a positive blood culture for yeast is a grim prognostic sign, being associated with a mortality of 85 percent. Treatment with parenteral antifungal agents (amphotericin B, miconazole) should be instituted as early as the diagnosis can be established. Solomkin has demonstrated the efficacy of low doses of amphotericin B in the treatment of *Candida* peritonitis and has avoided the toxicity sometimes associated with higher doses of this agent.

While immunosuppressed patients, particularly those with cancer or those receiving chronic steroids, may be prone to develop peritonitis due to yeast, all patients who have bowel surgery and receive broad-spectrum antibiotics are at risk for this complication. Overgrowth of *Candida* within the lumen of the intestine usually precedes the development of invasive infection. The oral administration of antifungal agents (nystatin, ketoconazole) to all patients at risk is beneficial in reducing the incidence of intestinal colonization.

OTHER GRANULOMATOUS PERITONEAL INFECTIONS. These are very rare diseases that occur under special circumstances. The organisms involved may be *Histoplasma* (fungus), ameba, or *Strongyloides* (parasite). Amebic peritonitis usually follows rupture of a hepatic amebic abscess, but a few cases have been due to perforation of amebic colitis. The prognosis is grave, but operative debridement results in a better outcome than nonoperative management.

IATROGENIC GRANULOMATOUS PERITONITIS. Peritoneal inflammation, exudation, formation of granulomas, and healing by formation of dense adhesions all may follow contamination of the peritoneal cavity by glove lubricants (talc, lycopodium, mineral oil, cornstarch, rice starch) or cellulose fibers from disposable gauze pads, drapes, and gowns. The reaction, particularly that to rice starch, is largely a hypersensitivity response.

The clinical features include migratory abdominal pain, fever, physical signs of peritonitis, and, often, the presence of an abdominal mass, all developing within 3 weeks after an otherwise uncomplicated abdominal operation. The surgical wound may appear normal or may be moderately indurated. Plain abdominal films are nonspecific. The total white blood cell count is normal; eosinophilia of 4 to 9 percent sometimes is identified.

Grant and colleagues have suggested the use of an intradermal skin test in the diagnosis of granulomatous starch peritonitis. While a positive response may be difficult to assess visually, microscopic changes are demonstrable on biopsy of the skin test site in a majority of patients and may obviate the need for an operation to establish the diagnosis. While no false-positive results with the skin-test delayed hypersensitivity response were reported, 20 percent of patients had false-negative tests.

When the diagnosis remains unclear, laparoscopy may be helpful. If recognized with assurance, reoperation may be avoided and corticosteroids administered. Eventually, the acute peritonitis resolves. If laparotomy is undertaken because the diagnosis is obscure, a thickened peritoneum studded with white nodules is found. Histologically, those nodules that contain starch granules are doubly refractile under polarized light and are surrounded by granulomatous foreign body inflammation.

The cornerstone of management of this problem is prevention. Current techniques of wiping and washing gloves do not remove all the starch from their surface. Nonetheless, gloves should be washed or wiped off before gloved hands are put into the peritoneal cavity, and care should be taken to avoid spillage of glove contents should a glove be torn during an operation. The search for a more acceptable glove lubricant continues. Sodium bicarbonate has been used successfully as a gloving agent but requires special sterilization measures; silicones also have been suggested.

SPONTANEOUS (PRIMARY) BACTERIAL PERITONITIS

Spontaneous bacterial peritonitis is an infection of ascitic fluid without any apparent intraabdominal source. It can be a life-threatening illness, particularly in patients with cirrhosis. The spectrum of bacteria causing this syndrome and the population primarily affected have changed during the last decade. Spontaneous bacterial peritonitis is now more common in adults than in children and shows no differential sex incidence. Children with nephrosis, formerly the group most commonly affected, have been replaced by adults with cirrhosis or systemic lupus as the population primarily affected. While gram-positive organisms formerly caused the majority of these infections, gram-negative enteric bacteria are more common today.

It appears that impairment of body immunological defense mechanisms is related to development of spontaneous peritonitis. The prevalence previously was reported to be about 8 percent in cirrhotics with ascites, but has now risen to about 18 percent. Preexisting ascites is a predisposing factor in the majority of cases, particularly if the protein concentration in the ascites is low. The mortality risk is of the order of 48 to 70 percent in cirrhotic adults but is lower in nephrotic children.

The relevance of preexisting ascites is not clear; ascites certainly provides an ideal culture medium. Any abnormal fluid collection appears to be at risk to develop infection in patients who are constitutionally predisposed; both spontaneous empyema and pericarditis have been reported in association with spontaneous peritonitis. On the other hand, adult patients have been described who have had no preceding ascites, and the great majority of patients who develop spontaneous peritonitis in childhood do not have ascites.

This form of peritonitis is a monomicrobial infection; i.e., there is only a single species of bacteria present, in contrast to the polymicrobial infection of typical suppurative (secondary) peritonitis. Though pneumococci formerly were the most frequent infecting organisms, coliform organisms now are the chief pathogens, accounting for 70 percent of the infections, with *E. coli* being the most common isolate. Gram-positive cocci account for 10 to 20 percent of cases and anaerobes are seen in 6 to 14 percent.

The route by which bacteria are transmitted to the peritoneal cavity is not known. Evidence favoring transmural migration of bacteria from the intestine is derived from the fact that systemic endotoxemia and the presence of endotoxin in ascitic fluid can be demonstrated by limulus assay in many decompensated cirrhotics, even though no bacteria are present in the ascites and the patients do not have clinical evidence of peritonitis. Evidence favoring the hematogenous route stems from the frequent clinical association of spontaneous peritonitis with urinary tract infections harboring the same organisms, and from cases of simultaneous spontaneous empyema and pericarditis associated with spontaneous peritonitis.

Clinical symptoms usually are of short duration in children; the onset of symptoms is more insidious in ascitic adults. Most patients complain of some abdominal pain and distention; vomiting, lethargy, and fever are more prominent in children. Diarrhea is usual in neonates but seldom seen in adults. Bowel sounds are variable. Leukocytosis usually is present. Free air usually is not seen on abdominal x-rays. All in all, the clinical picture may be quite desultory.

A peritoneal tap is the most useful diagnostic test. Fluid is examined for polymorphonuclear cell count and pH; a Gram's stain should be done and a specimen sent for culture. The polymorphonuclear cell count has the highest sensitivity and specificity in making the diagnosis. A polymorphonuclear cell count greater than 250/mm^3 is considered positive for the diagnosis. Recent studies of ascitic fluid in patients suspected of having spontaneous peritonitis have shown that a high arterial-ascitic fluid pH gradient also correlates with a positive diagnosis. Ascitic fluid pH is significantly lower in spontaneous bacterial peritonitis than in sterile ascitic fluid.

Only about a third of patients will have organisms seen on a Gram's stain of the centrifuged fluid that is subsequently culture positive. If the Gram's stain shows only gram-positive cocci, the presence of spontaneous peritonitis is strongly suggested. If a mixed flora, gram-positive and gram-negative bacteria, is present, intestinal perforation is likely and laparotomy is necessary. The presence of gram-negative bacteria only on the Gram's stain is consistent with either spontaneous peritonitis or secondary peritonitis. Antibiotic therapy should be started and the patient managed initially nonoperatively.

When the diagnosis of spontaneous bacterial peritonitis is confirmed by any of the above criteria, antibiotic therapy should be started. Usually, a cephalosporin or ampicillin plus an aminoglycoside are appropriate since 90 percent of the organisms causing spontaneous peritonitis are sensitive to these antibiotic regimens.

OTHER FORMS OF PERITONITIS

PERITONITIS RELATED TO PERITONEAL DIALYSIS. A resurgence in the use of peritoneal dialysis for patients with chronic renal failure has occurred. The major cause of morbidity in this group is associated peritonitis which is also the largest single cause of patient failure on chronic ambulatory peritoneal dialysis. Peritonitis occurs more frequently in patients undergoing continuous ambulatory peritoneal dialysis (CAPD) than in those who undergo intermittent peritoneal dialysis. Catheter-related infection is the most common complication. There appears to be no correlation between the occurrence of peritonitis and the duration of catheter placement. Other causes of peritonitis in CAPD patients are tunnel infections and cuff extrusion. The bacteriology and treatment of dialysis-related peritonitis are considerably different from those of patients with other types of peritoneal infections; fungal infections are more common in this group than in other forms of septic peritonitis.

The diagnosis is established when any of the following have occurred: (1) positive culture form the peritoneal fluid; (2) a cloudy dialysate effluent; (3) clinical signs of peritonitis. The Gram's stain of dialysis effluent is frequently negative in dialysis catheter-related peritonitis. Attention to sterile technique, use of topical povidine-iodine about the catheter wound, and use of sterile dialysate prepackaged in plastic bags all seem to reduce the incidence of infection.

In contrast to other causes of septic peritonitis, dialysis-related peritonitis usually is due to a single organism. Two-thirds of patients with positive cultures will have a gram-positive coccus as the causative organism, usually *Staph. aureus* or *Staph. epidermidis*. Gram-negative bacteria usually are found only in patients with recurring episodes of peritonitis, which may reflect a change in flora related to antibiotic administration for prior episodes. Patients with dialysis-related peritonitis rarely have a positive blood culture in contrast to patients with other causes of peritonitis who have a 30 percent incidence of bacteremia. Anaerobes rarely are cultured. The presence of anaerobes or a mixed flora suggests intestinal perforation or other intraabdominal disease, e.g., diverticulitis or cholecystitis, as the cause of peritonitis. Yeasts and tubercle bacilli rarely have been found as causative agents. The incidence of culture-negative peritonitis in dialysis patients ranges from 10 to 27 percent.

The initial treatment of dialysis-related peritonitis is administration of antibiotics and heparin in the dialysate, as well as an increase in the dwell time of the dialysate fluid. The indications for catheter removal include persistence of peritonitis after 4 to 5 days of treatment, the presence of fungal or tuberculous peritonitis, fecal peritonitis, or a severe skin catheter site infection.

A related form of peritonitis, due to infection of a ventriculoperitoneal shunt, exhibits clinical signs and symptoms similar to those of peritoneal dialysis catheter peritonitis. Peritonitis should be suspected in any patient having such a shunt who develops any abdominal symptoms.

Patients with chronically implanted peritoneal catheters may develop sclerosing encapsulating peritonitis; it is not a frequent occurrence, with a reported incidence of 1 to 6 percent. The etiology is unknown. Affected patients usually have had frequent bouts of peritonitis. Treatment is directed at complications such as bowel obstruction.

DRUG-RELATED PERITONITIS. A number of cases have been reported of patients who developed striking thickening of the visceral peritoneum weeks to months after treatment with beta-blocking drugs. The most frequent clinical presentation is with a typical small-bowel obstruction, often insidious in onset, associated with profound weight loss and with a prominent abdominal mass on physical examination. The operative findings are strik-

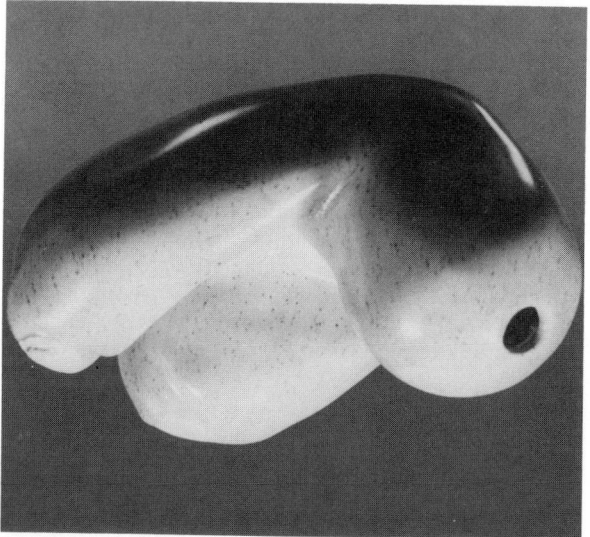

Fig. 34-4. Plaster model of peritoneal cavity recesses into which infected fluid may collect by gravity. Dependent areas are subdiaphragmatic, paravertebral, and pelvic. (From: *Monk and Wilson, 1966, with permission.*)

ing: the whole of the small bowel usually is caught up in a thick sac, which sometimes can be lifted as a single mass from the peritoneal cavity. The agglomeration of small intestine produces the mass that is palpable preoperatively.

Administration of isoniazid and erythromycin estolate has been reported to cause acute abdominal symptoms mimicking clinical peritonitis, but not development of true peritonitis.

PERIODIC PERITONITIS. Recurrent episodes of abdominal pain, fever, and leukocytosis occur in certain population groups in and around the Mediterranean basin, notably in Armenians, Jews, and Arabs. The disease appears to be familial. The major point for the surgeon is that the episodes do not require laparotomy; so the diagnosis should be kept in mind if dealing with patients from the Levant. Laparotomy often is performed for the first episode, since an acute intraabdominal process requiring surgical cure cannot be ruled out. At operation, the peritoneal surfaces may be inflamed and there is free fluid, but smears and cultures reveal no bacteria. Even though it is normal, the appendix should be removed to eliminate the possibility of acute appendicitis in the differential diagnosis of future episodes. Colchicine is highly effective in preventing recurrent attacks, and, in fact, a favorable response to chronic administration of colchicine is a definitive diagnostic test.

INTRAABDOMINAL ABSCESSES

BASIC CONSIDERATIONS. An intraabdominal abscess is a localized collection of pus walled off from the rest of the peritoneal cavity by inflammatory adhesions between the

parietes, loops of bowel, and other intraabdominal viscera, the mesenteries, or omentum. An abscess may be solitary or multiple and may be intraperitoneal, retroperitoneal, or visceral. Intraperitoneal abscesses arise during resolution of generalized peritonitis, following complications of spontaneous intraabdominal diseases (appendicitis, diverticulitis, perforated ulcer), are secondary to intraabdominal operations, or follow abdominal trauma. An abscess usually develops only when host peritoneal defenses are able to localize peritonitis. Abscesses within solid viscera usually arise following hematogenous or lymphatic dissemination of infection to these organs from a septic focus elsewhere in the body. Retroperitoneal abscesses typically arise as a consequence of primary infection or inflammation of one of the retroperitoneal viscera, followed by secondary bacterial contamination.

Resolution of peritonitis with formation of a pelvic or subphrenic abscess is a reflection of the anatomy of the peritoneal cavity (Fig. 34-4). The upper part of the abdomen is divided nearly in half by the vertebral column. Both the pelvis and the subphrenic spaces on either side form deep and dependent cavities into which infected material is directed by gravity. In addition, the suction effect of respiration tends to draw infected peritoneal fluid up under the diaphragm. In a clinical investigation conducted in patients undergoing cholecystectomy or appendectomy, Autio found that x-ray contrast media injected at the operative site became widely disseminated within a few hours after operation. Whether the contrast material originally had been placed in the upper or lower part of the abdomen seemed to make little difference in its ability to spread; material was noted to move initially along the paracolic gutters in both directions and to collect primarily in the pelvis and in the subphrenic spaces.

Intraabdominal abscesses generally are polymicrobic (Table 34-3). Anaerobic organisms usually are the predominant flora, with *Bacteroides* and *Peptostreptococcus*

Table 34-3. BACTERIOLOGY OF
SUBPHRENIC ABSCESS

	Percent of recovery of organisms	
	1950–1970 *(60 patients)*	*1970–1975* *(24 patients)*
Aerobes:		
E. coli	60	96
Streptococci	49	67
Staphylococci	31	8
Klebsiella	17	21
Proteus	11	38
Pseudomonas	8	8
Anaerobes:		
Bacteroides spp.	11	83
Anaerobic cocci	0	50
Clostridia	6	50
Fusobacteria	0	38
Eubacteria	0	8

SOURCE: From Wang and Wilson, 1977.

species being found most commonly. In part, the predominance of anaerobes in intraabdominal abscesses is related to the metabolic conditions existing within an abscess cavity but also may be a reflection of the fact that aerobic organisms previously present in a more generalized peritoneal infection have been reduced in numbers or eradicated as a result of interactions of antibiotics and host defense mechanisms.

SYMPTOMS, SIGNS, INVESTIGATIONS. Symptoms of an intraabdominal abscess often are desultory, particularly early in the clinical course or with deep-seated infections. Paralytic ileus, abdominal distention, and anorexia are frequent symptoms, and sometimes there is vomiting. Recurring or persisting fever is seen in nearly all patients, typically intermittent or spiking in character at first, then progressively more persistent as the abscess matures. The fever spikes, which often are accompanied by chills and tachycardia, are the result of transient episodes of bacteremia from the abscess. Although fever is the most common finding, it may be absent in the very young, the elderly, and in malnourished or immunocompromised individuals. In these cases, hypothermia may be present. Also, patients on antibiotic therapy may not develop much fever. On occasion, septicemia may be sufficiently persistent that septic shock ensues.

The intensity of symptoms may be modified by administration of antibiotics that tend to suppress the infection, although antibiotic therapy rarely achieves a cure once a phlegmonous infection has proceeded to the formation of fluid pus. Continued administration of antibiotics may only lead to a process that smolders for many weeks. Because continued administration of antibiotics may hamper diagnosis of an abscess, it often is preferable to discontinue antibiotic therapy when the presence of an intraabdominal abscess is suspected, and direct efforts toward establishing a precise diagnosis of the location of the abscess.

Abdominal tenderness and pain may be present with a visceral or midabdominal abscess but are less commonly seen with subphrenic or retroperitoneal abscesses. Pain involving the anterior abdominal wall usually is absent with a pelvic abscess. When present, signs of pain and tenderness tend to be geographically related to the location of the abscess. Recurring or worsening jaundice also is an important clinical hallmark of the presence of an intraabdominal abscess. Progressive, multiple organ system failure also may occur.

Patients harboring an abscess usually have leukocytosis which invariably is accompanied by a left shift in the differential white cell count. Blood cultures will document episodes of septicemia and may identify one or several of the organisms involved in the abscess.

Radiologic techniques continue to play an important role in the diagnosis of intraabdominal abscess. Newer radiologic techniques also have come to play an important role in abscess drainage. The plain abdominal film and chest x-ray may give valuable information. Basal atelectasis and pleural effusion may be seen on the chest x-ray in the presence of a subphrenic abscess. Abnormal gas outside the bowel lumen or air-fluid levels may be seen on the plain abdominal film. Contrast studies remain useful for showing perforation, leak, obstruction, or organ displacement. An intravenous pyelogram may indicate malfunction or displacement of genitourinary structures when the abscess is located in the retroperitoneum.

Computer-assisted tomography is the most useful radiographic study in the diagnosis of intraabdominal abscess with respect to specificity, sensitivity, and accuracy. Combined with ultrasound, computerized tomography is able to diagnose accurately greater than 90 percent of intraabdominal abscesses. The reported difficulty is with inability to differentiate tumors, hematomas, cysts, and seromas, all of which may mimic abscesses.

Ultrasound is a valuable diagnostic modality but is adversely affected by obesity, excessive bowel gas, and the presence of drains or bandages on the abdominal wall. It is the procedure of choice for identifying a pelvic abscess in the presence of pelvic inflammatory disease. Radioisotope scanning with gallium (^{67}Ga) or indium-111 oxine is useful on some occasions. Gallium collects and persists in areas of inflammation. The reported accuracy of a gallium scan ranges from 54 to 82 percent, but its usefulness as a diagnostic test has been limited by the long delay required between injection and imaging, poor image resolution, collection of radioisotope within the colon if colonic emptying is delayed, and localization in the surgical incision or any other site of inflammation. It has poor resolution in leukopenic patients and may not be able to distinguish between abscess, phlegmon, or tumor. Indium-111-labeled leukocytes also collect in areas of inflammation and may be useful in localizing an intraabdominal abscess. The specificity of the indium scan is reported to be slightly better than that of gallium.

MANAGEMENT. Treatment of a suspected intraabdominal abscess by antibiotic therapy without drainage usually fails. Such therapy may be successful in a proportion of cases if instituted at that earlier time when there is only a localized phlegmonous inflammation and before the appearance of fluid pus. But, in the later stages of evolution of an abscess, most antibiotics are ineffective because of poor penetration into the abscess, destruction by enzymes in the abscess, and the low redox potential in the abscess that obviates the oxidative metabolic processes in bacteria necessary for antibiotic uptake, membrane transport, and intracellular action.

Once a localized collection of pus is formed, it must be drained. If not, the risk of complications due to delayed rupture of the abscess increases markedly. Secondary abscess rupture may result in recurrent generalized peritonitis, dissection through the diaphragm with production of an empyema or bronchopleural fistula, rupture into an adjacent hollow or solid viscus with marked worsening of the clinical state of the patient, and, on occasion, necrosis of a major blood vessel with consequent exsanguination. Once an abscess forms, failure to drain only produces a prolonged course of illness that nearly always increases the risk of death. Since many patients suffering an intraabdominal abscess are nutritionally depleted and septic, judicious though urgent preparation with attention to fluid resuscitation, parenteral nutrition, administration of antibiotics, and appropriate monitoring measures should be instituted prior to drainage.

Percutaneous Drainage. Percutaneous needle aspiration and closed catheter drainage, using computed tomographic and ultrasound guidance, is now preferred to operative drainage of most intraabdominal abscesses. The technical aspects of the procedure are well described in the radiologic literature. Usually, computed tomography is used to localize the abscess and to find a "window" for needle and catheter insertion. The "window" is that portion of the abscess in contact with the abdominal wall without the presence of intervening viscera. Ultrasound is then used to guide successive percutaneous placement into the abscess of a needle, guidewire, and "pigtail" catheter. The success rate of this method of drainage is about 80 percent. When the rate of complications, episodes of inadequate drainage, and duration of drainage were compared retrospectively between operative and percutaneous drainage, the percutaneous method was as successful as operative drainage.

The advantages of the percutaneous catheter drainage method appear to be a lack of contamination of the remainder of the peritoneal cavity, avoidance of a general anesthetic, and, perhaps, a lower incidence of inadequate drainage. The disadvantages are the relatively longer period between initiation of drainage and complete resolution of the abscess, occasional erosion of the drainage catheter into adjacent viscera, and failure of the method in most patients in whom the abscess is related to cancer, pancreatitis, or a bowel fistula. The place of percutaneous versus traditional open surgical drainage remains to be more accurately defined as experience is gained with this new method. It appears to be a major contribution to the management of intraabdominal abscess though it may not be curative in all cases. It may be an appropriate temporizing measure in some situations.

Percutaneous drainage of an intraabdominal abscess is usually successful if the following criteria are met: (1) there must be a well-established, unilocular fluid collection; (2) a safe percutaneous route of access must be available, and this often means location of the abscess adjacent to the body wall; (3) patients should be jointly evaluated by a surgeon and a radiologist; (4) there must be immediate operative backup in case of failure or complications.

Open Surgical Drainage. The indications for open surgical drainage are failure of percutaneous drainage, inability to safely drain percutaneously, the presence of a pancreatic or carcinomatous abscess, or an abscess associated with a bowel fistula. Additionally, exploration and open drainage are undertaken whenever the presence of an abscess is suspected clinically but cannot be localized by computed tomography or ultrasound. Abscesses in the pelvis often can be drained through the rectum or vagina, obviating the need for an abdominal operation.

If the abscess is in contact with the abdominal parietes or the diaphragm, a direct and, insofar as possible, extra-peritoneal approach is preferred. If exploration of the abdomen is being done to find an occult abscess, a midline approach is more efficient. The initial exploration should be limited to the area above or below the transverse colon and mesocolon, the choice depending on clinical suspicion of the origin of infection.

As the pyogenic membrane is encountered during exploration, confirmation of the presence of pus is obtained by needle aspiration. It is essential to obtain specimens of the abscess contents for Gram's stain, and for aerobic and anaerobic culture and sensitivity studies. All of the abscess contents should be evacuated by suction. The cavity should be thoroughly explored and all loculations within it broken down to create a single residual space. The cavity is irrigated and debrided of nonviable tissue. Multiple soft (Penrose) drains then should be brought from the abscess cavity to the exterior as directly and dependently as possible. If the abscess cavity is particularly large, or if thorough dependent drainage cannot be established, sump-suction drains should be employed in addition to soft drains.

Drains are left in place until external drainage stops or is clear. The drainage tract should then be irrigated, and a sinogram obtained to document collapse of the cavity before the drains are moved. It may take several weeks for a large cavity to become small enough to permit drains to be slowly advanced, allowing the drainage tract to seal as they are withdrawn.

An alternative approach called "controlled open drainage" has been suggested by Bradley and colleagues. This requires use of a plastic intestinal bag or surgical glove packed with gauze placed into the abscess cavity and brought out through a separate stab wound. This allows removal of the packing without relaparotomy. Improvement in overall mortality was reported, but there is limited experience with this technique of open drainage. Open packing of the abdomen and frequent relaparotomy using a zipper to facilitate the operative approach also have enjoyed a recent vogue.

Antibiotic Therapy. Antibiotics should be continued following either percutaneous or operative abscess drainage, guided by the sensitivity studies obtained from the intraoperative specimen. Antibiotic administration should continue until all systemic signs of sepsis have resolved and the patient's appetite and sense of well-being have returned. It is not, however, necessary to continue antibiotic therapy simply because drains remain in place. In the usual case, antibiotics can be stopped no later than 48 to 72 h after drainage has been established.

Right Subphrenic Abscess. The right subphrenic space is only a potential space between the liver and the diaphragm, lying above the attachments of the coronary and triangular ligaments to the posterior parietes and extending anteriorly to the costal margin. Because the potential space is so limited in vertical dimension, right subphrenic abscesses tend to be localized to only a portion of the total potential space, loculating either anteriorly or posteriorly. Abscesses within this space are most frequently secondary to rupture of a hepatic abscess or to operations on the stomach or duodenum; less frequently, they are due to contamination of the subphrenic space during the course of a generalized peritonitis, and, least frequently, right subphrenic abscesses are related to operations on the appendix or biliary system.

Clinical signs and symptoms may be quite minimal. Pain is occasionally reported in the upper part of the abdomen or lower part of the chest, sometimes referred to the back or to the right shoulder. Chest x-rays show a pleural effusion or platelike atelectasis in the right lower lung in 9 out of 10 patients, and the diaphragm is elevated and shows reduced motion on sniffing in two out of three patients. An air fluid level can be demonstrated in about 25 percent of patients, and establishes the diagnosis.

The surgical management of right subphrenic abscesses was confused for years by a misunderstanding of the relevant anatomy. Barnard had described the triangular and coronary ligaments of the liver as arising from the dome of the diaphragm. This error, perpetuated by surgical authors for the next half century, resulted in the recommendation that abscesses loculated in the posterior part of the right subphrenic space should be drained posteriorly through the bed of the twelfth rib. This anatomic error was corrected by Boyd, who pointed out that the coronary and triangular ligaments attach posteriorly rather than superiorly. It should be emphasized that abscesses in the right subphrenic space cannot be drained through a posterior approach unless the route of drainage transgresses the pleural space, a step that obviously is not desirable.

Right subphrenic abscesses preferably are drained using a lateral subcostal approach (Fig. 34-5). The advantage of the lateral approach is that it is possible to drain all the subphrenic and subhepatic spaces while avoiding contamination of the remainder of the peritoneal cavity.

Right Subhepatic Abscess. The right subhepatic space lies under the liver, is bounded inferiorly by the hepatic flexure and the transverse mesocolon, medially by the duodenum and hepatoduodenal ligament, and laterally by the body wall. The most posterior (deepest) part of this space is called "Morison's pouch."

Gastric surgery, especially an emergency operation for complications of ulcer disease, is the most common antecedent event. Biliary tract procedures are second in frequency. Appendicitis has now declined in importance and accounts for only 8 percent of cases of right subhepatic abscesses. Complications of colonic surgery are increasing in importance. A right subhepatic abscess usually produces some tenderness in the right upper quadrant, and the patient may complain of pain, particularly exacerbated by coughing or similar activities that produce visceral motion in the region.

Left Subphrenic Abscess. Formerly uncommon, these are now the most common variety of upper abdominal abscess residual after peritonitis or leakage from a viscus. Left subphrenic abscess follows splenectomy, particularly when the splenic fossa is drained inappropriately; they also are a consequence of pancreatitis. The physical signs are costal tenderness on the left, sometimes pain in the shoulder (Kehr's sign), the presence of a left pleural effusion, and limitation of diaphragmatic motion noted by x-ray. Unlike the subdiaphragmatic space on the right, which is divided by the liver into suprahepatic and subhepatic spaces, on the left side all these areas are contiguous.

A left subphrenic abscess is best drained through a lateral extraserous approach, using fundamentally the same technique as recommended on the right side. Alternatively, abscesses in the left subphrenic space may be drained posteriorly through the bed of the twelfth rib (Fig.

Fig. 34-5. Drainage of a left subphrenic abscess through the bed of the twelfth rib. Resecting the rib greatly improves exposure but is not essential; if the twelfth rib is not excised, the incision is carried deeply along its inferior margin. The pararenal space is entered and the dissection continued bluntly upward and medially on the undersurface of the diaphragm to locate and enter the abscess cavity.

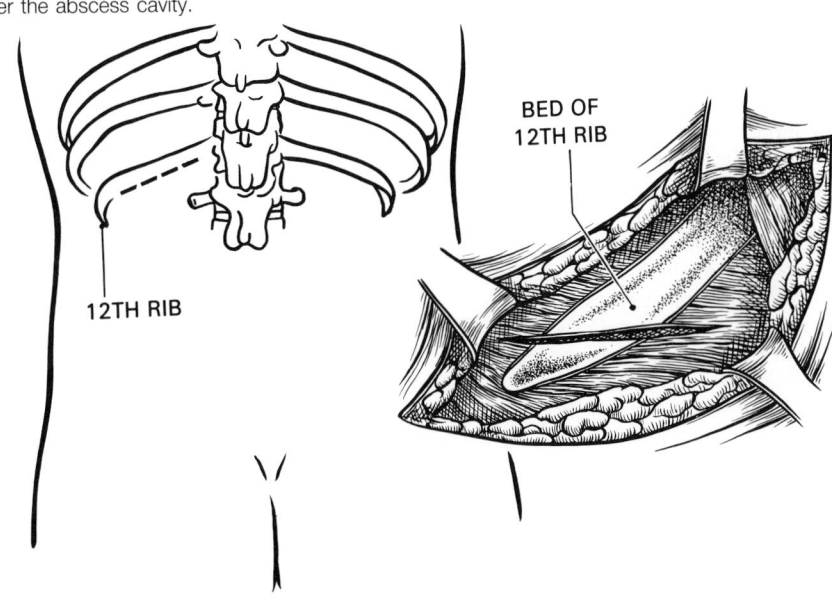

12TH RIB

BED OF 12TH RIB

34-5). Via either route, the point at which the abscess is encountered during dissection is usually much deeper than might be expected. It is important in approaching a left subphrenic abscess to avoid injury to the spleen, should it still be present, and to ensure that the entire space has been explored by palpating the aorta, the esophagus and the region of the esophageal hiatus, the caudate lobe of the liver, and the anterior margin of the left lobe of the liver during exploration; such anatomic identification by palpation of the structures at the borders of the left subphrenic space will assure that no loculation of pus goes undrained to form residual or recurrent abscess.

Right subphrenic, subhepatic, and left subphrenic abscesses are all amenable to percutaneous drainage. If they are unilocular (perhaps bilocular) and a safe percutaneous route is available, this may be attempted as an initial diagnostic and possibly therapeutic procedure. If the procedure is unsuccessful, or drainage is inadequate or the patient's signs of sepsis persist, then open surgical drainage is indicated via a transperitoneal or extraperitoneal approach. Overall, the success rate for cure and drainage of these abscesses is about 85 percent. Appropriate antibiotic therapy is an important adjunct in therapy for open or percutaneous drainage.

Lesser Sac Abscess. Technically, this is a variety of left subhepatic-subphrenic abscess, since the lesser peritoneal sac anatomically is a portion of the left subhepatic space. However, the anatomic features of this form of abscess, and the surgical maneuvers required for drainage, are distinctly different, hence its consideration as a separate entity. Lesser sac abscesses are an unusual complication of diseases of the stomach, duodenum, or pancreas. The most common cause is a pancreatic abscess or a secondarily contaminated pancreatic pseudocyst that involves the lesser sac by direct extension. Perforation of a gastric ulcer or, less commonly, of a duodenal ulcer also may result in formation of a lesser sac abscess. Occasionally, rupture of an ulcerating malignant gastric tumor produces an abscess in the lesser sac.

Clinical diagnosis of a lesser sac abscess can be extremely difficult, since much of this space is overlapped anteriorly by the liver. Tenderness to palpation in the midepigastrium usually is present but is such a nonspecific sign that it is not diagnostically very helpful. Ultrasonography is a most useful diagnostic test. Radiographic studies may show displacement of the stomach but often appear quite normal; very occasionally, plain radiographs show fine gas bubbles within the lesser sac, indicative of the presence of purulent material.

Because of its anatomic location, extraperitoneal drainage of this variety of abscess is impossible. Percutaneous drainage requires placement of the catheter through the substance of the left lobe of the liver. Since this usually is not a desirable maneuver, operative drainage of a lesser sac abscess is preferred. The abscess should be approached through an upper abdominal incision, either vertical or transverse. If a transverse incision is chosen, it should be confined within the rectus sheath; rectus muscle should not be transected, only retracted. Drainage should be accomplished as dependently as possible. The-

oretically, this would involve placement of drains inferior to the stomach, above the transverse mesocolon. It is usual for the lower portion of the lesser sac to be obliterated in cases of lesser sac abscess, with the stomach densely adherent both to the transverse mesocolon and to the pancreas; attempts at dissection are fraught with considerable difficulty. The commonly utilized route of drainage is along the superior border of the antrum, the drains being exteriorized through the operative wound.

Lesser sac abscesses have been associated with a poorer prognosis than abscesses located in other portions of the abdominal cavity. It is important that these abscesses be drained adequately, and their location often dictates the use of suction drains as dependent drainage may not be established.

Interloop (Midabdominal) Abscess. These abscesses arise as loculations between loops of bowel, mesentery, the abdominal wall, and omentum. The transverse mesocolon acts as a barrier to superior extension so that, as a group, interloop abscesses do not involve the upper part of the abdomen. Quite commonly, they may be associated with a simultaneous abscess in the pelvis.

Diagnosis of a midabdominal abscess is one of the most difficult exercises in abdominal surgery. There are no reliable symptoms or signs. Huge abscesses containing more than a liter of pus may occur without any significant physical findings. The surgeon must suspect the possible presence of an interloop abscess whenever the clinical context is appropriate, i.e., a preceding episode of peritonitis with incomplete clinical resolution and recurring signs of sepsis. Occasionally, abdominal films may show either edema in the wall of loops of bowel involved in the loculation, or separation or fixation of involved structures. Very occasionally an interloop abscess may produce a palpable, enlarging abdominal mass.

Halasz emphasized the serious problem of failure to recognize synchronous or multiple abscesses and recommended transperitoneal exploration as preferable to more limited exploration. In his series of 43 patients, one-fourth had synchronous abscesses elsewhere in the abdomen. Failure to find and drain the concomitant abscess resulted in therapeutic failure. Our indications for use of a transabdominal exploration in the management of intra-abdominal abscesses are limited to those situations in which the presence of an abscess in the midabdomen or in the lesser sac is suspected, and to those situations in which the geographic location of the abscess is obscure. Whenever a well-localized pelvic, subphrenic, or subhepatic abscess is diagnosed, a percutaneous or direct operative approach for drainage should be made. The expectation is that the patient will promptly improve; should this not occur, consideration should be given to transabdominal exploration to find and drain additional abscesses. Such a program will keep the risks of contamination of the general peritoneal cavity as a consequence of abscess drainage at a minimum, and yet should not result in excess mortality due to lingering, undrained, unrecognized abscesses.

Midabdominal interloop abscesses are multiple more often than not. Because of the need for general exploration, and because extraserous drainage cannot be arranged in any case, transabdominal exploration is utilized. All abscesses should be opened, aspirated, and debrided. Unless the abscess cavity is in contact with the abdominal wall, insertion of drains is not indicated. Rather, reliance is placed on thorough debridement and irrigation of the peritoneal cavity with copious amounts of saline solution followed by antibiotic irrigation, as outlined above in the management of suppurative peritonitis. Recurrence is common, and clinical evidence of such an event should be sought and treated vigorously.

Pelvic Abscess. These abscesses most often follow a ruptured colonic diverticulum, pelvic inflammatory disease, ruptured appendix, or drainage into the pelvis during resolution of generalized peritonitis. Unless the abscess involves the anterior abdominal wall, few symptoms or physical signs are present on examination of the abdomen. The patient may complain of poorly localized, dull, lower abdominal pain. Irritation of the urinary system and the rectum produces symptoms of urgency and frequency or diarrhea and tenesmus.

Localized purulent collections in the pelvis are the easiest of intraabdominal abscesses to diagnose. The abscess usually can be palpated directly by rectal or vaginal examination. The typical pelvic abscess bulges as a tender mass into the anterior rectal wall. It is important to distinguish between an inflammatory mass involving the pelvic organs and a true pelvic abscess. In general, pelvic inflammatory masses involving the fallopian tubes do not bulge into the rectum, and tend to become less tender and to resolve on serial examination, whereas a true pelvic abscess tends to enlarge and finally to rupture.

Drainage should be accomplished through either the rectum or the vagina. Incision for drainage should be delayed until formation of the pyogenic membrane has effectively excluded all of the small bowel and other intraabdominal viscera. If serial examinations have been done, readiness for drainage is apparent when the most prominent aspect of the abscess presenting vaginally or rectally begins to soften. Using a speculum or anoscope, the abscess should be exposed and the presence of pus confirmed by needle aspiration. The needle is left in place as a guide; sharp incision with a knife is made into the abscess cavity. The abscess cavity should be explored digitally, loculations broken down, and the cavity thoroughly irrigated. Drains are difficult to retain in a pelvic abscess cavity. To ensure continued drainage and obliteration of the cavity, daily dilations of the tract digitally or with an instrument should be done until the cavity becomes obliterated over the following few days.

Pancreatic Abscess. Acute pancreatitis is the antecedent cause of pancreatic abscess in the majority of cases. Secondary infection of a pancreatic pseudocyst and abdominal trauma with pancreatic injury are other important causes. Abdominal pain, nausea, vomiting, distention, and absent bowel sounds are frequently present. Abdominal tenderness along with a temperature greater than 39°C is also very commonly present.

Pancreatic abscesses are polymicrobial in nature, the common organisms being aerobic representatives of the fecal flora, predominantly *E. coli* and aerobic hemolytic streptococci. Staphylococci usually are not involved in

primary pancreatic abscesses but are frequently recovered in those abscesses that follow inadvertent early abdominal exploration in the presence of pancreatitis.

Antibiotic therapy alone is associated with nearly 100 percent mortality. Pancreatic abscesses are not amenable to percutaneous drainage; therefore, open surgical drainage is necessary. The approach is transperitoneal and consists of radical debridement with removal of all necrotic debris. This is followed by irrigation with saline and placement of large-bore sump suction and soft drains as essential features of therapy. Despite aggressive supportive therapy with antibiotics and fluids, mortality remains high. Recently, major pancreatic resection with packing of the abscess cavity has been advocated and appears to show some improvement in overall mortality.

Retroperitoneal Abscess. Abscesses within the retroperitoneal spaces are not common occurrences. Anatomically, they may be classified according to location: (1) perinephric; (2) upper retroperitoneum; (3) pelvic; (4) combined upper retroperitoneum and pelvis; and (5) musculoskeletal involving the iliacus, psoas, or gluteal muscles. Abscesses located in the upper retroperitoneum are usually secondary to infections of the pancreas and are discussed above. Abscesses in the remaining sites may be caused by primary or secondary infections of the kidneys, ureters, or colon, or osteomyelitis of the spine.

Retroperitoneal abscesses in these locations are usually insidious in onset, thereby causing a delay in diagnosis and therapy. They commonly present with fever, and tenderness may be present over the involved site. Computerized tomography is very helpful in defining the anatomic location and extent of the abscess. Treatment consists of intravenous antibiotic therapy and surgical drainage, preferably via an extraperitoneal approach. Percutaneous catheter drainage with CT or ultrasound guidance may be attempted. This may serve as a temporizing measure in patients who are not considered candidates for prompt open surgical drainage. Despite aggressive therapy, overall mortality remains greater than 50 percent in the presence of multiple organ system failure.

Bibliography

Peritoneum

Ahrenholz DH, Simmons RL: Fibrin in peritonitis: 1. Beneficial and adverse effects of fibrin in experimental *E. coli,* peritonitis. *Surgery* 88:41, 1980.

Allen L, Vogt E: Mechanism of lymphatic absorption from serous cavities. *Am J Physiol* 119:776, 1937.

Cascarano J, Rubin AD, et al: Metabolically induced permeability changes across mesothelium. *Am J Physiol* 206:373, 1964.

Courtice FC, Simmonds WJ: Physiological significance of lymph drainage of the serous cavities and lung. *Physiol Rev* 34:419, 1954.

Ellis H: Wound repair. Reaction of the peritoneum to injury. *Ann R Coll Surg Eng* 60:219, 1978.

Flessner MF, Dedrick RL, et al: A distributed model of peritoneal-plasma transport: Theoretical considerations. *Am J Physiol* 246:R597, 1984.

Hau T, Payne WD, et al: Fibrinolytic activity of the peritoneum during experimental peritonitis. *Surg Gynecol Obstet* 148:415, 1979.

Krediet RT, Berkinshaw K, et al: Clinical aspects of peritoneal permeability. *Neth J Med* 28:424, 1985.

Merlo G, Fausone G, et al: Fibrinolytic activity of the human peritoneum. *Eur Surg Res* 12:433, 1980.

Monk RS, Wilson SD: The abdominal cavity: An observation. *Am J Surg* 111:854, 1966.

Nolph KD: Peritoneal clearances. *J Lab Clin Med* 94:519, 1979.

Northover JMA, Williams EDF, et al: The investigation of small vessel anatomy by scanning electron microscopy of resin casts. A description of the technique and examples of its use in the study of the microvasculature of the peritoneum and bile duct wall. *J Anat* 130:43, 1980.

Raftery AT: Regeneration of parietal and visceral peritoneum, a light microscopical study. *Br J Surg* 60:293, 1973.

Raftery AT: Regeneration of peritoneum: A fibrinolytic study. *J Anat* 129:659, 1979.

Renvall SY: Peritoneal metabolism and intra-abdominal adhesion formation during experimental peritonitis. *Acta Chir Scand* 503(suppl):1, 1980.

Tsilibary EC, Wissig SL: Lymphatic absorption from the peritoneal cavity: Regulation of patency of mesothelial stomata. *Microvasc Res* 25:22, 1983.

General Responses in Peritonitis

Avila A, Warshawski F, et al: Peripheral lymph flow in sheep with bacterial peritonitis: Evidence for increased peripheral vascular permeability accompanying systemic sepsis. *Surgery* 97:685, 1985.

Cerra FB, Siegel JH, et al: The hepatic failure of sepsis: Cellular versus substrate. *Surgery* 86:409, 1979.

Duff JH, Groves AC, et al: Defective oxygen consumption in septic shock. *Surg Gynecol Obstet* 128:1051, 1969.

Fry DE, Ratcliffe DJ, et al: The effects of acidosis on canine hepatic and renal oxidative phosphorylation. *Surgery* 88:269, 1980.

Kukral JC, Riveron E, et al: Plasma protein metabolism in patients with acute surgical peritonitis. *Am J Surg* 113:173, 1967.

Lang CH, Bagby GJ, et al: Cardiac output and redistribution of organ blood flow in hypermetabolic sepsis. *Am J Physiol* 246:R331, 1984.

Renvall SY, Niinikoski J: Intraperitoneal oxygen and carbon dioxide tensions in experimental adhesion disease and peritonitis. *Am J Surg* 130:286, 1975.

Renvall S, Järvinen M: Energy metabolism of the peritoneal membrane in silica-induced peritonitis. A biochemical and enzyme histochemical study. *Acta Chir Scand* 146:177, 1980.

Renvall S, Niinikoski J: Effects of peritonitis on oxygen consumption by various tissue and peritoneal fluid cells. *Acta Chir Scand* 146:493, 1980.

Richmond JM, Walker JF, et al: Renal and cardiovascular responses to nonhypotensive sepsis in a large animal model with peritonitis. *Surgery* 97:205, 1985.

Skarstein A: The diagnosis of peritonitis. *Scand J Gastroenterol* 100:16, 1984.

Acute Suppurative Peritonitis

Bohnen J, Boulanger M, et al: Prognosis in generalized peritonitis. Relation to cause and risk factors. *Arch Surg* 118:285, 1983.

Crawfurd E, Ellis H: Generalized peritonitis—the changing spectrum. A report of 100 cases. *Br J Clin Pract* 39:177, 1985.

Rivlin ME, Hunt JA: Surgical management of diffuse peritonitis complicating obstetric/gynecologic infections. *Obstet Gynecol* 67:718, 1986.

Interaction of Bacteria and the Peritoneum

Altemeier WA: The pathogenicity of the bacteria of appendicitis peritonitis. *Ann Surg* 114:158, 1941.

Autio V: The spread of intraperitoneal infection: Studies with roentgen contrast medium. *Acta Chir Scand* 321(suppl):5, 1964.

Davis JH, Yull AB: A toxic factor in abdominal injury, II. The role of the red cell component. *J Trauma* 4:84, 1964.

Dunn DL, Barke RA, et al: Mechanisms of the adjuvant effect of hemoglobin in experimental peritonitis. VII. Hemoglobin does not inhibit clearance of *Escherichia coli* from the peritoneal cavity. *Surgery* 94:487, 1983.

Dunn DL, Barke RA, et al: The adjuvant effect of peritoneal fluid in experimental peritonitis. Mechanisms and clinical applications. *Ann Surg* 199:37, 1984.

Gorbach SL, Thadepalli H, et al: Anaerobic microorganisms in intraabdominal infections, in Balows A (ed): *Anaerobic Bacteria: Role in Disease*. Springfield, IL, Charles C Thomas, 1972, chap 32.

Lorber B, Swenson RM: The bacteriology of intraabdominal infections. *Surg Clin North Am* 55:1349, 1975.

Meleney FL: Bacterial synergism in disease processes. *Ann Surg* 94:961, 1931.

Nichols RL, Smith JW, et al: Peritonitis and intraabdominal abscess: An experimental model for the evaluation of human disease. *J Surg Res* 25:129, 1978.

Pruett TL, Rotstein OD, et al: Mechanisms of the adjuvant effect of hemoglobin in experimental peritonitis: VIII. A leukotoxin is produced by *Escherichia coli* metabolism in hemoglobin. *Surgery* 96:375, 1984.

Pruett TL, Rotstein OD, et al: Mechanisms of the adjuvant effect of hemoglobin in experimental peritonitis: IX. The infection-potentiating effect of hemoglobin in *Escherichia coli* peritonitis is strain specific. *Surgery* 98:371, 1985.

Stone HH, Kolb LD, et al: Incidence and significance for intraperitoneal anaerobic bacteria. *Ann Surg* 181:705, 1975.

Pathophysiology of Sepsis

Baue AE: Multiple, progressive, or sequential systems failure. *Arch Surg* 110:779, 1975.

Clowes GHA Jr, Hirsch E, et al: Septic lung and shock lung in man. *Ann Surg* 181:681, 1975.

Dunn RL, Simmons RL: The role of anaerobic bacteria in intra-abdominal infections. *Rev Infect Dis* 6(suppl 1):S139, 1984.

Eisman B, Beart R, et al: Multiple organ failure. *Surg Gynecol Obstet* 144:323, 1977.

Esteban A, Fernandez-Segoviano P, et al: Radiographic findings for the adult respiratory distress syndrome in patients with peritonitis. *Crit Care Med* 11:880, 1983.

Fry DE, Pearlstein L, et al: Multiple system organ failure: The role of uncontrolled infection. *Arch Surg* 115:136, 1980.

Hasselgren P, James JH, et al: Reduced muscle amino acid uptake in sepsis and the effects in vitro of septic plasma and interleukin-1. *Surgery* 100:222, 1986.

Hinshaw LB, Benjamin B, et al: Responses of the baboon to live Escherichia coli organisms and endotoxin. *Surg Gynecol Obstet* 145:1, 1977.

Iberti TJ, Rand JH: Thrombocytopenia following peritonitis in surgical patients. *Ann Surg* 204:341, 1986.

Jeppsson B, Freund HR, et al: Blood-brain barrier derangement in sepsis: Cause of septic encephalopathy? *Am J Surg* 141:136, 1981.

Lam C, Schulz F, et al: Opsonic activity of the alternative complement pathway in infected human intraabdominal fluid. *Infection* 13:8, 1985.

Lava J, Rice CL, et al: Pulmonary dysfunction in sepsis: Is pulmonary edema the culprit? *J Trauma* 22:280, 1982.

Pine RW, Wertz MJ, et al: Determinants of organ malfunction or death in patients with intraabdominal sepsis. *Arch Surg* 118:242, 1983.

Polk HC, Shields CL: Remote organ failure: A valid sign of occult intraabdominal infection. *Surgery* 81:310, 1977.

Postel J, Furtado D, et al: Effect of prolonged bacteremia on leukocyte bactericidal function. *Surgery* 81:180, 1977.

Shires GT, Davis JM: Intraabdominal infection: The disease. *Clin Ther* 6(suppl A):1, 1984.

Shuck JM: New concepts in intraabdominal infection. *Am Surg* 51:304, 1985.

Siegel JH, Cerra FB, et al: Physiological and metabolic correlations in human sepsis. Invited commentary. *Surgery* 86:163, 1979.

Smith-Erichsen J: Serial determinations of platelets, leukocytes and coagulation parameters in surgical septicemia. *Scand J Clin Lab Invest* 178(suppl):7, 1985.

Solomkin JS, Brodt JK, et al: Suppressed neutrophil oxidative activity in sepsis: A receptor-mediated regulatory response. *J Surg Res* 39:300, 1985.

Solomkin JS, Brodt JK, et al: Degranulation inhibition. A potential mechanism for control of neutrophil superoxide production in sepsis. *Arch Surg* 121:77, 1986.

Solomkin JS, Cotta LA, et al: Regulation of neutrophil superoxide production in sepsis. *Arch Surg* 120:93, 1985.

Stephen M, Loewenthal J: Generalized infective peritonitis. *Surg Gynecol Obstet* 147:231, 1978.

Sugarman HJ, Austin GL, et al: Thrombocytopenia in progressive lethal canine peritonitis. *Surg Gynecol Obstet* 154:193, 1982.

Townsend MC, Hampton WW, et al: Effective organ blood flow and bioenergy status in murine peritonitis. *Surgery* 100:205, 1986.

Vary TC, Siegel JH, et al: A biochemical basis for depressed ketogenesis in sepsis. *J Trauma* 26:419, 1986.

Vincent JL, Puri VK, et al: Acute respiratory failure in patients with generalized peritonitis. *Resuscitation* 10:283, 1983.

Management of Suppurative Peritonitis

Agrama HM, Blackwood JM, et al: Functional longevity of intraperitoneal drains. An experimental evaluation. *Am J Surg* 132:418, 1976.

Altemeier WA: The cause of the putrid odor of perforated appendicitis with peritonitis. *Ann Surg* 107:634, 1938.

Anderson ED, Mendelbaum DM, et al: Open packing of the peritoneal cavity in generalized bacterial peritonitis. *Am J Surg* 145:131, 1983.

Burnett WE, Brown GP Jr, et al: The treatment of peritonitis using peritoneal lavage. *Ann Surg* 145:675, 1957.

Busutill RW, McGrattan MA, et al: A comparative study of cefmandole versus gentamicin plus clindamycin in the treatment of documented or suspected bacterial peritonitis. *Surg Gynecol Obstet* 158:1, 1984.

Condon RE: Antibiotics in the management of peritonitis, in Condon RE, Gorbach SL (eds): *Surgical Infections: Selective Antibiotic Therapy.* Baltimore, Williams & Wilkins, 1981, pp 83–90.

DeMaria A, Heffernan JJ, et al: Naloxone versus placebo in treatment of septic shock. *Lancet* 1:1363, 1985.

Dougherty SH: Role of amikacin in the management of intraabdominal sepsis. *Am J Med* 79:28, 1985.

Duff JH, Moffat J: Abdominal sepsis managed by leaving abdomen open. *Surgery* 90:774, 1981.

Faden AL, Holaday JW: Experimental endotoxin shock: The pathophysiologic function of endorphins and treatment with opiate antagonists. *J Infect Dis* 142:229, 1980.

Galland RB, Heine KJ, et al: Reduction of surgical wound infection rates in contaminated wounds treated with antiseptics combined with systemic antibiotics: An experimental study. *Surgery* 91:329, 1982.

Groeger JS, Carlon GC, et al: Naloxone in septic shock. *Crit Care Med* 11:650, 1983.

Gupta S, Jain PK: Low-dose heparin in experimental peritonitis. *Eur Surg Res* 17:167, 1985.

Guthy E: Surgical aspects in the management of peritonitis. *Scand J Gastroenterol* 100:49, 1984.

Hagan B: Drainage after cholecystectomy. *Ann R Coll Surg Engl* 62:392, 1980.

Hann EA: Efficiency of peritoneal drainage. *Surg Gynecol Obstet* 131:983, 1970.

Hau T: Management of peritonitis. *Curr Surg* 41:165, 1984.

Hau T, Ahrenholz DH, et al: Secondary bacterial peritonitis: The biological basis of treatment. *Curr Probl Surg* 16:1, 1979.

Hau T, Nishikawa R, et al: Irrigation of the peritoneal cavity and local antibiotics in the treatment of peritonitis. *Surg Gynecol Obstet* 156:25, 1983.

Hau T, Simmons RL: Heparin in the treatment of experimental peritonitis. *Ann Surg* 187:294, 1978.

Hauser CJ, Shoemaker WC, et al: Oxygen transport responses to colloids and crystalloids in critically ill surgical patients. *Surg Gynecol Obstet* 150:811, 1980.

Hedderich GS, Wexler MJ, et al: The septic abdomen: Open management with Marlex mesh with a zipper. *Surgery* 99:399, 1986.

Hinshaw LB, Archer LT, et al: Survival of primates in LD_{100} septic shock following steroid/antibiotic therapy. *J Surg Res* 28:151, 1980.

Hinshaw LB, Archer LT, et al: Escherichia coli shock in the baboon and the response to adrenocorticosteroid treatment. *Surg Gynecol Obstet* 147:545, 1978.

Hudspeth AS: Radical surgical debridement in the treatment of advanced generalized bacterial peritonitis. *Arch Surg* 110:1233, 1975.

Hunt JL: Generalized peritonitis. To irrigate or not to irrigate the abdominal cavity. *Arch Surg* 117:209, 1982.

Hughes GS Jr, Porter RS, et al: Naloxone and septic shock. *Ann Intern Med* 98:559, 1983.

Jennings WC, Wood CD, et al: Continuous postoperative lavage in the treatment of peritoneal sepsis. *Dis Colon Rectum* 25:641, 1982.

Jones FE, Malangoni MA, et al: Antibiotic management of intraabdominal sepsis. *Infect Surg* 1(suppl 6):15, 1987.

Lally KP, Trettin JC, et al: Adjunctive antibiotic lavage in experimental peritonitis. *Surg Gynecol Obstet* 156:605, 1983.

Lennard ES, Minshew BH, et al: Stratified outcome comparison of clindamycin-gentamicin vs. chloramphenicol-gentamicin for treatment of intraabdominal sepsis. *Arch Surg* 120:889, 1985.

Lucas CE, Ledgerwood AM, et al: Impaired pulmonary function after albumin resuscitation from shock. *J Trauma* 20:446, 1980.

Malangoni MA, Condon RE, et al: Treatment of intraabdominal infections is appropriate with single-agent or combination antibiotic therapy. *Surgery* 98:648, 1985.

McAvinchey DJ, McCollum PT, et al: Towards a rational approach to the treatment of peritonitis: An experimental study in rats. *Br J Surg* 71:715, 1984.

Nichols RL: Intraabdominal infections: An overview. *Rev Infect Dis* 74(suppl):S709, 1985.

Noon GP, Beall AC Jr, et al: Clinical evaluation of peritoneal irrigation wtih antibiotic solution. *Surgery* 62:73, 1967.

Peters WP, Friedman PA, et al: Pressor effect of naloxone in septic shock. *Lancet* 1:529, 1981.

Platt J, Jones RA, et al: Intraperitoneal antiseptics in experimental bacterial peritonitis. *Br J Surg* 71:626, 1984.

Polk HC Jr, Fry DE: Radical peritoneal debridement for established peritonitis: The results of a prospective randomized clinical trial. *Ann Surg* 192:350, 1980.

Price J: Surgical intervention in cases of general peritonitis from typhoid fever and acute gonococcus infection. *Am Med* 9:769, 1905.

Rock P, Silverman H, et al: Efficacy and safety of naloxone in septic shock. *Crit Care Med* 13:28, 1985.

Silenas R, O'Keefe P, et al: Mechanical effectiveness of closed peritoneal irrigation in peritonitis. *Am J Surg* 145:371, 1983.

Sindelar WF, Brower ST, et al: Randomized trial of intraperitoneal irrigation with low molecular weight povidine-iodine solution to reduce intraabdominal infectious complications. *J Hosp Infect* 6(suppl A):103, 1985.

Spiegel CA, Malangoni MA, et al: Gas-liquid chromatography for rapid diagnosis of intra-abdominal infection. *Arch Surg* 119:28, 1984.

Sprung CL, Caralis PV, et al: The effects of high-dose corticosteroids in patients with septic shock. A prospective, controlled study. *N Engl J Med* 311:1137, 1984.

Stone HH, Mullins RJ, et al: Ceftriaxone versus combined gentamicin and clindamycin for polymicrobial surgical sepsis. *Am J Surg* 148:30, 1984.

Tally FP, Gorbach SL: Therapy of mixed anaerobic-aerobic infections. Lessons from studies of intraabdominal sepsis. *Am J Med* 78:145, 1985.

Torek F: The treatment of diffuse suppurative peritonitis following appendicitis. *Med Rec* 70:849, 1906.

Virgilio RW, Rice CL, et al: Crystalloid vs colloid resuscitation: Is one better? *Surgery* 85:129, 1979.

Washington BC, Villalba MR, et al: Cefmandole-erythromycin-heparin peritoneal irrigation: An adjunct to the surgical treatment of diffuse bacterial peritonitis. *Surgery* 94:576, 1983.

Weissglass IS: The role of endogenous opiates in shock: Experimental and clinical studies in vitro and in vivo. *Adv Shock Res* 10:87, 1983.

Yates JL: An experimental study of the local effects of peritoneal drainage. *Surg Gynecol Obstet* 1:473, 1905.

Aseptic (Chemical) Peritonitis

Carter R, Gosney WG: Abdominal apoplexy: Report of 6 cases and review of the literature. *Am J Surg* 111:388, 1966.

Cochran DQ, Almond CH, et al: An experimental study of the effects of barium and intestinal contents on the peritoneal cavity. *Am J Roentgenol* 89:883, 1963.

Dale G, Solheim K: Bile peritonitis in acute cholecystitis. *Acta Chir Scand* 141:746, 1975.

Dinner M: Biliary peritonitis due to idiopathic perforation of the common bile duct. *S Afr J Surg* 13:207, 1975.

Garfinkle SE, Chiu GW, et al: Spontaneous perforation of the neurogenic urinary bladder. *West J Med* 124:64, 1976.

Grobmyer AJ III, Ketlan RA, et al: Barium peritonitis. *Am Surg* 50:116, 1984.

Hamilton JE, Harbrecht PJ: Growing indications for vagotomy in perforated peptic ulcer. *Surg Gynecol Obstet* 124:61, 1967.

Kent SJ, Menzies-Gow N: Biliary peritonitis without perforation of the gallbladder in acute cholecystitis. *Br J Surg* 61:960, 1974.

Krizek TJ, Davis JH: Acute chylous peritonitis. *Arch Surg* 91:253, 1965.

Michas CA, Pollak EW, et al: Hemoperitoneum due to spontaneous gastroepiploic artery rupture. *JAMA* 237:2526, 1977.

Moore TC: Massive bile peritonitis in infancy due to spontaneous bile duct perforation with portal vein occlusion. *J Pediatr Surg* 10:537, 1975.

Yamamura M, Nishi M, et al: Barium peritonitis. Report of a case and review of the literature. *Dis Colon Rectum* 28:347, 1985.

Zheutlin N, Lasser EC, et al: Clinical studies on effect of barium in the peritoneal cavity following rupture of the colon. *Surgery* 32:967, 1952.

Granulomatous Peritonitis

Cromartie RS III: Tuberculous peritonitis. *Surg Gynecol Obstet* 144:876, 1977.

Grant JBF, Davies JD, et al: Diagnosis of granulomatous starch peritonitis by delay hypersensitivity skin reactions. *Br J Surg* 69:197, 1982.

Lintermans JP: Fatal peritonitis, an unusual complication of strongyloides stercoralis infestation. *Clin Pediatr* (Phila) 14:947, 1975.

Monga NK, Sood S, et al: Amebic peritonitis. *Am J Gastroenterol* 66:366, 1976.

Singh MM, Bhargava AN, et al: Tuberculous peritonitis: An evaluation of pathogenic mechanisms, diagnostic procedures and therapeutic measure. *N Engl J Med* 281:1091, 1969.

Solomkin JS, Flohr AB, et al: The role of Candida in intraperitoneal infections. *Surgery* 88:524, 1980.

Sturdy JH, Baird RM, et al: Surgical sponges, A cause of granuloma and adhesion formation. *Ann Surg* 165:128, 1967.

Tinker MA, Burdman D, et al: Granulomatous peritonitis due to cellulose fibers from disposable surgical fabrics: Laboratory investigation and clinical implications. *Ann Surg* 180:831, 1974.

Warshaw AL: Management of starch peritonitis without the unnecessary second operation. *Surgery* 73:681, 1973.

Spontaneous (Primary) Peritonitis

Clark JH, Fitzgerald JF, et al: Spontaneous bacterial peritonitis. *J Pediatr* 104:495, 1984.

Crossley IR, Williams R: Spontaneous bacterial peritonitis. *Gut* 26:325, 1985.

Murray HW, Marks SJ: Spontaneous bacterial empyema, pericarditis, and peritonitis in cirrhosis. *Gastroenterology* 72:772, 1977.

Pinzello G, Virdone R, et al: Is the acidity of ascitic fluid a reliable index in making the presumptive diagnosis of spontaneous bacterial peritonitis? *Hepatology* 6:244, 1986.

Reynolds TB: Rapid presumptive diagnosis of spontaneous bacterial peritonitis. *Gastroenterology* 90:1294, 1986.

Runyon BR: Low-protein-concentration ascitic fluid is predisposed to spontaneous bacterial peritonitis. *Gastroenterology* 91:1343, 1986.

Stassen WN, McCullough AJ, et al: Immediate diagnostic criteria for bacterial infection of ascitic fluid. Evaluation of ascitic fluid polymorphonuclear leukocyte count, pH, and lactate concentration, alone and in combination. *Gastroenterology* 90:1247, 1986.

Taraok SOK, Moroi T, et al: Detection of endotoxin in plasma and ascitic fluid of patients with cirrhosis: Its clinical significance. *Gastroenterology* 73:539, 1977.

Other Forms of Peritonitis

Eisenberg ES, Leviton I, et al: Fungal peritonitis in patients receiving peritoneal dialysis: Experience with 11 patients and review of the literature. *Rev Infect Dis* 8:309, 1986.

Eltringham WK, Espiner HJ, et al: Sclerosing peritonitis due to practolol: A report on 9 cases and their surgical management. *Br J Surg* 64:229, 1977.

Gandhi VC, Kamadana MR, et al: Aseptic peritonitis in patients on maintenance peritoneal dialysis. *Nephron* 24:257, 1979.

Hubschmann OR, Countee RW: Gram-positive peritonitis in patients with infected ventriculoperitoneal shunts. *Surg Gynecol Obstet* 149:69, 1979.

Knight KR, Polak A, et al: Laboratory diagnosis and oral treatment of CAPD peritonitis. *Lancet* 2:1301, 1982.

Kvale PA, Parks RD: Acute abdomen. An unusual reaction to isoniazid, *Chest* 68:271, 1975.

LaFerla G, McColl KE, et al: CSF induced sclerosing peritonitis: A new entity? *Br J Surg* 73:7, 1986.

Reimann HA: Periodic peritonitis—heredity and pathology. Report of seventy-two cases. *JAMA* 154:1254, 1954.

Reimann HA: Colchicine for periodic peritonitis. *JAMA* 231:64, 1975.

Robinson RJ, Leapman SB, et al: Surgical considerations of continuous ambulatory peritoneal dialysis. *Surgery* 96:723, 1984.

Rubin J, Rogers WA, et al: Peritonitis during continuous ambulatory peritoneal dialysis. *Ann Intern Med* 92:7, 1980.

Intraabdominal Abscesses

Ascher NL, Forstrom L, et al: Radiolabeled autologous leukocyte scanning in abscess detection. *World J Surg* 4:395, 1980.

Barnard HL: Address on surgical aspects of subphrenic abscess. *Br Med J* 1:371, 1908.

Boyd DP: The subphrenic spaces and the emperor's new robes. *N Engl J Med* 275:911, 1966.

Bradley SJ, Jurkovich GJ, et al: Controlled open drainage of severe intraabdominal sepsis. *Arch Surg* 120:629, 1985.

Crepps TJ, Welch JP, et al: Management and outcome of retroperitoneal abscesses. *Ann Surg* 205:276, 1987.

DeCosse JJ, Poulin TL, et al: Subphrenic abscess. *Surg Gynecol Obstet* 138:841, 1974.

Dobrin PB, Gully PH, et al: Radiologic diagnosis of an intraabdominal abscess. Do multiple tests help? *Arch Surg* 121:41, 1986.

Froelich JW, Swanson D: Imaging of inflammatory processes with labelled cells. *Semin Nucl Med* 14:128, 1984.

Fry DE, Garrison RN, et al: Determinants of death in patients with intraabdominal abscess. *Surgery* 88:517, 1980.

Gerzof SG, Robbins AH, et al: Percutaneous catheter drainage of abdominal abscesses: A five-year experience. *N Engl J Med* 305:653, 1981.

Halasz NA: Subphrenic abscesses: Myths and facts. *JAMA* 214:724, 1970.

Hickey NM, Tao HH: A modified procedure for percutaneous abscess and fluid drainage using the Malecot catheter-Stamey needle technique. *J Can Assoc Radiol* 35:220, 1984.

Johnson WC, Gerzof SG, et al: Treatment of abdominal abscesses: Comparative evaluation of operative drainage versus percutaneous catheter drainage guided by computed tomography or ultrasound. *Ann Surg* 194:510, 1981.

Liavag I: Intraabdominal abscesses, diagnosis and treatment. *Scand J Gastroenterol* [suppl] 100:40, 1984.

Lundstedt C, Hederström E, et al: Prospective investigation of radiologic methods in the diagnosis of intraabdominal abscesses. *Acta Radiol Diag* 27:49, 1986.

Mueller PR, vanSonnenberg E, et al: Percutaneous drainage of 250 abdominal abscesses and fluid collections. *Radiology* 151:343, 1984.

Olak J, Christou NV, et al: Operative vs. percutaneous drainage of intraabdominal abscesses. *Arch Surg* 121:141, 1986.

Owens BJ III, Hamit HF: Pancreatic abscess and pseudocyst. *Arch Surg* 112:42, 1977.

Pruett TL, Rotstein OD, et al: Percutaneous aspiration and drainage for suspected abdominal infection. *Surgery* 96:731, 1984.

Ranson JHC, Spencer FC: Prevention, diagnosis and treatment of pancreatic abscess. *Surgery* 82:99, 1977.

Serrano A, Dahl EP, et al: Eclectic drainage of subphrenic abscesses. *Arch Surg* 119:942, 1984.

Simon GL, Geelhoed GW: Diagnosis of intra-abdominal abscess. A review, *Am Surg* 51:431, 1985.

Stone HH, Strom PR, et al: Pancreatic abscess management of subtotal resection and packing. *World J Surg* 8:340, 1984.

Stone HH, Mullins RJ, et al: Extraperitoneal versus transperitoneal drainage of the intraabdominal abscess. *Surg Gynecol Obstet* 159:549, 1984.

vanSonnenberg E, Ferrucci JT Jr, et al: Percutaneous radiographically guided catheter drainage of abdominal abscesses. *JAMA* 247:190, 1982.

vanSonnenberg E, Ferrucci JT Jr, et al: Percutaneous drainage of abscesses and fluid collections: Techniques, results, and applications. *Radiology* 142:1, 1982.

Wang SMS, Wilson SD: Subphrenic abscess: The new epidemiology. *Arch Surg* 112:934, 1977.

Chapter 35

Abdominal Wall, Omentum, Mesentery, and Retroperitoneum

James T. Adams

ANTERIOR ABDOMINAL WALL

General Considerations

The abdominal parietes contain and protect the abdominal viscera. Topographically, the anterior abdominal wall

is bounded by the flare of the costal margins and the xiphoid process of the sternum above and by the iliac crests, inguinal ligaments, and pubis below. The principal structures that comprise the anterior abdominal wall are the rectus, external and internal oblique, and transversus abdominis and lower intercostal muscles together with their enveloping fascial sheaths and aponeuroses. The linea alba, a tendinous raphe formed by a blending of the aponeuroses of the oblique and transversus muscles in the midline, divides the anterior abdominal wall into two parts and thus restricts the medial extension of pathologic processes that may arise within it. Deep to the muscles is the continuous transversalis fascia, considered to be the strongest layer of the abdominal wall, and peritoneum.

The blood supply is furnished by the superior and inferior epigastric, lower intercostal, lumbar, and iliac circumflex arteries. The venous drainage corresponds to the arteries. Lymphatics in the upper half of the abdominal wall drain to the axillary nodes and those in the lower abdomen to the inguinal and thence to the iliac nodes. Lymph flow around the umbilicus may also ascend around the ligamentum teres (obliterated umbilical vein) to reach the porta hepatis. The nerve supply is via the intercostal and upper lumbar nerves.

In addition to protecting the abdominal viscera, the muscles function as an accessory respiratory apparatus and also aid in defecation by increasing intraabdominal muscle pressure with contraction.

Surgical diseases of the anterior abdominal wall include (1) hernia, (2) infection, (3) primary and metastatic tumors of soft tissue and muscle, (4) rectus sheath hematoma, and (5) desmoid tumor. With the exception of rectus sheath hematoma and desmoid tumor, these conditions are covered in other chapters of this textbook.

Rectus Sheath Hematoma

Bleeding into the rectus sheath produces a clinical picture that may simulate the acute surgical abdomen. The

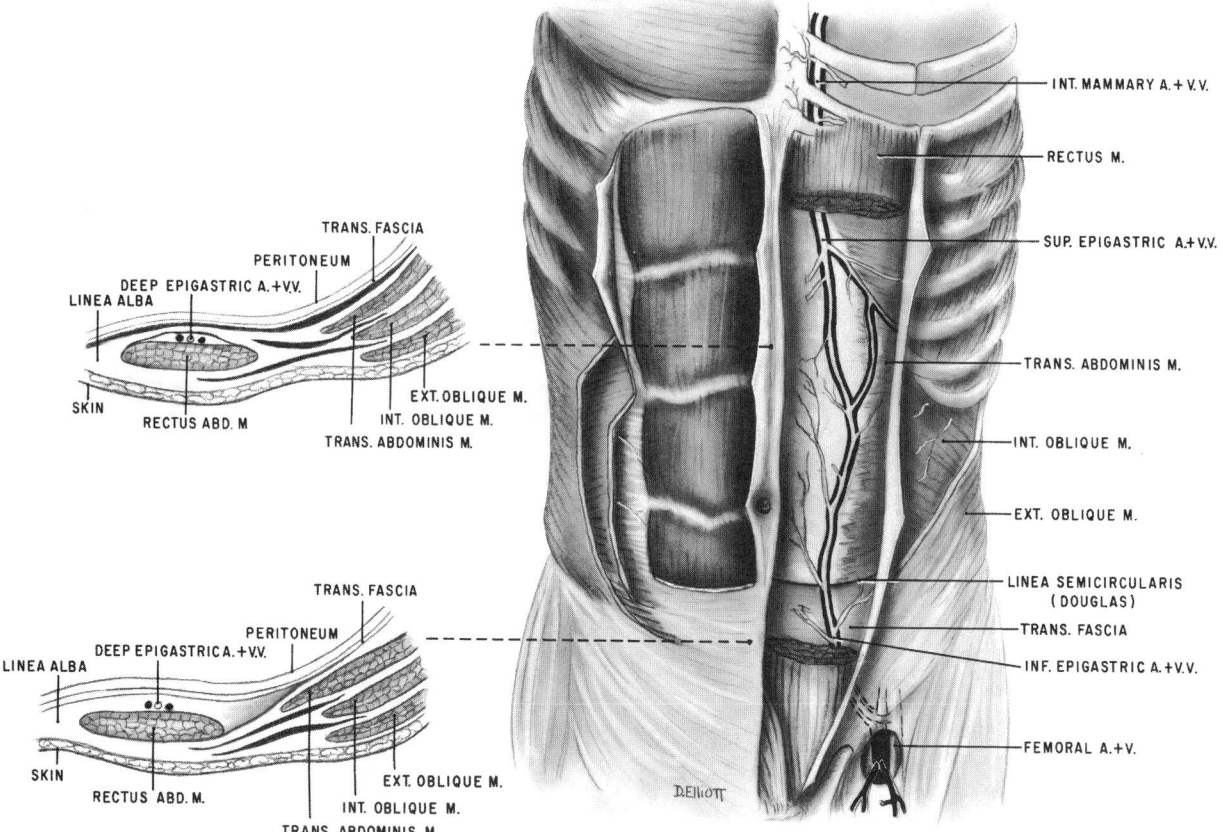

Fig. 35-1. Rectus abdominis muscle and rectus sheath. From the rib margin to a point midway between the umbilicus and the pubis (linea semicircularis of Douglas), the posterior sheath is made up of the posterior leaf of the internal oblique aponeurosis, the aponeurosis of the transversus abdominis muscle, and the transversalis fascia. Below this level, the posterior wall is formed by transversalis fascia alone. The deep epigastric arteries and veins course along the posterior surface of the rectus muscle so that below the linea semicircularis they are separated from the peritoneum by only transversalis fascia.

bleeding is usually the result of rupture of the epigastric artery or veins rather than a primary tear of the rectus muscle fibers. It is most often a self-limiting condition but if not recognized can lead to an unnecessary emergency surgical procedure.

ANATOMY. (Fig. 35-1). The rectus abdominis muscle is crossed by three transverse tendinous intersections on its anterior aspect, so that its contractile force is divided into three parts. The lowermost part is the longest, and hence its shortening with contraction is the greatest. There may be a difference of as much as 18 cm in length between extreme contraction and relaxation.

A strong fascial sheath, made up of the aponeuroses of the oblique and tranversus abdominis muscles and transversalis fascia, contains the muscle. Anteriorly, the sheath is complete throughout; however, midway between the umbilicus and the pubis, the posterior sheath ends, forming an arched border, the linea semicircularis (of Douglas). Cephalad to this level, the internal oblique aponeurosis splits into two leaves, one passing on either side of the rectus, while below it no such division takes place, and, together with the aponeurosis of the transversus abdominis, it passes anteriorly. This leaves the rectus muscle below the linea semicircularis separated from the abdominal viscera only by transversalis fascia and peritoneum. The anterior leaf of the sheath is adherent to the transverse tendons and also to the lateral and medial mar-

gins of the muscle, while posteriorly the muscle is free. As a consequence of this anatomic arrangement, when there is bleeding within the rectus sheath below the umbilicus, the free blood may lie against the peritoneum, producing irritation and pain suggesting an acute intraabdominal disease.

The blood supply to the rectus muscle is from the superior and inferior epigastric arteries. The superior epigastric enters the rectus sheath from above as a terminal branch of the internal mammary artery and passes caudad behind the muscle to anastomose with the larger inferior epigastric artery coming from below. The inferior epigastric artery, a branch of the external iliac artery, enters the rectus sheath just above the inguinal canal and courses upward along the posterior surface of the rectus muscle. Both arteries give off numerous muscular branches. Two veins accompany each artery. As the rectus muscle contracts, the epigastric vessels must glide beneath it to avoid injury.

ETIOLOGY. Rectus sheath hematoma may follow direct trauma to the epigastric blood vessels or occur spontaneously in association with several diseases. It has also been noted following a convulsive seizure. Spontaneous bleeding from the smaller muscular arteries has been reported in (1) infectious diseases, notably typhoid fever, (2) debilitating diseases, (3) collagen diseases, (4) blood dyscrasias such as hemophilia and leukemia, and (5) patients on anticoagulation therapy.

Frequently, however, bleeding occurs without obvious trauma or disease. In these patients the hematoma usually follows minor straining as in coughing or sneezing. Presumably the underlying factor is an inelasticity of the artery or vein that prevents the vessel from accommodating itself to the sudden marked variation in length that the rectus muscle undergoes during contraction and relaxation. Spontaneous rectus hematoma has also been described in pregnancy and in the puerperium. It is not known whether the hematoma is due to venous or arterial bleeding. Stretching of the epigastric vessels by a distended abdomen during pregnancy or sudden relaxation after delivery are probably factors causing vessel injury. In the elderly, atheroma of an epigastric artery may predispose the vessel to rupture following minor exertion.

CLINICAL MANIFESTATIONS. Rectus sheath hematoma is three times more frequent in women than in men. The condition is rare in children and has a peak age incidence in the fifth decade. A prior history of trauma, sudden muscular exertion, generalized vascular disease, or anticoagulation suggests the diagnosis. Hematomas related to anticoagulation therapy usually become apparent 4 to 14 days after treatment is instituted. The first symptom is pain. This is sudden in onset, sharp, and progressively severe. The pain is felt in the side of the abdomen where the bleeding occurs and remains localized, since the hematoma in the rectus muscle is limited by the confines of its sheath. Usually this is the lower abdomen and more often on the right side. Anorexia, nausea but rarely vomiting, tachycardia, low-grade fever, and a moderate leukocytosis are frequent findings. With severe bleeding, signs of peripheral vascular collapse may develop. This is more apt to occur with bleeding below the linea semicircularis, where the peritoneum is only loosely adherent to the rectus muscle and thus cannot tampon the ruptured epigastric vessel. Tenderness and spasm are frequently present over the site of the hemorrhage. The bowel sounds are usually not altered. There may or may not be a palpable mass, depending on the extent of the bleeding. If present, the mass is tender, does not usually cross the midline, and remains palpable when the patient tenses the rectus muscle (Fothergill's sign). A bluish discoloration of the overlying skin is virtually diagnostic; however, this finding does not usually occur until 3 or 4 days after the patient is first seen.

Rectus sheath hematoma has been mistaken clinically for almost every acute disease of the abdomen. Prior to the advent of ultrasonography and computerized tomography, a correct preoperative diagnosis was made in fewer than 30 percent of cases. Utilizing these scanning techniques, the condition can now be diagnosed in most patients by the demonstration of a cystic or complex mass lesion within the confines of the rectus sheath (Fig. 35-2). Above the linea semicircularis, the hematoma is limited medially by the linea alba and confined to one side; below this level, the mass may project across the midline.

TREATMENT. If the diagnosis is made and the rectus hematoma is not causing severe symptoms, the condition may be managed nonoperatively with bed rest and analgesics. Anticoagulants should be discontinued. It is rarely necessary to reverse a coagulation deficit when operation is not undertaken. Surgical intervention occasionally is necessary to relieve symptoms of the hematoma or, if the

Fig. 35-2. Rectus sheath hematoma. CT scan of lower abdomen showing an elliptical complex lesion in the left rectus muscle (arrowhead). The asymmetry of the rectus muscles is an important clue to the diagnosis.

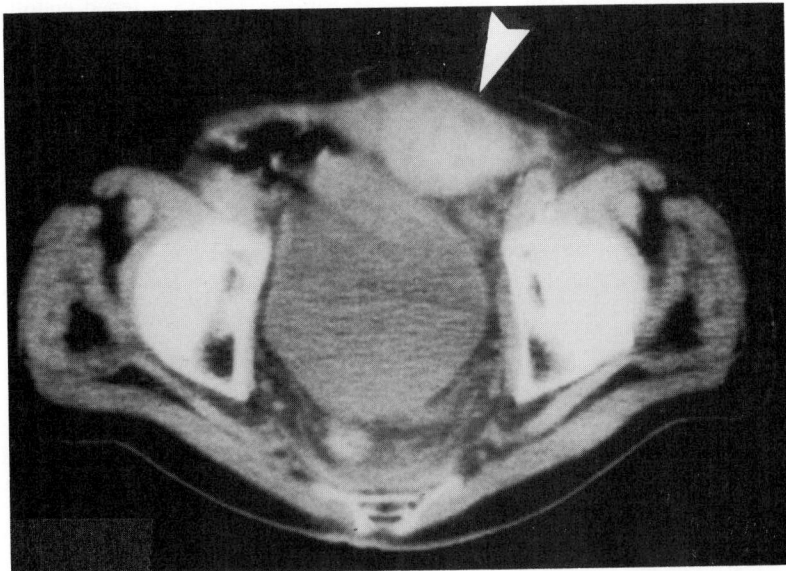

diagnosis is in doubt, to rule out other more serious diseases. With a paramedian incision, the situation will become obvious as soon as the rectus sheath is opened and free blood is found. The hematoma may be diffuse throughout the rectus muscle or may be a localized clot. Bleeding arteries may or may not be present. Ideally, the hematoma is evacuated without entering the peritoneal cavity. Bleeding points are then ligated and the wound closed without drainage. The prognosis is dependent upon the underlying or concurrent disease but is generally good, and a full recovery can be anticipated.

Desmoid Tumor

Desmoid tumors are essentially benign, hard fibromas. It is probable, however, that they are not true neoplasms but an aggressive variant within a group of conditions referred to as "fibromatoses." The tumor is of aponeurotic origin and usually is found within or deep to the flat muscles of the anterior abdominal wall. Extraabdominal desmoid tumors involving skeletal muscles of the extremities, chest, and buttocks have also been reported but occur less frequently.

Desmoid tumors account for 3 to 4 percent of all tumefactions (7 percent of benign tumors) of the anterior abdominal wall. They usually occur in women in the childbearing age group, often after a recent gestation.

ETIOLOGY. The cause of the tumor is unknown. It has been thought to be the result of hemorrhage following muscular injury from external trauma or sustained during pregnancy or parturition. Desmoids have also been reported arising in laparotomy scars. However, microscopic evidence of previous trauma, such as hemosiderin pigmentation, is usually absent. The finding of a high assay of gonadotropic substance in the tumor has prompted a sex-linked concept in explaining its cause. A genetic genesis of desmoid tumors is also evident from the frequent occurrence of the lesion in patients with familial polyposis coli (Gardner's syndrome), an inherited autosomal dominant trait.

PATHOLOGY. Desmoids are benign tumors that have the malignant property of local invasiveness. They grow slowly but progressively and can reach huge proportions. Rarely, they may penetrate the abdominal cavity or retroperitoneum and may even invade the periosteum of the pelvic bones. With such aggressive growth, they may not be totally resectable. Occasionally the tumor undergoes malignant transformation to a low-grade fibrosarcoma, but metastases from desmoids have never been reported. A striking feature of the tumor is its tendency to recur following local excision. The incidence of local recurrence is particularly high after excision of extraabdominal desmoids.

Grossly, the tumor is circumscribed or diffusely infiltrating yet characteristically unencapsulated and it invades as well as compresses muscle. It has a hard rubbery consistency that cuts with a creaking sensation and has a glistening whitish pink color. The microscopic appearance varies from an acellular fibroma to that of a cellular, low-grade fibrosarcoma. Masses of fibrous tissue can be seen that infiltrate, compress, and often destroy muscle

bundles. In this respect, the tumor differs from the more commonly occurring benign fibroma of soft tissue. The absence of mitotic figures and the well-differentiated fibrous tissue are features that differentiate it from the malignant fibrosarcoma.

CLINICAL MANIFESTATIONS. There are no special clinical features characteristic of desmoid tumors. They usually present as a painless, deeply situated mass that is solitary and may be fixed. Its deep location allows it to assume a large size before it is recognized. Usually the tumor is located in the lower abdomen and rarely crosses the midline. It must be differentiated from other tumors of soft tissue and muscle, particularly sarcomas.

TREATMENT. The ideal treatment of desmoid tumors is wide surgical excision. This often necessitates resection of a large portion of the abdominal wall including skin, muscle, and peritoneum. The resulting defect may require fascia, skin, or a sliding muscle graft for closure. The excision, however, should not sacrifice major blood vessels, nerves, or an extremity. Even though recurrences are frequent, they can sometimes be successfully treated by reexcision. In spite of its tendency to recur, the tumor is rarely fatal. Attention has been directed toward metabolic or hormonal manipulation of the tumor. Nonsteroidal, anti-inflammatory drugs such as sulindac (Clinoril), and antiestrogen agents such as tamoxifen (Nolvadex) have been reported to affect tumor regression. The mechanisms of action are unclear. Indomethacin, a drug that inhibits prostaglandin synthesis, together with ascorbic acid has also been shown to retard tumor growth. The value of irradiation therapy has been disputed but an occasional good response is reported.

DISEASES OF THE OMENTUM

General Considerations

The greater omentum consists of a double sheet of flattened endothelium; between the folds the epiploic vessels, lymphatics, and nerves pass in areolar tissue enmeshed with a variable amount of fat. The structure hangs in a double fold, or sling, between the greater curvature of the stomach and the transverse colon. At birth, an agglutination of the two layers occurs, creating an apronlike shield overlying the intestinal coils. The right border attaches to the pylorus or first portion of the duodenum, while the left border forms the gastrosplenic ligament. The right side is usually longer and heavier and may possess tonguelike processes extending into the pelvis. Occasionally, accessory omenta exist attached to the main portion. The size of the greater omentum is related to the amount of fat that it contains, so that often it is huge in obese individuals and very thin and small in emaciated persons. The omentum in infants is usually underdeveloped and may be almost nonexistent. With growth of the individual, there is elongation and thickening of the organ due to the deposition of fat within its layers.

As a peritoneal fold, the omentum assumes the mechanical function of a mesentery, that is, the fixation of viscera and the transmission of a vascular supply. It is otherwise not a vital organ. Furthermore, it can be removed without appreciable disturbance to the individual.

It has long been held that the omentum possesses an inherent motility which allows it to seek out and arrest trouble that may arise within the peritoneal cavity. In this regard, it has been referred to as the "policeman of the abdomen." While it is true that the omentum is often found at the site of an intraabdominal pathologic condition, yet objective evidence, summarized by Rubin, shows that it has no spontaneous or ameboid activity and that displacement occurs as a result of intestinal peristalsis, diaphragmatic excursions, and postural changes of the individual. The areolar tissue is rich in macrophages that have been shown to rapidly remove injected bacteria or foreign particles. Draper and Johnston concluded that the usefulness of the omentum in inflammatory processes is related to its bactericidal and absorptive properties and also its ability to form adhesions.

Surgical diseases of the omentum include torsion, infarction, cysts, and solid tumors.

Torsion of the Omentum

Torsion of the omentum is a condition in which the organ twists on its long axis to an extent causing vascular compromise. This may vary from mild vascular constriction producing edema to complete strangulation leading to infarction and frank gangrene. For torsion to occur, two situations must exist: first, a redundant and mobile segment and, second, a fixed point around which the segment may twist.

ETIOLOGY. Omental torsion has been classified as primary or secondary. Primary, or idiopathic, omental torsion is relatively rare. It was first described by Eitel in 1899, and since then less than 250 cases have been reported in the literature. The cause is obscure. Leitner et al. group the causes of primary torsion into predisposing factors and precipitating factors. Among the suggested predisposing factors are a variety of anatomic variations including tonguelike projections from the free edge of the omentum, bifid omentum, accessory omentum, a large and bulky omentum with a narrow pedicle, and obesity associated with irregular distribution of fat within the organ. Venous redundancy relative to the omental arterial blood supply has also been cited as a predisposing factor. The omental veins are larger and more tortuous than the arteries, allowing venous kinking and thus offering a point of fixation around which twisting may occur. The higher incidence of right-sided omental torsion is related to the greater size and mobility of the right omentum.

Precipitating factors are those which cause displacement of the omentum. These include heavy exertion, sudden change in body position, coughing, straining, and hyperperistalsis with overeating. Primary omental torsion is always unipolar in that there is only one locus of fixation.

Secondary omental torsion is that which is associated with adhesions of the free end of the omentum to cysts, tumors, foci of intraabdominal inflammation, postsurgical wounds, or scarring, or to internal or external hernias. It is more common than the primary type and is usually bi-

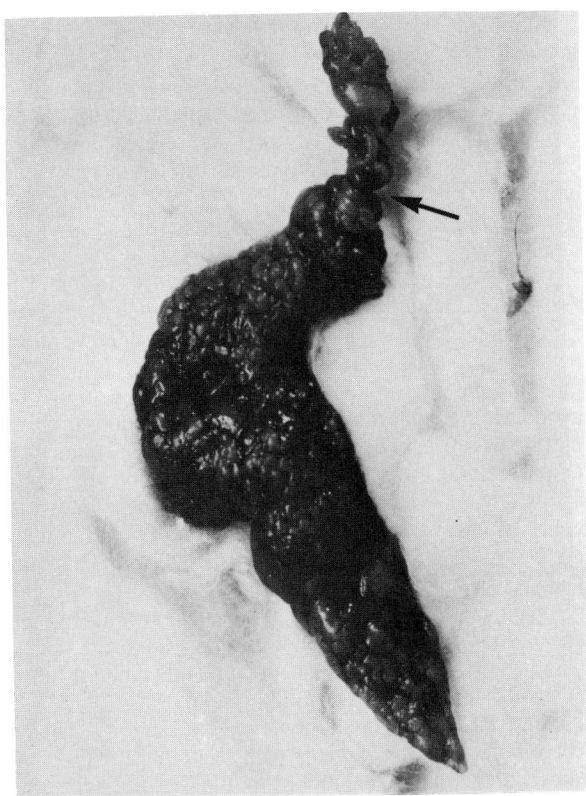

Fig. 35-3. Surgical specimen of primary torsion of the omentum. A small segment of normal-appearing omentum can be seen above the pivotal point (arrow), where it has twisted several times. The omentum below this is congested and hemorrhagic.

polar; that is, torsion of the central portion occurs between two fixed points. About two-thirds of these cases are found in patients with hernias, usually of the inguinal variety. The precipitating factors that incite secondary torsion are the same as those for primary torsion.

PATHOLOGY. The omentum in both the primary and secondary varieties twists a variable number of turns around a pivotal point, usually in a clockwise direction (Fig. 35-3). Either the whole omentum or more often a small portion may undergo torsion. The right side is involved more frequently. Venous return is restricted, and the distal omentum becomes congested and edematous. Hemorrhagic extravasation results in a characteristic serosanguineous effusion into the peritoneal cavity. If the process is of sufficient duration, acute hemorrhagic infarction and eventual necrosis of the segment occur. If not excised, the mass becomes atrophied and fibrotic, and on rare occasions is autoamputated.

CLINICAL MANIFESTATIONS. The clinical features of primary and secondary omental torsion are similar. The condition usually occurs in the fourth or fifth decades of life. Males are affected twice as frequently as females. Pain is the initial and predominant symptom. The onset of pain is usually sudden, and it is constant with a gradual increase in severity. Occasionally the pain is first experienced in the periumbilical region or is generalized. However, invariably it becomes localized to the right side of the abdomen, usually the right lower quadrant. This is in keeping with the more frequent involvement of the right side of the omentum. Movement intensifies the pain. Nausea and vomiting occur in less than half the patients. There is a moderate leukocytosis and a fever that rarely exceeds a rise of 1°C. Tenderness is invariably present, and rebound tenderness and voluntary spasm are also frequent findings. A mass may be palpable if the involved omentum is sufficiently large.

The symptoms and signs are not usually sufficient to allow an accurate preoperative diagnosis. Computerized tomography has been used in diagnosing omental pathology. This can be a sensitive modality for showing an omental mass but is not usually specific for making a diagnosis of omental torsion. Secondary torsion of the hernial type, however, can be suspected if a tender mass is palpable in the groin. The clinical impressions, in order of frequency, are acute appendicitis, acute cholecystitis, and twisted ovarian cyst. Actually, a preoperative diagnosis is of academic interest only, since the clinical manifestations usually warrant exploration. The finding of free serosanguineous fluid at the time of laparotomy in the absence of a pathologic condition in the appendix, gallbladder, or pelvic organs should alert the surgeon to the possibility of omental torsion.

TREATMENT. Treatment consists of resection of the involved omentum. In patients with secondary torsion, the underlying etiologic condition, that is, hernia, cysts, adhesions, etc., should also be corrected. The operative mortality and morbidity are virtually nil.

Idiopathic Segmental Infarction of Omentum

Idiopathic segmental omental infarction is an acute vascular disturbance of the omentum of unknown cause. The criteria for diagnosis of this condition are that it not be accompanied by omental torsion, that there be no associated cardiovascular disease or local intraabdominal pathologic condition, and that there be no history of external abdominal trauma, situations that produce secondary omental infarction. The condition is rare, less than 120 cases having been reported.

ETIOLOGY AND PATHOLOGY. The condition is precipitated by thrombosis of omental veins secondary to endothelial injury. Halligan and Rabiah summarized the several proposed causes of endothelial damage and thrombosis. These include (1) stretching or primary rupture of the omental veins by a sudden increase in intraabdominal pressure as with coughing, sneezing, or lifting, especially after the ingestion of a heavy meal; (2) gravitational pull of an extremely fatty omentum on the omental veins, causing their rupture; and (3) an anatomic peculiarity of the venous drainage of the omentum that predisposes to thrombosis.

The right lower segment of the omentum, which is the most mobile and richest in fat, is the portion usually involved. The area of infarction may vary from 2 to 20 cm in its greatest diameter. Grossly, the involved segment is well demarcated, edematous, and hemorrhagic or gangrenous. It is usually closely adherent to the parietal peritoneum or adjacent abdominal viscera. A variable amount of serosanguineous fluid in the free peritoneal cavity is a constant finding. Microscopically, the picture is that of a hemorrhagic infarction with thrombosis of the omental veins and infiltration of the omentum with inflammatory cells.

CLINICAL MANIFESTATIONS. The majority of patients are young or middle-aged adults, and there is a 3:1 predilection for males. The clinical features are nonspecific. Most patients present with a gradual onset of abdominal pain that is steady and virtually always on the right side of the abdomen. Anorexia and nausea are frequent, but vomiting is rare. Diarrhea or constipation is unusual. There is always tenderness and often rebound tenderness over the region of infarction. Voluntary guarding and, occasionally, spasm are also common. The infarcted segment, if large enough, may be palpable. A slight fever (rarely over 38.5°C) and a moderate leukocytosis are usual. The diagnosis can be suspected by the demonstration of finely infiltrated fat giving a "smudged" appearance to the omentum on computerized tomography.

TREATMENT. Treatment of this condition is resection of the infarcted area to prevent the possible complications of gangrene and adhesions. A correct preoperative diagnosis is unusual, and most patients are explored for acute appendicitis or acute cholecystitis. The finding of serosanguineous fluid in the abdomen and a normal appendix or gallbladder should make the surgeon suspect disease in the omentum. The operative mortality is nil.

Cysts of the Omentum

PATHOLOGY. Cysts of the omentum are rare. The pathogenesis of these lesions is unclear, but presumably most true cysts are caused by obstruction of lymphatic channels or by growth of congenitally misplaced lymphatic tissue that does not communicate with the vascular system. They contain serous fluid and may be unilocular or multilocular. The cysts have an endothelial lining similar to cystic lymphangiomas found elsewhere. Their size may vary from a few centimeters to over 30 cm in diameter. Dermoid cysts, which are very rare, are lined with squamous epithelium and may contain hair, teeth, and sebaceous material.

Pseudocysts of the omentum result from fat necrosis, trauma with hematoma, or foreign body reaction. These have a fibrous and inflammatory lining and usually contain cloudy or blood-tinged fluid.

CLINICAL MANIFESTATIONS. True omental cysts are discovered most frequently in children or young adults but have been reported in the aged. Small cysts are generally asymptomatic and discovered incidentally at laparotomy or at autopsy. Large cysts present as a palpable abdominal mass or produce diffuse abdominal swelling. These may cause symptoms of heaviness or pain or manifestations of possible complications of omental cysts such as torsion, infection, rupture, or intestinal obstruction. Complications are more frequent in children and often produce a clinical picture of an acute surgical condition of the abdomen. The uncomplicated omental cyst usually lies in the lower midabdomen and is freely movable, smooth, and nontender.

Plain radiographs sometimes show a circumscribed soft tissue haziness in the abdomen, or, following a barium meal, there may be displacement of intestinal loops with pressure on adjacent bowel. The presence of bone or teeth is diagnostic of dermoid cyst.

Ultrasonography or computerized tomography shows a fluid-filled mass that often contains internal septations.

Differential diagnosis includes cysts and solid tumors of the mesentery, peritoneum, and retroperitoneal region. An absolute diagnosis can be made only at the time of exploratory surgical procedures. Treatment consists of local excision.

Solid Tumors of the Omentum

The most common solid tumor of the omentum is metastatic carcinoma, which generally involves the omentum by tumor implant. The primary source is usually the colon, stomach, pancreas, or ovaries. Frequently there is associated ascites, presumably from "weeping" of serous or blood-tinged fluid from the metastatic implants. Diffuse neoplastic infiltration of the greater omentum produces a distinctive computed tomographic scan of a soft tissue mass ("omental cake") separating the colon or small intestine from the anterior abdominal wall (Fig. 35-4).

Primary solid tumors of the omentum are exceedingly rare. They may be benign or malignant. Stout et al. recorded only 24 seen over a 55-year period at a major tumor institution. Most are tumors of smooth muscle, and about one-third are malignant. Benign tumors consist of lipomas, leiomyomas, fibromas, and neurofibromas. The malignant tumors spread by direct extension or tumor

implants and kill by involvement of vital abdominal organs.

The only treatment is surgical excision. Primary malignant tumors are highly invasive and often require resection of adjacent organs as well as total omentectomy. The prognosis for these is very poor. Resection of benign tumors is curative, and recurrences have not been reported. Palliative omentectomy for metastatic tumor implants in the omentum has been suggested to control any associated ascites.

MESENTERY AND MESENTERIC CIRCULATION

Anatomy

The mesentery is essentially a reflection of the posterior parietal peritoneum onto the surface of the intestine, where it becomes visceral peritoneum. It connects the intestine to the posterior abdominal wall and carries blood vessels and nerves.

The mesentery proper serves primarily as a suspensory ligament of the jejunum and ileum. It is fan-shaped, its root extending downward and obliquely from the ligament of Treitz (duodenojejunal flexure) at the level of L_2 to the right sacroiliac articulation (ileocecal junction) (Fig. 35-5). The entire root is only about 6 in. long and allows free motion of the small intestine in any direction, limited only by the length of the mesentery. Within its two fused layers of peritoneum run the intestinal branches of the superior mesenteric artery and accompanying vein. It also contains lymph vessels, mesenteric lymph nodes, visceral nerve fibers, and a variable amount of adipose tissue.

Following the embryonic formation of a distinct intestinal loop, torsion of the loop takes place about the superior mesenteric artery. At about the third or fourth fetal

Fig. 35-4. Omental metastases from ovarian carcinoma. CT scan shows the characteristic soft tissue mass involving the greater omentum ("omental cake") (arrowhead).

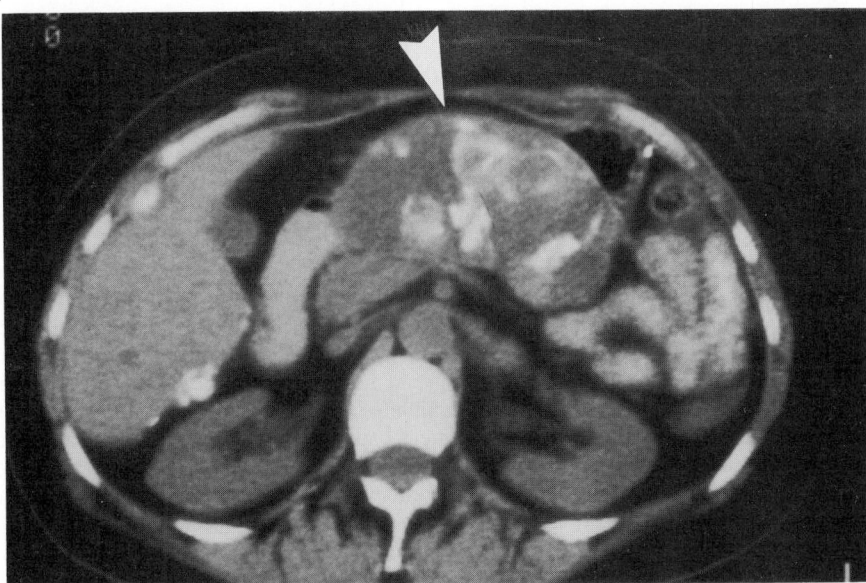

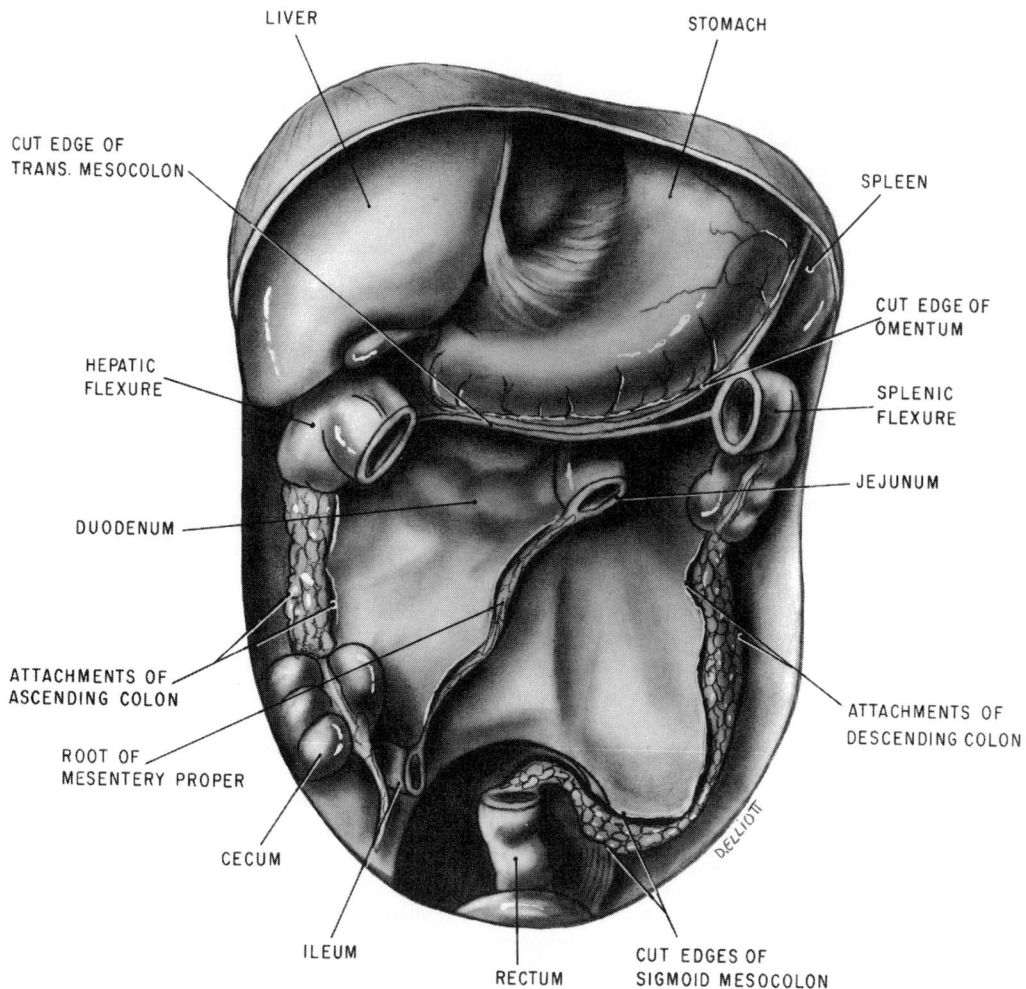

Fig. 35-5. Attachments of the mesenteries. The jejunum, ileum, and ascending, transverse, and descending colons have been removed.

month, posterior peritoneal fixation of the colon takes place. The leaves of the mesentery to the ascending colon fuse with the right parietal peritoneum, and those to the descending colon fuse with the left parietal peritoneum. The lateral posterior parietal peritoneum then passes directly from the abdominal wall over the ascending and descending colon respectively toward the midline and the root of the mesentery proper. For this reason, the mesentery to these portions of the large intestine is usually short or nonexistent. These fusions, however, form surgical cleavage planes allowing bloodless mobilization of the colon with its vascular supply. Within the embryonic mesentery to the ascending colon are the colonic arteries and veins from the superior mesenteric vessels, while those to the descending colon are derived from the inferior mesenteric vessels. On occasion, posterior fusion of the ascending or descending colon is incomplete or does not occur, leaving a well-developed mesentery and allowing free mobility of the bowel segment. This anomaly is more frequent with the right colon, thus predisposing to torsion with resulting intestinal obstruction.

The mesenteries of the transverse colon and sigmoid colon, in contrast to those of the ascending and descend-

ing colon, do not fuse with the posterior parietal peritoneum. These remain well developed and are referred to as the "transverse mesocolon" and "sigmoid mesocolon," respectively. The segment to the transverse colon extends obliquely across the posterior abdominal wall just below the pancreas, remaining fixed at the hepatic and splenic flexures of the bowel (Fig. 35-5). The fixation of the splenic flexure is higher than that of the hepatic flexure because of the presence of the liver on the right side. The mesocolon allows the transverse colon to hang over the small intestine. This sagging may be so marked that the transverse colon occasionally reaches the symphysis pubis. Within the transverse mesocolon run branches of the middle colic artery and accompanying vein. Fusion between the mesocolon and the undersurface of the greater omentum from the stomach offers stability that prevents the transverse colon from undergoing torsion.

The sigmoid mesocolon originates at the end of the descending colon in the left iliac fossa and has an inverted V-shape course (Fig. 35-5). It runs diagonally upward along the left iliac artery toward the aortic bifurcation and then bends directly downward into the pelvic fossa, where it is reflected off the rectum. It contains sigmoid vessels and branches of the superior hemorrhoidal vessels from the inferior mesenteric artery and vein. The length of the sigmoid mesocolon determines the location and mobility of the pelvic colon. If the sigmoid mesocolon is long, the bowel may cross the midline. Such a mobile pelvic colon may twist upon itself. The sigmoid colon is the most frequent site of torsion producing volvulus of the intestinal tract.

The lateral fixations of the ascending and descending colon and the superior origin of the transverse mesocolon serve to confine the small intestine within the midabdomen. The transverse mesocolon and greater omentum also restrict the small bowel from entering the upper abdomen to become adherent to inflammatory lesions of the stomach, duodenum, gallbladder, or liver.

Defects in the mesenteries are potential sites for internal hernia. Most defects are created inadvertently by the surgeon during the course of intraabdominal operations. On rare occasions congenital defects occur in areas of the mesentery that are thin and avascular. These are usually found in the mesenteries of the lower ileum, the sigmoid mesocolon, and the transverse mesocolon, the last through a wide avascular space just to the left of the middle colic artery (space of Riolan).

The mesenteries share with the omenta bactericidal and absorptive properties as well as the ability to form adhesions. In this regard, they function to localize and combat intraperitoneal infection and to seal off intestinal perforations.

MESENTERIC CIRCULATION

In addition to serving as a system for the transport of nutriments, the mesenteric vascular bed is of major importance in the maintaining of bodily homeostasis. Under resting conditions, the splanchnic (visceral) vascular bed receives 25 to 30 percent of cardiac output and contains as much as one-third of total blood volume. It has been suggested that this reservoir of blood produces a mechanism for "autotransfusion" during periods of hypovolemia, when a relatively large volume of blood can be rapidly released into the circulation by active constriction of the splanchnic vessels. Control of the mesenteric vascular bed is primarily neural via sympathetic autonomic elements carried by the splanchnic nerves. These nerves accompany the celiac, superior mesenteric, and inferior mesenteric arteries that contain both alpha- and beta-adrenergic receptors. Stimulation of the splanchnic nerves produces vasoconstriction, with an increase in regional resistance. The mesenteric vasculature is also responsive to a number of pharmacologic agents. Norepinephrine, an alpha-adrenergic stimulator, produces vasoconstriction, and epinephrine elicits a classic dose-dependent beta- or alpha-adrenergic response, low concentrations producing vasodilatation and higher concentrations producing vasoconstriction. Isoproterenol, a beta-adrenergic stimulator, effects a dilator response that can be blocked by propranolol. Tolazoline

hydrochloride and papaverine hydrochloride elicit a direct vasodilatory effect, and the digitalis glycosides have been shown to produce mesenteric vasoconstriction, also presumably by a direct action on the mesenteric vasculature.

Knowledge of the anatomy of the mesenteric circulation is important in the performance of safe and adequate operations on the intestine and in the management of patients with occlusive mesenteric vascular disease and portal hypertension. In resections for malignant lesions, it is necessary to excise a wide segment of adjacent mesentery in order that real or potential sites of tumor spread to the mesenteric lymphatics and lymph nodes are removed.

ARTERIES. With the exception of the stomach and duodenum and the distal rectum, the arterial supply to the entire intestinal tract is derived from the superior and inferior mesenteric arteries.

The superior mesenteric artery arises from the aorta just below the celiac artery opposite the level of L_2. It passes behind the neck of the pancreas but in front of the uncinate process and crosses in front of the third portion of the duodenum to enter the root of the mesentery proper. The acute angle that the superior mesenteric artery makes at its origin from the aorta may compress the transverse portion of the duodenum between it and the aorta, causing partial intestinal obstruction, a condition referred to as the "superior mesenteric artery compression syndrome."

As the superior mesenteric artery continues downward between the two leaves of the mesentery, it gives off 12 or more major branches from its left side that supply the jejunum and ileum (Fig. 35-6). These jejunal and ileal arteries divide and then reunite within the mesentery to form groups, or arcades. Two to five such anastomotic arches are formed and allow collateral pathways for blood to reach the intestinal wall should occlusion of short arterial segments occur. The arcades become more numerous as the terminal ileum is reached. From the terminal arcades, straight branches (vasa recta) alternately pass to opposite sides of the jejunum and ileum. Within the intestinal wall, the vessels run parallel to the circular muscle coat and perpendicular to the direction of the lumen traversing successively the serous, muscular, and submucosal layers. Each of these terminal arteries supplies only 1 or 2 cm of bowel length. For this reason, they must be preserved as close to the cut margins of the intestine as is technically possible when performing a bowel resection to avoid necrosis and breakdown of the subsequent anastomosis. The terminal straight arteries do not anastomose until reaching the submucous plexuses, where their ramifications anastomose freely. This situation predisposes to serious compromise of the blood supply to the antimesenteric border of the intestine following segmental small bowel resection. Therefore, to ensure adequate circulation to the antimesenteric portion, it is customary to transect the small intestine obliquely rather than at a right angle (Fig. 35-7).

Arising from the right side of the superior mesenteric artery is the inferior pancreaticoduodenal artery and then successively, the middle colic, the right colic, and the

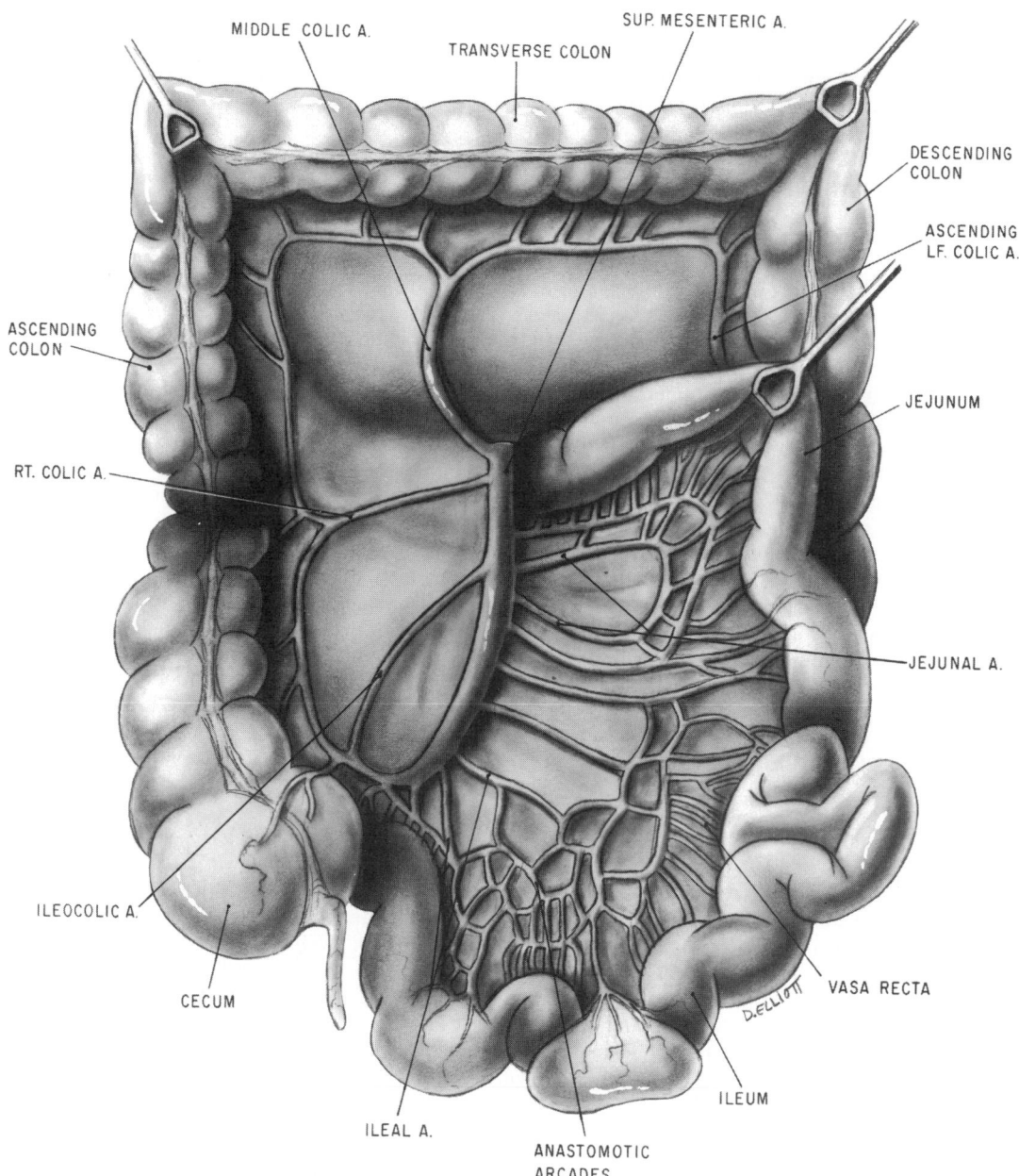

Fig. 35-6. Superior mesenteric artery and its branches. The artery supplies the distal duodenum, jejunum, ileum, ascending colon, and proximal two-thirds of the transverse colon.

ileocolic arteries (Fig. 35-6). Except for the ileocolic artery, these vessels do not form anastomotic arcades until nearly reaching the bowel wall.

The middle colic artery arises below the pancreas, enters the transverse mesocolon, and passing to the right divides into a right and left branch. The right branch connects with the superior branch of the right colic artery and the left branch with the ascending branch of the left colic artery from the inferior mesenteric. It supplies the transverse colon. The location of the main arterial trunk to the right of the midline allows the left side of the transverse mesocolon to be opened through a relatively avascular area (space of Riolan) when performing a retrocolic gastrojejunal anastomosis.

The right colic artery arises just below the middle colic and passes to the right just behind the peritoneum. On reaching the midascending colon, it divides into superior and inferior branches, which anastomose, close to the bowel wall, with branches from the middle colic and ileocolic arteries, respectively. The right colic artery supplies the ascending colon.

The ileocolic artery is the terminal branch of the superior mesenteric artery. It supplies the distal few inches of the ileum, the cecum, the appendix, and the lower portion of the ascending colon. It terminates by dividing into as-

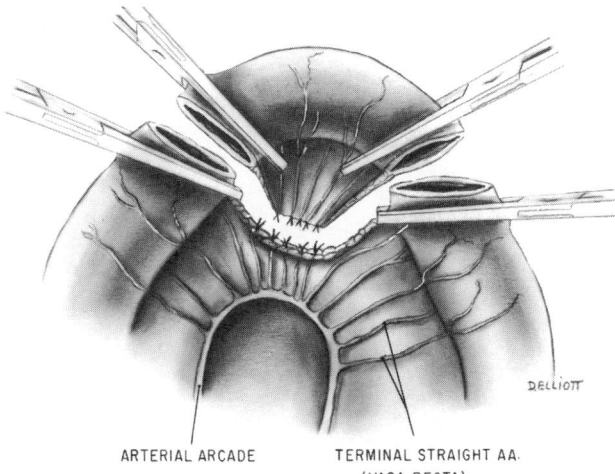

ARTERIAL ARCADE   TERMINAL STRAIGHT AA.
(VASA RECTA)

Fig. 35-7. Straight arteries (vasa recta) entering the wall of the small intestine perpendicular to the direction of its lumen. The arteries alternately pass to either side of the intestinal wall. In performing a segmental resection of the small intestine, transecting the bowel obliquely, as indicated, ensures an adequate blood supply to the antimesenteric border.

cending and descending branches. The ascending branch anastomoses with the inferior branch of the right colic artery, while the descending branch forms secondary and tertiary arcades by anastomosing with terminal branches of the superior mesenteric artery within the mesentery proper. From these arcades arise the appendicular artery to the appendix, and cecal and ileal branches.

The superior mesenteric artery supplies the intestinal tract from the third portion of the duodenum to the midtransverse colon. Collaterals between the inferior pancreaticoduodenal artery and the superior pancreaticoduodenal artery from the gastroduodenal, a secondary branch of the celiac artery, enable the third part of the duodenum and proximal 4 or 5 in. of jejunum to survive when the superior mesenteric artery is occluded.

The inferior mesenteric artery supplies the left transverse colon, descending colon, sigmoid colon, and proximal part of the rectum. It arises from the anterior aorta opposite the body of the third lumbar vertebra and passes downward and to the left, entering the pelvis as the superior hemorrhoidal artery (Fig. 35-8). As it descends, it gives off the left colic and sigmoidal arteries. The left colic artery is the principal branch. It divides into ascending and descending limbs that anastomose with branches from the middle colic and sigmoid arteries, respectively. The sigmoid artery passes into the sigmoid mesocolon and divides into branches that anastomose with one another, forming several arcades. The lowest sigmoid arcade joins with arcades from the superior hemorrhoidal artery. The superior hemorrhoidal artery continues downward behind the rectum, where it communicates with branches from the middle and inferior hemorrhoidal arteries from the internal iliac artery, giving the rectum a dual source of arterial supply.

The anastomoses between primary branches of the superior and inferior mesenteric arteries form an arcade that passes along the margin of the colon and is referred to as the "marginal artery of Drummond" (Fig. 35-8). It is situated about $\frac{1}{2}$ in. from the margin of the bowel and extends from the end of the ileum to the end of the sigmoid colon. Through its anastomoses, it is capable of supplying the bowel even though one of the major arteries is ligated.

VEINS. The venous drainage of the small intestine and colon is through tributaries of the inferior and superior mesenteric veins, which in turn ultimately terminate in the portal vein (Fig. 35-9). The portal circulation begins within the mucosa of the intestine. Small venules coalesce, and the confluent veins pass through the wall of the intestine, emerging alternately in a similar manner to that of the straight arteries entering the bowel wall. These then converge to form a system of venous arcades within the mesentery from which blood enters the main tributaries to the superior and inferior mesenteric veins.

The inferior mesenteric vein is a continuation of the superior hemorrhoidal vein. It passes upward to the left side of the inferior mesenteric artery, receiving tributaries that correspond in name and location to the branches of the artery. However, the main trunk of the vein does not accompany the artery but rather courses over the duodenojejunal flexure just lateral to the ligament of Treitz and, passing over the body of the pancreas, joins with the splenic vein (Figs. 35-8 and 35-9). It drains the left side of the large intestine from the upper rectum to the left midtransverse colon. A plexus of anastomoses around the midrectum between the superior hemorrhoidal vein and the middle and inferior hemorrhoidal veins to the internal iliac veins forms a collateral pathway between the portal and systemic circulation.

The superior mesenteric vein runs within the mesentery proper lateral to the superior mesenteric artery. It receives tributaries that accompany corresponding branches of the superior mesenteric artery and that drain the entire small intestine and right half of the colon. As it passes over the third portion of the duodenum and behind the neck of the pancreas, it receives the confluence of the inferior mesenteric and splenic veins to become the portal vein (see Chap. 30).

The venous drainage from the entire gastrointestinal tract passes through the liver via the portal circulation before returning to the heart. Together with the mesenteric lymphatics, it represents the sole means by which ingested food products find their way into the circulation. The normal portal venous pressure is between 12 and 15 cm of water; that within the inferior vena cava (systemic pressure) varies between a postitive pressure of about 3 cm during the expiratory phase of respiration to a negative pressure of 1 to 3 cm during inspiration. Like the vena cava, the portal system does not contain valves, and therefore the blood can flow in the direction of reduced venous pressure.

MESENTERIC LYMPHATICS AND LYMPH NODES. The lymph drainage of the small intestine and colon follows the course of the main blood vessels. Those accompanying the inferior mesenteric artery drain to periaortic nodes and thence to the superior mesenteric nodes before entering the cisterna chyli of the thoracic duct. Those accom-

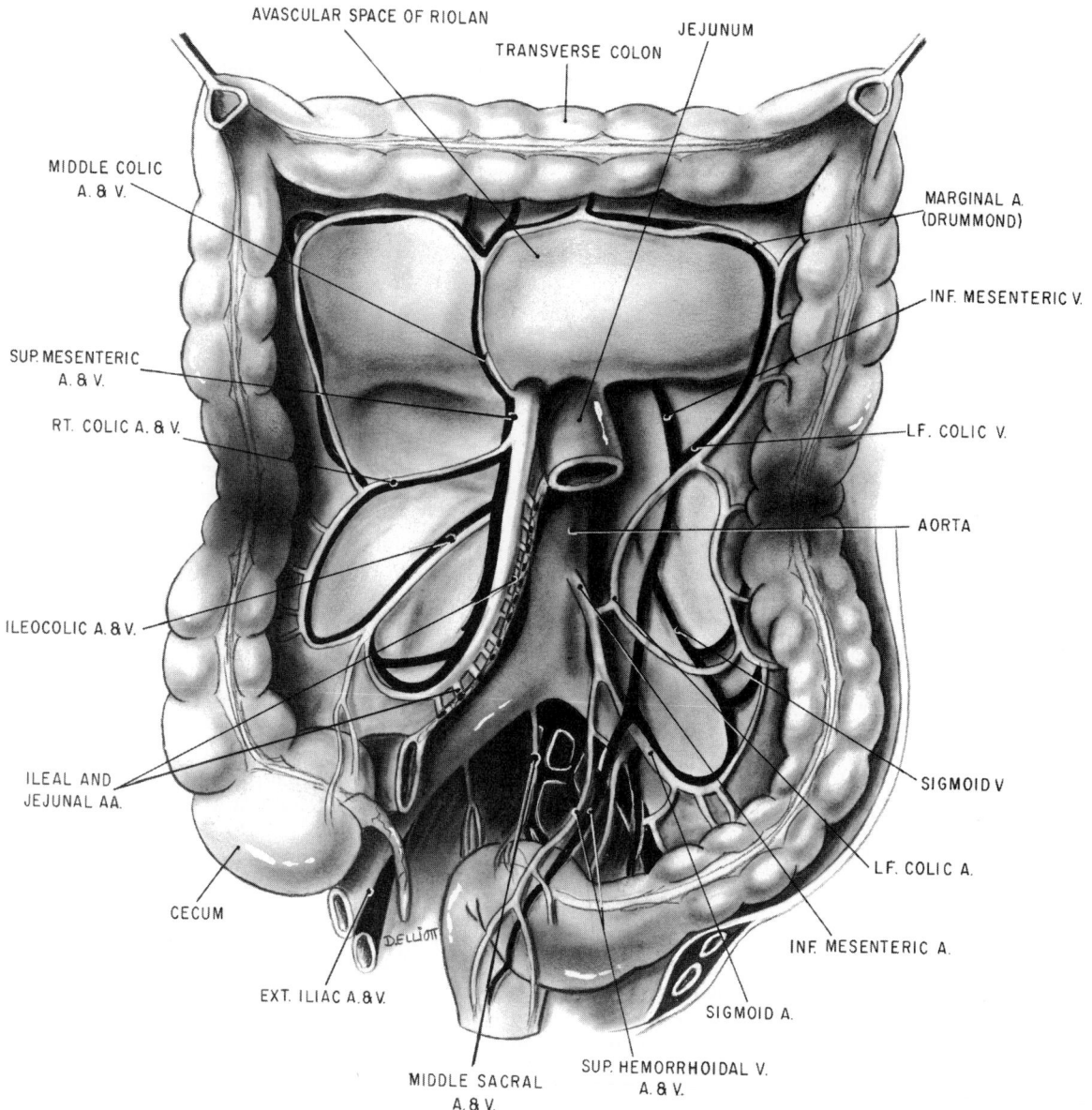

AVASCULAR SPACE OF RIOLAN
JEJUNUM
TRANSVERSE COLON
MIDDLE COLIC A. & V.
MARGINAL A. (DRUMMOND)
INF. MESENTERIC V.
SUP. MESENTERIC A. & V.
RT. COLIC A. & V.
LF. COLIC V.
AORTA
ILEOCOLIC A. & V.
ILEAL AND JEJUNAL AA.
SIGMOID V
CECUM
LF. COLIC A.
INF. MESENTERIC A.
EXT. ILIAC A. & V.
SIGMOID A.
MIDDLE SACRAL A. & V.
SUP. HEMORRHOIDAL V. A. & V.

Fig. 35-8. Blood supply to the large bowel. An arterial arcade, formed by anastomoses between branches of the colic arteries, runs along the margin of the large intestine and is referred to as the *marginal artery of Drummond*. This vessel is the major collateral supplying blood to the colon when a main stem mesenteric or colic artery is occluded.

panying branches of the superior mesenteric artery drain into the mesenteric glands within the mesentery proper, where they are closely related to the vascular arcades. The mesenteric nodes are distributed in three locations: (1) juxtaintestinal, at the last anastomotic branch of the mesenteric arteries before they enter the intestines; (2) intermediate, in the region of the larger anastomosing branches; and (3) central, at the root of the mesentery near the origin of the main mesenteric artery. The nodes are more numerous in the right half of the mesentery, and they increase in size and number as they approach its root. These nodes are the usual site for mesenteric adenitis, tuberculosis, and other inflammatory as well as neoplastic conditions. From the mesenteric nodes, lymph drains into the superior mesenteric and celiac nodes and then to the thoracic duct.

Mesenteric Vascular Disease

Mesenteric vascular disease is not a single entity but rather a syndrome that includes (1) complete occlusion or stenosis of mesenteric arteries by embolism, thrombosis, or obliterative disease; (2) thrombosis of mesenteric (portal) veins; (3) extraluminal obstruction of mesenteric arteries by aortic aneurysm, dissecting aneurysm, fibrous and ligamentous bands, or tumors; (4) aneurysms of the splanchnic arteries; and (5) traumatic injury to visceral vessels. These conditions produce vascular insufficiency

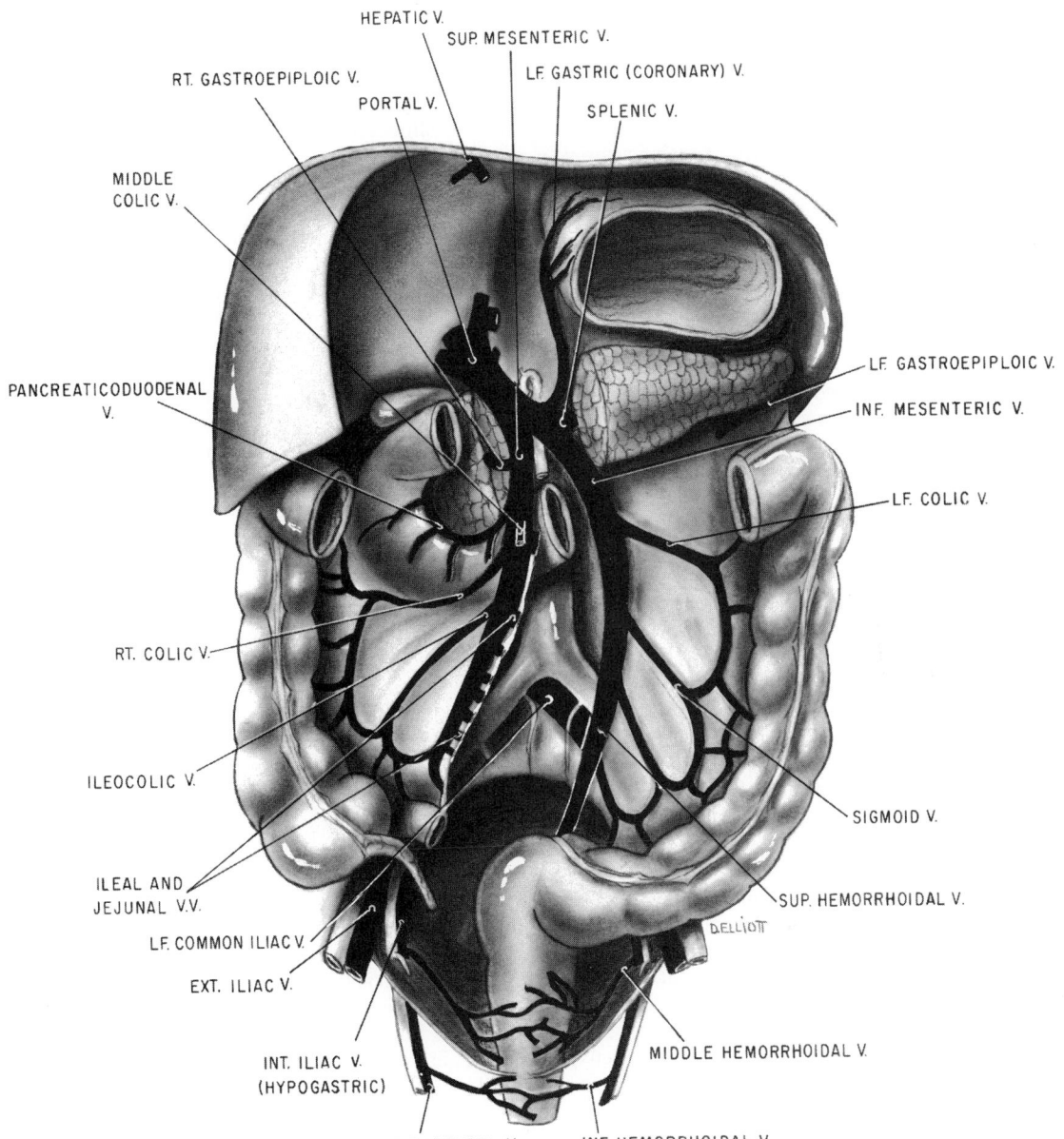

Fig. 35-9. Mesenteric (portal) venous circulation, showing the communication with the systemic circulation through the middle and inferior hemorrhoidal veins. A similar communication (not shown) exists between the left gastric vein and the azygos system of veins.

or infarction of the affected intestine. Intestinal disease due to impaired circulation is relatively uncommon when compared with the more frequently occurring mechanical obstructions of the mesenteric vessels by adhesive bands, strangulated hernia, or intestinal volvulus.

Occlusions of the mesenteric arteries may be acute and complete (those due to emboli or thrombosis), gradual and partial (those due to obliterative arterial disease), or acute and complete superimposed upon a previously narrowed or stenotic vessel. The superior mesenteric artery at its origin or close to the takeoff of its middle colic branch is the usual site of both acute and chronic mesenteric arterial occlusions. Complete occlusion of the inferior mesenteric artery produces symptoms only if there is compromise of collateral blood flow from the superior mesenteric or internal iliac (hypogastric) arteries. Clinically apparent venous occlusions are sudden and complete and invariably due to thrombosis. Partial mesenteric venous occlusion is usually due to external compression and is asymptomatic.

The relative incidence of mesenteric arterial as opposed to venous occlusions is not known. When intestinal infarction occurs, it is not unusual to find thrombosis of both sides of the splanchnic circulation at laparotomy or autopsy, since initial occlusion of one eventuates in clot formation in the other. The clinical distinction between the two is often difficult. It has been variously estimated that 15 to 20 percent of all clinically significant mesenteric vascular accidents are due to primary venous thrombosis and approximately 50 percent to primary arterial occlusion. In the remaining 30 to 35 percent of cases, intestinal infarction occurs in the absence of major arterial or venous occlusion.

ACUTE OCCLUSION OF SUPERIOR MESENTERIC ARTERY

ETIOLOGY. Embolism. Sudden, complete occlusion of the superior mesenteric artery is due more often to an embolus than to thrombosis. The anatomic characteristics of this artery make it more susceptible than the inferior mesenteric artery to symptomatic embolic occlusion. Its main stem leaves the aorta at an acute angle that runs parallel to the aorta, thus maintaining a straight-line connection with the heart. The smaller orifice of the inferior mesenteric artery allows only small emboli to enter it, and when this occurs, lodgment is more likely at a site beyond the division of the artery into its major branches.

Most emboli come from the heart, either from a mural thrombus in a patient with early postcoronary heart disease or from an auricular thrombus in a patient with atrial fibrillation. Less frequently, vegetative endocarditis, thrombi at the site of atheromatous plaques within the aorta, or dislodgment of atheromatous plaques during translumbar or retrograde femoral arteriography are the sources of the emboli. The embolus may occlude the main orifice of the artery, particularly if it has been previously narrowed by an atheromatous plaque. More often, however, it lodges near a major branch where the artery narrows, usually at the egress of the middle colic artery. It may then remain at its initial location or fragment and be carried more distad. The initial effect of the embolus on the artery is to cause spasm of its distal branches. This and the rapid closure of the main trunk do not usually allow time for the development of a collateral circulation. Secondary thrombosis of the distal artery then occurs, probably within a few hours. Frequently the artery proximal to the embolus dilates. Sudden occlusion of the main stem superior mesenteric artery produces ischemia of the entire small intestine distal to the ligament of Treitz and also ischemia of the proximal half of the colon. Only rarely, when there are exceptional collateral channels through the celiac axis and inferior mesenteric artery, does the bowel survive. Acute occlusion of short arterial segments or of smaller branches may or may not eventuate in infarction, depending on the status of the collateral circulation.

Thrombosis. Acute, complete thrombosis of the superior mesenteric artery nearly always occurs in an artery partially occluded by atherosclerosis. Less frequently, it is superimposed on a vessel narrowed by aortic aneurysm or involved by thromboangiitis obliterans or periarteritis nodosa. A sudden decrease in cardiac output, as occurs in acute congestive failure or myocardial infarction, often precedes the final thrombotic episode. The extent of intestinal ischemia or infarction is dependent on the site of thrombosis and the status of collateral channels. Sudden thrombosis of the main stem artery, as in embolic occlusion, usually results in infarction of the entire small intestine and right colon. Slowly developing stenosis may allow time for the development of adequate collaterals so that bowel viability is preserved when acute occlusion supervenes. In inflammatory vascular diseases, the smaller visceral branches are usually affected, and intestinal infarction occurs in shorter segments.

PATHOLOGY. Sudden, complete arterial occlusion first causes an ischemic infarct in which the bowel is pale. This is the result of intense vasospasm of the intramural vessels, and it produces mucosal ulceration. At this stage, the bowel becomes hypertonic and contracted. Within 1 to 2 h, the initial vessel spasm subsides, and the capillaries in the anoxic bowel wall become engorged with blood. As subsequent thrombosis of the artery beyond the site of occlusion occurs, the intestinal musculature becomes fatigued, and contractility is lost. Thrombosis of the visceral veins follows, and the bowel wall becomes inert, boggy, and cyanotic as a result of regurgitant flow from the veins or seepage of blood into the mural tissues of the ischemic intestine. As the infarction progresses to full-thickness necrosis of the intestine, the bowel wall becomes blood-soaked and cyanotic, and "weeps" serosanguineous fluid into the peritoneal cavity. The appearance is that of hemorrhagic infarction and is the end result of either primary arterial or venous occlusion.

CLINICAL MANIFESTATIONS. Sudden, complete occlusion of the superior mesenteric artery presents as a surgical emergency with all the manifestations of paralysis of the peristaltic mechanism as well as loss of viability of the affected intestine. The result is a form of strangulated intestinal obstruction and includes all the hazards associated with this condition (see Chap. 24).

The clinical features are usually the same whether occlusion is the result of embolism or thrombosis. Males are affected more often than females. The peak age incidence is in the fifth and sixth decades. Frequently the patient has coronary artery disease, with or without atrial fibrillation, and other manifestations of generalized atherosclerosis. A prior history of repeated episodes of cramping abdominal pain following the ingestion of food (intestinal angina) may be elicited from as many as one-third of these patients.

The most striking and constant complaint is extreme abdominal pain, often unresponsive to narcotics and initially out of proportion to the physical findings. The pain comes on suddenly and is first colicky but soon becomes steady and continuous. The early localization of the pain is to the segment of bowel involved. With acute main stem artery occlusion, the pain is first experienced in the midabdomen or epigastrium but later becomes generalized. Vomiting follows, is protracted, and may contain blood. Diarrhea and later constipation occur, and often the stool contains occult or gross blood. A peculiar, mottled cyanosis of the abdomen and flanks has been observed in about one-fifth of patients, a manifestation of low cardiac output accompanying extensive bowel infarction. The abdomen does not usually become distended until late. Voluntary and involuntary muscle spasm will be present, but the rigidity is almost never boardlike. Tenderness and rebound tenderness become severe as intestinal infarction occurs and are most marked over the ischemic segment of bowel. The presence of a mass is more usual with infarction of short intestinal segments. Bowel sounds are at first hyperactive, but within a short time the abdomen becomes silent. At the onset, temperature, pulse, and blood pressure may not be significantly altered. As infarction of the intestine progresses, the patient becomes febrile, the pulse rate increases, and the patient becomes hypotensive. Not infrequently, main stem artery occlusion initially produces acute circulatory collapse that is readily reversible but then recurs as gangrene of the bowel with peritonitis supervenes. Once bowel necrosis and perforation occur, the findings are those of generalized peritonitis and sepsis.

A correct clinical diagnosis is difficult to make, especially with occlusions of short arterial segments. The most important early diagnostic feature is the severity of the abdominal pain relative to the physical findings and its unresponsiveness to narcotics. This finding in a patient with a recent myocardial infarction or atrial fibrillation or in one who has previously suffered emboli to extremity arteries should make the physician highly suspicious of an acute mesenteric vascular accident.

DIAGNOSTIC STUDIES. The leukocyte count may be normal early in the course of the disease but is increased to over 20,000 as hemorrhagic infarction occurs. Most patients have normal or high hematocrit levels. Often the serum amylase level is elevated. This has been related to seepage of the enzyme through the ischemic bowel wall. Radiographs of the abdomen are not often of significant diagnostic value. Frequently they show moderate to slight distention of both small and large intestine. The presence of gas in the right half of the colon that stops abruptly in the midtransverse colon has been considered a valuable finding; however, this is infrequent and occurs late. Suspicion of the diagnosis of acute mesenteric ischemia is of itself an indication for obtaining an immediate mesenteric angiogram. In addition to demonstrating emboli, thrombosis, and mesenteric vasoconstriction, the arteriogram will ascertain the adequacy of the splanchnic circulation. The angiographic catheter also provides a route for the intraarterial administration of vasodilating agents. Embolic occlusion of the main superior mesenteric artery usually shows on the arteriogram as a sharp cutoff in the artery just below the origin of the middle colic artery. At times, an embolus will fragment and be seen as multiple filling defects in the peripheral branches of the artery. When the arteriogram is performed immediately after the onset of abdominal pain, emboli appear as discrete round filling defects, but if the study is delayed for several days, secondary thrombosis builds up proximally as well as distally. Acute occlusion of the superior mesenteric artery by thrombosis occurs most often at its immediate takeoff from the aorta where it is most severely involved by atherosclerotic narrowing.

TREATMENT. The essential treatment of acute mesenteric vascular occlusion is early surgical intervention, preferably before gangrene and perforation of the intestine has occurred. Prior to the 1950s, the only surgical procedure considered was resection of the ischemic intestine. Isolated reports then appeared on revascularization of the superior mesenteric artery together with intestinal resection. In 1957, Shaw and Rutledge reported the first successful superior mesenteric artery embolectomy not requiring associated bowel resection, and shortly thereafter Shaw performed a successful thromboendarterectomy for acute thrombosis. Yet, the number of patients who present with a situation amenable to arterial reconstruction is small. This is because, to be successful, embolectomy (or emergency thrombectomy) must be performed within a few hours after the acute occlusion, before irreversible changes have occurred.

Boley et al. outlined an aggressive radiological and surgical approach to the problem of acute mesenteric ischemia. Immediate mesenteric arteriography is the keystone of their approach and is obtained while efforts are made to improve the general cardiovascular condition of the patient, when indicated, by the replacement of plasma volume, relief of acute congestive heart failure, and correction of cardiac arrhythmias. If the arteriogram demonstrates an embolus or mesenteric vasoconstriction, an infusion of papaverine hydrochloride, a vasodilating agent, is begun through the angiographic catheter positioned within the superior mesenteric artery. The papaverine is infused at a rate of 30 to 60 mg/h by a constant-infusion pump. The use of papaverine is based on the association of mesenteric vasoconstriction with acute occlusion of the superior mesenteric artery by embolus or thrombosis. An occasional patient can be treated successfully by papaverine infusion alone without operation. Patients so treated are followed by clinical response and serial arteriograms. Treatment is continued if the abdominal pain subsides and the arteriogram shows progressive dilatation of the mesenteric arteries with perfusion of the intestine.

The great majority of patients will require an operation and are taken to the operating room while receiving intraarterial papaverine. At laparotomy, the ischemic intestine will be pale and thin (anemic infarction) or more often in the stage of hemorrhagic infarction. If the occlusion is limited to a branch of the superior mesenteric artery or to the superior mesenteric artery distal to the origin of the ileocolic artery, the relatively short segments of affected intestine are best handled by resection with a primary end-to-end anastomosis. From previous experience, it has been learned that as much as 70 percent of the small intestine can be removed without creating serious digestive disturbances.

In the situation where the main stem superior mesenteric artery is occluded, the decision to establish arterial flow is based on whether the process in the ischemic intestine is reversible. Although outwardly appearing nonviable, the deeply cyanotic and dull surface of the intestinal wall is at times deceiving. Intestine that initially appears infarcted may show surprising recovery following arterial reconstruction. An attempt should be made to stimulate peristalsis, since its presence is indicative of viable and potentially salvageable bowel. If the intestines are clearly gangrenous, the only surgical procedure that can be considered is resection. This will usually require removal of the entire small intestine distal to the ligament of Treitz and resection of the right half of the colon. Although this extensive a resection is associated with a high operative mortality and late morbidity, it is worthy of consideration in an otherwise hopeless situation, and with the use of parenteral central hyperalimentation postoperatively, some patients can be salvaged.

If there is any question of the reversibility of the ischemia of all or part of the intestine, an attempt at arterial reconstruction is indicated. The superior mesenteric artery is traced proximally and location of the embolus or thrombus determined by finding a bounding pulse proximal to the occlusion with no pulsation distad. The artery is isolated between vascular tapes, and the occluding lesion is removed through a longitudinal arteriotomy incision. An embolus can usually be easily extracted using a Fogarty balloon catheter while a thrombus within a sclerotic vessel will require a thromboendarterectomy. Proximal ''milking'' of the distal vessels may be necessary if fresh thrombus is present. The incision in the artery is then closed using a patch graft, preferably of autogenous vein. With resumption of arterial flow, pulsations will be felt in the mesenteric vessels and color will return to the bowel within a few minutes provided the ischemia is reversible. Revascularization with a bypass venous graft between the aorta and distal superior mesenteric artery will be necessary if adequate antegrade blood flow is not restored after removal of an embolus or thrombus.

Following completion of the revascularization procedure the entire gastrointestinal tract should be visualized for 10 to 15 min. A significant factor limiting the successful surgical management of patients with acute intestinal ischemic conditions is the difficulty at operation to accurately predict intestinal recovery. Clinical assessment, such as return of intestinal color and arterial pulsations and the presence of visible peristalsis, is usually reliable in determining that a segment of revascularized intestine will remain viable. The intraoperative use of the Doppler ultrasonic flowmeter to detect pulsatile mural blood flow can give added objective confirmation. Intravenous infusion of a vital dye, usually fluorescein, has also been advocated to define intestinal recovery. This technique involves injecting 1 g of sodium fluorescein into a peripheral vein and then examining the intestinal loops in a darkened room with a hand-held ultraviolet (Wood's) light. Viable intestine will show as a yellow fluorescent glow indicative of vascular perfusion. In a controlled study by Bulkley and associates, the fluorescence pattern provided a useful adjuvant to the clinical assessment of intestinal viability and proved to be significantly more reliable than either clinical judgment or the use of the Doppler flowmeter in borderline cases.

All obviously nonvascularized intestine and short segments of questionably viable intestine are resected. If there is any question about the viability of long segments of intestine, it is best to leave them and then reexamine them at a planned second operation 24 to 36 h later. The advantage of this two-stage approach is not only to allow a clear definition between dead and live intestine to take place but also to permit time for the institution of supportive measures that may render more of the intestine viable. The decision to perform a second-look operation is made at the initial laparotomy and is not routinely done if the intestine appears adequately arterialized.

The preoperative preparation and postoperative care of patients with acute mesenteric infarction is particularly important. Most of these patients will have a depleted circulating blood volume resulting from loss of plasma and whole blood into the bowel lumen, bowel wall, and peritoneal cavity. This loss can be considerable and rapid replacement should be started while readying the patient for operation. Added intravenous fluids are necessary postoperatively to combat the reactive hyperemia that occurs after revascularization of the intestine. Since the ischemic bowel wall allows passage of bacteria into the peritoneal cavity even before frank necrosis has occurred, broad-spectrum antibiotics should be administered in large doses beginning preoperatively and continuing throughout the postoperative period. Papaverine infusion via the superior mesenteric artery catheter is continued postoperatively and a repeat arteriogram obtained at 24 h to ascertain the success of a vascular reconstructive procedure. Anticoagulation, preferably with heparin, has also been recommended for patients who have had arterial reconstruction. Nasogastric decompression of the stomach and intestine is necessary until bowel function returns.

The overall mortality following sudden occlusion of the mesenteric artery varies between 56 and 85 percent. Using their aggressive radiographic and surgical approach, Boley et al. were able to decrease the mortality to 45 percent. Mortality is higher following acute occlusion by thrombosis compared with embolism. The cause of death is usually peritonitis with septicemia. Frequent atherosclerotic involvement of the heart, kidney, and other organs contributes to the high mortality rates.

NONOCCLUSIVE MESENTERIC INFARCTION

ETIOLOGY. In about 30 percent of patients with mesenteric infarction, careful examination will reveal no gross arterial or venous occlusion. Ottinger and Austen found this situation to be the most frequent cause of intestinal gangrene on a circulatory basis. It produces diffuse intestinal necrosis and is invariably fatal. It has been related to a sustained decrease in cardiac output such as in prolonged circulatory collapse and hypoxic states that may accompany septicemia, congestive heart failure, cardiac arrhythmia, acute myocardial infarction, and profound hypovolemia. The common denominator appears to be a low cardiac output state. Very frequently it is a terminal event in these illnesses. Its occurrence has been explained on the basis of persistent compensatory splanchnic vasoconstriction that becomes intractable. Sludging of blood due to erythrocytic agglutination follows as blood flow through the small arterioles slows down, and ultimately intestinal anoxia and infarction occur. Vasopressor therapy for shock may prolong the vasoconstriction and hasten the onset of gangrene. Additionally, the majority of patients presenting with nonocclusive mesenteric infarction have received digitalis, an agent that has been shown to induce mesenteric vasoconstriction. The genesis of acute nonocclusive mesenteric infarction has been explained by applying the law of Laplace. According to this law, the tension in the wall of the vessel must be less than the hydrostatic pressure exerted by the column of blood, or the vessel will collapse. It has been shown in dogs that when the blood pressure in the vasa recta drops below 15 mmHg with a blood flow below 10 mL/100 g of intestinal tissue for eight consecutive hours, irreversible ischemia develops.

PATHOLOGY. The gross pathologic picture seen in patients with nonocclusive mesenteric infarction is essentially that of hemorrhagic necrosis. The mucosa is ulcerated and edematous, and the submucosal vessels are grossly dilated and packed with erythrocytes. The outer surface of the bowel is initially mottled with segmental areas of cyanosis distributed throughout the length of the intestine. In the late stages of the disease, gangrenous changes become advanced and lead to perforation.

CLINICAL MANIFESTATIONS. The clinical picture may be identical to that of patients with acute arterial or venous mesenteric occlusions. The patients, however, are usually older, and the infarction develops slowly over a period of several days, during which time there may be prodromal symptoms of malaise and vague abdominal discomfort. Associated congestive heart failure, with or without arrhythmia, is frequent. An unusually large number of patients have been found to be overdigitalized. Infarction of the intestine is heralded by the sudden onset of severe abdominal pain and vomiting. The patient usually becomes acutely hypotensive and develops a rapid pulse. Watery diarrhea is frequent, and the stools may be grossly bloody. The abdomen becomes diffusely tender and rigid. Bowel sounds are diminished and later absent. Fever and leukocytosis are usual, and frequently there is a thrombocytopenia related to intravascular thrombosis. A characteristic early laboratory finding is a markedly elevated hematocrit, which is apparently due to "trapping" of serum in the bowel wall and seepage into the peritoneal cavity.

In disorders in which the splanchnic circulation is thought to be diminished, unexplained abdominal signs and symptoms should be viewed with the possibility of mesenteric vascular insufficiency and intestinal necrosis in mind. The single most important aid in establishing the diagnosis is abdominal angiography. A diagnostic selective superior mesenteric arteriogram will demonstrate patent major vessels with multiple segmental areas of narrowing of both small- and medium-sized branches and diminution or absence of a mural intestinal circulation.

TREATMENT. The initial approach to the treatment of this condition is to correct the underlying disorder producing the low flow state. At the same time, it has been suggested that an attempt be made to improve mesenteric artery flow. This can be accomplished by direct infusion of vasodilating drugs such as isoproterenol, tolazoline hydrochloride, or papaverine hydrochloride into a cathe-

ter positioned in the superior mesenteric artery, or by a continuous epidural block. The response can be assessed by obtaining sequential mesenteric angiograms. Antibiotics have been shown to delay or diminish loss of intestinal viability and should be administered early and in large doses.

If, despite mesenteric vasodilatation, the abdominal signs and symptoms persist or reappear, operation is mandatory. With intractable hypotension and congestive failure, the gangrenous changes in the bowel wall are usually segmental; areas of anemic infarction are found interspersed with those of hemorrhagic infarction. Pulses can be felt in the superior and inferior mesenteric arteries and their major branches extending almost to the bowel wall. Serosanguineous fluid is a constant finding in the peritoneal cavity. The process usually extends throughout the entire large and small intestine and may also involve the stomach. For this reason, resection is not usually feasible. With involvement of lesser portions of the intestine, primary resection with end-to-end anastomosis should be attempted, although too often the remaining intestine will subsequently become infarcted in the immediate postoperative period. Massive fluid replacement and support of cardiac function combined with interruption of splanchnic vasoconstriction by continuous epidural block have been recommended postoperatively to help prevent progression following intestinal resection. The reported mortality rates are upwards of 80 percent, a reflection primarily of the frequent occurrence of this type of mesenteric infarction in terminal illnesses.

CHRONIC OCCLUSION OF VISCERAL ARTERIES (INTESTINAL ANGINA)

Three possible sequelae may follow gradual occlusion of the main stem visceral arteries: (1) establishment of an adequate collateral circulation; (2) intestinal infarction; and (3) intestinal ischemia without infarction, due to collateral blood supply sufficient for life but not for function of the affected bowel. The last of these three sequelae produces a now well-recognized syndrome termed "intestinal angina." This entity is analogous to angina pectoris and intermittent claudication due to, respectively, arterial insufficiency to the heart and to the extremities.

ETIOLOGY. Collateral anastomoses among the three main gastrointestinal arteries from the aorta (celiac axis, superior mesenteric, and inferior mesenteric) provide for maintenance of intestinal viability and function when one of these branches is gradually occluded. For this reason, most patients with isolated chronic occlusion of the superior mesenteric artery are completely asymptomatic. However, when blood flow through one of the surviving vessels then becomes (or has been) compromised, the now relatively ischemic intestine is unable to respond to the demands of digestion for an increased blood supply. This explains the "food-pain" sequence that characterizes intestinal angina.

A rare cause of intestinal angina is isolated partial occlusion of the celiac artery by fibers of the median arcuate ligament, a condition referred to as the *median arcuate ligament syndrome*. The basis of the constriction appears to be due either to a high origin of the celiac artery, with resultant compression as it passes beneath the median arcuate ligament, or an abnormally low crossing of the ligament causing compression of a normally located artery. It has been inferred that the pain is related to intestinal ischemia, but true, chronic ischemia of the gastrointestinal tract generally requires interference with the blood flow in at least two of the three major visceral arteries.

As a major visceral artery becomes critically narrowed, the others dilate in order to carry more blood. This finding is of practical significance when the inferior mesenteric artery must be sacrificed in patients undergoing surgical treatment for aortic aneurysm or colon resection for carcinoma. In these circumstances, patency of the superior mesenteric artery should be ascertained before an unusually large inferior mesenteric is sacrificed. Otherwise, infarction of the intestine may be precipitated when the latter vessel is ligated. This complication can be prevented either by reimplanting the inferior mesenteric artery into the aortic graft or by restoring blood flow through the superior mesenteric artery.

PATHOLOGY. Chronic occlusion of the major visceral arteries is most often due to atherosclerosis. The atheromatous plaques are invariably located at or near the origin of these large vessels, thus in a segment that anatomically is suitable for arterial reconstruction. Most of these patients also have evidence of generalized arteriosclerosis. Less frequently, the stenosis is due to compression of the celiac axis by a celiac ganglion or arcuate ligament of the diaphragm, by involvement of the arteries in an expanding aortic aneurysm or dissecting aneurysm, or by thromboangiitis obliterans or periarteritis nodosa.

CLINICAL MANIFESTATIONS. The dominant clinical feature of intestinal angina is generalized cramping abdominal pain that comes on soon after eating and lasts as long as 3 h. The severity and duration of the distress depends on the amount of food ingested. Occasionally it is merely a sense of distention, or bloating, with a constant abdominal ache. If the pain is severe, nausea and vomiting often occur. Initially the patient will complain of constipation and later of diarrhea. There is usually a steady progression in the frequency and duration of symptoms. The food-pain relationship soon leads to a reluctance on the part of the patient to eat. The subsequent rapid and severe weight loss characterizes the syndrome. As the intestinal ischemia progresses, a form of malabsorption syndrome occurs that contributes to the weight loss and is manifest by bulky, foamy stools high in fat and protein content. Symptoms of intestinal angina may exist for months or years before the visceral circulation becomes critically curtailed. Morris et al. estimate that histories of prodromal symptoms of intestinal angina may be obtained from as many as one-third of patients with mesenteric infarction.

On physical examination, weight loss will be obvious. Usually there are varying degrees of disability associated with generalized arteriosclerosis. A bruit is often heard over the epigastrium, although this may be transmitted

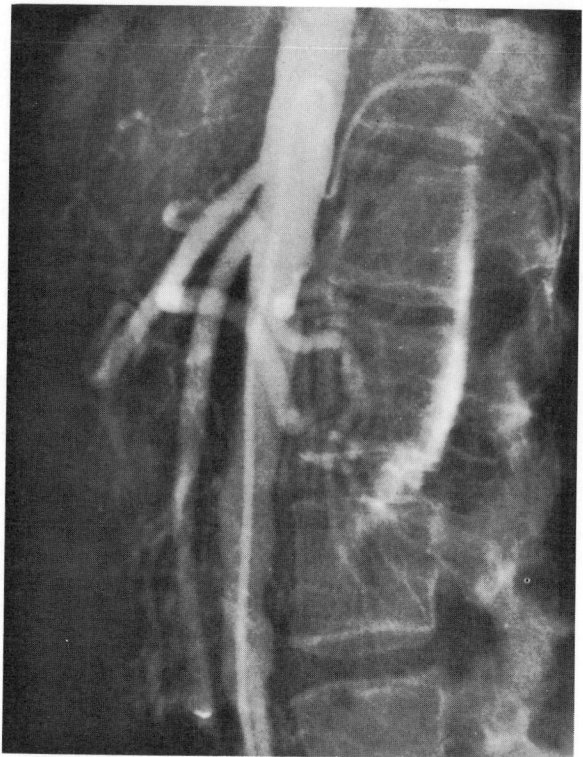

Fig. 35-10. Lateral view of a retrograde visceral arteriogram showing a normal celiac axis and superior mesenteric artery.

from the aorta or sites other than the stenotic visceral artery. Laboratory studies and routine radiographic studies are not often contributory except to rule out other abdominal conditions. The differential diagnosis includes peptic ulcer disease, cholecystitis, abdominal neoplasm, and pancreatitis.

An awareness of the syndrome is perhaps the most important factor in making the diagnosis, which is then best confirmed by a selective visceral angiogram using a Seldinger catheter (Fig. 35-10). Lateral views are essential, because the standard anteroposterior view does not show the origin of the celiac or mesenteric arteries. The catheter is passed via a femoral artery puncture to a level just above the origin of the celiac axis. After a small test dose has established the proper position of the catheter, 30 to 40 mL of 50 percent Hypaque is injected rapidly while taking multiple films using a rapid cassette changer. This outlines both the celiac axis and superior mesenteric arteries. Diagnostic arteriograms will show stenosis or complete occlusion of one or both of these vessels, usually within 1 cm of the aortic orifice (Fig. 35-11). The catheter is then repositioned just above the origin of the inferior mesenteric artery and the arteriogram is repeated. The demonstration of a markedly dilated and elongated inferior mesenteric artery that fills the superior mesenteric artery through collaterals is indicative of a superior mesenteric artery occlusion (Fig. 35-12).

For diagnosing the median arcuate ligament syndrome, the lateral arteriogram characteristically will show eccen-

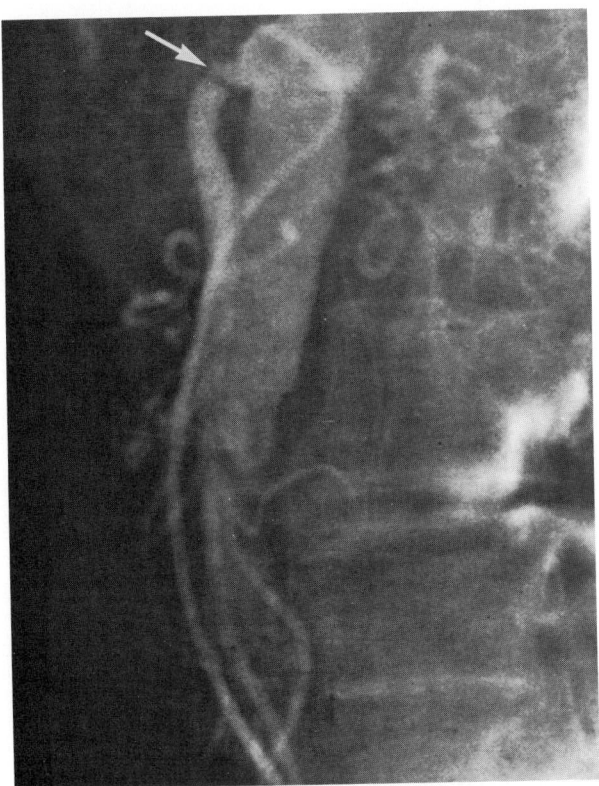

Fig. 35-11. Lateral view of retrograde visceral arteriogram showing a high-grade stenosis (arrow) of the superior mesenteric artery close to its origin from the aorta. (Compare with Fig. 35-10.)

Fig. 35-12. Left: Retrograde inferior mesenteric arteriogram showing a prominent marginal artery of Drummond filling from a dilated and tortuous inferior mesenteric artery. Right: Later film showing filling of the superior mesenteric artery (arrow) through collaterals. The patient had complete occlusion of the celiac axis and superior mesenteric artery at their origins from the aorta.

tric compression of the celiac artery along its superior border with caudal displacement of the artery so that it lies adjacent to the superior mesenteric artery. Occasionally the displacement results in compression of the superior mesenteric artery, but in the true syndrome the superior mesenteric, as well as the inferior mesenteric, artery is of normal caliber radiographically.

TREATMENT. Once stenosis of the celiac and mesenteric arteries has been demonstrated in a symptomatic patient, surgical correction is advised if the patient will tolerate the procedure. Arterial reconstruction not only corrects the symptoms of intestinal angina but also prevents the eventual progression to intestinal infarction. At laparotomy, critical stenosis of the involved arteries is obvious, because there will be weak or no palpable pulsations distal to the stenosis. Surgical treatment may be one of three types: (1) thromboendarterectomy; (2) synthetic or autogenous vein bypass graft circumventing the stenotic segment; or (3) excision of the stenotic segment and reimplantation of the superior mesenteric artery into the aorta. Since exposure of the origins of the superior mesenteric and celiac arteries is difficult, most surgeons prefer improving the circulation with a bypass graft. For a lesion in the celiac artery, the graft is inserted between a major branch of the celiac artery, usually the splenic, and the aorta. Occasionally, the splenic artery itself may be mobilized and anastomosed to the side of the aorta. Bypass of a superior mesenteric artery stenosis is best handled by inserting a graft to the side of the artery just beyond the egress of the middle colic artery and to the aorta below the origin of the renal arteries.

Most patients with the median arcuate ligament syndrome can have normal blood flow restored in the celiac artery by merely transecting the constricting ligament. Direct arterial reconstruction may be necessary if the stenosis persists and the patient remains symptomatic after division of the ligament.

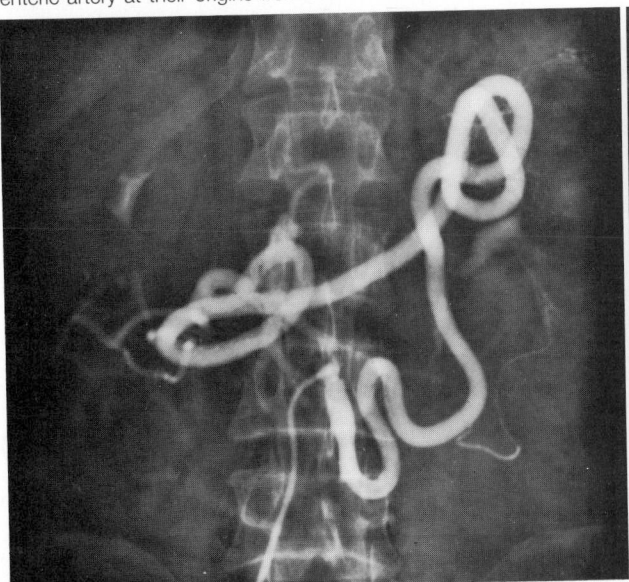

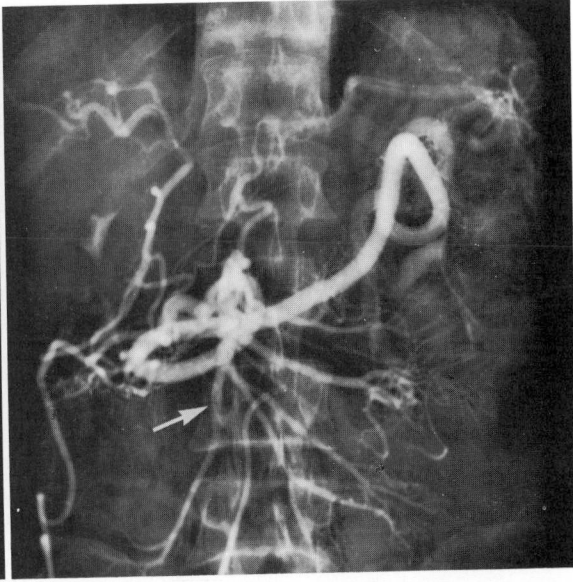

OCCLUSION OF INFERIOR MESENTERIC ARTERY

ETIOLOGY. Sudden occlusion of the inferior mesenteric artery is usually due to thrombosis superimposed on an atheromatous plaque and less often to embolism or a dissecting aneurysm. External compression by an expanding aortic aneurysm or involvement by atherosclerosis produces gradual occlusion. On occasion, obliterative arteritis, as associated with thromboangiitis obliterans and periarteritis nodosa, will involve the main artery or its branches.

Normally, the inferior mesenteric artery can be ligated at any point without interfering with bowel function or producing symptoms. This is because the extensive collateral circulation through anastomoses with branches of the middle colic artery (superior mesenteric) and lower hemorrhoidal arteries (internal iliac) are able to sustain the left colon. When infarction of the descending colon follows thrombosis or ligation of the inferior mesenteric artery, there is almost always preexisting inpairment of this collateral network. Usually this is due to advanced atheromatous narrowing or thrombosis of the superior mesenteric and internal iliac arteries. Such an event occasionally occurs when the inferior mesenteric artery is sacrificed during operations on the aorta for occlusive disease or aneurysm. Previous left colectomy with interruption of the marginal artery also predisposes to colon ischemia following occlusion of the inferior mesenteric artery.

CLINICAL MANIFESTATIONS. Circulatory infarction of the descending colon usually has a more insidious onset than infarction of other portions of the intestine. Since the inferior mesenteric supplies a shorter segment of bowel, occlusion produces less extensive disruption of circulating blood volume and fluid balance than when the superior mesenteric artery is occluded. Steady, slowly progressive lower abdominal pain is usually followed by loose, bloody stools and then constipation. The abdomen becomes distended and tender over the course of the descending colon. Occasionally a tubular mass may be felt in the left side of the abdomen. Some degree of circulatory collapse occurs. This is initially mild but becomes profound as the bowel becomes necrotic. The temperature and white blood cell count are only moderately elevated unless perforation has occurred. Radiographs of the abdomen may show an absence of gas in the descending colon, suggesting a mechanical obstruction of the transverse colon. Edema, cyanosis, and ulceration of the mucosal membrane of the sigmoid colon can often be detected by sigmoidoscopy. Unexplained diarrhea, with or without rectal bleeding, which comes on after operations on the abdominal aorta, suggests vascular impairment of the left colon and prompts immediate sigmoidoscopic evaluation.

TREATMENT. Early recognition of the intestinal ischemia and prompt surgical intervention is important for survival. Treatment consists of resection of the infarcted colonic segment. A temporary proximal end colostomy is safer than a primary anastomosis. The preexisting generalized arteriosclerotic disease afflicting most of these patients renders them poor operative risks. The overall mortality rate is about 70 percent.

MESENTERIC VENOUS OCCLUSION

ETIOLOGY. When occlusion of a visceral vein produces symptoms, they are almost always due to acute thrombosis. Mesenteric venous thrombosis may be idiopathic or evolve secondarily as a complication of several clinical disorders. The predisposing factors in secondary mesenteric venous thrombosis are (1) infection, usually intraabdominal suppuration such as appendicitis, diverticulitis, or pelvic abscess; (2) hematologic conditions such as polycythemia vera, the postsplenectomy state, and the hypercoagulability associated with oral contraceptives; (3) local venous congestion and stasis, as with hepatic cirrhosis with portal hypertension or extrinsic obstruction of portal venous radicles by tumor masses; and (4) accidental or operative trauma to the mesenteric veins, particularly during or following a portacaval surgical procedure. In approximately 25 percent, no associated factor may be implicated; these cases are classified as primary, or idiopathic. A significant number of patients in this last group will give a past history of peripheral thrombophlebitis, suggesting a common cause.

PATHOLOGY. Sudden occlusion of the main stem superior mesenteric vein in the dog leads to rapid sequestration of splanchnic venous circulation, stagnation shock, and hemorrhagic infarction of the bowel progressing to necrosis and gangrene. In human beings, ligation of the portal vein or superior mesenteric vein does not produce infarction unless secondary thrombosis extends to the bowel wall and involves the venous arcades and vasa rectal. Primary thrombotic occlusion of the visceral veins usually begins in the smaller tributaries. Depending on the extent and location of the propagating clot, the bowel lesion may be represented by small localized areas or extensive segments of infarction. With extensive venous occlusion, thrombosis of the arterial side of the splanchnic circulation often follows, so that it becomes impossible to determine accurately whether the occlusion was initially arterial or venous.

Phlebitis secondary to inflammatory disease of the bowel may extend to involve the entire portal system (pyelophlebitis) or give rise to septic emboli that lodge within the liver, causing intrahepatic abscess. This complication of mesenteric venous thrombosis has become less frequent with the advent of antibiotics, and the bowel symptoms are usually overshadowed by those due to the infection.

Acute thrombosis of mesenteric veins is followed promptly by hyperemia, edema, and subserosal hemorrhages in the affected segment of intestine. The bowel wall becomes markedly thickened and cyanotic, and the lumen fills with dark bloody fluid. Serosanguineous fluid seeps from the surface of the congested mesentery and also from the intestinal loop. The picture is that of hemorrhagic infarction.

CLINICAL MANIFESTATIONS. The clinical manifestations are similar to those following acute visceral artery occlusion. Not infrequently, the patient complains of vague abdominal discomfort, anorexia, and change in bowel habits a few days or even weeks prior to the onset of severe symptoms. This prodromal period is more evident when the venous thrombosis is idiopathic. The early symptoms are then followed by sudden severe abdominal pain, vomiting, and circulatory collapse. Narcotics usually do not relieve the pain. Bloody diarrhea is more frequent than with arterial occlusions. The bowel sounds will be hypoactive or absent. Generalized abdominal tenderness, guarding, and distention are usual; however, true rigidity is not present unless gangrene and perforation of the bowel have occurred. A marked leukocytosis and elevated hematocrit are characteristic findings in venous thrombosis. The latter reflects the trapping of plasma in the occluded bowel segment as arterial blood continues to flow into a splanchnic bed without adequate venous drainage. Plain radiographs of the abdomen usually show dilated loops of small bowel with air fluid levels that are not specific. Abdominal paracentesis invariably yields serosanguineous fluid, which, if foul-smelling, makes immediate laparotomy mandatory.

TREATMENT. The definitive treatment of mesenteric venous infarction is surgical. Without operation the mortality approaches 100 percent. Preparation of the patient for operation includes correcting the usually severe circulating volume deficit with blood and a balanced salt solution and decompression of the stomach via a nasogastric tube. Broad-spectrum antibiotics and penicillin in large doses should be started and should be continued in the postoperative period.

As soon as possible and when the condition permits, the patient is taken to the operating room. In contrast to acute mesenteric arterial occlusion, venous thrombosis tends to occur more frequently in peripheral tributaries than in the main stem vessel. For this reason, shorter segments of intestine are usually involved than if occlusion is primarily arterial. All devitalized intestine is resected and a primary end-to-end anastomosis is performed. Frequently the thrombosis extends beyond the limits of gross infarction. Therefore, resection should include adjacent normal bowel and mesentery until all grossly thrombosed veins are encompassed. Otherwise, extension of residual clot postoperatively will lead to subsequent infarction. Intestinal infarction associated with acute thrombosis of the portal vein is usually not amenable to resection because of the wide extent of involved intestine.

Anticoagulation with heparin should be started immediately, even during the operation, and continued for 6 to 8 weeks. Naitove and Weismann reported no deaths in their cases of idiopathic mesenteric venous thrombosis in which anticoagulants were administered, in contrast to a 50 percent mortality in the group in which the drugs were not used. A second-look operation 24 to 36 h later should be performed in this form of mesenteric infarction because of the frequent recurrence of thrombosis or extension of residual clots. In general, the prognosis is somewhat better than in mesenteric infarction due to arterial occlusion. This is probably a reflection of the shorter bowel segments usually involved, which make it more amenable to surgical treatment. The most important factor in prognosis is early operative intervention before extensive thrombosis has occurred throughout the splanchnic venous circulation.

ANEURYSMS OF THE SPLANCHNIC ARTERIES

Aneurysms of the splanchnic arteries are rare. The great majority are asymptomatic and remain undetected until they rupture, producing signs of intraabdominal hemorrhage. In the past, the term "abdominal apoplexy" was applied to the situation of massive abdominal bleeding from spontaneous rupture of visceral blood vessels. It is now recognized that the source of bleeding in most cases was rupture of a splanchnic artery aneurysm.

ETIOLOGY. The pathogenesis of splanchnic artery aneurysms is varied. Four major etiologies have been identified: (1) arteriosclerosis; (2) medial degeneration; (3) disorders of connective tissue, including necrotizing arteritis characteristic of periarteritis nodosa; and (4) mycotic embolization. Arteriosclerosis is the usual etiologic factor in older patients while congenital or acquired defects in the medial wall of the artery are more often incriminated in the young. Most patients with splanchnic artery aneurysms have hypertension that is believed to be of etiologic significance.

PATHOLOGY. The most common aneurysms of the splanchnic vessels are of the splenic artery, comprising about 60 percent in most large series reported. The majority occur in women, and in about 40 percent of patients the aneurysms are multiple. The usual cause is arteriosclerosis, but the relatively high incidence of splenic artery aneurysms in women who have had multiple pregnancies has incriminated gestational disorders. Alteration of the elastic tissue and ground substance in the media of the splenic artery has been shown to occur regularly during pregnancy, and the predilection for the artery to become aneurysmal may also be a reflection of excessive splenic arteriovenous shunting in the third trimester of pregnancy. Hepatic artery aneurysms make up 16 to 20 percent of all splanchnic artery aneurysms. Although the exact incidence is unknown, few go undetected because of their great propensity to rupture and thus become symptomatic. The majority involve the extrahepatic portion of the artery, and arteriosclerosis is the usual cause. Aneurysms of the celiac artery and of the superior mesenteric artery and its branches each account for about 3 percent of splanchnic artery aneurysms. Most are due to arteriosclerosis, but a relatively large number of aneurysms of the superior mesenteric artery result from mycotic involvement or necrotizing arteritis.

The size of splanchnic artery aneurysms varies. The majority are less than 2 cm in diameter but aneurysms of the splenic artery measuring up to 10 cm have been reported. Aneurysms of the superior mesenteric artery and its branches are typically very small, and when rupture occurs, frequently no site of bleeding can be found at laparotomy or at autopsy despite the loss of several liters of blood. In contrast to aneurysms of the abdominal aorta, size does not predict the risk of rupture. It has been estimated that only about 2 to 10 percent of splenic artery aneurysms rupture while the risk of rupture of hepatic, celiac, and superior mesenteric artery aneurysms is high, approximating 50 percent of patients.

Bleeding from ruptured splanchnic artery aneurysms initially may be intraperitoneal or, by extending between the leaves of the mesentery, retroperitoneal. The latter situation often secondarily produces a tear in the peritoneum, thus giving the picture of both retroperitoneal and intraperitoneal bleeding. On occasion, erosion with rupture occurs into an adjacent viscus such as the stomach, intestine, bile duct, or pancreas.

CLINICAL MANIFESTATIONS. Prior to rupture, most splanchnic artery aneurysms are asymptomatic and typically are diagnosed as an incidental finding on abdominal aortography. The presence of curvilinear, ringlike calcification in the left upper abdomen on plain x-ray film suggests splenic artery aneurysm, a finding in about one-half of patients with this lesion. Patients with large splenic artery aneurysms may complain of left upper quadrant pain and often a bruit can be heard, but this is not diagnostic of an aneurysm since it may arise from a very tortuous splenic artery. Patients with hepatic artery aneurysms infrequently complain of pain in the right upper quadrant mimicking cholecystitis or present with symptoms of extrahepatic obstructive jaundice. Celiac and superior mesenteric artery aneurysms are rarely symptomatic prior to rupture, but fever may be present when the aneurysm is of mycotic origin. Occasionally an aneurysm of the main stem superior mesenteric artery will interfere with blood flow to the intestinal tract, in which case the patient may experience postprandial abdominal pain characteristic of intestinal angina.

When rupture occurs, the major symptoms are related to signs of acute blood loss. With confined retroperitoneal bleeding, clinical features will include steady back or testicular pain, pallor, tachycardia, and occasionally vomiting. When bleeding is into the peritoneal cavity, there is sudden, severe abdominal pain rapidly followed by circulatory collapse. The pain is generalized and often referred to the left shoulder. Abdominal distention, spasm, and generalized tenderness are present. Bowel activity will be depressed or absent. The temperature is usually normal but generally the white blood cell count is increased. The hematocrit may or may not be low, depending on whether hemodilution has taken place. The vital signs following the initial bleed may improve for a period of several hours and then be followed by a second, usually massive episode of bleeding that is fatal without prompt intervention. On rare occasion, a splenic artery aneurysm will rupture into the adjacent stomach or pancreatic duct causing massive gastrointestinal bleeding. Erosion of a hepatic artery aneurysm into the bile duct is an unusual cause of hemobilia with the classic triad of gastrointestinal bleeding, biliary colic, and jaundice.

Rupture of a splanchnic artery aneurysm must be differentiated from such abdominal catastrophes as perforated peptic ulcer, hemorrhagic pancreatitis, strangulated intestinal obstruction, ruptured abdominal aortic aneurysm, and acute mesenteric vascular occlusion. Abdominal paracentesis with recovery of nonclotting blood is diagnostic of intraabdominal bleeding from any source. However, the definitive study for the diagnosis of splanchnic artery aneurysms both before and after rupture is selective mesenteric arteriography. Preoperative aortography is especially useful when the source of bleeding is from a small hepatic, celiac, or superior mesenteric artery aneurysm. Surgical exploration in these cases may not identify the source of bleeding and failure to do so will result in a high operative mortality rate. Unfortunately, the urgency of the situation is such that time is often not available to obtain an arteriogram.

TREATMENT. Since rupture occurs in fewer than 10 percent of patients with splenic artery aneurysms, a conservative approach is justified for the asymptomatic patient with a small aneurysm. However, there is an increased hazard of rupture during pregnancy, notably during the third trimester, with an associated high maternal and fetal mortality rate. For this reason, surgery is indicated for all women of childbearing age once the diagnosis of splenic artery aneurysm has been made by mesenteric arteriography. The preferred treatment is proximal and distal ligation of the aneurysm with obliteration of all feeding vessels in order to avoid splenectomy. If this is not feasible, resection of the aneurysm and splenectomy will be necessary. Because the risk of rupture of other splanchnic artery aneurysms is high, asymptomatic patients should undergo surgical correction as soon as the aneurysm is recognized and prior to the development of complications. Ideally, the hepatic artery or main stem superior mesenteric artery should be reconstructed with an autogenous vein graft following excision of the aneurysm. Aneurysms of the celiac artery can usually be safely treated by excision without reconstruction. Definitive treatment of branch aneurysms of the superior mesenteric artery involves excision with or without segmental bowel resection depending on whether blood flow to the intestine has been compromised.

Patients who present with ruptured aneurysms and intraabdominal or gastrointestinal blood loss require immediate resuscitation with fluid and blood and surgical intervention as soon as the patient's condition allows. At times the bleeding may be so brisk that it will be necessary to take the patient to the operating room while still in shock. The chances of finding the open vessel are better if the blood pressure can be elevated. If time allows, preoperative localization by arteriography should be carried out. When the patient's condition is critical and preoperative studies are not advisable, an operative aortogram may aid in localization of the site of bleeding if it is not obvious at the time of exploration. In the case of a ruptured splenic artery aneurysm, the urgency of the situation usually necessitates a splenectomy to facilitate exposure for the ligation of the ruptured artery. Rupture of a celiac artery aneurysm can be treated by ligation, and although most hepatic artery aneurysms can also be treated safely by ligation, an attempt should be made to reconstruct the hepatic artery with a graft. When it is necessary to ligate the hepatic artery, protection should be afforded the liver with large doses of broad-spectrum antibiotics postoperatively. Rupture of a main stem superior mesenteric artery aneurysm will require replacement with a graft, preferably of autogenous vein, following excision. Most ruptured aneurysms of the smaller visceral arteries can be treated by ligation. However, adequate circulation to the bowel must be assured and all obviously ischemic intestine resected. If there is a question of viability of a long segment of intestine, a second-look operation in 24 to 36 h may avoid an extensive resection.

The operative mortality for elective treatment of non-ruptured splanchnic artery aneurysms is less than 5 percent. The mortality rate is considerably higher once the aneurysm has ruptured and is related to the artery involved. Overall mortality following rupture of a splenic artery aneurysm is about 25 percent with a 65 percent maternal and 95 percent fetal mortality if rupture occurs during pregnancy. The mortality subsequent to rupture of a celiac or superior mesenteric artery aneurysm is between 40 and 60 percent, while rupture of a hepatic artery aneurysm is associated with a 70 percent mortality rate. Death is the result of massive blood loss complicated by effects of systemic arteriosclerosis, which many patients have.

TRAUMA TO VISCERAL BLOOD VESSELS

ETIOLOGY. Mesenteric arteries and veins may be injured by either penetrating or nonpenetrating abdominal trauma or accidentally during abdominal operations. In most cases, the vessels are lacerated. Less frequently, contusion of an artery by blunt trauma eventuates in thrombosis or later aneurysmal formation with rupture.

Most penetrating injuries of the mesenteric vessels are due to stabbings or gunshot wounds. In these circumstances, associated injury to other organs is frequent. Isolated injury to mesenteric vessels following blunt abdominal trauma is rare and usually involves vessels in the mesentery proper or porta hepatis.

CLINICAL MANIFESTATIONS. Depending on the size of the vessel lacerated, the rapidity of the bleeding, and associated organ injury, the patient will present with varying degrees of shock, abdominal pain, tenderness, distention, and spasm. Pain referred to the left shoulder is a particularly valuable diagnostic symptom. X-rays of the abdomen are not helpful unless associated visceral rupture has occurred, in which case free air may be seen.

TREATMENT. It is generally held that all gunshot wounds of the abdomen and most stab wounds should be explored early regardless of the physical findings. In nonpenetrating injury, a paracentesis yielding nonclotting blood prompts early surgical intervention. Basically, treatment consists of controlling the bleeding vessel. Lacerations of the inferior mesenteric artery or smaller mesenteric arteries and most mesenteric veins can usually be successfully treated by ligation. In the past, few patients with injury to the main trunk of the superior mesenteric artery survived. Most died from infarction of the intestine or because of complications arising from associated organ injury. Today, if the patient can be resuscitated and reaches the operating room, arterial repair may be possi-

ble. This can be accomplished by either primary suture or interposition of a vascular graft between the severed ends of the vessel. Every attempt should also be made to repair lacerations of the hepatic artery or portal vein. Whether treatment is by ligation or reconstruction, it is important that adequate circulation to the intestine be established and any obviously ischemic bowel resected before closing the abdomen. Long segments of small intestine that are of questionable viability are best left in place and reexamined at a second operation 24 h later.

Nonspecific Mesenteric Lymphadenitis

Nonspecific mesenteric lymphadenitis is one of the common causes of acute abdominal pain in young adults and children. Its existence as a distinct clinicopathologic entity is now well accepted, although the condition received little attention in early medical texts following its initial description by Wilensky and Hahn in 1926. An extensive review of the disease has been reported by McDonald.

Since the condition is invariably self-limiting and can be accurately diagnosed only at laparotomy, its true incidence is unknown. Yet, it is probably the most common cause of inflammatory enlargement of abdominal lymph glands, far surpassing that due to tuberculosis, with which it has been confused in the past. Consideration of the disease is important because of its clinical similarity to several abdominal conditions requiring surgical intervention, notably acute appendicitis.

PATHOLOGY AND PATHOGENESIS. The lymph nodes primarily involved in nonspecific mesenteric lymphadenitis are those that drain the ileocecal region. The stasis of intestinal contents in the terminal ileum favors absorption of toxic or bacterial products from the bowel lumen, agents that may have a bearing on the pathogenesis of the disease.

The nodes are enlarged, discrete, and soft and pink at first; later they may become firm and white. It is uncertain whether calcification ever occurs in nontuberculous adenitis, and suppuration is rare unless specific bacterial infection is present. Histologically, the involved nodes present a pattern of reactive hyperplasia similar to that found in inflammatory and allergic affections of lymph nodes in other parts of the body. The nodes, with rare exception, prove to be sterile on culture or on animal inoculation.

It seems likely that nonspecific mesenteric adenitis represents a reaction to some type of material absorbed from the small intestine. The stimulating substance could reach the nodes via either lymph channels or the bloodstream, although the usual absence of generalized lymphadenopathy would make the latter route unlikely. The possibility that the disease represents a hypersensitive reaction to a foreign protein has also been suggested.

CLINICAL MANIFESTATIONS. The disease most commonly occurs in patients under eighteen years of age. There is no sex predilection. The clinical signs and symptoms are not particularly characteristic. Very often there has been a recent sore throat or upper respiratory tract infection. Pain is usually the first symptom. It varies in intensity from an ache to a severe colic. The mechanism responsible for producing pain is not completely understood. Lymph nodes have not been shown to have sensory innervation, and therefore enlargement of the node by itself should not produce pain. It is probable that the pain is referred from the mesentery, which has an abundance of sensory end organs that are stimulated when the mesentery is stretched during peristalsis. The initial pain is usually in the upper abdomen, but it may also begin in the lower right quadrant or be generalized. Eventually the pain localizes to the right side; however, an important point in differentiating the disease from acute appendicitis is that the patient is unable to indicate the exact site of the most intense pain. Between spasms of colic, the patient feels well and moves about without difficulty. Nausea and vomiting occur in about one-third of patients, while malaise and anorexia are inconstant symptoms.

The patient often appears flushed, and an associated rhinorrhea or acute pharyngitis is not unusual. Approximately 20 percent of patients will have lymphadenopathy elsewhere, most often in the cervical region. The usual finding on examination of the abdomen is tenderness in the lower aspect of the right side, which is somewhat higher and more medial and considerably less severe than in acute appendicitis. The point of maximal tenderness often varies from one examination to the next. An appreciable number of patients will have diffuse or periumbilical tenderness as well. Rebound tenderness may or may not be demonstrated. Voluntary guarding is sometimes present; however, true muscular rigidity is rare. Early in the attack, the temperature is moderately elevated, to 38 or 38.5°C, and at least half of the patients will have leukocyte counts over 10,000/mm^3.

DIFFERENTIAL DIAGNOSIS. The disease is most often confused with acute appendicitis but must also be differentiated from regional enteritis, intussusception, specific bacterial and granulomatous adenitis, and other forms of mesenteric glandular enlargement such as with infectious mononucleosis or lymphoma. The clinical similarity to acute appendicitis is such that, in several large series, as many as 20 percent of patients coming to the operating room for appendectomy were found to have nonspecific mesenteric adenitis and a normal appendix. Important differentiating factors are the more localized and constant location of the pain and tenderness, the presence of muscle rigidity, and the frequent occurrence of nausea and vomiting in children with appendicitis.

Differentiation from *acute regional ileitis* is at times difficult. Mesenteric adenitis is an almost constant feature of regional ileitis, and indeed the adenitis is often nonspecific in this disease. Inflammatory edema or induration of the serous coat of the ileum with thickening and induration of the mesentery are characteristic of regional enteritis.

The low incidence of lymphadenopathy in other parts of the body and the brief course of nonspecific mesenteric adenitis are factors in excluding lymphomas and infectious mononucleosis. A peripheral blood smear and a Paul-Bunnell test for sheep red cell agglutinins are also helpful.

TREATMENT. The prognosis of nonspecific mesenteric adenitis is excellent, and complete recovery from an individual attack can be expected without specific treatment. Death from the disease is extremely rare and occurs only when secondary specific bacterial infection, usually caused by hemolytic streptococci, causes suppuration of the nodes with rupture leading to abscess or peritonitis.

If the condition is mistaken for acute appendicitis, as it frequently is, laparotomy should be undertaken. In such an instance, it is far safer to find a normal appendix than to run the risk of allowing acute appendicitis to go on to rupture. The diagnosis is readily established at the time of operation with the finding of enlarged mesenteric nodes in the absence of disease in the appendix or elsewhere in the intestinal tract or abdomen. In view of the tendency for recurrence and the difficulty of differentiating it from appendicitis, appendectomy should be performed.

Mesenteric Panniculitis

"Mesenteric panniculitis" is a term applied by Ogden et al. in 1960 to describe a process of extensive thickening of the mesentery by a nonspecific inflammatory process. It has also been variously designated "retractile mesenteritis," "mesenteric lipodystrophy," "lipogranuloma of the mesentery," and "mesenteric manifestations of Weber-Christian disease." Many consider it a variant of retroperitoneal fibrosis.

ETIOLOGY AND PATHOLOGY. The cause of the condition is unknown; however, the process apparently results from an insult to the fatty tissue of the mesentery. Trauma, allergy, and subacute infection have all been implicated. The process usually involves the mesenteric root of the small bowel. Grossly, the normal fat lobulations of the markedly thickened and firm mesentery are lost. Scattered throughout are irregular areas of discoloration, which vary from reddish brown plaques to pale yellow foci resembling fat necrosis. The superior mesenteric vessels, though surrounded by the tumorlike mass of tissue, pass through it unaltered. Histologic sections show inflammatory involvement of the fibroadipose tissue with round cells, foam cells, and giant cells and various degrees of necrosis, fibrosis, and calcification.

CLINICAL MANIFESTATIONS. Men are affected more often than women. It is rarely described in children, in whom mesenteric fat is usually scant. The clinical features are nonspecific; they include recurrent episodes of moderate to severe abdominal pain, nausea, vomiting, and malaise, usually in the right side of the abdomen. Radiographs are helpful only if the mass displaces or compresses viscera. Computerized tomography demonstrates mesenteric panniculitis as a localized fat-density mass containing areas of increased density representing fibrosis.

TREATMENT. Laparotomy is necessary to establish the diagnosis and to rule out other tumefactions of the abdomen. The widespread involvement of the mesentery precludes doing more than obtaining a biopsy. Since neoplasms of the mesenteric lymph nodes may present a similar gross appearance, several biopsies from different sites should be obtained. Rarely, colostomy or bypass will be necessary to relieve symptoms of obstruction. Treatment of the disease with steroids and irradiation has been suggested. However, the benefits from these are difficult to evaluate, because the inflammatory process is self-limiting and seldom causes any serious complications.

Tumors of the Mesentery

Tumors originating between the leaves of the mesentery are quite rare. In contrast, malignant implants from intraabdominal or pelvic tumors or metastases to mesenteric lymph nodes are relatively common. Tumors arising from mesenteric lymph nodes occur; however, these are not generally included in a discussion of primary mesenteric tumors.

PATHOLOGY. Primary tumors of the mesentery may be cystic or solid. Of these, cystic growths occur more frequently than solid ones in a ratio of 2:1. A variety of tissues, including lymphatic, vascular, nervous, and connective tissue, are the source of these tumors. In addition, cystic tumors may arise from embryonic rests (enteroceles or dermoids), from developmental defects (chylous or serous retention cysts), or following trauma (hemorrhagic cysts). A classification of these tumors is shown in Table 35-1.

The majority of cystic mesenteric tumors are benign. Rare exceptions are lymphangiosarcomas, which are true neoplasms arising from lymph channels, and malignant teratomas arising from multipotential embryonic rests. Rankin and Major contend that chylous or lymphatic cysts are the most frequently encountered benign mesenteric masses. These are thought to arise from developmental defects in mesenteric lymphatics creating closed spaces within which fluid accumulates. They may be unilocular or multilocular, have an endothelial lining, contain a grossly cloudy fluid resembling chyle, and often grow to extremely large size. A similar cause has been ascribed to serous cysts, which are differentiated from chylous cysts in that they contain clear fluid, are invariably unilocular, and may or may not have an endothelial lining. Lymphangioma of the mesentery is apparently a true neoplasm of lymphatics similar to those found in other parts of the body (cystic hygroma). Grossly and histologically, it is often difficult to differentiate this tumor from a chylous cyst, and in many series the two are grouped in a single category. Traumatic cysts follow external or surgical injury to the mesentery. They are lined with fibrous tissue and usually contain bloody fluid. It is probable that many serous retention cysts are in reality traumatic cysts that have evolved from disruption of mesenteric lymph channels. Enteric cysts are lined with intestinal mucosa and represent duplications of the intestinal tract that do not communicate with the bowel lumen. These and dermoid cysts of the mesentery are exceedingly rare.

Benign solid tumors of the mesentery are more common than malignant ones, and of these, lipomas and fibromas predominate. However, recurrence after incomplete excision of histologically benign mesenteric tumors has been reported and malignant degeneration also suggested. Moreover, histologically benign tumors can kill by local

Table 35-1. CLASSIFICATION OF PRIMARY MESENTERIC TUMORS

Origin	Benign	Malignant
Cystic tumors:		
Developmental		
defects	Chylous cyst	
	Serous cyst	
Lymphatic tissue	Lymphangioma	Lymphangiosarcoma
Trauma	Traumatic cyst	
Embryonic rests	Enteric cyst	
	Dermoid	Malignant teratoma
Solid tumors:		
Adipose tissue	Lipoma	Liposarcoma
Fibrous tissue	Fibroma	Fibrosarcoma
Nerve elements	Neurilemoma	Malignant schwannoma
	Neurofibroma	
Smooth muscle	Leiomyoma	Leiomyosarcoma
	Fibromyoma	Fibromyosarcoma
Vascular tissue	Hemangioma	Hemangiopericytoma

invasion with mechanical compression of adjacent viscera. The benign tumors of nerve elements and smooth muscles are uncommon. Vascular tumors of the mesentery are very rare, and of these, hemangiopericytomas dominate the picture. Ackerman states that liposarcoma is the most frequently encountered malignant tumor of this area, whereas Yannopoulos and Stout report leiomyosarcoma to be the most frequent. Few malignant mesenteric tumors have embolic metastases until very late. They spread by local extension or by peritoneal implants, which occur most often with leiomyosarcomas. As a rule, the malignant solid tumors arise near the root of the mesentery, whereas solid benign tumors have a greater tendency to develop peripherally near the intestine.

Approximately two-thirds of mesenteric tumors, either cystic or solid, are located in the mesentery of the small intestine, usually that of the ileum. Less frequently, they arise in the transverse or sigmoid mesocolon or in the gastrohepatic ligament. In the greater number of cases, the tumor is located peripherally in the mesentery, where it is often adherent to the adjacent intestine. The mobility of the mesentery permits both benign and malignant tumors to grow to very large sizes before causing symptoms.

CLINICAL MANIFESTATIONS. The early clinical features do not usually differentiate benign tumors from malignant ones. There is an equal sex incidence, although benign cystic tumors are somewhat more common in women and malignant tumors occur more frequently in men. These tumors have been described in children and also the very aged; however, the average age of patients with benign tumors is forty-five years, while those with malignant tumors average fifty-five years old.

The manifestations of mesenteric tumors are dependent upon the size, location, and mobility of the growth. In the vast majority of patients, symptoms are few or nonexistent, and the tumor is detected during a routine examination. Symptoms appear sooner when the tumor is situated in the periphery of the mesentery near the intestine than when it is located at its root. The patient may merely experience a sensation of fullness or pressure in the abdomen, particularly after eating. Less frequently, there are frank abdominal complaints. About one-half of patients with malignant tumors complain of abdominal pain, weakness, and weight loss, and one-third have diarrhea, cramps, anorexia, and nausea. Only rarely will the patient present with symptoms of complete intestinal obstruction or symptoms resulting from complications of the tumor per se such as torsion, hemorrhage, or infarction of the tumor mass. In the absence of intestinal obstruction or these complications, the sole clinical finding will be the presence of a nontender, intraabdominal mass, usually in the lower right part of the abdomen. The mass varies in size from a few inches in diameter to one that may literally fill the entire abdomen. The extremely large masses are usually cystic, in which case they are tense and fluctuant. Both cystic and solid tumors of the mesentery are mobile; they can be easily moved from side to side but only slightly in an upward and downward direction.

The differential diagnosis takes into consideration all tumefactions of the abdominal cavity and retroperitoneum. Contrast radiographs are helpful only when the mesenteric mass is sufficiently large to cause compression and displacement of the bowel or ureters (Fig. 35-13). They do not differentiate a benign tumor from a malignant one, and in most instances the x-ray studies are not helpful. Calcification in the mass is suggestive of a dermoid or teratoma.

Imaging techniques are the most useful means for diagnosing both cystic and solid mesenteric tumors. On ultrasonography, a mesenteric cyst appears as a well-outlined, sonolucent transonic abdominal mass. Computerized tomography demonstrates a simple mesenteric cyst as a nonenhancing near-water-density mass with a thin wall (Fig. 35-14).

TREATMENT. Surgical excision is the only treatment for both benign and malignant lesions. All mesenteric cysts of a size sufficient to be palpated should be removed if at all possible, since even benign lesions eventually cause pain and compression of neighboring structures. Benign cystic tumors can be removed by enucleation or local excision, although resection in continuity with the adjacent intestine is often necessary because of possible compromise to the vascularity of the bowel or difficulty in separating the tumor from the intestine. Wide excision together with resection of adjacent intestine are recommended for benign solid tumors, since these have a tendency toward local recurrence and malignant degeneration. Prognosis after adequate excision of both cystic and solid benign tumors of the mesentery is excellent.

The outlook for malignant mesenteric tumors is dependent upon whether complete removal is possible and is generally poor. Since malignant growths tend to occur in the root of the mesentery and often involve the great vessels and vasculature to most of the small intestine and colon, curative resection is usually prohibitive. Resectable lesions invariably will require removal of a portion of bowel; however, fewer than one-third of the malignant tumors are totally resectable. Nevertheless, since these growths may enlarge slowly and embolic metastases occur late, it is worthwhile to partially remove them to relieve obstructions, and prolonged survival has been recorded in a few instances. Irradiation therapy offers little if any benefit, since the tumors are invariably radioresistant. Few patients with malignant primary mesenteric tumors are alive after 5 years. Death results from invasion with obstruction of the gastrointestinal tract leading to perforation and hemorrhage or from metastases to liver and lung.

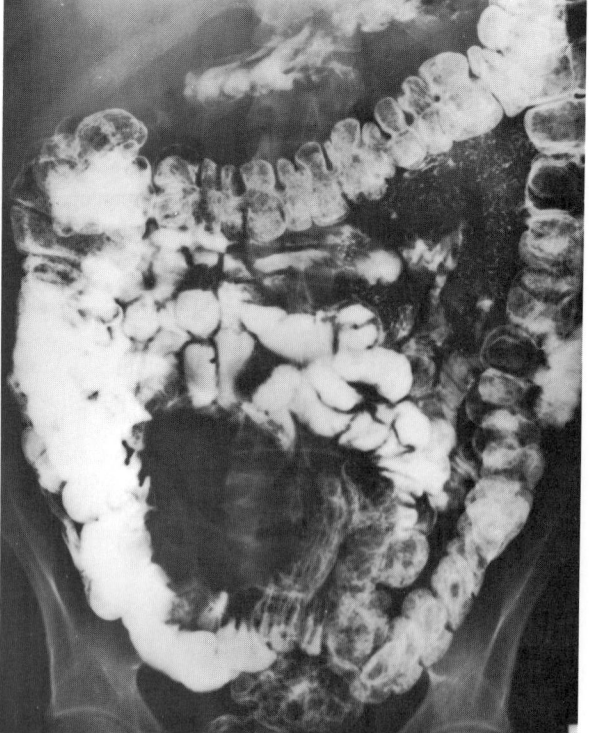

Fig. 35-13. Small intestinal series showing displacement of bowel loops by a mass lesion in the lower right side of the abdomen. The patient proved to have a large benign fibroma in the mesentery of the terminal ileum. (From: *Adams J, Kutner F: Am J Surg 111:735, 1966, with permission.*)

RETROPERITONEUM

General Considerations

The retroperitoneum consists of that portion of the body that is bounded anteriorly by the peritoneum, posteriorly by the spine and psoas and quadratus lumborum muscles, superiorly by the twelfth ribs and attachments of the diaphragm, and inferiorly by the brim of the pelvis. The lateral margins of the space correspond to the lateral borders of the quadratus lumborum muscles. These limits define both an actual and a potential space, the actual space containing solid organs and major blood vessels while the potential space includes soft tissues, nerve elements, and small blood vessels. Since there are no ana-

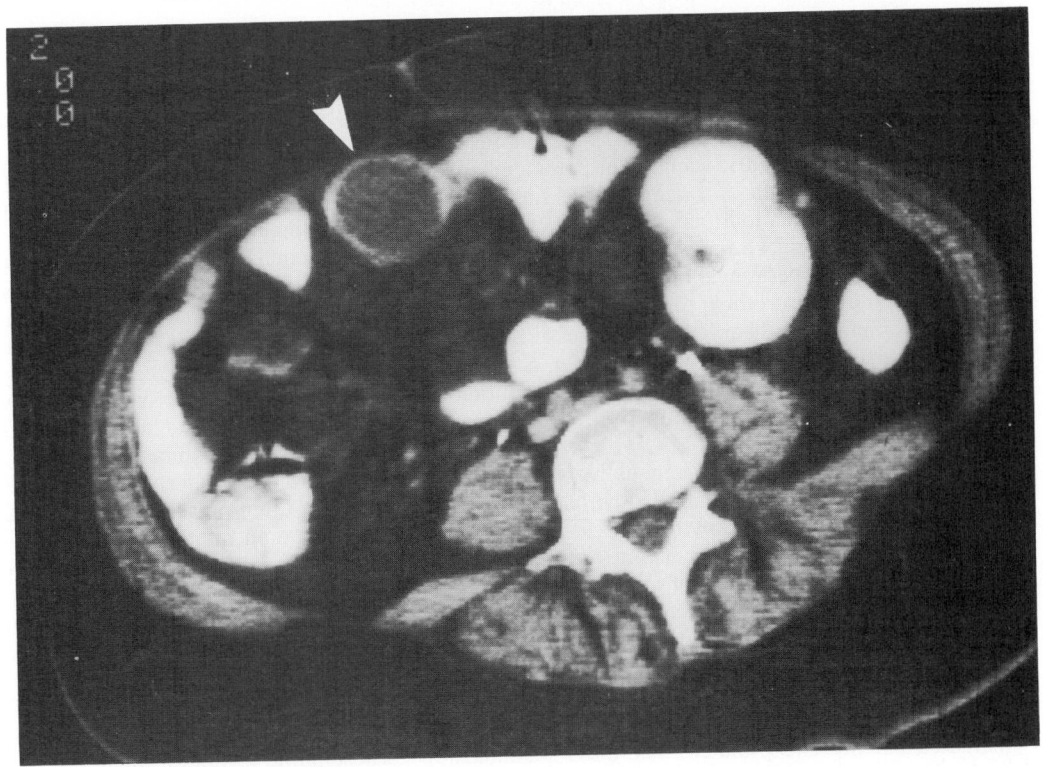

Fig. 35-14. Mesenteric cyst. CT scan shows a nonenhancing low-density, encapsulated mass in the transverse mesocolon (arrowhead).

tomic barriers in this area, pathologic processes may extend easily throughout it and therefore are often bilateral.

Contained within the retroperitoneum are the kidneys, ureters, adrenal glands, portions of the autonomic and peripheral nervous systems, pancreas, abdominal aorta, inferior vena cava, spermatic or ovarian vessels, lymphatics and lymph nodes, and certain portions of the intestinal tract, notably the duodenum. The space also contains fatty and areolar tissue and fibrous connective tissue.

The diagnosis of diseases involving the retroperitoneum has been enhanced by the application of such radiographic studies as pyelography, venography, arteriography, ultrasonography, and computerized tomography. Nevertheless, it remains an obscure area of the body, enabling pathologic processes to become advanced before producing symptoms.

The multiplicity of structures within the retroperitoneum gives rise to a variety of pathologic conditions. This chapter will deal with the relatively uncommon entities of (1) idiopathic retroperitoneal fibrosis and (2) primary tumors of the retroperitoneal space.

Idiopathic Retroperitoneal Fibrosis

Idiopathic retroperitoneal fibrosis is a nonspecific, nonsuppurative inflammation of fibroadipose tissue of unknown cause that produces symptoms by the gradual compression of the tubular structures in the retroperitoneal space. It is currently believed that the disease represents one of the manifestations of a widespread entity termed "systemic idiopathic fibrosis." Idiopathic mediastinal fibrosis, Riedel's struma, sclerosing cholangitis, mesenteric panniculitis, Peyronie's disease, pseudotumor of the orbit, and perhaps desmoid tumor are other fibromatoses that are considered to be localized forms of systemic idiopathic fibrosis. A factor common to all these diseases is an inflammatory fibrotic process involving areolar and adipose tissue.

Retroperitoneal fibrosis was first described in 1905 by Albarran, a French urologist, who performed ureterolysis for ureteral compression produced by the disease. The first report in English is credited to Ormond in 1948. It has since been referred to as Ormond's syndrome but has also been labeled "idiopathic fibrous retroperitonitis," "periureteritis plastica," and "sclerosing retroperitonitis." Retroperitoneal lipogranulomatosis (xanthogranulomatosis), which can produce a similar clinical picture, may be a granulomatous, prefibrotic stage of retroperitoneal fibrosis.

ETIOLOGY. Attesting to the obscure etiology of retroperitoneal fibrosis are the many theories that have been advanced to explain its origin. Hackett, in finding hemosiderin deposits in biopsy specimens, felt that the cause might be previous trauma that produced a retroperitoneal hematoma that subsequently underwent organization. The possibility that extravasated urine might cause a fibrotic reaction in the retroperitoneum was mentioned by Ormond, and both he and Hackett also suggested that an abortive infection elsewhere, only partially treated with antibiotics, might later start an inflammatory reaction in the lymphatic and perivascular tissues of the retroperitoneum. Others have speculated that the disease may be an autoimmune reaction to interstitial protein. Hache et al. proposed the concept that the fibrosis was the end result of an ascending lymphangitis, adenitis, or periadenitis in the retroperitoneum with the infection arising from chronic or recurrent genitourinary infections or inflammatory diseases of the gastrointestinal tract or pelvic organs. Reports of retroperitoneal fibrosis occurring in patients taking the antiserotonin drug methysergide for headache prompted the theory that the disease may be due to a hypersensitivity reaction to the drug. Suby reported a reversal of the fibrotic process after discontinuing the medication and speculated that other drugs may be similarly at fault.

It is probable that no single factor is responsible for causing the disease in all cases and that perhaps multiple factors may be implicated in any one case.

PATHOLOGY. The gross appearance of retroperitoneal fibrosis is usually that of a plaque of woody, white fibrous tissue that is distributed along the course of the periaortic lymphatics. In about one-third of the cases, it is bilateral. The diseased tissue, which may be 2 to 12 cm thick, extends from the sacral promontory to the renal pedicles and laterally to cover the iliopsoas muscles. It is sharply demarcated but not encapsulated. The mass surrounds and constricts but does not invade the regional structures in the retroperitoneum, primarily the blood vessels, nerves, and ureters to which it becomes adherent.

A localized form has been observed as a circumscribed fibrous reaction surrounding only the ureters, and extensive involvement of the entire retroperitoneum with compression of the duodenum, common bile duct, and pancreas has also been seen. A similar fibrotic process has been described penetrating the diaphragm along the great vessels into the mediastinum causing superior vena cava obstruction and also extending into the root of the mesentery, causing intestinal obstruction.

Microscopically, the pattern varies from a subacute cellular process with polymorphonuclear cells, lymphocytes, fibroblasts, and fat cells to a completely hyalinized, relatively acellular sclerosis. Eosinophils, foreign body giant cells, and small areas of calcification may also be present. Suppuration with abscess formation does not occur. The amount of fat and cellular infiltration and the degree of fibrosis vary between patients and in different biopsy specimens from the same patient. The more cellular picture is usually seen in the early stages of the disease, when there may be systemic signs of inflammation, whereas the dense fibrotic process is found late.

CLINICAL MANIFESTATIONS. Retroperitoneal fibrosis is two to three times more common among men than among women. It may occur in children and also the aged; however, about two-thirds of the patients are between forty and sixty years old.

The protean manifestations of the disease are related to the phase and extent of the process and the structures secondarily involved. Ormond divided the natural history of the disease into three periods: (1) the period of incidence and development; (2) the period of activity, that is, spread of the cellular and fibrotic process to envelopment of the retroperitoneal structures; and (3) the period of contraction of the fibrotic mass with compression of the involved structures. The disease is apparently self-limiting once the fibrotic stage is reached, a factor of major importance in considering types of therapy.

Early symptoms are vague and nonspecific, but the first complaint is invariably pain. This is dull, noncolicky, and insidious in onset. It usually originates in the flank or low back and often radiates to the lower abdomen, groin, genitalia, or anteromedial aspect of the thigh. The pain is unilateral at first but may become bilateral later, as the fibrotic process spreads. Anorexia, nausea, diarrhea, generalized malaise, and weight loss variably occur in the early and late phases of the disease. Features of a subacute inflammation such as lower abdominal or costovertebral tenderness, moderate fever, and leukocytosis are often present early. Invariably the erythrocytic sedimentation rate is elevated. A transabdominal or pelvic mass is palpable in about one-third of the patients during some phase of the disease.

Symptoms due to compression of the tubular retroperitoneal structures may follow the initial complaints by 1 month to 2 years and reflect the late fibrotic phase of the disease with sclerotic contraction. The major structures involved are the ureters, aorta, and inferior vena cava. These all lie within the same fascial compartment. However, the aorta is resistant to compression, and the inferior vena cava has abundant collaterals, so that the symptoms are generally related to ureteral involvement. Partial or complete ureteral obstruction occurs in 75 to 85 percent of patients. The usual site of obstruction is in the lower third of the ureter. The ureteral obstruction is usually functional, rather than organic, as a consequence of cessation of peristalsis in the incarcerated ureteral segment. In the majority of cases, a ureteral catheter can still be passed in a retrograde manner.

Dysuria, frequency of urination, and chills and fever occur with secondary infection of a hydronephrotic kidney. These symptoms may be intermittent for years, or a single attack may culminate in sudden anuria from bilateral obstruction. As many as 40 percent of patients will have oliguria or anuria with laboratory evidence of azotemia. Clinically, the enlarged kidneys may be palpable, and the urine, if infected, will contain white blood cells and bacteria. Hematuria, in the absence of infection, is rare.

Lower extremity edema, presumably from lymphatic as well as venous obstruction, occasionally occurs and may be unilateral. The level of obstruction in most cases will correspond to that of the ureteral obstruction and can be demonstrated on phlebograms.

Arterial insufficiency due to fibrous constriction of the aorta or iliac arteries is uncommon but can occur and may constitute the major problem. The intermittent claudication, rest pain, and limb ischemia are indistinguishable clinically and radiographically from those of atherosclerotic occlusion.

Rarely, the fibrotic process will involve the retroperitoneal duodenum and common bile ducts, causing duodenal and biliary obstruction. Mechanical or functional intestinal obstruction due to extension into the root of the mesentery or sigmoid mesocolon is also a rare manifestation.

The diagnosis of retroperitoneal fibrosis is usually suggested by the contrast radiographs of the urinary tract. Gray-scale ultrasonography and computerized axial tomography have also been utilized for the diagnosis of the entity as well as for follow-up management. A characteristic CT scan shows a homogeneous, soft tissue mass enveloping the ureters, aorta, and inferior vena cava. In contrast to malignant retroperitoneal adenopathy, with which retroperitoneal fibrosis is often confused, there is no anterior displacement of the great vessels. Intravenous pyelography is probably the most definitive noninvasive diagnostic test. A triad that is highly suggestive of retroperitoneal fibrosis on the pyelogram is (1) hydronephrosis with a dilated, tortuous upper ureter; (2) medial deviation of the ureter; and (3) extrinsic ureteral compression. The medial deviation of the ureter is in contrast to lateral displacement that is characteristically associated with retroperitoneal tumors. Since a variety of conditions can produce a similar picture, final confirmation of the diagnosis can be made only following exploratory surgical procedures and biopsy of the fibrotic mass. The differential diagnosis includes the primary retroperitoneal tumors, notably the malignant lymphomas, and metastatic tumor from the kidneys, pancreas, or pelvic organs. Inflammatory conditions to be excluded include tuberculosis, pancreatitis, and intraabdominal inflammation of the intestinal tract.

TREATMENT. Once the diagnosis is established, the patient should be carefully followed and surgical intervention timed properly. Improvement may be anticipated in some patients with supportive measures alone. However, with the onset of urinary infection or depression of renal function, surgical intervention becomes necessary.

The discontinuance of methysergide is sometimes followed by a reversal of the fibrotic process with an improvement in symptoms. Steroids, antibiotics, and x-ray therapy have been used with inconsistent results. The self-limiting nature of the disease and the reports of spontaneous resolution in untreated patients make it difficult to evaluate the results of any of these therapeutic modalities. Steroids are of theoretical use in the early inflammatory stages to diminish the generation of fibrosis or control a hyperimmune reaction if one exists. For patients in the prefibrotic stage of the disease with renal insufficiency and prominent constitutional symptoms, steroid-induced regression of the inflammatory edema may reestablish urinary patency and thus facilitate elective, rather than emergency, surgery. However, usually an advanced stage of fibrosis has been reached before the diagnosis is made.

Surgical treatment is directed toward relief of the tubular obstructions, which are usually urinary, less often vascular, and rarely intestinal. Since the disease is fundamentally a midline process that is often bilateral, a midtransabdominal approach offers the best exposure. Several deep biopsies of the mass should be obtained to rule out the possibility of an underlying neoplasm, since these may produce a similar picture, particularly tumors of lymphatic origin. The aorta, inferior vena cava, small bowel mesentery, and sigmoid mesocolon as well as the ureters should be adequately examined for possible involvement.

Ureterolysis with intraperitoneal transplantation is currently the most effective means of relieving obstruction of the involved ureter. This consists of freeing the ureter from the enveloping mass of fibrous tissue and transferring it into the peritoneal cavity, closing the posterior peritoneum behind it. Lateral reposition of the ureter within the retroperitoneal space has been reported to yield equally good results. A preliminary nephrostomy may be indicated if bilateral ureteral obstruction has resulted in severe renal impairment with uremia. On rare occasion, it will be necessary to reimplant the mobilized ureter into the bladder or, if this is not technically possible, to perform renal autotransplantation. Aortic or iliac artery obstruction are best treated by arteriolysis or bypass with a synthetic vascular graft.

Symptoms due to venous obstruction are best treated with elevation and elastic support to the lower limbs until a sufficient collateral venous system develops. The extent of any permanent venous insufficiency will depend upon the availability of collateral pathways and the competency of deep vein valves. Release of the obstructed vein from its fibrous encasement may be difficult and hazardous, and bypass procedures for obstruction of the inferior vena cava have been uniformly unsuccessful.

The prognosis of the disease is generally good, provided that appropriate treatment has been instituted prior to the development of irreversible renal damage. Ormond, in 1960, reviewed 64 cases and reported 10 deaths, most from renal failure secondary to unrecognized obstructive uropathy that presumably could have been corrected with earlier diagnosis. In 1977 a combined series of 481 cases reported by Koep and Zuidema showed the cumulative mortality to be 9 percent.

Retroperitoneal Tumors

Primary tumors of the retroperitoneum include those neoplasms arising from tissues that occupy the potential retroperitoneal space. These tumors develop independently and have no apparent connection with any organs or major vessels except by areolar tissue. Tumors of the retroperitoneal solid organs, such as the pancreas, adrenal, or kidney, and tumefactions of the great blood vessels, therefore, are not included in this category.

The first description of retroperitoneal tumors is credited to Morgagni in 1761. Several large series have been reported by Ackerman, Braasch, Melicow, and Pack and Tabah. Although they are uncommon, nonetheless, they are not rare and must always be considered in the differential diagnosis of an unexplained abdominal mass. The majority occur in the fifth or sixth decades with a peak incidence at about sixty years, although approximately 15 percent are found in children under ten years of age.

PATHOLOGY. Tumors in this locale may arise from fat, areolar connective tissue, fascia, muscle, vascular tissue, somatic and sympathetic nervous tissue, and lymph vessels and lymph nodes. Less frequent neoplasms are smooth muscle tumors, complex teratomas, embryonal

Table 35-2. CLASSIFICATION OF RETROPERITONEAL TUMORS

Tissue type	Benign tumors	Malignant tumors
Lymphatic tissue	Lymphangioma	Lymphangiosarcoma
Lymph nodes		Lymphosarcoma
		Hodgkin's disease
		Reticulum cell sarcoma
Adipose tissue	Lipoma	Liposarcoma
Fibrous tissue	Fibroma	Fibrosarcoma
Smooth muscle	Leiomyoma	Leiomyosarcoma
Nerve elements	Neurilemoma	Malignant schwannoma
	Neurofibroma	
	Ganglioneuroma	Sympathicoblastoma
		(neuroblastoma)
		Chordoma
Striated muscle	Rhabdomyoma	Rhabdomyosarcoma
Mucoid tissue	Myxoma	Myxosarcoma
Vascular tissue	Hemangioma	Malignant hemangiopericytoma
Mesothelial tissue		Mesothelioma
Mesenchyme		Mesenchymoma
Extraadrenal chromaffin tissue	Benign pheochromo-cytoma	Malignant pheochromocytoma
Gland tissue	Adenoma	Carcinoma
Embryonic remnants	Nephrogenic cysts	Urogenital ridge tumor
Cell rests	Dermoid	Teratoma
Miscellaneous	Xanthogranuloma	Synovioma
	Aggressive	Dysgerminoma
	fibromatosis	Undifferentiated malignant tumor

carcinomas, and certain bizarre cysts of unknown origin. These rarer tumors are believed to arise from remnants of the embryonal urogenital apparatus, which includes tissue of both epithelial and mesothelial origin. A classification of the benign and malignant tumors according to tissue type is given in Table 35-2.

Malignant tumors are four times more prevalent than benign tumors; the most common are malignant lymphomas or lymphosarcomas, comprising about one-third of the cases in most large series. Other malignant tumors, in order of frequency, are fibrosarcomas, liposarcomas, undifferentiated sarcomas, leiomyosarcomas, and rhabdomyosarcomas. Neurogenic sarcomas, which include sympathicoblastoma and neuroblastoma, also comprise a large group of malignant tumors. Of the benign tumors, the most frequent are lipomas, lymphatic or chylous cysts, cysts of urogenital origin, dermoids, and enterogenous cysts.

The tumors may be solid, cystic, or a combination of both. Their color varies from white (fibroma), yellow (lipoma), or pinkish to red (sarcoma), depending on the predominant tissue. They may be single or multiple and vary in size from small outgrowths to tumors weighing as much as 40 lb. As a rule, the predominantly cystic tumors are benign, whereas the solid tumors are usually malignant.

CLINICAL MANIFESTATIONS. Early symptoms of retroperitoneal tumors are characteristically vague or lacking. The loose retroperitoneal areolar tissue allows the tumor to grow unrestricted in all directions except posteriorly. For this reason, it may attain an extremely large size before producing symptoms. As the tumor grows, it compresses, obstructs, or invades adjacent organs or structures, so that the presenting symptoms are often referable to these organs.

The initial manifestations include an enlarging abdomen, backache, a sense of fullness or heaviness, and vague indefinite pain that later may become severe and radicular. Nausea, vomiting, change in bowel habits, and other symptoms suggestive of bowel obstruction result from the compression of portions of the gastrointestinal tract. Later, the malignant tumors cause anorexia, weight loss, weakness, fever, and, less frequently, hematemesis. Genitourinary complaints include hematuria, dysuria, urgency, and frequency of urination. Rarely, there is oliguria or anuria. Pain radiating into one or both thighs is usually late and due to involvement of lumbar and sacral nerve routes; it invariably denotes a malignant tumor. Swelling and varicosities of the lower extremities are usually due to obstruction of lymphatics and venous return. Hormonally active tumors of extraadrenal chromaffin tissue (pheochromocytoma) produce symptoms referable to hypertension. Rarely, hypoglycemia and its associated symptoms may be seen with retroperitoneal sarcomas.

The predominant physical finding is the presence of an abdominal mass. This is usually nontender and may fill the entire abdomen. A fixed, hard mass suggests malignancy, whereas a soft or tense and ballottable one may be a benign neoplasm or cyst. The mass usually occupies the midline and extends into one or both flanks or may be deep-seated in the pelvis, where it can be felt through the rectum. Ascites due to compression of the portal or hepatic veins, edema of the lower extremities, scrotal varicosities, and dilated superficial abdominal veins are infrequently present. Enlarged hemorrhoids or rectal tenesmus are symptoms in patients with presacral neoplasms.

The diagnosis of primary retroperitoneal tumors is mainly one of exclusion of other abdominal tumefactions. Differential diagnosis includes lesions of the kidney, such as hydronephrosis, polycystic disease, or hypernephroma; pancreatic cysts and tumors, splenomegaly, neoplasms of the liver, tumors of the gastrointestinal tract, ovarian tumors, abdominal aortic aneurysms, and cysts of the omentum and mesentery.

With the use of computerized tomographic scanning and ultrasonography, retroperitoneal tumors can often be detected early and distinguished from neoplasms arising from specific organs located in the retroperitoneum. The CT scan can demonstrate the contours of the tumor mass, its size and its relationships, as well as its effect on adjacent viscera and other tissues (Fig. 35-15). This information is useful in determining resectability of the tumor and in planning a surgical approach. Ultrasonography will differentiate between solid and cystic tumors. Percutaneous needle biopsy directed by computerized tomography or ultrasonography can also be utilized to obtain a preoperative histologic diagnosis and for the detection of treatment failures and early recurrences.

The main value of a gastrointestinal series and barium enema is the exclusion of gastrointestinal tumors. Calcification is not unusual in certain retroperitoneal tumors, while the finding of teeth or other recognizable bony structures is diagnostic of teratoma.

Aortography should be an essential part of the work-up of patients with a suspected or diagnosed retroperitoneal tumor. Aortography not only will help define tumor size and location but also can give useful information regarding variations in normal vascular anatomy. Lowman and associates reported in detail the diagnostic use of retroperitoneal angiography. The lumbar arteries supply a large segment of the retroperitoneal space, and stretching or displacement of these vessels or displacement of the aorta by the tumor mass can give precise localization of the tumor and exclude primary visceral tumors (Fig. 35-16). Neovascularity often indicates malignant disease, but most retroperitoneal tumors lack this feature.

TREATMENT. Some retroperitoneal tumors are benign and can be cured by simple excisions; some are histologically benign but clinically malignant; others grow slowly but tend to recur and invade locally; and still others are rapidly malignant from the start.

Treatment of these growths consists of surgical or irradiation therapy, or a combination of the two. With the exception of lymphomas, chemotherapy has only limited therapeutic application. Surgical treatment is the most effective and offers the greatest prospect for cure. In some cases, it is imperative because of intestinal or urinary obstructions or because of hemorrhage.

As many as one-third of patients with malignant tumors may be inoperable because of distant metastases to liver, lung, and bone, in order of frequency.

In operable patients, initial biopsy of the tumor with frozen section will usually determine its malignant or benign nature. A cure may be anticipated following complete resection of benign tumors. On occasion, however, a tumor previously considered benign will recur, and this is especially true of retroperitoneal lipomas, which may undergo sarcomatous change.

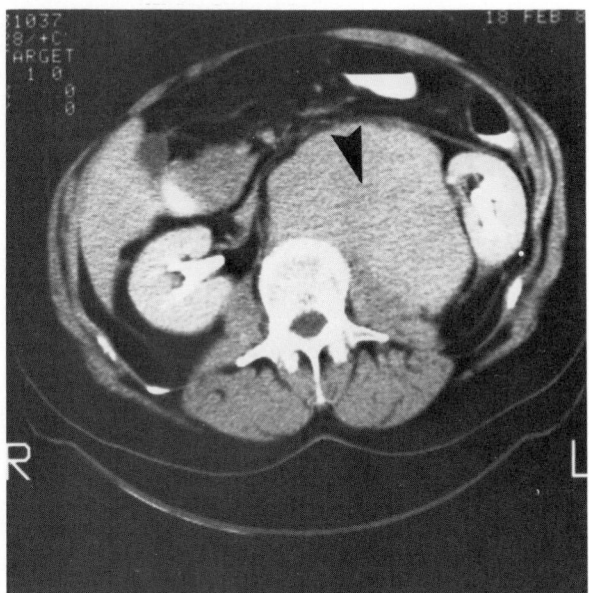

Fig. 35-15. Computerized tomography of abdomen showing a large, left retroperitoneal fibrosarcoma (arrow) that has displaced the left kidney laterally and invaded the left ileopsoas muscle.

For a malignant tumor, the initial operation offers the best chance for cure. These tumors are quite invasive and often become adherent to vital organs or structures. Adequate exposure is extremely important to enable safe dissection of the tumor and avoid injury to major blood vessels. For this reason, a generous transperitoneal abdominal incision is preferred over an extraperitoneal flank approach. Since major blood loss may occur during the operation, multiple units of blood and fresh frozen plasma should be available. It is estimated that fewer than 25 percent of malignant tumors can be completely resected with anticipation of cure. Fixation of the tumor to the parietes does not contraindicate an attempt at resection, since partial excision can often give satisfactory palliation. At times, nephrectomy or partial intestinal resection may be required. Operative mortality is high, with reports varying between 10 and 25 percent.

Malignant retroperitoneal tumors have a high recurrence rate, from 30 to 50 percent in most large series. The tumors become more malignant with each recurrence, and reoperation becomes more hazardous. Nevertheless, long-term survival has been reported after multiple resections.

Radiotherapy, although rarely curative, may relieve pain and obstruction and prolong life. As many as 75 percent of patients will benefit from irradiation therapy even though most retroperitoneal tumors are not radiocurative. Indications for irradiation include (1) inoperable tumors; (2) tumor recurrence following previous resection; (3)

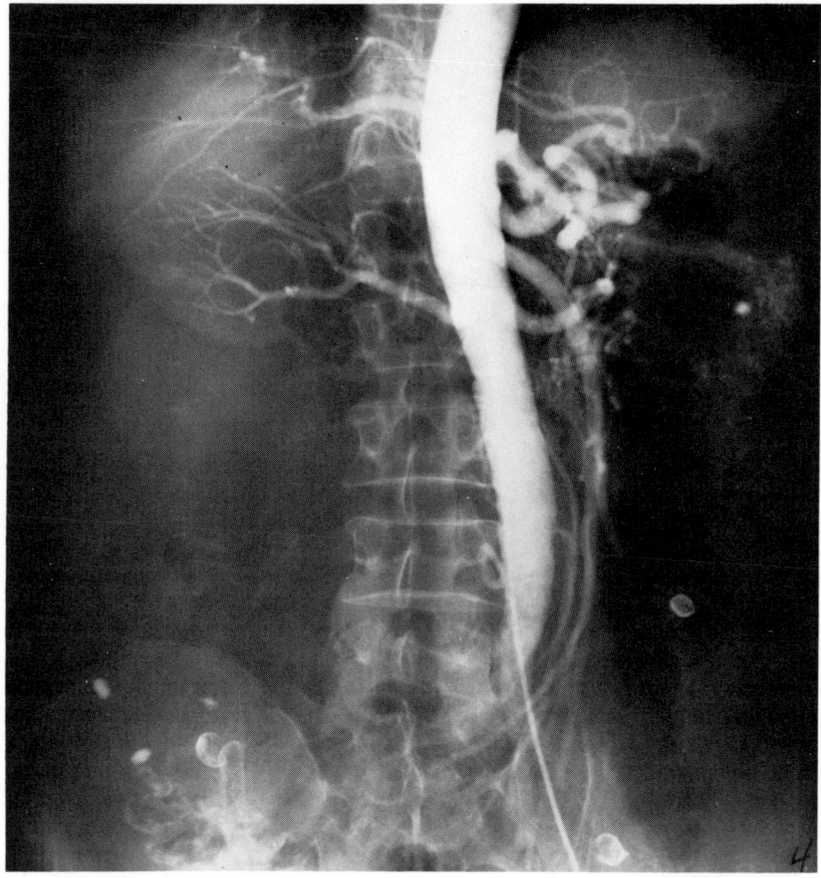

Fig. 35-16. Abdominal aortogram showing lateral displacement of the aorta and lumbar arteries by a large right retroperitoneal tumor.

residual tumor following partial surgical resection; (4) certain radiosensitive tumors, particularly the malignant lymphomas; and (5) as an adjunct to surgery for some malignant tumors such as neuroblastomas, liposarcomas, rhabdomyosarcomas, and undifferentiated anaplastic sarcomas. Radiotherapy and/or chemotherapy is the treatment of choice for malignant lymphomas, since the multicentric origin of these tumors makes surgical extirpation difficult.

The overall prognosis for malignant retroperitoneal tumors is poor. Five-year survival free of tumor is less than 10 percent and can be anticipated only in those patients in whom complete surgical removal is possible. Rare cures following irradiation therapy of neuroblastoma or lymphosarcoma have also been reported. Since many of the tumors are slow-growing or responsive to irradiation, long-term survival with existing tumor is possible in as much as 15 percent of patients. Neuroblastoma and liposarcoma offer the best prognosis with average survivals of 4 and 5 years, respectively. Most patients with other malignant retroperitoneal tumors are dead in 2 years, death resulting from widespread metastases, intestinal or urinary obstruction, or hemorrhage from invasion of major blood vessels.

Bibliography

Abdominal Wall

Allen PW: The fibromatosis: A clinicopathologic classification based on 140 cases. *Am J Surg Pathol* 1:255, 1977.

Belliveau P, Graham AM: Mesenteric desmoid tumor in Gardner's syndrome treated by Sulindac. *Dis Colon Rectum* 27:53, 1984.

Das Gupta TK, Brasfield RD, O'Hara J: Extra-abdominal desmoids: A clinicopathological study. *Ann Surg* 170:109, 1969.

Gocke JE, Maccarthy RL, Foulk WT: Rectus sheath hematoma diagnosed by computed tomography scanning. *Mayo Clin Proc* 56:757, 1981.

Hildreth D: Anticoagulant therapy and rectus sheath hematoma. *Am J Surg* 124:80, 1972.

Jones IT, Jagelman DG, et al: Desmoid tumors in familial polyposis coli. *Ann Surg* 204:94, 1986.

Khorsand J, Karakousis CP: Desmoid tumors and their management. *Am J Surg* 149:215, 1985.

Kiel KD, Suit HD: Radiation therapy in the treatment of aggressive fibromatoses. *Cancer* 54:2051, 1984.

Manier JW: Rectus sheath hematoma: Six case reports and a literature review. *Am J Gastroenterol* 57:443, 1972.

Stiles QR, Raskowski HJ, Henry W: Rectus sheath hematoma. *Surg Gynecol Obstet* 12:331, 1965.

Titone C, Lipsius M, Krakauer JS: "Spontaneous" hematoma of the rectus abdominis muscle: Critical review of 50 cases with emphasis on early diagnosis and treatment. *Surgery* 72:568, 1972.

Waddell WR, Gerner RE: Indomethacin and ascorbate inhibit desmoid tumors. *J Surg Oncol* 15:85, 1980.

Wyatt GM, Spitz HB: Ultrasound in the diagnosis of rectus sheath hematoma. *JAMA* 241:1499, 1979.

Omentum

Basson SE, Jones PA: Primary torsion of the omentum. *Ann R Coll Surg Engl* 63:132, 1980.

Baxter NS, Storey DJ, et al: Infarction of greater omentum. Exclusive cause of acute abdominal pain. *Postgrad Med* 79:141, 1986.

Beahrs OH, Judd EJ Jr, Dockerty MB: Chylous cysts of the abdomen. *Surg Clin North Am* 30:1081, 1950.

Cooper C, Jeffrey RB, et al: Computed tomography of omental pathology. *J Comput Assist Tomogr* 10:62, 1986.

Crofoot DD: Spontaneous segmental infarction of the greater omentum. *Am J Surg* 139:262, 1980.

Draper JW, Johnston RK: The pathologic omentum. *JAMA* 88:376, 1927.

Eitel GG: A rare omental tumor. *Med Rec* 55:715, 1899.

Halligan EJ, Rabiah FA: Primary idiopathic segmental infarction of the greater omentum. *Arch Surg* 79:738, 1959.

Leitner MJ, Jordan CG, et al: Torsion, infarction and hemorrhage of the omentum as a cause of acute abdominal distress. *Ann Surg* 135:103, 1952.

Mainzer RA, Simoes A: Primary idiopathic torsion of the omentum. *Arch Surg* 88:974, 1964.

Rubin IC: The functions of the great omentum. *Surg Gynecol Obstet* 12:117, 1911.

Stout AP, Hendry J, Purdie FJ: Solid tumors of the great omentum. *Cancer* 16:231, 1963.

Walker AR, Putnam TC: Omental, mesenteric and retroperitoneal cysts. *Surgery* 178:13, 1973.

Mesentery

Abdu RA, Zakhour BJ, et al: Mesenteric venous thrombosis—1901 to 1984. *Surgery* 101:383, 1987.

Ackerman LV: *Surgical Pathology.* St Louis, Mosby, 1964.

Adams JT, Kutner FR: Pure fibroma of the mesentery. *Am J Surg* 111:734, 1966.

Bergan JJ, Dean RH, et al: Revascularization in treatment of mesenteric infarction. *Ann Surg* 182:430, 1975.

Boley SJ, Feinstein FR, et al: New concepts in the management of emboli of the superior mesenteric artery. *Surg Gynecol Obstet* 153:561, 1981.

Britt LC, Cheek RC: Nonocclusive mesenteric vascular disease: Clinical and experimental observations. *Ann Surg* 169:704, 1969.

Bulkley GB, Zuidema GD, et al: Intraoperative determination of small intestinal viability following ischemic injury: A prospective controlled trial of two adjuvant methods (Doppler and fluorescein) compared with standard clinical judgement. *Ann Surg* 193:628, 1981.

Busuttil RW, Brin BJ: The diagnosis and management of visceral artery aneurysms. *Surgery* 88:619, 1980.

Carey JP, Stemmer EA, Connolly JE: Median arcuate ligament syndrome. *Arch Surg* 99:441, 1969.

Caropreso PR: Mesenteric cysts, a review. *Arch Surg* 108:242, 1974.

Clark RA, Gallant TE: Acute mesenteric ischemia; angiographic spectrum. *Am J Radiol* 142:555, 1984.

Collins G: Hypercoagulability in mesenteric venous occlusion. *Am J Surg* 132:390, 1976.

Connelly TI, Perdue GD, et al: Elective mesenteric revascularization. *Am Surg* 47:19, 1981.

Crawford ES, Morris GC, et al: Celiac axis, superior mesenteric artery and inferior mesenteric artery occlusion: Surgical considerations. *Surgery* 82:856, 1977.

Durst AL, Freund H, et al: Mesenteric panniculitis: Review of the literature and presentation of cases. *Surgery* 81:203, 1977.

Fogerty TJ, Fletcher WS: Genesis of nonocclusive mesenteric ischemia. *Am J Surg* 111:130, 1966.

Fowler EF: Primary cysts and tumors of the small bowel mesentery. *Am Surg* 27:653, 1961.

Graham JM, McCollum CH, Debakey ME: Aneurysms of the splanchnic arteries. *Am J Surg* 140:797, 1980.

Grendell JH, Ockner RK: Mesenteric venous thrombosis. *Gastroenterology* 82:358, 1982.

Habbooshe F, Wallace HW, et al: Nonocclusive mesenteric vascular insufficiency. *Ann Surg* 180:819, 1974.

Handelsman JC, Shelly WM: Mesenteric panniculitis. *Arch Surg* 91:842, 1965.

Hollister LN: Surgical management of chronic intestinal ischemia. *Surgery* 90:940, 1981.

Jaxheimer EC, Jewell ER, et al: Chronic intestinal ischemia. The Laney Clinic approach to management. *Surg Clin North Am* 65:123, 1985.

Keehan M, Kistner R, Banis J Jr: Angiography as an aid in extraenteric gastrointestinal bleeding due to visceral artery aneurysms. *Ann Surg* 187:357, 1978.

Khodadadi J, Rozencwajg J, et al: Mesenteric vein thrombosis: The importance of a second-look operation. *Arch Surg* 115:315, 1980.

Kleinsasser LJ: Abdominal apoplexy: Report of two cases and review of the literature. *Am J Surg* 120:623, 1970.

Kurtz RJ, Heimann TM, et al: Mesenteric and retroperitoneal cysts. *Am Surg* 203:109, 1986.

Laufman H, Nora PF, Mittelpunkt AI: Mesenteric blood vessels: Advances in surgery and physiology. *Arch Surg* 88:1021, 1964.

Lawson JD, Ochwner JL: Median arcuate ligament syndrome with severe two-vessel involvement. *Arch Surg* 119:226, 1984.

Levinsky RA, Lewis RM, et al: Digoxin induced intestinal vasoconstriction: The effects of proximal arterial stenosis and glucagon administration. *Circulation* 52:130, 1975.

McDonald JC: Nonspecific mesenteric lymphadenitis. *Surg Gynecol Obstet* 116:409, 1963.

McNamara MF, Griska LB: Superior mesenteric artery branch aneurysms. *Surgery* 88:625, 1980.

Madore P, Kahn DS, et al: Nonspecific mesenteric lymphadenitis. *Can J Surg* 5:59, 1962.

Marable SA, Kaplan MF, et al: Celiac compression syndrome. *Am J Surg* 115:97, 1968.

Morris GC, Crawford ES, et al: Revascularization of the celiac and superior mesenteric arteries. *Arch Surg* 84:95, 1962.

Naitove A, Weismann RE: Primary mesenteric venous thrombosis. *Ann Surg* 161:516, 1965.

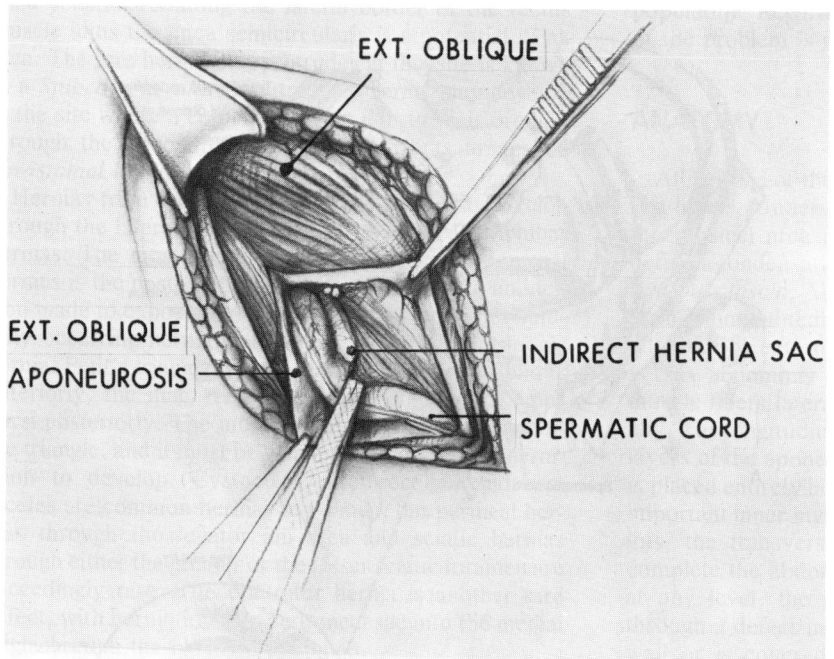

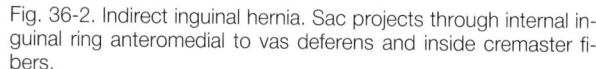

Fig. 36-2. Indirect inguinal hernia. Sac projects through internal inguinal ring anteromedial to vas deferens and inside cremaster fibers.

makes incarceration unusual in direct inguinal hernia. When incarceration does occur, it is usually at the level of the external inguinal ring in those rare situations where a direct sac passes through this area. With a large direct hernia it is not unusual for a portion of the wall of the urinary bladder to be incorporated in a sliding fashion in the medial portion of the sac.

The third groin hernia, the femoral type (Fig. 36-5), also depends for its development upon a defect in the transversalis fascia in Hesselbach's triangle. In this type of hernia, however, there is a peritoneal sac that passes under the inguinal ligament into the femoral triangle rather than following the course of the direct hernia anteriorly into the inguinal canal. The inguinal ligament stretches as a tight band from the anterior superior iliac spine to the pubic tubercle, and beneath it the femoral vessels enter the thigh. Medial to the femoral vein is a small empty space through which a femoral hernia may project. The resulting sac will have, perforce, a very narrow neck. Once the sac enters the thigh, however, it may

assume quite large proportions in the loose connective tissue. It may even double back on top of the external oblique aponeurosis, coming to lie over the groin, where it can be mistaken for an inguinal hernia. Because of the narrow neck in this type of hernia, incarceration with strangulation of the contents of the hernia is a strong possibility.

Umbilical Region

During the embryonic period before completion of intestinal rotation there is a herniation of abdominal contents through the umbilicus into the extraembryonic coelomic cavity. At about the tenth week of fetal life the viscera normally return to the abdominal cavity, the intestine completing its rotation in the process. The defect in the abdominal wall closes slowly during subsequent

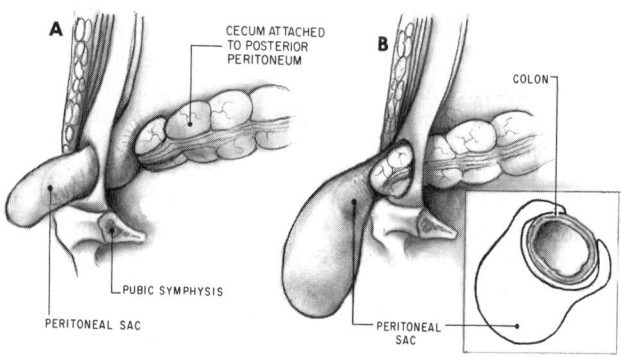

Fig. 36-3. Evolution of sliding hernia. *A*. Leading peritoneal sac "pulls" mobile cecum or sigmoid. *B*. Sliding hernia is established with colon or cecum as part of wall of sac.

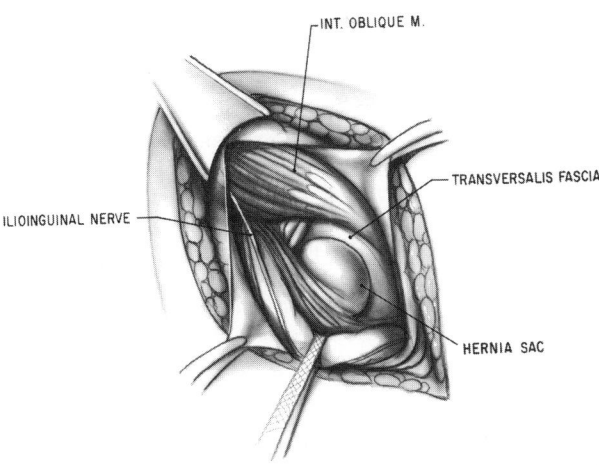

Fig. 36-4. Direct inguinal hernia. Weakness involves medial inguinal canal floor and lies behind structures of spermatic cord.

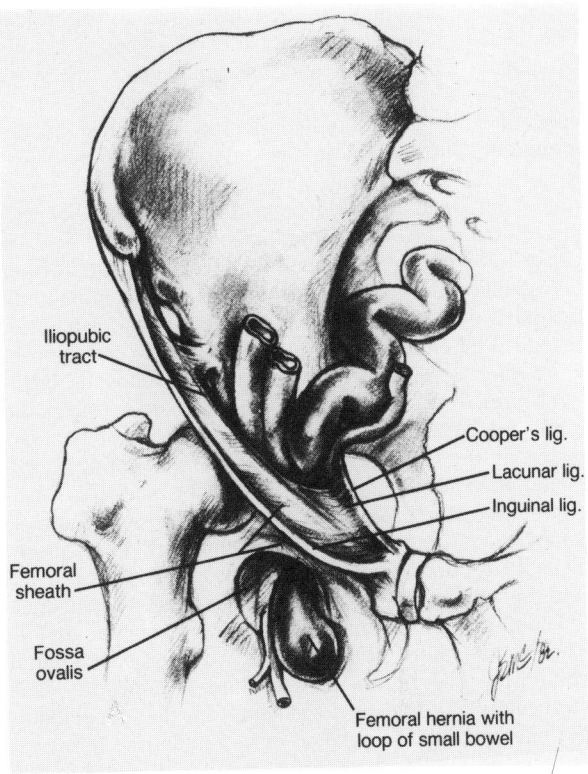

Fig. 36-5. Femoral hernia. Although sac projects beneath inguinal ligament into femoral triangle, basic defect making hernia possible is weakness in attachment of transversalis fascia and transversus abdominis aponeurosis to Cooper's ligament.

fetal development, until at birth only the space occupied by the umbilical cord remains patent. Following ligation of the cord, the umbilical stump heals by granulation and organization, with epithelialization from the margins of the defect. Abdominal wall closure at this level thus consists of the fusion of skin, a single fascial layer, and peritoneum.

At birth many infants will show a small umbilical hernia (Fig. 36-6) because this process has not been carried through to completion. In most of these children spontaneous closure of the fascial defect occurs within the first four years of life in a fashion identical with that described above. An umbilical hernia that is still present in a four-year-old will usually persist, but bowel strangulation in these congenital umbilical defects is unusual.

Occasionally, however, the process of abdominal wall closure is much less complete at birth, and several interesting congenital anomalies may be encountered. An omphalocele is present when at birth there is a defect at the umbilicus covered only by a peritoneal sac. Within such a sac virtually any abdominal organ may be encoun-

tered, but small bowel, colon, and liver are the most common viscera present.

If the embryologic duct from small bowel to yolk sac remains attached to the umbilical cord at birth, it is likely to be included in the tie placed by the obstetrician. This duct, although extremely narrow, amounting to no more than a cord, may be lined with bowel epithelium. When the umbilical remnant sloughs later under these circumstances, a fistula into the small gut is created. This anomaly is known as a patent omphalomesenteric or vitelline duct. On occasion the fibrous cord is not lined with epi-

Fig. 36-6. Umbilical hernia. Peritoneal sac is attached directly to underside of umbilical skin, with only thin attenuated fascia covering sac.

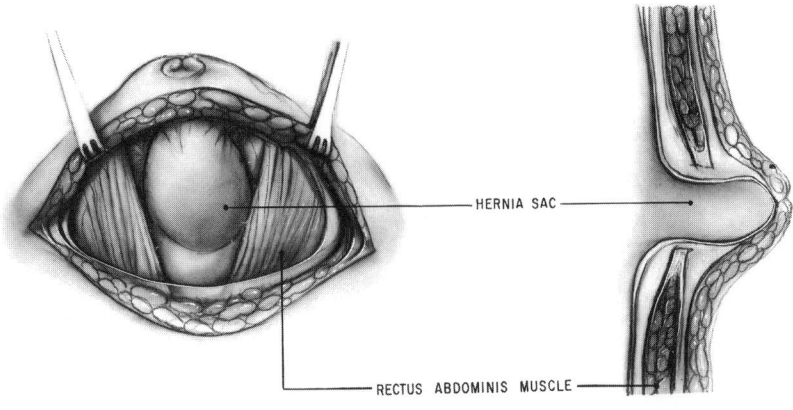

thelium, and the umbilicus then heals normally after ligation, usually without an umbilical hernia. The cord, however, may persist, connecting the umbilicus to the small gut, and it may be encountered in later life as one of the congenital bands leading to volvulus and intestinal obstruction. One patient in the author's experience was found to have a thin band of this type at abdominal exploration during adult life. The patient had never experienced drainage from the umbilicus, but the band was excised. A fecal fistula promptly developed. On further investigation it was evident that this band contained an epithelial lining at its intestinal end, although it had not extended far enough toward the umbilicus to create problems when cord ligature was performed following birth.

The urachus, a sinus tract from the bladder, enters the umbilical area from below, between the umbilical arteries, during fetal life. This tract, the remnant of the cephalic portion of the embryonic urinary bladder, is usually obliterated before birth, but should it remain patent, it may become incorporated in the umbilical cord ligature. Thus a later draining umbilical sinus may represent a patent urachus as well as a patent omphalomesenteric duct.

Umbilical hernias may also develop during adult life. This occurs more commonly in women, usually after childbirth. The hernia may become a large one, and strangulation of intestine or omentum within the defect is not uncommon. The surgeon must be cautious about repairing an umbilical hernia in an adult with portal hypertension. In these patients herniorrhaphy may compromise collateral circulation and cause bleeding varices.

ETIOLOGY

Hernias may result from congenital anomalies or may develop secondarily during later life. Although congenital umbilical hernias are more common in black infants, other congenital hernias occur with equal frequency in blacks and whites. Inguinal hernias are more common in males, and femoral hernias occur primarily in females. When a hernia develops secondarily in later life, it is sometimes the result of trauma. Hence it is compensable if the injury occurs when the patient is at work. It should be pointed out, however, that the traumatic explanation for these hernias is not entirely satisfying. In many instances, for example, the patient is not aware of any specific event that precipitated the hernia. Rather, a bulge develops gradually after years of hard work. In other circumstances, a similar hernia may develop in sedentary individuals who have not changed their habits before herniation occurs. In any case, many adults never develop a hernia despite a lifetime of vigorous physical activity. In evaluating the direct hernia of later life, Zimmerman and Anson concluded that this lesion also results from a congenital anatomic defect—the absence of adequate muscular support for the lower portion of the inguinal canal. They find the lowermost fibers of the internal oblique lacking, so that a larger triangle without muscular reinforcement is present in the individual who is prone to hernia formation. On the other hand, Condon concluded

from his dissections that a direct hernia resulted from the lack of adequate reinforcement of transversalis fascia in Hesselbach's triangle.

In considering the development of a hernia in the groin during middle life, it is wise to remember that increased intraabdominal pressure is at least as important a predisposing factor as external trauma. Chronic cough or symptoms of genitourinary tract or gastrointestinal tract obstruction may precede herniation. Benign prostatic hypertrophy and carcinoma of the left colon are two important entities that should be considered in an adult seeking medical attention because of a hernia. Cirrhosis of the liver with ascites, massive splenomegaly, and uterine enlargement during pregnancy are other possible etiologic factors of this type.

Recently, several investigators have suggested that a connective tissue abnormality may be involved in adult-onset hernias. Abnormalities in the ultrastructure and the physicochemical properties of collagen in patients with direct hernias suggest that the hernia is one manifestation of a generalized abnormality in collagen metabolism.

From the legal point of view a hernia is an important condition about which a physician must frequently testify, and the wording or interpretation of a workmen's compensation law can be important. Many young adult males first discover a hernia after some vigorous physical labor; this type of hernia is usually indirect. The physician is aware that such a defect is almost always congenital, and it would be difficult to testify that the traumatic incident produced the hernia. On the other hand, it is hard to convince a young man that the hernia has been present all his life and that he was unaware of it because no intraabdominal organ had previously entered the sac. This uncomfortable situation is satisfactorily avoided in jurisdictions where exacerbation of preexisting disease is sufficient evidence of a compensable injury. In these circumstances the surgeon can bear witness that the patient has a hernia and that the presenting symptoms may be related to the injury in question.

SYMPTOMS AND SIGNS

A hernia may be an asymptomatic defect, discovered incidentally during a routine physical examination. The individual may or may not have been aware of its presence. The usual reducible hernia produces no symptoms of importance other than pain. The type and degree of pain vary considerably from one individual to another. If the hernia is first recognized after an acute traumatic episode, local pain of a muscular type may be quite severe for several days. This pain occurs when, in the presence of a preexisting patent processus vaginalis, sudden enlargement of the internal inguinal ring permits development of a true hernia.

In a few days the discomfort subsides without specific treatment. In a long-standing hernia occasional twinges of local discomfort may be present, usually in association with straining or with the temporary entry of an intraperitoneal organ into the sac. Another type of discomfort may occur when a loop of small intestine enters the hernia. Epigastric or paraumbilical pain may then develop, representing visceral pain in the superior mesenteric distribution as a result of mesenteric stretching.

The physical signs of an uncomplicated hernia vary with the contents of the sac. When there are no peritoneal contents present, the sac is collapsed and its presence is difficult to identify. It is said that the opposing peritoneal surfaces may be rubbed one over the other to detect a sensation of gliding, but this is an unreliable sign. When an organ occupies the sac, the findings vary with the organ involved. If bowel is present, crepitation will be noted on palpation because of the presence of gas and fluid within the lumen. If a solid organ such as an ovary is present, a movable firm regular mass will be felt. When omentum is within the sac, an ill-defined irregular rubbery mass will be palpable. When an organ enters an inguinal hernia sac, reduction may be attempted by gentle pressure with a finger through the invaginated scrotal skin. This should be done with the patient supine and relaxed. If the organ is not readily reduced, a sliding hernia should be expected, especially if the bulge is a large one.

A solid mass palpable within a hernia in a female infant is usually a normal ovary. The ovary is simply returned to the abdominal cavity before the hernia repair is completed. However, Carmichael and Vorse point out that any gonad found in a labial hernia sac that appears abnormal or resembles a testis should be biopsied. This situation may occur in a patient with testicular feminization, a syndrome in which normal female genitalia are encountered in a 46, XY male. Despite the female genitalia, these patients have testes rather than ovaries, and over half of them have inguinal hernias. Biopsy of the testis encountered during herniorrhaphy is one step in establishing the diagnosis. Since malignancy is a frequent development in these gonads later in the patient's life, early diagnosis is an important guide to appropriate therapy.

On rare occasions males will be encountered with two normal testicles in one scrotal sac and an undeveloped scrotum on the opposite side. A number of patients with this syndrome, known as transverse testicular ectopia, are pseudohermaphrodites. Almost all of them have an indirect inguinal hernia on the side with the two testicles. Herniorrhaphy and repositioning of the ectopic testicle can be done as part of one operative procedure.

A hernia may be particularly difficult to identify in an infant, who cannot cooperate during examination. If the mother gives a suggestive history and no hernia can be found, she should be instructed to bring the infant back when a bulge is obvious or to return later with the youngster for a second examination under any circumstance. If a hydrocele of the cord is present in an infant, an indirect hernia is almost invariably present as well, and it should be repaired at the time of hydrocelectomy.

If no hernia is obvious when examination is begun, one may become apparent if the patient is requested to strain. A sustained contraction of the muscles of the abdominal wall is more effective than the traditional cough as a method of raising intraabdominal pressure, thus demonstrating the hernia. Position during the examination is important. When a ventral hernia is suspected, the supine patient should be asked to raise head and shoulders from the bed. When a male is being examined for a groin hernia, he should be standing in a relaxed position, and the physician should invaginate the scrotum with the examining finger. The finger should be introduced through the external ring into the inguinal canal while the patient strains. It is harder to examine a female for a groin hernia. She should be standing and the labia majora examined while she strains. A definite bulge and mass should be palpated before the diagnosis of a hernia can be considered secure. The presence of a dilated external inguinal ring is of no significance per se as regards the presence of a hernia and does not predispose to the later development of a hernia. With groin hernias the location of the mass should be helpful in distinguishing the femoral hernia, because the bulge from a femoral hernia should be found below the inguinal ligament, which runs between the anterior superior iliac spine and the pubic tubercle.

It is important to realize that an obese individual may be unaware of a hernia in the groin. If such a patient presents with intestinal obstruction, the physician must rule out an incarcerated hernia as the cause for the problem.

The clinical distinction between direct and indirect hernia by physical examination is academic, since the operative approach for repair is the same for both. This is fortunate since accurate distinction is often difficult to make. When the examining finger has been advanced well into the inguinal canal, the indirect hernia should strike the fingertip and the direct hernia the ball of the finger—but this difference is frequently hard to appreciate. A thumb placed over the internal inguinal ring should keep an indirect hernia reduced when the patient strains while permitting a direct hernia to appear; again, it is not always possible to locate the internal ring accurately enough to make this technique foolproof. A hernia that enters the scrotum is almost always indirect, lying with the cord structures inside the cremaster muscle. Rarely a very large direct hernia extends through the external ring behind the cremaster.

The predominant finding with an incarcerated or strangulated hernia is a tender mass at one of the hernial sites. A testicular torsion may be mistaken for an incarcerated inguinal hernia and an acute femoral lymphadenitis for an incarcerated femoral hernia.

COMPLICATIONS

The risk is that an intraperitoneal organ may become incarcerated or strangulated within the hernia sac. The small intestine is the organ most frequently affected, and acute incarceration or strangulation within a hernia sac remains one of the two most frequent causes for small bowel obstruction. This complication changes a simple situation into one that may prove fatal. As noted above, a mass incarcerated in the inguinal hernia of a female infant is commonly an ovary, although incarceration of the appendix has been reported.

Occasionally only a portion of the antimesenteric wall

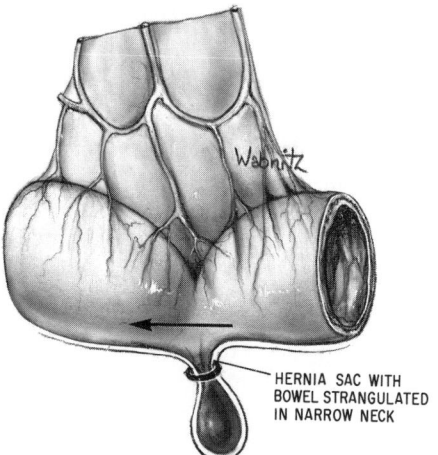

HERNIA SAC WITH
BOWEL STRANGULATED
IN NARROW NECK

Fig. 36-7. Richter's hernia. Strangulation of antimesenteric portion of the bowel may lead to abscess without intestinal obstruction.

of the intestine becomes strangulated within a hernia sac, producing a so-called Richter's hernia (Fig. 36-7). In this special situation there is not complete bowel obstruction, but the entrapped portion of bowel wall may become gangrenous. An abscess results if the strangulation is not recognized and treated early. An abscess of the medial thigh in an elderly female that, on incision and drainage, releases pus with a feculent odor suggests the presence of an obturator hernia with a partially strangulated bowel.

The development of complications in a hernia is not predictable. When complications do occur, an elective situation becomes an emergency, and a simple problem becomes more difficult. The rationale for elective herniorrhaphy is to prevent this situation. Paradoxically the small hernia may be more dangerous. Organs readily enter a larger hernia, but they reduce easily. Once an organ becomes trapped in a small hernial defect, the rapid development of edema may make reduction difficult or impossible.

Spontaneous rupture of an umbilical hernia in an individual with cirrhosis and ascites has been reported. This unusual event is accompanied by drainage of ascitic fluid through the site of rupture. Prolonged morbidity and significant mortality results even if the hernia is repaired on an emergency basis.

TREATMENT

General

A hernia may be approached in three ways: expectantly, nonoperatively, or by surgical repair. Expectant treatment is based on the hope of spontaneous cure; in most situations this is not realistic. However, with the congenital umbilical hernia spontaneous cure does occur in most children before the age of four. This is a natural process that is not enhanced by the use of adhesive strapping. The physician should not advise operation until the patient reaches age four unless the hernia has incarcerated—a most unusual event in a hernia of this type—or unless it is a very large defect of the proboscis type. Expectant management of uncomplicated groin hernias is also reasonable in patients severely ill from some other cause. In most other circumstances an expectant attitude is not warranted.

The nonoperative treatment of a hernia involves the use of some external device or truss to maintain hernial reduction. These devices are a nuisance to the patient, and they are expensive to construct and to fit. In the groin they are almost universally unsuccessful in maintaining satisfactory reduction. A properly fitting corset may be an excellent remedy, however, for a ventral hernia, particularly when a large defect develops in an abdominal wound that became infected following initial celiotomy. Surgical repair of these defects is difficult, and a trial with external support is certainly justified before operation is recommended. With this exception external support has little to recommend it. The injection of sclerosing solutions into the tissues around a hernia, at one time a popular method of therapy, is mentioned only to be condemned.

Once the decision is made to perform an elective herniorrhaphy, it is a general rule that the operation should not be delayed. However, the presence of some other illness, such as an infection of the upper respiratory tract or a recent myocardial infarction, justifies delay. With premature infants it is wise to wait until the child is making satisfactory progress nutritionally so that the risk of anesthesia is decreased. With other infants many surgeons would prefer not to operate before the infant is ten weeks of age, since by this time the hemoglobin level is returning from its postnatal dip. Whenever operation is delayed for any reason, however, it should be realized that there is always the possibility of strangulation, which changes an elective situation into an emergency. Elderly patients with hernias are just as prone to strangulation as younger, more vigorous individuals, and old age per se should not be considered a contraindication to an elective herniorrhaphy.

When the patient has no systemic signs such as fever or leukocytosis, one preoperative effort to reduce an acutely incarcerated hernia is permissible. An ice bag should be applied to the local area and an appropriate dose of morphine given parenterally. With a groin hernia the patient should be placed in the Trendelenburg position as well. After 30 to 40 min, gentle sustained pressure over the mass may effect reduction without undue difficulty. The sensation that some gas has moved within the intestine frequently presages successful reduction. No more than one such effort should be attempted prior to emergency operation, and the presence of systemic symptoms and signs contraindicates even this effort. Because of the small area below the inguinal ligament and medial to the femoral vein, reduction of an incarcerated femoral hernia is virtually impossible and should not be attempted. If these rules are followed, the reduction of a hernia en masse—that is, with the contained organ still strangulated—should not occur. The advantage of reducing an incarcerated hernia is that a repair 2 or 3 days later can be done at a time when edema has subsided, thus permitting a better herniorrhaphy. Also, if other medical problems are present, the patient's general condition may be improved preoperatively, thus permitting a safer operative and postoperative course.

Operative Repair

PRINCIPLES. In any herniorrhaphy there are two essential steps to consider: (1) the management of the peritoneal sac and its contents, and (2) the repair of the fascial defect. If the sac is a narrow-necked diverticulum, the proximal part of the sac is usually excised. Although the neck is usually closed, this step is not essential. There is no need to remove the entire distal portion of the sac. In a complete indirect inguinal hernia, removing that portion of the sac that is adherent to the testicle is contraindicated. Doing so may result in testicular damage. When the distal sac is left in situ, it is merely transected, leaving the cut end of the retained sac open. Closing the end invites the development of a hydrocele. If it is a broad-based bulge, the peritoneum is usually not opened; rather, it is reduced intact beneath the fascia and held there by the fascial repair. Management of the sac is complicated when a sliding hernia is present or when intraperitoneal organs are fixed within the sac by adhesions. If adhesions inside the sac are suspected, it is vital to make certain that the situation is not in reality a sliding hernia. Once the surgeon is convinced that adhesions are holding an organ *within* the peritoneal sac, these adhesions must be carefully divided to effect reduction of the incarcerated contents. The sac itself is then managed in the usual fashion. The presence of a sliding hernia requires that the organ forming part of the wall of the sac be returned to the abdomen before the sac is excised. If this condition is anticipated and recognized, direct reduction of the sliding organ from the groin through the fascial defect is usually possible. The peritoneal sac is then excised without injury to the bowel or its blood supply. Rarely, an adjacent separate incision into the peritoneal cavity may be required to reduce the viscus from above, but the need for this has been overemphasized in the literature (Fig. 36-8).

Once the peritoneal sac has been satisfactorily managed, attention is turned to the associated fascial defect. When the patient is a youngster with a congenital indirect inguinal hernia, the opening in the transversalis fascia around the internal inguinal ring may not be dilated, and repair may not be required. In almost all other circumstances, however, closing or decreasing the size of this defect is vital. In certain circumstances the fascial margins of the defect can be approximated satisfactorily after adequate mobilization; this technique is applicable to most umbilical hernias, congenital or acquired, that require repair. In other instances an adjacent fascial relaxing incision makes possible a primary closure that would not otherwise be feasible. In some circumstances, especially when a large defect is present, repair will require

the use of some substance introduced from elsewhere. An autogenous fascial graft, usually from the fascia lata, or an inert foreign body may be used for this purpose. A solid sheet of foreign material cannot be effectively organized by the body. Rather, it tends to become incorporated in a loose pocket or rejected altogether. Consequently, if an inert foreign material is selected, it should be in the form of a mesh that can be invaded and incorporated by the host's fibroblasts during the organization phase of wound healing. Formerly, screens of this type were constructed of a metal such as tantalum. Because metal screens fragment, current practice involves the use of a synthetic screen made from polypropylene (Marlex) or Dacron (Mersilene).

Following satisfactory repair of any hernia, it is traditional for the surgeon to advise against heavy lifting and other vigorous effort for 4 to 8 weeks. The rationale for this advice is to permit proper healing of the repaired tissues. Dunphy's studies indicate that collagen maturation and gain in tensile strength of the wound continue over many months, and this process is not complete within 4 weeks even under ideal circumstances. Studies by Lichtenstein and colleagues suggest that for at least the first 2 months strength of a repaired wound depends primarily upon an intact suture line. In their experiments, the sutured wound showed 70 percent of intact tissue strength immediately, and there was no appreciable gain in strength during the next 8 weeks. The 4-week period of inactivity is perhaps a satisfactory compromise, postponing vigorous effort until some degree of healing has occurred, but it should be recognized that the basis for the recommendation is empiric rather than scientific. Currently some surgeons who routinely employ mesh in the repair place no restriction on the patient's postoperative activities. Lichtenstein permits any activity with which the patient is comfortable.

STRANGULATED HERNIAS

When emergency operation is undertaken for a hernia with strangulated contents, it is vital that the operation be performed in such a manner that the contents of the sac can be inspected before reduction. To achieve this, it is necessary to open the sac early in the dissection and gain control of the structures within it. If operation has been done early enough, the prompt return of circulation to strangulated tissue indicates viability. Reduction is then effected and routine repair carried out. When gangrene has already developed, all gangrenous tissue must be resected. When strangulated intestine is present, this entails the construction of an anastomosis between normal bowel sections proximal and distal to the necrotic area. In some circumstances tissue viability is not so easily defined. Bowel of doubtful viability should be covered with a warm moist towel and reinspected after 5 min. Improved color of the bowel wall, passage of a peristaltic wave through the strangulated segment, or pulsation in the arcuate arteries usually indicate that the intestine will survive if returned to the peritoneal cavity. Intestine of

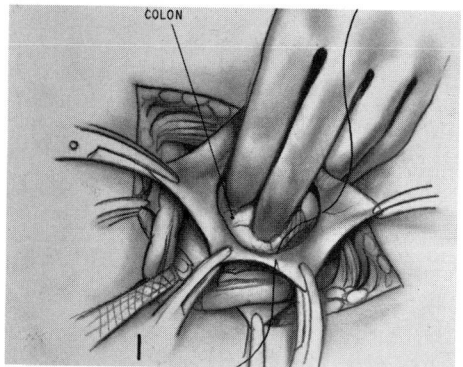

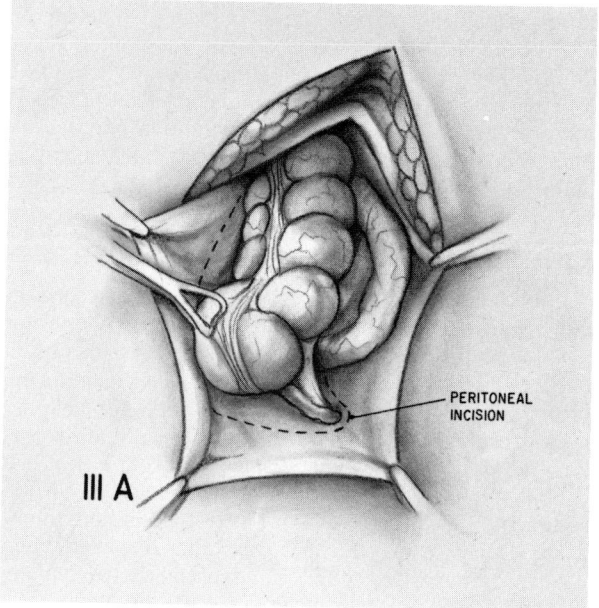

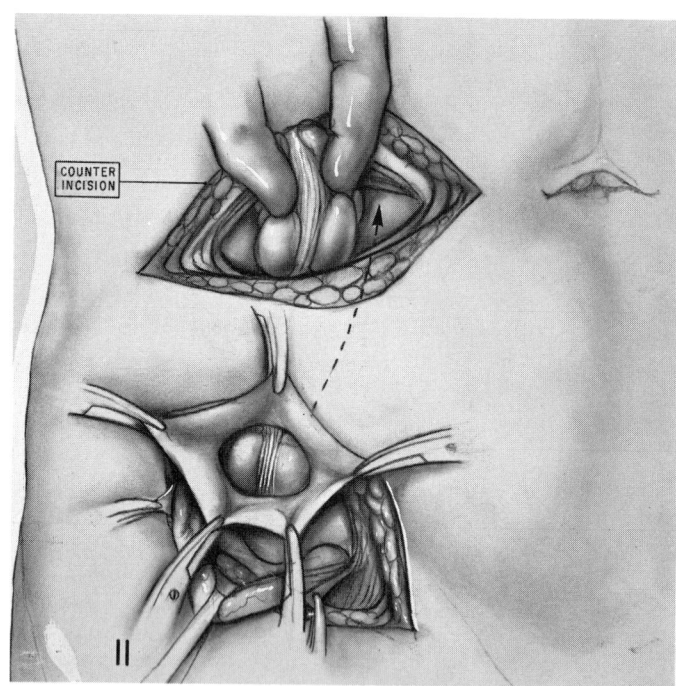

Fig. 36-8. Repair of sliding hernias. I. In simplest method, intestine, forming part of posterior wall of hernia sac, is directly reduced into abdomen, permitting closure of peritoneum and reconstruction of internal ring below it. II. Rarely, counterincision entering peritoneum above sac is needed to permit reduction of intestine by traction. III. *A,B,C.* Some surgeons free the sliding organ from the peritoneal sac *(A)*. The posterior surface of the organ is then peritonealized *(B)*, and the peritoneum is then closed at the internal ring *(C)*. This procedure seems time-consuming and unnecessary.

questionable viability should be resected, since reduction of bowel that is not viable may lead either to early perforation with peritonitis or to late stricture with intestinal obstruction. Unnecessary intestinal resection of poorly prepared bowel increases morbidity and mortality.

GROIN HERNIAS

Many surgeons make the mistake of performing the same operation for all hernias in the groin. A proper evaluation of the anatomy in the area makes it evident that indirect, direct, and femoral hernias are different anatomic problems requiring different repairs.

Groin hernias can be successfully repaired with general, spinal, or local anesthesia. Recently there has been increasing use of local anesthesia, and many herniorrhaphies are done successfully through ambulatory surgery centers. When local anesthesia is employed, preoperative sedation with diazepam is useful. The ilioinguinal and iliohypogastric nerves should be blocked just above and medial to the anterior superior iliac spine. The nerves lie deep to the external oblique aponeurosis at this level.

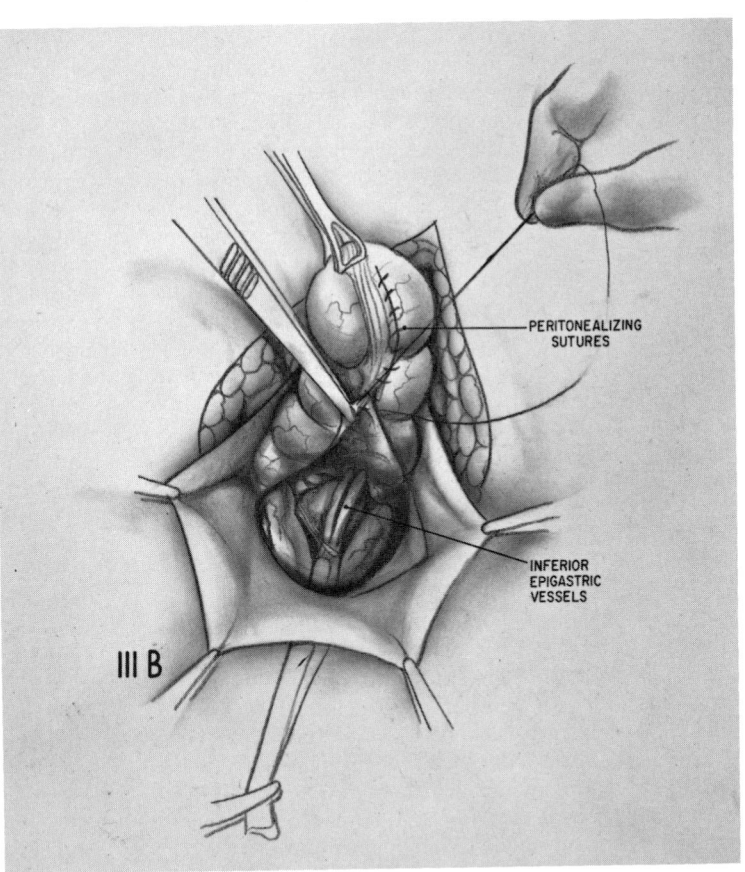

III B

PERITONEALIZING
SUTURES

INFERIOR
EPIGASTRIC
VESSELS

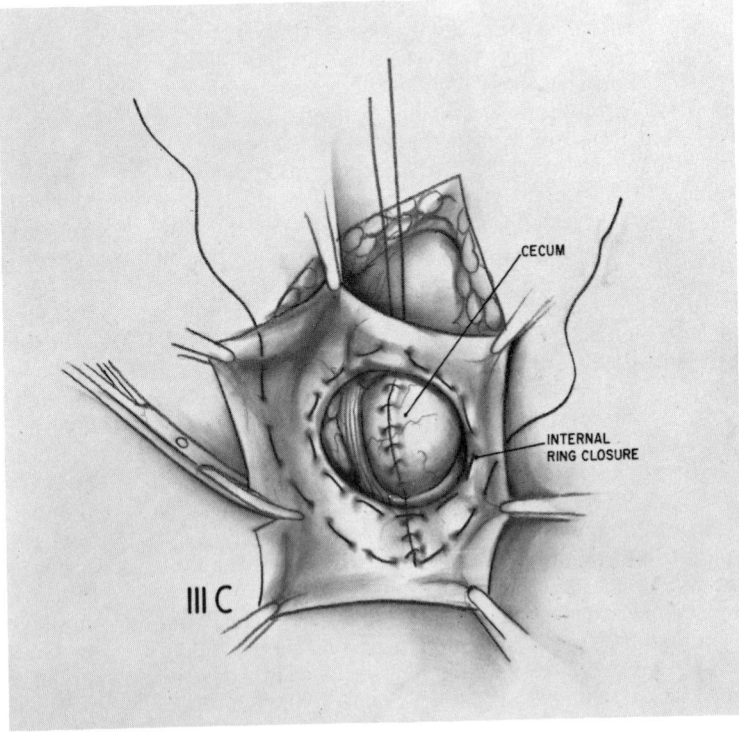

III C

CECUM

INTERNAL
RING CLOSURE

Fig. 36-8 III *B*, III *C*. Continued.

In addition, subcutaneous infiltration of the incision site and deeper injection of the area around the pubic tubercle are required. Xylocaine is an appropriate agent to employ. To avoid administering a possibly toxic dose, a 0.5% solution is used, and in most circumstances 30 to 40 mL of solution is adequate for the entire procedure. Unless the patient has cardiac disease making tachycardia undesirable, epinephrine in the anesthetic solution slows absorption and lengthens the time of effective anesthesia. At the end of the operation the field can be infiltrated with a long-acting anesthetic such as 0.25% bupivacaine to provide postoperative pain relief. Because bupivacaine takes effect slowly, it is not convenient to use it as the sole agent during the operation itself.

Certain authors suggest that the femoral hernia be repaired through a vertical incision over the femoral triangle. However, it is generally agreed that a better anatomic repair can be achieved through the groin. All groin hernias therefore should be approached through an incision above the inguinal ligament. Most frequently the incision is made above and parallel to the medial portion of the inguinal ligament; some surgeons extend this incision laterally almost to the iliac spine, but the lateral portion of the wound does not facilitate exposure and should be omitted. The subcutaneous tissue is incised and the external oblique aponeurosis exposed. The external oblique is then opened through the external inguinal ring, taking care not to injure the ilioinguinal nerve. The nerve is frequently adherent at the external ring; hence the aponeurosis should be opened from above downward to prevent nerve injury. Usually, the nerve is readily identified as a grayish white structure with a small red blood vessel on its surface, running parallel to the external oblique fibers. Moosman and Oelrich have found that the nerve lies inside the cremaster fibers in direct contact with spermatic cord structures in 35 percent of patients. By dividing those cremaster fibers that join the spermatic cord from the inguinal ligament, the cord is freed from the inguinal canal floor and a tape is passed around it at the level of the pubic tubercle. This step facilitates lifting the cord away from Hesselbach's triangle. The major portion of the cremaster muscle is then divided all the way around the cord at the internal inguinal ring, and it becomes possible to identify the type of hernia and isolate the structures required for fascial repair.

INDIRECT HERNIA. When an indirect hernia is present, the sac will be visible as a translucent white structure lying inside the cremaster fibers and anteromedial to the cord structures at the level of the internal inguinal ring. The sac may be obscured by a lobulated mass of fatty tissue, often incorrectly referred to as a "lipoma of the cord." In reality it represents a projection of fat from the retroperitoneal area. Typically the fat extends through the dilated internal inguinal ring lateral to the cord structures. Rarely, this retroperitoneal fat may be present without an associated peritoneal sac. In either instance it should be removed as part of the indirect hernia repair. Once the sac is identified, it is separated from the spermatic cord by sharp or blunt dissection back to the internal ring. If a sac is present extending through the external inguinal ring into the scrotum, it is neither necessary nor desirable to

remove the entire distal part of the sac. Rather, the sac should be transected at some convenient location along the inguinal canal. The distal sac is left in situ with its proximal end open. Leaving the distal sac in situ produces no problems and precludes injury to the testicle and cord structures secondary to dissection of the distal part of the sac. Wantz believes that this technique diminishes the possibility of postoperative ischemic orchitis and testicular atrophy. The vas deferens, which is usually adherent to the sac at the level of the internal ring, is the only cord structure that does not separate easily once the proper plane for dissection is entered. When the sac is adequately freed, it can be opened and any intraperitoneal contents reduced, with lysis of adhesions as necessary. If the hernia has a sliding component, it will form part or all of the posterior wall of the sac. This component should be manually replaced into the abdominal cavity before the hernia sac is excised.

A palpating finger can then be introduced into the peritoneal cavity through the open sac. The finger is brought up beneath the inguinal canal floor in Hesselbach's triangle to test the possibility of an associated direct hernia. Palpation beneath the inguinal ligament medial to the femoral vessels will disclose a femoral hernia if one is present. Directly behind this area the obturator membrane can be felt and an obturator hernia sought where the obturator artery and vein leave the true pelvis.

The sac is then transected at the level of the internal inguinal ring. In doing this it is well to remember that the parietal peritoneum is quite elastic and that by traction a good deal of peritoneum from the abdominal wall can be pulled through the ring. Depending upon the size of the peritoneal defect, it is usually closed with either a purse-string suture or a series of interrupted sutures of some nonabsorbable suture material. Some authors feel that no effort at closure of the neck of the sac is required.

Except in infants, in whom this step may be omitted because the internal ring is not dilated, the transversus abdominis aponeurosis below the spermatic cord should be reapproximated with a series of interrupted sutures (Fig. 36-9). This repair should be continued until it is barely possible to insert a small clamp through the internal ring alongside the cord. The external oblique muscle, subcutaneous tissue, and skin are then united over the cord, which occupies its usual location, passing obliquely through the inguinal canal. It is unnecessary to transplant the neck of the hernial sac superiorly beneath the abdominal muscles and unwise to move the cord into a subcutaneous location by closing the external oblique aponeurosis underneath it. If the medial inguinal canal floor is strong, this area should not be repaired. Indeed, Glassow suggests that in women direct recurrences may result from unnecessary dissection in Hesselbach's triangle during the initial operation. In closing the external oblique aponeurosis it is important to avoid passing a suture around the ilioinguinal nerve. Incorporating the nerve in a suture may lead to the development of a troublesome, painful neuroma.

When an indirect hernia has been neglected for a prolonged period, it may become very large, and the inferior epigastric vessels may be displaced medially all the way

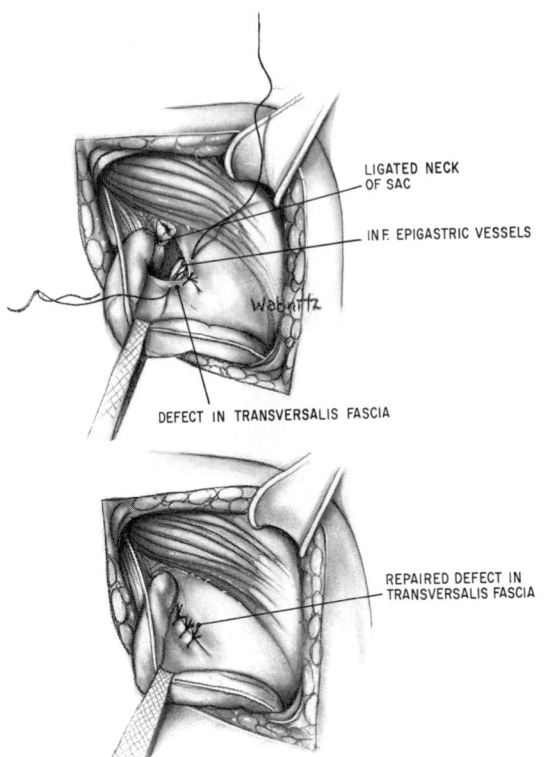

LIGATED NECK OF SAC

IN F. EPIGASTRIC VESSELS

DEFECT IN TRANSVERSALIS FASCIA

REPAIRED DEFECT IN TRANSVERSALIS FASCIA

Fig. 36-9. Indirect inguinal hernia repair. High ligation of sac is followed by closure of defect in transversus abdominis aponeurosis at internal inguinal ring.

to the pubic tubercle. In effect such a hernia is direct as well as indirect, and the area in Hesselbach's triangle should be managed in the manner adopted for a direct hernia. For large or recurrent indirect hernias it may be possible to achieve a more secure repair by dividing the cord at the internal ring and closing the defect completely at that level. Orchiectomy is usually performed along with cord transection. However, if the scrotum is not disturbed during operation and is handled gently after surgery, the testicle may be left in place with little likelihood that gangrene will occur.

SLIDING HERNIA. The most important step in operative management of a sliding hernia is recognition of the situation. On the right side the cecum and on the left the sigmoid colon or mesocolon may make up part of the posterior wall of an indirect sac, and failure to recognize this may lead to fecal contamination or to injury to colonic blood supply. The urinary bladder may be similarly involved in a direct sac, but since this type of sac is reduced unopened, the presence of bladder does not create a technical problem. Because a sliding component is present in only about 3 percent of groin hernias, the surgeon tends to forget the possibility. However, certain circumstances increase the likelihood of a sliding component. The surgeon should be wary when dealing with any hernia whose contents do not reduce readily. Any large indirect hernia, especially one of long standing in an elderly male, may be of the sliding type.

Most sliding hernias can be managed without undue difficulty. The peritoneal sac is identified and opened an-

teriorly away from the bowel or mesentery that makes up its posterior wall. The entire anterior portion of the sac is removed. Posteriorly as much sac as possible is removed without injuring the sliding bowel or its mesentery. The bowel is then reduced manually into its original retroperitoneal position and the defect in peritoneum is closed. The defect in the transversalis fascia at the internal inguinal ring is then closed in the same manner used for any indirect hernia, producing a snug internal ring. The herniorrhaphy is completed in whatever fashion is most appropriate to the remaining anatomic defect (Fig. 36-8I).

Rarely, when a long segment of colon is involved in the wall of the hernia, it may prove difficult to reduce the colon into its retroperitoneal position by manipulation from below. In these circumstances it is appropriate to enter the abdomen through a higher transverse incision so that the colon can be moved superiorly by traction from above, a procedure described by LaRoque. The abdomen may be entered through a fresh skin incision or by an extension of the groin incision, retracting the external oblique aponeurosis superiorly to facilitate the counterincision through the internal oblique, transversus abdominis, and peritoneum. In either event the colon is displaced from the internal ring by gentle traction and repair effected by excising the residual sac and carefully closing the internal ring (Fig. 36-8II).

Some surgeons consider it important to enter the abdomen in all cases and to dissect the herniated colon away from the peritoneal sac (Fig. 36-8IIIA). When the cecum is involved, these surgeons form a posterior peritoneal investment for this portion of the bowel by closing the margins of the peritoneal sac behind the cecum. In effect, this procedure makes an intraperitoneal organ out of one that previously lay retroperitoneally (Fig. 36-8IIIB). When the sliding hernia is on the left side involving the sigmoid, this procedure leaves a raw surface on the lateral aspect of the sigmoid mesocolon, and, again, closure of this area is advised. In addition, surgeons who advocate an abdominal approach to sliding hernias sometimes fix this freed colon higher in the abdomen by some kind of colopexy. Both these procedures are designed to decrease the incidence of recurrence when this type of hernia is repaired. However, both procedures are cumbersome, and the peritonealization of the posterior surface of the cecum is unsound anatomically. The hernia should not recur in any case if the internal ring is properly closed (Fig. 36-8IIIC).

DIRECT HERNIA. When a direct hernia is present instead of or in addition to an indirect hernia, a different type of repair is required. Here the weakness lies in the inguinal canal floor medial to the inferior epigastric artery. In most instances there is a general ballooning out in the area, and the peritoneum should be reduced beneath the reconstituted inguinal canal floor without being opened. In the unusual instances where a narrow-necked diverticulum of peritoneum is present, it should be managed in the same way as an indirect sac.

To restore the inguinal canal floor requires removal of attenuated fascia and reconstruction with a new and stronger layer. In some instances this layer can be developed from the strong aponeurotic portion of the transver-

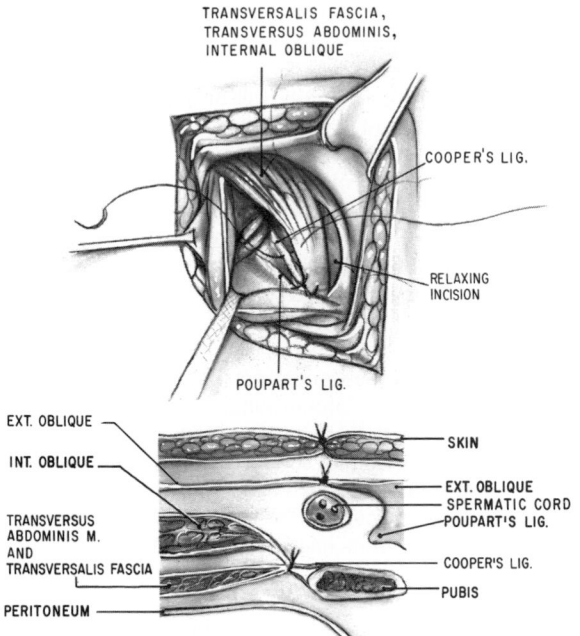

Fig. 36-10. Cooper's ligament repair. Cross section demonstrates level of repair; operative drawing shows placement of sutures in Cooper's ligament and relaxing incision in rectus sheath.

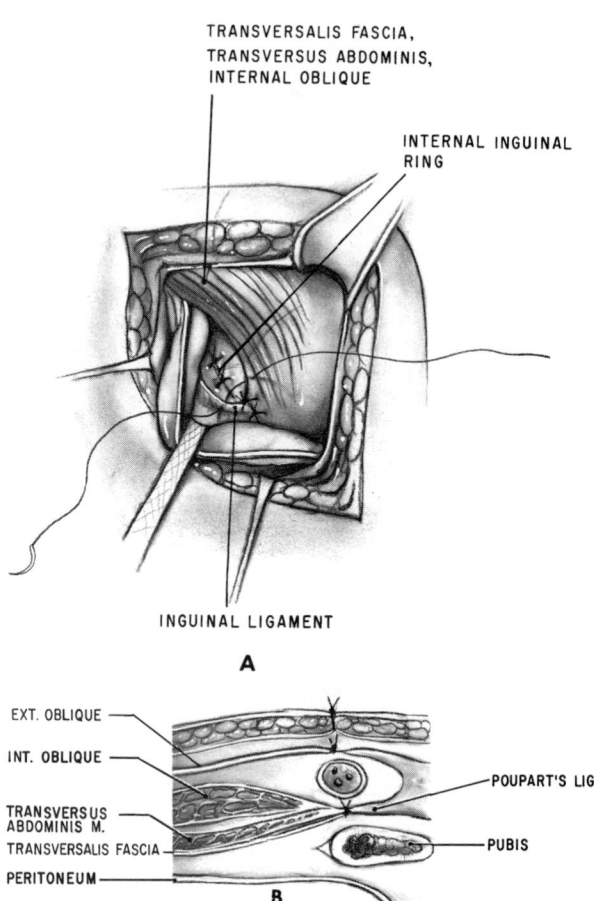

Fig. 36-11. Repair at level of inguinal ligament. Bassini operation remains standard against which other herniorrhaphies for direct inguinal hernia are judged; transversus abdominis aponeurosis as well as transversalis fascia should be incorporated in repair layer.

sus abdominis muscle which is found just superior to the weakness in the inguinal canal floor. If a curved relaxing incision is made in the inner layer of the rectus sheath where the internal oblique and transversus abdominis form a fused aponeurosis, it is usually not difficult to bring the transversus abdominis aponeurosis down across Hesselbach's triangle. This layer can then be approximated to Cooper's ligament (Fig. 36-10), to the iliopubic tract, an aponeurotic band superficial to Cooper's ligament, or to the shelving edge of Poupart's ligament (Fig. 36-11), depending upon the preference of the surgeon. If Poupart's ligament is used for the repair, there are several levels at which the spermatic cord may be placed. The cord lies beneath the repaired inguinal canal floor as far as the external inguinal ring in the Ferguson repair (Fig. 36-12) and in the later technique described by Halsted. In the Bassini herniorrhaphy (Fig. 36-11*B*) the cord lies on top of the repaired canal floor. In the Andrews operation (Fig. 36-13) the superior leaf of the incised external oblique aponeurosis is sutured to Poupart's ligament beneath the cord to reinforce the repair of the inguinal canal floor, and the inferior leaf of the external oblique is then sutured up over the cord. In the original Halsted operation (Fig. 36-14) the external oblique aponeurosis is closed underneath the cord as far laterally as the internal ring, thus transplanting the cord into the subcutaneous tissue. Halsted himself later abandoned this technique. Most of these operations are of historical interest only. Today the majority of surgeons employ some form of the Bassini operation. The Bassini repair involves bringing transversus abdominis aponeurosis rather than muscle fibers down to Poupart's ligament. Bassini emphasized

this point, although it has often been unwisely ignored by surgeons doing this type of repair. Bassini's technique—the first modern herniorrhaphy, originally described in 1887—has stood the test of time and remains today the standard against which the repair of direct inguinal hernias is judged.

Fig. 36-12. Ferguson operation. Spermatic cord is placed deep to reconstructed inguinal canal floor.

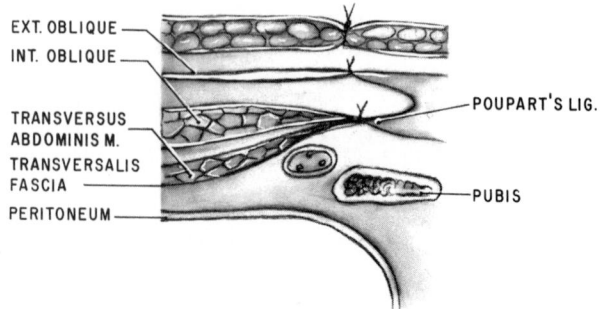

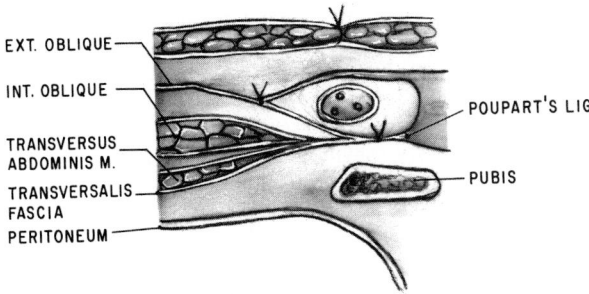

Fig. 36-13. Andrews operation. This involves suturing superior leaf of external oblique aponeurosis to shelving edge of Poupart's ligament beneath spermatic cord, with inferior leaf of external oblique sutured up over it.

McVay demonstrated that transversalis fascia normally attaches to Cooper's ligament, and theoretically transversalis fascia should be reapproximated to this ligament in direct hernia repairs. The procedure was first described by Lotheissen in 1898, and it is used in modified form by many surgeons today. However, this operation is technically more difficult than a repair to Poupart's ligament, and an adequate reconstruction based on Poupart's ligament will prevent recurrence of a direct hernia. Anatomically it is possible for a femoral hernia to develop below a Poupart's ligament repair, but if this actually occurs, it must be most unusual. If a Cooper's ligament repair is done, surgeons are faced with a problem when they reach the femoral vein, which passes in front of the ligament. From this point laterally the repair must be done at the more superficial Poupart's ligament level. Where the repair moves from Cooper's ligament to Poupart's ligament, there is a potential weakness, and recurrent herniation at this point is a distinct possibility. To prevent this weakness, McVay recommends suturing transversalis fascia to the medial side of the femoral sheath with one or two stitches as an intermediate step between the two levels of repair. The management of this area and the greater danger of injury to the femoral vein with a Cooper's ligament repair continue to be potential problems. Hence the majority of surgeons continue to prefer repair at the level of the inguinal ligament, and many good results have been

reported with this technique. Other surgeons feel that a Cooper's ligament repair for direct hernias is to be preferred whenever possible. A careful repair, beginning medially at the pubic tubercle and extending laterally to the internal ring, using strong tissue to cover the inguinal canal floor is probably more important than the level of the suture line. Glasgow emphasized excision of all weak tissue from the inguinal canal floor and the construction of a multilayered, overlapping floor repair using continuous sutures of an inert material. He believed that recurrent hernias could develop between stitches if interrupted sutures were used for the herniorrhaphy.

Whichever level is selected for repair, it must be remembered that the hernia developed through a weakened transversalis fascia initially. Therefore, although McVay does nothing further to the canal floor, many surgeons agree that the newly constituted transversalis fascia repair should be reinforced in some manner. The technique suggested by Zimmerman and Anson, employing the inferior portion of the incised external oblique aponeurosis as a pedicle flap brought underneath the cord and sutured to transversalis fascia superior to the free edge of the internal oblique muscle, is probably the best anatomically. Another technique involves turning down a flap from the inner layer of the rectus sheath beneath the cord and uniting it to Poupart's ligament, thus reversing the procedure advocated by Zimmerman and Anson. Still other surgeons prefer to place a free graft of autogenous fascia lata over the transversalis fascia repair. The graft is applied either as a single fascial sheet or as a mesh woven from fascial strips. In place of fascia lata, reinforcement can be done with a sheet of tantalum gauze or with a synthetic mesh sutured over the repaired Hesselbach's triangle beneath the cord. Because tantalum may break, leaving sharp metallic ends to traumatize neighboring structures, a synthetic material is preferred. Although synthetic mesh is relatively inert, there have been problems with its use. Increased morbidity and wound discomfort may be encountered when a mesh is employed. If a wound infection occurs, the patient may develop a draining wound sinus. Drainage may continue until the mesh is removed surgically. Under these circumstances the hernia is likely to recur. Despite these real and theoretic objections, the use of synthetic mesh is increasing. Lichtenstein believes that mesh should be used to bridge the defect in the inguinal canal floor and that no effort should be made to bring autogenous tissues together across the inguinal canal floor. He feels that this maneuver prevents the tension that may follow floor reconstruction with native tissue. However, most surgeons who use mesh employ it as a buttress to the floor repair. Once the inguinal canal floor is adequately repaired, the cord is replaced in the canal. External oblique aponeurosis, subcutaneous tissue, and skin are closed over it exactly as in the repair for indirect hernia.

FEMORAL HERNIA. The femoral hernia protrudes from the groin through the femoral ring underneath the inguinal ligament between the lacunar ligament medially and the femoral vein laterally. If transversalis fascia is strongly attached to Cooper's ligament, as is normally the case,

Fig. 36-14. Halsted's original repair. Spermatic cord is transplanted subcutaneously and inguinal canal closed beneath it. Halsted later abandoned this operation, and it is little used today.

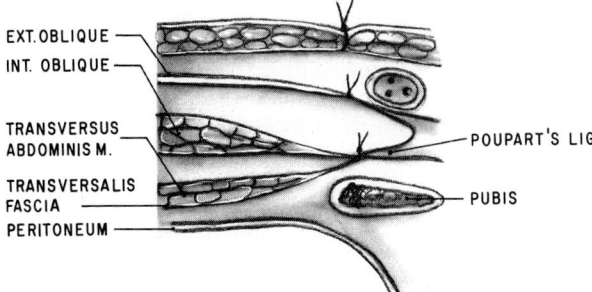

this creates a curtain that effectively prevents the peritoneum or any intraperitoneal structure from reaching the femoral ring. Thus the femoral hernia is a groin hernia and should be treated as such, with an incision above the inguinal ligament. When the inguinal canal is opened and the spermatic cord or the round ligament is retracted, a bulge will be evident beneath the transversalis fascia near the pubic tubercle. When the transversalis fascia is incised, the peritoneal neck of the hernia sac will be visible, and the surgeon thus has control of the sac and its contents. This is important especially when there may be strangulation of bowel in the sac, for the hernia should not be permitted to reduce before the viability of its contents has been ascertained. Attention may then be turned safely to the femoral triangle, where the peritoneal sac is dissected free from the subcutaneous tissues. Once the sac is freed, it is frequently possible to reduce it beneath the inguinal ligament by traction from above. Since the femoral ring is quite narrow, however, this reduction may not be possible without dividing the inguinal ligament transversely at the level of the hernia, thus releasing the sac. The continuity of the inguinal ligament is of little consequence, and it need not be restored.

After the contents of the sac are removed and returned to the peritoneal cavity, the sac itself is removed and its neck closed with a nonabsorbable purse-string suture. Anatomically, the best method of preventing recurrent herniation is to bring transversalis fascia down to Cooper's ligament exactly as described for the direct hernia. With the femoral hernia, transversalis fascia must be attached to Cooper's ligament rather than the inguinal ligament because herniation into the femoral triangle may recur beneath an inguinal ligament repair. Further reinforcement of the inguinal canal floor is then carried out, using the same approach described for the direct hernia.

Two other general methods for preventing recurrence of a femoral hernia have been advocated. In the first of these, the Moschcowitz technique, the femoral ring is obliterated by suturing Poupart's ligament to Cooper's ligament. In the second a pedicle of aponeurosis from the inferior margin of the external oblique incision is sutured down to Cooper's ligament. Both these methods effectively obliterate the femoral ring, but they do not strengthen the inguinal canal floor, so that development of a direct hernia through the weakened floor remains possible. Strengthening the inguinal canal floor through a femoral triangle incision is difficult or impossible; hence the incision above the inguinal ligament is preferred.

BILATERAL HERNIAS. It is possible to operate on bilateral groin hernias through two separate groin incisions as described above. Most surgeons feel that in adults it is better to stage these operations, rather than doing both simultaneously. The recurrence rate when bilateral repairs are done simultaneously in adults seems unacceptably high. If it is determined that both groins should be repaired at one time, it is more expeditious to use a Cheatle-Henry incision. In this approach a vertical lower-midline incision is made and carried down to the peritoneum, which is then reflected away from the lower abdominal wall. By traction upward on the abdominal wall it

is possible to dissect down to the inguinal triangle easily, and good exposure of Cooper's ligament is readily obtained. Transversalis fascia from the inner surface of the transversus abdominis can then be sutured down to Cooper's ligament under excellent direct vision to provide a satisfactory repair for either a direct or a femoral hernia. Reinforcement of the inguinal canal floor repair is not readily possible through this approach, and this represents a distinct disadvantage to its routine use. It is also somewhat more inconvenient, although not impossible, to deal with an indirect hernia. The major advantage of this approach is that bilateral hernias can be repaired much more rapidly. With a patient who is a poor anesthetic risk the resultant saving of time may be an important factor.

When an infant presents with a unilateral indirect inguinal hernia, there is perhaps 1 chance in 4 that a second undetected hernia is present on the opposite side. In the view of certain surgeons, this is sufficient reason for exploring the opposite side in all infants. Since right-sided hernias are somewhat more common than those on the left, this argument is advanced most strongly when a left-sided hernia is detected preoperatively. Since exploring the second side is a simple undertaking once the patient is under anesthesia, the argument seems superficially attractive. To carry out three negative explorations in the hope of finding one undetected hernia seems on reflection an unjustified meddling with normal tissues. Rather, a careful examination of both groins should precede any elective herniorrhaphy, and the second side should be explored only if there is reasonable suspicion of a defect on physical examination. It has been suggested recently that infant groin hernias may be identified preoperatively by injection of a radiopaque dye into the abdominal cavity followed by the exposure of an upright abdominal radiogram. Kiesewetter and Oh feel that the second side must be evaluated preoperatively and that herniography is an accurate procedure with few complications. Leape does not agree. He believes that positive herniography proves only a patent processus vaginalis and that many of these will close spontaneously without operative intervention.

UMBILICAL HERNIAS

When it has been decided that an umbilical hernia warrants surgical repair, a curved incision is made below the umbilicus and carried through subcutaneous fat to expose the anterior rectus sheath (Fig. 36-15). By dissecting superiorly toward the inferior margin of the defect, the surgeon delineates the peritoneal sac projecting through the fascial opening. Continued dissection at this level around the umbilicus defines the fascial defect and isolates the sac. The sac is then freed from the undersurface of the umbilical skin, and excess peritoneum is removed. Following closure of the peritoneum, the fascia above and below the defect is united by a series of nonabsorbable sutures. This repair is traditionally done by bringing the fascia above the defect down over the fascia from below to effect a two-layer closure—the so-called vest over

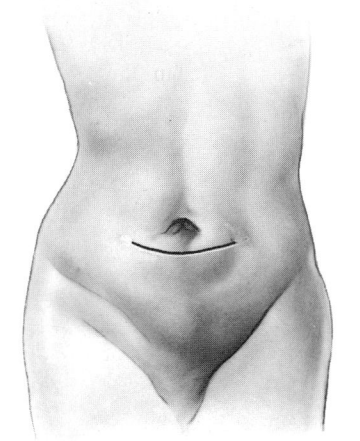

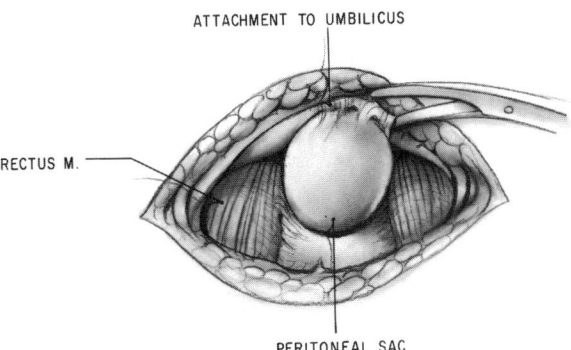

Fig. 36-15. Umbilical hernia repair. Curvilinear incision below the umbilicus gives excellent exposure. Sac must be freed by sharp dissection from undersurface of umbilicus.

pants type of repair (Fig. 36-16). These two fascial layers fuse, but there is no convincing proof that the resulting repair is any stronger than that produced by a careful approximation of fascial margins without undue tension. The umbilicus is then tacked down to the fascial repair

Fig. 36-16. Umbilical hernia repair. "Vest over pants" type of imbrication is traditionally used, but single layer, well apposed without imbrication, is equally effective.

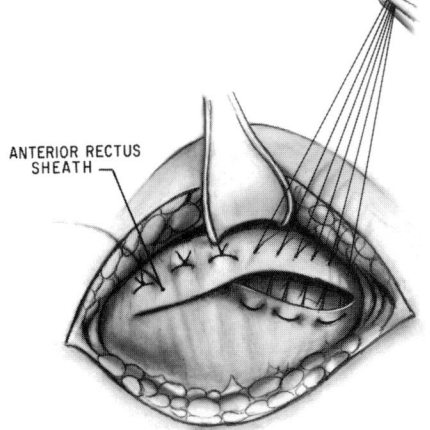

and the skin incision closed. When a large hernia has been repaired in an obese adult, it is desirable to drain the resulting dead space to prevent formation of a seroma in the incision; otherwise drainage is not employed. Formerly it was customary to excise the umbilicus during umbilical herniorrhaphy. This is unnecessary except when a proboscis-type defect is present, and the loss of the umbilicus is psychologically disturbing to many children and even to some adults. When, for technical reasons, removal of the umbilicus is desirable, the patient should be clearly informed of this preoperatively.

VENTRAL HERNIAS

The hernia that develops in an old operative incision may present a vexing problem in repair. Many hernias of this type can be successfully managed by a good external support. When operative repair is undertaken, the defect should be closed with local tissue if possible. The old operative scar can be excised or a fresh incision made perpendicular to it (Fig. 36-17A). In either event the first aim of the surgeon should be to dissect down to normal fascia all around the herniation. Dissection is then continued to separate the peritoneal sac from the margins of the fascial defect (Fig. 36-17B). The peritoneum is opened, the contents of the sac are appropriately managed, and excess peritoneum is removed. After closure of the peritoneal incision, the fascia is approximated to obliterate the hernia. If the initial defect was a small one, it may be possible to close it without undue tension by the use of interrupted sutures of some nonabsorbable material. With a larger defect, two relaxing incisions, one to either side of the original hernia, may make closure practical. This technique is particularly useful in the situation where the incisional hernia developed in a vertical midline or paramedian incision. The relaxing incisions are then made in the anterior rectus sheath, and midline approximation does not result in herniation laterally where the relaxing incisions were done (Fig. 36-17C). There is usually weak attenuated fascia surrounding the actual defect, and failure to extend the repair through this area is one of the common technical errors that frequently results in recurrence. Results with the repair of these hernias using local tissue have been poor. For this reason there has been increasing interest in the use of mesh. At one time a mesh of tantalum was used, but most surgeons now prefer a nonabsorbable synthetic such as polypropylene or Dacron. A mesh is used in preference to a solid sheet of material, because the mesh is incorporated by fibroplasia through the interstices while a solid sheet is usually rejected. Mesh is used either to bridge a gap in local tissue or to reinforce a repair constructed with weak scar tissue (Fig. 36-17D).

PARASTOMAL HERNIAS

A parastomal hernia is more apt to develop when the bowel is brought through the main abdominal incision. However, over time parastomal hernias develop with a large percentage of all permanent ileostomies or colostomies. Many of these defects are small and asympto-

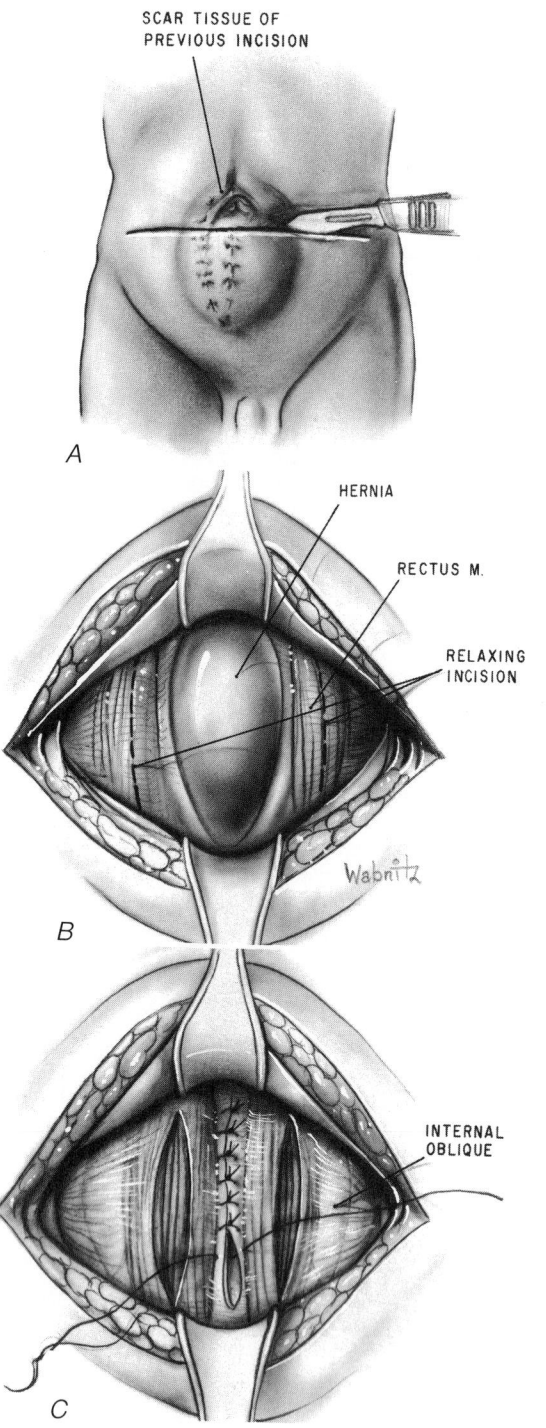

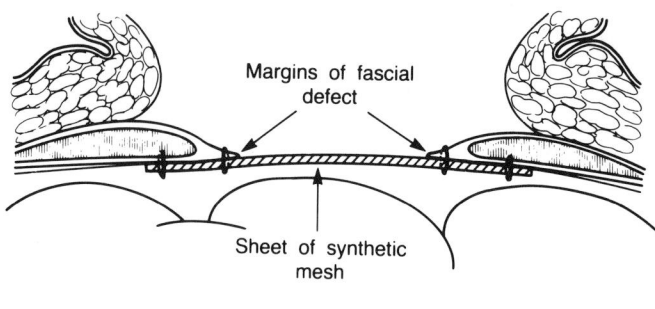

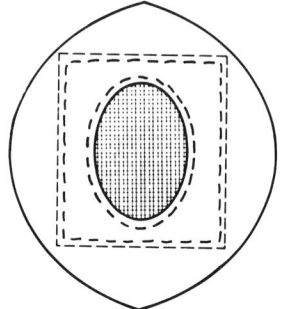

Fig. 36-17. Ventral hernia repair. *A.* It is frequently desirable to make fresh incision perpendicular to old hernia scar. *B.* Closure of fascial defect may be facilitated by making relaxing incision in rectus sheath to either side of hernia sac. *C.* Relaxing incisions permit good fascial approximation over defect without producing significant weakness in areas of relaxation. *D.* A piece of synthetic mesh placed below the fascial defect provides another method of repairing a large ventral hernia.

RESULTS

Uncomplicated herniorrhaphies have a negligible operative mortality, and results must be evaluated in terms of recurrence rate. Acutely incarcerated or strangulated hernias remain even today significant causes for morbidity and mortality.

The literature gives no basis for dogmatic statements about the results of herniorrhaphy. Most hernias can be satisfactorily treated, but a small number of recurrences can be expected. If patients undergoing herniorrhaphy are followed carefully for a long enough period of time, the number of known recurrences will, of course, increase.

As a general rule, hernias treated early yield better results, and recurrence following repair of an indirect inguinal hernia in an infant is quite unusual. Indirect hernias at any age have a lower recurrence rate than direct or femoral hernias. A rather high recurrence rate is to be anticipated following repair of postoperative ventral hernias, because they usually develop following some wound complication such as infection or dehiscence, with consequent weakness of the tissues available for repair.

matic. They may be satisfactorily managed by a well-made stoma belt. When operative repair is required, it is simplest to move the stoma to a new site and close the original defect completely. When this is not practical, Leslie describes a number of techniques, some involving the use of synthetic mesh, to repair the defect.

It is axiomatic that the first repair has the greatest chance of success and that recurrence is frequent following any secondary repair of a recurrent hernia. Glassow indicates that the recurrence rate for primary inguinal or femoral hernias in women should be less than 1 percent. On the other hand, the rate for recurrent femoral hernias after secondary surgery in women was 6.5 percent. Since one cause for recurrence is improper technique during the original operation, the importance of a proper initial approach is obvious. All too frequently a hernia is treated by a junior member of the staff without adequate supervision. No surgeon should undertake herniorrhaphy until thoroughly conversant with the anatomy of the area and the theory behind the technique of repair. When the hernia recurs months or years later, it is hard to blame a surgical error for the problem. On the basis of their experimental observations, Read and his associates claim that a direct inguinal hernia is a local manifestation of a generalized defect in collagen metabolism, either decreased production or increased destruction. Other workers have not accepted this hypothesis, and the etiology of those hernias which develop in adult life remains obscure.

Although McVay has reported recurrence rates as low as 0.6 percent for groin hernias, nationwide results do not approximate this degree of success. Zimmerman and Anson report from the literature recurrence rates varying between 2 and 30 percent for indirect hernias and between 4 and 33 percent for direct hernias. The recurrence rate for femoral hernias is harder to evaluate, but it probably approximates that for direct hernias. Certainly these results permit no ground for complacency. They emphasize the need for continued careful technique, with attention to detail and a proper evaluation of the type of repair appropriate for the hernia in question.

Complications of Herniorrhaphy

Most hernia repairs are straightforward operations with few complications. Wound infection is the most common problem. Infection may be confined to the superficial soft tissue with no side effects other than prolonged wound healing. A deeper infection or one that is neglected may result in recurrence of the hernia. An elective herniorrhaphy is a clean surgical procedure, and the administration of prophylactic antibiotics to prevent wound infection is not justified.

In any herniorrhaphy it is possible to injure bowel within the peritoneal sac. This is unlikely to occur unless the bowel is fixed in the sac by adhesions or forms part of the wall of the sac in a sliding hernia. Injury to bowel may occur while the surgeon is separating the intestine from the sac. A minor injury to bowel, if recognized and repaired, should cause little problem postoperatively. Exteriorization or bypassing of the injured intestine is not necessary.

The urinary bladder may be injured in a similar way when inguinal canal floor reconstruction is done for a groin hernia. The bladder lies directly behind Hesselbach's triangle and should be protected when this area

is undergoing repair. If the bladder is entered, the laceration should be closed appropriately. Suprapubic cystostomy is not necessary unless a bladder injury goes unrecognized at the initial operation.

In repair of a groin hernia it is possible to injure the testicle, the vas deferens, blood vessels, or nerves. If the testicle is delivered from the scrotum into the groin during operative manipulation, the organ is frequently swollen and tender postoperatively. Although this process may produce only prolonged postoperative discomfort, testicular atrophy may result. This is more common when the blood supply to the testis through the internal spermatic artery or vein is compromised. To prevent testicular injury, the surgeon should minimize manipulation of scrotal contents. There is no need to deliver the testicle from the scrotum into the groin during the operation, and it is not desirable to remove the peritoneal sac from the scrotum in a complete hernia.

It is possible but less likely that testicular problems will occur following injury to the internal spermatic vessels during the dissection of the spermatic cord. There is no need to divide these vessels while freeing the peritoneal sac from the structures of the cord, and vessel injury at this level is rare. On the other hand, the vas deferens is always in juxtaposition to an indirect hernia sac and must be separated from it. This dissection is carried out readily except at the level of the internal inguinal ring where the vas deferens is adherent to peritoneum and must be freed by sharp dissection. If the vas deferens is inadvertently divided, it should be repaired primarily with interrupted, fine, absorbable sutures.

In dissecting the inguinal canal floor it is possible to injure the inferior epigastric artery or vein along the lateral margin of Hesselbach's triangle. Damage to these vessels is not a problem if the surgeon recognizes the injury. The artery and vein can be divided and ligated without sequelae. Difficulty arises only if the injury is not recognized. Under these circumstances significant blood loss or secondary infection of a hematoma may occur.

Injury to the external iliac or common femoral vessels may occur when the surgeon is repairing the inguinal canal floor. This is most likely to happen when sutures are placed in the shelving edge of the inguinal ligament or the iliopubic tract at the level of the internal inguinal ring. At this point the major vessels are superficial, passing directly under the inguinal ligament into the thigh. A suture placed injudiciously may injure a vessel, the common femoral vein being in greatest jeopardy. If significant bleeding occurs when a suture is placed, the suture should be removed and pressure applied. If bleeding continues, the vessel must be exposed and repaired. Although major vascular injury is very rare after herniorrhaphy, severe intermittent claudication has been reported after unrecognized arterial injury during the operation.

An accessory obturator artery, a branch from the inferior epigastric artery to the posterior aspect of the pubis, is present in some patients. This artery is more superficially placed than the main obturator artery, a branch of the hypogastric artery with which it anastomoses. An accessory obturator artery may be injured by sutures repairing the medial inguinal canal floor. If the injury is recognized and the vessel ligated, no serious difficulties arise. Failure to control the bleeding may lead to a hematoma in the inguinal canal floor.

The iliohypogastric, ilioinguinal, or genitofemoral nerve may be injured during groin herniorrhaphy. Injury to the ilioinguinal nerve is most common since the nerve lies on the anterior surface of the spermatic cord. The nerve is frequently adherent to external oblique aponeurosis at the level of the external inguinal ring and is most vulnerable at that point. Division of the nerve is not a major problem, producing only loss of the cremasteric reflex and a small area of hypesthesia inferomedial to the incision. The sensory change is usually self-limited and regresses with time. Trapping the nerve, either by a suture or by heavy postoperative scarring, is a more serious problem. In these circumstances the patient may experience severe local pain. It is characteristically burning or lancinating and is aggravated by motion, radiating along the distribution of the nerve. The surgeon may be able to identify a trigger point during physical examination. Although repeated nerve blocks may control this discomfort, it is usually necessary to resect the involved nerve, leaving a proximal nerve stump away from the site of the neuroma in scar tissue. When the genitofemoral nerve is involved, it is simpler to approach the nerve through a lateral extraperitoneal incision.

SUMMARY

Hernias are among the most common afflictions of mankind. Although the operative results are not perfect, repair of an uncomplicated hernia prevents the possibility of intestinal obstruction or gangrene secondary to hernial incarceration. Both these complications remain potentially lethal and entail a prolonged convalescence at best. Therefore it is a general rule that—save for the congenital umbilical hernias, which are likely to close spontaneously, and for certain postoperative incisional hernias— all hernias of the abdominal wall should be subjected to prompt operative correction. When it is elected for medical reasons not to repair a hernia of the abdominal wall, it must be remembered that, with a poor-risk patient, the danger of emergency operation for strangulation is greatly increased. If good results are to be anticipated from operation, the surgeon must have a thorough knowledge of the involved anatomy and a respect for tissues. A repair that is appropriate to the type of defect present must be se-

lected, and the patients must be followed carefully so that the surgeon can profit from his or her mistakes.

Bibliography

Carlson RI: The historical development of the surgical treatment of inguinal hernia. *Surgery* 39:1031, 1956.

Carmichael DH, Vorse HB: Female inguinal hernias and testicular feminization. *South Med J* 74:772, 1981.

Condon RE: Surgical anatomy of the transversus abdominis and transversalis fascia. *Ann Surg* 173:1, 1971.

Dunphy JE: Wound healing, in Rob C, Smith R (eds): *Clinical Surgery,* vol 1. London, Butterworth, pp 219–232.

Gauderer MWL, Grisoni ER, et al: Transverse testicular ectopia. *J Pediatr Surg* 17:43, 1982.

Glassow F: Inguinal hernia repair, a comparison of the Shouldice and Cooper ligament repair of the posterior inguinal wall. *Am J Surg* 131:306, 1976.

Halverson K, McVay CB: Inguinal and femoral hernioplasty: 22-year study of authors' methods. *Arch Surg* 101:127, 1970.

Kiesewetter WB, Oh KS: Unilateral inguinal hernias in children. What about the opposite side? *Arch Surg* 115:1443, 1980.

Leslie D: The parastomal hernia. *Surg Clin North Am* 64:407, 1984.

Lichtenstein IL, Shore JM: Exploding the myths of hernia repair. *Am J Surg* 132:307, 1976.

McGregor DB, Halverson K, et al: The unilateral pediatric inguinal hernia: Should the contralateral side be explored? *J Pediatr Surg* 15:313, 1980.

Margoles JS, Braun RA: Properitoneal versus classical hernioplasty. *Am J Surg* 121:641, 1971.

Moosman DA, Oelrich TM: Prevention of accidental trauma to the ilioinguinal nerve during inguinal herniorrhaphy. *Am J Surg* 133:146, 1977.

Nyhus LM, Condon RE (eds): *Hernia,* 2d ed. Philadelphia, Lippincott, 1978.

Ralphs DNL, Brain AJL, et al: How accurately can direct and indirect inguinal hernias be distinguished? *Br Med J* 280:1039, 1980.

Ravitch MM, Hitzrot JM II: The operations for inguinal hernia. *Surgery* 48:439, 1960.

Read RC, White HJ: Inguinal herniation 1777–1977. *Am J Surg* 136:651, 1978.

Thompson W, Longerbeam JK, Reeves C: Herniograms, an aid to the diagnosis and treatment of groin hernias in infants and children. *Arch Surg* 105:71, 1972.

Wagh PV, Leverich AP, et al: Direct inguinal herniation in men: A disease of collagen. *J Surg Res* 17:425, 1974.

Wantz GE: Complications of inguinal hernia repair. *Surg Clin North Am* 64:287, 1984.

Zimmerman IM, Anson BJ: *The Anatomy and Surgery of Hernia.* Baltimore, Williams & Wilkins, 1953.

Chapter 37

Pituitary and Adrenal

Richard M. Bergland, Donald S. Gann, and Eric J. DeMaria

PITUITARY

(Richard M. Bergland)

Historical Background

Harvey Cushing, near the end of his career, wrote:

I was once told by Professor Kocher, who I suppose had his experiences with the thyroid in mind, that no satisfactions in medicine were so great as those which came from concentration upon and the mastery of a small subject, and that this necessitated an approach from all aspects; diagnostic, experimental, pathological, and therapeutic, not the least important part of which at one time or another in the history of the subject was likely to be surgical.

Cushing must have heeded Kocher's advice and could surely have been satisfied with his lifelong productive involvement with the pituitary gland. He was the first to describe the syndrome of chiasmal compression, the first to demonstrate the usefulness of radiographs in the diagnosis of pituitary tumors, the first to emphasize that the pituitary holds the dominant position in the endocrine orchestra, the first to describe the hyposecretion associated with chromophobe tumors and the hypersecretion of both eosinophilic and basophilic tumors, and the first surgeon to operate successfully on a large series of patients with pituitary problems.

Remarkably, Harvey Cushing proposed in 1910 that pituitary secretions were released into the ventricle. This proposal has not been generally accepted, but Cushing maintained this belief throughout his career and in 1930 studied the physiological effects of pituitrin injected into the ventricles of humans. The discovery of the tanycyte ependyma, coupled to the reassessment of the vascular anatomy of the pituitary, lends credibility to Cushing's hypothesis. If pituitary secretions are indeed secreted directly to the brain, most of what we now know about the pituitary, and about the brain, will require rethinking.

Cushing's contributions to the understanding of the pituitary are of eternal significance; no other surgeon has made such a profound and lasting impact on any other organ system. The biography of this remarkable man should be read by every student of surgery; predictably some students reading this chapter will enter surgical research and carry on the rewarding tradition passed from Kocher to Cushing.

Gross Anatomy

The pituitary and its parts are schematically illustrated in Fig. 37-1. Unfortunately, pituitary nomenclature is not well standardized, but that of Wislocki is recommended. In his terminology, the *neurohypophysis* is composed of three parts: the infundibulum (which is often termed the

median eminence), the infundibular stem (which is often termed the pituitary stalk), and the infundibular process (which is variably designated posterior lobe, posterior pituitary, or pars nervosa).

Wislocki separated the *adenohypophysis* into the pars distalis (often called the anterior lobe or anterior pituitary), the pars intermedia, and the pars tuberalis.

In clinical medicine the terms "median eminence," "pituitary stalk," "anterior pituitary," and "posterior

Fig. 37-1. A schematic illustration of the parts of the human pituitary, as well as the projection of parvicellular and magnocellular neurons into the neurohypophysis.

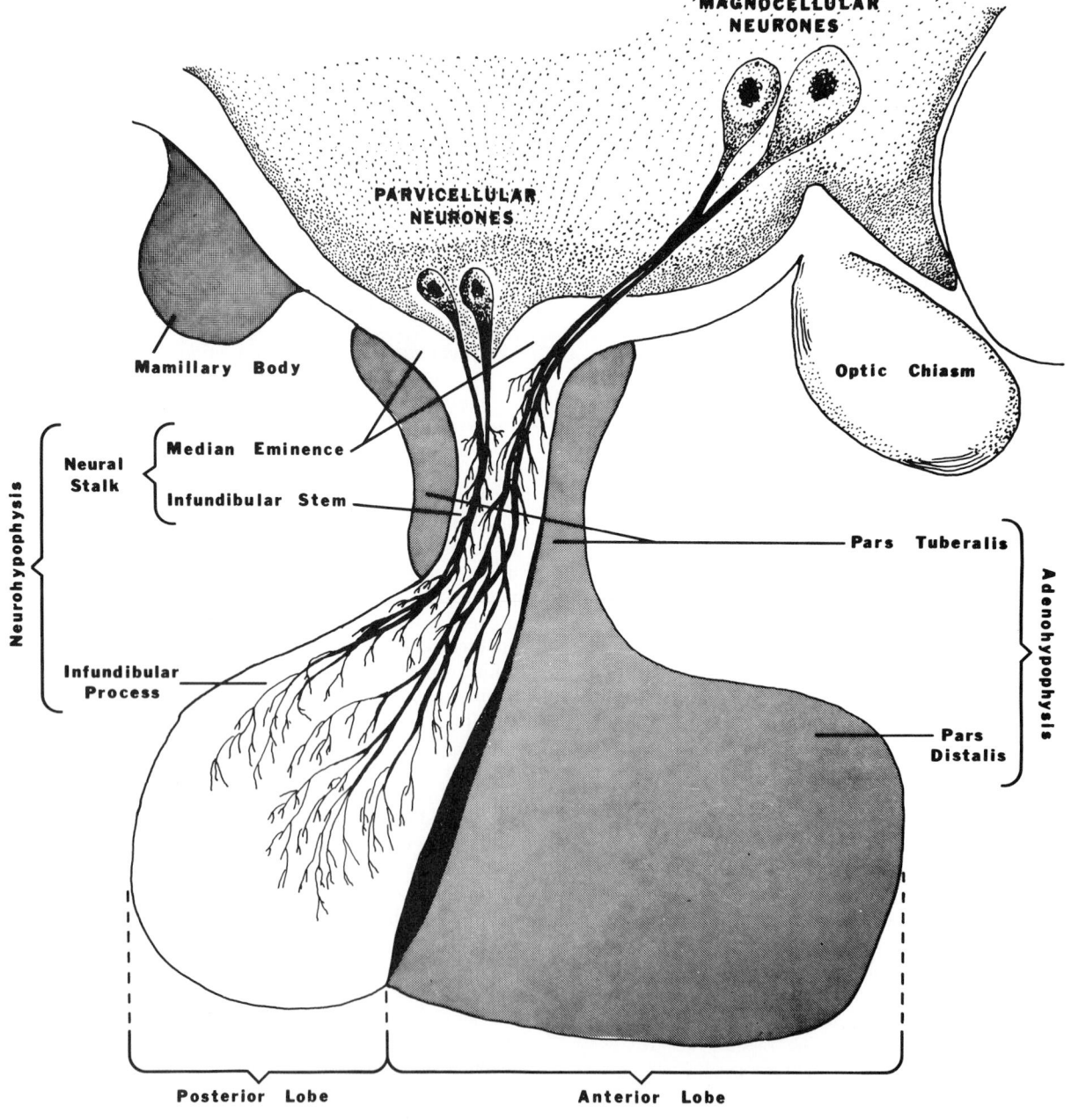

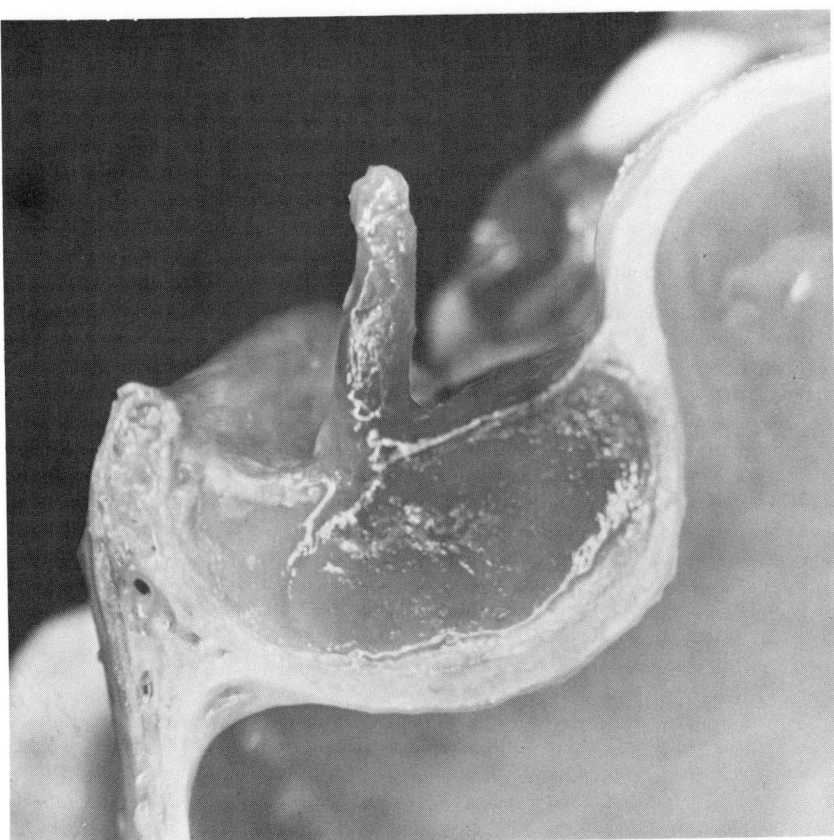

Fig. 37-2. A midline sagittal section of the human pituitary in situ within the sella. The height of the pituitary does not match the depth of the sella.

pituitary'' have gained general acceptance. But in basic research in other species, Wislocki's terminology is employed more often; an understanding of terms is essential if one is to apply laboratory observations to the understanding of clinical problems.

HUMAN ANATOMIC VARIATIONS. The adult human pituitary does not have a distinct pars intermedia (Fig. 37-2); the basophils that invade the human posterior pituitary might be considered the functional counterpart of the pars intermedia found in other species.

The pars tuberalis varies in human beings; sometimes the entire pituitary stalk is surrounded by secreting adenohypophyseal cells, but in other instances, the surface of the stalk is totally devoid of adenohypophyseal cells.

In 50 percent of human beings, the sella turcica is covered by the dura of the diaphragma sella, and the intrasellar space is thus separated from the intracranial space. In 40 percent of human beings, the opening in the diaphragma that surrounds the pituitary stalk is greater than 5 mm (Fig. 37-3), and in 10 percent of human beings, the diaphragma is extremely thin. Without the sturdy barrier of the diaphragma sella, a pituitary tumor may preferentially extend into the suprasellar region; with a sturdy, complete diaphragma, a growing tumor will preferentially enlarge and balloon the sella.

The height of the human pituitary does not match the depth of the sella (Fig. 37-2), and the width of the pituitary does not match the width of the sellar floor; thus plain x-rays permit assessment of the length of the pituitary but not of its height or its width.

Not infrequently the lateral margins of the pituitary are indented by the carotid arteries, and during pituitary procedures the carotids may be damaged. For this reason, most surgeons advocate careful preoperative study of carotid artery anatomy.

VASCULAR ANATOMY. The neurohypophysis is one of the seven areas of brain that does not have a blood-brain barrier. Its capillaries have a fenestrated endothelium (brain capillaries have no fenestrations) and are surrounded by a double basement membrane (brain capillaries have a single basement membrane). A distinct plane can be drawn between the neurohypophysis and the hypothalamus by the characteristics of the capillaries of each. No neuronal cell bodies are found within the neurohypophysis; all the axons projecting to the neurohypophysis are derived from hypothalamic neurons.

All the elements of the neurohypophysis (the median eminence, stalk, and posterior pituitary) are joined by a common capillary bed, and the direction of blood flow within that capillary bed is variable. The adenohypophysis does not receive a direct arterial supply; all blood reaching it must pass first through the capillary bed of the neurohypophysis.

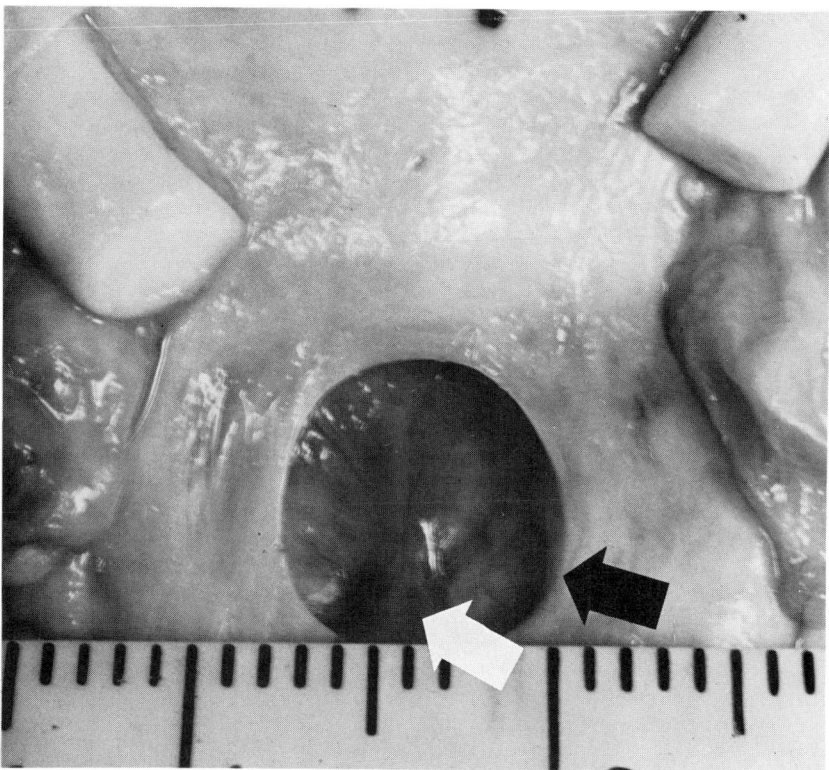

Adenohypophyseal capillaries resemble those of the neurohypophysis. No nerves terminate within the adeno-hypophysis, but neurosecretory material is conveyed by pituitary portal vessels from the neurohypophysis to the adenohypophysis. It has been established that some portal vessels carry adenohypophyseal secretions back to the neurohypophysis (Figs. 37-4 and 37-5).

Fig. 37-4. A vascular cast of the monkey pituitary. Very few connections are found between the capillary bed of the adenohypophysis (A) and the cavernous sinus (CS). This suggests that some blood must exit from the adenohypophysis via other routes.

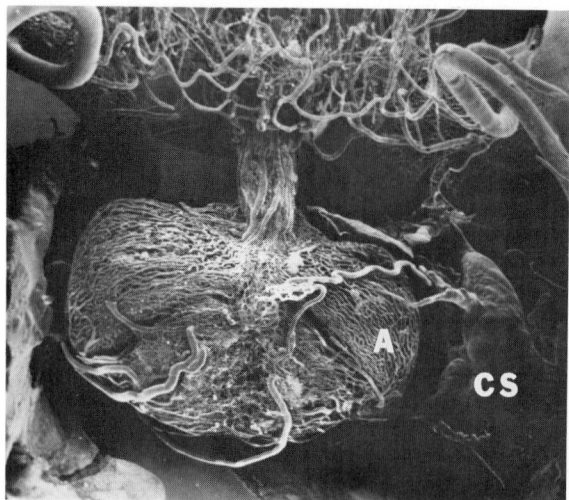

Fig. 37-3. The chiasm has been removed to expose the diaphragma sella. The opening in the diaphragm is about 7 mm in diameter (black arrow), much greater than the penetrating pituitary stalk (white arrow). In 40 percent of human beings, this opening is greater than 5 mm.

In other species the secreting cells within the pars intermedia have a limited capillary bed but are well innervated; in the human being those basophils that invade the posterior pituitary are also directly innervated.

The distortion of the normal vascular relationships of the pituitary by tumor growth may play an important role in the endocrine disturbances that develop with pituitary tumors, but the current techniques of angiography do not allow the visualization of pituitary vascular anatomy.

Cellular Physiology

THE NEUROHYPOPHYSIS

Hypothalamic neurons with large cell bodies (the *magnocellular neurons* of the supraoptic and paraventricular nuclei) project to the neurohypophysis, and most of them terminate near capillaries within the posterior pituitary (Fig. 37-1). The dense-core neurosecretory granules in these neurons measure about 2000 Å in diameter and are composed of small peptides coupled to the larger carrier protein neurophysin. At the nerve terminals the small peptides are uncoupled from neurophysin and released into the capillary bed of the neurohypophysis. Two kinds of small peptides are present: vasopressin and oxytocin. Vasopressin has many systemic actions, but most interest

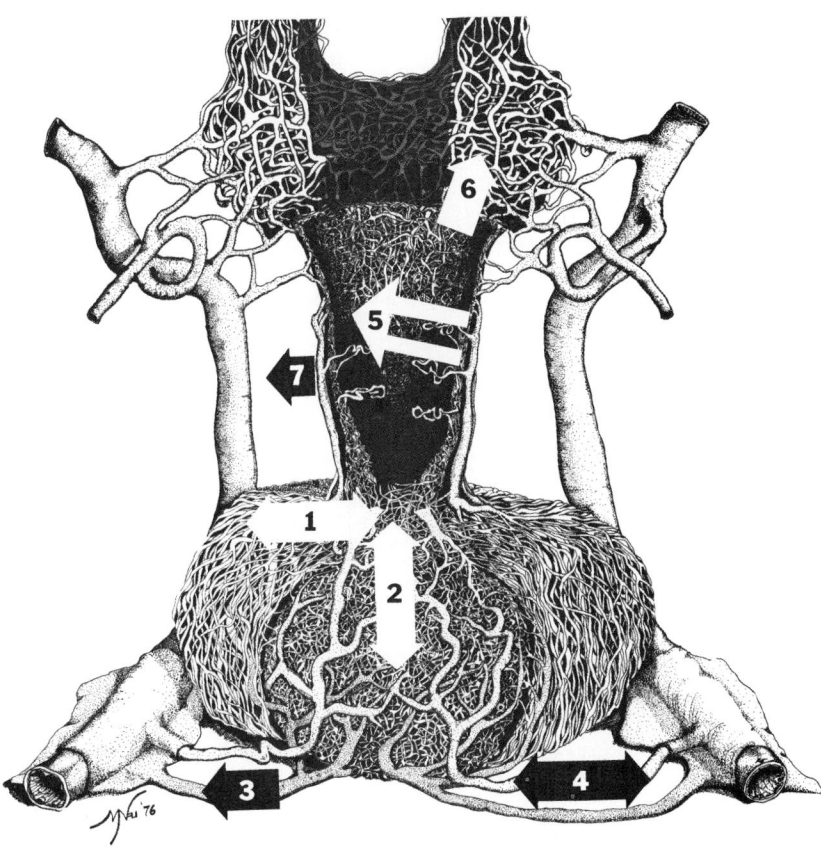

Fig. 37-5. The vascular relationships of the primate pituitary; arrows indicate the potential directions of blood flow. (1) In some portal vessels, flow may be *into* or *out of* the adenohypophysis. (2) Flow reversal may occur within the neurohypophysis. (3) Flow may occur from the posterior pituitary directly to the cavernous sinus. (4) Recent evidence suggests that flow reversal may occur in certain hypophyseal arteries. (5) Tanycytes may carry pituitary secretions into the ventricle. (6) Capillaries may carry hypophyseal blood directly to the hypothalamus. (7) Fenestrations within endothelial cells of the pituitary portal vessels may allow hormones access to the subarachnoid cerebrospinal fluid.

has focused on its antidiuretic effect. Oxytocin has few established physiological effects in the human male, but a profound effect on the pregnant uterus. Neurophysin is released into the neurohypophyseal capillary bed, but its physiological role is uncertain.

Hypothalamic neurons with small cell bodies (the *parvicellular neurons* of the arcuate and other hypothalamic nuclei) project to the neurohypophysis, and most of them terminate near capillaries within the median eminence (Fig. 37-1). The dense-core neurosecretory granules in these neurons are smaller (about 800 to 1000 Å in diameter) and are composed of releasing and inhibiting factors that are destined for the adenohypophysis. No carrier protein similar to neurophysin has been found for the releasing and inhibiting hormones. Many pituitary releasing and inhibiting substances have been isolated from hypothalamic extracts, and their chemical structure has been determined; five have been synthesized (TRH, GRF, somatostatin, GnRH, and CRF).

THE ADENOHYPOPHYSIS

It is appropriate to recall that the chromophobe/eosinophil/basophil cellular classification was introduced in 1892, preceding the birth of endocrinology. There was no need at that time to link the histological appearance of pituitary cells to their secretory function, but as the several secretory functions of the adenohypophysis were established, an effort was made to link cell structure to cell function. For many decades, both histochemistry and electron microscopy were employed in an effort to determine which cells secreted which hormones. These techniques were not very successful and produced a nomenclature of such complexity that clinicians had little choice but to employ the chromophobe/basophil/eosinophil system of classification.

The development of immunohistochemistry brought order to the study of pituitary histology, and for the first time, pituitary cells could be described according to their secretory function (Fig. 37-6). Remarkably, this technique has established that some pituitary cells secrete more than one hormone. The use of the functional classification of pituitary cell types allows the simultaneous consideration of the biochemistry and physiology of each different trophic hormone.

GROWTH HORMONE CELLS (SOMATOTROPES). Growth hormone-secreting cells are found in the lateral aspect of the adenohypophysis; these cells appear eosinophilic with traditional stains. Growth hormone (GH) is a large

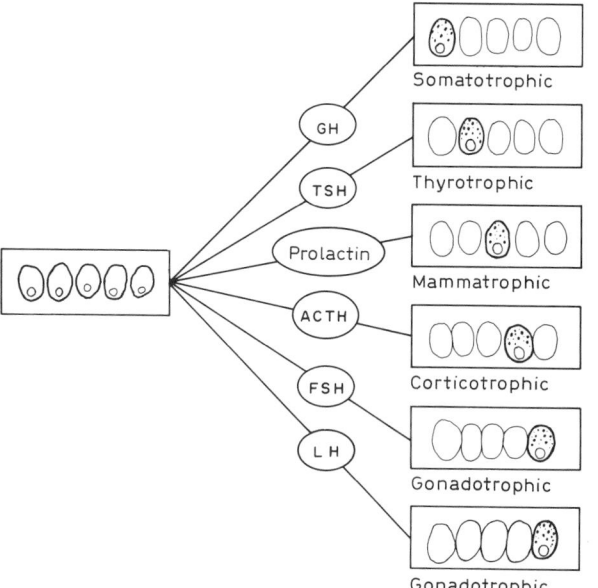

Fig. 37-6. A schematic illustration of the Nakane horseradish peroxidase immunohistochemical staining technique. Antibodies to specific trophic hormones are produced in vivo, harvested, and conjugated with horseradish peroxidase. Serial sections of the pituitary are obtained, washed with the various antibody-horseradish peroxidase conjugates, and reacted with lead. The lead precipitate (brownish-black) is visible over the cell containing the appropriate antigen. The technique allows a functional designation of pituitary cells, i.e., somatotrophic cell, thyrotrophic cell, etc. Note that follicle-stimulating hormone (FSH) and luteinizing hormone (LH) are formed in a common "gonadotroph." This technique may be employed with the light microscope or the electron microscope. GH, growth hormone; TSH, thyroid-stimulating hormone; ACTH, adrenocorticotrophic hormone.

peptide (191 amino acids) that effects the growth of bone, muscle, and visceral organs; it also elevates blood glucose level. GH is species-specific; human GH has been synthesized and is now produced by genetically altered bacteria in large quantities. For many decades patients were treated with growth hormone extracted from human pituitaries recovered at autopsy.

Between 5 and 10 percent of the weight of the adenohypophysis is accounted for by GH; the pituitary glands of children and adults have a similar GH content. The resting level of serum GH is 1 to 5 ng/mL, but secretory surges occur six to eight times daily; the largest surge occurs during sleep in the early morning hours. During adolescence the total amount of GH secreted per 24 h increases, largely because the secretory surges occur more frequently.

Secretions from the parvicellular hypothalamic neurons influence GH secretion; growth hormone-releasing factor (GRF) stimulates secretion, and growth hormone-inhibiting factor (somatostatin) limits secretion. GRF has been isolated from hypothalamic extracts, and its chemical structure has been determined. Somatostatin, found during the search for GRF, has been isolated, chemically identified as a tetradecapeptide, and synthesized. Somatostatin has other biological effects, including the inhibi-

tion of glucagon release from the pancreatic islet cells and the inhibition of gastrin secretion from the stomach; somatostatin is produced in the pancreas and the intestine as well as within the hypothalamus.

Exercise, stress, or hypoglycemia physiologically stimulate GH secretion. Insulin, arginine, epinephrine, L-dopa, and apomorphine can be infused pharmacologically to effect GH release.

PROLACTIN CELLS (MAMMOTROPES). Prolactin-secreting cells are also found in the lateral aspect of the adenohypophysis and also are eosinophils by traditional histochemical staining. Prolactin is a large peptide structurally similar in many ways to GH. In human beings, prolactin promotes lactation, but in lower species the hormone has many different and profound effects on behavior. Synthetic prolactin is not available for therapeutic use.

The normal daytime levels of prolactin are 15 to 25 ng/ mL; during sleep, prolactin levels increase two- or threefold by episodic surges of secretion. Men have circulating levels that equal those of nonpregnant women.

Hypothalamic control of prolactin secretion is achieved by the transport of prolactin-inhibiting factor (PIF) and prolactin-releasing factor (PRF) to the adenohypophysis. The net effect of the hypothalamic influence on prolactin secretion is inhibition. The chemical nature of PIF is not firmly established; most evidence suggests that dopamine may be PIF: for instance, L-dopa, the precursor of dopamine, limits prolactin secretion. No distinct prolactin-releasing factor (PRF) has been found, yet both TRH and somatostatin (along with their other established functions) increase prolactin levels, and either or both of them may serve as PRF.

Pregnancy, lactation, stress, and exercise are associated with high levels of prolactin; stimulation of the breast in both males and females activates reflex secretion of prolactin. Reserpine, synthetic TRH, and oral contraceptives all increase prolactin levels.

Prolactin levels are diminished by water loading and by administration of L-dopa, apomorphine, and bromergocryptine.

THYROID-STIMULATING HORMONE CELLS (THYROTROPES). The cells that make thyroid-stimulating hormone (TSH) are located in the central portion of the adenohypophysis and would be termed *basophils* by an older classification. TSH is a glycoprotein that increases thyroid growth and the synthesis of thyroid hormones.

Episodic secretory surges maintain a normal serum daytime level of TSH between 1 and 10 ng/mL; during the late stages of sleep (between 4 A.M. and 8 A.M.), a larger surge of secretion occurs that lasts 2 to 3 h.

Hypothalamic control of TSH secretion is achieved in part by the delivery of thyrotropin-releasing hormone (TRH) to the adenohypophysis; TRH is a tripeptide (perhaps the smallest peptide) that effects TSH release. Thyroid hormones also inhibit TSH release by a direct effect on thyrotropes.

Cold, stress, and electrical stimulation of the hypothalamus cause TSH release; TRH administration has become a convenient pharmacological way to increase TSH levels and to test TSH secretory reserve.

Age, hyperthyroidism, L-dopa, adrenal steroids, somatostatin, and bromergocriptine all result in diminished TSH levels.

ADRENOCORTICOTROPIC HORMONE CELLS (CORTICOTROPES). Adrenocorticotropic hormone (ACTH) is formed by cells within the adenohypophysis as well as by those basophils that have invaded the neurohypophysis. ACTH is a peptide (39 amino acids) that promotes growth of the adrenal cortex and the synthesis of the adrenal steroid hormones. ACTH is a fragment of pro-opiocortin (see below).

The biologic half-life of ACTH is about 10 min; throughout the day, from six to ten secretory surges occur, but circulating levels are highest during sleep. The nocturnal rise of ACTH is not the consequence of sleep and occurs in a circadian rhythm even in sleep-deprived subjects.

Hypothalamic stimulation, stress, fear, trauma, hemorrhage, and extreme cold cause ACTH release. The search for a hypothalamic corticotropin-releasing hormone ended in 1981 with the discovery of CRF, a peptide that contains 41 peptides. Since that discovery it has become more obvious that vasopressin is the most potent ACTH-releasing factor.

The feedback relationships between ACTH and the adrenal are discussed later in this chapter.

THE GONADOTROPES. Cells that produce follicle-stimulating hormone (FSH) and luteinizing hormone (LH) collectively have been termed *gonadotropes*. These cells would have been termed *basophils* by an earlier histological classification. Both FSH and LH are glycoproteins, and a single cell secretes both hormones. FSH promotes spermatogenesis in males and promotes the maturation of ovarian follicles and the production of ovarian steroids in females. LH stimulates the male's testes to produce testosterone and promotes the development of the corpus luteum in the female.

The basal levels of FSH and LH are maintained by small secretory surges that occur at hourly intervals. In the midcycle of menstruating women, a larger ovulatory surge of both hormones (the surge of LH is greater) occurs, which results in ovulation. During puberty, LH levels rise dramatically during sleep and are associated with REM (rapid eye movement) sleep.

The hypothalamus influences both FSH and LH secretion via a single releasing hormone that has been termed *gonadotropin-releasing hormone* (GnRH), a decapeptide that has been synthesized. Some have termed this substance *luteinizing hormone–releasing hormone* (LHRH), since its action is more pronounced on LH secretion than on FSH secretion.

The cyclical release of FSH and LH in females results from complex ovarian events, and although the hypothalamus controls gonadotropin release, the rhythm of the cycle is derived from cyclical changes in ovarian function. Gonadotropin secretion is increased by electrical stimulation of the hypothalamus, stress, certain visual or olfactory stimuli, and castration; in lower forms, dopamine causes FSH and LH release, but this has not been demonstrated in human beings. Synthetic GnRH can be employed to stimulate gonadotropin release and to test gonadotropin reserve.

FOLLICULAR CELLS. The pituitary gland in many species, including the human, contains stellate-shaped cells that form from PAS-positive follicles within the adenohypophysis. These cells are difficult to visualize with light microscopy, since their thin processes are below the level of optical resolution, but they are readily seen with the electron microscope.

To date, no function has been linked to follicular cells; they are the only cells within the pituitary that still must be designated by their structure rather than their function. Unfortunately, *follicular cells* (an anatomic designation) are often confused with *follicular-stimulating hormone cells* (a functional designation).

CELL RESTS. Frequently, large PAS-positive follicles or cysts are found in the cleft between the pars distalis and pars nervosa of the human pituitary; these cysts do not resemble the pars intermedia in lower species, and their function is unclear.

In the vicinity of the pars tuberalis, squamous cell rests are frequently found in the human being. These cells resemble those contained in a craniopharyngioma and may be the embryological remnant of Rathke's pouch.

PITUITARY ENDORPHINS. In 1975 endorphin and enkephalin, opiatelike peptides, were found in the brain. Almost immediately, it was recognized that these substances were produced in the pituitary as the prohormone beta-lipotropin (LPH). In 1978 it was verified that LPH was only part of a much larger prohormone that weighs 31,000 daltons. This substance, referred to as "31-K" or "pro-opiomelanocortin" (POMC), contains the amino acid sequence of several smaller peptides (see Fig. 37-7). More recently, it has been established that POMC is produced in the gut; thus it is one of many ubiquitous hormones.

In 1981 the structure of CRF was finally elucidated. This hypothalamic peptide contains 41 amino acids, and the control that it exerts over POMC in the brain, pituitary, and gut is only beginning to be understood.

The discovery of pituitary peptides in the brain has catalyzed an entire new branch of science that someday might be termed "endocrine neurology"; it recognizes that pituitary hormones and gut hormones are found throughout the brain and modify many aspects of behavior. The catalog of brain hormones grows longer each year but 35 brain hormones have already been found (see Fig. 37-8). Predictably, much that we know about the brain, the pituitary, and the gut will be radically revised in the next few years as the complex interrelationships of these hormones become understood.

Pituitary Disorders

TRAUMA

The pituitary stalk traverses the subdural space and may be partially or even totally disrupted during the deaceleration of head trauma. As many as 10 percent of patients with fatal head trauma have a divided pituitary

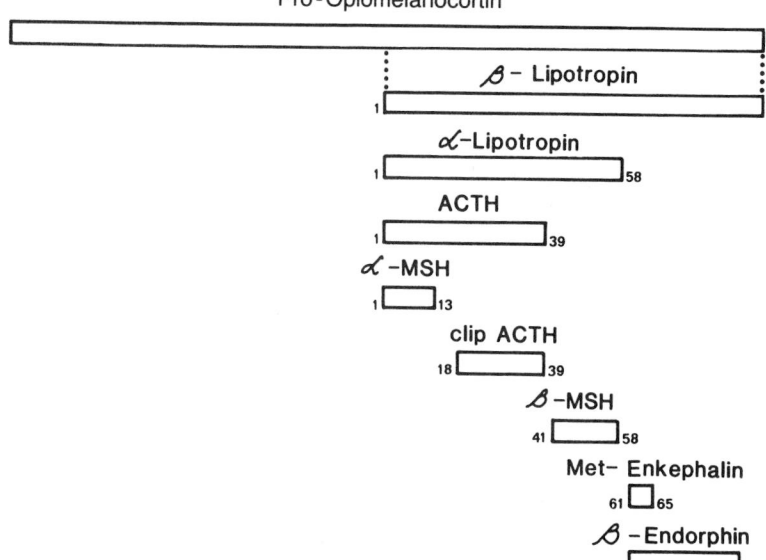

Fig. 37-7. A diagram of the peptide fragments that are contained in the prohormone pro-opiomelanocortin (POMC).

stalk. Since the adenohypophysis derives all of its blood supply from the pituitary portal vessels and has no independent arterial supply, pituitary necrosis and panhypopituitarism result.

POSTPARTUM PITUITARY ISCHEMIA

During pregnancy the weight of the pituitary increases by as much as 50 percent, and should postpartum hemorrhage result in shock, the pituitary becomes necrotic. This syndrome, variously described as Sheehan's syndrome or Simmonds' disease, generally results in panhypopituitarism. Treatment must focus on prevention, but once present, the condition can be treated with endocrine substitution therapy.

CHROMOPHOBE ADENOMAS

Nonsecreting pituitary tumors, first described by Cushing, are the most common kind of pituitary tumor; these tumor cells have very few cytoplasmic granules and are

Fig. 37-8. Brain hormones.

1.	ACTH	18.	oxytocin
2.	beta-lipotropin	19.	neurophysin
3.	beta-enkephalin	20.	neurotensin
4.	leu-enkephalin	21.	substance P
5.	met-enkephalin	22.	gastrin
6.	alpha-MSH	23.	cholecystokinin
7.	beta-MSH	24.	bombesin
8.	growth hormone	25.	insulin
9.	prolactin	26.	motilin
10.	TSH	27.	glucagon
11.	LH	28.	angiotensin II
12.	FSH	29.	bradykinin
13.	GNRH	30.	calcitonin
14.	CRF	31.	carnosine
15.	somatostatin	32.	sleep peptide
16.	TRH	33.	vasoactive intestinal peptide
17.	vasopressin	34.	avian pancreatic peptide
		35.	atrial naturetic peptide

commonly classified by the old nomenclature as *chromophobe adenomas*.

As chromophobe tumors enlarge, the adjoining secreting cells within the sella turcica are compressed, and diminished secretion results; most often growth hormone secretion is affected first, gonadotropic secretion next, thyrotropic secretion third, and ACTH secretion last. These functions are often lost in sequence, and patients who have lost adrenal function usually have had an earlier loss of thyroid and gonadal function. Despite the distortion of the neurohypophysis that is caused by chromophobe adenomas, diabetes insipidus seldom occurs.

The visual system may be distorted by larger chromophobe adenomas, and typically a bitemporal hemianopsia develops. Although large tumors may compress the inferior aspect of the optic nerves, optic chiasm, and optic tract, a horizontal altitudinal defect rarely ensues; the peculiarities of the vasculature of the chiasm (Fig. 37-9) make the central portion of the chiasm (containing the crossing fibers from the mesial retina) more vulnerable.

Rarely, chromophobe adenomas may enlarge laterally to compress those cranial nerves within the cavernous sinus (the oculomotor, the trochlear, the first division of the trigeminal, and the abducent); this is more commonly noted when the tumors outgrow their vascular supply and "pituitary apoplexy" results. This sudden hemorrhage within the tumor occurs in 5 percent of chromophobe adenomas, usually in large tumors, and is associated with sudden visual loss, severe headache, hyposecretion of trophic hormones, and subarachnoid hemorrhage.

The largest of the suprasellar chromophobe adenomas will extend into the third ventricle to cause hydrocephalus and/or hypothalamic dysfunction.

Although radiotherapy is effective in treating chromophobe adenomas, surgical procedures (via either a transfrontal or a transsphenoidal route) are generally indi-

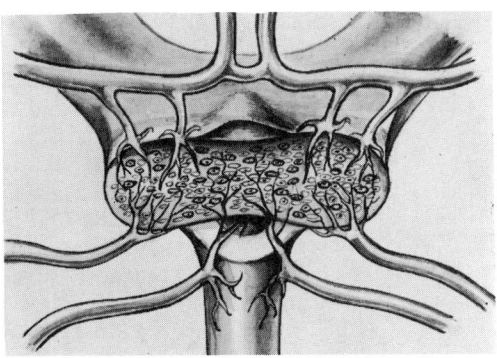
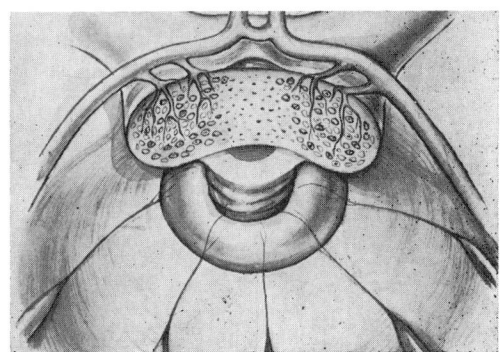

Fig. 37-9. *Left,* the normal arterial supply to the human optic chiasm. While the lateral portions of the chiasm receive a superior *and* an inferior arterial supply, the central portion of the chiasm receives only an inferior supply. *Right,* distortion of the inferior vascular supply by a pituitary tumor causes ischemia of the central portion of the chiasm, which results in a bitemporal hemianopsia.

cated, both to decrease the bulk of the tumor and to verify the histopathology. Surgery can be accomplished with a mortality rate of 1 percent.

ACROMEGALY

The hypersecretion of growth hormone results in gigantism in adolescents (before the epiphyses have closed) and acromegaly in adults (after the epiphyses have closed). Growth hormone causes excessive bone growth, excessive muscle growth (with weight gain), diabetes (with elevation of blood sugar level), and organomegaly. Enlargement of the face, hands, and feet often permits a bedside diagnosis (Fig. 37-10). The enlargement of the heart may result in valvular dysfunction and cardiomyopathy; patients with acromegaly commonly die of cardiac complications.

Some hypersecreting growth hormone tumors are large and cause hypofunction of other secreting cells, visual symptoms, and hydrocephalus. Although the first tumors associated with acromegaly were small eosinophilic microadenomas, the majority of acromegalic pituitary tumors removed at surgery are chromophobe tumors, not eosinophilic tumors. Even so, immunohistochemical analysis of the chromophobe tumors found in acromegaly will demonstrate GH within the cytoplasm of the tumor cells (Fig. 37-11).

The goal of therapy in acromegaly or gigantism is a reduced level of GH. In smaller, well-circumscribed tumors, the so-called microadenomas (Fig. 37-12), this can be accomplished by tumor removal alone, but in larger tumors a radical hypophysectomy is necessary, with postoperative endocrine replacement therapy.

The development of the proton beam, which has added a new dimension to the therapy of acromegaly, may supplant invasive surgical approaches.

CUSHING'S DISEASE

Hypersecretion of ACTH by the pituitary results in hypersecretion of steroid hormones from the adrenal cortex. Not all patients with excessive levels of adrenal ste-

roid hormones have ACTH-producing tumors; the cause of the steroid excess can be determined only by the measurement of pituitary and adrenal secretions and by manipulating the pituitary/adrenal axis with dexamethasone and/or metapyrone.

Many of the ACTH-producing tumors are small, and a normal-sized sella turcica does not exclude the presence of a pituitary tumor; patients with the signs and symptoms of Cushing's disease must have a variety of hormone determinations before a pituitary tumor is excluded. Many small ACTH-producing tumors have been removed from normal-sized sella turcicas.

Fig. 37-10. Patient with acromegaly. Note the large broad hands, stubby thumbs, thick lips, and prominent jaw. The classic full-blown features of acromegaly are seldom seen at present, since treatment is instituted at a much earlier stage than formerly.

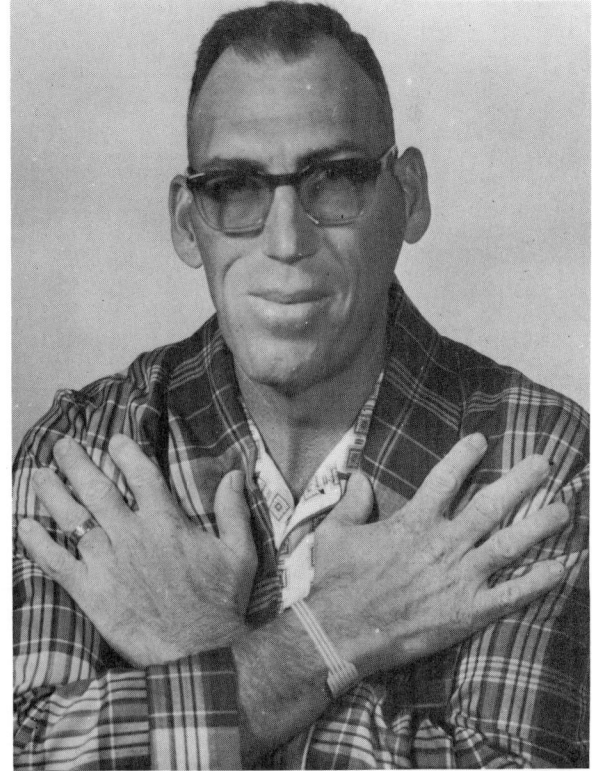

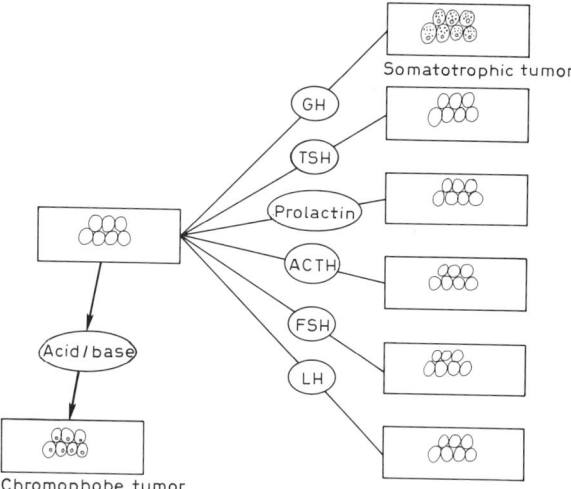

Fig. 37-11. Acidic-basic stains may show the tumor from an acromegalic patient to be chromophobic. The horseradish peroxidase immunohistochemical techniques can be used on serial sections of tumor tissue to reveal the presence of growth hormone within the cells. This allows a functional designation of the tumor, i.e., somatotrophic.

If excessive secretion of ACTH from a pituitary tumor is the cause of Cushing's disease, most investigators would agree that the pituitary tumor should be treated, rather than the adrenal hyperplasia.

The diagnosis and therapy of Cushing's disease is discussed more fully later in this chapter.

PROLACTIN-SECRETING TUMORS

Since a suitable assay for prolactin has been developed, it has been ascertained that 40 percent of all pituitary tumors originate in prolactin-secreting cells. Many of these grow to a large size and were previously termed *chromophobe adenomas*, but immunohistochemical analysis may demonstrate prolactin within the cytoplasm of the pale chromophobe cells.

In females, tumors that produce excessive prolactin cause amenorrhea as well as galactorrhea. The amenorrhea/galactorrhea syndrome (the "A/G syndrome") often results from microadenomas that do not enlarge the sella. With increasing frequency, surgeons are exploring the sella turcica to discover and remove small tumors that could not be visualized by radiography.

In males, excessive levels of prolactin may result in impotence; the removal of the offending prolactin-secreting tumor may return sexual function to normal.

Most patients with prolactin-secreting adenomas come to operation, and the surgical removal of a prolactin-secreting microadenoma can improve female fertility and give afflicted males a return of sexual vigor. Yet the systemic disturbances of prolactin excess are not known to be life threatening (in contrast to GH excess or ACTH excess), and a more conservative course often is indicated.

Bromocriptine, an ergot derivative with long-lasting dopaminergic activity, inhibits prolactin production and, indeed, reduces tumor bulk. In many clinics this drug has become the preferred treatment for prolactin-secreting tumors.

OTHER HYPERSECRETING TUMORS

Hypersecreting tumors of the gonadotropic cells or the thyrotropic cells are rare but have been reported.

Fig. 37-12. A microadenoma of the pituitary. These tumors may secrete large amounts of hormones, yet not enlarge the sella. Their presence may be determined by radioimmune assay; they are perhaps best removed by the transsphenoidal approach. *(Courtesy of Dr. J. Hardy.)*

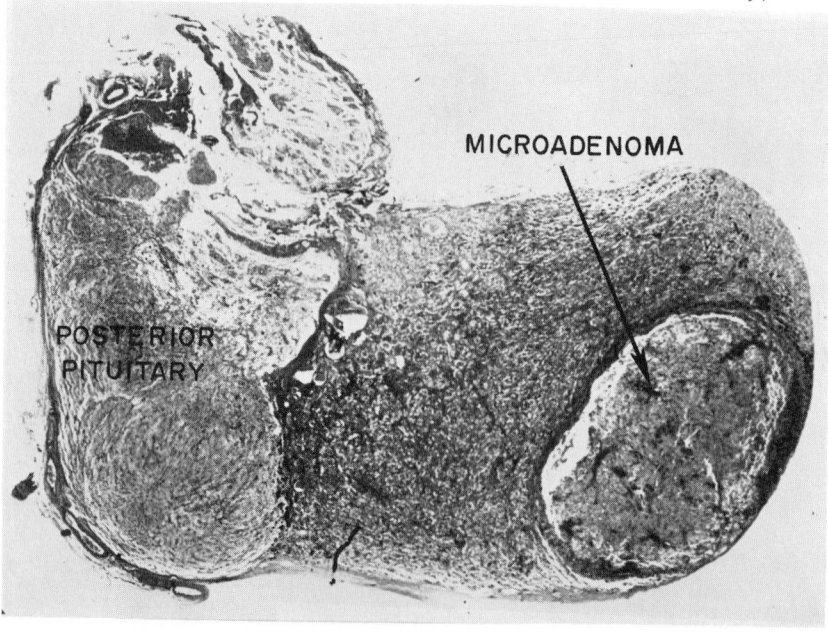

CRANIOPHARYNGIOMAS

In both children and adults, remnants of Rathke's pouch may produce a squamous cell tumor of the pituitary, which has been termed a *craniopharyngioma*. Those tumors that develop within the sella turcica result only in hypofunction of the adenohypophysis, but the majority of craniopharyngiomas develop above the diaphragma sella and affect the neurohypophysis, the hypothalamus, the visual system, and the ventricular system. This tumor is a common cause of dwarfism. Many of these tumors are cystic, and many are calcified; not all these tumors are well encapsulated.

Once recognized, craniopharyngiomas may be totally excised (if they are well encapsulated), but often cyst drainage with partial resection is preferable, and in some clinics this has become the therapy of choice. Palliation may be achieved by radiotherapy.

OTHER TUMORS

Meningiomas of the tuberculum sella, ependymomas, gliomas, and pinealomas may distort the hypothalamus and/or pituitary and cause signs and symptoms not easily distinguished from those produced by primary pituitary tumors.

Metastases to the pituitary are not infrequent. Since all blood reaching the pituitary initially passes through the neurohypophysis, most metastases occur in the neurohypophysis, not the adenohypophysis.

Diagnostic Studies

RADIOLOGIC PITUITARY STUDIES

Skull films should be obtained in patients whose signs and symptoms lead to the suspicion of a pituitary disorder. Lateral films will demonstrate the sagittal profile of the sella turcica, and anteroposterior films, properly taken, will demonstrate the floor of the sella. But only the posterior, anterior, and inferior aspects of the pituitary can be evaluated by these films. Tomograms provide a more certain assessment of the sella turcica and are especially helpful for the study of small microadenomas. CT and MRI scans (Figs. 37-13 and 37-14) are most helpful in the radiologic assessment of the pituitary.

Not all patients with enlargement of the sella turcica have pituitary tumors; fully 10 percent of this group has the empty sella syndrome, in which CT or MRI scans may demonstrate CSF within the sella. The etiology of this syndrome is unclear. Should endocrine studies point to a hypersecreting tumor, the sella nonetheless should be explored as a moderate number of microadenomas have been removed from so-called empty sellas.

FUNCTIONAL PITUITARY STUDIES

Increasingly, endocrine studies of pituitary function are replacing anatomical studies in the diagnosis of hypersecreting tumors. Since patients with pituitary disorders may have hyperfunction of some cell populations and hypofunction of other cell populations, a full battery of

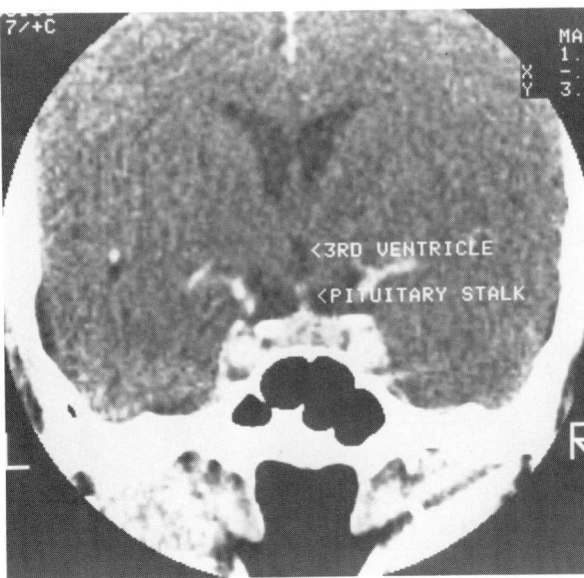

Fig. 37-13. A CT scan showing the brain and the ventricles. The pituitary is well visualized after contrast injection, and the pituitary stalk is clearly seen.

assays is usually essential to understand the functional derangements caused by the tumor.

Therapeutic Modalities

TRANSCRANIAL SURGERY

Before the era of antibiotics, surgeons were reluctant to open the frontal sinus to reach the pituitary; the intracranial route was via a lateral subfrontal or temporal approach. Antibiotics made it possible for surgeons to remove the frontal bone and, if needed, to open the frontal

Fig. 37-14. An MRI scan of a large cystic pituitary tumor. The elevated and flattened chiasm can be seen clearly.

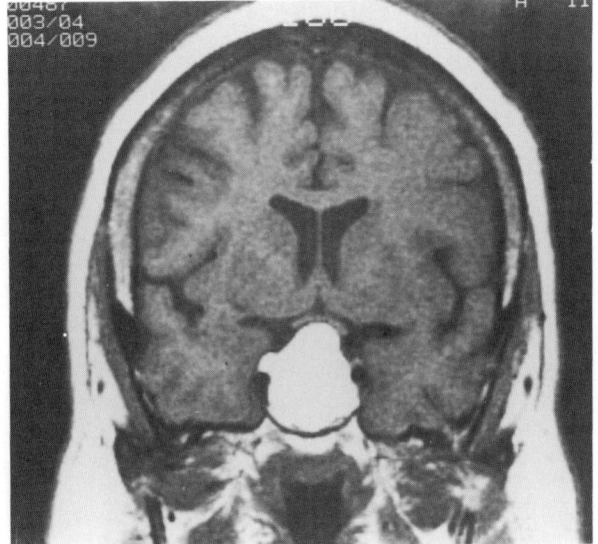

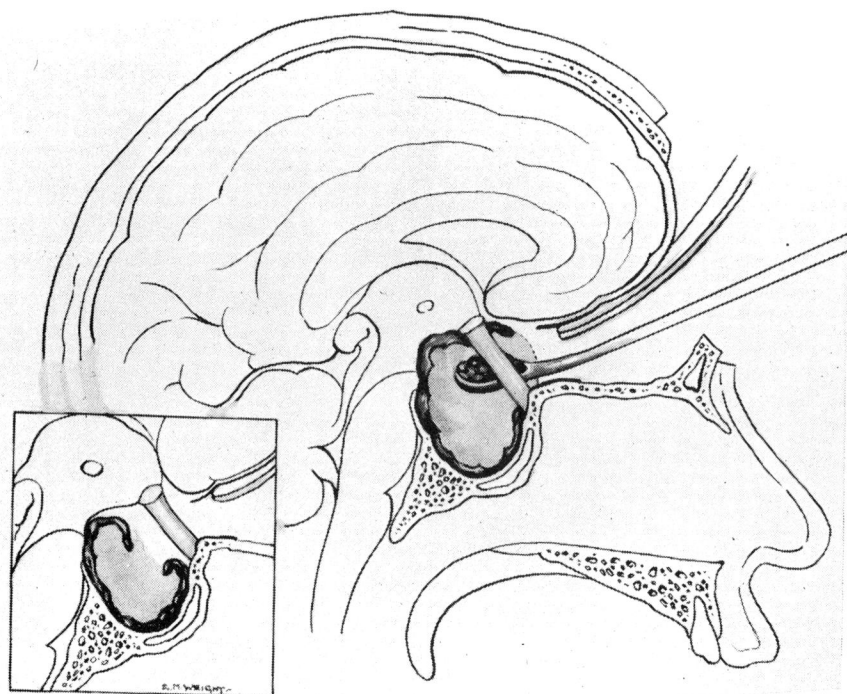

Fig. 37-15. An illustration from Cushing of the transcranial approach to the pituitary. Note the unopened frontal sinus; Cushing's efforts preceded the development of antibiotics, and meningitis often ensued if the frontal sinus was opened. Modern surgeons often open the frontal sinus, since the lower exposure provides better visualization of the pituitary.

sinus without fear of meningitis. Working through the frontal sinus (Fig. 37-15) permits less retraction of the frontal lobe and better exposure of the pituitary and chiasm; the unilateral anosmia that results is seldom noticed by patients.

Experienced surgeons can perform transfrontal pituitary surgery for hypophysectomy and for tumors with little morbidity or mortality. This approach allows the surgeon to visualize the anatomical variations that frequently surround the pituitary and to assay the distortions of the surrounding neural and vascular structures that result from tumor growth.

TRANSSPHENOIDAL APPROACHES

Early in the history of pituitary surgery, the advantages of the transsphenoidal approach to the pituitary were recognized; yet the high incidence of infection in the preantibiotic era worked against this approach. After the safety of opening the frontal sinus during pituitary surgery was established, the transnasal approach through the sphenoid sinus was again employed (Fig. 37-16).

Although this approach does not allow the surgeon to visualize intracranial anatomical variations or the variable distortions that occur with large tumors, it is cosmetically superior, since the incision is hidden in the gingival mucosa of the upper lip. Experience has verified that this approach to the pituitary is safe, and in recent years it has supplanted the transfrontal intracranial approach in most clinics. This procedure demands an operative microscope and intraoperative fluoroscopy.

By this approach the normal sella turcica can be opened and microadenomas that were not visible by x-ray but whose presence was ascertained by functional endo-

crine assays can be removed. The sella turcica can be explored, much as the abdomen or chest is explored in troublesome diagnostic cases.

STEREOTAXIC TECHNIQUES

Because the sella turcica is such a convenient radiographic target, the pituitary has been treated by a variety of stereotaxic techniques. Many of these techniques were developed for the purpose of hypophysectomy in the treatment of metastatic cancer, but in selected cases, the same techniques have been employed in the treatment of pituitary tumors.

In most instances, the cannula employed in stereotaxic pituitary surgery is introduced by the transsphenoidal or transethmoidal route. Radiographic control is essential, but these procedures can be performed under local anesthesia.

Radioactive gold, radioactive yttrium, cryosurgery, and radio-frequency generators have been employed with good success to destroy the normal pituitary and to treat certain pituitary tumors. A major problem with stereotaxic procedures has been the high incidence of cerebrospinal fluid rhinorrhea.

PROTON BEAM

The development of the linear accelerator led to efforts to treat certain pituitary diseases by the proton beam

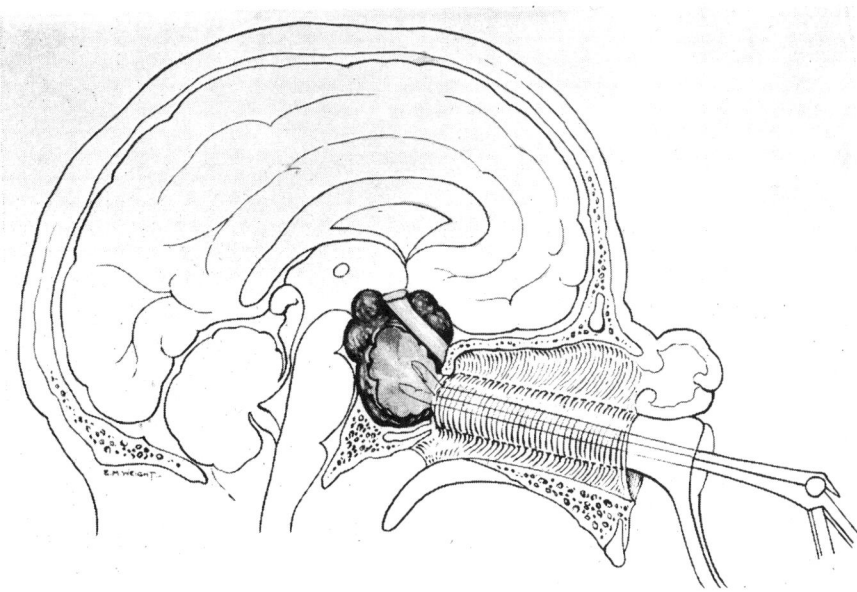

Fig. 37-16. Another illustration from Cushing of the transsphenoidal approach to the pituitary. Because of the high incidence of infection, Cushing gave up this approach. Since the advent of antibiotics, it has gained favor.

(only two clinics in this country have this capability). As in the stereotaxic procedures, the radiographic shadow of the sella turcica allows the surgeon to aim the proton beam at the pituitary and to destroy the normal pituitary or certain pituitary tumors. This procedure is performed without an incision and may be the first of many surgical procedures that will be done by noninvasive techniques.

HYPOPHYSECTOMY

The beneficial effect of oophorectomy for patients with metastatic breast cancer was known before the discovery of the endocrine system. The discovery that ovarian function was largely controlled by the pituitary, coupled to the realization that some estrogen was formed by the adrenals, suggested that hypophysectomy might be a more effective method for treating patients with far-advanced breast cancer. Since hypophysectomy also causes hypoadrenalism, it could not be employed until 1952, when adrenal replacement therapy became available.

There is little doubt that hypophysectomy is effective in the palliation of metastatic breast cancer (and prostatic cancer), but not all patients achieve a beneficial response and none is cured. Perhaps 40 percent of patients with metastatic breast cancer are benefited; their objective remission is usually measured in months, not years.

The demonstration of estrogen receptor sites in the pathological evaluation of the cancerous breast tissue has aided in predicting which patients will benefit from hypophysectomy, but proper selection of patients is still critical in the recommendation of hypophysectomy for breast cancer.

Hypophysectomy has also been employed in the therapy of diabetic retinopathy; the serendipitous observation

that retinopathy improved following postpartum necrosis of the pituitary led to this form of treatment. It has not been established which hormone is involved in the response, and selection of patients remains a problem; generally patients with hemorrhagic complications respond better than those with proliferative disease. It has been verified that the benefits of the procedure are enduring.

ADRENAL
(Donald S. Gann and Eric J. DeMaria)

Historical Background

The adrenal glands were first described in 1563 by Eustachius, but their function remained controversial for nearly 300 years. Then, in 1855, Thomas Addison first described the clinical syndrome of adrenal insufficiency and noted adrenal infarction at autopsy in these patients. Subsequently, Brown-Sequard performed unilateral and bilateral adrenalectomy in animals and determined that the adrenals were necessary to support life.

In human beings, the adrenal is composed of two endocrine tissues merged into a single gland. The cortex of the gland synthesizes and secretes the major glucocorticoid cortisol, the primary mineralocorticoid aldosterone, adrenal androgens, and small amounts of estrogen. The adrenal medulla synthesizes and secretes catecholamines including epinephrine, norepinephrine, and dopamine.

Diseases affecting the adrenal often involve either excessive or deficient secretion of hormones. Thus, the following brief historical overview is separated into categories based on hormonal syndromes. Although many areas of adrenal endocrinology and pathology are incompletely understood, future investigations will no doubt add to our understanding of the gland and its hormones.

ADRENAL CORTEX. Cushing's Syndrome. In 1912, Harvey Cushing first described the classic syndrome of patients with truncal obesity, hypertension, hirsutism, and purple abdominal striae that bears his name. Pituitary adenomas were found at autopsy in several of Cushing's cases. However, a long debate ensued as to whether pituitary or adrenal pathology caused the clinical syndrome. In 1935, Oppenheimer et al. demonstrated that basophilic pituitary adenomas were associated with Cushing's syndrome only in patients with adrenal hyperplasia, but they felt that the primary abnormality was in the adrenal. Eventually, the clinical features of all patients with Cushing's syndrome were demonstrated to be secondary to the hypersecretion of adrenal corticosteroids. Liddle and colleagues in 1963 carefully documented 13 cases of hypercortisolism as a result of nonpituitary neoplasms, demonstrating the distinct pathophysiologic entity now called the ectopic ACTH syndrome.

Aldosteronism. In 1949, Greep and Deane demonstrated that hypophysectomy led to atrophy of the zona fasciculata and zona reticularis of the adrenal cortex, but not of the zona glomerulosa. They hypothesized that the zona glomerulosa was the site of mineralocorticoid synthesis and secretion. In 1952, Tait and Simpson identified aldosterone. In 1955, Conn described the clinical syndrome of primary aldosteronism for the first time.

Virilizing Syndromes. In 1865, DeCrecchio first reported congenital adrenal hyperplasia occurring in a female pseudohermaphrodite. In 1887, Phillips reported four cases of female pseudohermaphroditism with adrenal hypertrophy and death probably from salt wasting. Marchand suggested that adrenal hyperplasia was a cause of pseudohermaphroditism, and in 1939 Butler postulated that salt wasting was due to adrenal insufficiency in these patients. Wilkins et al. in 1950 first demonstrated the therapeutic utility of cortisone in the treatment of congenital adrenal hyperplasia. Soon thereafter, Bartter, Albright, and colleagues demonstrated the role of ACTH hypersecretion in the adrenogenital syndrome based upon biochemical studies in patients treated with cortisone.

ADRENAL MEDULLA. Pheochromocytoma. In 1896, Frankel described the first case of pheochromocytoma.

The patient was an 18-year-old girl with recurrent attacks of palpitations, headaches, vomiting, pounding pulse, and retinitis. She was found to have bilateral adrenal neoplasms. Some years later, Manasse showed that tumors of the adrenal medulla stained with chronic salts, and Pick subsequently proposed the term pheochromocytoma for this reason. In 1923, Masson and Martin attempted surgical resection of a pheochromocytoma, but their patient died. Three years later, both Roux and Mayo reported the first successful resection of a pheochromocytoma.

In 1929, Rabin demonstrated that pheochromocytomas contained supranormal quantities of epinephrine and suggested that epinephrine was responsible for hypertension in patients with the disease. In 1937, Beer, King, and Prinzmetal demonstrated a circulating pressor agent that was assumed to be epinephrine during a hypertensive crisis in a patient with pheochromocytoma. In 1949, Holton reported the presence of norepinephrine in pheochromocytomas.

Embryology

The adrenal cortex and medulla arise separately during embryologic development. The adrenal cortex begins to develop during the fourth or fifth week of gestation. The fetal or primitive cortex develops from coelomic mesothelial cells that proliferate between the dorsal mesentery and the developing gonad (Fig. 37-17). A second group of mesothelial cells then proliferate and surround the cells of the primitive cortex to form the definitive cortex. Eventually, the primitive cortex degenerates and the definitive cortex develops into the functional adrenal cortex.

The adrenal medulla and sympathetic nervous system develop together. During the fifth week of gestation, ectodermal neural crest cells in the thoracic region migrate ventrally to lie on both sides of the spinal cord just behind

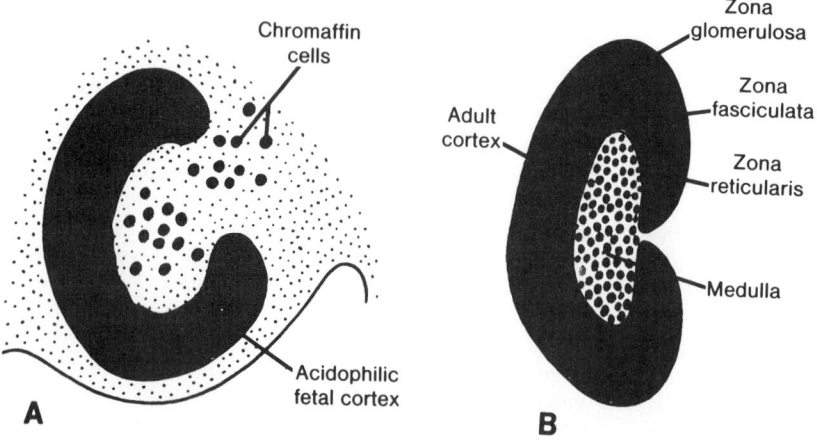

Fig. 37-17. *A.* Chromaffin (sympathetic) cells penetrating the fetal cortex of the adrenal gland. *B.* At a later stage of development, the definitive cortex surrounds the medulla almost completely. (From: *Sadler TW: Langman's Medical Embryology, 5th ed.* Baltimore, Williams and Wilkins, 1985, p 365, with permission.)

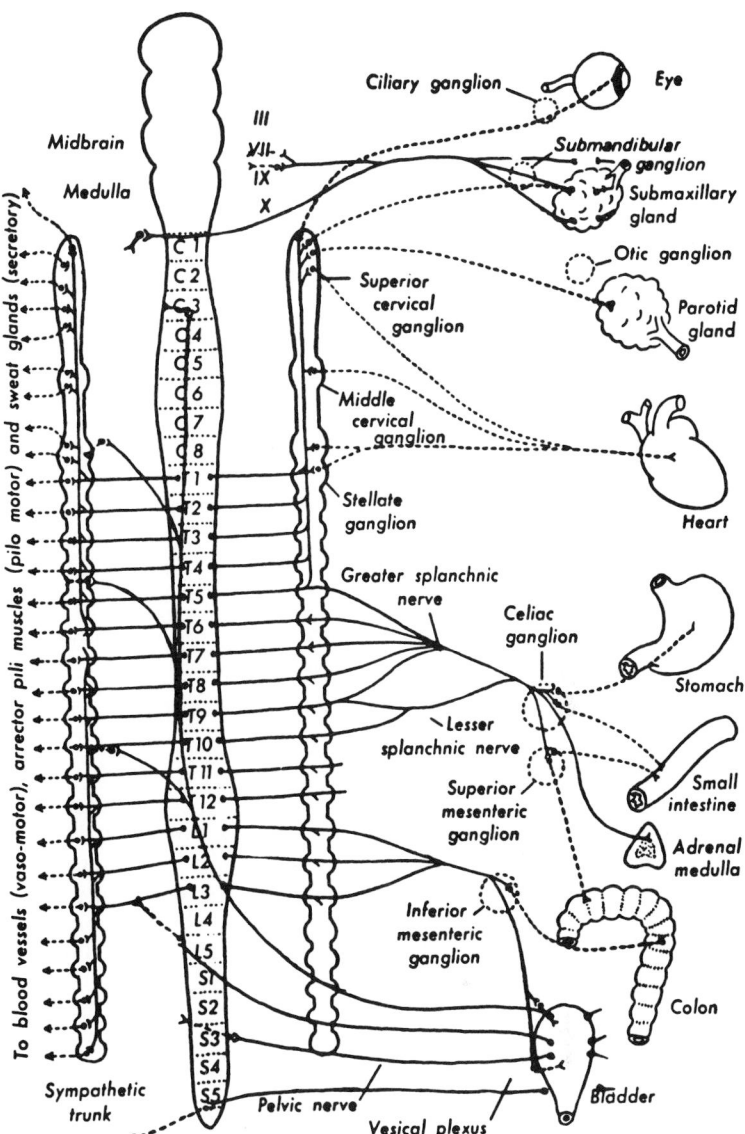

Fig. 37-18. Anatomic organization of the sympathetic nervous system. Solid lines represent preganglionic fibers and broken lines represent postganglionic fibers. (From: *Copenhaver WM, Kelly DE, Wood RD: Bailey's Textbook of Histology, 17th ed. Baltimore, Williams and Wilkins, 1978, p 287, with permission.*)

the aorta to form the primitive sympathetic ganglia. The preaortic celiac, renal, and mesenteric ganglia are formed by primitive neural crest cells that migrate to the anterior aspect of the aorta. Preganglionic nerve fibers from the spinal cord synapse on the developing neuroblasts, and postganglionic fibers from the ganglia innervate the heart, lungs, gut, brain, sweat glands, and peripheral blood vessels (Fig. 37-18). The primary neurotransmitter of sympathetic postganglionic fibers is norepinephrine.

While sympathetic ganglia are forming, small groups of cells become detached to form glandular elements along the vertebral column. Most of these chromaffin cell groups regress, with two notable exceptions. One cell group migrates along the adrenal vein, invades the adrenal cortex, eventually becomes surrounded by the primitive cortex, and forms the adrenal medulla. Analogous to the sympathetic ganglia, preganglionic sympathetic nerve fibers synapse directly on these developing adrenomedullary cells. The second cell group forms the aortic glands of Zuckerkandl located lateral to the aorta near the origin of the inferior mesenteric artery. Although the organs of Zuckerkandl usually atrophy during childhood, they are a frequent location of extraadrenal chromaffin tumors (Fig. 37-19). Neural crest cell derivatives are found in diverse locations including skin melanocytes, nerve sheaths, liver, visceral ganglia, endocrine glands, and connective tissues. Thus, neural crest cell tumors such as pheochromocytoma and neuroblastoma may occur in many locations.

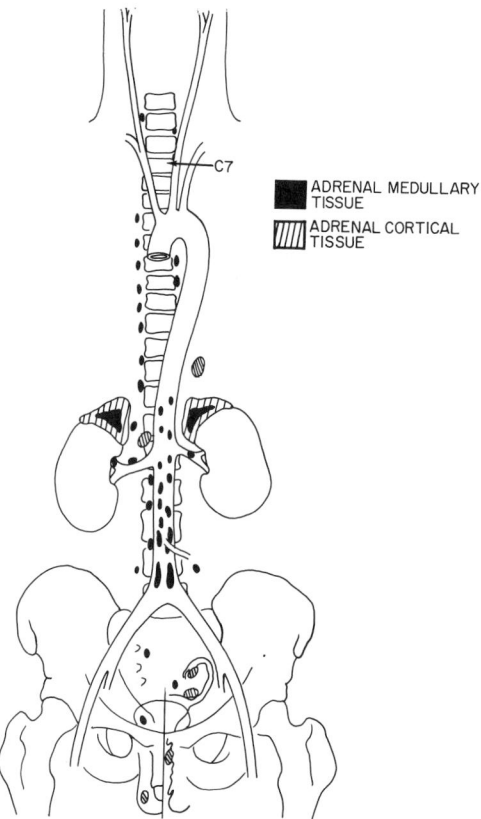

Fig. 37-19. Location of ectopic adrenal tissue. The location of ectopic adrenal medullary tissue is shown in black; cortical tissue is shown in the shaded areas. The incidence of extraadrenal medullary tissue is very high compared with the incidence of extraadrenal cortical tissue, and while functioning extraadrenal medullary tissue occurs in about 1 of every 8 cases of medullary hyperfunction, it occurs in fewer than 1 of 1000 cases of adrenocortical hyperfunction.

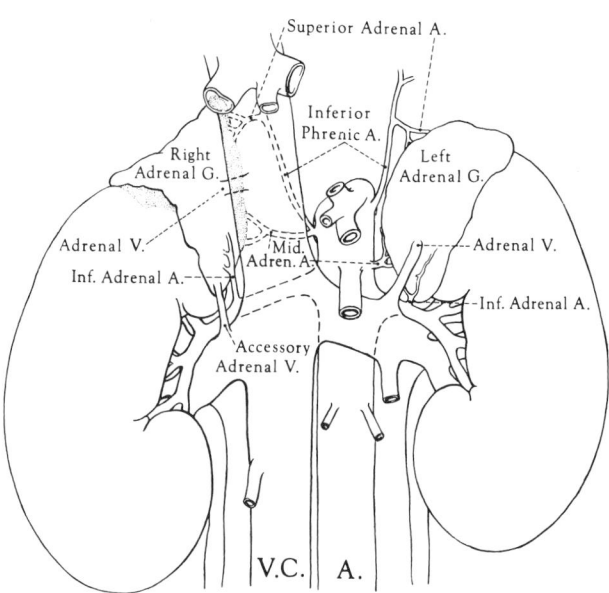

Fig. 37-20. Location and blood supply of the adrenal glands. There is great variation in the arterial blood supply of the glands, but this generally comes from three sources: a branch from the renal artery, a branch from the aorta, and a branch from the inferior phrenic artery. There is usually only one main vein on each side, the left adrenal vein opening into the left renal vein while the one on the right opens into the inferior vena cava. On occasion there may be very small accessory adrenal veins such as that illustrated for the right adrenal.

Anatomy

The adrenals are bilateral organs located near the superior pole of each kidney (Fig. 37-20). Each gland has a connective tissue capsule and is surrounded by areolar perirenal fat. The glands are small, normally weighing 3.5 to 5 g. In human beings the adrenals are 3 to 5 cm in length and width, but typically only 4 to 6 mm in thickness. The high lipid content of the glands makes them appear chrome yellow in color.

The right adrenal has a pyramidal shape and lies in contact with the hemidiaphragm posteriorly, the right kidney inferiorly, the inferior vena cava anteromedially, and the right lobe of the liver anterolaterally. The left gland is slightly larger than the right and has a crescent shape. The posterior surface of the left gland also rests against the hemidiaphragm. The anterosuperior surface is separated from the stomach by peritoneum, while the anteroinferior surface is not covered by peritoneum and rests against the pancreas, the splenic artery, and the renal vein.

Each adrenal gland is supplied by three main arteries: the superior suprarenal artery, a branch of the inferior phrenic artery; the middle suprarenal artery, arising from the aorta; and the inferior suprarenal artery, a branch of the renal artery. The arteries form a vascular plexus within the adrenal capsule that gives rise to three types of intraglandular vessels. The *arteriae capsulae* supply the capsule, the *arteriae corticis* form sinusoids in the cortical parenchyma and empty into medullary venous sinusoids, and the *arteriae medullae* traverse the cortex to supply the medullary tissue directly. Thus, the medullary blood supply is derived from both the *arteriae corticis* and *arteriae medullae* systems. The *arteriae corticis* system plays an important role in adrenal epinephrine secretion, because high cortisol concentrations flow directly to the medulla by this pathway to increase the activity of phenylethanolamine-*N*-methyltransferase, the enzyme that converts norepinephrine to epinephrine. Extraadrenal chromaffin tissues are not exposed to high cortisol concentrations and thus predominantly secrete norepinephrine.

The right adrenal vein exits the medial aspect of the gland and enters the posterior inferior vena cava. In contrast, the left adrenal vein exits anteriorly and joins the left renal vein. The lymphatic vessels draining from the glands are scarce and follow the arteries and vein. Preganglionic sympathetic neurons from the celiac and renal plexuses innervate the adrenal medulla via the splanchnic nerves. In human beings, the adrenal cortex has no known innervation.

Histologically, the adrenal cortex is made up of three distinct zones. The central zona fasciculata is the largest of the three, surrounded by the external zona glomeru- losa, and the internal zona reticularis. Accessory glands, or adrenocortical rests, usually contain only cortical tis- sue and are often found in the perirenal fat, and in or near the testis, ovary, broad ligament, kidney, or bladder.

Adrenal Cortex

Physiology

The adrenal cortex secretes corticosteroids, the andro- gens, and small amounts of estrogens. The corticoste-

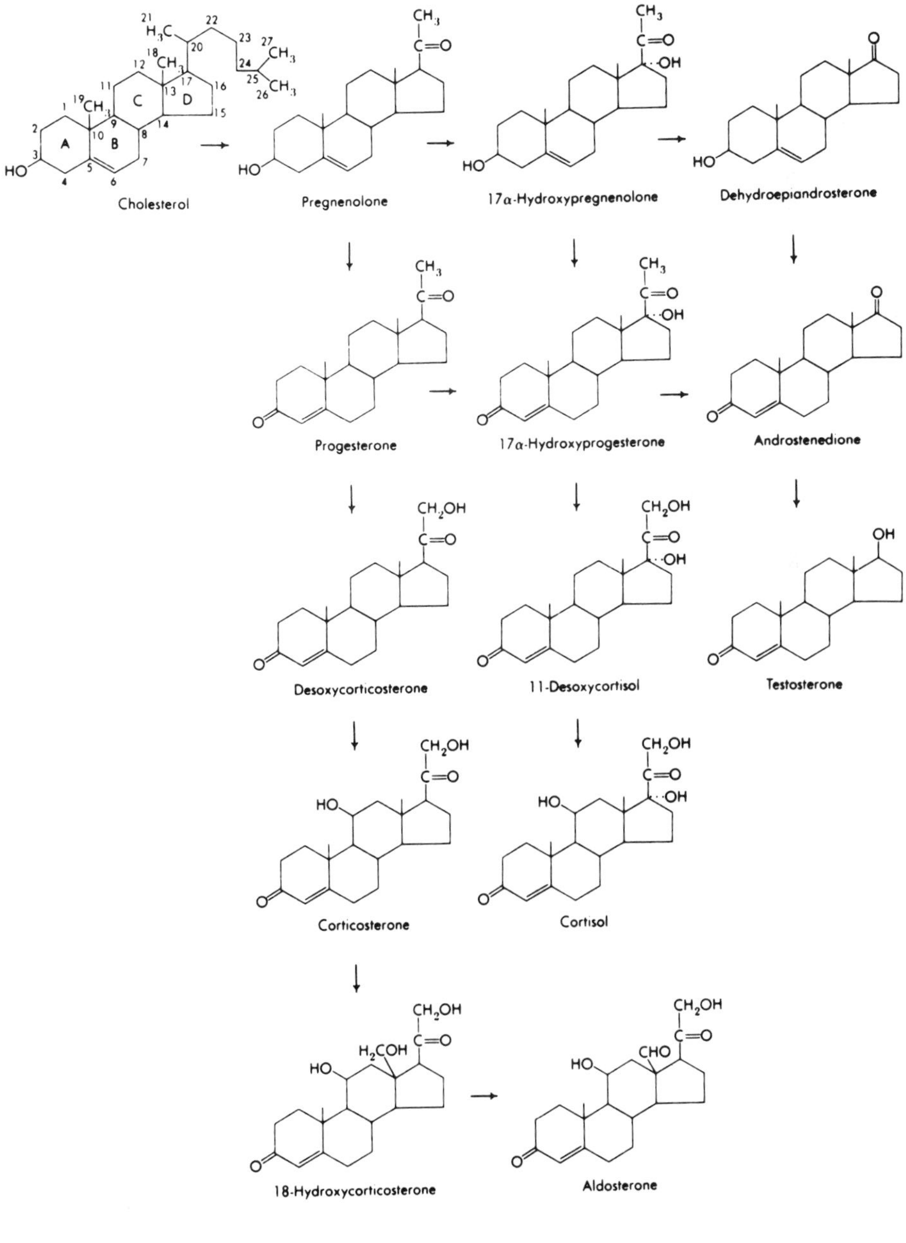

Fig. 37-21. Principal pathways for biosynthesis of adrenal cortico- steroids and adrenal androgens. (From: *Haynes RC, Murad F, in The Pharmacological Basis of Therapeutics, 6th ed. New York, Macmillan, 1980, chap 63, p 1472, with permission.*)

roids are 21 carbon compounds and include the primary glucocorticoid cortisol and the major mineralocorticoid aldosterone. The entire adrenal cortex contains 11- and 21-hydroxylating enzymes for cortisol synthesis, while only the zona glomerulosa contains the 18-oxidase re- quired for the aldosterone synthesis. The androgens are 19 carbon compounds, while the estrogens are C-18 ste- roids.

CORTISOL. Synthesis. Cholesterol is the basic precur- sor of all the adrenal steroids (Fig. 37-21). Cholesterol may be synthesized in the gland from acetate or supplied by the circulating blood. Cortical cells store only small amounts of finished hormone but do store large amounts of cholesterol in the esterified form. The rate-limiting, ini- tial step of steroid synthesis is cleavage of the isocaproyl

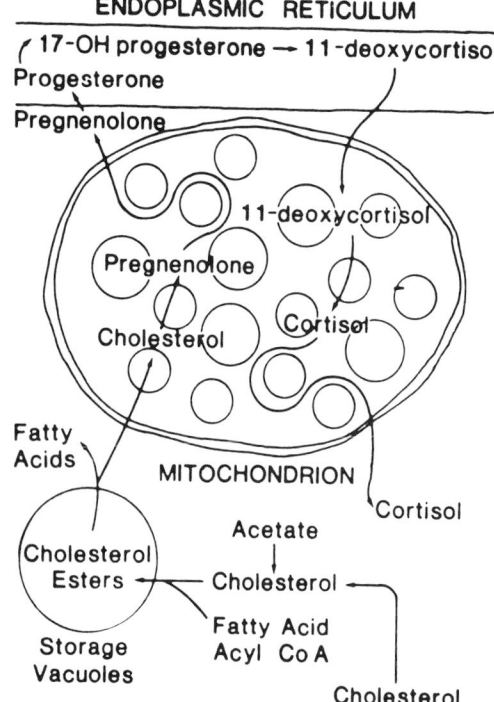

Fig. 37-22. Subcellular compartmentalization of the corticosteroid biosynthetic enzymes and the flow of biosynthetic intermediates. [From: *Harding BW, in DeGroot LJ, Cahill GF Jr, Martini L, et al (eds): Endocrinology. New York, Grune & Stratton, 1979, chap 92, p 1135, with permission.*]

sidechain from the steroid nucleus of cholesterol to form pregnenolone. This occurs in the mitochondria of adrenocortical cells and requires the presence of NADPH and oxygen.

From pregnenolone, a series of varied hydroxylation, dehydrogenation, and isomerization reactions occur in varied sequence to synthesize the corticosteroids, androgens, and estrogens. These reactions take place in the endoplasmic reticulum or mitochondria of adrenocortical cells, requiring that precursors move back and forth between these two subcellular areas (Fig. 37-22). Pregnenolone undergoes hydroxylation at the C-17 and C-21 positions to form 11-deoxycortisol. The enzyme 17-hydroxylase is not found in the zona glomerulosa where aldosterone synthesis occurs. Finally, hydroxylation of 11-deoxycortisol at the C-11 position yields cortisol.

Binding and Transport. Circulating cortisol in the bloodstream is protein-bound, unbound, or conjugated. Over 90 percent of cortisol is bound to plasma proteins under normal circumstances. Cortisol binding globulin (CBG or transcortin), an alpha-globulin synthesized by the liver, binds most of the circulating cortisol. CBG binds cortisol specifically and has a high affinity for the cortisol molecule. Small amounts of cortisol are also bound to albumin and other plasma proteins. CBG is increased in pregnancy, in patients taking estrogen supplements or oral contraceptives, and in hyperthyroidism. Low levels of CBG are found in patients with liver disease, multiple myeloma, obesity, or the nephrotic syndrome. Patients with congenital CBG deficiency have been reported. Free cortisol in plasma is the physiologically active form. Increases in cortisol secretion lead to saturation of the available protein binding sites and an increase in free cortisol.

Metabolism. Cortisol in plasma has a half-life of 70 to 120 min. The major site of cortisol metabolism is in the liver where a series of reduction reactions resulting in the production of tetrahydrocortisol inactivates the steroid (Fig. 37-23). Tetrahydrocortisol is then conjugated with sulfate or glucuronide at the C-3 position to yield a water-soluble product that is easily excreted in the urine. Seventeen-hydroxycorticosteroids and 17-ketosteroids formed by cleavage of the C-17 side chain are also excreted in the urine. Measurement of the urinary excretion of these corticosteroid metabolites is clinically useful in cases of suspected adrenal hypersecretory diseases.

Secretion. Adrenocorticotropin (ACTH) stimulates cortisol secretion by the adrenal gland. ACTH is a peptide fragment of a much larger pituitary protein called pro-opiomelanocortin (POMC) that consists of about 290 amino acids and contains the sequences of several peptides including beta-endorphin, melanocyte stimulating hormone, beta-lipotropin, and ACTH. The ACTH molecule is composed of 39 amino acids, although the active fraction of the molecule includes only amino acids 1 through 18. The adrenal cortex is very sensitive to ACTH. Adrenocortical cells store only small amounts of cortisol; thus ACTH must increase both the rate of steroid secretion and synthesis. ACTH that binds to membrane receptors on adrenocortical cells activates the intracellular enzyme adenyl cyclase to increase intracellular cyclic AMP, the second messenger that stimulates cortisol synthesis and secretion.

ACTH synthesis and secretion by the anterior pituitary is controlled by corticotropin releasing factors (CRFs). CRF-41 is a peptide synthesized by neurons in the paraventricular nucleus of the hypothalamus and secreted into the hypothalamohypophyseal portal vessels by neurons that terminate on vessels in the median eminence. CRF-41 stimulates the anterior pituitary to increase ACTH synthesis and secretion. Vasopressin secreted by neurons terminating in the median eminence also functions as a CRF, either alone or synergistically with CRF-41. Recent in vitro studies have suggested that interleukin-1 secreted by macrophages stimulates the release of ACTH from pituitary cells. Thus, control of the immune and endocrine systems may be closely interrelated, although the physiologic significance of this finding remains unproved.

The adrenal secretes cortisol in response to ACTH that in turn is released by a number of physiologic stimuli. Small changes in blood volume without hypotension cause cortisol secretion mediated by changes in afferent activity of atrial and cardiopulmonary stretch receptors. The rate and volume of blood loss determine the amount of ACTH released. Physical stimuli for cortisol release include tissue damage, hypoxia, deviations in body temperature, and hypoglycemia. Psychological influences including pain, anxiety, new surroundings, crowding, and restraint also activate cortisol secretion.

ACTH and cortisol responses to a stimulus are influenced by recent past stimuli. Administration of intravenous cortisol leads to inhibition of the adrenal response to subsequent stimuli. Continuous cortisol administration over prolonged periods results in persistent adrenocortical inhibition and eventual atrophy of the adrenal cortex. Cortisol inhibits its own secretion by blocking ACTH and CRF secretion and synthesis (Fig. 37-24). Feedback inhibition of cortisol release has been difficult to demonstrate with sequential physiologic stimuli. Repeated surgical trauma or hemorrhage cause an augmented release of ACTH and cortisol. Thus, the neuroendocrine system is activated after an initial stimulus causing facilitation rather than inhibition of the adrenal response to subsequent stimuli. This facilitation, termed "feedforward," provides a mechanism of increased hormonal release when recurrent stimuli threaten homeostasis.

Adrenal cortisol secretion follows a diurnal rhythm with peak cortisol secretion between 4 and 6 A.M. decreasing to a nadir in the evening between 8 and 12 P.M. Cortisol secretion is not continuous but occurs in episodic bursts of short duration. The purpose of the circadian rhythm of cortisol secretion is unclear, but it may help to maintain the sensitivity of target cells to cortisol's actions or avoid persistent exposure of cells to excessive, potentially harmful cortisol concentrations. The diurnal rhythm of cortisol secretion persists for 24 h in the absence of environmental stimuli.

Glucocorticoid Actions. The physiologic actions of cortisol are many and diverse. Although tolerance to stresses such as surgery and hemorrhage are seriously impaired in the absence of cortisol, it is unclear why the hormone is indispensable. Over the years, many investigators have formulated theories to explain the physiologic importance of cortisol. Seyle hypothesized that cortisol was important in what he termed the general adaptation syndrome,

METABOLISM OF CORTISOL

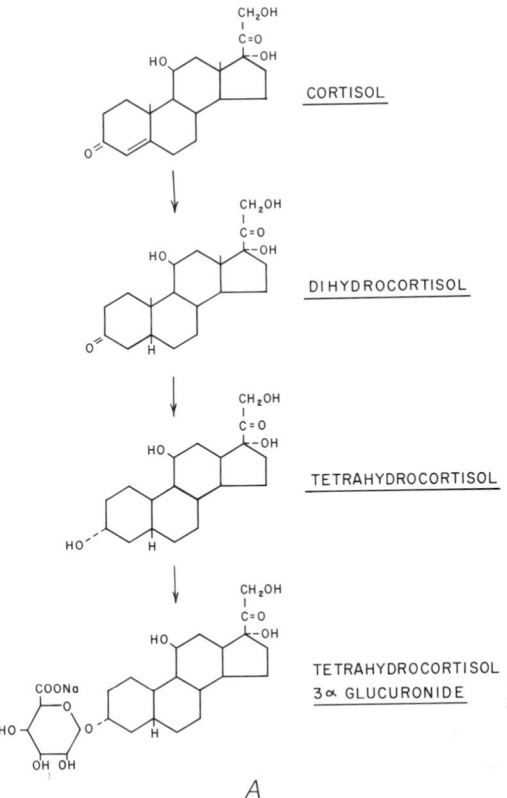

Fig. 37-23. Metabolism and excretion of cortisol. A. The degradation of cortisol takes place in the liver. In the first step dihydrocortisol is formed by a saturation of the double bond between carbons 4 and 5, adding a hydrogen to each of these carbon atoms. Further reduction takes place to the tetrahydrocortisol configuration by the substitution of a hydroxyl group on the 3 carbon atom. Some conjugation with sulfates also takes place. The conjugate tetrahydrocortisol is then excreted in the urine. B. The free cortisol excreted by the adrenal cortex becomes largely bound to transcortin, an alpha-globulin manufactured in the liver. This carrier protein prevents the rapid breakdown of cortisol but makes it available to the tissues as needed. As the cortisol passes through the liver, it becomes reduced and conjugated and thus inactivated. The conjugated corticosteroids are water-soluble and are excreted in the urine. A small amount of free cortisol is also excreted in the urine. At any given time the peripheral blood contains free, bound, and conjugated cortisol. If there is a marked increase in cortisol secretion, the transcortin-binding sites become saturated, and the amount of free cortisol increases greatly. In renal failure the conjugated corticosteroids are not excreted normally, and they pile up in the bloodstream. In hepatic failure there is very little conjugation of the corticosteroids, and a proportionately greater amount of free cortisol is present in the plasma.

EXAMPLES

	PLASMA μg %		URINE mgm/D	
	Free + Bound	Conj.	Free + Bound	Conj.
Normal	22	22	10	0.1
Liver Disease	22	2	3	0.1
Kidney Disease	22	900	2	0
Cushing's Disease	34	45	20	0.3

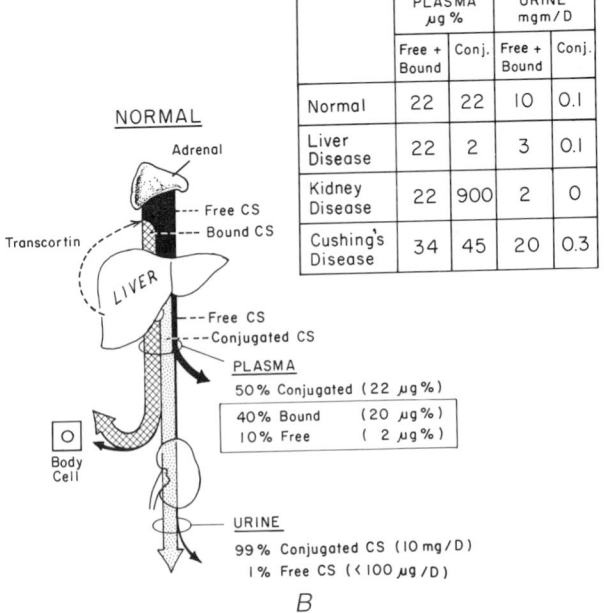

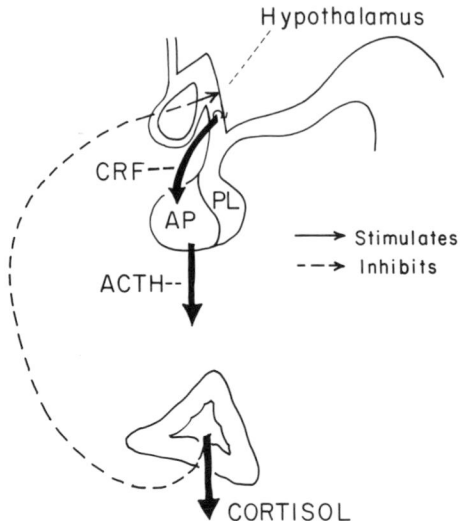

Fig. 37-24. Feedback regulation of cortisol secretion. CRF manufactured in the hypothalamus stimulates the anterior pituitary to release ACTH. ACTH stimulates the adrenal cortex to release cortisol and androgens. Cortisol, but not the androgens, act on the hypothalamus to inhibit release of CRF and thus of ACTH. In trauma the feedback mechanism is temporarily overcome as the hypothalamic centers secrete an increased amount of CRF leading to pituitary-adrenal stimulation and increased blood levels of cortisol.

which he defined as the sum of all systemic reactions to "stress." He predicted that diseases now known to be autoimmune phenomena (e.g., collagen vascular diseases) were caused by excessive responses to stress and thus cortisol, a stress hormone, would aggravate these conditions. The discovery of cortisol's anti-inflammatory effects contradicted Seyle's hypothesis.

The concept that cortisol confers resistance to stress was popular until the 1950s. Ingle and others postulated that cortisol performed a "permissive" function, wherein normal and stress-induced hormone responses required a basal circulating level of cortisol to permit an optimal response. This hypothesis failed to explain why severe stress mandated an increased cortisol response.

Excessive cortisol concentrations inhibit many normal immunologic functions. Although there is no convincing evidence that normal cortisol levels can influence the immune system, these findings have led some to question whether cortisol's effects are always beneficial. Munck and colleagues have attempted to incorporate the many diverse effects of cortisol on the immune system and inflammation into an intriguing hypothesis to explain why cortisol may be so important. They postulate that cortisol regulates the production of inflammatory mediators released in response to injury through inhibition of phospholipase A and, thus, thromboxane. Decreased synthesis of these mediators would, in turn, prevent these substances from harming the host. To date, this hypothesis remains unproved.

The known physiologic actions of cortisol can be divided into their effects on metabolism, effects on the immune system, and effects on blood volume restitution. Each area will be discussed briefly below.

Glucocorticoids influence metabolism of carbohydrates, proteins, and lipids. Although glucocorticoids block glucose uptake by most tissues, they do not interfere with glucose uptake by the liver, brain, or erythrocytes. They stimulate production of the catabolic hormone glucagon and inhibit insulin secretion synergistically with glucagon and catecholamines. The net effect of glucocorticoids is to mobilize glucose from peripheral tissues, while stimulating liver gluconeogenesis and glycogen deposition by activation of glycogen synthetase. Glucocorticoids block protein and nucleic acid synthesis in peripheral tissues while stimulating their degradation. The amino acids produced are utilized from hepatic gluconeogenesis. In contrast, glucocorticoids stimulate protein synthesis in the liver. Glucocorticoids also stimulate lipolysis and block lipid deposition in adipose tissue. Thus, glucocorticoids tend to cause hyperglycemia, negative nitrogen balance, and lipolysis. Peripheral tissues undergo catabolism while essential tissues such as the brain and liver are spared. The mobilization of metabolic energy substrates by cortisol in response to injury may aid the systemic injury response and facilitate subsequent tissue repair.

Many believe that the effects of glucocorticoids on the immune system and inflammation occur only at supraphysiologic cortisol concentrations. Thus, the physiologic significance of the glucocorticoid actions described below remains unclear. Patients treated with high doses of synthetic corticosteroids demonstrate more frequent infectious complications. Glucocorticoids inhibit nearly every aspect of the inflammatory response. They block interleukins, leukotrienes, histamine, and bradykinin, and inhibit the ability of these mediators to increase local vascular permeability that ordinarily delivers immune cells to an area of cell injury. Glucocorticoids block arachidonic acid and thromboxane release, and inhibit the local increase in vascular permeability caused by serotonin. Glucocorticoids also have been shown to interfere with nearly every component of the immune system. They inhibit macrophage and neutrophil chemotaxis, decrease complement levels, and suppress natural killer cell activity. Clearance of opsonized and nonopsonized material by the reticuloendothelial system is also inhibited. It is unclear whether glucocorticoids interfere with antibody responses.

The effects of glucocorticoids on the cardiovascular system are poorly understood. They may help to maintain capillary integrity and thereby regulate circulating blood volume or facilitate the action of catecholamines on the cardiovascular system. It is clear, however, that cardiovascular collapse occurs in patients with acute adrenocortical insufficiency and in animals subjected to hemorrhage after adrenalectomy. While intact animals deprived of water spontaneously restore their blood volume completely within 24 h after a moderate hemorrhage, adrenalectomized animals treated with only basal cortisol infusions are unable to do so. When cortisol infusion is increased to simulate the normal hypersecretion of cortisol after hemorrhage, restitution proceeds normally (Fig. 37-25). Restitution of blood volume is mediated by a shift of intracellular fluid to the interstitial compartment

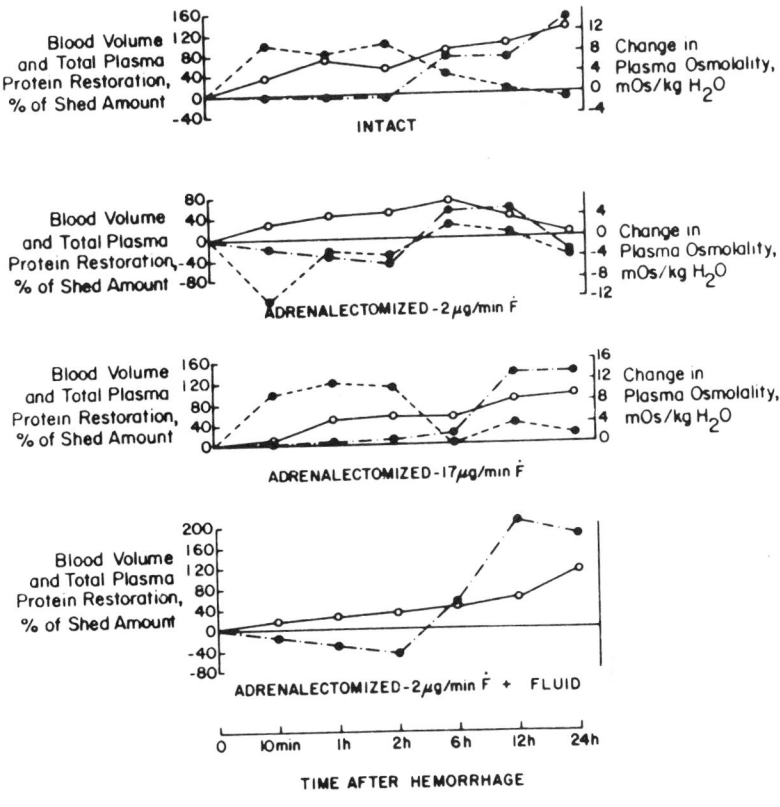

Fig. 37-25. Average changes in restoration of blood volume and plasma protein and in osmolality at various times in intact dogs (first panel), and in dogs subjected to adrenalectomy and infused with cortisol *(F)* at 2 µg/min (second panel), 17 µg/min (third panel), or 2 µg/min with glucose and saline added (fourth panel). (From: *Gann DS, Pirkle JC Jr: Role of cortisol in the resolution of blood volume after hemorrhage. Am J Surg 130:567, 1975, with permission.*)

caused by a transient increase in plasma osmolality. Protein and fluid from the expanded interstitium then replenish the intravascular volume. Thus, since cardiovascular stabilization after hemorrhage depends on the full restitution of blood volume, cortisol hypersecretion after injury is essential for cardiovascular stabilization and blood volume restitution.

ALDOSTERONE. Synthesis. Aldosterone is synthesized from progesterone formed by the C-3 dehydrogenation and isomerization of Δ-5-pregnenolone (Fig. 37-20). Hydroxylation of progesterone at the C-21 position of progesterone forms deoxycorticosterone, followed by C-11 beta-hydroxylation, yielding corticosterone. Corticosterone is hydroxylated at the C-18 position followed by oxidation of the C-18 hydroxyl group to an aldehyde to form aldosterone. The C-18 oxidation reaction is unique to the zona glomerulosa where aldosterone synthesis occurs.

Protein Binding. Although high fractions of other adrenal corticosteroids are protein-bound, only 55 percent of circulating aldosterone is bound to plasma proteins. Most aldosterone is bound to albumin. Unbound aldosterone is the physiologically active form in the circulation. Deoxycorticosterone, an intermediate compound in aldo-

sterone synthesis, is also a protein mineralocorticoid. Only 5 percent of circulating deoxycorticosterone is not bound to plasma proteins, and thus it has little physiologic activity.

Metabolism. Like cortisol, aldosterone is primarily metabolized in the liver by a series of reduction reactions. Aldosterone is a very active compound, and its concentrations in plasma and the amount excreted in the urine is much lower than the cortisol concentration. The half-life of circulating aldosterone is apparently 15 min.

Secretion. Aldosterone is synthesized and secreted by the adrenocortical cells of the zona glomerulosa. It is the most potent endogenous mineralocorticoid, 30 to 50 times more potent than deoxycorticosterone. Aldosterone secretion is stimulated by two physiologic stimuli: a decrease in circulating blood volume or an increase in serum potassium concentration (Fig. 37-26). Hemorrhage or hypovolemia stimulate aldosterone secretion leading to salt conservation that helps to conserve intravascular volume.

Angiotensin II and ACTH stimulate aldosterone secretion. Angiotensin II is a peptide hormone produced by a series of proteolysis reactions beginning with renin, a proteolytic enzyme secreted by renal juxtaglomerular cells. Renin cleaves angiotensinogen to form the decapeptide angiotensin I, which is subsequently cleaved by converting enzyme to form angiotensin II. Converting enzyme also inactivates bradykinin, and most of its activity is located in the lungs. Angiotensin II is a potent vasoconstrictor that plays a key role in blood pressure maintenance after hemorrhage. It is a transient substance with a plasma half-life of 1 to 2 min. Captopril is a competitive antagonist of converting enzyme with potent antihypertensive effects due to inhibition of angiotensin II production.

Renin secretion is stimulated by three physiologic stimuli (Fig. 37-26): (1) a decrease in arterial pressure in the renal afferent artery, (2) a decrease in chloride concentration in the renal tubules sensed by the macula densa, (3) stimulation of the renal sympathetic nerves via a beta-adrenergic mechanism. The half-life of renin in plasma is roughly 15 min.

Mineralocorticoid Actions. Aldosterone is an important regulator of electrolyte and fluid balance. It stimulates renal tubular sodium reabsorption and K, H^+, and $NH4^+$ secretion by a direct action on the tubule. Aldosterone also stimulates active sodium and potassium transport in other epithelial tissues such as sweat glands, gastrointestinal mucosa, and salivary glands. Experimental studies have shown that sodium reabsorption and potassium/hydrogen ion secretion are not coupled.

Increased aldosterone secretion due to increased renin secretion may complicate diseases associated with total body fluid overload due to a concomitant decrease in effective intravascular volume. In diseases such as congestive heart failure and hepatic cirrhosis, this so-called secondary hyperaldosteronism (Fig. 37-27) leads to further salt retention and increased fluid overload. Thus, therapy with the competitive aldosterone antagonist spironolactone has proved useful in the management of patients with these diseases.

CUSHING'S SYNDROME

Cushing's syndrome is caused by prolonged exposure to excessive cortisol concentrations. The most common cause is the chronic, iatrogenic administration of synthetic corticosteroids, whereas the spontaneous syndrome may be secondary to pathology in the hypothalamus, pituitary, or adrenal (Fig. 37-28). Additionally, some nonadrenal neoplasms secrete ACTH leading to adrenal cortisol hypersecretion. The signs and symptoms are similar regardless of the pathologic etiology of the syndrome.

ETIOLOGY. In contrast to Cushing's syndrome, Cushing's disease is specifically caused by a chronic hypersecretion of ACTH, which in turn leads to cortisol hypersecretion and hyperplasia of the adrenal cortex (Fig. 37-29). Pituitary tumors are responsible for ACTH hypersecretion in more than 90 percent of patients with Cushing's disease, most often a small unencapsulated basophilic adenoma. Alternatively, excessive CRF secretion or stimulation by some other factor with CRF activity (e.g., vasopressin) causes some cases of hypercortisolism. In

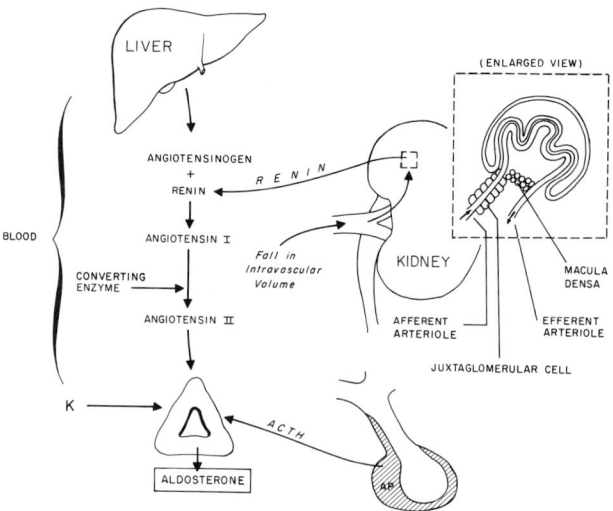

Fig. 37-26. Regulation of aldosterone secretion. A fall in blood volume, a fall in blood pressure, or vasoconstriction of the renal arteries due to norepinephrine produces a decrease in pressure in the afferent arteriole leading to a release of renin from the juxtaglomerular cells. The renin converts angiotensinogen manufactured in the liver to angiotensin I. This substance is further converted in the bloodstream by an enzyme in angiotensin II that stimulates the zona glomerulosa of the adrenal cortex to release aldosterone. Aldosterone, in turn, leads to sodium retention and a rise in blood pressure, which acts as a feedback mechanism to shut off the further release of renin. Secondary aldosteronism results when there is an obligatory secretion of renin as with an anatomic stricture of the renal arteries.

these cases, pituitary pathology usually reveals diffuse or adenomatous hyperplasia.

Primary adrenal pathology causes roughly 10 percent of all cases of Cushing's syndrome. Adrenal adenomas and carcinomas secrete cortisol independent of ACTH control. ACTH levels are low because of feedback leading to diffuse atrophy of nonneoplastic adrenocortical tissue. Adrenocortical carcinoma is more common than adenoma in children, while adenomas are more common in adults. Carcinoma is often diagnosed late in the course of the disease and fulminant cortisol hypersecretion may occur, especially when metastases are widespread. Documentation of local tumor invasion or metastatic spread is required to confirm malignancy because the usual histologic criteria for malignancy (e.g., pleomorphism and bizarre mitoses) do not correlate with malignant behavior.

Nonadrenal neoplasms may secrete ACTH leading to Cushing's syndrome. These tumors are infrequently identified, often because the patient rapidly deteriorates from the underlying malignancy. The so-called ectopic ACTH syndrome is responsible for roughly 15 percent of all cases of Cushing's syndrome. The patient may have severe hypercortisolism without the typical fat distribution of the disease because of cachexia related to malignancy. Hyperpigmentation due to hypersecretion of melanocyte stimulating hormone (MSH) in conjunction with ACTH is often present. Oat cell carcinoma of lung is the most common tumor causing the ectopic ACTH syndrome. Tumors of the parotid gland, liver, thymus, pancreatic islet cells,

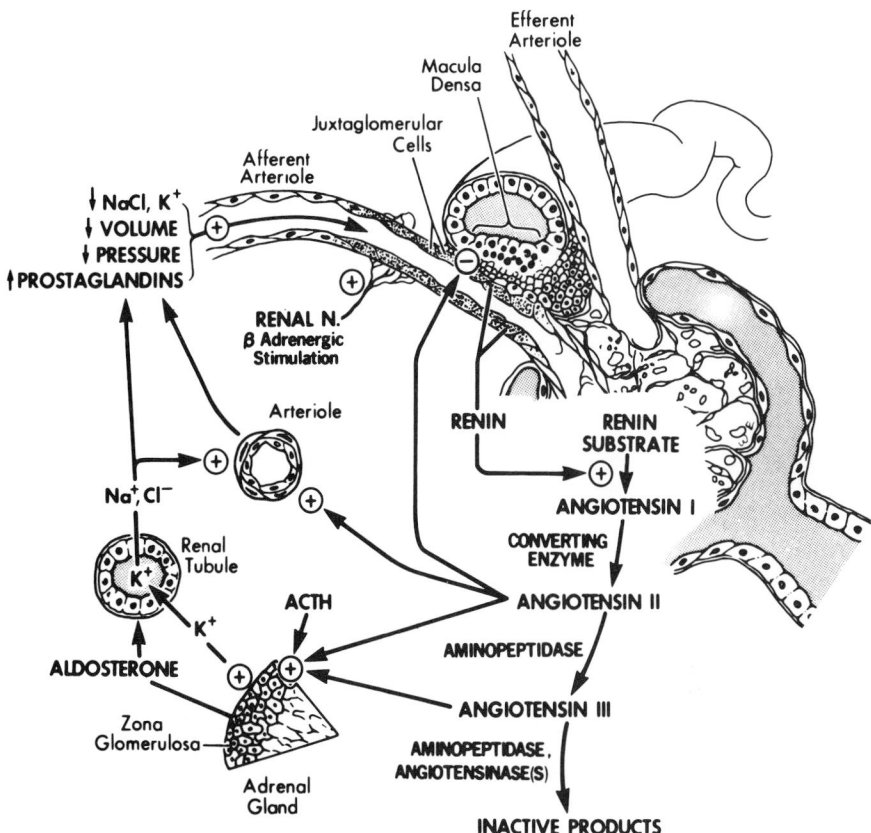

Fig. 37-27. Stimuli and pathways of activation of the renin-angiotensin system. +=stimulation, −=inhibition. [From: *Biglieri EG, Baxter JD, in Felig P, Baxter JD, Broadus AE, Frohman LA (eds): Endocrinology and Metabolism. New York, McGraw-Hill, 1981, chap 14, p 556, with permission.*]

SECONDARY ALDOSTERONISM | PRIMARY ALDOSTERONISM

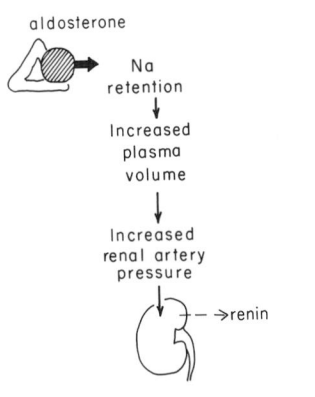

Fig. 37-28. Comparison of primary and secondary aldosteronism. In primary aldosteronism there is an obligatory secretion of aldosterone, which produces sodium retention, increased plasma volume, increased renal artery pressure, and inhibition of renin secretion. In secondary aldosteronism there is a primary decrease in renal artery pressure that stimulates the juxtaglomerular cells to secrete an increased amount of renin, thus leading to the production of angiotensin and stimulation of the adrenal cortex to produce increased amounts of aldosterone.

I. High aldosterone output

2. High renin output

I. High aldosterone output

2. Low renin output

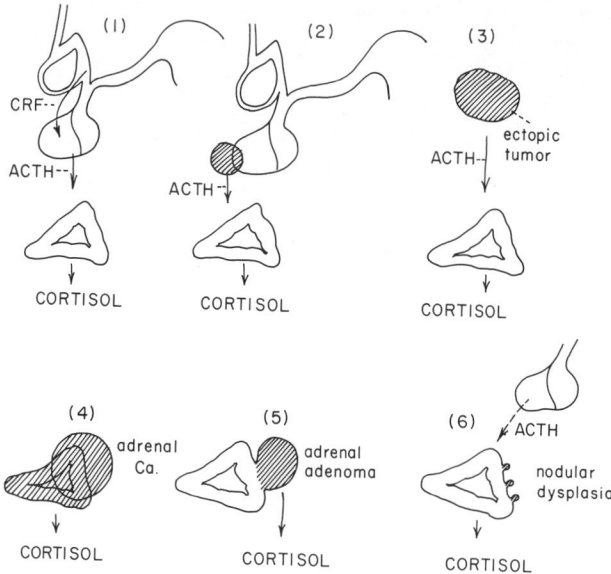

Fig. 37-29. Causes of Cushing's syndrome. Hyperplasia of the adrenal cortex is brought about by an increased secretion of ACTH that may result from a continual stimulation of the pituitary by CRF (1), an ACTH-secreting tumor of the anterior pituitary (2), or an ectopic malignant tumor secreting ACTH (3). The increased cortisol production can also come about as a consequence of an adrenal carcinoma (4), an adrenal adenoma (5), or nodular dysplasia (6).

esophagus, medullary carcinoma of the thyroid, and pheochromocytoma have also been reported in association with the ectopic secretion of ACTH.

Nodular dysplasia of the adrenal is an exceedingly rare cause of Cushing's syndrome (Fig. 37-30). In this disease, pathologic examination reveals numerous adrenal cortical nodules less than 2 mm in diameter containing large oval cells with small dark nuclei and granular eosinophilic cytoplasm.

CLINICAL MANIFESTATIONS. Females with Cushing's syndrome outnumber males four to one. The disease usually occurs in the third to fifth decade of life; however, cases in patients of all ages have been reported.

The common signs and symptoms of Cushing's syndrome are listed in Table 37-1. Truncal obesity with sparing of the extremities is classic, although generalized obesity is not uncommon. Fat deposition in the face and dorsocervical regions causes the classic "moon facies" and "buffalo hump," respectively (Fig. 37-31). Fat deposits also develop in the supraclavicular areas. Purple striae are often found on the lower abdomen and occa-

sionally on the trunk and upper legs. Hypertension, hirsutism, acne, and peripheral edema are common.

As the disease progresses, patients suffer marked muscle wasting. Many develop osteoporosis leading to vertebral compression fractures and spontaneous rib fractures. Arteriosclerosis and its sequelae are common. Patients frequently have a diabetic glucose tolerance curve or, occasionally, frank diabetes. Emotional lability and even psychosis have been reported. Hypokalemia is rare and suggests adrenocortical carcinoma or the ectopic ACTH syndrome as the cause of hypercortisolism.

DIAGNOSTIC TESTING. Diagnostic testing for Cushing's syndrome is divided into two categories. Initially, patients with suspected hypercortisolism undergo tests to confirm the diagnosis. Since treatment depends on the primary pathology, subsequent tests are performed to define whether the syndrome is a result of abnormal CRF or ACTH release, or autonomous cortisol secretion.

Fig. 37-30. Cushing's disease caused by nodular dysplasia: gross appearance of the gland.

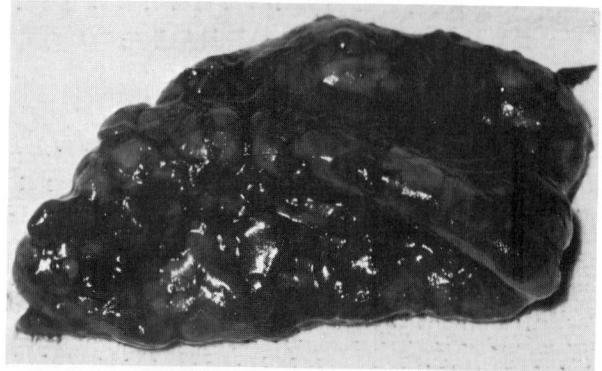

Table 37-1. CLINICAL MANIFESTATIONS OF CUSHING'S SYNDROME

	Percent (%)
Truncal obesity	95
Hypertension	85
Glucosuria and decreased glucose tolerance	80
Menstrual and sexual dysfunction	75
Hirsutism and acne	70
Striae	70
Muscle weakness	65
Osteoporosis	55
Easy bruisability	55
Poor wound healing	55
Psychiatric disturbances	50
Edema, hypokalemic alkalosis	40
Polyuria	15

SOURCE: Harrison TS, Gann DS, et al, 1975.

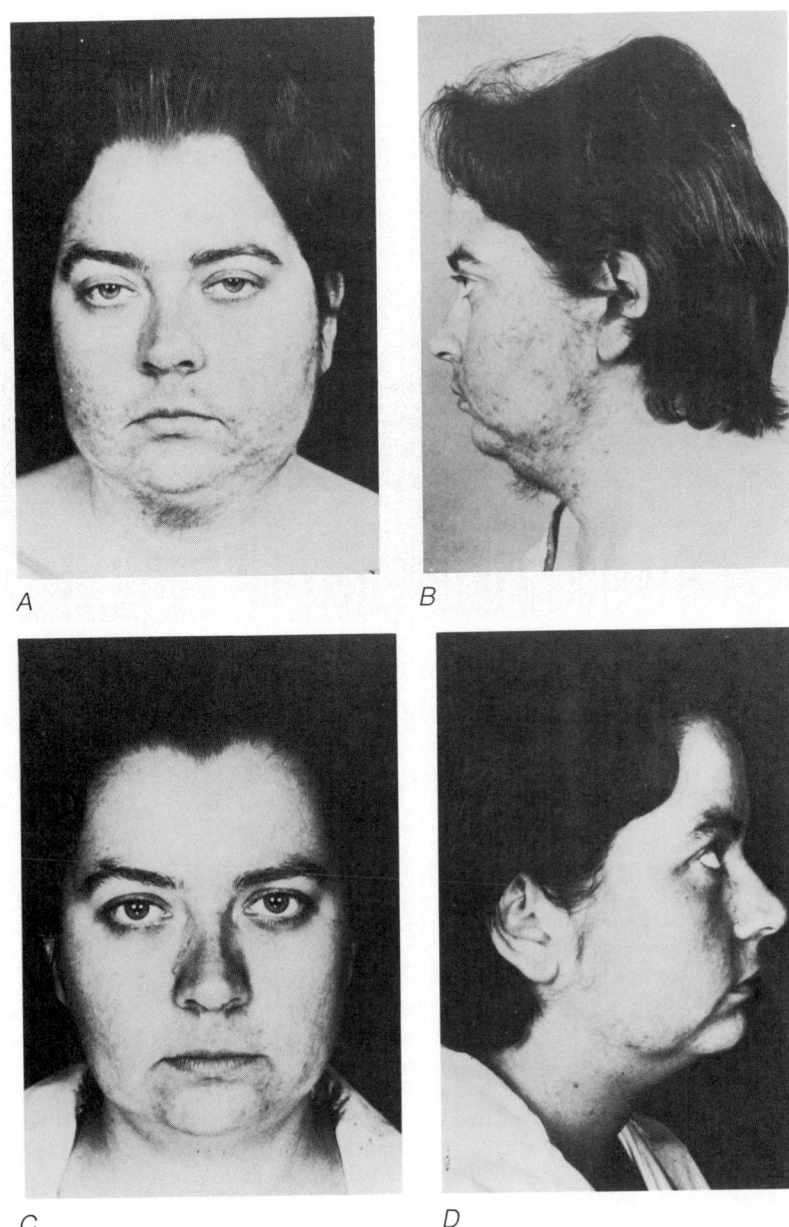

A *B*

C *D*

Fig. 37-31. Facial appearance of patient with Cushing's disease before *(A, B)* and after *(C, D)* remission was achieved by treatment with cyproheptadine. (From: *Hsu TH, Gann DS, et al: Cyprohepta-dine in the control of Cushing's disease. Johns Hopkins Med J 149:77, 1981, with permission.*)

Plasma Cortisol Levels. Measurement of the plasma cortisol concentration is usually not helpful in diagnosing Cushing's syndrome because it is possible to obtain normal plasma levels in patients with the disease. Furthermore, although the cortisol diurnal rhythm is usually abnormal, measurement of the cortisol nadir in the evening is rarely useful since there is large overlap between normal and abnormal values.

Urinary Cortisol Excretion. Determination of the excretion of free cortisol in a 24-h period is an important diag-

nostic test for Cushing's syndrome. Normally, urinary cortisol excretion is primarily in the form of conjugated cortisol metabolites and only a small amount of free cortisol is excreted. In Cushing's syndrome, the urinary free cortisol excretion is markedly elevated. Excretion of more than 100 μg of free cortisol in 24 h is considered abnormal and provides a nearly complete distinction between normal subjects and patients with Cushing's syndrome. Measurement of urinary free cortisol excretion is more accurate than measurement of 17-hydroxycorticosteroid or 17-ketosteroid urinary excretion. The incidence of false positive and negative results is less than 5 percent, and reliable patients may be tested on an outpatient basis.

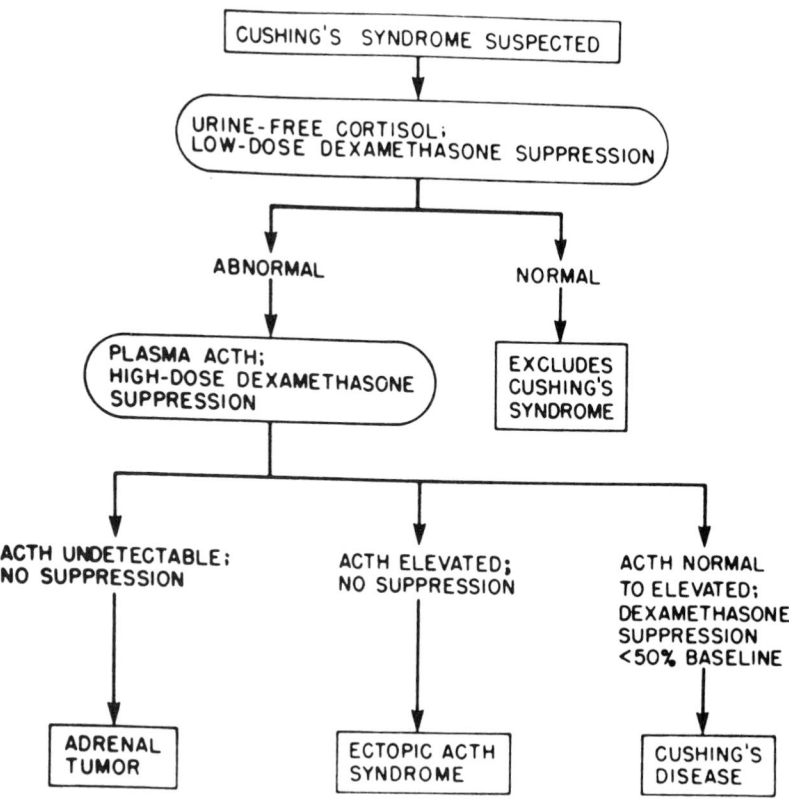

Fig. 37-32. Flow diagram for the evaluation of Cushing's syndrome. Boxes enclose clinical decisions and circles enclose diagnostic tests. [From: *Baxter JD, Tyrrell JB, in Felig P, Baxter JD, Broadus AE, Frohman LA (eds): Endocrinology and Metabolism. New York, McGraw-Hill, 1981, chap 12, p 475, with permission.*]

Dexamethasone Suppression Test. Dexamethasone is a synthetic corticosteroid that blocks ACTH release in normal subjects. Patients with Cushing's syndrome do not demonstrate suppressed cortisol concentrations after dexamethasone administration. Dexamethasone (1 mg) is administered orally to patients with suspected hypercortisolism at 11:00 P.M. and plasma cortisol is measured at 8:00 A.M. Patients who are obese, hospitalized, or chronically ill and those taking dilantin or estrogens have an increased risk of a false positive result compared with normal subjects. Additionally, the normal range for morning cortisol levels after dexamethasone suppression is wide, ranging from 3.5 to 10 μg/dL. Thus, utilizing both the 24-h urinary free cortisol excretion and overnight dexamethasone suppression together increases the accuracy of testing compared with one test alone (Fig. 37-32).

TESTS TO DETERMINE PRIMARY PATHOLOGY. Once the diagnosis of Cushing's syndrome is confirmed by the above tests, further work-up to determine the etiology of the syndrome is indicated. In order to direct therapy the etiology of Cushing's syndrome must be divided into (1) pituitary-dependent, (2) adrenal-dependent, or (3) ectopic ACTH-dependent categories.

Plasma ACTH Level. Measurement of the plasma ACTH concentration is useful in differentiating the cause of hypercortisolism. Patients with adrenal pathology usually have undetectable plasma ACTH levels. In contrast, patients with pituitary pathology or ectopic ACTH syndrome have normal to elevated ACTH levels. Usually, patients with the ectopic ACTH syndrome have the high-

est ACTH levels. Thus, measurement of the plasma ACTH often clearly separates patients with adrenal hypercortisolism from other causes, although in nodular dysplasia of the adrenal ACTH levels are often detectable. It is also difficult to distinguish between patients with a pituitary tumor and the ectopic ACTH syndrome because of the large overlap in ACTH levels found in these two groups.

High-Dose Dexamethasone Suppression Test. Suppression of cortisol excretion with a high dose of dexamethasone is useful in the differential diagnosis of Cushing's syndrome (Fig. 37-33), as compared with the low-dose dexamethasone suppression test used to diagnose hypercortisolism (Table 37-2). The 24-h urinary 17-hydroxycorticosteroid excretion is measured during the base line period and compared with the excretion while the patient takes 2 mg of dexamethasone orally every 6 h for 2 days. Nearly all patients with an adrenal tumor fail to suppress their 17-hydroxycorticosteroid output to 40 percent of base line during dexamethasone administration, whereas normal patients and those with pituitary tumors usually suppress to this level. This test again may not distinguish patients with pituitary and ectopic ACTH hypersecretion, since 25 percent of patients with the ectopic ACTH syndrome also suppress. Suppression does not occur in patients with nodular adrenal dysplasia.

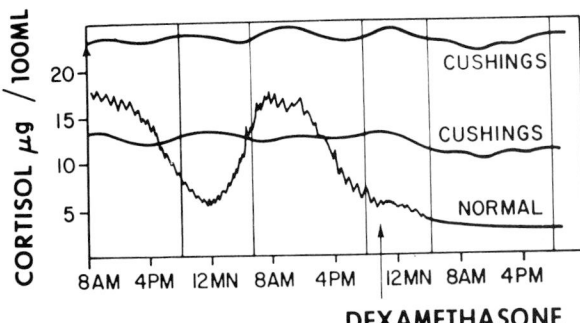

Fig. 37-33. A diurnal rhythm in cortisol secretion is present in a normal patient but lacking in two patients with Cushing's syndrome. A small dose of dexamethasone given at midnight suppresses the morning cortisol level in the normal subject but not in those with Cushing's syndrome.

Metyrapone Test. Metyrapone inhibits cortisol synthesis by blocking the final step in the cortisol synthesis pathway where 11-deoxycortisol is converted to cortisol by 11-hydroxylation. Administration of metyrapone to normal controls and in patients with a pituitary ACTH hypersecretion leads to a compensatory increase in plasma ACTH and a rise in urinary 17-hydroxycorticosteroid output when compared with the base line pretreatment value. Metyrapone usually causes a fall in urinary 17-hydroxycorticosteroid excretion in patients with an adrenal source of Cushing's syndrome due to a lack of compensatory increase in ACTH.

ACTH and CRF Stimulation Tests. Administration of ACTH intravenously to patients with adrenal cortical hyperplasia produces a greater rise in plasma cortisol than one would expect in normal patients. In contrast, adrenocortical adenomas have autonomous cortisol secretion and do not respond to ACTH increases. Although it is usually possible to differentiate between normals and patients with Cushing's syndrome, this test is not always capable of differentiating between hyperplasia and tumors.

With the recent isolation of CRF, a CRF stimulation test has been utilized with success in some centers to aid in the differential diagnosis of hypercortisolism. In particular, the response to CRF stimulation may aid in the differentiation of pituitary from ectopic sources of ACTH excess. In one recent clinical series, patients with ectopic ACTH syndrome did not respond with increased ACTH after CRF stimulation.

Other Tests. Differentiating patients with excessive ACTH from the pituitary versus an ectopic neoplasm may be particularly difficult. Patients with normal or increased ACTH plasma concentrations who suppress during high-dose dexamethasone suppression may have either disease. In patients with an obvious extraadrenal carcinoma, the answer is clear. In others, a careful search for lung carcinoma or other tumors may be required. Radiologic examination such as CT scanning and sellar radiography may reveal a pituitary lesion. Selective venous sampling from the inferior petrosal sinus may be helpful and a 2:1 central to peripheral ACTH gradient confirms the presence of a pituitary tumor. Pituitary exploration may also be thought of as a diagnostic test in some patients who have ACTH hypersecretion and no evidence for ectopic ACTH syndrome, since exploration of the pituitary may

Table 37-2. DEXAMETHASONE SUPPRESSION TESTS

Low-dose tests

Overnight test
  Dexamethasone, 1 mg p.o. at 11 P.M.; plasma cortisol at 8 to 9 A.M.
  Normal response—plasma cortisol <5 µg/dL

Two-day test
  Dexamethasone 0.5 mg p.o. q 6 h for 8 doses; plasma cortisol 6 h after last dose and 24-h urine-free cortisol and/or 17-OHCS during second day of dexamethasone

  Normal response—plasma cortisol <5 µg/dL; urine free cortisol <25 µg/24 h; urine 17-OHCS <4 mg/24 h or <1 mg/g urine creatinine

High-dose tests

Overnight test
  Dexamethasone 8 mg p.o. at 11 P.M.; plasma cortisol before and at 8 to 9 A.M. after dexamethasone

  Response—Cushing's disease; suppression of cortisol to <50% of base line; ectopic ACTH/adrenal tumors; no cortisol suppression

Two-day test
  Dexamethasone 2.0 mg p.o. q 6 h for 8 doses; plasma cortisol before dexamethasone and after last dose; 24-h urine-free cortisol and/or 17 OHCS before dexamethasone and during second day
  Response—Cushing's disease; suppression of plasma or urine steroids to <50% of base line; ectopic ACTH/adrenal tumors; no steroid suppression

SOURCE: Tyrrell JB, Baxter JD: Disorders of the adrenal cortex, in Wyngaarden JB, Smith LH Jr (eds): *Cecil Textbook of Medicine.* Philadelphia, Saunders, 1985, p 1308.

reveal a microadenoma in many patients despite normal preoperative radiologic studies.

TREATMENT. Termination of cortisol hypersecretion is the goal of all therapies for Cushing's syndrome, regardless of the syndrome's etiology. In the past, adrenalectomy was thought to be an appropriate therapy for all forms of Cushing's syndrome. Cases of ACTH hypersecretion were often treated with bilateral adrenalectomy, although the postoperative morbidity was high. Infectious complications were a frequent occurrence, presumably as a result of long-standing immunosuppression from prolonged exposure to high circulating concentrations of cortisol. Lifelong glucocorticoid and mineralocorticoid replacement was required with the associated complications of this therapy.

After bilateral adrenalectomy, many patients with Cushing's disease develop large ACTH-secreting pituitary tumors, called Nelson's syndrome. These tumors often developed years after adrenalectomy. Nelson's syndrome classically presents with marked hyperpigmentation of the skin. Visual disturbances are common when the pituitary tumor is large. Nelson's syndrome is a result of continued growth of the ACTH-secreting pituitary microadenoma that initially caused the syndrome. Some centers have reported success in preventing Nelson's syndrome by postoperative irradiation of the pituitary, although these results have been disputed. Alternatively, Nelson's syndrome may be treated by surgical resection; however, the tumors are often impossible to resect secondary to their large size and aggressive nature. Pituitary radiation therapy is usually a palliative measure. Fortunately, the incidence of Nelson's syndrome has decreased dramatically as bilateral adrenalectomy is no longer considered a primary therapy of Cushing's disease.

Pituitary Operations. The development of sophisticated techniques for pituitary microsurgery has revolutionized the treatment of Cushing's disease. Most patients with ACTH hypersecretion are best treated by pituitary exploration. Exploration of the gland may reveal an adenoma even if preoperative radiologic studies fail to demonstrate one.

Pituitary microadenectomy leads to cure in 50 to 90 percent of all cases of Cushing's disease. If no adenoma is discovered at exploration, corticotroph hyperplasia is likely on pathologic examination, presumably as a result of CRF hypersecretion. Total hypophysectomy is often curative in cases of CRF hypersecretion at the cost of panhypopituitarism.

Recurrence of Cushing's disease is common after pituitary microadenectomy. Krieger reported recurrence in 13 of 123 patients thought to have been cured. Recurrence may be precipitated by persistence of the factors responsible for the original ACTH hypersecretion, such as increased CRF secretion or corticotroph hypersensitivity to CRF. Fitzgerald has suggested that hypercortisolism results in all patients with successful treatment for Cushing's disease, and only patients who do not require postoperative steroid replacement are at risk for recurrence. The return of a normal response to dexamethasone sup-

pression and a normal ACTH response to insulin hypoglycemia occurs in patients cured by pituitary microsurgery. The diurnal rhythm of cortisol secretion is persistently abnormal months after apparent surgical cure in nearly half of patients.

Pituitary Irradiation. Conventional pituitary radiation therapy has largely been abandoned as initial therapy in patients with Cushing's disease in favor of pituitary microadenectomy. The success rate of irradiation varies between 15 and 83 percent in a number of reports, but a consistent favorable response rate of 80 percent has been reported in children with Cushing's disease. The major disadvantage of pituitary irradiation is the long interval between initiation of therapy and the clinical response, often 18 months or longer.

Neuropharmacologic Agents. Neuropharmacologic treatment of patients with Cushing's disease is not yet considered routine. Neuropharmacologic agents are primarily indicated in patients unresponsive to pituitary surgery or in cases of Cushing's disease proved secondary to CRF hypersecretion. Pathologic examination in the latter patients often reveals hyperplasia of pituitary corticotrophs rather than a single adenoma.

Cyproheptadine is effective in the management of some patients with Cushing's disease by blocking the release of CRF from the hypothalamus. Its primary action is via inhibition of central serotoninergic neurones, although it also blocks histaminergic, cholinergic, and dopaminergic pathways. Cyproheptadine does not affect the adrenal's response to ACTH but does block the normal circadian ACTH rhythm. Cyproheptadine causes remission in 30 to 50 percent of patients with Cushing's disease. Hyperphagia and somnolence are prominent side effects; however, these tend to decrease with continued administration of the drug. Treatment is begun with 4 mg orally three times daily and increased to 2 mg every 4 h over the first 2 weeks of treatment. A clinical response usually occurs after 2 to 3 weeks of therapy. Cyproheptadine may also be effective in some patients with ectopic ACTH syndrome. In these cases, cyproheptadine probably inhibits a CRF-like material produced by the tumor rather than the more common ectopic production of ACTH.

Bromocriptine is a dopamine antagonist that inhibits CRF secretion. Studies on the use of bromocriptine in the treatment of Cushing's disease have yielded conflicting results, and this drug is not recommended in the initial treatment of the disease.

Sodium valproate is an inhibitor of gamma-aminobutyric acid transaminase (GABA) that raises central nervous system levels of the inhibitory neurotransmitter GABA. Several reports have suggested that sodium valproate may be effective in blocking ACTH release when used along or in conjunction with diazepam, which facilitates GABA's activity.

Preliminary reports have suggested that opiate antagonists may be useful in the treatment of Cushing's disease. The site of action of these drugs in affecting ACTH release is unclear, but a central site of action on the hypothalamus or pituitary seems likely. Naloxone lowers plasma ACTH levels in patients with Nelson's syndrome and adrenal insufficiency. Although the long-acting metenkephalin analog FK-33824 decreases ACTH in normal subjects and in patients with adrenal insufficiency, its effectiveness in patients with Cushing's disease is controversial.

Adrenal Operations. A surgical procedure is the initial treatment of all patients with Cushing's syndrome secondary to adrenal adenoma or carcinoma. In the case of adrenal adenoma, preoperative radiologic studies should be performed to lateralize the tumor. This allows surgical resection of the tumor via a unilateral flank incision which has been shown to decrease the morbidity of surgery compared with a transabdominal approach.

CT scanning or iodocholesterol scintigraphy are the preferred tests for lateralization of adrenal adenomas. High-resolution CT scanning localizes 80 percent of adenomas. Nuclear scans, although not available in many centers, are quite useful. No iodocholesterol uptake is found on the side contralateral to an adenoma, while an adrenal carcinoma is likely in cases where no iodocholesterol uptake occurs bilaterally in a patient with presumed hypercortisolism of adrenal origin. CT scanning in adrenal carcinoma is useful to demonstrate the extent of invasive disease (Fig. 37-34).

Adrenal adenomas are treated and cured by unilateral adrenalectomy. Postoperatively, these patients should be treated with steroid replacement therapy until the contralateral, suppressed gland regains normal function, usually 3 to 6 months later.

Patients with adrenal carcinoma should be explored via a midline abdominal incision to allow radical resection of all tumor whenever possible since surgery offers the only hope for cure. Locally invasive and metastatic adrenal carcinomas should be removed when feasible, and repeated surgery to remove tumor tissue appears indicated in the treatment of recurrence. Postoperative adjunctive radiation therapy and chemotherapy with cytotoxic agents appears to improve survival.

Mitotane. Mitotane (*o,p'-DDD*) is a by-product of insecticide research that causes selective destruction of normal and neoplastic adrenocortical cells. Necrosis of the zona fasciculata, and eventually the zona reticularis, occurs with continued administration of the drug. Mitotane is the only chemotherapeutic agent that has proved of some value in the treatment of adrenal carcinoma. The adrenolytic effects usually occur over 2 to 4 months but may take as long as 16 months to develop. Adrenocortical insufficiency is the result of successful mitotane therapy, and patients require glucocorticoid and mineralocorticoid replacement therapy when prolonged mitotane chemotherapy has been utilized. The most common side effects of mitotane chemotherapy are anorexia and nausea, although diarrhea, vomiting, skin rashes, gynecomastia, memory loss, arthralgias, and leukopenia also may occur.

Mitotane chemotherapy has recently been used in the prophylactic treatment of nonmetastatic adrenal carcinoma after surgical resection of the primary tumor. Luton et al. have reported increased longevity in patients with adrenal carcinoma after surgical resection from an average of 10 months without chemotherapy to 47 months

with mitotane. Patients treated with mitotane before there was clinical evidence of metastases survived an average of 74 months. The combination of surgical resection with mitotane chemotherapy appears to offer the most promise for the future treatment of patients with adrenal carcinoma.

Ectopic ACTH Syndrome. Patients with the ectopic ACTH syndrome are best treated by complete resection of the primary neoplasm. However, surgical resection is often impossible in these patients. Oat cell carcinoma of the lung is responsible for more than 60 percent of all cases of the ectopic ACTH syndrome, and these tumors respond poorly to surgery. Occasionally, radiation therapy or chemotherapy may be beneficial. Debulking procedures may offer some palliation, and occasionally the response to debulking is improved with adjuvant radiation or chemotherapy.

Bilateral adrenalectomy may be considered in patients with ectopic ACTH syndrome and unresectable primary tumors that carry a fair prognosis for relatively long survival. A trial of chemotherapy with metyrapone or mitotane is warranted prior to consideration of bilateral adrenalectomy in these patients. If the response to these agents is good, bilateral adrenalectomy is not necessary. A rare patient with the ectopic ACTH syndrome develops profound hypokalemia unresponsive to medical management. These patients may require urgent bilateral adrenalectomy after preoperative stabilization.

ADRENOCORTICAL INSUFFICIENCY (ADDISON'S DISEASE)

Adrenocortical insufficiency is rare in the surgical patient. Although treatment is frequently successful, more often than not the diagnosis is only made at autopsy. A high index of suspicion is essential to diagnose adrenal insufficiency because the signs and symptoms are nonspecific.

In the perioperative period, adrenal insufficiency may occur in patients after adrenalectomy, in patients treated with chronic steroids, or in patients with metastatic cancer. Chronic adrenocortical insufficiency that is unrecognized before surgery also is a common cause of acute postoperative adrenal insufficiency. Acute adrenocortical insufficiency, or adrenal crisis, must be considered in any patient who develops sudden or progressive cardiovascular collapse or in patients with any acute illness that does not respond to appropriate therapy.

The actual incidence of postoperative adrenal insufficiency is uncertain. Alford and associates reviewed 5000 cardiothoracic surgery patients and found 5 patients with clinical evidence for adrenal insufficiency, an incidence of 0.1 percent. The incidence of adrenal hemorrhage in autopsy series ranges from 0.14 to 1.1 percent, but the incidence of clinical adrenal insufficiency in these patients is unknown.

ETIOLOGY. The most common cause of acute adrenocortical insufficiency is withdrawal of chronic steroid therapy. Chronic administration of supraphysiologic doses of glucocorticoids suppresses ACTH by feedback

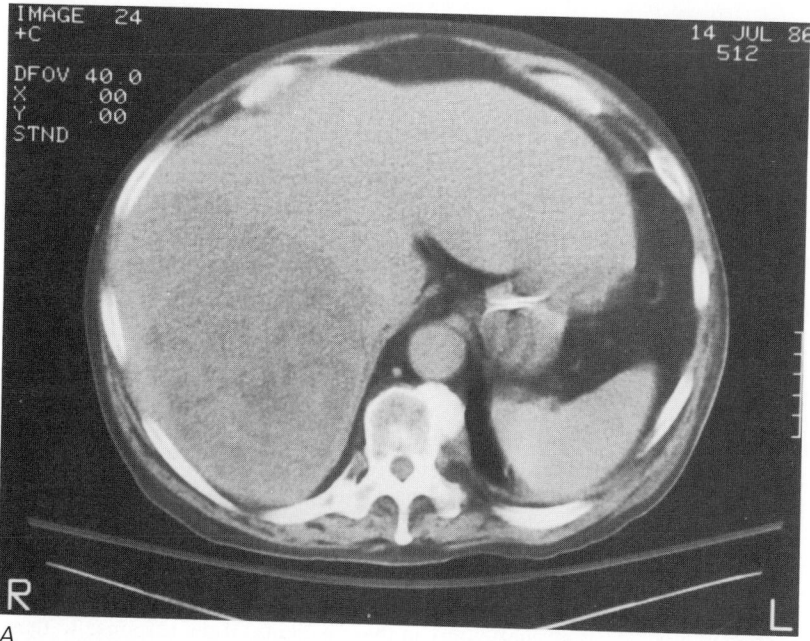

A

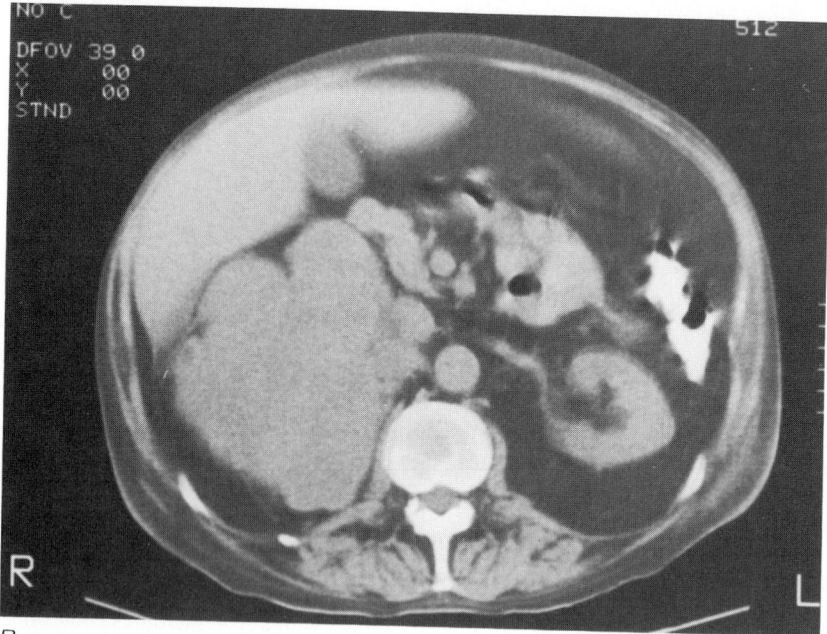

B

Fig. 37-34. CT scan of patient with locally invasive and metastatic adrenocortical carcinoma. The tumor is seen invading the right lobe of the liver (A) and the kidney and inferior vena cava (B). This patient was deemed inoperable and started on mitotane therapy in hopes of reducing the tumor burden enough to allow an attempt at resection.

at the pituitary and hypothalamus. The long-term result is adrenocortical atrophy. Patients treated with steroids for a variety of diseases are susceptible to acute adrenocortical insufficiency when steroids are abruptly discontinued. Thus, it is a common clinical practice to slowly taper the daily dosage of steroids to allow the pituitary-adrenal axis to recover its normal responsiveness.

More than 80 percent of spontaneous cases of adrenal insufficiency are secondary to autoimmune destruction of the adrenals. Antibodies against adrenocortical cells

occur in a high percentage of these patients, and adrenal histology usually reveals a lymphocytic infiltrate. Autoimmune adrenal insufficiency has a high association with other endocrinologic autoimmune diseases, called "Schmidt's syndrome." The most common associated disorder in patients with autoimmune adrenocortical insufficiency is hypothyroidism due to autoimmune thyroiditis, which occurs in up to 80 percent of patients. Other associated diseases include hyperthyroidism in 4 percent, diabetes in 12 percent, and hypoparathyroidism in 6 percent. Ovarian failure occurs in 25 percent of females with the syndrome.

Recent prospective studies have demonstrated an increased incidence of adrenocortical autoantibodies in the serum of patients with insulin-dependent diabetes and autoimmune thyroid disease. At least some of these patients develop clinical adrenocortical insufficiency within several years. Elevated levels of ACTH have been demonstrated in asymptomatic patients with adrenocortical autoantibodies despite normal plasma cortisol and aldosterone production. Thus, adrenocortical insufficiency appears to develop gradually in patients with autoimmune disease. These patients go through an interim period with normal cortisol and aldosterone production maintained by increased ACTH stimulation. The adrenal stress response may be impaired during this period and acute adrenal insufficiency precipitated by the stress of other illness. Although routine testing for adrenocortical antibodies in patients with autoimmune disorders does not appear cost-effective, these patients should be considered at increased risk of adrenal insufficiency during acute illness. More than 90 percent of the adrenal cortex must be destroyed before basal plasma cortisol levels decrease below normal.

In the past, tuberculosis was the most frequent cause of adrenocortical insufficiency and it remains an important cause in underdeveloped countries. Intraadrenal hemorrhage secondary to sepsis, anticoagulant therapy, or coagulopathy can cause acute adrenocortical insufficiency. Acute adrenal hemorrhage secondary to sepsis, the Waterhouse-Friderichsen syndrome, is usually caused by meningococcal septicemia in young children. Adults may also develop acute adrenal hemorrhage from meningococcal, pneumococcal, streptococcal, diphtherial, or fungal infection. Adrenal infarction secondary to arterial thrombosis or arteritis may occur but is uncommon.

Adrenal insufficiency has been reported in patients with advanced cancer secondary to adrenal metastases. Many patients with terminal malignancy have symptoms similar to the nonspecific symptoms of adrenal insufficiency, including weakness and fatigue, hyponatremia, fever, orthostatic symptoms, and oliguria. Furthermore, cancer patients are often treated with glucocorticoids for palliation, but it is unclear whether steroid treatment is beneficial in these patients due to replacement of deficient cortisol levels or the nonspecific euphoriant effects of corticosteroids. Cedermark and Sjoberg studied the incidence of adrenal insufficiency in a small series of patients with cancer and the effect of cortisol replacement in symptomatic, terminally ill cancer patients. They found no patients with suppressed plasma cortisol levels or a subnormal cortisol response to ACTH stimulation. Only three patients of 15 treated with corticosteroids had any clinical improvement, although diagnostic testing was normal in these patients. They conclude that symptoms suggestive of adrenal insufficiency infrequently reflect actual adrenal insufficiency in cancer patients.

CLINICAL MANIFESTATIONS. Patients with adrenocortical insufficiency often complain of weakness and fatigue, weight loss, and anorexia. Gastrointestinal symptoms are common including nausea, vomiting, and less commonly diarrhea. A diffuse hyperpigmentation or "bronzing" of the skin is a classic sign of the disease. Salt-craving, postural dizziness, dehydration, and amenorrhea in females are frequent symptoms.

Patients with acute adrenocortical insufficiency, or "adrenal crisis," may have some of the above chronic symptoms depending on the duration of the disease. Patients with acute adrenal hemorrhage or infarction often have other nonspecific symptoms including poorly defined upper quadrant abdominal or flank pain and fever. Anorexia, nausea, and vomiting are often pronounced in these patients. These patients are frequently subjected to surgery for suspected acute intraabdominal pathology, and the diagnosis often remains unclear even after exploration.

Changes in mental status such as lethargy, disorientation, and confusion often occur in adrenal crisis. Hypotension, hypoglycemia, and hyperkalemia are classic signs. Hyponatremia and hyperkalemia are due to associated mineralocorticoid deficiency. The characteristic normocytic, normochromic anemia of the disease may be masked by dehydration and hemoconcentration. Neutropenia, lymphocytosis, and, particularly, eosinophilia are common. Prerenal azotemia and mild metabolic acidosis may occur. Increased levels of serum calcium are common, but the mechanism of hypercalcemia is unclear.

The above signs with or without cardiovascular collapse in any intraoperative, postoperative, or critically ill patient should raise the suspicion of adrenocortical insufficiency. The diagnosis can only be made when clinicians maintain a high index of suspicion.

DIAGNOSTIC TESTING. Diagnostic tests to confirm the presence of adrenocortical insufficiency are undertaken only if the clinical condition of the patient is stable. If the patient's clinical condition is rapidly deteriorating, a blood sample for plasma ACTH and cortisol levels should be drawn and a 200-mg dose of a water-soluble corticosteroid such as cortisol hemisuccinate or cortisol sodium succinate is administered with the same needle. There is little risk in a short course of steroids, and, in this situation, corticosteroids are lifesaving. Further tests can be performed when the patient's condition has stabilized to confirm the diagnosis.

Plasma cortisol levels are often, but not invariably, depressed in patients with adrenal insufficiency. Seriously ill patients always have a random plasma cortisol level above 14 μg/dL, and it is often greater than 20 μg/dL. The morning cortisol level may be low and, less commonly, the evening nadir is depressed. ACTH concentration is usually elevated in the range of 250 to 400 pg/mL in cases of primary adrenocortical insufficiency. In adrenocortical insufficiency secondary to ACTH deficiency, plasma ACTH levels are low, ranging from 0 to 50 pg/mL.

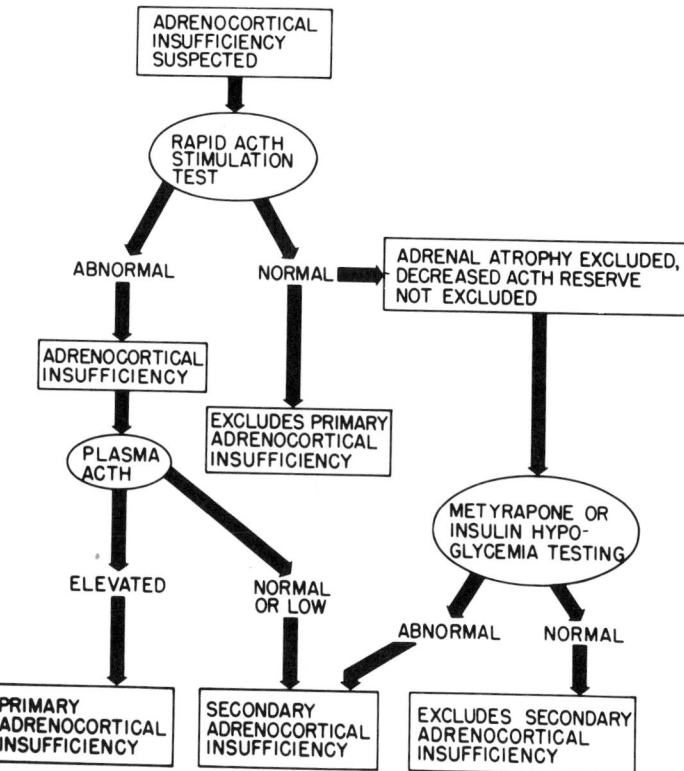

Fig. 37-35. Evaluation of a suspected primary or secondary adrenocortical insufficiency. Boxes enclose clinical decisions and circles enclose diagnostic tests. [From: *Baxter JD, Tyrrell JB, in Felig P, Baxter JD, Broadus AE, Frohman LA (eds): Endocrinology and Metabolism. New York, McGraw-Hill, 1981, chap 12, p 458, with permission.*]

Plasma cortisol levels do not prove the presence of adrenocortical insufficiency, as circulating levels may be normal despite an impaired stress response. The adrenal capacity to respond to ACTH stimulation must be evaluated to assess the stress response. The most useful test for this is the rapid ACTH stimulation test (Fig. 37-35). Plasma cortisol is measured immediately before and 15, 30, and 60 min after administration of 250 μg of ACTH intravenously. A peak cortisol increase of at least 7 $\mu g/dL$ is normal. The rare patient with secondary adrenocortical insufficiency will have a normal cortisol response due to ACTH deficiency, but these patients have a low basal level of ACTH as described above.

Recently, the isolation of corticotropin-releasing factor (CRF) has led to intravenous CRF administration as a diagnostic test for patients with adrenocortical insufficiency. This stimulation test appears particularly useful in patients with secondary adrenocortical insufficiency, separating these patients into two groups based on their ACTH response to CRF. Both groups have low basal ACTH levels, but the ACTH response to CRF is either diminished or augmented compared with normal subjects, presumably representing patients with primary pituitary or hypothalamic pathology, respectively.

Further tests to confirm the diagnosis are rarely required. Abdominal CT scanning and ultrasound can detect adrenal hemorrhage and alert the clinician to the possibility of adrenocortical insufficiency. Metyrapone or insulin hypoglycemia testing may be useful in patients with suspected secondary adrenocortical insufficiency with a normal cortisol response to ACTH stimulation. In addition, all patients with confirmed adrenocortical insufficiency should be tested for thyroid function to screen for Schmidt's syndrome. Menstrual problems in females with adrenocortical insufficiency should be evaluated with measurement of follicle stimulating hormone and luteinizing hormone to screen for associated ovarian failure.

TREATMENT. Adrenal Crisis. Therapy for acute adrenocortical insufficiency should be started immediately after the diagnosis is considered (Table 37-3). Administration of water-soluble corticosteroids and isotonic intravenous fluids for volume resuscitation are the mainstays of therapy. Initial steroid treatment should consist of an intravenous bolus of 200 mg of hydrocortisone. Additionally, 50 to 100 mg of cortisone acetate should be given intramuscularly in case intravenous access is compromised. After the initial bolus, steroids are administered in amounts three to ten times the usual endogenous cortisol production. Fifty to 100 mg of hydrocortisone may be given intravenously every 6 h, or a continuous infusion of hydrocortisone at 10 mg/h may be utilized.

Other treatment is directed at accompanying abnormalities. Hypoglycemia is corrected by using intravenous solutions that contain dextrose. Electrolyte disturbances must be addressed, but hypertonic solutions are not indi-

Table 37-3. THERAPY OF ADRENOCORTICAL INSUFFICIENCY

Acute crisis
1. Hydrocortisone, 100 mg I.V., every 6 h for 24 h. If stable, reduce to 50 mg every 6 h and then taper to oral maintenance in 4 to 5 days. Maintain or increase dose to 200 to 400 mg per 24 h if complications persist or occur.
2. Correct volume depletion, dehydration, hypotension, and hypoglycemia with intravenous saline and glucose.
3. Correct precipitating factors, especially infection.

Maintenance
1. Hydrocortisone 15 to 20 mg p.o. q A.M.: 5 to 10 mg at 4 to 6 P.M.
2. 9α-Fluorocortisol 0.05 to 0.1 mg q A.M. (primary)
3. Follow weight, blood pressure, and electrolytes
4. Educate patient and increase cortisol dosage during stress.

SOURCE: Tyrrell JB, Baxter JD: Disorders of the adrenal cortex, in Wyngaarden JB, Smith LH Jr (eds): *Cecil Textbook of Medicine.* Philadelphia, Saunders, 1985, p 1308.

cated to correct hyponatremia. Although inotropic and sympathomimetic agents are occasionally needed to support blood pressure early in the course of treatment, vigorous fluid resuscitation is preferred. The underlying cause of adrenal crisis also must be urgently addressed, particularly septicemia and coagulopathy. Administration of high doses of glucocorticoids provides adequate mineralocorticoid therapy since most glucocorticoids have salt-retaining actions.

Perioperative Treatment. Patients maintained on chronic corticosteroid treatment require steroid replacement therapy in the perioperative period, whether surgery is elective or emergent. An acceptable paradigm for perioperative steroid treatment is presented in Table 37-4. Patients currently taking steroids or those who have taken them within 2 years should be treated with steroids perioperatively.

Estimates of endogenous cortisol production in patients undergoing major surgery vary between 75 and 150 mg daily. Some authors have suggested that the usually recommended perioperative hydrocortisone dosage of 300 to 600 mg/day is excessive and potentially harmful owing to the potential for inhibition of wound healing, increased catabolism, electrolyte disturbances, and more frequent infectious complications described in patients treated with pharmacologic corticosteroid doses. Kehlet has proposed a low-dose regimen for perioperative steroid replacement, advocating administration of a 25-mg

intravenous bolus of hydrocortisone at the time of anesthesia induction followed by a total dose of 100 mg during the first 24 h after surgery. No ill effects were noted in a series of patients treated with this regimen.

Symreng and colleagues have utilized a preoperative ACTH stimulation test to assess the pituitary-adrenal axis in patients taking chronic steroids for a variety of nonadrenal diseases. They report that patients with a normal cortisol response to ACTH were treated successfully without steroids and suffered no circulatory instability. Six patients identified with a subnormal cortisol response to ACTH were treated with Kehlet's low-dose hydrocortisone replacement regimen and also suffered no ill effects.

Udelsman and colleagues reported that adrenalectomized monkeys undergoing cholecystectomy had increased hemodynamic instability and mortality if cortisol replacement was maintained at one-tenth physiologic levels, but did not find any difference in hemodynamics, wound healing, or mortality in monkeys treated with physiologic or ten times physiologic levels of cortisol replacement.

Although the above authors conclude that their results support low-dose perioperative steroid replacement, no study has demonstrated that complications are increased with daily steroid replacement three to ten times the usual endogenous steroid output that is recommended in most perioperative paradigms. In contrast, hemodynamic in-

Table 37-4. STEROID COVERAGE FOR SURGERY

1. Correct electrolytes, blood pressure, and hydration if necessary
2. Hydrocortisone phosphate or hemisuccinate, 100 mg I.M., on call to operating room
3. Hydrocortisone phosphate or hemisuccinate, 50 mg I.M. or I.V., in recovery room and every 6 h for the first 24 h
4. If progress is satisfactory, reduce dosage to 25 mg every 6 h for 24 h, then taper to maintenance dosage over 3 to 5 days. Resume previous 9α-fluorocortisol dose when patient is taking oral medications
5. Maintain or increase cortisol dosage to 200 to 400 mg per 24 h if fever, hypotension, or other complications occur

SOURCE: Baxter JD, Tyrrell JB, in Felig P et al (eds): *Endocrinology and Metabolism,* 2d ed. New York, McGraw-Hill, 1987, chap 12, p 596.

Table 37-5. BIOLOGIC ACTIVITY PROFILES
OF SYNTHETIC ANALOGS OF CORTISOL

Steroid	P Potency anti-inflammatory	P Equiv. dose (mg)	Sodium retention	Biol. t:½ (h)
Cortisol	1.0	20	1.0	8–12
9α-Fluorocortisol	10	—	125	—
Short-acting analogs				
Prednisolone	4	5	0.8	12–36
6α-Methylprednisolone	5	4	0.5	12–36
Triamcinolone (9α-F,16α-OH prednisolone)	5	4	0	12–36
Long-acting analogs				
Betamethasone (9α-F,16β-methylprednisolone)	25	0.6	0	36–54
Dexamethasone (9α-F,16α-methylprednisolone)	25	0.6	0	36–54

SOURCE: Tepperman J: *Metabolic and Endocrine Physiology*. Chicago, Year Book Medical Publishers, 1980, p 193.

stability and death are well-described consequences of inadequate steroid replacement. Thus, there are no apparent contraindications to the hydrocortisone replacement regimen described in Table 37-4, and the effectiveness of this regimen is well established.

Chronic Insufficiency. Chronic treatment of patients with adrenocortical insufficiency must include both glucocorticoid and mineralocorticoid replacement. After a period of adrenal crisis or acute illness, the doses of corticosteroids are usually tapered gradually over a period of days to prevent precipitation of further adrenal insufficiency until a maintenance level is reached.

Chronically, steroids are administered in a twice-daily fashion that roughly approximates the physiologic diurnal rhythm with a lower dose late in the day. Synthetic steroids and their relative anti-inflammatory and sodium-retaining potencies are listed in Table 37-5. Prednisone is frequently utilized for long-term treatment, and a representative dosage is 5 mg in the morning and 2.5 mg in the early evening. Mineralocorticoid replacement is also indicated, as this dosage of prednisone does not provide enough mineralocorticoid. Oral fluorohydrocortisone 0.1 to 0.2 mg daily is usually adequate mineralocorticoid replacement.

Patients must be educated that steroid therapy is continued for the rest of their lives and that failure to continue may lead to severe insufficiency and death. They should also wear an identification tag to alert medical personnel that immediate therapy with intravenous steroids is required when they become seriously ill. In addition, they should be instructed to seek early medical attention when they become ill or if they develop nausea, vomiting, or diarrhea, because intravenous corticosteroid therapy should be considered in these situations.

A novel idea for the long-term management of adrenal insufficiency has been reported by Saxe. He utilized implantable infusion pumps in dogs to administer a low-dose constant infusion of glucocorticoid and mineralocorticoid

replacement for prolonged time periods in adrenalectomized dogs. The results demonstrate the potential feasibility of long-term management of adrenal-insufficient patients with this technique. The low-dose regimen may also avoid many of the chronic effects of excess steroid administration on metabolism, wound healing, and the immune system. To date, however, no clinical studies have been reported.

PRIMARY HYPERALDOSTERONISM

Primary hyperaldosteronism is one of the few causes of hypertension that can be cured by surgery. Thus, the diagnosis should be considered in all patients with new-onset or worsening hypertension. Routine serum electrolytes should be measured in all hypertensive patients prior to initiating therapy, because spontaneous hypokalemia is suggestive of primary aldosteronism. Although all patients with hyperaldosteronism have hypertension, hyperaldosteronism is an uncommon cause of hypertension, occurring in less than 1 percent of all hypertensive patients.

ETIOLOGY. Primary hyperaldosteronism is caused by adrenocortical adenoma or hyperplasia. Eighty-five percent of all patients with the disease harbor a benign adrenocortical adenoma that autonomously secretes aldosterone (Fig. 37-36). The remaining 15 percent of patients have hyperplasia of the zona glomerulosa (idiopathic hyperaldosteronism). It is important to differentiate between adrenal adenoma and hyperplasia because the preferred treatments are different.

An interesting and important diagnostic difference between aldosteronomas and idiopathic hyperaldosteronism is that adenomas appear to be sensitive to ACTH while changes in angiotensin II influence aldosterone secretion in cases of bilateral hyperplasia. Although renin and angiotensin II are suppressed in both forms of hyperaldosteronism due to feedback, only patients with idio-

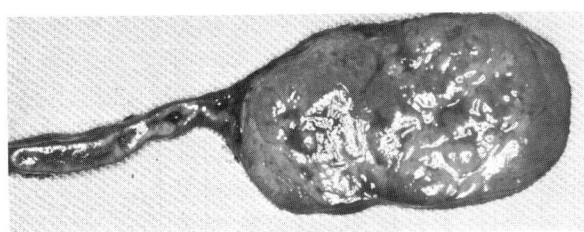

Fig. 37-36. Section cut through an aldosterone-producing tumor and a portion of the normal cortex. The tumor was a rather large one that was well circumscribed. The cut surface was bright yellow, and there was no atrophy of the normal adrenal cortex.

pathic hyperaldosteronism respond with further increases in aldosterone when the renin-angiotensin system is stimulated by postural changes. The reason for this difference is unclear, but a chronic increase in adrenal sensitivity to angiotensin II mediated by an unknown mechanism may be an important factor in the etiology of idiopathic hyperaldosteronism. Possible candidates for this aldosterone-stimulating factor include derivatives of the ACTH precursor molecule POMC including alpha-MSH, beta-MSH, gamma-MSH, beta-lipotropin, or beta-endorphin. Studies on aldosteronoma cells have revealed that fragments of POMC including the N-terminal fragment (16K), gamma$_3$-MSH, and beta-lipotropin stimulate aldosterone secretion by a mechanism similar to angiotensin II. More importantly, these factors potentiate the action of ACTH on aldosteronoma cells. Thus, one of these factors might contribute to the pathogenesis of primary aldosteronism.

CLINICAL MANIFESTATIONS. Patients with primary hyperaldosteronism classically have hypertension with spontaneous hypokalemia. Thus, all patients with new-onset hypertension should undergo serum electrolyte determination before treatment is begun. The serum sodium concentration is usually normal in patients with primary aldosteronism who are not taking diuretics.

Although many patients are asymptomatic, symptoms when they do occur are usually secondary to hypokalemia and, in general, nonspecific. Weakness, fatigue, paresthesias, tetany, and even paralysis may develop, particularly in patients treated for hypertension with thiazide diuretics that aggravate hypokalemia. Polyuria may develop secondary to vasopressin resistance from chronic hyperkaliuria. The resultant hypovolemia may lead to polydipsia and thus simulate untreated diabetes.

Primary hyperaldosteronism occurs more frequently in women and is most common in the third and fourth decades of life. Hypertension is always present, usually mild but occasionally severe. Long-standing hypertension with the sequelae of left ventricular hypertrophy, cardiomyopathy, or stroke may be present. Patients may have been treated for hypertension for prolonged periods before the diagnosis of hyperaldosteronism is made.

Hypertension or ecclampsia during pregnancy is common in women with primary hyperaldosteronism. A number of women also have menorrhagia, and Granberg reported that 25 percent of females had undergone hysterectomy before the diagnosis of hyperaldosteronism was made. Although the mechanism of menorrhagia is

unclear, a decrease in the amount of bleeding has been reported following adrenalectomy.

DIAGNOSTIC TESTING. Biochemical Determinations. Patients with hypertension and spontaneous hypokalemia should be evaluated for primary hyperaldosteronism. However, hypokalemia must be corrected with potassium replacement before diagnostic testing because hypokalemia inhibits aldosterone secretion and may lead to a false negative work-up (Fig. 37-37). During potassium replacement, the patient is also treated with salt loading because the diagnosis of primary hyperaldosteronism depends on the demonstration of elevated aldosterone levels with simultaneous suppression of plasma renin activity. Thus, salt loading is used to suppress renin. Nine grams of sodium chloride per day are given orally for 1 to 2 weeks before testing. Antihypertensive medications should also be withheld during evaluation. The treatment of severe hypertension after medications are withdrawn is best treated with the vasodilator hydralazine. After hypokalemia is corrected and salt loading has been completed, simultaneous measurement of plasma aldosterone and renin activity is performed. Elevated aldosterone levels with low plasma renin activity suggest primary hyperaldosteronism. Fluorohydrocortisone, a potent synthetic mineralocorticoid, is then administered in a dosage of 0.1 mg/day for 3 days to further inhibit plasma renin and angiotensin II. If the aldosterone level is still elevated after treatment with fluorohydrocortisone, the diagnosis of primary hyperaldosteronism is confirmed.

Subsequent tests are performed to establish the etiology of primary hyperaldosteronism. It is impossible to differentiate between idiopathic hyperaldosteronism and aldosteronoma by symptoms or degree of hypertension, although patients with aldosteronoma tend to have worse hypokalemia, alkalosis, and higher aldosterone levels.

The biochemical test of choice to differentiate between hyperplasia and adenoma is measurement of plasma aldosterone concentrations after changes in posture. Only patients with aldosteronoma experience a postural decrease in aldosterone. Plasma aldosterone is measured at 8 A.M. after overnight recumbency and again after 4 h of upright posture. A postural decrease in aldosterone level is not consistent with idiopathic hyperaldosteronism. This test yields an accuracy rate of 75 to 100 percent in differentiating aldosteronoma from idiopathic hyperaldosteronism. Postural changes in plasma renin and aldosterone concentrations typical of aldosteronoma, idiopathic hyperaldosteronism, and the rare aldosterone-producing adrenal carcinoma are presented in Fig. 37-38.

Localization. If the above tests suggest an aldosteronoma, surgical resection is indicated. Preoperative radiologic localization of the tumor should be performed prior to surgery. Lateralization of the adenoma allows surgical resection via posterior flank incision that is associated with lower postoperative morbidity compared with the transabdominal approach.

High-resolution CT scanning localizes approximately 75 percent of adenomas and is thus the best noninvasive test available. In the past, adrenal venography was an important imaging test in the work-up of adrenal adeno-

steronism, termed primary adrenal hyperplasia, with a good response to surgical therapy. However, this disease appears to be rare.

The therapy of choice for idiopathic hyperaldosteronism is medical management with spironolactone, a competitive antagonist of aldosterone. Correction of hypokalemia results from spironolactone therapy in almost all patients with idiopathic hyperaldosteronism. Two hundred to 400 mg a day in divided doses is usually effective in controlling hypokalemia. Hypertension is often not controlled with spironolactone alone, and other medications are often required. Amiloride is also useful in the management of these patients. Amiloride is a potassium-sparing diuretic that acts independently of aldosterone causing natriuresis. It is often effective in controlling hypertension in these patients and is often combined with spironolactone to increase the effectiveness of therapy. Cyproheptadine may also be useful in the medical management of patients with idiopathic hyperaldosteronism. This supports the hypothesis that hyperaldosteronism due to hyperplasia may be caused by an extraadrenal factor that increases the adrenal sensitivity to angiotensin. Calcium channel blockers such as nifedipine may be effective in controlling hypertension and decreasing plasma aldosterone levels in patients with idiopathic hyperaldosteronism or aldosteronoma, albeit by an unclear mechanism.

If medical management of hypokalemia or hypertension is unsuccessful in patients with idiopathic hyperaldosteronism, a surgical procedure may be required. Total or subtotal adrenalectomy is the surgical treatment of choice, and the response to therapy is often poor. Hypertension is cured by bilateral total adrenalectomy in one-third of patients and may be easier to control with medication in the remaining patients. The patients must be treated with lifelong steroid replacement. Thus, the long-term morbidity of total adrenalectomy may be high and its risks must be weighed against the risks of continued hypertension and hypokalemia due to persistent hyperaldosteronism.

Spironolactone should be administered for 6 to 10 days prior to surgery in all patients with adrenal adenomas to allow for the correction of hypokalemia and resultant cardiac arrhythmias. Preoperative spironolactone therapy also allows for normal fluid balance to be restored. The magnitude of the decrease in blood pressure with spironolactone therapy provides an indication of the blood pressure response that may be anticipated after adrenalectomy in patients with adenoma. Surgical resection of an aldosteronoma results in a return to normal blood pressure in roughly 50 percent of patients and a decrease in the need for antihypertensive medications in an additional 25 percent. Hypokalemia is almost always corrected by adrenalectomy. Hypertension recurs in as many as 40 percent of patients within 10 years after adrenalectomy; however, less medication is usually required to control arterial pressure in these patients.

An aldosteronoma must not be confused with a nonfunctioning adrenal nodule at the time of operation. Nonfunctioning nodules occur in as many as 20 percent of patients with hypertensive cardiovascular disease, increase in frequency with age, and may grow as big as 3 cm. Nonfunctioning nodules are usually multiple and characteristically pale in color, while aldosteronomas are usually single lesions, circumscribed, and the cut surface of the tumor is bright yellow.

ADRENOGENITAL SYNDROME

The adrenogenital syndrome is caused by adrenal androgen hypersecretion. The syndrome may be "pure" or "mixed" depending on whether the secretion of other adrenal hormones is increased, decreased, or unaffected. For example, patients may have virilization as well as signs of Cushing's syndrome due to cortisol hypersecretion. Although characteristics of masculinization are common with both Cushing's syndrome and hyperaldosteronism, androgen hypersecretion is the predominant finding in the adrenogenital syndrome.

ETIOLOGY. The adrenogenital syndrome may be diagnosed during the newborn period, infancy and childhood, or adulthood. In children and infants, a congenital enzyme deficiency in the pathways of cortisol biosynthesis and the resultant decrease in cortisol production causes hypersecretion of ACTH due to the loss of feedback inhibition. Secondary adrenocortical hyperplasia develops with overproduction of intermediary compounds in cortisol biosynthesis including the adrenal androgens. The incidence of congenital adrenocortical hyperplasia has been estimated at 1 in 15,000 live births. There are six variants of congenital adrenal hyperplasia, although the most common by far is a defect in C-21 hydroxylation. Females with C-21 hydroxylation defects are pseudohermaphrodites, while males have macrogenitosomia praecox. In newborns with a more complete hydroxylation defect, subnormal aldosterone secretion may occur, leading to salt wasting, vascular collapse, and death unless treatment with mineralocorticoids is promptly started.

A defect in C-11 hydroxylation causes virilization with hypertension because of the increased production of 11-deoxycortisol as well as adrenal androgens. Other enzymatic deficiencies are often associated with salt wasting and death. These include defects in 3-beta-hydroxysteroid dehydrogenase, C-20 hydroxylation, C-18 hydroxylation, and C-17 hydroxylation.

In postnatal children and adults, virilization is almost always caused by tumors of the adrenal. Adrenocortical carcinoma is the most common tumor causing virilization in both children and adults. Androgen-secreting adrenal adenomas are rare. Adrenocortical hyperplasia may occasionally cause virilization in adults.

CLINICAL MANIFESTATIONS. Androgen excess leads to masculinization in females and precocious puberty in young males. Symptoms may include acne, deepening of the voice, temporal baldness, increased strength, an increase in muscle mass, and amenorrhea. Hirsutism is the most classic symptom. Patients may also note an increase in sex drive.

DIAGNOSTIC TESTING. Patients with suspected adrenogenital syndrome should undergo a 24-h urine collection for 17-ketosteroids. The urinary excretion of 17-ketosteroids usually exceeds 30 to 40 mg in a 24-h period in patients with the syndrome. Plasma testosterone levels are increased in patients with syndrome due to peripheral conversion of adrenal androgens to testosterone.

Adrenal androgen secretion in cases of virilizing hyperplasia is sensitive to ACTH stimulation. Thus, failure of dexamethasone treatment to cause suppression of the urinary 17-ketosteroid excretion to normal ranges supports the diagnosis of an adrenal tumor causing virilization. Congenital adrenal hyperplasia is ruled out by the failure of dexamethasone suppression. To perform this test, dexamethasone is administered 0.5 mg four times a day for 7 days prior to urine collection. The diagnosis of adrenocortical carcinoma should also be suspected when the 24-h urinary 17-ketosteroid excretion exceeds 100 mg.

Ovarian tumors may also secrete testosterone and are important in the differential diagnosis of adrenogenital syndrome in adult females. Frequently the 24-h urinary 17-ketosteroid output is normal or only moderately elevated in patients with ovarian tumors, and excretion of more than 30 mg per 24 h is rare. Furthermore, ACTH inhibition with dexamethasone fails to suppress androgen and 17-ketosteroid urinary excretion in patients with ovarian tumors. Ovarian tumors may also be palpable on pelvic examination.

TREATMENT. Congenital Adrenocortical Hyperplasia. Congenital adrenocortical hyperplasia is treated with glucocorticoid administration to suppress ACTH. Surgical correction of abnormalities of the external genitalia in females is almost always required. These patients are usually operated on before the age of four years and sometime after the age of one. If the clitoris has not diminished significantly in size with medical management, resection and relocation of the enlarged clitoris as was originally described by Lattimer is preferable to amputation of the clitoris. Labial scrotal fusion is also corrected when present.

Tumors. Virilization caused by tumors of the adrenal are treated surgically. A transperitoneal approach is the procedure of choice. CT scanning and iodocholesterol scanning are utilized to localize the tumor preoperatively. The adrenal on the involved side should be resected along with locally metastatic disease when feasible. Some of these carcinomas are highly malignant and offer a very poor prognosis. Many times the carcinoma recurs several years after the initial resection. Monthly measurement of 17-ketosteroid urinary excretion may help to detect tumor recurrence. Mitotane may be used to treat recurrent tumors. Although no cures have been reported with mitotane, regression of metastases and a decrease in steroid production have been noted.

ADRENAL MASS

The wide application of high-resolution CT scanning has led to the incidental discovery of increasing numbers of asymptomatic masses of the adrenal. Glazer and colleagues reported incidentally discovered adrenal masses on 0.6 percent of upper abdominal CT scans. The appro-

priate management of these patients, with no clinical or biochemical evidence of adrenal disease, is controversial. Fine-needle aspiration with cytologic evaluation of the aspirate holds little promise for distinguishing benign from malignant adrenal lesions. Current techniques are unable to differentiate malignant and benign disease, and only invasion of local structures and the presence of distance metastases correlate with malignant behavior.

Various management strategies have been suggested for the asymptomatic mass. Prinz and colleagues emphasized the patient's age as an important factor, suggesting that a small nodule in an older patient was unlikely to be clinically significant. In patients under fifty years of age or with a nonfunctioning lesion greater than 3 cm in diameter, they felt surgical treatment was appropriate. Copeland has criticized this aggressive approach and advocates a conservative, nonoperative approach for adrenal masses less than 6 cm in size (Fig. 37-40). His recommendation was based on the observation that adrenal carcinomas are usually larger than 6 cm when initially detected. In various series, 92 percent of adrenal carcinomas were over 6 cm when first detected. Copeland recommended repeated CT scanning at regular intervals for small, solid masses with surgery only if the lesion increased in size.

Belldegrund and colleagues have advocated a more aggressive approach for the asymptomatic adrenal mass. They recommend that adrenal masses greater than 3.5 cm in diameter on CT scan deserve exploration to rule out malignancy. Like Copeland, they feel small lesions are safely observed with serial CT scans.

In summary, although the management of the asymptomatic adrenal mass is controversial, patients with this lesion should be evaluated for biochemical activity of an adrenal tumor with measurement of urinary free cortisol and catecholamine excretion, plasma renin activity, aldosterone, and androgen concentrations. If the tumor is found to be nonfunctional (using previously described criteria), it appears that careful management of the lesion with serial CT scanning may be appropriate. A young patient in good health may be better served by surgical exploration since the poor prognosis of carcinoma discovered at an advanced stage may outweigh the small risk of surgery.

Adrenal Medulla

PHYSIOLOGY

Synthesis. The human adrenal medulla synthesizes and secretes epinephrine, norepinephrine, and small amounts of dopamine. The enzymatic reactions of catecholamine synthesis are depicted in Fig. 37-41. Tyrosine is the precursor of all catecholamines. It is converted to dopa by tyrosine hydroxylase. Aromatic L-amino acid decarboxylase converts dopa to dopamine. The above reactions take place in the cytosol. Dopamine is then hydroxylated by dopamine beta-hydroxylase (DBH) to norepinephrine in the chromaffin granule where DBH is bound. Norepinephrine is then transported to the cytosol where the en-

with MEN IIB have medullary thyroid carcinoma, 31 percent have bilateral adrenal hyperplasia or tumors, and 81 percent exhibit marfinoid body habitus with skeletal deformities but without the characteristic aortic or ocular abnormalities. Ganglioneuromatosis of the gastrointestinal tract is common in MEN IIB. This may be diffuse, extending from lips to rectum, or segmental. Ganglioneuromatosis has a high genetic penetrance and may be the earliest sign of the MEN syndrome, often preceding the development of neoplasia.

CLINICAL MANIFESTATIONS. Pheochromocytomas occur in all age groups, although they are unusual in children less than six years old. The peak incidence is between the fourth and fifth decades of life. All races are equally affected and there is no sex predilection.

Symptoms from a pheochromocytoma are caused by catecholamine hypersecretion, the complications of hypertension, or, less commonly, the local effects of a space-occupying lesion. Fifty percent of patients have paroxysmal hypertensive episodes, and these patients often present with severe and dramatic symptoms. The severity of symptoms in patients with pheochromocytoma is related to rapid increases in circulating catecholamine concentrations rather than the absolute plasma levels. Patients with persistently elevated catecholamine concentrations become less responsive to their effects.

Patients with paroxysmal symptoms frequently describe attacks consistent in severity, composition, and order of symptom appearance. The duration of attacks may vary considerably lasting from minutes to hours and, rarely, days. Attacks may occur at night and awaken the patient and tend to occur more often over time. Occasionally, attacks disappear secondary to the development of sustained hypertension, spontaneous tumor necrosis, or tumor regression. A so-called acute pheochromocytoma presents with malignant hypertension and a rapid downhill course. Acute pheochromocytomas are rare.

Catecholamine hypersecretion in patients with pheochromocytoma may be precipitated by drugs that stimulate catecholamine secretion, mechanical deformation of the tumor, changes in body position, invasive tests, anesthesia, or increases in intraabdominal or intrathoracic pressure. Anxiety, anger, or any strong emotional response may precipitate an attack. Headache, generalized diaphoresis, and palpitations are the most common symptoms of pheochromocytoma. Headaches are usually of sudden onset and described as generalized with a severe "throbbing" sensation. The duration is usually brief, and these headaches are often ascribed to stress migraine. Diaphoresis may involve the face, neck, and upper torso. The extremities are often cool. Diaphoresis may be continuous, paroxysmal, or occurring only at the end of an attack. Other symptoms include facial pallor or flushing, a sense of anxiety, tremors, dizziness, and syncope. A more complete list of possible symptoms is presented in Table 37-7. Symptoms of pheochromocytoma may also be due to the complications of prolonged or severe hypertension including cardiovascular disorders, cerebrovascular disease, or renal failure. The initial presentation may be the sudden onset of severe hypertension or shock

due to vascular collapse in the course of pregnancy, invasive testing, or anesthesia. The mortality in this situation is high.

Hypertension is the most common sign of pheochromocytoma. Pheochromocytomas are responsible for hypertension in 0.1 to 0.2 percent of patients with sustained diastolic hypertension. Either sustained or paroxysmal hypertension with mild to severe elevations of systolic and diastolic blood pressures is possible, and arterial pressure is often normal between hypertensive episodes. Occasionally, hypotension may follow severe labile hypertension or alternate with hypertensive episodes secondary to excessive beta-adrenergic receptor stimulation by circulating catecholamines.

Decreased arterial pressure and tachycardia with postural changes in a hypertensive patient strongly suggest a pheochromocytoma. These postural changes in cardiovascular parameters may be secondary to volume contraction, impaired responsiveness to sympathetic reflexes, or a functional ganglionic blockade caused by sustained high levels of catecholamines. Thus, screening for pheochromocytoma should include screen for pheochromocytoma repeated arterial pressure and pulse recordings in the supine, sitting, and erect positions. The diagnosis should also be considered in hypertensive patients with poor control or wide fluctuations in arterial pressure under treatment with antihypertensives.

Table 37-7. SYMPTOMS AND SIGNS OF
PHEOCHROMOCYTOMA

	Approximate percent (%)	
	Adult	*Child*
Symptoms:		
Persistent hypertension	65	92
Paroxysmal hypertension	30	8
Headache	80	81
Sweating	70	68
Palpitation, nervousness	60	34
Pallor of face	40	27
Tremor	40	
Nausea	30	56
Weakness, fatigue	25	27
Weight loss	15	44
Abdominal or chest pain	15	35
Dyspnea	15	16
Visual changes	10	44
Constipation	5	8
Raynaud's phenomenon	5	
Convulsions	3	23
Polydipsia, polyuria		25
Puffy, red, cyanotic hands		11
Signs:		
BMR over +20 percent	50	83
Fasting blood sugar over 120 mg/100 mL	40	40
Glycosuria	10	3
Eye ground changes	30	70

SOURCE: From Hume DM, Astwood EB, Cassidy CE: Grune & Stratton, 1968.

Mottled cyanosis of the skin, mesenteric ischemia, claudication, Raynaud's phenomenon, or livedo reticularis may reflect peripheral vasomotor instability due to high circulating catecholamine concentrations in patients with pheochromocytoma. Low-grade fever, weight loss, and other signs of hypermetabolism may occur. Extreme catecholamine concentrations may induce myocarditis or even myocardial necrosis resulting in congestive heart failure. Catecholamines also lower the threshold for cardiac arrhythmias and may cause sudden death. Reflex bradycardia via a baroreceptor-mediated reflex in response to hypertension occasionally occurs. Although 95 percent of pheochromocytomas are intraabdominal, few are palpable on examination. An attack of hypertension during palpation of the abdomen or flank occurs in as many as half of cases.

Differential Diagnosis. Pheochromocytoma has been called the "great mimic" because of its diverse presentations and similarities to other illnesses. Difficulty arises in patients with mild or nonspecific symptoms. Table 37-8 lists illnesses that may be confused with pheochromocytoma.

Patients with mild or intermittent hypertension present the most difficult problem in screening for pheochromocytoma because the diagnosis is not suspected. The astute clinician will ask hypertensive patients about possible symptoms of pheochromocytoma and order the appropriate diagnostic tests.

Pheochromocytoma presenting as hypertension during pregnancy may be missed with disastrous consequences. Untreated pheochromocytoma carries a 50 percent mortality rate for both mother and fetus. Pheochromocytoma should be suspected in any pregnant female with paroxysmal or sustained hypertension. Although peripheral edema, hypertension, and proteinuria suggest ecclampsia, these symptoms also occur in pheochromocytoma. Suspicion of pheochromocytoma should be heightened if treatment for presumed ecclampsia with magnesium sulfate is not therapeutic.

Table 37-8. DIFFERENTIAL DIAGNOSIS OF PHEOCHROMOCYTOMA

Illness	Associated conditions
Hypertension	Essential hypertension, renovascular hypertension
Headaches	Migraine, cluster
Tachycardias	Paroxysmal atrial and nodal tachycardia
Endocrine abnormalities	Thyrotoxicosis, menopause, hypoglycemia, diabetes
CNS disorders	Diencephalic seizures, autonomic hyperreflexia, increased intracranial pressure due to tumors, infection, or stroke, lead poisoning
Tumors	Carcinoid, neuroblastoma
Pregnancy	Preeclampsia, eclampsia thyrotoxicosis or simple hypertension of pregnancy

Pheochromocytoma patients may have accompanying psychiatric symptoms ranging from anxiety to psychosis, although classically they experience only brief periods of apprehension and fear with intervening periods of normal affect. Simultaneous pheochromocytoma and depression has been reported.

Symptoms due to a carcinoid tumor may be confused with symptoms of pheochromocytoma. Carcinoids may secrete serotonin, kallikrein, bradykinin, histamine, or prostaglandins. Episodes of flushing with hypotension are prominent symptoms due to carcinoid tumors accompanied by diarrhea, hyperperistalsis, steatorrhea, wheezing, edema, pellagrous lesions, telangiectasis, or angiomata of the skin. Urinary levels of hydroxyindoleacetic acid are elevated in patients with a carcinoid and intravenous injection of small amounts of epinephrine or histamine induce flushing attacks. In contrast, small doses of catecholamine usually do not affect patients with pheochromocytoma. This test must be performed with care in the hospital, as histamine may cause catecholamines crisis in a patient with pheochromocytoma.

Neuroblastoma and ganglioneuroblastoma are usually seen in young patients and are usually asymptomatic. Patients with neuroblastoma usually have hepatomegaly and a palpable abdominal mass. Urinary norepinephrine, dopamine, metanephrines, homovanillic acid, VMA, and MHPG may be elevated. The presence of epinephrine in elevated levels strongly suggests pheochromocytoma, as almost all neuroblastomas secrete primarily norepinephrine or dopamine.

DIAGNOSTIC TESTING.   Urinary Catecholamine Excretion. Appropriate laboratory tests are necessary to confirm the clinical suspicion of a pheochromocytoma. Measuring the urinary excretion of free epinephrine, norepinephrine, or their metabolites is the test of choice. Most patients with pheochromocytoma have distinctly elevated levels of norepinephrine and epinephrine in 24-h urine collections. Measurement of the urinary metanephrines is the best screening test because of its high reliability and ease of performance. Measurement of the vanillymandelic acid content of urine is the least specific of all catecholamine excretion tests because of false-positive results in patients that consume products with high vanilla content such as coffee, tea, and raw fruits.

Plasma Catecholamines. Accurate measurement of plasma concentrations of epinephrine, norepinephrine, and the metanephrines is now possible. However, often catecholamine hypersecretion in patients with pheochromocytoma is intermittent and the plasma catecholamine concentration may be low in between secretory episodes. Thus, screening patients for a pheochromocytoma with these tests is inaccurate.

Provocative Tests. In the past, pharmacologic agents that induce catecholamine secretion in patients with pheochromocytoma have been utilized to supplement the diagnostic work-up. Administration of histamine, tyramine, and glucagon has been used to evoke catecholamine hypersecretion and induce an attack. Disadvantages of these tests include high false-positive and false-negative results. Significant morbidity and even death may result secondary to catecholamine crisis. Thus, provocative tests have no place in the initial evaluation of pheochromocytoma. These tests are occasionally useful in patients with negative biochemical tests if a strong clinical suspicion of pheochromocytoma persists. Phentolamine and antiarrhythmic agents should be immediately available when provocative tests are performed to abort a catecholamines crisis.

Significant hypotension in response to the alpha-adrenergic blocking agent phentolamine has been used to diagnose pheochromocytoma. This test is not useful as it lacks specificity and sudden death has been reported in several patients.

RADIOLOGIC STUDIES. Once the diagnosis of pheochromocytoma has been confirmed by biochemical testing, imaging procedures to localize the lesion are required. Radiographic tests also may reveal multifocal or bilateral adrenal disease and detect metastatic or locally invasive tumors. These tests may provide an estimate of tumor resectability as well as confirmation of the diagnosis. CT scanning and nuclear imaging with ^{131}I-metaiodobenzylguanidine (MIBG) have increased the amount of preoperative information available to the surgeon. In the past, adrenal angiography and venography were the primary preoperative studies for pheochromocytoma localization (Fig. 37-45); however, these tests are associated with significant morbidity and, occasionally, mortality. Frequent complications included adrenal infarction, periadrenal dye extravasation or hematoma, and the induction of catecholamine crisis. Complications with the current use of CT and MIBG scanning are virtually nonexistent, and these tests provide an accurate assessment of tumor location.

CT scanning localizes 90 to 95 percent of all pheochromocytomas greater than 1 cm in diameter. Multifocal, bilateral, and metastatic disease is often identified. The administration of intravenous contrast provides an estimate of tumor vascularity and renal function. CT scanning of the neck and thorax identifies most tumors in these locations, although dynamic CT scanning may be required to identify intrapericardial tumors. Today, the CT scan is available in most hospitals, whereas MIBG scanning is usually limited to research facilities. Thus, the CT scan is the mainstay of the preoperative work-up of pheochromocytoma. ^{131}I MIBG scanning is a recent advance in imaging studies for evaluation of pheochromocytoma. ^{131}I MIBG selectively accumulates in chromaffin tissues when administered intravenously, and it accumulates more rapidly in pheochromocytoma tissue than in normal chromaffin tissue. The MIBG scan is very sensitive in detecting pheochromocytomas. Rare false-negative and false-positive scans have been reported, usually with tumors in the renal hilum.

TREATMENT Surgical resection is the only curative procedure for both benign and malignant pheochromocytomas. Malignant disease may not be resectable for cure owing to local tissue invasion or invasion of the inferior

Fig. 37-45. A sixteen-year-old girl with episodic hypertension. *Left,* a subselective middle adrenal arteriogram showing a lesion of the inferior portion of the adrenal that displaces the normal gland superiorly. *Right,* a retrograde venogram at a slightly higher magnification showing a beautifully delicate outline of the right adrenal tumor's venous silhouette. The lesion measured 4 cm in diameter and was removed without difficulty. The patient's attacks have completely subsided. (From: *Harrison TS, Gann DS, et al: Surgical Disorders of the Adrenal Gland. New York, Grune & Stratton, 1975, p 102, with permission.*)

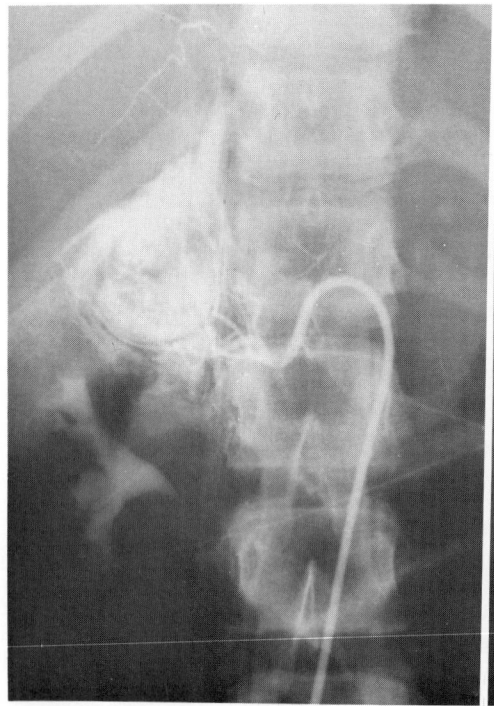
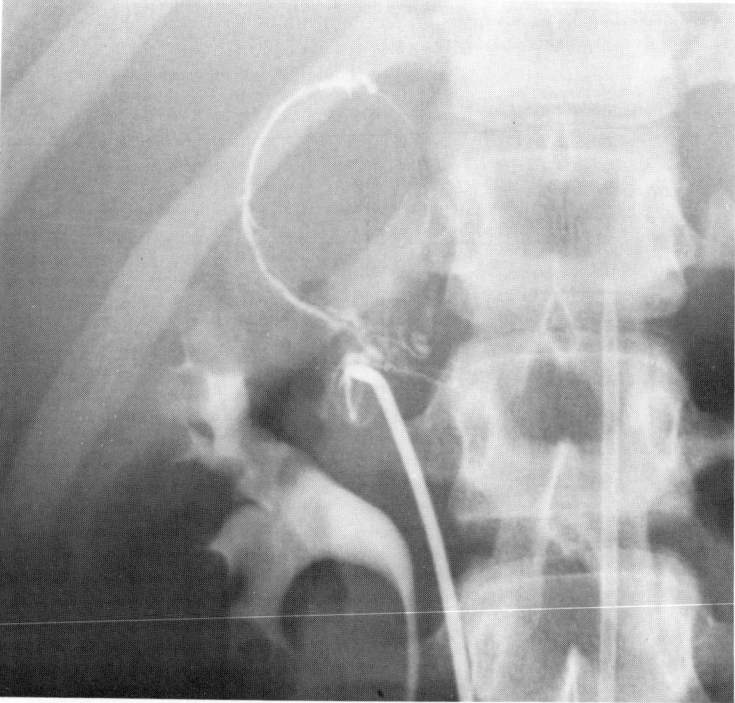

and adrenal carcinoma. The anterior approach is preferred in children and in all patients with associated intraabdominal disease that requires evaluation and possible surgical correction. In contrast, the posterior approach is used for adrenal adenomas and may be occasionally useful in patients with a pheochromocytoma that is localized to a single adrenal by ^{131}I MIBG scanning, although the scan is not available in many centers. The combined thoracoabdominal procedure is occasionally indicated for complete resection of large adrenal carcinomas, usually greater than 10 to 15 cm in diameter.

Bilateral adrenalectomy is rarely indicated, although 15 years ago this procedure was often used for the treatment of Cushing's disease. Today, pharmacologic ablation is preferable to resection. Cortisol synthesis inhibitors such as aminoglutethimide and metyrapone play an important role in the medical management of symptomatic hypercortisolism secondary to unresectable adrenal tumors and metastatic ectopic ACTH-producing neoplasms. Past authors have advocated bilateral adrenalectomy in the treatment of advanced breast cancer, but today cortisol synthesis inhibitors are used preferentially. Technologic advances in neurosurgery have made transphenoidal pituitary microsurgery feasible and replaced bilateral adrenalectomy in the management of Cushing's disease except in the rare resistant case of hypercortisolism. Furthermore, effective neuropharmacologic agents such as cyproheptadine and bromocryptine are also available for the treatment of Cushing's disease. If pituitary surgery, neuro-

pharmacologic agents, and medical adrenalectomy fail to control hypercortisolism, bilateral adrenalectomy may be performed as a last resort. Bilateral adrenalectomy is applicable for patients with bilateral pheochromocytoma.

POSTERIOR APPROACH. The patient is placed in a prone position and the table is flexed (Fig. 37-48). The chest and pelvis are supported with pillows to cause the intraabdominal contents to fall away from the retroperitoneal structures. A curvilinear skin incision is made from the level of the tenth thoracic vertebra inferiorly and laterally to the iliac crest. The incision is extended down through the subcutaneous fat and the latissimus dorsi muscle. The posterior lamella of the lumbodorsal fascia overlies the sacrospinalis muscle and is incised along its length. The sacrospinalis muscle is retracted medially and the lateral projections that insert on the posterior margin of the twelfth rib are divided for adequate mobilization. This maneuver exposes the anterior lamella of the lumbodorsal fascia and the lumbocostal ligament along the inferior border of the twelfth rib. The periosteum of the twelfth rib is divided longitudinally using the cautery, elevated with a periosteal elevator, and a subperiosteal rib resection is carried out as near to the midline as possible (Fig. 37-49). The anterior lamella is then divided along the length of the wound, starting in the bed of the twelfth rib and proceeding laterally to the edge of the quadratus lumborum muscle. The intercostal neurovascular bundle is handled with care and the vessels are clamped, divided, and ligated (Fig. 37-50). The twelfth intercostal nerve is spared and retracted inferiorly. The retroperitoneum has now been entered below the lower margin of the diaphragm with Gerota's fascia on its undersurface. The diaphragm is elevated off Gerota's fascia by blunt finger dissection and the diaphragm is separated from the pleura

Fig. 37-50. Starting in the bed of the twelfth rib, the anterior periosteum and the anterior lamella of the lumbodorsal fascia are divided. The twelfth intercostal artery and vein are ligated with 2-0 silk ligatures; the twelfth intercostal nerve is preserved and reflected inferiorly. The retroperitoneum is now entered.

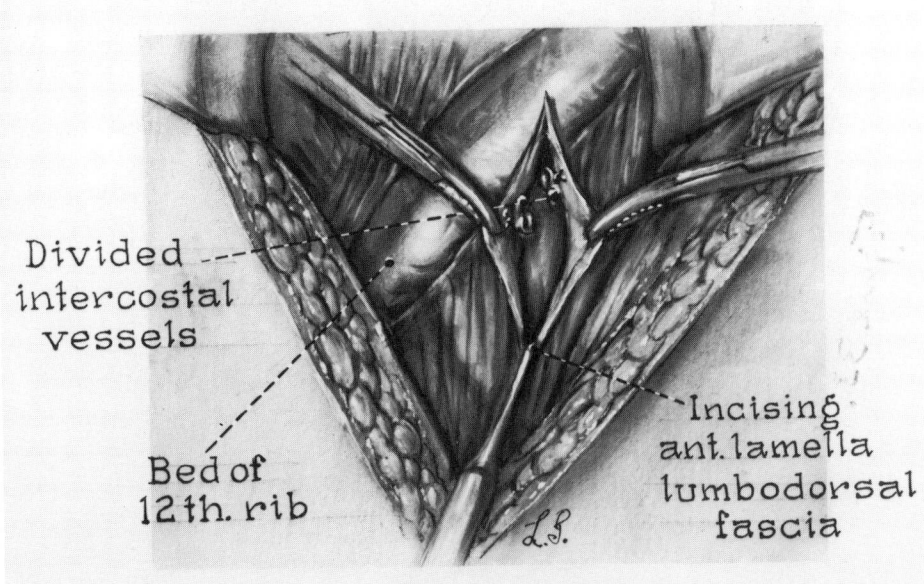

Divided intercostal vessels

Bed of 12th. rib

Incising ant. lamella lumbodorsal fascia

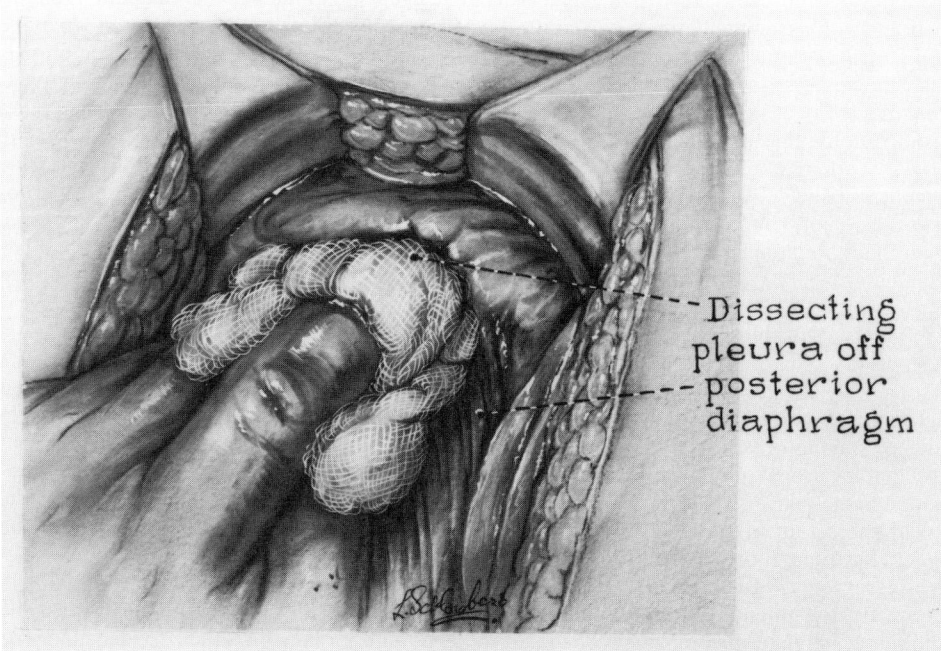

Fig. 37-51. The posterior reflection of the visceral pleura is dissected bluntly off the diaphragm with a sponge-covered finger.

using a sponge (Fig. 37-51). With the pleura safely out of harm's way, the diaphragm is divided between large clamps. Gerota's fascia is now clearly visible, incised, and the perirenal fat bluntly retracted to reveal the kidney and chrome-yellow adrenal gland. Downward traction on the kidney brings the adrenal into full view.

The adrenal is freed with blunt dissection initially on its superior, medial, and anterior aspects. The inferior and lateral attachments to the kidney are freed last to avoid retraction of the gland upward, which makes removal difficult. Small arterial feeding vessels are isolated with an angled clamp, tied with long silk sutures on the adrenal side, clipped, and divided (Fig. 37-52). The long 3-0 silk sutures on the adrenal side are used for countertraction during dissection because adrenal tissue is a loose, areolar tissue that tears easily with manipulation and mild

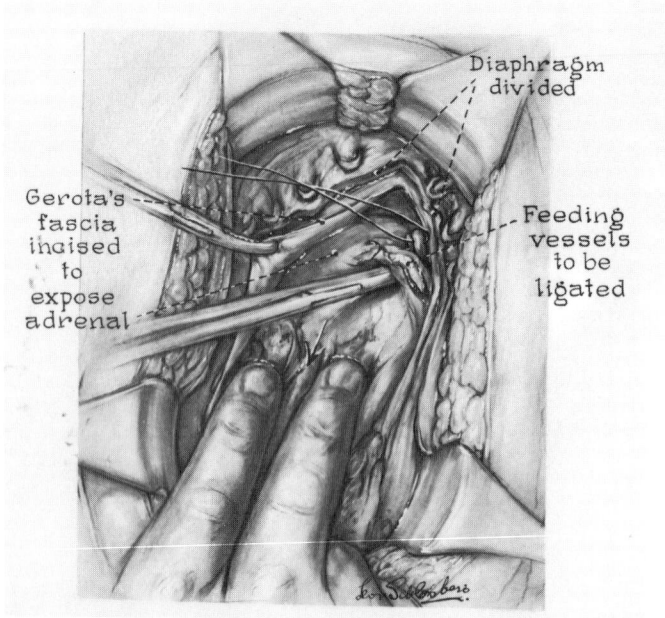

Fig. 37-52. Gerota's fascia has been divided and the kidney is retracted inferiorly. Feeding vessels are ligated with 3-0 silk ties and metallic clips.

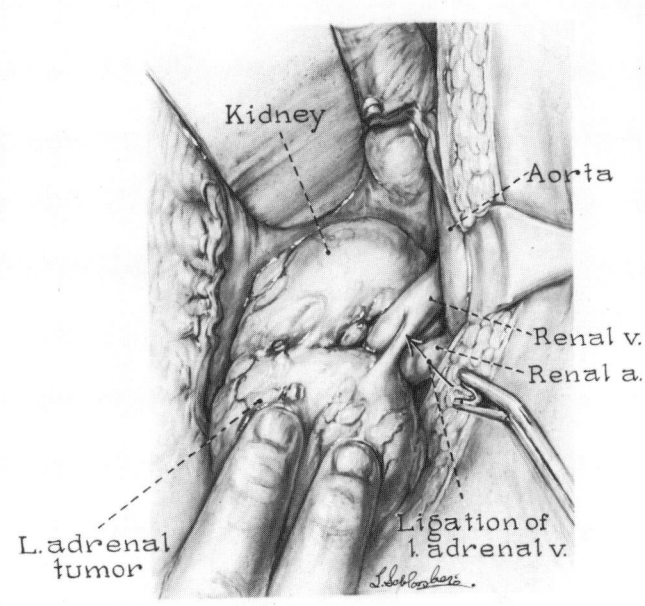

Fig. 37-53. The left adrenal vein is visualized where it enters the left renal vein. The adrenal vein is ligated twice with 2-0 silk ties, clipped, and divided. The aorta and left renal artery are located medially.

traction. Thus, only the vessels withstand the forces of countertraction without tearing. The dissection is continued until the left adrenal vein is seen clearly, emptying into the left renal vein on the anterior surface of the gland. The adrenal vein is tied twice with 2-0 silk ligatures, clip-

Fig. 37-54. To close the wound, first the anterior lamella and then the posterior lamella of the lumbodorsal fascia are approximated with continuous, running 0-vicryl sutures. The diaphragm is not re-approximated.

ped at its juncture with the left renal vein, and divided between the ligatures (Fig. 37-53). The adrenal is then removed.

It is not necessary to reapproximate the posterior diaphragm to close the wound. Closure is completed in three layers using a continuous running vicryl suture on both the anterior and posterior lamella of the lumbodorsal fascia (Fig. 37-54). The skin may be closed using a continu-

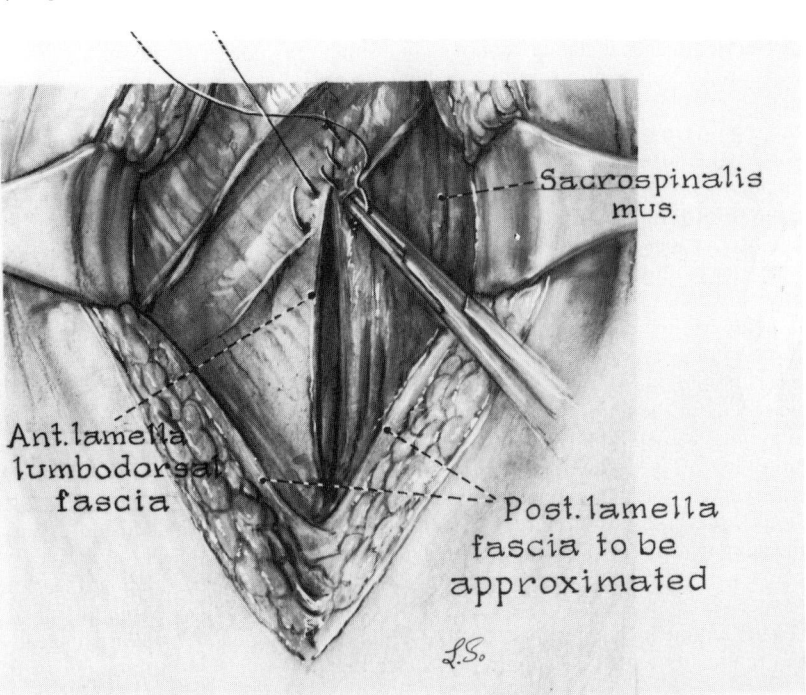

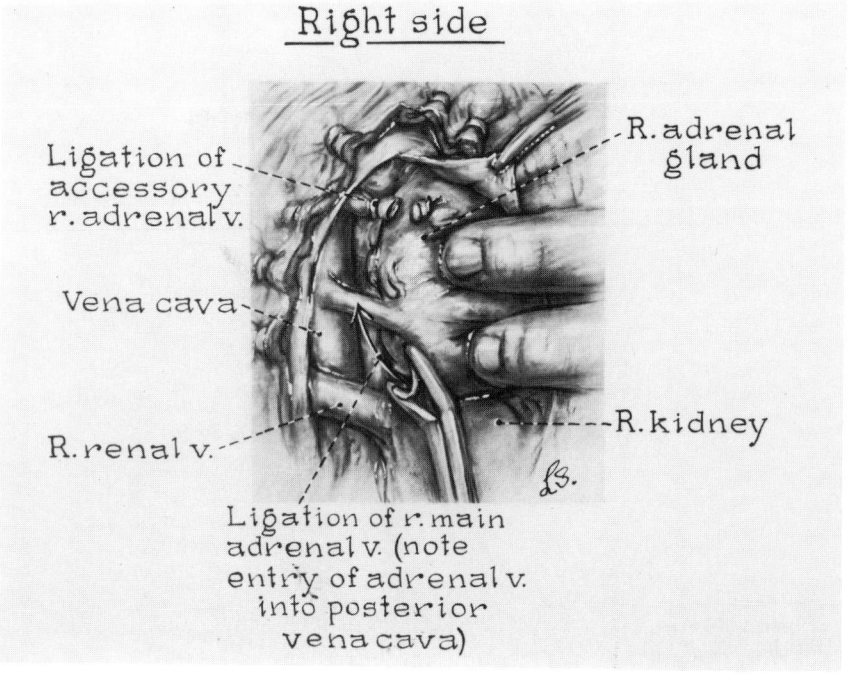

Fig. 37-55. In the posterior approach to right-sided adrenalectomy, the right adrenal has been dissected free from Georta's fascia. The adrenal vein exits from the medial aspect of the gland and enters the inferior vena cava posterolaterally. The adrenal vein is clipped flush with the inferior vena cava. Care must be taken not to injure the inferior vena cava and to search for an accessory right adrenal vein which has been divided in this figure.

ous absorbable subcuticular suture. Skin staples on this posterior wound may cause discomfort for the patient.

If the pleura was violated during the dissection, a large-caliber catheter is placed into the thoracic cavity prior to closure. Before complete closure of the skin, the lungs are hyperinflated by the anesthesiologist to expel any free pleural air and the catheter is quickly removed. The skin closure is then completed. A chest x-ray to evaluate any possible residual pneumothorax should always be obtained in the recovery room.

The right adrenal gland is removed in a similar fashion; the adrenal vein exits from the medial side of the gland and enters the posterior aspect of the vena cava instead of the renal vein (Fig. 37-55). Frequently, there is an accessory right adrenal vein on the superior aspect of the gland.

ANTERIOR APPROACH. A combination of reverse Trendelenburg position with an elevation of the right flank with a rolled towel and kidney support placed posteriorly at the level of the ninth rib allow proper positioning of the patient for the anterior approach to adrenalectomy. This positioning is less important for left-sided adrenal lesions but is helpful when exploration of the right adrenal is anticipated. In the anterior approach a variety of skin incisions may be suitable including bilateral subcostal incisions (as a large chevron), long midline incisions, and transverse upper abdominal incisions. A transverse incision is preferable in children. In adults, a long midline incision provides access to both adrenal glands, the organ of Zuckerkandl, and all areas of potential ectopic adrenal tissue.

The midline incision is made from the xiphoid to below the umbilicus and the abdomen is entered in the usual

manner. An abdominal exploration is performed to rule out bilateral and extraadrenal disease. In the case of left adrenalectomy, the small bowel is packed off medially and the splenic flexure of the colon is mobilized. The lesser sac is then opened by dividing the gastrocolic ligament. The phrenicocolic ligament is then clamped, divided, and tied with 2-0 silk ligatures (Fig. 37-56). Further blunt dissection and inferior retraction mobilizes the left colon. The posterior peritoneum parallel to the inferior border of the pancreas is incised to enter the retroperitoneal space. Blunt dissection is used to expose the left adrenal and to reflect the tail of the pancreas superiomedially. The left adrenal vein is isolated, ligated with 2-0 silk ties, and clipped at its junction with the left renal vein (Fig. 37-57). The vein is then divided, the remainder of the gland is dissected free, and the arterial supply is isolated and divided as previously described.

A pheochromocytoma should be manipulated as little as possible to avoid release of catecholamines. The adrenal vein should always be ligated first, although this is not as important if adequate administration of alpha-methyl-tyrosine or alpha and beta blockade have been started preoperatively. It is mandatory to explore both adrenal glands, the paraortic sympathetic chains, organ of Zuckerkandl, and each renal hilar area. If palpation of abdominal organs leads to elevations in blood pressure, a second tumor must be suspected. A 1-mg challenge of intrave-

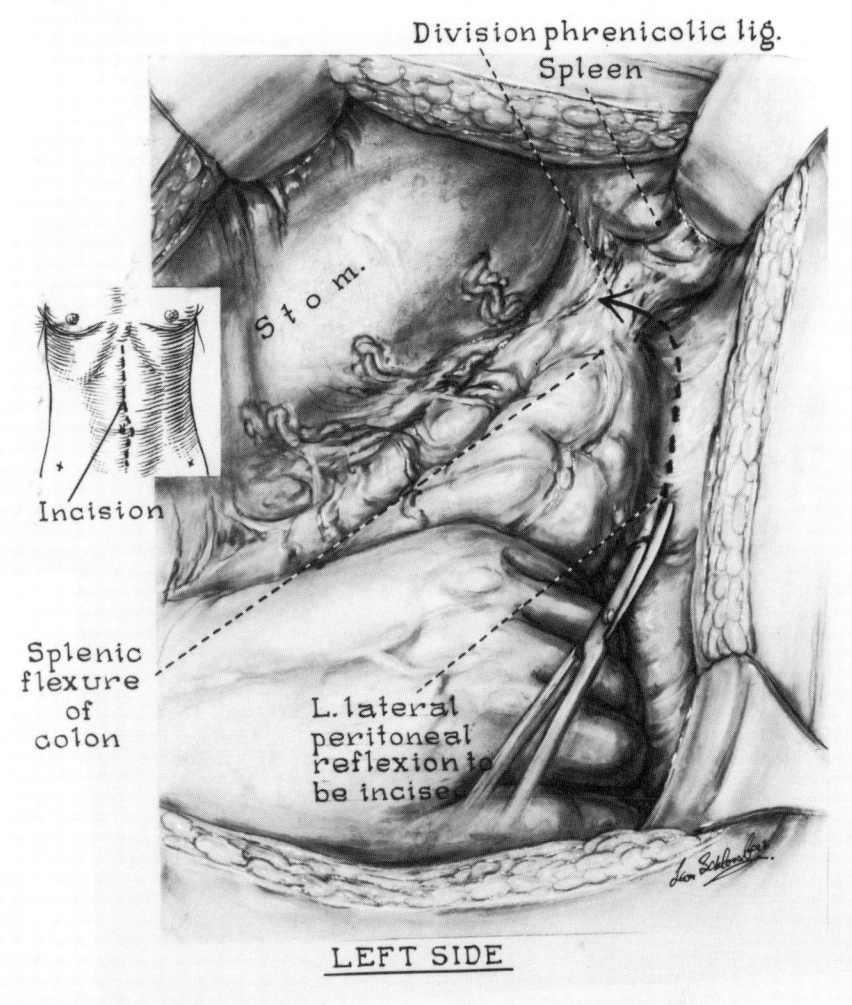

Fig. 37-56. The insert shows a standard, long midline incision for anterior adrenalectomy and abdominal exploration. To remove the left adrenal, the left colon is mobilized by dividing the left lateral peritoneal reflection, the phrenicocolic ligament, and the gastrocolic ligament.

nous glucagon may be administered to rule out a missed tumor. The response to glucagon will be hypertension or tachycardia if residual tumor is present.

Exposure of the right adrenal is obtained by mobilizing the hepatic flexure and right transverse colon. A generous Kocher maneuver is performed to mobilize the duodenum and stomach medially, whereas the right lobe of the liver is retracted superiorly. These maneuvers uncover the inferior vena cava, the right kidney, and the right adrenal. The medial and superior aspects of the right adrenal are dissected free first and arterial feeding vessels are ligated with 3-0 silk ties, clipped, and divided. The inferior vena cava is gently retracted medially with a vein retractor to expose its posterior-lateral surface with the right adrenal vein visualized emerging from the medial surface of the gland and entering the posterior aspect of the inferior

vena cava (Fig. 37-58). The vein is isolated, ligated with 2-0 silk ties, clipped flush with the inferior vena cava, and divided.

If an adrenal tumor cannot be dissected free of the kidney, a nephrectomy must be performed after the adrenal gland has been completely mobilized and all vessels divided. The adrenal, kidney, and Gerota's fascia should be removed en bloc.

THORACOABDOMINAL APPROACH. The thoracoabdominal approach to adrenalectomy is indicated for large adrenal carcinomas. The patient is placed in the supine position on the operating room table and the ipsilateral chest is elevated to 45° with pillows and the arms suspended from an ether screen. A transverse incision is made from the lateral border of the rectus muscle to the ipsilateral costal margin opposite the ninth inner space. The involved adrenal gland is exposed in the same manner as used in the anterior approach.

On the right side, the adrenal and tumor are mobilized from the under surface of the liver. If the tumor is resect-

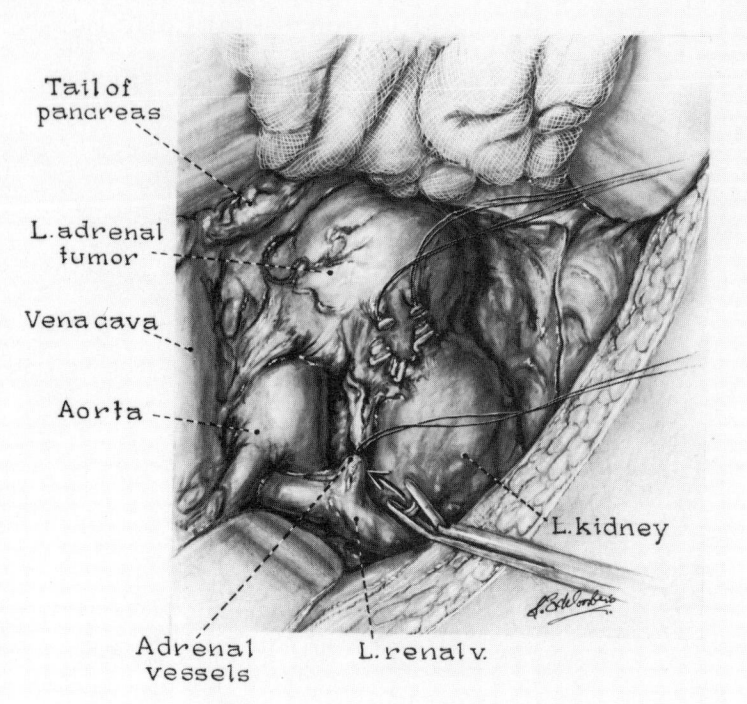

Fig. 37-57. The spleen and stomach are retracted superiorly and protected with large packs. The peritoneum along the inferior border of the pancreas has been incised revealing the left adrenal tumor and kidney. The aorta lies medially. The left adrenal vein is ligated above its junction with the left renal vein. Small feeding vessels have been divided.

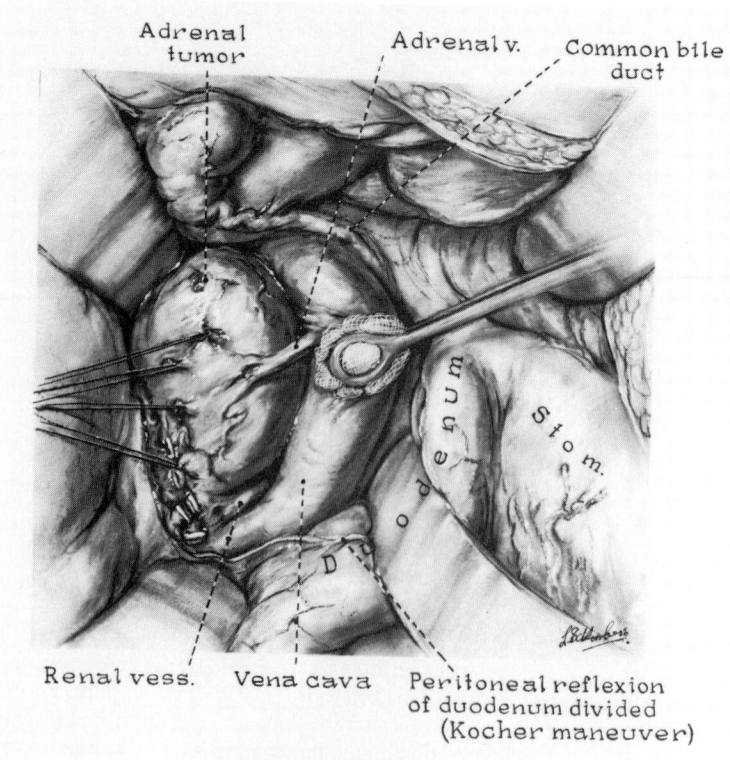

RIGHT SIDE

Fig. 37-58. The anterior transabdominal approach to the right adrenal requires mobilization of the right colon inferiorly, and the stomach and duodenum medially. Retraction of the liver superiorly brings the inferior vena cava, adrenal, and kidney into view. Gentle retraction of the inferior vena cava medially reveals the right adrenal vein entering the inferior vena cava posteriorly. The adrenal vein is divided between silk ligatures and clipped at its junction with the cava. The rest of the gland is resected as described previously for the left side.

able, the incision is extended across the ninth costal margin and along the ninth intercostal space to open the ipsilateral hemithorax. The inferior pulmonary ligament is divided between large clips and the diaphragm is incised in the direction of the thoracic incision. The phrenic nerve must be protected from injury. The liver is mobilized superiorly by dividing the triangular ligament. Thus, the superior extent of the adrenal tumor is completely exposed and dissection and division of vessels continue as previously described. In the case of a left adrenal tumor that involves adjacent organs, it may be necessary to perform a splenectomy, a distal pancreatectomy, or colon resection.

Bibliography

PITUITARY

Historical Background

Bergland RM, Davis SL, Page RB: Pituitary secretes to brain. *Lancet* 2:276, 1977.

Cushing H: Basophil adenomas of the pituitary body. *Bull Johns Hopkins Hosp* 50:137, 1932.

Cushing H: The reaction of posterior pituitary extract when introduced into the cerebral ventricles. *Proc Natl Acad Sci* 17:163, 239, 1931.

Cushing H, *Studies in Intracranial Physiology and Surgery*. Fair Lawn, NJ, Oxford University Press, 1926.

Cushing H: The functions of the pituitary body. *Am J Med Sci* 139:473, 1910.

Cushing H: *The Pituitary Body and Its Disorders*. Philadelphia, Lippincott, 1912.

Cushing H: The hypophysis cerebri: Clinical aspects of hyperpituitarism and hypopituitarism. *JAMA* 53:249, 1909.

Cushing H, Davidoff L: The pathological findings in acromegaly. Rockefeller Institute Monograph 22, pp 1–131, 1927.

Cushing H, Goetsch E: Concerning the secretion of the infundibular lobe of the pituitary body and its presence in cerebrospinal fluid. *Am J Phys* 27:60, 1910.

Fulton J: *Harvey Cushing, A Biography*. Springfield, IL, Charles C Thomas, 1946.

Henderson WR: The pituitary adenomata. *Br J Surg* 26:809, 1939.

Page RB, Munger BL, Bergland RM: Scanning microscopy of pituitary vascular casts. *Am J Anat* 146:273, 1976.

Rodriguez EM: Ependymal specializations. *Z Zellforsch* 102:153, 1969.

Gross Anatomy

Bergland RM, Ray BS, Torack RM: Anatomical variations in the pituitary gland. *J Neurosurg* 28:93, 1968.

Harris GW: Neural control of pituitary gland. *Physiol Rev* 28:139, 1948.

Lewis D, Lee FL: On the glandular elements in the posterior lobe of the human hypophysis. *Bull Johns Hopkins Hosp* 41:240, 1927.

Oliver C, Renon SM, Parter JC: Hypothalamic pituitary evidence vasculature: Evidence for retrograde blood flow in the pituitary stalk. *Endocrinol* 101:598, 1977.

Page RB, Bergland RM: The neurohypophyseal capillary bed. *Am J Anat* 148:345, 1977.

Wislocki GB, King LS: The permeability of the hypophysis and hypothalamus of vital dyes. *Am J Anat* 58:421, 1936.

Cellular Physiology

Bergland RM, Torack RM: An electronmicroscopic study of the human infundibulum. *Z Zellforsch* 99:1, 1969.

Bergland RM, Torack RM: An ultrastructural study of follicular cells in the anterior pituitary. *Am J Pathol* 57:273, 1969.

Bloom F, Segal D, et al: Endorphins: Profound behavioral effects in rats suggest new etiological factors in mental illness. *Science* 194:630, 1976.

deWied D, Bohus B: Retention of continued avoidance response in rats by treatment with pitressin or α-MSH. *Nature* (London) 212:1484, 1966.

Eipper BA, Mains RE: Structure and biosynthesis of proadrenocorticotropin. *Endo Rev* 1:1, 1980.

Goldstein A: Endorphins in pituitary and brain. *Science* 193:1081, 1976.

Hughes J, Smith TW, et al: Identification of two related pentapeptides from the brain with potent opiate agonist activity. *Nature* 258:577, 1975.

Martin JB, Reichlin S, Brown S: *Clinical Neuroendocrinology*. Philadelphia, Davis, 1977.

Nakane PK: Classifications of anterior pituitary cell types with immunoenzyme histochemistry. *J Histochem Cytochem* 18:9, 1970.

Phifer RF, Midgley AR, Spicer SS: Histology of human hypophyseal gonadotropin secreting cells, in Saxena BB, Beling CG (eds): *Gonadotropins*. New York, Wiley, 1972, pp 9–24.

Rasmussen AT: The percentage of different cells in male adult human hypophysis. *Am J Pathol* 5:263, 1929.

Roth J, LeRoith D, et al: The evolutionary origins of hormones, neurotransmitters, and other extracellular chemical messengers: Implications for mammalian biology. *N Engl J Med* 306:523, 1982.

Schonemann A: Hypophysis and thyreoida. *Arch Pathol* 129:310, 1892.

Snyder S: Opiate receptors in the brain. *N Engl J Med* 296:266, 1977.

Vale W, Spiess J, et al: Characterization of a 41-residue ovine hypothalamic peptide that stimulates secretion of a corticotropin and β-endorphin. *Science* 213:1394, 1981.

Pituitary Disorders

Bergland RM, Ray BS: The arterial supply of the human optic chiasm. *J Neurosurg* 31:327, 1966.

Ceballos R: Pituitary changes in head trauma. *Alabama J Med Sci* 3:185, 1966.

Hardy J: Transsphenoidal microsurgical removal of pituitary micro-adenoma. *Prog Neurosurg* (Karger) 6:200, 1975.

Hoff JT, Patterson RH: Craniopharyngiomas in children and adults. *J Neurosurg* 36:299, 1972.

Kjellberg RN, Kliman B: Bragg peak proton treatment for pituitary-related conditions. *Proc R Soc Med* 67:32, 1974.

Malarkey WB, Johnson JC: Pituitary tumors and hyperprolactinia. *Arch Intern Med* 136:40, 1976.

Ray BS, Horwith M: Surgical treatment of acromegaly. *Clin Neurosurg* 10:31, 1964.

Ray BS, Patterson RH: Surgical experience with chromophobe adenomas. *J Neurosurg* 34:726, 1971.

Rovitt R, Fein JM: Pituitary apoplexy: A review. *J Neurosurg* 37:280, 1972.

Sheehan HL, Whitehead R: The neurohypophysis in postpartum hypopituitarism. *J Pathol Bacteriol* 85:145, 1963.

Teears RJ, Silverman EM: Review of 88 cases of carcinoma metastatic to the pituitary gland. *Cancer* 36:216, 1975.

Young DG, Bohn RC, Randall RV: Pituitary tumors associated with acromegaly. *J Clin Endocrinol* 25:249, 1965.

Diagnostic Studies

Lee WM, Adams JE: The empty sella syndrome. *J Neurosurg* 28:351, 1968.

Therapeutic Modalities

Beatson GT: On the treatment of inoperable cases of carcinoma of the mamma. *Lancet* 2:104, 1896.

Fraser TR, Joplin GF: Subtotal or total pituitary ablation by implantation of radioactive rods. *Mod Treat* 3:189, 1966.

Luft R, Oliverona H: Experiences with hypophysectomy in man. *J Neurosurg* 10:301, 1953.

Maas H, Engel B, et al: Estrogen receptors in human breast cancer tissue. *Am J Obstet Gynecol* 113:377, 1972.

Mundinger F: Interstitial Curie-therapy in the treatment of pituitary adenomas. *Prog Neurol Surg* (Karger) 6:326, 1975.

Poulsen JE: Recovery from retinopathy in a case of diabetes with Simmonds' disease. *Diabetes* 2:7, 1953.

Rand RW, Dashe AM, et al: Stereotactic cryohypophysectomy. *JAMA* 189:255, 1964.

Ray BS: Intracranial hypophysectomy. *J Neurosurg* 28:180, 1968.

Ray BS, Pazianos AG, et al: Pituitary ablation for diabetic retinopathy. *JAMA* 203:79, 1968.

Weiss MH, Teal J, et al: Natural history of microprolactinomas: Six-year follow-up. *Neurosurgery* 12:180, 1983.

Weiss MH, Wycoff RR, et al: Bromocriptine treatment of prolactinosecreting tumors: Surgical implications. *Neurosurgery* 12:640, 1983.

Wilson CB: Transsphenoidal surgery for pituitary adenomas. *Anesthesiol Ref* 7:49, 1985.

Zervas N: Stereotaxic thermal hypophysectomy. *Prog Neurol Surg* (Karger) 6:217, 1975.

Zimmerman BR, Molnar GD: Prolonged followup in diabetic retinopathy. *Mayo Clin Proc* 52:233, 1977.

ADRENAL

Historical Background

Addison T: On the constitutional and local effects of disease of the suprarenal glands. Samuel Highley 32 Fleet Street, London, 1855, reprinted in facsimile by Dawson's 16 Pall Mall, London, 1968.

Bartter FC, Albright F, et al: The effects of adrenocorticotropic hormone and cortisone in the adrenogenital syndrome associated with congenital adrenal hyperplasia: An attempt to explain and correct its disordered hormonal pattern. *J Clin Invest* 30(3):237, 1951.

Brown-Sequard CE: Researches experimentales sur la physiologie et la pathologie des capsules surrenales. *Arch Gen Med* 2:385, 1856.

Cushing H: *The Pituitary Body and Its Disorders*. Philadelphia, Lippincott, 1912.

Cushing, H: The basophil adenomas of the pituitary body and their clinical manifestation (pituitary basophilism). *Bull Johns Hopkins Hosp* 1:137, 1932.

Eustachius B: Opuscula anatomica, printed by Vincentius Luchinus, Venice, 1563. Excerpts from an unpublished translation by William M. Klykylo.

Frankel F: Ein fall von doppelseitigem, vollig latent verlaufenen nebennieren tumor und gleich zeitiger nephritis mit verand erungen am circulation sapparat und retiuitis. *Virchows Arch* 103:244, 1886.

Kohn A: Das chromaffine gewebe. *Z Anat Entwicklungsgesch* 12:253, 1902.

Liddle GW, Island DP, et al: Nonpituitary neoplasma and Cushing's syndrome. *Arch Intern Med* 3:471–475, 1963.

Manasse P: Uber die hyperplastichen tumor en der nebennieren. *Virchows Arch* 133:391, 404, 1893.

Marchetti G: Beitrag zur kenntnis der pathologischen anatomie der nebennieren. *Virchows Arch* 177:227, 1904.

Pick L: Das ganglihoma embryonale sympathicum eine typische bosartige geschwuestform des sympathischen neurven system. *Berl Klin Wochenschr* 49:16, 1912.

Wilkins L, Lewis RA, et al: The suppression of androgen secretion by cortisone in a case of congenital adrenal hyperplasia: Preliminary report. *Bull Johns Hopkins Hosp* 86:749, 1956.

Embryology

Sadler TW: *Langman's Medical Embryology*, 5th ed. Baltimore, Williams and Wilkins, 1985.

ADRENAL CORTEX PHYSIOLOGY

Cortisol

Almli CR: Hyperosmolality accompanies hypovolemic: A single explanation steroid on menocyte function. *J Clin Invest* 54:1337, 1979.

Aschoff J: Circadian rhythms: General features and endocrinological aspects, in Krieger DT (ed): *Endocrine Rhythms*. New York, Raven, 1974.

Buckingham JC: Two distinct corticotropin releasing activities of vasopressin. *Br J Pharmacol* 84:213, 1985.

Butler WT, Rosen RD: Effect of corticosteroids on immunity in man: Decreased serum IgG concentration caused by three or five days of high doses of methylprednisolone. *J Clin Invest* 52:2629, 1973.

DeMaria EJ, Reichman W, Kenny PR: Septic complications of corticosteroid administration after central nervous system trauma. *Ann Surg* 202(2):248, 1986.

Eigler N, Sacca L, Sherwin RS: Synergistic interactions of physiologic increments of glucagon, epinephrine, and cortisol in the dog. *J Clin Invest* 63:114, 1979.

Fauci AS, Dale DC, Balow JE: Glucocorticosteroid therapy: Mechanisms of action and clinical considerations. *Ann Intern Med* 84:304, 1976.

Gann DS, Dallman MF, Engeland WC: Reflex control and modulation of ACTH and corticosteroids, in McCann SM (ed): *Endocrine Physiology III*. 1981, chap 4, p 157.

Gaunt R: History of the adrenal cortex, in *Handbook of Physiology*, Sec 7, *Adrenal Gland*. Washington, DC, American Physiology Society, 1975, vol 6, chap 1.

Hellman L, Nakada F, et al: Cortisol is secreted episodically by normal man. *J Clin Endocrinol Metab* 30:411, 1970.

Holbrook NJ, Cox WI, Horner HC: Direct suppression of natural killer activity in human peripheral blood leukocyte cultures by glucocorticoids and its modulation by interferon. *Can Res* 43:4019, 1983.

Ingle DJ: The role of the adrenal cortex in homeostasis. *J Endocrinol* 8:23, 1952.

Ingle DJ: Permissibility of hormone action: A review. *Acta Endocrinol (Copenh)* 17:172, 1954.

Keller-Wood ME, Dallman MF: Corticosteroid inhibition of ACTH secretion. *Endocr Rev* 5(1):1, 1984.

Morris DJ: The metabolism and mechanism of action of aldosterone. *Endocr Rev* 2(2):234, 1981.

Munck A, Guyre P, Holbrook NJ: Physiologic functions of glucocorticoids in stress and their relation to pharmacologic actions. *Endocr Rev* 5:75, 1984.

Pederson RC, Brownie AC, Ling N: Pro-adrenocorticotropin/endorphin-derived peptides: Coordinate action on adrenal steroidogenesis. *Science* 208:1044, 1980.

Pinehart JJ, Sagone AL, Balcerzak SP: Effects of corticosteroid on monocyte function. *J Clin Invest* 54:1337, 1979.

Pirkle JC, Gann DS: Restitution of blood volume after hemorrhage: Role of the adrenal cortex. *Am J Physiol* 230:1683, 1976.

Rivier C, Vale C: Interaction of corticotropin-releasing factor and arginine vasopressin on adrenocorticotropin secretion *in vivo*. *Endocrinology* 113:939, 1983.

Samuels LT, Nelson DH: Biosynthesis of corticosteroids, in Greep RP, Astwood EB (eds): *Handbook of Physiology, Sec 7, Endocrinology, vol VI: Adrenal Gland*. Washington, DC, American Physiology Society, 1975, pp 55–68.

Seyle H: The general adaptation syndrome and the diseases of adaptation. *J Clin Endocrinol Metab* 6:117, 1946.

Vale W, Spiess J, et al: Characterization of a 41-residue ovine hypothalamic peptide that stimulates secretion of corticotropin and B-endorphin. *Science* 213:1394, 1981.

Aldosterone

Aguilera G, Mendelsohn FAO, Catt KJ: Dopaminergic regulation of aldosterone secretion, in Martini L, Ganong WF (eds): *Frontiers in Neuroendocrinology*. New York, Raven, 1984, vol 8, chap 9.

Davis JO, Urquhart J, Higgins JT Jr: The effects of alterations of plasma sodium and potassium concentrations on aldosterone secretion. *J Clin Invest* 42:597, 1963.

Davis JO: Mechanisms regulating renin release. *Physiol Rev* 56:1, 1976.

Ganong WF, Barbieri C: Neuroendocrine components in the regulation of renin secretion, in Ganong WF, Martini L (eds): *Frontiers in Neuroendocrinology*. New York, Raven, 1982, vol 7, chap 9.

Peach MJ: Renin-angiotensin system: Biochemistry and mechanisms of action. *Physiol Rev* 57:313, 1977.

Reid IA, Morris BJ, Ganong WF: The renin-angiotensin system. *Ann Rev Physiol* 40:377, 1978.

Williamson HE: Mechanism of the antinatriuretic action of aldosterone. *Biochem Pharmacol* 12:1449, 1963.

CUSHING'S SYNDROME

General

Aron DC, Findling JW, Fitzgerald PA: Cushing's syndrome: Problems in management. *Endocr Rev* 3:229, 1982.

Flint LD, Jacobs EC: Belated recognition of adrenocorticotropic hormone-producing tumors in post-adrenalectomized Cushing's syndrome. *J Urol* 112:688, 1974.

Inura H, Matsukura S, et al: Studies on ectopic ACTH-producing tumors. II. Clinical and biochemical features of 30 cases. *Cancer* 35:1430, 1975.

Krieger DT: Physiopathology of Cushing's disease. *Endocr Rev* 4:22, 1983.

Meador CK, Bowdoin B, et al: Primary adrenocortical nodular dysplasia: A rare cause of Cushing's syndrome. *J Clin Endocrinol* 27:1255, 1967.

Montgomery D, Welbourn RB: Cushing's syndrome: Twenty years after adrenalectomy. *Br J Surg* 65:221, 1978.

Moore TJ, Dluhy RG, et al: Nelson's syndrome: Frequency, prognosis and effect of prior pituitary irradiation. *Ann Intern Med* 85:731, 1976.

Diagnostic Tests

Aron DC, Tyrrell JB, et al: Cushing's syndrome: Problems in diagnostic medicine. *Medicine (Baltimore)* 60:225, 1981.

Asfeldt WH: Simplified dexamethasone suppression test. *Acta Endocrinol* 61:219, 1969.

Burke CW, Beardwell CG: Cushing's syndrome: An evaluation of the clinical usefulness of urinary free cortisol and other urinary steroid measurements in diagnosis. *QJ Med* 42:175, 1973.

Chrousos GP, Schulte HM, Oldfield EH: The corticotropin-releasing factor stimulation test. An aid in the evaluation of patients with Cushing's syndrome. *N Engl J Med* 310:622, 1984.

Corrigan DF, Schaff M, Whaley RA: Selective venous sampling to differentiate ectopic ACTH secretion from pituitary Cushing's syndrome. *N Engl J Med* 296:861, 1977.

Crapo L: Cushing's syndrome: A review of diagnostic tests. *Metabolism* 28(9):955, 1979.

Cuerin CK, Wahner HW, Gorman CA: Computed tomographic scanning versus radioisotope imaging in adrenocortical diagnosis. *Am J Med* 75:653, 1983.

Eddy RL, Jones AL, Gilliland PF: Cushing's syndrome: A prospective study of diagnostic methods. *Am J Med* 55:621, 1970.

Thoren M, Sjoberg HE, Hall K: A rapid screening test for Cushing's syndrome. *Acta Med Scand* 198:303, 1975.

Thrall JH, Freitas JE, Beierwaltes WH: Adrenal scintigraphy. *Semin Nucl Med* 8:23, 1978.

Treatment

Bigos ST, Somma M, Rasio E: Cushing's disease: Management by transphenoidal pituitary microsurgery. *J Clin Endocrinol Metab* 50:348, 1980.

Doyle D, O'Donovan DK: More on cyproheptadine in Cushing's disease. *N Engl J Med* 296:576, 1977.

Gaillard AC, Grossman A, Smith R: The effects of a met-enkephalin analog on ACTH, B-OLPH, B-endorphin and met-enkephalin in patients with adrenocortical disease. *Clin Endocrinol* 14:471, 1981.

Hardy J: Transphenoidal microsurgical removal of pituitary microadenomas. *Prog Neurol Surg* 6:200, 1975.

Jennings AS, Liddle GW, Orth DN: Results of treating childhood Cushing's disease with pituitary irradiation. *N Engl J Med* 297:957.

Jones MT, Gilham B, Beckford U: Effect of treatment with sodium valproate and diazepam on plasma corticotropin in Nelson's syndrome. *Lancet* 1:1179, 1981.

Linfoot JA: Heavy-ion alpha-particle therapy of pituitary tumors, in Linfoot JA (ed): *Recent Advances in the Diagnosis and Treatment of Pituitary Tumors*. New York, Raven, 1975.

Luton JP, Mahoudeau JA, Bouchard P: Treatment of Cushing's disease by o,p'-DDD. *N Engl J Med* 300:459, 1979.

Misbin RI, Canary J, Willard A: Aminoglutehimide in the treatment of Cushing's syndrome. *J Clin Pharmacol* 16:374, 1967.

Orth DN, Liddle GW: Results of treatment of 108 patients with Cushing's syndrome. *N Engl J Med* 285:243, 1971.

Orth DN: Methyrapone is useful only as adjunctive therapy in Cushing's disease. *Ann Intern Med* 89:128, 1978.

Salassa RM, Laws ER, Carpenter PC: Transphenoidal removal of pituitary adenoma in Cushing's disease. *Mayo Clin Proc* 53:24, 1978.

Schteingard DS, Motazedi A, Noonan RA: Treatment of adrenal carcinomas. *Arch Surg* 117(9):1142, 1982.

Thompson NW, Allo MD: Management of acute hypercortisolism. *World J Surg* 6:748, 1982.

Tolis G, Jukier L, et al: Effect of naloxone on pituitary hypersecretory syndromes. *J Clin Endocrinol Metab* 54:780, 1982.

PRIMARY ALDOSTERONISM

General

Conn JW, Moriata R, Cohen EL: The changing clinical spectrum of primary aldosteronism. *Am J Med* 74:641, 1983.

Kotchen TA, Guthrie GGP Jr: Renin-angiotensin-aldosterone and hypertension. *Endocr Rev* 1:78, 1980.

ADRENAL INSUFFICIENCY

Albert SG, Wolverson MK, Johnson FE: Bilateral adrenal hemorrhage in an adult. Demonstration by computed tomography. *JAMA* 247(12)1737, 1982.

Alford WC Jr, Meador CK, et al: Acute adrenal insufficiency following cardiac surgical procedures. *J Thorac Cardiovasc Surg* 78(4):489, 1979.

Angeli A, Frairia R: Simultaneous diagnosis and treatment of acute adrenocortical insufficiency. Letter to the Editor. *Lancet* 2:1217, 1975.

Carpenter CJ, Solomon N, Silverberg SG: Schmidt's syndrome (thyroid and adrenal insufficiency): A review of the literature and a report of 15 new cases including 10 instances of coexistent diabetes mellitus. *Medicine (Baltimore)* 43:153, 1964.

Cedermark BJ, Sjoberg HE: The clinical significance of metastases to the adrenal glands. *Surg Gynecol Obstet* 152:607, 1981.

Clark OH: Postoperative adrenal hemorrhage. *Ann Surg* 182:124, 1975.

Danese CA, Viola RM: Adrenal hemorrhage during anticoagulant therapy. *Ann Surg* 179:70, 1974.

Irvine WJ: Autoimmunity in endocrine disease. *Proc Soc Med* 67:548, 1974.

Kaufman G: Adrenal cortical necrosis. An autopsy study. *Arch Pathol* 97:395, 1974.

Kehler H, Binder CHR: Adrenocortical function and clinical course during and after surgery in unsupplemented glucocorticoid-treated patients. *Br J Anaesth* 45:1043, 1973.

Liu L, Haskin ME, et al: Diagnosis of bilateral adrenocortical hemorrhage. *Ann Intern Med* 97(5):720, 1982.

Nerup J: Addison's disease—clinical studies. A report of 108 cases. *Acta Endocrinol* 76:127, 1974.

Nicholls MG, Espiner EA, Huges H: Primary aldosteronism. *Am J Med* 59:334, 1975.

Pham-Huu-Trung M, Bogyo A, et al: Effects of pro-opiomelanocortin peptides and angiotensin II on steroidogenesis in isolated aldosteronoma cells. *J Clin Endocrinol Metab* 61:467, 1985.

Schurmeyer TH, Tsokos GC, et al: Pituitary-adrenal responsiveness to corticotropin-releasing hormone in patients receiving chronic, alternate day glucocorticoid therapy. *J Clin Endocrin Metab* 61:22, 1985.

Scoggins BA, Coghlan JP: Primary hyperaldosteronism. *Pharmacol Ther* 9:367, 1980.

Xarli V, Steele AA, et al: Adrenal hemorrhage in the adult. *Medicine* 57(3):211, 1978.

Diagnostic Tests

Dunnick NR, Doppman JL, Gill JR Jr: Localization of functional adrenal tumors by computed tomography and venous sampling. *Radiography* 142:429, 1982.

Geisinger MA, Zelch MG, Bravo EL: Primary hyperaldosteronism: Comparison of CT, adrenal venography, and venous sampling. *Am J Roentgenol* 141:29, 1983.

Gross MD, Shapiro B, et al: The relationship of adrenal gland iodomethylcholesterol uptake to zona glomerulosa function in primary aldosteronism. *J Clin Endocrinol Metab* 57(3):477, 1983.

Rodrigues JA, Lopez JM, Biglieri EG: DOCA test for aldosteronism: Its usefulness and implications. *Hypertension* 3(Suppl II):102, 1981.

Streeten DHP, Anderson GH Jr: Simplified screening procedures for primary aldosteronism. Studies on the mechanism of the hyper-responsiveness to furosemide and standing. *Clin Exp Hypertens* A4:1663, 1982.

Treatment

Auda SP, Brennan MF, Gill JR: Evolution of the surgical management of primary aldosteronism. *Ann Surg* 191:1, 1980.

Banks WA, Kastin AJ, et al: Primary adrenal hyperplasia: A new subset of primary hyperaldosteronism. *J Clin Endocrinol Metab* 58:783, 1984.

Clarke D, Wilkson R, Johnston IDA: Severe hypertension in primary aldosteronism and good response to surgery. *Lancet* 1:482, 1979.

Granberg PO, Adamson U, Cohn KH: The management of patients with primary aldosteronism. *World J Surg* 6:757, 1982.

Mobley JE, Headstream JW, Melby JC: Primary aldosteronism: Preoperative preparation with spirolactane. *JAMA* 180:1056, 1962.

Nadler JL, Hsueh W, Horton R: Therapeutic effect of calcium channel blockage in primary aldosteronism. *J Clin Endocrinol Metab* 60:896, 1985.

Rerriss JB, Brown JJ, Fraser R: Results of adrenal surgery in patients with hypertension, aldosterone excess, and low plasma renin concentration. *Br Med J* 1:135, 1975.

Russell CF, Hamberger B, van Heerden, JA: Adrenalectomy: Anterior or posterior approach. *Am J Surg* 144:322, 1982.

ADRENOGENITAL SYNDROME

Migeon CJ: Diagnosis and treatment of adrenogenital disorders, in Degroot, LJ, Cahill CF, Odell WA (eds): *Endocrinology*. New York, Grune and Stratton, 1980, p 1203.

THE INCIDENTALLY DISCOVERED ADRENAL MASS

Belldegrun A, Hussain S, et al: Incidentally discovered mass of the adrenal gland. *Surg Gynecol Obstet* 163(3):203, 1986.

Copeland PM: The incidentally discovered adrenal mass. *Ann Intern Med* 98:940, 1983.

Didolkar MS, Bescher RA, et al: Natural history of adrenal carcinoma: A clinicopathologic study of 42 patients. *Cancer* 47:2153, 1984.

Glazer HS, Weyman PJ, et al: Nonfunctioning adrenal masses: Incidental discovery on computed tomography. *Am J Roentgenol* 139:81, 1982.

Prinz RA, Brooks MH, et al: Incidental asymptomatic adrenal mass detected by computer tomography scanning. Is operation required? *JAMA* 248:701, 1982.

ADRENAL MEDULLA PHYSIOLOGY

Ahlquist RP: A study of the adrenotropic receptors. *Am J Physiol* 153:586, 1948.

Albert SG, Wolverson MK, Johnson FE: Bilateral adrenal hemorrhage in an adult: Demonstration by computed tomography. *JAMA* 247(12):1737, 1979.

Alford WC, Meador CK, et al: Acute adrenal insufficiency following cardiac surgical procedures. *J Thorac Cardiovasc Surg* 78:489, 1979.

Boonaviroj P, Gutman Y: Alpha adrenergic stimulants, prostaglandins, and catecholamine release from the adrenal gland in vitro. *Prostaglandins* 10:109, 1975.

Burke WJ, Davis JW, et al: The effect of epinephrine on phenylethanolamine-N-methyltransferase in cultured explants of adrenal medulla. *Endocrinology* 103:358, 1978.

Clark OH: Postoperative adrenal hemorrhage. *Ann Surg* 182(2):125, 1975.

Critchley JAJH, Ungar A: Do the anterior pituitary and adrenal cortex participate in the reflex response of the adrenal medulla to arterial hypoxia? *J Physiol (Lond)* 239:16P, 1974.

Engeland WC, Dempsher DP, et al: The adrenal medullary response to graded hemorrhage in awake dogs. *Endocrinology* 109:1539, 1981.

Feuerstein G, Boonaviroj P, Gutman Y: Renin-angiotensin mediation of adrenal catecholamine secretion induced by haemorrhage. *Eur J Pharmacol* 44:131, 1977.

Guidotti A, Costa E: Involvement of adenosine 3'-5'-monophosphate in the activation of tyrosine hydroxylase elicited by drugs. *Science* 1979:902, 1973.

Himms-Hagen J: Sympathetic regulation of metabolism. *Pharmacol Rev* 19:367, 1967.

Holz RW: Evidence that catecholamine transport into chromaffin vesicles is coupled to vesicle membrane potential. *Proc Natl Acad Sci USA* 75:5190, 1978.

Kehlet H, Binder CHR: Adrenocortical function and clinical course during and after surgery in supplemented glucocorticoid-treated patients. *Br J Anaesth.* 45:1043, 1973.

Laduron P: Evidence for a localization of dopamine B-hydroxylase within chromaffin granules. *FEBS Lett* 52:132, 1975.

Liu L, Haskin ME, et al: Diagnosis of bilateral adrenocortical hemorrhage by computed tomography. *Ann Intern Med* 97(5):720, 1982.

Nerup J: Addison's disease—clinical studies. A report of 108 cases. *Acta Endocrinol* 76:127, 1974.

Palmer BQ, Watters JM, et al: Combined hormonal infusion simulates the metabolic response to injury. *Ann Surg* 200(3)264, 1984.

Petersen OH: The electrophysiology of gland cells. *Physiol Soc Monogr* 36, 1980.

Schurmeyer TH, Tsokos GC, et al: Pituitary-adrenal responsiveness to corticotropin-releasing hormone in patients receiving chronic, alternate day glucocorticoid therapy. *J Clin Endocrinol Metab* 61:22, 1985.

Udenfriendl S, Dairman W: Regulation of norepinephrine synthesis. *Adv Enzyme Regul* 9:145, 1971.

Ungar A, Phillips JH: Regulation of the adrenal medulla. *Physiol Rev* 63(3):787, 1983.

Winkler H: The composition of adrenal chromaffin granules: An assessment of controversial results. *Neuroscience* 1:65, 1976.

Winkler H: The biogenesis of adrenal chromaffin granules. *Neuroscience* 2:657, 1977.

Winkler H, Westhead E: The molecular organization of adrenal chromaffin granules. *Neuroscience* 5:1803, 1980.

PHEOCHROMOCYTOMA

General

Harrison TS, Gann DS, et al: *Surgical Disorders of the Adrenal Gland: Physiologic Background and Treatment.* New York, Grune and Stratton, 1975.

Manger WM, Gifford RW Jr: *Pheochromocytoma.* New York, Springer-Verlag, 1977.

Physiology and Inheritance

Baylin SB, Gann DS: Clonal origin of inherited medullary thyroid carcinomas and pheochromocytoma. *Science* 193:321, 1976.

Beierwalters WH: The spectrum of pheochromocytoma in hypertensive patients with neurofibromatosis. *Arch Intern Med* 142:2093, 1982.

Bravo EL, Tarazi RC, et al: Circulating and primary catecholamine in pheochromocytoma. Diagnostic and pathophysiologic implications. *N Engl J Med* 301:(13)682, 1979.

Cahill GF, Patter EM: Techniques involved in surgical removal of pheochromocytoma. *J Urol* 76:467, 1956.

Hoffman RW, Gardener DW, Mitchell FL: Intrathoracic and multiple abdominal pheochromocytomas in von Hipple-Lindau disease. *Arch Intern Med* V142:1962, 1982.

Diagnostic Tests

Francis IR, Glazer GM, et al: Complementary roles of CT and ^{131}I-MIBG scintigraphy in diagnosing pheochromocytoma. *Am J Roentgenol* 141:719, 1983.

Kaufman BH, Telander RL, et al: CT for pheochromocytoma diagnosis. *Am J Roentgenol* 134:277, 1980.

Machery D, Tippett PA, et al: New approach to the localization of pheochromocytoma imaging with iodine-131-meto-iodobenzyl-guanidine. *Br Med J* 288:1587, 1984.

Shapiro B, Sisson JC, et al: Malignant phaecochromocytoma: Clinical, biochemical and scintigraphic characterization. *Clin Endocrinol* 20:189, 1984.

Sisson JC: Scintigraphic localization of pheochromocytoma. *N Engl J Med* 305(1):12, 1981.

Small ME, Lawrence R, et al: Advances in the techniques of localization of adrenal tumors and their influence on the surgical approach to the tumor. *Br J Urol* 55:617, 1983.

Steward BH, Bravo EL, et al: Localization of pheochromocytoma by computed tomography. *N Engl J Med* 299:460, 1978.

Sutton H: Disseminated malignant pheochromocytomas localized with iodine-131-labelled meto-iodobenzyl guanidine. *Br Med J* 235:1153, 1982.

Thomas JL, Bernordiho ME, et al: CT of pheochromocytoma. *Am J Roentgenol* September 1980.

Treatment

Dawson B: Pheochromocytoma in the pediatric age group: Current status. *J Pediatr Surg,* 18(6):879, 1983.

McDougall IR: Malignant pheochromocytoma treated by I-131-MIBG. *J Nucl Med* 25(3):249, 1985.

Modlinger RS: Adrenergic blockage in pheochromocytoma. *Arch Intern Med* 143(12):2245, 1983.

Sisson JC: Radiopharmaceutical treatment of malignant pheochromocytoma. *J Nucl Med* 24:157, 1984.

Neuroblastoma

Akawari OE, Payne SW, et al: Dumbbell neurogenic tumors of the mediastinum. Diagnosis and management. *Mayo Clin Proc* 53:353, 1978.

D'Angio GJ, Evans AE, Koop CE: Special pattern of widespread neuroblastoma with a favorable prognosis. *Lancet 1:* 1046, 1971.

Evans AE: Staging and treatment of neuroblastoma. *Cancer* 45:1799, 1980.

Evans AE, Chatten J, et al: A review of 17 IV-S neuroblastoma patients at the Children's Hospital of Philadelphia. *Cancer* 45:833, 1980.

Evans AE, Baum E, Chaud R: Do infants with IV-S neuroblastoma need treatment? *Arch Dis Child* 56:271, 1981.

Evans AE, D'Angio J, Randolf J: A proposed staging for children with neuroblastoma. *Cancer* 27(2):374, 1971.

Finklestein JZ, Klemperer MR, et al: Multiagent chemotherapy for children with metastatic neuroblastoma: A report from Children's Cancer Study Group. *Med Pediatr Oncol* 6:179, 1979.

Gerson J, Evans AE, Rosen FS: The prognostic value of acute phase reactants in patients with neuroblastoma. *Cancer* 40:1655, 1977.

Hayes FA, Green AA: Neuroblastoma. *Pediatr Ann* 12(5):366, 1983.

MacManus M: The diagnosis and staging of neuroblastoma. *Clin Radiol* 34:523, 1983.

Patrick TR, Lee JY, et al: An analysis of neuroblastoma at a single institution. *Cancer* 53:2079, 1984.

Prodrasky AE, Stark DD, et al: Radionucleotide bone scanning in neuroblastoma skeletal metastases and primary tumor localization of ^{99}Tc-MDP. *Am J Roentgenol* 141:469, 1983.

Punt J, Pritchard J, et al: Neuroblastoma: A review of 21 cases presenting with spinal cord compression. Cancer 45:3095, 1980.

Rosen EM, Cassady RJ, et al: Influence of local-regional lymph node metastases on prognosis in neuroblastoma. *Med Pediatr Oncol* 12:260, 1984.

Russell CF, Hamberger B, et al: Adrenalectomy: Anterior or posterior approach. *Am J Surg* 1982.

Sandstedt B, Jereb B, Eklund G: Prognostic factors in neuroblastomas. *Acta Pathol Microbiol Scand* [c] 91:365, 1983.

Sawada T, Todo S, et al: Mass screening of neuroblastoma in infancy. *Am J Dis Child* 136:710, 1982.

Seeger RC, Siggel SE, Sidell N: Neuroblastoma: Clinical perspectives, monoclonal antibodies and retinoic acid. *Ann Intern Med* 97:873, 1982.

Sitarz A, Finklestein J, Grosfeld J: An evaluation of the role of surgery in disseminated neuroblastoma: A report from the Children's Cancer Study Group. *J Pediatr Surg* 18(2):147, 1983.

Stack DD, Brosch RC, et al: Current neuroblastoma: The role of CT and alternative imaging tests. *Radiology* 148:107, 1983.

Stark DD, Moss AA, et al: Neuroblastoma: Diagnostic imaging and staging. *Radiology* 148:101, 1983.

Stokes SH, Thomas PRM, et al: Stage IV-S neuroblastoma. *Cancer* 53:2083, 1984.

Wheeler MH, Austin TR, Lazarus JH: The management of the patient with catecholamine excess. *World J Surg* 6:735, 1982.

Young DG: Thoracic neuroblastoma/ganglioneuroma. *J Pediatr Surg* 18:1, 1983.

Young HH: A technique for simultaneous exposure and operation on the adrenals. *Surg Gynecol Obstet* 54:179, 1936.

Chapter 38

Thyroid and Parathyroid

Edwin L. Kaplan

THYROID

Historical Background

The thyroid gland, previously referred to as the "laryngeal" gland, was so named by Wharton in 1646 because of either its own shieldlike (*thyreos,* shield) shape or the shape of the thyroid cartilage, with which it is closely associated. Classic descriptions of *hyperthyroidism,* or *exophthalmic goiter,* were presented by Parry (1825), Graves (1835), and von Basedow (1840), and *hypothyroidism,* or *myxedema,* was described by Curling (1850) and Gull (1875). Schiff, in the middle of the nineteenth century, conducted experiments demonstrating the importance of the thyroid. Excision in dogs resulted in fatality that could be prevented by a previous graft of the gland. In 1882, Reverdin produced experimental myxedema by total or partial thyroidectomy. In the 1890s, Murray and Howitz successfully treated myxedema with thyroid extract. Although Billroth and his group successfully performed a number of thyroidectomies in the 1860s and thereafter, it is Theodor Kocher who is regarded as the father of thyroid surgery. He performed this operation in the later 1800s over 2000 times with only a 4.5 percent mortality. He also described "cachexia strumipriva," i.e., myxedema, which he noted as a sequel in 30 of his first 100 thyroidectomies. For his pioneering efforts in the field of thyroid surgery, he received the Nobel prize in 1909. The first successful transplantation of thyroid was reported by Payr in 1906, who transplanted a portion of the gland from a woman into the spleen of a myxedematous daughter with "successful" results. Isolation of the hormone thyroxine (T4) was accomplished by Kendall in 1914.

Anatomy

The thyroid gland, which has an average weight of 15 to 20 g, is convex anteriorly and concave posteriorly as a result of its relation to the anterolateral portions of the trachea and larynx, around which it is wrapped and to which it is firmly fixed by fibrous tissue. The lateral lobes extend along the sides of the larynx, reaching the level of the middle of the thyroid cartilage. They reside in a bed between the trachea and larynx mediad and the two carotid sheaths and the sternocleidomastoid muscles laterally. The thyroid gland is enveloped by a thickened fibrous capsule that sends septa into the gland substance to produce an irregular and incomplete pseudolobulation. No true lobulation exists. The deep cervical fascia divides into an anterior and posterior sheath, creating a loosely applied false capsule for the thyroid. Anteriorly, the thyroid lobes are in relation to the strap muscles. Situated on the posterior surface of the lateral lobes of the gland are the parathyroid glands and the recurrent nerves, which lie in a cleft between the trachea and esophagus just medial to the lateral lobes. The lateral lobes are joined by the isthmus that crosses the trachea. The pyramidal lobe is a long, narrow projection of thyroid tissue extending upward from the isthmus lying on the surface of the thyroid cartilage usually to the left of the prominence of that structure. It represents a vestige of the embryonic thyroglossal duct and can be demonstrated in about 80 percent of patients at operation.

The thyroid has an abundant blood supply. The four major arteries are the paired superior thyroid arteries, which arise from the external carotid arteries and descend several centimeters in the neck to reach the upper poles of each thyroid lobe where they branch, and the paired inferior thyroid arteries, which arise from the thyrocervical trunks of the subclavian arteries and enter the lower part of each thyroid lobe from behind. A fifth artery, the thyroidea ima, is sometimes present and arises from the arch of the aorta and enters the thyroid in the midline. A venous plexus forms under the capsule and contributes to confluences forming the superior thyroid vein at the upper pole and the middle thyroid vein in the middle of the lobe, both of which enter the internal jugular vein. Arising from the lower pole are the inferior thyroid veins, which drain directly into the innominate vein.

The gland receives its innervation from sympathetic and parasympathetic divisions of the autonomic nervous system. The sympathetic fibers arise from the cervical ganglion and enter with blood vessels, while the parasympathetic fibers are derived from the vagus and reach the gland via branches of the laryngeal nerves.

Microscopically, the thyroid is composed of follicles, or acini. The follicles are roughly spherical and have an average diameter of 30 μm. They represent storage depots that receive and store the products of the lining epithelial cells. These are usually cuboidal. Under the stimulation of the pituitary hormone, thyrotropin (TSH), the height of the cells increases, changing the shape to a columnar one, and the lumen decreases proportionately.

A second group of cells, called *C cells,* since they contain and secrete calcitonin, is also present. These cells are derived from neuroectoderm, and are part of the APUD series (i.e., *a*mine containing, *p*recursor *u*ptake, *d*ecarboxylase) described by Pearse. In fish, fowl, and amphibians, C cells are present in a separate ultimobranchial body, while in human beings these cells are incorporated embryologically into the thyroid gland as part of the lateral thyroid lobes.

The thyroid gland's relation to the recurrent laryngeal nerve and to the external branch of the superior laryngeal nerve is of major surgical significance. Riddell indicated that among cases in which surgeons "avoid" rather than expose the recurrent laryngeal nerve there is a 4 percent incidence of vocal cord damage. Hunt et al. reported the anatomy of the recurrent laryngeal nerves in 100 cases. The right recurrent laryngeal nerve resided in the tra-

cheoesophageal groove in 64 percent of cases, whereas the left nerve was similarly located on the left side in 77 percent of cases. The nerve was lateral to the trachea in 33 percent of cases on the right side and 22 percent on the left side. In six cases on the right side and four on the left, the nerve was anterolateral to the trachea and in danger of division during subtotal lobectomy. On one occasion on the right side, a direct (i.e., nonrecurrent) recurrent laryngeal nerve was given off in the neck without looping around the subclavian artery. The inferior thyroid artery is often used as a landmark for demonstration of the recurrent laryngeal nerve. The vessel was absent in five instances on the left and twice on the right in the above series. The recurrent laryngeal nerve passed anterior to the inferior thyroid artery in 37 percent of cases on the right side and 24 percent on the left. In 50 percent of cases, the nerve was embedded in the ligament of Berry, which is of importance because traction on the gland would put the nerve on stretch and make it subject to section. Damage to the recurrent laryngeal nerve results in paresis or paralysis of the intrinsic musculature of the larynx on that side, which results in vocal cord paralysis.

The external branch of the superior laryngeal nerves innervates the cricothyroid muscle. In most cases, the superior laryngeal nerves lie adjacent to the vascular pedicles of the superior poles of the thyroid glands, requiring that the vessels be ligated with care to avoid injury. In 18 percent of cases, the nerve is intimately related to the vessels lying parallel and just deep to them in the pretracheal fascia. In 7 percent, the nerve passes through the division of the superior thyroid vessels, coursing over the anterosuperior portion of the gland. In only 15 percent of cases does the superior laryngeal nerve enter the thyropharyngeal muscle before reaching the region of the superior pole of the thyroid gland, thus protecting it from manipulation by the surgeon.

ANOMALIES

The thyroid is embryologically an offshoot of the primitive alimentary tract, from which it later becomes separated. A median anlage arises from the pharyngeal floor in the region of the foramen cecum of the tongue. The main body of the thyroid descends into the neck from this origin (Fig. 38-1) and is joined by a pair of lateral components originating from the ultimobranchial bodies of the fourth and fifth branchial pouches. It is from these lateral components that the C cells enter the thyroid lobes (Fig. 38-2).

The median thyroid anlage may fail to develop, with the rare situation of athyreosis as a result, or it may differentiate in abnormal locations. The most common of these is the pyramidal lobe, which has been reported in as many as 80 percent of patients in whom the gland was surgically exposed. Usually the pyramidal lobe is small; however, in Graves' disease or in lymphocytic thyroiditis it is often enlarged and is clinically palpable. Other variations involving the median thyroid anlage represent an arrest in the usual descent of part or all of the thyroid-forming material to its normal location in front of the second to sixth

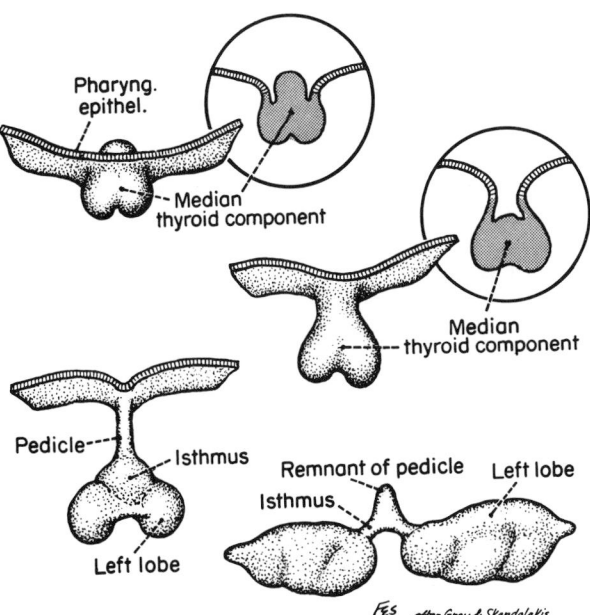

Fig. 38-1. Schematic representation of early thyroid gland development from midline floor of pharyngeal anlage with later downward growth and division into lobes connected by an isthmus. (From: *Sedgwick CE, Cady B: Surgery of the Thyroid and Parathyroid Glands. Philadelphia, Saunders, 1980, with permission.*)

Fig. 38-2. *A* and *B*. Schematic view of the shifts in location of thyroid, C cells, and parathyroid tissues. *C*. Approximates the adult location. (From: *Sedgwick CE, Cady B: Surgery of the Thyroid and Parathyroid Glands. Philadelphia, Saunders, 1980, with permission.*)

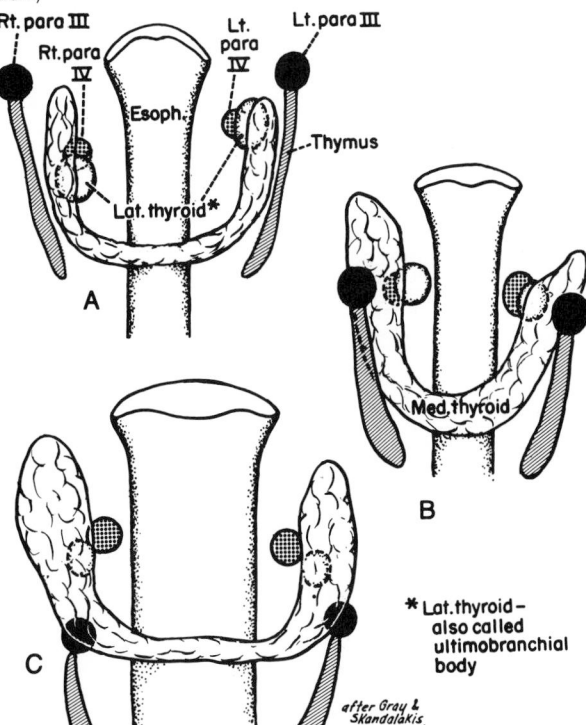

tracheal rings. These include the development of a lingual thyroid, suprahyoid, infrahyoid, and prethyroid tissue, and persistence of the thyroglossal duct, as a cyst, which is the most common of the clinically important anomalies of thyroid development. Infrequently, the entire gland or parts of it descend more caudad, which results in thyroid tissue located in the superior mediastinum behind the sternum, adjacent to the aortic arch or between the aorta and pulmonary trunk, within the upper portion of the pericardium, and even in the interventricular septum of the heart. Most intrathoracic goiters, however, are not true anomalies but rather extensions of pathologic elements of a normally situated gland into the superior or posterior mediastinum.

LATERAL ABERRANT THYROID RESTS. True lateral aberrant thyroid tissue is rare, since the lateral anlagen are normally incorporated into the expanding lateral lobes of the median thyroid anlage. It is now felt that the so-called lateral aberrant thyroid almost always represents papillary-follicular carcinoma that has metastasized from a primary thyroid cancer and has replaced a lymph node with tumor.

LINGUAL THYROID. Lingual thyroid, which is thyroid tissue at the base of the tongue, is relatively rare and estimated to occur in 1 in 3000 cases of thyroid disease. It does, however, represent the most common form of functioning ectopic thyroid tissue that achieves clinical significance. Lingual thyroids are associated with cervical athyreosis in 70 percent of cases and occur much more commonly in females.

Clinical Manifestations. The diagnosis may be made by discovery of an incidental posterior lingual mass in an asymptomatic patient. The mass may enlarge and cause dysphagia, dysphonia, dyspnea, or sensation of choking. Lingual thyroid has been known to cause complications during induction of anesthesia. Hypothyroidism is frequently present, but hyperthyroidism, which is unusual, can occur. The incidence of malignancy is extremely low, occurring in 4 of 144 patients with symptomatic lingual thyroid. The diagnosis should be suspected when a mass is detected in the region of the foramen cecum of the tongue. The diagnosis is readily established by scanning with ^{123}I or ^{99m}Tc.

Treatment. Unless there is immediate surgical indication, treatment should be instituted with replacement thyroid hormone to suppress the lingual thyroid and reduce its size. Radioactive ^{131}I may also be used to reduce the size and is particularly appropriate if there is associated hyperthyroidism.

Indications for surgical intervention include difficulty in swallowing, speech, or breathing; hemorrhage; degeneration and necrosis; uncontrolled hyperthyroidism; and, occasionally, the suspicion of malignancy. A preliminary tracheostomy may be indicated with large or hemorrhagic lesions to obviate the consequences of postoperative tracheal edema. The lingual thyroid may be removed by an intraoral route, by drawing the tongue forward and incising directly over the growth, which is completely or partially removed. Autotransplantation of the excised lingual thyroid has been recommended to avoid the development of hypothyroidism, and success has been reported by several writers.

Physiology

The thyroid gland has two physiologic functions—production of thyroid hormone and of calcitonin (thyrocalcitonin). Calcitonin, a 34 amino acid peptide, appears to be important physiologically in lower animals by preventing hypercalcemia. In human beings it has never been proved to play an important physiologic role. Its importance pharmacologically in the treatment of hypercalcemia and Paget's disease and as a tumor marker for medullary carcinoma of the thyroid will be discussed later in this chapter.

The principal function of the thyroid gland is to synthesize and secrete thyroid hormone, which is necessary for overall metabolism. This function is dependent upon an interplay between several processes, including (1) iodine metabolism, (2) the production, storage, and secretion of thyroid hormone by the thyroid gland, and (3) the effects of this hormone on various organ systems. The production of thyroid hormone is influenced by intricate regulatory mechanisms and responds to multiple and diverse physiologic, pathologic, and pharmacologic alterations.

IODINE METABOLISM. The formation of thyroid hormone depends upon the availability of exogenous iodine which is normally satisfied by dietary sources and is thus dependent upon the iodine content of water and soil. In-

gested iodine is rapidly absorbed from the gastrointestinal tract, usually within 1 h. It is then distributed through the extracellular space in the form of iodides and is progressively extracted from the plasma by both the thyroid and kidneys until essentially all the iodine is either bound in organic form within the thyroid or excreted as urinary iodides (Fig. 38-3). Ninety percent of the body iodine stores are present within the thyroid, predominantly in the organic form. Studies employing labeled iodine have demonstrated that approximately two-thirds of the administered dose ultimately appears in the urine, while the thyroid collects the remaining third. The partitioning of the ingested iodide between thyroid and kidney is complete within 48 h, and the plasma and tissues are almost cleared of iodide. The subsequent appearance of labeled iodine within the circulation is the result of the secretion of thyroid hormone. A small fraction of the iodine that had been removed from the extracellular fluid by the thyroid gland is ultimately secreted back into the circulation as inorganic iodide.

Fig. 38-3. The iodide cycle. Ingested iodide is trapped in the thyroid, oxidized, bound to iodotyrosines in thyroglobulin, and coupling of iodotyrosyl residues forms thyroxine and T3. Hormone secreted by the gland is transported in plasma, some T4 is deiodinated to T3, the hormone exerts its metabolic effect on the cell, is ultimately deiodinated, and the iodide is reutilized or excreted in the kidney. A second cycle goes on inside the thyroid gland, with deiodination of iodotyrosines generating iodide, which is reutilized without leaving the gland. (From: *DeGroot LJ, Stanbury JB: The Thyroid and Its Diseases, 4th ed. New York, Wiley, 1975, chap 2, with permission.*)

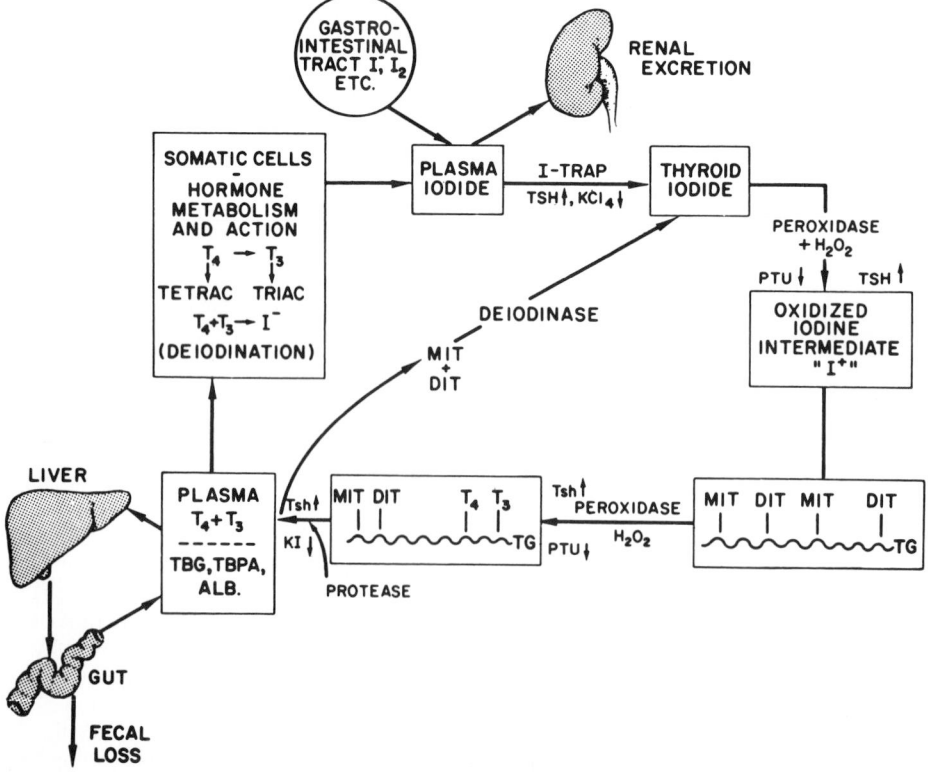

SYNTHESIS AND SECRETION OF THYROID HORMONE. The steps in the synthesis of thyroid hormone are (1) the concentration of iodide within the gland, (2) rapid oxidation of iodides to iodine, (3) the formation of precursor amino acids, 3-monoiodotyrosine (MIT) and 3-5-diiodotyrosine (DIT), and (4) the coupling of these inactive iodotyrosines to form the hormonally active iodothyronines, triiodothyronine (T3) and thyroxine (T4).

The production of thyroid hormone begins with the active transport of iodine from the plasma into the thyroid cells. A concentration gradient of iodine of 20:1 or more is found in normal individuals, while in Graves' disease, a form of thyrotoxicosis, gradients of 500:1 between the cells and the serum have been identified. The iodine transfer mechanism is influenced by thyroid-stimulating hormone (TSH), which stimulates every step in thyroid hormone synthesis and secretion, and is also modified by an internal autoregulatory system so that its responsiveness to TSH stimulation varies inversely with the glandular content of organic iodine. When iodine transport is defective, because of either pharmacologic inhibitors or spontaneous disease, goiter and/or hypothyroidism results.

The iodide that enters the thyroid remains in its free state only briefly before it is further metabolized. It is rapidly incorporated into thyroglobulin. Tyrosine radicals of protothyroglobulin molecules are iodinated to form MIT and DIT. Organic iodinations are conditioned to some extent by the stimulation of TSH and may be inhibited by a great number of pharmacologic agents, including the usual antithyroid drugs, or by defects in the organ-binding mechanism with resultant hypothyroidism and/or goiter. The coupling of two iodotyrosine molecules leads to the formation of iodothyronine, a process in which a variety of enzymatic systems have been implicated. T4 is formed by the coupling of two DIT radicals, while T3 is formed by the coupling of one MIT and one DIT radical. The proportion of T3 to T4 synthesized and secreted is dependent on the degree of iodination of intrafollicular thyroglobulin.

STORAGE, SECRETION, AND METABOLISM OF THYROID HORMONE. The hormonally active iodothyronines, T4 and T3, are held in peptide linkage with a specific thyroprotein, thyroglobulin, which forms the major component of intrafollicular colloid.

Release of the active hormones into the circulation involves hydrolysis of the thyroglobulin by proteases and peptidases, resulting in T4 and T3. The activity of these enzymes is enhanced by the administration of TSH. At the same time, some metabolically inert iodine amino acids enter the circulation and are deiodinized, and the iodine is reutilized in the metabolic cycle. The active thyroid hormones become attached to plasma protein, the best known of which is the thyroxine-binding globulin (TBG) and the more recently recognized thyroxine-binding prealbumin (TBPA).

In the plasma, the ratio of T4 to T3 is 10:1 to 20:1. T3 is bound less firmly to protein and thus enters the peripheral tissues more rapidly. It is three to four times more active than T4 per unit weight and accounts for approximately half the metabolic effect of the secreted hormone. The free hormone available to the tissue is responsible for its metabolic action. The half-life of T3 is about 3 days, while the half-life of T4 is about 7 to 8 days, and both hormones leave the blood in an exponential fashion. A significant amount of T4 is converted to T3, which may be the only active hormone intracellularly. As they lose iodine atoms, the iodine returns to the blood to reenter the metabolic pool. T3 and T4 are conjugated in the liver with glucuronic acid and excreted into the bile. In the intestine, these conjugates are disrupted, and a portion of the free hormones is resorbed. In human beings, less than 5 percent of the circulating T4 is involved in the enterohepatic circulation. Large amounts of hormone and iodide may appear in the milk of lactating females.

The metabolic impact of thyroid hormone on peripheral tissue is widespread and accompanied by an increased oxygen consumption and calorigenesis. Thyroid hormone stimulates protein synthesis and affects all aspects of carbohydrate metabolism. Thyroid hormone also influences the processes of lipid metabolism, as evidenced by the fact that the serum cholesterol and phospholipid vary inversely with the state of thyroid function. In general, thyroid hormone increases oxidative phosphorylation.

REGULATION OF THYROID ACTIVITY. The function of the thyroid gland is closely regulated by the central nervous system and by the level of circulating iodine. As a consequence of these regulatory mechanisms, thyroid activity responds to a variety of physiologic and pathologic changes as well as pharmacologic agents.

Anterior pituitary cells secrete TSH, which regulates thyroid function. Absence or reduction of TSH secretion is accompanied by decreased synthesis and secretion of thyroid hormone, flattening of the thyroid epithelium, and reduction in vascularity of the gland. Conversely, increased TSH secretion accelerates the production and release of thyroid hormone while anatomically increasing the cellularity and vascularity of the thyroid gland. TSH stimulates all processes leading to the synthesis and secretion of thyroid hormone. When the target gland is responsive, within a few hours of TSH administration there is an increase in the T4 and T3 secretion.

It is now known that the cerebral cortex acts on the hypothalamus, which secretes a thyrotropin-releasing hormone (TRH), which in turn acts on the anterior pituitary and induces the release of TSH. The secretion of TSH is also controlled in a "feedback" manner by the level of thyroid hormone in the blood (Fig. 38-4). TSH secretion is inhibited by an excess of circulating thyroid hormone and augmented by thyroid hormone deprivation. When hypothyroidism occurs for any reason, the pituitary responds by increasing TSH secretion with resultant hyperplasia and increased vascularity of the thyroid gland.

The concentration of intrathyroidal iodide inversely influences responsiveness to TSH, thus effecting an intrinsic regulatory system. When small doses of iodine are administered, there is an increase in thyroid hormone synthesis for a short time. With progressively larger doses, there is a biphasic response, at first increasing and

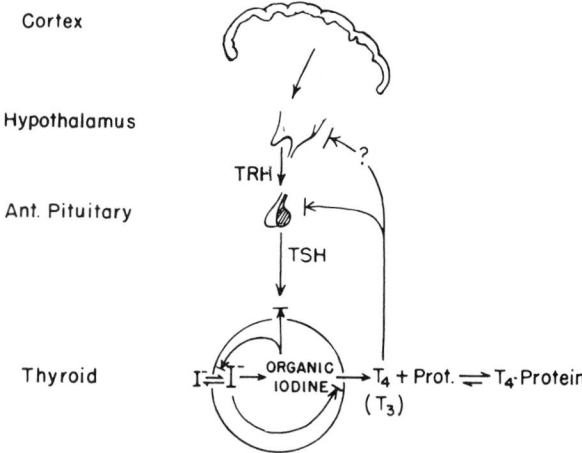

Fig. 38-4. Schema of the homeostatic regulation of thyroid function. Secretion of TSH is regulated by a negative feedback mechanism acting directly on the pituitary and is normally inversely related to the concentration of unbound hormone in the blood. Release of TSH is induced by TRH, secretion of which appears to set the level of the pituitary feedback mechanism. Factors regulating secretion of TRH are uncertain but may include the free hormone in the blood and stimuli from higher centers. Autoregulatory control of thyroid function is also shown. High concentrations of intrathyroidal iodide decrease the rate of release of thyroidal iodine. In addition, the magnitude of the organic iodine pool inversely influences the iodide transport mechanism and the response to TSH. [From: *Ingbar SH, Woeber KA: The thyroid gland, in Williams RH (ed): Textbook of Endocrinology, 4th ed. Philadelphia, Saunders, 1968, with permission.*]

then decreasing, due to a relative blockade in organic binding. With moderate or large doses administered repeatedly, the relative inhibition of organic binding eventually escapes, representing an adaptation phenomenon. Pharmacologic doses of iodide decrease the rate of release of glandular iodine and the formation of active hormone. The concentration of T4 in the serum is reduced, and thyrotoxicity in patients with diffuse toxic goiter is rapidly relieved. The vascularity and hyperplasia of the gland are reversed through the action of iodine on TSH, thus facilitating surgical excision.

In addition to these pharmacologic effects of iodine, the biosynthesis of thyroid hormone may be altered by agents known as *antithyroid drugs*. There are two major categories: The first, represented by perchlorate and thiocyanate, prevents the concentration of iodine by the thyroid. The second group of antithyroid drugs includes organic substances that prevent the binding of iodine to tyrosine radicals. The best known of this group are the thiourea derivatives propylthiouracil (PTU) and methimazole (Tapazole).

Evaluation of Patients with Thyroid Disease

One is generally asked to evaluate patients with two types of thyroid problems: (1) diseases of hyper- or hypofunctioning of the gland and (2) masses within the thyroid gland that may be suggestive of carcinoma. As in treating diseases of most other parts of the body, it is

appropriate to start with a careful history and physical examination.

Interview of the patient is directed at determining whether there is evidence of hyperfunction or insufficient function of the thyroid gland. The specific signs and symptoms of thyrotoxicosis and myxedema will be presented in subsequent sections of this chapter.

Symptoms related to pressure of the thyroid on neighboring structures in the neck include dysphagia, dysphonia, dyspnea, and a choking sensation. A change in one's voice may indicate recurrent laryngeal nerve dysfunction, usually the result of tumor invasion. When a thyroid mass is apparent, the duration, rate of growth, and presence of accompanying pain should be determined. A history of exposure to low-dose external ionizing radiation is probably the most important fact that can be ascertained when dealing with a mass lesion. In the patient with a nontoxic goiter, diet, possible ingestion of goiterogenic drugs, and family history are all relevant.

Physical examination requires a precise evaluation of the thyroid gland and adjacent cervical structures. The neck should be inspected while it is slightly extended. In thin patients, a normal thyroid, particularly in the region of the isthmus, may be visible. If the thyroid is visible, it will rise with swallowing. A goiter that fills the suprasternal notch may be seen to rise out of the chest with swallowing. Asymmetry and large masses within the gland may be apparent. Palpation should be performed from two vantage points, in front of and behind the seated patient, applying the tips of the fingers in a gentle fashion. In most thin people, it is possible to outline the gland, whereas the normal thyroid is not palpable in obese individuals and in those with short necks. Palpation of the cricoid cartilarge serves to orient the examiner, since the superior border of the isthmus lies just below this level.

The normal gland has a rubbery consistency. The diffuse goiter and hyperplastic gland is softer. In Hashimoto's disease the gland is firmer, while with carcinoma or Riedel's struma the thyroid may be stony hard. Nodules may be identified. In thyrotoxicosis, a bruit may be present because of increased blood flow but must be differentiated from murmurs transmitted from the base of the heart. The regional lymph nodes should be examined in the anterior triangles of the neck. A node, known as the Delphian node, may be palpable on the trachea just above the thyroid isthmus. This is frequently associated with malignant disease or thyroiditis.

THYROID FUNCTION TESTS

A variety of laboratory tests have been developed to assess thyroid function and thyroid lesions (Table 38-1). Each test has specific indications, none is uniformly reliable, and all are subject to alteration by exogenous and endogenous factors. The usefulness of these tests will become apparent as different disease states are discussed.

MEASURES OF T4 AND T3. A number of tests are available that directly or indirectly measure the supply of thyroxine (T4) and triiodothyronine (T3). Ideally, one would like to measure the *free T4*. However, these determina-

Table 38-1. PRINCIPAL DIAGNOSTIC TESTS OF THE THYROID

Direct and indirect measures of T4 and T3 supply	*Abbreviation*	*Normal values*
Serum T4	T4	4.9–12.0 μg/dL
Free thyroxine	RT4	2.8 ± 0.5 mμg/dL
Resin T3 uptake	RT3U	Varies with lab, 20–30%
Free thyroxine index	FTI or T7	Varies with lab, 6.4–10.5
Serum T3	T3	115–190 mμg/dL
Radioactive iodine uptake	RAIU	Varies with lab, <22%
Serum TSH	TSH	Varies with lab, 0–6 μU/mL
Thyroxine-binding globulin capacity	TBG	12–20 μg T4/100 mL ± 1.8 μg

Measures of autoimmunity

Antithyroglobulin antibodies	TGHA	Titer <1/20
Antimicrosomal antibodies	MCHA	Titer <1/20
Long-acting thyroid stimulator	LATS	Negative
Thyroid-stimulating immunoglobulins	TSI	

Measures of thyroid and pituitary responsiveness

T3 suppression test		Decrease 50% of control or to normal
TRH stimulation test		Peak TSH 10–30 μU/mL at 20–30 min
TSH stimulation test		Double RAIU or above 10%

Assessment of thyroid anatomy

Thyroid isotope scan	Scan	Homogeneous distribution; normal size, shape, and position
Ultrasonic scan		Determines presence of masses and whether solid or cystic

Assessment of thyroid histology

Core needle biopsy		
Aspiration biopsy with cytology (ABC)		

tions are difficult. Hence, most commonly one measures the *total T4 or T3*. These tests correlate well with disease states, but vary with the amount of thyroxine-binding globulin (TBG) that is present in the serum. Estrogens, increased when patients take oral contraceptive pills or during pregnancy, elevate the TBG values; thus, they also increase total T4; testosterone, anticonvulsants, and chronic illness decrease this level. The *T3 resin uptake test* quantitates the degree of saturation of the binding sites of TBG in the serum by T4 and T3. In most instances this test directly reflects the thyroid hormone concentration. The *free thyroxine index* (FTI), sometimes called the *T7 test,* is a test that controls for differences in TBG concentration. In most laboratories this index correlates very well with the patient's functional thyroid status and is one of the most useful tests. Another very sensitive test of thyroid function is the *serum TSH value*. When hypothyroidism is present, for example, the TSH value becomes elevated; when a patient is hyperthyroid, the circulating TSH level is low.

The *radioactive iodine uptake* (RAIU) by the thyroid is also an effective measure of thyroid function. In hyper-

thyroidism more iodine is trapped by the thyroid in a given period of time, and, hence, this value is elevated; in hypothyroidism, on the other hand, it is decreased. It must be remembered, however, that both thyroxine treatment and iodine administration will decrease this value and give falsely lowered results. The expansion of the body stores of iodine is probably the most common exogenous cause of lowering the thyroidal radioisotope uptake. This is seen following the administration of oral iodine but more commonly after organic iodinated dyes are used in radiologic studies, such as pyelography, cystography, arteriography, myelography, or computerized tomography. The effects of some of these dyes, especially the oil-based dyes used for myelography, may last for months and possibly even for years. The decreased RAIU that follows the administration of suppressive dosages of thyroid hormones is due to a decrease of secretion of TSH.

MEASURES OF AUTOIMMUNITY. Both circulating antithyroglobulin (TGHA) and thyroid antimicrosomal (MCHA) antibodies can be measured in the serum. High antibody levels are found primarily in individuals who

Table 38-2. ABSORBED DOSES FROM THYROID SCANNING AGENTS

Nuclide	Average dose of activity administered, μC	Maximal thyroid absorbed dose, rads	Total body absorbed dose, rads	Critical organ absorbed dose, rads
^{131}I	50	50	0.040	Thyroid
^{125}I	50	50	0.030	Thyroid
^{123}I	300	4.5	0.030	Thyroid
Pertechnetate-99m (Na ^{99m}TcO$_4$)	2500	1.0	0.030	Stomach ($\pm$1 rad)

SOURCE: From DeGroot LJ, Stanbury JB: *The Thyroid and Its Diseases.* New York, Wiley, 1975, p 232, with permission.

have either Graves' disease or chronic lymphocytic thyroiditis. Long-acting thyroid stimulator (LATS) or thyroid-stimulating immunoglobulins (TSI) are often detected in individuals with Graves' disease and may be the cause of the thyroid stimulation in this disease.

MEASURES OF THYROID AND PITUITARY RESPONSIVENESS. Suppression Test. Autonomy of thyroid function is present if the patient demonstrates a lack of suppression when T3 is administered in amounts that normally suppress TSH secretion. Seventy-five to 100 μg of T3 is given for 7 to 10 days. Normal individuals will suppress their RAIU values to normal or to 50 percent of control values. Nonsuppressibility occurs in Graves' disease, chronic lymphocytic thyroiditis, toxic adenomas, functioning carcinomas, and in so-called euthyroid Graves' disease.

TSH Stimulation Test. An RAIU test in the hypothyroid range might be the result of either primary thyroid failure or lack of pituitary TSH secretion. The administration of 5 units of TSH subcutaneously each day for 3 days will usually increase the RAIU of a patient with hypopituitarism to double the initial value or into the normal range. The response to TSH can also be detected by measuring increments in plasma concentrations of T4 and T3. If the disorder is due to primary thyroid destruction, TSH administration will have a lesser effect.

TRH Stimulation Test. This test measures the responsiveness of the pituitary to intravenously administered TRH, the hypothalamic stimulator of TSH. TRH is given in a dose of 400 μg/1.73 m^2 of body surface. In euthyroid individuals who have normal pituitary function, a prompt increase in TSH, which peaks at 20 to 30 min, is observed. In hypothyroid individuals, basal levels of TSH are elevated. Following TRH administration, the reaction is hyperresponsive; the TSH levels often reach 100 to 200 μU/mL at 30 min. On the other hand, patients with thyrotoxicosis or pituitary destruction or those taking thyroid hormone have blunted or absent TSH responses when TRH is given.

Other Factors. The serum cholesterol is usually increased in hypothyroidism when it is of a thyroid etiology. Characteristically this level is normal when hypothyroidism is due to pituitary failure.

THYROID SCANNING. Scintillation scanning localizes the site of radioiodine accumulation in the thyroid gland or in ectopic thyroid tissue. ^{131}I was the time-honored isotope utilized, but more recently this has been replaced by ^{123}I or by ^{99m}technetium (^{99m}Tc) as pertechnetate, because both of these isotopes result in a much lower dose of radiation to the thyroid (Table 38-2). The scan techniques employ either a mechanical device that moves a columnated detector back and forth and determines the location of activity (Fig. 38-5), or more recently a gamma camera is used.

Nodules of the thyroid may be classified as hyperfunctional, or "hot," that is, with more radioactivity than usual with the normal thyroid suppressed (Fig. 38-6); functional, or "warm," that is, nodules that concentrate radioactivity equal to the remainder of the gland (Fig. 38-7); finally, hypofunctional, or "cold," nodules that concentrate less activity than the remainder of the gland (Fig. 38-8). The scintillation scan also may be of value in determining the presence of abnormally positioned thyroid tissue, such as substernal thyroid (Fig. 38-9) or lingual thyroid.

After a total thyroidectomy for papillary or follicular cancer a total body scan is usually performed and can detect areas of metastases (Fig. 38-10).

THYROID BIOPSY. Biopsy of the thyroid is useful in establishing a diagnosis of thyroiditis and differentiating between benign and malignant thyroid nodules. A core biopsy may be obtained with a Vim-Silverman or a Trucut needle. More recently, thin needle aspiration biopsy with cytologic examination of cells obtained is gaining favor. The value of these techniques in the evaluation of a thyroid nodule will be discussed later in this chapter.

Thyrotoxicosis

Thyrotoxicosis refers to a spectrum of clinical manifestations that are related to primary excess secretion of active thyroid hormone. There are three main types of pathologic processes associated with thyrotoxicosis: Graves' disease (toxic diffuse goiter), toxic multinodular goiter, and a single toxic adenoma. In rare instances, the pathologic process is located in ectopic thyroid tissue such as lingual thyroid or struma ovarii, thyroid tissue in an ovarian teratoma. Other causes are listed in Table 38-3.

ETIOLOGY AND PATHOLOGY. Graves' Disease. The cause of Graves' disease is unknown. In general, this disorder is regarded as a systemic autoimmune disease in which hyperthyroidism, exophthalmus, and a der-

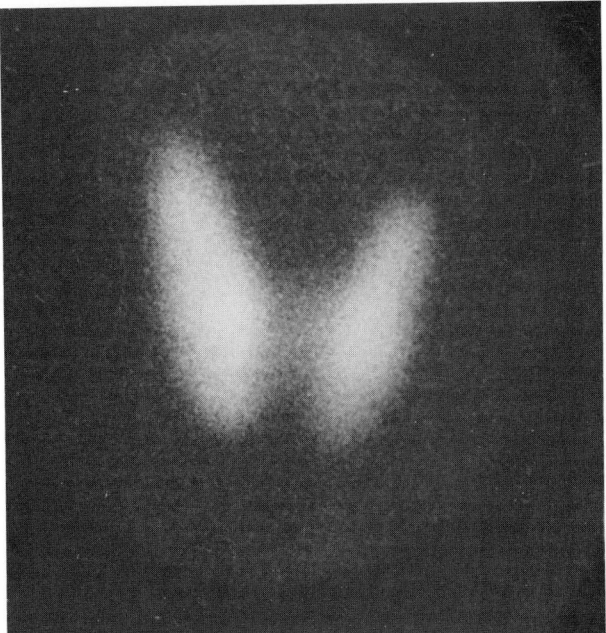

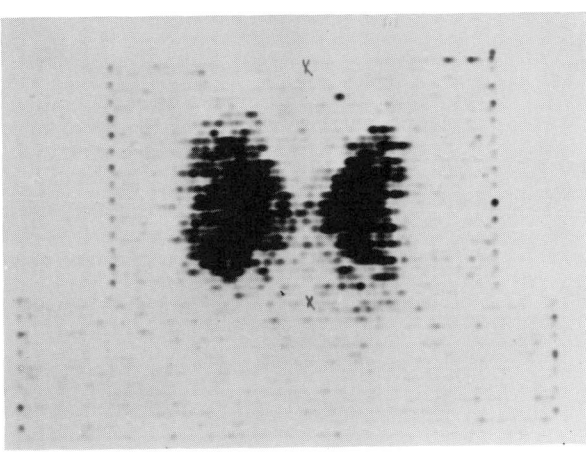

A

B

Fig. 38-5. Radioiodine scan. Normal thyroid. *A.* Obtained with a rectilinear scanner. *B.* Obtained with a gamma camera with pinhole collimator.

mopathy, called *pretibial myxedema*, are three parts of the same process. Hall and others believe that the hyperthyroidism results from antibodies to the TSH receptors that bind in the region of the receptor and thus stimulate thyroid function. Indeed, immunoglobulins called LATS (long-acting thyroid stimulator) and TSI (thyroid stimulating immunoglobulins) are detectable in many individuals with Graves' disease. Contributory factors include

heredity, sex, and emotional disturbances. There is a tendency for Graves' disease to be present in several members of the same family, and the incidence of thyroid disorders other than Graves' disease, particularly Hashimoto's thyroiditis, is also increased in these families. Some investigators have even reported a characteristic histocompatibility haplotype in Caucasians with Graves' disease. The incidence of females to males affected by Graves' disease is 6:1 to 7:1. The psychosomatic aspects have been stressed in many series, but although they

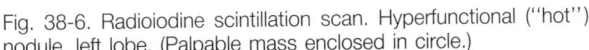

Fig. 38-6. Radioiodine scintillation scan. Hyperfunctional ("hot") nodule, left lobe. (Palpable mass enclosed in circle.)

Fig. 38-7. Radioiodine scintillation scan. Functional ("warm") nodule, left lobe. (Palpable mass enclosed in circle.)

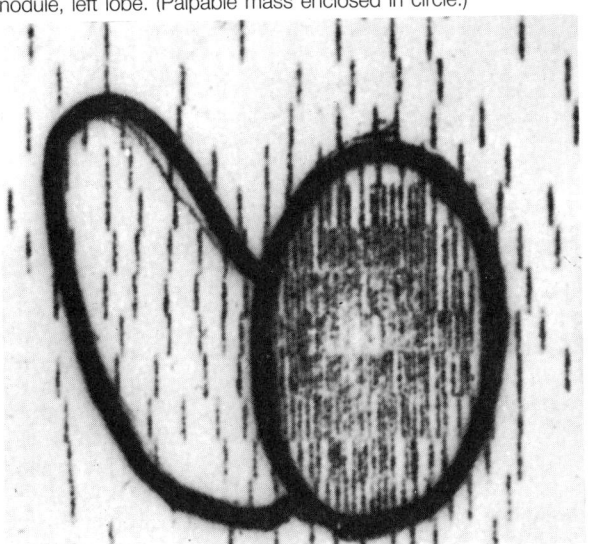

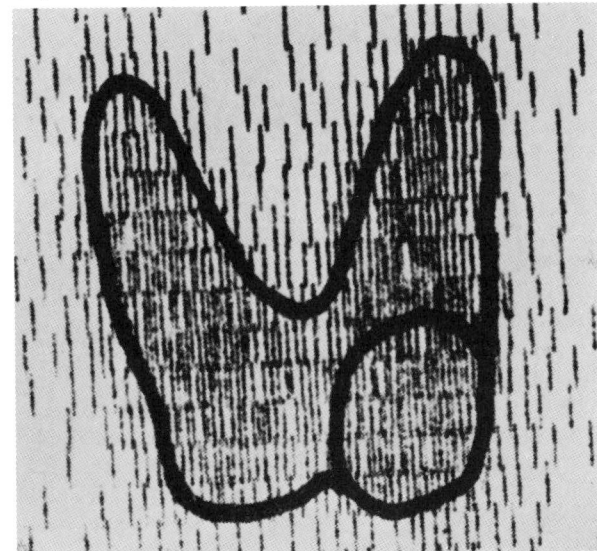

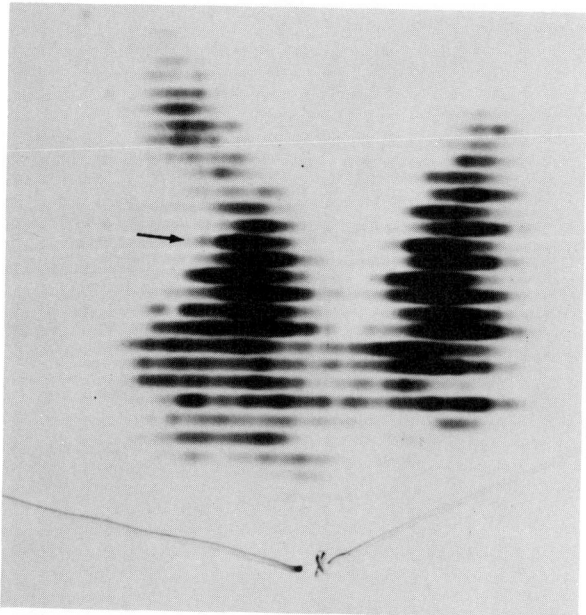

A

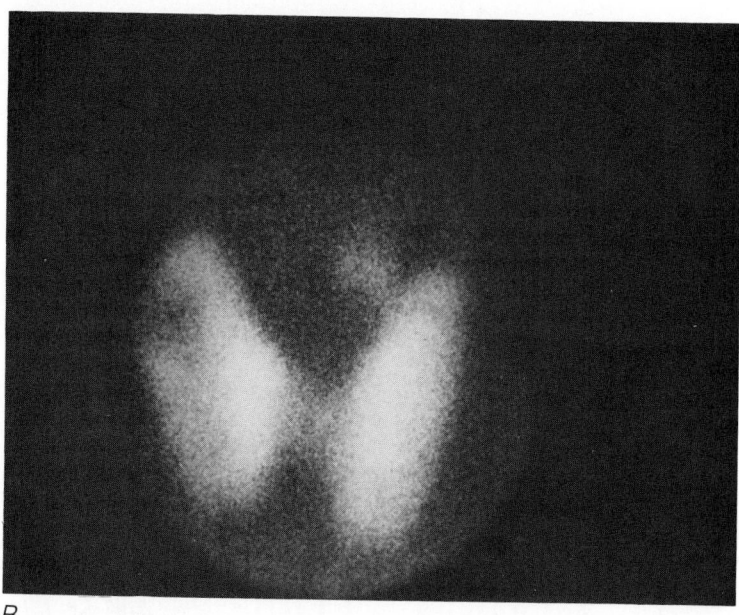

B

Fig. 38-8. Radioiodine scintillation scan. Nonfunctional ("cold") nodule, right lobe. *A.* Rectilinear scan. *B.* Obtained with a gamma camera with pinhole collimator.

modify the manifestations, their etiologic importance has not been defined.

In general the thyroid of the patient with Graves' disease is diffusely enlarged, and the surface is characteristically smooth but may be slightly nodular. Microscopically, the thyroid is hyperplastic, the epithelium is columnar, and only a minimal amount of colloid is evident in the gland. The nuclei may exhibit mitoses, and papillary projections of the hyperplastic epithelium are common. There may be aggregates of lymphoid tissue, and vascularity is markedly increased. These pathologic characteristics are associated with an overproduction of thyroid hormones.

Toxic Multinodular Goiter. This is usually superimposed on a long-standing nontoxic multinodular goiter. Grossly, the gland contains multiple nodules, many of which contain aggregates of irregularly large cells and scant amount of colloid. These areas are capable of function independent of stimulation by TSH; i.e., they are autonomously functioning nodules. The amount of overproduction of thyroid hormone is characteristically less than that associated with Graves' disease.

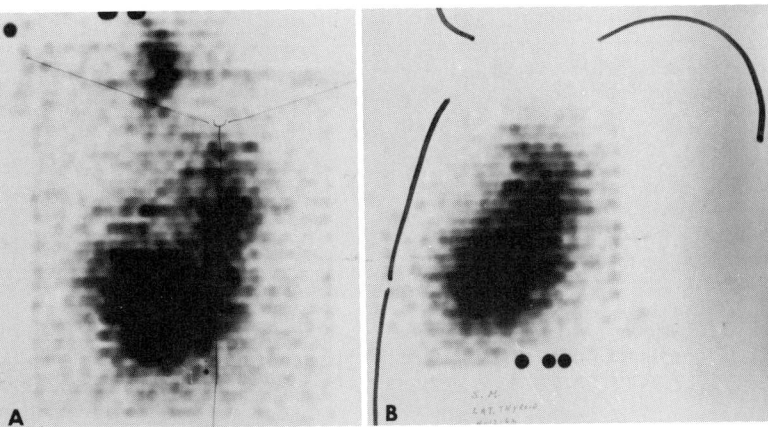

Fig. 38-9. ¹³¹I scintillation scan. Substernal thyroid. *A.* Anteroposterior. *B.* Lateral.

Toxic Adenoma. The solitary toxic adenoma is a follicular tumor. Like the multinodular toxic adenoma, it is capable of function independent of TSH, and the administration of exogenous thyroid fails to suppress the secretion of T3 and T4.

CLINICAL MANIFESTATIONS. The clinical manifestations of excessive secretion of thyroid hormone will be considered initially, since these pertain to Graves' disease, toxic multinodular goiter, and toxic adenoma, with minor individual variations.

Hyperthyroidism. The onset of symptoms and signs related to an excess amount of circulating thyroid hormone differs for the three main pathologic processes. Graves' disease most commonly becomes clinically apparent in young patients. Although the disease can occur at all ages from infancy on, it is rare before the age of ten and in the elderly patient. The male/female ratio of 1:6 pertains in all geographic areas. The thyrotoxicosis of toxic multinodular goiter usually becomes manifest after the age of fifty and is more common in women than in men. Toxic adenoma occurs in a younger age group, usually in the thirties to forties.

The patient feels warmer than other people in the same environment and becomes intolerant of heat. There is increased sweating and consequent thirst, owing to the need of dissipating the excess heat. As a result of increased calorigenesis, weight loss associated with an increased appetite is generally noted. At times the intake of food may be sufficiently increased to prevent this loss. These manifestations of increased calorigenesis are more marked in patients with Graves' disease than in those with toxic multinodular goiter or toxic adenoma.

By contrast, the cardiovascular manifestations of thyrotoxicosis are more prominent in the older patients with toxic multinodular goiters. These include marked tachycardia, frequent atrial fibrillation, congestive heart failure, and poor response to digitalis. Hyperthyroidism increases the force and rate of the heartbeat, perhaps

Fig. 38-10. ¹³¹I scintillation scan. Functional thyroid pulmonary metastases not demonstrated radiographically.

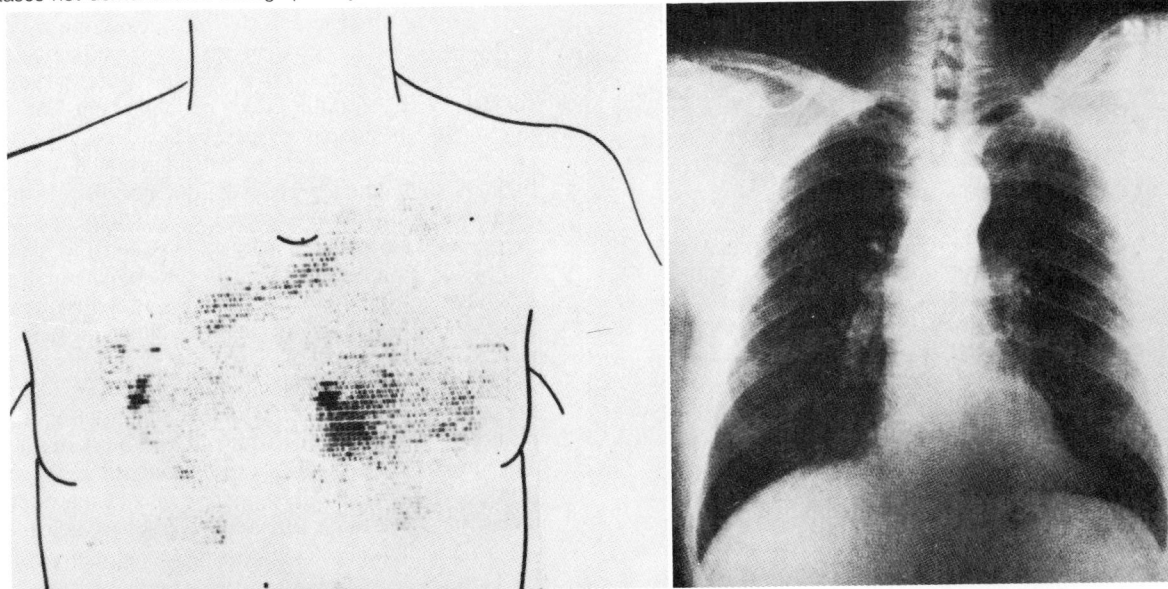

Table 38-3. CAUSES OF HYPERTHYROIDISM

Graves' disease and its variants
Toxic multinodular goiter
Toxic adenoma
de Quervain's thyroiditis
Silent thyroiditis
Postpartum hyperthyroidism
Disseminated thyroid autonomy
Jodbasedow syndrome
Thyrotoxicosis factitia
Hydatidiform mole and choriocarcinoma
Struma ovarii
Thyroid carcinoma
Iatrogenic hyperthyroidism (overtreatment of hypothyroidism)

because of a sensitization to adrenergic stimuli. Sleeping pulse rate is characteristically over 80, and marked tachycardia may be apparent during the physical examination. Patients commonly experience palpitations. The marked cutaneous and peripheral vasodilatation results in an increased pulse pressure. Atrial fibrillation initially may be paroxysmal but eventually becomes continuous and is a common finding among older patients. In this group, it may be the only clinically detectable sign of hyperthyroidism. Congestive heart failure with ankle edema and dyspnea is seldom seen unless there is an underlying heart disease.

Patients with thyrotoxicosis frequently are extremely excitable, restless, hyperkinetic, and emotionally unstable, and complain of insomnia. Frank psychosis may develop. Muscle wasting, muscle weakness, and fatigue are common manifestations of thyrotoxicosis. Myopathy af-

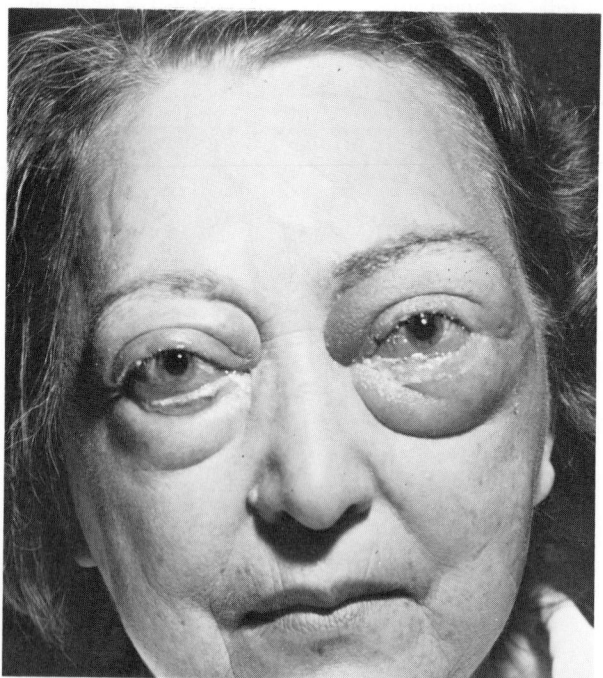

Fig. 38-11. Graves' disease with severe infiltrative ophthalmopathy. *(Courtesy of L. J. DeGroot.)*

fects men more frequently, and the clinical picture may be confused by the fact that thyrotoxicosis occurs in 3 to 6 percent of patients with myasthenia gravis. The muscle weakness is most evident in the proximal limb muscles. Physical examination of patients with hyperthyroidism may demonstrate a tremor of the extended and abducted fingers and hyperactive tendon reflexes. The emotional, neurogenic, and myopathic manifestations are more marked in patients with Graves' disease.

The changes of the skin and its appendages related to thyrotoxicosis include warm, moist skin, facial flushing, and perspiration. There also may be nail changes, which include softening, increased fragility, and separation of the distal margins from the nail bed. The hair is fine and readily falls out with combing. Pretibial myxedema occurs in 3 to 5 percent of patients with Graves' disease, is frequently present when the patient is euthyroid, and is almost always associated with eye signs. Gynecomastia occurs in 3 to 5 percent of males. Breast enlargement may be noted in females with diffuse toxic goiter. Menstrual periods are often scant or absent but return when thyroid function is controlled. Libido may be increased, but fertility is reduced, and the rate of miscarriages is reportedly high.

The effects on the gastrointestinal tract are variable. Diarrhea or increased frequency of defecation is the most characteristic symptom and may occur intermittently or chronically. Increased secretion of thyroid hormone results in increased bone turnover, which sometimes results in hypercalcemia. There is no increased incidence of renal calculi, however.

Graves' Disease. Clinically, Graves' disease is characterized by the classic triad of goiter, thyrotoxicosis, and exophthalmos. These features may occur singly or in any combination. The thyroid is nearly always diffusely enlarged and symmetric; the pyramidal lobe may be enlarged and palpable. The gland is characteristically smooth but may be irregular. The extreme vascularity is evidenced by an audible bruit, best heard over the superior poles on either side. In about 3 percent of the patients with Graves' disease and thyrotoxicosis, the thyroid is normal in size. The eye signs vary from minimal to severe and, fortunately, are mild in most patients. Excess thyroxine per se will not produce exophthalmos; rather it is due to the autoimmune aspects of Graves' disease. Severe thyrotoxicosis may be unaccompanied by exophthalmos, and, conversely, exophthalmos may be the only manifestation of Graves' disease. In about one-third of the cases, the ocular manifestations and the signs and symptoms of thyrotoxicosis begin coincidentally. Exophthalmos infrequently progresses after thyrotoxicosis has been relieved by surgical treatment or radioactive iodine.

The eye signs of Graves' disease include (1) spasm of the upper lid with lid retraction, (2) external ophthalmoplegia, (3) exophthalmos with proptosis, (4) supraorbital and infraorbital swelling, and (5) congestion and edema (Fig. 38-11). Spasm of the upper lid may be manifested by lid lag and excessively apparent sclerae. Weakness of the extrinsic ocular muscles is present in about 40 percent of patients with Graves' disease. Upper rotation is the most common abnormality, while lateral rotation also occurs frequently. The appearance of venous congestion and edema is a sign of severity and has been described as "malignant exophthalmos." It occurs more commonly in the male and is associated with increased lacrimation and pain in the eye. In extreme cases, the eyesight may be lost.

Toxic Multinodular Goiter. The thyroid in these patients contains several palpable nodules. On palpation, the characteristics of the goiter cannot be distinguished from those of nontoxic multinodular goiter. Symptoms related to obstruction of the trachea and/or esophagus occur more commonly than with Graves' disease. Exophthalmos is rarely present.

Toxic Adenoma. There is frequently a history of a slowly growing mass in the neck. Recent rapid growth may be associated with central necrosis and hemorrhage. Palpation reveals a solitary tumor within the thyroid. Thyrotoxicosis is uncommon unless the lesion is at least 3 cm in diameter. A toxic adenoma that undergoes hemorrhagic necrosis may be accompanied by spontaneous remission of the manifestations of thyrotoxicity. Exophthalmos is absent.

DIAGNOSTIC FINDINGS. Thyrotoxicosis is characterized by elevations of T4 and/or T3 levels as well as of the serum FTI (see the preceding section, Thyroid Function Tests).

Graves' Disease. The thyroidal radioiodine uptake is characteristically markedly elevated with 45 to 90 percent of the administered dose localizing in the gland. The T3 suppression test is occasionally applicable to the patient with an equivocal diagnosis. In normal patients the radioactive iodine uptake is decreased by 80 percent, and, for practical purposes, if the decrease is 50 percent or less, the diagnosis of hyperthyroidism can be made. About 1 percent of patients with Graves' disease have pernicious anemia, and 30 percent are reported to have circulating antibodies against gastric parietal cells. A high titer of thyroid autoantibodies is also found in many patients with Graves' disease.

Toxic Multinodular Goiter and Toxic Adenoma. In these patients, the RAIU is generally less than that in Graves' disease, 40 to 55 percent localizing in the functioning tissue. The diagnosis is often made by thyroid scan that demonstrates single or multiple "hot" areas, which often correspond to palpable nodules in cases of toxic multinodular goiter. In thyrotoxicosis due to a toxic adenoma, the scan demonstrates uptake of tracer in the area of the nodule, while the normal part of the gland is not visualized (see Fig. 38-6). If exogenous TSH is given, the remaining part of the gland will then take up isotope.

TREATMENT. Definitive treatment may be effected with antithyroid drugs, radioactive iodine, or surgical excision of thyroid tissue. The approach to a given patient must be individualized and depends on the patient's age, general health, and the pathologic process involved.

Antithyroid Drugs. The majority of the presently employed antithyroid drugs interfere with the organic binding of thyroidal iodine and inhibit the coupling of iodotyrosines. They have no effect on the underlying cause of disease, although there is recent evidence that propylthiouracil (PTU) treatment decreases thyroid-stimulating immunoglobulins. The drugs cross the placenta and inhibit fetal thyroid function and are also excreted in breast milk. Usually, some improvement in the degree of thyrotoxicosis is noted within the first 2 weeks of therapy, and a euthyroid state can be restored in 6 weeks. Treatment is generally regulated on a clinical basis, following the patient's weight and pulse. The T4 and/or T3 levels and FTI values are helpful in assessing treatment.

The majority of patients with Graves' disease are treated in the hope that a natural remission will occur after the patient is rendered euthyroid. In our experience, when individuals are treated for 6 months, and then the drugs are stopped, less than 40 percent have significant, long-lasting remissions. In most individuals thyrotoxicosis occurs again. This is especially true for those patients in whom a large goiter remains during treatment.

The drugs that are usually used in the United States are PTU and methimazole (Tapazole). Methimazole has a potency about ten times that of propylthiouracil, and therefore one-tenth the dose is required: 100 to 300 mg of propylthiouracil every 6 to 8 h or 10 to 40 mg of methimazole every 12 h. The side effects of drug therapy occur in 3 to 12 percent of patients and include skin rash, fever, peripheral neuritis, and polyarteritis. The serious complications of antithyroid drugs are agranulocytosis and aplastic anemia, which occur in less than 1 percent of the treated cases. When a significant reduction in the white blood cell count is noted, the drug should be stopped promptly, and the prognosis is good. Aplastic anemia is a much rarer complication, and the prognosis is poorer.

In order to be effective, the antithyroid pills must be taken every 6 to 8 h. Many of our patients are unreliable and do not take their medication faithfully. In such cases and in others in whom thyrotoxicosis recurs after the antithyroid drug is stopped, a definitive form of therapy—either radioactive iodine or surgery—is advised.

Radioactive Iodine. This represents the treatment of choice in many large series. The average dose for diffuse toxic goiter was 7 to 9 mC of ^{131}I and for toxic nodular goiter 12 to 15 mC. This is intended to deliver approximately 8500 rads to the thyroid. About 20 percent of patients treated in this manner with ^{131}I will require more than one dose. The advantages of radioactive therapy are the avoidance of a surgical procedure, with its attendant rare complications of recurrent nerve paralysis or hypoparathyroidism, and reduced cost. The major disadvantages of radioactive iodine treatment are the time required to gain control of the disease, the incidence of permanent myxedema, and the development of nodules. Remission rates ranging from 80 to 98 percent have been reported. In most series, the results have been less satisfactory for hyperthyroidism associated with nodular toxic goiter than with diffuse toxic goiter. Nofal et al. indicated a 70 percent incidence of hypothyroidism at the end of 10 years. The absence of a plateau in the slope of the curve suggests that hypothyroidism is a potentiality in almost 100 percent of the patients if they live long enough subsequent to therapy. Because of this very high incidence of progressive hypothyroidism, some groups have tried low-dosage radioiodine regimens. In several of the studies up to 50 percent required retreatment. It appears that hypothyroidism occurs even with these low-dose regimens.

It does not appear that thyroid cancer or bone leukemia is increased by this dose of radioiodine. Finally, the possibility of genetic abnormalities of the offspring following radioiodine treatment has been considered. This risk appears to be very minimal.

In the past, most centers restricted usage of radioiodine to women thirty-five years or older. Now there is a tendency to lower the age at which this agent is administered. Some even treat children with Graves' disease with radioiodine, although we do not favor this approach. Radioiodine must never be given to pregnant or lactating women because it crosses the placenta and is excreted in the milk and could ablate the fetal thyroid.

Preparation for Operation. Patients with active hyperthyroidism require preoperative preparation (Table 38-4). In mild cases of Graves' disease, iodine therapy alone can be utilized. In such instances a saturated solution of potassium iodide (SSKI) is given for several weeks in a dose of 5 drops, two or three times daily in orange juice. Usually, antithyroid drugs are used initially in order to establish a euthyroid state. Iodine is then added to the regimen 8 to 10 days prior to the operation, to decrease the vascularity of the gland. Sometimes thyroxine is added to this regimen to prevent hypothyroidism and to decrease the size of the gland. The beta-adrenergic blocker, propranolol, has added safety to the operation for Graves' disease. This drug decreases the pulse rate and the tremor of individuals with thyrotoxicosis, although they remain thyrotoxic. Some surgeons use 5 to 7 days of propranolol alone in preparation of Graves' patients for operation. Others use propranolol with iodine. We do not favor the use of propranolol alone or only with iodine for the routine preoperative preparation of our patients for it may not offer the same degree of safety as does the PTU and iodine regimen. Several cases of thyroid storm, fever, and tachycardia have been reported in patients who were taking propranolol. If used alone it is essential that propranolol be continued for several weeks after operation, for patients are still thyrotoxic immediately after operation.

Table 38-4. PREOPERATIVE TREATMENT REGIMENS FOR GRAVES' DISEASE

Iodine alone
PTU + iodine
PTU + thyroxine + iodine
PTU + propranolol + iodine
Propranolol + iodine
Propranolol alone

NOTE: Most of our patients are prepared for operation by the use of propylthiouracil (PTU) and iodine, with or without propranolol.

Results of Operation. The mortality rate associated with the procedure is extremely low. Gould et al. reported 1000 thyroidectomies for all causes with no deaths, while Colcock and King reported 1246 consecutive thyroidectomies with no mortality. In a collected review of major series, the mortality rate was less than 0.1 percent. Subtotal thyroidectomy provides rapid correction of the thyrotoxicotic state in over 95 percent of patients.

The incidence of complications varies with the series. Permanent recurrent laryngeal nerve paralysis has been reported in 0 to 3 percent of the cases. Damage to the parathyroid gland resulting in tetany has been reported in about 1 to 3 percent of patients subjected to thyroidectomy for thyrotoxicosis. In 10 to 30 percent of patients subjected to thyroidectomy for thyrotoxicosis, permanent hypothyroidism developed, while in 2 to 12 percent hyperthyroidism recurred. When hypothyroidism occurs following operation it usually is present within several years. The major advantages of surgical therapy are prompt control of disease and a lowered incidence of myxedema as compared with radioactive iodine therapy. Thyroidectomy also makes possible the simultaneous removal of any incidental papillary carcinomas. The patients usually leave the hospital 3 to 4 days postoperatively and resume work within 3 to 4 weeks.

Selection of Therapy. In young patients with Graves' disease and in others who are pregnant or lactating, antithyroid drug therapy is used initially. Radioactive iodine is usually employed in older patients. If prolonged drug therapy is required, or if recurrence of thyrotoxicosis follows the discontinuance of drugs, thyroidectomy or radioactive iodine is used. Subtotal thyroidectomy occasionally represents the treatment of choice in young adults with severe disease and large goiters or in patients in whom a rapid response is desirable. Radioactive iodine is the treatment of choice in some patients with toxic multinodular goiter, but in regions where goiter tends to be endemic, subtotal thyroidectomy may represent the procedure of choice. The preferable treatment for hyperfunctioning adenoma is surgical excision, especially in young individuals.

Hyperfunctioning thyroid tissue in the ovary should be treated by oophorectomy. Hyperfunctioning tissue within aberrant thyroid tissue, such as a lingual thyroid, may be treated by radioactive iodine or surgical excision. The uncommon situation of metastatic tumor with hyperfunctioning tissue is best treated by radioactive iodine.

TREATMENT OF EXOPHTHALMOS. The effects of treatment on the eye signs are variable. In general the eye disease appears to be independent of the treatment of the thyrotoxicosis. Lid retraction might lessen, however, following thyroidectomy. It is important to treat hypothyroidism if it occurs, since this appears to worsen the ophthalmopathy.

Severe exophthalmos is fortunately rare. The earliest signs and symptoms of development of the so-called malignant exophthalmos are increased lacrimation, venous congestion, and chemosis. Treatment is essentially symptomatic. The eyes should be protected against the wind and sun. The patients should sleep in a sitting position to reduce venous congestion. If chemosis is severe, tarsor-rhaphy to oppose the lids and prevent corneal ulceration may be indicated. Steroid eye drops or systemic steroids may offer benefit. External radiation to the retroorbital tissues is helpful, but cataract formation has occurred. In cases where the intraorbital pressure immediately threatens vision, surgical decompression of the orbit or its contents should be utilized.

Hypothyroidism

Hypothyroidism is the term applied to a failure of the thyroid gland to maintain an adequate plasma level of hormone. A brief discussion is included in this chapter for three reasons: (1) ablation of most of the thyroid by thyroidectomy or by radioactive iodine represents one of the causes of hypothyroidism, (2) some of the clinical manifestations of hypothyroidism mimic a variety of surgical diseases, and (3) a recognition of the hypothyroid state in the preoperative patient is important, since major surgical treatment in the grossly hypothyroid patient is associated with an increased mortality.

ETIOLOGY. Spontaneous hypothyroidism, or myxedema, may result from aplasia of the thyroid or replacement of the gland by nonfunctional goiter, adenoma, or thyroiditis. Rarely, hypothyroidism may be secondary to hypopituitarism. This is termed *pituitary myxedema.* Hypothyroidism following thyroidectomy or radioactive iodine therapy for hyperthyroidism accounts for about one-fourth of cases. Kocher recognized the importance of this disorder and referred to it as "cachexia strumipriva." In general, whenever most of the thyroid gland is resected, hypothyroidism will ensue unless thyroid hormone replacement is given. The occurrence is also related to the histologic state, being more common in patients with Hashimoto's disease and lymphadenoid changes. Autoantibodies against thyroid cytoplasm are frequently present in patients who become hypothyroid. The incidence varies inversely with the incidence of recurrent hyperthyroidism.

CLINICAL MANIFESTATIONS. Functional failure of the thyroid in the newborn is termed *cretinism.* This is not seen at birth because of the transplacental passage of hormone and becomes manifest later in infancy. Mental retardation is marked and frequently irreversible. Children demonstrate a poor growth pattern, are difficult to nurse, and present with a typical appearance that must be distinguished from mongolism and dwarfism. The remaining manifestations are similar to those which will be described below for adult hypothyroidism but are more pronounced.

Thyroid failure during childhood or adolescence is known as *juvenile hypothyroidism.* The child appears younger than his chronologic age. Intellectual performance is poor, but severe mental deficiency is not present. In children, abdominal distention, umbilical hernia, and prolapse of the rectum are all common.

Spontaneous hypothyroidism in the adult is frequently a manifestation of lymphocytic thyroiditis. Eighty percent of adults with spontaneous hypothyroidism are fe-

male. Both spontaneous hypothyroidism and hypothyroidism that follows ablative procedures on the thyroid gland have an insidiously progressive course in the adult, with protean manifestations. In mild cases, only tiredness and weight gain may be present. In severe cases there is increasing fatigue and apathy. Mental and physical processes are generally slowed. Intellectual function and speech may be impaired. Headaches occur frequently and dementia may develop. Weight gain is a characteristic feature. The skin becomes dry, thickened and puffy; the nonpitting bogginess of the skin is most apparent around the eyes, hands, and feet. The hair becomes dry and brittle, and tends to fall out. The tongue is enlarged and tends to fill the mouth, and the voice is hoarse. Muscle cramps are common and represent one of the early symptoms of hypothyroidism following ablative therapy.

The cardiovascular manifestations are related to a reduced cardiac output and hemodynamic alterations that resemble those of congestive heart failure. There is widening of cardiac dullness due to dilatation of the heart or pericardial effusion, and the heart sounds are distant. The resting pulse is slow, and at times the blood pressure is elevated to hypertensive levels. As the disease progresses, shortness of breath and pulmonary effusions become more common.

Abdominal symptoms may represent the outstanding complaint. Most frequently, these consist of constipation and changes in bowel habits. Abdominal distention due to intraintestinal gases or ascites may be present. When pain is present, it is generally of a dull, nonperistaltic character and occasionally colicky. Achlorhydria occurs in about half the patients. Pernicious anemia may be present in 12 percent of the cases.

In women, diminished libido, failure of ovulation, and menorrhagia may occur, and in men there may be decreased libido, impotency, and oligospermia.

DIAGNOSTIC FINDINGS. The hemogram may demonstrate anemia. The electrocardiogram is characterized by sinus bradycardia, diminished voltage, and inverted or flattened T waves; the electroencephalogram shows slow alpha activity and loss of amplitude. The tests of thyroidal function demonstrate decreased serum T4, T3, and FTI values; circulating TSH level is elevated, and the serum cholesterol is frequently in excess of 300 mg/dL.

TREATMENT. Treatment of adult hypothyroidism is extremely effective and is directed at producing a normal metabolic state. L-Thyroxine is most often used, and effectiveness of treatment can be ascertained by measurement of serum T4, FTI, or TSH levels. The approximate equivalence of biologic potency for the commonly used medications is 60 mg of thyroid extract = 100 μg of L-thyroxine = 25 μg of L-triiodothyronine.

The untreated patient with severe hypothyroidism is sensitive to small doses, and therefore caution is exercised in initiating replacement therapy. Treatment may be begun with L-thyroxine 50 μg once daily, and within several weeks this can be increased to 100 μg. The replacement therapy is augmented slowly to avoid cardiac problems related to an increased demand on the myocardium.

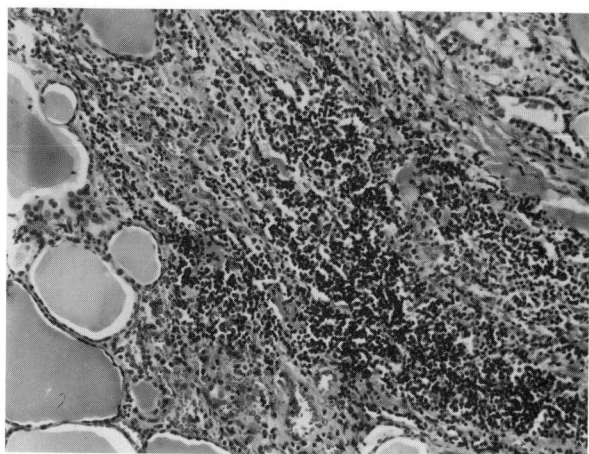

Fig. 38-12. Acute thyroiditis. Note infiltration of inflammatory cells.

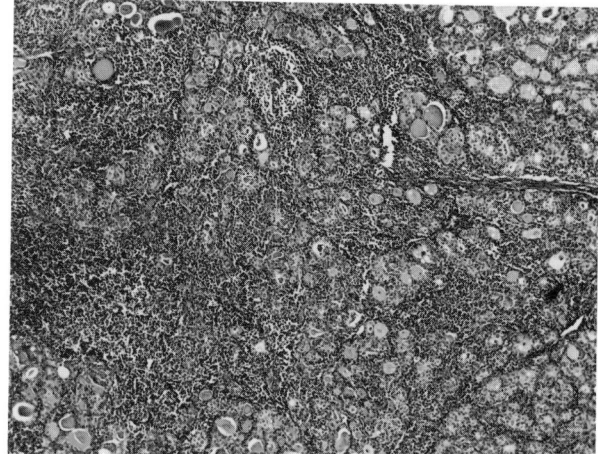

Fig. 38-13. Hashimoto's disease.

Thyroiditis

Inflammatory processes of the thyroid may be acute or chronic. Acute thyroiditis is further subdivided into the suppurative and nonsuppurative varieties. Chronic thyroiditis includes Hashimoto's disease, granulomatous (giant cell) thyroiditis, and Riedel's thyroiditis.

ACUTE SUPPURATIVE THYROIDITIS

Acute suppurative thyroiditis (Fig. 38-12) is the most uncommon form of thyroiditis. Acute suppurative thyroiditis, with abscess formation, almost invariably follows an acute upper respiratory tract infection. The disease is characterized by the sudden onset of severe pain in the thyroid and anterior neck, accompanied by dysphagia, fever, and chills. The suppurative process usually remains unilateral, but there may be extension into the deep spaces of the neck with invasion of the trachea and/or esophagus, or tracking into the chest. Treatment consists of drainage of the abscess. There is no persistent effect on thyroid function.

HASHIMOTO'S DISEASE (LYMPHADENOID GOITER)

Hashimoto's disease, or chronic lymphocytic thyroiditis, is the most common form of chronic thyroiditis, and the incidence apparently has been increasing. The disease occurs at least five to ten times more frequently than subacute thyroiditis.

ETIOLOGY. Hashimoto's disease is an autoimmune process in which the thyroid gland appears to be sensitive to its own thyroglobulin and cell constituents. In 1957, Doniach and Roitt first discovered antithyroid antibodies in the serum of most patients with this disease. Several of these antimicrosomal (MCHA) and antithyroglobulin (TGHA) antibodies can be measured in the patients' serum. Cell-mediated immunity may also play a role in the etiology of Hashimoto's disease. There is some evidence of genetic predisposition. Members of the families of patients with this disease have an increased incidence of Hashimoto's disease, goiter, spontaneous hypothyroidism, and thyrotoxicosis.

A statistically significant relationship has been demonstrated for the coexistence of papillary carcinoma of the thyroid and areas of lymphocytic involvement. The data of Hirabayashi and Lindsay suggest that these changes occur secondarily with papillary carcinoma and that there is a possibility that antigens from the neoplasm may be implicated in the formation of this localized form of thyroiditis.

PATHOLOGY. The thyroid is often symmetrically enlarged, pale, and semifirm. The enlargement, however, may be asymmetric, and the nodularity and firmness suggest colloid goiter and, at times, carcinoma. The disease is focal in the beginning but extends to involve one or both lobes and the isthmus. Lymphoid tissue predominates (Fig. 38-13). There is disruption of epithelial cells with degeneration and fragmentation of the follicular basement membrane. The remaining epithelial cells are larger and demonstrate oxyphilic changes (Askanazy cells). The lymphocytic infiltration may be focal or diffuse, and as the disease progresses, the thyroid tissue may degenerate or be replaced by fibrous tissue.

CLINICAL MANIFESTATIONS. The overwhelming majority of patients are women, and the disease occurs at an average age of fifty years. The most frequent complaints are enlargement of the neck with pain and tenderness in the region of the thyroid. There may be associated difficulty in breathing and swallowing caused by compression of the trachea and esophagus. Shortness of breath, increasing fatigue, and increase in weight are related to a hypothyroid state when this is present. Most individuals are euthyroid or hypothyroid when Hashimoto's thyroiditis is diagnosed. Recently, transient thyrotoxicosis has also been described. Palpation generally reveals a diffusely enlarged gland, and enlargement of the pyramidal lobe is common. In about 20 percent of cases, the gland is nodular rather than diffusely enlarged.

Several investigators have indicated an increased incidence of autoimmune diseases such as rheumatic fever and rheumatoid arthritis, disseminated lupus, hemolytic anemia, purpura, myasthenia gravis, and pernicious anemia in these patients. On occasion Hashimoto's disease is part of a generalized endocrine organ failure syndrome that may include idiopathic Addison's disease, diabetes mellitus, and ovarian or testicular insufficiency.

DIAGNOSTIC FINDINGS. Early in the course of the disease, tests of thyroidal function occasionally indicate thyroidal hyperfunction. As the disease progresses, the T4, T3, and FTI values reach subnormal levels. The RAIU uptake is usually low. In a majority of patients, however, tests of thyroidal function and clinical manifestations suggest a euthyroid state. Diagnosis is confirmed by demonstrating high titers of thyroid antibodies in the serum. Large-needle biopsy or needle aspiration with cytologic examination may be indicated in the case of asymmetric and nodular glands, to rule out the diagnosis of carcinoma.

TREATMENT. There is almost universal agreement that if the thyroid is symmetric and nonnodular and if there are no symptoms of compression, the patient should be managed with suppressive doses of thyroid hormone if there is evidence of a goiter. In the absence of a goiter and a euthyroid state, no therapy is necessary. Surgical intervention is indicated only if there are marked pressure symptoms, such as difficulty in swallowing, for suspected malignant tumor, and for cosmetic reasons, in the case of an extremely enlarged gland. The surgical procedure usually performed consists of subtotal thyroidectomy with clearing of the trachea. The treatment of a nodular form of Hashimoto's disease is controversial. Most writers prefer the use of suppressive hormone if carcinoma can be ruled out. If carcinoma is suspected, a lobectomy should be performed. Most carcinomas associated with Hashimoto's disease are of the papillary type. If a carcinoma is proved on frozen section, a near-total or total thyroidectomy should be performed. Suppressive therapy with thyroid hormone should be continued postoperatively.

SUBACUTE THYROIDITIS

In 1904, de Quervain described the pathology of subacute thyroiditis and reviewed the literature. Many synonyms, including granulomatous (giant cell), epidemic, and de Quervain's thyroiditis, have confused the diagnosis. In 1948, Crile clearly established subacute thyroiditis as an entity separate from Hashimoto's thyroiditis and Riedel's struma.

The disease occurs widely in over half of the United States but infrequently along the eastern seaboard, in England, and in Japan. The age of onset ranges from three to seventy-six, with a mean in the forties. Females outnumber males in every series, the proportion varying between 60 and 100 percent. Subacute thyroiditis is generally not felt to be of viral or autoimmune origin.

The gland is usually adherent to surrounding tissues but, unlike Riedel's struma, can be dissected free without difficulty. There is enlargement of the follicles with infiltration by large mononuclear cells, lymphocytes, and neutrophils. Giant cells of the epithelioid foreign body type containing many nuclei characterize the lesion.

Volpé et al. classified subacute thyroiditis into four stages:

Stage I—acute toxicity with a painful, swollen gland and thyrotoxic symptoms lasting 1 to 2 months.
Stage II—the transition or euthyroid stage with an enlarged, hard, nontender gland. The BMR is normal, but the sedimentation rate is still elevated.
Stage III—the compensation or hypothyroid phase, occurring 2 to 4 months after onset.
Stage IV—remission or recovery, which may occur in 1 to 6 months.

Almost all patients manifest thyroid swelling and pain that may radiate to parts of the head, neck, or anterior chest. The onset is usually sudden. About two-thirds of patients are febrile, and fatigue, weakness, malaise, menstrual irregularities, and weight loss are characteristic. White blood cell counts usually are normal, but the erythrocyte sedimentation rate (ESR) is almost always elevated during the first month. In the acute stage there is a characteristically low ^{131}I uptake. Needle biopsy or needle aspiration may aid in establishing the diagnosis.

ACTH and corticosteroids effectively relieve the symptoms but do not alter the disease. Therapy should be initiated with 40 mg of prednisone daily, tapering the drug over 1 to 2 months. Salicylates and thyroid hormone replacement have provided successful therapy.

RIEDEL'S (STRUMA) THYROIDITIS

Riedel's thyroiditis is a rare chronic inflammatory process involving one or both lobes of the thyroid, frequently extending to the surrounding fascia, trachea, muscles, nerves, and blood vessels. It is thought by some to be a terminal stage of Hashimoto's disease or granulomatous thyroiditis.

Microscopically, the follicles are small and few in number, and a dense fibrous tissue penetrates the gland (Fig. 38-14). There may be firm attachment to the trachea by scar tissue, resulting in constriction and narrowing of the tracheal lumen.

Fig. 38-14. Riedel's thyroiditis.

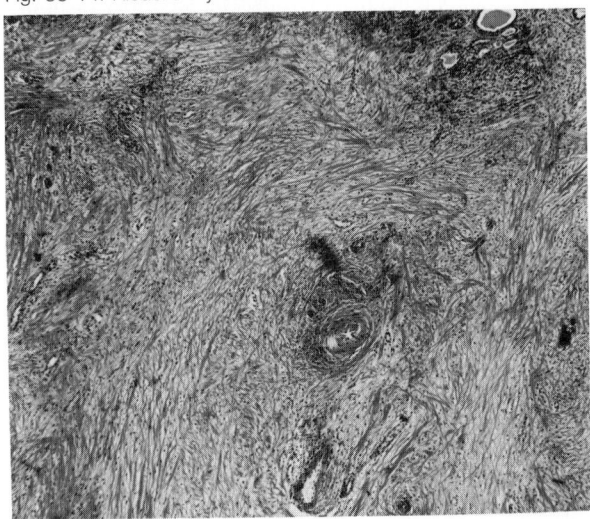

When involvement is unilateral, the disease is clinically indistinguishable from carcinoma. The disease occurs more frequently in women but not to the same extent as Hashimoto's disease. The average age of patients is about fifty. Symptoms are generally due to compression of the trachea, esophagus, and recurrent laryngeal nerve. Consequently, there is difficulty in swallowing and hoarseness. In advanced disease tests of thyroidal function may indicate hypothyroidism. Some patients have circulating thyroid autoantibodies, but this occurs less frequently and in lower titers than in patients with Hashimoto's disease.

Treatment consists of thyroid hormones. Surgical intervention is justified to relieve symptoms of tracheal or esophageal constriction. The operation may be dangerous, resulting in damage to the trachea, carotid sheath, or recurrent laryngeal nerve. When only one lobe is involved, unilateral lobectomy and isthmusectomy are indicated. When there is bilateral involvement, it has been recommended to remove the isthmus and as much of each lobe as possible. The prethyroid muscles are sutured to the lateral wall of the trachea to cover the severed ends of the lobe and prevent fibrous thyroid tissue from uniting. The medial borders of the "strap" muscles are then sutured together to prevent the trachea from becoming adherent to the skin.

Goiter

The term *goiter* is derived from the French word *goitre,* which in turn comes from the Latin *guttur,* meaning "throat." In general, the term is applied to benign enlargement of the thyroid gland.

ETIOLOGY. The development of a goiter may be related to a variety of factors, including inherited enzyme defects and extrinsic causes, or it may be idiopathic. Goiters associated with thyrotoxicosis, thyroiditis, and benign and malignant neoplasms are excluded from this discussion.

Familial Goiter. Goiters caused by inherited enzyme defects are usually associated with hypothyroidism, but many patients remain euthyroid. The inborn error in metabolism is generally inherited as an autosomal recessive trait, but inheritance as a dominant characteristic also has been reported. The metabolic defect may impair iodine accumulation, organification, coupling of iodotyrosine, or it may be related to a disorder affecting the serum iodoprotein.

Endemic Goiter. Endemic goiter is defined as thyroid enlargement affecting a significant number of inhabitants of a particular locale. Most major countries have goiter belts. In the United States, the prevalent regions used to be in mountainous areas, the upper northwest, and around the Great Lakes. The extrinsic factors implicated in the etiology include iodine deficiency and the ingestion of goitrogens. Genetic factors may play a contributory role. Iodine deficiency is particularly important, and in the endemic areas the iodine content of the drinking water is extremely low. The administration of iodine as prophylaxis prevents endemic goiter, and the preferable method

has been iodination of table salt. Today in the United States it is difficult to be iodine-deficient because table salt and most breads contain large amounts of iodine. Excess iodide given to patients with endemic goiter may lead to thyrotoxicosis, a condition known as Jodbasedow disease. Experiments in animals have demonstrated a goitrogenic property of yellow turnips, cabbage, kale, and other vegetables. However, the final proof implicating the goitrogenic factors in the etiology of endemic goiter in human beings is still lacking.

Sporadic Goiter. This term is applied to an enlargement of the thyroid for which a definite cause cannot be established. The diagnosis is one of exclusion in which thyroiditis and tumor and the possibility of endemic goiter are ruled out. Hypersecretion of TSH may lead to stimulation of glandular growth and morphologic changes.

PATHOLOGY. The thyroid gland may be diffusely enlarged and smooth, or it may be grossly nodular. In the early stages of development, the gland is hyperplastic. The hyperplastic state may be reversed by the ingestion of iodine. Subsequently, involution occurs forming enlarged follicles filled with colloid.

The nontoxic nodular goiter is grossly a multinodular structure in which the nodules vary in number and size. There is also variation in the histology, from nonfollicular areas to gelatinous colloid-rich nodules. Scattered between the nodules are areas of normal thyroid tissue. There may be gross or microscopic evidence of degeneration of the nodules with cyst formation, recent or old hemorrhage, or calcification.

CLINICAL MANIFESTATIONS. In totally goitrous endemic regions, there is no difference in incidence related to sex. However, as one proceeds to areas diminishing in intensity, the ratio of females to males increasingly rises until the ratio is 8:1. The age incidence varies with the amount of iodine available in the diet. In women, an increase in size may be noted during pregnancy with reduction in size after delivery to the antepartum level.

Most patients with goiter are asymptomatic. The manifestations of hospitalized patients are related to the physical effects of the goiter, associated symptoms, or psychologic effects.

The most common symptom related to the thyroid gland itself is an awareness of increasing size of the neck or the presence of a mass. Pressure effects may cause embarrassment of the respiration with tracheal compression or dysphagia due to pressure on the esophagus. The tracheal compression is frequently associated with a goiter extending into the thorax. Distention of the jugular veins in these cases is indicative of impedance of return of blood. Paralysis of the recurrent laryngeal nerve rarely is due to stretching across the surface of an expanding goiter and is more frequently related to a malignant tumor. Horner's syndrome is more suggestive of involvement by a neoplastic lesion. The patients may experience sudden pain in the neck associated with a rapid increase in size. This is generally related to hemorrhage into part of the goiter, either a cyst or a degenerating lesion.

The characteristic physical finding associated with an enlarged thyroid is a palpable mass that moves on swallowing. An enlarged thyroid in a patient who is euthyroid generally is softer than the gland in a patient with Graves' disease.

The history of a goiter and hypothyroidism that is manifest at birth or in childhood is evidence that some kind of inherited defect is present. If the patient has been deaf since birth and goitrous since infancy or middle childhood, the diagnosis of a genetic entity known as *Pendred's syndrome* can be made. In this group of patients, the audiogram reveals a characteristic loss of hearing for high tones in those who are not totally deaf, and the diagnosis is confirmed by showing that perchlorate will result in a discharge of the radioiodine accumulated within the thyroid during the first few hours after administration.

One-third of patients with endemic cretinism have appreciable enlargement of the thyroid gland. Some children are born with marked enlargement. Endemic cretins are usually not deaf-mute but are more likely to suffer from neurologic disorders causing spasticity.

Simple and nontoxic nodular goiters rarely progress to hypothyroidism. By contrast, thyrotoxicosis develops in a large percentage of patients with a long-standing history of goiter (toxic nodular goiter). In the series at the Mayo Clinic, 60 percent of patients with nodular goiter over the age of sixty were thyrotoxic. The average duration of goiter before the onset of thyrotoxicosis was 17 years. As indicated in the discussion of thyrotoxicosis, congestive heart failure and atrial fibrillation may dominate the picture.

DIAGNOSTIC FINDINGS. A radiogram of the chest and neck is important to visualize the trachea in order to establish its position and the diameter of the lumen. The study will also reveal whether the goiter has extended into the thorax. Barium swallowing is indicated only if the patient has dysphagia. In most patients with simple or endemic goiter, the T4, T3, and FTI values are normal.

TREATMENT. Diffuse (Nonnodular) Goiter. Goiters caused by inherited enzyme defects characteristically respond well to the administration of thyroxine. The drug eliminates hypothyroidism, if present, and diminishes the size of the gland by depressing TSH stimulation.

Treatment of drug-induced goiter requires the discontinuance of the offending drug, if possible. If continued drug therapy, such as para-aminosalicylic acid for tuberculosis, is required, thyroxine should be administered. Occasionally goiters in newborn children can be attributed to drugs taken by the mother during pregnancy. The enlargement disappears spontaneously during the first months of life. Endemic goiter is prevented by the administration of iodine. When endemic goiter is present, iodine therapy or thyroxine in replacement doses may result in a dramatic decrease in size. This is particularly true of the diffusely enlarged, nonnodular gland.

Low-lying goiters, intrathoracic goiters, and goiters that encircle the trachea are most likely to produce symptoms of respiratory obstruction. The rare circumstance of tracheal obstruction caused by congenital goiter in the newborn is best treated by resection of the thyroid isthmus rather than tracheostomy. Hemorrhage or rapid development of an intrathyroidal cyst may cause pain and an alarming mass. Crile has reported 50 patients treated with aspiration followed by administration of desiccated thyroid. There were only three failures. Others prefer surgical excision of the cyst and a rim of surrounding tissue. Surgical procedures for cosmesis must be individualized, but it is to be emphasized that partial thyroidectomy further restricts the ability of the gland to meet hormonal requirements. Therefore, whenever a significant segment of goiter is removed, supplemental hormone therapy is indicated.

Multinodular Goiter. The results achieved by suppressive therapy of thyroxine are variable. Astwood and associates noted reduction in size of multinodular goiters in over 50 percent of their cases, whereas most other investigators report favorable effects in less than one-quarter of the patients. The indications for operation, which have been considered in the treatment of nonnodular goiter, pertain to the nodular gland. The major argument concerning the management of the nodular thyroid is related to the likelihood that carcinoma is present within the gland.

Nodules

It is estimated that 4 percent of the population of the United States have thyroid nodules that are clinically palpable. The incidence of thyroid cancer, on the other hand, is 40 to 50 cases per million population per year, and deaths from thyroid cancer occur with an incidence of about 6 cases per million population per year. In the United States, about 1200 people die from thyroid cancer every year. This disease ranks thirty-fifth among deaths from cancers. However, cancer of the thyroid is much more important than its ranking indicates because of its morbidity and the difficulty in differentiating benign from malignant thyroid nodules.

HIGH-RISK GROUPS FOR CANCER. There are two groups of individuals who are at high risk for having carcinoma of the thyroid if a single nodule or multiple nodules of the thyroid gland are felt: (1) individuals who have been exposed to low-dose radiation to their head and neck regions, and (2) those in whom another family member has medullary carcinoma of the thyroid. The latter individuals are at great risk, since the familial medullary carcinoma syndrome is transmitted as an autosomal dominant trait and thus 50 percent of the offspring would be expected to have this disease. These groups will be discussed in greater detail.

Irradiation to the Head and Neck. Since the early 1950s it has been recognized that individuals exposed to *low-dose* irradiation to the head and neck have a much greater chance of having both benign and malignant nodules of the thyroid gland and elsewhere. It has been shown that as little as 6.5 rads of external irradiation to the thyroid bed leads to a statistically increased incidence of thyroid cancer many years later. This is especially significant when one considers that the unshielded thyroid gland receives up to 3.5 rads of exposure from a single panoramic film of the jaw and teeth.

It has now been demonstrated that there is a straight-line increase in the incidence of both benign and malignant thyroid nodules up to a dose of about 1500 rads, but only after a mean latency period of 25 years or longer. We have found new nodules of the thyroid that proved to be cancers even 40 to 50 years after exposure. In a recent group of unselected individuals with a known history of low-dose neck irradiation, Refetoff and associates reported that 25 percent had a palpable abnormality of the thyroid gland, and 6.8 percent of the total group were found to have thyroid cancer. Radiation treatment in these subjects was used for different purposes:

1. Enlarged thymus, in order to prevent "sudden crib death" which was thought to result from tracheal compression, from the large thymus. These infants received about 150 rads to their upper mediastinum.
2. Tonsils and adenoids, in order to prevent the need for tonsilectomy. These children, four to eight years of age, received up to 750 rads to the neck area.
3. Acne. These teenagers or young adults received up to 1500 rads to their face. Many others were irradiated for hemangiomas, scrofula, or other miscellaneous reasons.

Fortunately, the thyroid cancer that is associated with external irradiation exposure usually is the papillary type, which has an excellent prognosis, particularly in young adults. The cancer is sometimes small and is found along with benign nodules in the same gland. This has led some to discount these lesions as unimportant. In our series, however, they are equal in size to other papillary cancers found in patients without radiation exposure and more often show multicentric involvement within the thyroid gland and lymph node metastases. In our experience thyroid nodules were malignant in 14 percent of patients without a history of neck irradiation. When a history of irradiation was obtained, close to 40 percent of individuals who were operated upon had carcinoma within the gland.

Low-dose radiation exposure has also been associated with an increased incidence of basal and squamous cell skin cancers, benign and malignant brain and salivary gland tumors, and breast cancer. Even parathyroid adenomas appear to occur with greater frequency in those with previous external neck irradiation.

High-dose external irradiation, defined as greater than 2000 rads, was thought to be without risk to the thyroid. Recently, however, it has been shown that patients who received mantle irradiation for Hodgkin's disease and received 5000 rads to their thyroid glands have a higher prevalence of thyroid cancer than normal. This group also deserves special follow-up procedures.

The risk of exposure to the thyroid from radioisotopes is less clear, but radiation fallout has been implicated. A group of natives who accidentally received a high amount of radiation from nuclear fallout following an atomic bomb test at Bikini atoll in 1954 continues to have an increased prevalence of benign (39.6 percent) and malignant (5.7 percent) lesions. As a preventive action, many hospitals now use ^{123}I and ^{99m}Tc instead of ^{131}I for scanning, since the thyroid exposure is greatly diminished (see Table 38-2).

DIAGNOSTIC TESTS TO DIFFERENTIATE BENIGN AND MALIGNANT LESIONS. It is important to take a careful *history* and to conduct a complete *physical examination*. A history of low-dose irradiation to the neck is, perhaps, the most important fact that can be obtained. Recent onset of the nodule or rapid and painless growth also increases the suspicion of malignancy. On physical examination most cancers are felt to be hard and irregular lumps. Enlarged, abnormal lymph nodes in the lateral neck or adjacent to the thyroid strongly suggest malignancy, as do fixation of the gland, vocal cord paralysis, and a Horner's syndrome.

Thyroid function tests are not very useful as diagnostic tests since most patients with thyroid cancer are euthyroid. In the presence of hyperthyroidism, a nodule is less likely to be a cancer. *Radioactive scans* can be helpful. Most cancers of the thyroid appear to be "cold" on thyroid scan; however, so do most of the benign lesions. Thus, carcinomas are found in only a fraction of all cold nodules. *B-mode ultrasound* can be used to differentiate solid from cystic lesions. Since most cancers are solid, this can be helpful. Most cystic lesions are benign. However, some papillary cancers are also cystic. Finally, *needle biopsy* of the thyroid is helpful. Large-needle biopsy utilizing a Vim-Silverman or a Trucut needle yields a core of tissue that can be examined microscopically. More recently, cytologic evaluation of the aspirate of a nodule obtained by an 18- to 22-gauge needle is gaining greater usage. While these techniques are helpful, it should be pointed out that false-negative results have been obtained with the use of both core needle biopsies and needle aspiration cytology. False-positive results are rare, however. Needle aspiration with cytology can eliminate the need for operation of many colloid nodules. Papillary carcinoma of the thyroid is readily diagnosed as well. However, the differentiation of a follicular adenoma from a follicular carcinoma is difficult, since the capsule is not examined. Highly cellular follicular aspirates should therefore be placed in a "suspicious" category. The results of the Karolinska Hospital group are shown in Fig. 38-15.

In summary, of greatest concern are thyroid nodules that are solitary, recent in origin, found in young individuals or men of any age, and are cold on scan and solid on ultrasound. A prior history of low-dose irradiation to the head or neck should alert one to the fact that a cancer of the thyroid is likely even if the gland is multinodular. Finally, a definitive diagnosis of cancer can often be made preoperatively by needle aspiration of the nodule with cytologic evaluation.

THERAPEUTIC APPROACH. One diagnostic scheme utilized by many clinicians is shown in Fig. 38-16. Thyroid nodules are separated by scan into those that are "warm" or "hot" and others that are "cold." Warm or hot lesions on scan are less likely to represent carcinoma and thus might be observed or operated upon according to the evaluation of risk as assessed by the clinician. Cold nodules are more suspicious. If *cystic,* these are usually aspirated of their fluid. If a mass is no longer felt after aspiration, the nodule can be followed, for it is almost certainly

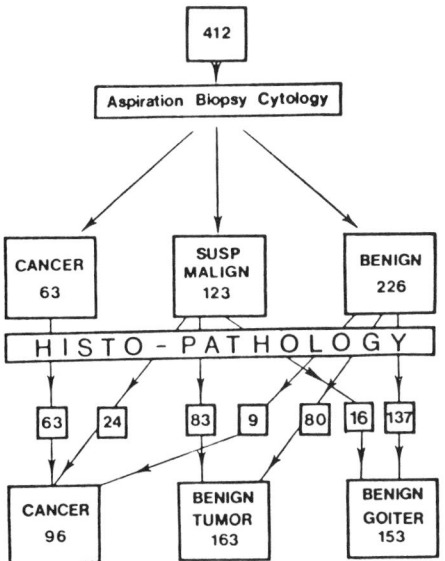

Fig. 38-15. Comparison of results obtained by aspiration biopsy and cytologic examination (ABC) versus thyroidectomy. (From: *Löwhagen T et al: Surg Clin North Am 59:3, 1979, with permission.*)

benign. Usually the fluid reaccumulates within several weeks of each aspiration; however, tetracycline injection may "cure" many cysts. If a lesion *cold* on scan is *solid* on ultrasound, this is a more suspicious group. These are either operated upon if clinically warranted, or occasionally suppressed with thyroxine. However, we are using needle aspiration with cytologic examination more and more in this group and have been pleased with the results.

Other groups have bypassed the use of ultrasound and isotope scanning for the most part, and rely primarily on the assessment of the nodule by aspiration cytology. Those lesions which are not operated upon must be followed clinically for evidence of change. Repeat aspiration biopsies should also be obtained if they are warranted.

The above criteria apply to those individuals without a history of irradiation to the head and neck. We believe that most patients with a history of radiation exposure who are found to have a single or multiple nodules should be operated upon.

Fig. 38-16. Diagnostic approaches to the solitary nodule. (*Courtesy of Orlo Clark.*)

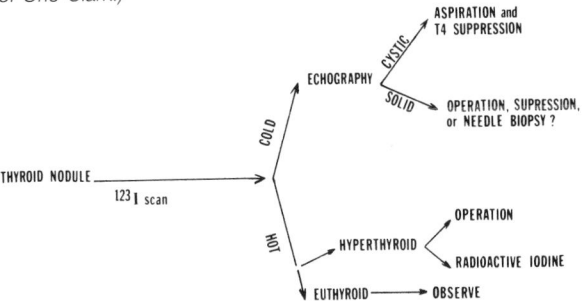

Benign Tumors

Benign adenomas of the thyroid are classified as embryonal, fetal, follicular, or microfollicular, according to their predominant histologic pattern. Grossly, the lesions are enveloped by a discrete capsule surrounded by a thin zone of compressed thyroid tissue. Microscopically, the architecture is orderly, mitoses are rare, and there is no lymphatic or blood vessel invasion. Several series have indicated that about 80 percent of surgical specimens that proved to contain a solitary nodule are benign tumors, while 20 percent are malignant growths.

CLINICAL MANIFESTATIONS. Patients usually present with a history of a slowly growing mass that must reach the size of 1 cm to be palpable. The lesions are rarely symptomatic. Bleeding into the mass is manifested by sudden onset of localized pain and a rapid increase in size. There is no evidence of cervical node involvement. Isotope scan may indicate concentration of iodine equal to, greater than, or less than normal thyroid tissue.

TREATMENT. Although some authors report treatment of solitary nodules with thyroid hormone, the majority have had no success with this approach. When malignancy cannot be ruled out, excisional biopsy is indicated. Usually a lobectomy and removal of the isthmus is performed if the lesion is at all suspicious. The specimen is submitted for frozen section analysis while the patient is asleep. If found to be benign, no further removal of thyroid tissue is necessary. The postoperative mortality approaches zero; the hospitalization is 3 to 4 days, and the postoperative morbidity is extremely low. After operation we prefer to treat most individuals with benign lesions with replacement doses of L-thyroxine, since this therapy appears to reduce the number of recurrent nodules.

Malignant Tumors

PATHOLOGY. The four major classes of thyroid cancers are (1) papillary, (2) follicular, (3) medullary, and (4) anaplastic. In addition, the thyroid may be involved with lymphosarcoma and metastatic carcinoma. The different types of thyroid carcinoma should be thought of as different diseases, which may have different etiologies, routes of spread, general virulence, and treatment requirements.

PAPILLARY CARCINOMA

Papillary and follicular carcinomas are referred to as *differentiated thyroid cancers*. They are derived from the thyroid epithelial cells. Papillary carcinoma is the most common of the malignant tumors of the thyroid, making up about two-thirds of all thyroid carcinomas. It accounts for approximately half the thyroid malignant tumors in adults and three-quarters of those in children. Over 90 percent of the radiation-induced carcinomas are papillary. Over half the cases are clinically manifest before the age of forty, with a peak incidence in the third and fourth decades. The tumors occur three times more frequently in females than in males.

PATHOLOGY. Papillary carcinoma is composed of columnar thyroidal epithelium arranged in papillary projections with connective tissue and vascular stalks. The nuclei have a characteristic vesicular appearance. The tumor may contain localized deposits of calcium arranged in concentric layers (psammoma bodies). Papillary carcinomas in this classification often contain both papillary and follicular elements.

Papillary carcinoma is the most slowly growing of the malignant tumors of the thyroid and has a tendency to become more malignant with advancing age. It has been suggested that anaplastic carcinoma may develop from a preexisting low-grade papillary carcinoma. There is some evidence that the growth of papillary carcinoma is dependent on TSH stimulation. Spread of the lesion is usually intraglandular and to pericapsular regional lymph nodes or lateral neck nodes. The so-called lateral aberrant thyroid rest is almost always papillary carcinoma that has replaced a lymph node. *Occult papillary carcinoma* refers to primary lesions less than 1.5 cm in diameter. *Minimal papillary carcinoma* refers to papillary carcinoma less than 1 cm in diameter. Within the thyroid gland itself, the tumor is found to be multicentric in up to 80 percent of cases if the gland is carefully examined. Although the carcinoma may persist in the neck for decades without further spread, distant metastases to the lungs and bones may occur. These may accumulate radioiodine, particularly if there is a follicular element. Thus, after total thyroidectomy has been performed, these can usually be treated with radioiodine therapy.

CLINICAL MANIFESTATIONS. The lesion usually presents as an asymptomatic nodule within the thyroid gland or as enlargement of the regional lymph nodes. Fixation of the thyroid, manifestations of pressure on adjacent structures, and distant metastases all occur late. A radiogram of the neck may reveal calcium flecks suggesting psammoma bodies. Isotope scan of the palpable nodule frequently demonstrates a lack of iodine uptake, and an ultrasonic scan usually suggests a solid lesion. A needle aspiration is usually diagnostic.

TREATMENT. All agree that the treatment of choice for contained lesions is surgical excision, but debate centers around the extent of resection. Some favor lobectomy; however, we and others feel that more radical surgical treatment is indicated if it can be safely done.

In *nonirradiated* patients, our approach is to excise the mass completely and widely, which almost always means performing a lobectomy; we then await the frozen section diagnosis while the patient is asleep. If the lesion is interpreted to be benign, no further resection of the thyroid is performed. If the tissue examined is clearly malignant and is other than a small sclerosing carcinoma, a near-total (or total) thyroidectomy is performed. In addition, any abnormal lymph nodes that are present in the tracheoesophageal groove or in the superior mediastinal areas are removed. If present, lymph nodes from the lateral neck that feel abnormal are biopsied. In general, a lymph-node biopsy is also taken from along the jugular chain for staging purposes, even if abnormal lymph nodes are not palpable. A modified radical neck dissection is performed only if

lateral nodes are found to be involved with tumor. A prophylactic lateral neck dissection should not be performed. A modified neck dissection might require dividing the sternocleidomastoid muscle, removing the nodes en bloc, and then reattaching it in men with large musculature. In women this is rarely necessary. The spinal accessory nerve is always preserved, and the internal jugular vein is also saved if nodes are not adherent to it. This procedure is quite satisfactory for thyroid cancer and creates a more favorable cosmetic result than does a classic radical neck dissection, especially if a transverse incision is made. We do not favor the so-called cherry picking operations where individual enlarged lymph nodes are removed.

In *irradiated patients* our overall operative approach is somewhat different. Here, for benign nodules a lobectomy is performed ipsilaterally and a contralateral subtotal thyroidectomy is usually done. If a carcinoma is diagnosed, generally, a near-total thyroidectomy or a total thyroidectomy is performed. The parathyroid glands can usually be left in situ. A parathyroid is transplanted only if it appears to be clearly devitalized and following histological confirmation of its identity. The recurrent laryngeal nerves are each identified, treated with care, and carefully preserved. A modified neck dissection is performed when indicated, as described for the nonirradiated patients.

We base this operative approach for the patient with papillary cancer first and foremost on the fact that such operations can be performed with no mortality and a very low morbidity. Papillary carcinoma has such an excellent prognosis that unless one can perform a near-total or total thyroidectomy with a very low morbidity, these procedures should not be attempted. Removal of most or all of the thyroid gland offers the following advantages:

1. Multicentricity of microscopic papillary tumor is present in up to 80 percent of cases, especially those with a history of radiation exposure. In approximately 7 to 10 percent of patients with an initial lesser procedure, clinical cancer of the remaining lobe develops. Often this portends widespread dissemination.
2. A fourth to a half of patients who die of thyroid cancer do so because of central neck disease.
3. Follow-up with isotope scans for metastases or treatment with radioiodine for disseminated disease is facilitated if the total thyroid, or most of it, has been removed.
4. The use of serum thyroglobulin levels as a tumor marker is facilitated. After total thyroidectomy the presence of measurable thyroglobulin indicates that metastatic disease is present.

Following thyroidectomy all individuals with papillary or follicular carcinoma should be placed on suppressive doses of thyroid hormone for life, whether or not the entire thyroid has been removed. Other ancillary modes of treatment, such as radioactive iodine, external irradiation, and chemotherapy, will be discussed later in this chapter.

PROGNOSIS. The prognosis for long-term survival of patients with papillary carcinoma is excellent. The prognosis is definitely worse in patients older than fifty, in whom papillary carcinoma is a much more aggressive disease. In the Mayo Clinic series, most patients received ipsilateral lobectomy and contralateral subtotal lobectomy. Neck dissections were performed in patients who had gross evidence of nodal involvement. Overall only 6 percent of patients with thyroid cancer died of their disease. Only four patients with occult papillary carcinoma died of tumor (i.e., primary lesions less than 1.5 cm). Lymph-node metastases in the young did not appear to worsen the prognosis, as long as the nodes could be removed. Patients with extrathyroidal disease, which means invasion into the trachea or esophagus or distant disease, did poorly. Many ultimately died of their papillary carcinoma.

In some aggressive cases, the originally dominant papillary elements become less prominent, and the histologic appearance becomes more anaplastic. Hirabayashi and Lindsay reported that 11 percent of their patients died of disease and that 40 percent of the deaths resulted from uncontrollable disease within the neck. At the Lahey Clinic, 12 percent of those treated for papillary carcinoma died of disease.

FOLLICULAR CARCINOMA

Follicular carcinoma is the predominant element of one-quarter of malignant tumors of the thyroid. The lesion tends to occur in older age groups, with a peak incidence in the fifth decade. It is three times more common in females than in males.

PATHOLOGY. Grossly, the tumor may appear encapsulated. Histologically, the lesion has follicles, but the cells are crowded and are recognizable as an adenocarcinoma. The lumen of the acini may be devoid of colloid. Capsular and vascular invasions are prominent features. Multicentricity is much less common than in papillary carcinoma.

The malignant potential exceeds that of papillary carcinoma. Although there may be spread to regional lymph nodes in about 15 percent of cases, hematogenous spread to distant sites such as bone, lung, and liver predominates and often occurs early.

CLINICAL MANIFESTATIONS. In many patients there is a long history of goiter with recent change in the gland, such as diffuse enlargement or the development of a single firm nodule. Usually, however, only a solitary nodule is present. Pain and invasion of adjacent structures are late manifestations. Regional lymph nodes are seldom enlarged, but distant metastases are frequent. In the Massachusetts General Hospital series, one-half of the patients had evidence of distant metastases at the time that the diagnosis was established. Pulmonary and bony lesions, which are usually osteolytic, represent the most frequent sites of metastases. The metastases usually possess an ability to concentrate iodine.

TREATMENT AND PROGNOSIS. Here too, there are differences of opinion concerning optimal surgical therapy. Some favor hemithyroidectomy with removal of the isthmus. We and others favor near-total or total thyroidectomy, not because of multicentricity but rather to facilitate later scanning of the body with radioiodine and treatment with ^{131}I if metastases are found. If local metastases are apparent, dissection includes these nodes. Since

lymph node metastases are less common than hematogenous spread, concomitant radical neck dissection is rarely indicated. Isolated metastases may be removed surgically.

Follicular carcinomas are more virulent than papillary cancers. Black et al. reported 10-year survival rate of 72 percent for follicular tumors. In those lesions without marked invasiveness, the 10-year survival rate was 86 percent, whereas when invasiveness was apparent, the 10-year survival rate was 44 percent.

OTHER TREATMENTS FOR DIFFERENTIATED CANCERS.
L-Thyroxine. Following surgical therapy for papillary or follicular cancers all patients are treated with enough L-thyroxine to suppress circulating TSH levels. This is done since in animal thyroid cancer models, growth of tumor is fostered by elevated TSH concentrations. In human beings, the usefulness of L-thyroxine therapy is not consistent; however, in some patients, regression of metastatic tumor has occurred simply with thyroxine treatment.

Radioiodine Therapy. At the University of Chicago hospitals, DeGroot and associates believe that it is appropriate to perform a total body scan with radioiodine on virtually all patients with differentiated thyroid carcinoma to ablate any uptake due to normal thyroid in the neck after thyroidectomy and to treat any distant metastases that are present with ^{131}I therapy. To facilitate this technique, thyroid hormone is stopped for 4 to 6 weeks and endogenous TSH level is permitted to rise, thus increasing the avidity of metastatic tumor for radioiodine. Treatment with 30 mC of ^{131}I will ablate most small remnants of normal thyroid in the neck, while doses of 150 mC or greater may be given for metastatic disease. As long as uptake of radioiodine is present, repeat treatment is given at intervals. One limiting factor is pulmonary fibrosis, which can result from treatment of lung metastases. Data accumulated by Beierwaltes and Mazzaferri strongly suggest that the prognosis of papillary carcinoma is improved when this regimen is followed. *External irradiation therapy* is useful primarily when thyroid cancer has invaded the trachea or esophagus or for the treatment of metastatic lesions that no longer take up radioiodine.

Chemotherapy. Widely metastatic lesions that no longer take up radioiodine have been treated with moderate success with systemic chemotherapeutic regimens. For most tumors, Adriamycin has been the single most effective agent.

HÜRTHLE CELL TUMORS

Hürthle cell (oxyphilic) tumors of the thyroid contain sheets of cells with eosinophilic cytoplasm. Some are obviously carcinomas and demonstrate capsular invasion, lymph node or distant metastases. Other lesions pose a problem for the pathologist and for the surgeon because occasionally, benign-appearing lesions will later metastasize. A second treatment problem relates to the fact that neither the primary tumor nor its metastases generally take up radioiodine. Therefore, this mode of therapy is not helpful for metastatic disease in most patients even after total thyroidectomy has been performed.

The Michigan group has advocated total thyroidectomy for all patients with Hürthle cell tumors. At the University of Chicago, 13.7 percent of these tumors have been diagnosed as being carcinomas either by their histologic appearance or by later metastatic spread. Only 1 in 40 (2.5 percent) benign-appearing lesions has later metastasized. Thus, we individualize treatment and perform total thyroid ablation for obvious carcinomas, for those with a history of external irradiation to the head and neck, for large lesions, for those with partial capsular infiltration, and when an associated differentiated carcinoma is also present. The minimal operation for other small, benign-appearing lesions with no risk factors should be a thyroid lobectomy.

MEDULLARY CARCINOMA

Medullary carcinoma of the thyroid is a C-cell, calcitonin-producing tumor. Calcitonin is a 32 amino acid polypeptide found in the thyroid gland of all mammals, including human beings. In lower animals—fish, birds, and amphibians—it is found in the ultimobranchial bodies. When injected into experimental animals it results in a lowering of the serum calcium concentration by an inhibition of bone resorption. In some mammalian species, calcitonin acts as a physiologic hormone that prevents hypercalcemia. In human beings, however, this function has never been proved.

Calcitonin is secreted by C cells (formerly called parafollicular, epifollicular, or light cells). These are derived from the neural crest and are part of the APUD series of polypeptide-secreting cells described by Pearse. In human beings, C cells migrate to the lateral thyroid lobes during embryologic development and are found in greatest number in the posterior-lateral areas of the upper and middle third of each lobe.

PATHOLOGY. Medullary carcinoma was first classified as a separate tumor by Hazard and associates in 1959. Prior to that time, such tumors were lumped together with anaplastic carcinomas. Microscopically, these tumors may present as clusters of cells separated by areas of collagen and amyloid, as sheets of cells that are round or polyhedral and resemble the cells of carcinoid tumors, or as spindle-shaped cells resembling immature fibroblasts. The finding of amyloid in the stroma of the tumor is diagnostic, since this is the only thyroid tumor that contains this substance. C-cell hyperplasia is thought to be a precursor of frank carcinoma.

Grossly, tumors may vary in size, from microscopic to 10 cm or greater in diameter. Bilateral multicentricity is the rule in familial cases, whereas in sporadic cases, single nodules are more common. Tumor spreads first to lymph nodes of the neck and superior mediastinum. Later, distal metastases may involve the lungs, liver, adrenals, bone (frequently osteoblastic), and other organ systems. Local invasion into the trachea and esophagus occurs in advanced cases.

CLINICAL FEATURES. With medullary cancer, there appears to be no predilection in regard to sex; 58 percent of the patients are female. In different series, these tumors make up 3.5 to 11.9 percent of all thyroid malignancies. This tumor has an occurrence ranging from children of two years of age to individuals in their eighties. In familial cases the median age is the early twenties. Most cases are sporadic; however, up to 27 percent of reported cases have been familial. Undoubtedly, the familial nature of many other cases has been overlooked. The familial type is inherited as an autosomal dominant. Thus, about 50 percent of offspring would be expected to have this tumor.

Patients present with a single nodule or with multiple thyroid nodules. Fifteen to twenty percent have cervical adenopathy when first recognized. Hoarseness or dysphagia is present in 10 percent. In addition, these patients may present with very distinctive symptomatology. Diarrhea is the most common complaint. Over 30 percent of patients with this tumor present with or develop diarrhea. Episodic flushing may also occur. Increased motility and impaired intestinal water and electrolyte fluxes may be responsible. Serotonin, calcitonin, or prostaglandins E_2 and $F_2\alpha$ have each been implicated. Calcium infusion and alcohol ingestion may trigger an attack.

Medullary carcinoma is the only thyroid tumor that is associated with Cushing's syndrome. From 2 to 4 percent of patients with this thyroid cancer have adrenal cortical hyperplasia. Ectopic production of ACTH by the medullary carcinoma has been demonstrated in most instances. Other patients may present with kidney stones and with symptoms of pheochromocytomas.

Familial Medullary Carcinoma Syndrome. Medullary carcinomas occur in families as part of a syndrome that has been called *multiple endocrine neoplasia, type II* (MEN-II); *familial medullary carcinoma syndrome;* and *Sipple's syndrome.* A further subdivision is appropriate, into MEN-IIA and MEN-IIB. MEN-IIA is the more common type. In its entirety it consists of multicentric medullary carcinoma or C-cell hyperplasia, pheochromocytomas or adrenal medullary hyperplasia, and hyperparathyroidism. MEN-IIB consists of medullary carcinoma; pheochromocytomas and mucosal neuromas of the lips, tongue, or conjunctiva; ganglioneuromas of the bowel; a typical facial appearance; and a Marfanlike habitus (Fig. 38-17). This unusual phenotypic expression may be found in families but more often is found in unrelated persons, presumably the result of a mutation. The medullary cancer of MEN-IIB patients is very virulent, and few patients live longer than 20 to 30 years.

In MEN-II, the adrenal medullary hyperplasia or pheochromocytomas are multicentric and bilateral in over 70 percent of cases, whereas only 8 to 10 percent of all pheochromocytomas are bilateral. Hypertension, sweating, and palpitations may occur; however, in some patients these tumors result in few symptoms. Various families have either medullary carcinomas or pheochromocytomas; however, about 50 percent of families have both of these lesions, either concomitantly or at different times. Ninety percent of adrenal pheochromocytomas are benign, but malignant lesions with metastases occur more frequently (46 percent) when the primary lesion is extraadrenal. Hypercalcemia is present in as many as 20

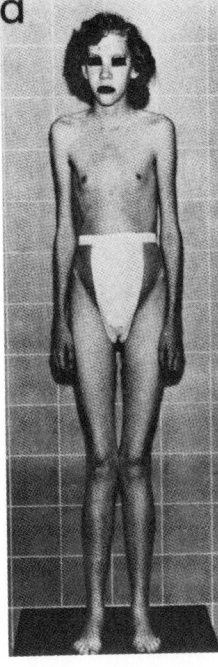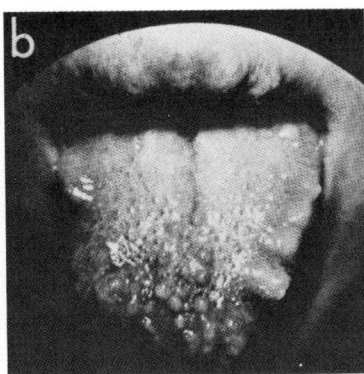

Fig. 38-17. An 18-year-old girl, who demonstrates the appearance typically associated with multiple endocrine neoplasia, type IIB (MEN-IIB), was found to have bilateral medullary carcinoma of the thyroid gland at operation. *a.* The Marfanlike body habitus and facial features typically present in patients with MEN-IIB are clearly seen. *b.* Multiple neuromas of the tongue and lips are demonstrated. *(Courtesy of Glen W. Sizemore.)*

percent of these patients; kidney stones occasionally occur. Hyperparathyroidism, when present, is usually due to chief cell hyperplasia. Elevated serum PTH or evidence of hyperparathyroidism at operation is found in 45 to 90 percent of patients with MEN-IIA. However, parathyroid disease rarely, if ever, is found in either sporadic medullary carcinomas or MEN-IIB. The role of calcitonin in the pathogenesis of parathyroid hyperplasia is largely discounted. Most authors favor a genetic origin or stimulation by an unknown factor.

DIAGNOSIS. An elevated serum calcitonin concentration, measured by radioimmunoassay, in a patient with a thyroid mass is virtually diagnostic of medullary carcinoma. However, some persons with this tumor or with C-cell hyperplasia have normal basal calcitonin concentrations but demonstrate abnormal responses to calcium infusion or to pentagastrin administration. The families of all patients with medullary carcinoma should be screened carefully and repeatedly. Affected children of MEN-IIB families often present with lymph-node metastases early in life. Their only chance of cure is early diagnosis during childhood and thyroidectomy. Any patient with the neuroma phenotype (MEN-IIB) should be assumed to have medullary carcinoma until proved otherwise. Carcinoembryonic antigen (CEA) is also elevated in most patients with this tumor. Pheochromocytomas should be searched for diligently. Serum calcium, adrenocortical and catecholamine function, 5-hydroxyindoleacetic acid, prostaglandins, and histaminase should be evaluated if possible.

In difficult diagnostic problems, selective catheterization, with venous sampling of blood for calcitonin, may aid in localization of metastases as well. Finally, the measurements have prognostic importance. Following the removal of all tumor, serum calcitonin and CEA values are no longer measurable; a return of elevated serum calcitonin or CEA concentrations signals the recurrence of tumor.

TREATMENT. Since medullary carcinomas are C-cell tumors, they do not respond to thyroxine therapy and do not concentrate radioiodine. Furthermore, they are relatively insensitive to external irradiation, although several groups are enthusiastic about results of high-dosage regimens for minimal disease. Therefore, surgery offers the best chance for cure. Total thyroidectomy should be performed because of the frequent multicentricity. Recurrences have been reported if thyroid tissue is left. More than 50 percent of patients will have positive lymph nodes at the time of initial exploration. Single or bilateral neck dissections should be performed if nodes are clinically involved or if elevated calcitonin concentrations pinpoint disease in these areas. A superior mediastinal dissection through a sternal splitting incision may be indicated in selected instances. Thallium scanning may help in locating areas of metastases.

In some cases of known metastatic disease, removal of the bulk of tumor is appropriate, since flushing, diarrhea, or Cushing's disease may be ameliorated. This is important, since patients with metastatic disease often survive for long periods. Chemotherapy with Adriamycin alone or with multidrug regimens often including streptozotocin has led to some remissions of medullary carcinoma and should be tried when metastatic disease is progressive.

Pheochromocytomas should be operated upon first, when found. Most favor bilateral, total adrenalectomy because of multicentricity and bilaterality of the lesions. Others feel that if the second adenal only has adrenal medullary hyperplasia and not a pheochromocytoma, it should be left in place and followed carefully because of the difficulties of adrenocortical hormone replacement in children. However, at least one viable parathyroid gland or a part of it should remain in the neck at the end of the procedure. In cases of normocalcemia the parathyroids need not be excised; in fact, they should be carefully preserved. When hypercalcemia is present, all four glands should be evaluated to determine the pathologic process. The enlarged parathyroid gland or glands should be removed with the thyroidectomy.

PROGNOSIS. In 128 patients who were operated on for cure at the Mayo Clinic, 63 had lymph node metastases at the time of surgery. The overall survival rate was 80 percent at 5 years and 57 percent at 10 years. In the group *without* lymph node metastases at the initial operation, the 10-year survival rate was 68 percent. Only 46 percent of those with initial lymph node involvement survived for 10 years. The overall 5-year survival rate of 169 patients who were followed at other institutions for 5 years or longer was 55 percent. The screening of families clearly leads to the diagnosis of medullary carcinoma in an earlier stage, when it is still curable.

ANAPLASTIC CARCINOMA

Undifferentiated carcinomas make up about 10 percent of malignant tumors of the thyroid and usually occur after the age of fifty. In some instances, the lesion represents a transformation of a low-grade differentiated tumor. Frazell and Foote reviewed 393 papillary tumors and reported 6 in which such a transformation occurred. Wychulis et al. reported 16 patients with mixed anaplastic and papillary carcinoma. The ratio of men to women is 1.3:1, and 50 percent are in the seventh and eighth decades of life, with an average age of sixty-six years.

Grossly, the tumor is unencapsulated and may extend widely outside the confines of the gland, invading adjacent structures. Histologically, the cell structure is variable, ranging from spindle-shaped to multinucleated giant cells. There are numerous mitoses. In some cases, areas of follicular or papillary carcinoma may be present.

Patients generally present with painful enlargement of the thyroid, which is often fixed and moves poorly on swallowing. Regional lymph nodes are frequently enlarged, and signs and symptoms of pressure effects are common. Metastases are usually located in the lungs rather than the bones. The disease is characterized by an extremely rapid progress. Total thyroidectomy and modified neck dissection is the treatment of choice, but in almost every patient the lesion is not resectable. In some cases removing some tissue to ensure an adequate airway or performing a tracheostomy is all that can be done. In others the diagnosis is made by needle biopsy, and ancillary treatment is started. In one series of 130 cases, resection was attempted in only 49, and only one patient was known to be alive at the time of the report. Seventy-five percent of the deaths occurred within 1 year. External radiation may afford palliation for pain. Radioactive iodine is ineffective, since the tumors do not concentrate the material. Chemotherapy with Adriamycin and combination drug regimens of vincristine, Adriamycin and chlorambucil have occasionally been helpful.

LYMPHOMA AND SARCOMA

The thyroid is a rare site for primary lymphoma. However, many lesions that were previously diagnosed as small cell anaplastic cancers are now known to be lymphomas. Mikal, in a review of the literature, indicated that 165 cases had been reported, with tumors arising from reticular cells, lymphoblasts, and lymphocytes. Only 13 cases of Hodgkin's disease arising primarily in the thyroid have been documented. Most lymphomas of the thyroid arise in thyroid glands of Hashimoto's thyroiditis.

Treatment is determined by the extent of disease, and patients are often staged to determine this as are other lymphoma patients. When the tumor is localized, a total or near-total thyroidectomy followed by deep x-ray therapy to the cervical nodes is indicated. In Stage I disease, 5-year survivals of 70 to 80 percent have been obtained. If the disease has metastasized to cervical nodes or invaded the capsule, a total thyroidectomy and radical neck dissection should be performed and followed by radiation.

Many times, if possible, debulking of the tumor followed by radiation is performed since the tumor invades into surrounding structures. Disseminated lymphoma is usually treated by multidrug chemotherapeutic regimens, depending upon the histologic type of the lymphoma and on institutional preferences. The prognosis is much poorer under these circumstances.

METASTATIC CARCINOMA

Metastases are present in the thyroid in 2 to 4 percent of the patients dying of malignant disease. Bronchogenic carcinomas account for 20 percent of secondary thyroid metastases. Three percent of all bronchogenic carcinomas autopsied demonstrate metastases to the thyroid. Wychulis et al. reported that among more than 20,000 surgical specimens 10 represented metastatic involvement of the thyroid gland. The most common primary lesion in that series was hypernephroma, with the average age of the patient fifty-six years. Freund reported two 5-year survivals following thyroidectomy in which there were metastatic lesions from bronchogenic carcinoma and lipomyxosarcoma.

Surgery of the Thyroid

Surgical treatment of the thyroid is performed (1) to establish the diagnosis in a patient with a mass within the thyroid gland, (2) to remove benign and malignant tumors, (3) as therapy for thyrotoxicosis, and (4) to alleviate pressure symptoms attributable to the thyroid.

OPERATIVE TECHNIQUE. The procedure (Fig. 38-18) is almost always performed under endotracheal anesthesia, although there was a time when local anesthesia was popular in some clinics. The patient's neck is extended by placing a roll beneath the shoulders. An equilateral low collar incision is made in the line of a natural skin crease approximately 1 to 2 cm above the clavicle. The incision is carried through skin, subcutaneous tissue, and platysma down to the dense cervical fascia that overlies the pretracheal muscles and anterior jugular veins. The upper flap is raised to the level of the upper border of the thyroid cartilage, with care to avoid cutting sensory nerves, in order to obviate unnecessary paresthesias during convalescence. The lower flap is elevated to the level of the manubrial notch. If dissection of the flap is performed in the plane between the platysmal muscle and the fascia overlying the strap muscles, the bleeding is minimal. The cervical fascia is then incised vertically in the midline from the upper margin of the thyroid cartilage to the manubrium.

Exposure of the superior and lateral aspects of the thyroid gland generally is achieved by retracting the sternohyoid and sternothyroid muscles or, occasionally, by dividing these muscles. Division of these muscles is associated with little or no disability, but is not necessary unless the gland is markedly enlarged. High transection is preferable, since the ansa hypoglossi nerve innervates the muscles from below. This diminishes the amount of muscle paralyzed.

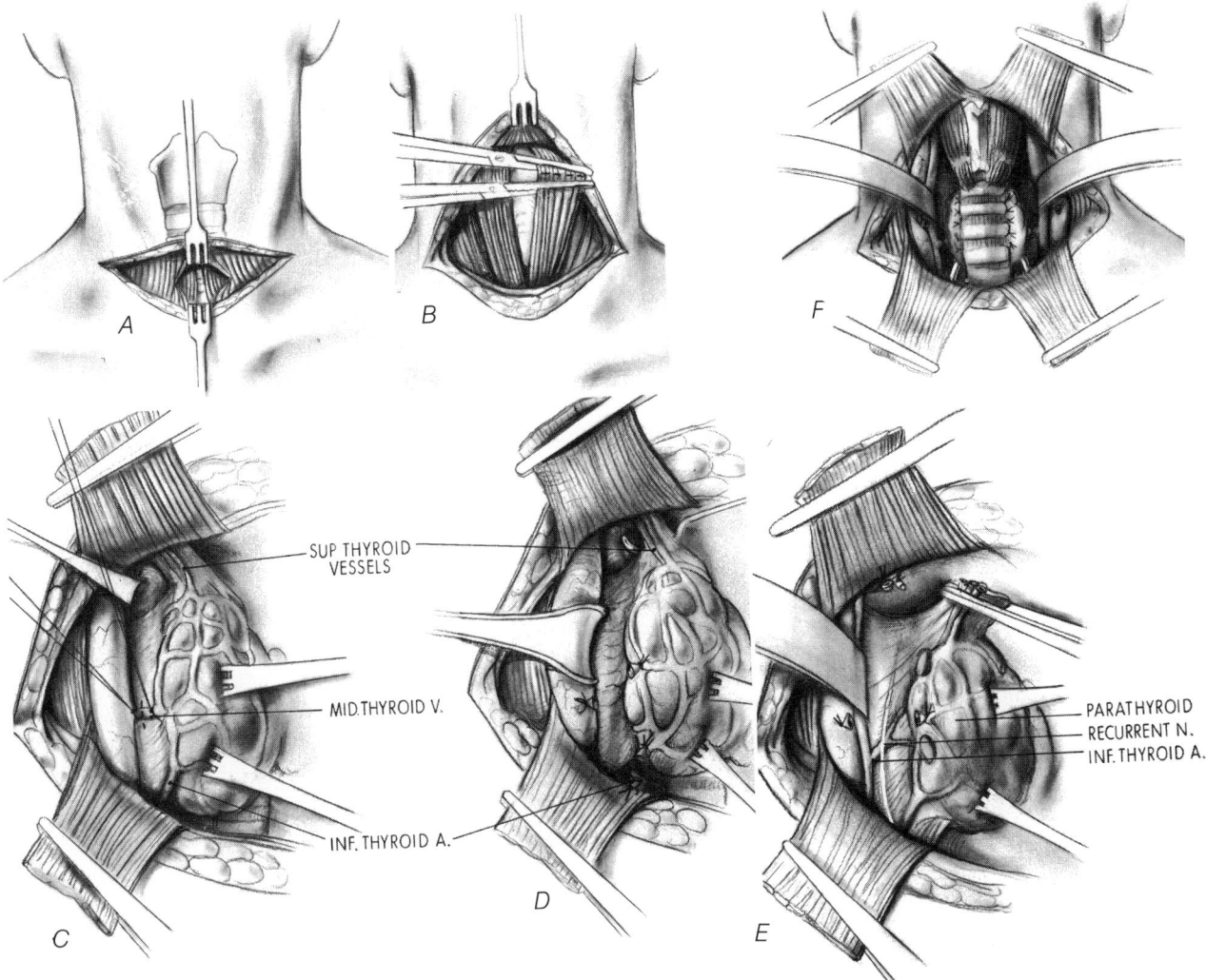

Fig. 38-18. Thyroidectomy. *A.* Collar incision made. Subplatysmal flaps developed. *B.* High transection of strap muscles, rarely done except for large goiters. *C.* Middle thyroid vein divided. *D.* Superior and inferior pole vessels divided. *E.* Identification of recurrent laryngeal nerve and parathyroids. *F.* Remnants of thyroid sutured to trachea to effect hemostasis in the case of subtotal thyroidectomy, as performed for Graves' disease. In total lobectomy the parathyroids are left with an intact blood supply and the entire lobe is removed.

Digital dissection frees the thyroid from surrounding fascia. We then prefer to rotate one lobe medially in order to identify the middle thyroid veins, which vary in number. These are doubly ligated in continuity and transected. This maneuver facilitates exposure of the superior and inferior poles of the thyroid. The suspensory ligaments are transected craniad to the isthmus, and the cricothyroid space is opened in order to separate the superior pole from surrounding tissue. During dissection of the superior lobe care is taken to avoid injury to the superior laryngeal nerve. The internal branch of the nerve, which provides sensory fibers to the epiglottis and larynx, is rarely in the operative field. It is the external branch,

which supplies motor innervation to the inferior pharyngeal constrictor and cricothyroid muscles, that must be protected. This is accomplished by trying to identify the nerve, and gently dissecting it away from the superior pole vessels. These vessels are then ligated separately very close to the thyroid lobe and divided.

The lobe is then retracted mediad to permit identification of the inferior thyroid artery and the recurrent laryngeal nerve. The inferior thyroid artery is isolated but is rarely if ever ligated laterally. Rather we choose to ligate and divide each arterial branch near the thyroid lobe after the parathyroid glands have been supplied. This technique, we feel, lessens the incidence of hypoparathyroidism. The recurrent laryngeal nerve is identified along its course, and is gently unroofed. At the junction of the trachea and larynx, in the area of the Ligament of Berry, it is in its most anterior position and most likely to be damaged. A total lobectomy may be performed at this point, as is indicated for tumor, or a remnant of approximately 2 to 4 g of posterior thyroid tissue may be left in those pa-

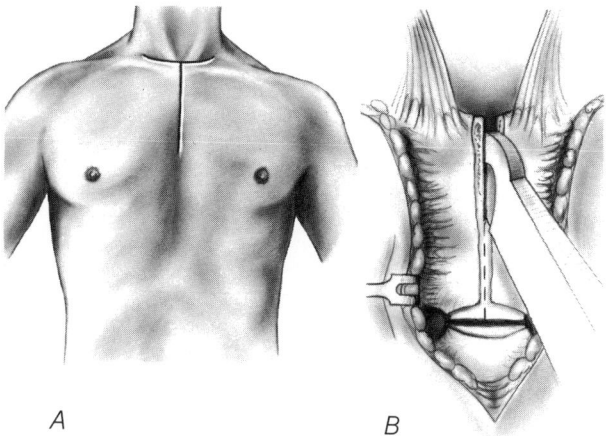

Fig. 38-19. Transsternal thyroidectomy. *A.* Incision. *B.* Transection of sternum. "T-ing" incision into second interspace.

tients in whom the operation is being performed for primary hyperthyroidism.

During exposure of the posterior surface of the thyroid gland, the parathyroids should be identified and preserved along with their vascular pedicle. Using sharp dissection, the lobe is then dissected clear from the lateral aspect of the trachea, and dissection is continued in order to separate the isthmus from the anterior trachea. If a pyramidal lobe is present, it is removed at this time. It is important that the entire anterior trachea be cleared in order to avoid development of a mass effect due to hypertrophy of the thyroid in this region. When the operation is being performed for a unilateral nodule that proved to be benign, it is terminated at this point by approximating the anterior and posterior aspects of the cut end of the medial portion of the remaining lobe. When subtotal or total thyroidectomy is performed, the remaining lobe is removed in the same manner.

If subtotal thyroidectomy is performed for Graves' disease, the remnants of thyroid are folded in and sutured to the trachea to complete hemostasis. The entire wound is inspected, and it is mandatory that the operative field show no evidence of bleeding. In most instances, a small suction catheter is utilized to drain the bed of the thyroid lobes. While it is conceded that rapid bleeding leading to respiratory distress cannot be decompressed by the small drain, the cosmetic results with this technique are far superior to those obtained when either no drainage or a Penrose drain is employed. The midline fascial incision is loosely closed, and if the sternothyroid and sternohyoid muscles were transected, they are reapproximated. We no longer suture the platysma muscle; we utilize a technique of approximating the dermis with 5-0 Vicryl subcuticular sutures and the epithelium with sterile skin tapes.

A tracheostomy set is left at the patient's bedside for 24 h, so that the wound can be opened rapidly if there is significant distention, or a tracheostomy can be performed if there is evidence of respiratory obstruction.

Intrathoracic Goiter. In about 1 percent of patients undergoing thyroidectomy, part or all of the thyroid tissue is intrathoracic. Intrathoracic goiter usually represents the extension of cervical thyroid tissue into the chest rather than aberrant glandular tissue. Since the lesion usually retains its connection to the cervical thyroid and receives its blood supply from the inferior thyroid artery, it generally can be removed through the conventional collar incision described above. In the case of a very large colloid goiter, the semiliquid colloid and degenerated portions may be evacuated to permit delivery of the remainder of the tissue and the capsule in the neck. The indications for transsternal or transpleural thyroidectomy include (1) an inability to remove the tumor totally through a cervical approach, (2) large masses with extensive blood supply within the mediastinum, (3) evidence of superior vena cava obstruction, and (4) undiagnosed superior mediastinal lesions.

If necessary, transsternal thyroidectomy (Fig. 38-19) can be performed as an extension of a cervical exploration by "T-ing" the cervical incision over the sternum. The sternum is transected horizontally at the level of the third interspace and vertically from the suprasternal notch down to the level of the horizontal transection. This permits extrapleural resection of the gland and provides excellent visualization of the recurrent laryngeal nerves and the vascular supply. Often a full sternotomy is necessary.

COMPLICATIONS

The mortality rate accompanying thyroidectomy is very low. Gould et al. reviewed 1000 patients, operated on consecutively by a large group of surgeons over a 5-year period, and reported no hospital deaths. The mortality rate reported by Colcock was 0.12 percent, with no deaths since 1954. The morbidity is about 13 percent when all complications, including those of the most minor types, are considered. Pulmonary problems and infections are relatively uncommon. Four major complications classically have been associated with thyroidectomy. These include (1) thyroid storm, which is related to the patient's thyrotoxicosis, (2) wound hemorrhage with hematoma formation, (3) recurrent laryngeal nerve injury, and (4) hypoparathyroidism. The latter three are regarded as complications of technique.

THYROID STORM. Thyroid storm occurs in patients with preexisting thyrotoxicosis who either have not been treated at all or have been treated incompletely. It usually occurs in patients with Graves' disease but may be related to toxic multinodular goiter. In the past, before adequate preparation with antithyroid drugs, surgical treatment was the most common precipitating factor. Presently thyroid storm is a rare complication of surgical treatment and is more frequently precipitated by trauma, infection, diabetic acidosis, or toxemia of pregnancy.

When thyroid storm is related to surgical treatment, the manifestation may develop during the operative procedure or in the recovery room. The patient becomes markedly hyperthermic with profuse sweating and tachycardia. Nausea, vomiting, and abdominal pain are common. Initial tremor and restlessness may progress to delirium with eventual coma.

Treatment is directed at inhibiting the production of thyroid hormone and antagonizing effects of the hormone. Large doses of sodium or potassium iodide, i.e., to 1 to 2.5 g, should be administered intravenously and supplemented with 100 mg of cortisol because of the danger of adrenal insufficiency. Oxygen and large amounts of glucose should be administered intravenously as therapy for the hypermetabolic state. Fluid and electrolytes must be maintained in view of the losses. A hypothermia blanket may be applied to reduce the temperature. Propranolol or other beta blockers are very important and have replaced guanethidine and reserpine to antagonize sympathetic effects. Large doses of propranolol may be needed in toxic patients, for tachycardia and early thyroid storm have been reported to occur in such individuals who were taking 40 mg every 6 h orally of this beta blocker when they developed a severe infection. The mortality rate for this complication is approximately 10 percent.

WOUND HEMORRHAGE. This is a problem of the early postoperative period, i.e., within the first few hours. It has been reported in 0.3 to 1 percent of consecutive thyroidectomies. Hemorrhage in the neck is a significant problem, since small amounts of blood in the deep space near the trachea may obstruct the airway and result in respiratory death. The complication is usually caused by bleeding from branches of the inferior thyroid or superior thyroid artery, and the rate of bleeding is such that the commonly employed drains do not afford protection.

The patients are rarely in shock. The initial manifestation is swelling of the neck and bulging of the wound, which demands immediate attention. If untreated, respiratory obstruction due to compression eventually ensues. Treatment consists of opening the incision, evacuating the clot, and securing the bleeding vessel. This constitutes an emergency procedure, and if it is deemed necessary, the wound should be opened and the clot evacuated at the bedside. Later the patient can be brought to the operating room. Tracheostomy is not required, and is in fact contraindicated, if the wound is decompressed early. Prolonged intubation is occasionally necessary. However, usually the crisis is totally relieved as soon as the hematoma is evacuated.

RECURRENT LARYNGEAL NERVE INJURY. Damage to the recurrent laryngeal nerve may be unilateral or bilateral and temporary or permanent. Injury occurs more commonly when thyroidectomy is being performed for malignant disease. In a series of 1011 thyroidectomies there were 28 examples of vocal cord paralysis, three of which proved to be permanent. The incidence of recurrent nerve injury in another series of 1000 patients reported by Gould et al. was 0.2 percent. Colcock and King, evaluating 1246 thyroid operations, noted one bilateral recurrent laryngeal nerve paralysis. Recently Thompson and Harness reported an incidence of 4.8 per-

cent for accidental unilateral nerve injury in total thyroidectomy for carcinoma.

Loss of function of the recurrent laryngeal nerve may result from excessive trauma to the nerve during exposure, inclusion of the nerve in a ligature, or an inadvertent sectioning of the nerve. Another uncommon cause is damage to the vagus nerve in the neck. Recurrent laryngeal nerve injury produces an abductor laryngeal paralysis, and the vocal cord assumes a median or paramedian position, which is identifiable on postoperative laryngoscopy. The involved cord or cords are initially flaccid, but with the passage of time the flaccidity is replaced by spasticity. If the injury is related to dissection and the nerve is intact, function should return usually within 3 to 6 months and invariably within 9 to 12 months. In the immediate postoperative period, cord paralysis results in narrowing of the glottic aperture, but this is not sufficient to produce obstruction of the airway unless it is accompanied by glottic edema due to hematoma in the cervical space or trauma to the larynx, or related to the cuffed endotracheal tube. Paralysis of one cord results in a huskiness of the voice with varying degrees of hoarseness.

Bilateral recurrent nerve injury is much more serious than a unilateral injury. A bilateral cord paralysis often results in problems related to coughing and respiratory toilet and, in the worst situations, to airway obstruction. Obstruction can worsen after several months or longer in such cases, for the cords move progressively toward the midline and the glottic aperture narrows.

The incidence of this complication can be markedly reduced by identifying the recurrent laryngeal nerves routinely during thyroidectomy. The recurrent laryngeal nerve is in greatest jeopardy at the level of the two upper tracheal rings, where the middle third of the thyroid lobe is in closest contact with it. The lobe is attached by a strong process of pretracheal fascia (the suspensory ligament of Berry) to the cricoid cartilage and trachea, which must be severed before the lobe can be removed. Although the recurrent laryngeal nerve usually runs posteriorly to this adherent connective tissue zone, in 25 percent of patients it courses through the ligament of Berry.

Asymptomatic unilateral paralysis does not require treatment. In rare instances, reexploration of the wound is indicated, since removal of a ligature often reestablishes function. Once the diagnosis of bilateral cord paralysis, a rarity, is established, tracheostomy should be considered and the patient watched carefully, since airway obstruction often occurs, frequently related to a respiratory tract infection. Subsequently the glottic aperture can be widened by arytenoidectomy or arytenoidopexy, which displaces the posterior portion of the vocal cord laterally. These procedures provide an adequate airway but cause further deterioration of the voice. Six to twelve months should be allowed to pass between the time of thyroidectomy and these procedures in order to be certain that there is no returning function. Direct repair of a transected recurrent laryngeal nerve should be performed at the time of thyroidectomy if it is recognized. Repair as late as 2 to 3 months postinjury has been successful in some cases. Splitting the vagus nerve and anastomosing it to the distal end of the recurrent laryngeal nerve or burying the nerve in the posterior cricoarytenoid muscle has rarely been successful. Likewise, implanting the omohyoid muscle with its nervous innervation into the cricothyroid muscle (Tucker procedure) is less commonly used. Finally, in unilateral cord injuries, Teflon injections into the paralyzed cord to move it to the midline can often improve the voice.

Injury to the external branch of the superior laryngeal nerve is not as serious as a recurrent laryngeal injury. It should be avoided because it results in a limitation of the force of projection of one's voice and impairs a singer's high tones. Not infrequently these disorders improve during the first 3 months after thyroidectomy.

HYPOPARATHYROIDISM. Overt manifestations of hypoparathyroidism occur in a minority of patients following thyroidectomy. This is usually a temporary syndrome related to dissection in the region of the parathyroid glands. There is an increased incidence of temporary hypoparathyroidism following thyroidectomy for hyperthyroidism and when a total thyroidectomy is performed. It is probably necessary to leave only one gland in situ with an adequate blood supply to avoid the complication. Postoperative permanent hypoparathyroidism occurred in 0.6 percent of the 1000 thyroidectomies reviewed by Gould et al. and in 2.8 percent of the total thyroidectomies in that series. Persik and Catz, in a review of 210 consecutive total thyroidectomies, noted that permanent hypoparathyroidism resulted in none of the patients with nonmalignant disease and in 9 percent of those with malignant disease. In the series of Thompson and Harness permanent hypoparathyroidism occurred in 5.4 percent of all patients undergoing total thyroidectomy for carcinoma, in 1.6 percent of those having primary procedures, and in 7.4 percent of those having secondary operations. An incidence of 8.2 percent was noted when there was an associated neck dissection. In a Mayo Clinic series, prior to 1970 total thyroidectomy for papillary thyroid carcinoma resulted in an incidence of permanent hypoparathyroidism of greater than 30 percent. This was reduced to only several percent when an ipsilateral lobectomy and contralateral subtotal lobectomy of the thyroid was performed.

Postthyroidectomy hypoparathyroidism may be due to the inadvertent removal of the parathyroid glands but more frequently is caused by damage to the blood supply. The parathyroid end arteries are very delicate and may be damaged during dissection. We do not ligate the inferior thyroid artery laterally because of the danger that this will decrease blood flow to the parathyroid glands when a lobectomy or a subtotal lobectomy is performed. Despite the care utilized by the surgeon in attempting to preserve the integrity and blood supply to the parathyroid glands, sometimes a parathyroid gland appears to be severely damaged or devascularized at the end of the lobectomy. In such cases, the parathyroid gland can be minced into 1- to 2-mm cubes, after the surgeon is certain of its identity by frozen section analysis, and then autotransplanted into small pockets in the sternocleidomastoid or the forearm

musculature utilizing the technique of Wells. Some surgeons routinely autotransplant one parathyroid gland in this manner at the time of total parathyroidectomy and feel that it reduces the incidence of permanent hypoparathyroidism. We prefer to individualize patients and only use this technique in the rare instance in which parathyroid function is deemed to be in jeopardy by the thyroidectomy.

The clinical manifestations of hypoparathyroidism usually occur within several days after operation. The initial symptoms are circumoral numbness, tingling of the fingertips, and intense anxiety. The Chvostek sign appears early, followed by Trousseau's sign and carpopedal spasm. As the disease progresses, muscle cramps and frank tetany develop. Prolonged hypoparathyroidism may cause cataracts, convulsive episodes, and psychoses. The diagnostic findings consist of reduced serum calcium, increased serum phosphorus, and decreased or absent calcium in the urine as evidenced by the Sulkowitch test.

Postoperative hypoparathyroidism must be differentiated from tetany caused by alkalosis associated with anxiety and hyperventilation. Hyperventilation causes a reduction in ionized calcium, but the manifestations can be promptly reversed by inhalation of carbon dioxide or breathing through an increased dead space. Another cause may be "bone hunger." In thyrotoxic patients bone turnover is increased. Following thyroidectomy, calcium ion may return to bone, causing hypocalcemia.

The treatment of hypoparathyroidism should be initiated promptly. When the diagnosis has been made, 10 mL of a 10% solution of calcium gluconate should be slowly administered intravenously and usually results in the immediate improvement of symptoms. Continuous intravenous infusions of calcium gluconate using 2 to 3 ampules of this agent every 8 h will abort most symptoms. Usually all hypocalcemia goes away in several days *(transient hypoparathyroidism)*, and the infusion can be stopped. For more prolonged hypocalcemia oral calcium therapy is started. The aim is to administer 1.5 to 2 g of calcium ion daily. This requires about 15 to 20 g of calcium gluconate daily, but lesser amounts of calcium carbonate. Vitamin D preparations are only used if prolonged hypocalcemia is present and *permanent hypoparathyroidism* is suspected. Starting doses of different vitamin D compounds include: Vitamin D_2 or D_3, 100,000 to 200,000 units/day; dehyrotachysterol, 2 to 4 mg/day; and $1,25\text{-}(OH)_2D_3$ (Rocaltrol), the active metabolite of vitamin D, 1 to 2 μg/day. The latter gives the fastest responses to therapy. It is important to follow the serum calcium and phosphorus levels closely during treatment, for hypercalcemia may occur. Furthermore, serum PTH concentrations should be repeatedly determined to be certain that permanent hypoparathyroidism is present. Maintenance doses of these vitamin D preparations are lower. The advantage of $1,25\text{-}(OH)_2D_3$ usage is a much faster onset of action, i.e., 2 to 4 days, and a much quicker return to normocalcemia if hypercalcemic crisis occurs from the administration of too much vitamin D. The intake of certain meat, fish and dairy products that

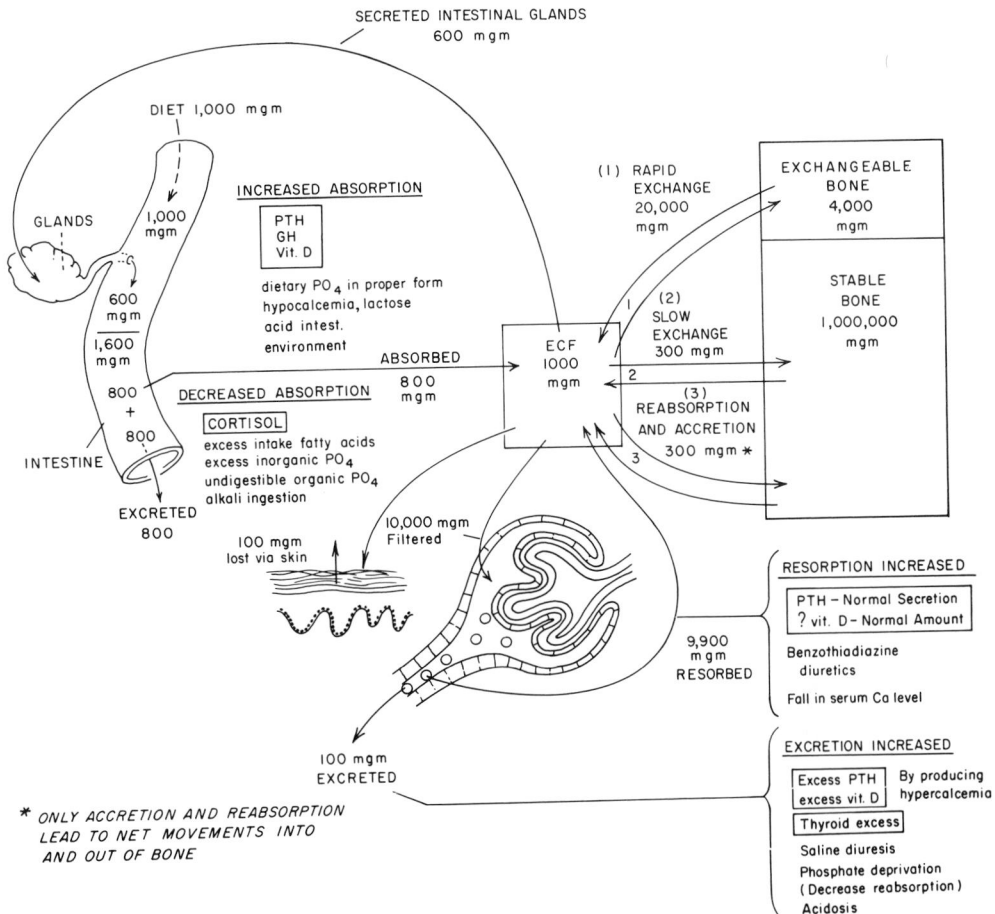

Fig. 38-26. Calcium metabolism. The diet contains approximately 1000 mg calcium each day. The intestinal glands secrete approximately 600 mg into the intestine. Of this 1600 mg, 800 is absorbed, and 800 is excreted in the feces. The extracellular fluid contains about 1000 mg calcium. This is constantly being exchanged with calcium in other pools. Each day 10,000 mg is filtered through the glomerulus, and 9900 mg of this is resorbed. There is a slow exchange from stable bone and a rapid exchange from exchangeable bone. Calcium is constantly being resorbed and added to bone, and this activity is under hormonal control.

form and is cleaved in the reticuloendothelial cells of the liver, primarily into N- and C-terminal fragments. The N-terminal fragment contains the biologic activity of the PTH molecule. As discussed later, measurement of the C-terminal fragment by radioimmunoassay is best for the diagnosis of primary hyperparathyroidism, since this fragment is slowly metabolized by the kidney, while the N-terminal fragment is rapidly degraded by liver and bone mechanisms.

Vitamin D. Many significant advances in vitamin D metabolism have been made in the last several decades. The natural form of vitamin D is called vitamin D_3, or cholecalciferol (Fig. 38-29). It is produced by the irradiation of 7-dihydrocholesterol in the skin. To be metabolically active, D_3 is first hydroxylated in the liver to 25-hydroxyvitamin D_3 (25-OH D_3). The 25-OH D_3 is further hydroxylated in the kidney to 1,25-dihydroxy-vitamin D_3 [1,25-$(OH)_2D_3$]. The latter metabolite is believed to be the metabolically active form of vitamin D that carries out the well-known functions of this substance—namely, mobilizing calcium and phosphorus from bone and enhancing intestinal absorption of calcium and phosphorus. Patients who have had their kidneys removed, for example, are insensitive to administration of both vitamin D_3 and 25-OH D_3, since they cannot convert this to the active 1,25-$(OH)_2D_3$ form.

It is now suggested that vitamin D acts as a physiologic hormone that has feedback control mechanisms. In the presence of parathyroid hormone, when serum calcium or serum phosphorus levels are low, there is an increased synthesis of 1,25-$(OH)_2D_3$, which then makes calcium and phosphorus available from the bone and intestines. Thus the serum calcium concentration returns toward normal. When the serum calcium concentrations are normal, less 1,25-$(OH)_2D_3$ and more 24,25-$(OH)_2D_3$ are produced. The latter metabolite is relatively inactive, and therefore less calcium and phosphorus are mobilized.

These findings are important clinically in the treatment of renal osteodystrophy and hypoparathyroidism. In both these conditions, microgram quantities of 1,25-$(OH)_2D_3$ have proved effective. 1,25-$(OH)_2D_3$ is commercially

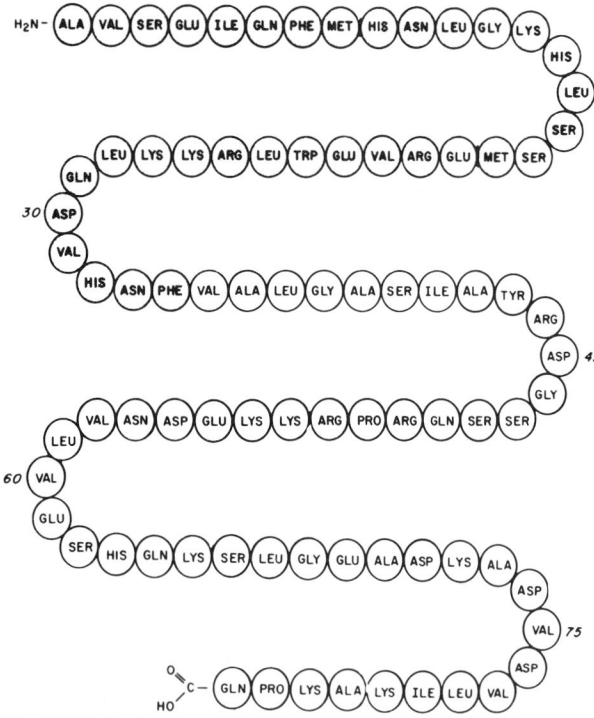

Fig. 38-27. Amino acid sequence of bovine parathyroid hormone. (From: *Potts JT Jr et al: Am J Med 50:639, 1971, with permission.*)

available. It is very effective in treating the renal osteodystrophy of dialysis patients and offers advantages in treating hypoparathyroidism as well.

Calcitonin (Thyrocalcitonin). Calcitonin was originally described by Copp (1962) and Hirsh and Munson (1963) as a calcium-lowering polypeptide. It was originally shown to be present in the epifollicular or parafollicular cells of the mammalian thyroid gland. These cells are now commonly referred to as *C cells*. It has now been demonstrated that C cells come from the neutral crest and are part of the APUD system of peptide- or amine-secreting cells described by Pearse. They migrate to the ultimobranchial bodies, glandular structures derived from the lowest branchial pouches embryologically. In human beings and other mammals these structures are vestigial; they fuse with and are incorporated into the lateral thyroid lobes during embryologic development. In lower animals C cells are found within the ultimobranchial bodies which remain as separate structures. Medullary carcinomas of the thyroid gland are C cell, calcitonin-producing tumors.

Calcitonin has been purified from the thyroid glands of pigs, sheep, and cows, from medullary carcinomas in human beings (called *calcitonin M*), and from salmon ultimobranchial glands. Each of these has a molecular weight of 3500 and 32 amino acids, and they have the same mo-

Fig. 38-28. Schema of the biosynthesis and metabolism of parathyroid hormone. (From: *Habener JF: Ann Rev Physiol 43:211, 1981, with permission.*)

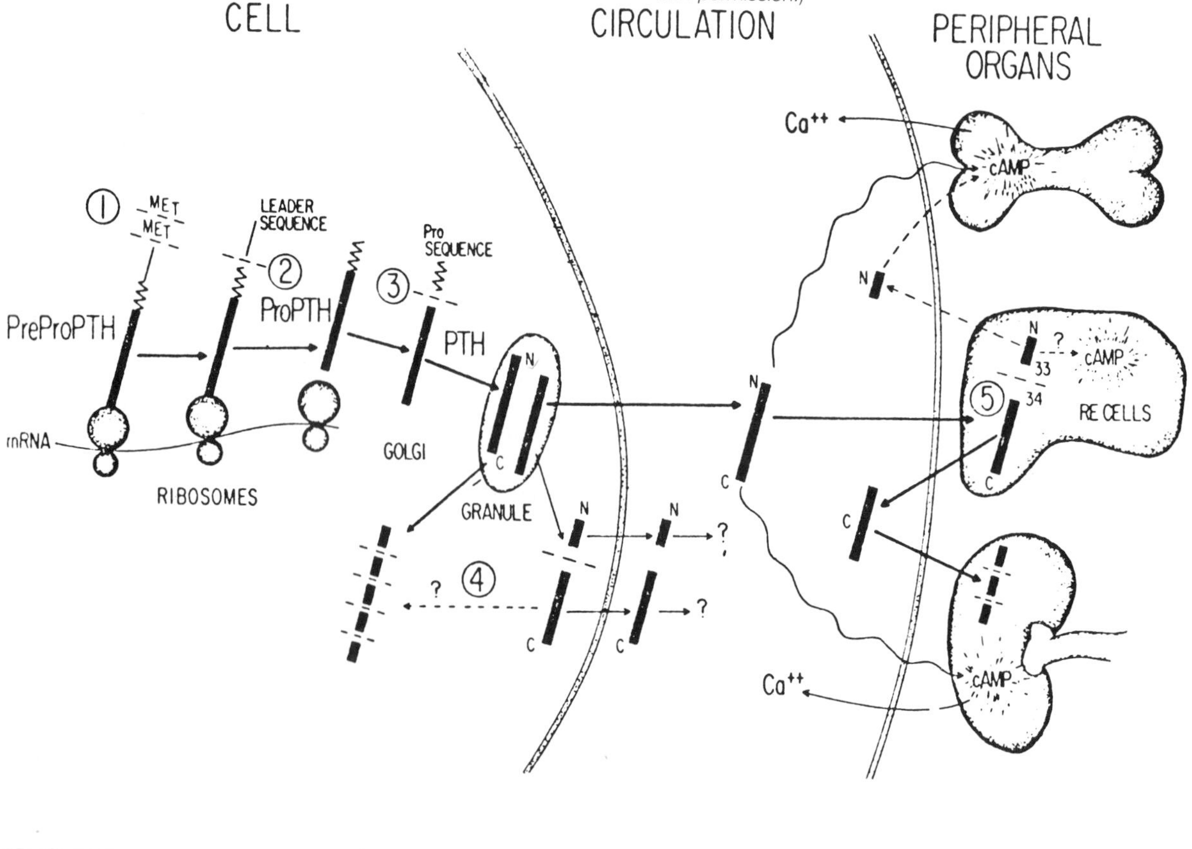

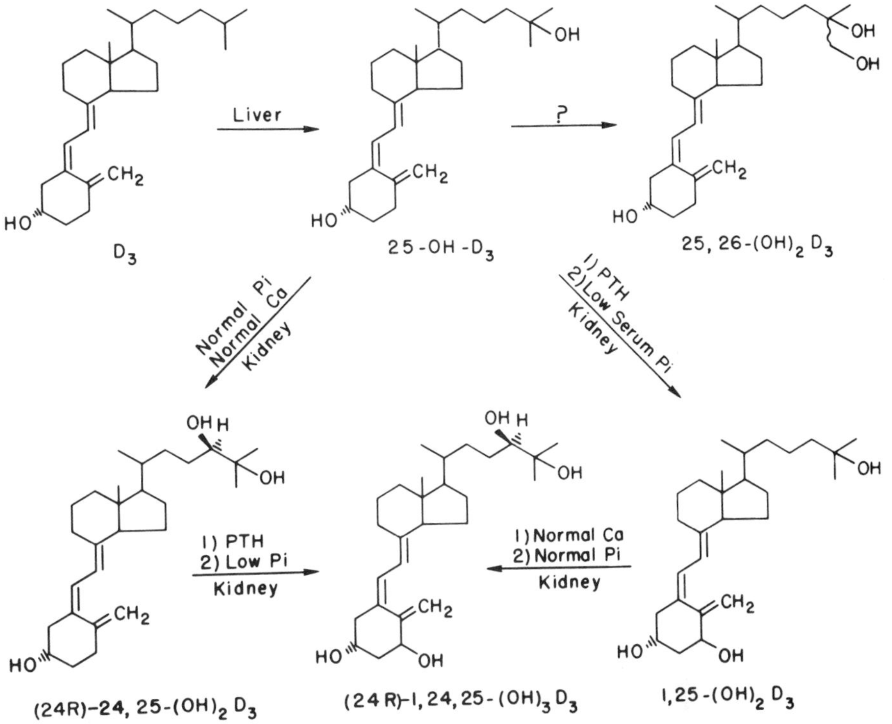

Fig. 38-29. Summary of vitamin D metabolism. (From: *DeLuca HF: Ann Intern Med 85:367, 1976, with permission.*)

lecular configuration. However, as shown in Fig. 38-30, wide variations of amino acid sequences occur within these molecules. Radioimmunoassay systems for measurement of the different calcitonins have added greatly to our knowledge of the physiology of calcitonin and are important in the diagnosis of occult medullary carcinoma of the thyroid in human beings.

Calcitonin lowers the serum calcium concentration in animals by inhibiting bone resorption. In pharmacologic doses, salmon calcitonin has been successfully utilized in the treatment of Paget's disease of bone.

Serum Calcium Homeostasis

Serum calcium concentration in human beings has long been recognized to vary only minimally from day to day (Fig. 38-31). Its regulation is primarily by the parathyroid glands through a negative feedback system. A fall in serum calcium (or serum magnesium) concentration stimulates secretion of PTH which results in a rise in $1,25(OH)_2D_3$. These then act peripherally to raise the serum calcium concentration to normal.

An elevation of the serum calcium level reduces both PTH secretion and also the formation of $1,25-(OH)_2D_3$. Both effects tend to lower serum calcium concentration. Calcitonin is important in the control of hypercalcemia in lower animals but has never been demonstrated to be physiologically important in this regard in human beings.

Hyperparathyroidism

PATHOLOGY. Parathyroid. Primary hyperparathyroidism may be due to a parathyroid adenoma, hyperplasia, or carcinoma of the parathyroid glands possibly from a nonparathyroid tumor that is producing a parathyroidlike substance. The symptoms are similar whatever the actual cause of the primary hyperparathyroidism. It is also possible for a patient with secondary hyperparathyroidism due to renal or bowel disease to develop hypercalcemia. This condition is referred to as *tertiary hyperparathyroidism* but perhaps is better named *severe secondary hyperparathyroidism*.

The relative frequency of entities producing primary hyperparathyroidism is shown in Table 38-6. Several points are important to note. Primary chief cell hyperplasia was described by Cope in 1958. Hence studies that include data prior to 1958 can be misleading, for at that time multiple enlarged glands were called "multiple adenomas" instead of *hyperplasia*.

It is apparent that the incidence of primary chief cell hyperplasia differs markedly as diagnosed in different institutions. While some authors believe that an increased incidence of primary hyperplasia is due to the fact that primary hyperparathyroidism is diagnosed and operated upon earlier, most others believe that these discrepancies are the result of nonuniformity of diagnostic criteria among different pathologists. Furthermore, it has been shown by Edis et al. that when more glands are removed by the surgeon at operation, the diagnosis of hyperplasia is more likely to be made. In those series in which a high

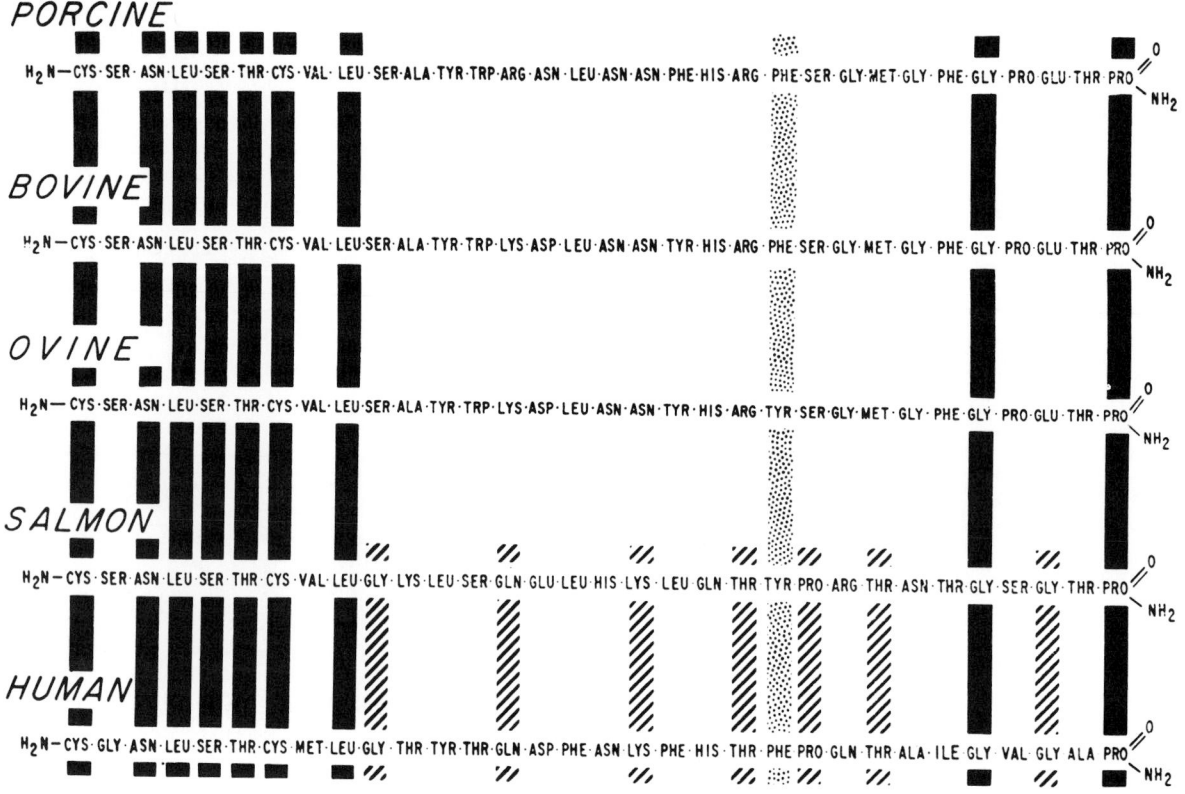

Fig. 38-30. Comparison of amino acid sequences of porcine, bovine, ovine, salmon, and human calcitonin. Solid bars indicate sequence positions homologous among all five molecules; cross-hatched bars indicate salmon and human calcitonin. [From: *Potts JT Jr et al, in Talmage RV, Munson PL (eds): Calcium Parathyroid Hormone and the Calcitonins. Proceedings of Fourth Parathyroid Conference, Excerpta Medica, Amsterdam, 1972, with permission.*]

incidence of primary chief cell hyperplasia is found, the surgeon usually practices subtotal parathyroidectomy as a routine procedure. When a single enlarged gland is removed by the surgeon it is most likely called an adenoma. The greatest differences of opinion relate to what constitutes *mild* hyperplasia. Some pathologists feel that normal-sized or mildly enlarged glands are hyperplastic if they do not contain enough extracellular fat. Others do not feel that these glands are abnormal and that the amount of *intracellular* fat is most important in this differentiation. Currently, most investigators believe that adenomas occur in 70 to 80 percent of patients, hyperplasia occurs in familial hyperparathyroidism and MEN syndromes, and carcinoma occurs in fewer than 1 percent of cases.

Knowledge of the normal development of parathyroid glands is imperative. From birth through three months of age, mean weight of the four parathyroid glands is 5 to 9 mg. There is then an almost linear increase in mean total parathyroid gland weight until the third to fourth decades, when it levels off at a mean of 117.6 mg for males and 131.3 mg for females. These changes in weight are accompanied by changes in histology of the gland. In children the gland is composed of fairly uniform sheets and cords of chief cells. The stroma has little or no mature fat cells, and oxyphil cells are absent. At puberty some mature fat cells appear. These increase in number through the remainder of life, and in older persons they may occupy 60

to 70 percent of the gland volume. Obese individuals have larger numbers of fat cells than one would expect for their age. Oxyphil cells also appear at puberty and show an increase with age. Chief cells and water-clear cells are thought to actively secrete PTH. Oxyphil cells have been thought of as inactive, but oxyphil adenomas certainly produce hypercalcemia.

To evaluate whether or not a parathyroid gland is normal, one must evaluate its size and weight, the number of chief cells, and the amount of fat that it contains in relation to the age of the individual.

The major problem for both the surgeon and the pathologist is to differentiate an adenoma from chief cell hyperplasia or single gland disease from multiglandular disease of the parathyroids. In general it is the surgeon who makes the diagnosis by recognizing whether one gland is enlarged (an adenoma) or multiple glands are enlarged (hyperplasia).

Adenomas. In the past the *sine qua non* for the diagnosis of a parathyroid adenoma was the presence of an enlarged hypercellular parathyroid gland with a rim or frag-

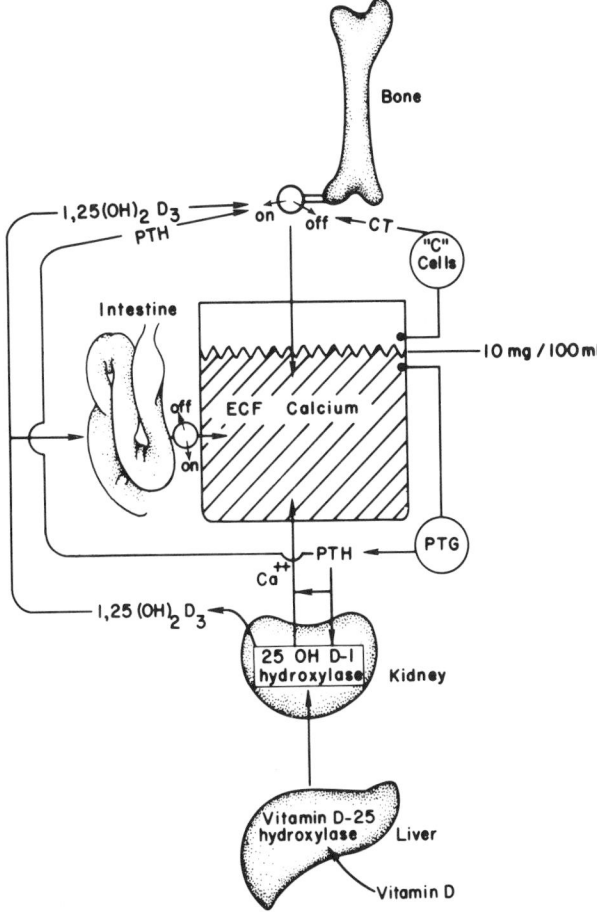

Fig. 38-31. Mechanism of calcium homeostasis. *Hypocalcemia* results in increased parathyroid hormone (PTH) secretion from the parathyroid glands (PTG). PTH acts directly on bone and on the kidney. PTH also results in an increase in the formation of 1,25-$(OH)_2D_3$ by the kidney, which acts on bone and promotes intestinal absorption of calcium as well. Each of these effects tends to raise the serum calcium concentration toward normal. *Hypercalcemia* results in a decrease in PTH secretion and a lesser production of 1,25-$(OH)_2D_3$. These changes tend to decrease serum calcium levels to normal. In human beings calcitonin secretion is not important in the physiologic control of hypercalcemia. (From: *DeLuca HF: Ann Intern Med 85:367, 1976, with permission.*)

ment of normal parathyroid that is being compressed by the adenoma. This is shown in Fig. 38-32. Currently the diagnosis is made by the recognition of a large hypercellular gland while the other parathyroid glands are normal.

Grossly adenomas are usually reddish brown, though they may be yellow-brown, particularly in older people. At times they may be very difficult to distinguish grossly from thyroid tissue, particularly when embedded in the thyroid. They are usually soft and smooth, and the surface is very vascular, bleeding easily when rubbed. They are generally not adherent to the surrounding structures. On occasion they contain cysts, hemorrhage, or areas of calcification.

Microscopically chief cell adenomas are composed of closely packed small cells that resemble the cells of the

normal parathyroid except that they are more tightly packed and there is little or no fat seen. A glandular pattern is sometimes seen.

The water-clear, or *wasserhellen*, adenomas have large vacuolated cells with clear cytoplasm arranged in a uniform pattern. Oxyphil adenomas have cells with a pink cytoplasm. Undoubtedly oxyphil cells can also secrete PTH, since adenomas of oxyphil cells can also cause hyperparathyroidism.

Hyperplasia. Although it is stated in most older texts that the most common type of hyperplasia is the water-clear cell type, this no longer is true. Almost all cases of hyperplasia are of the chief cell type. Primary chief cell hyperplasia cannot be differentiated by light microscopy from the chief cell hyperplasia that is always present in secondary hyperparathyroidism, although there are ultrastructural differences.

In water-clear hyperplasia, the glands may be very large, the total weight of all four glands ranging up to as much as 70 g. Their huge size plus the striking chocolate color makes them very easy to recognize.

Primary Chief Cell Hyperplasia. This condition was first described by Cope et al. in 1958. The incidence of this disease entity became more common as it was recognized that many cases thought to be multiple parathyroid adenomas were in reality chief cell hyperplasia. This disease entity is almost invariably encountered when surgical treatment of the parathyroid glands is carried out in patients with familial hyperparathyroidism and in patients with multiple endocrinopathies. (MEN syndromes).

It may sometimes be extremely difficult to differentiate chief cell hyperplasia from the typical parathyroid adenoma if only one gland is examined (Fig. 38-33). Roth and other pathologists believe that grossly and histologically a single hyperplastic gland is *indistinguishable* from an adenomatous gland. Classically, one expects each of the four glands to be enlarged; however, it is known that the size of glands may be very asymmetrical, and one or more glands may appear relatively normal. Thus, we think that it is wise to evaluate *all of the glands* of the neck before making a final decision.

Microscopically the cells appear identical to those of an adenoma (Fig. 38-34). There is a greater tendency, however, toward the appearance of many fibrous tissue septa, and the gland appears to have been composed of a number of nodules coalescing with each other. There are very few fatty cells.

The differentiation between chief cell hyperplasia and parathyroid adenoma is an important one, and can be made by inspecting all four parathyroid glands at operation for hyperparathyroidism, which is our practice.

Carcinoma. Carcinoma of the parathyroid is rare and probably represents no more than 1 percent of nonselected series. Many cases that have originally been thought to represent carcinoma have been discarded on review, since benign adenomas can sometimes have cells with bizarre nuclear patterns. Holmes et al. found 46 cases of hyperfunctioning parathyroid cancer and 4 cases of apparent nonfunctioning cancer when they reviewed the literature in 1969. In these 50 patients, 85 percent pre-

Table 38-6. RELATIVE FREQUENCY OF PARATHYROID ADENOMA, HYPERPLASIA, AND CARCINOMA IN REPORTED SERIES

Author and year	No. of patients	Adenoma %	Primary hyperplasia %	Carcinoma %
Goldman et al., 1971	300	96	3	1
Krementz et al., 1971	100	96	3	1
Hoehn et al., 1969	788	93	6	1
Davies, 1974	350	90	7	3
Palmer et al., 1975	250	90	9	<1
Satava et al., 1975	307	90	10	
Myers, 1974	185	82	11	1
Werner et al., 1974	129	84	14	1
Wang, 1976	431	82	14	4
Romanus et al., 1973	274	81	19	—
Block et al., 1974	121	80	20	—
Bruining, 1971	242	60	40	—
Haff and Armstrong, 1974	35	57	43	—
Esselstyn et al., 1974	100	51	49	—
Haff and Ballinger, 1971	74	50	50	—
Paloyan et al., 1973	84	33	65	2

SOURCE: Edis AJ: Surgical anatomy and technique of neck exploration for primary hyperparathyroidism. *Surg Clin North Am* 57:495, 1977, with permission.

sented with hypercalcemia. In fact 75 percent of patients with carcinoma have serum calcium concentrations greater than 14 mg/dL; only 9 percent of adenomas have serum calcium values over this level. Bone disease was present in 73 percent, a palpable neck mass in 52 percent, and renal disease in 32 percent. Thus, hypercalcemia and a palpable neck mass should alert one to the possibility of parathyroid carcinoma. Cervical metastases were found in 32 percent and distant metastases (liver, lung, bone, pancreas, and adrenal) in 21 percent. Cervical recurrences following surgery occurred in 65 percent of patients. Typically hypercalcemia recurred several months after surgery in many instances and was the first sign of recurrent tumor.

It is apparent that a diagnosis of malignant disease cannot be made by the histologic features of the tumor, a situation that also obtains in pheochromocytoma and other endocrine tumors. Very wild-looking tumors may

Fig. 38-32. Normal parathyroid compared with a chief cell adenoma. *A.* Photomicrograph of a normal parathyroid, below, adjacent to the thyroid gland, shown above. Note the abundant fat present in the normal gland. (×75.) *B.* Photomicrograph of a chief cell adenoma compressing the normal parathyroid beneath the capsule. The adenoma is the large mass shown to the right. The open spaces are blood vessels. The normal gland is the small rounded object shown to the left. The open spaces are fat cells. (×35.) *C.* Photomicrograph of a parathyroid adenoma shown below with the capsule separating it from the rim of normal parathyroid shown above. Note the fat in the normal parathyroid and the absence of fat cells in the adenoma. (×150.)

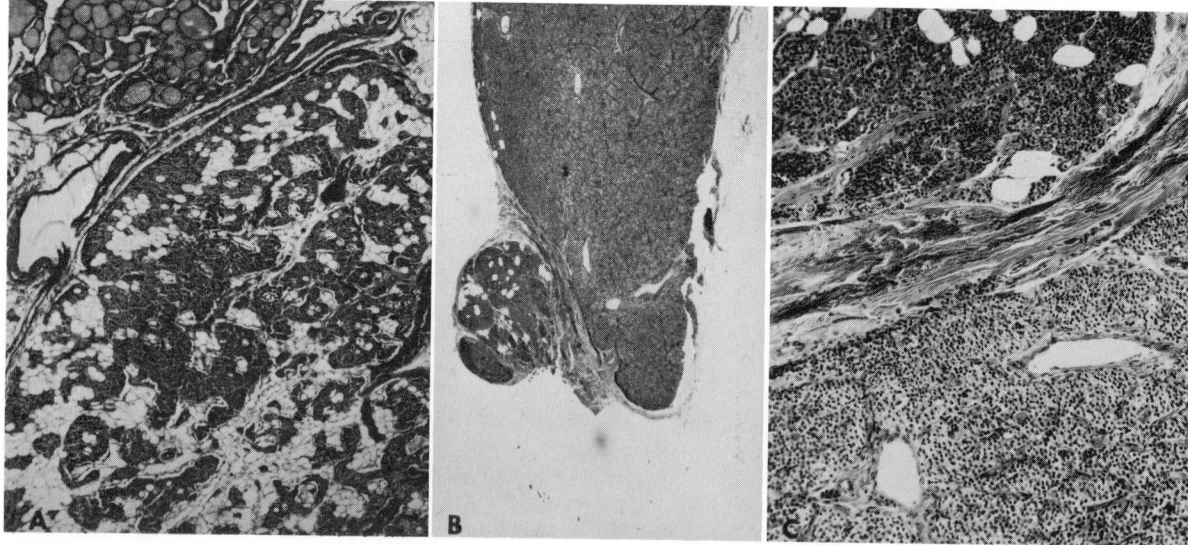

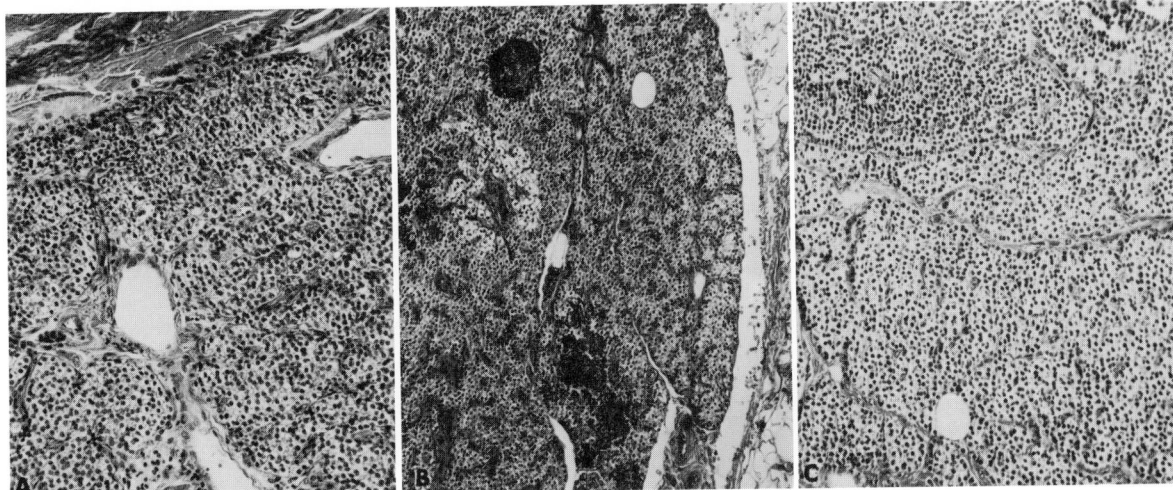

Fig. 38-33. Comparison of adenoma and hyperplasia. *A.* Detail of a chief cell adenoma adjacent to the capsule. Note the solid grouping of uniform chief cells, with absence of fat. (×200.) *B.* Chief cell hyperplasia. The cellular morphology is similar to that of the adenoma. Note the small focus of water-clear cells in the left central portion of the field. (×150.) *C.* Chief cell hyperplasia. Note the cords and small acinary groupings. (×200.)

pursue a completely benign course. The reverse is also true. Capsular infiltration is a particularly inadequate sign of malignancy, since this is often seen in benign adenomas. The only completely acceptable criteria for malignancy are recurrence of the tumor following removal, distant metastases, or invasion of adjacent structures. Some carcinomas can be identified grossly because they are attached to adjacent tissues by a thick fibrous capsule that gives the gland a whitish hue. Fifty percent of reported cases were adherent to or invading into adjacent structures at the time of surgery.

Death because of tumor growth and spread is rare. More commonly morbidity and mortality are related to the complications related to the persistent and progressive hypercalcemia, which is very difficult to control chronically. Because of this, Flye and Brennan recommend aggressive reoperation to try to totally excise or to debulk metastatic lesions. Schantz and Castleman collected 70 cases of proved parathyroid carcinoma in their review in 1973, and presently there are less than 100 cases in the literature. If the possibility of *carcinoma of the parathyroid gland* is entertained at operation, the lesion should be completely removed with an adequate margin of surrounding tissue, including the thyroid lobe on that side. Great care should be exercised *not* to enter the lesion or to spill tumor cells, since recurrent disease in the neck is very common. With good surgical technique and

Fig. 38-34. Comparison of water-clear and chief cell hyperplasia. *A.* Chief cell hyperplasia. The cells are small and uniform, with finely granular and transparent cytoplasm. (×400.) *B.* Water-clear cell hyperplasia. The tubules are well formed, and the cells are large and clear. (×200.) *C.* Water-clear cell hyperplasia: a higher magnification of *B.* (×400.) *(Photograph courtesy of Saul Kay.)*

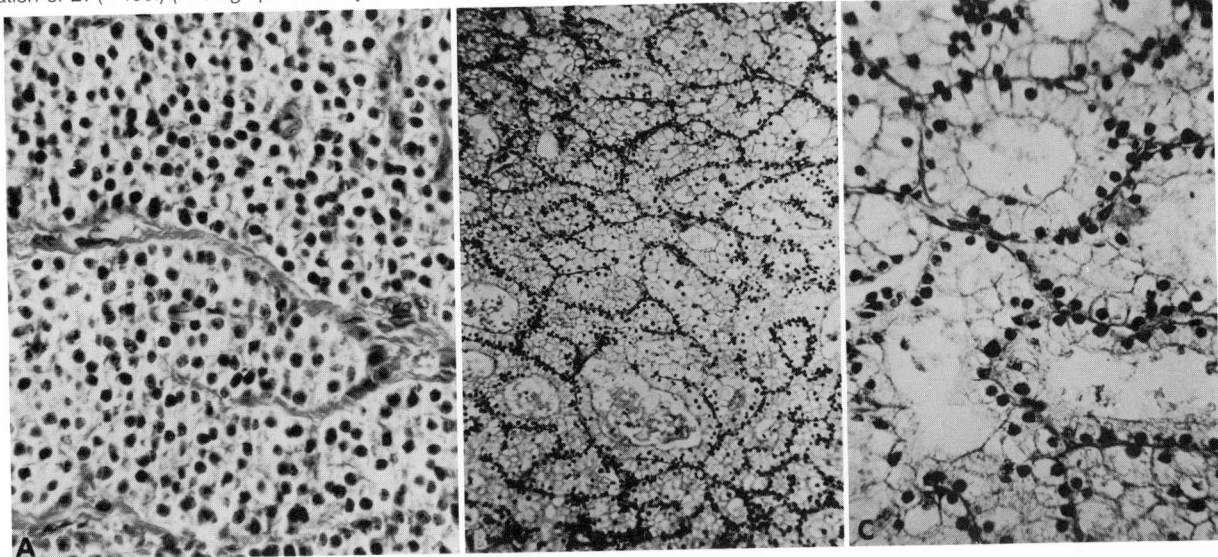

an en bloc resection much of this local recurrence is avoidable.

Hypercalcemia Associated with Nonparathyroid Malignancies. It has long been known that on occasion neoplasms can produce a variety of polypeptide hormones identical or biologically similar to ACTH, melanocyte-stimulating hormone (MSH), follicle-stimulating hormone (FSH), antidiuretic hormone (ADH), insulin, and chorionic gonadotropin. It is now clear that some tumors also produce PTH-like circulating hormones or prostaglandin E_2, each of which may result in hypercalcemia.

The most common cause of hypercalcemia of malignant disease is osseous metastasis. Normal radiographs do not always exclude the presence of bone metastases. Bachman and Sproul in a series of autopsies found that only one-half of the cases with histologically documented skeletal metastases had radiographic findings indicative of metastatic cancer. The use of bone scans has helped to diagnose some of these occult metastases.

One cause of hypercalcemia associated with malignant tumor without apparent skeletal metastases is the secretion of a PTH-like substance by the malignant tumor. This clinical syndrome of a nonparathyroid tumor associated with hypercalcemia and hypophosphatemia has been referred to as *pseudohyperparathyroidism*, or *ectopic hyperparathyroidism*.

Typically, the removal of tumors of this type has been associated many times with a prompt fall of serum calcium concentration to normal as demonstrated in the case of hypernephroma reported by Plimpton and Gelhorn. The reappearance of metastases may be associated with an elevation of the serum calcium level.

Although a number of tumors can produce ectopic hyperparathyroidism, the most common are squamous cell and small cell carcinomas of the lung, and hypernephromas. Other less common neoplasms include hepatoma and cancer of the ovary, stomach, pancreas, parotid gland, and colon.

The hypercalcemia of breast cancer has not been demonstrated to be due to ectopic hyperparathyroidism. It has been postulated, but never proved, that a *vitamin D-like sterol* is responsible for hypercalcemia in patients with this tumor in whom no bone metastases are found. Most cases of hypercalcemia of breast cancer do not have hypophosphatemia. When a low serum phosphorus level is present with hypercalcemia, one should consider the possibility of a coincident parathyroid adenoma. Samaan and coworkers recently reported that 35 percent of patients with different types of malignancy and hypercalcemia were subsequently proved to have *coexistent primary hyperparathyroidism*. Thus, this diagnostic possibility should not be excluded because the patient has a malignancy.

In addition to ectopic PTH secretion, several other humoral factors have been associated with the hypercalcemia of some malignancies. One factor is prostaglandin E_2. Seyberth and associates demonstrated that patients with various malignant tumors and hypercalcemia had elevated concentrations of metabolites of prostaglandins.

In several of their patients, treatment with aspirin or indomethacin (which decreases prostaglandin production) resulted in a lowering of the serum calcium levels to normal. Prostaglandin E_2 appears to result in hypercalcemia by stimulating bone resorption and may be an important causative agent for the hypercalcemia of malignancy in some patients.

Finally, Mundy and associates have described a factor that they call *osteoclast activating factor* (OAF). This is produced by myeloma and other lymphoid cells and causes bone resorption. It may be the cause of hypercalcemia in some patients with hematologic diseases. A great deal of investigation is continuing in the area of hypercalcemia in neoplastic diseases.

The differentiation of ectopic hyperparathyroidism from primary hyperparathyroidism due to parathyroid gland disease is often difficult. Lafferty suggests that ectopic hyperparathyroidism is more likely when the serum calcium concentration exceeds 14 mg/dL, when serum alkaline phosphatase activity is increased, when osteitis fibrosa is absent, and when there is a significant degree of anemia. Conversely, primary hyperparathyroidism is more likely with a long-standing history of repeated renal lithiasis or with radiographic evidence of osteitis fibrosa.

CLINICAL MANIFESTATIONS. Incidence. Hyperparathyroidism very rarely occurs under the age of puberty, although a very few instances of neonatal familial hyperparathyroidism have been reported. The most common age is between thirty and seventy. Women over sixty have the highest incidence in some series.

Hyperparathyroidism is more common in women than in men, in a ratio of at least 2:1. Originally, most patients were diagnosed as having primary hyperparathyroidism because they had severe bone disease. Later it was recognized that renal stones were more prevalent. More recently, hypertension, ulcer disease, pancreatitis, and mental disorders served as clues to this diagnosis. Primary hyperparathyroidism is being diagnosed in many relatively asymptomatic individuals who are found to have an elevated serum calcium level on routine multiphasic serum chemistry screening programs. The minimum incidence of primary hyperparathyroidism in the Rochester, Minnesota, area now exceeds 0.1 percent of the population. In other series, an incidence of primary hyperparathyroidism as high as 0.5 percent of the general population has been noted. Many patients in this recent group have only mild symptoms.

The incidence of hyperparathyroidism in patients who have had urinary calcium stones is variously estimated to be between 2.5 and 15 percent. The mean figure is somewhere around 5 percent.

Symptoms. When the disease of hyperparathyroidism was first recognized, it was thought to be a skeletal disease, and it was not until 7 years after the first patient had been operated upon that it was recognized that the disease could occur only with renal manifestations. Now the disease is seldom seen with marked skeletal involvement, because it is usually recognized long before this occurs. With the widespread application of multiphasic blood

Table 38-7. CLUES TO THE DIAGNOSIS OF HYPERPARATHYROIDISM IN THE FIRST 343 CASES AT THE MASSACHUSETTS GENERAL HOSPITAL

Clue	Number of cases
Renal stones	195
Bone disease	80
Peptic ulcer	27
Fatigue	10
Pancreatitis	9
Central nervous system signs	7
Hypertension	6
Mental disturbance	3
Multiple endocrine abnormalities	3
No symptoms (routine laboratory test)	2
Lump in neck	1

SOURCE: From Cope, 1966, with permission.

screening, more asymptomatic or mildly symptomatic (anxiety, depression, abdominal pain) patients are being discovered. In the Rochester, Minnesota, group, 49 percent had one or more of these serious complications possibly attributable to primary hyperparathyroidism: hypertension, 35 percent; renal stone disease, 25 percent; psychiatric symptoms, 21 percent; decreased renal function, 16 percent; and subperiosteal bone resorption, 5 percent.

The clues that first led to the diagnosis in 343 cases of the Massachusetts General Hospital series are shown in Table 38-7. As expected, renal stones head the list, with bone disease a distant second. Peptic ulcer and pancreatitis form a small but important minority, while 20 of the patients complained only of fatigue, mental disturbance, or central nervous system signs. Familial cases are sometimes diagnosed after diagnosis of one member of the family and subsequent screening of the kindred. A careful study of patients who are recurrent renal stone formers will establish the diagnosis of hyperparathyroidism in 2.5 to 12.5 percent of the cases. The causes of the symptomatology of hyperparathyroidism are shown in Table 38-8.

Renal Damage. The renal damage that occurs in this disease is a consequence both of the hypercalcemia and of the increased secretion of PTH. Hypersecretion of PTH results in increased excretion of phosphate and in relative urinary alkalosis, both of which may predispose to calcium precipitation. Urinary calcium excretion is also greatly increased. Kidney stones, nephrocalcinosis, polyuria, and polydypsia frequently occur.

Demineralization of the Skeleton. As a consequence of the increased bone resorption brought about by PTH the skeleton becomes demineralized and bone cysts, brown tumors, and pathologic fractures occur. Some degree of pathologic change in bone is present in virtually every case of hyperparathyroidism. This is frequently not detectable by the usual clinical means, however, and in many instances the patients do not have symptoms relating to the bones. The presence of demonstrable bony changes relates to the severity and the duration of the disease.

Cysts and tumors of the jaw are sometimes the presenting complaint. Vague pains in the back, hip, or shoulder, often thought by the patient to be arthritis, are sometimes present. In the more long-standing cases the stature may decrease, and a bowing of the spine and pathologic fractures may be apparent.

Joint Pains. Many patients also suffer from joint pains. This is due to *pseudogout,* a condition in which calcium pyrophosphate crystals are present in the joint fluid.

Table 38-8. CAUSES OF SYMPTOMS OF HYPERPARATHYROIDISM

Cause	Symptoms and signs
Hypercalcemia	Renal damage Mental: Depression, fatigue, delerium, coma Muscle: General muscle weakness and hypotonia, walking with cane, hypoactive reflexes Gastrointestinal: Peptic ulcer, constipation, gastric disturbance, loss of appetite, pancreatitis (?) Eye changes: Band keratitis, calcium in palpebral fissure Ectopic calcification Hypercalcemic crisis: Profound muscle weakness, nausea and vomiting, lethargy and drowsiness, confusion, bone pain, abdominal pain, thirst, polyuria, constipation, coma, hypertension, fever, ECG changes, short Q-T interval and nearly absent ST segment, azotemia with increased PO_4, and hypokalemia
Increased urinary calcium	Polyuria, polydipsia, and hypokalemia
Hypomagnesemia	Paresthesias, hyperreflexia
Direct action of PTH	Demineralization of the skeleton due to bone resorption: Bone pain, cysts, known tumors, fractures Renal damage Peptic ulcer (?) Pancreatitis (?)
Renal damage	Hypertension Renal stones, nephrocalcinosis

Often the arthritis-like symptoms improve after parathyroidectomy.

Peptic Ulcer (Questionable). Though it was originally thought that patients with primary hyperparathyroidism have a greatly increased incidence of peptic ulcers, this view has been challenged. It is well known that patients with severe ulcer diatheses and hyperparathyroidism are often markedly improved by parathyroidectomy and the return of their serum calcium level to normal. In these patients after parathyroidectomy, the gastric acid secretion falls dramatically and the ulcer may even heal. However, many of these individuals later prove to have a Zollinger-Ellison syndrome (gastrinoma) and their hyperparathyroidism is part of the multiple endocrine neoplasia, type 1, syndrome. If this group of Zollinger-Ellison patients with hypercalcemia is eliminated from consideration, it is difficult to demonstrate a truly increased incidence of peptic ulcer disease in patients with primary hyperparathyroidism.

Hypercalcemia acts to stimulate the parietal cells directly and also acts by increasing the serum gastrin levels. In patients with duodenal ulcer acid output rises to about 30 percent of maximal Histalog (beta-zole) stimulation. In Zollinger-Ellison patients, calcium-stimulated acid secretion equals that produced by maximal stimulation by Histalog. A marked increase of serum gastrin occurs as well. Calcium infusion with measurement of gastrin and gastric acid output is one of the most reliable provocative tests for Zollinger-Ellison tumors.

Patients with parathyroid disease and hypercalcemia without the Zollinger-Ellison syndrome have been demonstrated to have mildly elevated serum gastrin concentrations that return to normal after parathyroidectomy and restoration of normocalcemia. On the other hand, it has *not* been conclusively demonstrated that patients with primary hyperparathyroidism have statistically increased acid secretion as a group.

The incidence of peptic ulcer and hyperparathyroidism is probably somewhere around 10 percent. Incidences as high as this have been reported in some groups of normal population, and doubt has been expressed as to whether there really is an association between peptic ulcer and hyperparathyroidism.

Our view is that it is uncertain that hyperparathyroidism directly causes duodenal ulcer disease. In individuals who have an ulcer diathesis, however, this may be worsened by the hypercalcemia of parathyroid disease. Because 20 percent of patients with Zollinger-Ellison syndrome have associated parathyroid gland abnormalities, this islet cell tumor must be ruled out in any hypercalcemic individual with an ulcer by obtaining a serum gastrin determination and making other appropriate tests.

Pancreatitis (Questionable). The relation between hyperparathyroidism and pancreatitis seems less secure. If the relationship does exist, it is probably due to the effect of either hypercalcemia or PTH on the precipitation of calcium salts from the pancreatic juice. Although calcification of the pancreas occurs in some patients with hyperparathyroidism, it is frequently only an incidental finding. Pyrah et al. suggest that the cases in which pancreatitis and hyperparathyroidism are associated fall into six groups:

1. One or more attacks of acute pancreatitis following which the diagnosis of hyperparathyroidism is established. With removal of the parathyroid adenoma there are no further attacks of pancreatitis, and the serum amylase returns to normal.
2. Acute pancreatitis occurring as a complication of operation for the removal of a parathyroid adenoma.
3. Acute pancreatitis occurring as a complication of some unrelated operation in a patient with hyperparathyroidism, as, for example, the removal of a renal calculus.
4. Acute pancreatitis occurring as a complication of acute hypercalcemic crisis due to hyperparathyroidism.
5. Chronic pancreatitis manifested by recurring attacks of abdominal pain and associated with pancreatic calculi in patients with hyperparathyroidism.
6. Development of hypercalcemia (tertiary hyperparathyroidism) in a patient with known chronic pancreatitis, steatorrhea, and secondary hyperparathyroidism.

The incidence of pancreatitis associated with hyperparathyroidism has not been definitely established, but in the series reported by Mixter et al. it was about 7 percent. In carcinoma of the parathyroid and familial hyperparathyroidism the incidence of pancreatitis is somewhat higher.

Hypertension. Although the association of hypertension with hyperparathyroidism is well known, the mechanism is still uncertain. Some feel that it is likely that in almost all instances this is due to the renal damage brought about by the disease and not to any direct effect of PTH itself. A role of hypercalcemia, per se, as well as of serum renin in the pathogenesis of primary hyperparathyroidism has also been postulated. Urinary calcium excretion is also greatly increased. Kidney stones, nephrocalcinosis, polyuria, and polydypsia frequently occur.

Mental Changes. Patients with hypercalcemia frequently complain of mental symptoms consisting of depression, fatigue, listlessness, and occasionally confusion. The patients may be irritable or regressive, subject to crying spells, or simply depressed. In some individuals with severe hypercalcemia, delirium and even coma may occur, while others tolerate the same increase in serum calcium with few symptoms. Correction of the hyperparathyroidism and hypercalcemia results in a reversion to a normal mental state in many but not all persons.

Muscle Weakness. Generalized muscle weakness is common in hypercalcemia and is associated with hypotonia and hyporeflexia.

Eye Changes. Band keratitis and calcium in the palpebral fissure are seen in hypercalcemia of various causes.

Ectopic Calcification. Ectopic calcification occasionally occurs in primary hyperparathyroidism, almost always in association with gross pathologic changes in bone. It occurs in only a small percentage of patients and is not a particularly valuable sign of this disease.

Hypercalcemic Crisis. This is sometimes called "acute hyperparathyroidism," or "parathyroid crisis," but since the signs and symptoms are common to those of hypercalcemia of any origin (for example, breast cancer), it seems best to refer to it as *acute hypercalcemic crisis.* In hyperparathyroidism this usually does not eventuate until

Table 38-9. SYMPTOMS AND SIGNS IN 42 PATIENTS WITH HYPERCALCEMIC
CRISIS DUE TO HYPERPARATHYROIDISM

Symptoms	Percent of cases	Signs	Percent of cases
Muscular weakness	80	Hypotonia	44
Nausea and vomiting	80	Neck mass	42
Weight loss	65	Hypertension	35
Fatigue	65	Dehydration	31
Lethargy and drowsiness	65	Tachycardia	26
Confusion	57	Fever	22
Bone pain	55	Abdominal tenderness and distention	15
Abdominal pain	48	Band keratopathy	9
Polyuria	40	Tracheal deviation	4
Constipation	37		
Coma	26		
Polydipsia	24		
Renal colic	22		
Neck swelling	9		
Dysphagia and neck pain	4		

SOURCE: From Lemann and Donatelli, 1964, with permission.

the serum calcium level rises to 16 mg/dL or above. It is equally common in males and females, while hyperparathyroidism itself is twice as common in females as in males. It is much more apt to occur in the presence of severe renal damage, and at least 90 percent of the patients have some degree of renal failure. The patient has usually had a long-standing history of skeletal or renal involvement with more recent symptoms of loss of appetite and weight, nausea and vomiting, constipation, thirst and polyuria, and generalized muscular weakness. The relative frequency of the symptoms is shown in Table 38-9.

If the early symptoms of hypercalcemic crisis are ignored, they may progress to the more serious ones of lethargy and drowsiness, confusion, severe muscular weakness, prostration, and coma. The electrocardiographic changes of hypercalcemia do not usually make their appearance until the calcium levels are quite high, but they may be seen in hypercalcemic crisis and consist of a short Q-T interval and a nearly absent ST segment. Fever and tachycardia may be present. Occasionally there is an association of acute pancreatitis, and a rising blood urea nitrogen (BUN) level is common.

The mortality and morbidity of acute parathyroid crisis has been very high in the past, especially in the medically treated group. In recent years treatment with saline and lasix has facilitated both rehydration and a lowering of the serum calcium level. However, prolonged medical therapy continues to be associated with a high mortality. The optimal treatment therefore depends upon rapid resuscitation with saline and lasix, making a correct diagnosis of hyperparathyroidism as soon as possible, and early operation with correction of the hyperparathyroid state. Under these circumstances, mortality is low and the results are gratifying.

Patients whose severe hypercalcemia is not due to hyperparathyroidism should be treated by a medical regimen to lower the serum calcium concentration. Often

dramatic changes in their mental function occur as their serum calcium level returns to normal.

Physical Findings

It is seldom possible to palpate the parathyroid adenoma, except in patients with hypercalcemic crisis, where the adenoma is usually very large and can be felt in 40 percent of the cases. Apart from this circumstance, the adenoma can be felt in only about 5 percent of the cases or less. A large parathyroid malignant tumor may be palpable.

DIAGNOSTIC FINDINGS. Calcium, PTH, Phosphate, Alkaline Phosphatase, and Chloride Measurements. The diagnosis of hyperparathyroidism in most cases rests upon biochemical determinations. The most important of these is demonstrating an elevation of the *serum calcium level.* The normal range varies in different laboratories depending on the techniques used. In our own the normal range is generally considered to be between 8.5 and 10.2 mg/dL. The calcium level may be very close to the normal range or may fluctuate from the normal levels to slightly elevated levels. Measurements should be repeated over a period of months or even years in borderline cases until the diagnosis is firmly established. Bartter and associates have popularized the concept of "normocalcemic hyperparathyroidism" in which renal stones occur in patients with totally normal serum calcium concentrations. We agree that many patients with renal stones have only minimally elevated serum calcium values, but question whether or not those with perfectly normal values truly have primary hyperparathyroidism.

In order to interpret the calcium level adequately it is helpful to get a serum total protein determination or an ionized calcium value. It is well known that the protein-bound calcium varies with the serum protein concentration. Since it is only the *ionized calcium* that is physiologically active, it has been suggested that measurements of the ionized calcium would be more valuable than measurements of the total calcium. Ionized calcium has become much easier to measure because of the electrode systems that are available. Ionized calcium concentrations are occasionally elevated in primary hyperparathyroidism when total calcium is normal. It is of course essential to rule out other possible causes for the elevated serum calcium level before concluding that the patient has hyperparathyroidism.

The *serum phosphate level* is low in about 80 percent of cases. A normal value does not rule out primary hyperparathyroidism. Low values may occur, especially in malnutrition. Furthermore, it may rise considerably in patients with hyperparathyroidism in whom significant renal damage has developed.

The *serum alkaline phosphatase level* is elevated in hyperparathyroidism only when there is x-ray evidence of bone disease, and it is frequently elevated in other conditions. This has not proved to be a helpful diagnostic test in our experience.

Wills and McGowan have reported that the *plasma chloride level* is elevated in patients with primary hyperparathyroidism who do not have renal impairment and are not on diuretics. It was found to be higher than 102 meq/L in all except 1 of 33 patients with hyperparathyroidism, whereas it was less than 102 meq/L in all 28 patients with hypercalcemia due to other causes. The *chloride-to-phosphate ratio* is also helpful. When greater than 33, it is virtually diagnostic of primary hyperparathyroidism.

Plasma PTH Measurements. Measurement of PTH in serum by radioimmunoassay has been shown to be a very important and valuable tool for the diagnosis of hyperparathyroidism, since it provides a direct measurement of the hormone whose hypersecretion causes the disease. A patient who has hypercalcemia and an elevated serum PTH concentration has hyperparathyroidism—most often due to excessive parathyroid function in the neck but occasionally due to ectopic hyperparathyroidism.

Measurement of PTH by immunoassay proved to be difficult in the past. Circulating PTH in hyperparathyroidism is heterogeneous. At least three distinct fragments of PTH ranging in molecular weight from 4000 to 10,000 have been identified. The major ones are an N-terminal and a C-terminal fragment. Different antisera detect different parts of the PTH molecule and hence measure all or only some of the these PTH fragments. The amino (NH_2) terminal end of the PTH molecule confers the biological effects of parathyroid hormone. Antisera directed against this part of the molecule measure physiologic secretion rates. However, it has been clearly demonstrated that antisera directed against the carboxyl fragments (C-terminal) or the mid-molecular fragments of PTH are much better for diagnosing clinical primary hyperparathyroidism. This is because the C-terminal fragment is more slowly metabolized than the N-terminal fragment, which is short-lived in the serum.

An example of the value of direct measurement of plasma PTH is demonstrated in Fig. 38-35. Reiss and Canterbury were able to differentiate normal patients from those with primary hyperparathyroidism and others with hypoparathyroidism. In secondary hyperparathyroidism the serum PTH level is also elevated. In chronic renal failure, for example, circulating PTH varies inversely with the creatinine clearance; as renal function deteriorates, the PTH level rises to very high levels. Elevation of both the serum calcium and PTH levels is diagnostic of primary or tertiary hyperparathyroidism or less

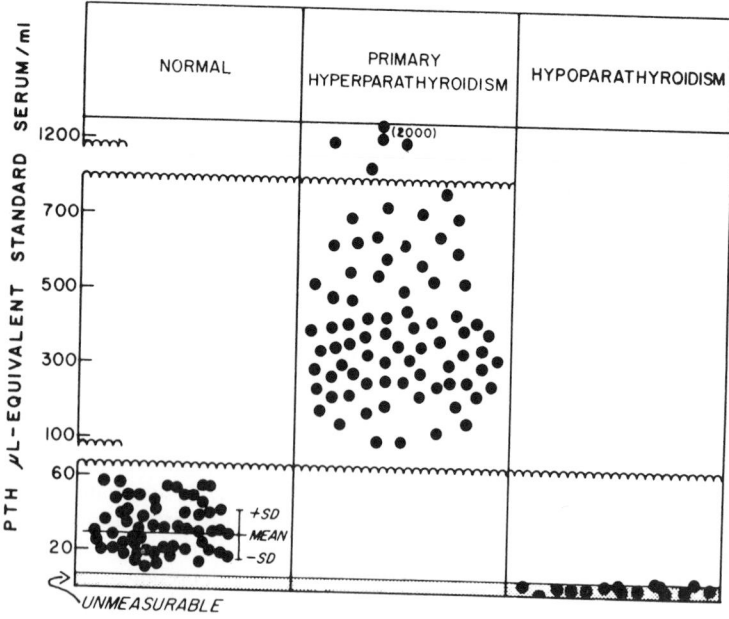

Fig. 38-35. Results of radioimmunoassay of PTH in normal subjects and patients with primary hyperparathyroidism and with hypoparathyroidism. The units of PTH in this figure relate the potency of test sera to that of an arbitrarily selected hyperparathyroid serum. In the hyperparathyroid group, the presence of disease was confirmed surgically in all instances. (From: *Reiss E, Canterbury JM: Am J Med 50:679, 1971, with permission.*)

commonly of ectopic secretion of PTH from a tumor; all other causes of hypercalcemia are associated with low PTH concentrations.

Urinary Calcium and Cyclic AMP Excretion. An elevated *urinary calcium level* is present in most cases of hyperparathyroidism but is certainly not diagnostic of this disease.

Cyclic AMP concentrations in the urine are elevated in about 80 to 90 percent of patients with primary hyperparathyroidism and fall to normal within 60 min after the hyperparathyroid state has been corrected. Several groups have used this measurement intraoperatively in difficult cases to predict that a cure has been achieved.

Tubular Resorption of Phosphate (TRP) Tests. One of the actions of PTH is to decrease the tubular absorption of phosphate. Thus, in selected cases the TRP is helpful in making a diagnosis of primary hyperparathyroidism. The formula for computing the TRP is

$$1 - \frac{UP \times SC}{SP \times UC} \times 100 = TRP$$

where UP = urinary phosphorus
SC = serum creatinine
SP = serum phosphorus
UC = urinary creatinine

The normal value is between 85 and 95 percent, whereas with hyperparathyroidism it falls to 35 to 85 percent. Although the TRP test is certainly not without error, it provides additional information that may help to confirm the diagnosis.

Cortisone Administration (Dent Test). The oral administration of 150 mg of cortisone daily for 10 days has been shown to reduce the serum calcium to normal levels in patients with hypercalcemia due to vitamin D intoxication or sarcoidosis, whereas the hypercalcemia of hyperparathyroidism is usually unaltered. Cortisone also usually reduces the hypercalcemia due to carcinomatosis and multiple myeloma.

Bone Biopsy. Even when no gross bone changes are discernible on x-ray, changes in the bone in hyperparathyroidism can almost always be detected on bone biopsy. A bone biopsy specimen can be taken from the iliac crest under local anesthesia. The findings may help to establish the diagnosis when added to all other evidence.

Bone Densitometry. Cameron and Sorenson introduced photon beam scanning of bone. This method appears to be very promising and is being tested in a number of centers. Changes in bone density as small as 5 to 10 percent may be measured by this means. In hyperparathyroidism there is frequently a loss of bone density that returns to normal after parathyroidectomy.

Radiography of Bones. The x-ray appearance of *advanced* hyperparathyroidism is characteristic. At times this will greatly aid in the diagnosis of primary hyperparathyroidism. X-rays of the skull may show the typical "moth-eaten" ground-glass skull of hyperparathyroidism (Fig. 38-36). In Paget's disease there is an overgrown fuzzy skull. In multiple myeloma there are many sharp,

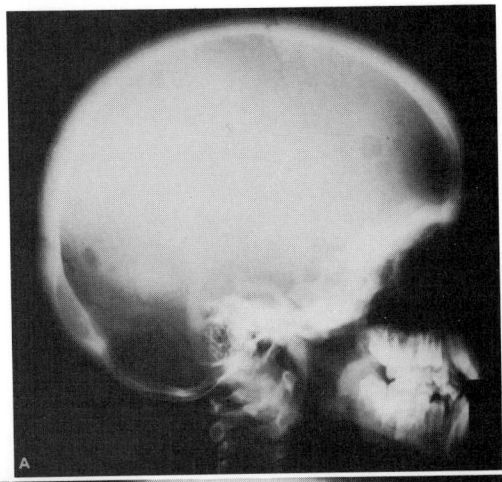
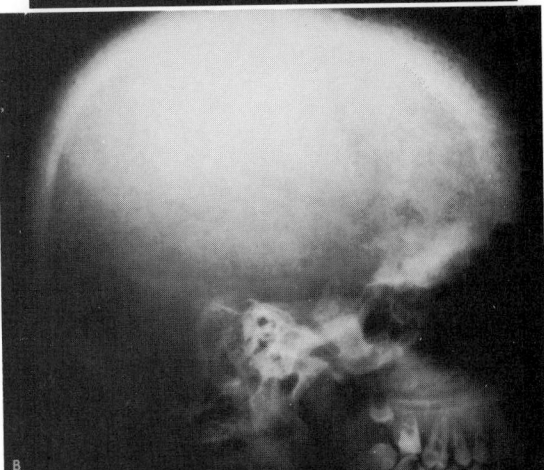
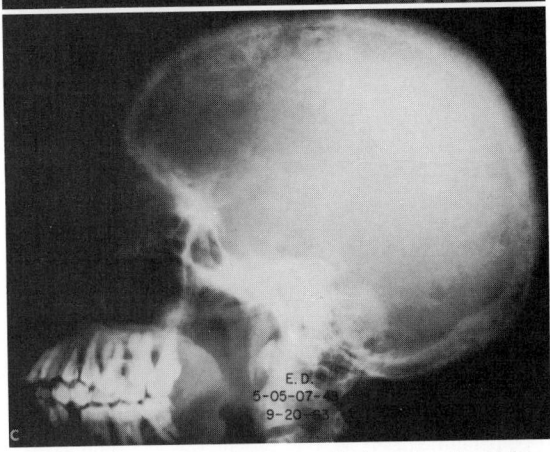

Fig. 38-36. Skull x-rays in patients with hyperparathyroidism. *A.* Lateral view of the skull in a child with secondary hyperparathyroidism due to renal failure. Note the punched-out lesions resembling multiple myeloma. *B.* Secondary hyperparathyroidism. Note the moth-eaten appearance of the skull. *C.* Primary hyperparathyroidism. Note the similarity between this and the patients with secondary hyperparathyroidism.

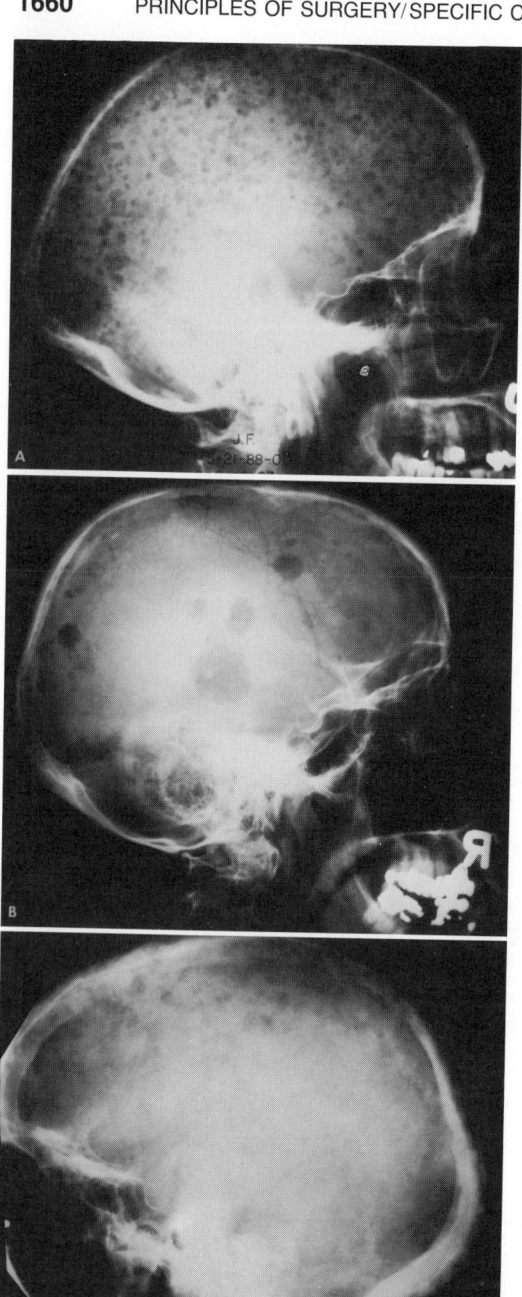

Fig. 38-37. Skull x-rays in patients with hypercalcemia but without hyperparathyroidism. *A.* This patient was admitted in a semi-comatose state with a serum calcium level of 21 mg/dL. The x-ray shows multiple small metastatic lesions. A bone biopsy showed metastatic squamous cell carcinoma. The metastases were ultimately demonstrated to have come from a squamous cell carcinoma of the esophagus. *B.* Skull metastases in carcinoma of the breast. *C.* Paget's disease. This disease is most often confused with hyperparathyroidism because of the bone changes. It can on occasion produce hypercalcemia.

punched-out areas, and metastatic cancer, especially that from the breast, can give a similar appearance (Fig. 38-37). Dental films often demonstrate an absence of the lamina dura, a line of calcification around each tooth, in patients with hyperparathyroidism.

In severe hyperparathyroidism, chest x-rays may show multiple bony lesions (Fig. 38-38*A*). X-rays of the clavicle often demonstrate a marked absorption of the distal third of the clavicle (Fig. 38-38*B*). The spine may show marked decalcification and wedging of the vertebrae (Fig. 38-39), resulting in kyphoscoliosis. The jaws are a favorite place for the development of osteoclastic bone tumors (Fig. 38-40*A*), and these may be seen in the metacarpals, metatarsals, and the ends of the long bones (Fig. 38-40*B*).

X-rays of the hands are particularly useful in diagnosis of hyperparathyroidism, since they may show the characteristic subperiosteal bone resorption in the middle and terminal phalanges of the fingers (Fig. 38-41). Soft tissue calcification is much more common in secondary than in primary hyperparathyroidism and still more common in vitamin D intoxication (Fig. 38-42).

In summary, in primary and secondary hyperparathyroidism bone changes may occur. Subperiosteal bone resorption of the middle and distal phalanges of the fingers and resorption of the distal end of the clavicle are the most common and useful diagnostic abnormalities noted. These abnormalities are pathognomonic of chronic, severe PTH excess.

Radiography of the Kidneys. A plain film of the kidneys will sometimes show renal calculi or nephrocalcinosis. Staghorn calculi may be present, as shown in Fig. 38-39. An example of nephrocalcinosis is shown in Fig. 38-43.

Localization of Hyperfunctioning Parathyroid Glands. A parathyroid adenoma is rarely palpable preoperatively. In about 5 percent of patients the hyperfunctioning gland is found in the chest, not in the neck at all. Furthermore, occasionally an enlarged parathyroid gland is difficult even for the experienced neck surgeon to find. For these reasons many attempts have been made to localize the enlarged overactive parathyroid gland or glands before operation. Until recently, most attempts have met with little success.

A chest x-ray will occasionally be helpful by demonstrating a mass in the mediastinum. On very rare occasions a barium swallow may demonstrate an indentation due to an enlarged parathyroid gland. Thermography has not proved to be useful. An isotope scan is an attractive idea; however, the use of [75]selenium methionine scanning, either preoperatively or at the operating table, has not proved to be of great value. We have recently visualized an adenoma using a gallium scan and another with a ^{99m}Tc scan. However, at present no isotope scan has great applicability. Ultrasonography has proved useful in locating enlarged parathyroid glands in the neck, and computerized tomography has localized about 50 percent of enlarged glands that are with the thymus gland in the chest. Other procedures utilizing PTH secretion have been of considerable help in some instances. Reiss has described the *parathyroid squeeze test.* Massage of the

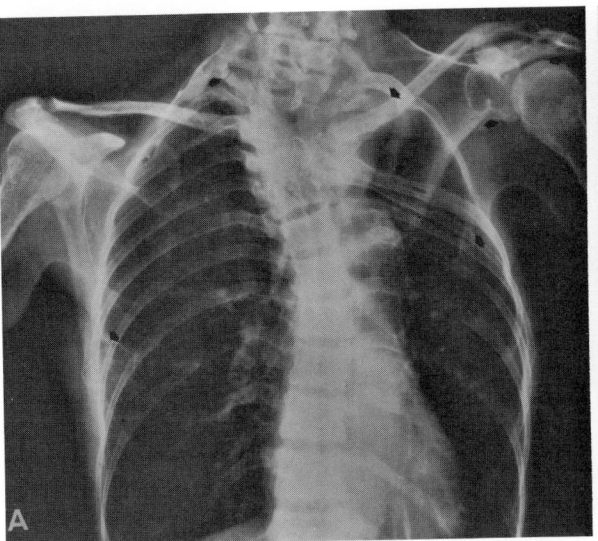
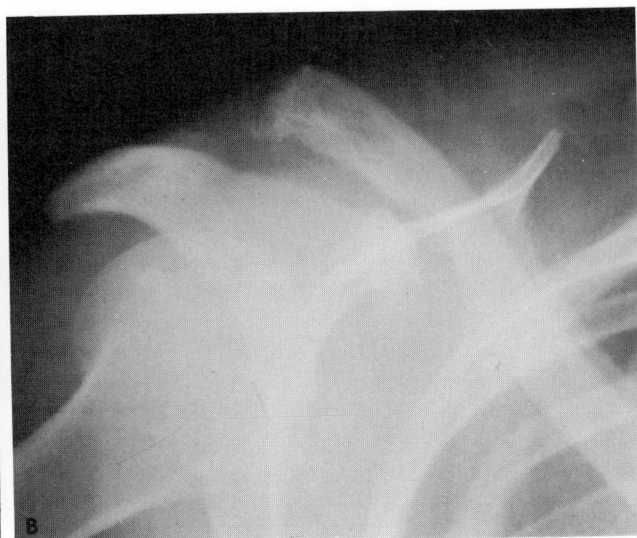

Fig. 38-38. Typical lesions of hyperparathyroidism. *A.* Multiple lesions of bones demonstrated on chest x-ray. Note the presence of scoliosis. *B.* Resorption of the outer end of the clavicle in a patient with secondary hyperparathyroidism. Similar lesions are seen in the primary disease.

Fig. 38-39. X-ray of the abdomen of a patient with primary hyperparathyroidism, showing bilateral staghorn calculi with severe osteoporosis, scoliosis, and splenic calcification. A parathyroid adenoma was removed, and this was followed by chemical and clinical improvement.

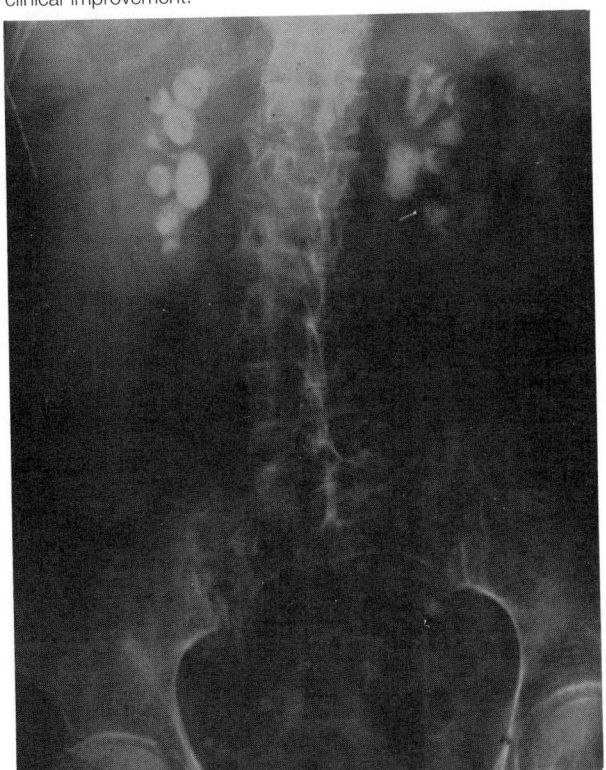

side of the neck harboring the parathyroid adenoma results in a rise of the peripheral serum PTH level. Massage of normal glands results in no change in serum PTH. In the presence of hyperplastic glands, a rise in peripheral serum PTH follows the massage of both sides of the neck, since this disease is bilateral. Catheterization of the large veins of the neck and mediastinum (the jugulars, innominate, and superior vena cava) with sampling of blood for serum PTH from various sites has successfully localized the site of abnormal parathyroid glands in some patients (Fig. 38-44). The serum PTH level will be highest at the site of drainage from a hyperfunctioning gland or glands.

A modification of this technique is more efficacious. The small veins draining the thyroid gland, as well as the large veins of the neck and chest, are catheterized and sampled for serum PTH (Fig. 38-45). An elevation of serum PTH on one side of the neck signifies an adenoma, while a gradient of PTH on neck veins of both sides signifies the presence of bilateral hyperplasia. Often this examination has been performed with arteriography (Fig. 38-46). Arteriography by itself may be helpful in localizing an enlarged parathyroid gland, since in some cases a vascular tumor blush is seen, or one inferior thyroid artery may be deviated from its normal position or may be larger than the other. However, several cases of hemiplegia and quadriplegia have followed highly selective inferior thyroid artery arteriography, presumably because of spinal cord injury. Hence, this technique should be used with the utmost of caution and only after careful consideration of alternative approaches.

Most endocrinologists and surgeons agree that venous catheterization studies and arteriography should *not* be done routinely on all patients before their initial parathyroid exploration. We reserve the use of this procedure for patients who have already had a negative neck exploration performed by a highly competent parathyroid surgeon. Its greatest potential usefulness is in the preoperative localization of a mediastinal parathyroid adenoma.

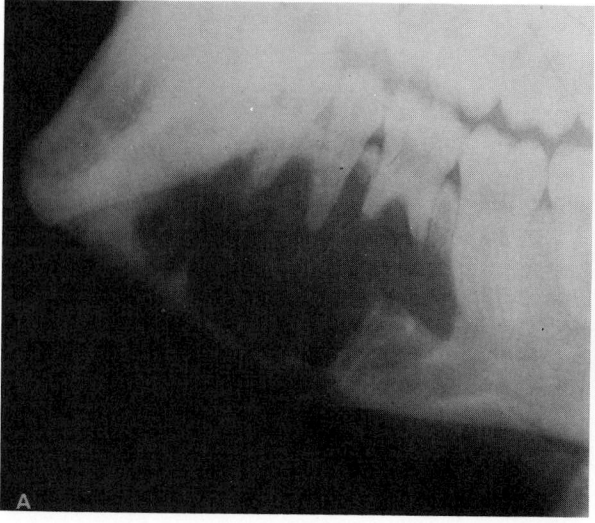
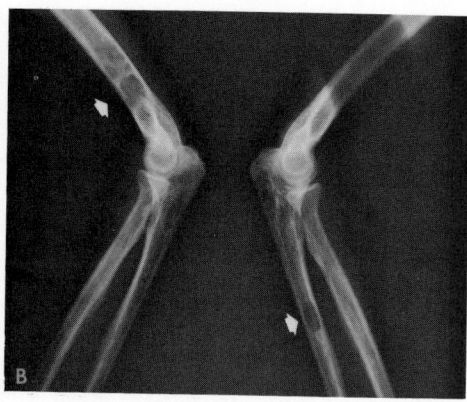

Fig. 38-40. Bone cysts and tumors in hyperparathyroidism. *A.* Bone cyst of the lower jaw. *B.* Cysts of long bones.

SPECIAL CONSIDERATIONS. Familial Hyperparathyroidism. The familial occurrence of hyperparathyroidism was first reported by Goldman and Smyth in 1936, who described a case in siblings. Since then a number of families have been reported in which more than one member has had hyperparathyroidism. Although the mode of inheritance has not been completely worked out, it has been assumed to be one of autosomal dominance with incomplete penetrance.

In familial hyperparathyroidism there is a high incidence of involvement of the glands by chief cell hyperplasia, and recurrence of the disease after operation is quite common. Occasionally, as in the cases reported by Stevens et al., however, the parathyroid involvement was by solitary adenomas in each case.

Familial hyperparathyroidism has been reported in conjunction with pancreatitis and with peptic ulceration. In one of the most convincing instances of familial hyperparathyroidism Cutler et al. reported a kindred involving 11 patients with hyperparathyroidism in two families in which the mothers were sisters and the fathers were brothers. In a recent study, in 11 percent of patients with primary hyperparathyroidism, other family members were proved to have this disease as well. Thus, a familial occurrence of primary hyperparathyroidism may be more common than previously considered.

Familial Hypocalciuric Hypercalcemia (FHH). In 1972, Foley and associates described a large family, many of whom had hypercalcemia, but none had complications of this abnormality. They called this condition *familial benign hypercalcemia.* In 1977, Marx and his group reported several other families with this condition, which they called *familial hypocalciuric hypercalcemia* (FHH) because there was no hypercalciuria in hypercalcemic members. Fifteen such kindreds have now been recognized.

The diagnosis is made by the recognition of hypercalcemia in many young family members, often before age ten—hypercalcemia without hypercalciuria and persistence of

hypercalcemia after standard subtotal parathyroidectomy. FHH is an autosomal dominant trait, with near 100 percent penetrance for all ages. While members often have fatigue, weakness, arthralgia, and polyuria, the incidence of nephrolithiasis or peptic ulcer is not increased over normal. These patients excrete very low amounts of calcium in their urine, usually less than 100 mg daily while eating a regular diet.

The diagnosis is important for the surgeon because standard subtotal parathyroidectomy is almost invariably followed by persistence of hypercalcemia. Total parathyroidectomy, on the other hand, leads to hypocalcemia. Thus, only a small amount of parathyroid tissue is capable of sustaining hypercalcemia.

Parathyroid surgery should be avoided unless symptoms or signs attributable to hypercalcemia are severe. If intervention is necessary, some recommend total parathyroidectomy with treatment of hypocalcemia if it occurs. Another possibility is total parathyroidectomy with parathyroid autotransplantation either immediately or after cryopreservation.

Surgeons should be especially wary of patients with primary hyperplasia who have not been cured by their initial operation.

Hyperparathyroidism in Children. Hyperparathyroidism is a rare occurrence before puberty. A few such cases have been reported, including neonates who have familial hyperparathyroidism.

The symptoms are the same as those recorded in the adult, including those referable to severe bone involvement. Duodenal ulcer has been reported, and joint abnormalities have occurred in 17 percent of the patients. Blindness was recorded in one case.

Acute hypercalcemic crisis has been recorded in neonates and in older children, with serum calcium values of over 20 mg/dL. The serum calcium values in children have generally been somewhat higher than those seen in adults.

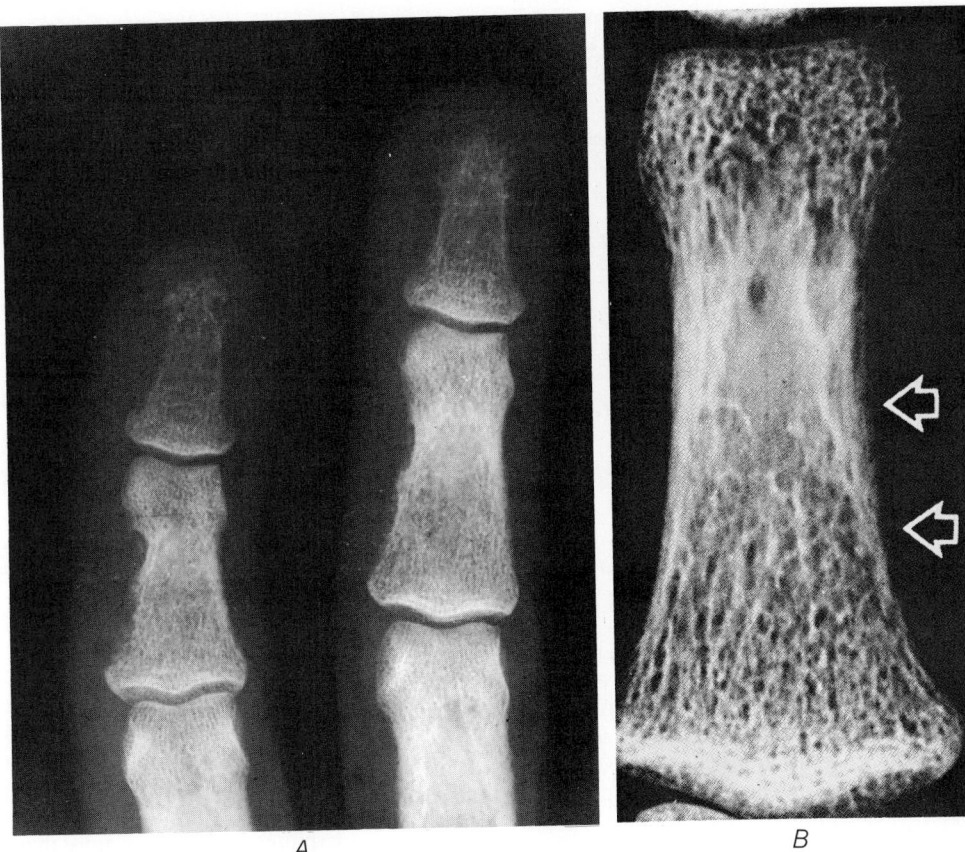

Fig. 38-41. X-rays of the fingers in primary and secondary hyperparathyroidism. *A.* Secondary hyperparathyroidism. Note the intense subperiosteal resorption of bone. This usually is most prominent on the radial side of the middle and distal phalanges of the index and middle fingers. *B.* Primary hyperparathyroidism. Many patients with primary hyperparathyroidism have normal hand films with conventional radiographic techniques. With *fine-detail* radiography, subtle cases of subperiosteal bone resorption can be recognized. Mild subperiosteal bone resorption (arrows) of middle phalanx in a patient with a parathyroid adenoma. (From: *Genant HK et al: Radiology 109:513, 1973, with permission.*)

Pregnancy. Fertility does not seem to be greatly depressed in hyperparathyroidism, and labor and delivery are not influenced by it. The birth weight of infants born to mothers who are suffering from hyperparathyroidism is low, being less than 3000 g in 50 percent of the cases. There is a high frequency of stillbirth, neonatal death, and neonatal tetany.

In 1962, Ludwig reviewed the literature and described the clinical course of 40 gestations of the 21 women who were recognized at that time as having primary hyperparathyroidism while they were pregnant. Serious fetal complications were noted in half these pregnancies. Stillbirths, spontaneous abortions, and neonatal deaths occurred in 31 percent and neonatal tetany in 19 percent of these instances. Delmonico and associates, analyzing the 15 pregnancies of 13 hyperparathyroid women reported since that time who were not operated upon, found that 80 percent of these gestations were complicated.

Spontaneous abortions and neonatal deaths occurred in 27 percent; 55 percent of the newborns suffered significant hypocalcemia soon after birth.

The diagnosis of primary hyperparathyroidism associated with pregnancy is rarely made. It is not uncommon, in fact, for this disease to be recognized in the mother only retrospectively following the appearance of hypocalcemia in the newborn infant. Even borderline high values of serum calcium obtained from the pregnant woman should be considered to be of utmost significance. Serial calcium concentrations should be performed as part of all routine prenatal care. The diagnosis of maternal primary hyperparathyroidism can be made with virtual certainty when an elevated serum calcium concentration is accompanied at the same time by an elevated serum parathyroid hormone level, since ectopic hyperparathyroidism from occult malignancy is rare in these young women.

When maternal hyperparathyroidism is diagnosed during pregnancy, Kaplan feels that the proper therapy is parathyroidectomy, optimally performed during the second trimester of pregnancy, since accidental abortion is lessened during this period. With correction of the hypercalcemic state at this early time, parathyroid development of the fetus can proceed normally.

The results in patients so managed are far better than those reported without operation. Only one instance of neonatal death and another of neonatal hypocalcemia occurred.

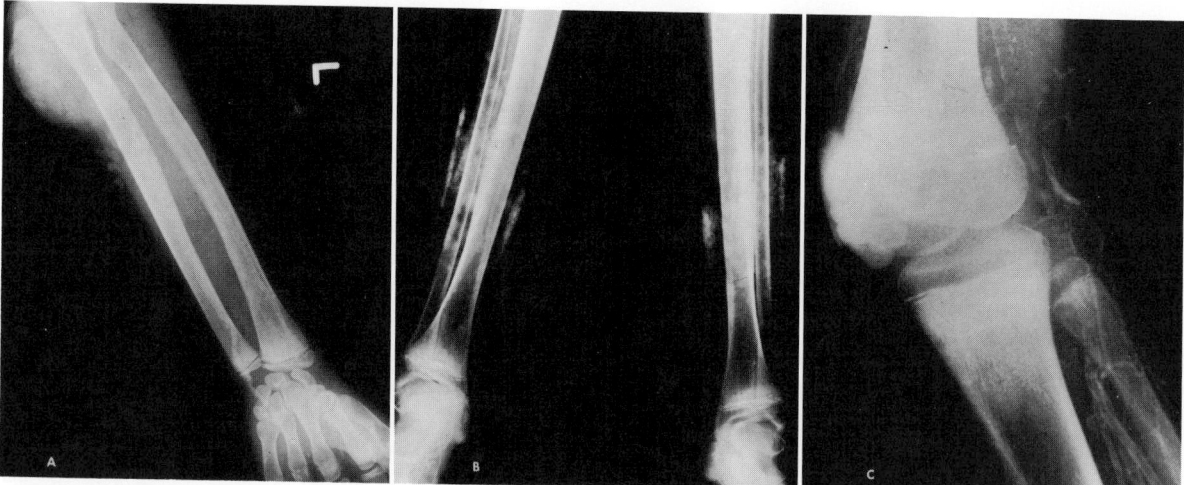

Fig. 38-42. X-ray studies of a child with chronic renal failure and vitamin D intoxication. Note the severe ectopic calcification in the soft tissues. *A.* The olecranon bursa and subcutaneous tissues of the left arm. *B.* The subcutaneous tissues and muscle of the lower leg. *C.* The patellar bursa and the popliteal and tibial arteries.

Multiple Endocrine Neoplasia, Type I. *General Considerations.* The first account of chronic polyglandular syndrome, type I, was given by Erdheim in 1903 and consists of a rather sketchy mention of a patient with acromegaly, eosinophilic adenoma of the pituitary, and four enlarged parathyroids. The first report of pituitary, parathyroid, and pancreatic islet cell tumors in combination was by Cushing and Davidoff in 1926; the first report of acromegaly and clinical hyperparathyroidism was in 1948. Involvement of pituitary, parathyroids, and islet cells occurs in 34 percent, pituitary and parathyroids in 25 percent, pituitary and islet cells in 19 percent, parathyroids and islet cells in 22 percent. Twenty-five percent of the patients have peptic ulcer due to the Zollinger-Ellison syndrome. An autosomal dominant inheritance pattern is

present in these patients. The glands involved in the MEN, type I syndrome are primarily the parathyroids, pancreatic islets, and the pituitary.

Hyperparathyroidism. These patients almost always have parathyroid chief cell hyperplasia if all glands are explored. Sometimes more than four glands are involved by this process. Recurrent hyperparathyroidism has occurred at a high rate following both subtotal parathyroidectomy and even after total parathyroidectomy with autotransplantation of parathyroid tissue into the arm muscles.

Pancreatic Tumors. Patients with MEN-I syndrome have islet cell tumors of the pancreas that are frequently multiple and located throughout the pancreas. These tumors secrete differing amines and peptides and can cause a number of clinical syndromes according to which hormone or combinations of hormones are released. These include the insulinoma syndrome (insulin), the glucagonoma syndrome (glucagon), the Zollinger-Ellison syndrome (gastrin), the watery diarrhea syndrome (vasoactive intestinal polypeptide), the carcinoid syndrome (serotonin, kinins, substance P), or the somatostatin syndrome. Other pancreatic islet tumors, such as those that secrete pancreatic polypeptide, give few if any symptoms or signs. When multiple islet cell tumors are found in the pancreas the possibility of a MEN-I syndrome should be entertained, for other manifestations of this syndrome can occur later.

Pituitary Tumors. While some pituitary tumors in the MEN-I syndrome can cause Cushing's syndrome or acromegaly, most of them appear to be nonfunctioning clinically. Many microadenomas of the pituitary that secrete prolactin have recently been discovered in such patients. Wilson believes that all patients with MEN-I syndromes eventually have evidence of pituitary, pancreatic, and parathyroid disease if these systems are studied.

Fig. 38-43. X-ray of the abdomen showing nephrocalcinosis. While this change sometimes occurs in hyperparathyroidism, it is not diagnostic of this condition.

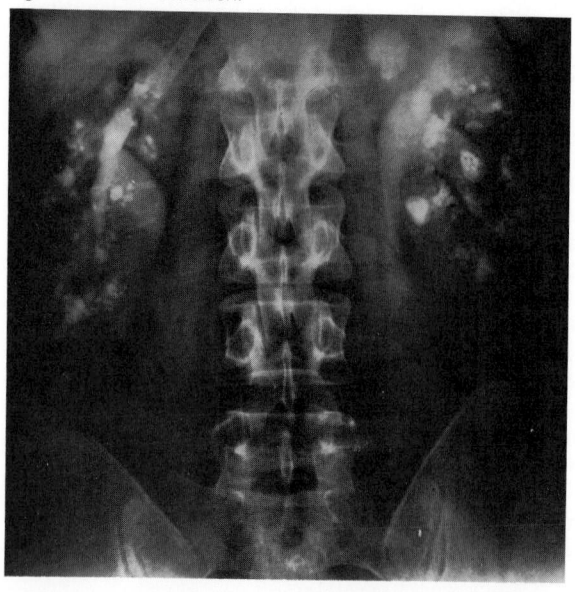

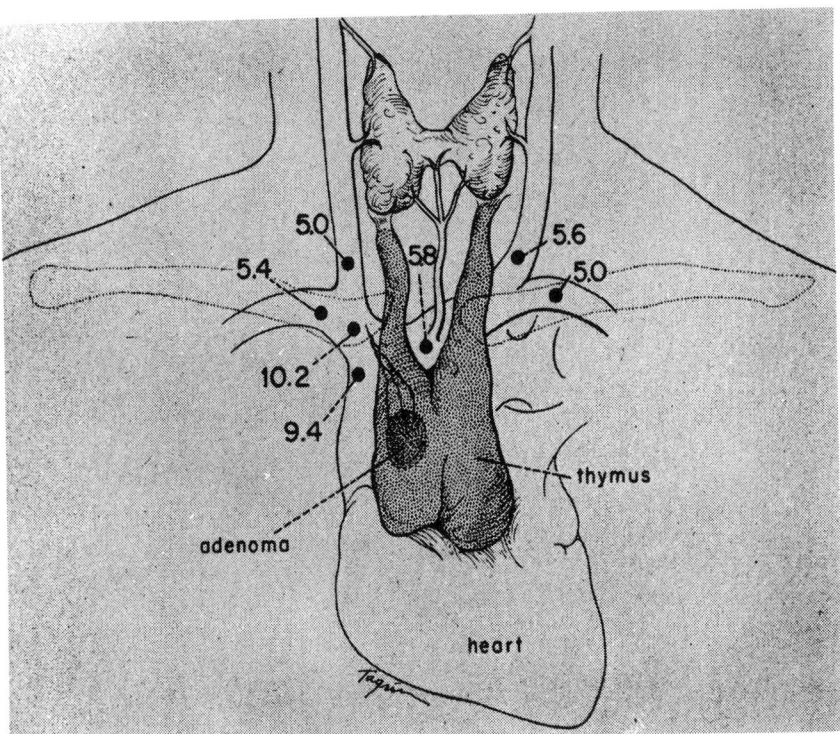

Fig. 38-44. Radioimmunoassay of blood samples obtained during venous catheterization of a patient with primary hyperparathyroidism. Localized increases in PTH values are demonstrated in the right innominate vein and the superior vena cava (10.2 and 9.4 mμg/mL). At operation a parathyroid adenoma was found in the thymus gland. Its venous drainage was to the right innominate vein and corresponded to the area of elevated PTH levels. (From: *Reitz RE et al: N Engl J Med 281:349, 1969, with permission.*)

Multiple Endocrinopathies, Type II. Medullary carcinoma of the thyroid or C-cell hyperplasia may be associated with all or part of a syndrome called multiple endocrine neoplasia, type IIA, familial medullary carcinoma syndrome, or sometimes Sipple's syndrome. In its entirety it consists of pheochromocytomas (often bilateral) or bilateral adrenal medullary hyperplasia and parathyroid gland abnormalities, usually chief cell hyperplasia. Occasional individuals with the MEN, type IIB subtype also have a Marfanoid habitus, neuromas of the tongue or conjunctiva, and ganglioneuromatous changes of the plexuses of Meissner and Auerbach. They have medullary carcinomas and pheochromocytomas as in the MEN-IIA group, but only rarely do they present with hyperparathyroidism.

Secondary Hyperparathyroidism. In primary hyperparathyroidism there is an oversecretion of PTH that does not cease even in the presence of an elevated serum calcium level. In secondary hyperparathyroidism there is also an increased secretion of PTH, but this is in response to a lowered blood calcium level often brought about by renal disease or malabsorption syndromes. These diseases are associated with abnormalities in vitamin D metabolism [lack of production of 1,25-$(OH)_2D_3$] and by poor calcium and vitamin D absorption from the intestines, respec-

Fig. 38-45. Plasma PTH concentrations in samples obtained at different points in the circulation. Veins are jugular (*J*), innominate (*I*), superior vena cava (*SVC*), superior thyroid veins (*STV*), and inferior thyroid veins (*ITV*). Samples also were obtained from the medial and lateral branches of the right inferior thyroid vein (*ITV—M* and *ITV—L*). Sites of sampling are indicated by ●; adjacent numbers indicate PTH concentration in mμg/mL. These data indicate an adenoma of the right lower parathyroid gland. Elevated PTH concentrations in samples from both sides of the neck indicate parathyroid hyperplasia. (From: *Potts JT Jr et al: Am J Med 50:639, 1971, with permission.*)

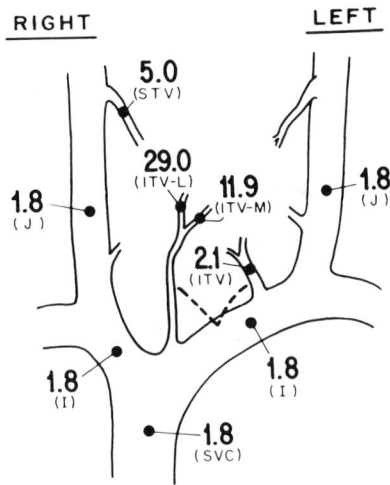

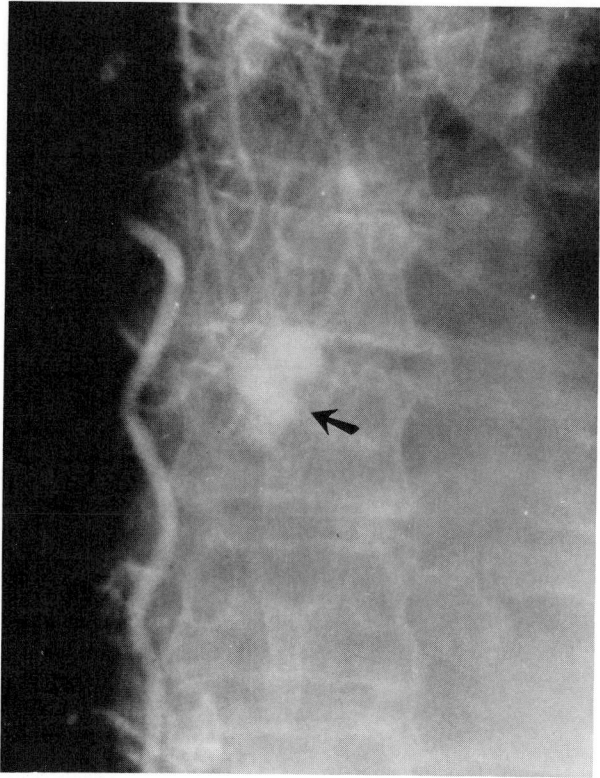

A

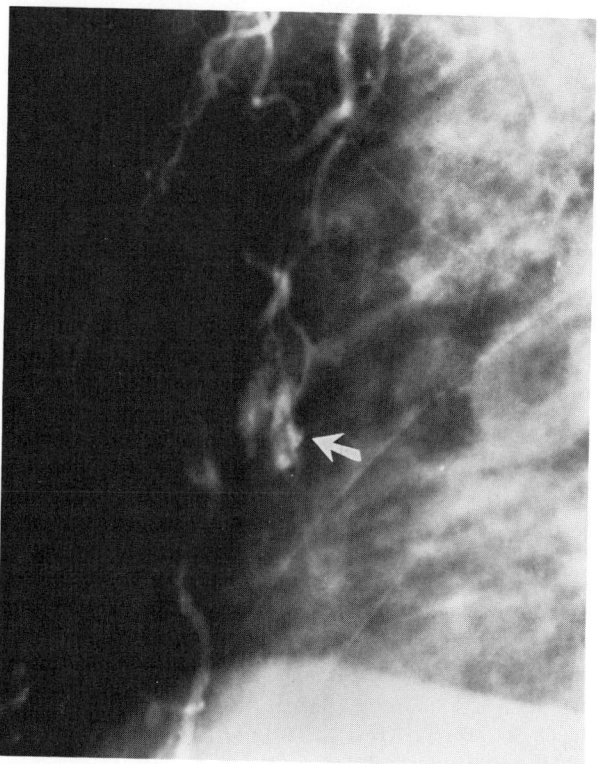

B

Fig. 38-46. Mediastinal parathyroid adenoma, fed by the right internal mammary artery, localized preoperatively by arteriography. *A.* AP view. *B.* Oblique view (arrows point to the adenoma). *(Courtesy of Chien-tai Lu.)*

tively. The response of the parathyroids is thus a compensatory one, as the body attempts to raise the serum calcium level to the normal range. In secondary hyperparathyroidism there is a chief cell hyperplasia of the parathyroids.

Other causes of secondary hyperparathyroidism include rickets and osteomalacia, where there is a deficient absorption of calcium from the intestine.

The skeletal changes of secondary hyperparathyroidism are identical to those of primary hyperparathyroidism except that ectopic calcification in the arteries, muscles, etc., is much more common in secondary hyperparathyroidism, especially if the patient has been given large doses of vitamin D (see Fig. 38-42). Today severe bone disease associated with hyperparathyroidism is rare in primary hyperparathyroidism but is not infrequently seen in patients with chronic renal failure maintained on chronic hemodialysis.

The bone disease in chronic renal failure, commonly called *renal osteodystrophy,* is caused by at least several factors: Hyperphosphatemia results in a decreased serum calcium. Hypocalcemia results in secondary hyperparathyroidism. Impaired calcium absorption due to vitamin D insensitivity results in osteomalacia. Systemic acidosis may also contribute to bone resorption.

Patients with chronic renal failure usually have an impaired ability to convert vitamin D_3 to its active metabolite $1,25\text{-}(OH)_2D_3$ because of the absence of a renal hydroxylase. This results in decreased calcium absorption from the intestine. In these patients, physiologic doses of vitamin D are usually ineffective, but improvement following administration of large pharmacologic doses of this vitamin may occur. In contrast, the $1,25\text{-}(OH)_2D_3$ metabolite is very effective in low doses. Administration of $1,25\text{-}(OH)_2D_3$ or other similar metabolites is often useful in the prevention and treatment of renal osteodystrophy. Medical therapy for the bone disease should be tried in all patients with secondary hyperparathyroidism before surgery is contemplated.

Parathyroidectomy is commonly utilized for patients in chronic renal failure with severe bone change who have developed intractable bone pain. The pain and severe itching, which is also sometimes present in patients on chronic dialysis, are often relieved in a dramatic fashion. Remineralization of the skeleton can be hastened by the administration of vitamin D and oral calcium supplements postoperatively.

Patients with secondary hyperparathyroidism due to chronic renal failure are dialyzed 1 day before surgery to reduce serum potassium. At operation four large hyperplastic parathyroid glands are usually found (Fig. 38-47). One of two operations is performed according to the preference of the surgeon: subtotal parathyroidectomy or total parathyroidectomy with autotransplantation of parathyroid tissue, usually to the arm. When subtotal parathy-

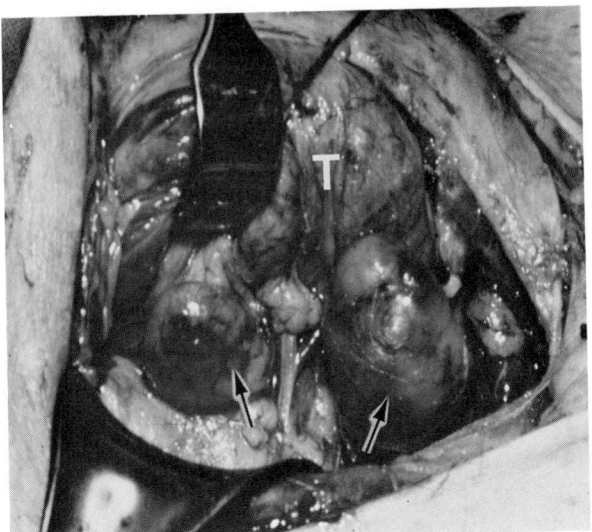

Fig. 38-47. Secondary hyperparathyroidism. Chief cell hyperplasia with four enlarged parathyroid glands was found in this patient with chronic renal failure and bone disease. Arrows point to two of the hyperplastic parathyroid glands. *T*, retracted thyroid lobe.

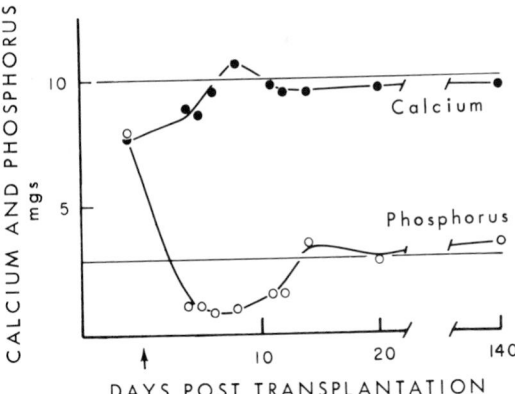

Fig. 38-48. Serum calcium and phosphate values in a patient with secondary hyperparathyroidism who received a kidney transplant. Preoperatively the serum calcium level was low and the phosphate level high. After an initial rise in calcium level and fall in phosphate level to levels outside the normal range the values quickly returned to normal levels. No parathyroid exploration was carried out.

roidectomy is done, about 60 to 100 mg of well-vascularized parathyroid tissue is left behind. Drains are always used. Postoperatively, the first dialysis is often accomplished with regional heparinization.

Tertiary Hyperparathyroidism. Tertiary hyperparathyroidism is the term that has been employed to describe the situation in which secondary hyperparathyroidism with chief cell hyperplasia appears to have become "autonomous." The diagnosis is made when an elevated serum calcium level develops in the patient with chronic renal failure and secondary hyperparathyroidism or in a patient with known intestinal malabsorption who previously had hypocalcemia.

When renal transplantation is carried out in a patient with renal failure and secondary hyperparathyroidism, three patterns are characteristically seen: In the first the phosphorus level falls and the serum calcium level rises for a short period of time, after which they both return to normal levels. This is illustrated in Fig. 38-48. In the second pattern the elevated calcium and lowered phosphorus levels may persist for several weeks before gradually returning to normal (Fig. 38-49A). In the third pattern, hypercalcemia with hypophosphatemia persists for long periods of time. In the patient illustrated in Fig. 38-49B a staghorn calculus developed in the transplanted kidney within 6 months. Parathyroidectomy was carried out at this point, and the function of the kidney has remained excellent up to the present time, 5 years after transplantation.

Recent studies suggest that true parathyroid autonomy rarely occurs in patients with so-called tertiary hyperparathyroidism. It has been demonstrated that the hyperplastic glands found in chronic renal failure do suppress their secretion but cannot completely shut off their secretion of PTH despite the presence of hypercalcemia. Because of their bulky size it may take a long time for them to involute. Johnson et al. have demonstrated that, following renal transplantation, PTH concentrations in these patients slowly return toward normal within several months if renal function is good (Fig. 38-50).

Some workers have a considerable fear that renal damage may occur very rapidly in the presence of hypercalcemia and advocate doing parathyroidectomy prior to renal transplantation in those patients suspected of having severe secondary or tertiary hyperparathyroidism. In view of the fact that in most of these cases normal serum calcium concentrations will return in a reasonable period after transplantation, it would seem a more appropriate policy to wait and watch the patient carefully posttransplantation for a period of time. Only rarely will parathyroidectomy be necessary. Subtotal parathyroidectomy was only necessary in 3 of 111 patients following transplantation in a Mayo Clinic series.

DIFFERENTIAL DIAGNOSIS. Some of the features of the differential diagnosis of hypercalcemia are shown in Table 38-10. If 100 consecutive patients with hypercalcemia are evaluated in a hospital setting, the greatest number will be found to have metastatic carcinoma with bone metastases, patients with primary hyperparathyroidism make up the next group, and thiazide therapy is the third most common cause. Many other causes of hypercalcemia have been recognized as well.

Metastatic Cancer. In metastatic cancer the phosphate level in the serum is usually not depressed. The cancer is usually of breast, kidney, lung, thyroid, or of prostatic origin. Serum PTH is low unless the tumor secretes ectopic parathyroid hormone-like fragments. The bony involvement usually can be detected by x-ray, but sometimes a bone scan is necessary. The plasma calcium level will usually fall in response to cortisone infusion. Sometimes the lesions in the bone may look quite similar to those seen with primary or secondary hyperparathyroidism as shown in Figs. 38-36 and 38-37.

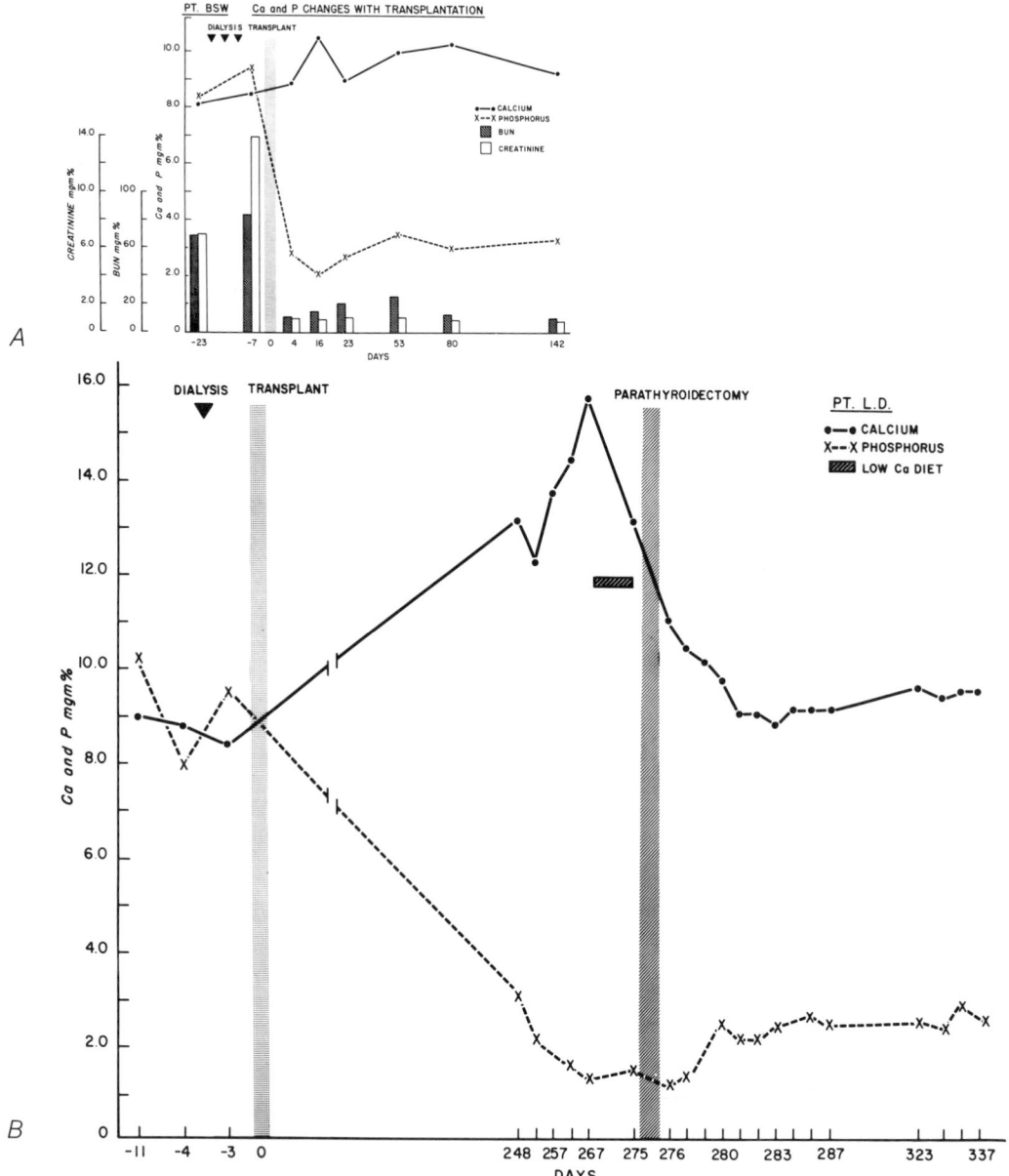

Parathyroid Disease versus Extraparathyroid PTH-Producing Tumor. It may be very difficult to make the differential diagnosis between a parathyroid adenoma and an extraparathyroid PTH-producing tumor, since the effects on the patient are identical. The known presence of tumors that are likely to produce this syndrome—bronchogenic or small cell carcinomas of the lung, hypernephromas, hepatomas, epidermoid cancer, bladder, ovary, uterus, vulva and pancreas—should suggest this possibility. This condition is rarely if ever seen in cases of breast cancer. Ectopic production of PTH-like fragments may be diagnosed by radioimmunoassay by certain antisera that react with these substances. Sometimes venous catheterization of neck veins with PTH analysis will result in the diagnosis of primary HPT, which can occur in some patients with other cancers.

Fig. 38-49. Serum calcium and phosphate values in patients with secondary hyperparathyroidism who received kidney transplants. *A*. Patient with secondary hyperparathyroidism whose serum phosphate level took somewhat longer to return to normal after renal homotransplantation. The calcium level remained in the high normal range for many days. *B*. Another patient with renal failure and secondary hyperparathyroidism. In this patient the preoperative serum calcium level was nearly in the normal range, whereas the phosphorus level was markedly elevated. After transplantation the serum calcium value steadily rose, while the phosphate value declined to abnormally low levels. No spontaneous return toward normal occurred, and it was apparent that tertiary hyperparathyroidism had developed. A parathyroidectomy was carried out on the 275th day after transplantation, and the patient was found to have chief cell hyperplasia with very large glands. By this time calcium deposits had developed in the walls of the calcyceal system of the transplanted kidney. After parathyroidectomy the serum calcium and phosphate values returned to normal. (From: *Hume DM et al: Ann Surg 164:352, 1966, with permission.*)

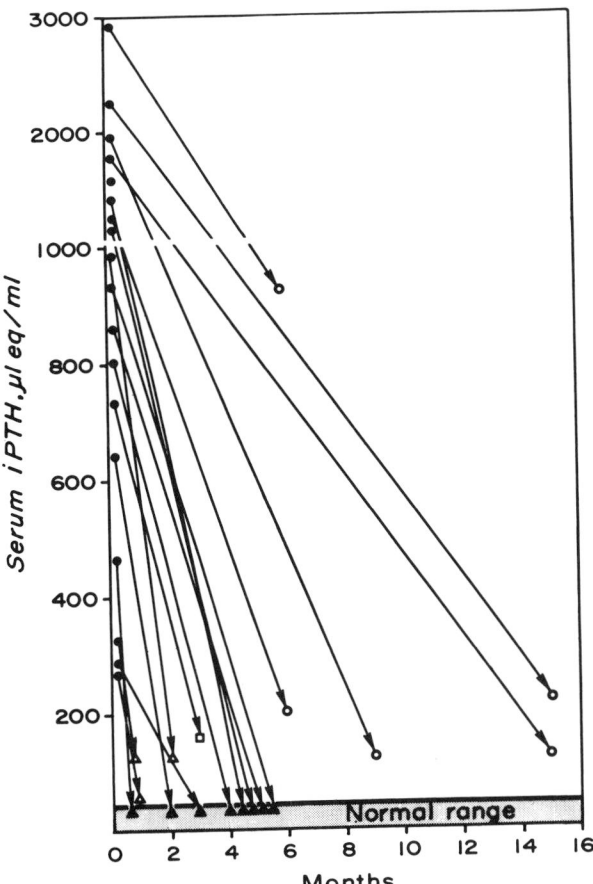

Fig. 38-50. Serum PTH concentrations before and after successful renal transplantation in patients with endogenous creatinine clearance of 60 mL/min/1.73 m² or greater. (From: *Johnson WJ et al: Med Clin North Am 56:961, 1972, with permission.*)

Thiazides. Hypercalcemia has been reported with increasing frequency in patients receiving benzothiadiazine diuretics. Hypercalcemia resulting solely from these diuretics is almost always mild. After cessation of the diuretic the serum calcium value usually returns to normal in several weeks. The thiazide diuretics can aggravate hypercalcemia in primary hyperparathyroidism. Thus when possible these diuretics should be stopped and the patient studied later.

Vitamin A and D Poisoning. Both vitamin A and D can cause hypercalcemia when taken in large doses. Vitamin D intoxication can be suspected when this vitamin has been administered in excess. The patients tend to have an increased, rather than decreased, phosphate level in the serum. Metastatic calcification is much more common in vitamin D intoxication than in hyperparathyroidism (see Fig. 38-42). It is somewhat more apt to occur in the presence of renal failure. In vitamin D intoxication small yellowish deposits may be present underneath the fingernails, along the outer borders of the lips, in the skin, and in the corneal conjunctiva. Serum PTH level is low.

Sarcoidosis and Other Granulomatous Diseases. Hypercalcemia in sarcoidosis was first described by Harrell and Fisher. It occurs in about a third of the cases. There ap-

pears instead to be a hypersensitivity to vitamin D in some individuals with sarcoid, and exposure to sunlight or administration of vitamin D will produce hypercalcemia in the patients manifesting this phenomenon. Since band keratopathy of the eyes, bone cysts, renal calculi, nephrocalcinosis, and polyuria can occur, the incorrect diagnosis of hyperparathyroidism is sometimes made.

The presence of an increased plasma globulin, hepatomegaly, and splenomegaly should suggest the correct diagnosis. The administration of 150 mg of cortisone daily for 10 to 14 days reduces the serum calcium to normal (Dent test). A positive diagnosis may be established by biopsy of the liver, lymph nodes, or, when present, skin nodules. Serum PTH level is low. Sarcoidosis and hyperparathyroidism may coexist in the same patient.

Recently, it has been shown that individuals with other granulomatous diseases such as tuberculosis or berylliosis can also develop hypercalcemia. The granuloma cells of sarcoidosis and these other diseases produce a hydroxylase that converts vitamin D to an active metabolite and thus results in increased calcium absorption from the gut and the production of hypercalcemia.

Multiple Myeloma. This entity usually shows sharp, punched-out areas of destruction in the bone, generally well seen in the skull. At times rather similar lesions can be produced by hyperparathyroidism (see Fig. 38-36). The Bence-Jones protein is present in about 50 percent of the patients, and the plasma globulin level is high. Plasma cells are present in the bone marrow. The alkaline phosphatase level is usually not elevated. Serum PTH is low and the plasma calcium level is decreased with cortisol infusion.

Hyperthyroidism. Hypercalcemia occurs on rare occasions in association with hyperthyroidism. It is thought to be the result of increased bone turnover. The serum calcium usually returns to normal when the hyperthyroidism is cured. Since hyperparathyroidism may coexist with hyperthyroidism, it is important to determine whether this may not be the cause of the hypercalcemia in any particular case.

Idiopathic Hypercalcemia of Infancy. This syndrome is believed to be due to a hypersensitivity to vitamin D, such as that seen in sarcoidosis. It occurs in infants who have mental retardation, an elevated serum cholesterol level, and hypercalcemia. The serum calcium level falls with the administration of cortisone.

The Milk-Alkali Syndrome. Burnett et al. described a syndrome in which hypercalcemia developed in patients ingesting large amounts of milk and absorbable alkali—such as sodium bicarbonate, usually for peptic ulcer. This is most apt to occur when there is some degree of renal insufficiency. The serum phosphate level is normal or elevated rather than low. Renal calculi and nephrocalcinosis may be present. Patients with primary hyperparathyroidism may develop renal failure, an elevated serum phosphate level, and peptic ulceration, at which point the picture may be difficult to distinguish from the milk-alkali syndrome. The history of ingestion of large amounts of milk and absorbable alkali, the improvement noted when these are stopped, and the absence of hypercalcinuria distinguish the latter condition. Serum PTH is low in this

Table 38-10. THE DIFFERENTIAL DIAGNOSIS OF SOME DISEASES PRODUCING HYPERCALCEMIA, HYPERCALCINURIA, OR BONE CHANGES

Disease	Serum			Urine		Special tests and criteria	Parathyroid hormone
	Calcium	Phosphate	Alkaline phosphatase	Calcium	Phosphate		
Primary hyperparathyroidism	Increased	Decreased*	Normal or increased	Increased	Increased	TRP measurements	Increased
Tertiary hyperparathyroidism (renal failure)	Increased	Increased	Increased	Decreased	Decreased	Chronic renal failure present	Markedly increased
Vitamin D intoxication	Increased	Increased	Decreased	Increased	Increased	Ectopic calcification present	Decreased
Metastatic carcinoma	Increased	Normal	Normal or increased	Increased	Normal	X-rays showing metastases	Decreased†
Multiple myeloma	Increased	Normal	Normal	Normal or increased	Normal or decreased	X-rays showing lesions Bence-Jones protein present Increased plasma globulin	Decreased
Sarcoidosis	Increased	Normal or decreased	Normal or increased	Increased	Increased	Increased plasma globulin Hepatomegaly—biopsy Splenomegaly	Decreased
Idiopathic hypercalcemia of infancy	Increased	Increased	Normal	Increased	Decreased	Presence of mental retardation Increased blood cholesterol Hypersensitivity to vitamin D	Decreased
Milk-alkali syndrome	Increased	Normal*	Normal	Normal or decreased	Normal or decreased	History of milk and alkali intake Renal insufficiency often present	Decreased*
Paget's disease	Normal or increased	Normal	Increased	Increased	Normal	Bone changes on x-ray Serum calcium reduced by mobilization	Normal or decreased
Idiopathic hypercalcinuria	Normal	Decreased	Normal	Increased	Normal or increased	Renal calculi may be present	Normal

* Increased when renal failure supervenes.
† In ectopic hyperparathyroidism, PTH is also elevated.

condition but might become increased if renal failure occurs.

Paget's Disease (Osteitis Deformans). Paget's disease may occasionally be associated with an elevated serum calcium level. X-rays will show the characteristic lesion, usually in the pelvis, lower extremities, or skull. The blood calcium concentration may be normal, but hypercalcemia can develop, particularly if the patient is immobilized.

Paget's disease and primary hyperparathyroidism may coexist, making it difficult to establish the latter diagnosis. The measurement of PTH (not elevated in Paget's disease) and the failure of cortisone and mobilization to reduce the blood calcium should suggest the correct diagnosis.

Idiopathic Hypercalcinuria. This syndrome is characterized by hypercalcinuria, hypophosphatemia, and stone formation in the presence of a normal serum calcium value. It occurs almost exclusively in men. The bones are normal, and the alkaline phosphatase level is not elevated. The cause is unknown. However, hyperabsorption of calcium from the intestine may be responsible for some cases. If an elevated serum calcium level develops, studies for hyperparathyroidism should be carried out. This condition has been treated successfully by thiazide administration, which lowers the urinary calcium output.

TREATMENT. Indications for Operation. Patients with primary hyperparathyroidism in whom the diagnosis has been established with relative certainty should definitely be subjected to parathyroid surgical treatment if they have either bony or renal manifestations of the disease, since these will almost inevitably become worse with time. The urgency is greater the higher the calcium level, the most impelling example being the patient with hypercalcemic crisis. Treatment is also indicated if peptic ulcer or pancreatitis is secondary to the hyperparathyroidism. Hypertension may or may not be benefited by parathyroidectomy, depending upon its relation to permanent renal damage that has been incurred by long-standing hypercalcemia.

As newer methods for establishing the diagnosis of hyperparathyroidism have developed, more and more cases are operated upon at an earlier stage. We have found that mild symptoms such as decreased appetite, arthritis, tiredness, and depression are common, especially in elderly patients, and that they are frequently helped by parathyroidectomy. The mortality and morbidity for this operation are so low that unless the patient presents an unusually poor risk, operation should be undertaken when any of the indications listed above present themselves.

Some completely asymptomatic patients with minimal hypercalcemia (serum Ca, 11 mg/dL) have been followed without surgery at the Mayo Clinic even though the diagnosis of primary hyperparathyroidism was definitively made. At the end of a 10-year study period, over 20 percent of these individuals required operation because of complications attributable to the disease or a rise in serum calcium levels to above 11.0 mg/dL. Another 20 percent were dropped from the study because of lack of cooperation in the follow-up program. Other patients requested the operation because of the uncertainty of being followed for this disease. No criteria are evident that would permit identification of those patients who will ultimately require a parathyroid operation. The Mayo group have concluded that surgical treatment is correct in this asymptomatic group in most cases. We follow this same recommendation.

The mainstay of preoperative management when the hypercalcemia is due to hyperparathyroidism is saline infusion and diuresis with furosemide (Lasix) (Table 38-11). No longer is parathyroidectomy necessary as an absolute emergency procedure. However, once the diagnosis is made and the patient's condition is stabilized, results are far better if a parathyroidectomy is performed without delay.

Table 38-11. USUAL DOSES OF HYPOCALCEMIC AGENTS

Drug	Route	Dosage	Reported complications	Contraindications
Sodium chloride solution (isotonic)	Intravenous	1 L every 3–4 h	Pulmonary edema	Congestive heart failure, renal insufficiency, hypertension
Furosemide	Intravenous	100 mg/h	Volume depletion, hypokalemia,	Renal insufficiency
EDTA	Intravenous	50 mg/kg body weight over 4–6 h	Renal failure, hypotension	Renal insufficiency
Cortisone	Oral or parenteral	150 mg/day	Hypercorticism	Emergency reduction of serum calcium required
Mithramycin	Intravenous	25 μg/kg body weight	Hemorrhage, thrombocytopenia, nausea, vomiting	Bleeding disorder, renal insufficiency, liver impairment
Phosphate	Oral	1–2 mM*/kg body weight daily	Diarrhea	
Calcitonin	Parenteral	1–5 MRC units/kg body weight daily	Nausea, vomiting	Thrombotic disorders

* 1 mM of phosphate is equivalent to 31 mg of phosphorus.
SOURCE: Modified from Suki WN, Yium JJ, et al: Acute treatment of hypercalcemia with furosemide. *N Engl J Med* 283:836, 1970, with permission.

EDTA therapy is rarely used and oral phosphate administration in very severe cases of hypercalcemia has been associated with calcium-phosphate crystallization and death.

Calcium and digitalis are synergistic in their effect on the myocardium and conducting system. Hence fully digitalized patients may manifest digitalis toxicity if they become hypercalcemic. Thus it may be necessary to reduce or stop digitalis. Similarly, if digitalization is necessary in a hypercalcemic patient, a lower dose is generally required.

Strategy of the Initial Parathyroid Exploration. The role of the surgeon in the first parathyroid exploration is to remove the parathyroid adenoma or hyperplastic glands appropriately and thus to cure the hyperparathyroid state. While Wang and Tibblin recommend unilateral neck exploration if one large gland (an adenoma) and a normal gland are found on the first side, and Paloyan has recommended subtotal parathyroidectomy for all patients, I think that a middle-ground approach is appropriate. Both sides of the neck should be carefully explored in all cases and the number of glands removed should fit the disease process.

In general, parathyroid surgery requires an unrushed, meticulous dissection with a bloodless field. Hence, try to keep the operative field as dry as possible. Neither methylene blue nor toluidine blue is used by most parathyroid surgeons in either primary or secondary neck explorations. Undoubtedly, the more thyroid or parathyroid operations that one performs, the more readily one will be able to recognize the parathyroid glands. Abnormal parathyroid glands are enlarged, more spherical and often have a darker color that can range from tan to reddish-brown. Normal parathyroid glands are usually more yellowish in color, they bleed more than fat when a small biopsy is taken, and sometimes they can be recognized by the small hematoma that often occurs within their substance following manipulation.

At neck exploration the surgeon must be a diagnostician as well as a therapist. In most cases, at the time of operation, it is up to him to recognize the pathologic process that is present. If one gland is enlarged and the others are normal, this is an adenoma. The adenoma should be removed and one or two normal glands should be biopsied. We no longer biopsy the fourth normal gland, because in our experience this practice leads to a greater degree of transient postoperative hypocalcemia.

If four glands are found to be enlarged, this is hyperplasia. In such cases a subtotal parathyroidectomy is necessary. Three glands and part of the fourth are excised, leaving a well-vascularized remnant of 50 to 80 mg of tissue. Each thymic tongue is also excised to be certain that more parathyroid tissue is not present therein. The partial resection of one parathyroid gland should always be performed first, so that one can see that the remnant remains well-vascularized before removing the other three glands. In cases of familial hyperparathyroidism or of the MEN syndrome one might consider doing a total parathyroidectomy with an autotransplant to the arm, as recommended by Wells.

When two parathyroid glands are enlarged and the others appear normal, this is probably a variant of hyperplasia (or multiglandular disease); others call this a double adenoma. In such cases, we have found that resection of the two enlarged glands and biopsy of the two normal glands has been curative. Always mark the remaining parathyroid remnant (or remnants) with a hemoclip or a nonabsorbable suture so that, if necessary, it can be found more readily in the future.

Operative Technique. Under general endotracheal anesthesia with the neck hyperextended, a transverse incision is made in the lower neck. The platysma muscle is elevated with the skin flap, and the superior flap is dissected to the hyoid superiorly and the upper border of the sternum inferiorly. The skin flaps may be held apart by a self-retaining retractor or by sutures, and the deep cervical fascia is divided longitudinally in the midline from the hyoid bone to the suprasternal notch. Others prefer to divide the sternohyoid and sternothyroid muscles routinely at the junction of the upper and middle third to facilitate exposure of the gland (Figs. 38-51 and 38-52); however, we usually do not find this necessary.

The thyroid gland is mobilized by dividing the middle thyroid veins and rolling the lobe of the thyroid anteriorly and mediad. The recurrent laryngeal nerve is then identified. The landmarks for this are the groove between the trachea and esophagus, and the inferior thyroid artery. The recurrent nerve may also be identified at the inferior cornu of the thyroid cartilage, as described by Wang. The best place to begin the search for a parathyroid adenoma is at the point where the recurrent laryngeal nerve crosses behind the inferior thyroid artery. The adenomas are frequently found under the lateral lobe of the thyroid in a space alongside the esophagus lying just slightly posterior to the groove between the esophagus and the trachea (Figs. 38-53 and 38-54). Tracing the branches of the inferior thyroid artery may sometimes be helpful in locating the hyperfunctioning parathyroid gland, since this vessel supplies the parathyroid adenoma with blood in nearly 90 percent of the cases (Figs. 38-55 and 38-56). After a preliminary search in this area the inferior parathyroid will usually be found just below the point at which the recurrent laryngeal nerve intersects the inferior thyroid artery. The superior parathyroid will often be found within 1 or 2 cm above this point, usually on a little prominence of the posterior surface of the thyroid.

An adenoma, particularly one of the lower gland, can be tucked well behind the thyroid or between the trachea and esophagus, so that it is not readily apparent until the thyroid has been rotated forward and the fatty tissue in this area has been gently teased away. The adenoma is not usually bound down to the surrounding tissues, however, and usually can be popped out of its hiding place. It is generally red-brown, at times yellow-brown, smooth, and with a surface that is vascular and bleeds easily when rubbed or cut. On rare occasions, particularly when it lies beneath the capsule of the thyroid, it may look extremely similar to thyroid tissue itself.

Once the provisional location of the glands has been established, the procedure is repeated on the other side.

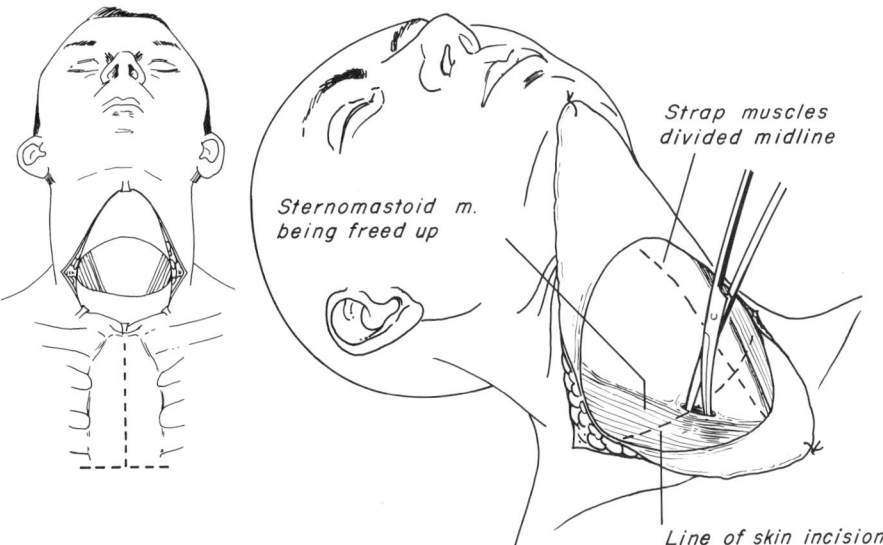

Strap muscles divided midline

Sternomastoid m. being freed up

Line of skin incision

Fig. 38-51. Incision for parathyroidectomy. The dotted lines indicate the extension of the incision used for mediastinal exploration. The deep fascia is divided in the midline, and the strap muscles are usually retracted.

We make it a policy to examine both sides of the neck and to evaluate all of the parathyroid glands that can be found before removing any of them. This is to protect against the circumstance in which three enlarged parathyroid glands are resected as they are encountered, only to find that the patient has no fourth gland. When all the parathyroids cannot be found adjacent to the thyroid gland, further search is facilitated by dividing the superior pole vessels on the side of the missing upper gland and performing the maneuvers described below.

When the operation is to be completed, the strap muscles are loosely opposed with several sutures. A small suction catheter is inserted. The dermis is approximated with interrupted subcuticular sutures and the epidermis with sterile skin tapes.

About 80 percent of all parathyroid adenomas are found near the thyroid. However, the others are located in ectopic sites. If an adenoma cannot be found in the usual locations at exploration the following procedures should be performed. Each normal parathyroid gland should be biopsied, and after positive identification as parathyroid tissue on frozen section, a diagram should be made of its location for later reference; each gland should be marked with a hemoclip. Do *not* remove normal parathyroid glands; this complicates the situation when the adenoma is ultimately found.

If three normal parathyroid glands are found and the fourth cannot be located, the surgeon should try to assess whether an upper or a lower parathyroid gland on that side is missing. If it is the lower parathyroid gland, as much of the thymus as possible should be pulled up into the neck and resected. Often the inferior adenoma will be found within the thymus.

Very frequently, it is an adenoma of the upper parathyroid gland that is overlooked. These fall down along the esophagus into the posterior-superior mediastinum. The mistake in this case is that the dissection was not carried out deep enough back to the prevertebral fascia of the neck. When this is done near the upper pole of the thyroid, a finger can be safely inserted behind the inferior thyroid artery and posterior to the recurrent laryngeal nerve. Not infrequently an adenoma will be palpable beside or behind the esophagus, and this gland can be pulled out and easily removed.

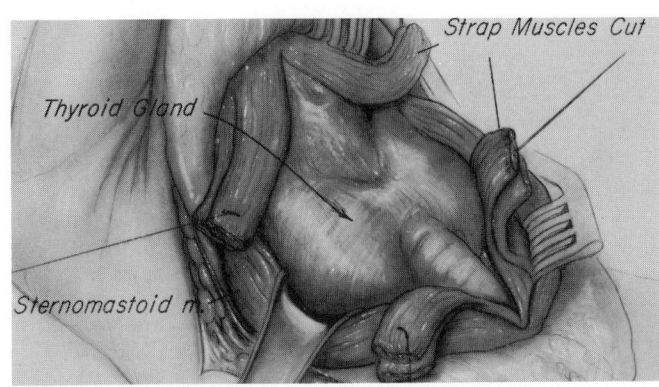

Strap Muscles Cut

Thyroid Gland

Sternomastoid m.

Fig. 38-52. When more exposure is necessary, the strap muscles may be divided. However, this is rarely necessary.

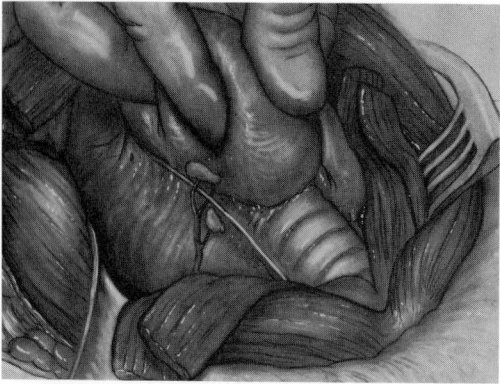

Fig. 38-53. The middle thyroid veins are divided, and the lateral lobe of the thyroid is retracted anteriorly and mediad. The recurrent laryngeal nerve is exposed in the tracheoesophageal groove, and the inferior thyroid artery is dissected out and preserved. The inferior parathyroid is usually located just below the intersection of these two structures and is supplied by a branch of the inferior thyroid artery.

If the parathyroid gland still cannot be found after these maneuvers, the dissection should be carried up in a cephalad direction to the hyoid bone where occasionally an "undescended" inferior adenoma will be found. Next, the thyroid lobe on the side of the missing gland should be carefully palpated. Any lump within the thyroid should be excised, for this might represent an intrathyroidal parathyroid adenoma. It is also important to remember that many patients, particularly those that have been exposed to low-dose external radiation in the past, have benign or malignant lesions of the thyroid gland that require proper surgical resection, along with parathyroidectomy. Even if no lump is present, a 'blind' subtotal excision of the thyroid lobe on the side of the missing gland should be performed. Sometimes a nonpalpable parathyroid adenoma will emerge. Others use a thyroidotomy and incise the lower pole of the thyroid rather than resecting it. Finally, the carotid sheath should be opened from the level of the clavicle upward. Occasionally, a parathyroid adenoma

that cannot be palpated because it is flattened out like a pancake will be found.

Even if four normal glands are found in the neck, the surgeon should search all of these ectopic sites for a fifth gland that is adenomatous. Similarly, if four hyperplastic glands cannot be found, these same sites should be explored.

Only rarely should a sternotomy and formal mediastinal dissection be done as part of the first exploration. This procedure is probably indicated only if the patient is extremely ill from hypercalcemia that cannot be adequately managed medically. The reasons for this approach are several: First of all, sometimes the diagnosis is in error. Second, occasionally hypercalcemia regresses or is eliminated by this first neck exploration despite the fact that no abnormal parathyroid tissue has been removed. This probably occurs when an adenoma is infarcted by accidental ligation of its arterial supply. Finally, it is well known that in most cases of persistent hyperparathyroidism, the offending gland or glands can later be removed through a neck incision, particularly if the first surgeon is not very experienced in this area. This fact is clearly demonstrated in the Mayo Clinic series in which, until 1970, 1000 parathyroid explorations were performed and only twelve required a sternotomy, an incidence of 1.2 percent. At the Massachusetts General Hospital 21 percent of cases of primary hyperparathyroidism involved ectopically placed parathyroid adenomas. However, almost all of these could be removed through a neck incision, and only 5 percent required a sternotomy. At the University of Chicago Hospitals, in a personal series of over three hundred cases, about two percent of cases required a sternotomy, and in each instance this operation was curative.

Management of Persistent or Recurrent Hyperparathyroidism. Persistent disease means that hypercalcemia remains after operation. This occurs when the diagnosis of hyperparathyroidism is incorrect, or when the hyperfunctioning gland or glands have not been adequately removed. In the hands of experienced neck surgeons, this should occur only infrequently, probably 5 percent of the

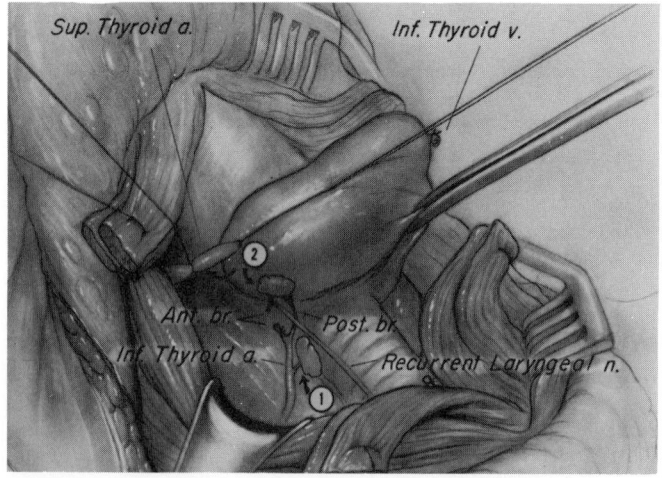

Fig. 38-54. It may be necessary to divide a branch of the inferior artery or to divide the superior thyroid artery to identify the upper parathyroid (2). The lower parathyroid gland (1) is not infrequently opposite the lower pole of the thyroid or below this in the thymus gland.

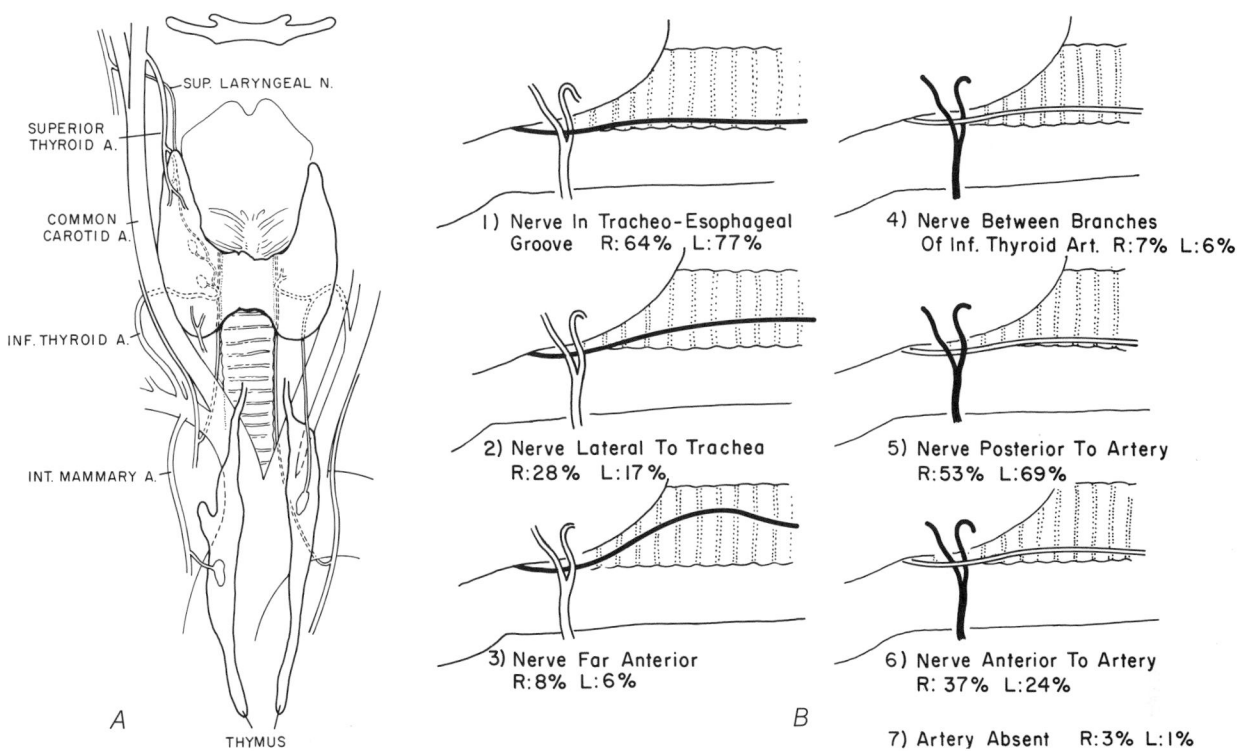

Fig. 38-55. *A.* Blood supply of the parathyroids. *B.* The relation of the inferior thyroid artery to the recurrent laryngeal nerve.

time or less for initial neck explorations. Recurrent disease means that the calcium returns to normal postoperatively but that months to years later, hypercalcemia due to hyperparathyroidism returns. This condition is relatively uncommon except in familial hyperparathyroidism or MEN, type I syndrome, and is most often seen if primary chief cell hyperplasia is not recognized and one or two enlarged glands are removed because they are diagnosed as adenomas. When recurrent hyperparathyroidism does occur, the parathyroid disease should be treated as hyperplasia with subtotal parathyroidectomy or a total resection of all glands with autotransplantation. A lesser

Fig. 38-56. Lateral view with the thyroid retracted anteriorly and mediad to show the surgical landmarks for locating the parathyroids.

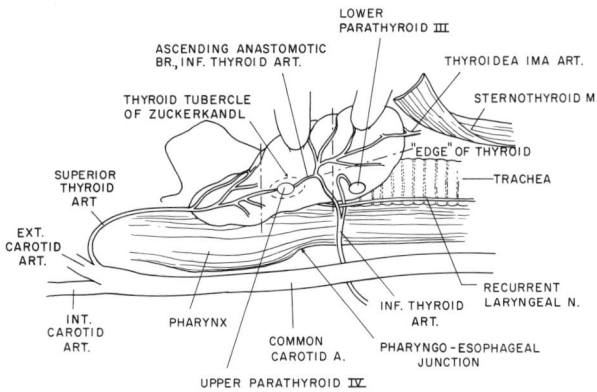

procedure will be once more doomed to failure. Hypercalcemia recurring several months after an apparently successful parathyroidectomy should alert the physician to the possibility of a parathyroid carcinoma, although inadequately treated hyperplasia is more likely. It is necessary to follow patients for many years following parathyroidectomy if the results of therapy are to be truly assessed.

Nine percent of recent patients referred for reexploration by the National Institutes of Health have been shown to have familial hypocalciuric hypercalcemia. This familial disease is probably a benign variant of hyperparathyroidism. Despite hypercalcemia and elevated parathyroid concentrations in most instances, these patients suffer few complications of their disease. The diagnosis is made by demonstrating a low urinary calcium output despite hypercalcemia and a calcium to creatinine clearance ratio of less than 0.01. Such patients will not benefit from parathyroidectomy since less than a total parathyroidectomy will not correct the hypercalcemia. Thus, if the correct diagnosis is made, a reoperation should not be contemplated.

Before reoperation, the operative note and the pathology report or slides should be carefully examined in order to find documentation of the number and location of normal or abnormal parathyroid glands that had been removed or biopsied. The location of each gland found at the initial operation and whether to expect an adenoma or hyperplasia are very helpful factors. Unfortunately, at times, it is very difficult to gain this information from the notes available. Localization tests are most applicable to this situation.

Strategy and Technique of Reoperation. Reoperations of the neck are more difficult because of the scarring, changes in anatomy, and loss of tissue planes that occur as a result of the first exploration, whether it was for a thyroid or parathyroid disorder. Frequently, for example, the strap muscles will be densely adherent to the anterior surface of the thyroid lobes, making entry into the usual anatomical planes more difficult. Furthermore, the recurrent laryngeal nerve is in greater jeopardy, first of all because it may be encased in scar tissue, but especially because it might lie immediately beneath the strap muscles if the thyroid lobe was previously removed. Finally, since one's knowledge of how many parathyroid glands remain in the neck after the first exploration is often limited, the chance of creating permanent hypoparathyroidism after removal of one or more abnormal parathyroid glands found at reexploration is increased. Usually there is not a rush to reoperate and it is better to allow some time to pass in order to permit the wound to heal, to reevaluate the diagnosis, and to assess the findings of the previous operation.

When reoperating, we always explore the neck again first unless an adenoma is localized to the mediastinum or an experienced parathyroid surgeon did the initial operation and was "certain" that the lesion was not in the neck. Only under these circumstances would a sternotomy be performed initially.

The prior transverse neck incision is used and subplatysmal flaps are elevated. The strap muscles are often adherent to the thyroid lobes; hence, instead of separating them in the midline, it is often easier to dissect the vertical plane between each sternocleidomastoid muscle and the strap muscles (see Fig. 38-51). Not infrequently this plane is totally unscarred and by retracting the carotid sheath laterally and the thyroid gland medially, a "fresh" area containing the recurrent laryngeal nerve and parathyroid glands will be entered. If this area is scarred, the dissection should be started as low in the neck as possible since this region is often untouched. Once the recurrent nerve is identified, it can be safely followed in a cephalad direction. If the adenoma was not localized beforehand, a bilateral neck exploration is usually necessary. In the case of either positive localization or retrospective determination of the side of the neck of the missing gland, the cervical dissection might be started there initially.

One of the most rewarding maneuvers that should be done early is to dissect the upper thyroid area posteriorly to the prevertebral fascia and to introduce one's finger downward behind the inferior thyroid artery along the esophagus into the posterior mediastinum as far as one can reach. Often the missing adenoma will be palpated here before it can be seen. This is the area in which many missing adenomas will be found because the initial dissection was not carried out deep enough.

If this is unsuccessful, all of the sites described above should be explored. This involves pulling up and dissecting the thymus on each side into the neck and removing all of the tissue down to the innominate artery, dissecting as high in the neck as the hyoid bone, removing a part of one or both thyroid lobes, and finally opening and exploring the carotid sheath areas. A careful neck reexploration in this manner wil almost always yield the missing adenoma or the elusive hyperplastic gland or glands that remain.

Before operation, consent for a possible sternotomy should be obtained, if that is your operative plan. Another approach used by many surgeons, however, is to plan to only reexplore the neck as carefully as possible, and to postpone the sternotomy for another time, especially if no localization studies were performed before the neck reexploration.

Either a partial sternotomy to the third intercostal space or a complete sternotomy can be performed. First the thymus and surrounding fat pads should be palpated. Several times we could feel a mass, which proved to be the missing adenoma and only a partial thymectomy was necessary. Otherwise, the entire thymus should be removed. If the parathyroid gland is not found therein, a posterior dissection should then be performed. Lesions have been found along the esophagus, between the aorta and pulmonary artery, and even very rarely in an intrapericardial location. Needless to say, these dissections can be very long and tedious.

When an adenoma is found in the neck or chest, it should be totally removed. If one additional normal gland was left after the first operation, the patient will have normal postoperative parathyroid function (thus, stressing the importance of *not* removing normal parathyroid glands during an unsuccessful initial operation). If hyperplastic glands are identified at reoperation, either a subtotal parathyroidectomy can be performed, or others prefer a total parathyroidectomy, arguing that if recurrence were to occur in a remnant that is left, this would necessitate a third neck operation. If total parathyroidectomy is used, or following removal of an adenoma when one thinks that no other parathyroid tissue remains, one has the option of either immediately autotransplanting some of the abnormal parathyroid to the arm or else cryopreserving the tissue and waiting to see whether or not hypocalcemia occurs postoperatively. If hypoparathyroidism occurs, a subsequent autotransplant to the arm could be employed, especially if the preserved tissue was shown to be suppressible. The frequency of recurrent hyperparathyroidism when part of an adenoma or of a hyperplastic gland is used as an autotransplant to the arm remains a fruitful area for study.

Postoperative Complications. Wound infections are rare following these procedures. *Hemorrhage and hematoma and damage to the recurrent laryngeal nerve* are potentially very serious complications. They are discussed earlier in the chapter under Complications of thyroidectomy. Hypoparathyroidism, the third serious complication, will be discussed later in this chapter.

RESULTS. Persistence of hyperparathyroidism occurs in less than 5 percent of patients who are operated upon by experienced parathyroid surgeons. In some series up to 98 percent are cured by their first operation. Recurrent hyperparathyroidism is low when an adenoma is found at the first operation. However, in patients with the multiple endocrine neoplasia, type I (MEN-I) or in others with familial hyperparathyroidism, recurrent disease occurs frequently—in 33 percent of patients in the review of Clark, for example. Recurrence in the latter patients occurs whether a subtotal parathyroidectomy or a total parathyroidectomy with the autotransplant to the arm is done. Long-term follow-up of patients is essential to know the true cure rates.

Recurrent laryngeal nerve injury is uncommon if the nerves are identified and handled with care at operation. Wound hematoma causing respiratory embarrassment is very uncommon but is a true emergency when it occurs.

Severe hypoparathyroidism may occur more frequently following subtotal parathyroidectomy than after lesser operations if great care is not exercised in performing this operation. When done by experienced surgeons, however, the incidence of permanent hypoparathyroidism necessitating vitamin D therapy is quite low.

Parathyroid Transplantation and Cryopreservation. Following subtotal parathyroidectomy for secondary hyperparathyroidism, the remnant of tissue is subjected to a continuing hypocalcemic stimulus. Thus, it is likely to hypertrophy and to cause symptoms again. To avoid reoperation in the neck, which is always more dangerous, Wells et al. have proposed that the parathyroid remnant be minced into small pieces and implanted into the muscles of the forearm. All other parathyroid tissues are removed. Total parathyroidectomy with autotransplantation of parathyroid tissue to the arm works effectively in almost all cases. Histologically viable parathyroid tissue can be biopsied in the arm, and the antecubital veins draining the grafted tissue have higher serum PTH levels than do veins of the opposite, nongrafted arm. If hyperparathyroidism recurs, some of the tissue can be removed from the forearm using local anesthesia (a much safer procedure).

Parathyroid cryopreservation can also be accomplished. This can be thought of as a "parathyroid bank," in which some of the minced parathyroid tissue is frozen in a specific manner and thus preserved. In the event of hypoparathyroidism, some of the patient's own parathyroid could be reimplanted.

Wells has suggested that patients with *primary* chief cell hyperplasia be treated by total parathyroidectomy, and transplantation of tissue to the arm; the same pertains to cases of familial hyperparathyroidism and MEN-1 syndromes.

Several immunosuppressed, aparathyroid patients received a parathyroid allograft from a patient who previously had been his renal transplant donor (Fig. 38-57). This technique has only limited application, however, since most patients do well with vitamin D therapy. Parathyroid graft rejection is a problem, as one would expect. Finally, parathyroid transplantation has been attempted in several aparathyroid infants with DiGeorge's syndrome, a condition in which the thymus and parathyroid glands do not develop. Such patients have limited or absent immune defenses. Thus, the graft would be expected to survive. Unfortunately, the infants died of infection before graft survival could be assessed.

Hypoparathyroidism

ETIOLOGY. The most common cause of hypoparathyroidism is surgical removal, trauma, or devascularization of the parathyroids either during parathyroid surgical treatment or, more commonly, during operations on the thyroid. Postoperative tetany after thyroidectomy for goiter was first described by Reverdin and Kocher in 1882, although of course it was not recognized that this was due to parathyroid deficiency. Primary idiopathic hypoparathyroidism is extremely rare and is usually first noted in patients under the age of sixteen.

Transient hypoparathyroidism can be noted after removal of a parathyroid adenoma or a resection of most of the tissue in parathyroid hyperplasia. This is made worse when the patient has some degree of renal disease that tends to lower the calcium level by itself or when the patient has serious bone disease, when the calcium tends to be deposited in the bone, thus producing hypocalcemia. This process is referred to as "bone hunger" and should be expected when the patient has a high alkaline phosphatase concentration preoperatively due to severe bone disease. In some instances the transient hypocalcemia is due to trauma to the remaining glands or to interference with the blood supply. Following parathyroidectomy, the serum calcium level is usually at its lowest on the second or third postoperative day when transient hypoparathyroidism is present.

Idiopathic hypoparathyroidism is an uncommon disease of unknown cause. Recent evidence would suggest that in some cases it is due to the presence of antibodies against parathyroid tissue. The patients may also have antibodies against adrenal, thyroid, and gastric parietal cells. One hypothesis is that the parathyroid disease is part of a generalized autoimmune disease. Other diseases sometimes associated with this include monilial infection, Hashimoto's thyroiditis, and steatorrhea.

CLINICAL MANIFESTATIONS. Symptoms. The symptoms of hypoparathyroidism are those of hypocalcemia and are related to the greatly increased neuromuscular excitability brought about by a decrease in the plasma ionized calcium. The most striking manifestation is tetany. This may consist of carpopedal spasm in which the fingers at the metacarpal phalangeal joint and the wrist are flexed and the elbow, legs, and feet are extended. Tonic and clonic convulsions and laryngeal stridor may be present and may even prove fatal. In the milder forms tingling of the fingertips and of the lips, muscle cramps, numbness, dysphagia, and dysarthria may be present. There may be some degree of anxiety. In chronic hypoparathyroidism cataracts and mental changes may occur.

Physical Signs. Chvostek's sign consists of a contraction of the facial muscles in response to a tap over the facial nerve in front of the ear. Occluding the circulation at the arm by inflation of a blood pressure cuff above the

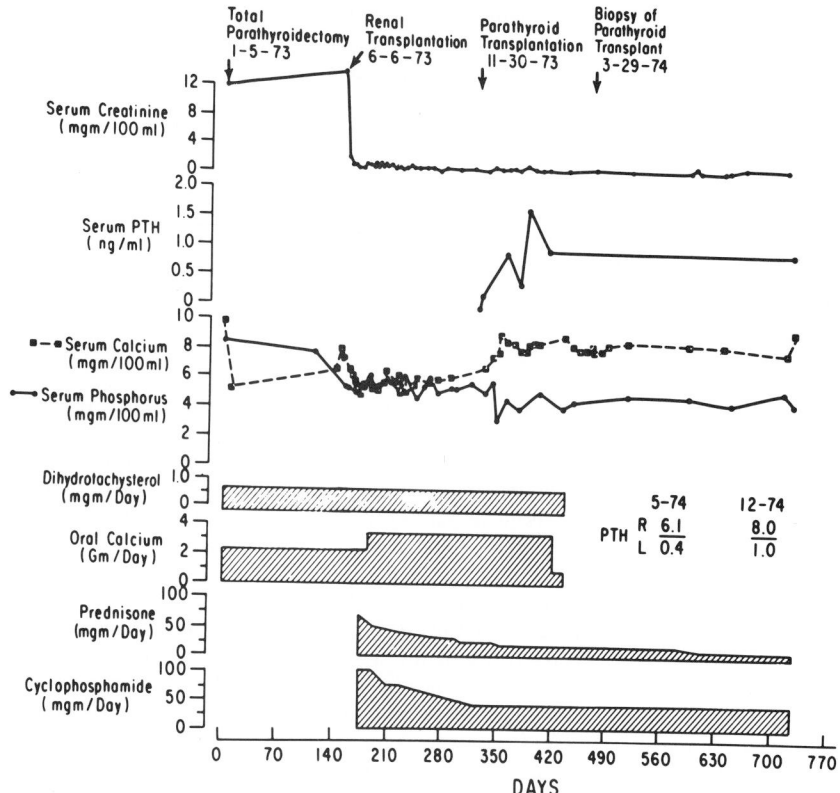

Fig. 38-57. The clinical course of a 19-year-old male who had undergone a total parathyroidectomy for severe bone pain in 1973 and then received a renal transplant 6 months later. Because of severe symptoms of hypocalcemia in the patient, two parathyroid glands were removed from his father (who had also contributed donor kidney) and implanted in the patient's forearm in November 1973. Thereafter serum calcium rose to normal values and calcium and vitamin D therapy was stopped. Serum PTH levels returned to normal and were higher in the antecubital veins on the side of the transplant. The patient remains on prednisone and cyclophosphamide (Cytoxan) therapy. (From: *Wells SA Jr et al: Surgery 78:34, 1975, with permission.*)

level of systolic pressure induces carpopedal spasm within 3 min. This is Trousseau's sign, a less reliable sign than Chvostek's sign.

The electrocardiogram shows a prolongation of the Q-T interval. The plasma calcium level is low, and the phosphate is increased.

Differential Diagnosis. Tetany can be caused by factors other than hypoparathyroidism. Alkalosis can produce tetany even in the presence of a normal blood total calcium level by lowering the ionized calcium level. Rickets in the child, osteomalacia in the adult, steatorrhea, and renal insufficiency all produce hypocalcemia. In rickets, osteomalacia, and steatorrhea there is a low plasma calcium level with a normal or low plasma phosphate level. This differentiates it from hypoparathyroidism, where the plasma phosphate level is generally elevated. Chronic renal insufficiency is associated with hypocalcemia with a markedly elevated plasma phosphate level—higher than that usually seen in hypoparathyroidism. This can further be distinguished from hypoparathyroidism by the elevated BUN level.

A low plasma magnesium level can also produce tetany. In some cases of tetany, hypomagnesemia and hypocalcemia are both present. The tetany often cannot be corrected until the circulating magnesium level is brought to normal.

TREATMENT. Postoperative Hypocalcemia. When mild, no treatment is needed, but careful, watchful waiting should be employed. Serum calcium levels should be determined every 12 h for the first few days and then daily

thereafter. If the patient becomes symptomatic, 1 g calcium gluconate can be given slowly intravenously, and then 1 to 2 g/8 h of this preparation may be dripped continuously in an intravenous bottle to alleviate all symptoms. Within several days all calcium therapy can usually be stopped. This condition is referred to as *transient hypoparathyroidism.*

For more persistent hypocalcemia, oral calcium is also begun in a dose of 1.5 to 2.0 g calcium ion per day. It is important to note that to provide 1 g elemental calcium one must administer 5.5 g hydrated calcium chloride, 8 g calcium lactate, or 11 g calcium gluconate. Calcium carbonate is usually preferred. The patient may be sent home on oral calcium therapy when asymptomatic, and this can usually be discontinued after several weeks. It is preferable not to add vitamin D to this early regimen unless one strongly suspects that permanent hypoparathyroidism has occurred (or unless a parathyroid transplant has been performed).

If *permanent hypoparathyroidism* has occurred, in addition to the oral calcium therapy the patient is started on vitamin D₃, 50,000 to 100,000 units/day (1.25 to 2.5 mg/day). Others prefer to use dihydrotachysterol, 0.125 to 1.0 mg/day. Larger initial doses of these compounds are often utilized. The use of 1,25 $(OH)_2D_3$, the active metabolite of vitamin D, is advantageous, since it is faster acting and more readily reversed if an overdose is given. Initial doses of 1 to 2 μg are given in divided doses. Maintenance doses are lower. The serum calcium concentration must be checked frequently, since some patients are insensitive to these preparations and need larger doses, whereas others develop vitamin D intoxication with severe hypercalcemia on relatively small dosages.

Serum PTH concentrations should be checked at intervals in patients being treated for permanent postoperative hypoparathyroidism. Several patients whom we have seen have been treated unnecessarily with vitamin D for many years because postoperative tetany had occurred. When serum PTH levels are detectable, vitamin D therapy should be slowly tapered and finally stopped if possible.

Other nonspecific factors may tend to influence the treatment of hypocalcemia. A diet high in phosphate or oxalate content should be avoided, since it may impair calcium absorption. Concomitant ingestion of anticonvulsants and tranquilizers may lower intestinal absorption of calcium both directly and by interfering with vitamin D metabolism. Estrogen and oral contraceptive therapy lower serum calcium level by suppressing bone resorption. Diuretics, such as furosemide, result in increased calcium excretion in the urine. Hypomagnesemia should be avoided since this leads to resistance to vitamin D therapy.

PSEUDOHYPOPARATHYROIDISM

Pseudohypoparathyroidism was first described by Albright et al. in 1942. This is a genetic disease in which the clinical and chemical features of hypoparathyroidism are present in association with the genetic stigmata of a round face, a short, thick body, and short, stubby fingers. There is a shortening of some of the metacarpal and metatarsal bones as a result of early epiphyseal closure, so that a dimple rather than a knuckle shows when the fist is clenched. Mental deficiency may be present, and there are sometimes areas of subcutaneous ossification. The manifestations are not due to lack of parathyroid secretion but to unresponsiveness of the end organ, the renal phosphaturic mechanism. The parathyroids are normal or hyperplastic, and serum PTH concentration is raised in these patients. Hypocalcemia and hyperphosphatemia are usually present. Patients with this syndrome may show evidence of increased bone resorption and even osteitis fibrosa cystica, since PTH appears to act appropriately on bone but not on the kidney.

Pseudohypoparathyroidism can be distinguished from hypoparathyroidism not only by the characteristic physical picture of the patient but also because individuals with hypoparathyroidism respond to parathyroid extract while those with pseudohypoparathyroidism usually do not. The Ellsworth-Howard test has been designed to demonstrate this difference. The patient is slowly given 200 units of parathyroid extract intravenously, and the urinary phosphate excretion is determined for 3 h before and 3 h after the administration. The parathyroid extract produces a fivefold increase in urine phosphate excretion in normal persons, a tenfold increase in patients with hypoparathyroidism, and less than a twofold increase in patients with pseudohypoparathyroidism.

Recently it has been demonstrated that patients with pseudohypoparathyroidism have a deficient renal adenyl cyclase system. This offers a new diagnostic test for differentiating patients with idiopathic hypoparathyroidism from those with pseudohypoparathyroidism. In the former group, PTH administration results in increased urinary cyclic 3'5'-AMP, while in pseudohypoparathyroid patients PTH gives no change or only a slight increase in urinary cyclic AMP.

A high concentration of calcitonin has been found in the thyroid gland of some patients with this disease. This, however, appears to be the result of the hypocalcemia rather than its cause.

The treatment of pseudohypoparathyroidism is the same as that for hypoparathyroidism: low-phosphate diet, alumina gel, and vitamin D or its new metabolites.

PSEUDOPSEUDOHYPOPARATHYROIDISM

Pseudopseudohypoparathyroidism is also a genetic defect, and these individuals have the same physical features as those with pseudohypoparathyroidism. It differs from pseudohypoparathyroidism in that the plasma calcium and phosphate levels are normal and Chvostek's and Trousseau's signs are absent. The administration of PTH in one patient resulted in a normal rise in urinary cyclic AMP.

Bibliography

Thyroid: Anatomy

Deane SA, Telander RL: Surgery for thyroglossal duct and branchial cleft anomalies. *Am J Surg* 136:348, 1978.

Fish J, Moore RM: Ectopic thyroid tissue and ectopic thyroid carcinoma. *Ann Surg* 157:212, 1963.

Hung W, Randolph JG, et al: Lingual and sublingual thyroid glands in euthyroid children. *Pediatrics* 38:647, 1966.

Katz AD, Zager WJ: The lingual thyroid. Its diagnosis and treatment. *Arch Surg* 102:582, 1971.

Moosman DA, DeWeese MS: The external laryngeal nerve as related to thyroidectomy. *Surg Gynecol Obstet* 127:1011, 1968.

Peters LL, Gardner RJ: Repair of recurrent laryngeal nerve injuries. *Surgery* 71:865, 1972.

Pollock WF, Stevenson EO: Cysts and sinuses of the thyroglossal duct. *Am J Surg* 112:225, 1966.

Riddell VH: Injury to recurrent laryngeal nerves during thyroidectomy. *Lancet* 2:638, 1956.

Wijetilaka SE: Non-recurrent laryngeal nerve. *Br J Surg* 65:179, 1978.

Thyroid: Physiology

Astwood, EB, Solomon DH: Mechanisms of action of an-tithyroid drugs, iodides, and other thyroid inhibitors, in Werner SC (ed): *The Thyroid.* New York, Harper & Row, Hoeber Medical Division, 1955, chap 6.

DeGroot LJ, Stanbury JB: *The Thyroid and Its Diseases,* 4th ed. New York, Wiley, 1975, chaps 2–4.

Miller LJ, Gorman CA, Go VLW: Gut-thyroid interrelationships. *Gastroenterology* 75:901, 1978.

Sterling K: Thyroid hormone action at the cell level (first of two parts). *N Engl J Med* 300:17, 1979.

Sterling K: Thyroid hormone action at the cell level (second of two parts). *N Engl J Med* 300:173, 1979.

Zellman HE: Iatrogenic and factitious thyroidal disease. *Med Clin North Am* 63:329, 1979.

Evaluation of Patients with Thyroid Disease

Boey J, Ilsn C, et al: A controlled trial of fine needle aspiration and drill biopsy of thyroid nodules. *World J Surg* 5:458, 1981.

DeGroot LJ, Stanbury JB: *The Thyroid and Its Diseases,* 4th ed. New York, Wiley, 1975, chap 5.

Frable MA, Frable WJ: Thin needle aspiration biopsy of the thyroid gland. *Laryngoscope* 90:1619, 1980.

Hamburger JB: Thyroid testing cost-benefit considerations. *J Nucl Med* 22:655, 1981.

Löwhagen T, Granberg P-O, et al: Aspiration biopsy cytology (ABC) in nodules of the thyroid gland suspected to be malignant. *Surg Clin North Am* 59:3, 1979.

Löwhagen T, Willems J-S, et al: Aspiration biopsy cytology in diagnosis of thyroid cancer. *World J Surg* 5:61, 1981.

Miller MJ, Hamburger JB, Kini S: Diagnosis of thyroid nodules: Use of fine needle aspiration and needle biopsy. *JAMA* 241:481, 1979.

Miller TR, Abele JS, Greenspan FS: Fine needle aspiration biopsy in the management of thyroid nodules. *West J Med* 134:198, 1981.

Task Force of Short-lived Radionuclides for Medical Applications: Evaluation of diseases of the thyroid gland with the in vivo use of radionuclides. *J Nucl Med* 19:107, 1978.

Walfish PG, Hazani E, et al: Combined ultrasound and needle aspiration biopsy in the assessment of hypofunctioning thyroid nodule. *Ann Intern Med* 87:270, 1977.

Hyperthyroidism

Beahrs OH, Ryan RF, et al: Surgical thyroidectomy in the management of exophthalmic goiter. *Arch Surg* 96:512, 1968.

Catz B, Perzik SL: Total thyroidectomy in the management of thyrotoxic and euthyroid Graves' disease. *Am J Surg* 118:434, 1969.

Cevalos JL, Hagen GA, et al: Low dosage ^{131}I therapy of thyrotoxicosis (diffuse goiters). A five-year follow-up study. *N Engl J Med* 290:141, 1974.

Dobyns BM: Prevention and management of hyperthyroid storm. *World J Surg* 2:293, 1978.

Eriksson M, Rubenfeld S, et al: Propranolol does not prevent thyroid storm. *N Engl J Med* 296:263, 1977.

Friedman JM, Fialkow PJ: The genetics of Graves' disease. *Clin Endocrinol Metab* 7:47, 1978.

Greer MA, Kammer H, Bouma DJ: Short-term antithyroid drug therapy for the thyrotoxicosis of Graves' disease. *N Engl J Med* 297:173, 1977.

Gwinup G: Prospective randomized comparison of propylthiouracil. *JAMA* 239:2457, 1978.

Hales IB, Rundle FF: Ocular changes in Graves' disease: A long-term follow-up study. *Quart J Med* 29:113, 1960.

Heimann P: Should hyperthyroidism be treated by surgery? *World J Surg* 2:281, 1978.

Hotem AL, Thomas CG, VanWyk JJ: Selection of treatment in the management of thyrotoxicosis in childhood and adolescence. *Ann Surg* 187:593, 1978.

Klementschitsch P, Shen K-L, Kapian EL: Reemergence of thyroidectomy as treatment for Graves' disease. *Surg Clin North Am* 59:35, 1979.

Lundstrom B, Hed J, et al: Thyroid function after subtotal thyroidectomy for hyperthyroidism related to some morphological and immunological features. *Acta Chir Scand* 143:215, 1977.

McGregor AM, Rees Smith B, et al: Prediction of relapse in hyperthyroid Graves' disease. *Lancet* I:1101, 1980.

Mitchie W, Pegg CAS, Bewsher PD: Prediction of hypothyroidism after partial thyroidectomy for thyrotoxicosis. *Br Med J* 1:13, 1972.

Munro DS, Dirmikis SM, et al: The role of thyroid stimulating immunoglobulins of Graves' disease in neonatal thyrotoxicosis. *Br J Obstet Gynaecol* 85:837, 1978.

Okita N, Row WW, Volpe R: Suppressor T-lymphocyte deficiency in Graves' disease and Hashimoto's thyroiditis. *J Clin Endocrinol Metab* 52:528, 1981.

Riley FC: Surgical management of ophthalmopathy in Graves' disease: Transfrontal orbital decompression. *Mayo Clin Proc* 47:986, 1972.

Rubenfeld S, Silverman VE, Welch KMA: Variable plasma propranolol levels in thyrotoxicosis. *N Engl J Med* 300:353, 1979.

Shapiro SJ, Friedman NB, et al: Incidence of thyroid carcinoma in Graves' disease. *Cancer* 26:1261, 1970.

Smith BR, Hall R: Thyroid stimulating immunoglobulins in Graves' disease. *Lancet* 2:427, 1974.

Teng CS, Yeung RTT, et al: A prospective study of the changes in thyrotropin binding inhibitory immunoglobulins in Graves' disease treated by subtotal thyroidectomy or radioactive iodine. *J Clin Endocrinol Metab* 50:1005, 1980.

Thompson NW, Dunn EL, et al: Surgical treatment of thyrotoxicosis in children and adolescents. *J Pediatr Surg* 12:1009, 1977.

Totten MA, Wool MS: Medical treatment of hyperthyroidism. *Med Clin North Am* 63:321, 1979.

Zonszein J, Santangelo RP, Mackin JF: Propranolol therapy in thyrotoxicosis. A review of 84 patients undergoing surgery. *Am J Med* 66:411, 1979.

Hypothyroidism

Kumar MS, Safa AM, et al: The relationship of thyroid-stimulating hormone (TSH), thyroxine (T4), and triiodothyronine (T3) in primary thyroid failure. *Am J Clin Pathol* 68:747, 1977.

Van Welsum M, Feltkamp TEW, et al: Hypoparathyroidism after thyroidectomy for Graves' disease: Search for an explanation. *Br Med J* 4:755, 1974.

Thyroiditis

Altemeier WA: Acute pyogenic thyroiditis. *Arch Surg* 61:76, 1950.

Crile G Jr, Hazard JB: Incidence of cancer in struma lymphomatosa. *Surg Gynecol Obstet* 115:101, 1962.

Greene JN: Subacute thyroiditis. *Am J Med* 51:97, 1971.

Hagan AD, Goffinet J, Davis JW: Acute streptococcal thyroiditis. *JAMA* 202:842, 1967.

Linden MC Jr, Clark JH: Indications for surgery in thyroiditis. *Am J Surg* 118:829, 1969.

Mulhern LM, Masi AT, Shulman LE: Hashimoto's disease: A search for associated disorders in 170 clinically detected cases. *Lancet* 2:508, 1966.

de Quervain F: Die akute, nicht eiterige thyroiditis. *Mitt Grenzgeb Med Chir* 2(suppl):1, 1904.

Rudman I, Novota OJ, Keener RL: Complications of Hashimoto thyroiditis surgery. *Arch Surg* 83:822, 1961.

Volpé R, Johnston MW, Huber N: Thyroid function in subacute thyroiditis. *J Clin Endocrinol Metab* 18:65, 1958.

Goiter

Crile G Jr: Treatment of thyroid cysts by aspiration. *Surgery* 59:210, 1966.

Glassford GH, Fowler EF, Cole WH: The treatment of nontoxic nodular goiter with dessicated thyroid: Results and evaluation. *Surgery* 58:621, 1965.

Jenny H, Block MA, et al: Recurrence following surgery for benign thyroid nodules. *Arch Surg* 92:525, 1966.

Benign Tumors

Ackerman LV: *Surgical Pathology*. St Louis, Mosby, 1964.

DeGroot LJ, Stanbury JB: *The Thyroid and Its Diseases*, 4th ed. New York, Wiley, 1975.

Malignant Tumors

Aldinger KA, Samaan NA, et al: Anaplastic carcinoma of the thyroid. A review of 84 cases of spindle and giant cell carcinoma of the thyroid. *Cancer* 41:2267, 1978.

Arganini M, Behar R, et al: Hürthle cell tumors: A twenty-five-year experience. *Surgery* 100:1108, 1986.

Block MA, Horn RC Jr: Medullary carcinoma of the thyroid: Surgical implications. *Arch Surg* 96:521, 1968.

Block MA, Jackson CE, Tashjian AH Jr: Medullary thyroid carcinoma detected by serum calcitonin assay. *Arch Surg* 104:579, 1972.

Boehm T, Rothouse L, Wartofsky L: Metastatic occult follicular thyroid carcinoma. *JAMA* 235:2420, 1976.

Cady B, Sedgwick CE, et al: Risk factor analysis in differentiated thyroid cancer. *Cancer* 43:810, 1979.

Carney JA, Sizemore GW, Tyce GM: Bilateral adrenal medullary hyperplasia in multiple endocrine neoplasia, type 2A: The precursor of bilateral pheochromocytoma. *Mayo Clin Proc* 50:3, 1975.

Charbord P, L'Heritier C, et al: Radioiodine treatment in differentiated thyroid carcinomas. Treatment of first local recurrences and of bone and lung metastases. *Annales de Radiologie* (Paris) 20:783, 1977.

Compagno J, Oertel JE: Malignant lymphoma and other lymphoproliferative disorders of the thyroid gland. A clinicopathologic study of 245 cases. *Am J Clin Pathol* 74:1, 1980.

Crile G Jr: The fallacy of the conventional radical neck dissection for papillary carcinoma of the thyroid. *Ann Surg* 145:317, 1957.

Crile G Jr: Lymphosarcoma and reticulum cell sarcoma of the thyroid. *Surg Gynecol Obstet* 116:449, 1963.

Crile G Jr: Struma lymphomatosa and carcinoma of the thyroid. *Surg Gynecol Obstet* 147:350, 1978.

Dobyns BM, Sheline GE, et al: Malignant and benign neoplasms of the thyroid in patients treated for hyperthyroidism: A report of the cooperative thyrotoxicosis follow-up study. *J Clin Endocrinol Metab* 38:976, 1974.

Doci R, Pilotti S, et al: Thyroid cancer in childhood. *Tumori* 64:649, 1978.

Durie BG, Hellman D, et al: High-risk thyroid cancer. Prolonged survival with multimodality therapy. *Cancer Clin Trials* 4:67, 1981.

Favus MJ, Schneider AB, et al: Thyroid cancer occurring as a late consequence of head- and neck-irradiation: Evaluation of 1,056 patients. *N Engl J Med* 294:1019, 1976.

Franssila KO: Prognosis in thyroid carcinoma. *Cancer* 36:1138, 1975.

Gétaz EP, Shimaoka K: Anaplastic carcinoma of the thyroid in a population irradiated for Hodgkin's disease, 1910–1960. *J Surg Oncol* 12:181, 1979.

Harada T, Ito K, et al: Fatal thyroid carcinoma. Anaplastic transformation of adenocarcinoma. *Cancer* 39:2588, 1977.

Harness JK, Thompson NW, et al: Differentiated thyroid carcinomas: Treatment of distant metastases. *Arch Surg* 108:410, 1974.

Hubert JP, Kiernan PD, et al: Occult papillary carcinoma of the thyroid. *Arch Surg* 115:394, 1980.

Kaplan EL, Peskin GW: Physiologic implications of medullary carcinoma of the thyroid gland. *Surg Clin North Am* 51:125, 1971.

Leeper RD, Crile G, et al: Final panel report. II. Thyroid carcinoma—natural history and relation to radiation and to therapy, in DeGroot LJ, Frohman LA, Kaplan EL, Refetoff S (eds): *Radiation-associated Thyroid Carcinoma*. New York, Grune & Stratton, 1977, p 497.

Lindahl F: Anaplastic thyroid carcinoma in Denmark, 1943–1968. *Dan Med Bull* 23:119, 1976.

Lindahl F: Follicular thyroid carcinoma in Denmark, 1943–1968. *Dan Med Bull* 23:107, 1976.

Marchetta FC, Sako K: Modified neck dissection for carcinoma of the thyroid gland. *Surg Gynecol Obstet* 119:551, 1964.

Mazzaferri EL: Thyroid carcinoma following therapeutic and accidental radiation exposure. in Cohen MP, Foa PP (eds): *Spec Topics Endocrinol Metab* 2:103, 1981.

Mazzaferri EL, Young RL: Papillary thyroid carcinoma: A 10-year follow-up report of the impact of therapy in 576 patients. *Am J Med* 70:511, 1981.

Nishiyama RH, Ludwig GK, Thompson NW: The prevalence of small papillary thyroid carcinomas in 100 consecutive necropsies in an American population, in DeGroot LJ, Frohman LA, Kaplan EL, Refetoff S (eds): *Radiation-associated Thyroid Carcinoma*. New York, Grune & Stratton, 1977, p 123.

Roudebush CP, Astersis GT, DeGroot LJ: Natural history of radiation-associated thyroid cancer. *Arch Intern Med* 138:1631, 1978.

Sampson RJ: Prevalence and significance of occult thyroid cancer, in DeGroot LJ, Frohman LA, Kaplan EL, Refetoff S (eds): *Radiation-associated Thyroid Carcinoma*. New York, Grune & Stratton, 1977, p 137.

Schachner SH, Hall A: Parathyroid adenoma and previous head-and-neck irradiation. *Ann Intern Med* 88:804, 1978.

Schneider AB, Favus MJ, et al: Salivary gland neoplasms as a late consequence of head and neck irradiation. *Ann Intern Med* 87:160, 1977.

Shimaoka K, Tsukada Y: Squamous cell carcinoma and adenosquamous carcinomas originating from the thyroid gland. *Cancer* 46:1833, 1980.

Sipple JH: The association of pheochromocytoma with carcinoma of the thyroid gland. *Am J Med* 31:163, 1961.

Swelstad J, Scanlon EF, et al: Thyroid disease following irradiation for benign conditions. *Arch Surg* 112:380, 1977.

Tollefsen HR, DeCosse JJ: Papillary carcinoma of the thyroid: Recurrence in the thyroid gland after initial surgical treatment. *Am J Surg* 106:728, 1963.

Wells SA Jr, Ontjes DA, et al: Early diagnosis of medullary carcinoma of the thyroid gland in patients with multiple endocrine neoplasia type II. *Ann Surg* 182:362, 1975.

Young RL, Mazzaferri EL, et al: Pure follicular thyroid carcinoma: Impact of therapy in 214 patients. *J Nucl Med* 21:733, 1980.

Surgery of the Thyroid

Block MA, Jackson CE, Tashjian AH: Management of parathyroid glands in surgery for medullary thyroid carcinoma. *Arch Surg* 110:617, 1975.

Doyle PJ, Everts EC, Brummett RE: Treatment of recurrent laryngeal nerve injury. *Arch Surg* 96:517, 1968.

Halsted WS, Evans HM: The parathyroid glandules: Their blood supply and preservation in operations upon the thyroid gland. *Ann Surg* 46:489, 1907.

Kaplan EL: Surgery of the thyroid gland, in DeGroot LJ, Larsen PR, et al (eds): *The Thyroid and Its Diseases*. New York, Wiley, 1984, chap 18.

Kaplan EL (ed): *Surgery of the Thyroid and Parathyroid Glands*. Edinburgh, Churchill Livingstone, 1983.

Kaplan EL, Fredland A: Surgery of the parathyroid glands, in Santen RJ, Manni A (eds): *Diagnosis and Management of Endocrine-Related Tumors*. Boston, Martinus Nijhoff, 1984, chap 9.

Lahey FH: Routine dissection and demonstration of recurrent laryngeal nerve in subtotal thyroidectomy. *Surg Gynecol Obstet* 66:775, 1938.

Thompson NW, Harness JK: Complications of total thyroidectomy for carcinoma. *Surg Gynecol Obstet* 131:861, 1970.

Thompson NW, Olsen WR, Hoffman GL: The continuing development of the technique of thyroidectomy. *Surgery* 73:913. 1973.

Parathyroid: Embryology and Anatomy

Gilmour JR: The embryology of the parathyroid glands, the thymus and certain associated rudiments. *J Pathol* 45:507, 1937.

Gilmour JR: The weight of the parathyroid glands. *J Pathol Bacteriol* 44:431, 1937.

Gilmour JR: The gross anatomy of the parathyroid glands. *J Pathol Bacteriol* 46:133, 1938.

Parathyroid Hormone: Chemistry

Brewer HB, Fairwell T, et al: Human parathyroid hormone: Amino-acid sequence of the amino-terminal residues 1–34. *Proc Natl Acad Sci USA* 69:3585, 1972.

Habener JF: Regulation of parathyroid hormone secretion and biosynthesis. *Ann Rev Physiol* 43:211, 1981.

Habener JF, Potts JT Jr, Rich A: Pre-preparathyroid hormone.

Evidence for an early biosynthetic precursor of proparathyroid hormone. *J Biol Chem* 251:3893, 1976.

Kemper B, Habener JF, et al: Pre-preparathyroid hormone analysis of radioactive tryptic peptides and amino acid sequence. *Biochemistry* 15:15, 1976.

Parathyroid: Vitamin D

DeLuca HF: Vitamin D endocrinology. *Ann Intern Med* 85:367, 1976.

Kodicek E: The story of vitamin D, from vitamin to hormone. *Lancet* 1:325, 1974.

Teitelbaum SL, Bone JM, et al: Calcifediol in chronic renal insufficiency. *JAMA* 235:164, 1976.

Calcitonin and Medullary Carcinoma of the Thyroid

Aliapoulios MA, Goldhaber P, Munson PL: Thyrocalcitonin inhibition of bone resorption induced by parathyroid hormone in tissue culture. *Science* 151:330, 1966.

Aliapoulios MA, Goldhaber P, et al: Radioimmunoassay for calcitonin: A preliminary report. *Proc Staff Meetings Mayo Clin* 43:496, 1968.

Chong GC, Beahrs OH, et al: Medullary carcinoma of the thyroid gland. *Cancer* 35:695, 1975.

Copp DH, Cameron EC, et al: Evidence for calcitonin: A new hormone from the parathyroid that lowers blood calcium. *Endocrinology* 70:638, 1962.

Copp DH, Cockcroft DW, Kueh Y: Calcitonin from ultimobranchial glands of dogfish and chickens, *Science* 158:924, 1967.

Gonzalez-Licea A, Hartmann WH, Yardley JH: Medullary carcinoma of the thyroid: Ultrastructural evidence of its origin from the parafollicular cell and its possible relation to carcinoid tumors. *J Clin Pathol* 49:512, 1968.

Hazard JB, Hawk WA, Crile G Jr: Medullary (solid) carcinoma of the thyroid: Clinicopathological entity. *J Clin Endocrinol Metab* 19:152, 1959.

Hirsch PF, Cauthier GF, Munson PL: Thyroid hypocalcemic principle and recurrent laryngeal nerve injury as factors affecting the response to parathyroidectomy in rats. *Endocrinology* 73:244, 1963.

Hirsch PF, Peskin GW: Physiologic implications of medullary carcinoma of the thyroid gland. *Surg Clin North Am* 51:125, 1971.

Melvin KEW, Tashjian AH Jr, Miller HH: Studies in familial (medullary) thyroid carcinoma. *Recent Prog Horm Res* 28:399, 1972.

Pearse AGE, Polak JM: Cytochemical evidence for the neural crest origin of mammalian ultimobranchial C cells. *Histochemie* 27:96, 1971.

Queener SF, Bell NH: Calcitonin: A general survey. *Metabolism* 24:555, 1975.

Samaan NA, Castillo S, et al: Serum calcitonin after pentagastrin stimulation in patients with bronchogenic and breast cancer compared to that in patients with medullary thyroid carcinoma. *J Clin Endocrinol Metab* 51:237, 1980.

Sizemore GW, Heath H III, Carney JA: Multiple endocrine neoplasia type 2. *Clin Endocrinol Metab* 9:299, 1980.

Wells SA Jr, Ontjes DA, et al: The early diagnosis of medullary carcinoma of the thyroid gland in patients with multiple endocrine neoplasia, type II. *Ann Surg* 182:362, 1975.

Wolfe HJ, Melvin KEW, et al: C-cell hyperplasia preceding medullary thyroid carcinoma. *N Engl J Med* 289:437, 1973.

Parathyroid: Pathology

Cope O, Keynes WM, et al: Primary chief-cell hyperplasia of the parathyroid glands: A new entity in the surgery of hyperparathyroidism. *Ann Surg* 148:375, 1958.

Flye MW, Brennan M: Surgical resection of metastatic parathyroid carcinoma. *Ann Surg* 193:425, 1981.

Holmes EC, Morton DL, Ketcham AS: Parathyroid carcinoma: A collective review. *Ann Surg* 169:631, 1969.

Roth SI: Recent advances in parathyroid gland pathology. *Am J Med* 50:612, 1971.

Roth SI: Marshall RB: Pathology and ultrastructure of the human parathyroid glands in chronic renal failure. *Arch Intern Med (Chicago)* 124:397, 1969.

Schantz A, Castleman B: Parathyroid carcinoma: A study of 70 cases. *Cancer* 31:600, 1973.

Utley JR, Black WC: Hyperparathyroidism: A clinicopathologic evaluation. *Am J Surg* 114:788, 1967.

Wermer P: Endocrine adenomatosis and peptic ulcer in a large kindred: Inherited multiple tumors and mosaic pleiotropism in man. *Am J Med* 35:205, 1963.

Primary Hyperparathyroidism

Arnaud CD, Tsao HS, Littledike T: Radioimmunoassay of human parathyroid hormone in serum. *J Clin Invest* 50:21, 1971.

Aurbach GD, Chase LR: Cyclic 3'5'-adenylic acid in bone and the mechanism of action of parathyroid hormone. *Fed Proc* 29:1179, 1970.

Ballard HS, Frane B, Hartsock RJ: Familial multiple endocrine adenoma-peptic ulcer complex. *Medicine (Baltimore)* 43:481, 1964.

Barreras RF, Donaldson RM Jr: Role of carcinoma in gastric hypersecretion, parathyroid adenoma and peptic ulcer. *N Engl J Med* 276:1122, 1967.

Bernstein DS: Hypercalcemia associated with sarcoidosis, hypernephroma, and parathyroid adenoma. *J Clin Endocrinol Metab* 25:1436, 1965.

Brennan MF, Brown EM, et al: Autotransplantation of cryopreserved parathyroid tissue in man. *Ann Surg* 189:139, 1979.

Brennan MF, Doppman JL, et al: Reoperative parathyroid surgery for persistent hyperparathyroidism. *Surgery* 83:669, 1978.

Bruining HA, van Houten H, et al: Results of operative treatment of 615 patients with primary hyperparathyroidism. *World J Surg* 5:85, 1981.

Cameron JR, Sorenson J: Measurement of bone mineral in vivo: An improved method. *Science* 142:230, 1963.

Chaves-Carballo E, Hayles AB: Parathyroid adenoma in children. *Am J Dis Child* 112:553, 1966.

Clark OH, Way LW: Hyperparathyroidism and management of the hypercalcemic patient, in Friesen SR, Bolinger RE (eds): *Surgical Endocrinology.* Philadelphia, Lippincott, 1978, pp 237–261.

Clark OH, Way LW, Hunt TK: Recurrent hyperparathyroidism. *Ann Surg* 184:391, 1976.

Clunie GJA, Gunn A, Robson JS: Hyperparathyroid crisis. *Br J Surg* 54:538, 1967.

Condon RE, Granville GE, et al: Hypercalcemic crisis and intractable gastrointestinal ulceration in a patient with endocrine polyglandular syndrome. *Ann Surg* 167:185, 1968.

Cope O: The study of hyperparathyroidism at the Massachusetts General Hospital. *N Engl J Med* 274:1174, 1966.

Cushing H, Davidoff LM: *The Pathological Findings in Four Autopsied Cases of Acromegaly with a Discussion of Their Significance,* Monograph 22. New York, The Rockefeller Institute for Medical Research, 1927.

Cutler RE, Reiss E, Ackerman LV: Familial hyperparathyroidism: A kindred involving eleven cases with a discussion of primary chief-cell hyperplasia. *N Engl J Med* 270:859, 1964.

Delmonico F, Neer RM, et al: Hyperparathyroidism during pregnancy. *Am J Surg* 131:328, 1976.

Edis AJ, Beahrs OH, et al: "Conservative" versus "liberal" approach to parathyroid neck exploration. *Surgery* 82:466, 1977.

Edis AJ, Evans TC Jr: High resolution, real-time ultrasonography in the preoperative location of parathyroid tumors. *N Engl J Med* 301:532, 1979.

Edis AJ, Sheedy PF, et al: Results of reoperation for hyperparathyroidism, with evaluation of preoperative localization studies. *Surgery* 84:384, 1978.

Farr HW: Hyperparathyroidism and cancer. *Cancer* 26:66, 1976.

Gaeke RF, Kaplan EL, et al: Successful treatment of maternal primary hyperparathyroidism of pregnancy by parathyroidectomy. *JAMA* 238(6):508, 1977.

Goldberg MF, Tashjian AH Jr, et al: Renal adenocarcinoma containing a parathyroid hormone-like substance and associated with marked hypercalcemia. *Am J Med* 36:805, 1964.

Graber AL, Jacobs K: Familial hyperparathyroidism. *JAMA* 240:542, 1968.

Heath H III, Hodgson SF, Kennedy MA: Primary hyperparathyroidism: Incidence, morbidity, and potential economic impact in a community. *N Engl J Med* 302:189, 1980.

Hellstrom J: Hyperparathyroidism and gastroduodenal ulcer. *Acta Chir Scand* 116:207, 1959.

Hellstrom J, Birke G, Edvall CA: Hypertension in hyperparathyroidism. *Br J Urol* 30:13, 1958.

Hillman DA, Scriver CR, et al: Neonatal familial primary hyperparathyroidism. *N Engl J Med* 270:483, 1964.

Jackson CE: Hereditary hyperparathyroidism associated with recurrent pancreatitis. *Ann Intern Med* 49:829, 1958.

Jackson CE, Boonstra CE: The relationship of hereditary hyperparathyroidism to endocrine adenomatosis. *Am J Med* 43:727, 1967.

Johansson H, Thoren L, Werner I: Hyperparathyroidism. *Upsala J Med Sci* 77:41, 1972.

Lafferty FW: Pseudohyperparathyroidism. *Medicine* 45:247, 1966.

Ludwig GD: Hyperparathyroidism in relation to pregnancy. *N Engl J Med* 267:637, 1962.

MacLeod WAJ, Holloway CK: Hyperparathyroid crisis: A collective review. *Ann Surg* 166:1012, 1967.

Mixter CG Jr, Keynes WM, Cope O: Further experience with pancreatitis as a diagnostic clue to hyperparathyroidism. *N Engl J Med* 266:265, 1962.

Mundy GR, Cove DH, Fisken R: Primary hyperparathyroidism: Changes in the pattern of clinical presentation. *Lancet* 1:1317, 1980.

Nathaniels EK, Nathaniels AM, Wang C-A: Mediastinal parathyroid tumors: A clinical and pathological study of 84 cases. *Ann Surg* 171:165, 1970.

Paloyan E, Lawrence AM, Straus FH: *Hyperparathyroidism.* New York and London, Grune & Stratton, 1973.

Plimpton CH, Gelhorn A: Hypercalcemia in malignant disease without evidence of bone destruction. *Am J Med* 21:750, 1956.

Raisz LG, Yajnik CH, et al: Comparison of commercially available parathyroid hormone immunoassays in the differential diagnosis of hypercalcemia due to primary hyperparathyroidism or malignancy. *Ann Intern Med* 91:739, 1979.

Romanus R, Heimann O, Hansson G: Surgical treatment of hyperparathyroidism. *Prog Surg* 12:22, 1973.

Scholz DA, Purnell DC: Asymptomatic primary hyperparathyroidism 10-year prospective study. *Mayo Clin Proc* 56:473, 1981.

Smallwood RA: Effect of intravenous calcium administration on gastric secretion of acid and pepsin in man. *Gut* 8:592, 1967.

Stevens LE, Bloomer A, Castleton KB: Familial hyperparathyroidism. *Arch Surg* 94:524, 1967.

Tisell L-E, Hansson G, et al: Hyperparathyroidism in persons treated with x-rays for tuberculous cervical adenitis. *Cancer* 40:846, 1977.

Underdahl LO, Woolner LB, Black BM: Multiple endocrine adenomas: Report of eight cases in which the parathyroids, pituitary and pancreatic islets were involved. *J Clin Endocrinol Metab* 13:20, 1953.

Werner P: Endocrine adenomatosis and peptic ulcer in a large kindred. *Am J Med* 35:205, 1963.

Wills MR, McGowan GK: Plasma-chloride levels in hyperparathyroidism and other hypercalcemic states. *Br Med J* 1:1153, 1964.

Wilson RE, Bernhard WF, et al: Hyperparathyroidism: The problem of acute parathyroid intoxication. *Ann Surg* 159:70, 1964.

Hypercalcemia: Differential Diagnosis

Berson SA, Yalow RS: Parathyroid hormone in plasma in adenomatous hyperparathyroidism, uremia, and bronchogenic carcinoma. *Science* 154:907, 1966.

Boonstra CE, Jackson CE: Serum calcium survey for hyperparathyroidism: Results in 50,000 clinic patients. *Am J Clin Pathol* 55:523, 1971.

Duarte CG, Winnacker JL, et al: Thiazide-induced hypercalcemia. *N Engl J Med* 284:828, 1971.

Knill-Jones RP, Buckle RM, et al: Hypercalcemia and increased parathyroid-hormone activity in a primary hepatoma: Studies before and after hepatic transplantation. *N Engl J Med* 282:704, 1970.

Lafferty FW: Pseudohyperparathyroidism. *Medicine (Baltimore)* 45:247, 1966.

Marx SJ, Attie MF, et al: The hypocalciuric or benign variant of hypercalcemia: Clinical and biochemical features in fifteen kindreds. *Medicine* 60:397, 1981.

Monchik JM, Doppman JL, et al: Localization of hyperfunctioning parathyroid tissue. Radioimmunoassay of parathyroid hormone on samples from the large veins of the neck and thorax and selectively catheterized thyroid veins. *Am J Surg* 129:413, 1975.

Reitz RE, Pollard JJ, et al: Localization of parathyroid adenomas by selective venous catheterization and radioimmunoassay. *N Engl J Med* 281:348, 1969.

Riggs BL, Arnaud CD, et al: Immunologic differentiation of primary hyperparathyroidism from hyperparathyroidism due to nonparathyroid cancer. *J Clin Invest* 50:2079, 1971.

Yendt ER, Gagne RJA: Detection of primary hyperparathyroidism, with special reference to its occurrence in hypercalciuric

females with "normal" or borderline serum calcium, *Can Med Assoc J* 98:331, 1968.

Ectopic Hyperparathyroidism

Benson RC Jr, Riggs BL, et al: Immunoreactive forms of circulating parathyroid hormone in primary and ectopic hyperparathyroidism. *J Clin Invest* 54:175, 1973.

Mundy GR, Luben RA, et al: Bone-resorbing activity in supernatant from lymphoid cell lines. *N Engl J Med* 290:867, 1974.

Seyberth HW, Segre GV, et al: Prostaglandins as mediators of hypercalcemia associated with certain types of cancer. *N Engl J Med* 293:1278, 1975.

Shaw JW, Oldham SB, et al: Urinary cyclic AMP analyzed as a function of the serum calcium and parathyroid hormone in the differential diagnosis of hypercalcemia. *J Clin Invest* 59:14, 1977.

Stewart AF, Horst R, et al: Biochemical evaluation of patients with cancer-associated hypercalcemia: Evidence for humoral and nonhumoral groups. *N Engl J Med* 303:1377, 1980.

Stewart AF, Vignery A, et al: Bone histomorphometry in humoral hypercalcemia of malignancy: Uncoupling of bone cell activity. *Clin Res* 29:423A, 1981.

Vichayanrat A, Avramides A, et al: Primary hyperparathyroidism and breast cancer. *Am J Med* 61:136, 1976.

Watson L, Moxham J, Fraser P: Hydrocortisone suppression test and discriminant analysis in differential diagnosis of hypercalcemia. *Lancet* 1:1320, 1980.

Treatment of Hypercalcemia

Kennedy BJ: Metabolic and toxic effects of mithramycin during tumor therapy. *Am J Med* 49:494, 1970.

Strauch BS, Ball MF: Hemodialysis in the treatment of severe hypercalcemia. *JAMA* 235:1347, 1976.

Secondary and Tertiary Hyperparathyroidism

Davies DR, Dent CE, Watson L: Tertiary hyperparathyroidism. *Br Med J* 3:395, 1968.

Easson LH, Faulds JS, Hartley JN: Van Recklinghausen's disease of bone associated with idiopathic steatorrhoea. *J R Coll Surg Edinb* 3:193, 1958.

Johnson WJ, Goldsmith RS, et al: Prevention and reversal of progressive secondary hyperparathyroidism in patients maintained on hemodialysis. *Am J Med* 56:827, 1974.

Mallick NP, Berlyne GM: Arterial calcification after vitamin-D therapy in hyperphosphatemic renal failure. *Lancet* 2:1316, 1968.

Sivula A, Kuhlback B, et al: Parathyroidectomy in chronic renal failure. *Acta Chir Scand* 145:19, 1979.

Slatopolsky E, Gray R, et al: The pathogenesis of secondary hyperparathyroidism in early renal failure, in Norman AW (ed): *Vitamin D Basic Research and Its Clinical Application.* New York, deGruyer, 1979, pp 1209–1215.

Slatopolsky E, Rutherford WE, et al: How important is phosphate in the pathogenesis of renal osteodystrophy? *Arch Intern Med* 138:848, 1978.

Hypoparathyroidism, Pseudohypoparathyroidism, and Parathyroid Transplants

Alvioli LV: The therapeutic approach to hypoparathyroidism. *Am J Med* 57:34, 1974.

Dubost CL, Drüeke T, et al: Hyperparathyroidie secondaire:

parathyroïdectomie subtotale ou totale avec autotransplantation parathyroïdienne. *Nouv Med* 9:2709, 1980.

Edis AJ, Linos DA, Kao PC: Parathyroid autotransplantation at the time of reoperation for persistent hyperparathyroidism. *Surgery* 88:588, 1980.

Franz AG, Lee JB: Pseudohypoparathyroidism: Assays of parathyroid hormone and thyrocalcitonin. *Proc Natl Acad Sci USA* 56:1138, 1966.

Kenney FM, Holliday MA: Hypoparathyroidism, moniliasis and Hashimoto's disease. *N Engl J Med* 271:708, 1964.

Kolb FO, Steinberg HL: Pseudohypoparathyroidism and secondary hyperparathyroidism and osteitis fibrosa. *J Clin Endocrinol Metab* 22:59, 1962.

Mozes MF, Soper WD, et al: Total parathyroidectomy and autotransplantation in secondary hyperparathyroidism. *Arch Surg* 115:378, 1980.

Wells SA Jr, Ellis GJ, et al: Parathyroid autotransplantation in primary parathyroid hyperplasia, *N Engl J Med* 295:57, 1976.

Wells SA Jr, Gunnells CJ, et al: The successful transplantation of frozen tissue in man. *Surgery* 81:86, 1977.

Williams E, Wood AOC: The syndrome of hypoparathyroidism and steatorrhea. *Arch Dis Child* 34:302, 1959.

Chapter 39

Pediatric Surgery

Philip C. Guzzetta, Kathryn D. Anderson, R. Peter Altman, Kurt D. Newman, Martin R. Eichelberger, and Judson G. Randolph

INTRODUCTION

Pediatric surgery has experienced the same rapid progress seen in other fields of surgery. New equipment, new diagnostic modalities, new support mechanisms for respiratory, metabolic, and nutritional needs of even the tiniest premature babies have brought success to surgical efforts undreamed 25 years ago. There is unique gratification from surgical efforts in behalf of infants and young children, unmatched by even the most triumphant operation on older subjects. Correction of atresia of the esophagus in a newborn infant, for example, not only offers a pleasing mechanical solution in a tiny subject, but there is special joy to be found, in Clatworthy's apt phrase, in "saving whole lifetimes."

GENERAL CONSIDERATIONS

The normal adaptive demands upon infants and young children are enormous. Illness and operations superimpose needs that require the most vigilant and meticulous care.

FLUID AND ELECTROLYTE BALANCE. In an infant or child the margin between dehydration and fluid overload is small. The infant is born with a surplus of body water, but within a few days this is excreted. At birth and for the first 10 days of life, fluid requirements are between 65 and 100 mL/kg (750 to 1000 mL/m^2). Maintenance fluids can be conveniently calculated at 100 mL/kg per 24 h. Calculation of fluid requirements based upon BSA (1500 mL/m^2 per 24 h) will vary only slightly. Fluid for maintenance is generally provided as 5% dextrose in $\frac{1}{4}$ or $\frac{1}{3}$ normal saline. For short-term intravenous therapy, sodium 5 meq/kg per day and potassium 2 meq/kg per day will satisfy the daily need. Fluid and electrolyte losses secondary to protracted vomiting or diarrhea are corrected by modifying this formula according to the measured losses. In the infant the normal serum osmolarity is between 280 and 290 mO/L. However, the immature kidney is unable to concentrate efficiently, and therefore, it is not always possible to utilize the urine osmolarity as a guideline for fluid replacement in neonates. For example, even in the dehydrated infant, the urine osmolarity rarely exceeds 400 mO/L. Hyperosmolarity is particularly hazardous in the neonate and can result in intracranial hemorrhage. Therefore, the administration of hypertonic solutions should be used only in extreme circumstances, and always must be carefully monitored.

Whatever the formula used to calculate fluid replacement for the infant or small child, there is no substitute for collecting and analyzing fluid losses and replacing the depleted constituents precisely.

ACID-BASE EQUILIBRIUM. Measurement of arterial blood gases permits the assessment of the status of alveolar ventilation and acid-base equilibrium. Just as in adults, these data are essential during the resuscitation of critically ill children and constitute an integral part of intraoperative and postoperative monitoring. Significant elevations of arterial P_{CO_2} usually indicate the need for endotracheal intubation and mechanical ventilation. Impaired arterial oxygenation as indicated by reduced Pa_{O_2} may be a consequence of compromised ventilation-perfusion secondary to pulmonary parenchymal disease or right-to-left shunting. From measurement of serum pH and P_{CO_2}, base deficits can be determined utilizing the standard Siggard-Anderson curve nomogram. Generally half the calculated requirement for sodium bicarbonate is administered, after which blood-gas measurements are repeated and then additional corrections are carried out. For infants requiring extensive metabolic manipulation

such as those with congenital diaphragmatic hernia, all intravenous sodium solution should be as sodium bicarbonate. This maximizes the amount of buffer provided while restricting sodium ion administration.

Fluid and electrolyte losses from the upper gastrointestinal tract in infants are generally equivalent to 0.45N saline solution. Adjustments for ileostomy or biliary losses are made when these are significant by analyzing the individual drainage.

BLOOD VOLUME AND BLOOD REPLACEMENT. A useful guideline for estimation of blood volume for the infant is 85 mL/kg of body weight. When packed red blood cells are utilized, the transfusion requirement is calculated as 10 mL/kg, which roughly is equivalent to a 500-mL transfusion for a 70-kg adult. In the child, coagulation deficiencies may rapidly assume clinical significance after extensive blood transfusion. It is advisable to have fresh frozen plasma and platelets available if more than 30 mL//kg have been transfused.

HYPERALIMENTATION AND NUTRITION. The physiologic nutritional demands imposed upon the growing infant are well recognized. When these are compounded by illness and the necessity to repair tissue and heal surgical wounds, the risks of protein calorie malnutrition are considerable. Thus, parenteral nutritional support has been integrated into the management of infants and children with surgical illness. When the gastrointestinal tract is not usable because of mechanical, ischemic, or inflammatory disorders, several options for nutritional support are available. Techniques for delivering calories by a central or a peripheral venous route have been refined to the stage that the caloric needs of all patients can be satisfied.

The original technique of parenteral nutrition made use of an indwelling central venous catheter for delivery of the nutritional substrate. The principle involved the provision of a source of calories (hypertonic glucose) in combination with the source of nitrogen (protein hydrolysate or amino acid solution). Essential fatty acid supplements, minerals, and vitamins are provided in the infusate, and long-term growth can be sustained even in the rapidly developing surgical infant. The risks of this technique are not trivial and include sepsis, caval thrombosis, pneumothorax, hydrothorax, and hypertonic crisis. For this reason alternatives to central venous alimentation have been developed. Peripheral alimentation, utilizing less concentrated but greater volume of solutions, in combination with intravenous lipid supplements has eliminated the need for central alimentation in many patients. In some centers peripheral alimentation techniques are employed almost exclusively. The infusion of all solutions utilized for alimentation and indeed any intravenous solution in an infant or small child should always be controlled by a properly alarmed, constant infusion pump. To prevent the development of trace metal deficiencies, supplementary copper, zinc, and iron are provided to patients receiving long-term parenteral nutritional support.

By utilizing these techniques, positive nitrogen balance can be accomplished for even premature infants. Refinements and advances in the techniques of parenteral nutrition have had an enormous impact on the survival of pediatric surgical patients.

THERMOREGULATION. Infants or children compromised by disease are extremely thermolabile. Premature infants are particularly susceptible to changes in environmental temperature. Because they are unable to shiver and lack stores of fat, their potential for thermogenesis is impaired. Since these patients lack adaptive mechanisms to cope with the environment, the environment must be regulated. Attention to heat conservation during transport of the infant to and from the operating room is essential. Transport units incorporating overhead radiant heating that is servo-controlled by a skin temperature probe is recommended. When this is not available, the simple expedient of wrapping the infant in aluminum foil during transportation will diminish radiant heat loss. In the operating room the ambient temperature should approach thermal neutrality for the patient 21°C (73°F). Supplementary heat is provided by means of direct warming lights during positioning and endotracheal intubation when much of the body surface is exposed. Irrigating solutions employed during operation should be warmed. Constant monitoring of inoperative temperature is essential.

LESIONS OF THE NECK

Cystic Hygroma

ETIOLOGY AND PATHOLOGY. Cystic hygroma occurs as a result of sequestration or obstruction of developing lymph vessels. Although the lesion can occur anywhere, the common sites are in the neck posterior to the sternocleidomastoid muscle axilla, groin, and mediastinum. The cysts are lined by endothelium and filled with lymph. Occasionally unilocular cysts occur, but more often there are multiple cysts "infiltrating" the surrounding structures and distorting the local anatomy. A particularly troublesome variant of cystic hygroma is that which involves the tongue, floor of the mouth, and structures deep in the neck (Fig. 39-1). Adjacent connective tissue may show extensive lymphocytic infiltration. The mass may be apparent at birth or may appear and enlarge rapidly in the early weeks or months of life as lymph accumulates. Occasionally cystic hygromas contain nests of vascular tissue. These poorly supported vessels may bleed and produce rapid enlargement and discoloration of the hygroma.

Infection within the cysts usually caused by streptococcus or staphylococcus may occur. In the neck this can cause rapid enlargement which may result in airway compromise. Rarely, it may be necessary to carry out percutaneous aspiration of an infected cyst to relieve respiratory distress.

TREATMENT. Surgical excision is the treatment of choice. Total extirpation may not be possible because of the extent of hygroma and its proximity and intimate relationship to adjacent nerves, muscles, and blood vessels. Radical ablative surgery is not indicated in this benign lesion. Conservative excision and unroofing of remaining cysts is advised with repeated partial excision of residual hygroma if necessary, preserving all adjacent crucial structures. Postoperative wound drainage is important

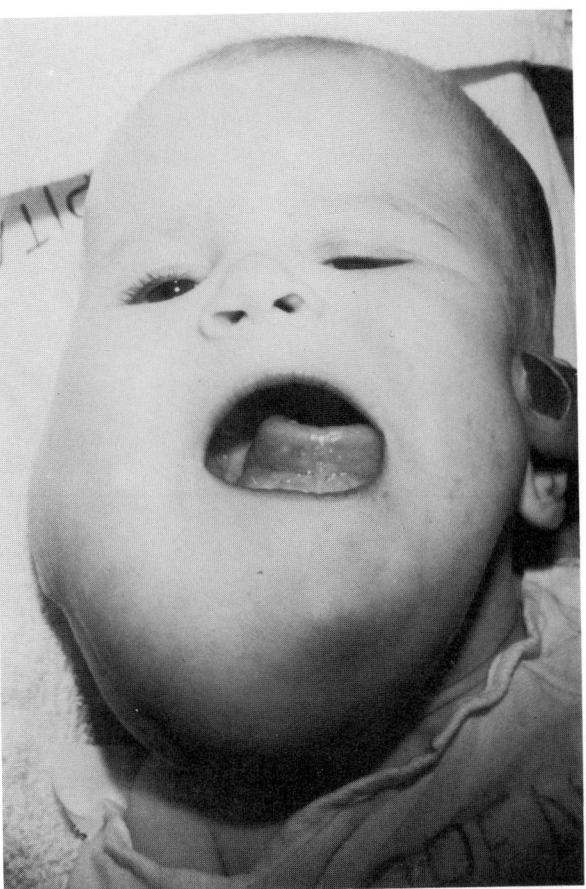

Fig. 39-1. Infant with cystic hygroma in the typical position in the neck.

and is best accomplished by closed-suction technique. In spite of this, fluid may accumulate beneath the surgically created flaps in the area from which the hygroma was excised, requiring multiple needle aspirations.

Thyroglossal Duct Remnants

PATHOLOGY AND CLINICAL MANIFESTATIONS. The thyroid gland begins as a foregut diverticulum at the base of the tongue in the region of the future foramen cecum at 3 weeks of embryonic life. With the development of the fetal neck the thyroid gradually assumes its normal position anterior and caudad. The "descent" of the thyroid is intimately connected to the development of the hyoid bone. Thyroid tissue left behind in the migration may persist and present in the midline of the neck as a thyroglossal duct cyst (Fig. 39-2). The mass is usually seen in the two- to four-year-old child when the baby fat subsides and irregularities in the neck are more readily apparent. Almost always the cyst is encountered in the midline at or below the level of the hyoid bone. Occasionally it presents as an intrathyroidal mass. Most thyroglossal duct cysts are asymptomatic. Infection may occur since the duct retains its connection with the pharynx; the resulting abscess will often need drainage, and a salivary fistula may be the result. Submental lymphadenopathy and mid-

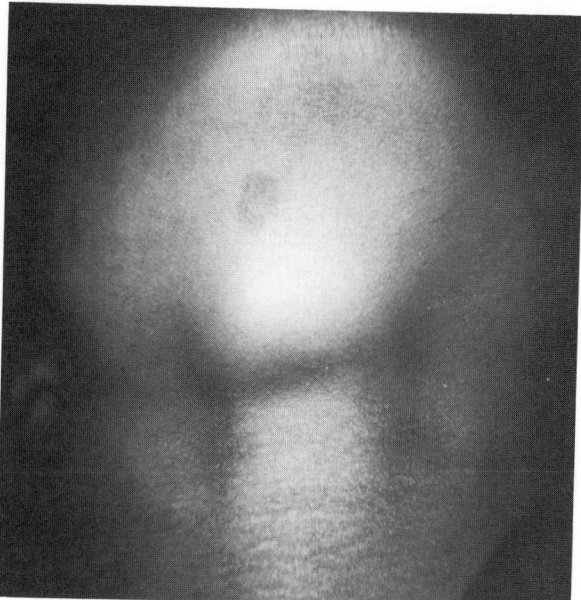

Fig. 39-2. Typical presentation of thyroglossal duct cyst as a midline mass.

line dermoid cysts can be confused with a thyroglossal duct cyst. Rarely, midline ectopic thyroid tissue masquerades as a thyroglossal duct cyst and may represent the patient's only thyroid tissue. Therefore, if there is any question regarding the diagnosis or if the thyroid gland cannot be palpated in its normal anatomic position, it is advisable to obtain a nuclear scan to confirm the presence of a normal thyroid gland.

TREATMENT. It is never advisable to carry out surgical excision through inflamed tissues; therefore, treatment with antibiotics and drainage of an abscess is initiated prior to surgical removal. Resection of the cyst, the central portion of the hyoid, and the tract into the pharynx is curative.

Branchial Cleft Anomalies

Branchial clefts are those embryologic grooves from which develop multiple structures in the lower part of the face and neck. The embryologic communication between the pharynx and the external surface may persist as a fistula (Fig. 39-3). This is most commonly seen with the second branchial cleft and extends from the anterior border of the sternocleidomastoid muscle superiorly, inward through the bifurcation of the carotid artery, and enters the posterolateral pharynx just below the tonsillar fossa. Other branchial cleft remnants may contain small pieces of cartilage and cysts, but internal fistulas are rare. Second branchial cleft sinus is suspected when clear fluid is noted draining from the external opening of the tract at the anterior border of the sternomastoid muscle in its lower third. The treatment is surgical, and complete removal of the cyst and tract is necessary for cure. Dissection of the sinus tract is facilitated by passing a fine lacrimal duct probe through the external opening into the tract and utilizing this as a guide for dissection. It is also useful to inject methylene blue dye into the ostium. A series of two or sometimes three small transverse "stair-step" incisions are preferred to a long oblique incision in the neck, which is cosmetically unacceptable (Fig. 39-4).

RESPIRATORY SYSTEM

Subglottic Stenosis

Congenital narrowing of the subglottic region usually occurs several millimeters below the level of the vocal cords (Fig. 39-5). The hallmark of upper airway obstruction is inspiratory and expiratory stridor. Congenital obstruction is usually a result of thickened subglottic tissues or abnormal cartilagenous overgrowth, such as complete tracheal rings. Acquired stenosis is seen more frequently

Fig. 39-3. Branchial cleft sinus tract opening at the anterior border of the sternocleidomastoid muscle.

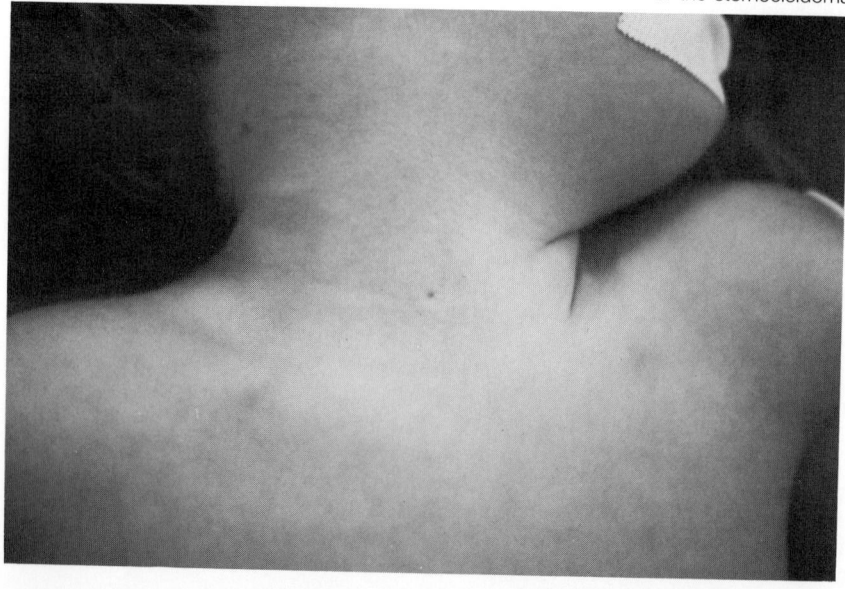

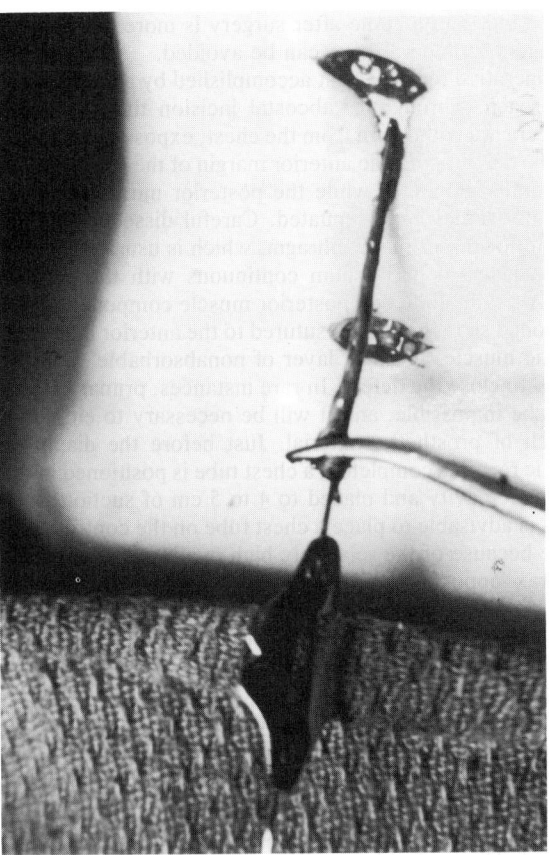

Fig. 39-4. "Stair-step" incisions for removal of branchial cleft sinus tract.

Fig. 39-5. Air tracheogram showing subglottic stenosis following protracted endotracheal intubation.

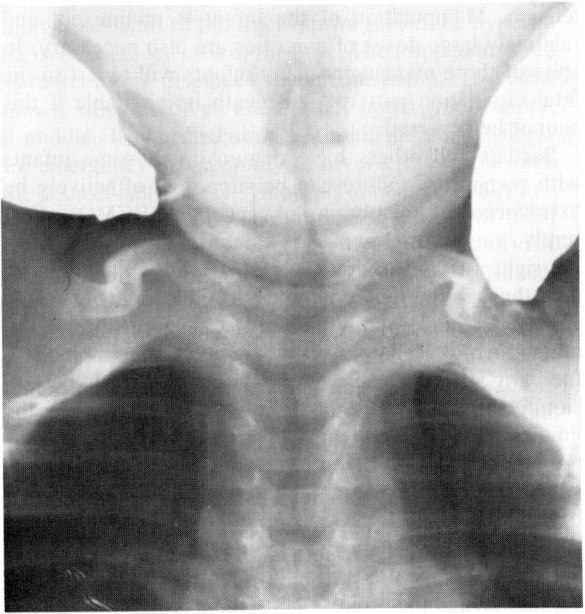

as infants are being sustained by ventilatory support requiring endotracheal intubation. Most patients with subglottic narrowing of the acquired type will outgrow the problem as the larynx enlarges. The occasional patient will require periodic stricture resections, commonly with a laser, to maintain airway patency. A tracheal split procedure or tracheoplasty using a costal cartilage to stent the upper airway is reserved for the most severe stenoses that do not respond to laser resection.

Subglottic Hemangioma

In an infant with inspiratory and expiratory stridor that is worsened with crying, suspect subglottic hemangioma. These children are usually female and present with dyspnea and difficulty feeding. Cutaneous hemangiomas are evident in many of the children who present usually before six months of age.

Endoscopy is the most reliable technique for diagnosis and usually reveals a bluish-tinged lesion in the subglottic region. Capillary hemangioma tends to enlarge early in life and regress with age. Unfortunately, respiratory obstruction may result. Systemic steroid therapy can diminish the size of the hemangioma. Present therapy is possible with a carbon dioxide (CO_2) or argon laser that permits treatment of these troublesome lesions. When the airway obstruction is critical, the child may require tracheostomy until the natural history of the hemangioma is completed.

Congenital Diaphragmatic Hernia (Bochdalek)

PATHOLOGY. During the formation of the diaphragm, the pleural and coelomic cavities remain in continuity via the pleuroperitoneal canal. This posterolateral communication is the last to be closed by the developing diaphragm. Failure of diaphragmatic development leaves a posterolateral defect known as Bochdalek hernia. This anomaly is more commonly encountered on the left.

Incomplete development of the posterior diaphragm allows the bowel to fill the chest cavity following its return to the abdominal cavity. The abdominal cavity is small and undeveloped and remains scaphoid after birth. The ipsilateral lung remains underdeveloped. Recently, prenatal ultrasound has been successful in making the diagnosis in the unborn child. Following delivery, the bowel fills with air, and the mediastinum is shifted to the opposite chest, compromising air exchange in the "good" lung. Respiratory failure will rapidly occur if the situation is not corrected. Chest x-ray will show loops of bowel in the chest (Fig. 39-6).

TREATMENT. While diaphragmatic hernia is acknowledged to be the most urgent surgical emergency in the newborn infant, it does not follow that the infants presenting earliest do best. In fact, the opposite is true. Infants with diaphragmatic hernia who develop respiratory distress after the first 24 h enjoy a better prognosis than those presenting with respiratory distress immediately after birth or within the first hours of life, presumably because the degree of pulmonary hypoplasia is less than in those infants who are distressed with their first breath.

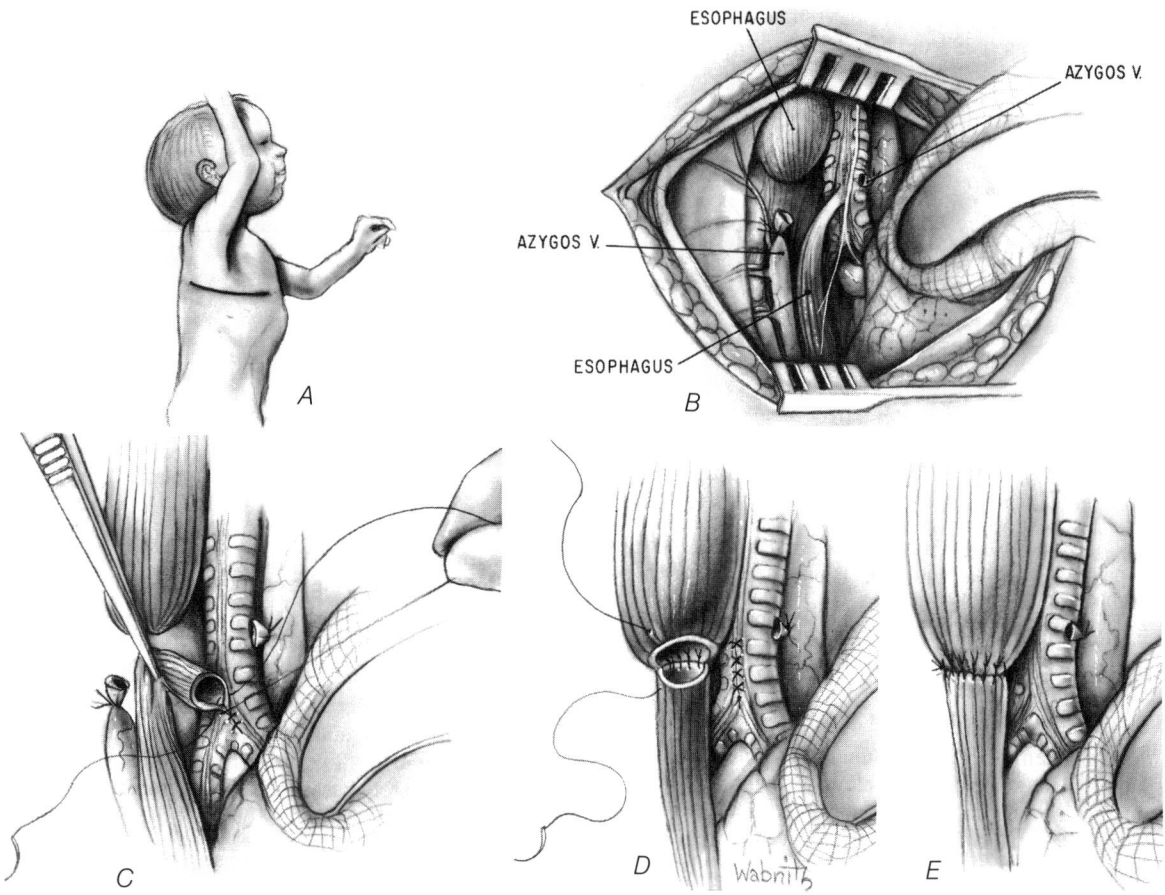

Fig. 39-10. Primary repair of type C tracheoesophageal fistula. A. Right thoracotomy incision. B. Azygos vein transected, proximal and distal esophagus demonstrated, and fistula identified. C. Tracheoesophageal fistula transected and defect in trachea closed. D. End-to-end anastomosis between proximal and distal esophagus (posterior row). E. Anastomosis completed.

The operative technique for primary repair is depicted in Fig. 39-10. The operation for primary repair of esophageal atresia and tracheoesophageal fistula has changed very little since its original description by Cameron Haight. Although the transpleural approach may reduce the operating time, most workers now agree that the retropleural approach is desirable. Exposure with this method is perfectly adequate, and the protection of the lung by maintaining its pleural envelope has a salutary postoperative effect. More important, an anastomotic leak will not communicate with the pleural cavity and can be drained directly from the mediastinum posteriorly with decreased morbidity or mortality.

Livaditis showed that incising the muscle of the upper pouch circumferentially produced remarkable lengthening without compromising blood supply. This approach is useful if the distance between the two pouches precludes anastomosis without producing undue tension.

Category B: Surgical Repair Following Short-Term Delay. If the infant has pneumonia or weighs less than 5 lb, surgery is deferred. A gastrostomy is always performed, sometimes under local anesthesia. Time is thus provided for stabilization and medical management of the pulmonary status. This method of management is useful for only a limited period, because reflux into the tracheobronchial tree via the tracheoesophageal fistula may occur in spite

of gastric decompression through the gastrostomy. Repair is carried out as described above when the infant's condition stabilizes and the risk of surgery has been reduced.

Category C: Staged Repair. In babies with serious coexisting anomalies, prematurity, low birth weight, or persistent pulmonary disease, survival is limited. The possibility of diminishing the mortality rate in compromised infants by staging the operative procedure has received considerable study. Although staged repair is used much less frequently today than a delayed primary repair, the approach has merit in selected patients, but staging of the operation has by no means led to universally acceptable results. The outstanding work of Dudrick and his coworkers in the field of parenteral nutrition has added a new dimension in the care of these difficult babies. It is now possible to provide nutritional support indefinitely for newborn infants by a central venous or even peripheral intravenous routes. This advance, coupled with the holding pattern provided by suction of the upper pouch and gastrostomy drainage, makes it possible to maintain infants with esophageal atresia and tracheoesophageal fistula indefinitely while growth and weight gain are achieved, pulmonary status is cleared, and other congenital anomalies are studied and corrected.

Correction of esophageal atresia with tracheoesophageal fistula leads to a satisfactory outcome with nearly normal esophageal function in most patients. Overall survival rates of greater than 90 percent have been achieved in patients classified in categories *A* and *B*. Infants classified in category *C* have an increased mortality (40 to 60 percent survival) because of the low birth weight, pulmonary complications, and potential fatal associated anomalies. The use of the staged procedure has increased the survival in these high-risk babies.

COMPLICATIONS. Although once considered fatal, a leak at the anastomosis can usually be dealt with satisfactorily, particularly if the pleural envelope has been maintained and drainage accomplished from the mediastinum via the retropleural route. Improved management of infection, nutrition, and respiratory support in infants has contributed to success in handling anastomotic leaks.

The mediastinal infection seen with esophageal disruption may cause recurrence of the tracheoesophageal fistula. This complication requires another operation to divide the tracheoesophageal fistula.

In the past decade it has become apparent that the necessary force applied to the esophagus to complete the anastomosis may alter the anatomy of the gastroesophageal junction, leading to gastroesophageal reflux. The clinical manifestations of this reflux are identical to those seen in other infants with primary gastroesophageal reflux.

ISOLATED ESOPHAGEAL ATRESIA

Among those babies born with esophageal anomalies, 8 percent have isolated esophageal atresia. Characteristically, infants with isolated esophageal atresia present with a scaphoid abdomen, since the gastrointestinal tract is devoid of air. The x-ray finding of a blind upper pouch and the absence of air below the diaphragm is pathognomonic of isolated esophageal atresia without fistula.

Prompt esophagostomy with the upper esophageal pouch brought to the skin of the left side of the neck allows drainage of saliva and prevents aspiration. A gastrostomy is performed and serves for feeding in the early months of life. Esophageal replacement with colon or gastric tube is then recommended at a year of age. Some authors have shown that the esophageal ends can be dilated over a period of several months, allowing end-to-end union and avoiding esophageal replacement.

ISOLATED (H-TYPE) TRACHEOESOPHAGEAL FISTULA

In rare instances (4 percent), an isolated congenital fistula connecting the trachea to the esophagus may exist. In this anomaly both the trachea and the esophagus are otherwise normal, with no narrowing or obstruction. Infants with this condition seem to swallow normally. The clinical features are subtle; weeks or months may elapse before a correct diagnosis is made. The presence of an H-type tracheoesophageal fistula is suggested by the following triad of symptoms: (1) choking when feeding, (2) gaseous distention of the bowel, and (3) recurrent aspiration pneumonia. Diagnosis can usually be confirmed by cine contrast x-ray studies or by bronchoesophagoscopy using a fiberoptic lens system. Definitive treatment consists of dividing the fistula. Surgical closure of the esophagus and trachea must be meticulous, and encroachment on the lumen of the trachea avoided. The fistula is usually accessible to surgical repair through an incision just above the clavicle.

Corrosive Injury of the Esophagus

Childproof containers, as well as better public education of the dangers of ingesting caustic agents, have lessened the incidence of esophageal injury. Nevertheless, toddlers will occasionally have access to commercial cleaners containing strong alkali or acid. Potassium or sodium hydroxide is extremely hygroscopic, attaches firmly to the moist epithelial surface of the mouth and esophagus, and may produce a full-thickness injury by protein coagulation. Children suspected of having swallowed corrosive materials should be admitted to the hospital and studied by esophagoscopy within 24 h of injury. The absence of mouth burns does not rule out esophageal injury. A burn will be seen as a whitish coagulum on the surface of the mucosa, surrounded by an area of hyperemia. Esophagoscopy is safely carried out to the level of the burn and no further. If the esophageal injury is circumferential, it has been our practice to perform a gastrostomy for feeding, and to insert a string for subsequent dilatation.

Steroids may decrease the incidence of stricture and are therefore administered for 3 weeks. Antibiotics are used routinely for 3 weeks. After this interval, esophageal dilatation is begun. Dilatations are continued as often as necessary to allow the child to eat a normal diet until the stricture is resolved or it becomes apparent that esophageal substitution is required. The latter decision is deferred for at least 6 to 12 months until scarring is complete and the full length of the esophageal stricture can be assessed.

Esophageal Substitution

Esophageal substitution is required in children for two major conditions: severe esophageal strictures and isolated esophageal atresia when deferred primary operation has failed. The colon has been the most widely used organ for esophageal substitution, reaching easily into the neck. The right colon can be used with a pedicle of the midcolic artery; the left colon is preferred by many using either the mid or left colic artery as its vascular supply. It can be placed in a substernal tunnel, in the left side of the chest behind the lung root (Fig. 39-11) or in the normal esophageal bed. Since the colon acts as an aperistaltic conduit, antiperistaltic and isoperistaltic segments function equally well. An alternative method of esophageal substitution gaining popularity is the reversed gastric tube. This

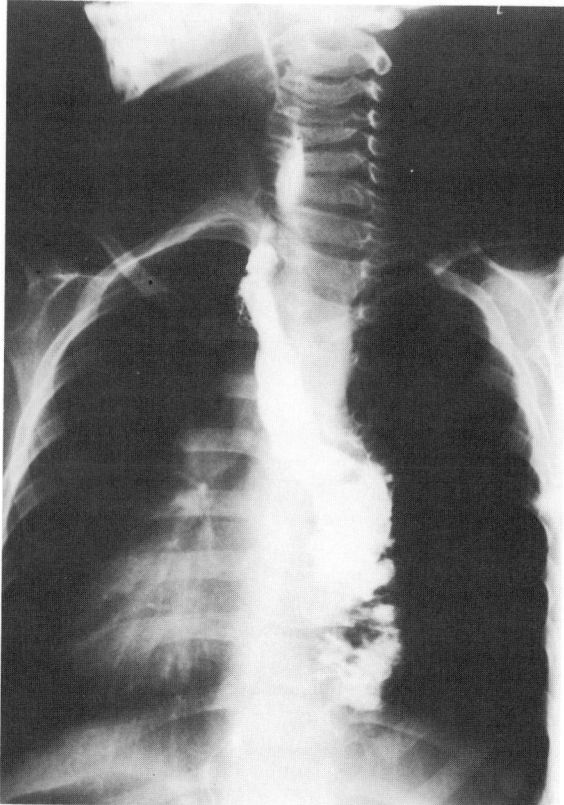

Fig. 39-11. Retrosternal coloesophagoplasty.

is fashioned from a flap cut from the greater curvature of the stomach, with a vascular pedicle based on the left gastroepiploic artery. The results of both these methods of esophageal substitution are satisfactory for normal growth and development. Long-term complications of ulcer formation and late anastomotic stricture are usually managed conservatively.

Gastroesophageal Reflux (GER)

In 1950, Berenberg and Neuhauser described a group of babies who vomited excessively and were demonstrated to have unimpeded gastroesophageal reflux. Their term, "chalasia" (relaxation at the cardia), became widely accepted, and the upright position that these workers advocated became the standard mode of therapy. A certain percentage of infants with "chalasia" were not controlled by the upright propping technique; in these babies persistent gastroesophageal reflux caused serious consequences in growth and development and in the respiratory tract. In the past two decades, pernicious gastroesophageal reflux, occurring without demonstrable hiatal hernia, has become recognized as a unique entity found in infants during their first year of life. Surprisingly, in this particular age group, the incidence of esophagitis and stricture is infrequent.

Failure to thrive is the usual presenting complaint in children with GER over one year of age. Esophagitis and

stricture development are most often seen in adolescents or in those children with mental retardation. Pulmonary complications of GER range from an asthma presentation to recurrent pneumonias. Some children present with a complex of GER, iron deficiency anemia (due to esophagitis), and apparent torticollis posturing to lessen reflux into the mouth, the Sutcliff-Sandifer syndrome. The association of gastroesophageal reflux following repair of esophageal atresia is reported with increasing frequency.

CLINICAL MANIFESTATIONS. History of repeated episodes of vomiting in an infant is the clearest indication of gastroesophageal reflux after obvious anatomic obstruction at or beyond the pylorus has been excluded. When the vomiting is associated with failure of normal development or chronic respiratory symptoms, the likelihood of pernicious gastroesophageal reflux is increased.

A child suspected of having GER is generally evaluated with a barium swallow to rule out an anatomic obstruction in the stomach or duodenum and a 24-h pH probe study to determine the severity of the reflux. The radioisotope "milk scan" and endoscopy with biopsies to prove esophagitis are utilized only in selected cases and do not significantly improve the accuracy of diagnosis of GER over the pH probe study done alone.

TREATMENT. After definitive diagnosis most patients are treated initially by conservative means. In the infant, propping and thickening the formula with rice cereal are generally recommended, although some authors prefer a prone, head-up position. The use of bethanacol or metaclopromide may be beneficial in some children resistant to position and feeding manipulations. Exceptions to a trial of medical therapy after establishing the diagnosis of gastroesophageal reflux in infants and children are as follows:

1. Life-threatening apneic spells related to the reflux
2. Congenital displacement of a major portion of the stomach in the chest
3. Significant esophagitis unaffected by medical therapy
4. Established stricture
5. Chronic pulmonary changes

Most infants and children respond favorably to one of the standard antireflux procedures. The Nissen fundoplication is probably the most widely used operation in younger patients, but partial wraps (Thal), Belsey Mark IV, and Boerema gastropexy all have been reported with success.

GASTROINTESTINAL TRACT

Pyloric Stenosis

CLINICAL MANIFESTATIONS. The typical infant with hypertrophic pyloric stenosis is 7 weeks of age, male, and the first-born child. Nonbilious vomiting, becoming increasingly projectile in nature, occurs over several days to weeks. Eventually the infant will not even hold down water and becomes severely dehydrated, showing a metabolic alkalosis and severe depletion of potassium and chloride ions. Potassium deficits may not be apparent until late stages since the serum potassium is maintained even after severe losses. Serum pH is high; urine pH is initially high but eventually drops as severe potassium deficit leaves only hydrogen ions for exchange with sodium ions in the distal tubule of the kidney.

The diagnosis of pyloric stenosis can usually be made on physical examination, the typical "olive" being palpable in the right upper quadrant. On occasion vigorous peristaltic waves can be seen passing from left to right across the epigastrium. Ultrasonography will accurately diagnose pyloric stenosis in 95 percent of those children in whom the hypertrophic pylorus cannot be palpated.

TREATMENT. Reversal of electrolyte abnormalities and metabolic alkalosis is essential before operation. For severe depletion a normal saline solution with added potassium (2 to 4 meq/kg over 18 to 24 h) at volumes sufficient to reverse dehydration and establish good urine flow (1 to 2 mL/kg per h) will be necessary. After resuscitation, a Fredet-Ramstedt pyloromyolotomy is performed (Fig. 39-12). Postoperatively, intravenous feedings are continued for several hours, after which small frequent feedings of dilute formula are offered with gradual increase to bolus feeds of full-strength formula. The infant can usually be discharged within 48 h of surgery.

Pneumoperitoneum

Pneumoperitoneum in the neonate is a surgical emergency. The commonest cause at this time is probably perforation of gangrenous bowel of necrotizing enterocolitis (see later). Also included in the differential diagnosis are idiopathic gastric perforation, perforation of the colon in Hirschsprung's disease, and occasionally breakthrough of mediastinal and retroperitoneal air in the infant with severe respiratory distress syndrome requiring high ventilator pressures.

Pneumoperitoneum itself can cause respiratory embarrassment by elevating the diaphragm and compromising lung volume. This can be alleviated by needle aspiration of the abdomen in the epigastrium before definitive surgical treatment of the underlying condition. If the diagnosis of pneumoperitoneum secondary to pulmonary air leaks can be established nonoperatively (such an infant would manifest no signs of peritonitis), repeated aspiration may be performed until ventilator pressures can be lowered.

Gastrostomy

The performance of a gastrostomy in an infant avoids the potential complications of an indwelling nasogastric tube, namely respiratory difficulty secondary to gastroesophageal reflux and aspiration, and blockage of the nares (infants are obligate nose breathers). Feeding by gastrostomy may be necessary for prolonged periods in small or sick infants and infants with orofacial anomalies or swallowing deficits. Such feedings can be performed safely by parents at home. Presence of a gastrostomy aggravates underlying gastroesophageal reflux; careful assessment to rule out reflux is undertaken for the chronically ill child prior to elective gastrostomy tube placement.

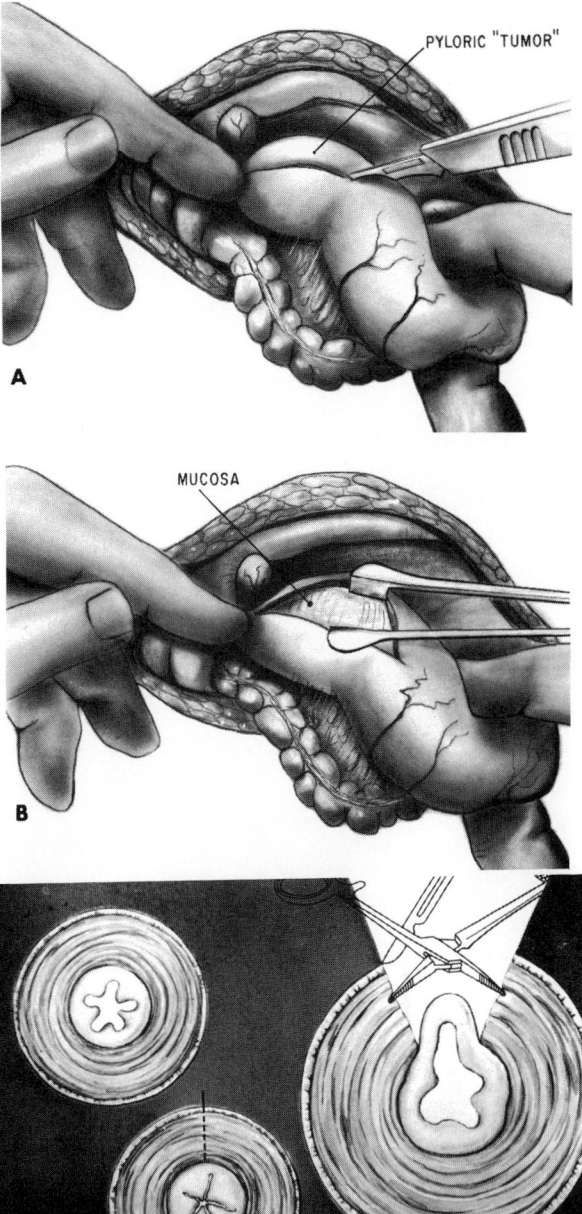

Fig. 39-12. Fredet-Ramstedt pyloromyolotomy. *A.* Pylorus delivered into wound and seromuscular layer incised. *B.* Seromuscular layer separated down to submucosal base to permit herniation of mucosa through pyloric incision. *C.* Cross section demonstrating hypertrophied pylorus, depth of incision, and spreading of muscle to permit mucosa to herniate through incision.

A Stamm gastrostomy is performed through a tiny vertical left upper quadrant incision. For emergency gastrostomies a Malecot catheter is inserted into the stomach and tied with a double purse-string suture and brought out through the wound. If prolonged use of the gastrostomy is anticipated, the catheter is brought out through a separate

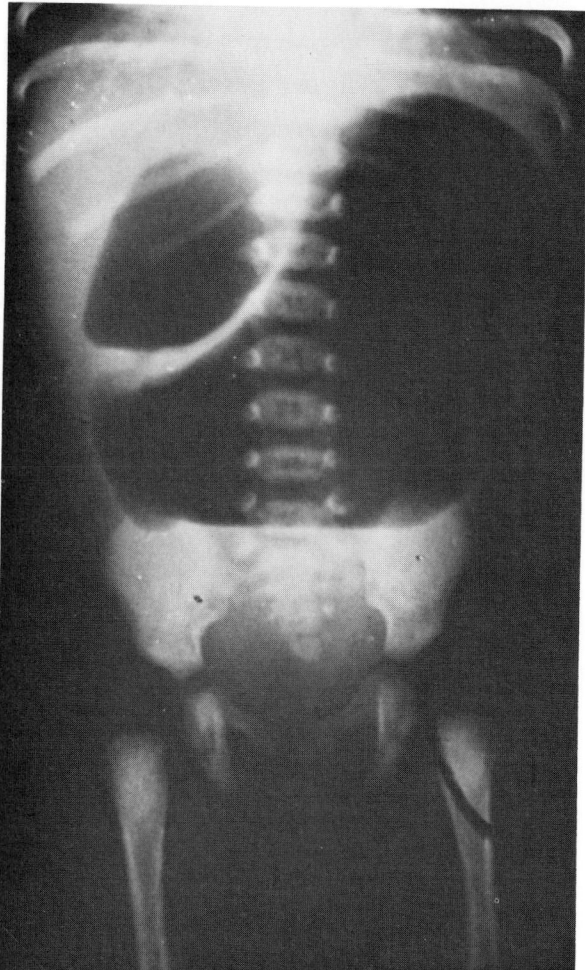

Fig. 39-13. Air-contrast study of an infant with congenital duodenal obstruction. Note size of stomach and distended duodenum, forming the "double bubble."

stab wound. It is important to suture the stomach to the abdominal wall to avoid intraperitoneal soilage by gastric contents. After the gastrostomy is no longer required, the Malecot catheter is removed and usually the stab wound will close spontaneously in a few days. Formal closure may be required if the gastrostomy has been in place for many months.

Intestinal Obstruction in the Newborn

Bilious vomiting is the most common manifestation of intestinal obstruction in the newborn. High obstruction such as duodenal and jejunal atresia produces early vomiting in the first 24 h of life. The later the onset of vomiting, the lower the obstruction is likely to be. Failure of passage of meconium is characteristic of lower ileal and colonic obstruction. The degree of abdominal distention is also correlated roughly with the level of obstruction. Distended loops of bowel, the number corresponding to

the level of the obstruction, and air-fluid levels on upright abdominal films are seen commonly and may be the only diagnostic studies necessary before surgery. Usually, 30 to 40 mL of air injected into the stomach is a satisfactory "contrast" material for high obstructions, and barium given from above is rarely necessary. Contrast enema may show a "micro" or unused colon in low obstruction.

DUODENAL MALFORMATIONS

Duodenal obstruction may be complete, as in duodenal atresia, or partial, as in duodenal web or stenosis, annular pancreas, and malrotation of the midgut. Anomalous entry of the common bile duct and pancreatic duct may be associated, requiring caution when anomalies are dealt with surgically by local plastic procedures on the duodenum. Although bilious vomiting is most often seen, entry of the bile duct distal to the site of obstruction may occur. In this case vomitus contains only clear gastric contents. The "double bubble" seen on an air-contrast upper gastrointestinal series is characteristic of duodenal atresia, with small amounts of air seen distally if obstruction is incomplete (Fig. 39-13).

The duodenum can be adequately decompressed via nasogastric tube so that surgical correction is relatively nonurgent. Time is needed to look for other anomalies (such as cardiac) in these infants because one-third of them with duodenal obstruction have trisomy 21. Surgery should not be deferred if malrotation is the cause of duodenal obstruction or if malrotation is present with intrinsic duodenal obstruction.

Congenital obstruction occurs almost exclusively in the second portion of the duodenum. The surgical treatment of duodenal obstruction is adapted to the anatomic situation found on exploration. Atresias, stenosis, and annular pancreas are bypassed via duodenoduodenostomy or duodenojejunostomy, performing the anastomosis between the most dependent portion of the proximal duodenum and the distal bowel in end-to-end (duodenum) or end-to-side (jejunum) fashion. Webs can be excised through a vertical duodenal incision, the mucosa oversewn, and the duodenotomy closed horizontally. Gastrostomy is performed routinely.

JEJUNOILEAL ATRESIA

There is good evidence, both experimental and clinical, that intestinal atresia is the result of interruption of the vascular supply to the bowel at the fetal stage of development. Tying off the end arterial branches in the mesentery of experimental fetal animals will reproduce all the variations of obstruction seen in the human infant. Bowel deprived of its blood supply may form a web, stenosis, or single or multiple atresias. The bowel and its mesentery may reabsorb, leaving a characteristic V-shaped mesenteric defect. The length of intestine remaining may be quite short, which can result in prolonged feeding difficulties characteristic of the "short-gut" syndrome. The most severe form of jejunoileal atresia seen is the so-called Christmas-tree deformity in which a single artery (usually the ileocolic) is all that remains of the superior mesenteric artery, supplying, in retrograde fashion, a very short ileum that arranges itself in reversing spirals around its blood supply.

The clinical presentation of newborn infants with jejunal or ileal atresia is similar to that found in other types of intestinal obstruction. Bilious vomiting is characteristic, and abdominal distention is progressive, being confined to the upper abdomen in high lesions, increasingly generalized the lower the obstruction. The number and distribution of obstructed loops on upright abdominal films offer some indication of the level of obstruction (Fig. 39-14).

If the obstruction is distal or if substantial loss of intestinal length has occurred, there is insufficient length of ileum distal to the atresia to produce "succus entericus" in sufficient quantity to dilate the colon to its normal neonatal size. A contrast enema will therefore show a "microcolon." Since the proximal distended loops cannot be adequately decompressed by nasogastric tube from above, accumulation of gas and fluid may be sufficient to produce perforation with resulting nonsterile peritonitis. In instances of prenatal perforation, the resulting meconium peritonitis may lead to characteristic calcifications on abdominal films.

Surgical correction of small bowel atresia is urgent. Disparity in lumen size (Fig. 39-15) between the proximal distended bowel and distal collapsed bowel has led to a number of innovative techniques of anastomosis of the atretic bowel. These include (1) end-to-back technique, fishmouthing the antimesenteric border of the distal loop; (2) tapering of the proximal distended loop to correspond

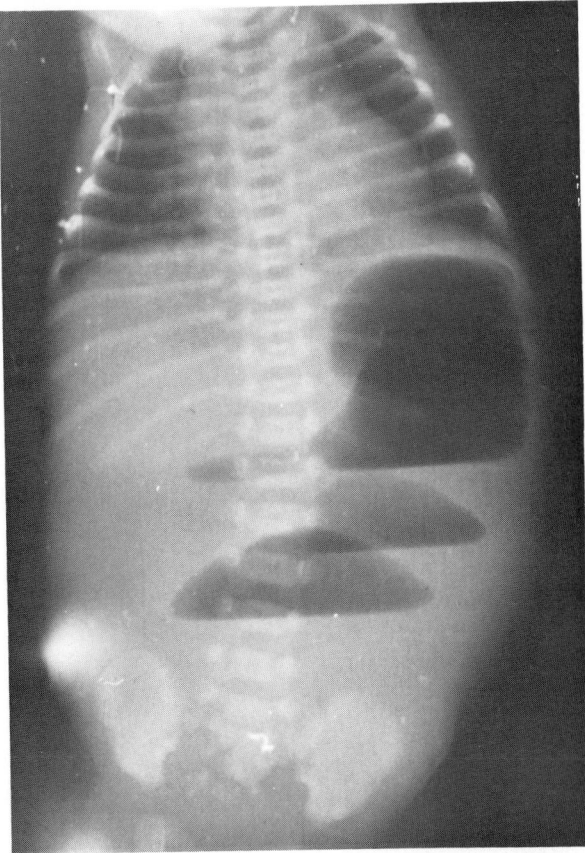

Fig. 39-14. Newborn intestinal obstruction showing several loops of distended bowel with air-fluid levels characteristic of jejunal atresia.

Fig. 39-15. Operative photograph of newborn with jejunal atresia. Note distended proximal portion; point of obstruction is seen just proximal of forceps.

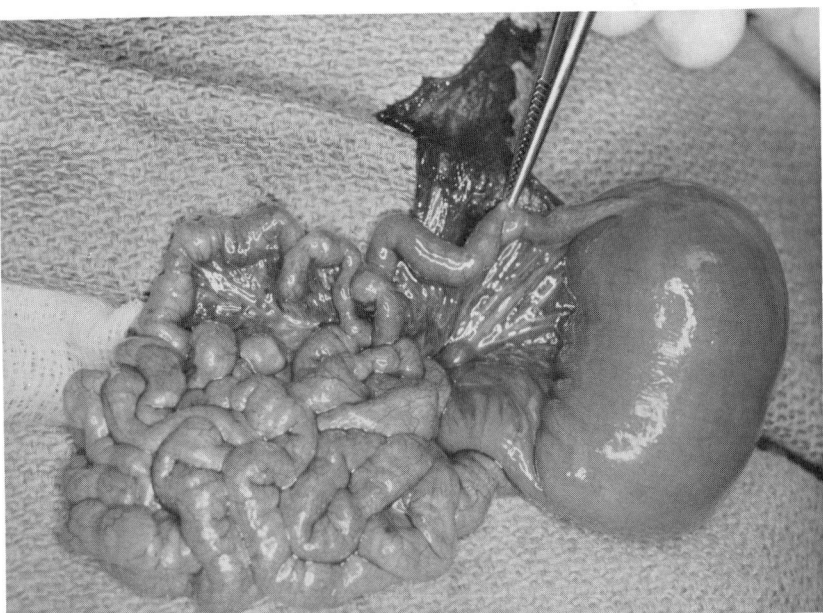

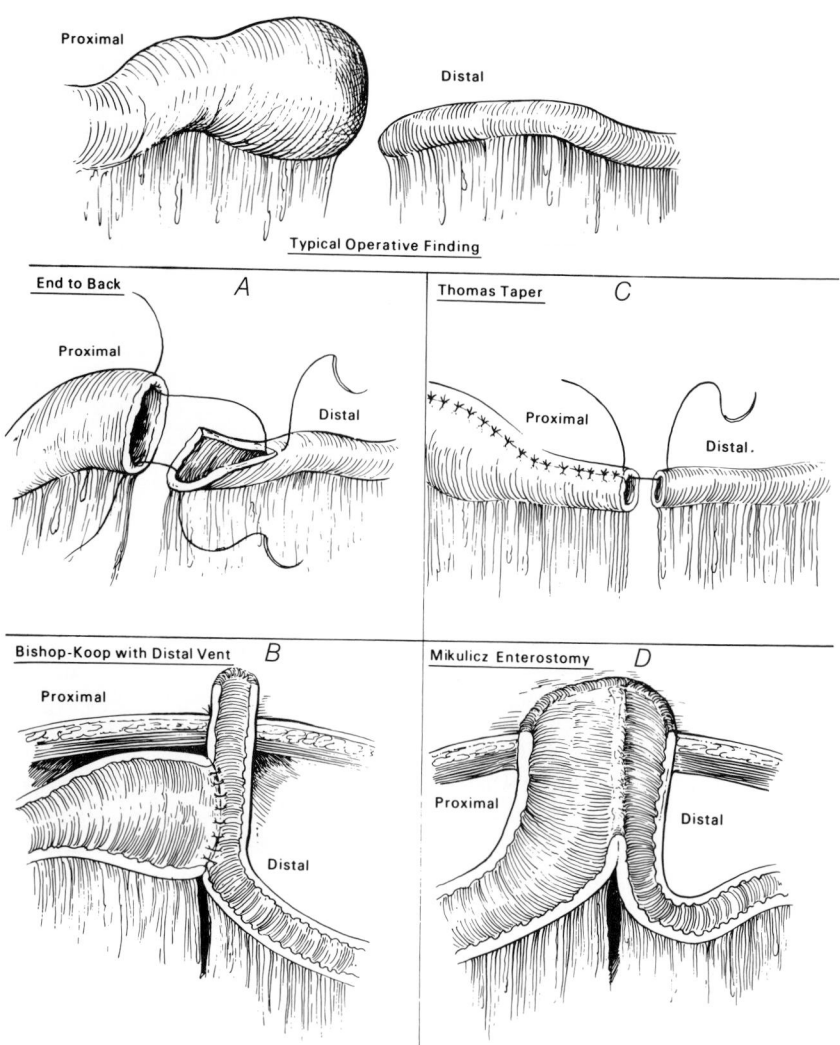

Fig. 39-16. Techniques of intestinal anastomosis for infants with small-bowel obstruction. (Typical operative findings: Proximal distention and discrepancy between ends of intestine to be anastomosed.) A. End-to-back distal limb has been incised, creating "fishmouth" to enlarge lumen. B. Bishop-Koop: proximal distended limb joined to side of small distal bowel, which is vented by "chimney" to the abdominal wall. C. Tapering: Portion of antimesenteric wall of proximal bowel excised, with longitudinal closure to minimize disparity in the limbs. D. Mikulicz double-barreled enterostomy is constructed by suturing the two limbs together, then exteriorizing the double stoma. The common wall can be crushed with a special clamp to create one large stoma. The stoma can be closed in an extraperitoneal manner.

to the distal loop with end-to-end anastomosis; (3) Bishop-Koop end-to-side union with exteriorization of the distal lumen; and rarely (4) Mikulicz exteriorization or (5) end ileostomies with delayed anastomosis (Fig. 39-16).

MALROTATION AND MIDGUT VOLVULUS

PATHOLOGY. During fetal development the intestine elongates too rapidly to be accommodated in the abdominal cavity. Around the sixth week the midgut, supplied by the superior mesenteric artery, prolapses into the umbilical cord and remains until the tenth week. As the midgut returns to the abdominal cavity, the developing cecum and the duodenum undergo a counterclockwise 270° rotation around the superior mesenteric artery, the final C-loop of the duodenum, and the transverse and ascending colon tracing the path of the rotation. The duodenum then becomes fixed retroperitoneally in its third portion, emerging at the ligament of Treitz, and the cecum is fixed by peritoneal bands to the right lateral abdominal wall. In addition, the takeoff of the branches of the superior mesenteric artery becomes elongated and fixed along a line

extending from the epigastrium to the right lower quadrant. If rotation is incomplete, the cecum remains high and the duodenum becomes shaped like a corkscrew to the right of the superior mesenteric artery. The clinical consequences of these events are (1) the bands (Ladd's bands) attempting to fix the cecum to the abdominal wall straddle the duodenum and may obstruct it, and (2) the mesenteric takeoff remains confined to the epigastric region. The entire midgut and its vascular supply are therefore suspended on a narrow pedicle that may twist. This

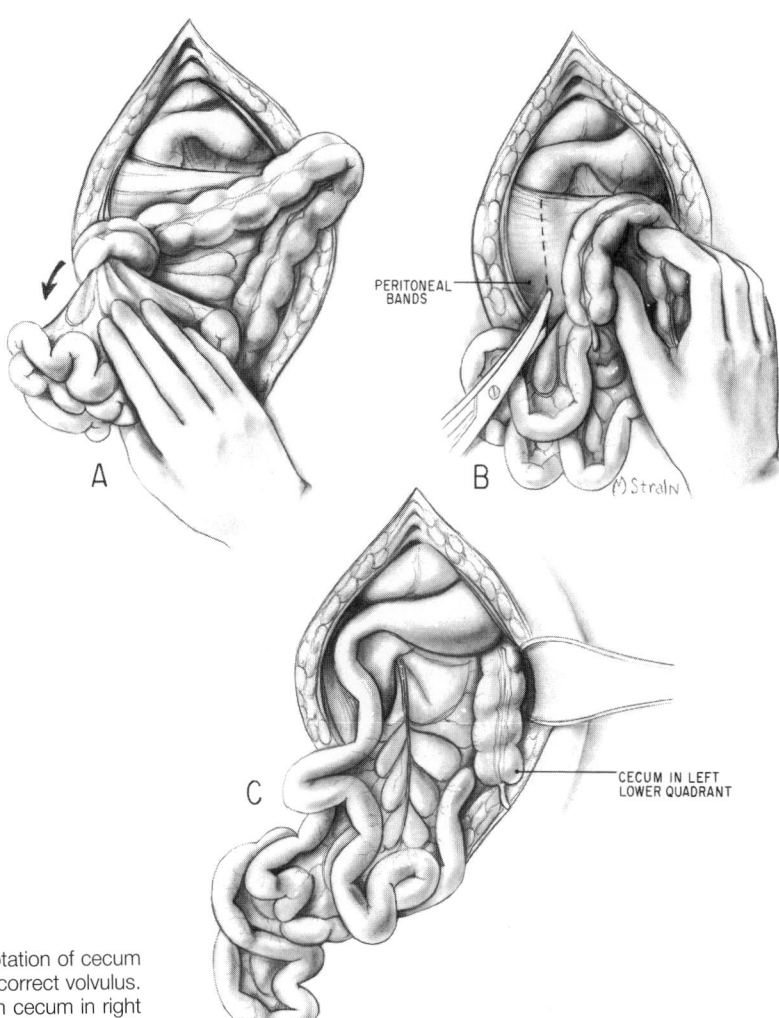

Fig. 39-17. Operative procedure for incomplete rotation of cecum and midgut volvulus. *A.* Unwinding of intestine to correct volvulus. *B.* Transection of peritoneal bands extending from cecum in right upper quadrant. *C.* Cecum relocated in left lower quadrant.

midgut volvulus results in high intestinal obstruction and midgut ischemia as the superior mesenteric blood flow is cut off.

CLINICAL MANIFESTATIONS. Such an infant presents with irritability and bilious vomiting with later manifestations of vascular compromise such as bloody stools. Abdominal signs are minimal early and may consist of mild upper distention and tenderness. As ischemia advances, erythema and edema of the abdominal wall and ultimately septic shock will signal gangrenous intestine and peritonitis. Abdominal films will show paucity of gas throughout the intestine with a few scattered air-fluid levels. A barium enema may show a displaced cecum, but an upper gastrointestinal series showing absent duodenal rotation makes a more reliable diagnosis.

TREATMENT. Early surgical intervention is mandatory if the ischemic process is to be reversed. The volvulus is untwisted counterclockwise followed by lysis of the bands between cecum and abdominal wall and between duodenum and terminal ileum to splay out the superior mesenteric artery and its branches. This procedure, origi-

nally described by Ladd, is still preferred. These maneuvers place the duodenum on the right and the cecum on the left of the abdomen (Fig. 39-17). The appendix is removed. It is not necessary to place any holding sutures in cecum or duodenum if the bands have been fully lysed. When the viability of the midgut is in doubt, the volvulus is reduced and all compromised bowel returned to the abdomen. A "second look" 24 to 36 h later will often show remarkable vascular recovery, and only irretrievably necrotic bowel is then resected.

MECONIUM ILEUS

The bowel obstruction in meconium ileus is a result of impaction of meconium in the distal ileum. Such infants have cystic fibrosis, and the accompanying lack of pancreatic enzymes in the intestine contributes to the viscous nature of the meconium. Bile vomiting is a late feature of this condition, which is characterized by progressive abdominal distention, failure of passage of meconium, and an upright abdominal film showing enormously distended

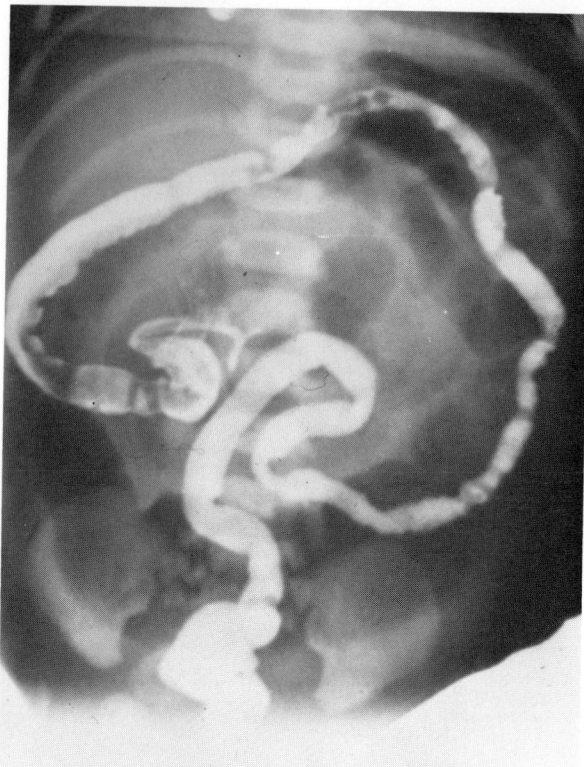

Fig. 39-18. Barium enema in an infant with meconium ileus. Microcolon is demonstrated. Colonic rotation is normal.

small bowel without air-fluid levels. Small bubbles of gas trapped in the inspissated meconium in the terminal ileum may produce a characteristic "ground-glass" appearance; a contrast enema will show a microcolon and terminal ileum filled with pellets of meconium (Fig. 39-18). The fetal reaction to prenatal perforation causes intraabdominal calcifications to form, producing an eggshell pattern on plain abdominal x-rays. Uncomplicated meconium ileus, i.e., that unassociated with perforation or vascular compromise of the distended ileum, can usually be resolved nonoperatively by a technique described by Noblett.

Dilute Gastrografin is advanced through the colon under fluoroscopic control into the dilated portion of the ileum. Since Gastrografin acts partially by absorbing fluid from the bowel wall into the intestinal lumen, maintaining adequate hydration of the infant during this maneuver is extremely important. The enema may be repeated at 12-h intervals over several days until all the meconium is evacuated per rectum. If surgical intervention is required because of failure of Gastrografin enemas to relieve obstruction, resection of the distended terminal ileum is performed, the meconium pellets are flushed from the distal small bowel by N-acetyl cysteine, and ileostomies or a Bishop-Koop anastomosis is performed. The microcolon can then be irrigated with saline or mineral oil to increase its lumen size, and anastomosis or closure of the Bishop-Koop chimney can be deferred for several weeks or months.

NECROTIZING ENTEROCOLITIS (NEC)

CLINICAL MANIFESTATIONS. Necrotizing enterocolitis is a disease of multifactorial origin that almost exclusively affects stressed premature infants. Common factors found in most infants with NEC include intestinal ischemia, bacterial colonization of the gut, and feedings of synthetic formulas. Clinically the first sign of NEC is formula intolerance, evident by vomiting or a large residual volume of a previous feeding in the stomach at the time of the next feeding. Abdominal distention and hematochezia are next signs of NEC and suggest ileus and mucosal ischemia, respectively. Invasion of the ischemic mucosa by gas-forming organisms causes pneumatosis intestinalis, which is the pathognomonic radiographic finding in NEC (Fig. 39-19). Development of hepatoportal venous gas suggests a particularly severe form of NEC. Some children, despite appropriate medical therapy, will develop a fulminant course with progressive peritonitis, acidosis, sepsis, disseminated intravascular coagulopathy, and death.

TREATMENT. Discontinuation of feedings, nasogastric decompression, and parenteral antibiotics are given to all babies suspected of having NEC. Free intraperitoneal air and signs of peritonitis are obvious indications for surgery. Children with significant acidosis (pH <7.20) after volume resuscitation and those with hepatoportal venous gas who do not promptly improve on medical therapy are also considered surgical candidates in our hospital. In equivocal cases, tapping the peritoneal cavity may aid in the decision to operate if the fluid withdrawn contains bacteria or intestinal contents. Resection of frankly gangrenous bowel should be carried out, and in the vast majority of cases, the intestinal ends are brought out as stomas. When massive intestinal involvement is present, marginally viable bowel is retained and a second look procedure is carried out in 24 h.

Total parenteral nutrition is maintained for at least 2 weeks postoperatively, after which oral feedings of small volumes of dilute formula are gradually introduced. Strictures develop in 20 percent of medically or surgically treated patients, and a contrast enema is mandatory before reestablishing intestinal continuity. If all other factors are favorable, the ileostomy is closed when the child is between 2 and 2.5 kg. Despite the severity of the illness in this premature population, survival rates for NEC approach 80 percent in many series.

Intussusception

Intussusception is a common cause of intestinal obstruction in the infant. It is most often observed in babies between 8 and 12 months of age and is slightly more common in males. The most frequent type is probably the result of hypertrophy of the Peyer's patches in the terminal ileum from an antecedent viral infection. The hypertrophied lymphatic patch becomes drawn into the lumen of the terminal ileum and is progressively moved into the ascending and transverse colon. Polyps, malignant tumors, such as lymphoma, and Meckel's diverticulum may act as lead points for intussusception; such intussuscep-

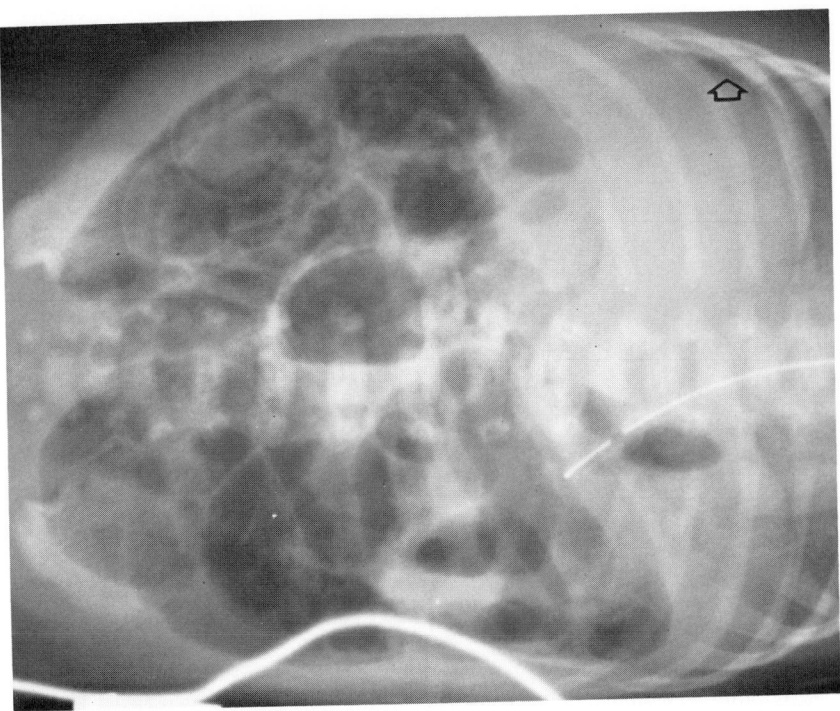

Fig. 39-19. X-ray study showing characteristic findings of necrotizing enterocolitis. There are distended, separated loops of bowel. Air is seen in the wall of the bowel (pneumotosis). The arrow depicts free air above the liver and below the diaphragm, signifying perforation.

tions are rarely reduced by barium enema, and thus the lead point is identified when operative reduction of the intussusception is performed.

CLINICAL MANIFESTATIONS. Since intussusception is frequently preceded by a gastrointestinal viral illness, the onset may not be easily discovered. Typically the infant develops paroxysms of crampy abdominal pain and intermittent vomiting. Between attacks the infant may act completely well, but as symptoms progress, increasing lethargy becomes apparent. Bloody mucus ("currant jelly stool") may be passed per rectum. Ultimately if reduction is not accomplished, gangrene of the intussusceptum occurs.

The pathognomonic physical finding is an elongated mass in the right upper quadrant or epigastrium with an absence of bowel in the right lower quadrant (Dance's sign). The mass may be seen on plain abdominal x-ray but is more easily demonstrated on barium enema. Barium outlines the leading portion of the intussusception, giving a "coiled-spring" appearance.

TREATMENT. The barium enema can also be used for hydrostatic reduction of the intussusception. Signs of peritonitis constitute a contraindication to barium enema reduction. The enema bag is suspended no higher than 1 m above the rectal catheter, and barium is allowed to enter the colon by gravity. Approximately 60 to 70 percent of the time, the barium column will push the intussusception before it and accomplish reduction. Free reflux into multiple small bowel loops and an infant who abruptly becomes well are characteristic of successful

reduction. Unless both of these signs are observed, it cannot be assumed that the intussusception is reduced, and preparations for exploration are made.

In some centers glucagon is injected intravenously in an effort to aid reduction by relaxing the smooth muscle of the intestine. A recent multicenter controlled study has not shown any increased success in children who received glucagon.

If hydrostatic reduction is successful, the infant is kept on intravenous fluids for 8 to 12 h before restarting oral fluids. The incidence of recurrent intussusception is 5 percent whether the intussusception is reduced by operation or by hydrostatic pressure. Failure to reduce the intussusception mandates surgery. Exploration is carried out through a right lower quadrant incision, delivering the intussuscepted mass into the wound. Reduction can usually be accomplished by gentle distal pressure, milking the bowel out of the intussuscipiens, never pulling it out. The blood supply to the appendix is often compromised, and appendectomy is performed. Resection of frankly gangrenous bowel is carried out without attempting reduction of the intussusception. As a rule, primary ileocolic anastomosis can be performed after resection.

Intravenous fluids are continued until peristalsis returns. If resection is necessary, prophylactic antibiotics are also administered for 72 h.

DUPLICATIONS, MECKEL'S DIVERTICULUM, AND MESENTERIC CYSTS

Duplications

Duplications can occur at any level in the gastrointestinal tract but are found most commonly in the ileum. They

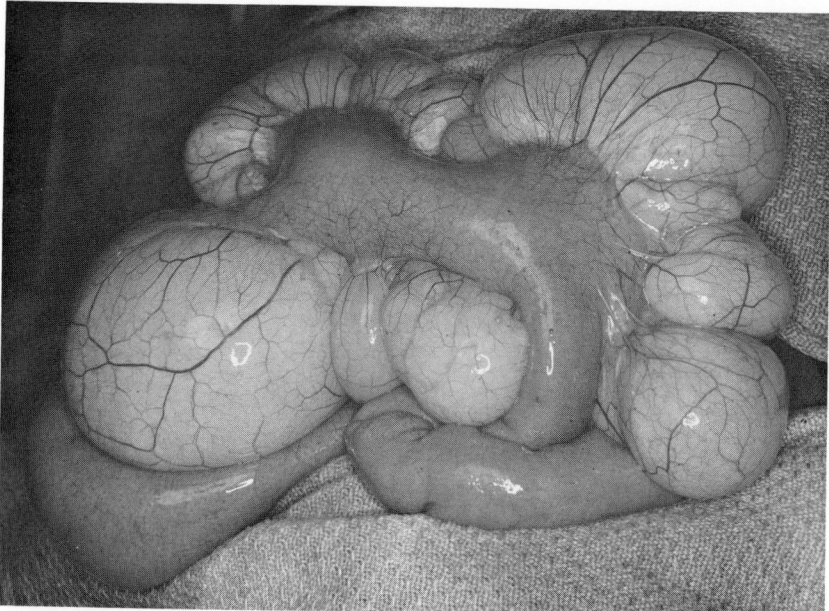

Fig. 39-20. Operative photograph depicting loops of ileum with a large chylous cyst in the mesentery. Note the relationship of the vascular supply to the bowel as it courses over the cyst. In most instances resection of the involved intestine is necessary.

may be long and tubular, but are usually cystic masses lying within the leaves of the mesentery and sharing a common wall with the intestine. Symptoms may include a palpable mass and/or frank intestinal obstruction. Torsion may produce gangrene and perforation, and subtle or massive bleeding may occur. This bleeding comes from ulceration in the duplication or adjacent intestine if the duplication contains ectopic gastric mucosa.

The ability to make a preoperative diagnosis of duplication usually depends on the presentation. Sonography and technetium pertechnatate scanning are the two most helpful diagnostic tests. For short duplications, resection of the cyst and adjacent intestine with end-to-end anastomosis is easily accomplished. If resection of long duplications would compromise intestinal length, multiple enterotomies and mucosal stripping in the duplicated segment will allow the walls to collapse and become adherent. An alternative method is to divide the common wall using the GIA stapler, forming a common lumen. This should not be done in duplications that contain ectopic gastric mucosa. In the patient with a very long duplication or multiple duplications, intraoperative nuclear medicine scanning will ensure complete excision of the ectopic gastric mucosa.

Meckel's Diverticulum

A Meckel's diverticulum is the persistence of a portion of the embryonic omphalomesenteric duct. It is located on the antimesenteric border of the ileum, usually a short distance (within 2 ft) from the ileocecal valve. It may be found incidentally at surgery or may present with inflammation masquerading as appendicitis. Like the duplication, ectopic gastric mucosa may produce ileal ulcerations that bleed and lead to the passage of maroon-colored stools. Diagnosis may be made by technetium

pertechnetate scans when the patient presents with bleeding. Surgical resection may be by wedge excision of the diverticulum and transverse closure of the ileum if the base is narrow. If wedge excision would compromise the ileal lumen, sleeve excision and end-to-end ileo-ileostomy are performed.

Mesenteric Cysts

Mesenteric cysts are similar to duplications in their location within the mesentery. However, they do not have any mucosa or muscular wall. Chylous cysts may result from congenital lymphatic obstruction (Fig. 39-20). Mesenteric cysts can cause intestinal obstruction or may present as an abdominal mass. Sonography may suggest the diagnosis. Surgical removal is accomplished by resection of the adjacent intestine, partial excision or marsupialization being reserved for cysts involving a large portion of the mesentery.

HIRSCHSPRUNG'S DISEASE

Hirschsprung's disease is characteristically a disease of the male infant. The defect is the absence of ganglion cells in the rectum and the rectosigmoid. The precursors of the ganglion cells are neural crest cells that migrate into the intestine from cephalad to caudad. The process is completed by the twelfth week of embryonic life, but the migration from midtransverse colon to anus takes 4 weeks. This increases the time period of vulnerability for failure of migration and accounts for the fact that most cases of aganglionosis involve the rectum and rectosigmoid. Longer segments of absent ganglion cells may also occur, and total colonic aganglionosis, although rare, is also seen. Sex incidence is equal in these cases of long-segment Hirschsprung's disease.

Aganglionic colon does not permit normal peristalsis to occur. Functional obstruction therefore supervenes, and the infant may present with complete colon obstruction or with a devastating enterocolitis. The presentation may, however, be much more subtle, with constipation and abdominal distention and sometimes, though not invariably, poor nutrition.

DIAGNOSIS. Infants with Hirschsprung's disease will usually fail to pass meconium in the first 24 h of life, although this history is often impossible to obtain. Added to this is the fact that it takes several weeks before the proximal colon containing ganglion cells hypertrophies and dilates enough to show the characteristic change in size of the aganglionic portion of the colon on barium enema. Barium enema is therefore often normal in the newborn infant. In older infants and children, barium enema will show the size contrast between the dilated ganglionic colon and the distal constricted rectal segment. The barium enema in total colonic aganglionous shows a markedly shortened colon, often in the form of a question mark.

Rectal biopsy makes the definitive diagnosis of Hirschsprung's disease. A suction biopsy technique is available that provides a small piece of mucosa and submucosa. The diagnosis may also be made by histochemical staining of cholinesterase in the ganglion-cell/nerve complex. Some surgeons have found the use of rectal manometry helpful, but it is not as accurate a diagnostic tool as is rectal biopsy.

TREATMENT. Treatment is surgical in all cases. Pull-through procedures have been performed in the newborn period in several centers. Most pediatric surgeons prefer to perform a colostomy in the newborn period and wait for a period of growth (to 10 kg) before doing definitive surgery. In the older infant and child who have been belatedly diagnosed it is important to allow the distended hypertrophied colon to return to a normal size before pulling it through the narrow pelvis. This is usually accomplished by waiting 3 to 6 months after a colostomy is performed.

Three pull-through procedures are currently in use for treating Hirschsprung's disease. The first of these is the original Swenson procedure, in which the aganglionic rectum is carefully dissected in the pelvis and removed down to the anus. The ganglionic colon is then anastomosed to the anus via a perineal approach (Fig. 39-21). Variations of Swenson's technique have been devised by Duhamel and Soave (Fig. 39-21). In the former, dissection outside the rectum is confined to the retrorectal space and the ganglionic colon anastomosed posteriorly just above the anus. Martin has modified this procedure by excising the anterior wall of the ganglionic colon and the posterior wall of the aganglionic rectum, using a stapling device. This avoids the accumulation of stool in the blind aganglionic rectum. In Soave's operation, dissection is

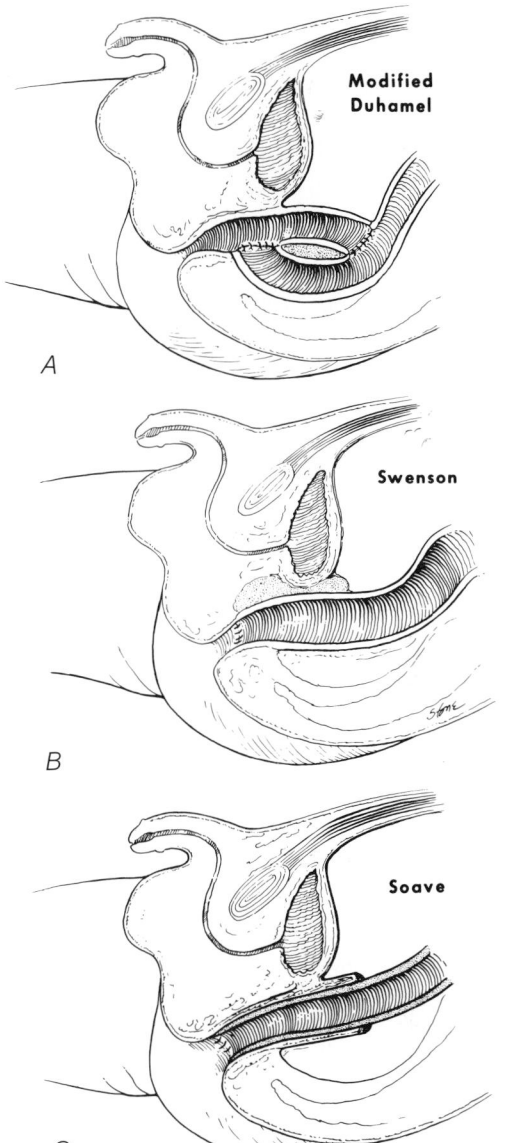

Fig. 39-21. The three basic operations for surgical correction of Hirschsprung's disease. *A.* The Duhamel procedure leaves the rectum in place and brings ganglionic bowel into the retrorectal space. The common wall, indicated by lines, is crushed to eliminate the septum. *B.* Classic Swenson operation (1948) is a resection with end-to-end anastomosis performed by exteriorizing bowel ends through the anus. *C.* The Soave operation is performed by endorectal dissection and removal of mucosa from the aganglionic distal segment and bringing the ganglionic bowel down to the anus within the seromuscular tunnel.

entirely within the rectum (Fig. 39-22). The rectal mucosa is stripped from the muscular sleeve, and the ganglionic colon is brought through this sleeve and later amputated at the anal level. Autoanastomosis is achieved by healing between the colon serosa and the circular muscle of the rectal sleeve. Boley performs a suture anastomosis between the distal colon and the anal mucosa and completes the operation in one stage. Long-term results with the

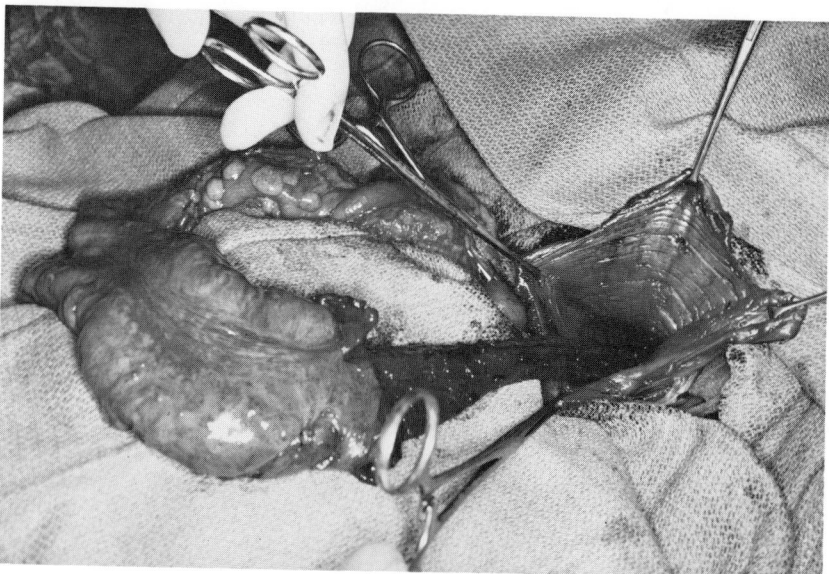

Fig. 39-22. Operative photograph of Soave procedure for Hirschsprung's disease. The seromuscular tunnel has been developed, and the circular muscle of the rectum is clearly seen. The mucosa has been stripped away from this tunnel and can be seen below the normally innervated sigmoid colon. The mucosal sleeve will be pulled through the rectum and the normal sigmoid colon drawn into the seromuscular tunnel for anastomosis at the anus.

three procedures are comparable and generally excellent in experienced hands. These three procedures can also be adapted for total colonic aganglionosis; the ileum is used for the pull-through.

IMPERFORATE ANUS

Imperforate anus affects males and females with equal frequency and occurs once in 20,000 live births. Failure of descent of the urorectal septum in embryonic life produces a variety of anorectal and cloacal anomalies. The level to which this septum descends determines the separation of the urinary and hind-gut systems. Broadly classified, the imperforate anus is characterized as "high" or "low" depending on whether the rectum ends above the levator ani muscle complex or partially descends through this muscle. The rectum usually ends in a fistula. In high imperforate anus in males the fistula usually ends in the prostatic urethra. In females the interposed vagina is the site of entry of the fistula. The low lesions have a fistula to the perineum. In males this is seen in the median raphe of the scrotum or penis, and in females the commonest perineal fistula ends at the posterior fourchette. Since the rectum has descended through the levator complex in low lesions, only a perineal operation is required; this situation occurs in 50 percent of males and 90 percent of females. Such children will be expected to be continent since the "muscle of continence," the levator ani muscle, and the rectum are in a normal relationship to each other.

Infants having high imperforate anus require a colostomy in the newborn period, with some kind of pull-through procedure performed after growth to about 10 kg, which makes the procedure easier. Careful assessment of the genital tracts in females and GU system in all patients with imperforate anus is imperative because of the very high incidence of associated anomalies, particularly in children with a high imperforate anus.

Diagnosis of imperforate anus is not difficult. The location of the fistula site may sometimes be a problem. Beading of mucus or meconium along the median raphe of the perineum and scrotum denotes a low imperforate anus in the male. Air in the bladder, voiding of gas or meconium, and retrograde urethrogram with contrast may demonstrate the urinary fistula of the high imperforate anus in the male. In the female, since most of the lesions are low, careful examination of the perineum, fourchette, and vestibule of the vagina will locate the fistula in most cases. A high fistula in the female may terminate in the vagina and will be harder to demonstrate. If a single perineal opening is seen in the female, a cloacal abnormality is present with urethra, vagina, and rectum opening into a common urogenital sinus. The "upside-down films" of Wangensteen and Rice are often confusing and not definitive and now are seldom used. The use of transperitoneal injection of contrast media, pelvic CT, ultrasound, or MRI has been advocated to define the anatomy in this anomaly. If there is any doubt of the level, it is much safer to perform a colostomy than ruin any chance for continence by an injudicious perineal operation.

A number of pull-through procedures have been developed for high imperforate anus. The hallmark of each of these operations is the location of the levator ani muscle, or so-called puborectalis portion of this muscle, and transposition of the rectum anterior to this muscle. The rectum is sutured to the skin of the perineum in the normal position of the anus. The Kiesewetter-Rehbein procedure utilizes an abdominal approach, with division of the fistula from above. The mucosa is then stripped from the imperforate rectum and the colon pulled through the mucosal sleeve to the perineum. In the Stephens approach, the dissection proceeds posteriorly through a transsacral approach. The chances of continence from each of these procedures have not proved to be very good, and mucosal anal prolapse has been a particular problem.

Recently Pena and DeVries have devised a posterior approach, dividing the levator ani and external sphincter complex in the midline posteriorly and bringing down the rectum after sufficient length is achieved. The muscles are then reconstructed and sutured to the rectum, which is tapered to fit into its new position. Initial reports of results with the posterior sagittal anorectoplasty have been encouraging for both the primary and secondary procedures for high imperforate anus as well as cloacal anomalies. Careful attention to detail is important to minimize complications utilizing this approach.

JAUNDICE—BILIARY ATRESIA

Neonatal jaundice is sufficiently common to be regarded as physiologic. In most cases, the jaundice resolves without treatment. Pathologic jaundice implies persistent (>2 weeks) elevation of bilirubin, particularly the direct fraction (>2 mg/dL), whether resulting from cholestasis or from obstruction. Biliary atresia affects not only the extrahepatic bile ducts but also the liver, which accounts for the biochemical overlap with many of the cholestatic syndromes. Biliary atresia occurs once in every 20,000 to 30,000 births, with an equal sex distribution. A familial occurrence has been reported.

ETIOLOGY AND PATHOLOGY. Originally biliary atresia was thought to be a developmental anomaly. There is evidence, however, that the cause of this condition may be infectious, presumably viral. REO-3 viral antibodies have been demonstrated in the sera of patients with biliary atresia while control sera were negative. Prospective epidemiologic and virologic investigations are in progress attempting to further elucidate the cause or causes of biliary atresia.

The developing bile ducts pass through a solid stage analogous to that of the intestine, becoming obliterated by epithelial concrescence or proliferation. In the course of normal development, this solid core becomes vacuolated, and the vacuoles coalesce to reestablish the lumen. An arrest in this solid stage affords the best explanation for the malformation, and innumerable anomalies are possible. The atretic segment may not be identifiable or may appear as a thin, fibrous cord. The obliterative process may involve the common duct, cystic duct, one or both hepatic ducts, and the gallbladder, in a variety of combinations. Approximately one-quarter of the patients have coincidental malformations including congenital heart disease, imperforate anus, duodenal atresia, mongolism, and, most commonly, urinary tract involvement.

CLINICAL MANIFESTATIONS. Jaundice, a constant finding, is usually present at birth or shortly thereafter but does not become marked until the child is two or three weeks old, after which it becomes progressively more intense. Initially, the growth and weight gains of the children are within normal limits, but in later stages of disease malnutrition and retarded growth may be apparent. Abdominal enlargement is frequent and may be related to hepatomegaly or, rarely, accumulation of ascites. In extended cases, the spleen also may be enlarged, and the anteroabdominal wall veins may be apparent, reflecting portal hypertension.

DIAGNOSIS. The urine is dark and positive for bile, and contains no urobilinogen. The stools are acholic with pasty consistency. The initial stool may have a normal green color, since it is formed at the fourth month of fetal development and the obstruction of the biliary tract may occur after that time. Later, the occasional appearance of a yellow color in the stool and a positive test for bile may be explained by the excretion of small amounts of pigment by the glands of the intestinal tract. The serum bilirubin progressively increases with ultimate establishment of extremely high levels. Weekly determinations for a period of 1 month are considered the single most valuable laboratory aid. High levels of alkaline phosphatase are common.

Most diagnostic tests are nonspecific but properly selected and combined will discriminate between cholestatic and obstructive jaundice. No single test or combination of studies is absolutely reliable. Usually the synthetic functions of the liver are unimpaired in the jaundiced infant. Thus, the serum albumin and clotting mechanism are normal. In many centers the nuclear scan using technetium 99m IDA (DISIDA), performed after pretreatment of the patient with phenobarbital, has proved the most accurate and reliable study. This examination, particularly when complemented by percutaneous needle biopsy of the liver, will establish a diagnosis with a high degree of certainty. If radionuclide appears in the intestine, extrahepatic bile duct patency is assured. If radiopharmaceutical is normally concentrated by the liver but not excreted despite treatment with phenobarbital, and the metabolic/infectious screens are negative, the presumptive diagnosis must be biliary atresia.

Complementary studies include the analysis of duodenal fluid for bile and abdominal ultrasound. The latter examination is reliable only when performed in the fasting patient. It should be emphasized that the presence of a gallbladder does not exclude the diagnosis of biliary atresia; in approximately 15 percent of these patients the distal biliary tract is patent although the proximal ducts are atretic. It is worth noting that the intrahepatic bile ducts are never dilated in the patient with biliary atresia.

DIFFERENTIAL DIAGNOSIS. Neonatal jaundice may also be due to (1) physiologic changes, (2) constitutional deficiency, (3) hemolytic disease, (4) sepsis, (5) neonatal hepatitis, (6) a-trypsin deficiency, or (7) the inspissated bile syndrome. Physiologic jaundice occurs in some full-term infants, more frequently in premature infants. It is due to the destruction of fetal red cells that are no longer required after birth, coupled with the normal functional immaturity of the liver at birth, which is unable to excrete the excessive load of pigment presented to it. The jaundice reaches its peak within 2 to 5 days after delivery and

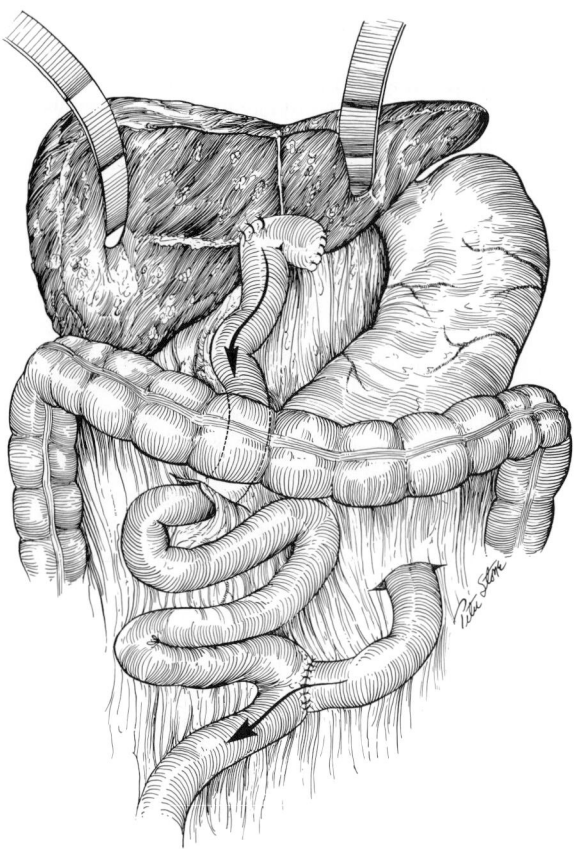

Fig. 39-23. Operative diagram of the Kasai portoenterostomy for biliary atresia. An isolated limb of jejunum has been brought to the porta hepatis and anastomosed to the transected ducts. The Roux en Y principle has been used to reconstitute intestinal continuity. The biliary conduit is usually vented externally.

then gradually disappears. The serum bilirubin levels rarely exceed 10 mg/dL.

Of the constitutional deficiencies causing hyperbilirubinemia, only the rare Crigler-Najjar syndrome is manifest early. The total serum bilirubin is usually over 10 mg/dL, and the greater proportion is unconjugated. There is always an associated hepatomegaly, and kernicterus is a common complication. The patients usually die early, although some may survive without neurologic deficit. Another hepatic disturbance with a familial tendency is related to the ingestion of lactose in infants with galactosemia. An obstructive type of jaundice appears after the first week of life and subsides immediately when lactose is removed from the diet. If the lactose is not withheld, the jaundice spontaneously subsides over a period of several weeks. Examination of the urine for reducing substances provides the diagnosis.

Hemolysis due to blood grouping incompatibility between fetus and mother may result in neonatal jaundice. Jaundice may intensify until death ensues or until a gradual recovery takes place in several weeks. The increase in the bilirubin is in the unconjugated portion, the urine con-

tains bilirubin and urobilinogen, and a positive Coombs test confirms the diagnosis for Rh incompatibility but may be negative with ABO incompatibility. Overwhelming sepsis can cause damage to the liver and jaundice. Recent interest has been directed toward cytomegalic inclusion disease, with jaundice occurring in the first week or later and accompanied by hepatomegaly and splenomegaly, microcephaly and mental retardation, motor disability, and petechiae.

Twenty-five percent of cases of prolonged obstructive jaundice in infancy have been ascribed to neonatal hepatitis. The usual clinical picture is that of a fluctuating jaundice that appears during the early weeks of life. Liver function tests contribute little to the differential diagnosis, but liver biopsy may be diagnostic by demonstrating the microscopic picture of local necrosis and large multinucleated liver cells. Neonatal jaundice may also be caused by the ''inspissated bile syndrome,'' which accounted for 15 percent of the cases in one large series. The term is applied to patients with normal biliary tracts who have had persistent signs of obstructive jaundice. Increased viscosity of bile and obstruction of the canaliculi are implicated as causes. Most cases are related to hemolytic disease, but in some instances no etiologic factor can be defined.

TREATMENT. Historically a variety of innovative surgical procedures have been attempted to promote bile flow from the liver in infants with biliary atresia. Only the hepatoportoenterostomy, developed by Kasai, has stood the test of time and demonstrated promise as a procedure that will not only provide relief of jaundice but also may result in cure. The procedure is based on Kasai's observation that the fibrous tissue at the portahepatis invests microscopically patent biliary ductules that, in turn, communicate with the intrahepatic ductal system. Transecting this fibrous tissue (just cephalad to the bifurcating portal vein) opens these channels, and bile will flow into a surgically constructed intestinal conduit, usually a Roux en Y limb of jejunum (Fig. 39-23). Operative success is usually precluded if the operation is delayed beyond the twelfth week of life. Surgical success is enhanced when the procedure is accomplished before the infant reaches eight weeks. Although bile drainage is anticipated when the operation is carried out early, decompression of the bile ducts does not necessarily imply cure. Hepatic fibrosis may progress even when bile drainage is achieved. Postoperative cholangitis continues to plague infants having successful protoenterostomy procedures. The incidence and severity of cholangitis are reduced by external venting of the surgically created biliary conduit or by incorporation of a valve within the conduit and by the long-term administration of antibiotics. Despite these measures, the problem of ascending infection has not been eliminated. Reoperation, with resectional debridement of the portoenterostomy anastomosis, has rescued selected children with intractable cholangitis. Cirrhosis and portal hypertension have emerged as new problems in some children, relieved of jaundice by functioning biliary conduits. Gastrointestinal hemorrhage from esophageal varices has been managed successfully by endoscopic sclerotherapy. Portosystemic shunting by selective and nonselective techniques has also proved successful. Nonshunt alternatives, including extensive paraesophageal and gastric devascularization and esophageal transection, are additional options. Percutaneous transhepatic embolization of varices after selective catheterization of the portal vein is also feasible as a temporary measure to control hemorrhage.

For the child afflicted with biliary atresia in whom the Kasai operation fails, or succeeds only temporarily, liver replacement by orthotopic transplantation remains the final hope for salvage. Biliary atresia has been the most common liver disease in pediatric recipients. Survival rates after liver transplantation have improved greatly since the introduction of cyclosporine-steroid immunosuppressant therapy. The 1-year survival rate now approaches 70 percent.

Biliary Hypoplasia

At the time of surgical exploration one may encounter in some infants a homogeneous smooth, chocolate brown liver, rather than the firm greenish liver characteristic of biliary atresia. In this circumstance, an operative cholangiogram will invariably demonstrate the gallbladder and extrahepatic biliary system to be patent, albeit diminutive, "biliary hypoplasia." Hypoplasia of the extrahepatic biliary system is associated with a wide range of hepatic paranchymal disorders that cause severe intrahepatic cholestasis. Included among these are α-antitrypsin deficiency and arteriohepatic dysplasia (Alagille's syndrome). The primary pathology resides within the liver and not the bile ducts; therefore, portal dissection and portoenterostomy are not indicated in these patients. Rather a generous liver biopsy is obtained and the operation terminated.

Choledochal Cyst

There have been numerous descriptions and classifications based upon the location and anatomy of the choledochal cyst. Among the most useful is Todani's modification of the classification proposed by Alonso Lej. The type 1 cyst characterized by fusiform dilatation of the bile duct into which the cystic duct enters is the most common. Choledochal cyst is most appropriately considered the predominant feature in a constellation of pathologic abnormalities within the pancreatic-biliary system. Frequently associated with choledochal cyst are anomalous junction of the pancreatic duct and common bile duct, distal bile duct stenosis, intrahepatic ductal dilatation, abnormal histology of the common bile duct, and hepatic histology ranging from normal to cirrhotic. These features are encountered in varying degrees and combinations and constitute the anatomic spectrum of the malformation. The etiology of choledochal cyst is controversial; one tenable accepted explanation is that proposed by Babbitt. He incriminated an abnormal pancreatic biliary duct junc-

tion with the formation of a "common channel" into which pancreatic enzyme secretions are discharged with resultant weakening of the bile duct wall by gradual enzymatic destruction leading to dilatation, inflammation, and finally cyst formation. It should be noted, however, that not all patients with choledochal cyst demonstrate an anatomic common channel.

Choledochal cyst is more common in females than in males (4:1). The so-called classic symptom complex of pain/mass/jaundice is actually encountered in fewer than half the patients. The more usual presentation is that of episodic abdominal pain often recurrent over months or years, generally associated with only minimal jaundice that may escape detection. If the condition persists unrecognized, sequelae including cholangitis, cirrhosis, and portal hypertension are almost inevitable.

DIAGNOSIS. Choledochal cyst has been demonstrated antenatally by maternal ultrasound. Ultrasonography and computerized axial tomography reveal the dimensions of the cyst and define its relationship to the vascular structures in the porta, as well as the intrahepatic ductal configuration. Endoscopic retrograde cholangiopancreatography (ERCP) is reserved for patients in whom confusion remains after evaluation by less invasive imaging modalities.

TREATMENT. The surgical options include internal drainage by cystenterostomy, and surgical excision. The morbidity from the former procedure has proved to be excessive. The cyst wall is composed of fibrous tissue and is devoid of mucosal lining. Anastomotic obstruction from scarring is inevitable. Further, the thick-walled fibrous cyst does not contract after drainage but rather persists as a receptacle for stagnant bile. The morbidity from complications relating to biliary stasis mitigates against internal drainage procedures. An additional and perhaps the most serious consequence of cyst retention is the development of malignancy arising within the cyst wall. The incidence of this aggressive and highly lethal neoplasm further supports the recommendation for cyst resection.

In most circumstances the caliber of the common hepatic duct cephalad to the choledochal cyst is normal. Successful resection of the cyst requires circumferential dissection, entering the posterior plane between the cyst and portal vein to accomplish removal. The pancreatic duct, which may enter the distal cyst, is vulnerable to injury.

For the patient in whom the anatomy of the porta is obscured and distorted by pericystic inflammation, an alternative technique is proposed. An arbitrary plane is entered within the posterior wall of the cyst that allows the inner lining of the back wall to be dissected free from the outer layer that directly overlies the portal vascular structures. The lateral and anterior cyst, as well as the internal aspect of the back wall, are removed. The outer posterior wall remains behind. In either circumstance cyst excision is accomplished, with reconstruction employing normal or near normal proximal bile duct and a mucosal union between the biliary system and intestinal tract. The likelihood of postoperative anastomotic stricture with atten-

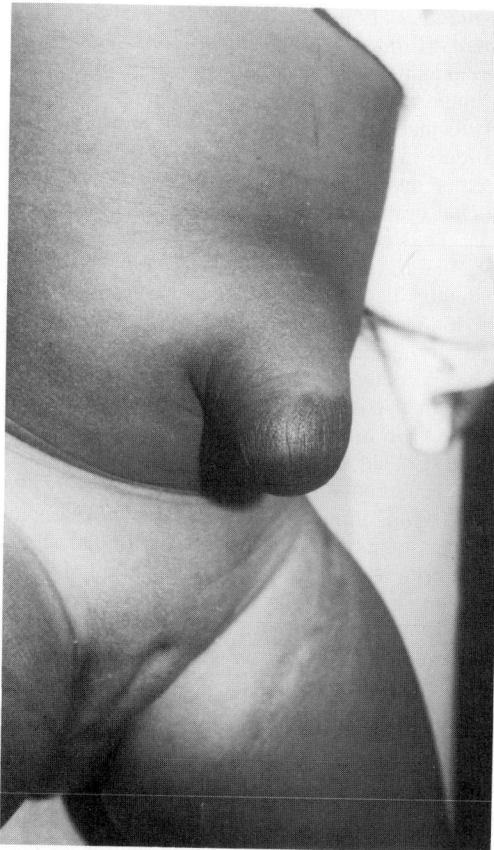

Fig. 39-24. One-year-old female with large umbilical hernia. Early repair indicated because of size.

dant sequelae is minimized. Further, the risk of malignancy is reduced although not completely eliminated.

DEFORMITIES OF THE ABDOMINAL WALL

Embryology

The abdominal wall is formed by four separate embryologic folds, cephalic, caudal, and right and left lateral folds, each of which is composed of somatic and splanchnic layers. Each of the folds develops toward the anterior center portion of the celomic cavity, joining to form a large umbilical ring that surrounds the two umbilical arteries, the vein, and the yolk sac or omphalomesenteric duct. These structures are covered by an outer layer of amnion, and the entire unit comprises the umbilical cord. Between the fifth and tenth weeks of fetal development the intestinal tract undergoes a rapid growth outside of the abdominal cavity within the proximal portion of the umbilical cord. As development is completed, the intestine gradually returns to the abdominal cavity. Contraction of the umbilical ring completes the process of abdominal wall formation. Duhamel has described failure of closure of any segment of the anterior abdominal wall as

celosomia. For example, (1) failure of the cephalic fold to close (upper celosomia) results in sternal defects (as congenital absence of the sternum or the pentalogy of Cantrell), (2) failure of the caudal fold to close (lower celosomia) results in exstrophy of the bladder and in more extreme cases, exstrophy of the cloaca. Interruption of central migration of the lateral folds results in omphalocele. Gastrochisis, originally thought to be a variant of omphalocele, probably results from a fetal accident in the form of intrauterine rupture of a hernia of the umbilical cord.

Umbilical Hernia

Failure of timely closure of the umbilical ring leaves a central defect in the linea alba. The resulting umbilical hernia is covered by normal umbilical skin and subcutaneous tissue, but the fascial defect allows protrusion of abdominal content (Fig. 39-24). Hernias less than a centimeter at the time of birth will usually close spontaneously by one to two years of life. Larger defects may require longer periods of time before spontaneous closure occurs. Some umbilical hernias never close spontaneously. Umbilical hernias are easily recognized as a protrusion of the umbilicus covered by normal skin. Sometimes the hernia is large enough that the protrusion is disfiguring and disturbing to both the child and the family. In such circumstances early repair may be advisable. When the defect is small and spontaneous closure likely, delay of surgical correction until four or five years of age is appropriate. Incarceration is rarely seen in an umbilical hernia. Unlike treatment for inguinal hernia of infants and young children, attempts at reduction of an incarcerated umbilical hernia are unwise. Repair of uncomplicated umbilical hernia is performed through a small curving infraumbilical incision that fits into the skin crease of the umbilicus. The fascial defect is repaired with permanent sutures in the midline. Fascial flaps or other complicated umbilical hernia repairs that have been recommended for adult patients are unnecessary in children. The umbilicus should never be excised in the repair of umbilical hernias in the childhood age.

Patent Urachus

During the development of the coelomic cavity, there is free communication between the urinary bladder and the abdominal wall through the urachus, which exits adjacent the omphalomesenteric duct. Persistence of this tract results in a communication between the bladder and the umbilicus (Fig. 39-25). The first sign of a patent urachus is moisture or obvious urine emission from the umbilicus. Recurrent urinary tract infection may result. The urachus may be partly obliterated, with a remnant remaining beneath the umbilicus in the extraperitoneal position as an isolated cyst, which may be identified by ultrasonography. Diagnosis of patent urachus is most reliably made by a cystogram in the lateral projection (Fig. 39-26). Surgical correction is carried out via extraperitoneal exposure of the infraumbilical area. Identification and excision of the

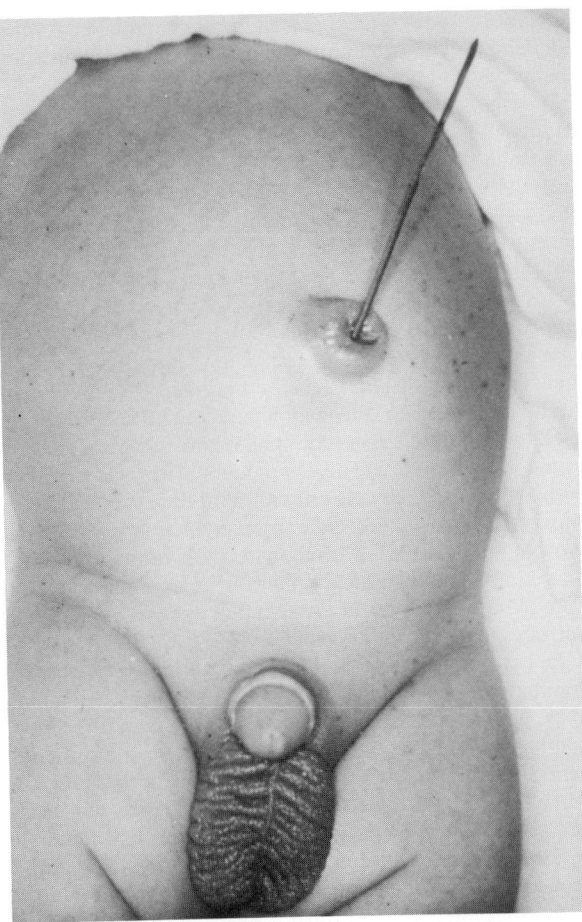

Fig. 39-25. Probe in opening of umbilicus. This defect could be patent urachus or patent omphalomesenteric duct.

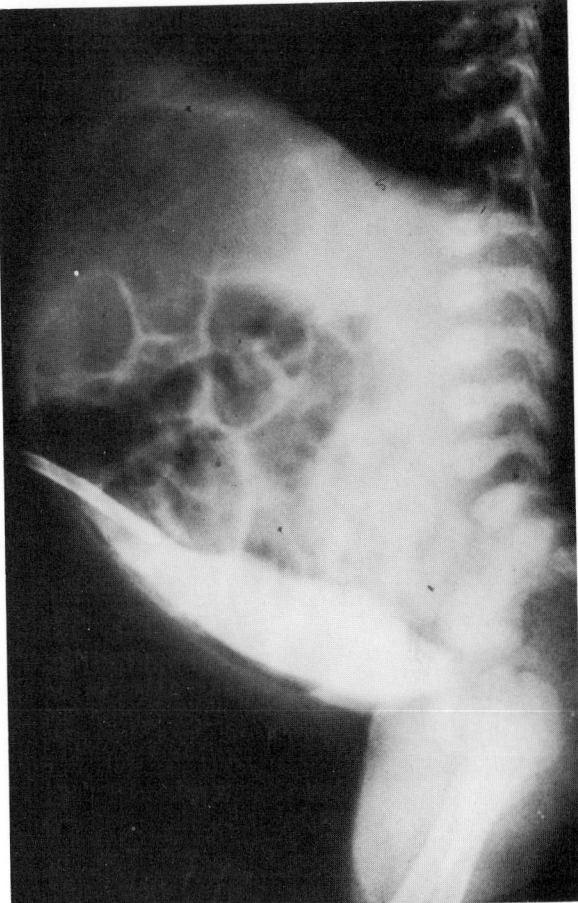

Fig. 39-26. Contrast material in urinary bladder introduced via catheter in umbilicus confirming patent urachus.

urachal tract with closure of the bladder is curative. Urachal cysts are also easily excised from this approach.

Patent Omphalomesenteric Duct

In fetal life, the omphalomesenteric duct is connected through the central wall of the coelomic cavity to the intestinal tract. Normally this duct involutes, but its persistence results in a tubular attachment between the ileum and the umbilicus (Fig. 39-27). Liquid ileal content refluxes through the umbilical defect, soiling the abdominal wall. Diagnosis of a congenital fistula at the umbilicus is made by inspection, probing of the tract, and introduction of radiopaque material into the ostium. Proper surgical treatment consists of elective abdominal exploration with closure of the fistula of the antimesenteric border of the ileum and total excision of the fistulous tract, including its attachment to the undersurface of the umbilicus. Though not an emergency, this procedure should not be postponed, since there is a potential for intestinal volvulus to occur around this intraabdominal structure. Occasionally the peristaltic activity of the bowel will cause eversion of the intestine through this patent duct. The

extruded intestine resembles a small ruptured omphalocele, and the lesion requires careful inspection at the neck of the defect to determine its true nature. In such cases the bowel has, in effect, turned inside out and prolapsed through the patent duct, forming an external intussusception. In this instance, immediate operation with reduction and correction is necessary.

Omphalocele

An omphalocele (Fig. 39-28) presents as a mass of bowel and solid viscera in the central abdomen, covered by translucent membrane. The size varies from about 1 cm in diameter to huge defects containing much or all of the abdominal viscera. In the latter forms, the bowel has lost its right of domain in the abdominal cavity, and temporizing techniques must be used until the abdominal cavity reaches a sufficient size to accommodate the bowel. The diagnosis is made by inspection. Babies born with omphaloceles are prone to other anomalies. Rickham collected reports from 11 large clinics whose combined experience yielded a 67 percent incidence of associated anomalies. Special syndromes such as exstrophy of

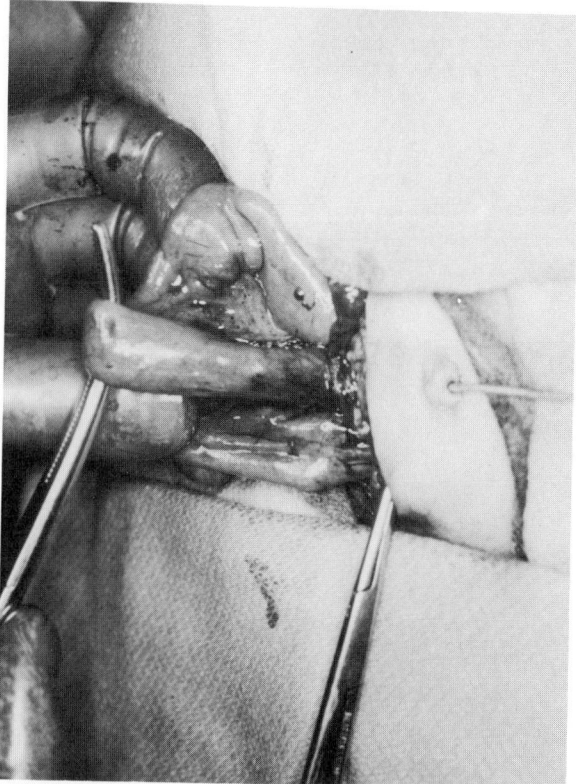

Fig. 39-27. Operative photograph depicting probe in umbilical defect passing directly into patent omphalomesenteric duct, which is connected to ileum.

Fig. 39-28. Infant with large omphalocele.

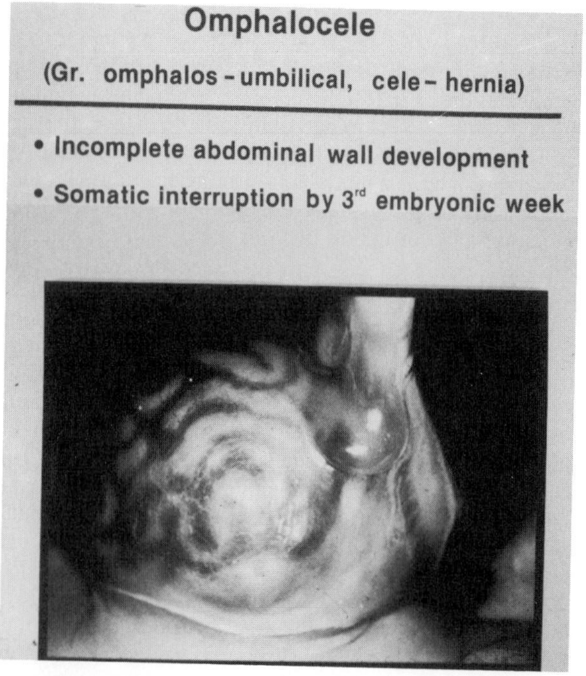

Omphalocele

(Gr. omphalos – umbilical, cele – hernia)

- **Incomplete abdominal wall development**
- **Somatic interruption by 3rd embryonic week**

the cloaca (vesicointestinal fissure) and the Beckwith-Wiedemann constellation of anomalies include omphalocele.

Emergency treatment immediately after delivery of an infant with omphalocele consists of covering the lesion with saline-soaked gauze and wrapping the trunk circumferentially. No pressure should be placed on the omphalocele sac in an effort to reduce its contents, because pressure can lead to rupture of the sac or may interfere with abdominal venous return, or impede respiratory effort. In 1957 Grob reported a conservative treatment for omphalocele using mercurochrome, to cause a thick eschar cover. This layer subsequently separated, and epithelization progressed from the periphery of the lesion, gradually covering the omphalocele. Although rarely used today, there are certain indications for this approach using betadine spray. These indications are (1) a newborn with a giant omphalocele and other life-threatening anomalies whose correction takes precedence over repair of the omphalocele, (2) the neonate with other anomalies that complicate a surgical repair of the omphalocele, and (3) newborns with severe associated anomalies that may not be consistent with survival.

In 1948 Gross described a technique whereby the abdominal wall was repaired in two stages. First wide skin flaps were developed that were closed over the intact omphalocele. A second stage was the correction of the ventral hernia at a much later date. Beginning in 1959, Schuster used prosthetic materials sutured to the fascia and covered with skin flaps to bring about a gradual enlargement of the abdominal cavity with staged operative procedures. Subsequently, Allen and Wrenn and Gilbert et al. suggested the use of a ''silo'' of silastic material sutured around the circumference of the defect as an exterior cover uncovered by skin (Fig. 39-29). This technique, refined over the years by many, has proved a basis for temporary coverage of large omphaloceles as well as the exposed bowel in gastroschisis. The main principle in

Fig. 39-29. Close-up of silastic prosthesis for temporary covering of gastroschisis. The remnant of the umbilicus is seen in the center of the photograph. A gastrostomy tube is seen.

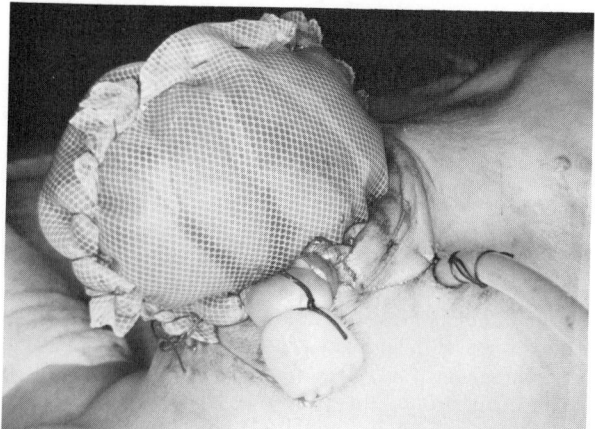

the use of the plastic material is steady pressure with gradual reduction of the plastic envelope over an interval of 5 to 14 days until the abdominal wall closure can be tolerated by the infant. Today most babies, even with large omphaloceles, can be salvaged. The persistent mortality rate of 20 to 30 percent from pediatric centers reflects the serious anomalies associated with this malformation.

Gastroschisis

Gastroschisis was once thought to be a form of ruptured omphalocele. It was incorrectly described in older literature as a defect of the abdominal wall separated from the umbilicus by a bridge of skin. In fact, the gastroschisis defect that permits escape of the intestines from the abdominal cavity occurs at the junction of the umbilicus and the normal skin. Shaw first suggested that gastroschisis is simply a hernia of the umbilical cord that ruptures after the complete development of the abdominal wall. Certainly this thesis is consistent with the findings. Babies with gastroschisis have a large amount of viscera on the surface of an intact abdominal wall that has a small defect at the right edge of the umbilicus that is still held in place by the two arteries and the umbilical vein (Fig. 39-30). The umbilicus has become partly detached, allowing free communication with the abdominal cavity. The intestine lying free outside of the abdominal cavity may be glistening, moist, and normal in appearance, suggesting that the rupture occurred immediately before or during delivery of the infant. More commonly, the intestine is thick, edematous, discolored, and covered with a shaggy exudate; it has been postulated that the intestine escaped from the fetal abdominal confines via the umbilical cord rupture weeks or even months before delivery, and, floating freely in the amnion, developed changes in the intestinal wall. Unlike babies born with omphalocele, associated anomalies seen with gastroschisis are confined to bowel atresia, further substantiating the mechanics of this abnormality.

TREATMENT. All infants born with gastroschisis should be taken to the operating room expeditiously. The intestine can be returned to the abdominal cavity and a secure surgical closure of the abdominal wall achieved primarily in many instances. Some authors report that mechanical stretching of the abdominal wall aids in successful primary closure. For others, particularly those infants whose intestine has become thickened and edematous, the construction of an extraabdominal compartment from silastic sheeting has proved beneficial (Fig. 39-29). As in the surgical correction of omphalocele, this allows gradual enlargement of the abdominal cavity as the intestines are accommodated and the silastic compartment gradually reduced. The latter process takes approximately 2 weeks and must be carried out carefully to assure that increased abdominal pressure does not cause caval compression that may impede venous return to the heart or diaphragmatic pressure preventing normal respiratory excursion. Intestinal function may not return for several weeks, and is especially delayed in shaggy edematous bowel. In these babies the advent of intravenous alimentation has been lifesaving. Although the condition was once uniformly fatal, gastroschisis patients can now usually be saved.

Fig. 39-30. Newborn with gastroschisis. The intestine has escaped through a defect just to the right of the umbilicus. The intestine is edematous and matted, indicating that these loops have been floating freely in the amnion for some time.

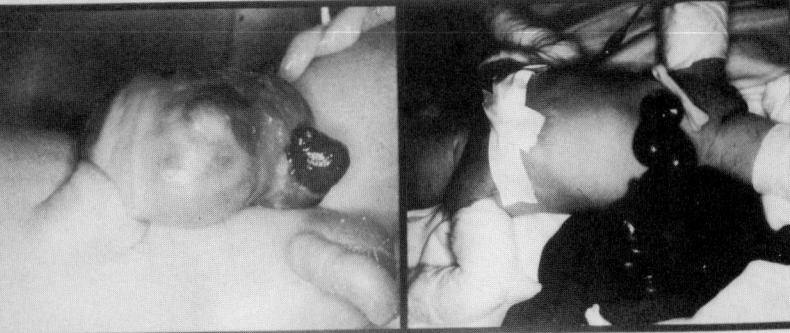

Gastroschisis
(Gr. Gaster·stomach, Schisis·split)

- A misnamed entity
- Originally misconstrued as a ruptured omphalocele
- Embryogenesis uncertain — possibly fetal accident involving hernia of the cord

Exstrophy of the Cloaca (Vesicointestinal Fissure)

Exstrophy of the cloaca represents one of the severest forms of embryologic derangement. In infants with cloacal exstrophy, the normal ventral closure of the pelvis and the wall is imperfect. Major components of the cloacal exstrophy are (1) omphalocele, (2) exstrophy of the bladder, (3) external intestinal fistula through the bladder (omphalomesenteric duct), (4) epispadias in the males, (5) imperforate anus, and (6) foreshortened colon. In addition there is often an associated orthopedic deformity of the distal leg and foot. The summation of these physical defects is such that many of the newborns are not hardy enough to survive.

Early surgical intervention in these patients becomes necessary when extensive intestinal prolapse through the fistula causes intestinal obstruction. In such circumstances an ileostomy is required. The colon is temporarily exteriorized as a mucous fistula. The omphalocele is closed primarily or treated with a topical agent that promotes epithelialization. There is no urgency about repairing the exstrophied bladder, and reconstruction of the urinary system need not be completed until the patient is two or three years of age. While most patients suffer a number of physical limitations, many have the potential for functional rehabilitation, which justifies aggressive surgical efforts on their behalf.

Congenital Deficiency of the Abdominal Musculature (Eagle-Barrett Syndrome; Prune-Belly Syndrome)

Congenital deficiency of the abdominal musculature is a rare anomaly occurring in males. In severely affected infants, there is marked wrinkling of the skin of the lower part of the abdomen and little or no muscular substance detectable beneath it (Fig. 39-31). In addition to the absent abdominal muscles, the bladder is large and the ureters are dilated and tortuous. The kidneys may be hypoplastic, but there is usually adequate renal parenchyma.

Aggressive therapy beginning in the newborn phase has led to marked improvement in the survival of these unfortunate children. Temporary urinary diversion with subsequent staged reconstruction of the draining system has given way in the recent past to conservative treatment of the deformed collecting system using long-term antibiotics. The dilated and tortuous ureters manage to convey urine to the bladder without obstruction. The urinary bladders are uniformly oversized in this syndrome, and reduction cystoplasty has proved useful in the rehabilitation of the urinary tract. Various surgical procedures have been devised to tighten the lax abdominal musculature and reduce the redundancy of the abdominal wall. In our

Fig. 39-31. Eagle-Barrett (prune-belly) syndrome. Baby with congenital absence of the abdominal musculature, showing lax, flaccid abdomen. This syndrome occurs in males and is associated with severe malformations of the urinary collecting system.

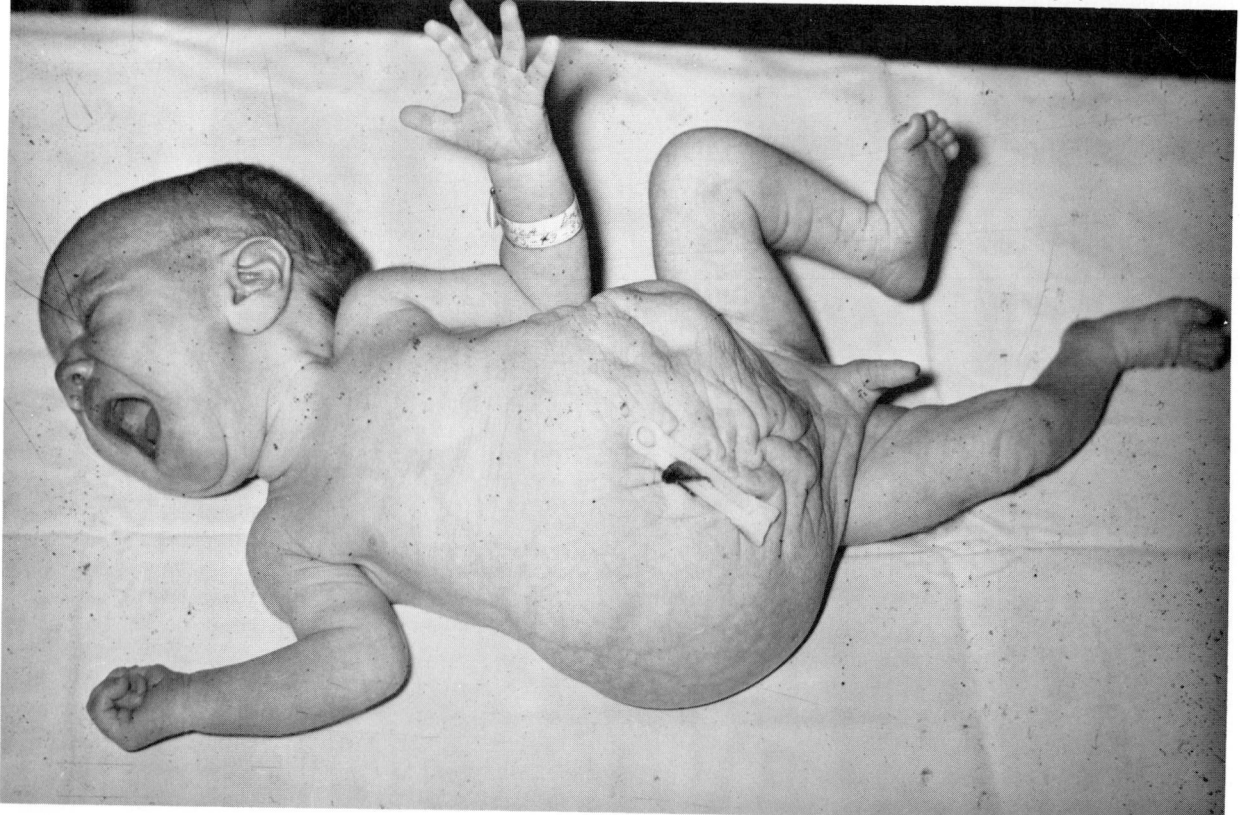

institution, we have employed a large curving transverse incision in the lower abdomen extending into the flanks. This is coupled with excision of the lower most redundant portion of the abdominal wall without sacrificing nerves and arteries supplying the remaining abdominal wall. This form of reconstruction has proved satisfactory in our hands and has produced improved cosmetic and functional results. Eighteen patients treated in this fashion over the past 15 years are currently being followed, and most have a vastly improved abdominal contour. Some older children are even able to partake of light athletic endeavors. Some patients require corsets to support the imperfect abdominal wall; others have needed treatment for scoliosis. The results are considerably different, however, from the dismal outlook these children faced two decades ago.

Inguinal Hernia

Inguinal hernia results from a failure of closure of the processus vaginalis, which is normally obliterated in males by two or three months of age. The processus is a fingerlike projection of the peritoneum that accompanies the testicle as it descends into the scrotum. Infants are at particular risk from incarceration of a hernia. The internal inguinal ring is narrow; therefore, intestine finding its way into the hernial sac in the inguinal canal can become trapped within the hernial sac. When there is diagnostic confusion between an incarcerated hernia and a hydrocele, a rectal examination with simultaneous abdominal palpation of the internal inguinal ring will delineate the structures passing through the internal ring into the inguinal canal. Using the vas deferens as a constant reference point, the presence of intestine adjacent to the vas between the examining fingers confirms the diagnosis of a hernia. Most often the hernia can be reduced. The infant is sedated, and moderate, bimanual pressure is applied by compressing the sac from below while a gentle counterforce downward is provided from the examiner's hand above the inguinal ring. Occasionally, these hernias will reduce spontaneously after sedation is given and the continuous struggling and crying are terminated. Following reduction of the incarcerated hernia, the child is admitted for observation and herniorrhaphy is performed within the next 24 to 48 h. If the hernia cannot be reduced or if intestinal obstruction is obvious, emergency operation, with reduction and repair, is necessary.

When the diagnosis of inguinal hernia is made in an otherwise normal child, operative repair should be planned since spontaneous resolution does not occur. Because of the frequency of bilateral hernias, contralateral groin exploration has been the subject of controversy over the years. In a very sensible approach, Rowe states, "After reviewing our own experience and that in the literature, we (now) explore the contralateral groin in all male infants under a year of age, girls at all ages, and infants and children who have excess peritoneal fluid as a result of ventriculoperitoneal shunts, peritoneal dialysis, or ascites."

An inguinal hernia in the female usually is indicated by the appearance of a nontender groin mass. The mass represents an ovary herniated into the patent sac. Although the gonad can usually be reduced into the abdomen by gentle pressure, it often prolapses in and out until surgical repair is carried out. In some patients the ovary and fallopian tube constitute one wall of the hernial sac (sliding hernia), and in these cases the ovary can be effectively reduced only at the time of operation.

Hydrocele is often associated with an inguinal hernia. The hydrocele may communicate with the peritoneal cavity via the patent processus vaginalis and therefore wax and wane in size. This is particularly noteworthy once children are upright; the hydrocele gains in size during the day and diminishes during sleep. Alternatively, the hydrocele may be persistent and confined to the scrotum or to the inguinal canal. It is not unusual for a hydrocele of the cord to be misdiagnosed as incarcerated hernia. In such circumstances one can usually differentiate the hydrocele of the cord from an inguinal hernia by using bimanual technique with concomitant rectal exam and abdominal examination at the inguinal ring. A simple hydrocele does not require prompt operation until it can be shown after months of observation that the hydrocele is persistent. Aspiration of a hydrocele is not effective, can be dangerous, and is not recommended.

GENITALIA

Cryptorchidism

The term "undescended testicle" describes that testicle which has been interrupted in its normal route of descent into the scrotum. Such a testicle may reside in the posterior abdomen, in the internal inguinal ring, in the inguinal canal, or even at the external ring, but is never in the scrotum. The testicle begins as a thickening on the urogenital ridge in the fifth to sixth week of embryologic life. In the seventh and eighth months the testicle descends along the inguinal canal into the upper scrotum, and with its progress the processus vaginalis is formed and pulled along with the migrating testicle. At birth approximately 95 percent of infants have the testicle normally positioned in the scrotum. The etiology of the testicle's failure to descend is unknown.

A distinction should be made between the undescended testicle and the ectopic testicle. An ectopic testis by definition is one that has passed through the external ring in the normal pathway and then has come to rest in an abnormal location either overlying the rectus abdominus or external oblique muscle, or the soft tissue of the medial thigh, or behind the scrotum in the perineum. A congenitally absent testicle results from failure of normal development or an intrauterine accident leading to loss of blood supply in the developing testicle.

CLINICAL MANIFESTATIONS. In most patients with a unilateral undescended testicle the testicle can be felt in the inguinal canal or in the upper scrotum. Occasionally, the testicle will be difficult or impossible to palpate, indicating either an abdominal testicle or congenital absence of the gonad. In patients with bilateral undescended testicles, it is appropriate to study the serum gonadotropin since the serum luteinizing hormone is elevated in patients without gonadal tissue.

Reasons for surgical placement of the testicle in the scrotum are (1) diminished spermatogenesis, (2) malignant degeneration, (3) increased trauma (to a testicle located at the pubic tubercle), (4) increased incidence of torsion, and (5) psychologic. The reason for malignant degeneration is not established, but the evidence points to an inherent abnormality of the testicle that predisposes it to incomplete descent and malignancy rather than a malignancy by an abnormal environment.

It appears that the male with bilateral undescended testicles is infertile. It is also suggested by most authors that the influence of the body temperature is significant in diminishing spermatogenesis. Mengel and coworkers studied 515 undescended testicles by histology and demonstrated a decreasing presence of spermatogonia after two years of age. Consequently it is now recommended that the undescended testicle be surgically repositioned by two years of age.

TREATMENT. Chorionic Gonadotropin. The use of chorionic gonadotropin has been occasionally effective in patients with bilateral undescended testes, suggesting that these patients are more apt to have a hormone insufficiency than children with unilateral undescended testicle. If there is no testicular descent after a month of endocrine therapy, operative correction should be undertaken.

Some patients who have an absent testis are greatly bothered by this anatomical deficiency. Gel-filled prostheses of all sizes are now available and can be simply inserted into the scrotum achieving normal appearance and a normal structure for palpation. Any patient who has an undescended testicle corrected surgically should be examined yearly by his surgeon until his midteen years. At that time the individual should undergo thorough explanation about the possibility of malignant degeneration and be instructed in self-examination, which should be carried out at least twice a year for life.

Ambiguous Genitalia (Intersex Syndromes)

Normal sexual differentiation occurs in the sixth fetal week. The testis-determining gene is probably located on the Y chromosome. In the recent past the HY antigen has been identified as a possible testis-determining factor. In every fetus, wolffian (male) and müllerian (female) ducts are present until the onset of sexual differentiation. The development of internal ducts into the male apparatus or the female anatomy is directed entirely by the fetal testis, which secretes both testosterone and müllerian inhibiting substance (Jost principle). Testosterone stimulates maturation of wolffian duct structures into epididymis, vas deferens, and seminal vesicles; simultaneously, the müllerian inhibiting substance produces regression of the female structures. In the absence of the fetal testis, the müllerian-inhibiting substance is not secreted and therefore the müllerian system proceeds to full maturation of female anatomy. Any disruption of the orderly steps in sexual differentiation may be reflected clinically as variants of the intersex syndromes. These may be classified as (1) true hermaphroditism (with ovarian and testicular gonadal tissue), (2) male pseudohermaphroditism (testicles only), (3) female pseudohermaphroditism (ovarian tissue only), and (4) mixed gonadal dysgenesis (usually undeveloped or imperfectly formed gonads). Most of these clinical forms present with ambiguous external genitalia, which may or may not be obvious at birth (Fig. 39-32).

Male pseudohermaphroditism is found in genotypic males with bilateral testes; however, the duct structures of many of these patients differentiate partly as phenotypic females. This group of disorders can result from defects in androsynthesis or incomplete müllerian regression. Female pseudohermaphroditism is most commonly found in those patients with congenital adrenal hyperplasia. These individuals are unable to synthesize cortisol; this deficiency causes ACTH to stimulate the secretion of excessive quantities of adrenal androgen which masculinizes the developing female. The rarest intersex form, that of the true hermaphrodite, is usually found with XX karyotype. These children have ambiguous genitalia and their gonad pattern may show an ovary and a testicle, or an ovotestis.

In the differential diagnosis of patients with intersexual anomalies, the following diagnostic steps are necessary: (1) evaluation of the genetic background and family history; (2) determination of biochemical factors in serum and urine; (3) assessment of the anatomical structures by physical examination and x-ray studies; (4) chromosome studies; and (5) when necessary, laparotomy and gonadal biopsy.

With refined diagnostic techniques, most infants with intersexual abnormalities can be accurately assessed in the first days of life, obviating errors in gender assignment. Subsequently, certain plastic surgical procedures are required to harmonize the external genitalia with the sex of rearing. Operations to reduce the size of the enlarged clitoris have been developed that spare the sensation and function of the clitoris. Plastic procedures to exteriorize the vagina or separate it from the urethra are necessary in patients born with a urogenital sinus. When the male assignment is appropriate for an infant with an ambiguous genitalia, hypospadius repair will be necessary. When contradictory gonads or ovotestes are present, removal of these structures is required to prevent the possibility of hormone secretion or malignant degeneration. For psychologic adjustment of some teenage male patients with inadequate or absent gonads, the insertion of a testicular prostheses may prove beneficial. Children with endocrine deficiency may require lifetime exogenous supplementation. Prompt recognition of infants with intersexual anomalies, followed by appropriate sex assignment and proper treatment, prevents the social and psychologic derangements that have occurred in the past because of delayed diagnosis or inappropriate gender assignment.

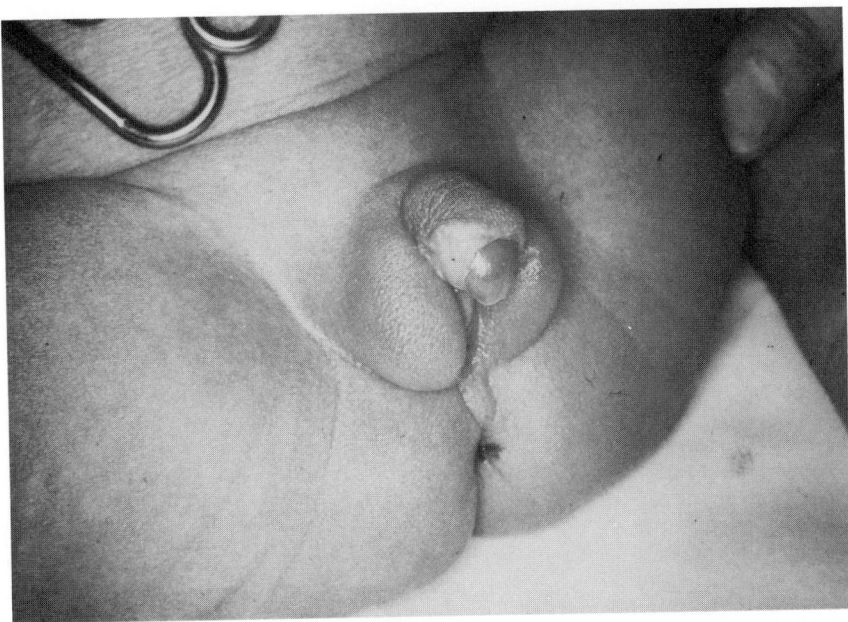

Fig. 39-32. Ambiguous genitalia, manifest as enlarged clitoris and labioscrotal folds in a baby with the adrenogenital syndrome. This configuration can be confused with a normal penis and undescended testicles.

NEOPLASTIC DISEASE

Cancer is the second leading cause of death in children one to fourteen years of age. Approximately 11 percent of the deaths of children in the United States are due to malignant diseases (Fig. 39-33). In the past 20 years there has been a marked increase in the survival of patients with childhood cancer. This improvement can be attributed to better diagnostic imaging techniques, new chemotherapy agents, collaborative approaches to surgery, chemotherapy, and radiation therapy, and multi-institutional studies evaluating new treatments and protocols. This unified approach to diagnosis, staging, and therapy has proved useful in the management of the more common pediatric solid malignancies, such as Wilms' tumor, hepatic tumor, rhabdomyosarcoma, neuroblastoma, and teratoma.

Wilms' Tumor

Approximately five hundred new cases of Wilms' tumors are diagnosed in the United States each year. Wilms' tumor is an embryonal neoplasm of the kidney and usually presents as an asymptomatic mass in the flank or upper abdomen. The peak age of incidence is between 1 and 3. This tumor has been associated with congenital anomalies such as aniridia, the Beckwith-Wiedemann syndrome, urinary tract defects, hemihypertrophy, and chromosomal deletion, suggesting a possible hereditary influence.

Prior to operation, all patients suspected of Wilms' tumor should be evaluated radiographically. The CT scan and ultrasound have supplanted the intravenous pyelo-

gram as mainstays of the work-up. The CT scan will usually show a large intrarenal mass (Fig. 39-34). Further, the scan has provided important preoperative data such as the status of the contralateral kidney and the presence of local or distant spread. The ultrasound provides comple-

Fig. 39-33. Most common sites of cancer in children.

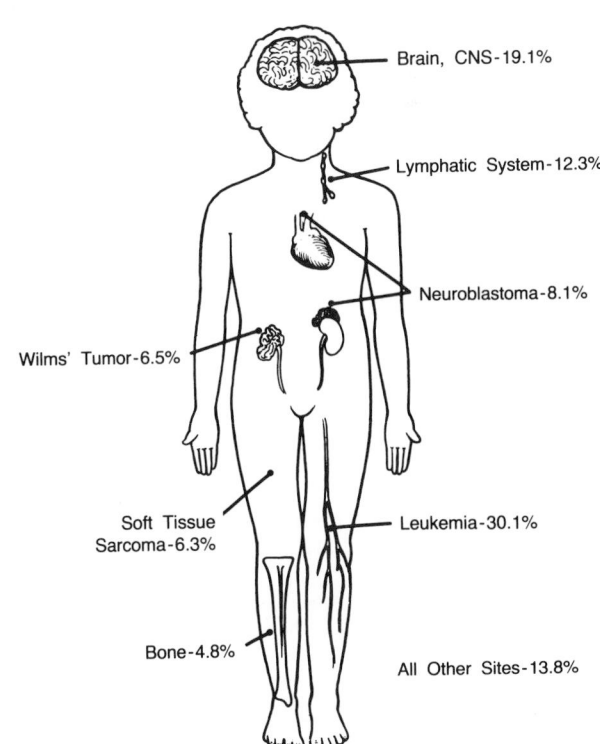

Brain, CNS-19.1%

Lymphatic System-12.3%

Neuroblastoma-8.1%

Wilms' Tumor-6.5%

Leukemia-30.1%

Soft Tissue Sarcoma-6.3%

Bone-4.8%

All Other Sites-13.8%

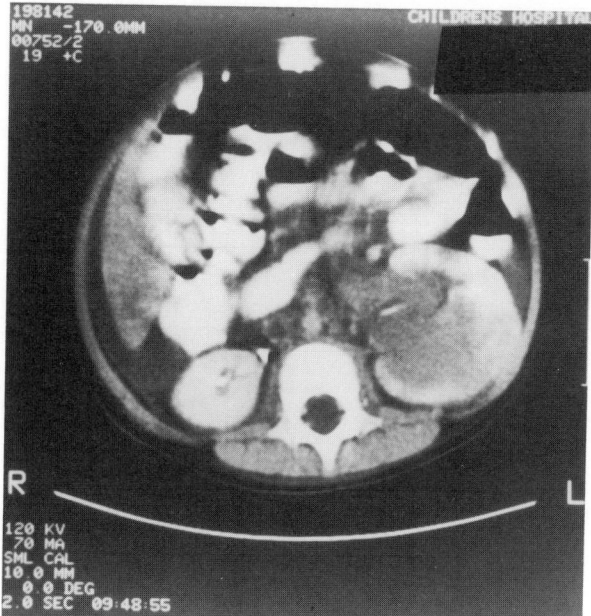

Fig. 39-34. CT scan from a patient with Wilms' tumor. Note the mass and distortion of the left kidney.

mentary information on involvement of the renal vein or vena cava.

The key to staging and treatment is surgical intervention. A generous transabdominal transverse incision is used to assure adequate exposure for removing the primary tumor, to evaluate the opposite kidney, and to inspect the rest of the abdomen. Whenever possible the renal vein should be clamped before the tumor is mobilized to prevent tumor emobilization. If there has been contiguous spread of the tumor into adjacent organs, the operation may be expanded to include part of the liver, spleen, diaphragm, pancreas, or stomach.

Following operative removal of a Wilms' tumor the need for chemotherapy and/or radiation therapy is determined by the histology of the tumor and the clinical stage of the patient (see Table 39-1). Patients with disease confined to one kidney, totally removed by surgery, receive only chemotherapy and can expect a 95 percent 2-year survival (2 years survival is tantamount to cure). Patients with tumor showing unfavorable histology or having a Stage II, III, or IV will receive a combination chemotherapy and often radiation therapy. Even in Stage IV, cure rates of 60 percent are being achieved. The survival rates are less favorable in the small percentage of patients considered to have unfavorable histology. Actinomycin-D and vincristine are the major chemotherapeutic agents used and Adriamycin is employed in advanced stages. Despite the enormous contribution of chemotherapy and radiation to improve survival, surgical excision remains the primary treatment.

Neuroblastoma

Neuroblastoma is the third most common pediatric malignancy, occurring in 9 children per million each year. Neuroblastomas arise from the neural crest cells and show different levels of differentiation. The tumor originates most frequently in the adrenal glands, posterior mediastinum, neck, or pelvis but can arise in any sympathetic ganglion. The clinical presentation is dependent on the site of the primary and the presence of metastasis. Ninety percent of patients present prior to nine years of age and 40 percent are less than two years old.

Two-thirds of these tumors are first noted as an asymptomatic abdominal mass. The tumor may cross the midline, and a majority of patients will already show signs of metastasis. The patient should be evaluated by CT scan and ultrasound, which usually show displacement of an intact kidney. Since these tumors derive from the sympathetic nervous system, catecholamines and their metabolites will be produced at increased levels and their measurement in serum and urine aid in the diagnosis and in monitoring adequacy of future treatment and recurrence.

Though CT scan, bone marrow biopsy, and radionuclide scans are important adjuncts to preoperative staging, surgical evaluation and excision when possible are essential. The main hope of cure is to resect the tumor completely, because chemotherapy and radiation therapy have not altered survival significantly in the last 20 years. Abdominal tumors are approached through a transverse incision, and every attempt is made to resect the tumor completely. Thoracic tumors may be approached through a posterolateral thoracotomy and often have an intraspinal component necessitating laminectomy and intraspinal removal. Staging can help predict survival and is useful in stratifying patients for treatment protocols (see Table 39-2).

Owing to variability in sites and in biologic behavior, the treatment of neuroblastoma must be individualized. Favorable survival may be realized even when there is metastatic spread to bone marrow, liver, or skin (Stage

Table 39-1. WILMS' TUMOR STAGING*

I Tumor limited to kidney and completely excised
II Tumor extends beyond kidney and is completely excised
III Residual tumor confined to the abdomen, nonhematogenous
IV Distant metastases
V Bilateral renal involvement

* Histologic type should be noted but does not change stage.
SOURCE: From National Wilms' Tumor Study Group.

Table 39-2. NEUROBLASTOMA-STAGING SYSTEM

I Tumor confined to structure of origin
II Tumor extends beyond structure of origin but not across midline
III Tumor extends contiguously across midline
IV Distant metastatic disease
IVs Patients who would otherwise be Stage I or II but have remote disease confined to one or more of these sites: liver, bone marrow, or skin

SOURCE: Adapted from Evans AE et al: *Cancer* 27:374, 1971, with permission.

Table 39-3. STAGING SYSTEM BY CLINICAL GROUP FOR RHABDOMYOSARCOMA*

Table 39-3. STAGING SYSTEM BY CLINICAL GROUP FOR RHABDOMYOSARCOMA*

I Localized disease, complete resected, no involved lymph nodes
II Localized or regional disease with total gross resection, lymph nodes may be involved
III Incomplete resection or biopsy with residual unresected disease
IV Distant metastatic disease at diagnosis

* Adapted from Intergroup Rhabdomyosarcoma study.
SOURCE: From Hays DM et al: *Curr Probl Surg* 23(3), 1986, with permission.

Table 39-4. INCIDENCE OF TERATOMA BY LOCATION

Head and neck	5.5%
Mediastinal	4%
Retroperitoneal and abdominal	5%
Sacrococcygeal	40%
Ovary	37%
Testicle	3%
Brain/spinal cord	3.5%
Other	2%

SOURCE: Adapted from Tapper D et al: *Ann Surg* 198:398, 1983, with permission.

IVs in infants). Over 85 percent of these patients if less than one year old will be completely and spontaneously cured. The spontaneous regression of tumor seen in many of these patients has led to much investigation of immunotherapy as a possible therapeutic tool. Though cure rates of greater than 80 percent have been achieved in Stages I and II, the poor survival in the higher stages is discouraging, which calls for new therapies and further research.

Rhabdomyosarcoma

Rhabdomyosarcoma is an embryonic tumor that can arise from a variety of mesenchymal tissues. The head and neck, extremities, and genitourinary tract are the most common sites of origin, although the tumor can arise virtually anywhere. The clinical presentation of the tumor is dependent on the site of origin. The diagnosis is confirmed by incisional or excisional biopsy after evaluation by radionuclide scans, CT scans of the chest, and bone marrow biopsy. The tumor grows locally into all surrounding structures and metastasizes widely to lung, regional lymph nodes, liver, brain, and bone marrow. The staging system for rhabdomyosarcoma is shown in Table 39-3.

Wide local excision with adequate margins is the optimal surgical treatment for localized forms of rhabdomyosarcoma. The potential mutilation of radical amputations or exenteration may be avoided because of progress with the use of chemotherapy and radiation therapy in the last two decades. The standard chemotherapy used is a combination of actinomycin-D, vincristine sulfate, and cyclophosphamide. The major determinants of outcome are the site of origin and the pathologic type. The prognosis in patients with embryonal pathology is much more favorable than alveolar histology. Three-year survival rates show an 86 percent survival in clinical group I, a 75 percent survival in clinical group II, a 66 percent survival in clinical group III, and a 33 percent survival in clinical group IV.

Teratoma

Teratomas are tumors comprised of tissue from all three embryonic germ layers. They may be benign or malignant, may arise in any part of the body, and are usually found in midline structures. Thoracic teratomas usually present as an anterior mediastinal mass. Ovarian teratomas present as an abdominal mass often with symptoms of torsion, bleeding, or rupture. Retroperitoneal teratomas may present as a flank or abdominal mass. The location incidence of teratomas in children is seen in Table 39-4. The goal of therapy is complete surgical excision because the success of chemotherapy and/or radiation therapy as seen in other pediatric tumors has not been realized in this group of tumors.

Sacrococcygeal Teratoma

Sacrococcygeal teratoma usually presents as a large mass extending from the sacrum in the newborn period. Many tumors have been diagnosed prenatally by ultrasound. The mass may be as small as a few centimeters in diameter or as massive as the size of the infant (Fig. 39-35). There is a form of tumor that does not present externally but grows in the presacral space. The differential diagnosis consists of neural tumors, lipoma, and myelomeningoceles.

Most of these tumors are benign, but with advancing age the potential for malignant degeneration is high. Complete resection of the tumor as early as possible is essential. The rectum and genital structures are often distorted by the tumor but can usually be preserved in the course of resection. The cure rate is excellent if the tumor is completely excised. With discovery of the tumor in older infants and children, the results are poor because of the high incidence of malignant degeneration.

Liver Tumors

More than two-thirds of all liver tumors in children are malignant. Hepatoblastoma is the most common malignancy of the liver in children, with 65 percent of these tumors diagnosed before two years of age. Hepatocellular carcinoma is the next most common lesion, with a peak age incidence between ten and fifteen years. Malignant mesenchymomas and sarcomas are much less common but constitute the remainder of the malignancies. Regardless of the tumor type, most children present with an abdominal mass that may be painful if a hepatocellular carcinoma but is painless if caused by another tumor.

The patients are rarely jaundiced but may complain of anorexia and weight loss. Most liver function tests are normal. Alphafetoprotein levels are elevated in 90 per-

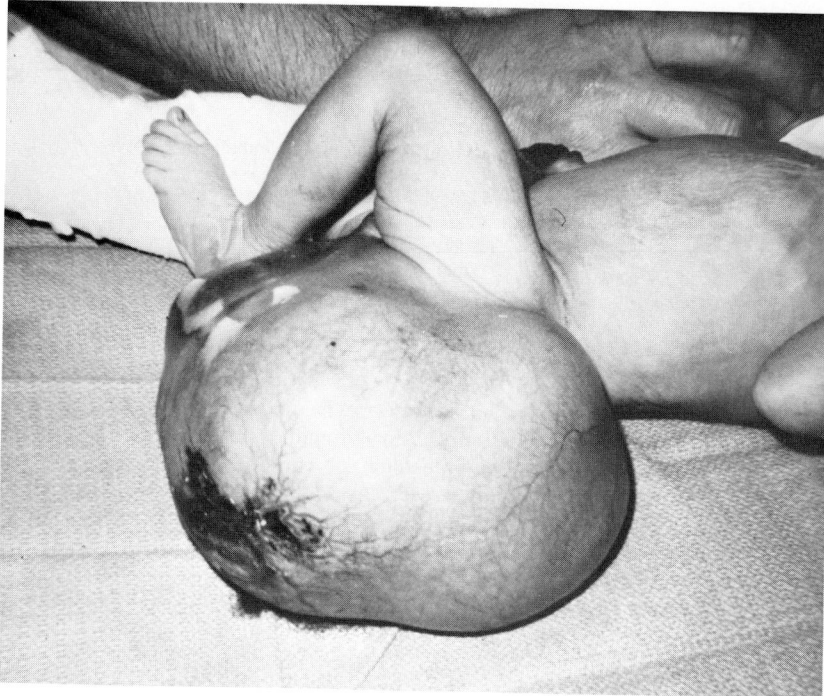

Fig. 39-35. Newborn with huge sacrococcygeal teratoma.

cent of children with hepatoblastomas but are increased much less commonly in other liver malignancies. Radiographic evaluation of these children should include a flat-plate abdominal radiograph, an ultrasound study, and a contrast-enhanced abdominal CT scan. Use of the liver-spleen scan is restricted to patients suspected of having a benign lesion that may pick up the radionuclide. Preoperative angiography is utilized in those patients in whom a major hepatic resection is contemplated and delineation of the hepatic vascular anatomy is desired.

Complete surgical extirpation of the tumor is essential for cure. Recent attempts to reduce the bulk of massive

Fig. 39-36. Operative photograph of hepatoblastoma in the right lobe of the liver in an eight-month-old child. Extended right hepatic lobectomy was curative.

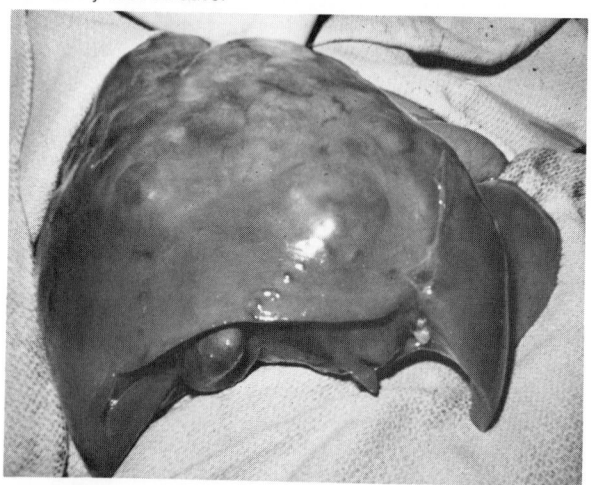

tumors by pretreatment with chemotherapy have met with limited success. The value of radiotherapy is also limited. Hepatic transplantation for unresectable primary lesions has been disappointing, with a high incidence of carcinomatosis and death. For hepatoblastoma, about half the patients have completely resectable lesions (Fig. 39-36) and about 80 percent of these can be cured with adjunct chemotherapy. Of all patients with hepatoblastomas, only about 30 percent are long-term survivors. Patients with hepatocellular carcinoma have a worse prognosis because fewer can be completely resected. The cure rate for all children with hepatocellular carcinomas is only 15 percent.

TRAUMA

The National Safety Council documents that 10 percent of individuals who die of accidental death are children below the age of fourteen. Accidents account for 46 percent of all pediatric deaths, more than cancer, congenital anomalies, pneumonia, heart disease, homicide, and meningitis combined. Motor vehicle accident is the most common cause of accidental death (20 percent) in children; drowning (8 percent), burns (5 percent), and firearms (1 percent) account for a significant segment of the remaining group. Not evident in the mortality statistics is the number of children who sustain injury and recover with a subsequent disability. In any given year, approximately 22 million children require the assistance of a physician as a consequence of accidents. Improved methods of communication, immediate prehospital care, and rapid transportation to regional centers increase the probability of survival following a major traumatic injury. Because of the complex requirements for resuscitation and treatment of the injured child, it is essential that each regional referral center establish a systematic approach to care of the young accident victim. Personnel trained in pediatric trauma are needed to plan, implement, and manage the injured child. Integration of the multidisciplinary human and material resources of each designated hospital is essential.

Management of the pediatric trauma patient requires immediate recognition and treatment of life-threatening injuries to the head, thorax, and abdomen. Recognition that the child with severe head injury manifests a different physiologic response from that of the adult forms the foundation for successful therapy. Aggressive therapy of elevated intracranial pressure results in improved survival; 9 percent of the childhood victims of serious head trauma die, 88 percent make a good-to-excellent recovery. Thoracic trauma occurs in a third to half of all children sustaining multiple trauma. Blunt abdominal trauma is common in the pediatric population; the spleen and liver are the most frequent intraabdominal organs sustaining injury. Nonoperative management is a reasonable approach in the child with blunt hepatic or splenic trauma with stable vital signs. Exploratory laparotomy is indicated for a physiologically unstable child despite appropriate fluid resuscitation. These children should undergo laparotomy for hemostasis, and an attempt at splenic salvage is warranted by splenorrhaphy if the child's condition permits.

Consideration of the unique requirements of the injured child during evaluation and therapy improves outcome and minimizes mortality. Aerophagia proceeding to gastric dilatation can compromise respiration or mimic an abdominal injury; therefore, nasogastric decompression is mandatory in all children with significant injury. The temperature of injured children must be monitored carefully because of the relatively large surface area to body mass ratio. Hypothermia potentiates the deleterious effects of shock. Hypovolemic shock with cellular hypoperfusion is treated with crystalloid infusion at a rate of 20 mL/kg, I.V. push. Urine output (1 mL/kg/h) in children should be maintained. Once initial assessment and resuscitation have been accomplished, diagnostic measures with conventional x-rays and CT scan may be important. Prompt movement to a pediatric intensive care unit is essential unless a decision for operation is necessary. Complete rehabilitation of the child and the family should be the ultimate goal of every pediatric trauma center.

Bibliography

General Considerations

Adamsons K Jr, Towell ME: Thermal homeostasis in the fetus and newborn. *Anesthesiology* 26:531, 1965.

Altman RP, Randolph JG: The applications and hazards of total parenteral nutrition in infants. *Ann Surg* 174:85, 1971.

Benner JW, Coran AG, et al: The importance of different calorie sources in the intravenous nutrition of infants and children. *Surgery* 86:429, 1979.

Coran AG: The long-term total intravenous feedings of infants using peripheral vein. *J Pediatr Surg* 8:801, 1973.

Coran AG: Parenteral nutrition in infants and children. *Surg Clin North Am* 61:1089, 1981.

Coran AG, Nesbakken R: The metabolism of intravenously administered fat in adult and newborn dogs. *Surgery* 66:922, 1969.

Filler FM, Eraklis AJ, et al: Long term parenteral nutrition in infants. *N Engl J Med* 281:589, 1969.

Goudsouzian NG, Morris RH, et al: The effect of a warming blanket on the maintenance of body temperature in anesthetized infants and children. *Anesthesiology* 39:351, 1973.

Groff DB: Complications of intravenous hyperalimentation in newborns and infants. *J Pediatr Surg* 4:460, 1969.

Karpel JT, Peden VH: Copper deficiency in long-term parenteral nutrition. *J Pediatr* 80:32, 1972.

Knutrud O: *The Water and Electrolyte Metabolism in the Newborn Child after Major Surgery.* Norwegian Monographs on Medical Science, Oslo, Scandinavian University Books, Universitets Forlaget, 1965.

Roe CF, Santulli TV, et al: Heat loss in infants during general anesthesia and operations. *J Pediatr Surg* 1:266, 1966.

Rowe MI, Lankau C, et al: Evaluation of methods to clinically monitor colloid oncotic pressure in the pediatric surgical patient. *Surg Gynecol Obstet* 139:889, 1974.

Wilmore DW, Dudrick SJ: Growth and development of an infant receiving all nutrients exclusively by vein. *JAMA* 203:860, 1968.

Lesions of Neck

Bill AH Jr, Sumner DS: Unified concept of lymphangioma and cystic hygroma. *Surg Gynecol Obstet* 120:79, 1965.

Bill AH Jr, Vadheim JL: Cysts, sinuses, and fistulas of the neck arising from the first and second brachial clefts. *Ann Surg* 142:904, 1955.

Brown PM, Judd ES: Thyroglossal cysts and sinuses: Results of radical (sistrunk) operation. *Am J Surg* 102:494, 1961.

Gross RE, Connerly ML: Thyroglossal cysts and sinuses. *N Engl J Med* 223:616, 1940.

Randolph JG: On the treatment of lymphangioma in children. *Surgery* 49:289, 1961.

Sistrunk WE: The surgical treatment of cysts of thyroglossal tract. *Ann Surg* 71:121, 1920.

Respiratory System

Adzick NS, Harrison MR, et al: Diaphragmatic hernia in the fetus: Prenatal diagnosis and outcome in 94 cases. *J Pediatr Surg* 20:357, 1985.

Bartlett RH, Andrews AF, et al: Extracorporeal membrane oxygenation for newborn respiratory failure: Forty-five cases. *Surgery* 9:425, 1982.

Bartlett RH, Gazzanig AB, et al: Extracorporeal circulation (ECMO) in neonatal respiratory failure. *J Thorac Cardiovasc Surg* 74:826, 1977.

Boix-Ochoa J, Peguro G, et al: Acid-base balance and blood gases in prognosis and therapy of congenital diaphragmatic hernia. *J Pediatr Surg* 9:49, 1974.

Boles ET, Schiller M, et al: Improved management of neonates with congenital diaphragmatic hernia. *Arch Surg* 103:344, 1971.

Collins DL, Pomerance JJ, et al: A new approach to congenital diaphragmatic hernia. *J Pediatr Surg* 12:149, 1977.

de Lorimier AA: Congenital malformations and neonatal problems of the respiratory tract, in Welch KJ, Randolph JG, Ravitch MM, O'Neill JA Jr, Rowe MI (eds): *Pediatric Surgery*. Chicago, Year Book Medical Publishers, 1986, pp. 639–640.

Ganitano ES, Pomerance JJ, et al: Successful surgical repair of iatrogenic lung perforation in the neonate. *J Pediatr Surg* 16:70, 1981.

Gans SL, Berci G: Advances in endoscopy of infants and children. *J Pediatr Surg* 6:199, 1971.

Grosfeld JL, Lemons JL, et al: Emergency thoracotomy for acquired bronchopleural fistula in the premature infant with respiratory distress. *J Pediatr Surg* 15:416, 1980.

Hall RT, Rhodes PG: Pneumothorax and pneumomediastinum in infants with idiopathic respiratory distress syndrome receiving continuous positive airway pressure. *Pediatrics* 55:493, 1975.

Healy GB, Fearon B, et al: Treatment of subglottic hemangioma with the carbon dioxide laser. *Laryngoscope* 90:809, 1982.

Hendren WH, McKee DM: Lobar emphysema of infancy. *J Pediatr Surg* 1:24, 1966.

Jones JC, Almond CH, et al: Lobar emphysema and congenital heart disease in infancy. *J Thorac Cardiovasc Surg* 49:1, 1965.

Kimura K, Mukohara N, et al: Tracheoplasty for congenital stenosis of the entire trachea. *J Pediatr Surg* 17:869, 1982.

Louhima I, Grahne B, et al: Acquired laryngotracheal stenosis in children. *J Pediatr Surg* 6:730, 1971.

Mattila MAK, Suutarinen T, et al: Prolonged endotracheal intubation or tracheostomy in infants and children. *J Pediatr Surg* 4:674, 1969.

Moodie DS, Telander RL, et al: Use of tolazoline in newborn infants with diaphragmatic hernia and severe cardiopulmonary disease. *J Thorac Cardiovasc Surg* 75:725, 1978.

Nakayama DK, Harrison MR, et al: Reconstructive surgery for obstructing lesions of the intrathoracic trachea in infants and small children. *J Pediatr Surg* 17:854, 1982.

Parkin JL: Laser use in otolaryngology and head and neck surgery, in Dixon JA (ed): *Surgical Application of Lasers*. Chicago, Year Book Medical Publishers, 1983.

Reynolds M, Luck SR, et al: The "critical" neonate with diaphragmatic hernia: A 21 year perspective. *J Pediatr Surg* 19:364, 1984.

Rowe MI, Uribe F: Diaphragmatic hernia in the newborn infant: Blood gas and pH considerations. *Surgery* 70:758, 1971.

Steele R, Metz JR, et al: Pneumothorax and pneumomediastinum in the newborn. *Radiology* 98:629, 1971.

Wilson AJ, Kraus HF: Lung perforation during chest tube placement in the stiff-lung syndrome. *J Pediatr Surg* 9:213, 1979.

Wilson JF, Decker A: The surgical management of childhood bronchiectasis. A review of 96 consecutive pulmonary resections in children with nontuberculous bronchiectasis. *Ann Surg* 195:354, 1982.

Wohl MEG, Grissom NT, et al: The lung following repair of congenital diaphragmatic hernia. *J Pediatr* 90:405, 1977.

Tracheoesophageal Fistula and Esophageal Atresia

Bishop PJ, Kelin MD: Transpleural repair of esophageal atresia without primary gastrostomy. *J Pediatr Surg* 20:823, 1985.

Dudrick SJ, Wilmore DW, et al: Long-term parenteral nutrition with growth, development and positive nitrogen balance. *Surgery* 64:134, 1968.

Fonkalsrud EW: Gastroesophageal fundoplication for reflux following repair of esophageal atresia. *Arch Surg* 114:48, 1979.

Gray SW, Skandalakis JE: *Embryology for Surgeons*. Philadelphia, Saunders, 1972.

Haight C, Towsley HA: Congenital atresia of the esophagus with tracheo-esophageal fistula. Extrapleural ligation of fistula and end-to-end anastomosis of esophageal segments. *Surg Gynecol Obstet* 76:672, 1943.

Holder TM, Cloud DT, et al: Esophageal atresia and tracheo-esophageal fistula. A survey of its members by the surgical section of the American Academy of Pediatrics. *Pediatrics* 34:542, 1960.

Holder TM, McDonald VG Jr, et al: The premature or critically ill infant with esophageal atresia. Increased success with a staged approach. *J Thorac Cardiovasc Surg* 44:344, 1962.

Ladd WE: The surgical treatment of esophageal atresia and tracheo-esophageal fistula. *N Engl J Med* 230:625, 1944.

Leven NL: Congenital atresia of the esophagus with tracheo-esophageal fistula. Report of successful extrapleural ligation of fistulous communication and cervical esophagostomy. *J Thorac Surg* 10:648, 1941.

Livaditis A: Esophageal atresia, a method of overbridging large segmental gaps. *Z Kinderchir* 13:298, 1973.

Louhimo J, Lindehl H: Esophageal atresia: Primary results of 500 consecutive treated patients. *J Pediatr Surg* 18:217, 1983.

Manning P, Coran A, et al: Fifty years' experience with esophageal atresia and tracheoesophageal fistula. *Ann Surg* 204:446, 1986.

Orringer MB, Kirsch MM, et al: Long-term esophageal function following repair of esophageal atresia. *Ann Surg* 186:436, 1977.

Randolph JG, Altman RP, et al: Selective surgical management based upon clinical status in infants with esophageal atresia. *J Thorac Cardiovasc Surg* 74:335, 1977.

Randolph JG, Tunnell WP, et al: Gastric division: A surgical adjunct in selected problems with esophageal anomalies. *J Pediatr Surg* 6:657, 1971.

Waterston DJ, Bonham-Carter RE, et al: Oesophageal atresia: Tracheo-esophageal fistula. A study of survival in 218 infants. *Lancet* 1:819, 1962.

Corrosive Injury of Esophagus

German JC, Waterston DJ: Colon interposition for the replacement of esophagus in children. *J Pediatr Surg* 11:227, 1976.

Haller JA, Andrews HG, et al: Pathophysiology and management of acute corrosive burns of the esophagus: Results of treatment in 285 children. *J Pediatr Surg* 6:578, 1971.

Reyes HM, Lin CY, et al: Experimental treatment of corrosive esophageal burns. *J Pediatr Surg* 9:317, 1974.

Webb WR, Koutras P, et al: An evaluation of steroids and antibiotics in caustic burns of the esophagus. *Ann Thorac Surg* 9:95, 1970.

Weisskopf A: Effects of cortisone on experimental lye burn of the esophagus. *Ann Otol Rhinol Laryngol* 61:681, 1952.

Esophageal Substitution

Anderson KD, Randolph JG: The gastric tube for esophageal replacement in children. *J Thorac Cardiovasc Surg* 66:33, 1973.

Moncrief JA, Randolph JG: Congenital tracheoesophageal fistula without atresia of the esophagus. A method for diagnosis and surgical correction. *J Thorac Cardiovasc Surg* 51:434, 1966.

Sherman CD Jr, Waterston D: Oesophageal reconstruction in children using intrathoracic colon. *Arch Dis Child* 32:11, 1957.

Gastroesophageal Reflux

Ashcraft KW, Goodwin CD, et al: Thal fundoplication: A simple and safe operative treatment for gastroesophageal reflux. *J Pediatr Surg* 13:643, 1978.

Ashcraft KW, Holder TM: The need for fundoplication as indicated by chronic respiratory distress in children. *Surg Rounds* 52:April 1986.

Berenberg W, Neuhauser FBD: Cardioesophageal relaxation (chalasia) as a cause of vomiting in infants. *Pediatrics* 5:414, 1950.

Foglia RP, Fonkalsrud EW, et al: Gastroesophageal fundoplication for the management of chronic pulmonary disease in children. *Am J Surg* 140:72, 1980.

Fonkalsrud EW: Gastroesophageal fundoplication for reflux following repair of esophageal atresia. *Arch Surg* 114:48, 1979.

Fonkalsrud EW, Ament ME, et al: Surgical management of the gastroesophageal reflux syndrome in childhood. *Surgery* 97:42, 1985.

Jolley SG, Johnson DG, et al: An assessment of gastroesophageal reflux in children by extended pH monitoring of the distal esophagus. *Surgery* 84:16, 1978.

Lilly JR, Randolph JG: Hiatal hernia and gastroesophageal reflux in infants and children. *J Thorac Cardiovasc Surg* 55:42, 1968.

Meyers WG, Roberts CC, et al: Value of tests for evaluation of gastroesophageal reflux in children. *J Pediatr Surg* 20:515, 1985.

O'Neill JA, Betts J, et al: Surgical management of reflux strictures of the esophagus in childhood. *Ann Surg* 196:453, 1982.

Orenstein SR, Whitington PF, et al: The infant seat as treatment for gastroesophageal reflux. *N Engl J Med* 309:760, 1983.

Ramenofsky MC, Powell RW, et al: Gastroesophageal reflux: pH probe-directed therapy. *Ann Surg* 203:531, 1986.

Randolph J: Experience with the Nissen fundoplication for correction of gastroesophageal reflux in infants. *Ann Surg* 198:579, 1983.

Wesley JR, Coran AG, et al: The need for evaluation of gastroesophageal reflux in brain-damaged children referred for feeding gastrostomy. *J Pediatr Surg* 16:866, 1981.

Gastrointestinal Conditions

Anderson DH: Cystic fibrosis of the pancreas and its relation to celiac disease: A clinical and pathologic study. *Am J Dis Child* 56:344, 1938.

Andrassy RJ, Mahaur GH: Malrotation of the midgut in infants and children. *Arch Surg* 116:158, 1981.

Berezim S, Schwartz SM, et al: Gastroesophageal reflux secondary to gastrostomy tube placement. *Am J Dis Child* 140:699, 1986.

Bergquist TH, Nolan NG, et al: Specificity of ^{99m}Tc-pertechnetate in scintigraphic diagnosis of Meckel's diverticulum. Review of 100 cases. *J Nucl Med* 17:465, 1976.

DeLorimier AA, Fonkalsrud EW, et al: Congenital atresia and stenosis of the jejunum and ileum. *Surgery* 65:819, 1969.

Filston HC, Kirks DR: Malrotation—the ubiquitous anomaly. *J Pediatr Surg* 16 N4(suppl 1):614, 1981.

Firor HV: The many faces of Meckel's diverticulum. *South Med J* 73:1507, 1980.

Grosfeld JL, O'Neill JA Jr, et al: Enteric duplications in infancy and childhood. *Ann Surg* 172:83, 1970.

Gross RE, Chisolm TC: Annular pancreas producing duodenal obstruction. *Am Surg* 119:759, 1944.

Haymond HE, Dragstedt LR: Anomalies of intestinal rotation. *Surg Gynecol Obstet* 53:316, 1931.

Jackson JM: Annular pancreas and duodenal obstruction in the neonate, a review. *Arch Surg* 87:379, 1963.

Kiesewetter WB, Smith JW: Malrotation of the midgut in infancy and childhood. *Arch Surg* 77:483, 1958.

Leonidas JC, Berdon WE, et al: Meconium ileus and its complications: A reappraisal of plain film roentgen diagnosis criteria. *Am J Roentgenol Radium Ther Nucl Med* 108:598, 1970.

Louw JH: Jejunoileal atresia and stenosis. *J Pediatr Surg* 1:8, 1966.

Martin LW, Zerella JT: Jejunoileal atresia: A proposed classification. *J Pediatr Surg* 11:399, 1976.

Nixon HH, Tawes R: Etiology and treatment of small intestinal atresia: Analysis of a series of 127 jejunoileal atresias and comparison with 62 duodenal atresias. *Surgery* 69:41, 1971.

Noblett HR: Treatment of uncomplicated meconium ileus by Gastrografin enema: A preliminary report. *J Pediatr Surg* 4:190, 1969.

Rowe MI, Furst AJ, et al: The neonatal response to Gastrografin enema. *Pediatrics* 48:29, 1971.

Santulli TV, Blanc WA: Congenital atresia of the intestine: Pathogenesis and treatment. *Ann Surg* 154:939, 1961.

Slovis TL, Klein MD, et al: Incomplete rotation of the intestine with a normal cecal position. *Surgery* 87:325, 1980.

Necrotizing Enterocolitis

Bell MJ, Shakelford P, et al: Hypothesis: Neonatal necrotizing enterocolitis is caused by the acquisition of a pathogenic organism by a susceptible host infant. *Surgery* 97:350, 1985.

Buras R, Guzzetta P, et al: Acidosis and hepatic portal venous gas: Indications for surgery in necrotizing enterocolitis. *Pediatrics* 78:273, 1986.

Kosloske AM: Necrotizing enterocolitis in the neonate. *Surg Gynecol Obstet* 148:259, 1979.

Kosloske AM, Burstein J, et al: Intestinal obstruction due to colonic stricture following neonatal necrotizing enterocolitis. *Ann Surg* 192:202, 1980.

Musemeche CA, Kosloske AM, et al: Comparative effects of ischemia, bacteria, and substrate on the pathogenesis of intestinal necrosis. *J Pediatr Surg* 21:536, 1986.

O'Neill JA, Holcomb GE: Surgical experience with neonatal necrotizing enterocolitis (NNE). *Ann Surg* 189:612, 1979.

Ricketts RR: Surgical therapy for necrotizing enterocolitis. *Ann Surg* 200:653, 1984.

Rothstein FC, Halpin TC, et al: Importance of early ileostomy closure to prevent chronic salt and water loss after necrotizing enterocolitis. *Pediatrics* 70:249, 1982.

Weber TR, Lewis JE: The role of second-look laparotomy in necrotizing enterocolitis. *J Pediatr Surg* 21:323, 1986.

Intussusception

Ein S: Leading points in childhood intussusception. *J Pediatr Surg* 11:209, 1976.

Hoy GR, Boles ET Jr, et al: Use of glucagon in the diagnosis and management of ileocolic intussusception. *J Pediatr Surg* 12:939, 1977.

Marks RM, Sieber WK, et al: Hydrostatic pressure in the treatment of the ileocolic intussusception in infants and children. *J Pediatr Surg* 1:566, 1966.

Ravitch MM: Intussusception, in Ravitch MM, Welch KJ, Benson CD, Aberdeen E, Randolph JG (eds): *Pediatric Surgery,* 3d ed. Chicago, Year Book Medical Publishers, 1979, vol 3, p 989.

Ravitch MM, McCune RM Jr: Reduction of intussusception by barium enema: A clinical and experimental study. *Ann Surg* 128:904, 1948.

Ravitch MM, McCune RM Jr: Intussusception in infants and children. *J Pediatr* 37:153, 1950.

Zachary RB: Acute intussusception in childhood. *Arch Dis Childhood* 30:32, 1955.

Hirschsprung's Disease

Asch MJ, Weitzman JJ, et al: Total colon aganglionosis. *Arch Surg* 105:74, 1972.

Boley SJ, Lafer DJ, et al: Endorectal pull-through procedure for Hirschsprung's disease with and without primary anastomosis. *J Pediatr Surg* 3:258, 1968.

Campbell PE, Noblett HR: Experience with rectal suction biopsy in the diagnosis of Hirschsprung's disease. *J Pediatr Surg* 4:410, 1969.

Carcassone M, Morrison-Lacombe A, et al: Primary operative correction without decompression in infants less than three months of age with Hirschsprung's disease. *J Pediatr Surg* 17:241, 1982.

Duhamel B: Retrorectal and transanal pull-through procedure for the treatment of Hirschsprung's disease. *Dis Colon Rectum* 7:455, 1964.

Harrison MW, Diets DM, et al: Diagnosis and management of Hirschsprung's disease. *Am J Surg* 152:44, 1986.

Huntley CC, Shaffner LD, et al: Histochemical diagnosis of Hirschsprung's disease. *Pediatrics* 69:755, 1982.

Martin LW: Surgical management of total colonic aganglionosis. *Ann Surg* 176:343, 1972.

Martin LW: Total colonic aganglionosis: Preservation and utilization of the entire colon. *J Pediatr Surg* 17:637, 1982.

Martin LW, Caudill DR: A method for elimination of the blind rectal pouch in the Duhamel operation for Hirschsprung's disease. *Surgery* 62:951, 1967.

Polley TZ, Coran AG, et al: A ten year experience with ninety-two cases of Hirschsprung's disease. *Ann Surg* 202:349, 1985.

Soave F: Hirschsprung's disease: A new surgical technique. *Arch Dis Child* 39:116, 1964.

Soper RT, Miller FE: Modification of Duhamel procedure: Elimination of rectal pouch and colorectal septum. *J Pediatr Surg* 3:376, 1968.

Swenson O, Bill AH Jr: Resection of rectum and rectosigmoid with preservation of the sphincter for benign spastic lesions producing megacolon: An experimental study. *Surgery* 24:212, 1948.

Swenson O, Sherman JO, et al: Diagnosis of congenital megacolon: An analysis of 501 patients. *J Pediatr Surg* 8:587, 1973.

Swenson O, Sherman JO, et al: Treatment and postoperative complications of congenital megacolon: A 25 year follow-up. *Ann Surg* 182:266, 1975.

Tamate S, Shiokawa C, et al: Manometric diagnosis of Hirschsprung's disease in the neonatal period. *J Pediatr Surg* 19:285, 1984.

Teich S, Schisgall RM, et al: Ischemic enterocolitis as a complication of Hirschsprung's disease. *J Pediatr Surg* 21:143, 1986.

Imperforate Anus

deVries PA, Pena A: Posterior sagittal anorectoplasty. *J Pediatr Surg* 17:638, 1982.

Fleming SE, Hall R, et al: Imperforate anus in females: Frequency of genital tract involvement, incidence of associated anomalies, and functional outcome. *J Pediatr Surg* 21:146, 1986.

Hendren WH: Repair of cloacal anomalies: Current techniques. *J Pediatr Surg* 21:1159, 1986.

Ikawa H, Yokoyama J, et al: The use of computerized tomography to evaluate anorectal anomalies. *J Pediatr Surg* 20:640, 1985.

Kiesewetter WB: Imperforate anus, II. The rationale and technique of the sacroabdominal operation. *J Pediatr Surg* 2:106, 1967.

Motovic A, Kovalivker M, et al: The value of transperineal injection for the diagnosis of imperforate anus. *Ann Surg* 190:668, 1979.

Nakayama DK, Templeton JM, et al: Complications of posterior sagittal anorectoplasty. *J Pediatr Surg* 21:488, 1986.

Pena A: Posterior sagittal anorectoplasty as a secondary operation for the treatment of fecal incontinence. *J Pediatr Surg* 18:762, 1983.

Pringle KC, Dunn V, et al: Magnetic resonance imaging (MRI) as an adjunct to planning an anorectal pullthrough. Presented at the Section on Surgery Program for Scientific Sessions, American Association of Pediatrics, Washington, DC, Nov 1–2, 1986.

Rehbein F: Imperforate anus: Experience with abdominal-perineal and abdominal-sacral-perineal-pull through procedures. *J Pediatr Surg* 2:99, 1967.

Santulli TV, Schullinger JN, et al: Imperforate anus: A survey from the members of the surgical section of the American Academy of Pediatrics. *J Pediatr Surg* 6:484, 1971.

Schuster SR, Teele RL: An analysis of ultrasound scanning as a guide in determination of "high" or "low" imperforate anus. *J Pediatr Surg* 14:798, 1979.

Stephens FD, Smith ED: *Anorectal Malformations in Children.* Chicago, Year Book Medical Publishers, 1971, p 139.

van der Putte SCJ: Normal and abnormal development of the anorectum. *J Pediatr Surg* 21:434, 1986.

Wangensteen OH, Rice CO: Imperforate anus: A method of determining the surgical approach. *Ann Surg* 92:77, 1930.

Jaundice

Abramson SJ, Treves S, et al: The infant with possible biliary atresia: Evaluation by ultrasound and nuclear medicine. *Pediatr Radiol* 12(1):1, 1982.

Alagille D, Odievre M, et al: Hepatic ductular hypoplasia associated with characteristics, vertebral malformations, retarded physical, menta, and sexual development and cardiac murmur. *J Pediatr* 86:63, 1975.

Altman RP: Portal decompression by interposition mesocaval shunt in patients with biliary atresia. *J Pediatr Surg* 11:890, 1976.

Altman RP: Results of re-operation for correction of extrahepatic biliary atresia. *J Pediatr Surg* 14:305, 1979.

Altman RP, Abramson S: Potential errors in the diagnosis and surgical management of neonatal jaundice. *J Pediatr Surg* 5:529, 1985.

Altman RP, Chandra R: Biliary hypoplasia consequent to alpha$_1$-antitrypsin deficiency. *Surg Forum* 37:377, 1976.

Altman RP, Chandra R, et al: Ongoing cirrhosis after successful porticoenterostomy in infants with biliary atresia. *J Pediatr Surg* 10:685, 1975.

Babbit DP: Congenital choledochal cysts: New etiological concept based on anomalous relationships of the common bile duct and pancreatic bulb. *Ann Radiol* 12:231, 1969.

Benner KG, Keefe EB, et al: Clinical outcome after percutaneous transhepatic obliteration of esophageal varices. *Gastroenterology* 85:146, 1983.

Bismuth H, Franco D, et al: Portal diversion for portal hypertension in children. *Ann Surg* 180:491, 1982.

Chandra RS, Altman RP: Ductal remnants in extrahepatic biliary atresia: A histopathologic study with clinical correlation. *J Pediatr* 93:196, 1978.

Chiba T, Kasai M: An attempt to determine surgical indication for biliary atresia by laboratory examination. *Tohoku J Exp Med* 115:345, 1975.

Flanigan DP: Biliary carcinoma associated with biliary cysts. *Cancer* 40:880, 1977.

Gordon RD, Shaw BW Jr, et al: Indications for liver transplantation in the cyclosporine era. *Surg Clin North Am* 6(3):541, 1986.

Howell CG, Templeton JM, et al: Antenatal diagnosis and early surgery for choledochal cyst. *J Pediatr Surg* 18:387, 1983.

Iwatsuki S, Shaw BW Jr, et al: Liver transplantation for biliary atresia. *World J Surg* 8(1):51, 1984.

Kasai M, Asakura Y, et al: Modifications of hepatic portoenterostomy to prevent postoperative ascending cholangitis. *Proc Pacific Assoc Pediatr Surg* 5:83, 1972.

Kasai M, Kimura S, et al: Surgical treatment of biliary atresia. *J Pediatr Surg* 3:665, 1968.

Kaufman BH, Luck SR, et al: The evolution of a valved hepatoduodenal intestinal conduit. *J Pediatr Surg* 16(3):279, 1981.

Lilly JR: Total excision of choledochal cyst. *Surg Gynecol Obstet* 146:254, 1978.

Lilly JR, Altman RP: Hepatic portoenterostomy (the Kasai operation) for biliary atresia. *Surgery* 78:76, 1975.

Majd M, Reba RC, et al: Hepatobiliary scintigraphy with ^{99m}Tc-PIPIDA in the evaluation of neonatal jaundice. *Pediatrics* 67(1):140, 1981.

Maksoud JG, Mies S: Distal splenorenal shunt (DDS) in children. *Ann Surg* 195:401, 1982.

Markowitz J, Daum F, et al: Arteriohepatic dysplasia. I. Pitfalls in diagnosis and management. *Hepatology* 3:74, 1983.

Morecki R, Glaser JH, et al: Detection of reovirus type 3 in the porta hepatis of an infant with extrahepatic biliary atresia: Ultrastructural and immunocytochemical study. *Hepatology* 4(6):1137, 1984.

Odievre M: Alpha$_1$-antitrypsin deficiency and liver disease in children: Phenotypes, manifestation, and prognosis. *Pediatrics* 57:226, 1976.

Ohi R, Hanamatsu M, et al: Reoperation in patients with biliary atresia. *J Pediatr Surg* 20(3):256, 1985.

Okada A, Yoshiro O, et al: Common channel syndrome—diagnosis with endoscopic cholangiopancreatography and surgical management. *Surgery* 93:634, 1983.

Stellen GP, Lilly JR: Esophageal endosclerosis in children. *Surgery* 98(5):970, 1985.

Todani T, Watanabe Y, et al: Portal hypertension after successful Kasai's operation for biliary atresia—special reference to esophageal varices. *Z Kinderchir* 34(3):240, 1981.

Todani T, Watanabe Y, et al: Congenital bile duct cysts. Classification, operative procedures, and review of thirty-seven cases including cancer arising from choledochal cyst. *Am J Surg* 134:263, 1977.

Voyles CR, Smadja C, et al: Carcinoma in choledochal cysts. Age-related incidence. *Arch Surg* 118:986, 1983.

Abdominal Wall Abnormalities

Allen RG, Wrenn EL: Silon as a sac in the treatment of omphalocele and gastroschisis. *J Pediatr Surg* 4:3, 1969.

Cantrell JR, Haller JA Jr, et al: A syndrome of congenital defects involving the abdominal wall, sternum, diaphragm, pericardium, and heart. *Surg Gynecol Obstet* 107:602, 1958.

Duckett JW: Prune belly syndrome, in Welch KJ, Randolph JG, Ravitch MM, O'Neill JA Jr, Rowe MI (eds): *Pediatric Surgery*, 4th ed. Chicago, Year Book Medical Publishers, 1986.

Filler RM, et al: Total intravenous nutrition, an adjunct to the management of infants with a ruptured omphalocele. *Am J Surg* 3:702, 1968.

Gray SW, Skandalakis JE: *Embryology for Surgeons*. Philadelphia, Saunders, 1972.

Gross RE: A new method for surgical treatment of large omphaloceles. *Surgery* 24:277, 1948.

Randolph JG, Cavett C, et al: Surgical correction and rehabilitation for children with "prune-belly" syndrome. *Ann Surg* 193:757, 1981.

Schuster SR: A new method for the staged repair of large omphaloceles. *Surg Gynecol Obstet* 125:837, 1967.

Schuster SR: Omphalocele, hernia of the cord, and gastroschisis, in Welch KJ, Randolph JG, Ravitch MM, O'Neill JA Jr, Rowe MI (eds): *Pediatric Surgery*, 4th ed. Chicago, Year Book Medical Publishers, 1986.

Shaw A: The myth of gastroschisis. *J Pediatr Surg* 10:235, 1975.

Exstrophy

Rosencrantz JG, Bailey WC, et al: Incomplete exstrophy of the cloaca. *J Urol* 91:549, 1964.

Inguinal Hernia

Rowe MI, Marchildon MD: Inguinal hernia and hydrocele in infants and children. *Surg Clin North Am* 61:1137, 1981.

Cryptorchidism

Bell AI: Psychologic implications of scrotal sac and testes for the male child. *Clin Pediatr* 13:838, 1974.

Fonkalsrud EW: Undescended testes, in Welch KJ, Randolph JG, Ravitch MM, O'Neill JA Jr, Rowe MI (eds): *Pediatric Surgery*, 4th ed. Chicago, Year Book Medical Publishers, 1986.

Mengel W, et al: Studies on cryptorchidism: A comparison of histological findings in the germinative epithelium. *J Pediatr Surg* 9:445, 1974.

Intersexual Abnormalities

Donahoe PK, Crawford JD, et al: Management of neonates and children with male pseudohermaphroditism. *J Pediatr Surg* 12:1045, 1977.

Donahoe PK, Crawford JD: Ambiguous genitalia in the newborn, in Welch KJ, Randolph JG, Ravitch MM, O'Neill JA Jr, Rowe MI (eds): *Pediatric Surgery*, 4th ed. Chicago, Year Book Medical Publishers, 1986.

Jost A: Sur la differenciation sexuelle de l'embryon de lapin. *CR Soc Biol* 140:461, 1946.

Randolph JG, Hung W, et al: Cliteroplasty for females born with ambiguous genitalia: A long-term study of 37 patients. *J Pediatr Surg* 16(6):882, 1981.

Wachtel S, Koo GC: H-Y antigen and abnormal sex differentiation. *Birth Defects* 14:1, 1978.

Neoplastic Disease

Altman RP, Randolph JG, et al: Surgical treatment of sacrococcygeal teratoma. *J Pediatr Surg* 9:389, 1974.

Beckwith JB, Palmer NF: Histopathology and prognosis of Wilms' tumor—results from the First National Wilms' Tumor Study. *Cancer* 41:1937, 1978.

Bishop H, Tefft M, et al: Survival in bilateral Wilms' tumor: Review of 30 national Wilms' tumor study cases. *J Pediatr Surg* 12:631, 1977.

Coldman A, Fryer C, et al: Neuroblastoma influence of age at diagnosis, stage, tumor site and sex on prognosis. *Cancer* 46:1896, 1980.

D'Angio GJ, Evans EA: The treatment of Wilms' tumor: Results of the National Wilms' Tumor Study. *Cancer* 38:633, 1976.

Evans AE: Staging and treatment of neuroblastoma. *Cancer* 45:1799, 1980.

Evans AE, D'Angio GJ, et al: The role of multimodel therapy in patients with local and regional neuroblastoma. *J Pediatr Surg* 19:77, 1984.

Evans A, D'Angio G, et al: Staging for children with neuroblastoma. Children's Cancer Study Group A. *Cancer* 12:374, 1971.

Evans AE, Land VJ, et al: Combination chemotherapy (vincristine, adriamycin, cyclophosphamide, and 5-fluorouracil) in the treatment of children with malignant hepatoma. *Cancer* 50:821, 1982.

Farber S: Chemotherapy in the treatment of leukemia and Wilms' tumor. *JAMA* 98:826, 1966.

Gauthier F, Valayer J, et al: Hepatoblastoma and hepatocarcinoma in children: Analysis of a series of 29 cases. *J Pediatr Surg* 21:424, 1986.

Gechen E, Glover F, et al: Prognostic factors in children with rhabdomyosarcoma. *Natl Cancer Inst Monogr* 56:83, 1981.

Grosfeld J, Smith J: Pelvic rhabdomyosarcoma in infants and children. *J Urol* 107:673, 1972.

Hays DM: Malignant solid tumors of childhood. *Curr Probl Surg* 23(3):161, 1986.

Hays DM, Soule E, et al: Bladder and prostatic tumors in the intergroup rhabdomyosarcoma study (IRS-I): Results of therapy. *Cancer* 50:1472, 1982.

Iwatsuki S, Gordon RD, et al: Role of liver transplantation in cancer therapy. *Ann Surg* 202:401, 1985.

Lampkin BC, Wong KY, et al: Solid malignancies: Children and adolescents. *Surg Clin North Am* 65:1351, 1985.

Leape C, Breslow N, et al: The surgical treatment of Wilms' tumor: Results of the National Wilms' Tumor Study. *Ann Surg* 187:351, 1978.

Leonard AS, Alyono D, et al: Role of the surgeon in the treatment of children's cancer. *Surg Clin North Am* 65:1387, 1985.

Mancini A, Dasgucle R, et al: IV-5 neuroblastoma: A cooperative study of 30 children. *Med Pediatr Oncol* 12:155, 1984.

Randolph JG, Altman RP, et al: Liver resection in children with hepatic neoplasms. *Ann Surg* 187:599, 1978.

Randolph JG, Guzzetta PC: Tumors of the liver, in Welch K, Randolph J, Ravitch M, et al (eds): *Pediatric Surgery,* 4th ed. Chicago, Year Book Medical Publishers, 1986.

Silverberg E, Lubera J: Cancer statistics. *CA* 36(1):9, 1986.

Sitarz A, Finkelstein J, et al: An evaluation of the role of surgery in disseminated neuroblastoma. *Cancer* 18:147, 1983.

Tapper D, Lack EE: Teratomas in infancy and childhood. A 54-year experience at the Children's Hospital Medical Center. *Ann Surg* 198:398, 1983.

Weinberg AG, Finegold MJ: Primary hepatic tumors of childhood. *Hum Pathol* 14:512, 1983.

Weinblatt ME, Siegel SE, et al: Preoperative chemotherapy for unresectable primary hepatic malignancies in children. *Cancer* 50:1061, 1982.

Wooley MM: Teratoma, in Welch K, Randolph J, Ravitch M, et al (eds): *Pediatric Surgery.* Chicago, Year Book Medical Publishers, 1986, chap 31.

Young JH, Miller RW: Incidence of malignant tumors in U.S. children. *J Pediatr* 86:254, 1975.

Trauma

Bruce DA, Abass A, et al: Diffuse cerebral swelling following head injuries in children: The syndrome of malignant brain edema. *J Neurosurg* 54:70, 1981.

Bruce DA, Genarali MD, et al: Resuscitation from coma due to head injury. *Crit Care Med* 6:254, 1978.

Bruce DA, Schut L, et al: Outcome following severe head injury in children. *J Neurosurg* 48:679, 1978.

Eichelberger MR, Anderson KA: Sequelae of thoracic injury to children, in Hix WR, Earon BL (eds): *Residue of Thoracic Trauma.* New York, Futura, 1987.

Eichelberger MR, Randolph JG: Abdominal trauma, in Welch KJ, Randolph JG, Ravitch MM, O'Neill JA Jr, Rowe MI (eds): *Pediatric Surgery,* 4th ed. Chicago, Year Book Medical Publishers, 1986.

Eichelberger MR, Randolph JG: Pediatric trauma: Initial resuscitation, in Moore EM, Eiseman B, Van Way CE (eds): *Critical Decisions in Trauma.* St Louis, Mosby, 1984.

Eichelberger MR, Randolph JG: Progress in pediatric trauma. *World J Surg* 9:222, 1985.

Eichelberger MR, Randolph JG: Thoracic trauma in children. *Surg Clin North Am* 61:1181, 1981.

West JG, et al: Systems of trauma care: A study of two countries. *Arch Surg* 114:445, 1979.

Urology

Irwin N. Frank

ANATOMY

Knowledge of the anatomy of the genitourinary system and adjacent structures is essential to the practice of urology. Accurate diagnosis and optimal therapy are often dependent upon this background information, since recognition of slight alterations in normal anatomy or anatomic relationships may indicate anomalies or disease states. Deviation of the renal axis, the course of the ureter, or configuration of the bladder contour may represent evidence of a pathologic condition in adjacent organs. Disease within the genitourinary system may manifest itself in the form of gastrointestinal, gynecologic, or pulmonary symptoms. Likewise, disease processes in these areas may result in genitourinary symptoms and signs. The importance of these anatomic relationships is obvious when surgery is contemplated, especially in the pelvis where the ureters and bladder are prone to iatrogenic injury.

KIDNEY. The kidneys are paired retroperitoneal organs that weigh approximately 160 g each in the healthy adult. They are situated within the fascia of Gerota, and a variable amount of perinephric fat is present between the cap-

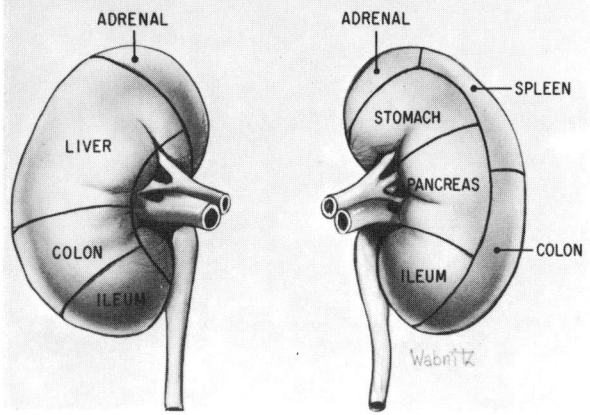

Fig. 40-1. Ventral (anterior) relationships of the kidneys to adjacent organs.

sule of the kidney and this fascial envelope. Further protection of the kidneys is provided dorsally (posteriorly) by their relationship to the lower ribs, the quadratus lumborum, and the psoas muscles. The ventral (anterior) relationships of the kidney are illustrated in Fig. 40-1. They lie beneath the diaphragm, with the right kidney usually 1 to 2 cm lower than the left kidney (Fig. 40-2).

The renal arteries originate from the aorta at the upper level of the second lumbar vertebra, and the right renal artery is longer than the left, since it crosses the midline behind the vena cava. About two-thirds of kidneys have a single renal artery. Multiple renal arteries do occur in normal kidneys, but are more prevalent in congenitally malformed or malpositioned kidneys. The main renal ar-

tery divides into five major branches, each of which represents an end artery supplying a renal segment. Partial occlusion of any branch produces ischemia, and complete occlusion produces infarction of the involved segment. The ureteral and capsular vessels, however, can provide significant blood flow in the presence of marked renal artery occlusion. The left renal vein crosses the midline ventral to the aorta after it has received blood from the left adrenal and gonadal veins. The renal lymphatics empty through hilar trunks in the region of the renal artery and vein. Capsular lymphatics travel through the perinephric fat to infradiaphragmatic periaortic nodes. The renal nerves, which receive contributions from T_4 to T_{12}, from the vagus nerve via the celiac axis, and from the splanchnics, contain vasomotor and pain fibers. Following total renal denervation, such as occurs with transplantation, no persistent abnormalities in renal function occur. The renal pelvis, which usually contains approximately 5 mL of urine, lies dorsal to the renal vessels and has a transitional cell epithelium. The kidney's position with respect to the vertebral bodies and the axis of a line drawn through the upper and lower calyces offers a clue to focal diseases of the kidney and adjacent organs. The axis of the kidney often parallels that of the psoas muscle edge as noted on x-rays of the abdomen (Fig. 40-2).

URETER. The ureters are muscular tubes that connect the renal pelvis to the bladder, traversing the retroperitoneal space in a linear course just lateral to the transverse processes of the lumbar vertebrae and crossing the common iliac arteries at their bifurcation. The lower ureter

Fig. 40-2. Tomogram from excretory urogram. Right kidney is lower than left. Axis of left kidney parallels left psoas margin, and right renal axis is slightly deviated because of the more dilated right renal pelvis.

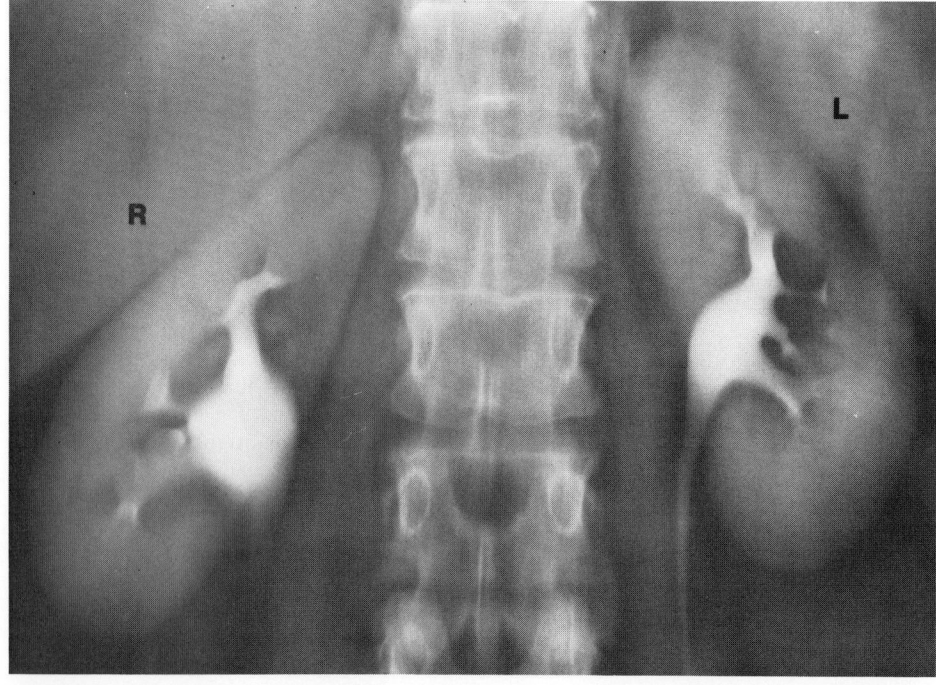

follows the contour of the pelvis and deviates laterally and then medially in a gentle curve to reach the trigone of the bladder above a line drawn between the spinous processes. The normal adult ureter is 28 to 30 cm long and about 5 mm in diameter and has an oblique course through the wall of the bladder. The ureteral orifice is an oblique slit in the trigone. The function of the ureter is to transmit the urine from the renal pelvis to the bladder. Ordinarily, urine is not modified in the ureter. Normally, there are about four peristaltic waves per minute developing pressures of about 30 mmHg. The ureteral blood supply originates from the renal, aortic, iliac, mesenteric, gonadal, vasal, and vesical arteries. Free intercommunication between these vessels permits extensive ureteral mobilization and transposition. Pain fibers refer stimuli to the T_{12} through L_2 segments, while the autonomic innervation is associated with intrinsic parasympathetic motor and sympathetic vasomotor ganglia. The lymphatic drainage is to segmental periaortic and caval nodes. The ureter may be drawn medially in retroperitoneal fibrosis and laterally as a result of enlargement of periaortic lymph node involvement with tumor or an aortic aneurysm. It is essential to be aware of the course of the ureter during aortic and pelvic surgery and in difficult dissections of adjacent organs.

BLADDER. The urinary bladder is a muscular pelvic organ lined with transitional cell epithelium. It is related to the peritoneum superiorly and posteriorly, the sigmoid colon and rectum in the male, and the uterus, cervix, and vagina in the female. In the male, the bladder is spherical, while in the female the uterus indents the dome. The smooth muscle (*detrusor*) is capable of stretching to a marked degree. The major blood supply originates from the superior, middle, and inferior branches of the hypogastric arteries. The lymphatics drain to the perivesical, hypogastric, and periaortic nodes. The autonomic nerve supply to the bladder is derived from the sacral cord and from the presacral and epigastric plexuses of nerves.

PROSTATE AND SEMINAL VESICLES. The chestnut-shaped adult prostate surrounds the proximal male urethra. It is firmly attached to the bladder neck and symphysis pubis. Posteriorly, the fascia of Denonvilliers intervenes between the rectal ampulla and the prostate and seminal vesicles (Fig. 40-3). Caudad, the prostate rests on the pelvic diaphragm, which contains the voluntary external sphincter. The blood supply derives from the inferior vesical, middle hemorrhoidal, and internal pudendal arteries, while the venous drainage communicates with an extensive pelvic plexus that empties into the hypogastric veins. This plexus also communicates with Batson's veins, thus explaining the frequently encountered metastatic spread of prostatic carcinoma to the bony pelvis and lumbar vertebral bodies. The prostate receives secretory and motor (parasympathetic) innervation from S_3 and S_4 and vasomotor (sympathetic) fibers from the hypogastric plexus. The lymphatics drain into the obturator nodes and the external, internal, and common iliac nodes and then to the periaortic nodes. The seminal vesicles lie behind the bladder, lateral to the ampullae of the vasa deferentia. They are closely related to the ureters. Their

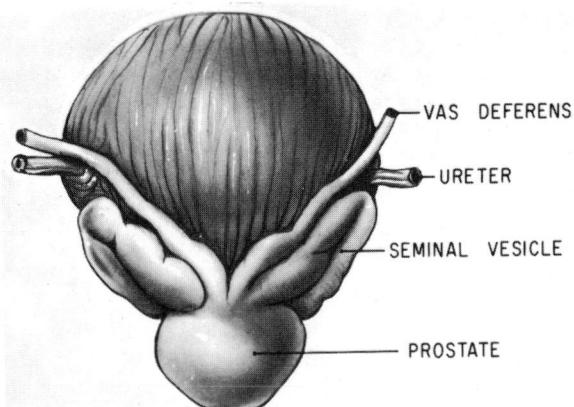

Fig. 40-3. Posterior relationships of prostate, seminal vesicles, ureters, and bladder.

secretions are rich in fructose, which may be of importance to survival of the spermatozoa.

PENIS AND URETHRA. The penis is composed of two lateral spongy erectile bodies (*corpora cavernosa*) and a single ventral body (*corpus spongiosum urethrae*) through which the urethra passes. The latter terminates in the glans penis, which is also composed of erectile tissue. As the urethra emerges from the pelvic diaphragm, it enlarges to become the bulbous urethra. The urethra continues as the pendulous urethra, which terminates in the tip of the glans penis. The female urethra corresponds to the prostatic and membranous urethra in the male. It averages 4 cm in length and 32 mm in circumference. The principal blood supply to the penis and urethra originates from the internal pudendal arteries. Somatic sensory innervation of the penis is from S_3 and S_4 via the ilioinguinal and genitofemoral nerves. Sympathetic vasomotor innervation derives from the hypogastric plexus, while the parasympathetic innervation originates from S_2, S_3, and S_4 via the nervi erigentes. The lymphatic drainage is to the superficial and deep inguinal nodes and then to the external iliac and hypogastric nodes.

TESTIS AND EPIDIDYMIS. The testis is an ovoid firm scrotal organ that measures $4 \times 2.5 \times 2.5$ cm. The left testis commonly resides lower in the scrotum than the right. The testis, which weighs approximately 20 g, is covered by a tough membrane, the *tunica albuginea*, except at its dorsal aspect where the epididymis and vascular pedicle are attached. The epididymis is a crescent-shaped body that curves around the dorsal portion of the testis. The *vas deferens* is a 4-mm thick-walled, firm tubular structure that originates at the inferior pole of the epididymis and follows a cranial course with the spermatic vessels. The arterial blood supply to the testis and epididymis originates from the aorta just below the renal arteries. The left spermatic vein empties into the left renal vein, while the right spermatic vein empties directly into the inferior vena cava. The primary lymphatic drainage from the testis is to the periaortic nodes in the vicinity of the kidney. Crossover from periaortic nodes to the opposite side may occur.

DIAGNOSIS

SEQUENCE IN UROLOGIC DIAGNOSIS. Accuracy of diagnosis is a characteristic feature of the practice of urology. In order to maintain the achievable degree of accuracy, it is essential that a clinical problem be approached in a logical sequence. When so conducted, diagnostic accuracy should approach the 95 percent level.

History

A variety of symptoms and signs are characteristic and often diagnostic of pathologic conditions involving the genitourinary system. The patient may spontaneously offer these clues, but in most instances it is necessary to ask the proper questions to obtain this information. A brief discussion of some of the more significant signs and symptoms follows, and suggestions for evaluating them are offered.

GROSS HEMATURIA. The presence of gross blood in the urine is a significant sign that is quite alarming to the patient and warrants further evaluation. Even small amounts of blood in the urine occurring on one occasion may be the only indication of a malignant process in the urinary tract. Intermittent bleeding is common; large tumors may manifest themselves with only a small amount of bleeding, while small tumors may produce considerable loss of blood. The bleeding originates from lesions that cause erosion or disruption of blood vessels or from inflammatory changes that in turn lead to erosions and diapedesis of red cells. The common causes are inflammation (including infections), tumors, calculi, and trauma.

In young individuals, gross hematuria is more likely to be the result of infection, while in older patients it is more likely to be related to tumors and prostatic disease. Older patients with unexplained *asymptomatic* gross hematuria should be evaluated for possible tumor.

It is important to determine whether hematuria appears at the beginning or end of voiding. Initial hematuria suggests lesions distal to the bladder neck, namely, the prostatic and membranous urethra. Predominantly terminal hematuria usually indicates involvement of the proximal urethra, bladder neck, or trigone. Uniform hematuria occurs with lesions of the bladder, ureter, or kidney. The passage of blood clots suggests that the bleeding is quantitatively great, since urine inhibits coagulation of blood by the presence of citrate. Long, wormlike clots suggest formation in the ureter. Reddish clots occur with recent bleeding, while brownish or grayish white clots indicate a time lapse between the bleeding episode and their passage.

ACUTE POSTRENAL RETENTION OF URINE. This term applies to an inability to empty a full bladder and is one of the most distressing symptoms. It should not be referred to as "anuria," since the latter indicates that urine is not being formed. The patient usually complains of lower abdominal distress, and the bladder is percussible or palpable as a tender suprapubic mass. A variety of afflictions may cause this condition.

Benign prostatic hypertrophy is the most common cause of acute retention in men. The vast majority have a long-standing history of increasing difficulty in voiding with gradually increasing nocturia. In contrast, *carcinoma of the prostate* is accompanied by a much shorter duration of symptoms. The history may be of months rather than years, and the urinary difficulties increase more rapidly. The patient with carcinoma of the prostate seldom presents with urinary retention when the lesion is early and amenable to surgical treatment. The presence of retention therefore suggests advanced disease, and symptoms of advanced malignancy such as malaise, weight loss, anorexia, and back pain are likely to be encountered. Carcinoma of the prostate usually coexists with benign prostatic hypertrophy. In young males, *prostatic inflammation* may cause acute retention. This results from acute urethritis and prostatitis that have not been promptly or effectively treated. There is usually an antecedent history of frequent urination and dysuria progressing to acute retention. Fever, chills, and symptoms of systemic infection are common, and abscess formation occasionally occurs. Acute urinary retention may be a manifestation of *urethral stricture* or may represent a recurrent problem related to the patient's unwillingness to undergo sufficiently frequent dilations, urethrotomy, or urethroplasty. These patients usually give an antecedent history of gonorrhea, transurethral instrumentation, trauma, or radiation therapy. Many will have noted a gradual decrease in the force of the stream.

Neurogenic bladder dysfunction may lead to progressive increase in residual urine and eventual complete retention. This may be the first indication of spinal cord disease. In other patients, the retention may be preceded by difficulty in initiating voiding and overflow incontinence related to changes in abdominal pressure exerting force on a markedly distended bladder. Acute retention on a neurogenic basis may follow trauma, pelvic surgery, the administration of general anesthetics, spinal anesthesia, or the administration of certain drugs that influence the innervation of the bladder, bladder neck, proximal urethra, or external sphincter. Acute urinary retention in women is unusual and may be caused by neurogenic and psychogenic factors or urethral obstructions secondary to carcinoma, stricture, vaginal lesions, or cervical fibroids. A cystocele is seldom the cause of acute retention.

INCONTINENCE. *True incontinence* is the situation in which a patient is unaware of the loss of urine until there is a sensation of wetness. The term is not a synonym for unintentional nocturnal bed wetting (*enuresis*) or urgency, where patients know they are going to wet themselves but are unable to reach a suitable place to empty their bladders before the bladder empties itself. A vesicovaginal, ureterovaginal, or vesicoperineal fistula may also produce incontinence. Occasionally an ectopic ureter will open into the vagina, and this also will produce a constant leakage of urine. *Stress incontinence* is the result of ineffective sphincter muscles that have been weakened by childbirth, stretched by an enlarged prostate, traumatized by surgical procedures, or denervated. *Overflow, or paradoxical, incontinence* represents a third type, in which the bladder retains a large amount of residual urine. With movement, the increased abdominal pressure may cause overflow of a small amount of urine from a distended bladder. This condition may accompany neurogenic diseases of the spinal cord, or it may be the result of long-standing obstructive uropathy with detrusor decompensation. These patients may never really void, intermittently passing small quantities of urine without control. Incontinence of urine is a common manifestation of various neurologic diseases and spinal cord trauma.

URETERAL COLIC. This is related to a sudden increase in pressure. Typically, there is sudden unilateral severe crescendo pain in the posterior subcostal region. The localization is frequently so precise that it can be defined by fingertip palpation. Obstruction at the ureteropelvic junction is associated with pain at the costovertebral angle, while obstruction lower in the ureter may have the added component of pain in the ipsilateral lower abdomen. With obstruction of the intramural ureter, pain may also be referred to the corresponding side of the scrotum or labia majora. Ureteral colic related to intramural obstruction is often associated with a sudden onset of urgency and frequency. Subsidence of these symptoms suggests that the stone has passed into the bladder and may be voided shortly. Narcotic addicts often simulate renal colic to procure drugs. Their deception may include fixing a radiopaque body to the skin in an appropriate area or placing blood from a finger prick in the urine sample.

FREQUENCY. This refers to the patient's voiding an excessive number of times. Frequency of urination should not be confused with polyuria where the patient excretes large volumes of urine at more frequent intervals than normal. The correct term for frequency of urination with small volumes is *pollakiuria*. Most normal well-hydrated individuals void four to six times daily and do not arise from sleep to empty the bladder. Frequency may be related to reduction in bladder capacity associated with inflammation of the urinary passages or effective reduction in functional bladder capacity by increased residual urine, such as occurs with obstructive prostatic hypertrophy. Frequency is also a symptom of psychologic stress.

When patients complain of frequency, it is essential to question them carefully regarding fluid and caffeine intake. It is sometimes of value to have the patient record accurately the time and volume of the amounts of fluid ingested as well as the amount excreted in a 24-h period. It is also essential to note the medications the patient is taking, since this may influence urinary frequency considerably. Further information regarding the relationship of urinary frequency to work, stress, weekend activity, and vacations is extremely helpful. Many patients have sought help from other physicians for this disturbing symptom, which may limit their activities because of the need to be close to a bathroom at all times. A careful history may lead to the information that will allow simple modification of habits, intake, and drug therapy to bring relief of this distressing and sometimes incapacitating problem.

NOCTURIA. Never normal, awakening at night to void

may be caused by consumption of an excessive amount of fluids prior to retiring, or it may be an expression of generalized restlessness. With cardiac decompensation, fluids that have accumulated in dependent portions of the body during the day are restored to the circulating blood when the patient maintains a horizontal position, thus causing nocturia. Patients with chronic renal disease who excrete large volumes because of an inability to concentrate the urine and patients on diuretics frequently experience nocturia. Prostatic hypertrophy and acute or chronic infection of the urinary tract cause nocturia by means of the same mechanisms described for frequency.

URGENCY. This is a symptom of vesical or vesical outlet inflammation and is most commonly due to prostatitis, urethritis, or cystitis. However, it may be a normal consequence of postponement of voiding for prolonged periods of time. The symptom may be so severe that the patient cannot restrain voiding, resulting in urgency incontinence.

DYSURIA. Difficult or painful urination is known as *dysuria*. The sensation is commonly described as burning and may be referred to the glans penis or perineum. The symptom may be caused by urinary infection and the passage of clots, calculi, or crystals. It may also result from passage of highly concentrated urine. Severe pain at the termination of, or subsequent to, voiding is referred to as a *strangury* and may be associated with presence of a bladder calculus or infection. Difficulty of urination is usually the result of an obstructive uropathy. *Hesitancy*, indicating delayed voiding in response to mental command, is another symptom of chronic obstructive uropathy or sphincter dyssynergia. *Intermittency* refers to the involuntary stopping and starting of the stream during voiding and may be a symptom of obstruction.

URINARY STREAM. The stream may lack force and have reduced projection in patients with obstructive uropathy. Stenosis of the meatus, which determines the caliber of the urinary stream, may be evidenced by a thin, deviated, or duplicated stream.

ERECTILE AND EJACULATORY DYSFUNCTION. History taking in this area may prove to be quite difficult for the physician who has had little training in dealing with these problems. A careful history regarding medications is essential, since certain drugs will produce erectile and ejaculatory disturbances. The etiology may be endocrinologic, vasculogenic, or neurogenic. In some situations, however, the underlying factor is situational or psychogenic, and this may become apparent during careful history taking. It is important to realize that in many instances patients wish to discuss their problems with a physician or have unsuccessfully attempted to do so before their present evaluation. In instances where physical or anatomic abnormality may be found to account for impotence, it may be correctable. In selected cases, insertion of a penile prosthesis may be indicated.

Physical Examination

RENAL AREAS. The kidney regions may first be examined with the patient in the upright position. Observation may reveal obvious bulging or asymmetry of the costovertebral region. Scoliosis may be present from guarding in the presence of unilateral pain. Herpetic lesions occasionally may be encountered on the skin surface of this area and may be a clue to the etiology of pain in this region. Gentle palpation of the costovertebral angle areas may be followed by sharp percussion, disclosing an underlying obstructed or infected kidney. If the patient complains of pain in the flank region prior to examination, it is wise to start the evaluation on the contralateral side. Further examination of the kidney areas should be carried out with the patient supine, knees flexed, and arms at the side.

The examiner should stand on the side being examined. The posterior hand is placed parallel to the twelfth rib and below it. The anterior hand is placed 4 cm below the anterior rib cage and parallel to the posterior hand. Renal and retroperitoneal masses can be ballotted between the two hands. In slender individuals, the lower pole of the right kidney is often palpable. In others, the kidney may be palpable with deep inspiration. With unusually mobile kidneys (*nephroptosis*) the organ may be more readily palpable in the upright position. Tenderness is usually related to obstruction or inflammation and is uncommon with uncomplicated tumors or cysts. The examiner again looks for evidence of asymmetry, rigidity of the costovertebral angle, tenderness, or bulging, which may suggest the presence of an underlying abscess, obstructed kidney, inflammation, or retroperitoneal extravasation of urine or blood.

URETERS. The deep retroperitoneal location of the ureters does not lend itself to palpation. It is unusual to be able to feel them when they are grossly dilated or to be able to localize a pathologic area within them.

BLADDER. The patient is examined in the supine position. The empty bladder is neither percussible nor palpable. In the markedly distended condition, occurring with chronic obstruction, the bladder may be visible as a large abdominal mass rising out of the pelvis. Under ordinary circumstances, the bladder is not percussible until it contains approximately 150 mL of urine. Persistence of a low abdominal mass following emptying of the bladder by catheterization documents the extravesical nature of the lesion.

PENIS. The penis may be examined with the patient in the upright position facing the examiner, who is sitting in a chair, or with the patient in a supine position on the examining table. If the patient is not circumcised, the foreskin should be retracted so that the underlying glans, urethral meatus, and inner aspect of the foreskin can be visualized. It is at this point in the examination that the patient may volunteer information regarding underlying fears, fantasies, or facts related to sexual dysfunction, erection, or impotence. If the patient does not do so, the examiner may utilize this opportunity to ask questions related to these topics. Further evaluation of the meatal caliber may be carried out with appropriate instrumentation, if indicated. A valid and recommended means of evaluating the presence of a meatal obstruction is observation of the patient voiding.

SCROTUM. Examination of the scrotum is carried out in conjunction with examination of the penis and with the patient in the positions noted above. Some patients are extremely sensitive to examination of this area, and the examiner may elicit a vasovagal response from the patient who is in the standing position. The examiner should be aware of this, since he may not appreciate that it is occurring while he is focusing his attention on the genital area. A knowledge of the normal scrotal contents and relationships is essential to the differential diagnosis of a variety of pathologic entities that occur in this area. Careful observation and palpation of this region and the use of a small flashlight to transilluminate lesions offer the best means of making an accurate diagnosis.

Scrotal Masses (Fig. 40-4)

As noted elsewhere in this text, an indirect *inguinal hernia* may present as a scrotal mass. The enlargement extends up into the inguinal region and may often be reduced with the patient in the supine position.

Epididymitis. Acute *epididymitis* is commonly a result of retrograde extension via the vas deferens from a focus of infection in the prostate, urethra, or bladder. It may follow prostatic massage or instrumentation. The patient is frequently febrile and has a typical straddling gait to minimize contact with the inflamed scrotal contents. The scrotum is exquisitely tender and may contain a mass. The overlying skin is red and edematous. *Nonspecific chronic epididymitis,* which is a result of incompletely resolved acute epididymitis, presents with an indurated mass that may or may not be tender. *Tuberculous epididymitis* is characteristically nontender, stony hard, and may be associated with irregular indurated beadings of the vas deferens. A *sterile or chemical epididymitis* may occur with the retrograde extravasation of fluid into the epididymis secondary to marked increase in intraabdominal pressure associated with heavy lifting while the bladder is distended. The urine is usually sterile in this situation, in contrast to the pyuria that is often present with acute epididymitis due to infection.

Varicocele. There is a predilection for the left side, because the left pampiniform plexus and spermatic vein drain into the left renal vein, which is usually a few centimeters higher than the point at which the right spermatic vein enters the inferior vena cava. Acute onset of a left varicocele after the age of forty suggests left renal vein occlusion, commonly related to renal tumor. A varicocele on the right side may be secondary to vena caval obstruction or occlusion. This occasionally occurs with tumor thrombus from a hypernephroma invading and involving the lumen of the vena cava. The usual type of left varicocele is observed best with the patient in the standing position facing the examiner. The characteristic "bag of worms" appearance and feeling of the scrotum is noted. With the patient in the supine position, the varicocele collapses and usually cannot be palpated. Failure of drainage in the supine position is suggestive of left renal vein occlusion as noted above. The presence of a varicocele in a patient who is being examined for infertility may be a sig

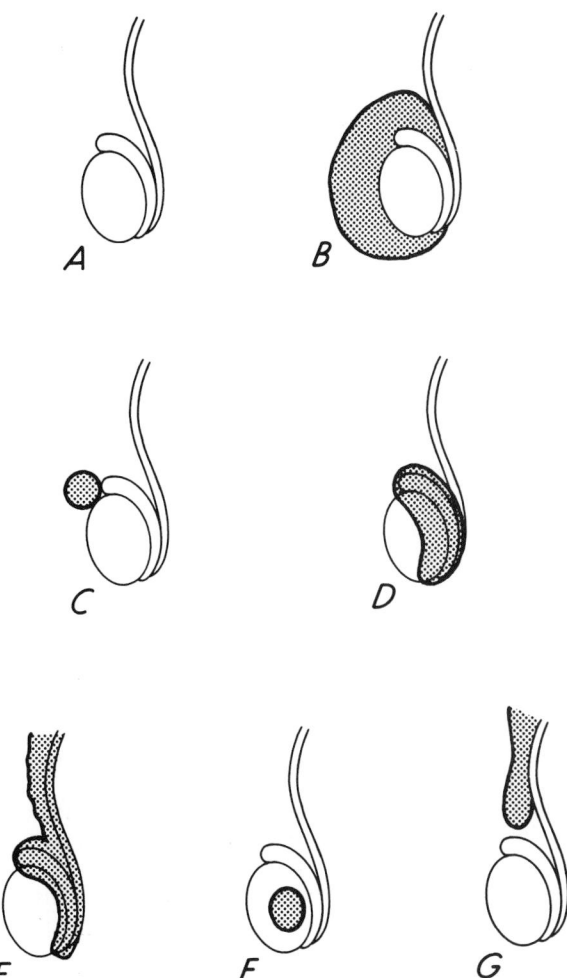

Fig. 40-4. Differential diagnosis of scrotal lesions. *A.* Normal. *B.* Hydrocele. *C.* Spermatocele. *D.* Epididymitis. *E.* Epididymovasitis. *F.* Testis tumor. *G.* Hernia.

nificant finding. This is especially true if the patient has a low sperm count with reduced motility of the sperm and changes in sperm morphology.

Hydrocele. *Primary idiopathic hydrocele* may be unilateral or bilateral and represents an increased collection of fluid between the tunica vaginalis and its contents. It is manifested as a nontender mass that is translucent and obscures palpation of the testis and epididymis. It is ventral, superior, and inferior to the testis and may become very large and symptomatic. *Secondary hydroceles* are the consequence of serous effusion in the vicinity of a disease process. Epididymitis, tuberculosis, trauma, and mumps are among the common causes. *Acute hydroceles* may be secondary to testicular tumors. Aspiration is contraindicated if tumor is suspected. A *communicating hydrocele* is present in a patient with a patent processus vaginalis. In this situation, the scrotal mass fills and empties with varying positions and, in small children, with crying.

Spermatocele. This is a cyst of an efferent ductule of the rete testis. It originates at the head of the epididymis and presents as a transilluminable cystic mass discrete from the testis. Spermatoceles are often bilateral and may be multiple. They are of no consequence except when they reach large proportions or become symptomatic.

Testicular Tumor. A palpable nodule within the testis represents a potential malignant tumor until proved otherwise. The lesion is usualy firm and nontender and is not transilluminable. It is often first noted by the patient or on a routine examination of this area. Ultrasonography of the scrotum may help in defining the size and location of the lesion. Prompt surgical exploration through an inguinal incision is indicated. One cannot stress enough the importance of being able to detect small lesions of the testis by careful palpation and the significance and urgency of proper management.

Mumps Orchitis. The lesion usually occurs in postpubertal males with acute parotitis. It commonly becomes apparent as the parotitis subsides, 7 to 10 days following the onset of the illness. Patients experience high fever, malaise, and marked testicular swelling which, unlike acute pyogenic epididymitis, is unaccompanied by scrotal edema. This condition is rarely encountered, but orchitis of viral etiology or orchitis associated with epididymitis may be seen.

Torsion of the Testis Appendages. "Torsion of the testis" generally refers to torsion of the spermatic cord with a characteristic rotation of the testis and often an anterior presentation of the epididymis. The patient presents with sudden onset of pain accompanied by scrotal enlargement and edema. The testis, which appears to be elevated because the cord is shortened by twisting, is exquisitely tender. The differential diagnosis between acute epididymitis and torsion of the testis may be difficult. Isotopic scanning of the testes may disclose the characteristic ischemia of the involved testis. Since prompt treatment is important to save the testis from infarction, it may be necessary occasionally to explore patients with acute epididymitis to prevent loss of testis in patients with torsion. Approximately 4 h of torsion appears to be the limit after which the testis is irreversibly damaged. Because of the high incidence of bilateral anatomic predisposition to torsion, bilateral orchidopexy should be performed when surgical treatment for unilateral torsion is undertaken.

Torsion of the testis can occur when there is a long mesorchium connecting it to the epididymis. In such a case, the testis, which is likened to a clapper in a bell, can twist inside the tunica vaginalis and undergo infarction. In this circumstance, the epididymis may lie in its normal position, and the testis, which is enlarged, tender, and hard, is not drawn up high in the scrotum. Another condition of torsion involves the appendix testis. This normally present embryologic remnant lies at the upper pole of the testis. When it undergoes torsion, the patient presents with a painful lump on the surface of the upper pole of the testis. Transillumination before major swelling occurs may reveal a characteristic "black dot" sign, which is visualization of the infarcted appendage. Since testicular tumors are rarely tender, they are not likely to be confused with torsion of the appendix testis.

PROSTATE. The gland can best be evaluated after the patient has emptied his bladder, and it is preferable for the patient to be bending forward over the examining table or bed during the examination. If the patient is unable to stand, he should be examined while lying on his side with knees flexed and facing the standing examiner. If the examiner is right-handed, the patient should lie on his right side. Rectal examination should be carried out carefully, with very little pressure exerted while passing the finger through the anus and while the examining finger is on the prostate gland. Furthermore, exertion of pressure in this area may produce considerable discomfort and limit the examination. The normal prostate is two fingerbreadths wide with a 0.5-cm-deep sulcus between the two lobes. It is about 3 to 4 cm from apex to base. However, rectal examination is inadequate to define the precise size and must be combined with cystoscopy.

The consistency of both the normal prostate and the prostate with benign hypertrophy is similar to that of the thenar eminence. In contrast, carcinoma of the prostate feels stony hard, similar to the interphalangeal joint. Crepitations are related to multiple prostatic calculi. With benign hyperplasia, the gland can be delineated from surrounding tissues, and the contours are smooth. With advanced carcinoma of the prostate, the surrounding tissues are frequently fixed to the gland, thus eliminating the usual discreteness of the prostatic contour. Extension of the tumor may proceed into the seminal vesicle area superior and lateral to the prostate. Since 90 percent of carcinomas arise in the posterior portion of the gland, they are readily detectable on rectal examination as induration or a nodular mass. Acute suppuration of the prostate is accompanied by tenderness or fluctuation and requires an atraumatic examination to avoid dissemination of the infection.

FEMALE URETHRA. Pelvic examination of the female patient in the lithotomy position is essential for evaluation of the lower urinary tract. Careful visualization and calibration of the urethral meatus can be carried out in this position. The presence of a cystocele or urethrocele can be determined with the patient bearing down. A urethral diverticulum may be detected by gentle pressure against the anterior vaginal wall, milking the urethra from the bladder to the meatus. Pressure in this region against the symphysis may result in release of purulent material or urine from a diverticulum of the urethra.

Urinalysis

A fresh two-glass specimen from the male or a catheterized specimen from the female provides optimal collections. However, a carefully obtained, clean-voided midstream specimen from the female is usually adequate. A midstream specimen from the circumcised male is usually satisfactory for culture and microscopic examination without any prior cleansing of the penis. The specimen should be examined while fresh, since refrigeration leads to sedimentation of phosphates and storage in a warm environment results in deterioration of formed elements and growth of bacteria.

A clear urine is usually normal. A cloudy urine may be normal if a few drops of dilute acetic acid render it clear, as in phosphaturia. The color may indicate disease, ingestion of certain foods, or administration of medications. Pyridium results in an orange-red color. Methylene blue incorporated in urinary medications leads to varying shades of green and blue. Pink urine may be due to beets or food dyes or to medications like Serenium. Various degrees of bluish gray and brown may be associated with acute porphyria, and bile is readily discernible. The degree and origin of bleeding can often be best estimated by examination of the gross urine specimen.

The odor is often characteristic. A mousy odor that accompanies *Escherichia coli* infection is related to formation of ammonia. A pungent odor is characteristic of either necrotic bladder tumors or calculous pyonephrosis. Certain medications, such as ampicillin, have a characteristic and readily identifiable odor in the urine.

Screening examination routinely includes test for the presence of blood, albumin, reducing sugars, acetone, and pH. Since there are no proteins in the secretions of the male genital organs, albuminuria cannot be ascribed to them. The various paper-dip tests are usually quite reliable and sensitive.

Casts, crystals, and clumps of epithelial cells are identified under low-power *microscopic examination,* while the nature of cells, crystals, and bacteria is determined under higher powers. When the urine sediment is heavy, both the centrifuged and uncentrifuged specimens should be examined. Staining with methylene blue facilitates the diagnosis of bacteriuria. Cytologic examination of urine for exfoliated cells may be helpful and may demonstrate clusters of cells with nucleocytoplasmic disparity characteristic of malignancy. Flow cytometry may add additional information regarding possible neoplastic changes. The identification of bacteria in an unspun urine specimen is strongly suggestive of the presence of a urinary tract infection rather than contamination and usually represents more than 100,000 bacteria/mL.

Genital Secretions

URETHRAL DISCHARGE. Collection is accomplished on a glass slide before the patient urinates. Noninfected urethral and prostatic secretions are usually whitish and opalescent; infected secretion is usually yellow and purulent in appearance. A heat-fixed and Gram's-stained specimen identifies organisms. Gonococcal urethritis is diagnosed by the presence of gram-negative intracellular diplococci. Examination of the wet specimen is helpful in identifying the presence of trichomonads. Confirmation of the presence of infection is established by adequate culture of the urethral discharge.

PROSTATIC SECRETION. The specimen is obtained by gentle massage of the gland. Examination of the normally opalescent fluid reveals three to five white cells per high-power field and tiny refractile cephalin bodies. Epithelial cells are present in small numbers. Seminal vesicle secretion presents as a gelatinous and fibrinous tree-shaped cast of the seminal vesicle containing strands and granules. In the presence of prostatic infection, the secretions become granular, and large clumps of white cells are readily seen. An increased amount of prostatic secretion with the presence of very few white blood cells is suggestive of prostatic congestion.

SEMEN ANALYSIS. For purposes of standardization, the specimen should be obtained by masturbation and collected in a dry container after 5 days of sexual abstinence. Examination, performed less than 1 h after ejaculation, normally reveals a volume of 3 to 5 mL with liquefaction complete within 1 h. There should be over 20 million spermatozoa per milliliter with at least 60 percent demonstrating motility and 80 percent appearing morphologically normal. More sophisticated studies of semen may be performed when indicated.

Instrumentation

The insertion of any foreign body or instrument into the urethra carries a risk of trauma, introduction of infection, sepsis, stricture formation, and the possibility of exacerbation of preexisting inflammatory or obstructive conditions. A variety of filiforms, followers, sounds, and catheters is available. Caliber of instruments is designated by the French numbering system relating to the circumference of the instrument in millimeters, i.e., a #24 French sound is 24 mm in circumference and has a diameter of approximately 8 mm.

CYSTOURETHROSCOPY. This investigative procedure should be performed in most cases of gross or microscopic hematuria and in selected cases of patients with symptoms of lower urinary tract obstruction or infection. It can often be performed as an office procedure. Instillation of a local anesthetic agent into the male urethra makes the procedure tolerable. The smallest caliber instrument that will provide adequate visualization of the bladder and urethra is used. No anesthetic is usually required for female cystourethroscopy. The presence of very small lesions of the bladder measuring 1 or 2 mm in diameter can readily be detected, as well as small calculi, the configuration and location of the ureteral orifices, prostate size, urethral strictures or valves, and other pathologic conditions that may be present in the bladder or the urethra.

URETEROPYELOSCOPY. The ureteral orifice can be dilated, and under direct vision the full length of the ureter and much of the renal pelvis and calyceal system can be visualized with special instruments. Stones can be manipulated and fragmented with ultrasonic probes, and lesions can be biopsied. This is performed under anesthesia.

THERAPEUTIC INSTRUMENTATION. An indwelling catheter affords temporary relief of obstruction. However, since maintenance for over 3 days is almost always attended by bacteriuria, external collection, such as condom drainage, is more appropriate to improve nursing care of the incontinent patient who has no obstruction. Relative contraindications to instrumentation include acute cystitis, urethritis, prostatitis, and a coagulopathy. In these instances, it is best to pretreat the patient for the infection or bleeding disorder. An exception to the rule is that if obstruction is the predisposing cause of infection, i.e., prostatic hypertrophy with retention and acute cystopyelitis, immediate instrumentation is necessary. Temporary drainage during the acute infection stage may be carried out by suprapubic tap and the insertion of a small polyethylene or plastic tube connected to constant drainage. Therapeutic instrumentation may be applied in the endoscopic removal of calculi or foreign bodies, biopsy or excision of tumors, cysts, or other obstructive lesions, drainage of prostatic abscesses, dilatation or incision of urethral strictures or valves, and transurethral removal of prostatic obstruction. Institution of catheter drainage may represent the most important therapeutic measure in obstructions secondary to prostatic hypertrophy or impacted ureteral calculus associated with cystopyelitis or pyelonephritis.

Catheterization should be performed with aseptic technique and minimal trauma. For routine stat catheterization, a #14 F or #16 F olive-tip coudé rubber catheter is the easiest to pass and the least traumatic. For indwelling drainage in the absence of gross bleeding or clots, a #16 F or #18 F Foley catheter is usually satisfactory. If one plans to allow the catheter to remain for several days, it should not be a tight fit which leads to ischemic changes of the urethra and subsequent stricture. Closed-system drainage should be instituted; periodic instillation of an antibacterial irrigating solution left in contact with the bladder mucosa may help prevent infection during this period of constant drainage.

The operator should wear sterile gloves or use a sterile clamp, and the patient should be prepped with Betadine or pHisoHex and draped. For dilatation or instrumentation of the male urethra, a topical anesthetic is instilled, and the catheter, which has been lubricated with a water-soluble lubricant, is inserted into the urethra. Resistance of the sphincter is best overcome by gentle pressure. In the case of acute retention, complete bladder decompression should be effected. With chronic and prolonged distention, rapid decompression of the bladder may lead to distressing vesical spasm and hemorrhage. Therefore, gradual decompression over a period of several hours is indicated.

Special Diagnostic Studies

EXCRETORY UROGRAPHY. Certain intravenously administered organic substances are filtered and excreted by the kidney. When rendered opaque by iodinization, they opacify the renal parenchyma and collecting system. Hypaque (sodium orthoiodohippurate) and Conray (meglumine iothalamate) are two examples. These agents are potent osmotic diuretics and may lead to dehydration, especially in children. Therefore, it is important to compensate for this effect by encouraging copious fluid intake following examination. Occasionally the study is followed by anuria and renal failure in elderly, dehydrated, debilitated patients who have evidence of renal dysfunction. Satisfactory hydration of these patients is essential to decrease the risk of this occurring, and the use of nonionic contrast media may decrease the incidence of complications in this high-risk population.

If time permits, a low-residue diet and oral laxatives should be administered to eliminate fecal and gas shadows. Also, the patient should ideally be dehydrated for 12 h prior to the examination to concentrate the opacified urine. Dehydration should not be carried out in the uremic patient, or in the instances previously stated. Patients with reduced renal function can excrete a sufficient concentration of opaque to give clinically useful information. Pyelograms with inadequate preparation may give useful information in emergencies, and visualization of the pelvocalyceal system is aided by tomography. Such studies may be adequate to determine the presence of obstruction, extravasation, or nonfunction.

Renal Size, Location, and Axis. The adult male kidney averages 13 by 6.2 cm on pyelography. The left kidney is usually a few millimeters longer and broader. The kidneys of females are approximately 5 mm smaller in both dimensions. The upper pole of the left kidney lies at mid T_{12}, while the right kidney is a half vertebral body lower. In the upright position, the kidney descends one vertebral body. If lines are drawn through the uppermost and lowermost calyces of the two kidneys, they should parallel the lateral margins of the psoas muscles (Figs. 40-2 and 40-5). Any deviation from this axis suggests the presence

Fig. 40-5. *A* and *B.* Excretory urogram showing complete left ureteral duplication and nonvisualizing upper segment. Axis of the left calyceal system BB is abnormal. *C* and *D.* Left retrograde pyelogram demonstrating the upper segment. Note correct axis of the right kidney AA and the corrected axis of the duplicated left pelvocalyceal systems.

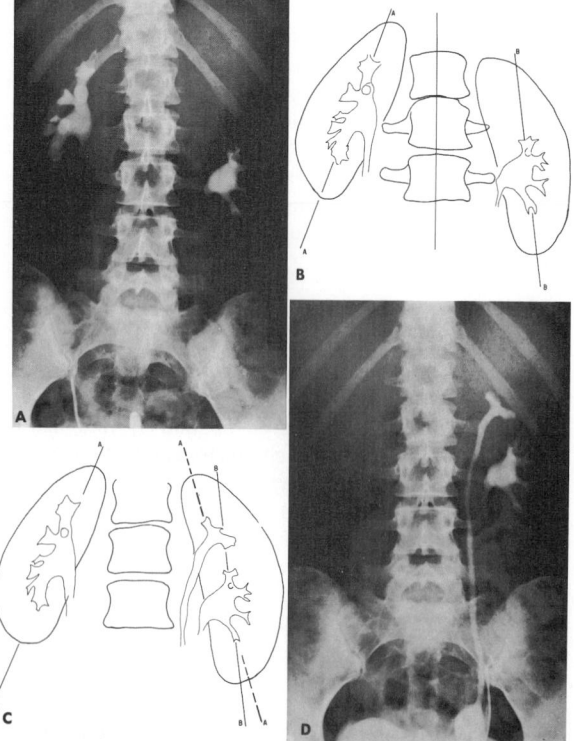

of a pathologic condition or a variant of normal. The calyces should be adequate in number and delicately cupped. The infundibulae are straight and fine. The pelvis points medially and describes a smooth curve without redundancy or tortuosity. There may be several areas of incomplete ureteral visualization due to peristalsis. The diameter of the ureter usually does not exceed 4 to 5 mm. Late upright films should demonstrate emptying of the collecting system and visualization of the urinary bladder. On supine films the contrast may pool in the fundus of the bladder and lead to the erroneous interpretation of an outlet filling defect. A postvoiding film is helpful in revealing the lower ureter and indicating the amount of residual urine.

NEPHROTOMOGRAPHY. More detailed and accurate visualization of the kidney and pelvocalyceal system is available by this technique. Several "slices" of the kidneys are obtained beginning posteriorly and advancing anteriorly. This eliminates the overlying gas and fecal material in the bowel. Lucent areas such as fat and cysts are more readily identifiable. The poorly prepared patient may be evaluated more satisfactorily (Fig. 40-2).

RETROGRADE PYELOURETEROGRAPHY. This study is indicated to further evaluate lesions of the pelvocalyceal system and ureter. "Filling defects" of these structures may not be evaluated adequately by excretory urography. Urine may be collected from the pelves for cytologic study and also to determine differential renal function. Instillation of contrast medium provides a more detailed visualization of these structures and is best done under fluoroscopic control. Improved techniques of excretory urography and nephrotomography have significantly decreased the need for retrograde pyeloureterography. But patients who manifest allergic response to intravenous contrast and patients with nonvisualizing or nonfunctioning kidneys can still be evaluated by this method.

CYSTOURETHROGRAPHY. The patient's bladder and urethra may be evaluated by antegrade or retrograde studies. Fluoroscopic examination of the patient voiding may reveal the dynamics of micturition and evidence of obstruction or reflux of urine. Voiding cystourethrography is a useful diagnostic tool in the evaluation of children with voiding problems or recurrent urinary tract infections. Isotopic cystograms may be employed for the evaluation of reflux in children and offer decreased radiation exposure.

ANTEGRADE PYELOGRAPHY. Percutaneous insertion of a small catheter into the pelvocalyceal system may be a valuable diagnostic and therapeutic tool. The procedure is performed with local anesthesia and with fluoroscopic or ultrasonic control. Once the small tube is placed properly within the drainage structures of the kidney, adequate drainage of an obstructed, infected pyohydronephrosis may be instituted and adequate x-ray visualization of the upper urinary tract may be obtained. Occasionally a ureter cannot be catheterized from below and may have to be visualized by this technique. It is an extremely valuable technique to use in the seriously ill, toxic patient. Adequate drainage may convert the situation from a surgical emergency to a relatively simple elective procedure in a nontoxic patient. Stone manipulations and ureteral dilatations may also be carried out. The percutaneous tract can be dilated and an instrument can be passed into the kidney allowing for direct-vision stone fragmentation (nephrostolithotripsy).

RENAL ARTERIOGRAPHY. Percutaneous, transfemoral renal arteriography is useful in the evaluation of possible renal vascular hypertension and therapeutic dilatation of narrow arteries can be performed (angioplasty). The technique can also demonstrate vascular lesions and thus define the surgical approach. With congenital anomalies of the kidney, arteriography is also helpful, since vascular anomalies frequently coexist and have an important bearing on surgical treatment. Arteriography is also applied to the differential diagnosis of renal masses; a characteristic neovasculature and pooling of opaque is noted in tumor vessels within the parenchyma, diagnostic for a hypernephroma. Therapeutic infarction of kidneys may also be carried out by this approach.

DIGITAL SUBTRACTION ANGIOGRAPHY. This technique provides a means of visualizing the arterial supply of the kidneys on an outpatient basis, with decreased morbidity as compared with standard renal arteriography. A bolus of contrast material is injected intravenously instead of intraarterially, and a computerized subtraction system provides clear visualization of the renal arteries and their branches, as well as of the aorta and other abdominal visceral arteries. Renovascular pathology, such as stenosis or anomalies, can be seen, as well as the presence of multiple renal arteries, which might preclude use of a kidney for donor transplantation (Fig. 40-6).

VENA CAVOGRAPHY. Percutaneous catheterization of the femoral vein with instillation of contrast material provides adequate visualization of the inferior vena cava. This study is particularly helpful in evaluating patients with carcinoma of the kidney and testicular neoplasms. Intrinsic involvement and obstruction of the vena cava and renal veins may be present with carcinoma of the kidney, and extrinsic compression of the vena cava may accompany enlargement of the periaortic nodes associated with metastatic testicular cancer. Preoperative evaluation with this study may help determine the most suitable type of surgical procedure for the patient.

LYMPHANGIOGRAPHY. Pedal lymphangiography may provide adequate visualization of the periaortic nodal drainage system as well as nodes of the pelvis. This study may be employed in evaluation of patients with testicular, bladder, or prostatic carcinomas. Computed tomography has almost completely replaced lymphangiography.

RENOGRAPHY AND RENAL PERFUSION SCAN. The ^{131}I hippurate renogram provides an isotopic evaluation of the

Fig. 40-6. Digital subtraction angiography. Intravenous injection of contrast, demonstrating aorta and renal arteries (arrows).

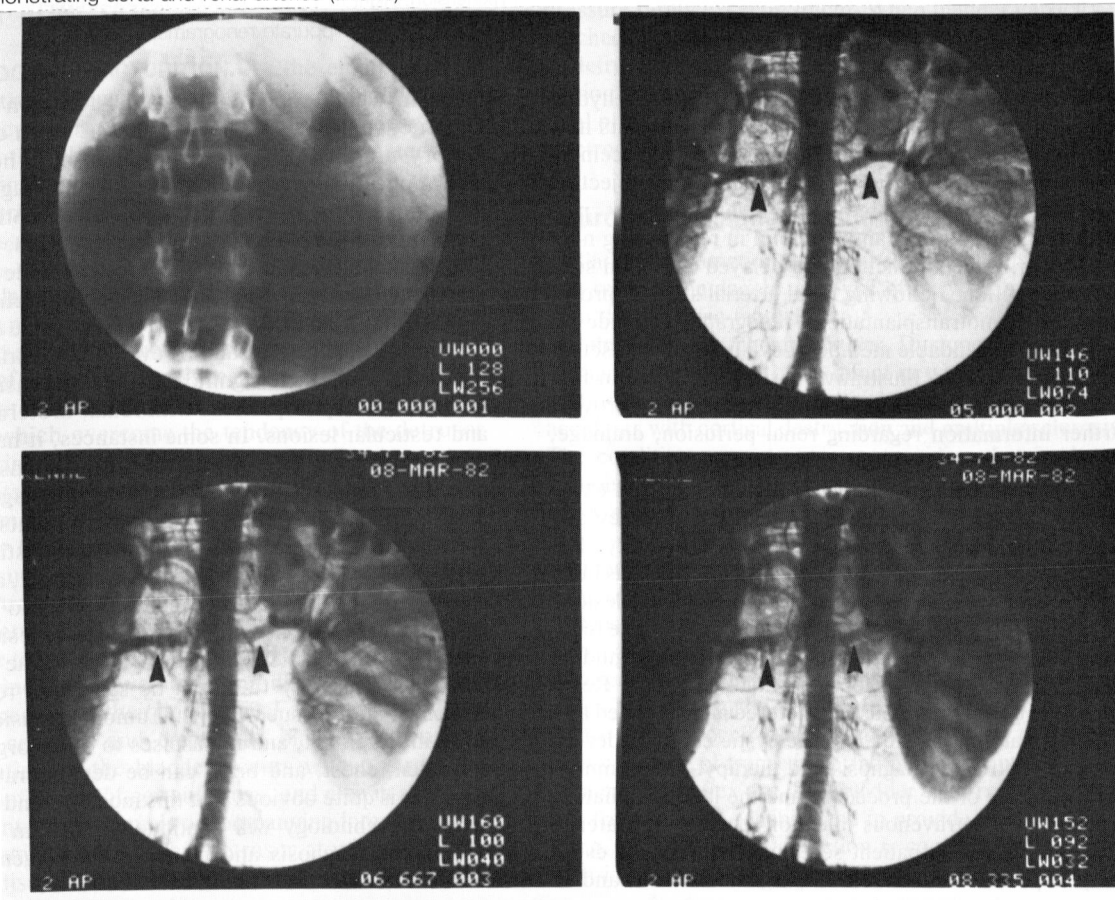

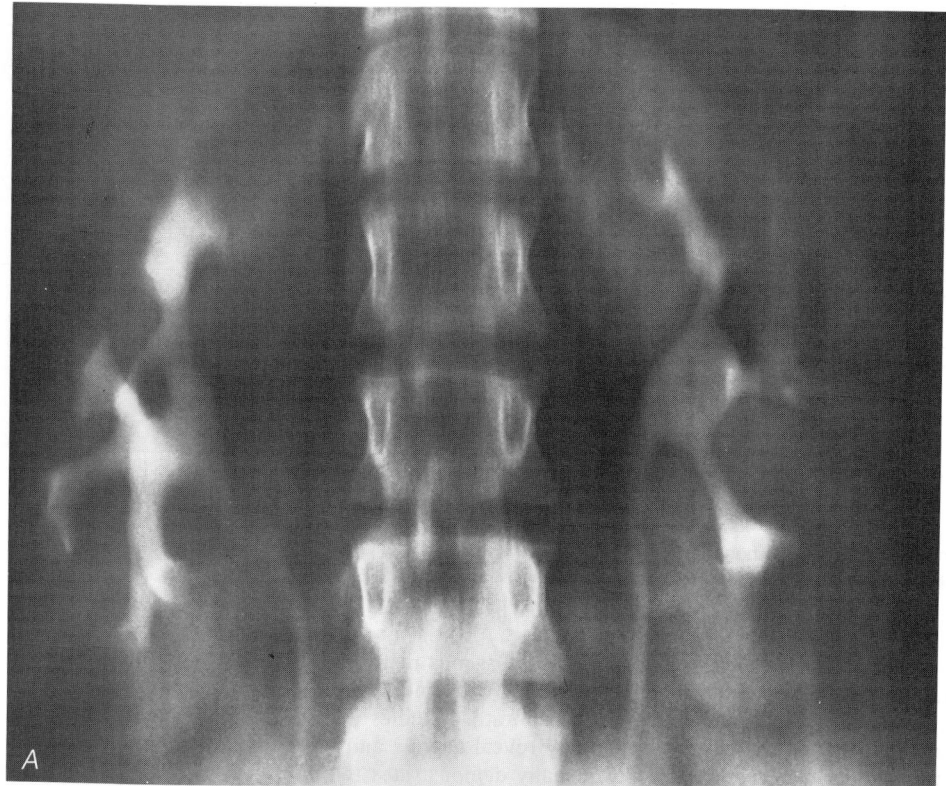

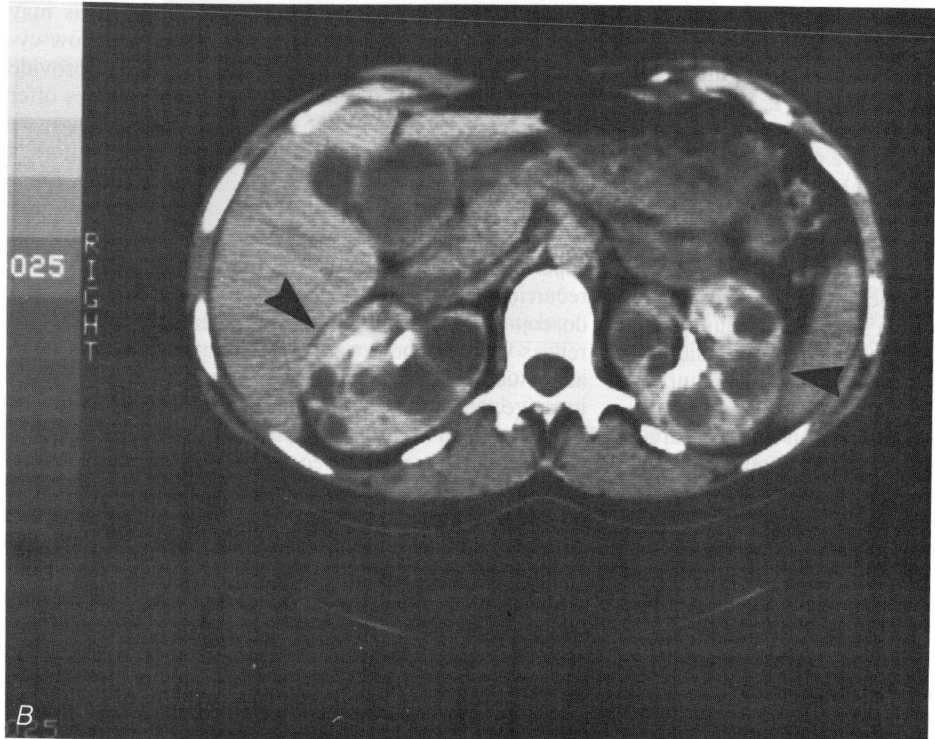

Fig. 40-18. Polycystic renal disease. *A.* Nephrotomogram of large kidneys with calyceal distortion. *B.* CT scan showing multiple cysts in both kidneys (arrows).

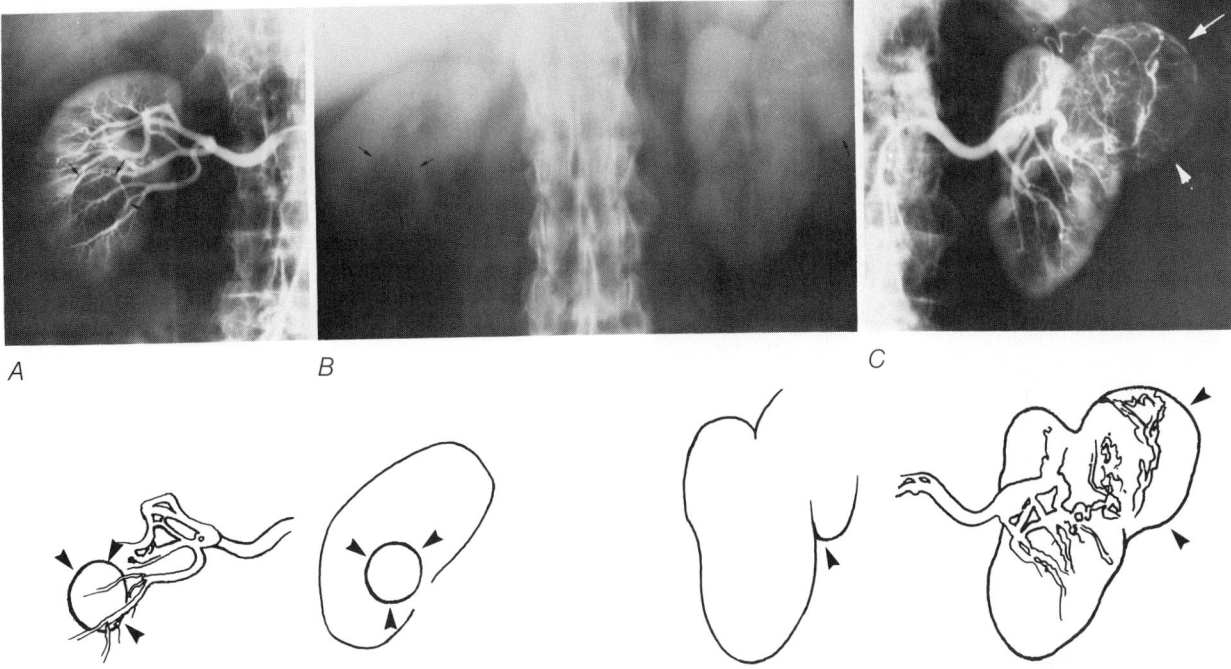

Fig. 40-19. Renal neoplasm and renal cyst. *A.* Selective right renal arteriogram showing an avascular lesion that proved to be a cyst. *B.* Nephrotomogram showing right renal cyst and a left upper pole renal carcinoma. *C.* Selective left renal arteriogram demonstrating a vascular renal neoplasm. Diagrams below demonstrate the pathology.

Fig. 40-20. Tumor involvement of vena cava. *A.* Renal vein tumor extending into lumen of vena cava. *B.* Direct extension of renal tumor into vena cava.

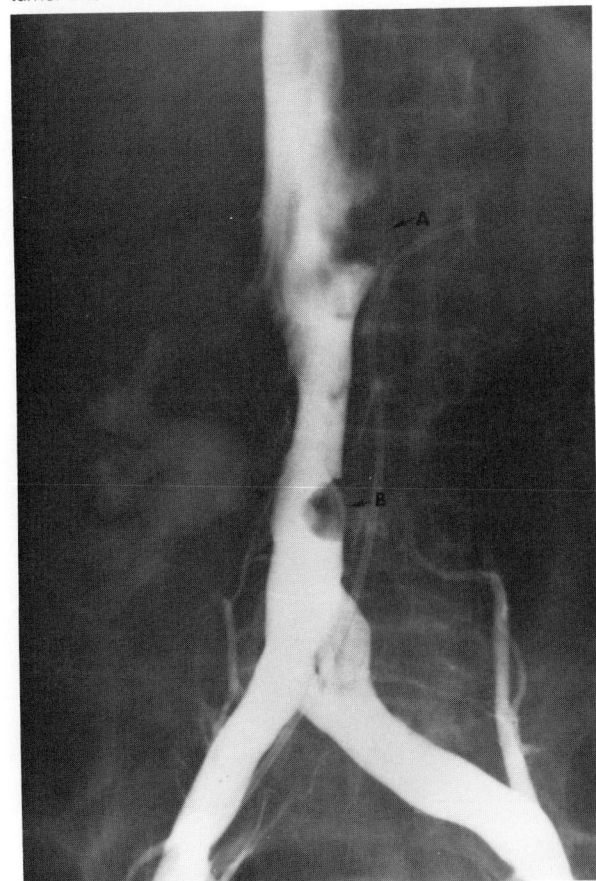

instilled at intervals, have destroyed superficial tumors and carcinoma-in-situ and decreased frequency of recurrence. The prognosis of a bladder tumor depends on the nature and extent of the tumor. Superficial, well-differentiated tumors have a better prognosis than do infiltrating, poorly differentiated lesions.

Prostatic Tumors

BENIGN PROSTATIC HYPERTROPHY

INCIDENCE AND ETIOLOGY. Benign prostatic hypertrophy (BPH) is a benign tumor that originates from the periurethral prostatic tissue. The lesion is rare before the age of forty and does not occur in eunuchs. After the age of fifty, approximately 50 percent of males manifest typical symptoms and lesions histologically, and after the age of eighty, 75 percent of males are so affected.

CLINICAL MANIFESTATIONS. The symptoms are related to mechanical obstruction. Although the initial symptoms consisting of diminished forcefulness and projection of the stream may be apparent, the onset of obstruction is usually so insidious that most patients are unaware of difficulty until it becomes more pronounced. Nocturia is a frequent symptom and is usually due to increased residual urine, but in the early stages the bladder capacity may be functionally reduced because of compensatory detrusor hypertrophy. Hematuria may result from straining to void

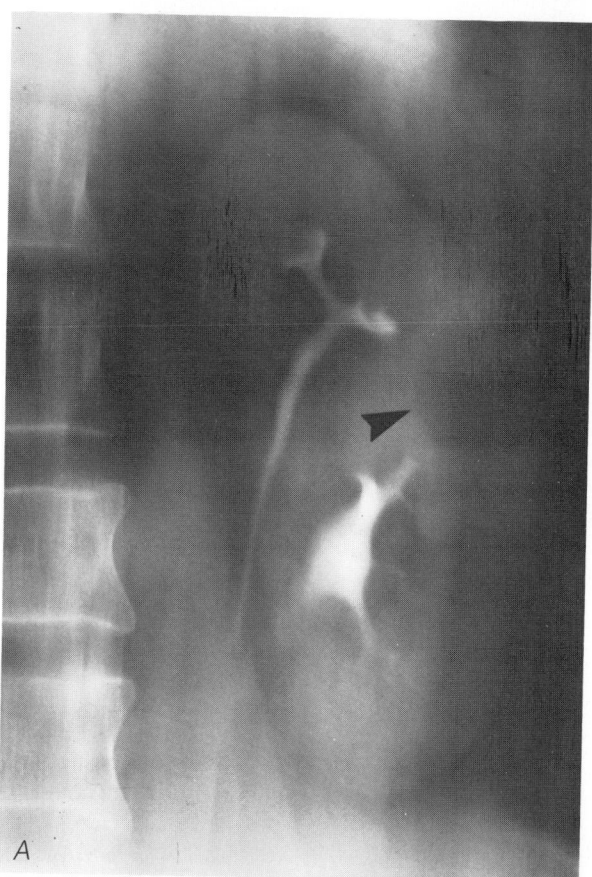

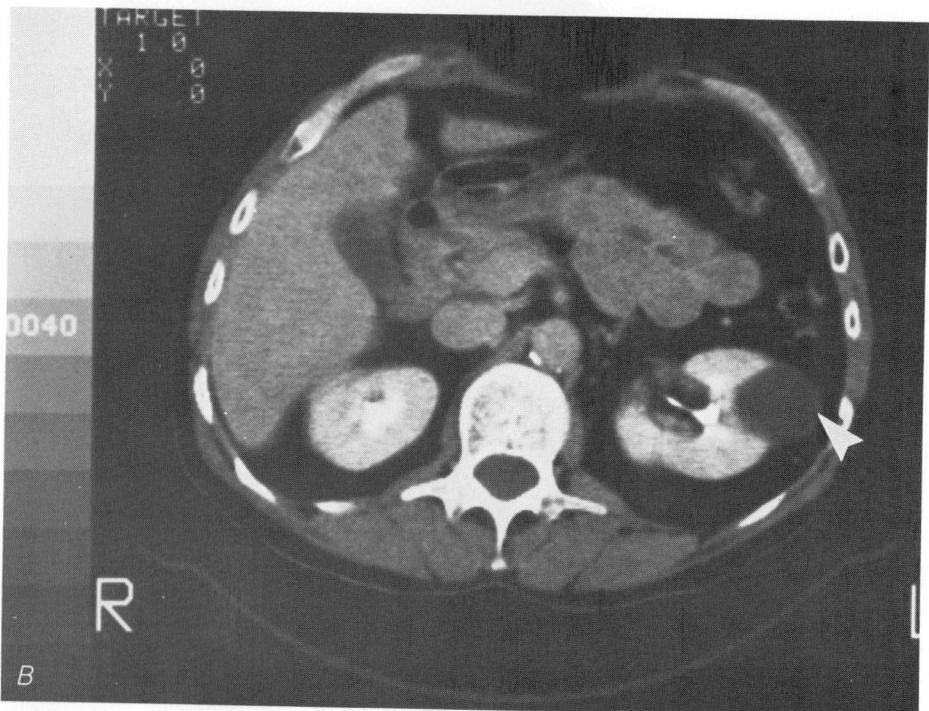

Fig. 40-21. Renal cyst. *A.* Tomogram of left kidney with nonopacifying lesion (arrow). *B.* CT scan shows lesion (arrow) is cystic, and density of lesion is same as water.

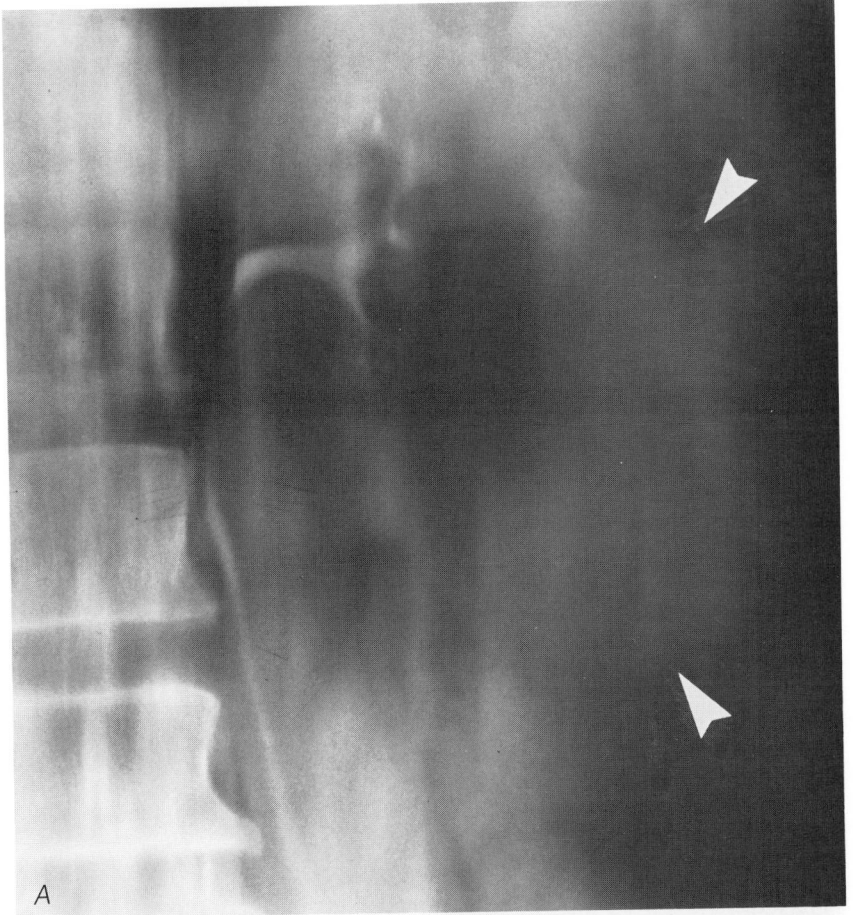

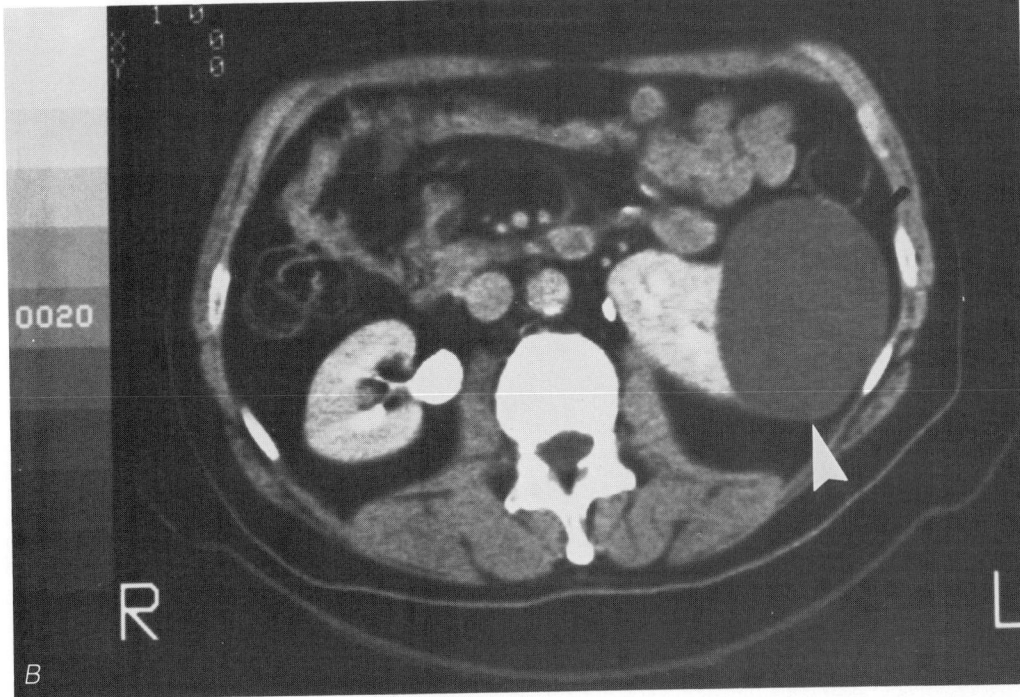

Fig. 40-22. Renal cyst. *A.* Tomogram of left kidney with large lower pole mass (arrows). *B.* CT scan defines mass (arrow), and density discloses water content.

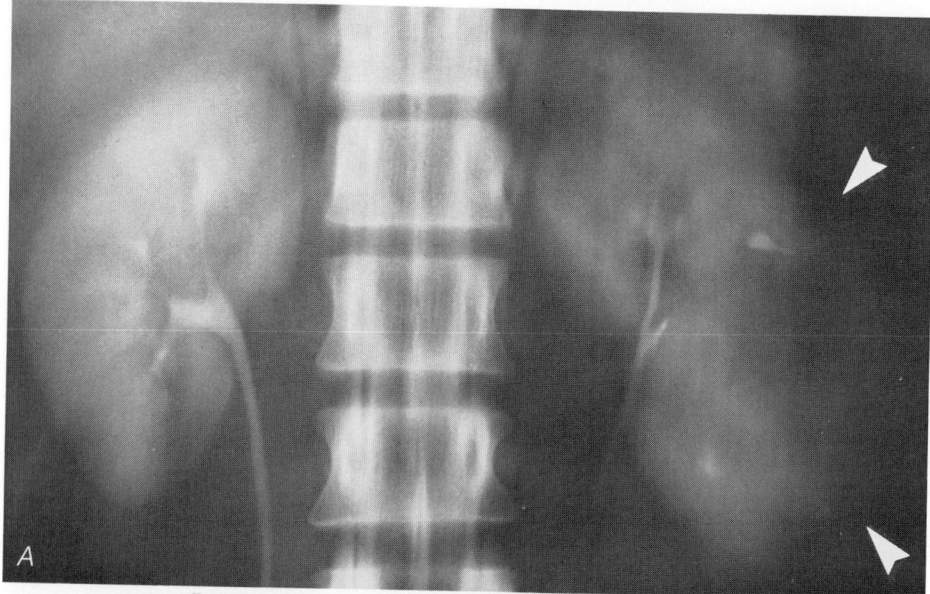

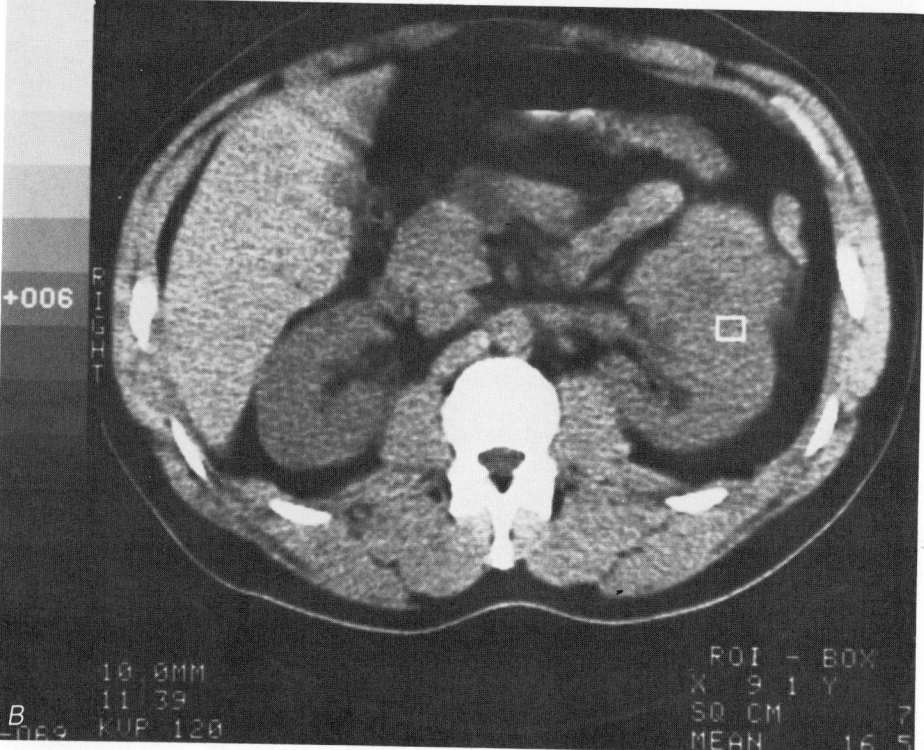

Fig. 40-23. Renal carcinoma. *A.* Tomogram shows left renal mass with calyceal distortion (arrows). *B.* CT scan showing solid left renal mass with irregular contour. Square on mass denotes area selected for density measurement. *C.* Selective left renal arteriogram reveals characteristic renal carcinoma hypervascularity (arrow).

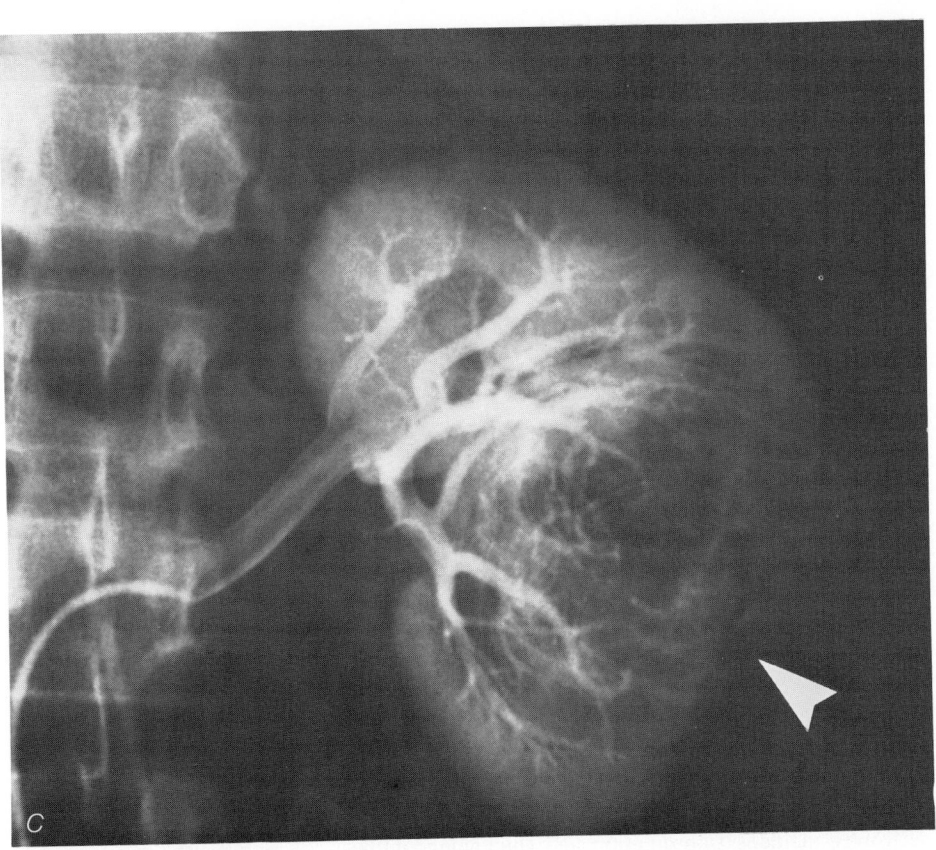

Fig. 40-23 *C.* Continued.

or from increased venous congestion and varicosities. Other causes of hematuria such as carcinoma or calculus should be excluded before a prostatic cause is accepted. Acute retention of urine is the consequence of detrusor decompensation and frequently is the symptom for which the patient first seeks medical assistance.

Fig. 40-24. Carcinoma of renal pelvis. *A.* Excretory urogram showing a filling defect in the right renal pelvis due to a transitional cell carcinoma. *B.* Tumor is indicated by arrow.

On examination, most patients demonstrate a smooth symmetrical enlargement of the prostate that has the consistency of the thenar eminence. Some patients with intravesical enlargement or a bladder neck median bar have a normal-feeling gland on rectal examination. A palpable, percussible bladder after voiding is indicative of retention of urine. Presence of bilateral direct inguinal hernia and/or external hemorrhoids of recent origin is often an indication of the degree of straining that the patient has expe-

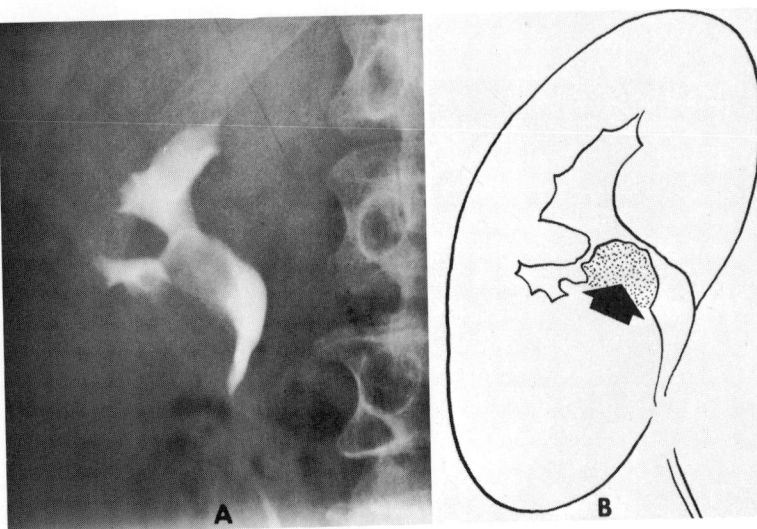

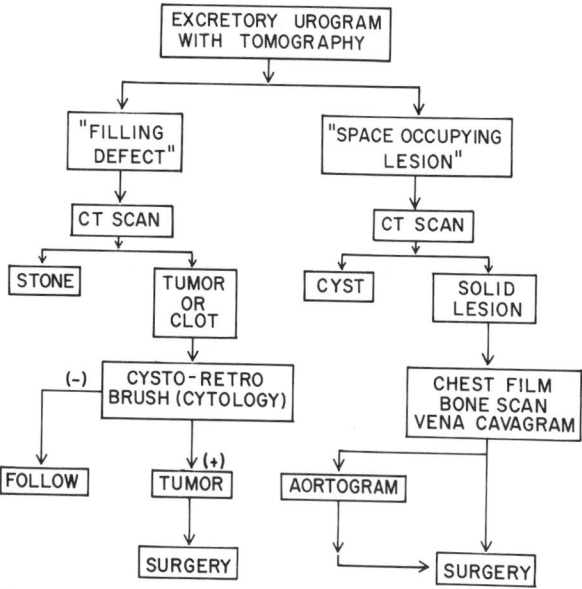

Fig. 40-25. Evaluation of a renal lesion. Plan shown may be altered subject to the age and general health of the patient.

rienced to pass his urine. Observation of the urinary stream will evaluate the degree of difficulty. In patients with prostatic obstruction, rates of less than 5 mL/s are common. Radiographic evidence of benign prostatic hypertrophy includes trabeculation and thickening of the bladder wall, increased postvoiding residual urine, formation of diverticula (Fig. 40-28), vesical calculi, ureteral

Fig. 40-26. Bladder carcinoma. Filling defect on right side of bladder due to papillary transitional cell carcinoma. Film is part of excretory urogram.

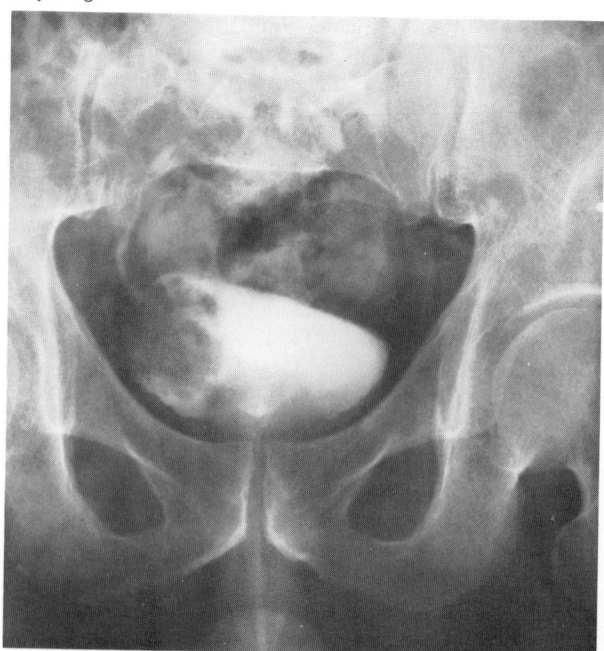

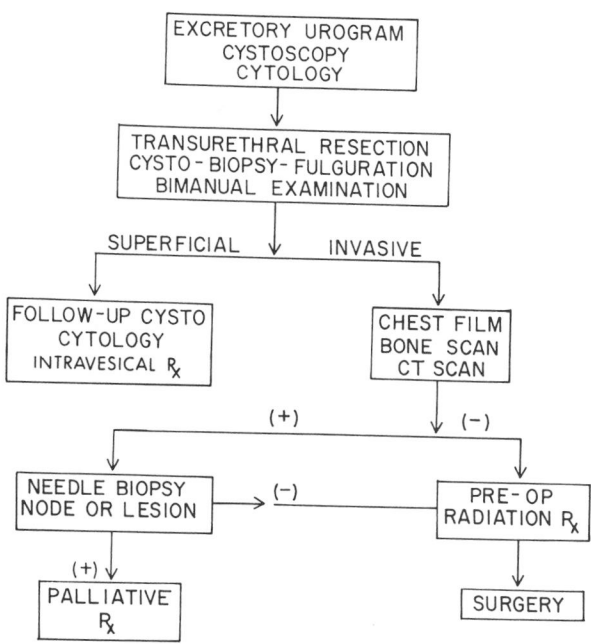

Fig. 40-27. Evaluation and treatment of a bladder lesion. Plan shown may be altered subject to the age and general health of the patient.

dilatation, and hydronephrosis. Cystoscopic examination confirms the prostatic enlargement, vesical changes, and increased residual urine.

RESIDUAL URINE. The amount of residual urine may be determined directly by catheterization after voiding or by indirect methods. Following voiding, the bladder is nor-

Fig. 40-28. Vesical diverticulum. Cystogram showing a large vesical diverticulum (arrow), an important cause of residual urine and persistent infection associated with prostatic hypertrophy.

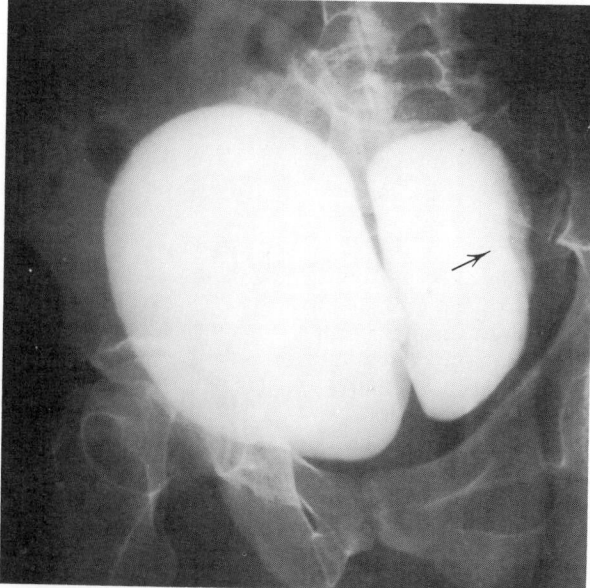

mally empty except for a few cubic centimeters of urine. A postvoiding film after an intravenous pyelogram may demonstrate the presence of residual urine.

Residual urine is the result of stretching of the detrusor muscle when the ability of the bladder to compensate and expel urine against an increased resistance is exceeded. As the degree of obstruction reduces the flow rate with maximal bladder pressures, the percent of bladder volume emptied with each voiding decreases. Thus, the residual urine volume increases. The formation of vesical diverticula and vesicoureteral reflux, which are consequences of the obstructive uropathy, also increases the amount of residual urine. The *functionally reduced bladder capacity* becomes manifest by the need for multiple voiding, particularly early in the morning. The patient soon learns that it is wiser to void when the need first becomes apparent, since procrastination compounds the difficulty. The patient with residual urine secondary to benign prostatic hypertrophy is always in danger of acute retention if he defers urination until the bladder is so distended that a detrusor contraction cannot be initiated. The diuretic and analgesic responses to alcohol and the effects of anesthesia and of anticholinergic and sympathomimetic drugs also increase the likelihood of acute retention.

The presence of residual urine favors formation of vesical calculi (Fig. 40-29). These may be associated with sharp twinges of pain, the "curbstone" symptom, when the patient descends a stairway or steps down from the curb. This is related to the calculi bouncing on the trigone. Following voiding, the patient may have severe strangury and terminal gross hematuria. Residual urine also predisposes to infection. The normally functioning bladder is capable of eliminating a heavy inoculum of bacteria, while the obstructed bladder remains infected.

TREATMENT. The obstructed and/or symptomatic patient who is a reasonable operative risk is best treated by prostatectomy. Circumstances may dictate a nonsurgical or an alternative surgical management. Patients with significant residual urine but without infection or compromised renal function can often be managed conservatively. Specific treatment of infection followed by long-term suppressive therapy is indicated. The patient should be instructed to avoid overdistention of the bladder and to void at the first indication of need. Caution is indicated against long automobile trips and ingestion of alcoholic beverages, anticholinergic and sympathomimetic medications, and diuretics. Hot tub baths and prostatic massages may effect symptomatic relief.

The patient with compromised renal function can be managed with an indwelling retention catheter until renal function returns to normal or stabilizes prior to surgical management. Patients who fail to tolerate the urethral catheter may be more comfortable with a suprapubic cystostomy performed under local or regional anesthesia. In either situation, the catheter care outlined previously should be adhered to. A leg bag for collection is convenient while the patient ambulates, whereas a floor bottle is preferred for night collection. This may represent definitive treatment for the poor-surgical-risk patient.

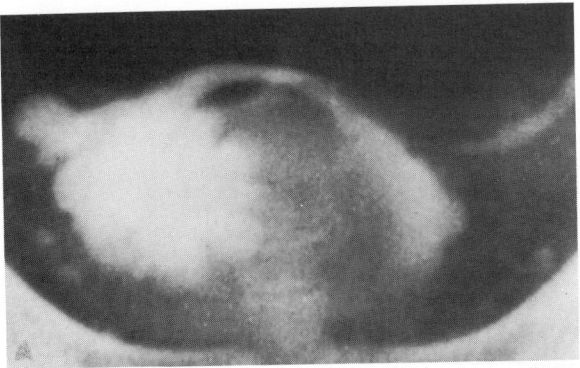

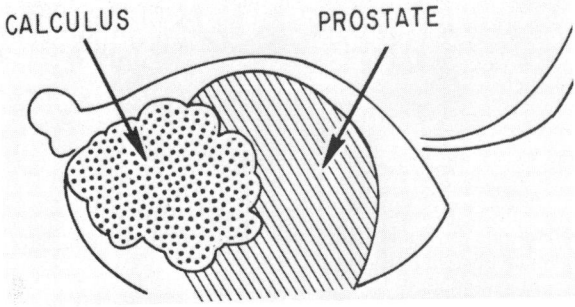

CALCULUS   PROSTATE

Fig. 40-29. Vesical calculus secondary to long-standing benign prostatic hypertrophy. Note intravesical intrusion of large middle lobe of prostate.

The indications for surgical intervention include significant residual urine, difficulty in voiding, and annoying frequency and nocturia, as well as the secondary effects of obstruction such as vesical diverticula, calculi, hydroureteronephrosis, and persistent infection. Presence of benign prostatic hypertrophy per se and symptoms of prostatitis do not constitute indications. As the size of the adenomatous mass increases, the true prostate is compressed. This portion remains after simple prostatectomy for benign prostatic hypertrophy. Although it is appreciated that carcinoma of the prostate may subsequently arise in the remaining gland, simple or partial prostatectomy is most appropriate, since it is attended by a low morbidity and mortality, and produces gratifying results with a low incidence of recurrence.

Transurethral Prostatectomy. This is performed by application of a high-frequency current to a tungsten wire loop and is the most commonly employed surgical means of relieving obstruction due to prostatic enlargement. Multiple fragments of the obstructive tissue are removed by successive cuts under direct endoscopic vision. Hemostasis is effected by sealing the vessels with the coagulating current. Because of low mortality and morbidity, transurethral resection is well tolerated by the elderly debilitated patient. It represents an excellent operation for the young patient who values sexual potency. Transurethral resection is particularly adaptable to a median bar prostatic hypertrophy and the removal of small or chronically inflamed glands that do not enucleate easily by the open route. The procedure can be combined with endoscopic *lithotripsy* (crushing and removal of a vesical

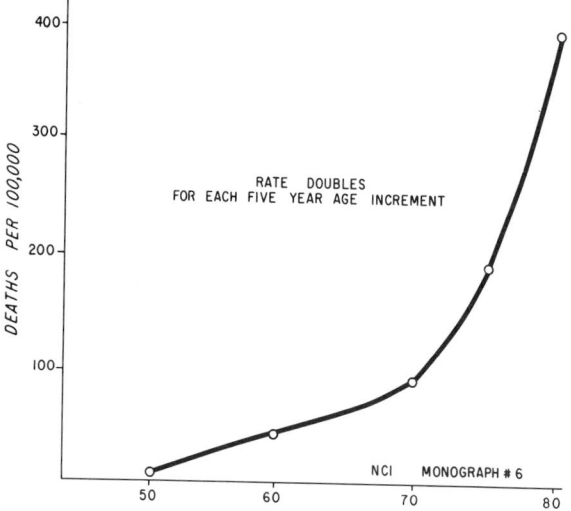

Fig. 40-30. Prostatic cancer death rate versus age.

calculus). The technique is also applicable for the relief of urinary obstruction due to carcinoma of the prostate that is not amenable to curative or palliative measures.

In view of the excellent results and low morbidity of transurethral resection, open surgical treatment of benign prostatic enlargement is seldom required. It is indicated for the enucleation of very large adenomas or when a cystotomy is also required to treat other associated bladder conditions such as calculi, diverticula, or tumors. With the suprapubic or retropubic approach, cleavage is developed with fingers or instruments so that the adenomas and attached prostatic urethra are removed. This leaves the entire prostatic fossa to reepithelialize from the bladder neck and urethral epithelium and from ducts of the acinar glands in the remaining surgical capsule.

Open prostatectomy is associated with greater morbidity and mortality than is transurethral resection. This is related to the increased bleeding problems, wound healing, and discomfort. The catheter drainage for open prostatectomy usually extends over 5 days, compared with 1 to 3 days for transurethral prostatectomy. The attendant increase in the risk of ascending epididymitis makes bilateral prophylactic vasectomy at the time of open prostatectomy advisable. The postoperative stay with transurethral resection usually is 3 to 5 days in contrast to approximately 7 days for open prostatectomy.

With either approach, adequate drainage to the catheter and appropriate antibacterial agents are indicated. Early ambulation should be encouraged and constipation prevented by oral laxatives. Enemas are usually best avoided, since they may initiate bleeding. Upon discharge, the patient should be cautioned that long, bumpy automobile trips, heavy lifting, straining during defecation, and inadequate hydration may lead to bleeding. Oral antibacterial agents are continued when urine cultures are positive. The patient is seen postoperatively at intervals to evaluate the character and frequency of voiding. The majority of patients who do light work may return to their work at about 2 to 3 weeks. Patients who do heavy labor require a longer convalescence.

PROGNOSIS. Over 90 percent of patients have improvement or complete relief of symptoms. Urethral stricture or contracture of the bladder neck may occur and must be treated. Many patients have persisting low-grade pyuria until reepithelialization is complete (6 to 8 weeks). Five-year results indicate that recurrent obstruction requiring additional surgical treatment develops in about 10 to 25 percent. It is important to appreciate the fact that carcinoma may develop in the remaining prostatic tissue.

CARCINOMA OF THE PROSTATE

INCIDENCE AND ETIOLOGY. The etiology of prostatic carcinoma is unknown. It does not occur in eunuchs and is rare below the age of fifty. The new case rate is estimated at 96,000 for 1987, with approximately 27,000 deaths that year. It is further estimated that approximately 5 million men in the United States are living with histologic cancer of the prostate, making it the second most common cancer in males in the United States. The tumor accounts for 10 percent of male cancer deaths. For each decade over fifty years, the deaths per 100,000 doubles, reaching 400 at age eighty (Fig. 40-30). Carcinoma of the prostate represents the most frequent malignant tumor in males over the age of sixty-five.

EARLY CARCINOMA. This represents the stage in which prostatic carcinoma is localized without extension or spread and is potentially curable. In most series, less than 10 percent of patients present as early cases; a vast majority are completely asymptomatic with the tumors detected on routine physical examination. Over 50 percent of prostatic nodules palpated on rectal examination are positive for carcinoma on biopsy. Following a positive biopsy, the patient should be evaluated for possible total prostatoseminalvesiculectomy. The patient's age and medical condition are major factors. In the radical operation, the bladder neck is sutured to the urethra, and the postoperative course is frequently less eventful than that following simple prostatectomy. An indwelling urethral catheter is necessary for several days, and constipation should be avoided to prevent straining and bleeding. A careful dissection with a nerve-sparing technique may preserve sexual function.

The diagnosis is established by transperineal or transrectal needle biopsy or aspiration. Induration of the prostate is also noted with prostatitis, calculus, benign prostatic hypertrophy, and carcinoma of the bladder and rectum with prostatic extension. The differential diagnosis of the blastic metastatic osseous lesions of the pelvis (Fig. 40-31) includes Paget's disease. The wavy, coarsened, trabecular pattern associated with cystic lesions is characteristic of Paget's disease. The distribution of bony metastases on a bone scan is characteristic for carcinoma of the prostate (Fig. 40-32). Elevation of the serum acid phosphatase level is also associated with hemolysis of the blood or the drawing of blood within 24 h subsequent to vigorous rectal examination. The alkaline phosphatase level is also elevated in other bone diseases such as Paget's, multiple myeloma, osteogenic sarcoma, and metastatic tumor. Obstructive lesions of the common bile duct also cause an increase in the serum alkaline phosphatase.

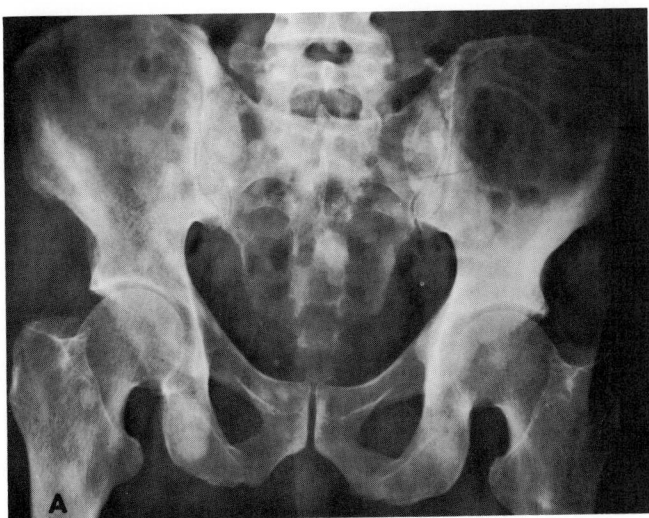

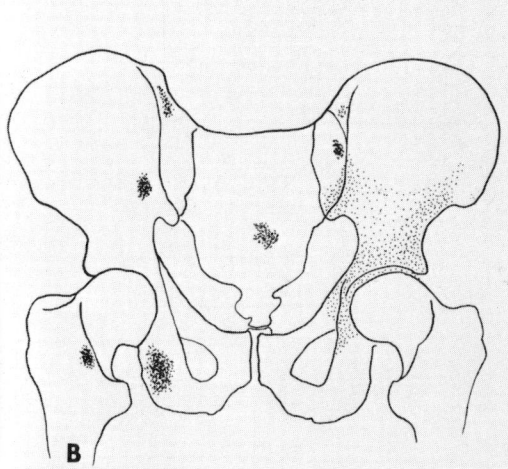

Fig. 40-31. Carcinoma of the prostate. Multiple focal osteoblastic pelvic metastases from prostatic carcinoma.

Histopathologically prostatic malignant tumors are adenocarcinomas, and the majority are well differentiated. Local extension of the tumor into perineural spaces is present in many cases. The prognosis is dependent on

the degree of differentiation of the tumor. Five- and 10-year survival rates also depend on the stage of the disease. If metastatic carcinoma is present, the figures are 20 and 10 percent, respectively. The 5-year survival for treated localized adenocarcinoma of the prostate is approximately 80 percent, with well-differentiated lesions yielding a better prognosis.

An alternative method of treatment for the patient with early carcinoma is radiation therapy. If the patient is not a

Fig. 40-32. Bone scan showing distribution of widespread bone metastases from carcinoma of the prostate. Dark areas represent increased uptake of radionuclide in metastatic sites.

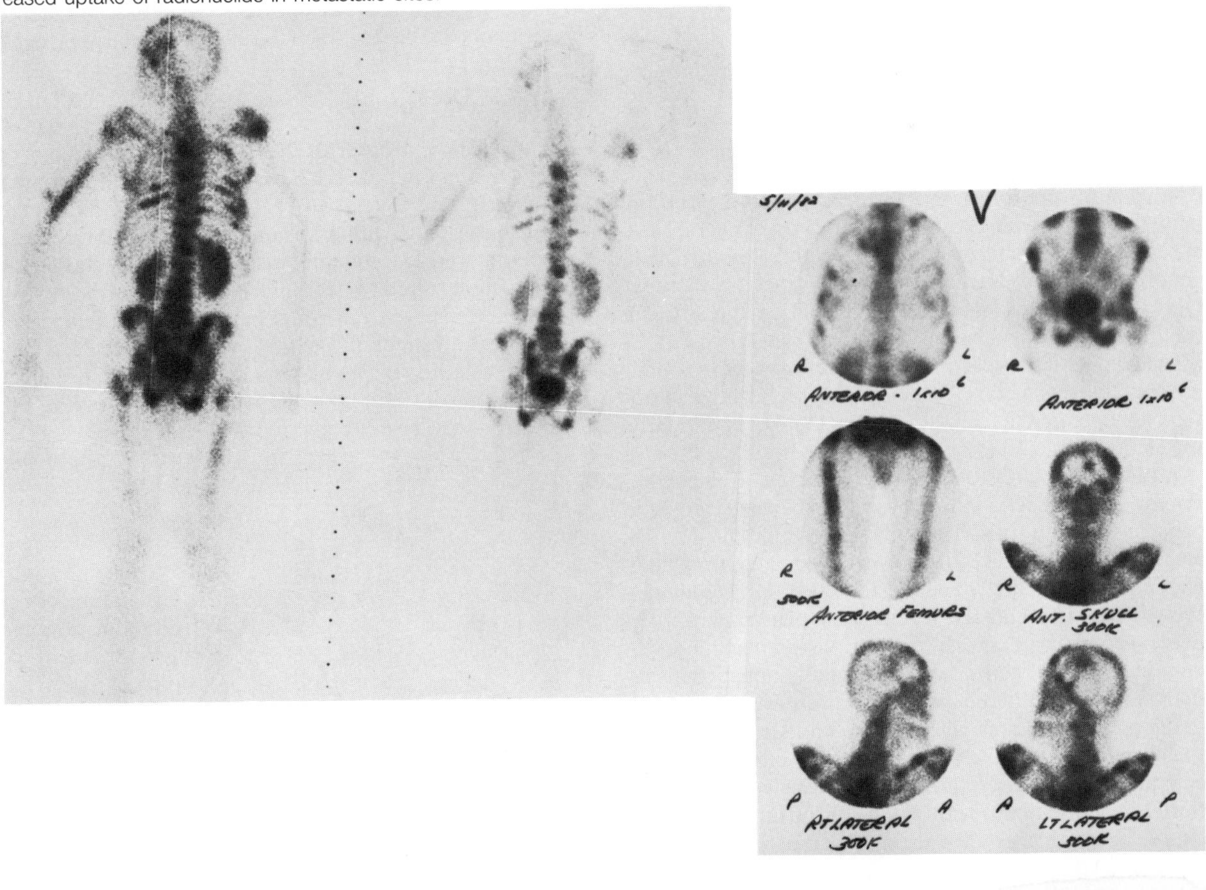

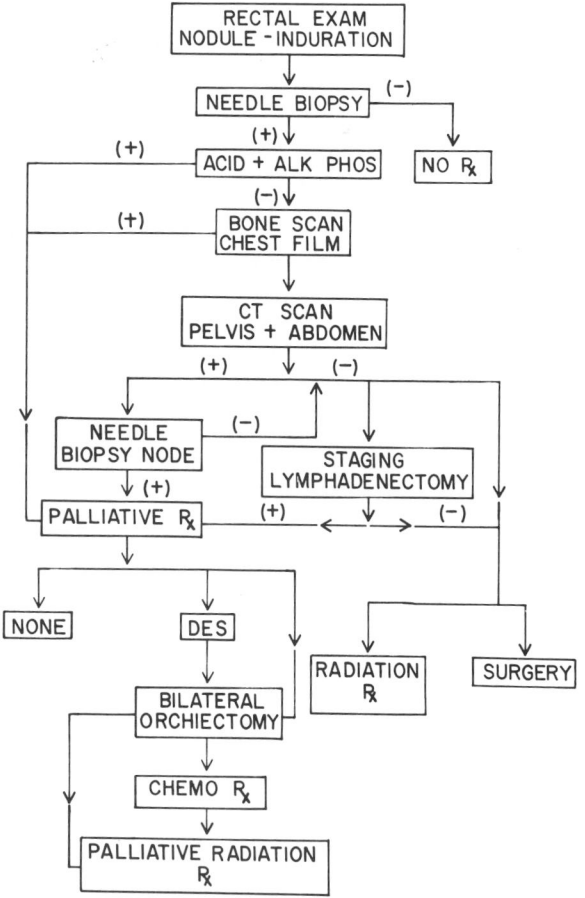

Fig. 40-33. Evaluation and treatment of carcinoma of the prostate. Plan shown may be altered subject to the age and general health of the patient.

candidate for radical surgery or for radiation therapy, he may be treated with estrogen therapy, other therapeutic agents to reduce androgen levels, or orchiectomy, or in some instances followed without any specific therapy. Only surgical excision or radical radiation therapy can offer a cure for this disease, and the 5- and 10-year rates associated with these forms of treatment are fairly similar in several series of cases. One can hope to achieve better than a 50 percent 5-year "no evidence of disease" status in selected cases.

ADVANCED CARCINOMA. The average age of the symptomatic patient who presents with advanced prostatic cancer is seventy-two. Typically, the symptoms are of a few month's duration with rapid progression of frequency and nocturia leading to acute retention in 28 percent. Weight loss is common, severe back pain occurs in 14 percent, and sciatica in 56 percent. Gross hematuria occurs in only 8 percent of patients, and lymphedema secondary to lymphatic obstruction is present in 4 percent. Rectal examination characteristically demonstrates a fixed, enlarged, nodular, stony hard prostate. The serum acid and alkaline phosphatase levels are elevated in two-thirds of the patients with extension of tumor or meta-

static disease. Combined osteoblastic and osteolytic bony metastases are present in 60 percent, while isolated osteolytic metastases are rare. Pulmonary metastases occur in some patients and may be miliary in appearance.

Treatment of symptomatic advanced carcinoma consists of androgen blockade therapy and/or orchiectomy. Reduction in serum testosterone to castration levels may be accomplished with administration of estrogens, ketoconazole flutamide, cyproterone acetate, amino glutethamide, and analogs of luteinizing hormone-releasing hormone (LHRH). This treatment rapidly improves pain and anorexia and gradually relieves the obstructive urinary symptoms. If a large residual urine persists, transurethral prostatic resection may be indicated. The endocrine therapy is accompanied by palliation in about 90 percent of patients. Diethylstilbestrol (1 mg daily) is generally adequate for long-term therapy and is not associated with significant thromboembolic complications. Increased dosage of stilbestrol may be necessary in the patient who has not had an orchiectomy. Recurrence of symptoms is attended by a poor prognosis. Symptomatic relief may be achieved by large doses of diethylstilbestrol diphosphate administered intravenously. X-ray therapy to isolated metastatic bone lesions is also palliative. Corticosteroids in large doses are symptomatically beneficial but have no direct effect on the tumor. Five- and ten-year survival rates depend on the stage of disease at the time of institution of therapy. There is no good chemotherapy regimen for advanced cases after endocrine therapy fails. An algorithm for the diagnosis and treatment of carcinoma of the prostate is shown in Fig. 40-33. It is dependent upon the age and general health of the patient.

Testicular Tumors

INCIDENCE AND ETIOLOGY. Testicular tumors account for 1 percent of cancers in the male, and the average age at diagnosis is thirty-two years (Fig. 40-34). The cause of human testicular tumors is unknown, but they occur eleven times more frequently in undescended testes and fifty times more often in abdominal undescended testes; they may be related to imperfect embryogenesis. Experimentally, intratesticular injections of zinc chloride result in teratomas, and systemic administration of estrogen produced Leydig cell tumors. Testicular cancer is infrequently seen in the black race.

Fig. 40-34. Age incidence of testicular tumors.

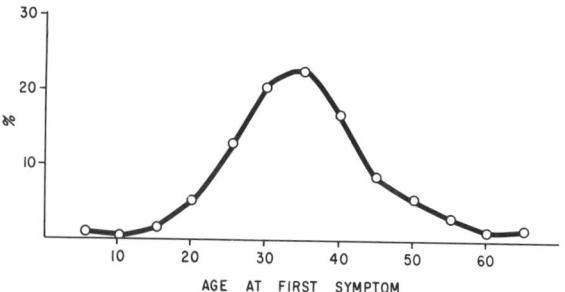

CLINICAL MANIFESTATIONS. Patients usually present with a nonpainful "lump" in the testis. On examination, the lesion is firm, nontender, and solid, and does not transilluminate. Occasionally tumors are misdiagnosed as simple hydroceles because of the formation of a secondary hydrocele. The diagnosis of epididymitis may be made erroneously in some situations and delay the appropriate diagnostic surgical intervention. In the patient with a testicular tumor, a large scrotal mass may also develop as a result of rupture of the tumor with formation of a hematocele. Late symptoms of metastatic disease include weight loss, fatigue, hemoptysis, and enlargement of the regional lymph nodes with associated ureteral obstruction.

DIAGNOSIS AND TREATMENT. If a testicular tumor is suspected, surgical exploration is indicated. Ultrasonographic evaluation may be helpful in localization of intrascrotal lesions. Measurement by radioimmunoassay of HCG and AFP markers may be useful but surgical treatment should not be delayed. If the lesion is confined to the testis on physical examination, an inguinal surgical approach is preferred. The spermatic vessels are occluded before the testis is exteriorized for inspection, in order to prevent the spread of tumor. Palpation of induration in the testis is indication for radical orchiectomy, and there is essentially no place for biopsy, since over 90 per-

cent of solid lesions of the testis in this age group are malignant. In patients with apparent lymphatic or pulmonary spread, the primary tumor should be resected for pathologic evaluation (Fig. 40-35). Seminomas represent about 40 percent of malignant testis tumors, embryonal cell carcinomas and teratocarcinomas about 25 percent each, and adult teratomas 8 percent; choriocarcinoma is limited to about 1 to 2 percent. Combinations of tumors are common, making the above figures difficult to arrive at. Benign tumors are very rare.

Subsequent therapy is dependent upon the histologic diagnosis. Additional surgical treatment is of little use with choriocarcinoma, since this tumor is associated with pulmonary metastases in 81 percent of cases. Pulmonary lesions are present in only 19 percent of cases with seminoma, but bilateral retroperitoneal lymph node resection appears unnecessary for this lesion, since it is extremely radiosensitive. Lymph node resection usually is indicated for adult teratomas, embryonal carcinoma, and teratocarcinoma without supradiaphragmatic spread. Lymphadenectomy in such patients increases the 5-year survival and aids in accurate staging of the disease.

The use of such chemotherapeutic agents as vinblastine, actinomycin, bleomycin, cisplatinum, and other drugs in combinations has markedly increased the survival of patients with advanced metastatic testicular tumors. These agents may cause severe hemopoietic changes, especially when combined with x-ray therapy.

Fig. 40-35. Testicular cancer. Chest film showing large metastatic pulmonary lesions from a primary nonseminomatous testis cancer (arrows).

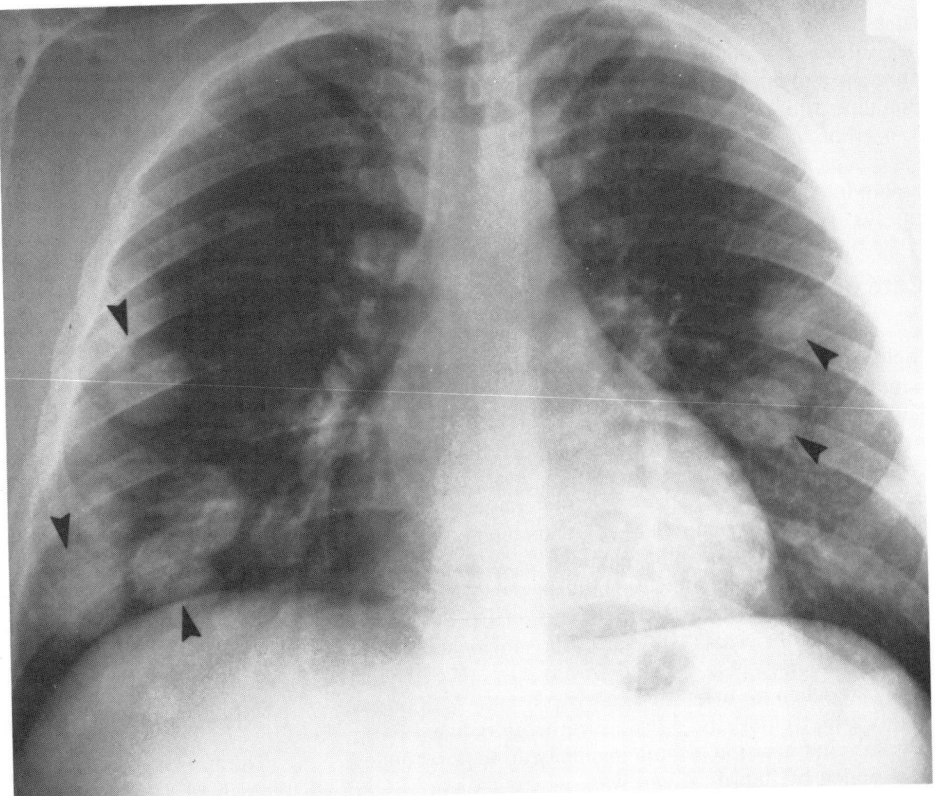

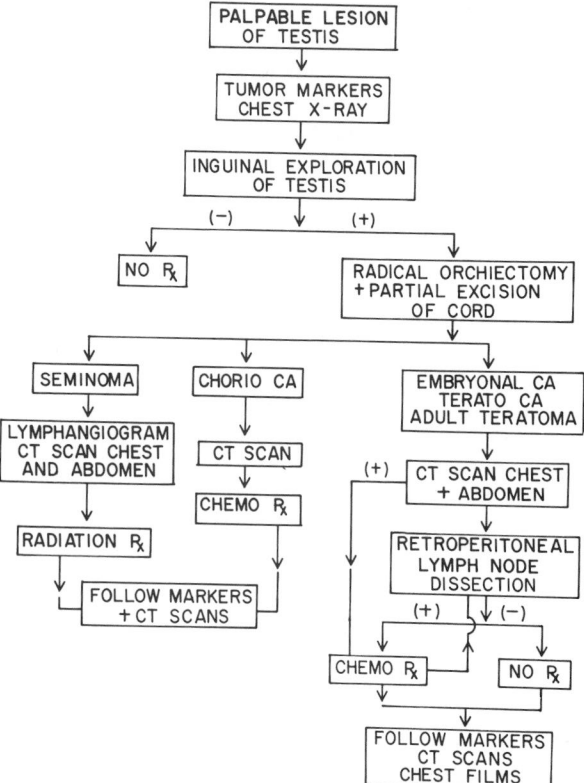

Fig. 40-36. Evaluation and treatment of testicular cancer.

The overall 5-year survival depends on the cell type and stage of disease at the time of diagnosis. Patients who have been free of disease for over 2 years usually are cured. Adjuvant chemotherapy has been responsible for doubling the number of long-term survivors with advanced disease. Tumor markers (HCG and AFP) are valuable aids in diagnosis and follow-up. Figure 40-36 offers a plan for the management of the patient with a lesion of the testis.

Carcinoma of the Penis

Carcinoma of the penis develops in the squamous epithelium of the glans and foreskin. The risk of squamous carcinoma of the penis is almost eliminated by circumcision in infancy, and the incidence is decreased when the procedure is carried out in adulthood. The lesion is uncommon in the United States, and the average age of onset is over sixty. Patients characteristically present with a sore that does not heal or a palpable nodule under the nonretractable foreskin (phimosis). Because of poor hygiene and associated infection the diagnosis may be difficult. Biopsy provides a definitive diagnosis. Squamous carcinoma of the glans is slow-growing, and local excision or x-ray therapy is associated with a 90 percent 5-year cure rate when no distant spread is present. With nodes involved by tumor, the 5-year survival is reduced to 32 percent, and excision of both inguinal and femoral nodes is attended by improved survival.

GENITOURINARY TRACT INJURIES

Renal Injury

A direct blow or crushing injury to the renal area represents the most frequent type of trauma. Knife and bullet wounds are less common. Change in momentum, such as accompanies a fall from a height, may result in a tear of the renal vessels. The patient frequently indicates pain in the renal area. Physical findings include local cutaneous ecchymoses, guarding, mass, and tenderness. Gross hematuria or microhematuria indicates a need for urologic evaluation. If either occurs without local findings or after trivial trauma, a predisposing renal lesion should be suspected. In children, 21 percent of renal injuries occur in abnormal kidneys involved with hydronephrosis or tumors that are enlarged to the extent that they are not protected by the rib cage.

Diagnosis of renal injury is confirmed by excretory urography or CT scan. The preinjection film may show obliteration of the psoas shadow, scoliosis with the concavity to the side of the injury, and displacement of intestinal gas. Postinjection films may demonstrate delayed, absent, or partial visualization of the injured kidney or extravasation of the contrast material. The contralateral kidney should be evaluated, particularly if nephrectomy is entertained. Arteriography, retrograde pyelography, computed tomography, and isotopic scans may be applicable and are of definite value if the kidney is not visualized. Abdominal computed tomography may be the single most important diagnostic test to evaluate the abdomen subjected to blunt trauma, to determine the type and extent of the injury, and to rule out liver or spleen involvement.

Patients with renal contusions and lacerations that do not result in extravasation of urine may be treated conservatively by bed rest and avoidance of strenuous activity until hematuria ceases and radiologic findings improve. When significant segments of the kidney fail to visualize on pyelography, CT scan, and arteriography or when there is extravasation, surgical treatment is considered. Preoperative evaluation for multiple internal injuries is important. At the time of surgical treatment, perinephric hematoma and necrotic renal parenchyma should be removed. The kidney can be reconstructed by suturing its torn capsule, and the perinephric tissues should be well drained. The transperitoneal approach facilitates exploration and early pedicle control. With massive trauma to the kidney, nephrectomy may be indicated to control the immediate situation but partial nephrectomy will often suffice if pedicle control has been achieved. Delayed bleeding, urinary extravasation, hypertension, or perinephric infection may require surgical intervention. Most cases of renal trauma can be treated conservatively.

Bladder and Urethral Injury

The full bladder is vulnerable to trauma especially in the patient who has recently had an excessive alcohol intake. Direct blows, penetrating injury by spicules of bone associated with pelvic fractures, stab wounds, and gunshot wounds may all result in rupture of the bladder. Direct blows without bony fracture usually cause intraperitoneal rupture, while pelvic fractures are more often associated with an extraperitoneal rupture. The patient may be unable to void, and either a low abdominal or anterior rectal mass may be palpable. The urine obtained by voiding or catheterization is grossly or microscopically bloody. If catheterization is not possible, this suggests that the urethra may have been injured or avulsed from the bladder, and retrograde urethrography is indicated. Cystography with postevacuation films defines the site of extravasation from the ruptured bladder. The presence of blood at the urethral meatus suggests urethral injury, and a retrograde urethrogram should be done before any instrumentation of the urethra.

Treatment for severe bladder trauma usually consists of surgical repair of the bladder and cystostomy drainage, which should be maintained for about 10 days, and a cystogram should be performed prior to removal of the catheter. In most cases of bladder injury, conservative management without an operation may prove satisfactory. This is especially true in the extraperitoneal rupture of the bladder, where catheter drainage may be all that is required in certain circumstances. If the urethra is avulsed, a splinting urethral catheter is inserted at the time of bladder repair. When urethral trauma is extensive or the patient's condition poor, cystostomy under local anesthesia may be adequate to allow the sites of rupture to heal themselves or to allow for a second-stage urethral repair at a later date. Differences of opinion exist regarding the surgical management. Some authors advocate simple suprapubic cystostomy drainage, while others suggest more extensive primary repair of the ruptured urethra.

Ureteral Trauma

Injuries to the ureter occur mainly as the result of trauma during surgery. If the injury is recognized at the time of the operation, a direct repair over an indwelling, splinting, ureteral catheter should be performed. If the condition is not recognized at operation, it may become manifest by anuria in the case of bilateral ligation or, more frequently, a urinary tract fistula or an expanding urinoma. At times, a unilateral ureteral ligation may produce no symptoms and result in a nonfunctioning kidney. Excretory urography frequently demonstrates obstructive changes at the site of the ureteral fistula or urinoma. Treatment of the sequelae of ureteral trauma consists of surgical repair with or without percutaneous nephrostomy drainage. The ureter occasionally may be injured by penetrating objects such as bullets and knives. This situation must be suspected when the patient who has sustained such an injury has microhematuria. There is a definite strong indication for an excretory urogram or CT scan on a patient who sustains a penetrating injury of the abdomen, and exploratory laparotomy is often mandatory to evaluate for and to correct injuries to other organs.

OPERATIONS ON GENITOURINARY ORGANS

Nephrectomy

The retroperitoneal approach to the kidney is the traditional route, since in the preantibiotic era a major proportion of renal operations were performed for pyogenic disease, and the avoidance of contamination of the peritoneum with urine was considered advantageous. Today, the flank or lumbar approach (Fig. 40-37A) remains popular but is supplanted on many occasions by the transabdominal route when early access to the renal vessels is required, as in renal tumor, trauma, or renal vascular disease.

Indications for the lumbar approach include inflammatory renal disease, calculi, perinephric abscess, hydronephrosis, and renal cystic disease. The disadvantages are a limited exposure for abdominal exploration, the fact that the position may be poorly tolerated by the patient, and that it precludes bilateral renal or adrenal exploration. In addition, the lumbar approach makes early control of the renal pedicle without manipulation of the kidney difficult and therefore it should not be applied for renal parenchymal tumors.

The lumbar approach may be carried out with the patient in the lateral flexed position, with the involved side

Fig. 40-37. Retroperitoneal nephrectomy (see text).

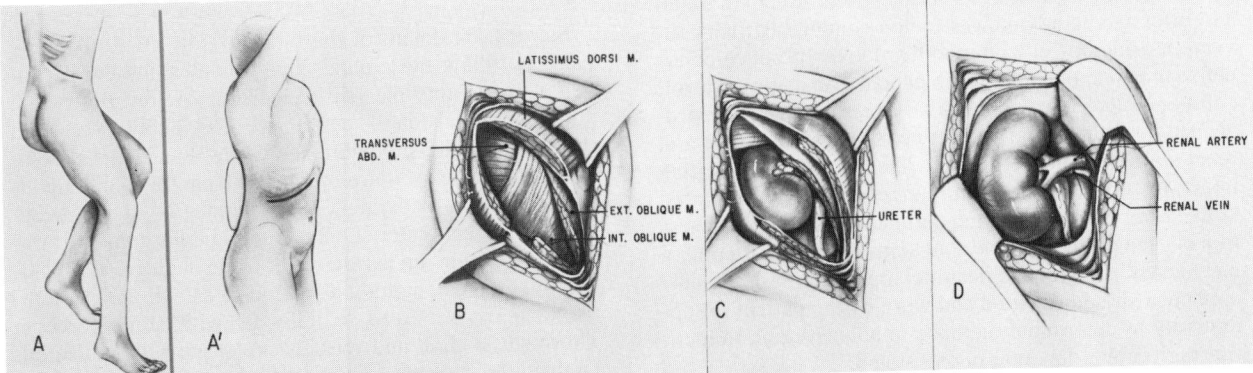

on stretch. A modified flank position can be utilized with a subcostal incision and by remaining retroperitoneal throughout the procedure (Fig. 40-37A'). The external and internal oblique muscles are divided in the line of the incision. The transversus muscle is separated, in the line of its fibers, the retroperitoneum is exposed, and the peritoneum is displaced medially. The fascia of Gerota is opened, thus exposing the kidney and the perinephric fatty tissue. The important structures within the renal pedicle are located anteriorly (ventrally). During mobilization of the kidney, particular care is necessary in the region of the upper pole because of the adrenal vessels and in the region of the lower pole because of aberrant arteries. Usually the renal artery and the vein can be dissected free of fatty areolar tissue, so that individual ligation may be applied. The vein is anterior to the artery, and the artery is ligated first if nephrectomy is performed. Under adverse circumstances, a renal pedicle clamp can be used to control bleeding and permit transection of the hilus. Suture ligature of the renal pedicle en masse may fail to control the bleeding and can lead to arteriovenous fistula. Absorbable sutures are often used when infection is present and drainage is instituted. The incision is closed in layers with chromic catgut or Vicryl, with the exception of the skin, which is closed with nonabsorbable sutures or staples. Nonabsorbable sutures with increased tensile strength, such as Prolene, may be used in the fascia to increase the strength of closure in debilitated patients or those in whom poor wound healing is expected. Nephrectomy for a renal carcinoma is carried out through a transperitoneal approach with vascular ligation before mobilization and without opening Gerota's fascia, and insertion of a drain is not required.

Cutaneous Ureteroileostomy (Ileal Conduit)

Currently, the most popular method of supravesical urinary diversion is cutaneous ureteroileostomy (Fig. 40-38). The major indications for this form of diversion are (1) required removal of the bladder and (2) impaired bladder detrusor function. The disadvantages of the procedure are the extent of the operation and the requirement of utilizing a meticulously applied external collection device. These disadvantages are offset by the advantages of the ileal conduit in providing a continuous unobstructed drainage of urine and its versatility in coping with varying anatomical situations. Colon is also used instead of ileum and offers some advantages (colon conduit). Urinary diversion using bowel with modifications to produce continence is also applicable (Koch pouch, Camay procedure).

Preoperative preparation is an integral part of any procedure, and the blood volume, cardiac, pulmonary, and renal status should be optimal. Treatment of preexisting infections or metabolic disturbances should be instituted at this time. Mechanical and antibacterial bowel preparation is used preoperatively, but some surgeons use only a mechanical prep for the ileal loop operation. The urinary appliance should be fitted and worn by the patient preoperatively to determine tolerance to adhesive and to identify the optimal location of the stoma.

The ileal loop is best performed through a midline abdominal incision. Prior to making this incision, it is preferable to create the abdominal wall defect for the ileostomy. This results in the creation of a tract through muscles that have not been distorted by the incision and avoids the problem of mechanical obstruction of the ileostomy. The abdomen is then entered. Appendectomy is performed. A segment of the ileum approximately 20 cm in length is selected for the formation of the conduit. A well-vascularized segment is essential. The ileum is divided at the selected sites, and the isolated segment is irrigated with saline solution. The continuity of the ileum is restored, and the isolated ileal segment is positioned posterior to the ileoileal anastomosis. The proximal end of the ileal segment to be utilized for the conduit is closed with a continuous inverting chromic catgut suture. The left ureter is brought through the sigmoid mesentery and mobilized to provide length and eliminate the possibility of kinking or obstruction. The full thickness of ureter is sutured to the ileal mucosa. If the left ureter is markedly dilated, an end-to-end ureteroileostomy is performed. Feeding tubes (#5 or #8) may be used to splint the anastomosis for a few days and to encourage good position of the ureters. The right ureter is anastomosed in a similar fashion over a catheter stent. The isolated segment of ileum and its mesentery are sutured to the posterior peritoneum to prevent an internal hernia. The distal end of the ileal conduit is brought to the previously prepared abdominal opening. The fascia is secured to the serosa of the ileum to prevent herniation. The ileostomy stoma is everted and sutured to the skin and itself. A 1-cm protuberant cuff under no tension is considered optimal. The wound is closed with catgut, Vicryl, or Prolene for the fascial layers and silk or staples for the skin. A nasogastric tube is usually necessary postoperatively for 3 to 5 days. Another variation of the procedure involves the joining of both ureters together with one large stoma, which is then anastomosed to the proximal end of the ileal loop as a "cap." This may provide a larger anastomotic opening between the ureters and the segment of ileum and decrease the incidence of the complication of stricture at this vital site. The stoma is usually placed on the right side but can be placed on the left side of the abdomen when indicated.

Cystostomy, Cystolithotomy

Surgical treatment of the bladder (Fig. 40-39) is facilitated by filling the organ, since this elevates the peritoneum out of the line of the incision. A low transverse abdominal incision 4 cm above the pubis is carried through the skin, subcutaneous tissue, and rectus abdominis fascia. The recti are mobilized from their midline attachments and separated. The bladder is easily recognized by its characteristic muscular and vascular pattern, and the peritoneum is reflected off the bladder. The bladder is entered longitudinally, and if calculi are present, they can be removed digitally or with stone forceps. Thorough digital and visual exploration is indicated. Drainage may be provided by a Malecot cystostomy cath-

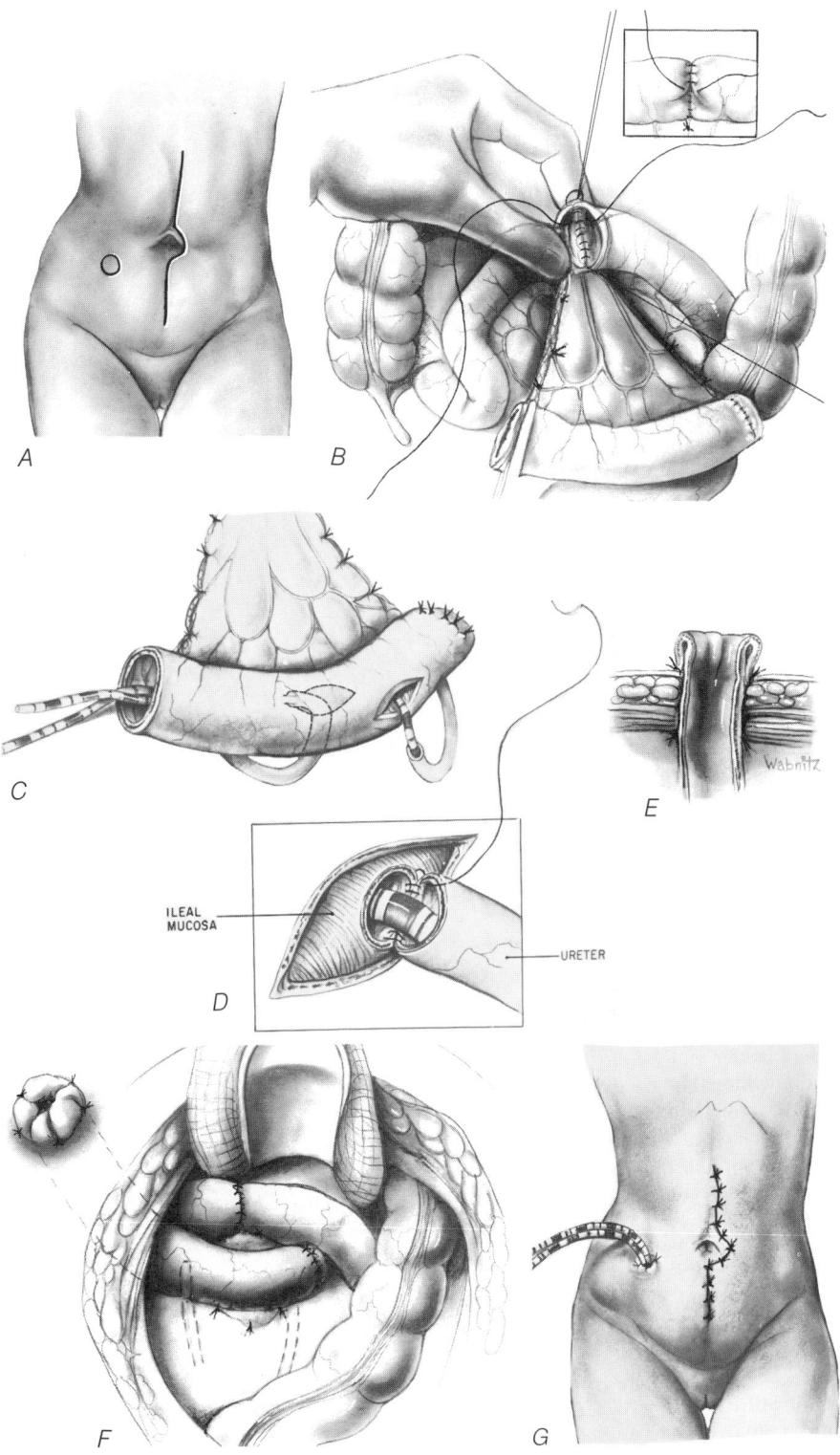

Labels within figure: ILEAL MUCOSA, URETER

A   B   C   D   E   F   G

Fig. 40-38. Cutaneous ureteroileostomy (ileal conduit).

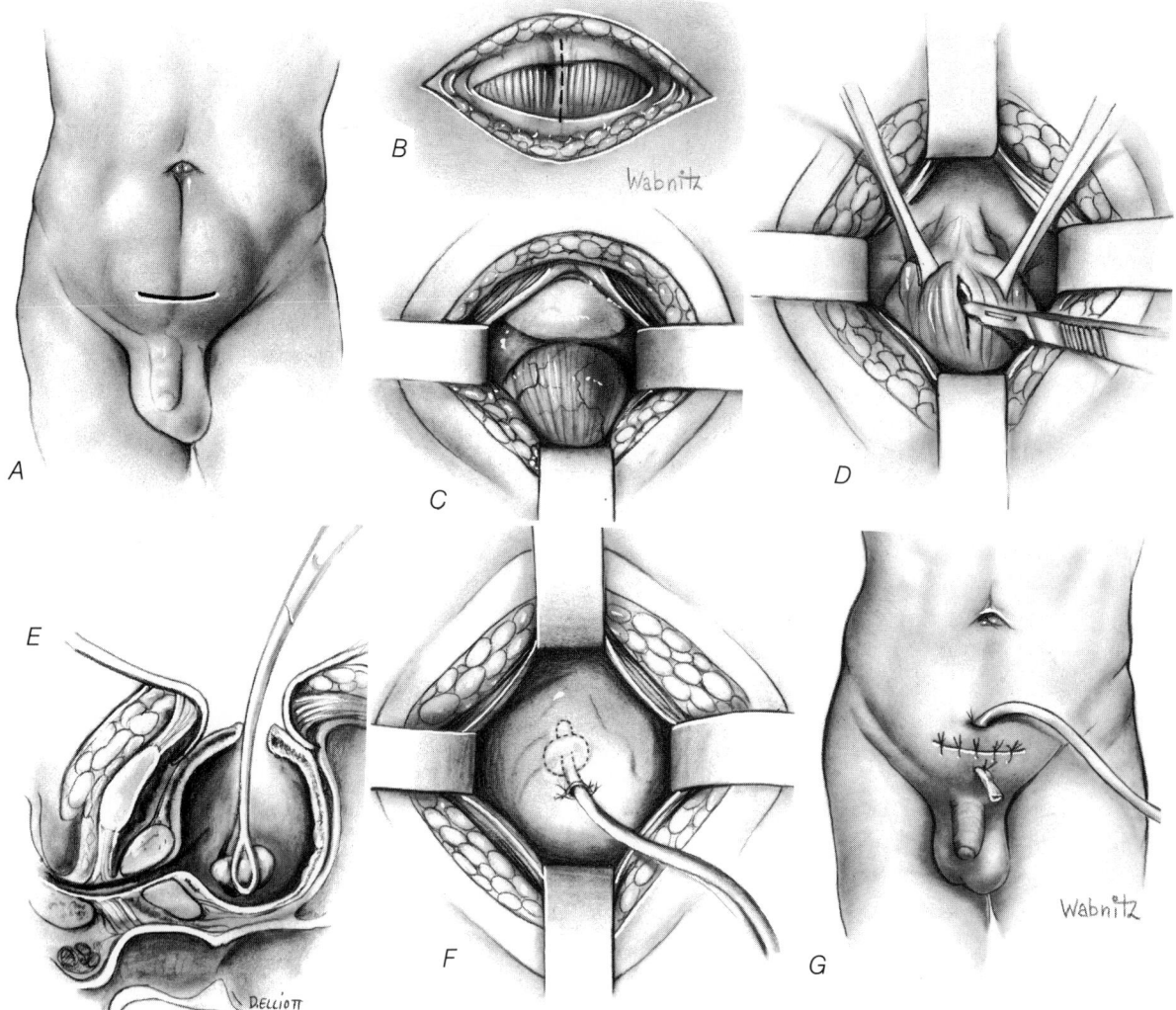

Fig. 40-39. Cystostomy, cystolithotomy (see text).

eter brought out through a stab wound above the incision, or the bladder may be closed primarily. A prevesical tissue drain should be used and brought out through a separate stab wound below the incision. The bladder is closed with a one-layer, continuous, zero chromic catgut suture that incorporates the seromuscular wall of the bladder. The rectus fascia is approximated with interrupted zero chromic catgut or Vicryl sutures. The subcutaneous fat may be approximated with 3-0 interrupted plain catgut sutures and the skin edges with nonabsorbable suture material, such as 4-0 silk, nylon, or staples.

Prostatectomy

TRANSURETHRAL PROSTATECTOMY. The most commonly employed operation for removal of prostatic obstruction is the endoscopic approach. Following adequate spinal or general anesthesia and dilatation of the urethra, the resectoscope sheath is inserted. Excellent visualization through the resectoscope allows for identification of the ureteral orifices, verumontanum, and external sphinc-

ter. With a cutting loop, the prostatic tissue is resected and hemostasis is secured with electrocoagulation. A catheter is inserted at the end of the procedure, and further hemostasis may be obtained by pulling the catheter bag against the bladder neck and prostatic fossa. This procedure is well tolerated by the patient, with minimal postoperative discomfort and early removal of the catheter. Contraindications to the transurethral resection are inability to place the patient in the lithotomy position, an excessively enlarged prostate gland, and the presence of other intravesical pathologic conditions that warrant open exploration. The skilled operator is able to avoid the complications of excessive bleeding, ureteral orifice injury, perforation, and injury to the external sphincter. The results of this procedure are gratifying, and it can be performed on elderly, debilitated patients with minimal morbidity and mortality.

SUPRAPUBIC PROSTATECTOMY (Fig. 40-40). This is performed through the cystostomy approach previously described. The compressed normal prostate represents

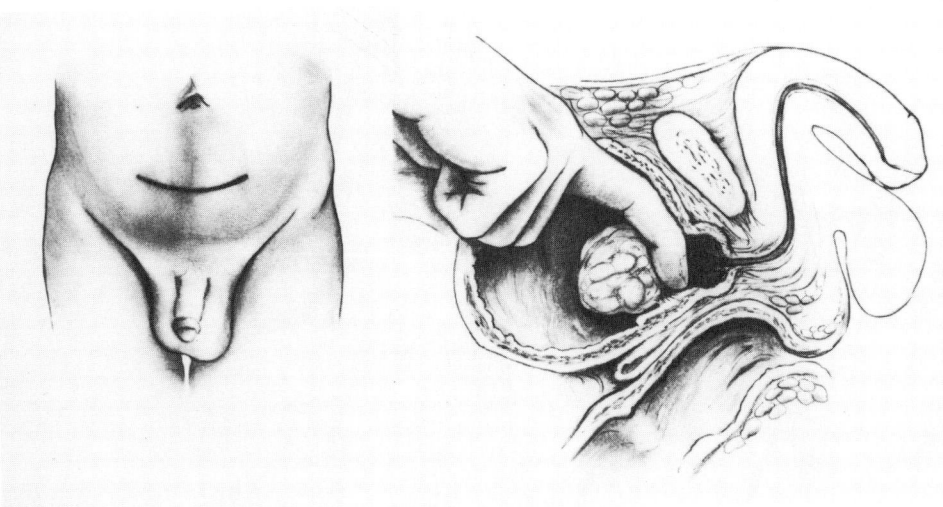

Fig. 40-40. Suprapubic prostatectomy.

the surgical capsule from which adenomatous tissue is mobilized and enucleated by finger dissection. The prostatic urethra and adenomas are removed together. The urethral attachment is transected, and the prostatic fossa is packed while the prostatic arteries that are located on either side of the posterior bladder neck are suture-ligated. Redundant mucosal fragments or small adenomas may be removed by sharp dissection. After the pack is removed, a #22 F, 30-mL urethral retention catheter is inserted. If oozing from the bladder neck or prostatic fossa occurs, gentle traction on the urethral catheter may effect hemostasis. A Malecot catheter and tissue drain are employed in similar fashion to that described for suprapubic cystostomy. The suprapubic tube is usually removed in 2 to 3 days and the urethral catheter in 5 to 7 days.

RETROPUBIC PROSTATECTOMY. This is also accomplished through the incision described for cystotomy. After the bladder wall is identified, the bladder is decompressed, and a 5-cm transverse incision is made 1.5 cm distal to the bladder neck. An alternative approach, known as a vesicocapsular prostatectomy, employs a vertical incision in line with the urethra and into the bladder and has the advantages of easier closure and avoidance of the anterior prostatic venous plexus. After the prostatic capsule is incised, the adenomas are mobilized by finger dissection. The distal urethra and bladder neck attachments are transected and hemostasis is effected by suture ligature. The prostatic capsule is closed with interrupted catgut sutures, and a watertight closure is desirable. The bladder is drained by a urethral retention catheter. Traction on the catheter following retropubic prostatectomy is not as effective for hemostasis as it is following transvesical prostatectomy and may interfere with closure of the capsule. If additional security against catheter obstruction is desired, a suprapubic cystostomy can be performed.

Hydrocelectomy (Fig. 40-41)

A vertical scrotal incision is usually employed. It is carried through the skin, dartos, and overlying coverings of the hydrocele sac. It is desirable to avoid opening the hydrocele until the sac is totally mobilized. The tunica vaginalis is then opened and the excess tunica excised. Hemostasis is secured with multiple ligatures or electrocoagulation of the small bleeders in the cut edge. The edges of the tunica may be sutured together behind the testis with a continuous 3-0 chromic suture. If hemostasis is satisfactory, this may not be necessary. A drain may be brought out through a stab wound in a dependent portion of the scrotum if the hydrocele is excessively large, but in most instances a drain is not required. The incision is then closed in layers with absorbable sutures. A scrotal suspensory provides an excellent dressing in the postoperative period, and the use of an ice bag decreases the swelling. Hydrocelectomy in children is carried out through an inguinal incision so that an associated hernia can be repaired at the same time.

Inguinal Orchiectomy (Fig. 40-42)

This approach is utilized when a testicular tumor is suspected. It provides access to the spermatic vessels prior to manipulation of the testis. The incision is identical to that performed for repair of a hernia, and the spermatic cord is identified at the external inguinal ring. After a rubber-shod or bulldog clamp has been applied to the cord at this level, the testis is mobilized from its scrotal attachments and exteriorized through the inguinal incision. The tunica vaginalis is opened to permit examination of the testis, and if the lesion looks or feels neoplastic, the cord is ligated and transected. Any solid lesion within the testis is considered potentially malignant, and biopsy is seldom performed. A metal clip is placed in the end of the remaining cord as a marker for future surgery or radiation therapy localization. After the testis has been

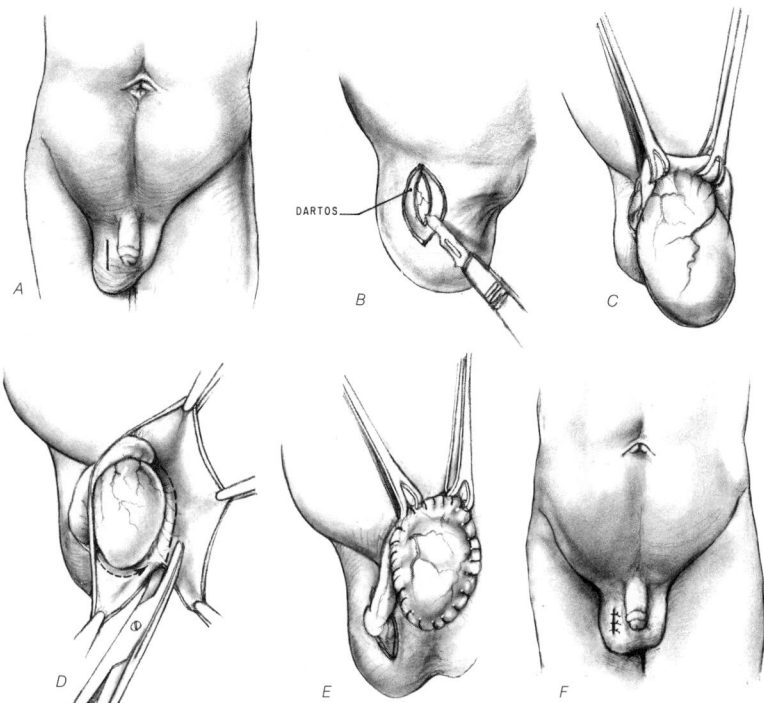

Fig. 40-41. Hydrocelectomy (see text).

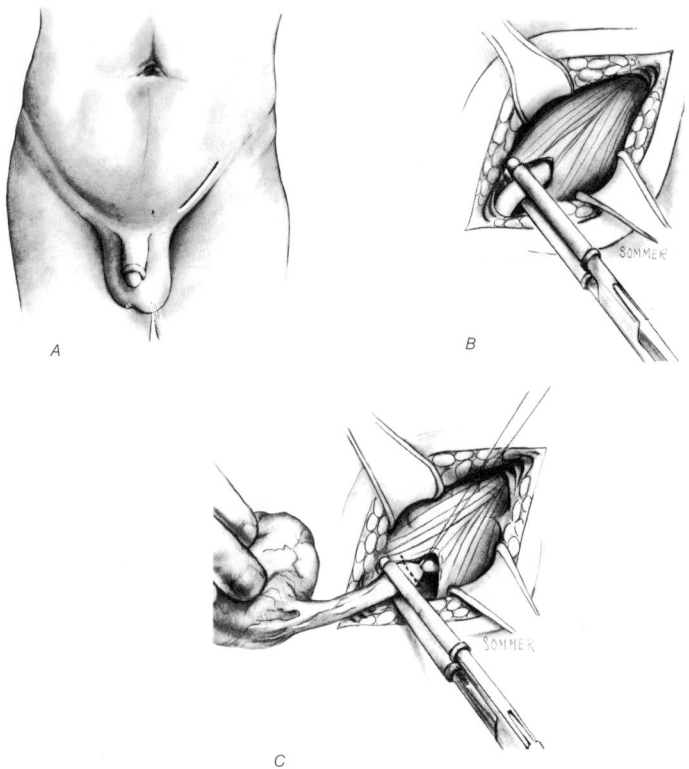

Fig. 40-42. Inguinal orchiectomy (see text)

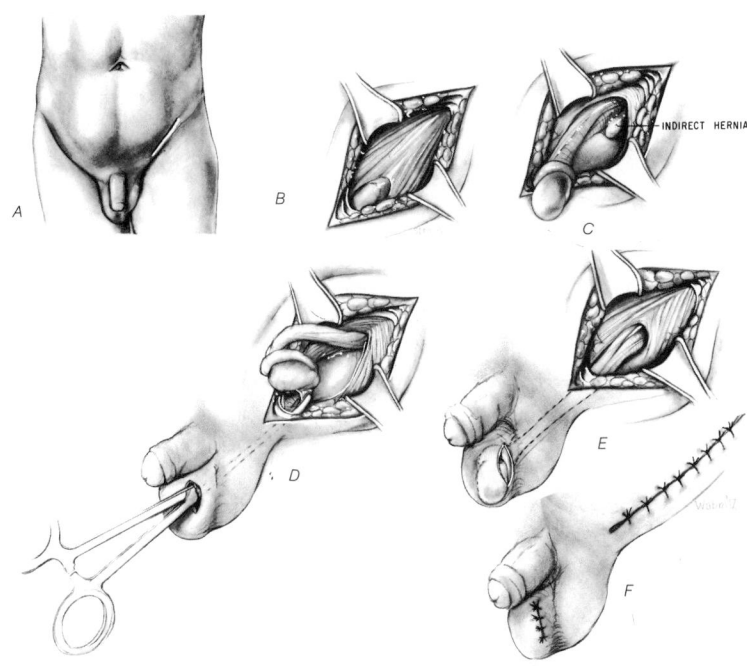

Fig. 40-43. Transseptal orchiopexy (see text).

removed, the inguinal incision is closed. The incision is *not* drained.

Transseptal Orchiopexy (Fig. 40-43)

The testis is identified through an inguinal incision that permits mobilization of the spermatic cord and correction of an indirect hernia that usually accompanies the undescended testis. After sufficient length of cord structures has been mobilized to permit placement of the testis in the scrotum, a small incision is made in the contralateral scrotum and a subdartos pouch is prepared to receive the cryptorchid testis. The scrotal septum is incised over a clamp, and traction is applied to the gubernaculum so that the testis is brought down through the scrotal septum into the contralateral scrotum. The septal defect may require a partial closure to prevent the testis from pulling back but should not be closed too tightly, since strangulation of the cord could occur. The testis may be brought down on the same side without using the transseptal method if there is absolutely no tension. The scrotal and inguinal incisions are closed, and the patient is usually able to leave the hospital the same day or a day later.

Bilateral Vasectomy (Fig. 40-44)

This male sterilization procedure usually is carried out under local anesthesia in an outpatient setting. Previous consultation with the patient and his wife has allowed for careful selection, instruction to the patient, and the signing of the required papers for sterilization and informed consent. The patient or his wife has been instructed to shave the scrotum on the night before the procedure, and

the patient brings a scrotal suspensory with him to the office. The procedure is carried out with the patient in the lithotomy or supine position. The vas on one side is isolated between thumb and index finger of the operator, and the overlying skin is infiltrated with 1% lidocaine or a similar local anesthetic agent. The underlying cord is also infiltrated. A towel clip is then used to isolate the vas. A small incision is made over the vas, and it is delivered into the incision. An Allis clamp is then used to pick up the vas and separate it from the surrounding cord structures. The vas is then mobilized for approximately 3 cm. A segment measuring approximately 1 to 2 cm is excised between clamps. The edges of the vas are then transfixed with sutures. Another suture is placed approximately 1 cm below the previous suture and tied. The end of that

Fig. 40-44. Vasectomy. *A.* Scrotal incision. *B.* Double ligation of vasa (see text).

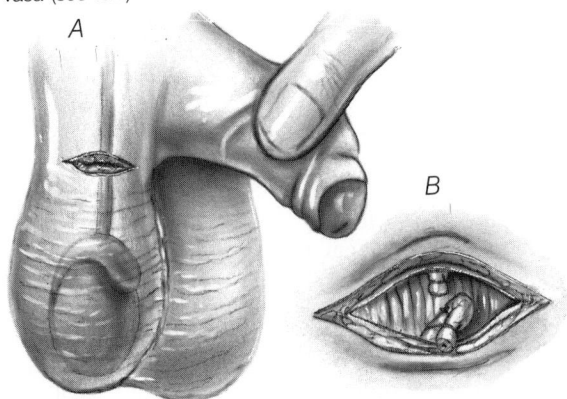

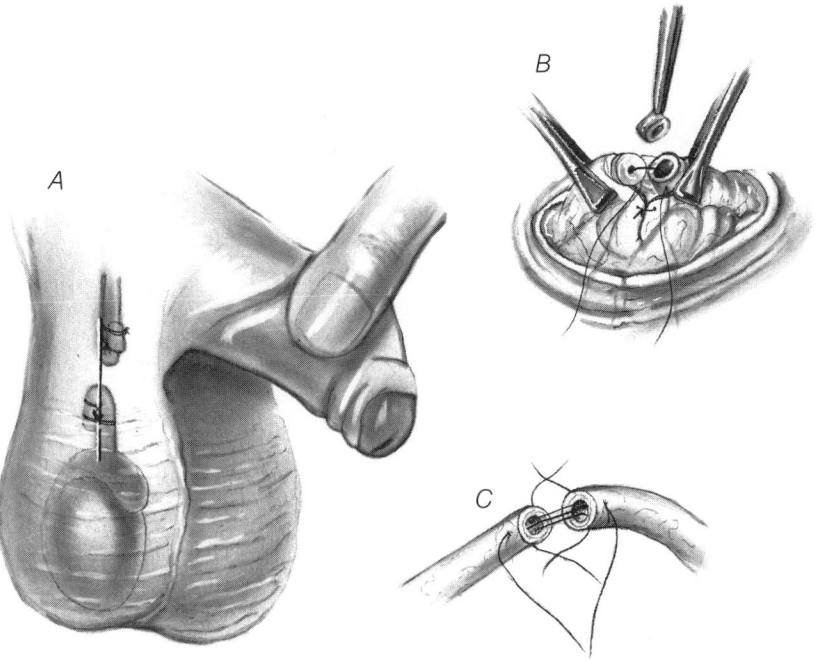

Fig. 40-45. Vasovasostomy. *A.* Scrotal incision. *B.* Excision of ligated (scarred) ends. *C.* Reanastamosis of ends, restoring continuity.

suture is then passed through the end of the vas and tied, producing a means of bending the vas back on itself so that the ends are no longer in close proximity. One of the ends can also be buried in the adjacent tissues to prevent recanalization. An alternative technique involving electrocoagulation of the lumen of each end is commonly employed. After satisfactory hemostasis has been secured, the ends of the vas are dropped back into the incision. The edges of the skin and underlying dartos are then approximated. A similar procedure is then carried out on the other side. Incorporating the underlying dartos in the skin closure provides excellent hemostasis. A collodion dressing is then applied, and the patient uses the scrotal suspensory over a small gauze dressing. He is instructed to use an ice bag on that area for the remainder of the day and returns to work wearing the scrotal suspensory the following day. He is advised to expect a minimal amount of discomfort, swelling, and ecchymosis. When he resumes intercourse, he continues contraception until an examination of his semen reveals no sperm. This usually requires a period of 6 weeks or at least 10 ejaculations to evacuate the remaining sperm that are distal to the anastomotic sites.

Vasovasostomy (Fig. 40-45)

This procedure is usually carried out on an in-hospital basis and with the patient under regional, general, or spinal anesthesia. An incision is made in the scrotum, and the underlying cord structures are delivered into view. The previous site of vasectomy is usually palpable unless a large segment of the vas has been excised. Magnifying lenses, or the use of the operating microscope, facilitate the operation and improve the results. Once the ends of

the vas have been isolated, they are excised back to a normal-appearing vas deferens. The lumen is dilated with lacrimal duct dilators. The ends are then carefully approximated and sutured with Prolene sutures. Finer suture material may be utilized when the operating microscope is employed. The lumen is usually reestablished by passage of some of the sutures through it. Care must be taken to prevent excessive tension on the completed anastomosis. Bleeding is minimal, and the reconstituted vas is then dropped back into the scrotum and the skin and dartos approximated. A similar procedure is then carried out on the other side. The patient is often able to leave the hospital the same day or the following day. Sperm may begin to appear in the ejaculate as early as 1 month following the procedure, but most often this does not occur until 2 or 3 months following the procedure, at which time the edema may subside enough to allow passage of sperm through the small lumen of the vas deferens. Satisfactory reconstitution with sperm in the ejaculate occurs in approximately 80 percent of cases. A higher percentage of success is reported when microsurgery is used. A satisfactory surgical result does not ensure that a pregnancy will result, since other factors such as sperm quality and antisperm antibodies may play a role in persistent infertility.

Bibliography

Bagshaw MA, Ray GR, Cox RS: Radiotherapy of prostatic carcinoma: Long- or short-term efficacy (Stanford University experience). *Urology* 25(suppl):17, 1985.

Byar DR: The Veterans Administration Cooperative Urological

Research Group's studies of cancer of the prostate. *Cancer* 32:1126, 1973.

Carson CC III, Segura JW, et al: Clinical importance of microhematuria. *JAMA* 241:149, 1979.

Chaussy C, et al: Extracorporeal shock wave lithotripsy for treatment of urolithiasis. *Urology* (special issue) 23:59, 1984.

Coe FL: Treated and untreated recurrent calcium nephrolithiasis in patients with idiopathic hypercalciuria, hyperuricosuria, or no metabolic disorder. *Ann Intern Med* 87:404, 1977.

Coe FL: Nephrolithiasis: Causes, classifications and management. *Hosp Pract* April 1981, p 33.

Coe FL, Favus MJ: Disorders of stone formation, in Brenner BM, Rector FC (eds): *The Kidney,* 2d ed. Philadelphia, Saunders, 1981, vol 2, pp 1950–2007.

D'Angio GJ, Evans A, et al: The treatment of Wilms' tumor: Results of the second national Wilms' tumor study. *Cancer* 47:2302, 1981.

De Kernion JB, Berry D: The diagnosis and treatment of renal cancer. *Cancer* 45:1947, 1980.

Donahue JP, Einhorn LH, et al: Cytoreductive surgery for metastatic testis cancer: Considerations of timing and extent. *J Urol* 123:876, 1980.

Eggleston JC, Walsh PC: Radical prostatectomy with preservation of sexual function: Pathological findings in the first 100 cases. *J Urol* 134:1146, 1985.

Einhorn LH, Donahue J: Cis-diaminodichloroplatinum, vinblastine, and bleomycin combination chemotherapy in disseminated testicular cancer. *Ann Intern Med* 87:293, 1977.

Fair WR, Fair WR III: Clinical value of sensitivity determinations in treating urinary tract infections. *Urology* 19:565, 1982.

Fowler J: Nonseminamatous germ cell cancer of the testis: Current management, future possibilities, in Stamey TA (ed): *1982 Monographs in Urology.* 1982, vol 3.

Frank IN: Urologic and male genital cancers, in Rubin P, Bakemeier RB (eds): *Clinical Oncology for Medical Students and Physicians: A Multidisciplinary Approach,* 6th ed. American Cancer Society, 1983, pp 198–219.

Glenn JF (ed): *Urologic Surgery,* 3d ed. Philadelphia, Lippincott, 1983.

Herr HW, Pinsky CM, et al: Long-term effect of intravesical bacillus Calmette-Guerin on flat carcinoma in situ of the bladder. *J Urol* 135:265, 1986.

Hricak H, Williams RD: Magnetic resonance imaging and its application in urology. *Urology* 23:442, 1984.

Javadapour N (ed): *Principles and Management of Urologic Cancer,* 2d ed. Baltimore, Williams & Wilkins, 1983.

Javadapour N (ed): The role of biological tumor markers in testicular cancer. *Cancer* 45:1755, 1980.

Javadapour N (ed): *Recent Advances in Urologic Cancer.* Baltimore, Williams & Wilkins, 1982, vol 2.

Kelalis PP, King LR, et al (eds): *Clinical Pediatric Urology,* 2d ed. Philadelphia, Saunders, 1985.

Klimberg IW, Wajsman Z: Treatment for muscle invasive carcinoma of the bladder. *J Urol* 136:1986.

McDonald MW: Current therapy for renal carcinoma. *J Urol* 127:211, 1982.

Meares EM Jr: Prostatitis syndromes: New perspectives about old woes. *J Urol* 123:141, 1980.

Murphy GP, Gaeta JF, et al: Current status of classification and staging of prostate cancer. *Cancer* 45:1889, 1980.

Pak YC: Medical management of nephrolithiasis. *J Urol* 128:1157, 1982.

Pak YC, Britton F, et al: Ambulatory evaluation of nephrolithiasis, classification, clinical presentation and diagnostic criteria. *Am J Med* 67:19, 1980.

Proceedings from a workshop symposium of the 14th International Congress of Chemotherapy. *Urology* 27(suppl):2, 1986.

Proceedings of symposium on prostatic carcinoma: Issues and debate. Part I. *Urology* 24(suppl):2, 1984.

Proceedings of symposium on prostatic carcinoma: Issues and debate. Part II. *Urology* 25(suppl):2, 1985.

Radwin HM: Radiotherapy and bladder cancer: A critical review. *J Urol* 124:43, 1980.

Resnick MI, Older RA: *Diagnosis of Genitourinary Disease.* New York, Thieme-Stratton, 1982.

Riehle RA Jr, Fair WR, Vaughan D Jr: Extracorporeal shock wave lithotripsy for upper urinary tract calculi: One year's experience at a single center. *JAMA* 255:2043, 1986.

Silverberg E: Cancer statistics, 1982. *CA* 37:2, 1987.

Skinner DG, de Kernion JB (eds): *Genitourinary Cancer.* Philadelphia, Saunders, 1978.

Solaway MS (ed): The role of intravesical therapy in the management of urothelial cancer. *Urology* 26(suppl):18, 1985.

Solaway MS: Intravesical and systemic chemotherapy in the management of superficial bladder cancer. *Urol Clin North Am* 11:623, 1984.

Solaway MS: Overview of treatment of superficial bladder cancer. *Urology* 26:18, 1985.

Stamey TA (ed): *Pathogenesis and Treatment of Urinary Tract Infections.* Baltimore, Williams & Wilkins, 1980.

Stamey TA (ed): Prostatitis. *1981 Monographs in Urology* 2:31, 1981.

Stamey TA (ed): Cancer of the prostate: An analysis of some important contributions and dilemmas. *1982 Monographs in Urology* 3:67, 1982.

Stamey TA, Wehner N, et al: The immunologic basis of recurrent bacteriuria: Role of cervicovaginal antibody in enterobacterial colonization of the introital mucosa. *Medicine* 57:47, 1978.

Vugrin D, Whitmore WF Jr: The role of chemotherapy and surgery in the treatment of retroperitoneal metastases in advanced nonseminomatous testis cancer. *Cancer* 55:1874, 1985.

Walsh PC, et al (eds): *Campbell's Urology,* 5th ed. Philadelphia, Saunders, 1985.

Walsh PC, Lepor H, Eggleston JC: Radical prostatectomy with preservation of sexual function: Anatomical and pathological considerations. *Prostate* 4:473, 1983.

Yendt ER, Cohanim M: Prevention of calcium stones with thiazides. *Kidney Int* 13:397, 1978.

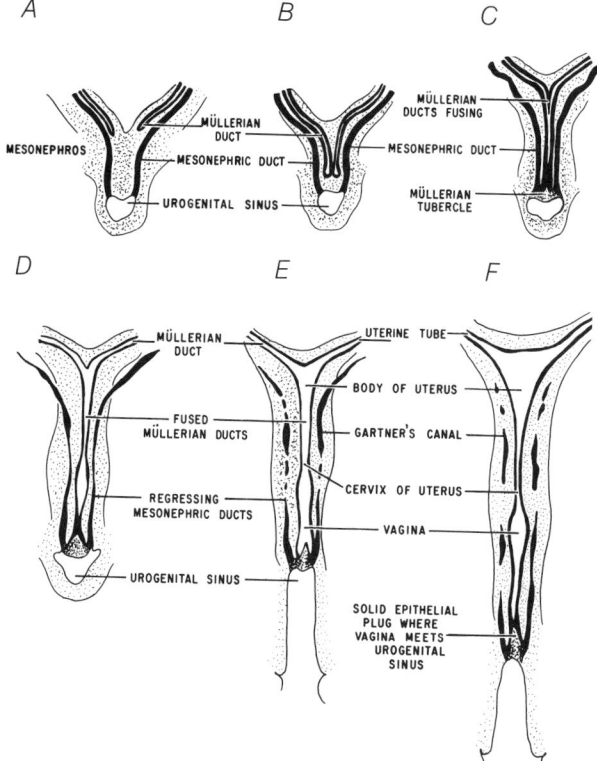

Fig. 41-1. Fusion of the müllerian ducts to form the uterus and vagina. *A.* 23 mm. *B.* 25 mm. *C.* 32.9 mm. *D.* 48 mm. *E.* 63 mm. *F.* 69 mm. *(Redrawn after Koff: Carnegie Contributions to Embryology, vol 24. 1933, with permission.)*

Fig. 41-2. Schematic diagram showing plan of developing female reproductive system. (From: *Patton BM: Human Embryology, 2d ed. New York, McGraw-Hill, 1953, with permission.*)

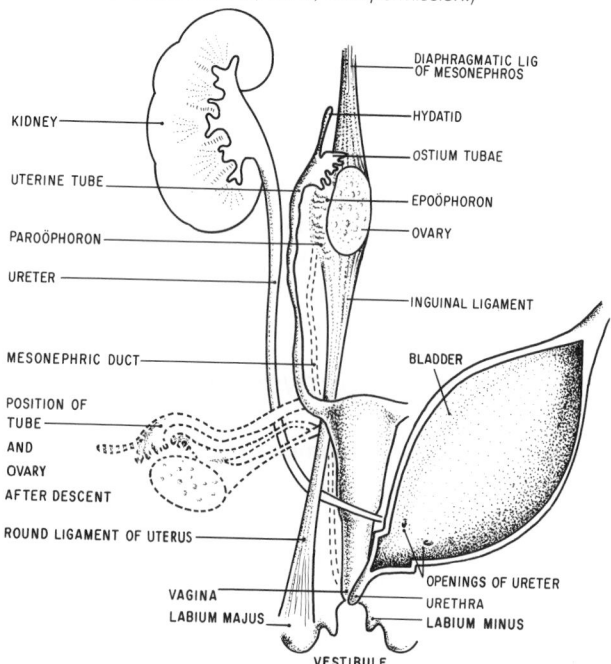

their lower two-thirds before the eleventh week of gestation; from this evolves the adult internal genital apparatus (Fig. 41-1). At the lower end it establishes communication with an entodermal derivative, the urogenital sinus, which, when fully differentiated, provides distinct and separate orifices for the urethra and vagina. The distal colon and anus lie well posterior.

In a classic set of experiments on the fetal rabbit, Alfred Jost contributed to our understanding of factors that affect the sexual dimorphism of the internal genital ducts. Bilateral castration of a male in early fetal development led to bilateral müllerian structures. Unilateral castration of a male produced müllerian development on the agonadal side and male (wolffian) development on the testis side. Bilateral castration of a male and administration of androgens led to both müllerian and wolffian development. The conclusions were (1) without a male gonad (or with a female gonad) müllerian structures arise; (2) androgens promote wolffian development; (3) a müllerian inhibiting factor (MIF) is produced by the testis which acts locally to prevent the development of müllerian structures.

The external genitalia begin as folds of ectoderm from the genital tubercle (clitoris), passing back on either side of the orifices and eventually forming the vulva with its major and minor labia (Fig. 41-2). The hymenal membrane partially occludes the vaginal canal at the level of the urogenital diaphragm, below the point of juncture between the urogenital sinus and the müllerian ducts. Although the male structures normally regress, remnants can often be seen as small cystic swellings near the ovaries (paraovarian cysts), as histologically recognizable rests in the broad ligaments or cervix, or as cystic tumors of the vagina (Gärtner's duct cysts).

A variety of anomalies of the tubes, uterus, cervix, and vagina have been described (Fig. 41-3). All are easily explained as improper müllerian duct development, either in partial or complete failure to fuse, in asymmetrical growth, or in unilateral or bilateral failure to develop. In approximately 10 percent of patients, müllerian anomalies are accompanied by renal (wolffian) abnormalities, including absent or malformed kidneys; therefore, an intravenous pyelogram (IVP) should be performed in individuals with these congenital uterine abnormalities. Abnormal development of the external genital structures usually takes the form of some degree of masculinization. There is enlargement of the clitoris and occasionally fusion of the labial folds caused by excessive androgen stimulation of the fetus in utero. When the hymen is imperforate, there is complete mechanical obstruction of the outlet of the vagina, usually resulting in a blood-filled pelvic mass, a *hematocolpos*, first noted months or years after menstruation should have started. Transverse fibrous ridges of the vagina and cervix, as well as distortions of the cavity of the uterus, have been described in association with intrauterine exposure to diethylstilbestrol (DES) and similar compounds. These presumably result from a disturbance in the development of the müllerian ducts; in the case of vaginal ridges, the urogenital sinus development may have been affected.

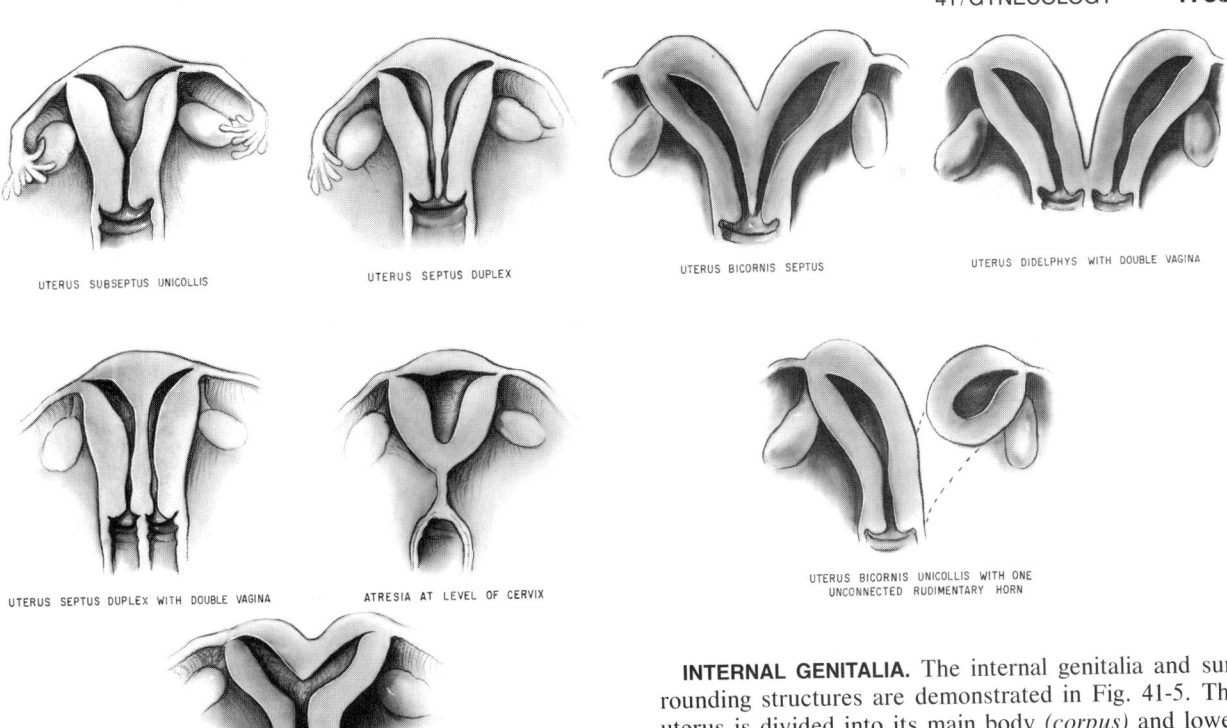

UTERUS SUBSEPTUS UNICOLLIS

UTERUS SEPTUS DUPLEX

UTERUS BICORNIS SEPTUS

UTERUS DIDELPHYS WITH DOUBLE VAGINA

UTERUS SEPTUS DUPLEX WITH DOUBLE VAGINA

ATRESIA AT LEVEL OF CERVIX

UTERUS BICORNIS UNICOLLIS WITH ONE UNCONNECTED RUDIMENTARY HORN

UTERUS BICORNIS UNICOLLIS

Fig. 41-3. Schematic diagram of various types of abnormal uteri.

Morphologic Anatomy

EXTERNAL GENITALIA. The external genitalia are shown in Fig. 41-4. The entrance to the vagina (introitus) is bounded laterally by two folds of skin, the external labia majora and the internal labia minora. The labia majora form the lateral boundary of the vulva. They meet anteriorly toward the lower abdomen and fuse in an area over the pubis known as the *mons veneris*. The posterior extensions of the labia meet in an area known as the *posterior commissure*. Just above the posterior commissure is the caudal part of the vaginal opening known as the *posterior fourchette*. The *vestibule* consists of that area into which the vagina and the urethra open and which is bounded laterally by the labia. The vulva includes both labia, the vestibular structures, and the clitoris. The clitoris lies immediately above the urethral meatus and is the analog of the male phallus. The *perineum* refers to the area between the rectum and the vagina, and it is through the tissues of this area that obstetric episiotomies are made.

Two types of glands can be considered with the external genitalia of the female. Skene's glands are located about the urethra and are important as a site of infection in cases of gonorrhea. Bartholin's glands are located immediately deep to the labia majora. The invasion of these glands by bacterial organisms results in acute bartholinitis and Bartholin's abscesses.

INTERNAL GENITALIA. The internal genitalia and surrounding structures are demonstrated in Fig. 41-5. The uterus is divided into its main body *(corpus)* and lower portion *(cervix)*. The fallopian tubes open into either side of the endometrial cavity of the uterus, traversing the wall of the uterus at the interstitial end of the tube. It exits the cornua of the uterus and becomes the isthmic portion of the tube. The tube widens throughout its course laterally to its ampullary, or infundibular, end. The ovaries are suspended immediately posterior to the tubes by a mesentery *(mesovarium)*. The round ligaments run laterally from the uterus through the inguinal ring in the anterior abdominal wall and end in the labia majora. They lie anteriorly to the fallopian tubes, a fact that is useful in orient-

Fig. 41-4. External genitalia of the female.

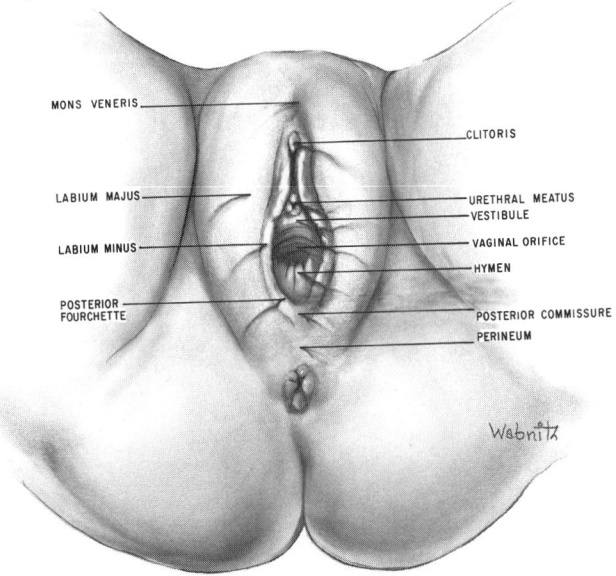

MONS VENERIS

CLITORIS

LABIUM MAJUS

URETHRAL MEATUS
VESTIBULE

LABIUM MINUS

VAGINAL ORIFICE

HYMEN

POSTERIOR FOURCHETTE

POSTERIOR COMMISSURE

PERINEUM

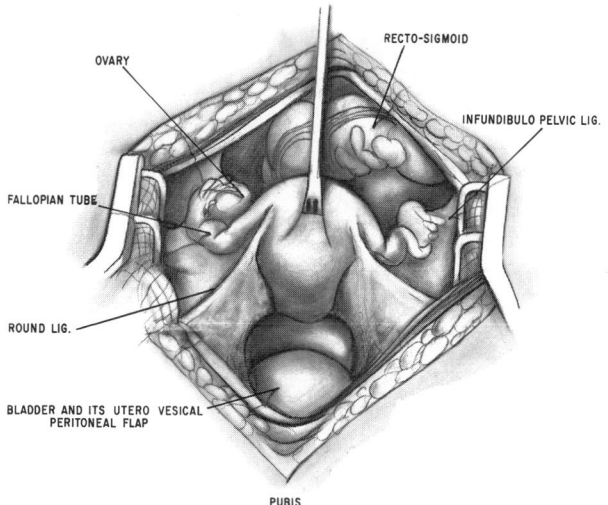

Fig. 41-5. Internal genitalia and surrounding structures.

ing surgical specimens. The round ligament forms the apex for the folds of peritoneum that contain the uterine blood supply (broad ligament). At the base of the broad ligament, running from the cervix to the lateral pelvic wall, are important supporting structures known as the ''cardinal'' (Mackenrodt's) ligaments. Posterior to these and running from the cervix to the sacrum are the utero-sacral ligaments. These ligaments and the relationship of the cervix to the bladder and the rectum with the spaces surrounding these structures are shown in Fig. 41-6.

The blood supply to the female pelvis is illustrated in Fig. 41-7, which shows the distribution of the common iliac, external iliac, and internal iliac arteries (hypogastric arteries). It should be noted that the posterior division of the internal iliac artery gives off its superior gluteal

branch and then continues farther to split into its varying visceral branches. The remainder of the hypogastric artery continues inferiorly into the pelvis and gives off the obturator artery and the obliterated internal iliac artery distal to the superior vesical branch, which runs to the bladder; other branches, including the uterine artery, run to the central pelvic organs. Each ureter enters the pelvis near the bifurcation of the common iliac artery. It passes medial to the internal iliac artery and runs immediately beneath the uterine artery, an important landmark in the anatomy of pelvic dissection (Fig. 41-32). The ureter then passes forward over the lateral aspect of the cervix and vagina to reach the bladder. Additional blood supply is contributed by the ovarian arteries which arise from the abdominal aorta just below the renal arteries and pass to the ovary on each side.

THE PELVIC ENVIRONMENT. Between the uterosacral ligaments anterior to the rectum and posterior to the cervix is a space known as the *cul-de-sac,* or *pouch of Douglas,* the most dependent extension of the free peritoneal cavity. This important area can be used for diagnostic exploration of the pelvis via the vagina. The uterosacral and cardinal ligaments form important stays for preventing prolapse of the uterus by helping to fix the position of the cervix back toward the hollow of the sacrum. Their effects can be demonstrated at the operating table by the great increase in mobility of the uterus and cervix after these ligaments are cut. The round ligament, though a firm structure, does not prevent *descensus,* i.e., downward motion of the uterus and cervix in the plane of the vagina. Changes in the length of the round ligaments do

Fig. 41-7. Anterior and superior view of the arterial system of the pelvis showing the named primary arteries and their relationships to the bony and ligamentous structures.

Fig. 41-6. Diagrammatic cross section of the pelvis to show the concentration of connective tissue forming ligamentous bands, the junction with the cardinal ligament (Mackenrodt's ligament), and the spaces and tissue planes. (Adapted from: *Peham H, Amreich I: Gynakologische Operationslehre, Berlin, Verlag Von S. Karger, 1930, p 191, with permission.*)

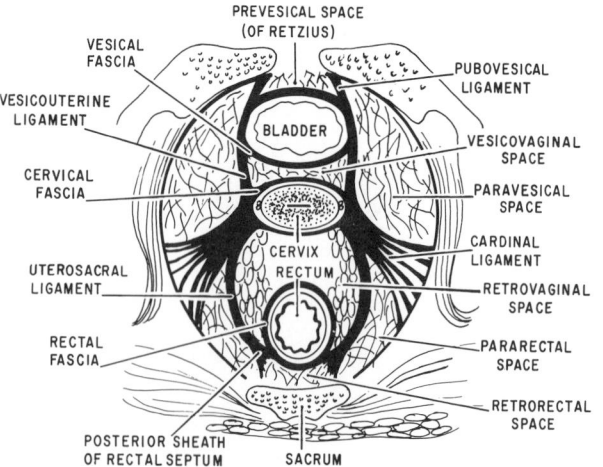

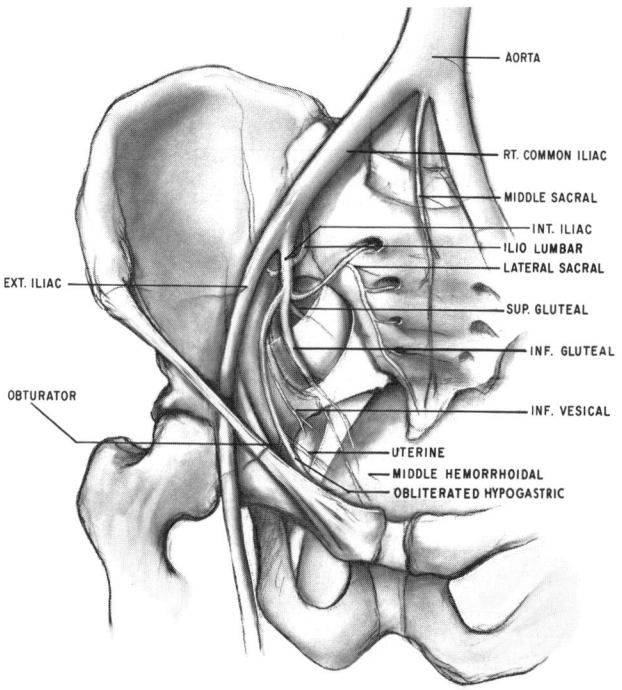

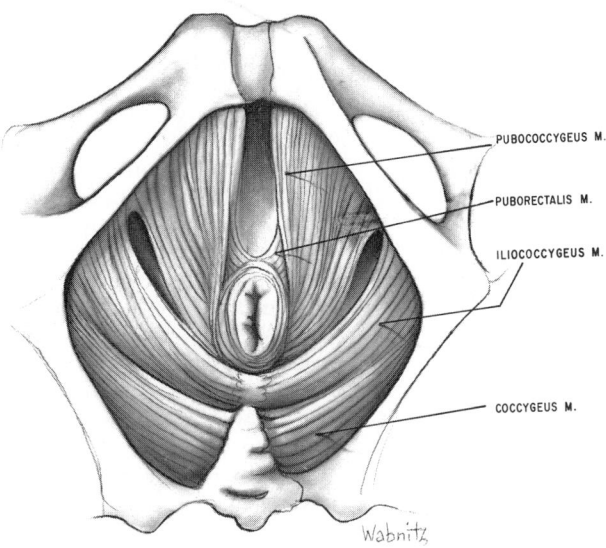

Fig. 41-8. Components of the levator muscles viewed from below.

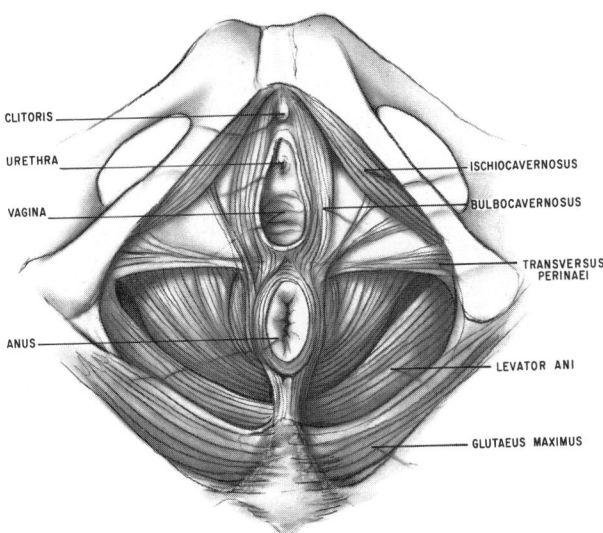

Fig. 41-9. Superficial layer of the urogenital diaphragm in the female.

appear to accompany changes in the anterior or posterior displacement of the uterus and cervix. Posterior displacement of the fundus is termed *retroversion,* a common finding in females during their reproductive years, especially following pregnancy. It is, in fact, so common that one should be extremely cautious before ascribing any pain or pelvic complaint to the existence of a retroverted uterus.

In addition to the ligamentous supports noted above, a firm and strong supportive shelf is provided by the levator ani muscles, as shown in Fig. 41-8. In the female this muscular complex is pierced by the urethra, vagina, and rectum, and these orifices provide a structural weakness for the start of herniation that may be seen in adult life. A second layer of reinforcement beyond the shelf of the levator ani muscles is provided by the muscles of the urogenital diaphragm, which is located between the ischial tuberosities and the pubis, as shown in Fig. 41-9. This secondary layer provides muscular support anteriorly to the main mass of the levator ani muscle. Thus it can be seen that in addition to the bony pelvis, the main support to the pelvic organs in the erect human female is provided by striated muscle, mainly of the levator ani complex, and partially by the urogenital diaphragm. The firm ligamentous attachments at the base of the cervix (the cardinal and uterosacral ligaments) stabilize the uterus at the apex of the vagina.

Weaknesses that give rise to various forms of herniation can occur in this area. Protrusion of the anterior vaginal wall, which includes the bladder, is referred to as a *cystocele,* while protrusion of the posterior vaginal wall, which includes the rectum, is referred to as a *rectocele.* The latter will occur especially after separation of the levator muscles following childbirth. If weakness develops in the area of the cul-de-sac, this portion of the vaginal wall descends, occasionally accompanied by the small bowel, resulting in an *enterocele.* A weakness can occur in the distal anterior vaginal wall with a bulging of the

urethra. This occurs after destruction of the fascial support of the urethra and the bladder neck, and urinary incontinence may accompany the hernia in these patients. Weakness can develop in the ligamentous support of the uterus as well as in the muscular support, and this results in varying degrees of uterine and cervical prolapse, as illustrated in Fig. 41-10.

ENDOCRINOLOGY

Hypothalamic Releasing Factors and Gonadotropic Hormones

Releasing factors are polypeptides that originate from the hypothalamus and travel via the portal system to the pituitary. A decapeptide, *luteinizing hormone-releasing factor* (LRF, or GnRH for gonadotropin-releasing hormone, which is synonymous with LRF) has been identified and seems to be associated with gonadotropin synthesis and release. LRF release is in turn modulated by

Fig. 41-10. Diagrammatic representation of first- and second-degree prolapses of the uterus.

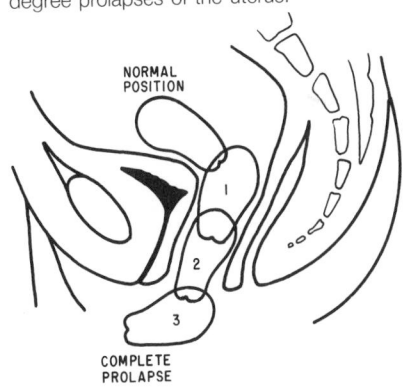

neurosecretory influences from above the hypothalamus. Various neurotransmitters, gonadal steroids, and, possibly, gonadal polypeptides, e.g., inhibin, also affect the synthesis and release of LRF. For example, norepinephrine-containing neuronal pathways seem to be stimulatory to LRF release, and dopaminergic pathways seem to be inhibitory.

Agonist and antagonist analogs of LRF have been synthesized. They have already begun to have clinical utility. For example, long-acting agonists might be used as contraceptives or for the treatment of precocious puberty.

FOLLICLE-STIMULATING HORMONES (FSH). In the female, FSH acts as a stimulator to follicular development, granulosa cell proliferation, and oocyte maturation. In the male, FSH seems to be synergistic with luteinizing hormone (LH) and testosterone in stimulating Leydig cell steroidogenesis. FSH also stimulates the germ cell elements of the testes to proliferate and undergo spermatogenesis.

LUTEINIZING HORMONES (LH). In women, LH is the predominant component of the midcycle FSH-LH surge. This surge is responsible for transformation of the ovarian follicle to a corpus luteum following ovulation. Low levels of LH in the luteal phase maintain the corpus luteum and support its production of progesterone and estrogen.

In the male, LH along with FSH stimulates testosterone secretion and initiates spermatogenesis.

HUMAN CHORIONIC GONADOTROPIN (HCG). This glycoprotein is normally secreted by the placenta during pregnancy. In the human being, HCG secretion is maximal at about 70 days gestation and declines thereafter. It is not detectable at approximately 2 weeks after delivery. Detection of HCG forms the basis of various pregnancy tests. Like FSH and LH, HCG consists of two noncovalently bound subunits designated alpha and beta. The alpha subunit of FSH, LH, HCG, and TSH (*thyroid-stimulating hormone*) is chemically similar and cannot be differentiated by immunoassays directed against it. However, assay of the beta subunit of HCG provides the basis of a sensitive and specific test by radioimmunoassay (RIA) or enzyme linked immunoabsorbent assay (ELISHA). Such assays can detect 5 international milliunits (ImU) per milliliter of serum or urine. This enables a pregnancy to be detected as soon as 72 h after implantation of the fertilized egg or about 10 days after the ovulatory surge of LH. Other less sensitive immunoassays include latex agglutination inhibition tube and slide tests. These will detect pregnancy as early as 5 to 6 weeks, respectively, from the last menstrual period.

HCG, like LH, is luteotropic and supports the corpus luteum during the first 5 to 6 weeks of pregnancy. After this time, placental production of steroids is sufficient to maintain the pregnancy. Ablation of the corpus luteum of pregnancy before 6 weeks can result in an aborted pregnancy.

HCG is also produced by trophoblastic tumors, making this molecule an extremely valuable tumor marker. Other neoplasms, such as germ cell tumors of the ovary and testis, gastric adenocarcinoma, and hepatoblastoma, may also produce HCG.

Steroid Hormones

A schema of steroid metabolism is shown in Fig. 41-11.

ESTROGENS

These female sex hormones are secreted primarily from the ovary with a small contribution from the adrenal. The mature testis also secretes estrogens. In the pregnant female, the placenta is the major source of both estrogens and progesterone. *Estradiol,* quantitatively the most potent estrogen in the nonpregnant female, is secreted throughout the menstrual cycle (Fig. 41-12).

Peripheral conversion of androgens to estrogens by the enzyme aromatase occurs in adipose tissue, muscle, liver, and other tissues. Particularly significant is the conversion of androstenedione to *estrone*. Hyperthyroidism, hepatic disease, aging, and obesity accelerate this conversion. Although obesity is a common accompaniment of endometrial carcinoma, a causal relationship between excessive estrogen production in obese subjects and endometrial cancer has not been established.

Estrogens are stimulatory to the uterus, fallopian tubes, vagina, and breast. The vaginal mucosa thickens with proliferation of the vaginal epithelium and cornification of surface cells under the influence of estrogen. Glycogen accumulates in the epithelial cells. This glycogen creates a favorable environment for lactobacilli that metabolize the glycogen to lactic acid. Thus, after puberty the pH of the vagina drops to about 4.5. This acid pH provides some measure of protection against infection.

Vaginal cytology can be used as a gauge to the hormonal environment in the patient. In the prepubertal, hypoestrogenic girl the predominant vaginal epithelial cell is the parabasal cell (Fig. 41-13A). In response to estrogen these cells mature, with the cytoplasm becoming thin and the nucleus becoming pyknotic, hyperchromatic, and lacking a fine chromatin pattern (Fig. 41-13B).

Estrogens (and other steroids) affect their response by combining with specific receptors in the cell. Messenger RNA (mRNA) is then produced, which directs specific protein synthesis. Measurement of these receptors in various malignancies such as breast and endometrial carcinoma has been useful in predicting hormone responsiveness of these tumors.

PROGESTERONE

Progesterone is secreted in significant quantities after ovulation and luteinization of the preovulatory follicle. Progesterone is thermogenic and also alters the endometrium. These changes are useful in detecting ovulation and include an increase in the basal body temperature of 0.5 to 1°F and/or transformation of a proliferative endometrium to a secretory endometrium (Figs. 41-12 and 41-14). The progestational support of the endometrium is necessary for continuation of pregnancy.

ANDROGENS

The *17-ketosteroids* (17-KS), *dehydroepiandrosterone* (DHA), *DHA sulfate* (DHAS), and *androstenedione* are

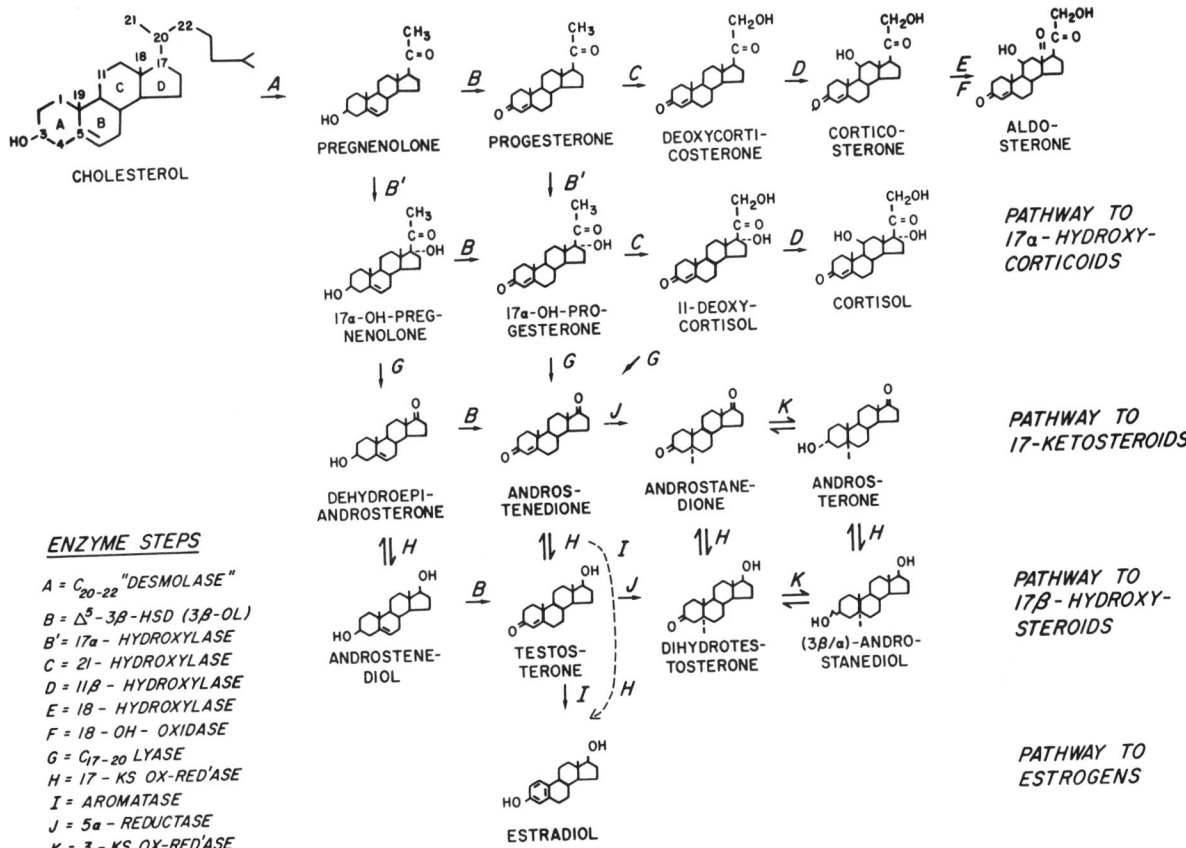

Fig. 41-11. Major pathways of steroid hormone biosynthesis from cholesterol. Relevant carbon atoms of cholesterol are designated by conventional numbers, and rings are indicated by letters. The flow of hormonogenesis is generally to the right and downward. Top line shows pathway from progesterone to mineralocorticoids; second line, pathway to glucocorticoids; third line, pathway to 17-KS; fourth line, pathway to potent androgens. Bottom line and dashed lines indicate those pathways to estrogen [long dashed line involves 17-ketoestrogen, estrone (not shown), as an intermediate]. HSD = hydroxysteroid dehydrogenase; OH = hydroxy. The terms *desmolase* and *lyase* are often used interchangeably, as are the terms *hydroxysteroid dehydrogenase* and *ketosteroid(oxido) reductase*.

the most abundant androgenic steroids secreted by women. However, they are relatively weak androgens. They are probably androgenic only by virtue of the extent to which they are converted to the circulating and target organ 17-β-hydroxysteroids (testosterone, androstenedione, dihydrotestosterone) shown in Fig. 41-11. Testosterone is the most important of the circulating androgens because of its biopotency.

The adrenal cortex secretes androgens as by-products of cortisol biosynthesis. Adrenal secretion normally accounts for the majority of 17-KS. About 90 percent of DHAS originates from the adrenal; hence evaluation of blood levels of this steroid have been used as an indicator of adrenal androgen production. About 25 percent of testosterone is secreted by the adrenal.

Androgens are obligate precursors of estrogens, hence their synthesis by the ovary. The ovary normally ac-

counts for about 25 percent of testosterone secretion and 50 percent of androstenedione production. Androgens are produced predominantly by the theca and interstitial compartments of the ovary in response to LH and FSH. Androgens are also produced by peripheral conversion of steroid precursors by nonendocrine organs. About 50 percent of plasma testosterone normally arises in this manner. Almost all (98 percent) of plasma testosterone is bound to testosterone-estradiol binding globulin (TEBG) and albumin. The biologically active portion of the plasma 17-β-hydroxysteroids appears to be the small proportion that is free from TEBG and albumin binding.

CHRONOLOGIC DEVELOPMENTAL FEMALE PHYSIOLOGY

The normal female infant is born with a small uterus, most of which is cervix. The ovaries and fallopian tubes are present but are much smaller than in the adult. The vaginal mucosa is thin, owing to lack of estrogen stimulation, and as a result is more susceptible to trauma and infection. Because of the high levels of estrogens immediately preceding parturition, the estrogen-dependent organs of the newborn infant may be transiently stimulated. This is the origin of breast milk (witch's milk) that may occasionally be seen in the newborn.

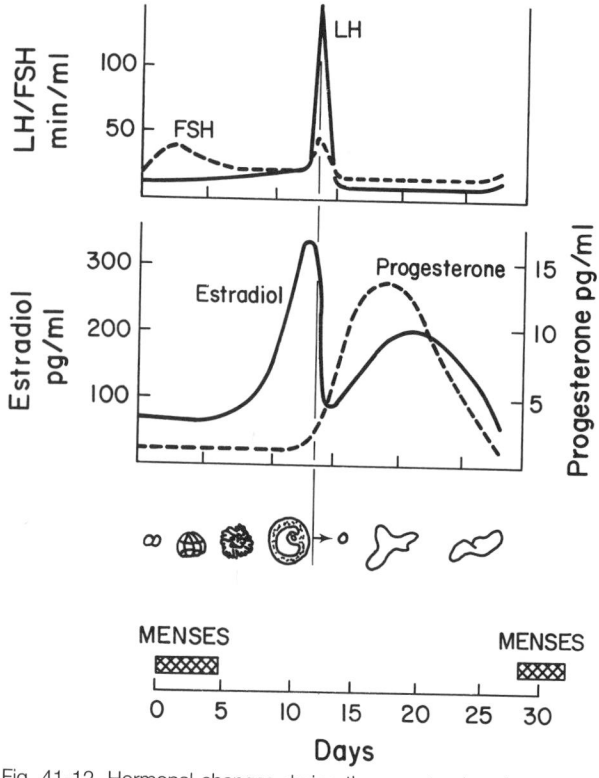

Fig. 41-12. Hormonal changes during the menstrual cycle.

Puberty

The first anatomic evidence of puberty is *thelarche,* or breast budding, which occurs on average at ten and a half years of age. Shortly thereafter the *adrenarche,* or development of pubic and axillary hair in response to adrenal androgen secretion, occurs. Subsequently there is a rapid increase in height which usually takes place at about age twelve years, 6 to 12 months prior to the start of menstruation. Ninety-five percent of females will have had menarche between nine and a half and sixteen years of age (average twelve and three-quarter years). The physiologic mechanisms that initiate puberty in the human being are not known. In laboratory animals, an increasing gonadal sensitivity to LH occurs preceding puberty. In human beings, sleep-induced spikes of LH secretion that stimulate ovarian steroidogenesis have been observed. The pituitary becomes more responsive to LRH, and the exquisite negative feedback between ovarian steroids and pituitary gonadotropins that characterizes the immature state diminishes, and positive feedback mechanisms mature, leading to cyclic ovarian-pituitary activity.

Menstrual bleeding usually follows the development of the secondary sexual characteristics already described. Initial bleeding is usually anovulatory and irregular. Ovulatory cycles, which may occur at 4- to 6-week intervals, begin in about 1 year. Their onset is often heralded by pelvic pain occurring at the time of menses. The average volume of blood loss during a normal menstrual cycle is estimated to be from 35 to 150 mL, and the bleeding will usually last from 3 to 6 days with much individual variation. An interval between menses of 6 to 8 weeks is not uncommon.

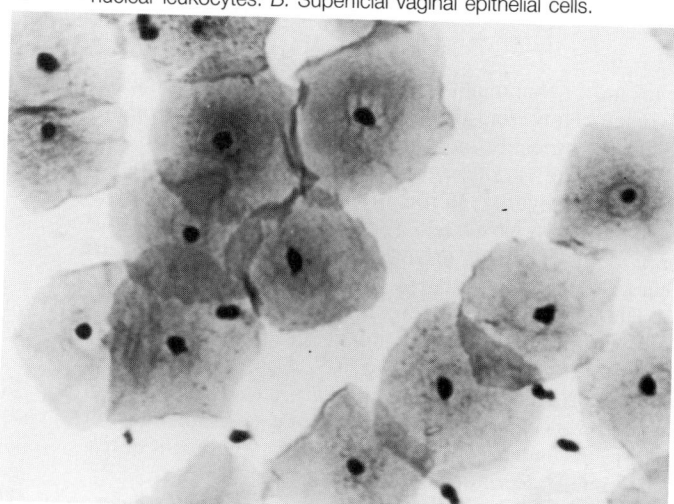

Fig. 41-13. *A.* Parabasal cells. In the background are polymorphonuclear leukocytes. *B.* Superficial vaginal epithelial cells.

A

B

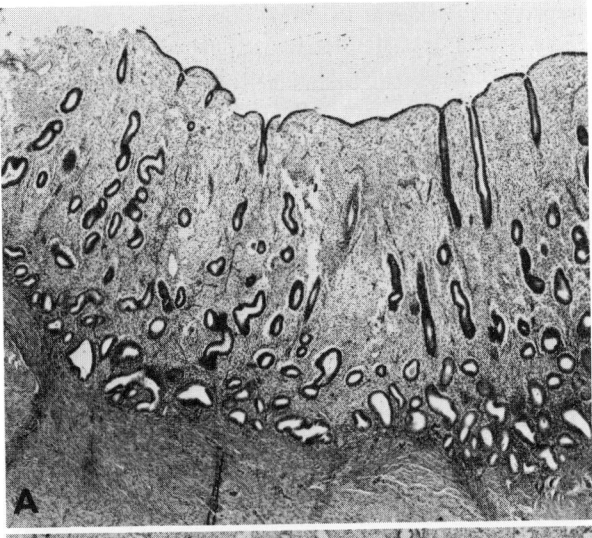

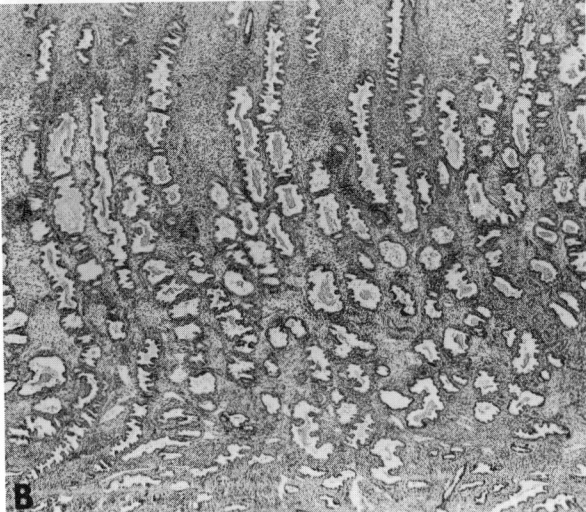

Fig. 41-14. *A.* Proliferative endometrium. *B.* Secretory endometrium.

Reproductive Life

The menstrual cycle in the mature female may be divided into proliferative and secretory phases. The *proliferative phase* begins with the onset of menses (day 1) and continues to ovulation. The *secretory, or luteal, phase* lasts from ovulation to the onset of the subsequent menstrual period. The luteal phase is usually constant at about 12 to 15 days. During the latter part of the luteal phase and early follicular phase (Fig. 41-12) FSH causes five to six follicles to mature and their granulosa cells to proliferate. Estradiol secreted by granulosa cells is synergistic to this stimulating process. One follicle becomes dominant and the others regress. The theca cell layer of cuboidal cells surrounds the granulosa cell layer, begins to develop, and contributes to the steroidogenic capacity of the ovary. Further biosynthesis of estrogen leads to a surge of LH with a smaller increase in FSH (positive feedback mechanism). Coincident with the LH surge,

progesterone begins to be secreted from the preovulatory follicle. Ovulation with extrusion of the ovum occurs 16 to 24 h after the LH surge, after which the follicle is transformed into a corpus luteum, with its enhanced capacity to secrete progesterone. The corpus luteum is programmed to last approximately 14 days.

The released oocyte will usually begin to undergo degeneration in about 24 h after ovulation unless fertilization occurs. After fertilization and zygote formation occur within the fallopian tubes, the zygote enters the uterus about 3 days after conception and spends another 3 to 4 days within the uterine cavity before implantation. HCG, which is then detectable in the serum, stimulates the corpus luteum, preventing its demise and thereby maintaining pregnancy.

During menstruation the superficial layers of endometrium are cast off, leaving the stratum basalis and much of the stratum spongiosum, which lies superficial to the basalis, in situ and ready to begin regeneration during the cycle. Estrogen stimulation during the first part of the menstrual cycle causes mitoses in the endometrial glands and stroma resulting in a proliferative endometrial pattern (Fig. 41-14*A*). During this proliferative phase of the cycle the endometrium increases in thickness. As the middle of the cycle approaches, estrogen output from the ovary increases (Fig. 41-12). Ovulation occurs, and corpus luteum formation resulting in progesterone secretion follows. Progesterone stimulates coiling of the glands of the endometrium, which become filled with fluid, resulting in a secretory pattern (Fig. 41-14*B*).

The cervical mucus and vaginal cytologic features are also altered during the menstrual cycle. In the proliferative phase the cervical mucus forms a fernlike pattern when it is allowed to dry. At ovulation the volume of cervical mucus greatly increases. It becomes tenacious and can be drawn into a long thread (*Spinnbarkheit* phenomenon). At this time the mucus is maximally receptive to sperm and thus ideally suited to fertilization of the recently released ovum. The cervical mucus then decreases in volume, and because of the influence of progesterone, loses its ability to fern. Serial examination of the vaginal smear during the proliferative phase of the cycle shows a gradual increase in the number of superficial cornified cells. After ovulation these cells are less prevalent because of the influence of progesterone. Thus, a rough estimate of hormonal status can be gained by examining the cervical mucus and vaginal smear during the menstrual cycle.

Menopause

The average age at the onset of menopause is fifty years. Menopause results from a depletion in ovarian follicles with the loss of estrogen-producing capacity. In response to hypoestrogenism, negative feedback mechanisms in the hypothalamic-pituitary complex cause increased secretion of gonadotropins, which are at greatly elevated levels during menopause. Chemically and clinically the transition to menopause is gradual. Ovulation has been documented months after elevated gonadotropin levels have been measured in certain patients. Menopausal bleeding is characterized by skips and delays. If menses is absent for more than 6 months, any subsequent vaginal bleeding should be considered abnormal and deserves further investigation. During menopause the vaginal pH becomes more alkaline because of a decrease in glycogenation of the vaginal epithelium and decreased action of the Doderlein bacillus. The vaginal mucosa becomes thinner and is more prone to secondary infection.

Some postmenopausal women have elevated levels of estrogen present. The bulk of this estrogen consists of estrone, which is derived from peripheral conversion of androstenedione that originates from the adrenal. Estrone levels are higher in obese subjects due to conversion in adipose tissue. Age seems to be another factor that leads to increased conversion of androstenedione to estrone. These two factors may be involved in an increased incidence of endometrial carcinoma in obese postmenopausal women. Estrogen withdrawal in postmenopausal (or castrated) women may lead to typical "hot flashes." These are sensations of heat beginning in the face and then migrating to the neck, chest, and entire body. They last about 3 min, and perspiration accompanies them. The flashes can be controlled with small dosages of estrogen. One regimen is the oral administration of 0.625 mg of conjugated estrogens or 10 μg of ethinyl estradiol from the 1st to the 25th of each month. The dose is adjusted so that the lowest possible effective dosage is given. Progestins such as medroxyprogesterone acetate may be given at 5 mg daily for the last 10 days in an attempt to diminish the putative cancer-producing side effects of the estrogen (see below). Biochemical evidence suggests that progestins should be given for at least 10 days for the complete progestin-induced changes in the endometrium to occur. One complication of prescribing progestins in addition to estrogens is that vaginal bleeding may occur. That can be difficult to distinguish from abnormal bleeding due to endometrial pathology. Endometrial sampling can be done to provide additional information about endometrial histology. Additionally, estrogens appear beneficial in preventing osteoporosis that may otherwise occur after the menopause. Additional risk factors for osteoporosis include Caucasian race, thin body build, smoking, and inactivity. An adequate calcium intake is also beneficial in the prevention of osteoporosis.

GYNECOLOGIC EXAMINATION

The gynecologic history includes careful attention to all the details of menstrual and reproductive function, such as onset and frequency of menstruation, length and amount of menstrual bleeding, and the dates of the two most recent menstrual periods. If pain is a problem, when does it occur? Is it related to the menstrual cycle? Where is it? How severe is it? Does it radiate? What relieves it, and what, if anything, makes it worse? Are there any urinary or gastrointestinal symptoms? Physical examination includes pelvic examination, which is most comfortably done with the patient in the lithotomy position, suitably

draped and always accompanied by a nurse chaperone. The external genitalia are first visualized, special note being made of hair distribution, the size of the clitoris, the patency of the hymen, and any enlargements or inflammations, such as may be associated with Bartholin's glands. Skin lesions, such as may be seen with venereal infection, and vaginal discharges are also noted. The cervix is exposed with a water-lubricated speculum. Surgical jelly is not used because it will interfere with cytologic sampling (Pap smear). After cytologic sampling is complete, a bimanual examination is carried out and palpation performed, as illustrated in Fig. 41-15. First the uterus is felt; its position, its size, and the contour of the surface are noted. Leiomyomas (fibroids) cause smooth irregularities in the uterine surface that may vary in size from a few millimeters to several centimeters. A smooth indentation at the apex of the fundus may suggest a bicornuate or arcuate uterus. The left and right adnexal regions are then carefully palpated bimanually. The patient is asked to cough, and the support of the pelvis is carefully noted. If there is a weakness in the anterior wall (cystocele), the support of the urethra is carefully examined, and the patient is evaluated for stress incontinence. Separation of the levators will develop a weakness and herniation of the posterior vaginal wall (rectocele), and occasionally these may become sufficiently severe to lead to a complaint of constipation. Such patients may have to reduce manually the rectocele in order to defecate. Herniation near the apex of the vagina between the uterosacral ligaments usually contains small bowel (enterocele) and frequently is seen in patients with pelvic relaxation. If the ligamentous attachment and levator supports of the uterus and cervix should become weakened, descensus will be noted, and occasionally the cervix may even be seen to protrude through the introitus. Finally a rectal examination is performed, both to confirm the findings of the vaginal examination and also to palpate carefully the uterosacral ligaments, the back of the cervix and uterus, and the contents of the cul-de-sac (pouch of Douglas). These areas are often sites of nodularity and tenderness in cases of endo-

Fig. 41-15. *A.* Bimanual abdominovaginal palpation of the uterus. *B.* Bimanual abdominovaginal palpation of the adnexa.

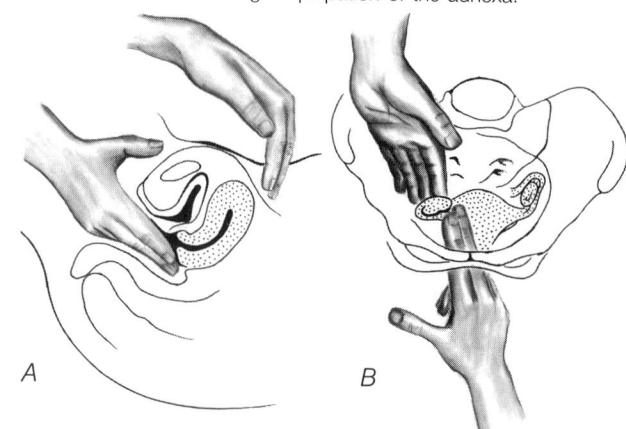

A   *B*

Tumors of the fallopian tubes rarely cause inter-menstrual bleeding. There may be an intermittent mucous or serous discharge with the bleeding or staining, *hydrops tubae profluens*. This occurs presumably as a result of blockage of the tube by a tumor. The tumor can occur at any age but is usually seen in older women and often occurs postmenopausally. Similarly, carcinoma of the endo-metrium is primarily a disease of postmenopausal women but may cause nonmenstrual bleeding in a younger woman.

Brisk bleeding can occur in early pregnancy. It may accompany implantation of the blastocyst a few days after fertilization. It is not unusual to have a small amount of bleeding or staining during the first few weeks of pregnancy. If the patient has bleeding during early pregnancy, the diagnosis is threatened abortion. If, however, tissue is passed, abortion is considered to have taken place. Ectopic pregnancy can cause irregular bleeding early in pregnancy. *Although there is no characteristic history obtained with an ectopic pregnancy,* many patients will complain of a delay in menses followed by scanty bleeding or staining, often in association with pelvic pain. There may or may not be symptoms of pregnancy. Finally, irregular bleeding early in pregnancy, especially if the uterus is larger than anticipated by the menstrual history, suggests trophoblastic disease.

Postmenopausal bleeding frequently is caused by an endometrial or endocervical polyp or atrophic vaginitis. Carcinoma of any part of the reproductive tract or prema-lignant change in the endometrium may exist in the post-menopausal female. In all cases of vaginal bleeding, the bladder and rectum must be ruled out as origins of the blood.

Endocrine-Related and Reproductive Problems

AMENORRHEA AND ABNORMAL SEXUAL DEVELOPMENT

Primary amenorrhea may be defined as the failure to initiate menstruation prior to age sixteen years in patients without secondary sex characteristics or age eighteen in those with secondary sexual characteristics. *Secondary amenorrhea* is the absence of menstrual periods for 6 months in those with regular monthly menses or perhaps after 1 year in those with infrequent periods. The incidence of amenorrhea is approximately 6 percent among college-aged women, a relatively common problem. In order for normal menstruation to occur, an intact CNS-hypothalamic-pituitary-ovarian-outflow tract axis must exist. Disorders leading to amenorrhea will therefore result if there is a disturbance in one of these areas. It is also convenient to characterize patients as having normal secondary sexual characteristics, absent secondary sexual characteristics, or ambiguous genitalia. The following schema and evaluation of amenorrhea classifies patients in these categories. Because disorders of sexual development are frequently associated with primary amenorrhea they will be considered together.

CNS-HYPOTHALAMIC-PITUITARY DISORDERS. Serious disease of any sort may cause amenorrhea. The point of affliction of the reproductive axis is usually at the CNS-hypothalamic-pituitary level. The initial history and physical examination are often sufficient to diagnose a serious illness, a severe psychiatric disease such as anorexia nervosa, or starvation, any of which may be reflected in menstrual dysfunction. Additional endocrine causes of amenorrhea are pituitary tumors or suprasellar tumors, thyroid or adrenal disease. Hypothyroidism classically is associated with menorrhagia, and as the disease becomes chronic, amenorrhea may ensue. Hyperthyroidism is usually initially associated with *hypomenorrhea,* or menses becoming more scant and less frequent. Amenorrhea is a frequent accompaniment of Cushing's syndrome, the mechanism possibly being excessive secretion of androgens that feed back to the hypothalamus-pituitary to decrease gonadotropin secretion.

Stress, probably through altered neurotransmission from the CNS to the hypothalamus, can be reflected in decreased GnRH secretion, and hence amenorrhea. For example, a study in Uppsala County, Sweden, demonstrated a significant association of bereavement or frustration regarding family, sexual partner, work, or divorce in an amenorrheic population as compared with controls. There was also a statistically significant increase in use of tranquilizers in the amenorrheic women. Low body weight, low body fat, or weight loss may be associated with amenorrhea. McArthur and Frisch have suggested that a critical amount of body fat is necessary for menstruation. Endocrine derangements in low-weight amenorrhea are similar to but less profound than that found in complete anorexia nervosa. The pituitary is less responsive to GnRH in simple low-weight amenorrhea but less so than that found in anorexia nervosa. Women athletes who undergo significant endurance-type training frequently become amenorrheic. One study found 30 percent of women who ran 40 miles per week to be amenorrheic.

Sheehan's syndrome, or postpartum pituitary necrosis, is panhypopituitarism resulting from infarction of the pituitary following obstetric hemorrhage such as abruptio placentae. Failure to lactate and failure to resume menses are early clues to the diagnosis. Eventually, loss of body hair, pallor, secondary hypothyroidism, and hypoadrenalism ensue. Treatment involves replacement of thyroid and adrenal hormones.

Pituitary tumors may interfere with LH and FSH release. The most common are prolactinomas that give rise to amenorrhea by their excessive secretion of prolactin. The precise mechanism is not clear, but prolactin levels much above the normal range of 25 mμg/mL have a deleterious effect on gonadal function, giving rise to amenorrhea. Galactorrhea may be also present. Inhibition of prolactin secretion is dependent upon tonic secretion by the hypothalamus of a prolactin-inhibiting factor (PIF). There is evidence that PIF is a dopamine-type substance. Any anatomical condition that interferes with the integrity of the hypothalamic pituitary connections, such as a hypothalamic tumor or meningitis in that area, can lead to a decrease in PIF, and hence to hyperprolactinemia. Certain drugs such as phenothiazines also may cause hyperprolactinemia probably by combining with dopamine receptors in the pituitary, hence blocking the action of dopamine. Primary hypothyroidism may be also associated with hyperprolactinemia and should be considered when hyperprolactinemia and/or galactorrhea are found. Non-prolactin-secreting pituitary tumors such as chromophobe adenomas may also cause amenorrhea.

GONADAL DEFECTS. Gonadal defects giving rise to amenorrhea may be placed in two categories: (1) polycystic ovarian syndrome and other conditions giving rise to hyperandrogenemia and (2) inherited reproductive defects in which often the genetic material is abnormal, being reflected in decreased or absent germ cells in the ovary. Polycystic ovarian disease usually does not cause amenorrhea but rather oligomenorrhea, and this will be discussed separately.

INHERITED REPRODUCTIVE DEFECTS

GONADAL DYSGENESIS. Genetic material is transmitted via the chromosomes, of which the normal human complement is 46, i.e., 23 pairs. These can be studied morphologically and arranged according to size in a karyotype. There are 22 autosomes and two sex chromosomes designated X and Y. The presence of two or more chromosome complements in an individual is termed a *mosaic*. In the female, there are normally two X chromosomes, and one of these chromosomes is believed to be the basis of a discrete bit of chromatin material in the nucleus of many female cells. This is referred to as the *Barr body* (Fig. 41-18). In general, the number of X chromosomes is one greater than the number of Barr bodies seen. Thus, if there are three X chromosomes, there would be two Barr bodies present in most cells examined. In the normal male (X-Y), Barr bodies are present in less than 2 percent of cells and in the normal female more than 20 percent.

Most commonly in cases of gonadal dysgenesis the ovaries are replaced by streaks of fibrous tissue devoid of oocytes. The karyotype usually is 45,X. One in approximately 2700 liveborn female infants is 45,X, with the percentage being much higher in abortuses; 45,X is the commonest karyotype abnormality in spontaneous abortion. Clinically, patients with 45,X (Turner's syndrome) have short stature, sexual infantilism, and a variety of somatic abnormalities, including web neck (pterygium colli), widely spaced nipples, cubitus valgus, micrognathia with a high arched palate, and epicanthal folds. Neonatal congenital lymphedema of the hands and feet occurs in 30 to 40 percent of affected infants. Various structural abnormalities of the kidney are also found in about 50 percent, coarctation of the aorta in 10 to 20 percent, and osteoporosis, diabetes mellitus, and Hashimoto's thyroiditis may occur. With absent sex steroid secretion from the ovaries, serum gonadotrophin levels are elevated.

Approximately 20 percent of patients with the typical syndrome of gonadal dysgenesis will have more than 20 percent Barr bodies. The karyotypes of these patients have either mosaicism involving an XO cell line or a structural rearrangement of the X chromosome. Such

mosaics may include XO/XX, XO/XXX, and XO/XY, and patients with a normal cell line (such as 45,X, 46,XX) may have partial ovarian function with resulting pubescence, secondary sexual characteristics, and ovulation. Pregnancy has been reported in these patients. However, premature menopause often occurs. If a Y chromosome is present in the karyotype, gonadectomy is indicated because of the propensity for such gonads to develop malignancy, chiefly gonadoblastoma. The term *pure gonadal dysgenesis* applies to those individuals with normal 46,XX or 46,XY karyotypes who have streak ovaries. Either the gonadal tissue has been destroyed by an unknown mechanism very early in development or undiagnosed mosaicism exists. Those who have 46,XY karyotypes may have an abnormality in expression in the H-Y antigen (a Y-linked material present on cells that causes differentiation of a gonad into a testis). Typically, patients with pure gonadal dysgenesis are somatically normal but

Fig. 41-18. Sex chromatin masses in cells of human skin (left) and vaginal mucosa (right). *A.* Normal female: XX. *B.* Klinefelter's syndrome with mental deficiency: XXXY. *C.* Eunuch with microorchism and mental deficiency: XXXXY. The finding of duplicate Barr bodies suggests the presence of a mosaic of an undetected third stem line, such as XXX or XXXY. (From: *Sohval AR: Am J Med 31:397, 1961; Barr ML, Carr DH: Can Med Assoc J 83:979, 1960, with permission.*)

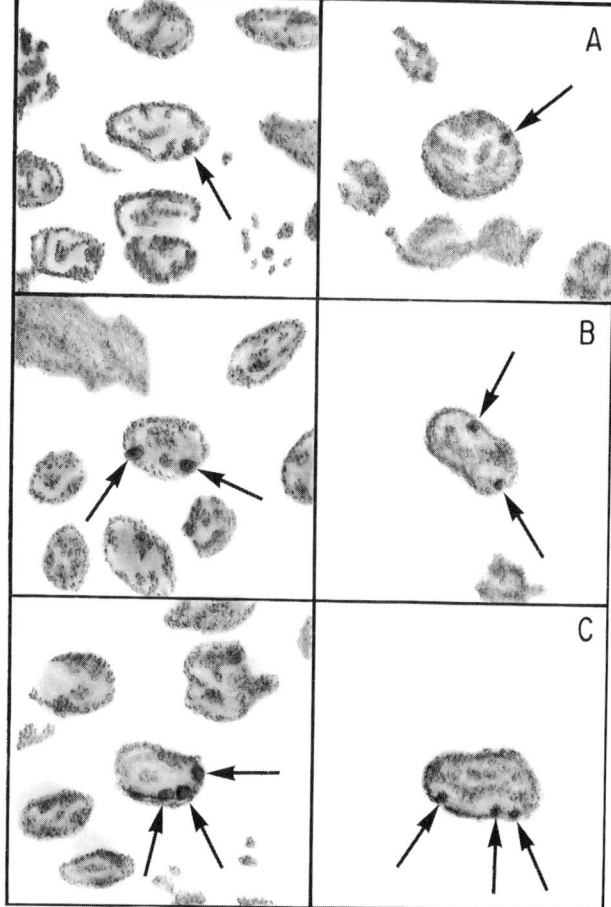

fail to develop normal secondary sex characteristics at the time of puberty. They are hence sexually infantile and may be tall and eunuchoidal. Those with a Y chromosome may have clitoromegaly.

Therapy for gonadal dysgenesis is directed toward cyclic estrogen and progesterone replacement. One regimen utilizes 0.625 mg of conjugated estrogens from days 1 to 25 of the month with the addition of medroxyprogesterone acetate 10 mg daily, days 16 to 25. An increased incidence of endometrial carcinoma has been reported in patients with gonadal dysgenesis who received estrogen replacement therapy alone. Progesterone supplementation for at least 10 days each cycle should decrease this risk.

Mixed gonadal dysgenesis refers to those with a unilateral streak gonad and a testis or germ cell tumor on the other side. The commonest karyotype is 45,X/46,XY. These individuals are usually raised as a female, but some have been raised as males, depending upon the appearance of the external genitalia at birth. Pubertal virilization is severe in those with a testis. Exploratory laparotomy and gonadectomy is indicated as soon as the presence of testicular tissue is detected. Appropriate sex steroid replacement therapy is then undertaken.

TRUE HERMAPHRODITISM. This implies the presence of both ovarian and testicular tissue, in either the same or opposite gonads. The most common peripheral blood karyotypes are 46,XX and 46,XY in that order. The diagnosis is uncommon, there having been something over 300 cases reported in the literature. The clinical manifestations are highly variable, depending upon the contribution of sex steroids from the ovary or testis. In the majority of cases the genitalia are ambiguous. About 75 percent of these patients have been raised as males. Internal genital development is also variable and depends upon the contribution from the corresponding gonad. The duct adjacent to the ovary is always a fallopian tube and that adjacent to a testis is always a vas deferens. The ovotestis is the most common gonad found and is usually associated with a fallopian tube, but there may be a vas. The testicular material is usually dysgenetic and should be surgically removed. Spermatogenesis is rare. The ovarian tissue present in true hermaphrodites may function normally, and pregnancy has been reported.

FEMALE PSEUDOHERMAPHRODITISM. Female pseudohermaphrodites have ovaries but are masculinized, usually from androgens present during fetal development, leading to the development of ambiguous genitalia (clitoromegaly, labioscrotal fusion, or a fully masculinized external genitalia with a single orifice at the end of a phallus). The degree of masculinization correlates with the degree of androgen excess. The primary sources of excess androgens are (1) exogenous drug ingestion during pregnancy, such as of certain progestins that have androgenic properties and (2) congenital virilizing adrenal hyperplasia (CAH), fetally derived. CAH accounts for most cases of female pseudohermaphroditism, and results from autosomal recessive inherited enzymatic deficiencies in the biosynthesis of cortisol. Hence, ACTH secretion is increased, and there is an increased production of cortisol

precursors, many of which are androgenic. The most common defect is 21-hydroxylase deficiency. This results in an increased secretion of 17-OH progesterone and 17-ketosteroids, including dehydroepiandrosterone and dehydroepiandrosterone sulfate (DHAS). In mild cases, female infants may be phenotypically normal, and the disease may not become manifest until during childhood or peripubertally when virilization with clitoromegaly, voice deepening, acne, and rapid growth results. The diagnosis should be suspected in any infant with a family history of CAH, in any infant with ambiguous genitalia, and in all apparent cryptorchid males. Any children who undergo rapid growth or female children who begin to grow large should be suspected of CAH. Aldosterone deficiency in infants is suspicious when hypokalemia or hyponatremia occurs.

The treatment of CAH involves replacement with glucocorticoids and mineralocorticoids. This replacement decreases ACTH, which in turn relieves the adrenal of the stimulus for increased adrenal androgen production. Females born with ambiguous genitalia should have a repair made prior to twelve months of age, providing a simple surgical reduction of the clitoris leads to a more normal appearing phallus. Extensive vaginal reconstruction, however, is not attempted at this time.

MALE PSEUDOHERMAPHRODITISM. Male pseudohermaphroditism implies that testicular tissue is present but that the patient expresses only partial masculinization (sometimes even to complete feminization). It may be broadly divided into two categories: (1) inadequate production of testosterone by the testis and (2) normal testosterone production but inadequate response to androgen at the end organ level.

Inadequate testosterone production is rare, and may result from inadequate LH or HCG receptors on the Leydig cell or errors of testosterone biosynthesis, analogous to CAH. Clinically, these individuals have inadequate masculinization of the external genitalia, and if not diagnosed in infancy may present with primary amenorrhea. A 46,XY karyotype and abnormality in steroid hormone production are diagnostic.

SYNDROMES OF ANDROGEN RESISTANCE. These individuals have a 46,XY karyotype with testes that have a normal capacity to secrete testosterone. The commonest of these is the syndrome of testicular feminization. These patients are raised as females and at puberty undergo normal breast development. However, they have scant to absent axillary and pubic hair and fail to menstruate. The vagina ends in a shallow pouch. The testis may be present either intraabdominally in an inguinal hernia or in the labia majora. The pathophysiologic basis of the disease has been determined to be a lack of responsiveness to testosterone in areas that are normally testosterone-sensitive. Hence, the external genitalia are completely feminine, there are no Wolffian ducts, and the breasts undergo normal physiologic increases in size at the time of puberty. The disorder seems to be inherited as an X-linked recessive trait.

Incomplete testicular feminization has been described. These individuals have a 46,XY karyotype, gynecomastia at puberty, bilateral testis, no müllerian structures, and inheritance as an X-linked recessive trait. There is a spectrum of masculinization from clitoromegaly with a lined pouchlike vagina to those with more masculine development consisting of perineoscrotal hypospadias and gynecomastia. The latter are raised as males and are infertile. The diagnosis of incomplete testicular feminization is suggested in patients who have 46,XY karyotype but do not have elevated steroid precursors, as seen in errors of testosterone synthesis. Laparotomy with inspection of the testis may have to be done to differentiate incomplete androgen resistance from true hermaphroditism. If diagnosed in infancy, the patient should probably be raised as female despite the possibility of substantial virilization at puberty. Gonadectomy is indicated due to the propensity for malignant change.

5-Alpha reductase deficiency is caused by an autosomal recessive defect of 5-alpha reductase that precludes normal conversion of testosterone to dihydrotestosterone. Since testosterone, in many androgen-sensitive tissues, is converted to dihydrotestosterone at the intracellular level, these XY patients are androgen-deficient. They have ambiguous genitalia at birth with normal testis, normal internal male ducts, and absence of müllerian structures. Many of the infants are raised as females, but at puberty, they undergo a striking metamorphosis with virilization including phallic enlargement, male muscular pattern, voice deepening, descent of testes, and the development of spermatogenesis. Those signs of masculinization that the patients fail to develop are dihydrotestosterone-dependent.

OUTFLOW TRACT OBSTRUCTION. The two most commonly encountered situations are the imperforate hymen and the complete absence of the vagina. In the case of the imperforate hymen, a pelvic mass is usually noted in either the pubertal or newborn female. In the newborn infant such a tumor may be produced by secretions trapped behind the hymen. The infant should be catheterized to rule out bladder distention. Before any newborn female is explored abdominally for a pelvic mass, an imperforate hymen or transverse vaginal septum should be ruled out, for these conditions can be treated quite simply by a hymenotomy or incision of the septum with release of the trapped fluid.

If no vagina exists, one can be constructed surgically. After an adequate space is created, split-thickness skin grafts are placed and held with a vaginal mold. This is usually carried out in the patient's late teens or early twenties when she has sufficient psychosexual maturity and also is able to keep the mold in situ and change it by herself. The mold must be used unless the patient is having frequent intercourse. An alternative is the daily use of graduated cylindrical dilators to give pressure at the vaginal dimple. This can lead to the development of an adequate vagina over many months.

Asherman's syndrome, or intrauterine synechiae, most often is a result of a postpartum or postabortal curettage or elective abortion accompanied by endometritis. The diagnosis may be suspected from such a history. Attempts at hysterosalpingogram or hysteroscopy make the diagnosis. Lysis of adhesions with the hysteroscope is probably the best method of treatment.

Cervical stenosis may follow a dilatation and curettage (D and C) or conization. Symptoms may be dysmenorrhea, amenorrhea, and infertility. Dilatation and opening of the cervix is necessary.

Evaluation and Treatment of Amenorrhea

The first obligation of the physician is to rule out serious disease. It should be remembered that pregnancy is the most common cause of amenorrhea.

Hyperprolactinemia is seen in about 15 percent of patients with long-standing amenorrhea, and a serum prolactin is always obtained in the evaluation. If the prolactin is at elevated levels, further work-up is necessary to search for a prolactin-secreting pituitary tumor, drug usage, or primary hypothyroidism, to name the most common conditions.

A progestin challenge test with 100 to 200 mg progesterone in oil I.M. or 20 mg medroxyprogesterone acetate orally for 5 days is used to test for adequate levels of estrogens. If present, a positive response with vaginal bleeding will occur within 10 days. Vaginal bleeding confirms that there is (1) a functional outflow tract including endometrium that has been adequately primed with estrogen, (2) functioning ovaries that are capable of producing estrogen, and (3) an intact CNS-hypothalamic-pituitary system capable of delivering gonadotropins to the ovary. Hence, a positive progestin challenge indicates that the patient most likely has simple anovulation or very infrequent ovulatory periods. Periodic progestin withdrawal may be prescribed to prevent heavy dysfunctional bleeding and endometrial atypia.

If there is no bleeding in response to a progestin challenge, there is a defect at either central, ovarian, or outflow tract level. The outflow obstruction has been discussed. To determine whether amenorrhea is due to central or ovarian pathology, measurement of serum FSH is useful. If the FSH is elevated (greater than 40 ImU/mL or 1000 mμg/mL), ovarian failure is likely. The ovarian failure process may be spread out over time. Ovulation sometimes occurs months after elevated levels of gonadotropins have been documented. If the patient is less than age thirty-five, a karyotype is obtained. If a Y chromosome is present, gonadectomy is indicated.

If the FSH is low or normal, a central cause of amenorrhea is most likely. The commonest is hypothalamic amenorrhea. The patient should be evaluated for stress or weight loss. Rarely a non-prolactin-secreting pituitary tumor can occur. A simple lateral skull film of the sella turcica is sufficient for the diagnosis of a large, nonfunctioning chromophobe adenoma.

Hirsutism and Masculinization

Most hirsute patients have elevated androgen levels. If urinary 17-KS are measured, only 15 percent of hirsute women will have elevated values. If total plasma testosterone is measured, 40 percent of hirsute patients are found to have an elevated value. If the total plasma levels of several androgenic hormones and prehormones such as testosterone, dihydrotestosterone, DHAS, androstenedione are determined, approximately 90 percent of patients will have elevated values of one or more of these. Plasma-free testosterone is at elevated levels in about 50 percent more cases than the total plasma testosterone. When free-plasma concentrations of both testosterone and the entire group of 17-β-hydroxysteroids are measured, 85 percent of hirsute women will have an elevated value of one or more. The reason that plasma-free androgen levels are elevated more often than total androgen concentration is that TEBG levels are often depressed in hyperandrogenemic states.

Because of episodic glandular secretion, a single plasma androgen value may not be representative of average levels throughout the day. Hence, if normal values are initially obtained, they may be elevated upon repeated sampling.

In hirsute women, androgens originate from either the adrenal gland or the ovary or from peripheral conversion of prehormones. To test the origin of excess secretion dexamethasone, 0.5 mg four times a day, may be given for 1 week to suppress adrenal androgen production. Elevated androgens after a dexamethasone suppression may be assumed to be of a predominantly ovarian source. *Ovarian hyperandrogenemia* most commonly results from the polycystic ovary syndrome (PCO). In this condition the ovaries are bilaterally enlarged with multiple follicular cysts and luteinized theca. *Hyperthecosis,* a more severe form of polycystic ovaries, is characterized by luteinized cells within the ovarian stroma. Patients with PCO are generally anovulatory and have rather consistent secretion of increased quantities of androstenedione and testosterone with steady-state levels of estrogens. Corpus luteum formation with progesterone production occurs infrequently, if at all, in these patients. Therefore, the endometrial lining is exposed to consistent estrogen stimulation.

It should be noted that obese patients occasionally have high levels of androgens, even in the absence of hirsutism. The mechanism for this is not known, but obese anovulatory hyperandrogenemic patients may have regular menstrual cycles and normal androgen levels with ovulation following loss of excess weight.

In approaching the hirsute patient, we recommend measuring two androgens, testosterone and DHAS. Androgen-producing tumor should be suspected with high levels of androgens, i.e., testosterone greater than 200 mμg/mL and DHAS greater than 800 μg/dL. Virilization (e.g., clitoromegaly, temporal balding, male muscular pattern, deepening of the voice) is indicative of high androgen levels that may be seen with tumor. A rapid onset of hyperandrogenemia and virilization is another clue of the presence of tumor. The use of adrenal ultrasound or computed tomography (CT scanning) has been helpful in diagnosing adrenal tumors. Clinical and laboratory signs of ovarian tumor coupled with an adnexal mass demand exploration. It should be remembered that some ovarian tumors are small and may escape detection on pelvic examination. Adrenal-ovarian vein catheterization with measurement of androgen level has been a useful method of detecting small androgen-secreting tumors.

If simple hirsutism is the patient's complaint and she is interested in fertility, induction of ovulation is usually successful. Cosmetic treatment for hirsutism may be undertaken with combined low-dose oral contraceptives. (Those contraceptive agents containing norgestrel are not recommended for the treatment of hirsutism as that compound is excessively androgenic.) This therapy places the ovary at rest and reduces ovarian secretion of androgens. At least 6 months are required before an improvement is seen. If the patient has dexamethasone-suppressible hyperandrogenemia, therapy may be used with very low dose dexamethasone, i.e., 0.5 mg/day. An alternative to oral contraceptive agents and glucocorticoid is the use of antiandrogens. Cimetidine and spironolactone are two agents that have been reported to be beneficial in the treatment of hirsutism. While all of the above pharmacologic agents may be beneficial in preventing further hair growth, electrolysis is the only method that permanently removes hairs that have already been established.

Disorders of Reproductive Capacity

A couple is not usually evaluated for infertility unless there has been 1 year of deliberate effort to conceive.

PROOF OF OVULATION. Since there is no proof except pregnancy, circumstantial evidence is used. A biphasic basal body temperature, an elevated serum progesterone level, and a secretory endometrial biopsy obtained in the luteal phase of the cycle can be considered as a reasonable indication of ovulation. As shown in Fig. 41-19, anovulatory patients who respond to a progestin challenge with vaginal bleeding, i.e., whose ovaries are producing adequate amounts of estrogens, are candidates for induction of ovulation with clomiphene citrate. Ovulation can successfully be induced about 80 percent of the time, with most of those achieving pregnancy if no other cause for infertility is present. Clomiphene failures and those with hypothalamic amenorrhea (who have low estrogens) are candidates for receiving human menopausal gonadotropins or GnRH to induce ovulation. Gonadotropin therapy is complicated and expensive, but the ovulation rate is 90 percent, with the pregnancy rate reported to vary from 40 to 70 percent. Results of GnRH therapy are preliminary, but the agent holds promise as a means to induce ovulation and to avoid some of the complications of gonadotropin therapy such as ovarian hyperstimulation.

THE TUBAL FACTOR. The patency of the tubes must be established. The passage of CO_2 through the tubes (Rubin's test) is recorded by alterations in CO_2 pressure during the test. Confirmation of passage of CO_2 is noted by shoulder pain in the erect patient a few minutes after the completion of the procedure. Since the test does not permit visualization of the tubes, it is possible that only one tube could be open. Direct visualization of the tubes can be obtained radiologically by a uterotubogram (hysterosalpingogram). In such cases the endometrial cavity is outlined, and tubal patency is established. Laparos-

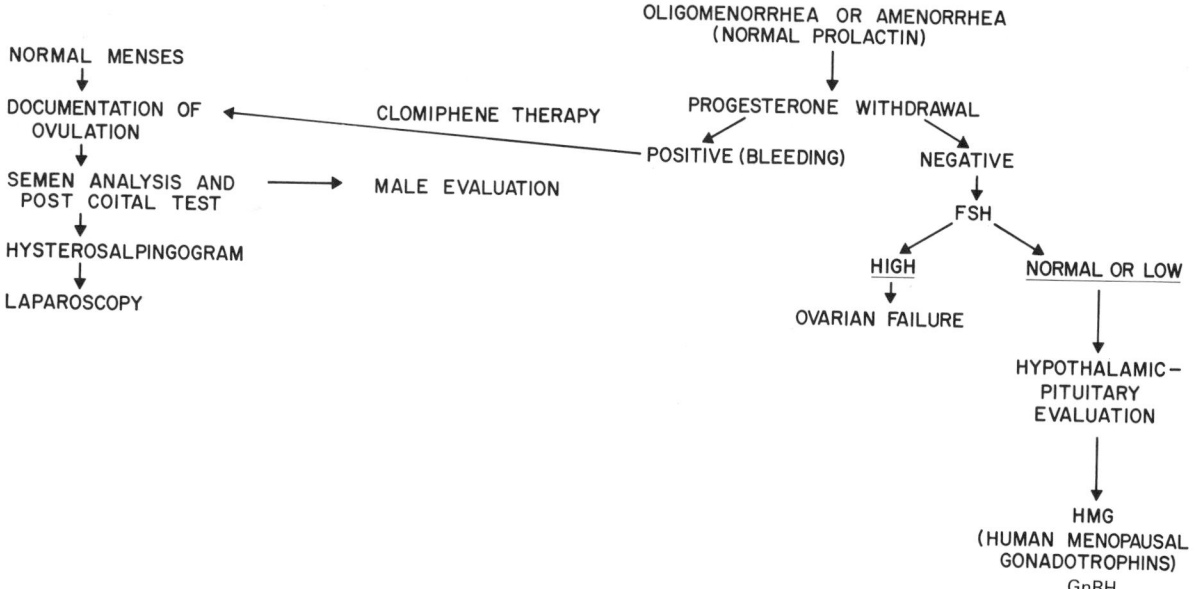

Fig. 41-19. Infertility evaluation.

copy (Fig. 41-16) is an essential step in the evaluation. When laparoscopy is performed, the tubes can be lavaged with a dye, such as indigo carmine, at the time of the surgical procedure; efflux of the dye through the fimbriate ends of both tubes proves patency. At the same time, the pelvic organs are inspected for other pathologic changes, including peritubal adhesions, endometriosis, etc. The success rate of tubal surgery depends upon the type of damage to the fallopian tubes. With distal (fimbrial) obstruction, which is usually associated with a history of pelvic inflammatory disease, the prognosis is poor. If there has been extensive endosalpingeal damage of the tubal mucosa with a resultant poorly physiologically functioning tube, the prognosis for pregnancy is less than 5 percent. Less extensively damaged tubes, as reflected by the maintenance of a delicate rugal pattern in the endosalpinx, carry a better prognosis.

The success in surgically reversing a tubal ligation depends on the location of the occlusion and degree of tubal destruction. Pomeroy, fallope ring, Uchida, Irving, and even cautery procedures can be reversed if more than 4 cm of distal tube remains along with a small proximal stump. Patency rates of nearly 95 percent and pregnancy rates of 70 to 80 percent have been reported. In these cases of end-to-end anastomosis, the operating microscope with 4- to 12-power magnification has proved useful.

Adhesions that bind the fallopian tube to the ovary, posterior aspect of the uterus, broad ligament, pelvic side wall or bowel may prevent ovum pick by the fimbria. Appendicitis, pelvic surgery, pelvic inflammatory disease, or the normal process of ovulation with extrusion of a small amount of blood may be etiologic. If there is no associated tubal damage, a 60 percent rate has been achieved following lysis of adhesions.

In all cases of infertility surgery, attention is paid to fine anatomical approximation and the avoidance of adhesions by eliminating rough tissue handling and utilizing

precise and complete hemostasis. Irrigation rather than sponging is used to clear the operative field of blood. Fine-tipped cautery instruments and nonreactive sutures are employed. It has been suggested that intraperitoneal instillation of 32% dextran-70 at the conclusion of the procedure and systemic corticosteroids may be helpful in the prevention of adhesions.

PROBLEMS OF IMPLANTATION. This includes an evaluation of the adequacy of the size and shape of the uterus, particularly in patients who have repeated first trimester pregnancy losses. Such patients may be found to have a bicornuate uterus, uterine septum, or large submucous fibroids that can distort the endometrial cavity. Although the presence of these conditions does not necessarily mean that the patient will abort, repeated abortions are an indication for surgical correction.

THE MALE FACTOR. The postcoital (PCT, PK, or Huhner's) test and a semen analysis evaluate the factor. The patient is instructed to have coitus with her husband about the time of midcycle, because it is at this time that the cervical mucus is most plentiful and most receptive to sperm. The mucus is then examined, optimally within 2 h after coitus, at which time there should be numerous motile active sperm in a high-powered field (hpf). The number will vary depending upon the time the test is done and the amount of cervical mucus present. Usually 15 or more active sperm per hpf are seen. When the PCT contains this many sperm per hpf, the semen analysis will usually be at least 30 million sperm per cubic milliliter. When the PCT is less than that, repeated semen analyses should be done. The minimum accepted value is 20 million sperm per cubic milliliter, and a normal range is 40 million to 100 million sperm per cubic milliliter. A few pregnancies have been conceived by patients with counts as low as 10 million sperm per cubic millimeter. If a period of continence is followed by frequent intercourse, a gradual lowering of the sperm count can result.

Therapy of the infertile couple depends on the causative factor. If anovulation is the problem, this should be treated according to the previously mentioned outline. In cases of uterine distortion, a myomectomy, reunification of a bicornuate uterus (Strassmann procedure), or removal of the uterine septum is usually necessary to achieve term pregnancy. If pelvic adhesions are present, chances for pregnancy can be improved if they are lysed, provided that ovulatory and sperm functions are normal. Areas of endometriosis should be resected. Tuboplastic procedures are performed to correct occlusion of the tube. Such surgical procedures should be avoided in cases of severe tubal destruction and are contraindicated in cases of tuberculosis. A few pregnancies will result from tuboplasty procedures, but in most cases the results have been disappointing.

In vitro fertilization (IVF) is an accepted procedure for cases of tubal blockage not amenable to tuboplasty. Clinics are reporting pregnancy rates of up to 25 percent per ovarian cycle. IVF has also been used as therapy for nontubal causes of infertility such as male factor, inadequate cervical mucus, and cases of unexplained infertility. Results in these cases are often less satisfactory than when tubal blockage is the indication.

Intrauterine insemination (IUI) of washed, concentrated spermatozoa is currently popular in the treatment of inadequate cervical mucus and unexplained infertility. Pregnancy rates of 5 to 70 percent have been reported, the vast majority of the studies being uncontrolled.

In evaluating studies on infertility, it is important to remember that the incidental pregnancy rate in infertile populations is substantial. In infertile couples in whom no obvious cause of sterility can be identified (such as tubal obstruction or azoospermia) who have been unsuccessfully trying to achieve pregnancy for a year, 50 percent will conceive over the next year if no therapy at all is done.

Pregnancy and Its Disorders

Amenorrhea in the reproductive years is most frequently caused by pregnancy. During the first weeks of normal pregnancy, the cervix becomes blue and soft. The cervicouterine junction softens, and the fundus of the uterus becomes boggy, especially near the implantation site. The cervical vessels enlarge and are easy to palpate. Enlargement of the uterus may be noted as early as 2 to 3 weeks after the first missed menstrual period. Uterine enlargement continues, and by the tenth week the fundus can be felt just above the symphysis. Usually the patient will notice fetal movement (quickening) by the sixteenth to eighteenth week of gestation. The examiner may hear the fetal heart as early as the seventeenth to twentieth week of gestation, depending upon the size of the patient. The fundus reaches the umbilicus by about the twentieth week of gestation and extends to the xiphoid of the sternum by the thirty-sixth week.

A small amount of staining early in the first trimester of pregnancy is not uncommon. However, if bleeding is severe and is unaccompanied by the passage of tissue or dilatation of the os, the diagnosis of *threatened abortion*

is made. The uterine size is usually consistent with the dates of gestation. The test for chorionic gonadotropin remains positive. If tissue has been passed through a dilated cervical os, usually some products of conception remain in the uterus. Under such circumstances, the diagnosis of *incomplete abortion* is made, and a curettage, usually performed with a suction apparatus, is indicated to prevent further hemorrhage and also to prevent infection from the retained products of conception. Occasionally, in the first trimester of pregnancy, the entire products of conception are passed, and the complete sac of the total pregnancy can be identified. These complete abortions do not require further surgical therapy.

Induced (therapeutic) abortions are frequently performed for a variety of indications, including the preference of the patient. Usually, under local anesthesia, the products of conception are removed by suction curettage after the cervix has been dilated. It is preferable to perform the procedure prior to the twelfth week of pregnancy. It may be performed later, but the risk of hemorrhage and complications is increased.

Some first trimester pregnancy losses are complicated by infection. These are almost invariably due to instrumentation to induce abortion. The patient usually presents with lower abdominal pain, fever, and occasionally cervical discharge. The uterus is tender, and there is pain on cervical motion. The white cell count is elevated. In severe cases, septicemia and septic shock may ensue. The patient becomes moribund and is unable to maintain her blood pressure. There is then decreased or absent urinary output.

Therapy of septic abortion is initiated by high doses of intravenous antibiotics. The treatment of septic shock is discussed in Chap. 4. Once the infection appears controlled and the patient stabilized, gentle evacuation of the uterus is carried out. A vigorous curettage should not be done, as bacteremia and septic shock can result from excessive surgical manipulation. If the patient does not respond to gentle evacuation of the uterus, or if there is persistent shock and decreased urinary output, or if there is a history of the intrauterine injection of a powerful chemical toxin such as soap, detergent, or lysol, then a hysterectomy may be required as a lifesaving procedure. In such cases it is important to remove both the tubes and ovaries, since these are often areas of microabscesses and toxic products that have accumulated as a result of sepsis.

A diagnosis of *missed abortion* is applied if the fetus does not remain viable and there is no sign of external bleeding or loss of the pregnancy. The uterus shrinks in size, and there is necrosis of the fetus and placenta. The chorionic gonadotropin test becomes negative. If the uterus is smaller than a 12-week size, it can usually be safely evacuated by a curettage. In very rare cases, a hysterotomy is necessary.

ECTOPIC PREGNANCY

Implantation of the fertilized ovum outside the endometrial cavity, usually in the tube or, occasionally, on the surface of the ovary or in the abdomen, results in an ectopic pregnancy. It occurs in less than 1 percent of pregnancies. Tubal ectopic pregnancy is believed to result from the improper transport of the fertilized ovum through the tube, either because of a congenital defect in the tube, as the sequela of infection, or as a complication of tubal surgery. It has been noted in many cases of ectopic pregnancies that the corpus luteum of pregnancy will exist in one ovary while the ectopic pregnancy is found to exist in the tube on the opposite side. Thus, there may have been transmigration of the fertilized ovum from one ovary to the contralateral tube; the time involved in this passage resulted in abnormal implantation into the tube rather than into the endometrial cavity. Patients who have had an ectopic pregnancy on one side are predisposed to the same problem in the opposite tube.

This is a disease of diagnostic surprises. There may be symptoms associated with early pregnancy, such as breast tenderness, nausea, vomiting, and a delay in menses. There may be some bleeding or staining that follows a previously scanty period. The uterus often grows, but if an increase in size is noted, it will usually be less than expected for pregnancy, the duration of which is estimated from the menstrual history. Pain and cramps are often present. On physical examination, in addition to change in uterine size, an adnexal mass is palpable 50 percent of the time. Pain on cervical motion does occur and is usually localized to the side of the ectopic pregnancy. About 50 percent of the time urine slide pregnancy tests are negative but newer antibody assays specific for HCG are sufficiently sensitive that they are usually positive. If the test for pregnancy is a serum radioimmunoassay for β-HCG with positive values greater than 35 mI.U./mL, 95 percent will be positive. If the serum β-HCG test is precisely quantitated, most of those showing a positive test will have low levels of HCG for the expected date of gestation.

Occasionally, a patient will present with the pregnancy ruptured from the tube or extruded from the tip of the tube into the peritoneal cavity. The symptoms will then be of local peritoneal irritation due to the presence of blood. Characteristically, the patient complains of pain in the shoulder due to diaphragmatic irritation. In advanced cases, shock occurs because of heavy blood loss. Most ectopic pregnancies should be diagnosed before a vascular emergency occurs, but shock may be seen.

Ruptured ovarian cysts and pelvic inflammatory disease present with similar findings. Culdocentesis may aid in establishing the correct diagnosis. In most cases, the diagnosis can be made by laparoscopy. If this procedure is not feasible and the diagnosis is suspected, an abdominal exploration is indicated.

The treatment of ectopic pregnancy consists of removal of the products of conception at the time of laparotomy. If the tube has ruptured and is extensively damaged, salpingectomy is indicated. If the pregnancy has distended the fallopian tube to 3 cm or less, a conservative approach utilizing a linear salpingostomy, evacuation of the products of conception, and microsurgical hemostasis may be done. If feasible, this conservative procedure may be done through the laparoscope. In terms of subsequent pregnancy, comparable results have been reported in both the conservatively treated and salpingectomy groups, 50 percent pregnancy and 10 percent recurrent ectopic rates.

ABNORMAL PREGNANCY GROWTH

Occasionally the products of conception will undergo abnormal growth and even malignant degeneration.

Trophoblastic Disease

Most cases of trophoblastic disease are benign hydatidiform moles that can be removed by curettage or hysterotomy. Following evaluation of a molar pregnancy, β-HCG is followed to be certain it returns to normal levels, usually within 3 months. Generally the patient is advised not to become pregnant for 1 year. Locally invasive trophoblastic disease has been referred to as *chorioadenoma destruens;* a malignant appearing tumor is referred to as *choriocarcinoma.* One cannot accurately predict the malignancy of trophoblastic disease from histologic appearance. The term *trophoblastic disease* is more generally applied to all of these disorders, and the malignant type is classified as *metastatic* or *nonmetastatic gestational trophoblastic neoplasia,* depending upon its location within or outside the uterus. The disease occurs rarely and in the United States appears in approximately 1 out of every 2000 pregnancies. There is a higher incidence in Asia, where there is approximately 1 case per 200 to 250 deliveries. The clinical picture is one of persistent bleeding and staining in early pregnancy with a uterus that is much larger than indicated by the menstrual history. Multiple pregnancies can be confused with this disease. Chorionic gonadotropin determinations often reveal levels higher than seen in normal pregnancy, while human placental lactogen (HPL) titers are lower. These can be measured in the patient's serum by radioimmunoassay. The use of ultrasonography aids in establishing the diagnosis of a normal or an abnormal pregnancy.

Placental polyp is not a true polyp but a term applied to a focally retained part of the placenta. There is necrosis, inflammation, and occasional bleeding. Hertig classifies a placental polyp as being potentially malignant. It may have neoplastic trophoblast at its base. On the other hand, syncytial endometritis, which histologically can be confused with choriocarcinoma, is probably a benign lesion from the placental site that contains many inflammatory cells.

Trophoblastic neoplasia commonly metastasizes to the lungs, vagina, brain, and liver, in decreasing order of occurrence. Antitumor agents provide excellent treatment; methotrexate, actinomycin D, and Velban have been the most commonly used chemotherapeutic agents. It has been estimated that there is complete remission in most cases following the use of methotrexate or actinomycin D in the treatment of trophoblastic neoplasia, and the overall cure rate approaches 100 percent for low-risk nonmetastatic cases. In certain cases, surgical intervention is necessary, either to control hemorrhage or infection or to eradicate a solitary site that has been refractive to chemotherapy.

CONTRACEPTION

ORAL CONTRACEPTION. Birth control pills are the most widely used method of contraception; one-third of all couples utilizing contraceptive methods choose oral contraceptives. Combination oral contraceptives consist of an estrogen, either ethinyl estradiol or mestranol, and a progestin. The progestins are either derivatives of 19-nor testosterone or derivatives of 17-alpha acteoxy progesterone. Naturally occurring estrogens or progesterone cannot be used orally because after absorption from the gastrointestinal tract and passage to the liver via the portal system they are metabolized to inactive forms.

The primary contraceptive action of the birth control pill is prevention of the LH and FSH surge that would otherwise induce ovulation. Also the progestin portion of the pill causes the cervical mucus to become more viscous and scant, retarding sperm penetration. In addition, the endometrium becomes somewhat atrophic, with diminished glandular glycogen making it hostile to implantation by the fertilized egg. If they are used properly the pregnancy rate with oral contraceptives is about 0.2 per 100 woman-years of use.

Although a large experience with oral contraception has demonstrated its effectiveness and safety in the vast majority of users, the side effects are numerous, and some are potentially serious. Several studies have confirmed that users have an increased risk of deep vein thrombosis (relative risk approximately 5.7 times greater than controls). Thromboembolic phenomena that can occur also include superficial vein thrombosis (1.5 times relative risk), neurovascular accidents (2 to 3 times relative risk), and myocardial infarction (2 to 6 times relative risk). The mortality from thromboembolic disease associated with the use of hormonal contraceptives has been estimated to be about 3 per 100,000 women per year of use. Increased coagulability results from an increase in clotting factors produced by the liver, a decrease in antithrombins, and increased platelet adhesiveness. Still, oral contraceptive use is less of a health risk than pregnancy.

Nearly every organ system is affected by oral contraceptives. There is an association toward carbohydrate intolerance with increased peripheral resistance to insulin. Levels of serum lipids, mainly of triglycerides, are elevated. Twenty percent of users show an increase in alkaline phosphatase. The relative risk of developing cholelithiasis is 2.0. Very rarely, benign adenomas of the liver have been identified in pill users. These are vascular and may rupture, with subsequent hemorrhage. Renin substrate is increased and about 5 percent of oral contraceptive users develop hypertension after 5 years, about 2.5 times greater than the expected incidence. Combination oral contraceptives are not associated with an increased incidence of malignant neoplasia in any tissue. A decreased incidence of benign breast tumors has been reported. Absolute contraindications to the use of oral contraceptives include estrogen-dependent neoplasia, thromboembolic disorders (a past history of deep vein thrombosis, cerebral vascular accidents, myocardial infarction), undiagnosed abnormal uterine bleeding, and pregnancy. Relative contraindications are congenital hyperlipidemia, hypertension, diabetes mellitus, migraine headaches, uterine leiomyomata, and seizure disorders. The pill should not be given to women over age forty. When there are other risk factors for thromboembolic phenomena (e.g., cigarette smoking, family history), oral contraceptives are an additional risk. In such women, consideration should be given to curtailing their use after age thirty-five.

The most serious side effects of the pill are estrogen-related. Therefore, the lowest effective dosage of estrogen should be used. Formulations that contain 50 μg of ethinyl estradiol or mestranol or less are recommended.

INTRAUTERINE DEVICE (IUD). The presence of a foreign body in the uterus elicits an inflammatory reaction, which renders the endometrium hostile to implantation by a fertilized egg. The effectiveness of the IUD is slightly less than that of oral contraceptives (2 pregnancies per 100 woman-years of users). Impregnating the device with copper or progesterone increases the effectiveness. Advantages of the IUD are (1) there are no further actions by the patient needed after insertion; (2) it can be removed, i.e., the method is reversible; and (3) most patients are relatively free of side effects. These side effects include expulsion (10 per 100 woman-years), bleeding (10 per 100 woman-years), cramps (5 per 100 woman-years), and pelvic inflammatory disease (overall relative risk is estimated to be 3). The latter side effect is the most serious. The risk seems to be higher in nulligravid patients.

In the spring of 1986, G.D. Searle, the manufacturers of the "Copper-7" (Cu-7) IUD, which had been the most widely used IUD, withdrew their product from the market because of excessive litigation. At the time of this writing, the authors are suggesting that this form of contraception not be used, except in those women who already have an IUD in place and are asymptomatic.

BARRIER METHODS. The condom has a theoretical effectiveness of 2.5 pregnancies per 100 woman-years. Because of patient noncompliance the real effectiveness is probably about 15 pregnancies per 100 woman-years. The condom, however, is the only known method of contraception that significantly decreases the transfer of venereal disease from one partner to another. The pregnancy rate with diaphragms is similar. Barrier methods are more effective in individuals who are more highly motivated to use them properly. Their great advantage is that they are free of side effects.

RHYTHM. This system of birth control is based upon a knowledge of the fact that in normally menstruating women, ovulation occurs at midcycle and that the viability of spermatozoa and oocytes is limited to about 72 and 24 h, respectively. According to the rhythm theory, if a woman has regular menstrual cycles and intercourse is performed only shortly after her period or before the onset of the next expected period, pregnancy should be avoided. However, even if educated, motivated couples utilize only rhythm, the pregnancy rate has been about 20 pregnancies per 100 woman-years. If the female partner uses a basal body temperature chart and is aware of cervical mucus, which is increased in quantity around the time of ovulation, the effectiveness of the method can be increased.

PERMANENT METHODS. In recent years, there has been an increase in the number of women choosing permanent sterilization as a method of contraception. In 1975, tubal sterilization was the third most frequently performed surgical procedure on fifteen- to forty-four-year-old women, 1 percent of all such women having had a tubal ligation. The operation may be done at the postpartum period via a small subumbilical incision. At an interval after pregnancy the procedure may be done through a small laparotomy incision or with the laparoscope. If the laparoscope is used, each tube is cauterized or has a small plastic ring placed on it. The failure rate is approximately 1 in 500. Because of increased expense and morbidity, hysterectomy is not recommended for sterilization.

SPECIFIC GYNECOLOGIC DISEASES

Infections and Discharges

During childhood, a whitish discharge, *leukorrhea,* may develop. At birth this increased vaginal secretion is usually due to maternal hormones and is entirely physiologic. A similar discharge may be seen in the pubertal female with the onset of estrogen stimulation. Severe leukorrhea during childhood is usually the result of infection and irritation caused by a foreign body in the vagina. If infection is present, a coliform organism is usually the offender. Occasionally pinworm infection is the cause. The correct diagnosis can be established by direct visualization of the foreign body and culturing for pathologic organisms, or by doing a Scotch-tape test for pinworms (*Enterobius vermicularis*). With the onset of menarche, a distinctive group of organisms can be implicated as the cause of a discharge. Discussion of specific infections follows.

TRICHOMONAS VAGINALIS INFECTION. This discharge is caused by a parasite. The trichomonad can be identified by its very active flagella, which can be seen beating when the vaginal discharge mixed with a drop of saline solution is examined microscopically. The parasite flourishes in an alkaline pH. It often causes a strawberry red inflammatory reaction of the cervix and is usually accompanied by a green and extremely odorous discharge that is often worse at the time of menstruation because of the alkalinity of the menstrual discharge. Treatment is carried out with a trichomonacidal drug, metronidazole. Vinegar douches are occasionally of symptomatic help. The male carries the infection asymptomatically and should be treated when there is recurrent infection in the female.

MONILIA VAGINITIS (*CANDIDA ALBICANS*). This fungous infection can occur at any time but is often seen during pregnancy, after the use of antibiotics, and frequently in diabetics. It flourishes in an acid environment. The fungus can be cultured on Nickerson's medium, but this is usually unnecessary to make the diagnosis. Mycelial budding can be seen on direct examination of the vaginal secretion which has previously been treated with 10% potassium hydroxide to lyse epithelial cells. Grossly, the discharge looks like a thick white cottage cheese. It is extremely irritating, and the patients usually complain of marked itching. Local antifungal agents are effective. Alkaline douches occasionally help, and gentian violet staining of the vagina may also provide relief. Anti-inflammatory agents such as cortisone can be used for the irritated vulva.

HAEMOPHILUS (GARDNERELLA) VAGINALIS. When vaginitis was present in the absence of *trichomonas vaginalis* or *Candida albicans,* the diagnosis of nonspecific vaginitis was formerly made. It is now known, however, that in these circumstances, *Haemophilus (Gardnerella) vaginalis* is the offending organism in the majority of cases. Anaerobes (bacteroides species, peptococcus, and peptostreptococcus) can usually be found in association with *Haemophilus* if appropriate culture techniques are used. For practical purposes, however, this is not necessary, as leukorrhea due to *Haemophilus* has a distinctive clinical picture. The discharge is malodorous and has a characteristic gray, homogeneous, creamy texture. The vaginal pH is between 5 and 6. Saline smears demonstrate vaginal epithelial cells covered with small coccoid bacteria (clue cells). Gram's stain demonstrates their gram-negative character. Metronidazole is effective against *Haemophilus* vaginitis. The safety of using metronidazole frequently against common vaginidities has not been established.

ATROPHIC VAGINITIS. This occurs in the elderly female or in the young patient after removal of the ovaries. The vaginitis is usually of a bacterial origin and results from secondary invasion of the atrophic vaginal tissues which have lost their thickness as well as their acid protection. Vinegar douches are occasionally helpful, and small doses of estrogen, either locally or orally, can restore the integrity of the vaginal mucosa.

BARTHOLINITIS. Infection of Bartholin's duct may lead to obstruction and eventual dilatation, with the formation of a Bartholin's cyst. Occasionally these are asymptomatic and require no treatment. If the cyst is acutely inflamed, drainage by marsupialization is usually successful; in cases of recurrent infection, removal of the cyst and gland may become necessary.

VENEREAL INFECTIONS AND PELVIC INFLAMMATORY DISEASE

SYPHILIS. This disease should be suspected in any genital lesion. Serologic screening (VDRL) tests can be done. Definitive diagnosis is made by dark-field examination of scrapings of ulcers to demonstrate the spirochetes or fluorescent treponema antibody absorption (FTA-ABS) blood tests. The diagnosis may be made by examination of the spinal fluid in more advanced cases. Treatment is with penicillin.

CHANCROID. This is a painful ulcer of the vulva caused by the organism *Haemophilus ducreyi,* which can be cultured from the ulcer and responds to sulfonamide or streptomycin therapy.

GRANULOMA INGUINALE. This is a chronic inflammatory disease. The offending *Donovania granulomatis* bacteria cause inclusion bodies to occur in the cells obtained from the ulcerating area (Donovan bodies). There are usually nontender ulcers, and tetracycline, streptomycin, or chloramphenicol therapy is usually effective.

LYMPHOPATHIA VENEREUM. This disease, which infiltrates the lymphatics and spreads to regional nodes causing a severe adenitis, is caused by *Chlamydia trachomatis.* The groins, perineum, and lower gastrointestinal tract can be involved. The diagnosis is made by skin test (Frei test) or by measurement of an antibody titer that remains elevated permanently, and therapy is effective with tetracycline. Scarring in the region of the anorectum can become so severe that colostomy may be necessary. Treatment is with tetracycline.

CONDYLOMA ACUMINATA. Condyloma acuminata typically occur as warts on the perineum but may arise in the vagina, cervix, anus, or urethra. They are caused by the human papilloma virus (HPV). When found on the cervix they are usually flat and often associated with cervical intraepithelial neoplasia (CIN). For this reason condyloma on the cervix should always be biopsied. Moreover, patients with HPV in association with neoplasia of the cervix are often younger than those with dysplasia alone. Application of dilute acetic acid to suspicious areas causes the lesions to become white and more prominent. Treatment can be with laser, cryosurgery, electrocautery, or local excision. 5-Fluorouracil (5-FU) cream has been used. Smaller lesions confined to the perineum may be treated with chemical therapy such as podophyllin or trichloroacetic acid. They frequently recur. Acidifying the vagina with boric acid suppositories or vinegar water douches may be helpful in preventing recurrences. As HPV is thought to be a venereal disease, examination and treatment of the male is essential. Condoms should be used during the healing phase.

HERPES VULVITIS. Genital herpes simplex infections caused by *Herpes simplex* virus type II are becoming more prevalent. They begin as painful vesicles, which over a period of several days undergo ulceration, pustular formation, encrustation, and eventually resolution. Inguinal adenopathy, fever, and malaise may accompany the attack. Emollient creams, ointments, and heterocyclic dyes with incandescent light have been tried as treatment, all without proved effect. Keeping the area dry with talcum powder and avoiding tight clothing may be helpful in reducing pain. Local anesthetic agents have occasionally been used. At times therapy for secondary bacterial infection with antibiotics is needed. Acylovir (an antiviral agent) may shorten the duration of attacks and reduce the frequency of recurrences. The long-term consequences of prolonged therapy with this drug are unknown.

GONORRHEA. This common disease is caused by bacteria of the genus *Neisseria gonorrhoeae.* The diagnosis may be established by examining the purulent discharge from the cervix, urethra, or Skene's gland. In 50 percent of culture-proved cases of gonorrhea, polymorphonuclear leukocytes containing gram-negative intracellular diplococci can be demonstrated on Gram's stain. The organisms can be cultured from the secretions, but the culture must be done immediately, since the organisms die soon after exposure to air, and a false-negative culture can result. Penicillin is the primary mode of therapy, but resistant strains of the organism are being detected. For the female with asymptomatic cervical gonorrhea, 4.8 million units of aqueous procaine penicillin plus 1 g of probenecid usually is given, and the dose is repeated if the culture remains positive. For patients allergic to penicillin, tetracycline can be used. Tetracycline can be given orally; after a loading dose of 1.5 g, 0.5 g is given four times daily for 4 additional days. Ampicillin, 3.5 g given orally as one dose, or spectinomycin, 4 g intramuscularly, may be used. Combined therapy with amoxicillin, 3.0 g orally; ampicillin, 3.5 g orally; or procaine penicillin 4.8 million units I.M. (all in combination with 1 g probenecid orally) may be given in combination with tetracycline 500 mg four times daily orally, or doxycycline 100 mg twice daily orally. Such therapy is effective against gonorrhea and any coexisting chlamydial infection. It is important to evaluate the patient about 5 days after treatment to ensure that symptomatic pelvic inflammatory disease (PID) has not developed. The cervix is recultured at this time. About 25 percent of patients with gonococcal pelvic inflammatory disease will have a recurrence. It is therefore important to treat all sexual contacts of the index case and reculture the index case. If adnexal pain and tenderness are present, indicating pelvic inflammatory disease, but the clinical picture does not warrant hospitalization (no fever, peritonitis, leukocytosis, or elevated erythrocyte sedimentation rate), therapy should be continued for 1 week, i.e., ampicillin or tetracycline 500 mg four times daily. If there is a question about the patient's status, she should be admitted to the hospital.

CHLAMYDIA. Infection with *Chlamydia trachomatis* seems to be becoming more prevalent. *Chlamydia* may be associated with salpingitis (see below) or the acute urethral syndrome. When *Chlamydia* is present in the female reproductive tract it is usually associated with a mucopurulent cervicitis. The mucus from the cervix is yellow or green when viewed with a cotton-tipped swab (positive swab test). A negative swab test is fairly good evidence against *Chlamydia* infection. Acute urethral syndrome is defined as dysuria, frequency, pyuria (greater than 10 leukocytes per high-power field of urine sediment), and a negative gram-stained smear of unspun urine. The treatment of uncomplicated chlamydial infections is with tetracycline. The treatment of pelvic inflammatory disease is discussed below.

PELVIC INFLAMMATORY DISEASE. Neisserian infection is frequently the initial cause of pelvic inflammatory disease in many patients. About 15 percent of patients with *Neisseria gonorrhoeae* cultured from the cervix will develop symptomatic pelvic inflammatory disease (PID). However, nongonoccal infection of the adnexa and pelvic tissue can follow gonococcal infection, once endosalpingeal damage has occurred. The infection is polymicrobial in nature with anaerobes (bacteroides species, peptococcus, peptostreptococcus) and aerobes, including coliforms, present. There is an increased risk of developing pelvic inflammatory disease if an IUD is present. Recently *Chlamydia trachomatis* has received attention as an etiologic agent in pelvic inflammatory disease. For example, in Sweden, *Chlamydia* was recovered from fallopian tube isolates in 30 percent of patients hospitalized with pelvic inflammatory disease. Studies thus far in the United States have indicated about a 10 percent recovery rate.

The patients characteristically present with acute diffuse lower abdominal pain and high fever, which may reach 103 to 104°F. There is severe pain on even slight motion of the cervix. The vagina is hyperemic and extremely warm. The tenderness noted on pelvic examination usually is bilateral because of the presence of a diffuse cellulitis. There may be some minor gastrointestinal complaints, but normal bowel sounds are usually present. The white blood cell count is elevated out of proportion to the degree of morbidity. In many cases, it is not possible to culture the pathogenic organism, but certainly an attempt should be made to rule out gonorrhea. Acute lower abdominal pain may also suggest appendicitis, ectopic pregnancy, twisted or ruptured ovarian cyst, or occasionally involvement of the urinary tract or the lower gastrointestinal tract.

Treatment consists of antibiotics and bed rest. Suitable antibiotic regimens include Clindamycin plus an aminoglycoside such as gentamycin and ampicillin doxycycline and a third generation cephalosporin, or doxycycline and metronidazole. The response is usually rapid. If an IUD is present, it should be removed. There is danger that a focus of chronic infection will exist in the pelvis and that repeated attacks will predispose to infertility. Therefore, complete and adequate therapy may require hospitalization. Occasionally, acute attacks are followed by scarring in the pelvis. This may then result in chronic pain and menstrual irregularity. In such patients, blocked tubes, sterility, and adnexal adhesions may then develop. The infertility rate of patients with a single episode of pelvic inflammatory disease has been estimated to be about 15 percent; after three episodes, about 75 percent. In certain cases, the secretions from the lining of the tube are trapped in the tube, and hydrosalpinx develops. In more advanced cases, an abscess develops between the tube and the ovary (TOA). About 50 percent of patients with TOA will come to surgery. This usually requires total abdominal hysterectomy and bilateral salpingo-oophorectomy, although if a unilocular abscess points in the cul-de-sac, it may be drained there. If the abscess has leaked or ruptured, there will be signs of generalized peritonitis, and prompt surgical therapy should be instituted. Total hysterectomy with bilateral salpingo-oophorectomy is the treatment of choice for ruptured tuboovarian abscesses. Occasionally, massive doses of antibiotics and supportive therapy with blood replacement and plasma must precede surgical procedures in order to bring the patient into optimal preoperative condition.

TUBERCULOUS PELVIC INFECTION

Tuberculosis is an uncommon cause of chronic pelvic inflammatory disease in the United States. It is generally associated with irreversible infertility. Tuberculosis is usually not a primary infection of the genital tract and is of either pulmonary or gastrointestinal origin. The diagnosis is usually made by curettings obtained at the time of menstruation and stained, cultured, and inoculated into guinea pigs. Chemotherapy with antituberculous drugs is the preferred treatment. Attempts to restore fertility by corrective surgical procedures in these cases have uniformly met with poor results.

Endometriosis

The growth of endometrial glands and stroma in areas outside the uterus is known as endometriosis. Such areas may undergo cyclic changes during the menstrual cycle, although histologically the changes do not necessarily mimic that of the endometrium. The sites of occurrence are wide and varied, and may be anywhere in the pelvis. The uterosacral ligaments are typical locations for this disease, and tender nodularity felt along these ligaments is diagnostic. Endometriosis is commonly found on the ovaries, where it exists as large chocolate cysts, or endometriomas. Posterior cul-de-sac peritoneal implants are very common, and multiple 2- to 3-mm nodules are often seen in this area. Endometriosis may be on the vulva or vagina and may undergo cyclic changes during the menstrual cycle that can be directly observed. Endometrial implants on the bowel can be the cause of cyclic lower gastrointestinal tract bleeding, and cases of cyclic hemoptysis have been reported from lesions in the lung.

Many theories have been proposed to explain the origin of endometriosis. None has been proved. One widely held theory postulates that implantation of endometrium occurs at the time of menstruation as a result of reflux of endometrial tissue into the peritoneal cavity through the fallopian tubes. The reflux theory is given some support by the fact that implantation of endometrial tissue can occur in cesarean section scars. Embryologic changes have also been suggested as a cause for endometriosis. It has been postulated that a change occurs in the coelomic epithelium, which gives rise to endometrial cell nests. This assumes that the cells with the potential of undergoing change to endometriosis are present at birth and transform during the reproductive years. Such a theory is given strength by endometrial implants found, not only on the bowel, but also in the lung and in other places in the body at a distance from the pelvis. Other theories have been advanced, but none can claim any greater acceptability.

A patient with endometriosis may have no symptoms or may complain of severe dysmenorrhea that becomes increasingly debilitating with the passage of time. Severe dysmenorrhea is usually seen in a patient in her late twenties who has never been pregnant, although endometriosis can occur in an older patient who has not been pregnant for years. The origin of the pain is uncertain but is probably due, in part, to cyclic bleeding into the sites of endometriosis at the time of menstruation. Large endometrial implants are often asymptomatic, while millimeter-size nodules are often associated with severe pain. Although it cannot be stated that endometriosis per se will cause infertility, it is generally accepted that patients with endometriosis will have a smaller chance of becoming pregnant than the general population.

Clinically, the diagnosis can be confirmed by direct visualization of the endometriosis at either laparotomy or laparoscopy. In order to make a microscopic diagnosis of endometriosis, endometrial glands, endometrial stroma, or blood should be demonstrated. The blood may appear in the form of hemosiderin. If two of these three diagnostic criteria are present, the histologic diagnosis of endometriosis is justified.

Many patients with endometriosis have no symptoms and require no special therapy. Spontaneous regression in some cases has been documented. Since there is an increased incidence of infertility in these patients, pregnancy preferably should not be delayed. If this is not possible and the patient is symptomatic, hormonal treatment with progestational agents accompanied by estrogen (pseudopregnancy) has been suggested to induce long periods of amenorrhea. This may decrease the size of endometrial nodules, but endometriosis may recur following such long-term therapy. Since growth of endometriosis is dependent on ovarian steroids, particularly estrogens, attempts have been made to treat the disease by drugs that inhibit ovarian function. Danazol, an expensive hormonal treatment, has been reported to be successful. The mechanism of danazol is not known, but the induction of a "pseudomenopause" with lack of an LH surge has been suggested. It also has some androgenic side effects that may contribute to decreased ovarian function. Long-acting analogs of GnRH, which by down regulation bring FSH to low levels with subsequent ovarian quiescence and reduction of estradiol, have also been suggested as a possible treatment for endometriosis and will probably be used more widely for that purpose.

In certain cases, surgical treatment must be performed. Conservative surgical measures consist of complete removal of as much of the endometriosis as possible, taking care to preserve normal anatomic structures, especially in the areas of the tubes and ovaries. A presacral neurectomy may be performed by a complete dissection between the hypogastric vessels, with careful identification of both ureters, and removal of the bundle of presacral nerves. In cases where the endometriosis can be completely excised, excellent results are obtained, and the patients usually remain pain-free. In general, the pregnancy rate after medical or surgical treatment is about the same—50 percent, depending on the severity of the disease. Whenever the disease is more severe than simple ovarian and cul-de-sac implants, i.e., when significant tuboperitoneal adhesions are present, medical therapy is usually not sufficient to restore fertility, and surgery must be done. The recurrence rate for conservatively treated endometriosis, by drugs or surgery, is about 40 percent.

If symptomatic endometriosis exists in an older patient who no longer desires to have children, a total hysterectomy with bilateral salpingo-oophorectomy can be considered. By surgical castration, the endogenous hormonal support of the endometriosis is removed, and the disease is cured.

Intrauterine DES Exposure

Clear cell adenocarcinomas of the vagina and cervix have been observed in young women whose mothers were treated with DES and similar compounds during pregnancy. Fortunately these cancers are rare among the exposed. They have been noted to occur primarily after puberty, with a peak incidence at age nineteen. Through age twenty-four, the risk of cancer is estimated to be 1:1000 or less. Since most of the exposed population is under forty years of age, it is not known what effect, if any, the exposure may have on these women as they age.

In spite of the apparent low risk of malignancy, DES-exposed females should have a complete gynecologic evaluation once they begin to menstruate or reach the age of fourteen, in order to rule out the presence of malignancy as well as to detect the common nonneoplastic changes that have been found in their vaginas and cervixes. These changes include vaginal adenosis; the presence of columnar tissue or its mucinous products in the vagina; cervical eversion (or ectropion); the presence of columnar epithelium or its mucinous products on the cervix; and transverse vaginal and cervical fibrous ridges. The ridges are found in about 20 percent of the exposed; while vaginal adenosis occurs in about one-half (depending upon the time in pregnancy when DES was started) and cervical eversion occurs commonly among the unexposed population, vaginal adenosis and transverse ridges are rare in the absence of intrauterine DES exposure.

Adenosis appears to be a benign lesion that is usually found near the vaginal clear cell adenocarcinoma. Current evidence suggests that adenosis does not require therapy. The columnar epithelium of vaginal adenosis and cervical eversion is usually physiologically replaced by squamous epithelium (metaplasia). Occasionally neoplastic, squamous epithelium develops (dysplasia, carcinoma in situ), as is discussed under Malignant Disease of the Uterus. Squamous malignancies have not been demonstrated to occur with increased frequency in the exposed, although there is concern about such a risk due to the large areas of squamous metaplasia found in the vagina and on the cervix.

The complete evaluation consists of careful palpation, direct visualization, and cytologic sampling of the vagina and cervix. This is usually followed by colposcopy to study transformation areas of metaplasia, followed by an iodine stain to delineate the extent of the nonglycogenated epithelium. Biopsies are taken from the areas or nodules that are suggestive of malignancy. In the case of abnormal Pap smears, biopsies are taken under colposcopic direction from the most abnormal areas.

It has been observed that the uteri of some DES-exposed females are deformed when they are examined by hysterosalpingogram. Alterations include small uterus

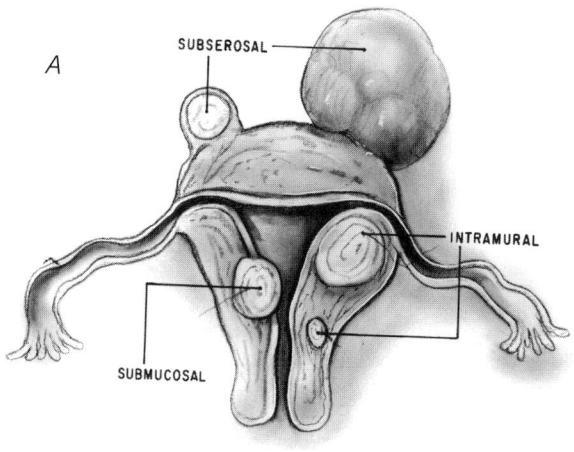

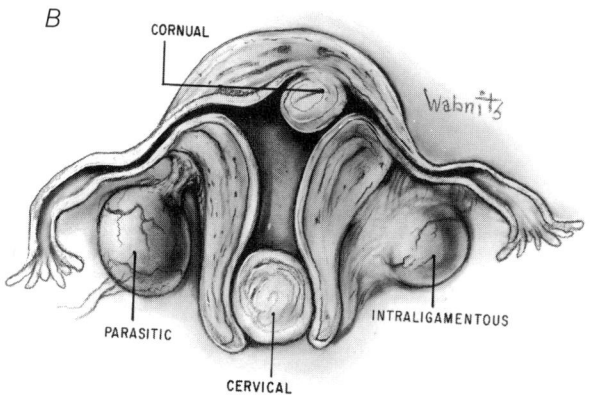

Fig. 41-20. Uterine fibroids. *A.* Types. *B.* Various locations.

(hypoplasia), T shape, "constriction ring," etc. Evaluation of reproductive performance has shown an increase of pregnancy loss, including premature birth, ectopic pregnancy, and miscarriage. Some of those who have experienced premature birth have had a successful pregnancy after cervical circlage. This operation is only performed in the DES-exposed when the usual obstetrical indications exist, such as midpregnancy loss or premature dilations of the cervix in the absence of labor. Current data indicate that over 80 percent of DES-exposed females who desire children have successfully achieved a live birth.

Benign Disorders of the Uterus

CORPUS

Fibroids

Fibroids *(leiomyoma)* are extremely common, occurring in perhaps 50 percent of women. They are collections of whorls of interlacing, smooth muscle fibers. Fibroids vary tremendously in size, being as small as a few millimeters or growing sufficiently large to fill the entire pelvis. They are usually named by their location, as shown in Fig. 41-20, where *subserosal, intramural,* and *submucous fibroids* are illustrated. Occasionally, a subserosal fibroid develops with a large stalk attached to the fundus of the uterus, in which case it is referred to as a *pedunculated fibroid*. This is easily confused on physical examination with an adnexal mass or ovarian tumor. The origin of these benign tumors is unknown, but there appears to be a definite hormonal influence, as the tumors are rarely seen prior to the age of twenty and are known to involute after the menopause. In addition, leiomyomas can be stimulated to grow by administering estrogens. Therefore, estrogen-containing medication, such as oral contraceptives, must be used judiciously in the presence of these tumors.

Their presence is not in itself an indication for any treatment. The therapy of leiomyomas is dependent upon the symptoms and problems that are associated with them. Fibroids are associated with four major problems. These are bleeding, pain, increase in size, and reproductive wastage.

Bleeding. An increase in menstrual flow or prolongation of the menstrual period sufficient to cause anemia can be associated with submucous fibroids. The endometrial cavity is markedly enlarged and distorted, and there is incomplete endometrial regeneration over the surface of the fibroid, leading to continuous oozing or bleeding and sometimes hemorrhage.

Pain. This is not a common symptom. It occurs primarily when there is degeneration, which usually results when one of these large tumors outgrows its blood supply. It may also occur when a pedunculated fibroid twists and becomes infarcted. Rarely pain is associated with a large leiomyoma that has impinged or caused pressure on local adjacent viscera, and the discomfort would be referred to the involved organ.

Growth. Fibroids do grow during the reproductive years. Usually the growth is at a slow rate, unless there is excessive hormonal stimulation as a result of medication or in association with pregnancy. Since malignancy occurring in a fibroid is an exceedingly rare event, malignant change need only be considered if the growth of the fibroid is extremely rapid, especially during the menopausal years.

Reproductive Wastage. In habitual abortion and possibly in infertility, fibroids may be etiologic.

A submucous fibroid will occasionally extrude through the cervix and present as a bleeding and infected mass attached by a stalk to the endometrial cavity. These fibroids are safely treated by removing the stalk, followed by a few weeks' rest period to allow infection to clear from the pelvic lymphatics prior to undertaking further surgical treatment. Attempts at surgical procedures without this waiting period usually result in a high incidence of postoperative complications and wound sepsis. In general, the surgical therapy of fibroids consists of either hysterectomy or myomectomy.

Adenomyosis

Adenomyosis is a growth of endometrial tissue in the myometrium of the uterus and is sometimes referred to as *endometriosis of the uterine corpus*. The condition occurs primarily during the reproductive years and leads to a thickening of the myometrial wall with subsequent uterine enlargement. Adenomyosis usually occurs in women who have had a number of pregnancies. Occasionally patients with adenomyosis will complain of dysmenorrhea, and some present with increased uterine bleeding and heavy menstrual flow. However, a number of patients with adenomyosis in hysterectomy specimens have been asymptomatic. Therefore, the association of adenomyosis with heavy menstrual bleeding and dysmenorrhea is questionable.

Polyps

Endometrial polyps can occur at any time after puberty. A polyp is a local hyperplastic growth of endometrial tissue that usually causes postmenstrual or postmenopausal bleeding or staining, which is cured by polyps removal at curettage. The polyps are usually benign, but cases of adenocarcinoma of the endometrium arising in a polyp have been reported.

Endometritis

Occasionally patients with menstrual irregularity and postmenstrual staining are found to have endometritis. Histologically, the lesion demonstrates massive inflammatory cell infiltration of the stroma of the endometrium. The infiltration is greater than that normally seen at the time of menstruation and is usually accompanied by plasma cells. Antibiotics and curettage usually are sufficient treatment. Instrumentation or procedure such as obtaining a tubogram should not be performed in the presence of endometritis, since a severe exacerbation of diffuse pelvic inflammation could result.

CERVIX

Common benign conditions of the uterine cervix include inflammation, Nabothian cysts, and polyps. *Cervical polyps* cause the same symptoms as *endometrial polyps*. Since they are often quite small and are visible at the external os, they often can be removed as an outpatient procedure followed by cauterization of the base of the polyp. *Nabothian cysts* are mucous inclusion cysts of the cervix. They are occasionally associated with chronic inflammation and can easily be removed with a cautery. However, they are harmless, usually asymptomatic, and generally do not require therapy.

During reproductive years the portio of the cervix is covered primarily with glycogenated squamous epithelium, and columnar epithelium is normally found centrally near the external os in most women. This exposed columnar epithelium is termed *ectropion,* or *eversion,* and usually is bright red. Unless accompanied by inflammation and a purulent discharge (cervicitis), it requires no treatment. During adult life, the columnar epithelium is usually replaced by squamous metaplasia, and this physiologic process occurs in the transformation zone at the interface of squamous and columnar epithelium. After menopause the squamous columnar junction is usually in the endocervical canal.

Malignant Disease of the Uterus

CARCINOMA OF THE CERVIX

Carcinoma of the cervix formerly was the most common malignant tumor of the female reproductive tract. Recently, carcinoma of the endometrium has become the most common. Carcinoma of the cervix comprises approximately 40 percent of genital tract cancers. Most of the tumors are epithelial cell or squamous cell carcinomas, while approximately 5 to 10 percent are adenocarcinomas. The tumor occurs more frequently in women who have started to bear children at an early age. The malignant change develops at the squamocolumnar junction, and this area is also involved with inflammatory changes following pregnancy. Squamous cell carcinomas are not often seen in the virgin female. There is a possibility that a male factor may be etiologically related, and the disease appears to have a venereal association. Although a specific etiologic agent has not been identified, viruses, especially human papilloma virus (HPV) types 16 and 18, and *herpes simplex* virus type II (HSV-II), have been found in association with the tumor.

SYMPTOMS. Carcinoma of the cervix may be discovered in a patient who has no symptoms or complaints. She may have intermenstrual bleeding or staining and may complain of bleeding that occurs following douching or intercourse. Any bleeding of an irregular nature that is not associated with menstruation is a danger signal in the female of reproductive years. Postmenopausal bleeding also may be caused by cervical carcinoma, but it occurs more commonly with endometrial malignancy. Pain is a late manifestation of this disease, as is general malaise.

DETECTION AND DIAGNOSIS. The advent of the Papanicolaou smear has offered the possibility of screening large segments of the population for cervical tumor by methods that are approximately 95 percent accurate. The smear is usually taken by direct aspiration or scraping from the cervix. The stained smear can then be categorized as showing normal, suspicious, or malignant changes. Although malignancy can be suggested by the Papanicolaou smear, the diagnosis of cervical carcinoma can be made only on biopsy. Even in the presence of malignant disease, a benign smear may be obtained, especially where there is a great deal of secondary infection accompanying the tumor. Therefore, a malignant tumor of the cervix is not definitely ruled out by a benign Papanicolaou smear, and grossly suspicious areas should be biopsied. A suspicious Papanicolaou smear or report of malignant cells in the smear also requires further investigation by biopsy.

By helping the examiner identify abnormal epithelial and vascular patterns in the transformation zone, the col-

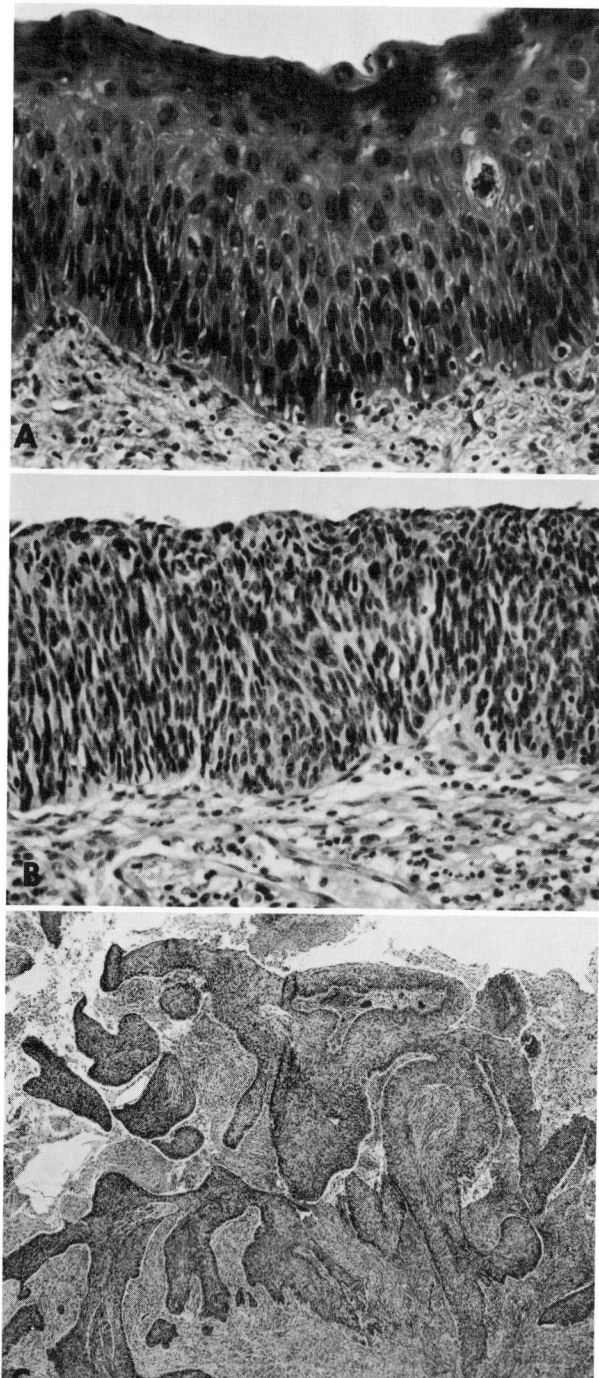

Fig. 41-21. *A.* Cervical dysplasia. *B.* Carcinoma in situ of cervix. *C.* Invasive squamous cell carcinoma of cervix.

Schiller's or Lugol's iodine stain can also be used as a nonspecific guide for biopsy. Nonglycogenated epithelium will usually appear grossly normal but does not stain with iodine. These suggestive areas are then biopsied, although such areas may contain only nonneoplastic or inflammatory changes.

The Papanicolaou smear is particularly important in that it not only can detect the cells of a frankly malignant condition but also can detect changes in the cervical epithelium that are potentially malignant. These changes are termed *anaplasia* (dysplasia) or *carcinoma in situ,* depending upon the severity of the alterations in the cervical epithelium. Alternately these are designated as cervical intraepithelial neoplasia (CIN I—mild dysplasia, CIN II—moderate dysplasia, CIN III—severe dysplasia or carcinoma in situ).

Colposcopy, which consists of the examination of the cervix with a low-power microscope and built-in light source, has recently gained popularity. It is a technique that aids in differentiating neoplastic processes and other atypical lesions.

Dysplasia. Figure 41-21 shows an area of dysplasia of the cervix in which the architecture of the squamous epithelium has been disturbed and there is progressive loss of differentiation of the squamous epithelial cells. Dysplasia is a premalignant change and can be treated successfully by cauterization, cryosurgery, or laser. Local destruction of this premalignant change will eradicate it, provided the entire area of atypicality is treated. Patients with dysplasia must be thoroughly investigated and followed to make sure that a more serious cervical change does not exist or develop in the future.

Carcinoma in Situ. The lesion consists of malignant epithelium that is confined to the surface of the cervix (Fig. 41-21*B*). There is no invasion of the deep layers of the cervix by malignant cells. In spite of its malignant potential, the lesion does not metastasize. Carcinoma in situ is considered a precursor of invasive carcinoma for the following reasons:

1. The peak rate of occurrence of carcinoma in situ precedes by approximately 10 years in age distribution the peak occurrence of invasive carcinoma of the cervix. In situ lesions are seen at about the age of thirty-eight, while invasive carcinoma occurs most frequently at age forty-eight, and both diseases occur at approximately the same rate, with the 10-year span separating them.
2. There is a similar racial and ethnic distribution. The disease is uncommon in Jewish women when compared with non-Jewish women and is more frequently seen in blacks than in whites.
3. It is common in cases of carcinoma of the cervix to note microscopically coexisting, adjacent areas of carcinoma in situ.
4. A few patients with carcinoma in situ have been known to develop invasive carcinoma later.

Once the question of malignancy of the cervix has been raised, either by Papanicolaou smear or by biopsy, carcinoma in situ must be differentiated from invasive carcinoma of the cervix, since these lesions can coexist. Colposcopy is used to identify the most abnormal areas. It is vital to rule out invasive cancer, and hospitalization for diagnostic conization of the cervix is occasionally re-

poscope aids in directed biopsy of the most suggestive areas. It is important that the entire transformation zone be visible on the portio of the cervix for a satisfactory colposcopy to be performed. If colposcopy is unsatisfactory, a diagnostic conization of the cervix will usually be necessary to rule out the presence of invasive carcinoma.

quired if an adequate evaluation cannot be obtained by colposcopy and biopsy.

THERAPY. Treatment is determined by the nature of the lesion and most particularly by the extent of involvement.

Carcinoma in Situ. If the diagnosis of carcinoma in situ without invasion can be made, adequate therapy consists of conization or a total abdominal hysterectomy. The cervix and vagina may be stained with Schiller's solution prior to surgical treatment to detect any parts that do not take Schiller's stain, and these parts are included with the specimen.

All patients treated for carcinoma in situ should be followed by yearly vaginal smears, since the remaining squamous epithelium of the vagina can undergo malignant changes in future years. Patients with carcinoma in situ in whom preservation of reproductive function is desired can be treated by a therapeutic conization of the cervix. Some investigators have utilized locally destructive procedures such as cryosurgery, cauterization, or laser to treat carcinoma in situ, with good results. The follow-up of these patients is particularly important, since future premalignant epithelial change can occur in both the vagina and retained cervix.

Invasive Carcinoma. Carcinoma of the cervix is a locally invasive tumor (Fig. 41-21C). It spreads over the surface of the adjacent epithelium of the cervix and may invade the underlying muscular walls and disseminate via lymph channels. Parametrial areas and paracervical areas are prime sites for the spread of the disease. The first metastases are usually found in the lymph nodes of the pelvis and often in the parametrium and paracervical tissues. The tumor spreads to the pelvic wall along the hypogastric vessels and then to the areas of the external and common iliac arteries. The tumor will extend outside the true pelvis as a late manifestation. In untreated cases, death can result from hemorrhage due to major vessel erosion or from urinary tract obstruction that leads to subsequent uremia while the disease may be confined to the pelvic cavity.

STAGING. In order to determine the proper therapy of carcinoma of the cervix, the precise extent of the disease must be defined. This is accomplished by diagnostic x-rays, sigmoidoscopy, cystoscopy, and pelvic examination under general anesthesia. The tumor spread is classified according to international agreement that divides the various categories into the stages depicted in Fig. 41-22.

Stage I refers to invasive carcinoma that is confined to the cervix. If invasive tumor is not clinically evident and a small focus is discovered microscopically, microinvasion or preclinical carcinoma is diagnosed and assigned to Stage IA. The diagnosis of microinvasive carcinoma is usually made if invasion is 3 mm or less and vascular or lymphatic involvement is absent. All other Stage I carcinomas then are assigned to Stage IB. *Stage II* refers to carcinoma that extends beyond the cervix but has not yet reached the pelvic wall and is confined to the upper two-thirds of the vagina. The stage is subdivided by most clinics into Stage IIA, which indicates involvement only of the vagina, and Stage IIB, which indicates involvement beyond the vagina, into the parametrial and paracervical

areas. *Stage III* refers to involvement of either the lower third of the vagina or the extension of tumor to the pelvic wall. If tumor has caused hydronephrosis or a nonfunctioning kidney as determined by intravenous pyelogram, the tumor is assigned to Stage III. *Stage IV* represents either spread of tumor outside the pelvis or invasion of the mucosa of the bladder or rectum by malignant disease.

CHOICE OF THERAPY. Radical surgical procedures and radiation therapy both provide effective treatment for carcinoma of the cervix. The modality of therapy will depend upon the extent of the tumor, the condition of the patient, and the capabilities of the clinic. There are a large number of cases that can be treated successfully by either method with similar likelihood of cure. Although attempts have been made to measure the patient's responsiveness to radiation by studying the histology of cervical tumor following external radiation and by examining the cellular components of the smear, there is no available test that permits one to separate those cases that will best respond to surgical treatment from those that will do better with radiation.

State I and II-A. Most patients with Stage I carcinoma of the cervix or early Stage IIA lesions can be treated equally satisfactorily by either radical surgery or radiation. If radical surgery is performed, ovarian function occasionally can be preserved. Patients with local inflammation or pelvic infection should be treated surgically, since massive sepsis can result if radiotherapy is undertaken. The development of a wide en bloc dissection is an integral part of adequate surgical therapy for this disease, and the extent to which an adequate dissection can be done is illustrated in Fig. 41-23. It can be seen that wide areas of the parametrial and paracervical tissues can be removed. Many investigators feel that microinvasive carcinoma (Stage IA) can be effectively treated with total (extrafascial) hysterectomy.

RADIATION CONSIDERATIONS. Adequate radiation therapy requires the delivery of tumoricidal doses of radiation to all areas that either are or can be affected by tumor. The dose of radiation delivered is inversely proportional to the distance between the source and the point being treated. In addition, the tissue absorption of radiation is inversely proportional to the wavelength of the administered dose. Thus, by lowering the wavelength, one increases penetration of the radiation. This can be done by raising the therapeutic voltage, as for example, with the million-electron-volt machines, or it can be accomplished by using filters to eliminate the longer wavelengths. Time and volume factors are important. When a given dose is administered over a long period of time, the tissue reaction is less than if it is given in a short interval. Similarly, a dose that is distributed throughout a large volume causes greater tissue damage than one that is confined to a small volume. The unit of exposure in radiation is usually expressed as the rad, which is equivalent to the transfer of 100 ergs of energy per gram of tissue. For practical purposes, this is equivalent to 1 rad. Thus, 10,000 rads given to the cervix is a dose that can be tolerated, while the same dose given to the entire pelvis would

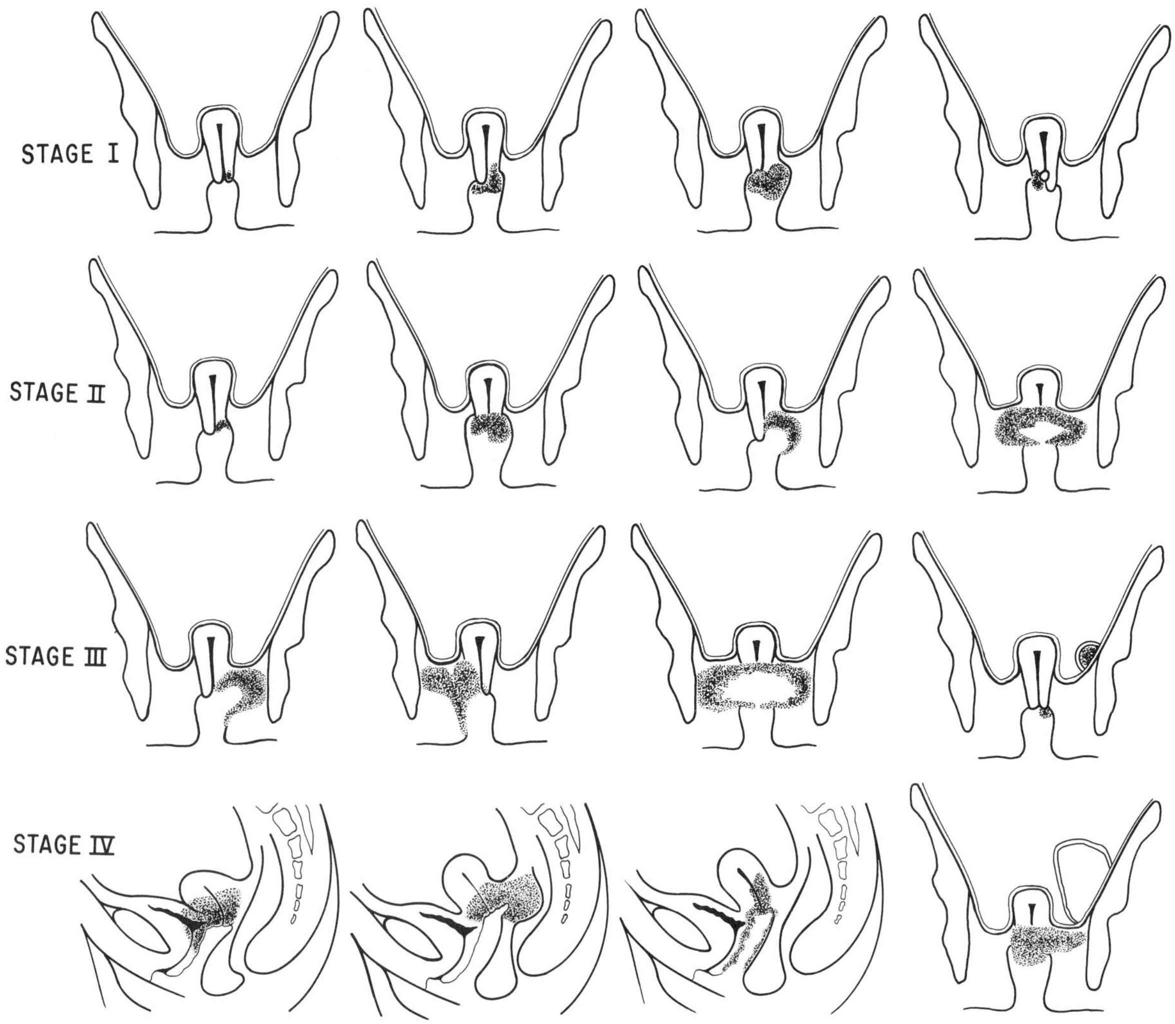

STAGE I

STAGE II

STAGE III

STAGE IV

Fig. 41-22. Clinical stages of cervical cancer (International Classification).

Fig. 41-23. Radical hysterectomy section.

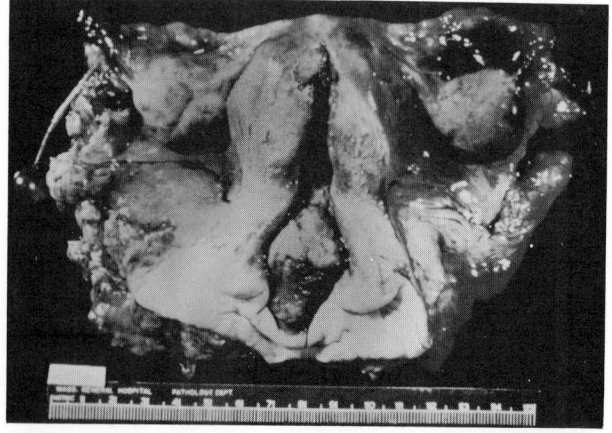

cause necrosis of normal tissue. Occasionally, radium or cesium doses are expressed in terms of milligram-hours, a quantity determined by multiplying the milligrams of radium used by the number of hours it is in place. However, this gives no indication of the overall effect or distribution of the dose in relation to surrounding tissue. For convenience, two standard reference points, identified as A and B, are used to specify the dose of radiation given. Point A is 2 cm superior to the fornix and 2 cm lateral to the uterine canal. Point B lies in the same plane but is located 5 cm laterally.

The radiosensitivity of a tissue is proportional to its reproductive capacity and degree of differentiation. Since neoplastic tissues are generally poorly differentiated and have increased mitotic activity, they are, as a rule, more sensitive to radiation than normal tissue. The radiosensitivity of a tumor is an expression of its ability to respond to radiation, and this is not necessarily the same as its ability to be cured by radiation. The radiocurability of a tumor depends upon the ability to deliver sufficient radiation to destroy the tumor completely and eliminate it from the host. The presence in the pelvis of vital structures immediately adjacent to the anatomic distribution of the tumor limits the amount and dose of radiation that can be given, just as it limits surgical treatment. Local irradiation is usually done in two applications separated by 2 to 3 weeks. By dividing the application, the tumor is given a chance to shrink following the first local application, and a better application can be accomplished the second time. The treatments are supplemented with external therapy to the entire pelvis, usually with shielding of the midline. Treatment may be initiated with external therapy followed by use of local (intracavitary) sources. As a rule, 6000 to 8000 rads are delivered to Point A and approximately 5000 rads to Point B. Afterloading devices, utilizing a central stem and side ovoids (Fletcher-Suit applicator), permit the appliance without radiation exposure to medical personnel. An x-ray film of the application is taken and dosimetry calculated on a computer, depending upon the arrangement of stem and ovoids.

Stages IIB, III, and IV. In cases of extensive Stage IIB carcinomas of the cervix or in Stage III or IV lesions, external radiation is usually initially employed. Since intracavitary treatment is effective only for local cervical disease, external therapy permits treatment of the entire bulk of the tumor before concentrating on the small central part. Following preliminary external radiotherapy, radium application usually can be more effectively completed. If Stage IV lesions involve the bladder or rectum but not the pelvic wall, then a radical surgical procedure removing the bladder (anterior exenteration) or rectum (posterior exenteration) is used, since radiation cure of these lesions is usually less than 5 percent and fistulas can result from radiation treatment. However, preliminary external radiotherapy can be useful to reduce the size of the tumor as well as secondary infection. Smaller doses of radiotherapy are used when future surgical therapy is planned.

PROBLEMS OF SURGERY AND RADIATION. The immediate problems concerned with radiation therapy relate to discomfort of the patient as a result of gastrointestinal upset. Nausea, vomiting, or diarrhea are frequently encountered. However, long-term complications can also occur, and these usually relate to bleeding or inflammation of the lower bowel or chronic irritation of the bladder. Radiation proctitis or cystitis can occasionally become extremely debilitating. Fistulas may result either between the bowel and the vagina or between the bladder and the vagina, especially where extremely heavy doses of radiation have to be used. With recent refinements in radiation techniques, these complications are occurring less frequently.

Surgical complications usually occur early and relate to damage of either the genitourinary tract or the bowel. Urinary fistula is the most common severe complication and occurs in approximately 1 percent of cases treated by radical hysterectomy. Some of these close spontaneously, but a few require further surgical treatment, such as repair of a damaged ureter or removal of the affected kidney.

RESULTS OF THERAPY. The curability of carcinoma of the cervix is directly related to the extent of the disease at the time therapy is initiated. Comparable results have been obtained following the effective use of surgical and radiation therapy. Average approximate 5-year survival rates for the various stages are as follows: Stage I, 85 percent; Stage II, 50 percent; Stage III, 25 percent; Stage IV, 10 percent. In Stage I lesions with negative nodes, the 5-year survival approaches 90 percent. When the nodes are positive, the rates drop to 45 percent.

Recurrent Cervical Carcinoma. Carcinoma of the cervix can metastasize to any part of the body, but most recurrences are found in the pelvis. If the patient has pelvic recurrence after primary surgical therapy, then radiation can be tried to treat local disease. If recurrence occurs after primary therapy with radiation, then only by radical removal of the contents of the pelvis is there hope of curing the patient. This usually requires removal of both the lower bowel and bladder (total exenteration), and this procedure is reserved only for those cases where there is some hope of cure. It is occasionally done for palliation. In properly selected cases, a 30 to 40 percent 5-year survival can be obtained by using exenteration for therapy of recurrent carcinoma of the cervix. Chemotherapy is occasionally palliative for those with recurrent disease not treatable by radiation or operation.

Carcinoma of the Cervix in Pregnancy. In general, the therapy of carcinoma of the cervix that occurs during a pregnancy follows the same principles that would pertain if the patient were not pregnant. Consideration for the viability of the fetus is important only in the latter stages of pregnancy and should not be allowed to change treatment in a way that will diminish the chances of curing the mother. In the first trimester of pregnancy, therapy for early Stage I lesions can be accomplished either by radical hysterectomy or by radiation therapy. The latter is followed by spontaneous delivery of the products of conception. In the second and third trimesters the fetus has become sufficiently large that the size of the uterus becomes a technical problem. In the third trimester, cesarean section is usually performed once the fetus reaches viability. For patients diagnosed in the second trimester, therapy can be initiated with external irradiation, but there is concern about risk of hemorrhage if a sizable fetus delivers through a friable cervix, so preliminary hysterotomy may be required. For the advanced Stage II and III cases, radiation therapy remains the treatment of choice. Results of therapy indicate that for each stage the survival following treatment for carcinoma of the cervix in pregnancy is much the same as it is in the nonpregnant patient, except that the prognosis tends to be worse for lesions diagnosed later in pregnancy.

TUMORS OF THE CORPUS OF THE UTERUS

Endometrial Carcinoma

Most malignant tumors of the corpus of the uterus arise in the glands of the endometrium. Adenocarcinoma (Fig. 41-24*C*) is the most frequently found tumor, although a

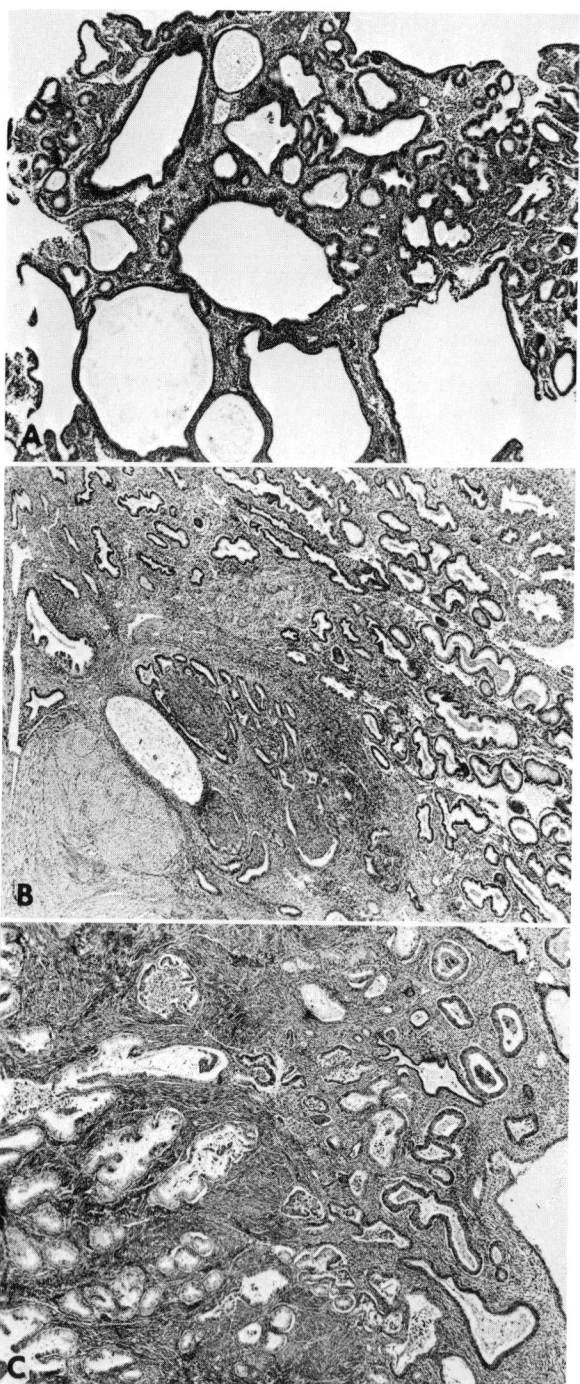

Fig. 41-24. *A.* Endometrial hyperplasia (cystic and adenomatous). *B.* Carcinoma in situ. *C.* Adenocarcinoma of endometrium.

few adenocarcinomas with squamous tissue elements (adenocanthoma) are seen. These tumors are histologically different but appear to have a similar clinical behavior.

Carcinomas of the endometrium are becoming more common, especially among Caucasians. They are the most common tumor seen in the female reproductive tract. Most cases occur in the sixth decade of life and are associated with nulliparity or late childbirth. There is also an increased incidence of endometrial carcinoma in patients who are obese, diabetic, and hypertensive. Thus, these patients will generally present a markedly different social history, reproductive history, and somatic appearance than patients with carcinoma of the cervix.

The endometrium is exquisitely sensitive to hormonal stimulation, and it appears that abnormal stimulation of the endometrium could play a part in the development of certain endometrial carcinomas. It has been observed that there is an increased incidence of endometrial carcinomas in cases of prolonged and excessive estrogen stimulation, such as with estrogen-secreting tumors, as well as among individuals receiving menopausal estrogen replacement therapy (see under Endocrine-Related and Reproductive Problems for discussion of estrogen plus progestin therapy).

A scheme of development of malignancy has been suggested that begins with a local hyperplastic growth of endometrial glands in the form of an endometrial polyp; then cystic hyperplasia develops, followed by both cystic and adenomatous hyperplasia (Fig. 41-24*A*), and finally carcinoma in situ (Fig. 41-24*B*) of the endometrium. This sequence of changes might occur in a fashion similar to that already described for carcinoma of the cervix, although the stimuli are evidently quite different. Patients who have had prolonged anovulatory cycles and continuous estrogen stimulation without progesterone appear to be prime candidates for the development of hyperplastic changes and endometrial carcinoma.

Corpus carcinoma can be staged as follows:

Stage I—the carcinoma is confined to the corpus
    IA—the uterus sounds to 8 cm or less
    IB—the uterus sounds to more than 8 cm
Stage II—the carcinoma involves the corpus and cervix
Stage III—the carcinoma extends outside the uterus but is confined to the true pelvis
Stage IV—the carcinoma extends outside the true pelvis or involves the mucosa of the bladder or rectum

The grade of endometrial carcinoma is also important. Three grades (G1, G2, G3) are usually assigned, with the latter identifying the least differentiated lesion.

Initially, carcinoma of the endometrium invades the myometrium and then the lymphatics. When the tumor is low in the uterus and involves the cervix, the paths of spread are the same as those for cervical carcinoma. In contrast, spread of tumor from the upper part of the fundus goes directly to the aortic or inguinal nodes, which are sites outside the limits of radical pelvic surgical therapy.

THERAPY. The primary method for carcinoma of the endometrium is surgical therapy. This usually consists of a simple total hysterectomy when the carcinoma is well differentiated and confined to the fundus. Regional lymph nodes and occasionally para-aortic lymph nodes are sampled to delineate potential spread of the disease outside the uterus. To reduce the incidence of vaginal recurrence, a postoperative vaginal application containing radioactive sources is usually done in 4 to 6 weeks. In those cases where the cervix also is involved, therapy is best carried out in accordance with the principles outlined under the discussion of carcinoma of the cervix. External radiation therapy is employed in cases of spread to lymph nodes or for less well-differentiated tumors and for those that invade deeply into the myometrium. Radiotherapy alone is used for patients who are unable to tolerate surgical therapy. These patients are then given additional radium therapy.

RESULTS OF THERAPY. The results of therapy in cases of carcinoma of the endometrium will vary with the extent of the lesion originally treated. For tumors confined to the fundus and treatable by surgical methods, approximately 70 to 80 percent will be alive and free of disease 5 years following treatment. For those who are not, because of medical reasons or spread of tumor, able to be treated by primary surgical procedures, the 5-year survival is markedly reduced. The overall salvage is approximately 50 to 60 percent.

PROBLEMS OF RECURRENCES. Recurrences of carcinoma of the endometrium are most frequently seen in the vagina, especially in the suburethral area or at the vaginal apex. They occasionally occur in the pelvis. Distant metastases are most commonly found in the lung and in the liver. Occasionally, there are intraperitoneal, nonpelvic sites of metastatic disease, but these are less common. Therapy for recurrence of endometrial carcinoma depends upon its location and extent of tumor. In cases where there is a local recurrence in the pelvis, either in the vagina or intraperitoneally, radiation is the treatment of choice. Occasionally, local vaginal radium applications are possible. If there is a large recurrence located centrally within the pelvis and especially if there has been prior radiation therapy, radical pelvic surgical therapy should be considered. However, as in the case of carcinoma of the cervix, exenteration is generally considered for cure of a patient who is in good medical condition. Distant metastases of carcinoma of the endometrium have been successfully treated by high doses of progestational agents. Delalutin (17-hydroxyprogesterone caproate), Depo-Provera (medroxyprogesterone), and Megace (megestrol acetate) have been employed and in some cases have resulted in regression of metastatic nodules, particularly in the lung. Well-differentiated tumors respond most favorably, while highly undifferentiated tumors or those which have been previously irradiated have a less satisfactory response. An overall response rate of about 25 percent has been obtained.

Sarcomas

These are rare tumors, comprising less than 5 percent of uterine malignant disease. They primarily occur in the postmenopausal female. The following types are those most frequently encountered.

Mixed Müllerian Tumor. These tumors contain adenocarcinoma and sarcomatous elements. If the sarcomatous portion arises from cells normally found in the uterus (smooth muscle, fibrous, etc.), the term *homologous* is used, and if they arise from cells found at other sites (car-tilage, striated muscle) the term *heterologous* is used. The prognosis is frequently poor.

Endolymphatic Stromal Myosis. This refers to an endometrial tissue infiltration into the myometrium. It is a form of low-grade stromal sarcoma. The more mitoses noted in these tumors, the more malignant is the behavior.

Leiomyosarcoma. This category is the most common variety of sarcoma. These tumors generally arise from the myometrium and may be either smooth muscle leiomyosarcomas or may contain more fibrous tissues in the form of fibrosarcoma. Occasionally, one encounters malignant degeneration in a fibroid, but this is a rare occurrence. The prognosis is believed to be better if the sarcomatous change is confined to a leiomyoma.

Stromal Sarcoma. This is a sarcoma that arises from a stromal cell of the endometrium, which then invades the myometrium. It is the more malignant expression of endolymphatic stromal myosis. There are pleomorphic endometrial cells with occasional giant cell formation present inside the tumor. Many of these tumors appear to arise in patients who have had previous radiation. These tumors are usually found in the older age group and are seen primarily in the postmenopausal female. Many of them are associated with pyometrium, since the endocervix becomes closed and there is some accumulated secretion and infection behind it developing into purulent contents contained within the endometrial cavity. It has been estimated that approximately 2 to 4 percent of all patients with uterine cancer, regardless of the histologic features, may be found to have pyometrium.

THERAPY. The primary therapy of sarcoma of the fundus is surgery, consisting of total simple hysterectomy. In general, the prognosis for all these tumors is poor unless they are detected early and confined to the uterus. Radical surgical treatment generally has not been successful. Although some sarcomas have been found to be radiosensitive, they have not, as a rule, been radiocurative. Some additional palliation has been obtained by the use of chemotherapeutic agents, primarily with combinations containing Adriamycin (doxorubicin).

Disorders of the Vulva

BENIGN AND PREMALIGNANT CHANGES

The vulva is an area that is readily accessible to examination and treatment. Therefore, much attention has been focused on the local changes that precede the development of malignancy. Whitish areas have been noted to coexist with vulvar malignancy, and in many cases these white areas have existed prior to tumor development. Such areas have been termed *leukoplakia* (white patch). However, confusion has arisen, since many white areas of the vulva are associated with pruritic irritations that bear no relationship to malignancy and are without malignant potential. The correct diagnosis of a white vulvar lesion can be made only by biopsy, and this examination should be performed for lesions that are not temporary irritations.

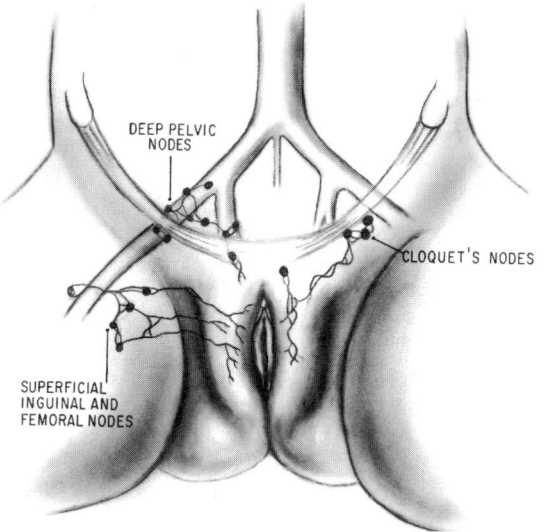

Fig. 41-25. Routes of lymphatic spread in carcinoma of the vulva.

Although the term *leukoplakia* is often used for any white patch of the vulva, it is properly reserved for areas that show histologically atypical epithelial activity. These alterations may precede the development of malignant changes. In many instances chronically irritated and itchy white areas of the vulva will show sclerosing atrophy of the skin (*lichen sclerosus et atrophicus*). Lichen sclerosus et atrophicus is a pruritic lesion that does not appear to be premalignant. Hyperplastic lesions termed *hypertrophic dystrophies* are found that may be benign (epithelial hyperplasia) or may show atypia, in which case dysplastic changes can be observed. The pruritic symptoms can be helped by topical application of corticosteroids. Testosterone has also been beneficial, especially for the atrophic changes (lichen sclerosus et atrophicus).

Noninvasive malignant change of the surface squamous epithelium of the vulva occurs in the same way that has been described for the cervix. Carcinoma in situ of the vulva, both histologically and clinically, behaves like carcinoma in situ of the cervix. The changes are confined to the squamous elements of the vulva, and the condition is sometimes referred to as "Bowen's disease." In certain instances, the apocrine glandular elements of the vulva are involved in association with an intensely pruritic area. Histologically, large, foamy Paget's cells are seen, similar to those noted in the breast, although invasive carcinoma occasionally can accompany Paget cells. Both Bowen's disease and usually Paget's disease are considered part of the carcinoma in situ complex of the vulva and are adequately treated by wide local surgical excision that consists of a simple vulvectomy. The laser also is used to treat these lesions locally.

VULVAR MALIGNANCY

Most malignant tumors of the vulva are of the squamous cell variety. These tumors make up approximately 5 percent of all gynecologic malignant tumors and occur primarily in elderly patients. The average age of a patient treated for this disease is about sixty-one years, and the incidence of vulvar carcinoma increases in each decade. As with carcinoma of the endometrium, vulvar carcinoma tends to occur in obese patients and in nulliparous patients, and the incidence of diabetes is increased in those with this disease. In addition, as many as 10 percent of these patients may have malignant tumors at other sites.

As a rule, the carcinoma arises unilaterally and may be present on any part of the vulva. It may be multicentric in origin. The disease spreads via the lymphatics and in spite of the unilaterality of the primary lesion the lymphatics carry the tumor to both sides. Initially, metastases occur from the vulva to the superficial inguinal and femoral nodes. Then spread progresses to the deep pelvic nodes of the external iliac group (Fig. 41-25). Vulvar carcinomas tend to be slow-growing, locally spreading tumors with distant metastases occurring as late manifestations of the disease.

The rate of cure of this tumor formerly was poor because of attempts at treatment by simple local excision. The recent advent of a wide surgical en bloc resection (Fig. 41-26) has markedly improved the survival rate of these patients. Adequate therapy usually consists of a radical vulvectomy combined with bilateral superficial groin node dissection (Fig. 41-26B). Dissection usually includes both groins, even though the tumor is confined to one side of the vulva, because of the high incidence of bilateral spread through the rich supply of anastomosing vulvar lymphatics. Occasionally, separate groin incisions are used to reduce the frequency of skin slough and wound infection. If the superficial nodes are involved the deep nodes are usually removed surgically or treated with radiation.

Approximately half the patients treated in this fashion are cured of the carcinoma. If the lymph nodes are uninvolved with tumor, the cure rate rises to 80 or 90 percent. Even if the lymph nodes are involved, almost half the patients treated by radical vulvectomy and bilateral node dissection can be salvaged. Involvement of the deep nodes markedly diminishes the prognosis. Radiotherapy as sole treatment has not proved to be as satisfactory as surgery, especially since the vulvar skin becomes chronically irritated and pruritic after radiation. Recently, however, preoperative radiation has been used as an adjuvant in the case of large vulvar lesions that encroach on the anus or urethra.

Tumors other than epithelial carcinomas can occur in the vulva. Basal cell carcinomas are treated by simple excision. The vulva is a common site for malignant melanoma, and approximately 8 percent of melanomas that occur in females are noted in this region. However, they constitute only about 2 percent of all vulvar malignant tumors. Melanomas occur at any time but are usually noted in later years. Vulvar melanoma is treated similarly to epithelial cell carcinoma, i.e., by radical vulvectomy and bilateral superficial and deep node dissection.

Carcinomas of Bartholin's glands have been reported,

A

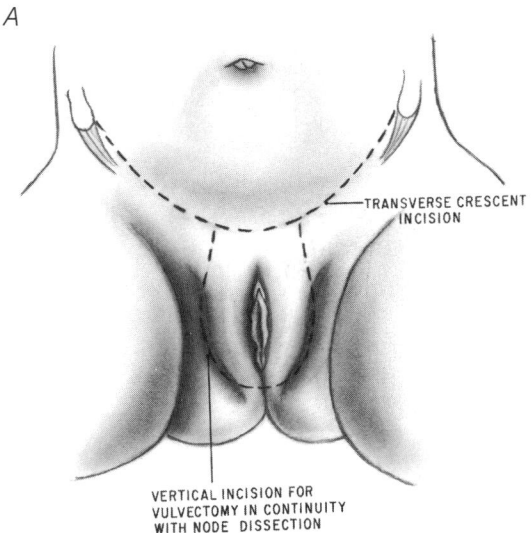

—TRANSVERSE CRESCENT INCISION

VERTICAL INCISION FOR VULVECTOMY IN CONTINUITY WITH NODE DISSECTION

B

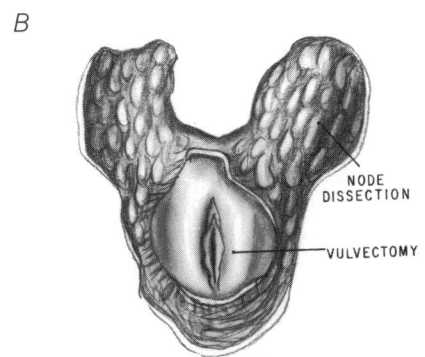

NODE DISSECTION

VULVECTOMY

Fig. 41-26. Radical surgical treatment for carcinoma of the vulva. *A.* Incision for a one-stage approach to radical vulvectomy in continuity with bilateral groin and deep pelvic lymph node dissections. *B.* Final operative specimen.

but these are exceedingly rare. Since the tumors are often diagnosed late in the course of the disease, they have generally disseminated through lymphatics. The results of therapy have been poor, although a wide local resection with node dissection would appear to offer the best opportunity for eradication.

Finally, tumors of sweat gland origin are seen in the vulva. These are referred to as *hidradenomas*. There is some disagreement as to whether or not these tumors can occur as carcinomas. However, they are locally invasive, and therefore minimum adequate therapy consists of wide local excision.

Malignant Tumors of the Vagina

Although the vagina is frequently a site of extension from vulvar, cervical, or endometrial tumors, it is the rarest site for the origin of a malignant tumor in the female genital tract, with the exception of the fallopian tube. Usually vaginal malignant tumors occur in postmeno-

pausal females around the age of sixty. One exception to this is the *sarcoma botryoides,* which is a tumor of young children. This malignant sarcoma usually presents as a mass in young infants. It is a bulky, polypoid tumor that is radiation-resistant, and the only hope of cure lies with radical surgical therapy.

Most primary cancers of the vagina are *squamous cell carcinomas.* Their clinical behavior depends upon the location in the vagina. Those that occur in the upper vagina usually behave as cervical tumors and therefore are treated by the same criteria used in therapy of carcinoma of the cervix. If a squamous cell carcinoma appears to be primarily occupying the vagina but is also on the cervix, it must be classified as a primary cervical tumor. For tumors located in the anterior vagina, either radiotherapy or an anterior exenteration will provide adequate therapy. For those lying in the posterior or upper vagina, either a posterior exenteration or radiotherapy must be considered. The tumors involving the lower vagina are treated as vulvar tumors, since the lymphatic spread in these instances is similar to that noted for vulvar carcinoma.

Adenocarcinomas of the vagina and cervix have been noted in young women in their late teens and early twenties, many of whose mothers took diethylstilbestrol and similar hormones during pregnancy (see section on disorders of bleeding). Histologically, the tumors consist of clear cells containing glycogen and so-called hobnail cells. Therefore, they are called *clear cell carcinomas,* although they also have been called *mesonephromas.* Benign glandular infiltration of the vagina (vaginal adenosis) often accompanies these tumors, and transverse vaginal septa occasionally are seen, presumably resulting from in utero exposure to diethylstilbestrol. Diagnosis is made by vaginal examination. Although vaginal cytology occasionally can detect the tumor, the smear sometimes is negative with tumor present. Thus a complete pelvic examination including inspection of the walls of the vagina is necessary to rule out this malignancy. Therapy is accomplished by the usual considerations governing the treatment of malignancy in this area. Both operative resection and irradiation have been effective in eradicating these tumors. The operative approach is favored for young patients with early resectable lesions. A few small vaginal tumors have been treated with local radiation with preservation of ovarian and uterine function. When recurrences occur, they are most frequently noted locally, in the lungs, and in supraclavicular nodes. The results with chemotherapy have been disappointing.

Ovarian Tumors

DIAGNOSIS. Many types of ovarian tumors can occur in both benign and malignant forms, and a few tumors cannot be classified until their clinical behavior has been clarified by following the patient for a number of years. This multipotential behavior of ovarian tumors necessitates the consideration of benign and malignant lesions together. Ovarian malignant tumors occur less frequently than those from either the cervix or the endometrium. In general, there is an increased incidence of malignancy in ovarian tumors with advancing age.

In an infant or child, ovarian tumors may present as large pelvic masses. Adequate evaluation requires an intravenous pyelogram to rule out the urinary tract as the cause of the mass (Wilms' tumor). Patency of the hymen and vagina should be checked to rule out hydrocolpos, and the patient should be catheterized to be sure the mass is not a urine-filled bladder. An ovarian tumor in these young patients is most likely to be a teratoma, usually of the cystic variety (dermoid), or a follicle cyst. Ovarian malignant tumors do occur in the young age group, but they are rare.

During puberty and the reproductive years, ovarian tumors become more common. There is little need for concern about an enlargement unless it has become 5 cm or larger. Most 5-cm tumors in this age group are benign follicle cysts and may be followed through two menstrual periods. If the lesion persists for this length of time or appears to be enlarging, diagnosis through direct visualization is indicated. Depending upon the size and location of the mass and the age of the patient, this may be accomplished by laparoscopy or abdominal exploration. For patients who are over age forty or in the menopausal years the ovarian masses estimated to be 5 cm or larger should be explored.

Since ovarian enlargements are often asymptomatic, there can be significant spread of an ovarian tumor before the diagnosis is made. Common subjective symptoms consist of lower abdominal discomfort occasionally accompanied by the feeling of distention. Pain is rare unless there is advanced disease. In about one-third of the cases, the patient may complain of abnormal vaginal bleeding, and in a few cases urinary or intestinal complaints may be elicited.

NONNEOPLASTIC CYSTS

By definition a cystic enlargement of the ovary should be at least 2.5 cm in diameter to be termed a cyst. Some of the more common cysts are as follows.

FOLLICULAR CYSTS. These are unruptured, enlarged graafian follicles. They may grossly resemble true cystomas which are described in the following section. They can rupture, causing acute peritoneal irritation, may undergo torsion and infarction of the ovary or infarction of the tube and ovary, or may spontaneously regress.

CORPUS LUTEUM CYSTS. At times these cysts may become as large as 10 to 11 cm. They can rupture and lead to severe hemorrhage and occasionally vascular collapse from blood loss. The symptoms and physical findings of these cysts may mimic those of ectopic pregnancy, and they are thought by some to be associated with delayed menses and spotting.

ENDOMETRIOMAS. These account for most "chocolate cysts" and are simply cystic forms of endometriosis of the ovary.

WOLFFIAN DUCT REMNANTS. These are not ovarian cysts but often cannot be distinguished clinically from tumors of the ovary. They are small unilocular cysts. Occasionally, they enlarge and may twist and infarct. In most instances, they are incidental findings at laparotomy and cause no difficulties or symptoms.

MÜLLERIAN DUCT REMNANTS. These can appear as paraovarian cysts or as small cystic swellings at the fimbriated end of the fallopian tube (hydatids of Morgagni).

NONFUNCTIONING TUMORS

Cystadenomas

Many of the common, benign, cystic tumors of the ovary are believed to arise from the surface germinal epithelium. Some of these tumors, referred to as *serous cystadenomas,* appear as cysts with thin, translucent walls containing clear fluid and lined by simple ciliated epithelium. They frequently are on a pedicle and may undergo torsion leading to pain and infarction. When encountered surgically, they are adequately treated by simple salpingo-oophorectomy. Many serum-containing cystic tumors of the ovary are also accompanied by papillary projections and are known as papillary serous cystadenomas. Because of epithelial variation in these tumors, it is often difficult to be sure where they fit in the spectrum of benign to malignant disease. A similar problem of malignant potential exists for the mucinous cystadenoma, which is a cystic tumor containing sticky, gelatinous material. These mucinous tumors are less likely to be malignant than the serous cystadenomas. About 20 percent of the serous tumors and 5 percent of the mucinous tumors are bilateral.

It is not always possible to be sure by gross inspection whether cystic tumors with solid components are benign or malignant. It is usually necessary to excise the involved ovary completely, even though there is no definite evidence of malignancy. The malignant potential of the cystoma is then determined by histologic examination. Some cystomas are classified as *borderline tumors,* or adenocarcinomas of low malignant potential. These (grade 0) carcinomas are usually associated with an excellent prognosis and if they are unilateral may be treated by unilateral adnexectomy for women in their reproductive years. However, borderline tumors can escape the confines of the ovary, in which case therapy as described below for ovarian carcinoma is considered. In those in whom childbearing is not an issue, therapy for ovarian cancer is performed even if the borderline lesion is confined to one ovary. Frozen-section examination of the tumor at the time of surgical intervention is necessary to determine the proper course of therapy for patients in the reproductive age group. The opposite ovary should be examined for a lesion and may be bivalved.

Occasionally, a condition known as *pseudomyxoma peritonei* is encountered; it is a locally infiltrating tumor composed of multiple cysts containing thick mucin. These tumors arise either from ovarian mucinous cystadenomas or from mucoceles of the appendix, both of which commonly coexist. Histologically, they are benign, but by local spread and infiltration they compromise surrounding vital structures. Localized tumors should be completely excised, if possible. Both ovaries and the appendix are removed even though they grossly appear to be normal.

Primary Carcinomas

Primary carcinomas of the ovary most commonly are serous, mucinous, or endometroid cystadenocarcinomas. These are malignant variations of the previously discussed cystadenomas and of endometriosis. A useful method of staging these tumors is as follows:

Stage I—tumor confined to the ovaries
Stage II—tumor confined to the true pelvis
Stage III—tumor extends to peritoneum outside pelvis
Stage IV—spread beyond the abdominal cavity or intrahepatic
    metastases

Stages III and IV tumors have a markedly poorer prognosis than in those cases with malignancy confined to the ovary.

It is common to see seedings on both peritoneum and serosal surfaces of bowel. Giant masses can develop and slowly spread to fill the entire peritoneal cavity encasing the bowel but rarely invading the lumen. Fluid retention occurs, and both ascites and hydrothorax may be present. Lower leg edema may be seen secondary to abdominal lymphatic obstruction. The patient may experience an increase in abdominal girth and, possibly, weight gain accompanied by wasting of the extremities, loss of appetite, and reduction in muscle mass. Increase in fluid retention and in the size of the abdomen continues with the growth of the intraabdominal tumor.

Surgical intervention is the primary therapy for ovarian malignancy and consists of hysterectomy and bilateral salpingo-oophorectomy. If ascites is present, ascitic fluid is examined cytologically for malignant cells. If there is no obvious extension of tumor outside the ovaries, peritoneal saline washings are examined for malignant cells. The omentum is also excised, and suspiciously enlarged pelvic and paraaortic nodes are sampled. An attempt should be made to remove all sites of the tumor, including local peritoneal metastases. Resection of bowel is performed to allow complete removal of the tumor, and the patient should have a preoperative bowel prep. In widespread cases, however, radical pelvic surgical treatment with removal of the bladder or the rectum has generally not proved to be helpful. Therefore, if a few discrete peritoneal metastases exist, it is wise to remove them and it is generally accepted that maximum tumor reduction surgery is beneficial if it does not seriously expose the patient to the risk of life-threatening complications. Reduction of tumor mass appears to be helpful in improving the response to chemotherapy or irradiation.

Chemotherapy has been effective in treatment of ovarian carcinoma. Combination chemotherapy is usually utilized for advanced disease, using cis-platinum and an alkylating agent as parts of one combination regimen. These potent agents interfere with rapidly growing cells and thus particularly affect the bone marrow and gastrointestinal tract as well as the tumor. Nausea, vomiting, diarrhea, and loss of hair can accompany their use. Blood indices must be carefully observed since leukopenia and thrombocytopenia may occur, especially in patients who have received radiotherapy. The dosages are adjusted to maintain a slight leukocyte depression with the white blood cell count kept in the range of 3500 to 5000 cells per cubic millimeter. Other agents have been effectively used including Adriamycin, hexamethyl-melamine as well as methotrexate and 5-fluorouracil (5-FU). Combinations and dosages are adjusted depending upon toxicity and patient status.

Intraperitoneal instillation of radioactive material has been utilized as adjunctive therapy for cases of carcinoma with positive peritoneal washings or ascites when gross disease has been removed. Agents such as ^{32}P are effective since they emit primary beta radiation and this is effective for approximately 1 month. One must be careful in using intraperitoneal instillations, since there is often loculation of fluid between areas of tumor and bowel that can cause a high local concentration, and bowel perforation can result. Efforts have been made recently to improve results with intraperitoneal chemotherapy, particularly using higher doses of cis-platinum.

Radiotherapy can also be used to treat ovarian carcinoma when gross disease remains after surgery. However, multiple-agent chemotherapy is more frequently used as initial therapy at most centers in the United States.

The ovary is a site for metastases from tumors originating elsewhere in the body. Solid ovarian tumors containing malignant disease that is usually metastatic from the stomach are known as *Krukenberg tumors*, identified histologically by the presence of signet cells. However, ovarian metastases from other intestinal malignant tumors are more common. In cases where a Krukenberg tumor can be diagnosed, it is felt by some that oophorectomy may offer a palliation to the patient, even though the primary malignant tumor cannot be found. The ovary is also a common site for metastases from breast carcinoma.

Dysgerminoma

This germ cell tumor is most often seen in females in the age group of ten to thirty years. It often occurs in pseudohermaphrodites. Dysgerminomas are often found during pregnancy, perhaps because they occur most frequently during the reproductive years. Histologically (Fig. 41-27C), the tumors contain masses of germ cells infiltrated with lymphocytes. If the tumor is unilateral and has not broken through its capsule, a simple oophorectomy is usually sufficient therapy. If it has broken through its capsule but has not spread beyond the ovary and the contralateral ovary is normal, preservation of the contralateral ovary with radiation to the side of the surgically removed specimen may be considered. If the tumor has spread or metastasized locally in the pelvis, the prognosis is poorer. The tumor is sensitive to radiation, resembling the seminoma of the male.

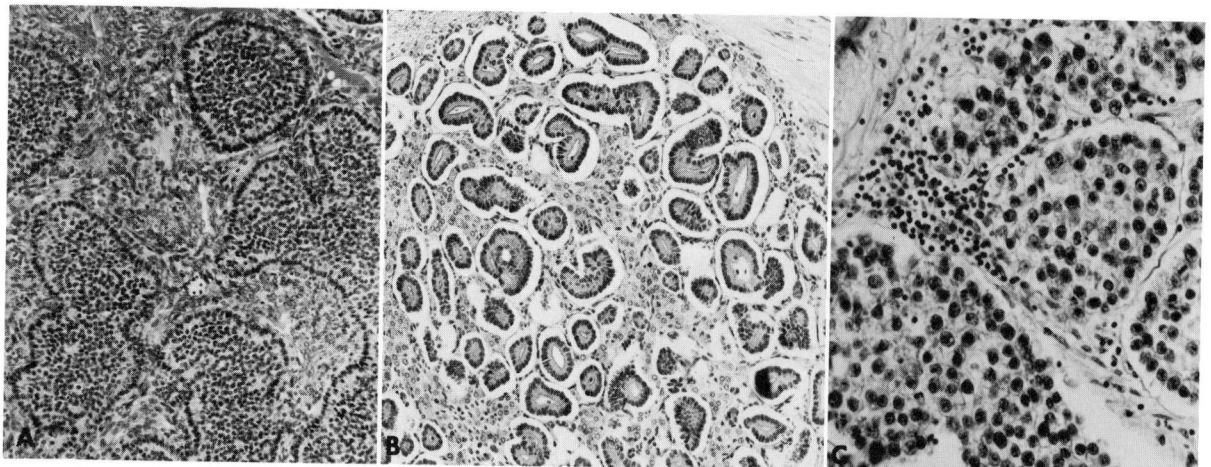

Fig. 41-27. *A.* Granulosa-theca cell tumor. *B.* Arrhenoblastoma. *C.* Dysgerminoma.

Teratoma

These germ cell tumors are thought to arise from the totipotential germ cells of the ovary. The tumors often contain calcified masses, and occasionally either teeth or pieces of bone can be seen on abdominal x-rays. Teratomas occur at any age but are more frequent in patients between twenty and forty years. They are usually benign dermoid cysts but occasionally are solid and then are usually malignant (solid malignant teratomas; immature teratomas).

If a cystic teratoma (dermoid) is encountered in a young woman, it is preferable to shell it out from the ovarian stroma, preserving functioning tissue in the affected ovary. Usually these cysts contain ectodermal, mesodermal, and entodermal tissues, in addition to a thick, greasy, fatty material. If this material is spilled during surgery, a chemical peritonitis may result, and, therefore, it is important to remove these tumors intact. The opposite ovary should be inspected but no further operative procedure performed if the opposite ovary appears normal. In approximately 12 percent of the cases these tumors are bilateral. Immature teratomas are treated as a carcinoma of the ovary by hysterectomy and bilateral salpingo-oophorectomy.

Brenner Tumor

These are fibroepithelial tumors that are rare and usually do not secrete hormones. Histologically, the epithelial elements are similar to Walthard rests and are believed to arise from these. These tumors occur primarily in later life and have a small malignant potential. Simple oophorectomy is usually sufficient therapy, and the prognosis is excellent.

Clear Cell Carcinomas

These epithelial carcinomas account for as many as 5 percent of primary carcinomas of the ovary. Histologically they consist of clear cells containing glycogen and "hobnail" cells. In most cases the ovaries and uterus are removed since the tumors predominantly occur in older women.

Meigs' Syndrome

This pertains to ascites with hydrothorax, seen in association with benign ovarian tumors with fibrous elements, usually fibromas. It is more common to see fluid accumulation with ovarian fibromas that are more than 6 cm in size. The cause of the condition is unknown, but the ascitic fluid may originate from the tumor, as a result of lymphatic obstruction of the ovary. Frequently, this clinical picture is encountered with other ovarian tumors, especially ovarian malignancy, which can produce a cytologically benign pleural effusion; in such cases it is termed a "pseudo-Meigs" syndrome. Meigs' syndrome can be cured by excising the fibroma.

FUNCTIONING TUMORS

Granulosa-Theca Cell Tumor

Pure theca cell tumors (thecomas) are benign, but those with granulosa cell elements may be malignant. It is often impossible to predict their behavior from the histologic features (Fig. 41-27*A*), and prolonged follow-up is necessary in order to judge the nature. Usually, granulosa cell tumors elaborate estrogen, but some of these tumors have no hormone production. In the young girl they are characteristically manifested by precocious puberty, and in the elderly female they are sometimes associated with endometrial carcinoma. The tumor can occur at all ages from childhood to the postmenopausal period but are most common in later life, with maximal occurrence between the ages of forty and sixty. If the tumor is discovered in the reproductive years and confined to one ovary without signs of surface spread or dissemination, a simple oophorectomy may be sufficient therapy. If it is discovered in later life, removal of both ovaries with the uterus is indicated.

Sertoli-Leydig Cell Tumors (Arrhenoblastomas)

These are rare but potentially malignant tumors that are associated with androgen output and masculinization. Rarely, they elaborate estrogen. They usually occur in the reproductive age group and appear to contain tubular structures as well as Leydig-type cells (Fig. 41-27B). In young patients with a singly involved ovary, unilateral oophorectomy is adequate therapy, provided there is no extension of the tumor. For older patients or for those with bilateral involvement, total hysterectomy and bilateral salpingo-oophorectomy are performed.

Hilus Cell Tumors

These are also rare tumors and consist of nests of cells resembling the hilus cells of the ovary. They are characteristically associated with masculinization. They occur primarily in the later years of life and often in the menopausal female. None of the reported cases was malignant.

Struma Ovarii

This term refers to the presence of grossly detectable thyroid tissue in the ovary, usually as the predominant element in dermoid cysts. This tissue occasionally may produce the clinical picture of hyperthyroidism.

Choriocarcinoma

These very rare primary tumors of the ovary elaborate chorionic gonadotropin, and the therapy follows similar considerations already outlined for the trophoblastic disease, but the therapeutic results for the ovarian tumors have been disappointing.

Adrenal Rest Tumors (Lipoid Cell Tumors)

These are also very rare tumors of the ovary that may occur at any age and are not always associated with hormonal activity. Those with adrenal tissue usually show masculinization and are, as a rule, benign. Although most of the signs of masculinization regress after surgical therapy, some of the effects, such as enlarged clitoris, may remain.

Tumors of the Fallopian Tube

BENIGN TUMORS

Tumors of the fallopian tube are rare. Occasionally one sees a tube with thick nodularities at its proximal end. This benign condition is referred to as *salpingitis isthmica nodosa,* and although its origin is not definitely known, it is thought to be a sequela of tubal inflammation. It is associated with infertility due to blockage of the tubes. In cases of infertility, a tuboplastic procedure can be attempted, often in the hope of restoring tubal patency, but the prognosis is poor.

Another type of benign lesion is referred to as *adenomatoid tumor.* These are small gland-containing enlargements of the tube that are usually located in the tubal muscularis and are often incidental findings at the time of surgical intervention. Other enlargements of the tube secondary to inflammation or associated with pregnancy are discussed in previous sections of the chapter.

MALIGNANT TUMORS

Primary malignant tumors of the tube are the least frequently seen cancers of the female genital tract. There may be an association between previous tubal inflammation and subsequent development of carcinoma in the tube. Usually these tumors are papillary adenocarcinomas. They may present as a pelvic mass. Occasionally, the tumors block the distal end of the fallopian tube and cause a bloody, mucous vaginal discharge. These tumors are occasionally seen during the reproductive years but occur more often in the postmenopausal age group. Because of the paucity of symptoms and physical findings associated with them, tumors of the fallopian tube are difficult to diagnose early. They may metastasize locally and occasionally spread to the inguinal nodes. Primary therapy is by surgical excision, preferably removal of the tumor and of the uterus and opposite tube and ovary as well. In cases where there appears to be some lymphatic spread of the tumor in the area of the cervix, a radical hysterectomy may effect a cure. The 5-year survival ranges between 10 and 40 percent. Radiotherapy or chemotherapy may be tried as palliation or as adjunctive therapy.

TECHNICAL CONSIDERATIONS OF GYNECOLOGIC OPERATIONS

Dilatation and Curettage

Dilatation and curettage (D and C) are frequently indicated in a variety of clinical problems. In patients of reproductive age it is often advisable to perform a curettage after a first-trimester pregnancy loss. In such circumstances, as has been noted in this chapter, an incomplete abortion may have occurred, and curettage is advisable both to prevent further blood loss and to reduce the incidence of postabortal infection. These considerations apply only to cases of spontaneous noninfected abortion. In those cases where instrumentation or sepsis have supervened, a curettage should not be carried out until the patient is adequately treated with antibiotics. Any manipulation of a pregnant uterus should be carried out with extreme care because of the high risk of uterine perforation. In addition, only the major products of conception need be removed. Excessively vigorous curettage at this time can denude the uterine cavity of regenerative tissue, which may result in postcurettage intrauterine synechiae (Asherman's syndrome).

A curettage may also be indicated during reproductive years for excessive bleeding and hemorrhage not associated with pregnancy. The procedure may be combined with hysteroscopy. In such instances, it is important to carry out a meticulous exploration of the endometrial cavity to be sure that neither endometrial polyps nor sub-

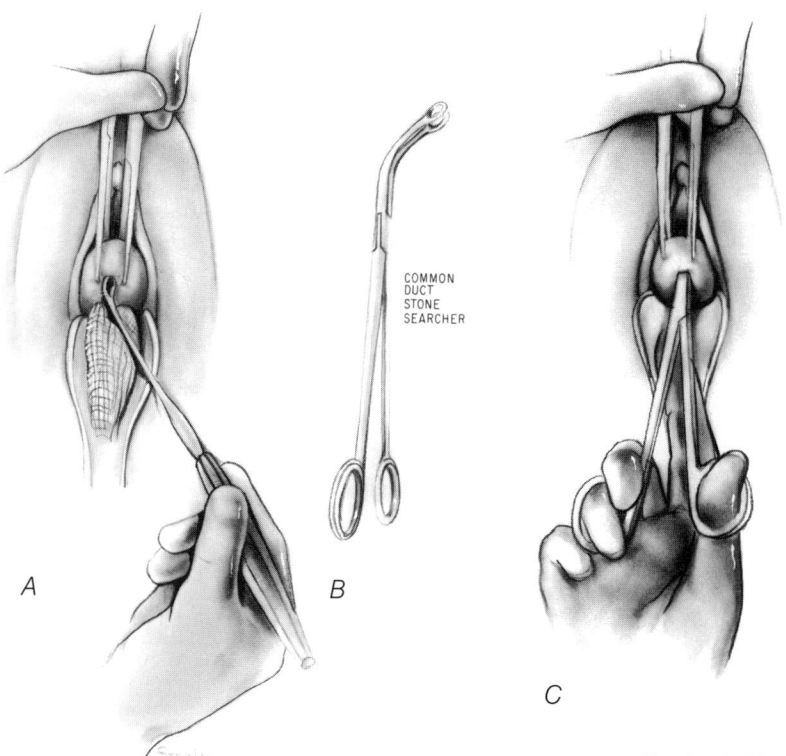

COMMON
DUCT
STONE
SEARCHER

A   *B*

C

Fig. 41-28. Dilatation and curettage. (See description in text.)

mucous fibroids are present. During the menopause, excessive bleeding may necessitate a curettage for diagnostic as well as therapeutic reasons. In these circumstances, a thorough curettage of the endometrial cavity is mandatory, not only to remove all foci that might harbor malignancy, but also to denude the cavity of excess endometrial tissue that may be the cause of the bleeding. A thorough curettage is also required in cases of postmenopausal bleeding. In such cases, a "fractional" curettage is accomplished by first curetting the cervix and then dilating the cervix and curetting the uterine fundus. In this way separate endocervical and endometrial specimens are submitted for pathologic examination. If endometrial carcinoma is discovered, the presence or absence of endocervical involvement is immediately determined, and therapy is planned accordingly (see section on therapy of endometrial carcinoma). In all cases a thorough pelvic examination should be performed, since the anesthetized patients provide the physician with an excellent opportunity to find previously unsuspected intrapelvic pathologic conditions.

TECHNIQUE (Fig. 41-28). The cervix is grasped with a tenaculum. Dilatation of the cervix following abortion is not necessary, and in other cases a dilatation is carried out with graduated dilators of increasing diameter. A blunt curet is gently introduced into the cervix and endometrial cavity using only minimal force. Extra pressure on the curet is avoided during this time. The curet is then withdrawn, scraping sharply against the sidewalls of the uterus. Firm pressure on the curet is applied during the withdrawal stroke. The cavity is further explored with a

common duct stone searcher in order to remove any large masses of tissue. A sharp curet is often unnecessary in cases associated with pregnancy but is used routinely when a diagnostic or therapeutic curettage is being performed in the nonpregnant uterus.

There are numerous surgical procedures that can be performed vaginally. The uterus can be removed by this route in cases of pelvic relaxation, and many disorders of pelvic support can be corrected by a vaginal operation. A few general guidelines are worth considering: exposure at all times should be adequate, small bites of tissue should be taken under direct vision, and a meticulous dissection should be carried out. An enlarged uterus or adnexal mass may preclude a safe vaginal dissection; under these circumstances the abdominal route is used. The excess blood loss that all too frequently accompanies vaginal surgical procedures must be avoided. Damage to surrounding structures, including bladder, ureter, and rectum, can be prevented by adhering to these principles.

Abdominal Gynecologic Procedures

Laparoscopy

The two most common diagnostic indications for pelvic laparoscopy are infertility and pelvic pain. Laparoscopy has proved useful in the early diagnosis of ectopic pregnancy. Therapeutically, sterilization by tubal interruption is commonly done through the laparoscope. The procedure usually is done with the patient in lithotomy position under general anesthesia with endotracheal intubation, but local or conduction anesthesia may be used (Fig. 41-16). Insufflation of the abdomen with 3 to 5 L of CO_2 through a needle with a blunt, hollow stylet, such as a Veress needle, is usually accomplished through a subumbilical puncture. At the same location the trocar is aimed at the hollow of the pelvis in order to bypass the promontory. It is pushed slowly, steadily, and firmly with a slight twisting motion into the peritoneal cavity. After the optical device is inserted through the sleeve of the trocar, the accessory trocar is inserted under direct vision over the suprapubic crease after the bladder has been emptied.

Contraindications are low pulmonary capacity, gross abdominal distention from generalized peritonitis, dilated small or large bowel, ileostomy or colostomy, and advanced gestation. Umbilical hernia is a contraindication to using the subumbilical area for puncture. Relative contraindications include previous lower abdominal midline laparotomy and obesity.

Incisions

The lower abdomen may be conveniently entered through a transverse or vertical incision. For most gynecologic procedures, either a midline or paramedian incision will provide good exposure. The right paramedian incision is frequently used when there is a pathologic condition in the right lower quadrant, especially in cases where the appendix or right adnexal structures could be involved. If a paramedian incision is used, the rectus abdominis muscle is retracted laterally away from the midline. If a midline approach is used, both the right and left rectus sheaths are opened and then resutured at the close of the procedure, since approximation prevents postoperative diastasis and adds to the long-term strength of the wound. Permanent suture material or heavy absorbable suture material can be used to reapproximate the anterior rectus fascia, since this is the layer that provides the main strength of the wound closure.

In certain instances, where surgical treatment is performed on young patients, a Pfannenstiel incision may be used. This incision provides a better cosmetic result, and although there may be slight decrease in exposure, this usually poses no problem. The incision can provide adequate exposure for operations confined to the uterus or to the adnexa. The risk of hematoma formation and subsequent sepsis is somewhat higher in a Pfannenstiel incision. The incision is placed transversely just above the pubic hairline and extends beyond the border of both rectus abdominis muscles (Fig. 41-29*A*). The subcutaneous tissue is divided, and the rectus fascia is split transversely (Fig. 41-29*B*). With traction placed on the lower rectus

Fig. 41-29. Pfannenstiel incision. (See description in text.)

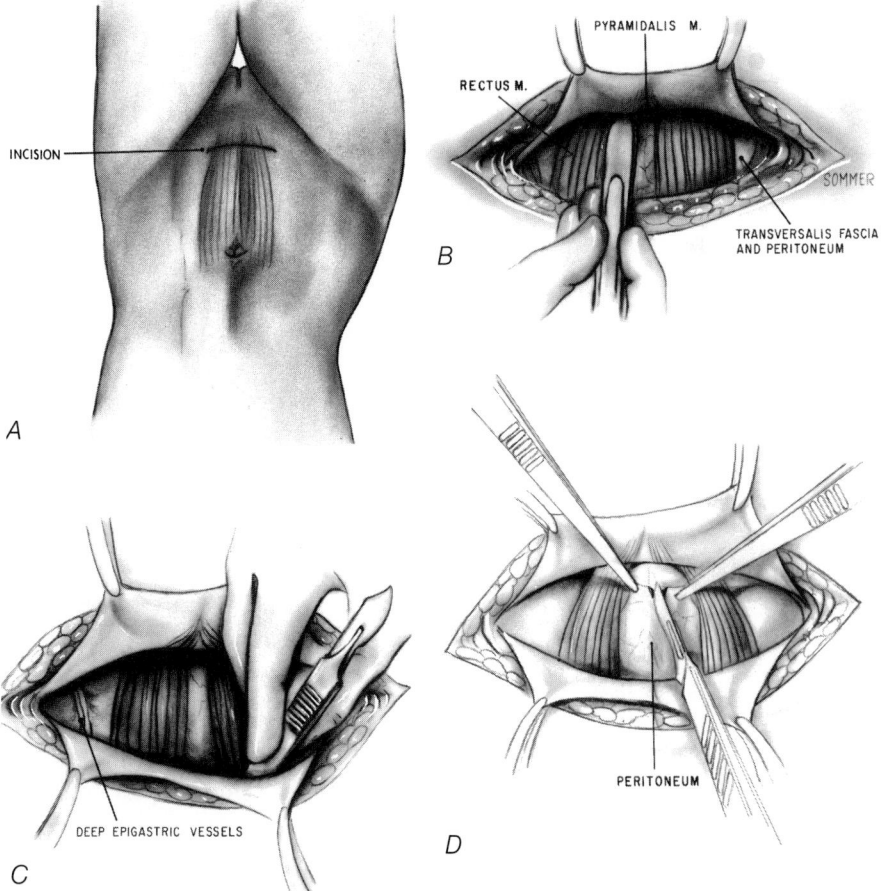

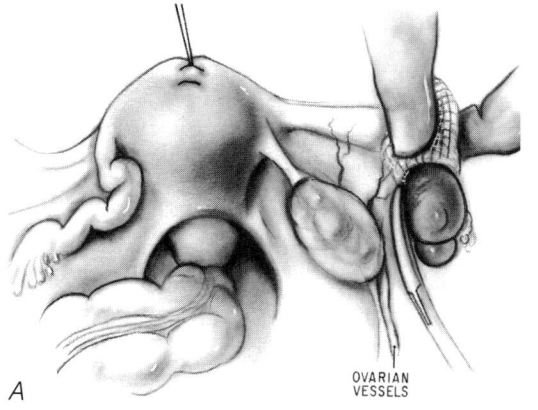

A

OVARIAN
VESSELS

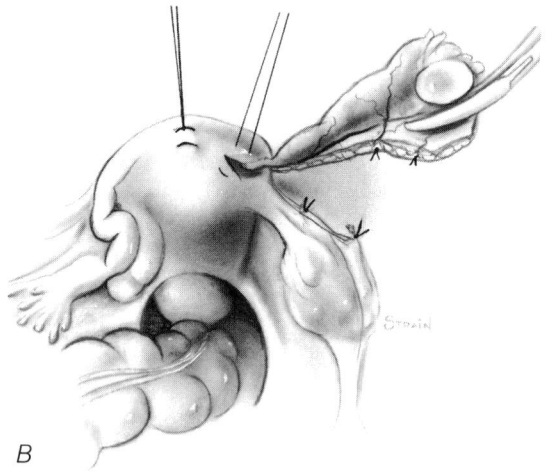

B

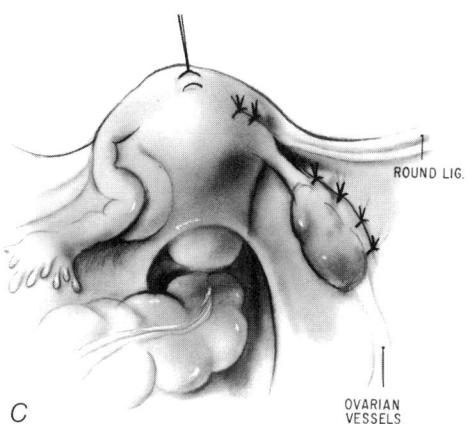

C

ROUND LIG.

OVARIAN
VESSELS

Fig. 41-30. Salpingectomy. (See description in text.)

fascia it is separated from the rectus muscle, and the pyramidalis muscle is preserved on its fascial attachment. After the inferior border of the incision has been delineated, the upper segment of the incision of the anterior

rectus fascia is also freed from the underlying muscles (Fig. 41-29*C*). The rectus abdominis muscles are separated in the midline, and the peritoneum is entered in a vertical fashion (Fig. 41-29*D*). After the conclusion of the procedure, the peritoneum is reapproximated in the midline. The muscles are then reapproximated with loose interrupted sutures, and then the rectus sheath is reapproximated in a transverse direction. The skin and subcutaneous tissues are closed in routine fashion.

OPERATION FOR ECTOPIC PREGNANCY

Death from intraperitoneal hemorrhage can occur, and rapid entry into the abdomen through a vertical incision may be necessary. In most cases, the architecture of the tube is destroyed. In rare circumstances the tube may be left in situ. Unfortunately a second ectopic pregnancy is a significant risk in these patients.

The question of prophylactic removal of the ipsilateral ovary with the tube in cases of ectopic pregnancy has received a great deal of attention due to the introduction of the theory of transmigration, discussed previously in this chapter. Therefore, it has been suggested that the removal of both the tube and the ovary on the same side may prevent a future ectopic pregnancy in the remaining opposite tube. However, this practice is not routinely adopted in younger patients whose reproductive life is just beginning and who do run the risk of a pathologic condition developing in the opposite ovary. This is consistent with the general concept of retaining normal tissue in conservative operations on the reproductive tract.

TECHNIQUE. A traction suture is placed on the uterus, which is retracted to the side opposite the tube. The tube is brought up into view, and the mesentery of the tube is divided (Fig. 41-30*A*). After the tube has been freed from its mesentery, it is placed on traction, elevated, and dissected free at its base, in order to be sure that the cornual end of the tube is removed (Fig. 41-30*B*). This prevents the occurrence of future cornual pregnancy. A mattress suture placed in the cornual end of the tube prior to cornual resection helps control hemorrhage. The uterus is repaired, and the mesentery of the ovary is brought to the posterior edge of the broad ligament in order to cover any remaining raw surface (Fig. 41-30*C*).

With the aid of diagnostic laparoscopy, more ectopic pregnancies are being diagnosed earlier, before tubal rupture has occurred. In order to optimize future fertility, conservative tubal surgery, i.e., salpingotomy, evacuation of the products of conception, and either primary or secondary closure of the tube has been advocated. The results in most series of conservative surgery vs. salpingectomy are the same: approximately 40 percent subsequent intrauterine pregnancy rate and 10 percent recurrent ectopic rate. Thus when ectopic tubal pregnancy occurs in a patient with only one fallopian tube or if the contralateral tube is diseased, conservative surgery would appear worthwhile. Under appropriate conditions, a conservative procedure may be performed through the laparoscope. Quantitative HCG titers should be followed

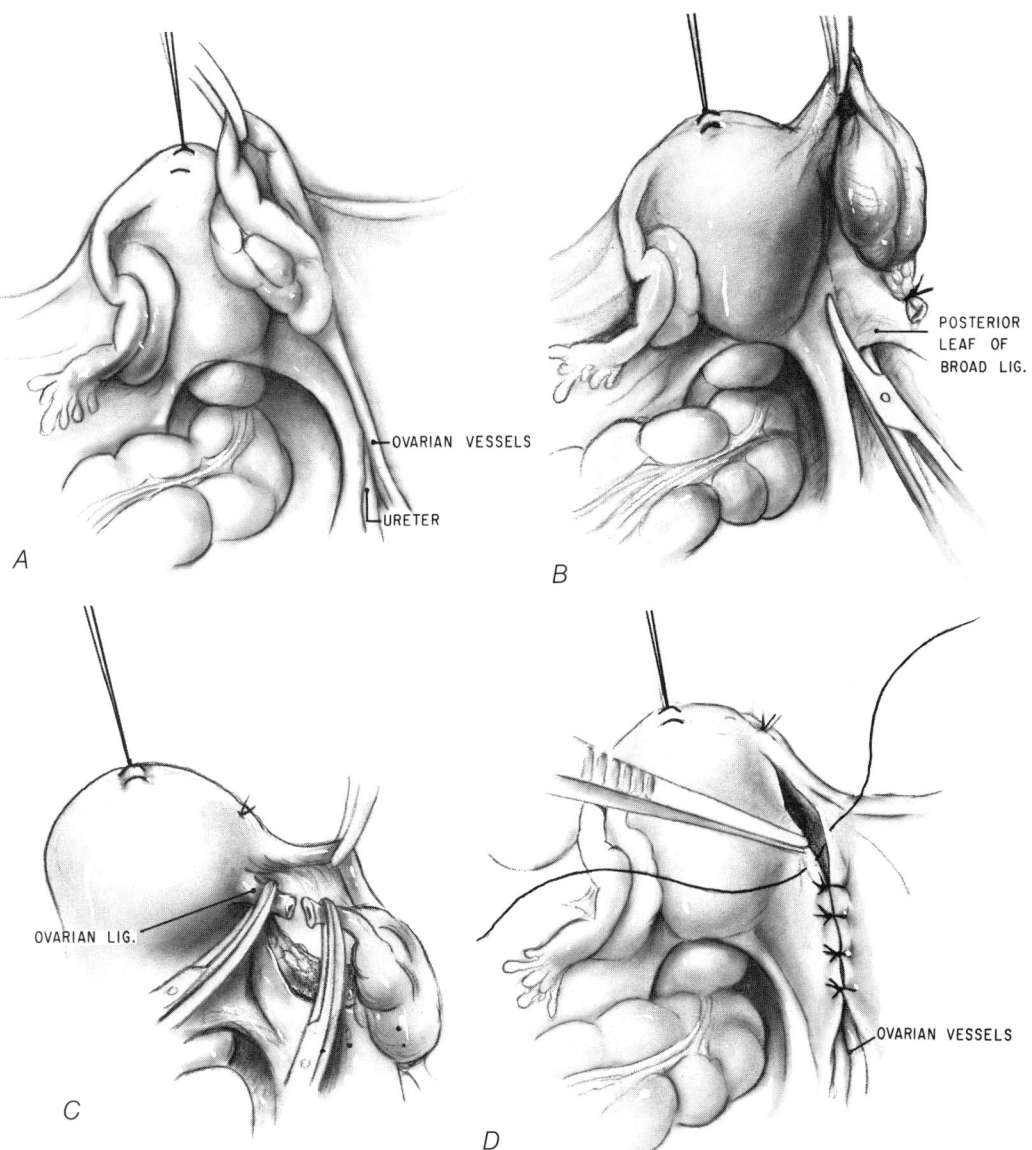

OVARIAN VESSELS

URETER

A

POSTERIOR LEAF OF BROAD LIG.

B

OVARIAN LIG.

C

OVARIAN VESSELS

D

Fig. 41-31. Salpingo-oophorectomy. (See description in text.)

to ensure that all of the products of conception have been removed.

SALPINGO-OOPHORECTOMY

In cases of large ovarian tumors or with torsion of the adnexa, the architecture of the tube and ovary may be destroyed. In this instance, unilateral removal of both is performed. First the infundibulopelvic ligament is divided after the ovarian vessels are sutured (Fig. 41-31A). The broad ligament is divided and dissection carried to the insertion of the tube into the uterus near the origin of the round ligament (Fig. 41-31B). The ovarian branch of the uterine artery is ligated (Fig. 41-31C). The cornual end of the tube is excised (as in Fig. 41-30B), and the defect in the peritoneum is closed (Fig. 41-31D).

ABDOMINAL HYSTERECTOMY

In cases of ovarian or endometrial malignancy, the ovaries and tubes are removed with the hysterectomy specimen. In younger patients who are undergoing surgical treatment for other diseases, ovarian conservation may be practiced. The ureter, bladder, and adjacent intestine can be injured during the course of hysterectomy unless careful surgical technique and adequate exposure are maintained (Fig. 41-32). The ureters are particularly prone to injury in the areas of uterosacral ligaments and the uterine artery, since they pass close to these structures. In cases where there is any doubt, the ureter should be visually identified.

TECHNIQUE. The uterus is placed on tension by a tenaculum in the fundus. The anterior leaf of the broad liga-

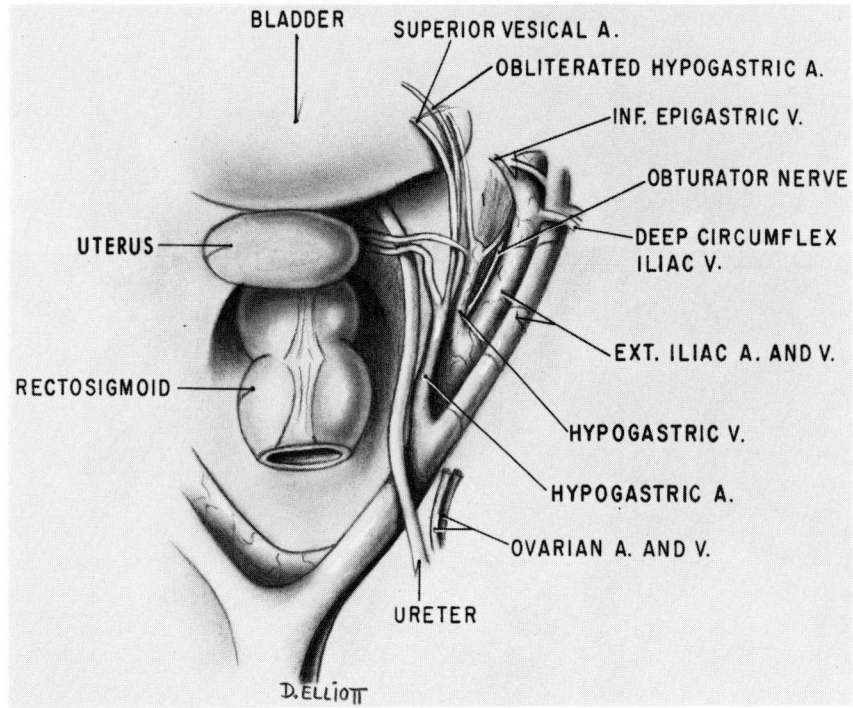

Fig. 41-32. Surgical anatomy of pelvis.

ment is opened (Fig. 41-33A), and the peritoneum above the bladder is separated away from the anterior portion of the uterus (Fig. 41-33B). The bladder is then advanced off the uterus and cervix (Fig. 41-33C), with the peritoneal sheath kept on tension during the course of this dissection in order not to injure the dome of the bladder.

If the ovaries are to be preserved, the ovarian vessels with the fallopian tube are ligated approximately 1 in. lateral to the uterus (Fig. 41-33D). If the ovaries are to be removed, the technique is similar to that shown in Fig. 41-31. The round ligament is then divided, and the anterior and posterior leaves of the broad ligaments are separated. The uterine vessels lie at the base of the broad ligament, and the ureter can be palpated as it passes beneath the uterine vessels (Fig. 41-33E). The uterosacral liga-

ments are next divided, and once again careful attention should be paid to the location of the ureter (Fig. 41-33F). After both uterosacral ligaments have been divided, the posterior peritoneum is separated from the back of the specimen, and care is taken to ensure that the rectosigmoid is separated from the posterior part of the dissection. In this fashion, the posterior wall of the vagina is exposed, and the uterus is separated from its peritoneal attachment.

The uterine vessels are then secured. Clamps should be applied under direct vision (Fig. 41-33G). The branches of the uterine artery and vein run close to the cervix and cervicouterine junction, and hemostasis must be obtained at the lateral edge of the cervix and lower portion of the

Fig. 41-33. Hysterectomy. (See description in text.)

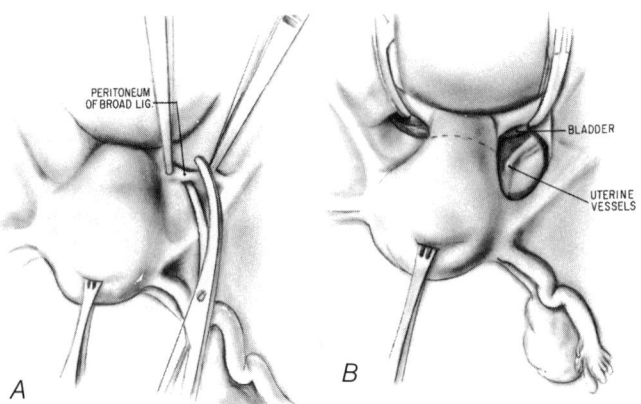

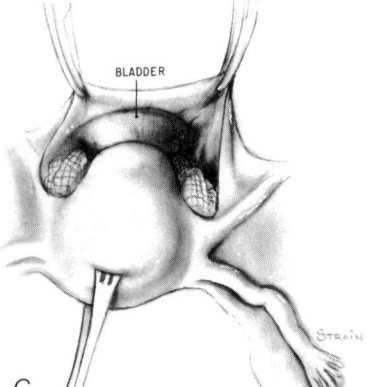

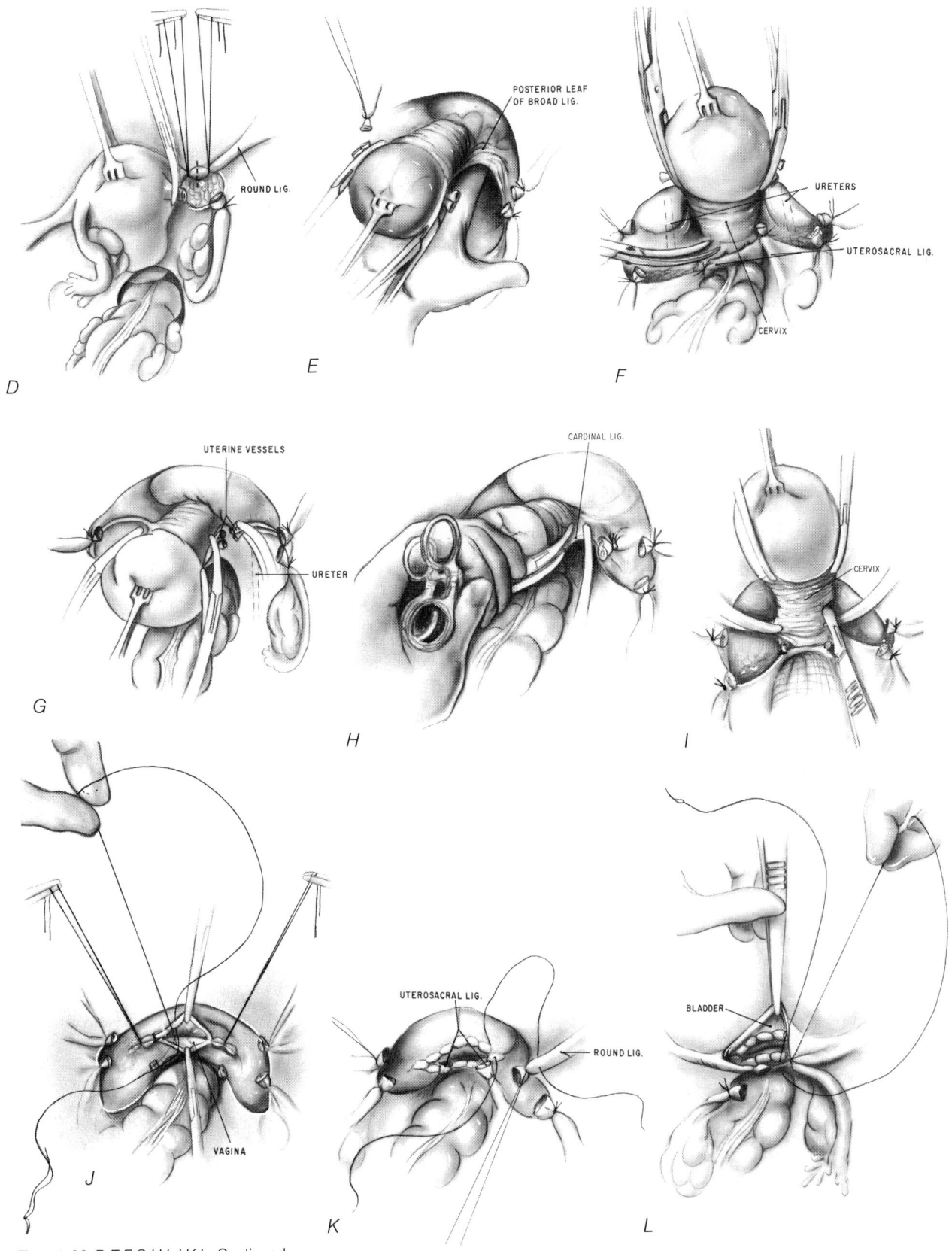

Fig. 41-33 *D,E,F,G,H,I,J,K,L.* Continued.

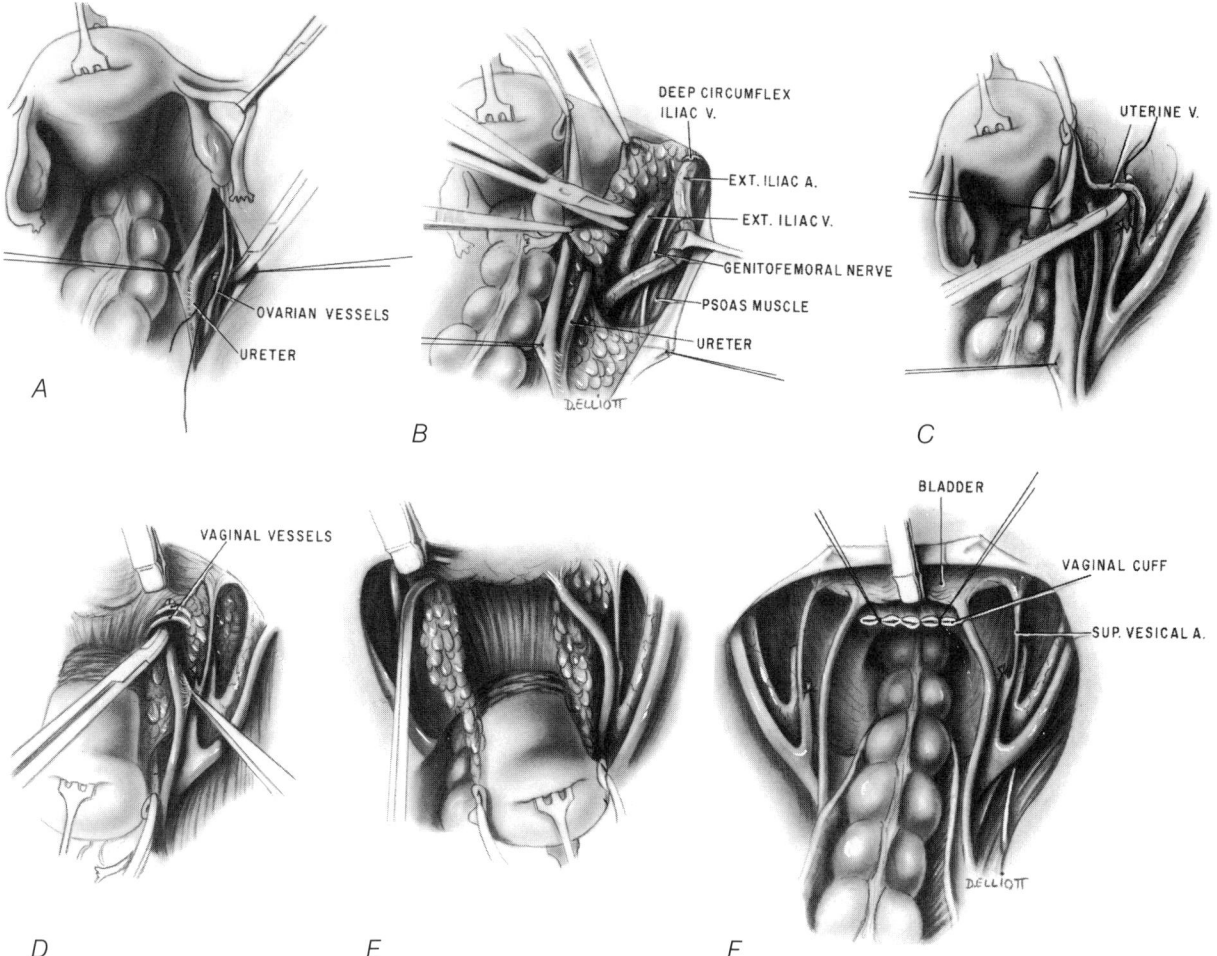

Fig. 41-34. Wertheim hysterectomy with pelvic lymphadenectomy. (See description in text.)

uterus. Traction is placed on the fundus, and the uterine vessels are clamped. A second clamp is added to protect against back-bleeding. The vessels are divided, and an additional clamp is placed to ensure against loss of control of the uterine vessel pedicle. The vessels are ligated, removing the lateral clamp first, following which a second suture is placed.

The bladder is mobilized anteriorly to free it completely from the vagina in the area of the cervix. The cardinal ligament is divided and sutured (Fig. 41-33*H*). It may be necessary to accomplish this step in a number of small bites. The vagina is then entered. This can be accomplished by elevating the uterus and placing clamps at the lateral corners of the vagina. The tissue above the clamps is then divided (Fig. 41-33*I*). The specimen is removed by dividing the vaginal tissue under direct vision. Sutures are placed at each angle of the vagina to ensure hemostasis, and the vaginal tissue is then repaired by a running atraumatic chromic catgut suture placed around the apex, which is then left open for improved drainage (Fig. 41-33*J*).

The pelvis is reconstructed by suturing the uterosacral ligaments to the posterior vaginal wall (Fig. 41-33*K*). This provides important support to the vagina. The round ligaments are then brought to the corners of the vagina (Fig. 41-33*L*). Although this maneuver does not add to the permanent support of the vagina, it does aid in reperitonealization of the pelvis. The procedure is completed by bringing together the edges of the remaining peritoneum in order to leave a smooth operative field (Fig. 41-33*L*).

Wertheim Hysterectomy with Pelvic Lymphadenectomy

This operation is performed primarily for cancer of the cervix when the disease appears to be confined to the cervix itself or the immediately adjacent vaginal wall. It has also been performed for treatment of cancer of the endometrium. The operation removes the contents of the pelvis from one obturator fossa to the other, including the lymph nodes in the common iliac, hypogastric, external iliac, and obturator artery areas. The ureters are identified through their entire course from bifurcation of the aorta to entrance into the bladder. Complete mobilization of the bladder and ureters from the vagina permits removal of all the tissue extending from the side wall of the pelvis to the paracervical and paravaginal area. The entire uterus, the adnexa, and a wide block of lymphatic tissue are removed in one piece, together with a large segment of vagina.

TECHNIQUE. The operation is performed through a low abdominal vertical incision. Most of the points of technique enumerated for hysterectomy apply; those specifically applicable to the Wertheim hysterectomy are outlined in this discussion. The ureter is initially identified at a point where it crosses the common iliac artery (Fig. 41-34*A*); the ovarian arteries are dissected free of the ureter and underlying common iliac artery. The ovarian vessels are then divided. The bladder flap is then developed as in the technique of total hysterectomy. The round ligament and broad ligament are transected. The uterus is then retracted medially to permit exposure of the areolar tissue overlying the external and internal iliac arteries. Dissection begins lateral to the artery on the psoas muscle and continues down along its medial surface to enter the upper portion of the obturator space. The genitofemoral nerve lies on the psoas and should be preserved. This dissection exposes the lateral and inferior surface of the external iliac vein and mobilizes all areolar tissue toward the midline (Fig. 41-34*B*). The common iliac lymph nodes and the external iliac lymph nodes are freed. Dissection of this areolar tissue mass permits exposure of the pubic ramus. The obturator and internal iliac nodes are also dissected free. In the course of this dissection, the obturator nerve is identified and spared. The uterine vein is identified at a point where it enters the internal iliac vein and is transected (Fig. 41-34*C*). The same dissection is carried out on the opposite side up to this point.

Attention is next directed to the original side, and freeing of the ureter continues. The ureter is dissected down to its entrance into the bladder. The ureter must be cleared from its tunnel along the anterior vaginal wall to permit excision of the paracervical and paravaginal lymphatics. A plexus of vaginal veins lies above and below it, and these must be transected (Fig. 41-34*D*). The ureter is now completely free from its bed, and the junction with the bladder can be identified. This permits dissection of an adequate length of vagina and paravaginal tissue.

The rectum is then separated from the posterior vaginal wall. All posterior attachments of the uterus are transected, and attention is directed to the anterolateral attachments. The uterus is drawn sharply back toward the promontory of the sacrum, and the bladder and ureters are carefully elevated so that dissection can begin beneath the bladder, freeing it laterally first on one side and then on the other. This represents the most important area of dissection; in order to avoid risk of recurrence, it is imperative that a wide block of tissue containing the paravaginal lymphatics be removed (Fig. 41-34*E*). This maneuver permits demonstration of the vaginal wall and allows transection and removal of one-half of the vagina. Complete dissection clears both iliac areas and the obturator fossa of all intervening lymphatic tissue. The bladder and ureters lie mobile above the closed vaginal stump (Fig. 41-34*F*). The vaginal cuff is oversewn, and the area is reperitonealized.

Bibliography

General

Droegemuller V, Herbst AL, et al: *Comprehensive Gynecology.* St Louis, CV Mosby, 1987.

Glass R: *Office Gynecology,* 2d ed. Baltimore, Williams & Wilkins, 1981.

Parsons L, Sommers SC: *Gynecology,* 2d ed. Philadelphia, Saunders, 1978.

Gynecologic Procedures and Techniques

Cibils LA: *Gynecologic Laparoscopy.* Philadelphia, Lea & Febiger, 1975.

Kolstad P, Stafl A: *Atlas of Colposcopy,* 2d ed. Oslo, Scandinavian University Books, 1977.

Mattingly RF, Thompson JD: *TeLinde's Operative Gynecology,* 6th ed. Philadelphia, Lippincott, 1985.

Parsons L, Ulfelder H: *An Atlas of Pelvic Operations,* 2d ed. Philadelphia, Saunders, 1968.

Related Texts of Special Interest

Blaustein A (ed): *Pathology of the Female Genital Tract,* 2d ed. New York, Springer-Verlag, 1981.

Coppelson M (ed): *Gynecologic Oncology.* Edinburg, Churchill Livingstone, 1981.

DeGroot LJ: *Endocrinology.* New York, Grune & Stratton, 1979.

Herbst AL, Bern HA (eds): *Development Effects of Diethylstilbestrol (DES) in Pregnancy.* New York, Thieme-Stratton, 1981.

Jones HW Jr, Scott W: *Hermaphroditism: Genital Anomalies and Related Endocrine Disorders,* 3d ed. Baltimore, Williams & Wilkins, 1971.

Speroff L, Glass RH, Kase NG: *Clinical Gynecologic Endocrinology and Infertility,* 3d ed. Baltimore, Williams & Wilkins, 1983.

Chapter 42

Neurologic Surgery

Dennis D. Spencer, Douglas Chyatte, William F. Collins, Charles C. Duncan, Laura Ment,
Joseph M. Piepmeier, Franklin Robinson, and Kimberlee J. Sass

GENERAL CONSIDERATIONS

Consciousness and cognition are prime signs of the working brain, and loss of these functions can result from many conditions, for the function of the brain is dependent not only upon controlled excitability in many interrelated and interconnected neurons and the integrity of their supporting glia but also upon adequate function in the rest of the organism. Normal central nervous system function presupposes adequate cardiac output of oxygenated blood with normal ionic and molecular constituents and intact vascular channels for perfusion. Loss of consciousness as a presenting symptom requires not only consideration of central nervous system pathology but evaluations of cardiac output, blood vessel competence, serum chemistry aberrations, possible circulating toxic substances, alterations in body temperature, and the myriad causes of each.

To address the issue of consciousness, neurophysiology has shown that small lesions placed in the mesencephalic reticular formation of experimental animals produce a state of coma. Sudden isolation of the spinal cord from descending influences of the reticular core of the brainstem by transsection at the cervical medullary junction or more caudad in the spinal cord produces areflexic paralysis or spinal shock distal to the section, followed by mass withdrawal reflexes when spinal shock ceases. Isolation of the brainstem reticular formation from descending hemispheric impulses by a section at the upper midbrain produces facilitation of antigravity musculature, or the state known as *decerebrate rigidity*. Removal of the cerebellum in the midbrain-sectioned animal decreases the extensor tone, while sensory stimuli of any sort enhance it.

Electrophysiologic studies have shown that the reticular core is activated by all sensory stimuli and, conversely, that with total sensory deprivation, i.e., section of all sensory nerves, a sleep record is obtained from the electroencephalogram that is altered or "activated" by stimulation within the reticular core. For this reason the ascending cortical influences of the reticular core of the brainstem have been called the *reticular activating system*. The reticular core is more than this. Its network of neurons influences cortical and subcortical function in the broadest sense in that consciousness and gnosis (recognition of sensation), and motor function are all dependent upon its integrity. For these reasons small lesions in the reticular core of the brainstem can cause loss of consciousness, as seen with contusions of the brainstem or infarcts following thrombosis of perforating branches of the basilar artery. These lesions also can alter motor function and motor tone and muscle tone from areflexic paralysis to decerebrate rigidity.

Fig. 42-1. Angiograms of thick longitudinal sections of the midline brainstem. *A.* Normal specimen with demonstration of the basilar artery and its paramedian branches. *B.* Specimen from a case with an expanding supratentorial mass. Caudal displacement of the brainstem has occurred with longitudinal shortening of the brainstem and an increase in the anteroposterior dimension. There are several paramedian arteries that have been ruptured with the demonstration of parenchymal hemorrhages. (From: *Hassler O: Neurology 17:368, 1967, with permission.*)

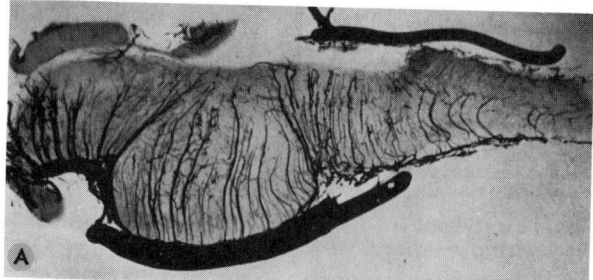

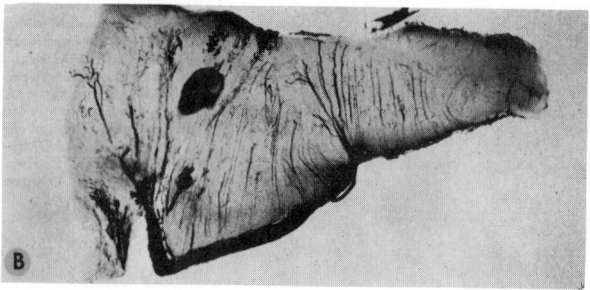

Surgical diseases of the nervous system are most frequently manifestations of space-occupying lesions, be they tumor, hemorrhage, abscess, edema, spinal fluid, or foreign body. The technique of their removal or the control of their effects, as well as an understanding of the mechanisms causing malfunction in the nervous system, makes neurologic surgery a specialty. The fact that the intracranial space and the spinal canal are confined spaces determines a set of mechanical conditions basic to many considerations of the effect of mass lesions on the nervous system. The intracranial space, compartmentalized by the falx and tentorium cerebri, has communication to the spinal space through the incisura of the tentorium and the foramen magnum of the skull. This represents its only major extracranial communication. The brainstem passes through these areas of communication, i.e., from the incisura of the tentorium through the posterior fossa to the foramen magnum. Rostrally it is continuous with the diencephalon and the internal capsule of each hemisphere, where the medial portion of the temporal lobes has immediate lateral relation to the upper brainstem, with a portion of the circle of Willis, the subarachnoid space, and the oculomotor nerve between them. Caudad it is continuous with the cervical spinal cord, where at the foramen magnum it lies immediately anterior to the inferior portion of the ansiform lobes of the cerebellum, more commonly known as the *cerebellar tonsils*.

Central nervous system (CNS) tissue has many of the properties of a fluid; that is, it is deformable but not compressible, and when deformed it flows in the course of least resistance. Deformation over months or years causes loss of substance, mainly of myelin, but rapid deformation varying with the imposed pressure causes flow toward sites of decompression, the incisura of the tentorium and the foramen magnum. While the tissue is not compressible, the lumen of its blood supply is, and obstruction of veins, capillaries, and arteries occurs with deformation. The lethal factors of the flow toward decompression areas are in part the limitation of the accommodation allowed by the semirigid infolded meningeal structures of the falx and the tentorium, the sheer stress at their edges, and the unyielding character of the bony rim of the foramen magnum. In addition, the axial as well as lateral shift of the brainstem is functionally limited by the mobility of the circle of Willis, fixed by the carotid arteries where they pierce the dura. The circle of Willis and the basilar arteries (Fig. 42-1) supply blood to the brainstem by vessels that enter perpendicular to its surface. With progressive axial shift the normally lax vessels become straightened and eventually tether the brain. With continuing shift there is collapse of the vessels with infarction and rupture of the smaller vessels with hemorrhage. At the foramen magnum compression of the medulla by the decompressing (herniating) cerebellar tonsils causes the same phenomena, but failure of perfusion of this area more commonly causes a cardiorespiratory death before gross visible changes occur.

The situation of a noncompressible tissue nurtured by vessels whose lumens are compressible allows the compressing force to set in motion a cycle that includes production of further mass by edema with consequent increase of the size and compressing force of the original mass. The incisural syndrome of altered consciousness followed by loss of function of the oculomotor nerve, decerebrate rigidity, and death reflects the cycle in supratentorial mass lesions. At the foramen magnum, altered consciousness, followed by depression of respiration requiring the stimulus of increased blood CO_2, or Cheyne-Stokes respiration, depression of reflexes, cessation of respiration, and death represent progression of the cycle. The early recognition of any portion of these patterns is necessary if the lethal effects of intracranial masses are to be reversed. Their recognition and treatment is a sine qua non of neurologic surgery.

It is beyond the scope of this section to review all the neurodiagnostic techniques (and their indications) that can or should be used to investigate neurologic diseases requiring neurosurgical intervention. With the recognition that the central nervous system requires a degree of homeostasis in the patient in order to function normally, it becomes obvious that a complete history, physical examination, neurologic examination, and basic laboratory studies are requisites for any evaluation of neurologic disease. The history should be carefully done, since there is a high probability of its indicating the cause of the condition being studied. In contrast, neurologic examination indicates the area or areas of the central nervous system involved, and when combined with the history will define the questions to be answered by special diagnostic studies.

DIAGNOSTIC STUDIES. Much of the recent growth in the clinical neurosciences and patient care is directly attributed to the rapid advancements in neuroimaging. The past 10 years have witnessed a tremendous growth from the first-generation computed tomographic (CT) scanners that allowed us our first noninvasive picture of the central nervous system. Now third- and fourth-generation CT scanners and magnetic resonance imaging (MRI) devices, as they are also called, have revolutionized our diagnostic abilities and clearly enhanced preoperative preparation. These tests, as with skull x-rays and electroencephalography, are noninvasive and benign save for allergic reactions to iodine dye. Other special studies can carry a higher risk such as arteriography, myelography, or the infrequently performed pneumoencephalography. The accuracy of the special studies depends not only on the technical skill with which they are performed but also on knowing what question is being asked of the test and what answers can be gained. This latter aspect, as well as knowing what the risks of the test are, is why as much knowledge of the patient as a whole should be gained before using the tests and why their use in neurological evaluation is restricted to physicians knowledgeable in nervous system disease.

X-rays of the skull can be helpful in the diagnosis of neurologic disorders, although less frequently ordered since they are generally only a prelude to CT or MRI scanning, both of which will answer most questions more completely. Nevertheless they may reveal many clues. Increased intracranial pressure may be reflected in springing of the sutures in the infant or decalcification of the sella turcica in the adult. A calcified pineal gland that defines the posterior position of the third ventricle may be shifted from its usual midline position by a supratentorial mass. Many tumors contain radiopaque calcification that may be visible in skull x-rays. Meningiomas may contain calcification but usually are recognized, because they evoke hyperostosis in the adjacent bones of the skull. Other stigmata of brain tumor in skull x-rays are erosions of the internal auditory meatus with an eighth nerve tumor or erosion of the optic foramen or anterior clinoid with an optic nerve tumor.

Special diagnostic studies can indicate the position, the size, and the blood supply of the tumor, and also may give information as to the amount of brain shift. The studies that involve no risk to the patient are CT and MRI scanning, positron emission tomography, ultrasound, nuclear brain scan, electroencephalography, and electromyography.

Computerized Axial Tomography. Computerized axial tomography (CT) is a major advance in radiological diagnosis whose unique attributes are particularly advantageous for diagnosis of intracranial disease. Conventional x-rays use photographic film to measure the relative amount of x-ray absorbed by the structures through which the beam has passed. Limitations of conventional x-ray include the fact that with photographic film, quantitative definition of the amount of x-ray absorbed is poor and slanted toward high-absorption matter such as bone, and the resulting image is only two-dimensional. In the early 1970s, Geoffrey Houndsfield, a British engineer, developed a technique of a carefully controlled small beam of x-ray, a focused crystal scintillation counter, to measure accurately the amount of x-ray remaining after the beam passed through an object, and computer technology along with matrix mathematics and pattern storage techniques to produce a three-dimensional array in a computer of the object being studied, which he called *computerized axial tomography*. The small x-ray beam is passed through the object being studied through multiple directions, and the matrix is formed in the computer so that by simultaneously solving a number of equations, the amount of x-ray absorbed in each portion of the matrix is determined. The size of the area in each point is determined by the size of the matrix; with recent scanners, the image resolution is approximately 1 mm in diameter. Since brain, cerebrospinal fluid, and bone have different x-ray absorption coefficients, with the technique of computerized axial tomography, the amount and position of each of these structures can be determined, and with the use of radiopaque compounds, areas of abnormal vascularity or breakdown in the blood-brain barrier can be accurately determined. The ability to show enlarged ventricles, altered cortical surfaces, tumors, and abscesses has allowed accurate diagnosis of many neurologic conditions without any significant risk to the patient.

With the addition of a water-soluble contrast agent such as metrizamide (Amipaque, Winthrop Labs), which carries with it the slight risk of irritation of the nervous system, CT scanning can define the surfaces of the cen-

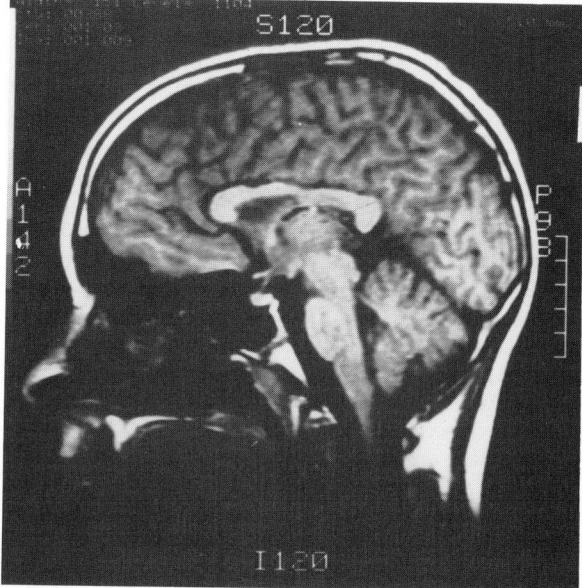

Fig. 42-2. This represents a normal midsaggital MRI of the adult. Note the clear gray-white matter demarcation and the anatomic detail afforded of such structures as the brainstem, pituitary, and corpus callosum.

tral nervous system including the spinal cord, the brainstem, and intracranial cerebral spinal fluid cisterns. Alterations in position or shape of these structures can be used in diagnosis of CNS problems. Since 1974, when Ambrose at the Atkinson Morley Hospital in England demonstrated the value of CT scanning in neurologic diagnosis, continued improvement in instrumentation and computer technology has made CT scanning the principal

Fig. 42-3. This axial MRI illustrates a right temporal cystic astrocytoma with a nodule. The anatomic relationships of the medial temporal lobe, brainstem, and tumors are clearly demarcated.

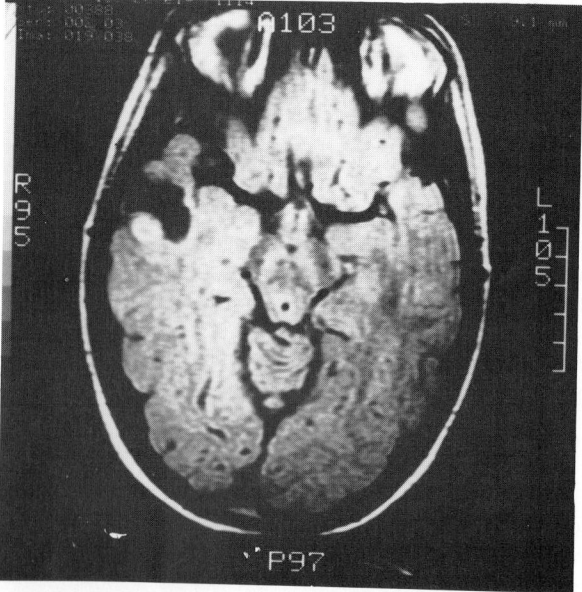

radiologic diagnostic tool in neurologic disease. It has completely displaced pneumoencephalography and is displacing myelography in the diagnosis of intervertebral disc disease. It also adds considerable information in cases of cranial and intervertebral bony abnormalities.

Magnetic Resonance Imaging (MRI). The majority of present-day images depend on the magnetic polar alignment of hydrogen protons. The signal is monitored by a radiofrequency pulse that knocks these protons out of alignment and measures in three planes their return. The image of the brain (Fig. 42-2) created reveals startling anatomic precision and has extended our ability to diagnose such diseases as multiple sclerosis, cerebrovascular disease, primary brain tumor (Fig. 42-3), syringomyelia, and many others. At the present time MRI and CT scanning are complementary for many diseases, but certain conditions such as pituitary tumors are best diagnosed and followed by the MRI.

Electroencephalography. The electroencephalogram, or EEG, is the recording of the electrical activity of the brain by amplification of potentials obtained from electrodes placed on the scalp. Its interpretation is based on knowledge of the ''normal'' cerebral electrical activity and the significance of alterations in symmetry, form, frequency, and amplitude of the potentials in nervous system disorders. Its most frequent use is in the diagnosis of epilepsy, with changes in the form of the potentials and the presence of focal or diffuse paroxysmal activity as important aspects of the interpretation. Focal slowing is seen in the area of tumors of the cerebral hemisphere, and formerly EEG was a frequently used diagnostic test in evaluating patients suspected of having a brain tumor. Because of the accuracy of the information and the increased amount of information obtained with CT and MRI scanning, these modulities have replaced EEG in such evaluation, just as they have in other conditions such as intracranial hemorrhage and stroke.

Ultrasonography. Ultrasound uses a reflection of ultrasonic waves to localize structures and abnormalities within the cranium. The presence of the intact skull limits the procedure in children and adults to the determination of the position of large or high echo characteristic structures such as ventricles or the pineal gland. In infants with an open fontanelle or a patient with a skull defect, ultrasound can give considerable information concerning not only ventricular size and position, but also presence of hemorrhage, tumor, or foreign bodies. Its advantages, particularly for the infant, are that such information can be obtained without exposing the patient to x-ray and that the equipment is portable, allowing studies to be done without moving critically ill patients.

Advances in technology and instrumentation have also allowed neurosurgeons to take ultrasound into the operating theater. Portable modules with small hand pieces are now used over the surface of the brain and spinal cord to localize intracerebral masses for biopsy or excision, to identify the lateral ventricles for catheter placement, to outline a syringomyelia cavity, and to check for retained disc fragments during discectomy.

Nuclear Brain Scan. The brain scan uses radioactive materials such as mercury 203 or technetium 99 that will not cross the intact blood-brain barrier. Since most brain tumors are not included within the barrier, an abnormal amount of radioactive material will be present in the area of the tumor and can be localized by counting this radioactive material with a scintillation counter. This counter localizes the abnormal activity through the intact skull, producing a graphic display. Since there are many causes for breakdown of the blood-brain barrier, positive brain scans can be found in conditions that are not caused by tumors, such as in vascular occlusion, infection, or trauma. The problem of false-negative studies of lesions contained within the blood-brain barrier further limits the value of the study.

Single Photon Emission Tomography. Single photon emission tomography (SPECT) is another imaging device that potentially may provide cerebral physiologic studies. It is not readily available but is much less expensive than positron emission tomography and may become more widely used to study cerebral metabolism, blood flow, and neurotransmitters. New radiopharmaceutical agents such as $^{99m}T_c$-hexamethylpropyleneamine oxime (HM−PAO) may be particularly useful for the measurement of cerebral blood flow.

More invasive neuroradiologic diagnostic studies that have some risk to the patient include pneumoencephalography, angiography, and myelography. Their use is determined by the need for information balanced against the risk involved, and therefore, they are rarely used unless a neurologist or neurosurgeon has determined that they are required.

Pneumoencephalography. Pneumoencephalography, or the x-ray study of the brain with air, utilizes the difference in the absorption of x-rays between air, brain, and fluid. As mentioned earlier, this test is rarely performed today. Occasionally a small amount of air may be introduced into the spinal subarachnoid space and allowed to percolate into the cerebellar pontine angle and internal auditory meatus to help define by using CR on a small suspected acoustic neuroma. MRI is rapidly replacing even this usage. There is also the occasional need to introduce air or contrast media into one of the lateral ventricles by ventricular puncture or via an existing shunt system. This is usually performed to evaluate the CSF flow dynamics between the two lateral ventricles and their relationship to the third ventricle.

Cerebral Angiography. Cerebral angiography, or what is more commonly called carotid or vertebral arteriography, is the x-ray study of the intracranial circulation as demonstrated by the injection of contrast material. These studies can define the position of the arteries and the presence or absence of abnormal vasculature, and thereby often define not only the presence of a brain tumor but also its blood supply and how it has affected the adjacent structures. Angiography is the main method of demonstrating vascular lesions such as arteriovenous malformations, aneurysms, and vascular occlusive disease. The most common method for performing angiography is by a transfemoral artery puncture, fluoroscopic positioning of a catheter into the aortic arch, carotid arteries, or vertebral arteries, and serial x-rays of the injection of contrast material. The x-rays are taken at intervals to demonstrate arterial, capillary, and venous filling. With injection of a single vessel, such as the internal carotid or vertebral, and with subtraction techniques and various timings of the serial x-rays, information necessary for the surgical approach to tumors, for repair of vascular malformations, or for reestablishing blood supply to the nervous system is obtained. The major danger is a cerebrovascular accident secondary to manipulation of the vessels or in response to injection of the contrast material. Recent computer techniques combined with fluoroscopy, called *digital enhanced angiography,* have decreased the risk by decreasing the amount of contrast material injected. A number of centers now offer therapeutic angiographic techniques including microballoon occlusion of carotid cavernous fistula and small-particle embolization of surgically inaccessible arteriovenous malformations. These new embolization materials such as polyvinyl alcohol can also be used preoperatively in vascular tumors or in staging some AVM resections.

Myelography. Myelography is the radiologic study of the spinal canal, whereby a radiopaque contrast material is placed in the spinal subarachnoid space by a lumbar puncture or a lateral C_1-C_2 cervical puncture. The contrast agent is then positioned by fluoroscopy, obstructions to flow are delineated, and the spinal cord, spinal roots, and soft tissue of the spinal canal are outlined. The study is used to diagnose ruptured intervertebral discs, spinal cord tumors, and arterial venous malformations of the spinal cord. CT scanning with and without contrast is now used frequently to diagnose spinal disease and is probably the best modality for bony relationships. Of the two procedures, however, CT following myelography with water-soluble agents remains one of the best ways to evaluate the spinal subarachnoid space. MRI has been most helpful in dramatically revealing syrinx cavities in exacting detail. Within the past few years, the water-soluble x-ray contrast materials that have been developed have decreased the complication of arachnoiditis that was seen with nonsoluble agents such as pantopaque. The water-soluble contrast materials can irritate the cerebral cortex, causing seizures. Another possible complication of this study is an increasing neurologic deficit in tumors of the spinal cord or other lesions that block the flow of spinal fluid. The cause is alteration in relative pressures on each side of the blocking lesion after a subarachnoid puncture. For these reasons, the study is done only when the neurologic problem requires the information that can be obtained, and it is always done with supervision of persons trained in nervous system diagnosis and treatment. In patients suspected of having a spinal fluid block immediate neurosurgical care to treat precipitate deterioration in function should be available following such an exam.

HEAD INJURY

Included within the term "head injury" are injuries of the scalp, skull, and brain. The immediate care of patients with head injury is no different from that of any injured patient. Primary consideration must be given to the establishment of adequate respiratory exchange, control of hemorrhage, and maintenance of peripheral vascular circulation. Physicians caring for the patient with traumatic injury to the nervous system too often forget these cardinal necessities or blame apparent respiratory difficulty or peripheral vascular collapse on central nervous system factors that they feel unable to alter. During the initial period of treatment of a patient with head injury, as measures are instituted for the control of the vital functions, a preliminary evaluation of the nervous system function is essential and should be followed as soon as possible by careful repetitive neurologic examinations. Repetitive neurologic examinations are necessary to detect deterioration or improvement in neurologic function. Management decisions are made based on the information obtained from these examinations and the findings on diagnostic x-rays.

Scalp

Although the scalp consists of five layers, from a surgical point of view its two important layers are the dermis and the galea. The principles in the care of scalp lacerations are the same as in the care of any laceration, that is, to change a contaminated open wound into a closed clean wound, but some unique problems arise because of the structure of the scalp and its anatomic relationships. The unyielding character of the scalp with its major blood supply lying between the galea and the dermis has a tendency to hold blood vessels open following laceration with the possibility of considerable loss of blood. Hemostasis of the scalp is easily obtained, if the skull is intact, by compression of the scalp against the skull either in a circumferential fashion at the base of the scalp or by direct pressure on the wound edges. When the skull is not intact, traction on the galea by a clamp that grasps the galea, pulling it back over the dermis, will usually control the hemorrhage. The minor hemorrhage of contusions lying between the galea and the skin rarely causes any significant difficulty, but hematomas of the scalp that lie beneath the galea can attain considerable size, causing elevation of a major portion of the scalp from the skull. These hematomas may make up a significant percentage of the circulating blood volume in infants. Early control of such hemorrhage sometimes can be accomplished by pressure and a firm dressing. Such subgaleal hematomas may take weeks to absorb, but with intact skin over them they are best treated by allowing natural absorption to occur. However, if the hematoma is of significant size to embarrass circulation of the scalp or if there is a question of infection as manifested by heat, swelling, and fever, evacuation of the hematoma is indicated. This should be done under sterile conditions, the hematoma totally evacuated, and any dead space obliterated by a compression dressing.

The approximation of the scalp to the skull not only allows lacerations to occur with blunt injury but also causes increased morbidity with infections of the scalp. Infections of the scalp may spread into the intracranial epidural space through the connecting emissary veins in the diploic spaces of the skull and into the veins on the surface of the brain. With these channels for spread of infection, epidural abscess, subdural abscess, cerebral thrombophlebitis, cerebritis, or brain abscess can occur.

Finally the galea not only is a strong fascial layer that is firmly attached to the skin by numerous fascial bands but is also the attachment of the occipitalis and frontalis muscles. These muscles tend by their contraction to separate any weak area of the galea. The problem of such contraction is that any laceration of more than a few centimeters in size will have a tendency to pull open unless the galea is closed at the time that the dermis is closed; any large laceration of the scalp that is allowed to remain open for more than 5 to 6 days may show a significant amount of contraction with fibrosis, so that it cannot be closed without special surgical techniques.

Thus, care of a scalp wound must be thorough and include shaving of hair in the immediate vicinity, debridement of all the devitalized tissue, and removal of any foreign body. The wound closure must include closure of the galea, either as a separate layer or as a layer included within the dermis. If the laceration is of a large size with separation of a major portion of the galea from the subgaleal tissue, a compression dressing will make the patient more comfortable and decrease the chances of a subgaleal hematoma and infection.

Skull

ANATOMY. The skull is divided into the cranium, which contains and protects the brain, and the facial bones. The cranium consists of eight bones: two parietal and temporal bones and one frontal, occipital, ethmoid, and sphenoid bone. The superior, or rounded, portion of the skull is called the *vault,* and its bones are formed as membranous bone. In the adult the bone consists of firm inner and outer tables with cancellous bone, or diploë, lying between them. The skull contains within the frontal, ethmoid, and sphenoid bones mucous membrane-lined sinuses that connect to the nasal cavities. The basilar, or petrous, portion of the temporal bones contains the middle ear and mastoid air cells, which also connect to the nasopharynx via the eustachian tube.

CLASSIFICATION OF SKULL FRACTURE. The clinical term "skull fracture" is used for fractures of the cranium. Such fractures are described by using a term describing the pattern of the fracture (linear, stellate, comminuted), by using the term "depressed" to denote an inward displacement of a portion of the vault, by naming the bone involved, by including the term "basilar" for fractures traversing the base of the skull, and by describing a break in the scalp or mucous membrane over such a fracture with the term "compound fracture." Thus, a compound comminuted depressed fracture of the left parietal bone states that there is a scalp laceration over a fracture of the parietal bone on the left that consists of multiple fragments of bone driven beneath the surface of the cranial vault.

Fractures of the skull may occur in any area of the skull and have a tendency to radiate from the point of contact into the weaker areas of the skull, e.g., basilar or temporal areas. Most skull fractures require no treatment in themselves, but compound and depressed fractures must be treated. A compound fracture of the cranial vault should be cleansed and debrided, and the wound closed. Replacement of large skull fragments in the area of a compound fracture requires surgical judgment and depends upon the degree of contamination, intactness of the dura, the area of the skull involved, and the ability to watch the patient closely after injury. If the surgeon is in doubt in any of these respects, it is always wisest to remove all fragments of a compound fracture.

With depressed fractures the rule is to elevate all of them, but again this should be based on surgical judgment of the size of the depressed segment, the depth to which it is depressed, and the area of the skull depressed, and the ability to be certain that the dura has not been torn. Any fragment that has been depressed more than a centimeter, a fragment that is over the motor strip, and most small fragments that appear sharp on x-ray usually should be elevated, since they may tear the dura and cause damage to the brain. The combination of a depressed and compound fracture will always require elevation to be certain that contamination has not been driven through the dura into the subarachnoid space or the brain.

Another type of compound skull injury, one that is not as obvious as a penetrating injury, is the injury in which a fracture of the skull traverses one or more of the paranasal sinuses, the mastoid air cells, or the middle ear. The indication that this type of open head injury has occurred is the presence of cerebrospinal fluid drainage from the nose or ear. It signifies a rupture of the protective meningeal coverings of the brain and requires observation and prophylactic antibiotics to be certain that infection of the subarachnoid space or brain does not occur. The post-traumatic cerebrospinal fluid fistula of the ear almost always heals within a few days, but healing of rhinorrhea may be more difficult. It is important in both injuries that the patient remain under medical supervision until such drainage ceases, and usually if either otorrhea or rhinorrhea continues for more than 10 to 14 days, surgical repair of the dural tear is necessary.

Brain

MECHANISMS OF INJURY. The immediate damage that results from head trauma is dependent upon the energy absorbed by the brain tissue. This damage can be caused by direct disruption of brain tissue from a penetrating object or more commonly by distortion of the tissue from rapid deceleration of the brain against the rigid skull. A more generalized injury can result in neurologic deficits in regions of the brain that are distant from the point of impact. When brain tissue receives a traumatic injury, it responds by an alteration in intracellular and extracellular fluid content, hemorrhage, alterations in cerebral blood flow, and swelling. These events can contribute to further injury by direct compression of surrounding tissue or by increasing the pressure within the skull to transmit injury to distant parts of the brain. These injuries can be compounded by alterations in cerebrovascular vasomotor tone and the loss of autoregulation of blood flow that further compromise the brain's blood supply. The dependency of the brain on continuous supply of glucose and oxygen mandates a rapid intervention when these substrates are compromised in order to prevent further injury and permit the recovery of viable tissue.

An important part of understanding the mechanisms of brain injury is an adequate perception of the historic events concerning the injury. These include information about the mechanism of injury, the status of the patient immediately following the trauma, and a detailed description of the patient's neurologic function. For example, head trauma following a motor vehicle accident should be described in terms of the speed of the vehicle, the status of the automobile, the patient's position in the car, the status of the windshield, and whether a seat belt was used. The status of the patient at the scene of the accident will provide further information about the additional complicating factors of hypoxia or ischemia. An appreciation of the importance of the mechanisms of injury will facilitate the management of the patient and alert the surgeon to the potential for complications.

Care of the Head-Injured Patient

The care of the head-injured patient can be divided into temporally sequential aspects. These are resuscitation; evaluation; diagnostic studies; treatment; prevention, recognition, and treatment of complications; and rehabilitation. The mortality and morbidity of head trauma can be improved by knowledgeable and effective care throughout the course of the illness. In general, a patient's recovery will be improved with the rapid intervention by surgeons skilled in the management of these patients. Consequently, hospitals with specialized centers for neurosurgical patients should be utilized as soon as it is feasible to transfer the patient. When possible, it is best to triage patients to these facilities directly from the scene of the accident.

RESUSCITATION. The importance of adequate respiration and control of hemorrhage cannot be overstressed. The head-injured patient is particularly susceptible to the deleterious effects of hypoxia, hypercarbia, and ischemia. It is not uncommon to see a patient's neurologic status improve remarkably when hypoxia and ischemia are reversed. Because the control of oxygen and carbon dioxide in the blood is of primary importance, endotracheal intubation of a severely head-injured patient should be frequently performed. Even in patients who appear to be adequately exchanging, intubation provides protection from delayed airway compromise and may be necessary for transportation to another facility. In any evaluation of a patient with multiple traumatic injuries attention must be directed toward the possibility of spinal injury or occult bleeding in the chest or abdomen. A failure to detect these injuries in an unresponsive patient also can result in drastic consequences.

EVALUATION. Following the initial resuscitation and stabilization of the patient's vital signs, a detailed neuro-

Table 42-1. LEVELS OF CONSCIOUSNESS

Responds to spoken word, is alert, cooperative, and oriented.
Responds to spoken word, is confused, and obeys simple commands.
Responds to spoken word only after receiving painful stimuli of supraorbital pressure; obeys commands only while receiving painful stimuli.
Does not respond to auditory stimuli before or while receiving painful stimuli but has purposeful, effective motor response to painful supraorbital and sternal pressure.
Responds to painful supraorbital and sternal pressure with purposeful but noneffective motor movements.
Responds to painful supraorbital and sternal pressure with nonpurposeful movement.
Responds to painful stimuli only with alteration in pulse and respiratory rate or with decerebrate posturing.
No response to painful stimuli, but cough and gag reflexes are present.
No response to stimuli.
Lowest level is unconsciousness; the only step below this is death.

logic evaluation should be performed. The most important part of this evaluation is a description of the level of consciousness. Terms such as "comatose" or "semicomatose" are not helpful. The evaluation of the level of consciousness is obtained by describing the patient's responses to various stimuli and the amount of stimuli necessary to elicit that response. If the stimulus and response are described, the evaluation can be repeated for later comparison. Table 42-1 illustrates examples of the level of consciousness that can be determined by this method.

By comparing the patient's response to stimuli over time it is not difficult to detect a deterioration in the patient's neurologic status. This method can alert the surgeon to subtle changes in status that may be the early signs of impending problems. For example, an alert, oriented patient who later requires a painful stimulus to elicit an appropriate response has demonstrated a change in the level of consciousness, and this deterioration is sufficient to warrant an investigation for a cause.

While most physicians can evaluate a conscious patient, the unconscious patient who does not generate speech or follow instructions requires more expertise. When a verbal response or appropriate motor response cannot be detected, the examiner must rely on brainstem function to determine what level of the brain is compromised. This is best obtained by a series of tests for brainstem reflexes. Table 42-2 gives an illustration of these

Table 42-2. BRAINSTEM REFLEXES

Pupil reaction to light	Midbrain
Decorticate posture	Midbrain
Corneal reflex	Pons
Oculocephalic reflex	Pons
Decerebrate posture	Pons
Caloric stimulation	Pons
Spontaneous respiration	Medulla
Cardiovascular function	Medulla

tests and the level of the brainstem being tested. For example, the patient who does not generate speech or follow commands and who also does not show a pupillary constriction to light and shows decorticate posturing to a noxious stimulus has clear evidence of midbrain dysfunction. Because a permanent injury to the midbrain may result in a persistent vegetative state, rapid evaluation and intervention are required to salvage the patient.

Another method frequently used to evaluate head-injured patients is the Glasgow coma scale (Table 42-3). By evaluating a patient on three parameters (motor response, verbal response, and eye opening), a numerical score can be obtained. Patients with a score of 5 or less have a mortality of greater than 50 percent. This scale is helpful in demonstrating that a measure of these parameters can be correlated with mortality rates. Although it is valuable in comparing the outcomes of large numbers of patients with various forms of treatment, this scale is not sufficient by itself to manage the individual trauma victim.

DIAGNOSTIC STUDIES. The rapidity with which diagnostic studies must be performed is dictated by the patient's neurologic condition. It should be remembered that regardless of what test is to be done, the traumatized patient should not leave the emergency room if the vital signs have not been stabilized. The only reason for an unstable patient to be transported is the need for an emergency procedure necessary to save the patient's life. It should also be remembered that patients require frequent evaluations in order to detect changes in neurologic function.

In general, patients who demonstrate a marked alteration in consciousness, a deterioration in neurologic function, or evidence of brainstem dysfunction require a rapid evaluation for intracranial mass that would require an operation. The term "mass effect" refers to an increase in blood (hematoma) or brain (edema) volume, or both, that causes a shift of brain tissue away from the area of injury and an increase in pressure inside the skull. The best method for evaluating the traumatized brain for mass effect is by CT scanning. The surgical management of these masses will be discussed in a later section of this

Table 42-3. GLASGOW COMA SCALE

Best motor response	Obeys	M6
	Localizes	5
	Withdraws	4
	Abnormal flexion	3
	Extensor response	2
	Nil	1
Verbal response	Oriented	V5
	Confused conversation	4
	Inappropriate words	3
	Incomprehensible sounds	2
	Nil	1
Eye opening	Spontaneous	E4
	To speech	3
	To pain	2
	Nil	1

NOTE: The coma scale score is the sum of the sectional scores. See text for details.

chapter. In addition to CT scanning, other testing such as angiography may be necessary in patients who are suspected of having an injury to a major extracranial or intracranial blood vessel.

Stable patients with less severe head trauma do not require immediate radiographic testing. They may first receive skull x-rays in search of a skull fracture, intracranial air, or a foreign body. As a general rule, a patient who has any alteration in the level of consciousness following trauma should receive a CT scan of the brain. Skull fractures are also detectable by CT scanning, and this test can preclude the need for skull x-rays. Despite the sensitivity of CT scans in detecting intracranial hemorrhage and masses, no test should replace clinical observation.

There is no reason to perform a lumbar puncture as part of the initial evaluation of a trauma patient. The risk of altering spinal fluid pressure when the possibility of a mass lesion exists in the calvarium far outweighs any information gained. A lumbar puncture may be necessary at some time in the patient's care to evaluate the possibility of meningitis or may be helpful in deciding that an unconscious patient without a history has had a subarachnoid hemorrhage or meningitis instead of head trauma. A CT scan, however, should be performed before the lumbar puncture is performed.

TREATMENT. Treatment for a head-injured patient begins as soon as the diagnosis has been made. Maintaining an airway and reversal of shock are considered important parts of this treatment. The general principles to be followed include adequate oxygenation and brain circulation, removal of mass effect, control of intracranial pressure, prevention of infection, and rehabilitation. Frequent monitoring of vital signs, arterial blood gases, and fluid intake and output is a routine necessity. The principles of surgical decision making are beyond the scope of this text. As a rule, a focal mass from hemorrhage of swelling that alters the patient's level of consciousness should be removed. This operation may include not only removing a hematoma, but also the removal of damaged brain.

An important part of treatment includes the control of intracranial pressure (ICP). Because the skull is a closed compartment, any increase in intracranial volume will result in an increase in pressure inside the skull unless there is a compensatory decrease in volume. Posttraumatic swelling of brain tissue can cause such raised ICP that cerebral perfusion is compromised, and most episodes of inadequate cerebral perfusion are caused by repetitive episodes of transient waves of pressure. These "plateau waves" may be caused by changes in the diameter of intracranial blood vessels in the absence of autoregulation. Since cerebral blood flow passively follows systemic arterial pressure, it can be measured by the equation

$$CBF = \frac{(SAP - ICP)K}{VR}$$

where CBF = cerebral blood flow
     SAP = systemic arterial pressure
     ICP = intracranial pressure
     VR = vascular resistance
     K = perfusion constant

One method of measuring ICP is by the use of an intraventricular catheter or by commercially available pressure devices. These are inserted into the brain and give a continuous digital readout of the pressure by a transducer. These monitors can alert the surgeon to changes in the pressure and can be valuable as a warning of an evolving mass inside the brain. Intervention can then be performed as indicated. Control of intracranial pressure is obtained by the removal of mass. Operative intervention has already been addressed as one method. Additional methods of ICP control include deliberate hypocarbia, removal of spinal fluid, osmotic diuresis, and avoidance of fluid overload and hyponatremia. Carbon dioxide is a potent cerebral vasodilator. Deliberate hypocapnia (P_{CO_2} 25 to 30 torr) will result in cerebral vasoconstriction and a resultant decrease in intracranial blood volume. This is a reliable method for immediate ICP reduction. Spinal fluid can be removed by an intraventricular catheter which precludes the danger of a pressure cone from the intracranial cavity through the foramen magnum. Hyponatremia and fluid overload increase the risk of cerebral edema by increasing the extracellular water volume. This is particularly important in patients with the inappropriate secretion of antidiuretic hormone (SIADH) which causes reabsorption of fluid by the kidney and a concomitant decrease in serum sodium. A restriction of water intake may be necessary to maintain a normal serum sodium. Osmotic diuretics such as mannitol provide a method to temporarily reduce extracellular fluid by osmotically pulling fluid into the intravascular space to be diuresed. If these methods prove to be inadequate, the patient can be given high doses of barbiturates to reduce the cerebral metabolic rate and cerebral blood flow. In addition neuromuscular blockage for pharmacologic paralysis will eliminate resistance to blood flow from muscular activity. The latter methods also obviate the neurologic exam as a monitoring method and should be used only when high ICP has failed other forms of treatment. Following a severe brain injury, the methods of ICP control may be required for several days to a few weeks. During this period of time attention to pulmonary hygiene, venous stasis, and skin care will help to prevent the complications of pneumonia, pulmonary embolism, and skin breakdown that complicate patient management.

Intracranial Hemorrhage

Progressive neurologic deficit, the most common being progressive loss of consciousness, following head trauma should always be assumed to be due to intracranial hemorrhage until proved otherwise. The patterns of neurologic change vary with the type of hemorrhage, but all have as a major component the neurologic deficit of progressive loss of consciousness.

The most common intracranial hemorrhage following head trauma is subarachnoid hemorrhage. It has little significance and usually causes signs of meningismus or stiff neck and headache. It may, in the young male, produce maniacal behavior. It has little significance surgically, because the blood is rapidly diluted by the cerebrospinal fluid and flows throughout the subarachnoid space, so that no significant localized mass effect occurs. It may have significance as a late complication of head injury, causing progressive communicating hydrocephalus. This complication is rare, occurring weeks or months after injury, and presents as a progressive dementia with motor apraxia, usually most marked as a gait disturbance. The mechanism is thought to be obstruction of the arachnoid villi and/or basal cisterns so that the absorption of cerebrospinal fluid is altered. The treatment is the same as for infantile hydrocephalus with the construction of an artificial path for the absorption of cerebrospinal fluid. This is done with a shunt from the lateral ventricle to the superior vena cava or peritoneum using a valve to prevent blood reflux and to stabilize the pressure in the ventricle at 50 to 70 mmH$_2$O.

Surgically significant intracranial hemorrhages are best classified by their anatomic positions, i.e., subdural hematoma, epidural hematoma, and intracerebral hematoma. While they are relatively rare, unrecognized and untreated posttraumatic intracranial hematomas have almost a 100 percent mortality rate. Since most of this mortality can be averted by surgical treatment, early and accurate diagnosis is important.

SUBDURAL HEMATOMA

One of the most common types of posttraumatic intracranial hemorrhage is subdural hematoma. It is caused either by rupture of the veins traversing the subdural space from the brain to the dural sinuses or by a laceration of the brain that has torn the overlying piarachnoid. The symptoms may appear as early as within the first few minutes or as late as 6 to 8 weeks after injury. The pattern of symptoms, the findings, the treatment, and the prognosis vary with the rapidity of formation of the hematoma, so that it is logical to consider the syndrome of subdural hematoma as three different types: acute subdural, subacute subdural, and chronic subdural. Subdural hematomas and epidural and intracerebral hematomas are the common surgically important intracranial hemorrhagic complications of trauma. Although each has a different symptom pattern, all have somewhere in their history the finding of decreased level of consciousness out of proportion to focal neurologic deficit. Portions of the basic patterns are usually present in all patients with subdural hematoma, but at times discovering them can tax the most astute clinician. The following descriptions are to be taken as outlines of patterns commonly presented by the patient with the different types of intracranial hematoma, but the reader should always keep in mind the protean signs and symptoms possible in a patient with intracranial hematoma.

Acute Subdural Hematoma

Acute subdural hematomas are defined as hematomas that cause significant progressive neurologic deficit within 48 h of injury. They almost always occur following severe head trauma, and since they may have both arterial and venous sources for bleeding, the progression of the neurologic deficit can be rapid, often in terms of min-

utes or hours. The source of the arterial bleeding is frequently a laceration of the brain, and therefore focal neurologic deficit such as a hemiparesis is common.

Clinical Manifestations. When first seen, the patient is usually unresponsive with a focal neurologic deficit. Progressive decrease in sensorium with or without progressive focal neurologic deficit is the warning of increasing intracranial mass. Without treatment the brainstem will be compressed by hemorrhage, edema, and herniation until death results. Death may occur within hours, with cessation of respiration, maintenance of pulse and blood pressure for a short time, and then peripheral vascular collapse as the medulla fails. Diagnosis is made by always considering the possibility of acute subdural hematoma in the severely head-injured patient who shows any deterioration in neurologic status. Aid in the diagnosis and in determining the site of major hemorrhage can be gained by the localization of any focal neurologic deficit, and by CT. CT also can define adjacent intracerebral hematomas, a common concomitant of acute subdural hematomas, making surgical approach to the hemorrhage more accurate and effective. More than half of acute subdural hematomas are bilateral, so that evaluation of both subdural spaces is indicated.

Treatment. Treatment consists of removal of the hematoma through a large craniotomy with control of bleeding areas, decompression by excision of large areas of the skull and relaxation of the compressing dura, and, when necessary, internal decompression by excision of portions of the frontal or temporal lobes. The methods of controlling edema and a secondary injury from loss of effective cerebral perfusion pressure, as outlined in a preceding section, have decreased, but not eliminated, the need for such decompressive procedures and decreased both the problem of shift of the brain and the damage that can occur as an area of brain protrudes through a decompression site, as well as the later need for repair of surgical defect in the skull. Drainage of the hematoma through perforator openings is never satisfactory, since the major portion of the hematoma is solid clot and the problem is a combination of mass from clot and reaction of the brain to severe trauma. Without prompt surgical care mortality is 100 percent, and even with the best care it can be quite high.

Subacute Subdural Hematoma

Subacute subdural hematomas are complications of head trauma that cause significant neurologic deficit more than 48 h but less than 2 weeks after injury. They are usually caused by venous bleeding into the subdural space.

Clinical Manifestations. The basic pattern of symptoms and signs is a history of head trauma with unconsciousness, gradual improvement in the first few days followed by lack of improvement, fluctuation in levels of consciousness, and then decompensation with progressive loss of consciousness and often partial loss of hemispheric function. The patients are usually not as severely injured as are the patients with acute subdural hematomas. The phase of fluctuation in level of consciousness often heralds that significant shift of the intracranial contents has occurred, and patients may change from relatively alert to difficult to arouse even with painful stimuli and back to their alert status within a few hours. Herniation of the medial temporal lobe through the incisura of the tentorium and compensation of the midbrain to the pressure of such herniation is a possible mechanism of such fluctuation in levels of consciousness. The presence of a third nerve paresis with dilatation of the pupil is often a warning that midbrain decompensation is imminent. The computerized scanner may not identify subacute subdural hematomas, since they can become isodense within the first 10 to 12 days after injury (i.e., the x-ray absorbed is approximately the same as brain). If the hematoma is unilateral or asymmetrical, the shift of the ventricular system as seen on computerized scanning will suggest the location of the hematoma. If the clinical history and signs suggest subdural hematoma, even without confirmation by CT scanning, the diagnosis should be confirmed or excluded by multiple perforator openings, by angiography or by MRI.

Treatment. Treatment is dependent upon how critical the patient's condition is, how much liquid clot there is, and whether significant temporal lobe herniation has occurred. The patient with solid clot, unresponsive from uncal herniation, requires craniotomy, removal of the clot, and elevation of the temporal lobe herniation with or without incision of the tentorial edge. In the less critically ill patient and in the patient with considerable liquefaction of the hematoma the removal of a major portion of the clot through a small craniectomy and multiple perforator openings followed by external drainage of the subdural space may be all that is required. As with acute subdural hematomas, these hematomas are commonly bilateral, and exploration of both subdural spaces is indicated unless the CT scan or angiograms have ruled out the presence of bilateral hematomas.

Chronic Subdural Hematoma

Although the initial cause of the chronic subdural hematoma is usually rupture by head trauma of one of the veins traversing the subdural space, the symptoms are caused by the increasing mass effect of the hematoma surrounded by a semipermeable membrane. Within 7 to 10 days after bleeding has occurred in the subdural space the blood is surrounded by a fibrous membrane. As the blood cells within the membrane break down, fluid is osmotically pulled into the hematoma, causing an increase in its volume. This may cause further bleeding from tears in the membrane or by rupturing other traversing veins with the reestablishment of the same process and an increasing size of the semiliquid-filled membrane.

Clinical Manifestations. Chronic subdural hematomas may occur at any age but are most frequent in the infant or the elderly. The causative trauma, particularly in the elderly, may be so slight that the patient does not remember it and gives no history of trauma. The symptoms and signs are best classified as a progressive alteration in

mentation and level of consciousness of 4 to 6 weeks duration out of proportion to the focal neurologic deficit. Therefore, any patient presenting with a progressive change in mental faculties and fluctuation or decreasing level of consciousness should be considered a subdural hematoma suspect.

Treatment. Since the hematoma is liquid, drainage through perforator openings is usually all that is required. In the past many neurosurgeons have felt that removal of the membranes is required, since they may be quite thick. However, experience has shown that there is increased mortality and morbidity from craniotomy removal of membranes and no improvement in the long-term results over those achieved by simple drainage of chronic subdural hematomas.

Subdural Hygroma

Although subdural hygromas are not a part of intracranial hemorrhage, they can produce similar symptoms. Subdural hygroma is usually caused by a tear in the piarachnoid that acts as a one-way valve with leakage of cerebrospinal fluid into the subdural space. The hygroma can increase in size quite rapidly and therefore can mimic an acute or subacute subdural hematoma. Perforator openings of the skull with external drainage is the treatment of choice, but at times formation of an artificial fistula between the subarachnoid space and the subdural space must be made in order to control continued formation of the hygroma.

EPIDURAL HEMATOMA

Epidural hematomas may be caused by either venous or arterial bleeding. They lie between the skull and the dura. The most common cause is venous bleeding, but the surgically important epidural hematomas most frequently are formed by arterial bleeding. Occasionally the patient with a skull fracture may have a significant venous epidural, the removal of which allows decrease in intracranial pressure or release of focal compression of the brain, but generally venous epidural hematomas are limited by the firm adherence of the dura to the inner surface of the skull. The central point of the venous epidural is almost always at the site of a fracture.

The epidural hematoma from arterial bleeding commonly occurs from rupture of the middle meningeal artery. This may be caused by a fracture of the temporal bone where the artery is in close proximity to the bone or by a tear of the middle meningeal artery when a blow causes angular acceleration of the head or sudden decrease or increase in any diameter of the skull. The tear may occur at the foramen spinosum, where the artery enters the skull, or anywhere along its branches.

CLINICAL MANIFESTATIONS. The basic historical pattern of the epidural hematoma is a young adult who has received a relatively minor blow causing momentary alteration in consciousness, followed by a lucid interval extending from a few minutes to a few hours. This interval terminates by rapid progressive loss of consciousness, dilatation of the pupil on the side of the epidural hematoma, evidence of compression of the upper midbrain, by either the production of a hemiparesis or decerebrate rigidity, and then evidence of compromise of the entire brainstem and death. The frequency of the hematoma being over the temporal area, the direct pressure onto the temporal lobe and therefore the maximal chance of herniation of the medial temporal lobe through the incisura, and the arterial pressure as a source of bleeding are the main reasons for the rapidity with which the entire syndrome can be completed.

TREATMENT. Treatment consists of early recognition, a temporal craniectomy, evacuation of the hemorrhage, and control of the bleeding artery either at the foramen spinosum or at the point of tear in the dura. With early surgical intervention, the mortality from epidural hemorrhage can be dramatically reduced.

INTRACEREBRAL HEMATOMA

Posttraumatic intracerebral hematomas are most often seen in patients with severe head trauma, often mimic the symptom patterns of an acute or subacute subdural hematoma, and frequently are found in conjunction with them. In some series of posttraumatic intracranial hemorrhage intracerebral hematomas are as frequent as subdural hematomas, especially if the series includes many patients injured in high-speed vehicle accidents. The hematoma usually presents either beneath a cortical laceration or as a confluence of small hemorrhages in a contused area of the brain. Intracerebral hematomas are most commonly found in the anterior third of the temporal lobe where the temporal lobe may strike the sphenoid bone, and less frequently in the tips of the frontal or occipital lobes. They can be seen in any area of the cerebrum. The symptoms of clinically significant posttraumatic intracerebral hematomas are similar to the symptoms of an acute or subacute subdural hematoma. There are many intracerebral hematomas that do not alter the clinical course of a patient, are not diagnosed, and resolve by liquefaction, phagocytosis, and gliosis. The surgically significant intracerebral hematomas present with progressive decrease in consciousness and/or progressive focal neurologic deficit. Most frequently, focal deficits are third nerve palsy and hemiparesis. These symptoms may develop within a few hours or a few days of the injury. As with acute subdural hematomas, CT accurately diagnoses, localizes, and determines the extent of intracerebral hematomas.

TREATMENT. The only effective treatment of surgically significant posttraumatic intracerebral hematomas is craniotomy or craniectomy with incision into the hemisphere at the most superficial area of the hematoma and evacuation of the clot. Simple aspiration of the lesion is not adequate since the majority of the hemorrhage is usually solid clot. The evacuation often must include excision of part of the lobe involved in order to remove devitalized brain and to obtain effective decompression of the injured cerebrum.

REHABILITATION. Rehabilitation of head-injured patients starts with initial care and finishes when their function is stabilized at its highest possible level. The rehabilitation of the brain-injured patient is a specialty in itself,

but fortunately few patients require retraining or reconstructive surgical procedures to overcome their neurologic deficits. A majority of head-injured patients require only the support and care of a knowledgeable physician. Special problems of the head-injured patient during convalescence fall within three categories: psychologic problems, convulsions, and problems with cerebrospinal fluid circulation.

Psychologic Problems. Changes in personality and mood during the period of convalescence are one of the most common and often one of the most difficult symptoms for both patient and physician. The symptoms usually fall into the broad psychiatric category of a reactive depression with an overlay of anxiety. Complaints of headache, fatigue, loss of memory, excessive difficulty with performing tasks, transient despondency, and overreaction to emotional stimuli demonstrate a mixture of possible organic and psychologic bases for the symptoms. On the organic side is the suggestion of temporal and frontal lobe malfunction, while on the psychologic side is the reaction to physical and mental fatigue with a superimposed anxiety from the fear that the change may be permanent.

Gradually increasing physical activity in a planned fashion with limited goals that can be reached in reasonable periods of time and a planned return to increasingly difficult mental tasks is usually the best method for overcoming the problem. The settlement of any pending litigation is important when psychologic problems become paramount, for unnecessary delay can make a psychologic cripple of the patient. The physician should not abandon these patients or allow them to become dependent but rather insist that they get psychiatric help when necessary and that they work toward any physical and mental goals that seem possible. The best method of giving such support is for the physician to see the patient at planned intervals and during the visits to evaluate the neurologic progress of the patient to be certain that a portion of the problem is not coming from seizures or altered cerebrospinal fluid circulation.

Convulsions. Approximately 30 to 45 percent of patients with a compound injury that involves a laceration of the brain will have seizures if they are not on anticonvulsive medication. In contrast, the incidence of convulsions in the closed-head-injury patient is much lower. It is difficult to obtain any significant figures on the incidence of convulsion in the closed-head-injury patient, for in large series it varies from 0.5 percent to as high as 10 percent. In general it is safe to assume that a patient who has had less than 4 h of either markedly altered consciousness or focal neurologic deficit will have no significant chance of convulsions developing late in the convalescence that relate to the head injury. In the group with more serious head injuries there remains a small but persistent percentage in whom convulsions will develop that appear to relate to the head injury. The period in which convulsions may develop extends over many years. It is often difficult to recognize that focal or partial seizures are occurring, but they always should be considered when any paroxysmal symptoms occur, that is, symptoms of relatively brief duration that end with excessive fatigue. Electroencephalograms may be of help in diagnosing the cause of such symptoms as seizures, but at times trials of anticonvulsants are necessary to rule them out. Control of posttraumatic seizures with Dilantin or phenobarbital is usually sufficient, but occasionally resection of the damaged area is necessary for control with anticonvulsant drugs.

SPINAL CORD INJURIES

The primary objectives in the treatment of traumatic spinal cord injuries are to prevent further injury, optimize the conditions for recovery of function, stabilize the spinal column, and rehabilitate patients in an attempt to return them to a productive life.

MECHANISM OF INJURY. The majority of nonpenetrating injuries are caused by a fracture and dislocation of the vertebral segments resulting in an acute compression of the cord. The cervical spine is the site of most frequent injury comprising 50 to 60 percent of all cases. The next most common region of trauma is the thoracolumbar junction (20 to 30 percent). The remainder of the injuries are located in the lumbar and the thoracic cord. A fracture dislocation of the spine that reduces the diameter of the canal causes a mechanical distortion of the cord tissue and frequently a compromise of the anterior and posterior spinal arteries.

Experimental laboratory spinal cord injuries in animals have demonstrated that acute compression sets into motion a series of pathologic changes that evolve over hours to days. These delayed changes are called secondary injuries and, in certain cases, may contribute to the failure of recovery of function. These secondary injuries include a central gray matter hemorrhage followed by an expanding ischemia and edema that will involve the surrounding white matter fiber tracts. In addition, loss of membrane ionic gradients, cation shifts, and the release of vasoactive compounds may contribute to the evolution of cord destruction. Experimental treatment methods in the laboratory have been primarily developed to prevent these secondary injuries, and many have been demonstrated to improve neurologic recovery and to prevent the delayed hemorrhagic necrosis. Despite the laboratory success, no treatment method has been shown to improve the recovery of neurologic function in spinal cord injured humans.

Any patient with multiple trauma is at risk of a spinal cord injury. Motor vehicle accidents are the most frequent cause of injury followed by diving into shallow water and falls. Males outnumber females by 3:1. A majority of the patients are between the ages of fifteen and thirty.

Approximately 50 percent of the injuries will result in an immediate and total loss of function below the level of injury. The remainder of the patients will demonstrate some preservation of sensory and/or motor function when initially examined by a physician. Because the chances of recovery are directly related to the amount of retained function, careful management is mandatory.

Penetrating Injuries. The majority of penetrating injuries is the result of gunshot wounds, followed by stabbings and foreign bodies from explosions. The management of the spinal cord injury is similar to that of nonpenetrating injuries with a few exceptions. Because of the concussive energy delivered to the cord following a gunshot wound, the chances of recovery of function are extremely small. The initial patient management should be directed toward other injuries caused by the bullet that may be life-threatening. Surgical debridement of the spinal cord is indicated in a stable patient for prevention of infection, closure of CSP leaks, and stabilization of an unstable spine.

Spinal Cord Injury Syndromes. The topographic orientation of fiber tracts in the spinal cord permits a description of the anatomy of the injury based upon the neurologic exam.

Transverse Injury. A transverse or complete injury results in the total loss of neurologic function below the level of injury. Immediately following trauma, there is a loss of reflex activity and autonomic function as well as motor and sensory activity (spinal shock). A return of deep tendon reflexes and some of the autonomic activity occurs within days to weeks.

Central Cord Syndrome. Because the destruction of spinal cord tissue starts as a hemorrhage in the central gray matter and spreads in a centrifugal pattern toward the white matter, lesions that do not destroy the entire cross section of the cord will preserve the peripheral white matter tracts. As a result, the sacral fibers of the lateral corticospinal and spinothalamic tracts will be preserved. This will result in sacral sparing. For example, a cervical injury that preserves the lumbar and sacral fibers will result in retained motor power and pin and temperature sensation in the legs and sacral area with plegia and anesthesia in the arms and the thorax.

Brown Sequard Syndrome. A lesion that destroys the lateral half of the cord will produce plegia and loss of vibration and position sensation ipsilateral to the injury with a contralateral loss of pain and temperature sensation. This syndrome is most commonly seen in lateral cord compression or penetrating knife wounds.

Anterior Spinal Artery Syndrome. The anterior spinal artery supplies the majority of the spinal cord's blood supply and around two-thirds of the cross-sectional area of the cord. This includes all the gray matter except for the dorsal horns and most of the lateral funiculus and anterior funiculus. Interruption of this blood supply causes motor plegia and loss of pain and temperature sensation with preservation of vibration and position sensation.

PATIENT MANAGEMENT. Any patient who is at risk for a spinal cord injury should be immobilized on a long board or firm surface and with a cervical collar and/or sandbags. A detailed neurologic exam that evaluates motor power, sensory function, and reflex activity will provide the information necessary to localize the area of injury. Sensory functions are represented in anatomically distinct fiber tracts, and pin sensation, vibration and position, light touch, and deep pressure should be tested. Based upon the results of this examination, the appropriate x-rays of the spine can be obtained.

Cervical injuries may require reduction of a dislocation, and this can be accomplished by traction using skull tongs. In order to obtain a direct axial force for reduction,

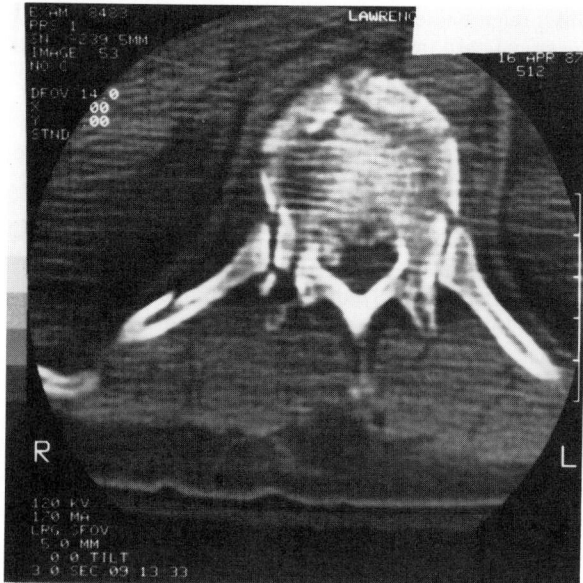

Fig. 42-4. CT of a compression of the T_{12} vertebral segment demonstrating posterior displacement of bone fragments into the right side of the canal resulting in paraplegia. Note the excellent resolution of the fractures in the right pedicle, facet, rib, and multiple fragments of the body.

the tongs should be inserted directly above the mastoid tips. An initial weight of 5 to 10 lb (2.265 to 4.53 kg) can be used to immobilize the head. Additional weights added at 5-lb (2.265-kg) increments are then used in an attempt to realign the canal. A maximum weight of 40 to 50 lb (18.22 to 22.65 kg) should not be exceeded except in un-

usual circumstances. Care must be taken to prevent further injury by distraction or further dislocation during this process. This is best performed by repeating the neurologic exam and a lateral C-spine x-ray whenever the weights are changed or there is a deterioration in the exam. Thoracic or lumbar injuries cannot be reduced with skull traction, and these injuries are best treated by immobilization on a firm surface.

Radiologic Examination. AP and lateral x-rays of the area of injury are very important in order to evaluate the severity of the fracture and the amount of dislocation. Additional x-ray views may be helpful in order to complete this examination. Following attempted reduction of a dislocation, high-resolution CT scanning with a small amount of water-soluble intrathecal contrast material will indicate the extent of the injury, the severity of the fractures, the amount of cord compression, and the presence of extradural masses. MRI may also be useful but, at this time, it is not universally available. Reconstruction of the CT images in a sagittal plane is also very helpful (Figs. 42-4, 42-5, 42-6).

TREATMENT. Despite an aggressive surgical approach by many neurosurgeons, decompression of bone, disc, or hematoma has not been demonstrated to improve the neurologic recovery in patients with an acute and complete loss of distal spinal cord function. While most surgeons will emergently remove the source of continued compression in patients with some retained neurologic function, this also has not been convincingly demonstrated to improve neurologic recovery. Early stabilization of an unstable injury and removal of residual compression probably enables the patient to avoid many of the complications of prolonged immobilization. Addi-

Fig. 42-5. CT of the same injury with intrathecal contrast material that outlines the left side of the spinal cord. The right side of the canal does not fill with contrast because of cord swelling and displaced bone.

Fig. 42-6. Sagittal reconstruction of the area of injury along the dotted line reveals a markedly swollen cord. Contrast material in the subarachnoid space outlines the spinal cord.

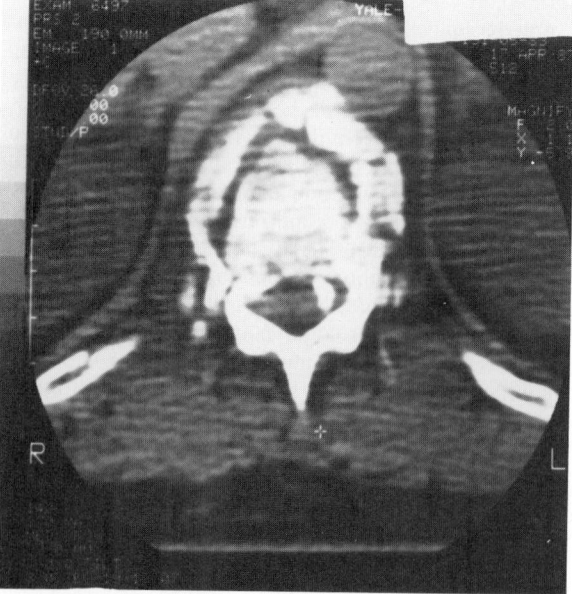

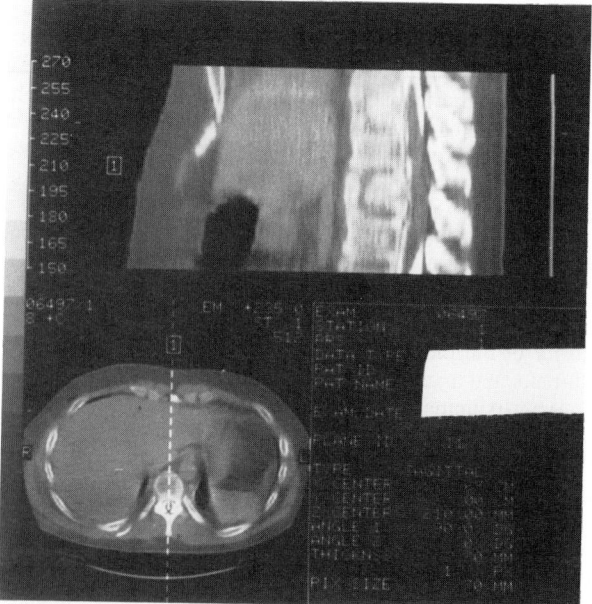

tional problems including loss of bowel and bladder control, skin ulceration, respiratory compromise, and cardiovascular instability also require constant attention.

PROGNOSIS. The most important factor that can be used to predict the recovery of neurologic function following traumatic spinal cord injury is the severity of the injury at the moment of trauma. Patients with acute transverse lesions that demonstrate no retained motor or sensory function generally do not recover. If preserved sensory perception of motor activity can be detected, the chances of recovery of useful function increase dramatically. It is very important to properly manage these patients in order to prevent the loss of retained function and to avoid causing a deteriorating or ascending level. If a patient is noted to lose neurologic function, it is necessary to reevaluate the area of injury for increased dislocation, movement at the fracture site, or hematoma formation. Rapid intervention then may prevent further damage.

PERIPHERAL NERVE INJURIES

Acute peripheral nerve injuries are uncommon in the civilian practice of medicine. Peripheral nerve injuries may occur in a variety of ways. Low-energy penetrating wounds such as those created by a knife or a piece of glass may result in laceration of a peripheral nerve; high-energy penetrating wounds such as those produced from gunshot can result in more extensive nerve disruption; compressive or stress injuries may produce damage over a long segment of nerve as can electrical injuries; and finally poorly placed drug injections can result in chemical damage to the nerve. Pathophysiologically nerve injuries can be grouped into three types. Although certain mechanisms favor certain types of neuronal damage, most peripheral nerve damage injuries represent a composite of these three types of neuronal injury. *Neuronapraxis,* the least severe of these injuries, commonly occurs after compression injury to the peripheral nerve. The partial peroneal nerve deficit commonly called "Saturday night palsy," which occurs when the legs are crossed an excessive time, is a common example of such an injury. Typically the neurologic deficit is incomplete, with motor loss typically being more prominent than sensory loss. When present, sensory loss occurs in the large fiber-mediated sensory modalities of touch and proprioception. Although the exact mechanism of neuronal dysfunction is unclear in neuronapraxis, it is believed to occur as a result of the inability of the axons to reestablish their membrane potentials rather than because of axonal loss itself. Typically, neurologic recovery is complete by 6 weeks and again occurs in a fashion that cannot be adequately explained by axonal regrowth. *Axonotmesis* occurs when there is both axonal and myelin loss in the injured nerve. The connective tissue scaffolding of the peripheral nerve remains inviolate. Typically, there is a complete motor and sensory neurologic loss. Recovery occurs in a proximal to distal fashion as axonal regrowth occurs. *Neurotmesis* occurs when the peripheral nerve is partially or completely severed. This commonly occurs

after penetrating injuries and at least anatomically represents the most severe form of injury.

Competent evaluation of the nerve injuries requires an accurate knowledge of the anatomy and function of the injured nerve, an understanding of the mechanism of the injury, and an understanding of the type of injury that has resulted. Therapeutic decisions are further based on the comparative prognoses of the various forms of therapy available.

TREATMENT. Appropriate treatment for peripheral nerve injuries may include careful serial observation and monitoring of neuronal healing alone, suture repair of the nerve, resection and reconstruction of damaged neuronal segments, or no specific treatment of the nerve itself but reestablishment of function of the limb utilizing other muscles and internal and external supports. Selection of the appropriate treatment and its timing is often a difficult decision; however, a rational treatment is based on several principles.

As mentioned above, neuronapraxis may cause complete functional loss of a nerve without anatomic disruption, and return occurs within 6 weeks. Therefore, although immediate surgical repair gives the best functional results for more severe nerve injuries, little is lost by a delay of 3 to 6 weeks if the nerve is thought to be in continuity. After disruption and reapproximation of a nerve the axons require about 3 weeks to grow across the suture line and then grow about 3 cm per month. In general, counting the delay across the suture line and the time for reinnervation of muscle end plates or peripheral end organs an estimated functional growth of 1 in. per month is usually accurate. Following denervation the muscle end plates atrophy and muscle fibers progressively degenerate so that within 20 to 24 months no significant muscle contraction can be expected from reinnervation. While muscle tone reappears and some movement will occur up to that time, significant strength in a muscle rarely can be regained past 15 months. Since functional nerve regeneration proceeds approximately 1 in. per month, a nerve suture that is more than 15 in. from the deinnervated muscle cannot be expected to give significant motor return, and tendon transplants, joint fixations, or bracing should be considered as treatment for the motor loss. Tone in facial muscles will return up to 24 months past deinnervation, but as the end of the 24-month period approaches no movement of expression can be expected.

All nerve injuries are painful, and pain will continue with varying intensity for many months. Narcotics have no place in the treatment of chronic pain and therefore should not be used after the immediate wound pain has ceased. Functional use of the extremity is the best therapy for the pain and is an important reason for using passive and active motion and functional bracing as soon as possible. It is also a major reason for not waiting for an improbable result, such as reinnervation of a muscle too distant from the point of suture, before using other reconstructive methods. In contrast to the time limits on return of motor function, sensory function of a significant degree can help in relieving the discomfort as well as in providing protection of an extremity. This is especially true of the protection offered by the sensory reinnervation of the foot.

In many instances, segmental loss of 8 to 10 cm of nerve can be bridged by proximal and distal dissection to release the nerve from surrounding tissue and by positioning of the nerve or the extremity to minimize distance across joints. This may require wide dissection and positioning of more than one joint of the extremity. When neurorrhaphy is planned, skin preparation and draping should allow for such maneuvers. Despite these maneuvers, if the nerve ends cannot be reapproximated without tension, interpositional neuronal grafts such as a sural nerve graft may be necessary. Present evidence indicates interfascicular repair, when possible, gives better results than epineural repair.

EVALUATION. The evaluation of peripheral nerve injuries is in part similar to the evaluation of central nervous system injuries, for comparison of serial observations and recognition of progressive neurologic deficit or improvement often determine the type of therapy required. The treatment differs from that for central nervous system injuries in that regeneration with reinnervation can occur and therefore the treatment of peripheral nerve injury includes neurorrhaphy, or the surgical repair of the nerve. Since comparison of later examinations with the initial one is important in therapy, it is essential to have an accurate examination that includes the sensory and motor function of all nerves thought to be injured. Peripheral nerve injuries often occur as part of more extensive injuries, and since an accurate examination can be done only on a cooperative patient, all patients suspected of nerve injury should be reexamined when well enough to cooperate.

Nerve injuries are a relatively rare experience for the civilian physician, and the accuracy even of an experienced neurosurgeon can be enhanced by reviewing the anatomy and functions of nerves suspected of injury.

EVALUATION OF FUNCTIONAL RECOVERY. In the evaluation of the injured nerve, evidence for functional recovery of the nerve is important, for it determines the success or failure of the therapy. Evidence that the nerve functions is not the same as functional recovery, for nerve function means only that some portion of the nerve has anatomic continuity. Definite evidence of functional recovery consists of

1. Voluntary motor function of a muscle innervated by the nerve distal to the injury. This means that a major number of the motor fibers have reinnervated the muscle and that with time increase in strength will occur, either through increased strength of the individual reinnervated muscle fibers or by further innervation.
2. Muscle contraction on electrical stimulation of the nerve distal to the point of injury when performed more than 7 days after injury. Since the distal segment of a divided nerve will conduct impulses for only 5 to 6 days, evidence of ability to conduct later than 7 days after injury indicates functional continuity or regeneration. Muscle contraction following the stimulation means a major portion of the motor fibers are conducting. Direct electrical stimulation of the muscle does not give evidence of functional recovery, since contraction with this type of stimulation will occur until atrophy of the muscle is complete.

3. Recovery of sensation in an autogenous area of innervation. There are few such areas for individual nerves. The distal phalanx of the index finger for the median nerve and the distal phalanx of the little finger for the ulnar nerve are the only two in the upper extremity. The distal phalanges of the middle three toes of the foot are autogenous for the sciatic nerve but only if both peroneal and tibial divisions are involved.

Evidence of anatomic continuity but not of prognostic significance for functional recovery consists of

1. Tinel's sign distal to the site of injury. Tinel's sign is elicited by percussing the nerve and obtaining paresthesia referred to the superficial area of skin innervation. Although the absence of Tinel's sign is clear evidence that neuronal regeneration is not occurring, its presence is more difficult to interpret. Eliciting Tinel's sign requires the activation of only a small number of small fibers that may have been spared by the initial injury or may have since regenerated. Tinel's sign therefore may be present under circumstances that may not necessarily favor functional recovery. A distal migration of Tinel's sign over time coupled with matched evidence of sensory reinnervation does, however, suggest significant neuronal recovery.
2. Alteration in electromyographic activity with attempted voluntary motion or nerve stimulation. As with Tinel's sign, the activation of far fewer fibers than is necessary for functional return of a muscle is required to elicit alteration in the recorded electromyographic activity.

Evidence that indicates neither anatomic nor functional continuity of an injured nerve consists of

1. Shrinkage of the area of sensory loss. The marked overlap of sensory innervation in all areas of the body has been alluded to with the description of the very few autogenous zones of peripheral nerve innervation. Decrease in an area of sensory loss after nerve injury can occur from recovery of the nerve function, but even without reinnervation adjacent nerves reestablish sensation in the area. The mechanism appears to be both utilization of fibers that function with the damaged nerve but that without the spatial summation of the damaged nerve activity do not reach consciousness, and branching of the superficial nerve fibers of the remaining nerves with growth into the denervated area.
2. Improved use of the extremity. The adaptability of the child to use any remaining function to accomplish coordinated tasks is a major example, but use of gravity, momentum, and muscles with remaining function to simulate the lost function must not be confused with reinnervation.

Illustrative Cases

The application of these concepts is most easily understood in relation to examples of the three major groups of peripheral nerve injury, laceration, or focal sharp injury, focal contusion, and compression or stretch injury.

Focal Laceration. An example of focal sharp injury is a knife wound of the upper extremity at approximately the midhumeral level, resulting in loss of median nerve function. Motor loss would consist of paralysis of all flexors of the wrist and fingers except the flexor capri ulnaris and the ulnar portion of the flexor digitorum profundus. The latter two muscles would give wrist flexion with ulnar deviation and flexion of the ring and little fingers. Sensory loss would consist of loss of superficial sensation of the palmar surface of the hand extending to the thumb and first two fingers and the radial half of the ring finger. Deep as well as superficial sensation would be lost in the distal phalanx of the index finger.

Immediate repair is indicated *except* when any of the following apply: (1) The nerve appears contused for more than a few millimeters on either side of the injury. (2) There is blood loss from arterial injury that would jeopardize the life of the patient in undergoing a long (2- to 3-h) operation for repair of the artery and nerve. (3) The wound is older than 5 to 6 h, and dissection might spread contamination. (4) The surgeon is not certain of the ability to perform adequate neurorrhaphy.

If inadequate repair is done so that regeneration does not occur (no matter what the reason), it will take approximately 6 months, or the time it takes the nerve to grow 6 in. to the flexor muscles of the forearm, before the inadequacy of the repair is recognized. Since the opponens of the thumb is beyond the distance where significant strength can be expected to be regained, as soon as the flexor muscles of the forearm are reinnervated, tendon transplant of one of the flexors to strengthen the apposition of the thumb is indicated.

Focal Contusion. The most common focal contusion of nerve is that secondary to a gunshot wound, and the treatment of a gunshot wound of the midthigh resulting in loss of sciatic nerve function is an example of such an injury. Immediate repair of the nerve is not indicated, since the damage extending up and down the nerve cannot be determined by inspection and after a high-velocity-missile injury it is always present in varying degrees.

The wound is treated to prevent infection, and the patient is fitted with a short leg brace for stabilization of the ankle. Stabilization is necessary, since motor function in all flexors, extensors, evertors, and invertors of the foot, as well as in the intrinsic muscles of the foot will be lost. The patient is ambulated with a brace as soon as possible and taught to inspect the skin of the foot three or four times a day in order to protect it from unrecognized injury in the anesthetic area. Four to five weeks later, if no function has returned or if only minimal function in one portion of the sciatic nerve has returned, exploration is indicated. By this time fibrosis or neuroma formation will define the area of injury. Resection and resuture may be indicated. Three weeks after repair, when the anastomosis is secure, active use of the leg with the same precautions that were observed preoperatively should be started. Fifteen months later the stability of the ankle should be evaluated, and internal stabilization or arthrodesis may be indicated because of failure of adequate reinnervation.

Stretch or Compression Injury. The problem of the nerve with stretch or compression injury is more difficult. The segment of injury is often longer than can be bridged by any technique, and the loss is usually incomplete, so that even if the area might be bridged by surgical technique, comparison of the deficit from the injury with what might be obtained by resection and suture is essential in the decision for treatment. A common area of stretch injury is the brachial plexus, as might be seen following a shoulder injury. Careful recording of all sensory and motor loss is necessary, and if the pattern of loss suggests a radicular pattern, that is, loss of root function such as at C_5 and C_6, myelography or the fluoroscopic study of the spinal

arachnoid space with radiopaque substance may be useful. Rupture of the arachnoid root sleeve with formation of a traumatic meningocele or pouching of the arachnoid through the intervertebral foramen may be demonstrated, indicating avulsion of the roots from the cord. Root avulsions are not repairable, and reconstructive measures such as fusion of the shoulder and triceps transplantation for elbow flexion are indicated rather than surgical exploration of the area of injury.

BRAIN TUMORS

Brain tumors constitute almost 10 percent of all benign and malignant tumors requiring hospitalization for surgical removal, and nearly 1 percent of all deaths are caused by primary intracranial neoplasms. Because the initial symptoms of a brain tumor may be diverse and confusing, the diagnosis is too frequently delayed until there is a profound loss of neurologic function. Recent evidences in noninvasive diagnostic imaging have provided the means for accurate localization of these lesions and when properly utilized can improve the early detection of brain tumors.

CLASSIFICATION AND CHARACTERISTICS. The classifications of brain tumors are at best confusing, partly because the naming of tumors has usually been on the basis of cellular characteristics. The difficulties of such classifications arise not only from the many different names that can be applied to the same tumor in different situations but also from the difficulty of describing the different characteristics of even the same cell type within a tumor. Clinically, a useful classification of brain tumors is the one proposed by Kernohan and Sayre based on naming the tumors for the cells present in the adult nervous system, vascular tissue, and developmental defects, combined with a grading of the malignancy of the tumor from grade I to grade IV, with IV the most malignant (Table 42-4). Although the Kernohan and Sayre grading system is still commonly used, astrocytic tumors are more accurately classified into three major groups. This system is based upon specific histologic characteristics including cell density, pleomorphism, neovascularity, and necrosis and classifies these tumors as astrocytomas, anaplastic astrocytomas, and glioblastomas.

Certain types of tumors are more frequent at certain ages and occur with greater frequency in those ages in different areas of the brain. For example, 70 percent of adult tumors are supratentorial, that is, in the middle or anterior fossa, while 75 percent of childhood tumors occur in the posterior fossa. The most common primary tumor of the brain in the middle-aged and elderly is a malignant astrocytomas, while the most common tumor of childhood is the astrocytoma of the cerebellum. Malignant astrocytomas are by far the most common primary brain tumor in adults, followed by meningiomas, pituitary tumors, and neurilemmomas, while in childhood the most common tumors are the relatively benign astrocytomas of the posterior fossa, followed very closely by the highly malignant medulloblastomas, and then by ependymomas

Table 42-4. BRAIN TUMORS

	Percent
Gliomas	40–50
Astrocytoma, grade I	5–10
Astrocytoma, grade II	2–5
Astrocytoma, grades III and IV	
(glioblastoma multiforme)	20–30
Medulloblastoma	3–5
Oligodendroglioma	1–4
Ependymoma, grades I–IV	1–3
Meningioma	12–20
Pituitary tumors	5–15
Neurolemmomas (mainly eighth nerve)	3–10
Metastatic tumors	5–10
Blood vessel tumors	
Arteriovenous malformations	
Hemangioblastomas	
Endotheliomas	0.5–1
Tumors of developmental defects	2–3
Dermoids, epidermoids, teratomas	
Chordomas, paraphyseal cysts	
Craniopharyngiomas	3–8
Pinealomas	0.5–0.8
Miscellaneous	
Sarcomas, papillomas of the choroid plexus,	
lipomas, unclassified, etc	1–3

and craniopharyngiomas. Tumors of childhood occur characteristically near the midline of the brain, as with the tumors of developmental defects, the medulloblastomas, and the astrocytomas of the brainstem and cerebellum. Gliomas in adults occur at a frequency that is related to the volume of the brain itself and therefore are more common in the cerebral hemispheres. Meningiomas have a predilection for areas of arachnoid villi and arachnoid invaginations that contain cells similar to those seen in the meningioma. These areas of predilection are along the sagittal sinus, the sella, the olfactory groove, the tentorium, and the petrous ridges.

PATHOPHYSIOLOGY. The basic pattern is one of progressive neurologic deficit. This deficit can be a progressive focal deficit or a progression in the neurologic dysfunction that occurs secondary to increased intracranial pressure. Since these clinical patterns are a continuum, the historical examination of the patient must include the factor of time and its relationship to the development of the symptoms and signs. Their development may vary within the basic patterns because of the different mechanisms by which tumors disturb normal function, the different positions the tumor may occupy within the skull, and the diverse growth potentials of the different tumor types. These variables, when combined with the concepts discussed in the opening portion of this chapter, namely, the anatomic confinement within compartments of the skull of a deformable but relatively noncompressible brain and the changes in neural function that occur from compression of the brainstem passing through the incisura of the tentorium and the foramen magnum, explain in part the diversity of the presenting symptoms produced by brain tumors. With so many combinations of variables

possible, learning the symptoms for the different types of tumors in their different clinical stages is almost an endless task unless it is related to functional anatomy of the brain, the mechanisms used by tumors in producing signs and symptoms, and a classification of the tumors by frequency of occurrence and growth potential.

Tumors of the central nervous system manifest themselves most frequently by effects caused by one or more of the following mechanisms:

1. Compression of neural tissue
2. Infiltration or direct invasion with destruction of neural tissue
3. Alteration in the blood supply to neurons
4. Alteration in neuronal excitability
5. Increase in mass within the skull
6. Alteration in cerebrospinal fluid circulation.

CLINICAL MANIFESTATIONS. Direct compression of neural tissue produces a progressive focal neurologic deficit that is the most easily recognized sign of brain tumor. The deficit will vary depending upon the area of the brain involved and is usually partial rather than complete. Thus, hemiparesis rather than hemiplegia is more frequently seen, and sensory loss is more commonly a partial rather than a total deficit.

Progressive focal neurologic deficit can be produced by other mechanisms, such as direct destruction of neural tissue by malignant cells and loss of neural function by alteration in local blood supply. Direct destruction of neural tissue by involvement of malignant cells is uncommon, but alteration in local blood supply does occur and particularly may be seen in the older patient with a highly malignant glioma. Interference with arterial blood supply by tumor usually manifests itself as an acute loss of function, suggesting primary vascular disease, and only the later focal progression from increasing mass effects, or further involvement of local blood supply, completes the pattern of progressive focal neurologic deficit, indicating the diagnosis of brain tumor.

Compression, invasion, and altered blood supply may also cause altered neuronal excitability that is manifested by seizures. Seizures are paroxysmal episodes of uncontrolled neural activity, and since the neurons of the cerebral cortex have a low threshold for such paroxysmal activity, seizures caused by tumors are commonly seen in lesions adjacent to or within the cerebral cortex. A focal seizure in an adult may indicate the localization of a lesion and is strongly suggestive of a brain tumor.

The signs and symptoms of generalized increase in pressure are cloudy mentation and consciousness, headache, papilledema, vomiting, bradycardia, and systolic hypertension. It is rare to have all these findings except as terminal events. More commonly, a patient's family will notice a change in behavior, a loss of recent memory, inattention to details, and personality alterations. Increased intracranial pressure from brain tumors can result from mass, impaired cerebrospinal fluid circulation, or a combination of these.

The increase in mass may result from a number of factors. There is the neoplastic growth itself and edema formation. Malignant tumors especially produce edema in the adjacent brain. The cause of this edema is not understood, but it can result in massive swelling at considerable distances from the tumor. Some tumors form cysts that have osmotic gradients that cause an enlargement of the cyst by absorption of fluid. Infrequently rapid enlargement may result from hemorrhage within a tumor. Changes may occur in the surrounding nervous tissue, such as edema from venous obstruction or edema from breakdown of the integrity of the blood-brain barrier, secondary to either arterial or venous insufficiency.

The increased intracranial pressure caused by alteration in cerebrospinal fluid circulation usually occurs from obstruction of the passage of cerebrospinal fluid from the lateral ventricles to the subarachnoid space. This can occur when tumors arise within the ventricular system. Obstruction in the flow of cerebrospinal fluid may also occur when there is a shift of the brainstem so that the aqueduct of Sylvius is compressed or the outlets of the fourth ventricle are blocked. Tumors in the basal cisterns may also obstruct cerebrospinal fluid reabsorption.

There are compensatory intracranial mechanisms for altering the effects of increased mass and pressure. Most of them require days or months to be effective and therefore are best utilized in controlling pressure from a slowly growing, benign tumor. These mechanisms include decreases in intracranial blood volume, cerebrospinal fluid volume, intracellular fluid volume, and parenchymal cell numbers.

EVALUATION. The primary necessity in the diagnosis of brain tumor is the suspicion that should be initiated by the patient's history of a progressive neurologic deficit. The more knowledgeable physicians are of the functional anatomy of the brain, the more accurately they will recognize progressive neurologic deficit. While hemiparesis and hemisensory loss or lack of motor function in a cranial nerve are easily recognizable, a change in behavior, slow progressive dementia, decrease in pituitary function, or progression in the severity of seizures are more difficult neurologic deficits to recognize as indicating brain tumor.

It is beyond the scope of this section to review the diagnostic investigation that should be completed in evaluating a patient suspected of having a brain tumor, but complete physical and neurologic examinations are the minimal requisites to the use of special diagnostic tests that have been described in the opening section of this chapter. CT scanning (Figs. 42-7 and 42-8) has become the major method of diagnosing brain tumors. MRI has become an important tool for the diagnosis. Arteriography is used as an aid in making surgical decisions and, in combination with CT scanning and MRI imaging, aids considerably in the final judgment of what should be done with a brain tumor (Figs. 42-9, 42-10).

TREATMENT. The primary goal of tumor therapy is cure, and surgical excision is the method most likely to accomplish a cure. Unfortunately, in the case of brain tumor surgical removal is not always possible or even desirable, since the resulting neurologic deficit may leave a patient so impaired that saving life is of no significance. The treatment of brain tumors therefore is not just their surgical removal, and it requires experience and knowl-

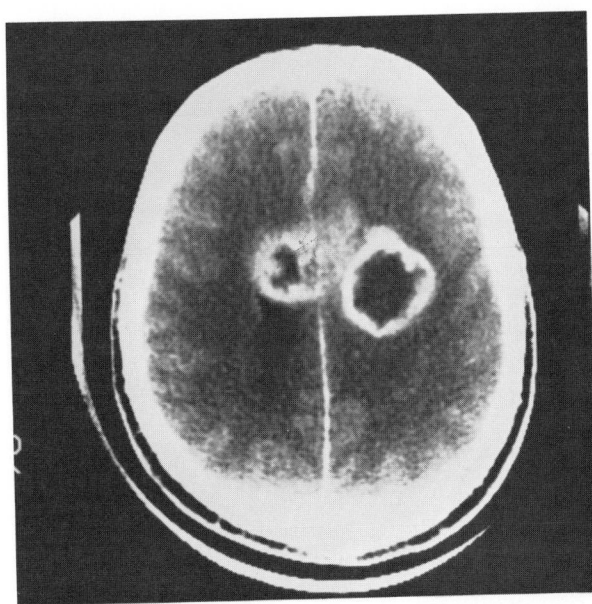

Fig. 42-7. A forty-eight-year-old woman with rapid onset of dementia with symptoms of increased intracranial pressure. A contrast-enhanced CT scan showed left frontoparietal tumor extending across the corpus callosum to the right parietal area. On biopsy this was a glioblastoma.

edge combined with surgical skill in order to obtain the maximal functional result. At times the repetitive use of these special diagnostic tests and evaluation over a period of time are necessary to be certain of what would be the optimal therapy.

The spread of malignant cells in the cerebrospinal fluid (meningeal carcinomatosis) is common in aggressive cancers and frequently causes hydrocephalus, cranial nerve

Fig. 42-8. A fifty-four-year-old right-handed male with temporal lobe seizures and postictal dysphasia. Contrast-enhanced CT scan showed a large middle fossa tumor. At surgery this was a lateral sphenoid wing meningioma.

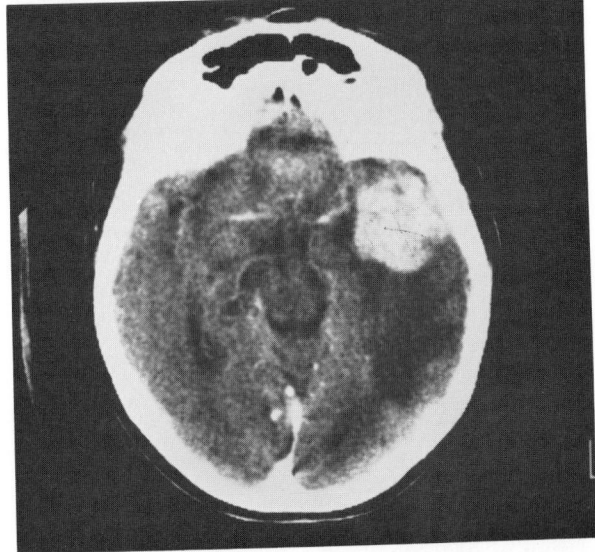

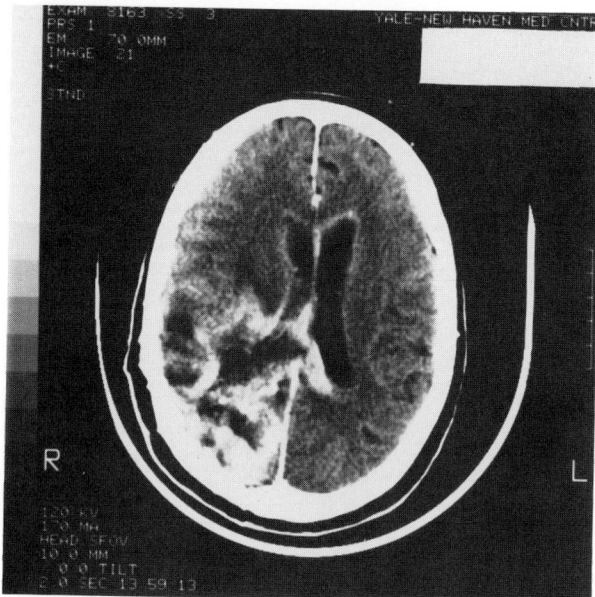

Fig. 42-9. CT of the brain in a patient with a right hemisphere glioblastoma. Contrast enhancement outlines a central low-density area of necrosis. Tumor extension is clearly demonstrated throughout the parietal and occipital lobes and across the midline to the left occipital lobe.

palsies, as well as evidence of increased intracranial pressure. This is generally treated with intrathecal chemotherapy (methotrexate) delivered by lumbar puncture or an indwelling catheter (Ommaya).

Benign tumors such as meningiomas or schwanomas can be cured if totally removed. Even benign tumors can

Fig. 42-10. MRI of the same tumor in a T$_2$ weighted scan. The white areas in the right parietal and occipital lobes represent the extension of the tumor and surrounding white matter edema.

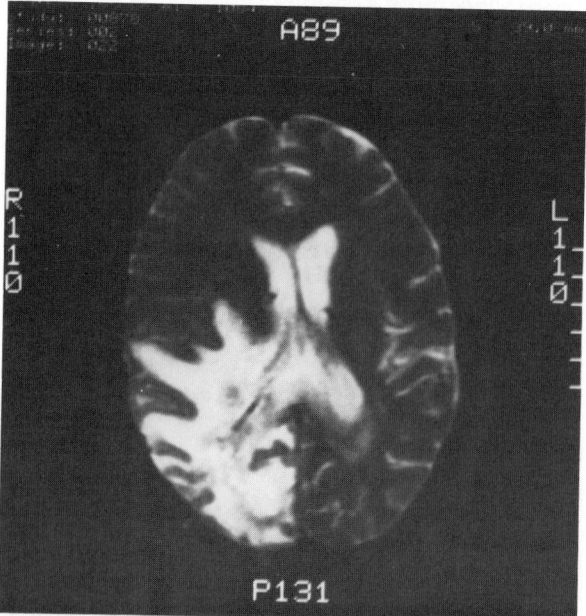

be located in areas adjacent to vital brain structures that preclude total removal. In general, single metastatic tumors are considered for surgery if they are located in an accessible area of the brain and the patient's cancer is under control or treatable. Primary malignant tumors are, as a rule, not curable, but significant palliation may be obtained with surgery, irradiation, and chemotherapy. Recent observations concerning immunotherapy may be important for the future treatment of these lesions.

Pituitary Tumors

The pituitary gland lies within the base of the skull in the sella turcica or hypophyseal fossa. In the human being it is divided into two portions that have separate embryological origins, the posterior or neural lobe and the anterior or glandular lobe. The posterior lobe arises from an infundibular process of the diencephalon, while the anterior lobe develops from Rathke's pouch, the cephalad portion of the alimentary tube. The anterior lobe constitutes about 70 percent of the pituitary gland. The posterior lobe retains its neural connection to the hypothalamus via the infundibulum. The epithelial remnants of Rathke's pouch form a vestigial, apparently nonfunctioning intermediate lobe between the anterior and posterior lobes. The pituitary gland is covered by the dura of the diaphragm superiorly, the dura of the pituitary fossa inferiorly, anteriorly, and posteriorly, that of the cavernous sinuses laterally, and the circular venous sinuses anteriorly and posteriorly. The surrounding important structures that may be subject to compression by an enlarging pituitary tumor are the optic chiasm and nerves lying above the diaphragm in the suprasellar cistern and the contents of the lateral cavernous sinuses. The cavernous sinuses contain the carotid arteries, oculomotor, trochlear, and abducens nerves, and the ophthalmic division of the trigeminal nerves. The arterial blood supply consists of numerous small vessels emanating directly from the carotid arteries. The hypophyseal-portal circulation is a separate venous blood supply along the infundibulum connecting the hypothalamus and the anterior lobe as a pathway for hormone transportation.

The pituitary hormones are polypeptides regulated by the hypothalamus and feedback from target endocrine glands. The hormones of the anterior pituitary are adrenocorticotropin (ACTH), thyrotropin (TSH), growth hormone (GH), prolactin (PR), and the gonadotropins, luteinizing hormone (LH), and follicle-stimulating hormone (FSH). The hormones of the posterior pituitary are vasospressin, or antidiuretic hormone (ADH), and oxytocin.

PATHOLOGY AND PATHOPHYSIOLOGY. Pituitary tumors are often classified as brain tumors since the pituitary lies intracranially, and their mass effect can cause neurologic loss. Pituitary tumors are rarely of neural origin. The majority of pituitary tumors are adenomas in the anterior lobe. Pituitary tumors are almost always benign and cause symptoms by overproduction of hormones, mass effect, loss of anterior pituitary gland function, or a combination of these mechanisms. Formerly, pituitary adenomas were classified by the histologic affinity to aniline dyes, with chromophobe adenomas having little or no affinity, eosinophilic adenomas having an affinity for acid dyes, and basophilic tumors having an affinity for basic dyes. They are better classified as endocrine-active or -inactive, with identification of the hormone or hormones produced, and described by their size or growth characteristics since both methods correlate with the symptoms they produce and relate to the therapy effective in their control.

Endocrine-active tumors may produce prolactin (PR), growth hormone (GH), adrenocorticotrophic hormone (ACTH), thyroid stimulating hormone (TSH), or luteinizing and follicular stimulating hormone (LSH-FSH). Prolactin-secreting adenomas are the most common endocrine-active tumors, followed by growth hormone and the much less frequent ACTH-producing tumors. TSH- and LSH-TSH-producing tumors are extremely rare. Endocrine-inactive tumors are the second most common pituitary adenoma, occurring with frequency between prolactin- and growth hormone–producing tumors. The other description of pituitary adenomas is on the basis of size and/or evidence of invasive growth. Tumors less than 1 cm in diameter are called microadenomas, while those greater than 1 cm are called macroadenomas. The latter may have suprasellar or parasellar extension, and when they invade the skull base and paranasal sinuses or the cavernous sinus, they are termed invasive adenomas. Thus, a patient may have a prolactin-secreting invasive macroadenoma with suprasellar extension, signifying a large endocrine-active tumor that produces prolactin that has destroyed part of the base of the skull or invaded the cavernous sinus with extension out of the sella.

DIAGNOSIS. The diagnosis of pituitary tumor should be considered when endocrine symptoms and/or parasellar neurologic deficits are found by history or examination. The endocrine symptoms depend on the hormone produced and/or destruction of the anterior pituitary. Rarely do pituitary tumors cause the posterior pituitary lobe dysfunction of diabetes insipidus except when suprasellar extension damages the hypothalamus. The most common parasellar neurologic deficit is caused by compression of the crossing fibers of the optic chiasm that arise from the nasal portion of the retina causing a bitemporal visual field loss (bitemporal hemianopsia) (Fig. 42-11). Depending on the size and rapidity of growth of the tumor, optic nerve dysfunction, extraocular motor loss, hypothalamic dysfunction, or frontal or medial temporal lobe signs and symptoms may occur. Recognition of a progressive endocrinopathy that includes more than one system, such as hypothyroidism followed by hypogonadism and adrenal insufficiency, should suggest a pituitary tumor.

The most common endocrine symptoms result from an excess production of prolactin. In the female the excess production causes menstrual irregularities or amenorrhea, infertility, and galactorrhea. The same hyperproduction in the male causes decrease in potency and fertility, and since these symptoms are often not reported or recognized, the prolactin tumors of male patients are usually larger, causing hypopituitarism and neurologic deficit before being diagnosed.

The next most common endocrine symptom is hypopi-

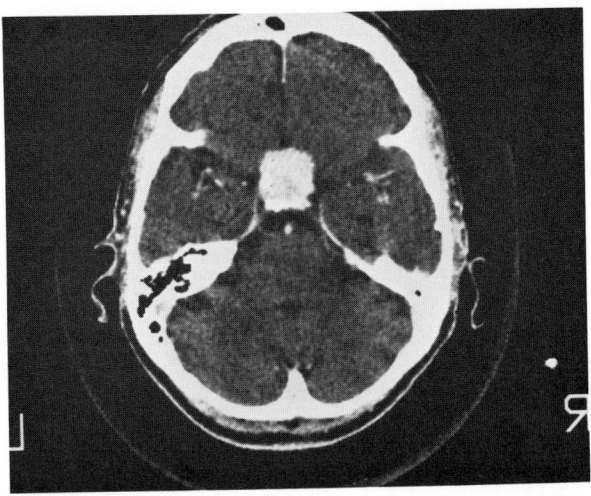

Fig. 42-11. A fifty-six-year-old woman with hypopituitarism and bitemporal hemianopsia. Contrast-enhanced CT scan showed a suprasellar tumor. On surgical exploration this was a pituitary adenoma.

tuitarism, which can be caused by endocrine-inactive tumors and large endocrine-active tumors. Endocrine-inactive tumors present usually in the fifth or sixth decade and are of considerable size with no sexual predominance. The most common symptoms are early menopause or lack of fertility in the female and lack of potency in the male. The patients may also complain of excessive fatigue, intolerance to temperature extremes, decrease in hair growth, and pallor. Headache may be referred to either the vertex or the retroorbital region. The most common neurologic sign is a variation of bitemporal visual field loss and/or decrease in visual acuity. The diagnosis is confirmed by evaluating pituitary function and CT and/or MRI scanning. The second most common endocrine-active tumor produces growth hormone. Excess growth hormone produces gigantism in the young and acromegaly in the patient who has finished growing. Acromegaly literally means enlargement of the distal parts, e.g., hands, feet, jaw, nose, etc. Excess growth hormone also alters glucose and fat metabolism, and the patients have a high incidence of diabetes mellitus and atherosclerosis along with changes in facial features and enlargement of the hands and feet. This alteration in glucose and fat metabolism will shorten their life span because of cardiovascular and cerebrovascular disease. Patients with pituitary tumors that produce growth hormone have a high incidence of elevated prolactin, and females with acromegaly may have galactorrhea and menstrual dysfunction. Both prolactin-secreting tumors and growth hormone–secreting tumors can be diagnosed by direct radioimmunoassay of the circulating levels of the respective hormone, and the size of the tumors can be determined by x-ray studies of the sella including polytomography, CT, and MRI scanning. Growth hormone–producing tumors are usually not subtle on CT or MRI, and a fasting GH serum level greater than 15 mg/mL confirms the diagnosis. A somatomedin C level above 2.0 is also diagnostic.

A glucose tolerance test suppresses GH levels and intravenous TRH stimulates GH.

ACTH-producing tumors are infrequent and produce Cushing's disease, that portion of Cushing's syndrome of hypercortisolism caused by hypothalamic pituitary dysfunction. Recent series of Cushing's disease indicate that very small, 1 to 2 mm in diameter, or larger adenomas of the pituitary are the etiological factor of the disease in 85 to 90 percent of patients. Hypercortisolism causes signs and symptoms of weakness, centripetal weight gain, easy bruisability, psychologic changes, excess body hair, oligoamenorrhea, muscle wasting, thin skin, ecchymosis, telangiectasis, facial plethora, stretch marks and acne, impotence, congestive heart failure, and edema. ACTH tumors are small and infrequently seen on CT scanning. Low doses of dexamethasone administered over 2 days will not suppress an abnormal cortisol of >5 mg percent. Higher doses will cause suppression separating the pituitary tumor from other ACTH tumor sources such as some ectopic tumors and the adrenal glands. Many surgeons believe exploration of the sella, with a search for such tumors, is indicated when Cushing's disease is diagnosed by endocrine testing despite lack of x-ray evidence of the presence of pituitary tumor. The average length of life of a patient with severe Cushing's syndrome is approximately 5 years, and thus radical treatment such as exploration of the sella or adrenalectomy is indicated.

TSH-producing and LSH-FSH-producing pituitary adenomas usually are seen in patients with thyroid gland or gonadal insufficiency and often will respond with decrease in size when the hormone deficiency is replaced with exogenous hormone.

TREATMENT. Prolactin is the only anterior pituitary hormone that is mainly under a suppressive effect by the hypothalamic neurons. The inhibitory factor is either dopamine or a dopamine-like substance, and dopamine agonists such as bromocryptine decrease the production of prolactin and often decrease the size of prolactin-secreting tumors of the pituitary. Normalization of prolactin levels between 20 and 100 ng/mL is common with this drug but uncommon when the prolactin rises above 300 ng/mL. The most successful surgical cure rates (60 to 70 percent) of this tumor are by transnasal transsphenoidal microsurgical excision when the lesion is a microadenoma and the prolactin level less than 200 ng/mL. Bromocryptine also can suppress production of growth hormone in growth hormone–producing tumors but has been less successful in decreasing the size of growth hormone–producing tumors. The success of bromocryptine in treating pituitary tumors, both the endocrinopathy and mass effect, has led to the search for other drugs that may control pituitary tumors, but the major effective therapies remain surgery and x-ray therapy.

In the past two decades, the reestablishment of the transnasal and transsphenoidal operation for tumors of the sella turcica combined with microsurgical techniques and the operating microscope has markedly decreased the mortality and morbidity of pituitary surgery and allowed the removal of microadenomas without damage to the remaining pituitary gland. In larger tumors, it has allowed the removal of the major mass without the risk of craniotomy, and when this surgery is followed by x-ray therapy, it has allowed control of the pituitary adenoma in 80 to 90 percent of patients for as long as 10 years. Surgical treatment in the form of biopsy or excision is also indicated for tumors adjacent to the pituitary that cause the patient to present with symptoms and signs of hypopituitarism and mass effect. Such tumors are craniopharyngiomas, meningiomas, gliomas, germinomas, chondromas, chondrosarcomas, and chordomas.

Urgent surgical intervention is often required in the condition of pituitary gland infarction called pituitary apoplexy. This syndrome of hemorrhagic infarction can extend from no symptoms at all through severe neurologic loss, subarachnoidal hemorrhage, and death. This most often occurs in large pituitary adenomas and presents with acute headache, oculomotor paresis, visual loss, and decreased consciousness that can lead to death.

In many autopsy series, 20 percent or more of pituitary glands studied contained adenoma, and as far as can be ascertained from the hospital charts, without premortem endocrine symptoms. This may indicate that many pituitary adenomas have little or no growth potential and result from the activity of the hypothalamic pituitary releasing substances, aging, and/or the propensity for all glandular tissue to form adenoma. No technique has been devised that can differentiate between pituitary adenomas that have growth potential and those that do not. The high incidence of adenoma formation in the pituitary, along with clinical experience, indicates that the presence of pituitary adenoma that is not causing endocrinopathy is probably not an indication for surgical removal, and since a clinically significant adenoma may require 5 to 10 years to develop symptoms, there is need for long-term follow-up of any patient suspected of or diagnosed as having a pituitary adenoma.

SUMMATION. In summary, it is the evidence of a progressive neurologic deficit that should raise the suspicion of diagnosis of a brain tumor, for progressive neurologic deficit is the most common presenting symptom of brain tumor. This deficit may be of a focal nature that varies according to the area of the brain involved or may be a more generalized type secondary to increased intracranial pressure. The focal neurologic deficit may be a loss of function or can be altered excitability. Loss of neural function secondary to brain tumor is most frequently incomplete, and altered excitability usually presents as a convulsion. The effects of generalized increased intracranial pressure can be secondary to increased mass, alteration in cerebrospinal fluid circulation, or a combination of these. The deficits seen in brain tumor have a common denominator, that is, evidence of progression in symptomatology and signs over a period of time. A knowledge of the functional anatomy of the brain, classification of brain tumors, their frequency of occurrence and growth potential, and the mechanisms by which tumors manifest themselves will facilitate a high degree of accuracy in suspecting brain tumors, thereby allowing the physician to have the aid of the specialist in diagnosing and treating the tumor.

SPINAL CORD TUMORS

The term *spinal tumors* includes all tumors encroaching on the spinal cord. Primary tumors of the spine are approximately one-sixth as common as intracranial tumors but have a much better prognosis, since almost 60 percent are benign and a high percentage of the remainder respond to therapy, so that prolonged functional palliation can be expected. Metastatic spinal tumors are reported to present as often as primary spinal tumors. Any malignant tumor may metastasize to the bones of the spinal column or to the spinal epidural space, but the most common are from lung, breast, lymphoid tissue, prostate, kidney, and thyroid. Metastatic spinal tumors usually cause pain, followed by neurologic deficit. Since these tumors rarely cause death, palliation by surgical and radiation therapy is indicated in order to preserve neurologic function and decrease suffering during a terminal illness.

CLASSIFICATION AND CHARACTERISTICS. The symptoms, the type of tumor, and the prognosis correlate with where the tumor is in relation to the dura and spinal cord. Therefore, the classification of tumors into extradural and intradural groups and the subdivision of the intradural group into extramedullary and intramedullary has significance from both a clinical and pathologic point of view. Ninety percent of extradural tumors are malignant, while 60 percent of intradural tumors are benign. Seventy-five to 80 percent of extradural tumors are metastatic, while 98 percent of intradural tumors are primary tumors. The common clinical course of extradural tumors is one of rapid compression of the spinal cord, either by the tumor itself or from collapse of involved vertebrae. The patient may present with rapidly progressing paraparesis and sensory loss that requires rapid recognition and surgical decompression in order to have significant palliative effect. The common clinical course of the intradural tumor is usually much slower and may extend over months or years with the patient presenting with spastic paraparesis and partial sensory loss.

Knowledge of the types of tumors, their potential for growth, and their mechanisms of production of symptoms is the means by which the finer aspects of diagnosis of spinal cord tumor are best attained, but the clinician should always consider the diagnosis of spinal cord tumor when any bilateral progressive neurologic loss occurs below any transverse level of the body. The value of such constant suspicion is the high degree of functional return and the high percentage of cure or palliation of symptoms resulting from the early surgical treatment.

EVALUATION. A suspected spinal cord tumor is localized by utilizing the findings of the neurologic examination, the bony changes in spinal x-rays, and the results of spinal contrast studies, or myelography with CT scanning or MRI.

CLINICAL MANIFESTATIONS. The diagnostic neurologic examination findings are of two types, local signs and tract signs. The local signs are segmental changes and localize the lesion along the rostral-caudal axis. The local motor signs are weakness and loss of reflexes with normal above and normal or hyperactive reflexes below the level, fasciculations over a segmental distribution, and atrophy in a myotome pattern. These indicate involvement of the anterior motor horn cells or the anterior spinal roots. Local sensory signs are localized pain and spinal tenderness, radicular or radiating pain, and loss of sensation over a dermatome pattern, indicating involvement of the dorsal root or dorsal root entry zone. Segmental loss of pain and temperature with preservation of touch (sensory dissociation) is also a local sign and indicates involvement of the crossing fibers in the anterior commissure of the spinal cord from an intramedullary lesion of the cord.

Tract signs only indicate that the lesion must be cephalad to the highest point of involvement, and the motor changes may vary from increased tone and reflexes to flaccidity with absent reflexes. The difference usually relates to the timing of onset, since with rapid loss of spinal cord function spinal shock with flaccid, areflexic paralysis may result whereas spastic paraparesis is more common with the slow, progressive loss of motor function. The other tract signs may relate to involvement of any portion of the spinal cord and thus can consist of loss of pain and temperature (anterolateral fasciculus); loss of position and vibratory sense (dorsal column); weakness, spasticity, hyperreflexia, and Babinski signs (posterolateral fasciculus).

DIAGNOSTIC STUDIES. Radiographs are of diagnostic aid if they are taken of the correct area. When doubt exists or when there is a question of multiple levels, the entire spinal column should be visualized. Diagnostic findings in the radiographs relate to the type of tumor present. With malignant tumors areas of invasion and destruction, particularly of the vertebral body and pedicles, may give localization. With benign or slowly growing tumors, widening of the interpedicular and anteroposterior diameter of the neural canal, erosion of a pedicle or of a body, and enlargement of the intervertebral foramina are diagnostic.

Definitive localization, however, is done by myelography. It is usually best to do the lumbar puncture and obtain fluid at the time that myelography is done. Prompt surgical intervention may be required with lumbar puncture or myelography, since increase in deficit may follow removal of spinal fluid below the level of the lesion. For this reason none of these should be done unless the patient is in an area where definitive neurosurgical care is available and the patient is under the observation or care of a neurosurgeon. High-resolution CT scanning with the use of water-soluble contrast agents will provide detailed pictures of intraspinal detail and frequently will outline the spinal mass. Magnetic resonance imaging is becoming more universally accepted as a noninvasive test for evaluating the entire spinal axis. The images on machines with 1.5-T magnets are of a quality of resolution comparable with CT studies.

Extradural Tumors

The different types of patterns of symptoms and the local and tract signs are best remembered in relation to the different types of spinal cord tumors, namely, extradural, intradural-extramedullary, and intradural-intramedullary.

Aside from a rare extradural meningioma, neurofibroma, and benign osteoma of the vertebra, extradural tumors are malignant with rapid growth and a tendency to destroy the spinal column. The symptom pattern of the extradural tumor is one of pain, both localized to the area of involvement and radiating over the dermatome level of the adjacent spinal roots (local sign). This is followed by rapidly progressive transverse loss of spinal cord function (tract sign). The local pain is frequently more severe at night and at rest, while the radicular pain relates to movement, coughing, and straining. Both types of pain may be present for weeks or months before spinal cord involvement. The progressive transverse loss of spinal cord function can be as rapid as a few hours or as slow as a few days, and effective palliation is possible only if surgical decompression is done before total loss of spinal cord function has occurred.

Since these tumors frequently involve the adjacent vertebrae, x-rays of the spine with particular attention to the integrity of the vertebral body and pedicles will often suggest the diagnosis before as well as after the onset of progressive neurologic deficit in the spinal cord. Because the majority of these tumors originate in the vertebral body and compress the anterior and/or lateral aspect of the cord, they are best removed through an anterior or posterior-lateral approach rather than by a laminectomy. The excision is almost always followed by treatment with irradiation.

Intradural-Extramedullary Tumors

Approximately 65 percent of all intradural tumors are extramedullary, and 90 percent are either neurofibromas or meningiomas. Neurofibromas are slightly more common and often are multiple. They have no sex predilection and are more common in the cervical and thoracic areas, while meningiomas are more frequent in females and more common in the thoracic region. It has been stated that the frequency of occurrence of both these tumors in the thoracic areas is in the same ratio as the length of the thoracic spine to the length of the spinal column.

Angiomas are also common in the thoracic area. They are arteriovenous malformations and not true tumors but may at times present like an extramedullary tumor. This is particularly true during the last trimester of pregnancy. Other tumors that occur in the extramedullary-intradural area are epidermoids, dermoids, and lipomas. The basic pattern of symptoms of the extramedullary-intradural tumor is similar to the extradural tumors, namely, local pain and radicular pain (local sign), followed by progressive spinal cord malfunction (tract sign). The course is slower, and the development of the spinal cord deficit is often prolonged so that partial patterns of loss are seen.

Intramedullary Tumors

Over 95 percent of intramedullary tumors are gliomas. In contrast to intracranial gliomas they tend to be more benign histologically and to have a more benign course. This is in part because of the low grade of their malignancy and in part because of their frequently nonlethal position in the spinal cord. Except for the preponderance of ependymomas occurring in the conus medullaris and the filum terminale, they occur equally frequently in all areas of the spinal cord. Approximately one-half of intramedullary tumors are ependymomas, and 45 percent are astrocytomas, with a few oligodendrogliomas, hemangioblastomas, and ganglioneuromas making up the remainder. Arterial venous malformations and syringomyelia may present as intramedullary spinal cord tumors but are developmental abnormalities and not neoplasms.

The basic pattern of symptoms for the intramedullary tumor is different from the extradural and extramedullary tumor in that radicular or radiating pain is rare and the complaint of local pain is uncommon. These tumors tend to grow into the central part of the spinal cord and to destroy crossing fibers and neurons of the gray matter. The destruction of crossing fibers causes segmental loss of pain and temperature sensation with preservation of touch (sensory dissociation), resulting in damage to peripheral skin areas because of lack of protection of pain and temperature sensation (local sign). Trophic changes with alteration in vasomotor control and sweating may cause symptoms that resemble Raynaud's phenomenon. Alteration in the function of descending motor pathways or ascending sensory pathways is usually late in appearance, but alteration in sexual function and bladder function may occur early (tract sign). Segmental lower motor neuron destruction is common, and the signs of such destruction, namely, weakness, atrophy, loss of reflex, and fasciculations, should always be searched for in these patients, since they have localizing value (local sign). The ability of neurosurgeons to remove intramedullary tumors has increased because of newer surgical techniques. These include the use of the laser, ultrasonic aspiration, and ultrasound. As a consequence, the total removal of these lesions can often produce prolonged palliation or a cure.

SUMMATION. In summary, spinal cord tumors have a good prognosis if treated early. It is important to keep in mind that a progressive decrease in spinal cord function must always be considered to indicate a spinal cord tumor until proved otherwise. Early diagnosis, accurate localization, and surgical therapy can be expected to give a large percentage of cures with good functional result and in the remainder to give considerable and prolonged palliation of symptoms.

VASCULAR DISEASES OF THE NERVOUS SYSTEM

ETIOLOGY. Diseases affecting the vascular supply of the central nervous system may produce cerebral ischemia, intracranial hemorrhage, or less commonly other neurologic disturbances. Despite a declining incidence in the last several decades, disorders that produce cerebral ischemia by interrupting the blood supply to the brain continue to be a leading cause of morbidity and mortality.

Most commonly, ischemia is linked to atherosclerosis involving major arterial trunks. Disorders of small vessels, such as those related to hypertension, diabetes, arteritis and infection, cardioembolic events, and even blood dyscrasias may be responsible.

Nontraumatic intracranial hemorrhage may occur exclusively in the cerebrospinal fluid space such as a subarachnoid hemorrhage or intraventricular hemorrhage. Hemorrhage within the brain parenchyma may also occur and form an intracerebral hematoma. Often a structural lesion such as a saccular aneurysm, arteriovenous malformation, mycotic aneurysm, or even a neoplasm may be the source of hemorrhage; however, other hemorrhages may be related to hypertension, small-vessel disease, or coagulopathies.

ANATOMY. The major arterial supply to the brain consists of paired internal carotid and vertebral arteries. The internal carotid arteries begin in the neck at the division of the common carotid artery into the external and internal carotid arteries. The internal carotid arteries can be divided into cervical, petrous, cavernous, and intradural portions. The cervical portion has no branches, but the remaining portions have branches that can be significant in collateral blood supply to the brain following obstruction in the internal or common carotid artery. Branches of the petrous portion that anastomose with the internal maxillary artery are the caroticotympanic and pterygoid canal arteries. These are relatively small branches and rarely have significant anastomotic capacity. In the cavernous portion are branches to the cavernous sinus, the hypophysis, semilunar ganglion, meninges, and orbit. The semilunar and meningeal arteries can have significant anastomosis with the meningeal branches of the internal maxillary artery, and the ophthalmic artery is commonly a significant anastomotic channel with the terminal branches of the external maxillary artery. The cavernous sinus branches may be a source of communication between the carotid artery and the cavernous sinus, a carotid cavernous fistula, when they are ruptured by trauma or disease. The intradural branches of the internal carotid artery are the anterior cerebral, the middle cerebral, the posterior communicating, and the choroid arteries. The posterior communicating artery forms an anastomosis with the posterior cerebral artery, and the anterior cerebral artery with the anterior communicating and the opposite anterior cerebral artery to complete the anterior portion of the circle of Willis. The vertebral arteries in their cervical or extradural portion have anastomotic branches with the thyrocervical trunk of the subclavian artery and with the posterior branches of the external carotid. After traversing the dura, they join to form the basilar artery giving branches to the brainstem. The division of the basilar artery into the posterior cerebral arteries completes the posterior portion of the circle of Willis.

There are, therefore, extensive anastomoses between the vertebral basilar system and the carotid system. The collateral circulation can be divided into the extracranial, extracranial-intracranial, and intracranial. The extracranial anastomoses consist of posterior branches of the external carotid and the vertebral and the thyrocervical trunk of the subclavian, the internal maxillary branch of the carotid through the meningeal branches of the internal carotid, and between terminal branches of both external carotid arteries. Most of these anastomoses are normally small but have the capacity to enlarge following proximal or distal occlusion of a carotid or vertebral artery. For example, after obstruction of the cervical common carotid artery below the bifurcation, anastomosis through the external carotid arteries can result in retrograde flow in the ipsilateral external carotid artery to its origin and consequent forward flow in the internal carotid artery to the brain, bypassing the obstruction. Extracranial-intracranial collaterals are principally by anastomosis of the external carotid artery to the intracranial circulation by the ophthalmic artery and by collaterals developed between meningeal vessels and the intracranial arteries of the pia on the convexity of the cerebral hemispheres. The major intracranial anastomosis is the circle of Willis. In only 18 percent of brains is the circle of Willis fully developed, there being various degrees of hypoplasia in one or more vessels in the majority of cases. Extensive anastomoses of branches of the anterior, middle, and posterior cerebral arteries have been demonstrated by arteriography following occlusion of major intracerebral vessels. Although these anastomoses are, in general, not important normally, they develop rapidly following vascular compromise and may in part, explain neurologic recovery following major vessel occlusion. All the anastomoses, but particularly the larger extracranial-intracranial and intracranial anastomoses, play a significant role in the protection of the brain against neurologic dysfunction in vascular disease and major occlusion.

PHYSIOLOGY. The brain is one of the most metabolically active organs in the body, requiring a constant supply of oxygen and glucose and, therefore, constant blood flow. Intracerebral blood flow has been calculated by several techniques with variations between 44 and 80 mL/100 g of brain per minute, but the generally accepted value in the adult normal brain is approximately 50 to 55 mL/100 g of brain per minute, or approximately 750 mL of blood per minute in the adult. Thus, the brain, representing only 2 percent of the body weight, ordinarily receives between 17 and 18 percent of the heart's output and consumes nearly 20 percent of the oxygen supply of the body. Gray matter blood flow has been measured at 80 mL/100 g of brain per minute, while that of the white matter is 20 mL/100 g of brain per minute or roughly one-fourth of the gray matter, contrasting the metabolic activity of the two areas. Under normal conditions, global cerebral blood flow remains relatively constant over a wide range of systemic blood pressures through a process called autoregulation. In experimental animals, autoregulation occurs between systolic blood pressures of 80 and 180 mmHg. In human beings this range may vary depending on the degree of preexisting hypertension. Global cerebral blood flow increases via vasodilatation with increasing P_{CO_2} and decreasing P_{O_2}. Alterations in pH cause similar flow changes as P_{CO_2}. Local regulation of cerebral blood flow appears to be linked to the regional metabolic needs of the brain. Although the mechanisms of this coupling remain controversial, it appears to be mediated, at least in part, by extracellular products of neuronal activity such as hydrogen and potassium ions and adenosine and by direct neuronal innervation of cerebral blood vessels.

The cerebral hemispheric arterial circulation can be divided into two general types of arteries: (1) the conducting vessels, consisting of the internal carotid artery and its named branches, which then divide into a network of interlacing and anastomosing smaller arteries on the surface of the brain; and (2) the penetrating or nutrient arterioles that arise on the surface of the brain from the conducting vessels and enter the parenchyma. In human beings, there is only a 10 to 15 percent decrease in perfusion pressure between the origin of the internal carotid artery and the penetrating vessels. The conducting vessels can be regarded as a pressure-equalizing reservoir modulated in part by the sympathetic nervous system. Modulation of cerebral blood flow and autoregulation probably occur at the level of the penetrating arterioles which in part are innervated by neurons residing in the brainstem. These arterioles must be supplied with an adequate perfusion pressure to function normally. As perfusion pressure falls, these arterioles maximally dilate and lose the ability to autoregulate. When cerebral blood flow falls below a critical threshold, neuronal function is lost and eventually cell death occurs. The critical flow required to maintain normal electrical activity appears to be higher than the critical flow required to maintain basic cellular metabolism so that even with a state of physiologic paralysis cell death may not occur for a variable period of time and recovery is possible. Normal adult intracerebral blood flow is approximately 50 to 55 mL/100 g of brain per minute. The ischemic tolerance of neuronal tissue appears to be proportional to both the severity and duration of the flow reduction; however, the precise duration of time that these reduced flows can be tolerated before cellular injury occurs is unknown. Although biologic variation occurs in the critical flow needed to support electrical activity and undoubtedly variation exists for the critical flow required to maintain cell viability, the studies of Boysen et al. suggest that the critical flow for the former is 15 to 20 mL/100 g/min and laboratory studies suggest that the critical flow for the latter is 10 to 15 mL/100 g.

Because ischemic regions of the brain may be physiologically paralyzed but still viable, some ischemic neurological deficits may in part be reversible. Initial therapy may be directed at expanding intravascular volume and enhancing cardiac output in an effort to improve regional cerebral blood flow in the dysautoregulated region of the brain. Some patients show dramatic clinical improvement after these therapeutic maneuvers are made. Efforts to improve regional cerebral blood flow and consequently neurologic outcome by surgical revascularization, although physiologically appealing, remain a source of controversy.

CLINICAL MANIFESTATIONS. The temporal profile of neurologic dysfunction is fundamental in the evaluation of all neurologic disease. Cerebrovascular disease, unlike degenerative diseases or tumors of the central nervous system, usually presents with an abrupt change in neuro-

logic function. Ischemic disease is almost always characterized by a sudden deterioration and, for epidemiologic purposes, has been divided into three groups based on the duration of neurologic dysfunction. A "transient ischemic attack" (TIA) begins abruptly and is soon followed by full recovery. By definition, neurologic dysfunction must have completely resolved by 24 h. A "reversible ischemic neurologic deficit" (RIND) is eventually followed by full recovery as is a TIA, but by definition, recovery occurs more than 24 h but before 7 days after the onset. "Infarction" occurs if the neurologic dysfunction fails to clear completely and the patient is left with a residual neurologic deficit. TIAs, RINDs, and infarctions are all produced by similar mechanisms. These mechanisms may remain active after the initial event and impose future risk of ischemia and neurologic dysfunction. Because of this, the erroneous interpretation of infarction as a "completed" event rather than a manifestation of a potentially still active disease can be the prelude to catastrophe. Vascular disease that produces intracranial hemorrhage is also associated with an abrupt onset of signs and symptoms. Hemorrhagic diseases, unlike ischemic diseases, except for some embolic strokes, are usually associated with headache. The sudden onset of a severe headache with or without associated changes in consciousness or neurologic function is typical of subarachnoid hemorrhage. Headache, progressive neurologic dysfunction, and later depressed consciousness is often produced by an enlarging intracerebral hematoma.

Occasionally the patient with an abrupt history typical of cerebrovascular disease, on more complete work-up, proves to have a tumor or other intracranial mass lesion. Conversely, the progressive subacute neurologic deficit that has caused a patient to be suspected of having a tumor turns out to be recurrent or progressive ischemic vascular disease.

Surgical strategies are designed to manage elevated intracranial pressure or local mass effect caused by cerebrovascular disease as well as reduce, prevent, or lessen the risk of future ischemic or hemorrhagic difficulties. The decision to choose surgical rather than medical management in a particular situation is based on an understanding of the natural history of the disease process, the individual circumstances of that patient, the risks and benefits of each treatment alternative, and the availability of an experienced neurovascular surgical team. Surgical intervention may be indicated in

Increased intracranial pressure or local mass lesion
    Intracranial hemorrhage
    Cerebellar infarction
    Aneurysm
Prevention of future ischemia or hemorrhage
    Aneurysm
    Arteriovenous malformation
    Large-vessel occlusive disease

Cerebral Ischemia and Infarction

Cerebral infarction is the third leading cause of death and disability in the United States and accounts for the disability of some 2 million persons today. Management strategies are based on identification of individuals at risk for future ischemia and disease mechanism that may remain active. Appropriate therapeutic intervention can be made to lower subsequent risk.

Cerebral ischemia may result from cardiac disorders, disorders of the small cerebral blood vessels, hematologic disorders, and large-vessel occlusive disease. Aside from some cardiac operations, surgical intervention designed to lower the risk of future cerebral ischemia is appropriate only for patients with large-vessel occlusive disease.

The sites of atherosclerosis are generally bifurcations of major vessels. In decreasing order they are the carotid bifurcation in the neck; the vertebral basilar junction; the middle cerebral (MCA), posterior cerebral (PCA), and anterior cerebral (ACA) arteries; and the major ascending vessels from the aorta. Hypertension increases the predilection for atherosclerosis at each of these sites. Most ischemic episodes are believed to be the result of large-vessel to large-vessel emboli. Fibrin-platelet emboli form on thrombogenic areas of arteriosclerotic plaques or in areas of slow flow produced by stenotic plaques. Less commonly, cholesterol or calcified bits of plaque may serve as emboli. These emboli are carried downstream until they eventually become lodged in blood vessels through which they are too large to pass. Large-vessel thrombosis or high-grade stenosis may embarrass cerebral perfusion if collateral sources of blood are inadequate and produce cerebral ischemia on a "hemodynamic" basis.

For example, the syndrome of "middle cerebral artery occlusion," described as a hemiparesis most severe in the arm with cortical sensory dysfunction, a partial visual field defect, and, if the hemisphere involved is the dominant hemisphere, dysphasia, does not necessarily require occlusion of the middle cerebral artery. It may result from narrowing of proximal vessels, the common sites being in the internal carotid artery at its origin in the neck or intracranially in its cavernous portion. In contrast, an individual may have a clinically silent carotid occlusion with maintenance of normal cerebral function distal to it because of adequate perfusion of the vessels by segments of the circle of Willis. Such a patient may eventually present with a "middle cerebral artery" syndrome when the opposite internal carotid has become sufficiently narrowed by atheromas to impair the adequacy of collateral flow. Thus, the effects of ischemia may be first apparent in the most distant reaches of the circulation on the side of the originally silent carotid occlusion. Anomalies and imperfections of the circle of Willis may remove its safety factor for some and make them early victims of arteriosclerosis, for they are less likely to have been protected from the effects of the loss of individual vessels.

Active cerebrovascular disease often presents with a transient ischemic attack (TIA), defined as focal neurologic signs or symptoms of less than 24 h duration about half the time. TIAs are usually associated with active embolic disease and herald an infarction in one-third of patients within 5 years. The best available evidence suggests that about half of patients with cerebral infarction

may not experience any warning TIAs, while others may have only one or two warning spells. Patients with crescendo TIAs appear to be at especially high risk for cerebral infarction. TIA symptoms in the carotid distribution include hemiparesis, hemisensory disturbance, and, commonly, decrease or loss of vision in the eye of the involved side (anaurosis fugax). Vertebrobasilar TIA symptoms include cranial nerve palsies, diplopia, quadraparesis, and drop attacks. Vertigo occurring alone by strict definition is not considered a vertebrobasilar TIA but nevertheless should be approached with caution by the clinician. The previous conclusion that vertebrobasilar TIAs less frequently herald future infarction than do carotid TIAs does not appear to be valid.

The evaluation of patients with TIAs should begin with a history and physical examination, including auscultation for a focal bruit over the suspected vessel—the carotid in hemispheric lesions, the subclavian or vertebral in brainstem disease. A blood count, erythrocyte sedimentation rate, chest x-ray, and ECG are useful screening tests to identify hematologic, cardiac, or inflammatory disease causing cerebral ischemia. A head CT scan can exclude intracranial mass lesions that may present with transient symptoms. If large-vessel disease is suspected, the extracranial carotid arteries can be evaluated with a variety of noninvasive techniques such as ultrasound, Doppler, and oculoplethysmography. Although useful as low-risk, low-cost screens, noninvasive studies are limited by their sensitivity and specificity as well as their inability to evaluate the vertebrobasilar and intracranial carotid circulations.

Cerebral angiography remains the only reliable method of imaging pathologic vascular anatomy. Conventional intraarterial angiography is associated with about a 1 percent risk of transient or permanent cerebral ischemia. Digital intravenous angiography eliminates the risks associated with intraarterial injection and intraarterial catheter manipulation, but requires a cooperative patient and a much larger dye load and has limited resolution, particularly in evaluating the vertebrobasilar circulation. Techniques to noninvasively measure cerebral blood flow and neuronal metabolic activity such as xenon clearance, emission tomography, and MRI spectroscopy promise to provide a more complete understanding of ischemic cerebrovascular disease; however, these techniques have not evolved sufficiently to provide widespread clinical utility.

Commonly, a stenosis of the cervical internal carotid artery near its origin will be found. Although antiplatelet agents, anticoagulates, and carotid endarterectomy may all lower the risk of future cerebral ischemia in such a situation, the data suggest that in the hands of an experienced neurovascular team, carotid endarterectomy may be superior to medical therapy, at least for significant stenoses. Non- or minimally stenotic ulcerated lesions are best managed nonsurgically; however, rarely endarterectomy may be appropriate if recurrent ischemic episodes occur despite adequate medical therapy. The management of intermediate degrees of symptomatic carotid stenosis continues to be a source of controversy. Sundt analyzed 1145 consecutive carotid endarterectomies and found an overall operative mortality of 1.5 percent, major morbidity of 1 percent, minor morbidity of 1 percent, and transient neurologic dysfunction of 2 percent. Intraoperative embolization and postoperative hyperperfusion syndromes were the most common source of neurologic complications. Risk of surgery was increased in patients with angiographically determined risk factors or major medical risk factors but was highest in patients who were neurologically unstable before surgery. Long-term follow-up of endarterectomized patients shows an ischemic stroke rate of 2 percent per year with two-thirds of the stroke ipsilateral to the endarterectomy. The risk of developing late postoperative ischemia appears to be highest in patients whose cerebral blood flow remains less than 40 mL/100 g brain per minute following endarterectomy. Long-term ischemic stroke morbidity is less than would be expected for a comparable group of patients with TIAs who were not treated with endarterectomy. Long-term mortality following endarterectomy is 3 percent/year, and the percentage of deaths from cardiac causes is greater than expected, owing to a relative shift from stroke mortality to cardiac mortality.

At Yale, carotid endarterectomies are routinely performed under general anesthesia with simultaneous EEG and evoked cortical response monitoring. If the EEG or evoked responses change with carotid occlusion, a temporary bypass shunt is placed, thus restoring cerebral perfusion while the endarterectomy is performed. We routinely repair the carotid artery with a saphenous vein patch graft rather than direct suture repair of the arteriotomy because we believe that this substantially reduces the immediate and late postoperative occlusion rate. Using these techniques, we are able to perform endarterectomies at minimal risk with our results similar to those reported by Sundt.

Extracranial and intracranial focal vascular lesions that may not be remedial to direct surgical repair occur in a substantial number of symptomatic patients. Lesions inaccessible to direct surgical repair include most vertebrobasilar lesions, intracranial ICA or MCA stenosis, and complete ICA occlusion. In 1967, Donaghy and Yasargil successfully anastomosed the superficial temporary artery (STA) to a cortical branch of the middle cerebral artery (MCA) in two patients with inaccessible vascular disease. Recently, enthusiasm for the STA-MCA bypass procedure has been eclipsed by the realization that risks for future ischemia in most patients previously believed to be candidates for bypass are similar whether these patients are treated with surgery or antiplatelet therapy (aspirin) alone. Most patients with symptomatic large-vessel occlusion disease not amenable to direct surgical repair should be managed medically. Extracranial-intracranial bypass should, however, be considered in patients who continue to have episodes of hemodynamic ischemia despite adequate medical therapy. At Yale we have favored using saphenous vein interposition grafts rather than STA grafts in some situations because the high flows provided by vein grafts represent an advantage over STA grafts.

The value of emergency surgical revascularization by extracranial endarterectomy, extracranial-intracranial bypass, and intracranial embolectomy or endarterectomy for static or progressive cerebral ischemia remains a source of continued debate. An incomplete understanding of the natural history of specific vascular lesions, the inability to identify those patients who will improve with medical therapy alone, those who will improve only with surgical revascularization, and those patients who will never improve underlies this controversy. The recent report of the Japanese Cooperative Study of Ischemic Cerebrovascular Disease of poor prognosis following middle cerebral artery occlusion represents an initial step in understanding and rationally managing this set of disorders. Preliminary experience from North America suggests that patients with a fluctuating rather than fixed neurologic deficit or those with angiographically demonstrated collaterals may fare the best following emergency surgical revascularization.

Once cerebral infarction has occurred, management goals include support of cerebral perfusion in areas of the brain that may be ischemic but still viable and limitation of secondary neuronal damage that may occur from the mass effect of ectematous infarcted tissue. The ability to autoregulate is lost in ischemic areas of the brain, and as a consequence, imprudent hypotension, hypertension, or intravascular volume depletion should be avoided. Experimental and preliminary human experience suggests that hemodilutional volume expansion may increase perfusion in ischemic areas of the brain. Whether or not this therapy will prove to be useful at the bedside remains to be seen. Experimental evidence also suggests that hyperglycemia may also contribute to delayed neuronal loss. It has been suggested, therefore, that during the periischemic period only glucose-free intravenous solutions be given to patients and that hyperglycemia be aggressively treated with insulin. The value of this approach remains speculative, and no data exist to support its widespread clinical use. As edema increases in infarcted tissue, intracranial pressure may rise and contribute to secondary neuronal injury. Management of elevated intracranial pressure with head of bed elevation, fluid restriction, diuretics, and hyperventilation has met with varying success. Steroids do not appear to be of significant benefit in the management of edema associated with cerebral ischemia. Efforts to surgically manage elevated intracranial pressure by debulking large areas of infarcted brain have been disappointing and at best only contribute to the survival of severely neurologically impaired patients. Cerebellar infarction is a notable exception. As edema develops, the ischemic cerebellar hemisphere may directly compress the brainstem as well as produce hydrocephalus by obstructing the fourth ventricle. Surgical removal of the infarcted cerebellum can decompress the brainstem and relieve hydrocephalus. Loss of a large portion of the cerebellar hemisphere may be associated with only minimal functional deficit.

Cerebral and Cerebellar Hemorrhage

Although intracranial hemorrhage may result from underlying structural abnormalities in the blood vessels or blood dyscrasias, hypertensive hemorrhagic vascular disease remains a common but decreasing cause. In patients succumbing to hypertensive intracranial hemorrhage, the larger arteries show hypertrophic and degenerative changes in their media and intima; the arterioles demonstrate thickness of the vessel walls and reduction in lumen caliber secondary to hypertrophy of the intimal lining; and only minor structural changes are present in the capillaries. Whether or not microaneurysms develop in these arterioles as previously believed is not clear. The pathogenesis of hypertensive hemorrhage is unclear and thought to involve many factors. The blood pressure fluctuates in hypertension and, during periods of decreased systolic pressure, ischemia of tissue supplied by these diseased vessels and/or the arteries themselves may occur. The lack of arterial support from surrounding tissue (evidenced by ''état lacunaire'') and weakness in the vessel wall result in hemorrhage when the increased intraluminal pressure returns to the damaged segment. Arterial spasm with distal ischemia and decreased tonus may be significant mechanisms with hemorrhage resulting at the devitalized or necrotic channel after relaxation of the spasm.

The most common sites of hypertensive hemorrhages are in the regions of the lentiform nucleus, deep white matter or cerebellar hemispheres, pons, and midbrain. Hemorrhage into the basal ganglion can be divided into lateral and medial involvement. The latter arises medial to the putamen and destroys the hypothalamus, it may result in death; however, the lateral group are in the putamen, external capsule, and claustrum and often are compatible with survival. In contrast to hemorrhagic infarction in which all tissue in the area is destroyed, hemorrhage has a tendency to track along axonal planes, separating or splitting axonal fibers rather than destroying the nervous tissue. This phenomenon is especially true when the hematoma has its origin in white matter and may result in relatively minor permanent neurologic deficit. Amyloid angiopathy may also present as an intracerebral hemorrhage.

CLINICAL MANIFESTATIONS. Initial symptoms of intracranial hemorrhage may include headache, dizziness, paresthesia, or mild speech disturbances. These symptoms are followed by a rapidly developing paresis, severe headache, severe speech disturbances, vomiting, and/or loss of consciousness. The space-occupying hemorrhage may continue to enlarge and result in herniation of brain, secondary brainstem hemorrhage, and death. Computerized cranial tomography rapidly establishes the diagnosis and location of the intracerebral hemorrhage. In many instances, surgical evacuation of the hemorrhage may be lifesaving and be followed with almost complete neurologic recovery. Smaller hemorrhages may not pose an immediate life threat, and neurologic recovery may occur without surgical intervention. Other patients may be so devastated by the initial ictus that consideration of surgery is not appropriate. Management decisions are made after considering the patient's neurologic function, size and location of hemorrhage, age and premorbid function, and medical status. Like cerebellar infarction, cerebellar hemorrhage can produce brainstem compression and obstructive hydrocephalus. Early recognition and management of cerebellar hemorrhage are important in optimizing management results.

Aneurysms

Most cerebral aneurysms are asymptomatic, do not cause clinical disease, and are often incidental findings at autopsy. Intracranial hemorrhage from rupture of an aneurysm, however, initiates a morbid train of events. Nearly one-third of all patients who suffer an aneurysmal subarachnoid hemorrhage will die before they receive medical attention. Of those who reach hospitals, only half will survive and recover in a functional state despite the best available treatment. Overall management outcome is closely linked to initial neurologic function. Most patients who are alert with a normal neurologic exam when admitted to the hospital following aneurysmal subarachnoid hemorrhage will usually survive and have an excellent functional result. Patients who have a major alteration in sensorium and major focal neurologic deficit on admission survive and have an excellent functional result substantially less often. Most morbidity and mortality is a direct result of the initial hemorrhage. Delayed cerebral ischemia from chronic cerebral vasospasm that occurs as intracranial conducting arteries narrow in response to the subarachnoid blood produces most of the morbidity and mortality in those patients who survive the initial ictus. Half of all surviving patients will develop clinically significant delayed cerebral ischemia. Symptomatic vasospasm usually begins insidiously 5 to 20 days after hemorrhage and may be heralded by a subtle alteration in cognition. As ischemia progresses, major focal neurologic deficits, depressed sensorium, and death may rapidly follow. Aneurysmal rebleeding, although associated with 40 to 50 percent mortality, occurs substantially less often than delayed cerebral ischemia. Nearly half of all patients who will rehemorrhage do so in the first 3 days; however, a lesser risk peak occurs 7 to 12 days following the initial hemorrhage. The risk of rebleeding gradually decreases and eventually stabilizes at about 3 percent per year in patients who have not received specific treatment for their aneurysm.

Most intracranial aneurysms arise at the branch points of the conducting arteries of the circle of Willis and the vertebrobasilar system. Intracranial arteries have a thin, poorly developed, adventitial layer, a media that is partially or completely devoid of elastic fibers, and an intima consisting of an elastic lamella and thin collagenous tissue covered by an endothelial lining. Hemodynamic factors as well as errors in vessel wall construction that occur where vessels branch probably contribute to the development of aneurysms.

The most common sites of intracranial aneurysms are the internal carotid artery (42 percent), anterior cerebral artery (43 percent), and middle cerebral arteries (20 percent), with 6 percent of aneurysms arising from the vertebrobasilar system in the posterior fossae. The majority of aneurysms are single; however, 20 percent of patients have multiple aneurysms. When two aneurysms are present, they have a proclivity either for being symmetric in location or for arising from the same parent vessel.

The immediate cause of rupture of aneurysms usually cannot be determined, but the coincidence of hypertension and aneurysms appears to increase the possibility of rupture no matter what the cause of hypertension. In young patients with coarctation of the aorta with hypertension ruptured aneurysms are common. There also seems to be a correlation between systolic hypertension and rupture of the aneurysm. Silent aneurysms are seen with approximately the same incidence in patients with or without hypertension, while rupture is more frequent in patients with hypertension.

CLINICAL MANIFESTATIONS. The explosive onset of a severe headache should be considered a subarachnoid hemorrhage until proved otherwise. Focal neurologic deficit may occur, but headache, meningeal signs, and altered consciousness are usually much more prominent. Other aneurysms may enlarge without rupturing and present with cranial nerve or neuronal dysfunction produced as the aneurysm compresses nearby structures. Rarely thrombosis may develop within the aneurysm and cause thromboembolic ischemia.

TREATMENT. Elimination or reduction of the risk of rebleeding and minimizing the wastage produced by delayed cerebral ischemia form the cornerstone of aneurysmal subarachnoid hemorrhage management. Initially, rebleeding risks can be reduced with antihypertensives and sedatives while the patient is stabilized and the aneurysm identified with cerebral angiography. Epsilon-aminocaproic acid does reduce the risk of rebleeding; however, it is associated with thromboembolic complication and an increased risk of delayed cerebral ischemia. Direct surgical repair of intracranial aneurysms eliminates the risk of rebleeding and in the hands of an experienced neurovascular team can be accomplished with minimal risk in most instances. Occasionally, direct aneurysm repair is not possible, but the risks of rebleeding can be reduced in some situations by occlusion of a parent vessel. Wrapping or coating aneurysms may also decrease the risk of rebleeding.

Arteriovenous Malformations

Arteriovenous malformations are congenital lesions in which the arterial system drains directly into the venous system without a capillary bed interposed. Such malformations tend to enlarge with time and may present in a variety of ways. Because the nearby cerebral tissue may be chronically ischemic, neurologic symptoms and signs include focal loss of neurologic function and altered excitability. For this reason focal neurologic deficits of a minor or major nature and seizures are frequently seen in these patients. Arteriovenous malformations also are causes of subarachnoid, intracerebral, and intraventricular hemorrhages.

Subarachnoid hemorrhge due to arteriovenous malformation occurs generally at a younger age than that due to aneurysm. The majority of cases occur between twenty and forty-nine years of age without a peak incidence,

whereas with aneurysm the majority occur between forty and sixty-four years of age with a peak incidence between fifty and fifty-four years.

Intracerebral hematoma resulting from "cryptic" vascular malformations is probably more common than generally appreciated and is frequently mistaken for hypertensive hemorrhage. These small arteriovenous malformations are usually clinically silent and may be more common than the classic arteriovenous anomaly. The cryptic anomaly may be destroyed by the hematoma and its pathogenesis impossible to determine. In contrast to hypertensive hemorrhage, hematomas secondary to arteriovenous anomalies tend to occur outside the basal ganglion in the cerebral hemisphere white matter and may be present in the cerebellum, spinal cord, and brainstem.

TREATMENT. Because each arteriovenous malformation is unique and each patient has specific individual needs, appropriate treatment should be selected on an individual basis. A malformation that has produced a life-threatening intracerebral hematoma requires urgent clot evaluation and surgical removal. On the other hand, the decision to surgically treat a malformation that has produced no or only minor symptoms requires consideration of the long-term risks associated with not treating that particular malformation and the risks of therapies. Complete surgical excision remains the cornerstone of treatment. Transfemoral intraarterial embolization may be useful in high-flow, high-shunt malformations alone or as a preoperative adjunct to decrease flow. In lesions not amenable to surgical excision or embolization, some evidence suggests that high-energy irradiation may decrease the long-term risk of hemorrhage. Balloon occlusion of intracranial aneurysm using superselective transferral catheters is possible in some instances. Efforts to reconcile the worry of aneurysmal rebleeding and the risk of precipitating delayed cerebral ischemia by performing a craniotomy soon after a subarachnoid hemorrhage have stimulated discussion concerning the timing of aneurysm repair. Using modern techniques, surgery soon after subarachnoid hemorrhage appears to be safe and technically feasible and should be considered for some patients. Chronic cerebral vasospasm, once established, appears to be an irreversible vasculopathy rather than a reversible prolonged active contraction of the vessel wall as its name suggests. Ischemia associated with vessel narrowing may be lessened by increasing cerebral perfusion with intravascular volume expansion, induced hypertension, or increased cardiac output. These maneuvers, although helpful, do not always halt the relentless progression of delayed cerebral ischemia, and it continues to be a major source of morbidity and mortality. Preliminary human trials suggest that certain anti-inflammatory agents and some calcium channel blockers may improve management outcome by lessening vasospasm.

EPILEPSY

Epilepsy is perhaps the oldest recorded neurologic disorder. Its history traces a fascinating path from mysticism to accurate descriptions of cortical physiology and pathology. Although its study has provided insight into cerebral pathways and cortical functional localization, the cure or control of this disorder continues to frustrate the physician devoted to caring for seizure victims. Epilepsy affects at least 1 in 200 people. Therefore, the population of epileptics in the United States today totals more than 1 million. Of course, more than 600,000 have partial seizures, e.g., having focal origin. Two-thirds of patients with seizures have their initial seizure before the age of twenty. The older the patient, however, at the onset of epilepsy, the more likely a focal etiologic cause will be found. In patients presenting with their first seizure after age twenty, between 10 and 25 percent will have a focal lesion (such as a tumor or arteriovenous malformation) demonstrated on a complete neurologic work-up.

The cornerstone of seizure control is medical therapy for those patients without obvious cerebral pathologic change. Anticonvulsant drugs will control seizures in more than half of the patients with epilepsy and achieve partial to almost complete control in another 25 percent. It is estimated that there are approximately 200,000 patients with uncontrolled focal epilepsy in the United States. Forty-five thousand to 100,000 of these patients are potential surgical candidates. Surgical therapy is reserved for patients whose seizures are not well controlled with medication and whose history, description of the seizures, neurologic examination, or electroencephalogram suggests a focal cerebral origin. Success of surgical treatment correlates best with accurate identification of these patients with focal seizures, precise localization of the point of origin, and careful surgical excision of the area. Accurate localization of the area and identification of any motor, sensory, or intellectual deficit that may be caused by excision of the focus require a team approach, utilizing the neurosurgeon, neurologist, electroencephalographer, neuroradiologist, and neuropsychologist, as well as the proper electrophysiologic equipment and techniques.

The evaluation of a patient being considered for surgical treatment consists of four phases. In phase 1, the patient has a careful physical and neurologic examination with evaluation of past medication and additional medical trials if medication has not been used adequately. When the decision is made to continue the surgical work-up, the aims are to establish scalp localization if possible and to exclude those with EEG and clinical evidence of multifocal disease. This requires continuous electroencephalographic monitoring in order to record spontaneously the electrical seizures. Audiovisual monitoring is essential to provide behavioral correlation with electrical evidence of seizure events. To enhance the opportunity of recording spontaneous seizures, the patient may undergo sleep deprivation, and anticonvulsant medication is often stopped or markedly decreased. This methodology, of course, requires constant observation by specially trained nursing and medical personnel. The patient also undergoes investigation to document other localizing findings. Structural central nervous system abnormalities are searched for, which might lead directly to surgery, circumventing additional work-up. The patient undergoes CT, MRI, cerebral angiography, examination of the cerebral spinal fluid, neuropsychologic evaluation, and formal visual fields. At the time of arteriography, a short-acting barbiturate,

Amytal, is injected selectively into each internal carotid artery, and behavioral testing is carried out by the neuropsychologist and neurologist to determine speech dominance and the memory capacity of each temporal lobe (modified WADA test). If a mass lesion is identified and its position is compatible with another noninvasive localizing phenomenon, the patient may be able to proceed directly to surgery and excision of the mass and surrounding gliotic brain. Sometimes the mass lies close to the primary cortical regions of movement, sensation, or language or the epileptogenic region surrounding the mass needs better definition. In that case flexible electrode grids may be placed over the lesion and surrounding brain in order to map function by electrical stimulation and/or to record seizures. If a space-occupying mass lesion is not identified during this phase but there is continued evidence of focal epilepsy, the patient enters phase 3, which aims to establish definitive localization or to exclude those patients with multifocal disease or surgically inaccessible disease by the use of depth electrodes. In this phase, electrodes are implanted stereotactically and the patient again undergoes prolonged, continuous audiovisual electroencephalographic recording. In a special nursing unit, medication is again withdrawn if necessary to precipitate ictal clinical and subclinical seizures, and at least three such events are recorded before a decision is reached regarding the patient's appropriateness for surgical treatment. There is still a great deal of controversy regarding the use of scalp versus depth electrodes to localize focal cerebral epilepsy. We have reviewed the accumulated literature on depth and scalp localization. In this review, depth EEG identified some candidates who had localized depth EEG recordings but unlocalized scalp EEGs. This increased the number of operative candidates by 36 percent of the patients reported. Conversely, there were patients who had scalp localization but in whom the depth EEG was unlocalized, and these patients were excluded from surgical consideration. Thus, the depth EEG seemed to alter surgical plans in more than 50 percent of patients where scalp and depth patterns could be compared.

At Yale 100 patients have recently been evaluated regarding the success of surgery and our ability to localize the seizure focus. Forty-one patients had unlocalized scalp electroencephalography. Depth electrodes were localized and allowed surgical treatment in 44 percent of these patients. Fifty-nine patients had focal scalp EEG abnormalities, but 12 percent of these were found to be unlocalized or multifocal using depth monitoring and an additional 17 percent were localized to a different lobe of the brain than the scalp EEG indicated. Altogether when the depth studies reproducibly show multiple ictal events from the same location, surgery can provide an 85 to 90 percent chance of cure or diminishing the seizure by 90 percent. Most patients falling in the surgical success category had temporal lobe foci. Those with less good control were determined to have predominantly frontal lobe or multifocal onset of their seizure disorder. A frontal lobe focus usually indicates more diffuse pathology and has been one of the most frustrating groups with which to deal surgically. Of patients without radiographic lesions, neuronal dropout and astrocytosis were the most common pathologic findings at surgical excision being seen in all cases. At the present time the excised tissue is undergoing a scrupulous anatomic-biochemical analysis including neuronal quantification, neuropeptide and neurotransmitter immunohistochemistry and radioimmunoassay, ganglioside survey, in vitro electrophysiology, and nuclear magnetic resonance (NMR) spectroscopy. The purpose of this search is to elucidate anatomic and biochemical disruption responsible for initiating and propagating focal seizures. All patients are maintained on their anticonvulsants for at least 5 years postoperatively, and if they remain seizure-free, the drugs may then be tapered. Thus, patients with well-localized complex seizures, especially in the temporal lobe, may do very well following cortical excision. However, this leaves a number of patients who are localized to either the frontal, parietal, or occipital lobe who do less well, perhaps because their disease process is more diffuse and sometimes because complete resection is impossible without an unacceptable neurologic deficit.

Those patients who present with radiographic mass lesions, such as tumors or calcifications, are an exception to this rule. Of 171 patients followed at Yale for medically intractable partial epilepsy, 15 percent were ultimately found to have an intracranial mass. These masses included 16 neoplasms and 9 nonneoplastic structural lesions (2 calcified arteriovenous malformations, 3 arachnoid cysts, 1 granuloma, and 3 calcifications of unknown etiology). Although any treatment directed at the mass lesions, such as biopsy and radiation in unresectable neoplasms, gave good results in terms of reduction of uncontrolled seizures, patients undergoing lobectomy consistently showed more than 95 percent reduction in seizures, regardless of the cerebral lobe involved.

This leaves a group of patients with multifocal epilepsy who are much more difficult to treat. Their seizure disorder may emanate from a diffuse process in one hemisphere or may have bilateral cortical onset. It is in this group of patients that more experimental forms of treatment are being attempted, such as stereotactic subcortical radiofrequency ablations, cerebellar stimulation, and, perhaps most promising, limited or complete section of the corpus callosum. The latter surgical procedure has been found most efficacious in those patients presenting with form fruste congenital infantile hemiplegia whose seizures originate diffusely from the affected hemisphere. Division of the corpus callosum confines the abnormal electrical activity to the bad hemisphere and stops secondary generalization and, therefore, loss of consciousness in the majority of patients. Although all the indications for this operation are not clearly defined, the prospect for this being a standard and recommended operative procedure in some patients is clearly evident.

INTRACRANIAL INFECTIONS

Infections of the central nervous system and its coverings have surgical significance if they produce a mass, hydrocephalus, or osteomyelitis, or are the result of a break in, or absence of, continuity of the nervous system coverings.

A mass can be caused by pus, as in abscess or empyema, by the edema of the reaction of the nervous system to infection, by the edema of venous occlusion, or by an effusion in the subdural space. Hydrocephalus may be caused by the interruption of cerebrospinal fluid flow by blockage at the villi or basal cisterns, or within the ventricular system. Osteomyelitis of the skull and spine has surgical significance because of the propensity for the infected bone to become necrotic and sequester, forming the nidus for chronic inflammation, abscess, and progressive infection of adjacent bone and intracranial contents.

Surgical therapy of infections of the nervous system falls into one or more of the following categories: excision of infected bone, drainage or excision of abscess or empyema, decompression to relieve the effects of edema, shunting to relieve obstruction of cerebrospinal fluid circulation, and the repair or establishment of anatomic barriers to infection. This last category may involve surgical procedures as diverse as repair of a congenital heart lesion, eradication of a chronic middle ear infection, or removal of a pituitary tumor that has eroded into the sphenoid sinus.

Osteomyelitis of the Skull

Infections of the skull are relatively rare. The pathogenesis of osteomyelitis of the skull includes three major avenues of origin: (1) direct extension of preexisting infection in a paranasal sinus, middle ear, or mastoid air cells; (2) infection from a wound of the scalp that extends into or below the subgaleal space; and (3) hematogenous spread from elsewhere in the body. Any organism can be the causative agent, but by far the most common are *S. aureus* and the gram-negative contaminants of ear infection, such as *Bacillus proteus* and *B. pyocyaneus*. Once the infection is established, it usually spreads through the diploic spaces and the epidural space. Although spread under the outer periosteal layer or pericranium does occur, the pericranium is so firmly attached to the skull that it limits this as an important avenue of spread. This same attachment of the pericranium sometimes gives a false impression of the extent of the skull infection. Part of the mechanism of spread of the infection includes damage to the blood supply of the skull, and therefore necrosis and sequestration of the bone is common.

CLINICAL MANIFESTATIONS. The signs and symptoms of pyogenic infection of the skull are those of generalized infection, that is, fever, malaise, and leukocytosis, with focal tenderness and swelling. At times the infection can be indolent and manifest itself first by drainage through an area of the scalp, but more often it is highly virulent with spread into the intracranial structures, resulting in irritation and inflammation of the brain.

TREATMENT. The only effective treatment is excision of the involved bone and drainage of the area. Care must be taken to be certain that no infection remains in the epidural space to strip away the dura or in the diploic spaces to further necrose and infect adjacent bone. Appropriate antibiotics are helpful in protecting the bone edges and epidural space from further spread of the infection but are of little help without surgical excision of infected necrotic bone.

Epidural Abscess

Intracranial epidural abscesses are most commonly seen adjacent to infections of the skull and therefore are common near the middle ear, mastoid air cells, and nasal sinuses. Although the dura is a good protective barrier against inward spread of infection and although many epidural abscesses are discovered as incidental findings of surgical treatment for mastoid and sinus infection, they should not be considered benign processes. The infection can and often does break through the dural barrier, meningitis being the most common result and brain abscess the next most common. As already mentioned, the epidural space is an avenue for progression of osteomyelitis of the skull.

CLINICAL MANIFESTATIONS. The symptoms of epidural abscess are quite similar to skull infections, except that seizures and focal neurologic deficits are more common. These are commonly secondary to thrombophlebitis of superficial cortical veins.

TREATMENT. Treatment of epidural abscess is trephination, drainage, excision of infected bone, and the use of appropriate antibiotics. The excision of any infected bone and the drainage of any infected sinus or mastoid air cells are mandatory if the infection is not to recur.

Subdural Empyema

Although intracranial spread of paranasal sinus, ear, and mastoid infections to the epidural and subarachnoid spaces is more common, the high rate of morbidity and mortality seen with delayed or inadequate treatment with spread to the subdural space requires that this possibility always be kept in mind. Infections of the paranasal sinuses are the most common source of subdural empyema, and the spread of the infection to the subdural space is felt to include direct extension along emissary veins and via dural sinuses.

CLINICAL MANIFESTATIONS. The symptom complex of subdural empyema is related to five factors: First is the pathogenicity of the organism. Although staphylococci, *B. proteus,* and *B. pyocyaneus* are common chronic infecting agents of the sinus, ear, and mastoid areas and may cause subdural empyema, the infection is more often caused by staphylococci or streptococci that are acutely superimposed on a chronic infection. With these highly pathogenic organisms the course of subdural empyema may proceed to serious neurologic deficit in hours and to death within days. Second, there is no natural barrier to spread of the infection within the subdural space. Because of this the surface of an entire hemisphere may be involved within a very short period of time, and progression beneath the falx to the opposite hemisphere may occur as soon as significant pus has accumulated. Third, the veins traversing the subdural space from cortex to the dural sinuses are particularly vulnerable to inflammatory

response from the infection, with progressive thrombosis of the cortical veins and dural sinuses resulting. Fourth, the reaction in the subarachnoid space and surface of the hemisphere through the thin piarachnoid causes a sterile meningitis and an acute encephalitis. Finally, there is the mass effect, mainly secondary to the inflammatory reaction and the occlusion in venous drainage but also in part secondary to the volume of pus.

The first factors relate to rapidity of onset and the involvement of the entire hemisphere within a short period of time, while the last three explain in part the high incidence of seizures, signs of meningitis, neurologic deficit, and massive edema. Thus the symptom pattern of a patient with subdural empyema may vary but is best characterized as follows: A patient with a history of chronic sinusitis or chronic ear infection has an acute upper respiratory tract infection. Two or three days later when he should be making an uneventful recovery, he has a sudden secondary rise in temperature, shaking chills, and a convulsion. On regaining consciousness he complains of severe lateralized headache and of mild weakness or numbness on the opposite side of the body. Within a short period of time, a few moments to a few hours, he has another convulsion and then progressive decrease in his sensorium. At this point he is frequently either brought to a hospital or seen by a physician. Initial examination reveals an acutely ill patient with signs of meningitis. Lumbar puncture shows increased cellular response, but the spinal fluid sugar is within normal limits, and the microscopic smears fail to reveal any evidence of bacteria.

Within a few hours the patient can be in severe difficulty, often with total loss of function in the involved hemisphere, evidence of herniation of the temporal lobe with a dilated pupil on the side involved, and the beginning of decerebration.

TREATMENT. Treatment varies with the severity of the symptoms at the time that the patient is seen and the rapidity with which they have progressed. However, early trephination and drainage alone would be a satisfactory treatment only if the patient shows no sign of increased intracranial pressure, major alteration of conscious level, or shift of the midline structures. If the patient already shows any of these signs, drainage of the subdural space, external decompression by removal of a major portion of the skull on the side involved, and opening of the dura to allow expansion of the hemisphere are mandatory if the patient is to survive with good neurologic function. Although this appears to be a rather heroic treatment, the fact that the major deficit is secondary to inflammation and venous occlusion allows a degree of recovery to occur that is most gratifying, provided the treatment is started before the upper brainstem becomes irreversibly damaged.

Brain Abscess

Intracerebral pyogenic infection can be categorized as acute, subacute, or chronic. The symptoms and signs of suppuration within the brain encompass a range that extends from rapidly progressive focal neurologic deficit with a systemic response indicative of severe infection to

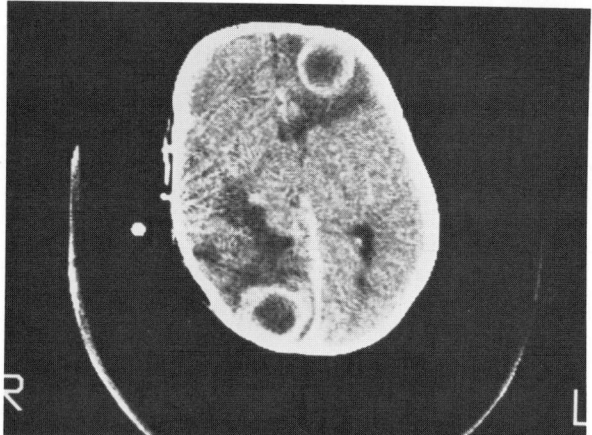

Fig. 42-12. A two-year-old male with cyanotic congenital heart disease and recent onset of seizures and decreased level of consciousness. Contrast-enhanced CT scan showed multiple abscesses.

evidence of an expanding intracranial mass with no suggestion of infection. In the former, the symptoms usually relate to a focal pyogenic encephalitis with little or no frank pus that will either resolve into an abscess or cause death if it continues to spread unchecked, while in the latter the abscess has a well-formed capsule of fibrous tissue and glial reaction.

The brain is resistant to infection by bacteria. Experimentally it is difficult to produce an abscess or focal encephalitis within the brain unless the area in which bacteria are placed is damaged beforehand, as by trauma, hemorrhage, or anoxia. Although the brain initially responds to infection in the same fashion as any tissue, its ability to wall off the infection by granulation and glial tissue is so effective that it often isolates the infection not only from the brain but even from significant contact with the systemic blood supply. For this reason the contents of a localized brain abscess usually cannot be sterilized by systemic antibiotics.

The pathogenesis of brain abscess includes, in the order of frequency of occurrence, three main routes of entry of the infecting organism: by direct extension from middle ear, mastoid, and paranasal sinus infections; through the blood supply to the central nervous system; and by direct traumatic penetration. Posttraumatic brain abscess is now rare, since adequate surgical care of the wound and antibiotic protection are excellent preventives. The ear is three or four times more common as a source of the infection for brain abscess than are the sinuses, and the temporal lobe and cerebellar hemispheres are the more common sites for abscesses secondary to these infections. Hematogenous abscesses can occur following any bacteremia but are more commonly seen with lung abscess, infected bronchiectasis, and cyanotic heart disease. In the patient with cyanotic heart disease the presence of a right-to-left heart shunt with the loss of the lung as a filter to remove blood-borne bacteria is felt to be the mechanism responsible for the high frequency of occurrence of brain abscess. Since in cyanotic heart disease

one of the most common causes of cerebral dysfunction is abscess, a patient with symptoms of cerebral disease, either seizures or neurologic loss, should have a contrast CT scan to rule out abscess. The organisms commonly seen in brain abscess are streptococci, pneumococci, and staphylococci. The most common streptococci are the anaerobic strains.

CLINICAL MANIFESTATIONS. The symptom complex of brain abscess will vary according to whether the infection is acute, subacute, or chronic. As was noted earlier, in the chronic walled-off brain abscess there may be no signs of systemic reaction to infection, that is, no fever or leukocytosis. Brain abscess should be considered as a possible diagnosis in any patient with progressive focal neurologic deficit and increasing mass with a short, that is a 2- to 3-week, history. Often with questioning a source of possible brain abscess or an episode suggestive of bacteremia can be found in the recent past. Acute pyogenic encephalitis has a course quite similar to a subdural abscess, from which it is often difficult to differentiate.

The subacute abscess varies between these two extremes, so that the combination of signs of inflammation, progressive focal neurologic deficit, and increasing mass effect not only suggests the presence of a brain abscess but also frequently from the neurologic signs localizes it. A CT scan is the most accurate method to identify the presence of a brain abscess, to differentiate cerebritis from abscess, and to demonstrate the presence or absence of a capsule, and it is the mandatory test when brain abscess is suspected (Fig. 42-12).

TREATMENT. Although in the past it was taught that suppurative intracranial encephalitis could not be treated surgically, decompression, removal of portions of the infected brain, and the use of antibiotics may be lifesaving and function-saving when applied to the critically ill patient in the acute stage. Usually the patient can be carried through the acute stage by the use of antibiotics and anti-inflammatory agents, such as steroids, and by careful control of fluids. The progress of the treatment can be monitored by repeated CT scans, and the formation of a capsule demonstrated. This usually takes 10 to 12 days.

Once localization has been accomplished, drainage of the abscess by intermittent tapping through a perforator opening, by constant drainage, or by excision of the abscess will give a high percentage of cures. In hematogenous abscesses more than half will be multiple, and care must be taken to be certain that an abscess is not missed. The major dangers to the patient with abscess of the brain are (1) the early acute edematous response the brain has to pyogenic infection, (2) the continued problem of a mass lesion from both the edema and the suppuration itself, and (3) the continued possibility of rupture of the abscess into the ventricular system. The latter complication can be rapidly fatal. With the advent of antibiotics and anti-inflammatory agents such as steroids, brain abscess should have low mortality and, depending upon its location, low morbidity rates. However, failure to diagnose its presence until late in its course, failure to realize the dangers of mass effects from the abscess, the surrounding reaction of the brain, and the concurrence of cardiac disease and systemic infection have kept the mortality rate in most reported series between 35 and 45 percent.

PAIN

Pain, the symptom that most commonly brings a patient to a physician, can be both the protector and the debilitator. As a protector it calls for diagnostic inquiry, but when it no longer has protective value, it can be a disease in itself. The best treatment of pain is the removal of its cause. When this is not possible or must be delayed, drugs, and particularly opiates and their derivatives, can be used for relief. All potent analgesics, however, have addicting qualities and therefore decreasing effectiveness with continued use, so that if more than a few months of pain relief is required, drugs not only are ineffective but also can contribute to physical deterioration and mental depression. The need for prolonged effective control has been the impetus for surgeons to devise surgical means for relieving pain. Horsley's resection of the gasserian ganglion (1891), section of dorsal roots by Bennett and Abbe (1889), and Martin's incision into the anterolateral portion of the spinal cord (1911) were milestones in this quest. Lack of knowledge still exists not only in the spheres of anatomy and physiology but even in defining pain. Is pain a sensory modality with its own anatomic and physiologic correlates, or is it a learned response to environmental alteration that threatens the organism? Is pain an emotional reaction evoked with or without stimuli, or is it the recognition that a central nervous system pathway or area has been activated, indicating that a portion of the organism has reached or exceeded its functional limits? There is justification for the concept that pain contains some or all of these attributes.

A mark of a good clinician is the ability to separate pain caused by stimulation of peripheral nerves from complaints of pain that signify a psychologic or psychiatric disorder. The major cause for failure of any treatment of pain is the failure to differentiate pain from suffering. Even in the face of obvious disease that can cause pain, such as cancer, the complaints of pain may relate more to depression over the disease and its progress than to nerve stimulus. Failure to treat both aspects will give little relief, and denervating the offending part may increase suffering by reinforcing the patient's concept of progressive deterioration. Drugs given for anxiety may increase the depression and increase suffering. Careful evaluation of the situation and the response to each therapeutic maneuver is necessary to obtain maximum benefit of any treatment for pain. In general, patients with a life expectancy of 2 months or less are best treated with drugs. The treatment should include drugs of sufficient potency and in sufficient amounts to relieve pain. Such treatment, while a blessing to a terminal patient because of the changes in sensorium, does not allow a patient with longer life expectancy to enjoy the remaining time. Surgical interruption of pain pathways can both relieve the pain and allow a drug-free existence and should be considered in any patient with severe pain that cannot be relieved by medi-

cation. Surgical intervention for the relief of pain of benign origin should be employed only after a concerted multidisciplinary approach has failed. Accurate diagnosis, careful evaluation of functional status, and neuropsychologic assessment are essential before dealing with drug dependence or attempting behavioral modification. Some preliminary therapeutic techniques that may be of help include physiotherapy, nerve blocks, transcutaneous electrical stimulation, hypnosia, and acupuncture, with varying degrees of effectiveness in any given case.

Surgical Relief of Pain

Empiric observations combined with physiologic studies have given neurosurgeons effective methods for surgically relieving pain. These approaches fall into one of five general categories:

1. Section of the peripheral nerve pathway: neurectomy, splanchnicectomy, dorsal rhizotomy
2. Section of central nervous system pathways: anterolateral cordotomy, trigeminal tractotomy, and dorsal root entry zone (DREZ) lesioning.
3. Procedures to alter affective response to pain: thalamotomy, lobotomy, cingulotomy
4. Section of the efferent arc of the vasomotor reflex: sympathectomy
5. Suppression by nonablative techniques: stimulation of peripheral nerve, spinal, deep brain, intraspinal drug infusion

Despite many variations in technique and many claims for various procedures, clinical experience has demonstrated that all the procedures for relief of pain from lesions of the nervous system fall into one of the first four categories and that each category has its area of application, its inherent rate of success, and its complications. Application of the correct procedure at the correct time to a suitable patient is the most difficult aspect of the surgery for pain.

SECTION OF THE PERIPHERAL PATHWAY. Section of the peripheral pathway for pain causes loss of all sensation distal to the area of section. From what is presently known, transmission of nociceptive information from the periphery appears to be by way of small myelinated (A delta) and unmyelinated (C) fibers from cells of origin in the dorsal root ganglia. Although there are specific receptor types for different sensory modalities, free nerve endings probably are the receptors for pain stimuli. These afferent nerve fibers (A delta and C) then terminate centrally and arborize within the superficial neuronal cell layers of the dorsal horn of the spinal cord which seems to function as a processing station for nociceptive signals. The axons from some of the cell layers of the dorsal horn decussate anterior to the central canal of the spinal cord and project centrally as the epinothalamic tract.

It has been shown recently that the ventral roots of several species, including human beings, have significant numbers of unmyelinated fibers, up to 30 percent, and that some of these originate in the dorsal root ganglion. These afferent fibers are believed to project to the same superficial dorsal horn neurons as well. This potential for ventral root nociceptive transmission has been proposed as the basis for the return of pain that may follow dorsal root rhizotomy in some patients.

This concept has been further supported by the observation that dorsal root ganglionectomy may relieve pain in those patients who experienced return of pain following dorsal rhizotomy. Dorsal root ganglionectomy is effective for the relief of persistent chest wall pain following thoracotomy, disabling flank pain after renal surgery, and painful monoradiculopathy that may follow lumbar disc surgery. Accurate assessment of specific levels of pain medication may be made with differential somatic paravertebral anesthetic blocks for determining the extent of ganglionectomy. In patients with painful monoradiculopathy following lumbar disc surgery, ganglionectomy is of significant benefit in 60 percent of patients. Annoying dysesthesias are experienced by 50 percent of patients postoperatively, but they usually subside after 2 to 3 months.

Any procedure that damages primary sensory neurons gives subjective sensory loss, which can have as a complication painful paresthesia or spontaneous pain in the anesthetic area. This may be explained by altered excitability of the DREZ neurons. Since further pain pathway interruption usually intensifies the pain, a more logical explanation appears to be that in this group of patients the subjective sensation of sensory loss signifies something wrong with the area and is painful. Any further alteration in sensation increases the pain. The psychologic basis of this may be that anything painful is abnormal, and therefore anything abnormal is painful. Stressing the lack of significance of such feelings at times helps, but alteration in affective response by either psychotherapeutic drugs or surgical intervention sometimes is the only recourse when the paresthesia becomes unbearable.

Section of multiple dorsal roots is seldom considered for relief of pain in a functioning limb, since loss of position sense, gamma afferents, and sense of touch leave the limb useless. It is of value in the thoracic area or where only one root is directly involved. In the former, touch and position senses are not of functional significance, and in the latter, sensory overlap of adjacent roots makes the peripheral sensory loss minimal. This sensory overlap of adjacent roots makes section of at least two and usually three roots necessary for effective deafferentation of any peripheral area.

Rhizotomy of the trigeminal nerve is used to control pain of malignant tumors of the face and trigeminal neuralgia. It can be performed by direct section of the trigeminal roots in the middle or posterior fossa or stereotaxically in the middle fossa with a radiofrequency electrode through the foramen ovale. Trigeminal neuralgia, or tic douloureux, is a painful condition of the trigeminal nerve of uncertain cause, characterized by paroxysms of pain over one or two adjacent divisions of the fifth cranial nerve. The paroxysms are often initiated by any stimulus in localized areas of the division involved, known as "trigger zones." Section of the postganglionic fibers of the trigeminal nerve or of the descending trigeminal tract in the brainstem permanently controls the pain, but as with peripheral nerve section painful paresthesia may arise.

An earlier observation by Dandy that patients with trigeminal neuralgia frequently have vascular compression of the trigeminal rootlets as they enter the pons led Jannetta to postulate altered conduction and excitability at the root entry zone of the brainstem as the cause of the syndrome. Jannetta also has suggested that other paroxysmal disorders of cranial nerves, such as glossopharyngeal neuralgia and facial tic, have the same cause. Compression of the trigeminal nerve more distally does not correlate with the syndrome, and decompression of the vascular trigeminal rootlets has achieved a relief of pain without significant sensory loss in a high percentage of patients.

Peripheral pathway section was the first procedure used for relief of pain, but because of the annoyance of the feeling of numbness, the incidence of paresthesia, nerve regeneration, and the availability of other procedures, it is now rarely used except in the extremely debilitated for denervating trigger areas in the control of trigeminal pain by avulsion of the supraorbital, or infraorbital, or the inferior alveolar nerve.

Splanchnicectomy effectively denervates the upper abdominal viscera and is used for relief of intractable pain of the upper abdomen. Although the splanchnic nerves are part of the sympathetic nervous system, it is the interruption of the visceral afferent fibers coursing within the sympathetic nerves that gives the relief of pain. Their cells of origin are in the dorsal root ganglion, as are the cells of all peripheral sensory nerves, but since they have no surface innervation and paresthesia of denervation is always referred to the surface, painful paresthesia is not seen following their interruption. When malignant disease of the upper abdomen involves somatic sensory fibers in the intercostal nerves, dorsal root section or cordotomy may be more effective than splanchnicectomy. Absolute alcohol and phenol in glycerin given by subarachnoid injection with appropriate technique are effective neurolytic agents for selective rhizotomy, chiefly for the control of pelvic pain due to advanced cancer as an alternative to open sacral rhizotomy.

SECTION OF CENTRAL NERVOUS SYSTEM PATHWAYS. When Martin in 1911 made an incision in the anterolateral quadrant of a patient's spinal cord, the era of surgical control of intractable pain commenced. Anterolateral cordotomy remains an effective means of controlling intractable pain, and many surgeons have contributed their skill and knowledge to modify Martin's original procedure so that it is a simple and reliable method for production of analgesia. Cordotomy may be performed by the conventional open surgical approach in the upper thoracic or high cervical region, or as a percutaneous stereotactic radiofrequency (RF) procedure at the C_1–C_2 level with preliminary electrical stimulation to confirm correct positioning in the spinothalamic tract. This technique has the obvious advantage over open cordotomy in avoiding a major surgical procedure. Monitoring the patient closely under local anesthesia permits the RF lesion to be made precisely, reducing the risk of ipsilateral motor weakness. Bilateral high cervical cordotomy carries the risk of sleep-induced apnea, which may be fatal. Section of the tract in the spinal cord causes no subjective sensory loss and therefore rarely causes dysesthesia or paresthesia, but it has limitations. Since the fibers projecting to the anterolateral quadrant of the spinal cord ascend three to four segments before crossing in the spinal cord, incision of the quadrant gives loss of pain and temperature sensation on the opposite side of the body three or more segments below the level of the cordotomy. Thus, even a perfectly performed high cervical cordotomy fails to block pain in the upper arm, shoulder, or neck; therefore the procedure is best used for control of pain below the upper thoracic level. Approximately 10 percent of patients subsequently develop pain on the side opposite to that initially experienced, and a second-stage contralateral cordotomy at an adjacent level may be required, with increasing risk for lower-extremity paresis, ataxia, and/or sphincter dysfunction. The loss of pain, although marked, can be demonstrated to be incomplete, and with time islands of pain perception appear, and with them the original pain may return. This may take a year or more to occur and limits in part the usefulness of the procedure for pain from benign conditions.

Commissural myelotomy, a procedure that involves section of the decussating nociceptive fibers in the anterior commissure of the spinal cord over several segments, is useful for the relief of midline or bilateral pain of malignant disease in the lower abdomen, pelvis, and perineum, and for the pain associated with chronic adhesive arachnoiditis. Although transient paresthesia of the lower extremities and bladder dysfunction may follow the procedure, persisting complications are generally infrequent and the success rate for appreciable improvement is seen in 60 to 70 percent of patients.

Lesions of the DREZ of the spinal cord, produced by thermal coagulation either with RF electrode or with a laser, have been shown to relieve chronic intractable pain associated with brachial and lumbar plexus avulsion and spinal cord trauma in approximately 65 to 70 percent of patients. As theorized, neuronal hyperactivity in the DREZ follows traumatic deafferentation in spinal cord injury and plexus avulsion, and the syndrome that develops has the characteristics of central pain. The pain may occur spontaneously or may be triggered by mere touch of the affected part inducing extremely intolerable dysesthesia. Further understanding of the pathophysiologic basis of the DREZ in deafferentation pain syndromes awaits correlative histopathologic studies of patients who have undergone therapeutic DREZ lesions.

Lesions further cephalad in the spinothalamic tract, that is, at the midbrain, although causing loss of pain without subjective sensory loss may also cause dysesthesia or the sensation of pain from nonpainful stimuli. The cause of this dysesthesia is unknown.

Section of the descending, or spinal, tract of the trigeminal nerve in the medulla causes loss of pain and temperature sensation in the ipsilateral face. Since the operation has a higher morbidity and mortality than postganglionic section of the trigeminal nerve in the middle fossa, it is usually used only when it is feared a patient would not tolerate anesthesia of the face or when paralysis of the motor portion of the trigeminal on the opposite side is already present. In the latter condition the danger of bilat-

eral paralysis of the muscles of mastication by approaching the nerve distad is higher than the morbidity of medullary tractotomy.

Stereotaxic lesions have been placed in the posterior medial thalamus in the area of the centramedian and nucleus parafascicularis, structures suggested by electrophysiologic and axonal degeneration studies as projections of the medial spinal reticular tracts. These procedures have been reported to relieve pain without any loss of pinprick or temperature sensation in the periphery, but their effectiveness is short-lived. It can be hoped, however, that with more basic information lesions for control will be devised that either interrupt major projections of the impulses defining a stimulus as noxious or increase the blockade of such impulses as they attempt to pass each controlled synaptic junction.

PROCEDURES TO ALTER AFFECTIVE RESPONSE TO PAIN. On a basis of the work in primates of Fulton and Jacobson, Egas Moniz in 1935 persuaded his neurosurgical colleague Lima to perform a prefrontal lobotomy on a psychiatric patient with marked anxiety as part of the basis for the psychiatric problem. The success of the procedure prompted many other surgeons to try prefrontal lobotomy for psychiatric illness. Altered affect, particularly in response to peripheral stimuli, and relief of anxiety were seen in the patients just as they had been seen in the animals, and it seemed probable that the reaction of the patients to pain might be similarly altered. Van Wagenen in 1942 performed bilateral prefrontal lobotomies on a mentally ill patient who had phantom limb pain, and his success in altering the patient's complaint prompted other surgeons to use the same procedure in patients with intractable pain. Experience with this procedure has shown that the lobotomy patient is unconcerned with the pain but when questioned still reports the pain as present. This lack of concern is no different for pain than it is for other stimuli, and therefore the procedure alters not only the response to pain but the entire affect of the patient. Lesions of the nonspecific nuclei of the thalamus, as in the dorsal median nucleus, lesions of the limbic system, such as cingulotomy, or excisions of gyri in the prefrontal cortex produce the same response with varying degrees of affective change.

The major limitation of these procedures is this change in personality. The same effect can be obtained with psychotherapeutic drugs, such as chlorpromazine, but with drugs it can be reversed. For this reason, the procedures for altering affective response to pain are rarely used but still should remain a part of the physician's armamentarium for care of the terminally ill patient whose fears make the situation and the pain unbearable for the patient and the family alike, and for the occasional patient where relief of anxiety will make it possible to resume a more normal life.

SECTION OF THE EFFERENT ARC OF THE VASOMOTOR REFLEX. Pain that occurs in diseases that cause alteration in blood flow of an extremity, such as Raynaud's syndrome or erythromelalgia, or conditions that cause marked vasospasm, such as causalgia following nerve injury, and the pain of obstruction of the major vessels in an extremity where circulation can be reestablished by dilatation of collateral vessels will respond to sympathectomy. Much has been written about possible sensory function in the sympathetic nervous system; however, aside from the visceral afferent fibers in the splanchnic nerves, no evidence of sensory function has been demonstrated. The clinical experience that sympathectomy does not relieve pain unless evidence of altered blood flow is present before sympathectomy bears this out. The occasional exception experienced by surgeons is more likely related to the placebo effect of any form of therapy rather than to alteration in peripheral afferent pathways.

Surgical treatment for pain is a useful adjunct to the care of patients and can be effective in prolonging useful life in many situations. An understanding of what it can and cannot do and an awareness of its limitations are an important aspect of its use. The striking relief afforded a patient with intractable pain of malignant pelvic tumor and the return of such a patient to normal interpersonal relationships provide an experience that can demonstrate to any physician the effectiveness of cordotomy. The failure of ablative surgical procedures for pain in patients using pain as a means of removing themselves from an intolerable situation should demonstrate just as strikingly to the physician that no therapy should be applied just because a symptom is present.

SUPPRESSION OF PAIN BY NONABLATIVE TECHNIQUES. Counterstimulation, such as acupuncture, based on theories foreign to most Western neurophysiologic concepts has been used for centuries. Unfortunately, scientific evaluation of the results is not available, and allegorical reports not recognizing placebo effects, emotional factors, and the striking immediate effect of one pain to suppress a less severe pain are the only evidence available for evaluation. More recently, electrical stimulation applied to peripheral nerves, dorsal columns of the spinal cord, and various subcortical cerebral structures has been used for a variety of intractably painful states with varying clinical results.

Although the initial rationale for using these techniques was based on physiologic concepts, the development of the techniques appears to be more empirically than theoretically based. Stimulation of peripheral nerves is done for painful dysesthesia limited to an area innervated by a single nerve. The technique is based on electrophysiologic evidence that the larger nonpainful fibers of peripheral nerves inhibit the subsequent spinal cord activity secondary to smaller fibers, the latter being essential for pain conduction. Stimulation of nonpainful myelinated fibers by implanted cuff electrodes on peripheral nerve has had limited success in alleviation of pain, and the method is limited to painful entities in a single nerve distribution. It has been more effective in the upper extremity than in the lower extremity.

Electrical stimulation of the spinal cord dorsal column by percutaneously implanted epidural electrodes has been used for more diffuse intractable pain, particularly of the lower extremities. A theoretic basis for this type of stimulation includes increasing descending inhibition in the dorsal root entry zone, and experimental evidence that such stimulation inhibits the central conduction of smaller fiber activity has been demonstrated. Using nonpainful paresthesia to determine the threshold, implanted dorsal column stimulators have had effective short-term results for relief of intractable pain in some patients.

Evidence of the production of effective analgesia in rats by stimulation of the raphe's nuclei of the brainstem, the presence of opiate receptors in the paraventricular and brainstem gray matter in vertebrates, and the identification of endogenous polypeptides, called endorphins, with opiate properties have led to techniques for stimulating the medial thalamic and upper brainstem nuclei to control pain. These techniques consist of stereotaxically placed electrodes and implanted self-contained stimulators that the patient can control with a radiofrequency generator placed over the implanted stimulator antenna. Evidence that a system relating to the action of endogenous opiates is being activated by such stimulation includes the blocking of analgesic effects with nalaxone, an opiate antagonist. Initial reports of this technique are encouraging, but long-term results are not yet available and evaluation of complications awaits further experience.

The neurophysiologic and pharmacologic basis for spinal opiate analgesia was extensively reviewed by Yaksh, to which the reader is referred. Opiates intrathecally administered, with action restricted to the spinal cord, markedly inhibit spinal nociceptive neuronal discharge and do not affect tactile perception or motor function. High levels of opiate binding have been demonstrated within the substantia gelatinosa, the superficial layer of the dorsal horn, where A delta and C fibers terminate and morphine exerts inhibition of nociceptive neuronal discharge.

Chronic intraspinal narcotic analgesia is an effective method for control of intractable cancer pain that has gained increasing acceptance during the past decade as an alternative to a major neuroablative procedure. Low doses of morphine are delivered either intrathecally or epidurally by implanted pump or by intermittent bolus through a subcutaneously implanted reservoir. Effective control of pain is achieved with intrathecal doses of morphine, initially 0.5 mg/day and up to 7 mg/day maintenance, whereas with epidural administration doses are higher, 4 to 6 mg/day initially and up to 50 mg/day maintenance. Clinical trials to control chronic pain of benign origin, i.e., phantom limb pain, chronic arachnoiditis, failed back surgery, with intraspinal infusion of narcotid drugs have been uniformly unsuccessful.

STRUCTURAL ABNORMALITIES OF THE AXIAL SKELETON

General Considerations

ANATOMY. The vertebral column with its ligaments and musculature serves two functions: the support of body weight and protection of the neuraxis. The same dual role is played by the basiocciput, which may be considered from an embryologic and functional standpoint as an extension of the spine. In health, the spine is a sturdy yet flexible weight-bearing structure. Most of its weight-bearing property is provided by the vertebral bodies and intervertebral discs. The neural arch formed by the pedicles and laminae complete a bony ring at each vertebral level defining the vertebral canal, while the articular processes and attached facets bridge the intervertebral spaces posterolaterally, providing further support and protection. The spinous and transverse processes of the neural arch serve as attachments for the spinal musculature. The ligamentum flavum and the posterior atlantooccipital ligament, both thick elastic structures, complete the bony and ligamentous tube that extends from the foramen magnum to the lowest part of the sacrum. In the normal skeleton there is ample room within the foramen magnum and the vertebral canal for the contained neural and vascular elements, and the intervertebral foramina provide unrestricted pasage of the nerve roots and blood vessels.

There is a considerable discrepancy between the cross-sectional area of the vertebral canal and that of the spinal cord at all levels, the additional space being occupied by the cerebrospinal fluid-filled subarachnoid space and the fat-filled epidural space. The fluid and fat suspend and cushion the neuraxis and, because they are displaceable, provide room for lateral and anteroposterior movement of the neuraxis that must take place with normal motion of the axial skeleton. Radiologic and postmortem studies have shown that the spinal cord and nerve roots also undergo grossly perceptible axial movement when the spine is flexed or extended. The spinal cord and roots must, therefore, be free to move up and down the vertebral canal, and the stress applied to the nerve roots through the movement of the peripheral nerves must be relieved by movement within the intervertebral foramina.

PATHOPHYSIOLOGY. Structural abnormalities that markedly decrease the dimensions of the foramen magnum, the vertebral canal, or the intervertebral foramina may damage or irritate the nervous system. The mechanism of injury is primarily that of direct compression of nervous tissue, although in some instances concomitant interference with blood supply may be a factor. Injury to the nervous system may be caused by acute angulation of the vertebral axis, subluxation of one part of the axial skeleton upon another, or encroachment of a mass upon the vertebral canal or intervertebral foramina. Both the degree and rate of compression are important. Angulation of the spine, for example, in idiopathic scoliosis may be extremely severe but rarely causes neurologic deficit because of the ability of the cord and roots to accommodate gradual distortion. In contrast, less pronounced angulation from an acute process such as collapse of vertebra in an osteoporotic spine may result in complete destruction of the spinal cord.

The causes of structural abnormalities of the spine that affect the nervous system are extremely diverse. The bones, joints, and associated muscles of the axial skeleton are subject to the same diseases as they are elsewhere in the body. They may be congenital or acquired, local or diffuse. Symptomatic abnormalities often result from a combination of these factors. As an example, the foramen magnum and the vertebral canal in achondroplasia is malformed and disproportionately small as compared with the normal size of the spinal cord. A relatively minor degree of disc protrusion or scoliosis in these patients often causes severe neurologic deficit. It is becoming increasingly apparent as careful measurement of the spinal canal becomes more prevalent that individual differences in reponse to structural disease in the general population can, at least in part, be accounted for by congenital differences in the size of the vertebral canal. Those persons with congenitally small but undistorted vertebral canals are much more liable to major neurologic deficit in response to degenerative spondylosis or disc disease or relatively minor spine trauma.

It is not the intention of this section to discuss all the etiologic agents that may result in structural abnormalities of the spine. What will be emphasized are the often misunderstood structural lesions occurring at the craniovertebral border and the common lesions resulting from disease of the intervertebral discs.

Abnormalities of the Craniovertebral Border

Structural abnormalities involving the basiocciput and the cephalic portion of the cervical spine are uncommon as compared with those of the remainder of the axial skeleton. Frequently they may produce profound neurologic dysfunction, which may be misinterpreted or misdiagnosed. Craniovertebral abnormalities are usually congenital but may be acquired. Anatomically these lesions divide into two basic categories, those that affect the basiocciput and those that primarily involve the first and second cervical vertebrae. Both limit the space available for the cervicomedullary junction and may produce neurologic dysfunction.

PATHOLOGY. Maldevelopment of the occipital bone resulting in an abnormally small and irregularly shaped foramen magnum occurs in achondroplasia and occasionally in craniosynostosis. More common deformities of the basiocciput are those termed *platybasia (platys,* flat) and *basilar impression.* To accommodate the cerebellum and the brainstem, which lie in approximately the same axis as the spinal cord, the level of the floor of the posterior fossa is normally well below that of the anterior and middle fossae. In platybasia, the entire floor of the posterior fossa appears elevated. As seen in a lateral x-ray of the skull, the angle formed by the floor of the anterior fossa and the posterior border of the clivus approaches 180°, and the posterior fossa is therefore extremely shallow. In basilar impression the margins of the foramen magnum are indented as if the weight of the head had caused it to sink toward the vertebral column. This may in fact be the mechanism in acquired basilar impression associated with rickets and Paget's disease. In both platybasia and basilar impression the capacity of the posterior fossa is reduced, and the dimensions of the foramen magnum, especially the anteroposterior diameter, are decreased. In accommodating to the small and abnormally shaped posterior fossa, the hindbrain may be distorted and compressed, especially on its ventral surface. Thus the lower cranial nerves and the cervicomedullary junction may be compressed directly or stretched. Hydrocephalus can result from local obstruction to cerebrospinal fluid pathways.

Atlantoaxial dislocation is one of the most severe disturbances of the upper cervical spine still compatible with life. This can occur for a variety of reasons. As with dislocations at other levels, it may be the result of trauma, infection, or degenerative bone disease. It most commonly, however, occurs in association with maldevelopment of the atlas. The atlas may be fused to the base of the occiput, and the odontoid, which represents the body of the atlas, may be maldeveloped. Failure of fusion of the odontoid process to the body of the axis may occur without other abnormalities. In occipitalization of the atlas, the head can no longer flex and extend at the atlantooccipital joint, and the added stress on the ligaments holding the odontoid process in place may eventually produce a dislocation. The same ventral dislocation of the atlas on the axis may occur if the odontoid process is rudimentary or ununited to the atlas. With atlantoaxial dislocation the upper cervical spinal cord may be compressed between the odontoid process and the posterior arch of the atlas or foramen magnum. The lower medulla may become compromised as well.

CLINICAL MANIFESTATIONS. Structural abnormalities of the craniovertebral border frequently remain asymptomatic until adult life, and then frequently symptoms are precipitated by relatively minor trauma. Cranial nerve signs include disassociated sensory loss over the face (descending trigeminal tract) and palatal and vocal cord weakness. Nystagmus and spastic weakness of the extremities are common, and the patient may have loss of position sense, ataxia, bladder dysfunction, and atrophy of the shoulder musculature and small muscles of the hand. Examination may reveal a short neck and restriction of head movement and the diagnosis is confirmed by x-ray studies. Myelography, CT, and MRI are useful in defining the relationships of the neuronal and structural tissues.

TREATMENT. Immobilization of the neck may be usefull for patients with minor degrees of impairment. If the dysfunction is progressive or is already severe, decompression of the craniovertebral border may be indicated. If hydrocephalus is found, CSF drainage with a ventriculoperitoneal or ventriculoatrial shunt may stabilize or reverse the neurologic dysfunction. In other cases, the distortion and direct compression of the cervicomedullary junction must be relieved by anterior or posterior surgical decompression of this region. Often a bony fusion is also necessary. If a syrinx or hydromyelia is present, drainage and shunting may be required.

Degenerative Disease of the Intervertebral Disc

Degenerative disease of the intervertebral disc is one of the most common, yet one of the least understood and often one of the most mistreated, disorders of the spine (see Chap. 43). Although many patients have benefited from removal of herniated portions of an intervertebral disc compressing neural tissue, too many have been crippled by ill-advised operation for symptoms mistakenly interpreted as being due to this same cause. Just as not all right lower quadrant abdominal pain is caused by appendicitis, not all neck and low back pain is caused by surgical disease of the intervertebral disc.

ANATOMY. The intervertebral disc is well suited for its task of supporting and cushioning considerable weight while still allowing flexibility of the spine. It is classically and practically described as consisting of two parts: a tough yet slightly flexible outer ring, the annulus fibrosis, which joins the periphery of adjacent vertebral bodies to one another; and a semisolid center, the nucleus pulposus, interposed between the hyaline cartilage faces of the vertebral bodies. The anterior and posterior longitudinal ligaments reinforce the disc on their respective sides and extend the entire length of the spine. Actually, the intervertebral disc is a composite structure in which three zones grading into one another may be recognized. The outer zone, which may be regarded as the capsule, is composed of lamellae of interlacing bundles of fibrous tissue that blend with the longitudinal ligaments. Beneath this fibrous capsule and intimately adherent to it lies a thick envelope of fibrocartilage that in turn surrounds and attaches to the less dense nucleus pulposus. The latter substance is composed primarily of collagenous fibrils and cartilage cells suspended in a fluid matrix. In younger persons remnants of the notochord may be found here as well. Motion between vertebral bodies is allowed by the flexibility of the outer layers, the more fluid center responding to variations in weight distribution by flowing into areas of least pressure within the confines of the annulus.

ETIOLOGY AND PATHOLOGY. Although the intervertebral disc may be damaged by infection, collagen disease, and severe trauma, it is, in comparison with other weight-bearing structures, particularly liable to early degenerative changes. Knowledge of the basic cause of this deterioration, which secondarily involves surrounding bone as well, is lacking, but it is at least presumably in part a response to the trauma of daily normal activity. It is more prevalent in men than in women and in laborers than in sedentary workers. Degenerative changes occur most frequently in portions of the spine where there is a transition between a relatively mobile segment and a less mobile one, namely, in the lower cervical and lower lumbar region. This distribution again implicates trauma as a causative factor, since there is relatively more motion and therefore more stress at these levels.

Pathologically there is thinning of the fibrous layers of the annulus, destruction of fibrocartilage, and dehydration of the nucleus pulposus. The interspace becomes narrowed, and there is frequently new bone formation (osteoarthritis) at the margins of the interspace. These changes often remain relatively asymptomatic, producing only transient local pain and the progressive loss of spine mobility usually taken as a matter of course with advancing age. Under certain circumstances, however, essentially the same degenerative processes may have more serious consequences. The nucleus pulposus may herniate through the weakened annulus and/or large bony spurs may develop to project into the vertebral foramina. Of the two processes, herniation of the nucleus pulposus is a much more common cause of neurologic dysfunction and occurs at an earlier age. Approximately three-quarters of symptomatic herniations of the nucleus pulposus occur between the ages of thirty and fifty years. Neurologic disability resulting from osteoarthritis occurs predominantly in the individuals fifty years of age or older.

The effects of herniation of the nucleus pulposus depend on its location, both in respect to the transverse plane and the disc involved, its size, rate of development, and individual differences in surrounding structures. Herniation of the nucleus pulposis through the annulus may be asymptomatic. It most commonly occurs at its weakest portion just lateral to the posterior longitudinal ligament near the intervertebral foramen. Herniation into the center of the vertebral canal is relatively uncommon. When it does occur, however, it may result in compression of the spinal cord or of multiple nerve roots if it is below the conus medullaris. The size of the herniated mass varies considerably; it ranges from a protrusion still covered by thinned-out annulus to complete extrusion of the nucleus pulposus as well as the fibrocartilage layers of the annulus into the vertebra canal. The largest intervertebral discs are those in the lumbar region, and, as might be expected, the largest herniated masses occur there. Herniations of the same size are better tolerated in the lumbar area than in other regions, since the spinal cord ends at the thoracolumbar junction, and the lumbar vertebral canal and the intervertebral foramina are larger.

Occasionally in response to severe trauma, especially flexion injuries, an acute rupture of the annulus occurs with massive herniation of the nucleus pulposus and immediate onset of severe neurologic deficit. In the vast majority of patients, however, signs and symptoms resulting from herniation of the nucleus pulposus are more chronic. Although patients often relate their disability to a recent event, such as bending, turning, or lifting, they almost invariably also give a history of past neck or back pain with or without symptoms of nerve root compression. Herniation of the nucleus pulposus is therefore usually a gradual and intermittent process. Signs and symptoms appear when surrounding pain-sensitive structures, such as the annulus, longitudinal ligaments, and dura, are stimulated or nervous tissue, usually roots, is compressed. Anatomic and pathologic adjustments then often occur, and the symptoms regress, perhaps to reappear when the mass enlarges or anatomic relationships change.

CLINICAL MANIFESTATIONS. The clinical picture produced by the common posterolateral disc herniation is characteristic. Diagnosis often can be made by history alone. Signs and symptoms are primarily those of extradural mass: pain over the distribution of the nerve root involved and evidence of lower motor neuron functional loss. Complaints of sensory disturbance over the peripheral distribution of the nerve root involved is commonly of a "pins and needles" type or just a slightly numb feeling. While weakness may be a symptom, it is much less common. The other root signs are loss or decrease in the deep tendon reflex and weakness and atrophy. Examination of the involved area of the spine reveals muscle spasm that may cause loss of normal lumbar or cervical lordosis. In lumbar lesions scoliosis is frequently present, the convexity usually occurring on the side of the lesion. Motion in the affected portion of the spine is limited and painful, especially on lateral flexion toward the lesion. Palpation over the major nerve trunks produces pain. Maneuvers such as straight-leg raising that increase the tension of the nerve roots are painful.

DIAGNOSTIC FINDINGS. Plain x-rays may be normal or reveal distortion of alignment of the spine produced by muscle spasm. They may, however, show narrowing of the interspace, lipping of the margins of the vertebral bodies bordering on the disc, and osteoarthritic spurs. X-rays also serve to rule out bone erosion that may be present with spinal neoplasms and congenital bony anomalies such as spondylolisthesis. CT defines the cross-sectional diameter of the spinal canal including osteoarthritic and facet hypertrophy encroachment on the spinal canal and intervertebral foramen. In cases of myelopathy secondary to stenosis, CT scans both can be diagnostic and can outline, in combination with positive contrast, the extent of spinal cord compression. The later-generation CT scanners can be used to diagnose ruptures of intervertebral discs. Myelography or high-resolution MRI is often recommended to complement CT so that an intraspinal tumor is not inadvertently misdiagnosed as a disc herniation.

HERNIATED LUMBAR DISC

The highest incidence of symptomatic herniation of the intervertebral disc is in the lumbar region. Ninety-five percent of lumbar herniations occur at the last two interspaces. The relative frequencies of herniations at these two interspaces are approximately equal. Most of the remainder of the herniated lumbar intervertebral discs occur at the third lumbar interspace. The vast majority of herniations in the lumbar as well as in other locations are unilateral. The disposition of the nerve roots in the lumbar space is such that posterolateral herniation does not usually compress the nerve existing at the corresponding intervertebral foramen but rather impinges on the root that crosses the disc in its course of the foramen immediately caudad.

CLINICAL MANIFESTATIONS. Herniation at the interspace between the fourth and fifth lumbar vertebral bodies usually compresses the fifth lumbar roots, and herniation at the disc located at the lumbosacral junction produces signs and symptoms referable to the first sacral roots. The fifth lumbar root serves as a major supply to the anterior crural muscles, which dorsiflex the foot, and the peroneal muscles, which evert and plantar-flex the foot. The dermatome served by the fifth lumbar root includes the anterolateral aspect of the leg and crosses anteriorly at the ankle to supply the medial aspect of the foot including its dorsum. Compression of the fifth nerve root by a herniated nucleus pulposus may produce a foot drop. Usually the motor deficit is less severe and the most common finding is weakness of dorsiflexion of the great toe. Hypesthesia and hypalgesia are usually most evident on the dorsum of the foot between the great and second toes. The first sacral nerve root supplies some innervation to the gluteal and hamstring muscles but gives a large supply to the muscles of the calf and the small muscles of the foot. Its sensory distribution covers a narrow strip on the posterior aspect of the leg and the lateral aspect of the foot. Weakness may be brought out by having patients attempt to walk on their toes. In addition, the ankle reflex is diminished or absent, and sensory deficit is found on the lateral aspect of the foot.

TREATMENT. For the majority of patients with herniated lumbar intervertebral discs the appropriate treatment includes a regimen of strict bed rest on a firm mattress, local heat, and analgesics. Pain usually subsides in 1 to 2 weeks, and the patient may then be mobilized and started on a graded program of exercises designed to strengthen the back musculature. The patient should be instructed to refrain from heavy lifting and from activities that involve sudden bending or twisting of the lumbar spine. Early operation is reserved for those patients who have evidence of major neurologic dysfunction such as a foot drop or bowel and bladder disturbances that indicate a massive disc protrusion. If the patient has not responded to conservative management in a few weeks or is losing considerable time from work each year from repetitive episodes, operation should be considered. Back pain alone is not an indication for operation. The aim of the operation, done through a partial hemilaminectomy, is to relieve nerve root compression by excision of the mass of herniated nucleus pulposus. Relief of signs and symptoms referable to such compression is usual, but many of the patients have residual low back pain or a phantom of the previous radiculopathy. In our experience, fusion of the vertebrae does not often prevent postoperative back pain.

HERNIATED CERVICAL DISC

The lower cervical region is the next most common site of herniated discs. Approximately 90 percent of the herniations in this region occur at the interspaces between C_5 and C_6 and between C_6 and C_7 with the lower level predominating. In contrast with the lower lumbar region, cervical nerve roots are short and almost horizontal.

CLINICAL MANIFESTATIONS. Relatively small herniations are often symptomatic, usually lying just beneath the corresponding roots as they enter the intervertebral foramen. It is fortunate that large or medially placed herniations are rare, for when they do occur, they often result in quadriparesis.

With lateral herniations at the lower cervical levels, patients complain of neck pain radiating into the corresponding shoulder and arm. Referred interscapular pain is common. Localization of the compressed roots by history and physical signs is important. Compression of the sixth cervical roots by posterolateral herniation at the C_5–C_6 interspace usually results in clinically evident weakness of the biceps muscle, depression or absence of the biceps

tendon reflex, and sensory loss on the dorsal and lateral aspect of the thumb and radial aspect of the hand often including the index finger. The syndrome of the seventh cervical roots includes weakness of the triceps muscle and wrist extensors, decrease or absence of the triceps reflex, and sensory deficit of the distal portions of the corresponding dermatome, which is medial to that of the sixth cervical dermatome. It usually includes both the dorsal and palmar aspects of the index and middle fingers.

TREATMENT. The rationale of treatment of cervical disc herniation is similar to that in the lumbar region. Signs and symptoms in the majority of patients will regress with conservative management. Operation is indicated only in patients with evidence of spinal cord compression and those with root compression not responding to conservative measures. Central herniations are best removed through the interspace from the anterior aspect of the spine. The common lateral herniations can be removed effectively either from the same anterior approach or by partial hemilaminectomy.

HERNIATED THORACIC DISC

Disc herniation in the thoracic region is rare. When it does occur, it is usually in the lower thoracic spine and is apt to produce a major neurologic deficit. This lesion may be suspected on the basis of a past history of trauma to the thoracic spine, but it is usually clinically indistinguishable from the more common neoplasms occurring in this region. Diagnosis is made by x-ray studies. There may be narrowing of an interspace and, in contrast to disc disease in other regions, calcification in the interspace. Myelography complemented with CT is essential for diagnosis. MRI promises to be a useful tool for evaluating thoracic myelopathy. Results of operation by the classic approach, i.e., laminectomy, are in general poor with no improvement or with increased deficit in about one-half of the patients reported in larger series. The reasons for these poor results include the fact that most of these lesions are anterior to the cord and are firm and partially calcified. Their removal with a posterior exposure therefore often necessitates major retraction of an already compressed spinal cord. Removal of the herniated disc by approach through the interspace, either by removing the adjacent ribs and transverse processes or by going through the chest cavity, has been more effective in relieving the myelopathy and safer.

SPONDYLOSIS

Hypertrophic bone changes are not infrequently associated with disc herniation even in younger individuals. They are especially prevalent in cervical herniations in which spurs of bone projecting into the intervertebral foramina are often a contributing cause of nerve root compression. In relation to its almost uniform presence in the elderly, hypertrophic bony change alone as a cause of significant neurologic dysfunction is uncommon. However, in some patients with advanced hypertrophic bone disease of the cervical spine, often termed *spondylosis,* major spinal cord and nerve root dysfunction develop.

This entity, which usually affects two or more lower cervical interspaces, is characterized by narrowing of the interspaces and extensive bony proliferation on the lips of the vertebral bodies adjacent to the discs, producing transverse ridges that project into the vertebral canal. The corresponding intervertebral foramina are narrowed, and in advanced disease minor degrees of subluxation of one vertebra on another may exist.

Why many persons tolerate advanced cervical spondylosis without significant disability while in others a severe spastic quadriparesis may develop is largely unknown. It has been demonstrated that a greater number of patients with symptomatic spondylosis have congenitally narrow cervical vertebral canals than those without spinal cord signs. A simple compressive mechanism, however, does not entirely suffice to explain the problem, since return of function often does not follow seemingly adequate decompression that includes extensive laminectomy combined with removal of bony spurs and fusion from the anterior approach. Chronic vascular insufficiency resulting from a combination of such factors as arteriosclerosis, compression of a long segment of spinal cord, and compression of the arterial supply entering through the intervertebral foramina may in part explain these sometimes disappointing results. Irreversible neuronal loss from long-standing myelopathy may also contribute to lack of improvement following surgery.

CLINICAL MANIFESTATIONS. The clinical picture of symptomatic cervical spondylosis varies considerably. Neck pain radiating bilaterally into the shoulders is frequently but not invariably present. Examination reveals evidence of compression of multiple cervical nerve roots and signs of cervical spinal cord compression. The course of the disease is also variable. Occasionally there is rapid progression that may lead to a severe spastic quadriparesis within a year or less. More often the onset of signs is insidious, and progression is slow. Spontaneous regression of neurologic deficit is rare, but on the other hand progression of deficit may halt at any point.

TREATMENT. Surgical therapy is reserved for those patients who have persistent or progressive pain or neurologic deficit believed to be caused by spondylitic disease. Surgical decompression of the cord and roots may be performed by a posterior or anterior approach. Selection of the procedure to be performed is based on the patient's neurologic deficit, the morbid anatomy, and the number of spinal levels involved. Despite surgical relief of cord compression, about a third of all patients with cervical myelopathy continue to progress. Another third will experience neurologic stabilization, while the remaining patients may improve.

PEDIATRIC NEUROSURGERY

Children with neurologic and cranial disorders present in most instances a distinct group of problems. The presentation, examination, and care of the young further require different approaches as one progresses from the fetus to the preterm infant, neonate, toddler, and school-aged child. The patterns of the adolescent, in terms of presentation and range of disease processes, more closely follow those of the young adult than those of the child.

FETUS. Aggressive high-risk obstetrics and real-time ultrasound have provided a means for the diagnosis and treatment of a wide range of congenital lesions of the nervous system including hydrocephalus, dysraphism, and other brain anomalies. Decisions regarding the fetus with congenital CNS anomalies may now be made before birth, with several options available to the parent. Previous to these capabilities, such problems required that decision in most instances be made in the delivery room or during the immediate newborn period.

With prenatal diagnosis, potential options include termination of the pregnancy, early delivery, fetal shunting, cephalocentesis, or no intervention. Which option is chosen is dependent upon the particular findings of a case and parental decision. As yet, no data exist as to improved outcome with aggressive fetal therapy for hydrocephalus or early delivery and shunting.

PRETERM INFANT. The preterm (PT) infant weighing less than 1500 g has a 40 percent risk of intraventricular hemorrhage (IVH), and the PT weighing less than 1250 g has a 50 percent incidence of IVH. Bleeding occurs in most instances in the germinal matrix region, which by this point in development represents a watershed area of cerebral blood flow. Such hemorrhage has significant influence on the infant's neurodevelopmental outcome.

Diagnosis was carried out earlier by CT scan and more recently by real-time ultrasound. The incidence of hydrocephalus requiring shunting varies considerably from center to center. The use of serial ultrasounds and lumbar punctures appears to decrease dramatically the incidence of hydrocephalus requiring shunt. Some of the PT infants may block their aqueduct with clot and require earlier shunting. More frequently, communicating hydrocephalus develops from the decreased absorption of CSF at the level of the arachnoid granulations. With time, in the majority of these children, the error in CSF absorption diminishes and the hydrocephalus resolves.

INFANT. For the PT and full-term infant, neurologic evaluation in a meaningful fashion is quite different from that of the older child and adult. Initially, the only cortical function observed is whether the infant is able to fix and follow a visual stimulus. The remainder of the examination is subcortical. Several pediatric neurology texts detail the examination in this age group. For brief repetitive objective examinations by all levels of personnel, the Neonatal Arousal Scale is useful. The scale is based on the infant's response to sound, light, and motor response and may be used from 26 to 52 weeks postconceptual age (Table 42-5).

Pediatric neurosurgery in this group is primarily directed toward congenital anomalies, although acquired disorders may rapidly appear that would include posthemorrhagic hydrocephalus, subdural hematoma, and depressed fractures. Additionally, occasional tumors may present very early.

Myelomeningocele. Dysraphisms along the entire neuraxis may occur. Myelomeningocele is the most common

Table 42-5. NEONATAL AROUSAL SCALE

Best response to bell	
Facial and extremity movements	5
Grimaces/blinks	4
Increase in RR/HR	3
Seizures/extensor posturing	2
No response	1
Best response to light	
Blink and facial/extremity movements	4
Blink	3
Seizures/extensor posturing	2
No response	1
Best motor response	
Spontaneous	
Periods of activity alternating with sleep	6
Occasional spontaneous movements	5
Sternal rub	
Extremity movements	4
Grimace/facial movements	3
Seizures/extensor posturing	2
No response	1
Total	3–15

SOURCE: Copyright 1980 Charles Cecil Duncan, MD, and Laura Rowe Ment, MD.

of these and provides an approach to these disorders. With myelomeningocele an incomplete closure of the neural tube occurs between 21 and 25 days postconception. Diagnosis in early stages of pregnancy may be suspected by an elevated maternal serum alpha-fetoprotein (AFP) or diagnosed with amniocentesis and AFP measurement or real-time ultrasound. Hydrocephalus occurs in 80 to 90 percent of cases, with the exception of the lipomyelomeningocele where hydrocephalus occurs only rarely. Virtually 100 percent of patients with myelomeningocele have Arnold Chiari Type II malformations as well, which means that the structures of the posterior fossa are caudally displaced, such that the cerebellar tonsils, medulla, and IV ventricle are in the cervical canal.

Treatment of these patients has been the subject of extended controversy in neurosurgical literature for many years. The accepted approach for most pediatric neurosurgeons in the United States is for aggressive treatment if there is any significant chance for survival. Closure of the back does not improve lower extremity function. Rather, it protects the neural placode and the nervous system from mechanical trauma and infection. The neurodevelopmental outcome of children with myelomeningocele is significantly better than that of unselected cases of hydrocephalus. The care of patients with myelomeningocele is a multidisciplinary approach that must continue throughout the patient's life.

Craniosynostosis. Abnormalities of head shape, or craniosynostoses, are also recognized in the early postnatal weeks. The development of a normal head shape requires two primary factors. The first is the growth of normal brain beneath the skull, and the second is functional cranial sutures that permit increase in head size. When craniosynostosis occurs, the brain continues to grow but not in the place of the abnormal suture. Total craniosynostosis is quite rare. Other causes of microcephaly are far more common and result from lack of brain growth. Urgent opening of the suture is required in the rare case of total craniosynostosis.

For the more usual cases of metopic, sagittal, coronal, and lambdoidal synostosis, the appearance of the infant's head usually yields the diagnosis. Plane films show the anomalous suture in less than half the cases. Although other investigations, including xeroradiographs and bone scans, may be advocated for diagnosis, the clinical evaluation is the most reliable. With coronal and lambdoidal synostosis, sutures in the skull base are more likely to be involved than with sagittal synostosis.

Patients with sagittal synostosis have very long, narrow heads and usually a prominent ridge along the saggital suture. Coronal synostosis presents with a narrow anterior portion of the cranial vault and orbits that are angled such that their lateral portion is much more posterior then the medial. Metopic synostosis presents with a similar picture and a prominent midline forehead ridge. Lambdoidal synostosis presents with the ipsilateral occipital being quite flat, the ear on that side protruding and anteriorly placed with respect to the contralateral. As well, the ipsilateral forehead protrudes more than the opposite side. Therapy is directed toward providing an artificial suture in the form of a linear craniectomy coated with silastic film and maximal time for brain growth to reshape the head. Coronal and metopic synostosis, which frequently involves the anterior skull base, requires forward displacement of the lateral superior orbital rims for a good cosmetic result.

Operations such as these for a single fused suture are basically for appearance. In order for the surgery to be as effective as possible, the operation should be carried out quite early in life. As a result, major surgery is carried out in infants on an elective basis. Such operations should be done with maximally experienced anesthesia, pediatric, and pediatric neurosurgical personnel to assure that the safest procedure possible is being done.

Further complex varieties of craniofacial anomalies and incompletely treated patients with simpler synostosis at an older age are beyond the scope of this discussion and frequently require specialized multidisciplinary operative teams.

YOUNG CHILDREN. Trauma. Trauma is the most frequently encountered neurosurgical problem in this age group. Preventive measures, such as suitable restraints for automobiles, instruction regarding roadways, household and play safety, bicycle helmets, and the identification of children at risk for abuse, are far more effective lifesaving maneuvers than any particular neurosurgical intervention.

Formal neurologic examination of this group theoretically should be like that of older individuals, but it must be couched in play and patience to be effective. With a few notable exceptions, disease processes of a congenital origin will continue to be found in younger adults. Similarly, some symptoms in patients of this age group are quite different from those of older and younger individuals.

Trauma in the young presents three major distinctions from older populations. In this group head injury is likely to be a cause of shock. The intracranial compartment with a partially closed head with a fontanelle that may bulge and sutures that will separate is sufficient to contain enough blood to result in hypovolemic shock. CT has provided a means for rapid accurate assessment of intracranial pathology. In the instance of trauma even with a widely open fontanelle, real-time ultrasound is not an appropriate diagnostic approach because of the difficulty of visualizing peripheral lesions. A second distinction is the relation of skull fracture to subsequent intracranial pathology. With the malleability of the young skull, dural vessels, for example, may be torn and other significant intracranial injury can occur without fracture. As well, detailed neurologic examination may be very difficult to carry out following head injury. As a consequence, most children sustaining loss or alteration of level of consciousness should be carefully observed in hospital. The third distinction relates to child abuse. Any child who has an injury the cause of which is not clearly understood should be considered as having sustained potential abuse. Care should involve clarifying the mechanism of injury, checking for associated recent or old injury, and giving appropriate follow-up.

Tumors. In this age group headache should be considered the most dramatically different symptom from older populations. While in adolescents and adults this may be one of the most frequently found complaints, in young children such a complaint requires serious consideration. With the availability of computerized axial tomography, appropriate work-up may be carried out with minimal risk and reasonable expense. Tumors in this age group usually present as headache and not as seizure. As the children become older, seizure becomes a more likely presenting symptom. Conversely, seizure was rarely thought to be a heralding event for an intracranial structural lesion in the young. However, as computerized axial tomography has become widely available, far more structural lesions in this age group are found than were previously expected.

Tumors tend to be midline. These include medulloblastoma and ependymoma in the IV ventricle and pinealomas, craniopharyngiomas, and neuroentodermal tumors supratentorially. Other tumors may present laterally. Choroid plexus papilloma, which is the classic example for the overproduction of CSF, usually occurs in the lateral ventricle. A vast variety of other intracranial masses also occur.

Vascular malformations and aneurysms occur in these age groups as well. The general approach is as in older individuals. Aneurysms, while unusual at this age, may have a tendency toward a higher and more rapid rebleed rate that encourages earlier operative care.

OLDER CHILDREN AND ADOLESCENTS. From the surgical standpoint the care of these patients begins to approach that of the young adult. Dealing with the adolescent and older school-aged child may be quite difficult. The problem is not so much a different category of diseases, or a different type of neurologic examination; instead, the problem is how to deal with these patients on an appropriate level such that trust, honesty, and rapport are developed.

Reye syndrome is the most significant distinctive disease process in this age group. It frequently follows a recent or resolving viral illness, especially chicken pox or influenza B, and is characterized by an altered level of consciousness with elevated values of arterial ammonia. When the altered level of consciousness approaches coma, aggressive control of the intracranial pressure is required.

Hydrocephalus

Much of pediatric neurosurgery deals with the shunt for hydrocephalus. In a number of large hospitals in the United States the shunt is likely to be the second or third most commonly performed operation in the hospital. Similarly, the children requiring this care are likely to be inpatients in essentially all of the age groups of the pediatric service. Hydrocephalus is not a primary problem; rather it is a second-order manifestation of some other process. The primary processes include aqueductal stenosis, dysfunction of the arachnoidal granulation, scarring of the subarachnoid spaces over the cerebral convexities or base, block of the flow of CSF by tumor, and overproduction of CSF from a choroid plexus papilloma. Situations such as arachnoidal granulation, dysfunction, and scarring of the subarachnoid spaces may result from bleeding, infections, or tumor. Enlargement of the ventricular system to produce hydrocephalus is the result of these processes.

By convention hydrocephalus has been divided into two broad categories: communicating and noncommunicating hydrocephalus. In noncommunicating hydrocephalus there is an obstruction to the flow of CSF from inside the ventricular system. In communicating hydrocephalus the obstruction is outside the ventricular system.

In most instances, therapy of hydrocephalus requires the placement of a pressure-regulated shunt system. This consists of the insertion of a catheter into the ventricular system, a valve, and a distal catheter to an area where CSF is absorbed. A wide range of distal sites have been tried and used. At the present time most shunts are ventricular-peritoneal. The distal catheter lies free in the peritoneal cavity where fluid absorption takes place.

Shunt systems have many disadvantages, but none can compare with the usual devastation of untreated hydrocephalus. The shunt crosses enormous anatomic barriers, the plastic does not grow, and the valve system treats a volume transfer problem by pressure regulation. These situations indicate the need for continued care of these patients as well as the need for advances in treatment modalities.

The outcome of these patients has steadily improved over the past two decades. Follow-up studies carried out in the 1960s indicated that approximately one-third of these children would have a normal intelligence. Follow-up studies in the 1970s indicated that close to two-thirds may have a normal intelligence. In the 1980s follow-up studies indicate that these children have a mean IQ of 90 ± 19. These figures are significantly below the general population. Some of these children do very poorly and may require special education; some are very bright. Overall shunted patients do not perform as well in sibling matched control groups. To some extent how well an individual performs depends upon the basic disease process. Performance also depends on several variables such as the prevention of ventriculitis and maintenance of shunt function.

NEUROPSYCHOLOGY

CLINICAL NEUROPSYCHOLOGIC EXAMINATION. Traditional neuropsychologic examination is essentially a refined mental status examination, but methods are strictly standardized, data are quantified, and evaluation is through statistical contrast with normative standards for nonpatient and patient populations. These techniques exploit the lateralized cerebral dominance for motor and sensory processes, language and language-mediated memory and intellectual functions, and nonverbal memory and intellectual functions to localize focal CNS dysfunction. Through consultation of normative standards, absolute levels of performance can be established as well, facilitating examination of patients with diffuse or mild CNS dysfunction. Neuropsychologic examination has diagnostic utility when the nature of a disease process prevents its identification by diagnostic imaging techniques. Examples of such diseases include epilepsy, normal pressure hydrocephalus, and degenerative diseases. Examination before and after surgery is also useful in determining the functional recovery of the patient and establishing the morbidity of the surgical procedure.

Familiar examples of traditional assessment materials include the IQ examination and MMPI. These measures, derived from standard clinical psychologic practices, are often supplemented by procedures used more routinely in cognitive and psychophysiologic psychology (e.g., binocular viewing, dichotic listening, and electrophysiologic techniques). When determination of surgical risks is contingent upon the identification of the memory capacities exclusive of one hemisphere, language dominance or the location of centers mediating specific language functions within the dominant hemisphere, the intracarotid amytal procedure and/or intraoperative stimulation are conducted.

REMEDIATION. Impaired higher cortical functioning often follows CNS diseases and their surgical treatment. Some spontaneous recovery is almost always noted. Persisting liabilities may be addressed through techniques that exploit functional areas of brain in the performance of those that are impaired.

This practice, referred to as "cognitive remediation," has been divided into three subtypes. Type I techniques

are directed toward development of formal intellectual processes (e.g., deductive and inductive reasoning) and executive capabilities (e.g., organization, self-monitoring). Type II techniques address specific behavioral systems (e.g., attention deployment, visuomotor skills, perception, memory, communication). Type III techniques focus upon aspects of specific behaviors that require development. A wide range of rehabilitation personnel may be involved in the development and instruction of these restorative techniques. Deficits in motor control are the province of physical therapists. Speech therapists address disorders of speech and language. Perceptual and intellectual abilities required for activities of daily living (e.g., balancing a checkbook, planning meals) are typically addressed by the occupational therapist. A broader range of intellectual disturbances, disorders of memory, and emotional or behavioral problems are addressed by the neuropsychologist.

The treatment of some central nervous system diseases may result in significant improvements in higher cortical functioning. However, such gains may not themselves lead to improved adaptive functioning. Long-standing diseases may be associated directly or indirectly with personality disorders and a restricted range of social or occupational skills. When these deficiencies are targeted through cognitive remediation and psychotherapy, improved neurologic functioning may more often result in improved adaptive functioning.

Bibliography

General Considerations

Dooms GC, Hecht S, et al: Brain radiation lesions: MR imaging. *Radiology* 158:149, 1986.

Daniels DL, Pech P, et al: Magnetic resonance imaging of the cavernous sinus. *AJR* 144:1009, 1985.

Jefferson G: *Selected Papers*. London, Pitman Medical Publications, 1960.

Kelly PJ, Kall BA, et al: Computer-assisted stereotaxic laser resection of intra-axial brain neoplasms. *J Neurosurg* 64:427, 1986.

Mullan S: *Essentials of Neurosurgery*. New York, Springer, 1961.

Naidich TP, Tomita T, et al: Direct coronal computer tomography for presurgical evaluation of posterior possa tumors. *J Comput Assist Tomogr* 9:1065, 1985.

Plum F, Posner J: *The Diagnosis of Stupor and Coma*. Philadelphia, FA Davis, 1972.

Head Injury, Mechanisms of Injury, Care of Head-Injured Patient

Adams JH: *The Neuropathology of Head Trauma: Handbook of Clinical Neurology*. Amsterdam, North-Holland, 1975, pp. 35–65.

Jennett B, Teasdale G, et al: Severe head injuries in three countries. *J Neurol Neurosurg Psychiatry* 40:291, 1977.

Johnson RT, Yates PO: Brain stem haemorrhages in expanding supratentorial conditions. *Acta Radiol (Stockh)* 46:250, 1956.

Langfitt TW, Gennarelli T: Can the outcome from head injury be improved? *J Neurosurg* 56:19, 1982.

Lindenberg R: Compression of brain arteries as a pathogenetic factor for tissue necroses and their areas of predilection. *J Neuropathol Exp Neurol* 14:223, 1955.

Miller JD, Butterworth JF, et al: Further experience in the management of severe head injury. *J Neurosurg* 54:304, 1981.

Piepmeier JM, Wagner FC: Delayed post-traumatic extracerebral hematomas. *J Trauma* 22:455, 1982.

Ward AA: Physiological basis of concussion. *J Neurosurg* 15:129, 1958.

Young B, Rapp RP, et al: Early prediction of outcome in head-injured patients. *J Neurosurg* 54:300, 1981.

Spinal Cord Injuries

DeLaTorre JC: Spinal cord injury: Review of basic and applied research. *Spine* 6:315, 1981.

Norrell H: The early management of spinal injuries. *Clin Neurosurg* 27:385, 1980.

Piepmeier JM: The management of the cervical fracture, in Long D (ed): *Current Therapy in Neurological Surgery*. BC Decker, 1985.

Piepmeier JM, Thibodeau L: Spinal cord injury research: Pathways for the future in Mall K (ed): *Advances in Trauma*. Chicago, Year Book Medical Publishers, 1986.

Schneider RC, Crosby EC, et al: Traumatic spinal cord syndromes and their management. *Clin Neurosurg* 20:424, 1973.

Wagner FC: Management of acute spinal cord injury. *Surg Neurol* 7:346, 1977.

Young JS, Dexter WR: Neurological recovery distal to the zone of injury in 172 cases of closed traumatic spinal cord injury. *Paraplegia* 16:39, 1978–1979.

Peripheral Nerve Injuries

Lyons WR, Woodhall B: *Atlas of Peripheral Nerve Injuries*. Philadelphia, Saunders, 1949.

Millese H, Meissl G, Berger A: Further experiences with interfascicular grafting of the median, ulnar and radial nerves. *J Bone Joint Surg* 58-A:209, 1976.

Smith JW: Microsurgery of peripheral nerves. *Plast Reconstr Surg* 33:317, 1964.

Sunderland S: Advances in diagnosis and treatment of root and peripheral nerve injury. *Adv Neurol* 22:271, 1979.

Woodhall B: Surgical repair of acute peripheral nerve injury. *Surg Clin North Am* 30:1369, 1951.

Young JZ: The functional repair of nervous tissue. *Physiol Rev* 22:318, 1942.

Brain Tumors

Kernohan JW, Sayre GP: *Tumors of the Central Nervous System*, sec X, fasicles 35, 37. Washington, Armed Forces Institute of Pathology, 1952.

Rose F, Fields W (eds): *Neuro-oncology*. Basel, Karger, 1985.

Russell D, Rubenstein L: *Pathology of Tumors of the Nervous System*. Baltimore, Williams & Wilkins, 1963.

Vick N, Bigner D (eds): *Symposium on Neuro-oncology, Neurologic Clinics*. Philadelphia, Saunders, 1985.

Pituitary Tumors

Felig P, Baxter J, Broadus A, Frohman L (eds): *Endocrinology and Metabolism*, 2d ed. New York, McGraw-Hill, 1987.

Martin JB: *Clinical Neuroendocrinology*. Philadelphia, FA Davis, 1977.

Tindall GT, Collins WF: *Clinical Management of Pituitary Disorders*. New York, Raven, 1979.

Spinal Tumors

Dodge HW Jr, Keith HM, Campagna MJ: Intraspinal tumors in infants and children. *J Int Coll Surg* 26:199, 1957.

Garrido E, Stein B: Microsurgical removal of intramedullary spinal cord tumors. *Surg Neurol* 7:215, 1977.

Kennady JC, Stern WE: Metastatic neoplasms of the vertebral column producing compression of the spinal cord. *Am J Surg* 104:155, 1962.

Sundaresan N, DiGiacinto G, Hughes J: Surgical treatment of spinal metastases. *Clin Neurosurg* 33:503, 1985.

Woltman HW, Kernohan JW, et al: Intramedullary tumors of spinal cord and gliomas of intradural portion of filum terminale. *Arch Neurol Psychiatry* 65:378, 1951.

Surgical Aspects of Central Nervous System Infections

Evans W: The pathology and aetiology of brain abscess. *Lancet* 1:1231, 1931.

Vascular Disease of the Nervous System

Blackwood W et al (eds): *Greenfield's Neuropathology*. Baltimore, Williams & Wilkins, 1963, chap 2.

Boysen G: Cerebral hemodynamics in carotid surgery. *Acta Neurol Scand* 52(suppl):1, 1973.

Crawford T: Some observations on the pathogenesis and natural history of intracranial aneurysms. *J Neurol Neurosurg Psychiatry* 22:259, 1959.

Drake CG: Progress in cerebrovascular disease. Management of cerebral aneurysm. *Stroke* 12:273, 1981.

EC/IC Bypass Study Group: Failure of extracranial-intracranial arterial bypass to reduce the risk of ischemic stroke: Results of an international randomized trial. *N Engl J Med* 313:1191, 1985.

Meyer FB, Piepgras DG, et al: Emergency embolectomy for acute emboli occlusion of the middle cerebral artery, in Little JR (ed): *Clinical Neurosurgery*. Baltimore, Williams & Wilkins, 1984, vol 32, chap 9.

Millikan CH, McDowell FH: Progress in cerebrovascular disease. Treatment of progressing stroke. *Stroke* 12:397, 1981.

Moskowitz MA, Coughlin SR: Current concepts of cerebrovascular disease—Stroke: Clinical applications of prostaglandins and their inhibitors. *Stroke* 12:882, 1981.

Report on the cooperative study of intracranial aneurysms. *J Neurosurg* 24:782, 24:789, 24:792, 24:807, 24:922, 24:1034, 25:98, 25:219, 25:321, 25:467, 25:574, 25:593, 25:660, 25:683, 1966.

Russell DS: The pathology of spontaneous intracranial hemorrhage. *Proc R Soc Med* 47:689, 1954.

Sundt TM, Kobayashi S, et al: Results and complications of surgical management of 809 intracranial aneurysms in 722 cases. Related and unrelated to grade of patient, type of aneurysm, and timing of surgery. *J Neurosurg* 56:753, 1982.

Sundt TM, Sharbrough FW, et al: Correlation of cerebral blood flow and electroencephalographic changes during carotid endarterectomy: With results of surgery and hemodynamics of cerebral ischemia. *Mayo Clin Proc* 56:533, 1981.

Yasargil MD: *Microneurosurgery Applied to Neurosurgery*. New York, Academic, 1969.

Yoshimoto T, Ogawa A, et al: Clinical course of acute middle cerebral artery occlusion. *J Neurosurg* 65:326, 1986.

The Surgery of Epilepsy

Bailey P, Gibbs FA: The surgical treatment of psychomotor epilepsy. *JAMA* 145:365, 1951.

Commission for the Control of Epilepsy and Its Consequences: Plan for Nationwide Action of Epilepsy, DHEW Publication No. (NIH) 78-311, p 314, 1978.

Goldring S: A method for surgical management of focal epilepsy, especially as it relates to children. *J Neurosurg* 49:344, 1978.

Mattson RH: Value of intensive monitoring, in Wada JA, Penry JK (eds): *Advancement in Epileptology: The Xth Epilepsy International Symposium.* New York, Raven, 1980, pp 43–51.

Penfield W, Jasper H: *Epilepsy and the Functional Anatomy of the Human Brain.* Boston, Little, Brown, 1954.

Rasmussen T: Cortical resection in the treatment of focal epilepsy, in Purpura DP, Penry JK, Walter AD (eds): *Advances in Neurology. Neurosurgical Management of the Epilepsies.* New York, Raven, 1975, vol 8, p 139.

Soloway SS, Williamson PD, et al: Surgery for epilepsy: Role of depth electroencephalography. *Conn Med* 44(2):70, 1980.

Spencer DD, Spencer SS, et al: Intracerebral masses in patients with refractory partial epilepsy. *Neurology* 34:432, 1984.

Spencer DD, Spencer SS, et al: Access to the posterior medial temporal lobe structures in the surgical treatment of temporal lobe epilepsy. *Neurosurgery* 15:667, 1984.

Spencer SS: Depth electroencephalography in selection of refractory epileptic patients. *Ann Neurol* 16:686, 1985.

Spencer SS, Spencer DD, et al: The localizing value of depth electroencephalography in 32 refractory epileptic patients. *Ann Neurol* 12:248, 1982.

vanBuren JM, Ajmone-Marsan C, et al: Surgery of temporal lobe epilepsy, in Purpura DP, Penry JK, Walter RD (eds): *Advances in Neurology. Neurosurgical Management of the Epilepsies.* New York, Raven, 1975, vol 8, p 155.

Wada J: A new method for the determination of the side of cerebral speech dominance. A preliminary report of the intracarotid injection of sodium amytal in man. *Igaku Seibutsugaku (Med Biol)* 14:221, 1949.

Williamson PD: Corpus callosum section for intractable epilepsy: Criteria for patient selection, in Reeves A (ed): *Epilepsy and the Corpus Callosum.* New York, Plenum, 1985.

Intracranial Infections

Booss J, Esiri MM: *Viral Encephalitis: Pathology, Diagnosis, and Management.* Oxford, Blackwell, 1986.

Booss J, Thornton GF: Infectious Diseases of the Central Nervous System. *Neurol Clin* 4:1, 1986.

Klastersky J, Kahan-Coppens L, Brihaye J: Infections in neurosurgery, in Krayenbuhl H (ed): *Advances and Technical Standards in Neurosurgery.* New York, Springer-Verlag, 1979, vol 6.

Mollman HD, Haines SJ: Risk factors for postoperative neurosurgical wound infection. *J Neurosurg* 64:902, 1986.

Thompson RA, Green JR: *Infectious Diseases of the Central Nervous System.* New York, Spectrum, 1984.

Vinken DJ, Bruyn GW: *Infections of the Nervous System,* vol 1; *Handbook of Clinical Neurosurgery,* vol 33. Amsterdam, North Holland, 1978.

Pain

Bessou P, Perl ER: Response of cutaneous sensory units with unmyelinated fibers to noxious stimuli. *J Neurophysiol* 32:1025, 1969.

Bowsher D: Termination of the central pain pathway in man: The conscious appreciation of pain. *Brain* 80:606, 1957.

Jannetta PJ, Sweet WH: Trigeminal neuralgia, in Wilson CB, Hoff JT (eds): *Current Neurosurgery.* New York, Churchill Livingstone, 1980, chap 22.

Keele KD: *Anatomies of Pain.* Oxford, Blackwell, 1957.

Knighton RS, Dumke PR: *Pain.* Boston, Little, Brown, 1966.

Melzack R, Wall P: Pain mechanisms in a new theory. *Science* 150:971, 1965.

Nashold BS Jr, et al: Dorsal root entry zone lesions for pain relief, in Wilkins RR, Rengachary SS (eds): *Neurosurgery.* New York, McGraw-Hill, 1985, chap 328.

Stookey B, Ransohoff J: *Trigeminal Neuralgia: Its History and Treatment.* Springfield IL, Charles C Thomas, 1959.

Wang JS, et al: Pain relief by intrathecally applied morphine in man. *Anesthesiology* 50:149, 1979.

White JC, Sweet WH: *Pain and the Neurosurgeon: A Forty-Year Experience.* Springfield, IL, Charles C Thomas, 1969.

Yaksh TH: Spinal opiate analgesia: Characteristics and principles of action. *Pain* 11:293, 1981.

Young RF, et al: Electrical stimulation of brain in treatment of chronic pain: Experiences over five years. *J Neurosurg* 62:389, 1985.

Structural Abnormalities of the Axial Skeleton

Hinck VC, Sachdev NS: Developmental stenosis of the cervical spinal canal. *Brain* 89:27, 1966.

List CF: Clinical syndromes of craniovertebral anomalies. *Arch Neurol Psychiatry* 45:577, 1941.

Spurling RG: *Lesions of the Lumbar Intervertebral Disc.* Springfield IL, Charles C Thomas, 1953.

Spurling RG: *Lesions of the Cervical Intervertebral Disc.* Springfield IL, Charles C Thomas, 1956.

Wilkinson M: The morbid anatomy of cervical spondylosis and myelopathy. *Brain* 83:589, 1960.

Pediatric Neurosurgery

Epstein F, Hoffman H: *Anomalies of the Developing Nervous System.* Boston, Blackwell Scientific, 1986.

Matson DD: *Neurosurgery of Infancy and Childhood,* 2d ed. Springfield IL, Charles C Thomas, 1969.

McLaurin R, Schut L, et al: *Pediatric Neurosurgery,* 2d ed. Orlando FL, Grune & Stratton, 1987.

Menkes JH: *Textbook of Child Neurology,* 2d ed. Philadelphia, Lea & Febiger, 1980.

Ment LR, Duncan DD: *Perinated Neurocology.* Orlando FL, Grune & Stratton, 1987.

Milhorat TH: *Pediatric Neurosurgery,* Contemporary Neurology Series, vol. 16. Philadelphia, FA Davis, 1978.

Neuropsychology

Ben-Yishay Y: *Working Approaches to Remediation of Cognitive Deficits in Brain Damaged Patients.* New York, New York University Medical Center, IRM Rehabilitation Monograph No. 62, 1981.

Chapter 43

Orthopaedics

Robert B. Duthie and Franklin T. Hoaglund

Manifestations of Musculoskeletal Disorders

PAIN

Pain, defined by Sherrington as "the physical adjunct of an imperative protective reflex," is a sensation one feels when injured. The afferent nociceptive impulses produced by injurious agents stream into the central nervous system, where they are given meaning by the emotional state of the individual based upon the past and present experience.

Anatomy and Physiology

PAINFUL STIMULUS. Stimulation of peripheral receptors by noxious agents produces a spatiotemporal pattern of nervous impulses that is interpreted as pain within the higher cerebral centers. Such patterns of nervous activity may be produced by many physical phenomena such as pressure, puncturing, squeezing, and tension; by alteration in temperature; or by chemical effects, such as the alteration in pH or the concentration of histaminelike substances, serotonin, bradykinin, and other polypeptide compounds. Prostaglandins, particularly E_2, are known to lower the pain threshold for various physical and chemical stimuli. These local hormones are derived from lipid breakdown via arachidonic acid. Inflammation, accompanied by local acidosis, may convert normal stimuli into stimuli with certain patterns of nervous activity that will be interpreted as pain.

SENSORY END ORGANS. Most cutaneous sensory nerve endings are unmyelinated fibers which, when stimulated, may produce sensations of pressure, touch, or pain, depending upon the impulse pattern invoked, rather than the excitation of specific fibers beyond their normal threshold. Similar networks of unmyelinated nerve fibers are found in the walls of blood vessels, particularly arteries, in periosteum, in bone, in synovium, and in joint capsule. In muscles, a similar role is conducted by small myelinated fibers. Cartilage has no sensory end organs.

SENSORY PATHWAYS. The conduction velocity and frequency of impulses in afferent nerve fibers is dependent upon fiber diameter (Table 43-1). The afferent fibers are carried within the peripheral nerves to spinal root ganglia and then to the cord, where they synapse within one or two segments of the dorsal column before crossing the midline to form the contralateral lateral spinothalamic tract. At the site of dorsal column synapse, the pathway of pain fibers is regulated by fibers descending in the ipsilateral corticospinal tract. There is a controlling mechanism acting at every junction at which nerve impulses are relayed from one neuron to the next on their cerebral ascent. Melzack has described five links in the path by which pain reaches the cerebrum (Fig. 43-1):

1. The spinothalamic tract, excitatory in function and carrying the majority of pain impulses.
2. The central tegmental tract, inhibitory in function. Division increases pain sensitivity.
3. The central gray pathway. Division decreases pain sensitivity.
4. The ascending reticular system, which alerts the entire brain.
5. The medial lemniscal tract, for proprioception and light touch.

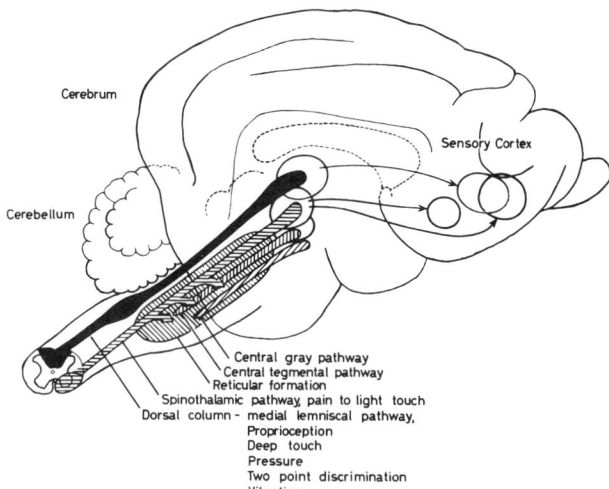

Fig. 43-1. Major pathways along which pain reaches the brain. *(After Melzack, 1961. Taken with permission from Scientific American, 1961.)*

The first three of these pathways are depressed by analgesic agents, while the fifth maintains the function of spatial awareness.

An encephalic neurotransmitter or modulator mechanism inhibits the impulses of the gelatinosa substantiae in the midbrain area. In addition, in the hypothalamus as well as in the intermediate lobe of the pituitary, there is a neurohormone called endorphin that also contains an encephalinlike complex with opiatelike effects.

Characteristics

Pain may be expressed in many ways. A deep boring ache is characteristic of tension, whereas a "burning" pain with paresthesias, especially if accompanied by vasomotor phenomena (sweating or redness), indicates a sympathetic as well as a somatic sensory involvement.

Sites

Pain may be described as localized, diffuse, radicular, or referred.

Local Pain. Local pain is felt at the site of pathologic processes in superficial structures and is usually associated with local tenderness on palpation or percussion.

Diffuse Pain. Diffuse pain appears to be more characteristic of deep-lying tissues and has a more or less segmental distribution.

Radicular Pain. Radicular pain, as seen in sciatica and brachalgia, is characterized by its radiation from the center to the periphery in a strict anatomic sense. It is often associated with paresthesia and tenderness along the nerve root. Clinical examination frequently reveals neurologic deficits such as sensory loss, reflex depression, and muscle paresis or paralysis.

Referred Pain. Referred pain occurs with injury to, or disease affecting, deep structures such as the spine or the

Table 43-1

Type	Velocity	Fiber diameter	Fiber function
A	120 m/s	15–25 μm	Proprioceptive afferents from the skin and joints
B		Less than 2 μm	Unmyelinated pain afferents accompanying sympathetic fibers from muscle and bone
C	10 m/s	5–15 μm	Afferents from muscle and tendon
D			Myelinated fibers in association with visceral nerves

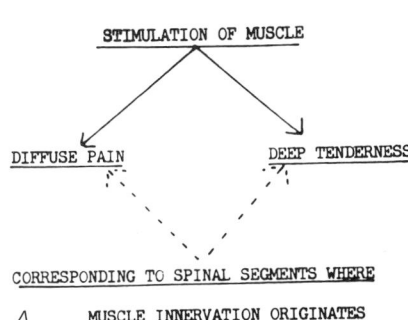

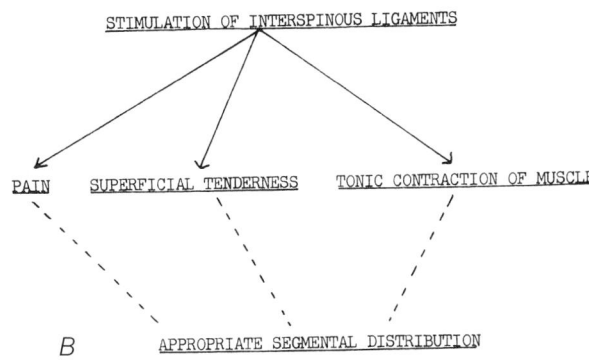

Fig. 43-2. *A.* Characteristics of muscle pain when stimulated by injected saline solution. *B.* Characteristics of ligament pain when stimulated. *[After Kellgren, 1943. Taken with permission from Duthie RB, Bentley JB (eds): Orthopaedic Surgery. London, Edward Arnold, 1982.]*

viscera and is a result of misplaced pain projection caused by cortical misrepresentation (Fig. 43-2).

The experiments of Kellgren and Samuel have demonstrated some characteristics of referred pain. Pain resulting from the injection of 6% saline solution into muscle was diffuse and referred into the spinal segments from which the muscle receives its motor innervation. Pain resulting from injection into deep fascia, periosteum, ligament, or tendon was more accurately localized when these tissues were close to the body surface (Fig. 43-3). When the structures were deeper, the pain was more diffuse and had minimal segmental distribution.

Feinstein et al. demonstrated that similar injection of muscle and intervertebral articulations produced gripping, boring, and cramplike pain, often accompanied by muscle spasm and autonomic effects such as hypotension, nausea, and bradycardia. There was less segmental distribution of pain because of extensive arborization of nerve endings and excitation within the internuncial pools, which resulted in extensive overflow into neighboring segments.

Tissue Patterns

BONE PAIN. Pain originating in bone is carried by small myelinated and unmyelinated fibers from the periosteum and small blood vessels. It has a characteristic deep, boring quality usually attributable to the stimulus of internal tension. The deep, boring night pain of osteoarthritis is probably of vascular origin. Pain of a similar boring nature but of a somewhat diffuse character occurs in generalized osseous diseases such as osteomalacia, osteoporosis, and hyperparathyroidism or metastatic lesions. Bone pain associated with fracture has quite a different character. It is often described as sharp or piercing and is characteristically relieved by rest.

MUSCLE AND TENDON PAIN. Muscle pain may be the result of direct injury or the effect of chemical irritants such as lactic acid and other products of tissue anoxia. That due to direct injury is usually described as "tearing"

and is followed by a soreness aggravated by movement, whereas that consequent upon anoxia is described as a "cramplike" pain. Such a cramplike pain is characteristic of intermittent claudication secondary to atherosclerosis, Volkmann's ischemia, and the anterior tibial syndrome. The pain is aggravated by muscle movement.

Muscle spasm refers to sustained muscular contraction and is felt as deep, diffuse, persistent pain. Characteristically, in sciatica it produces a scoliosis and in brachialgia a torticollis due to lumbar and cervical nerve root irritation. It is accompanied by local tenderness and a feeling of hardness of the muscles.

Fig. 43-3. *A.* Distribution of pain in the trunk when the interspinous ligaments between various vertebrae were stimulated. *B.* Distribution of pain in the lower extremities when interspinous ligaments were stimulated. *[After Kellgren, 1943. Taken with permission from Duthie RB, Bentley JB (eds): Orthopaedic Surgery. London, Edward Arnold, 1982.]*

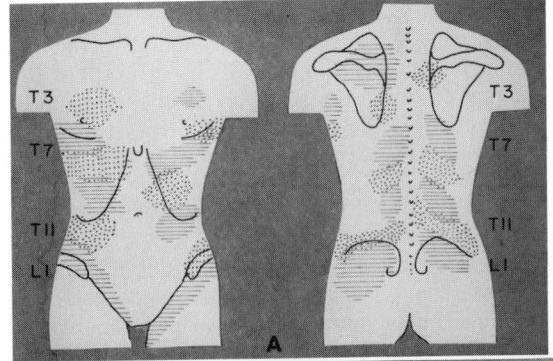

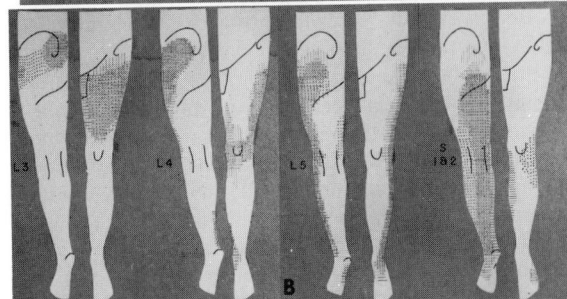

Paroxysmal cramplike pain accompanied by rigidity or excessive muscle spasm is seen in tetany, which is due to increased sensitivity of the neuromuscular unit consequent upon hypocalcemia or alkalosis. Muscle cramps are also noted with sodium depletion due to hypermotility of muscle cells, a condition rapidly reversed by restoration of the electrolyte balance. Peripheral neuritis may also present cramping of muscle masses as well as paresthesia. Pain is rare in muscular dystrophies and myotonic disorders and common in the inflammatory myopathies. The pain and accompanying tenderness of fibrositis are related to a specific muscle group, but the pathology is not understood. Morgan-Hughes has emphasized how rare muscle pain is in the muscular dystrophies and in myotonic disorders; pain is common in the inflammatory myopathies such as polyarthritis nodosa or in polymeralgia rheumatica where there is rapid destruction of muscle cells, involvement of intramuscular blood vessels, and defects in the muscular energy metabolism.

Joint pain may be attributable to a number of factors: (1) hyperemia, of both the synovium and bone; (2) joint effusion, producing capsular distention and ligamentous laxity; (3) joint instability, producing traction on capsular structures; (4) asymmetry of the joint surfaces, particularly in the presence of exposed subchondral bone or cyst formation with tension; and (5) muscle spasm. Cartilage is avascular and aneural and, therefore, insensitive to stimuli.

PERIPHERAL NERVE PAIN. Peripheral nerve fibers may be subject to (1) external pressure—neuralgia, (2) ischemia, (3) infection—herpes zoster, (4) metabolic disturbance—avitaminosis neuritis, and (5) toxins—lead or arsenic.

The pain of neuralgia is usually paroxysmal and radicular in type. Paresthesia is common, and examination frequently reveals changes in reflexes, loss of sensation, and muscle atrophy. The pain of neuritis, however, tends to be continuous until relief of the disease process or total destruction of neural tissue ensues. The special pain of herpes zoster or Guillain-Barré syndrome is accompanied by hyperesthesia, with or without sympathetic vasomotor changes.

PAIN ARISING FROM THE VERTEBRAL COLUMN AND/OR ITS CONTENTS. Lesions of the Cord. Intraspinal lesions tend to be progressive without periods of remission. The pain is not relieved by rest, and any progression of the intramedullary compression will produce a rapid loss of motor power in the extremities and loss of sphincter control. Benign nerve sheath tumors and meningiomas are much more common than tumors of the spinal cord itself, i.e., metastatic carcinoma, glial and ependymal tumors, and, more rarely, connective tissue tumors. Infections involving the spinal cord such as poliomyelitis, meningitis, and the Guillain-Barré syndrome tend to produce lancinating peripheral pain due to the involvement of the internuncial pool cells by the virus. The conditions of amyotrophic lateral sclerosis, multiple sclerosis, subacute combined degeneration of the cord, and tabes dorsalis will all present with lancinating pain radiating to the extremities. Loss of reflexes is commonly found. Syrin-

gomyelia can usually be diagnosed by the loss of both pain and temperature sensations.

Lesions of the Vertebrae and/or Joints. Primary and secondary neoplasms, osteoporosis with pathologic fractures, and tuberculous and pyogenic infections affecting bones of the spine will produce severe local pain with local tenderness on palpation and percussion. Radicular pain does not occur unless the peripheral nerves are involved by the lesion. Carcinoma metastases to the skeletal structures may produce significant symptoms before there are visible radiographic changes.

Coccygodynia is deep, throbbing pain in the vicinity of the lower end of the sacrum and coccyx aggravated by sitting. It tends to be progressive and to last several months, but without any radicular expression or involvement of sphincteric function. It can be traumatic in origin, from arthritis involving the sacrococcygeal joint or from a disc protrusion at the lumbosacral junction. Localized tenderness on rectal examination is present, and radiographic changes of the joint may be noted. Treatment is usually conservative and consists of application of local heat and cushioned sitting. Rarely does the patient require excision of the coccyx.

Lesions Involving Peripheral Nerves. Peripheral nerves may be compressed in the intervertebral foramina by such conditions as neurofibromas, trauma, osteophyte formation associated with osteoarthrosis, and intervertebral disc protrusions. The pain is usually radicular over the area supplied by the nerve roots involved.

Pain in the Upper Limbs

SHOULDER-SCAPULAR AREA. This will arise from cervical disc protrusion, diseases of the cervical vertebrae, and affections of the shoulder joint, e.g., supraspinatus tendonitis and subacromial bursitis, or it may be referred visceral pain arising from disease of the heart, lungs, or pleura.

VICINITY OF THE ELBOW. This may result from local conditions such as arthritis of the radiohumeral articulations or lateral epicondylitis ("tennis elbow"), or it may be referred pain with involvement of the fifth, sixth, or seventh cervical vertebrae or associated discs.

WRIST AND HAND. This may be the result of local lesions such as tendon sheath disease, e.g., Quervain's disease, radiocarpal arthritis, neoplastic or infective diseases of the bones, or compression of the median nerve within the carpal tunnel. Radicular pain may be due to compression of the ulnar nerve at the elbow or of the brachial plexus at any point from the roots at the intervertebral foramina or in the thoracic outlet; these conditions will be accompanied by other signs of neurologic deficit such as paresthesia, muscle atrophy, reflex changes, and overlying skin changes. Associated vasomotor trophic changes suggest Sudeck's atrophy or the shoulder-hand syndrome.

BRACHIALGIA (BRACHIAL NEURALGIA)

This pain involves the neck, shoulder, or upper extremity; i.e., it is distributed within the brachial plexus dermatome and sclerotome. It may be characterized by: upper extremity pain, either unilateral or bilateral; paresthesia, in a dermatome with altered sensation; deep tendon reflex changes in the jaw and/or in the upper extremity; muscle weakness, with atrophy and possibly fibrillation; and vertebral artery or sympathetic plexus disturbance with giddiness, tinnitus, or visual disturbance. The disease process may involve the motor neuron, the pyramidal tract, the root, or the surrounding vertebrae.

Radiography (AP and lateral, as well as oblique views), lumbar puncture to show the presence of some degree of block on jugular compression, examination of cerebrospinal fluid for changes in protein and other chemical constituents, and a cell count should be carried out. Computer tomography (CT scan) and magnetic resonance imaging (MRI) are now routine to visualize transverse sections in two-dimensional slices from 0.8 to 1.2 cm thick. The size and volume of soft tissue, as well as bony masses, can be seen as well as their relationships (dimensions of spinal cord, position and size of intervertebral disc nucleus pulposus in relationship to the peripheral nerve, and tumors). This is a safer procedure than myelography, particularly in the cervical spinal region. The differential diagnosis of brachialgia includes (1) tumors of the cord and its membranes or of the vertebral column, e.g., ependymoma, neurofibroma, or neurolemmoma, (2) infections, such as acute tuberculosis, osteomyelitis, actinomycosis, (3) prolapsing intervertebral disc, or degenerative disc with arthritis, (4) Pancoast's tumor of the apex of lung, (5) congenital anomalies of the cord, e.g., syringomyelia, and (6) atlantoaxial dislocation.

CERVICAL COMPRESSION SYNDROME (CERVICAL DISC DISEASE)

Maximal movement of flexion or extension and static curvature occur at the level of C_4 to C_6. Maximal stress is to be expected at this level, and this is the most common site for herniations of the cervical intervertebral discs.

A prominence of disc protrusion or an osteophyte in the midline will compress the whole spinal cord and the anterior nerve roots that emerge at this level, but a bulge to one side of the midline will cause unilateral cord compression with a Brown-Séquard type of syndrome. The most common variety of protrusion is that arising from the lateral portion of the disc in relation to the nerve root and is either dorsolateral or intraforaminal in location. An intraforaminal lesion may also be the result of narrowing of an already small intervertebral foramen by osteophytic lipping of the margins of the neurocentral joints of Luschka.

Protrusion of a cervical intervertebral disc can produce (1) nerve root compression alone, with pain down the arm, (2) compression of the spinal cord structures, (3) a combination of both, and (4) local and referred pain in the absence of nerve root compression.

CLINICAL MANIFESTATIONS. Occasionally, there is a history of trauma, but usually it is minor in nature. Symptoms of nerve root compression, when present, usually constitute the chief complaint. The majority of patients have only symptoms of local and referred pain as a consequence of the disc degeneration. A form of precipitating injury may be an unexpected and abrupt forward jerk of the head as with sudden acceleration or deceleration of an automobile when hit from behind or in a head-on collision.

The predominant feature of nerve root compression from a laterally placed protrusion is persistent aching pain distributed according to the level of the disc lesion and the nerve root involved. A disc herniation at a particular level will compress the nerve root immediately below it; e.g., a sixth cervical disc will compress a seventh cervical nerve root. Lesions of the sixth cervical nerve produce pain and paresthesia over the radial aspect of the forearm, thumb, and index finger. There is wasting, weakness, and loss of biceps reflex. Involvement of the seventh cervical nerve root will produce pain and paresthesia referred to the dorsal aspect of the forearm and wrist and to one or all of the three middle fingers. On the left side, involvement of the seventh cervical nerve root frequently produces chest pain, which may be misdiagnosed as a coronary thrombosis.

There is usually a reduction of mobility in the cervical spine in both lateral and anteroposterior flexion, but even in the presence of marked neurologic signs, cervical movements may sometimes be quite unrestricted.

The compression test of steady downward pressure on the vertex of the skull or forehead from behind with flexion and extension toward the affected side will often produce severe radicular pain, whereas suspension of the head may relieve the pain. Localized tenderness in muscle at the affected level is common, as is tenderness in areas of the shoulder girdle and the upper limb secondary to localized muscle spasm caused by anterior rami irritation.

Neurologic signs such as selective wasting of muscles, reduction or abolition of deep tendon reflexes, e.g., the biceps, triceps, or brachioradialis, and sensory changes in an area of dermatome distribution may be present.

Radiologic examination will reveal absence of the normal cervical lordosis and narrowing of the involved intervertebral space. Oblique views of the cervical spine may reveal narrowing of the anteroposterior diameter of the intervertebral foramina by osteophytes or by osteoarthritic changes of the lateral articulations. Myelography may show a partial block, and the protein content of the cerebrospinal fluid may be increased.

Cervical Myelopathy

This condition will present as weakness and spasticity in one or both legs, with associated exaggerated reflexes and an extensor plantar response. There may be weakness and wasting, which may be limited to a single root distribution or confined to the small muscles of the hand on one side or both or may be generalized throughout the arm with fasciculation. Sphincter disturbances occur in about a third of the patients but are not severe and consist mainly of hesitancy or urgency of micturition. Incontinence is unusual. Compression of the spinal cord and its fibers may be the mechanism responsible for neurologic signs in cervical myelopathy. Most probably the cause of cord damage is interference with the blood flow in the anterior spinal artery and branches brought about either by intermittent compression or by frictional injuries of the vessel during neck movement.

The differential diagnosis of cervical compression or irritative lesions includes (1) spinal cord tumors and syringomyelia, (2) osteoarthritis of the cervical spine, (3) direct injury producing laminar fractures, (4) thoracic inlet syndrome, cervical rib, (5) scalenus anticus syndrome, and (6) pancoast tumor (superior pulmonary sulcus tumor).

TREATMENT OF THE CERVICAL COMPRESSION SYNDROME. If the pain persists for more than a few weeks, strict recumbency and immobilization of the neck in cervical traction are indicated with adequate sedation and physiotherapy. Once the pain has subsided, or in less severe attacks, the patient may be placed in a cervical collar during the period of the spasm.

Active resistance exercises should be carried out to elongate the soft tissues within their normal range and reduce periarticular fibrous contracture. If there is progression of the neurologic deficit or cord structure compression, surgical intervention is indicated. In cases with a centrally situated lesion, laminectomy is necessary. Fusion of the spine may be required, particularly if an extensive laminectomy has been necessary. Some prefer the use of a light Minerva plastic jacket with both chest and back pieces extending up to form a head halter.

Low Back Pain

"Low back syndrome" refers to a disease or injury of the lumbosacral spine with or without an underlying predisposing condition. The condition may be acute, producing a temporary or permanent change in the physical state of the individual, or may be a chronic condition, exhibiting variable degrees of frequency, duration of symptoms, and degress of physical deterioration.

Rowe described the varying conditions that can produce the low back syndrome. These are presented in Table 43-2, which does not include lumbosacral pain consequent to visceral disease or psychosomatic disorder.

CLINICAL MANIFESTATIONS. The low back syndrome usually occurs in the third, fourth, or fifth decades of life as an acute low back pain associated with muscle spasm. The pain may be aggravated by coughing, sneezing, defecation, or any other maneuver that raises the intrathecal pressure, but it is rarely of true radicular nature and is usually relieved by lying down with the knees flexed.

In evaluating the clinical history of low back pain, it is important to assess the type of pain, its site, whether it is referred, its duration, its mode of onset, its relationship to activity and to rest, and its association with symptoms relevant to other systems such as the genitourinary, gynecologic, and alimentary organs.

In disease processes such as neoplasm, tuberculosis, and various types of osteomyelitis of the spine, the pain is usually severe, localized, and not relieved by rest. In mechanical lesions, rest usually relieves the pain, except

Table 43-2. CAUSES OF LOW BACK PAIN

A. Structural defects
  1. Segmentation defects
    a. Six lumbar vertebrae
    b. Four lumbar vertebrae
    c. Transitional lumbosacral junction
  2. Ossification defects
    a. Spina bifida
    b. Spondylolysis
    c. Spondylolisthesis
  3. Facet abnormalities
    a. Asymmetry (tropism)
    b. Anteroposterior lumbosacral facets
  4. Increased lumbosacral angle
B. Functional defects
  1. Lateral imbalance (leg-length discrepancy, scoliosis, work or postural attitudes, etc.)
  2. Anteroposterior imbalance (pregnancy, potbelly, flexion contracture of hips and knees, etc.)
C. Infections
  1. Bone and joint
    a. Arthritis
    b. Tuberculosis
    c. Brucellosis
    d. Osteomyelitis
  2. Soft tissue
    a. "Myositis"
    b. "Fibrositis"
D. Degenerative processes
  1. Osteoarthritis
  2. Senile osteoporosis
  3. Degenerative disc disease
E. Neoplastic processes
  1. Primary
    a. Multiple myeloma
    b. Hemangioma
    c. Giant cell tumor, eosinophilic granuloma, osteogenic sarcoma
  2. Metastatic
    a. Prostate and breast
    b. Lung, kidney, thyroid, gastrointestinal tract
F. Traumatic
  1. Compression fracture
  2. Vertebral process fracture (faces, transverse, and spinous process)
  3. Sprain and strain
  4. Ruptured disc

SOURCE: From Rowe ML: *J Occup Med* 2:219, 1960, with permission.

in the presence of severe root irritation. Diurnal variation of the pain and associated stiffness are important. Ankylosing spondylitis is characterized by early morning pain, relieved as activity increases. Pain due to intervertebral disc lesions or lumbar spondylosis is usually relieved by bed rest and aggravated by activity.

The patient is examined standing; posture, weight, muscular development, the state of lumbar lordotic curve, and the presence of any structural or "discogenic" scoliosis are noted. There may be tenderness in the lumbrospinal angle or of the spinous processes and interspinous ligaments. Ranges of flexion, extension, and lateral flexion of the lumbar spine are determined, especially if there is restriction because of spasm or pain.

The patient is then examined supine. The abdomen is palpated for any mass or tenderness. Particular attention is paid to the presence or absence of peripheral pulses. Joints of the lower limbs are put through the range of movement, and then the straight-leg-raising test is carried out. In this test the patient's straight leg is flexed at the hip and can, under normal circumstances, be lifted to almost 90° depending on the tightness of the hamstrings. Limitation of this movement is usually present in low back pain and sciatica. When dorsiflexion of the foot (Bragard's test) is superimposed upon straight-leg raising, the pull on the sciatic produces sciatic pain. With straight-leg raising, there is a 4-mm excursion of the L_4, L_5, S_1, and S_2 nerve roots within the intervertebral foramen. This is restricted by adhesion formation, by tumor, or by prolapse of an intervertebral disc. A comprehensive neurologic examination is carried out, with assessment of the reflexes, the presence of sensation, and motor power. A rectal and prostatic examination of the male and a gynecologic examination of the female are essential.

RADIOLOGIC FINDINGS. Anteroposterior, lateral, and oblique views of the lumbosacral spine including cone views of the lumbosacral junction are necessary in a patient complaining of back pain. Radiologic examination may show narrowing of the L_4, L_5, or S_1 disc spaces with some associated lumbar spondylosis or posterior facet joint subluxation (Fig. 43-4). Radiographic evidence of such underlying lesions should not be taken as necessarily indicative of the causative pathologic condition.

TREATMENT. The treatment of low back syndrome should be essentially conservative, with adequate bed rest in a low Fowler position, sedation, and some type of superficial heat to relieve the muscle spasm. When the pain improves, knee-to-chest flexion exercises or lumbar flexion and hanging exercises may be beneficial. In some cases, the restriction of back movements by the use of a corset or brace will help both to relieve symptoms and to prevent recurrence.

SPONDYLOLISTHESIS AND SPONDYLOLYSIS

The term "spondylolisthesis" was first used by Kilian in 1853 to describe the condition of forward subluxation of one vertebral body upon another. The condition is not limited to any specific segment of the vertebral column, but most commonly the term refers to displacement of the fifth lumbar vertebra on the body of the first sacral vertebra. The term "spondylolysis" is used to describe a bony defect of the neural arch, a condition that is felt to be one of the predisposing factors in the production of spondylolisthesis.

There is some evidence that this condition is genetically inherited with an increased penetrance caused by inbreeding. The incidence obviously varies throughout the world and is higher in certain races or occupations. (White male/female = 6.4/2.3 percent; black male/female = 2.8/2.3 percent.)

PATHOLOGY. Spondylolisthesis usually results from a structural defect in the fifth lumbar vertebra, the defective vertebra being divided into two separate parts by a deep bilateral defect in the pars interarticularis of the neu-

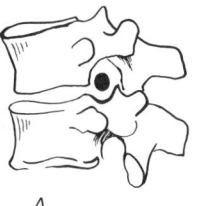 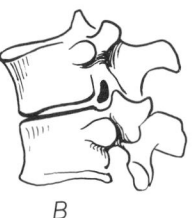

Fig. 43-4. Narrowing of lumbar disc space with a reversed spondylosis and deformation of the peripheral nerve. [*After Rowe, 1960. Taken with permission from Duthie RB, Bentley JB (eds): Orthopaedic Surgery. London, Edward Arnold, 1982.*]

ral arch. The anterior segment of the vertebra is composed of the body, pedicles, transverse processes, and superior articular facets, while the posterior fragment includes the spinous process, the laminae, and the inferior articular facets. There is no certainty as to the manner by which the defect develops, although it does not appear to be congenital. Wiltse described the etiology of spondylolisthesis as resulting from a defect in the pars interarticularis due to (1) an inherited dysplasia in the cartilaginous arch of the affected vertebra; (2) the physical forces resulting from the erect position and the curvature of the lumbar spine acting on a weakened pars interarticularis. He believes that bone reabsorption results, rather than any new-bone-formation defect. In his series, the condition was never present at birth and seldom present below the age of four, and the greatest incidence of slipping was seen between the ages of ten and fifteen years. Spondylolysis, however, is not the only cause of spondylolisthesis, which can occur in the absence of any defect of the neural arch. Newman has described the following types of spondylolisthesis:

1. Infantile spondylolisthesis
   a. Facet deficiency or subluxation
   b. Attenuation of the pars interarticularis
   c. Loss of continuity of the pars interarticularis (spondylolysis)
2. Adult spondylolisthesis
   a. Stress fracture in mature bone
   b. Facet deficiency due to degenerative joint disease

CLINICAL MANIFESTATIONS. In children the condition is usually painless, although the parents may notice an unduly prominent abdomen and buttock. In adolescents and adults, backache may be the presenting symptom. It is usually intermittent, coming on after exercise or strain, and in some cases there may be sciatica as a consequence of root pressure. Probably the most commonly experienced pain is that which arises in the disc adjacent to the unstable vertebrae as a consequence of altered spine mechanics and increased forces on the disc.

Spondylolisthesis can be completely asymptomatic and may be found during examination for other complaints. Spondylolisthesis in an asymptomatic individual is not a reason to deny employment. Many patients first appear for treatment in the middle or late decades of life, but they have probably had the defect since early childhood.

Spondylolisthesis may be seen as a characteristic deformity that is the result of forward displacement of the involved vertebra and the vertebrae above. The spinous process above form a "step" kyphosis in contrast to the "angular" kyphosis of tuberculous disease. The pelvis is rotated about a transverse axis passing through the hip joints so that the anterosuperior iliac spines are raised to the same level as the posterosuperior iliac spines. This rotation may be so great that the thighs are not in a straight line with the trunk even when they are fully extended. Consequently the patient must stand with the trunk thrust forward if the legs are vertical or with the hips and knees flexed if the trunk is held erect. As the trunk is shortened by the downward displacement accompanying the forward slip, the ribs overlap or approach the iliac crest, and transverse creases appear above the waist.

RADIOLOGIC FINDINGS. In the early stages of disease, especially in cases of simple spondylolysis, a simple translucency may be seen in the pars interarticularis. The lateral radiograph will show the presence of any spondylolisthesis (Fig. 43-5), but doubtful cases are best shown by an oblique view of the pars interarticularis. Under normal circumstances the pars interarticularis and the superior articular facet form the outline of a "Scottish terrier." In the condition of spondylolysis without slip, the terrier is seen to wear a collar of translucency as compared with the rest of the bone, whereas in spondylolisthesis, when there has been movement forward of the superior articular facet, the terrier is seen to be decapitated.

TREATMENT. The initial treatment is conservative, i.e., exercises to strengthen abdominal muscles, corset, or, even better, rest. In patients not responding to an adequate course of nonoperative treatment, surgical treatment may be indicated. If nerve root impingement is present, decompression by removal of the posterior fragment (Gill procedure) is indicated with exploration of the nerve roots. For patients with back pain without radiculopathy, fusion of the involved segments above and below the slip can be done. The actual method of lumbosacral fusion varies. The fusion can be a posterolateral one uniting the transverse processes of the proximal vertebrae or the involved vertebrae to the normal vertebrae below. An alternative method is anterior interbody fusion which gives immediate stability.

Fig. 43-5. Radiograph showing a spondylolisthesis of the fifth lumbar upon the first sacral vertebra, with an obvious defect in the pars interarticularis.

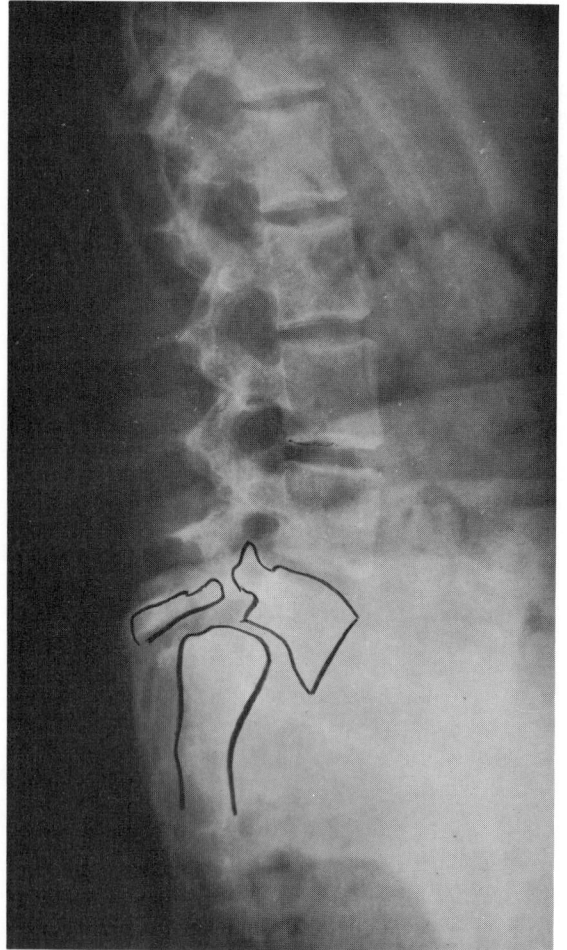

SCIATICA

Sciatica is a symptom and not a disease. It is a term used to describe pain of a radicular nature occurring in one or both lower limbs consequent to inflammation or pressure on one or more nerve roots involved in the formation of the lumbosacral plexus.

Causes of Sciatica

A. Nerve root compression
  1. Intraspinal compression. This may be due to a prolapsed intervertebral disc, an intraspinal tumor, or an intraspinal abscess.
  2. Compression with the intervertebral foramen. This may arise through a tumor of the nerve roots, such as neurofibroma, or a narrowing of the foramen due to a spondylolisthesis, spondylosis, or osteoarthritis of the posterior apophyseal joints.
  3. Compression within the pelvis or buttock. This may arise as a result of intrapelvic or gluteal abscess, or a tumor in one or the other of these sites.
B. Inflammation of nerve and nerve roots
  1. Toxic
    a. Alcoholism
    b. Diabetic neuritis
    c. Arsenical poisoning
    d. Lead poisoning
  2. "Infective"
    a. Focal sepsis
    b. Rheumatism
    c. Syphilis

Of all the causes of sciatica listed above, intervertebral disc protrusion is by far the most common.

LUMBAR AND INTERVERTEBRAL DISC PROTRUSION

ANATOMY. Intervertebral discs, which unite the bodies of successive vertebrae from the second cervical vertebra to the sacrum, form a series of amphiarthrotic, or slightly movable, joints with no synovial cavity. Structurally, intervertebral discs consist of three parts: the cartilage end plate, the annulus fibrosus, and the nucleus pulposus.

The cartilaginous end plate is a thin layer of hyaline cartilage adherent to the trabeculae of cancellous bone making up the major portion of the vertebral body.

The nucleus pulposus constitutes the central portion of the intervertebral disc; it is a soft, semifluid mass containing over 80 percent water by weight, the water being bound to mucopolysaccharides as in myxoid tissue. Because it contains so much water, the nucleus is virtually incompressible and inelastic. Surrounding the nucleus pulposus is the annulus fibrosus, composed of laminas, fibrocartilage, and fibrous tissue, and containing more cells, a greater abundance of collagen, and a lesser amount of mucopolysaccharide ground substance than the nucleus. The annulus is somewhat elastic; it bends with the overlying spinal ligaments, its fibers running obliquely from vertebra to vertebra, continuous with the fibrils in the cartilaginous end plates and ossified epiphyseal rings in the vertebral bodies. The function of the annulus fibrosus would appear to be twofold: to restrict and regulate movements of the vertebral column and to enclose and retain the nucleus pulposus.

The two components of the intervertebral discs, the annulus fibrosus and the nucleus pulposus, are avascular except for the most peripheral fibers of the annulus, which receive a small blood supply from adjacent vessels. Fine unmyelinated nerve fibers have been found in the posterior longitudinal ligament and in the annulus fibrosus. None are in the nucleus pulposus. The ligamentous and articular structures of the vertebral column have a considerable sensory innervation from the nervus sinuvertebralis of Luschka.

MECHANISM OF HERNIATIONS AND PROTRUSIONS OF THE INTERVERTEBRAL DISC. With aging, the collagen increases and becomes coarser. The elasticity, viscosity, and water-binding capacity of the ground substance decrease. The proportion of water decreases from 90 percent in childhood to less than 70 percent in old age.

The nucleus is constantly under compression, and the turgid nucleus, bounded laterally by the strong elastic laminas of the annulus and vertically by the cartilaginous end plate, may burst through either one of these barriers. Spontaneous herniation of an intervertebral disc may take place either vertically into the spongiosa of the vertebral body or horizontally. Prolapse of nuclear substance cannot occur in older people whose nuclei pulposi have undergone desiccation.

Vertical prolapse of an intervertebral disc into the vertebral bodies produces the phenomenon known as "Schmorl's nodes." It is of no clinical importance. Horizontal prolapse is of considerable clinical importance. Two forms of horizontal prolapse may occur, namely, nuclear herniation and annular protrusion (Fig. 43-6). In nuclear herniation the nucleus usually displaces posteriorly, but in annular prolapse there is convex bulging of the relaxed annulus fibers in all directions.

Most of these posterior herniations lie to one side of the midline, because the posterior longitudinal ligament prevents direct posterior herniation. Consequently, neuro-

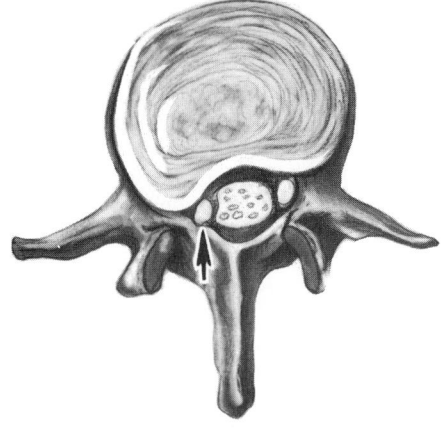

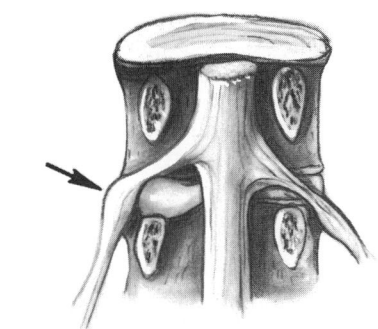

Fig. 43-6. Posterolateral herniation, or prolapse, with deformation of the peripheral nerve. [From: *Duthie RB, Bentley JB (eds): Orthopaedic Surgery. London, Edward Arnold, 1982, with permission.*]

logic symptoms caused by direct pressure on the neural tissues tend to be unilateral. Annular protrusions follow the narrowing of the disc space resulting from desiccation or vertebral prolapse of the nucleus, and the relaxed annulus fibers are squeezed outward. It is these anterolateral protrusions of the fibers of the annulus that account for the common and well-known form of osteophytosis or spondylosis of the vertebral columns.

PATHOLOGY OF NUCLEAR PROTRUSIONS. Posterolateral herniation of nuclear material may enlarge and may impinge on neighboring nerve roots, producing symptoms and signs similar to any other space-occupying lesion in the intraspinal canal. There may be irritation of the nerve root by compression, or by stretching, or by friction, an occlusion of its vasa nervorum, or a combination of all these factors. A nerve root may be stretched tautly over a nuclear protrusion in close proximity to the ligamentum flavum. On straight-leg raising there is an excursion of 4 mm of spinal roots at L_4–L_5 and S_1–S_2. Therefore, any pressure from a nuclear protrusion on such a nerve root will interfere with its range of movement. This is the basis of the restricted straight-leg-raising test. If the pressure is severe and prolonged, impairment of axonal conductivity will occur in the nerve root, producing symptoms and signs of motor and sensory loss in the lower limb.

CLINICAL MANIFESTATIONS. Fifty percent of cases of intervertebral disc protrusion present initially as low backache followed later by radicular sciatic pain, whereas about one-third of patients may give a history of sciatica preceding the backache. In the remainder, sciatica and backache commence simultaneously.

The onset may be acute following a minor degree of trauma such as a fall in the sitting position or the lifting of a heavy weight in the stooping position, but in many cases there is no evidence of any traumatic incident. In some cases the first attack may be the most severe one, followed by a series of perhaps minor but annoying exacerbations, but in others the reverse sequence of presentation may be the case. Characteristically the pain of sciatica is usually described as a dull ache or a shooting pain radiating from the lower lumbar limb. The actual pain is referred to the dermatome of the involved nerve root and is a valuable method of localizing the site of the occlusion.

It is most important also to ask the patient whether there is any loss of sensation or motor power. It is quite common to find that there is subjective loss of motor power when no such loss is detectable on clinical examination. Inquiry as to urgency or frequency of micturition is most important, since this is an early sign of the rare but serious condition of central protrusion which embarrasses the cauda equina.

Examination of the patient is first carried out with the patient standing and undressed. Special note is taken of the presence of any alterations of the spinal curvature with respect to both lumbar lordosis and the presence of any discogenic scoliosis; then movements of flexion, extension, and lateral flexion to either side are assessed. Where these initially appear to be normal, attention should be paid to the rhythm of flexion and extension of the lumbar spine. It is also important to make sure that what appears to be relatively normal lateral flexion on one side or the other is actually being carried out at the lumbar spine and not at the thoracolumbar junction.

With the patient in the supine position the effect of straight-leg raising, or the possible presence of a positive Lasègue sign, is then assessed. In the presence of a protrusion, the straight-leg raising test will aggravate the pain and may actually aggravate the radiation to the extremity. The greater the restriction of straight-leg raising, the larger the protrusion. Such symptoms are aggravated in the straight-leg-raising position by forced dorsiflexion of the foot and then are known as Lasègue's sign.

A neurologic assessment with respect to reflexes, motor power, and sensation is carried out on the lower limbs. Impairment of sensation may be found along the dermatome of the nerve root involved, especially along the outer thigh, the calf, and the foot. Examination for motor power may reveal weakness of the long extensor or flexor of the great toe (fifth lumbar root) and occasionally of the gluteal muscles, where the symptom must be assessed with the patient in the prone position. In the presence of a severe protrusion at the L_5–S_1 disc space the ankle jerk (1 and 2 roots) may well be diminished. The absence of a knee jerk (1, 2, 3, and 4 roots) indicates a higher prolapse than usual.

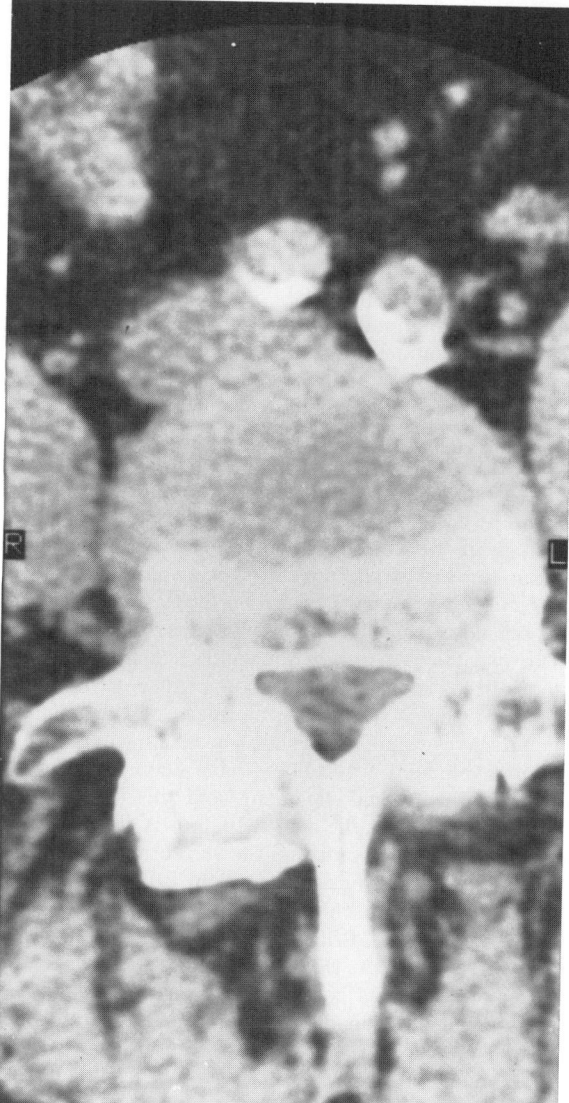

Fig. 43-7. CT scan of spinal stenosis at L_4–L_5.

SPECIAL EXAMINATIONS. Radiography. Anteroposterior and lateral views of the lumbosacral spine and similar cone views of the lumbosacral junction are taken routinely. The major purpose of these x-rays is to exclude diseases of a more sinister nature. They also help to assess the possible presence of discogenic scoliosis and the state of the intervertebral discs. The lumbar disc spaces normally show progressive widening in a caudal direction, the space between L_2 and L_3 being wider than the one above. The lateral view may show diminished disc spaces, but a normal space does not always exclude a small disc protrusion at this level.

Computerized Tomography. Thin cross-sectional x-rays are an invaluable aid in the diagnosis of all patients with spinal disease. In the low back area, CT scans can delineate the size of the spinal canal and neural foramen, local-

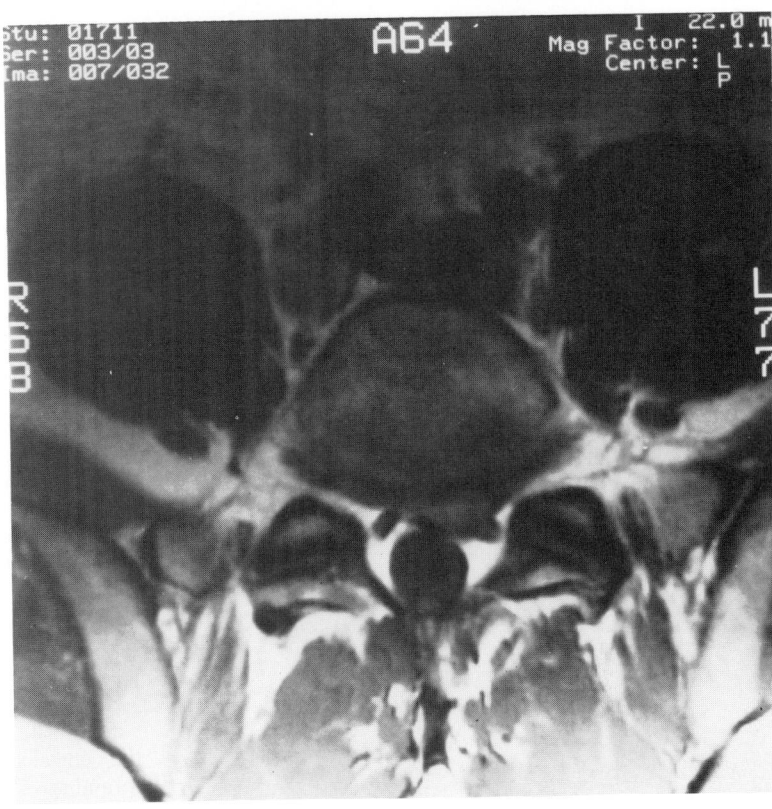

Fig. 43-8. MRI showing disc prolapse at L_5–S_1. *(Courtesy of Dr. David W. Stoller.)*

ize single or multiple disc protrusions, and define nerve root encroachment, especially when it is lateral to the myelographic dye column. Localization of nerve root impingement is enhanced by combining metrizanide myelography with CT scans (Fig. 43-7). More recently MRI has been applied (Fig. 43-8).

Myelography. Myelography is a valuable additional radiographic investigation to exclude other conditions and to help localize the site of the intervertebral disc protrusion (Fig. 43-9). It is especially valuable where the diagnosis is in doubt, as in the presence of an intraspinal tumor. But it is not always necessary as a preliminary to operative removal of the disc protrusion, because neurologic assessment of the level of the herniation, even without myelography, is highly reliable.

Water-soluble radiopaque material is helpful in outlining the dural sleeves around the peripheral nerve roots as they come out of the cauda equina in order to define deformation of normal anatomical course. Other tests, such as spinal venography outlining the spinal veins, epidurography by injecting material into the cauda space, or discography by injecting the radiopaque material into the disc space itself, all contribute to the final diagnosis. CT scan is of great value in outlining the dimensions of the spinal cord and the extent of soft tissue spread from either tumor or intervertebral disc material.

Since the process of myelography involves lumbar puncture, the opportunity should be taken to test the dynamics of the cerebrospinal fluid as well as to obtain a specimen for biochemical assessment.

DIFFERENTIAL DIAGNOSIS. Although most cases of backache and sciatica are a result of a prolapsed intervertebral disc, it is most important in all cases to exclude the possibility of tuberculosis or tumors of the vertebral column, meninges, or nerve roots, and especially secondary deposits. In a prolapsed intervertebral disc the complaint is usually episodic, whereas in most other conditions of tumor or infection the symptoms and signs tend to be constant and progressive.

TREATMENT. Nonoperative Treatment. With few exceptions conservative treatment is recommended initially in all cases of prolapsed intervertebral discs; in about 80 percent of cases this may effect complete and permanent relief. The ideal method of instituting conservative treatment is to advise strict recumbency for a period of at least 3 weeks, and, if the attack is severe, up to 6 weeks. This forced bed rest should be accompanied by adequate sedation, simple analgesics, and the use of heat. When the symptoms have subsided to some degree, and in some cases as a primary method of treatment, immobilization of the lumbar spine in a plaster jacket that permits the patient to remain mobile is useful. Recurrence of the intervertebral disc protrusion may be prevented by instructing the patient to avoid stooping and lifting as far as possible. A back brace or a lumbosacral corset is of value in limiting motion of the lumbosacral spine, decreasing

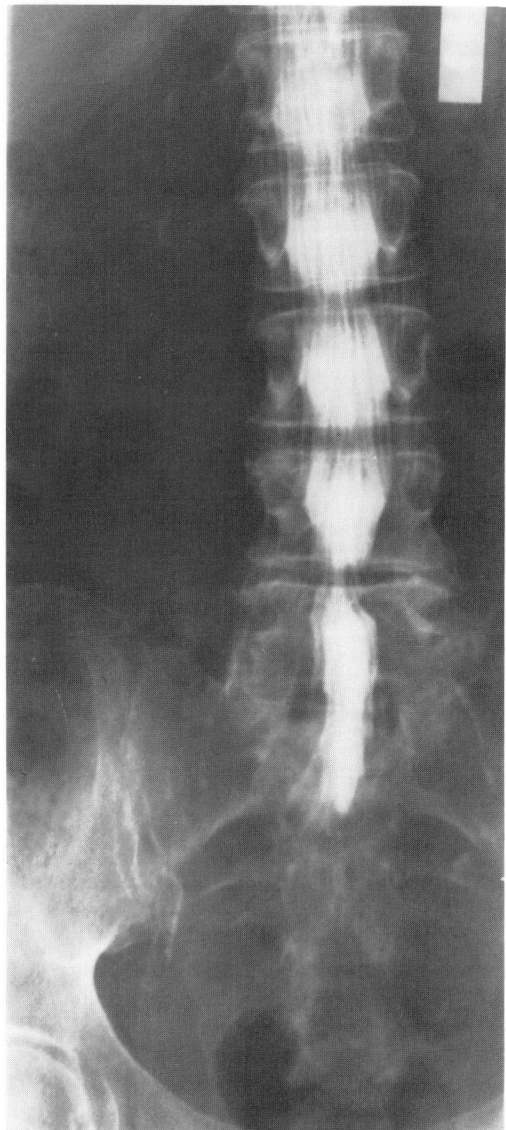

Fig. 43-9. Metrizamide myelogram shows disc prolapse at L_4–L_5 (left). *(Courtesy of Dr. David W. Stoller.)*

lordosis, and providing counterpressure for the abdominal wall when abdominal muscles are weak. Patients are instructed in Williams' exercises to strengthen the lumbar spine flexors, especially the abdominal muscles and the gluteus maximus.

Surgical Treatment. Operative removal of a herniated intervertebral disc is indicated if the attacks are severe, disabling, frequent, or persisting in spite of a well-planned conservative regimen of treatment. In a few cases, a sudden paraplegia or very severe nerve root compression with paralysis or paresis of muscle groups, or bladder and bowel disturbance, demands an emergency operation.

The operative procedure for removal of the herniated nucleus pulposus is one of disc fenestration rather than a laminectomy in which a small portion of the lamina and ligamentum flavum is removed at the site of the protrusion, the embarrassed nerve root retracted, and the prolapsed and herniating nucleus material removed. Concomitant spinal fusion is necessary only if there has been an extensive laminectomy, if there is associated degenerative disease of the intervertebral column or a congenital malformation, or when the patient is to return to very heavy manual labor.

Therapeutic Disc Injections. In many patients with recurrent disc symptoms, an epidural injection of cortisone, which can be given on an outpatient basis, will relieve back and leg pain. Presumably, the mechanism of action is to reduce local inflammation and provide space for the nerve root.

Chymopapain. This plant enzyme, which is proteolytic when injected into discs, causes breakdown of the chondromucoprotein of the nucleus to reduce the size of a bulging disc. Severe anaphylactic reactions to the enzyme and rare cases of transverse myelitis occur, reducing the safety of this drug.

DISORDERS OF THE LUMBOSACRAL JUNCTION

Lumbar Spinal Stenosis

Spinal stenosis, broadly defined, includes narrowing of the central spinal canal, lateral recesses, or intervertebral foramina. The etiology may be congenital or acquired. Included in the congenital type is achondroplasia. The most common acquired types include degenerative disease in which there is concomitant degenerative disc disease and hypertrophy of the ligamenta flava. In postoperative disc disease, encroachment on the canal may occur as a result of postoperative scarring or bone graft and fusion hypertrophy. Quantification of the stenosis in the past has depended upon plane film x-rays, lateral tomograms, and myelography. The present techniques of CT scanning or MRI can quantify and qualify both soft tissue and bony anatomy accurately.

CLINICAL MANIFESTATIONS. The clinical history and physical findings depend upon the area of the lumbar spine involved.

Patients have pain in the back or legs or both. Pain may be constant, intermittent, or similar to the intermittent claudication associated with vascular disease. Symptoms may be brought on by walking a short or long distance, and relieved by rest or changing the position of spinal posture.

Physical findings include slight to severe restriction of spine motion, positive straight-leg-raising tests, and sensory and motor deficits. Perhaps the most classic finding is the loss of reflexes or a sensory loss that is brought on by the patient walking or assuming an extreme position of the spine. A helpful examination is to test motor power in muscles supplied by the lumbar roots with the patient in the "jackknife" position (in which patients sit and attempt to touch their toes with knees extended). Reflexes may change remarkably in this stretched position or after walking one or two blocks.

CT scans of the involved area of spine alone or in combination with metrizamide myelography may be diagnostic.

TREATMENT. Initially, patients may be helped by engaging in an abdominal strengthening exercise program or using a lumbar spine flexion orthosis. By placing the spine in moderate flexion, more space is available in the spinal canal. Epidural methylprednisolone acetate (Depo-medrol) may provide a period of short- or even long-term relief. In patients not responding to conservative treatment, surgical decompression of the involved areas can be done. This may involve laminectomies and facetectomies over the involved area. An alternative technique is anterior interbody fusion, which both eliminates motion and increases space in the spinal canal by increasing disc height with a properly-placed bone graft.

SPINAL OSTEOARTHRITIS AND SPONDYLOSIS

Osteoarthritis is a disease of synovial diarthrodial joints such as the posterior apophyseal joints of the vertebral column. It must be distinguished from spondylosis, which depends upon degeneration of the intervertebral discs, which are amphiarthrotic, and less-movable joints possessing no synovial cavity or synovial membrane. Osteoarthritis of the facette joints can occur in the absence of disc disease or in association with it. The processes of osteoarthritis and degenerative disc disease are separate but frequently may coexist in the older patient.

TUMORS OF THE VERTEBRAL COLUMN

Certain types of primary bone tumors including aneurysmal bone cysts and benign osteoblastomas predominate in the vertebral column, and one primary bone tumor, i. e., the chordoma, occurs exclusively in the axial skeleton. However, most types of primary bone tumors, including giant cell tumor, osteogenic sarcoma, chondrosarcoma, and fibrosarcoma, occur less frequently in the spine than in other parts of the skeleton. Metastatic tumors commonly involve the spine and account for the majority of cases in any series of vertebral tumors in adults. The most common primary tumors affecting the vertebral column are multiple myeloma, fibrosarcoma, Hodgkin's disease, hemangioma, giant cell tumor, chondroma, and chondrosarcoma.

A classification of tumors of the vertebral column includes:

A. Primary tumors
 1. Malignant
  a.Myelomatosis
  b.Chordoma
  c.Giant cell tumor
  d.Ewing's tumor
  e.Chondrosarcoma
  f.Osteogenic sarcoma
  g.Fibrosarcoma
  h.Hodgkin's disease
 2. Benign
  a.Angioma
  b.Aneurysmal bone cyst
  c.Benign osteoblastoma
B. Secondary tumors
 1. Metastatic carcinoma

CLINICAL MANIFESTATIONS. The symptoms produced by vertebral tumors depend upon their site, the speed of their growth, and the degree of involvement of cord and/or of nerve roots. In the early stages back pain is the most common symptom, and clinical signs may be restricted to tenderness over the area in which the disease process is present. Later, when the nerve roots or cord are involved, neurologic signs become manifest. Evidence of the *lower motor neuron* lesion is weakness or paralysis of individual muscles, decrease in muscle tone, reduction in tendon and cutaneous reflexes, which help to delineate the level of involvement, and wasting of muscle. *Upper motor neuron* disease of the pyramidal tract is characterized by loss of voluntary movement with spasticity, increased tendon reflexes, sensory changes, and an increased plantar reflex or a positive Babinski sign. The posterior columns of the posterior nerve roots or the peripheral nerve may also be involved. Autonomic system involvement may be evidenced by increased sweating with vasomotor and pilomotor reactions as well as a Horner syndrome when the inferior cervical ganglion is involved. Incontinence or retention of urine, or constipation or incontinence of feces, may be present.

LABORATORY FINDINGS. Biochemical investigations are also important in recognizing myelomatosis, which has an abnormal electrophoretic pattern of the serum proteins, with a Bence Jones proteinuria. In metastatic prostatic carcinoma the serum acid phosphatase level may be elevated. Occasionally in osteoblastic lesions, such as a metastatic carcinoma of the prostate or of the lung, the serum alkaline phosphatase level may be elevated. Radiologic examination and biopsy are important aids to diagnosis.

TREATMENT. With circumscribed and presumably benign lesions, surgical excision is usually the treatment of choice, and this is a procedure that provides the histologic diagnosis. When, however, there is clinical uncertainty about the possibility of malignancy and when some other treatment such as radiotherapy is contemplated, elective biopsy must be undertaken in order to establish the nature of the lesion. Open surgical biopsy is the most desirable procedure, but this is not always possible, because of inaccessibility of the deep-seated vertebrae. In such cases, aspiration biopsy by the special techniques described by Ottolenghi and by Schajowicz may be used.

PYOGENIC OSTEOMYELITIS OF THE VERTEBRAL COLUMN

The most common organism responsible for this condition is *Staphylococcus aureus,* which spreads hematogenously from infective foci, such as boils, septic teeth, tonsilitis, otitis media, or the urinary tract. Pyogenic osteomyelitis in the vertebral column may occur at any age, but it is most common during adolescence and in young adulthood and considerably more common in males than in females.

The levels most commonly affected are the lumbar, thoracic, and cervical regions, in that order, and the actual site of infection is usually in the metaphyseal portion of the vertebra. It often rapidly spreads across the periphery of the disc to involve the metaphysis of the adjacent vertebra above or below, and sometimes two separate pairs of vertebrae are affected, or even three in succession. Marked collapse of the bodies with gibbus formation as in tuberculosis is uncommon in pyogenic vertebral osteomyelitis, as is large paravertebral abscess formation. Pus will spread along normal cleavage planes in the tissues to present in the retropharyngeal space in the cervical region, the mediastinum in the thoracic region, and the retroperitoneal space in the lumbar region with perirenal, psoas, and pelvic abscess formation. Occasionally the pus may track backward to form an epidural abscess with compression of the spinal cord.

CLINICAL MANIFESTATIONS. The acute fulminating type is most common in young patients and may be accompanied by very severe and intense toxemia. The chronic type, which seems to be somewhat more common in the adult, usually presents as malaise, fever, and very severe spinal pain, which is aggravated by movement and not relieved by rest. Unrelieved or increasing back pain after posterior laminectomy should immediately raise the question of a disc space infection. Examination of these patients reveals marked tenderness over the spinous processes of the involved vertebrae and severe muscle spasm and rigidity of the vertebral column. If the symptoms are of long standing, an abscess may be detected, and if there has been involvement of the spinal cord, signs of partial or complete paraplegia may be evident.

There is a marked polymorphonuclear leukocytosis and a raised sedimentation rate. A positive blood culture is helpful for both obtaining the organism and determining its sensitivity.

RADIOLOGIC FINDINGS. Radiologic evidence of the lesion may take from 10 days to 2 weeks to appear, although a small paravertebral abscess may be apparent before evidence of bony destruction. One of the earliest signs is slight haziness and loss of definition of bone structure in the end plates adjacent to the disc space. Later a more localized lesion becomes visible with destruction of adjacent vertebral bodies, new bone formation, and disc-space narrowing.

Radionuclide Scan. An intravenous injection of 15 mL of ^{99m}Tc-methylene diphosphate is given 2 to 3 h before the bone scan is carried out. A whole body rectilinear scanner or gamma camera is used to conduct the scan. Radionuclide scan is particularly useful in diagnosing osteolytic or osteoblastic lesions within the spine and determining viability of bone.

TREATMENT. This is based upon the three principles of treating bone infection, i.e., immobilization of the patient, both local and general, the use of the appropriate antibiotic, and surgical drainage of abscesses with debridement if at all possible.

Immobilization is best achieved by means of a plaster bed. Chemotherapy is selected from the results of culture of blood, urine, or pus aspirated from any localized abscess. In general, when surgical debridement is indicated, it is best carried out by an anterior approach to the spine with or without bone grafting.

Pain in the Chest Wall

Such pain may be referred or from local disease of the thoracic structures, i.e.,

1. In the spinal cord and its membranes from tumors or inflammation
2. In the posterior root ganglion from herpes zoster or tabes dorsalis
3. From disease of the vertebrae, such as tumor, tuberculosis, spondylolysis, osteophyte formation
4. From peripheral nerve lesions
5. From visceral disease of underlying lung, pleura, mediastinum, heart
6. From Tietze's syndrome involving the costochondral junctions

DISORDERS OF MUSCLE

Anatomy

A single skeletal muscle consists of long cylindrical fibers collected together in many bundles, collections of which form the muscle as a whole. The muscle fibers are supported by fibrous connective tissue containing capillaries, nerve fibers, fibroblasts, histiocytes, and mast cells. A supporting fibrous connective tissue surrounds each individual muscle as the endomysium, from which it extends to enclose fiber bundles as the perimysium, and finally it extends to ensheathe the entire muscle to become the epimysium (Fig. 43-10).

Definitions of Function

The following are some of the definitions used when describing muscle function:

1. A *motor unit* consists of a single motor neuron, its axon, and a group of muscle fibers innervated by this single axon.
2. A *twitch response* is a brief phasic contraction of a muscle fiber or fibers of a muscle unit resulting from a single impulse. It is followed by depolarization of these muscle fibers.
3. *Tetanus* is maximal contraction in the fibers of a motor unit resulting from a series of stimuli or summation of responses from a single stimulus.
4. An *isotonic contraction* is one in which there is shortening of the fibers of the muscle under a constant tension, and work is done.

Fig. 43-10. The various parts of muscle mass, a muscle fiber, and a myofibril. [From: *Duthie RB, Bentley JB (eds): Orthopaedic Surgery. London, Edward Arnold, 1982, with permission.*]

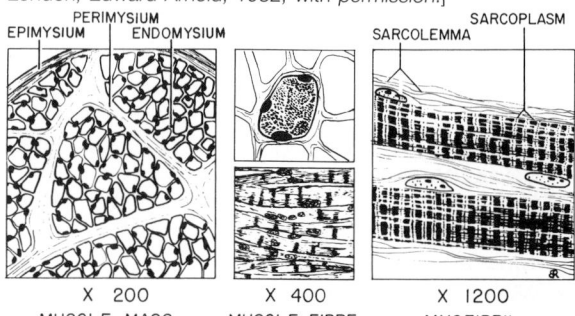

| X 200 MUSCLE MASS | X 400 MUSCLE FIBRE | X 1200 MYOFIBRIL |

5. An *isometric contraction* is one in which there is no shortening of the muscle fibers and in which no external work is done, but tension is maintained.
6. The *equilibrium length* of a muscle is the length of the relaxed muscle at which the resting tension is zero.
7. The *resting, or optimal, length* of a muscle is that length at which maximal contraction tension develops.
8. *Latency relaxation* is the period between the stimulus and the contraction.
9. *Stress relaxation* is the slow loss of tension after a muscle is suddenly stressed and placed under a constant strain. The accompanying slow lengthening is called "creep."

Muscle Paralysis and Spasticity

BASIC CONSIDERATIONS

Motor paralysis is the loss of voluntary muscle power either resulting from interruption of the motor or lower motor neuron pathways controlling it or due to some deficiency of the muscle itself, making it incapable of responding to nervous control. As a result of muscle paralysis, there will be changes in muscle tone, tendon reflexes, and the physical mass of the muscle or muscles involved.

MUSCLE TONE. The term "muscle tone" is used differently by the physiologist and the clinician. The physiologist defines it as a state of partial tetanus of the muscle that is maintained by an asynchronous discharge of impulses in motor neurons supplying it. It is reflexly produced from afferent nerve endings situated within the muscle itself and profoundly influenced by supraspinal mechanisms. Muscle tone provides the background of posture in which active movements occur and is an important element in the coordination of movement.

Clinicians commonly estimate tone by the passive manipulation of limbs. This gives them a sense of the degree of tension, or elastic resistance, in the muscle. In lesions of the lower motor neuron muscle tone is abolished; this condition is called "flaccidity," or "flaccid paralysis." In lesions of the upper motor neuron muscle tone is increased, a condition of spasticity that occurs when the pyramidal tract is involved; when there is rigidity, the extrapyramidal tract is involved.

TENDON REFLEXES. The tendon reflexes are short-lived stretch reflexes elicited by tapping the tendon of the muscle, which evokes stimulation of the intrafusal muscle fibers of the muscle spindles. When muscle tone is increased, as in lesions of the upper motor neuron, the response to the tendon tap is increased, and the tendon jerk is thus increased in both amplitude and duration. Sometimes sudden stretching of the muscle will result in a repetitive jerk known as "clonus." The tendon reflex will be completely abolished by any interruption of the lower motor neuron reflex arc system on either the afferent or efferent loop.

PHYSICAL MASS OF MUSCLE. In upper motor neuron lesions the actual physical mass of the muscle remains unchanged, but in lower motor neuron lesions rapid wasting of the affected muscles will occur.

ATAXIA. "Ataxia" may be defined as imperfectly controlled or uncoordinated voluntary movements. It may be

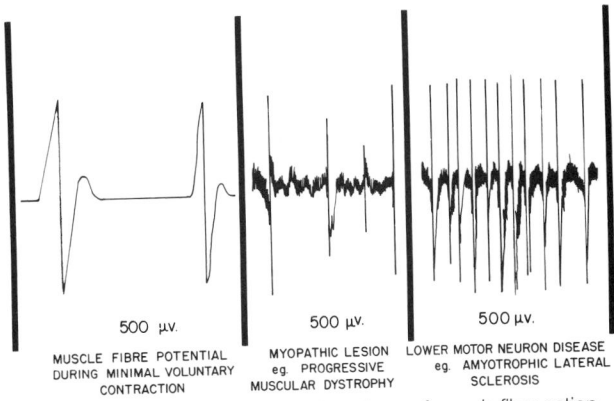

Fig. 43-11. Three electromyographic patterns of muscle fiber action potential showing normal potential curves (left), a myopathic lesion (middle), and lower motor neuron disease (right). [From: *Duthie RB, Bentley JB (eds): Orthopaedic Surgery. London, Edward Arnold, 1982, with permission.*]

(Figure labels: MUSCLE FIBRE POTENTIAL DURING MINIMAL VOLUNTARY CONTRACTION — 500 μv. / MYOPATHIC LESION eg. PROGRESSIVE MUSCULAR DYSTROPHY — 500 μv. / LOWER MOTOR NEURON DISEASE eg. AMYOTROPHIC LATERAL SCLEROSIS — 500 μv.)

due to lesions of the cerebellum or the vestibular system. A sensory ataxia may arise from involvement of the pathways of proprioceptive and position sense, i.e., as seen in tabes dorsalis and in Friedreich's ataxia.

ELECTRICAL DIAGNOSIS AND ASSESSMENT OF MUSCLE DENERVATION. The method of obtaining the electrical "reaction" of muscle by faradic or galvanic stimulation applied to a muscle and its motor nerve has given way to more precise methods of greater complexity such as the intensity duration curve, electromyography, and nerve conduction velocity tests.

Intensity Duration Curve. Intensity duration curves are obtained by stimulating the muscle mass with pulses of known duration and intensity that produce characteristic patterns of contraction.

Electromyography. Electromyography (Fig. 43-11) is carried out with needle electrodes inserted into a muscle by means of which recordings are made of action potentials picked up within the muscles. The potential patterns reveal the presence or absence of denervation and of certain stages of regeneration of nerve.

Nerve Conduction Tests. Nerve conduction velocity tests are chiefly of value in defining peripheral nerve conduction interruption and, together with electromyography, form a useful basis in distinguishing among true motor neuron disease, peripheral nerve disease, and myopathy.

Intrinsic Diseases of Muscle

CLASSIFICATION

A. Muscular dystrophies
   1. Progressive muscular dystrophy of Duchenne
   2. Fasciascapulohumeral dystrophy of Landouzy-Déjerine
   3. Dystrophia myotonica, or Steinert's disease
B. Periodic diseases
   1. Myasthenia gravis
   2. Familial periodic paralysis
C. Other diseases of muscle
   1. Benign congenital hypotonia of Oppenheim-Walton

2. Glycogen storage diseases of muscle
    a. Type 5, or McArdle-Schmid-Pearson disease
    b. Type 6, or Hers' disease
3. Myotonia congenita, or Thomsen's disease
4. Central core disease
D. Developmental defects of muscle
    1. Hypoplasia and aplasia
    2. Arthrogryposis
E. Constitutional disorders of muscle
    1. Neuromuscular atrophies
        a. Poliomyelitis
        b. Progressive muscular atrophy of Duchenne-Aran
        c. Infantile muscular atrophy of Hoffman-Werdnig
        d. Peroneal muscular atrophy (Charcot-Marie-Tooth disease)
        e. Amyotrophic lateral sclerosis
        f. Syringomyelia
        g. Myelodysplasia
    2. Endocrine and metabolic disturbances
        a. Thyrotoxic myopathy
        b. Adrenal insufficiency
        c. Cushing's syndrome
        d. Hyperinsulinism
        e. Hyperkalemia and hypokalemia

In distinguishing the true myopathies from other causes of muscular paralysis, one must take into consideration the early age of onset, the familial history, and the progressive wasting of muscle groups without anatomic relation to any particular nerve supply. Other factors are the absence of fibrillation and the presence of normal tendon reflexes in the face of severe muscle wasting, and if necessary more specific data can be obtained by electromyography, muscle biopsy, and biochemical tests for serum aldolase and urine creatinine levels.

MUSCULAR DYSTROPHIES

PSEUDOHYPERTROPHIC MUSCULAR DYSTROPHY (DUCHENNE). The Duchenne type of muscular dystrophy is a progressive muscular disease that is usually manifested during the first 3 to 6 years, although it may be present in infancy or not recognized until adolescence. It affects boys primarily and is genetically determined by a sex-linked recessive gene. The presenting complaint is difficulty or instability in standing or walking. There may be an awkward waddling gait. The child gets up from the floor in a characteristic manner using the arms to get up on the legs to attain the upright posture. The child stands with increased lordosis, is weak, and usually has enlarged bulky muscles. The enlargement is conspicuous in the calves, the deltoids, and the quadriceps. The hands and the forearms usually are not involved. With progression, the pelvic musculature, erector spinae, and intercostals may be involved. Contractures occur early in the course of the disease and are first seen as equinovarus deformity of the foot. The cardiac muscle may be involved late in the course of the disease and may be responsible for death. Most patients are dead by the age of twenty years.

FASCIOSCAPULOHUMERAL TYPE OF MUSCULAR DYSTROPHY (LANDOUZY-DÉJERINE). This type of muscular dystrophy presents with facial and shoulder girdle involvement and is the most common form of muscular dystrophy in adults.

The facial muscles are involved early and may present in childhood or late adolescence. The cheeks droop, the lips pout, and the facies are immobile. Shoulder girdle involvement causes abnormal shoulder posture and difficulty in raising arms. Pelvic musculature is rarely involved. The heart may be affected, but life span is usually not shortened. The disease is transmitted by an autosomal dominant gene and may affect either sex.

LIMB GIRDLE TYPE OF MUSCULAR DYSTROPHY (ERB). This type of muscular dystrophy is much less common than Duchenne's and occurs later in life, usually in the second decade. Pseudohypertrophy is uncommon. The involvement begins first about the shoulder and pelvic girdles with involvement of the upper arm and thigh. The atrophy of the involved muscles produces striking contrast in the size of the arm, forearm, thigh, and leg in a typical case. The course is progressively downhill until there is involvement of all muscles and is more rapid, with earlier onset. Both sexes are involved. Inheritance is by an autosomal recessive gene.

OCULAR MUSCULAR DYSTROPHY. This is a dystrophic process involving first the levator palpabrae superioris and later the external ocular muscles. There may be weakness and wasting of other muscles about the face, head, and neck. Sexes are affected equally. Inheritance is by autosomal dominant gene.

PATHOLOGY OF MUSCULAR DYSTROPHY. The pathologic features of the various forms of muscular dystrophy are similar. The involved muscle is pink or gray and more whitish than normal. Microscopically there is greater variation of individual fiber size, from 10 to 200 mμ. On cross section, fibers are rounded instead of polygonal, lose striation, and appear hyalinized in longitudinal section. There is no attempt at muscle regeneration. Fat and connective tissue replace degenerating muscle fibers. Sarcolemmic nuclei may be increased. The deformity of scoliosis can derange the posture of standing or sitting. Correction with internal rodding and wiring and immediate ambulation can be achieved, but recognize that prolonged bed rest or immobilization is destructive to these patients.

DIAGNOSIS. Early in the course of the disease, the diagnosis may be confused with polymyositis, since it may respond to medication. Serum enzymes, electromyography, and muscle biopsy are helpful in making the diagnosis of dystrophy, although the clinical features must be considered to distinguish the type of dystrophy.

In the Duchenne type of muscular dystrophy, the serum aldolase or creatine phosphokinase levels are invariably extremely high. Late in the disease, they may approach normal after muscle destruction has been complete. In the other dystrophies serum aldolase and creatine phosphokinase levels are raised according to the degree of muscle involvement, and the elevations are usually much lower than in the Duchenne type. Levels of creatine in the urine are increased above normal, while there is a reduction in the urinary excretion of creatinine that is probably related to a decrease in muscle mass. Urinary excretion of amino acid is also increased.

Electromyography of an involved muscle shows lower potentials and polyphasic pattern during voluntary contraction.

The value of the muscle biopsy depends upon the selection of abnormal muscle, careful technique, and adequate tissue preparation. The selected muscle should be a muscle that is abnormal but not severely involved. The site of biopsy should be away from the insertion of the muscle where there is variation in the fiber size. A specimen at least $1\frac{1}{2}$ cm long and 1 cm wide is required for adequate study. The specimen should be gently stretched to the necessary length with ends fastened on a card or held in a special muscle clamp, placed in saline solution for 30 min, and then fixed in formalin. The basic lesion in Duchenne's appears to be loss of integrity of the muscle cell membrane.

TREATMENT. There is no specific curative therapy for muscular dystrophy. Treatment is symptomatic. Exercise is valuable in maintaining the patients's ability to ambulate and remain functional. The orthopaedist should be aware that procedures that confine a patient to bed rest tend to accelerate the muscle weakness. Patients should not be confined to a wheelchair prematurely. Parents are instructed in stretching exercises of the lower extremities, hamstrings, spinal extensors, and gastrocnemius, and encouraged in a program of muscle strengthening exercises against active resistance.

Short and long leg braces for the lower extremities are used to keep the child standing and ambulating as long as possible. When equinus contractures are severe, heel cord lengthening may be carried out. The child should be fitted with a brace postoperatively and encouraged to ambulate within a few days. When spinal extensor and abdominal flex or weakness is severe and a wheelchair is required, the application of a torso body plaster may be of value in maintaining sitting posture.

MYOTONIAS

MYOTONIC DYSTROPHY. This is a rare disorder in which there is a myopathy in combination with other abnormalities. The disorder is inherited as an autosomal dominant. The onset may be at any time during the first three decades of life. The onset commonly starts with dystrophy in the distal musculature and the muscles of the face and neck. Myopathic facies are common. Progress is slow, and proximal muscles may be involved much later. Percussion of a muscle or electric stimulation results in prolonged contraction of the muscle. Gonadal atrophy, cataracts, and frontal baldness occur in males with this disorder.

MYOTONIA CONGENITA OR THOMSEN'S DISEASE. This is a rare hereditary disorder transmitted as an autosomal recessive or dominant gene. In all voluntary muscles there is difficulty in starting movement following rest. Symptoms may begin at infancy but usually appear between the ages of five and ten years. The patient gives the appearance of excessive muscle mass and muscular overdevelopment. Following repeated motion, the initial weakness improves to where muscle strength may be normal. Percussion of the muscle results in a myotonic sustained contraction. The disease is compatible with normal life expectancy.

PATHOLOGY AND DIAGNOSIS OF MYOTONIA. Histologic examination of a myotonic muscle reveals the presence of long chains of centrally placed nuclei in otherwise intact muscle fibers. Characteristically, some muscle fibers are enlarged. On cross section, the peripheral myofibrils have degenerated and surround a central group of normal fibrils. There is no regeneration, and connective tissue does not replace the muscle, thus accounting for the absence of contractures.

On electromyography, a characteristic shower of electric activity occurs spontaneously after stimulation. Serum enzyme levels may be similar to those in the dystrophies other than Duchenne's, which has a marked elevation of creatine phosphokinase and serum aldolase levels.

TREATMENT. There is no effective treatment for myotonic dystrophy. However, patients with Thomsen's disease can be improved by the use of procainamide, prednisone, and quinine.

Inflammatory Disease

Myositis, or inflammation in muscles, may be due to specific etiologic agents such as a virus, parasite, bacterium, or spirochete. Myositis occurs in diseases of unknown cause such as the collagen vascular diseases, dermatomyositis, lupus, scleroderma, and rheumatoid arthritis. The term "polymyositis" is used to describe the changes in muscle associated with these conditions as well as those found in association with malignant tumors.

The clinical course of polymyositis is variable and may present as an insidious chronic muscle weakness, or it may begin with acute symptoms of high fever, marked muscle pain, spasm, and weakness. The heart muscle may be involved in any of these conditions. Skin changes associated with the primary diagnosis, i. e., lupus or scleroderma, will assist in making the diagnosis. The course of the disease is variable and may be rapidly progressive, resulting in death, or it may persist with episodes of remission and exacerbation. Spontaneous arrest may occur.

Electromyography of the involved muscle reveals spontaneous fibrillation potential in the relaxed muscle, distinguishing polymyositis from muscular dystrophy. There is degeneration and necrosis of muscle fibers associated with infiltration by chronic inflammatory cells, both interstitially and about blood vessels.

TREATMENT. The treatment of polymyositis is directed at diagnosis of the primary condition. In elderly patients presenting with polymyositis, an unrecognized malignant tumor should be suspected. Most patients with polymyositis may be controlled dramatically with the use of cortisone preparations or ACTH. General treatment requires supportive care, physiotherapy in the form of exercise to maintain existing muscle power, appropriate bracing, and occasionally surgical treatment for contractures. Orthopaedic treatment is directed at control of deformities by appropriate bracing or surgical arthrodesis of neurotrophic joints.

POLIOMYELITIS

Poliomyelitis is an acute infectious disease caused by the poliomyelitis virus. The virus is present in the pharynx and feces of infected patients during the preparalytic and postparalytic stages. Invasion of the central nervous system is thought to take place by virus traveling proximally along the peripheral nerve to the spinal cord. Once established in the central nervous system, the virus causes anterior horn cell destruction that results in a flaccid paralysis. With loss of innervation, the motor unit muscle fibers atrophy. Paralysis or deformity and leg-length discrepancies are the result.

CLINICAL COURSE OF THE DISEASE. In about one-third of patients with poliomyelitis infection an initial febrile illness develops consisting of headache, malaise, and low-grade fever, lasting 48 h. Such a patient may recover completely or go on to a second, acute phase after 4 or 5 days of apparent good health. The acute phase may develop in the absence of the initial symptoms.

The acute phase lasts from a few days to a week and also may resolve without paralysis. The illness is characterized by meningeal symptoms including headache, fever, stiff neck, and muscle spasms in the spine or extremities. "Nonparalytic poliomyelitis" describes those patients who do not progress to the paralytic stage.

About the third or fourth day of the acute illness, paralysis may develop. There may be loss of deep reflexes, muscle spasm of the erector spinae, and even signs of bulbar paralysis. The lower limbs are involved twice as frequently as the upper extremities. Death may result from bulbar paralysis, due to respiratory insufficiency.

The convalescent stage begins after the acute illness and ends up to 2 years later at a point where there is no significant recovery in muscle power.

The residual stage occurs following changes in muscle recovery. Children will continue to improve in the residual stage because of their improved coordination.

TREATMENT. In the acute stage, treatment is directed at isolation of patients with the disease, general nursing care, and the treatment of respiratory difficulty by the use of mechanical respirators.

In the early stages of convalescence, treatment is directed at eliminating deforming tendencies, restoring joint motion, and training and protecting recovering muscles. Later on, the patient is fitted with suitable protective braces and taught resistance exercises to develop residual muscle power. Muscle spasm is treated to prevent asymmetrical muscle tightness and soft tissue contractures. Trained therapists apply hot packs and give passive range-of-motion exercises. The patients must be nursed in the proper position, to prevent overstretching of para-

lyzed muscles and joint contractures. Appropriate splints are utilized, depending upon muscle weakness.

The patient is taught muscle reeducation to reestablish control of the extremities and joints as early as possible, when acute symptoms subside. When the patient is ambulatory, orthotic devices to protect and assist control of the paralyzed extremities are utilized.

Treatment in the residual stage requires orthopaedic surgical procedures to correct joint contractures, to improve joint power and function by appropriate muscle and tendon transfers, to stabilize joints by arthrodesis, and to correct leg-length inequality.

Tendon transfer is utilized to restore muscle balance to a joint, to restore lost function, and to increase active power of joint motions. Before undertaking tendon transfer, an expandable muscle of suitable strength and excursion must be available for transfer about a joint with a normal passive range of motion.

Grade	Muscle power
0	Complete paralysis
1	Flicker of contraction without joint excursion
2	Muscle power to effect partial range of motion
3	Muscle power to effect a full range of joint motion against gravity
4	Less than normal strength but full range of joint motion against resistance
5	Normal muscle strength

A muscle will lose one grade of strength following transfer, so that its power must be grade 4 or better. The muscle selected should have sufficient excursion to replace the lost function. Muscles from synergistic groups provide better results by making muscle reeducation more complete. Joint contractures should be corrected and a passive range of joint motion established prior to tendon transfer. The tendon connecting the new origin and insertion should be as straight as possible to improve the efficiency of muscle action and should be placed in an area where gliding is possible.

BONY STABILIZATION. When muscle power is insufficient to protect or move the joint or when sufficiently expandable muscles are not available for transfer, *arthrodesis* of the joint will provide stability, prevent deformity, and even permit transfer of local muscles for other functions. A prerequisite of arthrodesis is the presence of adjacent mobile joints to compensate for the lost motion.

Joint contractures are corrected by judicious stretching by a physiotherapist or by braces incorporating dynamic stretching. The joints may be gradually stretched into the corrected position by successive plaster-cast changes or plaster-cast wedging. Leg-length discrepancy may be corrected by bone lengthening or shortening procedures. A 1-in. difference in leg length is usually of no practical significance.

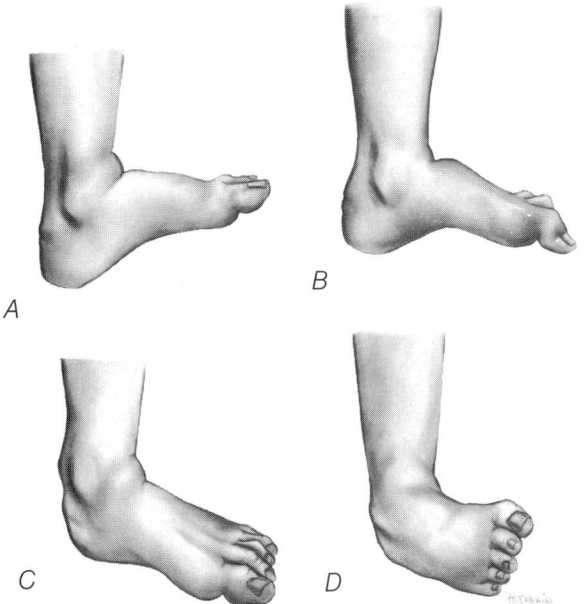

Fig. 43-12. Paralytic deformities of the foot. *A.* Calcaneal deformity. *B.* Cavus (claw) foot. *C.* Valgus deformity. *D.* Varus deformity.

Treatment of Deformities

Foot Paralysis. (Fig. 43-12). Deformities are treated by proper bracing to maintain stability and prevent deformity until maximal recovery has occurred. When maximal recovery has occurred, tendon transfers or bony stabilization procedures are indicated. Bony stabilization other than the Grice extraarticular arthrodesis of the subtalar joint is not performed until bony maturity is achieved at age twelve to fifteen.

Valgus deformity is due to muscle imbalance, from weakness or absence of functioning invertors, that results in pronation of the forefoot and eversion of the calcaneus. The extraarticular arthrodesis of the subtalar joint (Grice) is an effective means of controlling this until bony maturity. (Fig. 43-13*A*). Varus deformity is due to muscle imbalance with paralysis of the peroneal muscles. Treatment is directed at restoring eversion power and strength. The anterior tibial may be transferred laterally to reduce its varus deforming force and improve eversion. The posterior tibial tendon may be released from its tendon sheath and allowed to ride in front of the medial malleolus.

Calcaneus Deformity. Calcaneus deformity is the result of paralysis of the calf muscles. The unopposed dorsiflexors pull the foot into dorsiflexion, and the calcaneal foot results. This is a difficult deformity to control with bracing. The posterior or peroneal tendons may be transferred into the calcaneus, effecting partial improvement in plantar flexion power. Alternatives are tenodesis of the Achilles tendon, which will provide the fulcrum for pushoff. At age twelve to fifteen years, triple arthrodesis may be required (Fig. 43-13*B*).

Equinus Deformity. Equinus deformity results from paralysis of the anterior tibial tendon, causing foot drop.

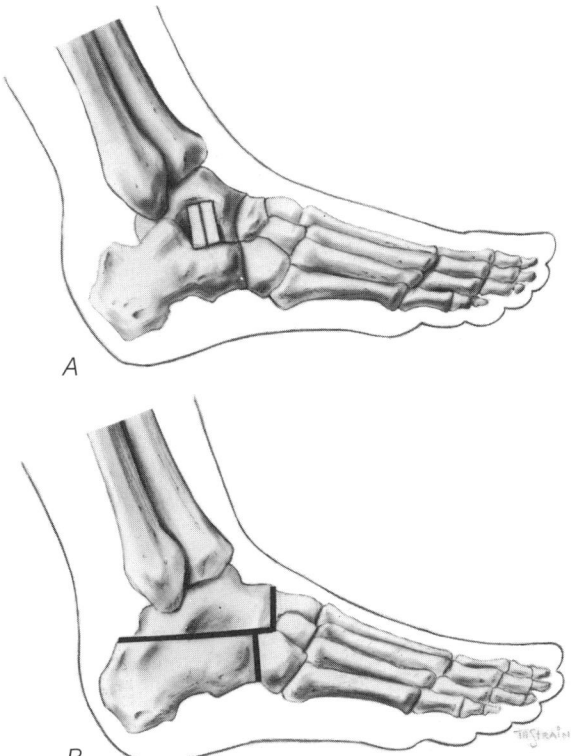

Fig. 43-13. *A.* Grice procedure with a strut of tibial bone graft wedged between talus and calcaneus. *B.* Triple arthrodesis.

This deformity may be controlled with a foot drop short leg brace. Forward transfer of the peroneals for dorsiflexion, combined with triple arthrodesis, may be accomplished at bony maturity. A triple arthrodesis may be effective in the absence of functioning peroneal muscles.

Claw Hallux Deformity. Extension of the metatarsophalangeal (MP) joint of the great toe with flexion of the interphalangeal (IP) joint commonly occurs with paralysis of the tibialis anterior. The overpull of the extensor hallucis longus results in dorsiflexion of the MP joint and clawing. Depression of the first metatarsal shaft is due to the unbalanced pull of the peroneus longus. This deformity can be effectively treated by the Jones procedure. This consists of transplantation of the extensor hallucis longus into the neck of the first metatarsal shaft, combined with stabilization of the IP joint by arthrodesis.

PARALYSIS ABOUT THE KNEE JOINT. Patients with isolated paralysis of the quadriceps get along satisfactorily if there is adequate power in the gastrocnemius and gluteus maximus to stabilize the knee in extension. Transplantation of the biceps combined with semitendinosis transfer to the patella may be indicated.

PARALYSIS ABOUT THE HIP. Paralytic deformity of the hip results in severe disability through the disturbance of gait. The indications for treatment depend upon the availability of function in adjacent muscles and the degree of disability. A posterior transfer of extensor fascia lata, lateral transfer of the iliopsoas (Mustard procedure), or erector spinae transfer for gluteus maximus paralysis give variable results. In properly selected patients, a small gain in stability may result in great benefit by relieving fatigability of gait and pelvic stabilization. If a painful hip, subluxation, or frank dislocation due to muscle imbalance develops, arthrodesis may be necessary.

PARALYSIS IN THE UPPER EXTREMITY. Shoulder. Paralysis of the deltoid and rotator cuff in the presence of remaining power in the scapular stabilizing muscles—trapezius, rhomboids, serratus anterior—may be treated by arthrodesis of the glenohumeral joint in the appropriate position. The resulting stabilization allows shoulder stability, adequate motion, and power from the function of scapulothoracic muscles.

Elbow. Surgical procedures to improve power across the elbow are directed primarily at restoring elbow flexion in paralysis of the biceps and brachialis. If normal power exists in the flexors of the wrist and fingers, proximal transfer of the common flexor origin will improve elbow flexion power. Alternative methods include transfer of the inferior portion of the pectoralis major or the sternocleidomastoideus attached to a free tendon graft.

Paralytic Hand. Paralysis of wrist extensors may be treated by dorsal transfer of the flexor carpi ulnaris or pronator teres into the extensor carpi radialis longus and brevis. Loss of thumb extension is treated by insertion of the flexor carpi radialis into the abductor pollicis longus and extensor pollicis brevis. The palmaris longus may be inserted into the extensor pollicis longus. Paralysis of the extensor digitorum communis may be treated by transfer of the flexor carpi ulnaris dorsally.

Loss of opposition of the thumb is a common finding in the paralytic hand due to poliomyelitis. Various procedures are available to restore opposition, including transfer of the flexor digitorum superficialis to the ring finger routed about a pulley on the flexor carpi ulnaris and inserted into the base of the thumb.

Wrist arthrodesis may provide stability of the hand and make available expendable tendons for transfer.

CEREBRAL PALSY

Cerebral palsy occurs in about 3 births for every 100,000 population.

ETIOLOGY. Cerebral palsy may be caused by a number of factors including head trauma at birth, head injury in childhood, anoxic brain damage (only 10 to 14 percent can be attributed to postnatal conditions), vascular accidents following treatment of brain tumor, involvement of the central nervous system from encephalitis, and other viral diseases, e.g., measles, cytomegalic inclusion body. The pathologic lesions in the brain have not been well documented, and little information has been correlated between pathology and symptoms.

CLINICAL MANIFESTATIONS. Fifty percent of all new patients are spastic, 25 percent are athetoid, 5 percent are ataxic, 5 percent are rigid, and the remainder have the mixed-type lesion.

Spasticity is due to an upper motor neuron lesion, involving the pyramidal tract. Clinical examination reveals hyperactive stretch reflexes. Sudden passive motion of a joint produced by spastic muscles activates this reflex, and clonus results. Weakness may be present in antagonistic muscle groups and contributes to the development of joint flexion contractures.

Cerebral spastic patients are of four types: 60 percent of all spastics are hemiplegic with paralysis of ipsilateral arm and leg; the patient with left-sided hemiplegia is more likely to have better preservation of intellectual function. The second most common type is the diplegic with symmetrical spastic involvement in the lower extremities and less severe involvement in the upper extremities. Paraplegic patients are uncommon, having involvement only of the lower extremities. The quadriplegic patient tends to have symmetrical involvement of all four extremities.

Athetosis is characterized by involuntary repetitive motion of a muscle group or extremity resulting in severe dysfunction. Athetotic motions may be worsened by sudden stress, tension, weight bearing, and even sudden changes of light. Joint contractures are rare with this manifestation.

Ataxia is related to lesions of the cerebellum, causing deficient postural reflexes. There is commonly a voluntary tremor, hypotonia, and easy fatigability. The child walks with a staggering, broad-based gait. Reflexes are decreased and contractures uncommon.

Rigidity results from diffuse cerebral involvement, commonly from birth ataxia.

In *mixed types of cerebral palsy* spasticity commonly coexists with athetosis. Not infrequently, children at age two to four with spasticity show evidence of coexisting athetosis as they grow older.

TREATMENT. Successful treatment is directly related to the intelligence of the child. About two-thirds of cerebral palsied children have IQs below 70. Physiotherapy for muscle strengthening, gait training, and effective bracing are needed. Orthopaedic surgical correction of deformities is important but is the least frequently required therapeutic approach.

Orthotics. Orthoses are necessary (1) to prevent contractures from muscle imbalance and spasticity; (2) to provide stability in the lower extremities, because of muscle weakness; (3) to minimize purposeless motion; and (4) to provide evaluation prior to performing stabilization procedures.

Braces have their greatest application to the lower extremities to control varus or valgus deformities of the foot, provide stability in walking and standing, and assist in preventing contractures. In the spastic child with the tendency to equinus contractures of the foot or flexion deformities of the knees, posterior plaster splints or bivalved plaster casts will assist in overcoming these deformities. Long leg braces are applied to assist in preventing knee flexion contractures and valgus deformities and provide stability in the upright position. Bilateral long leg braces with a pelvic band provide additional stability at the hip joint. Upper extremity bracing assists in holding the hand in the position of function and preventing flexion contractures at the wrists and fingers, or adduction deformities of the thumb.

THERAPY FOR SPECIFIC AREAS. Hip. Adductor spasticity with weakened abductors results in a valgus deformity of the femoral neck that can lead to lateral displacement of the hips. Tenotomy, and neurectomy, a subtrochanteric varus osteotomy with internal fixation, may become necessary (Fig. 43-14). Rotational deformity is corrected at the same time.

Knee. If a contracture has developed, it may be corrected by plaster-cast wedging. When this is unsuccessful, posterior capsulotomy or hamstring lengthening by Z-plasty may effectively relieve the contracture. In the child walking in a crouched position with hips and knees flexed, surgical release of the hamstrings will assist in bringing both hip and knee to extension and improve the erect posture and gait. If there has been long-standing stretching of the anterior patellar retinacula and lengthening of the patellar ligament, effective quadriceps power can be improved by division of the posterior component of the patellar retinacula; this allows any quadriceps power to be applied effectively to the stretched patellar ligaments.

Foot. If an equinovarus contracture can be demonstrated with the knee extended but not with the knee flexed, contracture of the gastrocnemius is the cause, and its release is required.

Orthopaedic Surgical Treatment

An operation is used for

1. Weakening spastic muscles by tendon lengthening
2. Improving joint motion by tendon transplantation
3. Stabilizing deformed or contracted joints by arthrodesis
4. Correcting deformity by osteotomy and correction of leg-length inequality

If children with cerebral palsy are put to bed for surgical procedures, their motor abilities deteriorate at least temporarily. For the athetoid child, surgical intervention is rarely indicated. Correction of the deformity at one level results in expression of the disorder at a more proximal level. Most surgical procedures are applied in the treatment of the spastic. Procedures that require stabilization are more likely to be successful, since muscle re-education and patient cooperation are not required. When tendon transfers are indicated, good sensation, a higher IQ, and higher motor age are prerequisites.

UPPER EXTREMITY. Surgical treatment of the upper extremity is rarely indicated and is done to improve appearance and position of the hand, wrist, and forearm. Arthrodesis of the wrist is done in extension and moderate ulnar deviation in order passively to improve thumb abduction. By eliminating wrist motion, finger power and control are improved. An alternative method is transfer of the flexor carpi ulnaris tendon around the ulnar side of the forearm and insertion into radial wrist extensor tendons. This will improve wrist extension, though there is little effect on supination power. Stabilization of the thumb by an iliac bone graft between the first two metacarpals may be necessary.

LOWER EXTREMITY. For flexion adduction deformity of the hip, the infant is splinted with an abduction splint, and

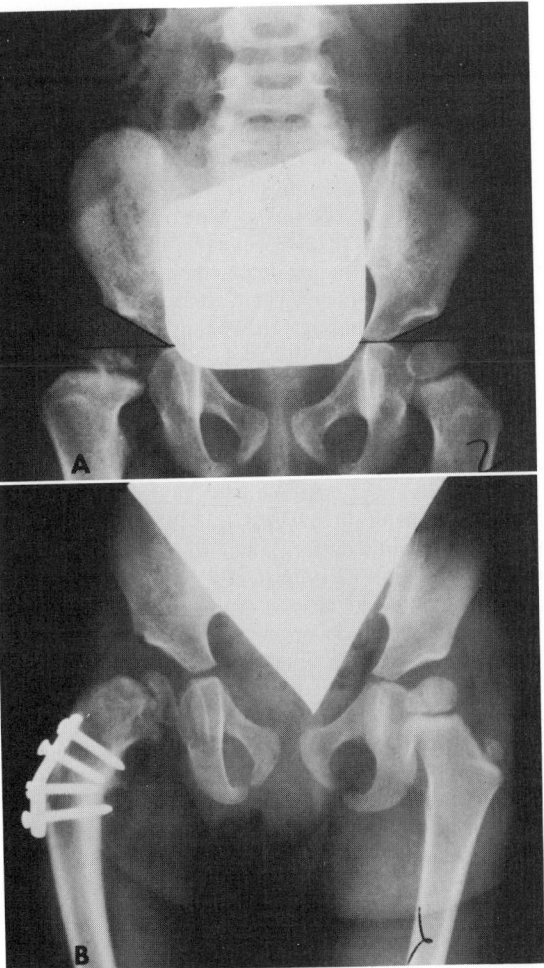

Fig. 43-14. Hip subluxation in spastic diplegia. *A.* AP of the pelvis showing lateral displacement of the right hip. *B.* AP of the pelvis showing maintenance of the head in the acetabulum following varus derotation osteotomy.

daily passive stretching is carried out to minimize deformity. Adductor tenotomy dividing the major adductor origins from the pelvis may be indicated. Flexion deformity of the knee due to muscle spasm may be corrected by plaster wedging. When contracture is established and there is a weakened quadriceps or an overstretched patellar tendon with upward migration of the patella, the best procedure is posterior capsulotomy of the knee and Z-plasty lengthening of the hamstrings. In the foot, the common equinus deformity may be treated by division of the nerve supply to the gastrocnemius or soleus muscles, or by lengthening of the Achilles tendon or gastrocnemius. When bony maturity is reached, varus and vagus deformities may be treated by triple arthrodesis.

MYELODYSPLASIA (SPINAL DYSRAPHISM)

Myelodysplasia describes a developmental defect in the vertebral column with associated peripheral neurologic lesions. "Spinal dysraphism" refers to congenital defects of the lumbosacral regions with failure of fusion of midline structures. The vertebral lesion may be present without involvement of the cord, i.e., as spina bifida occulta. Spina bifida may be associated with meningocele, myelomeningocele, or myeloschisis, an open neural plate. Hydrocephalus is frequently associated with these lesions. Antenatal screening for the alphafetoprotein (AFP) can aid in the diagnosis of neural tube defects.

CLINICAL MANIFESTATIONS. Spina bifida occulta is frequently an incidental finding detected by x-ray and is not usually associated with neurologic abnormality. An occasional patient may have detectable muscle imbalance or sensory abnormalities of the foot that are quite localized.

Meningoceles (cystic enlargement of the lower meninges), myelomeningoceles (cystic enlargement of meninges and intradural contents), or myeloschisis (a frank open neural plate) may occur with spina bifida resulting in severe deformities of the lower extremity. Early surgical closure may prevent deterioration of the distal neurologic function. The neural sac is closed by mobilization of fascial flaps and full-thickness skin coverage. Associated hydrocephalus, which occurs in 80 percent of these patients, should be treated simultaneously. The prognosis for a child with these developmental abnormalities of the central nervous system will depend upon the degree of resultant lower extremity paralysis as well as neurologic abnormalities of the bladder and urinary tract. The cases with bad prognoses manifest gross limb paralysis in a thoracic lumbosacral lesion and scoliosis or kyphosis, evidence of hydrocephalus, intracerebral injury, or cardiac abnormality.

ORTHOPAEDIC MANAGEMENT. The deformities of the lower extremities are related to the level of spinal involvement, which may be complete or spotty in distribution. If a complete lesion occurs at the first lumbar segment, flaccid paralysis is the result; treatment is directed at obtaining weight-bearing attitude in the lower extremities. When the level is between L_3 and L_4, hip adduction and flexion is present, whereas hip abduction and extension are absent, with resulting potential paralytic hip dislocation. The management of such paralytic deformities is similar to that of deformities that occur as a result of flaccid paralysis of poliomyelitis.

Talipes equinovarus is the most common foot deformity resulting from muscle imbalance, although calcaneal valgus or varus also may occur. Management is directed at maintaining the weight-bearing position. If deformity is already present, plaster-cast correction of the foot is carried out and followed by short leg braces to control the muscle imbalance. Lack of sensation makes the possibility of pressure sores a chronic problem for these patients. For the valgus foot, the Grice procedure may be required. When bony maturity has been reached, triple arthrodesis is performed to stabilize the foot.

When a complete lesion occurs at the levels of L_3 and L_4, quadriceps function remains in the absence of the hamstring function, and hyperextension of the knee results. In such a patient, the deformity is managed by plaster casts, splints, and long leg braces to prevent recurvation of the knee. Osteotomy may be necessary to correct rotational deformities.

When a complete lesion occurs between L_3 and L_4, coxa valga and subluxation of the hip occur. It is important to recognize this deformity before actual dislocation results. Management is directed at restoring the muscle balance responsible for the deformity. Sharrard's lateral transfer of the iliopsoas through the wing of the ilium will improve hip abduction and extension and has given satisfactory results. Varus osteotomy and derotational osteotomy of the femur may also be necessary.

DEGENERATIVE DISEASES OF THE NERVOUS SYSTEM WITH SKELETAL DEFORMITY

Peroneal Muscle Atrophy (Charcot-Marie-Tooth Muscular Atrophy)

Peroneal muscular atrophy is a hereditary degenerative process beginning in the peroneal nerve and resulting in peroneal muscular weakness. As the disease progresses, nerve trunks supplying the distal parts of the extremities are involved. Degenerative changes may occur in the spinal nerve roots in pyramidal tracts.

CLINICAL MANIFESTATIONS. The disease usually manifests itself in the first or second decade and may occur as late as the third. The initial complaint is varus deformity of the feet, such that the child walks on the outer borders of the feet. With progressive involvement of the anterior tibial group and foot drop, the patient develops a slapping gait.

Neurologic examination reveals a decrease in reflexes of muscles supplied by involved nerve roots. Anesthesia may accompany the muscle atrophy. The disease is found in several generations and is transmitted as a dominant, recessive, or sex-linked recessive.

Treatment does not affect the slow progressive changes. Short leg braces may control the varus deformity.

Friedreich's Ataxia

Friedreich's cerebellar ataxia is a familial disease in which there is degeneration of spinocerebellar tracts, corticospinal tracts, and posterior columns of the cord.

CLINICAL MANIFESTATIONS. There is usually evidence of the disease in previous generations. It affects males more commonly than females. The onset is usually insidious in childhood, the first abnormality being one of gait or a tendency to fall easily. Later on, there is incoordination, followed by nystagmus and speech disturbances. Thoracic scoliosis and pes cavus with claw toes are seen very commonly. The disease runs a steadily downhill course. Early in the course of this disease, orthopaedic bracing procedures, or even tendon transfers or bony stabilization, may be indicated to maintain ambulation.

Syringomyelia

Syringomyelia is a degenerative condition of the spinal cord in which there is destruction of neurons in the central portion and proliferation of glial elements resulting in the formation of a cavity. It is usually related to defective development, but similar cavities may occur following vascular processes or trauma.

The sexes are affected with equal frequency. The onset usually is in the second or third decade. Rarely are symptoms severe before the age of twenty. The small muscles of the hands are frequently involved early in the course, with deformity and wasting of the hands a result. Disturbances in sensibility with loss of pain sense result in trophic disturbances about the hands and upper extremities. There is progressive atrophy of the muscle supplied by the area of the cord, commonly the cervical area, less commonly the bulbar or lumbar area. Skeletal deformities such as kyphosis, scoliosis, and pes cavus may be evident. The diagnosis depends on finding the associated anesthesia with muscle wasting and skeletal deformity.

If the disease occurs early in life, the prognosis is relatively serious. The disease may progress very slowly, and the patient may function for many years.

Orthopaedic treatment is directed at control of deformities by appropriate bracing or surgical arthrodesis of neuropathic joints. Laminectomy may be required to relieve rapidly expanding cavities of the spinal cord.

ORTHOPAEDIC MANAGEMENT OF STROKE

EARLY TREATMENT. Rehabilitation of the stroke patient begins at the earliest possible time, usually on the third or fourth day after the stroke. In the flaccid state the patient is in urgent need of external stimuli, to replace the proprioceptive impulses produced by movement of limbs. This deficiency of motion may be corrected by a trained physical therapist. Placing the patient in a wheelchair is far preferable to confining him or her to bed. Correct positioning in bed by the use of a foot board may prevent equinus, and the use of a rolled blanket between the greater trochanters to roll the legs may prevent external rotation deformity and flexion of the knees. Correct support of the upper limbs by the use of a pillow in the axilla will maintain shoulder abduction and prevent "frozen shoulder."

Frequent change of position is also of vital importance to prevent hypostatic pneumonia and pressure sores. At each change of position the joints of the limbs are placed through a range of motion and positioned to maintain or increase their range of movement. The prone position should also be used to provide good drainage of secretions and to prevent hip flexion and knee flexion deformities.

ASSESSMENT. Pseudomotor changes are of value in assessing motor control deficits, and it may be possible to predict whether the involvement is bilateral.

The involvement of the extrapyramidal system is of importance, because of its potential reversibility. The classical signs of facial immobility, failure of accommodation, and flexor rigidity in the neck muscles are much later occurrences. In the early stages the most reliable sign of cog wheel rigidity is the test of internal/external rotation of the shoulder and, to a lesser extent, of the hip joint.

Difficulties in balance are often overlooked; it is essential to evaluate patients in the upright position when attempting to assess their ability to walk. Only very occasionally does a stroke disturb the central control of balance. More frequently the inability to stand erect is related to a disturbance of the patient's body image, resulting from a lesion in the nondominant hemisphere of the brain.

Patients with a distorted body image will make no attempt to support or otherwise accommodate for the weight of that side, and thus fall toward the involved side without making any effort to protect themselves. Techniques to stimulate body awareness, walking aids, and braces are possible means of overcoming this inadequacy.

CONTROL OF SPASTICITY. The ideal method of controlling spasticity would decrease excessive muscle tone permanently without associated loss of motor control and without loss of sensation. The most useful method is a peripheral muscle release, but this has the disadvantage of associated muscle weakness.

Peripheral nerve block with phenol reduces or abolishes spasticity for a comparatively short period of time; it begins to return at the second or third month. Intramuscular alcohol is injected in the approximate locus of the motor point used. Its effect lasts about 3 months.

SURGICAL CORRECTION OF DISABILITIES. Lower Limb Problems. The most common site of deformity in the stroke patient is the foot and ankle equinus. This deformity, whether due to actual contracture or to spasticity, is relieved by elongation of the Achilles tendon. In order to control the varus deformity of the foot that is frequently associated with spasticity or contracture of the gastrocnemius and soleus, the tibialis anterior tendon transfer is a useful adjunct. Release of the hamstrings by sectioning at the musculotendinous junction corrects the knee flexion deformity. Hip adduction contracture may be released by adductor division, or, in the case of spasticity, by obturator neurectomy.

The painful frozen shoulder is a major impairment to rehabilitation. Mild spasticity in the internal rotator adductor group at the shoulder is noted frequently in the third and fourth months following a stroke. Active assisted exercises combined with a positioning program may maintain or help restore a good range of shoulder movement.

Severe spasticity of the flexors of the elbow does not respond to exercising and positioning programs and may result in a flexion contracture. Release procedures in the antecubital fossa are rarely called for, and the surgeon must be prepared to release or lengthen the biceps tendon, brachialis, brachioradialis, the forearm flexor muscles, and the elbow joint capsule.

Spasticity and poor motor control are common in the hemiplegic forearm and hand. If a patient with an apparent flexion deformity of the wrist and fingers is able to extend the wrist and fingers selectively following a nerve block, then a flexor slide procedure will be of value to weaken the spastic flexor pronators.

POSTURE

Posture is the basis of all movement. The regulation of normal posture in an intact animal depends upon the integrated activity of many reflex mechanisms. The maintenance of posture is thought to be exclusively a function of reflex arcs that have centers in the pons, medulla, and midbrain.

Tonic neck reflexes appear in infants between the fourth and twelfth week, but it is not until the twenty-eighth week that an infant is able to raise his or her head and control it. By the fifth month the child can roll over, but is usually only creeping or moving forward in the prone position by the tenth month. By the thirty-sixth week he or she will be able to stand still for a short while without support but usually will not walk unaided before the age of twelve months.

When assessing any disturbance of posture, one must inspect children while they are standing, sitting, and lying and determine the presence or absence of any abnormal movements or response to movements. In addition, one should look for any laxity of joints or hypertonia of muscles. When the child stands erect, changes in the spinal column occur with the development of a cervical lordosis, a thoracic kyphosis, and a lumbar lordosis.

Postural deformities resulting from habit, occupational attitudes, or body carriage in movement must be differentiated from static forces, which are concerned with bodies at rest, or the equilibrium of weights that are not moving. A postural deformity is dynamic in origin, whereas a static deformity occurs because of weakened musculature.

Disturbances in Gait (Limping)

REQUIREMENTS FOR EFFICIENT LOCOMOTION. These are

1. Stability of joints, normal bone length, normal skeletal relationships
2. Normal joint range of movement and normal muscle power
3. Cortical control of voluntary muscle action
4. Normal muscle tone, including coordination as well as postural tone
5. Normal sensory modalities
6. Cerebellar control of muscle action, and intact ocular and auditory balance mechanism

Abnormal, or disturbed, gait of mechanical origin must be clearly distinguished from ataxic and other gait patterns of neurologic origin. This requires examination of the joints to determine normal range of motion and detect fixed flexion contractures. Abnormalities of the foot and ankle should be searched for and neurologic disorders evaluated.

NEUROLOGIC DISORDERS

Ataxic gait consists of an uncoordinated, awkward, unbalanced, wide-based gait with poor symmetry and repetition pattern. It may result from

1. Disturbances of the cerebellum, such as thrombosis of the cerebellar artery, or tumors of the posterior cranial fossa

2. Lesions involving the posterior columns such as disseminated sclerosis, the Guillain-Barré syndrome, and Friedreich's ataxia
3. Lesions, involving peripheral sensation and proprioceptive modalities, such as tabes dorsalis, or neuritis and subacute combined degeneration of the cord, which give a characteristic high-stepping gait

A spastic paraplegic gait is characterized by scissoring of the legs, which are held stiff in extension and adducted. If adduction deformity, which is common in cerebral palsy, is severe, the degree of pelvic rotation and elevation may be markedly exaggerated. In hemiplegia the flail, or spastic, leg is used as a prop until the good leg can be brought forward for the propulsion phase.

MECHANICAL DISORDERS

Among the numerous joint abnormalities that may produce gait disturbances are congenital dysplasia, congenital dislocation of the hip, slipped upper femoral epiphysis, Legg-Calvé-Perthes disease, and knee conditions such as juvenile arthritis, osteochondritis dissecans, discoid menisci, congenital genu valgum or varus, and congenital metatarsus varus, flatfoot, or congenital talipes equinovarus (clubfoot). Leg-length discrepancy may result in abnormal gait. Among the muscular disorders resulting in abnormal gait are those secondary to anterior poliomyelitis, cerebral palsy, nerve injury, spina bifida, myelodysplasia, primary motor neuron disease, and muscular dystrophy.

Spinal Deformities

The convexity of the thoracic and sacral curves, the primary curves of the vertebral column, results from the shape of the vertebral bodies, whereas the secondary, lordotic curves of the cervical and lumbar regions are due more to the shape of the intervertebral discs, which are wider anteriorly than posteriorly. In addition, the contour of the vertebral column is dependent upon the integrity of its supporting ligaments and the sacrospinalis and anterior abdominal musculatures.

The intervertebral discs, like arterial walls, reflect the age and tone of the body tissues. With increasing age, the nucleus pulposus loses its elasticity and fluid content, and the fibers of the annulus fibrosus lose their definition. These changes are very marked in those engaged in heavy work, but they are a feature of all aging spines. Alterations in the normal anteroposterior curvature of the spine occur in both the young and the old and are the consequence of affections of bones, intervertebral discs, or spinal muscles.

KYPHOSIS

"Kyphosis" refers to an increase in the normal posterior convexity of the thoracic spine, involving a number of vertebral bodies, if not the entire thoracic column. On the other hand, "gibbus" refers to an acute angular deformity resulting from a disease such as tuberculosis or from a fractured vertebral body.

Kyphosis of Adolescence

MUSCULAR TYPE. The muscular type of adolescent kyphosis is seen in children of poor physical development and is characterized by a thoracic kyphosis, or "round shoulders." Such children are often slow and clumsy in their movements, i.e., uncoordinated. In the early stages, spinal movements are normal, but later the mobility of the spine decreases, and the kyphosis becomes fixed. Pain is not a common feature of the condition, but postural strain on ligaments may produce backache or pain in the feet or legs.

Early treatment aimed at improving musculature by exercise, swimming, deep breathing, and posture training produces dramatic improvement. External support by braces is not recommended.

OSSEOUS TYPE. This usually results from developmental disturbances such as arachnodactyly, osteochondral dystrophy, or acquired lesions such as tuberculosis. Tuberculosis as a result of bony destruction tends to produce an acute gibbus rather than a smooth kyphosis.

DISCOGENIC TYPE, OR TRUE ADOLESCENT KYPHOSIS (SCHEUERMANN'S DISEASE; VERTEBRAL EPIPHYSITIS). This condition occurs in both sexes between the ages of twelve and seventeen and is seen as marked thoracic kyphosis with round, drooping shoulders and a flat, narrow chest with prominent scapulae. The cause of this condition, which is familial, is unknown.

Early active treatment in the form of spinal traction followed by hyperextension and spinal exercises can limit the progress of this deformity. Once spinal growth is complete at the age of sixteen to eighteen years, no further progression will occur.

"TRUE" SENILE KYPHOSIS. Especially in those engaged in heavy occupations, degeneration of the anterior portion of the annulus fibrosis leads to final disintegration of the intervertebral discs. This results in wedging of the anterior aspects of the vertebral bodies until they touch, by osteophyte formation as well as bony absorption.

SENILE OR POSTMENOPAUSAL OSTEOPOROSIS. In this condition, although the degree of osteoporosis of the vertebral bodies varies, it is evenly distributed throughout the vertebral column. There is absorption of the bony trabeculae, but the intervertebral discs remain normal or even tend to bulge into the atrophied spongy tissue of the vertebral body.

In the earliest phase the patient has great difficulty in carrying out extremes of movement, and there is often a history of attacks of "lumbago." Pain may never completely disappear. The individual loses stature and the carriage is stooping, the head and shoulders thrust forward. This loss in height must be differentiated from Paget's disease, Kümmel's disease, multiple myeloma, and secondary malignant deposits.

SCOLIOSIS

When the spine is viewed from the back, any deviation from the normally straight spine to one side or the other, i.e., a lateral deviation, constitutes scoliosis.

Classification of Scoliosis (Modified by Ponsetti and Freedman)

I. Postural scoliosis
II. Structural scoliosis
   A. Idiopathic
      1. Cervicothoracic
      2. Thoracic
         a. Infantile—age of onset birth to three years
         b. Juvenile—age of onset four to nine years
         c. Adolescence—age of onset ten years to the end of growth
      3. Thoracolumbar
      4. Lumbar
      5. Combined thoracic and lumbar
   B. Osteopathic
      1. Congenital vertebral anomalies
      2. Thoracogenic following thoracoplasty or empyema
      3. Osteochondrodystrophy
   C. Neuropathic
      1. Congenital
      2. Postpoliomyelitis
      3. Neurofibromatosis
      4. Other neuropathies
         a. Syringomyelia
         b. Charcot-Marie-Tooth syndrome
         c. Friedreich's ataxia
         d. Cerebral palsy
   D. Myopathic
      1. Congenital scoliosis
      2. Muscular dystrophies

Postural Scoliosis

Postural scoliosis is seen most commonly in adolescent girls. The curve is usually slight, single, and characteristically a long left thoracolumbar scoliosis, without vertebral rotation, which disappears when the child hangs from a bar or bends forward. In recumbency, the spine appears straight, and when tested for lateral flexion it will bend equally well to both sides. A short leg will cause a compensatory scoliosis convex to the side of the depressed pelvis, but correcting the shortening with a lift under the shoe, thus leveling the pelvis, will correct the scoliosis. Treatment of postural scoliosis is the same as for poor posture in general, i.e., improvement in musculature by general spinal exercises.

Structural Scoliosis

CONGENITAL SCOLIOSIS. Congenital scoliosis is associated with demonstrable vertebral anomalies. There may be one hemivertebra or more involved with congenital absence of discs or fusions of vertebral bodies and ribs. In general, isolated vertebral anomalies have a good prognosis, but there are cases, particularly in the thoracic region, in which a long vertebral segment is involved and in which a gross scoliosis develops. It is preferable to determine and to treat surgically at a young age those with an anomalous vertebral development in association with undifferentiated posterolateral bony bars. Congenital scoliosis is more likely than other forms of scoliosis to lead to paraplegia, usually in the later years of growth, and for this reason must remain under observation until the end of the growth period.

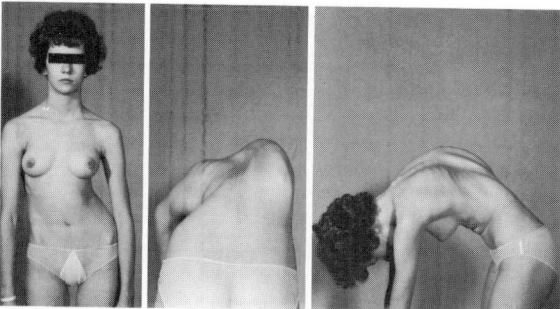

Fig. 43-15. Features of an idiopathic scoliosis in a girl with a right thoracic curve.

PARALYTIC SCOLIOSIS. This most commonly results after anterior poliomyelitis and can be prevented or minimized by adequate initial management. In the young patient with paralytic poliomyelitis and asymmetrical involvement of trunk musculature, asymmetrical soft tissue contractures and subsequent disturbances of vertebral growth may develop.

The various curve patterns of paralytic scoliosis have been divided into high thoracic, thoracic, thoracolumbar, lumbar, and combined thoracic and lumbar scoliosis, and a telescoping spine. The prognosis in paralytic scoliosis is less dependent on the localization of the primary curve than in idiopathic scoliosis. A more important prognostic factor is the age at which the disease first occurs, because the longer the imbalance of muscle affects vertebral growth, the greater the distortion.

Idiopathic Scoliosis

PATHOLOGY. The true pathologic basis of idiopathic scoliosis is unknown. Idiopathic scoliosis will progress during growth in the majority of cases. Therefore, the two important factors in deciding the prognosis of this condition are the *age of onset* and the *site of the curve.*

Completion of ossification of the iliac apophysis coincides with completion of spinal growth. Therefore, any growth after this is minimal, as is deterioration in the curve. Thoracic curves beginning before the age of ten years carry a very poor prognosis and usually result in a severe deformity. Deterioration occurs during two main periods: shortly after diagnosis at the age of two to four years, when it is related to the midgrowth spurt, and, second, at the age of six to nine in boys and six to ten in girls. Although the infantile idiopathic scoliosis makes up only 10 percent of all cases of scoliosis, it is exposed to the total effects of growth throughout its natural history and because of this has an extremely poor prognosis, producing the most progressive and severe of all curvatures.

In general, to prognosticate for any particular case of idiopathic scoliosis, the following observations are required:

1. The site of the curve
2. The age of onset
3. The skeletal or physiologic age rather than the chronological age
4. The state of ossification of the iliac apophysis
5. The developmental age in relation to puberty

CLINICAL FEATURES OF IDIOPATHIC AND OTHER FORMS OF STRUCTURAL SCOLIOSIS. There is rarely a complaint of backache or fatigue. However, in adult life, particularly in lumbar scoliosis, pain due to secondary degenerative changes may produce symptoms. Idiopathic scoliosis develops insidiously. Later complications of severe scoliosis include reductions in the vital capacity of the lungs and the development of cor pulmonale.

The most common type of idiopathic scoliosis is a right thoracic curve, which occurs predominantly in girls (Fig. 43-15). The curvature of congenital scoliosis due to abnormal vertebral development is usually a short, sharp curve that is rigid and associated with much less rotational prominence of the posterior rib cage or lumbar area than the idiopathic and paralytic curves. An angular but short scoliosis in the presence of café au lait spots and subcutaneous nevi indicates neurofibromatosis.

The shoulder girdles, the thoracic and lumbar areas of the trunk, and the iliac crests are assessed for asymmetry. The height of the iliac crest and the posterosuperior iliac spines is determined to note whether the pelvis is level. On forward flexion of the spine a rotational prominence of the transverse processes will be noted, particularly on the convex side of the curve. The mobility of the spine is tested by traction applied to the head manually as well as by lateral bending in the erect position and lateral bending in the recumbent position. A complete radiologic survey of the entire spine is essential including an anteroposterior view with the patient bending to the right and to the left. Lateral views of the spine are also required to assess any degree of congenital anomaly.

The primary curve is defined as

1. The longest curve with the greatest degree of angulation
2. The least flexible curve as determined by clinical and radiologic examination
3. The curve toward which the trunk lists

The degree of angulation is measured on the radiograph. Perpendicular lines are erected to the superior surface of the proximal vertebra and the inferior surface of the distal vertebra involved. The angle formed by these two intersecting lines is the angle of the curve (Fig. 43-16).

Treatment of Scoliosis

CONSERVATIVE TREATMENT. The object of treatment is to obtain correction and to prevent any further increase in the deformity. In idiopathic scoliosis in particular, treatment requires regular clinical, radiographic, and photographic examination to observe and to record progress of the curvature during growth. General exercises are prescribed to obtain good posture and to maintain mobility of the spine.

With respect to external supports, Moe or other braces (Fig. 43-17), which relieve pressure of the vertebral epiphyses on the concave side of the curve, are the most efficient appliances available. The efficient use of these braces permits the postponement of surgical treatment until final correction, and spinal fusion can be carried out at the age of ten years or more. An alternative form of treatment is the use of an external muscle stimulator that

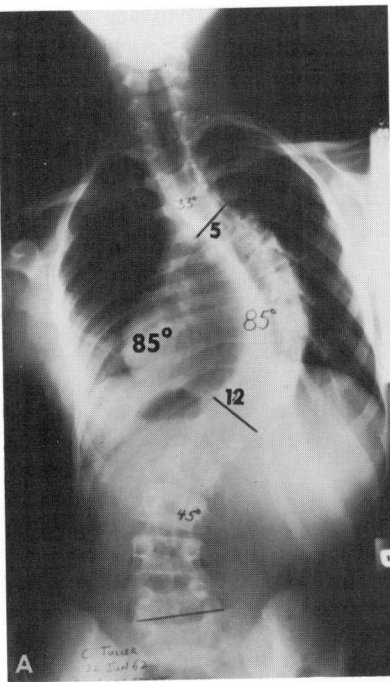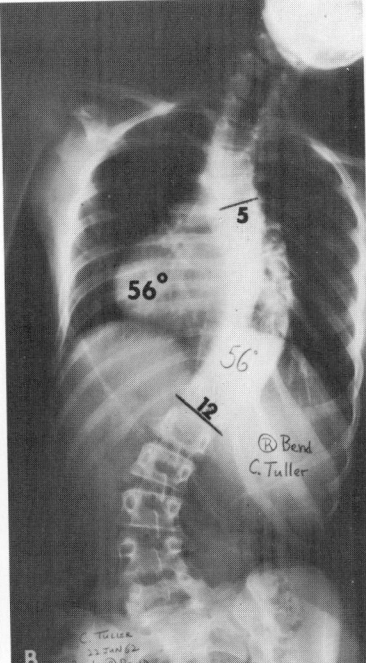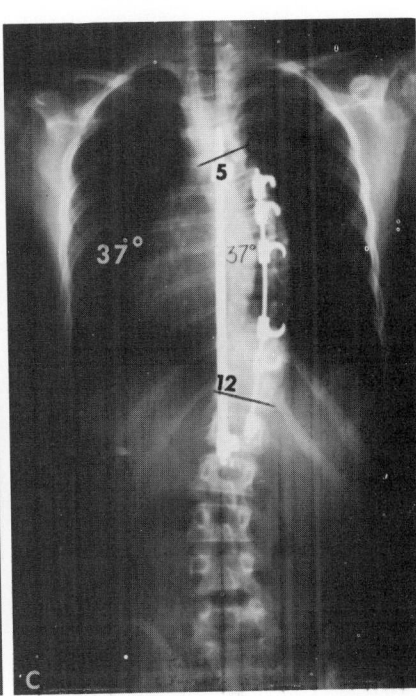

Fig. 43-16. Idiopathic scoliosis treated by Harrington rod and massive bone graft. Goldstein technique. *A.* 85° right thoracic primary curve between T_5 and T_{12}. *B.* Lateral bend to the right corrects curve to 56°. *C.* Postoperative correction following Harrington rod instrumentation and bone grafting with massive autogenous cancellous bone. The curve is corrected to 37° and is fused to T_1.

is applied at night. The muscles on the convex side of the curve are electrically stimulated, providing dynamic curve correction.

Paralytic scoliosis is treated more aggressively than idiopathic curvatures during development of the deformity. Initially in the very young child prolonged recumbency is advocated, and stretching exercises are instituted to maintain good spinal mobility and to prevent soft tissue contractures. Bent plaster shells are used intermittently to counteract any deforming attitude in recumbency, and once correction is obtained, the vertebral column must be supported with a removable plaster jacket or a Milwaukee brace.

SURGICAL TREATMENT. Surgical treatment is required when the deformity cannot be controlled by the use of the Milwaukee brace or a thoracic lumbar sacral orthosis (TLSO) and in the case of any correctable deformity at or after maturity that is accompanied by pain. As a general rule, curves under 40° can be controlled by an orthosis, but when progression of the curve occurs, correction and spinal fusion is indicated. With progression of a paralytic scoliotic curve and instability of the trunk due to muscle imbalance, stabilization of the spine is indicated. In cases of congenital scoliosis where there is a definite undifferentiated bony bar in the concavity of the curve, early fusion over a short segment of the involved vertebrae is mandatory, since the curve will relentlessly progress without it. Congenital curves should be watched closely and fused early if there is progression. Specific indications for operation include a curve over 60° or one involv-

ing the thoracic or thoracolumbar spine. A more conservative approach may be adopted for double major curves, which are usually balanced. Operative intervention is rarely required in adults unless there is severe pain.

The usual operative measures are those of posterior spinal fusion utilizing cancellous bone and some form of internal and external splintage after adequate correction has been obtained. The Harrington rod has added greatly to the ability to improve correction and, when utilized with sound spine fusion techniques, has lowered the rate of pseudarthrosis and loss of correction postoperatively. When Harrington rod and posterior spine fusions are carried out, patients are immobilized postoperatively in a plaster cast extending from the chin and occiput to the groin. External immobilization is usually required for 9 to 12 months after surgery. The Dwyer or Zielke techniques involve an anterior approach to the vertebral bodies, interbody fusion, and correction of the curve by the swaged cable fixed to screws attached to the vertebral bodies. For some types of rigid curves and severe thoracolumbar curves this technique is a definite advantage.

Knee Deformities

GENU VALGUM

This deformity is characterized by an abnormal increase in the distance between the two medial malleoli when the extended knees are just touching each other. It may arise from disturbances of the epiphyseal plate, epiphysis, or ligamentous structures of the knee joint and after fractures of the lateral tibial or the lateral femoral condyle. A common cause used to be deficiency rickets with disturbance of the mineralization process in endochondral ossification. Rachitic deformities may still arise

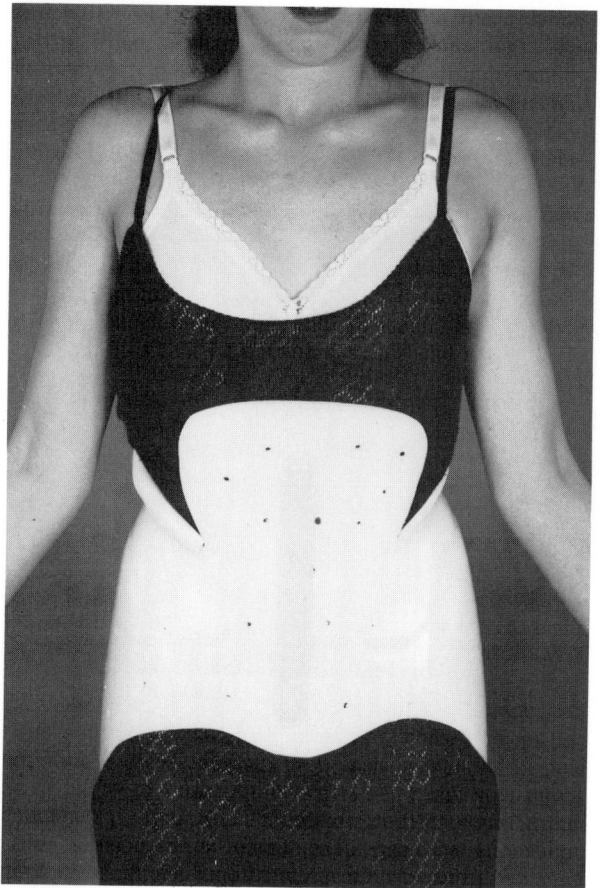

Fig. 43-17. Boston brace treatment for idiopathic lumbar scoliosis.

Fig. 43-18. Idiopathic genu valgum deformity.

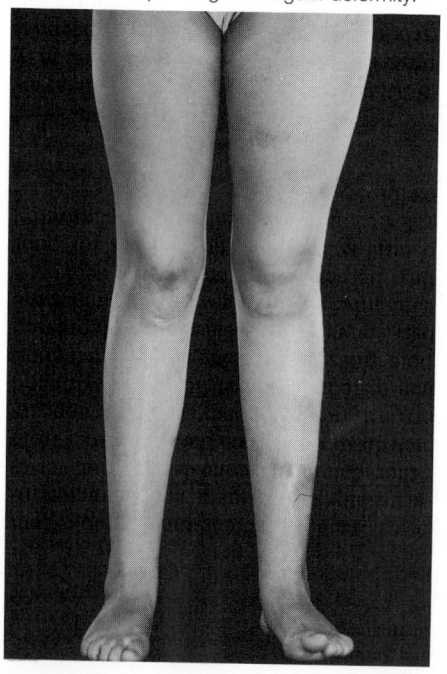

from congenital renal insufficiency such as Fanconi's syndrome or vitamin D–resistant rickets. Genu valgum is not an uncommon complication of rheumatoid arthritis, in which there is gradual attenuation of the medial ligament and collapse of the lateral tibial condyle. Similarly it may complicate postmenopausal osteoporosis.

However, the most common type of genu valgum, or knock-knee, is that seen in young children and is considered to be postural, or idiopathic, in type (Fig. 43-18). It is so common during infancy that it might be considered a normal phase of development. The deformity arises because the line of weight transmission from the femur falls within the lateral side of the center of the knee joint, so that the lateral condyles of both the femur and the tibia bear more weight than their medial counterparts.

TREATMENT. Genu valgum in infants and children below the age of seven can be safely ignored if not excessive and in the absence of underlying causes. It may be advisable in certain cases to raise the inner edge of the heel by $\frac{1}{8}$ to $\frac{3}{16}$ in., especially as a measure of reassurance to the anxious parents.

Active treatment is occasionally necessary in the form of Jones walking genu valgum braces or mermaid night splints. In severe cases, some of which commence posturally and have been aggravated by obesity, operative

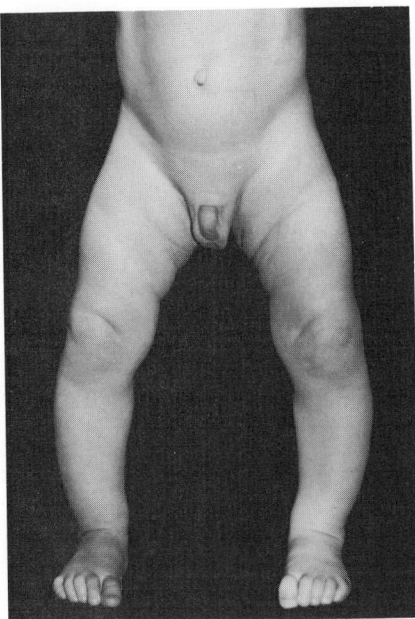

Fig. 43-19. Genu varum deformity in an infant boy mainly arising from the tibiae.

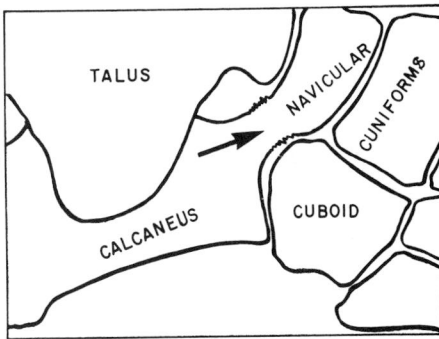

Fig. 43-20. Calcaneonavicular bar.

niques such as tomograms or CT scans are necessary to demonstrate the abnormal osseous anatomy. There are three common sites for such osseous coalescence between tarsal bones:

1. A calcaneonavicular bar (Fig. 43-20)
2. A talocalcaneal bar (Fig. 43-21)
3. A calcaneocuboid bar

Conservative treatment in the form of manipulation and the use of braces offers little chance of success. An operation is usually indicated. In young children if a bar can be demonstrated, simple resection may be successful, but usually the diagnosis is not made until adolescence or early adulthood when tarsal arthritis supervenes, necessitating triple arthrodesis.

Acquired Flatfoot

Acquired flatfoot may be divided into three pathologic types:

1. Osseous type, due to bony distortion produced by trauma or disease processes
2. Ligamentous type, which may follow rupture or avulsion of the ligamentous attachments of the foot, or sprain
3. Muscular imbalance, as in anterior poliomyelitis and cerebral palsy

The muscle hypotonia following recumbency accompanying long illness places the full strain of weight bearing and walking upon the bony and ligamentous structure of the arch. Stretching of these ligaments, which form the segmental ties of the archlike structure, will result in flat-

correction in the form of supracondylar femoral osteotomy may be required.

GENU VARUM

The pathogenesis of genu varum is similar to that outlined above for genu valgum. The idiopathic, or postural, variety in infancy is the most common clinical form of presentation.

A minor degree of the deformity is quite common in children up to three years of age, and the deformity is usually restricted to the tibia (Fig. 43-19). Occasionally the deformity may be more apparent than real—a manifestation of an abnormal arc of rotation in the hips, or of persistent fetal alignment, in which there is excess of internal rotation over external rotation due to marked anteversion of the femoral neck. As in genu valgum, most postural, idiopathic types without any evidence of underlying metabolic or congenital epiphyseal disorders regress spontaneously and require no treatment.

Foot and Ankle Deformities

FLATFOOT (PES PLANUS; PES VALGUS)

Peroneal Spastic Flatfoot

Although this condition may be produced by inflammatory and traumatic affections of the tarsal joints, the most common cause is an abnormal coalescence between two or more of the tarsal bones. In young children tarsal coalescence cannot be seen on x-ray, because it is cartilaginous and ossification does not occur until the age of nine or ten. Even in adulthood, special x-ray views and tech-

Fig. 43-21. Talocalcaneal bar.

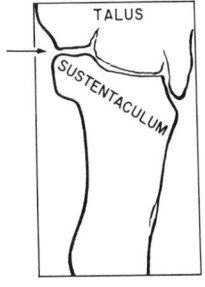
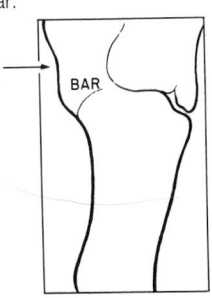

A.   B.

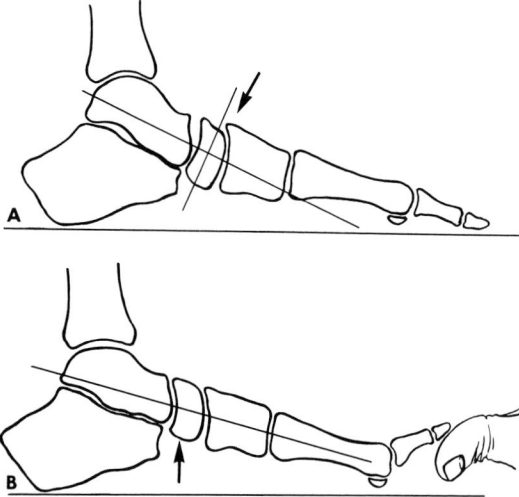

Fig. 43-22. *A.* Line drawing of the lateral aspect of the foot to show the break occurring at the talonavicular and naviculocuneiform joints. *B.* Line drawing of the lateral aspect of the foot showing the correction of the talonavicular and naviculocuneiform joints, so that a straight line can be drawn through the axes of the talus, navicular, medial cuneiform, and metatarsals. *(After Jack, 1953, with permission.)*

tening of the foot. Relative muscular insufficiency as another factor in the development of acquired flatfoot is seen with sudden increases in body weight.

PATHOLOGY. If the calcaneonavicular ligament gives way, the talus deviates downward and mediad, and the head of the talus and the tuberosity of the navicular come to form prominences on the medial aspect of the foot.

In the normal weight-bearing foot a straight line can be drawn through the axis of the talus, the middle of the navicular, the medial cuneiform, and the metatarsals. A break at the talonavicular joint or at the naviculocuneiform joint, or at both these joints combined, will produce the so-called vertical talus deformity (Fig. 43-22*A*). Jack demonstrated that dorsiflexion of the great toe restored the arch, particularly in cases of navicular cuneiform break, but not when the break occurred at other joints (Fig. 43-22*B*).

CLINICAL MANIFESTATIONS. Four types of flatfoot may present:

1. Foot strain, or incipient flatfoot. This is the earliest stage, the period when pressure is first being exerted upon the ligaments. There is no evidence of deformity but simply symptoms of tenderness and pain.
2. Mobile flatfoot.
   a. Due to faulty postural activity of muscles. This is seen in the very young child in whom there has been no development of postural tone.
   b. Due to short calcaneus tendon. In these patients, the malalignment disappears on tiptoeing, but when the foot is correctly aligned, it is noted to be in planus.
3. Voluntary flatfoot. This corresponds to the stage in which flattening of the arch has occurred but secondary adaptive changes have not yet ensued and the leg muscles, though they have lost their postural tone, can be used for volitional restoration of the arch.

4. Rigid flatfoot. In these cases marked degenerative changes have occurred in the subtaloid and midtarsal joints, and the deformity has become fixed.

TREATMENT. The absolute indications for treatment are pain and impaired function. The existence of flatfoot per se does not necessarily mean that treatment is required. The ideal objectives of treatment, if indicated, are

1. To correct the abnormal center of gravity in the foot so that the body weight is transferred to the outer side
2. To remove pressure symptoms

Treatment of Acute Foot Strain. Treatment of acute foot strain usually resolves itself into palliative measures, such as contrast footbaths, faradic footbaths, and foot exercises. Attention should also be directed toward the use of correct footwear.

Gait instruction and foot exercises are usual adjuncts in the management of foot strain from any cause. The patient should be taught to walk with the feet parallel, as the muscles supporting the arch are then activated and facilitate correction of the arch. Moreover, the heel-and-toe gait also brings into play the strong leg muscles which indirectly support the bony architecture of the foot.

Exercises, both active and against resistance, should be carried out twice daily. The rationale of these exercises is to stretch shortened structures such as the Achilles tendon and the soft parts of the lateral side of the foot and to strengthen relaxed muscles so that they are in a better condition to play their part in supporting the arch.

At the stage of voluntary flatfoot, in which there is still some possibility of volitional correction of the arch by muscle strength, exercises play a great part. While the muscles are being redeveloped, arch supports are often helpful in relieving symptoms. In the rigid and permanent types, however, the degenerative changes in the tarsal joints necessitate either triple arthrodesis or less extensive talonavicular fusions.

CONTRACTURE

The seventeeth-century term "contracture" means "a drawing together or becoming smaller." It implies, in pathologic terms, a permanent shortening and rigidity of muscles, joints, and fascial structures. Contractures may be congenital or acquired.

Characteristic examples of congenital contractures are talipes equinovarus (clubfoot), sternocleidomastoid tumor (congenital torticollis), and the deformities associated with arthrogryposis multiplex congenita. Acquired contractures of muscle, fascia, and ligaments involve disturbances of many tissue types, and it is therefore best to consider acquired contractures as primary or secondary with respect to their pathogenesis and tissue involvement. Primary muscle contracture includes primary muscular disorders such as progressive muscular dystrophy, the ischemia of Volkmann's contracture, and posttraumatic fibrosis. The classic primary, fascial type of contracture is that of Dupuytren's deformity affecting the palmar fascia and producing contractures of the fingers. It is occasionally seen in association with chronic barbiturism and may involve the plantar aponeurosis. Many types of arthritic disorder such as rheumatoid arthritis, osteoarthritis, hemophilic arthropathy, and infective and traumatic disorders of joints may result in contractures involving the intraarticular or periarticular structures, or both. Secondary contractures may be defined as contractures of muscles and joints as the result of primary disorders of nervous tissue such as anterior poliomyelitis, cerebral palsy, and many other types of neurologic disorder that produce paresis of muscle groups and unbalanced muscular activity.

Dupuytren's Contracture (See Chapter 45)

Volkmann's Ischemic Contracture

In 1875 Volkmann described a contracture of the forearm muscles following the tight bandaging of an arm after fracturing the bones of the elbow. Such a contracture is due to ischemia of the muscles and is a common hazard in children following injuries about the elbow, particularly supracondylar fracture. Simultaneous damage to the brachial artery by inducing spasm or by thrombosis may produce segmental arterial spasm with severe ischemia of both muscle and nerves. Hemophilia with a bleed into the anterior forearm muscles and associated muscle death can produce this lesion.

PATHOLOGY. The gross pathologic picture is one of muscle infarction in an elliptoid zone that has its axis near the anterior interosseous artery and its central point a little above the middle of the forearm. The greatest damage is usually to the flexor digitorum profundus and flexor pollicis longus, these being the deepest muscles lying in close relation to the anterior interosseous artery. The median nerve running near the anterior interosseous artery may also be involved in the ischemic process, and in very severe cases the ulnar nerve may be involved as well.

In the center of the ischemic mass the muscle fibers lose their nuclei and cross striations, and fuse into a homogeneous mass with little more than a defining membrane separating them. This picture is in contrast to muscle degeneration from other causes, such as denervation and sepsis, in which the appearance is one of diffuse interfibrillar fibrosis.

CLINICAL MANIFESTATIONS. The symptoms of pain, pallor, paralysis, and loss of radial pulse occur within a few hours of the injury, and usually intense pain is associated with either passive or active attempts to extend the fingers. Active and passive finger extension should be specifically checked in every patient with an elbow or forearm injury, since inability to extend in association with pain is the earliest sign of a Volkmann's ischemic contracture. Ultimately all voluntary motion is lost. Most of the damage occurs within the first few hours, so that initial treatment is urgent. After this period swelling gradually subsides, the muscles become hard and fibrotic, and as the fibrosis increases, a characteristic deformity of the

wrist and hand develops. When the wrist is flexed, extension occurs at the MP joints and flexion at the IP joints, while the forearm is often pronated and the elbow flexed.

PROPHYLAXIS. The circulatory and neurologic condition of the forearm and hand must be carefully watched in the early stage of treatment of all injuries or fractures about the elbow or forearm. If there is a suggestion of a compartment syndrome, compartment pressures should be measured with a Wick catheter. When pressures are elevated or borderline, surgical decompression of the compartment muscles and exploration of the brachial artery are mandatory. It is inadvisable to treat fractures about the elbow, such as supracondylar fractures in children, with splints or bandages applied in a circular fashion.

TREATMENT. In the acute stage it is important to reestablish circulation before irreparable damage is done. The limb must be elevated, any circular bandages removed, and mild external warmth applied.

In established cases, prevention of contracture and maintenance of joint mobility can be obtained by splintage and physiotherapy of the fingers and thumb. Once maximal recovery is attained, operative procedures are necessary to remove the fibrotic muscular tissue. Occasionally if the median nerve has been irreparably damaged and the ulnar nerve is intact, the latter has been used successfully as a pedicle nerve graft to restore maximal sensation to the hand.

EPIPHYSEAL DISORDERS (OSTEOCHONDRITIS)

General Considerations

The epiphysis is concerned with the growth in length of a bone. It also forms a part of joints and acts as an attachment for muscles and tendons. There are three types of epiphysis: (1) pressure epiphysis, which transmits weight from one bone to another, (2) traction epiphysis, or apophysis, which is situated at the point of attachment of muscles, and (3) atavistic epiphysis, which represents a part of the skeleton that has lost its function.

The cartilage lying between the bony tissue and the diaphysis is known as the "epiphyseal cartilage." It does not ossify until bone growth has ceased, nor does the epiphysis become joined to the body of the bone until that time.

The term "osteochondritis," or "epiphysitis," is used to signify a derangement of growth at various ossification centers.

Areas Involved with Epiphysitis

Primary centers of ossification:
Vertebral body (Calvé)
Carpal scaphoid (Preoser)
Semilunar, adult (Kienböck)
Patella (Köhler)
Talus (Mouchet)
Tarsal navicular (Köhler)

Secondary centers of ossification:
   Vertebral epiphysis (Scheuermann)
   Head of humerus (Hass)
   Capitellum of humerus (Panner)
   Head of radius (Brailsford)
   Pubic symphysis (Van Neck)
   Ischiopubic junction (Oldsberg)
   Head of femur (Legg)
   Patella (Sinding-Larsen)
   Tubercle of tibia (Osgood-Schlatter)
   Calcaneus (Sever)
   Metatarsals (Freiberg)

ETIOLOGY. The causes of epiphysitis have not been agreed upon. The theory presently favored is that a vascular disturbance, possibly following trauma, results in an avascular necrosis. The traumatic factor is supported by a frequent history of injury, by the greater frequency of the condition in boys, and by the more usual location either in weight-bearing joints, such as the hip, or in epiphyses that are subjected to great strain. There is increasing evidence that these various lesions or osteochondroses may be the result of a constitutional disease, i.e., an inherent disease resulting from an inherited genotype characteristic that involves the whole body rather than being confined to one area.

A relationship between osteochondritis and skeletal growth has been described. It should be noted that the condition appears clinically (1) soon after the appearance of ossification, e.g., Legg-Calvé-Perthes disease at four years and Osgood-Schlatter disease at eleven years; (2) during or immediately after the midgrowth, or adolescent spurt, e.g., Scheuermann's disease, which is aggravated by adolescent growth spurt; and (3) earlier in girls than in boys, because the latter are slower in maturation.

CLINICAL MANIFESTATIONS. The affection may be bilateral or unilateral. The onset is usually gradual in a patient with good health who may offer a history of trauma. The local effects of the disease are similar to those of early tuberculosis and include slight pain, limp in a weight-bearing joint, limitation of the movement, and at times muscle spasm. The symptoms are usually mild. Many cases are asymptomatic and discovered only when deformities develop.

RADIOGRAPHIC FINDINGS. The radiographic appearance is usually much more severe than the clinical picture would suggest. There is early osteoporosis with subsequent signs of repair. The epiphysis becomes fissured, fragmented, broadened, and irregular in outline. Areas of dense necrotic bone become evident. The process may involve both the epiphysis and metaphysis, and the former may be compressed and flattened. In the stage of regeneration, there is a gradual loss of osteoporosis with absorption of the dense necrotic bone in the epiphysis. This is followed by slowly advancing replacement of the necrotic bone by new bone until there is complete bony restitution.

Legg-Calvé-Perthes Disease

Osteochondritis of the hip, also known as "coxa plana," is essentially a disease of boys, occurring usually between the ages of five and nine, but may become manifest between two and eighteen years of age. It is bilateral in about 10 percent of the cases.

CLINICAL MANIFESTATIONS. There are three main stages: (1) the prodromal stage, (2) the active stage, and (3) the restoration stage. During the prodromal stage, the most constant early sign is a limp, which may or may not be accompanied by pain. Muscular spasm may be present in early stages of the disease. During the active stage, the spasm tends to disappear but leaves a residual limitation of mobility. The pain and tenderness also usually disappear. The limping may remit for short periods or may be marked with a completely fixed and painless hip in a position of slight flexion and adduction. The affected hip joint shows limitation of abduction, medial rotation, and flexion, initially because of spasm of adductive muscles and at a later stage because of true shortening of these muscles. Still later, the deformation of the femoral head results in a mechanical condition that prevents full degree of motion. The muscles on the affected side are usually atrophied, but, in spite of the considerable degree of deformity at the head of the femur, there is little if any shortening.

During the restoration stage, the subjective and objective signs gradually diminish, until the function of the hip is restored. Trochanteric thickening and limitation of range of abduction, however, persist through life.

RADIOGRAPHIC FINDINGS. Radiographs (Fig. 43-23) of the femoral head progressively demonstrate flattening, flattening plus fragmentation, flattening with fusion in the disorganized nucleus, and finally an expanded flattened

Fig. 43-23. Legg-Calvé-Perthes disease.

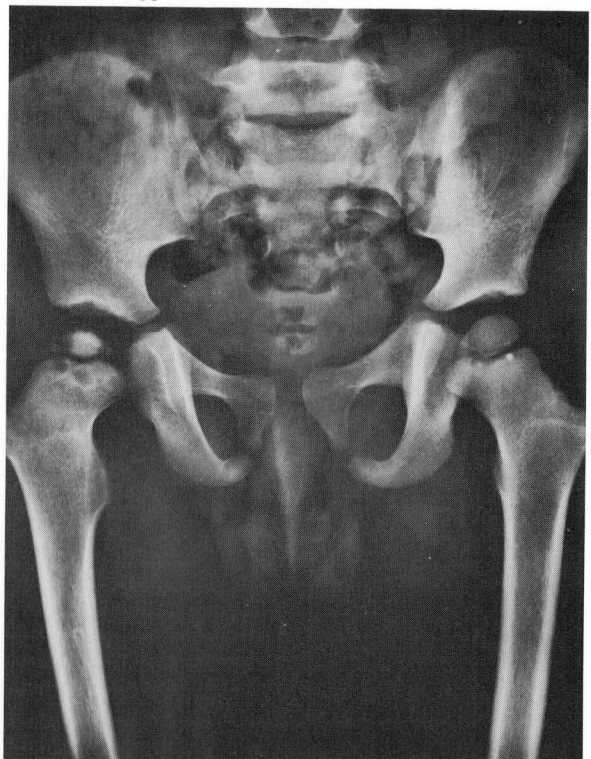

head. Although the expression fragmentation is commonly used, the actual histology is one of irregular ossification in an abnormal cartilage, i.e., a dyschondrosis. The head is at first slightly reduced in its vertical diameter with no appreciable increase in its lateral extent. Later, there is a uniform increased radiodensity of the nucleus with irregular ossification. As fragmentation develops, there is some breaking up of the bony nucleus of the epiphysis with radiolucency apparent. At the same time, the head usually becomes more flattened and expands out of the acetabulum. The onset of the healing stage is marked with fusion changes. The bony fragments join, and the density of the epiphysis diminishes until the shadow becomes not only uniform but comparable with that of the other side. The head, however, remains flattened. Even after the lesion has healed, deformity of the head persists, usually throughout life. In rare cases in which there has been no weight bearing on the joint, the normal contour may be preserved.

In the neck of the femur, deformity can develop early in the disease, even before the head has demonstrated osteoporosis. The upper part of the neck is expanded, and its metaphyseal ends become rounded off. At the same time, the neck becomes progressively shorter. In the acetabular cavity, the distance between the medial pole of the head and the floor of the socket increases early in the disease. This may reach such a degree that the shadows of the head and the ischial bone no longer overlap but leave a gap. This sign may be caused by a grossly swollen ligamentum teres resulting in excavation of the acetabular roof by pressure. In 68 cases of Perthes' disease, there were 58 patients who exhibited acetabular changes; 51 had concomitant abnormality of the triradiate cartilage such as irregular ossification. Associated lesions in the spine of a Scheuermann's type may well indicate that this lesion is a generalized one like an osteochondrosis rather than a localized vascular one as commonly thought. An arthrogram may show whether the cartilaginous outline is nearly normal and can be used to determine the efficacy of treatment.

TREATMENT. It is generally agreed that no systemic measures are successful in modifying the pathologic process. The aim of treatment is to contain the softened revascularizing femoral head in the acetabulum and to try to preserve its normal contour. When first seen, if the patient has considerable spasm of hip musculature, a preliminary period of skin traction is indicated. After 5 to 10 days of bed rest and skin traction, the patient is usually comfortable. The patient may then be placed in bilateral, long-leg walking casts fixed with two transverse bars to maintain both hips in 45° of abduction and 5° to 10° of internal rotation.

The child is allowed to walk with crutches, bearing full weight on the two casts. Plaster casts are changed at intervals of 3 to 4 months and continued until radiographs indicate that mature bone has replaced the avascular epiphysis. Total plaster time averages 19 months. A similar approach can be carried out using the Toronto brace. In order to reduce the long period of abduction immobilization to provide containment of the femoral head, a rotational-varus osteotomy of the upper femoral component

may be performed, or a Salter osteotomy in which acetabular coverage is increased may be applied.

Prognosis depends upon the degree of involvement of the femoral epiphysis, as well as the age and sex of the child. In general, with less involvement of the epiphysis, children under four and boys have a better prognosis. In patients followed into adult life, the overall results of treatment have been disappointing. Failure of growth of the femoral neck with resultant shortening also may be a complication.

Osgood-Schlatter Disease (Tibial Tubercle Epiphysitis)

CLINICAL MANIFESTATIONS. Osgood-Schlatter disease occurs usually in patients from thirteen to fifteen years of age, and the history may suggest injury as a causative factor. The onset of pain and local tenderness is insidious. The patient first complains of some aching in the front of the knee after exercise. In many cases, the overexertion is the only history of trauma obtained. The pain is increased by full voluntary extension of the joint, since the affected epiphysis is pulled on by the contracted quadriceps muscle. There is also pain on passive complete flexion, because the epiphysis is dragged by the quadriceps stretch. The epiphysis itself is tender, and in many cases there is localized swelling and increased temperature.

The radiographic appearance is characteristic (Fig. 43-24). The tibial tubercle is irregular in contour and even

Fig. 43-24. Osgood-Schlatter disease: tibial tubercle osteochondritis.

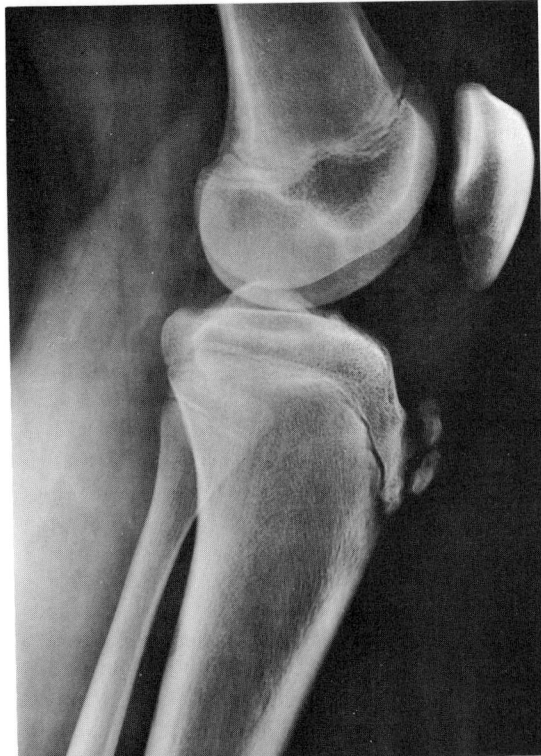

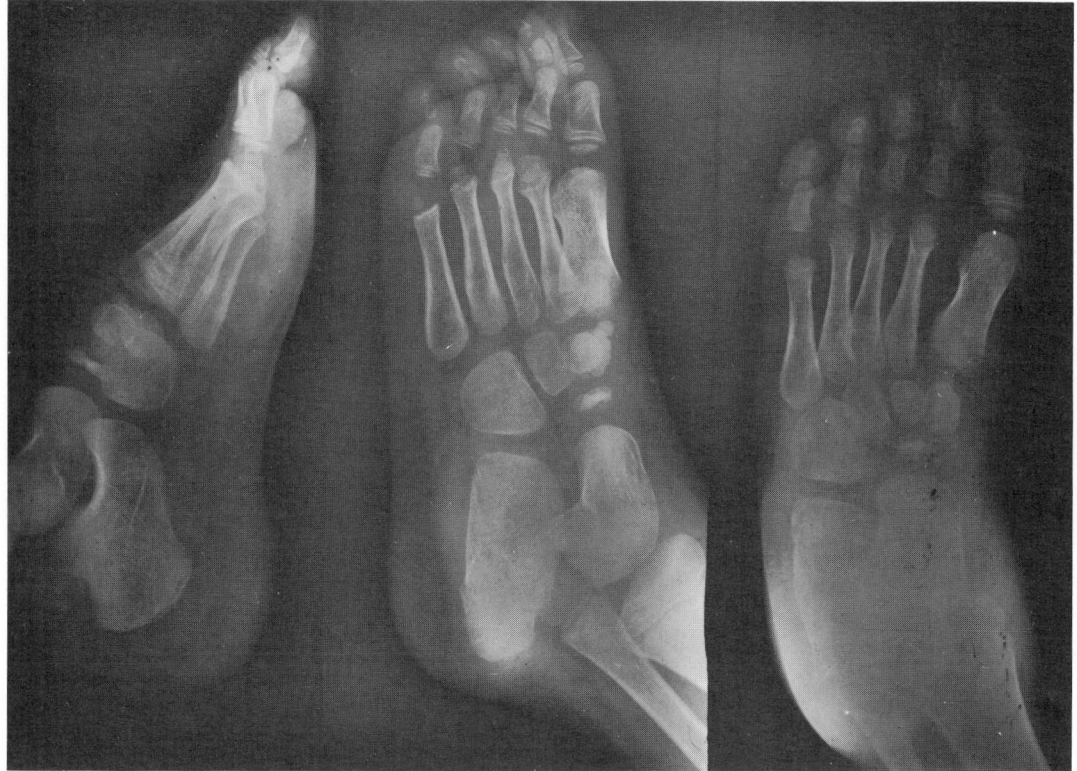

Fig. 43-25. Osteochondritis of the tarsal navicular: Köhler's disease.

fragmented. There may be localized haziness in the adjacent tibial metaphysis.

Osgood-Schlatter disease must be differentiated from osteomyelitis, sarcoma of the head of the tibia, bone cysts, and infrapatellar bursitis. It must also be differentiated from partial separation of the tuberosity associated with trauma, which is mainly caused by violent contraction of the quadriceps muscles in males between the ages of sixteen and eighteen.

TREATMENT. The condition is treated in a fashion similar to that used for an epiphyseal separation with severe symptoms. A cylinder plaster cast is applied initially for 6 weeks, during which time weight bearing is permitted. Following removal of the cast the knee is mobilized and the patient's activities modified, i.e., no contact sports or hard running are allowed for a number of months. When symptoms are mild, simple restriction of heavy athletic activity and running is usually sufficient to get the patient through the growth period without immobilization of the extremity. The end result of Osgood-Schlatter disease is usually a prominent tibial tubercle that persists into adulthood. A rare complication is that of genu recurvatum.

Köhler's Disease of the Tarsal Navicular

As is true of the other forms of epiphysitis, Köhler's disease is probably an osteochondritis, but the cause has not been definitely established. It is analogous to Kienböck's disease, which affects the semilunar bone of adults. The navicular is the last bone of the foot to ossify, and since it forms the keystone of the long arch, it is subjected to considerable strain while in the cartilaginous state. Köhler's disease usually occurs in young children, especially between the ages of three and six.

CLINICAL MANIFESTATIONS. The symptoms and signs are often minimal, usually consisting of pain and swelling in the region of the tarsal navicular. The pain is exaggerated by weight bearing, and the affected region is sensitive to movement and may be tender. The condition is usually diagnosed by radiographs that reveal definite changes in the bone (Fig. 43-25). These consist of sclerotic narrowing in the anteroposterior diameter with no fragmentation of the bony nucleus. The joint spaces remain clear, and the neighboring tarsal and metatarsal bones are normal in appearance.

TREATMENT. The treatment is relatively simple, and symptomatic recovery usually occurs in a few months. A plaster cast should be applied to hold the foot in a slight varus position, and weight bearing is prevented by the use of crutches. After a few weeks the plaster is removed, and adhesive strapping is used to support the ankle and midtarsal region. The shoe is then fitted with a Thomas heel, i.e., with the medial half of the heel extended forward toward the sole, and sponge-rubber pads are inserted to relieve strain on the longitudinal arch, and, more particularly, on the navicular.

Congenital Orthopaedic Deformities

Deformities Resulting from In Utero Position

Congenital Dysplasia and Dislocation of the Hip

Congenital Dislocation of the Knee (Congenital Genu Recurvatum)

Congenital Pseudoarthrosis of the Tibia

Congenital Talipes Equinovarus (Clubfoot)

Congenital Convex Pes Valgus (Vertical Talus)

Arthrogryposis Multiplex Congenita (Myodystrophia Fetalis)

Congenital High Scapula

Congenital Short Neck (Klippel-Feil Syndrome: Brevicollis)

Cleidocranial Dysostosis Syndrome

Congenital Wryneck (Torticollis)

Congenital Radioulnar Synostosis

Madelung's Deformity

Congenital Aplasia and/or Dysplasia of Long Bones
Absence of the Radius
Absence of the Ulna
Absence or Dysplasia of the Fibula
Shortening of the Femur

Stevenson has described three categories of congenital and/or hereditary disorders: (1) those malformations which are seen at birth but which have arisen during intrauterine life, i.e., true congenital malformations; (2) disorders or diseases determined by a single gene substitution or mutation; and (3) disease in which the genetic contribution is made more complex by the presence of environmental factors or prenatal influences. Malformations due only to environmental causes are infrequent, e.g., viral infection of rubella or syphilis and the use of aminopyrine (amidopyrine) drugs and thalidomide. These produce teratogenic changes in the fetus, particularly during the first 4 weeks of pregnancy when the fetus is undergoing marked cellular differentiation. By considering embryonic development and its susceptibility to multiple factors it is possible to make a timetable (Fig. 43-26) of the appearance of various congenital malformations. A survey of 56,760 live births showed a total incidence of malformations 5 years after birth of 23.08 per 1000. Talipes was found in 4.44 per 1000, spina bifida and other spinal defects were noted in 3 per 1000, and dislocation of the hip appeared in 0.67 per 1000.

DEFORMITIES RESULTING FROM IN UTERO POSITION

The in utero position has often been implicated as a deforming force, particularly of the lower extremities. The optimal time for a detailed musculoskeletal examination is between the third and fourth weeks. Several moderately severe conditions are seen shortly after birth, but these can usually be treated by simple conservative measures:

1. Metatarsus adductus of one or both feet.
2. Everted, or valgus, foot.
3. Talipes equinovarus deformity with one or more of four characteristics: forefoot adduction, inversion of the hind part of the foot, equinus of the whole foot at the ankle joint, and/or torsion of the tibia.
4. Unilateral externally rotated leg with an everted foot, the other leg being either in a neutral position or in internal rotation.
5. Bilateral internally rotated tibiae, which are aggravated by the prone position.
6. Adducted thigh and hip with some external rotation of the leg as a whole. This type of deformity has to be closely differentiated from congenital dysplasia or dislocation of the hip.

Resistance to achieving the full range of passive movements of the hip, knee, ankle, or midtarsal joints must be corrected by passive stretching exercises and by correc-

Fig. 43-26. Etiological timetable of some congenital malformations.

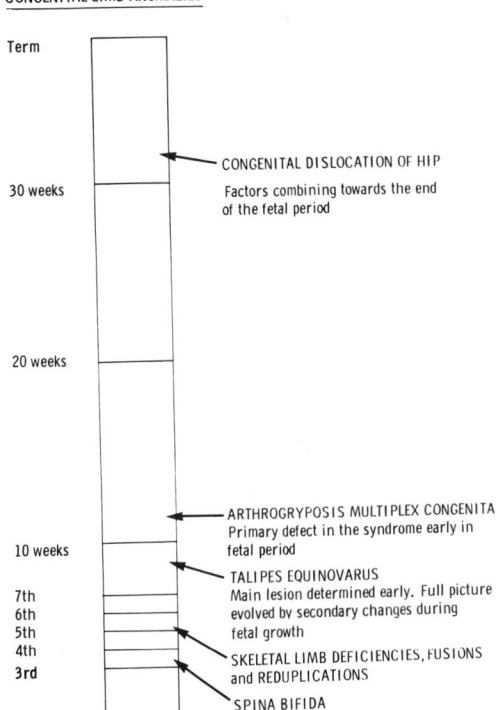

COMPOSITE TIMETABLE FOR DEVELOPMENT OF
CONGENITAL LIMB ANOMALIES

Term

30 weeks — CONGENITAL DISLOCATION OF HIP
Factors combining towards the end of the fetal period

20 weeks

ARTHROGRYPOSIS MULTIPLEX CONGENITA
Primary defect in the syndrome early in fetal period

10 weeks — TALIPES EQUINOVARUS
Main lesion determined early. Full picture evolved by secondary changes during fetal growth

7th
6th
5th
4th — SKELETAL LIMB DEFICIENCIES, FUSIONS and REDUPLICATIONS
3rd — SPINA BIFIDA

0

tive appliances. The postural deformity must be treated before the development of a static deformity with a structural disorder. If soft tissue contractures develop and passive stretching cannot produce an anatomic position after about 6 weeks of treatment, corrective plaster-of-paris casting may be necessary.

CONGENITAL DYSPLASIA AND DISLOCATION OF THE HIP

Congenital dislocation of the hip consists of a partial or complete displacement of the femoral head from the acetabulum. It is very common, particularly in certian racial and ethnic groups such as the northern Italian, the American Navaho Indian, and the Japanese. It is distinctly uncommon in the Hong Kong Chinese. It occurs once in a thousand births in the Caucasian male, with a higher incidence in the Caucasian female.

PATHOLOGY. The acetabulum is shallower than normal; later its rounded shape disappears, and it becomes triangular with the base in front and below and the apex above and behind. X-ray examination shows that the outer surface of the ilium and the floor of the acetabulum lie in an almost straight line. Instead of containing the head of the femur, the acetabulum becomes occupied by an overgrowth of fibrocartilage and the remains of the ligamentum teres, and is covered over by adherent capsule.

Fig. 43-27. *A.* Trendelenburg sign: left buttock rises slightly when the patient stands on her good right leg and the trunk is vertical. *B.* Same patient, standing on the side of the dislocated left hip. Right buttock drops, and the trunk now leans over the dislocated hip.

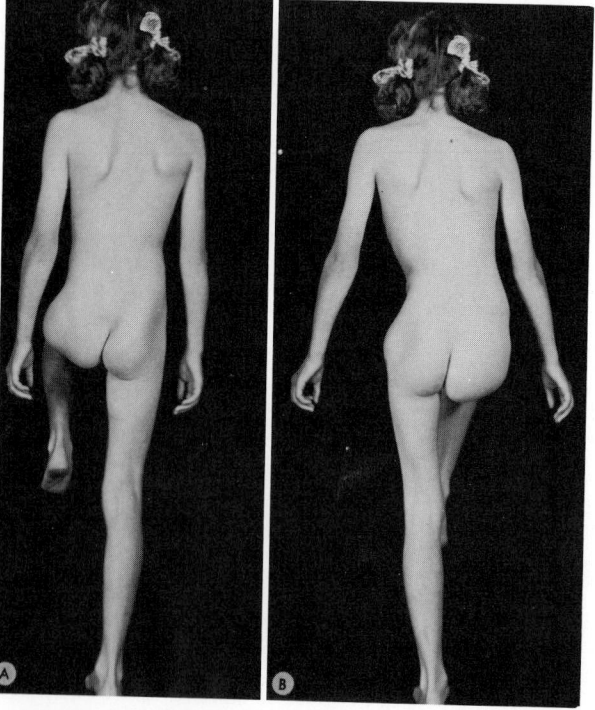

Above the acetabulum there is a depression on the ilium—a false acetabulum lined with periosteum—in which the head of the femur lies with a fold of the capsule intervening between the ilium and the head.

Ossification of the *head of the femur* is delayed and there is usually femoral neck anteversion so that the normal anteversion is increased, until, in late cases, it may be almost 90°; i.e., the neck appears to project forward from the shaft. When there is a bilateral dislocation, the *pelvis* is tilted forward and the normal lumbosacral lordosis increased.

The *capsule* often becomes hourglass-shaped, one cavity containing the head, the other covering the acetabulum; the constriction is caused by the crossing iliopsoas tendon. The ligamentum teres is usually attenuated and may be altogether absent, although in certain cases hypertrophy of the ligamentum teres occurs and blocks reduction. There is shortening of the adductors, the hamstrings, and the gracilis, sartorius, tensor fasciae latae, pectineus, and rectus femoris muscles. There is elongation of the obturators, the quadratus femoris, and the psoas tendon, with alteration in the function of the gluteal group. The degree of primary hypoplasia affecting the cartilaginous roof of the acetabulum is probably the most important etiologic factor. Its ability to contain the head and to ossify in response to a correctly reduced head will determine the final result.

CLINICAL MANIFESTATIONS. All babies must be examined at birth to determine the presence of congenital hip dysplasia, as successful treatment depends upon immediate diagnosis. Diagnosis at birth depends upon detection of the classic signs of dysplasia, which are (1) snap or click (Ortolani's sign) elicited when the head rides over the acetabular rim by abducting the flexed hip, (2) limitation of hip abduction with the knees and hips flexed to 90° with the child on its back, and (3) apparent shortening of the thigh with the hip and knee flexed to 90°.

All children at follow-up examinations at six weeks and three months should be specifically examined for congenital hip dysplasia. If the click sign is no longer present, the only positive finding may be limitation of the symmetric abduction of both hips. If both hips are dysplastic, symmetric abduction may be present, in which case one should suspect dysplasia if adduction is limited to 75° or less. If the hip progresses to a dislocation, the diagnosis will be apparent when the child begins to walk. The gait becomes abnormal, i.e., a ducklike waddle. Leg shortening is evident, and lordosis often is noticeable, especially in bilateral cases. A Trendelenburg sign is seen when the child stands first on one foot and then on the other. In unilateral cases, when the child stands on the sound side, the buttock of the opposite side rises slightly, for the gluteus medius contracts in order to raise the pelvis and bring the trunk more directly above the limb that is sustaining the body weight (Fig. 43-27*A*). When the child stands on the dislocated side, the opposite buttock drops, for the gluteus medius is relatively inefficient and the pelvis therefore cannot be raised or even kept horizontal (Fig. 43-27*B*). In bilateral cases, the phenomenon is present on both sides. The Trendelenburg test is not pathognomonic of congenital dislocation of the hip but occurs whenever the action of the gluteus medius is interfered with—e.g., in poliomyelitis and in coxa vara. Other signs are the position of the femoral artery, buttock creases, etc.

Symptoms attributable to hip joint with moderate dysplasia and a chronically subluxing hip resulting from inadequate diagnosis or treatment may appear in the early teens, depending upon the degree of anatomic distortion. The results of closed reduction depend upon the ability to restore a congruent stable hip joint relationship, and this depends upon the age at which treatment is started. It is clear that maximal short-term and late results of congenital hip dysplasia depend upon early diagnosis and adequate treatment.

RADIOLOGIC FINDINGS. X-ray examination is essential to establish the diagnosis, but in the young baby it must be realized that the cartilaginous structures involved are not visible on radiographs.

The relation of the head to the acetabulum can be established by Hilgenreiner's lines: the epiphyseal nucleus should be inside a vertical line drawn from the acetabular margin (Perkins line) and below the horizontal line drawn through the Y cartilages (Fig. 43-28A).

The slope of the osseous roof may be measured from the acetabular angle; the normal inclination is 22°, but in congenital dislocation it may be increased to 30 or 40°. The outline of the femoral head should be noted, and it will be seen that the femur is displaced outward and upward. The epiphyseal shadow is usually smaller than normal and displaced outward in relation to the neck (Fig. 43-28B). The neck is foreshortened and may be anteverted. An arthrogram reveals the extent of the cartilaginous roof in subluxation and in dislocations confirms the interposition of the limbus between the head and socket.

Fig. 43-28. Congenital dislocation of the hip. *A.* The right hip is held in the position of adduction compared with the left. The line parallel with the roof of the acetabulum intersecting Hilgenreiner's line indicates an acetabular index of 38° on the right and acetabular dysplasia. The dotted perpendicular line dropped from the outer margin of the acetabulum shows the proximal capital femoral epiphysis to be laterally displaced, indicating dislocation. The normal left side shows the dotted line at the outer margin of the proximal capital femoral epiphysis. *B.* Right proximal capital femoral epiphysis is much smaller than the left and is laterally displaced.

TREATMENT. Predislocation. Infants with congenital hip dysplasia without subluxation or with initial subluxation stages diagnosed in the neonatal period of life are treated by simple abduction in a Freijka pillow splint, a Von Rosen splint, or a Pavlik harness (Fig. 43-29). Hips recognized at birth usually need only 3 to 6 months of splinting until x-rays show normal acetabular and hip joint development.

Subluxation. If the femoral head is badly subluxated or dislocated, there is associated tightness of the adductor muscles that must be overcome before reduction is possible. Reduction by overhead traction or traction on a modified abduction frame followed by retention in a Batchelor-type plaster is preferred to manipulation under anesthesia. Frame reduction is a gradual process, but in the average case the head can be brought down and opposite the acetabulum in less than 3 weeks. Children under six years of age may be treated on the abduction frame, but reduction becomes increasingly difficult after the age of four.

Following successful reduction on the frame, the hips must be protected until ossification of the acetabular roof provides a more stable socket. Plaster is applied under general anesthesia, and hips are flexed to more than 90° and in a position of about 45° abduction, the so-called human position. The duration of treatment depends upon the development of the acetabulum and is usually less than 1 year. Children are readmitted for plaster changes under anesthesia at 2- to 3-month intervals.

In younger children the subluxation is reduced on the frame and the reduction maintained by abduction plaster until ossification of the cartilaginous roof increases. Mobilization is then permitted, unless a marked degree of anteversion persists, in which case correction by derotation osteotomy of the femur should be carried out in order to maintain reduction and provide concentric stimulus to development of the osseous roof.

Dislocation. Dislocation implies complete displacement of the head and loss of contact with the articular surface of the original cartilaginous acetabulum. Differentiation between subluxation and dislocation may prove difficult in some cases without the aid of arthrography, ultrasonography, or MRI. Dislocation should be treated by con-

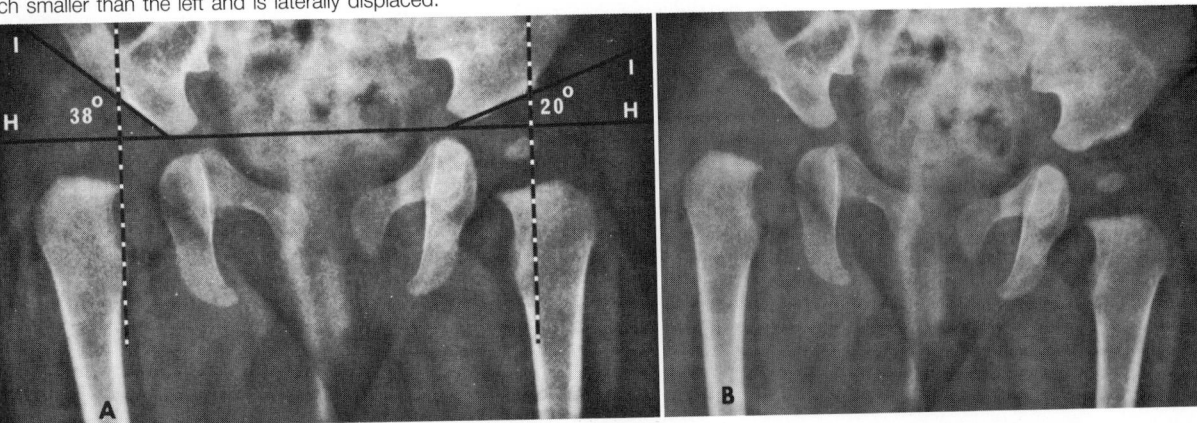

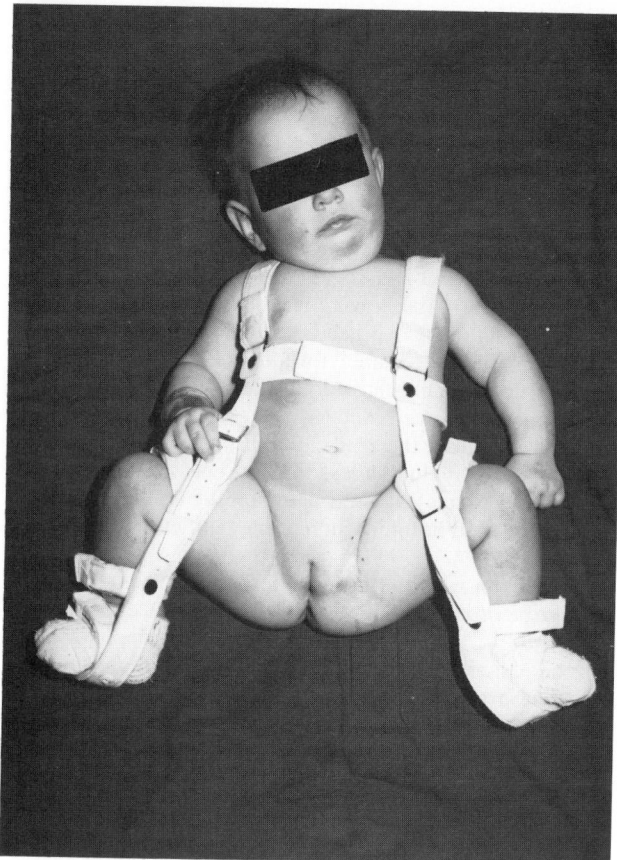

Fig. 43-29. Pavlik harness orthosis for hip maintenance in congenital hip dysplasia. Abduction position.

servative methods, provided the head appears accurately centered following frame reduction and application of abduction plasters. Any tendency of the head to stand out from the acetabulum after reduction, or when freedom is permitted, indicates the probable presence of an obstruction and requires open reduction.

Operative Treatment. Open reduction of the dislocated hip is usually not required before the age of one year. Open reduction is usually carried out in association with procedures to improve coverage of the head by some type of acetabuloplasty or redirection of the acetabulum (Fig. 43-30). Any soft tissue mass within the acetabulum, such as an inverted limbus, hypertrophied ligamentum teres, or fibrofatty pad, is looked for and, if found, turned outward and upward. The head is then rotated inward and the limb abducted to locate the head concentrically.

Innominate osteotomy is usually carried out in conjunction with open reduction. It involves cutting the innominate bone immediately above the acetabulum and levering down (anteriorly and laterally) the acetabulum with its attached rami. The point of fulcrum for this rotation is at the symphysis pubis. A wedge of bone from the anterior crest of the ilium is wedged into the osteotomy defect between the upper ilium bone graft and the acetabular portion of the innominate bone, and fixed with two K-wires.

In an attempt to restore a congruent relationship between the femoral head and the acetabulum in the presence of anteversion of the proximal femur, a derotation osteotomy of the femur is occasionally indicated. Osteochondritis deformans juvenilis, which is due to avascular necrosis of the femoral head, may develop after reduction of a dislocated hip, but its occurrence in the normal hip in unilateral cases has also been recorded.

Palliative operations are reserved for cases in which reduction is no longer possible by either closed or open methods. They are designed to improve stability, decrease lordosis, and control pain arising from the hip or lower back. Palliative procedures fall into two categories: (1) arthrodesis and (2) osteotomy.

Total hip reconstruction may be considered in middle-aged patients with pain as the main presenting feature.

CONGENITAL DISLOCATION OF THE KNEE (CONGENITAL GENU RECURVATUM)

There are three types:

1. The developmental type, which is the most common and is considered to be due to malposition in utero. The legs may be caught by the chin or axilla with the knees extended.
2. A primary embryonic defect, accompanied by other defects, such as harelip, cardiac defects, spina bifida, and congenital

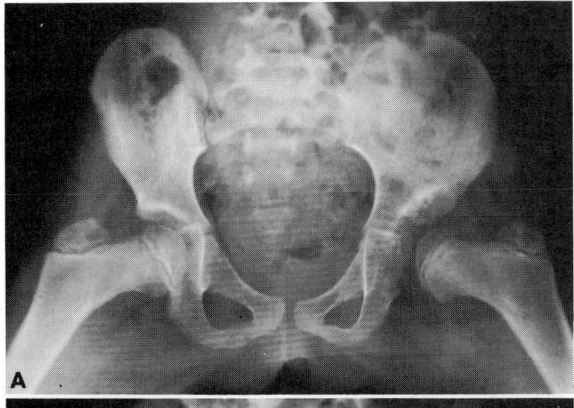

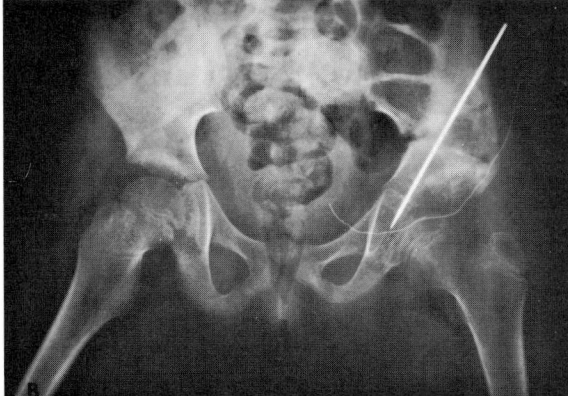

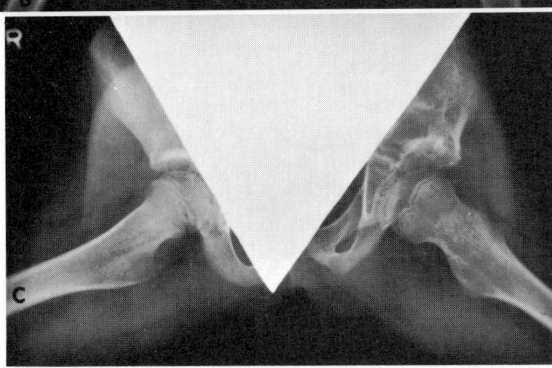

Fig. 43-30. Congenital hip dysplasia, diagnosed at age five. *A.* Position of abduction showing left acetabular dysplasia and subluxation of the femoral head. *B.* Ten weeks after innominate osteotomy with Steinmann's pin in place. *C.* One year following surgical treatment with maintenance of the head in the acetabulum and satisfactory acetabular coverage.

dislocation of the hip. It is fortunate that this type is uncommon, since it is much more difficult to treat and usually requires operation.

3. Contracture of the quadriceps extensor muscle due to arthrogryposis.

CLINICAL MANIFESTATIONS. The knee is fixed in hyperextension with a varying degree of subluxation or dislocation of the tibia forward on the femoral condyles, and the skin over the anterior aspect of the joint shows several transverse creases. The patella is small or absent. On the posterior aspect of the joint, the hamstring muscles are palpable as tense cords, and the femoral condyles are felt projecting in the popliteal fossa.

TREATMENT. It may be possible to stretch the shortened quadriceps and replace the tibia in mild cases at birth. In more severe cases manipulation will be insufficient to overcome the contracture. Operative division or lengthening of the quadriceps and its lateral expansion—and occasionally of the iliotibial tract—will permit replacement. After operation, the corrected position is maintained by a splint or light plaster cast.

CONGENITAL PSEUDOARTHROSIS OF THE TIBIA

This is situated at the junction of the middle and lower thirds of the tibia, with sclerosis of bone ends and a gap between the fragments occupied by fibrous tissue. The leg is shorter. This lesion results from aplasia of a portion of the tibial shaft. A definite association with neurofibromatosis has been described.

TREATMENT. Treatment has been unsatisfactory, especially since the child may present after several attempts to obtain union and may never have walked on the limb. Treatment of the pseudoarthrosis is by some form of bone grafting, including vascularized fibula technique.

CONGENITAL TALIPES EQUINOVARUS (CLUBFOOT)

Congenital talipes equinovarus is a deformity involving four elements: flexion of the ankle, inversion of the foot, adduction of the forefoot, and medial rotation of the tibia (Fig. 43-31). The idiopathic type may arise from such environmental factors as increased intrauterine compression because of change in the size of the uterus or reduction in the amount of amniotic fluid, e.g., oligohydramnios, or from intrinsic anatomic disturbances in the talocalcaneal joint and in the innervation of the peroneal

Fig. 43-31. Characteristic deformities of talipes equinovarus, or clubfoot.

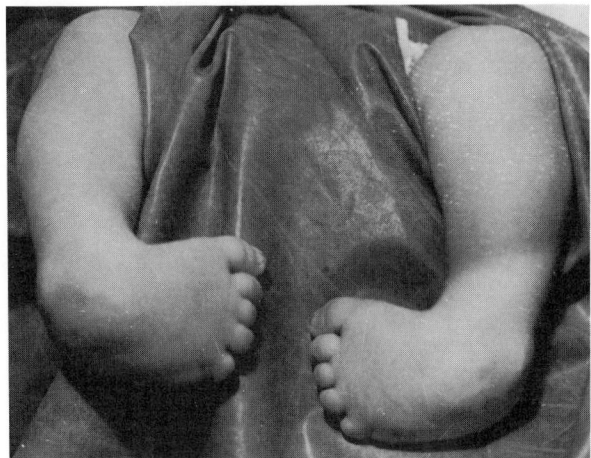

muscles with segmental changes in the spinal cord. As to genetic factors, Wynne-Davies has studied over 100 patients and their first-degree relatives. This deformity occurred in 2.9 percent of siblings. No significant observations were possible concerning consanguinity, age of parents, birth order, etc. Twin studies show a high concordance in monozygous twins and a low rate in the dizygotic; the latter have the same incidence as that found in the nontwin sibling. There is really no recognizable or acceptable inheritance pattern as yet. There is, however; 1:800 chance of any individual having this deformity; 1:35 chance of having it if any siblings have the deformity; and 1:3 chance if an identical twin is involved.

PATHOLOGIC ANATOMY. The essential features are plantar flexion of the talus, inversion of the calcaneus (and with it the other tarsal bones), and adduction of the forefoot. At birth the bones of the foot are normal in shape but altered in position. Over the skin on the outer part of the foot there are usually dimples that may be so marked as to resemble scars. The lateral malleolus is prominent; the medial malleolus appears flattened and poorly developed.

PROGNOSIS. Without treatment, the deformity increases, the gait becomes more unsightly, and the foot becomes more troublesome on account of calluses and ulceration. With early, effective, and continued treatment, all cases of clubfoot should be cured and a useful and properly shaped foot obtained.

TREATMENT. There are two objects of successful treatment: correction of the deformity and development of sufficient muscular power of the limb to maintain the correction. The deformity of the hind part of the foot, which is the keystone to the function of such a deformed foot, must be brought into a vertical plane before the equinus deformity is corrected.

Treatment of a clubfoot should begin while the child is still in the newborn nursery. The most effective treatment is application of serial corrective plaster casts to include the leg and foot. It is extremely important to correct the forefoot adduction first, then the hindfoot varus, and not begin to dorsiflex the foot at the ankle until both forefoot adduction and hindfoot varus are completely corrected.

An alternative method is to manipulate the foot and then strap the foot in some type of L splint, e.g., a Denis-Browne splint. If it becomes apparent after some months that the equinus deformity has not been completely overcome, it is occasionally necessary to do a heel cord lengthening and a posterior capsulotomy of the ankle joint.

Treatment of Old and Relapsed Cases. However early and thoroughly congenital clubfoot is treated, in a certain percentage of cases, because of rigidity or a constant tendency to relapse, manipulative treatment will not suffice. To ensure a good result in this type of case, an operation is necessary to release the contracted ligaments between the tarsal bones, especially on the medial side of the foot. It is also necessary to release the talus in the ankle joint. Lateral transfer of the tibialis anterior tendon insertion has been recommended in addition to ligamentous and soft tissue release in order to remove a deforming force.

If the talipes equinovarus is due to arthrogryposis, the only consistently successful procedure to overcome this deformity is an astragalectomy, which allows positioning of a plantigrade foot.

In the adult, no manipulation, tenotomy, or muscle operation is likely to be of benefit; operation on the bone is necessary in most cases. Cuneiform tarsectomy is the more certain and satisfactory operation.

CONGENITAL CONVEX PES VALGUS (VERTICAL TALUS)

This condition goes under a variety of names, including *congenital vertical talus* and *congenital rocker-bottom flatfoot*. The pathology involves a primary dislocation of the talonavicular joint. The navicular articulates with the dorsal aspect of the talus, which is in a plantar-flexed or vertical position. The dorsal talonavicular ligament and the anterior aspect of the deltoid are both contracted, as is the calcaneal cuboid ligament. The muscles of the anterior compartment, peroneus brevis, and triceps surae are contracted.

CLINICAL MANIFESTATIONS. The deformity can be diagnosed at birth because of a rigid flatfoot. The sole of the foot has a rocker-bottom configuration. The head of the talus can be palpated on the medial plantar aspect of the foot. The forefoot is abducted. The hindfoot is in equinovalgus, and the heel cord is tight. The child is able to walk on the foot without pain, although the gait may be awkward.

TREATMENT. Treatment is directed at early manipulative stretching and plaster correction of the forefoot into plantar flexion, inversion, and adduction. If manipulation and plaster cast immobilization can reduce the talonavicular dislocation, it is pinned with percutaneous K wires. If this is unsuccessful, open reduction is indicated at three months of age with a simultaneous tendoachilles lengthening. The calcaneal fibular ligament is also sectioned and posterior capsulotomy of the ankle and subtalar ligaments performed as necessary. Triple arthrodesis may be necessary in the older child.

ARTHROGRYPOSIS MULTIPLEX CONGENITA (MYODYSTROPHIA FETALIS)

There is marked muscular wasting with loss of mass, increased fibrous tissue around the joints, loss of mobility, and characteristic deformities without progressive neurologic disease. Bone changes are usually secondary to the overlying soft tissue changes. There may be unilateral or bilateral clubfoot and clubhand with marked rigidity of joints.

For the characteristics and treatment of the individual lesions that arise in myodystrophia fetalis, see the discussions of congenital dislocation of the hip, congenital dislocation of the knee, and congenital talipes equinovarus earlier in the chapter.

CONGENITAL HIGH SCAPULA

Congenital high scapula (Sprengel's shoulder) consists of an abnormally high and permanent elevation of the shoulder and is frequently associated with other deformities, such as congenital scoliosis, absence of vertebrae, fusion of ribs, or cervical rib, bony bridge to the spine, and errors in segmentation or position of the cervical spine.

PATHOGENESIS. This deformity is the result of deranged descent of the shoulder girdle. The muscles suffer in their normal development, undergoing degeneration and necrosis at an early embryonic stage and becoming fibrous. The scapula may be of normal shape or broadened. It lies at an unusually high level and may be attached to the vertebral column or the occipital bone by a band of imperfect muscle tissue or by fibrous tissue, or even by a bar of cartilage called the *omovertebral mass.* The atlas may be in two halves, one or both of which may be fused to the occipital condyles.

CLINICAL MANIFESTATONS. The scapula on one or both sides is 1 to 4 in. higher than usual. It is also tilted forward, so that the shoulder appears to be displaced upward and forward. When the arm is raised, the scapula does not move laterally, nor does its lower angle rotate when the arm is raised above the horizontal. The deformity of the shoulders rather than any functional disability of the arm attracts attention. Torticollis is present in about 10 percent of cases. Cranium bifidum and spina bifida are often present. Congenital kyphosis affecting the thoracic region almost invariably accompanies the deformity, while scoliosis is quite frequently present as well. The x-ray appearances are characteristic, the films showing the unduly high situation of the scapula. Other congenital defects in the neighborhood may also be apparent (Fig. 43-32).

TREATMENT. Mild cases need no operation, although more severe cases can be improved at least cosmetically. Surgery is usually not done until the patient is three years old. Best results occur in the three-to-six age group, when associated deformities about the shoulder are fewer and there is a longer period of growth to adjust to the new position of the scapula. The omovertebral bone is removed and the band of fascia to the scapula tenotomized or excised. In severe deformities release of the multiple muscles attached to the scapula is necessary.

CONGENITAL SHORT NECK (KLIPPEL-FEIL SYNDROME: BREVICOLLIS)

The trapezius muscles are tense and produce a winglike appearance, which has given rise to the name *congenital webbed neck,* with a torticollis of muscular or bony origin. The posterior hairline of the scalp is so low that it reaches the upper part of the thoracic wall. Scoliosis, elevation of the scapula, and other congenital anomalies may be present. Varying degrees of the deformity occur. In the typical extreme case there is a fusion of the lower cervical vertebrae and usually the thoracic vertebrae into a solid

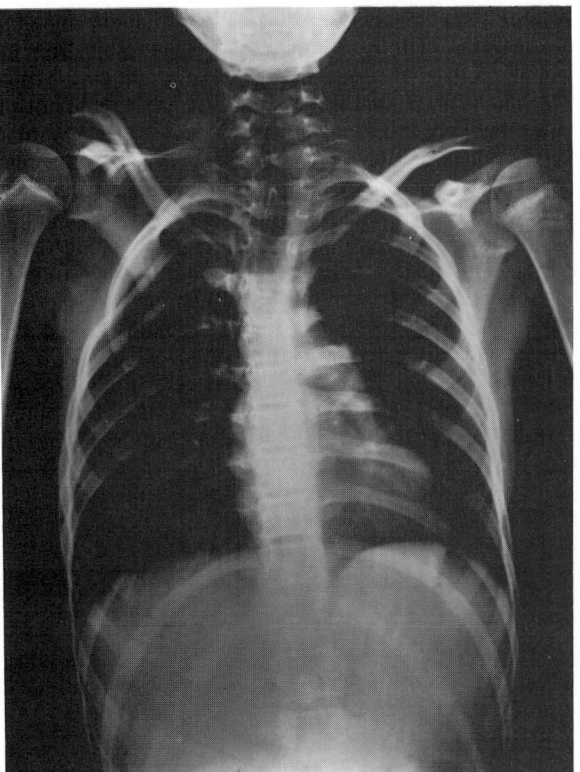

Fig. 43-32. Radiograph showing the abnormal high situation of the right scapula in Sprengel's deformity.

mass. Cervical spina bifida is usually present. Occasionally mental retardation is present. Treatment as a general rule is not indicated, but for patients with an extensive fold of skin a plastic operation may produce marked improvement.

CLEIDOCRANIAL DYSOSTOSIS SYNDROME

The syndrome consists of (1) aplasia of the clavicles, (2) exaggerated development of the transverse diameter of the cranium, and (3) delayed closure of the fontanelles. Hereditary transmission is by a dominant expression affecting both sexes equally, although several cases have been reported with neither a familial nor a hereditary history.

Where the scapula is absent in addition, the deformity must be regarded as an aplasia of the whole shoulder girdle rather than a dysostosis. The deformities of the clavicles are always accompanied by variations in the muscles.

CLINICAL MANIFESTATIONS. There is an apparently ununited fracture, defect in the midclavicle, or complete absence of the clavicle, and the patient can usually approximate the tips of his shoulders to each other below the chin. As a rule there is little or no disability or discomfort with abnormal mobility.

CONGENITAL WRYNECK (TORTICOLLIS)

This is a deformity characterized by lateral inclination of the head toward the shoulder, accompanied by torsion of the neck and dysplasia of the face. It is caused by unilateral contracture of the sternocleidomastoid, with secondary shortening of the fasciae and the other muscles of that side of the neck. It is generally believed that trauma is the primary cause of this deformity, producing a temporary acute obstruction of the veins followed by patchy intravascular clotting in the obstructed venous tree.

CLINICAL MANIFESTATIONS. The condition first becomes evident in the early months of life, when the mother notices an elongated swelling in the lower half of the sternocleidomastoid muscle. Every patient should be x-rayed to exclude any vertebral anomaly that may be the primary error. This swelling is at first tender, especially if the muscle is stretched. Gradually the swelling and the tenderness subside, but by the end of the first year of life the muscle becomes tense, pulling the head into the characteristic attitude, so that the ear on the affected side appears to be pulled down toward the sternoclavicular joint of the same side while the face is rotated toward the opposite side. If the deformity is not corrected, a gradual atrophy of the face on the affected side becomes increasingly evident with the growth of the child.

TREATMENT. The treatment should be begun at an early stage, as the development of the deformity can be arrested in mild cases by traction or by a collar.

In later and mild cases, however, traction and exercises are sufficient. Manipulation can be carried out daily, and there will probably be little or no evidence of contracture at the end of a few months. When the child is not seen until the age of two or three years, operation is usually indicated. The muscular heads are divided. During the operation the head is gradually manipulated into the correct position, in order to bring any shortened structures into prominence. The aftertreatment, which is of great importance, should be continued for about 6 months. It consists of active and passive movements to prevent any recurrence of the deformity.

CONGENITAL RADIOULNAR SYNOSTOSIS

One or both forearms are fixed at birth in a position midway between pronation and supination as a result of fusion of the proximal ends of the radius and ulna. In some cases the condition is inherited, and it is equally common in both sexes.

In the *true congenital radioulnar synostosis,* the upper end of the radius is imperfectly formed, being fused by bone to the ulna for a distance of several centimeters, and appears to grow from its upper end. The shaft of the radius angles forward more than usual and is longer and stouter than that of the ulna. The lower ends of the bones are almost invariably separate. Primary synostosis is usually bilateral; in over 80 percent of the recorded cases both forearms have been affected. There may be congenital dislocation of an ill-formed head of the radius, the radius and ulna being anchored at some point a short way distal to their upper extremities, usually in the region of the coronoid process, by a short, thick interosseous ligament.

TREATMENT. Although operation on the bony bridge would seem to be the obvious treatment, the soft tissues are not normally developed, and because of this, the recorded results of operation are disappointing. In the type of condition associated with dislocation of the head of the radius, where the soft parts are more normal, the prospect of intervention is more hopeful. If the pronation is extreme, it can be reduced by osteotomy.

MADELUNG'S DEFORMITY

In this congenital condition the radial shaft is bowed backward, the interosseous space is increased, and the lower end of the ulna is subluxated backward. The deformity is often bilateral, is most common in females, and appears frequently for the first time in adolescence. The hand and wrist are weak, and while flexion may be increased, other movements are restricted and may be painful. The wrist appears enlarged, and dorsiflexion of the hand is impaired. In severe cases pronation and supination are limited. Operation is occasionally indicated and consists of an osteotomy of the lower end of the radius.

CONGENITAL APLASIA AND/OR DYSPLASIA OF LONG BONES

These uncommon deformities, consisting of absence of an organ or part, are not recognized as inherited. Various maternal disturbances, e.g., thalidomide toxicity or rubella, can produce such changes.

Frantz and O'Rahilly have classified these various complex and poorly named abnormalities under the general heading of "congenital skeletal limb deficiencies," using a combination of the following terms: *melia,* limb; *podia,* foot; *dactylia,* finger; *preaxial,* the thumb or big toe border of the limb; *postaxial,* the opposite border; and *terminal,* either transverse or longitudinal. For example, an absence of the fibula and distal ray of the foot would be called *preaxial fibular hemimelia,* and the absence of the radius would be *radial preaxial hemimelia.*

Absence of the Radius

Absence of the radius is a rare developmental error but important because it is the commonest cause of clubhand, in which the hand is permanently deviated from the normal axis of the forearm. In less than half the cases the deformity is bilateral. The condition is sometimes hereditary and frequently coexists with other forms of congenital anomaly, notably harelip, cleft palate, and certain forms of congenital clubfoot.

Usually the whole radius is absent, but when a small portion of it remains generally at the upper end. When a small fragment of radius is present, the ulna may be fused to it, giving rise to a form of radioulnar synostosis. The carpus often shows associated abnormalities, including absence of the scaphoid or fusion of that bone with neighboring carpal bones. More rarely the lunate is absent.

When the radius is totally absent, the biceps is usually inserted into the lacertus fibrosus, though in some cases the muscle is either completely absent or fused with the brachialis anterior or the coracobrachialis. Other disturbances in the brachialis, the extensor carpi radialis longus and brevis, the extensor digitorum communis, the extensor pollicis longus, the flexor pollicis longus, and the pronator quadratus are frequently seen. The radial nerve usually terminates at the elbow, and there is often no radial artery.

CLINICAL MANIFESTATIONS. Generally the affected arm shows some degree of atrophy, but this is most marked in the forearm, which is invariably short, stubby, and bowed with a posterior convexity. The hand is small and atrophic. It is also deviated to the radial side and slightly palmar-flexed—"radiopalmar clubhand." The thumb is occasionally absent. Despite these deformities the limb may retain a surprisingly good function, although grasping power is usually impaired.

TREATMENT. The treatment is aimed at relieving the deformity, weakness, inability to use the arm, and limitation of certain movements, such as dorsiflexion.

The aim should be to overcome the deformity as early as possible by splintage or by operative removal of the bony anlage that is producing the bowing defect as well as growth disturbance of the intact ulnar bone. Every attempt should be made to stabilize the carpus and hand to the ulnar bone in order to obtain stretching of muscle and any available growth.

Absence of the Ulna

This is a much more uncommon lesion than the absence of the radius and is most difficult to differentiate from the latter lesion.

Absence or Dysplasia of the Fibula

This is a relatively uncommon condition. The whole limb is seen to be shortened in length and reduced in girth. The tibia appears bowed in an anterior direction with the hind part of the foot in the equinovalgus position, and there may be absence of part of the lateral forefoot and toes. There is obvious soft tissue atrophy and development of contractures. There may be bilateral involvement in about 30 percent of the cases. Radiography will show varying degrees of hypoplasia throughout the bones with delay in the appearance of their ossification centers.

TREATMENT. Because manipulation, casting, tendon lengthening, osteotomy of the tibia, etc., have been unsuccessful, early amputation, such as a Syme amputation of the foot, with fitting of a below-knee prosthesis, may be preferred.

Shortening of the Femur

Unlike the fibula, the dysplasia appears to affect mainly the proximal end of the femur rather than its center aspect. As growth proceeds, the deformity becomes more severe with marked leg length discrepancy due to disturbance in all bones of the lower extremity. Often these children never put weight on the involved limb.

Treatment is directed toward providing some means of ambulation through an ischial-bearing, weight-relieving brace. Although bracing allows ambulation, it does not provide for the normal stimulation to growth or weight bearing, and, therefore, as well as the aplastic or dysplastic elements, the remaining "normal" components of bone fail to grow and develop. Thus, if the main disturbance is in the more distal components, early amputation with a prosthesis is indicated.

Generalized Bone Disorders

Bone
Composition
Ossification
Remodeling

Classification of Generalized Bone Disorders

Developmental Disorders of Bone
Achondroplasia (Chondrodystrophia Fetalis)
Dyschondroplasia (Ollier's Disease)
Multiple Enchondromas
Metaphyseal Aclasis
Polyostotic Fibrous Dysplasia
    Monostotic Fibrous Dysplasia
Osteogenesis Imperfecta
Osteopetrosis
    Melorheostosis

Metabolic Diseases
Calcification
Scurvy
Rickets
    Celiac Rickets (Gluten-Sensitive Enteropathy)
    Renal Osteodystrophy
    Hypophosphatasia
Osteomalacia
Parathyroid Osteodystrophy
Osteoporosis
Pituitary Disturbances
    Pituitary Short Stature
    Hyperpituitary Syndromes
Congenital Hypothyroidism
Mucopolysaccharidoses

Osteitis Deformans

Reticuloses

Reticuloendothelial System
    Lipoid Granulomatosis
    Eosinophilic Granulomatosis
    Letterer-Siwe Disease
Lymphatic System
    Hodgkin's Disease

Hematopoietic System

Leukemia
Multiple Myeloma
Hemolytic Anemia

BONE

Composition

Bone is made up of organic and inorganic materials, and water.

ORGANIC PHASE. This is made up of osteogenic cells—i.e., the osteoblast, the osteocyte, and the osteoclast—the cartilage cell, or chondroblast, and the intercellular matrix, as well, which consists of approximately 89 percent collagen, 1 percent amorphous mucopolysaccharide complexes, and other proteins (Fig. 43-33).

Abnormalities of collagen have been described in such conditions as Ehlers-Danlos syndrome, which is a hydroxylysine deficiency disease, and some forms of osteogenesis imperfecta, in which there is lack of type I collagen. Chondroitin sulfate, keratin sulfate, and dermatan sulfate make up the sulfated glycosaminoglycans. These are very important structures for the elasticity and resilience of cartilage, particularly when load is applied.

The intercellular matrix, or ground substance, *osseomucoid,* is common to all connective tissues and contains protein, crystalloids, metabolites, and gases similar to plasma. It forms the final diffusion or circulatory pathway for the exchange of nutritional substances from blood to the osteogenic cells through the various lacunae and canalicular systems. Osseous mucoid substance consists of (1) proteoglycans and (2) glycoproteins containing chondroitin sulfate, all having a great capacity for binding metal with various radionuclides and possibly calcium.

INORGANIC PHASE. In this phase, bone contains 99 percent of the total calcium and 90 percent of the phosphorus of the human body. It is made up of calcium, phosphate, hydroxyl, carbonates, and magnesium.

WATER. Eight to 9 percent of the bone matrix, even in the fully mineralized state, is water in the form of either interstitial or extracellular fluid, or within the hydration shell of the apatite crystals. There is much water in the organic phase of mucopolysaccharide complexes, in collagen, in the inorganic component of bone, and in the marrow and osteocytic spaces of bone.

CITRATE. This represents 70 percent of the total body citrate. As well as being concerned with the metabolic, oxidative processes of carbohydrate, fat, and protein in mammals, it forms soluble but complex compounds with calcium to facilitate absorption from the intestine, diffusion, and hence deposition of calcium into bone. In vitamin D deficiency rickets, the serum citrate level is low even when the calcium level remains normal; the administration of citrate as the sodium salt is followed by healing of the rachitic lesion of bone.

ENZYMES. Bone cells contain the normal complement of enzymes similar, for example, to those found in liver cells. Bone cells have an active metabolism, the rate of oxygen consumption reaching 50 percent of that of liver cells. Bone differs from other tissues in relying largely on glycolysis for energy production. Certain enzymes and enzyme systems have special importance in bone tissue.

Glycolytic Enzymes in Osteoclasts. These enzymes transform glucose into pyruvate with concomitant formation of adenosine triphosphate (ATP), which is used by the cell in various synthetic reactions. The pyruvate can then be metabolized further to lactate or to citrate. The production of lactic acid is an important factor in bone resorption, and the metabolism of osteoclasts is primarily glycolytic or anaerobic, which promotes lactate formation.

Acid Hydrolases. An example is cathepsin D, a protease with optimal activity at a pH of 3.6. The acid hydrolases are normally found within the lysosome. Thus, the extrusion or breakdown of the lysosomes in cells leads to the digestion of cells and their surrounding matrix when bone is resorbed by osteoblasts.

Collagenases. Bone contains enzymes that will specifically degrade collagen, a property that few proteases exhibit. Such enzymes are important in the breakdown of the organic matrix of bone during resorption.

Alkaline Phosphatase. The serum level is altered in certain disorders of the skeletal and hepatobiliary systems (see Table 43-3). It is considered to be concerned with the preosseous cellular metabolism and with the subsequent elaboration of bone matrix before the crystallization of calcium and phosphate ions. It is detectable in the serum of adults with normal levels of 35 to 80 I.U./L and is also present in calcifying cartilage, intestinal mucosa, liver, and kidneys.

Phosphorylase and Glycolytic Enzyme Systems. These are concerned with converting glycogen via the hexophosphopyruvates into excess phosphate ions.

Acid Phosphatase. This is present in high levels in the osteoclasts and cells of the prostate. Serum levels in both sexes are very low under normal conditions.

Fig. 43-33. Organic components of bone. [From: *Mercer W, Duthie RB (eds): Orthopaedic Surgery. London, Edward Arnold, 1974, with permission.*]

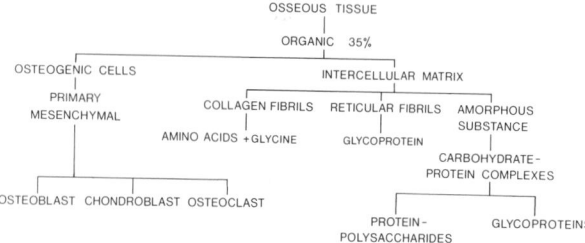

Table 43-3. ALKALINE PHOSPHATASE LEVELS

Alkaline phosphatase levels	Skeletal disease	Hepatobiliary disease
Increased	Rickets and osteomalacia	
	In calcifying cartilage	
	Paget's disease	
	Osteosarcoma	
	At site of disease	
	Carcinoma, osteoblastic metastases	Intra- and extra-hepatobiliary obstructions
Normal	Osteoporosis	Metastases
	Osteopetrosis	Thorazine toxicity
	Healing fracture	
	Increase in phosphatase locally	
	Osteosclerosis	
	Fibrous dysplasia	
	Variable level	
Decreased	Achondroplasia	
	Deposition of radioactive substances in bone	
	Hypophosphatasia	
	Arrest of skeletal growth with decreased osteoblastic activity	
	Cretinism	
	Scurvy	

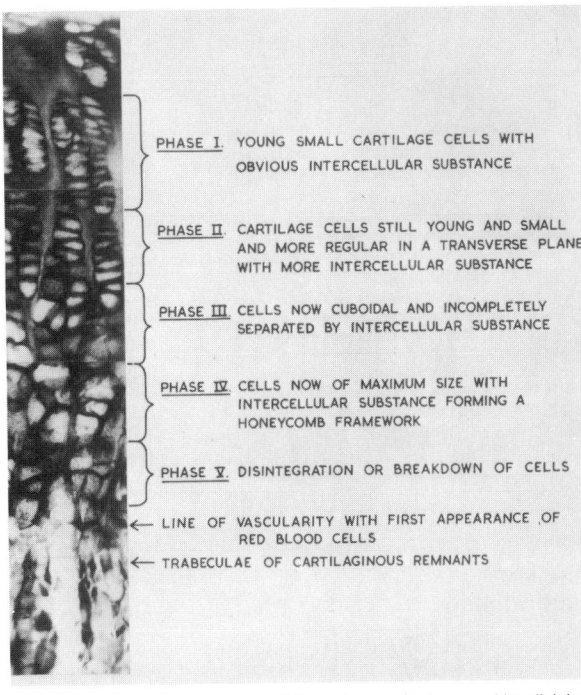

PHASE I. YOUNG SMALL CARTILAGE CELLS WITH OBVIOUS INTERCELLULAR SUBSTANCE

PHASE II. CARTILAGE CELLS STILL YOUNG AND SMALL AND MORE REGULAR IN A TRANSVERSE PLANE WITH MORE INTERCELLULAR SUBSTANCE

PHASE III. CELLS NOW CUBOIDAL AND INCOMPLETELY SEPARATED BY INTERCELLULAR SUBSTANCE

PHASE IV. CELLS NOW OF MAXIMUM SIZE WITH INTERCELLULAR SUBSTANCE FORMING A HONEYCOMB FRAMEWORK

PHASE V. DISINTEGRATION OR BREAKDOWN OF CELLS

← LINE OF VASCULARITY WITH FIRST APPEARANCE OF RED BLOOD CELLS
← TRABECULAE OF CARTILAGINOUS REMNANTS

Fig. 43-34. Photomicrograph of the epiphyseal plate and its division into Streeter's five phases. [From: *Mercer W, Duthie RB (eds): Orthopaedic Surgery. London, Edward Arnold, 1974,* with permission.]

in length, further cartilage cells are added to the epiphysis from the juxtaepiphyseal apparatus or the perichondral ring of Lacroix. Streeter has described the classic five phases of the epiphyseal plate with the characteristic appearance of the cartilage cells (Fig. 43-34).

Accompanying such longitudinal and accretional growth there is remodeling to produce the tubular shape of bone as a result of cellular activity. In the five normal processes of endochondral ossification there are three main phases that can undergo disturbance:

1. Disturbance in the actual growth and differentiation of cartilage, such as in achondroplasia
2. Disturbance in the osteogenic-osteolytic balance, such as in osteoporosis, osteosclerosis, and osteitis fibrosis
3. Disturbance in the deposition of the calcium phosphate crystals in the cartilage matrix and/or osteoid, such as in rickets or osteomalacia

INTRAMEMBRANOUS OSSIFICATION. This form of ossification occurs without any preformed cartilage model and is seen particularly in the development of the calvarium. The cells are developed from the germinal layers, and at a certain stage of differentiation the mesodermal cells condense and begin to proliferate in the area where bone will be formed. In this area the cells elaborate increased cytoplasm with an eosinophilic staining reaction and, at the same time, begin to secrete a metachromatic intercellular substance, as well as collagen fibrils. These cells soon become osteoblasts that continue to secrete much intracellular substance, or osteoid, which mineralizes to form bone. From such centers of ossification the process spreads.

Ossification

ENDOCHONDRAL OSSIFICATION. The long bones of the skeleton, with the exception of the clavicle, are all laid down primarily as hyaline cartilage in recognizable anatomic form. In the center of this cartilage model, at a certain stage, the cells undergo hypertrophy and accumulate glycogen. Phosphorylases and other enzymes with their glycolytic action appear in the cells and cartilage matrix to form the osseous centrum. Such changes in the cartilage are accompanied by ossification in the perichondrium and an ingrowth of vascular connective tissue that replaces the hypertrophied cartilage cells. Osteoblasts derived from this connective tissue then begin to lay down osteoid and fetal bone on the cartilage matrix. Hematopoietic cells appear from the invading tissues, and red marrow is soon identified.

The process extends up and down the shaft until the level of the future growth plates is reached at the epiphyseal-metaphyseal junction. Here the replacement of the cartilage model ceases, and the cartilage organizes into the proliferative epiphyseal growth plate.

During fetal and childhood osteogenesis, the endochondral growth of bone continues in the epiphyseal plate areas, as well as within the epiphysis. To maintain growth

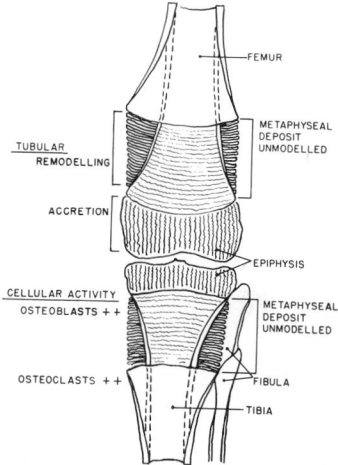

Fig. 43-35. Tubular remodeling and accretion of a long bone. *[After Keith, taken with permission from Mercer W, Duthie RB (eds): Orthopaedic Surgery. London, Edward Arnold, 1974.]*

Remodeling

This consists of extensive but constructive resorption and deposition of new bone which, although most marked during growth and development, continues in the mature skeleton. With resorption there is the shift of both mineral and organic matrix into a fluid phase. During growth at the epiphyseal plate area the remodeling process is essential to change the shape and function of the bones, both in the longitudinal and in the circumferential planes and within the spongiosa of the medullary cavity (Fig. 43-35) in order to produce the normal tubular shape of the shaft. There is a morphologic remodeling process in the periosteal area, adjacent to the juxtaepiphyseal area or the perichondral ring of Lacroix, which contains large numbers of osteoclasts. There is a constant remodeling process taking place within the basic structure of bone, i.e., in the osteon itself. The marrow cavity is also widened during remodeling by osteoclastic activity on the endosteal surfaces of cortex and spongiosa.

CLASSIFICATION OF GENERALIZED BONE DISORDERS

I. *Developmental disorders* involving the organic phase of bone, i.e., collagen and cartilage matrix formation, calcification, and remodeling
   A. Achondroplasia
   B. Chondroosteodystrophy
   C. Dyschondroplasia
   D. Multiple enchondromas
   E. Metaphyseal aclasis
   F. Osteogenesis imperfecta
   G. Polyostotic fibrous dysplasia
   H. Osteopetrosis
II. Metabolic disorders
   A. Deficiency in inorganic constituents of bone
      1. Insufficient absorption of calcium or phosphates
        a. Low intake
           (1) Starvation
           (2) Rickets
           (3) Osteomalacia

        b. Defective absorption
           (1) Vitamin D deficiency
           (2) Defective fat absorption
              (a) Biliary deficiency
              (b) Pancreatic deficiency
              (c) Celiac disease
           (3) Chronic diarrhea
      2. Excessive secretion of calcium or phosphates
        a. Renal rickets, or osteodystrophy
           (1) Total renal insufficiency
           (2) Tubular insufficiency
              (a) Lignac-Fanconi syndrome
              (b) Hyperchloremic acidosis
              (c) Vitamin D–resistant rickets, or "phosphate rickets"
        b. During pregnancy, via placenta and breast
           (1) Osteomalacia
        c. Hyperparathyroidism
      3. Decreased phosphate excretion
        a. Hypoparathyroidism
   B. Deficiency in organic constituents of bone
      1. Decreased intake
        a. Starvation
        b. Chronic diarrhea
      2. Excessive utilization or loss
        a. Chronic infection
        b. Renal disease
        c. Liver disease
        d. Hormonal
           (1) Hyperthyroidism
           (2) Postmenopausal osteoporosis
           (3) Disuse atrophy
           (4) Stress
           (5) Cushing's disease
III. *Hormonal disorders*—normal, excessive, or deficient secretion, the effect being seen in a *child* as altered rate of epiphyseal growth and skeletal maturation and in an *adult* as alteration in the balance of osteolytic and osteoblastic activity
   A. Pituitary
   B. Sex glands
   C. Thyroid
   D. Adrenals
   E. Parathyroids
IV. *Reticulosis*—disease of bone marrow constituents such as
   A. Reticuloendothelial system
      1. Histiocytic granulomatosis
        a. Letterer-Siwe disease
        b. Eosinophilic granuloma
        c. Hand-Schüller-Christian disease
      2. Lipoid granulomatosis
        a. Gaucher's disease
        b. Niemann-Pick disease
        c. Xanthomatosis with hypercholesterolemia
   B. Lymphatic system
      1. Hodgkin's disease
      2. Lymphosarcoma
   C. Hematopoietic system
      1. Leukemia
        a. Lymphoblastic
        b. Myeloblastic
      2. Multiple myeloma
      3. Hemolytic anemia
        a. Mediterranean, or Cooley's anemia
        b. Sickle cell anemia
        c. Erythroblastosis foetalis
V. *Vascular disorders*
   A. Paget's disease
   B. Osteodystrophy or Sudeck's atrophy
   C. Massive osteolysis, or "disappearing bones"

DEVELOPMENTAL DISORDERS OF BONE

The common developmental diseases of bone apart from the obvious endocrine errors can all be arranged in two groups:

1. Errors in the proliferation and calcification of the cartilage model
   a. Achondroplasia
   b. Chondroosteodystrophy
   c. Dyschondroplasia
   d. Metaphyseal aclasis
   e. Multiple enchondromas
   f. Polyostotic fibrous dysplasia
2. Errors in the collagen and matrix formation
   a. Osteogenesis imperfecta
   b. Osteopetrosis

The epiphyseal cartilage proliferates normally in columnar fashion and in due course undergoes maturation, degeneration, and calcification. If the chondroblast is defective, multiple pathologic lesions may occur as a result of failure or irregularity in the maturation and calcification of the cartilage cells. If the failure of maturation and calcification is diffuse, the lack of the zone of preliminary calcification will result in delay of epiphyseal ossification and dwarfism.

A central chondroblast, if it continues to proliferate, will form an enchondroma that gives the bone a cystic appearance; if peripheral, this will result in an ecchondroma, or an exostosis may result instead of calcification to give a fibrous tissue mass. In general the following conditions are produced:

Achondroplasia—dwarfism
Metaphyseal aclasia—exostoses
Dyschondroplasia—cyst formation
Multiple chondromas—enchondromas
Chondroosteodystrophy—combination of all

Achondroplasia (Chondrodystrophia Fetalis)

The basic disturbance is in the calcification and remodeling of cartilage. Membranous bones, e. g., ribs and sternum, are formed, and all develop normally. The severity can vary, and in very severe cases the fetus dies in utero. Achondroplasia is inherited as a dominant expression in the majority of those individuals who survive and reproduce. The most evident histologic feature is the absence of cartilage proliferation and the columnar formation of cartilage. Ossification is irregular. Bone accretion at the periosteal surface is attached to the growth cartilage and may deposit a layer of compact bone over part of the metaphysis.

CLINICAL MANIFESTATIONS (Fig. 43-36). At birth, the typical infant with achondroplasia has a normal-sized body, very short, fat, flabby limbs, and a large head, with a characteristic depression at the root of the nose. Smallness in stature due to the absence of growth of the extremities becomes increasingly evident during childhood. A dwarf results. Walking occurs at the usual age, and dentition is normal.

When the patient stands erect, the tips of the fingers may only reach the great trochanter of the iliac crests,

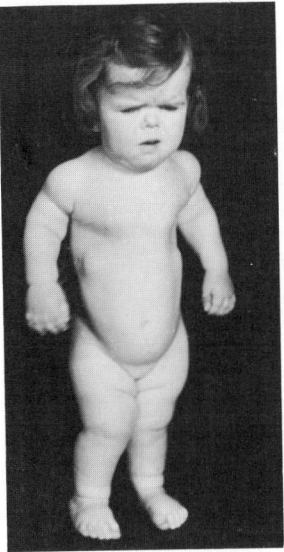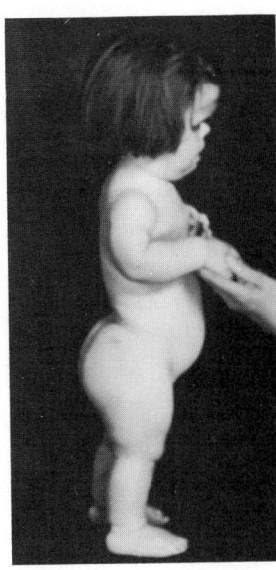

Fig. 43-36. Achondroplastic girl showing the decreased limb growth with foreshortening of the stature but normal trunk height.

instead of normally reaching the lower part of the thigh. The achondroplastic hand is short and broad, with the fingers of equal length, e.g., *main en trident*. The short limbs, especially the lower, are often curved, in contrast to the trunk, which is virtually normal. The sacrum is tilted, and, as a consequence, contracture of the pelvic inlet follows.

The head is enlarged, rounded, and markedly brachycephalic. The face is broad, and at the root of the short nose is a characteristic depression or indentation. The upper alveolar processes protrude, and prominence of the lower jaw results in prognathism. Persons with achondroplasia usually have normal intelligence.

Although the vertebral column is of normal length, the centers of ossification of the bodies may be smaller than normal. Often there is a long regular kyphosis at the lumbodorsal region. The most striking feature is the early synostosis between the body and the arch, which in some cases is so severe as to lead to marked diminution in the caliber of the vertebral canal. The prognosis varies with the degree of the affection, but an achondroplastic individual may live to a considerable age.

Dyschondroplasia (Ollier's Disease)

In 1899, Ollier first described this condition of varying degrees of ossification of abnormal metaphyseal cartilage formation. Dyschondroplasia is more commonly diffusely unilateral or bilateral, but occasionally it may be confined to a single bone.

The typical changes are in the ends of the diaphysis of long bones—humerus, femur, radius, etc.—or in the long bones of the hands and feet, where growth is most rapid. The metaphysis is usually broadened and cystic with trabeculae running in parallel lines in the long axis of the bone. Occasionally small exostoses project from the surface, and foreshortening is evident. In the short long bones, multiple enchondromas may form. The ilium, ischium, and pubis may appear stippled and varying in bone density because of the presence of small rounded areas of cartilage. Dyschondroplasia may be associated with cavernous hemangiomas and phleboliths of the soft tissue, a syndrome described by Maffucci.

The prognosis for normal life expectancy appears to be good, but deformity and secondary arthritis are constant sequelae. Surgical intervention is indicated only when there is mechanical interference with joint function and after epiphyseal growth has ceased.

Multiple Enchondromas

This is a disturbance of growth in which multiple cartilaginous tumors are present in the shafts of the short long bones of the hands and feet. The lesion may be a variant of dyschondroplasia.

The bone may be grossly expanded, and the expansion may be regular, with faint body striations along the periphery of the expanded area. As the chondromatous tissue grows, more and more of the bone is destroyed, until little of the affected bone may remain save a few scattered bony fragments embedded in irregular striped masses of exuberant chondromatous tissue. Pathologic fractures may occur and require bone grafting.

Metaphyseal Aclasis (Multiple Exostoses, Diaphyseal Aclasis, Hereditary Deforming Dyschondroplasia)

The disease affects only those bones arising from cartilage and is inherited in an autosomal dominant form. The basic defect is in a failure of remodeling of the metaphysis with the formation of multiple outgrowths or exostoses from the surface of the shaft of long bones, leading to some stunting of skeletal growth.

PATHOLOGY. The membrane bones of the skeleton, the tarsal and carpal bones, are not involved. The condition affects those parts of the long bones in which tubular remodeling is active, i.e., the distal end of the femur, the proximal ends of the tibia and fibula, the distal ends of the radius and ulna, and the proximal end of the humerus. It is also seen at the medial and lateral ends of the clavicle, the vertebral border of the scapula, and occasionally at the neurocentral synchondroses of the vertebrae. The metaphysis is increased in diameter, with roughly parallel sides. Irregular projections—exostoses—appear on the surface.

There is usually well-marked interference with growth in length of the affected bones with irregularity of the ossification at the epiphyseal plate. It is essentially a failure of maturation of the cartilage cells. In the leg, growth of the fibula lags behind that of the tibia.

Two occasional complications of metaphyseal aclasis occur:

1. Formation of a *chondroma* that projects from the surface of the bone near the epiphyseal cartilage and can become chondrosarcomatous
2. Osteogenic sarcoma or *chondrosarcoma,* which may arise in one of the exostoses

In the diffuse type there may be extensive distortion. The stature is short or even dwarfed. In addition the limbs may show deformities of the nature of bowing or genu valgum. Fracture from slight trauma is common, but the fragments unite as readily as in normal individuals.

The most typical feature is the presence of numerous exotoses. These are most common at sites of active growth, such as the knee and shoulder. The projections are hard, the skin overlying them is normal, and the soft tissues move easily on them. They may be associated with pain if the tumor presses on a peripheral nerve or a nerve root or if the process is inadvertently fractured. They are also liable to interfere with the free play of associated tendons or may even act as a mechanical obstruction to joint movement in which event they may give rise to considerable disability. A bursa may form over the projection and from time to time become inflamed.

Radiologic examination shows an irregularly expanded metaphyseal mass, with little or no compact cortical bone. The normal cancellous tissue is replaced by a mass of less dense tissue, in which islands of normal ossification may be observed.

The disease has no effect on the general health, but there may be disability as a result of nerve pressure or interference with joint movement. The only treatment indicated is the removal of exostoses that are giving rise to symptoms or that have become malignant.

Polyostotic Fibrous Dysplasia (Osteodystrophy Fibrosa, Unilateral Recklinghausen's Disease, Albright's Syndrome)

The disease usually appears in childhood or puberty as cyst formation in the diaphysis or metaphysis, but rarely in the epiphysis, of long bones. The bones most frequently involved are the femur, tibia, humerus, and radius. Bending deformities of the weight-bearing bones and pathologic fractures with slow union or nonunion are frequent occurrences. On biopsy, there is usually a distinctive appearance of bony trabeculae formation in a stroma of fibrous tissue.

The x-ray shows expansion of the bone and thinning of the cortex with numerous trabeculated cystic areas. It is usually a unilateral disease affecting multiple long bones. When it affects only one bone, it is known as *monostotic fibrous dysplasia*. The treatment is of the deformities, and prognosis is good, as this is a self-limiting disease. Certain lesions may require curettage and autogenous grafting.

Albright's syndrome is a variation of polyostotic fibrous dysplasia occurring in a female and accompanied by sexual precocity and flat pigmented areas of skin.

MONOSTOTIC FIBROUS DYSPLASIA

In this condition a single bone is the site of partial replacement of its substance by fibrous tissue, with or without the additional presence of osteoid. Any bone may be involved. The clinical findings are local swelling where the bone is superficial and pain if the lesion is near a joint.

The condition may represent a disturbance of the normal bone reparative process following trauma.

Osteogenesis Imperfecta

Osteogenesis imperfecta, in which extreme fragility of bones is present, originates in fetal life. In the autosomal, dominant inherited form the stature is stunted, the joints are hypermobile, the sclera is blue, and deafness frequently appears after adolescence. Among adults with blue sclera 60 percent have associated fragile bones, and 60 percent have associated deafness.

The basic defect of osteogenesis imperfecta is a diffuse defect of the primitive mesenchymal cells, which fail to produce normal collagen. The bones are extremely fragile, because of the absence of a well-formed cortex, the sparse and widely separated trabeculae, and the nature of the osseous substance, which is less compact than the ordinary laminated bone. The bone is liable to undergo osteoclastic absorption and also, in late cases, appears to undergo spontaneous disintegration. The raised serum alkaline phosphatase level is frequently elevated because of compensatory activity of bone repair.

CLINICAL MANIFESTATIONS. In the *fetal form*, the disease is severe, and the child is stillborn or survives only a very short time as a result of brain injury. There are multiple fractures, some healed at birth, while the cranium shows grossly imperfect ossification and consists merely of a membranous bag with a few plaques of poor bone embedded in it.

In the *infantile form*, the disease is less severe. At birth there may be some stunting and evidence of fractures, but the ossification of the skull is more advanced. The child survives for a year or two, but the bones are fragile and break at a touch. The skull may assume a globular shape and may appear large in proportion to the rest of the body. True hydrocephalus may develop.

In the *adolescent type*, often called *osteogenesis imperfecta tarda*, the child may appear normal at birth and during childhood. The only disturbance observed may be a special liability to fractures from comparatively minor injuries. The ossification of the skull may be normal, but one or two soft areas may be found on examination. As time passes, the tendency to fracture decreases.

The disease may on rare occasions be encountered first in adult life, when a case that was slight at birth and during adolescence becomes active or when a case that has regressed spontaneously is reactivated.

Prominent features are

1. Stunting of growth.
2. Fractures from trivial trauma. The fractures are often subperiosteal and unite readily, often more so than in normal bone, and the callus is often more dense than in normal bone. The fractures are distinctive in that they cause little or no pain or tenderness—largely because they are subperiosteal.
3. Blue sclera.
4. Characteristic skull, showing broadening of the forehead, angular projections above the zygoma, a downward tilting of the axis of the orbit, the ear, and the auditory canals, and an underhung jaw.

Radiologic Findings. In severe types the bones may show almost complete absence of cancellous texture, the cortex appearing as a faintly penciled line. The bones are shorter than normal and occasionally broader. In less severe types the long bones are stunted, are diffusely rarefied, and may have expanded club-shaped extremities. Fractures or old deformities following fractures are often apparent. In adult cases the shafts of the bones appear to shrink and have a dense, relatively thick cortex with no medulla. The ends of the bones are expanded and contain coarse cancellation with poor density. Ultimately the long bones may appear as two poorly calcified end bulbs joined by a slender rod of denser bone.

The ribs are usually bent sharply downward at their angles, and the thorax is therefore greatly deformed. This may be accentuated by scoliosis. The pelvis is asymmetric with irregular deformity. The skull has irregular ossification, with islands of denser bone in a poorly calcified matrix—the so-called Wormian bones.

PROGNOSIS AND TREATMENT. In the majority of cases early death is the outcome. Occasionally adult life is reached, but the constant occurrence of fractures and the repeated confinement to bed produce real disability. Protective pneumatic prostheses may prevent fractures or osteoporosis. No specific treatment is known. When fractures occur, they are treated along the usual lines. When healing takes place with deformity, osteotomy may be carried out.

Osteopetrosis (Albers-Schönberg Disease, Marble Bones, Osteosclerosis Fragilis Generalisata, Congenital Osteosclerosis)

Albers-Schönberg, in 1904, described this rare bone disease associated with increased density of the skeleton. Fewer than 40 cases have been described. The condition has occasionally affected several members of a family as an autosomal recessive inheritance.

The characteristic change is the increased density and thickness with loss of trabeculation of the affected bone, in symmetric fashion, most commonly in the metaphysis. The most marked changes are found in the most rapidly growing extremities of the long bones—the lower end of the femur and radius, and the upper end of the tibia and humerus.

The ribs are similarly affected—thick, dense, and apparently structureless. The vertebrae may be uniformly dense, or a dense zone at the upper and lower thirds of the body may be separated by a zone of normal density in the middle, indicating that the process is affecting the bone laid down from the cartilage end plates of the body. The skull may be so dense that no detail of its architecture can be made out. The bones of the carpus and tarsus are ringed by layers of dense bone, the result of peripheral accretions. These so-called marble bones are liable to fractures, especially in the adolescent.

In the absence of true ossification or any lamellar system by osteoblastic activity, much of the sclerosis is due to excessive calcification of osteoid tissues.

The progressive sclerosis of the long bones gradually reduces the medullary cavity and the bone marrow to a degree incompatible with normal hematopoiesis, producing a true aplastic anemia, sometimes with enlargement of the liver and spleen. In the skull the thickening is apt to restrict the size of the foramina, leading to pressure on, and paralysis of, the cranial nerves, to give blindness, nystagmus and ocular palsies, hydrocephalus, and occasionally signs of hypopituitarism.

MELORHEOSTOSIS

The condition was first reported by Léri in 1922. Its distinguishing features are (1) that the sclerotic changes are confined to one limb, (2) that the outline of an affected bone is definitely distorted, (3) the presence of pain, often severe, and (4) limitation of movement in the joints formed by the affected bone.

A portion of the cortex of one of the limb bones is irregularly enlarged, sufficiently to give rise to a swelling with an undulating surface. Between one undulation and another, a linear band of increased density may extend that has been likened to a "flow" of hyperostosis resembling "candle drippings."

METABOLIC DISEASES

Calcification

This process consists of two phases, or systems: first, cellular differentiation to form a suitable medium of ma-

trix osteoid, collagen fibrils, etc., and second, the process of mineralization.

Osteoblasts secrete the organic matrix, or *osteoid*, which is made up of collagen fibers and an interfibrillar cement substance.

Sulfation first appears at the cell membrane along with prefibrillar collagen formation, and then the matrix contains the sulfated mucopolysaccharide chondroitin sulfate. This sulfation is defective in vitamin C scurvy. Any failure of alkaline phosphatase, of sulfation, or of vitamin C may alter the formation of osteoid and hence its calcification. Calcification involves the precipitation of mineral salts, i.e., calcium phosphate.

Scurvy

The absence of vitamin C from the diet gives rise to the clinical condition of scurvy. The disease occurs most commonly in infants from six to eight months of age who have been fed exclusively on artificial food which has had its vitamin content destroyed. It also occurs in adults who are deprived of fresh food. The cardinal feature of scurvy is a defect in the formation of intercellular substances which results in hemorrhage—from the gums, from the alimentary tract, from the subcutaneous tissues, and in bone. The hemorrhage is capillary in origin and occurs at sites at which new capillaries are sprouting, e.g., in bone, at the most actively growing metaphyses and beneath the periosteum. In very extreme cases, the hemorrhage may be sufficient to disrupt the growing area, with separation of the epiphyses. The subperiosteal hemorrhages are often extensive, the periosteum being stripped from the shaft for a considerable distance, with abnormal ossification.

CLINICAL MANIFESTATIONS. The child may or may not appear ill-nourished. The earliest features are restlessness and fretfulness, with one or more of the extremities not used. Handling of the parts produces extreme pain.

On examination there may be obvious swelling, fluid in character, in relation to the shaft of one or more of the long bones. The joints may appear swollen and are exquisitely sensitive to touch, appearing like an infective condition. The immobility of the parts may stimulate paralysis, and this feature is often known as the *pseudoparalysis of scurvy*. Hemorrhages may also occur into and beneath the skin, and the gums may be swollen and spongy. The typical x-ray appearances are seen in Fig. 43-37.

TREATMENT. The administration of vitamin C in any of its forms leads to rapid cure. Within 24 h pain and crying cease, and in a few days hemorrhages are beginning to heal. It is some months, however, before the bone remodeling occurs. Rest in bed is indicated in the early stages, and, later, exercises may be usefully employed to augment muscle tone. Unprotected weight bearing should be relieved by caliper until there is radiographic evidence of a return of bony structure, to prevent deformities.

Rickets

Rickets and osteomalacia in modern civilizations are usually due to primary metabolic abnormalities that are

Fig. 43-37. X-ray of the lower limbs of a baby with scurvy showing the epiphyseal disturbance and calcifying periosteal hematoma formation.

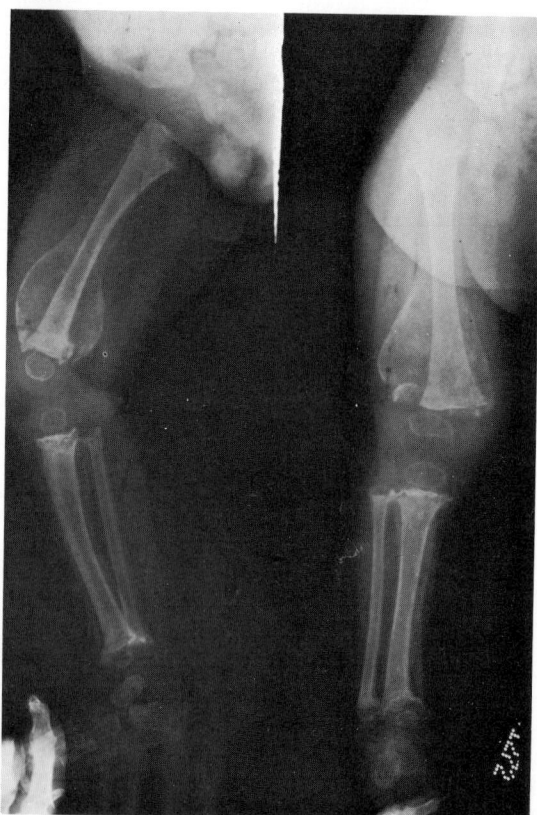

genetically determined. Most of the cases now appearing, although clinically similar to environmental or nutritional rickets, are vitamin D–resistant rickets, with or without an abnormality of renal tubular function but requiring massive dosages of vitamin D for cure. The primary defect of vitamin D deficiency intake or effect leads to a state of hypophosphatemia because of the decreased renal tubular resorption of phosphate.

The most common type of the disease begins during the early years of infancy and is extremely rare after the age of four. It is known as *infantile rickets*. Comparable disturbances may arise at other age periods and are known as *late rickets and osteomalacia*.

PATHOLOGY. The normal epiphyseal line is a well-defined narrow strip of cartilage 2 mm deep, but in rickets it forms a wide irregular band, and the metaphysis is broad and irregular from excessive proliferation of the cells of the epiphyseal line. Mineralization is patchy in distribution and uniformly deficient. The cartilage in the proliferating zone is hyperplastic, but instead of the normal palisade arrangement of the cells, the proliferated cells are arranged irregularly. Associated with this is a poor development of the bone marrow. In the metaphysis the bony trabeculae are thinned with connective tissue hyperplasia, so that the extremity of the bone appears misshapen and unmodeled—particularly in the costochondral junctions. These changes are most marked in the most actively growing part of the bones.

CLINICAL MANIFESTATIONS. When the child is able to crawl or to walk, the femur becomes bowed anteriorly and to the lateral side. The neck-shaft angle of the femur may be diminished (coxa vara), the tibia may be bowed, or the knee may assume a valgus attitude. The whole pelvis may be flattened, or it may assume a trefoil shape as in osteomalacia causing obstetric difficulties. The skull is broadened, the forehead square, and bosses of new bone may form in the parietal and frontal regions. The vertebral column may assume exaggerated curvatures.

Cardinal manifestations include (1) restlessness associated with fear on moving limbs, (2) recurrent diarrhea and constipation, (3) evidences of irritability of the central nervous system, such as convulsions, laryngismus, or other types of spasmophilia, (4) large head, open fontanels, and craniotabes, (5) prominent abdomen, (6) narrow chest and rachitic rosary of costochondral junctions, (7) enlarged and tender epiphyses, (8) bowing of the long bones, (9) delayed dentition, with irregular, soft, decaying teeth, and (10) poorly developed muscles, with delay in walking.

Radiologic Findings. In the *acute stage,* the epiphysis is widened and lacks radiodensity, with delay in appearance of centers of ossification. The metaphysis is splayed out (Fig. 43-38). The periosteum is thickened, with fractures of the long bones frequently seen. In the *chronic stage,* bowing occurs with the cortical part of the affected bone thickened on the side of the concavity (Fig. 43-39).

TREATMENT. Nutritional, or vitamin D deficiency, rickets may be cured by administration of one of the vitamin D–containing foods or by one of the standard preparations of the vitamin (e.g., calciferol, 3000 I.U./day). The effect of this is enhanced by the addition of a cal-

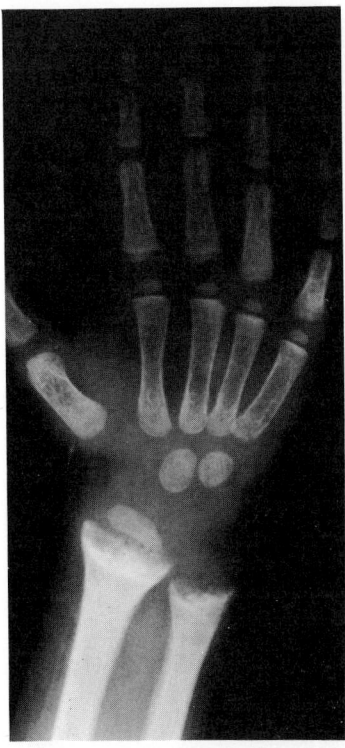

Fig. 43-38. X-ray of the hand and wrist of a three-year-old rachitic child showing the delay in the appearance of the carpal ossification center and the widening of the epiphysis with loss of bone density. *(Courtesy of Dr. R. C. Alcheson.)*

cium preparation (calcium carbonate or calcium phosphate).

Prevention of Deformity. When the bones are so soft, the child's movements should be so controlled that little or no pressure is exerted upon the limbs and physiotherapy should be administered in bed. For difficult children it is often advisable to fit rickets splints.

Treatment of the Established Deformity. Splinting is used where the deformity is slight and the disease still active and is most useful for deformities of the lower limb. Osteotomy should never be carried out until the radiograph shows eburnation, clearness, and regularity of outline. If corrective operations are attempted before this period, nonunion is likely to occur.

CELIAC RICKETS (GLUTEN-SENSITIVE ENTEROPATHY)

There is increased sensitivity to the gluten of wheat with marked atrophy of the villi in the small intestine; therefore, the standard doses of vitamin D will not reverse the rachitic changes until the diet is made free of gluten. The absorption of calcium, though greatly diminished, appears to be sufficient to calcify the fragile bones of celiac disease so long as there is little or no growth, but when considerable growth appears, this defective absorption results in the development of rickets.

Bone changes appear only in late and long-established cases, i.e., after the age of seven years, and are similar to those of rickets. The zone of calcified cartilage is narrow, with poor calcification and ossification.

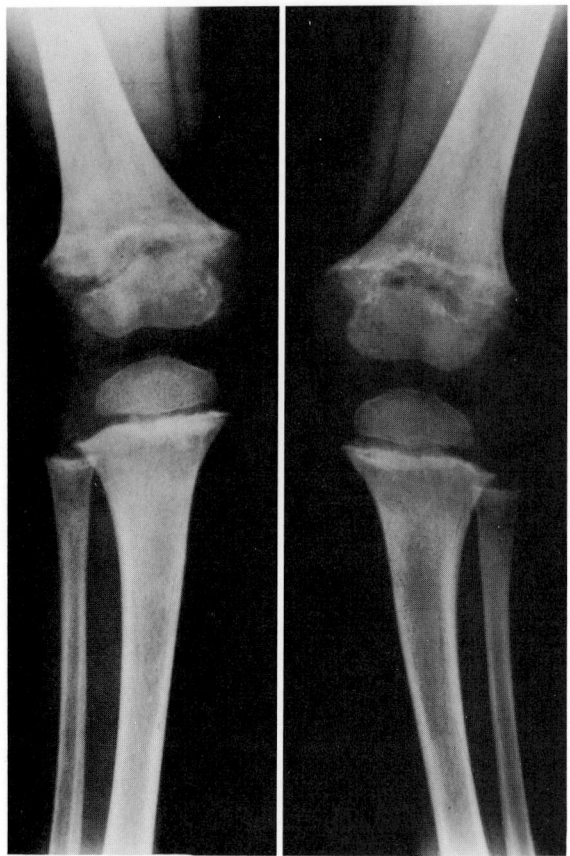

Fig. 43-39. X-ray of both knee areas during the healing phase of rickets showing the increasing ossification of the epiphyses but obvious valgus deformity of the knees and a tibia vara deformity.

There are the characteristic appearances of celiac disease—pallor, cachexia, muscular hypotonicity, and abdominal swelling. In addition there is stunting and skeletal deformity. Genu valgum is a common feature. Enlargement of the distal ends of the radius and ulna are also frequent signs. Enlarged costochondral junctions, Harrison's sulcus, kyphosis, coxa vara, or bowleg may be noted. Fractures may occur with mild trauma. There is invariably a lowered serum calcium content and decreased fat absorption. X-ray of the whole bone is usually fragile and porotic. The epiphyseal cartilage is broad and irregular with transverse striations of denser bone. Treatment is based upon high dosages of vitamin D and special diets.

RENAL OSTEODYSTROPHY

In addition to the mainfestations of the renal lesion, features of disturbance in growth include stunting in growth, often to a degree not equaled by any other form of infantilism. The body weight is correspondingly small, though malnutrition is not present, and the mental development is normal. Genu valgum is common with enlargement of the epiphyses at the wrist and ankles, a costochondral rosary, Harrison's sulcus, or bowleg. The

average age of recognition of deformity is between five and seven years.

Fanconi's Syndrome. Fanconi in 1931 described a case of renal diabetes in which there was retardation of growth. The features of Fanconi's syndrome are resistant and intractable rickets, hypophosphatemia, renal glycosuria, acidosis, and in some cases calcinosis. It is an affection of early life usually beginning within the first two years due to an autosomal recessive gene.

The Lignac-Fanconi Syndrome. The primary lesion appears to be an impaired resorption of glucose and phosphate because of some failure of phosphorylation in the tubules. The children exhibit rickets as well as dwarfism and usually die before puberty. Massive dosages of vitamin D may improve the skeletal disorder. Abnormal deposition of cystine crystals in the cornea, spleen, and lymph nodes gives the syndrome the name *cystinosis*.

Renal, or Hyperchloremic, Acidosis. In this condition, the primary defect is in the distal tubules, which fail to resorb water and to secrete ammonium. The skeletal changes of either osteitis fibrosa or rickets are caused by the excessive mobilization of calcium from bone in response to the acidosis. This condition can be improved by administering excessive alkalizing salts, such as ammonium or calcium chlorides, and vitamin D.

Vitamin D–Resistant Rickets, or "Phosphate Diabetes." This is characterized by a failure of phosphate resorption with a marked hyperphosphaturia and hypophosphatemia. Accompanying this, there is also excessive fecal loss of calcium leading to the typical changes of rickets in children or osteomalacia in adults. Unlike vitamin D deficiency rickets, this form requires massive doses of vitamin D (i.e., 50,000 to 100,000) units.

HYPOPHOSPHATASIA

This is an inherited rachitic disease that was first described by Rathbun in 1948 as a markedly impaired mineralization of the long bones and skull. The blood shows increased calcium, phosphorus, and nonprotein nitrogen levels, but a reduced alkaline phosphatase level. There is a large urinary excretion of phosphoethanoline without the other amino acids commonly seen in renal rickets. The occurrence of bone deformities is itself grave, and the average duration of life after their appearance is said to be less than 2 years.

In hyperchloremic renal acidosis and nephrocalcinosis, an organic acid such as citric acid should be given in conjunction with sodium citrate to aid absorption of calcium from the intestines. Vitamin D should also be given in those cases to help calcification of the skeleton. In the active stage of the osteodystrophy, weight bearing should be prevented, and splints may be applied to limit deformity until spontaneous remission of the disease occurs.

Osteomalacia

Osteomalacia is a metabolic disease of adult bone in which there is a deficient mineralization of the bony matrix due to the lowered concentration of calcium or phosphorus or both in the body fluids. The diagnosis should be suspected in any patient with radiographic changes of osteoporosis or reduced skeletal mass. Reduced serum calcium or phosphorus may result from reduced dietary intake, impaired absorption from the gastrointestinal tract, increased renal excretion, or lack of vitamin D. Accompanying such change there is a generalized increase in the amount of osteoid, i.e., uncalcified, tissue. Osteomalacia may develop as a consequence of pregnancy with increased demands for calcium or in circumstances in which there is a reduction of the amount of available calcium, i.e., starvation or steatorrhea.

All the bones of the skeleton show decrease in bone density and strength. Frequently the bones are grossly deformed. The trabeculae are attenuated or absent, and the interstices of the spongy bone are filled with vascular or fibrofatty connective tissue, or osteoid tissue. Osteoclastic activity is marked and Howship's lacunae enlarged. The skeleton may become deformed, but bones subjected to muscular strains or to the influence of posture or gravity are the most grossly disturbed. The lower limb bones are therefore more affected than the arm bones, and curvatures of the femur and tibia, i.e., coxa vara, are common. Kyphosis is also frequent. Changes in the pelvis result from pressure of the femoral heads medially with displacement of the acetabula. The angle of the pubic symphysis therefore becomes more acute, and the pubis projects as a sharp beak. The sacral promontory rotates forward under the body weight to assume a trefoil shape. The rib deformities are similar to those of rickets. In some cases multiple almost symmetric radiotranslucent bands of diminished density resembling fractures appear in the cortex of the bone. A characteristic x-ray finding is that of Looser's zones or pseudofractures which are commonly seen in the tibia, in the ribs, or in the pelvic rami as translucent lines extending a short distance through the cortex.

Parathyroid Osteodystrophy (Osteitis Fibrosa, or Von Recklinghausen's Disease)

The disease is caused by an increased secretion of parathormone, which stimulates the excretion of phosphate so that the serum phosphate level falls and the serum calcium level rises with mobilization of calcium phosphate from the bones. The excess of calcium is excreted along with the phosphate in the urine, and more calcium phosphate is resorbed from the bones. Parathormone also acts directly on the osteoclastic activity of bone. Many of the clinical features of hyperparathyroidism are discussed in Chap. 38, but certain aspects of the skeletal involvement will be discussed in this section.

The most common initial skeletal feature is increasing bone pain and tenderness felt especially in the lower limbs and back. Usually the pain is associated with general weakness and accompanied by pallor and debility. Hypotonia and muscular weakness are common. There may be a fracture from trivial injury, taking a long time to heal, often in a position of deformity. Occasionally, the development of a "brown tumor," in the maxilla or the mandible, may be the earliest evidence.

The radiologic appearance consists chiefly of irregular diffuse osteoporosis with absorption of the compact bone and cystlike degeneration. In the skull the bones show a well-marked stippling, but the opaque areas are pinhead in size, distinguishing them from the grosser mottling of Paget's disease. The vertebrae are less dense and show central collapse, the upper and lower surfaces being concave, and bulging of the intervertebral discs. The pelvis shows coarse striations among which large, clear cystlike spaces are usually visible. The earliest changes occur in the hand, the skull, and the outer end of the clavicle.

The femur shows loss of trabeculation. Deformity is common—coxa vara, bowing, and cystlike spaces may be present at the extremities and in the middle of the shaft. Over the cysts the bone may show a slight fusiform enlargement in the long as well as the short bones of the hand and foot. Loss of the lamina dura around the teeth and severe demineralization of the distal ends of the clavicles, and tufts of the fingers are characteristic though not irreversible changes.

TREATMENT. Parathyroidectomy is the treatment of the basic disorder. Following this procedure the prognosis is generally good with immediate relief of bone pain and gain in weight and in strength of the bones. Orthopaedic treatment is directed toward adequate protection of the softened bones with reduction in all deforming stresses and strains. After the disease has been arrested and recalcification of bone has taken place, any established deformity can be corrected by osteotomy or other measures.

Osteoporosis

This condition is a disorder of protein metabolism characterized by a structural change in bone whereby the supporting tissue is reduced in amount but remains highly mineralized. The metabolism of calcium is normal, and the trabeculae present are normally calcified.

Osteoporosis is a response of the bony skeleton to a variety of factors such as immobilization, protein deficiency, or endocrine abnormalities. Osteoporosis may accompany Cushing's syndrome, hyperparathyroidism, myxedema, or thyrotoxicosis. The most frequently indicted endocrine abnormality is postmenopausal estrogen deprivation. Pathologic fractures, especially of the femoral neck, commonly arise because of this condition.

Pain is in the nature of a lumbar backache that radiates around the trunk or down the lower limbs. It is aggravated by movement or jarring, and although suggestive of a nerve root compression, this is rarely seen. Acute sudden onset of pain with localized tenderness in the chest or back is most suggestive of a pathologic fracture of a rib or vertebral body.

Loss of height may have been noted by the patient, with the appearance of a thoracic kyphosis and an approximation of the rib margin to the iliac crests.

Radiologic Findings. The involved bone has a "ground glass" appearance (a late manifestation) because of loss of definition of the trabeculae. In the spine, the vertebral bodies become flattened but biconcave with increase in

fracture, extending from the joint surface through the bony epiphysis to the plate and then along the plate to the periphery. Accurate reduction is necessary to minimize articular deformity. The prognosis is good if the blood supply to the fractured portion has not been compromised.

Type IV is also an intraarticular epiphyseal injury. The fracture line extends through the joint surface across the bony epiphyseal plate and through a portion of the metaphysis. The commonest Type IV injury is a fracture of the lateral condyle of the humerus. Anatomic reduction and usually open reduction are required to prevent union across the epiphyseal plate at the fracture site and growth abnormality.

Type V epiphyseal plate injuries are those in which severe crushing damages the epiphyseal plate. Displacement is not common, and the initial severity may go unrecognized. Because of crushing injury to the proliferating cartilage cells, growth disturbances may occur.

With any injury or suspected injury to an epiphyseal plate, the parent of the child should be cautioned that growth abnormalities are possible. Type IV and Type V injuries are more likely to cause growth disturbances. Injuries that interfere with the blood supply to the epiphysis or damage proliferating cells will result in greater deformity in the young child. If neither of these occurs, the younger child has greater remodeling potential where accurate reduction cannot be obtained.

Fractures in Children

A fracture in a child presents different problems from those of a similar fracture in the adult. Nonunion is almost unheard of in children. Fracture healing is more rapid with the younger patient. The challenge in handling children's fractures is in recognizing and understanding what degree of fracture site angulation, displacement, and shortening will be corrected, in relation to remaining growth potential. The presence of healing fracture callus in the neighborhood of an epiphysis causes epiphyseal stimulation. If a displaced femoral shaft fracture is reduced anatomically, overgrowth and leg length inequality will ensue. If rotational deformity at a fracture site involving a long bone is not corrected, permanent deformity results. However, certain degrees of angulation, displacement, and shortening will be corrected and remodeled depending upon the age of the child. Shaft fractures in the long bones must not be opened because of the hazard of infection or epiphyseal growth disturbance and deformity. Certain articular and epiphyseal fractures must be recognized and anatomically reduced.

Closed Reduction versus Open Reduction

The optimal method for handling a specific fracture should (1) permit rapid union, (2) reestablish length and alignment of the injured extremity, (3) restore complete painless range of motion of adjacent joints, and (4) return the patient to gainful functional activity, with as little morbidity and hazard to the patient as possible.

The closed treatment of fractures has the advantages of little or no risk of infection or subsequent interference with local blood supply to the fracture site. Closed treatment requires prolonged traction or immobilization that may cause restriction of joint motion, and accurate anatomic restoration of length and alignment may not be possible.

In order to obviate the difficulties of prolonged immobilization and overcome the problems of inaccurate reduction, open reduction and internal fixation have been proposed. Open reduction carries the risks of local infection and delayed union resulting from compromise of local blood supply to fracture fragments. Despite the disadvantages of each technique, closed treatment is frequently indicated for some situations, while open reduction is mandatory for others.

Application of Plaster Casts

External immobilization for fractures and dislocations is obtained by the application of plaster or fiberglass casts. Plaster consists of anhydrous calcium sulfate, which solidifies with hydration. Plaster, to which water is added, sets up in minutes but does not completely dry for 36 to 48 h. Postinjury patients in plaster casts should have the extremity elevated.

COMPLICATIONS OF PLASTER CAST TREATMENT. The most serious complication associated with plaster casts is the development of vascular insufficiency due to unrelieved swelling. The cast will not shrink, but it may restrict soft tissue swelling to the point of gangrenous necrosis. Unrelieved pain, pulselessness, pallor, and sensory or motor paralysis are signs of this complication. Unrelenting pain should be investigated immediately and not allowed to progress to the point where other signs are present. Narcotics are administered with great caution to patients in plaster. Unrelieved pain beneath the cast should be treated by splitting the cast with parallel cuts on the opposite sides of the extremity, to allow anteroposterior swelling. The cast is split down to include the underlying padding, since blood-soaked padding may be as resistant as plaster and not allow sufficient expansion. Leg casts are split medially and laterally in their entirety, and forearm casts split along the radial and ulnar borders of the arm.

Patients who complain of burning pain at a localized site in the cast should be suspected of a pressure point from the plaster. This commonly occurs over the site of a bony prominence. This is investigated by cutting an appropriate window and inspecting the underlying skin. Skin necrosis may result and be associated with pain relief due to damage of sensory receptors. When a point of pressure is detected, the cast window should be hollowed out and sufficient padding applied to relieve the pressure. Windows in the cast should always be replaced, or local swelling will occur through the window and cause pressure on the skin at the window margins.

TYPES OF CAST. Casts for fractures should immobilize the joint above and the joint below the fracture. Plasters that include the ankle are extended to the bases

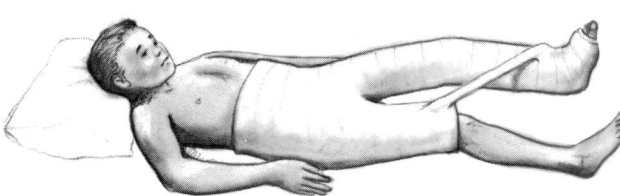

Fig. 43-47. A 1½ hip spica.

of the toes to prevent swelling, edema, and irritation of the forefoot. A long leg cast extends from the bases of the toes to include the knee and thigh as high as possible. A boot cast extends to the level of the tibial tubercle. A cylinder cast is a circular cast that extends from just above the ankle to include leg, knee, and thigh. It is used for immobilization of the knee.

A hip spica is a plaster designed to immobilize the hip. A single hip spica extends from the nipple line or upper abdomen to include the pelvis and one thigh and lower leg. A double hip spica immobilizes the pelvis and extends to include both thighs and lower legs. A 1½ hip spica extends only as far as the knee on one side (Fig. 43-47).

A short arm cast extends from below the elbow to the proximal palmar crease, leaving the entire thumb free. A gauntlet cast is similar but includes the thumb. A long arm cast extends from the proximal palmar crease, leaving the thumb free to include the elbow and arm as far as the axilla. A shoulder spica is a body jacket with the plaster immobilizing the shoulder and elbow.

Body casts are applied for immobilization of the spine and extend to the groin and as high as the sternum, anteriorly. They may be applied with plaster straps across the shoulders. A scoliosis cast, or localizer cast for scoliosis correction, extends to the groin anteriorly, to the sacrum posteriorly, and as far proximally as to provide a distracting force on the chin and occiput. Distally, the distracting force is applied by well-molded pressure areas across the crest of the ilia.

External Fixation

Fracture immobilization can be obtained by inserting pins above and below the fracture site and fixing these to a rigid outrigger (Fig. 43-48). The pins are inserted percutaneously usually through both long bone cortices. This type of fixation is helpful with open fractures where there has been extensive soft tissue loss. It allows inspection of the wound along with good control of the fracture. Pin site infection is a common complication. Less common are injuries to peripheral nerves from pin injury. Infections at pin sites and delayed or nonunion can be minimized by pin removal as soon as there is fracture stability (4 to 6 weeks).

Traction

Traction is used in orthopaedics:

1. To overcome muscle spasm and apply reducing force in fractures of the long bones

2. To provide immobilization of long bone fractures
3. To provide immobilization and distracting force for painful and diseased joints
4. To correct joint deformities or contractures

Skin traction is applied by tapes attached to the skin and skeletal traction by pins or screws affixed to bone. The maximal weight tolerated by adhesive tapes to the skin is about 10 lb. In children, skin traction is usually sufficient to overcome muscle pull in the reduction and treatment of fractures. The most common form of skin traction is Buck's traction, in which tapes with attached weights are applied to the leg and thigh (Fig. 43-49). This is commonly used prior to surgical treatment in the immobilization of intertrochanteric hip fractures. Skin traction is used with Russell's traction (Fig. 43-50), which is designed to apply traction to the femoral shaft with the knee flexed. A femoral shaft fracture in a small child may be treated with Bryant's traction. In this technique, skin traction is attached to both legs, which are suspended from the bed.

Skeletal traction is usually applied to a Steinmann pin or Kirschner wire driven percutaneously across the distal

Fig. 43-48. The Oxford external fixator. Percutaneous pins attached to the external fixation device can be used to stabilize an open fracture tibia with soft tissue loss.

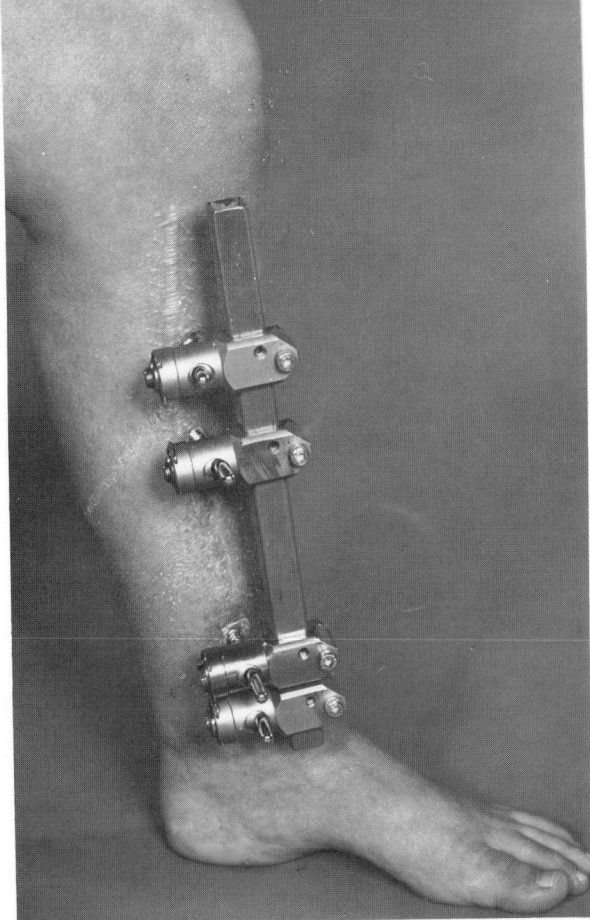

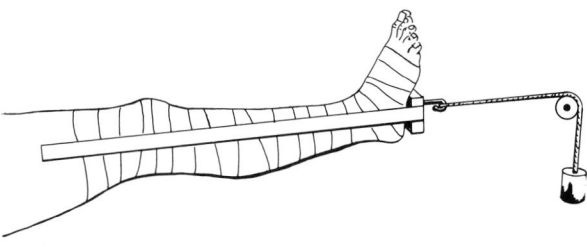

Fig. 43-49. Buck's traction.

femoral shaft or proximal tibia. A traction bow is affixed to the metal wire and weight applied. Kirschner wires drilled across the olecranon may be used for supracondylar or humeral shaft fractures. Crutchfield tongs affixed to the outer table of the skull and the halo device, which has a similar purchase on the skull, are other forms of skeletal traction.

Electrical Stimulation of Ununited Fractures

Basic investigations combined with some clinical research studies but no controlled trials under the leadership of Bassett and by Brighton have shown that electricity can stimulate nonunions to heal. Mechanically stressed bones will generate electronegative potentials in areas of compression and electropositive potentials in areas of tension. The underlying mechanism by which electrical stimulation facilitates union is still unknown. The technique can be used for treating nonunions.

Three months of electrical stimulation is required. Patients are followed subsequently with further cast immobilization depending upon the radiographic signs of healing. The overall success rate is in the region of 75 percent proved in large numbers of fractures, many of which have been ununited for years. A bone scan is done in order to detect the presence of a synovial pseudoarthrosis, which will preclude healing. Only fracture nonunions with a longitudinal gap less than half the diameter of the bone are selected for this treatment.

Fig. 43-50. Russell's traction.

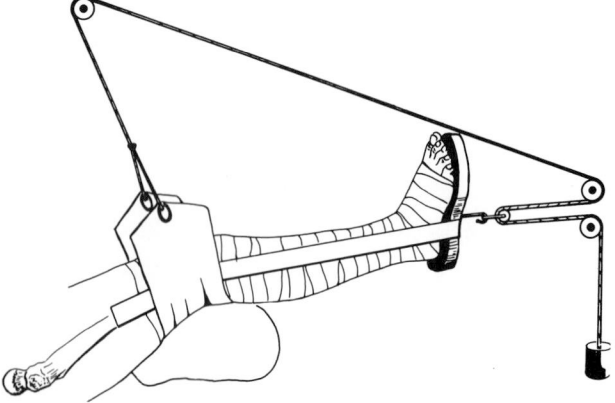

FRACTURES AND JOINT INJURIES IN THE UPPER EXTREMITY

SHOULDER MOTION. The act of moving the hand from the anatomic position to a position of full abduction requires normal function in the glenohumeral joint, the acromioclavicular joint, the sternoclavicular joint, and the scapulothoracic joint. Interference with any of these joints will limit full shoulder motion. The rotation of the scapula involves motion of the sternoclavicular and the acromioclavicular joints. As the arm is elevated, elevation of the clavicle occurs at the sternoclavicular joint. It is almost complete during the first 90° of arm elevation. For every 10° of elevation of the arm, there are 4° of elevation of the clavicle. Motion at the acromioclavicular joint is approximately 20° and occurs during the first 30° of abduction and after 135° of elevation. On the long axis of the acromioclavicular joint during the position of 60 to 180° of elevation of the arm, 40° of clavicular rotation occurs. It is apparent, from this anatomic description, that fusion or disruption of any one joint will interfere with the elevation of the arm.

Sternoclavicular Joint Injuries

Injuries to the sternoclavicular joint occur from direct lateral force to the shoulder applied in an axial direction to the clavicle. Dislocations are commonly anterior, but in some cases, when posterior and lateral forces are applied, retrosternal dislocation of the sternoclavicular joint occurs.

Reduction is necessary in retrosternal dislocations, because of compression of neurovascular structures. When closed manipulation and lateral traction are not sufficient, open reduction is indicated. With interior dislocation, reduction is not critical. For best results, closed reduction and maintenance of position are required. Old, unreduced dislocations, if symptomatic, require excision of the proximal end of the clavicle.

Fractures of the Clavicle

Fractures of the clavicle occur at any age from direct downward force to the shoulder or from forces applied indirectly as in falling on the extended arm. Fractures may occur at any level but are most common at the junction of the middle and distal thirds (Fig. 43-51). In older age groups, fractures of the distal tip of the clavicle are more common.

CLINICAL MANIFESTATIONS. The patient presents supporting the affected extremity by the opposite hand, with the head tilted to the affected side, and chin rotated away. There is local swelling and direct tenderness at the site of the fracture. Any motion of the extremity causes pain. The diagnosis is confirmed by x-ray.

TREATMENT. The clavicle is difficult to immobilize, because of its anatomic location and muscle attachments. In spite of this, nonunion is rare (about $\frac{1}{2}$ percent) with conservative treatment. The weight of the shoulder causes the distal fragment to be inferiorly angulated or

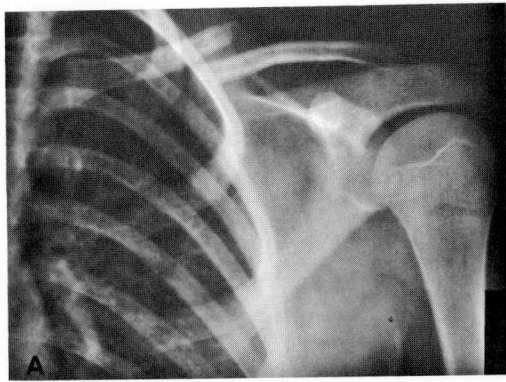
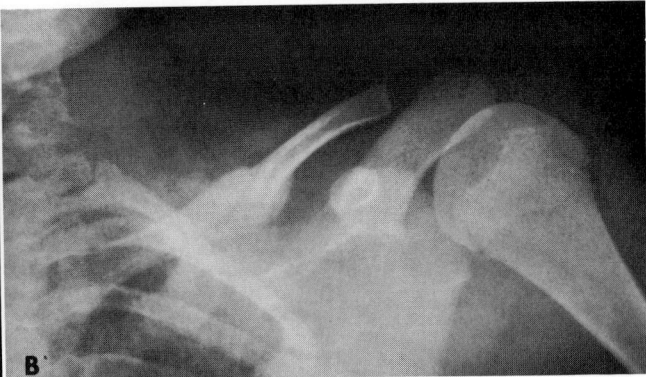

Fig. 43-51. *A.* Fracture of the middle third of the clavicle with complete displacement and overriding. *B.* Healing of a clavicle fracture in 6 weeks with internal callus formation.

depressed, while the proximal fragment is superiorly angulated by the pull of the sternocleidomastoid and upper fibers of the trapezius.

Children. Both shoulders are drawn back and elevated by a figure-of-eight apparatus, which may be constructed of felt padding covered with stockinet (Fig. 43-52). Warning is given about swelling in the hands from venostasis. This is relieved by having the patient lie supine while elevating the arms overhead. Fracture reduction in children is not important. Bayonet overriding is accepted and will remodel with age. The figure-of-eight is left in place for 2 weeks in infants and until the fracture is clinically solid in older children, 4 to 6 weeks if necessary.

Adults. When growth of the clavicle has been completed, accurate reduction and maintenance of position is required to prevent cosmetic deformity. It is difficult to maintain a displaced fractured clavicle in the reduced position with any ambulatory apparatus. In men and older women, a figure-of-eight apparatus for 6 weeks would provide sufficient immobilization for union but may leave a cosmetic deformity. In women who desire a cosmetic result, supine bed rest with a small sandbag placed in the interscapular area and lateral traction on the abducted arm are required for 4 to 6 weeks. Open surgical reduction with intramedullary fixation will minimize angular deformity at the fracture site but leaves a scar and may result in nonunion.

Acromioclavicular Injuries

The acromioclavicular joint is injured by forces applied downward from the point of the shoulder. Such injuries occur frequently in football or ice hockey and in all contact sports. Acromioclavicular joint injuries may occur in the elderly, but fractures of the distal third of the clavicle are more common in this age group, with the same type of trauma. The integrity of the acromioclavicular joint is primarily dependent upon the coracoclavicular ligaments, the conoid and trapezoid, which run upward, backward, and laterally from the base of the coracoid process to the inferior surface of the clavicle. Superior and inferior acro-

mioclavicular ligaments contribute little to the stability of the joint.

CLINICAL MANIFESTATIONS. Signs of acromioclavicular joint injury include local swelling and tenderness over the acromioclavicular joint and palpable deformity. The patient cocks the head to the affected side to relax the sternocleidomastoid and supports the arm with the opposite hand to relieve the weight of the shoulder distracting the joint.

When the patient is examined lying supine, a subluxation may reduce spontaneously, making diagnosis difficult. In the upright position or in the obese patient, or with sufficient local swelling, the diagnosis may not be readily apparent. The diagnosis is made by obtaining comparable AP x-rays of both acromioclavicular joints with the patient standing. With a subluxation, it may be necessary to have the patient suspend a 10-lb weight in the affected hand to distract a partially disrupted acromioclavicular articulation.

TREATMENT. The treatment of minor sprains or subluxations is symptomatic. It is accomplished by a sling on the affected side, supporting the weight of the arm. Complete dislocation of the acromioclavicular joint will not be corrected with less than open reduction. In treating complete dislocations of the acromioclavicular joint, consideration

Fig. 43-52. Figure-of-eight for treatment of a fractured clavicle. The axillae are padded with gauze pads over which a figure-of-eight of felt and stockinet is applied.

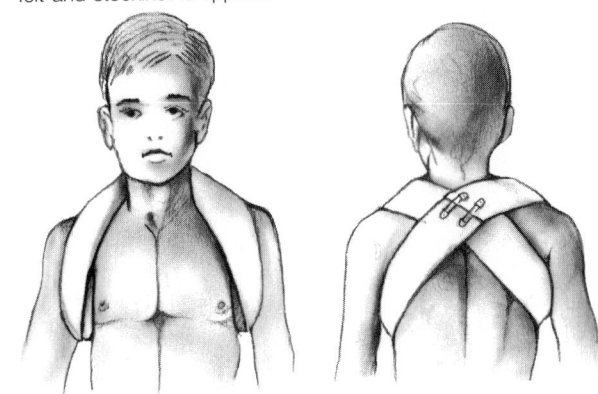

should be given to the patient's age and occupation. There is no significant improvement in results whether conservative treatment (sling) or open surgical reduction is used. Surgical treatment may be indicated in severe displacements or as delayed treatment when symptoms persist. Open reduction is also indicated for young women who will accept the surgical scar in the place of a permanent high-riding clavicle. For older patients symptomatic treatment for the initial dislocation is all that is necessary. In any patient with persistent symptoms from a subluxed or painful acromioclavicular joint, excision of the distal end of the clavicle generally provides good results.

Fractures of the Scapula

Fractures of the body of the scapular and glenoid are invariably the result of severe trauma, to either pedestrians or automobile occupants. Such injuries are usually associated with injuries to the brachial plexus, fractured ribs, and cardiopulmonary trauma. Treatment of such patients is aimed primarily at the associated injuries. Symptomatic immobilization of the shoulder is usually preferable to open reduction.

Dislocations of the Shoulder

ACUTE ANTERIOR DISLOCATIONS

The humeral head may be dislocated from the glenoid in any direction. For superior dislocation to occur, fracture of the overlying acromion must be present. Anterior dislocations include subglenoid and subcoracoid dislocations. The humeral head is dislocated anteriorly when an extension force is applied to the abducted arm. The initial injury is typically one involving a fall with the arm in the abducted position or direct trauma to the abducted arm as may occur with football injuries. Less force is required to dislocate the shoulder when there is a congenital defect in the labrum or with paralysis of shoulder musculature. The humeral head is driven anteriorly, tearing the anterior shoulder joint capsule and detaching the labrum from the glenoid, producing a compression fracture in the posterior lateral aspect of the humeral head, as it is wedged between the anterior-lying subscapularis tendon and the anterior rim of the glenoid.

CLINICAL MANIFESTATIONS. The patient holds the arm in slight abduction and is unable to bring the elbow to the side. There is flattening of the normal deltoid prominence with a depression laterally beneath the acromion. The humeral head creates a prominence anteriorly, although in the obese person these findings may be difficult to define. Any attempt at arm motion causes severe pain. In a small percentage of cases, injury to the axillary nerve is incurred, as it is stretched around the neck of the humerus. This diagnosis may be made before reduction by localizing an area of sensory loss overlying the deltoid muscles and supplied by the superficial branch of the axillary nerve. Postreduction, weakness or loss of power in the deltoid may be demonstrable.

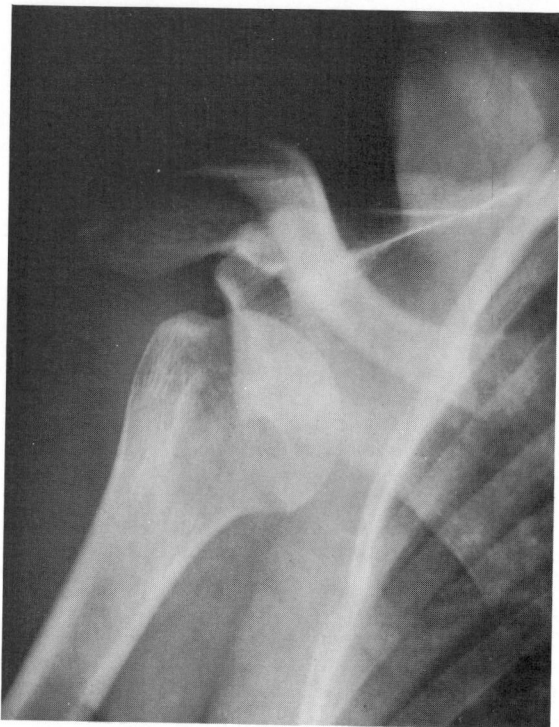

Fig. 43-53. Anterior subcoracoid dislocation of the shoulder. The articular surface of the humeral head can be seen medial to the glenoid fossa and inferior to the coracoid process.

Anteroposterior x-rays of the shoulder will reveal the head displaced medially into the subcoracoid or subglenoid position (Fig. 43-53).

TREATMENT. The dislocation should be reduced immediately. Closed reduction can be accomplished within the first 2 to 3 weeks, but open reduction may be required when dislocations are neglected for longer periods.

Over 90 percent of acute anterior dislocations may be reduced by a modification of the Milch maneuver (Fig. 43-54). Under mild analgesia, the patient is placed supine on a stretcher with the elbow extended and the arm in the position of 90° forward flexion, hanging off the side of the stretcher. A pail of water is attached to the arm with an Ace bandage. Water can gradually be added to the bucket and traction increased. A few minutes of this traction is sufficient for the shoulder to reduce gradually, but in more muscular individuals 30 min may be required. In some instances, it is necessary to rotate the humeral head internally while maintaining traction. In the few instances where this treatment is insufficient, general anesthesia and a Hippocratic maneuver is accomplished by applying manual traction with countertraction applied by the stockinged foot of the operator to the axilla. Postoperative management is as important as the closed reduction. The arm is bound to the side with the elbow flexed at 90° across the abdomen. A sling and swath are applied and are not disturbed for 3 to 4 weeks in young individuals. In patients over fifty, 2 weeks is sufficient.

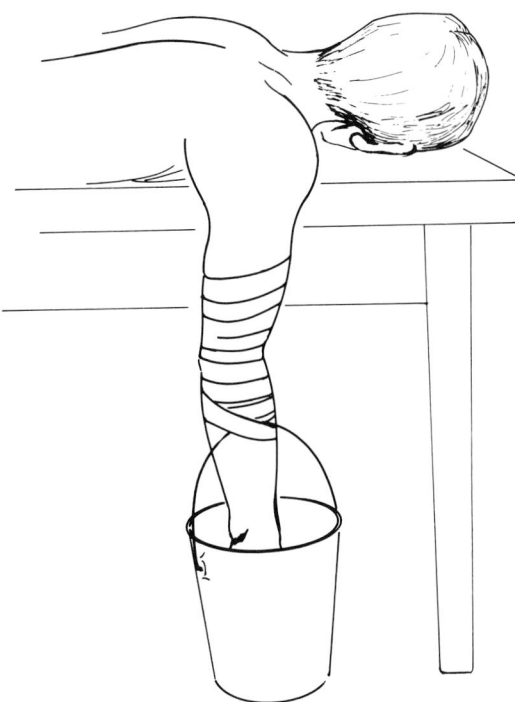

Fig. 43-54. Reduction technique for anterior dislocation of the shoulder. With the patient in the prone position and the arm in the position of forward flexion, water is added to the bucket, and traction is gradually increased.

bile accidents in which the arm is axially loaded in the position of forward flexion. Any patient complaining of shoulder pain following a convulsion should be considered to have a dislocated shoulder until proved otherwise. Clinical findings on examination reveal prominence of the humeral head posteriorly, loss of the anterior shoulder contour, limitation of full abduction, and complete loss of external rotation.

Routine AP x-rays may reveal the diagnosis, but an axillary x-ray will confirm the location of the humeral head posterior to the glenoid fossa. On the AP x-ray, the humeral head will appear smaller than the opposite side, since it is closer to the x-ray film (Fig. 43-55). In the normal shoulder, there is an overlap of the shadow of the humeral head on the posterior lip of the glenoid, which gives a *sharp* half-moon shadow. When the head is dislocated posteriorly, this half-moon shadow will be blurred or absent. Proof of posterior dislocation is by an axillary x-ray. Frequently, the lesser tuberosity is fractured at the time of the dislocation. The presence of this finding should suggest a posterior dislocation or a reduced posterior dislocation.

TREATMENT. Reduction is accomplished by the modified Milch maneuver under analgesia or general anesthesia or by direct traction. Following reduction, the shoulder is immobilized in 30° of abduction, in external rotation, with a modified shoulder spica. This permits adequate healing of the posterior capsule in the shortened position.

RECURRENT ANTERIOR DISLOCATIONS

With adequate initial treatment and postreduction immobilization, the majority of patients will not redislocate unless subjected to significant trauma. However, redislocations occur when the initial dislocation is not immobilized in sufficient time and may do so with minor trauma. Some patients abducting the arm in getting dressed or reaching out to open a door may incur a recurrent dislocation. There is a group of patients who have recurrent anterior subluxations and have as much difficulty as those with dislocations. The subluxed humeral head impinges on the glenoid but patients can invariably reduce the subluxation by themselves. A number of surgical repairs are used in the treatment of recurrent dislocations. Before instituting any of these, it is mandatory to document the direction of the dislocation. All repairs are directed at repairing and/or shortening the structure of the anterior shoulder and capsule with subscapularis.

CHRONIC DISLOCATIONS. In patients with chronic complete anterior dislocation, arthrodesis of the shoulder at 45° of abduction, 15° of internal rotation, and 20° of forward flexion will eliminate pain and restore shoulder function.

POSTERIOR DISLOCATIONS

The shoulder dislocates posteriorly during epileptiform convulsions, during electroshock therapy, and in automo-

Fig. 43-55. Posterior dislocation of the shoulder. AP x-ray shows an indistinct border of the humeral head, superimposed upon the glenoid rim. There is also compression fracture in the region of the lesser tubercle.

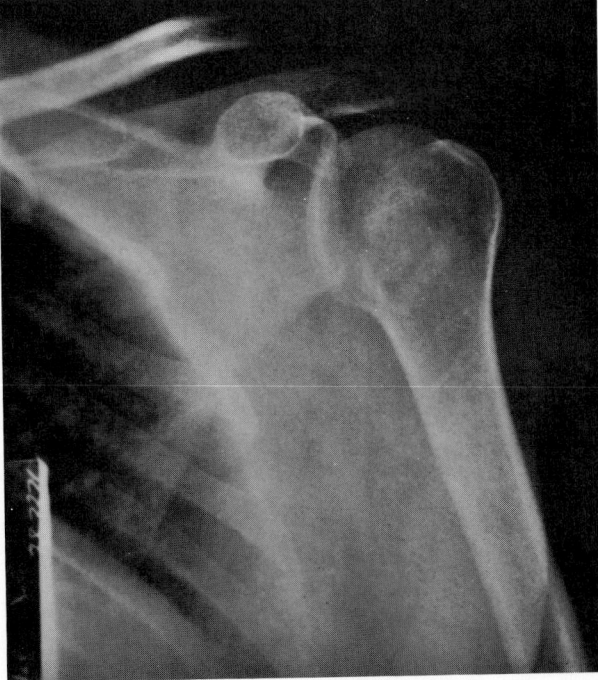

A few posterior dislocations are recurrent. Treatment of posterior recurrent dislocations is accomplished by a bone block applied to the posterior glenoid or reefing of the infraspinatus tendon.

FRACTURE-DISLOCATIONS OF THE SHOULDER

A fracture of the neck of the humerus may occur in combination with an anterior dislocation. The initial treatment is the same but generally requires closed reduction and manipulation under general anesthesia. Traction is applied in the long axis of the shaft of the humerus in the position in which it lies. Direct counterpressure is applied in a posterior direction over the head of the humerus. If the dislocation can be reduced, subsequent treatment is the same as for fractures of the humeral neck. In the young, when it is not possible to reduce such fracture-dislocations, open reduction and internal fixation of the fracture or prosthetic replacement is indicated.

Fractures of the Proximal Humerus

The most common fracture of the proximal humerus is a fracture of the surgical neck. It is prevalent in older individuals but may occur at any age. In children, a similar injury results in a fracture of the anatomic neck, with epiphyseal displacement, usually of Type II of the Salter and Harris classification. The treatment of such an injury in a child is by closed reduction with manual traction, followed by hanging cast immobilization. Moderate degrees of displacement may be accepted if there is sufficient growth potential remaining in the epiphysis (Fig. 43-56). It may be necessary to place the arm at full abduction in a shoulder spica, to hold position.

Fractures of the surgical neck of the humerus have a varus deformity at the fracture site. A sling and swath are sufficient to hold reduction of most fractures of the surgical neck. When manual reduction and sling and swath are unsuccessful in maintaining reduction, skin traction applied to the adducted arm will maintain position. In some patients, open reduction and internal fixation may be necessary.

Fractures of the greater tuberosity should be reduced anatomically to maintain normal function. If this cannot be obtained by closed means, open reduction and screw fixation of the fragment are necessary. In all fractures of the proximal humerus in elderly patients, it is necessary to begin shoulder motion as early as 7 to 10 days.

Fractures of the Humeral Shaft

Fractures of the humeral shaft (Fig. 43-57) occur from direct blows to the humerus, which cause transverse or comminuted fractures, or by indirect force, i.e., torsional stress, as in falling on the elbow. On physical examination, there is swelling, ecchymosis, and deformity, with inability to elevate the arm because of painful instability. It is necessary to determine the presence or absence of associated neurovascular injuries, which are common, especially with serious traumatic forces. The radial nerve is the most commonly injured nerve, but any of or all the major nerves may be stretched or interrupted with either closed or open fractures. Radial nerve injury is commonly encountered with an oblique fracture at the junction of the middle and distal thirds of the humerus.

TREATMENT. Various methods of treatment have been devised for this injury, but the most successful has been to reduce the fracture with gentle longitudinal traction, injecting 2% Xylocaine at the fracture site as necessary. With the patient in a sitting position, a coaptation plaster splint is applied to the medial surface of the arm, as high in the axilla as possible, encompassing the elbow and continuing over the lateral surface of the arm with a small extension of the plaster over the superior surface of the shoulder. While the plaster is hardening, it is circumferentially wrapped to the arm with a soft bandage roll. The elbow is flexed 90° across the abdomen, and the entire arm is bound to the side with a Velpeau, or sling and

Fig. 43-56. Fracture of the proximal humerus in a twelve-year-old girl. The fracture is an epiphyseal separation with a large metaphyseal fragment attached to the epiphysis. *A.* Initial fracture position. *B.* Slight improvement after closed reduction. *C.* Healed fracture with remodeling changes at 1 year postinjury. The patient has a normal range of shoulder motion.

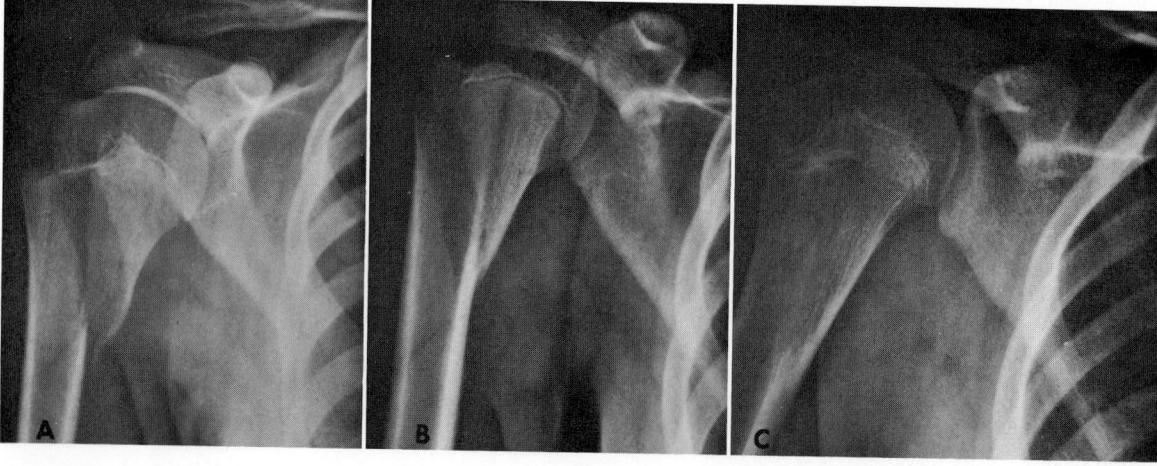

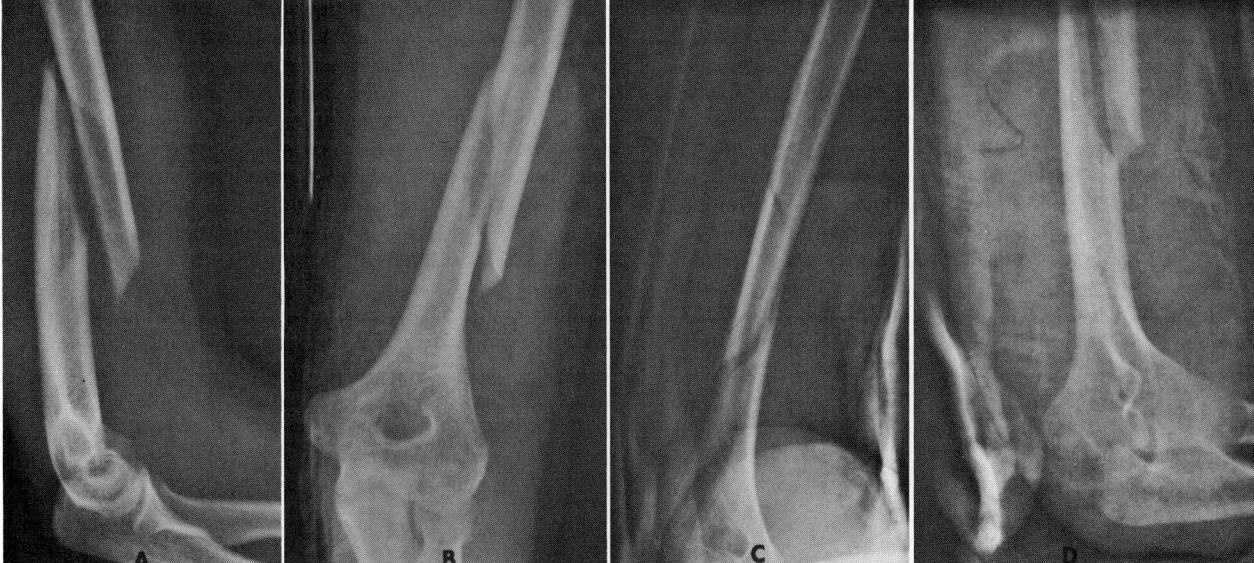

Fig. 43-57. Spiral fracture at the junction of the middle and distal thirds of the humeral shaft. *A.* Lateral x-ray showing displacement with angulation. *B.* AP x-ray. *C* and *D.* AP and lateral x-rays showing postreduction positions after closed reduction and the application of coaptation splints. The patient had a complete radial nerve palsy (axonotmesis) from which there was complete recovery in 8 months.

swath, dressing. The weight of the arm in this situation acts like a hanging cast to apply gentle traction for the fracture.

Spontaneous recovery ensues in over 95 percent of the patients with associated traction injuries to the radial nerve. The presence of such a lesion is not an indication for open reduction or primary exploration of the nerve.

When primary repair of a brachial artery is required, internal fixation of the humeral shaft is necessary. This is accomplished by plate and screw fixation but may also be effected by an intramedullary rod. Primary open reduction of the closed humeral shaft fracture is indicated when it is not possible to get bony apposition because of marked displacement or interposition of soft tissue. In all humeral shaft fractures, it is necessary to get biplanar check x-rays at intervals during the first 3 weeks and make traction or plaster adjustments as necessary.

Fractures and Dislocations about the Elbow

The motions at the elbow joint are flexion and extension from the hinge joint between the distal end of the humerus and the proximal radius and ulna, and pronation and supination of the forearm, which requires motion of the proximal radioulnar joint and radiohumeral joint. Significant injury to any area of these articulations may interfere with both forearm and elbow motion. This complex articulation is less able to withstand minor degrees of anatomic distortion. Injuries involving the elbow have a propensity for stiffness if immobilized too long and for production of new periosteal bone or myositis ossificans

if irritated during the immediate postinjury period. Because rather minor injuries can produce subtle fractures, it is imperative not only to have standard AP and lateral x-ray views of the elbow joint but also oblique x-rays; in difficult diagnostic situations comparable views of the opposite normal side should be obtained. With children, in the presence of incompletely or unossified bony epiphyses, interpretation of x-rays following trauma is difficult. Therefore comparably positioned x-rays of the normal side are indicated.

FRACTURES OF THE RADIAL HEAD AND NECK

Fractures of the head of the radius usually occur from falls on the outstretched hand. This force drives the head of the radius against the capitellum, causing various degrees of cartilage contusion on the capitellum or head of the radius or fractures of the radial head.

CLINICAL MANIFESTATIONS. Patients with isolated fractures of the radial head may notice immediate stiffness of the elbow. As the hematoma and effusion increase, further limitation is noted, and pain becomes constant and severe. There is localized tenderness over the radial head, with painful limitation of motion.

TREATMENT. Successful treatment of radial head fractures is dependent upon the establishment of early joint motion. The initial treatment consists of aspiration of the joint hematoma and instillation of 2 to 3 mL of 2% Xylocaine. Following this, the patient should have improved motion and comfort. The patient is treated with a sling, and active motion within the range of pain tolerance is encouraged. After 3 weeks, the sling is discarded, but the patient is instructed to refrain from lifting heavy objects for 6 weeks. For some comminuted fractures excision of the radial head is indicated, because of mechanical block. Immediate range of motion is started following excision of all fragments of the radial head.

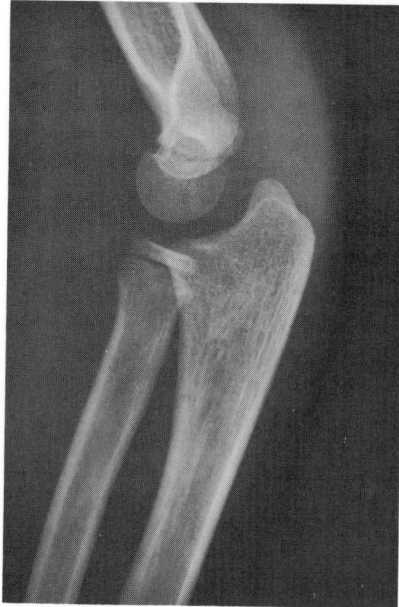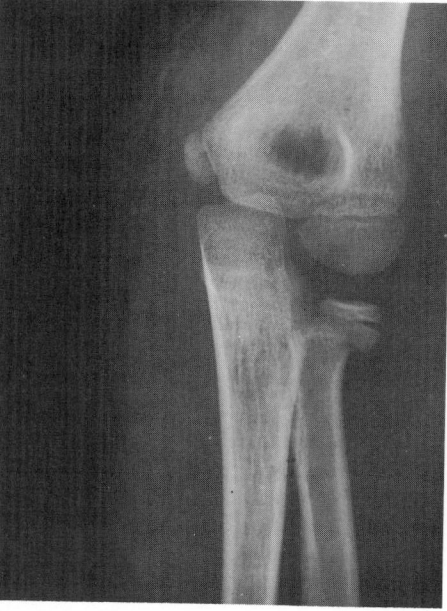

Fig. 43-58. AP and lateral x-rays of a fracture of the radial neck in a child.

FRACTURES OF THE RADIAL NECK IN CHILDREN

The mechanism of injury causing a fracture of the radial head in adults produces a fracture of the radial neck (Fig. 43-58) in young children. This fracture is reduced by manipulation. The elbow is angulated into varus, while direct digital pressure is applied to the valgus-angulated radial head.

If less than 45° of angulation is present, the end result will be excellent; if residual angulation is more than 45°, open reduction during the first week is indicated. After 3 weeks open reduction is not justified. The radial head should never be excised in a child, because of the resultant deformity that will develop from loss of the proximal radial epiphysis.

FRACTURES OF THE PROXIMAL ULNA

Isolated fractures of the olecranon occur most commonly in adults and are very infrequent in children. They are caused by forced flexion of the elbow against the actively contracting triceps, as when a patient falls on an outstretched hand. The olecranon is avulsed by the triceps.

In children, the fractures are, as a rule, undisplaced and can be treated with immobilization in extension. When the fracture is displaced in adults, operation is invariably indicated if local skin condition is satisfactory. For noncomminuted fractures, open reduction and internal fixation of the fracture with a tension band wire is the treatment of choice. For very comminuted fractures, it may be necessary to excise the olecranon fragments and resuture the triceps aponeurosis to restore active extension.

SUPRACONDYLAR FRACTURES OF THE HUMERUS

The supracondylar fracture (Fig. 43-59) accounts for the majority of fractures sustained about the elbow in children; in adults this fracture occurs less commonly. It is usually caused by a fall upon the extended elbow; a small percentage of these fractures occur with the elbow flexed and should be recognized, so that the treatment and immobilization can be applied in extension.

A supracondylar fracture is the most hazardous fracture treated by the orthopaedist, because of the complication of a compartment syndrome or of Volkmann's ischemic contracture. As the humeral condyles are driven back into extension, the brachial artery may be stretched, contused, or lacerated over the distal end of the proximal fragment during the initial injury. An injury to the brachial artery may cause collateral vasospasm, producing swelling with ischemia to the flexor forearm muscles and resulting Volkmann's contractures.

CLINICAL MANIFESTATIONS. Children with displaced supracondylar fractures present with marked swelling about the elbow, deformity, and ecchymosis when initially seen. Undisplaced fractures may have considerable swelling and symptoms of pain, but without deformity. Before instituting treatment, it is necessary to determine the presence of circulation to the hand and the presence or absence of a radial pulse. A small percentage have injuries to the radial or median nerves in the presence of normal circulation. If the radial pulse is absent, it is imperative to reduce the fracture immediately.

TREATMENT. Manipulation reduction can be accomplished after local anesthetic infiltration of the fracture site with 2% Xylocaine or using general anesthesia. With countertraction applied to the axilla, one hand of the operator grasps the biceps, placing the thumb over the distal fragment. Traction is applied to the forearm with the opposite hand, and when the fracture fragments have been disengaged by slight hyperextension, the elbow is brought into the position of maximal flexion. While holding the

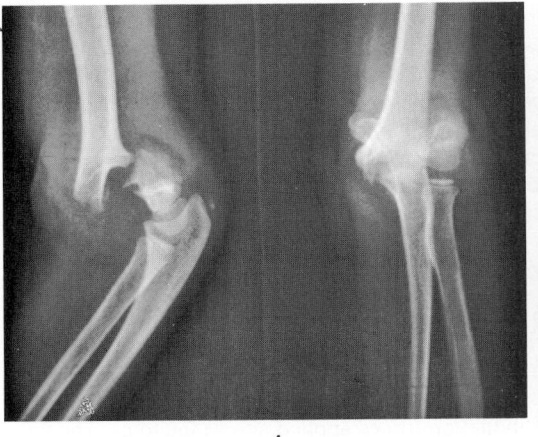
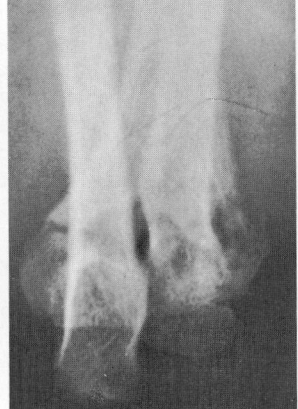
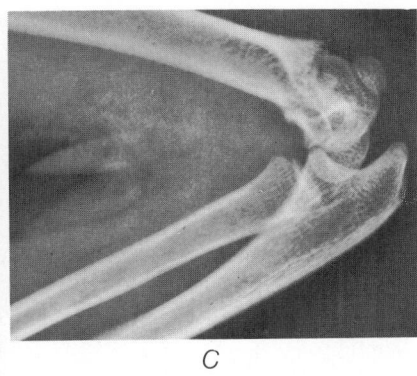

A   *B*
                                          C

Fig. 43-59. Displaced supracondylar fractures of the humerus in a child. *A*. AP and lateral x-rays on initial examination. *B* and *C*. AP and lateral x-rays obtained following closed manipulation after the local instillation of 1% Xylocaine.

elbow in maximal flexion, x-rays are obtained to determine the accuracy of reduction. If reduction is satisfactory and the radial pulse is present or has returned, the arm is immobilized at 90° with the forearm in neutral or slight pronation, in a collar and cuff, with plaster splints. All patients with supracondylar fractures should be hospitalized so that possible changes in circulation and signs of compartment syndromes can be monitored.

If the radial pulse disappears with maximal flexion, the elbow is brought toward a right angle into a position in which the pulse is present but with as much flexion as possible. If the pulse does not return and there is good capillary circulation to the hand, the patient has no pain and can fully extend the fingers without discomfort, it is sufficient to temporize and evaluate these findings every 1 or 2 h. If at any time circulation to the hand is in doubt or in the presence of pain or inability to extend the fingers painlessly, exploration of the brachial artery where it crosses the fracture site is indicated, along with release of the forearm fascial compartments.

If fracture reduction and its maintenance are not possible, the patient should be placed in a traction device (Fig. 43-60). A Kirschner wire is driven across the crest of the ulna, 1 in. distal to the tip of the olecranon process, and a traction bow is attached. With the patient lying supine in bed and the arm in forward flexion of 90°, enough weight is suspended overhead to reduce the fracture with the elbow at 90° of flexion and the forearm suspended in an overhead sling. The accuracy of reduction is determined by aligning the bony prominences with the distal humerus and comparing it with the opposite side. X-ray check is made to determine the degree of apposition and rotation of fracture sites, but alignment is best determined by the visual method. Traction is removed at 14 days, and the arm is placed in a long arm cast. Reversal of the carrying angle, or so-called gunstock deformity, results when medial angulation of the distal fragment is not corrected. It also may be due to stimulation of the lateral condylar epiphyses from the fracture itself, since late deformities have been noted following undisplaced fractures.

FRACTURES OF THE LATERAL EPICONDYLE IN CHILDREN

These injuries occur from hyperextension of the elbow with a valgus force. The child complains of pain with minimal swelling. If adequate x-rays are not taken and compared with the opposite side, this fracture may be overlooked. The fracture is either undisplaced or pulled from its normal location (Fig. 43-61) and rotated into the joint by the extensor muscles of the forearm attached to the fragment.

Fig. 43-60. Position of skeletal traction (Smith) for supracondylar fracture of the humerus.

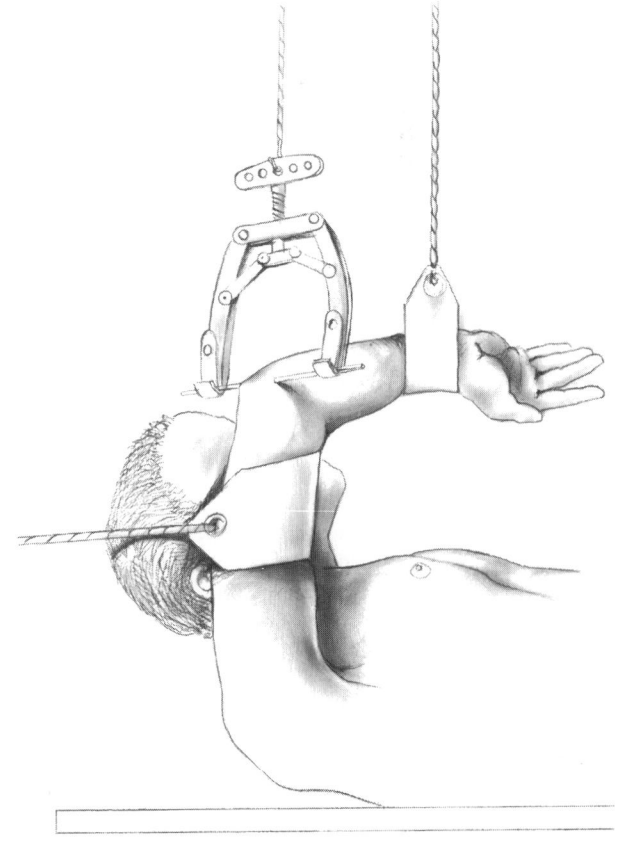

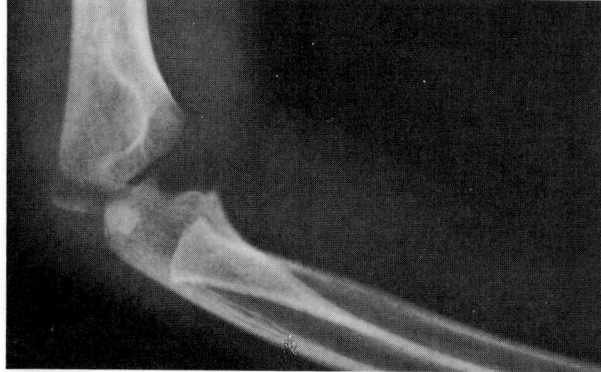

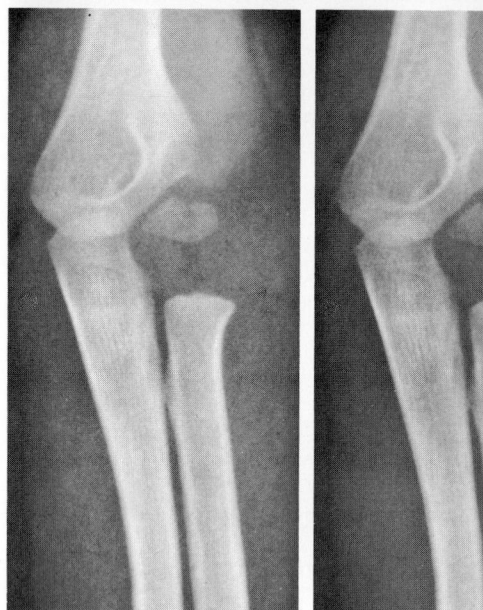

Fig. 43-61. AP, lateral, and oblique x-rays showing Type IV epiphyseal fracture of the lateral epicondyle with displacement and rotation.

TREATMENT. This is a Type IV epiphyseal injury of the Salter and Harris classification, and requires anatomic reduction. Even if reduction is successful and the elbow is placed in acute flexion, when muscle tone is recovered following anesthesia, the fragment will be displaced again. As a rule, only undisplaced fractures do not require surgical treatment.

FRACTURES OF THE MEDIAL EPICONDYLE IN CHILDREN

A sudden valgus strain of the elbow in a child may avulse the medial epicondylar apophysis. Minor degrees of displacement need not be anatomically reduced. If there has been a temporary dislocation of the joint with avulsion and incarceration of fragments in the joint or if ulnar nerve symptoms are present, open reduction and pinning of the fragments are required.

COMMINUTED FRACTURES OF THE DISTAL HUMERUS

Comminuted fractures of the distal end of the humerus are uncommon and usually result from a direct fall on the elbow or automobile collisions. Open reduction and internal fixation carried out through a posterior approach is the treatment of choice. If sound fixation can be obtained, early elbow motion at 7 to 10 days is started. If secure internal fixation cannot be anticipated, traction through an olecranon pin is used, followed with motion as soon as callus can be demonstrated. Residual disability from such an injury is painless loss of motion.

DISLOCATIONS OF THE ELBOW

A posterior dislocation of the elbow without associated fracture is more likely to occur in a child than an adult but is not a common injury. The injury is caused by falling on an outstretched arm with extension confined by adduction or abduction forces applied across the joint. The entire anterior capsule is torn with damage to medial and lateral ligaments of the elbow. These patients have severe pain and marked swelling. In contrast to fractures of the supracondylar region, the dislocation is quite stable. The treatment is immediate reduction and splinting with the elbow at 90°.

FRACTURE-DISLOCATIONS OF THE ELBOW

In addition to a posterior dislocation of the elbow, there may be a fracture of the coronoid process, the head of the radius (Fig. 43-62), or the lateral condyle. In the coronoid process it is usually a small chip fracture and is caused by the insertion of the brachialis, avulsing this portion of the bone during the dislocation. Its significance is that postreduction position of the elbow is more unstable, and immobilization is continued for a longer interval (3 weeks). If the radial head is fractured, the elbow is treated in the same manner as a posterior dislocation (reduction and immobilization). If motion does not return, radial head excision is indicated.

Monteggia's Deformity

Monteggia described a deformity in which there was a dislocation of the radial head with a fracture of the proximal third of the ulna (Fig. 43-63). In 85 percent of the cases the radial head is dislocated anteriorly, and in 15 percent, posteriorly. The deformity may be caused by a direct blow on the ulna, fracturing it and driving the radial head anteriorly. Whenever an x-ray reveals a fracture of one bone of the forearm or dislocation of one end, the concomitant injury to the adjacent bone should be ruled out by x-rays of the entire forearm.

If reduction of the ulna can be maintained, closed reduction of the radial head is usually possible by maintaining the arm in supination. If the ulnar fracture is displaced, intramedullary fixation (except in children) is required. After stabilization of the ulna, supination of the forearm and direct pressure over the radial head will accomplish its reduction. If the radial head is still not reduced, open reduction and suture of the annular ligament are carried out. If the radial head is anterior, the elbow is reduced and maintained in flexion. If the radial head is posterior, reduction and immobilization are carried out in full extension with the forearm in supination. Following

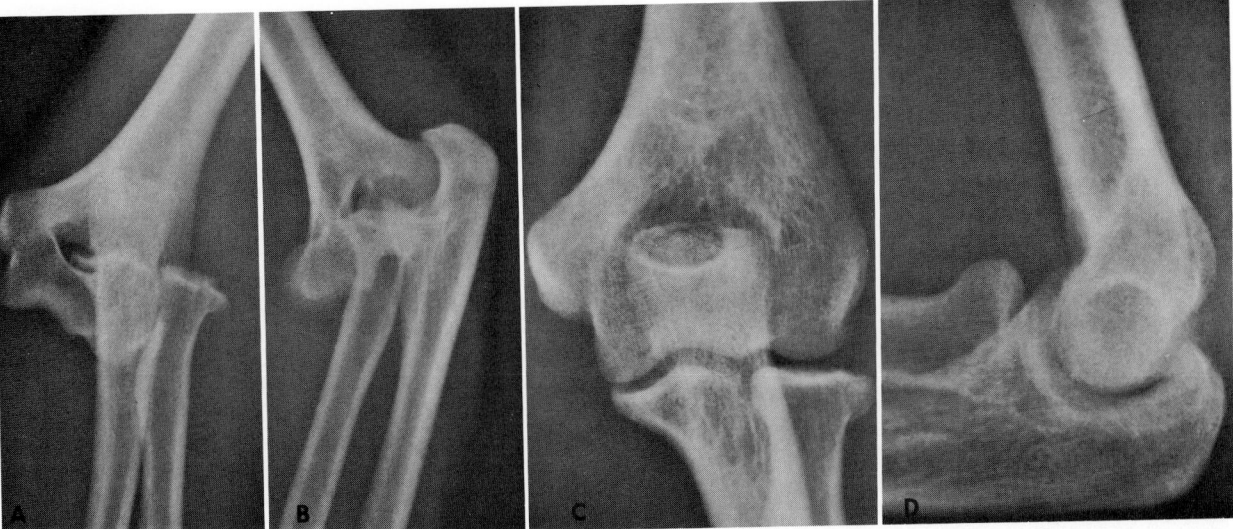

Fig. 43-62. Posterolateral dislocation of the elbow with a fracture of the radial head. *A* and *B.* AP and lateral x-rays prior to reduction. *C* and *D.* Postreduction x-rays showing satisfactory reduction with a minimally displaced small fracture of the radial head.

reduction, immobilization is maintained with a circular plaster cast.

SUBLUXATION OF THE RADIAL HEAD IN CHILDREN

One of the most common injuries of children under the age of five is the "nursemaid's elbow," or "pulled elbow." The usual history is that the child's hand is suddenly pulled, forcing the elbow into extension and causing the sudden onset of pain in the elbow. The child avoids motion of the arm. Passive, painless elbow flexion

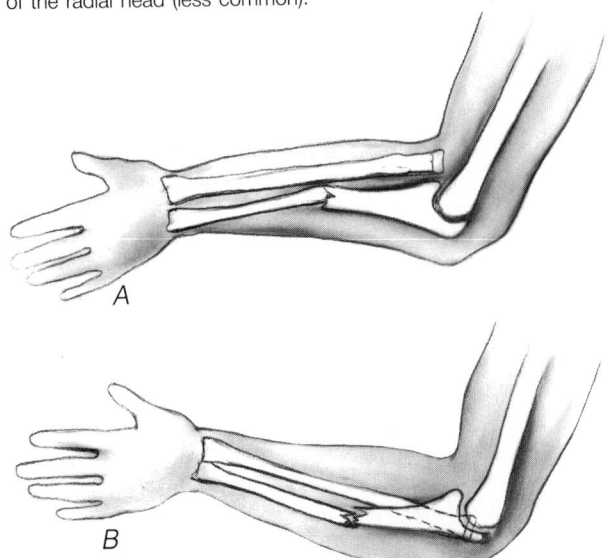

Fig. 43-63. Monteggia's deformity. *A.* Midshaft ulna fracture with anterior bowing and anterior dislocation of the radial head. *B.* Midshaft ulna fracture with posterior bowing and posterior dislocation of the radial head (less common).

is possible from 30 to 120°. X-rays of the elbow are negative.

The thin distal attachment of the annular ligament to the periosteum of the radial neck is torn when traction is applied to the pronated radius. The radial head escapes beneath the anterior part of the annular ligament, which is caught between the joint surfaces.

Treatment is effected by the maneuver of firm supination with the elbow held at 90° flexion. The arm may be in a sling 1 week, and the parents should be cautioned against repeated traction injury to the elbow.

FRACTURES OF THE CAPITELLUM

Fractures of the capitellum may occur in the same manner as fractures of the radial head. The patient complains of pain with any attempt at motion, and flexion is limited, depending upon the degree of displacement of the fracture.

TREATMENT. In some cases, closed reduction is sufficient. This is accomplished by extending the elbow while applying adduction force to the elbow joint. While traction is maintained, local digital pressure is applied to the fragment. The elbow is then maintained in marked flexion for 3 to 4 weeks, at the end of which time active motion is begun. If closed manipulation fails, the elbow is exposed through a lateral Kocher approach. If the fragment is small, it is excised; if large, reattachment may be possible with a Kirschner wire or screw fixation. When the capitellar fracture is recognized after 4 weeks, excision and early motion are necessary.

Fractures of the Forearm

Fractures of the forearm are most common in children, but occur at any age from falls on the outstretched arm or direct trauma. Clinical findings include deformity, local swelling, tenderness, and instability. Anteroposterior and lateral x-rays are obtained of both bones and should include views of the elbow and wrist. If only one bone is

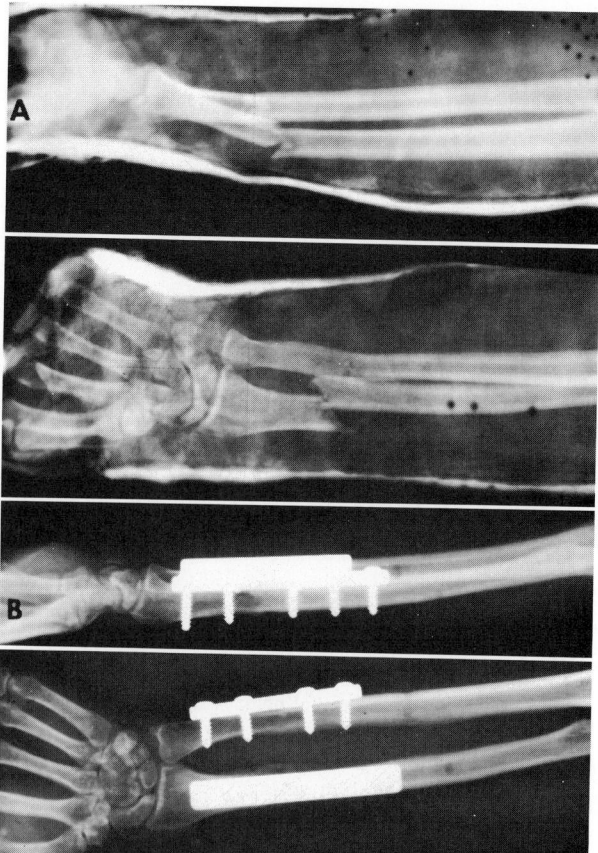

Fig. 43-64. Fracture of both bones of the forearm with open reduction and internal fixation. *A.* AP and lateral x-rays following closed reduction, showing displacement of distal radial fragment. *B.* AP and lateral x-rays showing anatomic position following open reduction and fixation with compression plates.

fractured, dislocation of the proximal or distal joint should be suspected.

ANATOMIC CONSIDERATIONS. The radius has both a slight lateral bow and a posterior bow. The ulna has less medial bow but also has a slight dorsal curve. Any loss of this anatomic feature or compression of the interosseous space will interfere with rotation.

The pronator quadratus attached to the distal radius tends to pull it ulnaward and encroach upon the interosseous space. Both supinators act upon the proximal radial fragment. In fractures of the proximal third, the proximal radius will usually be in supination. The attachments of the pronator teres and the brachioradialis act to shorten the deformity and increase the lateral bow of the radius. Interference with the interosseous membrane from scarring will interfere with rotation.

In other diaphyseal fractures, axial alignment is the only consideration. In fractures of both bones of the forearm, because of the interrelationship required for rotation, anatomic restoration is required for normal function. If this can be accomplished by the closed method, there will be less scarring from surgical trauma, and the patient is more likely to have normal function. If the anatomic

features cannot be restored by closed means, open reduction is indicated.

TREATMENT. General anesthesia or axillary block anesthesia is required for reduction of forearm fractures. With the elbow flexed 90°, traction is applied to the long axis of the forearm by grasping the thumb and index finger of the patient and applying countertraction to the humerus. This may be done with the help of an assistant or by suspending the thumb and index finger with traction and adding weight over the humerus proximal to the flexed elbow as countertraction. When length has been regained, the fracture fragments are grasped by the operator, angulation increased, displacement corrected, and the fracture reduced.

If there is more than one fracture, reduction of the transverse fracture is accomplished first. Using the length gained from this reduction, reduction of the adjacent bone is then effected. The arm is immobilized in a position in which stability is greatest. For proximal-third fractures, this is supination, and for distal-third fractures, pronation, although there are exceptions to this rule. A well-molded, minimally padded plaster from the proximal palmar crease to the axilla, with the elbow at 90° flexion, is used. X-rays are obtained to determine accuracy of reduction. Interpretation may require comparison with the normal side. It is necessary to take check x-rays at intervals during the first 3 weeks to be certain that position is maintained. When position is lost, open reduction may be necessary.

The fractures most often requiring open reduction are displaced fractures of the proximal third and oblique fractures of the radius. Segmental fractures also require open reduction and internal fixation (Fig. 43-64).

FOREARM SHAFT FRACTURES IN CHILDREN

Operative reduction of shafts of both bones is almost never indicated in the young child. Treatment of these injuries is by closed reduction and immobilization in plaster. However, in children twelve years of age and older (i.e., close to epiphyseal maturity), there will be minimal remodeling, and operative reduction may be required.

Greenstick fractures with angulation (Fig. 43-65) should be manipulated to correct the deformity and at the same time break the unbroken cortex. Otherwise, deformity will occur in the cast. The apex of the deformity is deftly snapped over the operator's knee, a maneuver that will usually correct the deformity.

The principles of reduction of displaced fractures in children are the same as for displaced fractures in adults. If both bones are displaced, one bone is reduced, and using this as a lever the adjacent bone is reduced. The forearm is then immobilized with the elbow at 90° and in the position of greatest stability: supination for proximal-third, pronation for distal-third, and neutral position for midshaft fractures. Check x-rays are obtained immediately postreduction and at 7 to 10 days to be certain that reduction is maintained. If it is not possible to hold both bones reduced, skin traction is applied to the fingers and attached to an outrigger splint from the cast. Experience

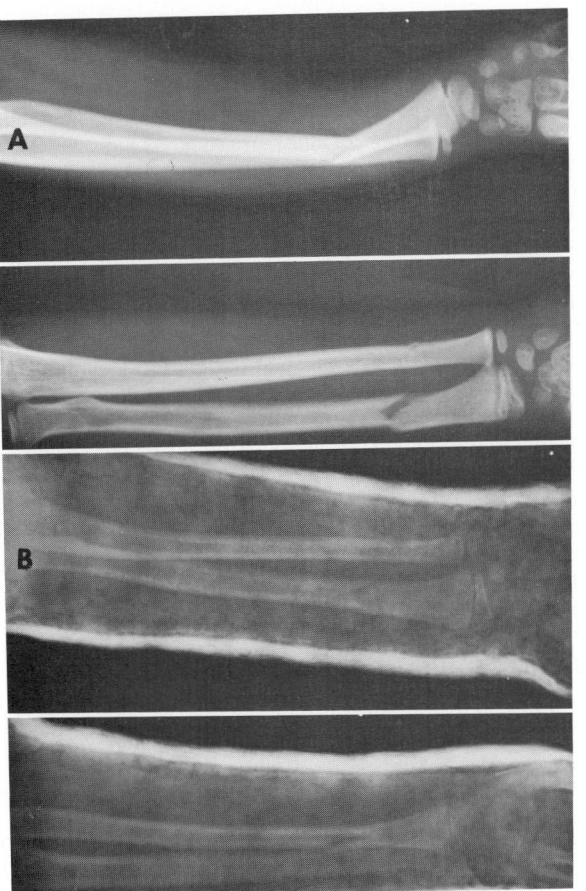

Fig. 43-65. *A.* Greenstick fracture of the radius with torus fracture of the ulna. *B.* Satisfactory position following manipulation and application of plaster.

is required in judging what degrees of angulation will be corrected with remodeling. The closer the fracture to the growing epiphysis, the greater remodeling possible. In general, 30° of shaft angulation in an infant will correct itself. This should not be accepted in the older child.

Fractures of the Distal Radius

COLLES FRACTURE

A fracture of the distal radius with dorsal angulation produces a typical dinner fork deformity, as was described by Abraham Colles in 1814. Since Colles was describing a clinical deformity before the use of x-ray, the use of the term *Colles fracture* has come to mean dorsally-radially angulated fractures of the distal radial metaphysis with an associated fracture of the ulnar styloid (Fig. 43-66) and not fracture of the distal ulnar shift, which occurs in children.

CLINICAL MANIFESTATIONS. Distal radial fractures usually occur in patients over the age of fifty, more commonly in women, and are produced by a fall on the outstretched hand. The term "dinner fork" offers an appropriate clinical description. Depending upon the degree of comminution, there may be considerable instability, tenderness, and swelling about the wrist. Palpation of the wrist will reveal a more proximal position of the tip of the radial styloid. On examination, it is important to rule out the presence or absence of a concomitant median nerve injury. X-ray examination should include AP, lateral, and both oblique views. A carpal dislocation can clinically simulate this deformity.

TREATMENT. The aim of treatment of this injury is to obtain a functional hand and wrist and, second, to minimize cosmetic deformity. In the past, many operative skeletal traction methods have been used in an attempt to improve the cosmetic deformity. Unfortunately, immobilization of the hand required of these methods compromises hand function. The best results in this fracture have

Fig. 43-66. Colles fracture in a twenty-five-year-old woman. *A.* AP and lateral x-rays postinjury. *B.* AP and lateral x-rays after closed reduction under local anesthesia and cast immobilization.

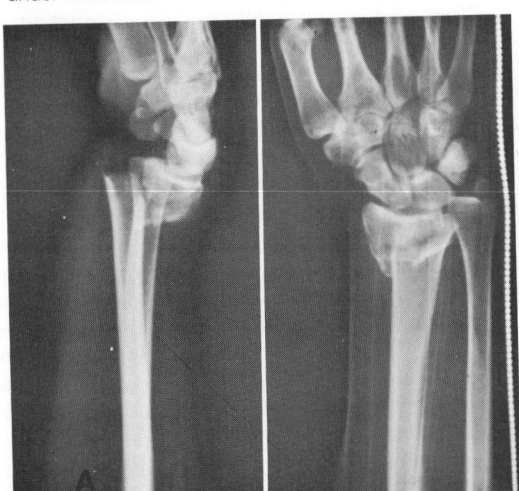

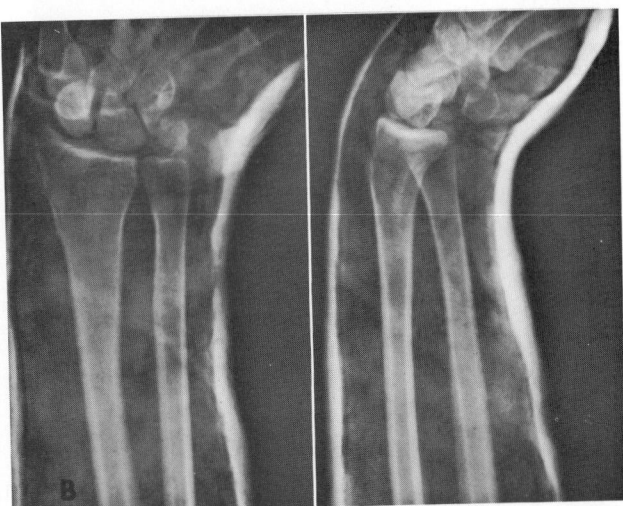

been obtained by closed reduction and plaster immobilization.

The easiest method of reduction is traction in which the thumb, index, and long finger are hung up with Chinese finger traps with a counterweight applied to the humerus (elbow at 90°). If reduction is not satisfactory, manipulation is carried out. With an assistant applying countertraction to the humerus and with the elbow flexed, traction is applied to the radial side of the hand for disimpaction of the distal radial fragment, which is displaced and angulated in a radial and dorsal direction.

While traction is maintained, the operator grasps the distal radial fragment between thumb and index finger and displaces it anteriorly to correct the displacement. At the same time, counterpressure is applied in a dorsal direction, with the opposite hand applied to the anterior surface of the forearm. Simultaneously, the wrist is brought into maximal flexion and ulnar deviation while pronating the forearm.

Over two layers of sheet wadding a well-molded plaster cast is applied which includes the elbow, with the wrist in

Fig. 43-67. Fracture of the navicular-scaphoid. *A.* AP x-ray 1 day postinjury is negative for fracture. *B.* Patient was persistently tender over the navicular tuberosity. X-ray at 3 weeks reveals fracture at the junction of the proximal and middle thirds. Fracture subsequently healed without avascular necrosis.

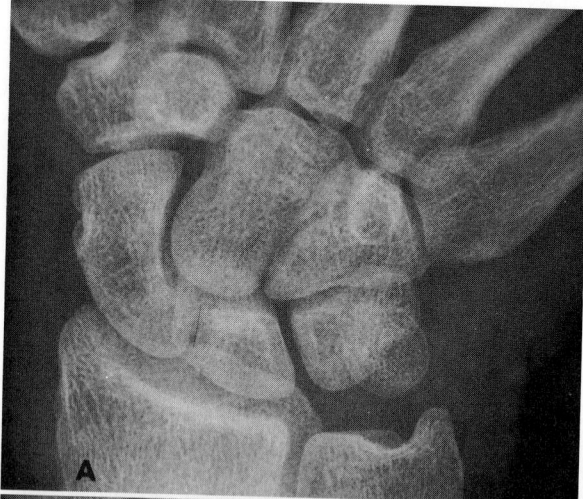

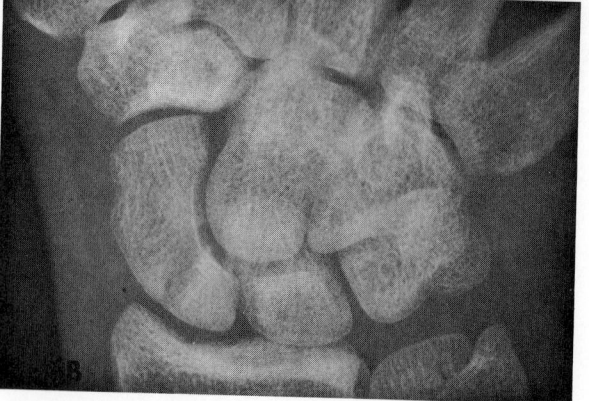

maximal ulnar deviation, 30° of palmar flexion. Check x-rays are obtained immediately and at 7 to 10 days to be certain that reduction has been maintained.

The patient should be encouraged to keep the hand elevated for 2 or 3 days or until swelling has subsided. The patient is instructed in exercises to maintain a full range of motion of all interphalangeal (IP) and metaphalangeal (MP) joints. The patient should maximally flex the IP joints with the MP joints in extension and flex the MP joints with the IP joints in extension. Patients who are able to do this have little difficulty in mobilizing the wrist following 6 weeks of plaster immobilization. Patients should do range-of-motion shoulder exercises daily. This prevents the occasional episodes of shoulder stiffness that accompany Colles fractures. Shoulder stiffness may be due to traction on the shoulder joint from the weight of the cast or from a primary capsular injury at the time of initial injury. If the wrist is placed in maximal palmar flexion, median nerve compression in the carpal tunnel may ensue. If median nerve paresthesias occur, decrease in the amount of wrist flexion is necessary. If unrelieved, the flexor retinaculum is incised surgically.

SMITH FRACTURE

A fall on the dorsum of the wrist may cause a reversed Colles fracture (called Smith fracture). In such fractures position is difficult to maintain because of comminution. Plaster immobilization in the position of dorsiflexion of the wrist is required. If this will not maintain position, continuous skeletal traction to the thumb matacarpal or open reduction plate and screw fixation are necessary.

Injuries to the Wrist

A person falling on the outstretched wrist may sprain the anterior radial carpal ligament, with resulting synovial effusion and wrist pain, and limitation of motion. It is important to distinguish this from a fractured navicular or dislocation of the lunate, which have similar signs.

FRACTURES OF THE NAVICULAR—SCAPHOID

Young adults who fall on the outstretched hand frequently fracture the navicular (Fig. 43-67) against the unyielding anterior radial carpal ligament. In elderly patients, a Colles fracture occurs, because the distal radius is the point of least resistance. There is tenderness to direct pressure over the tuberosity of the navicular, with limitation of wrist flexion and extension. With any wrist injury, it is imperative to rule out a fractured navicular by x-ray examination.

In addition to AP, lateral, and oblique x-rays of the carpal bones, with the wrist in neutral position, a special 17° angled AP x-ray view of the wrist is needed. If the patient has tenderness over the tuberosity of the navicular and x-ray examination is negative, the patient is presumed to have a fractured navicular, treated as such, and then re-x-rayed when there has been some resorption at the fracture site (3 weeks). At 3 weeks, if clinical and x-ray examinations are still negative, the wrist is mobilized.

There is little or no displacement with fractures of the navicular. Arterial supply enters the distal third of the bone constantly. The proximal-third blood supply may be only by communication in the bone from the vessels entering distally. Fractures transecting the waist or proximal third may interrupt the entire circulation to the proximal third. Because of this, nonunion or avascular necrosis of the proximal fragments is not uncommon.

TREATMENT. When there is little or no displacement and the injury is diagnosed accurately, the optimal treatment is by plaster cast immobilization. Plaster is applied from the tip of the thumb to include the elbow. By immobilizing the elbow, pronation-supination, which causes motion at the fracture site, is prevented.

Most navicular fractures require 16 weeks of adequate plaster immobilization. The patient is seen at monthly intervals and the cast replaced, if loose, without disturbing the position of the wrist. X-rays out of plaster are obtained at 8 weeks and at subsequent 4-week intervals. When all tenderness from direct pressure over the tuberosity of the navicular has disappeared and x-rays show obliteration of the fracture site, plaster immobilization is discontinued. In some situations, 6 months or longer is necessary.

When a patient has an acute fracture in which displacement cannot be corrected, the best treatment is open reduction and screw fixation. This is preferable to accepting a possible nonunion or the long delay necessary for union of the displaced fracture. Displaced fractures usually occur as the result of, and in combination with, perilunar dislocation of the carpus. When the interval between trauma and diagnosis is less than 6 months, prolonged plaster immobilization (6 to 9 months) will usually result in union.

NONUNION OF NAVICULAR-SCAPHOID FRACTURES. With a simple nonunion of navicular fractures, without avascular necrosis and without degenerative arthritis at the wrist, an autogenous bone graft is indicated. Techniques using electrical stimulation should also be considered. In patients with significant degenerative changes adjacent to the nonunion, excision of the radial styloid may give satisfactory pain relief and maintenance of wrist power.

DISLOCATIONS OF THE LUNATE

Dislocations of the lunate are uncommon but occur from trauma causing hyperextension of the wrist. Patients complain of pain, swelling, and limitation of motion. Median nerve symptoms are frequent. The diagnosis is made by AP and lateral x-rays. On the lateral x-ray of the wrist, the semilunar shape of the lunate is displaced anterior to the distal radial articular surface. On the AP x-ray, the normal quadrilateral shape of the lunate appears triangular and larger than on the opposite side.

TREATMENT. Treatment is by closed reduction and plaster immobilization. Reduction is accomplished by hyperextending the wrist and applying direct pressure of the operator's thumb over the dislocated lunate. After it is reduced, the wrist is brought into the flexed position.

There is a high incidence of avascular necrosis following this injury, for which lunate excision is indicated. Kienböck's disease, which is avascular necrosis of the lunate, may occur without known trauma. The onset of symptoms, which include wrist pain, stiffness, and local swelling, is insidious. Treatment is excision or surgical shortening of the ulna.

A similar mechanism of injury may produce a perilunar dislocation of the carpus with or without fracture of the scaphoid or rotatory subluxation of the scaphoid— so-called traumatic instability of the wrist. The diagnosis of the former is obvious radiographically, but attention should always be directed at the scaphoid-lunate relationship to detect subtle signs of scaphoid subluxation.

Fractures and Dislocations in the Hand

METACARPAL FRACTURES

Metacarpal fractures occur from direct violence to the hand, as in crushing injuries, although the most common mechanism is by striking the hand against an opponent. Fractures of the necks of fourth and fifth metacarpals invariably occur in young men as a result of altercations. There is local swelling involving the fracture site that minimizes the actual degree of anterior angulation of the head of the metacarpal. Therefore, the degree of angulation can be determined only by x-ray. Rotational deformity of such a fracture must be determined clinically. Each finger, when flexed individually into the palm, points to the navicular, and any deviation from this is an indication of rotational deformity of the finger or its metacarpal shaft.

TREATMENT. Treatment of the acute metacarpal neck fractures is by closed manipulation, making certain that rotational deformity is corrected. The finger is then splinted with the MP and the IP joints in 45° of flexion and with the tip pointing toward the navicular. It is not always possible to hold the fracture by this method, and some cosmetic deformity of the knuckle may persist. Since there is mobility at the carpometacarpal joints of the fourth and fifth fingers, the grip will not be compromised.

Metacarpal shaft fractures that are oblique or spiral usually require nothing more than anterior splinting for 2 to 3 weeks. Anterior angulated fractures of the second and third metacarpals that do not have carpometacarpal mobility must be protected against anterior angulation, or interference with grasp will result. Multiple fractures of metacarpal shafts may require intramedullary fixation. This is done by inserting a single intramedullary wire percutaneously from distal to proximal direction, starting on the lip of the metacarpal head and avoiding the articular surface. Comminuted fractures of the metacarpal heads involving the articular surface are difficult to treat because of the extensive damage to the articular surface. Such fractures should be immobilized in a position of function over a metal splint and motion started at 2 to 3 weeks.

Fracture-dislocations of the carpometacarpal joint occur very rarely. A typical mechanism of injury is severe

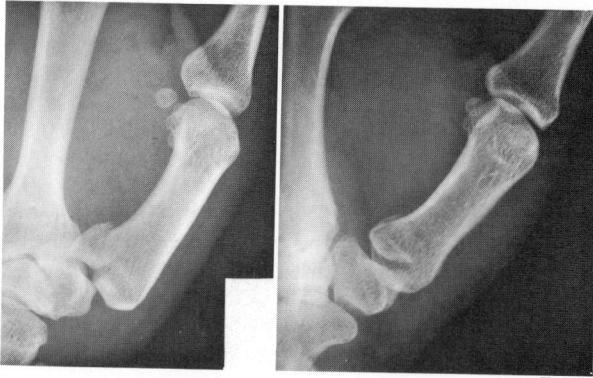

Fig. 43-68. Bennett's fracture. Two views showing intraarticular fracture of the base of the proximal first phalanx with displacement. Such an injury requires reduction and maintenance of position by plaster or open reduction.

force applied to a hyperextended wrist. It is preferable to carry out closed reduction of a carpometacarpal fracture-dislocation. There may be interposition of tendons and soft tissue, necessitating open reduction. Kirschner wire fixation across the carpometacarpal junction is used to maintain the reduction.

BENNETT'S FRACTURE

Bennett's fracture is an intraarticular fracture involving the base of the carpometacarpal joint of the thumb (Fig. 43-68). Such an injury is the result of forcible abduction

Fig. 43-69. *A.* Lateral x-ray of the dorsal dislocation of the proximal interphalangeal joint of an index finger. *B.* After closed reduction under local anesthesia, postreduction position was maintained on a metal splint in the position of function.

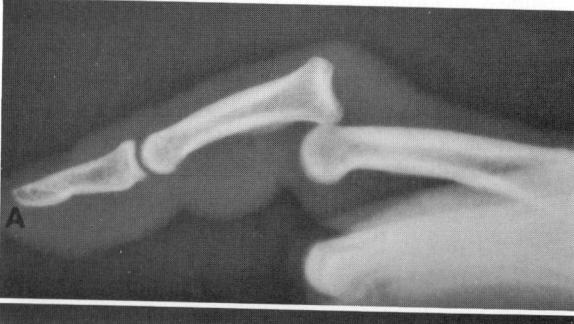

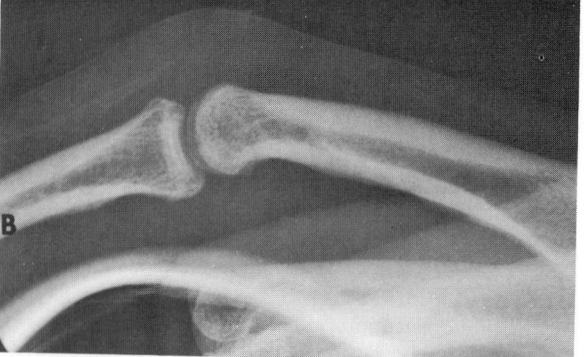

on the thumb. There is an oblique fracture that involves the base of the metacarpal and transects the proximal articular surface. The resulting instability causes subluxation of the shaft and the remaining articular surface. If such a fracture is unreduced, the normal range of abduction and carpometacarpal joint motion will be compromised.

Closed methods may hold reduction of minimally displaced and undisplaced fractures. Traction is applied to the axis of the shaft of the metacarpal, which is then brought into abduction, while direct adduction pressure is applied over the base of the carpometacarpal joint. If displacement persists, closed reduction and percutaneous wire fixation of the first carpometacarpal joint will hold the fracture. If this is not sufficient, open reduction and Kirschner wire fixation across the fracture is indicated.

PHALANGEAL FRACTURES

Undisplaced fractures of phalangeal shafts require splinting with the MP joints in 70° flexion and IP joints in slight flexion. The finger is placed on a metal splint and taped in this position without traction. If the fracture is displaced, it is manipulated into position and placed on a metal splint as for undisplaced fractures.

A small chip fracture involving an IP joint is treated symptomatically by the use of a splint for 2 weeks followed by early motion. Interphalangeal dislocations (Fig. 43-69) require closed reduction and splinting in a position of function. Open reduction with fine K-wire fixation is rarely necessary.

Distal Phalanx

A crushed fingertip with resultant fracture of the distal phalanx is one of the most common injuries seen in an emergency room. Initial treatment is aimed at cleansing the skin and relieving the pain by splinting the finger. There is usually no intraarticular involvement, and position of fragments is rarely a consideration.

Mallet Finger

When the distal phalanx is forcibly flexed against the taut extensor tendon, avulsion of the extensor tendon may occur with or without a fragment of bone from its insertion on the distal phalanx. This causes a characteristic dropped finger; the last 15 to 20° of active extension is lost, although full passive extension is possible. There is local tenderness and swelling over the dorsal aspect of the distal interphalangeal (DIP) joint.

Many types of treatment have been tried for this lesion. If the tendon has been avulsed without a bone fragment, the finger is splinted over a metal splint with the DIP joint in maximal extension or hyperextension and with the proximal interphalangeal (PIP) joint in 60° of flexion. The splint needs to be repeatedly inspected and adjusted. Care should be taken not to cause skin necrosis by excessive pressure over the DIP joint. If active extension is not gained in 6 weeks, splinting should be continued for another 2 or 3 weeks. Incomplete extension is not always

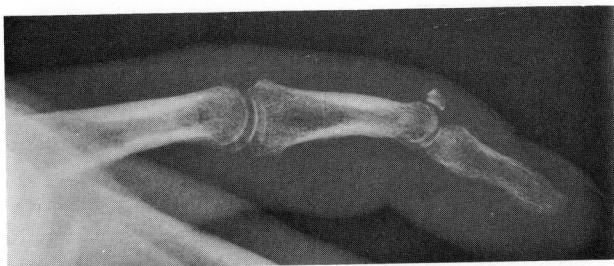

Fig. 43-70. Mallet finger. Lateral x-ray of a finger with avulsion of the extensor tendon at its bony insertion with minimal subluxation.

associated with disability. If the patient shows symptoms, surgical reefing of the lengthened extensor tendon is indicated.

When avulsion occurs with a fragment of bone (Fig. 43-70) involving one-third of the distal articular surface, open reduction and Bunnell pullout wire fixation are required. If the bone chip is small or does not involve the articular surface, the treatment may be the same as with a pure tendon avulsion.

In crush injuries of any IP joint with severe comminution of articular surface the phalanges should be splinted in a position of function at 45° of flexion and consideration given to early arthrodesis, if symptoms are evident. Compound fractures involving the hand invoke the same principles as those applied to other compound fractures.

FRACTURES AND JOINT INJURIES IN THE LOWER EXTREMITY

Fractures of the Proximal Femur

Fractures of the proximal femur are a challenge to everyone responsible for the care of patients with such injuries. Prior to the introduction of internal fixation, such fractures were treated by bed rest and traction, with a much higher mortality rate. The age of most patients with fractures of the proximal femur is in the sixties or seventies. Complications of immobility imposed by this fracture in this elderly age group are responsible for a significant mortality. Operative fixation will allow early mobility and relief of pain and is the treatment of choice. Only in the occasional younger individual with this injury can bed rest and traction be tolerated.

FEMORAL NECK FRACTURES

Femoral neck fractures usually occur in the elderly but may occur in young adults or children when severe trauma is involved. Fractures are commonly produced by a fall, although the history may suggest that the fracture occurred from a twist or indirect type of force and the patient fell as the fractured femoral neck gave way.

CLINICAL MANIFESTATIONS. The patient is usually unable to stand on the side of the affected hip and has increasing pain as a tense hemarthrosis develops. The affected leg may be slightly shorter and held in a position of external rotation of 30 to 40°. Attempts at motion cause excruciating pain. There may be ecchymosis over the trochanter, but local swelling is not prominent.

Anteroposterior and tube lateral x-rays demonstrate interruption between the trabeculae of the head and neck. The head is rotated into varus with posterior angulation. There are varying degrees of comminution of the posterior neck at the fracture site.

CLASSIFICATION. Garden has classified femoral neck fractures according to displacement and comminution (Fig. 43-71): Type I fractures are incomplete fractures; Type II, complete fractures without displacement; Type III, partially displaced fractures; Type IV, complete displacement. This classification is useful in evaluating therapy, since displaced fractures have a higher rate of nonunion and avascular necrosis.

TREATMENT. The prognosis of this fracture depends upon the attainment of union, without development of avascular necrosis. In adults, the blood supply to the femoral head is via the metaphyseal vessels (which are interrupted by the fracture), the artery of the ligamentum teres, and the lateral epiphyseal vessels. The location of a fracture site high on the neck with associated displacement may damage the lateral epiphyseal vessels. If the artery of the ligamentum teres provides insufficient circulation, avascular necrosis may ensue.

The periosteum on the neck has no cambium layer, so that external callus does not develop. The absence of external callus and the precarious circulation contribute to the high incidence of nonunion.

Despite the apparent medical contraindication for surgical treatment in these patients, operative treatment is

Fig. 43-71. Types of subcapital fracture (Garden; see text).

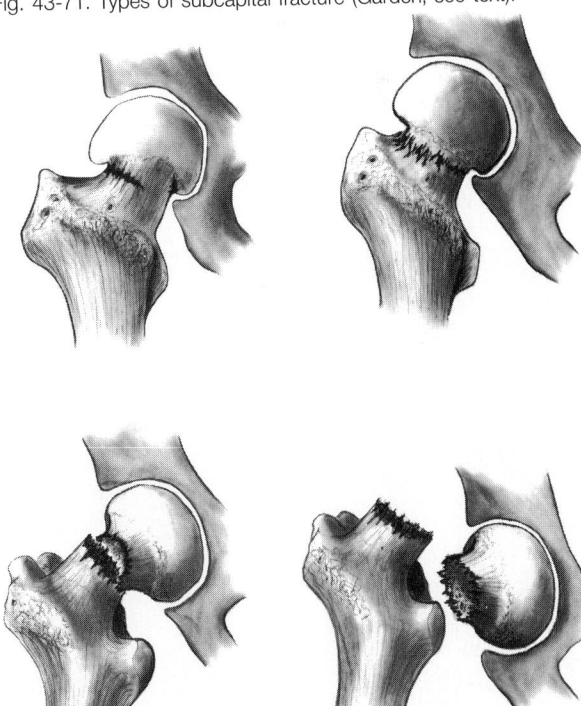

MEISENZAHL

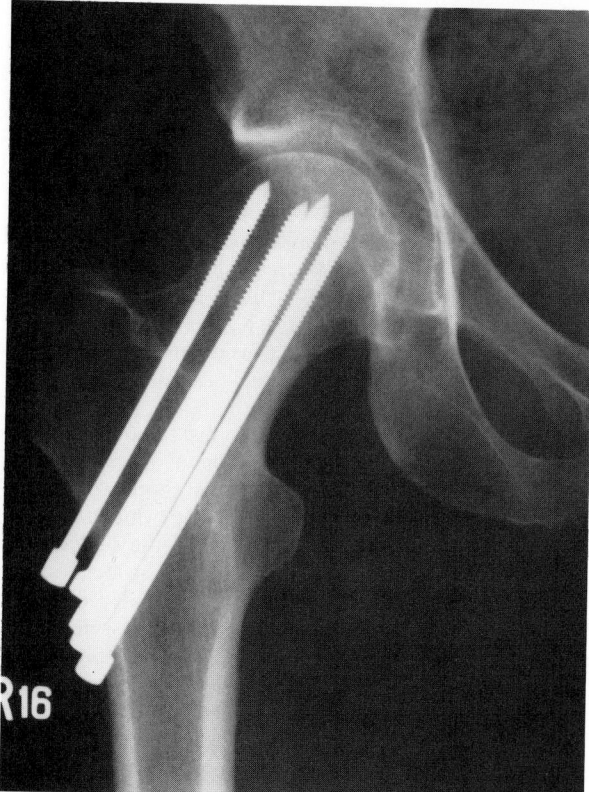

Fig. 43-72. Subcapital fracture fixed with multiple Knowles pins.

necessary to allow early mobilization and thus to reduce the morbidity and mortality associated with bed rest in the elderly. In general, internal fixation is indicated in younger patients and prosthetic replacement, using a bipolar prosthesis, in the more elderly.

Fig. 43-73. *A.* Fracture of the femoral neck in a nine-year-old boy with varus deformity. *B.* AP x-ray showing united fracture 1 year postinjury in satisfactory position. Russell's traction was the method of treatment.

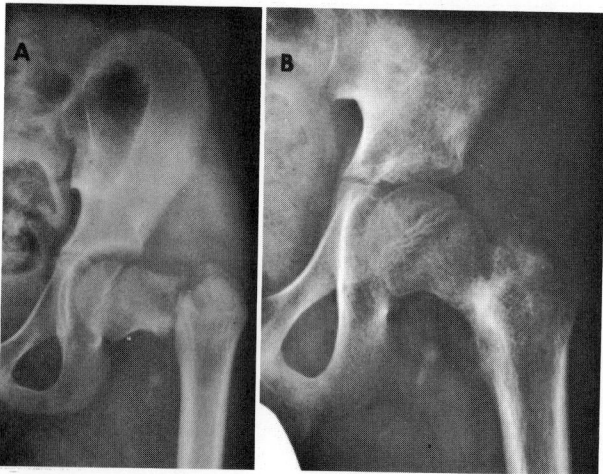

Impacted Femoral Neck Fractures

Type I (Garden) subcapital fractures or Type II fractures that are impacted may be treated conservatively. Some patients have walked with the fracture by the time of examination. If the fracture is impacted in slight valgus with less than 15 to 20° of anterior angulation at the fracture site, it is worthwhile to attempt nonoperative management. The patient is instructed not to bear weight or use leverage with the leg. The patient is kept in bed until he or she can actively control the leg without discomfort. This usually takes from a few days to a week. The few impacted fractures that subsequently become displaced occur within the first 10 days. If displacement occurs, closed reduction and internal fixation are indicated (Fig. 43-72).

Postoperative Management. Postoperatively, patients are mobilized as rapidly as possible. They are encouraged to get out of bed the following day and mobilized to use crutches without weight bearing as soon as possible. Check x-rays are obtained at intervals to follow the progress of healing. Approximately 4 to 6 months is required for sufficient healing across the fracture site. Unprotected weight bearing is not allowed until union is solid.

If nonunion exists in the presence of a viable head, reconstructive surgical treatment, with bone grafts, or osteotomy may be required. In elderly patients, excision of the femoral head and insertion of a prosthesis is a satisfactory solution when this complication occurs.

Insertion of Femoral Head Prosthesis

Because nonunion and avascular necrosis are problems, attempts have been made to obviate these difficulties by the insertion of a primary femoral head prosthesis. Such measures taken on a routine basis do not give as good results as hip nailing. Hinchey and Day list spastic hemiplegia, severe arthritis of the fractured hip, pathologic fracture, the need for ambulatory care because of blindness, extreme age, or poor general health, contraindicating a second operation as indications for a primary prosthesis. If the complications of avascular necrosis or nonunion develop in the aged patient, a femoral head replacement prosthesis is indicated.

Femoral Neck Fractures in Children

Fractures of the femoral neck occur in children (Fig. 43-73) only after severe trauma, such as in pedestrian injuries or in falls from a great height. If satisfactory reduction can be obtained by Russell's traction, it is continued until union is sound, usually for 10 to 16 weeks, depending upon the age of the child. If union is not sound, a hip spica will not protect against loss of position into varus. If closed reduction is not satisfactory, operative internal fixation treatment, as in adults, is indicated. The fracture should be pinned with three parallel Knowles pins. There is a high incidence of avascular necrosis of both the head and neck in children.

INTERTROCHANTERIC AND SUBTROCHANTERIC FRACTURES

Intertrochanteric and subtrochanteric fractures occur very commonly in the elderly from a direct fall onto the hip. They also occur from severe traumatic forces in younger individuals as in automobile accidents or crush injury. There is considerably more instability to this type of fracture than intracapsular fractures of the femoral neck. There is shortening and external rotation, which may be 90°, and swelling about the anterior and proximal thigh.

In treatment of this type of fracture in the elderly patient indications for open reduction are the same as in intracapsular fractures. The main aim of treatment is to relieve pain and mobilize the elderly patient to prevent the complications of immobility. In younger individuals who can tolerate bed rest, the conservative treatment, such as Russell's traction or skeletal traction and balanced suspension, will maintain reduction if there are contraindications to surgical treatment. If traction is decided upon, it must continue until union is solid, which may require 16 weeks or longer with bed rest. Surgical treatment involves closed or open reduction on a fracture table, combined with internal fixation using a compression screw device. Subtrochanteric fractures should have a sufficiently longer fixation on the shaft than intertrochanteric fractures. There should be at least three to four screw holes below the lowest point of the subtrochanteric fracture.

Postoperative care should include attention to early mobilization, proper hydration, and pulmonary hygiene. Prophylactic coumadin, dextran, or graduated elastic stockings or external pneumatic compression, which have been shown to prevent embolic complication, should be considered. The medical aspects of the patient's condition are a challenge to the surgeon and are at least as important as the technique and insertion of internal fixation devices. Since most of these fractures in the middle-aged or elderly are related to osteoporosis, treatment of the underlying bone problem is a basic consideration.

Fractures of the Femoral Shaft

Femoral shaft fractures occur at any age, from severe violence, but injuries in children may occur from less severe indirect torsional stress applied to the leg. When major trauma is involved, associated injuries of the chest, head, and abdomen are common and should be the first consideration. When a patient with a fractured femur is in shock, other injuries requiring immediate attention should be suspected, although hemorrhage into a thigh may produce severe hypotension.

CLINICAL MANIFESTATIONS. Patients with a fractured femoral shaft have severe pain with any attempt at motion of the extremity. There is usually rotational deformity, shortening of the affected leg, with prominent swelling of the thigh.

The most important immediate local consideration with fractures of the femoral shaft is whether there has been damage to the femoral or popliteal vessels. If the patient has good pedal pulses, with normal sensation and motor power in the foot, major arterial injury is unlikely. When signs of ischemia are present or cannot be ruled out, arteriography and/or exploration of the vessels are indicated.

TREATMENT. Emergency treatment at the scene of the accident should include splinting the leg to the adjacent extremity or, optimally, traction applied to the foot over a Thomas splint. If the wound is compound and the bones are protruding, they should not be repositioned until proper debridement has been carried out.

Femoral shaft fractures in children are treated exclusively by closed methods. Internal fixation is contraindicated because of potential damage to the epiphyseal plate and growth disturbances of the femur. Anatomic reduction is not required (Fig. 43-74). With a displaced femoral shaft fracture in a child, 1 cm of overriding is acceptable as long as there are no more than a few degrees of angulation and rotational deformity has been completely corrected. The epiphyseal stimulation provided by the presence of healing callus will make up 1 cm of shortening. In the very young child, where a maximum of 2 lb can be used to reduce the fracture. Bryant's traction provides an effective means for reduction without compromise to the blood flow. The child's ability to dorsiflex the great toe should be repeatedly inspected to be certain that an anterior compartment syndrome or vascular compromise is not developing in either lower extremity. Russell's traction is used for older children. Repeat check x-rays are obtained at intervals to be certain that position and reduction are maintained. Reduction must be accomplished in a few days, because by 10 days most fractures in children are clinically firm. When the fracture is clinically stable and nontender and callus is present by x-ray, the child is placed in a $1\frac{1}{2}$ hip spica. Progressive weight bearing between crutches is started when bony union is solid. Treatment of shaft fractures in adults may be accomplished by either closed methods or operative intramedullary nailing.

Closed intramedullary nailing is superior to that in which the fracture site must be opened. The incidence of infection with blind nailing is much less than with exposure of the fracture site. This may be nearly as safe as the treatment with skeletal traction. The operator must be familiar with the technique and be equipped with a fracture table as well as an image intensifier for accomplishing the closed reduction and blind nailing.

If closed treatment is utilized, skeletal traction is necessary. Traction is applied to a threaded Steinmann pin placed across the supracondylar area or proximal tibia. When there is associated knee injury, it is best to insert the Steinmann pin through the supracondylar area and not to apply skeletal traction across the injured knee.

When the fracture is stable and firm, i.e., with no tenderness at the fracture site, and shortening does not occur when traction is removed, the patient is ready for immobilization in a hip spica if the fracture is high at the junc-

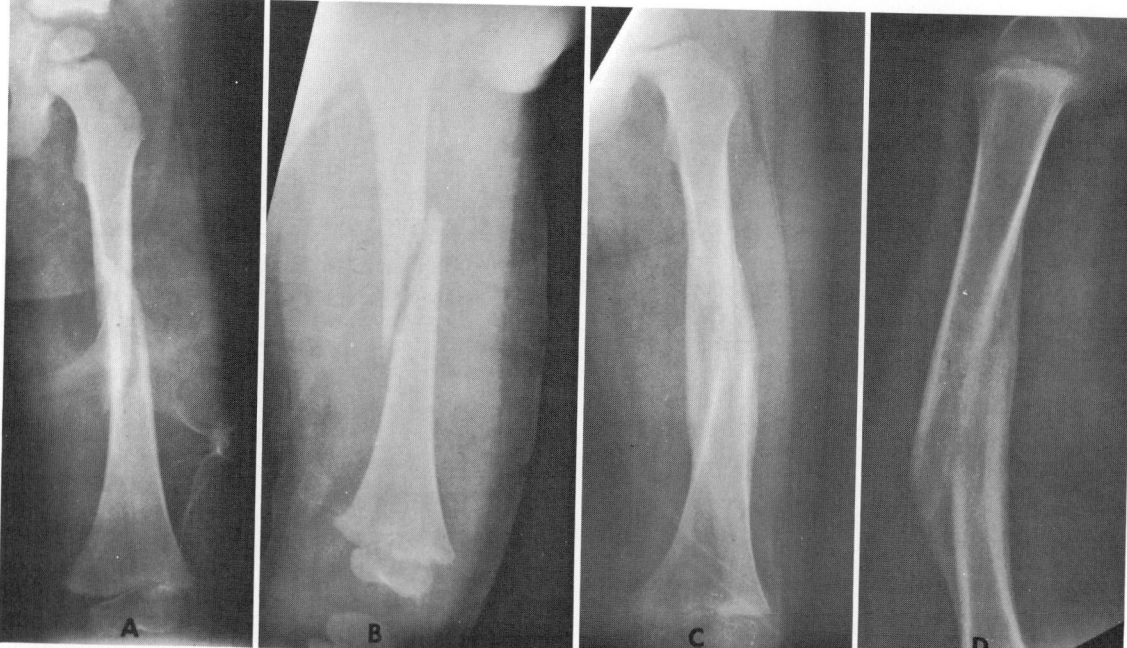

Fig. 43-74. Femoral shaft fracture in a child treated by traction. *A* and *B*. AP and lateral x-rays in satisfactory position in skin traction. *C* and *D*. AP and lateral x-rays of healed fracture showing satisfactory position. The anterior angulation of the fracture site will remodel itself.

tion of the upper and middle thirds. A cast brace is applied and weight-bearing treatment instituted if the fracture is in the middle or distal third of the femur.

Cast brace treatment for fractures of the midshaft and distal one-third of the femur treated initially with skeletal traction allows more rapid mobilization of the patient and results in more rapid union and better functional return of knee motion than with spica cast immobilization. It may be possible to mobilize some fractures in a cast brace as early as the first or second week postinjury.

Supracondylar Fractures

Supracondylar fractures of the femur and Y or T intracondylar fractures occur in all age groups from trauma occurring in automobile accidents, pedestrian injuries, falls, and various other accidents. Patients with this injury present with the usual signs of fracture, i.e., local swelling, instability, deformity. In some cases, the patient will appear to have only a knee effusion. Supracondylar fractures are intraarticular fractures, since they communicate with the suprapatellar pouch of the knee. Scarring in this region may obliterate the suprapatellar pouch and interfere with knee motion. Treatment of these difficult fractures is usually by open reduction and internal fixation or by skeletal traction.

TRAUMATIC EPIPHYSEAL SEPARATION OF THE DISTAL FEMUR

This injury occurs from forced hyperextension of the knee, in the adolescent child. Treatment should be immediate closed reduction and plaster immobilization. Open reduction of this injury may be indicated when the fracture is causing circulatory embarrassment.

Ligamentous Injuries of the Knee Joint

Injuries to the ligamentous supporting structures of the knee occur in all types of athletic endeavors but are especially common in sports utilizing cleats where the foot becomes fixed to the ground and direct or indirect force is applied to the knee joint. A similar mechanism occurs in skiing, where the long lever arm of the ski applies torque or stress to the knee joint, resulting in ligamentous damage. Determination of ligamentous damage is dependent upon clinical examination, and routine x-rays add little information.

MEDIAL COLLATERAL LIGAMENT INJURY

The medial collateral ligament consists of a superficial portion on the medial aspect of the tibia beneath the pes anserinus. In addition to the medial collateral ligament are capsular ligaments that form a half-sleeve medially extending from the popliteal space behind to the patellar tendon in front. The anterior portion is represented by the anterior knee capsule with a contribution from the vastus medialis retinaculum. The anterior capsular ligament is tight when the knee is flexed and relaxes as the knee is extended. The middle portion of the capsular ligament is also referred to as the deep layer of the medial ligament and is attached to the medial femoral condyle. The middle one-third is taut in all positions of flexion. The posterior part of the medial capsular ligament is a portion of the posterior capsule. When the knee is extended, the posterior ligament tightens; it slackens as the knee is flexed.

With increasing valgus stress to the knee and usually with simultaneous external rotation of the tibia upon the femur, medial capsular ligaments rupture, followed by rupture of the tibial collateral ligament. If the force continues, rupture of the anterior cruciate may occur (Fig. 43-75).

CLINICAL MANIFESTATIONS. With an acute injury to the medial ligamentous structures, symptoms and findings will vary according to the degree of damage. With a mild sprain without complete disruption of any of the components, the patient may only complain of pain and have a mild hemarthrosis. Occasionally, there is no hemarthrosis as the bleeding is external to the capsule. If clinical examination of the knee does not reveal instability or increased motion as compared with the opposite knee, the injury can be treated as a sprain with temporary immobilization and restriction of activity. When the force results in complete disruption of the ligaments, the findings are usually obvious, and there is no difficulty in deciding upon the need for surgical repair.

The real difficulty lies in moderate degrees of instability on clinical examination. If there is any doubt as to the integrity of the ligaments, the examination should be repeated under anesthesia and surgical exploration carried out as necessary. The uninjured knee is examined first and all examinations repeated on the injured side and compared with the normal. The knee joint is flexed 20° to relax the posterior capsule, and valgus stress is applied to the knee. Opening up of the medial joint space is abnormal and indicates ligamentous discontinuity.

AP stability is tested with the knee at 20° of flexion (the Lachman test). Excessive forward motion of the tibia indicates anterior cruciate injury either isolated or in association with other collateral or capsular injuries. The knee is then flexed to 90° and AP stability tested by pulling the tibia forward on the femur. This is carried out with the tibia in internal rotation, external rotation, and neutral rotation. Motion of the medial tibial condyle greater than 5 mm is abnormal and is a sign of rotational instability with damage to the medial capsular ligament. Forward motion of both condyles is an indication of anterior cruciate damage. When varus stress applied to the knee in 20° of flexion causes greater opening up of the lateral joint than the normal, it indicates lateral collateral and iliotibial band disruption. Valgus and varus testing is carried out on the extended knee to determine the integrity of the posterior capsule. Instability in this position indicates posterior capsule damage in addition to medial or lateral collateral ligament injury.

ANTERIOR CRUCIATE LIGAMENT RUPTURE

The anterior cruciate ligament may be ruptured in association with complete tears of the medial collateral ligaments. Isolated tears occur as the result of hyperextension or internal rotation of the tibia on the femur but may be due to a direct blow on a flexed knee. Determination of anterior cruciate rupture depends upon demonstrating forward displacement of both tibial condyles on the femur usually of more than 5 mm when compared with the op-

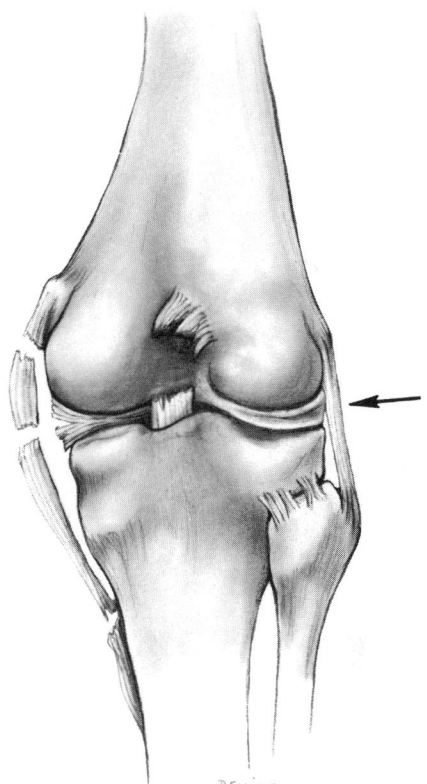

Fig. 43-75. Knee ligament injuries from valgus force. Anterior cruciate is interrupted near its femoral origin. Medial collateral may avulse at the upper and lower ends of rupture in the middle as well as be disrupted from its meniscal attachment. *(After O'Donoghue, with permission.)*

posite uninjured knee. This test is best carried out with the knee in near-extension. Interpretation of the findings is subjective, and great experience is necessary in this examination.

TREATMENT OF MEDIAL COLLATERAL AND CRUCIATE LIGAMENT INJURIES. Mild sprains of the medial collateral ligament when there is no evidence of instability are treated symptomatically. A tense hemarthrosis may be aspirated with considerable relief. The limb is splinted in a position of extension with a compression bandage or a posterior plaster splint. The patient is started on immediate isometric quadriceps exercises performed hourly. The patient may bear partial weight between crutches with the quadriceps set and the knee in full extension. It is helpful to reevaluate the knee in a few days in order to confirm the findings of stability.

Complete tears of the medial collateral ligaments, medial capsular ligaments, or anterior cruciate may require surgical repair. This should be carried out as soon as possible but certainly within 2 weeks. A detached ligament may be retracted from its attachment with resultant healing in a lengthened or lax position. Complete tears in the substance of the anterior cruciate ligament will require reconstruction with a semitendinosus tenodesis or other technique. For isolated tears of the anterior cruciate liga-

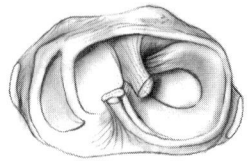 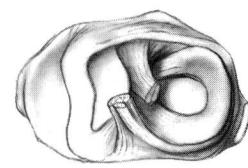

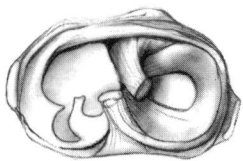 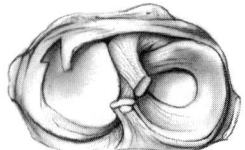

Fig. 43-76. Types of meniscal injury. Top left, complete bucket-handle tear; top right, complete detachment of the meniscus from its peripheral margin; lower left, posterior tab tear; lower right, anterior tab tear of the medial meniscus.

ment, repair and/or reconstruction will depend on the age, occupation, and athletic needs of the patient.

INJURIES TO THE LATERAL COLLATERAL LIGAMENT

The lateral collateral ligament is interrupted when a varus force is applied to the knee. The lateral popliteal nerve, by virtue of its location and fixation as it winds around the neck of the fibula, is commonly stretched by the same injury. The treatment of this acute injury requires open exploration repair of the avulsed ligament from the femoral condyle or head of the fibula. The iliotibial band crossing the knee joint is commonly ruptured and requires repair. The nerve should be examined at the time of surgical treatment, but since this is usually a stretch injury, delayed repair depending upon follow-up evaluation is necessary. Injuries to the posterior cruciate ligament occur rarely as isolated injury but may accompany medial lateral collateral ligamentous injuries. Repair of the posterior cruciate can be attempted.

CHRONIC LIGAMENTOUS INJURIES TO THE KNEE

Persistent laxity of the collateral ligamentous structures or cruciate ligaments results in knee joint instability. Such injuries, if severe, are disabling and may require the competitive athlete to discontinue competition. With minor degrees of instability, symptoms may be apparent only with vigorous athletics. When severe, the knee may be chronically effused, painful, and unstable with normal activity. Patients give a history of pain, locking, sudden giving way, or feeling of instability.

Reconstruction of the chronically unstable knee is difficult and is not always successful in returning a patient to athletics. Reefing the posterior medial capsule, shortening the medial collateral structures, and pes anserinus transfer are of value for medial collateral instability. Similar procedures are available for the lateral side. It is occasionally difficult to separate medial from lateral instability in the chronically unstable knee, in which case stress x-rays should be obtained.

INJURIES OF KNEE MENISCI

The tibia rotates laterally upon the femur as the knee joint goes from flexion to extension, and medial with the opposite motion. If this simultaneous rotation is interfered with or forcibly reversed, the semilunar cartilage may be injured. A common injury occurs when the football player catches a cleated shoe while weight is applied to the flexed knee. Similarly, a person squatting with knees fully flexed and suddenly twisting the knee without simultaneous movement into extension will suffer an acute meniscus tear. Helfet believes that only the fibrotic medial meniscus of the elderly is actually torn by pressure grinding between the femoral and tibial surfaces.

In the young adult, rotation without flexion or extension causes the cartilage to straighten out. If the force is excessive, the cartilage is unable to accommodate, and a tear occurs at its inner free border, usually about the midpoint. The cartilage may be detached from its attachment to the anterior cruciate or be split longitudinally to produce a bucket-handle tear, or it may be injured in its posterior portion by detachment from its posterior capsular attachments (Fig. 43-76). The medial meniscus is injured at least nine times as commonly as the lateral in the Caucasian, although lateral meniscal tears are more common in the Oriental. The medial meniscus is fixed to the capsule and is relatively immobile, whereas the lateral meniscus is not fixed to the capsule and has the popliteus muscle to assist in controlling its position.

CLINICAL MANIFESTATIONS. Meniscal injuries are commonly found in young men who use the knee vigorously, either for athletics or vocationally. Such injuries are less common in women.

The injury causes acute pain, which may subside rapidly. If the cartilage is undisplaced, there may be no immediate interference with motion. A joint effusion, with associated discomfort and stiffness, gradually develops in response to the injury. This will occur sooner and more severely if the meniscal damage is at its peripheral attachment, where blood vessels may be interrupted.

The diagnosis of a torn meniscus will depend on an accurate history, which should include the position of the knee and the direction of the rotational force at the time of the injury. The patient should be questioned about locking, instability, episodes of giving way or buckling, and previous injuries to the knee.

Examination of the knee after an acute injury may reveal varying degrees of joint effusion. There is local tenderness over the meniscus, which is greatest at the site of injury. Stability of the knee ligaments should be examined by valgus, varus, and anteroposterior stress.

The knee motion is examined with special emphasis on testing for synchronous rotation as the knee goes into full extension. By grasping both heels, both knees are passively brought to full extension and any limitation determined. Normally, the tibial tubercle in full extension aligns with the lateral border of the patella. If rotation has been compromised, the tibial tubercle will align with the central axis of the patella. In carrying out extension motions, there is localization of pain to medial or lateral aspects of the joint, at the site of the injury to the meniscus. Palpation of the joint line may indicate displacement of the meniscus. The test described by McMurray to delineate meniscal tears is occasionally helpful. The maneuver is elicited by extending and rotating the flexed knee of the supine patient. The foot is gradually externally rotated, while abduction stress is applied to the knee as it is gradually brought into extension. A displaced portion of the medial meniscus, catching between the femur and tibia, will cause a definite click and pain.

The diagnosis of acute meniscus injury may be difficult. Unless there is definite evidence of locking or displacement of the meniscus, the patient should be treated conservatively and reevaluated when the acute symptoms subside. Knee effusion, if severe, is aspirated, and the knee is brought to maximal extension and immobilized in a splint or compression bandage. The patient is allowed to bear weight between crutches with the quadriceps taut. The patient is reevaluated at weekly intervals and meniscectomy carried out only when the diagnosis is certain.

Arthrography is helpful when the diagnosis is not absolutely certain but the more recent technique of MRI defines the pathology exactly. The technique of arthrography is demanding and requires exact positioning of the knee at the time of x-ray and experience in interpreting the arthrograms.

Diagnostic arthroscopy can improve the accuracy of diagnosis of interarticular lesions, such as torn menisci and torn cruciate ligaments, and locate specific areas of cartilage damage, synovial disease, or tumors by allowing the accurate inspection of all intraarticular cartilage and synovial surfaces. In this technique a small telescope (arthroscope) is inserted percutaneously through puncture wounds in the knee joint. Diagnostic arthroscopy is employed routinely whenever meniscectomy is being considered.

The newer noninvasive technique of MRI will give accurate information on cruciate ligamentous and meniscal injuries and osteochondral fractures.

TREATMENT. Surgical Arthroscopy. When pathology has been located with the diagnostic arthroscope, intraarticular surgery can be done with arthroscopic surgical techniques. Procedures include synovial biopsy, removal of loose bodies, shaving of damaged articular cartilage, meniscorresis, and removal of torn or degenerative menisci. The specific advantage of arthroscopic meniscectomy is the shortening of the postoperative rehabilitation time. By avoiding a large capsular incision patients can move their knees sooner and have less morbidity. A theoretical advantage over conventional meniscectomy is the ability to remove only the offending portion of the meniscus. The possibility exists that there will be less degenerative change when partial meniscectomy is done compared with complete meniscectomy. However, the result

from removal of only the bucket-handle tear portion of a torn meniscus is the same with conventional arthrotomy techniques as when the entire meniscus is excised. When the tear is within the peripheral one-third of the meniscus (where circulation for healing exists), meniscal repair is the treatment of choice if the anterior cruciate ligament is intact.

Fractures of the Patella

Patellar fractures are usually due to direct trauma to the patella but also occur with sudden forced flexion of an actively contracting quadriceps. Fractures are more commonly transverse or comminuted but may take any direction. As the patella is an integral part of the extensor mechanism, separation at the fracture site is an indication that the adjacent patellar retinacula have been interrupted and active extension will not be possible (Fig. 43-77). Treatment is aimed at restoring a smoothly gliding extensor mechanism.

TREATMENT. Undisplaced fractures require a plaster cylinder cast for 6 to 8 weeks to prevent separation of the fragments. Check x-rays in plaster should be obtained at 7 to 10 days to be certain that displacement has not occurred. The patient is instructed in quadriceps exercises and may bear partial weight between crutches.

Transverse fractures with separation of the fragments require operative intervention to restore continuity of the extensor mechanism. Although some surgeons advocate circumferential wire suture to hold the fragments together, there is usually enough comminution in the region of the subchondral surface of the patella that an irregular articular surface of the patella will remain. For this reason, excision of the smaller fragments, usually the lower half, is indicated, combined with reattachment of the patellar ligament through drill holes on the raw fracture sur-

Fig. 43-77. Comminuted fracture of patella. *A,* AP and *B,* lateral x-rays showing comminuted patella with separation of the upper and lower major fragments indicating interruption of the extensor mechanism.

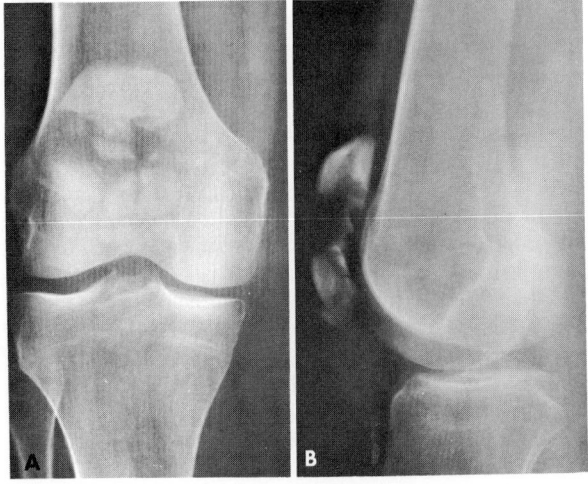

face of the proximal fragment. At the same time, the patellar retinaculum is surgically repaired.

For grossly comminuted fractures of the patella, immediate excision of all fragments is carried out and the quadriceps mechanism repaired. Postoperatively, the limb is maintained in extension, and quadriceps exercises are immediately instituted. At 4 weeks, the cast is removed and beginning range-of-motion exercises started. At 6 weeks, active flexion is begun. The same principles apply to open fractures of the patella.

The quadriceps may be ruptured or the patellar ligament avulsed from its insertion on the patella when acute flexion forces are applied to the contracting extensor mechanism. Immediate diagnosis and surgical repair are required.

Recurrent Dislocation of the Patella

The patella may be dislocated in any direction. Upward dislocation is the result of rupture of the patellar ligament. Medial dislocation is uncommon but may occur from severe injury or, rarely, after poliomyelitis. Lateral dislocation is the most common type. This may occur with severe injury or poliomyelitis but is most commonly seen in young women or girls after minor trauma. It is related to the increased valgus angle of the female knee but may also be the result of hypoplastic development of the external condyle of the femur, congenital abnormalities of the patella, or congenital contractures of the vastus intermedius.

The patient complains of the knee's giving way as the patella momentarily slips laterally over the lateral femoral condyle and spontaneously reduces. In more severe cases the patella may become lodged lateral to the femoral condyle, requiring manipulative reduction. Following spontaneous relocation of the patella, the patient has symptoms of mild synovitis and effusion.

Initial treatment for the acutely dislocated patella is manual reduction followed by immobilization of the knee in full extension in plaster and rehabilitation of quadriceps muscle power. It is necessary to treat the initial dislocation by plaster immobilization of the knee, or the medial patellar retinaculum will heal with capsular laxity, allowing subsequent dislocation. By maintaining the tone of the vastus medialis, there may be sufficient muscle power to prevent subsequent dislocation. With recurrent dislocations, surgical treatment is usually necessary. Before epiphyseal closure, the Roux-Goldthwait operation may be done. This consists of transposing the lateral half of the patellar ligament at its insertion medially beneath the undisturbed medial insertion. At the same time, an ellipse of capsule and medial patella retinaculum is excised and the capsule reefed to hold the patella medially. After the age of fourteen a modification of the Hauser procedure in which the bone containing the tibial tubercle is moved medially and distally, and elevated anteriorily is utilized. With recurrent dislocation, the progression of chondromalacia to severe damage to the undersurface of the patella rarely necessitates patellectomy and quadricepsplasty.

Fractures of the Tibial Plateau

Fractures of the tibial plateau are more common in the middle-aged or elderly. Fractures of the lateral tibial plateau occur when there is a sudden valgus stress to the knee joint, when there is an axial load applied to the femoral shaft. Common causes involve an automobile bumper striking the knee joint of a pedestrian or a worker falling from a scaffolding. The medial collateral ligament may be ruptured, concomitantly.

Types of fractures are (1) a simple split fracture of the lateral tibial plateau, (2) severe comminution of the lateral tibial plateau, and (3) fractures of both condyles with a vertical fracture line into the region of the tibial spines.

TREATMENT. If the medial collateral ligament is ruptured, surgical repair is indicated. If there is severe displacement of the lateral tibial plateau, open reduction in an attempt at elevation of the depression may be required.

Many fractures with minimal depression can be handled by the method of Weissman and Harold. Large hemarthroses are aspirated. The knee is splinted in extension for 1 week during which time hourly quadriceps and straight-leg-raising exercises are instituted. When normal quadriceps muscle power has been regained, flexion exercises are started; a posterior splint is reapplied between exercises. The splint is gradually discontinued as power and motion improve. Partial weight bearing is permitted between 4 and 6 weeks, and full weight bearing at about 8 to 10 weeks. A fracture with significant condylar depression and displacement will require open treatment.

Tibial Shaft Fractures

Fractures of the tibial shaft occur from direct trauma and may occur when an automobile passenger strikes a leg against the dashboard or when the leg of a pedestrian is struck by a car bumper (Fig. 43-78). Fractures also may occur by indirect torsional forces as with sports injuries, such as in skiing. Some fractures of the tibia occur from simple falls.

Tibial shaft fractures occur at any age. About 70 percent of such fractures are closed and 30 percent open. Indirect torsional forces cause oblique or spiral fractures, whereas direct trauma may result in transverse, segmental, or comminuted fractures of the tibial shaft. There is no difference in the rate of healing of tibial shaft fractures according to the location of the fracture or the plane of the fracture surface. Rate of healing is correlated with the severity of trauma. Fractures caused by high-energy trauma from automobile accidents with or without open wounds have the longest rate of healing. The presence of an intact fibula results in a more rapid rate of union.

CLINICAL MANIFESTATIONS. Undisplaced fractures may have only tenderness and swelling at the site of fracture, but patients are unable to put weight on the affected extremity. Undisplaced spiral fractures occur in the very young. Such fractures may be quite stable, and diagnosis is suggested by the fact that the child will not use the affected leg. Displaced fractures result in deformity with

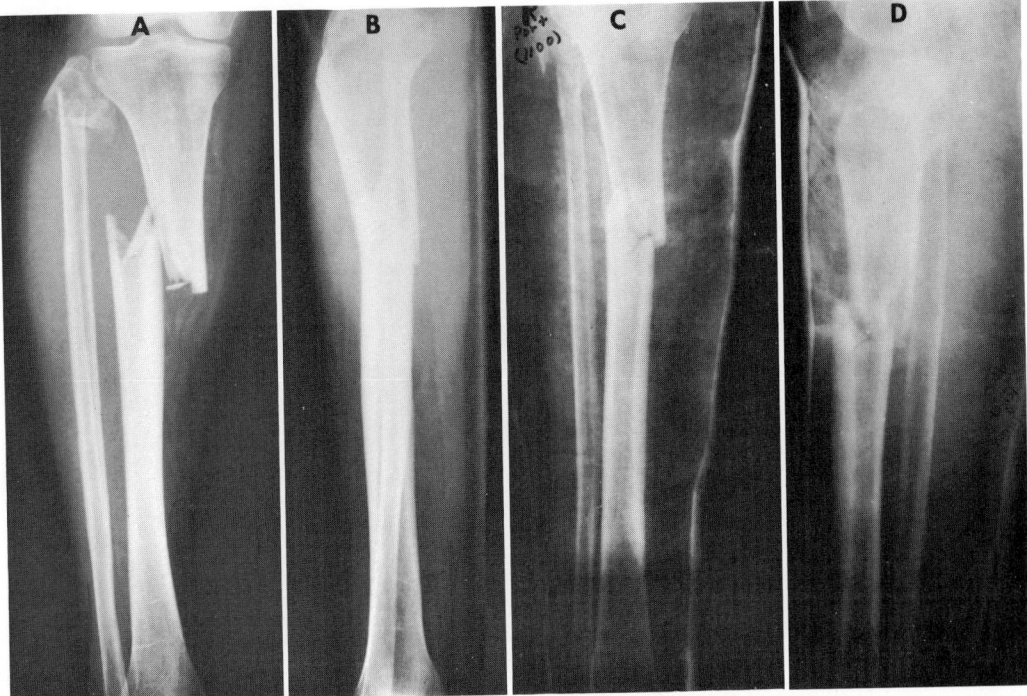

Fig. 43-78. Fracture of the proximal tibia shaft with fracture of the neck of the fibula incurred by an automobile bumper's striking a pedestrian. *A* and *B*. AP and lateral x-rays postinjury. *C* and *D*. AP and lateral x-rays showing postreduction position in a long leg cast.

swelling and ecchymosis. Anteroposterior and lateral x-rays will characterize the fracture.

TREATMENT. Closed tibial shaft fractures are best handled by closed conservative measures (Fig. 43-79) using plaster methods and allowing early weight bearing.

Technique of Closed Reduction

With the patient under analgesia or local anesthesia to the fracture site and lying supine with both legs flexed at the knees, hanging over the end of the table, most tibial shaft fractures can be realigned and deformity corrected by gentle manipulation. The opposite leg is used as a guide to determine correction of rotation and deformity.

Over one layer of stockinet and one layer of sheet wadding, a well-molded plaster cast is applied to the knee with the foot in 10 to 15° of plantar flexion or, if possible, at a right angle. When the plaster has hardened, the knee is brought to full extension and the plaster extended to include the thigh. The reduction is checked by AP and lateral x-rays. The patient is hospitalized with the leg elevated and ice applied over the region of the fracture site. Circulation to the foot and the patient's ability to dorsiflex and plantar flex toes comfortably is checked every 2 h to be certain that vascular insufficiency or compartment syndromes are not occurring. If necessary, the cast is split to relieve swelling.

When the patient is comfortable and can actively control the affected extremity, the patient is allowed up on crutches to bear as much weight as pain tolerates. The patient may continue in the long leg cast until union is complete, or at 3 weeks the plaster may be changed to a below-knee cast appropriately molded about the tibial condyles and patellar ligament to control rotation.

Any type of fracture including transverse, comminuted, or oblique spiral fractures may be treated in this fashion. Approximately a ½-cm shortening can be anticipated from the weight-bearing treatment in addition to whatever shortening is present at the time of the closed reduction. If this seems unacceptable, pins may be placed above and below the fracture site to control length and weight bearing not allowed. In some fractures, because of inability to control position and in some polytrauma patients, blind intramedullary nailing may be necessary. Open reduction and plating is contraindicated because of the severity of problems if infection occurs.

Management of Compound Fractures. Compound fractures must be immediately debrided and fractures immobilized. Depending upon the kind of wound and adequacy of debridement, the skin may be closed, but the indications for this are extremely rare. Secondary closure of the wound may be carried out or the wound left open to granulate beneath a weight-bearing plaster cast. The use of internal fixation in open fractures is not justified because of the hazard of infection, skin loss, and nonunion. Administration of antibiotics is continued until the wound is healed and followed with appropriate check x-rays during the first month to make certain that position is being maintained. Cast wedging or remanipulation may be required to restore alignment.

Compartment Syndromes. After fractures, soft tissue injury, prolonged limb compression (as in drug-overdosed patients), and arterial operations, progressive muscle

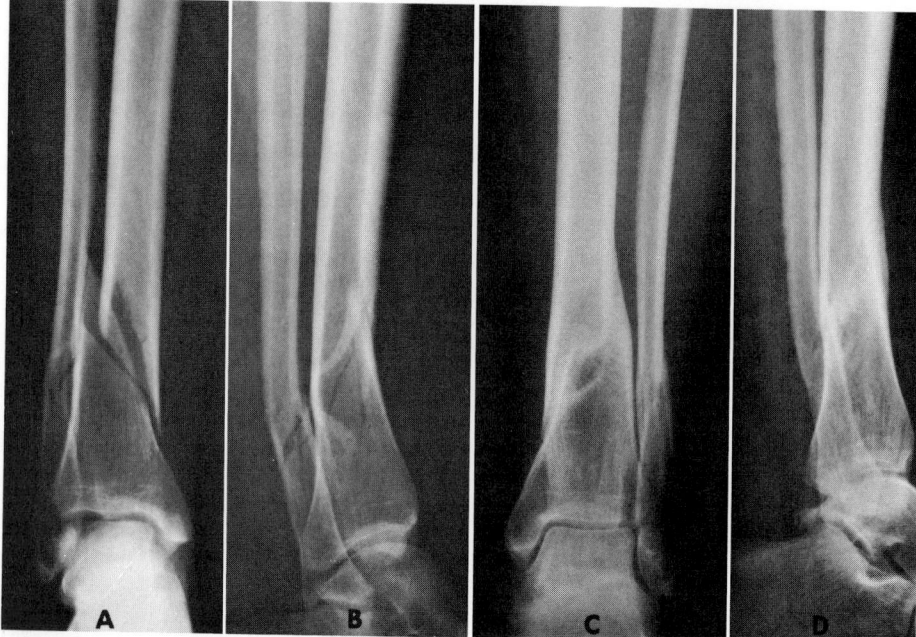

Fig. 43-79. Fracture of the distal tibia and fibula shafts. *A* and *B*. AP and lateral x-rays postinjury. *C* and *D*. AP and lateral x-rays showing healed fracture in satisfactory position.

ischemia may occur in any of the fascial compartments of the limbs. In the upper extremity this includes the anterior compartments of the forearm, and in the lower extremity the four anterior and posterior compartments. The mechanism involved is unrelieved swelling in the tight osseofascial compartments. The arteries may continue to pulsate while the ischemia is developing, since the latter occurs when the capillary filling pressure is exceeded. Hence the clinical signs depend upon detection of change in muscle function, i.e., loss of motor power or extreme pain with passive stretch. Patients should also be observed for ischemic pain (severe pain at rest) or pain not responding to analgesics. Distal pulses of the extremity are usually present early in the course and may persist until complete and irreversible necrosis has occurred.

Prevention of sequelae depends upon early recognition and surgical decompression of the individual compartments. Compartment pressures can be determined by direct measurement, as with the Wick catheter, but when in doubt surgical exploration (and decompression) is indicated. It is important to consider the possibility that compartment syndromes may develop after open fractures or during elective tibial osteotomies. In those instances compartments should be decompressed prophylactically.

Ankle Injuries

ANATOMY. Motion of the tibiotalar joint is pure flexion and extension. Inversion and eversion of the foot is accomplished at the subtalar and midtarsal joints. The upper surface of the talus is dome-shaped in the anteroposterior plane, with a narrower articular surface, poste-

riorly. The talus is without muscular origin or insertion and is attached to its related articulations by capsule and ligaments. The ankle mortise is formed by the downward medial and lateral projections of malleoli grasping the dome of the talus. Maintenance of the normal mortise is a prerequisite for painless ankle motion. Stability of the talus in the mortise is dependent on the distal tibiofibular ligaments and interosseous membrane, as well as the anterior and posterior talofibular ligaments, calcaneofibular ligaments laterally, and a strong deltoid ligament medially.

MECHANISMS OF INJURY. Ankle injuries are caused by a sudden application of force that exceeds the strength of the ligaments or malleoli. Applied across the ankle joint, the force rotates the foot into inversion-eversion, or adduction-abduction in relation to the tibia, or rotates the tibia similarly in relation to the fixed foot. Athletic injuries account for a large proportion of ankle injuries, although a simple fall or sudden misstep may be sufficient to cause a severe fracture-dislocation. All combinations of ligamentous injuries and fractures are possible, depending upon the severity and direction of force.

The injured ankle should be carefully examined for the location of tenderness, swelling, and deformity. If the patient was able to walk on the ankle immediately after the injury, this indicates stability but does not rule out undisplaced fracture. Caution should be applied in diagnosing injuries on the football field before all signs have had time to develop.

The ankle can be splinted with an air splint or with a pillow splint until x-ray examination is complete. Three x-ray views are necessary for x-ray evaluation of the ankle joint. Standard AP and lateral x-rays are required and, in addition, a 30° medial oblique view to determine the competence of the mortise.

LIGAMENTOUS INJURIES

The most common ankle injury that involves portions of the lateral collateral ligaments is caused by a sudden inversion force applied to the foot. The anterior talofibular ligament is usually involved. There is local tenderness and ecchymosis at the midpoint or attachments of the anterior talofibular ligament or calcaneofibular or posterior talofibular ligaments. If the patient has minimal swelling and tenderness on examination, can walk with minimal discomfort, and x-rays are normal, it is sufficient to treat the injury as a sprain by adhesive strapping for 2 to 4 weeks. Patients with more pain may require crutches or plaster casting up to 6 weeks.

Distal Tibiofibular Diastasis

With eversion injuries to the ankle, there may be interruption of the ligamentous continuity of the distal tibiofibular joint, resulting in a diastasis of the ankle mortise. The patient's ankle is unable to bear weight, and marked swelling occurs in the region of the tibiofibular joint.

It is rarely possible to maintain reduction without operative intervention. A 1½-in. vertical incision is made over the distal fibula and the periosteum elevated from the fibula, proximal to the level of the tibiotalar articulation. A lag screw is inserted across an overdrilled hole in the fibula to close the diastasis. This is accomplished with the ankle at 90° and not with the foot in plantar flexion. When the foot is in plantar flexion, the narrowest portion of the talus is in contact with the tibia, and permanent limitation of dorsiflexion will result. At 8 weeks, the cast is removed and the screw excised at a second operation.

FRACTURES AND DISLOCATIONS

Undisplaced fractures of malleoli require immobilization in plaster for 8 weeks. The most common isolated malleolar fracture is an oblique fracture of the lateral malleolus caused by an external rotation injury. If the ankle mortise is not involved, a well-molded plaster cast is applied with the foot in neutral varus-valgus position and maintained for 6 weeks. Check x-rays are obtained to be certain that reduction has not been lost. If there is a fracture of the lateral malleolus with lateral displacement of the talus, this is corrected by manipulation under local or general anesthesia and the hind part of the foot placed in maximal inversion with the ankle at 90° of dorsiflexion. If the mortise cannot be restored to normal by closed techniques, open reduction and internal fixation is indicated.

Medial Malleolar Fractures

Undisplaced fractures of the medial malleolus with an intact mortise are treated by plaster immobilization. Bimalleolar ankle fractures with dislocation require accu-

rate reduction until union is solid. The usual mechanism of injury of a bimalleolar fracture is by external rotation and eversion. If the talus is displaced laterally, reduction is necessary. Most fractures can be handled by closed reduction.

Technique of Closed Reduction. With local or general anesthesia and the leg hanging over the end of the table, traction is applied to the hind part of the foot in the long axis of the leg. With traction maintained, the hind part of the foot is gradually brought into inversion, to correct the lateral displacement, while lateral countertraction is applied to the medial subcutaneous surface of the tibia. Simultaneously the foot, which is resting on the knee of the operator, is brought into 90° of dorsiflexion. The reduction should be stable when the foot is held at 90° of dorsiflexion at maximal inversion. A well-molded cast is applied over one thickness of stockinet and one thickness of sheet wadding. The cast is then extended to include the knee. Check x-rays are obtained and the patient admitted to the hospital for evaluation of circulation. If the medial malleolus fracture extends to the point where the vertical and horizontal articular cartilage meet at the distal end of the tibia, sufficient medial buttress will not be present to hold a closed reduction, and open reduction will be required. Closed reduction or open reduction and internal fixation with screws or plates is carried out on the fibular malleolus (Fig. 43-80). Failed closed reduction of malleolar fractures implies the interposition of periosteum flap and requires elevation and screw fixation.

Posterior Malleolar Fractures

The posterior malleolus is usually fractured in combination with medial or lateral malleolar fractures. The importance of the posterior malleolus is to maintain anteroposterior stability of the ankle joint. When 30 percent of the tibial articular surface is involved in the posterior malleolar fracture, instability will ensue if anatomic reduction is not obtained.

Anatomic reduction of a large posterior malleolar fragment can be maintained only with internal fixation. The posterior malleolar fragment is fixed with a screw to the major tibial fragment. Trimalleolar fractures with small posterior fragments and good anteroposterior stability require maintenance of reduction of the mortise, and the posterior fragment can be disregarded (Fig. 43-81).

Fractures involving the anterior articular surface occur from severe trauma, as in falls from heights and in automobile injuries. The anterior portion of the distal tibial articular surface may be fractured or crushed, but usually this is in association with adjacent malleolar fractures. Such injuries are serious, because there is an associated crush injury to the articular cartilage that may cause difficulty, regardless of the reduction.

Attempts should be made to realign the articular surface by closed manipulation. In some cases, it may be possible to perform open reduction, although when comminution is severe, subsequent ankle arthrodesis may be necessary.

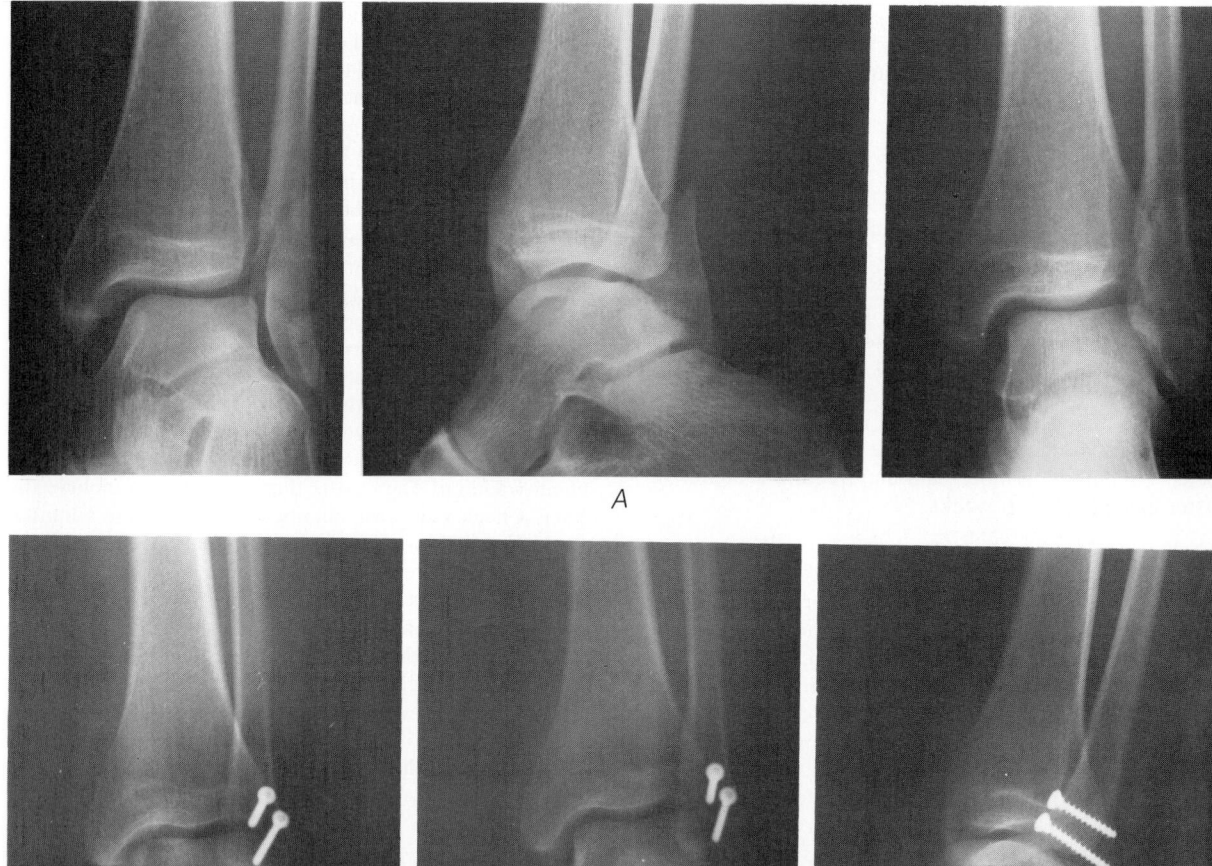

Fig. 43-80. *A.* Fractured fibular malleolus with torn deltoid and wide ankle mortise (supination external rotation type fracture). *B.* Open reduction and screw fixation of the fibula fracture was carried out. The deltoid ligament was opened and sutured.

Fractures and Dislocations of the Foot

FRACTURES AND DISLOCATIONS OF THE TALUS

The talus is fractured in its distal portion, through the neck or body. Neck fractures account for the majority of talus injuries. Fractures of the neck occur from forcible dorsiflexion of the foot, such that the neck is driven against the anterior margin of the distal tibia.

If the vertical force continues, a subtalar dislocation may complicate the fracture. Still greater force is associated with fractures of the neck of the talus, subtalar dislocation, and posterior displacement of the body from the ankle joint. Such fracture-dislocations are commonly compound. In some cases, the patient presents with the posterior body of the talus having been driven out through the wound and left at the scene of the accident.

The subtalar joint may be dislocated by maximal inversion stress in the position of plantar flexion. In such a case, the foot is dislocated medially, beneath the body of the talus. Greater force results in dislocation of the talus from the ankle joint, resulting in total dislocation of the talus.

If there is sufficient damage across the neck of the talus, avascular necrosis of the body may ensue. In one series, avascular necrosis developed in 69 percent of neck fracture-dislocations and 50 percent of body fractures.

TREATMENT. Fractures of the neck are treated by closed reduction and plaster cast immobilization until bony union is complete. Displaced fractures with dislocation are reduced by closed manipulation carried out with the foot in the talipes equinus position. If accurate closed reduction cannot be accomplished, open reduction is indicated. Care is taken not to devitalize soft tissue attach-

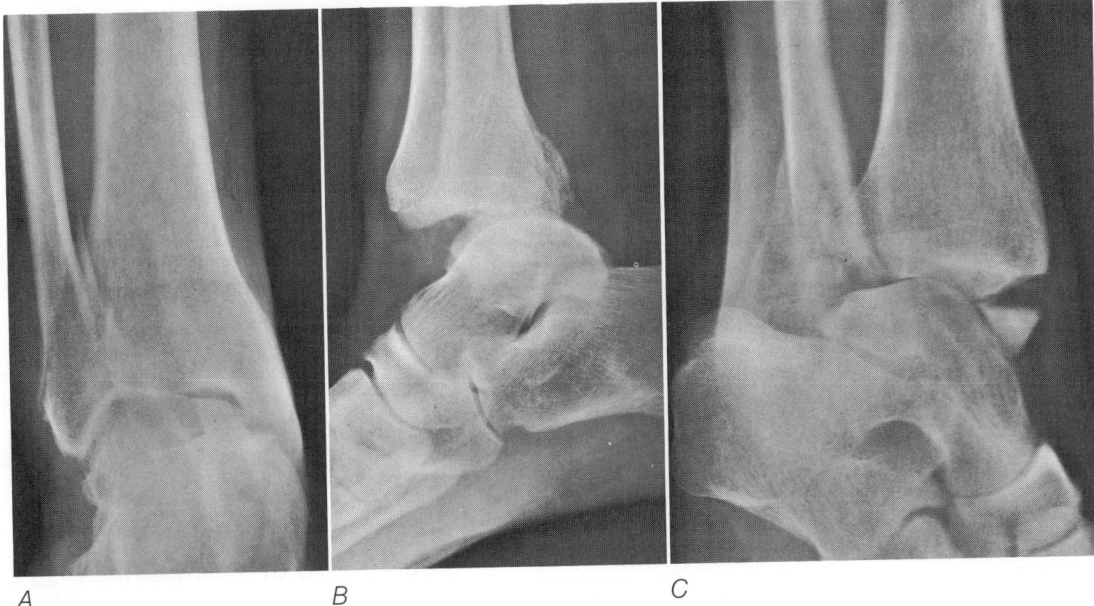

Fig. 43-81. Trimalleolar ankle fracture-dislocation. *A, B,* and *C.* AP, lateral, and oblique x-rays showing posterior dislocation of the talus and fractures of the medial malleolus, the lateral malleolus, and a small fragment from the posterior malleolus.

ments. Kirschner wires are used for internal fixation. Postoperative plaster immobilization is continued for 3 months or longer until union is evident.

Undisplaced fractures of the body of the talus may be treated by immobilization in neutral position. For severe compression fractures, primary tibial-talar fusion using the method of Blair may be indicated. Avascular necrosis, which develops in the majority of cases, is not a deterrent to a good result if immobilization is continued until union is solid and weight bearing is prevented until revascularization occurs.

Complete talar dislocations or subtalar dislocations are reduced by placing the foot in maximal inversion and, with direct pressure over the talus, bringing the calcaneus and forefoot into eversion. Considerable force and general anesthesia may be necessary to accomplish reduction of the completely dislocated talus. The foot is then immobilized until soft tissue healing is complete.

FRACTURES OF THE CALCANEUS

Fractures of the calcaneus commonly occur from falls in which the maximal force is applied to the calcaneus. Involvement of the posterior articular facet is least likely to occur when the foot is in maximal pronation. The main fracture line is oblique, creating two major fragments, an anteromedial fragment and a posterolateral fragment. Fractures of the anterior portion of the calcaneus or the tuberosity also may occur.

A suitable classification of fractures of the calcaneus has been described by Dart and Graham (Fig. 43-82). Type I isolated fractures include beak fractures of the tuberosity or fractures of the anterior part of the calcaneus with minimal calcaneocuboid joint involvement.

Type II includes fractures of the body without joint surface involvement. Type IIIa consists of depressed fractures of the posterior facet with minimal depression of Böhler's angle. Böhler's angle (tuberosity joint angle) is the angle formed by the axis of the subtalar joint and the superior surface of the tuberosity. Type IIIb is severe depression of Böhler's angle. Type IV fractures are grossly comminuted fractures, involving subtalar and calcaneocuboid joints. Type V consists of avulsions of the tendocalcaneus with a portion of bone from the posterior portion of the calcaneus.

Fractures that involve the posterior facet joint are of two types, the joint depression type and tongue type. Both types arise in the medial cortex of the os calcis and divide the bone into a superomedial fragment and a lateral fragment. The identification of the fracture type is impor-

Fig. 43-82. Types of fracture of the calcaneus. *(After Dart and Graham, with permission.)*

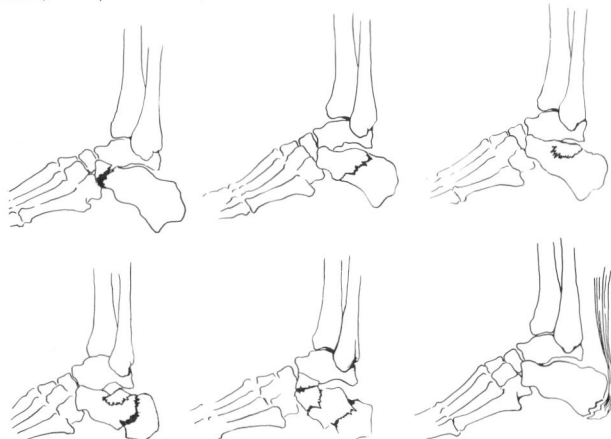

tant because careful reconstitution of this medial wall by open reduction and derotation of the superomedial fragment can restore the subtalar joint.

Approximately 25 percent of patients presenting with fractures of the calcaneus have associated injuries, including compression fractures of the spine, pelvic fractures, or fractures in the lower extremities.

TREATMENT. The patient should be hospitalized; regardless of what course of treatment is decided upon, the limb must be immediately elevated to prevent swelling and minimize hematoma formation. Types I and II are treated by bed rest, elevation, and early range-of-motion exercises. Patients are allowed to ambulate with crutches after 2 to 3 weeks, and weight bearing is prevented for 3 months. In Type III fractures, of the tongue or joint depression type, open reduction of the superomedial fragment through the medial approach and fixation with a three-pronged staple as described by McReynolds gives excellent results. Patients are allowed to walk in a short leg cast postoperatively. Plaster is removed at 5 to 8 weeks.

One may elect the same type of treatment for Type IV fractures, although rest, elevation, and early mobilization without weight bearing is an alternative method for both Types III and IV fractures. For Type V fractures, the fragment should have open reduction and screw fixation of the tendocalcaneus insertion.

METATARSAL FRACTURES

Fractures of the Fifth Metatarsal

The base of the fifth metatarsal may be fractured during inversion injuries of the foot. The attachment of the peroneus brevis to the base of the fifth metatarsal avulses this portion of the bone during sudden, forceful inversion. The patient may sustain an associated sprain of the anterior talotibular ligament at the same time. On examination, there is local tenderness over the base of the fifth metatarsal. The patient may be unable to bear weight because of discomfort.

Treatment of this injury is symptomatic. For some individuals, taping of the foot and ankle to provide immobilization in the position of eversion is all that is necessary. Most patients, however, are best managed with a short leg walking plaster that will provide stability and comfort for a 4- to 6-week period.

Multiple Metatarsal Fractures

Fractures of the metatarsal shafts may occur with severe traumatic or crush injuries to the foot. Isolated fractures of the necks of fourth and fifth metatarsals may also occur. Stress fractures of the shafts of the second and third metatarsals should be suspected when the patient complains of insidious pain, without acute injury.

Fracture-dislocations occur at the tarsometatarsal junction, with associated fractures of the bases of metatarsals. Such injuries occur from severe trauma, such as cycling injuries or crush injuries to the feet. There is commonly associated severe soft tissue damage with or without compounding. In closed fractures, reduction should be accomplished by closed efforts, but in some instances Kirschner wire fixation is required. The handling of multiple fractures of the metatarsal shafts should include an attempt at alignment to restore painless weight bearing.

PHALANGEAL FRACTURES

Fractures of the phalanges of the toes may occur at any age from direct trauma to the forefoot, as in the dropping of heavy objects upon the toes or striking the toes against a door or foot of the bed. Such an injury may dislocate MP or IP joints as well.

Treatment of phalangeal fractures is directed at alignment and relief of pain. Reduction should be accomplished and the toes splinted to adjacent toes with adhesive tape. The patient may be allowed to walk if symptoms are tolerated.

PELVIC AND SPINE INJURIES

Acetabular Fractures and Hip Dislocations

Dislocation of the hip with or without associated fracture of the acetabulum is caused by force applied to the proximal femur. Such injuries may result from automobile collisions, pedestrian injuries, or falls from a great height. The type of fracture and dislocation is dependent upon the position of the hip and the direction of the force at the moment of impact. Force applied to an abducted femur may result in an anterior hip dislocation without fracture. Striking the knee on a dashboard of a car with the hip in a position of adduction and flexed at 90° may result in a posterior dislocation (Fig. 43-83) with or without a fracture of the posterior acetabular rim. Direct trauma to the trochanter with the hip in various positions will result in inner wall or bursting fractures of the acetabulum, including central dislocation.

Patients with fracture-dislocations about the hip may have other, more serious injuries, as with any fractures of the pelvis. Regardless of the type of dislocation, reduction should be accomplished as soon as possible, to minimize the chance of avascular necrosis of the femoral head.

ANTERIOR HIP DISLOCATIONS

Such injuries occur from extreme abduction or trauma applied anteroposteriorly to an abducted thigh. Patients with this dislocation have the thigh held in abduction, flexion, and external rotation. Reduction is accomplished by applying force to the anesthetized patient in the direction of the deformity. When muscle resistance has been overcome and the femoral head has been pulled laterally to the rim of the acetabulum, the leg is adducted in flexion and internally rotated. Check x-rays are obtained to be certain that bone fragments are not displaced into the acetabulum. If bone fragments are obstructing reduction, open excision of the fragments must be accomplished.

The patient is maintained in traction, with the hip in

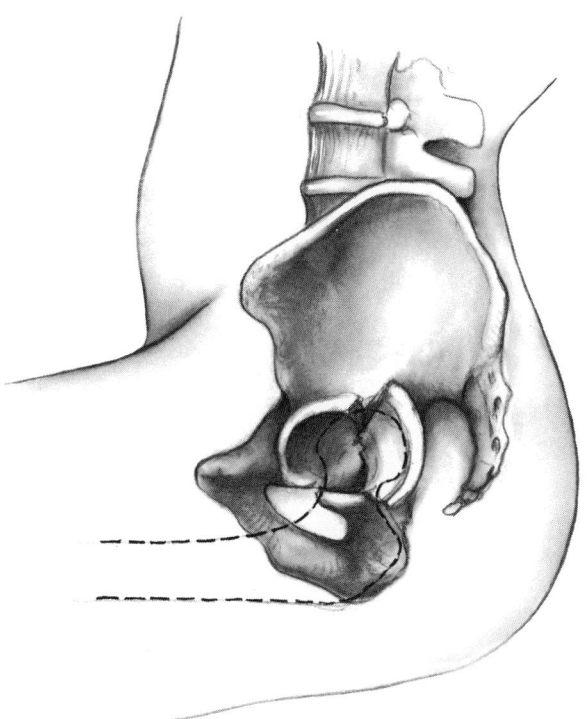

Fig. 43-83. Posterior dislocation of the hip with fracture of the posterior acetabular rim. Axial force applied to the femur drives the femoral head from the acetabulum and the posterior rim of the acetabulum along with it. Such injuries are common to automobile passengers.

extension for 10 to 14 days, following which active range of motion is carried out. Crutch walking with partial weight bearing is continued for 6 weeks, and then full weight bearing is allowed.

Fig. 43-84. Posterior dislocation of the hip with fracture of the acetabular rim. *A.* AP x-ray postinjury showing the femoral head, which appears smaller than that of the opposite side and is superiorly displaced. *B.* AP x-ray showing the relocation of the femoral head with persistent displacement of the acetabular fragment. *C.* AP x-ray following open reduction and screw fixation of the acetabular fragment.

POSTERIOR HIP DISLOCATIONS

Posterior hip dislocations occur when axial force is applied to the flexed, adducted femur. The hip may be dislocated through a rent in the posterior capsule or with the posterior rim of the acetabulum driven off by the femoral head (Fig. 43-84). The diagnosis is usually apparent on clinical examination. The clinical deformity reveals the hip in a position of flexion adduction and internal rotation. Careful examination for sciatic nerve integrity is essential. Attempts to lower the limb to the table are met with severe resistance and anguish from the patient. Reduction of a dislocation should be accomplished immediately, but not before x-rays define the lesion. A standard AP x-ray of the pelvis is required, but a lateral x-ray of the hip joint may be necessary to demonstrate the dislocation accurately.

TREATMENT. Before moving the patient from the x-ray table, reduction should be accomplished. Most patients can be reduced under mild analgesia or with local anesthesia to the hip joint, but a few require general anesthesia. The basic principle is to pull the dislocated femoral head back through the rent in the capsule. If a large fragment has been fractured from the acetabulum, reduction may not be difficult. It is imperative to rule out intraarticular fractures and displaced fragments by CT.

Technique of Reduction. With the patient lying supine and with countertraction exerted across the pelvis, traction is applied to the long axis of the femoral shaft, with the knee flexed, and with the hip in a position of flexion, adduction, and internal rotation. When the femoral head has been brought to the level of the posterior acetabular rim, the femur is gradually abducted, externally rotated, and placed in extension. If this cannot be accomplished gently or if the hip does not reduce with a sudden click, it should not be forced, or fracture of the femoral neck may occur. The stability or tendency to redislocation should be estimated after reduction, to decide whether screw fixation of this fragment is indicated. Anteroposterior, oblique, and lateral check x-rays or a CT scan are obtained to delineate the position of the posterior rim of the acetabulum to be certain that fragments are not displaced intraarticularly and that the posterior acetabular rim has

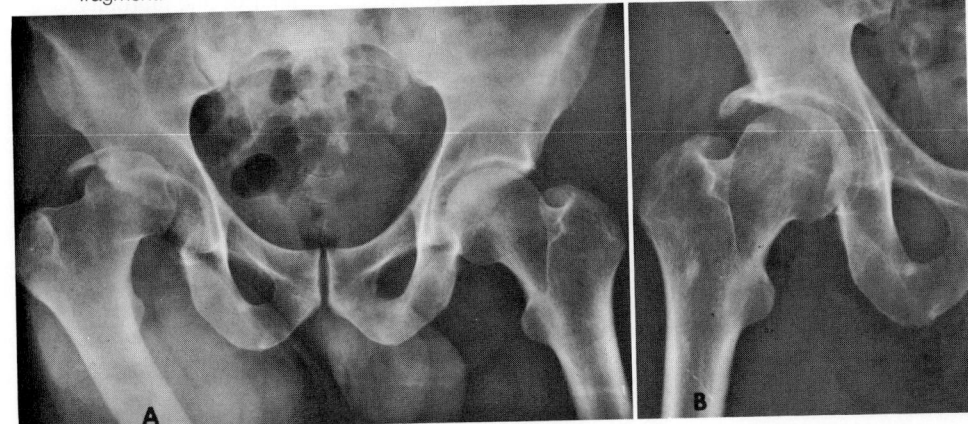
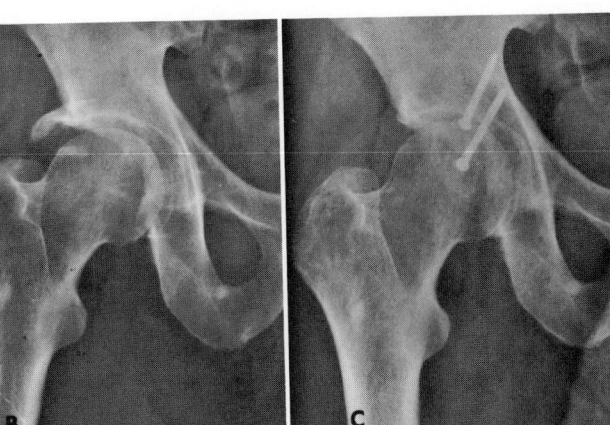

A   B   C

been satisfactorily reduced. As a general rule, the acetabular rim requires open reduction. It is important to reduce the dislocation promptly and carry out open reduction of the acetabular rim when the patient's condition warrants, usually within the first week.

The uncomplicated dislocation is reduced, the patient is placed in skin traction of 10 lb for 10 to 14 days, and weight bearing is prevented for an additional 4 weeks. Aspirin is administered to minimize progression of the cartilage injury sustained at the time of dislocation. All patients with hip dislocations should be followed indefinitely after this injury, because of the incidence of avascular necrosis and degenerative arthritis. Avascular necrosis, the incidence of which is directly related to the delay of reduction, develops in about 20 percent of patients and is usually clinically apparent by the 2-year interval. Traumatic arthritis occurs in about 50 percent of patients and may occur as late as 5 years postreduction. When a sciatic nerve lesion is diagnosed, open reduction is indicated.

FRACTURES OF THE INNER WALL OF THE ACETABULUM

Fractures of the inner wall of the acetabulum represent the most common type. If there is a central dislocation of the femoral head and the superior dome of the acetabulum is intact, reduction of the dislocation should be accomplished by manipulation and maintained with skeletal traction for 8 weeks. The femoral head must be reduced into a normal relationship with the intact superior weight-bearing portion of the acetabulum. Active motion of the hip is then begun. Protected weight bearing between crutches is not allowed until the fractures are consolidated, about 4 months after injury.

Fractures of the Superior Acetabulum

Bursting or superior wall fractures have the worst prognosis of acetabular fractures. The ultimate result will depend upon the severity of comminution of the superior dome, as well as the restoration of the superior dome relationship to the femoral head. Attempts should be made to restore this relationship by closed or conservative methods. In some instances, open reduction through an anterior approach or even a combined anterior and posterior approach is necessary.

Pelvic Fractures

The pelvic ring, composed of the coxae and sacrum, provides protection for the pelvic viscera, attachments of muscles, and the transmission of weight-bearing forces from the lower extremities. Only the posterolateral wings, which connect the acetabula with the sacrum, function in the transmission of weight.

Injuries to the pelvic ring may occur at any age and from various types of violence. Elderly patients with osteoporosis who fall may sustain isolated fractures of the pubic rami or undisplaced fractures of the acetabula, the coccyx, or even the sacrum but usually do not have disruptions of the weight-bearing segments. The most com-

mon cause of the pelvic fracture is automobile collision. Newer techniques of CT and MRI provide better definition of actual pathology.

CLINICAL MANIFESTATIONS. Patients with acute fracture of the pelvis are unable to bear weight without discomfort. If this is an isolated fracture of the pubic ramus, weight bearing on the affected side causes pain in the groin. There may be local tenderness and swelling at the site of the fractured pubic ramus.

The examiner should test the stability of the pelvis by anterior compression with direct pressure over the symphysis and should determine lateral stability by compressing the pelvis in a frontal plane and applying direct pressure over both iliac wings. Both hips should be put through a range of motion. Any pain associated with these maneuvers requires AP, lateral, and oblique x-ray views of the pelvis to delineate fractures and displacement.

TREATMENT. The treatment of the acute pelvic fracture is first directed at the detection and treatment of associated injuries to the pelvic viscera or abdominal viscera, as well as treatment for shock. One-third of patients with pelvic fractures die as a result of local hemorrhage. Patients with severe retroperitoneal or pelvic hemorrhage complain of abdominal or back pain. There may be signs of hemorrhage into the scrotum or buttocks. If there is any doubt of intraabdominal hemorrhage, laparotomy is indicated. The risk of laparotomy is far outweighed by the hazard associated with missing an intraabdominal lesion. Ten to twelve percent of patients with pelvic fractures, especially bilateral pubic rami fractures, have an associated injury to the bladder or urethra. Therefore, a large indwelling catheter should be inserted immediately and retrograde cystograms obtained. Lesions of the lumbosacral plexus also should be suspected.

Isolated fractures occurring in elderly patients from a single fall are treated by bed rest for a few days, until acute symptoms subside. The patient is then gradually mobilized, and weight bearing is allowed as it is tolerated. Since the anterior arch is not contributing to weight bearing, there is no problem of pelvic stability. Thrombophlebitis and ileus with urinary retention are common complications.

Bilateral fractures of the pubic rami (Fig. 43-85) have the highest incidence of associated injuries and mortality of any pelvic fractures. Some degree of immobilization of bilateral pubic rami fractures can be obtained by bed rest and a pelvic sling.

Symphysis pubis separations account for a small percentage of all pelvic fractures. The main complication is damage to the urethra and bladder. There may be an associated subluxation or dislocation of one sacroiliac joint (Fig. 43-86). Reduction is accomplished by placing the patient in the lateral position on the sound side and, with direct downward and forward pressure, rotating the displaced hemipelvis into position. The patient may then be nursed in a pelvic sling, or an external fixator may be applied.

It is not always possible to reduce these fractures anatomically. Every attempt should be made to restore the

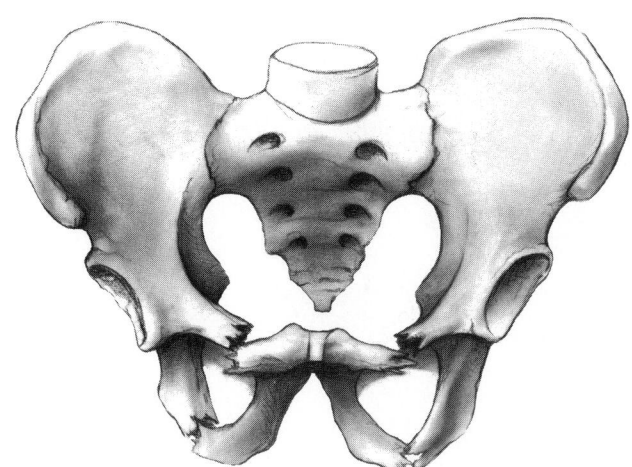

Fig. 43-85. Displaced fracture of all pubic rami, suggesting injury to the pelvic viscera.

pelvic outlet in young women of childbearing age. Open reduction is rarely indicated.

Isolated fractures of the iliac wing are usually the result of a direct blow to the crest of the ilium. If the major portion of the iliac wing is intact, weight bearing will not be affected. Fractures of the sacrum may occur from direct trauma or in association with fractures of the hemipelvis. Fractures of the coccyx occur from a direct blow to the coccyx as in a fall to a sitting position. Patients are treated by having them sit on a support beneath the thighs to take the direct pressure from the coccyx. In refractory situations, the coccyx may be excised.

Fractures and Dislocations of the Spine

Fractures and dislocations involving the cervical, thoracic, or lumbar spine are most commonly the result of injuries sustained by pedestrians, motorcyclists, or automobile occupants but may occur with any severe trauma. The prognosis in these injuries is dependent on whether there is associated cord injury. Fractures or dislocations without cord damage can result in normal function.

MANAGEMENT OF THE ACUTE INJURY. Any patient complaining of neck or back pain from an automobile collision or serious fall should be presumed to have an unstable spine until completely examined both clinically and radiologically by a competent physician. Patients sustaining a neck injury with or without acute cord damage should be placed supine on a stretcher with sandbags beside the head to hold it in neutral position. Since half of the cervical spine fractures occur from hyperextension, the neck should be positioned midway between flexion and extension.

Patients with thoracic or lumbar spine injuries should be transported in a position to minimize motion of the spine. The patient is placed supine or prone on a board or rigid stretcher, which can be moved to the x-ray table so that repositioning is not necessary. If the patient has other injuries, including chest, head, or abdominal hemorrhage, these should be treated first with the establishment of airway, resuscitation, and blood replacement.

A neurologic examination and record is carried out as soon as possible. Appropriate AP and lateral x-rays of the cervical, thoracic, or lumbar spine are obtained before

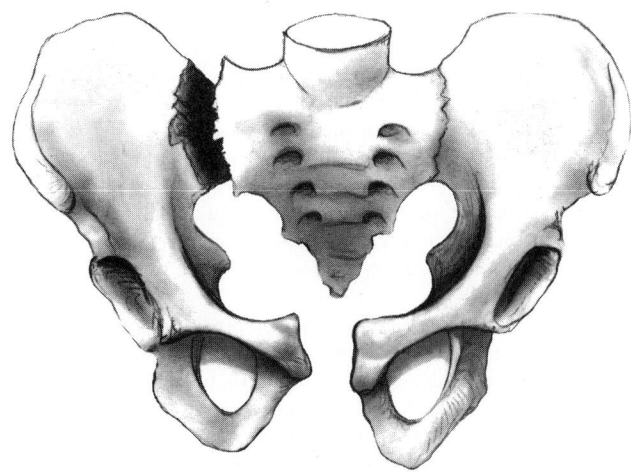

Fig. 43-86. Disruption of the hemipelvis by separation of symphysis pubis and sacroiliac joint.

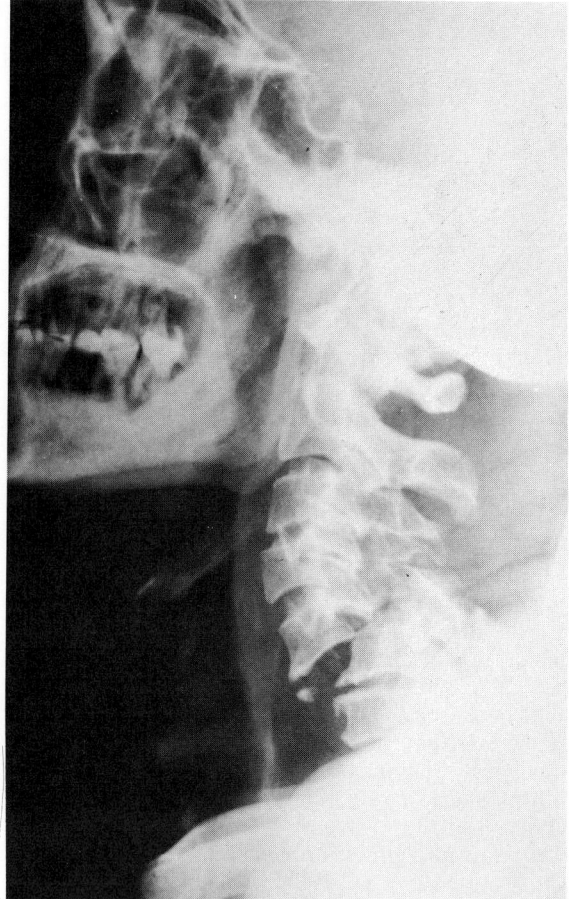

Fig. 43-87. Fracture-dislocation of C$_5$ upon C$_6$. Lateral x-rays show complete displacement of C$_5$ with fracture of the neural arch. The patient was paraplegic immediately following his injury.

moving the patient from the stretcher. A CT scan of the appropriate area of the spine will show the pathologic anatomy in detail. If x-rays indicate stability of the spine, oblique x-rays of the cervical spine may be obtained to supplement the AP and lateral x-rays. Immediate and continued immobilization is indicated if there is any question of instability.

CERVICAL FRACTURES AND DISLOCATIONS

Flexion injuries of the cervical spine occur when there is acute forcible flexion of the head upon the neck. With this type of injury, the first lesion to occur is compression of the vertebral body, resulting in an anterior wedge compression fracture of the vertebral body. The common areas are the lower three cervical vertebrae. The x-ray must include the entire cervical spine and the relationship between C$_7$ and T$_1$.

As the flexion force continues, the posterior longitudinal ligament may be ruptured, and one or both facets may be subluxated or dislocated. A unilateral facet dislocation results in only forward displacement of less than one-fifth the anteroposterior diameter of the vertebra. With bilateral facet dislocations, forward displacement may be greater than one-half the anteroposterior diameter. Cord injuries occur when the neural canal is compromised by forward dislocation and are more common with bilateral dislocations of the facets.

When a compression force (vertical load) is applied to the cervical spine, a bursting fracture of a vertebral body may occur. This may result in backward displacement of the posterior portion of the vertebral body, resulting in impingement upon, and damage to, the spinal cord. Combinations of flexion, compression, and rotation may occur, resulting in pedicle or lamina fractures, causing dislocation with or without cord damage (Fig. 43-87).

Patients from automobile accidents may present with a contusion of the forehead, and x-rays may reveal forward displacement of an upper vertebra upon the one below it. As the upper cervical spine is driven into extension, the anterior longitudinal ligament is ruptured, causing a compression force at the facet joints. As the force continues and the head is driven back, secondary flexion and forward displacement of an upper vertebra occurs upon the adjacent lower vertebra. Lateral x-rays reveal horizontal facet fracture or fracture of the anteroinferior border of the cervical spine body. Care must be taken in these injuries not to hyperextend the neck, or subsequent cord damage may result. Hyperextension injuries may result without a facet or body fracture and spontaneously be reduced. The cord is driven back against the sharp edge of the lamina, resulting in cord damage. With the head brought into neutral position, the dislocation may be spontaneously reduced, and the x-rays may appear normal, although the patient is paraplegic.

Injuries of the transverse process in the cervical spine are rare and represent avulsion fractures. Fractures of the spinous processes may also occur and have been characterized as the clay shoveler's fracture. A sudden stress on the supraspinous ligament pulls off the tip of the spinous process. Also, a direct blow to the spinous process may cause fracture.

Fractures of the atlas occur when compression force is applied to a thin posterior ring by downward force on the head (Jefferson's fracture).

Fractures of C$_2$, involving the odontoid or posterior elements, may occur from flexion and extension or rotational forces. In children under the age of six, injuries to the odontoid result in an epiphyseal displacement and associated subluxation or dislocation of atlas upon the axis.

MANAGEMENT OF CERVICAL SPINE FRACTURES AND DISLOCATIONS WITHOUT NEUROLOGIC INJURY. Unstable fractures must be immobilized and dislocations or subluxations reduced. Patients arriving at the emergency room are placed in a cervical halter traction, which will provide immediate stability, while appropriate x-rays or associated conditions are managed. For the long-term immobilization of these injuries, skeletal traction is required. This is accomplished by the use of a halo apparatus. The halo purchases with four pins inserted under local anesthesia onto the outer table of the skull. To this skeletal traction device 5 lb is added for upper cervical lesions and as much as 30 lb for lower cervical lesions.

Dislocations with fractures are reduced with skeletal traction. When the dislocation or fracture is reduced, the halo device is connected to either a plaster body jacket or a vest orthosis and the patient is allowed to walk until stability has ensued, a period of approximately 12 weeks. The patient is then immobilized in a four-poster cervical brace for an additional period. Before immobilization is discontinued, flexion and extension films are obtained to determine stability. When stability cannot be anticipated with immobilization alone, spine fusion is carried out after a 6-week interval.

In some undisplaced fractures, such as a pedicle or lamina fracture, where stability is certain, an initial halo vest may be employed. If there is uncertainty about stability, skeletal traction, followed by application of a halo vest, is the safest procedure.

Twelve percent recurrent instability following the conservative management of unstable fractures and dislocations has been reported. For this reason, early posterior spine fusion with wiring of spinous processes has been recommended. The procedure is to resolve the acute general injuries, during which time skeletal traction is maintained and is then continued during posterior spine fusion. The technique is to wire together the spinous process of the affected adjacent vertebrae. Autogenous iliac bone is applied to the roughened posterior lamina and spinous processes. If satisfactory stability is obtained by wiring, the patient is kept in a four-poster cervical spine brace until bone union is solid (12 to 16 weeks).

CERVICAL FRACTURES AND DISLOCATIONS WITH ASSOCIATED NEUROLOGIC INJURY. There is little disagreement that patients who present with minimal neurologic findings and have progressive neurologic deficits require immediate laminectomy and exploration. Another indication is unsuccessful reduction and persistence of bone fragments in the spinal canal. Proponents of the nonexploration attitude argue that irreparable damage has been done from the time of the initial injury and will not be influenced by decompression and subsequent exploration, which in themselves are life-threatening procedures. Also, if the lesion is partial, surgical procedures may further endanger the cord. The operative school base their indications on the fact that occasionally a displaced disc or fragment of bone will compress the cord and unrelieved swelling may further damage a cord capable of recovery.

THORACOLUMBAR FRACTURES AND DISLOCATIONS

Fractures and dislocations involving the upper thoracic and midthoracic regions are uncommon because of the stability afforded by the adjacent rib cage. The principles involved in treatment of such injuries are the same as in thoracolumbar spine fractures.

Flexion force applied to the thoracolumbar spine results in anterior wedge compression fractures that are stable by virtue of intact posterior structures and longitudinal ligaments (Fig. 43-88). Wedge compression fractures may occur in any osteoporotic spine from relatively minor trauma. Wedge compression fractures also occur in

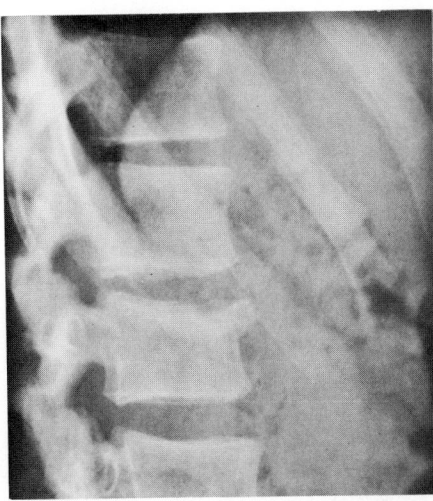

Fig. 43-88. Wedge compression fracture L$_2$. Lateral x-ray shows compression wedging of the upper portion of L$_2$.

normal spines from severe flexion forces common in mine cave-ins, automobile collisions, and falls from a height.

When rotation is combined with flexion, the posterior ligaments rupture or the articular processes fracture, and a wedge-shaped fracture may occur through the upper border of the lower vertebral body, resulting in a fracture-dislocation (Fig. 43-89). Extension injuries may cause dislocation with rupture of the anterior longitudinal ligaments and may cause posterior dislocation. This is rare in the lumbar region. When compression force (vertical load) is applied to the line of vertebral bodies, especially at the thoracolumbar area and upper lumbar spine, the result is a bursting fracture with the posterior fragments displaced into the spinal canal.

MANAGEMENT OF ACUTE INJURIES OF THE THORACOLUMBAR SPINE. Patients with acute traumatic injury to the spine should be presumed to have an unstable situation and potential paraplegia until proved otherwise. They should be placed prone or supine on a stretcher and not moved until AP and lateral x-rays delineate the lesion.

The patient should be inspected for signs of impact, abrasion over one shoulder causing flexion and rotation, etc. If the supraspinous ligaments are ruptured, a defect between the spinous processes will be evident. With any compression fracture, there is tenderness over the affected vertebrae. Flexion injury causing compression wedging will be evident on the lateral x-ray but not on the AP x-ray. When the ''slice wedge'' fracture of the upper part of the lower vertebrae is seen on both AP and lateral x-rays without dislocation, instability should be suspected. Such fractures are so unstable that they are reduced just by placing the patient supine. Any displacement in the lumbar spine is an indication of instability.

Treatment of fractures of the thoracolumbar spine will depend on the degree of instability caused by the trauma. Patients are confined to bed rest until symptoms allow mobilization. The patient should be watched for paralytic ileus. When patients are comfortable, they are taught hyperextension exercises, which are continued for 6 to 12

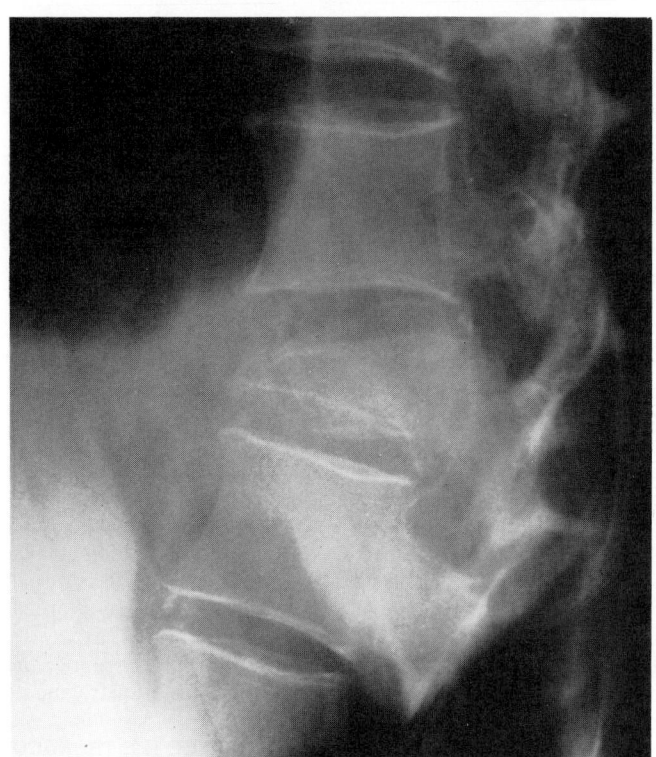

A

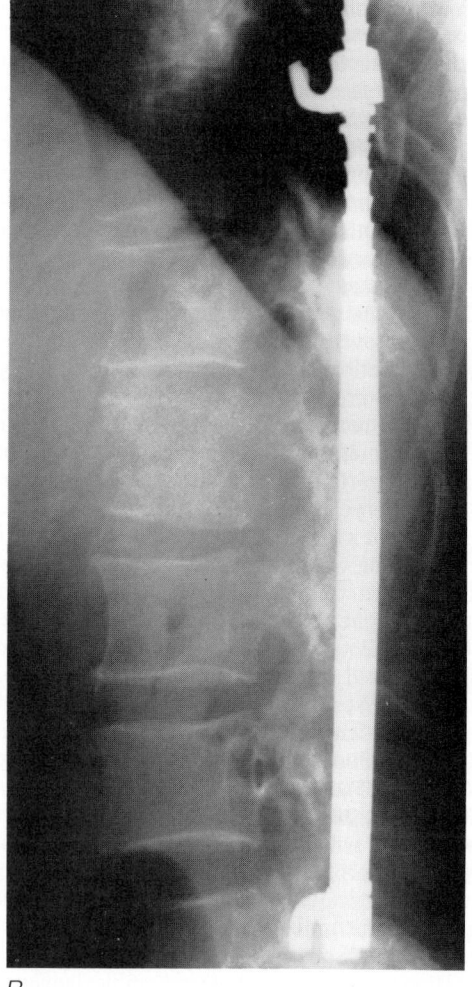

B

Fig. 43-89. *A.* Burst compression fracture L$_1$. *B.* Harrington rod reduction and fixation shows correction.

weeks. No reduction for a stable wedge compression fracture is necessary, since the deformity rarely causes disability. Bursting fractures are usually stable. A CT scan of the spine will allow accurate determination of fractures and a reasonable judgment of stability and the need for surgical stabilization. Stable fractures are immobilized in plaster, and spontaneous fusion across the involved disc will usually result. If instability is present or questionable, the patient is treated by localized posterior spine fusion and fixation with a Harrington rod. Pure dislocations in the thoracolumbar region are rare; when they occur they require spine fusion.

A different situation exists when injury to the cauda equina is associated with this rotational fracture-dislocation. The fracture must be adequately reduced to free the nerve roots from pressure. Immobilization must be maintained to prevent recurrent injury during the early postfracture period. The best method for stabilization is the use of Harrington rods. For this reason, some advise early stabilization above and below the site of injury. Others feel that exploration is not indicated and Foster frame reduction and immobilization are sufficient.

Diseases of Joints

The problem of joint injury or disease is common. An estimated 2 to 8 percent of the population has rheumatic complaints at some time in their lives. Virtually everyone over the age of fifty years has sufficient degenerative changes in joints to have some restriction of some joint motion, although only a small percentage show symptoms. Injuries frequently involve joints; the immobilization imposed by every fracture or injured extremity results in restriction of joint motion either temporarily or in some cases permanently.

ANATOMY

Joints are either fibrous or cartilaginous. A fibrous joint, or synarthrosis, consists of two bones united by fibrous tissue, such as the syndesmoses or sutures of the skull.

Cartilaginous joints consist of bones united by either hyaline cartilage or fibrocartilage. An example of a primary cartilaginous joint is an epiphyseal plate. Examples of fibrocartilaginous joints are the pubic symphysis and the intervertebral discs.

Diarthrodial joints are movable joints in which the cartilage-covered bone ends are united by a capsule lined with synovium (Fig. 43-90).

The plane or planes of motion occurring in the synovial joint characterize the joints as uniaxial, i.e., ginglymus (hinge), trochoid (pivot), biaxial, or multiaxial. The motion permitted in a diarthrosis depends upon the configuration of the articular surface, adjacent capsule, and supporting musculature, and upon the unique properties of articular cartilage.

ARTICULAR CARTILAGE. Normal articular cartilage is blue-white, has a smooth surface, and is slightly compressible. The thickness of articular cartilage varies in different locations of specific joints.

Articular cartilage is composed of chondrocytes, which are embedded in a network of collagen fibers, surrounded by a matrix of proteoglycans. It is separated from the underlying supporting subchondral bone by a thin layer of calcified cartilage. Cell reproduction does not occur in normal healthy adult articular cartilage. After injury and in degenerative disease of articular cartilage, the rate of

Fig. 43-90. Schematic drawing of synovial joint structures.

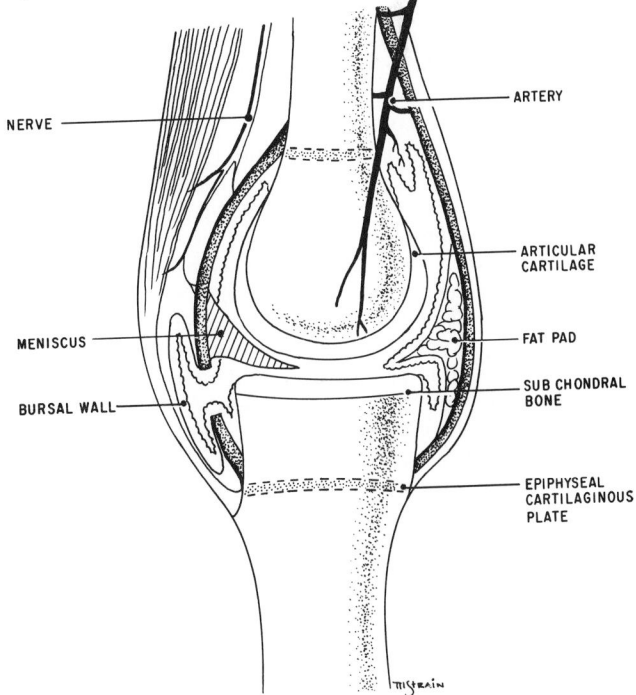

NERVE

ARTERY

ARTICULAR CARTILAGE

MENISCUS

FAT PAD

BURSAL WALL

SUB CHONDRAL BONE

EPIPHYSEAL CARTILAGINOUS PLATE

deoxyribonucleic acid (DNA) synthesis is increased, indicating cell replication.

The cartilage cells produce the intercellular substances composed of matrix, or ground substance, and collagen fibers. The matrix, proteoglycan, is a complex substance and contributes to the maintenance of the water content and resiliency of the cartilage. Articular cartilage being composed of water forms a gel in combination with glycoaminoglycans. The amount of water declines with increasing age and is increased in osteoarthrosis cartilage as a response to cartilage damage.

The collagen of articular cartilage is different from that of bone. The collagen fibers have a definite arrangement. In the depths of the cartilage, the fibers are at right angles to the surface of the subchondral bone. At the articular surface, the fibers curve to run parallel with the surface. The resulting network is called Benninghoff's arcades. In the adult, cartilage is nourished by diffusion of substances from the synovial fluid on the surface and in the immature animal before the basal layer calcifies, also by diffusion from the underlying capillaries on the subchondral bone.

The synovial membrane is composed of secretory and phagocytic cells, which are arranged in depths of one to three cells over subsynovial connective tissue. Over ligaments, the synovium is quite thin, while in regions of the fat pads and loose capsule there is considerable areolar tissue beneath the synovium. Circulation to the synovium comes from the main blood vessels about the joint that first supply the fibrous capsule. The synovium is much more vascular, with a large plexus immediately beneath the synovial surface. The blood vessels in the synovia are continuous and communicate with metaphyseal and epiphyseal blood vessels.

The secretory cells produce the hyaluronate of the synovial fluid. In addition, electrolytes and certain plasma proteins diffuse from the synovial capillaries into the joint space. Normal synovial fluid is a weakly alkaline, viscous, clear, pale yellow nonclottable fluid. The viscosity is dependent upon the presence of hyaluronate; when hyaluronate is depolymerized, the viscosity is reduced.

Normal synovial fluid contains up to 200 nucleated cells consisting of polymorphonuclear leukocytes, lymphocytes, and monocytes. Electrolytes and glucose are present. Nonprotein nitrogen and uric acid concentrations are approximately the same as in serum.

The synovium contains two plexuses of nerve fibers, a superficial plexus lying in close proximity to the capsule and a deeper one in the synovial villi. This plexus is intimately related to blood vessels that carry within their tunica media many unmyelinated sensory fibers.

The capsule has a rich supply of sonatic sensory fibers and proprioceptive fibers in the form of specialized Golgi apparatus, Vater-Pacini corpuscles, and Ruffini-like endings. Its connection with joint pain appreciation was demonstrated by Leriche, who showed that local anesthetic injected into the capsule was more effective than a simple intraarticular injection.

Coomes produced patterns of pain around the hip, depending upon the aspect of the capsule stimulated. Stimulation of the anterior capsule produced pain in the groin, buttock, anterior thigh, and knee, whereas posterior capsule stimulation produced pain in the buttock, posterior aspect of the thigh, and heel.

The nerve supply of each synovial joint is by articular twigs from nerves supplying muscles responsible for the control of motion of that joint. The distribution and location of these branches is quite variable, making complete denervation of a joint difficult. The capsule and ligaments are the most pain-sensitive structures in a joint. Synovium also contains free nerve endings, but the areas of pain sensation are variable and ill defined.

Nerve fibers accompany arteries into bone, and this may be the basis for bone pain in certain inflammatory conditions about joints. The pain from the joint is difficult to localize and is often referred distally. There are proprioceptive endings in the capsule and joint ligaments that are sensitive to stretch and are indicators of joint position. Articular cartilage is without sensation.

EXAMINATION

The diagnosis of joint disease is dependent upon the following:

1. Clinical history of joint symptomatology
2. Clinical examination of all joints
3. Bone and joint imaging
4. Synovial fluid analysis
5. Serologic tests

The patient is questioned about the specific onset of the joint complaint and any relation to trauma. Information about aggravation and relief of pain, and history of previous joint complaints, morning stiffness, locking, giving way, swelling, erythema, and symptoms related to other joints are necessary.

CLINICAL EXAMINATION. The involved joint or joints should be inspected for signs of swelling and effusion, and evidence of erythema and local skin temperature increase. In unilateral involvement, the opposite side is used for comparison. The ligaments responsible for stability are examined and ranges of joint motion recorded. Active motion is examined by asking the patient to put the joint through a range of motion. Passive motion is measured by putting the joint through the maximal range of motion with muscles relaxed. The proximal and distal joints are always examined to be certain that the complaint is not due to referred pain. Muscle girth is determined by measurement, and muscle power is graded. Clinical examination is incomplete without evaluation of all joints in both upper and lower extremities, as well as a complete physical examination.

RADIOGRAPHIC EXAMINATION. Standard biplanar x-rays of the involved joints are necessary. The x-rays should clearly show the margins of the joint, as well as the adjacent bone metaphysis. In many situations, CT or MRI are necessary to delineate the adjacent bone and specific lesion. X-rays may be required in positions of flexion and extension to test for subluxation and dislocation. In certain traumatic situations, i.e., ankle and knee injuries, x-rays may be required with stress applied to the joint to determine the continuity of ligaments. Arthrography with the injection of radiopaque dyes is useful in delineating the shoulder capsule and rotator cuff, as well as soft tissue structures involved in congenital dislocation of the hip, and damage to menisci of the knee.

SYNOVIAL FLUID EXAMINATION. The examination of synovial fluid may give a specific diagnosis in pyogenic arthritis, tuberculous arthritis, gout, and pseudogout, and may add valuable diagnostic information in most other types of arthritis, including degenerative and rheumatoid arthritis, and in traumatic injuries. The technique of aspiration of a joint will depend on an accurate knowledge of anatomy of the specific joint to be aspirated. The fluid is collected in (1) a culture tube, (2) a tube with a few crystals of EDTA, and (3) an empty tube.

The synovial fluid is examined for color, appearance, and viscosity. Bacterial culture, Gram's stain examination, mucin clot test, white blood cell count, crystal examination, and glucose concentration determination are made.

Color, Turbidity, and Viscosity. Normal synovial fluid is slightly straw-colored. In gout, the fluid may be white or yellow, depending upon the concentration of urate crystals. Septic joint fluid may be gray, thin, and watery or white, purulent, and thick.

A tube of normal joint fluid is completely clear, and newsprint can be read through it. When the white cell count is increased or crystals are present, turbidity is increased. Viscosity is tested by spreading a drop of fluid between the thumb and index finger. It is usually possible to spread the stringy viscous fluid for 2 in. before it separates. In conditions of inflammation, hyaluronic acid is depolymerized, and viscosity is reduced.

Mucin Clot Test. The mucin clot test is an indication of the character of the protein polysaccharide complex of the synovial fluid. The simplest test is the Ropes test, which is performed by adding a few drops of synovial fluid to a small test tube containing 10 mL of 5% acetic acid. A good clot is a firm, ropey clot that on agitation will not separate or fragment. These characteristics are dependent upon normal polymerization and normal concentration of mucin. A good clot is present in normal joints and with degenerative arthritis. A poor clot is one that is small and fragments immediately with agitation. Poor clots occur in the presence of inflammation such as rheumatoid arthritis, gout, or septic arthritis.

Fluid removed at the bedside should be cultured aerobically and also plated on anaerobic media such as chocolate agar if gonococcal arthritis is suspected. Aspirates should be cultured in hypertonic growth media in order to detect the presence of atypical bacterial forms. Routine cultures for tuberculosis as well as guinea pig inoculation may be carried out if tuberculous arthritis is suspected.

Cell Count and Other Determinations. A total cell count is carried out on the fluid, to which EDTA has been added. If normal white cell counting solution is used, the acidity will precipitate the mucin and make the count inaccurate. The joint fluid is diluted with saline solution to which a drop of methylene blue is added, and a routine count is done in a white cell counting chamber. A differential white blood cell count is done on smears of this fluid stained with Wright's stain.

Joint fluid is examined for the presence of urate or calcium pyrophosphate crystals. It is important not to perform this on fluid to which oxylate or EDTA has been added. The fluid is first centrifuged to concentrate the white blood cells. Supernatant is removed and the sediment examined under polarized light. Urate crystals will be rod-shaped with rounded ends and exhibit strongly negative birefringence under polarized light. Calcium pyrophosphate crystals are rodlike or rhomboid with sharp ends. Under polarized light, they show weakly positive birefringence. If there is doubt about the type present, uricase is added to dissolve the urate crystals.

Glucose determination is performed on the synovial fluid. At the same time, a fasting blood glucose is determined. In conditions with a high white cell count, such as rheumatoid arthritis or infection, the gradient between blood and joint fluid may be 50 mg/dL or greater. In the normal, there is 10 mg/dL less glucose in joint fluid than in blood.

PYOGENIC ARTHRITIS

If the diagnosis of septic arthritis can be made very early, the chances of restoring a normal joint are excellent. If the diagnosis is missed and the purulent destructive process goes unchecked, disability due to chronic arthritis is the end result.

PATHOGENESIS. Joints may become infected by

1. Hematogenous spread from septicemia
2. Direct infection by traumatic wounds or at surgical treatment
3. Extension of an adjacent osteomyelitis

In hematogenous infection, a nidus of bacteria is lodged in the synovium and if not destroyed erupts into the joint space. Inflammatory response results in passage of plasma proteins, fibrinogen, and plasminogen into the joint space because of the increased capillary permeability. Leukocytes are attracted into the joint fluid by chemotaxis. The end result of this inflammation is an abscess in the joint space. This abscess is no different from an abscess in other areas of the body, with the exception that the lining or synovial wall may be more permeable to systemic antibiotics. Proteolytic enzymes from the lysozymes of disintegrating white blood cells and activated plasminogen degrade the proteoglycan of the articular cartilage, exposing collagen fibers. The collagen fibers are then subject to degradation by white blood cell enzymes.

Staphylococcus aureus and hemolytic streptococci are the two most common organisms producing a pyogenic arthritis. The actual incidence is not important, since the bacterial type in each infection must be determined. Coliform organisms, *Hemophilus influenzae,* pneumococci, meningococci, and *Brucella,* may be the etiologic agents.

CLINICAL MANIFESTATIONS. Septic arthritis may occur at any age but has higher incidence in patients with debili-

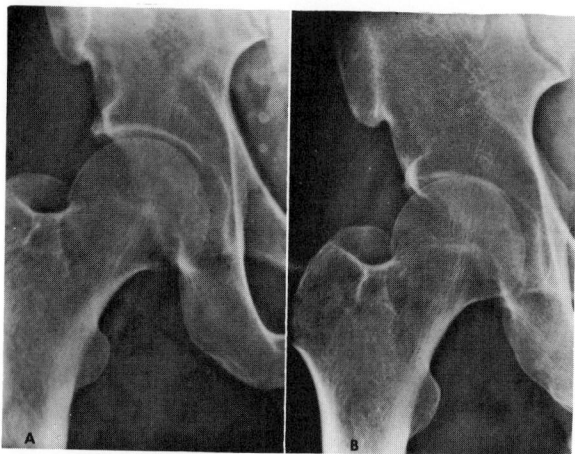

Fig. 43-91. Pyogenic hip joint. *A.* AP x-ray of hip joint taken 48 h after onset of acute hip pain associated with minor hip injury. Joint space is normal. No bone changes are seen. *B.* Three and one-half weeks later there is complete loss of joint space with no bone changes. Cartilage destruction was due to *Hemophilus influenzae* septic arthritis.

tating disease and/or on cortisone therapy, or in those with rheumatoid arthritis. Premature infants have a high incidence of septic arthritis of the hip joint.

Patients with hematogenous spread may have more than one joint involved, although localization is commonly confined to one large joint. The patients complain of malaise, chills, fever, and general lassitude. An increase in the white blood cell count with increased polymorphonuclear leukocytes is usually noted. In some patients, an elevated sedimentation rate may be the only abnormality.

Examination of the involved joint will reveal the classic signs of inflammation, local tenderness, erythema, swelling, and extreme pain with attempts at motion. The joint will assume a position that is influenced by muscle spasm and pressure/volume relationship. For the knee joint, this is about 20° of flexion. Usually, the patient will not allow complete examination of the joint because of the excruciating pain. In some low-grade infections the range of joint motion may be close to normal early in the course of the disease.

X-rays of a septic joint will show only tissue swelling and joint effusion. Bone changes will not be present on the initial x-ray examination (Fig. 43-91). In a child with lax joint capsule and ligaments, the shoulder or hip joint may be subluxed or dislocated as a result of the pressure from the synovial abscess.

DIAGNOSIS. The diagnosis of pyogenic arthritis is made by joint aspiration and synovial fluid analysis. The physician should be cautioned to be reasonably certain that the joint is infected and that the symptoms are not coming from an overlying cellulitis. This problem occurs in children in whom an infected prepatellar bursitis develops with secondary effusion of the knee joint. If ill-advised aspiration is done through an overlying bacteria, the joint may be directly inoculated with bacteria. If there is doubt, however, the joint should be aspirated away from the area of superficial infection. At the time of aspiration, every attempt is made to evacuate the joint completely by compressing fluid into the suprapatellar pouch, from which it is aspirated. Gram's stain examination is carried out on the synovial fluid as well. If organisms are seen in the fluid and the culture is positive, this is diagnostic of sepsis. A poor mucin clot, a white blood cell count between 23,000 and 250,000 with 90 percent polymorphonuclear leukocytes, and a blood/synovial fluid glucose gradient of more than 40 mg/dL are consistent with the diagnosis of septic arthritis.

TREATMENT. The treatment of septic arthritis begins with complete aspiration of the joint. If the Gram's stain is positive, immediate antibiotic treatment is instituted. If the Gram's stain is negative and the diagnosis is still strongly suspected, antibiotic therapy should be started. For children, antibiotic coverage for *H. influenzae* should be included; ampicillin is appropriate. For an adult patient with suspected staphylococci, one of the cephalosporins should be included in the antibiotic regimen.

Surgical Drainage. Surgical drainage is the treatment of choice, but daily aspiration and systemic antibiotic treatment are occasionally indicated. With joints previously damaged by rheumatoid arthritis and where it is possible to evacuate the joint completely by aspiration, or with streptococcal infections where complete daily aspiration is possible, omission of surgical drainage may be appropriate. When it is not possible to evacuate the joint completely because of loculated collections of fluid, surgical drainage should be undertaken as soon as the diagnosis is certain. All infections of the hip must be drained, since the surrounding musculature makes it difficult to monitor the adequacy of needle aspiration drainage. For the knee joint, two parapatellar incisions are necessary, while the hip joint usually requires one well-placed posterior incision. Septic hips of children should always be drained surgically in order to minimize the chance of dislocation from pressure of the intraarticular abscess.

In the case of the knee or hip joint, skin traction is applied to the leg for purposes of immobilization, and an attempt is made to minimize cartilage compression at the point of contact. Where traction is not possible, i.e., for the elbow or wrist, a posterior plaster splint is applied to the joint for immobilization in a position of function.

Antibiotic therapy is continued for a minimum of 4 weeks or until the sedimentation rate returns to normal. If the septic arthritis is an extension of adjacent osteomyelitis, antibiotic treatment is indicated until osteomyelitis has been successfully controlled, i.e., 6 weeks or longer.

If the joint has been treated by closed methods, i.e., aspiration and antibiotics, when the joint remains dry and asymptomatic, early active range-of-motion exercises are started. If treated by surgical drainage, joint motion is not begun until the wounds are granulating or completely closed. Early motion is important in giving a good result.

If damage to the articular cartilage occurs, patients may have residual stiffness, deformity, and a painful joint. Depending upon the severity of symptoms, reconstructive procedures including arthrodesis, arthroplasty, or osteotomy may be necessary.

BONE AND JOINT TUBERCULOSIS

General Considerations

Skeletal tuberculosis is now an uncommon infection in the United States, although it is still a major problem in parts of Asia and Africa. Tuberculosis involving the spine or peripheral joints is always secondary to infection elsewhere in the body. The primary infection is usually pulmonary.

PATHOLOGY. The most common site of skeletal involvement with tuberculosis is the spine. The highest incidence occurs in the vertebral bodies opposite the kidney. Once infection starts in a vertebral body, it may spread across the disc space margin to involve the adjacent vertebrae by tracking beneath the anterior longitudinal ligament. It may spread through Batson's plexus of veins to other vertebral bodies. Infection in the dorsal spine usually is contained beneath the anterior longitudinal ligament, but in the lumbar spine the intimate origin of fibers of the psoas muscle results in spread into the psoas and formation of a psoas abscess.

Peripheral joint tuberculosis involves synovial membrane, bone, and cartilage. Tuberculous synovitis with tubercle formation and synovial pannus develops, which gradually covers the cartilage and invades the underlying subchondral bone. The cartilage is the last structure to be involved. In contrast to pyogenic joints that have increased leukocytic protease activity, the cartilage in tuberculous joints is destroyed by interference with its underlying circulation. The end result of this process is complete destruction of the joint. Fibrous ankylosis of adjacent surfaces is a common sequel, but spontaneous bony ankylosis is rare.

CLINICAL MANIFESTATIONS. Any chronic monarthritis should be suspected of being tuberculous. There is fre-

quently a history of pulmonary disease, although tuberculous monarthritis may be the first presentation of the systemic illness. Any of the large joints may be infected. Tuberculous arthritis may occur at any age but is more common in children in Asia and Africa.

The clinical course is insidious, and patients have symptoms for weeks or months prior to seeking consultation. Low-grade pain occurring at night is common. Limitation of joint motion with local synovial swelling is present. Examination of the joint reveals local synovitis out of proportion to the content of synovial fluid. There may be limitation of joint motion and signs of higher local temperature over the joint, but erythema is uncommon. Frequently, in children, the onset of tuberculosis of the hip is suggested by a limp and a history of pain and night crying.

RADIOGRAPHIC FINDINGS. Early in the course of the infection, there may be radiographic evidence of soft tissue swelling and adjacent osteoporosis. As the disease progresses, marginal erosion occurring at the cartilage synovial junction may be seen on both sides of the joint (Fig. 43-92). The joint space commonly maintains its integrity because cartilage destruction occurs late in the course of the disease. In children with long-standing tuberculous synovitis, there may be enlargement of the adjacent growing epiphyses due to chronic inflammation. In long-standing disease in adults, the joint may be completely destroyed with areas of necrosis secondary to undermining, and "kissing" sequestra develop.

DIAGNOSIS. The specific diagnosis of tuberculous arthritis is dependent upon the recovery of organisms from the joint or demonstration of organisms in granulomas on pathologic section. The demonstration of pulmonary lesions or other joint infections as well as positive Mantoux test results are helpful but are not pathognomonic. Joint aspiration, smear, and culture or guinea pig inoculation with the synovial fluid should be carried out in all suspected cases. Synovial fluid analysis will reveal a leukocytic response of less than 20,000 and a poor mucin clot. If the diagnosis cannot be made by joint fluid aspiration,

Fig. 43-92. Tuberculosis of the knee joint. *A* and *B*. AP and lateral x-rays of the knee showing erosion of the margins of the medial tibial plateau and medial femoral condyle. There is only minimal joint space narrowing. *C* and *D*. Postsurgical arthrodesis of the knee.

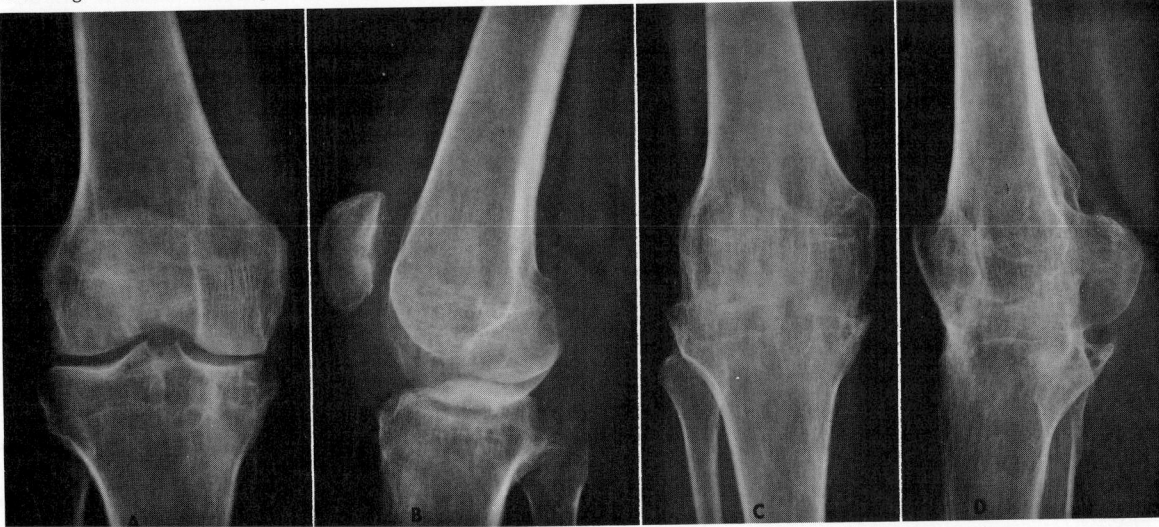

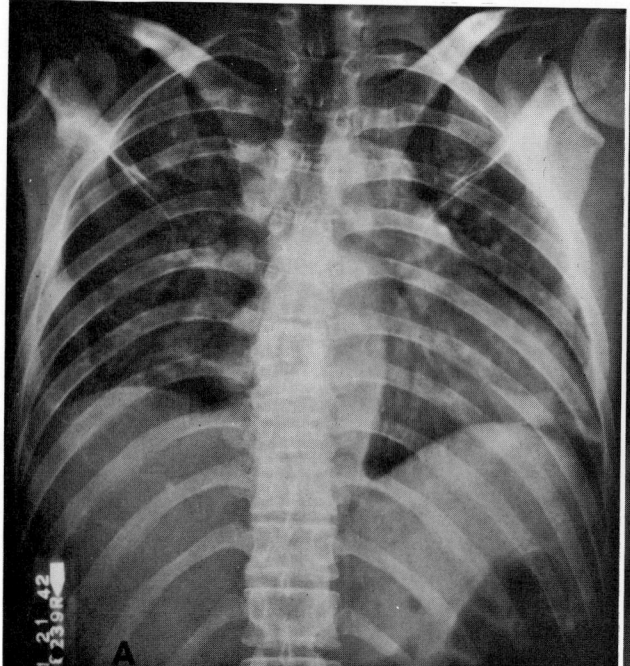
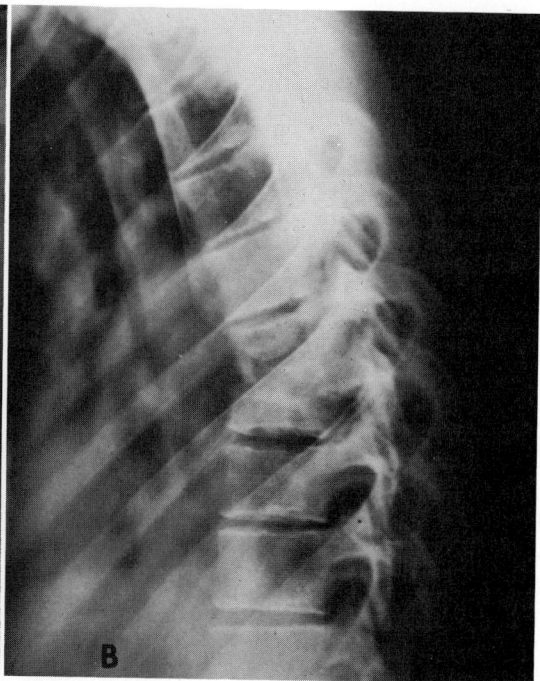

Fig. 43-93. Spinal tuberculosis (Pott's disease). *A.* AP x-ray of thoracic spine showing large paravertebral abscess. *B.* Lateral x-ray of thoracic spine showing disruption of the $T_7–T_8$ interspace with kyphotic deformity.

open biopsy should be done without hesitation, since early treatment is mandatory.

TREATMENT. Treatment of skeletal tuberculosis includes (1) general supportive measures, (2) chemotherapy, (3) local treatment of the involved joint or joints, (4) surgical treatment.

General supportive measures include adequate protein and caloric intake, hydration, and proper rest. Patients are started on antituberculous chemotherapy. If the chemotherapy is started before significant necrosis and caseation or walling off has occurred, treatment is associated with a high success rate.

Patients are started on triple-drug therapy until culture reports of the specific organisms are available. Rifampicin daily, combined with INH and ethenbutol, is the more modern regimen and need only be continued for 6 months. If necessary, the latter two should be continued for 1 year. Ethenbutol has largely replaced PAS and streptomycin, which can produce VIII cranial nerve toxicity.

The treatment of the specific joint involves immobilization by traction, plaster splinting, or casts, combined with bed rest. If the infection is diagnosed early, local immobilization combined with chemotherapy may be sufficient. If the joint does not respond to these measures or if the disease has already progressed to involve subchondral bone, surgical joint clearance including synovectomy and excision of tuberculous foci is necessary. Joint debridement with the excision of involved tissues may be quite successful in controlling the local infection and still allow a partially mobile joint. If the joint is totally destroyed, arthrodesis of the involved joint is the treatment of choice.

Tuberculosis of the Spine

Tuberculous spondylitis (Pott's disease) is the most common form of skeletal tuberculosis (Fig. 43-93). The infection is located in the anterior border of the vertebral body, commonly in the thoracic region. Multiple areas may be involved. The infection spreads across the disc space to involve the adjacent upper or lower vertebrae. The disc space is lost because of loss of fluid from the disc. Actual destruction of the disc does not occur early, because of lack of proteolytic enzymes. The disc may be sequestrated into the paraspinal abscess that develops if treatment is delayed. If there is sufficient destruction of the involved vertebrae, damage to the posterior-lying spinal cord may occur from the pressure of abscess formation or from angular deformity at the site of infection.

Symptoms of Pott's disease include back pain, limitation of spinal motion, paraspinal muscle spasm, and the systemic signs of infection, as well. With cord involvement, the patient will have neurologic signs and symptoms involving the lower extremities.

The x-ray findings of tuberculous spondylitis and staphylococcal disc space infection are the same. The diagnosis rests on the recovery of organisms or characteristic histologic evidence from the site of infection. The direct anterior approach to the spine, as described by Hodgson and Stuck, provides an effective means for early diagnosis and stabilization of the spine at the same time.

Patients suspected of having spinal tuberculosis are started on triple-drug chemotherapy and bed rest in anterior and posterior plaster shells. After adequate chemotherapy has been established, the spine is exposed by the anterior approach and biopsy material obtained. All infected disc and bone are excised and the adjacent vertebral bodies stabilized with autogenous rib or iliac bone grafts. Where such operations are impracticable, drug therapy with P.O.P. body jackets can be used for 6 to 12 months.

Postoperatively patients are nursed in plaster shells until consolidation has occurred at the site of bone grafting. If paraplegia is present, immediate decompression of the spinal cord is mandatory via the same anterior approach or, occasionally, costotransversectomy. Laminectomy is contraindicated, because it decreases posterior spine stability and allows the anterior-lying abscess, which is not drained, to increase pressure on the dural contents.

Tuberculosis of the Hip

When the diagnosis of tuberculosis of the hip is made early, bed rest with skin traction to the hip, combined with antituberculous chemotherapy, may suffice. If the infection cannot be controlled, open arthrotomy through the Smith-Petersen approach and joint debridement should be carried out to remove the necrotic material. Postoperatively, the patient is kept in traction until the wound is healed. Chemotherapy is continued, and early active motion of the joint is instituted. With severe destruction of the hip joint, surgical arthrodesis may be required.

GONOCOCCAL ARTHRITIS

Gonococcal arthritis occurs in females secondary to gonococcal cervicitis or vaginitis. Since the clinical manifestations of the primary cervical infection are relatively occult, treatment may not be effected, and the patient is subject to gonococcal septicemia and gonococcal arthritis. By contrast, the male with gonococcal urethritis has symptoms, seeks early medical treatment, and rarely presents with a gonococcal joint infection.

CLINICAL MANIFESTATIONS. Symptoms usually begin with migratory polyarthralgia, followed by localization in one or two joints. The knee, elbow, and wrist are common sites of infection. A variable febrile course may occur concomitantly with the joint infection.

DIAGNOSIS. The diagnosis is dependent upon the recovery of gonococcal organisms from the septic joint. Cultures of joint fluid are performed on chocolate agar and incubated in 10% carbon dioxide. Aspirates should be cultured in hypertonic broth media to detect the presence of bacterial L forms. It is important to inoculate the culture medium at the bedside and to withhold antibiotics until the culture has been taken.

Synovial fluid analysis will reveal white cell counts in the region of 20,000, with poor mucin and depressed glucose content, which are not in themselves diagnostic of gonococcal infection. X-rays early in the course of the disease will show only soft tissue swelling.

TREATMENT. Intramuscular penicillin G, 1 to 2 million units/day for 2 weeks, or fludoxicillin, is sufficient to eradicate the primary focus and the intraarticular infections completely. With a patient failing to respond to penicillin therapy, resistant gonococci or other organisms, Reiter's syndrome, or early rheumatoid arthritis should be considered. Local treatment of the joint by aspiration and then immobilization is required and provides additional symptomatic relief. With early adequate penicillin treatment, recovery of a normal joint is the rule.

LYME ARTHRITIS

Lyme disease is a tick-borne illness caused by a spirochete *Borrelia bungdorferi*. The disease has a characteristic skin lesion that starts as a red macule and progresses to a bright-red annular ring with a clearing center. The skin eruption may herald the onset of a rheumatic syndrome resembling rheumatoid arthritis or juvenile rheumatoid arthritis, especially of the aligoarticular presentation. Cardiac and neurologic manifestations also occur. Patients with suspected rheumatoid arthritis should be questioned for a history of tick bites and the characteristic skin rash. Penicillin or tetracycline therapy is effective in overcoming the infection, at least early in the illness.

RHEUMATOID ARTHRITIS

General Considerations

Rheumatoid arthritis is a systemic disease affecting any organ of the body including those of the cardiovascular, respiratory, nervous, and musculoskeletal systems.

PATHOLOGY. The pathologic features of rheumatoid arthritis are found in the diarthrodial joints as well as in adjacent tissues, tendons, tendon sheaths, and bursa. The synovium is congested and edematous with fibrin exudates on the surface or diffusely dispersed throughout the synovium itself. The articular cartilage may be covered by the synovial granulation tissue called pannus. At the cartilage synovial junction, the synovial granulation tissue invades the subchondral bone, causing erosive changes, which are visible by x-ray. New periosteal bone formation develops in the region of the capsular attachments, and subchondral bone becomes osteoporotic.

As the granulation tissue and pannus increase, the articular cartilage is eroded. The area of calcified cartilage increases in thickness, effectively diminishing the thickness of the uncalcified cartilage. Radiographically, the joint space is narrower, because of the advancement of calcified cartilage as well as the loss of surface contour. The end result of the cartilage destruction and synovial inflammation may be complete disintegration of the joint and instability, with or without superimposed degenerative changes. The joint may undergo fibrous or bony ankylosis.

In about 25 percent of patients subcutaneous nodules develop commonly over the subcutaneous border of the ulna, olecranon process, dorsal aspects of the fingers, or any area receiving recurrent trauma. Similar nodules occur in the tenosynovial lining of tendons. Ruptures, due to attrition or invasion by the rheumatoid process, may result.

Skeletal muscle commonly has scattered foci of chronic inflammatory cells. Aggregations of lymphocytes and chronic inflammatory cells may be present in the endoneurium and perineurium of peripheral nerves. The granuloma-like lesions resembling the subcutaneous nodules may occur in valve leaflets or any of the layers of the heart. Pericarditis is present in about 40 percent of cases of rheumatoid arthritis. Granulomatous lesions also occur in the lungs. Rheumatoid arthritis patients may demonstrate uveitis or episcleritis. There may be involvement of lacrimal and salivary glands with lymphoid infiltration.

CLINICAL MANIFESTATIONS. Rheumatoid arthritis affects two or three females to one male and occurs at any age with the peak incidence in the thirties and forties. Involvement of joints may be sudden but is usually insidious without antecedent cause. Patients commonly have stiffness of the hands or affected joints in the morning or after inactivity. Muscular weakness and atrophy occur and may be related to the joint pain but are also due to lymphocytic infiltration of the muscles.

DIAGNOSIS. The diagnosis of a patient with long-standing classic rheumatoid arthritis and deformity is not difficult, but in the early stages and with unusual presentations the diagnosis may be quite difficult. There is no specific histopathologic character, since the pathologic findings in the arthritis associated with lupus, dermatomyositis, or periarthritis may be indistinguishable from classic rheumatoid arthritis. Laboratory tests such as the sheep cell agglutination test and latex fixation test are not specific and are positive in other diseases. Because of the

difficulty and confusion associated with this diagnosis, the committee on diagnosis of the American Rheumatism Association set up criteria to aid in this diagnosis. The following features of the disease should be considered:

1. Morning stiffness present for longer than 15 min
2. Pain with motion or direct tenderness in at least one joint
3. Swelling unrelated to bony overgrowth of at least one joint for at least 6 weeks
4. Swelling observed in a second joint within a 3-month interval
5. Symmetric joint swelling excluding distal interphalangeal (DIP) joints
6. Presence of subcutaneous nodules over bony prominences
7. X-ray changes consistent with rheumatoid arthritis
8. Positive sheep cell agglutination test or latex fixation test
9. Poor mucin clot on synovial fluid analysis
10. Characteristic histopathologic changes in the synovial membrane on biopsy
11. Characteristic histopathologic changes in nodules
12. Elevated sedimentation rate
13. Iritis

Classic rheumatoid arthritis would have seven of the above criteria with continuous joint swelling for 6 weeks. A definite diagnosis requires five criteria with continuous joint swelling for at least 6 weeks. A "probable rheumatoid" has three of the above criteria and joint symptoms for at least 4 weeks.

Rheumatoid arthritis is excluded if a diagnosis of lupus, polyarteritis nodosa, or erythema nodosum can be made. Similarly, rheumatic fever, gout, tuberculous arthritis, Reiter's syndrome, hypertrophic pulmonary osteoarthropathy, ochranosis, multiple myeloma, or lymphomas may simulate the joint findings.

LABORATORY FINDINGS. A normochromic or hyperchromic, normocytic anemia of moderate severity occurs with rheumatoid arthritis. The sedimentation rate is elevated and is a good index of the activity of the disease.

In the serum of 90 percent of adult patients with rheumatoid arthritis the anti-γ-globulin factor called *rheumatoid factor* is present. Only 20 percent of juvenile patients with rheumatoid arthritis have positive results of tests for rheumatoid factor. Rheumatoid factor is measured by the sheep cell agglutination test or latex fixation test. Analysis of synovial fluid from a rheumatoid joint will reveal a poor mucin clot, decrease in synovial fluid glucose, joint fluid leukocytosis reaching 50,000 or more, and decreased viscosity.

RADIOGRAPHIC FINDINGS. The radiographic findings (Fig. 43-94) in the extremities of early rheumatoid arthritis are related to the presence of destructive influences of the hyperplastic synovia. As the disease progresses, degenerative or responsive changes in the joint may be superimposed upon the rheumatoid process. The earliest x-ray changes are best identified in the involved hands. Similar processes and changes may occur in any joint.

The earliest finding is soft tissue swelling. This fusiform swelling may be about the proximal interphalangeal (PIP) joint, metatarsophalangeal (MP) joints, or radiocarpal joint. The presence of persistent synovial swelling causes osteoporosis in the ends of the bones adjacent to the inflammation. With long-standing arthritis, osteoporosis is

Fig. 43-94. X-ray changes in rheumatoid arthritis: severe destruction of radiocarpal articulation with subluxation and ulna deviation at the wrist; loss of ulna styloid bilaterally due to the rheumatoid process; dislocation of the PIP joint of the left thumb and dislocation of the right fourth and fifth finger MP joints and left MP joint; diffuse joint space narrowing of many IP joints.

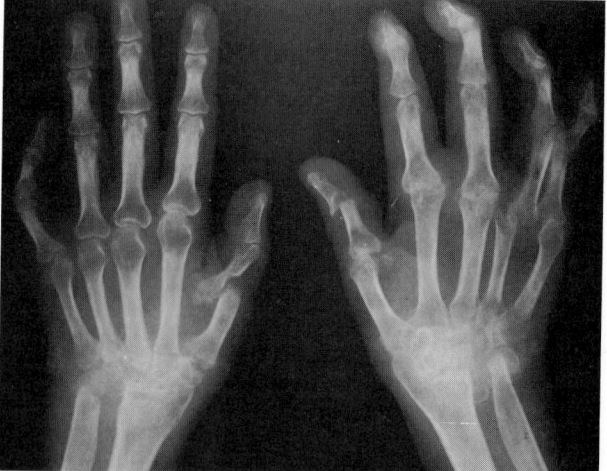

a common finding and is in part related to disuse atrophy of the bone.

The presence of synovial and capsular inflammation produces new periosteal bone in the region of capsular attachment. This is noted particularly in the region of capsular attachments about the PIP and MP joints. Proximal to the capsular attachment, there may be cortical involvement with irregularity produced by osteoclastic resorption. The presence of rheumatoid synovium causes erosion at the cartilage synovial junction and on the so-called bare area of bone. Erosions occur commonly on the metacarpal heads, PIP joints, radial margin of the navicular, ulnar styloid, and ulnar aspect of the triquetrum. The damage caused by the synovium when seen in profile appears to be a pseudocyst. The presence of vascular tenosynovium in the region of the radial styloid or on the dorsal aspect of the first metacarpal may cause resorption of bone resulting in irregularity of the bone cortex.

Joint space narrowing may occur quite early in the disease or late. The presence of joint space narrowing in the absence of sclerosis or degenerative changes is indicative of an inflammatory process of the rheumatoid type. With progression of the rheumatoid process, joint subluxations, ulnar deviation at the MP joints (Fig. 43-95), and dislocation may occur. If the patient is actively using this hand, superimposed degenerative changes may occur.

In the juvenile, the presence of rheumatoid synovitis causes soft tissue swelling and osteoporosis. Increased local vascularity results in circumferential enlargement and change in shape of the epiphyses. Leg length inequality may occur as a result of unilateral epiphyseal stimulation. Juvenile rheumatoid arthritis is more likely to go on to ankylosis in comparison with the erosion and instability that predominates in adults.

Management

Ideally, a team should consist of a rheumatologist, orthopaedist, physiotherapist, occupational therapist, and social worker. Only by combining the efforts and interests of these individuals can maximal therapy be rendered to the arthritic. The orthopaedic surgeon should be involved in the care of every rheumatoid patient. The basic aim of treatment is to halt the progressive destruction caused by this disease, to relieve the patient's pain, and to allow him or her to continue functioning without the hazard of progressive deformity. This is not possible for all patients, but the progress of the disease usually can be minimized with adequate medical and physical therapy and well-timed surgical intervention.

MEDICAL MANAGEMENT. Medical management includes administration of anti-inflammatory drugs and analgesics, as well as physical and emotional supportive treatment. The drugs now available for treating this form of arthritis are numerous, but Huskisson has suggested a simple classification:

1. Simple analgesics, e.g., aspirin in small doses (2 mg daily), paracetamol, codeine

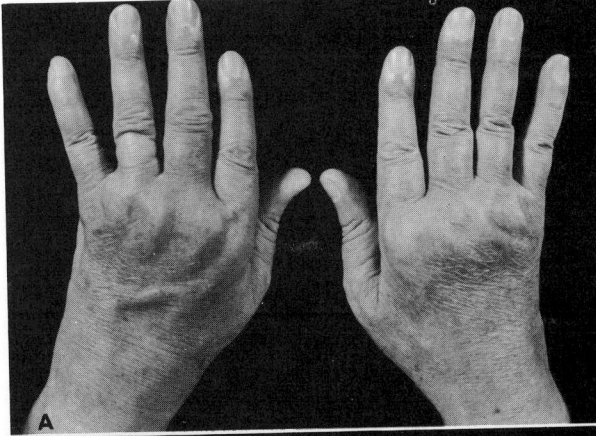

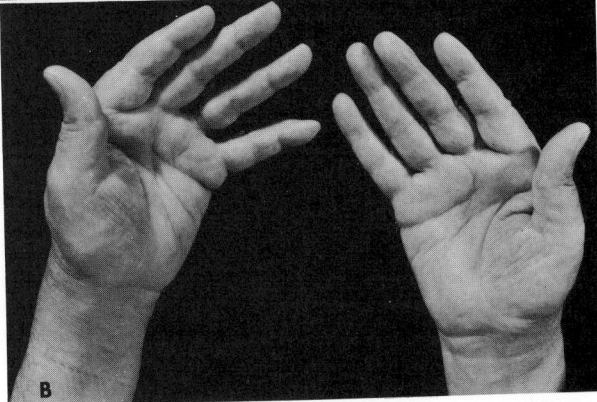

Fig. 43-95. A rheumatoid arthritic hand showing a mild degree of ulnar deviation with MP joint swelling.

2. Analgesics with minor anti-inflammatory properties, e.g., ibuprofen, naproxen, nefenamid acid
3. Analgesics with major anti-inflammatory properties, e.g., indomethacin, phenylbutazone, aspirin (at least 3.6 g daily)
4. Pure anti-inflammatory drugs, e.g., corticosteroids, corticotropin
5. "Slow-acting" drugs, e.g., gold, penicillamine, the antimalarials, and immunosuppressives such as azothiaprine, or cyclophosphamide

Corticosteroids have a place in the management of rheumatoid arthritis, especially in life-threatening situations of vasculitis or severe exacerbations of the disease, but are contraindicated as routine treatment.

ORTHOPAEDIC MANAGEMENT

PHYSICAL THERAPY. The patient should be informed about deforming forces on inflamed joints. For example, patients with MP joint involvement should understand that grasping heavy objects between thumb and forefingers or grasping objects over long periods which requires excessive force will put undue strain on the inflamed capsule, contributing to subluxation and ulnar drift. Patients with acutely swollen knees should be cautioned about putting excessive stress on the knees when arising from a chair, walking, or standing for long periods. Patients with hip disease should be cautioned to use crutches during acute flare-up of the joint disease.

Inflamed joints should be protected against mechanical trauma that aggravates and complicates the inflammatory destruction. An inflamed joint assumes the position in which the greatest volume of fluid can be accommodated in the joint with the least capsular pressure. In the knee, this is about 20° of flexion. If a contracture in the position of 20° flexion occurs, the patient will have difficulty walking and will superimpose mechanical trauma on the joint inflammation. Wrists go into flexion, which weakens grip. Metatarsophalangeal joints drift into flexion and ulnar deviation, weakening grasp and function.

Splinting is recommended for wrists in 30° dorsiflexion, knees in full extension, and ankles at 90°. Splints are always worn at night and may be worn continuously during the acute episode.

It is extremely important for patients with joint disease to maintain active muscle power. Patients are instructed to carry out daily range-of-motion exercises. This should be done without putting undue force on the capsule of the joint. Knee joints should be exercised while the patient is sitting or lying without body weight applied. Patients should do isometric exercises in a position of function, i.e., full extension for the knees. Patients with cervical spine involvement are urged to maintain a range of full extension. Inflamed hips will develop flexion deformities that can be minimized by passive stretching daily. The patient accomplishes this by lying in a prone position for 15 to 20 min twice a day.

The surgeon should be prepared to fit patients with lower extremity braces as well as wrist splints. The patient who must continue to work and walk with severely involved knees can be helped by the use of a long leg brace with the knee locked in full extension. Valgus and varus deformities involving ankle and subtalar joints can be stabilized by the use of below-knee orthoses.

SURGICAL TREATMENT. At the present time, when proper joint rest, modification of activity, and systemic anti-inflammatory medications are unable to control the rheumatoid process, early synovectomy is indicated. If this is carried out before there is significant joint space narrowing and bony collapse, it can protect against joint destruction and effectively relieve pain. As reported in multicenter trials, after 3 years, knees treated by early synovectomy were less painful and tender than those treated by conservative measures and had less effusion. This procedure did not halt the irreversible changes in all treated joints but significantly slowed the development of further pathologic changes in some knee joints. The results from metacarpophalangeal joints when treated by synovectomy showed no advantage over control joints at 3 years, either clinically or radiographically. Synovectomy is particularly applicable when synovitis is concentrated in a few joints. When the synovitis is generalized, early synovectomy is indicated, especially in the knees.

Knee

If the rheumatoid process has progressed to the point where cartilage substance has been lost, there is concomitant relative lengthening of the collateral ligaments and, therefore, instability. There may be a varus or valgus deformity associated with the cartilage destruction. Synovectomy alone at this stage of the disease is not sufficient to relieve pain and provide knee stability. Such patients require total knee replacements.

Over the past decade, total knee replacements have evolved to the point of success approaching that of total hip replacement. The total knee replacement is important in the treatment of painful unstable rheumatoid knees, especially since the alternative of fusion is frequently contraindicated because of multiple joint involvement.

The incidence of the dread complication of wound infection varies from less than 1 to as high as 10 percent, which has been reported with constrained knee replacement. Treatment of this infection, if recognized early, is the insertion of large-bore tubes that permit closed ingress/egress irrigation with antibiotics or by immediate debridement and prosthesis exchange. Other acute complications include patellar tendon rupture and peroneal nerve injuries. The most common complication of total knee replacement is loosening of the tibial component. The incidence may approach 10 percent after 2 years. A loose painful prosthesis usually requires surgical revision.

Hip

At the present time, there has been insufficient experience with prophylactic synovectomy in the rheumatoid hip with early involvement. However, for the patient with moderate or severe hip disease with disabling pain, total hip replacement is the treatment of choice. (See Total Hip Replacement, under Osteoarthritis.) When there is failure of total hip replacement or infection, the Girdlestone pseudarthrosis will provide pain relief and good hip mobility.

Ankle and Foot

Most rheumatoid deformities about the ankle and hind part of the foot can be controlled by adequate bracing techniques. An occasional patient will require bony stabilization with correction of deformity at the ankle or subtalar joints. The insertion of a total ankle in which the damaged joint surfaces are replaced with metal and polyethylene has not been proved successful.

Forefoot

The rheumatoid process occurs almost as frequently in the MP joints of the toes as in the hands. Claw toes with dislocation of the MP joints and flexion of the IP joints is the resultant deformity. The patient is unable to displace forefoot weight between the toes and the metatarsal heads. With the loss of fat pad beneath metatarsal heads and increased weight over this area, painful calluses develop, and difficulty in ambulation occurs. The Hoffman operation, which consists of proximal partial phalangectomy of all MP joints and excision of the metatarsal heads, will give great relief to the patient and improve gait (Fig. 43-96).

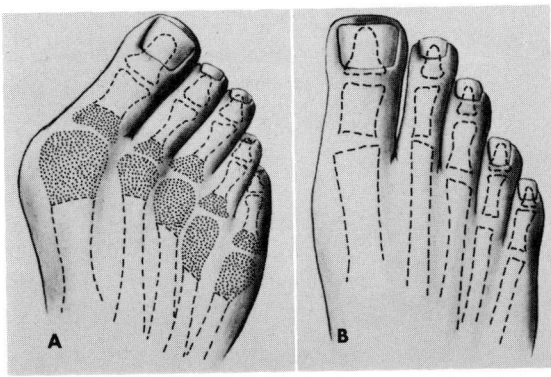

Fig. 43-96. Hoffman operation used in rheumatoid deformities of the forefoot to relieve metatarsal head pressure and improve toe function and alignment. Metatarsal head and proximal portions of phalanges are excised through transverse dorsal incision.

Hand

The rheumatoid process commonly involves the PIP joints, MP joints, carpal joints, and the tenosynovium of the flexor and extensor tendons about the wrist. The rheumatoid synovitis of the MP joints causes capsular distention and laxity of collateral ligaments (Fig. 43-95). As the disease progresses, the MP joints sublux anteriorly and ulnaward, causing ulnar drift of the fingers. The extensor tendons are dislocated into the gutters between the metacarpal heads, accentuating the deformity.

Joint involvement of the MP joints as well as rheumatoid disease involvement of the intrinsic muscle mass may produce flexion contracture of the MP joints, hyperextension of the PIP joints, and flexion of the DIP joints. This is the so-called swan-neck deformity of the intrinsic-plus hand. Involvement of the PIP joint may result in rupture of the central slip of the extensor tendon crossing the PIP joint, which allows the lateral bands to sublux anteriorly, and a typical boutonnière flexion deformity of the PIP joint develops.

With synovial distention of the MP joint of the thumb, lateral instability occurs, usually with a flexion deformity due to damage or attrition of the extensor pollicis brevis as it inserts into the proximal phalanx. Synovitis may similarly injure the interphalangeal joint of the thumb. Destruction of the carpometacarpal joint may interfere with opposition.

Synovial inflammation of the carpal joints will result in limitation of wrist dorsiflexion and cause anterior subluxation of the wrist. Involvement of the distal radioulnar joint may cause dorsal dislocation of the ulna, interference with wrist rotation, flexion, and extension.

Tenosynovitis occurs about the extensor tendons, and rheumatoid nodules may develop in the tendons themselves. The tendon may stretch or rupture because of the tenosynovial inflammation process or because of mechanical erosion from the involved distal radioulnar joint. The common tendon ruptures occur in those tendons crossing the distal radioulnar joint, the extensor tendons to ring and small finger, and the extensor digiti minimi proprius. The extensor pollicis longus may be involved

along its path across the dorsum of the wrist. Flexor tenosynovitis is commonly overlooked because of the deep position of these structures. With sufficient tenosynovitis, there may be compression of the median nerve in the carpal tunnel. Tenosynovitis of the flexor tendons will cause limitation of active motion of the fingers in the absence of MP or IP joint involvement. If an intrinsic-plus deformity is present, Littler releases in addition to MP joint synovectomy are carried out.

Arthroplasty. When there is subluxation or dislocation of the MP joint that cannot be corrected by crossed intrinsic muscle transfer, MP arthroplasties are indicated. The technique of arthroplasty using an implant described by Swanson or Niebauer is recommended.

Tenosynovial Involvement of Extensor Tendons? Unrelieved tenosynovitis of the dorsum of the wrist will result in attrition or destruction of tendons. Early dorsal tenosynovectomy should be carried out when possible. At the same time, the distal ¾ in. of the ulnar shaft and styloid should be excised with adjacent diseased synovium of the distal radioulnar joint.

Tendon Ruptures. The extensor tendons of the ring and small fingers are commonly ruptured with any long-standing process in the dorsum of the wrist. The extensor pollicis longus may also rupture. When rupture has occurred, tenosynovectomy is indicated, during the repair of the tendons. The tendons are repaired by attaching the distal stumps to the intact extensors of the index and long fingers. In the case of the extensor pollicis longus, a new motor tendon is attached to the distal stump. This is best supplied by the extensor indicis proprius.

Flexor Tenosynovitis and the Carpal Tunnel Syndrome. In rheumatoid arthritic patients, flexor tenosynovitis may encroach on the available space for the median nerve as it passes through the carpal tunnel. The patient complains of pain in the thumb, index finger, or long finger with weakness of grasp due to thenar muscle weakness. The patient is commonly awakened at night and shakes the hand in an attempt to relieve the discomfort. On examination, there may only be minimal swelling due to the flexor tenosynovitis. A positive Tinel sign, thenar weakness, and atrophy and numbness in the median nerve distribution may be present in varying degrees. Frequently there is only a history of night pain with paresthesia in the median distribution.

Flexor tenosynovitis may limit active flexion of the fingers with or without median nerve compression. The patient should always be examined for the ability to flex fingers actively to the same degree as that achieved in passive motion. When passive motion is significantly increased over active, flexor tenosynovitis is the diagnosis.

Thumb Deformities. With sufficient destruction of the MP or IP joint, the functioning of the hand may be severely limited. Instability is corrected by MP arthrodesis (Fig. 43-97) in the position of 15 to 20° of flexion. The pulp of the thumb should be rotated into the position of opposition. In some instances, it may be necessary to fuse the IP joint. Painful involvement of the carpometacarpal joint with subluxation or limitation of motion will require an arthroplasty by excision of the trapezium.

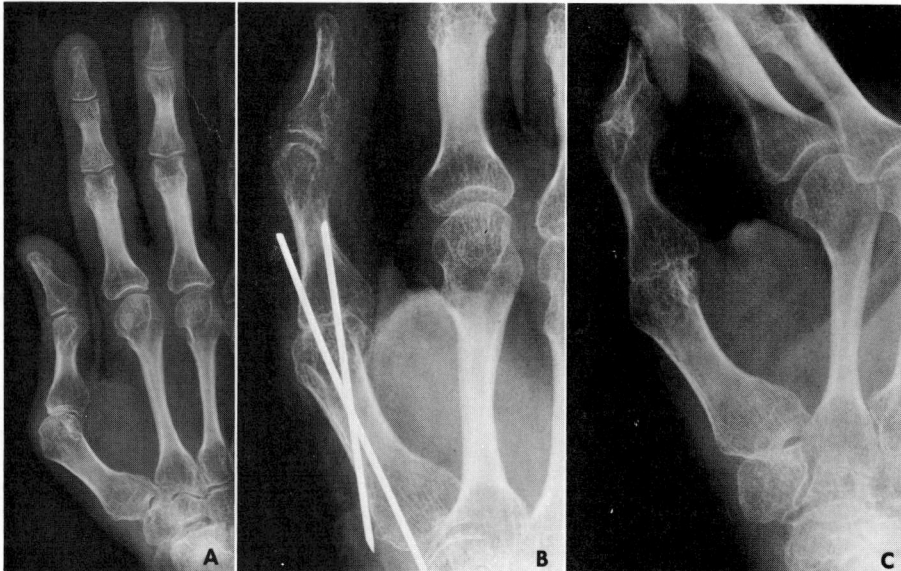

Fig. 43-97. Flexion deformity of the thumb in a patient with long-standing juvenile rheumatoid arthritis, treated by arthrodesis of the MP joint. *A.* Joint space narrowing of the MP joint with inability to extend the thumb beyond 45° flexion. *B.* Crossed Kirschner wire fixation following excision of articular surfaces. *C.* Eight months postfusion with solid arthrodesis in functional position.

Other Upper Extremity Deformities

The rheumatoid process may cause severe painful instability of the elbow. Pain is controlled by proper splinting of the elbow, which is usually sufficient. If ankylosis of the elbow occurs bilaterally or flexion is limited bilaterally, so that patients cannot feed themselves, an arthroplasty may be necessary. This is carried out by excision of the distal humerus and proximal ulna and radius with interposition of fascia lata. Total elbow replacement has not been successful. Rheumatoid disease of the glenohumeral joints is quite difficult to manage. Local injection of cortisone may be helpful in managing the acute state. Persistent pain with restricted motion may require shoulder arthroplasty.

OSTEOARTHRITIS

Osteoarthritis is a term used to describe degenerative changes in diarthrodial joints. The primary change is in the articular cartilage, which is characterized by softening, fibrillation, and abrasion of the articular surface. Since inflammation is not a primary mechanism, *osteoarthrosis* or *degenerative joint diseases* are, perhaps, more accurate terms. Degenerative joint changes occur secondarily in joints previously damaged by inflammation or trauma.

PATHOLOGY. The first recognizable changes in osteoarthritic joints occur in the articular cartilage. There is a loss of metachromasia followed by fissuring in the surface of the cartilage. On gross examination, the cartilage appears softer and yellower than its normal blue-gray color. As the process progresses, flaking of the articular cartilage and fibrillation of its surface occur. The earliest changes, since they are present only in the articular cartilage, are not demonstrable by x-ray until there has been some joint space narrowing, usually in the weight-bearing area.

With loss of cartilage, the underlying subchondral bone may be exposed and eburnated. Osteophytes occur at the margins of the articular surfaces or in the capsule and ligamentous attachments at the joint margins. The osteophytes on the joint margins are usually covered with a layer of hyalin or fibrocartilage. The earliest radiographic change may be sharpening of the normally smooth, rounded marginal contours of the subchondral bone. Bone proliferates in the area below cartilage fibrillation and accounts for sclerosis, which is manifested radiographically by increased density in the subchondral region.

Cysts may develop in the subchondral bone. In this situation, the marrow has undergone mucoid degeneration; trabeculae are lost and sclerotic new bone encircles the cystic rarefied area. The zone of calcification of the base of the articular cartilage advances into the uncalcified cartilage, which accounts for further loss of joint space seen by x-ray.

Concomitant with changes in the underlying bone, the subsynovial layers develop increasing amounts of fibrous tissue with capsular scarring. There may be moderate degrees of villous synovitis if the joint has been repeatedly injured.

Joints deranged by any process will develop secondary osteoarthritic changes. Secondary osteoarthritis is particularly common in the hip following congenital dysplasia, Legg-Calvé-Perthes disease, slipped capital femoral epiphysis, aseptic necrosis of the femoral head, or fractures involving the acetabulum. In joints damaged by crystal deposition, such as in gout or pseudogout, by ochronosis, or by hemophilia and neurogenic lesions, secondary osteoarthritis develops. When there is no predisposing cause for the articular cartilage change, the osteoarthritis is considered primary. There is no known cause of primary osteoarthritis. Primary osteoarthritis leads to affect the large weight-bearing joints—hips or knees (Fig. 43-98). Osteoarthritis without underlying trauma or other inflammatory joint disease only rarely involves elbows, wrists, or MP joints.

Primary generalized osteoarthritis occurs mainly in females, with onset during menopause, and involves multiple joints to include the DIP, in which Heberden's nodes develop. Heberden's nodes are osteophytic growths on the proximal aspects of the distal finger phalanges. The symptoms in this type of arthritis tend to be more acute, with clinical evidence of local inflammation at the articular sites.

Certain factors predispose to specific joint osteoarthritis. Trauma or repetitive stress to a joint may be a contributing factor, but hereditary factors as yet unknown are also implicated. Patients with obesity have a significantly higher incidence of osteoarthritis of the knees. Elbows of pneumatic drill operators are frequently involved. Population and genetic studies indicate a higher incidence of affected relatives with osteoarthritis in patients who have Heberden's nodes.

CLINICAL MANIFESTATIONS. Although radiologic and pathologic studies indicate that the incidence of osteoarthritic joints increases with age, only a small percentage have symptoms related to the joint pathology. It is estimated that only 5 percent of all individuals past fifty have clinical symptoms, and the percentage increases to 20 to 30 percent after the age of sixty. Clinical manifestations are more common in women, although pathologic changes are found with equal incidence in both sexes.

The onset of osteoarthritis symptoms is commonly insidious; at the time of presentation the x-ray changes indicate that bone and joint abnormality has long been present. Except in primary generalized osteoarthritis there are no systemic manifestations. Local symptoms include pain with motion, relieved by rest. Stiffness occurs after rest and resolves after the joint has been repetitively exercised. Muscle atrophy is not common. On examination, there is restriction of joint motion.

There are no specific laboratory examinations to prove the diagnosis. The synovial fluid is normal. X-ray findings may be quite normal in the very early stages of cartilage change. As the disease progresses, joint space narrowing, subchondral bone sclerosis, osteophyte formation, and subchondral bone cysts are present in varying degrees (Fig. 43-99). The presence of such x-ray signs should not be interpreted as the cause of the patient's symptoms, since these x-ray findings may exist without symptoms.

CONSERVATIVE TREATMENT. Most patients with osteoarthritis can be treated by conservative measures. The patient should understand the differences between osteoarthritis and rheumatoid arthritis, etc., and be given reassurance of a good prognosis. Immobilization of a painful osteoarthritic joint is dramatic in its relief of pain. Frequently, protection of a painful joint for a few days or weeks is sufficient to alleviate symptoms, and the patient can return to previous activity.

All factors adding to stress across the symptomatic

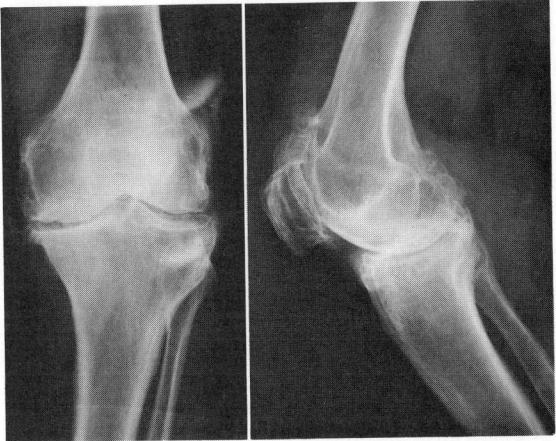

Fig. 43-98. Primary osteoarthritis of the knee. AP and lateral x-rays showing varus deformity of the knee with joint space narrowing, osteophyte production on medial, lateral, and posterior aspects of the tibia, on anterior aspects of femoral condyles, and on both upper and lower poles of the patella. There is minimal cyst formation and sclerosis of subchondral bone of the medial joint space.

joint or joints should be minimized or eliminated. Obese patients should be put on a reducing diet. One pound of body weight is calculated to produce 2 ft-lb/in.^{2} through the hip joint. Muscle power that will stabilize the damaged joint should be strengthened. The patient should be instructed to rest the joint when minor symptoms return so as to prevent the pain–muscle-spasm–limitation-of-motion cycle. In some situations, weight-relieving calipers or braces or splints will effectively protect the joint. Daily and occupational activities should be evaluated and activities modified, if possible. Range-of-motion and muscle-strengthening exercises may be helpful because of the protective stabilizing effect to a deranged joint.

Analgesic drugs are helpful in controlling symptoms, but under no circumstances should the patient be started on narcotic or habit-forming drugs. Aspirin, in addition to its analgesic action, has a direct anti-inflammatory effect

Fig. 43-99. Bilateral osteoarthritis of the hips showing marked osteophyte formation, sclerosis, acetabular cysts, obliteration of joint space, and partial subluxation.

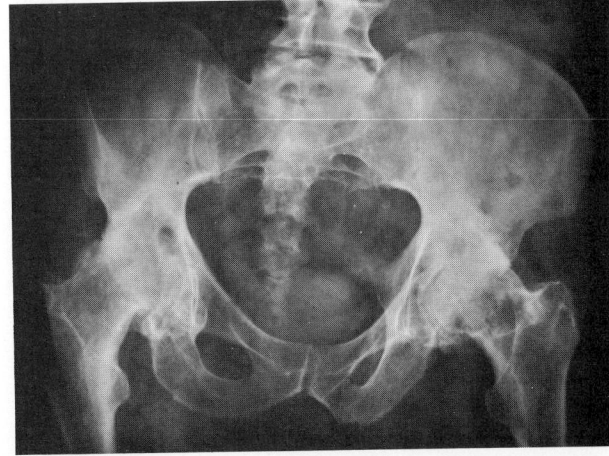

on cartilage, as well as on periarticular structures. Non-steroidal anti-inflammatory drugs are also helpful. The local instillation of hydrocortisone into a painful joint may afford relief if conservative splinting and local rest measures fail, but there have been reports of neurotropic joints developing following excessive injections.

ORTHOPAEDIC MANAGEMENT. Surgical treatment of osteoarthritis is indicated when conservative measures fail to control pain or when joint motion is significantly limited and symptomatic. Procedures available for relief of pain of an osteoarthritic joint include arthrodesis, arthroplasty, osteotomy, pseudarthrosis, and neurectomy.

Arthrodesis eliminates motion and relieves the irritation of pain-producing structures. Arthroplasty and pseudarthrosis provide increased mobility of a joint but may be less effective in relieving the discomfort. Osteotomy is effective in correcting deformity and realigning joints and has the added benefit of pain relief by mechanisms incompletely understood at the present time. Neurectomy is indicated in rare situations, but because of the gross overlap of articular innervation, complete denervation of a joint is difficult.

Thumb Carpometacarpal Joint

In clothing workers, seamstresses, and surgeons, osteoarthritis of the carpometacarpal joint of the thumb may develop. The patients have pain with any motion of the thumb and marked interference with grasp, due to pain. Painful DIP joints afflicted with osteoarthritis are rarely unstable. Conservative treatment will usually suffice, and rarely arthrodesis or flexible implant arthroplasty of one of these joints may be indicated.

Wrist, Elbow, and Shoulder

Surgical treatment is infrequently required for wrist, elbow, and shoulder osteoarthritis, which usually result from injuries. Wrist pain due to posttraumatic arthritis not responding to conservative measures may be treated by arthrodesis of the radiocarpal and intercarpal joints. Management of the painful posttraumatic elbow may require excision of the radial head because of radiohumeral joint subluxation. In sedentary individuals and office workers, a fascia lata arthroplasty will allow motion, although it will increase instability. For laborers who are unable to change occupations, arthrodesis of the elbows in the correct position will provide pain relief and stability. Posttraumatic symptomatic acromioclavicular and sternoclavicular joints may be treated by arthroplasty. In the case of the acromioclavicular joint, the distal 1 in. of the clavicle is removed, and for the sternoclavicular joint, the proximal 1 in. of the clavicle is excised. The rare patient with osteoarthritis of the shoulder may be treated by total shoulder replacement.

Hip

Osteoarthritis of the hip may be primary or secondary as a result of abnormalities of the acetabulum or shape and alignment of femoral head and neck. Patients with significant acetabular dysplasia, post-Legg-Calvé-Perthes disease with femoral head enlargement, and slipped epiphyses tend to become symptomatic a decade sooner, in their forties and fifties, than patients with primary osteoarthritis of the hip.

The presenting complaint with osteoarthritis of the hip is invariably pain. In the early symptomatic stages, pain is intermittent with episodes occurring after excessive activity and followed by asymptomatic remissions. Pain is aching in character, referred to the groin, the lateral aspect of the thigh, and frequently as far distally as the medial aspect of the knee. Pain is more severe with activity following joint rest, either in the morning or after sitting. With increased activity, the symptoms are less severe. Later in the course of the disease, pain may be severely aggravated by activity, followed by rest pain lasting a few hours.

Patients with osteoarthritis of the hip are usually unaware of restriction of motion early in the disease. As the disease progresses, restriction may be severe. The earliest loss of motion is that of internal rotation but also with associated loss of abduction and extension. Patients may present with an adduction–external-rotation flexion contracture. Patients walk with a characteristic hip limp of the Trendelenburg type or an abductor lurch.

Treatment. Conservative treatment should be attempted. It may be sufficient to allow the patient to continue activities with modification, and while conservative treatment is in progress, the physician can evaluate the patient's cooperation and motivation prior to undertaking reconstructive surgical procedures.

Rest in bed with skin traction to the leg or non-weight-bearing crutch walking during acute episodes are helpful when the pain is severe. The simple maneuver of having the patient carry a cane in the opposite hand to relieve weight load across the contralateral hip may dramatically relieve symptoms. Nonsteroidal anti-inflammatory drugs are administered. Often, modification of the patient's activities and job requirements will allow continued working. If conservative measures fail, surgical procedures are available, each with advantages and disadvantages but all requiring a patient who is a good operative risk (Fig. 43-100).

Arthrodesis. For the young individual who experiences repetitive stress to a hip and who must stand for long periods, hip arthrodesis (Fig. 43-100A) may be the procedure of choice. The most frequent indications are sepsis (pyogenic or tuberculous) and cases in which implant arthroplasty is contraindicated. Surgical arthrodesis requires a patient who is physiologically young enough to undergo this treatment, and who will tolerate the plaster cast immobilization and bed rest for 3 to 6 months. Patients with previous back injuries or disease are not suitable candidates for this procedure because of the added stress to the lumbar spine. Patients with bilateral hip disease or involvement of other joints in the lower extremities should be considered for other surgical procedures.

Femoral Osteotomy. The displacement osteotomy (Fig. 43-100B) described by McMurray may provide dramatic pain relief and allow hip joint mobility. In young patients

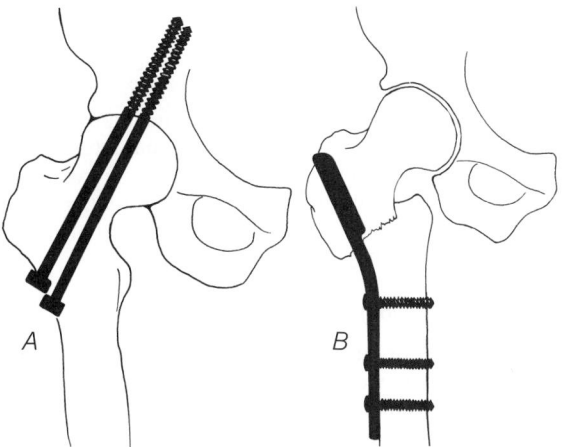

Fig. 43-100. Surgical treatment of hip disease. *A.* Arthrodesis. *B.* Displacement osteotomy.

with early osteoarthritis, before bone collapse, and with 90° of hip flexion, displacement osteotomy is a good procedure with a high rate of pain relief and minimal risk to the patient. In the early stages of osteoarthritis, this procedure can provide complete pain relief and a mobile hip, which can be expected to last for many years. Compared with hip arthrodesis, there is less risk to the patient in this procedure, and if unsuccessful (10 to 20 percent of patients) anatomy is not distorted, and other procedures may be undertaken. Bombelli (1984) has rejuvenated the interest in osteotomy for the young patient by extending Panwell's mechanical analysis of sheer forces around varus, valgus angular deformities of the femoral neck as well as acetabular abnormalities.

Total Hip Replacement Arthroplasty. All reconstructive procedures on the adult hip must be evaluated in the light of the superior results being obtained with total hip replacement arthroplasty. The total hip replaces both sides of the joint with a prosthetic femoral head and prosthetic acetabular component. Total hip replacement surgery has been utilized for various types of disabling hip diseases such as osteoarthritis, primary or secondary, and rheumatoid arthritis. It is also used for reconstruction of previously unsuccessful hip surgery such as osteotomy or cup arthroplasty and in any type of joint disorder where infection is not present. The operation has the best short- or medium-term results of any type of hip reconstructive operation. The uncertainties, of course, are whether the fixation of the component parts to bone can be maintained, how long the bearing surfaces will wear, and whether there is any long-term toxicity to the cement or wear debris. A 26 percent revision rate has been reported after 5 years. Newer prostheses made with porous surfaces to allow ingrowth of bone from the host may reduce this incidence.

The most serious complication of total hip replacement is a wound infection. This may occur as an acute postoperative complication or as a delayed phenomenon months or years after primary wound healing. Prevention of wound infection from total hip replacement requires scrupulous operative technique on the part of operating personnel. Surgery is often carried out in operating theaters equipped with positive-pressure rapid air changes with high-efficiency particle filters. Penicillinase-resistant antibiotics are administered preoperatively, intraoperatively, and postoperatively. Infection rates in total hip replacement series are approximately 1 percent.

Thrombophlebitis and pulmonary embolism are complications of any type of hip surgery, and total hip replacement is no exception. Prophylactic measures against thrombophlebitis are indicated, such as administration of Coumadin or low-molecular-weight dextran. Both lower extremities should be elevated postoperatively. Patients should be cautioned against sitting for even short periods until hip motion and activity have been restored.

The prosthesis can be dislocated. The incidence of this is about 1 percent and can be minimized by accurate positioning of the prosthetic components and positioning of the operative extremity until soft tissue healing has occurred. Loosening of the prosthetic components is a late complication and may be evident if the patient begins to experience pain in the characteristic hip distribution. Loosening can be determined by unusual resorption of bone at the bone-cement interphase. It may be necessary to do an arthrogram or bone scan for diagnosis.

Ninety percent of the patients maintain excellent results. Preoperative range of motion was improved in all patients, and there was no tendency to decrease motion with increasing time of follow-up. Late mechanical failures occur in about 1 percent of patients. The overall infection rate is 4 percent, 2 percent in late infections. The average degree of acetabular prosthesis wear varied from 1 mm in 5 years to absence of wear at 7 years postsurgery.

Chondromalacia of the Patella

Chondromalacia of the patella represents degeneration, or the first stage of osteoarthritis, involving the cartilage surface of the patella. Changes in this cartilage are common by the age of thirty, although symptomatology is infrequent. The earliest changes occur on the medial facet of the patella. The cause of chondromalacia is unknown, but trauma of an incongruent relationship of the patella with the femoral condyle may play a role. In teenagers, especially girls, mild degrees of recurvatum and valgus knees are associated with subluxing patella with attendant chondromalacia. Symptomatic chondromalacia is not uncommon after immobilization of a fractured femur for prolonged periods.

The onset may be insidious; the patient is aware only of minor discomfort in the knee with acute flexion or in descending stairs or kneeling. Often the onset is acute following a direct blow to the knee. Chondromalacia frequently presents with symptoms of subluxation or even frank dislocation of the patella. The patient may be aware of crepitus. Physical examination will demonstrate tenderness if the patella is pressed distad in its groove while the quadriceps is actively contracted. By displacing the patella, medial, the undersurface can be palpated and also may reveal tenderness.

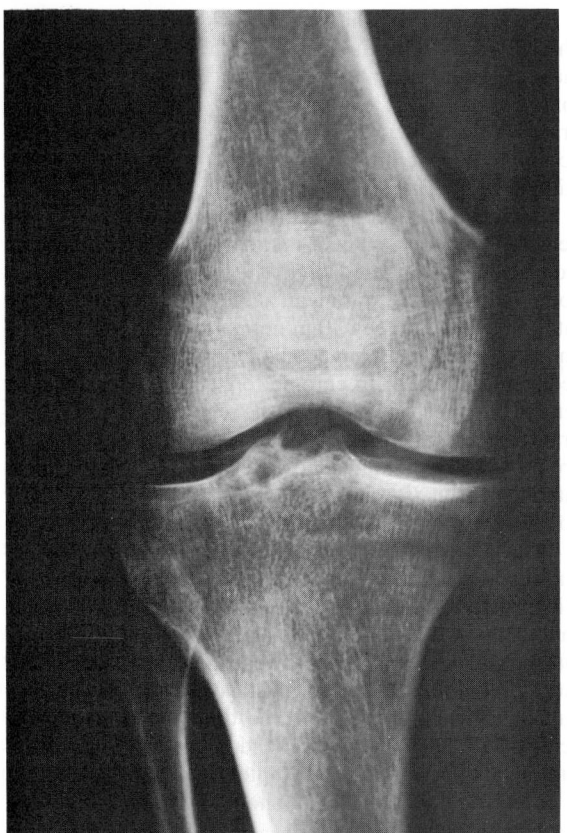

Fig. 43-103. Calcification of knee menisci in a patient with pseudo-gout.

The onset may be acute, with symptoms increasing in a joint over 1 to 2 days in contrast to the more abrupt onset of gout. The joint most commonly involved is the knee joint. It is quite uncommon in the MP joint of the great

Fig. 43-104. Hemophilic arthritis. AP and lateral x-rays of the knee joint showing enlargement of epiphyses of the knee, joint space narrowing, with irregularity and squaring of the lower end of the patella. Note also the soft tissue swelling about the knee. *A*. AP x-rays. *B*. Lateral x-rays.

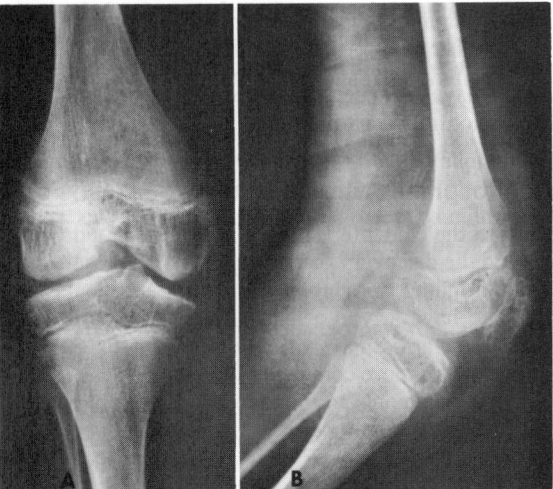

toe. Patients with acute attacks have asymptomatic intervals. One-third of such patients have an elevation of the serum uric acid level. A small percentage of patients will have continuous acute attacks, but the most frequent pattern is that of progressive chronic arthritis of large joints. Hypertension and diabetes are associated with one-fourth to one-half of patients with pseudogout. The patients complain of acute pain in the involved joint with stiffness, local swelling, tenderness, and erythema overlying the joint. In the chronic presentation, the joint may resemble a degenerative arthritis.

The diagnosis is dependent upon finding calcium pyrophosphate crystals in the synovial fluid or in leukocytes of synovial fluid. Polarized light microscopy reveals the crystals to show weakly positive birefringence. X-rays reveal crystalline deposits in the articular cartilage as well as in fibrocartilaginous structures as menisci (Fig. 43-103) and ligaments in joint capsules. The distal radioulnar joint and symphysis pubis, as well as glenoid and acetabular labra, may show calcification. The calcification of the articular cartilage is in the midzonal layer and appears as a radiopaque line, paralleling the subchondral bone.

Treatment of an acute attack is by aspiration of the synovial effusion and the local injection of cortisone. Systemic phenylbutazone and salicylates may be helpful, but colchicine is not. At present, there is no means of halting the progressive deposition in joints.

HEMOPHILIC ARTHRITIS

The major problem confronting the hemophiliac between episodes of acute bleeding is disability due to hemophilic arthropathy. Duthie et al. have shown spontaneous bleeding occurs only with 0 percent circulating factor VIII; severe bleeding after minor injury occurs when factor VIII is between 1 and 5 percent, and excessive bleeding after minor injury or operation at 5 to 25 percent of normal. Repeated hemorrhage into growing joints results in progressive deterioration and chronic arthritis.

CLINICAL MANIFESTATIONS. In the severe hemophiliac, bleeding into one of the large joints occurs spontaneously or with mild trauma. The most common joint of involvement is the knee, followed by elbow, ankle, and shoulder, with joint hemorrhage in any joint a possibility. If unchecked by coagulation therapy, hemarthrosis becomes acute, and the joint assumes that position which accommodates the greatest volume of fluid and comfort, i.e., 20° of flexion for the knee or adduction and external rotation for the hip joint. The patient will not move the joint because of pain and associated muscle spasm.

The hemorrhage tends to run in cycles, one or two joints being repeatedly affected, followed by other joints with recurrent episodes. In the chronic stage, with sufficient joint destruction and arthritis, there is limitation of motion, fixed contracture, and deformity.

In the acutely involved joint, x-ray findings may show only soft tissue swelling and the presence of effusion. With repeated hemorrhage, adjacent epiphyses enlarge and change the configuration. The characteristic findings in the knee joint (Fig. 43-104) are a squared-off lower pole of the patella, enlargement of femoral condyles, and increase in size of the intercondylar notch. Osteoporosis may be marked, and joint space is narrow. In the chronic state, the residual changes in epiphyseal configuration are superimposed with sclerosis and osteophytes of degenerative change.

TREATMENT. If joint hemorrhage can be minimized, the chronic arthritis will not ensue. Patients with the first sign of hemorrhage into the joint should be treated with appropriate coagulation factors, i.e., factor VIII. The joint is splinted with a compression bandage until effective blood clotting ensues. Weight-bearing joints are protected with crutches until the range of motion of the joint returns and the joint effusion resolves. Joints subjected to repeated hemorrhage must be protected with bracing to limit motion and prevent recurrence. The short leg brace preventing ankle motion is used for the ankle, and a light plastic splint is used for repeated hemorrhage into the knee.

If contractures have developed, these are corrected by reversed dynamic traction. When the contracture has been corrected, an immobilizing brace is applied. Ischial weight-bearing braces may be required for serious involvement of the hip joints. With adequate prophylaxis and early treatment, severe deformity can be prevented. Reconstructive surgery, total hip replacement, arthrodesis, surface replacement, etc., for joint deformities are now being carried out in specialized centers where the clotting factor deficiency can be reversed for the healing and rehabilitation phases.

SYNOVIAL LESIONS

Pigmented Villonodular Synovitis

Pigmented villonodular synovitis is an inflammatory process of unknown cause that occurs in monarticular form in young adults. The peak incidence of this condition is in the thirties, with men more frequently involved than women.

Patients present with symptoms of pain and swelling that may be intermittent and are frequently of long duration. The most commonly involved joint is the knee, but any single large joint may be involved. On examination there is usually evidence of synovial thickening with effusion. Joint aspiration characteristically reveals bloody or dark brown sanguineous fluid. X-ray evaluation may reveal soft tissue swelling, occasionally cystic erosion of joint margins, and loss of articular space.

The pathologic finding is a villous, thickened, brownish proliferation of synovial tissue that has nodules and pedicles of synovium projecting into the joint. Microscopic examination reveals proliferated synovial cells with large, round, stromal connective cells beneath the surface. Hemosiderin and cholesterol are diffused throughout the synovium in the intercellular space and in multinucleated giant cells.

Treatment of this condition depends upon its early recognition and removal by synovectomy. If there is recurrence after synovectomy, repeat surgical treatment is required and is usually successful. The same process may

occur as a localized nodular form, and a similar pathologic condition may occur in a bursa or as a localized nodular tenosynovitis.

Synovial Chondromatosis

Synovial chondromatosis is a condition occurring in synovium, bursa, or tendon sheaths in which metaplastic cartilage growth occurs. Such growth may ossify and persist in the synovium or become detached and displaced into the joint cavity as a loose body. The condition occurs as a monarticular arthritis in middle-aged adults. The knee is most commonly involved, but any large joint may be affected. Clinical examination reveals signs of inflammation with effusion. X-rays show evidence of calcified bodies in the synovium or joint space. The remainder of the joint may be normal or secondarily degenerative because of mechanical trauma from the loose body. Synovectomy is the treatment of choice.

Ankylosing Spondylitis

Ankylosing spondylitis is one of the group of seronegative spondyloarthropathies (others being Reiter's disease, psoriatic arthritis, and enteropathic arthritis). These are characterized by the disease of sacroiliitis and an increased HLA B27 positivity. It occurs in 1:1000 of the male population, and there is an increasing awareness of tendonitis, large joint involvement, plantar fasciitis particularly in the younger age group. There may well be a genetic predisposition (reflected by the high incidence of HLA B23), but an environmental influence, e.g., the presence of a gut bacteria Klebsiella is also implicated.

Conservative treatment of the spine consists of correction of abnormal posture by P.O.P., bed, physiotherapy, and the administration of indomethacin or other anti-inflammatory agents. When the ankylosis becomes bony and painful, lumbar osteotomy for the spine or total joint replacement for hip or knee may be indicated. Prevention of ectopic bone formation postoperatively may require radiotherapy or the administration of diphosphonates.

Acute Synovitis of the Hip in Childhood

Children in the Legg-Calvé-Perthes age group, age three to ten years, may present with an acutely painful hip. The mother may note a hip limp of several days' duration in the child. In other situations, the discomfort is acute enough so that the child will not bear weight. X-rays of the hip may reveal soft tissue swelling of the hip in the absence of bone changes of the capital femoral epiphyses. Ultrasound investigation is now very useful in demonstrating the fluid in the joint.

Immediate evaluation should attempt to rule out acute septic arthritis by hip joint aspiration. Acute synovitis of the hip is a diagnosis of exclusion. If an initial sepsis can be ruled out, the child is placed at bed rest with the leg in Buck's traction. When the acute symptoms resolve, the child is allowed to ambulate with non-weight-bearing crutch walking. Repeat x-rays are obtained in 6 weeks to be certain that Legg-Calvé-Perthes disease is not developing. In the absence of signs of Legg-Calvé-Perthes disease, the child is allowed weight-bearing ambulation.

SLIPPING CAPITAL FEMORAL EPIPHYSIS

Slipping capital femoral epiphysis is a disease in which one or both proximal femoral epiphyses slip from their anatomical location gradually or acutely. It affects adolescent males from ages twelve to fifteen and girls from ages ten to thirteen. The disease is quite uncommon. It occurs in boys five times more frequently. The etiology is unknown, but some evidence suggests that immunologic mechanisms may be involved.

PATHOLOGY. Separation of the proximal capital femoral epiphysis occurs in the region just above the zone of calcified cartilage. By virtue of the muscular forces across the hip, the capital epiphysis is displaced both medially and posteriorly. The synovium may be inflamed during the acute stages, raising the possibility of a primary inflammatory process in the synovium. The slip of the epiphysis results in the metaphysis becoming prominent anteriorly and laterally, which contributes to joint incongruity and subsequent degenerative arthritis.

CLINICAL MANIFESTATIONS. The most common presentation of a slipping capital femoral epiphysis is pain in the distribution associated with hip disease. Not uncommonly pain is referred from the hip and localized to the knee region. Trochanteric and groin pain are common. Patients may walk with an antalgic gait and are comfortable only at rest. On physical examination patients usually have some pain on motion of the hip, but the most common finding is the loss of the normal internal rotation as a consequence of the deformity created by the capital epiphyseal displacement. When the deformity has been present for some time, atrophy from disuse of thigh muscles may be present.

Diagnosis depends upon biplane radiography. Since the condition is bilateral in 25 percent of cases the contralateral hip should be carefully examined for x-ray signs of preslip. These include widening and irregularity of the epiphyseal plate with radiolucency in the juxtaepiphyseal areas. When a minimal slip has occurred, the most obvious sign with the AP x-ray is the medial displacement of the capital epiphysis such that a line projected along the superior neck does not interrupt the epiphysis (as occurs normally). Lateral or frog-leg x-rays will usually leave no doubt about the posterior displacement of the epiphysis. If the process has been present for some time, prominence of the anterior femoral metaphysis with a hump will be present anteriorly. New bone formation or callus occurs inferior and posterior to the junction of the head and neck where the periosteum has been displaced.

TREATMENT. The principles of treatment of a slipping capital femoral epiphysis are to prevent progressive slip since results depend upon minimizing the degree of deformity created by the slip. As soon as the diagnosis is made in mild and moderate slips, an operation is carried out to fix the existing head and neck relationship. With symptoms shorter than 10 days due to a significant slip

(an acute slip), a closed reduction followed by Knowles pinning is carried out. In severe subacute or chronic slips alternative procedures include an osteotomy to realign the proximal femur. Other procedures include a cuneiform osteotomy through the femoral neck or surgical epiphyseolysis, both of which may be complicated by avascular necrosis. Acute chondrolysis occurs in patients treated for slipping capital femoral epiphysis usually after surgical treatment. If pins had been allowed to penetrate the articular cartilage, the incidence would reach 50 percent. Blacks and females, for unknown reasons, have the highest incidence of this complication. The greater the deformity, the earlier the patients will have secondary degenerative changes.

HYPERTROPHIC PULMONARY OSTEOARTHROPATHY

Hypertrophic pulmonary osteoarthropathy is a syndrome affecting bone and joints of the extremities and occurring in association with intrathoracic pathologic conditions. Patients develop insidious asymptomatic clubbing of the fingers, which is an increased nail bed convexity with loss of the normal angle between the proximal nail beds and the distal covering of the dorsal surface of the phalanx. The nail may be brittle and striated with an underlying vascular engorgement. Associated with the clubbing may be a synovitis of a peripheral joint. X-ray examination of the extremities may reveal new periosteal bone along the shafts, including distal phalanges. This is responsible for the clubbing effect.

The exact cause is unknown, but is thought to be associated with changes in tissue oxygenation or arteriolar blood flow as a consequence of lung disease. Treatment depends upon diagnosis and treatment of the underlying lung condition. It is not uncommon to excise a pulmonary neoplasm and have peripheral joint symptoms completely resolve.

NEUROPATHIC, OR CHARCOT, JOINTS

A neuropathic joint, or Charcot joint, is a condition that occurs as a consequence of various neurologic diseases. Tabes dorsalis, syringomyelia, leprosy, or diabetes may be associated with the development of neuropathic joints. Neuropathic joints have also been described in association with insensitivity due to peripheral nerve lesions and in rare situations where no neurologic lesion is evident.

The prevailing opinion as to the mechanism of destruction in such joints has been repeated trauma on structures rendered insensitive by sensory interruption. However, some patients do have pain associated with these lesions, suggesting that other factors may be responsible.

CLINICAL MANIFESTATIONS. There may be minor discomfort in a weight-bearing joint—hip, knee, ankle, or tarsus—with diffuse swelling about the joint, but medical aid may not be sought until gross instability and deformity are present. The knee joint may have a massive effusion with gross instability of all ligamentous-supporting structures. Associated with this may be varying degrees of edema and swelling involving the leg. In the case of the tarsal joints, swelling with erythema and valgus or varus deformity are common presentations.

Radiographic findings (Fig. 43-105) include extreme dissolution of bone ends with frank dislocation, enlarged joint space, and large collections of bone fragments deposited in the enlarged synovial cavity. A rapid rate of change by x-ray, with bone loss and destruction, is suggestive of a neuropathic joint. Infection frequently complicates the diagnosis of neuropathic joints, due to diabetes.

TREATMENT. The rate and degree of destruction of bone ends with marked ligamentous instability make conservative treatment difficult. A well-fitting ischial weight-bearing brace may benefit a patient with a Charcot knee or hip joint. If this is not tolerated, surgical arthrodesis of the knee, or hip arthrodesis, is indicated.

In the insensitive foot of the diabetic, plaster cast immobilization has resulted in spontaneous fusion. Molded orthopaedic shoes with contoured arch supports and metatarsal bars have been used for diabetics and lepers with severe neurotropic destruction of the tarsal joints. The end result in the diabetic is usually below-knee amputation.

PAINFUL SHOULDER

Spontaneous pain or pain after minor strains of the shoulder are extremely common after the age of thirty-five. The most common lesion responsible for shoulder pain in this age group is that of lesions of the rotator cuff, bicipital tendonitis, subacromial bursitis, or impingement syndrome. Before ascribing the diagnosis to a local lesion, it is mandatory to rule out disease of the cervical spine and central nervous system, as well as lesions of the brachial plexus, caused by Pancoast's tumor, and referred pain from the heart, lungs, or other upper abdominal subdiaphragmatic disease.

Lesions of the Rotator Cuff

The rotator cuff consists of the common tendinous insertion of supraspinatus, infraspinatus, and teres minor muscles as well as the subscapularis tendon. These tendons form a continuous fibrous sheath, which is intimately adherent to the underlying shoulder capsule. When the shoulder is moved from the anatomic position to the position of full elevation or abduction, the rotator cuff comes in contact with the undersurface of the coracoacromial ligament and is subject to mechanical irritation, *producing an impingement lesion.* Bursitis may develop in the intervening subacromial bursa, which separates the undersurface of the acromion and coracoacromial ligament from the rotator cuff. With progression, degeneration of the tendon leading to rupture may occur. A deposition of calcium may occur in the worn and degenerative tendon, as well as in the subacromial bursa.

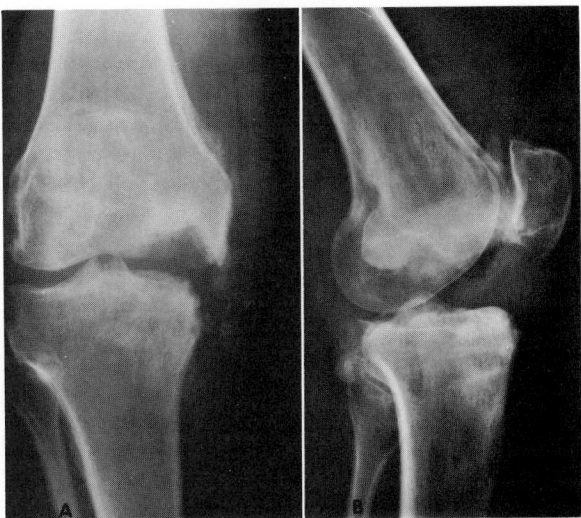

Fig. 43-105. Neuropathic knee due to tabes dorsalis showing marked destruction of medial femoral condyle. Clinically there was marked synovial swelling and effusion with marked instability due to the loss of bone substances.

CLINICAL MANIFESTATIONS. In the absence of preexisting symptomatology, a patient may note the spontaneous acute onset of severe unrelenting pain in the shoulder and in the region of the glenohumeral joint, occasionally referred into the arm and elbow. The onset may occur after unusual vigorous exercise or sports activities in the patient over thirty-five years. The patient may awaken with minor discomfort in the shoulder, which gradually increases in severity. The pain is unimproved by position and may require narcotics for relief.

On examination, there is local tenderness over the greater tuberosity of the humerus. Any motion of the shoulder causes pain. Routine x-rays of the shoulder may be negative or show a calcium deposit in the subacromial bursa or supraspinatus tendon or arthritis of the acromioclavicular or glenohumeral joints. The distinction between this lesion and bursitis or impingement syndrome will require diagnostic arthrography.

TREATMENT. Untreated, the lesion will take about 5 to 10 days for relief of symptoms. If the patient is seen when symptoms are resolving, sling immobilization combined with analgesia may be sufficient. In the acutely painful situation, the bursa should be needled, 2% Xylocaine injected, and an aspiration of the bursa contents attempted. One milliliter of cortisone is then introduced. The results of this treatment are often dramatic. After injection, the shoulder is immobilized until pain relief is complete: then gradual shoulder-motion exercises of the pendulum type are instituted. If the shoulder symptoms do not completely resolve, repeat cortisone injection is considered.

IMPINGEMENT SYNDROME

If patients continue to have symptoms not relieved by injection and continue to have a painful arc of motion in the midrange of abduction, an impingement syndrome with or without a rotator cuff tear should be suspected.

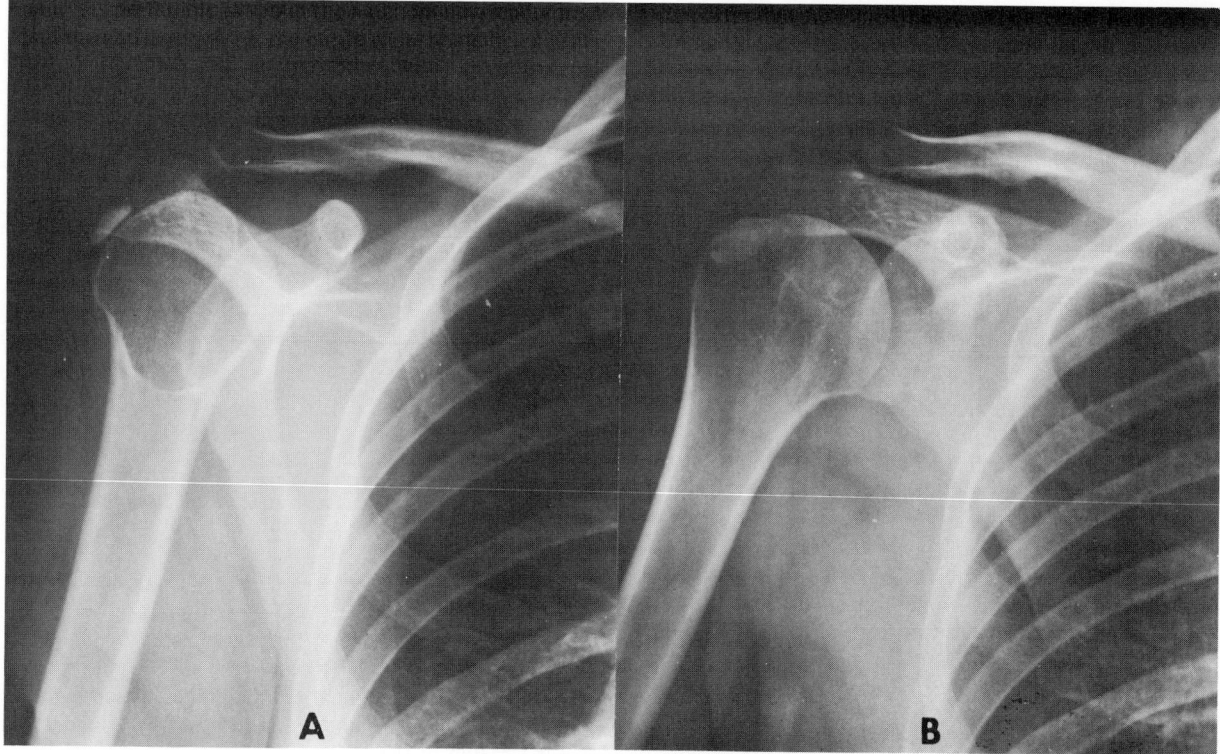

Fig. 43-106. Calcific supraspinatus tendonitis. *A.* AP x-ray of the shoulder with internal rotation shows calcium deposit in the region of the supraspinatus tendon. *B.* External rotation shows calcific shadow superimposed over the greater tuberosity.

Such patients may be helped by an anterior acromioplasty in which half of the acromion and the attached coracoacromial ligament is excised.

CHRONIC SUPRASPINATUS TENDONITIS

The presentation of degenerative lesions of the rotator cuff is often insidious. The patient complains of low-grade discomfort in the shoulder with sudden motion and with certain positions, such as full internal rotation and the extremes of abduction. These may be aggravated by increase in shoulder activity.

X-ray examination in such instances is more likely to show evidence of calcification in the supraspinatus tendon (Fig. 43-106). The treatment of this lesion should start with conservative therapy. The shoulder is immobilized in a sling and swath for 10 days to 2 weeks until relief from pain is complete. Then gradual range-of-motion exercises are started. If this does not produce a response, cortisone is injected into the shoulder, or the shoulder is treated with diathermy or ultrasound.

RUPTURES OF THE ROTATOR CUFF

A rupture of the rotator cuff occurs commonly in middle age but may also occur in late adolescence and in the elderly. Occupation has no relationship to incidence. Minor strain or injury will cause a rupture in a previously degenerated tendon. The patient may have had preexisting chronic low-grade shoulder symptoms. The patient has difficulty in achieving full active shoulder motion, although there is no contracture on examination.

If radiopaque solution is injected into the shoulder, the solution will enter subdeltoid bursa if there is discontinu-

ity in the rotator cuff. X-ray evidence of fracture of the greater tuberosity indicates that the tendon has been avulsed. If the rupture has been present for a few weeks, the muscles involved, such as the supraspinatus, may show evidence of atrophy. If a calcium deposit is present, it is unlikely that rupture has occurred.

TREATMENT. Since 25 percent of shoulders at postmortem, in the absence of previous symptoms, have had evidence of torn or degenerated cuffs, immediate surgical treatment is not indicated. Most patients will recover with conservative treatment. The acute symptoms are treated by immobilization in a sling. When pain is resolved, gradual range-of-motion exercises are instituted. If symptoms do not resolve within a few months with this type of treatment, open surgical repair, as described by McLaughlin, is done.

BICIPITAL TENDONITIS

Shoulder symptoms resembling supraspinatus tendonitis may be due to a bicipital tendon that has become irritated and inflamed in its groove and long passage through the shoulder joint. The symptoms are quite similar, but differentiation may be made on the basis of pain and tenderness extending farther distad over the bicipital groove. Treatment is by conservative means—cortisone, shortwave diathermy, immobilization—followed by return of motion. An occasional patient will require surgical exploration.

Tumors of the Musculoskeletal System

Biologic Properties

Classification of Bone Tumors

True Bone Tumors

Osteoma
Osteoid Osteoma
Osteosarcoma (Osteogenic Sarcoma)
　　Osteosarcoma in Paget's Disease
　　Parosteal Sarcoma
Chondroma
Benign Chondroblastoma (Codman's Tumor)
Chondrosarcoma
Fibroma
Fibrosarcoma
Osteoclastoma (Giant Cell Tumor)

Nonosteogenic Tumors of Bone

Unicameral (Solitary) or Juvenile Bone Cyst
Periosteal Fibrosarcoma
Ewing's Tumor
Reticulum Cell Sarcoma

Blood Vessel Tumors

Tumors Arising from Included Tissues

Malignant Tumors of Soft Tissues

Metastatic Tumors of Bone

B. Tumors arising from tissues normally found in bone but not participating in bone formation
　　1. Tumors arising from fibrous tissue
　　　　a. Periosteal fibroma
　　　　b. Periosteal fibrosarcoma
　　2. Tumors arising from bone marrow
　　　　a. Myeloma
　　　　b. Reticulum cell sarcoma
　　　　c. Hodgkin's disease of bone
　　　　d. Lymphosarcoma
　　　　e. Ewing's tumor
　　3. Tumors from blood vessels
　　　　a. Hemangioma
　　　　b. Hemangioblastoma
　　　　c. Aneurysmal bone cyst
　　　　d. Angiosarcoma
　　4. Tumors arising from adipose tissue
　　　　a. Lipoma
　　　　b. Liposarcoma
　　5. Tumors arising from nerves
　　　　a. Neurilemmoma
　　　　b. Neurofibroma
C. Tumors arising from included tissue
　　　　a. Chordoma
　　　　b. Adamantinoma
D. Metastatic tumors

TRUE BONE TUMORS

Osteoma

This small, sessile, rare tumor is found in the orbit, nasal sinuses, external auditory meatus, and oral side of the mandible. The tumor is dense and hard and is termed

BIOLOGIC PROPERTIES

In relating the site of origin of musculoskeletal tumors to the cellular activity in that area (Fig. 43-107), Johnson has shown that the giant cell tumor commonly arises in the juxtametaphyseal area, where there is much osteoclastic activity, required for remodeling; the osteogenicosteolytic sarcoma is seen just below this area, whereas the fibrosarcoma is in relation to the endosteum and the round cell sarcoma occurs within the medullary cavity.

The relative age incidence shows the first peak of mortality between the ages of fifteen and twenty years and a secondary peak from the age of thirty years up to about seventy-five years. The first peak is due mainly to the primary malignant tumors of bone, e.g., osteogenic sarcoma, whereas the second peak is due to malignant neoplasia in such preexisting conditions as Paget's disease.

CLASSIFICATION OF BONE TUMORS

A. True bone tumors — neoplasms arising from cells of mesenchymal origin, whose function is primarily skeletal bone formation. These tumors fall into four main groups according to the predominant cell type present.

Fig. 43-107. Common sites of origin of bone tumors. *(Used with permission of LC Johnson, 1953.)*

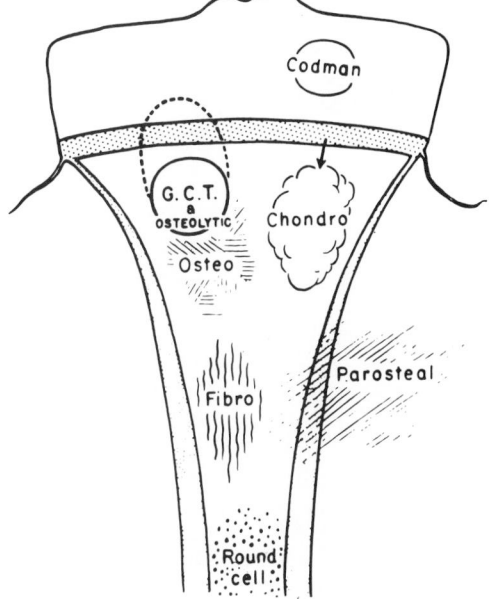

ivory exostosis.   Bone may form from abnormal growth or imperfect remodeling, and a variety of names have been given depending on the site and etiology. *Irritative exostosis* results from lesions causing a proliferation of fibroblasts or granulation tissue with ossification. *Traumatic osteomas* are most frequently seen on the femur in relation to the adductor magnus (the so-called ''rider's bone'') or in relation to the medial collateral ligament of the knee joint (Pellegrini-Stieda disease).

Osteoid Osteoma

This lesion occurs in young males between the ages of ten and thirty years, particularly in the bones of the lower extremities. There is doubt as to whether this is a true tumor. The patient presents with pain, frequently felt during the night and not aggravated by exercise or position but often relieved specifically, although empirically, by salicylates. On radiography, a zone of bony sclerosis is seen surrounding a radiolucent nidus (Fig. 43-108). This condition has to be distinguished from (1) the sclerosing nonsuppurative osteomyelitis of Garre, (2) Brodie's abscess, (3) osteogenic sarcoma, (4) Ewing's tumor, (5) nonossifying fibroma.

Three characteristic regions have been described by Jaffe: (1) an inner region of vascular granulation tissue containing osteoblasts and (2) a zone of calcification and osteoid formation that is surrounded by (3) a zone of trabecular formation of bone in various stages of reorganization.

Complete resection, if possible, will provide cure, but partial removal of the sclerotic bone and the nidus is often sufficient for symptomatic improvement.

Fig. 43-108. Tomographs of a patella showing an osteoid osteoma in the right upper quadrant. [From: *Mercer W, Duthie RB (eds): Orthopaedic Surgery. London, Edward Arnold, 1974, with permission.*]

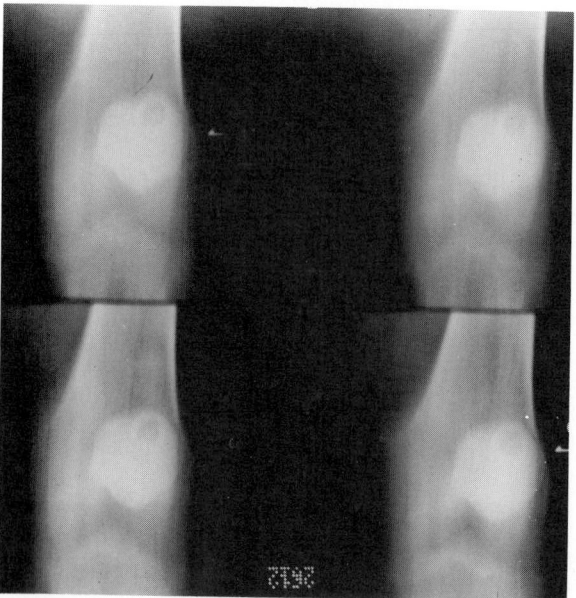

Osteosarcoma (Osteogenic Sarcoma)

These tumors arise from cells concerned with bone formation. There are various forms, or types, including myxosarcoma, pseudomyxoma, and osteochondrosarcoma. Osteosarcoma is rare, about 2.8 in 1,000,000 of the population, with a predilection for the second decade. The tumor occurs in the metaphysis of the femur (52 percent), in the upper end of the tibia (20 percent), and in the humerus (9 percent). Less usual sites are the radius, the ulna, the ilium, and the scapula. The short long bones are rarely affected.

The tumor may originate beneath the periosteum or more centrally in the shaft of the bone and extend in two directions: (1) toward the medulla and (2) to the subperiosteal area, with destruction of bone trabeculae. Initially the periosteum is a barrier and is raised off the bone with new bone formation to produce a fusiform swelling.

The tumor may be soft, fleshy, vascular, and destructive, or it may be grayish white, containing cartilage or bone. The new bone may be arranged as scattered islands throughout the tumor that impart a gritty sensation on cutting, and in the form of spicules radiating from the periosteum, giving the ''sun ray'' appearance on radiography. On the diaphyseal side of the tumor the periosteum is often raised for a short distance, with new bone formation, triangular in shape, and is called Codman's triangle. Pathologic fractures may occur.

Histologically, cells are small and spindle-shaped, with hyperchromatic nuclei with great variation in cell form and shape. The degree of pleomorphism is most marked in the extremely anaplastic tumors in which there are often giant multinucleated cells of bizarre shapes. Mitosis is evident. The intercellular substance may be scanty in amount and in character, being myxomatous, cartilaginous, osteoid, or osseous, according to the degree of differentiation and metaplasia taking place. Blood vessels are thin-walled and numerous.

Pain, especially at night, is usually the first symptom and is caused by periosteal irritation. Such pain in the long bone (41 percent—femur, 16 percent—tibia, 15 percent—humerus) of a young adult should arouse suspicion of sarcoma. While the lymphatic stream occasionally plays a definite role, spread by the blood vessels is predominant. Pulmonary metastases are the most frequent. The first clinical signs of these lesions are usually those of a diffuse bronchitis, but occasionally the cough, dullness, fever, and leukocytosis suggest a diagnosis of pneumonia. Dilated veins may be evident at an early stage.

Pathologic fracture is not typical of osteogenic sarcoma, since the swelling and pain usually keep the patient from walking. There may be some initial pain and effusion into the nearest joint, but movement is free and painless.

The x-ray appearances (Fig. 43-109) have been categorized:

1. The sclerotic type, usually found at puberty, where dense new irregular bone occurs in the metaphysis and there may be a few spicules projecting from its surface.
2. The osteolytic type, usually metaphyseal. An eccentric trans-

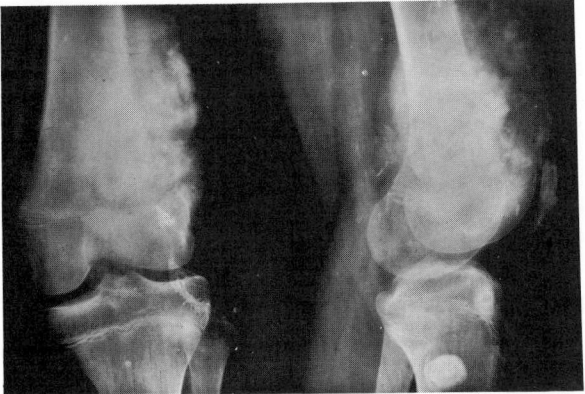

Fig. 43-109. Osteogenic sarcoma of the femur. The films show characteristic bone destruction, soft tissue mass, new bone formation, and sclerosis limited to the metaphysis of the lower femur.

lucent gap is found and at its edges a gradual increase of density compared with that of the normal bone.
3. The radiating spicule type, the least common, usually found at puberty in the metaphyseal region.

The standard treatment has been intensive irradiation with delayed amputation, giving a 5-year survival of about 20 percent. Primary amputation with chemotherapy is now producing over 50 percent survivals.

Attempts have been made to enhance the host's immune mechanisms either by specific antibodies to the tumor-specific antigen or by sensitized lymphocytes. Morton et al. reported management of extremity, skeletal, and soft tissue sarcomas with preoperative intraarterial chemotherapy and radiation therapy, radical surgical resection, and postoperative chemotherapy or immunotherapy. Some patients in whom bone was resected and replaced with cadaver allografts remained free of disease with functional extremity for over 5 years.

OSTEOSARCOMA IN PAGET'S DISEASE

In 10 percent of cases of Paget's disease sarcomatous changes occur. The histologic appearance is similar to that arising de novo in younger patients. The tumor is more diffuse in character and can arise simultaneously at multiple sites; i.e., it can be polyostotic. Osteosarcoma in Paget's disease has the lowest rate of survival of any of the tumors of the sarcoma series.

PAROSTEAL SARCOMA

This occurs in older age groups and presents as a painful tumor mass, near the knee joint. It is juxtacortical and usually is densely ossified with areas of less ossified or calcified cartilage. There are usually no periosteal reactions, or "sun rays." Growth is slow, but eventual destruction of the cortex with invasion of the medullary cavity by malignant bone and osteoid tissue with malignant connective tissue stroma occurs. Parosteal sarcoma has a better prognosis than osteosarcoma, particularly when treated with a primary amputation. There is now a 50 to 95 percent survival.

Chondroma

Chondroma is a benign tumor arising from the cartilaginous elements of developing bone with slow growth. Calcification frequently occurs in the fibrous septums dividing the lobules. Microscopically there is a chondroid matrix containing cartilage cells; encapsulation and lobulation are present. When ossification does occur, the lesion is known as *osteochondroma*.

If malignancy develops, it does so after the age of thirty-five and occurs most commonly in tumors of the large long bones. If this type of tumor presents as a centrally placed mass of such a bone or of a flat bone, e.g., the ilium or scapula, one must seriously consider a low-grade chondrosarcoma. Radiologic features include a dense shadow, with a feathery outline composed of calcified spicules.

Solitary cystic enchondroma occurs in the short long bones of the hand and foot in the metaphyseal region of a proximal phalanx or metacarpal. The tumor arises asymptomatically and is brought to attention by trauma or even a pathologic fracture. If cortical expansion or pathologic fracture occurs, the cyst should be curetted with bone grafting. When the cyst wall is thick and asymptomatic, it should be left alone. *Cartilaginous hypertrophy* always arises from existing cartilage; when it occurs mainly in the confines of bone, it is known as *enchondroma* and when on the surface, *ecchondroma*. The common sites are the epiphyseal plates, the cartilaginous parts of ribs (Fig. 43-110), and the symphysis pubis. Such lesions may be part of a generalized chondroosteodystrophy. They rarely, if ever, become malignant and may be multiple, especially in the short long bones of the hand and foot. The well-formed fibrous capsule enables the tumor in most cases to be cleanly excised.

Multiple enchondromas occur in childhood and affect

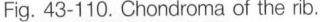

Fig. 43-110. Chondroma of the rib.

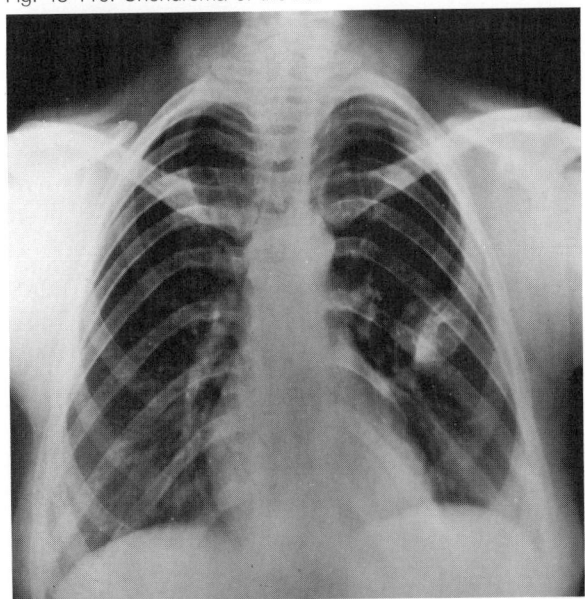

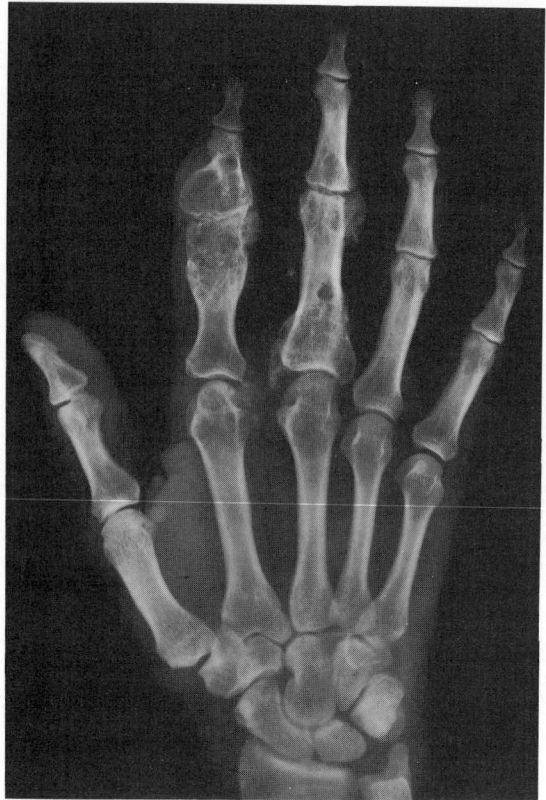

Fig. 43-111. Multiple enchondromas of the hand.

Fig. 43-112. Benign chondroblastoma (Codman's tumor) of the humerus.

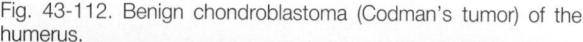
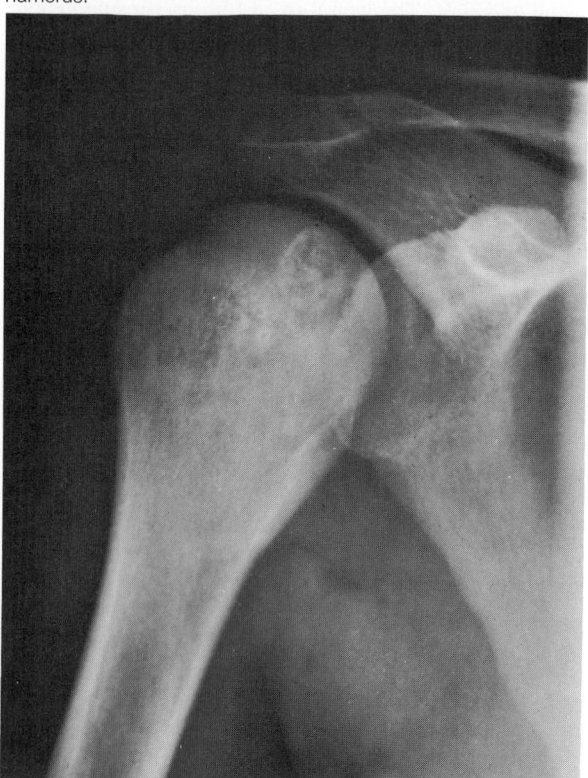

the short long bones of the hand and foot, so that the part may be distorted and appear to be of excessive size. They arise in the center of the shaft as a collection of cartilage cells that, in the process of growth, gradually expand the surrounding cortex (Fig. 43-111). Operative treatment is indicated when the tumors are rapidly growing and have become unsightly or a source of inconvenience. Complete excision, with curettage and autogenous bone grafting, is the treatment of choice.

Benign Chondroblastoma (Codman's Tumor)

The lesion occurs in the first and second decades, when the epiphyseal line has not yet closed. There is often a long history of a painful swelling with loss of joint function. On x-rays (Fig. 43-112) the typical lesion in the epiphysis is an osteolytic one that contains calcium deposits. Extension into the metaphysis and articular cartilage may occur, but the margin is always discrete and demarcated by a zone of sclerotic or condensed bone.

The lesion is very vascular and gritty. There is much chondroid material with "chondroblastic"-appearing cells, which exhibit strong metachromasia and a positive periodic acid–Schiff reaction. Osteoid tissue and calcified areas are seen. Treatment consisting of adequate curettage and cancellous bone grafting gives excellent results.

Chondrosarcoma

This tumor occurs mainly between the ages of twenty and sixty years. It occurs as a primary malignant tumor in the earlier age groups but as secondary malignant change in such conditions as an osteochondroma, in Paget's disease, or diaphyseal aclasia.

The bones most commonly involved are the pelvis, the ribs and sternum, and the femur. The nearer a cartilaginous tumor is to the axial skeleton and the larger it is, the more likely it is to be malignant. *Secondary chondrosarcoma* arises in a preexisting chondroma, osteochondroma, multiple exostoses, and Ollier's disease, occurring mainly in the pelvis, the vertebrae, the femora, and the humeri.

On x-ray (Fig. 43-113), there is often frank destruction of trabecular bone and cortex with an expanding lesion that contains irregular flecking or mottling of calcified tissue. Periosteal new bone formation often extends outward. The sarcomatous mass appears as grayish, translucent, fairly vascular tissue. Varying degrees of pleomorphism, hyperchromatism, mitotic figures of cartilage cells, and chondroid formation with calcification and ossification are seen.

Thomson and Turner-Warwick have divided this tumor into three types of malignancy:

1. *Low-grade,* a well-differentiated tumor, in which the cells are cartilaginous in type although increased in number, with the matrix well formed. Nearly three-quarters of these patients were alive 10 years after treatment.
2. *Average-grade,* in which there is a reduction in the amount of matrix and an increase in the cellularity, the cells varying in size and shape with nuclear irregularities. Less than half the patients were alive at 5 years, and only one-third were alive at 10 years.

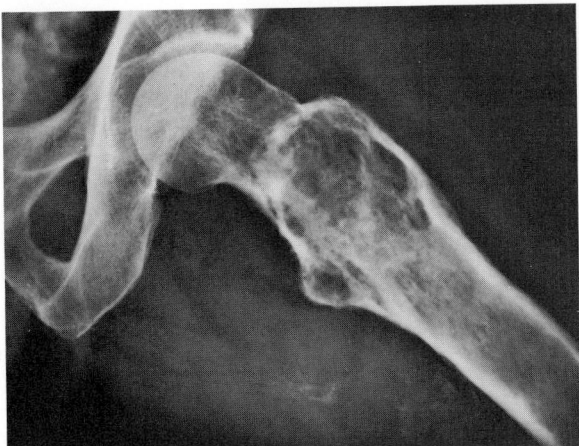

Fig. 43-113. Chondrosarcoma of the upper femur showing an expanding lesion with irregular mottling of calcified tissue. No definite periosteal reaction or spiculation is seen.

3. *High-grade,* a poorly differentiated cartilaginous pattern with anaplastic cells common, frequent mitoses, and only occasional islands of cartilage seen. This type of tumor behaves similarly to osteosarcoma; i.e., only 1 of 10 patients survived 3 years. Treatment should be excision, using a wide margin, or amputation, especially if recurrence takes place after resection. Chondrosarcoma is radioresistant.

Fibroma

Benign fibrous tumors of bone are rare lesions and closely allied to the fibrous dysplasia.

The cellular and collagenous fibrous content varies but is usually arranged in whorls. Growth is slow and unlimited with mucoid and necrotic degeneration. Ossification is also common but differs in that the bone is laid down in an irregular manner without the organized compact bone of a true osteoma (Fig. 43-114). Included in this group is the *nonosteogenic fibroma* (nonossifying fibroma).

These lesions are usually discovered incidentally by x-rays in children. Radiographically they present as small cortical areas of translucency in the metaphysis. During growth some will disappear. However, a few are displaced toward the center of the bone, where they may grow large, with thinning of the sclerotic cortex.

The tissue is fibrous, containing both fibroblasts and "small" giant cells in a relatively large amount of collagenous fibrous tissue in which rarely there are delicate trabeculae of bone that help to differentiate these lesions from fibrous dysplasia. Curettage or local resection is indicated.

Fibrosarcoma

Medullary fibrosarcomas are characterized by definite collagen formation as the predominant feature, and early destruction of bone. These tumors appear to have a much more favorable prognosis than osteosarcoma, with a 26 to 34 percent 5-year survival rate by radical surgical treatment or x-radiation and local excision. Thomson and Turner-Warwick differentiate fibrosarcoma from a spin-

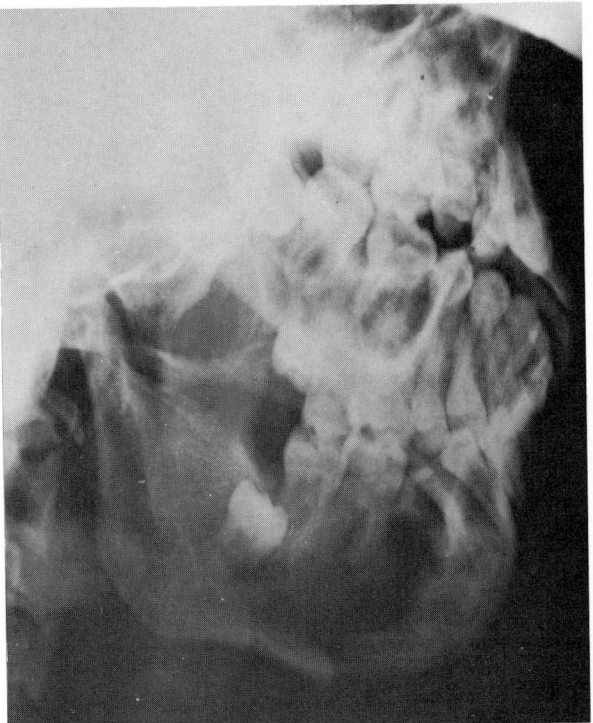

Fig. 43-114. Ossifying fibroma of the mandible in a fourteen-year-old boy with a 1-year history of gradual, painless swelling.

dle cell sarcoma, which is distinguished by the complete lack of intercellular substance, by its occurrence in a younger age group, and by its greater radiosensitivity.

Fibrosarcomas have been reported at all ages and as a secondary malignant degeneration in Paget's disease of the skull, etc. They usually occur in long bones around the knee joint, as a central lesion that expands and partially destroys the cortex (Fig. 43-115).

Osteoclastoma (Giant Cell Tumor)

The typical osteoclast is a large cell containing a variable number of centrally placed but distinct nuclei, which are identical in vesicular appearance, ovoid, and basophilic on staining with hematoxylin and eosin. These cells are commonly found in areas where bone is being remodeled, in recesses named *Howship's lacunae.* They also follow hemorrhage into the marrow or during cyst formation and are particularly prominent in hyperparathyroidism or osteitis fibrosa cystica during the formation of the "brown tumor." They are also found in such bone lesions as nonosteogenic fibroma, unicameral bone cysts, aneurysmal bone cyst, fibrous dysplasia, chondroblastoma, osteosarcoma, and histocytic granulomatosis, but these must be clearly differentiated from a giant cell tumor.

The critical feature of this tumor is the vascular and cellular stroma, which is made up of oval-shaped cells containing a small, elongated, darkly stained nucleus with little eosinophilic cytoplasm on staining with hematoxylin and eosin. The stroma cells show a varying degree of malignancy with the typical features of mitotic activity, pleo-

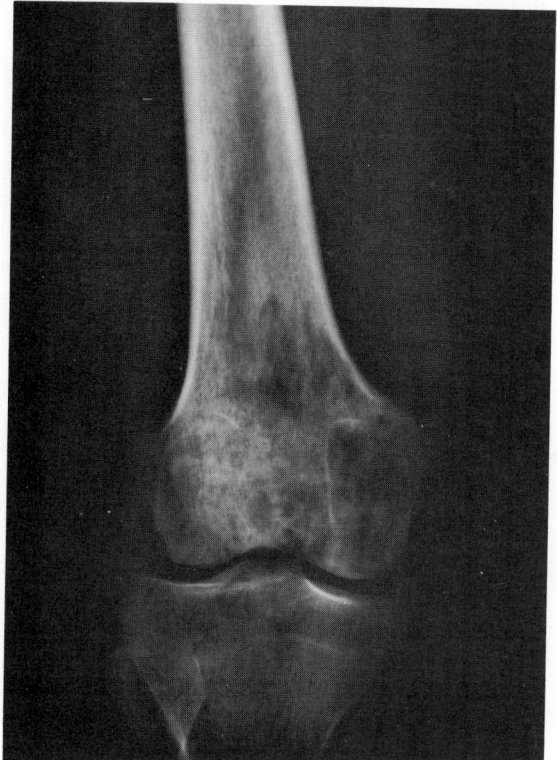

Fig. 43-115. Fibrosarcoma of the lower femur. The films show a lytic lesion apparently of medullary origin on the distal end of the femur. The lesion is destroying cortex. There is no evidence of sclerosis and new bone formation or any definite soft tissue mass.

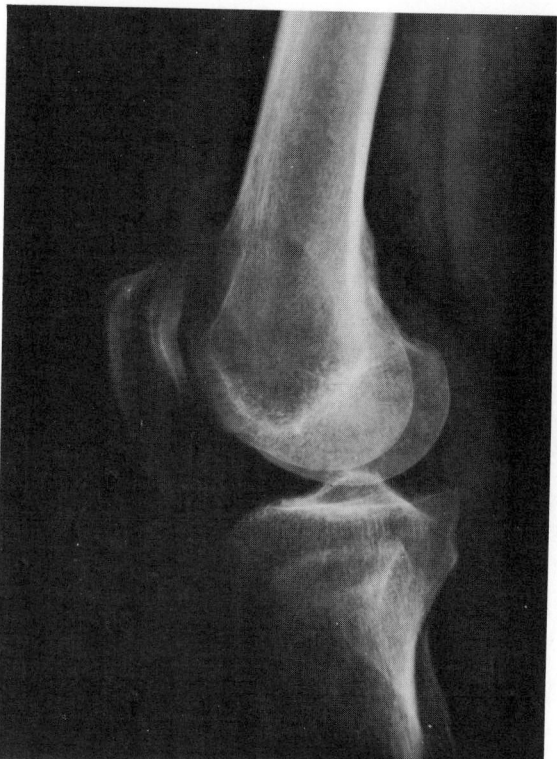

Fig. 43-116. Benign giant cell tumor of the lower femur. The films show a sharply demarcated area of decreased density in the lateral condyle of the femur, extending through the cortex. Some soft tissue swelling around the lesion is visible.

morphism, and hyperchromatism. In the more frankly malignant giant cell tumors, the giant cells become anaplastic, with areas of necrotic material and hemorrhage. These true neoplasms occur primarily in the second and third decades with an equal sex distribution. They are seen mainly in the ends of long bones, particularly in the vicinity of the knee and at the lower end of the radius. They commonly arise in the metaphyseoepiphyseal area and are related to the usual osteoclastic activity of remodeling in this area.

On x-rays, the metaphyseoepiphyseal areas are seen to be enlarged and occupied by a clear cystic tumor (Fig. 43-116). The cortex is thin and may sharply limit the tumor from the surrounding soft tissues, with a sharp line of demarcation between the tumor and the unaffected shaft in contradistinction to sarcomas and bone cysts. The expanding osteolytic lesion can continue to destroy the cortex, although usually it leaves some external rim. The tumor grows eccentrically to destroy the epiphyseal cartilage, and it may penetrate the articular cartilage; but rarely does it extend into a joint. Pathologic fractures occur.

Clinically these patients present because of pain and loss of function around the joint, which may even suggest a possible inflammatory lesion or a swelling of an asymmetric nature.

Although in the past these tumors have been regarded as relatively benign, up to 30 percent behave with malignant characteristics despite a benign histologic appearance. There are varying degrees of malignancy of this tumor; because of this, excision is indicated. With curettage there is up to a 50 percent local recurrence rate. Treatment is therefore directed to a complete and total local resection if at all possible. Amputation is occasionally indicated. Radiotherapy has not been shown by Dahlin's group to decrease the recurrence rate, and 10 percent of tumors given such treatment underwent sarcomatous degeneration.

Malignant giant cells are found in osteosarcomas. These are found especially in the more anaplastic lesions and contain a variable number of nuclei but seldom so many as in the osteoclast. The cells and nuclei are irregular in form and size. These features serve to differentiate such malignant giant cells from the osteoclast.

NONOSTEOGENIC TUMORS OF BONE

Unicameral (Solitary) or Juvenile Bone Cyst

This lesion occurs during the years of active bone growth, particularly in the metaphyseal area of long bones, such as the upper end of the humerus and femur. It usually presents because of a pathologic fracture without previous symptoms except for a minor injury.

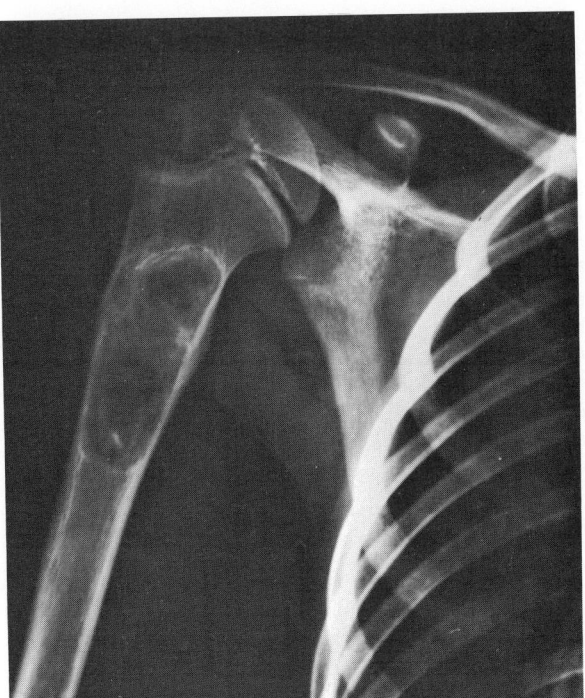

Fig. 43-117. Simple bone cyst of the humerus.

On x-ray (Fig. 43-117) a characteristic expanding lesion is seen in the metaphysis with thinning of the cortex as a shell, but rarely, if ever, penetrates or passes through the still open epiphysis like a giant cell tumor. It is loculated with relatively large cystlike areas.

On biopsy, these cysts are seen to contain a clear, viscous fluid with a fine fibrous framework that is relatively avascular. Histologically, the thin fibrous framework is in continuity with the fibrous wall, but there is little cellular activity unless a pathologic fracture has occurred.

This lesion must be differentiated from:

1. *Osteitis fibrosa cystica,* either the generalized form of von Recklinghausen's disease or the localized form. The latter usually occurs during adolescence in the metaphysis, but it tends to spread down the shaft more often. On biopsy, the obvious feature of vascular connective tissue invading cortex and cancellous bone, with degeneration and cyst formation, is observed.
2. *Hydatid disease.* This usually occurs in the long bones of adults, in which there are localized "solid" masses of hydatid material replacing the marrow, cancellous, and cortical components of bone to extend into the soft tissues.
3. *Tumors.* Giant cell tumors in older age groups, and although the x-ray appearance may be similar, the histologic character is obviously different. Chondromas, myelomas, sarcomas, neurofibromatosis, and secondary metastases must also be differentiated. In sarcoidosis, also to be considered, the tumors are usually multiple, involving the short, miniature bones, such as the metacarpals or phalanges.

Treatment is surgical and directed toward total obliteration of the cavity by a guttering and curetting procedure or collapsing down of the surrounding and thinned cortex by compression. Bone grafting, to restore continuity, is then carried out with both autogenous cancellous bone and overlying cortical matchstick grafts. More recently the injection of hydrocortisone intraarticular solution under pressure into these simple bone cysts has produced significant diminution in the amount of the bone cavity with new bone formation.

Periosteal Fibrosarcoma

This tumor originates in the outer nonosteogenic fibrous layer of the periosteum. It is a fascial sarcoma and similar in character to those arising in other sites in the soft tissues. It is extracortical and neither invades nor infiltrates the bone. The tumor remains encapsulated for a long time; as it grows, it pushes aside the soft tissues but rarely infiltrates them.

Secondary changes eventually appear in the underlying bone, but they result from the pressure and the contact of the tumor. Saucer-shaped erosions may occur where the cortex is in contact with the tumor and areas of new periosteal bone formation at the periphery.

The tumor may appear to be encapsulated, but the capsule merely consists of the condensed surrounding tissues. It remains localized for a considerable time, but ultimately, as the vascularity and cellularity increase, it becomes more malignant. At this state secondary metastases usually occur in the lungs.

Histologically the tumor is a spindle cell fibrosarcoma with a variable degree of collagen formation. There is no true ossification, but calcification can occur.

Radical removal of the tumor is the operation of choice, with a favorable prognosis when the tumor is encapsulated. If the operation is incomplete, it may be followed by local recurrence and general metastases. The operation should be supplemented by a prolonged course of deep x-ray therapy, although its beneficial effects are questionable.

Ewing's Tumor

In 1921 Ewing described a rare lesion of bone characterized by the development of a tumor from the endothelial marrow of the diaphysis of the long bones, occurring in childhood and associated with febrile attacks. The tumor rapidly involved other parts of the skeleton and was radiosensitive. Willis demonstrated that many of the cases diagnosed clinically and radiologically as "Ewing's tumor," because the histologic pattern demonstrated a rosette formation, were really neuroblastomas, and a primary tumor could be found in the adrenal. Ewing's tumor must also be differentiated from reticulum cell sarcoma and from chronic osteomyelitis.

Ewing's tumor usually appears between the ages of five and fifteen. The bones most commonly affected are the tibia, the fibula, the humerus, and the femur. Regional lymph glands may be involved, and polyostotic lesions may be present.

The tumor begins in the diaphyseal marrow; it is grayish white with areas of necrosis and hemorrhage causing destruction of trabeculae and suggesting osteomyelitis. From the medulla the tumor extends to the periosteum, where new bone formation occurs. This has been aptly described as "onion layers."

The tumor is very cellular; the cells are small, round or polyhedral, and arranged in solid cords or sheets with little intercellular substance. The nuclei are always prominent, and mitosis is frequent.

Many tumors show a rosette arrangement, and within the center of the rosette, by special staining methods, fibrils can sometimes be demonstrated, similar to those of a neuroblastoma. The vessels of both the tumor and the lymphatics may contain obvious emboli, for the tumor spreads by the blood and lymphatic systems.

CLINICAL MANIFESTATIONS. A history of trauma may be elicited, and chronic pain may occur. There may be febrile attacks and leukocytosis. X-rays demonstrate a circumscribed osteoporotic area in the center of the shaft, extending for a considerable distance. Later, the periosteum shows onion-skin layers parallel to the shaft and rather like osteomyelitis, or more commonly small spicules appear (Fig. 43-118). Pathologic fracture seldom occurs. When the vertebrae are involved, there is severe root pain or paralysis. Death usually results from meta-

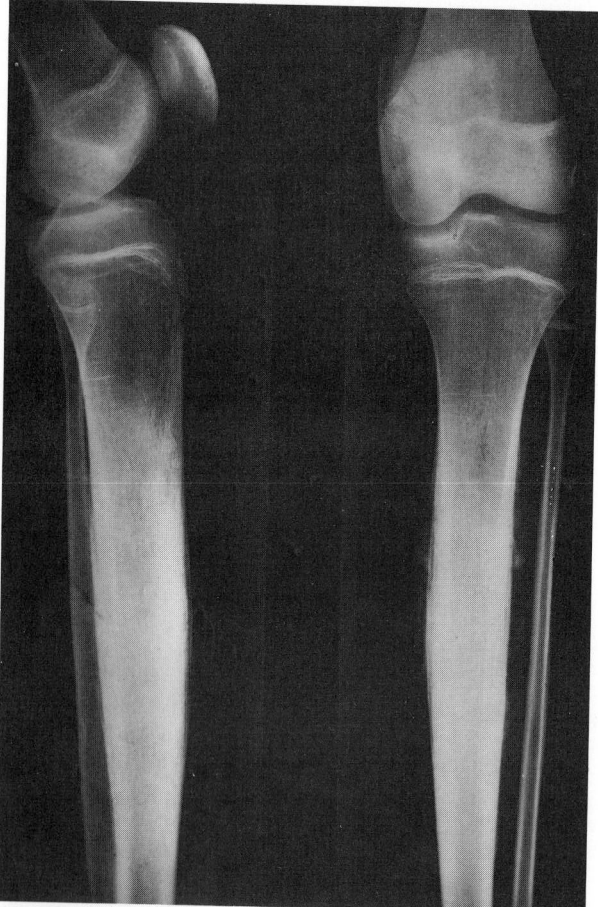

Fig. 43-118. Ewing's tumor of the tibia. The films show diffuse bone reaction with periosteal lifting and onion-skin thickening of the cortex plus some spiculation.

static involvement of the lungs. Twenty-five percent have metastasis at the time of clinical presentation.

TREATMENT. Deep x-ray therapy may cause the local lesion to disappear, but subsequent local recurrence is the rule. Accordingly it has been the practice to follow primary radiation with amputation. Such treatment will not affect the ultimate prognosis in those cases where the tumor has metastasized. Survival is usually about 2 years, and it is commonly stated that the lesions of the so-called 5-year survivors have been misdiagnosed and have really been radiosensitive reticulum cell sarcoma. Dahlin et al. reviewed their experience of Ewing's sarcoma treated at the Mayo Clinic and emphasized that the 5-year survival rate of 133 patients was only 15 percent, 95 patients having died within 2 years of the time of diagnosis. Recently, chemotherapy has been used in conjunction with surgery, with better results.

Reticulum Cell Sarcoma

This tumor occurs in patients between twenty and forty years of age and particularly affects the femur, tibia, and humerus. Pain is often the first complaint, preceding the formation of a tumor that may invade a large part of the shaft.

Radiologically there is an osteolytic lesion in the end of the diaphysis that later extends throughout the length, and pathologic fracture may occur.

The tumor is made up of a pinkish gray granulation tissue, and the cells are larger than a lymphocyte and have round, oval, indented, or lobulated nuclei with considerable cytoplasm. Delicate reticulum fibers pass between the cells, which often show a large number of mitotic figures.

Although the initial response to radiation is good, local recurrence may take place, and therefore radiation should be followed by amputation or radical resection.

BLOOD VESSEL TUMORS

ANEURYSMAL BONE CYST. The lesion occurs in the metaphyses of long bones in young people. X-rays show a characteristic lesion of an eccentrically placed osteolytic expansion of the cortex, with some extension into the surrounding soft tissues, and periosteal new bone formation. On biopsy, there is a mass of blood spaces filled with frank blood. Histologically, the characteristic feature consists of cavernous spaces built by fibrous tissue containing some osteoid tissue, but rarely an endothelial lining. Giant cells may be present, particularly in the more cellular areas of the tumor. Stroma cells are usually fibroblastic and have to be differentiated from those of a giant cell tumor. Local curettage, with or without bone grafting, may give an adequate result, but local resection may be required for recurrence.

HEMANGIOMA. Vascular tumors of bone are rare, but the most common sites for these lesions are in the skull and vertebral column. In the vertebral column when the body is affected, the appearance may suggest tuberculosis, secondary neoplasm, or Paget's disease. Collapse of the vertebral body occurs with pressure on the cord.

These tumors are benign in a majority of instances. Treatment is difficult on account of the location of the tumor, but should the lesion be peripheral, radical excision has been advised.

ANGIOSARCOMA (ANGIOENDOTHELIOMA). This is *extremely* rare and must be differentiated from the reticulosarcoma, which may mimic it closely because of the potential endothelial function of reticular cells.

TUMORS ARISING FROM INCLUDED TISSUES

ADAMANTINOMA. Adamantinoma, or adamantine epithelioma, occurs in the jaw and more rarely in the tibia. The long-bone tumors may not be related to adamantinomas of the jaw, since no enamel has been found in them. Pain accompanied by tenderness is commonly the first symptom.

It is a slow-growing tumor the origin of which is unknown. This epithelial tumor may be a basal cell or squamous cell carcinoma. Microscopically it consists of solid strands, sheets, or whorls of dark-staining polygonal or spindle-shaped cells, often with a tendency toward a synctial character. It shows a tendency to form clefts and cysts, and in most cases there are collections of cuboidal cells arranged in irregular acini. The treatment of choice is amputation, preferably through the more proximal bone. Metastasis has been proved by biopsy in several cases, further emphasizing the need for radical surgical treatment, especially with local bone destruction.

NEURILEMMOMA. This is a type of nerve sheath tumor that may grow in bone. Clinically the tumor may present as a cystic swelling, and the x-rays show a destruction of the bone. The common and often only symptom is the physical presence of a tumor. This is always single and circumscribed. The clinical course appears to be benign, and local removal appears to be adequate.

CHORDOMA. Chordoma is a rare malignant neoplasm found at either end of the spinal axis. It is generally accepted as originating from embryonic remnants of the notochord. Although in the adult remnants of the notochord persist in the intervertebral disks in the form of the nucleus pulposus, the majority of chordomas arise in either the sphenooccipital or sacrococcygeal region. Sixty percent occur in the latter area. The physical presence of a tumor is usually the first symptom, though there is often pain in the back with sacral tumors. The tumors are locally invasive and tend to recur after removal.

The radiograph usually shows destruction of bone with an expanding soft tissue shadow (Fig. 43-119). There is nothing characteristic in the bony erosion, and the diagnosis, though it may be guessed at from the site, is usually made by biopsy. The tumor is slow-growing but malignant and kills by invasion of vital structures.

Microscopically chordomas are distinguished with difficulty from atypical chondromas and mucoid, or signet-ring cell, carcinomas arising in the gastrointestinal tract. Myeloblastomas originating in the sacrococcygeal region

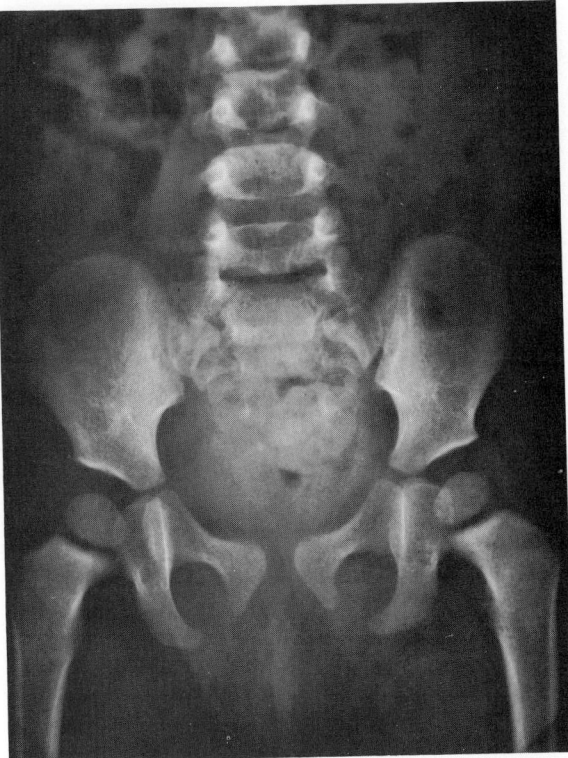

Fig. 43-119. Chordoma destroying the coccyx of an infant.

are usually interpreted as chordomas. The chordoma cells are more epithelial in appearance than cartilage and more variable in size. There is a great tendency for vacuolization and variability in the size of the nuclei.

An attempt at complete surgical extirpation must be made, since these growths are radioresistant.

MALIGNANT TUMORS OF SOFT TISSUES

FIBROSARCOMA OF MUSCLE. These are of two types: differentiated fibrosarcoma with malignant fibroblasts and malignant fibrosarcoma with anaplastic cells. Both usually infiltrate widely, and the patient presents with a painful and large tumor mass, particularly in the thigh.

LIPOSARCOMA. This occurs in the soft tissues of the extremities and is one of the more common malignant soft tissue tumors. It presents in the middle age groups with little difference between the sexes. It occurs commonly in the thigh, in the popliteal area as well as in the inguinal and gluteal regions. It does not appear to arise in simple lipomas. Like the fibrosarcoma, these tumors are of two types, well-differentiated and anaplastic. Curative treatment is directed toward wide surgical excision, because their radiosensitivity varies.

RHABDOMYOSARCOMA. This is a malignant tumor involving the striated muscle cells. It occurs commonly in infants and young adults. It has a high incidence of blood metastasis with rapid growth and fungation. Histologically it is characterized by giant rhabdomyoblasts with

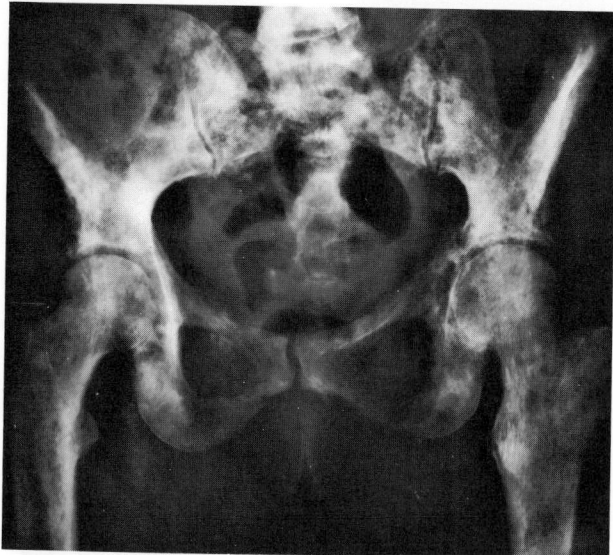

Fig. 43-120. Osteoblastic metastases from carcinoma of the breast.

multiple nuclei that attempt to form myofibrils. It is rarely radiosensitive.

SYNOVIAL SARCOMAS. These occur in subcutaneous tissue as well as in deeply placed muscle layers and have no obvious continuity with joint tissue, although it is supposed that they arise from embryologically sequestered "synovioblastic cells." They infiltrate and spread locally. Total radical local excision should be carried out and should include the main muscle mass involved.

RETICULUM CELL SARCOMA. This also arises in subcutaneous as well as in muscle layers and develops at any age, growing rapidly and infiltrating widely with metastasis via the bloodstream to the lungs. These tumors have to be differentiated from Ewing's sarcoma.

MALIGNANT GIANT CELL TUMORS. These tumors can arise in subcutaneous tissues as well as joint structures, tendons, and tendon sheaths. Their malignancy is variable and can be evaluated by their histologic pattern.

DESMOID TUMOR. This appears to be a very low-grade fibrosarcoma that is locally invasive but does not tend to metastasize by blood. It occurs in the deep muscle masses as a painful tumor or swelling. It has a much better prognosis than a fibrosarcoma, even though it occurs in young people, but it can recur following inadequate resection. Therefore, it is advisable to remove the involved muscle mass in its entirety.

GENERAL PRINCIPLES OF TREATMENT OF SOFT TISSUE MALIGNANT TUMORS. Usually no capsule surrounds the malignant cells but by rapid growth the surrounding soft tissues may be compressed to form a pseudocapsule. Therefore, if the malignant tumor is only enucleated, a shell of neoplastic cells will be left behind. The entire muscle bundle surrounding the sarcoma must be removed from its point of origin to its insertion, by sharp dissection as well as ligation of all major tributaries. Amputation is indicated when the anatomic location requires it.

Although heroic attempts have been made to reduce the mortality and morbidity of malignant tumors in the upper aspect of both extremities, by such operations as the forequarter and hindquarter amputations, for such tumors as osteosarcoma, Ewing's tumor, etc., these procedures have proved of little value in prolonging life. Their main indication appears to be the need to prevent fungation or ulceration and to relieve local symptoms, except in malignant tumors of soft tissues arising high in the buttock or thigh, such as liposarcoma, fibrosarcoma, or secondary chondrosarcoma. Modification of the classic hemipelvectomy has been described by Sherman and Duthie in which there is less deformity and dysfunction but still an adequate tumor excision. With operation it is possible to obtain a 30 to 40 percent 5-year survival rate. Enneking, using modern techniques of CT and MRI, has emphasized the compartmental nature of these tumors and provided a basis for planning excision.

METASTATIC TUMORS OF BONE

The skeleton is one of the most common sites for metastases, accounting for more than half the cases of malignant bone tumors. Their actual incidence is probably higher than that recorded, since the skeleton is inadequately examined at necropsy. The carcinomas that commonly metastasize to bone arise in the breast (about 30 percent; Fig. 43-120), prostate, thyroid, kidney, and lung, as well as from adrenal neuroblastoma. Skeletal metastases have been found in virtually all types of malignant tumors including melanomas, carcinoids, and testicular, ovarian, and intestinal tumors.

METHOD OF SPREAD. Bone may be involved as a result of direct spread from an overlying tumor such as from squamous carcinoma of the skin in the facial bones and in the calvarium and in the ribs from bronchogenic and mammary carcinoma. The usual route is via the bloodstream. This may be the systemic circulation with the cells entering veins in the tumor, passing through the pulmonary circulation to the arterial bloodstream, and then to the capillary beds. This does not explain the selective distribution of skeletal metastases in the dorsal and lumbar spine, pelvis, rib cage, skull, and proximal end of the femur.

In an attempt to explain the high incidence of metastases in the axial skeleton, Batson described an alternative route for the dissemination of malignant cells. He showed that the vertebral venous system, which contains no valves, communicates freely with venous channels of the chest wall and the intrathoracic and abdominal viscera. When the intrathoracic or intraabdominal pressure rises as in coughing or sneezing, the flow of blood in the venous vertebral system can be reversed. By this method malignant cells may be carried into the bodies of the vertebrae or reach the central nervous system.

DIAGNOSIS. Conventional methods of diagnosing skeletal metastases are inaccurate. Of 86 patients with advanced mammary carcinoma, all of whom had skeletal metastases evident on x-ray, only 65.1 percent complained of pain at any stage of the disease, tenderness was elicited in only 16 percent, and the alkaline phosphatase level was raised in only 66 percent. Pain may be localized to a few sites and is not associated with every metastasis.

The serum phosphorus level is raised only when there is associated renal failure with phosphate retention. The serum acid phosphatase concentration is usually elevated in patients with skeletal metastases from prostatic carcinoma.

X-rays also are unreliable. Metastases start growing in the medulla and from there involve the cortex. It has been shown that at least 50 percent of the medulla must be destroyed before a lesion will be seen radiologically. Tomograms are more sensitive.

Radioisotopes may be more sensitive than x-rays for the early detection of skeletal metastases. The use of ^{99m}Tc has proved most valuable not only in indicating the severity of the metastatic spread, but also in the response of the bone to various forms of therapeutic agents. CT scans or MRI give much greater morphologic detail of both the bone lesion and the surrounding soft tissue involvement. The vast majority of skeletal metastases evoke an osteoid reaction by the invaded bone. The degree of osteoid and new bone formation varies from tumor to tumor. It is most marked in prostatic carcinoma. Because this osteoid has an increased avidity for the bone-seeking isotopes, they can be used for the early detection of skeletal metastases.

The separation of skeletal metastases into lytic or sclerotic, depending on their radiologic appearance, is reinforced by histologic examination. In all metastases there is a combination of destruction due to the tumor and new bone formation caused by the reaction of the bone to the lesion.

Hypercalcemia is found particularly in association with bronchogenic and mammary carcinoma. It is usually produced as a result of the destruction of the skeleton by metastases. As the bone is destroyed, the calcium is released into the circulation. If the kidneys are functioning, the calcium is excreted in the urine as a hypercalcinuria. However, if the kidneys are unable to excrete the increased load, the serum calcium level rises to produce hypercalcemia.

TREATMENT. Treatment of skeletal metastases is essentially palliative, although there have been cases described where a solitary metastasis from a hypernephroma has been removed, after the primary tumor was treated, with apparent cure (Fig. 43-121). As many patients may live for months or years with skeletal metastases, it is important to relieve their symptoms.

Pain may occur only in association with hypercalcemia. Once the hypercalcemia has been treated, the pain will be relieved. It may be associated with a pathologic fracture; again, the pathologic fracture must be treated. Large lytic metastases with impending fracture may also produce pain and require treatment. If the patient has a hormonally dependent tumor such as carcinoma of the breast or prostate, the pain is often relieved by hormonal therapy. In carcinoma of the prostate, therapy with diethylstilbestrol diphosphate (stilbestrol), orchidectomy, or a combi-

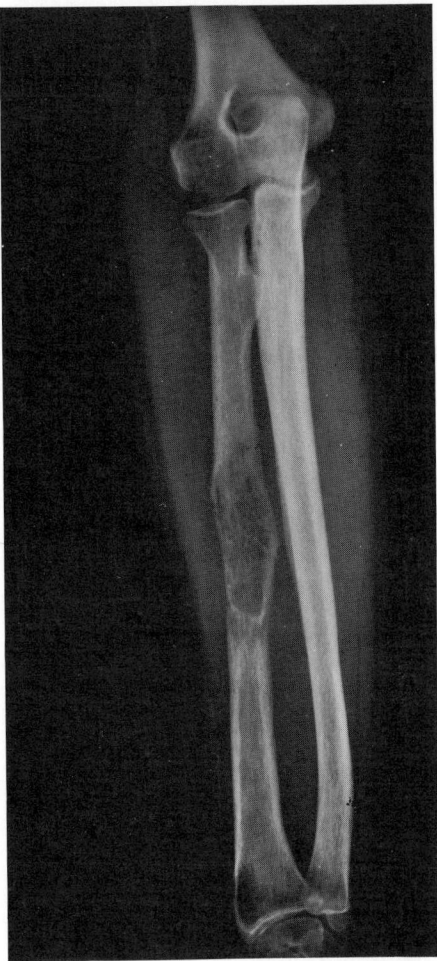

Fig. 43-121. Solitary metastasis in the radius from hypernephroma. The lesion characteristically involves the more proximal bones such as the humerus and femur.

nation of both frequently relieves pain. In mammary carcinoma approximately 27 percent of patients respond objectively to hormonal therapy. In the premenopausal woman this usually consists of an oophorectomy. In the postmenopausal woman diethylstilbestrol is usually given. In both groups when the primary treatment fails to produce a remission, androgens, progestogens, or corticosteroids have been tried; if these fail, endocrine ablative surgery is usually indicated. This includes procedures such as adrenalectomy, hypophysectomy, or pituitary ablation using rods of yttrium 90.

Where hormonal therapy is not indicated or not effective, radiotherapy to a localized area of pain will frequently produce relief. Where the pain is not controlled by radiotherapy or hormonal therapy, analgesics must be given without concern over drug addiction. Interruption of the nerve supply to the painful area is sometimes indicated. This may take the form of phenol blocks, rhizotomies, and even a spinothalamic tactotomy.

Large lytic lesions with impending fracture should be internally fixed after excision of the malignancy and its replacement by methylacrylic cement. They usually occur in the shafts of the femur or humerus or in the neck of the femur. Lesions in the shafts should be fixed with a closed nailing using a Küntschner nail. For lesions in the neck of the femur a Massie nail pin and plate are required. Following internal fixation the area is irradiated. Where radiotherapy is given prior to internal fixation, a pathologic fracture may occur, making treatment more difficult.

More than 50 percent of patients in whom a pathologic fracture occurs die of the disease within 3 months, although survivals of 6 years or more after pathologic fracture have been known. Without treatment the fracture will not heal. Since the most common site is the femur, the patient will become bedridden.

When several vertebrae have collapsed, some form of brace may be required. Occasionally compression fractures may be associated with involvement of the spinal cord or cauda equina with sensory, motor, or bladder disturbances. Laminectomy and decompression is urgently indicated, since once paraplegia is established, it is very rarely relieved by surgery. Radiotherapy is very useful for treating pain but usually does not improve an established paraplegia. If a laminectomy is carried out, it is imperative to stabilize the spine by Harrington rods to prevent complete collapse and instability of the spinal column.

Bibliography

Manifestations of Musculoskeletal Disease

Adams RD, Brown D, Pearson C: *Disease of Muscles.* New York, Hansen and Broether, 1962.

Baker LD, Hill LM: Foot alignment in cerebral palsy patient. *J Bone Joint Surg [Am]* 46A:1, 1964.

Bergofsky EH, Turino GM, Fishman AP: Cardiorespiratory failure in kyphoscoliosis. *Medicine* 38:263, 1959.

Boskey AL: Overview of cellular elements and macromolecules implicated in the initiation of mineralization, in Butchers WT (ed): *The Chemistry and Biology of Mineralized Tissues.* Birmingham, AL, Ebsco Media, Inc, 1985, pp 80–94.

Buchthal F, Knappies GG, Lindhard J: Bie Struktur der quergestreisten, legenden Muskelfaser des Frosches in Ruhe und wahrend der Kontraktion. *Scand Arch Physiol* 73:163, 1936.

Burleigh MC: Degradation of collagen by nonspecific proteinases, in Barrett AJ (ed): *Proteinases of Mammalian Cells and Tissues.* Amsterdam, North Holland, 1977, pp 285–309.

Campbell AM, Phillips DG: Cervical disk lesions with neurological disorder: Differential diagnosis, treatment, and prognosis. *Br Med J* 5197:481, 1960.

Duthie RB: The significance of growth in orthopaedic surgery. *Clin Orthop* 14:7, 1959.

Duthie RB, Houghton GR: Constitutional aspects of the osteochondroses. *Clin Orthop Rel Res* 158:19, 1981.

Eggers GWN, Evans EB: Surgery in cerebral palsy, instructional course lecture. American Academy of Orthopaedic Surgeons. *J Bone Joint Surg [Am]* 45A:1275, 1963.

Fischer LW: The nature of the proteoglycans of bone, in Butchers WT (ed): *The Chemistry and Biology of Mineralized Tissues.* Birmington, AL, Ebso Media, Inc, 1985, pp 188–197.

Fleisch H, Felix R: Diphosphonates. *Calcif Tissue Int* 27:91, 1979.

Gaze RM, Gordon G: Representation of cutaneous sense in thalamus of cat and monkey. *Q J Exp Physiol* 39:279, 1954.

Genant HK: Computed tomography of the lumbar spine: Technical considerations, in Genant HK, Chafetz N, Helms CA (eds): *Computed Tomography of the Lumbar Spine.* Berkeley, University of California Press, 1982, p 23.

Gill GG: Facetectomy for the relief of intraforaminal compression of the fifth lumbar nerve root at the collapsed lumbosacral disk. *Clin Orthop* 119:159, 1976.

Goldner JL: Reconstructive surgery of the hand in cerebral palsy and spastic paralysis resulting from injuries of the spinal cord. *J Bone Joint Surg [Am]* 37A:1141, 1955.

Green WT, Banks HH: Flexor carpi ulnaris transplant and its use in cerebral palsy. *J Bone Joint Surg [Am]* 44A:1343, 1962.

Grice DS: Further experience with extra-articular arthrodesis of the subtalar joint. *J Bone Joint Surg [Am]* 37A:246, 1955.

Harris RI, Beath T: Etiology of peroneal spastic flat foot. *J Bone Joint Surg [Br]* 30B:624, 1948.

Hayes JT, Gross HP, Dow S: Surgery for paralytic defects secondary to meningomyelocele and myelodyspasia, instructional coarse lecture, American Academy of Orthopaedic Surgeons. *J Bone Joint Surg [Am]* 46A:1577, 1964.

Haythorn SR: Pathological changes found in material removed at operation in Legg-Calvé-Perthes disease. *J Bone Joint Surg [Am]* 31A:599, 1949.

Helms CA, Vogler JB: in Genant HK, Chafetz N, Helms CA (eds): *Computed Tomography of Spinal Stenoses and Arthroses.* Berkeley, University of California Press, 1982.

Hicks JH: Foot as support. *Acta Anat (Basel)* 25:34, 1955.

Hueston JT, Wilson WF: Knuckle pads. *Aust NZ J Surg* 42:274, 1973.

Hyman G: Children's footwear. *Br Med J* 1:1189, 1959.

Inman BT, Ralston HJ, Todd F: *Human Walking.* Baltimore, Williams & Wilkins, 1981.

Jack EA: Naviculo-cuneiform fusion in the treatment of flat foot. *J Bone Joint Surg [Br]* 35B:75, 1953.

James JIP: Idiopathic scoliosis: Prognosis, diagnosis, and operative indications related to curve patterns and age at onset. *J Bone Joint Surg [Br]* 36B:36, 1954.

Johnson IC: Histogenesis of avascular necrosis, Proceedings of the Conference on Aseptic Necrosis of the Femoral head, St Louis, Missouri, United States Public Health Service, p 55.

Kanis JA: Osteoporosis, in Butchers WT (ed): *The Chemistry and Biology of Mineralized Tissues.* Birmingham, AL, Ebsco Media, Inc, 1985, pp 398–408.

Keith A: Bone growth and bone repair. *Br J Surg* 5:685, 1918.

Khalili AA, Betts HG: Peripheral nerve block with phenol in the management of spasticity. *JAMA* 200:1155, 1968.

Killgren JH, Samuel EP: The sensitivity and innervation of the articular capsule. *J Bone Joint Surg [Br]* 32B:84, 1950.

King ESL: Localized rarefying conditions of bones as exemplified by Legg-Perthes disease, Osgood-Schlatter disease, Kümmell's disease and related conditions. London, Edward Arnold, 1935.

Lam SF, Hodgson AR: A comparison of foot form among the non-shoe- and shoe-wearing Chinese population. *J Bone Joint Surg [Am]* 40A:1058, 1958.

Langenskiöld A, Michelsson JE: Experimental progressive scoliosis in the rabbit. *J Bone Joint Surg* 43B:116, 1961.

McLeod JG: The representation of the splanchnic afferent pathways in the thalamus of the cat. *J Physiol* 140:462, 1958.

Mair WGP, Druckman R: Aberrant regenerating nerve fibers in injury to spinal cord. *Brain* 6:448, 1953.

Melzack R: The perception of pain. *Sci Am* 204:41, 1961.

Miller EJ: Recent information on the chemistry of the collagens, in Butchers WT (ed): *The Chemistry and Biology of Mineralized Tissues*. Birmingham, AL, Ebsco Media, Inc, 1985, pp 80–94.

Mooney V, Frykman G, McLamb J: Present status of intraneurol phenol injections. *Clin Orthop* 63:122, 1969.

Morgan-Hughes JA: Painful disorders of muscle. *Br J Hosp Med* 22:360, 1979.

Morley AJM: Knock-knee in children. *Br Med J* 2:976, 1957.

Nachemson A: The mechanical properties of the lumbar intervertebral discs and their clinical implications. *J Bone Joint Surg* 54B:195, 1972.

Newman PH: Sprung back. *J Bone Joint Surg [Br]* 30B:30, 1952.

Newman PH: Spondylolisthesis: Its cause and effect. *Ann R Coll Surg Engl* 16:305, 1955.

Ottolenghi CE: Diagnosis of orthopaedic lesions by aspiration biopsy: Results of 1061 punctures. *J Bone Joint Surg [Am]* 37A:443, 1955.

Outland T, Sherk HH: Congenital vertical talus. *Clin Orthop* 16:214, 1960.

Petrie JG, Bitenc I: The abduction weight-bearing treatment in Legg-Perthes' disease. *J Bone Joint Surg [Br]* 53B:54, 1971.

Pheasant HC, Dyck P: Failed lumbar disk surgery: Cause, assessment, and treatment. *Clin Orthop* 167:93, 1982.

Phelps WM: Prevention of acquired dislocation of the hip in cerebral palsy. *J Bone Joint Surg [Am]* 41A:440, 1959.

Ponsetti IV, Friedman B: Prognosis idiopathic scoliosis. *J Bone Joint Surg [Am]* 32A:381, 1950.

Ramirez F, Chu ML, de Wet W: Genetic defects and clinical manifestations in osteogenesis imperfecta, in Butchers WT (ed): *The Chemistry and Biology of Mineralized Tissues*. Birmingham, AL, Ebsco Media, Inc, 1985, pp 391–398.

Rowe ML: Newer concepts of low back pain. *J Occup Med* 2:219, 1960.

Rumbold C: Industrial back prevention. *J Occup Med* 2:132, 1960.

Russell RGG, Smith R: Diphosphonates: Experimental and clinical aspects. *J Bone Joint Surg [Am]* 55B:66, 1973.

Seddon HJ: Volkmann's contracture: Treatment by excision of infarct. *J Bone Joint Surg [Br]* 38B:152, 1956.

Sharrard WJW: Posterior ilio-psoas transplantation in treatment of paralytic dislocation of the hip. *J Bone Joint Surg [Br]* 46B:426, 1965.

Shepstone BJ: Bone scintigraphy with a view. *S Afr J Hosp Med* 1:215, 1978.

Smith CF: Current concepts review, tibia vara (Blount's disease). *J Bone Joint Surg* 64A:630, 1982.

Smith GW, Robinson RA: The treatment of certain cervical-spine disorders by anterior removal of the intervertebral disc and interbody fusion. *J Bone Joint Surg [Am]* 40A:3, 607, 1958.

Splithoff CA: Lumbo-sacral junction: Roentgenographic comparison of patients with and without backaches. *JAMA* 152:1610, 1953.

Stamp WG: Bracing in cerebral palsy, instructional course lecture, American Academy of Orthopaedic Surgeons. *J Bone Joint Surg [Am]* 44A:1457, 1962.

Strayer LM: Gastrocnemius resection five year report of cases. *J Bone Joint Surg [Am]* 40A:1019, 1959.

Thomasen E: *Myotonia: Thomsen's Disease, Paramyotonia,* *Dystrophia, Myotonia*. Aarhus, Denmark, Universities Forloget, 1948.

Thompson CF: Fusion of the metacarpals to the thumb and index finger to maintain functional position of the thumb. *J Bone Joint Surg* 24:907, 1942.

Vignos PJ, Watkins MP: The effect of exercise in muscular dystrophy. *JAMA* 197:843, 1966.

Walmsley T: The articular mechanics of diarthrosis. *J Bone Joint Surg* 10:40: 1928.

Weinstein S, Zavala DC, Ponsetti IB: Idiopathic scoliosis. Long-term followup and prognosis in untreated patients. *J Bone Joint Surg* 63A:702, 1981.

Whitty CWM, Hockaday JM: Patterns of referred pain in the normal subject. *Brain* 90:481, 1967.

Wiltse LI: The etiology of spondylolisthesis. *J Bone Joint Surg [Am]* 44A:539, 1962.

Wuthier RE, Register TC: Role of alkaline phosphatase. A polyfunctional enzyme in mineralizing tissues, in Butchers WT (ed): *The Chemistry and Biology of Mineralized Tissues*. Birmingham, AL, Ebsco Media, Inc, 1985, p 113.

Congenital Orthopaedic

Coleman SS: *Congenital Dysplasia of the Hip*. St Louis, Mosby, 1978.

Crabbe WA: Aetiology of congenital talipes. *Br Med J* 2:1060, 1960.

Denis-Browne R: Congenital postural scoliosis. *Proc R Soc Med* 49:395, 1956.

Duthie RB, Townes PL: The genetics of orthopaedic conditions. *J Bone Joint Surg [Br]* 49B2, 1967.

Frantz CG, O'Rahilly R: Congenital skeletal limb deficiencies. *J Bone Joint Surg [Am]* 43A:1202, 1961.

Fuller DJ, Duthie RB: The timed appearance of some congenital malformations and orthopaedic abnormalities, American Academy of Orthopaedic Surgery, Instructional Course Lectures. St Louis, Mosby, 23:53, 1974.

Gentry JT, Parkhurst E, Bulin GV Jr: An epidemiological study of congenital malformations in New York State. *Am J Public Health* 49:497, 1959.

Goldner JL: Congenital talipes equinovarus: Fifteen years of surgical treatment in Adams JP (ed): *Current Practice in Orthopaedic Surgery*. St Louis, Mosby, 1969, vol 4, p 61.

Green WT: The surgical correction of congenital elevation of the scapula (Sprengel's deformity). *J Bone Joint Surg [Am]* 39A:1439, 1957.

Green WT, Rudo N: Pseudoarthrosis and neurofibromatosis. *Arch Surg* 46:639, 1943.

Heyman CH, Herndon CH, Strong JM: Mobilization of the tarsometatarsal and intermtatarsal joints for the correction of resistant adduction of the fore part of the foot in congenital club-foot or congenital metatarsus varus. *J Bone Joint Surg [Am]* 40A:299, 1958.

Hummer CD, MacEwen GD: The coexistence of torticollis and congenital dysplasia of the hip. *J Bone Joint Surg [Am]* 54A:1255, 1972.

Kite JH: *The Clubfoot*. New York, Grune & Stratton, 1964.

MacKenzie JJG, Seddon HJ, Trevor D: Congenital dislocation of the hip. *J Bone Joint Surg [Br]* 42B:689, 1960.

McKeown J, Record RG: Malformations in a population observed for five years after birth in Wolstenholme GEW, O'Conner CM (eds): *Ciba Foundation Symposium on Congenital Malformations*. 1960, p 2.

Neibauer JJ, King DE: Congenital dislocation of the knee, *J Bone Joint Surg [Am]* 42A:2, 1960.

Norton PL: Pediatric orthopedics. *Med Clin North Am* 37:1427, 1953.

Record RG, Edwards JH: Environmental influences related to the aetiology of congenital dislocation of the hip. *Br J Prevent Social Med* 12:8, 1958.

Salter RB: Innominate osteotomy in the treatment of congenital dislocation and subluxation of the hip. *J Bone Joint Surg [Br]* 34B:518, 1961.

Salvatti EA, Wilson PD Jr: Treatment of irreducible hip subluxation by Chiari's illiac osteotomy. *Rev Hosp Spec Surg* 1:49, 1971.

Sanders JW: The proximo-distal sequence of origin of the parts of the chick wing and the role of the ectoderm. *J Exp Zool* 108:363, 1948.

Scott JC: Frame reduction in congenital dislocation of the hip. *J Bone Joint Surg [Br]* 36B:372, 1953.

Stevenson AC: Frequency of congenital and hereditary disease: With special reference to maturation. *Br Med Bull* 17:3, 1961.

Symposium of the Swedish Orthopaedic Association: Prevention of congenital dislocation of the hip joint in Sweden: Efficiency of early diagnosis and treatment. *Acta Orthop Scand Suppl* 130, 1970.

Tachdjian MO: Congenital convex pes valgus, in Symposium on Current Pediatric Problems. *Orthop Clin North Am* 3:131, 1972.

Thompson TC, Straub LR, Arnold WD: Congenital absence of the fibula. *J Bone Joint Surg [Am]* 39A:1229, 1957.

Turco VJ: Resistant congenital club foot—one-stage posteromedial release with internal fixation. A follow-up report of a fifteen-year experience. *J Bone Joint Surg [Am]* 61:805, 1979.

Wynne-Davies R: Acetabular dysplasia and familial joint laxity: Two etiological factors in congenital dislocation of the hip. A review of 589 patients and their families. *J Bone Joint Surg [Br]* 52B:704, 1970.

Wynne-Davies R: Family studies and the cause of congenital clubfoot: Talipes equinovarus, talipes calcaneovalgus and metatarsus varus, *J Bone Joint Surg [Br]* 46B:445, 1964.

Generalized Bone Disorders

Albers-Schönberg W: Roentgenbildung einer seltenen Knochenerkrakung. *Munch Med Wochenschr* 51:365, 1904.

Albers-Schönberg W: Einer seltener bisher nicht bekannter Structuranomalie des Skellets. *Fortschr Geb Roentgenstr Nuklearmed* 23:174, 1915.

Avioli LV: *The Osteoporotic Syndrome*. New York, Grune & Stratton, 1983.

Bailey JA: Orthopedic aspects of achondroplasia. *J Bone Joint Surg [Am]* 52A:1285, 1970.

Bauer CCH, Carlsson A, Lindquist B: Bone salt metabolism in human rickets studied with radioactive phosphorus. *Metabolism* 5:573, 1956.

Brailsford JF: *The Radiology of Bones and Joints*. London, J & A Churchill, 1964.

Compere EL, Johnson WE, Coventry MB: Vertebra Plana (Calvé's disease) due to eosinophilic granuloma. *J Bone Joint Surg [Am]* 36A:969, 1954.

Dixon TF, Perkins HR: The chemistry of calcification, in Bourne GH (ed): *Biochemistry and Physiology of Bone*. New York, Academic Press, 1956, chap 10.

Duthie RB, Barker AN: Autoradiographic study of mucopoly-

saccharide and phosphate complexes in bone growth and repair. *J Bone Joint Surg [Br]* 38B:304, 1955.

Fanconi G, Girardet P: Familiärerpersistierender Phosphatidiabetes mit D-Vitamin-resistenter Rachitis. *Helv Paediatr Acta* 7:14, 1952.

Fleisch H: Mechanism of calcification: Inhibitory role of pyrophosphate. *Nature* 195:911, 1962.

Fleisch H, Russell RGG, et al: Influence of pyrophosphate on the transformation of amorphous to crystalline calcium phosphate. *Calcif Tissue Res* 2:49, 1968.

Fraser D, Leeming JM, et al: Studies of the pathogenesis of the high renal clearance of phosphate in hypophosphatemic vitamin-D refractory rickets of the simple type. *Am J dis Child* 98:586, 1959.

Glimcher MJ: Calcification in Biological systems. *Symp Am Assoc Adv Sci Washington 1958* 64:421, 1960.

Gutman AB, Yü TF: A concept of the role of enzymes in endochondral calcification. *Metab Interrelations Trans conf 2d.* 2:167, 1950.

Harrison HE: The interrelation of citrate and calcium metabolism. *Am J Med* 20:1, 1956.

Hass GM: Studies of cartilage: Morphologic and chemical analysis of aging human costal cartilage. *Arch Pathol* 35:275, 1943.

Jackson SF: The fine structure of developing bone in the embryonic owl. *Proc R Soc Lond [Biol]* 146:270, 1957.

Keith A: Bone growth and bone repair. *Br J Surg* 5:685, 1918.

Lacroix P: Radiocalcium and radiosulphur in the study of bone metabolism at the histological level. *Proc Radioisotope Conf 2d, Oxford Engl* 1:134, 1954.

Mercer W, Duthie RB: Histiocytic granulomatosis. *J Bone Joint Surg [Br]* 38B:279, 1956.

Milkman LA: Pseudofractures (hunger osteopathy, late rickets, osteomalacia): Report of case. *Am J Roentgenol* 24:29, 1930.

Neuman WF, Neuman MW: The nature of the mineral phase of bone. *Chem Rev* 53:1, 1953.

Nordin BEC: Osteomalacia, osteoporosis and calcium deficiency. *Clin Orthop* 17:235, 1960.

Rathbun JC: "Hypophosphatasia": New developmental anomaly. *Am J Dis Child* 75:822, 1948.

Reddi KK, Nörstrom A: Influence of vitamin C on utilization of sulphate labelled with sulphur-35 in synthesis of chondroitin sulphate of costal cartilage of guinea pig. *Nature (Lond)* 173:1232, 1954.

Robinson RA: Crystal-collagen-water relaionships in bone matrix. *Clin Orthop* 17:69, 1960.

Sheldon H, Robinson RA: Electron microscope studies of crystal collagen relationships in bone. IV. The occurrence of crystals within collagen fibres. *J Biophys Biochem Cytol* 3:1011, 1957.

Siffert RS: Role of alkaline phosphatase in osteogenesis. *J Exp Med* 93:415, 1951.

Smith R, Francis MIO, Houghton GR: *The Brittle Bone Syndrome Osteogenesis Imperfecta*. London, Butterworths, 1983.

Snapper I, Nathan DJ: Rickets and osteomalacia. *Am J Med* 22:939, 1957.

Vincent YJ, Haumont S: Autoradiographic identification of metabolic osteones after the administration of CA 45. *Rev Fr Etud Clin Biol* 5:348, 1960.

Fractures and Joint Injuries

Adler JB, Shaftan GW: Radial head fractures: Is excision necessary? *J Trauma* 4:115, 1964.

Aegerter E, Kirkpatrick JA: *Orthopaedic Diseases*. Philadelphia, Saunders, 1964.

Amstutz HC: Arthroplasty of the hip: The search for durable component fixation. *Clin Orthop* 200:343, 1985.

Anderson LD: Compression plate fixation and the effect of different types of internal fixation on fracture healing, instructional course lecture, American Academy of Orthopaedic Surgeons. *J Bone Joint Surg [Am]* 47A:191, 1965.

Barnard L, Stubbins SG: Styloidectomy of the radius in the surgical treatment of non-union of the carpal navicular: A preliminary report. *J Bone Joint Surg [Am]* 30A:98, 1948.

Basset CAL, Mitchell SN, Gaston SR: Treatment of un-united tibial diaphysial fractures with pulsing electromagnetic fields. *J Bone Joint Surg [Am]* 63A:511, 1981.

Beatson TR: Fractures and dislocations of the cervical spine. *J Bone Joint Surg [Br]* 45B:21, 1963.

Bedbrook GM: Fracture dislocation of the spine with and without paralysis. The case for conservativism and against operative techniques, in Leach RE, Hoaglund FT, Reseborough EJ (eds): *Controversies in Orthopaedic Surgery*. Philadelphia, Saunders, 1982.

Bergman BR: Antibiotic prophylaxis in open and closed fractures: A controlled clinical trial. *Acta Orthop Scand* 53:57, 1982.

Blount WP: *Fractures in Children*. St Louis, Mosby, 1955.

Bohlman HH: Acute fractures and dislocations of the cervical spine: An analysis of 300 hospitalized patients and review of the literature. *J Bone Joint Surg* 61A:119, 1979.

Bowes DN, Hohl M: Tibial/condylar fractures, evaluation of treatment and outcome. *Clin Orthop* 171:104, 1982.

Bradford DS, Akbarnia BA, et al: Surgical stabilization of fracture dislocation of the thoracic spine. *Spine* 2:185, 1977.

Brighton CT, Pollack SR: Treatment of recalcitrant nonunion with a capacitively coupled field. *J Bone Joint Surg* 67A:577, 1985.

Brown PW, Urban JG: Early weight-bearing treatment of open fractures of the tibia: An end-result study of 63 cases. *J Bone Joint Surg [Am]* 51A:59, 1969.

Cann CE: Low-dose CT scanning for quantitative spinal mineral analysis. *Radiology* 140:813, 1981.

Cann CE, Genant K, et al: Spinal mineral loss in oophorectomized women. *JAMA* 244:2056, 1980.

Clawson DK: Trochanteric fractures treated by the sliding screw plate fixation method. *J Trauma* 4:737, 1964.

Coleman DA, Blair WF, et al: Resection of the radial head for fracture of the radial head: Long-term follow-up with 17 cases. *J Bone Joint Surg* 69A:385, 1987.

Crawford HB: Conservative treatment of impacted fractures of the femoral neck: A report of 50 cases. *J Bone Joint Surg [Am]* 42A:471, 1960.

Dart DE, Graham WD: Treatment of the fractured calcaneum. *J Trauma* 6:362, 1966.

DeHaven KE: Diagnosis of acute knee injuries with hemiarthrosis. *Am J Sports Med* 8:9, 1980.

DeHaven KE: Peripheral meniscus repair: An alternative to meniscectomy. *Orthop Transplant* 5:399, 1981.

Dekel S, Francis MJO: The treatment of osteomyelitis of the tibia with sodium salicylate. *J Bone Joint Surg [Br]* 63B:178, 1981.

Dimon JH, Hughston JC: Unstable intertrochanteric fractures of the hip. *J Bone Joint Surg [Am]* 49A:440, 1967.

Dunne LR, Jacobs B, Campbell RD: Fractures of the talus. *J Trauma* 6:443, 1966.

Ellman H, Hanker G, et al: Repair of the rotator cuff: End result of factors influencing reconstruction. *J Bone Joint Surg* 68A:1136, 1986.

Evans EM: Pronation injuries of the forearm with special reference to the anterior monteggia fracture. *J Bone Joint Surg [Br]* 31B:578, 1949.

Flesch JR, Leider LL, et al: Harrington instrumentation and spine fusion for unstable fractures and fracture-dislocation of the thoracic and lumbar spine. *J Bone Joint Surg* 59A:143, 1977.

Forsythe HF: Extension injuries of the cervical spine, instructional coarse lecture, American Academy of Orthopaedic Surgeons. *J Bone Joint Surg [Am]* 46A:1792, 1964.

Garden RS: Stability and union in subcapital fractures of the femur. *J Bone Joint Surg [Br]* 46B:630, 1964.

Gossling HR, Pellegrini VD: Fat embolism syndrome: A review of the pathophysiology and physiological basis of treatment. *Clin Orthop* 165:68, 1982.

Gillquist J, Oretorp N: Arthroscopic partial meniscectomy: Technique and long-term results. *Clin Orthop* 167:29, 1982.

Griffiths LL: The management of acute circulatory failure in an injured limb. *J Bone Joint Surg [Br]* 30B:280, 1948.

Gustilo RB, Anderson JT: Prevention of infection in the treatment of one thousand and twenty-five open fractures of long bones: Retrospective and prospective analysis. *J Bone Joint Surg* 58A:453, 1976.

Helfet AJ: *The Management of Internal Derangements of the Knee*. Philadelphia, Lippincott, 1963.

Hoaglund FT, Shiba R, et al: Diseases of the hip: A comparative study of Japanese oriental and American white patients. *J Bone Joint Surg* 67A:1376, 1985.

Hoaglund FT, States JD: Factors influencing rate of healing in tibial shaft fractures. *Surg Gynecol Obstet* 124:71, 1967.

Hohl M, Larson RI: Fractures about the knee, in Rockwood CA, Green DE (eds): *Fractures*. Philadelphia, Lippincott, 1975, chap 16.

Holdsworth FW: Fractures, dislocations, and fracture-dislocations of the spine. *J Bone Joint Surb [Br]* 45B:6, 1963.

Holstein A, Lewis GB: Fractures of humerus with radial nerve paralysis. *J Bone Joint Surg [Am]* 45A:1382, 1963.

Hughston JC: Fracture of the forearm in children, instructional course lecture, American Academy of Orthopaedic Surgeons. *J Bone Joint Surg [Am]* 44A:1678, 1962.

Inman VT, Saunders JB, Abbott IC: Observations on the function of the shoulder joint. *J Bone Joint Surg [Am]* 26A:1, 1944.

Ishikawa H, Ohno O, et al: Synovectomy in rheumatoid patients: Long-term results. *J Bone Joint Surg* 68A:198, 1986.

Jacobs B, Wade PA: Acromioclavicular joint injury and end result study. *J Bone Joint Surg [Am]* 48A:475, 1966.

Johnson LC, Stradford HT, et al: Histogenesis of stress fractures. *Armed for Inst Pathol Annu Lec* 1963.

Jones KG: Reconstruction of the anterior cruciate ligament using the central one-third of the patellar ligament. *J Bone Joint Surg [Am]* 45A:925, 1970.

Karlan A: Congenital fibrosis of the vastus intermedius muscle. *J Bone Joint Surg [Br]* 46B:488, 1964.

Keene JS, Goletzth, et al: Diagnosis of vertebral fractures: A comparison of conventional radiography, conventional tomography, and computed axial tomography. *J Bone Joint Surg* 64A:586, 1982.

King KF, Rush J: Closed intramedullary nailing of femoral shaft fractures: A review of 112 cases by the Kuntscher technique. *J Bone Joint Surg [Am]* 63A:1319, 1981.

Kort JS, Schink MN, et al: Congenital pseudoarthrosis of the tibia: Treatment with pulsing electromagnetic fields. The international experience. *Clin Orthop* 165:124, 1982.

Lacey T III, Crawford HB: Reduction of anterior dislocation of the shoulder by means of milch abduction techniques. *J Bone Joint Surg [Am]* 34A:108, 1952.

Lange-Hansen N: Fractures of the ankle. Combined experimental-surgical and experimental-roentgenologie investigation. *Arch Surg* 60:957, 1950.

Letournel E: Acetabular fractures: Classification and management. *Clin Orthop* 151:82, 1980.

Ma G, Griffith T: Percutaneous repair of acute closed ruptured achilles tendon. *Clin Orthop* 128:247, 1977.

McCarroll JR, Braunstein TW, et al: Fatal pedestrian automobile accidents. *JAMA* 180:127, 1962.

McKibbin B: The biology of fracture healing in long bones. *J Bone Joint Surg* 60B:150, 1978.

McReynolds IS: The case for operative treatment of fractures of the oscalcis, in Leach R, Hoaglund TF, Riseborough E (eds): *Controversies in Orthopaedic Surgery*. Philadelphia, Saunders, 1982, pp 232–256.

Maquet P: Unbalanced patella: II. Biomechanical back motion: Review of surgery and orthopaedics. *Chir Orthop* 66:209, 1980.

Marshall JL, Rubin RM: Knee ligament injuries—a diagnostic and therapeutic approach. *Ortho Clin North Am* 8:641, 1977.

Mears DC, Fu F: External fixation and pelvic fractures. *Orthop Clin North Am* 11:465, 1980.

Mercer W, Duthie RB: *Orthopaedic Surgery*, 6th ed. London, Edward Arnold, 1964.

Milford L: Tendon injuries, in Crenshaw AH (ed): *Campbell's Operative Orthopaedics*, 7th ed. St Louis, Mosby, 1987, vol I, pp 149–182.

Miller WE: Comminuted fractures of the humerus in the adult, instructional coarse lecture, American Academy of Orthopaedic Surgeons, *J Bone Joint Surg [Am]* 46A:6444, 1964.

Miller GK, Drennan DD, Maylahn DJ: Treatment of displaced segmental radial head fractures. *J Bone Joint Surg [Am]* 63A:712, 1981.

Mooney V, Nickel VL, et al: Cast-brace treatment for fractures of the distal part of the femur. *J Bone Joint Surg [Am]* 52A:1563, 1970.

Morris HD: Hand WL, Dunn AW: The modified Blair fusion for fractures of the talus. *J Bone Joint Surg [Am]* 53A:1289, 1971.

Mubarak SJ, Owen CA, et al: Acute compartment syndromes. Diagnosis and treatment with the aid of the Wick catheter. *J Bone Joint Surg [Am]* 60A:1091, 1978.

Muller ME, Allgower M, Willenegger H: *Technique of Internal Fixation of Fractures*, 2d ed. New York, Springer-Verlag, 1979.

Nachemson AL: Advances: Low back pain. *Clin Orthop* 200:266, 1985.

Neer CS: Four-segment classification of displaced proximal humeral fractures, instructional course lectures, American Academy of Orthopaedic Surgeons. *J Bone Joint Surg* 24:160, 1975.

Nicoll EH: Fractures of the tibial shaft: A survey of 705 cases. *J Bone Joint Surg [Am]* 46B:373, 1964.

O'Donoghue DH: Surgical treatment of fresh injuries to the major ligaments of the knee. *J Bone Joint Surg [Am]* 32A:721, 1950.

Olerud S, Karlstrom: The spectrum of intramedullary mailing of the tibia. *Clin Orthop* 212:101, 1986.

Osmond-Clark H: Habitual dislocation of the shoulder: The Putti-Platt operation. *J Bone Joint Surg [Br]* 30B:19, 1948.

Post M: Current concepts in the diagnosis of management of acromioclavicular dislocations. *Clin Orthop* 200:234, 1985.

Protzman RR: Anterior instability of the shoulder. *J Bone Joint Surg* 62A:909, 1980.

Ray RD, Sankaran B, Fetro KO: Delayed union in non-union fractures, instructional course lecture, American Academy of Orthopaedic Surgeons. *J Bone Joint Surg [Am]* 46A:627, 1964.

Reckling FW: Unstable fracture dislocations of the forearm: Montegia and galiazzi lesions. *J Bone Joint Surg* 64A:857, 1982.

Rogers WA: Treatment of fracture dislocation of the cervical spine. *J Bone Joint Surg [Am]* 24:245, 1942.

Rowe CR, Patel D, Southmayd W: The Bankert procedure. A long-term end-results study. *J Bone Joint Surg [Am]* 60A:1, 1978.

Rowe CR, Lowell JD: Prognosis of fractures of the acetabulum. *J Bone Joint Surg [Am]* 43A:30, 1961.

Salter RB, Harris RW: Injuries involving the epiphyseal plate, instructional coarse lecture, American Academy of Orthopaedic Surgeons. *J Bone Joint Surg [Am]* 45A:587, 1963.

Salter RB, Harris RW: Injuries involving the shoulder joint, instructional course lecture, American Academy of Orthopaedic Surgeons. *J Bone Joint Surg [Am]* 45A:587, 1963.

Salter RB, Zaltz C: Anatomic investigations of the mechanism of injury and pathologic anatomy of "pulled elbow" in young children. *Clin Orthop* 77:134, 1971.

Sarmiento A: A functional below-the-knee cast fr tibial fractures. *J Bone Joint Surg [Am]* 49A:885, 1967.

Scheck M: The significance of posterior comminution in femoral neck fractures. *Clin Orthop* 152:138, 1980.

Scott GA, Jolly BL, et al: Combined posterior incision and arthroscopic intraarticular repair of the meniscus and examination of the factors affecting healing. *J Bone Joint Surg* 68A:847, 1986.

Scuderi CS: Operative indications in fractures of both bones of the forearm, instructional course lecture, American Academy of Orthopaedic Surgeons. *J Bone Joint Surg [Am]* 44A:1671, 1962.

Seddon HJ: Three types of nerve injury. *Brain* 66:237, 1943.

Sherk HH: Fractures of the atlas and odontoid process. *Orthop Clin North Am* 9:973, 1978.

Sledge CB, Walker PS: Total knee arthroplasty in rheumatoid arthritis. *Clin Orthop* 182:127, 1984.

Slocum DB, James SL, Lanson RL: Clinical test for anterolateral instability of the knee. *Clin Orthop* 118:659, 1976.

Slocum DB, Larson RL: Rotatory instability of the knee: Its pathogenesis and a clinical test to demonstrate its presence. *J Bone Joint Surg [Am]* 50A:211, 1968.

Smith L: Deformity following supracondylar fractures of the humerus. *J Bone Joint Surg* 42A:235, 1960.

Soreff J, Axdorphf G, et al: Treatment of patients with unstable fractures of the thoracic lumbar spine. *Acta Orthop Scand* 53:369, 1982.

Stewart MJ, Milford LW: Prevention of disability after traumatic dislocation of the hip, and end result study. *J Bone Joint Surg [Am]* 36A:315, 1964.

Tachakra SS, Sevin S: Hypoaxemia after fractures. *J Bone Joint Surg* 57B:197, 1975.

Thoren O: Os calcis fractures. *Acta Orthop Scand Suppl* 70, 1964.

Trueta J, Harrison MH: The normal vascular anatomy of the

femoral head in adult man. *J Bone Joint Surg [Br]* 35B:442, 1953.

Watson-Jones Sir Reginald: *Fractures and Joint Injuries,* 4th ed. Baltimore, Williams & Wilkins, 1956, vol II, chap 28, p 813, chap 29, p 862.

Waugh W: Tibial osteotomy in the management of osteoarthritis of the knee. *Clin Orthop* 210:55, 1986.

Weaver JK, Dunn HK: Treatment of acromioclavicular injuries, especially complete acromioclavicular separation. *J Bone Joint Surg* 54A:1187, 1972.

Welch RB, Taylor LW, et al: Results with the cemented hemiarthroplasty for displaced fractures of the femoral neck and hip. *Proceedings of the Fifth Open Scientific Meeting of the Hip Society.* St Louis, Mosby, 1977, p 87.

Weissman SL, Harold ZH: Fractures of the tibial plateau. *Clin Orthop* 33:194, 1964.

White AA, Panjabi MM: *Clinical Biomechanics of the Spine.* Philadelphia, Lippincott, 1978, pp 143–151.

Wroblewski DM: Fifteen twenty-one year results of Charnley low-friction arthroplasty. *Clin Orthop* 211:30, 1986.

Yosipovitch Z, Robin GC, et al: Open resection of the unstable thoraco-lumbar spinal injuries and fixation with harrington rods. *J Bone Joint Surg* 59A:1003, 1977.

Diseases of Joints

Atprup T, Sjolini KE: Thromboplastic and fibrinolytic activity of human synovial membrane in fibrous capsular tissue. *Proc Soc Exp Biol* 92:852, 1958.

Arthritis and Rheumatism Council and British Orthopaedic Association: Controlled Trial of Synovectomy of Knee and Metacarpophalangeal Joints in Rheumatoid Arthritis. *Ann Rheum Dis* 35:437, 1976.

Charnley J: The long-term results of low friction arthroplasty of the hip performed as a primary intervention. *J Bone Joint Surg [Br]* 54B:61, 1972.

Charnley J, Baker SL: Compression arthrodesis of the knee: A clinical and histological study. *J Bone Joint Surg [Am]* 34A:187, 1952.

Chung SMK, James JM: Diffuse pigmented villonodular synovitis of the hip joint. *J Bone Joint Surg [Am]* 47A:239, 1965.

Clawson BK, Dunn AW: Management of common bacterial infections of bones and joints, instructional course lecture, American Academy of Orthopaedic Surgeons. *J Bone Joint Surg [Am]* 49A:164, 1967.

Clayton ML: Surgery of the thumb in rheumatoid arthritis. *J Bone Joint Surg [Am]* 44A:1376, 1962.

Curtiss RH, Klein L: Destruction of articular surfaces in septic arthritis. I. In vitro studies. *J Bone Joint Surg [Am]* 45A:797, 1963.

Curtiss RH: Changes produced in the synovial membranes and synovial fluid by disease, instructional course lecture, American Academy of Orthopaedic Surgeons. *J Bone Joint Surg [Am]* 46A:873, 1964.

Duthie RB, Bentley JB: *Mercer's Textbook of Orthopaedic Surgery.* London, Edward Arnold, 1983.

Duthie RB, Matthews JM, et al: *The Musculoskeletal Problems in the Haemophilics.* Oxford, England, Blackwell Scientific Publications, 1972.

Ford DK: Gonorrheal arthritis, in Hollander JL (ed): *Arthritis and Allied Conditions.* Philadelphia, Lea & Febiger, 1966.

Girdlestone GR: Acute pyogenic arthritis of the hip. *Lancet* 1:419, 1943.

Griffith MJ, Seidenstein MK, et al: Eight year results of

Charnley arthroplasties of the hip with special reference to the behavior of cement. *Clin Orthop* 137:36, 1978.

Harris NH, Kirwan E: The results of osteotomy for early primary osteoarthritis of the hip. *J Bone Joint Surg [Br]* 46B:477, 1964.

Henderson MS: Tuberculosis of joints with special reference to knee. *Aust NZ J Surg* 6:27, 1936.

Hoaglund FT: Osteoarthritis. *Orthop Clin North Am* 2:3, 1970.

Hodgson AR, Stuck FE: Anterior spine fusion for the treatment of tuberculosis in the spine. *J Bone Joint Surg [Am]* 42A:295, 1960.

Hodgson AR, Wong W, Yau A: *X-Ray Appearances of Tuberculosis of the Spine.* Springfield, IL, Charles C Thomas, 1969.

Hoffman P: An operation for severe grades of contracted or claw toes. *J Orthop Surg* 9:441, 916.

Huskisson EC: Report on rheumatic diseases. No. 54, Arthritis and Rheumatism Council, London, 1974.

Jaffe HL, LIchtenstein L, Seutro CJ: Pigmented villonodular synovitis, bursitis, and tenosynovitis. *Arch Pathol* 31:731, 1941.

Johnson JTH: Neuropathic fractures and joint injuries: Pathogenesis and rationale of prevention and treatment. *J Bone Joint Surg [Am]* 49A:1, 1967.

Keller WL: Surgical treatment of bunions and hallux valgus. *NY Med J* 80:741, 1904.

Kellgren JH, Moore R: Generalized osteoarthritis and Heberden's nodes. *Br Med J* 1:181, 1952.

Kelly WN, Harris ED, et al: *Textbook of Rheumatology.* Philadelphia, Saunders, 1981.

Kettelkamp DB: Current concepts: Review management of patellar malalignment. *J Bone Joint Surg [Am]* 63A:1344, 1981.

Kettelkamp DB, Wenger DR, et al: Results of proximal tibial ostectomy: The effects of tibiofemoral angle, stance-phase flexion-extension and medial plateau force. *J Bone Joint Surg* 58A:952, 1976.

King EJS: On some aspects of the pathology of hypertrophic charcot's joints. *Br J Surg* 18:113, 1930.

Littler JW: Basic principles of reconstructive surgery of the hand. *Surg Clin North Am* 40:383, 1960.

McBride ED: Hallux valgus, bunion deformity: Its treatment in mild, moderate, and severe stage. *J Int Coll Surg* 21:99, 1954.

McCarty DJ: Pseudogout: Articular chondrocalcinosis calcium pyrophosphate crystal deposition disease, in Hollander JL (ed): *Arthritis and Allied Conditions.* Philadelphia, Lea & Febiger, 1966, chap 16.

McLaughlin H: Rupture of the rotator cuff, instructional course lecture, American Academy of Orthopaedic Surgeons. *J Bone Joint Surg [Am]* 44A:979, 1962.

Mankin HJ: Biochemical and metabolic aspects of osteoarthritis. *Orthop Clin North Am* 2:19, 1971.

Maquet P: *Biomechanics of the Knee.* New York, Springer-Verlag, 1976.

Milone FP, Copeland MM: Calcific tendonitis of the shoulder joint: Presentation of 136 cases treated by irradiation. *Am J roentgenol Radium Ther Nucl Med* 85:901, 1961.

Murray WR, Lucas DB, Inman VT: Femoral head and neck resection. *J Bone Joint Surg [Am]* 46A:1184, 1964.

Neer CS, Watson KC, Stanton FJ: Recent experience in total shoulder replacement. *J Bone Joint Surg [Am]* 64A:319, 1982.

Phemister DB: The effect of pressure on articular surfaces in pyogenic and tuberculosis arthritides and its bearing on treatment. *Ann Surg* 80:481, 1924.

Seegmiller JE, Howell RR, Makowista SE: The inflammatory

reaction to sodium urate: Its possible relationship to the genesis of acute gouty arthritis. *JAMA* 180:469, 1962.

Sledge CB, Ewald FC: Total knee arthroplasty experiences at the Robert Brigham Hospital. *Clin Orthop* 145:78, 1979.

Smyth CJ: Rheumatism and arthritis: Sixteenth rheumatism review. *Ann Intern Med* 61(suppl 6):3, 1964.

Sokoloff L: Pathology of rheumatoid arthritis and allied diseases, in Hollander JL (ed): *Arthritis and Allied Conditions*. Philadelphia, Lea & Febiger, 1966.

Stecher RM, Hersh AH, Solomon WM: The heredity of gout and its relationship to familial hyperuricemia. *Ann Intern Med* 31:595, 1949.

Steere AC, Grodzicki RL, et al: The spirochetal etiology of Lyme disease. *N Engl J Med* 308:733, 1983.

Tumors of the Musculoskeletal System

Abrams HL: Skeletal metastases in carcinoma. *Radiology* 55:534, 1950.

Batson OV: The role of the vertebral veins in metastatic processes. *Ann Intern Med* 16:38, 1942.

Dahlin DC: *Bone Tumours*. Springfield, IL, Charles C Thomas, 1980.

Dahlin DC, Coventry MB, Scanlon PW: Ewing's sarcoma: A critical analysis of 165 cases. *J Bone Joint Surg [Am]* 43A:185, 1961.

Dahlin DC, Henderson ED: Chondrosarcoma, a surgical and pathological problem: Review of 212 cases. *J Bone Joint Surg [Am]* 38A:5, 1956.

Edelstyn GA, Gillespie PJ, Grebbell FS: The radiological demonstration of osseous metastases: Experimental observations. *Clin Radiol* 18:158, 1967.

Enneking WF, Spanier SS, et al: A system for surgical staging of musculoskeletal sarcoma. *Clin Orthop Rel Res* 153:106, 1980.

Enneking WF: *Musculoskeletal Tumour Staging*. New York, Churchill Livingstone, 1983.

Grimes BJ, Fisher B, et al: Steroid-resistant hypercalcemia and parathyroid hyperplasia in non-osseous cancer. *Acta Endocrinol (Kbb)* 56:510, 1967.

Jaffe HL: "Osteoid-osteoma": Benign osteoblastic tumour composed of osteoid and atypical bone. *Arch Surg* 31:709, 1935.

Jaffe HL: *Tumors and Tumorous Conditions of the Bones and Joints*. Philadelphia, Lea & Febiger, 1968.

Johnson LC: A general theory of bone tumours. *Bull NY Acad Med* 29:2, 1953.

Lichtenstein L: *Bone Tumors*, 4th ed. St Louis, Mosby, 1982.

McKenna RJ, Schwinn CP, et al: Sarcomata of the osteogenic series (osteosarcoma, fibrosarcoma, chondrosarcoma, parosteal osteogenic sarcoma, and sarcomata arising in abnormal bone): An analysis of 552 cases, *J Bone Joint Surg [Am]* 48A:1, 1966.

Marcove RC, Miké, V, et al: Osteogenic sarcoma under the age of 21: A review of 145 operative cases. *J Bone Joint Surg [Am]* 52A:411, 1970.

Marsh B, Flynn L, Enneking W: Immunological aspects of osteosarcoma and their relationship to therapy. *J Bone Joint Surg [Am]* 54A:1367, 1972.

Morton DL, Eilber FR, et al: Limb salvage from a multidisciplinary treatment approach for skeletal and soft tissue sarcomas of the extremity. *Ann Surg* 184:268, 1976.

Plimpton CH, Gelhorn A: Hypercalcemia in malignant disease without evidence of bone destruction. *Am J Med* 21:5, 1956.

Pritchard DJ: Is adjuvant chemotherapy of osteosarcoma of proven value?, in Wiemer P (ed): *Controversies in Oncology*. New York, Wiley, 1982.

Sherman CD, Duthie RB: Modified hemipelvectomy. *Cancer* 13:1, 1960.

Sissons HA, Duthie RB: *British Surgical Practice: Surgical Progress*. London, Butterworth, 1959.

Spjut HJ, Dorfman H, et al: *Tumors of Bone and Cartilage*, ser 2. Washington, Armed Forces Institute of Pathology, 1971.

Thomson AD, Turner-Warwick RT: Skeletal sarcomata and giant-cell tumour. *J Bone Joint Surg [Br]* 37B:266, 1955.

Chapter 44

Amputations

Seymour I. Schwartz and Franklin T. Hoaglund

GENERAL CONSIDERATIONS

Indications

The indications for amputation of part or all of an extremity include (1) trauma that is sufficiently extensive to preclude repair; (2) tumor of the bone, soft tissue, muscles, blood vessels, or nerves; (3) extensive infection that does not respond to conservative measures or contributes to septicemia; and (4) a variety of peripheral vascular diseases. Refinement in surgical technique as applied to blood vessels and peripheral nerves has markedly reduced the indications for amputation following trauma and has permitted reimplantation of totally amputated extremities.

Presently, more than two-thirds of the amputations on civilians in Western society are performed for peripheral vascular disease in patients over the age of fifty.

AMPUTATION OF ISCHEMIC LIMBS

Amputations are performed for four main categories of vascular disease: (1) arteriosclerosis obliterans, (2) arteriosclerosis obliterans with diabetes, (3) thromboangiitis obliterans, and (4) miscellaneous conditions such as embolic occlusion, peripheral aneurysm, vascular trauma, and venous obstruction. The specific indications for amputation in these patients are severe arterial insufficiency with necrosis of all or part of an extremity, intractable and severe pain that disables the patient, and infection that is spreading or unresponsive to therapy. In a few patients, extrarenal azotemia and hyperkalemia secondary to tissue necrosis constitute specific indications for amputation.

Amputation performed on a patient with compromised circulation requires special consideration. The patients are generally more brittle and require more intensive preoperative preparation. The compromised vascular supply within the limb necessitates meticulous and somewhat refined techniques, as described below. It is more difficult to achieve healing of the stump, and even after it has healed, breakdown related to the trauma of a prosthesis may occur. The patients are generally less vigorous and less adept at handling prostheses.

Selection of Site

Several factors contribute to the decision concerning level of amputation. When amputation is performed for malignant disease, the principal factor is wide excision of grossly apparent tumor. In the case of amputation subsequent to trauma or for peripheral vascular disease, the major factor determining the optimal level is usually the extent of healthy tissue. Other factors include the length of the stump sufficient for function of a prosthesis and the cosmetic effect of a prosthesis.

In general, the longer the amputation stump, the more functional the limb and the better control the patient has of the prosthesis. For traumatic amputations with irregular damage to the skin, grafting procedures and mobilization of flaps are indicated to maintain as much of the bony length as possible. In a long-term follow-up review of causes of death in World War II veterans by Ryder, patients with amputations at or above the knee (AK), had 1.4 times the mortality rate due to cardiovascular disease as that of distal amputees. The implication is that walking ability and beneficial exercise is better with the presence of a functional knee. AK amputees expend about twice as much energy to ambulate as BK amputees. Regarding the upper extremity, as much length as possible should always be saved, even if there is only a very short below-elbow or humeral stump. There are exceptions to the general rule of ''the longer, the better.'' For the lower extremity, proximal to the Syme amputation, the best level below the knee as far as prosthetic fitting is concerned is at the gastrocnemius musculotendinous junction. Every effort should be made to preserve the knee joint. A below-knee (BK) prosthesis can be fitted to a 2-in. stump. The knee should be preserved even if skin coverage requires grafting, since the prosthetist can fit virtually any stump regardless of the scars. A knee disarticulation is preferable to a long AK stump because it permits a prosthesis with end-weight-bearing characteristics should the patient lose the other limb. Ambulation is more likely if the initial amputation was below the knee or there was an end-bearing stump. Proximal to knee disarticulation, an amputation that removes at least 4 in. of the distal femur is indicated, so that a prosthetic knee joint can be fitted with less difficulty. For children, disarticulation is frequently the procedure of choice in order to save the growing epiphysis and minimize the problem of distal bone overgrowth.

Other factors that contribute to selection of amputation site are the patient's general condition and, particularly, the feasibility of rehabilitation. More proximal amputations are indicated for bedridden patients who require nursing care, since these procedures are associated with a higher incidence of primary healing. If there is established contracture, it is usually preferable to plan to amputate above the level of contracture, to permit rehabilitation.

At all levels, healing ability is a function of nutritional skin blood flow. The status of the skin circulation may be evidenced by the extent of skin circulation. The clearance of radioxenon, measured at the anterior incision line, has been shown to correlate well with the healing of amputations. In one series no patient with a flow exceeding 0.6 mL/100 g tissue per minute failed to heal because of ischemia, and no patient with a lower flow was able to heal a BK amputation. Quantification of skin fluorescein delivery by fiberoptic fluorometry also has predicted the healing of an amputation site.

A correlation has been reported between the healing of both digital and transmetatarsal amputations and the presence of peripheral pulses. In patients with a palpable popliteal pulse, healing at this level occurred twice as effectively as in those in whom only femoral pulse was demonstrated. The presence of a popliteal pulse has been associated with a 97 percent success rate for BK amputations, while 82 percent of patients with absent popliteal pulses also healed amputation sites at this level. In another study, when the femoral pulse was absent, 79 percent of BK amputations failed. When the femoral pulse was palpable, only 29 percent wound breakdown occurred. When the popliteal pulses were present, the failure rate was 10 percent. The value of Doppler systolic blood pressure and arterial waveform analysis using the segmental plethysmograph in the selection of BK and forefoot amputation sites has been assessed by Nicholas et al. A calf systolic pressure greater than 70 torr was associated with a 97 percent success rate for BK amputations. However, because of a high false-negative rate, a patient should not be denied a BK amputation on the basis of this determination. The ankle systolic pressure has not proved valuable in predicting the healing of forefoot amputations. An assessment of Doppler ultrasound and digital plethysmography concluded that they are imprecise indices of the healing of amputations for arterial insufficiency.

The recent advances in rehabilitation and the application of the immediate prosthetic fitting have increased the indications of BK amputations and reduced the incidence of AK amputations. In selecting between these two sites, there are two additional factors that have to be assessed, the patient's general condition and the prospect for rehabilitation. There has been a significant improvement in the mortality and wound complication rates for BK amputations in diabetics.

Preoperative Management

Amputations for massive trauma should be performed early to reduce the extent of contamination and the potential for infection. Atelectasis, pneumonia, and decubiti must be prevented in elderly bedridden patients. This can be accomplished by frequently turning the patients and providing them with a trapeze that can also be used to condition muscles to be used postoperatively. If the patient is diabetic, it is generally preferable to convert to a regimen of crystalline insulin rather than long-acting medications, since this is easier to regulate on the day of the operation and postoperatively.

Care of the ischemic extremity and also the contralateral extremity, which is frequently compromised, involves strict avoidance of injuries to areas of deficient circulation. The strength of wasted muscles and the motion of the critical joints must be preserved or, frequently, restored. Efforts should be made to heal necrotic or infected lesions, and only after direct arterial reconstruction and occasionally sympathectomy have failed to evidence improvement of the lesion is amputation indicated. The leg is usually kept in a slightly dependent position, and Buerger's exercises may be applied to improve the circulation. In the face of infection, drainage and local wet dressings of warm saline solution coupled with the appropriate antibiotic are employed. Antibiotics have been shown to have a beneficial effect in patients with a diminished or absent femoral pulse undergoing AK amputations. Wrapping of the extremity in towels impregnated with antiseptic materials for 12 h prior to operation has been advised as a method of reducing the incidence of wound infection. Foot care is administered to all areas without open lesions and to the uninvolved extremity. In some instances of digital gangrene, spontaneous amputation will occur, and this is frequently preferable to an operative procedure.

Refrigeration may be used preliminary to amputation to improve the condition of the patient by decreasing the metabolic by-products of the necrotic limb and also decreasing the absorption of these products and infectious material. Refrigeration also relieves pain, but the technique should not be employed if there is any hope of salvaging the extremity. The technique involves the placement of ice bags below the proposed level of amputation and may require use of mild narcotics.

Principles of Technique

The three general classes of amputations are (1) the standard or conventional amputation, (2) the osteomyoplastic or myodesis amputation, and (3) the provisional, or open (guillotine), amputation.

The conventional amputation is performed by constructing curved skin and fascial flaps that have their base at the level of amputation. The muscles, major blood vessels, and bone are divided at the level of amputation, while the major nerves are put on slight stretch and transected so that they retract approximately 1 in. proximal to the level of amputation. The muscles may be tapered so that not too much soft tissue remains over the bone end, and the distal inch of periosteum may be removed to avoid leaving a detached segment that can cause bone spur formation. After the amputation has been completed, the deep and superficial fascia are approximated over the bone, and the skin is loosely closed. The wound may be closed without drainage, or drainage may be established by soft rubber tubes or preferably a catheter connected to a closed section suction apparatus.

The osteomyoplastic amputations and myodesis provide for improved function and have been employed with increasing frequency when immediate postsurgical prosthetics (IPOP) are applied. Skin and fascial flaps are prepared in a manner similar to that used during conventional amputation, and the nerves and blood vessels are also divided in a routine fashion. In the osteomyoplastic technique, the muscles are divided 2 in. distal to the level of bone transection, and, prior to amputation of the bone, an osteoperiosteal flap is developed so that it may be sutured to the opposing periosteum in order to cover the bone and plug the marrow cavity. Then, with the remaining extremity in neutral position, i.e., extension for BK amputation and hip extension for AK amputation, the antagonistic muscles are sutured across the bone ends. Closure and drainage is similar to that employed in conventional amputations. In the case of myodesis, the distal ends of the transected muscle are attached to the bone by suturing through drill holes through the distal end. The muscles should be attached at a point that will put them under moderate tension so that they will become fixed along their normal pathway in a position slightly beyond rest length and therefore capable of providing maximal function.

Open, or provisional (guillotine), amputations should be regarded as drainage procedures and are still occasionally indicated. They are of historical interest in that they represent the most commonly employed procedures prior to the age of modern surgery. The procedure is still employed to release a person whose extremity is caught under an immovable object and is used for severely ill and toxic patients who are considered unable to tolerate a definitive amputation. All tissues are cut circularly, but the bone is transected higher than the fascia, which, in turn, is cut higher than the skin, in the hope that the soft tissue will ultimately cover the bone end with the help of traction. A large scar, which adheres to bone, often results, and revision of the wound is often required. It has been shown, however, that guillotine ankle amputation followed by BK amputation for the nonsalvageable infected lower extremity is associated with a lower amputation failure rate than primary definitive amputation.

AMPUTATIONS FOR PERIPHERAL VASCULAR DISEASE

Under no circumstance should a tourniquet or constricting bandage be applied, and throughout the procedure undue trauma should be avoided. Short skin and fascial flaps with minimal undermining are employed.

For patients who are to be fitted with an IPOP, the technique is modified. The anterior incision is made at the level of the anticipated bone division, and no anterior flap is constructed. Skin coverage is achieved with a thick posterior flap that includes subcutaneous tissue and fascia. Extreme gentleness is used throughout the procedure. Careful hemostasis is necessary to prevent hematoma formation and subsequent infection. If there is any question of compromised blood supply at the level of amputation, that site of amputation is abandoned and a higher site immediately used.

Postoperative Management

The conventional postoperative care has been directed toward providing an adequate period of rest for tissues by splinting, firm compression over the injured tissue to prevent postoperative edema, exercises and positioning to prevent contracture, and rehabilitation to provide the patient ultimately with a prosthesis compatible with his or her vocational demands and ability.

A lightly compressive dressing is applied to the stump immediately after the operation and until the sutures are removed. Following this, elastic bandages are repeatedly applied to minimize the postoperative edema. Contractures are prevented by stump exercises and stretching the proximal joint in the hope of achieving full motion of the remaining joints of the amputated extremity. Rehabilitation requires the services of an experienced physiotherapist, occupational therapist, and prosthetist. In the case of lower extremity amputees, the sequence progresses from balance to crutch walking to use of temporary prosthesis with eventual application of permanent prosthesis. The upper extremity amputee frequently requires intensive training in the activities of daily living and of his or her specific vocation.

IPOP have achieved popularity in the management of extremity amputees. In this situation, a rigid dressing is applied at the operating table. The stump is covered with a sterilized sock and elastic plaster of paris bandages, and a prosthetic unit that includes socket attachment flaps may be applied immediately after the rigid dressing has dried. The patient is then encouraged to walk between parallel bars 24 h after the operation, and weight bearing is increased daily. At 48 h, a window may be cut in the plaster of paris to permit removal of the drain, and the material removed to provide the window is immediately replaced with plaster bandage. The rigid dressing is kept in place for approximately 2 weeks, at which time the sutures are removed and a new socket is applied without delay. Ten days later the second socket is removed, and at that time stump measurements and a cast are made for permanent prosthesis. Another temporary socket is provided until the permanent prosthesis is available. With both IPOP and the conventional management, shrinkage of the stump occurs in time and may necessitate a new socket for use with a permanent prosthesis.

Prognosis, Morbidity, and Mortality

The operative mortality for amputations performed for isolated tumor, trauma, or infection is less than 3 percent. The mortality rate doubles in patients who exhibit signs of arteriosclerotic disease and is increased twofold by postoperative complications. Diabetes does not significantly influence the mortality rate. The mortality rates are generally higher for more proximal amputations in the lower extremity. This could be related to the greater frailty of patients subjected to more proximal procedures. The results of recent series are more encouraging, with mortality rates of 3 percent and failure rates of 4 percent. The most frequent causes are cardiac (52 percent) and pulmonary (26 percent) complications.

Phantom limb pain occurred relatively infrequently in most series, and the incidence has been reduced by avoiding the incorporation of nerve in scar tissue of the stump and by IPOP. In a series of 130 patients with unilateral amputation, 70 received prostheses and 84 percent of these had successful rehabilitation. Of the total group of those receiving unilateral amputations, only 30 percent of the AK group were successfully rehabilitated, while 66 percent of the BK group walked on prosthesis. In those patients with bilateral amputations, 30 percent have had successful rehabilitation, and this required that at least one of the amputation sites be at the BK level. The IPOP group had a reduction of time from amputation to fitting of a permanent prosthesis, and an increased rate of rehabilitation.

AMPUTATIONS OF THE LOWER EXTREMITY

The overwhelming majority of amputations in the lower extremity (Fig. 44-1) are performed for ischemia. A variety of eponyms have been applied to specific levels of amputations and refinements of technique, but the most commonly employed procedures are AK and BK amputations. Transmetatarsal and digital amputations are less frequently applicable in patients with peripheral vascular disease. The Syme amputation, knee disarticulation, hip disarticulation, and hemipelvectomy are usually reserved for malignant and traumatic lesions. At each level, the operative procedure and postoperative management are directed at achieving primary healing, a painless stump that will withstand the pressures of a prosthesis, and relatively unrestricted ambulation.

Toe Amputation

Amputation of one or more toes may be performed for gangrene or osteomyelitis. The procedure is rarely indicated for deformity, because excision of a toe results in deviation of adjacent toes. A transphalangeal level may be used if necrosis is distal to the proximal interphalangeal (PIP) joint and if there is absence of cellulitis, necrosis, and edema in the skin to be used for the flaps. If a more proximal amputation is required, transmetatarsal resection with removal of the head is preferable to disarticulation. The latter is associated with an increased incidence of breakdown, since the stump is bulky, and in the face of infection or poor vascular supply the exposed cartilage resists infection less effectively than bone. The incidence of healing at both the transphalangeal and transmetatarsal level has been relatively poor, with reports ranging from 40 to 60 percent. A direct relationship has been demonstrated between healing at these levels and the presence of popliteal and pedal pulses, suggesting that

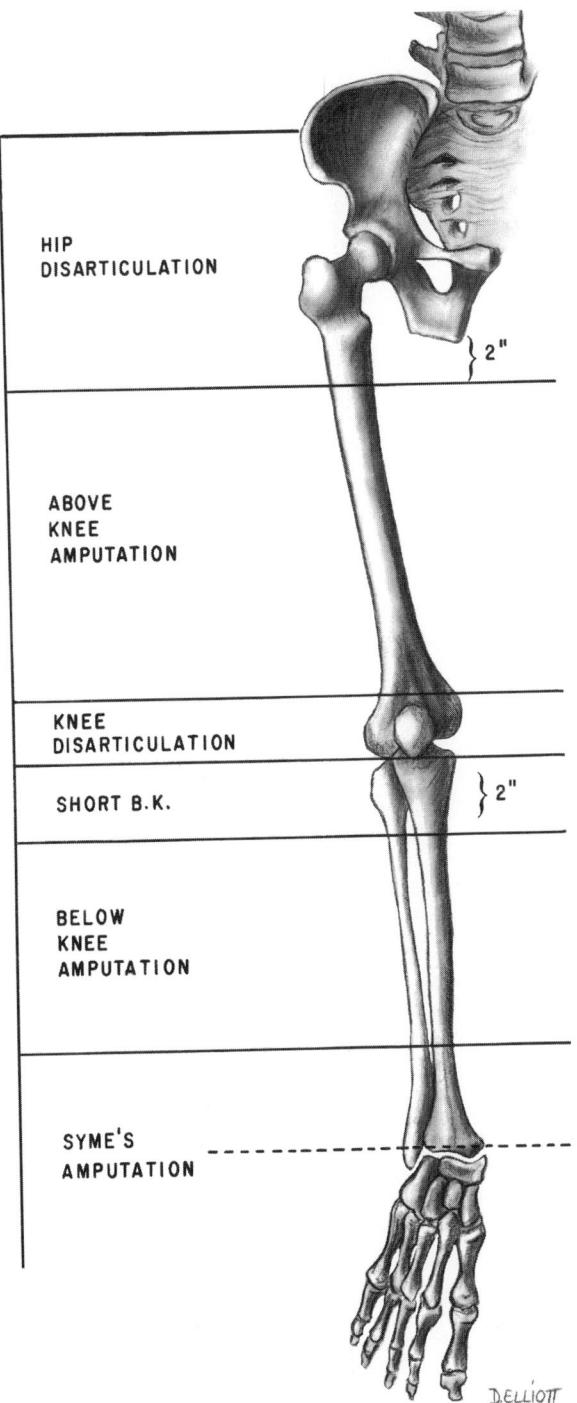

Fig. 44-1. Levels of amputations in the lower extremity.

the poor results have been related to poor selection of amputation sites.

TRANSPHALANGEAL AMPUTATION

Either lateral or anteroposterior flaps may be used, and in either instance they should be sufficiently long to cover anticipated bone length. If an anteroposterior flap is em-

ployed, the plantar flap should be longer, so that the scar is placed dorsad. After the flaps have been established, the tendons and nerves are placed under slight tension and transected to permit retraction. The bone is transected and the skin and subcutaneous tissue closed loosely.

TRANSMETATARSAL AMPUTATION (Fig. 44-2)

A racquet incision is usually employed. In the case of a second, third, and fourth toe, the long limb is positioned on the dorsum of the foot, whereas it is placed on the medial and lateral surface for the great and small toes, respectively. Skin and subcutaneous tissue flaps are developed, and the head and neck of the metatarsal is amputated. Excessive skin is removed, and a closure without tension is accomplished.

The foot should be elevated in the immediate postoperative period, and ambulation may begin as soon as the incision is healed. There is no need for a special shoe.

Transmetatarsal Foot Amputation

The indications for this procedure include necrosis proximal to the PIP joint but distal to the level of the transmetatarsal incision. Necrosis in the interdigital creases constitutes a relatively frequent indication. In one series, primary healing was achieved in 54 percent of patients with absent pedal pulses. Prior lumbar sympathectomy apparently did not alter the rate of healing.

TECHNIQUE (Fig. 44-3). Skin incisions and subcutaneous flaps are established so that the plantar flap is longer than the dorsal flap in order to maintain the thicker skin and permit placement of the scar on the distal surface. The plantar incision extends to within a centimeter of the crease between the base of the toes and the ball of the foot, and this flap is left as thick as possible, while the dorsal incision is developed directly to the bone and not established as a flap. Metatarsals are divided just proximal to the level of the dorsal incision, the specimen is removed, and the skin and fascia are closed in layers.

POSTOPERATIVE MANAGEMENT. The amputation provides a good stump, and preservation of the tibialis anterior tendon and intrinsic flexors and the fat pad help to maintain the short arch. The patients generally walk within 3 weeks after the operation, using a shoe with a pad of cotton in the toe.

Syme Amputation

This procedure is usually performed when most of the foot has been destroyed by trauma. Terminal arterial disease involving the distal part of the foot constitutes one of the few peripheral vascular disorders for which the Syme amputation is indicated. Functionally, it represents an excellent level for amputation since it maintains the length of the extremity, and preservation of the heel skin provides an excellent weight-bearing stump. The prosthesis is more difficult to fit, and because it is bulky, a BK amputation is preferable for females.

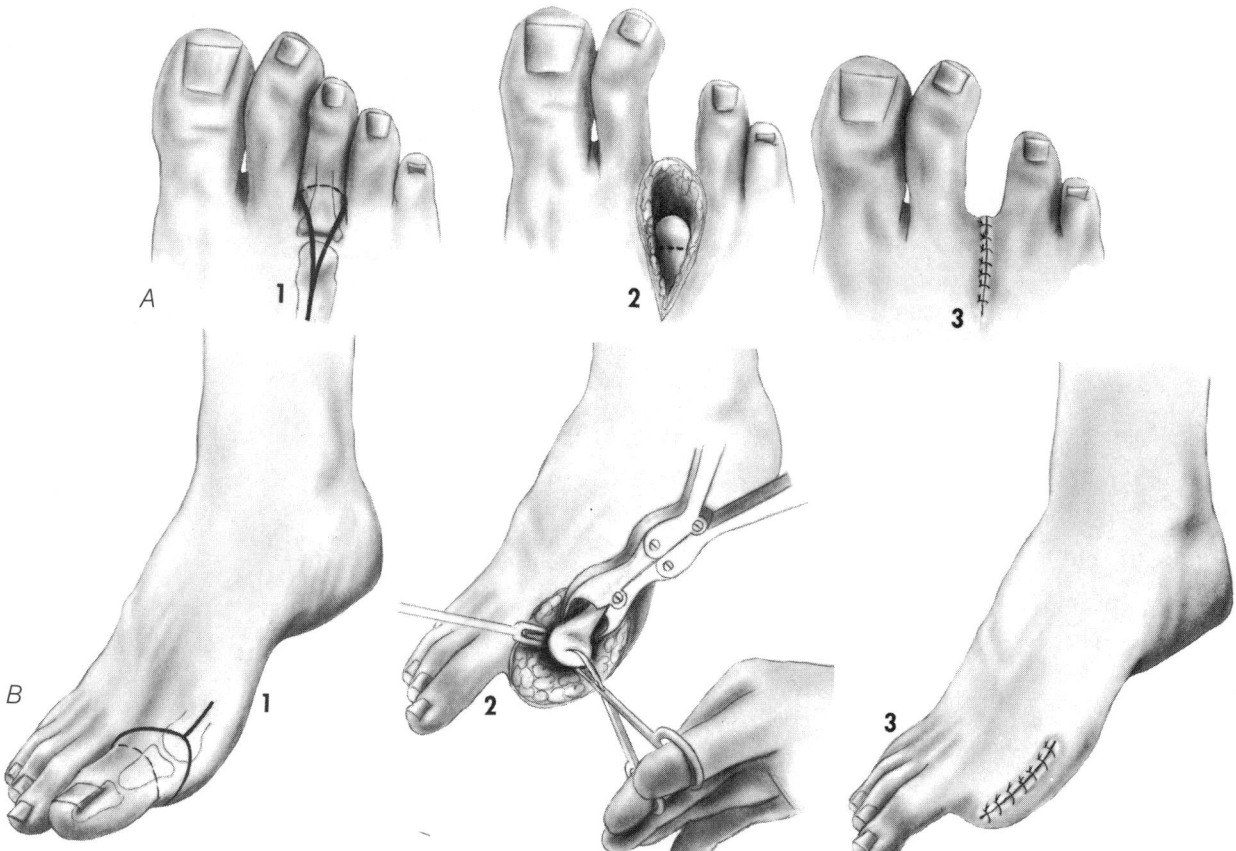

Fig. 44-2. Transmetatarsal toe amputation. *A.* Technique for amputation of any of the middle three toes. 1. Racquet incision made. 2. Toe disarticulated and line of transection of the head of the metatarsal indicated. 3. Skin closure. *B.* Transmetatarsal amputation of the great or little toe. 1. Racquet incision with long limb on the side of the foot. 2. Toe disarticulated and the head of the metatarsal resected. 3. Lateral skin closure.

TECHNIQUE (Fig. 44-4). The incision extends from the anteroinferior border of the medial malleolus around the sole to the lateral malleolus and around the anterior aspect of the ankle to complete the circumference. The soft tissue is incised in a line down to the bone, avoiding trauma to the posterior tibial artery and its branches. The talus is removed and the calcaneus is dissected from the skin and shelled from its attachments to permit removal of the foot. The tibia and fibula are then cleared and transected proximal to the flare of the tibial malleolus. The long plantar flap is sutured to the anterior portion of the incision, with care to center the heel flap.

POSTOPERATIVE MANAGEMENT. In the conventional approach, the position of the heel pad is supported by tape. Since weight bearing occurs at the end of the stump, healing should be advanced and the heel flap firmly fixed to the end of the stump before the patient is permitted to walk either on the stump or on the prosthesis. The Canadian Syme prosthesis, which incorporates a SACH (solid ankle cushion heel) foot and ankle and an end-bearing socket on foam rubber, is one that is frequently employed. Excellent results have been obtained with immediate fitting of a prosthesis following the Syme procedure. Some of the weight-bearing load is transferred to the patellar tendon and the flares of the tibial condyles, and it is not necessary to immobilize the knee joint. Weight bearing is then begun within 24 h when the stump is mature

and stable, measurements for a permanent prosthesis are made, and the stump is replaced in a plaster bandage until the prosthesis is available. The permanent prosthesis is usually applied earlier with this approach than with the conventional management.

Below-the-Knee Amputation (BK)

This level is being employed with increasing frequency since the advent of IPOP. Major functional advantages of the BK amputation over the AK level are the ability to provide a more functional prosthesis for complete rehabilitation, the ability of the patient to move more easily in and out of bed, and a reduction in energy expenditure and in the incidence of phantom limb pain. Even a BK stump that is too short to accept a BK prosthesis is superior to an AK stump and can be fitted with a bent-knee prosthesis. BK amputations constitute the level of choice for ischemic lesions of the foot that do not extend above the malleoli but are generally not applicable if the gangrene extends in continuity above the ankle. Ischemic rigor of

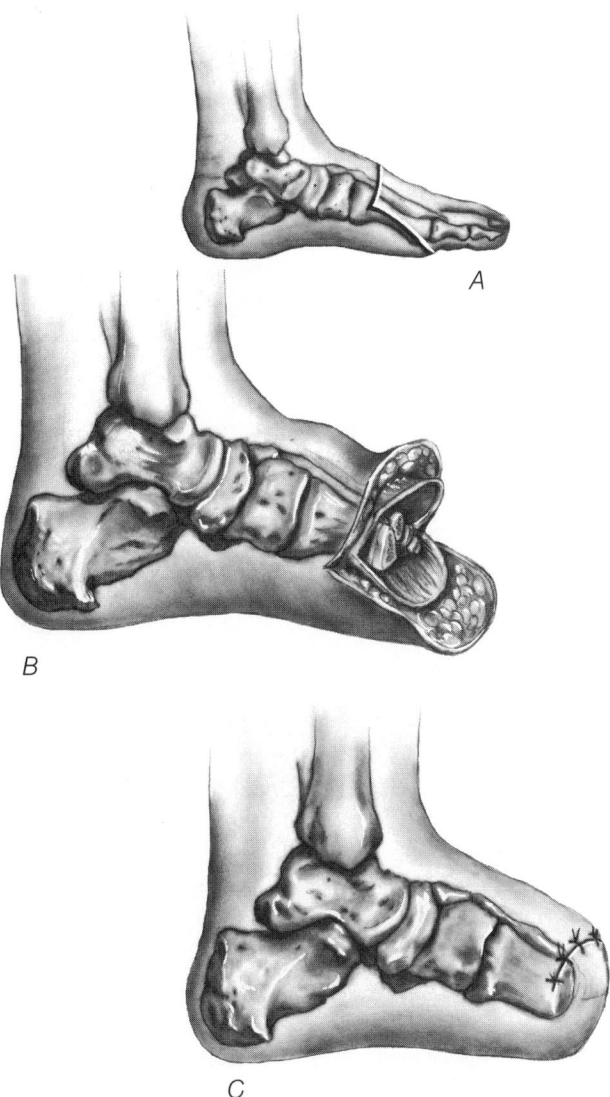

Fig. 44-3. Transmetatarsal foot amputation. *A*. Skin incision is outlined. Note the short dorsal flap and longer plantar flap. *B*. Distal part of the foot has been removed, and the head of the metatarsals have all been amputated. *C*. Fascia and skin have been closed so that the scar is located dorsad.

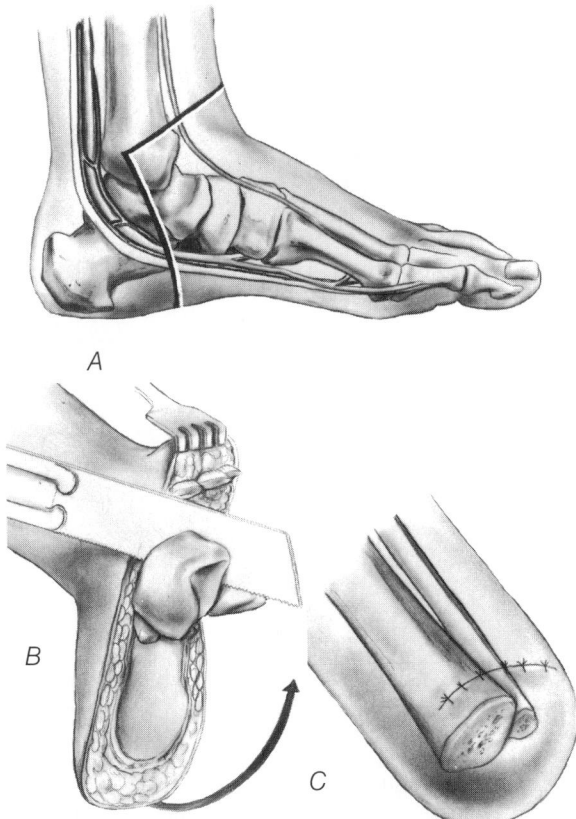

Fig. 44-4. Syme amputation. *A*. Incision is outlined. *B*. Foot has been amputated by disarticulating the calcaneus. Tibia and fibula are transected proximal to the flare of the tibial malleolus. *C*. The long plantar flap is sutured to the anterior part of the incision, with care to center the heel flap.

the calf muscles is another contraindication. Contracture of the knee or hip represents a relative contraindication, since it negates the functional advantages of this level.

The choice between the BK and AK amputation is determined by the patient's general health and potential for rehabilitation and an evaluation of the vascular status at the proposed level of amputation. No essential difference in healing rate was noted in patients with or without palpable popliteal pulses but the absence of a femoral pulse was associated with a high failure rate for BK amputations. Healing was not influenced by the presence or absence of diabetes. Healing of BK amputations has been reported in 68 to 90 percent of cases in large series as compared with healing rates of 82 and 98 percent, respectively, for AK amputations. By contrast, considering the

relative general status of the patients, a higher percentage of BK amputees walk on prostheses. The range of reported figures for rehabilitation of BK amputations in patients with ischemia is from 50 to 90 percent.

TECHNIQUE (Fig. 44-5). The amputation should be performed proximal to the lower third of the tibia, since the preponderance of tendinous structures distal to this area predisposes to poor circulation and an unstable, painful stump. Equally short anterior and posterior flaps may be made, or a longer posterior flap may be combined with a short anterior flap. When possible, the skin flaps are fashioned so that they are longer to permit an even closure, but if there is compromised circulation, short skin and subcutaneous flaps are used. The posterior incision is beveled to reduce the bulk of muscle in order to provide a better stump. The tibia is usually transected 2 in. above the distal level of the skin flap, and the fibula is transected approximately 1 in. above the tibial level. The tibia may be beveled approximately 45° both anteriorly and mediad to provide a better stump. The nerves are pulled down gently and transected so that they are allowed to retract, and the vessels are ligated above the level of the end of the tibia. If a myodesis is performed (see Fig. 44-5*B*), the muscles are sutured to the tibia by drilling small holes

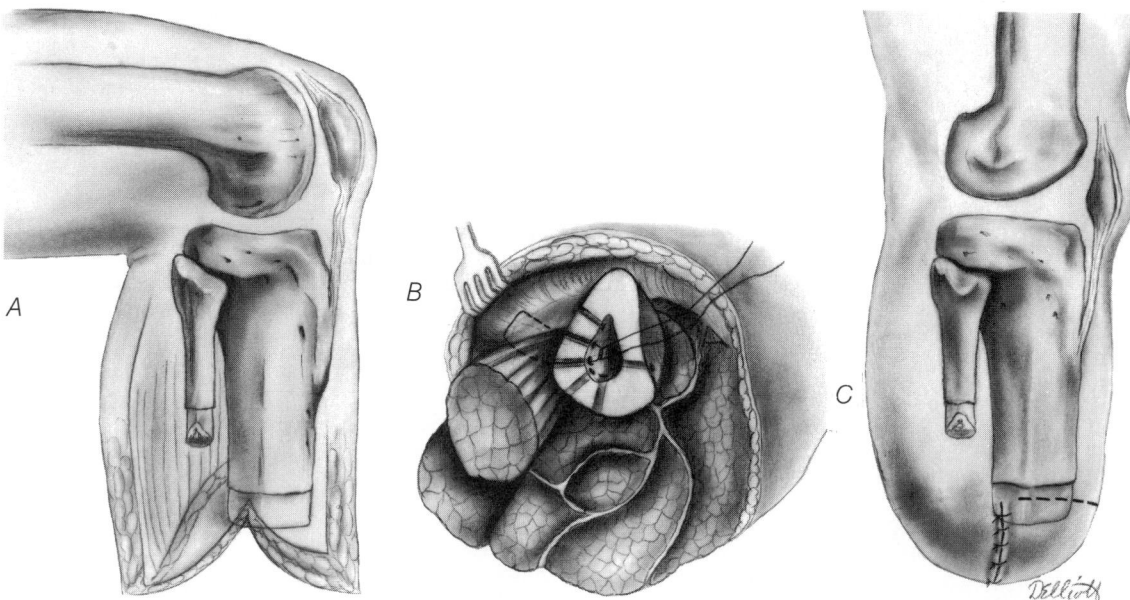

Fig. 44-5. BK amputation. *A.* Equally short anterior and posterior flaps have been made (a long posterior flap may be combined with a very short anterior flap). The muscles have been beveled, and the fibula is transected approximately 1 in. above the tibia. The periosteum has been removed from the distal portion of the bones. *B.* Myodesis: individual muscle fibers are sutured to the tibia through small drill holes. *C.* Fascia and skin are closed (dotted lines indicate skin closure when a long posterior flap is used).

through the bone into the marrow and suturing the muscles so that they are attached under moderate tension along their normal pathways, in a position slightly beyond rest length. The fascia and skin are loosely closed, and either a through-and-through drain or a catheter that will be connected to suction apparatus may be used for 2 days.

Fig. 44-6. Postoperative rehabilitation for BK amputation. Left. BK stump. Right. Prosthesis fitted.

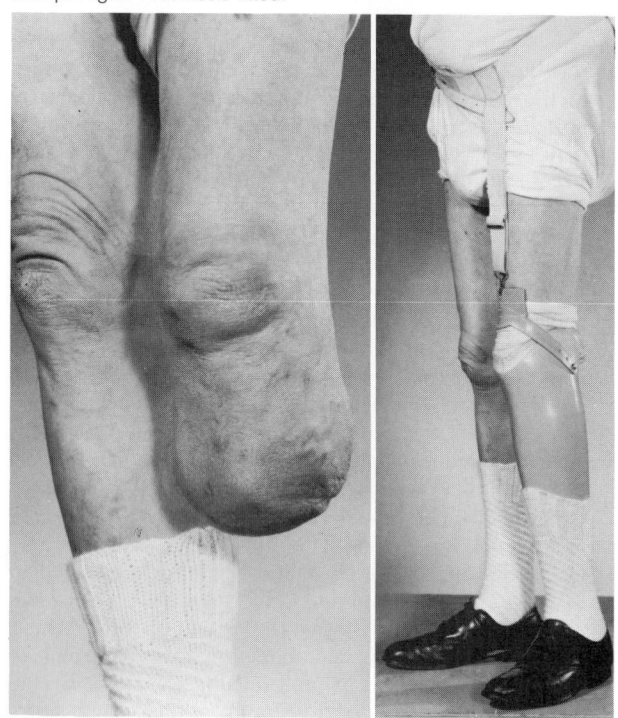

POSTOPERATIVE MANAGEMENT (Fig. 44-6). With the conventional management, a small splint is applied in the operating room to prevent flexion of the knee joint. The splint is usually removed on the second day, and joint motion is then begun. Measurements for a temporary prosthesis may be made on the second day, and walking on this temporary prosthesis, with which the weight is borne on the ischium, may be performed within 3 days. When the patient is physically capable and the stump is well healed, a permanent prosthesis with which the weight is borne on the patellar tendon and tibial flares is provided. Walking on this permanent prosthesis should be possible about the fourth postoperative week.

IPOP may be applied, in which case the patient is encouraged to stand and bear weight on the first postoperative day and activity is rapidly increased. A permanent prosthesis can usually be applied at the time of the second cast change, i.e., at 3 weeks when the stump is sufficiently mature. In a series of cases, the use of IPOP at this level has not been associated with a single incidence of sustained phantom limb pain.

Knee Disarticulation

This is most commonly employed in children in whom there is a reason for maintaining the epiphysis for bone growth. Other advantages of the disarticulation are that it provides maximal length and good end bearing and lends itself to a good fit between stump and socket. The disadvantages are that the end of the stump is bulky and has bony prominences that make prosthesis fitting more difficult. The procedure is rarely indicated when there is impaired circulation.

TECHNIQUE. The skin incision is placed about 1 in. above the stump end posteriorly, and the anterior flap is fashioned approximately 4 in. distal to the inferior border of the patella. The skin and subcutaneous tissue are reflected together. The femoral condyles and patella are usually not disturbed. If the patella is displaced or damaged by disease, it should be excised, leaving the quadriceps tendon or patellar ligament intact. Myodesis is easy to perform at this level. If the patella has been left in place, the patellar tendon is then sutured to the cruciate ligaments posteriorly. If the patella has been removed, the remaining tendon and quadriceps tendon are brought down through the intercondylar notch and sutured to the cruciate ligaments posteriorly. The hamstring tendons may also be brought down through this notch and sewn to the cruciate ligaments.

POSTOPERATIVE MANAGEMENT. The postoperative care and the application of a prosthesis is similar to that which is described below for the AK amputations.

Fig. 44-7. AK amputation. *A.* Outline of short anterior and posterior flaps. *B.* Amputation completed with muscles beveled. Note that the sciatic nerve has been cut after tension had been applied in order that it retract proximal to the bone end. *C.* Skin closure that does not interfere with fitting of prosthesis.

Above-the-Knee Amputation (AK)

This level has generally been selected when gangrene extends above the level of the malleoli. Absolute indications for the procedure include extension of skin gangrene above a level that would permit BK amputation and rigor of the calf muscles. Peripheral gangrene coupled with contracture of the knee or hip constitutes a relative indication, since there is no advantage to a BK amputation.

The AK amputation is associated with the highest healing rates in patients with peripheral vascular disease, between 84 and 100 percent. The rate of reamputation is lower; this is an important consideration in elderly and debilitated patients. These characteristics contribute to the fact that the mortality rate is higher than that reported for other levels of amputation of the lower extremity.

TECHNIQUE (Fig. 44-7). Anterior and posterior skin flaps are fashioned of equal length, and if there is any question of compromised vascular supply short skin flaps are used. The skin and subcutaneous tissue are reflected together, taking care not to compromise the circulatory status. When possible, the adductor and hamstring muscles are beveled to provide a cylindrical stump rather than a bulbous one, but if there is a severe vascular problem, beveling is contraindicated. The vascular bundles are divided individually at the level of proposed transection of the femur, and gentle traction is applied to the sciatic

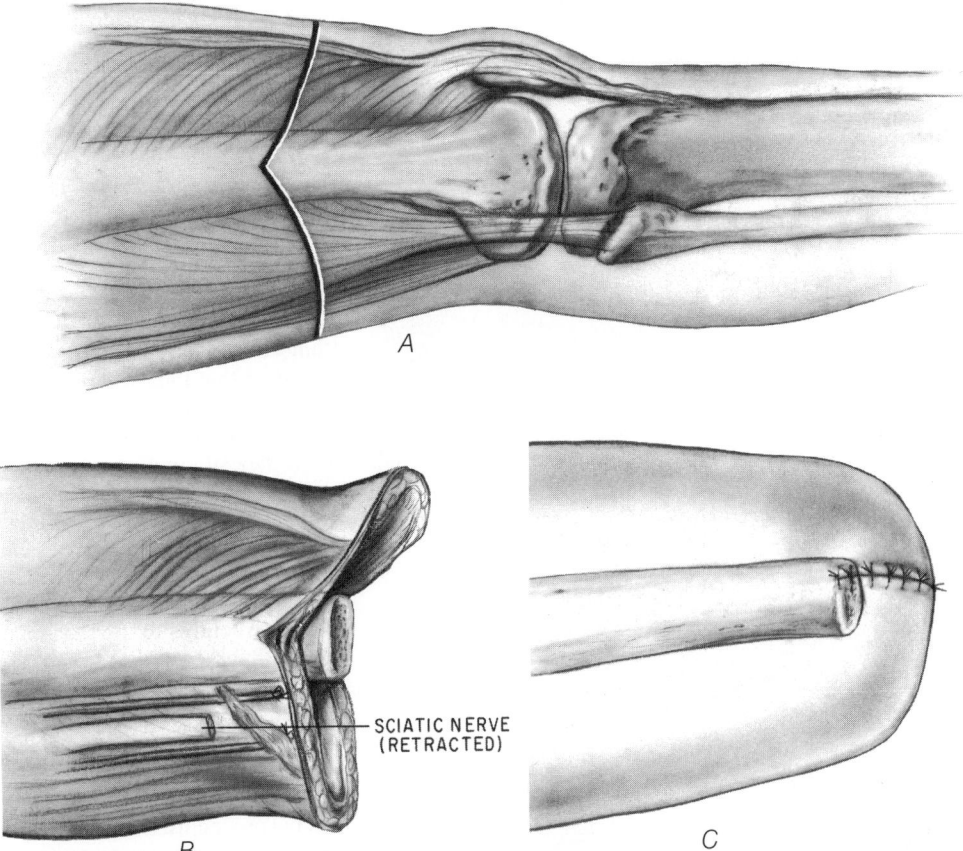

SCIATIC NERVE
(RETRACTED)

A

B

C

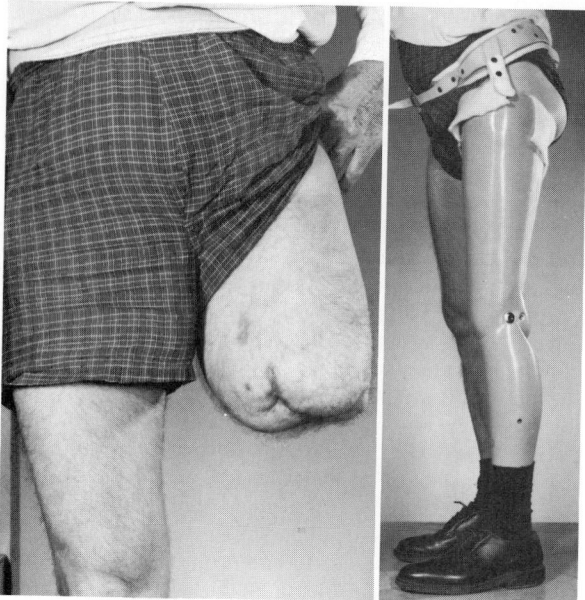

Fig. 44-8. Rehabilitation for AK amputation. *A.* Healed AK stump. *B.* Prosthesis for AK amputation. Note that the weight is not borne on the end of the stump.

nerve. The nerve is transected so that it retracts proximal to the stump of the femur. The periosteum of the femur is incised circularly and scraped to avoid leaving detached periosteum in the stump and consequent bone formation. The femur is transected at a level proximal to the condyles at a distance approximately equal to one-half the anteroposterior diameter of the thigh proximal to the most distal point of the skin flap. The edge of the bone is beveled to provide a smooth radius.

Fig. 44-9. Rehabilitation following hip disarticulation. *A.* Healed amputation site. *B.* Patient fitted with special Canadian prosthesis.

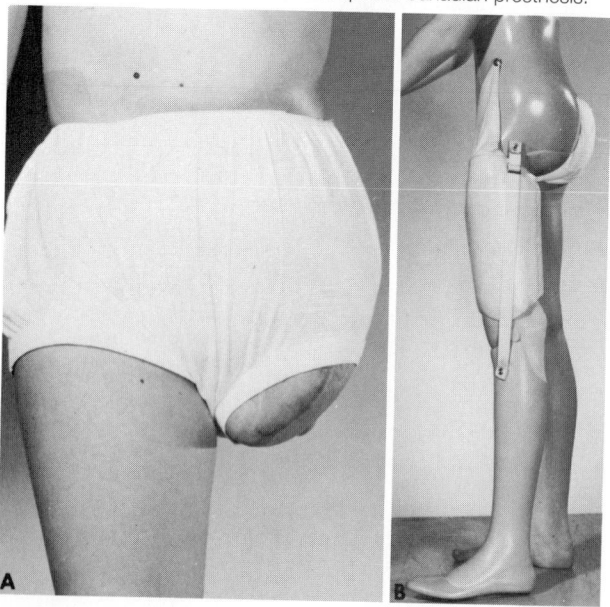

If myodesis is performed (see Fig. 44-5*B*), the muscles are attached through several small holes extending through the bone to the marrow, approximately 1 in. proximal to the distal end of the bone. Slight tension is applied to the anterior, medial, and posterior muscle groups, and these are sutured individually to the bone. The muscle should be able to effect maximal contraction and provide good function for the use of a prosthesis. Subcutaneous tissue and skin flaps are loosely approximated.

POSTOPERATIVE MANAGEMENT. With conventional management, a small dressing and stockinet are employed. The patient is positioned in bed so that there is no hip flexion and is turned frequently to the prone position. Sitting in a chair or bed is prohibited until the patient is able to hyperextend the stump. Measurements may be performed for a temporary prosthesis as early as the second day. The body weight is borne by total contact of the prosthesis on the ischial tuberosity. Fitting of the permanent prosthesis may take several months because of stump shrinkage but may occur as early as 4 to 6 weeks after amputation. A total contact suction socket may be used for younger patients with long stumps, but a suspension apparatus (Fig. 44-8) with a purchase across the iliac crest is more frequently employed. The incorporation of a constant friction knee or a hydraulic mechanism that incorporates swing phase control depends upon the degree of rehabilitation required. A SACH foot and ankle are usually incorporated.

If an IPOP is used, a rigid dressing is applied in the operating room in such a fashion that the ischial tuberosity is resting on the posterior brim incorporating a waist belt and harness for suspension. The patient is encouraged to stand as soon as possible after the first postoperative day and to progress rapidly toward ambulation. Rehabilitation toward ambulation usually requires more time than with BK amputations.

Hip Disarticulation

The indications usually include bone tumors, soft tissue tumors, and extensive traumatic injuries. Flaps are fashioned so that they will come together anteriorly, and the posterior flap is constructed so that it forms a unit of skin, fascia, and muscle to swing forward in order that the patient may sit comfortably in the socket of the prosthesis. The femoral vessels are ligated anteriorly, and after the posterior dissection is completed, the femur is disarticulated. The sciatic nerve is cut high and tied in order to prevent bleeding from vasa nervorum. The undersurface of the gluteal muscle is tapered to facilitate approximation of the structures to the lower abdominal wall. Prostheses are available to permit ambulation, and have been applied to this level. A specially constructed Canadian Hip Disarticulation prosthesis is used for these patients (Fig. 44-9).

Hemipelvectomy

This procedure has been used in the treatment of malignant tumors of the upper thigh, particularly those of soft

Table 44-1. COMMON PROSTHETIC PRESCRIPTIONS FOR LOWER LIMB AMPUTEES

	Active AK amputee with long stump	*Elderly AK amputee*	*Young adult knee disarticulation*	*Below-knee adult*
Socket	Quadrilateral total contact	Quadrilateral open-end socket	End-bearing	PTB or PTS
Suspension	Suction socket	Pelvic band with hip joint	Leather thigh corset soft insert, air cushion	Cuff or wedge suspension
Knee	UC-BL 4-bar knee with pneumatic swing-phase control	3P23 Otto Bock with extension assist	External hinges Dupaco hydraulic swing phase	
Foot	SACH or Greissinger	SACH or 2-way ankle	SACH	SACH

tissue and bone, when it is felt that hip disarticulation would give a questionable margin of clearance around tumor. Modification of the classic procedure by dividing the ileum through the greater sciatic notch requires less surgical manipulation and results in less shock. The adjustment to a prosthesis is better when a leaf of the ileum and pubic rami are left as supporting points for the socket. Following this procedure, patients have also been permitted to ambulate with a special Canadian prosthesis.

Prosthetics for the Lower Limb Amputee (Table 44-1)

The artificial limb should provide gait symmetry for maximal walking efficiency and cosmesis, which is important psychologically to the patient. A properly designed prosthesis will lower the energy requirements for walking when compared with the alternative of crutch walking. An exception is the diabetic AK amputee who can walk faster with crutches and be more efficient per meter of distance but has an increased minute energy cost.

The lower extremity prosthesis requires (1) a socket to interface with the residual limb (the stump) and (2) a suspension device to maintain the relationship with the stump and suitable prosthetic joints to simulate lost joint function (Fig. 44-10).

SOCKET CONSTRUCTION. The most critical aspect of the prosthesis is a properly fitting, comfortable socket, across which residual limb forces are transmitted to the prosthesis. In general, the longer the residual stump, the greater the surface area over which forces can be transmitted to minimize excessive stump pressures. Socket design is best constructed to broaden total surface area contact. Pressure distribution in the socket should distribute maximum loads where the soft tissues are tolerant and minimize it in sensitive areas. The socket must accommodate the stump during stance and swing phases of gait but be fashioned to allow other postures such as sitting.

Above-Knee Sockets (Fig. 44-10*A, B*). The quadrilateral total contact socket is the most common design for the AK amputee. A suction socket facilitates suspension and minimizes pistoning during the swing phase of gait by permitting atmospheric pressure to overcome the negative internal socket pressure as the prosthetic foot leaves the ground. The quadrilateral design and the exact shape and direction of the brims for ischial bearing are designed to provide appropriate relief for muscle function and to maintain the stump in a socket when leverage is applied. It is aligned so that gluteus medius hip musculature is at resting length for maximum function. The technique of check socket construction, in which a transparent socket is made to best detect points of excessive pressure, should be utilized in some patients.

Below-Knee Sockets. The patellar-tendon-bearing-type socket (Fig. 44-10*C, D, E, F*) developed by the University of California Biomechanics Laboratory provides optimal total contact for the BK amputee. A hard socket may be constructed or it may be used with a soft liner. The main points of pressure are on the patellar tendon and the medial flare of the proximal tibial condyle. Relief for the hamstring tendons is necessary, and proper curve of the popliteal flare is required for maximal comfort. Variation on the PTB (patellar-tendon-bearing) socket are the PTS (patellar tendon supracondylar) or PTS/SP (patellar-tendon-bearing supracondylar/suprapatellar socket). These devices have flares about the condyles and patella for added stability and suspension.

SUSPENSION SYSTEMS. For AK, long, and good musculature stumps, total-contact suction devices are sufficient to keep the prosthesis suspended in relationship to the stump. With shorter or flabby stumps, auxiliary suspension such as a Silesian bandage or a pelvic belt with a metal hip joint may be necessary. Suspensions for a BK patellar-tendon-bearing prosthesis may be achieved with a small supracondylar cuff strap. The PTS type has larger flares medially and laterally for a wedge insert above the femoral condyle to provide suspension. For patients with extremely short stumps, or in some elderly patients, a leather corset is added to the thigh to which hinges are attached for the below-knee prosthesis. In this device, the corset acts as a suspension device but can be tightened to relieve weight or to minimize below-knee stump pressures.

PROSTHETIC KNEE MECHANISMS. The prosthetic knee simulates the normal knee mechanism in allowing for gait symmetry and smoothing the forward motion of the

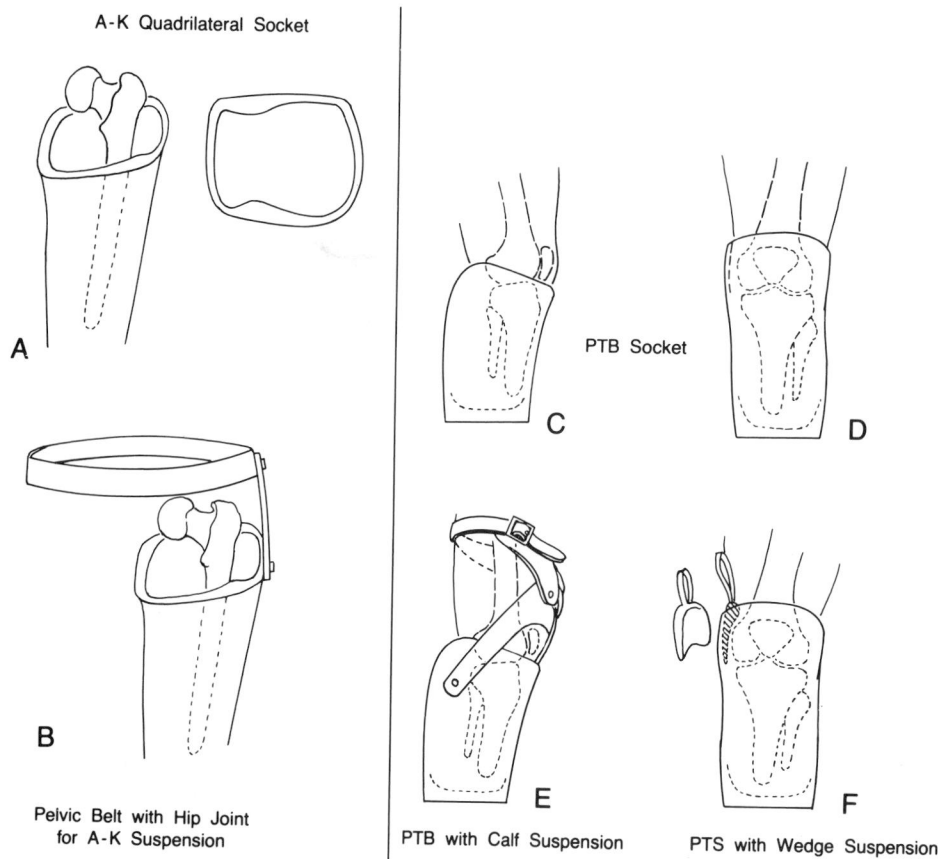

Fig. 44-10. Examples of above-knee and below-knee sockets and suspensions.

body's center of gravity. The knee mechanism can provide control over both stance phase and the swing phase of gait. The simplest mechanism is a single-axis hinge. Simply by locating the single-axis hinge anterior to the trochanteric-knee-ankle axis (the TKA) the knee will have alignment stability at the point of heel strike. This, however, necessitates more effort to initiate the swing phase. By adding a constant-friction device to the single axis, resistance to both the flexion and extension swing phases is accomplished.

Devices such as hydraulic units or pneumatic units attached to the knee can provide both independent flexion and extension swing-phase control. The resistance provided by the hydraulic unit controls the forceful swing of the shank and foot of young, vigorous, fast-walking AK amputees.

The elderly AK amputee with less muscle control or balance needs stability during the stance phase. A device with an extension assist or one that locks in extension may be required. The simplest concept of this type is an elastic extension strap applied over the anterior aspect of the AK prosthesis. An optimal device for the elderly AK amputee is an endoskeletal device that is light in weight and has extension stability to provide the necessary control of the knee at heel strike.

Another concept for the knee is a polycentric device in which the center of rotation changes as the knee goes from flexion to extension. The best example of this type is the UC-BL 4-bar knee mechanism (Fig. 44-11). The center of rotation is proximally located with the knee in extension and moves distally as the knee flexes (Fig. 44-12). The effect of this polycentric mechanism is to increase the lever arm force of the AK stump when the knee is in a position of 20 to 30° flexion. Thus, the AK amputee in going up or down ramps or stairs can initiate flexion or extension at the correct instant without excessive effort. This device has an increased range of flexion that allows the amputee to kneel and sit back on the heels, which is not possible with most AK prosthetic knees. The additional flexion makes it easier for the amputee to get in and out of cars. The UC-BL 4-bar knee mechanism has a pneumatic unit for swing-phase control that allows independent adjustment for both flexion and extension.

Prosthetic Foot and Ankle Assemblies

Ankle and foot mechanisms were originally designed with a single-axis ankle mechanism with rubber stops for plantar and dorsiflexion of a solid foot. An improvement on this design is the five-way Greissinger mechanism in which a rubber pivot is provided at approximately the location of the normal ankle joint and allows dorsiflexion,

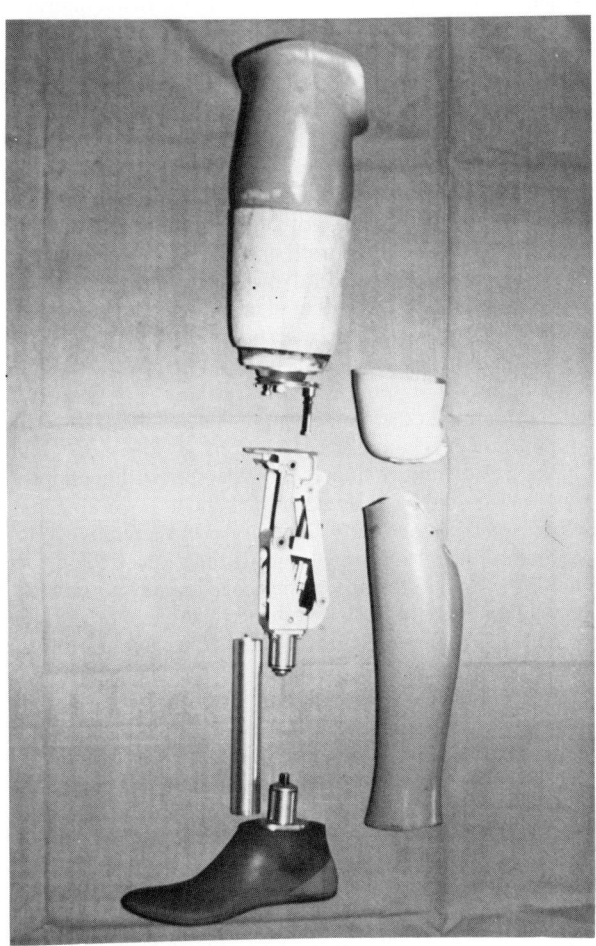

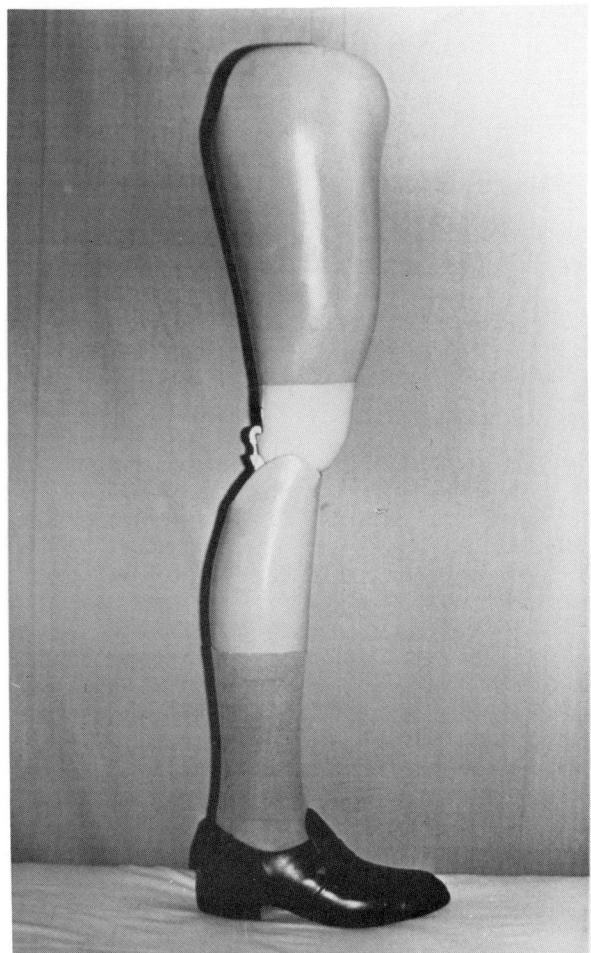

A

B

Fig. 44-11. *A.* Component parts of AK prosthesis with UC-BL 4-bar knee mechanism. *B.* Assembled AK prosthesis with 4-bar knee. *(Constructed by Leigh Wilson.)*

plantar flexion, inversion, eversion, and some rotation. The most commonly used foot/ankle assembly is the SACH foot. This device, which has a cushion heel, collapses at the point of heel strike and simulates the normal plantar flexion (Fig. 44-13). As the shank of the prosthesis approaches midstance, the body weight rolls over a solid forefoot simulating pushoff. This device has the advantage of being maintenance-free. The selection of the appropriate heel-cushion stiffness in relationship to body weight is necessary to provide gait symmetry and avoid interference with correct prosthetic knee motion.

AMPUTATIONS OF THE UPPER EXTREMITY

In most instances, upper extremity amputations (Fig. 44-14) are performed for trauma. Malignant disease represents the second most common indication. Peripheral vascular disease, particularly thromboangiitis obliterans, constitutes a rare indication.

In all circumstances, the treatment is directed at conserving as much viable tissue as possible and, with more distal amputations, maintaining the function of the hand as a grasping organ. The latter requires preservation of intrinsic muscle-tendon systems of the hand and the longer and more powerful flexors and extensors originating in the arm. The technique employed for amputations in the upper extremity is directed at producing minimal scar tissue, and the procedure is planned so that the scar is in an area as far removed as possible from bones, tendons, nerves, and points of external contact. Above the level of the metacarpals, opposing tendons should be fixed in order to preserve muscle length and tone.

In view of the precise nature of surgical technique, tourniquets are frequently employed to provide a bloodless field and facilitate identification of critical structures. They are best tolerated high in the upper arm with the cuff inflated to 280 mmHg. Digital tourniquets, such as rubber bands, should not be used, because of the danger of thrombosis. Anesthesia is frequently best accomplished by the use of regional block, particularly since many of the patients present with multiple injuries and a full stom-

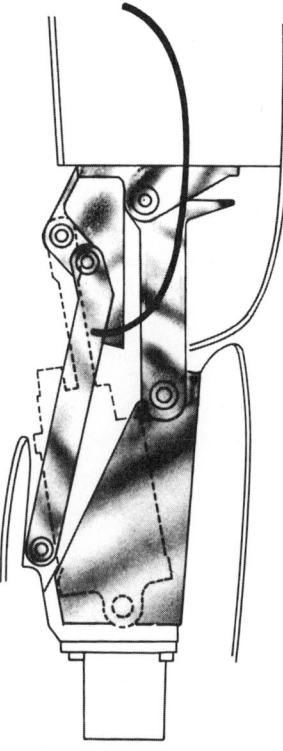

Fig. 44-12. UC-BL 4-bar knee mechanism for above knee amputees. Heavy line represents change in center of rotation as knee goes from extension to flexion.

ach and cannot tolerate general anesthesia at the preferred time for operation.

Amputation in the Hand (See Chap. 45)

AMPUTATION OF DIGITS

When part or all of the distal phalanx requires amputation, an attempt should be made to create a longer volar flap and a shorter dorsal flap, so that the scar may be positioned dorsad away from pressure. Neither bone nor viable soft tissue should be sacrificed to produce an ideal flap. If the amputation removes less than one-half the nail, it is preferable to retain the nail bed, but if more than half the nail is removed, the entire root should be excised.

When it is necessary to disarticulate at the distal interphalangeal joint, the cartilage should be removed from the head of the middle phalanx, and the flexor digitorum profundus tendon should be withdrawn, transected, and allowed to retract.

Amputations of fingers distal to the PIP joint should leave pinching and finer movements. Amputations through the middle phalanx result in little alteration of extension when only the more distal portion of the dorsal expansion of the extensor digitorum communis tendon is cut. By contrast, the flexor digitorum superficialis tendon has a long insertion on either side of the phalanx, and if a significant portion of this insertion cannot be left intact, disarticulation may be necessary. Whenever possible, amputation through the proximal phalanx is preferable to disarticulation at the metacarpophalangeal joint, since the stump, however short, has function.

When one or more fingers must be removed in entirety, attention should be directed at the hand as a working unit. When the long and ring fingers are both removed, the adjoining fingers may continue to function perfectly, or they may deviate toward each other, and deviation weakens flexion. If only the long or ring finger is removed, it is best also to remove the head of its metacarpal to allow the adjoining metacarpals to approximate each other. This tends to prevent adjoining fingers from rotating and crossing toward each other. As a secondary procedure, the index (in the case of amputation of the long finger) or the little finger (in the case of amputation of the ring finger) may be moved over by resecting the metacarpal of the missing finger through the proximal third of its shaft and shifting the adjoining finger on to the stump (Fig. 44-15).

When the middle finger plus either the index or little finger are removed together, the heads of the metacarpals should be obliqued to produce a smooth contour. When the index finger has been disarticulated, the metacarpal should be partially excised to improve the final appearance of the hand and to avoid interference with function. In the case of the little finger, it is preferable not to resect the whole metacarpal because the extensor and flexor carpi ulnaris tendons are attached to the base.

The thumb is the most important of the digits, and every bit should be saved, since even the smallest stump is preferable to a prosthesis. When only the thumb and small finger remain, a rotation osteotomy of the metacar-

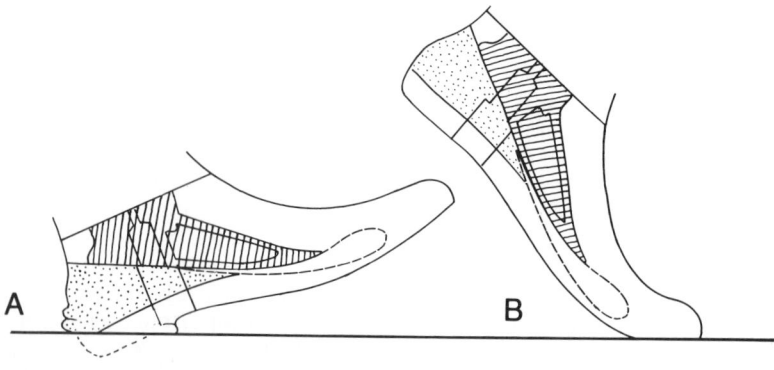

Fig. 44-13. SACH foot prosthesis. *A.* Position at heel strike. *B.* Position at toe off.

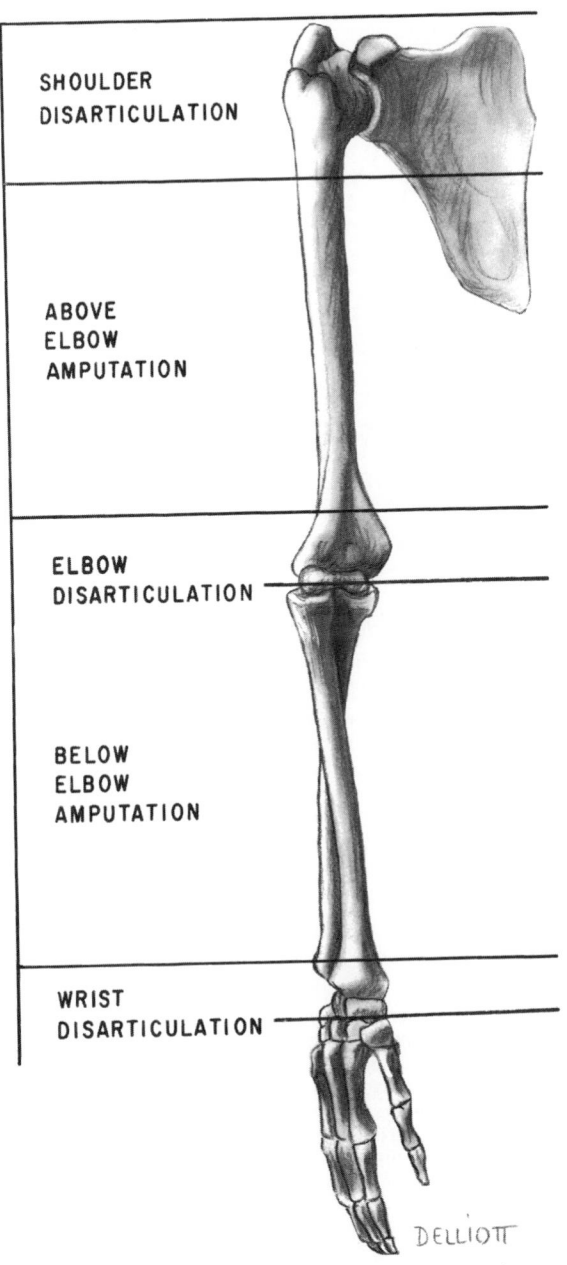

SHOULDER
DISARTICULATION

ABOVE
ELBOW
AMPUTATION

ELBOW
DISARTICULATION

BELOW
ELBOW
AMPUTATION

WRIST
DISARTICULATION

DELLIOTT

Fig. 44-14. Levels of amputation in the upper extremity.

pal of the thumb may be performed to permit approximation and grasping.

A variety of prostheses are available for more major amputations of the digits. These include functional terminal devices, such as hooks and cosmetically acceptable plastic hands. The selection of the prosthesis is dependent upon the patient's individual needs.

AMPUTATION THROUGH THE CARPOMETACARPAL LEVEL

After dorsal and volar skin and subcutaneous tissue flaps have been established, the digital extensor tendons are pulled down, transected, and allowed to retract, while

the tendons of the carpal extensors are separated from their attachments to the metacarpal bases and left long so that they may be inserted into the carpal bone. The thenar and hypothenar muscles are tapered to make a smoothly rounded stump. The long flexor tendons are transected after applying gentle traction so that they will retract. After the metacarpals have been disarticulated from the carpals and the synovial cartilage has been removed from the distal carpals, the flexor carpi radialis and the tendons of carpal extension are sutured to the carpal bones. The skin and subcutaneous tissue is then closed. The stump should be capable of more motion than a forearm stump, since there is more pronation and supination and good flexion and extension at the wrist. It accepts prostheses to provide a cosmetic hand and also more versatile and functional hooks.

Wrist Disarticulation

This level preserves greater length and provides better prosthetic control than amputations proximal to the wrist joint. The tendons of the hand should be transected with the muscles at rest length, so that they may be sutured to the ligaments and periosteum in order to prevent retraction and atrophy. The brachioradialis should not be disturbed. The styloid processes should be removed to permit a smoother fit for the prosthesis. The articular cartilage should also be removed and covered with a fascial flap to prevent limitation of pronation and supination by scar formation.

Although the stump is less strong and less versatile than when the carpal bones are left in, a less conspicuous prosthesis can be used. In women, amputations are generally carried a little higher in order to reduce the size of the prosthetic wrist by removal of the bulbous mass of bone at the end.

Forearm Amputation

In order to avoid excessive scarring and immobility of skin, skin flaps should not be dissected extensively from the fascia. The long flexor and extensor muscles and tendons are dissected and tapered so that they adhere to underlying tissue. After the bones have been transected, about $\frac{1}{2}$ in. of periosteum should be removed to prevent spur formation, and the fascia should be closed over the end so that muscle length is maintained.

With longer stumps, the actions of pronation and supination should be preserved, and the tendinous muscles and bones are therefore treated atraumatically to prevent fibrosis. Even if only a short stump can be achieved, this is superior to an above-elbow amputation. The formation of a functioning stump through the upper forearm can be successful if there is only a short segment of either radius or ulna that may be preserved distal to the tuberosity. This can be lengthened secondarily with a bone graft or flap.

The biceps and pectoralis muscles have been used in cineplastic operations as prime movers of artificial limbs in this situation. The plastic procedure is usually performed secondarily after the stump has healed. An in-

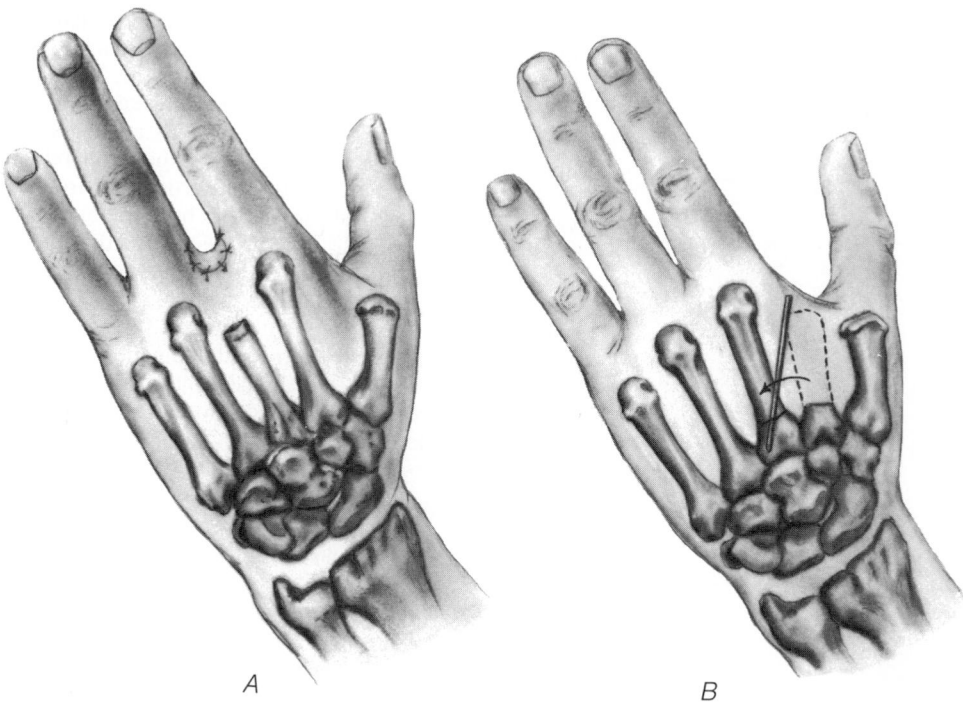

A

B

Fig. 44-15. Shifting of finger. *A.* Middle finger has been amputated at a transmetacarpal level. *B.* The remaining portion of the shaft of the middle finger metacarpal has been resected, and the metacarpal of the index finger has been transected and the distal portion secured to the base of the metacarpal of the middle finger by means of a Kirschner wire.

verted skin flap is formed and sutured into a tube and drawn through a tunnel of muscle in the biceps. The biceps tendon is divided at the midpoint and skin graft applied to cover the defect from the inverted flap (Fig. 44-16). The biceps can then transmit its force externally, while the brachialis muscle remains as a flexor of the forearm. The transmission of force is accomplished by attaching the rod through a muscle to a cable that exercises power over a hook.

The Krukenberg operation may be used in the forearm when amputation is performed on a blind patient. With

Fig. 44-16. Cineplastic procedure for forearm amputation. *A.* Amputation has healed, and an inverted skin flap has been fashioned into a tube. *B.* Dermal tube has been brought through a tunnel of biceps muscle, and the biceps tendon is divided at the midpoint. A skin graft is then applied to cover the defect on the inverted flap. *C.* Prosthesis fitted. The transmission of force is accomplished from the biceps muscle to the cable that powers the hook.

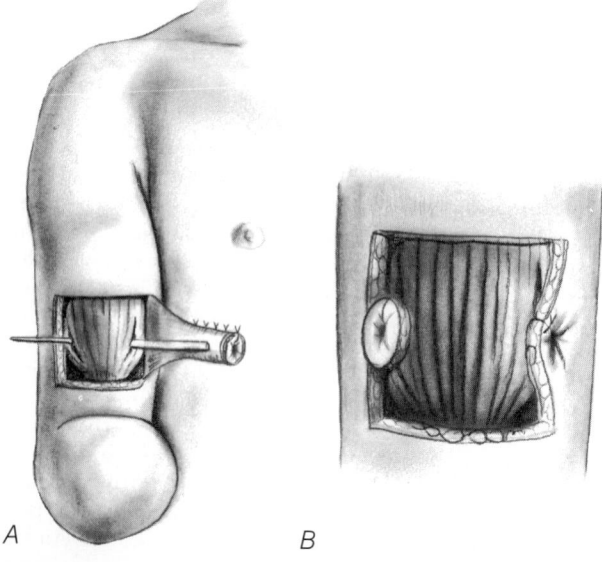

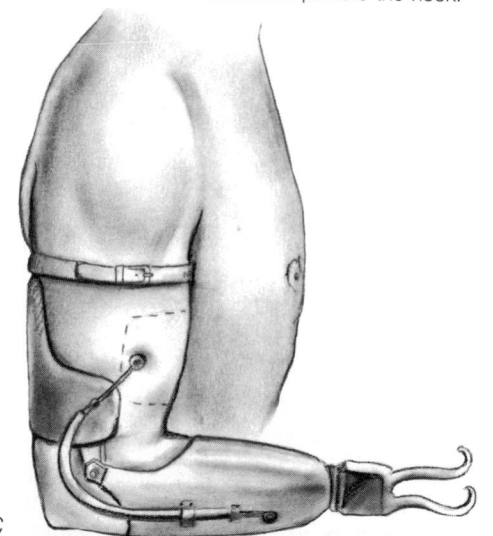

A

B

C

this procedure, a cleft is constructed between the radius and ulna to provide a grasping terminus that possesses tactile sensation.

Elbow Disarticulation

Flaps are created as in the case of forearm amputations so that the closure of skin and fat will not lie directly over the fascial incision. In order to obviate a bulky stump, the epicondyles are removed, and the cartilage is excised from the end of the bone. The tendons of the biceps, brachialis, and triceps muscles are sutured over the end at rest length. A cineplastic procedure to develop power for a functional terminal device may be performed secondarily.

Amputation through the Humerus

Every attempt should be made to preserve as long a stump as possible, since the longer the stump, the greater the applicability of subsequent cineplastic procedures for functional prosthesis. If a high amputation is necessary, it is preferable to preserve the head of the humerus, since this maintains the width of the shoulder and acts as a support for a prosthesis.

After anterior and posterior flaps are developed, the muscles are transected so that there is sufficient length of biceps and brachialis tendons and triceps muscle so that these muscles can be joined over the end of the bone to avoid retraction. In the case of shorter stumps, the biceps and triceps may be fixed to the humerus in a fashion similar to that described for myodesis procedures in the lower extremity. The skin and muscles are then closed loosely.

As soon as the stump is mature, it can be fitted with a prosthesis with a terminal device operated by a shoulder cable and with an elbow that can be fixed at varying degrees of flexion. The type of elbow joint utilized depends upon the type of function required by the patient. The most functional terminal devices are hooks that may be voluntarily opened. In the case of the adult unilateral amputee, the prosthesis usually functions only as an aid for the contralateral hand.

Disarticulation of the Humerus and Forequarter Amputation

The former procedure is usually performed for extensive trauma, whereas the latter operation may be indicated for malignant disease of the proximal upper extremity.

In most instances, care must be taken in individually ligating the vessels and nerves. In the case of disarticulation of the humerus, the flaps are fashioned to provide covering of the glenoid fossa, and the deltoid muscle is retained to be incorporated in this closure. Forequarter amputation includes excision of the scapula and clavicle followed by closure of the chest and back muscles over the chest wall and coverage with previously established skin flaps. A prosthetic device operated by the opposite shoulder may be applied.

Upper Extremity Prostheses

There are three main groups of upper extremity prostheses: (1) passive prostheses that are primarily for cosmesis but have some degree of useful function; (2) prostheses controlled by movements of the remaining body segment; and (3) externally powered prostheses. These main categories may be combined to produce a single prosthesis. The passive devices are designed to enable the stump to hold an object or a tool. Aesthetic prostheses have achieved high quality and near normal appearance. Active devices provide one or more movements, and are structured according to individual needs of the patient.

EXTREMITY REPLANTATION

The first report on reattachments of a fully amputated hand, with return of useful function, was in 1963. In the ensuing 25 years, refinements in microvascular techniques have resulted in an increasing success rate.

There remains difficulty assessing results because of a lack of a precise definition of functional recovery. A summary of the experiences from China, Switzerland, and the United States noted that overall, one-third of the patients had excellent functional recovery, one-third had good results, and one-third had fair-to-poor results.

No shoulder replantation achieved excellent or good functional results. Good function resulted with replantation above the elbow in 0 to 40 percent of cases. Replantation at the proximal forearm was associated with excellent to good functional results in 0 to 70 percent. Much better results were noted when replantation was carried out at the distal forearm, with success rates ranging between 50 and 83 percent. At the wrist, the success rate was approximately 80 percent, at the palm between 25 and 70 percent, the thumb between 32 and 90 percent, the fingers proximal to the PIP joint, about 70 percent, and distal to the PIP joint, almost 100 percent.

Guillotine injuries were associated with a higher degree of success following replantation than were compression or crush injuries, and the worst results occurred in avulsion injuries. Reasonable success rates were achieved if the duration of anoxia was less than 20 h; the success rate dropped sharply when anoxia periods were greater than 20 h.

The essential structures of the dismembered extremity must be intact and the severed limb reasonably well preserved if the reimplantation is to be attempted. Following thorough debridement, the bones are repaired before the circulation is reestablished. A main vein is anastomosed prior to the arterial repair. The muscles, tendon, and nerves are then repaired and skin coverage is provided. Decompressive fasciotomy is frequently indicated.

Bibliography

General Considerations

Aitken GT: Surgical amputations in children. *J Bone Joint Surg [Am]* 45A:1735, 1963.

Burgess EM, Romano RL: Immediate postsurgical prosthesis fitting. *Bull Prosthetic Res* 10(4): 1965.

Amputations of the Lower Extremity

Baker WH, Barnes RW: Minor forefoot amputation in patients with low ankle pressure. *Am J Surg* 133:331, 1977.

Baker WH, Barnes RW, et al: Healing of below-knee amputations: Comparison of soft and plaster dressings. *Am J Surg* 133:716, 1977.

Barnes RW, Thornhill B, et al: Prediction of amputation wound healing: Roles of Doppler ultrasound and digit photoplethysmography. *Arch Surg* 116:80, 1981.

Couch NP, David JK, et al: Natural history of the leg amputee. *Am J Surg* 133:469, 1977.

Fearon J, Campbell DR, et al: Improved results with diabetic below-knee amputations. *Arch Surg* 120:777, 1985.

Harris PD, Schwartz SI, DeWeese JA: Midcalf amputation for peripheral vascular disease. *Arch Surg* 82:381, 1961.

Hoaglund FT, Jergesen HE, et al: Evaluation of problems and needs of veteran lower limb amputees in the San Francisco Bay during the period of 1977–1980. *J Rehab Res Dev* 20:57, 1983.

Jergesen HE, Hoaglund FT, et al: The University of California Biomechanics Laboratory four-bar polycentric knee linkage: A clinical trail in 20 above-knee amputees. *Clin Orthop* 204:184, 1986.

McIntyre KE, Bailey SA, et al: Guillotine amputation in the treatment of nonsalvageable lower-extremity infections. *Arch Surg* 119:450, 1984.

Moore WS: Determination of amputation level: Measurement of skin blood flow with xenon-133. *Arch Surg* 107:798, 1973.

Moore WS, Hall AD, Lim RC Jr: Below the knee amputation for ischemic gangrene. *Am J Surg* 124:127, 1972.

Nicholas GG, Myers JL, et al: The role of vascular laboratory criteria in the selection of patients for lower extremity amputation. *Ann Surg* 195:469, 1982.

O'Dwyer KJ, Edwards MH: The association between lowest palpable pulse and wound healing in below knee amputations. *Ann R Coll Surg Engl* 67:232, 1985.

Radcliffe CW: The University of California 4-bar linkage knee for the above-knee amputee. Presented at the Fourth International Symposium on External Control of Human Extremities, Yugoslavia. 1972.

Ryder RA: Amputations of extremities in cardiovascular disease. *Bull Prosthetics Res* 16(2):21, 1979 (Veterans Administration Department of Medicine and Surgery, Washington, DC).

Sherman CD, Duthie RB: Modified hemipelvectomy. *Cancer* 13:51, 1960.

Silverman DG, Roberts A, et al: Fluorometric quantification of low-dose fluorescein delivery to predict amputation site healing. *Surgery* 101:335, 1987.

Squires JW, Johnson WC, et al: Cause of wound complications in elderly patients with above-knee amputations. *Am J Surg* 143:523, 1982.

Stahlgren LH, Otteman MG: Review of criteria for the selection of the level for lower extremity amputation of arteriosclerosis. *Ann Surg* 162:886, 1965.

Staros A, Goralnik B: Lower limb prosthetic systems, in *Atlas of Limb Prosthetics: Surgical and Prosthetic Principles.* American Academy of Orthopaedic Surgeons, St Louis, CV Mosby, 1981, chap 20, pp 277–314.

Warren R, Kihn RB: A survey of lower extremity amputations for ischemia. *Surgery* 63:107, 1968.

Waters RL, Perry J, et al: Energy cost of walking amputees: The influence of level of amputation. *J Bone Joint Surg [Am]* 58A:42, 1976.

Amputations of the Upper Extremity

Burnham PJ: Amputation of the upper extremity. *Clin Symp* 11:107, 1959.

Burnham PJ: Regional block at the wrist of the great nerves of the hand. *JAMA* 167:847, 1958.

Chase RA, Laub DR: The hand: Therapeutic strategy for acute problems. *Curr Probl Surg* 1966.

Law HT: Engineering of upper limb prostheses. *Orthoped Clin North Am* 12:929, 1981.

Extremity Replantation

Ahong-Wei C, Meyer VE, et al: Present indications and contraindications for replantation as reflected by long-term functional results. *Orthoped Clin North Am* 12:849, 1981.

The Hand

Richard I. Burton

The philosophic exaltation of the hand by scholars of antiquity is equaled by the profound regard for its complexity and versatility held today by functional anatomists and surgeons. The hand is composed of material of dexterity, strength, sensitivity, and refinement—all in the most complex array and condensed into a unit weighing significantly less than 1 kg. With this amazing tool we implement the desires of the human brain, whether requiring the speed and precision of the fingering hand of a concert violinist or the brute power grasp needed to wield a sledgehammer. With the hands the laborer supports a family, the parent loves and cares for a baby, the musician plays a sonata, the blind ''read,'' and the deaf ''talk.''

This essential organ, the hand, is often crippled by injury, by disease, or by birth defects. As the general surgeon Sterling Bunnell aptly summarized in 1943, ''To recondition these members successfully is difficult. Surgical reconstruction of the hand requires special careful technique . . . . It is a composite problem requiring the correlation of various specialties—orthopaedic, plastic, and neurologic surgery—the knowledge of any one of which alone is inadequate for repairing the hand . . . . As the problem is composite, the surgeon must also be . . . . The surgeon must face the situation and equip himself to handle any and all tissues of a limb.''

George Omer stated in 1978 ''Modern surgery of the hand is not a limited regional specialty. No medical or surgical specialist treats a greater variety of pathologic entities than the hand surgeon. The armamentarium of the hand surgeon includes the established procedures of the orthopaedic surgeon and the plastic surgeon, plus innovative techniques such as tendon implants for the severe injury or rheumatoid arthritis. The technical skills of the neurosurgeon and vascular surgeon are modified for microsurgery such as the replantation of amputated digits. Pediatric studies are utilized by the hand surgeon in the medical and surgical management of the congenital upper extremity anomaly.''

As reported by Kelsey et al. in the epidemiologic study done by the Yale University School of Medicine in 1980, hand problems are enormously common and often first present to the family physician, general surgeon, internist, or emergency room. They quote the following statistics. One-third of all injuries involve the upper extremities, numbering approximately 16 million each year in the United States. This results in 50,000 inpatient hospitaliza-

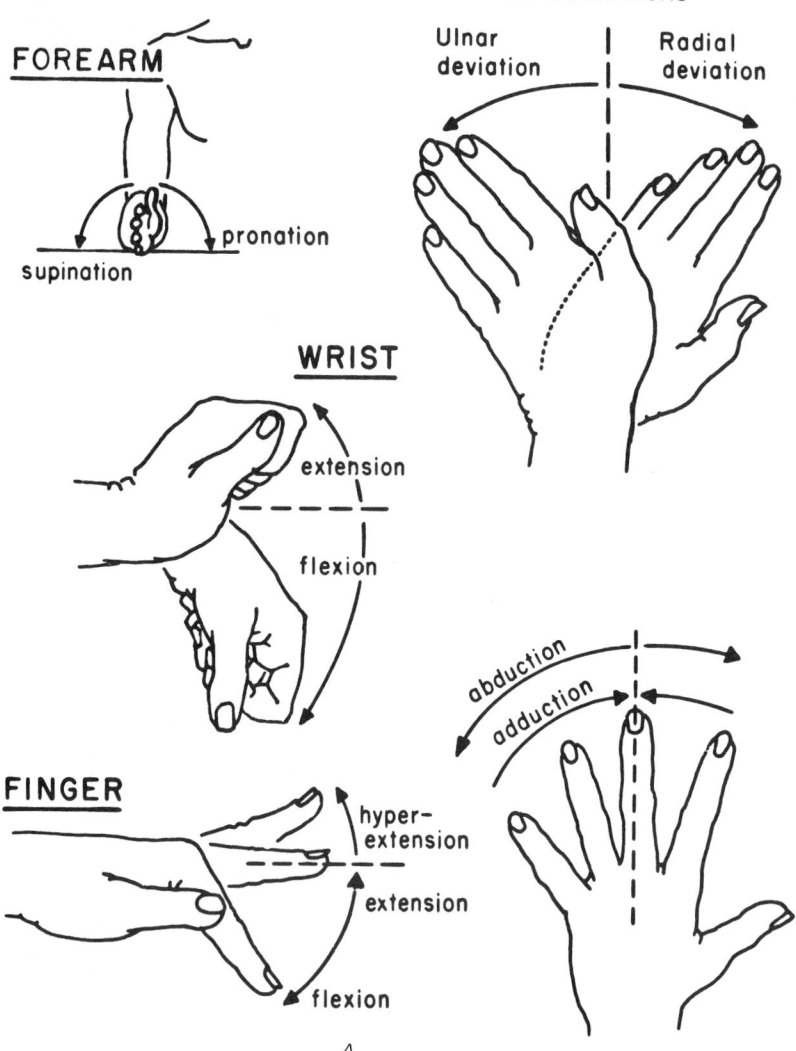

Fig. 45-1. Common terminology as used in describing hand mobility. (From: *American Society for Surgery of the Hand: The Hand: Examination and Diagnosis.* Edinburgh, Churchill-Livingstone, 1983, with permission.)

tions, 6 million visits to hospital emergency rooms, and 12 million visits to physicians' offices each year. Sixteen million days are lost from work yearly. If the 25 million people with arthritis are combined with the large number of upper extremity disorders from stroke, paralysis, congenital anomalies, various neurologic disorders, and the residuals of trauma, the total number of involved patients is enormous. The total cost of upper extremity disorders in the United States in 1980 was estimated by Kelsey to be over 10 billion dollars. A majority of people with hand disorders are afflicted during their wage-earning years.

BASIC PRINCIPLES

Clinical Assessment

HISTORY. The treating physician must know the *injured patient's* age, occupation, hand dominance, history of previous hand impairment or injury, time interval since injury, location and conditions under which the patient

was injured (e.g., environment clean or dirty), mechanism of injury (e.g., crush, thermal), and previous treatment administered. The elderly steroid-dependent arthritic patient with a laceration several hours previous on a garden tool presents an entirely different problem from the healthy teenager with a laceration sustained carving a pumpkin with a recently washed kitchen knife. The numb fingertip of the concert violinist and that of the heavy construction worker have far different occupational implications.

For *nontraumatic* problems additional information is required about pain, sensory changes, swelling, loss of mobility, impairments of occupation or routine activities of daily living, similar problems in other areas of the body, activities making symptoms worse or better, etc.

PHYSICAL EXAMINATION. It is essential that a standard terminology be used in describing results of the examination (see Fig. 45-1). There are two basic tenets in examination of the hand: *(a)* the entire involved upper extremity should be exposed for complete examination; *(b)* the hand should be examined "by systems"—(1) circulatory,

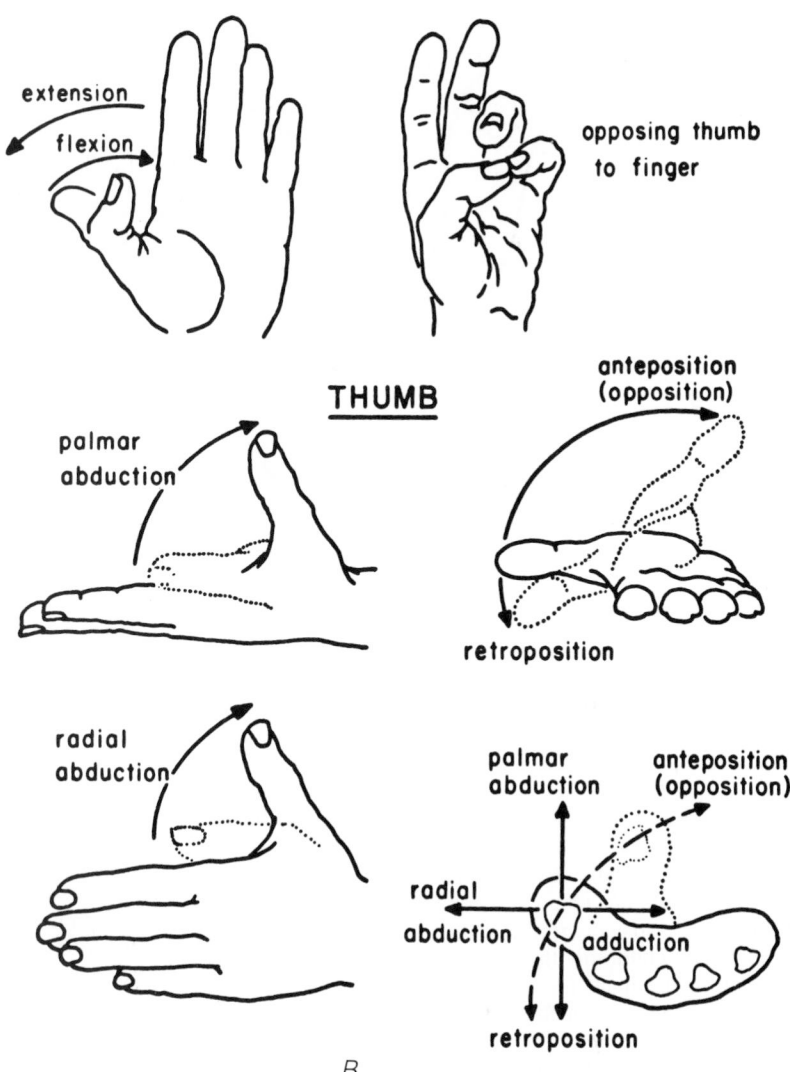

extension
flexion

opposing thumb to finger

THUMB

palmar abduction

anteposition (opposition)

retroposition

radial abduction

palmar abduction | anteposition (opposition)

radial abduction | adduction

retroposition

Fig. 45-1 *B.* Continued.

B

(2) sensibility, (3) coverage, (4) bone, (5) joints and ligaments, (6) flexor tendons, (7) extensor tendons, and (8) intrinsic muscle function.

Circulation. The presence or absence of edema, cyanosis, and pallor should be noted. Radial and ulnar pulses should be checked as well as the Allen test performed. Capillary filling is a very helpful indicator of perfusion. Arterial and venous insufficiencies are particularly important to document now that microsurgery has made realistic their reconstitution.

Sensibility. It is absolutely essential that the patterns of anesthesia be carefully examined and clearly documented following any type of injury before any local anesthetic agent is used in the wound or as a peripheral nerve block. Following acute injury, the most accurate assessment of sensibility is provided by light touch with a wisp of cotton. Particularly in the frightened child or in the apprehensive adult, this is far more reliable than the use of pinprick testing. In the assessment of the noninjured patient, light touch and two-point discrimination are the two most valuable sensory tests.

There is considerable cutaneous overlap. However, there are certain autonomous zones: the median nerve on the flexor surface of the terminal segment of the index finger, the ulnar nerve on the flexor aspect of the terminal segment of the little finger, and the radial nerve on the dorsal web space of the thumb.

Coverage. In cases of open injury, the nature of the wound and the loss of soft tissue must be carefully noted. In the nonacute case, the quality of the soft tissue coverage (e.g., scleroderma) is important.

Bones. In any case of suspected bone injury, tumor, or infection, adequate radiographic examination is essential. This requires an AP and true lateral of the part involved. The customary oblique x-ray of the hand with the fingers gently flexed, which is the standard x-ray exposure, is of little value. Lateral x-rays of the fingers must not be taken with the digits superimposed—either the digits must be fanned, or separate laterals must be taken for each digit.

Joints and Ligaments. Joint and/or ligamentous injuries are extremely common in the hand. There is no such diagnosis as "jammed finger," any more than a physician

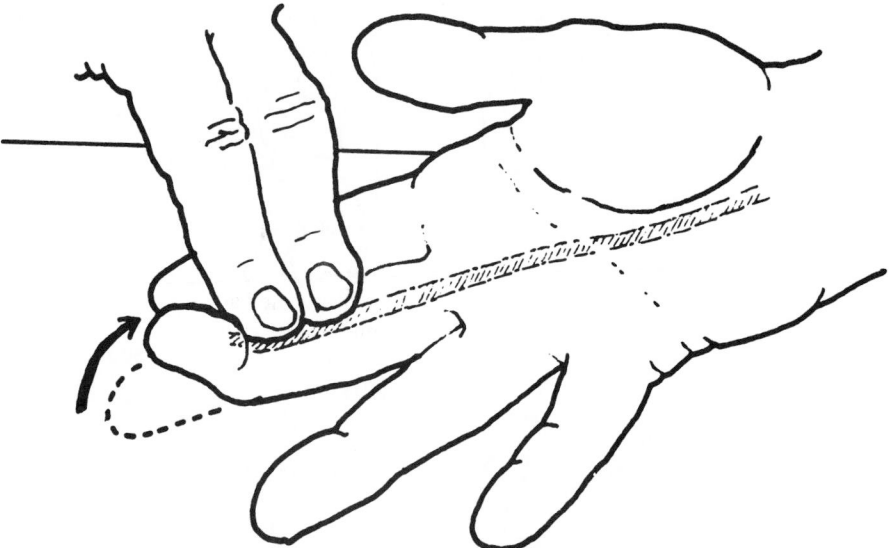

Fig. 45-2. Test for flexor digitorum profundus function. (From: *American Society for Surgery of the Hand: The Hand: Examination and Diagnosis. Edinburgh, Churchill-Livingstone, 1983, with permission.*)

would diagnose a "jammed knee" or "jammed ankle." Accurate AP and lateral x-rays of the involved joint are necessary to rule out fracture, subluxation, dislocation, or fracture-dislocation. Ligamentous avulsion injuries are common. For certain injuries, stress x-rays are very helpful. The specific areas of tenderness must be localized relative to the various ligamentous structures, and the ranges of both active and passive motion must be recorded. Stability and instability must be noted. It must be recalled that frequently the ligaments in children are stronger than the epiphyseal plate, and it is this latter structure in close proximity to the joints that is frequently injured in children—thus contraindicating joint stress testing in the hand for children in most circumstances.

Flexor Tendons. The flexor digitorum profundus musculotendinous units and the flexor pollicis longus flex the terminal segments of the digits (Fig. 45-2). The flexor digitorum superficialis primarily flexes the proximal inter-

phalangeal joints (PIP). They operate independently of one another, and thus if the profundus tendon is check-reined by holding adjacent digits in extension, the ability to flex the finger in question at the PIP level requires intact flexor digitorum superficialis function (Fig. 45-3).

Extensor Tendons. The extensor digitorum communis tendons passing to each of the four fingers, the extensor digit minimi (to the little finger), and the extensor inducis proprius (index) are the prime extensors of the metacarpophalangeal joints of the fingers. Theoretically, transection of the extensor tendon to a single digit will result in

Fig. 45-3. Test for flexor digitorum superficialis function. (From: *American Society for Surgery of the Hand: The Hand: Examination and Diagnosis. Edinburgh, Churchill-Livingstone, 1983, with permission.*)

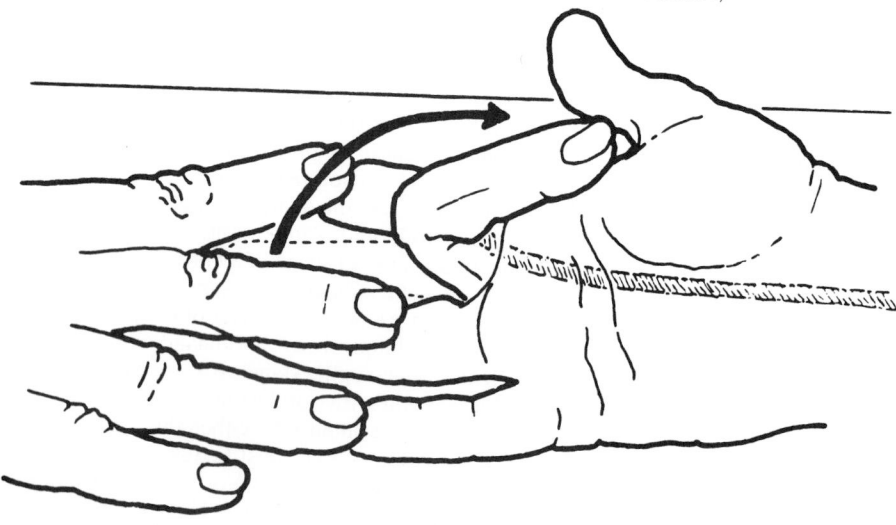

an extensor lag of that finger at the metacarpophalangeal joint level. The intertendinous bridges (juncturae tendonae) on the dorsum of the hand and the double tendons passing to the index and little fingers may cause diagnostic confusion.

Intrinsic Musculotendinous Function. The thenar muscles, hypothenar muscles, lumbrical muscles, and interossei muscles have their entire musculotendinous course within the hand itself. There is considerable variation in the innervation of these muscles. The classic pattern is for median nerve innervation to the intrinsics of the thenar eminence on the radial side of the flexor pollicis longus (abductor pollicis brevis, opponens pollicis, and superficial head of flexor pollicis brevis) as well as the first two lumbricals. The ulnar nerve innervates the hypothenar muscles, the interossei muscles, the ulnar two lumbricals, and the remainder of the thenar muscles (ulnar head of the flexor pollicis brevis) and the adductor

pollicis. The median nerve is tested by palmar abduction of the thumb and opposition (see Fig. 45-1*B*). The ulnar innervated intrinsics are responsible for finger abduction and adduction (see Fig. 45-1*A*). The intrinsic muscles flex the metacarpophalangeal joints and extend the interphalangeal joints.

Distal Block Anesthesia Techniques

Two specific block techniques may be of great value in the emergency room—(1) median, radial, and/or ulnar nerve at the wrist; and (2) digital block at the base of the individual finger.

To block the median nerve (Fig. 45-4*A*) the needle is inserted either to the ulnar or radial side of the palmaris longus tendon at the level of the wrist flexion crease, with the needle angled 20° distally. The ulnar nerve block (Fig. 45-4*B*) is inserted just to the dorsal aspect of the flexor carpi ulnaris tendon, in a plane perpendicular to the long axis of the forearm and parallel to that of the palm. The needle is introduced to a depth of 1 cm; it is essential to aspirate to be certain the tip of the needle is not within the ulnar artery. The radial sensory nerve (Fig. 45-4*C*) is best blocked three finger breadths proximal to the radial styloid along an imaginary line drawn between the radial styloid and the lateral epicondyle. It is at this point that the radial nerve emerges from beneath the brachioradialis tendon but has not yet split into its many branches.

Fig. 45-4. Common distal regional blocks as used for hand disorders. The radial, median, and ulnar nerves are easily blocked at the wrist. Epinephrine should never be used with the local anesthetic agents for these blocks because of the risk of arterial spasm and digital loss. For median block, ulnar block, or radial block, 5 to 6 mL is required at the wrist level, and for digital block, 2 to 3 mL is required. The use of a #25 needle is recommended. Injection should not be into the nerve but adjacent to the nerve. If the patient complains of paresthesia at the time of needle introduction, the needle must be redirected. [From: *Burton RI: Acute joint injuries of the hand, in Wolfort (ed): Acute Hand Injuries: A Multispecialty Approach. Boston, Little, Brown, 1980, with permission.*]

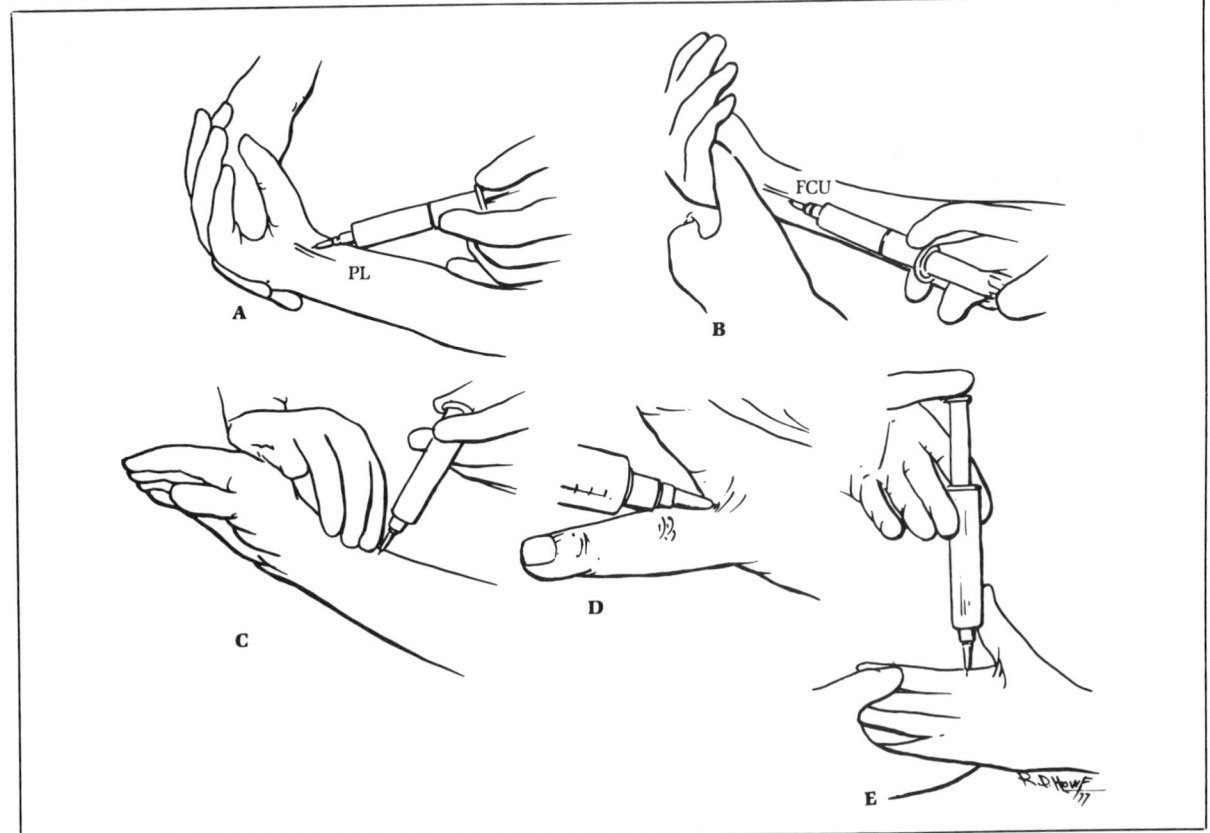

The digital block (see Fig. 45-4D and E) is best done by injecting a few milliliters in the web space on both sides at the base of the involved digit. This is much less traumatic, much easier, and much safer than a ring block around the base of the digit. The ring block should never be used, because it is painful, it will increase venous pressure within the digit, and it may compromise digital vascularity. To block the radial border of the index finger and the ulnar margin of the little finger, the appropriate proper digital nerve is easily located in the subcutaneous fatty tissue just anterior to the corresponding metacarpal head.

The physician must recall that the wrist block will paralyze the intrinsic musculature, unlike the digital block, and therefore the digital block should be used if pain relief is required to adequately assess active digital movement following injury (rather than wrist block).

This author prefers 1% mepivacaine (Carbocaine), or 2% lidocaine (Xylocaine), using a 1-cm 25-gauge needle.

Because of possible disastrous irreversible vascular complications, epinephrine should *never* be combined with any anesthetic agent used for digital or wrist block anesthesia.

Treatment of the Acutely Injured Hand

Several principles merit emphasis.

1. Injuries to the hand are extremely important.
2. The majority of hand injuries occur to the otherwise young and healthy individual and thus have enormous implications for occupation, home life, and/or future career choices.
3. The quality of the primary care, more than anything done subsequently, will determine the final result. The best example of this is the patient with a flexor tendon injury. No secondary reconstruction, no matter how skillfully done and sophisticated, can recover the function irrevocably lost by inappropriate primary treatment.
4. Acute wounds should *not* be explored or probed for diagnostic purposes in the emergency room setting. There is a desire by inexperienced surgeons to look directly into the wound "to see if nerves and/or tendons are lacerated." To the contrary, much more can be ascertained by covering the wound and performing an organized gentle and systematic examination of the forearm and hand distal to the injury, testing separately for each appropriate tendon and nerve function.
5. All examinations must be conducted in an organized fashion, including each of the systems listed above.
6. Control of hemorrhage is with local gentle pressure. Vigorous bleeding from the hand rarely, if ever, requires clamping. The patient who presents with a bleeding laceration of the hand should be asked to lie down. The hand is elevated and the wound supported with a gentle sterile dressing. The bleeding is usually stopped within a few minutes. The well-intentioned "clamping a bleeder" in the lacerated hand must be avoided if at all possible. Previously undamaged vital structures such as nerve and tendon are unfortunately all too often inadvertently crushed and irretrievably damaged by such well-intentioned but unnecessary maneuvers. If necessary, a brachial tourniquet can be applied after the limb has been exsanguinated with a rubber bandage or Ace bandage; under the appropriate sterile and avascular conditions, the offending vessel can be carefully dissected free from adjacent vital structures, clamped, and ligated—or repaired if recommended.
7. Primary versus secondary wound closure must be carefully considered. The great majority of civilian injuries are classified as "tidy" wounds for which primary closure is indicated after the appropriate deeper tendon, nerve, and/or bone re-

constructions. However, experiences with highly contaminated wounds, such as military injuries and farm injuries, emphasize that the principles of secondary wound closure that are applicable elsewhere in the body are also pertinent to the hand. In such wounds, the initial debridement is accomplished and the hand carefully dressed. After the initial debridement, the hand is reevaluated 2 to 4 days later in the operating room, and further debridement performed or definitive closure obtained (direct suture, skin graft, or flap).

Reconstructive Hand Surgery

1. To a large measure, the success or failure of reconstructive hand surgery following trauma is predetermined by the quality of the primary care rendered.
2. In many types of reconstructive hand surgery, whether following injury or for nontraumatic problems such as rheumatoid arthritis, the functional result is enormously improved by a prompt and intensive program of preoperative exercises to make joints limber and to strengthen the musculotendinous units present.
3. Preoperative and postoperative serial measurements of range of motion (active and passive), strength, and sensibility (two-point discrimination) are essential.
4. The goal of reconstructive hand surgery is not cosmesis but function. What is function for the patient with one type of occupation may not be for another. In this connection, note that cosmesis is function for certain occupations. For example, a deformed hand may ruin the career of a ballerina or model.
5. Most reconstructive hand procedures require staging.
6. In assessing the hand for reconstruction, it is helpful to divide it into three zones: the wrist, the thumb, and the fingers.
7. In planning reconstruction, each of the tissues involved must be considered, usually in the following sequence: (1) coverage, and with coverage, excellent circulation (many cases of chronic osteomyelitis are dramatically improved with good soft tissue coverage and circulation); (2) stability of the skeletal framework; (3) joint reconstruction for mobility with stability, or joint arthrodeses in favorable positions for stability; (4) reconstitution of the musculotendinous units by either tendon transfers, tendon grafting, or in certain situations free muscle transfer; (5) repair of innervation, either by direct neurorrhaphy or by fascicular nerve grafting.
8. In planning a staged program of hand reconstruction, two "rules of three" are very helpful. The first is that there are five basic structures to be considered—coverage, bone, joint, musculotendinous, and nerve. If *three* of these five require reconstruction, consideration may need to be given to amputation of that digit as an alternative to staged reconstruction. This is *not* applicable for the thumb or for the entire hand. The second "rule of three" is that any series of staged operations on the hand should if possible be kept to *three* or less. Should a series of more than three reconstructive surgeries be required, it is best for the surgeon to rethink the functional deficit and proposed reconstruction to see if a simpler and more effective surgical plan may be designed.
9. When there is a carefully directed postoperative program of hand therapy, the postoperative convalescence of almost all patients requiring reconstructive hand surgery will be significantly shortened and impressively smoothed, and there will be a definite improvement in the final result. Such a program requires a close professional working relationship among the hand therapist, the surgeon, and the patient. It cannot be managed with simple requisitions and telephone requests, but requires direct person-to-person contact. The hand therapist is not a physical therapist or an occupational therapist, but is an interested individual who has had training in physical therapy and/or occupational therapy, with additional training in the specific techniques of hand therapy.

Tourniquet Use

The use of a tourniquet to ensure a bloodless field is essential in hand surgery, whether for trauma or for reconstruction. As Sterling Bunnell is oft-quoted, "A watchmaker cannot repair a watch at the bottom of an inkwell." A tourniquet should be applied as far proximal on the upper arm as possible, over adequate Webril padding, smoothly applied to the arm without wrinkles, and of proper length. Tourniquets designed for leg use that need to be wrapped several times around the upper extremity should never be used. The 16- to 18-in. lengths are best except for children. Small pediatric cuffs are available. The limb should be exsanguinated before tourniquet inflation, either by rubber or Ace bandage or by elevation. The better the exsanguination, the longer the tourniquet will be tolerated. With axillary block anesthesia the tourniquet will cause minimal or no discomfort for 1 to $1\frac{1}{2}$ h. With distal regional anesthesia, the tourniquet ischemia is well tolerated by the patient for approximately 20 min. Rubber-band tourniquets at the base of digits should *never* be used. A well-padded $\frac{3}{4}$- to 1-in. Penrose drain can be used at the base of the digit, secured with a clamp.

Incisions

Hand incisions, whether they are extensions of lacerations for adequate treatment following primary injury or whether they are for secondary reconstruction, must adhere to certain simple principles but may be very complex in design. It is a paradox that a small ill-conceived incision can be very disabling, and yet the hand can be liter-

ally taken apart through complex but proper incisions with little or no late disability. All incisions must be very accurately placed and must be designed so that they may be extended proximally and/or distally if needed for additional exposure either at the time of primary surgery or during subsequent reconstruction. The incisions on the volar palm, digit, and dorsum of the hand each must adhere to certain principles (Fig. 45-5).

Incisions on the palm in general parallel the skin creases or cross them obliquely. In order to locate deeper structures and plan the flaps, it is very helpful to recall that an imaginary line drawn from the intererminential point to the midline base of a digit will overlie the flexor tendons, and a comparable line drawn to the interdigital cleft will overlie the lumbrical canal with its neurovascular structures.

Digital incisions on the side of a digit must be midaxial, not midlateral. The abrupt change in the normal character of dorsal and volar skin is helpful. It is better to err to the dorsal rather than the volar in the placement of incisions on the side of a digit, especially in children. A midlateral incision in a child will tend to migrate volarly with growth and may form a bridling scar. A second principle for digital incisions is that those which transgress the flexor side must avoid the shaded areas shown in Fig. 45-5A. These diamonds are the areas where the palmar skin from one phalanx will contact that of another in maximum digital flexion, not unlike the pages of a book. These diamond-shaped areas of skin contact have maximum mobility with

Fig. 45-5. Common volar and dorsal incisions for the hand. [From: *Burton RI: The hand, in Goldstein LA, Dickerson RC (eds): Atlas of Orthopaedic Surgery. St Louis, CV Mosby, 1981, with permission.*]

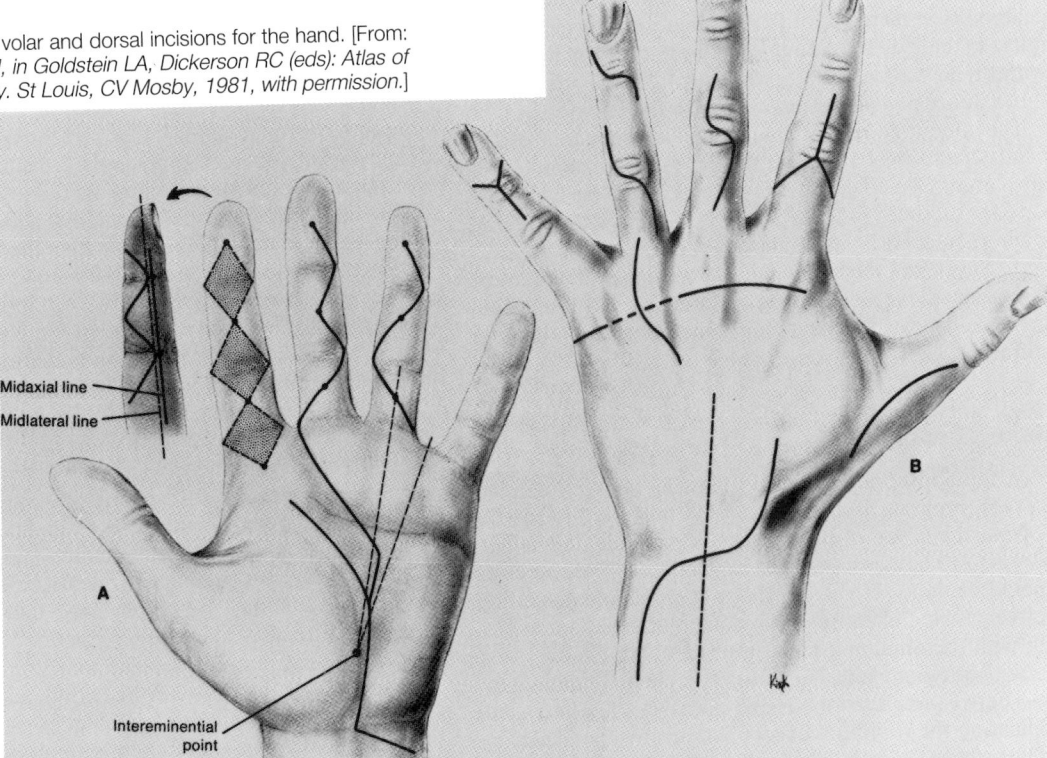

Midaxial line
Midlateral line
Interereminential point

digital flexion and extension, and any longitudinal or oblique scars transgressing into these areas will be predisposed to subsequent scar contracture. Thus a great variety of incisions can be designed on the digit as shown in Fig. 45-5*A*.

Dorsal skin incisions (Fig. 45-5*B*) should cross skin creases transversely or obliquely, with the exception that for surgery on the rheumatoid wrist the dorsal skin incision should be longitudinal or minimally curved. The usual bayonet incision, which is best for the nonrheumatoid, may lead to slough of a distal-based flap in the rheumatoid, often necessitating a subsequent abdominal pedicle flap for closure.

Dressings and Splints

A hand dressing and/or splint is an integral part of any hand surgical procedure, not to be delegated. An ill-conceived or poorly applied hand dressing may destroy the purpose of the surgical procedure. The layer applied to the skin or wound should be conforming and absorptive, not occlusive. The use of Telfa or Vaseline gauze is to be discouraged. A well-contoured, moist, smooth gauze sponge or a single layer of xeroform is excellent. The subsequent layers of the dressing should be soft, longitudinally applied, absorptive gauze sponges (never the type with paper or fiber filling). Next, a Kling type of gauze is applied, followed by Webril, plaster splints, and an overlying roll of plaster. It is essential that no pressure be applied over the dorsum of the wrist since to do so will decrease venous drainage from the hand.

The hand must be immobilized in the "safe position"—the wrist in 20 to 30° of extension, the metacarpophalangeal joints in 60 to 90° of flexion, and the interphalangeal joints extended. The thumb should project from the hand, with the metacarpal shaft projecting from the wrist in the three dimensions it assumes when a fist is made.

The uninjured and/or unoperated components of the hand should be left free from the immobilization. It is absolutely essential that the patient keep the hand elevated at all times following surgery or injury—on pillows when recumbent, "with elbows on the table for meals," and "Statue of Liberty" when ambulating. A sling is to be discouraged except in young children, as it will not hold the hand above the heart and tends to cause shoulder stiffness.

Hand Therapy

At the appropriate interval following injury, the hand therapy program is commenced. Details of this are far beyond the scope of this book. Six principles merit emphasis. (1) The exercises must be gentle. (2) The exercises should be done actively by the patient, supplemented by active assisted exercises, also done by the patient assisting with the uninjured hand. (3) The entire exercise and activity program must emphasize antiedema measures. (4) There is *no* place for passive exercises. (5) There is *no* indication for whirlpool except perhaps for the cleansing of burns. (6) There are rarely, if ever, indications for heat.

Dependency, heat, and whirlpool will all tend to produce swelling and therefore retard the convalescence.

TRAUMA

Common Fractures and Joint Injuries

COLLES FRACTURE. This is a fracture of a distal radius with dorsal angulation such that the distal radial articular surface faces dorsally, usually associated with a fracture of the ulnar styloid (not combined with fracture of a distal ulnar shaft as is commonly seen in children). This fracture most commonly occurs in women over the age of fifty who fall on the outstretched hand. Depending upon the amount of displacement and comminution, there may be considerable tenderness, swelling, and instability. The dorsally displaced distal fragment can usually be palpated in a more proximal position relative to the ulnar styloid when compared with the opposite normal wrist (see Fig. 43-66).

At the time of examination it is essential to rule out the presence or absence of coexistent median nerve injury before any anesthetic or treatment is given. The x-ray examination should include an AP and lateral of the wrist. The radial head at the elbow should be carefully checked for tenderness and x-rayed if any question exists to rule out fracture of this radial head.

The goal of treatment is to obtain a functional hand and wrist and secondarily to minimize cosmetic deformity. Many operative and skeletal traction techniques have been devised, but usually the best results are obtained by closed reduction with external immobilization, although in certain severe fractures other techniques are necessary.

Manipulative Technique. It is essential to have good muscle relaxation either by sedation combined with local anesthesia, by regional block technique, or by general anesthesia. An assistant applies countertraction to the humerus, and with the elbow flexed traction is applied to the radial side of the hand steadily and firmly to disimpact the distal radial fragment. While the traction is maintained, the operator grasps the distal radial fragment between the thumb and index finger of the free hand, reducing the displaced distal fragment anteriorly in alignment with the radius. The reduction is maintained by bringing the wrist into maximum ulnar deviation and then gentle flexion. If reduction has been successful, the tip of the radial styloid will be approximately 1 cm distal to the ulnar styloid and there will be no apparent deformity. It may be necessary to repeat the manipulation if check x-rays do not show satisfactory reduction. The two most essential components to the reduction are adequate muscle relaxation and adequate traction before the attempted reduction. It must be emphasized that repeated unsuccessful attempts at closed reduction without adequate traction and muscle relaxation may cause iatrogenic crumpling of the dorsal cortex, thus making the final reduction far less inherently stable.

Immobilization is obtained with a well-molded plaster cast or with dorsoradial and volar ulnar splints, holding the wrist in (1) maximal ulnar deviation and (2) 25° of palmar flexion. Many prefer that the immobilization be extended above the elbow to control pronation and supination in approximately 45° pronation. Check x-rays are obtained immediately in plaster and again at 7 to 10 days to be certain that the reduction is maintained.

The patient must be encouraged to keep the hand elevated for the first 1 to 2 weeks or until the swelling subsides. The patient must be carefully observed for any signs of median nerve compression. Should median nerve paresthesia occur, the position of wrist flexion in the cast must be reduced. If the nerve compression is unrelieved, the flexor retinaculum must be released for the acute carpal tunnel syndrome.

The patient must be instructed on an exercise program to maintain full range of motion of all interphalangeal (IP) and metacarpophalangeal (MCP) joints. The patient should maximally flex the IP joints with the MCP joints in extension, and maximally flex the MCP joints with the IP joints in extension. Range-of-motion exercises must also be done daily for the shoulder.

SMITH'S FRACTURE. A fall on the dorsum of the wrist may cause the "reversed Colles" or Smith's fracture. Reduction is analogous, but with immobilization with the wrist in some extension.

In certain very comminuted or unstable fractures, it is not possible to maintain the reduction with external immobilization by plaster and/or splint techniques. For these patients it may be necessary to resort to more complex techniques. These may involve the percutaneous placement of a pin through one of the fragment(s), the insertion of pins into the index metacarpal and the proximal ulna or midradius with the use of external rigid framing or plaster incorporating the pins, or various types of plates with screws.

Regardless of the technique used, the assessment of the adequacy of the reduction must include length of the radial styloid, volar tilt of the distal articular face of the radius, and congruity and alignment of the articular surfaces of both the distal radius to the carpus and the distal radius to the distal ulna.

LIGAMENTOUS INJURIES OF THE WRIST. The multiple carpal bones are interconnected with an incredibly complex array of interosseous ligaments. Disruption of these ligaments can be caused by many types of significant wrist trauma with or without associated fractures. Ligament injury diagnosis is difficult and may require multiple special x-ray techniques. The most common involve the ligaments between the radius, scaphoid, and lunate, resulting in scapholunate dissociation and rotatory instability of the scaphoid. With this injury, the two most common x-ray findings are an increase in the gap between the scaphoid and lunate on anteroposterior x-ray ("Terry Thomas sign") and a decrease in the scaphoid height on the anteroposterior x-ray taken in the neutral position such that the scaphoid looks round rather than oval (signet sign). Another interosseous disruption is that of the lunatotriquetral joint. Satisfactory results from treatment of this condition are rare unless the ligaments are repaired acutely.

FRACTURES OF THE SCAPHOID. Young adults who fall on the outstretched hand frequently fracture the scaphoid (see Fig. 43-67). The most consistent physical finding is that of tenderness over the scaphoid in the anatomic snuffbox. With any wrist injury, it is imperative to rule out a fractured scaphoid, as delay in treatment may well result in nonunion. The arterial supply to the scaphoid enters the distal third, most commonly the proximal third blood supply being only by intraosseous vascular channels. Fractures that transect the waist or proximal third may often interrupt the entire circulaton to the proximal pole, resulting not only in nonunion, but in avascular necrosis of this proximal third.

In addition to the standard AP, lateral, and oblique x-rays of the wrist, a special 17° angled AP x-ray view (scaphoid view) is needed. Note that if the patient has a history of recent trauma, with well-localized tenderness over the scaphoid, the patient must be presumed to have a fracture of the scaphoid even if the x-ray examination is negative. This patient should be immobilized in plaster as if the scaphoid were fractured, and then re-x-rayed at 3 weeks. At this time, if a fracture is present, the resorption at the fracture site will usually be apparent. Occasionally, marked tenderness will persist in spite of repeat normal x-rays; if this is the case, three more weeks of immobilization are advised with another set of x-rays after that. At 6 weeks, if no fracture is seen but the tenderness persists, another source of pain must be sought.

With undisplaced fractures of the scaphoid, the optimal treatment is plaster immobilization from the tip of the thumb to include the elbow. By immobilizing the elbow, pronation-supination (which will cause motion at the fracture site) is prevented.

Most scaphoid fractures will heal with 4 months of adequate plaster immobilization. The patient is usually seen at monthly intervals for skin care and cast change. X-rays out of plaster are usually obtained at 6 weeks and subsequently at 4-week intervals. When all tenderness from direct pressure over the tuberosity of the scaphoid has disappeared *and* x-rays show obliteration of the fracture site, plaster immobilization is discontinued. In some situations, 6 months is required for bony union. If nonunion occurs, bone grafting is necessary. If the interval between trauma and diagnosis is less than 4 months, in certain situations prolonged plaster immobilization will result in union without bone grafting.

In displaced fractures of the scaphoid that are not reduced by gentle positioning of the wrist, open reduction and internal fixation of the scaphoid may be necessary.

LUNATE AND PERILUNATE DISLOCATIONS. These injuries must be considered in any patient who falls on the outstretched hand with secondary wrist hyperextension. The diagnosis is made by x-ray. On the normal lateral x-ray, the radius, lunate, and capitate are axially aligned. Disruption of this alignment with the lunate anterior, or the capitate dorsal, is diagnostic (Fig. 45-6).

Treatment of the acute injury is closed reduction and plaster immobilization. Reduction is accomplished by traction and manipulation. The wrist must be carefully checked clinically and by x-ray after reduction for intercarpal instability. If intercarpal instability is present, ligamentous repair is advised.

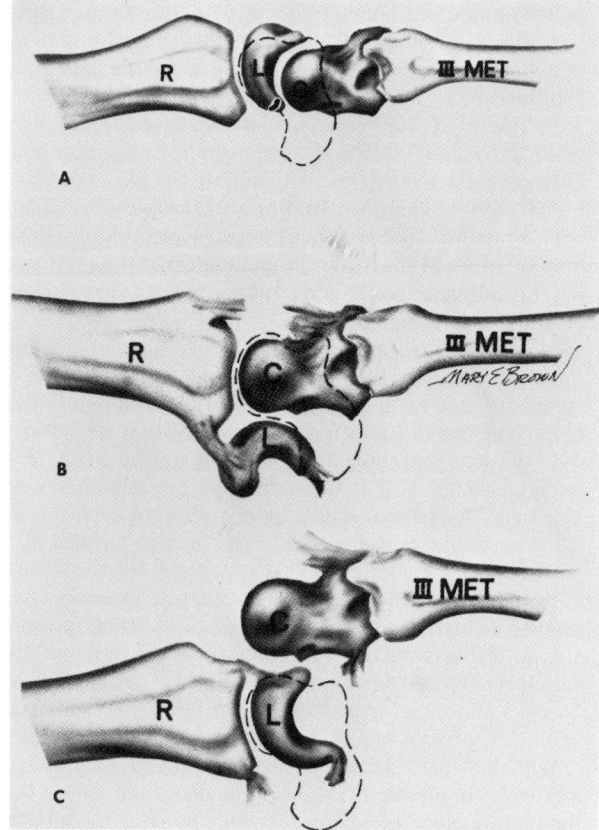

Fig. 45-6. *A.* Normal lateral view of the radius (R), lunate (L), capitate (C), and scaphoid (dotted outline B). *B.* Dislocated lunate. Note position of lunate relative to the radius and capitate. *C.* Perilunar dislocation. Note position of capitate relative to the radius and lunate. (From: *Hill NA: Fractures and dislocations of the carpus. Orthop Clin North Am 1:275, 1970, with permission.*)

It may be very difficult to reduce these dislocations when seen late, even with surgical exploration. It is therefore essential, when reviewing the lateral wrist x-ray of a patient with a history of trauma, to be certain that the radius, lunate, and capitate are in normal alignment.

METACARPAL FRACTURES. Metacarpal fractures are very common, most often occurring when the hand strikes against an opponent (so-called boxer fracture). These are more common for the ring and little fingers than the index and long. The diagnosis is suspected by local swelling and tenderness over the distal metacarpal, combined with some loss of knuckle prominence. Any lacerations associated with these should be assumed a human bite until definitely established otherwise, and treated accordingly. The degree of angulation may be masked by the amount of swelling and can be determined only by accurate *lateral* x-ray. The rotational deformity of these fractures must be carefully assessed clinically to avoid grotesque rotational malunions. Each finger, when flexed individually into the palm, should point to the scaphoid.

Treatment of the acute metacarpal neck fracture is by closed reduction of both the angulation and any rotational deformity that might be present. Up to 35 to 40° of angula-

tion of the metacarpal neck can be accepted for the ring and little fingers if rotation is normal, but only 10 to 15° for the index and long fingers. The digit is immobilized with the metacarpophalangeal joint flexed 60 to 70° and the interphalangeal joints in full extension. An adjacent digit should be included in the immobilization to facilitate control of rotational alignment. Should the fracture be unstable in this position, or should multiple metacarpal fractures be present, intermedullary fixation is often required. This is done in the operating room environment by inserting a single intramedullary wire percutaneously from distal to proximal, starting on the margin of the metacarpal head and avoiding the articular surface.

Any such percutaneous Kirschner wire fixation serves only as an internal support and *must* be combined with the use of external plaster immobilization. Pins and cast are discontinued after the fracture has healed. Oblique, spiral, or transverse metacarpal shaft fractures should be similarly reduced and immobilized, and also may require percutaneous internal fixation if unstable in the anteroposterior, lateral, or rotatory planes. Occasional metacarpal fractures require plate and/or screw fixation.

CARPOMETACARPAL JOINT DISLOCATIONS. Carpometacarpal joint dislocations of the digits are most easily diagnosed on an accurate lateral x-ray of the involved area. It is often possible to reduce these closed, but percutaneous internal fixation is usually necessary. Not infrequently these injuries require open reduction and internal fixation.

BENNETT'S FRACTURE. Bennett's fracture is an intraarticular fracture at the base of the thumb metacarpal (see Fig. 43-68). Essentially, it is an avulsion fracture with the strong joint ligaments remaining attached to the small bone fragment and with the abductor pollicis longus subluxing the metacarpal shaft laterally. This results in an unstable fracture with joint incongruity.

These fractures often can be reduced closed, but usually are unstable. Traction is applied to the axis of the shaft of the metacarpal, which is then brought into abduction while direct adduction pressure is applied to the base of the metacarpal. Percutaneous wire fixation of the metacarpal to the trapezium and adjacent carpus (not attempting to transfix the small fragment) will usually maintain the adequate reduction. Assessment of the reduction must include the alignment of the metacarpal shaft on the trapezium and restoration of the articular contour of the metacarpal base. If this is not the situation, open reduction and internal fixation with a Kirschner pin are indicated.

THUMB METACARPOPHALANGEAL JOINT. One of the most common injuries to the hand is an abduction force applied to the thumb with disruption of the ulnar collateral ligament system at the metacarpophalangeal joint. This is a common acute injury in skiing and in football. It also may follow repetitive low-grade force, as originally described in gamekeepers who used their thumb to dislocate rabbit necks—hence the term "gamekeeper's thumb." The diagnosis is made by valgus instability of the joint (Fig. 45-7, bottom). In a high percentage of cases, the ruptured ligament, with or without an avulsed

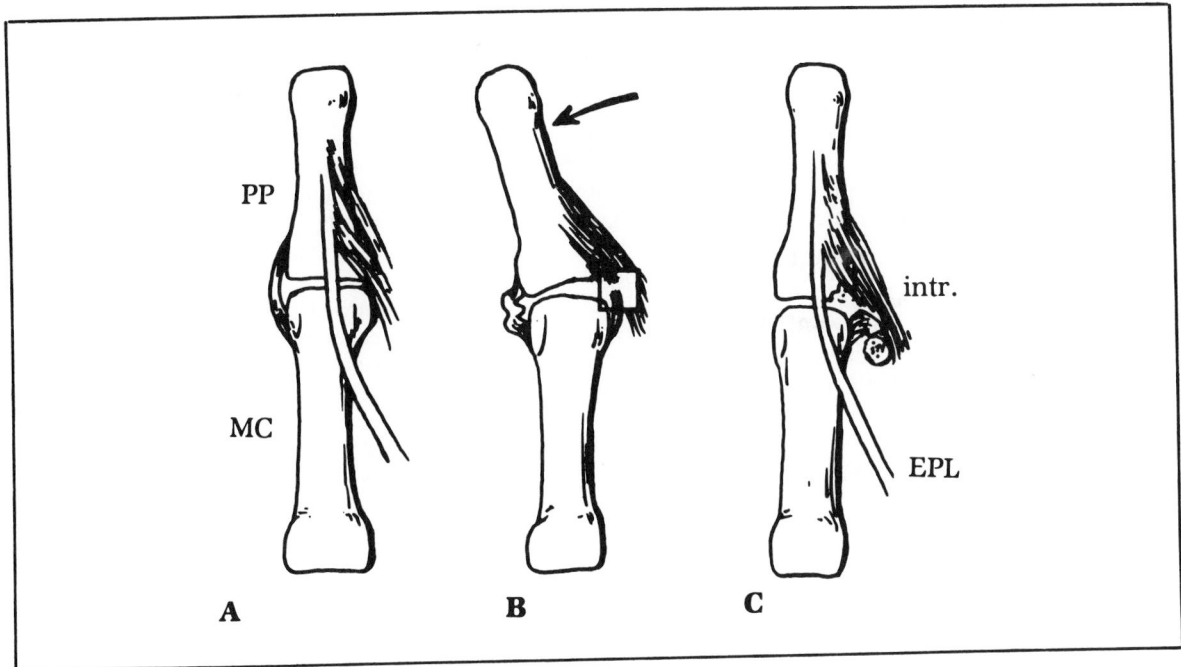

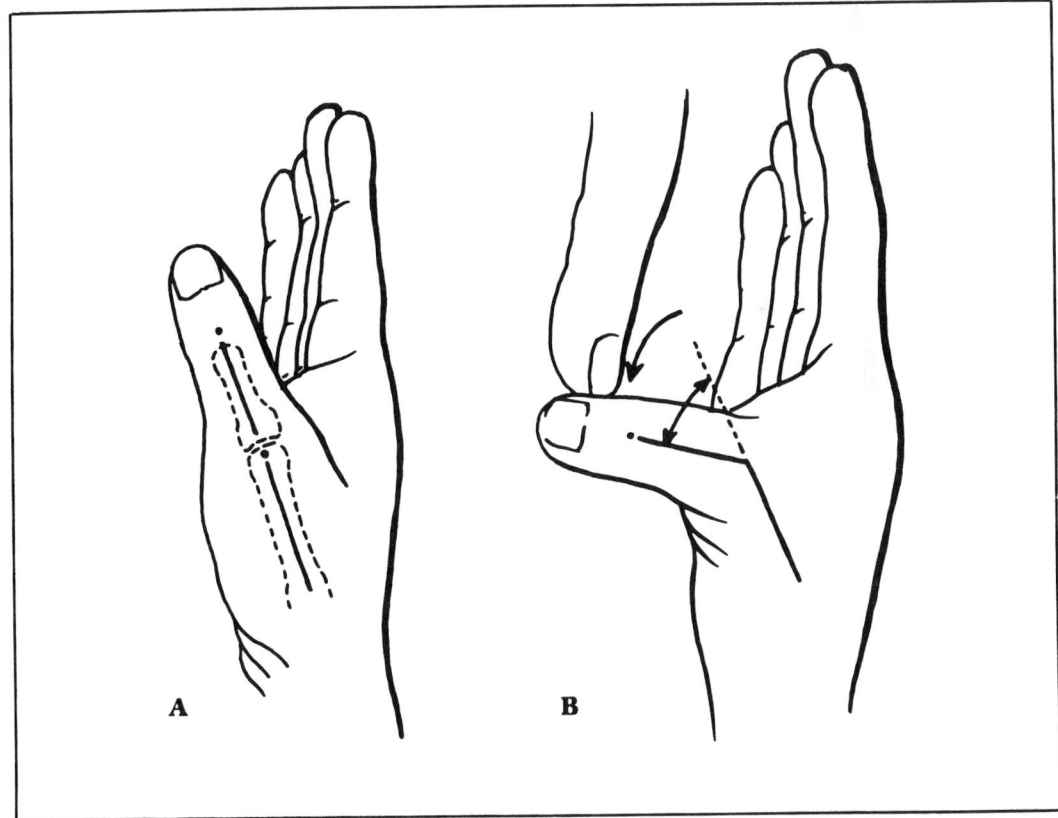

Fig. 45-7. *Top,* disruption of the ulnar collateral ligament mechanism of the metacarpophalangeal joint of the thumb is common. It may be with or without an avulsion fracture. The ligament is held in its displaced position by the adductor tendon expansion. *Bottom,* clinical diagnosis is made by a valgus stress test. This test should not be performed if a fracture is suspected or if the patient is a child with suspected epiphyseal injury. [From: *Burton RI: Acute joint injuries of the hand, in Wolfort FG (ed): Acute Hand Injuries: A Multispecialty Approach. Boston, Little, Brown, 1980, with permission.*]

bony fragment, is held in a displaced position by the interposed adductor and flexor brevis tendon expansion (Fig. 45-7, top). If valgus instability of the joint is present, open repair of the ligament system is indicated.

PROXIMAL PHALANGEAL FRACTURES. Fractures of the proximal phalanx of the fingers are common and potentially very disabling. There is an essential joint for digital function at either end of the bone. This phalanx is surrounded by tendons, the extensor mechanism on the dorsum and each side and the flexor tendon volarly. These tendons are directly adjacent to the periosteum. Because of the critical joints at each end of the bone and the tendon on all four sides, reduction of these fractures must be precise if disability is to be minimized. If the fracture is unstable in the "safe position," percutaneous fixation with a Kirschner pin(s) may be necessary. The pin(s) should be placed in an operating room environment after the appropriate aseptic technique to minimize the risk of secondary infection. External plaster immobilization in the safe position is necessary for 3 to 4 weeks with or without the Kirschner pin. The percutaneous fixation serves only as an internal strut, and its use will be fraught with complications if it is not combined with external immobilization as well.

PROXIMAL INTERPHALANGEAL JOINT. The proximal interphalangeal joint is frequently injured. Incomplete collateral ligament tears can be treated with *dorsal* splinting for 2 weeks followed by "buddy taping." Dorsal dislocations are common, and once reduced, are usually stable because the collateral ligaments remain intact (Fig. 45-8). These dislocations should be protected with a *dor-*sal splint in 20° of flexion for 3 weeks followed by 2 additional weeks of "buddy taping." Dorsal dislocations/subluxations with avulsion fractures from the volar base of the middle phalanx can be treated as simple dislocations if the fragment is small. If the fragment involves over 20 percent of the articular surface, the joint may be very unstable and require open treatment (Fig. 45-8).

MIDDLE PHALANX. These fractures are common and usually respond to closed reduction with external immobilization.

DISTAL PHALANX. Crushing injuries of the terminal segment occur frequently. They are often associated with significant nail and nail matrix injuries. Injuries to the nail matrix must be repaired. If the nail matrix and nail plate are intact, but a subungual hematoma is present, this can be drained by drilling through the nail plate with a hot paper clip heated on a Bunsen burner or by a #11 blade. This should be done after sterile preparation, as it will compound the fracture. If a fracture of a distal phalanx is displaced and associated with nail matrix injury, it is important to explore the fracture site to be certain that no nail matrix is interposed, as this will predispose to chronic osteomyelitis. The nail matrix must then be very precisely repaired with 6-0 or 7-0 absorbable sutures, using magnification.

Fig. 45-8. Lateral view of the finger showing the common types of proximal interphalangeal joint injuries. Dorsal dislocations without intraarticular fracture are usually stable once reduced. Similarly, small avulsion fragments are stable, but with a large fragment the dislocation is unstable (see text). [From: *Burton RI: Acute joint injuries of the hand, in Wolfort FG (ed): Acute Hand Injuries: A Multispecialty Approach. Boston, Little, Brown, 1980, with permission.*]

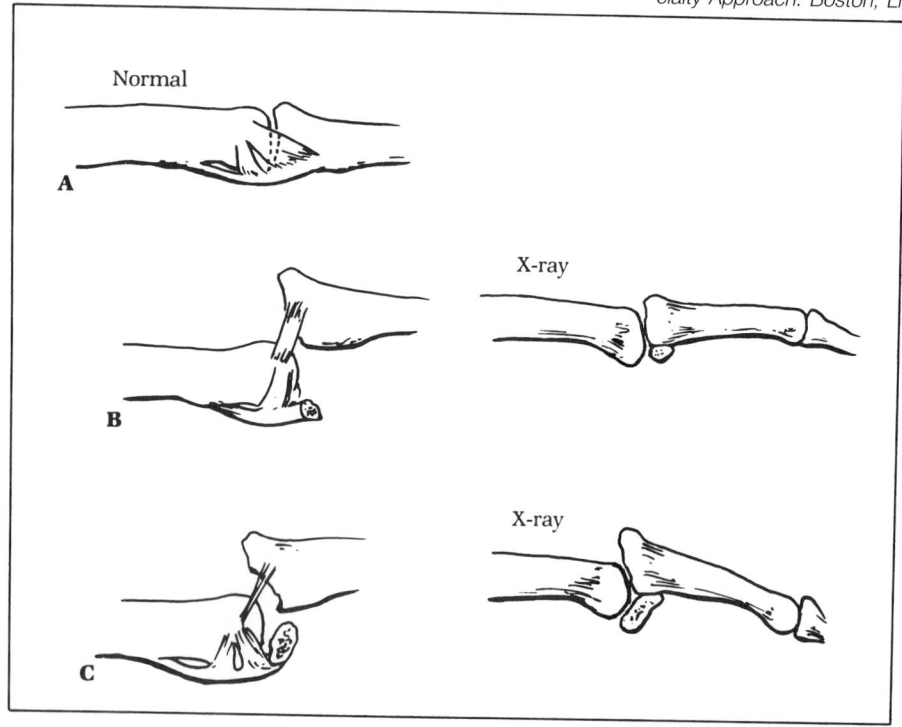

Tendon Injuries

The healing of tendon is a dynamic event depending upon local cellular activity. There is debate over whether the tendons possess the necessary metabolic activity for inherent healing, or whether healing depends upon cellular ingrowth from the sheath and other adjacent tissues. Both are probably possible. Because of the relatively avascular nature of tendons, the slow metabolism of the very few cells within the tendon substance, and the great reactivity of the vascular pedicle (mesotendon) and the layering of the covering structures, tendon healing is relatively slow and prone to scarring and adhesions to adjacent structures. Clinical results are facilitated if the intratendinous healing predominates, and the operation and postoperative care must assume this.

The ideal goal of tendon surgery is to place unmolested tendon surface into an untraumatized bed. The ultimate goal is good tendon strength with remodeling of the tendon callus to allow the differential development of healed tendon substance with a smooth surface to allow gliding capability. Repair of a traumatized tendon is technically very difficult, requires special training, and must bring cut tendon ends into precise coaptation without interfering seriously with the physiologic elements important for healing. Technical finesse is necessary to minimize scar formation. Unfortunately, there remain many situations where unavoidable adhesions will negate good technical

surgery. In certain secondary reconstructive procedures, silicone rods are used to create channels for tendon sliding of the subsequent second-stage flexor tendon graft.

FLEXOR TENDON INJURIES. The management of lacerations of flexor tendon injuries of the forearm, wrist, hand, and fingers has been the subject of debate for many years. There are no absolute rules for correct treatment, but several facts must be considered. Any injury that involves tendons, nerves, vessels, fascia, joints, and soft tissue will heal as a single wound. Tendons with repairs adjacent to each other are likely to become adherent to each other as healing progresses. Similarly, a tendon repair that is adjacent to a fixed fibrous structure, such as palmar fascia, transverse carpal ligament, or flexor tendon pulleys, may become fixed to that adjacent tissue by scar tissue, thus obviating the goal of flexor tendon surgery. Better understanding of the anatomy and physiology, combined with significant technical advances during the past several years, has improved the prognosis for these injuries.

It should be noted that the intrinsic musculotendinous units (interossei and lumbricals) do flex the metacarpophalangeal joints (see Fig. 45-9). The goal of extrinsic flexor tendon repair is to reestablish interphalangeal joint flexion.

The long flexor tendons (superficialis and profundus) in each digit pass through a rigid tunnel of fascia that extends from the distal palmar crease to the distal portion of

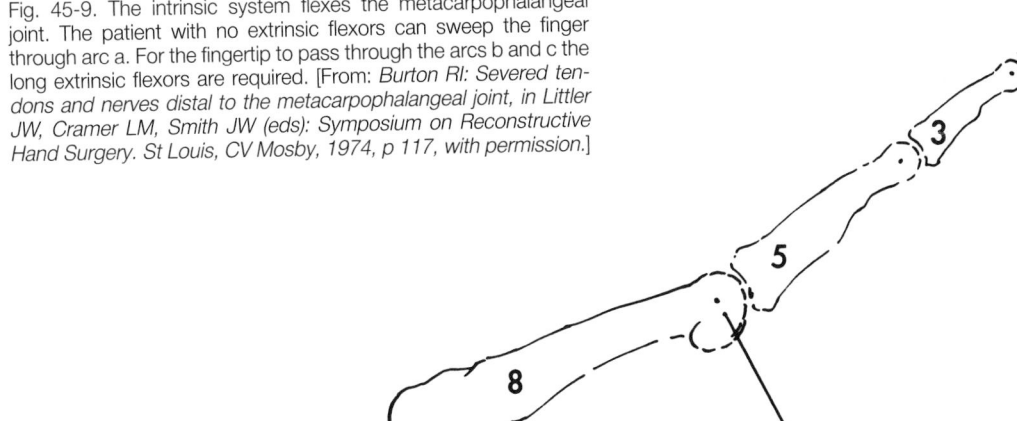
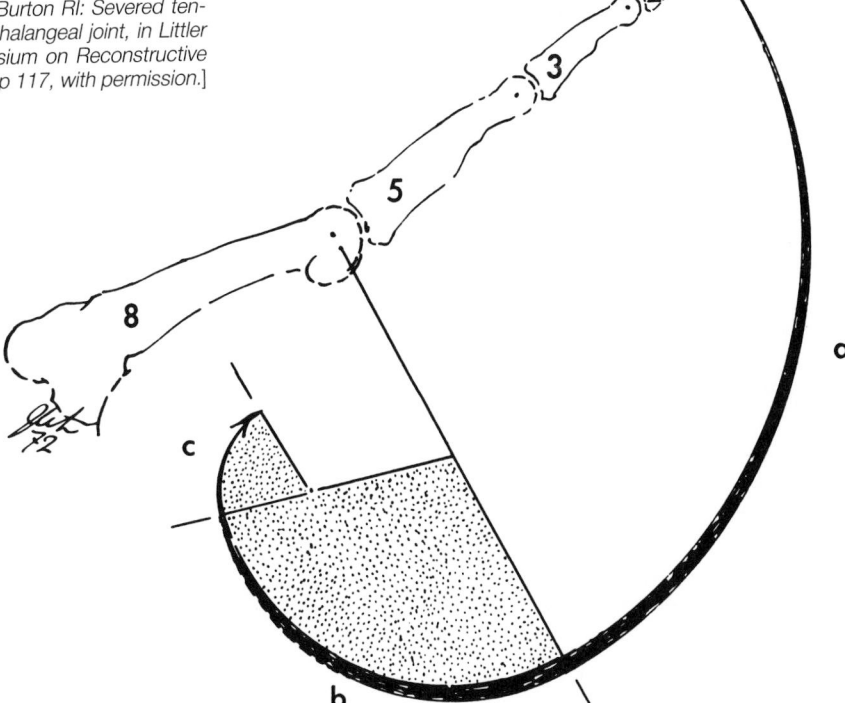

Fig. 45-9. The intrinsic system flexes the metacarpophalangeal joint. The patient with no extrinsic flexors can sweep the finger through arc a. For the fingertip to pass through the arcs b and c the long extrinsic flexors are required. [From: *Burton RI: Severed tendons and nerves distal to the metacarpophalangeal joint, in Littler JW, Cramer LM, Smith JW (eds): Symposium on Reconstructive Hand Surgery. St Louis, CV Mosby, 1974, p 117, with permission.*]

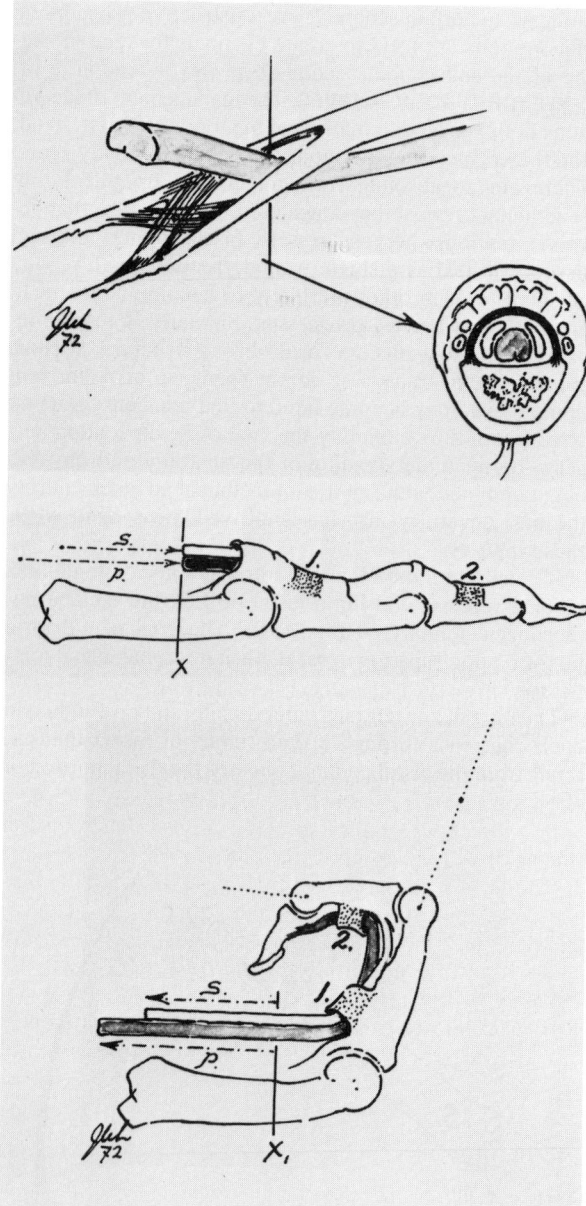

Fig. 45-10. A fibroosseous tunnel extends on the flexor aspect of the digit from the metacarpophalangeal joint level to the base of the terminal phalanx. There are two strategic areas of thickening, one at the proximal end of the proximal phalanx and one at the midportion of the middle phalanx, although a total of seven pulleys are well described in the literature. There is a significant excursion of the flexor tendons within this sheath, that for the profundus being greater than that for the superficial flexor. Note that the profundus passes through a decussation in the superficial flexor at the proximal phalangeal level. (From: *Burton RI, Littler JW: Dynamics of normal hand function, in Nontraumatic Soft Tissue Afflictions of the Hand. Current Problems in Surgery. Chicago, Year Book Medical Publishers, 1975, with permission.*)

the middle phalanx. There are four annular pulleys and three cruciate pulleys; the annular restraint at the base of the proximal phalanx and the annular restraint at the midportion of the middle phalanx are the two essential structures to prevent ventral bowstringing of the tendons during active digital flexion (Fig. 45-10). In addition, at the wrist the thick fibrous flexor retinaculum that constitutes the roof of the carpal tunnel is a major pulley mechanism.

Verdan (Fig. 45-11) has designated six zones of the hand where lacerations correlate with prognosis. It must be emphasized that it is the level of tendon laceration, not the location of the skin laceration, that determines the zone. If the laceration occurs with the digits in flexion, as when grabbing the blade of an assailant's knife, the level of tendon laceration may be several centimeters from the level of skin laceration when the digit is in the extended position. Zone 1, distal to the digital fibroosseous tunnel, is an area where prognosis is good. Repair of the profundus tendon can be performed primarily at this level. In Zone 6, the wrist area, only the profundus tendon is usually repaired. In Zone 5, the palm, both superficial and profundus tendons are often repaired.

Tendon lacerations in Zone 2 (no-man's land), the region of the digital fibroosseous tunnel, remain controversial in terms of treatment. For children, all surgeons agree on primary repair of the profundus tendon or the flexor

Fig. 45-11. Zones of flexor tendon injury as described by Verdan. Note that the level refers to that of tendon injury, not of skin laceration.

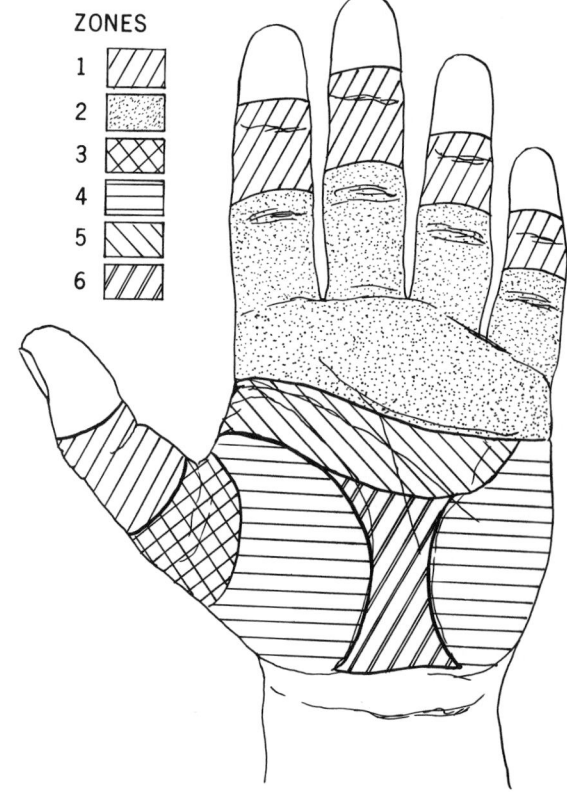

ZONES
1
2
3
4
5
6

pollicis longus. Many will repair the flexor digitorum superficialis as well. In adults, the trend is toward primary repair of the profundus tendon in the digit, provided the laceration is clean, there is minimal associated injury with at least one intact digital nerve, and the initial wound treatment is prompt. The term "primary repair" is used by some surgeons to refer to repair within 4 to 6 h. Many surgeons prefer to do primary repair as follows: directly after the injury, the wound is copiously irrigated and meticulously closed, the hand placed in a bulky protective dressing, the patient given antibiotics, and the hand kept elevated. The sutures are removed at approximately 2 days. If there is no evidence of infection, the primary flexor tendon repair is done within the first 7 days following injury. It must be emphasized that primary repair of flexor tendons is a technically demanding surgical procedure and must be done by surgeons with special training and experience. There must be proper attention to technique, good wound care, and early and proper intensive hand therapy in order to produce adequate results. There are many different techniques of tendon repair (Fig. 45-12); types A, B, C, and D are those most often selected for flexor tendon repair.

As an alternative procedure, thorough wound irrigation and primary skin closure with digital nerve repair if necessary is performed. This is particularly applicable if the laceration is jagged, treatment is delayed, or the wound is heavily inoculated. After the digit has been mobilized passively and after there has been a suitable delay for wound healing, a free tendon graft is performed. One repair site is placed in the palm and the other at the insertion on the distal phalanx, both favorable sites for tendon repair without fixed adjacent structures.

EXTENSOR TENDON INJURIES. Extensor tendon lacerations in the forearm or over the dorsum of the hand have a favorable prognosis because of the tendon location within loose areolar tissue and skin that are usually as mobile as the physiologic excursion of the extensor tendon at that level, thus rarely restricting function. This is not the case over the dorsum of the wrist, where the tendons may adhere to the extensor retinaculum. At this site it is often advisable to transpose the repair tendon into the subcutaneous plane, closing the retinaculum deep to the repaired tendon with inverting sutures.

BOUTONNIERE DEFORMITY. Disruption of the central tendon near its insertion into the dorsal base of the middle phalanx is accompanied by tears in the lateral extensions into the two lateral bands. The lateral bands then displace palmar to the axis of PIP joint rotation, causing these lateral band tendons to lose extensor function at the PIP joint and to become actually PIP joint flexors (Fig. 45-13). Thus the joint has lost both intrinsic and extrinsic extensors and must assume an attitude of flexion. Acutely, after injury, the patient will usually be able to sustain the joint in full extension once it is passively placed in that position, but will be unable to initiate full extension from the flexed position. With time in the untreated patient, the joint becomes fixed in the flexed position. Repeated attempts by the patient to actively extend the PIP joint will bypass that joint and will be transmitted to the distal joint through the lateral bands, causing hyperextension of the DIP joint.

The acute injury may be a laceration or may be a closed injury. In either, if the proximal interphalangeal joint is immobilized with a dorsal splint holding it in 0° of extension for 6 to 8 weeks, the tendon will heal satisfactorily and chronic deformity is prevented. The MCP joint and DIP joint may be left free to move. Following the weeks of immobilization, the joint motion is started in the hand therapy unit, with a dorsal splint to be used between the exercise sessions until motion has been regained. Some surgeons prefer to repair the tendon laceration surgically. If surgery is selected, the sutures must be very accurately placed and the exact same splinting program followed. The surgery does not shorten the postinjury splinting or exercise program. The length and tension in the repaired tendon must be accurate within 1 mm if the exquisitely balanced tendon mechanics are to be maintained.

MALLET FINGER. Injuries of the extensor insertion into the dorsal base of the distal phalanx are common. These injuries are usually closed and caused by blunt trauma to the tip of the digit with resultant avulsion of the insertion of the extensor mechanism, with or without a fracture fragment (Fig. 45-14). X-rays must be taken to determine the presence or absence of the avulsion fracture. If blunt trauma caused the mallet, the PIP joint must also be carefully examined clinically and by x-ray to rule out the frequent associated injuries at that level. If the fracture fragment is small with a minimal amount of the joint surface involved, the treatment is the same as for simple tendon avulsion without fracture using a dorsal splint, holding the terminal joint at 0° with the PIP joint free. This splinting must be continued for 8 weeks, with the splint removed daily for skin care; the DIP joint must be supported at 0° whenever the splint is off. If the fracture involves more than one-third of the articular surface and is displaced, particularly if there is volar subluxation of the terminal phalanx, a procedure of open reduction and internal fixation is often recommended.

Nerve Injuries

Injury to a specific peripheral nerve will result in a specific pattern of distal sensory and motor loss. The ultimate final recovery of any complex injury may depend to a large measure upon the proper surgical management of the injured nerve(s). Nerve injuries may involve stretching or compression (neuropraxia) or nerve transection (axonotmesis or neurotmesis).

Stretching or compression injuries that do not transect the nerve have a better prognosis with a faster and more complete recovery than those involving transection. Electromyography and nerve conduction studies may be helpful in diagnosis and in assessment of recovery.

Following complete nerve transection, operative repair is required. There has been much debate over whether nerves should be repaired primarily at the time of initial wound therapy or secondarily after a short delay, but it is generally agreed that nerve repair is definitely progressively less effective after 6 months following injury. Al-

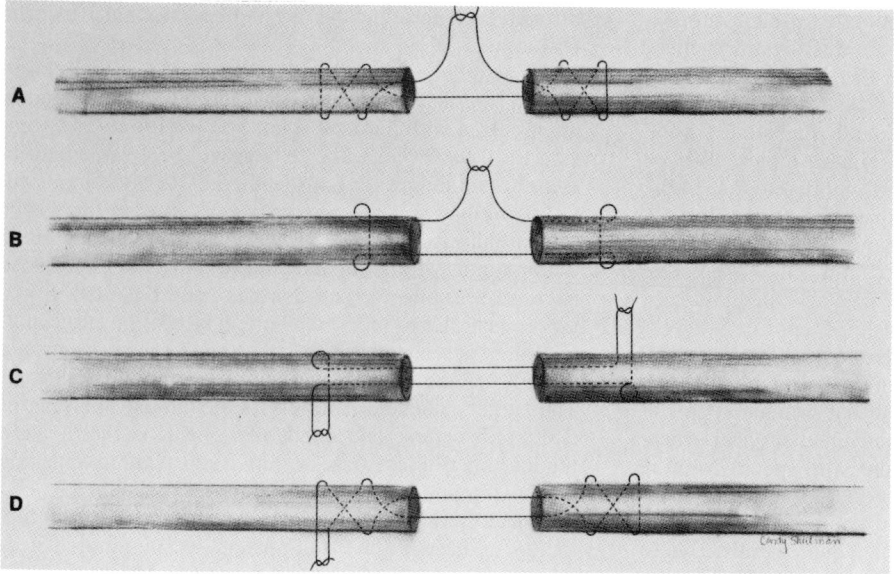

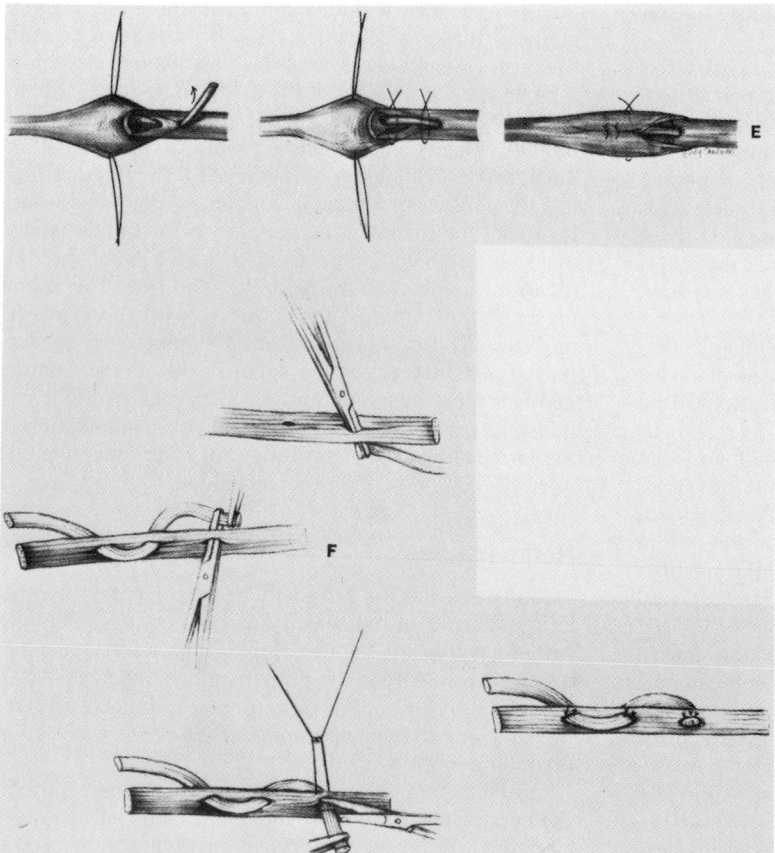

Fig. 45-12. Common types of suture used for tendon repair. *A* to *D* illustrate types used for tendons of equal diameter; *E* and *F* illustrate repairs for tendons of significantly dissimilar diameters. [From: *Burton RI: The hand, in Goldstein LA, Dickerson RC (eds): Atlas of Orthopaedic Surgery. St Louis, CV Mosby, 1981, with permission.*]

though results are generally poor with repair delayed over 2 years, exceptions may occur, especially in children.

Whether repaired at the time of initial wound treatment or shortly thereafter, a precise repair with careful realignment of the fascicles (orientation aided by realigning the small blood vessels found on the nerve surface) is best done with 4 to 15 power magnification and 8-0 to 11-0 nylon suture material. The repair should be under minimal or no tension. Careful epineural repair is generally favored (Fig. 45-15).

Recovery after successful nerve repair progresses in a predictable manner. Sensibility returns, starting proxi-

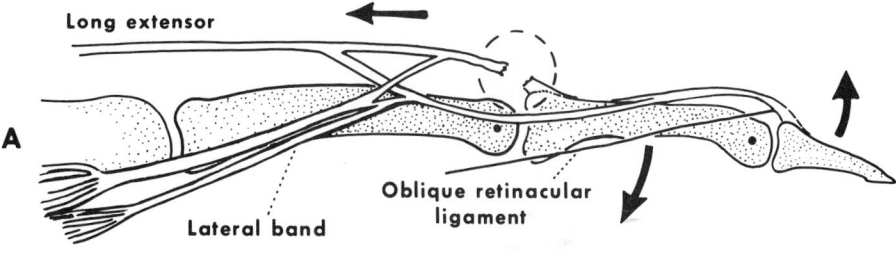

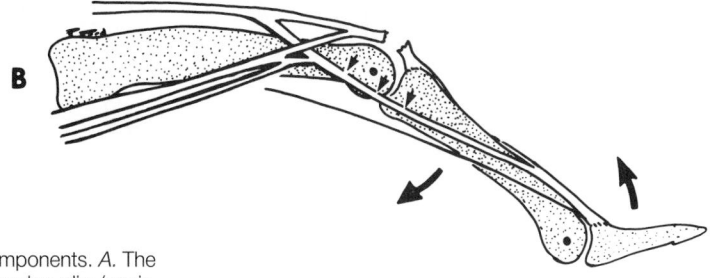

Fig. 45-13. Boutonniere deformity has several components. *A.* The acute lesion involves disruption of the central tendon slip (encircled). The proximal interphalangeal joint then drops into flexion, and the extensor mechanism shifts proximally and volarly. *B.* The lateral bands are then anterior to the axis of PIP joint motion (small arrows). If the extensor mechanism heals in this position, the lateral bands and oblique retinacular ligaments will tether the PIP joint in flexion and the DIP joint in extension. (From: *Burton RI, Eaton RG: Hand injuries in the athlete. Orthop Clin North Am 4:809, 1973, with permission.*)

mally and moving distally as the axons regenerate and grow down the sheath. Regeneration will proceed on the average of 1 mm per day and will be faster and more complete in young children than in adults. Regeneration may be followed clinically by observation of the distal progression of the Tinel's sign (an electriclike sensation perceived by the patient with percussion over the regenerating nerve), specific sensibility testing, careful distal motor examination, electromyography, nerve conduction velocities, and sudomotor testing.

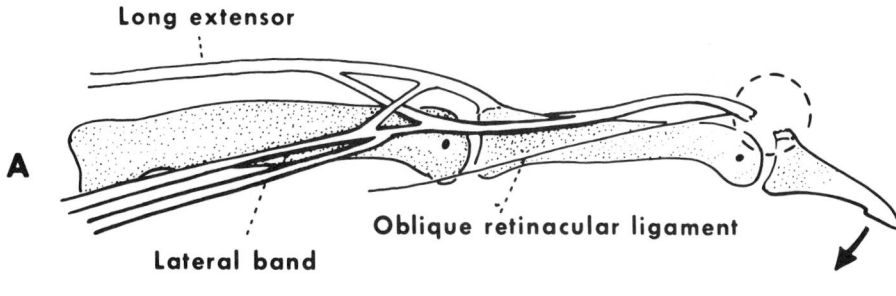

Fig. 45-14. The mallet deformity results from a disruption of the insertion of the extensor mechanism into the dorsal base of the distal phalanx by tendon avulsion *(A)* or by fracture *(B, C).* The lesions of *A* and *B* are treated closed, but *C* requires open reduction and internal fixation because of joint incongruity and volar subluxation of the terminal phalanx. (From: *Burton RI, Eaton RG: Hand injuries in the athlete. Orthop Clin North Am 4:809, 1973, with permission.*)

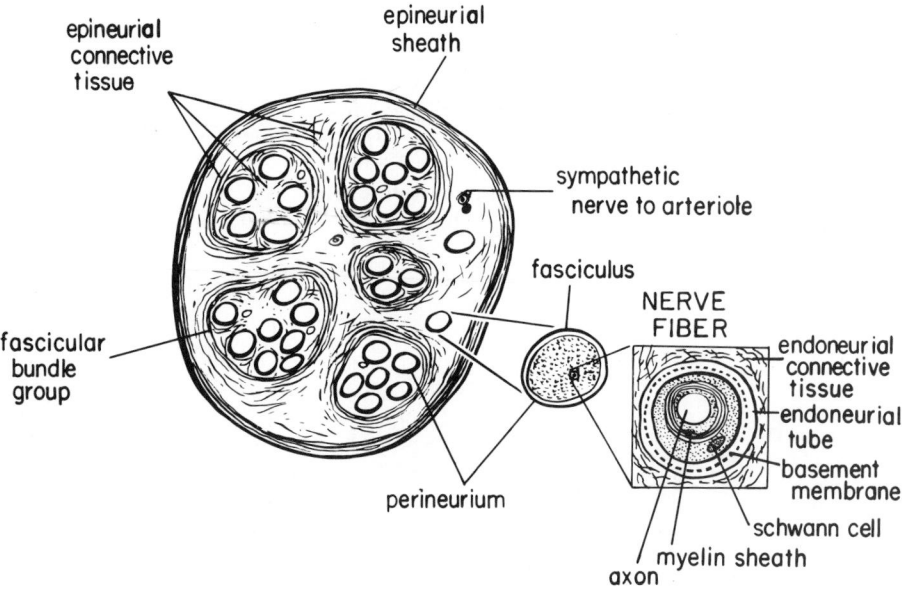

Fig. 45-15. Cross-sectional anatomy of nerve. [From: *Tupper JW: Fascicular nerve repair, in Omer GE, Spinner M (eds): Management of Peripheral Nerve Problems. Philadelphia, Saunders, 1980, with permission.*]

In late (secondary) cases of nerve repair, or in acute injuries with loss of nerve substance, there is a gap in the nerve. The nerve must be repaired without tension. Techniques to accomplish this include the proximal and distal immobilization of the nerve, sometimes with rerouting of the nerve to gain additional length. Care must be taken not to devascularize the nerve. Fascicular nerve grafting is being done with increasing frequency in these difficult problems to avoid tension on the repair site; if the nerve does not easily come together with 8-0 suture, the tension is probably excessive.

Fingertip Injuries

Simple lacerations should be meticulously debrided and closed as soon as possible. If the nail matrix or nail bed is injured, it should be carefully approximated with 6-0 absorbable suture material. To do this, it may be necessary to remove the nail plate for adequate exposure. When severe crush injury is involved, or mangling injuries, conservative terminal amputation may be indicated. Distal transverse amputations are best closed with a thin split-thickness skin graft. If the absent tissue contained the pulp, thus leaving bone or tendon exposed, a cross-finger flap can be considered. If adequate pulp remains to cover the bone (as seen with a tangential amputation of the tip), a free full-thickness skin graft will give a good result. Fractures of the tuft of the distal phalanx rarely require internal fixation, but if displaced, should be carefully checked to rule out interposed nail matrix. Badly comminuted open tuft fractures with insufficient soft tissue cover are best treated by shortening, with available local tissue or free skin graft.

Excellent results, particularly in young children, can be obtained by careful wound toilet and dressing to allow epithelialization, *if* there is no exposed bone or tendon.

Infections

The vulnerability of the hand to frequent wounding makes it a common portal of entry for bacterial invasion. This, coupled with the superficial location of bone, joints, and the concentration of relatively avascular tendons, sets the stage for grave local infections. The potential spaces of the bursa and moist synovial sheaths with the constant massaging motion augment the problem (Table 45-1).

In taking the history, particular note must be made of influencing diseases, such as diabetes, arthritis, cardio-pulmonary or renal disorders, and drug addiction. The amount and the quality of pain are important. Severe pain is ominous, but the absence of pain can be misleading. Injuries that are particularly susceptible to subsequent infection are those with crush, those occurring in a filthy environment (meat-cutting plants, farmyards, certain types of manual labor), puncture wounds with contaminated foreign bodies, and the injection of human saliva. There is an ever-increasing incidence of severe and exotic hand infections in drug addicts. As the proximal veins become obstructed and thrombosed, the addict turns to the digital veins as a portal of entry. At this site, the extravasation of contaminated materials may lead to disastrous infections. At the time of physical examination for suspected infection, the regional examination must include not only the local findings but also possible lymphangitis or lymphadenopathy.

When an area shows signs of early inflammation and possible infection, the differential diagnosis must include chemical or metabolic synovitis, gout, rheumatoid arthritis, Reiter's syndrome, and nonspecific tenosynovitis.

Table 45-1. DIFFERENTIAL DIAGNOSIS OF HAND INFECTION

	Paronychia	Terminal pulp infection	Acute cellulitis
Time of presentation from onset	2–5 days	4–5 days	12–24 h
Cause	Nail biting Manicuring	Puncture wound	Prick or not known
Organism	Mixed	Staphylococcus	Streptococcus
Symptoms	Tender swelling around nail fold	Throbbing pain confined to the end of the finger increasing daily and preventing sleep	Hot red finger. Malaise, shivering, and tenderness up arm to axilla
Physical signs	Fluctuant swelling of nail fold Often subcuticular pus	Hot, red, tense, and tender pulp. Often subcuticular pus. Rest of the finger normal	Hot red finger. Not very swollen
Movements	Full. Painless	Full. Painless	Practically full. Painless
Temperature	Normal	Normal	Raised
Lymphangitis	No	No	Yes
Differential diagnosis	1 Early acute cellulitis 2 Lateral pulp infection 3 Late subungual hematoma	1 Acute cellulitis 2 Early paronychia 3 Hematoma of pulp following trauma	Early pulp infection, especially apical infection

	Tendon sheath infection	Boil or carbuncle	Palmar and web infection	Infective arthritis
	6–36 h	2–3 days	2–3 days	1–3 days from onset infection. Up to 3 weeks from time of original injury
	Midline injury with sharp instrument	Often not known	Puncture wound—often splinter	Cut or puncture over dorsum of the joint
	Streptococcus	Staphylococcus	Staphylococcus	Mixed
	Hot, red, swollen finger. Extremely painful especially on movement. Malaise. Tenderness up arm to axilla	Painful swelling on the back of the hand or fingers. History of previous boils	Throbbing pain in the palm and gross swelling of the back of the hand	Painful swelling all round the infected joint and discharging wound on the dorsum
	Whole finger hot, red, and swollen. Maximal on dorsum. Tenderness along course of the sheath maximal in proximal compartment in the palm	Cellulitis and edema of dorsum, with triangular spread to the wrist. Later, discharging lesion	Infected puncture wound in palm brawny, red, and tender. Swelling and pitting edema of dorsum. In web infections fingers separated. Best seen from the dorsum	Cellulitis of whole finger. Swelling tenderness maximal all round the infected joint. Discharging wound on dorsum
	Extremely painful, especially extension	Full	Slight limitation by pain in fingers	Flexion and extension limited and painful. Lateral movement increased and crepitus present
	Raised	Slightly raised	Slightly raised	Normal
	Yes	Sometimes	Sometimes	No
	1 Acute cellulitis 2 Middle or proximal space infection 3 Fascial infection	Palmar or web infection	1 Early carbuncle 2 Tendon sheath infection involving proximal compartment	1 Infected laceration not involving the joint 2 Neglected acute paronychia 3 Mallet finger

Many of the common and less serious infections can be treated on an ambulatory basis. If pus is localized in a subcutaneous abscess or paronychia, drainage can be done in the emergency department or physician's office. The need for a bloodless field to ensure accuracy is critical, even for the most seemingly insignificant drainage procedure. The brachial cuff tourniquet is preferred, but some physicians commonly use a digital tourniquet for fingertip procedures. A rubber band should never be used as a digital tourniquet, as the pressure is difficult to control and may injure the digital nerves, and the band might easily be left in place accidentally. A soft Penrose rubber tubing held in place with a large clamp is preferable. Inducing ischemia by distal to proximal wrapping as is done for elective clean surgery is contraindicated, as this will encourage proximal spread via synovial sheaths or lymphatics and thus enhance the spread of infection.

Postoperative care of these ambulatory cases consists of rest, constant elevation with the hand higher than the heart, absorptive and nonconstrictive dressing in a position of function, antibiotics, and follow-up evaluation at 24 and 48 h to observe the patient's response. A specific culture sensitivity will determine subsequent continuation or change of antibiotic. For the more seriously ill patient, immediate hospitalization may be needed. Prompt surgery may be necessary. Intravenous antibiotic therapy is usually required. All incision and drainage operations for these complex deep infections should be done in the operating room. The prompt judicious use of antibiotics is important, and urgency may necessitate initiating the appropriate agent on the basis of smear and the characteristics of the clinical picture before the receipt of culture and sensitivity reports.

Staphylococci are present in nearly 80 percent of hand infections; over one-half are penicillinase-producing. Beta-hemolytic streptococci, *Escherichia coli,* Proteus species, and Pseudomonas account for the remainder. *Eikenella corrodens* is common in human bite wounds. Over one-third of hand infections will have a mixed flora. Tuberculous tenosynovitis and atypical mycobacterial infections do occur in the hand as well as do various fungus infections.

Despite the possibility of encouraging a superinfection, for the seriously infected hand, it is best to "overtreat" a patient initially and be able to withdraw a possibly unnecessary antibiotic when the culture information is available, rather than have the infection progress rapidly because of delay.

Special note should be made of infections from human bites caused when the fist strikes the tooth of an opponent. In this situation there is not only crush of tissue, but inoculation of organisms in the metacarpophalangeal joint, and frequently into the metacarpal head itself. These wounds should be debrided and irrigated, not sutured, and aggressive antibiotic therapy is indicated.

There are many potential sites for infection (Fig. 45-16). Some of the more common ones will be considered in turn. For all of these, it must be emphasized that should the infection be a cellulitis *without* localization, antibiotics and the proper dressing, combined with elevation, are the best treatment. Drainage procedures should be reserved to decompress loculations of purulence and "decompress pus under pressure." There is no need to "drain a cellulitis" in the hand.

SUBCUTANEOUS ABSCESS. These abscesses are common, usually on the flexor surface of the digits or palm. They often follow a needle or thorn prick, blistering from hard manual work, and usually present in the stage of cellulitis with diffuse redness and swelling. It is essential to differentiate this from some of the deeper and more dangerous infections. The tenderness is generally confined at the area of abscess and cellulitis. Treatment with rest, elevation, and antibiotics may abort the process, but if the abscess is localized, drainage is required. Note that

Fig. 45-16. *A.* Diagram of the locations of common infections showing spreading and pointing. 1. Dorsal subcutaneous abscess. 2. Paronychia. 3. A vesicle or pustule indicative of felon beneath. 4. Felon. 5. Abscess in volar fat pad; this can point in a palmar direction or track to the dorsum before pointing; the flexion creases frequently act as barriers to spread. 6. Abscess in palmar fat pad may spread by perforating dorsad, by passing the flexion crease barrier through bacterial action and going proximally to the subcutaneous tissue in the palm, or by spreading via the lumbrical canal to a palmar space. *B.* The collar-button abscess. This advanced lesion, with abscess cavities on both the palmar and dorsal aspects, is common in the area of the metacarpophalangeal joint. It has the potential for spreading beneath the palmar fascia or into the dorsal compartment opposite the web space, or it may fill the web space and extend along the tendons into the midpalmar space or to the thenar space.

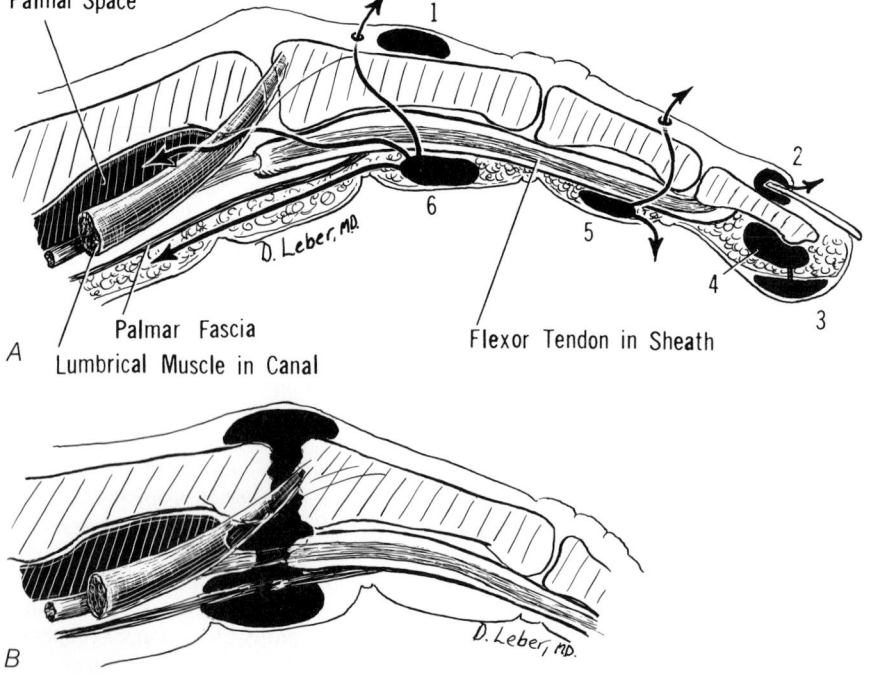

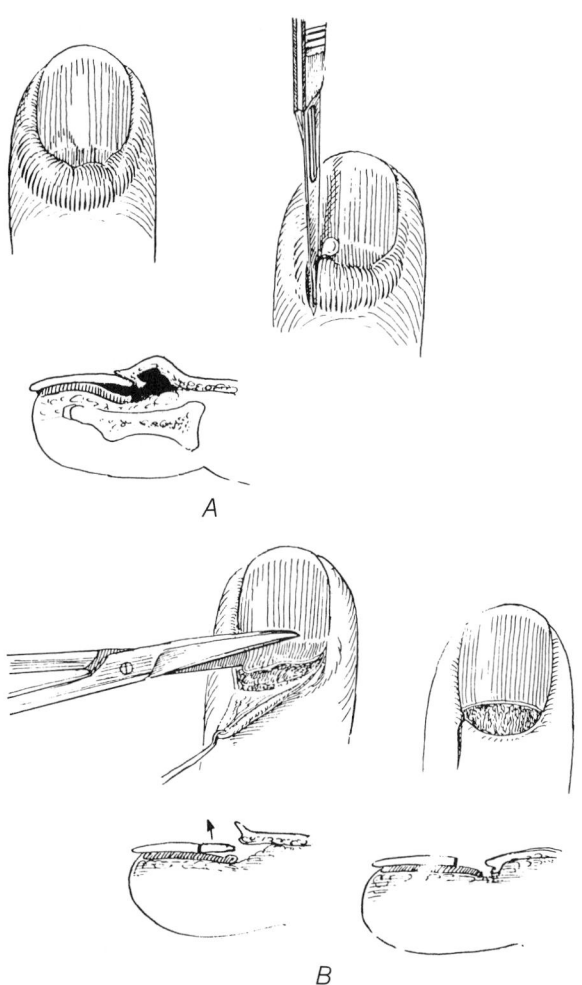

A

B

Fig. 45-17. *A*. Surgical drainage of the paronychial abscess is best performed through an incision proximal to the corner of the involved nail. *B*. If the abscess extends around the nail base or lateral margin, the base or margin should be excised to assure adequate drainage and removal of nonviable nail that serves as a foreign body. The fingernail will regenerate from the nail bed.

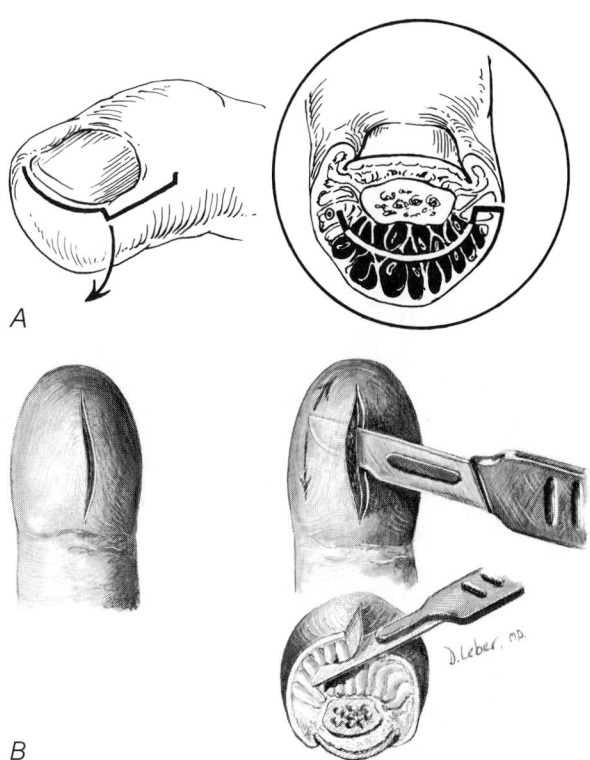

A

B

Fig. 45-18. *A*. Incision and drainage of felon with preservation of sensory digit pulp. (From: *Chase RA, Laub DR: The hand: Therapeutic strategy for acute problems, in Current Problems in Surgery. Chicago, Year Book Medical Publishers, 1966, with permission.*) *B*. A centrally located incision permits excellent drainage and decompression. This alternate incision lies between innervation areas but does leave a scar in the finger pad.

the abscess may point in a palmar direction but may take the path of least resistance and present dorsally in the looser areolar tissues. This situation, if not treated promptly with antibiotics and drainage, can lead to acute suppurative tenosynovitis, acute suppurative arthritis, osteomyelitis, and occasionally even gangrene.

PARONYCHIA. This infection occurs around the margin of the nail plate. The initiating cause may be hangnails, ingrown nails, manicure trauma, steel-wool slivers, or other small foreign bodies. Staphylococcus is usually the offending organism. If presenting early as a simple cellulitis, antibiotics and soaks are sufficient. Should a small abscess have formed, drainage is necessary, often requiring removal of a portion of the nail plate (Fig. 45-17).

FELON. Infection of the digital pulp of the terminal segment has certain important characteristics. The fibrous septa to the skin compartmentalize the pulp and limit

swelling, resulting in a buildup of pressure in the pulp spaces. If untreated, this results in deep ischemic necrosis and severe deep infection and can progress to osteomyelitis and/or pulp necrosis and slough. This entire process will occur before the abscess points and drains spontaneously. Severe pain out of proportion to the amount of swelling, erythema, and exquisite tenderness characterize the felon. The pulp space must be incised and drained before the tissue necrosis occurs (Fig. 45-18).

BACTERIAL TENOSYNOVITIS. The synovial sheath compartment is characterized by a poor natural resistance to infection with the presence of a nearly avascular tendon. It takes little disruption to convert this living tendon into a collagenous foreign body with its tendency to augment the infectious process. The anatomy of the tendon sheaths will vary significantly from patient to patient, but the most common pattern should be known as it often predicts routes of natural extension for the infection (Fig. 45-19). For example, a little finger felon that extends to the flexor sheath will take a natural anatomic route to the ulnar bursa, thence to the radial bursa, and finally into the thumb flexor tendon sheath. Thus, with the classic anatomic pattern, the little finger infection is more apt to extend to the thumb than to the adjacent ring finger.

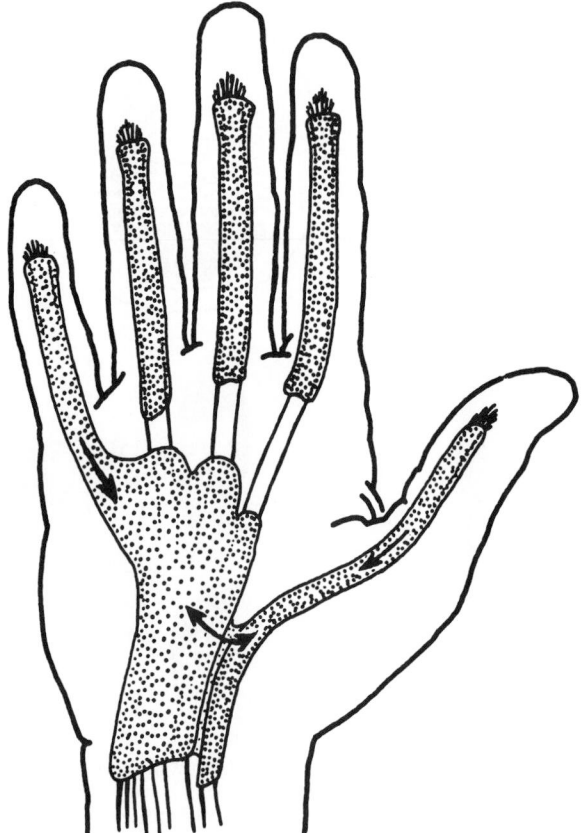

Fig. 45-19. Anatomy of synovial sheaths and deep spaces of the hand. (From: *American Society for Surgery of the Hand: The Hand: Examination and Diagnosis.* Edinburgh, Churchill-Livingstone, 1983, with permission.)

The digit with a flexor tendon sheath infection assumes a posture of mild flexion at all joints. Active or passive finger extension elicits local pain. Tenderness will be present along the sheath, and the digit is uniformly swollen. The differential diagnosis between bacterial tenosynovitis and acute rheumatoid tenosynovitis can be difficult.

Proper therapy for bacterial tenosynovitis is surgical drainage (Fig. 45-20) and the administration of appropriate intravenous antibiotics. The tendon sheath must be adequately opened with a midaxial (along the axis of joint motion) incision. Should the finger be decompressed via a midaxial incision, the wound is best left open for drainage. If the incision is truly midaxial, the healing will result in a fine scar. Should any anterior incision be selected, even if zigzag, it must be closed to avoid unacceptable risk of bridling scar formation.

A more recent technique for these flexor sheath infections that has been most effective is the use of an incision in the distal palm over the proximal sheath at the level of the distal palmar crease, and a second incision that is midaxial at the distal end of that sheath at the DIP joint. Small catheters (infant feeding tubes or intravenous catheters) are used to thoroughly irrigate the sheath at the

time of operation. These catheters are then sutured in place and used postoperatively to continue antibiotic irrigation into the sheath until the tubes seal off (usually at 48 h).

Even with prompt control of these tendon sheath infections by antibiotics and by proper surgery, stiffness of the digit is a significant risk. Early hand therapy and motion exercises are essential as soon as the acute phase of the wound has subsided. This usually occurs earlier with the catheter technique.

PALMAR SPACE INFECTIONS. The deep spaces of the hand are located between the deep flexor tendons and the metacarpals in the palm. This subtendinous palmar area is divided into a thenar space and the midpalmar space. Serious deep infection may occur in one of these deep spaces. Localized swelling, redness, and tenderness are present. These spaces must be surgically drained in accordance with the general principle of hand incisions (Fig. 45-5).

ACUTE SUPPURATIVE ARTHRITIS. When the hand or wrist joints are involved with sepsis, acute suppurative arthritis most commonly occurs secondary to a penetrating wound or to the spread from adjacent abscess or osteomyelitis. With the increasing incidence of venereal disease, hematogenous monarticular gonococcal arthritis is becoming much more common. Except for the gonococcal arthritis that usually responds to intravenous antibiotics, septic joints are best treated by surgical drainage combined with intravenous antibiotics. Some function is usually preserved, but the prognosis for a normal joint is guarded. Differential diagnosis includes gout, pseudogout, and acute rheumatoid arthritis.

UNUSUAL INFECTIONS. A group of severe infections that must be carefully watched for includes tuberculosis, atypical mycobacteria, fungi, acute streptococcal hemolytic gangrene, necrotizing fasciitis, streptococcal myositis, clostridial cellulitis, gram-negative, anaerobic cutaneous gangrene, and progressive bacterial synergistic gangrene. Although these severe soft tissue infections fortunately occur infrequently, early recognition is essential to prevent progressive destruction either from continuing bacterial action or from ischemic necrosis induced by increasing tissue pressures.

Burns

Burns of the hand are common. They may be secondary to heat, frostbite, radiation, or electricity. Particularly in severe thermal burns, a tragedy occurs when a severely burned patient is saved by heroic treatment only to be left helpless because the hands are grossly deformed and do not work, leaving the patient totally dependent upon others.

It is important to initiate treatment of the burn on the first day. This obviously must include an accurate assessment of the depth and extent of the burned hand. There is rarely a full-thickness skin loss to the palm or proximal flexor surface of the digits in the absence of contact, chemical, or electrical burn. Full-thickness destruction of the flexor surface of the digital tip and the entire dorsum

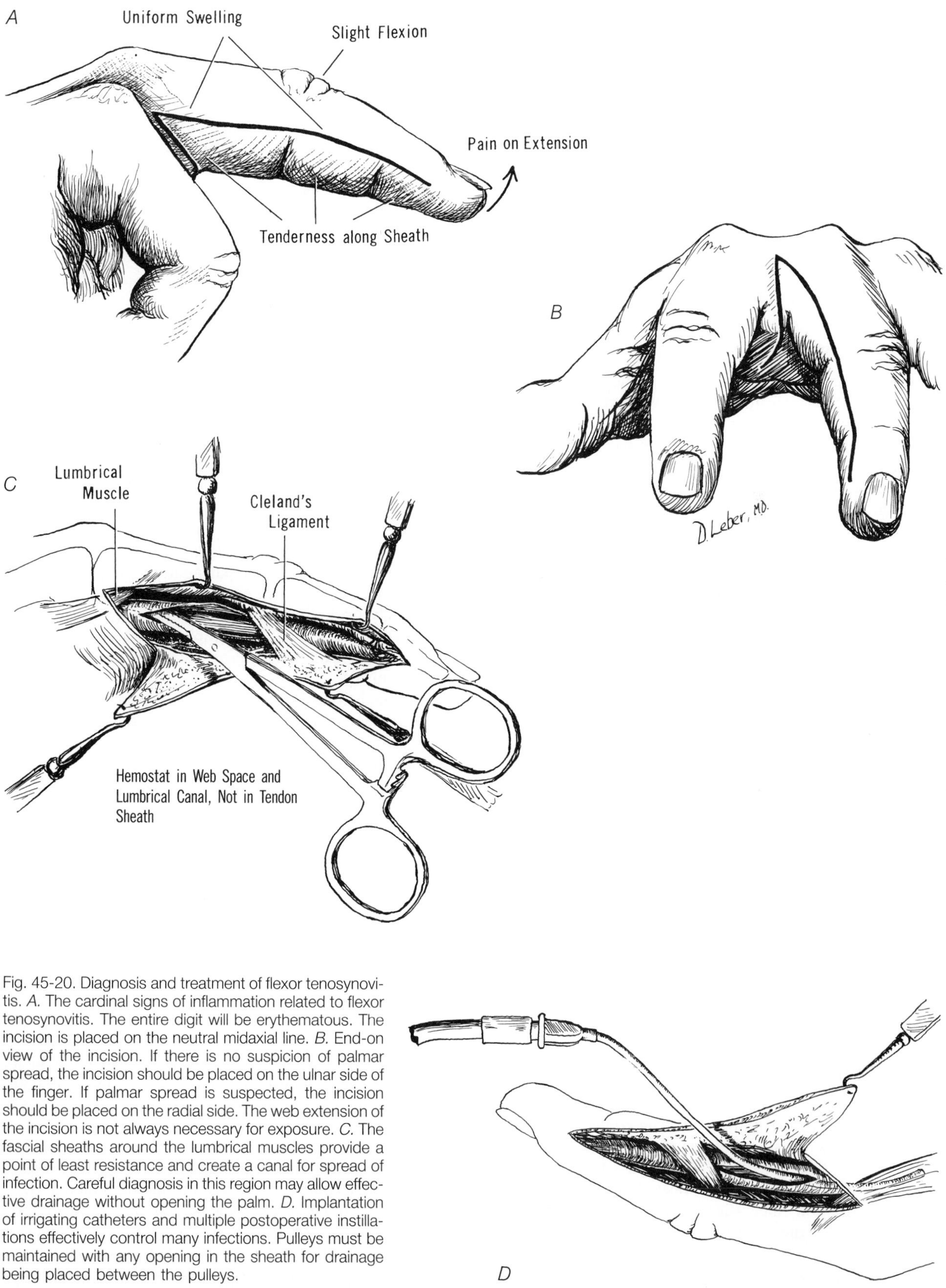

A

Uniform Swelling

Slight Flexion

Pain on Extension

Tenderness along Sheath

B

D.Leber, MD.

C

Lumbrical
Muscle

Cleland's
Ligament

Hemostat in Web Space and
Lumbrical Canal, Not in Tendon
Sheath

Fig. 45-20. Diagnosis and treatment of flexor tenosynovitis. *A.* The cardinal signs of inflammation related to flexor tenosynovitis. The entire digit will be erythematous. The incision is placed on the neutral midaxial line. *B.* End-on view of the incision. If there is no suspicion of palmar spread, the incision should be placed on the ulnar side of the finger. If palmar spread is suspected, the incision should be placed on the radial side. The web extension of the incision is not always necessary for exposure. *C.* The fascial sheaths around the lumbrical muscles provide a point of least resistance and create a canal for spread of infection. Careful diagnosis in this region may allow effective drainage without opening the palm. *D.* Implantation of irrigating catheters and multiple postoperative instillations effectively control many infections. Pulleys must be maintained with any opening in the sheath for drainage being placed between the pulleys.

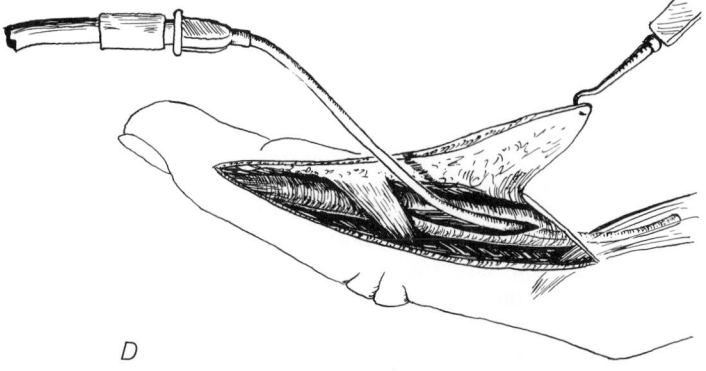

D

of the hand frequently occurs. In addition, the delicate central tendon of the extensor mechanism over the proximal interphalangeal joint is frequently destroyed either by direct thermal injury or by secondary bacterial digestion. If the thermal injury results in tendon destruction, the joint must be fused in an appropriate position, because the unopposed pull of the flexor muscles will impose a flexion contracture.

The early treatment of the burned hand includes the appropriate splinting in the safe position with the proper dressings. Partial-thickness burns are well debrided of their necrotic superficial tissue using whirlpool. Deep second-degree burns and third-degree burns of the hand are well treated by early excision with skin grafting.

Wringer Injuries

Home wringer injuries (from washing machines) are very common, particularly in children, with crushing of the hand and upper extremity. These must be distinguished from the severe crush injuries seen in industrial or farm machinery accidents that are usually complicated by deep tissue destruction, impending ischemia, components of avulsion injuries, and usually fractures. Industrial rollers may be heated as well, adding further complication.

In those patients injured in the home washing machine, friction burns occur most severely at points of increasing size of the extremity—the metacarpophalangeal joint level, the thenar area and base of hand, the proximal forearm and elbow region, and the shoulder. Neuropraxia is common. Edema and hematoma formation occurs, and the patient must be carefully observed for impending compartment syndrome.

Hospitalization is recommended for careful observation. Experienced examination of the skin, nerves, and vascular supply is required. X-rays are necessary only if there are signs of a fracture. Lacerations are sutured. Absorptive noncompressive dressings are applied to the areas of burn. The elbow and wrist are immobilized in extension.

Those patients with severe industrial or farm machinery injuries frequently require early radical wound debridement with primary or staged coverage with grafts or flaps. Fasciotomies are commonly needed. Definitive tendon, nerve, and bone surgery is delayed except for the stabilization of evident unstable bony fragments. Obviously if major blood vessels are damaged, they must be repaired initially by either suture or graft.

Crush Syndromes

An increasing and easily overlooked problem consequent to the growing number of drug addicts is the appearance of the crush syndrome occurring in the comatose patient. The weight of the patient's body upon an extremity will compromise the vascularity, result in erythema, induration, ulceration, vesiculation, and paralysis. Swelling of the limb may or may not occur early. There is usually a matching area on the body or thigh of the patient to correspond in size to that of the involved limb. An early reliable sign of impending muscle damage is increased turgor in the muscle compartment with pain on passive muscle stretch. Myoglobinemia and myoglobinuria should be tested for. Nerve involvement is common, both sensory and motor. The peripheral pulse is usually normal to palpation. If the patient is still comatose, compartment pressure measurements may be helpful. Recognition of this crush syndrome is critical because prompt replacement of fluid deficits and careful renal management will diminish the threat of renal shutdown, and early fasciotomy may preserve function of the involved limb by decreasing the severity of damage to the involved nerves and muscles.

Compartment Syndromes

In 1881 Volkmann described a contracture of forearm musculature that he attributed to tight bandaging of an arm following a fracture at the elbow. This condition is well described now following a multitude of causes: supracondylar fractures, fractures of the forearm, brachial artery puncture for obtaining arterial gases or for arteriography, subfascial intravenous infiltration, hemophilia, crush injuries, drug overdose, following periods of ischemia (i.e., after replantation), gunshot wounds, etc.

The basic cause is that of increasing tissue pressure within the deep flexor compartment of the forearm from whatever cause, initially occluding the venous return and ultimately occluding the arterial inflow. This deep compartment is particularly vulnerable because it is nourished by the anterior interosseous artery with no significant collateral inflow.

The final clinical state of the untreated patient is a complete replacement of the deep forearm musculature with heavy yellow fibrous tissue, giving a severe fixed flexion contracture of the wrist and fingers. A "strangulation neuropathy" of the median and ulnar nerves occurs as they pass through the fibrous tissue, resulting in a hand without intrinsic muscle function that is completely numb in the median and ulnar nerve distributions.

DIAGNOSIS. The classic four P's of pain, pallor, paralysis, and pulselessness are totally *inadequate*. Indeed the radial artery does *not* pass within this compartment at all and usually remains patent. Most patients with late established Volkmann's will still have a bounding radial pulse.

Early diagnosis is contingent upon an alert physician with an index of suspicion. Induration and local tenderness over the muscle bellies with increasing pain on gentle passive finger extension are the two most valuable clinical findings. Paresthesia and hypesthesia in the distribution of the median or ulnar nerves are helpful. If the clinical diagnosis is uncertain, the intracompartmental pressure should be measured.

TREATMENT. In the acute stage it is essential to make an early diagnosis and to promptly perform a fasciotomy. The incision should start near the medial epicondyle at the elbow, course distally and obliquely toward the pronator teres insertion at the radial margin of the forearm at the junction of the mid and proximal thirds, gently curve again ulnarward to reach the ulnar border of the forearm at the junction of the distal and midthird of the forearm, and thence gently curve in a radial direction and distally to the midportion of the wrist flexion crease. A complete fasciotomy should be performed from elbow to wrist. Each of the individual muscle bellies should have an epimysiotomy. The median and ulnar nerves should be carefully explored and freed from points of constriction, the median nerve particularly at the pronator teres and at the proximal yoke of the flexor digitorum superficialis, and the ulnar nerve particularly as it passes through the two heads of the flexor carpi ulnaris. In established late cases, treatment involves major reconstructive surgery, with excision of the entire fibrotic muscle infarct, neurolysis and epineurolysis of the median and ulnar nerves from the elbow to the hand, and multiple tendon transfers.

Complex Injuries

The care of the patient with a complex hand injury involving multiple systems—bone, joint, tendon, nerve, and coverage—requires in-depth knowledge and experience in hand surgery. The primary care is essential. All obviously devitalized tissue is debrided. Nothing that is viable is discarded in hopes it may later prove useful in reconstruction. Indeed, the early preliminary formulation of a staged reconstruction starts at the time of primary debridement.

The initial goals are to obtain bone and joint stability with adequate soft tissue coverage. The principles of primary and secondary wound closure apply to the hand as elsewhere in heavily contaminated wounds. Tendon and nerve reconstructions can be done as secondary procedures. Obviously the reestablishment of adequate arterial inflow and venous return is a primary consideration, one that has been enormously enhanced by microsurgical techniques and the skills and surgical disciplines involved in replantation.

Replantation

With the advent of small artery and vein repair using microsurgical techniques, replantation is technically possible for some traumatic amputations. These technical triumphs present the need to establish sensible indications for the use of that technology. Sound reasoning is necessary to establish prudent indications and significant contraindications. To achieve survival of a part by reestablishing its blood supply only to have that part remain useless or even detrimental—to survive as a nonfunctioning parasite—represents a serious breach of the doctrine "First, do no harm." For many years it has been possible for surgeons to operate successfully upon bones, joints, tendons, and nerves and to achieve soft tissue coverage and closure. With these techniques, certain principles of surgery in the care of the patient with the acutely injured hand have evolved and withstood the test of time. The simple ability to repair a small vessel does not justify abandonment of the sound principles involved in returning some function to an injured hand.

Certain principles in replantation surgery are becoming well established:

1. The goal of the surgical procedure is function.
2. There are risks to the patient in the form of a long anesthesia and risks also to uninjured parts of the same extremity or hand. The age of the patient and the presence or absence of significant preexistent systemic illness or simultaneous injury (i.e., head injury, ruptured spleen, etc.) obviously must be considered.
3. Patients with a history of heavy smoking, diabetes mellitus, hypertension, or Raynaud's phenomenon in general make very poor candidates for attempted replantation.
4. The interval since injury must be considered. Was the part cooled? In proximal amputations with significant amounts of muscle in the part, perfusion to that muscle must be reestablished within 4 h. In more distal amputations where there is no significant avascular muscle, the cooled part will tolerate the ischemia for as long as 24 h. Note that these times are to the reestablishment of perfusion, not to the initiation of the surgical procedure.
5. The mechanism of injury is important. Guillotine injuries are far easier to reattach surgically than avulsion injuries.
6. It is essential to have a team of surgeons trained in these techniques before undertaking this type of surgery. This surgery cannot be done by a single surgeon without special training.

Certain guidelines concerning the amputation must be considered:

1. An entire hand or an entire thumb should be a candidate for replantation unless definite contraindications exist.
2. Rarely is there an indication for replantation of a single finger, except in children.
3. Rarely is there an indication for replantation of one or two fingers where the level of amputation is through no-man's land.
4. Amputation of a guillotine nature through the wrist or low forearm of a young healthy person is an ideal situation to attempt replantation, all other things being equal.
5. Amputation may be considered above the elbow, particularly in children, even if it is anticipated that the hand will not function. Subsequent elective amputation through the forearm with prosthesis may be decided upon, thus salvaging a functional elbow by the replantation effort and making rehabilitation by prosthesis far better than the amputation through the original level.

If the patient is considered for transfer to a replantation center, certain treatments are necessary. The patient should be evaluated for other significant injuries. Antibiotics should be given intravenously. Tetanus toxoid and antitoxin should be given if necessary. Low-molecular-weight dextran and aspirin are indicated. The part itself should not be perfused. It should be kept clean in a sterile dressing that in turn is placed in a plastic bag. This plastic bag is then placed in ice water at 4° C. The part should *not* be frozen. The part should not be immersed in fluid unprotected, and should not be in direct contact with the ice. The wound at the amputation site should be gently cleansed and a sterile dressing applied. Any bleeding can be controlled with pressure. If possible, no clamping should be done in the wound because of the risk of damage to adjacent nerves. X-rays of the stump and the part are helpful.

The referring physician should contact the replantation center and discuss the patient directly with a member of the team, to be certain that the team is available and not operating upon another replantation effort at the same time. Furthermore, this provides for a smooth transition. The initially treating physician should not give the patient false hopes about the possibility of a replantation effort. Should replantation be attempted and should the part survive, many, many months of hand therapy will be necessary for that patient to obtain whatever function is to be regained.

Amputations

Amputations within the hand must follow a careful assessment of the critical levels of function for the hand of

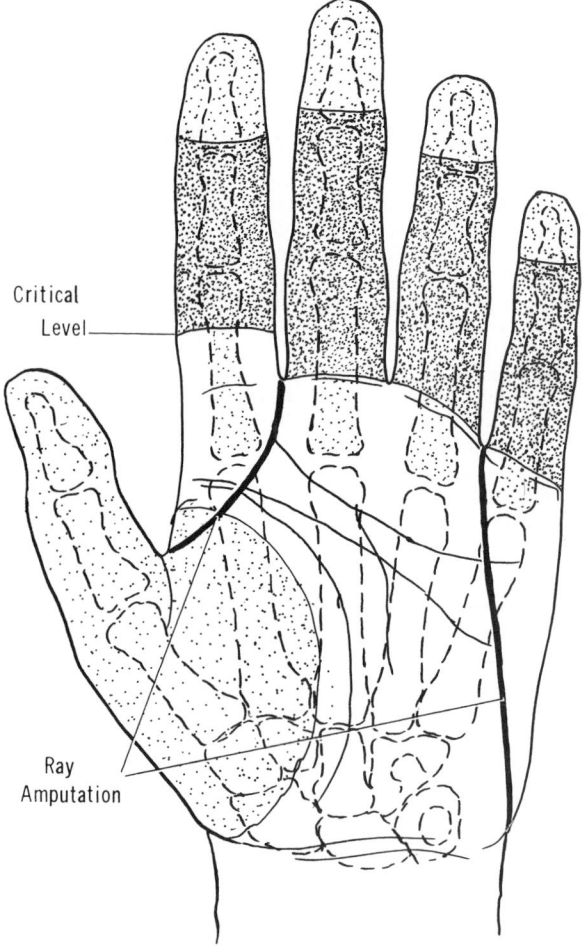

Fig. 45-21. The recommended levels for elective amputations or for completion of traumatic amputations.

Critical
Level

Ray
Amputation

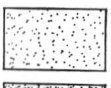 Save all possible length, unless crushed

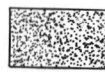 Can be shortened for good coverage

that patient and for the appearance of each digit (Fig. 45-21). It is important to consider the handedness, age, and occupation of the patient. What is suitable for the typist may not be suitable for the laborer. Preservation of bony architecture to encourage strong grasp is preferable for manual laborers (Fig. 45-22A), while people requiring dexterity and/or who are primarily concerned with appearance have different functional and aesthetic needs (Fig. 45-22B). The thumb is the most important digit, having the mobility to oppose each of the fingers and the strength to withstand their combined force. Any length of the thumb that can be salvaged by conservative surgical management should be preserved. When an injury results in loss of soft tissue with an excess of bone, the protruding bone may be salvageable by immediate coverage with vascularized soft tissue from either local or distant pedicle flap or even a primary vascularized island pedicle flap or a free flap. Usually the primary coverage is by skin graft if possible, to minimize risk of infection. These complex techniques are performed secondarily when wounds are closed and healed.

With injuries to many digits, normally less important fingers or partial digital lengths will obtain prime importance. If border fingers (index and little) are significantly shortened, they may be best treated by ray resection (amputation through the proximal metacarpal), especially if there is any damage to the MCP joint. Although the index finger is important and versatile and functions primarily in pinch and manipulation with its pulp opposed to that of the thumb, the hand functions very well without an index finger, with a normal middle finger assuming the role of primary pinch. Note that any amputation of an index finger proximal to the PIP level leaves insufficient length for useful pinch function, although the digit will remain useful in grasp. Therefore, all possible lengths should be saved in the index finger with amputations distal to the PIP joint; with injuries proximal to the PIP joint, immediate closure by further shortening may be done, with consideration in the early rehabilitative phase for ray resection.

Even when the central fingers (middle and ring) are amputated, the stumps will contribute to efficient handling of small objects as long as a portion of the proximal phalanx remains. Note that an amputation at the metacarpophalangeal joint level of the two center fingers leaves a space between the digits where the hand is cupped or in a fist. If this creates a palmar incompetence that allows small objects to fall through the space, transfer of the adjacent peripheral finger with its metacarpal should be considered.

Amputation of all fingers and the thumb at the metacarpophalangeal joint level leaves a stump with little function. Later reconstruction to increase function should include a deepening of the space between the thumb metacarpal and the rest of the hand, and occasionally toe transfers to the hand.

In patients with complete traumatic loss of the thumb, late reconstruction of a thumb by either digital transposition or toe transfer can be considered.

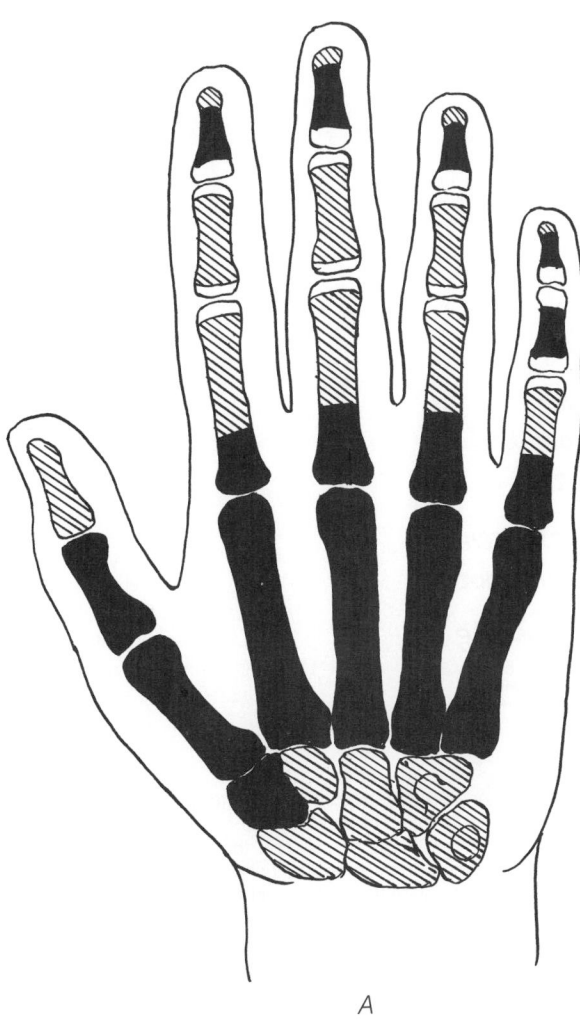

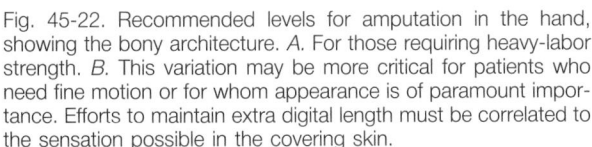

A

■ Preserve

▨ Less important

□ Amputate

B

Fig. 45-22. Recommended levels for amputation in the hand, showing the bony architecture. *A*. For those requiring heavy-labor strength. *B*. This variation may be more critical for patients who need fine motion or for whom appearance is of paramount importance. Efforts to maintain extra digital length must be correlated to the sensation possible in the covering skin.

NONTRAUMATIC CONDITIONS AND RECONSTRUCTION

Entrapment Syndromes of the Retinacular Restraining Systems

Carpal Tunnel Syndrome

Carpal tunnel syndrome is a neurapraxia of the median nerve from compression within the carpal canal. This condition was first described by Paget (1853), later reported on by Omerod (1883), and more recently popularized in the United States by Phalen and Lipscomb. It is seen in women more often than in men, especially post-

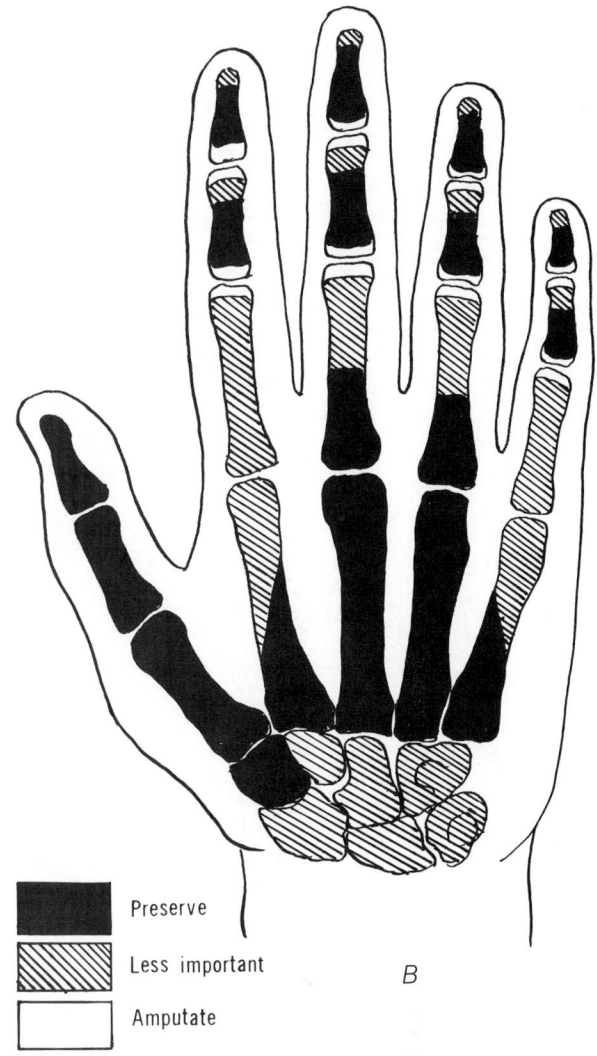

menopausal, and usually is of idiopathic etiology. The median nerve is subject to this compression where it passes through the carpal tunnel along with the nine extrinsic digital flexor tendons (Fig. 45-23).

Most commonly it is of nontraumatic origin. A chronic flexor tenosynovitis may be present. This condition is seen following Colles fracture, Smith's fracture, or lunate or perilunar dislocations. It has been described with ganglia, lipomas, or anomalous muscle bellies (lumbrical or flexor digitorum superficialis) within the canal. Carpal tunnel syndrome may be seen as a presenting syndrome of, or in conjunction with, rheumatoid arthritis, gout, diabetes mellitus, hypothyroidism, and amyloidosis. More proximal sites of nerve entrapment must be ruled out—at the cervical spine level, Pancoast's tumor at the apex of the lung, or where the nerve passes through the two heads of the pronator teres (pronator teres syndrome).

Patients present with pain and numbness of the median nerve distribution, particularly nocturnal, often referred

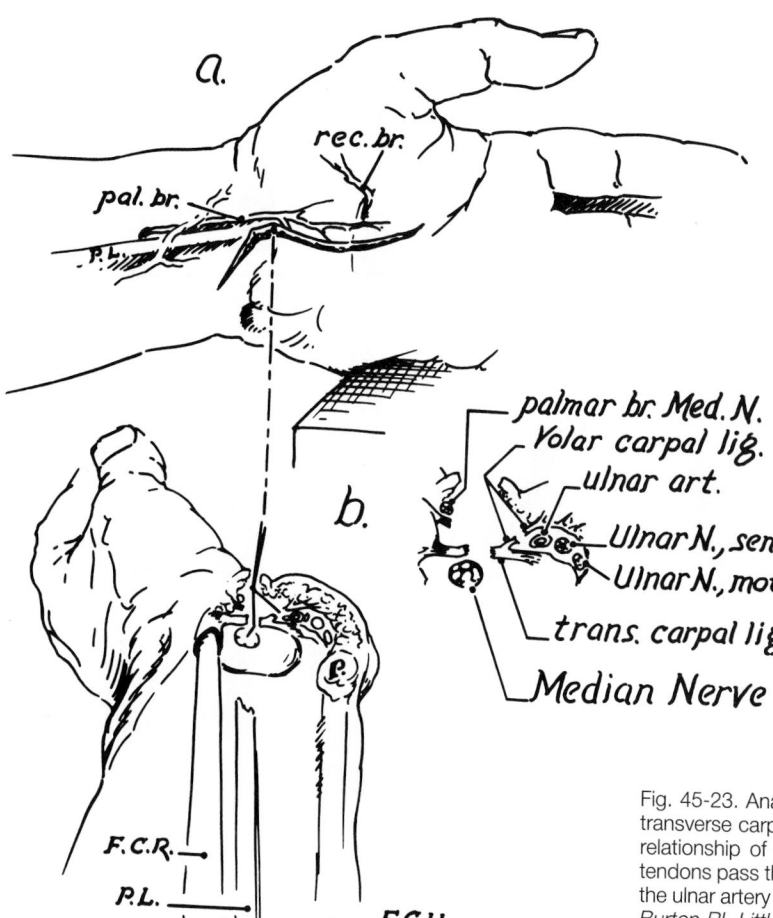

a.

rec. br.

pal. br.

P.L.

b.

palmar br. Med. N.
Volar carpal lig.
ulnar art.
Ulnar N., sen.
Ulnar N., mot.
trans. carpal lig.
Median Nerve

F.C.R.
P.L.
F.C.U.

Fig. 45-23. Anatomy of carpal tunnel. Note the relationship of the transverse carpal ligament and the volar carpal ligament. Note the relationship of the median nerve and the ulnar nerve. The flexor tendons pass through the carpal tunnel with the median nerve, and the ulnar artery through the ulnar tunnel with the ulnar nerve. (From: *Burton RI, Littler JW: Entrapment syndromes of the retinacular or restraining systems of the hand, in Nontraumatic Soft Tissue Afflictions of the Hand. Current Problems in Surgery. Chicago, Year Book Medical Publishers, 1975, with permission.*)

to the shoulder and neck. Findings on examination include hypesthesia in the median nerve distribution, thenar atrophy, a positive Tinel's sign over the nerve at the wrist, and increased symptoms with forced wrist flexion. Electromyograms and nerve conduction tests may be helpful to substantiate the diagnosis and rule out more proximal nerve entrapment.

Treatment in the early stages includes splinting, nonsteroidal anti-inflammatory agents, and possibly a single injection of cortisone preparation into the canal. The presence of atrophy or weakness and the failure to respond to conservative treatment are considered indications for operative intervention. If the epineurium is thick, it may require longitudinal release by dissection. Frequently the motor branch needs to be decompressed as it passes through the fascia into the thenar musculature. In cases of advanced thenar atrophy, the nerve decompression can be combined with primary opponens tendon transfer.

Other Nerve Entrapment Syndromes. The ulnar nerve may also become entrapped at the wrist (Fig. 45-23). This is seen in association with carpal tunnel syndrome, or may occur with conditions such as ulnar artery thrombo-

sis, fractured hook of the hamate, or repeated trauma to the hypothenar area (such as occurs in people riding a 10-speed bicycle in the down position on the handlebars for long periods). The median nerve may become entrapped at the level of the pronator teres, the ulnar nerve medial to the elbow (so-called tardy nerve palsy), and the radial nerve beneath the supinator at the level of the radial head.

Tendon Entrapment Syndrome of First Extensor Compartment (deQuervain's Disorder)

The abductor pollicis longus and extensor pollicis brevis tendons can develop an entrapment syndrome within the first extensor compartment at the wrist. This was first described by deQuervain in 1895. This idiopathic tenosynovitis causes significant pain over the radial styloid at the wrist, proportional to use. On physical examination local tenderness is present, usually with some swelling. Asking the patient to grasp his or her own thumb within the clenched fist and then ulnar-deviate the wrist will usually increase the pain (Finkelstein's test). The differential diagnosis includes nonunion of a scaph-

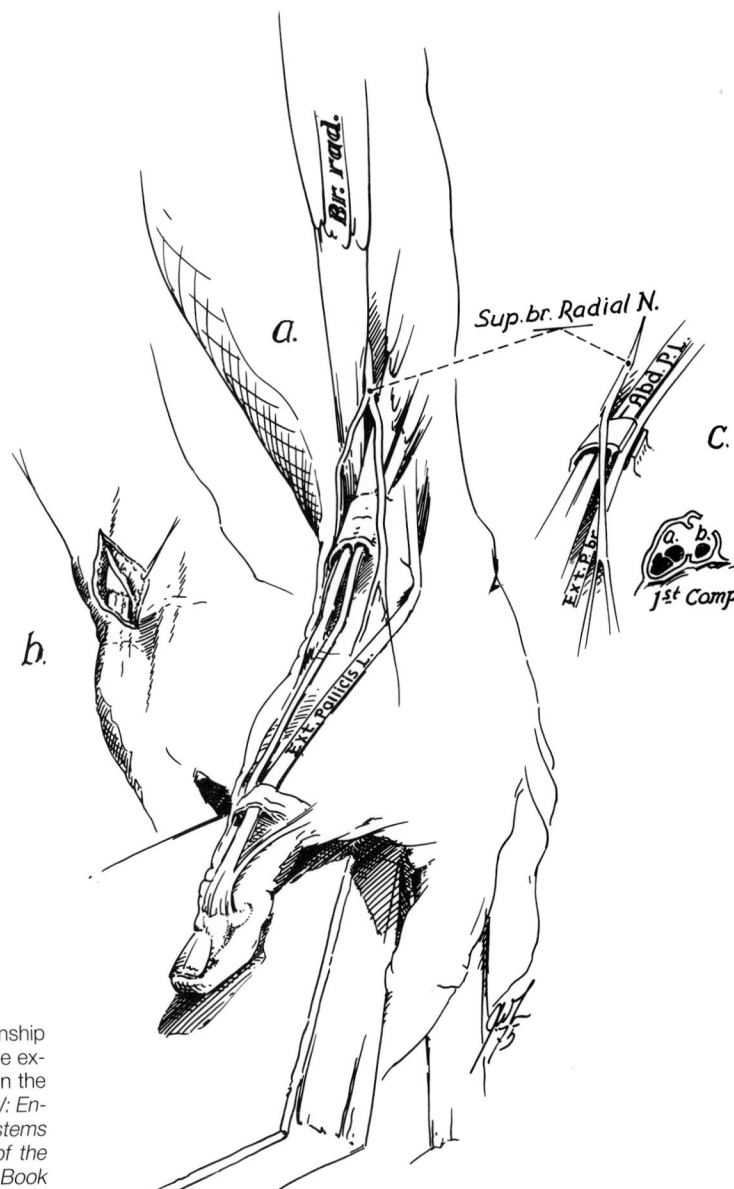

Fig. 45-24. Anatomy of deQuervain's. Note the relationship of the radial sensory nerve. Note the relationships of the extensor pollicis brevis and abductor pollicis longus within the first extensor compartment. (From: *Burton RI, Littler JW: Entrapment syndromes of the retinacular or restraining systems of the hand, in Nontraumatic Soft Tissue Afflictions of the Hand. Current Problems in Surgery. Chicago, Year Book Medical Publishers, 1975, with permission.*)

oid fracture, arthritis on the radial aspect of the wrist or at the base of the thumb, and atypical carpal tunnel syndrome. It is particularly important to rule out coexistent arthritis at the base of the thumb, as the symptoms and physical findings from this condition so closely mimic those of deQuervain's tenosynovitis.

Treatment of the tenosynovitis is with splinting and nonsteroidal anti-inflammatory drugs, combined with a change in pattern of hand use. Failure of response to conservative treatment is an indication for surgical decompression (Fig. 45-24). It is essential to be aware of the radial sensory nerve and its branches, for to damage those by transection or heavy traction will result in a radial sensory neuroma or neuritis far more symptomatic than the original tenosynovitis. Failure of response to surgical decompression is most commonly secondary to

incomplete decompression, as the abductor pollicis longus often has three to four separate tendon slips, some of which may have been overlooked. It is important to incise the retinaculum dorsally, so as to leave a volar cuff of retinaculum to prevent volar tendon prolapse with wrist flexion.

Stenosing Tenovaginitis (Trigger Finger and Trigger Thumb)

The flexor tendons pass through a fibroosseous tunnel extending from the distal palm to the distal finger joint (see Fig. 45-10). Slight fusiform swelling or minimal tenosynovitis of these flexor tendon systems may result in a painful "snapping" sensation as the enlarged tendon forces its way beneath the pulley system. In the extreme

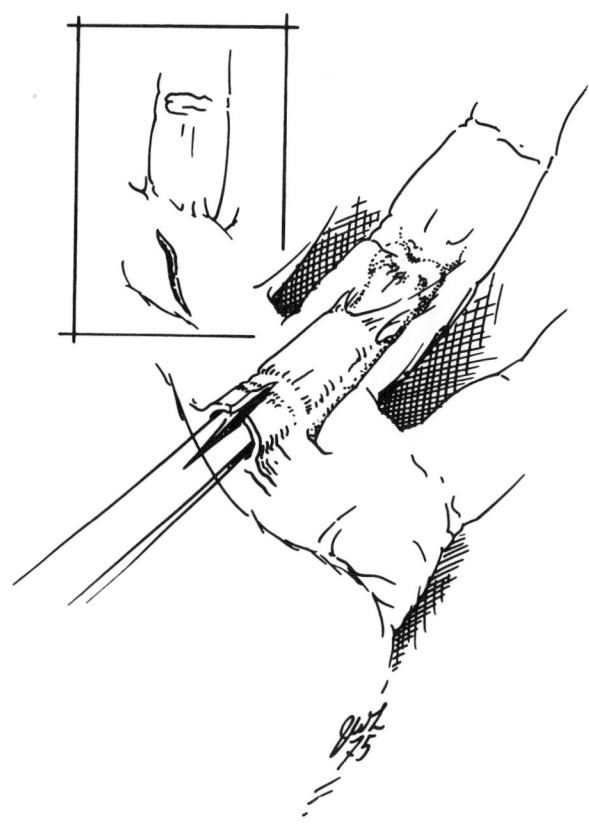

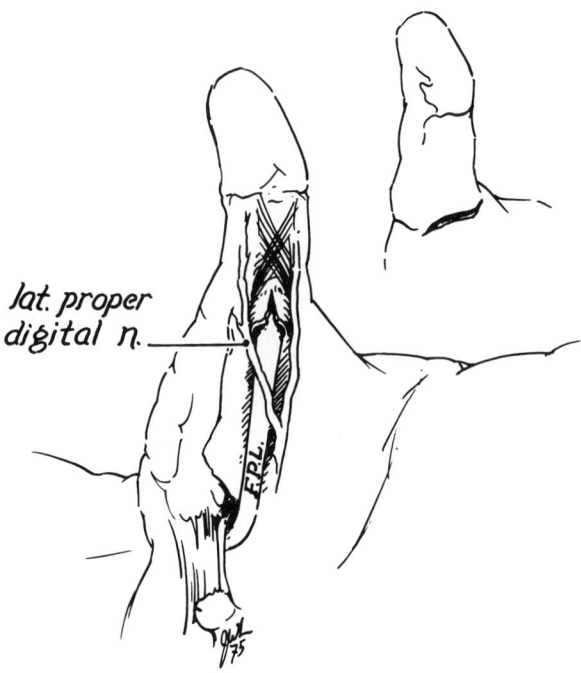

Fig. 45-25. Release of proximal portion of pulley for relief of trigger digit. Only enough is released to allow for full digital mobility without triggering. Complete pulley release will result in tendon bowstring. See Fig. 45-10. (From: *Burton RI, Littler JW: Entrapment syndromes of the retinacular or restraining systems of the hand, in Nontraumatic Soft Tissue Afflictions of the Hand. Current Problems in Surgery. Chicago, Year Book Medical Publishers, 1975, with permission.*)

situation, this can cause a locking of the digit and either flexion or extension. Differential diagnosis includes tendon rupture (if locked) and loose bodies within the finger joints. Treatment is with nonsteroidal anti-inflammatory drugs and steroid injection or surgical intervention. If surgery is elected, it should be done with wrist block anesthesia to allow active patient digital flexion and extension to assure complete decompression (Fig. 45-25). Complications are inexcusable damage of an adjacent digital nerve (also at risk in the thumb), tendon prolapse from ill-conceived excess pulley release, or persistent symptoms from inadequate release. There is a congenital trigger thumb condition that is usually first noticed by parents when the infant is six months of age, and for which surgery is best deferred until the age of one year.

Dupuytren's Contracture

This condition was first described by Dupuytren in 1832, who demonstrated that it was a contracture of the palmar aponeurosis.

INCIDENCE AND ETIOLOGY. Dupuytren's contracture afflicts people primarily of northern European genetic origin, males twice as often as females. Frequency increases with age. Although it would appear to be an autosomal inheritance, to assume a single gene is the cause is probably too simplistic an approach. The expression of the gene appears to be determined by other endogenous and exogenous factors such as hand injury, alcoholism,

liver disease, pulmonary disease, and chronic bowel disease. The condition is commonly seen in epileptics on medications. The condition does not appear to be occupational.

PATHOLOGY. The earliest change is that of nodule formation within the palmar fascia in line with the pretendinous bands. There will be some thickening with fixation of the skin to the pretendinous band, resulting in dimpling of the skin. The pretendinous bands, vertical septae, and natatory ligaments become involved with gradually increasing contracture resulting at both metacarpophalangeal and proximal interphalangeal joint levels (Figs. 45-26 and 45-27).

CLINICAL MANIFESTATIONS. Heuston describes four clinical types:

1. Senile type. This is seen in the older patient, usually male. This type consists of single, pretendinous bands that cause contracture most commonly in the ring or little finger, is slowly progressive, and usually does not involve other portions of the hand.
2. Middle-age type. Patients with the middle-age type have multifocal nodules with developing bands, often bilateral, that may involve more than one digit.

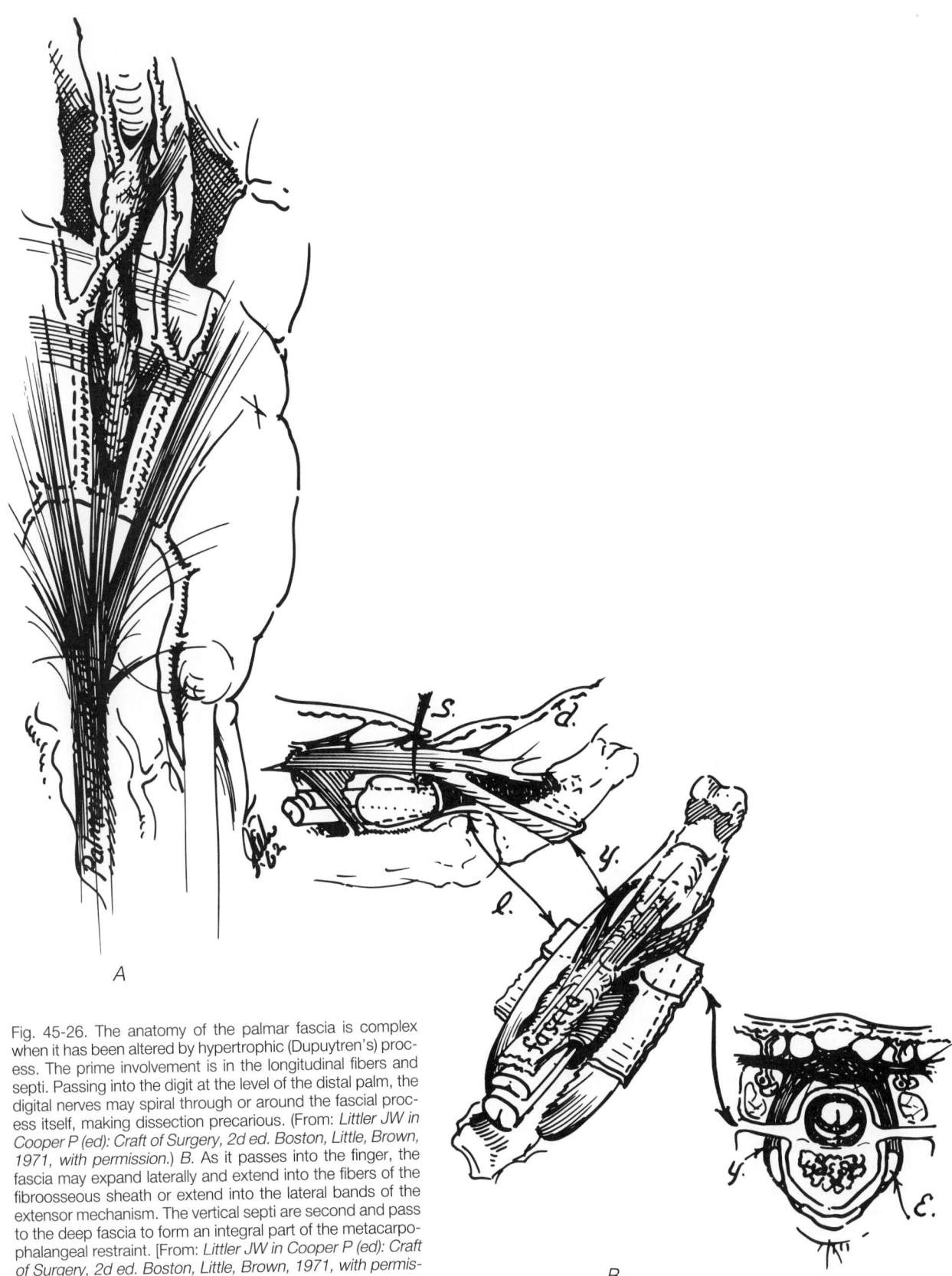

A

Fig. 45-26. The anatomy of the palmar fascia is complex when it has been altered by hypertrophic (Dupuytren's) process. The prime involvement is in the longitudinal fibers and septi. Passing into the digit at the level of the distal palm, the digital nerves may spiral through or around the fascial process itself, making dissection precarious. (From: *Littler JW in Cooper P (ed): Craft of Surgery, 2d ed. Boston, Little, Brown, 1971, with permission.*) *B.* As it passes into the finger, the fascia may expand laterally and extend into the fibers of the fibroosseous sheath or extend into the lateral bands of the extensor mechanism. The vertical septi are second and pass to the deep fascia to form an integral part of the metacarpophalangeal restraint. [From: *Littler JW in Cooper P (ed): Craft of Surgery, 2d ed. Boston, Little, Brown, 1971, with permission.*]

B

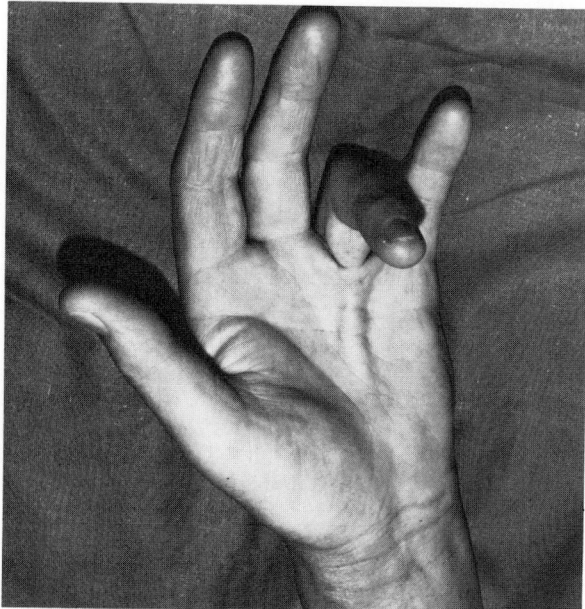

A

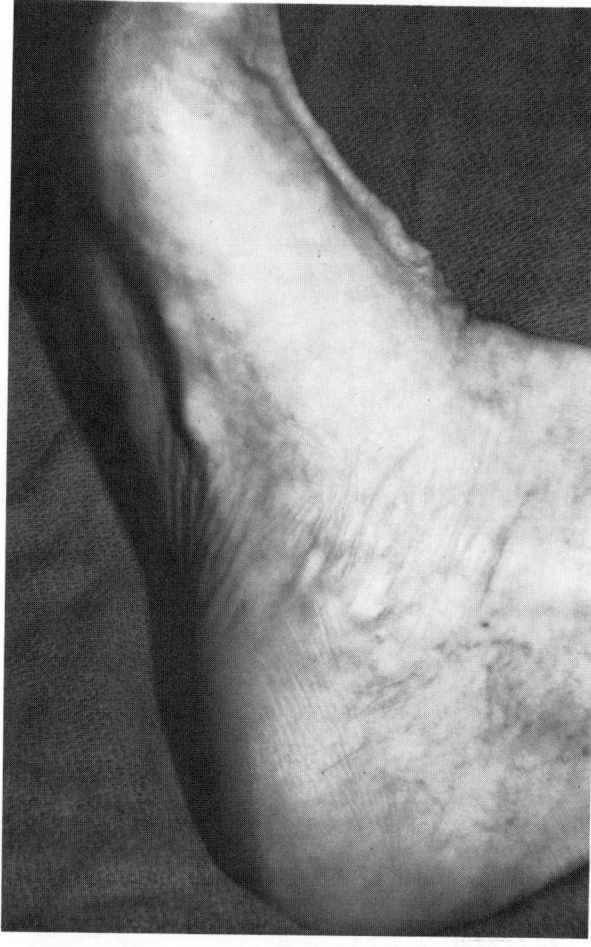

B

Fig. 45-27. *A.* Typical clinical appearance of the hand of a patient with Dupuytren's. *B.* Dupuytren's may involve the foot and present as nodules on the sole. Note that microscopically this material has the exact appearance of low-grade fibrosarcoma. Should the material from the sole be excised, the pathologist must be alerted to the presence of Dupuytren's to avoid a potentially disastrous mis-reading of the microscopic slide with the obvious tragic consequence.

3. Young fulminating type. Patients with this type have tender palmar fascia, and their hands are often pink and warm, may have increased sweating, and frequently have knuckle pads (subcutaneous nodules over the dorsum of the proximal interphalangeal joints). These patients are usually quite young. The prognosis for this type is extremely poor, with or without surgery.

4. Feminine. This type demonstrates long-standing localized palmar fascia nodularity without contracture. There may be slender pretendinous bands attached to these small nodules, usually quite superficial, and resulting in minimal deformity. This "feminine" type is occasionally seen in men with delicate hand structure.

TREATMENT. There is no known nonoperative treatment that will influence the course of the Dupuytren's contracture. Patients should avoid the use of power equipment that causes excessive vibration (air guns on assembly lines, power sanders, etc.). The use of this type of equipment in the patient who already has the Dupuytren's may well accelerate the process.

Choice of surgical procedure will depend upon the nature and severity of the contracture and on the patient's general condition. The alternatives are open fasciotomy, with or without interposed skin grafting, radical excision of the palmar fascia, including the vertical septae, natatory ligaments, etc., with or without skin grafting, and partial palmar fasciectomy with or without skin grafting. Some surgeons prefer zigzag incisions, and others Z-plasties or Y-V advancement flaps in order to obtain closure once the correction has been obtained.

Complications of the surgical procedures include hematoma, damage to the digital nerves that are often intimately related to the fascial bands, and, rarely, loss of the digit from digital artery involvment. Recurrences are uncommon, and are most often seen in the young fulminating type, younger patients of any type, and women. The longer the patients are followed after operation, the greater the recurrence rate.

The ultimate result may well depend as much on the postoperative treatment splinting program and hand therapy program combined with patient cooperation, as it does on the actual operative procedure.

Tendon Graft

Flexor tendon grafting is frequently required in the secondary reconstruction of the injured flexor tendon system of the hand. This is often the situation in the reconstruction following complex injuries involving not only the tendon systems, but also fractures and nerve injury. The purpose of the flexor tendon graft is to interpose an intact tendon through the area of soft tissue injury, placing the juncture sites at favorable locations. The site of proximal tendon repair is usually in either the palm or the forearm, and the distal repair site at the insertion into the volar base of the terminal phalanx. These surgical procedures are technically demanding and may well require simultaneous pulley reconstruction. The tendon graft itself must be handled with a no-touch technique to minimize the risk of scarring. The donor tendon may be harvested from the palmaris longus, plantaris, or various other sites, depending upon the clinical situation. If the bed for the proposed tendon graft requires reconstruction, particularly of pulleys, or if the bed is heavily scarred, a two-stage grafting procedure is performed. At the initial stage a silicone rod is placed as a passive spacer around which the body forms a smooth bursal sheath. Approximately 6 weeks later the tendon graft is then inserted down this preformed sheath.

Nerve Graft

Nerve Gaps

Patients frequently present with a history of nerve injury with a gap in nerve substance either from segmental nerve loss or from nerve retraction. If the gap is small, it is sometimes possible to mobilize the nerve proximally and distally and do a secondary direct repair. This is not an effective technique if the repair is done under tension. As a general guideline, if the repair cannot be accomplished with 8-0 or 10-0 suture material, there is too much tension.

Millesi et al. have made a recent major contribution by demonstrating that when injury results in loss of nerve substance, the best results are achieved if the nerve gap is overcome by accurate interposition of fascicular nerve autografts. The key to their successes, well corroborated by other authors, is first and foremost the absence of any tension upon the proximal or distal suture lines. The importance must be emphasized of (1) meticulous surgical technique, (2) microscopic magnification, (3) use of fine nerve instruments, and (4) use of 8-0 or 10-0 suture material. The results are much superior to those previously achieved by rerouting peripheral nerves and positioning joints to gain enough length in a nerve to overcome large nerve gap.

Because nerve homografts (allografts) are not successful, the patient must exchange one deficit for another. The donor nerve most commonly used is the sural. The deficit on the lateral aspect of the foot and ankle is usually not troublesome to the patient, and because of peripheral ingrowth eventually leaves the patient usually with a fairly small area of anesthesia in a noncritical area. Unfortunately, allografts of nerve, notoriously unsuccessful in the past, remain so despite efforts to decrease their antigenicity by immunosuppressive agents.

Neuroma

When a peripheral nerve is left unrepaired, the sprouting axons at the proximal cut end form a tumor mass with local fibroblasts. This neuroma is tender to palpation and percussion, and electric-shock-like sensations interpreted as coming from the area previously innervated are bothersome to the patient. The best treatment is nerve repair, thus allowing the axons to progress peripherally. When this cannot be accomplished, the cut nerve ends should be placed deep into soft tissue or into bone away from the superficial scar and away from sites where trauma would occur from ordinary daily use of the extremity. This protection from repeated trauma may serve to relieve the symptoms.

Alternative Methods for Sensibility Restoration

When peripheral nerve repair or grafting is impossible, alternative measures for restoring sensibility may be considered. The best technique is that of transfer of a nerve together with its patch of innervated soft tissue on a neurovascular pedicle. The versatility of such innervated and vascularized islands of skin and subcutaneous tissue is great. The radial arrangement of digital vessels and nerves lends itself to this method. For example, a prime digit such as a thumb may be resurfaced and reinnervated with simultaneous correction of skin and sensory deficit using a neurovascular island pedicle flap from the ulnar border of the terminal two segments of the ring finger. The transferred sensibility is precise and immediate, although the switch does result in misidentification of the source of a stimulus—that is, a touch to the resurfaced thumb may be interpreted by the patient as a touch to the ring finger. Usually this can be "relearned" or reoriented by the patient.

Musculotendinous Transfers

When there is irreversible paralysis of muscles innervated by a peripheral nerve not suitable for nerve grafting, some muscles still innervated by intact motor units may be transferred to replace the lost function. Several factors must be considered in planning such transfers.

1. The donor motor unit must be carefully selected. Factors to be considered include the deficit remaining at the site from which the motor unit is harvested, the strength of the motor unit and the power that it will be able to impart at its new insertion, and the amplitude of that muscle belly contraction that will determine the excursion imparted to the new tendon recipient.
2. The pathway that the transferred motor unit will take is important as it will predetermine the angle of approach to its new insertion.
3. The bed through which the transferred musculotendinous unit must pass should be as free from scar as possible.
4. Consideration needs to be given to pulley formation to "fine-tune" the angle of approach for the transfer.
5. The insertion must be carefully considered—bone, tendon, etc.
6. As has been emphasized by Littler, it is essential to simplify the polyarticulated digital system with selected fusions, combined with the tendon transfers, if adequate function is to be obtained. This is a very complex type of reconstructive surgery, and a few examples of the various types of transfers available are given below (these examples are in no way intended as a complete list).

Median Nerve Palsy

Median nerve loss at the wrist will result in paralysis of those muscles needed for thumb abduction and opposition. The important functional deficit is inability to position the thumb for proper pulp-to-pulp pinch against the fingers. The tendon of the unparalyzed ring finger digitorum superficialis can be transferred to the insertion of the abductor pollicis longus. Should the median nerve loss be at the elbow, however, the superficialis to the ring finger cannot be used, as it will also be denervated. In this situation, one alternative is a transfer of the ulnar innervated abductor digiti minimi across the palm as an opponens substitute.

Ulnar Nerve Palsy

If the ulnar nerve is lost at the wrist level, all the intrinsic muscles of the hand except for the thenar thumb positioning muscles innervated by the median nerve will be paralyzed. A claw deformity occurs in the ring and little fingers because the metacarpophalangeal extensors are unopposed. As the metacarpophalangeal joints are pulled into hyperextension, the long flexors cause a clawing or intrinsic minus position of the fingers. In this situation, the flexor digitorum superficialis to the ring finger can be transferred to the base of the proximal phalanx of the ring and little fingers to reestablish active metacarpophalangeal joint flexion.

If the ulnar nerve is interrupted as it enters the forearm, the flexor digitorum profundus to the ring and little fingers is also denervated. This will result in a less severe claw deformity for the ring and little fingers, but also means that the superficial flexor cannot be used as a motor unit, for to do so would leave that digit without an active extrinsic flexor. In this situation one transfer that is used is that of the extensor carpi radialis longus divided into four separate tails, prolonged with tendon grafts, and routed anterior to the axis of motion at the metacarpophalangeal joint to be inserted into the lateral bands of the fingers. Transfers are also required to replace first dorsal interosseous function and thumb adductor function to improve pinch power.

Radial Nerve Palsy

A common radial nerve interruption occurs over the mid or distal humerus and results in loss of active wrist extension, metacarpophalangeal joint finger extension, and thumb abduction extension. The most common transfer used for reconstitution of this is the pronator teres to the extensor carpi radialis brevis, the flexor carpi ulnaris to the extensor digitorum communis, and the palmaris longus to the extensor pollicis longus.

POSTOPERATIVE CARE. Obviously the postoperative dressing, hand therapy, and exercise and splinting program are critical to the success of this type of surgery.

Bony Nonunion

Nonunions in the hand and wrist are fortunately uncommon except for the scaphoid and occasionally a meta-carpal that has sustained a segmental loss from something such as a gunshot wound.

For nonunions of the scaphoid, the bone grafting technique most often preferred is that of the Russe technique with the bone harvested either from the distal radius or from the ilium.

For nonunions of metacarpals with segmental defects, the most common source of bone graft material is the ilium with a small block of bone being interposed into the defect.

For nonunions of the forearm, the most common technique currently used is that for compression plate fixation combined with iliac medullary bone grafting. For long segmental defects in the forearm, vascularized fibular bone grafts have provided the best results. As an alternative, a single bone form can be created.

Congenital Anomalies

The genetic and environmental factors cited as etiologic agents in other congenital anomalies also apply to upper limb deficiencies. Anomalies have no fixed pattern and may involve supernumerary parts, failure to differentiate, failure of formation, hypertrophy, or atrophy. Note that the limb bud forms within the first 6 weeks of gestation, and therefore the physician must carefully look for other congenital abnormalities, especially cardiac and renal.

Syndactyly

Webbing of the fingers is the most common of all congenital abnormalities. It may involve simply a thin-skinned web between otherwise normal digits to a fusion of bony elements with a common distal nail. Syndactyly is characterized by phenotypic variability and genetic heterogeneity. There may be dominant autosomal inheritance. Syndactyly is an integral part of many different syndromes such as Poland's syndrome and Apert's syndrome (acrocephalosyndactyly). Commonly, both hands and feet are involved. Males are affected more frequently than females. X-ray examination may be helpful in assessing skeletal involvement, but recall that in the young child much of the skeletal framework is still cartilaginous.

The best timing for surgical intervention is a subject of debate. Most surgeons agree that when digits of different growth rates are involved with a syndactyly involving distal bony junctures, separation of these distal components is recommended before one year of age in order to prevent growth retardation of the longer digit and thus prevent progressive deviation of the longer digit toward the shorter. After this has been attended to, or if there is no concern for a growth differential problem, it is advisable to wait until the end of the second or third year of life for surgical intervention. Surgical correction must be carefully planned to avoid the creation of skin scar contractures. If syndactyly release is done before the age of one, there will frequently be a bridling scar with recurrence of the webbing.

The operation for separation will involve the creation of interdigitating skin flaps on the adjacent sides of the

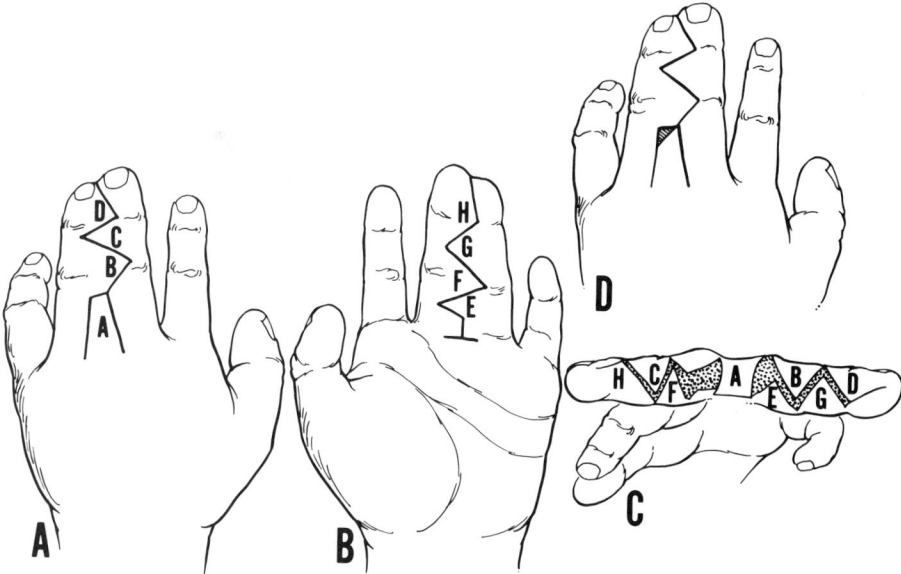

Fig. 45-28. Common type of syndactyly repair. [From: *Dobbins J, Wood V, et al: Congenital anomalies, in Green D (ed): Operative Hand Surgery. New York, Churchill-Livingstone, 1982, with permission.*]

two involved digits (Fig. 45-28). If more than two digits are involved, it is essential to stage the release with at least 6 months between operations. To release both sides of any single digit will seriously endanger its blood supply. The flaps of skin and subcutaneous tissue are designed to interdigitate to re-form the web cleft and to re-surface a portion of the released fingers. Note that the skin envelope required for the conjoined fingers will be deficient to ensheath the two separated digits. Full-thickness skin grafting will be required, most commonly harvested from the lateral inguinal crease. The more medial groin, with its potential for future pubic hair, should be avoided as a donor site to the hand.

Polydactyly

Extra digits may appear as a supernumerary phalanx or duplication of an entire extremity—or any variation between these extremes. The most common form of polydactyly is a rudimentary digit extending from the radial or ulnar margin of the hand. If this is simply a nubbin, it is removed without difficulty. However, the duplication may be much more complex. For example, duplications of the thumb are most common, and it is occasionally difficult to tell which is the prime digit and which is vestigial.

Such supernumerary digits must be amputated precisely and with great surgical judgment. Care must be taken to preserve tendons and sensory nerves to the digit left in situ. It may be necessary to do selected tendon transfers from the amputated digit to make more normal the digit that remains. Should the supernumerary digit arise at a joint level, ligament reconstructions of that joint are essential if long-range joint instability is to be avoided.

Circumferential Grooves

Circumferential grooves in the extremity are common, and may be shallow or deep. If shallow, they will not threaten the survival of a part and may be either ignored or treated by Z-plasty for cosmetic improvement. In some situations the constriction is so severe that the survival of the part is threatened from poor distal venous return. Surgical release with Z-plasty reconstructions then becomes more urgent.

Missing Parts

Children are frequently born with missing parts of the hand or arm. There are many combinations, but a few are common enough to merit emphasis. Absence of segments of the forearm such as congenital absence of the radius or ulna may be found in combination with incomplete preaxial or postaxial hand formation. The most common is that of the radial club hand with an absent radius, deficient radial carpal bones, and absent thumb.

Isolated absence of a thumb is very disabling, as it prevents good prehensile grasp (see Thumb Reconstruction below).

Thumb Reconstruction

Hand function is severely compromised in the absence of a thumb. Thumb loss may be congenital or traumatic.

In the congenital absence of a thumb, if the child has four normal digits, pollicization of the index finger is a reasonable procedure (Fig. 45-29). The index finger is rotated into the thumb position and shortened to the appropriate length by resection of the majority of the metacarpal, bringing with it intact sensation and circulation. A basal joint is reconstructed using the metacarpophalangeal joint. Various tendon transfers are performed to redistribute the index finger tendons into the positions needed for abductor pollicis longus, extensor pollicis

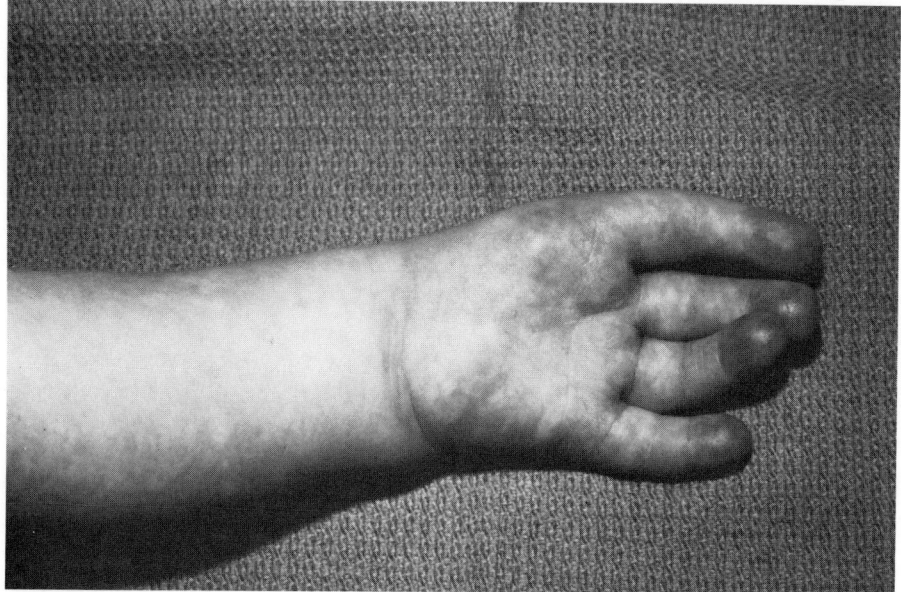

A

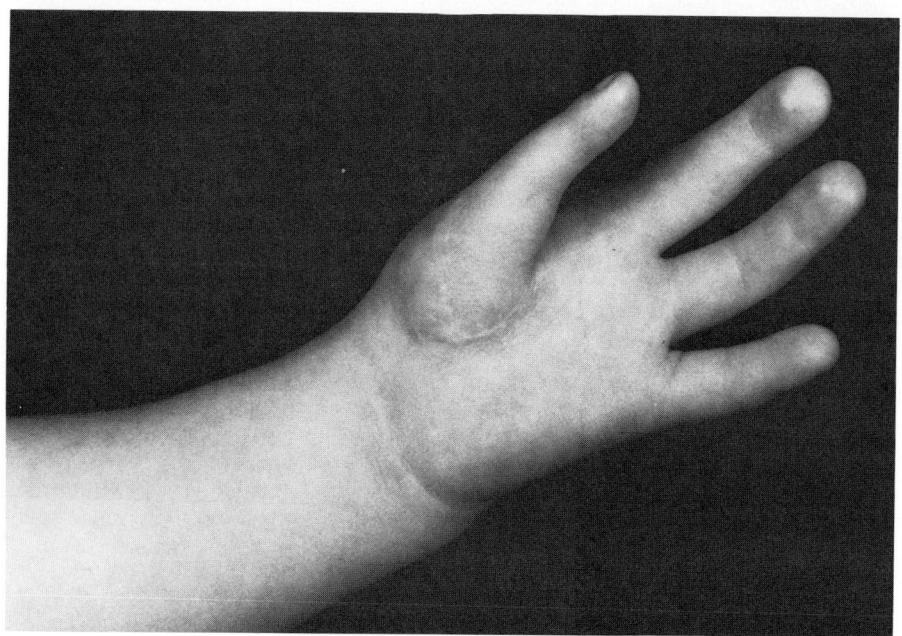

B

Fig. 45-29. Thumb reconstruction for congenital absence by pollicization of index finger into thumb position. *A.* Preoperative photograph. *B* and *C.* Postoperative result with excellent function. (From: *Burton RI, 1983, with permission.*)

brevis, and extensor pollicis longus, and, using the interossei, to reconstruct the muscles of the thenar eminence. The skin incisions and flaps must be carefully designed to accommodate this increased bulk. This procedure is best and most safely performed at the ages of three to five years, before the child enters school. Some surgeons prefer to carry out the procedure in the first year of life.

Thumb reconstruction following traumatic loss can be done by one of two means. The first is a pollicization analogous to that used in the congenital situation. However, this is usually somewhat simpler as a basal joint,

and proximal metacarpal usually remains. As an alternative, a toe may be placed in the thumb position as a free transfer.

Tumors

Tumors of the hand are common, fortunately most often benign. The malignant tumors may be bony or fas-

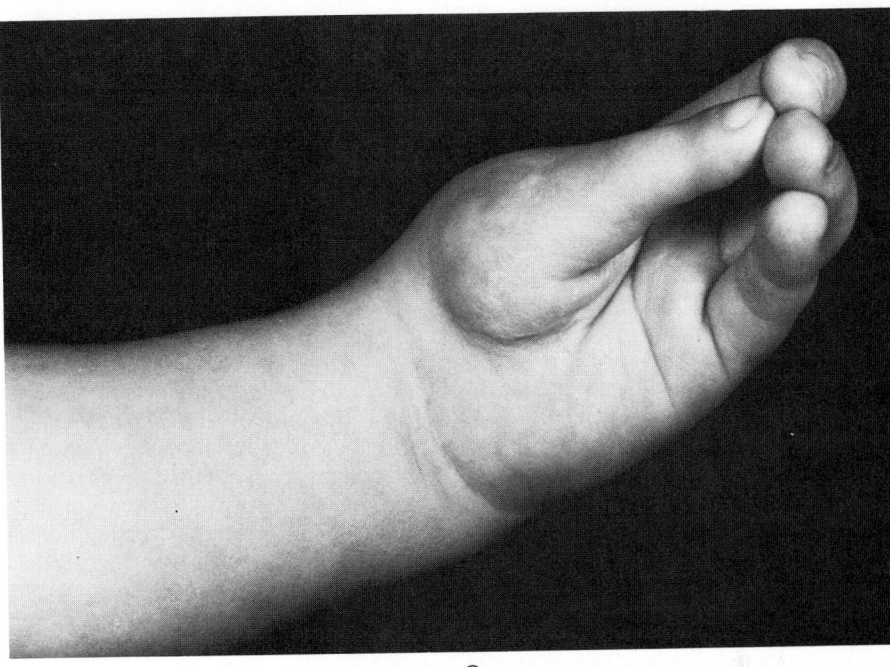

C

Fig. 45-29 *C*. Continued.

cial in origin, but those which occur in the hand are most apt to be either squamous cell carcinoma or malignant melanoma.

Ganglion

The ganglion is the most common soft tissue tumor in the hand. It is commonly seen in four locations.

1. The ganglion that occurs on the dorsum of the wrist usually has a stalk that extends to the joint, most commonly into the area of the scapholunate joint. This ganglion may be painful when impinged beneath the wrist extensor tendons.
2. Ganglia that occur on the flexor side of the wrist are usually adjacent to the flexorcarpi radialis tendon and may have a stalk extending to the pantrapezial joints. In this situation the ganglion may be secondary to a basal joint arthritis of the thumb. The stalk, as an alternative, may extend toward the carpal canal to take origin from the flexor side of the wrist, and may be associated with a carpal tunnel syndrome.
3. Ganglia may arise from the flexor sheath and usually present as small tender BB-sized nodules at the base of the digit.
4. A ganglion that arises from the distal interphalangeal joint is called a mucous cyst. This structure originates from the joint with a stalk that extends in the interval between the extensor tendon insertion and a marginal osteophyte. As emphasized by both Eaton and Kleinert, it is necessary to remove the cyst, the stalk, and the offending osteophyte. Skin grafting is rarely, if ever, necessary. Note that these lesions are commonly seen in association with osteoarthritis. The skin over the lesion may have become very thin in the past with a blisterlike appearance. Nail deformity from the lesion is not uncommon. Should the lesion extend close to the eponychial margin, rupture at the time of manicure is not uncommon. With rupture, infection can occur and may extend into the distal joint in the form of a septic arthritis.

Giant Cell Tumor of Tendon

Giant cell tumor of tendon is a common benign tumor, characteristically multilobular, and it appears to originate from the short vinculum of the flexor tendons near interphalangeal joints. The tumor will characteristically involve both tendon and tendon sheath and may secondarily erode into bone or the adjacent joint. The tendon will lie deep to the neurovascular bundles with the digital nerve splayed over its surface. This condition is treated by operation.

Inclusion Cyst

Pathology is an implantation of epithelium with or without a foreign body. The cyst appears as a fibrous capsule with a squamous epithelial lining containing a creamy white pastelike substance. The cysts are seen on the flexor aspect of the palm and fingers.

Other Benign Lesions

Other tumors include lipomas, which are most commonly seen around the thenar eminence, sebaceous cysts, which most commonly occur on the dorsum of the hand, vascular tumors, and glomus tumors. The latter lesions usually present as severely painful lesions deep to the nail plate or in the paronychial area.

Arthritis

Arthritic involvement of the hand and wrist is very common and may be one of several types—rheumatoid arthritis, osteoarthritis, gout, pseudogout, or traumatic—or it may involve avascular necrosis of bones (Kienbock's, Preisser's).

Rheumatoid Arthritis

The treatment of patients with rheumatoid arthritis must be multidisciplinary. A *team* ideally will include the hand surgeon, a rheumatologist, a hand therapist, a social worker, the support of a good family unit, and the patient. It is essential to understand that this is a *systemic* disease not only involving multiple joints of upper and lower extremity, but also having cardiac, pulmonary, and renal manifestations.

Nonoperative treatment must include the appropriate anti-inflammatory medications regulated by the internist or the rheumatologist, the appropriate splints, and a carefully designed exercise program. These exercises should include not only range of motion, but also stretching exercises for the contracted musculotendinous units, such as the ulnar intrinsics.

The patient must be informed in detail about patterns of hand use in the activities of daily living and various aids for this. For example, the patient with involvement at the metacarpophalangeal joints of the fingers must understand that grasping heavy objects between the thumb and forefinger or excessive pinch activities will put undue ulnar-deforming force on the inflamed capsule, helping to potentiate the speed of ulnar drift deformity. Similarly these patients must be cautioned about not pushing up out of a chair, which also puts ulnar-deviating forces on those fingers. Patients with lower extremity involvement should use platform crutches rather than axillary crutches.

Operative procedures for the hand of the patient with rheumatoid arthritis should only be done after the lower extremity reconstruction has been completed. Surgical procedures can be grouped into those performed at the wrist level, those on the thumb, and those on the fingers. Rheumatoid arthritis will involve any and all of the tendon systems and joints of the wrist and hand. Frequently the first presentation of rheumatoid arthritis is in the hand (see Figs. 43-94 and 43-95). No surgical procedure should be undertaken unless the patient is following a well-regulated program of anti-inflammatory medications and has had a preoperative course of night splinting to control factors such as ulnar deviation, in conjunction with an exercise program (see Fig. 45-30).

Surgery at the wrist involves surgery on the extensor tendons, the flexor tendons, and the joint itself. Unrelieved tenosynovitis on the dorsum of the wrist frequently results in attrition and rupture of the extensor tendons, most commonly over the distal ulna. If dorsal tenosynovitis does not respond to 6 months of conservative management, tenosynovectomy should be performed. Tendon ruptures, if present, will require tendon transfers rather than repair, as the substance of the tendon at the site of rupture is usually severely attenuated and infiltrated with synovium.

The wrist joint itself is usually significantly involved with the arthritic process. Underlying bony irregularities, particularly Lister's tubercle and the distal ulna, may be contributory to the tendon ruptures. If rupture of the tendon transfers is to be avoided, it is frequently necessary to operate upon the wrist joint itself.

The surgery on the wrist joint is done through the same dorsal incision as that for the tendons. Depending upon the findings in the joint, the surgery may involve synovectomy, wrist fusion, or total wrist replacement. It is

rare that simple excision of the distal ulna (Darrach procedure) is indicated as a solitary procedure because of the risk of late ulnar angulation and translocation of the carpus upon the distal radius. Excision of the distal ulna must be combined with other reconstructive procedures to provide wrist stability.

A flexor tenosynovitis at the wrist is also common in the patient with rheumatoid arthritis, and may present with carpal tunnel syndrome, trigger digits, or flexor tendon ruptures. Flexor tenosynovectomy in the carpal canal area frequently needs to be combined with flexor tenosynovectomy in the distal palm and in the fingers as well.

Thumb deformities are complex. They may involve the basal joint, the metacarpophalangeal joint, and/or the interphalangeal joint. The deformities may involve multiple joints. Surgery for correction of these deformities usually involves a combination of joint fusions, joint arthroplasties, and tendon transfers.

Finger deformity in rheumatoid arthritis is common. Such deformities usually involve joint destruction at the metacarpophalangeal joint level with anterior subluxation/dislocation combined with extensor lag and ulnar drift (Fig. 45-30). The interphalangeal joints are often afflicted, resulting in either the boutonniere or swan neck deformities.

At the metacarpophalangeal joint level, implant arthroplasty is often necessary. This involves resection of the destroyed joint remnants, ligamentous and volar plate releases, and Littler intrinsic musculotendinous release on the ulnar aspect of the finger, sometimes combined with crossed intrinsic transfers, implant insertion, capsuloplasty, and reconstitution of the extrinsic extensor tendon mechanisms.

The postoperative exercise and splinting program is of critical importance. Following surgery, in order to maintain the corrections gained, the splinting and exercise programs are often continued for 6 months, and indeed the splinting program may be necessary at night for several years.

Surgery on these swan neck deformities and boutonniere deformities is most complex and usually involves a combination of joint fusions and joint arthroplasties.

Osteoarthritis

Osteoarthritis very commonly inflicts multiple joints in the hand, particularly in the postmenopausal female. Those joints most often involved are the interphalangeal joints of the fingers and thumb, and the basal joint of the thumb. The osteophytic overgrowth at the distal joint is known as Heberden's nodes and that at the proximal interphalangeal joints Bouchard's nodes (Fig. 45-30). Involvement at the terminal digital joint if associated with severe pain and deformity is best treated by arthrodesis. Involvement of the proximal interphalangeal joints of the fingers is often managed by implant arthroplasty if the symptoms are not controlled by conservative measures such as nonsteroidal anti-inflammatory drugs and aids for activities of daily living.

The arthritis involving the basal joint of the thumb is

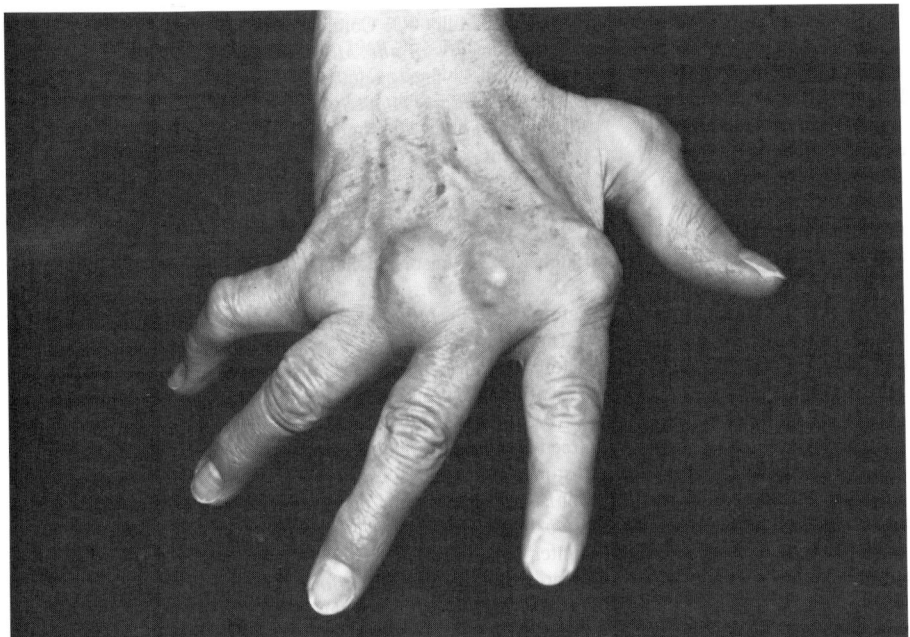

A

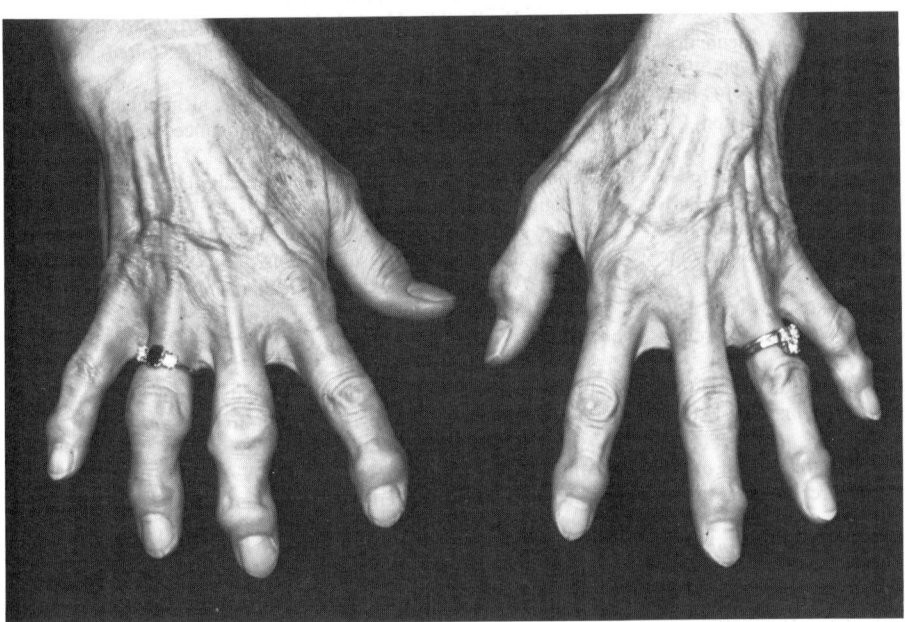

B

Fig. 45-30. *A.* Classic clinical appearance of rheumatoid arthritis in hand. Note radial deviation of wrist, extensor lag, and ulnar drift at the MCP level. *B.* Classic clinical appearance of osteoarthritis in hand. Note the involvement of IP joints with Heberden's and Bouchard's nodes with sparing of MCP joints.

the most disabling. In its later stages it renders the thumb almost useless because of the severe pain, often combined with a severe adduction deformity of the thumb metacarpal. In the young laboring hand, arthrodesis may be the procedure of choice. Most surgeons prefer arthroplasty of the basal joint for this condition. Some favor

implant arthroplasty, and others fascial arthroplasty. Implant arthroplasty has been associated with some problems including prosthesis failure, bone resorption, and/or instability. Fascial arthroplasty has been associated with some residual weakness.

New techniques of ligament reconstruction combined with various types of soft tissue interposition arthroplasty have produced excellent results in the basal joint of the osteoarthritic hand, even in the hand requiring demanding use.

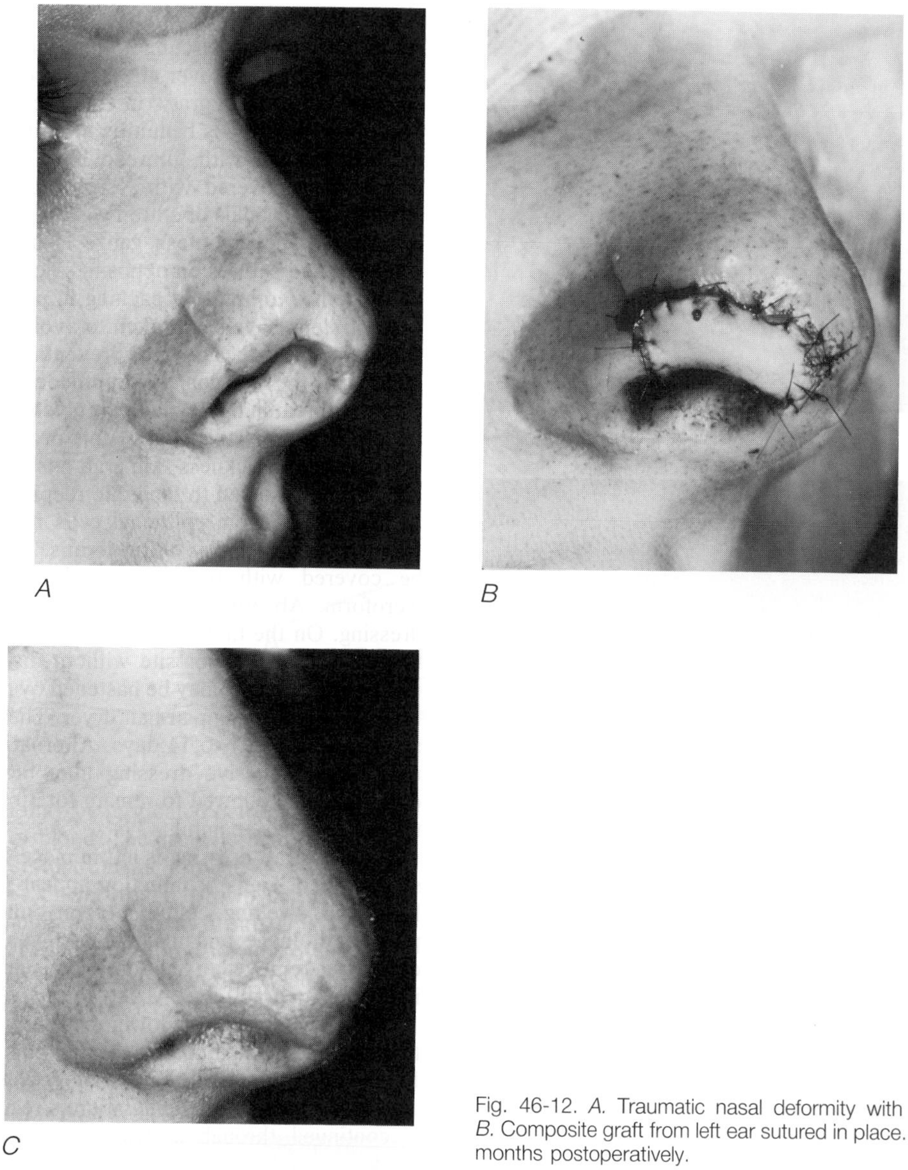

Fig. 46-12. *A.* Traumatic nasal deformity with loss of alar rim. *B.* Composite graft from left ear sutured in place. *C.* Appearance 6 months postoperatively.

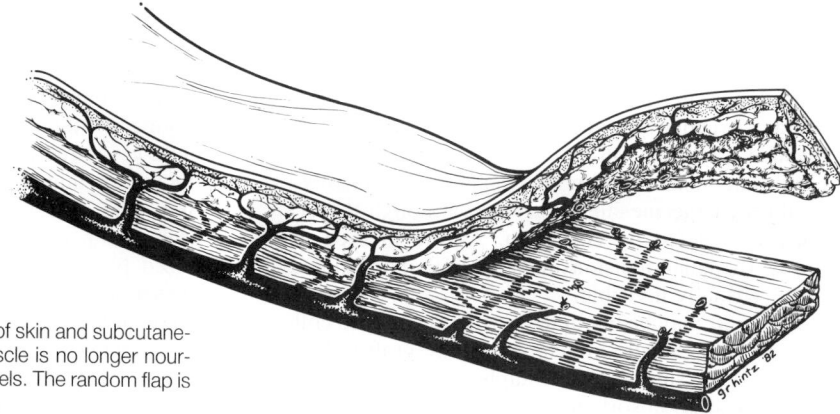

Fig. 46-13. Random skin flap. The segment of skin and subcutaneous tissue elevated from the underlying muscle is no longer nourished by musculocutaneous perforating vessels. The random flap is supplied by a subdermal plexus of vessels.

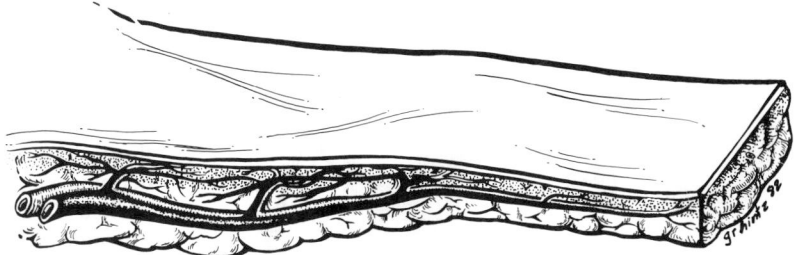

46-14. Axial pattern flap. This flap is supplied by a defined cutaneous artery and vein. Examples of the axial pattern flap include the groin flap, deltopectoral flap, and forehead flap.

usually take if no portion of it is more than 1 cm from the vascular bed. Revascularization occurs by processes similar to those seen in other skin grafts.

The next great advance in skin grafting may well be the use of a living skin equivalent. Skin equivalents have been developed in experimental animals. The material consists of dermal and epidermal elements made with cells taken from the graft recipient. It holds the promise of providing skin coverage in patients with limited donor sites.

Flaps

Use of a tissue flap is an important technique in management of the difficult wound. In general, the cutaneous flap used in plastic surgery is composed of skin and associated tissues attached to the body through a vascular or skin pedicle. This pedicle contains nutrient vessels and draining veins. A well-chosen flap can promote healing of a wound as well as improve the functional and aesthetic result.

A skin flap is classified as either random, axial pattern, musculocutaneous, or fasciocutaneous depending upon the nature of its blood supply. The *random pattern skin flap* receives blood through its dermal-subdermal plexus (Fig. 46-13). This plexus is supplied by musculocutaneous vessels and nourishes the flap through its pedicle. In contrast to the random flap, the *axial pattern skin flap* is vascularized by a direct cutaneous artery (Fig. 46-14). A *fasciocutaneous flap* consists of skin and the fascia deep to it. This type of flap receives its blood supply from the vascular plexus contained in the deep fascia. The plexus sends branches to the overlying skin. The fasciocutaneous flap is better vascularized and survives at a greater length-to-width ratio than does a comparable random pattern flap.

RANDOM FLAPS. The *Z-plasty* is a particularly useful application of random skin flaps. The *Z-plasty* may be employed to lengthen a straight scar, break the line of a linear scar, and position a scar within the lines of minimal tension. The classic Z-plasty consists of two triangular flaps of skin and subcutaneous tissue. The sides of both triangles are equal in length and the angles are 60° (Fig. 46-15). Special requirements in individual patients may

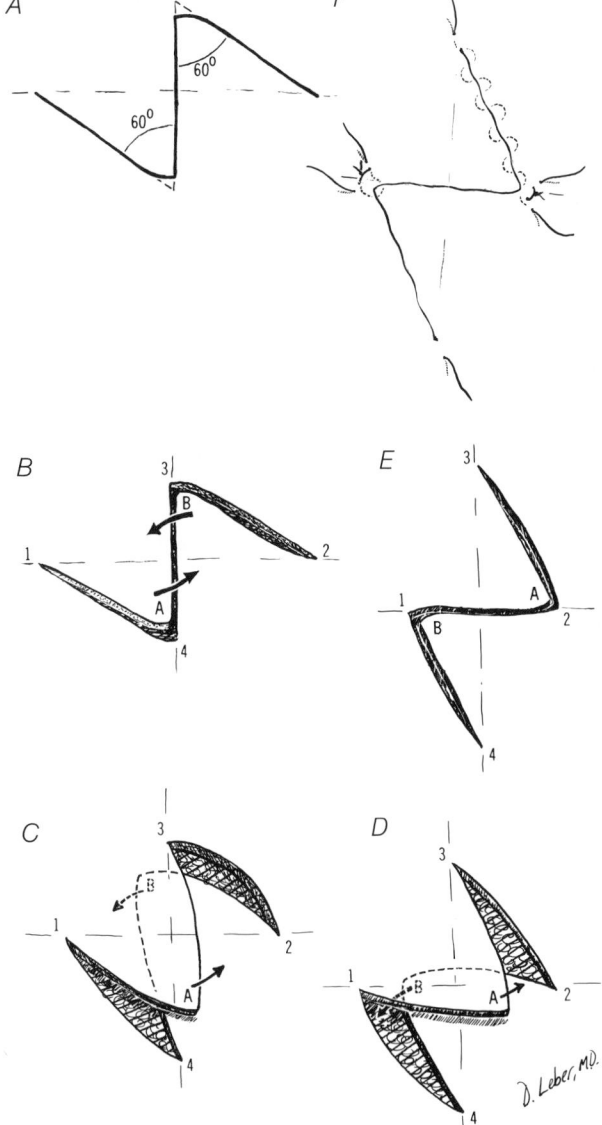

Fig 46-15. The Z-plasty. Construction of two identical equilateral triangles based on any scar line creates two triangular flaps that together constitute a parallelogram. Interchanging these two flaps will lengthen the original scar line, exchanging the short diagonal of the parallelogram for the long diagonal.

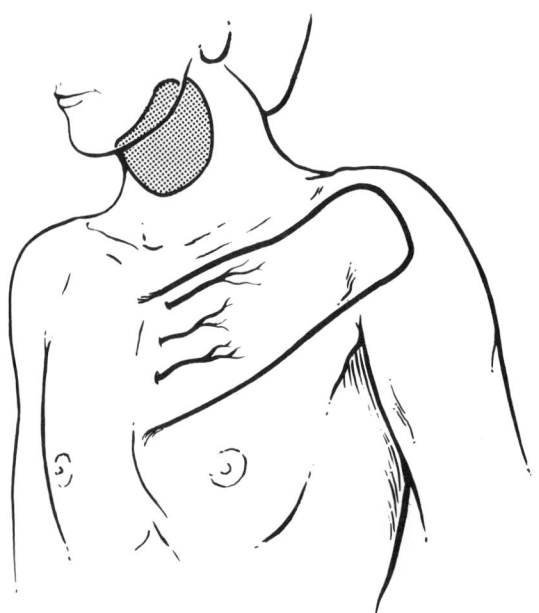

Fig. 46-23. Deltopectoral flap. This axial pattern flap, as illustrated, is being used to close a defect in the neck. Blood supply comes from perforating branches of the internal thoracic artery.

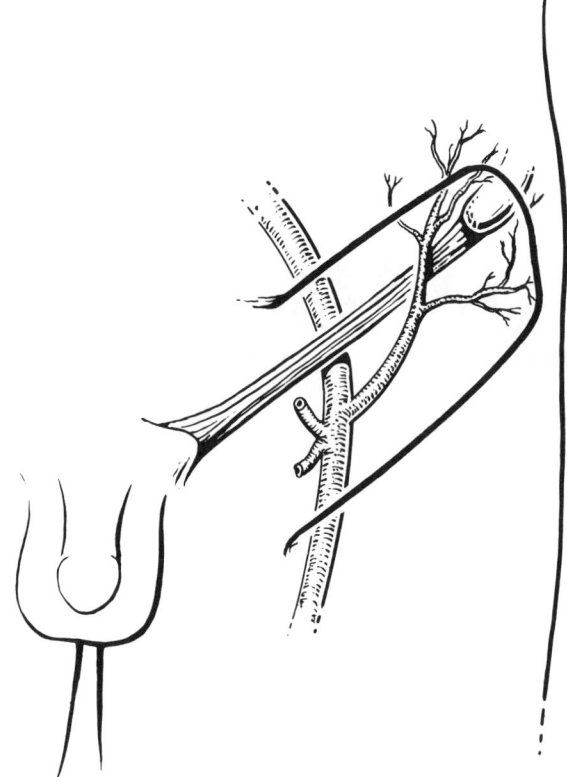

Fig. 46-24. Groin flap. The superficial circumflex iliac artery nourishes this flap in an axial pattern; the diameter of the artery is exaggerated for purposes of illustration.

Fig. 46-25. Omental flap. *A.* The greater omentum is dissected free of the stomach and transverse colon. The blood supply is provided via the left gastroepiploic vessels. *B.* A left chest wall defect is filled with the omentum and a split-thickness skin graft applied.

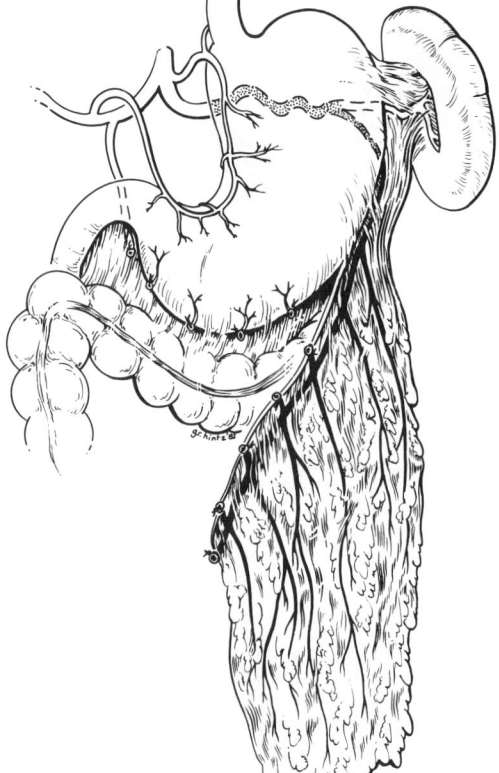

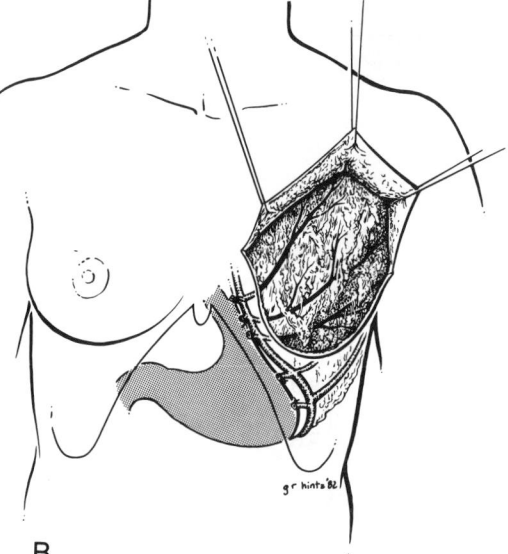

A

B

fourth anterior perforating branches of the internal mammary artery (Fig. 46-23). This flap is particularly helpful in reconstructing head and neck wounds. The *groin flap*, nourished by the superficial circumflex iliac artery, allows coverage of hand and forearm wounds (Fig. 46-24).

The omentum is dissected from the greater curvature of the stomach and sustained as an axial pattern flap on the right or left gastroepiploic vessels. It may be transferred to satisfy a defect of the abdominal or chest wall (Fig. 46-25). After the defect is filled, the omentum may be covered with a meshed split-thickness skin graft.

The *island flap* is of the axial pattern type. Its pedicle consists of the nutrient vessels without a bridge of skin or subcutaneous tissue (Fig. 46-26). A sensory nerve may be included in the pedicle. These flaps have been used for hand and face reconstruction (Fig. 46-27).

FASCIOCUTANEOUS FLAPS. Elevation of a skin flap with the underlying fascia provides a well-vascularized flap that survives to a greater length than the random pattern variety. The fasciocutaneous flap has found application in management of difficult wounds of the trunk and extremities (Fig. 46-28).

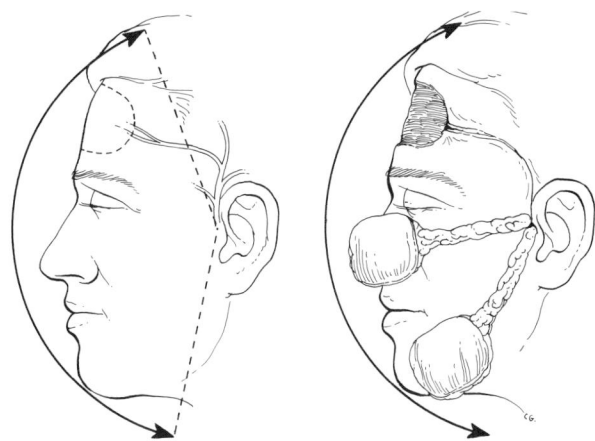

Fig. 46-26. Island pedicle flap. A vascularized island of composite tissues may be transferred over a wide area when carried solely on the temporal vessels.

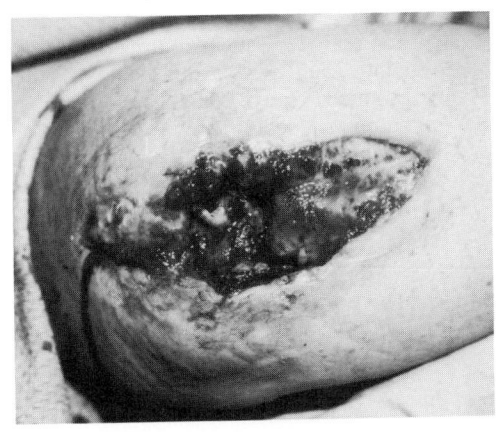

A

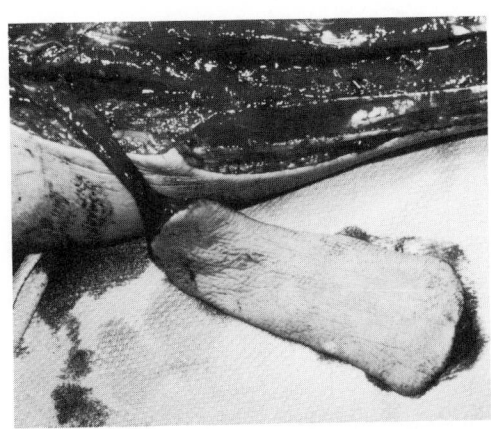

B

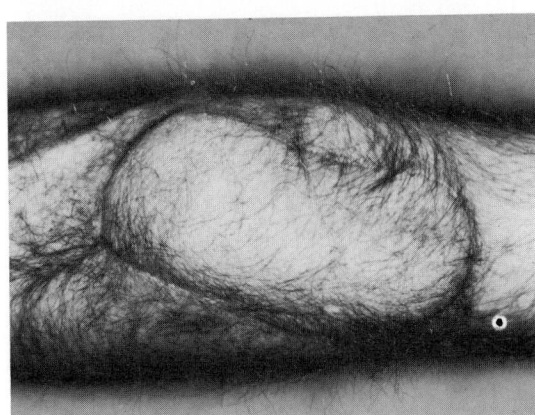

C

Fig. 46-27. Application of island pedicle flap. *A.* Osteoradionecrosis of olecranon. *B.* Radial forearm island flap raised. *C.* Elbow wound healed.

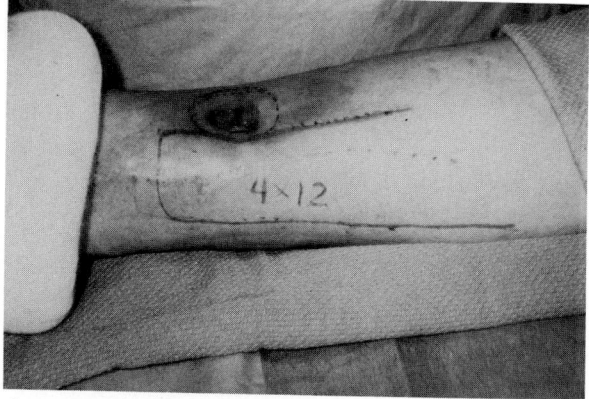

A

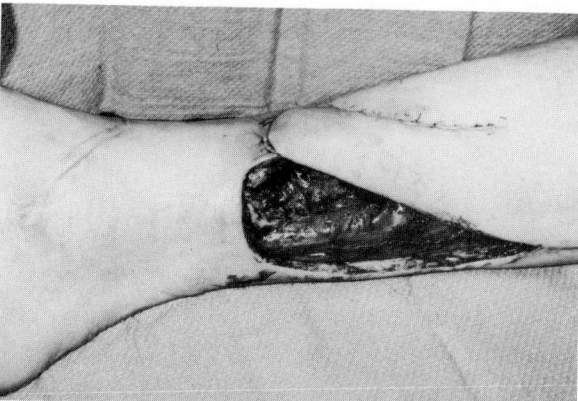

B

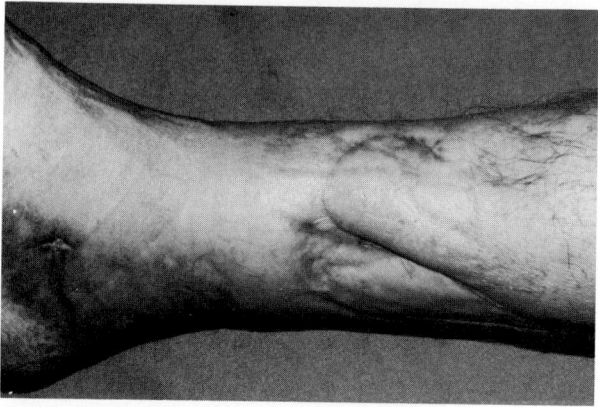

C

Fig. 46-28. Fasciocutaneous flap. *A.* Flap outlined before transposition to cover calf defect. *B.* Flap elevated. *C.* Wound healed 7 months postoperatively.

MUSCLE AND MUSCULOCUTANEOUS FLAPS. Muscle transposition is an extremely valuable reconstructive technique. This tissue has a vigorous blood supply and, when transferred into a poorly vascularized wound, can

promote healing. Although described by Manchot in a doctoral thesis (1897), it has only recently been appreciated that the skin receives much of its blood supply from the underlying muscle. In clinical practice, an island of overlying skin can be transferred with certain muscles as a single, musculocutaneous unit (Fig. 46-29). A musculocutaneous flap helps solve many difficult reconstructive and aesthetic problems where replacement of missing skin and deeper tissues is required.

FREE TISSUE TRANSFER. Most musculocutaneous and axial pattern flaps and some fasciocutaneous flaps have a single, anatomically consistent vascular pedicle. It is often possible to elevate the flap, divide the vascular pedicle, and anastamose the vessels to a recipient artery and vein at a distant site. Microvascular surgical instruments and techniques have been developed that permit anastamosis of vessels whose internal diameter is in the range of 0.8 mm. Free tissue transfer has permitted closure of some otherwise irremediable wounds and expanded the utility of many flaps (Fig. 46-30).

Tissue Expansion

Skin and subcutaneous tissue has the capacity to stretch or expand under the influence of gradually increasing pressure. After the pressure is relieved, the skin tends to return to its previous dimensions. This characteristic of skin can be observed in the abdominal distention and subsequent return to near normal seen in pregnancy and postpartum states. Whether new skin is produced or existing skin is simply stretched remains to be determined.

Popularized by Radovan, the tissue expander was developed to increase the surface area of skin adjacent to a

Fig. 46-29. Musculocutaneous flap. The muscle is nourished by its anatomic blood supply. The overlying skin survives on perforating vessels from the muscle.

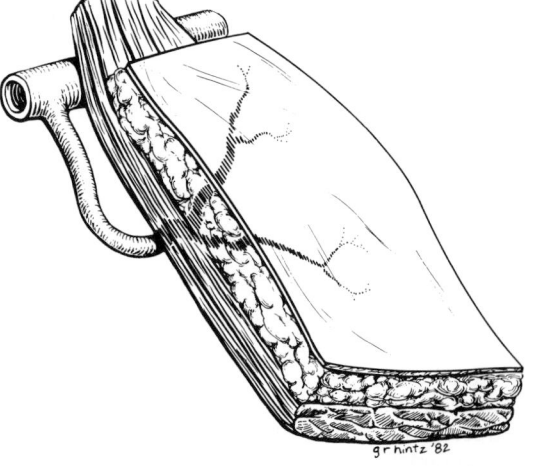

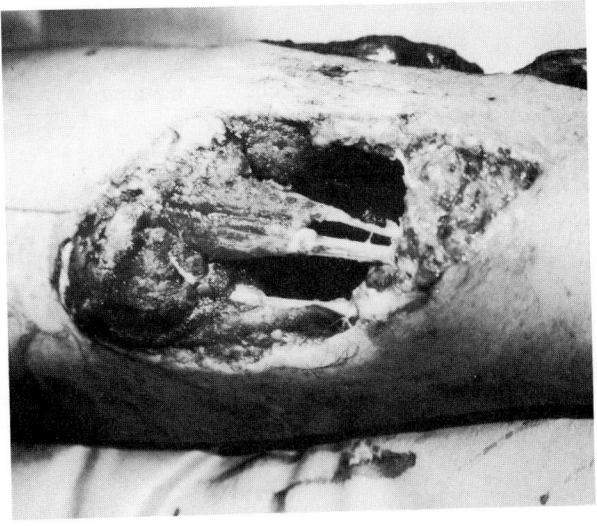

A

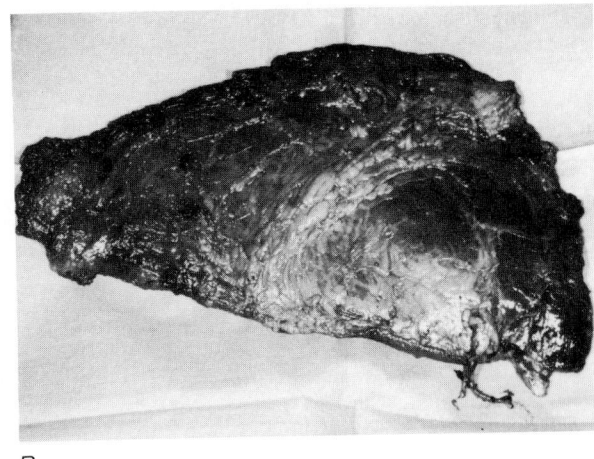

B

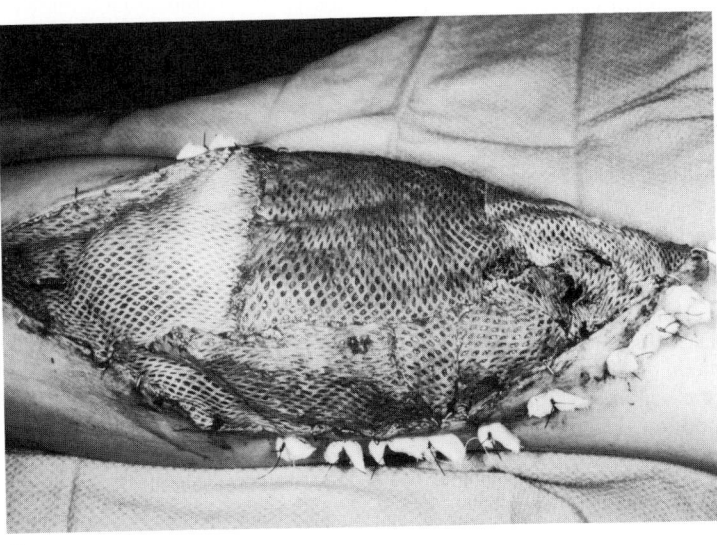

C

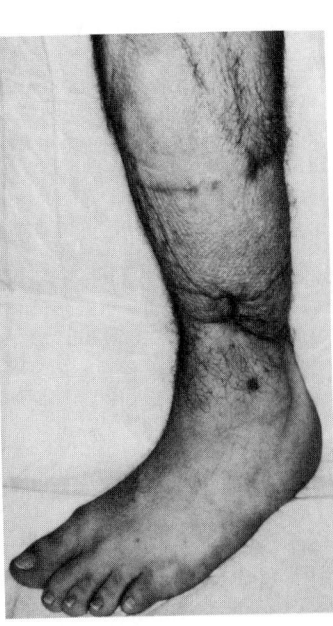

D

Fig. 46-30. Free tissue transfer. *A.* Through-and-through gunshot wound of leg with massive soft tissue loss. *B.* Latissimus dorsi muscle harvested with vascular pedicle. *C.* Muscle transposed with meshed split-thickness skin graft applied. *D.* Wound healed 3 months postoperatively.

defect and permit closure by skin flap transposition. A collapsed plastic bag of varying shape and maximal volume is attached to a self-sealing reservoir by means of a silicone rubber tube, forming a "tissue expander" (Fig. 46-31). This expander is inserted through a small incision and the wound allowed to heal. After 3 weeks, the reservoir is entered percutaneously and sterile saline injected. With repeated fillings over several weeks time, the plastic bag enlarges and expands the overlying skin. When the process is complete, the expander is removed and the ad-

jacent defect to be reconstructed is closed by transposition of the expanded skin. Tissue expansion has proved particularly useful in scalp and breast reconstruction (Fig. 46-32).

Tissue Transplantation

Autogenous tissue may be transplanted to restore contour or provide structural support to a specific area. The tissue to be transplanted is separated entirely from its

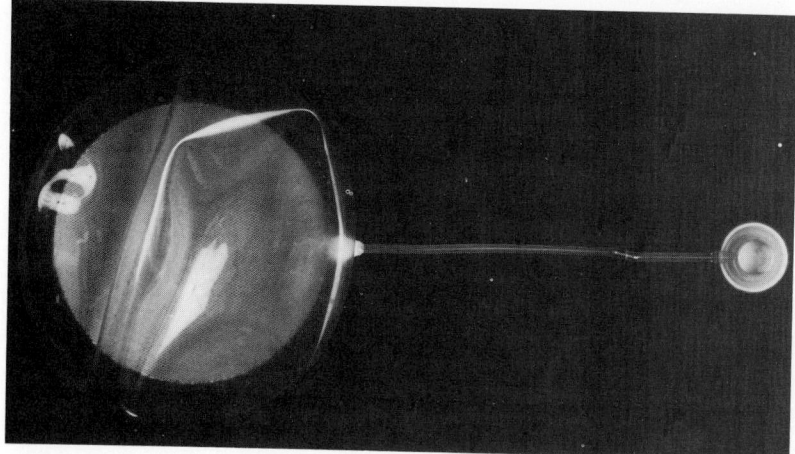

Fig. 46-31. Tissue expander. The smaller reservoir is a self-sealing injection port where saline is introduced into the expander.

blood supply, moved to a new location, and revascularized through gradual ingrowth of blood vessels at the recipient site. To ensure healing, a transplant must be stabilized securely during the postoperative period and infection, hematoma, and seroma must be prevented.

Many autogenous tissues have been used as transplants. Dermis harvested from the infragluteal fold can be used to augment a depressed area. Fat has been employed in a similar fashion. Both dermis and fat tend to be absorbed over time. Rib, iliac crest, ulnar, and cranial bone are useful in providing support. They also undergo gradual, although incomplete, resorption. Nasal septal, ear, and costal cartilage have found wide application, although the amount of autogenous cartilage is limited. Tendon and fascia both serve as successful autografts. Homograft collagen compounds can be injected intradermally or subdermally to elevate a depressed area. These compounds are also gradually resorbed but can provide prolonged variable relief from deformity.

Synthetic Materials

Synthetic materials are used in plastic surgery if autogenous tissues are unsuitable or in short supply. Various plastics and metals are available. The most commonly used tissue substitutes are fabricated from silicone elastomers. These compounds are long chains of dimethylsiloxane units that are provided in the forms of silicone fluids and silicone rubber. The mammary implant is a silicone elastomer shell filled with a silicone gel. Bone substitutes are being used both experimentally and clinically.

Microsurgery

Plastic surgical procedures requiring an operating microscope and specialized techniques fall in the category of microsurgery. Improvements in microsurgical equipment have permitted reliable anastomosis of vessels. Microsurgery has made possible the transfer of free flaps and replantation of traumatic amputations. In selected cases, microsurgical neurorrhaphy yields a superior result.

Liposuction

Liposuction, or suction-assisted lipectomy, is a technique recently developed for the removal of localized fat deposits. Metal cannulae of varying size have been designed with one or more sharpened side holes near the tip. A cannula is attached by tubing to a suction device capable of developing a high vacuum. The cannula is passed through a small skin incision and advanced into the area of fat deposition. When the vacuum device is activated, fat is drawn into the cannula's side hole. By moving the cannula back and forth, fat is cut off and aspirated through the tubing into a reservoir. This technique finds application in the removal of localized fat of the face, neck, breasts, abdomen, and extremities.

RECONSTRUCTIVE SURGERY

Breast

MACROMASTIA. *Macromastia* is an abnormal enlargement of the breasts caused by hormonal factors or obesity. On examination, the nipple and areola are displaced inferiorly. The skin of the breast is present in excess. Volume of the breast fat or parenchyma is increased. The patient experiences a feeling of heaviness or pain in the breasts, particularly before a menstrual period. Pain is often present in the shoulders, neck, and back. Skin irritation (intertrigo) occurs in the submammary fold.

Evaluation of a patient with macromastia requires a careful breast examination, including mammography for patients over thirty-five years of age or with a family history of breast cancer. Obesity is a common finding, and the patient is advised to lose weight before considering surgery. *Reduction mammaplasty* relieves macromastia. Before undergoing operation, the patient is informed of the intended postoperative result and complications including the possibility of hematoma, nipple necrosis, and hypertrophic scar formation. The patient must have an understanding of the location of the scars. She is told that lactation and breast feeding may not be possible after re-

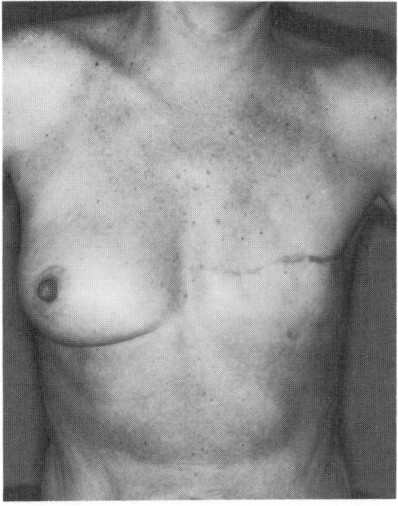

A

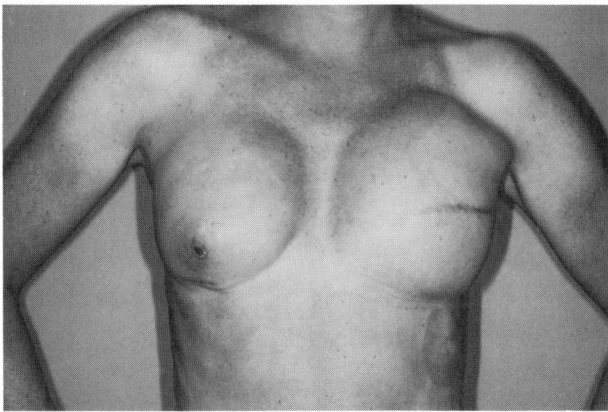

B

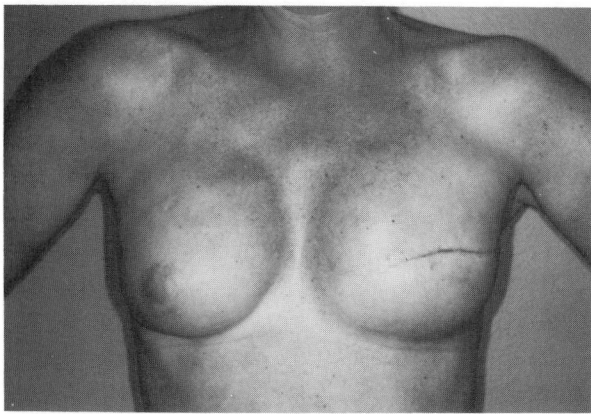

C

Fig. 46-32. Breast reconstruction by tissue expansion. *A.* Patient following left modified radical mastectomy for carcinoma of the breast. *B.* Expander maximally inflated. *C.* Expander exchanged for permanent prosthesis.

duction mammaplasty. Some women experience a decrease in nipple sensibility postoperatively and must be warned of this occurrence.

The various reduction mammaplasty operations are designed to address the same component problems of macromastia. Repositioning of the nipple and areola, usually with reduction of areolar diameter, is important. Blood supply to the nipple and areola is preserved through a dermal-fat pedicle that is nourished by perforating vessels from the internal mammary artery, pectoralis major muscle, intercostal arteries, and lateral thoracic artery. Excess breast skin is removed, forming a new skin brassiere. A subtotal resection of the breast fat and parenchyma is done in such a way as to provide a natural breast mound about which the skin is draped. Meticulous skin closure completes the procedure.

Outlining the proposed incisions is done preoperatively with the patient awake and in a sitting or standing position. The new site for the nipple and areola is selected. The nipple is centered at the level of the inframammary fold, usually 20 to 24 cm from the sternal notch and 11 to 13 cm from the midsternum. The inframammary fold is marked and remains in a constant position throughout the procedure. The remaining lines are drawn on the skin of the breast.

Selection of an operative technique from among the many available is made on the basis of breast size and the surgeon's experience. A patient with extreme hypertrophy is best treated by a free nipple graft and removal of excess skin and breast tissue. This operation involves raising the nipple-areolar complex as a full-thickness graft, performing a reduction of breast skin and parenchyma, and placing the defatted nipple-areolar graft in an appropriate position. A large volume of parenchyma can be removed and operating time minimized. A satisfactory contour is achieved. Disadvantages of this procedure include sacrifice of lactating function and nipple sensibility. The nipple often loses pigment and projection.

Less severe enlargement is usually managed by the inferior pedicle technique employing a keyhole pattern of skin excision and an appropriate parenchymal reduction (Fig. 46-33). The nipple and areola will survive consistently when carried on an inferiorly based vascularized dermal-fat pedicle. The postoperative result improves the patient aesthetically and relieves the symptoms of macromastia (Fig. 46-34).

PTOSIS. *Ptosis of the breast* exists when the nipple has descended below the level of the inframammary crease. It is usually present in patients with macromastia but may occur alone. Ptosis is caused by weight loss, aging, and atrophy in the postpartum or postmenopausal period. Nipple repositioning is achieved with excision of varying amounts of breast skin. A new nipple site is selected and the appropriate vertical and horizontal skin redundancy excised (Fig. 46-35). The maximum amount of breast tissue is preserved (Fig. 46-36). Breasts that are small can be augmented simultaneously using subpectoral silicone gel implants. The patient whose nipples are at or above the inframammary fold may still have apparent ptosis. This ptosis is caused by hypoplasia of the upper breast quad-

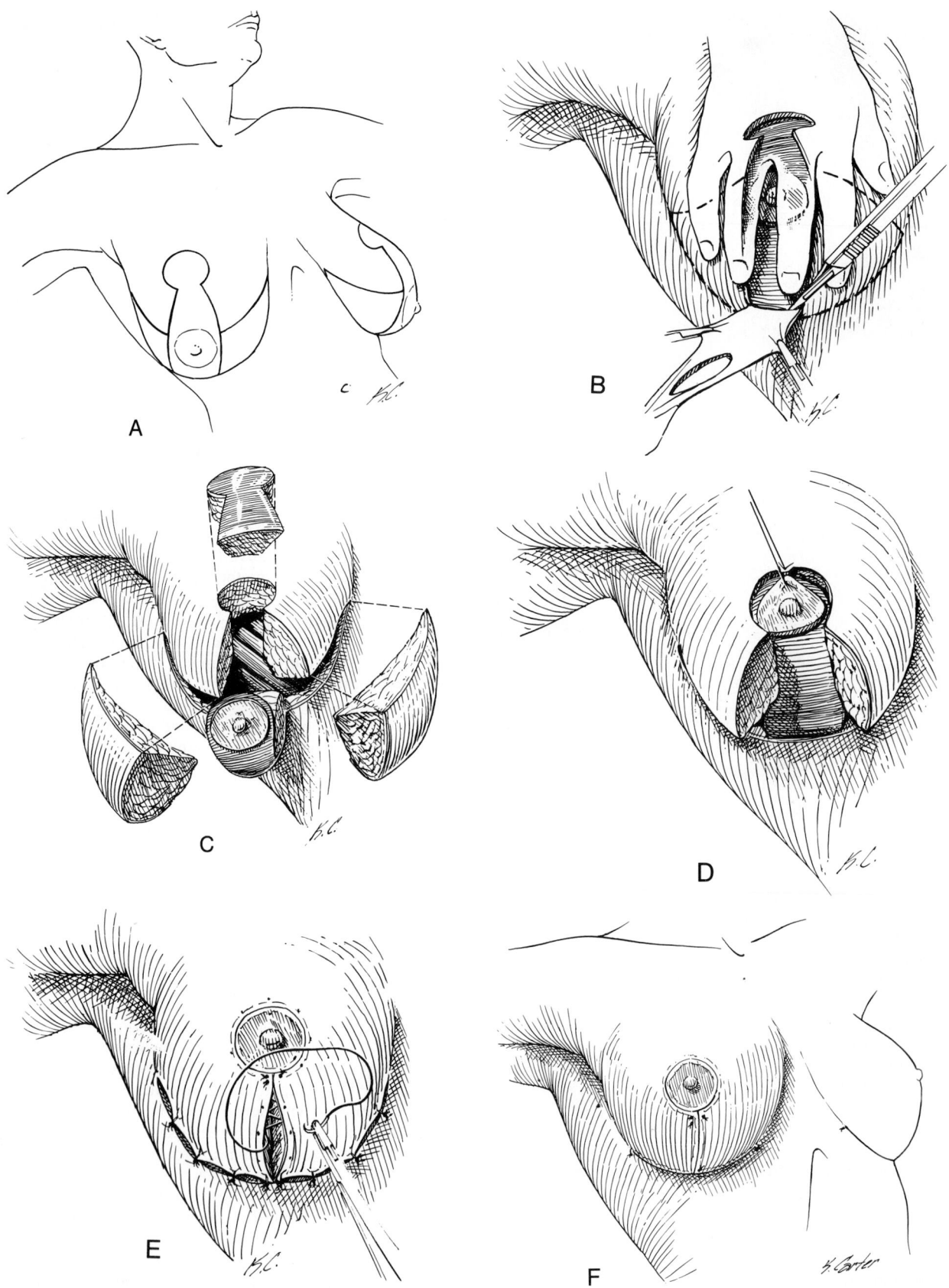

A

B

C

D

E

F

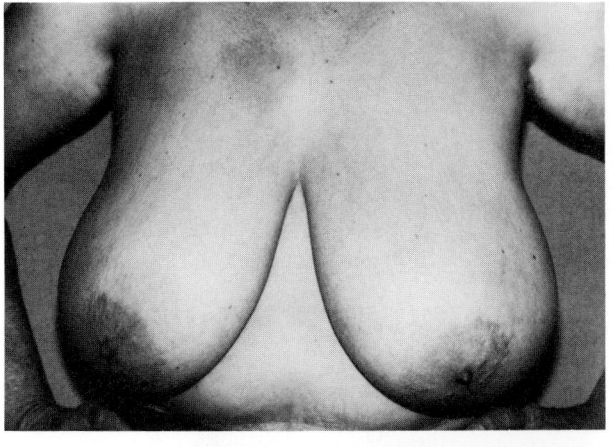
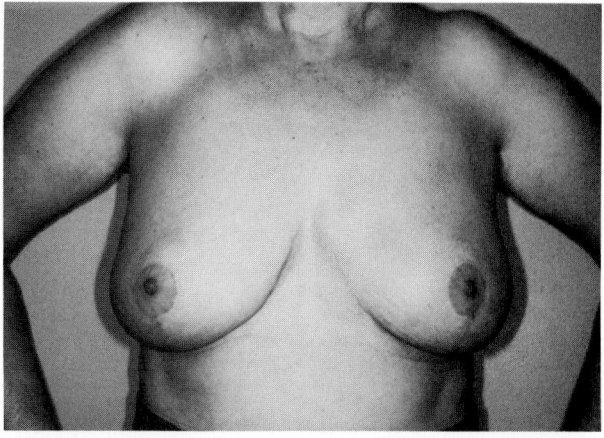
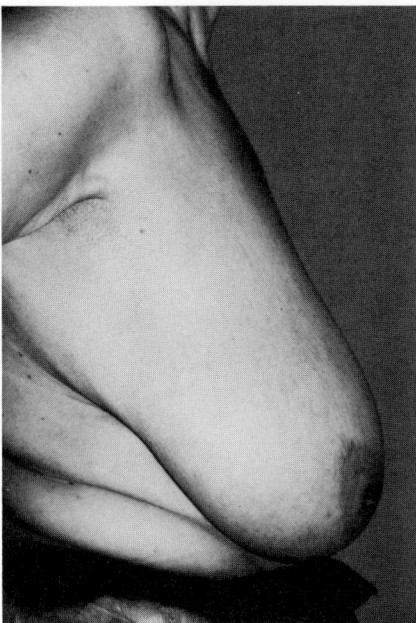
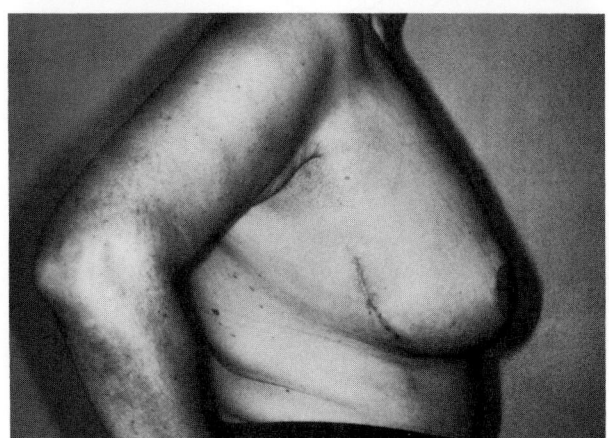

Fig. 46-34. Reduction mammaplasty. The patient is shown preoperatively (left, upper and lower) and postoperatively (right, upper and lower) following reduction mammaplasty using an inferior pedicle technique.

rants, descent of the remaining breast tissue, and redundant skin. The preferred treatment is *augmentation mammaplasty*.

HYPOMASTIA. *Hypomastia* is present when there is insufficient volume of one or both breasts. Patients with hypomastia request augmentation mammaplasty to improve self-image and facilitate clothing fit (Fig. 46-37).

Numerous different prosthesis designs are available. Most breast prostheses consist of a silicone elastomer

◀ Fig. 46-33. Reduction mammaplasty. *A.* The proposed lines of skin incision are drawn. *B.* The pedicle bearing the nipple is deepithelialized. *C.* Wedges of skin and breast tissue are removed, leaving the nipple on an inferiorly based pedicle of subcutaneous tissue, fat, and breast tissue. This pedicle is nourished by perforating vessels from the pectoralis muscle and the subdermal plexus. *D.* The nipple is brought into place. *E.* Subcuticular closure is begun. *F.* The breast is shown in its immediate postoperative state.

shell filled with a dimethylsiloxane polymer gel. This may be enclosed in a second bag inflated with varying amounts of saline. Some prostheses are coated with polyurethane to alter the tissue's reaction to the implant.

The breast prosthesis is inserted under local or general anesthesia. Either an axillary, periareolar, or inframammary incision is made. A pocket is created in the submammary position or in the submuscular plane deep to the pectoralis major and serratus anterior muscles. Whatever position is selected, the pocket is opened adequately to accommodate the prosthesis. The pocket is irrigated with an antibiotic solution prior to insertion of the implant.

RECONSTRUCTION AFTER MASTECTOMY. Reconstruction of the breast after mastectomy for cancer provides the patient with an improved body image and relieves the necessity of wearing an external prosthesis. The ideal candidate for breast reconstruction is a woman who had a

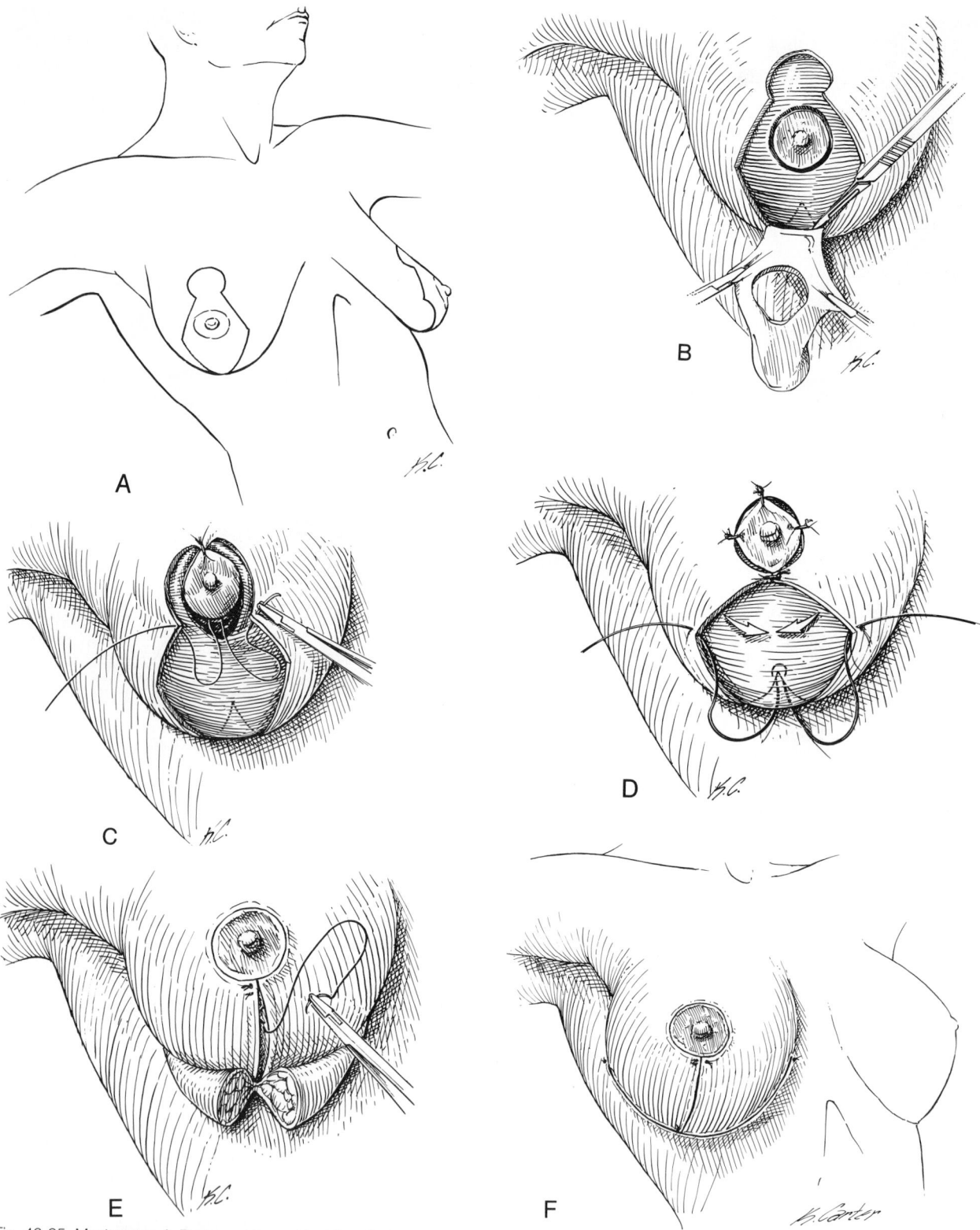

Fig. 46-35. Mastopexy. *A.* Proposed lines of incision. *B.* Appropriate area of breast skin deepithelialized. *C.* Nipple elevated to proper level. *D.* Closure of skin begun. A minimum of breast tissue is excised to facilitate closure. *E.* Subcuticular closure begun. The wedges of redundant skin and breast tissue in the inframammary fold are removed, creating a short horizontal scar. *F.* Appearance of the breast at the completion of the procedure. *(Modified from Goulian D: Dermal Mastopexy. Clin Plast Surg 3:171, 1976, with permission.)*

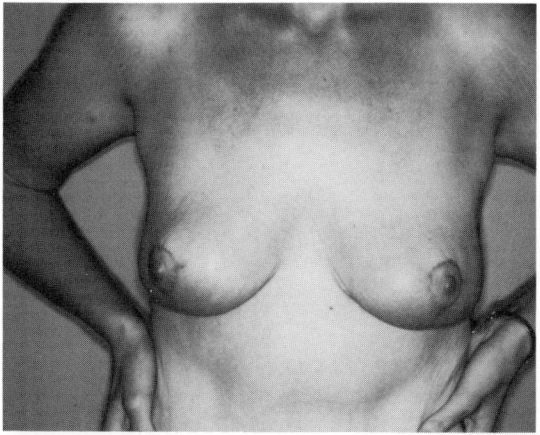

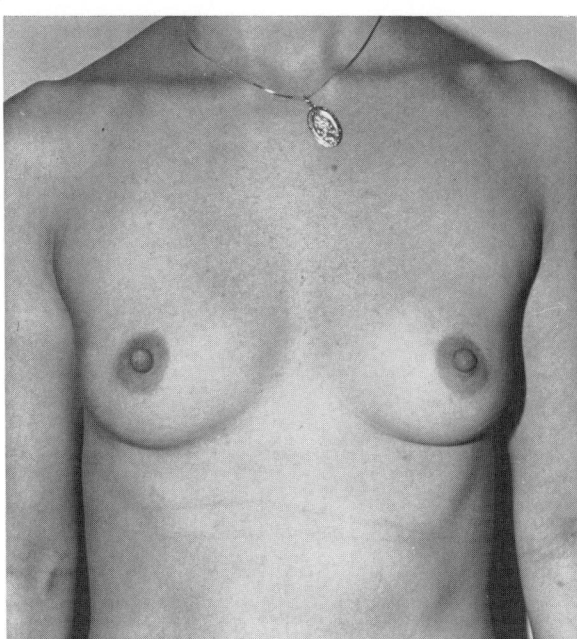

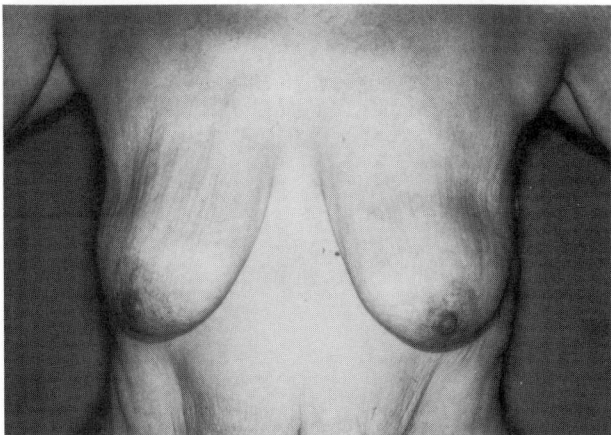

Fig. 46-36. Mastopexy. The volume of the breast is only slightly decreased postoperatively (top) from the preoperative state (bottom).

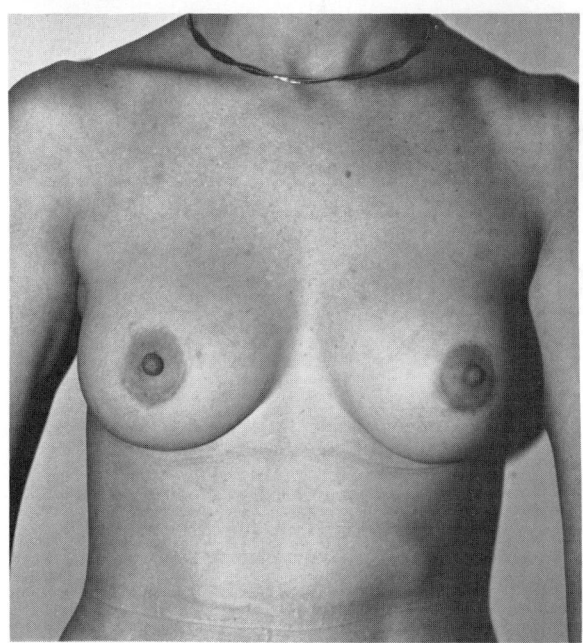

Fig. 46-37. Augmentation mammaplasty. These breast implants were placed in a subpectoral position (preoperative, top; postoperative bottom).

small tumor with no nodal metastases and has little chance of local recurrence or distant spread. Nevertheless, advancing age and even the presence of well-controlled systemic metastases are not absolute contraindications to reconstruction. If chemotherapy or radiation therapy are required, reconstruction is usually delayed until completion of these treatment modalities.

Many of the currently available breast reconstructive techniques use the silicone gel prosthesis to fashion a breast mound. If sufficient skin and subcutaneous tissue exist in the anterior chest after mastectomy, reconstruction can be accomplished by incising through a portion of the mastectomy scar and developing a pocket deep to the pectoralis major muscle and, in some cases, the serratus anterior muscle and anterior rectus sheath. A prosthesis is inserted in the pocket and the wound closed. The aesthetic result is satisfactory, although the reconstructed breast often lacks any element of ptosis (Fig. 46-38).

In some patients, owing to a lack of chest wall skin, it is not possible to place a prosthesis large enough to restore

a breast of adequate volume or to match the opposite unoperated breast. This situation can be approached by placing the largest implant possible, closing the wound, and allowing the site to heal and stretch. After several months, the implant is removed and a larger permanent one placed. Another alternative is to increase the available skin in two operations through the use of a tissue expander (Fig. 46-32).

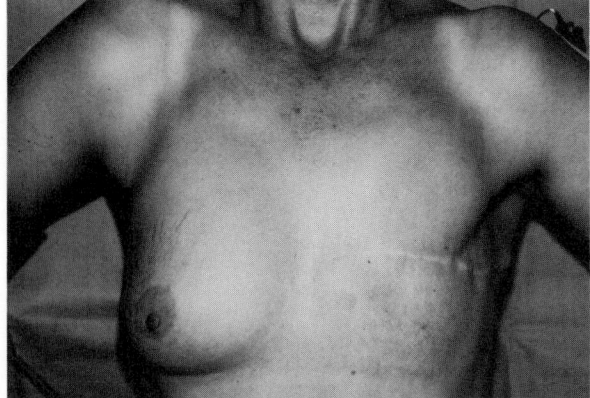

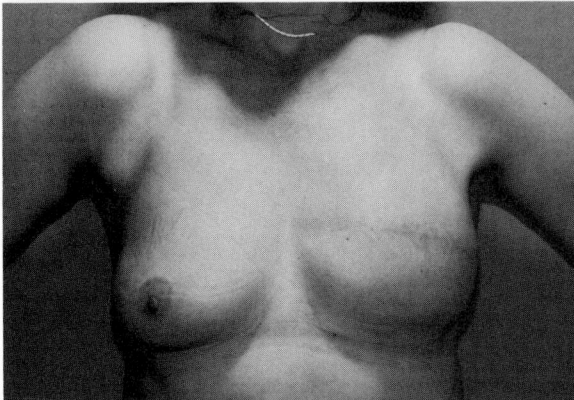

Fig. 46-38. Breast reconstruction after modified radical mastectomy. Above, the pectoralis major muscle and an adequate amount of skin remain after the mastectomy to allow reconstruction of a breast mound using a silicone gel implant. Below, postoperative appearance.

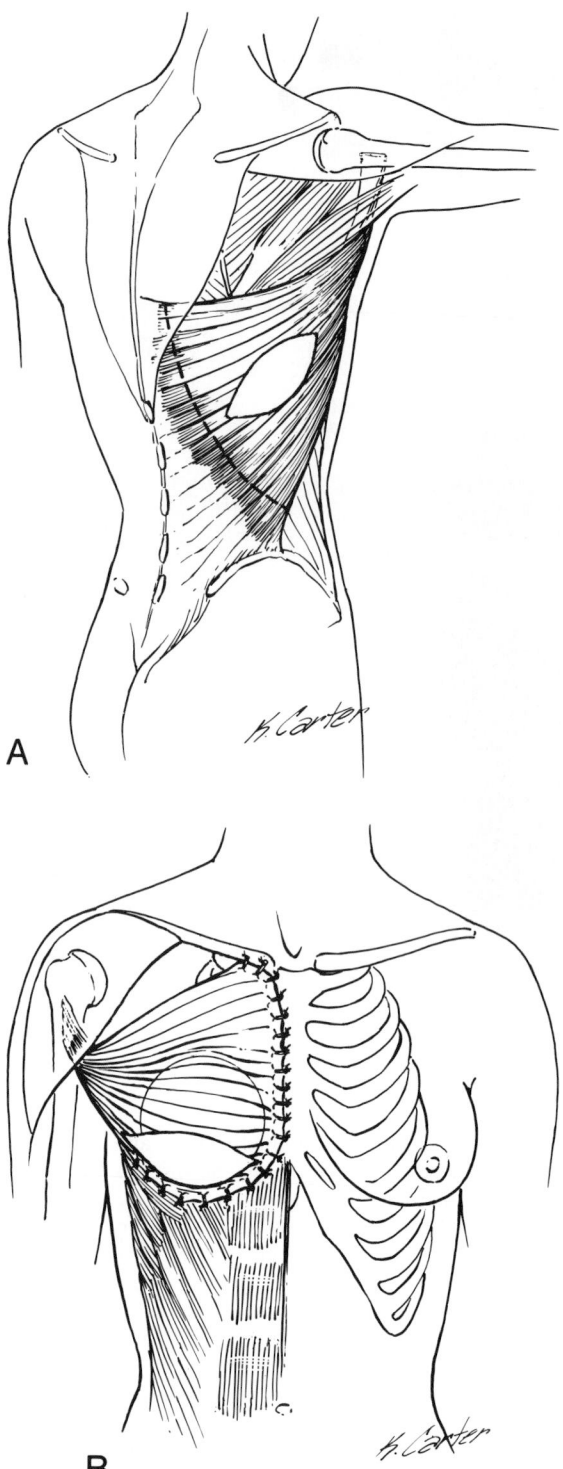

A

B

Fig. 46-39. Breast reconstruction using latissimus dorsi musculocutaneous flap. A. A skin island and suitable amount of latissimus dorsi muscle are elevated. B. The musculocutaneous flap is transposed into the anterior chest wall defect and sutured into place. The skin island is positioned to lie along the inferior aspect of the reconstructed breast, without regard for the mastectomy scar. A silicone gel breast prosthesis is placed deep to the latissimus dorsi muscle, providing a breast mound.

In the presence of marked skin deficiency, additional skin and soft tissue for breast reconstruction can be provided by transposition of a latissimus dorsi musculocutaneous flap (Fig. 46-39). A prosthesis is positioned simultaneously beneath the latissimus dorsi muscle to produce a breast mound (Fig. 46-40). In all cases, nipple reconstruction is delayed for 3 to 6 months after breast restoration.

Operative treatment of the opposite breast is often indicated at the same time as or within a few months of breast reconstruction. Following physical examination and mammography to assess the other breast, either a reduction mammaplasty, mastopexy, or augmentation may be performed to achieve symmetry. If the patient has a high risk of developing cancer in the previously unoperated breast, a simple mastectomy or subcutaneous mastectomy with immediate reconstruction should be considered.

Following breast reconstruction with a silicone gel prosthesis, complications including hematoma formation and infection do infrequently occur. The risk of capsular contracture related to the prosthesis with firmness of the

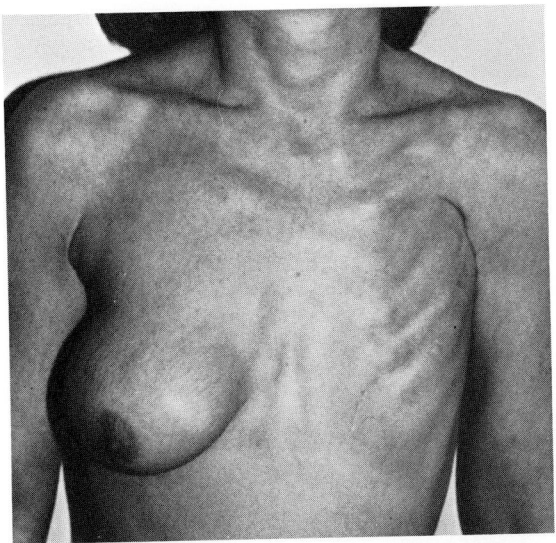

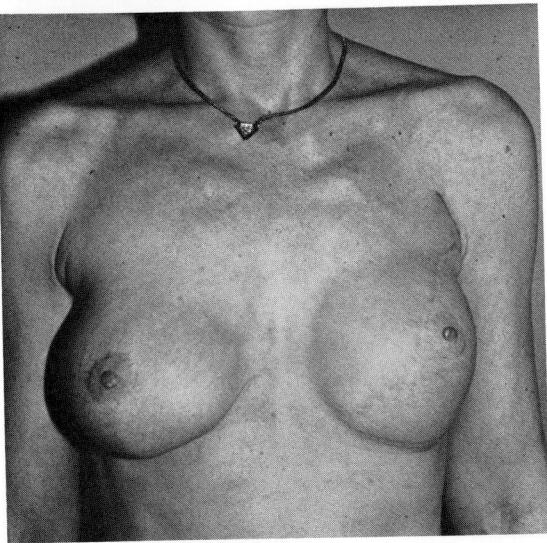

Fig. 46-40. Latissimus dorsi breast reconstruction. Preoperatively (top) the patient has had a radical mastectomy. Postoperatively (bottom) she has undergone a left latissimus dorsi breast reconstruction, left nipple reconstruction, and mastopexy of the right breast. *(Photographs used by permission from Bostwick J: Aesthetic and Reconstructive Breast Surgery. St Louis, CV Mosby, 1982.)*

breast ranges from 5 to 20 percent or more, depending upon the type of reconstruction selected.

As an alternative to the use of a prosthesis, breast reconstruction can be accomplished using the transverse rectus abdominis musculocutaneous (TRAM) flap (Fig. 46-41). Skin of the upper and lower abdomen receives a portion of its blood supply from perforating vessels that originate in the rectus abdominis muscles and pass through the anterior rectus sheath. A skin island designed over one or both rectus abdominis muscles can be raised with it as a musculocutaneous flap, leaving the muscle attached caudally to its major blood supply (superior epigastric vessels). This musculocutaneous flap is passed

beneath the skin of the upper abdomen and used to reconstruct the absent breast. A breast prosthesis is rarely required since the skin, subcutaneous tissue, and muscle provide sufficient bulk for reconstruction (Fig. 46-42). The risk of capsular contracture about a silicone gel prosthesis is avoided. Breast reconstruction by the TRAM flap method does require more operating time than other techniques and recovery is more prolonged. Abdominal wall weakness rarely occurs and the incidence of postoperative ventral hernia formation has been low.

Subcutaneous mastectomy is sometimes indicated in patients who have a high risk of developing cancer of the breast or refractory mastodynia. Prior to undergoing this procedure, the patient must understand that the removal of breast tissue is never complete, and a small risk of developing breast cancer remains. Following subcutaneous mastectomy, the breast is reconstructed by submuscular augmentation with a prosthesis. Reconstruction is either performed simultaneously with the mastectomy or delayed until pathology reports are available and healing is complete. The results of reconstruction after subcutaneous mastectomy are usually satisfactory (Fig. 46-43). A reconstructed breast is rarely confused with a normal one, as distortion of the contour or nipple-areolar complex often occurs.

GYNECOMASTIA. *Gynecomastia* is an enlargement of the male breast secondary to increase in ductal tissue. Numerous causes for gynecomastia have been described. The most common form occurs in adolescence and is of unknown etiology. A testicular tumor may cause gynecomastia in the prepubertal patient. Male breast enlargement is seen in association with certain endocrine disorders including hyperthyroidism, hypothyroidism, pituitary chromophobe adenoma, acromegaly, and adrenal tumors. Males with Klinefelter's syndrome usually have gynecomastia. Liver disorders, especially cirrhosis, are associated with breast enlargement as well as drugs such as digitalis, estrogens, and cimetidine. In addition, cannabis drug abuse will cause gynecomastia.

The treatment of gynecomastia in adolescents is expectant, as the process usually resolves within 2 years. If the enlargement is excessive or lasts over 2 years, operative treatment is considered. Resection for gynecomastia is performed through a periareolar incision. Excess breast tissue is excised, and care is taken to bevel the tissues at the periphery. A thick nipple flap is preserved to reduce the chance of nipple necrosis. There is a variable amount of fat deposition in gynecomastia. Suction-assisted resection of such fat deposition is of help in treating this disorder.

Chest and Abdominal Wall

Defects of the chest and abdominal wall may result from trauma, tumor resection, radiation necrosis, congenital abnormalities, and infection. These defects are repaired to protect vital organs, enhance respiratory function, eradicate infection, and improve appearance. The goal of therapy is to provide a stable, healed wound without herniation of abdominal or thoracic organs. Ide-

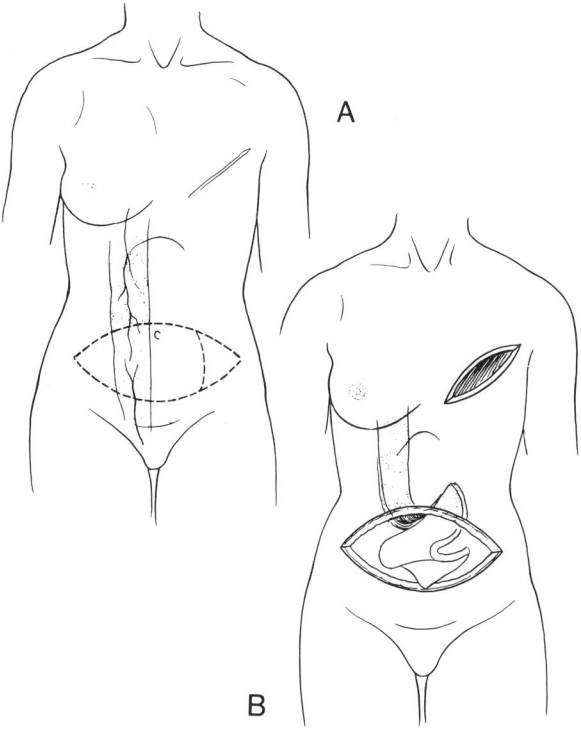

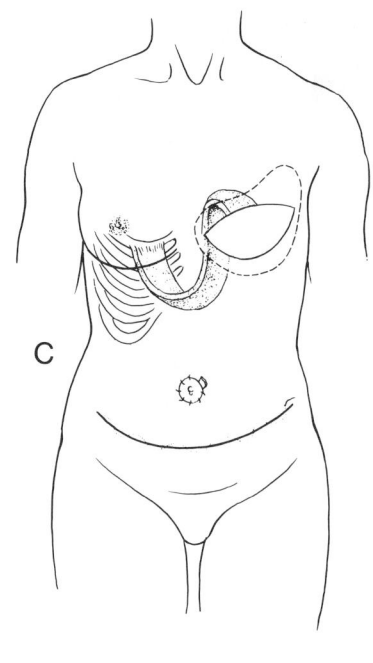

ally, coverage is provided by flaps of uninvolved tissue. Structural integrity is restored when necessary using fascia, synthetic material, or bone. A single-stage procedure is preferred.

Muscle and musculocutaneous flaps find application in the treatment of chest and abdominal wounds. The pectoralis major muscle is particularly useful in managing the infected median sternotomy. Branches of the thoracoacromial, lateral thoracic, and internal mammary arteries supply the pectoralis major. After debridement of the

Fig. 46-41. Transverse rectus abdominis musculocutaneous (TRAM) flap. *A.* Skin of the lower abdomen receives a significant portion of its blood supply from the rectus abdominis muscles. The skin island outlined will survive based on the left rectus abdominis muscle. *B.* TRAM flap elevated and being transposed. *C.* Skin island positioned for right breast reconstruction.

Fig. 46-42. Breast reconstruction using TRAM flap. *A.* Patient following left modified radical mastectomy for carcinoma of the breast. *B.* Appearance one year after left breast and nipple reconstruction and right breast reduction.

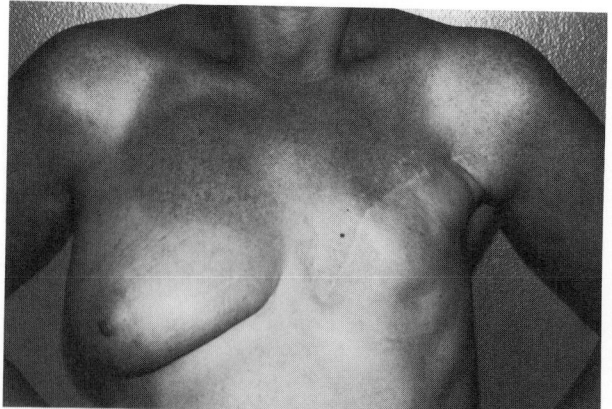

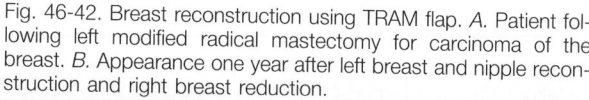

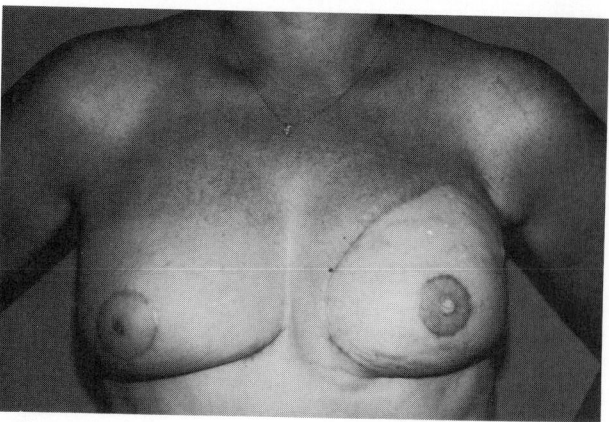

A

B

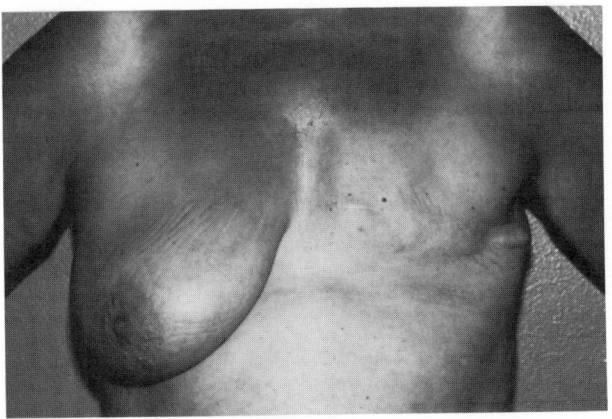
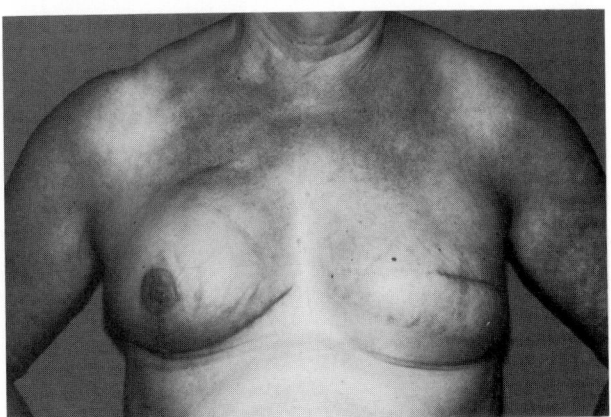

A   *B*

Fig. 46-43. Subcutaneous mastectomy and immediate reconstruction. *A.* Patient following left modified radical mastectomy for breast cancer. *B.* Appearance 3 months after right breast subcutaneous mastectomy and immediate reconstruction and left breast reconstruction.

sternum, the pectoralis major is mobilized based on one vascular supply and transposed into the defect (Fig. 46-44). Frequently, the dead space in the caudal portion of the wound is filled by transposition of a rectus abdominis muscle.

The latissimus dorsi can be mobilized as a muscle or musculocutaneous flap based on its major pedicle (thoracodorsal vessels) and transposed to cover defects of the anterior, lateral, and posterior chest. This muscle can also be used in a "reverse" fashion, receiving its blood supply from posterior branches of the intercostal vessels. Designed in this manner, the flap can be extended to close wounds in the posterior lumbar region (Fig. 46-45).

A patient may experience sustained pressure to a part of the body because of unconsciousness, rigid casting, physical restraint, or spinal cord injury with paralysis. The risk of tissue damage due to pressure is minimized by periodic pressure relief in areas at risk, control of spasticity, meticulous skin care, and the avoidance of shear forces. Unrelieved pressure will eventually result in skin ulceration.

Cursory examination of a pressure sore reveals a skin ulcer usually located over a bony prominence. This ulcer belies a more extensive wound involving the underlying subcutaneous tissues, fascia, muscle, and often bone itself. Long-standing pressure sores contain a partially epithelialized cavity, or bursa, which retards spontaneous healing.

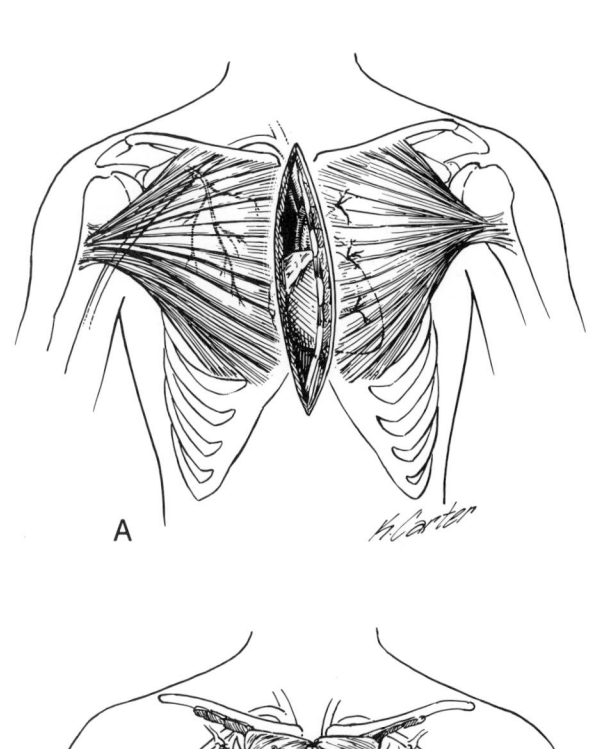

A

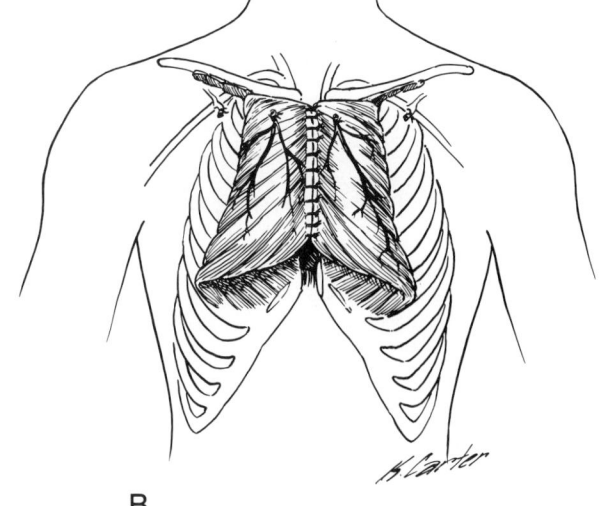

Fig. 46-44. Pectoralis major muscle coverage of infected sternal wound. *A.* The infected sternal wound is debrided, exposing the mediastinal structures. The pectoralis major muscle receives blood from perforating branches of the internal mammary artery and from a branch of the thoracoacromial artery. The muscle can survive on either source alone. *B.* The pectoralis major muscles are separated from their humeral attachments, the thoracoacromial branches are divided, and the muscles are sutured to one another in the midline to cover the defect. Usually, enough laxity is present in the chest wall skin to allow direct closure.

B

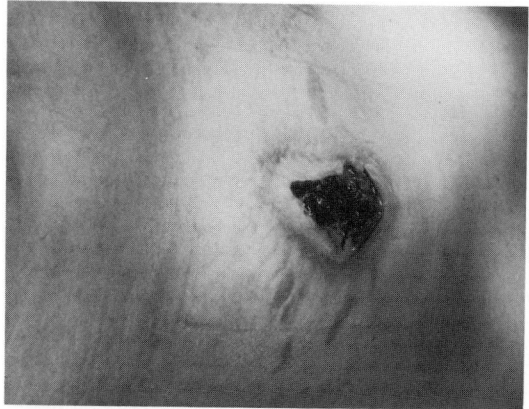

A

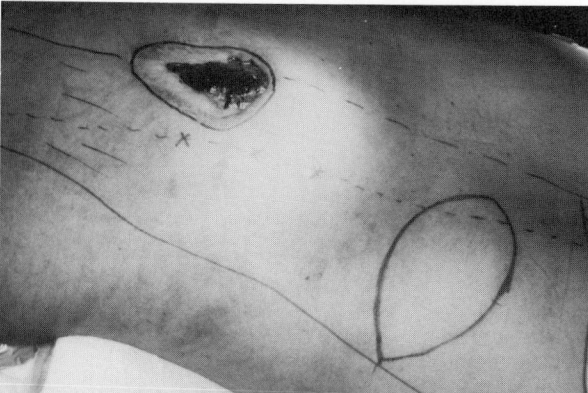

B

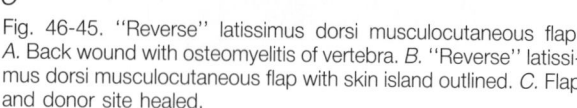

C

Fig. 46-45. "Reverse" latissimus dorsi musculocutaneous flap. *A.* Back wound with osteomyelitis of vertebra. *B.* "Reverse" latissimus dorsi musculocutaneous flap with skin island outlined. *C.* Flap and donor site healed.

Basic care of the patient who has, or is at risk of developing, a pressure sore is directed at the avoidance of pressure. In attempting to heal the pressure sore, the body expends considerable energy. Therefore, the patient's nutrition must be vigorously maintained.

Once a pressure sore becomes established, surgical treatment is necessary. Although a superficial sore will often heal spontaneously with avoidance of pressure, a deeper sore requires operative therapy. The wound is completely excised, including the epithelialized bursa. Any underlying bony prominence is removed, along with all granulation tissue covering the exposed bone. The resultant defect is either closed directly or filled with vascularized tissue. Small local flaps are unreliable. The transposition of muscle and musculocutaneous flaps results in more secure healing initially and in a more durable wound.

Selection of the appropriate flap depends upon location of the ulcer. A sacral sore is best treated using a transverse back flap or a gluteus maximus musculocutaneous flap. The greater trochanter sore is usually treated with the tensor fascia lata musculocutaneous flap. An ischial sore is closed using a gluteus maximus island, musculocutaneous flap (Fig. 46-46), hamstring musculocutaneous flap, or posterior thigh flap.

Lymphedema

Lymphedema is an abnormal accumulation of lymph in the intercellular spaces of a part of the body, usually the upper or lower extremity. It may result from removal or destruction of the regional lymph nodes or from a congenital defect in the lymphatic vessels. A patient with persistent lymphedema suffers permanent changes in the extremity. Fibrosis develops in the connective and subcutaneous tissues, the skin thickens, the region swells, and nonpitting edema appears. Lymphangiosarcoma may arise in areas of chronic lymphedema.

The nonoperative management of lymphedema includes compression and elevation of the extremity. Care is taken to avoid infection, particularly by β-hemolytic streptococcus, as each episode worsens the edema. Diuretics are useful adjuncts.

Operation is reserved for patients in whom medical therapy has failed. Excision of the involved skin and subcutaneous tissues, with split-thickness or full-thickness skin grafting of the area is often successful. The use of a pedicled omental flap inset into the extremity to drain lymph has not been uniformly effective. Microvascular lymphaticovenous anastomoses offer some promise. A satisfactory therapeutic compromise is staged, subtotal excision of the involved tissues beneath local skin flaps. All operations must be followed by sustained elastic compression of the extremity.

Lower Extremity Defects

Wounds of the lower extremity are incurred through trauma, venous stasis, arterial insufficiency, diabetes, and the extirpation of cancer. Infections of the soft tissue and bone of the leg present difficult management problems.

Small soft tissue defects less than 1 cm² in area can be expected to heal spontaneously. Skin grafts promote healing in larger defects that are adequately vascularized

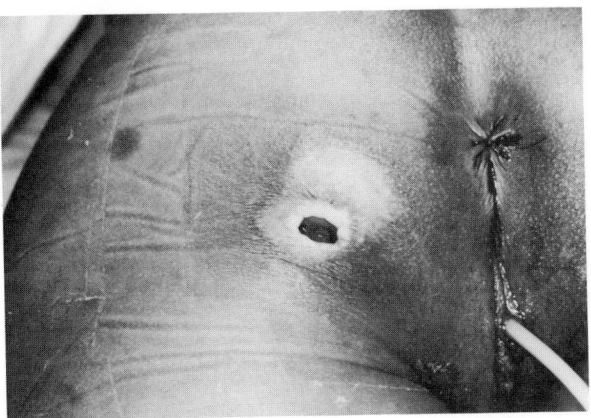

A

Fig. 46-46. Ischial pressure sore management. *A.* Right ischial pressure sore. *B.* Gluteus maximus island musculocutaneous flap outlined. *C.* Sore debrided and flap interpolated. *D.* Wound healed 3 months postoperatively.

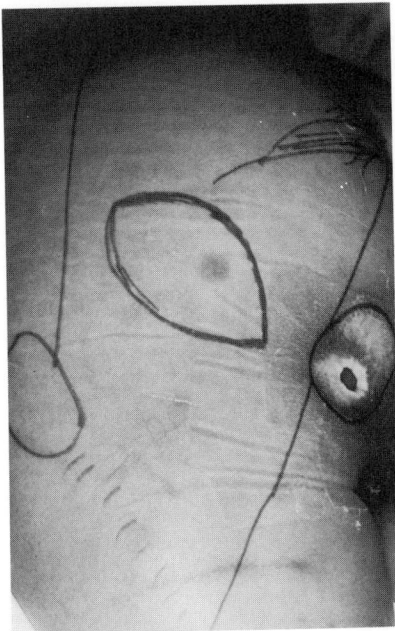

B

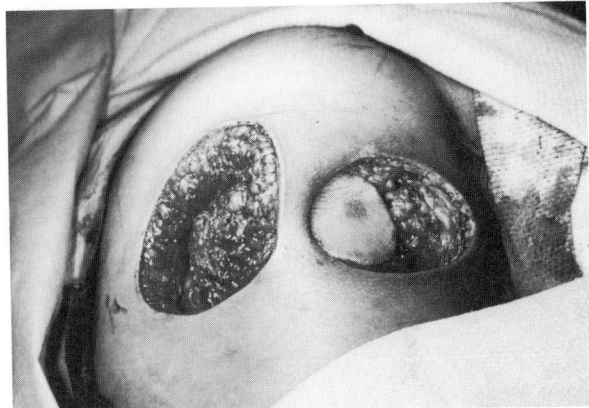

C

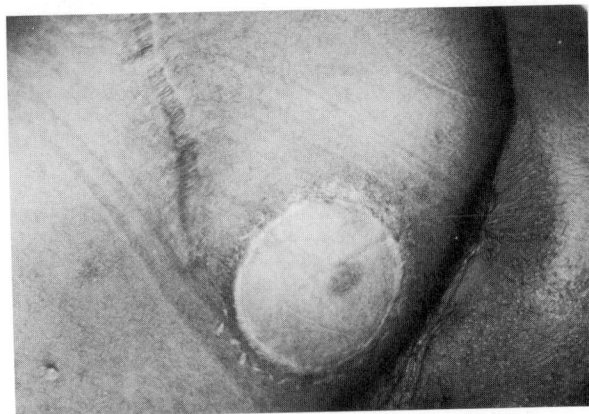

D

and do not involve exposed tendon or devitalized bone. Ulcers that occur in association with arterial insufficiency heal after restoration of blood flow to the extremity.

Venous stasis ulcer appears in the patient with chronic venous insufficiency of the lower extremity. Venous insufficiency is treated first. The ulcers are then allowed to heal by epithelialization or are managed by excision and skin grafting. Free microvascular tissue transplantation has been unsuccessful in treating venous stasis ulcers. After the ulcers are controlled, the patient must persist in wearing compression hose.

A patient whose wound involves a large segment of exposed bone with minimal surrounding skin and soft tissue injury can be treated using a fasciocutaneous, muscle, or musculocutaneous flap. This principle applies to most injuries of the thigh, both bony and soft tissue. A compound fracture of the tibia with extensive soft tissue injury is best managed by debridement, bone reduction and fixation, and coverage with a muscle or musculocutaneous flap. Local muscle transposition is preferred in such a wound except in the distal third of the tibia, where free microvascular muscle transfer is indicated. Chronic osteomyelitis of the tibia can be successfully treated by serial debridement and closure with a local muscle or musculocutaneous flap in the upper two-thirds of the bone and a free tissue transfer in the lower one-third (Fig. 46-47).

Genitourinary System

Hypospadias occurs when the urethral meatus opens on the ventral surface of the penis, on the scrotum, or in the perineum. Most patients with hypospadias have chordee, a ventral curvature of the penis that becomes more obvious during erection. Chordee is caused by tissue extending between the urethral meatus and glans penis. In evaluating the patient with hypospadias, obtaining an IVP has been suggested because of an increased incidence of renal abnormalities.

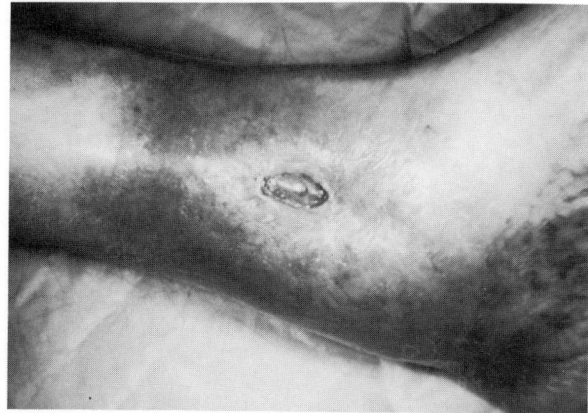

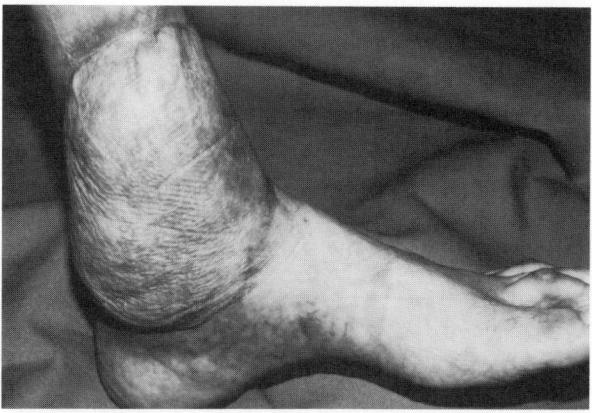

Fig. 46-47. Latissimus dorsi muscle free flap. Preoperatively (left), the patient is seen with long-standing osteomyelitis of the tibia. Postoperatively (right), a latissimus dorsi muscle free flap is transferred and skin graft applied after thorough debridement of the tibia. A healed wound has resulted.

The goals of hypospadias management are the relief of chordee, a sexually adequate penis, placement of the urethral meatus at the tip of the glans penis, and restoration of normal urination. Consideration of treatment begins soon after birth with the avoidance of circumcision. An intact foreskin is useful in subsequent reconstruction.

Two-stage techniques of hypospadias repair start with the operative relief of chordee as early as age one and a half years. A urethroplasty is done as a second stage at age four to nine years.

Numerous single-stage techniques for hypospadias have been described. The procedure developed by Horton and Devine is useful for hypospadias with any meatal position. The chordee is released and a "flip-flap" of skin and soft tissue of the glans penis is fashioned to form the distal urethral meatus (Fig. 46-48). If the meatus is located far proximally, a full-thickness skin graft is tubed and used to reconstruct the urethra.

Fig. 46-48. "Flip-flap" repair of hypospadias. *A.* The lines of incision are outlined. *B.* The incisions are made in the glans and shaft of the penis. An incision is made to release the prepuce. *C.* The V flap is sutured to the dorsal aspect of the urethra. *D.* Excess skin of the prepuce is removed. *E.* The closure is completed. *(Modified from Horton CE, Devine CJ: Hypospadias, in Converse JM: Reconstructive Plastic Surgery, Philadelphia, Saunders, 1977, with permission.)*

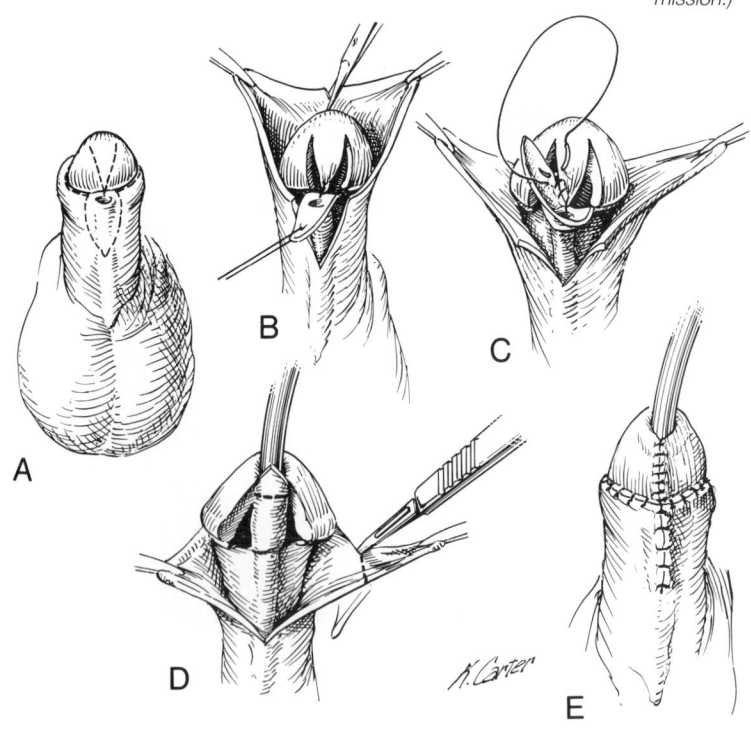

The success rate for hypospadias repair is approximately 85 percent. Complications include initial failure to make the proper gender assignment, hematoma, infection, flap necrosis, stricture, and fistula formation. If a urinary fistula occurs postoperatively, it is repaired after a 6-month interval.

In the patient with *epispadias,* the urethral meatus opens on the dorsum of the penis. Epispadias is commonly associated with exstrophy of the urinary bladder. Exstrophy is characterized by the bladder opening anteriorly on the abdominal wall, failure of pubic symphysis fusion, and midline diastasis of the abdominal wall muscles. The primary treatment objective in patients with epispadias and exstrophy of the bladder is the establishment of unobstructed renal function. If the bladder can be closed, it should be. Otherwise, the bladder should be excised and a urinary diversion procedure carried out for ureteral drainage. Repairs of the epispadias resemble those of hypospadias. Intrinsic to the repairs is reconstruction of the bladder neck, including urinary sphincters.

The patient suffering loss of the scrotum or penis often seeks reconstruction. Both the penis and scrotum have been restored using local abdominal flaps and gracilis musculocutaneous flaps. Alternatively, the testes may be covered with split-thickness skin grafts or buried in subcutaneous pockets of the abdomen or thighs. Testes so buried will retain hormonal function, but because of the higher temperature in this heterotopic site, aspermia may result.

Vaginal agenesis may be idiopathic or may result from testicular feminization syndrome, adrenogenital syndrome, and gonadal dysgenesis. Treatment involves the dissection of a perineal pocket and insertion of a split-thickness skin graft to create a vagina. The graft is tailored and held in place by a stent until healing is complete. It has been demonstrated that an adequately capacious vagina can result from simple progressive dilatation by vaginal bougies.

Removal of the vagina and vulva for cancer creates a large defect. Successful perineal and vaginal reconstruction has been achieved using local skin flaps or gracilis musculocutaneous flaps.

AESTHETIC SURGERY

Facial Aging

A desire to look younger or simply to improve facial appearance can motivate a patient to seek consultation for aesthetic surgery. Before undergoing an operation, the patient needs to understand the proposed procedure, the potential result, and the possible complications. The patient must have realistic goals in order to be satisfied with the postoperative results.

The *rhytidectomy* (facelift) is performed under local or general anesthesia. After the proposed sites of incision are marked with methylene blue, the areas to be incised are infiltrated with $\frac{1}{4}$% lidocaine with 1:400,000 epineph-

rine. The incision begins in the hairline above and anterior to the ear, continues in front of the ear, and curves posteriorly around the lobe to terminate approximately 6 cm posterior to the mastoid process (Fig. 46-49). Appropriate undermining is performed medially to free the skin from the underlying structures. A fibrous tissue layer of varying thickness known as the *superficial musculoaponeurotic system* (SMAS) lies between the skin and facial muscles. This tissue extends from the frontalis muscle in the upper face to the platysma below. The SMAS transmits the pull of the facial muscles to the overlying skin. Tightening the SMAS by plicating it to itself or by removing a portion and suturing it to fascia anterior to the ear and tissue overlying the mastoid bone gives additional support to the facelift operation. After the SMAS is secured, an appropriate amount of skin is excised from the skin flap, and the wound is closed. Drains are sometimes used. A firm head dressing helps prevent hematoma formation.

The submental region and neck often require special attention. A submental lipectomy through a separate incision may be required to remove fat deposits beneath the chin. Suction lipectomy can also be used to remove this fat. Suturing and/or repositioning of the platysma muscle have been advocated to improve the contour of the neck.

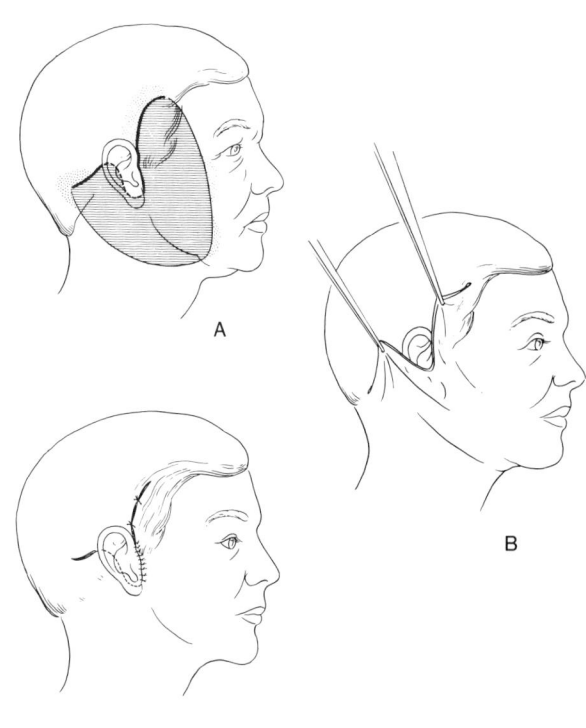

Fig. 46-49. Facelift. *A.* Planned facelift incision and area of undermining. *B.* Excess skin is estimated and removed. *C.* Wound closed at end of procedure.

Serious complications following rhytidectomy are unusual. Significant hematomas beneath the skin flap requiring operative evacuation occur in approximately 4 percent of patients. Should preauricular or postauricular skin necrosis develop, these areas are debrided and allowed to heal secondarily. The scars are revised later if needed. Less than 1 percent of patients experience injury to a major branch of the facial nerve.

Dermabrasion improves the appearance of fine wrinkles, particularly in the perioral region. Superficial acne scars and other minor surface irregularities are smoothed using dermabrasion. A power-driven rotary device is preferred. The wound following dermabrasion is cleansed several times a day and dressed with antibiotic ointment. Protection against direct sunlight while the wound is red to pink in color reduces the chance of developing local hyperpigmentation.

Chemical face peel is used to flatten fine wrinkles and tighten the skin. This technique involves creation of a superficial chemical burn that, when healed, relieves wrinkling. It is sometimes difficult to control the burn depth, and unsatisfactory scarring has resulted. Hyperpigmentation, particularly in dark-skinned individuals, occasionally complicates this procedure. Many patients find it necessary to wear cosmetics after chemical peel to camouflage irregularities in pigmentation.

Eyelid

The appearance of baggy eyelids is due to drooping of the eyebrows, redundance of eyelid muscle and skin, and bulging of intraorbital fat. The patient desires relief from a perpetual "tired look" about the eyes. Caution is exercised when considering surgery for a patient with a history of thyroid disease or chronic "dry eyes," as symptoms may worsen postoperatively.

Blepharoplasty involves removing a variable amount of skin and obicularis oculi muscle from the upper and lower eyelids. If excess intraorbital fat is present, a subtotal excision of the fat decreases bulging of the lids. Eyebrow ptosis is relieved by a browlift using either a supraciliary or coronal incision and skin resection.

Nose

A perceived nasal deformity and the desire for improved appearance stimulate the patient to request reconstruction. Complaints include a nasal hump, nasal tip deformity, unsatisfactory nasolabial angle, broad alar rims, broad nasal bridge, and deviation of the nose from the midline. This is often accompanied by nasal airway obstruction due to deviation of the cartilagenous or bony septum.

A rhinoplasty is done under local or general anesthesia. The nasal cavity may be packed initially with cotton soaked in a cocaine or epinephrine solution to reduce bleeding. The nose is usually injected with a local anesthetic containing epinephrine. Surgical incisions can be confined to areas inside the nose to minimize visible scar-

ring. In the average rhinoplasty, the alar cartilages are exposed and reshaped by judicious excision or scarring.

The skin of the nose is undermined and the bony and cartilagenous hump is removed. The nasal bones are separated from the maxilla with an osteotome and subsequently placed in the desired position. If nasal obstruction is present, resection or repositioning of the nasal septum deep to the mucous membrane and perichondrium of the septal cartilage completes the procedure. The nasal cavities are packed lightly, and the external nose is supported with adhesive paper strips and a rigid split. Several weeks are required for swelling of the soft tissue to disappear and the nose to assume its final shape (Fig. 46-50).

Abdomen

Weight loss, parturition, and aging can result in sagging of the abdominal skin. This may be accompanied by striae formation, subcutaneous fat deposits, and diastasis of the rectus abdominis muscles.

Abdominoplasty is used to treat the more moderate excesses of skin and fat. A shield-shaped segment of abdominal skin and fat is removed from the lower abdomen and discarded. The umbilicus is left attached to the abdominal wall. If a diastasis recti or ventral hernia is present, it is repaired. After undermining the abdominal skin flap superiorly, the patient is placed in a sitting position, the upper flap is advanced to the inguinal level, and the wound is closed (Fig. 46-51). Underclothing conceals the scar. More modest fatty excess of the abdomen may be treated by suction lipectomy. The massive abdominal panniculus is managed by amputation and primary closure without skin undermining.

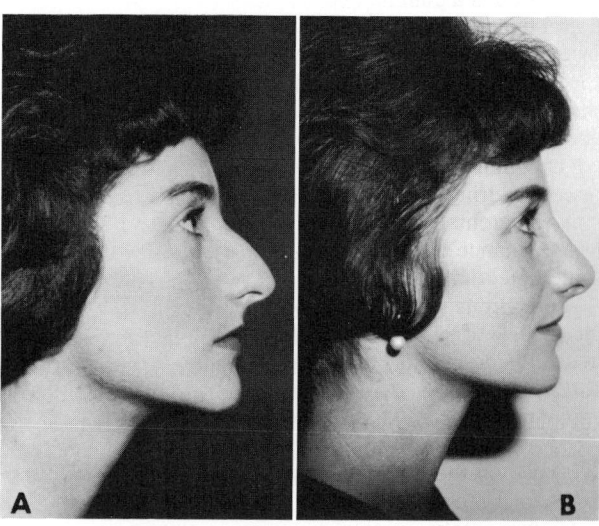

Fig. 46-50. Aesthetic rhinoplasty. *A.* Preoperative photograph. *B.* Postoperative result.

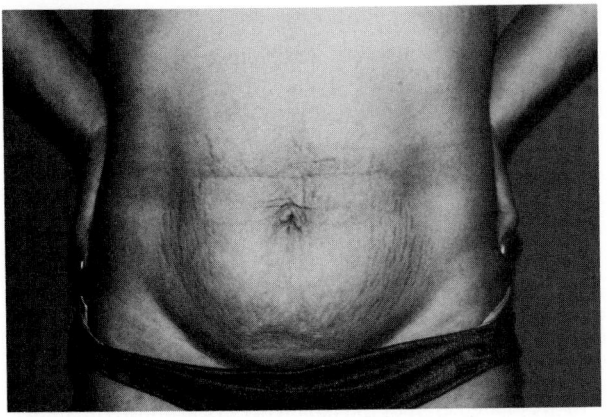

A

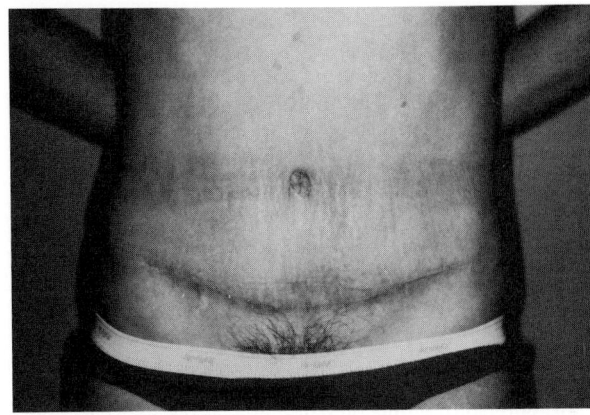

B

Fig. 46-51. Abdominoplasty. *A.* Laxity and excess of abdominal skin. *B.* Appearance of abdomen one year after abdominoplasty.

Thighs, Buttocks, and Upper Arms

A patient often notes skin redundancy of the thighs, buttocks, and upper arms following massive weight loss. This is particularly common in the individual who has undergone an intestinal or gastric bypass for morbid obesity. Removal of the redundant skin can be done to improve contour in the affected area. However, the resultant scars are often prominent and difficult to conceal.

HEAD AND NECK SURGERY

Congenital Deformities

CLEFT LIP

Cleft lip is a common genetic abnormality occurring in approximately one out of every 1000 live births. Genetic factors that influence the development of cleft lip include race and sex. A cleft lip deformity is seen more commonly among Orientals than among Caucasians or blacks, and occurs more often in males. Environmental factors contributing to the development of cleft lip are maternal disease during pregnancy, teratogenic drugs, and advanced parental age. If a parent or older sibling has a cleft lip the chance of a subsequent child being born with the same defect is higher.

A cleft lip may be *unilateral* or *bilateral*. It is said to be *incomplete* if a bridge of skin connects the cleft and noncleft sides. If no skin bridge exists, the cleft is termed *complete* (Fig. 46-52). Deformity of the nose usually accompanies the cleft lip. The nasal defect is represented by a distortion of the alar cartilage and displacement of the alar base on the involved side.

When the child is old enough to tolerate an elective procedure safely, surgical repair is done. In general, the surgical date is selected by the "rule of tens." That is, the

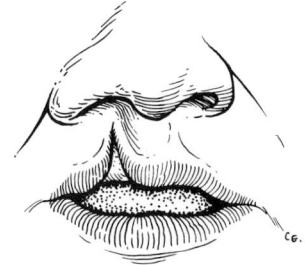

A

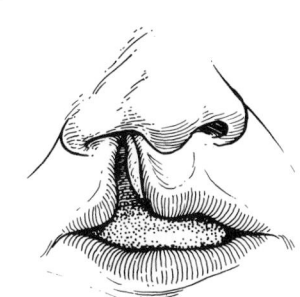

B

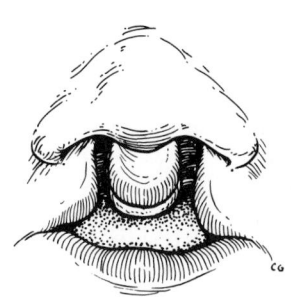

C

Fig. 46-52. Cleft lip types. *A.* Incomplete cleft lip. *B.* Complete cleft lip, unilateral. *C.* Complete cleft lip, bilateral.

child must be at least 10 weeks of age, weigh 10 lb, and have a hemoglobin of 10 gm%. By that time, the tissues are large enough to allow accurate repair.

The goal of every cleft lip operation is to approximate the normal state. Existing lip elements are rearranged to achieve the desired result. The operation is done under general anesthesia. Lines of incision are marked with indelible ink, the lip is infiltrated with dilute epinephrine solution to provide vasoconstriction and attendant hemostasis, and the procedure is performed. The technique described by Millard and in common use today closes the lip defect and assists in proper positioning of the involved nasal cartilage (Fig. 46-53). Many plastic surgeons advocate primary rhinoplasty at the time of cleft lip repair, with mobilization and repositioning of the alar cartilage. After cleft lip repair, pressure of the lip on the alveolar ridge narrows an associated cleft palate (Fig. 46-54). Fur-

ther correction of the nasal deformity, often with simultaneous revision of minor lip irregularities, is done when the child is older.

Bilateral clefts of the lip are repaired in one or two stages. Before operation, the central portion of the lip and maxilla (prolabium and premaxilla) often protrude excessively. This protrusion has been corrected using external pressure applied through adhesive tape or a specially designed bonnet that molds the central segment into an anatomic position.

CLEFT PALATE

An isolated cleft of the palate occurs in approximately 4 out of every 10,000 live births. The incisive foramen divides the normal palate into the primary palate anteriorly

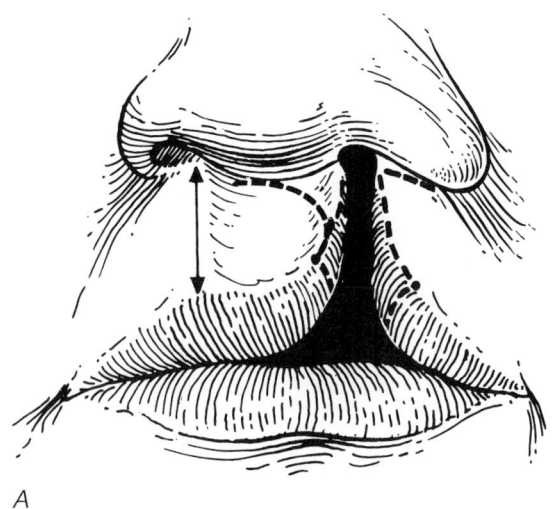

A

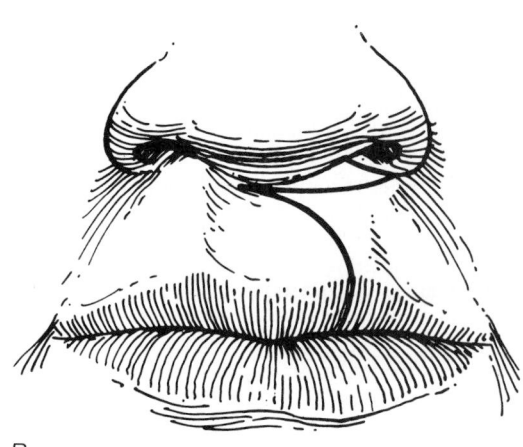

B

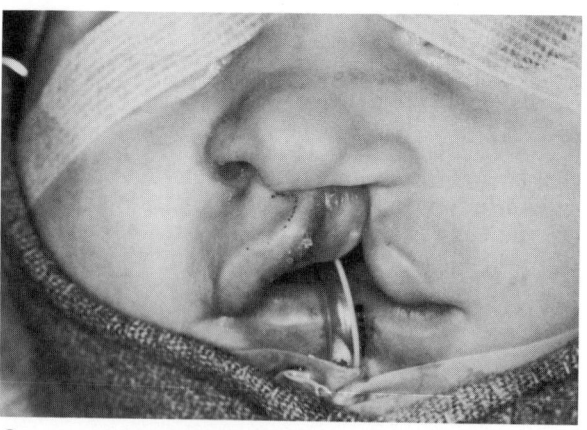

C

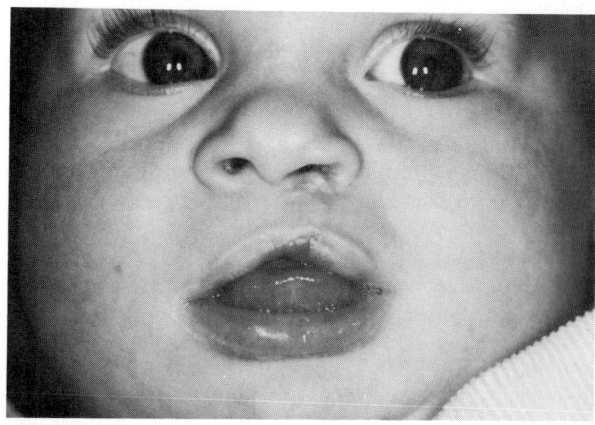

D

Fig. 46-53. Millard rotation-advancement repair of unilateral complete cleft lip. *A.* Preoperatively, the lines of incision are marked. *B.* Postoperatively, the flaps are interdigitated to close the lip and improve the position of the nasal alar base on the left. *C.* Preoperative photograph. *D.* Postoperative photograph.

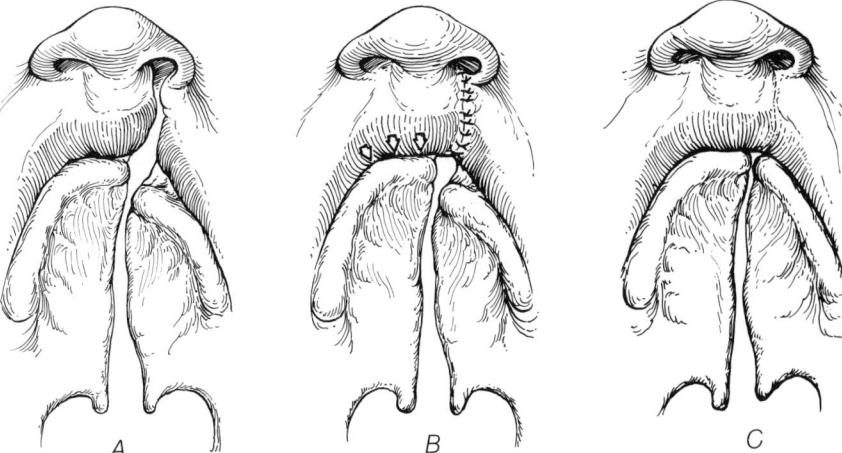

Fig. 46-54. Effect of lip closure on alveolar dental arch. *A.* Complete cleft of the lip and primary palate on the left end of the secondary palate. *B.* Closure of the lip defect brings pressure to bear on the anterior alveolar ridge. *C.* Alveolar ridge in more anatomic position.

and the secondary palate posteriorly. A *unilateral cleft of the primary palate* extends from the incisive foramen anteriorly and obliquely to the right or left to terminate in a fissure between a canine and its adjacent incisor. Primary palatal clefts are occasionally *bilateral.* A *cleft of the secondary palate* occurs in the midline and extends posteriorly from the incisive foramen to involve the posterior aspect of the bony palate, the soft palate, and the uvula. Clefts of the primary and secondary palates may occur together or independently (Fig. 46-55). If the defect does not extend to the incisive foramen, the cleft is termed incomplete. At an early stage, the patient with a cleft palate should be evaluated and a treatment plan outlined by a team of specialists including a plastic surgeon, orthodontist, oral surgeon, speech therapist, and otologist.

In clefts of the primary and/or secondary palate, the soft palate often appears short. The palatal muscles are abnormally inserted into the posterior margin of the hard palate. In normal speech the palate moves superiorly and posteriorly during speech and swallowing. This action intermittently and accurately blocks the nasopharynx and is termed *velopharyngeal closure.* Owing to numerous influences, probably including malpositioning of the palatal muscles and palatal shortening, the cleft palate patient often suffers from insufficient velopharyngeal closure. The result is *hypernasal speech.* Mild feeding difficulties are common in the infant with a cleft palate. Middle ear infections occur frequently and, if inadequately managed, result in hearing loss.

Timing of the cleft palate repair is variable, depending upon the plastic surgeon's training and experience. The palate can be repaired in one or two stages from age three months to four years. It appears that speech results can be optimized if the palate is closed entirely by age twelve

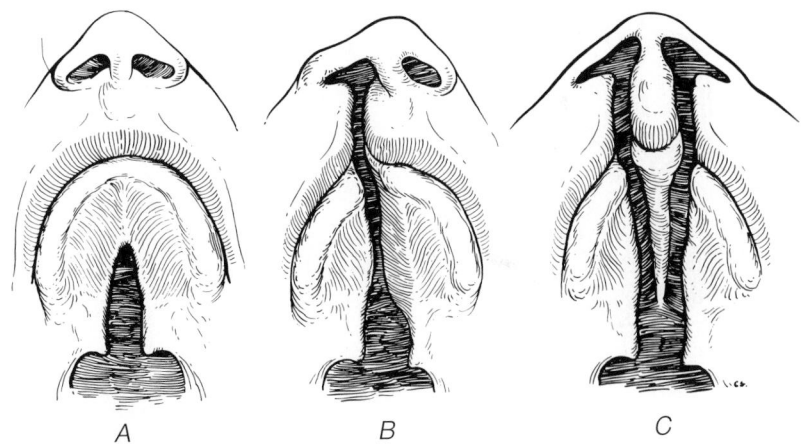

Fig. 46-55. Cleft palate types. *A.* Complete cleft of the secondary palate. *B.* Complete cleft of the secondary palate with complete cleft of lip and primary palate on the right. *C.* Complete cleft of the secondary palate and complete bilateral cleft of the lip and primary palate.

to fourteen months. With early closure, 75 percent of patients develop good to excellent speech. Early cleft palate closure has been implicated in growth disturbances of the palate and maxilla, although the influence of operative procedures remains to be defined.

Cleft palate repair is done under general endotracheal anesthesia. The technique we employ requires elevation of two mucoperiosteal flaps based on the greater palatine vessels (Fig. 46-56). The free margins of the cleft are also incised. Misplaced muscle fibers of the levator and tensor veli palatini are freed from the posterior aspect of the hard palate. The nasal mucosa is closed directly or through the use of mucoperichondrial flaps from the vomer. End-to-end approximation of the palatal muscles is followed by closure of the free margins of the cleft. The bare areas of the hard palate can sometimes be covered by direct suturing, although they heal quickly by secondary intention.

Velopharyngeal insufficiency that presents after palate repair or as an isolated phenomenon is evaluated by speech testing, cineradiography, and nasal endoscopy. If speech therapy is unsuccessful, operative procedures have a place in reducing hypernasality. These procedures produce a static or dynamic reduction in the cross-sectional area of the nasopharynx and improve velopharyngeal competence.

CRANIOFACIAL ANOMALIES

Craniofacial anomalies are relatively rare disorders resulting in abnormal facial contours and often a grotesque appearance (Fig. 46-57). Paul Tessier pioneered the accurate description and treatment of these deformities. Craniofacial anomalies may be divided into rare facial clefts and craniosynostosis.

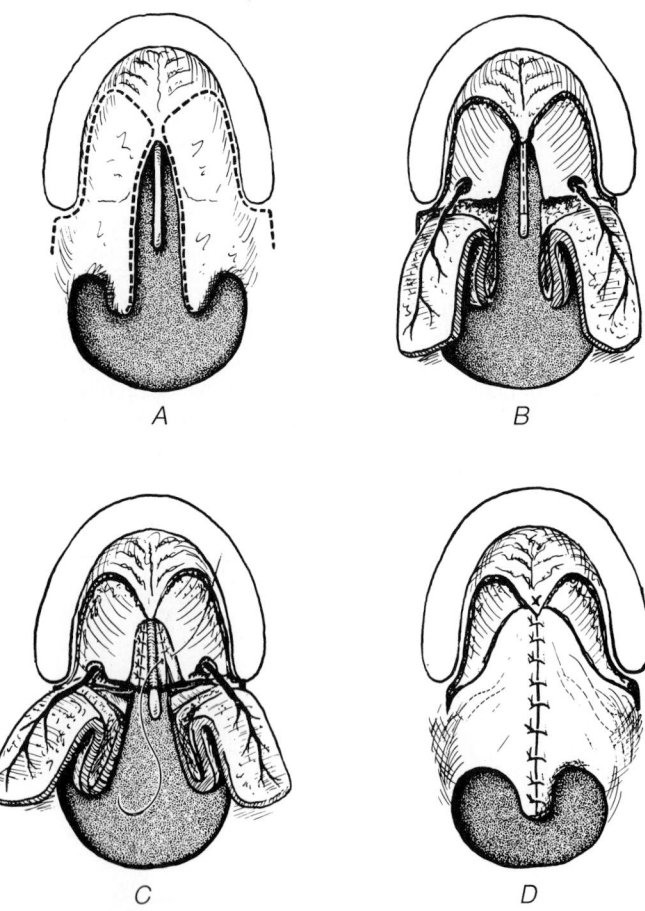

A

B

C

D

Fig. 46-56. Cleft palate repair. *A*. Proposed lines of incision. *B*. Elevation of mucoperiosteal flaps from the hard palate, based on the greater palatine arteries. A line of incision is made along the vomer, for development of mucosal flaps. *C*. Nasal mucosa being sutured to mucosal flaps from vomer. The palatine muscles are separated from their abnormal attachments to the hard palate and sutured across the midline. *D*. Closure of the oral mucosa completed. The exposed areas of hard palate close secondarily.

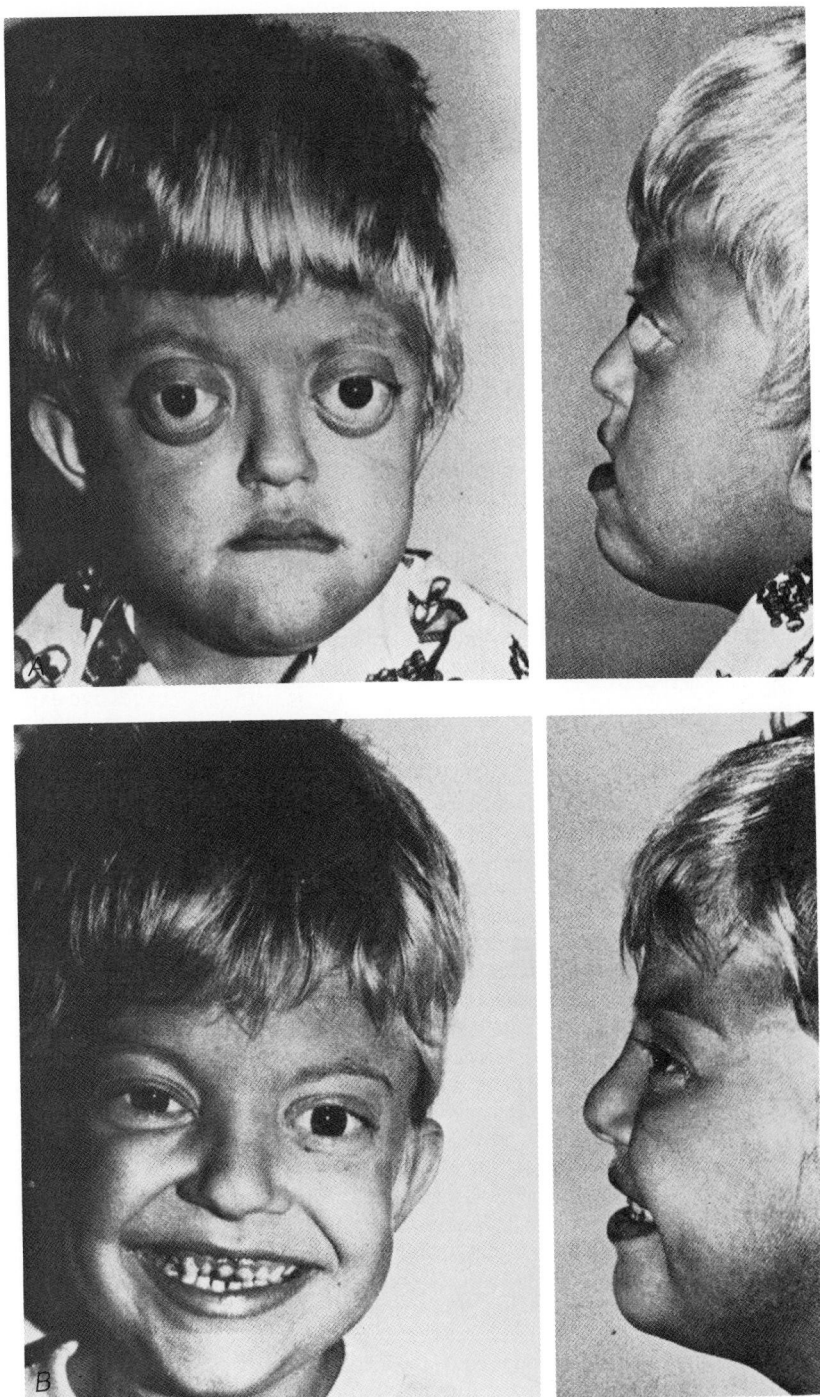

Fig. 46-57. *A.* Crouzon's disease in a four-year-old boy. The disorder is characterized by malformation of the skull (scaphocephaly), midface retrusion and stenosis, and bilateral exorbitism. *B.* Amelioration of the disorder by craniofacial osteotomies and bone grafting. *(Photographs courtesy of Robert G. Brown, M.D.)*

Unusual facial clefts are described anatomically, with the orbit as a center of reference. *Craniofacial microsomia* is the most common of these clefts. The deformity is usually unilateral, but may be bilateral. A groove is present in the cheek from the oral commissure to the ear, producing macrostomia. The ear is deformed and preauricular tags are usually present. The trigeminal and facial nerves on the affected side and the muscles supplied by them are often involved, producing occlusal abnormalities and weakness in facial expression. The zygomatic bone and vertical elements of the mandible on the involved side are hypoplastic.

Craniosynostosis is a pathologic process caused by premature closure of one or more cranial sutures. *Crouzon's syndrome* is characterized by early closure of the coronal suture with a hypoplastic, retruded midface. The orbits are shallow and the globe protruberant. The eyelids are often unable to close over the cornea, and ulceration results. Some degree of ocular hypertelorism is common. The children with this defect are generally of normal intelligence.

Apert's syndrome is a more severe form of craniosynostosis and also involves the coronal suture. The forehead is tall and depressed. Orbital hypertelorism is common, along with midface hypoplasia and clefting of the palate. Syndactyly is frequently seen, usually involving the central three digits. Most children with Apert's syndrome have some mental retardation.

Surgical repair of these anomalies is achieved using extracranial and intracranial approaches to the cranium and facial bones. The involved bones are separated, repositioned, and supported with bone grafts and interosseous wiring.

MAXILLOMANDIBULAR DISPROPORTION

An abnormality in the shape, size, or position of the mandible or maxilla can result in malocclusion of the teeth with difficulty in chewing. Associated with a bony disproportion may be significant aesthetic deformity. In analyzing the patient with maxillomandibular disproportion, the plastic surgeon must consider the relative position of the mandible to the maxilla and the relationship of facial bones to the cranial base. Evaluation of such a patient includes taking dental impressions and construction of models as well as examination of cephalograms for proper analysis. Frequently, the less severe case of maxillomandibular disproportion can be treated successfully by orthodontia. The more severe deformity requires operative management.

In retrognathia, the mandible is of normal size but is located posterior to its normal position. *Micrognathia* is manifest by a small mandible. The mandible appears recessed in the patient with retrognathia or micrognathia. In both cases, the operative technique for treating the deformity involves splitting the mandibular rami bilaterally in the sagittal plane. The mandible is advanced and held in position by plates, screws, or intermaxillary fixation. There is some risk of damage to the inferior alveolar nerve during the procedure.

The patient with mandibular *prognathism* suffers from a prominent, overdeveloped mandible. This is corrected operatively by a sagittal split of the mandibular rami, removal of a segment of bone on the external surface of the mandible along the margin of the osteotomy, and repositioning of the jaw posteriorly. An alternative approach is through a vertical osteotomy beginning at the sigmoid notch and carried to a point just posterior to the

mandibular angle. The mandible is then set back, allowing the bones to overlap at the osteotomy site. With both the sagittal split or vertical osteotomy, the patient is placed in intermaxillary fixation for 10 to 12 weeks or the segments are stabilized internally using interosseous plates and screws.

A patient may have a mandible of normal dimensions, but suffer from a chin that lacks projection. A small chin can be augmented with a silicone prosthesis. The more severe case is treated by a horizontal osteotomy and repositioning of the mentum.

A common deformity of the maxilla is *hypoplasia,* often seen in the patient with cleft lip and palate. *Hyperplasia of the maxilla* is manifest by a long face and excessive exposure of the gingiva when smiling. The operative treatment of hypoplasia of the mandible involves a LeFort I osteotomy. A mucosal incision is made in the upper gingivobuccal sulcus exposing the maxilla above the tooth roots. By means of an air-driven reciprocating saw, an osteotomy is cut along the outer wall of the maxilla from the pyriform aperture to the pterygopalatine suture bilaterally. This isolated lower segment of the maxilla is then repositioned and stabilized.

Vertical maxillary excess is manifest by a long face and excessive exposure of the gingiva when smiling. This deformity is also treated by Le Fort I osteotomy with removal of a vertical segment of maxilla, allowing the lower portion to shift upward into a more normal position.

EAR DEFORMITIES

Microtia is characterized by a congenitally small, malformed ear. Often all that remains is a malpositioned ear remnant. A hearing deficit is almost always present in the involved ear. Repair of microtia begins at age five to six years and is performed in stages. The first stage is implantation of a framework fashioned from a rib cartilage. Carving this cartilage requires considerable artistic ability. Subsequent stages include lobule rotation, elevation of the ear, deepening of the concha, and a formation of a tragus (Fig. 46-58).

Prominent ears are congenital deformities characterized by lack of definition of the antihelical fold and increase in projection of the conchal cartilage. This results in ears that project from the skull excessively. The goal of operation is to recreate an antihelical fold and decrease conchal prominence. To achieve this, the surgeon takes advantage of cartilage's tendency to bend away from the side where it is scratched or scored. The operative procedure is carried out by elevating the skin from a portion of the exterior surface of the ear cartilage, scoring the cartilage, including the anterior perichondrium, and removing a skin ellipse from the posterior aspect of the ear. A more natural contour is assumed immediately (Fig. 46-59).

An eqally satisfactory technique involves recreation of an antihelical fold by exposing the ear cartilage posteriorly and placing of horizontal mattress sutures to fold the ear into the desired shape. At the same time, the conchal cartilage is shaved on its medial surface to diminish its prominence.

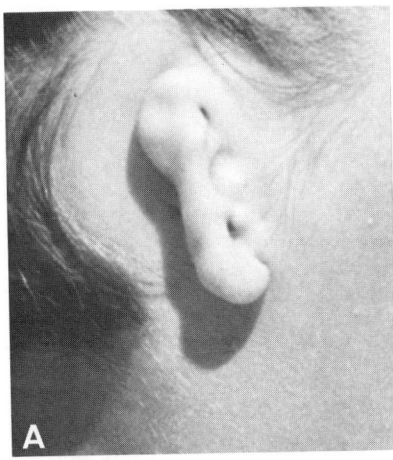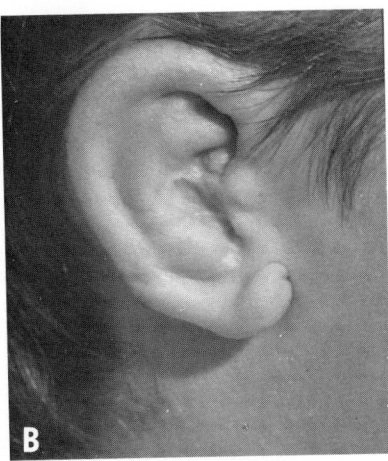

Fig. 46-58. Microtia reconstruction. *A.* Preoperative photograph. *B.* Ear reconstructed using cartilage framework.

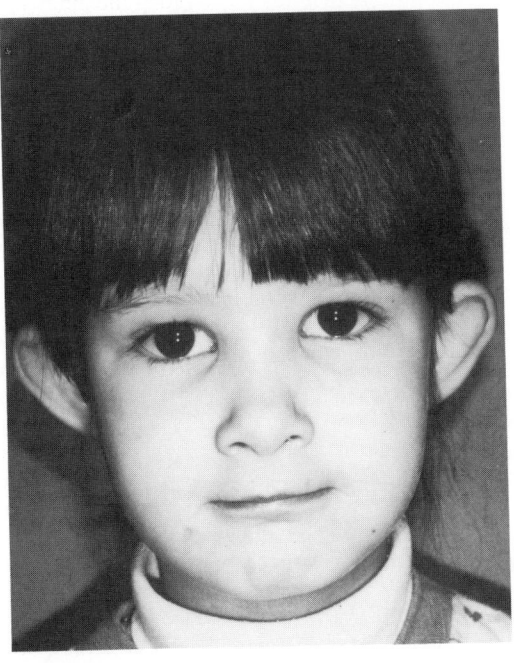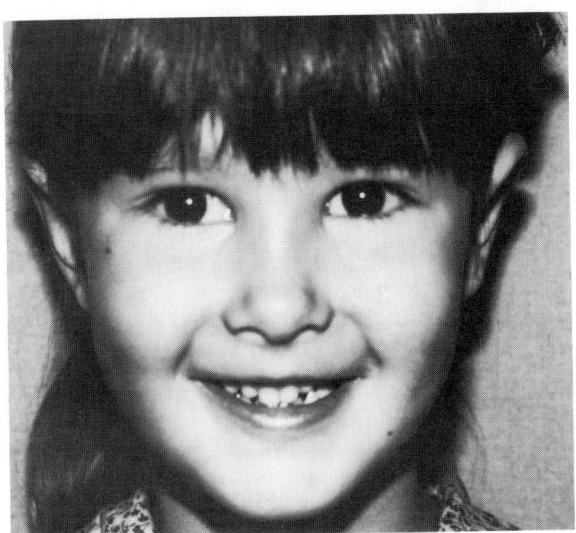

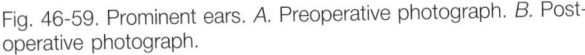

Fig. 46-59. Prominent ears. *A.* Preoperative photograph. *B.* Post-operative photograph.

HEMANGIOMA AND LYMPHANGIOMA

The *capillary hemangioma* is a common disorder in the pediatric age group. It represents an abnormal accumulation of small vessels in the subepidermal and deep dermal layers. A *port wine stain* is a form of capillary hemangioma that is flat and uniformly dark red in color. Port wine stains do not resolve spontaneously and are present at birth. Treatment is by excision, laser cauterization, tattooing, and application of cosmetics. The *strawberry hemangioma* is also a form of capillary hemangioma. This lesion is raised and bright red. It may not be prominent at birth but becomes apparent within 1 to 3 weeks after birth. A strawberry hemangioma usually grows rapidly for the first 6 months of life, then stabilizes in size and may begin to disappear. Therapy initially consists of observation, as the majority of strawberry hemangiomas resolve spontaneously by age 10 years. Surgical excision or treatment with a laser is done in selected cases when obstruction of vision or respiration is imminent. The systemic or local use of steroids hastens regression.

In the *cavernous hemangioma,* cell organization is more mature and deeply situated in the tissues. Location in the head and neck is common. This lesion is blue, swollen, and present from birth. Gigantism of the affected part can occur. The cavernous hemangioma with numerous venovenous communications seldom involutes, and complete cure is rare. Management is by palliative, and often subtotal, excision. If excision is indicated, intraoperative bleeding can be minimized by preoperative embolization of vessels supplying the hemangioma.

The *arteriovenous malformation* is an accumulation of communicating arteries and veins. This lesion consists of abnormal arteriovenous connections. It may be congenital or arise from trauma to a single artery and vein. Arteriography may be important in defining the extent of the lesion. The traumatic arteriovenous fistula is controlled by closing the fistula between the artery and vein. Cure of the congenital arteriovenous fistula is difficult. Operation is hazardous and usually palliative. Selective arterial embolization shows promise as an adjunctive and perhaps curative procedure.

A *lymphangioma* consists of a mass of immature lymphatic channels. The *cystic hygroma* is a form of lymphangioma with cellular and cystic components. This lesion is distributed through a particular region without regard to tissue planes. Most often seen in the head and neck, the cystic hygroma swells when the patient contracts an upper respiratory infection. This swelling can cause difficulty in breathing. Some cystic hygromas will involute unless there is a hemangiomatous component. If operation is required, it may be possible only to debulk the lesion and remove it completely.

THYROGLOSSAL DUCT AND BRANCHIAL CLEFT ANOMALIES

The embryonic thyroglossal duct gives rise to the thyroglossal duct cyst and fistula (Fig. 46-60). A thyroglossal duct cyst presents as a midline mass in the anterior neck. If the duct is open to the skin, it is termed a fistula. Both the cyst and fistula can become infected. If infection is present, incision and drainage are performed. Once infection is controlled, the lesion is treated by complete excision, usually with removal of the central portion of the hyoid bone. A preoperative thyroid scan is essential.

The branchial cleft cyst, sinus, and fistula are remnants of the first or second branchial cleft or pouch (Fig. 46-61). Both first and second branchial cleft fistulas are located adjacent to cranial nerves, the first close to the facial nerve and the second associated with the hypoglossal nerve. A branchial cleft fistula has both an internal and an external opening. The fistula that opens onto the skin between the external auditory canal and the submandibular area originates from the first branchial cleft. The internal opening of the second branchial cleft fistula is usually in the posterior tonsillar pillar, while the external one is found along the anterior border of the sternocleidomastoid muscle (Fig. 46-62). The branchial cleft sinus has either an external or internal opening but not both. The branchial cleft cyst is closed at both ends. These structures sometimes become infected and require drainage. When the infection has cleared, complete excision is indicated. In the case of a second branchial cleft fistula this may require several incisions in a "stepladder" fashion, progressing upward from the external opening to expose the entire length of the fistula or sinus.

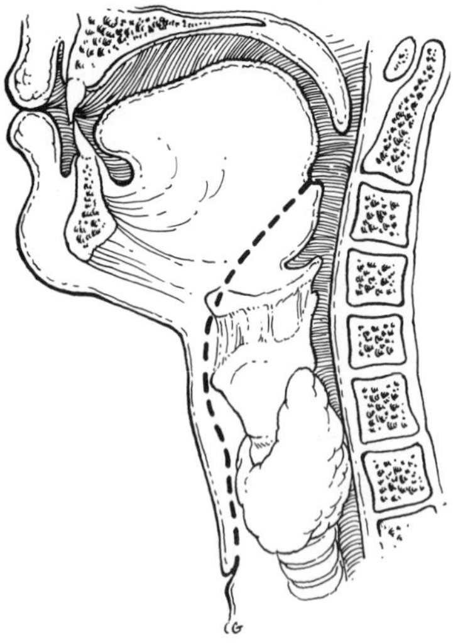

Fig. 46-60. Thyroglossal duct fistula. The thyroglossal duct originates at the foramen cecum, passes through the hyoid bone in the midline, and opens onto the skin at the suprasternal notch.

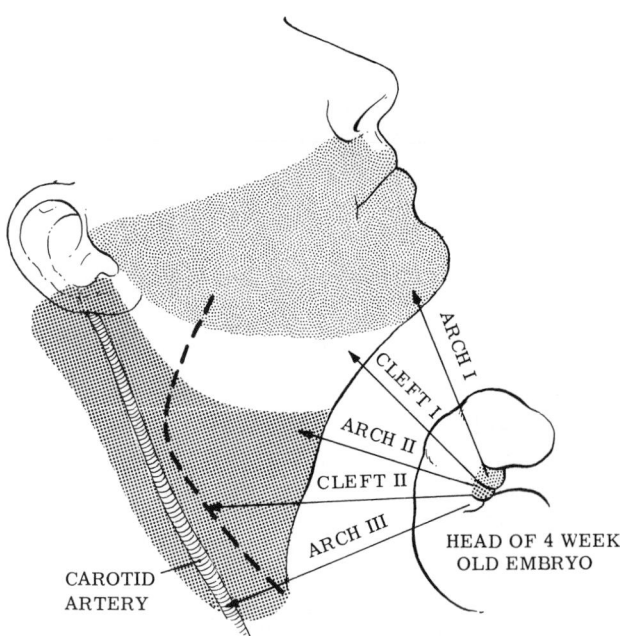

Fig. 46-61. Contributions of the embryonic branchial arches and clefts to the adult face.

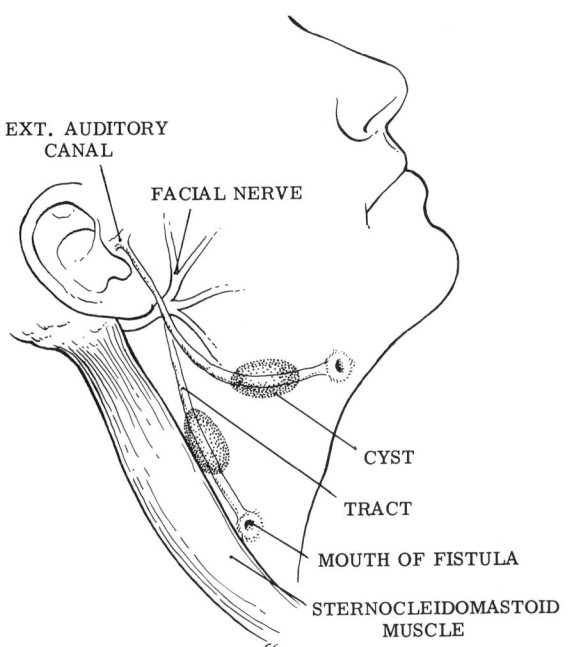

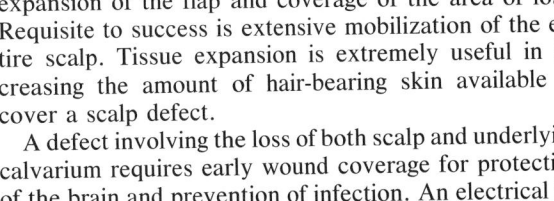

Fig. 46-62. Consequences of incomplete dissolution of the first and second branchial clefts.

Acquired Deformities

SKULL AND SCALP DEFORMITIES

Injuries that involve large areas of scalp loss are treated in several ways. Avulsion of the scalp has been successfully treated by replantation using microvascular techniques. If replantation is impossible, application of a split-thickness skin graft allows the wound to heal. Later, the skin graft is excised serially to reduce the size of the defect. Orticochea has described a technique for management of larger wounds of the scalp. This procedure involves the use of three or four scalp flaps that are transposed into the defect. The underside of each flap is scored with multiple parallel incisions through the galea to allow expansion of the flap and coverage of the area of loss. Requisite to success is extensive mobilization of the entire scalp. Tissue expansion is extremely useful in increasing the amount of hair-bearing skin available to cover a scalp defect.

A defect involving the loss of both scalp and underlying calvarium requires early wound coverage for protection of the brain and prevention of infection. An electrical injury sometimes results in such a full-thickness loss. If the bone is charred, debridement is carried down to the meninges. A small defect can be covered by a transposition flap. The larger wound can be managed temporarily by application of a split-thickness skin graft to the dura. Given the difficulty of removing a mature skin graft from dura, a better solution is immediate coverage using a free tissue transfer. If reconstruction of the calvarium is required at a later date, split-rib grafts or alloplastic material may be placed beneath the healed wound cover.

EYELID AND EYEBROW RECONSTRUCTION

A full-thickness defect of the eyelid may result from trauma, infection, and tumor excision. The upper eyelid is the more important of the two lids. It is the principal protector of the cornea and functions best when it is mobile. A loss of one-fourth or less of either eyelid is closed directly. Larger defects of the upper eyelid are reconstructed using composite tissue from the lower eyelid. Local flaps of tissue from the adjacent cheek or a portion of the upper lid can be used to recreate the lower lid. When conjunctiva is lost, it can be provided by a mucosal graft from the nasal septum, with or without cartilage.

Laceration through the eyebrow requires careful approximation (Fig. 46-63). Loss of the eyebrow is treated using hair-bearing tissue from the scalp. This tissue is transferred as a free graft (Fig. 46-64) or an island flap (Fig. 46-65).

EYELID PTOSIS

When the eye opens voluntarily, the upper eyelid elevates through contraction of the levator muscle (CN III innervated) and Mueller's muscle (sympathetically innervated). The work of muscular contraction is transmitted to the eyelid through a fibrous tract called the levator

Fig. 46-63. Avoidance of alopecia during repair of eyebrow laceration. *A.* Oblique laceration of eyebrow hairs creates eyebrow alopecia at the wound site unless revised parallel to the hair follicles. *B.* Laceration crossing the eyebrow. Precise realignment of eyebrow elements is important.

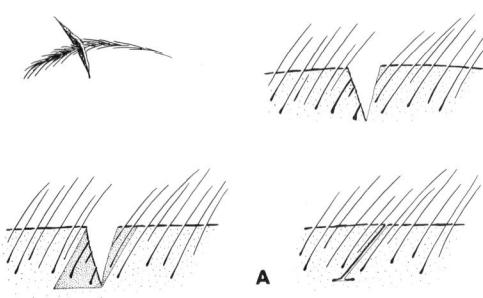

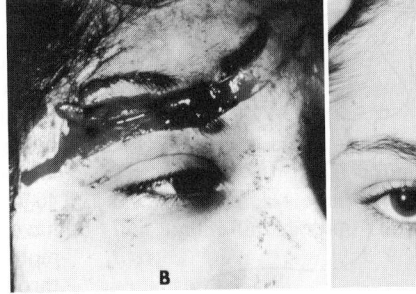

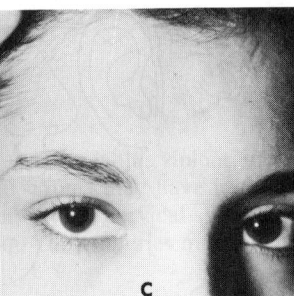

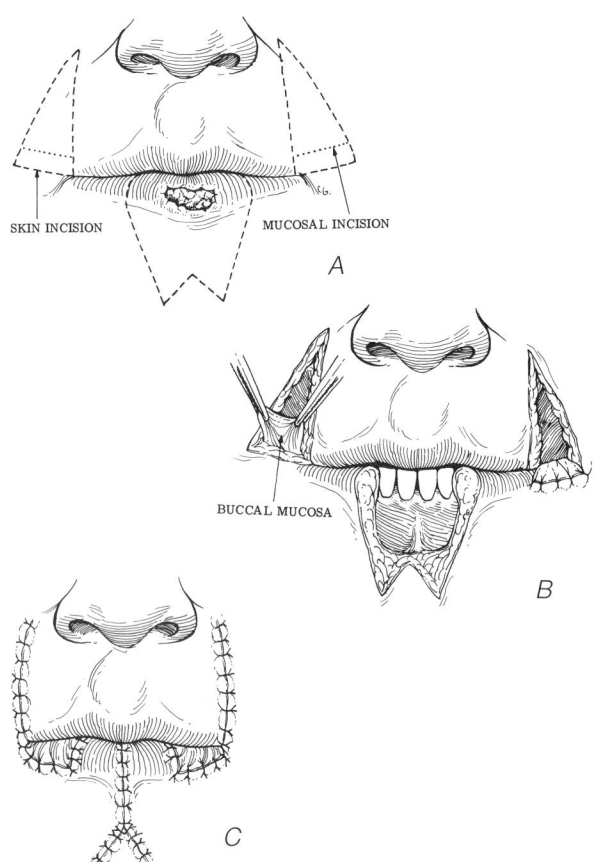

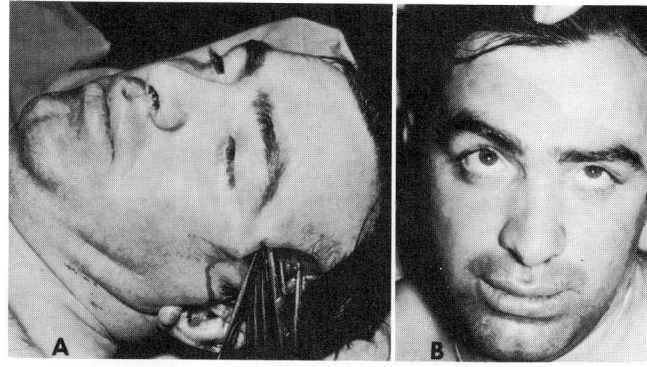

Fig. 46-69. Facial nerve injury. *A.* Laceration of temple with bleeding controlled by multiple hemostats. *B.* Paralysis of left forehead due to injury of facial nerve, temporal branch. The paralysis may have been the result of the laceration or the attempts at achieving hemostasis.

Fig. 46-67. Bernard procedure. *A.* Outline of skin incisions for removal of tumor and mucosal incisions for excision of nasolabial triangles. *B.* Tumor and nasolabial triangles removed and buccal mucosa turned down into lower lip. *C.* Incisions closed.

Fig. 46-68. Abbe flap. *A.* Incisions outlined. *B.* Tumor excised and flap developed, based on the labial artery. *C.* Flap healed in place. *D.* Pedicle of flap divided and wound revised.

Fig. 46-70. Facial nerve injury. *A*1. Laceration of submandibular region. *A*2. Injury of marginal mandibular branch of facial nerve, producing paralysis of lower lip on the right. *B*1. Stab wound anterior to mastoid process. *B*2. Result of complete division of facial nerve.

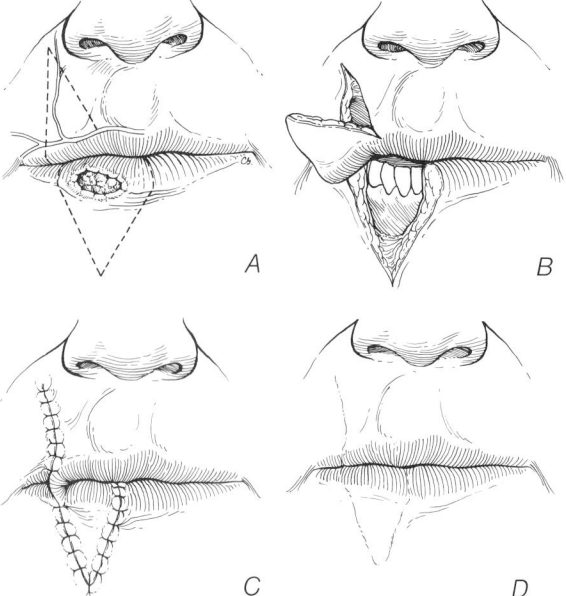

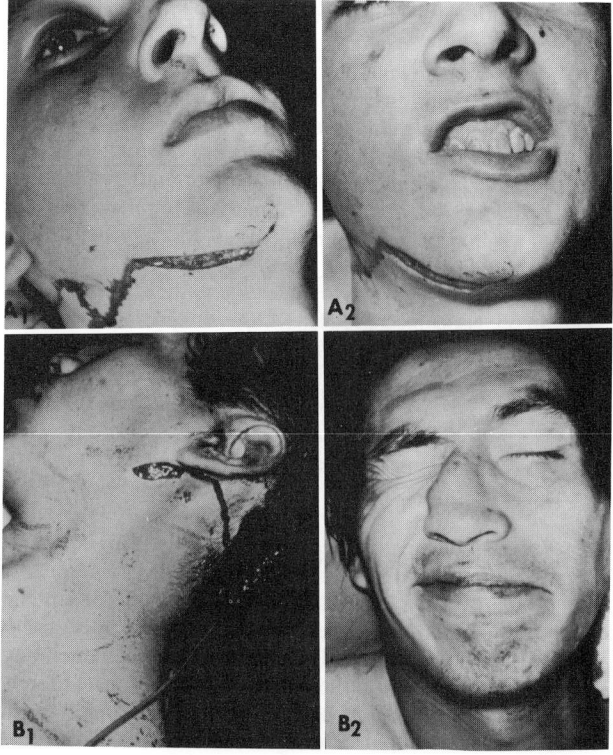

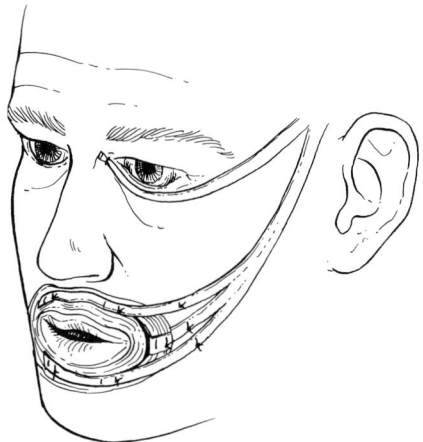

Fig. 46-71. Facial palsy treated by fascia lata slings to lower eyelid and mouth.

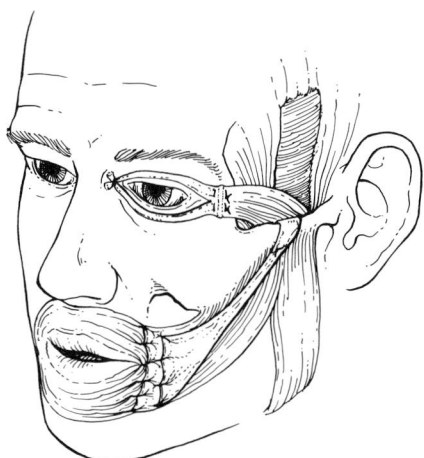

Fig. 46-73. Facial palsy treated with transfer of temporalis muscle and a static sling to the zygomatic arch.

Fig. 46-72. Gillies's procedure to establish motor power for eyelids. *A* and *B.* Temporalis muscle reflected forward with strips of its own fascia passed through the upper and lower lids to the medial canthal ligament. *C* and *D.* Preoperative eyelid paralysis. *E* and *F.* After Gillies's operation.

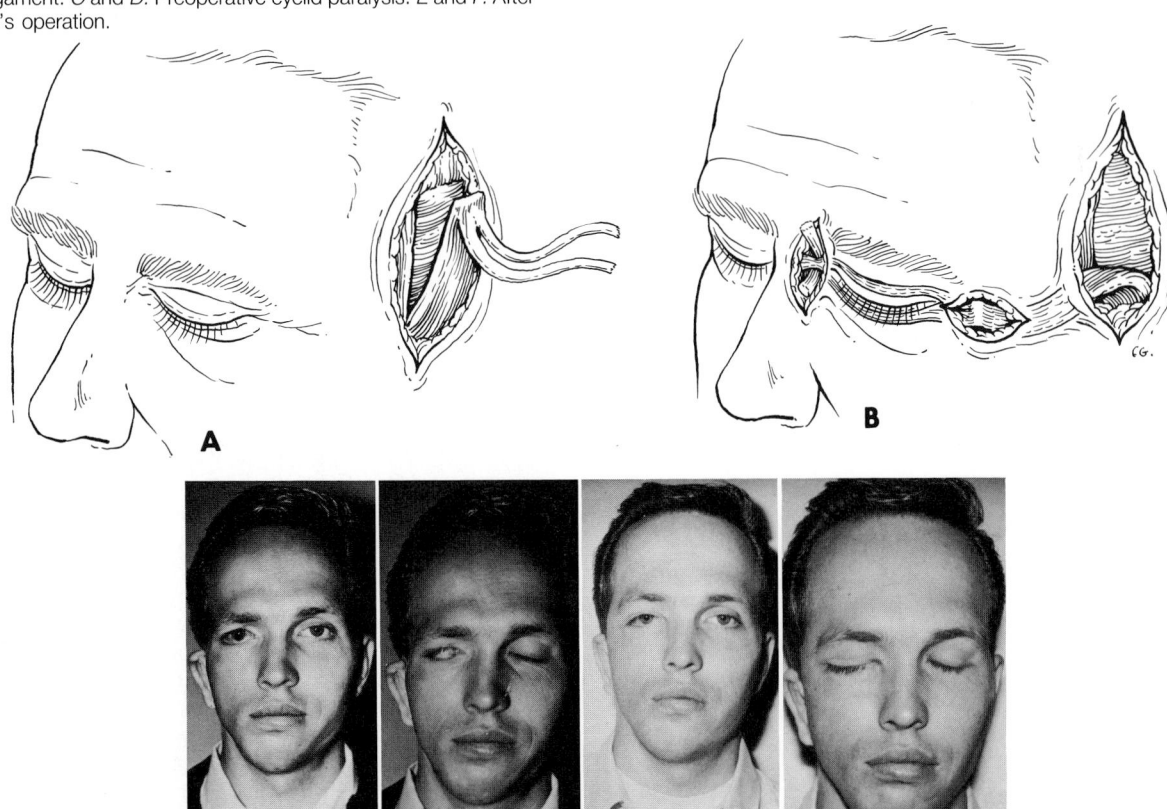

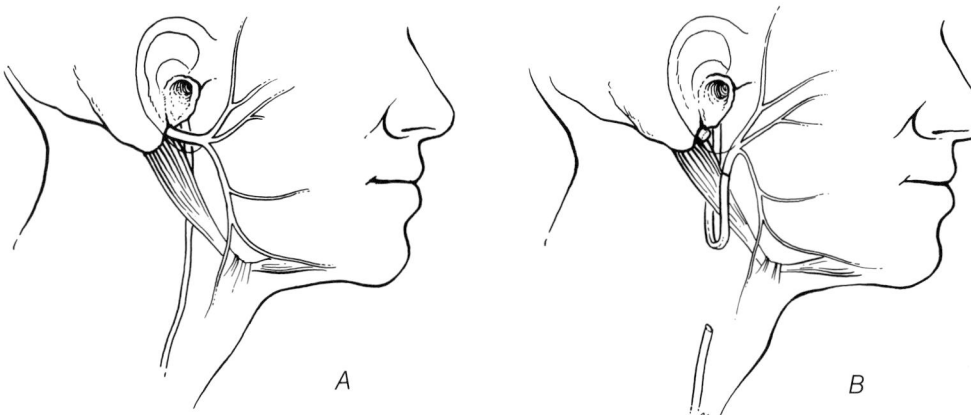

Fig. 46-74. Facial nerve graft using hypoglossal nerve. *A.* Normal relationship between descendens hypoglossi and facial nerves. *B.* Nerve graft from proximal descendens hypoglossi to distal facial nerve.

Examination of the facial skeleton proceeds from the upper to lower face (Fig. 46-76). The forehead is palpated for signs of depressed fracture or frontal sinus injury. Orbital margins are checked for any irregularity. Ophthalmologic examination is pursued for evidence of enophthalmos, inferior displacement of the globe, and intrinsic damage to the eye. The nose is observed for asymmetry or depression and the septum examined for hematoma. The zygomatic arches and malar eminences are palpated to reveal any deformity. Dental occlusion is noted. The maxillary bones are examined intraorally and extraorally. Midface stability is checked by grasping the upper incisors and alveolar ridge and gently attempting to displace the structures anteriorly or posteriorly. Intraoral and extraoral palpation of the mandible completes the bony examination. Numbness of the nasolabial region or chin implies injury to the infraorbital or inferior alveolar nerve.

Fig. 46-75. Surface projection of the parotid duct, on a line between the earlobe and nasal alar base. The oral entry is found at the bisection of this line by a vertical line from the lateral canthus of the eye.

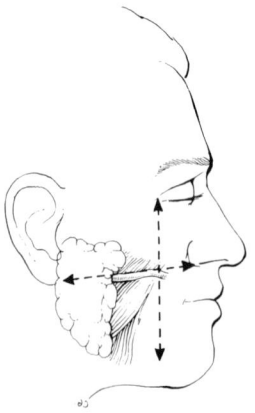

A thorough radiologic examination is necessary for the proper diagnosis of a facial fracture (Table 46-1). This examination requires manipulation of the patient. Therefore, the status of the cervical spine first must be determined radiographically. Appropriate x-rays include a posterior-anterior, lateral, and Water's view of the facial bones (Fig. 46-77). A nasal fracture can be confirmed by lateral film of the nose. Oblique, lateral, and Towne's views of the mandible are useful if a mandibular fracture is suspected. A Panorex roentgenogram exposes most of the mandible except the mentum and is helpful in localizing fractures. Submental vertex films of the zygomatic arches may be necessary to demonstrate a fracture in this area. Suspected fractures within the bony orbit are diagnosed by tomography. Computerized tomography is becoming increasingly important in diagnosing facial fractures.

Treatment of a mandibular fracture is dictated by its location and extent of displacement (Fig. 46-78). The pull of the muscles of mastication contribute to displacement of the fracture. The mandibular condyle is the single area most often fractured, although it is not uncommon for the mandible to break in more than one place.

The principles of management of a mandibular fracture are early reduction with the restoration of normal dental occlusion, firm immobilization, and control of infection with antibiotics. Intermaxillary fixation (IMF) is a basic technique of immobilization. Metal bars are ligated to the upper and lower rows of teeth using stainless steel wire. The upper and lower bars are joined by rubber bands to achieve occlusion, with the mandible held tightly against the maxilla. Open reduction and internal fixation (ORIF) of the mandibular fraction using plates and screws is becoming accepted as a means of providing accurate reduction and early resumption of eating.

Fractures of the various anatomic regions of the mandible are managed individually. A fracture in the parasymphyseal region is treated by open reduction and internal

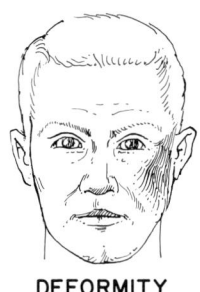

DEFORMITY

FACIAL FRACTURE DIAGNOSIS

(CLINICAL)

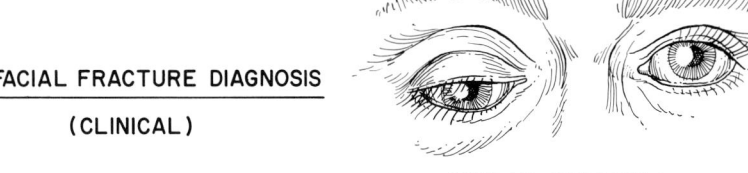

OCULAR DISPARITY

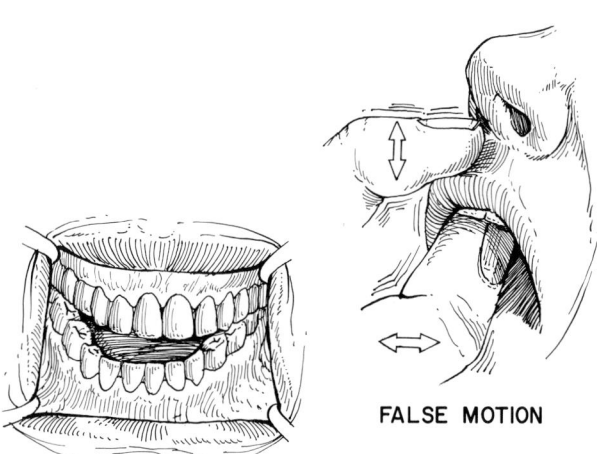

FALSE MOTION

MALOCCLUSION

Fig. 46-76. Common physical findings in facial fractures.

FACIAL FRACTURE DIAGNOSIS
(X-RAY)

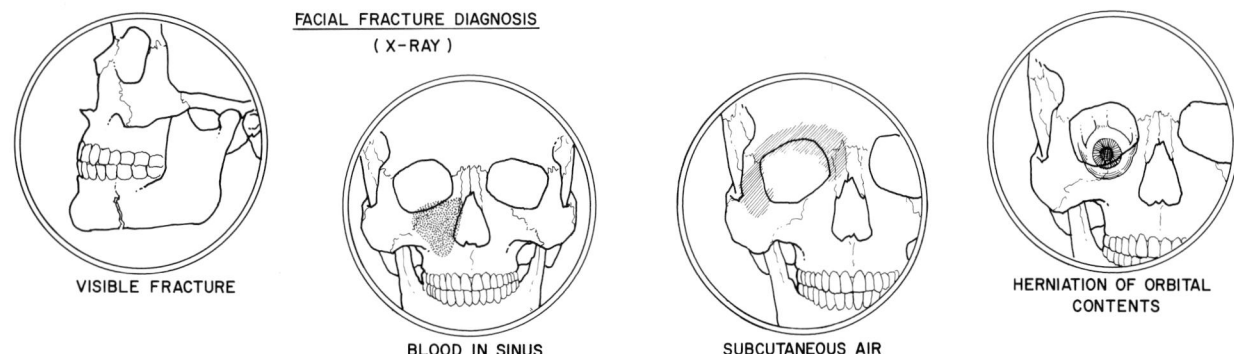

VISIBLE FRACTURE

BLOOD IN SINUS

SUBCUTANEOUS AIR

HERNIATION OF ORBITAL
CONTENTS

Fig. 46-77. Common radiographic findings in facial fractures.

Table 46-1. CHART FOR X-RAY FOR FACIAL FRACTURES

Bone	X-Ray
Mandible:	
Condylar and coronoid processes	Right and left lateral obliques of mandible
Ascending ramus and body	
Symphysis, parasymphyseal	
Body and ascending rami	Posterior-anterior of mandible
Condyle and condylar neck	Towne's (modified)
	Anterior-posterior of base of skull
Anterior arch	Occlusal of anterior mandible
Maxilla & Zygoma	Water's (posterior-anterior oblique)
	Anterior-posterior of face
	Lateral of face
Zygomatic arch	Submental-vertex
Orbital Floor	Water's
	Stereo Water's
	Laminography
Nasal Bone	Superior-inferior of nose
	Lateral of nose

fixation of the fragments, followed by IMF. When a fracture occurs in the body of the mandible and a full complement of teeth is present, ORIF or IMF alone is used. A body fracture of the edentulous mandible is treated by performing open reduction and internal fixation, combined with IMF using dentures or dental splints. An alternative in the case of an edentulous body fracture is application of an external fixation device. Fractures of the ramus, coronoïd process, and condylar process are splinted with IMF. An alveolar ridge fracture is stabilized by ligating the involved and adjacent uninvolved teeth to themselves or to an arch bar.

A zygomatic bone fracture is often displaced, resulting in depression of the malar eminence (Fig. 46-79). The lateral canthus of the eye is displaced laterally and inferiorly (Fig. 46-80). If significant deformity has occurred, open reduction and internal fixation are mandatory.

Certain fractures inside the bony orbit are sustained as a result of a blow to the eye. The sudden increase in intraorbital pressure causes collapse of the floor or medial wall of the orbit (Fig. 46-81). These "blowout" fractures are accompanied by a herniation of orbital fat into the maxillary, or ethmoid, sinus. The patient often complains of double vision. Acute enophthalmos is sometimes noted. An orbital floor fracture can sometimes trap the tissues adjacent to the inferior rectus muscle and prevent upward gaze on the injured side (Fig. 46-82). Blunt trauma to the extraocular muscles is sufficient to impede their function. True mechanical entrapment of the extraocular muscles is best assessed by the forced duction test. Local anesthetic drops are instilled into the inferior fornix and the insertion of the inferior rectus muscle is grasped with forceps. Traction on the muscle at this point and observation of the globe's mobility confirm the presence or absence of entrapment.

The indications for operation in blowout fracture are entrapment on forced duction, significant enophthalmos, and the presence of a large fracture on x-ray examination. The surgical procedure involves exposure of the orbital floor and return of the herniated tissue to the orbit. Often the bony fragments of the orbital floor are stable after anatomic reduction. If not, a silastic or absorbable synthetic sheet is used to reinforce the floor of the orbit. Alternatively, a thin bone graft or cartilage segment may be used.

A nasal fracture is frequently accompanied by depression of the nasal bones, asymmetry, and nasal obstruction. Nasal roentgenograms are of limited value. An obvi-

Fig. 46-78. The common mandibular fracture sites. (*After Dingman RO, Natvig P: Surgery of Facial Fractures. Philadelphia, Saunders, 1964, with permission.*)

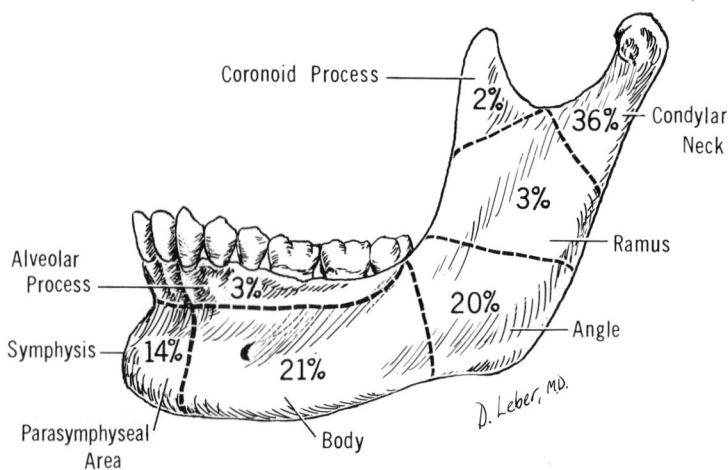

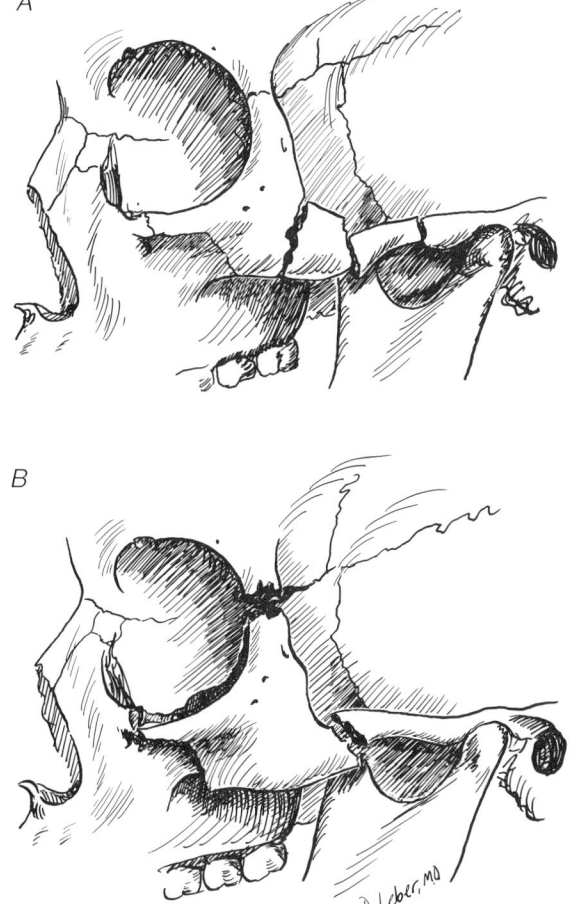

A

B

Fig. 46-79. Zygomatic bone fractures. *A.* Depressed fracture of the zygomatic arch. This fracture may impinge upon the mandible, producing pain (trismus) and difficulty in opening the mouth. *B.* Displaced fracture of the zygomatic bone. The zygomaticofrontal, zygomaticotemporal, and zygomaticomaxillary sutures are separated. The orbital floor and lateral orbital wall are always involved in this fracture.

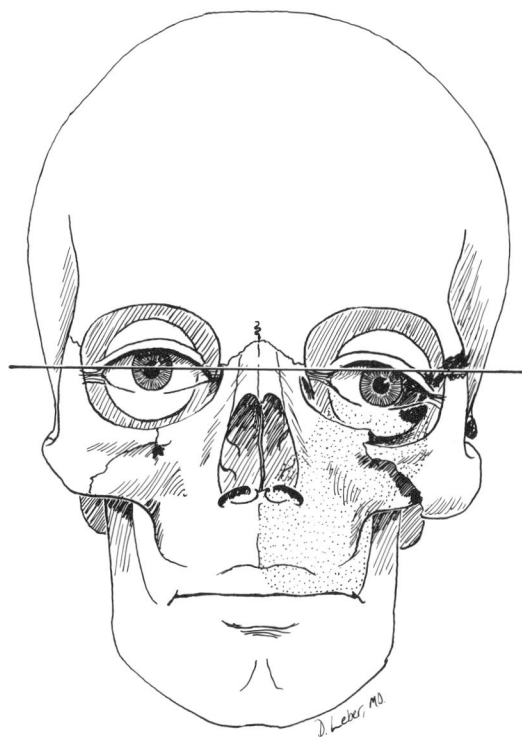

Fig. 46-80. Fracture-dislocation of the zygoma, with rotation of the fragment, lateral and inferior displacement of the lateral canthus, and subscleral hematoma. Note the surface representation of anesthesia due to infraorbital nerve injury.

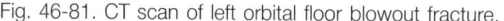

Fig. 46-81. CT scan of left orbital floor blowout fracture.

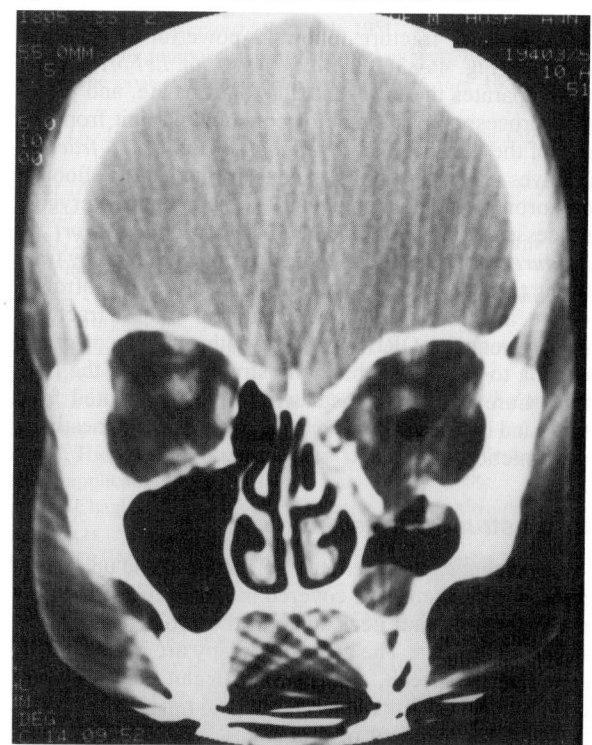

ous deformity is corrected immediately under local or general anesthesia. If the nose is swollen, reduction of the nasal fracture is delayed several days until the swelling subsides and accurate reduction of the fracture is possible. If a displaced fracture is allowed to completely heal without reduction, the resultant deformity often requires operative correction. A hematoma of the nasal septum occasionally complicates a fracture of the nose. This hematoma must be drained immediately and the nose packed. An untreated hematoma is prone to infection, which can lead to septal perforation or collapse.

Complex nasoorbital fractures involve the frontal sinus, root of the nose, and ethmoid sinuses. These fractures are best managed by repair under direct vision. Exposure is obtained through an associated laceration or a transcoronal incision.

Weiland AJ, Phillips JW, Randolph MA: Bone grafts: A radiologic, histologic, and biomechanical model comparing autografts, allografts, and free vascularized bone grafts. *Plast Reconstr Surg* 74:368, 1984.

Reconstructive Surgery

Arnold PG, Irons G: The greater omentum: Extensions in transportation and free transfer. *Plast Reconstr Surg* 67:169, 1981.

Bostwick J: Breast reconstruction: A comprehensive approach. *Clin Plast Surg* 6:143, 1979.

Bostwick J: Repairs in the lower abdomen, groin, or perineum with myocutaneous or omental flaps. *Plast Reconstr Surg* 63:186, 1979.

Bostwick J, Scheflan M: The latissimus dorsi musculocutaneous flap: A one-stage breast reconstruction. *Clin Plast Surg* 7:71, 1980.

Burget GC, Menick FJ: Nasal reconstruction: Seeking a fourth dimension. *Plast Reconstr Surg* 78:145, 1986.

Byrd HS, Cierny G, Tebbetts JB: The management of open tibial fractures with associated soft-tissue loss: External pin fixation with early flap coverage. *Plast Reconstr Surg* 68:73, 1981.

Carlson, H. E.: Spicer TE, Cierney G: Management of open tibial fractures. *Plast Reconstr Surg* 76:719, 1985.

Constantian MB: *Pressure Ulcers: Principles and Techniques of Management*. Boston, Little, Brown, 1980.

Courtiss EH, Goldwyn RM: Reduction mammaplasty by the inferior pedicle technique. *Plast Reconstr Surg* 59:500, 1977.

Dingman RO, Argenta LC: Reconstruction of the chest wall. *Ann Thorac Surg* 32:202, 1982.

Dinner MI, Labandter HP, Dowden RV: The role of the rectus abdominis myocutaneous flap in breast reconstruction. *Plast Reconstr Surg* 69:209, 1982.

Ger R: Muscle transposition for treatment and prevention of chronic post-traumatic osteomyelitis of the tibia. *J Bone and Joint Surg* 59:A:784, 1977.

Gong-Kang H, Ru-Qi H, et al: Microlymphaticovenous anastomosis in the treatment of lower limb obstructive lymphedema: Analysis of 91 cases. *Plast Reconstr Surg* 76:671, 1985.

Goulian D: Dermal mastopexy. *Clin Plast Surg,* 3:171, 1976.

Hartrampf CR, Scheflan M, Black PW: Breast reconstruction with a transverse abdominal island flap. *Plast Reconstr Surg* 69:216, 1982.

Hartrampf CR, Scheflan M, Bostwick J: The flexor digitorum brevis muscle island pedicle flap: A new dimension in heel reconstruction. *Plast Reconstr Surg* 66:264, 1980.

Hurteau JE, Bostwick J, et al: V-Y advancement of hamstring musculocutaneous flap for coverage of ischial pressure sores. *Plast Reconstr Surg* 68:539, 1981.

Jurkiewicz MJ, Bostwick J, et al: Infected median sternotomy wound. *Ann Surg* 191:738, 1980.

Kernahan DA, Thomson HG, Bauer BS: *Symposium on Pediatric Plastic Surgery*. St Louis, CV Mosby, 1982.

Larson DL, McMurtrey MJ: Musculocutaneous flap reconstruction of chest-wall defects: An experience with 50 patients. *Plast Reconstr Surg* 73:734, 1984.

Leighton WD, Johnson ML, Friedland JA: Use of the temporary soft-tissue expander in post-traumatic alopecia. *Plast Reconstr Surg* 77:737, 1986.

Leighton WD, Halls MJ, Simon SR: Free microvascular muscle flap with skin graft reconstruction of extensive defects of the foot: A clinical and gait analysis study. *Plast Reconstr Surg* 75:627, 1985.

May JW, Gallico GG, Lupash FN: Microvascular transfer of free tissue for closure of bone wounds of the distal lower extremity. *N Engl J Med* 306:253, 1982.

Mustarde JC: *Plastic Surgery in Infancy and Childhood*. Edinburgh, Churchill Livingstone, 1979.

Nahai F: Muscle and musculocutaneous flaps in gynecologic surgery. *Clin Obstet Gynecol* 24:1277, 1981.

Nahai F, Silverton JS, et al: The tensor fascia lata musculocutaneous flap. *Ann Plast Surg* 1:372, 1978.

Pendergrast WJ, Bostwick J, Jurkiewicz MJ: The subcutaneous mastectomy cripple: Surgical rehabilitation with the latissimus dorsi flap. *Plast Reconstr Surg* 66:554, 1980.

Regnault P: Breast ptosis. *Clin Plast Surg* 3:193, 1976.

Reiffel RS, McCarthy JG: Coverage of heel and sole defects: A new subfascial arterialized flap. *Plast Reconstr Surg* 66:250, 1980.

Robbins TH: A reduction mammaplasty with the areola-nipple based on an inferior dermal pedicle. *Plast Reconstr Surg* 59:64, 1977.

Russell RC, Pribaz J, et al: Functional evaluation of latissimus dorsi donor site. *Plast Reconstr Surg* 78:336, 1986.

Scheflan M, Nahai F, Bostwick J: Gluteus maximus island musculocutaneous flap for closure of sacral and ischial ulcers. *Plast Reconstr Surg* 68:533, 1981.

Schwartz WM, Mears DC: The role of free-tissue transfers in lower-extremity reconstruction. *Plast Reconstr Surg* 76:364, 1985.

Stevenson TR, Rohrich RJ, et al: More experience with the "reverse" latissimus dorsi musculocutaneous flap: Precise location of blood supply. *Plast Reconstr Surg* 74:237, 1984.

Stone HH, Fabian TC, et al: Management of acute full-thickness losses of the abdominal wall. *Ann Surg* 193:612, 1981.

Aesthetic Surgery

Baker TJ: Patient selection and psychological evaluation. *Clin Plast Surg* 5:3, 1978.

Baker TJ, Gordon HL, Mosienko, P: Rhytidectomy. *Plast Reconstr Surg* 59:24, 1977.

Baker TJ, Gordon HL, Mosienko P: Upper lid blepharoplasty. *Plast Reconstr Surg* 60:692, 1977.

Castanares S: Blepharoplasty for herniated intraorbital fat. *Plast Reconstr Surg* 8:46, 1951.

Connell BF: Contouring the neck in rhytidectomy by lipectomy and a muscle sling. *Plast Reconstr Surg* 61:376, 1978.

Courtiss EH: *Male Aesthetic Surgery*. St Louis, CV Mosby, 1982.

Courtiss EH: Suction lipectomy of the neck. *Plast Reconstr Surg* 76:882, 1985.

Courtiss EH: Suction lipectomy: A retrospective analysis of 100 patients. *Plast Reconstr Surg* 73:780, 1984.

Diamond HP: Rhinoplasty technique. *Surg Clin North Am* 51:317, 1971.

Dingman RO, Natvig P: The deviated nose. *Clin Plast Surg* 4:145, 1977.

Dingman RO, Natvig P: Surgical anatomy in aesthetic and corrective rhinoplasty. *Clin Plast Surg* 4:111, 1977.

Goldwyn RM: *Long-term Results in Plastic Surgery*. Boston, Little, Brown, 1980.

Grazer FM, Klingbeil JR: *Body Image: A Surgical Prospective*. St Louis, CV Mosby, 1980.

Guerrero-Santos J: The role of the platysma muscle in rhytidoplasty. *Clin Plast Surg* 5:39, 1978.

Lemmon ML, Hamra ST: Skoog rhytidectomy: A five-year experience with 577 patients. *Plast Reconstr Surg* 65:283, 1980.

Meyer R, Kesselring UK: Sculpturing and reconstructive procedures in aesthetic and functional rhinoplasty. *Clin Plast Surg* 4:15, 1977.

Millard DR, Garst WP, et al: Submental and submandibular lipectomy in conjunction with a facelift, in the male or female. *Plast Reconstr Surg* 49:385, 1972.

Mitz V, Peyronie M: The superficial musculo-aponeurotic system (SMAS) in the parotid and cheek area. *Plast Reconstr Surg* 58:80, 1976.

Mosienko P, Baker TJ: Chemical peel. *Clin Plast Surg* 5:79, 1978.

Peck GC: Aesthetic rhinoplasty, in Grabb WC, Smith JW: *Plastic Surgery.* Boston, Little, Brown, 1979.

Pitman GH, Teimourian B: Suction lipectomy: Complications and results by surgery. *Plast Reconstr Surg* 76:65, 1985.

Sheen JH: *Aesthetic Rhinoplasty.* St Louis, CV Mosby, 1978.

Spira M: Lower blepharoplasty—A clinical study. *Plast Reconstr Surg* 59:35, 1977.

Spira M, Dahl C, et al: Chemosurgery—A histological study. *Plast Reconstr Surg* 45:247, 1970.

Stark RB: *Aesthetic Plastic Surgery.* Boston, Little, Brown, 1980.

Vinas JC, Caviglia C, Cortinas JL: Forehead rhytidoplasty and brow lifting. *Plast Reconstr Surg* 57:445, 1976.

Congenital Head and Neck Deformities

Bardach J, Morris HL, Olin WH: Late results of primary veloplasty: The Marburg Project. *Plast Reconstr Surg* 73:207, 1984.

Brent B: The correction of microtia with autogenous cartilage grafts: I. The classic deformity. *Plast Reconstr Surg* 66:1, 1980.

Brent B: The correction of microtia with autogenous cartilage grafts: II. Atypical and complex deformities. *Plast Reconstr Surg* 66:13, 1980.

Brent B, Byrd HS: Secondary ear reconstruction with cartilage grafts covered by axial, random, and free flaps of temporoparietal fascia. *Plast Reconstr Surg* 72:141, 1983.

Brent B, Upton J, et al: Experience with the temporoparietal fascial free flap. *Plast Reconstr Surg* 76:177, 1985.

Habib Z: Genetic counselling and genetics of cleft lip and cleft palate. *Obstet Gynecol Surv* 33:441, 1978.

Hagerty RF, Mylin WK: Facial growth and arch symmetry in the surgical prosthetic treatment of cleft lip and palate. *Plast Reconstr Surg* 68:682, 1981.

McCarthy JG, Epstein F: Early surgery for craniofacial synostosis: An 8-year experience. *Plast Reconstr Surg* 73:521, 1984.

McComb H: Primary repair of the bilateral cleft lip nose: A 10-year review. *Plast Reconstr Surg* 77:701, 1986.

McComb H: Primary correction of unilateral cleft lip nasal deformity: A 10-year review. *Plast Reconstr* Surg 75:791, 1985.

McWilliams BJ, Glaser ER, et al: A comparative study of four methods of evaluating velopharyngeal adequacy. *Plast Reconstr Surg* 68:1, 1981.

Maue-Dickson W, Dickson DR: Anatomy and physiology related to cleft palate: Current research and clinical implications. *Plast Reconstr Surg* 65:83, 1980.

Millard DR: Refinements in rotation-advancement cleft lip technique. *Plast Reconsr Surg* 33:26, 1964.

Millard DR: Extensions of the rotation-advancement principle for wide unilateral cleft lips. *Plast Reconstr Surg* 42:535, 1968.

Orticochea M: A review of 236 cleft palate patients treated with dynamic muscle sphincter. *Plast Reconstr Surg* 71:180, 1983.

Psillakis JM, Grotting JC, et al: Vascularized outer-table calvarial bone flaps. *Plast Reconstr Surg* 78:309, 1986.

Stenstrom SJ: A simple operation for prominent ears. *Acta Otolaryngol* 224(suppl):393, 1967.

Tessier P: The definitive plastic surgical treatment of the severe facial deformities of craniofacial dysostosis. *Plast Reconstr Surg* 48:419, 1971.

Tessier P: Orbital hypertelorism: I. Successive surgical attempts. Material and methods. Causes and mechanisms. *Scand J Plast Reconstr Surg* 6:135, 1972.

Tessier P, Guiot J, Derome P: Orbital hypertelorism: II. Definite treatment of orbital hypertelorism (Or.H.) by craniofacial or by extracranial osteotomies. *Scand J Plast Reconstr Surg* 7:39, 1973.

Thompson H: Hemangioma, lymphangioma and arteriovenous fistula, in Grabb WC, Smith JW (eds): *Plastic Surgery.* Boston, Little, Brown, 1979.

Zide B, Grayson B, McCarthy JG: Cephalometric analysis: Part I. *Plast Reconstr Surg* 68:816, 1981.

Zide B, Grayson B, McCarthy JG: Cephalometric analysis for upper and lower midface surgery: Part II. *Plast Reconstr Surg* 68:961, 1981.

Zide B, Grayson B, McCarthy JG: Cephalometric analysis for mandibular surgery: Part III. *Plast Reconstr Surg* 69:155, 1982.

Acquired Head and Neck Deformities

Carraway JH, Vincent MP: Levator advancement technique for eyelid ptosis. *Plast Reconstr Surg* 77:394, 1986.

Converse JM: *Reconstructive Plastic Surgery.* Philadelphia, Saunders, 1977.

Converse JM, Smith B: Naso-orbital fractures and traumatic deformities of the medial canthus. *Plast Reconstr Surg* 38:147, 1966.

Cruse CW, Blevins PK, Luce EA: Naso-ethmoid-orbital fractures. *J Trauma* 20:551, 1980.

Dingman RO, Natvig P: *Surgery of Facial Fractures.* Philadelphia, Saunders, 1964.

Duncan MJ, Manktelow RT, et al: Mandibular reconstruction in the radiated patient: The role of osteocutaneous free tissue transfer. *Plast Reconstr Surg* 76:829, 1985.

Gruss JS, Mackinnon SE: Complex maxillary fractures: Role of buttress reconstruction and immediate bone grafts. *Plast Reconstr Surg* 78:9, 1986.

Gruss JS, Mackinnon SE: Naso-ethmoid-orbital fractures: Classification and role of primary bone grafting. *Plast Reconstr Surg* 75:303, 1985.

Jones NF, Sekhar LN, Schramm VL: Free rectus abdominis muscle flap reconstruction of the middle and posterior cranial base. *Plast Reconstr Surg* 78:471, 1986.

Jones NF, Grivas A, et al: Studies on enophthalmos: II. The measurement of orbital injuries and their treatment by quantitative computer tomography. *Plast Reconstr Surg* 77:203, 1986.

Jones NF, Crawley WA, et al: Midface fractures: Advantages of immediate extended open reduction and bone grafting. *Plast Reconstr Surg* 76:1, 1985.

Kawamoto HK: Surgery of the jaws in Lesavoy MA: *Reconstruction of the Head and Neck.* Baltimore, Williams & Wilkins, 1981.

Index